Body Mass Index

Height (inches)	Normal						Overweight					Obese										Extreme Obesity														
BMI	19	20	21	22	23	24	25	26	27	28	29	30	31	32	33	34	35	36	37	38	39	40	41	42	43	44	45	46	47	48	49	50	51	52	53	54
	Body Weight (pounds)																																			
58	91	96	100	105	110	115	119	124	129	134	138	143	148	153	158	162	167	172	177	181	186	191	196	201	205	210	215	220	224	229	234	239	244	248	253	258
59	94	99	104	109	114	119	124	128	133	138	143	148	153	158	163	168	173	178	183	188	193	198	203	208	212	217	222	227	232	237	242	247	252	257	262	267
60	97	102	107	112	118	123	128	133	138	143	148	153	158	163	168	174	179	184	189	194	199	204	209	215	220	225	230	235	240	245	250	255	261	266	271	276
61	100	106	111	116	122	127	132	137	143	148	153	158	164	169	174	180	185	190	195	201	206	211	217	222	227	232	238	243	248	254	259	264	269	275	280	285
62	104	109	115	120	126	131	136	142	147	153	158	164	169	175	180	186	191	196	202	207	213	218	224	229	235	240	246	251	256	262	267	273	278	284	289	295
63	107	113	118	124	130	135	141	146	152	158	163	169	175	180	186	191	197	203	208	214	220	225	231	237	242	248	254	259	265	270	278	282	287	293	299	304
64	110	116	122	128	134	140	145	151	157	163	169	174	180	186	192	197	204	209	215	221	227	232	238	244	250	256	262	267	273	279	285	291	296	302	308	314
65	114	120	126	132	138	144	150	156	162	168	174	180	186	192	198	204	210	216	222	228	234	240	246	252	258	264	270	276	282	288	294	300	306	312	318	324
66	118	124	130	136	142	148	155	161	167	173	179	186	192	198	204	210	216	223	229	235	241	247	253	260	266	272	278	284	291	297	303	309	315	322	328	334
67	121	127	134	140	146	153	159	166	172	178	185	191	198	204	211	217	223	230	236	242	249	255	261	268	274	280	287	293	299	306	312	319	325	331	338	344
68	125	131	138	144	151	158	164	171	177	184	190	197	203	210	216	223	230	236	243	249	256	262	269	276	282	289	295	302	308	315	322	328	335	341	348	354
69	128	135	142	149	155	162	169	176	182	189	196	203	209	216	223	230	236	243	250	257	263	270	277	284	291	297	304	311	318	324	331	338	345	351	358	365
70	132	139	146	153	160	167	174	181	188	195	202	209	216	222	229	236	243	250	257	264	271	278	285	292	299	306	313	320	327	334	341	348	355	362	369	376
71	136	143	150	157	165	172	179	186	193	200	208	215	222	229	236	243	250	257	265	272	279	286	293	301	308	315	322	329	338	343	351	358	365	372	379	386
72	140	147	154	162	169	177	184	191	199	206	213	221	228	235	242	250	258	265	272	279	287	294	302	309	316	324	331	338	346	353	361	368	375	383	390	397
73	144	151	159	166	174	182	189	197	204	212	219	227	235	242	250	257	265	272	280	288	295	302	310	318	325	333	340	348	355	363	371	378	386	393	401	408
74	148	155	163	171	179	186	194	202	210	218	225	233	241	249	256	264	272	280	287	295	303	311	319	326	334	342	350	358	365	373	381	389	396	404	412	420
75	152	160	168	176	184	192	200	208	216	224	232	240	248	256	264	272	279	287	295	303	311	319	327	335	343	351	359	367	375	383	391	399	407	415	423	431
76	156	164	172	180	189	197	205	213	221	230	238	246	254	263	271	279	287	295	304	312	320	328	336	344	353	361	369	377	385	394	402	410	418	426	435	443

Source: Adapted from National Heart, Lung, and Blood Institute: Clinical Guidelines on the Identification, Evaluation, and Treatment of Overweight and Obesity in Adults: the Evidence Report.
See http://www.nhlbhi.nih.gov/guidelines/obesity/bmi_tbl.pdf

![CONN'S logo]

CONN'S
CURRENT
THERAPY
2022

CONN'S CURRENT THERAPY 2022

RICK D. KELLERMAN, MD
Professor and Chair
Department of Family and Community Medicine
University of Kansas School of Medicine–Wichita
Wichita, Kansas

DAVID P. RAKEL, MD
Esther Millard Endowed Professor & Chair
Department of Family Medicine and Community Health
University of Wisconsin School of Medicine and Public Health
Madison, Wisconsin

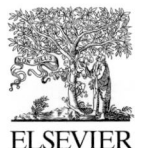

ELSEVIER

ELSEVIER
1600 John F. Kennedy Blvd.
Ste 1600
Philadelphia, PA 19103-2899

CONN'S CURRENT THERAPY 2022

ISBN: 978-0-323-83378-3

Notice

Practitioners and researchers must always rely on their own experience and knowledge in evaluating and using any information, methods, compounds or experiments described herein. Because of rapid advances in the medical sciences, in particular, independent verification of diagnoses and drug dosages should be made. To the fullest extent of the law, no responsibility is assumed by Elsevier, authors, editors or contributors for any injury and/or damage to persons or property as a matter of products liability, negligence or otherwise, or from any use or operation of any methods, products, instructions, or ideas contained in the material herein.

ISBN: 978-0-323-83378-3

Senior Content Strategy: Charlotta Kryhl
Senior Content Development Manager: Katie DeFrancesco
Publishing Services Manager: Catherine Jackson
Senior Project Manager: Kate Mannix
Design Direction: Renee Duenow

Printed in India

Last digit is the print number: 9   8   7   6   5   4   3   2   1

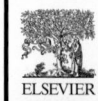

Working together
to grow libraries in
developing countries

www.elsevier.com • www.bookaid.org

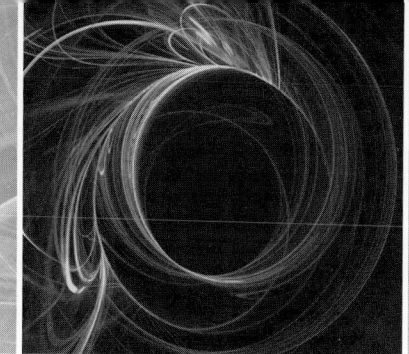

Contributors

Mustafa Abdul-Hussein, MD, MSCR
Department of Gastroenterology and Hepatology, St. Anthony Hospital, Oklahoma City, Oklahoma
Gastroesophageal Reflux Disease (GERD)

Sunil Abhyankar, MD
Professor of Medicine, Midwest Stem Cell Therapy Center and the Hematological Malignancy, Cellular Therapy Program, University of Kansas Medical Center, Kansas City, Kansas
Stem Cell Therapy

Rodney D. Adam, MD
Professor of Pathology and Medicine, Aga Khan University, Nairobi, Kenya; Professor Emeritus, University of Arizona Health Sciences Center, Tucson, Arizona
Giardiasis

Paul C. Adams, MD
Professor of Medicine, University of Western Ontario; Gastroenterologist, University Hospital, London, Ontario, Canada
Hemochromatosis

Nelson Iván Agudelo Higuita, MD
Associate Professor, Department of Internal Medicine, University of Oklahoma Health Sciences Center, Oklahoma City, Oklahoma
Plague

Omar G. Ahmed, MD
Clinical Faculty, Otolaryngology-Head and Neck Surgery, Houston Methodist Hospital, Houston, Texas
Obstructive Sleep Apnea; Rhinitis

Lee Akst, MD
Director, Johns Hopkins Voice Center, Assistant Professor of Otolaryngology–Head and Neck Surgery, The Johns Hopkins Medical Institute, Baltimore, Maryland
Hoarseness and Laryngitis

Kelley P. Anderson, MD
Adjunct Clinical Professor of Medicine, University of Wisconsin School of Medicine and Public Health, Madison, Wisconsin; Department of Cardiology, Marshfield Clinic, Marshfield, Wisconsin
Heart Block

Paul Andre, MD
Assistant Professor, Department of Internal Medicine, University of New Mexico School of Medicine, Albuquerque, New Mexico
Tachycardias

Gregory M. Anstead, MD, PhD
Staff Physician, Audie L. Murphy Memorial Veterans Affairs Hospital; Professor, Department of Medicine, University of Texas Health, San Antonio, Texas
Coccidioidomycosis

Ann M. Aring, MD
Clinical Assistant Professor of Family Medicine, College of Medicine and Public Health, The Ohio State University; Associate Program Director, Family Medicine Residency, OhioHealth Riverside Methodist Hospital, Columbus, Ohio
Drug Hypersensitivity Reactions; Rhinosinusitis

Arash Arshi, MD
Interventional Cardiology, Cardiovascular Disease, OhioHealth, Columbus, Ohio
Valvular Heart Disease

Danny Avalos, MD
Assistant Professor, Gastroenterology, Herbert Wertheim College of Medicine–Florida International University, Miami, Florida
Inflammatory Bowel Disease

Cecilio M. Azar, MD
Associate in Medicine, Division of Gastroenterology, Department of Internal Medicine, American University of Beirut Medical Center, Beirut, Lebanon
Bleeding Esophageal Varices

Amir Azarbal, MD
Cardiology Fellow, Fletcher Allen Health Care, Burlington, Vermont
Pericarditis

Zachary J. Baeseman, MD, MPH
Associate Medical Director, ThedaCare Physicians, Wild Rose and Appleton, Wisconsin; Adjunct Professor of Family Medicine, Department of Family Medicine, Medical College of Wisconsin, Milwaukee, Wisconsin; Adjunct Faculty of Family Medicine, University of Wisconsin School of Medicine and Public Health, Madison, Wisconsin
Vaginal Bleeding in Pregnancy

Justin Bailey, MD
Associate Professor of Family Medicine, University of Washington School of Medicine; Director, Procedures Institute, Family Medicine Residency of Idaho, Boise, Idaho
Gaseousness, Indigestion, Nausea, and Vomiting; Palpitations

Mandeep Bajaj, MD
Professor of Medicine, Baylor College of Medicine, Houston, Texas
Hyperlipidemia

Vladimer Bakhutashvili, MD
West Virginia University School of Medicine, Morgantown, West Virginia
Nonalcoholic Fatty Liver Disease

Federico Balagué, MD
Médecin agree, Rheumatology, HFR Fribourg-hôpital cantonal, Fribourg, Switzerland
Spine Pain

Matthew Banti, MD
Physician, Department of Urology, University of Kansas Medical Center, Kansas City, Kansas
Hematuria

Bradley E. Barth, MD
Associate Professor, Department of Emergency Medicine, University of Kansas Medical Center, Kansas City, Kansas
Burns

Gina M. Basello, DO
Assistant Clinical Professor, Family and Social Medicine, Albert Einstein College of Medicine; Vice Chair, Department of Family Medicine, Director, Family Medicine Residency Program, Associate Director, Palliative Medicine, Jamaica Hospital Medical Center, New York, New York
Fever

Renee M. Bassaly, DO
Associate Professor, Female Pelvic Medicine and Reconstructive Surgery, Department of Obstetrics and Gynecology, Division Director and Fellowship Director, University of South Florida, Tampa, Florida
Urinary Incontinence

Adel Bassily-Marcus, MD
Associate Professor, Surgical Critical Care, The Mount Sinai Hospital, New York, New York
Targeted Temperature Management (Therapeutic Hypothermia)

Julie M. Baughn, MD
Consultant, Sleep Medicine, Mayo Clinic, Rochester, Minnesota
Pediatric Sleep Disorders

Aleksandr Belakovskiy, MD
Assistant Professor, Family Medicine, University of Michigan, Ann Arbor, Michigan
Erectile Dysfunction

Ronen Ben-Ami, MD
Head, Infectious Disease Unit, Tel Aviv Sourasky Medical Center, Tel Aviv, Israel
Cat Scratch Disease

Hassan Bencheqroun, MD
Assistant Clinical Professor, Pulmonary and Critical Care, University of California Riverside School of Medicine, Riverside, California
Pruritus

David I. Bernstein, MD
Professor Emeritus of Medicine, Division of Immunology, Allergy, and Rheumatology, Department of Internal Medicine, University of Cincinnati College of Medicine, Cincinnati, Ohio
Hypersensitivity Pneumonitis

Jonathan A. Bernstein, MD
Department of Internal Medicine, Division of Immunology, Rheumatology and Allergy, University of Cincinnati College of Medicine, Cincinnati, Ohio
Anaphylaxis

Caroline Beyer, MD
Resident, Family Medicine Residency of Idaho, Boise, Idaho
Palpitations

Kristin Schmid Biggerstaff, MD
Associate Professor, Ophthalmology, Baylor College of Medicine; Glaucoma Staff, Eye Care Line, Michael E. DeBakey Veteran's Affairs Medical Center, Houston, Texas
Glaucoma

Mitchell Birt, MD
Assistant Professor, Department of Orthopaedic Surgery, University of Kansas Medical Center, Kansas City, Kansas
Osteomyelitis

William Blum, MD
Professor and Director, Acute Leukemia Program, Winship Cancer Institute of Emory University, Atlanta, Georgia
Acute Leukemia in Adults

Diana Bolotin, MD, PhD
Associate Professor, Director of Dermatologic Surgery, Section of Dermatology, University of Chicago, Chicago, Illinois
Nonmelanoma Cancer of the Skin

Rachel A. Bonnema, MD, MS
Associate Professor of Medicine, University of Nebraska Medical Center, Omaha, Nebraska
Contraception

David Borenstein, MD
Clinical Professor of Medicine, The George Washington University Medical Center, Washington, DC
Spine Pain

Christopher Bossart, MD
Assistant Professor, Department of Emergency Medicine, University of New Mexico, Albuquerque, New Mexico
Osteoarthritis

Dee Ann Bragg, MD
Clinical Assistant Professor, Department of Family and Community Medicine, The University of Kansas School of Medicine–Wichita; Faculty, Via Christi Family Medicine Residency Program, Wichita, Kansas
Rubella and Congenital Rubella

Scott Bragg, PharmD
Associate Professor, Clinical Pharmacy and Outcomes Science, Medical University of South Carolina College of Pharmacy; Department of Family Medicine, Medical University of South Carolina, Charleston, South Carolina
Osteoporosis

Sylvia L. Brice, MD
Clinical Professor of Dermatology, University of Colorado, Denver, Colorado
Viral Diseases of the Skin

Allyson M. Briggs, MD
Chief Resident, Department of Emergency Medicine, University of Kansas Medical Center, Kansas City, Kansas
Burns

John Brill, MD, MPH
Vice-President, Population Health, Advocate Aurora Health, Milwaukee, Wisconsin
Gonorrhea

Patricia D. Brown, MD
Professor of Medicine, Department of Internal Medicine, Division of Infectious Diseases, Wayne State University School of Medicine; Associate Chief of Staff for Medicine, John D. Dingell VA Medical Center, Detroit, Michigan
Pyelonephritis

Rachel Brown, MBBS
Professor and Chair, Psychiatry and Behavioral Sciences, University of Kansas School of Medicine–Wichita, Wichita, Kansas
Autism

Peter F. Buckley, MD
Dean, School of Medicine, Virginia Commonwealth University; Executive Vice President for Medical Affairs, VCU Health, Richmond, Virginia
Schizophrenia

Sarah Burns, DO, MS
Assistant Professor, Division of Hospital Medicine, Department of Internal Medicine, University of New Mexico School of Medicine, Albuquerque, New Mexico
Acute Kidney Injury

Kenneth Byrd, DO
Assistant Professor, Division of Hematologic Malignancies and Cellular Therapeutics, Department of Internal Medicine, University of Kansas Medical Center, Kansas City, Kansas
Disseminated Intravascular Coagulation

Diego Cadavid, MD
Affiliate Instructor in Neurology, University of Massachusetts Medical School; Senior Vice President of Clinical Development, Fulcrum Therapeutics, Worchester, Massachusetts
Relapsing Fever

Thomas R. Caraccio, PharmD
Clinical Pharmacist and Toxicologist, Pharmacy Department, New York University Winthrop Hospital, Mineola, New York
Medical Toxicology

Peter J. Carek, MD, MS
Professor, Department of Family Medicine, Medical University of South Carolina; Campus Dean, MUSC AnMed Health Clinical Campus, Director of Medical Education, AnMed Health, Charleston, South Carolina
Osteoporosis

Andres F. Carrion, MD
Associate Professor of Medicine, Division of Digestive Health and Liver Disease, University of Miami, Miami, Florida
Cirrhosis

Amanda S. Cass, PharmD
Clinical Pharmacist Specialist, Thoracic Oncology, Department of Pharmaceutical Services, Vanderbilt Ingram Cancer Center, Vanderbilt University Medical Center, Nashville, Tennessee
Lung Cancer

Donald O. Castell, MD
Professor of Medicine, Division of Gastroenterology and Hepatology, Medical University of South Carolina, Charleston, South Carolina
Gastroesophageal Reflux Disease (GERD)

Anthony Peter Catinella, MD, MPH
Associate Professor of Family Medicine, Texas Tech University Health Science Center; Chair, Department of Family Medicine–Transmountain, Paul L. Foster School of Medicine, El Paso, Texas
Pulmonary Hypertension

William E. Cayley Jr., MD, MDiv
Adjunct Clinical Professor, University of Wisconsin School of Medicine and Public Health; Prevea Family Medicine Residency, Augusta and Eau Claire, Wisconsin
Chest Pain

Sonia Cerquozzi, MD
Clinical Assistant Professor, Division of Hematology and Hematologic Malignancies, University of Calgary, Calgary, Alberta, Canada
Polycythemia Vera

Alvaro Cervera, MD, PhD
Consultant Neurologist, Royal Darwin Hospital, Northern Territory, Australia
Ischemic Cerebrovascular Disease

Filomena Cetani, MD
Endocrine Unit, University Hospital of Pisa, Pisa, Italy
Hyperparathyroidism and Hypoparathyroidism

Rachel Chamberlain, MD
Assistant Professor, Department of Family and Community Medicine, Associate Program Director, Primary Care Sports Medicine Fellowship, University of New Mexico, Albuquerque, New Mexico
Osteoarthritis

Lawrence Chan, MD
Professor, Departments of Medicine, Molecular and Cellular Biology, Biochemistry and Molecular Biology, and Molecular and Human Genetics, Baylor College of Medicine, Houston, Texas
Hyperaldosteronism; Hyperlipidemia; Hyperprolactinemia

Miriam Chan, PharmD
Family Medicine Residency Program, Director of Pharmacy Education, Riverside Methodist Hospital, Columbus, Ohio
Drug Hypersensitivity Reactions; Popular Herbs and Nutritional Supplements

Zenas Chang, MD, MS
Assistant Professor, Gynecologic Oncology, Indiana University School of Medicine, Indianapolis, Indiana
Ovarian Cancer

Jimmy Chen, MD
Assistant Professor of Pediatrics, Department of Pediatrics, Division of Hospital Pediatrics, University of Florida–Jacksonville, Jacksonville, Florida
Parenteral Fluid Therapy for Infants and Children

Lin Yee Chen, MBBS, MS
Professor, Cardiovascular Division, Department of Medicine, University of Minnesota Medical School, Minneapolis, Minnesota
Atrial Fibrillation

Shingo Chihara, MD
Section of Infectious Diseases, Virginia Mason Medical Center, Seattle, Washington
Anthrax

Meera Chitlur, MD
Professor of Pediatrics, Central Michigan University; Pediatric Hematology/Oncology, Children's Hospital of Michigan; Barnhart-Lusher Hemostasis Research Endowed Chair, Department of Pediatrics, Wayne State University, Detroit, Michigan
Hemophilia and Related Conditions

Saima Chohan, MD
Clinical Assistant Professor, Department of Internal Medicine, Division of Rheumatology, University of Arizona College of Medicine, Phoenix, Arizona; Clinical Assistant Professor, Division of Clinical Education, Arizona College of Osteopathic Medicine, Glendale, Arizona
Gout and Hyperuricemia

Jacob Christensen, DO
Family Medicine, University of Mexico, Albuquerque, New Mexico
Osteoarthritis

Kuang-Yuh Chyu, MD, PhD
Health Sciences Clinical Professor of Medicine, University of California; Associate Director, Coronary Intensive Care Unit, Department of Cardiology, Cedars Sinai Medical Center, Los Angeles, California
Acute Myocardial Infarction

Joaquin E. Cigarroa, MD
Professor of Medicine, Clinical Chief, Knight Cardiovascular Institute; Division Head, Cardiology, Oregon Health & Science University, Portland, Oregon
Congenital Heart Disease

Paul Cleland, MD
Clinical Assistant Professor, Department of Family and Community Medicine, University of Kansas School of Medicine–Wichita; Associate Director, University of Kansas School of Medicine–Wichita Sports Medicine Fellowship, Wichita, Kansas
Heat-Related Illness

Matthew K. Cline, MD
Affiliate Professor, Medical University of South Carolina, Charleston, South Carolina
Antepartum Care

Laura C. Coates, MBChB, PhD
Associate Professor, Nuffield Department of Orthopaedics, Rheumatology and Musculoskeletal Sciences, University of Oxford, Oxford, Great Britain
Psoriatic Arthritis

August Colenbrander, MD
Affiliate Senior Scientist, Rehabilitation Engineering Research Center, Smith-Kettlewell Eye Research Institute, San Francisco, California
Vision Rehabilitation

Tracie C. Collins, MD, MPH, MHCDS
Dean and Professor, College of Population Health, University of New Mexico, Albuquerque, New Mexico
Peripheral Artery Disease

Ryan M. Commins, MD
Internal Medicine, Georgetown University Medical Center, Washington, DC
High Altitude Illness

Christine Conageski, MD
Associate Professor, Obstetrics and Gynecology, University of Colorado, Aurora, Colorado
Vulvar Neoplasia

John M. Conly, MD
Professor of Medicine and Microbiology, Immunology & Infectious Diseases, University of Calgary, Calgary, Alberta, Canada
Methicillin-Resistant Staphylococcus aureus

Carlo Contini, MD
Full Professor of Infectious Diseases, Director of Infectious Diseases Unit, Department of Medical Sciences, University of Ferrara, Ferrara, Italy
Toxoplasmosis

Ashley Cooper, MD
Assistant Professor of Medicine, Tulane School of Medicine, New Orleans, Louisiana
Juvenile Idiopathic Arthritis

Stacy Cooper, MD
Assistant Professor, Department of Oncology, Johns Hopkins School of Medicine, Baltimore, Maryland
Acute Leukemia in Children

Allison K. Cormier, MD
Assistant Professor of Medicine, Tulane School of Medicine, New Orleans, Louisiana
Human Immunodeficiency Virus: Treatment and Prevention

Burke A. Cunha, MD
Professor, State University of New York School of Medicine, Stony Brook, New York; Chief, Infectious Disease Division, Winthrop–University Hospital, Mineola, New York
Babesiosis; Viral and Mycoplasmal Pneumonias

Cheston B. Cunha, MD
Medical Director, Antimicrobial Stewardship, Infectious Disease Division, Alpert School of Medicine, Brown University, Providence, Rhode Island
Babesiosis; Viral and Mycoplasmal Pneumonias

Amy E. Curry, MD
Clinical Associate Professor, Department of Family and Community Medicine, University of Kansas School of Medicine–Wichita; Via Christi Family Medicine Residency, Wichita, Kansas
Pelvic Inflammatory Disease

Julia Dai, MD
Associate Professor, Director of Dermatologic Surgery, Section of Dermatology, University of Chicago, Chicago, Illinois
Nonmelanoma Cancer of the Skin

Cori L. Daines, MD
Professor, Division Chief, Director, Pediatric Pulmonary and Sleep Medicine Center, Tucson Cystic Fibrosis Center; Director, Pediatric Pulmonary Center, The University of Arizona College of Medicine, Tucson, Arizona
Cystic Fibrosis

Oriana M. Damas, MD
Assistant Professor, Director of Translational Studies for the Crohn's and Colitis Center, Division of Gastroenterology, Department of Medicine, University of Miami Miller School of Medicine, Miami, Florida
Inflammatory Bowel Disease

Beth A. Damitz, MD
Associate Professor, Family and Community Medicine, Medical College of Wisconsin, Milwaukee, Wisconsin
Immunization Practices

Nandini Datta, PhD
Physician, Department of Child and Adolescent Psychiatry, Stanford University, Stanford, California
Eating Disorders

Natalie C. Dattilo, PhD
Director of Psychology, Department of Psychiatry, Brigham and Women's Hospital, Boston, Massachusetts
Generalized Anxiety Disorder; Posttraumatic Stress Disorder

Raul Davaro, MD
Associate Professor of Clinical Medicine, University of Massachusetts, Worcester, Massachusetts
Smallpox; Whooping Cough (Pertussis)

Kevin A. David, MD
Associate Professor of Medicine, Rutgers Robert Wood Johnson Medical School; Member, Rutgers Cancer Institute of New Jersey, New Brunswick, New Jersey
Non-Hodgkin Lymphoma

André de Leon, MD
Family Medicine/Sports Medicine, OhioHealth Primary Care and Pediatric Physicians, Delaware, Ohio
Chronic Diarrhea

Tate de Leon, MD
Faculty, Family Medicine, Eisenhower Family Medicine Residency, Rancho Mirage, California
Acute Diarrhea

Alexei O. DeCastro, MD
Associate Professor, Department of Family Medicine, Medical University of South Carolina, Charleston, South Carolina
Osteoporosis

Katharine C. DeGeorge, MD, MS
Associate Professor, Department of Family Medicine, University of Virginia, Charlottesville, Virginia
Bacterial Pneumonia; Asthma in Children

Thomas G. DeLoughery, MD
Professor of Medicine, Pathology, and Pediatrics, Oregon Health & Science University, Portland, Oregon
Hemolytic Anemias

Atul Deodhar, MD, MRCP
Professor of Medicine, Division of Arthritis & Rheumatic Diseases, Oregon Health & Science University, Portland, Oregon
Axial Spondyloarthritis

Urmi Desai, MD, MS
Assistant Professor of Medicine, Center for Family and Community Medicine, Director, Foundations of Clinical Medicine Clerkships, Columbia University Irving Medical Center, New York, New York
Vulvovaginitis

Clio Dessinioti, MD, MSc, PhD
Dermatologist, Andreas Sygros Hospital, Athens, Greece
Parasitic Diseases of the Skin

Michael P. Diamond, MD
Leon Henri Charbonnier Endowed Chair in Reproductive Endocrinology, Professor of Obstetrics and Gynecology, Associate Dean for Research, Medical College of Georgia; Senior Vice President for Research, Augusta University, Augusta, Georgia
Infertility

Catherine Do, MD
Assistant Professor of Medicine, University of New Mexico, Albuquerque, New Mexico
Chronic Kidney Disease

Geoffrey A. Donnan, MD
Department of Neurology, University of Melbourne Faculty of Medicine, Dentistry, and Health Sciences; Florey Neuroscience Institutes, Carlton South, Victoria, Australia
Ischemic Cerebrovascular Disease

John N. Dorsch, MD
Professor Emeritus, Department of Family and Community Medicine, University of Kansas School of Medicine–Wichita, Wichita, Kansas
Red Eye

Chad Douglas, MD, PharmD
Assistant Professor of Family and Preventive Medicine, Medical & Didactic Education Director, University of Oklahoma Health Sciences Center; Department of Family and Preventive Medicine, Medical Director–OU Physicians Health and Wellness Clinic, Oklahoma City, Oklahoma
Erythema Multiforme

Dar Dowlatshahi, MD, PhD
Professor, Department of Medicine (Neurology), University of Ottawa; Senior Scientist, Ottawa Hospital Research Institute, Ottowa, Ontario, Canada
Intracerebral Hemorrhage

Shannon Dowler, MD
Adjunct Associate Professor, Department of Family Medicine, University of North Carolina Chapel Hill, Asheville, North Carolina
Nongonococcal Urethritis

Douglas A. Drevets, MD
Professor and Chief, Section of Infectious Diseases, University of Oklahoma Health Sciences Center; Staff Physician, Veterans Affairs Medical Center, Oklahoma City, Oklahoma
Plague

Samuel C. Dudley Jr., MD, PhD
Professor, Department of Medicine, Division of Cardiology, University of Minnesota, Minneapolis, Minnesota
Atrial Fibrillation

Peter R. Duggan, MD
Associate Clinical Professor of Medicine, University of Calgary, Calgary, Alberta, Canada
Polycythemia Vera

Kim Eagle, MD
Albion Walter Hewlett Professor of Internal Medicine, Director, Cardiovascular Center, University of Michigan Health System, Ann Arbor, Michigan
Angina Pectoris

Leigh M. Eck, MD
Associate Professor of Medicine, Program Director–Internal Medicine Residency Program, Vice Chair of GME–Department of Internal Medicine, The University of Kansas Health System, Kansas City, Kansas
Thyroiditis

Genevieve L. Egnatios, MD
Dermatologist, Scottsdale Skin Boutique and Dermatology, Scottsdale, Arizona
Contact Dermatitis

Wissam El Atrouni, MD, MSc
Associate Professor, Division of Infectious Diseases, University of Kansas Hospital, Kansas City, Kansas
Osteomyelitis

Dirk M. Elston, MD
Professor and Chairman, Department of Dermatology and Dermatologic Surgery, Medical University of South Carolina, Charleston, South Carolina
Diseases of the Hair

John M. Embil, MD
Professor, Departments of Internal Medicine (Section of Infectious Diseases) and Medical Microbiology, Consultant, Infectious Diseases, Director, BSc(Med) Program, University of Manitoba; Medical Director, Infection Prevention and Control Unit, Health Sciences Centre and Winnipeg Regional Health Authority, Winnipeg, Manitoba, Canada
Blastomycosis

Scott K. Epstein, MD
Dean for Educational Affairs and Professor of Medicine, Tufts University School of Medicine, Boston, Massachusetts
Acute Respiratory Failure

Susan Evans, MD
Assistant Professor, Department of Family Medicine, University of Nebraska Medical Center
Iron Deficiency Anemia

Andrew M. Evens, DO, MSc
Professor of Medicine, Rutgers Robert Wood Johnson Medical School; Associate Director for Clinical Services, Rutgers Cancer Institute of New Jersey; Director, Lymphoma Program, Division of Blood Disorders, Medical Director, Oncology Service Line, RWJBarnabas Health, New Brunswick, New Jersey
Non-Hodgkin Lymphoma

J. Barry Fagan, MD
Service Chief, Specialty Medicine, Central Ohio VA Healthcare System, Columbus, Ohio
Chronic Obstructive Pulmonary Disease

Mark Fairweather, MD
Associate Surgeon, Brigham and Women's Hospital, Boston, Massachusetts
Tumors of the Stomach

Marni J. Falk, MD
Professor, Department of Pediatrics, University of Pennsylvania Perelman School of Medicine; Executive Director, Mitochondrial Medicine Frontier Program, Division of Human Genetics, Department of Pediatrics, The Children's Hospital of Philadelphia, Philadelphia, Pennsylvania
Mitochondrial Disease

Anna Faris, MD
Resident Physician, Department of Urology, University of Michigan, Ann Arbor, Michigan
Trauma to the Genitourinary Tract

Anthony J. Faugno III, MD
Instructor in Medicine, Department of Medicine, Division of Pulmonary, Critical Care and Sleep, Tufts Medical Center, Boston, Massachusetts
Acute Respiratory Failure

Kinder Fayssoux, MD
Center for Family Medicine, Eisenhower Medical Associates, La Quinta, California
Bacterial Infections of the Urinary Tract in Women

Dorianne Feldman, MD, MSPT
Medical Director, Inpatient Rehabilitation, Department of Physical Medicine and Rehabilitation, Johns Hopkins University School of Medicine, Baltimore, Maryland
Rehabilitation of the Stroke Patient

Terry D. Fife, MD
Director, Otoneurology and Balance Disorders, Barrow Neurological Institute, Phoenix, Arizona
Ménière's Disease

David J. Finley, MD
Co-Director, Complex Airway Program, Surgeon, Thoracic Service, Memorial Sloan Kettering Cancer Center, New York, New York
Pleural Effusions and Empyema

Jonathon Firnhaber, MD, MAEd, MBA
Residency Program Director, Department of Family Medicine, East Carolina University, Greenville, North Carolina
Diseases of the Nail

Lynn Fisher, MD
Assistant Professor, Family & Community Medicine, University of Kansas School of Medicine-Witchita, Wichita, Kansas
Red Eye

William E. Fisher, MD
Professor, Clinical Vice-Chair and Chief, Division of General Surgery, George L. Jordan, MD Chair of General Surgery, Vice Chair, Clinical Affairs, Director, Elkins Pancreas Center, Michael E. DeBakey Department of Surgery, Chief, Surgery Service Line, Baylor St. Luke's Medical Center, Houston, Texas
Acute and Chronic Pancreatitis

Maria Fleseriu, MD
Professor of Medicine and Neurological Surgery, Director of Pituitary Center, Oregon Health & Science University, Portland, Oregon
Adrenocortical Insufficiency; Hypopituitarism

Donald C. Fletcher, MD
Adjunct Associate Professor, Department of Ophthalmology, University of Kansas School of Medicine, Kansas City, Kansas
Vision Rehabilitation

Jeffrey Michael Foster, DO
Clinical Assistant Professor of Anesthesiology, University of Missouri at Kansas City; Anesthesiology and Interventional Pain Medicine, Saint Luke's Hospital of Kansas City, Kansas City, Missouri
Fibromyalgia

Jennifer Frank, MD
Chief Medical Officer, Clinically Integrated Network, Theda Care Physicians, Neenah, Wisconsin
Syphilis

Ellen W. Freeman, PhD
Research Professor, Obstetrics/Gynecology, Perelman School of Medicine, University of Pennsylvania, Philadelphia, Pennsylvania
Premenstrual Syndrome

David A. Frenz, MD
Adjunct Clinical Assistant Professor, Department of Family Medicine & Community Health, University of Minnesota, Minneapolis, Minnesota
Alcohol Use Disorders

Ruchi Gaba, MD
Endocrinology, Diabetes and Metabolism, Baylor College of Medicine, Houston, Texas
Hyperaldosteronism

Melissa Gaines, MD
Cox Senior Health, Geriatrics Division, Springfield, Missouri
Constipation

Mark E. Garcia, MD
Department of Internal Medicine, Division of Cardiology, University of New Mexico, Albuquerque, New Mexico
Congestive Heart Failure

Marc G. Ghany, MD, MHSc
Clinical Research Section, Liver Diseases Branch, National Institute of Diabetes and Digestive and Kidney Diseases, National Institutes of Health, Bethesda, Maryland
Hepatitis A, B, D, and E

Muhammad Ahmad Ghazi, MD
Family Physician, Jacksonville, Florida
Pruritus Ani and Vulvae

Geoffrey Gibney, MD
Co-Leader Melanoma Program, Lombardi Comprehensive Cancer Center, Medstar Georgetown University Hospital, Washington, DC
Melanoma

Donald L. Gilbert, MD, MS
Professor of Pediatrics and Neurology, Cincinnati Children's Hospital Medical Center, Cincinnati, Ohio
Gilles de la Tourette Syndrome

Karissa Gilchrist, MD
Assistant Professor, Department of Family and Community Medicine, University of Kansas School of Medicine–Wichita, Wichita, Kansas
Bacterial Diseases of the Skin

Erin A. Gillaspie, MD, MPH
Assistant Professor of Thoracic Surgery, Head of Thoracic Surgery Robotics, Vanderbilt University Medical Center, Nashville, Tennessee
Lung Cancer

Tarvinder Gilotra, MD
Department of Infectious Disease, Kenmore Specialty Center, Kenmore, New York
Intestinal Parasites

Mark T. Gladwin, MD
Jack D. Myers Distinguished Professor and Chair, Department of Medicine, Director, Pittsburgh Heart, Lung, Blood and Vascular Medicine Institute, UPMC and the University of Pittsburgh School of Medicine, Pittsburgh, Pennsylvania
Sickle Cell Disease

Stephen J. Gluckman, MD
Professor of Medicine, Perelman School of Medicine, University of Pennsylvania, Philadelphia, Pennsylvania
Myalgic Encephalomyelitis/Chronic Fatigue Syndrome

Andrew W. Goddard, MD
Professor of Psychiatry, University of California, San Francisco; Fresno Medical Education & Research Program, San Francisco, California
Generalized Anxiety Disorder

Kyle Goerl, MD
Clinical Assistant Professor, Department of Family and Community Medicine, University of Kansas School of Medicine-Wichita, Wichita, Kansas; Team Physician, Kansas State University Athletics; Sports and Family Medicine, Lafene Health Center, Kansas State University, Manhattan, Kansas
Bursitis and Tendinopathy

Mark S. Gold, MD
Professor, Department of Psychiatry, Washington University School of Medicine, St. Louis, Missouri
Drug Use Disorders

Amy Goldstein, MD
Associate Professor, Department of Pediatrics, University of Pennsylvania Perelman School of Medicine; Clinical Director, Mitochondrial Medicine Frontier Program, Division of Human Genetics, Department of Pediatrics, Children's Hospital of Philadelphia, Philadelphia, Pennsylvania
Mitochondrial Disease

Marlís González-Fernández, MD, PhD
Associate Professor, Departments of Physical Medicine and Rehabilitation and Orthopaedic Surgery, Vice Chair, Clinical Affairs, Department of Physical Medicine and Rehabilitation, The Johns Hopkins University School of Medicine, Baltimore, Maryland
Rehabilitation of the Stroke Patient

Gregory Goodwin, MD
Assistant Professor of Pediatrics, Harvard Medical School; Senior Associate Physician in Pediatrics, Boston Children's Hospital, Boston, Massachusetts
Diabetes Mellitus in Children

Aidar R. Gosmanov, MD, PhD, DMSc
Chief, Endocrinology Section, Stratton Veterans Affairs Medical Center; Associate Professor of Medicine, Division of Endocrinology, Albany Medical College, Albany, New York
Diabetic Ketoacidosis

Luigi Gradoni, PhD
Research Director, Unit of Vector-Borne Diseases, Department of Infectious Diseases, Istituto Superiore di Sanità, Rome, Italy
Leishmaniasis

Timothy P. Graham, MD
Program Director, Mount Carmel Family Medicine Residency; Chair, Department of Family Medicine, Mount Carmel St. Ann's Hospital, Westerville, Ohio
Hypertension

Jane M. Grant-Kels, MD
Professor of Dermatology, Pathology and Pediatrics, Founding Chair Emeritus and Vice Chair, Department of Dermatology, Director, the Cutaneous Oncology Center and Melanoma Program, University of Connecticut Health Center, Farmington, Connecticut
Nevi

Kristine Grdinovac, MD
Assistant Professor, Endocrinology, Metabolism and Genetics, The University of Kansas Healthcare System, Kansas City, Kansas
Diabetes Mellitus in Adults

Leslie A. Greenberg, MD
Associate Professor of Family and Community Medicine, University of Nevada Reno School of Medicine; Assistant Program Director, University of Nevada Reno Family Medicine Residency Program, Reno, Nevada
Keloids

William M. Greene, MD
Associate Professor, Addiction Medicine Division, Department of Psychiatry, University of Florida College of Medicine, Gainesville, Florida
Drug Use Disorders

Joseph Greensher, MD
Professor of Pediatrics, Stony Brook University Medical Center School of Medicine, Stony Brook, New York; Medical Director and Associate Chair, Department of Pediatrics, Long Island Regional Poison and Drug Information Center, Winthrop-University Hospital, Mineola, New York
Medical Toxicology

David S. Gregory, MD
Assistant Clinical Professor of Family Medicine, Virginia Commonwealth University School of Medicine, Richmond, Virginia; Associate Clinical Professor of Family Medicine, University of Virginia School of Medicine, Charlottesville, Virginia; Faculty Physician, Virginia Tech–Carilion Clinic Family Medicine Residency, Roanoke, Virginia
Resuscitation of the Newborn

Justin Greiwe, MD
Clinical Assistant Professor of Medicine, Division of Immunology, Allergy, and Rheumatology, University of Cincinnati, Cincinnati, Ohio
Anaphylaxis

Melissa Hague, MD
Clinical Associate Professor, Obstetrics and Gynecology, University of Kansas School of Medicine–Wichita, Wichita, Kansas
Female Sexual Dysfunction

Rebat M. Halder, MD
Professor Emeritus and Chair Emeritus, Department of Dermatology, Howard University College of Medicine, Washington, DC
Pigmentary Disorders

Alan M. Hall, MD
Associate Professor of Internal Medicine and Pediatrics, Divisions of Hospital Medicine and Hospital Pediatrics, Departments of Internal Medicine and Pediatrics, University of Kentucky College of Medicine, Lexington, Kentucky
Parenteral Fluid Therapy for Infants and Children

Lynn E. Harman, MD
Clinical Associate Professor of Ophthalmology, University of South Florida Morsani College of Medicine, Tampa, Florida
Dry Eye Syndrome; Uveitis

Kari R. Harris, MD
Associate Professor, Department of Pediatrics, University of Kansas School of Medicine–Wichita, Wichita, Kansas
Adolescent Health

Taylor B. Harrison, MD
Associate Professor, Neuromuscular Division, Program Director, Clinical Neurophysiology Fellowship, Department of Neurology, Emory University, Atlanta, Georgia
Myasthenia Gravis

Adam L. Hartman, MD
Program Director, Division of Clinical Research, National Institute of Neurological Disorders and Stroke, National Institutes of Health, Bethesda, Maryland
Epilepsy in Infants and Children

James W. Haynes, MD
Professor and Chair, Department of Family Medicine, The University of Tennessee Health Sciences Center College of Medicine–Chattanooga; Family Medicine, Erlanger Health System, Chattanooga, Tennessee
Uterine Leiomyoma

Joel J. Heidelbaugh, MD
Clinical Professor, Departments of Family Medicine and Urology, Medical Education and Clerkship Director, Department of Family Medicine, Director, Patients and Populations Branch, University of Michigan Medical School, Ann Arbor, Michigan
Erectile Dysfunction

Molly A. Hinshaw, MD
Associate Professor of Dermatology, Section Chief of Dermatopathology, Director of Dermatology Nail Clinic, University of Wisconsin School of Medicine and Public Health, Dermatopathology Laboratory, Madison, Wisconsin
Connective Tissue Disorders; Cutaneous Vasculitis

Brandon Hockenberry, MD
Sports Medicine Physician, Renown Sports Medicine, Reno, Nevada
Sports-Related Head Injuries

Raymond J. Hohl, MD, PhD
Director, Penn State Cancer Institute, Hershey, Pennsylvania
Thalassemia

Therese Holguin, MD
Assistant Professor of Dermatology, University of New Mexico, Albuquerque, New Mexico
Fungal Infections of the Skin

Sarah A. Holstein, MD, PhD
Associate Professor, Department of Internal Medicine, University of Nebraska Medical Center, Omaha, Nebraska
Thalassemia

Michael Holyoak, MD
St. Luke's Clinic–Idaho Endocrinology, Meridian, Idaho
Thyroid Cancer

Gretchen Homan, MD
Associate Professor, Department of Pediatrics, University of Kansas School of Medicine–Wichita, Wichita, Kansas
Pediatric Failure to Thrive

Kevin Hommema, BSME
Principal Research Scientist, Battelle, Columbus, Ohio
Biologic Agents Reference Chart; Toxic Chemical Agents Reference Chart

Laurie A.M. Hommema, MD
Associate Program Director, Family Medicine Residency, Riverside Methodist Hospital; Medical Director, Provider and Associate Well-Being, Quality and Patient Safety, OhioHealth, Columbus, Ohio
Biologic Agents Reference Chart; Toxic Chemical Agents Reference Chart

Leora Horn, MD, MSc
Ingram Associate Professor of Cancer Research, Associate Professor of Medicine, Vanderbilt Ingram Cancer Center, Vanderbilt University Medical Center, Nashville, Tennessee
Lung Cancer

Ahmad Reza Hossani-Madani, MD, MS
Dermatologist, Kaiser Permanente, Upper Marlboro, Maryland
Pigmentary Disorders

Steven A. House, MD
Professor, Department of Family and Geriatric Medicine, Program Director, University of Louisville/Glasgow Family Medicine Residency, Glasgow, Kentucky
Pain; Palliative and End-of-Life Care

Sarah Houssayni, MD
Clinical Associate Professor, Department of Family and Community Medicine, University of Kansas School of Medicine–Wichita; Pediatrics, Via Christi Family Medicine Residency, Wichita, Kansas
Encopresis

William J. Hueston, MD
Associate Provost for Education, Senior Associate Dean for Medical Education, Medical College of Wisconsin, Milwaukee, Wisconsin
Hyperthyroidism; Hypothyroidism

Alison N. Huffstetler, MD
Assistant Professor of Family Medicine, Virginia Commonwealth University, Richmond, Virginia
Bacterial Pneumonia

Oyetokunbo Ibidapo-Obe, MD
Assistant Professor, Director of Women's Health, Department of Family Medicine, University of Texas Medical Branch, Galveston, Texas
Infective Endocarditis

Gretchen M. Irwin, MD, MBA
Associate Professor, Department of Family and Community Medicine, Associate Dean for Graduate Medical Education, University of Kansas School of Medicine–Wichita, Wichita, Kansas
Otitis Media

Daniel Isaac, DO
Assistant Professor of Medicine, Division of Hematology/Oncology, College of Human Medicine, Michigan State University, East Lansing, Michigan
Chronic Leukemias

Gerald A. Isenberg, MD
Professor of Surgery, Director, Surgical Undergraduate Medical Education, Sidney Kimmel Medical College; Program Director, Colorectal Surgery Residency, Thomas Jefferson University Hospitals, Philadelphia, Pennsylvania
Tumors of the Colon and Rectum

Alan C. Jackson, MD
Professor, Section of Neurology, Internal Medicine, University of Manitoba, Winnipeg, Manitoba, Canada
Rabies

Kurt M. Jacobson, MD
Associate Professor of Medicine, Cardiovascular Medicine Division, University of Wisconsin School of Medicine and Public Health, Madison, Wisconsin
Mitral Valve Prolapse

Jose A. Jaller, MD
Department of Medicine, Division of Dermatology, Albert Einstein College of Medicine, Bronx, New York
Venous Ulcers

W. Ennis James, MD
Assistant Professor, Pulmonary and Critical Care Medicine, Medical University of South Carolina, Charleston, South Carolina
Sarcoidosis

Xiaoming Jia, MD
Instructor, Medicine, Baylor College of Medicine, Houston, Texas
Hyperlipidemia

Casey R. Johnson, MD, MS
Resident Physician, Department of Pediatric and Adolescent Medicine, Mayo Clinic, Rochester, Minnesota
Obesity in Children

Lisa M. Johnson, MD
Associate Professor, Department of Family Medicine, University of Cincinnati College of Medicine, Cincinnati, Ohio
Acne Vulgaris; Rosacea

Joshua S. Jolissaint, MD
Department of Surgery, Brigham and Women's Hospital, Boston, Massachusetts
Atelectasis; Pancreatic Cancer

Marc A. Judson, MD
Chief, Division of Pulmonary and Critical Care Medicine, Albany Medical College, Albany, New York
Sarcoidosis

Tamilarasu Kadhiravan, MD
Additional Professor of Medicine, Jawaharlal Institute of Postgraduate Medical Education and Research, Puducherry, India
Typhoid Fever

Rachna Kalia, MD
Clinical Assistant Professor, Department of Psychiatry and Behavioral Sciences, University of Kansas School of Medicine–Wichita, Wichita, Kansas
Obsessive-Compulsive Disorder

Sagar Kamprath, MD
Associate Professor, Family Medicine, University of Texas Medical Branch, Galveston, Texas
Post-COVID Syndrome

Jessica Rachel Kanter, MD
Fellow, Reproductive Endocrinology and Infertility, Hospital of the University of Pennsylvania, Philadelphia, Pennsylvania
Infertility

Dilip R. Karnad, MD
Consultant in Critical Care, Jupiter Hospital, Thane, Maharashtra, India
Tetanus

Rudruidee Karnchanasorn, MD
Associate Professor, Internal Medicine, The University of Kansas Medical Center, Kansas City, Kansas
Thyroid Cancer

Andreas Katsabas, MD, PhD
Professor of Dermatology, University of Athens School of Medicine, Athens, Greece
Parasitic Diseases of the Skin

Ben Z. Katz, MD
Professor of Pediatrics, Northwestern University Feinberg School of Medicine, Chicago, Illinois
Infectious Mononucleosis

Rebecca Katzman, MD
Clinical Assistant Professor, Family Medicine, University of Washington, Seattle, Washington
Palpitations

Andrew M. Kaunitz, MD
Professor and Associate Chairman, Department of Obstetrics and Gynecology, University of Florida College of Medicine–Jacksonville; Medical Director and Director of Menopause and Gynecologic Ultrasound Services, University of Florida Women's Health Specialists–Emerson, Jacksonville, Florida
Menopause

B. Mark Keegan, MD
Professor of Neurology, Mayo Clinic College of Medicine, Division Chair, Multiple Sclerosis and Autoimmune Neurology, Rochester, Minnesota
Multiple Sclerosis

Rick D. Kellerman, MD
Professor and Chair, Department of Family and Community Medicine, University of Kansas School of Medicine–Wichita, Wichita, Kansas
Chikungunya; Zika Virus Disease

Scott Kellermann, MD, MPH
Faculty, University of San Francisco, San Francisco, California; Founder, Bwindi Community Hospital, Buhoma, Uganda
Chikungunya; Zika Virus Disease

Christina M. Kelly, MD
Assistant Professor, Family Medicine, Uniformed Services University of the Health Sciences, Bethesda, Maryland
Ectopic Pregnancy

Sheevaun Khaki, MD
Assistant Professor, General Pediatrics, Medical Director, Mother Baby Unit, Director of Pediatric Electives, Oregon Health & Science University, Portland, Oregon
Infant Hyperbilirubinemia

Arthur Y. Kim, MD
Associate Professor of Medicine, Harvard Medical School; Division of Infectious Diseases, Massachusetts General Hospital, Boston, Massachusetts
Hepatitis C

Haejin Kim, MD
Senior Staff Allergist, Division of Allergy and Clinical Immunology, Department of Internal Medicine, Henry Ford Health System, Detroit, Michigan
Hypersensitivity Pneumonitis

Robert S. Kirsner, MD, PhD
Chair & Harvey Blank Professor, Dr. Phillip Frost Department of Dermatology & Cutaneous Surgery, University of Miami Miller School of Medicine, Miami, Florida
Venous Ulcers

Sonam Kiwalkar, MBBS
Assistant Professor, Elson S. Floyd College of Medicine, Washington State University, Spokane, Washington
Axial Spondyloarthritis

Janice Knoefel, MD, MPH
Professor, Departments of Internal Medicine (Geriatrics) and Neurology, Memory & Aging Center, New Mexico Alzheimer Disease Research Center, University of New Mexico, Albuquerque, New Mexico
Alzheimer's Disease

Amanda Kolb, MD
Instructor, Department of Family Medicine, University of Virginia, Charlottesville, Virginia
Asthma in Children

Bhanu Prakash Kolla, MD, MRCPsych
Assistant Professor of Psychiatry and Psychology, Mayo Clinic College of Medicine; Senior Associate Consultant, Center for Sleep Medicine, Department of Psychiatry and Psychology, Mayo Clinic and Foundation, Rochester, Minnesota
Sleep Disorders

Frederick K. Korley, MD
Robert E. Meyerhoff Assistant Professor of Emergency Medicine, The Johns Hopkins University School of Medicine; Staff, The Johns Hopkins Medical Institutions, Baltimore, Maryland
Disturbances Due to Cold

Adrienne N. Kovalsky, DO, MPH
Assistant Professor of Medicine, Department of Hospital Medicine, Georgetown University Hospital, Washington, District of Columbia
High Altitude Illness

Megan Krause, MD
Assistant Professor, Division of Allergy, Clinical Immunology, and Rheumatology, University of Kansas School of Medicine, Kansas City, Kansas
Rheumatoid Arthritis

Eric H. Kraut, MD
Professor of Medicine, Director, Benign Hematology, Division of Hematology, The Ohio State University, Columbus, Ohio
Platelet-Mediated Bleeding Disorders

Lakshmanan Krishnamurti, MD
Professor of Pediatrics, Division of Hematology/Oncology, Children's Hospital of Pittsburgh, University of Pittsburgh Medical Center, Pittsburgh, Pennsylvania
Sickle Cell Disease

Kumar Krishnan, MD
Assistant Professor of Medicine, Harvard Medical School; Division of Gastroenterology, Massachusetts General Hospital, Boston, Massachusetts
Dysphagia and Esophageal Obstruction

Zachary Kuhlmann, DO
Clinical Associate Professor, Residency Program Director, Department of Obstetrics and Gynecology, University of Kansas School of Medicine–Wichita, Wichita, Kansas
Endometriosis

Roshni Kulkarni, MD
Professor Emerita, Michigan State University Center for Bleeding and Clotting Disorders, Department of Pediatrics and Human Development, College of Human Medicine, Michigan State University, East Lansing, Michigan
Hemophilia and Related Conditions

Seema Kumar, MD
Professor of Pediatrics, Chair, Division of Pediatric Endocrinology and Metabolism, Program Director, Pediatric Endocrinology Fellowship, Department of Pediatrics, Mayo Clinic, Rochester, Minnesota
Obesity in Children

Mary R. Kwaan, MD, MPH
Health Sciences Associate Clinical Professor of Surgery, David Geffen School of Medicine at University of California, Los Angeles, Los Angeles, California
Hemorrhoids, Anal Fissure, and Anorectal Abscess and Fistula

Robert A. Kyle, MD
Professor of Medicine, Laboratory Medicine, and Pathology, Mayo Clinic College of Medicine, Rochester, Minnesota
Multiple Myeloma

Lucius M. Lampton, MD
Clinical Associate Professor, Family and Community Medicine, Tulane University School of Medicine, New Orleans, Louisiana; Clinical Professor, Family Medicine, William Carey University College of Osteopathic Medicine, Hattiesburg, Mississippi
COVID-19; Yellow Fever

Richard A. Lange, MD, MBA
President, Texas Tech University Health Sciences Center El Paso; Dean, Paul L. Foster School of Medicine, El Paso, Texas
Congenital Heart Disease

Fabienne Langlois, MD
Assistant Professor, Division of Endocrinology, Department of Medicine, Universite de Sherbrooke, Fleurimont, Quebec, Canada
Adrenocortical Insufficiency; Hypopituitarism

Jerome Larkin, MD
Assistant Professor of Medicine, Infectious Diseases, Alpert Medical School, Brown University, Providence, Rhode Island
Severe Sepsis

Christine L. Lau, MD
George Minor Professor of Surgery, University of Virginia Health System, Charlottesville, Virginia
Atelectasis

Susan Lawrence-Hylland, MD
Clinical Assistant Professor, Rheumatology Section, University of Wisconsin Hospital and Clinics, Madison, Wisconsin
Connective Tissue Disorders; Cutaneous Vasculitis

Lydia U. Lee, MD
Clinical Lecturer, Department of Family Medicine, University of Michigan, Ann Arbor, Michigan
Postpartum Depression

Jerrold B. Leikin, MD
Clinical Professor of Medicine, Pritzker School of Medicine, University of Chicago, Chicago, Illinois; Director of Medical Toxicology, NorthShore University, HealthSystem–OMEGA, Glenbrook Hospital, Glenview, Illinois
Disturbances Due to Cold

Scott Leikin, DO
Critical Care Medicine Fellow, Icahn School of Medicine at Mount Sinai, New York, New York
Targeted Temperature Management (Therapeutic Hypothermia); Disturbances Due to Cold

Alexander K.C. Leung, MBBS
Clinical Professor of Pediatrics, University of Calgary, Calgary, Alberta, Canada
Nocturnal Enuresis

Martin M. LeWinter, MD
Professor of Medicine and Molecular Physiology and Biophysics, University of Vermont Larner College of Medicine; Attending Cardiologist, University of Vermont Medical Center, Burlington, Vermont
Pericarditis

Jennifer Lewis, MD, MPH
Assistant Professor of Medicine, Vanderbilt Ingram Cancer Center, Vanderbilt University Medical Center; VA Quality Scholars Fellow, Geriatric Research Education and Clinical Center, VA Tennessee Valley Healthcare System, Nashville, Tennessee
Lung Cancer

Ming Li, MD, PhD
Section of Endocrinology, Phoenix VA Health Care System; Department of Internal Medicine, University of Arizona, College of Medicine at Phoenix, Phoenix, Arizona
Hyperprolactinemia

Tyler K. Liebenstein, PharmD
Clinical Pharmacy Specialist, William S. Middleton Memorial Veterans Hospital, Madison, Wisconsin
Human Immunodeficiency Virus: Treatment and Prevention

Albert P. Lin, MD
Assistant Professor, Ophthalmology, Baylor College of Medicine; Staff Physician, Eye Care Line, Michael E. DeBakey Veterans Affairs Medical Center, Houston, Texas
Glaucoma

Jeffrey A. Linder, MD, MPH
Michael A. Gertz Professor of Medicine, Chief, Division of General Internal Medicine and Geriatrics, Northwestern University Feinberg School of Medicine, Chicago, Illinois
Influenza

James Lock, MD, PhD
Professor of Psychiatry, Stanford University, Stanford, California
Eating Disorders

M. Chantel Long, MD
Clinical Assistant Professor, Department of Family and Community Medicine, University of Kansas School of Medicine–Wichita
Condylomata Acuminata; Warts (Verrucae)

Colleen Loo-Gross, MD, MPH
Assistant Professor, Department of Family & Community Medicine, University of Kansas School of Medicine-Wichita, Wichita, Kansas
Amenorrhea

Ronda Lun, MD
Resident Physician, Department of Medicine: Division of Neurology, The Ottawa Hospital, Ottawa, Ontario, Canada
Intracerebral Hemorrhage

David A. Mahvi, MD
Surgical Resident, Brigham and Women's Hospital, Boston, Massachusetts
Tumors of the Stomach

Uma Malhotra, MD
Clinical Associate Professor, Infectious Diseases, University of Washington; Department of Medicine, Section of Infectious Diseases, Virginia Mason Medical Center, Seattle, Washington
Ebola Virus Disease

Emily Manlove, MD, MPH
Adjunct Clinical Assistant Professor, Family Medicine, IU Health Southern Indiana Physicians, Bloomington, Indiana
Cough

JoAnn E. Manson, MD, DrPH
Professor of Medicine, Michael and Lee Bell Professor of Women's Health, Harvard Medical School; Chief, Division of Preventive Medicine, Department of Medicine, Brigham and Women's Hospital, Boston, Massachusetts
Menopause

Meghna P. Mansukhani, MD
Associate Professor, Center for Sleep Medicine, Mayo Clinic and Foundation, Mayo Clinic College of Medicine, Rochester, Minnesota
Sleep Disorders

Claudio Marcocci, MD
Professor of Endocrinology, Department of Clinical and Experimental Medicine, University of Pisa; Head, Endocrine Unit 2, University Hospital of Pisa, Pisa, Italy
Hyperparathyroidism and Hypoparathyroidism

Curtis E. Margo, MD, MPH
Clinical Professor, Departments of Pathology and Cell Biology and Ophthalmology, University of South Florida Morsani College of Medicine, Tampa, Florida
Dry Eye Syndrome; Uveitis

Jason E. Marker, MD, MPA
Associate Director, Memorial Hospital Family Medicine Residency; Clinic Director, E. Blair Warner Family Medicine Center, South Bend, Indiana
Neurofibromatosis (Type 1)

Paul Martin, MD
Chief, Division of Digestive Health and Liver Disease, Mandel Chair in Gastroenterology, University of Miami, Miami, Florida
Cirrhosis

Samuel E. Mathis, MD
Assistant Professor, Family Medicine, University of Texas Medical Branch, Galveston, Texas
Infective Endocarditis

Kristine Matson, MD, MPH
Clinical Associate Professor, Division of Infectious Diseases, University of Wisconsin Hospital and Clinics, Madison, Wisconsin
Travel Medicine

Mark A. Matza, MD, MBA
Department of Rheumatology, Massachusetts General Hospital, Boston, Massachusetts
Polymyalgia Pneumatica and Giant Cell Arteritis

Pinckney J. Maxwell IV, MD
Associate Professor of Surgery, Division of Gastrointestinal and Laparoscopic Surgery, Medical University of South Carolina, Charleston, South Carolina
Tumors of the Colon and Rectum

Danica May, MD
Assistant Professor, Department of Urology, University of Kansas Medical Center, Kansas City, Kansas
Malignant Tumors of the Urogenital Tract

Marshall Mazepa, MD
Department of Medicine, Division of Hematology, Oncology and Transplantation, University of Minnesota Medical School, Minneapolis, Minnesota
Porphyrias

Molly McClain, MD, MPH, MS
Assistant Professor, Program Director, Department of Family and Community Medicine, University of New Mexico, Albuquerque, New Mexico
Gender Affirming Care

Christopher McGrew, MD
Departments of Family and Community Medicine and Orthopedics and Rehabilitation, Sports Medicine Division, University of New Mexico Health Sciences Center, Albuquerque, New Mexico
Sports-Related Head Injuries

Christopher C. McGuigan, MB, ChB, MPH
Consultant in Public Health Medicine, Health Protection, NHS Fife, Cameron Hospital, Leven, Fife, United Kingdom
Psittacosis

Michael McGuigan, MD
Medical Director, Long Island Regional Poison and Drug Information Center, Winthrop-University Hospital, Mineola, New York
Medical Toxicology

Meetal Mehta, MD
Nutrition Support Service Attending Physician, Obesity Medicine Physician, Brigham and Women's Hospital, Harvard Medical School, Boston, Massachusetts
Parenteral Nutrition in Adults

Mick S. Meiselman, MD
Director of Advanced Therapeutic Endoscopy, Central Coast Gastroenterology, San Luis Obispo, California
Calculous Biliary Disease

Moises Mercado, MD
Director, Experimental Endocrinology Unit, Hospital de Especialidades, Centro Medico Nacional Siglo XXI, Institute Mexicano del Seguro Social, Mexico City, Mexico
Acromegaly

Ryan Merrell, MD
Clinical Assistant Professor, Neurology, NorthShore University HealthSystem, Evanston, Illinois
Brain Tumors

Steven L. Meyers, MD
Vice Chair, Quality and Informatics, Neurology, NorthShore University Health System, Evanston, Illinois
Acute Facial Paralysis

Brian J. Miller, MD, PhD, MPH
Professor, Department of Psychiatry, Augusta University, Augusta, Georgia
Schizophrenia

Timothy M. Millington, MD
Assistant Professor, Department of Surgery, Dartmouth-Hitchcock Medical Center, Lebanon, New Hampshire
Pleural Effusion and Empyema

Moben Mirza, MD
Associate Professor, Residency Program Director, Division of Urologic Oncology, Department of Urology, University of Kansas Medical Center, Kansas City, Kansas
Hematuria; Malignant Tumors of the Urogenital Tract

Kriti Mishra, MD
Department of Dermatology, University of New Mexico, Albuquerque, New Mexico
Fungal Infections of the Skin

Howard C. Mofenson, MD
Professor of Pharmacology and Toxicology, New York College of Osteopathic Medicine, Old Westbury, New York; Professor of Pediatrics and Emergency Medicine, Stony Brook University Medical Center School of Medicine, Stony Brook, New York
Medical Toxicology

Kris M. Mogensen, MS
Team Leader, Dietitian Specialist, Department of Nutrition, Brigham and Women's Hospital, Boston, Massachusetts
Parenteral Nutrition in Adults

Michael L. Moritz, MD
Professor of Pediatrics, Division of Nephrology, Department of Pediatrics, The University of Pittsburgh School of Medicine, Children's Hospital of Pittsburgh, Pittsburgh, Pennsylvania
Parenteral Fluid Therapy for Infants and Children

Rami Mortada, MD
Endocrine Center of Kansas, Wichita, Kansas
Diabetes Insipidus

Parisa Mortaji, MD
Department of Medicine, University of Colorado, Aurora, Colorado
Tuberculosis and Other Mycobacterial Diseases

Scott E. Moser, MD
Professor of Family and Community Medicine, Associate Dean for Curriculum, University of Kansas School of Medicine–Wichita, Wichita, Kansas
Attention-Deficit/Hyperactivity Disorder

Heather E. Moss, MD, PhD
Assistant Professor, Departments of Ophthalmology & Neurology and Neurological Sciences, Stanford University, Stanford, California
Optic Neuritis

Judd W. Moul, MD
James H. Semans, MD Professor of Surgery, Urologic Surgery, Duke University, Durham, North Carolina
Benign Prostatic Hyperplasia

Martha L. Muller, MD, MPH
Professor, Department of Pediatrics, University of New Mexico, Albuquerque, New Mexico
Bacterial Meningitis

Heidi E.K. Mullen, DO
Dermatologist, Northeast Dermatology Associates, Portsmouth, New Hampshire
Contact Dermatitis

Natalia Murinova, MD
Clinical Associate Professor, Department of Neurology, University of Washington, Seattle, Washington
Migraine

Michael Murphy, MD
Professor of Dermatology, University of Connecticut School of Medicine; Attending Dermatopathologist, Department of Dermatology, UConn Health, Farmington, Connecticut
Nevi

Arjun Muthusubramanian, MD, MPH
Physician, MedExpress Urgent Care, Richmond, Virginia
Bacterial Pneumonia

Alykhan S. Nagji, MD
Assistant Professor, Associate Program Director, Cardiothoracic Surgery Residency Program, University of Kansas, Kansas City, Kansas
Atelectasis

Moniba Nazeef, MD
Department of Medicine, Division of Hematology/Oncology, University of Wisconsin School of Medicine and Public Health, UW Carbone Cancer Center, Madison, Wisconsin
Venous Thromboembolism

Viswanathan K. Neelakantan, MD
Senior Professor of Medicine and Tropical Medicine, Sri Manakula Vinayagar Medical College Hospital, Pondicherry, India
Foodborne Illnesses

Donald A. Neff, MD
Assistant Professor, Department of Urology, University of Kansas School of Medicine, Kansas City, Kansas
Urinary Tract Infections in the Male

Tara J. Neil, MD
Associate Professor, Department of Family and Community Medicine, University of Kansas School of Medicine–Wichita; Senior Associate Director, Via Christi Family Medicine Residency, Wichita, Kansas
Postpartum Care

William G. Nelson, MD, PhD
Marion I. Knott Professor of Oncology, Director of the Sidney Kimmel Comprehensive Cancer Center, The Johns Hopkins University School of Medicine, Baltimore, Maryland
Prostate Cancer

David G. Neschis, MD
Clinical Associate Professor of Surgery, University of Maryland School of Medicine, Baltimore, Maryland; Maryland Vascular Center, Glen Burnie, Maryland
Aortic Disease: Aneurysm and Dissection

Theresa Nester, MD
Professor of Laboratory Medicine, University of Washington Medical Center; Medical Director of Integrated Transfusion Service Laboratories, Bloodworks Northwest, Seattle, Washington
Blood Component Therapy and Transfusion Reactions

Tam T. Nguyen, MD
Assistant Clinical Professor, Family and Community Medicine, University of California, Davis, Sacramento, California; Clinician and Instructor, Family Medicine, Washington Township Medical Group, Fremont, California
Papulosquamous Eruptions

Andrea L. Nicol, MD, MSc
Associate Professor, Department of Anesthesiology, University of Kansas School of Medicine, Kansas City, Kansas
Fibromyalgia

Lucybeth Nieves-Arriba, MD
Assistant Professor, Gynecology Oncology, Zimmer Cancer Center, Wilmington, North Carolina
Cancer of the Uterine Cervix

Andrei Novac, MD
Clinical Professor of Psychiatry, Director, Traumatic Stress Program, University of California–Irvine School of Medicine, Irvine, California
Depressive, Bipolar, and Related Mood Disorders

Enrico M. Novelli, MD
Associate Professor of Medicine, Chief, Section of Benign Hematology, Director, Adult Sickle Cell Program, Department of Medicine, Division of Hematology/Oncology, Vascular Medicine Institute, Pittsburgh, Pennsylvania
Sickle Cell Disease

Lauren Nye, MD
Assistant Professor of Internal Medicine, Division of Medical Oncology, Breast Cancer Prevention and Survivorship Research Center, University of Kansas Medical Center, Kansas City, Kansas
Benign Breast Disease; Breast Cancer

Andrea T. Obi, MD
Section of Vascular Surgery, Department of Surgery, University of Michigan, Ann Arbor, Michigan
Venous Thrombosis

Jeffrey P. Okeson, DMD
Professor and Interim Dean, Department of Oral Health Science, University of Kentucky College of Dentistry, Lexington, Kentucky
Temporomandibular Disorders

Carlos R. Oliveira, MD, PhD
Assistant Professor, Yale School of Medicine, Division of Pediatric Infectious Diseases, Yale Child Health Research Center, New Haven, Connecticut
Lyme Disease and Post-Treatment Lyme Disease Syndrome

Peck Y. Ong, MD
Associate Professor of Clinical Pediatrics, Keck School of Medicine, University of Southern California/Children's Hospital Los Angeles, Los Angeles, California
Atopic Dermatitis

Daniel S. Oram, MD
Clinical Lecturer, Department of Family Medicine, Women's Health Fellow, Department of Obstetrics and Gynecology, University of Michigan Medical School, Ann Arbor, Michigan
Postpartum Depression

Sabah Osmani, BA
Medical Student, University of New Mexico School of Medicine, Albuquerque, New Mexico
Fungal Infections of the Skin

Bulent Ozgonenel, MD
Associate Professor in Pediatric Hematology/Oncology, Central Michigan University/Children's Hospital of Michigan, Wayne State University, Detroit, Michigan
Hemophilia and Related Conditions

Karel Pacak, MD, PhD, DSc
Senior Investigator, Chief, Section on Medical Neuroendocrinology, Eunice Kennedy Shriver National Institute of Child Health and Human Development, National Institutes of Health, Bethesda, Maryland
Pheochromocytoma

José A. Padin-Rosado, MD
Associate Professor, Department of Neurology, University of New Mexico School of Medicine, Albuquerque, New Mexico
Seizures and Epilepsy in Adolescents and Adults

Tanyatuth Padungkiatsagul, MD
Attending Physician, Department of Ophthalmology, Faculty of Medicine, Ramathibodi Hospital, Mahidol University, Bangkok, Thailand; Visiting Scholar, Department of Ophthalmology, Stanford University, Palo Alto, California
Optic Neuritis

Heather L. Paladine, MD, MEd
Assistant Professor of Medicine at Columbia University Medical Center, Center for Family and Community Medicine, Columbia College of Physicians and Surgeons, New York, New York
Vulvovaginitis

John E. Pandolfino, MD
Hans Popper Professor of Medicine, Feinberg School of Medicine, Northwestern University, Chicago, Illinois
Dysphagia and Esophageal Obstruction

Deval Patel, MD
Division of Hospital Pediatrics, Nemours Children's Specialty Care–Jacksonville; Associate Program Director, University of Florida Pediatric Residency Training Program–Jacksonville, Jacksonville, Florida
Parenteral Fluid Therapy for Infants and Children

Simon Patton, MD
Female Pelvic Medicine and Reconstructive Surgery, Via Christi Health, Wichita, Kansas
Urinary Incontinence

Gerson O. Penna, MD, PhD
Full Researcher, Tropical Medicine Center, University of Brasilia, Fiocruz School of Government, Brasilia, Brazil
Leprosy

Maria Lucia Penna, MD, PhD
Professor, Department of Epidemiology and Biostatistics, Federal University Fluminense, Rio de Janeiro, Brazil
Leprosy

Allen Perkins, MD, MPH
Professor and Chair, Family Medicine, University of South Alabama, Mobile, Alabama
Marine Poisonings, Envenomations, and Trauma

Leah Peterson, MD
Clinical Assistant Professor, Department of Family and Community Medicine, University of Kansas School of Medicine–Wichita, Wichita, Kansas; Smoky Hill Family Medicine Residency, Salina, Kansas
Hypertension in Pregnancy

Contributors

Georg A. Petroianu, MD, PhD
Professor & Chair, Department of Pharmacology & Therapeutics, College of Medicine–Khalifa University, Abu Dhabi, United Arab Emirates
Hiccups

Vesna M. Petronic-Rosic, MD, MSc, MBA
Professor and Founding Chair, Department of Dermatology, Georgetown University School of Medicine; Physician Executive Director, Dermatolog, Washington, DC
Melanoma

Hanna Phan, PharmD
Clinical Associate Professor, Department of Clinical Pharmacy, The University of Michigan College of Pharmacy; Clinical Pharmacist Specialist, Ambulatory Care–Pediatric Cystic Fibrosis, Michigan Medicine, C. S. Mott Children's Hospital, Ann Arbor, Michigan
Cystic Fibrosis

Mark Pietroni, MD, MBA
Medical Director, Gloucestershire Hospitals NHS Foundation Trust, Gloucester, United Kingdom
Cholera

Susan M. Pollart, MD, MS
Ruth E. Murdaugh Professor, Family Medicine, University of Virginia School of Medicine, Charlottesville, Virginia
Asthma in Children

Andrew S.T. Porter, DO
Clinical Associate Professor, Department of Family and Community Medicine, University of Kansas School of Medicine–Wichita; Director, University of Kansas School of Medicine–Wichita Sports Medicine Fellowship, Wichita, Kansas
Common Sports Injuries

Charles R. Powell, MD
Associate Professor, Department of Urology, Indiana University School of Medicine–Indianapolis, Indianapolis, Indiana
Prostatitis

Margaret Pusateri, MD
Emergency Medicine Physician, US Acute Care Solutions, Pittsburgh, Pennsylvania
Sports-Related Head Injuries

James M. Quinn, MD
Associate Professor of Medicine, Uniformed Services University of the Health Sciences, Bethesda, Maryland; Associate Program Director, Allergy/Immunology, San Antonio Uniformed Service Health Education Consortium, San Antonio, Texas
Allergic Reactions to Insect Stings

Peter S. Rahko, MD
Professor of Medicine, Cardiovascular Medicine Division, University of Wisconsin, Madison, Wisconsin
Mitral Valve Prolapse

S. Vincent Rajkumar, MD
Edward W. and Betty Knight Scripps Professor of Medicine, Division of Hematology, Mayo Clinic, Rochester, Minnesota
Multiple Myeloma

Anand Rajpara, MD
Associate Professor of Dermatology, Residency Program Director, Kansas University Medical Center, Kansas City, Kansas
Autoimmune Bullous Diseases; Pyoderma Gangrenosum

David P. Rakel, MD
Professor and Chair, Department of Family and Community Medicine, University of New Mexico School of Medicine, Albuquerque, New Mexico
Severe Sepsis

Kalyanakrishnan Ramakrishnan, MD
Professor, Department of Family and Preventive Medicine, University of Oklahoma Health Sciences Center, Oklahoma City, Oklahoma
Necrotizing Skin and Soft-Tissue Infections

Julio A. Ramirez, MD
Professor of Medicine, University of Louisville School of Medicine; Chief, Division of Infectious Diseases, Department of Veterans Affairs Medical Center, Louisville, Kentucky
Legionellosis (Legionnaires' Disease and Pontiac Fever)

Jatin Rana, MD
Assistant Professor of Medicine, Division of Hematology/Oncology, College of Human Medicine, Michigan State University, East Lansing, Michigan
Chronic Leukemias

Matthew A. Rank, MD
Professor of Medicine, Division of Allergy, Asthma, and Clinical Immunology, Mayo Clinic Alix School of Medicine, Mayo Clinic, Scottsdale, Arizona
Asthma in Adolescents and Adults

Didier Raoult, MD, PhD
Unite de recherche sur les maladies infectieuses tropicales, Aix-Marseille Universite, Marseille, France
Q Fever

Alwyn Rapose, MD
Assistant Professor, Department of Medicine, University of Massachusetts; Department of Infectious Diseases, Reliant Medical Group, Worcester, Massachusetts
Toxic Shock Syndrome

Rachel E. Rau, MD
Assistant Professor of Pediatrics, Baylor College of Medicine, Houston, Texas
Acute Leukemia in Children

Anita Devi K. Ravindran, MD
Faculty of Medicine, Atma Jaya Catholic University of Indonesia, Jakarta, Indonesia
Foodborne Illnesses

Jared Regehr, MD
Clinical Instructor, Department of Family and Community Medicine, University of Kansas School of Medicine, Wichita, Kansas
Fatigue

Ian R. Reid, MD
Distinguished Professor of Medicine and Endocrinology, University of Auckland, Auckland, New Zealand
Paget's Disease of Bone

Elissa Rennert-May, MD, MSc
Clinical Lecturer, University of Calgary, Alberta Health Services Calgary, Calgary, Alberta, Canada
Methicillin-Resistant Staphylococcus aureus

Karl T. Rew, MD
Associate Professor of Family Medicine and Urology, University of Michigan Medical School, Ann Arbor, Michigan
Erectile Dysfunction

Mona Rezapour, MD, MHS
Clinical Instructor, Gastroenterology, University of California, Los Angeles, Los Angeles, California
Inflammatory Bowel Disease

Amanda Rhyne, MD
Clinical Assistant Professor, Department of Family and Community Medicine, University of Kansas School of Medicine–Wichita, Wichita, Kansas
Serum Sickness

Martha Riese, MD
Clinical Instructor, Department of Family and Community Medicine, University of Kansas School of Medicine–Wichita, Wichita, Kansas
Varicella (Chickenpox)

David C. Robbins, MD
Bud and Sally Cray Professor of Medicine, Director, University of Kansas Diabetes Institute, Department of Medicine, University of Kansas Medical School, Kansas City, Kansas
Diabetes Mellitus in Adults

Amy Robertson, PharmD
Clinical Assistant Professor, Departments of Pharmacy Practice and Family and Community Medicine, University of Kansas School of Pharmacy; Clinical Pharmacist, Wesley Family Medicine Residency Program, Wichita, Kansas
Serum Sickness

Malcolm K. Robinson, MD
Associate Professor of Surgery, Harvard Medical School; Vice Chair for Clinical Operations, Department of Surgery, Director, Nutrition Support Service, Brigham and Women's Hospital, Boston, Massachusetts
Parenteral Nutrition in Adults

William P. Roche, MD
Neuromuscular Division, Emory University, Atlanta, Georgia
Myasthenia Gravis

Tessa E. Rohrberg, MD
Assistant Professor, Family and Community Medicine, University of Kansas School of Medicine–Wichita, Wichita, Kansas
Delirium

Candice Rose, MD, MS, RD
Assistant Professor of Medicine, University of Kansas Medical Center, Section of Endocrinology, Kansas City, Kansas
Diabetes Mellitus in Adults

Peter G. Rose, MD
Case Western Reserve University School of Medicine; Section Head, Gynecologic Oncology, Women's Health Institute, Cleveland Clinic, Cleveland, Ohio
Cancer of the Uterine Cervix

Stephen Ross, MD
Professor and Vice Chair, Department of Neurology, Penn State University, Hershey, Pennsylvania
Nonmigraine Headache

Alan R. Roth, DO
Assistant Professor, Department of Family and Social Medicine, Albert Einstein College of Medicine, Bronx, New York; Chairman, Department of Family Medicine, Ambulatory Care and Community Medicine, Jamaica Hospital Medical Center, Queens, New York
Fever

Anne-Michelle Ruha, MD
Professor, Departments of Internal Medicine and Emergency Medicine, University of Arizona College of Medicine-Phoenix; Chair, Department of Medical Toxicology, Banner–University Medical Center Phoenix, Phoenix, Arizona
Spider Bites and Scorpion Stings

Kristen Rundell, MS, MD
Associate Professor, Department of Family Medicine, The Ohio State University, Columbus, Ohio
Drug Hypersensitivity Reactions; Mumps

Adnan Said, MD, MS
Associate Professor of Medicine, Gastroenterology, and Hepatology, University of Wisconsin School of Medicine and Public Health; Chief, Gastroenterology and Hepatology, Director, Liver Transplant, William S. Middleton VAMC, Madison, Wisconsin
Nonalcoholic Fatty Liver Disease

Tomoko Sairenji, MD, MS
Assistant Professor of Family Medicine, University of Washington, Seattle, Washington
Acute Bronchitis and Other Viral Respiratory Infections

Susan L. Samson, MD, PhD
Associate Professor, Baylor College of Medicine, Houston, Texas
Hyponatremia

Carlos E. Sanchez, MD
Interventional Cardiology, Structural Heart Disease, Cardiovascular Diseases, Riverside Methodist Hospital, Columbus, Ohio
Valvular Heart Disease

Sandeep Sangodkar, DO
Assistant Professor of Clinical Medicine, University of California, Riverside School of Medicine; Cardiologist, Cardiology Specialists Medical Group, Riverside, California
Hypertrophic Cardiomyopathy

Arelis Santana, MD, MPH
Assistant Professor, Division of Infectious Diseases, University of New Mexico School of Medicine, Albuquerque, New Mexico
Salmonellosis

Ravi Sarode, MD
Professor, Pathology and Internal Medicine (Hematology/Oncology), Director, Division of Transfusion Medicine and Hemostasis, Southwestern Medical Center, Dallas, Texas
Thrombotic Thrombocytopenic Purpura

Michael Schatz, MD, MS
Clinical Professor, Department of Medicine, University of California San Diego School of Medicine; Department of Allergy, Kaiser Permanente, San Diego, California
Asthma in Adolescents and Adults

Alex Schevchuck, MD, MS
Associate Professor, Internal Medicine/Cardiology, University of New Mexico, Albuquerque, New Mexico
Congestive Heart Failure; Tachycardias

Lawrence R. Schiller, MD
Attending Physician, Gastroenterology Division, Baylor University Medical Center, Dallas, Texas
Malabsorption

Sarina Schrager, MD, MS
Professor of Family Medicine, University of Wisconsin, Madison, Wisconsin
Abnormal Uterine Bleeding

Dan Schuller, MD
Chair and Professor, Department of Internal Medicine–Transmountain, Texas Tech University Health Sciences Center, Paul L. Foster School of Medicine, Dallas, Texas
Lung Abscess; Pulmonary Hypertension

Justin Seashore, MD
Assistant Professor, Department of Pulmonary and Critical Care Medicine, University of Texas Medical Branch, Galveston, Texas
Post-COVID Syndrome

Amy Seery, MD
Assistant Professor, Department of Family and Community Medicine, University of Kansas School of Medicine–Wichita; Associate Director of Pediatrics, Via Christi Family Medicine Residency, Wichita, Kansas
Normal Infant Feeding

Steven A. Seifert, MD
Professor of Emergency Medicine, University of New Mexico School of Medicine, Albuquerque, New Mexico
Venomous Snakebite

Jeffery D. Semel, MD
Head, Section of Infectious Diseases, NorthShore University Healthsystem, Evanston, Illinois
Clostridioides difficile Colitis

Saeed Kamran Shaffi, MD, MS
Associate Professor, Internal Medicine/Nephrology, University of New Mexico, Albuquerque, New Mexico
Primary Glomerular Diseases

Beejal Shah, MD
Endocrinologist, Bay Pines VA HealthCare System, Bay Pines, Florida
Hyponatremia

Meera Shah, MBChB, MRCP (Edin)
Consultant, Division of Endocrinology, Diabetes and Nutrition, Mayo Clinic, Rochester, Minnesota
Obesity in Adults

Prediman K. Shah, MD, MACC
Professor of Medicine, University of California, Los Angeles, Cedars-Sinai Medical Center; Shapell and Webb Chair in Clinical Cardiology, Director, Oppenheimer Atherosclerosis Research Center and Atherosclerosis Prevention and Treatment Center, Smidt Heart Institute, Cedars-Sinai Medical Center, Los Angeles, California
Acute Myocardial Infarction

Samir S. Shah, MD, MSCE
Professor, Department of Pediatrics, University of Cincinnati College of Medicine; Director, Division of Hospital Medicine, James M. Ewell Endowed Chair, Cincinnati Children's Hospital Medical Center, Cincinnati, Ohio
Viral Meningitis

Shenil Shah, MD
Cardiovascular Medicine, University of Wisconsin School of Medicine and Public Health, Madison, Wisconsin
Mitral Valve Prolapse

Jamile M. Shammo, MD
Professor of Medicine and Pathology, Division of Hematology, Oncology and Stem Cell Transplantation, Rush University Medical Center, Chicago, Illinois
Myelodysplastic Syndromes

Eugene D. Shapiro, MD
Professor of Pediatrics (General Pediatrics) and Epidemiology (Microbial Diseases), Vice Chair for Research, Department of Pediatrics, Deputy Director, Investigative Medicine PhD Program, Co-Director of Education, Yale Center for Clinical Investigation, New Haven, Connecticut
Lyme Disease and Post-Treatment Lyme Disease Syndrome

Ala I. Sharara, MD
Professor, Division of Gastroenterology, American University of Beirut Medical Center, Beirut, Lebanon; Consulting Professor, Duke University Medical Center, Durham, North Carolina
Bleeding Esophageal Varices

Sonal Sharma, MD
Attending Physician, Mitochondrial Medicine Frontier Program, Division of Human Genetics, Department of Pediatrics, Children's Hospital of Philadelphia, Philadelphia
Mitochondrial Disease

John P. Sheehan, MD
Department of Medicine, Division of Hematology/Oncology, University of Wisconsin School of Medicine and Public Health, UW Carbone Cancer Center, Madison, Wisconsin
Venous Thromboembolism

Kamille S. Sherman, MD
Assistant Professor, Family and Community Medicine, University of North Dakota School of Medicine and Health Sciences, Grand Forks, North Dakota
Sunburn

Laura Elyse Shevy, MD
Associate Professor, Department of Infectious Diseases, University of New Mexico Health Sciences, Albuquerque, New Mexico
Tuberculosis and Other Mycobacterial Diseases

Sable Shew, MD
Department of Urology, Naval Medical Center San Diego, San Diego, California
Urethral Stricture Disease

Victor S. Sierpina, MD
Professor, Family and Integrative Medicine, University of Texas Medical Branch, Galveston, Texas
Post-COVID Syndrome

Karlynn Sievers, MD
Faculty Physician, St. Mary's Family Medicine Residency, Grand Junction, Colorado
Trigeminal Neuralgia

Hugh Silk, MD, MPH

Professor, Department of Family Medicine & Community Health, UMass Medical School; Learning Communities Mentor, Blackstone House; Part-time Lecturer, Harvard School of Dental Medicine, Boston, Massachusetts; Medical Director, Primary Care Wellness Center/Community, Healthlink Center for Integration of Primary Care and Oral Health, Worcester, Massachusetts
Trigeminal Neuralgia; Diseases of the Mouth

Lisa Simon, MD, DMD

Fellow in Oral Health and Medicine Integration, Oral Health Policy and Epidemiology, Harvard School of Dental Medicine, Boston, Massachusetts
Diseases of the Mouth

Aaron D. Sinclair, MD

Associate Professor, Department of Family and Community Medicine, Wesley Family Medicine Residency, University of Kansas School of Medicine–Wichita, Wichita, Kansas
Diverticula of the Alimentary Tract

Dawd S. Siraj, MD, MPH&TM

Professor of Medicine, Associate Program Director, Infectious Diseases Fellowship, Director, Global Health Pathway, Department of IM; Director, International Travel Clinic, Division of Infectious Diseases, University of Wisconsin-Madison, Madison, Wisconsin
Travel Medicine

Zachary L. Smith, DO

Assistant Professor of Medicine, Case Western Reserve University School of Medicine; Division of Gastroenterology and Liver Disease, University Hospitals Digestive Health Institute, Cleveland, Ohio
Calculous Biliary Disease

Rupal Soder, PhD

Project Director, Midwest Stem Cell Therapy Center, University of Kansas Medical Center, Kansas City, Kansas
Stem Cell Therapy

John Sojka, MD

Associate Professor, Department of Orthopaedic Surgery, University of Kansas Medical Center, Kansas City, Kansas
Osteomyelitis

William J. Somers, MD

Urology Department, Veteran Affairs Ambulatory Care Center, Columbus, Ohio
Nephrolithiasis

Mihae Song, MD

Assistant Professor, Department of Gynecologic Oncology, Rutgers Cancer Institute of New Jersey, New Brunswick, New Jersey
Ovarian Cancer

Nestor Sosa, MD

Chief, Infectious Disease Division, Department of Internal Medicine, University of New Mexico School of Medicine, Albuquerque, New Mexico
Malaria

Timothy Sowder, MD

Associate Professor, Department of Anesthesiology, University of Kansas School of Medicine, Kansas City, Kansas
Fibromyalgia

Linda Speer, MD

Professor and Chair, Family Medicine, University of Toledo, Toledo, Ohio
Dysmenorrhea

Abby L. Spencer, MD, MS

Vice Chair of Education–Medicine Institute, Associate Professor of Medicine, Cleveland Clinic Lerner College of Medicine, Cleveland, Ohio
Contraception

Todd Stephens, MD

Clinical Associate Professor, Department of Family and Community Medicine, University of Kansas School of Medicine–Wichita; Associate Director, Via Christi Family Medicine Residency, Wichita, Kansas
Genital Ulcer Disease: Chancroid, Granuloma Inguinale, and Lymphogranuloma

Erik Kent St. Louis, MD, MS

Associate Professor, Neurology, Mayo Clinic College of Medicine, Rochester, Minnesota
Sleep Disorders

Constantine A. Stratakis, MD, PhD

Head, Section on Endocrinology and Genetics, Scientific Director, National Institute of Child Health and Human Development, National Institutes of Health, Bethesda, Maryland
Cushing's Syndrome

Daniel Stulberg, MD

Professor and Vice Chair of Education, Department of Family and Community Medicine, University of New Mexico School of Medicine, Albuquerque, New Mexico
Premalignant Skin Lesions

José Antonio Suárez, MD

Clinic Research Unit, Instituto Conmemorativo Gorgas de Estudios de la Salud, Panama City, Panama
Malaria

Masayoshi Takashima, MD

Professor and Chairman, Department of Otolaryngology–Head and Neck Surgery, Houston Methodist Academic Institute, Houston, Texas
Obstructive Sleep Apnea; Rhinitis

Varun Takyar, MD

Staff Hepatologist, Department of GI/Liver, Sutter Health East Bay Medical Foundation, Berkeley, California
Hepatitis A, B, D, and E

Carolina Talhari, MD, PhD

Associate Professor of Dermatology, State University of Amazonas; Dermatologist, Alfredo da Matta Foundation for Dermatology, Manaus, Amazonas, Brazil
Leprosy

Jie Tang, MD

Associate Professor, Division of Kidney Diseases and Hypertension, Alpert Medical School, Brown University, Providence, Rhode Island
Hypokalemia and Hyperkalemia

Jessica Tate, MD

Assistant Professor of Neurology, Wake Forest University School of Medicine, Winston-Salem, North Carolina
Parkinson Disease

Kim Templeton, MD
Professor of Orthopaedic Surgery, Department of Orthopaedic Surgery, University of Kansas Medical Center, Kansas City, Kansas
Osteomyelitis

Joyce M.C. Teng, MD, PhD
Professor of Dermatology and Pediatrics, Stanford University School of Medicine; Lucile Packard Children's Hospital at Stanford, Stanford, California
Urticaria and Angioedema

Joanna Thomson, MD, MPH
Associate Professor, Department of Pediatrics, University of Cincinnati College of Medicine; Pediatric Hospitalist, Cincinnati Children's Hospital Medical Center, Cincinnati, Ohio
Viral Meningitis

William Tillett, MBChB, PhD
Consultant Rheumatologist, Royal National Hospital for Rheumatic Diseases; Senior Lecturer, Pharmacy and Pharmacology, University of Bath, Bath, United Kingdom
Psoriatic Arthritis

Paresh J. Timbadia, MD
Staff Pulmonologist, Chalmers P. Wylie VA Ambulatory Care Center, Columbus, Ohio
Chronic Obstructive Pulmonary Disease

Kenneth Tobin, DO
Clinical Assistant Professor, Director, Chest Pain Center, University of Michigan, Northville, Michigan
Angina Pectoris

Theodore T. Tsaltas, MD
Tri-Star Summit Medical Center, Hermitage, Tennessee; OB Hospitalist Group, Chattanooga, Tennessee
Uterine Leiomyoma

Sebastian H. Unizony, MD
Assistant Professor of Medicine, Massachusetts General Hospital; Instructor in Medicine, Massachusetts General Hospital Rheumatology, Allergy and Immunology Division, Harvard Medical School, Boston, Massachusetts
Polymyalgia Rheumatica and Giant Cell Arteritis

Mark Unruh, MD, MS
Chair, Department of Internal Medicine, University of New Mexico School of Medicine, Albuquerque, New Mexico
Chronic Kidney Disease

Locke Uppendahl, MD
Clinical Instructor, Obstetrics and Gynecology, Division of Gynecologic Oncology, University of Kansas School of Medicine–Wichita, Wichita, Kansas
Cancer of the Endometrium

Anusha Vallurupalli, MBBS
Assistant Professor of Medicine, Division of Hematologic Malignancies and Cellular Therapeutics, University of Kansas Medical Center, Kansas City, Kansas
Hodgkin Lymphoma; Pernicious Anemia/Megaloblastic Anemia

George Van Buren II, MD
Associate Professor of Surgery, Michael E. DeBakey Department of Surgery, Baylor College of Medicine, Houston, Texas
Acute and Chronic Pancreatitis

David van Duin, MD, PhD
Associate Professor of Medicine, University of North Carolina, Chapel Hill, North Carolina
Histoplasmosis

Daniel J. Van Durme, MD, MPH
Professor and Chair, Family Medicine and Rural Health, Florida State University College of Medicine, Tallahassee, Florida
Acne Vulgaris; Rosacea

Elena V. Varlamov, MD
Assistant Professor, Departments of Neurological Surgery and Medicine, Northwest Pituitary Center, Oregon Health & Science University, Portland, Oregon
Adrenocortical Insufficiency; Hypopituitarism

Christopher Vélez, MD
Center of Neurointestinal Health, Massachusetts General Hospital, Boston, Massachusetts
Dysphagia and Esophageal Obstruction

Gregory Vercellotti, MD
Professor, Department of Medicine, University of Minnesota, Minneapolis, Minnesota
Porphyrias

Kyle Vincent, MD
Clinical Associate Professor, Department of Surgery, University of Kansas School of Medicine–Wichita, Wichita, Kansas
Gastritis and Peptic Ulcer Disease

Donald C. Vinh, MD
Associate Professor, Department of Medicine, Divisions of Infectious Diseases and Allergy and Clinical Immunology, Departments of Medical Microbiology and Human Genetics, Director, Infectious Disease Susceptibility Program, McGill University Health Centre–Research Institute, Montreal, Quebec, Canada
Blastomycosis

Jatin M. Vyas, MD, PhD
Associate Professor of Medicine, Division of Infectious Disease, Massachusetts General Hospital, Boston, Massachusetts
Rat-Bite Fever

Tamara Wagner, MD
Associate Professor, Department of Pediatrics, Oregon Health & Science University, Portland, Oregon
Bronchiolitis

Thomas W. Wakefield, MD
Stanley Professor of Surgery, Section of Vascular Surgery, Department of Surgery, University of Michigan, Ann Arbor, Michigan
Venous Thrombosis

Arnold Wald, MD
Division of Gastroenterology and Hepatology, University of Wisconsin School of Medicine and Public Health, Madison, Wisconsin
Irritable Bowel Syndrome

Ellen R. Wald, MD
Chair, Department of Pediatrics, University of Wisconsin School of Medicine and Public Health, Madison, Wisconsin
Urinary Tract Infections in Infants and Children

Robin A. Walker, MD
Clinical Assistant Professor, Department of Family and Community Medicine, University of Kansas School of Medicine – Wichita, Northwest Family Physicians, Wichita, Kansas
Epididymitis and Orchitis

Ernest Wang, MD
Clinical Professor of Emergency Medicine, Evanston Hospital, NorthShore University HealthSystem, Evanston, Illinois
Disturbances Due to Cold

Jennifer Wang, DO
Assistant Professor, Critical Care Medicine, The Mount Sinai Hospital, New York, New York
Targeted Temperature Management (Therapeutic Hypothermia)

Koji Watanabe, MD, PhD
Staff Doctor, AIDS Clinical Center, National Center for Global Health and Medicine, Tokyo, Japan
Amebiasis

Ruth Weber, MD, MSEd
Clinical Associate Professor, Department of Family and Community Medicine, Medical University of South Carolina, Charleston, South Carolina
Pharyngitis

Cheryl Wehler, MD
Assistant Professor, Department of Psychiatry and Behavioral Sciences, University of Kansas School of Medicine–Wichita, Wichita, Kansas
Panic Disorder

Alice C. Wei, MD, MSc
Associate Attending Surgeon, Memorial Sloan Kettering Cancer Center; Associate Professor of Surgery, Weill Medical College of Cornell University, New York, New York
Pancreatic Cancer

Jane A. Weida, MS, MD
Professor, Family, Internal and Rural Medicine, Interim Department Chair, Director of Clinical Affairs, University of Alabama College of Community Health Sciences, Tuscaloosa, Alabama
Measles (Rubeola)

David N. Weissman, MD
Director, Respiratory Health Division, National Institute for Occupational Safety and Health, Morgantown, West Virginia
Pneumoconiosis: Asbestosis and Silicosis

Robert C. Welliver Sr., MD
Professor of Pediatrics, Chief, Division of Pediatric Infectious Diseases, Children's Hospital Foundation Hobbs-Recknagel Endowed Chair in Pediatrics, The Children's Hospital at University of Oklahoma Health Sciences Center, Oklahoma City, Oklahoma
Viral Respiratory Infections

Rebecca M. Wester, MD
Adjunct Associate Professor, Family Medicine-Geriatrics, University of Nebraska Medical Center, Omaha, Nebraska
Pressure Injury

Ryan P. Westergaard, MD, PhD, MPH
Associate Professor, Division of Infectious Diseases, University of Wisconsin School of Medicine and Public Health; Chief Medical Officer and State Epidemiologist for Communicable Diseases, Wisconsin Department of Health Services, Madison, Wisconsin
Human Immunodeficiency Virus: Treatment and Prevention

Randell Wexler, MD MPH
Professor, Vice Chair, Clinical Services, Department of Family Medicine, The Ohio State University, Columbus, Ohio
Premature Beats

Katarzyna Wilamowska, MD, PhD
Research Volunteer, Center for Memory and Aging, University of New Mexico, Albuquerque, New Mexico
Alzheimer's Disease, Premalignant Skin Lesions

Kimberly Williams, MD
Assistant Professor, Department of Family and Community Medicine, University of Kansas School of Medicine–Wichita, Wichita, Kansas; Program Director, Smoky Hill Family Medicine Residency, Salina, Kansas
Otitis Externa

Tracy L. Williams, MD
Associate Professor, Department of Family and Community Medicine, University of Kansas School of Medicine–Wichita; Via Christi Family Medicine Residency, Wichita, Kansas
Chlamydia trachomatis

Boris Winterhoff, MD
Assistant Professor, Obstetrics, Gynecology, and Women's Health, University of Minnesota, Minneapolis, Minnesota
Cancer of the Endometrium

Jennifer Wipperman, MD, MPH
Clinical Associate Professor, Department of Family and Community Medicine, University of Kansas School of Medicine–Wichita, Wichita, Kansas
Dizziness and Vertigo

Robert Wittler, MD
Professor of Pediatrics & Pediatric Infectious Diseases, University of Kansas School of Medicine–Wichita, Wichita, Kansas
Tickborne Rickettsial Diseases (Rocky Mountain Spotted Fever and Other Spotted Fever Group Rickettsioses, Ehrlichioses, and Anaplasmosis)

Katherine I. Wolf, BS
Postbaccalaureate IRTA Fellow, Eunice Kennedy Shriver National Institute of Child Health and Human Development, National Institutes of Health, Bethesda, Maryland
Pheochromocytoma

Gary S. Wood, MD
Professor and Founding Chair, Dean's Chair in Cutaneous Research, Geneva F. and Sture Johnson Professor Emeritus, Department of Dermatology, University of Wisconsin–Madison
Cutaneous T-Cell Lymphomas, Including Mycosis Fungoides and Sézary Syndrome

Scott Worswick, MD
Associate Clinical Professor of Dermatology, Keck Hospital of the University of Southern California; Director of Inpatient Dermatology, Los Angeles County Hospital; Co-Program Director, USC Dermatology Residency Program, Los Angeles, California
Stevens-Johnson Syndrome and Toxic Epidermal Necrolysis

Dominic J. Wu, MD
Physician, Department of Dermatology, University of Kansas Medical Center, Kansas City, Kansas
Autoimmune Bullous Diseases; Pyoderma Gangrenosum

Steve W. Wu, MD
Associate Professor, University of Cincinnati College of Medicine; Assistant Professor, Cincinnati Children's Hospital Medical Center, Cincinnati, Ohio
Gilles de la Tourette Syndrome

Hadley Wyre, MD
Assistant Professor of Urology, University of Kansas Medical Center, Kansas City, Kansas
Urethral Stricture Disease

Steven J. Yakubov, MD
John H. McConnell Chair of Advanced Structural Heart Disease, System Chief, OhioHealth Structural Heart Disease, Columbus, Ohio
Valvular Heart Disease

Xinghong Yang, PhD
Infectious Diseases and Pathology, University of Florida, Gainesville, Florida
Brucellosis

Kenneth S. Yew, MD, MPH
Faculty, Gundersen Medical Foundation Family Medicine Residency Program, Gundersen Medical Center, La Crosse, Wisconsin
Tinnitus

Yooni Yi, MD
Assistant Professor, Department of Urology, University of Michigan, Ann Arbor, Michigan
Trauma to the Genitourinary Tract

James A. Yiannias, MD
Professor of Dermatology, Mayo Clinic, Scottsdale, Arizona
Contact Dermatitis

Natawadee Young, MD
Adjunct Professor, Clinical Director, Family Medicine, AnMed Health Family Medicine Residency Program, Anderson, South Carolina
Antepartum Care

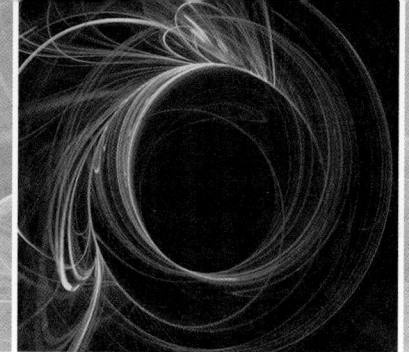

Preface

At the time of this writing, we are almost 2 years into the COVID pandemic that has taken the life of 1 out of every 500 Americans. The delta variant has knocked us back on our heels and drained us of emotional reserves.

In the face of these challenges, there is always a glimmer of light in the dark that results in progress. Health care has changed more in the past year than any other time in modern history. The pandemic has made telemedicine a norm, improving patient access. A traditionally conservative industry has learned to quickly adapt, improving testing and the rapid dissemination of evidence and vaccines. The virus also revealed significant health inequities that have encouraged insight into the importance of allocating resources and health delivery strategies to our most vulnerable populations.

These realities are echoed throughout the pages of the 2022 edition of *Conn's Current Therapy*. In this 74th printing, we have removed chapters on conditions that are less common and included those that meet the needs of our current medical challenges. We continue to devote a chapter to COVID-19 and have included one on Post-COVID Syndrome. We have also added chapters on emerging therapies, including Gender Affirming Care, Stem Cell Therapy and Non-Alcoholic Fatty Liver Disease. Every one of the 328 chapters has been reviewed and revised with inclusions of how the pandemic has touched many of the conditions we manage.

An annual text such as this cannot happen without the help of many dedicated and talented partners. In 2020, we lost Joan Ryan who was the content development specialist for *Conn's Current Therapy* and an Elsevier employee of 21 years. In 2021, we lost Peggy Rakel, wife and editorial assistant of Robert Rakel, who was editor of *Conn's Current Therapy* for 26 years. Peggy would communicate with authors, offering support and kind reminders to submit manuscripts. She was also a talented writer, able to help with editing and offering her important perspective as a nurse. We will miss Joan and Peggy greatly.

The two "heavy lifters" for *Conn's Current Therapy* who deserve special recognition are Kathryn "Katie" DeFrancesco and Miriam Chan, PharmD. Katie is the Senior Content Development Manager who organizes the whole editorial process, communicating regularly with us and the authors. She is dependable, gifted, and kind. She is the glue that binds the book together. As pharmacy editor, Dr. Chan reviews dosing accuracy and FDA approval of every drug mentioned in the text. This is a large task for 328 chapters! She does it with an exacting grace. We are grateful to partner with you both.

Our editorial leader and Senior Content Specialist is Charlotta "Lotta" Kryhl who offers guidance and support as we review the table of contents each year. Lotta also provides data on chapter utilization that helps us understand which chapters are being read the most and which ones we can let go of. This helps us keep current and pragmatic for the practicing clinician. Kate Mannix, Senior Project Manager, organizes the book in the final stages of production and is a talented "finisher" of the layout you see before you. She works with Renee Duenow, Senior Book Designer, for the beautiful form and feel.

We would like to dedicate this 74th printing, 2022 edition of *Conn's Current Therapy* to you, the clinician who has had to adapt, manage, and work beyond personal limits to bring care to patients, neighbors, and friends during this unprecedented time. We hope the information in this text provides guidance and support for the vital work you provide your community. This pandemic has created medicine's greatest generation. Thank you for being the light in the dark.

Gratefully,
Rick D. Kellerman, MD
David P. Rakel, MD

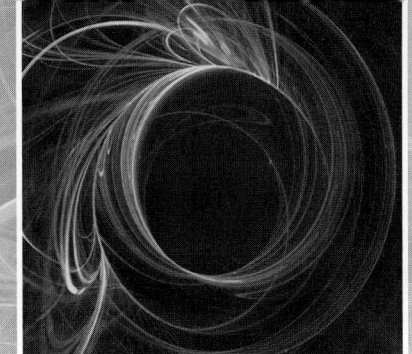

Contents

Contents

xxx

Contents

xxxiii

Contents

xxxiv

Contents

xxxv

***Conn's Current Therapy 2021* uses a standardized system of footnotes:**

1. Not FDA approved for this indication.
2. Not available in the United States.
3. Exceeds dosage recommended by the manufacturer.
4. Not yet approved for use in the United States.
5. Investigational drug in the United States.
6. May be compounded by pharmacists.
7. Available as dietary supplement.
8. Orphan drug in the United States.
9. Available as homeopathic remedy.
10. Available in the United States from the Centers for Disease Control and Prevention.

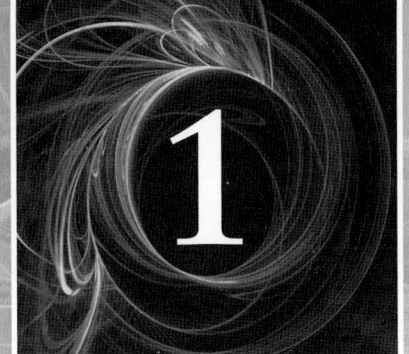

Symptomatic Care Pending Diagnosis

CHEST PAIN

Method of
William E. Cayley Jr., MD, MDiv

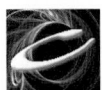

CURRENT DIAGNOSIS

- Initial evaluation of chest pain should include evaluation of clinical stability, a concise history and physical, and a chest x-ray and electrocardiogram (ECG) unless the cause is clearly not life threatening.
- Chest pain described as exertional, radiating to one or both arms, similar to or worse than prior cardiac chest pain, or associated with nausea, vomiting, or diaphoresis indicates high risk for acute coronary syndrome (ACS). ECG identifies ST-elevation myocardial infarction (STEMI); cardiac biomarkers are essential for further evaluation of suspected chest pain in the absence of STEMI.
- The Wells, Geneva, and Pisa clinical prediction rules as well as the Pulmonary Embolism Rule-out Criteria (PERC) can help stratify a patient's risk of pulmonary embolism (PE).
- Aortic dissection is an uncommon cause of chest pain, but patients with abrupt or instantaneous chest pain that is ripping, tearing, or stabbing should be evaluated for dissection with chest x-ray, computed tomography (CT), or magnetic resonance imaging (MRI).
- Esophageal rupture may be suspected in patients with pain, dyspnea, and shock following a forceful emesis, and prompt imaging with CT or esophagram is essential.
- Patients who have suspected tension pneumothorax and who are clinically stable should have a chest x-ray for confirmation before needle decompression is attempted.

CURRENT THERAPY

- Patients with STEMI require urgent reperfusion, and those with unstable angina or non–STEMI (NSTEMI) require admission for further monitoring and evaluation.
- Most patients with PE require admission for monitoring and anticoagulation, although outpatient treatment may be possible for low-risk patients after initial evaluation and anticoagulation.
- Prompt surgical consultation is required for patients with confirmed or suspected aortic dissection or esophageal rupture.
- Clinically unstable patients with suspected tension pneumothorax need immediate needle decompression.

Epidemiology

Chest pain is the chief complaint in 1% to 2% of all outpatient primary care visits. More than 50% of emergency department (ED) visits for chest pain are due to serious cardiovascular conditions such as acute coronary syndrome (ACS) or pulmonary embolism (PE), but these account for less than 15% of outpatient primary care encounters for chest pain, and up to 15% of chest pain episodes never reach a definitive diagnosis. Other potentially life-threatening etiologies for chest pain include PE, dissecting aortic aneurysm (AA), esophageal rupture, and tension pneumothorax. In outpatient primary care, the most common causes of chest pain are musculoskeletal, gastrointestinal, angina due to stable coronary artery disease (CAD), anxiety or other psychiatric conditions, and pulmonary disease.

Initial Assessment

In initial evaluation of chest pain, it is important to obtain a clear history of the onset and evolution of the pain, especially details such as location, quality, duration, and aggravating or alleviating factors. Initial physical examination should include vital signs, assessment of the patient's overall general condition, and examination of the heart and lungs. If there are any clinical signs of instability (altered mental status, hypotension, marked dyspnea, or other signs of shock), initial stabilization and diagnosis must be addressed simultaneously, consistent with current guidelines for emergency cardiovascular care. Unless the history and physical examination suggest an obviously nonthreatening cause of chest discomfort, most adults with chest pain should at least have basic diagnostic testing with an ECG and a chest x-ray. Several clinical prediction rules are available to help confirm or exclude some common causes of chest pain (Box 1).

Diagnosis and Treatment

Acute Coronary Syndrome

ACS includes acute myocardial infarction (MI) (ST-segment elevation and depression, and Q wave and non–Q wave) and unstable angina. Findings on the history and physical examination that increase the likelihood of ACS include radiation of pain to the right arm or shoulder, to both arms or shoulders, or to the left arm; pain associated with exertion, diaphoresis, nausea, or vomiting; pain described as pressure or as "worse than previous angina or similar to a previous MI"; or the presence of hypotension or an S3 on cardiac auscultation. Elements of the history and examination that decrease the likelihood of ACS are pleuritic, positional, or sharp chest pain; pain in an inframammary location; pain not associated with exertion; pain lasting just seconds or lasting more than 24 hours; or chest pain reproducible with palpation. The Marburg Heart Score (MHS) and the Interchest Clinical Prediction Rule can both help exclude CAD in primary care patients with chest pain, and use of the MHS when evaluating primary care patients with chest pain has been shown to improve clinical diagnostic accuracy (Table 1). Recent studies have demonstrated that the presence or absence of typical cardiac risk factors (e.g., diabetes, hypertension, smoking, high cholesterol, or family history) have little diagnostic value for determining the likelihood of ACS in patients over 40 years of age.

An ECG should be obtained promptly for any patient with suspected ACS. ST-segment elevation in two or more contiguous leads, or presumed new left bundle branch block, is diagnostic of ST-elevation MI (STEMI) and requires urgent revascularization with thrombolysis or angioplasty at an appropriate facility. Ischemic ST-segment depression more than 0.5 mm, dynamic T-wave inversion with chest discomfort, or transient ST-segment

Acute Coronary Syndrome

- Diagnosing cardiac ischemia with exercise treadmill testing: Duke treadmill score: https://www.mdcalc.com/duke-treadmill-score
- What is the risk of a major cardiac event in the next 6 weeks? HEART Score: https://www.mdcalc.com/heart-score-major-cardiac-events
- What is the risk of ACS in someone with chest pain? Marburg Heart Score: https://www.mdcalc.com/marburg-heart-score-mhs
- What is the risk of ACS in someone with chest pain? Interchest Clinical Prediction Rule: https://www.mdcalc.com/interchest-clinical-prediction-rule-chest-pain-primary-care
- Assesses long-term risk in those with ACS: GRACE ACS risk calculator: http://www.outcomes-umassmed.org/grace/
- Estimates mortality for patients with unstable angina and non-ST elevation MI: TIMI risk score: http://www.timi.org/

Pulmonary Embolism

- Geneva score for predicting risk of pulmonary embolism: https://www.mdcalc.com/geneva-score-revised-pulmonary-embolism
- Pisa clinical model for predicting the probability of PE: https://ebmcalc.com/PulmonaryEmbRiskPisaCXR.htm
- Wells scoring system for risk of pulmonary embolism: https://www.mdcalc.com/wells-criteria-pulmonary-embolism
- Pulmonary Embolism Rule-out Criteria: https://www.mdcalc.com/perc-rule-pulmonary-embolism

Thoracic Aortic Dissection

- Aortic Dissection Detection Risk Score (ADD-RS): https://www.mdcalc.com/aortic-dissection-detection-risk-score-add-rs

Pneumonia

- Diehr diagnostic rule for pneumonia in adults with acute cough: http://www.soapnote.org/infectious/diehr-rule/

TABLE 1 | Marburg Heart Score

FINDING	POINTS
Woman >64 years, man >54 years	1
Known CAD, cerebrovascular disease, or peripheral vascular disease	1
Pain worse with exercise	1
Pain not reproducible with palpation	1
Patient assumes pain is cardiac	1

CAD, Coronary artery disease. Approximately 97% of patients with an MHS score of 2 or less will not have CAD. Approximately 23% of patients with an MHS score of 3 or more will have CAD.

Adapted from Haasenritter J, Bösner S, Vaucher P, Herzig L, Heinzel-Gutenbrunner M, Baum E, Donner-Banzhoff N: Ruling out coronary heart disease in primary care: External validation of a clinical prediction rule. *Br J Gen Pract* 62(599):e415–e421, 2012. https://doi.org/10.3399/bjgp12X649106. http://www.ncbi.nlm.nih.gov/pmc/articles/PMC3361121/.

elevation of 0.5 mm or more is classified as unstable angina or non-STEMI (NSTEMI). However, none of these findings is sensitive enough that its absence can exclude MI, and patients whose chest pain is not low risk still require further assessment for ACS.

In patients with high-risk chest pain who do not have STEMI, elevated cardiac biomarkers distinguish NSTEMI from unstable angina. Cardiac troponins T and I are more sensitive for detecting NSTEMI than creatine kinase (CK) or the MB isoform (CK-MB).

TABLE 2 | Simplified Wells Scoring System for Pulmonary Embolism

CLINICAL FINDING	SCORE
Symptoms of DVT	3.0
No alternative diagnosis more likely than PE	3.0
Heart rate >100 beats/min	1.5
Immobilization greater than 3 days or surgery in past 4 weeks	1.5
Previous objectively diagnosed DVT or PE	1.5
Hemoptysis	1.0
Malignancy	1.0
Probability of PE: <2 points = low, 2–6 points = moderate, >6 points = high	

DVT, Deep vein thrombosis; *PE,* pulmonary embolism.

Adapted from Miniati M, Bottai M, Monti S: Comparison of 3 clinical models for predicting the probability of pulmonary embolism. *Medicine (Baltimore)* 84:107–114, 2005; Torbicki A, Perrier A, Konstantinides S, et al: ESC Committee for Practice Guidelines (CPG): Guidelines on the diagnosis and management of acute pulmonary embolism. *Eur Heart J* 29:2276–315, 2008. http://eurheartj.oxfordjournals.org/content/29/18/2276.long.

High-sensitivity troponins will be coming into use with an even greater sensitivity (negative predictive values Σ 99.5%).

Initial management of NSTEMI includes hospital admission for antiplatelet, antithrombin, and antianginal therapy. Patients with unstable angina should also be hospitalized for observation, and those with either NSTEMI or unstable angina require risk stratification using the Thrombolysis in Myocardial Infarction Study Group (TIMI) or Global Registry of Acute Coronary Events (GRACE) risk scores (see Box 1). Patients with chest pain suspicious for CAD but no definite initial diagnosis of STEMI or NSTEMI on initial presentation are often admitted to hospital for overnight observation and serial cardiac biomarker measurements to "rule out MI." However, use of the History, ECG, Age, Risk factors, Troponin (HEART), TIMI, or GRACE scores may help determine who is at sufficiently low risk of major adverse cardiac events to allow discharge for close follow-up. Recent evidence suggests that the HEART score may outperform TIMI and GRACE in determining which patients are at low risk (see Box 1), and the combination of a low-risk HEART score plus a single normal Troponin value may predict sufficiently low risk of ACS to allow discharge from emergency care with short-term outpatient follow-up.

Patients at low risk for ACS or MI can usually defer further testing unless there are other risk factors in their family or past medical history markedly increasing the likelihood of CAD. Current recommendations are that all other patients with chest pain suggestive of CAD should have further noninvasive testing within 7 days; however, a study of 4181 patients in an ED chest pain unit found that a reasonable alternative may be to test troponin levels twice over a 6-hour interval, with no stress testing if both values are normal. Patients who can exercise and have no left-bundle-branch block, preexcitation, or significant resting ST-segment depression on an ECG can be evaluated with an exercise stress ECG, and the Duke treadmill score can then be used to further quantify cardiac risk (see Box 1). Patients with baseline ECG abnormalities should have perfusion imaging performed along with a stress ECG, and those who cannot exercise may be evaluated with a pharmacologic stress or vasodilator test (e.g., dobutamine [Dobutrex][1] or adenosine [Adenocard][1]). Patients at high risk for CAD or those with NSTEMI should generally proceed directly to angiography, which enables definitive assessment of the coronary artery anatomy.

---

[1]Not FDA approved for this indication.

TABLE 3	Pulmonary Embolism Rule-out Criteria
Criteria (Excludes PE if all criteria are met and pretest probability is estimated at less than 15%)	
Age <50 years	
Heart rate <100 beats/min	
Pulse oximetry on room air >95%	
No unilateral leg swelling	
No hemoptysis	
No surgery or trauma in the last 4 weeks	
No prior DVT or PE	
No hormone use	

DVT, Deep vein thrombosis; *PE,* pulmonary embolism.
Adapted from Kline JA, Mitchell AM, Kabrhel C, Richman PB, Courtney DM: Clinical criteria to prevent unnecessary diagnostic testing in emergency department patients with suspected pulmonary embolism. *J Thromb Haemost* 2(8):1247–1255, 2004. https://onlinelibrary.wiley.com/doi/full/10.1111/j.1538-7836.2004.00790.x.

Pulmonary Embolism

There are no individual symptoms or physical examination findings that reliably diagnose or exclude PE, but three clinical prediction rules have all been validated for use in determining likelihood of PE and therefore whether further testing is needed (see Box 1). The Pisa rule may be the most accurate, but it is also the most mathematically complicated and depends on clinical, ECG, and x-ray findings. The Geneva rule requires blood gas and chest x-ray findings. The Wells rule (Table 2) is based on the simplest combination of history and examination findings, and a comparison between the Wells and Geneva rules found that the Wells rule has a lower failure rate. With the Wells and Geneva prediction rules, the likelihood of PE is approximately 10% in the low-probability category, 30% in the moderate-probability category, and 65% in the high-probability category. If a patient is clinically suspected to be at low risk for PE (<15% pretest probability) and meets all of the PERC (Table 3), the risk of PE is less than 2% and no further testing is needed.

Routine tests done for patients with chest pain are not particularly helpful in diagnosing or excluding PE. The chest x-ray may be abnormal, but findings that typically occur with PE (atelectasis, effusion, or elevation of a hemidiaphragm) are nonspecific. ECG signs of right ventricular strain (S wave in lead I, Q wave and inverted T wave in lead III) may be helpful if present, but their absence does not exclude PE. Hypoxia may be present, but up to 20% of patients with PE have a normal alveolar-arterial oxygen gradient.

Additional tests recommended for evaluating patients with suspected PE include D-dimer testing, compression ultrasonography, and pulmonary imaging with ventilation-perfusion (VQ) scintigraphy or computed tomography (CT) angiography. While CT may be more sensitive than VQ scanning, CT is also associated with higher radiation doses; for younger patients with suspected PE and a normal chest x-ray, VQ scanning may be preferable to limit overall radiation exposure. The use of adjusted D-dimer levels based on age or clinical setting has been studied, but none of these approaches have been standardized. Patients with suspected high-risk PE (i.e., those with shock or hypotension) should have immediate imaging and treatment for PE if the imaging is positive, although an echocardiographic finding of right ventricular overload may be used to justify treatment for PE in the unstable patient with high clinical suspicion for PE when imaging is not available. Patients who have suspected PE and are not at high risk (i.e., no shock or hypotension) and have a high clinical probability (based on Wells, Geneva, or Pisa scoring) should also proceed directly to imaging, with appropriate treatment if the scan is positive. Patients with a low

clinical probability of PE (based on one of the validated clinical prediction rules) do not need further D-dimer testing or imaging. Patients with intermediate clinical probability should initially have D-dimer testing; further testing or treatment for PE is unnecessary if the D-dimer is negative, and imaging should be performed if the D-dimer is positive.

Anticoagulation, with thrombolysis in high-risk patients, is the foundation of treatment for PE. Patients with shock or hypotension are at high risk and require hemodynamic and respiratory support, thrombolysis, or embolectomy, followed by appropriate attention to anticoagulation. Normotensive patients with echocardiographic evidence of right ventricular dysfunction or serologic evidence of myocardial injury (no elevation of troponins or CK-MB) have intermediate risk and should be admitted for anticoagulation. Normotensive patients who have normal results on echocardiography and testing for myocardial injury are at low risk and often may be discharged early for management at home after initiation of anticoagulation. Anticoagulation for PE should be started at the time of diagnosis. Apixaban (Eliquis) or rivaroxaban (Xarelto) may be used without prior oral anticoagulation; alternatively, unfractionated heparin, low-molecular-weight heparin, or fondaparinux (Arixtra) may be started and continued for 5 to 10 days with simultaneous initiation of dabigatran (Pradaxa), edoxaban (Savaysa or Lixiana), or warfarin (Coumadin) titrated to maintain an international normalized ratio (INR) between 2.0 and 3.0.

Thoracic Aortic Dissection

Thoracic aortic dissection is a much less common cause of chest pain; prevalence estimates are 2 to 3.5 cases per 100,000 person-years. Up to 40% of patients die immediately, and 5% to 20% die during or shortly after surgery. Risk factors for acute thoracic aortic dissection include hypertension, presence of a pheochromocytoma, cocaine use, weightlifting, trauma or a rapid deceleration event, coarctation of the aorta, and certain genetic abnormalities. Pain due to acute aortic dissection is perceived as abrupt and severe in 84% to 90% of cases, and more than 50% of patients describe the pain as sharp or stabbing. No physical findings are sensitive or specific for detecting aortic dissection because approximately equal percentages of patients are hypertensive or normotensive or have hypotension or shock. The most common physical findings (a murmur of aortic insufficiency or a pulse deficit) occur in less than half of patients.

In any patient with severe chest pain that is abrupt or instantaneous in onset or has a ripping, tearing, or stabbing quality, acute thoracic aortic dissection should be suspected. Physical examination should assess for a pulse deficit, a systolic pressure differential between limbs of greater than 20 mm Hg, a focal neurologic deficit, or a new aortic regurgitation murmur. It is also important to ask about a family history of connective tissue disease (including Marfan syndrome), about any family or personal history of aortic dissection or thoracic aneurysm, and about any known aortic valve disease or recent aortic interventions. D-dimer testing has been proposed as a way to screen for aortic dissection, but it is more important to obtain prompt imaging and surgical intervention for those in whom dissection is confirmed. A low-risk Aortic Dissection Detection Risk Score (ADD-RS) can help exclude the diagnosis of aortic dissection, whereas patients with a high-risk score require further evaluation.

An ECG should be obtained in all patients with suspected aortic dissection to exclude STEMI (which can manifest with similar symptoms). In all low- and intermediate-risk patients, a prompt chest x-ray can help by either confirming an alternative diagnosis or confirming the presence of thoracic aortic disease. High-risk patients should have prompt imaging with CT or magnetic resonance imaging (MRI), and those who are in shock or clinically unstable may be evaluated by bedside transesophageal echocardiography. If thoracic aortic dissection is confirmed on imaging, urgent surgical consultation is required. Medical therapy should be started with intravenous β blockers. Patients with dissection of the ascending aorta require urgent surgery, whereas those with descending thoracic aortic dissection may be managed medically unless hypotension or other complications develop.

Esophageal Rupture

Esophageal rupture, or Boerhaave syndrome, has a high mortality rate. Esophageal rupture is rare; the most common cause is endoscopically induced injury, but it can happen in other settings as well. Common misdiagnoses include perforated ulcer, MI, PE, dissecting aneurysm, and pancreatitis. The "classic" presentation has been described as pain, dyspnea, and shock followed by forceful emesis, but the history and physical are commonly nonspecific. Diagnosis most commonly is made by contrast esophagram or CT scan of the chest.

Patients whose rupture is diagnosed less than 48 hours after symptom onset should be treated surgically (especially if sepsis is present) or endoscopically. Those who present more than 48 hours after symptom onset may be considered for conservative treatment with hyperalimentation, antibiotics, and nasogastric suction.

Tension Pneumothorax

Tension pneumothorax is relatively rare among patients presenting with chest pain, but it is potentially life threatening if not treated properly. Common symptoms and physical findings include chest pain, respiratory distress, decreased ipsilateral air entry, and tachycardia; hypoxia, tracheal deviation, and hypotension are less common.

Emergency needle decompression is usually recommended if tension pneumothorax is suspected, but this is ineffective in some cases and is associated with risks to the patient of pain, bleeding, infection, and cardiac tamponade. However, waiting for radiographic confirmation of the diagnosis is associated with up to a fourfold increase in mortality due to delay in decompression of the pneumothorax. Patients most likely to benefit from an immediate attempt at needle decompression are those with an oxygen saturation below 92% while on oxygen, a decreased level of consciousness while on oxygen, a systolic blood pressure less than 90 mm Hg, or a respiratory rate below 10 breaths/min. Patients without these signs of instability may be better managed by waiting for chest imaging to confirm or exclude the presence of a pneumothorax. Although plain chest x-rays have typically been used for diagnosing a pneumothorax, one study has found that pleural ultrasound may have higher sensitivity.

Other Causes of Chest Pain

A patient with chest pain and cough, fever, egophony, or dullness to percussion might have pneumonia, but none of these individual findings is specific enough to confirm the diagnosis. However, adults with an acute respiratory infection who have normal vital signs and a normal pulmonary examination are very unlikely to have community-acquired pneumonia. A large study in 1984 developed a decision rule (Table 4) using seven clinical findings to predict the likelihood of pneumonia. There is ongoing debate over the reliability of pneumonia diagnosis based solely on history and physical examination; chest x-ray is usually considered the reference standard. However, a recent Cochrane review found two trials suggesting that routine chest radiography does not affect the clinical outcomes in adults and children whose presentations are suggestive of a lower respiratory tract infection. Thus at least for clinically stable outpatients, treatment for pneumonia based on appropriate clinical findings alone may be reasonable.

Heart failure alone is an uncommon cause of chest pain, but it may accompany ACS or cardiac valve disease. A displaced apical impulse and a prior history of CAD support this diagnosis, and because virtually all patients with heart failure have exertional dyspnea, its absence is very helpful in excluding this diagnosis. An abnormal ECG and cardiomegaly on chest x-ray can increase the likelihood of heart failure among patients with chest pain, and B-natriuretic peptide (BNP) is now commonly used for detecting heart failure in patients presenting with acute dyspnea. One recent study also found that point-of-care ultrasound (POCUS) may have high sensitivity and specificity for diagnosing acute cardiogenic pulmonary edema.

A three-item questionnaire has been developed specifically to assess for panic disorder among patients with chest pain referred for cardiac evaluation (Table 5), and there is good evidence that

TABLE 4	Diehr Diagnostic Rule for Pneumonia in Adults with Acute Cough
SIGNS AND SYMPTOMS	
FINDING	**POINTS**
Rhinorrhea	−2
Sore throat	−1
Night sweats	1
Myalgia	1
Sputum all day	1
Respiratory rate >25	2
Temperature >100°F	2
INTERPRETATION	
SCORE	**PROBABILITY OF PNEUMONIA**
−3	5
−1	12
0	21
1	30
3	37

Adapted from Cayley Jr WE: Diagnosing the cause of chest pain. *Am Fam Physician* 72:2012–2021, 2005. http://www.aafp.org/afp/2005/1115/p2012.html.

TABLE 5	Evaluation for Chest Pain from Panic Disorder					
ITEM	**0**	**1**	**2**	**3**	**4**	**5**
When you are nervous, how often do you think "I am going to pass out"?		Never	Rarely	Half the time	Usually	Always
During the last 7 days, including today, how much have you been bothered by pains in the chest?		Not at all	A little bit	Moderately	Quite a bit	Extremely
To what degree is your chest pain tiring or exhausting?		None	Mild		Moderate	Severe

Approximately 76% of patients with a score of 4 or less will not have panic disorder (PD). Approximately 71% of patients with a score of 5 or more will have PD.
Adapted from Dammen T, Ekeberg O, Arnesen H, Friis S: The detection of panic disorder in chest pain patients. *Gen Hosp Psychiatry* 21(5):323–332, 1999. PubMed PMID: 10572773. http://www.ncbi.nlm.nih.gov/pubmed/10572773.

psychological interventions such as cognitive behavioral therapy (CBT) and breathing exercises can improve chest pain symptoms for patients with nonspecific chest pain who do not have CAD. However, even in patients with possible panic disorder, further cardiac testing should be done if there are significant cardiac risk factors.

Gastrointestinal disease can cause chest pain, but the history and physical examination are relatively inaccurate for diagnosing or excluding serious gastrointestinal pathology. However, if life-threatening cardiovascular or pulmonary causes of chest pain have been excluded, it is appropriate to try a short course of a high-dose proton pump inhibitor (omeprazole [Prilosec] 40 mg twice daily,[3] lansoprazole [Prevacid] 30 mg daily, or esomeprazole [Nexium] 40 mg twice daily[3]) to evaluate for undiagnosed gastroesophageal reflux disease (GERD) as the cause of chest pain (even for patients without typical GERD symptoms).

Chest wall pain can usually be diagnosed by history and examination if other etiologies have been excluded, and such pain is more likely if the patient's pain is reproducible by palpation. Measurement of the sedimentation rate is not generally helpful in making the diagnosis, although in unusual situations radiography may be helpful.

---

[3]Exceeds dosage recommended by the manufacturer.

References

Cao AM, Choy JP, Mohanakrishnan LN, et al: Chest radiographs for acute lower respiratory tract infections, *Cochrane Database Syst Rev* 12:CD009119, 2013.

Cayley Jr WE: Chest pain–tools to improve your in-office evaluation, *J Fam Pract* 63(5):246–251, 2014.

Cayley Jr WE: Diagnosing the cause of chest pain, *Am Fam Physician* 72:2012–2021, 2005.

de Schipper JP, Pull terGunne AF, Oostvogel HJ, van Laarhoven CJ: Spontaneous rupture of the oesophagus: Boerhaave's syndrome in 2008. Literature review and treatment algorithm, *Dig Surg* 26:1–6, 2009.

Eriksson D, Khoshnood A, Larsson D, et al: Diagnostic accuracy of history and physical examination for predicting major adverse cardiac events within 30 days in patients with acute chest pain, *J Emerg Med* 5;S0736–S4679(19):30828, 2019. https://doi.org/10.1016/j.jemermed.2019.09.044.

Harskamp RE, Laeven SC, Himmelreich JC, et al: Chest pain in general practice: a systematic review of prediction rules, *BMJ Open* 27;9(2):e027081, 2019.

Hendriksen JM, Geersing GJ, Lucassen WA, et al: Diagnostic prediction models for suspected pulmonary embolism: systematic review and independent external validation in primary care, *BMJ* 8(351):h4438, 2015.

Hiratzka LF, Bakris GL, Beckman JA, et al: 2010 ACCF/AHA/AATS/ACR/ASA/SCA/SCAI/SIR/STS/SVM guidelines for the diagnosis and management of patients with thoracic aortic disease: a report of the American College of Cardiology foundation/American Heart Association Task Force on Practice Guidelines, *Circulation* 121:e266–e369, 2010. Erratum in Circulation 2010;122(4):e410.

Kisely SR, Campbell LA, Yelland MJ, Paydar A: Psychological interventions for symptomatic management of non-specific chest pain in patients with normal coronary anatomy, *Cochrane Database Syst Rev* 6:CD004101, 2015.

Leigh-Smith S, Harris T: Tension pneumothorax–time for a re-think? *Emerg Med J* 21:8–16, 2005.

McConaghy JR, Sharma M, Patel H: Acute chest pain in adults: outpatient evaluation, *Am Fam Physician* 102(12):721–727, 2020.

Nienaber CA, Clough RE: Management of acute aortic dissection, *Lancet* 385(9970):800–811, 2015.

O'Connor RE, Al Ali AS, Brady WJ, et al: Part 9: acute coronary syndromes: 2015 American Heart Association guidelines update for cardiopulmonary resuscitation and emergency cardiovascular care, *Circulation* 132(18 Suppl 2):S483–S500, 2015.

Raja AS, Greenberg JO, Qaseem A, et al: Clinical Guidelines Committee of the American College of Physicians. Evaluation of patients with suspected acute pulmonary embolism: best practice advice from the clinical guidelines committee of the American College of Physicians, *Ann Intern Med* 163(9):701–711, 2015.

Reinhardt SW, Lin CJ, Novak E, Brown DL: Noninvasive cardiac testing vs clinical evaluation alone in acute chest pain: a secondary analysis of the ROMICAT-II randomized clinical trial, *JAMA Intern Med* 178(2):212–219, 2018.

Swap CJ, Nagurney JT: Value and limitations of chest pain history in the evaluation of patients with suspected acute coronary syndromes, *J Am Med Assoc* 294:2623–2629, 2005.

Wong BC: Is proton pump inhibitor testing an effective approach to diagnose gastroesophageal reflux disease in patients with noncardiac chest pain?: a meta-analysis, *Arch Intern Med* 165(11):1222–1228, 2005.

CONSTIPATION

Method of
Melissa Gaines, MD

CURRENT DIAGNOSIS

- Although constipation is a benign process, it is important to recognize signs of a serious condition.
- Classification of normal transit constipation, slow transit constipation, or pelvic floor dysfunction guides therapy.
- Clinical testing has low benefit, but colonoscopy or imaging can assess organic causes.

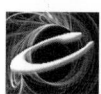

CURRENT THERAPY

- Initial therapy includes soluble dietary fiber to improve symptoms in chronic constipation.
- Osmotic laxatives are preferred while using stimulant laxatives as rescue agents.
- Surgery is reserved for pelvic floor dysfunction after optimal therapies have failed.

Epidemiology

Constipation is common, with a prevalence of 1.9% to 27.2%, but the description of symptoms is variable. A thorough history and focused physical examination aids diagnosis. Treatment is directed toward relief of symptoms, alleviation of precipitating factors, and prevention of recurrence. Although constipation is a benign process, it is important to recognize concerning signs for a more serious medical condition such as malignancy.

Risk Factors

Vulnerable populations include female, elderly, neurodegenerative disease, low-fiber diet, painful rectal disorders, hypothyroidism, and diabetes mellitus.

Pathophysiology

With aging, there is decreased rectal compliance, diminished rectal sensation, and decreased resting anal pressures, while colonic transit time is preserved. Normal transit constipation is a component of irritable bowel syndrome with normal transit time and stool frequency. Slow transit constipation is a condition with colonic dysmotility resulting from altered enteric nervous system. Defecatory disorders include structural disturbances of the pelvic floor. Pelvic floor dysfunction is the paradoxical contraction of the external anal sphincter and puborectalis muscles during defecation. Secondary causes of constipation are listed in Table 1.

Prevention

Provide an environment of privacy and comfort to allow for natural defecation. Prescribe an adequate fluid and fiber intake with specific amounts that vary depending on the patient's condition. Encourage physical activity, with a low to moderate level of exercise depending on the patient's functional status. Develop a routine for defecation with a prompt response to a call to defecate urgently. Recurrent fecal impaction can be prevented with polyethylene glycol (PEG, MiraLAX).

Clinical Manifestations

Patients will complain using qualitative terms of hard stools, a feeling of incomplete voiding, straining, prolonged time for laxation, the need for additional maneuvers, abdominal bloating, and abdominal pain (Table 2). A change in bowel habit differentiates the current complaint from a serious medical condition. Red flags include acute onset, weight loss, abdominal pain or cramping, rectal bleeding, nausea or vomiting, rectal pain, fever, or a change

TABLE 1	Causes of Constipation
Dietary	Low-fiber diet, dementia, depression, anorexia, dehydration
Metabolic	Diabetes mellitus, hypercalcemia, hypokalemia, hypothyroidism, systemic sclerosis
Neurologic	Parkinson disease, spinal cord disorder, multiple sclerosis, cerebrovascular disease (stroke)
Iatrogenic	Antacids, iron, anticholinergics, antidepressants, antipsychotics, opiates, antiepileptics
Painful anorectal condition	Anal fissure, hemorrhoids, abscess, fistula, pelvic floor dysfunction, malignancy

TABLE 2	Rome III Criteria
More than two present:	1. Straining in more than 25% of defecations
	2. Hard or lumpy stool in more than 25% of defecations
	3. Sensation of incomplete evacuation
	4. Sensation of anorectal blockage
	5. Manual maneuvers
	6. Fewer than three defecations per week
Loose stools are rare without laxative use	
Insufficient criteria for irritable bowel syndrome	
Symptoms for 3 months with onset 6 months before diagnosis	

TABLE 3	Drug Dosing and Adverse Effects				
CLASS	DRUG NAME (BRAND)	ADULT DOSING	MECHANISM OF ACTION	TIME TO ONSET (H)	ADVERSE EFFECT
Fiber	Bran Psyllium (Metamucil) Methylcellulose (Citrucel) Calcium polycarbophil (FiberCon)	1 cup/day 1 tsp 1 tbsp or 1 tab twice daily 2–4 tabs/day	Increase water content and bulk of stool decreasing transit time	Unknown	Bloating excessive gas
Hyperosmolar agent	Sorbitol 70% Lactulose (Chronulac)	15–30 mL twice daily	Disaccharide metabolized by colonic bacteria into acetic acid and short-chain fatty acids	24–48	Sweet tasting, transient abdominal cramps, flatulence
Hyperosmolar agent	PEG-ES (GoLytely,[1] CoLyte[1]) PEG (MiraLAX)	8–32 oz daily 17 g (1 tbsp) qd	Osmotic effect increasing intraluminal fluids	0.5–1	Incontinence
Guanylate cyclase-C agonist	Plecanatide (Trulance) Linaclotide (Linzess)	CIC and IBS-C: 3 mg once daily CIC: 72–145 mcg once daily IBS-C: 290 mcg once daily	Osmotic effect increasing intraluminal fluids, increase transit time	Cannot be calculated	Diarrhea Abdominal pain, diarrhea
Chloride channel activator	Lubiprostone (Amitiza)	CIC and OIC: 24 mcg twice daily IBS-C in women ≥18 y: 8 mcg twice daily	Increase intestinal fluid secretion and improve fecal transit	Unknown	Headache, nausea, diarrhea
Stimulant	Glycerin suppository Bisacodyl (Dulcolax) Senna (Senokot, Perdiem) Senna/docusate (Peri-Colace)	1 daily 10 mg suppository or 5–10 mg PO 3 times a week 2–4 tabs twice daily	Local rectal stimulation, secretory and prokinetic effect	8–12	Degeneration of Meissner and Auerbach plexus
Enemas	Mineral oil retention enema Tap water enema Sodium phosphate enema (Fleet)	199–250 mL daily PR 500–1000 mL PR 1 unit PR	Evacuation induced by distended colon and mechanical lavage	6–8 for a mineral oil enema 5–15 min for all other enemas	Mechanical trauma, incontinence, rectal damage
Opioid antagonist	Methylnaltrexone (Relistor)	8–12 mg 1 dose SC every other day as needed for OIC with advanced illness. 450 mg PO once daily or 12 mg SC once daily for OIC with chronic noncancer pain.	Opioid mu receptor antagonist in gut decreasing transit time	4	Diarrhea, intestinal perforation
Opioid antagonist	Naloxegol (Movantik)	12.5–25 mg PO daily	Same as Relistor	6–36	Abdominal pain, opioid withdrawal reported

[1]Not US Food and Drug Administration (FDA) approved for this indication.
CIC, Chronic idiopathic constipation; *IBS-C*, irritable bowel syndrome with constipation; *OIC*, opioid-induced constipation; *PEG-ES*, polyethylene glycol and electrolyte solution; *PO*, by mouth; *PR*, per rectum; *SC*, subcutaneously.

in stool caliber. Infants with abdominal distension and failure to pass meconium within 24 hours indicate Hirschsprung disease. Patients should be asked if they have had loose stools or bowel incontinence to assess for fecal impaction. A medication review is required (see Table 1). Classification of patients with normal transit constipation, slow transit constipation, or pelvic floor dysfunction/defecatory disorders guides therapy.

Diagnosis

Diagnostic criteria have been established because the symptoms can vary (see Table 2). Conduct a physical examination that includes an assessment of vital signs, weight, volume status, auscultation of bowel sounds, abdominal percussion for tympani, and abdominal palpation for tenderness or mass. A rectal examination can detect resting rectal tone, fecal impaction, anorectal disorders, or rectal mass. Defecatory disorders show an increased resistance to the insertion of the examiner's finger with an impaired relaxation of the sphincter complex and reduced perineal descent during a Valsalva maneuver. Conduct laboratory testing on electrolytes, hemoglobin, thyroid-stimulating hormone, and fecal occult after initial measures fail. Red flag symptoms require imaging with computed tomography (CT) of the abdomen and pelvis or an endoscopy to diagnose malignancy or fecal impaction. Anorectal testing with manometry and a rectal balloon expulsion test is appropriate for pelvic floor dysfunction or defecatory disorders. Hirschsprung disease is diagnosed with barium enema, rectal manometry, or a rectal suction biopsy. Colonic transit rates with radiopaque markers (Sitz) on serial abdominal radiographs over 4 to 7 days diagnose slow transit constipation disorders.

Treatment

Nonpharmacologic therapies have limited benefit. Unless there are signs of dehydration, increasing fluid intake is not indicated. Moderate-intensity exercise improves symptoms of irritable bowel syndrome. Probiotics are not beneficial.

There is moderate evidence for pharmacologic agents (Table 3). Normal transit constipation responds to soluble dietary fiber supplements (e.g., psyllium [Metamucil]); however, these should not be used in the case of slow transit constipation or drug-induced constipation. Osmotic agents with PEG (MiraLAX) or lactulose (Chronulac) can be dose increased for soft stools. Stimulant laxatives are used as rescue therapy if patients do not have a bowel movement for 2 days.

New classes of drugs to manage constipation include intestinal secretagogues, serotonin 5-HT$_4$ receptor antagonists, and opiate antagonists. Lubiprostone (Amitiza) requires a negative pregnancy test with contraception. Linaclotide (Linzess) is a 14–amino acid peptide similar to heat-stable enterotoxins that cause diarrhea. Lubiprostone and linaclotide are US Food and Drug Administration (FDA)-approved for chronic idiopathic constipation (CIC) and irritable bowel syndrome with constipation (IBS-C). Lubiprostone is also indicated for treatment of opioid-induced constipation (OIC). Plecanatide (Trulance) is an approved drug for treatment of CIC and IBS-C in adults. It is a guanylate cyclase-C agonist that increases fluid secretion into the upper intestine. Methylnaltrexone (Relistor) and naloxegol (Movantik) are opiate receptor antagonists that can cause laxation in patients on chronic opiate therapy with number needed to treat (NNT) of 5.

Pelvic floor dysfunction or defecatory disorders respond to biofeedback therapy by using manometry and visual or auditory feedback. Patients practice expelling a balloon and improve pelvic floor muscle coordination with Kegel exercises. Surgical intervention with subtotal colectomy with ileorectal anastomosis is indicated for slow transit constipation or defecatory disorders after failure of optimal medical management.

Complications

Fecal impaction is a complication and a large bowel obstruction with colonic perforation has high mortality. Pediatric and geriatric patients are most susceptible with signs and symptoms of fecal incontinence, abdominal pain, abdominal distention, anorexia, weight loss, and delirium. Treatments for adults include a large-volume tap-water enema (500 to 1000 mL), local anesthetics administered topically with abdominal massage, a colonoscopy, or surgery. The prevention of recurrence requires maintenance bowel regimen with osmotic agents such as PEG (MiraLAX).

References

Arshad A, Powell C: Easily missed? Hirschsprung's disease, *Br Med J* 345:e5521, 2012.

Barish DF, Crozier RA, Griffin PH: Long-term treatment with plecanatide was safe and tolerable in patients with irritable bowel syndrome with constipation, *Curr Med Res Opin* 1–5, 2018.

Bharucha AE, Pemberton JH, Locke GR: American Gastroenterological Association technical review on constipation, *Gastroenterology* 144:218–238, 2013.

Gallagher PF, O'Mahony D, Quigley EM: Management of chronic constipation in the elderly, *Drugs Aging* 25:807–821, 2008.

Gastroenterology: Rome criteria. Available at http://www.romecriteria.org/.

Higgins PD, Johanson JF: Epidemiology of constipation in North America: a systematic review, *Am J Gastroenterol* 99:750–759, 2004.

Larkin PJ, Sykes NP, Centeno C, et al: The management of constipation in palliative care: Clinical practice recommendations, *Palliat Med* 22:796–807, 2008.

McCallum IJ, Ong S, Mercer-Jones M: Chronic constipation in adults, *Br Med J* 338:b831, 2009.

Nee J, et al: Efficacy of treatments for opioid-induced constipation: a systemic review and meta-analysis, *Clin Gastroenterol Hepatol*, 2018 Jan 25.

Schoenfeld P, et al: Low-Dose linaclotide (72ug) for chronic idiopathic constipation: A 12-week, randomized, double-blind, placebo-controlled trial, *Am J Gastroenterol*, 2018, 113-105–114. https://doi.org/10.1038/ajg.2017.230.

Thomas J, Karver S, Cooney GA, et al: Methylnaltrexone for opioid-induced constipation in advanced illness, *N Engl J Med* 358:2332–2343, 2008.

Wald A: Management and prevention of fecal impaction, *Curr Gastroenterol Rep* 10:299–501, 2008.

Wald A: Constipation: Advances in diagnosis and treatment, *JAMA* 315(2):185–191, 2016 Jan 12.

COUGH

Method of
Emily Manlove, MD, MPH

CURRENT DIAGNOSIS

- Acute Cough
  - Noninfectious
    - Chronic obstructive pulmonary disease exacerbation
    - Asthma exacerbation
    - Congestive heart failure exacerbation
    - Pulmonary embolism
  - Infectious
    - Viral rhinosinusitis (the common cold)
    - Acute bacterial sinusitis
    - Acute bronchitis (chest cold)
    - Pneumonia
    - Pertussis (whooping cough)
    - Bronchiolitis (infants)
- Chronic cough
  - First, evaluate/rule out
    - Tobacco smoking and risk for lung cancer
    - Angiotensin-converting enzyme (ACE) inhibitor associated cough
  - Next, evaluate for the three most common etiologies
    - Chronic upper airway cough syndrome
    - Cough variant asthma/nonasthmatic eosinophilic bronchitis
    - Gastroesophageal reflux disease
  - Last, consider other causes and more advanced testing (bronchoscopy, high-resolution computed tomography [CT] scanning, referral) and consider earlier if history, physical, or chest x-ray suggests an alternative diagnosis
    - Oral pharyngeal dysphagia
    - Lung tumors
    - Interstitial pulmonary diseases
    - Bronchiectasis
    - Occupational and environmental exposures
    - Sarcoidosis
    - Tuberculosis
    - Somatic cough syndrome
    - Tic cough

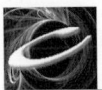
CURRENT THERAPY

- Acute cough due to viral rhinosinusitis
  - Dextromethorphan (Delsym) 30 mg PO every 6 to 8 hours × 1 week
  - Diphenhydramine (Benadryl) 25 mg PO every 4 hours × 1 week
  - Nasal saline irrigation twice daily × 1 week
- Acute or subacute cough caused by *Bordetella pertussis*
  - Azithromycin (Z-Pak)[1] 500 mg PO on day 1 followed by 250 mg PO daily on days 2 to 5
- Treatment of unexplained chronic cough
  - Multimodality speech pathology therapy
  - Gabapentin (Neurontin) 300 mg PO daily, can be titrated up to a maximum daily dose of 1800 mg a day in two divided doses (off label use)

[1]Not FDA approved for this indication.

Acute Cough

Acute cough is a cough that lasts fewer than 3 weeks. It is a common presenting complaint in the primary care physician's office and also in the emergency room. The key goal is to differentiate between those patients whose cough has a benign cause and those who may be at risk for more serious illness. Infectious causes of cough are most common, but noninfectious causes should also be considered. Exacerbations of preexisting pulmonary conditions such as asthma and chronic obstructive pulmonary disease (COPD) can be associated with cough, therefore a thorough medical history should be obtained. Cough can also be associated with decompensated heart failure; in fact, cough is present in 70% of congestive heart failure (CHF) exacerbations. Also, 30% to 40% of patients with acute pulmonary embolism (PE) have a new cough at presentation of symptoms, and the classic signs and symptoms of chest pain, dyspnea, and hypoxia may not always accompany the cough.

Upper respiratory tract infections are a common cause of benign acute cough. The common cold, also known as viral rhinosinusitis, is probably the most common cause of acute cough. The lung exam is normal. If fever is present it is low grade and is only present on the first or second day of illness. Most symptoms begin to resolve by 7 to 10 days, but cigarette smokers may be ill for twice as long. Symptomatic treatment is the mainstay of therapy. First-generation antihistamines combined with a decongestant and naproxen have been proven to reduce the length of cough. Second-generation antihistamines are not effective in the treatment of cough associated with viral rhinosinusitis; it is likely that first-generation antihistamines are effective because of their anticholinergic properties. Other treatments that may be helpful include nasal saline irrigation, nasal glucocorticoids, and nasal decongestants. It is necessary to distinguish viral rhinosinusitis from acute bacterial rhinosinusitis, which may also be associated with cough. Less than 2% of all rhinosinusitis has a bacterial cause. Acute bacterial rhinosinusitis should not be diagnosed in the first week of symptoms unless the patient displays severe symptoms such as high fever. Sinus imaging studies are unlikely to be helpful, as both viral and bacterial sinusitis will have radiologic evidence of inflammation.

It is also necessary to distinguish an acute cough caused by an upper respiratory tract infection and that caused by a lower respiratory tract infection. Furthermore, it is necessary to distinguish between acute bronchitis, which almost always has a viral cause, versus pneumonia, which has a bacterial cause. Both illnesses often have a presenting symptom of cough, which may be productive. If there is any derangement in vital signs or evidence of pulmonary consolidation on the lung exam, a chest x-ray should be performed. Infectious Diseases Society of America (IDSA) guidelines require the presence of consolidation on chest x-ray to diagnose pneumonia. Influenza should also be considered for those patients who have fever and cough during flu season. An elevated procalcitonin level may help guide the physician in his or her decision to prescribe antibiotics. Beta agonists should not be routinely used to alleviate cough in acute viral bronchitis, but may be helpful for the alleviation of wheezing and are more likely to benefit patients with airflow obstruction at baseline.

In pediatric patients, bronchiolitis should be considered as a cause of cough and fever. It is the most common cause of hospitalization in those less than 1 year old. The most recent guidelines recommend abstaining from lab testing (including viral swabs), radiographic imaging, and treatment with beta agonists, epinephrine, or glucocorticoids as these interventions do not change the course of illness. Exclusive breastfeeding for the first 6 months of infancy can decrease the morbidity of respiratory infections. *Bordetella pertussis* can cause severe illness with cough and apnea in infants. However, adults have subtle symptoms and lack the classic "whooping cough" and posttussive emesis seen in children. The physician should have suspicion for pertussis in patients who have a cough lasting longer than 2 weeks and paroxysms of coughing; the cough can last up to 2 months. The diagnosis can be confirmed with polymerase chain reaction (PCR). Antibiotics do not alter the course of illness but reduce the spread of infection; azithromycin (Zithromax)[1] should be given for 3 to 5 days. Vaccination rates remain low. Pregnant women should be vaccinated with each pregnancy and other adults should replace 1 dose of Td at the earliest convenience.

Chronic Cough

A chronic cough is a cough lasting more than 8 weeks. Patients may have a presenting symptom of a cough that has been present for more than 3 but fewer than 8 weeks; this is considered a subacute cough. In this case, the physician should illicit a history of respiratory infection; the patient is likely suffering from a postinfectious cough, which is related to inflammation of the airway epithelium, mucus hypersecretion, and/or increased cough reflex sensitivity. Inhaled corticosteroids may provide some benefit. If there is no history of recent infection, then the cough should be managed as a chronic cough. Chest x-ray can be considered during this time frame, but if no red flags are present (fever, unintended weight loss, night sweats, dysphagia, odynophagia, hemoptysis) the physician and patient together can decide to wait on radiography.

Chronic cough must be approached in a systematic manner, which is more likely to identify the causative agent of the cough and provide alleviation of symptoms. All of the common causes of chronic cough (see later) must be considered, as the associated symptoms and the patient's description of the cough do not alter the diagnostic algorithm. It is important to confirm compliance throughout the treatment course and identify barriers to compliance with the patient. Failure to respond to empiric treatment does not necessarily rule out a diagnosis, as the patient may have two diagnoses. Therefore, it is prudent to continue any partially effective treatment for chronic cough.

First, it must be determined if the patient smokes. If so, the differential diagnosis is altered. The physician must determine if the cough is a simple smoker's cough, chronic bronchitis, or possibly lung cancer; cough is the most common presenting symptom of lung cancer. Smokers are less likely to seek help for a cough and may not see a physician until a more serious problem has advanced. It is possible for a cough to worsen initially after smoking cessation, but a cough persisting more than 1 month after cessation should be investigated. Any change in a smoker's cough, a new cough, and cough with hemoptysis should be investigated. Physicians should consider low dose CT scanning as screening for lung cancer in qualifying smokers. The second factor to rule out in all chronic cough cases is cough induced by an angiotensin-converting enzyme (ACE) inhibitor. All patients with chronic cough should stop taking an ACE inhibitor. The medication is more likely to cause a cough if it was started in the prior year, and the cough should resolve within 1 month after cessation of

[1]Not FDA approved for this indication.

the ACE inhibitor. The next step to determining the cause of a chronic cough is to rule out the three most common causes of cough. Last, all patients with a cough lasting more than 8 weeks should be evaluated with chest radiography to identify any obvious causative factors.

Upper Airway Cough Syndrome

Upper airway cough syndrome (UACS), previously called post-nasal drip syndrome, is likely caused by activation of cough receptors in the hypopharynx or larynx and increased sensitivity of these receptors. It is likely the most common cause of chronic cough. UACS is almost always associated with rhinosinusitis, which can be caused by a number of factors (allergic rhinitis, postinfectious rhinitis, perennial nonallergic rhinitis, rhinitis resulting from chemical irritants, rhinitis medicamentosa, pregnancy-associated rhinitis, bacterial sinusitis, allergic fungal sinusitis, etc.). The patient may complain of frequently needing to clear the throat or a sensation of "dripping" in the back of the throat; however, absence of these symptoms does not rule out UACS, nor does a history of wheezing. Physical exam may reveal mucus in the posterior oropharynx and cobblestoning of the mucosa. If the cause of rhinitis is obvious, it should be specifically treated. Otherwise, a trial of a first-generation antihistamine should be started; improvement should be seen in 2 weeks. If the side effects of this therapy are intolerable, a nasal antihistamine, nasal anticholinergic, or nasal corticosteroid can be used. If the diagnosis of UACS is highly suspected but the patient does not respond to empiric therapy, sinus CT imaging may be necessary to guide diagnosis and treatment.

Cough Variant Asthma and Nonasthmatic Eosinophilic Bronchitis

Cough variant asthma and nonasthmatic eosinophilic bronchitis (NAEB) both primarily present with a cough, and the patient may have few other symptoms. Patients with cough variant asthma will have abnormal spirometry, whereas those with NAEB will not. When spirometry is performed, bronchoprovocation testing with methacholine should be performed as it increases the negative predicative value of the test. If spirometry is negative, the sputum should be evaluated for eosinophils, which are present in both diseases. Both diseases are treated as asthma; an inhaled corticosteroid should be started and leukotriene receptor antagonists can be considered. A positive response should be expected within 2 weeks.

Gastroesophageal Reflux Disease

Gastroesophageal reflux disease (GERD) is common, but not all patients with GERD have an associated cough; therefore, the presence of GERD does not ensure that it is the source of the patient's cough. However, those patients whose cough is clearly not caused by UACS, cough variant asthma, or NAEB are very likely to have a GERD-induced cough. Cough can be caused by acidic and nonacidic reflux, so a proton pump inhibitor (PPI) may not always be of benefit. A pH probe can be performed in cases when it is unclear whether reflux is occurring. All patients should utilize lifestyle changes to attenuate reflux, such as smoking cessation, avoidance of alcohol and acidic foods, weight loss, and treatment of sleep apnea. It may take 3 to 6 months of treatment to see improvement in cough. If the patient does not improve and GERD is highly suspected, referral to a surgeon may be necessary for fundoplication.

Other Causes of Chronic Cough

In those patients who still suffer from chronic cough and the above causes have been ruled out, further investigation should be sought. Referral to a pulmonologist may be necessary, in addition to high-resolution CT scanning and bronchoscopy. Causative factors may include oral pharyngeal dysphagia, lung tumors, interstitial pulmonary diseases, bronchiectasis, occupational and environmental exposures, sarcoidosis, and tuberculosis. Somatic cough syndrome (previously referred to as psychogenic cough)

and tic cough (previously referred to as habit cough) may be considered in some patients; hypnosis, suggestion therapy, and/or counseling may be beneficial. In patients who remain symptomatic, regardless of known or unknown causes, the diagnosis of "difficult to treat" cough is made. Assessing cough severity and quality of life with validated tools may be beneficial. Options do remain for these patients, including speech language pathology intervention, empiric gabapentin, and/or referral to a cough clinic.

References

Benich III JJ, Carek PJ: Evaluation of the patient with chronic cough, *Am fam physician* 2011 Oct 15 84(8), 887–92.
Côté A, Russell RJ, Boulet LP, et al: Managing chronic cough due to asthma and NAEB in adults and adolescents: CHEST guideline and expert panel report. *Chest.* 2020 Jan 20.
Irwin RS, French CL, Chang AB, et al: Classification of cough as a symptom in adults and management algorithms: CHEST guideline and expert panel report, *Chest* 2018;153(1):196–209.

DIZZINESS AND VERTIGO

Method of
Jennifer Wipperman, MD, MPH

CURRENT DIAGNOSIS

- Benign paroxysmal positional vertigo
  - Repeated, brief episodes lasting less than 1 minute
  - Triggered by changes in head position
  - Positive Dix-Hallpike or Supine Roll Test
- Vestibular neuritis
  - Single, severe, constant episode lasting days
  - Subacute onset
  - Positive head impulse test
  - Nystagmus is unidirectional and horizontal
- Vestibular migraine
  - Recurrent episodes lasting hours to days
  - Includes features of migraine headache
  - Responds to traditional migraine treatment
- Ménière's disease
  - Recurrent episodes of vertigo lasting hours
  - May have hearing loss, tinnitus, or ear fullness
- Red flags for stroke include:
  - Sudden onset
  - Risk factors for stroke
  - Bidirectional or purely vertical nystagmus
  - Abnormal HINTS exam
  - Focal neurologic signs
  - Inability to walk

CURRENT THERAPY

- Benign paroxysmal positional vertigo
  - The canalith repositioning procedure (Epley maneuver) is the most effective treatment.
  - Avoid vestibular suppressant medications
  - Observation with close follow-up is optional if a patient will not tolerate the canalith repositioning procedure and if symptoms are mild
- Vestibular neuritis
  - Brief symptomatic care with benzodiazepines, antiemetics, and antihistamines
  - Early vestibular rehabilitation speeds recovery.
  - Use of corticosteroids is controversial.

The "dizzy" patient is often a frustrating phenomenon in clinical medicine. However, after a careful history and physical examination, most patients can be diagnosed and serious causes excluded. Peripheral causes of vertigo are usually benign and include vestibular neuritis and benign paroxysmal positional vertigo (BPPV). Life-threatening central causes include stroke, demyelinating disease, and an intracranial mass. The first step in evaluating vertigo is differentiating among the four types of dizziness: near syncope or light-headedness, disequilibrium, psychogenic dizziness, and true vertigo. True vertigo is a false sense of motion, and patients often report that "the room is spinning." This chapter will focus on the two most common causes of episodic vertigo: BPPV and vestibular neuritis.

Epidemiology

Vertigo is a common office complaint. Every year, millions of Americans are evaluated for dizziness in ambulatory care settings, and approximately 50% of these cases are vertigo. BPPV and vestibular neuritis are two of the most common causes of vertigo seen in the office setting.

Risk Factors

BPPV is seven times more likely in individuals over age 60, and it is also more common in women. A history of prior head trauma and other vestibular disorders increases risk of BPPV. There are no identified risk factors for vestibular neuritis.

Pathophysiology

BPPV is thought to occur when calcium carbonate debris (otoconia) are dislodged and float freely in the semicircular canals of the inner ear. The posterior canal is most often involved. During head movement, loose otoconia move in the canal and cause a continued sense of motion for a few seconds until they settle. The pathophysiology of vestibular neuritis is uncertain. Limited evidence supports a viral infection, most likely HSV-1, which causes inflammation of the eighth cranial nerve. When hearing loss accompanies vertigo, the condition is called *acute labrynthitis*.

Clinical Manifestations

The history and physical examination are fundamental in the evaluation of vertigo. Key questions include the frequency and duration of attacks, triggers such as positional or pressure changes, prior head trauma, associated neurologic symptoms, hearing loss, and headache. A personal history of diabetes, hypertension,

and hyperlipidemia are risk factors for stroke. BPPV, stroke, and migraine can have a familial preponderance. Many medications, including anticonvulsants and antihypertensives, cause dizziness.

BPPV causes brief, recurrent episodes that last less than 1 minute and are brought on by changes in head movement or position. Nausea and vomiting may be associated. Vestibular neuritis usually has a subacute onset over several hours, peaks in intensity for 1 to 2 days, and then gradually subsides over the next few weeks. Symptoms of vertigo are constant, and nausea and vomiting can be severe during the first few days. Patients with vestibular neuritis may have difficulty standing and veer toward the affected side. Although changes in position worsen the vertigo in vestibular neuritis, vertigo is always present at baseline. In BPPV, patients have no vertigo between attacks.

General physical examination should include a thorough cardiovascular, ear, nose, throat, and neurologic examination. The neurologic examination can differentiate between benign (peripheral) and life-threatening (central) causes based on the ability to walk, type of nystagmus, results of the head impulse test, and presence of associated neurologic signs (Table 1).

Patients with vestibular neuritis may have difficulty walking, but the inability to walk is a red flag for a central lesion. Nystagmus is unidirectional (always beats in the same direction) and horizontal in vestibular neuritis, and is suppressed by visual fixation. Having a patient focus on an object in the room will stop the nystagmus, which reappears if a blank sheet of paper is placed a few inches in front of the patient's face. Nystagmus in central causes is not suppressed by visual fixation and may be direction-changing (nystagmus beats to the right when the patient looks right, and beats to the left when the patient looks left) or purely vertical. The head impulse test (Figure 1) is positive in peripheral causes like vestibular neuritis. The examiner holds the patient's head while the patient fixes her eyes on the examiner's nose, and then the examiner quickly moves the patient's head 10 degrees to the right and left. If a saccade (the eyes look away and then re-fixate on the examiner's nose) is found, this indicates a peripheral lesion on the side that the head is turned toward. Central lesions will not cause saccades, and the head impulse test will be negative. HINTS (Head Impulse test, Nystagmus, Test of Skew), which combines three physical examination findings, has been found to have a 97% sensitivity and 99% specificity for a central cause of vertigo in the acute setting and to be more accurate than MRI in the initial 24 hours after symptom onset. If one or more of the tests indicate a central cause, (e.g., a negative head

TABLE 1	Differentiating Peripheral and Central Causes of Vertigo		
	PERIPHERAL CAUSES		
	BPPV	**VESTIBULAR NEURITIS**	**CENTRAL CAUSES**
History	Brief, recurrent attacks of vertigo lasting less than 1 minute Triggered by positional changes No vertigo between attacks	Subacute onset Constant and severe vertigo lasting days Nausea and vomiting may be severe	Sudden onset Risk factors for stroke May have severe headache
Nystagmus	Up-beating and torsional	Horizontal and unidirectional	Bidirectional Pure vertical Pure torsional
Gait	Unaffected between episodes	May veer towards affected side	Unable to walk
Specialized physical examination tests	Positive Dix-Hallpike or Positive supine roll test	Positive head impulse test Visual fixation stops nystagmus	HINTS exam abnormal Visual fixation does not stop nystagmus
Additional neurologic signs	Rare	Rare	Common (e.g., dysarthria, aphasia, incoordination, weakness, or numbness)

Abbreviation: BPPV = benign paroxysmal positional vertigo.

impulse test, direction-changing horizontal nystagmus, or vertical eye misalignment grossly observed or detected on cover-uncover test), then the HINTS test is considered positive for a central cause and imaging should be obtained. A negative HINTS exam is an excellent rule-out test for stroke, with a negative likelihood ratio of 0.02.

The Dix-Hallpike maneuver is diagnostic of posterior canal BPPV (Figure 2). The patient should be warned that nausea and vomiting may occur. After the patient is placed in the head-hanging position, there is a 5- to 20-second latency period before the nystagmus and symptoms appear. Both the nystagmus and vertigo will increase in severity and then resolve within 60 seconds. The nystagmus observed is up-beating and torsional. If nystagmus is constant for as long as the head is in the hanging position, the patient should be evaluated for a central cause. The maneuver should be repeated with the head held to the opposite side. The side that elicits the symptoms and nystagmus diagnoses BPPV in the ipsilateral ear. If both sides elicit symptoms, the patient may have bilateral BPPV. If the test is negative and BPPV is strongly suspected, the patient should lie supine and the examiner can turn the head to each side (supine roll test; Figure 3). This maneuver will cause vertigo and nystagmus in patients with horizontal canal BPPV.

Diagnosis

BPPV and vestibular neuritis are diagnosed clinically. Further diagnostic testing is indicated if the diagnosis is uncertain or a central cause is suspected. Audiometry may be abnormal in Ménière's disease. MRI is the best imaging test for central lesions because it includes the posterior fossa and is most sensitive for stroke. Vestibular function testing is useful if the diagnosis is unclear or in cases of refractory vertigo. Vestibular function testing evaluates the ocular and vestibular response to position changes and caloric stimulation. Video-oculographic recordings of nystagmus can magnify the eye and allow for repeated viewings for further study. Some patients with BPPV may have additional vestibular disorders causing vertigo that vestibular function testing can elucidate.

Differential Diagnosis

Ménière's disease is suspected in patients with the triad of tinnitus, fluctuating hearing loss, and vertigo. Episodes usually last hours, are disabling, and are recurrent over years, over time leading to permanent dysfunction. Migrainous vertigo features episodes lasting hours to days in patients with other migraine symptoms such as headache, photophobia, phonophobia, or aura. Central lesions such as stroke or intracranial mass are most concerning. Red flags for stroke include sudden onset, risk factors for stroke, associated neurologic signs, inability to walk, abnormal HINTS exam, severe associated headache, and characteristic nystagmus. Posttraumatic vertigo may occur in patients after head trauma who present with vertigo, tinnitus, and headache. A perilymphatic fistula is rare, but may be suspected in a patient with episodic vertigo after head trauma, heavy lifting, or barotrauma. Pressure changes with sneezing or coughing trigger vertigo attacks. Postural hypotension should be ruled out in all patients. An acoustic neuroma presents with slowly progressive, unilateral sensorineural hearing loss and tinnitus. Many patients may have an unsteady gait, but true vertigo is rare.

Treatment

Posterior canal BPPV is best treated with the *canalith repositioning procedure (CRP)*, such as the Epley maneuver (Figure 2). Studies have shown the procedure is safe and effective with an odds ratio of 4.2 (95% CI. 2.3-11.4) for symptom resolution. Patients should be warned that nausea or vomiting may occur during the procedure, and may be pretreated with an antiemetic medication. The procedure can be repeated immediately if

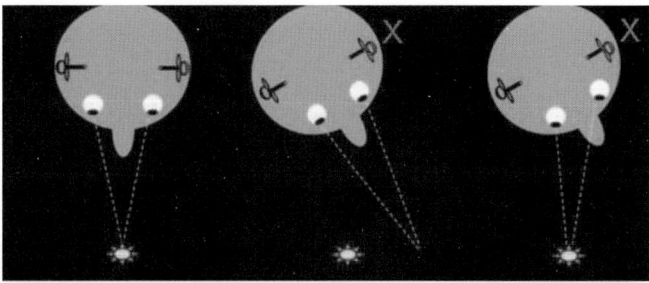
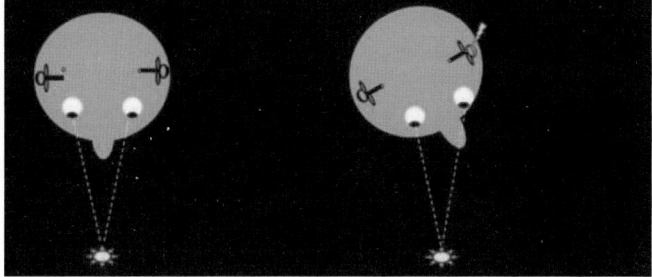

Figure 1 Head impulse test. Top panel shows a positive head impulse test. The examiner moves the patient's head quickly 10 degrees to the side, in this case to the patient's left. A catch-up saccade is observed when the patient looks away and then refixes on the visual target, indicating a peripheral lesion on the left. Lower figure shows a normal head impulse test. The patient maintains visual fixation during head movement. Adapted from Seemungal BM, Bronstein AM. A practical approach to acute vertigo. *Pract Neurol* 2008; 8:211–21.

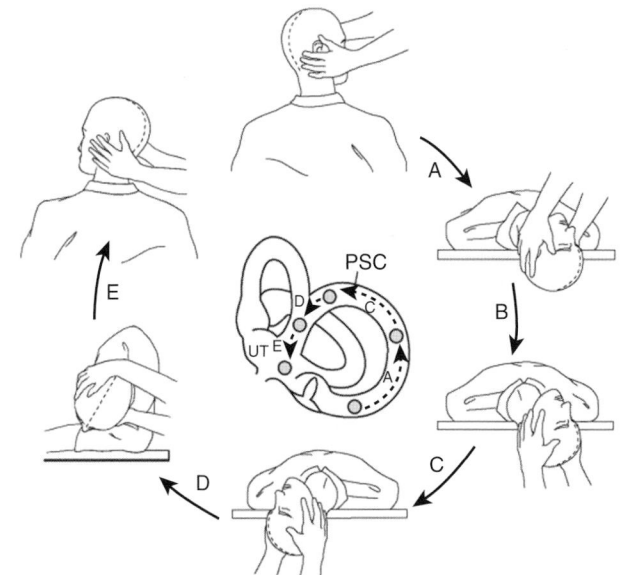

Figure 2 Treatment maneuver for posterior canal benign paroxysmal positional vertigo affecting the right ear. To treat the left ear, the procedure is reversed. The drawing of the labyrinth in the center shows the position of the particle as it moves around the posterior semicircular canal (PSC) and into the utricle (UT). The patient is seated upright, with head facing the examiner, who is standing on the right. **A**, The patient is rapidly moved to head-hanging right position (Dix-Hallpike test). This position is maintained until the nystagmus ceases. **B**, The examiner moves to the head of the table, repositioning hands as shown. **C**, The head is rotated quickly to the left with right ear upward. This position is maintained for 30 seconds. **D**, The patient rolls onto the left side while the examiner rapidly rotates the head leftward until the nose is directed toward the floor. This position is then held for 30 seconds. **E**, The patient is rapidly lifted into the sitting position, now facing left. The entire sequence should be repeated until no nystagmus can be elicited. After the maneuver, the patient is instructed to avoid head-hanging positions to prevent the particles from reentering the posterior canal. Reprinted with permission from Rakel RE. *Conn's Current Therapy 1995.* Philadelphia, WB Saunders, 1995, p 839.

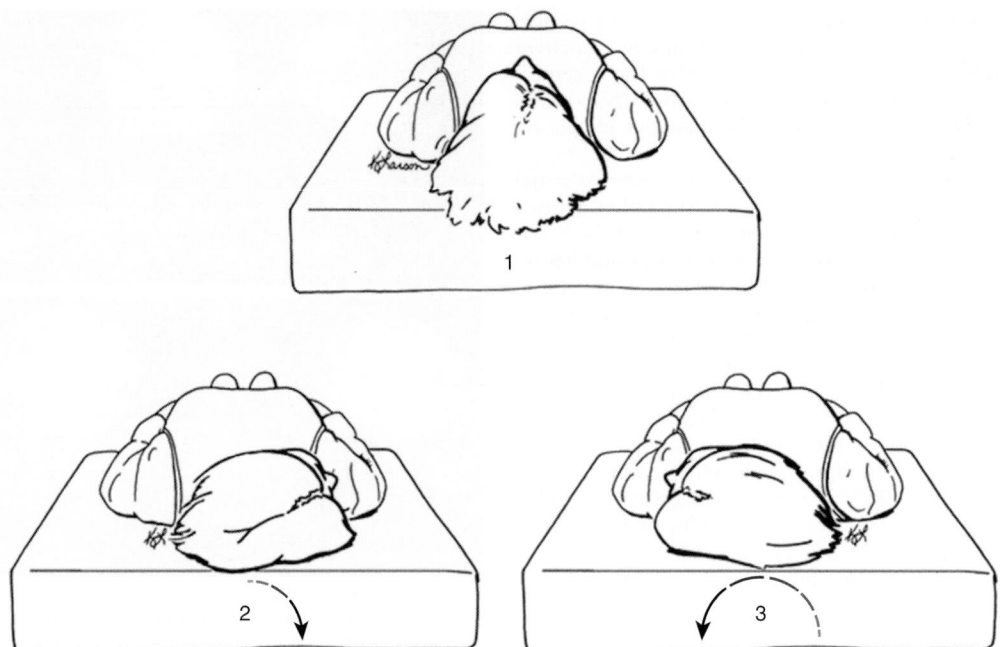

Figure 3 Supine roll test. Patient begins lying supine facing upward. The patient's head is rotated to one side laterally 90 degrees and the examiner observes for nystagmus and vertigo. Once symptoms resolve, the patient's head is rotated back to midline. Next, the patient's head is rotated 90 degrees laterally to the opposite side and the examiner observes for nystagmus and vertigo. The side with the worst symptoms indicates the involved ear. (From Kerber KA, et al: Benign paroxysmal positional vertigo in the acute care setting. NCL, Elsevier, 2015.)

unsuccessful, and the majority of patients will respond after three attempts. Posttreatment activity restrictions are unnecessary. Horizontal canal BPPV can be treated with the barbeque roll maneuver (Figure 4). Vestibular rehabilitation (VR) is a treatment option for BPPV but is significantly less effective than the canalith repositioning procedure. VR is helpful in patients with chronic, nonspecific dizziness after successful treatment with CRP and for improving gait stability in those with increased fall risk, such as the elderly. Observation is an option if symptoms are mild and if a patient will not tolerate the canalith repositioning procedure. However, time to resolution with observation is 1–3 months, and recurrence rates are higher compared to treatment with CRP. Vestibular-suppressant medications such as antihistamines and benzodiazepines are discouraged because they increase fall risk and treatment with CRP is effective. Surgery is rarely needed for BPPV, but may be helpful in refractory cases.

Vestibular neuritis is primarily treated with rest, vestibular suppressant medications, and vestibular rehabilitation. Patients may initially be hospitalized if symptoms, such as nausea and vomiting, are severe or if stroke is suspected. Treatment with antihistamines (dimenhydrinate [Dramamine][1] 50 mg every 6 hours), antiemetics (promethazine [Phenergan][1] 25 mg every 6 hours), or benzodiazepines (lorazepam [Ativan][1] 1 to 2 mg every 4 hours) may be used to treat severe symptoms. However, these should not be continued for more than 2 to 3 days because they inhibit central compensation. In vestibular neuritis, patients' vertigo improves not due to return of vestibular nerve function, but due to central compensation for the peripheral deficit. Using vestibular suppressants blocks central

compensation and lengthens the course of the disease. The use of corticosteroids is controversial; a 2011 Cochrane review concluded that there is insufficient evidence to recommend corticosteroids for the treatment of vestibular neuritis. Finally, antiviral medications have not been proven effective for vestibular neuritis.

For patients with vestibular neuritis, vestibular rehabilitation should be started as soon as symptoms improve and a patient can tolerate the exercises. Exercises include balance and gait training as well as coordination of head and eye movements. Vestibular rehabilitation hastens recovery and improves balance, gait, and vision by increasing central compensation for vestibular dysfunction. Exercises may be home-based for compliant patients with mild symptoms, whereas formal referral may be more beneficial for patients with severe symptoms, or for the elderly.

Monitoring
Patients diagnosed with BPPV should be reassessed in 1 month regardless of treatment. Failure to improve warrants further evaluation for other etiologies, including central causes. Similarly, patients with vestibular neuritis should slowly improve over several weeks, and failure to do so suggests alternative diagnoses.

Complications
Patients with BPPV are at increased risk for falls. Thirty percent of elderly patients with BPPV have multiple falls in a year. Thus patients should be assessed for fall risk, functional mobility, and balance. Home safety evaluation and home supervision should be considered. BPPV often recurs, with an estimated rate of 15% per year. Counseling patients about recurrence can lead to earlier recognition, earlier treatment, and avoidance of falls. Patients with vestibular neuritis are at increased risk for BPPV and Ménière's disease. Vestibular neuritis rarely recurs.

---

[1] Not FDA approved for this indication.

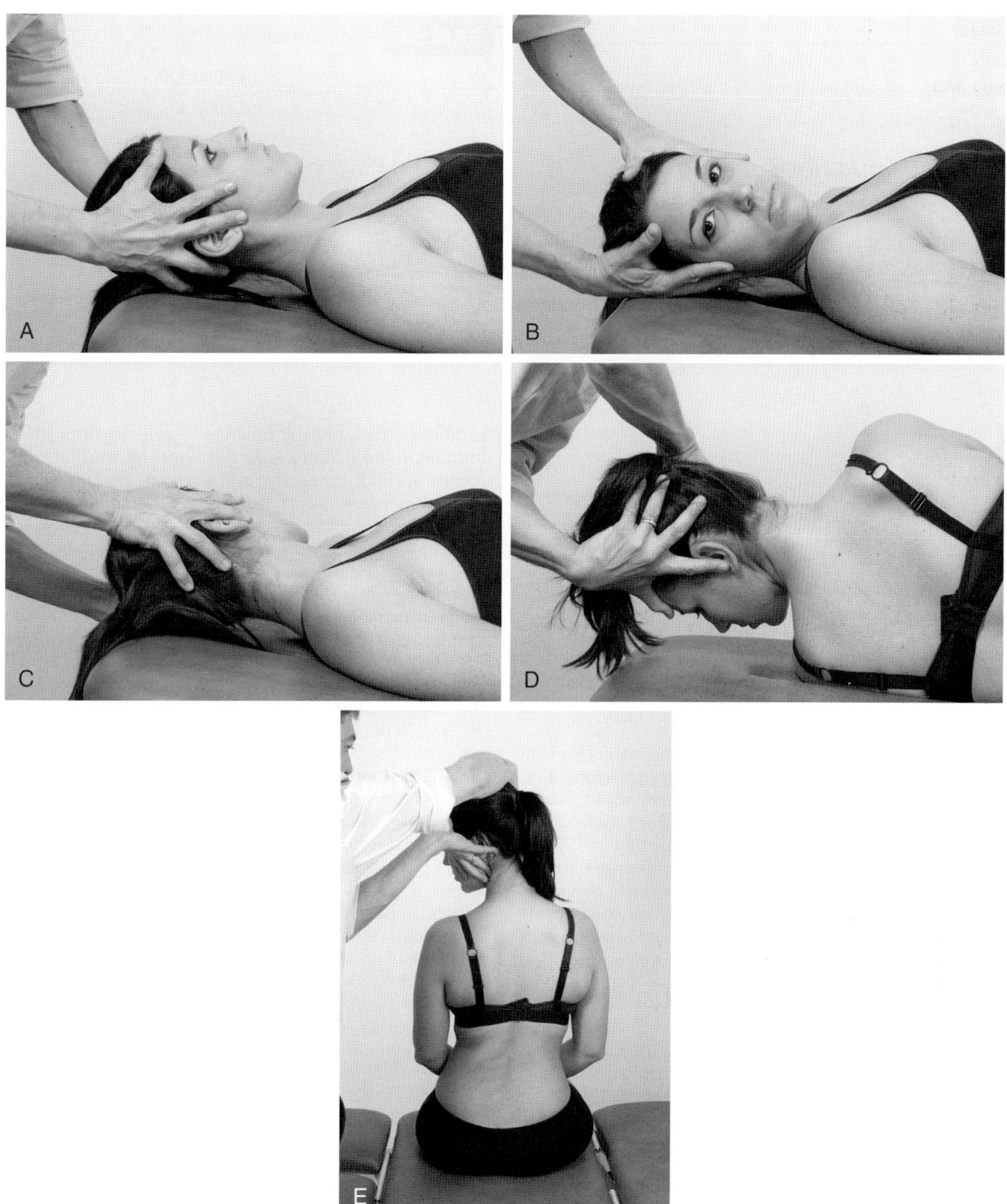

Figure 4 Barbecue roll (Lempert maneuver). Patient begins lying supine facing upward (A). Head is rotated laterally 90 degrees toward the affected ear (B). Next, the head is rotated another 90 degrees laterally back to midline (B). Next, the head is rotated laterally 90 degrees toward the opposite side (C). Next, the head is rotated laterally 90 degrees in the same direction (D). Finally, with the patient's head in the same position, the patient is brought into a seated position (E). Each position is held 30 to 60 seconds, long enough for symptoms to occur and then resolve. Once resolved, the patient is moved into the next position. (From Moseley L, Cueco RT: Essential guide to the cervical spine - Volume 2: Clinical Syndromes and Manipulative Treatment. Elsevier, 2016.)

References

Baloh RW: Vestibular neuritis, *N Engl J Med* 348:1027–1032, 2003.

Bhattacharyya N, Gubbels SP, Schwartz SR, et al: Clinical practice guideline: benign paroxysmal positional vertigo (update), *Otolaryngol Head Neck Surg* 156(Supp 3):S1–S47, 2017.

Chan Y: Differential diagnosis of dizziness, *Otolaryngol Head Neck Surg* 17:200–203, 2009.

Epley JM: The canalith repositioning procedure: for treatment of benign paroxysmal positional vertigo, *Otolaryngol Head Neck Surg* 107:399–404, 1992.

Fishman JM, Burgess C, Waddell A: Corticosteroids for the treatment of idiopathic acute vestibular dysfunction (vestibular neuritis), *Cochran Database Syst Rev 5*, CD008607, 2011. Review.

Hilton MP, Pinder DK: The Epley (canalith repositioning) manoeuvre for benign paroxysmal positional vertigo, *Cochrane Database Syst Rev 12*, CD003162, 2014.

Kerber KA: Vertigo and dizziness in the emergency department, *Emerg Med Clin North Am* 27:39–50, 2009.

McDonnell MN, Hillier SL: Vestibular rehabilitation for unilateral peripheral vestibular dysfunction, *Cochrane Database Syst Rev 1*, CD005397, 2015.

Newman-Toker DE, Kerber KA, Hsieh YH, et al: HINTS outperforms ABCD2 to screen for stroke in acute continuous vertigo and dizziness, *Acad Emerg Med* 20(10):986–996, 2013.

Seemungal BM, Bronstein AM: A practical approach to acute vertigo, *Pract Neurol* 8:211–221, 2008.

FATIGUE

Method of
Jared Regehr, MD

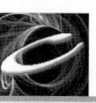

CURRENT DIAGNOSIS

- It is important to evaluate for potential causes of fatigue with a thorough history and physical exam. Basic lab work is also important to evaluate for organic etiologies of fatigue.
- Most cases of fatigue do not have an identifiable underlying etiology.
- A broad differential is important as clinicians evaluate patients with fatigue.

CURRENT THERAPY

- Identifying the underlying cause of fatigue is the most important step in treatment, and any discovered cause should be treated promptly.
- Good sleep hygiene, physical activity, regularly scheduled follow-up visits, and cognitive behavioral therapy have all been shown to improve symptoms of fatigue.
- Short naps are proven performance enhancers.

Epidemiology

Fatigue is a common concern for patients and is the primary complaint for 5% to 10% of patient encounters in the primary care setting. Certain risk factors predispose patients to fatigue. Female sex (1.5 times more likely to report fatigue than males), increased age, and coexisting depression are all associated with higher rates of fatigue. While fatigue can be a normal physiologic response to prolonged activity or stressors, pathologic fatigue has a significant negative impact on patients each year. Individuals with fatigue report decreased quality of life, along with social and emotional dysfunction. Furthermore, it is estimated that fatigue costs US employers $126 billion each year due to decreased production and lost work days.

Prevention

Prevention of fatigue is very similar to the treatment of fatigue. Good sleep hygiene, regular physical exercise, and stress reduction all help with preventing fatigue. Additionally, regularly scheduled follow-up for health maintenance examinations with primary care physicians helps patients avoid comorbidities that may exacerbate fatigue.

Clinical Manifestations

Patients with fatigue often present with lack of energy, delayed recovery after activity, poor muscle endurance, mental exhaustion, and nonrestorative sleep. There is a wide spectrum of severity of disease from a general nuisance to debilitating symptoms.

Diagnosis

Fatigue can be classified based on duration: recent (<1 month), prolonged (1–6 months), and chronic (>6 months). Notably, these timeframes are arbitrary based on the continuous nature of fatigue. For most clinicians, having a broad differential is more helpful in identifying a cause than categorizing fatigue based on time. Even so, identifying the underlying etiology of fatigue can be a challenging and frustrating diagnosis for primary care physicians to make because of vague symptoms and the overlap with comorbidities. A thorough history and physical examination along with appropriate laboratory tests can aid in the diagnosis. There is much debate about the extent of initial laboratory workup, but a reasonable approach includes a complete blood count, basic

TABLE 1	Common Causes of Fatigue: DEAD TIRED
D	Depression
E	Endocrine
A	Anemia, apnea
D	Diabetes
T	Thyroid, tumors
I	Infection, insomnia
R	Rheumatologic
E	Endocarditis/cardiovascular
D	Drugs

metabolic panel, hepatic function testing, erythrocyte sedimentation rate, thyroid-stimulating hormone, ferritin, pregnancy test in women of childbearing age, and screening for HIV and hepatitis C in at-risk populations. These tests are useful to help identify "can't miss" diagnoses, but results of laboratory studies only affect management in about 5% of cases. Therefore the importance of a thorough history and physical examination is paramount. It is essential to remember that the information collected from the patient does not need to be limited to the time spent together in the office; a symptom diary with close follow-up can be an extremely beneficial tool as the physician–patient dyad works to find a cause.

The causes of fatigue are extensive and oftentimes coexisting. The most common causes are encompassed in the mnemonic DEAD TIRED (Table 1). Most of these categories have multiple subcategories. As with all chief complaints, it is imperative to allow patients the opportunity to lead the physician to the diagnosis by letting them speak without interruption. Depression is a common cause of fatigue. Medically unexplained symptoms of fatigue are associated with depressive disorders in 50% to 75% of patients, and patients are nearly 11 times more likely to have a lifetime diagnosis of depression than nonfatigued individuals. Importantly, fatigue may be the first presenting symptom for patients who do not yet meet the *Diagnostic and Statistical Manual of Mental Disorders* (DSM) criteria for depression, so close monitoring for other depressive symptoms is vital for prompt recognition and treatment. In most of these cases, there are often other lifestyle factors that contribute to patients' feelings of fatigue. It is important to ask about sleep hygiene, physical exercise, and home/social stressors, as suboptimal functioning in these areas can exacerbate symptoms of fatigue.

Other common secondary causes of fatigue include anemia, endocrine abnormalities, sleep apnea, and medication use. If anemia is noted on initial laboratory evaluation, further workup is usually patient-specific. Markers such as mean corpuscular volume (MCV), ferritin, iron profile, B12, folate, lactate dehydrogenase, and haptoglobin can help guide decision making as clinicians consider causes of anemia. Gastrointestinal bleeding secondary to ulcers, colon cancer, inflammatory bowel disease, or diverticulosis are critical to rule out. Lack of sufficient dietary vitamin intake may be a simple reason for anemia. Endocrine abnormalities that can lead to fatigue include thyroid dysfunction, diabetes mellitus, and adrenal insufficiency. If patients describe persistent daytime sleepiness, evaluation for obstructive sleep apnea is useful, especially in the setting of risk factors (obesity, snoring, hypertension). Additionally, medication usage can cause fatigue. An in-depth review of the legion of medications that can cause fatigue is beyond the scope of this article, but prescription, over-the-counter, and illicit drugs should be considered in the evaluation of fatigue.

Infection is a cause of fatigue, and the most frequent infectious etiology associated with fatigue is of viral origin. Any one of several viruses can cause fatigue, including hepatitis A, B, and C; Epstein-Barr virus; human immunodeficiency virus; and as of recently, COVID-19. Certainly not every patient presenting with fatigue necessitates laboratory evaluation for each of these causes, but if the history or examination suggests an infectious cause, further workup is prudent. Even after recovery from COVID-19, 72.8% of patients report persistent fatigue, by far the most common long-term symptom reported by survivors of COVID-19. This is an important consideration even months after patients have otherwise recovered from the disease. Postinfluenza asthenia refers to the prolonged fatigue some patients experience after a bout of influenza.

Finally, rheumatologic, cardiovascular, and neoplastic causes should be considered when appropriate in the evaluation of fatigue. Although there are innumerable reports of fatigue in patients with rheumatologic, cardiovascular, oncologic, and hematologic disorders, isolated fatigue as the presenting complaint is not well documented in current medical literature. Additionally, multiple neurologic and autoimmune disorders can have associated fatigue. If the rest of the history and examination warrants further workup for these causes, then evaluation should be pursued. However, an extensive workup based on an isolated complaint of fatigue is not likely to yield beneficial results.

Therapy

Treatment for fatigue should be directed at managing the underlying cause of fatigue when an etiology can be identified based on the history, physical, and laboratory evaluation. However, when no organic cause is identified, there are still ways to help patients get relief. Importantly, ordering more tests is not one of them. In a systemic review of patients with fatigue in which there was a low level of clinical concern for serious illness, the degree of patient reassurance was not increased with additional laboratory testing. Instead, the clinician should start with having an honest conversation with the patient regarding ways to move forward. It is imperative to acknowledge the patient's symptoms and the negative effects on the patient's life, discuss consistent follow-up, and discuss assessment of any new symptoms that may develop. Additionally, there is evidence that sleep hygiene, physical activity, and cognitive behavioral therapy may be helpful in these settings of nondiagnostic fatigue. Short naps have also proven to be helpful and may be a possible solution for some patients.

Monitoring

Monitoring patients with persistent fatigue in the primary care setting can be accomplished by administering a Fatigue Severity Scale (FSS). This method assesses the impact of fatigue on patients' daily lives with a nine-item survey that incorporates a Likert-type rating scale. The FSS has been validated in multiple studies as a reliable tool to assess fatigue. Although there is no generally agreed upon timing for frequency of monitoring, it is reasonable to start with monthly assessments and utilize shared decision making with each patient to individualize a management plan.

References

Corfield E, Martin N, Nyholt D: Co-occurrence and symptomatology of fatigue and depression, *Compr Psychiatry* 71:1–10, 2016.
Finsterer J, Zarrouk-Mahjoub S: Fatigue in health and diseased individuals, *Am J Hosp Palliat Med* 31(5):562–575, 2014.
Friedberg F, Napoli A, Coronel J, et al: Chronic fatigue self-management in primary care: a randomized trial, *Psychosom Med* 75(7):650–657, 2013.
Kamal M, Abo Omirah M, Hussein A, Saeed H: Assessment and characterisation of post–COVID–19 manifestations, *Int J Clin Pract*, 2020. Available at: https://doi-org.proxy.kumc.edu/10.1111/ijcp.13746. Accessed December 31, 2020.
Morelli V: Toward a comprehensive differential diagnosis and clinical approach to fatigue in the elderly, *Clin Geriatr Med* 27(4):687–692, 2011.
O'Connor K, Wright J: Fatigue, *Med Clin North Am* 98(3):597–608, 2014.
Rosenthal T, Majeroni B, Pretorius R, Malik K. Fatigue: an overview. *Am Fam Physician.* 15;78(10):1173–1179
Valko P, Bassetti C, Bloch K, Held U, Baumann C: Validation of the fatigue severity scale in a swiss cohort, *Sleep* 31(11):1601–1607, 2008.
Zhang XY, Huang HJ, Zhuang DL, et al: Biological, clinical and epidemiological features of COVID-19, SARS and MERS and AutoDock simulation of ACE2, *Infect Dis Poverty* 9, 2020. Available at: https://doi.org/10.1186/s40249-020-00691-6. Accessed December 31, 2020.

FEVER

Method of
Alan R. Roth, DO; and Gina M. Basello, DO

CURRENT DIAGNOSIS

- Numerous endogenous and exogenous factors play a role in determining body temperature. Current standards define *fever* as an oral temperature of ≥100.4°F (≥38°C).
- Though temperature varies with measurement technique, in clinical practice, most recommendations refer to oral, rectal, and axillary temperature measurements, with rectal temperature being the standard of care in infants and young children.
- Tympanic thermometers should not be used in young children.
- Fever is not an illness. It is the body's physiologic response to a disease process and has beneficial effects in fighting infection.
- All neonates with a fever should be admitted to the hospital for a full sepsis evaluation. For infants between 1 and 3 months of age, evidence-based guidelines, along with clinical evaluation, determine the diagnostic and therapeutic approach.
- With widespread immunization use, the incidence of bacteremia and bacterial meningitis in young infants has significantly decreased, and UTI is now the most prevalent bacterial infection, with the most common etiologic pathogen being *E. coli.*
- The possibility of infection with the SARS-CoV-2 virus must be considered in all patients presenting with fever and tested for appropriately.
- Urine leukocyte esterase has emerged as a highly accurate diagnostic test for UTI in febrile infants with greater than 95% sensitivity.
- FUO requires a systematic, thoughtful, and thorough evaluation based on the age of the patient and the existing clinical evidence, with repeated clinical assessments being essential.
- Hyperthermia is an unregulated, significant elevation of core body temperature above the normal diurnal range due to failure of thermoregulation from a hypothalamic insult, not a pyogenic source, and is considered a medical emergency. It is not synonymous with fever and often requires immediate intervention to avoid deleterious central nervous system (CNS) effects.

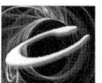

CURRENT THERAPY

- Treating a fever significantly increases the patient's level of comfort, activity, and oral feeding and fluid intake, in addition to decreasing the body temperature.
- Multiple randomized, controlled trials reveal that treating fever does not shorten or prolong the overall duration of illness or reduce the occurrence of febrile seizures.
- Many clinical recommendations state that a temperature less than 102.2°F (39°C) in healthy children does not require treatment. Antipyretics are known to provide comfort to children and their caregivers.
- Antipyretic treatment for children includes acetaminophen (Tylenol) 10 to 15mg/kg every 4 to 6 hours or ibuprofen (Advil, Motrin) 10mg/kg every 6 hours.
- Ibuprofen and acetaminophen have both been shown to reduce fever effectively and safely. Combination therapy has been shown in some studies to have an added benefit in both reduction of temperature and comfort without an increase in side effects, though caution should be taken to avoid dosing errors.

- Antipyretic therapy for adults and adolescents includes acetaminophen 650 to 1000 mg orally (PO) every 6 hours to a maximum of 3 g per day, ibuprofen 200 to 400 mg PO every 6 hours, or aspirin (ASA) 325 to 650 mg every 6 hours as needed (PRN) for fever.
- ASA should not be used in children due to the risk of Reye's syndrome.
- Sponge bathing should be done with tepid water and no alcohol. Recommendation: sponge bathing and other home remedies should not be used as sole treatment.

Fever is one of the most common clinical presentations encountered by primary care physicians and the most common complaint of acute visits for children in the ambulatory or emergency department setting. Fever is a symptom and one of the most reliable signs of illness rather than a disease process itself. Most causes of fever are secondary to acute viral illnesses such as upper respiratory infections (URIs), which account for 50 million visits to primary care providers annually. Less commonly, bacterial infections may cause pharyngitis, otitis, sinusitis, pneumonia, and urinary tract infections (UTIs). A cost-effective, evidence-based approach using clinical protocols, guidelines, and consensus recommendations to the diagnosis and management of febrile illness, including the appropriate use of antibiotic therapy, is the cornerstone of quality medical care for this presentation. Fever produces significant anxiety for patients, parents, and health care providers, which can lead to overtreatment. Typically, fever is transient and only requires treatment to provide patient comfort.

Definitions

The definition of fever is dependent on numerous endogenous and exogenous factors that play a role in determining body temperature, including age, time of day, site, and measuring device, as well as operator variables. Fever is an elevation of body temperature due to the adjustment of the hypothalamic-pituitary set point. This usually occurs in response to a pathologic stimulus. Fever is a beneficial physiologic mechanism that helps to promote an augmented immunologic response.

Despite individual variability, core body temperature is maintained at about 98.6°F (37°C). Diurnal variation results in lower body temperatures in the early morning and a temperature higher in the late afternoon or early evening, which is consistent with what is encountered in clinical practice.

In adults, a morning oral temperature of 98.9°F (37.2°C) or higher, or an evening temperature of 99.9°F (37.7°C) or higher defines a fever. Rectal temperatures are generally considered to be 0.7°F (0.4°C) higher than oral readings.

In infants and young children, rectal temperatures are still considered the standard of care and a rectal temperature greater than 100.4°F (38°C) is considered a fever.

Axillary temperatures of greater than 98.6°F (37°C) are regarded as a fever, though this measurement site is generally considered less accurate. An accurate measurement of body temperature is dependent on site, measuring device, and the clinical skills of the operator. Site selection should be determined by the age of the patient.

Young infants and older adults often have a diminished febrile response due to physiologic factors, thereby warranting the use of other clinical factors to guide diagnosis.

Recent technologic advances, including electronic devices, tympanic membrane scanning, and temporal artery scanning, have replaced the older mercury-in-glass thermometers. These devices offer faster results and minimal inconvenience to the patient and are becoming increasingly reliable. Chemical content or liquid crystal thermometers applied to the skin are neither accurate nor cost-effective.

Hyperthermia is an uncontrolled elevation of core body temperature that exceeds the body's ability to lose heat. In hyperthermia, the setting of the hypothalamic thermoregulatory center is unchanged, in contrast to fever. Hyperthermia requires urgent medical intervention because it could be rapidly fatal and does not respond to antipyretics. Common etiologies include heat stroke, neuromalignant syndrome, serotonin syndrome, malignant hyperthermia, endocrinopathy, and CNS damage.

Classic *fever of unknown origin* (FUO) is defined as a disorder with temperatures ≥100.9°F (38.3°C) that have persisted for at least 3 weeks, with no definitive cause elucidated after initial comprehensive inpatient or outpatient workup. The etiologies of FUO generally fall into four diagnostic categories: infectious, autoimmune or inflammatory, neoplastic, and miscellaneous.

Pathophysiology

Fever occurs as part of an inflammatory response to an inciting stimulus. The response includes the production of various cytokines that ultimately increase the production of prostaglandin E_2 (PGE_2), which resets the hypothalamic thermoregulatory set point at a higher level. Important pyogenic cytokines include interleukin-1 (IL-1), interleukin-6 (IL-6), tumor necrosis factor α (TNF-α), interferon-β (IFN-β), and interferon-γ (IFN-γ).

Risks and Benefits of Fever

Fever is known to enhance the immunologic response while suppressing the growth and replication of bacterial and viral infections. Though often uncomfortable for patients, caregivers, and health care providers, evidence supports the notion that fever is beneficial and ultimately protects against the development of asthma and other allergic disorders. In most instances, fever is not harmful. It does increase cardiac demand and metabolic needs, resulting in the common associated signs and symptoms of tachycardia, tachypnea, shivering, malaise, and diaphoresis.

The use of antipyretic agents has not been shown to either prolong or shorten the duration of illness. Febrile seizures cause significant anxiety for parents. They occur most commonly in children between the ages of 6 months and 6 years. Most febrile seizures are uncomplicated and have not been shown to be associated with significant bacteremia or to lead to the development of seizure disorder in older children. Antipyretic agents have not been shown to decrease the incidence of febrile seizures.

Diagnostic Evaluation of Fever

In most cases, the etiology of a febrile illness is a self-limiting viral infection. From 5% to 10% of fevers may be associated with a more serious bacterial infection such as pneumonia, UTI, bacteremia, meningitis, or bone and joint infections. At times, these conditions may be challenging to distinguish, and a thoughtful, systematic, evidence-based approach to the diagnostic evaluation will be most cost-effective while avoiding the inappropriate use of antibiotics.

Although the most common clinical presentation of COVID is fever with respiratory symptoms, a significant proportion of patients will present with fever alone or atypically. Considering this, COVID testing is indicated for all patients presenting with fever. All infants less than 28 days old with a fever should be admitted to the hospital for a full sepsis workup and empiric intravenous antibiotic therapy.

Young infants, 1 to 3 months of age, with a febrile illness can be especially challenging. Numerous studies addressing this challenging population have led to the development of multiple guidelines and clinical protocols that utilize risk stratification criteria. The use of these age-specific stratification criteria, along with clinical treatment guidelines, helps guide the clinician in the evaluation of febrile illness. Clinical judgment remains the cornerstone of good clinical care.

With the widespread use of *Haemophilus influenzae* type B (Hib) and pneumococcal vaccinations, the incidence of bacteremic illness has decreased significantly. UTI has emerged as the most prevalent bacterial infection. The increased use of rapid viral testing in the office and emergency department settings may alleviate the need for more invasive testing and antibiotic use because the risk of concurrent bacterial infection has been reported to be negligible.

In this age group, an initial workup that reveals a white blood cell (WBC) count of less than 5000 or greater than 15,000 indicates an increased likelihood of a significant bacterial illness (SBI). Blood cultures, urinalysis, urine culture, and cerebrospinal fluid (CSF) evaluation should then be obtained and accompanied by intravenous antibiotic therapy. When considering the use of inflammatory markers diagnostically, procalcitonin has emerged as the most accurate inflammatory marker, followed by (in descending order) C-reactive protein, absolute neutrophil count, and white blood cell count. Incorporating urine concentration when interpreting urine analyses can help in the differentiation of infants at higher risk of UTI.

Children age 3 to 36 months, who appear well and do not have any underlying medical history, require only a comprehensive clinical evaluation and do not warrant antibiotic therapy or diagnostic testing in most instances. Septic or ill-appearing children need a more aggressive evaluation, including complete blood count (CBC), inflammatory markers, urinalysis, urine culture, blood cultures, and a chest x-ray. High-risk children in this age group require empiric antibiotic therapy, and clinical judgment should guide the decision to hospitalize.

Classic FUO is defined as a disorder with temperatures greater than 100.9 °F (38.3 °C) that has persisted for at least 3 weeks with no clear etiology determined after 3 days of hospital evaluation or three outpatient visits. Common etiologic categories include infectious, neoplastic, inflammatory, and miscellaneous causes, of which drug fever has been shown to be the most prevalent.

The initial approach includes a thorough history, physical examination, and appropriate laboratory testing. The initial choice of imaging should be guided by clinical findings and most commonly includes a chest x-ray and a CAT scan of the abdomen and pelvis. If the etiology remains elusive, positron emission tomography (PET) scanning or invasive diagnostic testing should then be considered.

Differential Diagnosis

Hyperthermia is an unregulated, significant elevation of core body temperature above the normal diurnal range due to failure of thermoregulation from a hypothalamic insult, not a pyogenic source, and is considered a medical emergency. It is not synonymous with fever and often requires immediate intervention to avoid deleterious CNS effects. Since the hypothalamic set point remains unchanged, antipyretics are ineffective in hyperthermia. The most common etiology is the inability to regulate or dissipate excess body heat. Hyperthermia is a medical emergency that requires immediate treatment to prevent excessive morbidity and mortality.

Treatment

Though controversy exists regarding the necessity of lowering fever, antipyretics have been shown to effectively and safely reduce temperature and improve symptoms with minimal side effects. Acetaminophen (Tylenol) is available in many formulations. Dosing should be based on body weight and not age of the patient. The dose is 10 to 15 mg/kg every 4 to 6 hours, not to exceed 3 g daily or 2 g in patients with renal or hepatic impairment. Ibuprofen (Advil, Motrin) is a nonsteroidal antiinflammatory drug (NSAID) that has both antiinflammatory and antipyretic effects. Dosing is 10 mg/kg every 6 to 8 hours in children and 200 to 400 mg every 6 hours in adolescents and adults. Ibuprofen is also available in multiple formulations, including a newer intravenous preparation (ibuprofen [Caldolor]) that may be beneficial in oral-intolerant hospitalized patients. Some studies suggest that ibuprofen may be a more effective antipyretic agent than acetaminophen.

In adults, aspirin (ASA) remains a therapeutic alternative for lowering fever at a dose of 325 to 650 mg every 4 to 6 hours. It should not be used in children with a febrile illness due to the risk of Reye's syndrome.

A combination of acetaminophen and ibuprofen in alternating doses has been shown in some studies to have an added benefit in both reduction of temperature and comfort without an increase in side effects, though caution should be taken to avoid dosing errors.

Nonpharmacologic therapies such as sponge bathing with tepid water and other environmental measures to control temperature, including adjusting room temperatures and sipping cool fluids to avoid dehydration, are used commonly and do provide symptom relief and comfort. These measures should never be used as the sole therapy for fever reduction.

References

Cunha BA: Fever of unknown origin: focused diagnostic approach based on clinical clues from the history, physical examination, and laboratory tests, *Infect Dis Clin North Am* 21:1137–1187, 2007.

Dorney K, Bachur RG: Febrile infant update, *Curr Opin Pediatr* 29:280–285, 2017.

Hernandez D, Nguyen V: Fever in infants <3 months old: what is the current standard? *Pract J Pediatr Emerg Med* 16:1–15, 2011.

Herzog L, Phillips S: Addressing concerns about fever, *Clin Pediatr* 50:383–390, 2011.

Huppler AR, Eickhoff JC, Wald ER: Performance of low-risk criteria in the evaluation of young infants with fever: review of the literature, *Pediatrics* 125:228, 2010.

Jhavier R, Byington C, Klein J, Shapiro E: Management of the non-toxic appearing acutely febrile child: a 21st century approach, *J Pediatr* 159:181–185, 2011.

Makoni M, Mukundan D: Fever, *Curr Opin Pediatr* 22:100–106, 2010.

Pantell RH, Roberts KB, Greenhow TL, Pantell MS: Advances in the diagnosis and management of febrile infants: challenging tradition, *Adv Pediatr* 65(1):173–208, 2018.

Roth AR, Basello GM: Fever. In Paulman PM, Harrison JD, Paulman MD, et al, *Signs and Symptoms in Family Medicine*, Philadelphia, 2012, Mosby, pp 317–326.

Roth AR, Basello GM: Approach to the adult patient with fever of unknown origin, *Am Fam Physician* 68:2223–2228, 2003.

Struyf T, Deeks, Dinnes J, et al; Cochrane COVID-19 Diagnostic Test Accuracy Group: Signs and symptoms to determine if a patient presenting in primary care or hospital outpatient settings has COVID-19. *Cochrane Database of Systematic Reviews* 2021, Issue 2. Art. No.: CD013665.

Sullivan J, Farrar HC: Clinical report: fever and antipyretic use in children, *Pediatrics* 127:580–587, 2011.

Van den Bruel A, Thompson MJ, Haj-Hassan, et al: Diagnostic value of laboratory tests in identifying serious infections in febrile children; systematic review, *BMJ* 342:382, 2011.

GASEOUSNESS, INDIGESTION, NAUSEA, AND VOMITING

Method of
Justin Bailey, MD

Nausea is a vague, subjective feeling that vomiting (forceful expulsion of gastric contents) is imminent. Dyspepsia (based on Rome III criteria) can include postprandial fullness, early satiety, epigastric pain, burning, and reflux (return of gastric content to the lower esophagus or mouth, accompanied by a sour taste or "heartburn" sensation). Gaseousness can present with a variety of complaints, including belching, bloating, abdominal pain, or flatulence.

Epidemiology

Nausea and vomiting (ICD-10 Code R11.2) is one of the top reasons patients see a primary care provider. Infectious diseases causing nausea and vomiting, gastroenteritis, diarrhea, and dehydration are leading causes of death in developing countries, and of sick days and reduction of employee productivity in the United States. Nausea and vomiting postoperatively and during cancer chemotherapy add significant costs, pain, and discomfort to hospital and ambulatory treatment. Dyspepsia occurs in an estimated 25% of the US population every year, many of whom do not seek care. Gaseousness is ubiquitous in the population and is troubling to a small portion.

Risk Factors

Previous gastrointestinal (GI) surgery, certain medications, chemotherapeutic regimens, substance abuse, pregnancy, infectious diseases, medical conditions, and central nervous system disorders increase the risk for nausea and vomiting symptoms. Dyspepsia risk is increased significantly with ingestion of nonsteroidal anti-inflammatory drugs (NSAIDs), tobacco use, *Helicobacter pylori* infection, obesity, anxiety, somatization, neuroticism, depression, and unemployment. Increased upper GI gaseousness can be seen with air swallowing from gum chewing and eating quickly, as well as consumption of foods that relax the lower esophageal sphincter (e.g., chocolate, fats, mints). Ingestion of lactose, fructose, sorbitol, undigested starches (e.g., bran), and carbonated beverages can all increase the risk of bloating and flatulence.

Pathophysiology

The pathophysiologic regulation of nausea and vomiting is complex and incompletely understood. Multiple neurotransmitters are involved, including acetylcholine, dopamine, histamine, and serotonin. The therapeutic action of antiemetics is often based on blocking the action of these neurotransmitters. Neurologic regulation of nausea and vomiting involves the chemoreceptor triggers in the fourth ventricle, the nucleus tractus solitarius in the medulla, motor nuclei that control the vomiting reflex, and vagal afferent nerves from the GI tract. The sympathetic and parasympathetic nervous systems are involved in conjunction with the smooth muscle cells and the enteric brain within the wall of the stomach and intestine.

The pathophysiology of dyspepsia is unclear but probably has multiple causes. Delayed gastric motility can occur in up to 30% of patients with dyspepsia. In addition, decreased gastric compliance, alteration in gut microbiome, duodenal inflammation, and psychosocial dysfunction can also be associated with dyspeptic patients.

Sensations of lower tract gaseousness result from one of three different mechanisms: excess gas production, abnormal intestinal transit, and increased visceral sensitivity. Gas production caused by carbohydrate maldigestion, (e.g., lactose intolerance, poorly absorbed starches) results in bloating and a sensation of fullness. High-fiber diets, celiac disease, and small intestine bacterial overgrowth can increase gas production. Dysmotility associated with diabetes mellitus, scleroderma, amyloidosis, and endocrine disease may result in gastroparesis and chronic intestinal pseudo-obstruction. In addition, previous Nissen fundoplication, fat intolerance, and various familial conditions may cause dysmotility. Increased visceral sensitivity is thought to be a main cause of pain and fullness in patients with functional bowel disorders such as irritable bowel syndrome (IBS) and functional dyspepsia.

Prevention

Once the diagnosis has been established, appropriate treatment of the underlying cause of the symptoms can be instituted. When the cause of nausea and vomiting is related to medication, the dose can be adjusted or the medication changed as appropriate.

Upper GI bloating and fullness is almost exclusively caused by excess air swallow and can be improved with altering behaviors such as gulping food and gum chewing. Lower GI symptoms can be prevented by avoiding problem foods such as milk products in patients with lactose intolerance.

Clinical Manifestations

Nausea and vomiting are extremely common and are associated with many conditions. Associated symptoms are helpful in sorting out causes. Many common historical associations are listed in Table 1.

The diagnosis of dyspepsia is based mainly on clinical symptoms. The Rome III criteria are listed in the opening paragraph. Alarm symptoms that should raise suspicions for gastric cancer include unintended weight loss, persistent vomiting, progressive dysphasia, odynophagia, unexplained anemia, iron deficiency, hematemesis, palpable abdominal mass, lymphadenopathy, family history of gastric cancer, previous gastric surgery, or jaundice.

TABLE 1	Key Symptoms and Differential Vomiting, Dyspepsia, and Bloating
SYMPTOMS	**DIFFERENTIAL**
Abdominal Pain ± N/V • RUQ • Epigastric • RLQ • LLQ • Pelvic	Organic etiologies • Cholelithiasis, cholecystitis • Dyspepsia, pancreatitis, GERD, gastritis, MI • Appendicitis • Diverticulitis • PID, ovarian torsion, ectopic pregnancy
Abdominal pain + distention + N/V	Bowel obstruction
Abdominal distention associated with foods (lactose, wheat-based products, bran, legumes)	Lactose intolerance Celiac disease Carbohydrate malabsorption, Oligosaccharide fermentation (legumes)
Vomiting several hours after eating + succussion splash + N/V	Gastric obstruction Gastroparesis
Heartburn ± N/V	GERD, dyspepsia
Early morning + N/V	Pregnancy
Feculent vomiting + N/V	Intestinal obstruction Gastrocolic fistula
Vertigo + nystagmus + N/V	Vestibular neuritis
Dental erosions, parotid gland enlargement, lanugo-like hair, callus on dorsal surface of hands	Bulimia
Positional N/V	Neurogenic
N/V relieved with hot shower or bath	Cannabis hyperemesis

GERD, Gastroesophageal reflux disease; *LLQ*, left lower quadrant; *MI*, myocardial infarction; *N/V*, nausea and vomiting; *PID*, pelvic inflammatory disease; *RLQ*, right lower quadrant; *RUQ*, right upper quadrant.

Gaseousness usually presents with abdominal fullness and bloating. Pain associated with the fullness is often relieved with eructation or flatulence (see Table 1).

Diagnosis

The first step in the assessment of patients with abdominal complaints is complete history of the duration of symptoms, the frequency of episodes, work environment, recent travel, household member illness, association of symptoms with certain foods or beverages (i.e., pain relief or worsening with food), and determination of the success or failure of what the patient has tried to alleviate the symptoms, all of which may offer diagnostic clues. Focused inquiries into surgeries, sexual activity, and other elements of a review of symptoms may be helpful. A complete review of medication usage, with particular attention to GI-irritating medications such as NSAIDs and over-the-counter medications, illicit drugs, and herbal products is important. Physical examination and diagnostic work-up can help isolate the cause (Table 2).

In patients with acute (<24 hours) nausea and vomiting, a laboratory work-up is often unnecessary. Patients with the most commonly identified acute causes, such as acute gastroenteritis, vestibular neuritis, chemotherapy, medication, and alcohol ingestion, and those who are postoperative, can be started on symptomatic therapy. For persistent symptoms of nausea and vomiting, laboratory work-up is guided by the history and physical examination and can include a complete blood count and differential, serum chemistries, renal function, liver function

TABLE 2	Physical Examination: Nausea, Vomiting, Dyspepsia, and Gaseousness
FINDINGS	**POSSIBLE ETIOLOGY**
Fever	Infectious
Tachycardia, hypotension	Dehydration, volume depletion, sepsis (infectious), ectopic pregnancy, myocardial infarction, aortic aneurysm
Exophthalmos	Hyperthyroid
Papilledema	Increased intracranial pressure (tumors, subdural hemorrhage)
Bulging tympanic membrane	Otitis media, effusion
Thyromegaly	Hypothyroid
Lymphadenopathy	Infection, malignancy
Dry mucous membranes	Dehydration, volume depletion
Dental erosions	Bulimia
Abdominal distention	Obstruction, ileus, gastroparesis, irritable bowel, hepatic/splenic flexure syndrome, postoperative gas-bloat syndrome
Absent bowel sounds	Ileus, perforation
Sense of abdominal distention without bloating	Irritable bowel syndrome
Abdominal bloating	Irritable bowel syndrome, obstruction
RUQ abdominal pain/guarding	Cholecystitis, cholelithiasis
RLQ/LLQ abdominal pain/guarding	Appendicitis (RLQ), ovarian torsion, diverticulitis, ectopic pregnancy
Cervical motion tenderness	Pelvic inflammatory disease, endometriosis
Bladder tenderness	Urinary tract infection
Testicular pain	Torsion, epididymitis
Abnormal rectal examination	Fecal impaction, prostatitis, appendicitis, ovarian tumor, ectopic pregnancy, endometriosis
Delayed cap refill, poor skin turgor	Dehydration
Jaundice	Gallbladder disease, biliary obstruction

LLQ, Left lower quadrant; *RLQ*, right lower quadrant; *RUQ*, right upper quadrant.

TABLE 3	Differential Diagnosis for Nausea and Vomiting

Central Nervous System
Multiple sclerosis, tumor, intracranial bleeding, infarction, abscess, meningitis, trauma, labyrinthitis, Ménière disease, vestibular neuritis, motion sickness
Migraine headaches, seizure disorders
Gastrointestinal Disorders
Appendicitis, gastric bypass, gastroparesis, hepatobiliary disease, cholecystitis, hepatitis, neoplasia
Ileus
Crohn disease, ulcerative colitis
Irritable bowel syndrome
Ischemia: mesenteric, small bowel
Obstruction: scarring/adhesions from previous surgeries, small bowel obstruction, esophageal spasm
Pancreatitis
Peptic ulcer disease: esophagitis, gastritis, gastroesophageal reflux
Peritonitis
Endocrine
Addison disease, diabetes (ketoacidosis, gastroparesis), hyperthyroidism, hypothyroidism, hyperparathyroidism, hypoparathyroidism, porphyria
Genitourinary
Nephritis, nephrolithiasis, torsion (ovary, testicle), uremia, kidney stone
Infectious Etiologies
Bacterial: Campylobacter, Salmonella, Shigella, Enterogenic Escherichia coli
Viral: rotavirus, influenza
Otitis media: bacterial or viral
Sexually transmitted infection: cervicitis, epididymitis, pelvic inflammatory disease, prostatitis, urethritis; multiple organisms including gonorrhea and chlamydia
Urinary tract infection: lower (cystitis) or upper (pyelonephritis)
Pregnancy
Morning sickness, hyperemesis gravidarum, intrauterine and ectopic pregnancies

Psychiatric
Anorexia, anxiety, bulimia, depression
Medication Related
Acetaminophen (Tylenol)
Acyclovir (Zovirax)
Alcohol abuse
Antibiotics: azithromycin (Zithromax), sulfasalazine (Azulfidine), erythromycin, metronidazole (Flagyl), sulfonamides (e.g., sulfamethoxazole-trimethoprim [Bactrim]), tetracycline
Antidepressants: Selective serotonin reuptake inhibitors (SSRIs)
Antihypertensives: β-blockers (atenolol [Tenormin], metoprolol [Lopressor]), calcium channel blockers, diuretics (hydrochlorothiazide)
Cannabis
Chemotherapeutic agents: cisplatinum (Cisplatin [Platinol]), cyclophosphamide (Cytoxan), nitrogen mustard (Mustargen), dacarbazine (DTIC-Dome), methotrexate (Trexall), vinblastine (Velban)
Diabetes treatment: metformin (Glucophage), sulfonylureas
Digoxin (Lanoxin)
Ergotamines: dihydroergotamine (Migranal), methysergide (Sansert)[2]
Ferrous gluconate, ferrous sulfate
Gout treatment: allopurinol (Zyloprim)
Hormones: estrogen, progesterone, and oral and injected contraceptives
Levodopa (L-dopa), carbidopa (Lodosyn)
Nicotine (patch, gum, smokeless tobacco, cigarette/pipe/cigar)
Nonsteroidal antiinflammatory: aspirin, ibuprofen (Motrin), naproxen (Naprosyn)
Opioids: codeine, heroin, hydrocodone, oxycodone, morphine, buprenorphine/naloxone (Suboxone)
Prednisone
Seizure medications: phenobarbital, phenytoin (Dilantin)
Theophylline (Uniphyl)

[2]Not available in the United States.

tests, serum protein and albumin, thyroid-stimulating hormone, amylase or lipase, drug screen, and a pregnancy test in women of childbearing age. Imaging should not be routine but should be directed by the history and physical findings as well as pertinent laboratory results. Useful studies may include acute abdominal series (chest x-ray, flat and upright views of the abdomen), abdominal computed tomography (CT), and abdominal ultrasound.

Similarly, in patients with dyspeptic symptoms, laboratory tests should be obtained based on the history and physical examination. Many therapies, such as discontinuing offending medications (e.g., NSAIDs) or acid suppression in patients without alarm symptoms, may be started without a laboratory work-up. Blood count chemistries and *H. pylori* testing can be considered if warranted. Alarm symptoms may warrant further imaging or direct visualization with esophagogastroduodenoscopy (EGD).

In gaseousness and bloating, the most sensitive work-up is the history and physical examination. Further work-up should be directed by initial findings. Patients with alarm symptoms such as weight loss, diarrhea, abdominal pain, distention, and anorexia may benefit from a malabsorption work-up including lactose tolerance test, stool fat, ova and parasites, stool culture, *Clostridium difficile*, acute abdominal series, or EGD. A hydrogen breath test may be beneficial in selected patients to assess the relationship between specific foods and symptoms. Other blood work, tests, and imaging, such as CT, magnetic resonance imaging (MRI),

TABLE 4 Differential Diagnosis of Dyspepsia

Gastrointestinal Disorders	Medications
Functional or nonulcer (most common)	NSAIDs
Peptic ulcer disease	Antibiotics (macrolides and metronidazole)
Gastroesophageal reflux	Corticosteroids
Gastritis	Digoxin
Pancreatitis	Narcotics
Gastroparesis	Theophylline
Gastric cancer	**Respiratory**
Intestinal ischemia	Pneumonia
Esophageal rupture	**Cardiac**
Malabsorption	Myocardial ischemia or pericarditis
Lactase deficiency	**Musculoskeletal**
Celiac	Abdominal hernia
Infectious	**Psychiatric**
Parasite infection	Physical sexual abuse
Helicobacter pylori	
Pregnancy	

NSAIDs, Nonsteroidal antiinflammatory drugs.

TABLE 5 Differential Diagnosis of Bloating and Gaseousness

Upper Gastrointestinal	Gas-Producing Foods
Air swallowing	Beans, peas, lentils, broccoli, Brussels sprouts, cauliflower, cabbage, parsnips, leeks, onions, beer, coffee, pork
Small Bowel	
Pneumatosis cystoides intestinalis	
Carbohydrate Malabsorption	**Infectious**
Lactase deficiency	Parasites
Legumes (indigestible oligosaccharides)	*Helicobacter pylori*
Fructose malabsorption	Bacterial overgrowth
Undigested starch (bran)	**Malabsorption**
Irritable Bowel Syndrome	Celiac
	Crohn disease

and EGD are guided by availability of testing and the history, examination, and laboratory findings.

Differential Diagnosis

Tables 3, 4, and 5 summarize the wide differential diagnoses of nausea and vomiting, dyspepsia, and gaseousness.

Treatment

Antiemetics, hydration, and dietary changes are the first line treatments for acute episodes of nausea and vomiting. Controlling the symptoms is often all that is necessary in acute, self-limited bouts of nausea and vomiting symptoms. If patients are dehydrated, oral rehydration can be accomplished by encouraging the patient to take small amounts (6 ounces or less) of cool water or electrolyte solutions on a frequent basis. If patients are unable to accomplish this, parenteral rehydration and antiemetics may be warranted.

Table 6 lists the common antiemetics agent, indications, dosages, side effects, and relative cost of medications.

Location of the cause with directed treatment is most effective for gaseousness. If no cause is found, it can be difficult to treat. Avoiding foods that are contributory, such as those containing lactose, fructose, sorbitol, high fiber, and starches, may be all that is necessary. Symptoms associated with increased sensitivity to normal levels of gas (i.e., IBS) can be difficult to treat. Therapeutic relationships, education, and dietary modification are the mainstays of IBS treatment. For moderate to severe symptoms, short-term treatment with antispasmodics, tricyclic antidepressants, and antidiarrheal agents may have some benefit. Medical treatments for bloating are listed in Table 7.

For most patients with dyspepsia, information can be powerful. Validation of symptoms and working toward a goal of management rather than cure are therapeutic. In patients with dyspepsia in which a concern for *H. pylori* exists, a test-and-treatment strategy can be effective. In other patients, proton pump inhibitors, H-2 receptor antagonists, prokinetic agents, and peppermint oil are all effective short-term therapies.

TABLE 6 Medications for Nausea and Vomiting

DRUG	USE	SIDE EFFECTS	DOSAGE
Anticholinergics Act as antimuscarinic agents		Sedation, dry mouth, dizziness, hallucinations, confusion, exacerbate narrow angle glaucoma, blurred vision.	
Scopalamine	Nausea associated with motion sickness		1–1.5 mg patch TD q3d
Antihistamines		Sedation, dry mouth, confusion, urinary retention, blurred vision	
Diphenhydramine (Benadryl)	Nausea associated with motion sickness		50 mg PO q6h or 10–50 mg IV or IM
Doxylamine (Unisom)[1]	Nausea associated with pregnancy		5–10 mg PO qd
Hydroxyzine (Vistaril)[1]	Nausea associated with motion sickness		25–100 mg q6h
Meclizine (Antivert)	Nausea associated with motion sickness		25–50 mg q6h
Promethazine (Phenergan)	Nausea associated with motion sickness		12.5–25 mg (PO, IM, IV, PR) q4–6h
Benzamides: Prokinetic agents; work on peripheral and central dopamine, weak hydroxytryptamine type 3 (5-HT₃)		Sedation, hypotension, extrapyramidal effects, diarrhea, neuroleptic syndrome, supraventricular tachycardia, CNS depression	

TABLE 6	Medications for Nausea and Vomiting—cont'd		
DRUG	**USE**	**SIDE EFFECTS**	**DOSAGE**
Metoclopramide (Reglan)	Second line therapy for chemotherapy-induced nausea		10 mg (PO, IM, IV) q6h
Trimethobenzamide (Tigan)[1]	Chemotherapy-induced nausea		300 mg PO q6h
Butyrophenones: Dopamine antagonists		Sedation, hypotension, extrapyramidal effects, tachycardia, dizziness, QT prolongation and torsades de pointes, neuroleptic malignant syndrome	
Droperidol (Inapsine)	Postoperative nausea/vomiting		0.625–1.25 mg (IM, IV) q4h
Haloperidol (Haldol)[1]			0.5–5 mg (PO, IM, IV) q8h
Phenothiazines: Dopamine antagonists		Sedation, hypotension, extrapyramidal effects, neuroleptic malignant syndrome, cholestatic jaundice	
Chlorpromazine (Thorazine)	Generalized nausea		10–25 mg (PO, IM, PR) q6h
Prochlorperazine (Compazine)	Generalized nausea		10 mg (PO, IM, IV) q6h; 25 mg q12h PR
5-HT3: Serotonin Antagonists		Fever, constipation, diarrhea, dizziness, sedation, nervousness, altered liver function tests, headache, fatigue	
Dolasetron (Anzemet)	Chemotherapy-induced nausea		100 mg (PO, IV) q24h
Granisetron (Kytril)	Chemotherapy-induced nausea		2 mg (PO, IV) q24h
Ondansetron (Zofran)	Chemotherapy-induced nausea		4–8 mg (PO, IV) q8–12h
Palonosetron (Aloxi)	Prevention of chemotherapy-induced nausea		0.5 mg PO or 0.25 mg IV ×1
Neurokinin Receptor Antagonists		Headache, site reaction	
Aprepitant capsule (Emend)	Prevention of postoperative nausea and vomiting (POV)		40 mg PO × 1 prior to anesthesia
Fosaprepitant (Emend IV)	Prevention of chemotherapy-induced nausea		115 mg IV × 1, 125 mg PO ×1[3]
Steroids		GI upset, anxiety, euphoria, flushing, insomnia	
Dexamethasone (Decadron)[1]	Prophylaxis of chemotherapy-related nausea and vomiting		4 mg–10 mg (PO, IM, IV) q6–12h
Methylprednisolone (Medrol)[1]			40–100 mg (PO, IM, IV) q24h
Cannabinoids		Vertigo, xerostomia, hypotension, dysphoria	
Dronabinol (Marinol)	Chronic or chemotherapy-induced nausea and vomiting		5 mg/m^2 PO q2-4h; 4–6 doses per day
Miscellaneous			
Erythromycin[1]	Nausea associated with gastroparesis		250 mg PO q8h × 5–7 d
Ginger[7]	Nausea associated with pregnancy		250 mg PO q6h or 1 g qd
Pyridoxine (vitamin B6)[1]	Nausea associated with pregnancy (traditionally combined with doxylamine)		10 mg q6h
Aromatherapy-Isopropyl Alcohol[1]	Nausea	None	Swab held under nose and inhaled.

CNS, central nervous system; *IM*, intramuscular; *IV*, intravenous; *PO*, by mouth; *PR*, per rectum
[1]Not US Food and Drug Administration (FDA) approved for this indication.
[3]Exceeds dosage recommended by the manufacturer.
[7]Available as dietary supplement.

TABLE 7	Medications for Treatment of Gaseousness and Bloating	
MEDICATION	**INDICATION**	**DOSE**
Rifaximin (Xifaxan)[1]	Bloating (flatulence) from suspected bacterial overgrowth	200 mg PO tid × 7 days
Probiotics (multi-component)[7]	Bloating (flatulence)	Varies by preparation
Alpha-galactosidase (Bean-o)	Bloating associated with gas-producing foods	300–1200 mg with meals high in fermentable carbs
Simethicone	Bloating (flatulence) (indicated but not found to be effective)	80–120 mg qid prn
Bismuth subsalicylate	Odor from flatus	525 mg PO qid prn
Odor-neutralizing devices (briefs, pillows)	Odor from flatus	prn

[1]Not US Food and Drug Administration (FDA) approved for this indication.
[7]Available as dietary supplement

Monitoring

For patients who have complications related to nausea and vomiting, monitoring serum electrolytes, renal function, nutritional status, and other parameters may be necessary until hydration improves, electrolytes are replaced, and laboratory results and clinical status return to normal.

Further testing is needed in patients with dyspepsia and alarm symptoms; however, in patients without alarm symptoms, no further testing is needed.

Complications

The complications of prolonged nausea and vomiting are dehydration, electrolyte disturbances (e.g., hypokalemia, hypophosphatemia, and hypomagnesemia), depletion of vitamins and trace elements, metabolic alkalosis, and malnutrition. Usually these can be corrected with oral or intravenous hydration, correction of electrolyte deficiencies, and treatment of the underlying cause. In patients whose nausea and vomiting are accompanied by gastroenteritis, symptoms and clinical status may not return to baseline unless all electrolytes such as potassium, magnesium, phosphorus, and trace elements such as zinc are replaced.

Dyspeptic patients without alarm symptoms rarely have complications. In patients with chronic bloating, complications are uncommon.

References

Abraczinskas D: Intestinal gas and bloating. Available http://www.uptodate.com, December 2018. [Accessed 3 February 2020].
ACOG Practice Bulletin No: 189: American College of Obstetrics and Gynecology: nausea and vomiting in pregnancy, *Obstet Gynecol* 131:e15–e30, 2018.
Bailey J: Effective management of flatulence, *Am Fam Phys* 79:1098–1100, 2009.
Flake ZA, Linn B, Hornecker J: Practical selection of antiemetics in an ambulatory care setting, *Am Fam Phys* 91(15):293–296, 2015 Mar 1.
Kraft R: Nausea and vomiting. In Bope ET, Rakel RE, Kellerman R, editors: *Conn's Current Therapy 2010*, Philadelphia, 2010, Saunders, pp 5–9.
Lacy B, Parkman H, Camilleri M: Chronic Nausea and Vomiting, Evaluation and Treatment, *Am J Gastroenterology* 113:647–659, 2018.
Longstreth GF: Functional dyspepsia in adults. Available at http://www.uptodate.com, December 2019. [Accessed 3 February 2020].
Longstreth GF: Approach to the patient with dyspepsia. Available at http://www.uptodate.com, December, 2019. [Accessed 3 February 2020].
Owings S: Gaseousness and dyspepsia. In Bope ET, Rakel RE, Kellerman R, editors: *Conn's Current Therapy 2010*, Philadelphia, 2010, Saunders, pp 9–11.
Talley NJ, Vakil NB, Moayyedi P: 2005 American Gastroenterological Association technical review on the evaluation of dyspepsia, *Gastroenterology* 125:1756–1780, 2005.

HEMATURIA

Method of
Matthew Banti, MD; and Moben Mirza, MD

CURRENT DIAGNOSIS

- Hematuria is defined as the presence of red blood cells in the urine.
- Hematuria can be gross (readily visible) or microscopic (detected by dipstick or microscopy).
- In the adult population, any unexplained hematuria should be presumed to be of malignant origin until proven otherwise.
- Urologic evaluation of the upper and lower urinary tract is compulsory for patients with gross hematuria.
- Patients with asymptomatic microscopic hematuria (>3 RBC/HPF) should have a careful history and physical examination performed to rule out benign causes of hematuria as well as to assess overall risk of urologic malignancy.
- Following patient risk stratification, further diagnostic evaluation with repeat urinalysis, cystoscopy, and upper tract imaging (renal ultrasound or multiphasic computed tomography) may be indicated.
- Concurrent nephrologic evaluation should occur in select cases.

Epidemiology

Hematuria is a common clinical finding in adults. The prevalence of hematuria ranges from 2.4% to 31.1%. Prevalence varies based on age, gender, frequency of testing, threshold used to define hematuria, and study group characteristics. Transient microscopic hematuria may occur in up to 40% of patients; however, persistent microscopic hematuria in greater than three evaluated urine samples is limited to 2% of the population. A wide range of causes can result in hematuria. Transient hematuria may be caused by vigorous exercise, sexual intercourse, mild trauma, menstrual contamination, and instrumentation. Patients with underlying urinary tract disease can have transient or persistent hematuria. The difference between gross and microscopic hematuria is that the chances of finding significant pathology are higher in patients with gross hematuria. For example, approximately 5% of patients with microscopic hematuria in contrast to 40% of patients with gross hematuria are found to have urologic malignancy on evaluation. The most common cause of gross hematuria in adults older than age 50 is bladder cancer.

Risk Factors

Given the wide range of etiologies for hematuria, the risk factors are dependent on the etiology itself. The most concerning etiology of hematuria is urothelial malignancy. Smoking is the best-established and the most significant risk factor for the development of urothelial malignancies of the kidney, ureter, and bladder.

Pathophysiology

The presence of blood in the urine can be separated into glomerular and nonglomerular origin. Normal urine contains less than three red blood cells per high-power field. The kidney does not excrete red blood cells under physiologic conditions. Therefore presence of blood in the urine is due to pathology at the glomerulus (glomerular hematuria), allowing excretion of red blood cells into the urine or pathology in the urinary tract distal to the glomerulus (nonglomerular hematuria), which results in blood mixing into the already excreted urine. Nonglomerular hematuria can be further divided into medical and surgical disorders. Except for renal tumors, nonglomerular hematuria of medical/renal origin is due to tubulointerstitial, renovascular, or systemic disorders. Surgical nonglomerular hematuria or essential hematuria includes urologic tumors, stones, and urinary tract infections.

The urine dipstick commonly used for the detection of blood in the urine is dependent on the peroxidase-like activity of hemoglobin, which catalyzes the reaction and causes oxidation of the chromogen indicator. False positives can occur in states of hemoglobinuria and myoglobinuria, and microscopic examination of the urine for red blood cells can distinguish hematuria. Glomerular hematuria is suggested when dysmorphic erythrocytes, red blood cell casts, and proteinuria are present. Nonglomerular hematuria can be distinguished from glomerular hematuria in the presence of circular erythrocytes and the absence of erythrocyte casts. In the surgical and medical subcategories of nonglomerular hematuria, surgical hematuria is suggested by the absence of significant proteinuria.

Anticoagulation at normal therapeutic levels does not predispose patients to hematuria. Therefore patients who have hematuria while receiving anticoagulation therapy should undergo evaluation similarly to patients who are not receiving anticoagulation therapy. In fact, super therapeutic anticoagulation may serve to unmask underlying pathology.

Prevention

Hematuria can be caused by a spectrum of causes. Prevention can be achieved by the prevention of what results in the pathologic state. For example, smoking is a modifiable risk factor in urothelial malignancy. Patients who have never smoked are at low risk for bladder cancer. Smoking cessation can also reduce the risk of developing bladder cancer. Liberal fluid intake and balanced sodium and protein intake can help prevent urolithiasis. Urinary tract infections can also be prevented by good voiding habits, facilitation of complete bladder emptying, and use of vaginal estrogen cream[1] in postmenopausal women.

Clinical Manifestations

The presentation of hematuria is often dependent on the cause. Certain characteristics of the presentation can help in the investigation. Is the hematuria gross or microscopic? Is the hematuria associated with pain? Are there any irritative voiding symptoms? Is there a presence of blood clots? Is it related to exercise? Is there any family history? Is there a presence of rash, arthritis, hemoptysis, upper respiratory infection, or skin infection? Is there a history of radiation, diabetes, or analgesic abuse? Is there a history of smoking or occupational exposures? Table 1 highlights findings in etiologies of hematuria. Patients with bladder cancer generally present with gross painless hematuria.

Diagnosis

The diagnosis and evaluation of hematuria starts with a careful history, physical examination, and microscopic urinalysis. The cause in an adult patient is urologic malignancy until proven otherwise. Some important questions are outlined in the section

---

[1] Not FDA approved for this indication

Clinical Manifestation. The physical examination should focus on blood pressure, a cardiovascular examination, an abdominal examination, a palpable mass, costovertebral angle tenderness, and a complete genitourinary examination inclusive of a prostate examination in the male and vaginal examination in the female patient. The assessment should help rule out causes such as infection, menstruation, vigorous exercise, medical renal disease, viral illness, trauma, or recent urologic procedures.

The urine should be collected as a midstream sample, and patients should be instructed to discard the initial 10 mL. The sample should be collected in a sterile cup after gently cleaning the urethral meatus with a sterilization towelette. Uncircumcised men should retract the foreskin before collection. Female patients should be asked to spread the labia adequately to allow cleansing of the urethral meatus and avoid introital contamination.

The following patients may require catheterization for collection: menstruating women, obese patients, patient with a nonintact urinary tract, and patients who do intermittent catheterization or have an indwelling urinary catheter or suprapubic tube. Additionally, a urine sample with excessive squamous cells is a sign of contamination, and catheterization may be required for an adequate specimen. A urine dipstick can be performed in the office setting, but all samples should be sent for microscopic analysis. As mentioned previously, attention should be paid to dysmorphic erythrocytes, red blood cell casts, and the presence of protein. A urine culture should be performed based on the clinical presentation and findings of urinalysis. Urine cytology should not be used in the initial evaluation of microscopic hematuria but may have clinical utility in evaluating patients with irritative voiding symptoms or persistent microhematuria after a comprehensive urologic evaluation. The laboratory workup should include an evaluation of the serum creatinine. Additional helpful tests are serum electrolytes and a complete blood count.

Patients with a urinary tract infection should be treated appropriately and should have a urinalysis repeated in 2 to 6 weeks after treatment. Patients with an identified etiology such as urolithiasis should have a reevaluation of urine after the stone has been passed or treated.

A urologic evaluation of the upper and lower urinary tract is compulsory for patients with gross hematuria. Given the high prevalence of asymptomatic microscopic hematuria (>3 RBC/HPF) and lower rate of malignancy in this population, risk stratification should be performed to guide diagnostic evaluation and limit the potential for patient harm. Patients should be categorized as low, intermediate, and high risk based on factors in Table 2. Low-risk patients should undergo cystoscopy and renal ultrasound or repeat urinalysis within 6 months to assess for persistence of the microscopic hematuria. An abnormal repeat urinalysis should prompt reclassification as intermediate or high risk and full evaluation should be performed. Cystoscopy and renal ultrasound (intermediate risk) or multiphasic computed tomography (high risk) are indicated for the evaluation of these risk groups. While contrasted computed tomography is preferred for evaluation of the upper tracts, a contraindication may exist for some patients due to allergy or renal insufficiency. In this scenario, a urologist can determine whether magnetic resonance imaging or retrograde pyelography is appropriate.

Differential Diagnosis

The differential diagnosis of hematuria includes glomerular diseases, nonglomerular medical diseases, and nonglomerular surgical diseases. Table 1 shows a differential diagnosis for hematuria.

Hematuria is considered to be from a malignant source until proven otherwise.

Therapy, Monitoring, and Complications

Therapy, monitoring, and complications for hematuria are dependent on the etiology. It is important that hematuria not be ignored even when treated empirically. For example, it is important to recheck a urinalysis after a course of antibiotics for a presumed

TABLE 1 — Differential Diagnosis and Findings in Etiologies of Hematuria

DIAGNOSIS	FINDINGS	OTHER
Glomerular		
Familial hematuria	Abnormal urinalysis	Family history
Systemic lupus erythematous	Elevated C3, C4, ANA	Rash, arthritis
Goodpasture syndrome	Microcytic anemia	Hemoptysis, bleeding tendency
Poststreptococcal glomerulonephritis	Elevated ASO titer, C3	Recent upper respiratory infection, rash
IgA nephropathy	Normal ASO and C3, renal biopsy positive for IgA, IgG	Related to exercise
Nonglomerular Medical		
Exercise-induced hematuria	Abnormal urine analysis	After strenuous exercise
Papillary necrosis	Gross hematuria, absence of urolithiasis on CT	Flank pain, African American, analgesic abuse, diabetes
Medullary sponge kidney, polycystic kidney disease	Abnormal CT	Family history of renal cystic disease
Renovascular disease	Renal artery embolus, vein thrombus, AV fistula	Atrial fibrillation, dehydration, bruit
Nonglomerular Surgical		
Urinary tract infection	Urine dip with LCE, Nit. positive urine culture, elevated WBC	Dysuria, fever
Urolithiasis (renal, ureteral, or bladder stone)	Demonstrated on imaging such as CT, ultrasound, KUB	Flank pain, pelvic pain, vomiting, infection, renal obstruction
Urologic tumor (kidney, ureter, bladder, urethra)	Demonstrated on CT, cystoscopy, ureteropyeloscopy	Constitutional, irritative symptoms, pain if obstructed, blood clots
Enlarged prostate or benign prostatic hyperplasia	Enlarged prostate on examination or cystoscopy	Irritative and obstructive voiding symptoms
Radiation cystitis	Generally gross hematuria, friable tissue on cystoscopy	Irritative voiding symptoms, history of pelvic radiation
Urothelial strictures (ureter or urethra)	Demonstrated on ureteroscopy, pyelography, cystoscopy, or urethrography	Flank pain, renal insufficiency, bladder outlet obstruction

ANA, Antinuclear antibodies; *ASO,* antistreptolysin O; *AV,* atrioventricular; *CT,* computed tomography; *Ig,* immunoglobulin; *KUB kidney, ureter, bladder radiograph, LCE leukocyte esterase, WBC, white blood cell.*

TABLE 2 — Microhematuria Risk Stratification

LOW RISK (ALL OF THE FOLLOWING):	INTERMEDIATE RISK (ANY OF THE FOLLOWING):	HIGH RISK (ANY OF THE FOLLOWING):
• Women age <50 years • Men age <40 years • Never smoker or <10 pack-years • 3–10 RBC/HPF on one UA • No additional risk factors for urothelial cancer* • No prior episodes of microscopic hematuria	• Women age 50–59 • Men age 40–59 • 10–30 pack-years • 11–25 RBC/HPF on one UA • One or more risk factors for urothelial cancer[1] • Previously low risk, no prior evaluation, and 3–25 RBC/HPF on repeat UA	• Women and men age >60 years • >30 pack-years • >25 RBC/HPF on one UA • History of gross hematuria • Previously low risk, no prior evaluation, and >25 RBC/HPF on repeat UA

*Irritative voiding symptoms, history of cyclophosphamide or ifosamide chemotherapy, family history of urothelial carcinoma or Lynch syndrome, occupational exposures to benzene chemicals or aromatic amines, history of chronic indwelling foreign object in urinary tract
UA, Urinalysis.
Adapted from Barocas D, Boorjian S, Alvarez R, et al: Microhematuria: AUA/SUFU guideline, *J Urol* 204:778–786, 2020.

urinary tract infection. Often, the transient nature of hematuria fools clinicians into thinking that an intervention or observation without the appropriate workup is adequate. Unfortunately, this can result in significant morbidity from the progression of disease, especially in the case of urothelial malignancies.

References

Barocas D, Boorjian S, Alvarez R, et al: Microhematuria: AUA/SUFU Guideline, *J Urol* 204:778–786, 2020.

Davis R, Jones SJ, Barocas D, et al: Diagnosis, evaluation and follow-up of asymptomatic microscopic hematuria (AMH) in adults. AUA guideline, *J Urol* 188(Suppl 6):2473, 2012.

Gerber GS, Brendler CB: Evaluation of the urologic patient: History, physical, and urinalysis. In *Wein Campbell-Walsh Urology,* ed 10, Philadelphia, 2011, Saunders, pp 73–98.

Khadra MH, Pickard RS, Charlton M, et al: A prospective analysis of 1,930 patients with hematuria to evaluate current diagnostic practice, *J Urol* 163:524, 2000.

Masahito J: Evaluation and management of hematuria, *Prim Care* 37:461, 2010.

Sudakoff GS, Dunn DP, Guralnick ML, et al: Multidetector computerized tomography urography as the primary imaging modality for detecting urinary tract neoplasms in patients with asymptomatic hematuria, *J Urol* 179:862, 2008.

HICCUPS

Method of
Georg A. Petroianu, MD, PhD

Mechanistic Description

Hiccup (Latin, *singultus*) is caused by an involuntary, usually repetitive and rhythmic, spasmodic contraction of the diaphragm (or hemidiaphragm) and accessory inspiratory muscles followed shortly (within 35 msec) by the sudden closure of the glottis. The forcefully inspired air meeting a closed glottis causes the typical hiccup sound. Occasional hiccups are generally perceived as being "funny"; however, hiccupping of extended duration can be incapacitating. Its most common direct consequence is esophagitis, due to concomitant relaxation of the lower esophageal sphincter favoring reflux, but extended hiccupping can also lead to wound dehiscence, depression, weight loss, malnutrition, insomnia, and exhaustion. The possibility of developing tardive dyskinesia weighs against the routine use of this drug

Classifications

Most classifications use arbitrary time limits to categorize hiccupping. Generally hiccups lasting less than 1 day are considered transient (acute), those lasting less than 1 week are labeled persistent, and hiccupping for more than 1 week is described as chronic. A simplified categorization draws the line at 48 hours: any hiccupping episode lasting longer is described as chronic. The practical value of these classifications is questionable; by the time the practitioner sees the patient, almost invariably the case involves persistent or chronic hiccup forms requiring drug therapy. The exceptions (in terms of time between appearance and presentation) are hiccup forms presenting immediately postoperatively or in critical care units. Brief episodes of hiccupping, as experienced by the vast majority of people at some point in time, are certainly physiologic. The point of transition to a pathologic form is not well defined. The rule of thumb of hiccup therapy, however, is that the longer the duration of the hiccupping, the less amenable it will be to nonpharmacologic interventions.

Etiologic classifications are also fraught with problems. Hiccup is not a disease, but a symptom. Literally, there is no known disease that has not been associated with hiccups. Although the categories psychogenic, organic, and idiopathic are most commonly used in practice, the situation most commonly encountered is that of hiccup of unknown (idiopathic) origin. In this context, "idiopathic" describes one's inability to demonstrate, rather than the absence of, an organic origin.

Epidemiology

During intrauterine life, hiccups are universally present, their incidence peaking in the third trimester. They can also be seen regularly in the newborn, the frequency of occurrence decreasing slowly over the first year of life. In adults, occasional transient hiccup is also so frequent that it can be viewed as physiologic. Persistent and chronic idiopathic singultus, the pathologic forms, are rare, their prevalence being estimated at 1 in 100,000. Males are almost exclusively affected (the male-to-female patient ratio is approximately 80:1), suggesting a hormone (estrogen) protective effect. The incidence increases with age. The psychogenic form, though less frequent overall by one order of magnitude, is believed to be more prevalent in females, with an even distribution among all age groups; however, data to support this view are almost nonexistent.

Pathophysiology

The universality of hiccups during fetal life begs the question of purposefulness. As early as 1887, it was suggested that hiccups might represent a necessary and vital primitive reflex that would permit intrauterine training of the diaphragm without aspiration of amniotic fluid. During intrapartum and postpartum maturation, higher centers would then suppress this primitive reflex. Immaturity or damage to the central nervous system would favor the persistence or reappearance of the reflex. The putative reflex arch includes autonomic afferent fibers (the majority vagal fibers) from the digestive tract to a putative medullary hiccup center and motor efferent fibers via the phrenic nerve (diaphragm) and other branches of the vagus nerve to the intrinsic muscles of the larynx adducting the vocal cords. In an analogy with the vomiting center, the assumed role of the medullary hiccup center is to coordinate and fine-tune the sequence of events required for hiccupping; it is therefore a "pattern generator." The concept described, though useful for the purpose of designing a quasi-rational treatment protocol for hiccup, is neither proven nor generally accepted.

Another school of thought that questions the assumption that hiccupping is a reflex phenomenon suggests instead a similarity with cardiac arrhythmias: hiccups would therefore be due to arrhythmias of the breathing center. Still other researchers work on the assumption that hiccup is a myoclonic event, or that it represents brainstem seizures. These views are not necessarily mutually exclusive, because hiccup is not primarily a disease but a symptom, possibly representing different pathophysiologies.

Evaluation of the Hiccup Patient

Hiccup is a symptom associated with a multitude of pathologies. The practitioner must take the hiccupping patient seriously, and for the purpose of finding and treating hidden pathology, persistent and chronic hiccups should be investigated. No consensus exists, however, concerning the extent of such investigations. Even the most enthusiastic users of modern imaging technologies will in most cases end up with a working diagnosis of chronic idiopathic singultus. Nonetheless, a detailed history, a thorough physical examination, and basic laboratory and diagnostic procedures are essential.

History

Ask about previous episodes, as well as precipitating and alleviating factors. The patient who describes vomiting as a "cure" for previous hiccup episodes gives a telltale sign that acidity is an etiologic factor, and omeprazole is a drug to consider. If the patient indicates that hyperventilation is a "sure bet" to worsen his or her hiccups, you can assume that drugs lowering the excitability of the nervous system are likely to help. Elucidating present drug consumption (medical and recreational) is essential: aripiprazole (Abilify), benzodiazepines, barbiturates, alcohol, and steroids are well-known hiccup inducers.

Physical Examination

Foreign bodies in the external auditory canal can induce hiccups, so look in the ears. Examine neck, chest, and abdomen, looking for possible sources of irritation (infection, neoplastic processes, or both) to the vagus and phrenic nerves and the diaphragm. Perform a neurologic examination, keeping in mind the association of hiccup with multiple sclerosis and intracranial processes.

Laboratory and Diagnostic Procedures

An upright chest x-ray, together with complete blood count (CBC) with differential, will help exclude neoplastic or infectious disease. An electrocardiogram (ECG) will help exclude pericarditis and malfunctioning pacemakers, and electrolyte and urea determinations will exclude known metabolic causes (hyponatremia and uremia).

To what extent magnetic resonance imaging (MRI), ultrasound scanning, or endoscopic examinations are necessary is a judgment call, and no generalizations are possible; they might occasionally be indicated.

Nonpharmacologic Interventions

A multitude of nonpharmacologic interventions to terminate hiccup belong to the public-domain hiccup "mythology" or have been described in the medical literature as case reports. Though usually effective in terminating bouts of acute hiccup, they are mostly ineffective in cases of hiccupping that has been present for an extended period. The common denominator of these maneuvers (also used to terminate paroxysmal supraventricular tachycardia) is their ability to directly or indirectly increase efferent vagal activity; the increased parasympathetic tone has a limiting effect on hiccupping. Interestingly, estrogens are also considered to be parasympathomimetic, which offers a plausible explanation of why the singultus prevalence in females is much lower than in males.

Pharmacologic Interventions

Probably only a few drugs in the *Physician's Desk Reference* have not been tried in the therapy of singultus, and anyone who looks hard enough at the literature will be able to find anecdotal support for the use of almost any drug. However, prospective controlled studies to support the use of a particular therapy are very few and rare.

Conceptually, all drugs potentially successful in the therapy of chronic hiccups work either by decreasing the input from the gastrointestinal tract to a (putative) hiccup center or by decreasing the excitability of the nervous system and therefore the output from the (putative) hiccup center.

Sedative-Hypnotics

Both benzodiazepine and barbiturate γ-aminobutyric acid receptor type A ($GABA_A$) agonists have been tried for treatment of hiccups. The consensus is that these substances not only are ineffective but can actually worsen the clinical picture, producing a situation similar to the paradoxical excitation seen with the use of sedatives and explained by inhibitory effects on inhibitory centers.

Antiemetics

Following up on the analogy between the vomiting center and hiccup center as pattern generators, "setron"-class antiemetics (5-HT_3 receptor antagonists) have been tried, with no success. Anecdotal evidence hints at possible worsening of the hiccup under the influence of ondansetron (Zofran).[1]

Analeptics

The use of analeptics derives from the concept that hiccup is a suppressed primitive reflex. Analeptics potentiate the central suppression. Although some success has been reported with methylphenidate (Ritalin),[1] caffeine produced failure.

Anticonvulsants

Anticonvulsants (phenytoin [Dilantin],[1] carbamazepine [Tegretol],[1] valproate [Depacon][1]) have been used to try to suppress hiccups. Considering the multitude of pharmacodynamic effects of anticonvulsants, it is not surprising that some success was achieved.

Antipsychotics

Historically, chlorpromazine (Thorazine) has been the most widely used drug for treatment of hiccup, and it is the only drug approved by the FDA for the disorder. Aliphatic phenothiazines such as chlorpromazine have strong sedative, hypotensive, and anticholinergic properties and mild to moderate extrapyramidal effects. For hiccup control, results are mixed at best, and in view of the side effects, routine use is not warranted. Haloperidol (Haldol),[1] a butyropherone derivative, has also been used for hiccup control; again, results are mixed at best, and the possibility of developing tardive dyskinesia weighs heavily against the routine use of this drug.

Antidepressants

The tertiary amine tricyclic antidepressant amitriptyline (Elavil)[1] is one of the oldest players in the therapy of hiccup; its use was being suggested in the mid-1960s. As with anticonvulsants, considering the multitude of pharmacodynamic effects of tricyclic antidepressants, it is not surprising that some success was

achieved with these drugs. Their effectiveness is not related to their ability to inhibit monoamine uptake, but probably to their sodium channel blocking properties.

Calcium Channel Blockers

Nifedipine (Adalat)[1] is the dihydropyridine derivative most commonly used for hiccup control. Nimodipine (Nimotop)[1] has also been tried for the same purpose. Interestingly, anecdotal reports about the use of calcium for the same purpose also exist.

Sodium Channel Blockers

The local anesthetic class Ib antidysrhythmic lidocaine (Xylocaine)[1] and its oral analogue mexiletine (Mexitil)[1] have been used for hiccup control, with mixed results.

$GABA_B$ Agonists

Among the substances acting on the nervous system, baclofen (Lioresal)[1] has by far the best credentials in the treatment of chronic hiccup. It is one of the very few substances proven in clinical studies (albeit with small patient numbers) to be efficacious. This γ-aminobutyric acid receptor type B ($GABA_B$) agonist, normally used to lower an increased muscle tone (spasticity), has also been shown to suppress hiccups in an animal (cat) hiccup model. $GABA_B$ agonists, by reducing transmitter release, are generally able to depress complex reflexes.

Antacids

Lowering the acidity of the stomach using H_2-receptor blockers or proton pump inhibitors conceptually decreases the input from the gastrointestinal tract to the hiccup center. Omeprazole (Prilosec)[1] has been shown in a limited number of trials to be effective in hiccup treatment.

Gastrokinetic Drugs

One of the few reliable methods to induce a physiologic hiccup in humans is rapidly drinking an ice-cold can of beer on a hot summer day. Although it is highly debatable whether it has to be beer, stomach distention by carbon dioxide induces hiccups. Conversely, reducing stomach distention by using a gastrokinetic drug is helpful in alleviating hiccups. The strongest evidence available for the usefulness of a gastrokinetic drug was for cisapride (Propulsid); however, this selective serotonine 5-HT_4-receptor agonist was withdrawn from the market because of its propensity to prolong the QT interval and induce torsades de pointes. The available alternative is the related benzamide metoclopramide (Reglan),[1] a mixed dopamine receptor antagonist, 5-HT_4-receptor agonist, and cholinesterase inhibitor, with a long tradition in the treatment of hiccups, going back to the late 1960s. The possibility of developing tardive dyskinesia weighs against the routine use of this drug.

Physical Interventions
Phrenic Nerve Destruction

Irreversible surgical destruction of the phrenic nerve cannot be recommended. Even if hiccup relief is achieved after unilateral local anesthetic blockade of the phrenic nerve without serious compromise in respiratory function, the long-term effects of phrenic nerve destruction are unpredictable. Possible effects include both hiccup reappearance—even after bilateral phrenic nerve transection—and deterioration in respiratory function. More recently, diaphragmatic (phrenic) pacing has been described; however, experience is very limited.

Hypercapnia

Rebreathing in a paper bag is a well-known and reliable remedy for hyperventilation tetany. The increase in blood CO_2 levels (hypercapnia) thus induced leads to mild acidosis and thus to a liberation of calcium ions from the protein binding. The increase in plasma-free calcium decreases neuronal excitability,

---

[1]Not FDA approved for this indication.

[1]Not FDA approved for this indication.

thus terminating not only the tetany but possibly also hiccupping. It was suggested that abolishing the venous-arterial CO_2 gradient is required for efficacy of the method. A more high-tech version of this is the induction of normoxic hypercapnia in ventilated patients.

Positive End-Expiratory Pressure
Also practicable only in intubated patients is the application of high positive end-expiratory pressure (PEEP), a high-tech version of the Valsalva maneuver.

Nasogastric Tube
Gastric decompression via a nasogastric tube can terminate hiccups.

Treatment
The treatment algorithm described is based on the assumption that correctable organic causes have been excluded or treated.

We start therapy with omeprazole (Prilosec)[1] 20 to 40 mg orally (PO) daily. If after 7 days no satisfactory change has occurred, baclofen (Lioresal)[1] is introduced. With baclofen, a "start low, go very slow" approach is indicated in order to avoid excessive drowsiness, weakness, and fatigue. The maximum daily dose is 45 mg. Quite often, patients are already on a proton pump inhibitor (PPI) when presenting. In these cases, immediate introduction of baclofen and continuation of the PPI are recommended. In our experience, the time of response to the combination therapy omeprazole plus baclofen is unpredictable; however, all changes that we observed happened within the first 6 months, and the vast majority within the first 6 weeks. If the desired result is achieved, we continue therapy for another 6 months, after which a very cautious weaning from baclofen is attempted. In cases- where the combination therapy omeprazole plus baclofen is not (or not entirely) satisfactory, the addition of gabapentin (Neurontin)[1] or pregabalin (Lyrica)[1] "on the top" can be attempted. As with baclofen, with gabapentin or pregabalin a "start low, go slow" approach is indicated, the maximum dose of 400 mg three times daily or pregabalin 100 mg three times daily used in such cases being reached after 3 weeks. An inverse approach with PPI plus gabapentin or pregabalin as initial combination is also possible.

In addition to any pharmacologic therapy, the practitioner must convey to the patient the feeling that he or she understands and appreciates the seriousness of the condition. Compliance with the treatment is required from the patient, who must understand that success can take time. Lifestyle and habit changes are also required. The hiccup patient must limit the size of meals and avoid carbonated beverages and "gas-forming" foods.

The approach presented here represents our experience in the treatment of chronic singultus. The views expressed are neither guidelines nor regulations.

---

[1]Not FDA approved for this indication.

References
Jatzko A, Stegmeier-Petroianu A, Petroianu GA: Alpha-2-delta ligands for singultus (hiccup) treatment: three case reports, *J Pain Symptom Manage* 33:756–760, 2007.

Petroianu GA: Singultus, paper-bag ventilation, and hypercapnia, *J Hist Neurosci* 8:1–13, 2020.

Petroianu G: Idiopathic chronic hiccup (ICH): phrenic nerve block is not the way to go, *Anesthesiology* 89:1284–1285, 1998.

Petroianu G, Hein G, Petroianu A, et al: Idiopathic chronic hiccup: combination therapy with cisapride, omeprazole, and Baclofen, *Clin Ther* 19:1031–1038, 1997.

Petroianu G, Hein G, Petroianu A, et al: ETICS study: empirical therapy of idiopathic chronic singultus, *Z Gastroenterol* 36:559–566, 1998.

Petroianu G, Hein G, Stegmeier-Petroianu A, et al: Gabapentin "add-on therapy" for idiopathic chronic hiccup (ICH), *J Clin Gastroenterol* 30:321–324, 2000.

Petroianu G: Treatment of hiccup by vagal maneuvers, *J Hist Neurosci* 24:123–136, 2015.

HOARSENESS AND LARYNGITIS
Method of
Lee Akst, MD

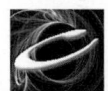

CURRENT DIAGNOSIS

- The general term to describe vocal difficulty is dysphonia. Hoarseness is a specific term for rough voice quality, which is one type of dysphonia. Laryngitis signifies laryngeal inflammation, which is one possible cause of dysphonia.
- An accurate history and physical examination guide the diagnosis of voice complaints. Although many portions of the examination for dysphonia can be done in a general setting, videostroboscopy is often necessary for diagnosis and may be available only in specialized laryngology offices.
- The most common cause of acute hoarseness is viral laryngitis. Symptoms are self-limited and usually resolve within 2 weeks.
- Dysphonia persisting for longer than 2 weeks suggests the possibility of another diagnosis, such as vocal cord paralysis, neoplasm, phonotraumatic lesion, or chronic laryngitis.
- Indications for referral of a patient with voice complaints to an otolaryngologist include dysphonia that persists for longer than 2 weeks, that is of acute onset during voicing, or that is accompanied by other symptoms such as otalgia, dysphagia, or difficulty breathing.

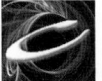

CURRENT THERAPY

- Appropriate treatment of voice complaints depends on accurate diagnosis.
- Supportive therapy is all that is necessary for most cases of acute laryngitis associated with viral upper respiratory tract infections.
- Laryngopharyngeal reflux is a common cause of chronic laryngitis, and appropriate therapy often requires twice-daily administration of proton pump inhibitors for at least 2 months.
- Microlaryngeal phonosurgery may be indicated for some patients with benign phonotraumatic lesions.
- Vocal cord medialization can rehabilitate the voice in a patient with unilateral vocal cord paralysis.
- Many patients with dysphonia benefit from voice therapy, alone or in combination with other treatment strategies.

Voice is an essential component of communication. Vocal difficulty is very distressing to patients and can have a negative impact on physical, social, and emotional qualities of life. To understand the pathophysiology, evaluation, and treatment of voice complaints, it is important to understand the anatomy and physiology of normal voice production. Looking first at how good voice quality is achieved makes it readily apparent how alterations in vocal fold vibration, symmetry, or closure can lead to various vocal difficulties.

To aid discussion of voice complaints, clarification of terminology is necessary. Although "hoarseness" is a term that most patients use to describe any type of voice complaint and "laryngitis" is the presumptive explanation that many patients provide for their symptoms, each of these terms has a more precise meaning. Dysphonia is the general term for vocal difficulty. Hoarseness implies a rough or raspy change in voice quality and is one type of dysphonia. Other categories include limited vocal projection, strained vocal effort, and change in pitch—each of which may occur with or without vocal roughness. The term "laryngitis" specifically describes inflammation of the larynx. This inflammation

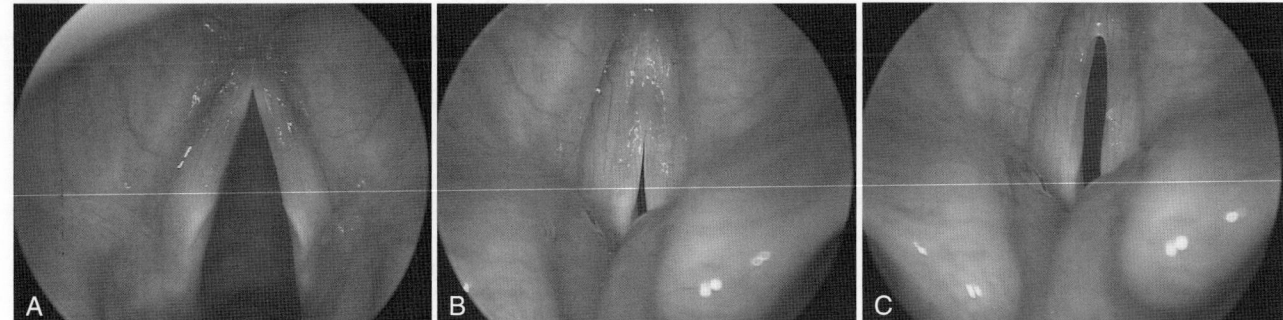

Figure 1 A, Normal vocal folds in abducted position for inspiration. B, Normal vocal folds in adducted position for phonation. C, Displacement of the vocal fold medial edges creates mucosal wave propagation during phonation and produces voice.

may be acute or chronic, and again it describes some but certainly not all cases of dysphonia. This distinction will be made clear as the evaluation and management of dysphonia are described.

Normal Laryngeal Function

The larynx plays a central role in voice production by serving as a vibrating instrument that turns airflow from the lungs into sound. The sound is shaped into intelligible speech through the resonating and articulating functions of the pharynx and oral cavity. The ability of the larynx to create vibration and serve as a sound source is a function of its complex, layered microanatomy. The deeper layers of the vocal fold include the thyroarytenoid muscle and the vocal ligament, which position the more superficial layers of the superficial lamina propria and epithelium during phonation. Compared with the fibrous nature of the vocal ligament, the superficial lamina propria is a loose gelatinous layer whose pliability allows for voice production.

During inspiration (Figure 1A), the vocal folds are abducted so that air can move past the larynx without resistance. During phonation (Figure 1B), the vocal folds are held in an adducted position while the lungs drive air toward the larynx. Air pressure builds in the subglottis, beneath the vocal folds, until it overcomes the forces of vocal fold closure, pushes past the vocal folds, and generates negative pressure in its wake as it moves past the larynx. A combination of the vocal folds' intrinsic viscoelasticity and the negative pressure created through Bernoulli's effect draws the vocal fold edges back together, allowing subglottic pressure to rebuild and the cycle to repeat. Repeated cycles of opening and closing at the level of the vocal fold edges generate a so-called mucosal wave, which travels from the inferior edge of each vocal fold up across the medial and superior edges (Figure 1C). These waves may repeat hundreds of times each second, depending on pitch. This cycled opening and closing of the vocal folds during phonation imparts pressure waves to the air column that moves the vocal folds, generating sound. The ability of vocal folds to vibrate easily and symmetrically in this very rapid fashion allows for clear, smooth voicing.

Evaluation of Dysphonia

Central to the evaluation of dysphonia is the understanding that any disruption of vocal fold closure, symmetry, or vibration impairs the ability of the vocal folds to generate a clear sound source. Most voice complaints arise from anatomic or functional limitations in glottal closure or mucosal wave formation, although other parts of the respiratory tree are also responsible for components of the voice. General points concerning evaluation of dysphonia are discussed in this section, with specific causes discussed afterward.

History

A careful history can provide many clues that point toward the proper diagnosis in patients with dysphonia. Although many patients offer the complaint of "hoarseness" as a general term, a careful historian distinguishes between complaints related to voice quality, vocal projection, vocal effort or strain, vocal fatigue, and so on. Two questions that can help a patient organize his or her own thoughts related to poor voice are "What abnormal things does your voice do now that it did not do before?" and "What normal things did your voice do before that it no longer can do?" The acuteness of onset, duration, severity, and progression of any complaint should be determined.

The history should also determine what other factors or events might have caused or exacerbated the dysphonia. Recent sources of laryngeal inflammation might include intubation, excessive voice use, or upper respiratory tract infection. Baseline conditions that foster chronic laryngeal inflammation include environmental allergies, rhinitis, and laryngopharyngeal reflux. Laryngopharyngeal reflux can exist in the absence of heartburn, with reflux-associated inflammation of the larynx and pharynx providing symptoms of globus pharyngeus, throat clearing, nonproductive cough, effortful swallowing, and even mild dysphagia in association with dysphonia.

Concerning the possibility of laryngeal malignancy, any patient with dysphonia should be asked about smoking and alcohol use, because these are risk factors for squamous cell carcinoma. Another important question in distinguishing inflammatory dysphonia from a mass lesion of the vocal fold concerns whether there are any periods of normal voice or the dysphonia is constant—inflammation may wax and wane, but dysphonia associated with mass lesions is usually progressive and unremitting. Finally, the history should elicit other possible head and neck complaints, including dyspnea, stridor, dysphagia, odynophagia, otalgia, sore throat, and pain with speaking (odynophonia). If hoarseness is associated with some of these symptoms for longer than 2 weeks, the suspicion of malignancy is increased.

Physical Examination

The physical examination for patients with dysphonia includes a complete head and neck evaluation with focus on the larynx and laryngeal function. Although much of the head and neck examination can be performed in a general setting, some portions of the laryngeal examination require specialized equipment found only in some otolaryngology offices that specialize in voice care. Routine head and neck evaluation should include systematic examination of the ears, nose, oral cavity, oropharynx, and neck.

Complaint of otalgia in the setting of an unremarkable ear examination suggests a possibility of referred pain from a lesion of the larynx or pharynx, and is concerning for possible malignancy. Edematous and erythematous nasal mucosa suggests rhinitis, with the possibility of postnasal drip contributing to laryngeal inflammation. Tremor of the tongue or palate might suggest neurologic disorder, whereas pharyngeal erythema and exudate suggest possible acute infection. Pachydermia (cobblestoning) of the posterior pharyngeal wall suggests the possibility of laryngopharyngeal reflux. Tenderness with manipulation of the hyoid bone suggests tension of the strap muscles and correlates closely with complaint of odynophonia and the possibility of muscle tension dysphonia. A neck mass might represent either metastatic lymphadenopathy from a laryngeal malignancy or a primary lesion which itself compresses the recurrent laryngeal nerve and causes paralytic dysphonia. Surgical scarring along the neck suggests the possibility that prior thyroid surgery, carotid endarterectomy, or anterior approach to the cervical spine might have led to vocal fold paralysis.

Laryngeal Examination

Beyond a general examination of the head and neck, there should be directed evaluation of the larynx and laryngeal function. The examiner should listen to the voice carefully, because vocal characteristics such as roughness, breathiness, strain, vocal breaks, and diplophonia (pitch instability, with two different pitches present simultaneously) can help guide the differential diagnosis of dysphonia. Visual examination of the larynx has many forms, ranging from mirror examination to flexible fiberoptic laryngoscopy to videostrobolaryngoscopy.

Mirror examination offers an adequate view of the vocal folds in many patients but may be limited by patient tolerance, physician inexperience, and the inherently limited ability of this technique to brightly illuminate the larynx or record the examination for later review. Flexible laryngoscopy is routinely available in almost all otolaryngology offices, is well tolerated by patients, and offers good views of the larynx that can be recorded with appropriate equipment. Mirror examination and flexible laryngoscopy are limited to observation of vocal fold motion and anatomy but cannot observe laryngeal function because they do not visualize vibration of the vocal folds. To examine vocal fold vibration, videostroboscopy uses a strobe light to create the impression of slow-motion analysis of mucosal waves. Stroboscopy is typically available only in selected otolaryngology practices in which laryngologists specialize in the treatment of voice disorders.

Other Testing

Videostroboscopic evaluation, combined with a thorough history and routine physical examination, can establish the diagnosis for almost all patients with voice complaints, but further testing is sometimes indicated. For instance, electromyography is used by some laryngologists for further evaluation of vocal fold paralysis or paresis. More commonly, radiographic studies are used for further evaluation of some voice complaints. Computed tomography (CT) scans are ordered most often in the evaluation of suspected laryngeal neoplasms and for patients with vocal fold paralysis.

In the case of neoplasm, CT scanning is useful to assess the extent of the primary lesion and to evaluate possible metastatic cervical lymphadenopathy. In patients with laryngeal malignancy, chest radiography is also important to assess for pulmonary metastases. For patients with vocal fold paralysis who do not have a clear history of surgical injury of the recurrent laryngeal nerve, a CT scan from skull base to thoracic inlet identifies possible lesions along the course of the recurrent laryngeal nerve. Central problems are less likely, but if they are suspected as a cause of vocal fold paralysis, then magnetic resonance imaging of the brain may be indicated as well.

Types of Dysphonia

Although not comprehensive, the conditions discussed here account for the vast majority of voice complaints. Some patients with voice complaints have more than one condition, and not every patient will fit neatly into a single category. Nevertheless, understanding how each of these conditions creates dysphonia, and knowing which particular history and physical examination findings might be associated with each cause, can help a physician to appropriately diagnose and manage voice complaints.

Acute Laryngitis

Acute laryngitis is the most common cause of hoarseness and dysphonia. It is most often viral in nature, and onset of laryngeal symptoms may be associated with other symptoms of upper respiratory tract infection, including fever, myalgia, sore throat, and rhinorrhea. Viral inflammation of the vocal folds leads to diminished and more effortful vocal fold vibration, yielding a voice characterized by increased effort and a harsh, strained quality with decreased projection. Characteristic findings on laryngoscopy include vocal fold edema and erythema with decreased amplitude of the mucosal wave. Treatment of acute viral laryngitis is supportive, with counseling for hydration, humidification, and mucolytics. Symptoms generally are self-limited and resolve within 2 weeks. During this time, patients should be instructed to

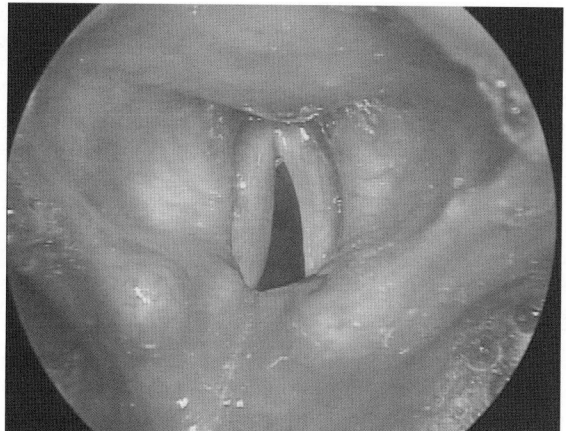

Figure 2 Vocal fold paralysis prevents the right vocal fold from closing to midline and creates dysphonia.

use the voice in a comfortable fashion, rather than straining or pushing to get loudness, because pushing behaviors may lead to the development of persistent muscle tension dysphonia.

Bacterial or fungal infections also cause acute laryngitis in rare cases. With appropriate physical findings and in the right clinical setting, antibiotic or antifungal therapy may be used to treat these conditions. Amoxicillin-clavulanate (Augmentin) is often the antibiotic of choice, and fluconazole (Diflucan) is a commonly used antifungal agent.

Chronic Laryngitis

Chronic laryngitis is the nonspecific condition of prolonged laryngeal inflammation; the term itself does not indicate an etiology for the inflammation. Among the many possible sources for this inflammation are mechanical irritation from traumatic coughing or prolonged speaking, chemical irritation from environmental irritants (e.g., smoking, inhaled medications), and irritation from postnasal drip or laryngopharyngeal reflux. More than one cause may exist simultaneously. Issues related to cigarette use, excessive voice use, medication effect, and rhinitis can be identified with careful history taking. Laryngopharyngeal reflux is a very common source of chronic laryngitis. It may manifest with several nonspecific symptoms, such as throat irritation, globus pharyngeus, frequent throat clearing, and nonproductive cough, with or without accompanying heartburn. Because vocal fold inflammation increases with continued mechanical trauma, the hoarseness of chronic laryngitis typically gets worse with prolonged voice use and improves with voice rest. Examination findings in chronic laryngitis include generalized laryngeal edema and erythema, and careful inspection may also reveal interarytenoid hyperplasia, subglottic edema, laryngeal ventricular obliteration, and an increase in thick glottic secretions.

Treatment of chronic laryngitis is tailored to the cause of the inflammation. Vocal hygiene with moderate voice use and instructions to reduce throat clearing and coughing may diminish mechanical irritation, and smoking cessation is recommended to any smoker with laryngeal complaints. Several studies have suggested that an appropriate trial of proton pump inhibitors for treatment of laryngopharyngeal reflux includes twice-daily therapy for at least 2 months, in contrast to the once-daily dosing often used for typical heartburn complaints. Lifestyle counseling to limit consumption of caffeine, carbonation, alcohol, and acidic foods can improve reflux, and attention to hydration and humidification decreases the viscosity of glottic secretions. For patients who are troubled by vocal difficulties associated with chronic laryngitis, referral to a speech–language pathologist for voice therapy can improve compliance with suggested lifestyle changes and help foster vocal improvement.

Vocal Fold Paralysis

The dysphonia in cases of vocal fold paralysis usually relates to poor vocal fold closure (Figure 2). The result is a breathy voice with limited projection and increased vocal effort. The farther from midline the immobile vocal fold, the more air leaks through the incompetent glottal valve without being turned into sound. Patients whose immobile vocal fold sits in a lateral position may have severely weak and breathy voices, whereas patients whose immobile vocal fold sits near midline may have a perceptually near-normal conversational voice and complain only of mild increase in effort, vocal fatigue, or problems with loud projection. Because of their glottal insufficiency, patients may complain of "running out of air" with prolonged speech. Impaired glottal closure may also decrease airway protection during swallowing, so patients with vocal fold paralysis need to be questioned about aspiration as well. Whereas rehabilitation of poor voice may be elective, patients with increased aspiration risk need prompt therapy.

Evaluation of vocal fold paralysis includes identification of the cause of paralysis. Surgical injury to the recurrent laryngeal nerve accounts for almost half of all cases of unilateral vocal fold paralysis, and cervical or thoracic neoplasm and idiopathic paralysis account for most of the remaining cases. In a patient without a clear surgical history explaining the paralysis, CT scanning from skull base to mediastinum can identify any possible lesions along the course of the recurrent laryngeal nerve. In those patients whose histories suggest other possible causes (e.g., central neurologic injury, Lyme disease), further investigations, such as magnetic resonance imaging of the brain or blood work may be indicated as well. Some physicians perform laryngeal electromyography to help with the prognosis of paralysis or to differentiate neurologic injury from cricoarytenoid joint fixation; however, this study is neither standardized nor routine in many practices. Although flexible laryngoscopy alone may be satisfactory to document vocal fold immobility, stroboscopy can be added to investigate the impact of glottal insufficiency on vocal cord vibration and possible vocal fold flutter.

Treatment of vocal fold paralysis might include any combination of voice therapy, injection laryngoplasty, transcervical medialization laryngoplasty, and laryngeal reinnervation. Depending on the cause of the paralysis, some patients experience gradual recovery with synkinetic reinnervation or recovery of purposeful vocal fold motion over a period of several months. Based on the degree of voice and swallowing handicap, treatment of patients with vocal fold paralysis may be optional rather than necessary. Voice therapy can help teach patients to produce a stronger voice despite the paralysis, but by itself will not help a paralyzed vocal cord to recover motion. Various medialization techniques have been developed to help reposition an immobile vocal fold in the midline, where the contralateral mobile vocal fold can provide for complete glottal closure and lead to improved voice and swallowing. Injection medialization can be performed in the office or in the operating room, with temporary or permanent materials; if recovery of vocal fold motion is thought possible, then temporary injection is preferred. Transcervical medialization is a permanent but reversible surgical technique performed by otolaryngologists that repositions an immobile vocal fold in the midline. Laryngeal reinnervation offers the possibility of midline positioning of the immobile vocal fold with restored tone and bulk of the vocal fold musculature; however, because results may not mature for several months, this technique is less commonly performed than either injection or transcervical medialization.

Phonotraumatic Lesions: Nodules, Polyps, and Cysts

During vibration, vocal folds are subject to the shearing stresses of vibration. Although vocal fold structure is designed to accommodate these stresses in most circumstances, patients with vocal abuse or excessive voice use are at risk for development of lesions as the result of cumulative phonotrauma. Depending on the location and nature of these lesions, they are categorized as nodules, polyps, or cysts.

Vocal fold nodules are areas of fibrovascular scarring that are located just beneath the epithelium, at the level of the basement membrane and superficial lamina propria. They are typically bilateral and symmetrical, sitting at the junction of the anterior one third and the posterior two thirds of each vocal fold. Polyps are typically unilateral lesions that may be edematous or fibrous in nature and

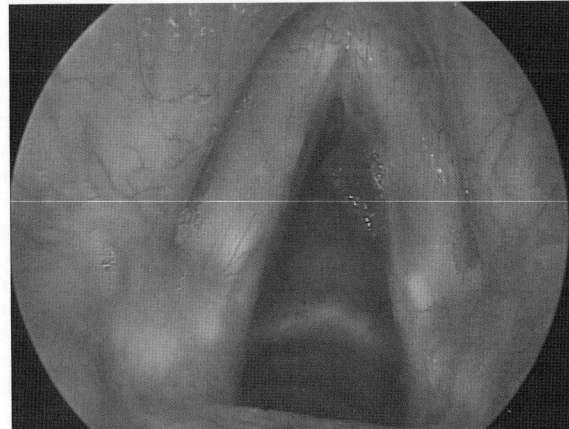

Figure 3 A large right hemorrhagic polyp, which can impair vocal fold vibration.

may contain hemorrhage (Figure 3). They usually are exophytic and extend outward from the vocal fold epithelium, although the fibrous base of a polyp may extend into the superficial lamina propria of a vocal fold. In contrast to an epithelial-based lesion such as a polyp, a vocal fold cyst is a subepithelial encapsulated lesion that sits entirely within the vocal fold; its size may exert a mass effect that deforms the medial edge of the involved vocal fold. These cysts are occasionally noted as congenital lesions in children, but in adults they are more often caused by traumatic occlusion of the ducts of the seromucinous glands within the larynx.

Nodules, polyps, and cysts cause dysphonia by disturbing vocal fold vibration, leading to rough voice quality. These lesions get larger as traumatic voice use accumulates, and vocal roughness usually becomes more severe and more constant as the lesions progress. Because vibration is more easily disturbed at high pitch, performers with these lesions may notice that high pitch is affected first. Effort of phonation often increases, but projection remains intact. Lesions large enough to limit vocal fold closure may also cause a slightly breathy voice quality. Because patients with excessive voice use are at risk for these lesions, a history of social and occupational voice demands is valuable in cases of suspected phonotrauma.

Treatment for these lesions always begins with voice therapy designed to modify the patient's voice use so as to diminish trauma. Voice therapy may be all that is necessary to allow resolution of some early traumatic changes, particularly in the case of edematous nodules. If dysphonia persists despite voice therapy and other conservative measures, surgery may be considered. Surgery with the goal of voice preservation and restoration (phonosurgery) is typically performed by otolaryngologists who specialize in the care of persons with vocal difficulties. The goal of phonosurgery for these lesions is to remove the lesion that impairs vibration while preserving as much of the remaining, pliable superficial lamina propria as possible, so that vocal fold vibration can be restored.

Reinke's Edema

Reinke's edema, also known as polypoid corditis, is a benign swelling of the vocal folds that is most commonly seen in patients with a long-term smoking history. The edema, a reaction to long-term irritation, accumulates within the superficial lamina propria. The edema is most often bilateral and occurs diffusely along the entire length of the vocal fold, rather than being limited to a more discrete area, as is seen with phonotraumatic polyps (Figure 4). As vocal fold mass increases with disease progression, the pitch of the voice decreases, and this is the change in voice most associated with Reinke's edema. A classic presentation of this condition is a female in her fifth or sixth decade of life who provides a long history of smoking and progressive deepening of her voice. In rare circumstances, the vocal folds gradually accumulate enough edema to compromise the airway, so breathing complaints should be evaluated as well.

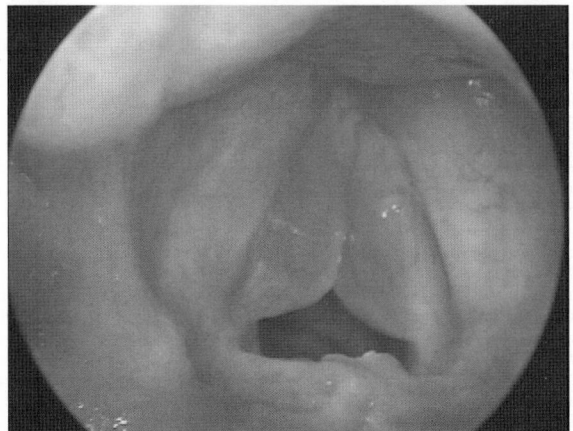

Figure 4 Symmetrical polypoid degeneration of the bilateral vocal folds, characteristic of Reinke's edema.

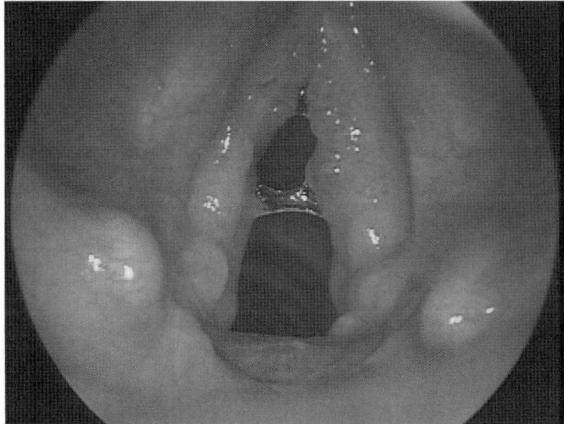

Figure 5 Recurrent respiratory papillomatosis, whose presence along each vocal fold medial edge disrupts sound production.

Because a significant smoking history is also a risk factor for vocal fold leukoplakia and malignancy, good visualization of the vocal folds is necessary to evaluate for other lesions in these patients. If benign edema of the vocal folds is truly the only lesion noted, management depends on the degree to which voice quality is disturbing to the patient or the degree to which the airway is narrowed. Smoking cessation can lead to stabilization of pitch at its current level, and phonosurgery to remove excess vocal fold mass can help lead to normalization of pitch and improve the airway. Phonosurgery may be performed with cold instruments or with the pulsed photoangiolytic lasers, an emerging therapy; in either case, there is a risk of creating a vocal fold scar that might limit vocal fold vibration even as vocal fold contours are improved.

Recurrent Respiratory Papillomatosis
Recurrent respiratory papillomatosis (Figure 5) is a benign laryngeal neoplasm that is caused by the human papilloma virus. It is the most common source of hoarseness in children, although adults also may be affected. As the lesions grow on the laryngeal epithelium, they create hoarseness and sometimes effortful voice by disrupting vocal fold vibration, particularly if the lesions are located along the medial edge of either vocal fold. Large and bulky lesions may lead to airway compromise, and advanced disease may spread throughout the mucosa of the upper aerodigestive tract rather than being limited to the larynx. Although accurate diagnosis depends on histopathologic analysis, a diagnosis of benign papilloma can be suspected from the characteristic appearance of the vascular fronds, which can be seen under magnified visualization in the office or in the operating room.

Treatment of recurrent respiratory papillomatosis is surgery, which is performed with a carbon dioxide laser, microdebrider,

cold instruments, or the emerging technology of pulsed potassium titanyl phosphate (KTP) laser. As its name implies, the condition is recurrent: Even though surgery may reduce or remove the papilloma temporarily, the tissue continues to harbor the papilloma virus, and the disease usually grows back. Because repeated surgeries are expected, the goal of any single procedure is to remove as much disease as possible while limiting surgical scarring of the vocal folds. Scarring created as a result of surgery is cumulative, and over time patients develop persistent dysphonia caused as much by repeated surgeries as by recurrence of the disease. An ability to treat epithelial lesions while limiting scarring at the level of the superficial lamina propria is one main advantage of pulsed laser photoangiolysis; that these pulsed laser procedures can be performed in the office as well as the operating room is another. To help limit the need for repeated surgical procedures, adjunct medical therapies such as interferon and cidofovir are sometimes used for treatment of advanced disease.

Vocal Cord Cancer
In 2008, an estimated 12,250 new cases of laryngeal cancer and 3,670 deaths attributable to laryngeal cancer occurred in the United States. The annual incidence of laryngeal cancer is 6.4 cases per 100,000 for men and 1.3 cases per 100,000 for women. Smoking is the single largest risk factor for laryngeal cancer, and excessive alcohol use has a synergistic effect as a risk factor as well. Survival rates for laryngeal cancer depend on the stage of the tumor at the time of diagnosis, which is a function of tumor size and possible tumor spread to the cervical lymph nodes or distant metastatic sites. Cancers that occur on the medial edge of the vocal fold produce dysphonia while still small, and many laryngeal cancers are diagnosed early.

The dysphonia associated with laryngeal cancer is constant, progressive, and unremitting, without the intermittent vocal improvement that may occur in inflammatory conditions. The presence of dysphagia, odynophagia, otalgia, hemoptysis, or unexplained weight loss further increases the index of suspicion for malignancy. Cervical lymphadenopathy is associated with advanced tumors. Diagnosis may be suspected on the basis of laryngeal examination and is confirmed with biopsy. The presence or absence of mucosal waves on the involved vocal fold on videostroboscopic examination can help predict the depth of the lesion. Both a CT scan of the neck and chest radiographs are indicated to assess for tumor size and spread. Early cancers are treated with surgery or radiation therapy, with similar cure rates. Emerging technologies such as pulsed photoangiolytic lasers may allow for surgical treatment of early disease with better preservation of surrounding normal tissue. More advanced tumors are usually treated with a combination of radiation therapy and surgery or chemotherapy.

Leukoplakia, or a raised white plaque on the epithelial surface, is a visual marker for the likely presence of dysplasia or carcinoma in situ. As a very early lesion, vocal fold leukoplakia may manifest with mild dysphonia or may be found incidentally on head and neck examination performed for other reasons. This early disease may take many years before progressing to invasive carcinoma, and recognition of leukoplakia presents an opportunity for early treatment to prevent progression of disease. Pulsed laser photoangiolysis has emerged as a state-of-the-art therapy for treatment of this epithelial lesion with preservation of the underlying vocal fold pliability.

Neurologic Disorders and the Voice
Neurologic conditions that affect the voice usually do so by causing poor coordination of vocal fold motion. Spasmodic dysphonia, for instance, leads to involuntary spasms that bring the vocal folds either tightly together (adductor spasmodic dysphonia) or apart (abductor spasmodic dysphonia) during phonation. These spasms lead to vocal breaks that are strained or breathy, respectively. Although the cause of spasmodic dysphonia is thought to lie within the central nervous system, the gold standard treatment of botulinum toxin is targeted at the end organ. Injection of

botulinum toxin (Botox)[1] into appropriate laryngeal muscles can weaken these muscles and diminish the spasm.

Vocal fold tremor is a neurologic disorder that is distinct from spasmodic dysphonia. Its hallmark is tremulous voice quality caused by tremor of the larynx, which may occur both during phonation and at rest. Vocal fold tremor may exist alone or as part of systemic tremor. Botulinum toxin[1] can decrease the amplitude of the tremor but may exacerbate the loss of projection that many tremor patients also have as a complaint. Medications such as anxiolytics or β-blockers that are used to treat systemic tremor may also improve the voice in patients with vocal fold tremor without worsening hypophonia.

Functional Voice Disorders

Functional dysphonia may exist by itself or in combination with an anatomic or neurologic source of dysphonia. The most common form of functional voice disorder is muscle tension dysphonia, which describes inappropriate hyperfunction of the supraglottic muscles. This hyperfunction often occurs in response to another source of hoarseness, as the patient tries to force out a strained voice with improved projection rather than accept the limited voice quality that may accompany the other disorder. The hyperfunction may then become an entrenched habit separate from the original pathology. In this sense, a classic scenario for muscle tension dysphonia is a patient who strains to speak more loudly during an acute laryngitis episode and whose strained, squeezed voice pattern persists even after the acute laryngitis has resolved. Patients with muscle tension dysphonia may complain of odynophonia as tension in the involved supraglottic muscles leads to muscular pain with prolonged speaking. Once other lesions have been evaluated, the treatment of muscle tension dysphonia is expert voice therapy with an emphasis on decreased hyperfunction.

Presbylaryngis

Presbylaryngis is the term that is used to describe the aging voice. It typically manifests in the seventh or eighth decade but can develop earlier. Acoustically, presbylaryngis results in a characteristic thinned voice, often with decreased projection and increased vocal strain. The condition occurs as cumulative voice use leads to traumatic thinning of the superficial lamina propria, particularly at the mid-cord level. This loss of superficial lamina propria leads to deficiency at the medial edge of each vocal fold, and a spindle-shaped defect in glottal closure may be noticed with close evaluation. Many patients with a complaint of presbylaryngis find that appropriate voice therapy to address breath support and vocal projection leads to satisfactory improvement in the voice without altering the vocal fold anatomy. For those patients who remain unsatisfied with their voice after therapy, vocal fold medialization procedures can restore straight vocal cord edges and may lead to improved projection; however, currently available injectables and implants that address contour defects cannot restore pliability.

Conclusion

Understanding the anatomy and physiology of normal voice production provides a framework through which dysphonia can be evaluated. Application of this knowledge during the history and physical examination guides the diagnosis of hoarseness and allows clinicians to distinguish among conditions as varied as acute laryngitis, benign phonotraumatic lesions, vocal fold paralysis, and laryngeal cancer as part of a differential diagnosis. Videostrobolaryngoscopy allows evaluation of vocal fold function as well as structure and can confirm diagnosis. As with any condition, accurate diagnosis directs appropriate therapy. Because no further evaluation or management is necessary for acute viral laryngitis, many patients with hoarseness require no more than a careful history and physical examination. However, if dysphonia persists for longer than 2 weeks or is accompanied by other laryngopharyngeal symptoms that are not thought to be related to an upper respiratory tract infection, referral should be made to an otolaryngologist for further evaluation.

References

Koufman JA, Aviv JE, Casiano RR, et al: Laryngopharyngeal reflux: Position statement of the committee on speech, voice, and swallowing disorders of the American Academy of Otolaryngology-Head and Neck Surgery, *Otolaryngol Head Neck Surg* 127:32–35, 2002.

Merati AL, Heman-Ackah YD, Abaza M, et al: Common movement disorders affecting the larynx: A report from the neurolaryngology committee of the AAO-HNS, *Otolaryngol Head Neck Surg* 133:654–665, 2005.

Swibel Rosenthal LH, Benninger MS, Deeb RH: Vocal fold immobility: A longitudinal analysis of etiology over 20 years, *Laryngoscope* 117:1864–1870, 2007.

Wilson JA, Deary IJ, Millar A, et al: The quality of life impact of dysphonia, *Clin Otolaryngol* 27:179–182, 2002.

Zeitels SM, Casiano RR, Gardner GM, et al: Management of common voice problems: Committee report, *Otolaryngol Head Neck Surg* 126:333–348, 2002.

Zeitels SM, Healy GB: Laryngology and phonosurgery, *N Engl J Med* 349:882–892, 2003.

PAIN

Method of
Steven A. House, MD

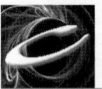

CURRENT DIAGNOSIS

- Always use history and physical examination and consider imaging or laboratory studies to rule out life- or function-threatening pathologies before merely providing symptomatic treatment.

Acute Pain
- Acute pain has a sudden onset, is usually nociceptive (somatic, visceral) in nature, and likely is due to apparent injury or medical condition.
- It can last up to 3 months and can demonstrate hypersympathetic signs of tachycardia, elevated blood pressure, dilated pupils, or diaphoresis.

Chronic Pain
- Chronic pain is usually gradual in onset, lasts more than 3 months, and rarely serves any purpose. It can manifest with hyperalgesia (hurts more than it should) or allodynia (hurts when it should not, e.g., light touch).
- Vegetative symptoms such as depression, fatigue, or anorexia may be present.
- A significant neuropathic component may be present.
- Psychiatric and social or socioeconomic issues may be exacerbating factors.
- Examples can include headaches, low back pain, osteoarthritis, and fibromyalgia.
- While opioids might be appropriate for some conditions or situations, in general, they are proving to be neither as safe nor as effective for chronic, non-cancer pain as had been believed.

Quality
- Quality of the pain (e.g., sharp, dull, radiating, deep, superficial, lancinating, tingling, burning) is an important factor in determining the best management modalities.
- Quality plays a role in ruling in or ruling out severe disease that can require urgent surgical or other interventions rather than analgesics or adjunctive medications or therapies.

Severity
- Severity of the pain can be rated on a variety of scales such as numerical (0 to 5, 0 to 10), analogue (marked on a line with a range from no pain to the worst possible pain), or facial expression (smiles to grimaces, available for children and the elderly or patients with dementia).
- Functional scales (fully satisfactory function to debilitated) may be more helpful in determining the impact of the pain on the person's life.

[1]Not FDA approved for this indication

CURRENT THERAPY

- Acute pain commonly responds to simple analgesics of the nonopioid, opioid, or combination varieties. Rest, ice, compression, and elevation (RICE) are helpful for acute inflammatory conditions and injuries.
- Chronic pain, because of its complexity, often requires multiple modalities. Pharmacologic options include nonopioid, opioid, adjuvant, or botanical medications. Nonpharmacologic options include physical therapy, chiropractic care, transcutaneous electrical nerve stimulation (TENS) unit, acupuncture, or surgical or anesthesia interventions.
- Adjuvant medications are drugs that are used for pain but do not have pain treatment as their primary indication, and they are often the most effective agents in neuropathic and/or chronic pain.
- Opioids are sometimes safer for long-term use, but the individual's risk for falls must be considered in the elderly, as opioids can increase this risk, and the risks of overdose and other adverse effects rise with increasing age and duration of exposure. For many chronic conditions such as low back pain, the evidence supporting the use of opioids is lacking, with efficacy often superseded by nonopioid medications. The risk of addiction MUST be considered before starting opioids on any patient. From 1999 to 2017, overdose death rates have increased from 8.2 to 29.1/100,000 in males and from 3.9 to 14.4 in females; 67.8% of the 70,237 drug overdose deaths in 2017 involved opioids, and the rates were highest in the 25 to 54-year-old age range. According to the CDC, nearly 2 million Americans above the age of 12 years abused or were dependent on opioids in 2014.
- Nonsteroidal antiinflammatory drugs (NSAIDs) carry a risk for GI and cardiac complications, especially in the elderly and those with a history of CAD or GI ulcers or gastritis.
- The patient *must* be involved in and cooperative with the treatment plan. Honesty and trust are necessary components of a therapeutic physician-patient relationship.
- Do not underestimate the placebo effect. If the patient feels that a harmless treatment is beneficial, take advantage of it.
- If the patient is not improving adequately, consult a surgeon if the source of pain is an operable condition, or consult a pain specialist if surgical intervention is not appropriate.

Epidemiology

Although estimates vary, approximately 50 million Americans experience chronic pain and incur costs and overall economic impact is estimated as high as $635 billion per year. Pain is the most common symptom that causes patients to pursue medical evaluation and management. The prevalence of several common pain syndromes including headaches, facial pain, abdominal pain, pelvic pain, and low back pain is slightly higher in women than in men because there are gender variations in the perception, coping, and reporting of pain. Pain tends to be undertreated in women, people of color, children, and the elderly, and it is underreported in nonverbal or cognitively impaired children and adults.

Risk Factors

Traumatic injury is a cause of acute pain and a risk factor for chronic pain. Patients who have mastectomy, laminectomy, thoracotomy, or amputations are at risk for pain syndromes. Chronic musculoskeletal conditions such as arthritis, spinal stenosis, degenerative disk disease, or fibromyalgia; infectious diseases including HIV or varicella zoster; neuropathies from diagnoses such as diabetes, B_{12} deficiency, or multiple sclerosis; treatment with certain chemotherapies or isoniazid (INH) without adequate vitamin B_6; psychiatric disorders such as depression, anxiety, or posttraumatic stress disorder (PTSD), especially as a consequence of domestic violence; or autoimmune disorders including lupus and rheumatoid arthritis can predispose the individual to chronic pain. Although the risk of pain increases with age, pain should not be considered a usual part of aging until it is appropriately evaluated. A motor vehicle accident or work-related injury or other condition where secondary gain is a possibility, especially if there is no apparent injury, raises the consideration of malingering.

Pathophysiology

Injury or potential injury is detected by nociceptors in the peripheral nervous system, and the signal is then transmitted through the dorsal horn of the spinal cord up to the brain for processing. The three primary classes of opioid receptors are the mu, kappa, and delta receptors, which are located in areas throughout the central and peripheral nervous system. Upon binding these receptors, opioids block calcium channels and modulate the nociceptive pathways. The hyperstimulation of chronic pain (often via the N-methyl-D-aspartate [NMDA] receptor and the resultant increase in intracellular calcium are neurotoxic due to lowering the neuronal firing threshold and increasing firing frequency. This neurotoxicity can lead to ongoing pain in the absence of physical insult. Additionally, NMDA receptor activation can increase pre- and post-synaptic substance P while downregulating the mu receptors. This can decrease the efficacy of mu-agonists, as there are fewer receptors to bind. Neuropathic pain can result from chronic pain or from physical or pathophysiologic injury or changes to the nerve, as in diabetic neuropathy or other neuropathies.

Prevention

The best prevention is a safe and healthy lifestyle. The combination of healthy diet and exercise has been demonstrated to improve pain in osteoarthritis better than either intervention alone, and maintaining a healthy weight can help prevent the arthritis in the first place. Smoking and obesity (odds ratio increasing with BMI) have been associated with chronic pain. Relative to people of normal weight, rates of recurring pain were 20% higher in the overweight, 68% greater with class I obesity, 136% more in class II obesity, and 254% more in the morbidly obese.

Regarding safety, wearing seat belts while driving or using appropriate safety equipment at work and during recreational activities can help reduce the severity of injuries should they occur. Proper body mechanics are important as well.

Clinical Manifestations

Manifestations of pain depend on the location and underlying cause. In the acute setting, the patient can have tachycardia, elevated blood pressure, or diaphoresis, whereas chronic pain can manifest with vegetative symptoms of depression, fatigue, anorexia, or insomnia.

Diagnosis

Pain is most commonly a symptom rather than a disease in and of itself, so it behooves the provider to pursue treatable causes, especially red flag conditions, in addition to providing symptomatic treatment. The history regarding onset (shorter or longer than 3 months), exacerbating or remitting factors, quality, radiation, severity, and timing of the pain (constant versus intermittent), in addition to any associated signs or symptoms such as fever, nausea, vomiting, or diarrhea, can help the provider in that regard. The physical examination is a key component in ruling out life- or function-threatening disorders. Is there tenderness, swelling, bruising, erythema, or deformity? Are strength, reflexes, and sensation intact? Does the patient demonstrate a consistent demeanor (grimace or other signs of pain) and gait (antalgic versus normal) when moving from the waiting area to the examination room and out to the parking lot? The choice to use laboratory studies or imaging is determined by the location of the pain and the structures or organs that might be in that area. When determining severity, "What does the pain keep you from doing?" (which uses function as the measure of impairment and treatment efficacy rather than a subjective pain score to guide therapy) may be a much more helpful question than "How bad is your pain?" If function is not improving, that could be considered a treatment failure, and medications and therapy should be adjusted rather than continuing the same regimen.

Differential Diagnosis

The differential diagnosis for all types of pain is far too extensive for the brevity of this chapter, but in addition to the plethora of physical diagnoses to be considered, the provider must consider that chronic fatigue, depression, and domestic abuse can manifest as a chronic pain syndrome.

Treatment

Nonpharmacologic

Physical therapy for chronic pain (for recent-onset low back pain, relief was statistically but not clinically significant as compared to usual care), TENS units, chiropractic care, and regular exercise have shown benefit in certain conditions. Cognitive behavioral therapy (CBT) and mindfulness training improve function more than pain, and CBT, acupuncture, and mind-body therapies (e.g., yoga, tai chi, mindfulness-based stress reduction) provide safer options that may be both beneficial and cost-effective. Surgery may be required, and interventions such as nerve blocks or epidural injections may also be of benefit. Kyphoplasty and vertebroplasty have fallen out of favor. Aerobic exercise and water therapy are helpful for fibromyalgia, but the patient must not overexert because this can exacerbate the pain.

Pharmacologic

Nonopioid Analgesics

Acetaminophen (Tylenol) is generally a safe and effective medication provided the total daily dose for adults remains less than 3 g/day. For osteoarthritis of the hips and knees, acetaminophen provides modest short-term benefit, and it is not generally effective for the management of low back pain. However, due to its relative safety as compared to other medications, it is certainly worth a try. Chronic use can increase the likelihood of transaminase elevations 4-fold, so this is a consideration when patients are using other potentially hepatotoxic medications. There is an IV preparation available (Ofirmev), but the only benefit of the IV over the oral preparations is shorter onset of action. Both the absorption and the action of acetaminophen are augmented by caffeine, so caffeine is utilized in multiple over the counter (OTC) and prescription medications (e.g., Excedrin or Fioricet).

Numerous NSAIDs are available, but none has been shown to be superior to another except for the convenience of dosing daily versus every 6 hours. All are generally safe in the acute setting but should be used with caution if needed long term, and they should be avoided altogether for long-term use in the elderly or patients with cardiovascular, renal, or peptic ulcer disease. This caution includes the cyclooxygenase (COX)-2-specific drugs. Naproxen seems to have the best cardiac profile while the COX-2 drugs tend to have the best GI profile. Misoprostol (Cytotec) or proton pump inhibitors can be used for GI prophylaxis.

Topical agents such as diclofenac (Flector 1.3% Patch, Voltaren 1% Gel), menthol, camphor, lidocaine, and capsaicin (Zostrix Cream, Qutenza 8% Patch) are effective in some patients.

Opioids (Table.1)

For patients with inadequate response to the nonopioid analgesics, opioids are an option (see Table 1). However, the proven efficacy for cancer pain and palliative care as well as some acute pain conditions cannot be extrapolated to chronic pain syndromes. The benefits of opioids in some conditions (e.g., chronic low back pain), and the overall safety of opioids have been called into question due to the dramatic increase in opioid abuse and opioid overdose deaths. Recent research has demonstrated a 2- to 3-fold increase in all-cause mortality with chronic opioid use and up to 11-fold increase if using more than 200 mg/day morphine equivalent dose (MED) and/or sustained-release or long-acting (methadone) preparations. Additionally, risk of overdose death is increased to 3.7- to 4.6-fold at doses of 50 to 100 mg/day MED and as high as 9-fold increased risk for MED >100 mg/day as compared to MED of less than 20 mg/day. After exceeding 200 mg/day MED, 1 in 32 dies. These risks are further escalated by co-administration of benzodiazepines or gabapentinoids. A prescription for naltrexone should be considered if the patient is using >50 mg MED per day, and it is highly recommended if using >100 mg MED per day. A useful calculator to calculate MED can be found at http://www.agencymeddirectors.wa.gov/calculator/dosecalculator.htm

According to the CDC, opioids were implicated in 71% of the pharmaceutical overdose deaths in 2013, and 60% were legally prescribed by a single provider. Opioids might be a safer option in the elderly as compared to NSAIDs, but they can increase fall risk. They should be avoided in patients with untreated sleep apnea because of increased risk for complications, especially in combination with benzodiazepines. This risk increases with age with as much as an eightfold increase for those older than 80 years of age. The risk of postoperative respiratory depression also increases with age. The risks of using chronic opioids likely outweigh the benefits in the management of headache, fibromyalgia, and chronic low back pain, according to a 2014 position paper from the American Academy of Neurology.

The risks and the adverse outcomes (abuse, addiction, overdose, and death) related to this class of medications culminated in the release of guidelines with twelve recommendations from the CDC in March 2016 for the prescribing of opioids for chronic pain. A brief summary of the author's recommendations: (1) Nonpharmacologic therapy and nonopioids are preferred for chronic pain. (2) Benefits of opioids on pain and function need to outweigh the risks. Screen for risk of dependence. (3) Establish treatment goals with the patient and discuss plan to discontinue opioids if treatment fails. (4) On initiation, use immediate release rather than ER/LA (extended release, long-acting) preparations. (5) Use the lowest effective dose, and reassess risks if dose is increased, especially if greater than 50 mg MED per day. (See Table 1 for equivalent doses.) (6) Acute pain should be treated acutely; less than 3 days usually but no more than 7 days. (7) Reassess within 1 to 4 weeks of initiation of treatment or dose escalation and at least every 3 months thereafter. Discontinue if benefits do not justify risk. (8) Consider prescribing naloxone if there is concurrent benzodiazepine use, a history of overdose, or MED >50 mg/day. (9) Use state drug monitoring programs at initiation and at least every 3 months. (10) Obtain a urine drug screen at initiation and at least annually. Nothing but the prescribed medications should be present. (Additionally, consider testing periodically for the presence of prescribed NSAIDs and adjuvant medications to assess compliance with the whole treatment plan rather than just the opioid.) (11) Avoid concurrent with benzodiazepines. (12) Offer or arrange evidence-based treatment for patients with opioid use disorder.

In addition to these steps, multiple drugs have been formulated with "abuse-deterrent" properties. Preparations that meet the FDA's Guidance for Industry regarding abuse-deterrent opioids include: OxyContin (oxycodone), Targiniq ER (oxycodone/naloxone), Embeda (morphine/naltrexone), Hysingla ER (hydrocodone), MorphaBond ER (morphine), Xtampza ER (oxycodone), Troxyca ER (oxycodone/naltrexone), Arymo ER (morphine), Vantrela ER (hydrocodone), and RoxyBond (oxycodone). Unfortunately, there are no generic opioids with FDA-approved abuse-deterrent labeling.

Tramadol (Ultram, ConZip) is a weak mu-agonist and an inhibitor of norepinephrine and serotonin uptake, a quality that

TABLE 1	Opioid Analgesics, Equianalgesic Table			
		ADMINISTRATION		
OPIOID		**PARENTERAL**	**ORAL**	**PROPERTIES**
Buprenorphine				
Butrans transdermal patch: 5, 7.5, 10, 15, 20 μg/h weekly patches Subutex* SL tab and film: 2, 8 mg Buprenex injection: 0.3 mg/mL		0.3 mg (IV) Patch: MED <30 mg/day= 5 μg/h patch 30–80 mg/day = 10 μg/h patch; >80 mg/day: do not use	Oral buprenorphine, with or without naloxone (Suboxone, Subutex) is limited to treatment of opiate addiction Requires training, approval, and new DEA number	Partial agonist Can cause QT prolongation C-III
Codeine				
Tablet: 15, 30, 60 mg Oral solution: 15 mg/5 mL		130 mg	180 mg	Prodrug converted by liver to morphine About 10% of population cannot convert, and some are rapid metabolizers, resulting in increased levels of morphine Ceiling dose is 60 mg/dose
Fentanyl				
Duragesic 72 h patch: 12, 25, 37.5, 50, 62.5, 75, 87.5, 100 μg/h		~100 μg/h	—	Patch for those who cannot swallow Patient *must* have subcutaneous fat, because drug is lipophilic
Actiq or Oralet lozenge: 200, 400, 600, 800, 1200, 1600 μg Fentora buccal tab or Abstral SL tab: 100, 200, 300, 400, 600, 800 μg Subsys sublingual spray: 100, 200, 400, 600, 800 μg/spray. Lazanda nasal: 100, 300, 400 mcg/spray. Fentanyl injection: 50 mcg/mL.		No conversion for lozenges or buccal tabs; various formulations are not bioequivalent, so use caution when switching from one formulation to another; *must* start at lowest dose and titrate	~½ × daily morphine dose, disregarding units, e.g., 200 mg morphine PO/day = 100 μg/h patch	Lozenge or buccal tab for transmucosal use No cheap forms available Buccal formulations *only* indicated for breakthrough cancer pain in the opioid tolerant; can be rapidly fatal in opioid naïve patients.
Hydrocodone				
Tab: 2.5, 5, 7.5, 10 mg with a max of 325 mg APAP per tablet (Norco, Lortab) as of 2014. (Lorcet no longer available) or with 200 mg ibuprofen (Vicoprofen 7.5/200; Ibudone 5/200, 10/200; Reprexain 2.5/200, 5/200, 10/200); Zohydro ER: 10, 15, 20, 30, 40, 50 mg/cap q 12 h; Vantrela ER: 15, 30, 45, 60, 90 mg tab q 12 h; Hysingla ER: 20, 30, 40, 60, 80, 100, 120 mg tabs q 24 h; Solution: with APAP 7.5/325, 10/325 per 15 mL.		N/A	20 mg	C-II as of 2014, so refills and phone orders are no longer allowed. Metabolized to hydromorphone and others
Hydromorphone (Dilaudid)				
Tab: 2, 4, 8 mg Liquid: 1 mg/mL Suppository: 3 mg SR† 24-h tab (Exalgo): 8, 12, 16, 32 mg Injection: 1, 2, 4, 10 mg/mL pre-filled syringes and 1, 2, 4 mg/mL vials.		1.5 mg	7.5 mg	Good alternative to morphine, especially if using SC by continuous infusion (>20 mg/h) Active glucuronide metabolites
Meperidine (Demerol)				
Tab: 50, 100 mg Syrup: 50 mg/5 mL		100 mg	300 mg	Indicated for *acute use only* (i.e., <48 h) Contraindicated with MAOI and/or renal disease: neurotoxic metabolite normeperidine can cause seizures and death
Methadone (Dolophine)				

Continued

TABLE 1 Opioid Analgesics, Equianalgesic Table—cont'd

OPIOID	ADMINISTRATION		PROPERTIES
	PARENTERAL	ORAL	
Tab: 5, 10, 40 mg Oral liquid: 1, 2, 10 mg/mL* 40 mg dispersible tab (Methadose)—restricted use in United States, mostly for detox or addiction maintenance dosing		Variable conversion ratios (see Table 2): converted by oral morphine equivalent dose	At least 3 mechanisms: mu agonist, NMDA receptor antagonist, norepinephrine–serotonin reuptake inhibition The longest-acting opioid Cheap: ~ 1¢ /mg Can cause QT prolongation Torsades de pointes is more likely with IV dosing STRONGLY consider risks before prescribing. Safety guidelines available from the American Pain Society.
Morphine			
Tab: 15, 30 mg Liquid: 10, 20, or 100 mg/5 mL (Roxanol) SR† 12-h tab (MS Contin): 15, 30, 60, 100, 200 mg SR† 12-h tab (Oramorph SR): 15, 30, 60, 100 mg SR† 24-h cap (Kadian): 10, 20, 30, 50, 60, 80, 100, 200 mg SR† 24-h cap (Avinza): 30, 45, 60, 75, 90, 120 mg SR† cap with naltrexone (Embeda): 20/0.8, 30/1.2, 50/2, 60/2.4, 80/3.2, 100/4 mg Suppository: 5, 10, 20, 30 mg	10 mg	30 mg	Numerous routes; very cheap, readily available; active metabolites, morphine-6-glucuronide 10 × more potent than morphine Avinza and Kadian capsules may be opened and beads sprinkled in applesauce, but the beads should not be crushed Avinza may be opened into apple juice and injected via gastric tube Kadian may be opened into water and given by gastric tube
Oxycodone			
Tab: 5, 10, 15, 20, 30 mg Liquid: 5 mg/5 mL or 20 mg/mL (OxyFast) SR† 12-h tab (generic, OxyContin): 10, 15, 20, 30, 40, 60, 80 mg SR† 12-h w/naltrexone (Troxyca ER caps): 10/1.2, 20/2.4, 30/3.6, 40/4.8, 60/7.2, 80/9.6 mg oxycodone/naltrexone Multiple combinations w/APAP (Percocet, Endocet, Tylox) SR† 12-h w/APAP 7.5/325 (Xartemis XR)	N/A	20 mg	Equal potency but a little more bioavailable than morphine Caution in liver disease: T½ extends up to 4 × normal. Metabolized to oxymorphone: 40 × more potent than oxycodone ER/LA. Opioids require REMS.
Oxymorphone			
Tab: 5, 10 mg (Opana); in opioid-naïve patients, starting dose > 20 mg/day is not recommended	1 mg	10 mg	Potentiated by cimetidine (Tagamet), MAOIs, and other CNS depressants 10% bioavailability Caution with CrCl < 50 or with liver impairment Take 1 h before or 2 h after food (food increases absorption)

*Only approved in the United States for the treatment of opioid dependence.
†Sustained-release formulations should never be crushed.

APAP, Acetaminophen (N-acetyl-*p*-aminophenol); *bid*, two times per day; *CNS*, central nervous system; *CrCl*, creatinine clearance; *IM*, intramuscular; *IV*, intravenous-*MAOI*, monoamine oxidase inhibitor; *MED*, morphine equivalent dose; *NMDA*, N-methyl-D-aspartate; *po*, by mouth; *pr*, per rectum; *prn*, as needed; *qw4h*, every four hours; *q6h*, every 6 hours; *q8h*, every 8 hours; *qAC*, before meals; *qd*, daily; *qHS*, at bedtime; *SC*, subcutaneous; *tid*, three times per day.

gives it a niche in the treatment of neuropathic and radicular pain.[1] It is the only opioid studied for fibromyalgia in a randomized trial. While it was found to be beneficial, this is likely due to its inhibition of serotonin and norepinephrine uptake rather than its weak mu-agonism. A study has demonstrated an increased risk for hypoglycemia, notably in the first 30 days of treatment with tramadol.

Codeine is a prodrug that must be converted to morphine to be effective, and about 10% of the population lacks the cytochrome P450 2D6 enzyme that makes the conversion, resulting in poor analgesic response. Owing to the need for conversion, doses exceeding 60 mg do not increase benefit because the enzyme system is saturated. Avoid prescribing codeine to children, as deaths have been reported, even with the use of age- and weight-appropriate dosages, as a result of the hypermetabolism of codeine to morphine.

Morphine is the prototype for the opioids. It is extremely versatile, it can be given via almost any route, and it is available in multiple dosages and preparations ranging from liquid to daily sustained release. Hydromorphone (Dilaudid, Exalgo) shares similar qualities but is more potent. Hydrocodone is only available in a sustained-release oral form (Zohydro ER,

[1]Not FDA approved for this indication.

TABLE 2	Morphine and Methadone Equivalents
MORPHINE (DAILY REQUIREMENT)	**METHADONE EQUIVALENT**
<500 mg	5:1
500–1000 mg	10:1
>1000 mg	20:1

Acute pain: methadone = morphine (1:1). Chronic pain: The above conversion is for illustration of the complexity of methadone use. A more detailed table should be referenced before prescribing, and methadone should be used with extreme caution because of the risk for cardiac complications and respiratory depression. Many sources recommend starting at 10% of the calculated equianalgesic dose of methadone.

Hysingla ER), and in combination with acetaminophen (Lortab, Norco, Vicodin). It was rescheduled by the DEA to schedule II in 2014. It had been the number-one prescribed medication in the United States for several years until the rescheduling, which led to >20% reduction in prescriptions and >16% reduction in tablets dispensed.

Methadone (Dolophine) is the longest acting of the opioids at a half-life of 23 hours, although the duration of action can be variable. It is active as an NMDA receptor antagonist, inhibits norepinephrine and serotonin uptake, and is an agonist at the mu receptor. Therefore, methadone can be effective when other opioids fail, especially in the case of chronic or neuropathic pain, where the NMDA receptor is more of a factor in pain control. It must be used with caution (Table 2) because it can prolong the QT interval and has an increased dose-dependent risk of respiratory depression as compared to other opioids.

Meperidine (Demerol) is relatively weak compared to morphine and others, and it is limited by poor oral bioavailability, a 48-hour acute pain indication, and the neurotoxicity of one of its metabolites, normeperidine (renally cleared, so it is contraindicated in renal patients). Other opioids are safer and more effective, so its use should be limited.

The mu agonists, other than codeine, meperidine, and tramadol, do not technically have a ceiling dose; however, the dose should be limited to the lowest effective dose (ideally <50 mg morphine equivalents per day), keeping in mind the possible adverse effects and increased risk of death with higher doses. In a 2020 study in the journal *Pain*, opioid dose escalation was not associated with improvements in chronic musculoskeletal pain. In the purely palliative or hospice patient, the dosage may be titrated to effect until the pain is relieved or side effects limit the dosage.

The mixed agonist-antagonists such as nalbuphine (Nubain), pentazocine (Talwin), and butorphanol (Stadol) tend to have a higher incidence of hallucination and confusion, and because they are agonists at kappa and delta receptors and antagonists at the mu receptor, they can produce withdrawal symptoms in patients who are routinely taking mu agonists. The partial agonist buprenorphine (Butrans patch, Subutex, Buprenex) is dose limited because it has a maximal effective dose as well as a potential to cause QT prolongation.

Patients who are taking opioids on a chronic basis should use a stimulant laxative such as senna with or without docusate, because fiber and dietary modification are usually inadequate for opioid-induced constipation, and fiber can aggravate the problem. Lubiprostone (Amitiza) can be used for opioid-induced constipation at the 24 mcg twice-daily dose. Naloxegol (Movantik), naldemedine (Symproic), and methylnaltrexone (Relistor) are peripheral rather than central mu antagonists, so they are indicated for managing opioid-induced constipation without negatively impacting pain control. Bisacodyl should not be used chronically due to its potential to damage the myenteric

plexus of the gut and cause severe and permanent impairment of colonic motility; however, for PRN use, it can be quite effective with the suppository having quicker onset of action than the tablet.

Adjuvant Drugs

Adjuvant medications are drugs that are useful in the management of pain but do not have pain treatment as an indication. Some adjuvant medications such as duloxetine (Cymbalta) and pregabalin (Lyrica) have received an FDA indication for diabetic peripheral neuropathic pain. Tricyclic antidepressants are useful for chronic pain and they have the benefit, unlike duloxetine, of working at the lowest doses rather than having to titrate to the maximum dose to gain benefit.

Several anticonvulsants have demonstrated efficacy in the management of pain, most notably gabapentin (Neurontin)[1], pregabalin (Lyrica), and carbamazepine (Tegretol)[1]. Others have been tested in trials, but these three have the most evidence to support their use. Gabapentin and pregabalin have the benefit of not requiring monitoring of blood levels or for marrow, liver, or renal toxicities. Gabapentin (Neurontin)[1] has been beneficial using a single dose of 1200 mg preoperatively, notably in combination with celecoxib (Celebrex)[1], in reducing postoperative opioid requirements in mastectomy, laminectomy, and thoracotomy patients. The benefits of the gabapentinoids, a.k.a. α-2-δ-ligand calcium channel blockers, in peripheral neuropathies have been inappropriately extrapolated to pain related to radiculopathy. Significant benefits in lumbar and cervical radiculopathy have not been demonstrated in randomized trials.

Corticosteroids can be beneficial in inflammatory conditions, nerve or spinal cord compression, or increased intracranial pressure due to neoplasms. Any can help, but blood pressure elevations and fluid retention can be problematic in all but dexamethasone (Decadron)[1], which lacks mineralocorticoid activity. Steroids also have the downside of elevating blood glucose and, in long-term use, causing osteoporosis and a host of other problems, including Cushing syndrome.

Muscle relaxants may be beneficial if muscle spasm is a source of pain, but there is insufficient evidence to determine relative efficacy or safety. Of these, two stand out: metaxalone (Skelaxin), which lacks the black-box warning for the operation of heavy equipment, and tizanidine (Zanaflex), which can antagonize α₁ receptors in the spinal cord to provide additional pain relief. In chronic use, the patient will need to be monitored for anemia and leukopenia with metaxalone and for liver abnormalities with tizanidine. Cyclobenzaprine (Flexeril) plus naproxen was not superior to naproxen alone for low back pain.

Calcitonin (Miacalcin)[1] has shown very modest benefit for pain due to osteoporotic vertebral compression fractures, but it shows no benefit for compression fractures due to bone metastasis.

Ziconotide (Prialt) has demonstrated benefit as well as safety for long-term pain management, but it is limited to only intrathecal use owing to gastrointestinal side effects.

Caffeine can modulate pain via action upon adenosine receptors that are involved in nociception. It is found in several over-the-counter analgesics, notably for migraine treatment. Regarding alternative medications, riboflavin,[7] butterbur,[7] and coenzyme Q10 (CoQ10)[7] are effective for migraine prophylaxis. Glucosamine,[7] S-adenosylmethionine (SAM-e),[7] methylsulfonylmethane (MSM),[7] and willow bark[7] are likely effective for arthritic and low-back pain.

Acetyl-L-carnitine (ALC)[7] had demonstrated efficacy in diabetic neuropathy at 2 to 3 g/day. Capsaicin 0.075% cream (Zostrix) and 8% patch (Qutenza) have demonstrated benefit

[1]Not FDA approved for this indication.
[7]Available as a dietary supplement

Controlled Substances Agreement Template

1. This agreement is provided to prevent misunderstandings about policies regarding medications designated by the DEA as "controlled substances" that you will be taking for pain management or other medical conditions.

2. I understand that my provider is consenting to treat me based on this Agreement.

3. I understand that if I break this Agreement, my provider might stop prescribing these medications, whether by tapering my medication, discontinuing the medication and prescribing another medication to treat the withdrawal symptoms, or discontinuing the medication and referring me to a detoxification program.

4. I will communicate fully and honestly with my provider about the character and intensity of my pain, the effect that my pain has on my daily life and how well the medication is helping to relieve my pain. I will take the medication ONLY as prescribed and for the treatment of my physical pain as opposed to emotional or psychological distress (i.e., to get high).

5. My physician may prescribe other medications (adjuvant medications) or non-pharmacological therapies (physical therapy, TENS unit, etc.) to help with certain aspects of pain such as muscle spasm, burning, tingling or radiating pain. I will comply with this treatment with the same diligence as is expected for my controlled medication.

6. I will not use ANY illegal substances or any legal medication not prescribed to me. Additionally, I understand that alcohol, although legal, should not be used in conjunction with my medication as the combination could be fatal.

7. I will not share, sell or trade my medications with anyone.

8. I will use only one provider and one pharmacy for my medications unless otherwise agreed upon with my provider.

9. I am responsible for my own prescriptions and medications. I will safeguard my written prescription and medications from loss or theft, understanding they will not be replaced. I will secure my medication in a lock box or safe out of the reach of children at all times.

10. I understand that refills of my prescriptions will be made at the time of an office visit or during regular office hours and never during evenings or weekends when the office is closed.

11. I authorize my provider and my pharmacy to cooperate fully with any city, state and/or federal law enforcement agency in the investigation of any possible misuse, sale or other diversion of my medications.

12. I agree to submit to a blood or urine test, if requested by my provider, in order to determine my compliance with my medication program.

13. I understand that the use of these medications may adversely affect my ability to drive, operate machinery or perform certain tasks, and I agree not to attempt these tasks under the influence of medication. Additional risks include low testosterone, depression, sleep disturbances, constipation, respiratory depression, and death.

14. I understand that smoking cessation and a healthy lifestyle can be helpful in achieving control of pain. I will strive toward smoking cessation, a healthy diet, and exercise as my condition allows.

15. I agree to these guidelines, and they have been fully explained to me. All of my questions and concerns regarding treatment have been adequately answered.

I agree to use _____ pharmacy, *and only this pharmacy*, for my prescriptions for controlled substances.

This Agreement entered on this date: _____

Patient / Parent / Guardian signature:_____

Provider signature:_____

Figure 1 Controlled substances agreement.

for peripheral neuropathy,[1] post-herpetic neuralgia, and HIV-associated neuropathy.[1]

Numerous medications in multiple drug classes have been studied for fibromyalgia, but many of the trials are small and/or of poor quality. Of these drugs, duloxetine (Cymbalta), pregabalin (Lyrica), and milnacipran (Savella) have received an FDA indication for fibromyalgia; gabapentin (Neurontin)[1], ondansetron (Zofran)[1], and naltrexone (Depade, Revia)[1] demonstrated modest benefit. The greatest benefit seems to be achieved by duloxetine and tricyclic antidepressants.

The use of cannabinoids has become legal in some states; however, their use for the management of pain is somewhat controversial, as the studies evaluating these drugs are often of low to modest quality. A 2015 systematic review and meta-analysis showed mild reductions in pain, but the comparison groups were placebo rather than standard care. Additionally, cannabinoids are not without adverse effects, including impacts on cognition, motivation, reaction time, and psychosis in a 2016 review. Negative impacts could be even greater as unintended consequences of medical and/or recreational use come to light. Isolation of the various compounds such as cannabidiol and β-caryophyllene from others like Δ9-tetrahydrocannabinol (THC) could improve benefit, including oral administration, while limiting adverse physical and psychological effects. The cannabinoids do show some promise, but they need to be studied further and subjected to the same scientific rigor as any other medication in the FDA approval process. A 2020 systematic review and meta-analysis did not demonstrate a benefit of adding cannabinoids to opioids for the management of pain related to advanced cancer.

Monitoring

Controlled-substance agreements are beneficial in setting the boundaries for the use of opioid pain relievers (Figure 1). Routine visits are necessary to document ongoing need for and adequate response to the prescribed regimen. Routine drug screening is beneficial for monitoring compliance with the opioid as well as nonopioid medications. However, the provider needs to be aware of the metabolites of the different drugs. Hydromorphone (Dilaudid) and oxymorphone (Opana) are metabolites of hydrocodone (Lortab, Norco) and oxycodone (Percocet, Endocet, OxyContin), respectively. All states except Missouri have prescription-monitoring programs that allow providers to monitor for the use of multiple providers and pharmacies to obtain controlled medications. Rules governing the prescribing and use of controlled substances vary among states, so the provider should be knowledgeable of local regulations as well as federal DEA requirements.

Complications

The Centers for Disease Control and Prevention (CDC) reported in 2011 that opioid pain relievers were involved in 73.8% of the 20,044 prescription drug overdose deaths. By 2017, overdose deaths increased to 70,237 with 47,600 (67.8%) involving opioids. Of the 47,600 overdoses, deaths were mostly driven by synthetic opioids other than methadone (i.e., fentanyl, fentanyl analogs, and tramadol [60%], followed by heroin [32.5%], natural and semi-synthetic, for example, hydrocodone and oxycodone [30.5%], and methadone [6.7%]. (Percentages do not equal 100% due to some deaths involving more than one drug.) There are over 130 opioid overdose deaths per day in the United States. From 1999 to 2017, overdose death rates have increased from 8.2 to 29.1/100,000 in males and from 3.9 to 14.4 in females, and the rates were highest in the 25- to 54-year-old age range. Medicaid populations are at greater risk of opioid overdose than non-Medicaid populations, and prescription drug overdose death rates are higher in the more rural and impoverished counties. A 2020 study demonstrated that more than 25%

of opioid overdoses in the United States involve children and adolescents.

In addition to the deaths, there is a significant cost burden of substance abuse treatment admissions, with the 2008 rates being six times the 1999 rate. Nonmedical use of opioids represents up to $78.5 billion in healthcare costs, lost productivity, addiction management, and legal and law enforcement involvement. Drug addiction is very real, and about 15% of patients may be genetically predisposed to addiction; therefore, clinicians should strongly consider this in their risk/benefit analysis before exposing a patient to these powerful medications. About 25% of opioid-managed chronic pain patients misuse the medications, and about 10% develop opioid use disorders. Using a tool such as the Opioid Risk Tool may be helpful in determining the risk of addiction in a particular individual.

Long-term safety of opioids has not been demonstrated, and chronic use has been associated with sleep disorders, adrenal suppression, and hypogonadism (and secondary erectile dysfunction and depression) among other problems.

References

Baratloo A, Rouhipour A, Forouzanfar MM, et al: The role of caffeine in pain management: a brief literature review, *Anesth Pain Med* 6(3):e33193, 2016, Published online March 26, 2016.

Boland EG, Bennett MI, Allgar V, Boland JW: Cannabinoids for adult cancer-related pain: systematic review and meta-analysis, *BMJ Support Palliat Care* 10:14–24, 2020.

Center for Behavioral Health Statistics and Quality (CBHSQ): *2017 National Survey on Drug Use and Health: Detailed Tables*, Rockville, MD, 2018, Substance Abuse and Mental Health Services Administration. 05.24.2019 https://www.samhsa.gov/data/nsduh/reports-detailed-tables-2017-NSDUH. Accessed 24 May 2019.

Chou R, Peterson K, Helfand M: Comparative efficacy and safety of skeletal muscle relaxants for spasticity and musculoskeletal conditions, *J Pain Sympt Manage* 28:140–175, 2004.

Dowell D, Haegerich TM, Chou R: CDC guideline for prescribing opioids for chronic pain—United States, *JAMA*, March 15, March 15.

Franklin GM: Opioids for chronic noncancer pain: a position paper of the American Academy of Neurology, *Neurology* 83:1277–1284, 2014.

Fritz JM, Magel JS, McFadden M, et al: Early physical therapy vs usual care in patients with recent- onset low back pain: a randomized clinical trial, *JAMA* 314(14):1459–1467, 2015.

Gomes T, Mandani MM, Dhalla IA, Paterson JM, Juurlink DN: Opioid dose and drug-related mortality in patients with nonmalignant pain, *Arch Intern Med* 171(6):686–691, 2011.

Hedegaard H, Minino A, Warner M: *Drug Overdose Deaths in the United States, 1999-2017. NCHS Data Brief, No. 329*, November 2018, 05.24.2019 https://www.cdc.gov/nchs/data/databriefs/db329-h.pdf.

Jellin JM, Gregory PJ, et al: *Pharmacist's Letter/Prescriber's Letter Natural Medicines Comprehensive Database*, ed 12, Stockton, CA, 2009, Therapeutic Research Faculty.

Jones CM, Lurie PG, Throckmorton DC: Effect of US Drug Enforcement Administration's rescheduling of hydrocodone combination analgesic products on opioid analgesic prescribing, *JAMA Intern Med* 176(3):399–402, 2016, https://doi.org/10.1001/jamainternmed.2015.7799.

Machado GC, Maher CG, Ferreira PH, et al: Efficacy and safety of paracetamol for spinal pain and osteoarthritis: systematic review and meta-analysis of randomised placebo controlled trials, *BMJ* 350:h1225, 2014. Accessed 20 April 2019.

Morasco BJ, Smith N, Dobscha SK, et al: Outcomes of prescription opioid dose escalation for chronic pain: results from a prospective cohort study, *Pain* 161:1332–1340, 2020.

Okifuji A, Hare BD: The association between chronic pain and obesity, *Journal of Pain Research* 8:399–408, 2015. https://doi.org/10.2147/JPR.S55598.

Onysko M, Legerski P, Potthoff J, Erlandson E: Targeting neuropathic pain: consider these alternatives, *J Fam Pract* 64(8):470–475, 2015.

Scholl L, Seth P, Kariisa M, Wilson N, Baldwin G. Drug and opioid-involved overdose deaths – United States, 2013-2017. *Morb Mortal Wkly Rep.* ePub: 21 December 2018.

Seth P, Scholl L, Rudd RA, Bacon S: Increases and geographic variations in overdose deaths involving opioids, cocaine, and psychostimulants with abuse potential—United States, 2015-2016, *MMWR Morb Mortal Wkly Rep.* ePub: March 29, ePub: March 29.

Volkow ND, Swanson JM, Evins AE, et al: Effects of cannabis use on human behavior, including cognition, motivation, and psychosis: a review, *JAMA Psychiatry* 73(3):292–297, 2016.

Vowles KE, McEntee ML, Julnes PS, Frohe T, Ney JP, van der Goes DN: Rates of opioid misuse, abuse, and addiction in chronic pain: a systematic review and data synthesis, *Pain* 156(4):569–576, 2015, https://doi.org/10.1097/01.j.pain.0000460357.01998.f1.

Whiting PF, Wolff RF, Deshpande S, et al: Cannabinoids for medical use: a systematic review and meta-analysis, *JAMA* 313(24):2456–2473, 2015.

PALLIATIVE AND END-OF-LIFE CARE

Method of
Steven A. House, MD

CURRENT DIAGNOSIS

- Any symptom can be in the realm of palliative care. Rapid identification and aggressive management of symptoms are important in maintaining the patient's quality of life.
- Palliative care is treatment that is focused on pain and symptom management, as well as quality of life for patients and their families. It can be rendered at any point in the course or treatment of illness, whether that illness is life limiting/threatening or not.
- Hospice is a philosophy and method of care that is completely focused on symptom management, quality of life for patients and families, and the transition at the end of life.

CURRENT THERAPY

- Recommend that all adult patients, regardless of current health status, execute advance directives (living will, power of attorney for healthcare, healthcare surrogate, etc.) to help ensure that their treatment wishes and end-of-life care goals are met.
- For patients with life-threatening (e.g., progressing cancer) or life-limiting (e.g., patients with severe chronic obstructive pulmonary disease [COPD] or heart failure, requiring dialysis, or residing in a nursing home) illness, consider a Physician Order for Life-Sustaining Treatment (POLST) or Medical Order for Scope of Treatment (MOST) form (the name varies by state). These forms are used to convert the salient points of advance directives into medical orders so that they are immediately actionable by nurses or emergency medical services if the situation arises.
- Advance care planning discussions are billable under Medicare: 99497 for the first 30 minutes and 99498 for each additional 30 minutes.
- The best palliative care involves an interdisciplinary approach by physicians, nurses, counselors, chaplains, and others for the optimal management of symptoms (whether the suffering is physical, emotional, spiritual, existential, or practical) and family support.
- Early addition of palliative care to the overall treatment plan can improve survival and quality of life.
- Cancer pain is an indication for opioid therapy because opioids have proven efficacy in this scenario. For detailed information on opioids, see Table 1 in chapter titled "Pain". Multiple modalities may be required for optimal pain control.
- For patients using opioids chronically, initiate a stimulant laxative such as sennosides (Senokot, Ex-Lax) or lubiprostone (Amitiza) as the opioid's companion. Peripheral mu antagonists such as methylnaltrexone (Relistor), naldemedine (Symproic), or naloxegol (Movantik) are indicated for refractory opioid-induced constipation.
- Control nausea because it can contribute to anorexia, weight loss, and functional decline. The antiserotonergic drugs (e.g., ondansetron [Zofran], granisetron [Kytril], palonosetron [Aloxi], dolasetron [Anzemet]) or the combination netupitant/palonosetron (Akynzeo) are superior to the other classes of antiemetics in the settings of chemotherapy administration and postanesthesia. For uncomplicated nausea, prochlorperazine (Compazine) was found to be superior to promethazine (Phenergan).

- Dyspnea can be improved by providing a fan, a cooler room, and a view to the outside and avoiding confined spaces. Opioids, benzodiazepines, and/or other agents, depending on the situation, might be required. Thoracentesis can be palliative when an effusion is the source of dyspnea.
- Delirium must be evaluated for potential causes. Delirium with or without agitation can occur in up to 80% of patients, depending on the underlying condition. Medications are common causes, but pain and multiple other conditions can cause it as well. Medications such as haloperidol (Haldol)[1], chlorpromazine (Thorazine, brand discontinued),[1] or olanzapine (Zyprexa, Zyprexa Zydis)[1] can be helpful in many patients, but haloperidol is by far the cheapest alternative and a good place to start.
- Chlorpromazine is the only medication with the US Food and Drug Administration (FDA) indication for hiccups.
- Feeding tubes do not improve outcomes in late-stage dementia and can contribute to suffering.

[1]Not FDA approved for this indication

Epidemiology

There Table 1 are more than 2.5 million deaths in the United States annually. The most recent year for which mortality data are available is 2017, and cardiovascular disease is the top cause of death, followed by all cancers combined, unintentional injuries, chronic obstructive pulmonary disease (COPD), congestive heart failure, cerebrovascular disease, chronic kidney disease, and chronic liver disease, among others. The ranking was unchanged from 2016. Any of these disease processes can have a significant symptom burden that worsens with disease progression.

Life has 100% mortality, so individuals should take the time to plan for it. The consequences of failing to plan for the transition to end-of-life care include increased psychological distress, medical treatments that are inconsistent with individual preferences, increased utilization of healthcare resources that have little therapeutic benefit while being very costly in dollars, as well as quality of life, and a more difficult bereavement for survivors.

Cardiopulmonary resuscitation has poor outcomes under the best of circumstances (~15%), but it is even worse in patients with late-stage cancer, with only approximately 2% surviving to hospital discharge. Outcomes are also poor for the other noncardiac diseases listed previously and decline further with age and comorbidities.

Risk Factors

Factors associated with worse pain or less symptom control are being female, elderly, or a child and race other than white. Historically, these groups have received less pain medication than white males for very similar diagnoses. These trends should be reversing. Lacking advance directives and failing to have such discussions with family members are related to receiving excessive and/or unbeneficial interventions/treatments.

Pathophysiology

A patient's symptoms can be caused by the underlying disease itself, mechanical encroachment on other organs and structures (e.g., bowel obstruction, neuropathic pain from nerve destruction, bone metastasis), becoming more sedentary or bedbound, medications, and/or tumor necrosis factor, neurokinin-1, and other inflammatory cytokines. Therefore symptoms may have different etiologies and pathophysiology depending on the underlying disease state. Such a review would be far too extensive for this section.

Prevention

Encourage all adult patients, regardless of current health status, to execute advance directives (living will, power of attorney for healthcare, healthcare surrogate, etc.) to help ensure that their treatment wishes and end-of-life care goals are met. These

TABLE 1	Coanalgesic and Adjuvant Treatments for Pain: Adult Dosages

Nonsteroidal Antiinflammatory Drugs

Celecoxib (Celebrex) 200 mg PO daily or 100–200 mg PO bid; maximum: 400 mg/d
Diclofenac sodium (Voltaren, Voltaren XR) 50–75 mg PO bid; injection (Dyloject) 37.5 mg IV q6h prn; maximum: 150 mg/d; Diclofenac
    epolamine topical (Flector patch 1.3%); apply 1 patch to most painful area bid
Ibuprofen (Motrin, Advil) 400–800 mg PO tid; maximum: 3200 mg/d
Ketorolac Nasal (Sprix) 15.75 mg/spray
<65 years old and <50 kg: 1 spray in one nostril q6h prn. Maximum: 4 sprays/d ×5 days
<65 years old and ≥50 kg: 1 spray in each nostril q6h prn. Maximum: 8 sprays/d ×5 days
Ketorolac Oral & Injection
10 mg PO q4h prn. Maximum: 40 mg/day ×5 days
Single dose: 30–60 mg IM or 15–30 mg IV
Multiple dose: if <65 years old and >50 kg, 30 mg IM/IV q6h prn. Maximum: 120 mg/d ×5 days
Or if >65 years old or <50 kg, 15 mg IM/IV q6h prn up to 60 mg/d ×5 days
Naproxen (Naprosyn, EC-Naprosyn) 250–500 mg PO bid prn; maximum: 1500 mg/d
Naproxen sodium (Aleve, Anaprox) 220–550 PO q12h prn: maximum: 1650 mg/d

Bisphosphonates—Usually Provide Analgesia Within a Week and Last Up to 3 Months

Pamidronate (Aredia)
    Malignant hypercalcemia: 60–90 mg (depending on the severity of hypercalcemia) IV ×1
    Osteolytic lesions (multiple myeloma) or bone metastases: 90 mg IV monthly
Zoledronic acid (Zometa)
    Malignant hypercalcemia: 4 mg IV ×1
    Osteolytic lesions (multiple myeloma) or bone metastases: 4 mg IV q3–4 weeks

Radiopharmaceuticals—usually provide analgesia within 1–2 weeks and lasting 1–6 months. Dosing determined by radiation oncologist.

Antidepressants

Tricyclics
Amitriptyline (Elavil)[1] 25–100 mg qhs. Can increase to 150 mg daily for pain.
Nortriptyline (Pamelor)[1] 25–100 mg qhs. Up to 150 mg/d.
    Start low and titrate as needed. Use with caution in the elderly.

Serotonin and Norepinephrine Reuptake Inhibitors

Duloxetine 60 mg/d; >60 mg rarely more effective for pain, but can titrate higher for comorbid anxiety and/or depression if needed
Venlafaxine (Effexor)[1] 37.5–225 mg daily. Start low and titrate.
    Selective norepinephrine reuptake inhibitors—can be used to improve coexisting anxiety and/or depression.

Antiepileptic Drugs

Gabapentin (Neurontin)[1] 300–1200 mg tid. Maximum: 3600 mg/d. Start 300 mg qhs ×2–3 days, then bid ×2–3 days, then tid. May start with
    100 mg qhs in the elderly.
Pregabalin (Lyrica) 50–300 mg bid. Maximum: 600 mg/d. Start low and titrate for effect, using the lowest effective dose.

General Anesthesia/Sedation

Ketamine (Ketalar)[1] 0.1–0.2 mg/min IV (no bolus). This dosage is an adjunct to opioid therapy for severe uncontrolled pain and NOT intended
    to achieve general anesthesia. However, the clinician should seek assistance from anesthesiology or palliative care specialists. Hospital policies
    may vary.

[1]Not US Food and Drug Administration approved for this indication.

bid, Two times per day; *IM*, intramuscular; *IV*, intravenous; *q4h*, every four hours; *q6h*, every 6 hours; *q8h*, every 8 hours; *qAC*, before meals; *qd*, daily; *qHS*, at bedtime;
    po, by mouth; *pr*, per rectum; *prn*, as needed; *SC*, subcutaneous; *tid*, three times per day.

discussions are billable under Medicare using CPT 99497 for the first 30 minutes face to face with patient, family members, and/or surrogate and 99498 for each additional 30 minutes. For patients with life-threatening (e.g., progressing cancer) or life-limiting (e.g., severe COPD or heart failure, dialysis-dependent, or nursing home residents) illness, consider a Physician Order for Life-Sustaining Treatment (POLST) or a Medical Order for Scope of Treatment (MOST) form (forms vary by state). They are used to convert the salient points of advance directives into medical orders so that they are immediately actionable by nurses, emergency medical services, and others if the situation arises.

Ascertain the patient's/family's goals of care, and assess whether those goals are realistic under the circumstances. Evaluate whether a particular intervention will help achieve that goal. For example, if a patient's goal is to take a child on a special vacation, this cannot be achieved if the patient remains in the hospital receiving chemotherapy that is not working. Another example is a nursing home resident with dementia whose family just wants them "to be kept comfortable" but is considering feeding tube placement. Placing a feeding tube in advanced dementia does not improve outcomes and might require physical restraints to keep the patient from removing the tube. Therefore feeding tube placement will negatively impact the goal of comfort.

When maintaining comfort and improving quality of life become the primary goals, assist patients and their families with the transition to hospice care. Hospice is grossly underused, with median and average lengths of service of only 24 days and 71 days, respectively. Referrals are too often made excessively late, with 28% of patients having 7 or fewer days of service; therefore all of the benefits of hospice cannot always be fully realized in such a short time.

Palliative and end-of-life care, like all medical care, needs to be influenced by all four major aspects of medical ethics: autonomy (patient/surrogate has the right to pursue aggressive treatment, as well as to refuse treatment, even if that treatment could be considered life sustaining), beneficence (do "good" for the patient), nonmaleficence ("do no harm"), and justice (appropriate distribution of finite resources to do the most good for the most people). These four ethics can come into conflict at times, especially with the emphasis on autonomy above the other three in the healthcare system in the United States. Hospitals and other medical facilities should have specific policies regarding medical futility, and ethics committees can be helpful in difficult or unusual cases.

Clinical Manifestations

Common symptoms in palliative care include pain, nausea with or without vomiting, dyspnea, delirium, constipation, dysphagia (cannot swallow food, fluids, or medications), and general functional decline (i.e., requiring more assistance with transfers, toileting, and self-care). Anorexia and lack of thirst are very common, notably in the last few hours to days of life, but anorexia can also be a side effect of medications. Intervening with intravenous (IV) fluids or nasogastric feeding can exacerbate symptoms (secretions, dyspnea, pain, nausea) and worsen outcomes. Weight loss is commonly observed. Medications for diabetes and other disorders can often be discontinued at this stage to help avoid side effects, drug interactions, and adverse reactions (e.g., hypoglycemia).

As patients enter the last hours of life, they might experience decreased level of consciousness, agitated delirium, mottling of the extremities beginning distally and moving proximally, changes in breathing (Cheyne-Stokes, rapid and shallow, Kussmaul, or agonal), decreased or absent oral intake, and/or skin cool to touch.

Diagnosis

Diagnosis and prognosis will vary widely depending on the underlying disease processes, but in palliative care, much of the diagnosis (symptom identification) is based on history. Any patient with symptom burden is a candidate for palliative care, whether the symptoms are physical, psychological, spiritual, or existential. The Edmonton Symptom Assessment Scale (https://www.centralhealthline.ca/healthlibrary_docs/ESASrevised.pdf) rates each of 11 different symptoms on a scale of 0 to 3, for a total score of 0 to 33. This scale gives an idea of overall symptom burden. The Karnovsky and Palliative Performance Scales (http://www.nprc.org/files/news/karnofsky_performance_scale.pdf) range from 0% (deceased) to 100% (fully functional) rated on ambulation, activity and evidence of disease, self-care, oral intake, and level of consciousness. A score of approximately 40% is often associated with appropriateness for hospice. Hospice eligibility in the United States is solely based on a life expectancy of 6 months or less if the disease progresses on its expected course. The National Hospice and Palliative Care Organization (NHPCO; https://www.nhpco.org/) has devised some prognostic criteria for a variety of diagnoses including dementia, amyotrophic lateral sclerosis (ALS), acquired immune deficiency syndrome (AIDS), congestive heart failure, end-stage liver or kidney disease, COPD, and so on. Although not fully validated, the criteria can help to guide the clinician in discussions with patients/families. "Hospice" is commonly associated with cancer; however, according to the NHPCO, only 27.2% of hospice patients in 2016 suffered from cancer (often referred late, as the median length of stay was only 19 days), followed by 18.7% cardiovascular and 18.0% dementia to round out the top three. There are various prognostic scoring systems for different disease states, and the Palliative Prognosis Score can help to determine the prognosis for patients with terminal cancer. In addition, the American Cancer Society (https://www.cancer.org/) has 5-year survival rates for various stages of numerous cancers on its website.

Differential Diagnosis

Because this chapter discusses management of symptoms for a plethora of different diseases, the differential diagnosis of all symptomatic disease processes is far beyond its scope. However, when assessing various symptoms, treatment options can be selected based on the probable source. Is the pain new or in a new location, or is it in the same area, radiating, or worsening? Are the nausea/vomiting due to chemotherapy, anesthesia, metabolic disorders, bowel obstruction, anxiety, increased intracranial pressure, or something else? Is the constipation opioid induced, due to poor intake, a result of using fiber without adequate fluid intake, or caused by another issue altogether? Is the dyspnea due to pleural effusion (may respond to thoracentesis far better than it would respond to medications), anxiety (could use selective serotonin reuptake inhibitors [SSRIs], hydroxyzine [Vistaril],

benzodiazepine, cognitive behavioral therapy), airway obstruction (might use bronchoscopy, suction, or bronchodilators rather than other medications), excessive secretions (could treat with anticholinergic medications such as glycopyrrolate [Robinul] or scopolamine), or other cause?

Therapy

To meet the needs of all forms of suffering (physical, emotional/psychological, spiritual, existential), an interdisciplinary approach using physicians, nurses, chaplains, counselors, social workers, and others is essential. For all patients entering palliative care, and especially hospice care, all of their medications should be evaluated for risk and benefit and then prioritized based on the goals of care. In one study, patients with a life expectancy of less than 1 year taking a statin for primary or secondary prevention were randomized to continue or stop the statin. The average number of days until death was 229 after discontinuation versus 190 for continuation; thus survival and quality of life improved at a lower cost. Consider discontinuing statins, some oral hypoglycemic agents (notably sulfonylureas due to risk of hypoglycemia), or oral anticoagulants such as warfarin (Coumadin), apixaban (Eliquis), or dabigatran (Pradaxa) if risks now outweigh benefits. As the end of life approaches, discontinue other medications that are not essential for symptom control or quality of life, have more risks than benefits, or contribute to symptom burden (e.g., cholinesterase inhibitors) at this advanced stage of the disease.

Clinicians might withhold or withdraw treatments, but they should never withdraw "care." Providers can change from "doing everything possible to cure a patient" to "doing everything possible to maintain comfort and quality of life." This is more than semantics. Consider turning off the defibrillator component of a pacer-defibrillator to avoid unnecessary shocks. The pacer can remain on because it can improve some symptoms while not prolonging life.

Pain

For a detailed review of medications used for pain, especially opioids, see chapter titled "Pain." This section will focus on cancer pain and end-of-life pain.

Pain of All Types

Opioids have demonstrated efficacy for cancer-related pain in numerous clinical trials. Methadone (Dolophine) can be effective when other opioids have failed, but it should be used with caution and by those familiar with its use due to variable pharmacokinetics and an increased risk of respiratory depression as compared to other opioids. A 2020 systematic review and meta-analysis did not demonstrate a benefit of adding cannabinoids to opioids for the management of pain related to advanced cancer. Additionally, medical cannabis did not improve insomnia in adults with chronic pain. Acupuncture and/or accupressure were associated with improved pain scores and reduction of opioid requirements in cancer patients.

Bone Pain

The bone pain due to metastatic lesions is partly due to prostaglandin release; thus coanalgesics such as nonsteroidal antiinflammatory drugs or adjuvant medications such as corticosteroids, (e.g., dexamethasone[1] or prednisone[1]) can be particularly helpful. Bisphosphonates such as zoledronic acid (Zometa) and pamidronate (Aredia) usually provide analgesia within a week that lasts up to 3 months. Monthly dosing may be required. In addition, radiopharmaceuticals such as strontium-89 (Metastron), samarium-153 (Quadramet), and phosphorus-32 (Phosphocol P-32) may be helpful for cancer-related bone pain, with analgesia usually beginning within 1 to 2 weeks and lasting 2 to 6 months. Their benefit is derived from significant uptake by areas of high bone turnover to provide internal, localized radiation. Radium-223 (Xofigo;

---

[1] Not FDA approved for this indication

indication limited to castration-resistant prostate cancer with bone metastasis) emits alpha radiation rather than the beta radiation of the three aforementioned agents, and it is more selective for metastatic lesions. External-beam radiation treatment (EBRT) achieves pain relief in more than 75% of patients with analgesia beginning in 1 to 2 weeks and lasting 2 to 6 months. The appropriateness and dosing of radiopharmaceuticals and EBRT are determined by a radiation oncologist. The radiation oncologist might choose a single large fraction of EBRT rather than multiple small fractions if survival is expected to be greater than 3 months or if prolonged treatment will present too much hardship (transportation, increased suffering, time off work for caregivers, etc.) on the patient/family.

Neuropathic Pain

Neuropathic pain can have multiple causes, such as nerve invasion/compression, medication toxicities, human immunodeficiency virus (HIV), and complications of diabetes. Adjuvant medications that have proven efficacy, but not necessarily an indication for use by the US Food and Drug Administration (FDA), include antidepressants such as amitriptyline (Elavil)[1], duloxetine (Cymbalta), and venlafaxine (Effexor)[1], anticonvulsants such as pregabalin (Lyrica) and gabapentin (Neurontin)[1], or, for highly refractory cases (due to significant risk, side effects, and/or legality), ketamine (Ketalar)[1] or cannabinoids[1]. Topical agents such as capsaicin (Capzasin-HP, Salonpas Gel Patch Hot) have evidence to support their use in diabetic neuropathy. Highly active antiretroviral therapy can decrease viral load and improve symptoms of AIDS, including those of HIV-related neuropathy.

Visceral Pain

Octreotide (Sandostatin) can be used for the severe abdominal cramping and diarrhea associated with carcinoid tumors (can overproduce serotonin) or VIPomas (overproduce vasoactive intestinal peptide) or off-label for abdominal pain and other symptoms related to malignant bowel obstruction. An interventional radiologist or pain specialist could provide additional options, such as celiac plexus blocks or thoracoscopic splanchnicectomy, for refractory abdominal pain, notably in patients with pancreatic cancer.

Dyspnea

Dyspnea is a sensation of breathlessness, and the only measure is a patient's self-report. It does not correlate well with respiratory rate, blood gas measurements, or pulse oximetry. The potential causes are many, and they should be considered before merely managing the symptom. The cause can determine the therapy. Anxiety can be managed with SSRIs or benzodiazepines. Airway obstruction could be relieved by suction or bronchoscopy. Hypoxemia has numerous causes that would have to be considered, but supplemental oxygen could help. Pleural or pericardial effusions could be drained. Pneumonia can be treated with antibiotics, pulmonary edema can be managed with diuretics and opioids, and pulmonary embolus can respond to anticoagulants. Transfusions can be helpful for dyspnea due to significant anemia (hemoglobin <7 g/dL) resulting from hemorrhage or myelosuppression. Bronchospasm usually responds to inhaled β_2 agonists. If underlying causes are addressed, either by management or recognizing that treatment would not achieve the goals of care, symptom control is appropriate. The use of pharmacologic interventions such as opioids, benzodiazepines, or other medications for breathlessness in advanced cancer is not supported by the evidence; however, for patients who have tried other options without relief, a trial of medications is appropriate. Nebulized morphine[1] is no better than saline. Excessive secretions can be managed with scopolamine or glycopyrrolate. The latter is preferred in the elderly because it does not cross the blood-brain barrier. For nonpharmacologic interventions, see Box 1.

Nausea/Vomiting

The treatment of nausea and vomiting depends on the underlying cause. For chemotherapy-related nausea/vomiting, the 5HT3

BOX 1	Nonpharmacologic Interventions for Dyspnea

- Reassure, work to manage anxiety.
- Behavioral approaches: relaxation, distraction, hypnosis.
- Limit the number of people in the room.
- Open window.
- Eliminate environmental irritants.
- Keep line of sight clear to outside.
- Reduce room temperature, but avoid chilling the patient.
- Introduce humidity.
- Reposition, elevate the head of the bed, keep patient turned.
- Educate and support the family.

receptor antagonists are far more effective than other classes of antiemetics. The 5HT3 class includes ondansetron (Zofran), granisetron (Sancuso, Sustol), dolasetron (Anzemet), and palonosetron (Aloxi). In addition, there is a combination of netupitant/palonosetron (Akynzeo), which combines a 5HT3 antagonist for acute-phase nausea/vomiting and a substance P/neurokinin-1 receptor antagonist (NK1RA) for the delayed phase, and it should be given with dexamethasone (Decadron)[1]. Its only indication is for prophylaxis of chemotherapy-related nausea/vomiting, especially with highly emetogenic chemotherapy. The combination demonstrated superiority over palonosetron alone. Rolapitant (Varubi), another NK1RA, has a longer half-life than netupitant, with fewer drug interactions. Aprepitant (Emend) is an NK1RA with fosaprepitant (Emend injection) as its IV alternative. Olanzapine (Zyprexa)[1] was more effective than aprepitant and noninferior to fosaprepitant in the setting of highly emetogenic chemotherapy, whereas it is far more cost-effective than either NK1RA and serves as a better acute antiemetic than metoclopramide (Reglan). Prochlorperazine (Compazine) was found to be superior to promethazine (Phenergan) for uncomplicated nausea/vomiting (Table 2).

Constipation

Constipation is quite common in palliative care, and it is easier to prevent than to treat. It is one of the primary side effects of opioids that does not attenuate with time. For routine constipation, almost any laxative will do. Polyethylene glycol 3350 (MiraLax, GlycoLax) daily with as-needed sennosides (Senokot) or bisacodyl (Dulcolax) is one example of a simple regimen. If the patient is taking medications that have constipation as a side effect, such as anticholinergic medications or calcium channel blockers, they should be discontinued if possible. Opioid-induced constipation is due to the interaction of opioids with the mu receptors in the gut, thus leading to poor motility. It can be prevented for the most part if a stimulant laxative is initiated simultaneously with the opioid. Senna is safe for long-term use, but bisacodyl can damage the myenteric plexus over time. The chloride-channel activator lubiprostone (Amitiza) and the guanylate cyclase activator linaclotide (Linzess)[1] increase intestinal fluid secretion and motility, and the peripheral mu antagonists methylnaltrexone (Relistor) and naloxegol (Movantik) are indicated for use by the FDA to treat refractory opioid-induced constipation. Alvimopan (Entereg)[1] is another peripheral mu antagonist, but its primary indication is for ileus, especially postoperatively. Fiber and bulking agents should be avoided because they can worsen the problem (Table 3).

Anxiety

There are numerous reasons for patients receiving palliative care to be anxious, whether undergoing painful/unpleasant but curative interventions, suffering uncontrolled pain or dyspnea, or progressing toward hospice. Fear and uncertainty about the future

---

[1] Not FDA approved for this indication

---

[1] Not FDA approved for this indication

TABLE 2	Antiemetics

Antipsychotics/Dopamine Antagonists

Chlorpromazine (Thorazine) 10–25 mg PO q4h prn. Can use 25–50 mg IM q3h prn, but change to PO as soon as possible. Also available as 25 mg or 100 mg (can be halved) suppositories that can be given every 6 hours as needed.

Haloperidol (Haldol) 0.5–5 mg PO/IV bid–tid prn (off-label for nausea/vomiting); maximum 100 mg/d, but use lowest effective dose. Good choice when also managing delirium.

Metoclopramide (Reglan) 5–10 mg PO/IV q6h prn

Olanzapine (Zyprexa) 5–10 mg PO daily–bid prn (off-label for nausea/vomiting)

Prochlorperazine (Compazine) 5–10 mg PO/IM/IV q6h prn; maximum 10 mg/dose, 40 mg/d. Suppository, 25 mg PR q12h prn

Antihistamines

Hydroxyzine (Atarax, Vistaril) 25–100 mg PO q6h prn or IM q4h prn

Meclizine (Antivert, Bonine) 25–100 mg/d PO divided bid–tid prn (off-label)

Promethazine (Phenergan) 12.5–25 mg PO/PR/IM/IV q4h prn. Use with caution IV: can cause necrosis and gangrene.

Antiserotonin (5HT3 Antagonists)

Dolasetron (Anzemet) 12.5 mg IV 15 min before ending anesthesia or at onset of postoperative nausea/vomiting; 100 mg PO ×1 within an hour before chemotherapy.

Granisetron (Granisol, Sancuso [transdermal], Sustol [sustained release SC injection]) 2 mg PO ×1 or 1 mg PO q12h ×2 doses given within an hour before chemotherapy. If IV, 10 mcg/kg IV ×1 within 30 min before chemotherapy. Transdermal, apply 1 patch (3.1 mg/24 h) ×1 24 h before chemotherapy and leave on for up to 7 days. If SC, 10 mg SC q 7 days (give with dexamethasone [Decadron][1]).

Ondansetron (Zuplenz, Zofran, Zofran ODT) 8 mg PO q8h for nausea/vomiting; 24 mg PO ×1 30 min before highly emetogenic chemotherapy.

Palonosetron (Aloxi) 0.25 mg IV ×1 or 0.5 mg PO ×1 30 min before chemotherapy.

Antineurokinin (NK1 RA)

Aprepitant (Emend), fosaprepitant (Emend injection) 125 mg PO ×1 day 1 of chemotherapy, then 80 mg PO daily ×2 days. Or 150 mg IV ×1 30 min before chemotherapy.

Netupitant/palonosetron (Akynzeo) 300/0.5 mg, 1 capsule 1 h before highly emetogenic chemotherapy.

Rolapitant (Varubi) 180 mg PO ×1, 1–2 h before chemotherapy.

Netupitant/palonosetron is already a combination, but all NK1RAs should be given with an HT3RA and dexamethasone before highly emetogenic chemotherapy.

Cannabinoid Receptor Agonists

Dronabinol (Marinol, Syndros) 2.5–10 mg PO bid prn. Syndros is available as a 5 mg/mL solution.

Nabilone (Cesamet) 1–2 mg PO bid prn; maximum: 2 mg PO tid

Both drugs are indicated for chemotherapy-related nausea/vomiting refractory to other drugs. Significant psychiatric adverse events are possible.

Unknown Mechanism

Trimethobenzamide (Tigan) 300 mg PO or 200 mg IM q6h prn

[1]Not US Food and Drug Administration approved for this indication.
bid, Two times per day; *IM*, intramuscular; *IV*, intravenous; *q4h*, every four hours; *q6h*, every 6 hours; *q8h*, every 8 hours; *qAC*, before meals; *qd*, daily; *qHS*, at bedtime; *po*, by mouth; *pr*, per rectum; *prn*, as needed; *SC*, subcutaneous; *tid*, three times per day.

TABLE 3	Laxatives

Osmotic

Lactulose (Kristalose) 10 g per 15 mL; 15–30 mL daily or BID, maximum 60 mL/day (40 g/day)

Magnesium citrate (1.745 g/30 mL) 195–300 mL/d PO daily or divided bid; maximum: 300 mL/d

Magnesium hydroxide (milk of magnesia), 400 mg/5 mL; 30–60 mL (2400–4800 mg) PO daily PRN. Maximum 60 mL/day, can be divided 2–4 doses per day.

Polyethylene glycol 3350 (MiraLax), 17 g in 8 oz. liquid PO daily

Stimulant

Bisacodyl (Dulcolax) 5 mg tabs 1–3 PO daily prn or 10 mg suppository PR daily prn

Sennosides (Senna) 8.6 mg tabs; 2–4 tabs PO bid; maximum: 4 tabs PO bid

Secretory

Linaclotide (Linzess)[1] 145 mcg PO daily. Stimulates cGMP production to increase intestinal fluid secretion and motility.

Lubiprostone (Amitiza) 24 mcg PO bid. Activates chloride channel to increase intestinal fluid secretion and motility.

Plecanatide (Trulance)[1] 3 mg PO daily. Stimulates cGMP production to increase intestinal fluid secretion and motility.

Peripheral Mu-Receptor Antagonists

Methylnaltrexone (Relistor) 8–12 mg SC qod prn (or 0.15 mg/kg SC qod prn). Maximum: 1 dose/24 h

Naldemedine (Symproic) 0.2 mg PO daily

Naloxegol (Movantik) 25 mg PO daily

[1]Not US Food and Drug Administration approved for this indication.
bid, Two times per day; *IM*, intramuscular; *IV*, intravenous; *q4h*, every four hours; *q6h*, every 6 hours; *q8h*, every 8 hours; *qAC*, before meals; *qd*, daily; *qHS*, at bedtime; *po*, by mouth; *pr*, per rectum; *prn*, as needed; *SC*, subcutaneous; *tid*, three times per day.

are common causes, and they can be related to physical, psychological, social, spiritual, or practical (finances, managing home responsibilities) issues. Excessive alcohol or caffeine use can exacerbate anxiety, which may present with agitation, insomnia, restlessness, sweating, tachycardia, hyperventilation, panic disorder, worry, tension, and/or psychosomatic symptoms. For patients with expectation of cure or longer survival, SSRI or serotonin and norepinephrine reuptake inhibitor (SNRI) antidepressants can be beneficial. Venlafaxine (Effexor ER) has the shortest half-life, and steady state can be reached in 4 to 7 days. Benzodiazepines are helpful for shorter life expectancy, or they can be used until the antidepressants take effect. Diazepam (Valium) has a long duration of action due to numerous active metabolites, but it is slower in onset, as is clonazepam (Klonopin)[1]. Alprazolam (Xanax) has very rapid onset but short duration of action. Lorazepam (Ativan) strikes a happy medium between speed of onset and duration of action. Counseling and cognitive behavioral therapy are effective, especially in combination with medications.

Delirium

Delirium is a waxing/waning state of confusion that can be characterized by anxiety, disorientation, cognitive dysfunction, and hallucinations. There is also a catatonic variety of delirium. This condition can be caused by many things, but a short list would include constipation/impaction, hypoxemia, infection, electrolyte abnormalities, medications (including benzodiazepines and opioids), and pain. If a cause is identified and corrected but the patient is still symptomatic, haloperidol (Haldol)[1], chlorpromazine (Thorazine)[1], or olanzapine (Zyprexa)[1] can be helpful; however, haloperidol is by far the cheapest alternative and a good place to start. It can be given intravenously or orally, or it can be given subcutaneously (off-label).

Hiccups

Hiccups (singultus) is a common nuisance that can become quite distressing, especially if persistent (>48 hours) or intractable (>1 month). For patients with pain in the chest or abdominal regions, hiccups can make pain difficult to control in addition to being a bothersome symptom that can significantly decrease quality of life. Chlorpromazine, at 25 to 50 mg PO up to four times per day prn, is the only FDA-approved medication for hiccups, but haloperidol[1] is a viable and much cheaper alternative, as is metoclopramide (Reglan)[1]. Gabapentin (Neurontin)[1] and phenytoin (Dilantin)[1] have been used with some success, notably in cases with a central nervous system etiology. Many other medications, including baclofen (Lioresal)[1], have been tried without much success (i.e., some improvement in symptoms but did not eliminate the hiccups). Nonpharmacologic methods (e.g., breath holding, hyperventilation, gargling) are worth trying, but evidence is lacking for any particular intervention.

Monitoring

Patients should be reevaluated routinely for the adequacy of pain and symptom control, as well as for their ability to cope with the underlying disease, symptom burden, and functional decline. The family needs to be assessed for additional stressors and coping mechanisms, as the family's adjustment, or lack thereof, can be detrimental to the patient's condition. If opioids or benzodiazepines are being used, the supply needs to be monitored for any signs of aberrant use by the patient and/or the family and visitors. In addition, patients can be monitored for excessive sedation or respiratory depression, especially when using methadone with or without a benzodiazepine. The FDA has issued a warning regarding coadministration of benzodiazepines and opioids as a cause of worsened respiratory depression, so these patients in particular should be monitored.

Palliative Sedation

For symptoms refractory to all other measures and with a life expectancy of less than 2 weeks, palliative sedation can be considered, after informed consent, without hastening death according to one study.

---

[1] Not FDA approved for this indication

Physician-Assisted Suicide

Although this practice has been legalized in several states, the American Medical Association's Council on Ethical and Judicial Affairs has determined that physician-assisted suicide (PAS), as opposed to "aid in dying," is the most accurate description of the practice and that the AMA's current policy forbidding PAS should be upheld. Similarly, in 2017 the American College of Physicians (ACP) also determined that PAS is contradictory to the physician's role in the physician–patient relationship. The NHPCO issued a statement opposing all forms of "Legally Assisted Death" in November 2018, citing numerous reasons for their rationale. Notable among these is that PAS does not meet the World Health Organization (WHO) definition of palliative care (i.e., "intends to neither hasten nor postpone death"). Conversely, the American Academy of Family Physicians (AAFP) and the American Academy of Hospice and Palliative Medicine (AAHPM) have taken a neutral stance.

Complications

Emergencies do exist within the palliative care and hospice settings. Spinal cord compression, hypercalcemia, superior vena cava syndrome, seizures, airway obstruction, hemorrhage, or acute worsening or crisis in pain or other symptom are examples. Management will depend on the patient's goals of care and stage of illness; however, uncontrolled symptoms should always be addressed. Having dark-colored linens and towels are good to have on hand for patients at risk for hemorrhage, because the blood does not appear as dramatic or traumatic for the patient and family as it would on white or light-colored materials.

References

2017 NHPCO Facts & Figures—NHPCO April 2018. Available at: https://www.nhpco.org/sites/default/files/public/Statistics_Research/2017_Facts_Figures.pdf. [accessed 05.24.2019].

Bath C. ASCO 2014: Stopping statins is safe and can improve quality of life for patients with cancer near the end of life. Available at: http://www.ascopost.com/News/16304. Posted 6/11/14. [accessed 05.24.2019].

Boland EG, Bennett MI, Allgar V, Boland JW: Cannabinoids for adult cancer-related pain: systematic review and meta-analysis, *BMJ Support Palliat Care* 10:14–24, 2020.

Davis MP: New therapies for antiemetic prophylaxis for chemotherapy, *J Community Support Oncol* 14:11–20, 2016.

Dowling R: Bill end-of-life discussion codes correctly, Med Econ March 10, 2016. Available at: http://medicaleconomics.modernmedicine.com/medical-economics/news/how-bill-end-life-discussion-codes-correctly. [accessed 05.20.2019].

Ebell MH: Determining prognosis for patients with terminal cancer, *Am Fam Physician* 72:668–669, 2005.

Farmer C. Fast facts and concepts #81. Management of hiccups. Updated June 2015. Available at: https://www.mypcnow.org/blank-mkw97. [accessed 05.20.2019].

Feliciano JL, Waldfogel JM, Sharma R, Zhang A, et al: Phamacologic interventions for breathlessness in patients with advanced cancer: a systematic review and meta-analysis, *JAMA Network Open* 4(2):e2037632, 2021.

He Y, Guo X, May BH, Zhang AL, et al: Clinical evidence for association of acupuncture and acupressure with improved cancer pain: a systematic review and meta-analysis, *JAMA Oncol* 6:271–278, 2019.

Murphy SL, Xu J, Kochanek KD, Arias E. Mortality in the United States, 2017. NCHS data brief No. 328, November 2018. Available at: https://www.cdc.gov/nchs/data/databriefs/db293.pdf. [accessed 05.30.2018].

NCCN clinical practice guidelines in oncology: *antiemesis, version 1*, National Comprehensive Care Network, 2015. AE2–6.

Planning the transition to end-of-life care in advanced cancer–health professional version (PDQ). Available at: http://www.cancer.gov/cancertopics/pdq/supportivecare/transitiontoEOLcare/healthprofessional. [accessed 05.20.2019].

Reisfield GM, Wilson GR: Fast facts and concepts #116. Radiopharmaceuticals for painful osseous metastases, Available at: https://www.mypcnow.org/blank-qfwwm. June 2015 [accessed 05.20.2019].

Rutter C, Johnstone C, Weissman DE. Fast facts and concepts #66. Radiation for palliation – part 1. Updated April 2016. Available at: https://www.mypcnow.org/blank-r9t7g. [accessed 05.20.2019].

Rutter C, Johnstone C, Weissman DE: Fast facts and concepts #67. Radiation for palliation – part 2, ed 2. Available at: https://www.mypcnow.org/fast-fact-61-120. [accessed 05.20.2019].

"NHPCO Statement on Legally Accelerated Death." https://www.nhpco.org/sites/default/files/public/communications/Legally_Accelerated_Death_Position_Statement.pdf. [accessed 05.24.2019].

Weinstein E, Arnold R: Fast facts and concepts #113. Bisphosphonates for bone pain, Available at: https://www.mypcnow.org/blank-ux03d; June 2015 [accessed 05.20.2019].

Yang J, Wahner-Roedler DL, Zhou X, et al: Acupuncture for palliative cancer pain management: systematic review, *BMJ Supportive & Palliative Care*. Epub ahead of print: January 13, 2021.

PALPITATIONS

Method of
Rebecca Katzman, MD; Justin Bailey, MD; and Caroline Beyer, MD

CURRENT DIAGNOSIS

- History and physical examination
- Electrocardiogram
- Complete blood count (CBC)
- Thyroid-stimulating hormone (TSH)
- Complete metabolic panel

CURRENT THERAPY

- Dependent on underlying etiology. See Table 5.

Palpitations are the unpleasant sensation or awareness of one's own heartbeat. Patients may feel a racing heart, skipped heartbeats, or pounding in the chest or neck. Palpitations have been described as a "flip-flop" or "fluttering" in the chest. Palpitations may be due to cardiac arrhythmia, nonarrhythmic cardiac disease, drugs, other medical conditions, or psychiatric disease. Cardiac arrhythmias and anxiety account for a majority of cases. Palpitations may be completely benign or a manifestation of a potentially fatal arrhythmia.

Epidemiology

Palpitations (ICD-10-CM R00.2) are a common presenting complaint in a primary care office or the emergency department. They affect all genders and ages. Up to 16% of patients in general medical settings report palpitations, and up to 18% of cardiology outpatient visits are for cardiac arrhythmias. The most common etiologies of palpitations are cardiac arrhythmias (43%) and anxiety/psychiatric (31%). In outpatient clinics psychiatric etiologies are slightly more common; in emergency department settings cardiac causes are increasingly likely. The underlying cause of palpitations in 15% of patients cannot be identified.

Nearly 90% of patients who have palpitations have recurrent symptoms. Overall, 1-year mortality does not appear to be significantly increased, but patients report a moderate impact on their quality of life.

Although arrhythmias are frequently found to be the underlying cause of palpitations, it is important to note that many patients with arrhythmias do not have any symptoms.

Differential Diagnosis

The differential for palpitations is broad but can generally be broken down into cardiac versus noncardiac causes. Cardiac causes may be further divided into structural or arrhythmic causes. Noncardiac causes include medications and drugs, high-output states, and certain medical conditions. Gastroesophageal reflux or esophageal spasm may present as a brief intermittent episode of tightness or pounding in the chest. See Table 1 for a full listing of causes.

Psychiatric causes may account for up to one-third of presentations; palpitations can occur with panic attacks, generalized anxiety, depression, and somatization. However, it is important to note that psychiatric illness can coexist with cardiac or other medical causes.

Cardiac arrhythmias often present as palpitations. Nearly any arrhythmia or change from a sinus rhythm can produce this sensation. A less common condition in otherwise healthy patients is inappropriate sinus tachycardia (IST), demonstrated by an elevated resting heart rate, an exaggerated heart rate response to exercise, or both. IST is thought to be due to abnormal autonomic control and response. Long-QT syndrome, both congenital/familial and medication-induced, may predispose to ventricular tachyarrhythmias, including the often-fatal torsades de pointes.

Risk Factors

Structural cardiac disease, including valvular disease, may predispose patients to arrhythmias and palpitations. Box 1 lists symptoms and risk factors that indicate an increased likelihood that palpitations are due to an underlying arrhythmia.

Pathophysiology

An arrhythmia is caused by the disruption of the normal electrical impulse that originates at the sinoatrial node and is conducted to the atrioventricular node, then through the His-Purkinje system to depolarize the ventricles. Disruption may occur anywhere along this pathway. Underlying structural disease, prior ischemia, congenital abnormalities in myocytes, or electrical pathways affect a normal electrical conduction pathway. Palpitations that are due to supraventricular or ventricular tachyarrhythmias often result from sympathetic stimulation and catecholamine surges.

Palpitations involving skipped or premature beats are often a sensation that results from the following episode of systole when stroke volume is increased secondary to the prolonged length of the preceding diastole and increased ventricular inotropy.

Clinical Assessment

The keys to evaluation are a history and physical, a 12-lead electrocardiogram (ECG), and a basic laboratory evaluation including an evaluation of the thyroid gland. Clinicians must identify which patients are more likely to have underlying arrhythmia and require further evaluation. A good clinical history includes age of onset, description of palpitations, frequency, duration, timing, position, and associated symptoms, including dizziness, presyncope, and syncope. The clinical history should include a thorough medication review, including over-the-counter medications, alcohol and tobacco use, and illicit substance use. An increasing number of medications are being found to cause QT prolongation, especially when used in combination, and may predispose the patient to ventricular arrhythmias (see Table 2 and Box 2). A physical examination should be performed but may be limited, as clinicians rarely have the opportunity to examine a patient during an episode of palpitations.

Diagnostic Testing

A 12-lead ECG should be performed in all patients. It is appropriate to do limited laboratory evaluation with a complete blood count (CBC), thyroid-stimulating hormone (TSH), and complete metabolic panel (CMP or Chem-14) to identify anemia, thyroid disease, and electrolyte abnormalities that predispose to arrhythmias. Etiology can be determined in 40% of patients from this limited evaluation (see Tables 3 and 4).

Traditionally, ambulatory cardiac monitoring has been done via a Holter monitor. Patients keep a diary of the time and characteristics of their symptoms. This method is appropriate for patients who have daily palpitations. The monitor is worn for 24 to 48 hours. If symptoms are not present during the time the monitor is being worn, the test will be unrevealing. In addition, Holter monitoring may uncover arrhythmias (most commonly benign ectopy) that are unrelated to patient symptoms.

If arrhythmia is suspected in a patient but 24 to 48 hours is insufficient time to record an event, it is recommended that the patient be evaluated with an event (loop) monitor or a patch monitor for at least 2 weeks. These ambulatory monitors record continuously but only save data from the specific interval when the patient or program settings activate the monitor (e.g., 2 min before and after an episode of palpitations). Some of these

TABLE 1 Differential Diagnosis for Palpitations

CARDIAC		NONCARDIAC	
Arrhythmias	Atrial fibrillation	*Medications*	Digoxin [Lanoxin]
	Atrial flutter		Beta agonists (e.g., albuterol [Proventil])
	Benign ectopy (premature ventricular contractions, premature atrial contractions)		Vasodilators
	Nonsustained ventricular tachycardia		Anticholinergics
	Supraventricular tachyarrhythmias (e.g., atrioventricular reentrant tachycardia)		Hydralazine
	Inappropriate sinus tachycardia		Over-the-counter nasal decongestants (e.g., pseudoephedrine [Sudafed])
	Long-QT syndrome	*Substances*	Caffeine
	Torsades de pointes		Alcohol
Structural abnormalities	Mitral regurgitations		Cocaine
	Aortic insufficiency		Amphetamines
	Mitral valve prolapse		Nicotine
	Hypertrophic obstructive cardiomyopathy	*Systemic conditions*	Hyperthyroidism
Other	Pericarditis		Pheochromocytoma
	Pacemaker-mediated tachycardia		Anemia
	Vasovagal syncope		Hypoglycemia
			Mastocytosis
			Gastroesophageal reflux
			Esophageal spasm
		High output states	Fever
			Pregnancy
			Paget's disease
			Extracardiac shunt
			Exercise
			Stress
		Psychiatric conditions	Panic attack
			Generalized anxiety
			Depression
			Somatization

BOX 1 Indicators of Arrhythmic Etiology of Palpitations

Increased Likelihood of Underlying Arrhythmia
Known structural or valvular cardiac disease
Visible neck pulsations
Palpitations that affect sleep
Palpitations that occur at work
Subjective feeling of irregular heart rate
Duration of palpitations more than 5 min
Male gender
Older age

Decreased Likelihood of Underlying Arrhythmia
Family history of panic disorder
Duration of palpitations less than 5 min

monitors transmit real-time information to a central monitoring system and others store data on the device itself for analysis after completion of the recording period. In patients with infrequent palpitations but known severe heart disease, an implantable loop recorder is an option. These monitors are implanted subcutaneously, typically in the left pectoral region, and usually are left in place for 1 year. As with other loop event recorders, they save data when activated by the patient or the device settings and transmit the information to an external system.

Panic disorder or anxiety is a diagnosis of exclusion. A patient with anxiety or other psychiatric illness may have a significant underlying arrhythmia. The catecholamine increase in patients with psychiatric disorder in times of stress or intense emotional experience may be proarrhythmogenic. These patients should undergo evaluation for arrhythmia, especially in the presence of risk factors, before having all of their symptoms attributed to their psychiatric illness.

TABLE 2 History and Physical Examination Clues to the Etiology of Palpitations

CLUES FROM HISTORY OR EXAMINATION	SUGGESTED DIAGNOSIS
Onset in childhood or adolescence	• AV nodal reentrant tachycardia • Wolff-Parkinson-White syndrome • Idiopathic ventricular tachyarrhythmia
Onset in older adult Description of irregular rate	Atrial fibrillation
Feeling of "fluttering"	Prolonged tachyarrhythmia
Pounding in the neck Exaggerated "a" wave in jugular venous pulse	AV dissociations
Midsystolic click followed by late systolic murmur	Mitral valve prolapse
Holosystolic murmur along left sternal border that increases with Valsalva	Hypertrophic obstructive cardiomyopathy Left ventricle outflow tract obstruction
Pale conjunctiva	Anemia
Exophthalmos Goiter	Thyrotoxicosis
Gravid abdomen	Pregnancy

AV, Atrioventricular.

BOX 2 Medications That Cause QT Prolongation

- Cardiac Antiarrhythmics
  - Amiodarone (Cordarone)
  - Disopyramide (Norpace)
  - Procainamide
  - Quinidine
  - Sotalol (Betapace)
  - Diuretics
  - Sympathomimetics
  - Vasodilators
- Antibiotics
  - Fluoroquinolones
  - Macrolides
- Psychiatric
  - Phenothiazines
    - Chlorpromazine (Thorazine)
    - Promethazine (Phenergan)
    - Prochlorperazine (Compazine)
    - Fluphenazine (Prolixin)
    - Trifluoperazine (Stelazine)
  - Selective serotonin reuptake inhibitors
  - Tricyclic antidepressants
  - Haloperidol (Haldol)
  - Amphetamines
  - Anticholinergics
  - Antihistamines
  - Protease inhibitors
  - Methadone (Dolophine)

TABLE 3 ECG Findings Suggestive of Diagnosis of Palpitations

ECG FINDINGS	SUGGESTED DIAGNOSIS
Irregularly irregular rhythm Absent P waves	Atrial fibrillation
Delta wave Short PR interval Widened QRS	Wolff-Parkinson-White syndrome
Short PR	AV nodal reentrant tachycardia
QT interval >460 m/s in women, >440 m/s in men	Predisposition to ventricular tachyarrhythmias, including torsades de pointes
Left ventricular enlargement with left atrial abnormality	May be a focus for atrial fibrillation

AV, Atrioventricular, ECG, electrocardiogram.

TABLE 4 Diagnostic Considerations in the Evaluation of Palpitations

FINDINGS	FURTHER EVALUATION
Arrhythmia or predisposition to arrhythmia seen on ECG	Echocardiogram to look for structural heart disease
Palpitations brought on by exertion	Exercise stress test (avoid dobutamine if suspect arrhythmia)
Suspected arrhythmia, but none identified on ECG	Ambulatory cardiac monitoring • Holter monitor (24–48 h) • Continuous loop event recorder • Patch recorder • Implantable loop recorder
Associated dizziness, syncope, presyncope	Referral to cardiologist for electrophysiology study
Known cardiac dysfunction, structural or valvular abnormality	Referral to cardiologist for electrophysiology study
Family history of sudden cardiac death	Referral to cardiologist for electrophysiology study

Patients who have palpitations associated with dizziness, presyncope, or syncope in whom the diagnosis is not apparent should be referred for evaluation by a cardiologist. This sort of palpitation is the kind most likely to be associated with ventricular tachycardia or other serious arrhythmia.

Palpitations may occur more frequently during pregnancy, which is a high-output state. Postpartum cardiomyopathy is a structural disease that is unique to this population. Because pregnant women also have an increased risk of new arrhythmias, including atrial fibrillation, persistent palpitations should be evaluated thoroughly.

TABLE 5	Treatment of Specific Causes of Palpitations
CAUSE OF PALPITATIONS	**TREATMENT**
Medication or drug	Stop offending agent
Premature atrial contractions	Decrease caffeine and alcohol Tobacco cessation Beta blockers may reduce symptoms of PAC
Ectopy (PVCs)	Beta blockers • *Metoprolol Succinate* [Toprol XL][1] 50 mg PO daily • *Atenolol* [Tenormin][1] 50 mg PO daily Nondihydropyridine calcium channel blockers • *Verapamil* [Calan SR][1] 240 mg/day PO • *Diltiazem* [Cardizem CD][1] 120 mg/day PO Antiarrhythmic agents have been shown to reduce PVCs but may increase mortality especially in patients with previous myocardial infarction.
AVNRT Orthodromic AVRT SVT of unknown etiology	Vagal maneuvers (carotid massage, Valsalva, dive reflex) *Adenosine* [Adenocard] 6 mg IV bolus over 1–2 s, increased up to 12 mg IV every 1–2 min as needed for two doses If ineffective can reasonably consider: • *Verapamil* [Isoptin] 5–10 mg IV over 2 min, repeated in 30 min as necessary, then infusion at 0.005 mg/kg/min *Diltiazem* [Cardizem], 0.25 mg/kg IV over 2 min, repeat bolus of 0.35 mg/kg 15 min later if first dose is tolerated but does not produce desired reduction in heart rate. Can then be run as a continuous infusion at a rate of 5–15 mg/h • *Metoprolol Tartrate* [Lopressor][1] 2.5–5 mg IV bolus over 2 min, repeated at 5 min intervals up to three doses *Esmolol* [Brevibloc] 500 mcg/kg IV bolus over 1 min, followed by 50 mcg/kg/min continuous infusion. Can titrate up in 50 mcg/kg/min increments every 4 min to maximum 200 mcg/kg/min with repeat bolus doses between each rate change.
Antidromic AVRT	*Procainamide*[1] 20–50 mg/min up to total 17 mg/kg
Focal atrial tachycardia or multifocal atrial tachycardia	*Metoprolol Tartrate* [Lopressor]1 2.5–5 mg IV bolus over 2 min, repeated at 5 min intervals up to three doses *Verapamil* [Isoptin] 5–10 mg IV over 2 min, repeated in 30 min as necessary, then infusion at 0.005 mg/kg/min
Atrial fibrillation/flutter with rapid ventricular response	*Metoprolol Tartrate* [Lopressor]1 2.5–5 mg IV bolus over 2 min, repeated at 5 min intervals up to three doses *Esmolol* [Brevibloc] 500 mcg/kg IV bolus over 1 min, followed by 50 mcg/kg/min continuous infusion. Can titrate up in 50 mcg/kg/min increments every 4 min to maximum 200 mcg/kg/min with repeat bolus doses between each rate change. *Verapamil* [Isoptin] 5–10 mg IV over 2 min, repeated in 30 min as necessary, then infusion at 0.005 mg/kg/min *Diltiazem* [Cardizem], 0.25 mg/kg IV over 2 min, repeat bolus of 0.35 mg/kg 15 min later if first dose is tolerated but does not produce desired reduction in heart rate. Can then be run as a continuous infusion at a rate of 5–15 mg/h
Preexcited atrial fibrillation	*Procainamide*[1] 20–50 mg/min up to total 17 mg/kg *Ibutilide* [Corvert] 0.01 mg/kg (<60 kg) or 1 mg (≥60 kg) IV over 10 minutes
Ventricular Tachycardia	Synchronized cardioversion

[1]Not FDA approved for this indication. AVNRT, Atrioventricular nodal reentry tachycardia; IV, intravenous; PAC, premature atrial contraction; PVC, premature ventricular contraction; PO, per os (by mouth); SVT, supraventricular tachycardia.

Treatment

Treatment should be focused toward the underlying cause of the palpitation.

Discussion of the management of specific causes of palpitations, including anemia, thyrotoxicosis, and hypoglycemia, can be found elsewhere. Chronic management of atrial fibrillation is also beyond the scope of this article.

Table 5 outlines the treatment of specific causes of palpitations.

Referral to a cardiologist is appropriate for patients with supraventricular tachyarrhythmias, long-QT syndrome, or palpitations associated with syncope/presyncope, as these are more likely to be ventricular arrhythmias.

Patients with potentially malignant ventricular tachyarrhythmias (e.g., frequent premature ventricular depolarizations, up to 3–10 per hour with some repetitive forms) are at increased risk for sudden cardiac death, but there is little evidence that treating with antiarrhythmics decreases mortality; in fact, some evidence suggests that these drugs actually increase mortality via proarrhythmic mechanisms. In these patients, consider a referral to a cardiologist for evaluation for an implantable cardiac defibrillator.

References

Abbott AV: Diagnostic approach to palpitations, *Am Fam Physician* 71:743–750, 2005.
Chan T, Worster A: The clinical diagnosis of arrhythmias in patients presenting with palpitations, *Ann Emerg Med* 57:303–304, 2011.
Crawford MH, Bernstein SJ, Deedwania PC, et al: ACC/AHA guidelines for ambulatory electrocardiography: executive summary and recommendations, *Circulation* 100:886–893, 1999.
Tayal U, Dancy M: Palpitations, *Medicine* 41:118–124, 2013.
Weber BE, Kapoor WN: Evaluation and outcomes of patients with palpitations, *Am J Med* 100:138–148, 1996.
Wexler AK, Pleister A, Raman S: Outpatient approach to palpitations, *Am Fam Physician* 84:63–69, 2011.

PHARYNGITIS

Method of
Ruth Weber, MD, MSEd

CURRENT DIAGNOSIS

- Patients prioritize symptom relief over microbiologic cure.
- Most pharyngitis is viral; microbiologic confirmation is required for group A β-hemolytic streptococcus pharyngitis diagnosis.
- In adults, throat culture is not necessary if rapid antigen detection test is negative.
- Stop presumptive antibiotic therapy if throat culture results are negative for group A β-hemolytic streptococcus.

CURRENT THERAPY

- Penicillin is the drug of choice for group A β-hemolytic streptococcus pharyngitis. A first-generation cephalosporin or macrolide is indicated if the patient is allergic to penicillin.
- Treatment is necessary for 10 days to eradicate group A β-hemolytic streptococcus from the pharynx.
- Amoxicillin can be substituted for penicillin. Patients older than 12 years may be treated with once-daily amoxicillin (Moxatag).
- Patients are not infectious after 24 hours of appropriate antibiotic treatment.

Epidemiology

Pharyngitis is common and has substantial medical and societal costs. "Sore throat" accounts for more than 7 million outpatient visits by children annually. The estimated total cost of pharyngitis in children is $540 million per year.

An estimated 30% of childhood pharyngitis is caused by group A β-hemolytic streptococcus (GABHS). In temperate climates, pharyngitis occurs in outbreaks during winter and early spring, predominantly involving children 5 to 15 years of age. GABHS is uncommon in preschool-aged children and in adults. Group C β-hemolytic streptococcus pharyngitis occurs mainly in college students and young adults.

Of other causes of pharyngitis (Table 1), gonococcal pharyngitis is most common in older adolescents and young adults. Transmission is by oral-genital contact. If gonococcal pharyngitis is diagnosed in a prepubertal child, sexual abuse must be considered.

Risk Factors

The major risk factors for GABHS pharyngitis are age and exposure such as in crowded schools or through household contacts. Oral sexual activity is implicated in gonococcal pharyngitis. Swimming pools have been implicated in transmission of group C and D β streptococcal pharyngitis.

Pathophysiology

Pathogenic strains of *Streptococcus pyogenes* can be differentiated by Lancefield antigens and by hemolysis on blood agar. The strain containing group A antigen and displaying β hemolysis causes pharyngitis (GABHS). The M protein is responsible for virulence. The M protein cross-reacts with cardiac myosin and laminin, potentially causing rheumatic heart disease. More than 100 M-protein serotypes have been identified. Some streptococcus strains produce erythrogenic toxins, causing the rash of scarlet fever. Patients develop lifelong immunity to one serotype after infection, but reinfection with a different serotype is possible.

TABLE 1 Pharyngitis: Distribution of Causative Organisms (All Age Groups)

PATHOGEN	PERCENTAGE OF POPULATION
Group A β-hemolytic streptococcus	15–30
Rhinovirus	20
Adenovirus	2–5
Coronavirus	2–5
Coxsackievirus	2–5
Group C β-hemolytic streptococcus	2–5
Herpes simplex virus	2–5
Influenza virus	2–5
Chlamydia trachomatis	< 1
Corynebacterium diphtheriae	< 1
Epstein-Barr virus	< 1
Human immunodeficiency virus	< 1
Arcanobacterium haemolyticum	< 1
Mycoplasma spp.	< 1
Neisseria gonorrhoeae	< 1

Prevention

GABHS is transmitted by droplet spread. No evidence supports other forms of transmission. Patients and household/close contacts should be educated on minimizing droplet spread to reduce the transmission of GABHS.

Phase I trials have been completed on a multivalent vaccine targeting streptococcus M proteins that cause pharyngitis, invasive disease, and rheumatic fever.

Clinical Manifestations

The type of pharyngitis cannot be identified by history and clinical findings. Microbiologic confirmation is necessary to diagnose GABHS pharyngitis.

Group A β-Hemolytic Streptococcal Pharyngitis

In patients age 3 years to adult, sudden onset of sore throat, pain on swallowing, and fever (101°F–104°F) suggest GABHS pharyngitis. Nausea and vomiting can also occur in school-aged children. Clinical signs can include tonsillar erythema with or without exudate, anterior cervical lymphadenitis, soft palate petechiae, red swollen uvula, and scarletiniform rash. Infants rarely present with exudative pharyngitis but have coryza with excoriation and crusting of the nares. Posttonsillectomy patients with GABHS can have milder symptoms and clinical signs.

Patients with suppurative complications of GABHS have unusually severe symptoms, with neck swelling, drooling, and "hot potato" voice. The clinician must look for peritonsillar abscess and infections in the parapharyngeal and submandibular spaces (Ludwig's angina).

Scarlet Fever

Some strains of GABHS produce a pyogenic exotoxin that causes scarlet fever in susceptible patients. The clinical signs and symptoms are identical to GABHS pharyngitis plus development of the characteristic rash within 24 to 48 hours of symptom onset. The fine, papular, bright red rash blanches with pressure, begins on the neck, and spreads to the extremities and trunk. It is more pronounced in creases and feels rough, with a goose-pimple appearance. The punctate rash spares the face, but patients have flushed cheeks and forehead with pallor around the mouth. The rash fades in 3 to 4 days and is followed by desquamation. After desquamation of an initial white coating, the tongue has a classical strawberry appearance caused by edematous papillae.

Poststreptococcal Glomerulonephritis
Renal symptoms of hypertension, edema, and hematuria can occur 1 to 3 weeks after GABHS pharyngitis. Glomerulonephritis is an autoimmune response to M proteins. It is not preventable by antibiotics.

Viral Pharyngitis
Coryza, hoarseness, cough, diarrhea, viral exanthem, anterior stomatitis, and conjunctivitis can indicate a viral etiology for pharyngitis. Adenovirus infections can cause fever for 7 days, and conjunctivitis can persist for 14 days. Adenoviral outbreaks are often associated with swimming pools.

Enterovirus pharyngitis (coxsackievirus, echovirus, enterovirus) occurs in summer and fall. Fever, cervical adenopathy, and erythema of the tonsils are common, but exudates are rare. Herpangina (Coxsackie virus A/B) manifests with fever and painful papulovesicular lesions in the posterior oropharynx that resolve in 7 days. Hand-foot-and-mouth disease (Coxsackie virus A-16) manifests with painful vesicles and ulcers in the mouth plus painful vesicles on the palms, soles, and occasionally trunk. Lesions resolve in 7 days.

Primary oral herpes simplex infection occurs in young children. It manifests as acute gingivostomatitis, with ulcerating vesicles on the anterior mouth and lips but not on the posterior pharynx. High fever with intense pain is common, and dehydration can occur. Symptoms last for 14 days.

Diagnosis
It is necessary to obtain microbiologic confirmation of infection before treating GABHS pharyngitis. If the clinical symptoms suggest GABHS pharyngitis, a throat culture or rapid antigen detection test (RADT) are indicated. If the clinical symptoms suggest viral pharyngitis, the pretest probability of GABHS infection is low, and a diagnostic test should not be performed.

Several methods for determining the probability of GABHS infection have been proposed. The Centor criteria (for adults) are widely accepted. A score of 1 is given for each of the following characteristics: tonsillar exudate, tender anterior cervical adenopathy, history of fever, and an absence of cough. A score of 3 or more indicates a positive predictive value for GABHS of 40% to 60%. A score of 0 to 1 indicates a positive predictive value for GABHS of 1% to 5%.

Throat culture is the gold standard for diagnosing GABHS infection. The tonsils and the posterior pharynx should be aggressively swabbed. Other areas of the mouth should not be touched when obtaining the culture. The culture should be obtained before beginning antibiotic therapy, because even a single dose of antibiotics can cause the culture to be negative. The swab is plated on a sheep's blood agar plate and incubated. The plate must be read at both 24 and 48 hours of incubation. When done correctly, the throat culture has 90% to 95% sensitivity. Although throat culture is considered the gold standard for diagnosing GABHS infection, it does not differentiate a carrier state from clinical infection.

RADT has high specificity but low sensitivity. The many tests available have different performance characteristics. In children aged 5 to 15, a throat culture should be performed if the RADT test is negative to identify patients who have a false-negative RADT result. In adults, throat culture is not necessary after a negative RADT because of the low incidence of GABHS and extremely low risk of acute rheumatic fever. The use of RADT has allowed clinicians to begin antibiotic therapy early in those with a positive test. This decreases the risk of spread of GABHS, allows earlier return to school or work, and modestly improves clinical signs and symptoms.

Streptococcal antibody testing has no value in the acute diagnosis of GABHS pharyngitis. Testing has some value in confirming prior GABHS infection in patients in whom acute rheumatic fever or acute poststreptococcal glomerulonephritis is suspected. The two antibodies that can be identified are antistreptolysin O (ASO) and antideoxyribonuclease B (ARB). Positive, elevated, or increasing titers are confirmation of recent GABHS infection. ASO titers rise within a week of infection and peak 3 to 6 weeks after infection. ARB titers rise within 1 to 2 weeks of infection and peak at 6 to 8 weeks. In some patients titers remain elevated for prolonged periods; therefore a doubling of the titer in 6 weeks is necessary for diagnosing prior GABHS infection.

Differential Diagnosis
Infectious Mononucleosis
Classically a triad of severe sore throat, lymphadenopathy, and fever (up to 104°F) in 15- to 25-year-olds, mononucleosis begins with a prodrome of chills, sweats, fever, and malaise. Clinical signs include enlarged tonsils; posterior and anterior cervical, axillary and inguinal adenopathy; and hepatosplenomegaly. Approximately 15% of patients present with jaundice and 5% with rash. Patients with mononucleosis who are treated with amoxicillin (Amoxil)[1] often develop a pruritic maculopapular rash. Complete blood count (CBC) shows an absolute lymphocytosis with greater than 10% atypical lymphocytes. Within 2 to 3 weeks, the heterophile antibody test (Mono Spot) becomes positive. The antibody test has a higher false-negative rate in children than in adults. If a false-negative test is suspected, an IgM antibody to viral capsid antigen is indicated to confirm the diagnosis.

Acute Retroviral Syndrome
Primary infection with HIV can manifest as a syndrome of fever, nonexudative pharyngitis, arthralgia, myalgia, and lymphadenopathy. Some 40% to 80% of patients develop a rash. HIV antibodies are negative. Assay for HIV type 1 RNA or p24 antigen is positive.

Neisseria gonorrhea
N. gonorrhea pharyngitis is usually asymptomatic and associated with oral sexual practices. The diagnosis is confirmed by isolating the organism on Thayer-Martin medium. All patients should be screened and treated for coinfection with chlamydia.

Lemierre's Syndrome
Lemierre's syndrome is a rare etiology of severe pharyngitis caused by *Fusobacterium necrophorum*. Infection spreads from the pharynx to include the surrounding tissues, with subsequent thrombophlebitis of the internal jugular vein.

Treatment
A major therapeutic decision is to determine if whether the patient needs an antibiotic in addition to symptomatic treatment.

The goal of treatment of viral pharyngitis is control of symptoms, especially relief of pain. Nonsteroidal antiinflammatory drugs are slightly superior to acetaminophen (Tylenol) for pain relief. No evidence supports the use of Chinese herbs for symptom relief. A single dose of corticosteroids (oral dexamethasone[1] 0.6 mg/kg—maximum dose 10 mg) may provide pain relief, for moderate to severe symptoms. Short term oral corticosteroid use is associated with an increased risk of sepsis, venous thromboembolism, and fracture in adults <65. The risk of recurrent dosing of corticosteroids has not been determined. Many patients mistakenly believe that antibiotic therapy relieves pain. Ancillary treatment options include rest, adequate fluid intake, and antipyretic medications.

The goals of antibiotic treatment of GABHS pharyngitis are to decrease infectivity and prevent suppurative and other complications, especially acute rheumatic fever. Symptoms generally improve within 3 to 4 days without treatment. Delay of treatment of GABHS pharyngitis for up to 9 days after symptoms begin does not appear to increase the risk of acute rheumatic fever,

---

[1]Not FDA approved for this indication.

and a delay of 24 to 48 hours while awaiting culture results does not increase the risk of acute rheumatic fever. Early treatment of GABHS pharyngitis does reduce infectivity, lessens morbidity, and promotes early return to normal activities. Nevertheless, criteria for initiating antibiotics remain controversial.

The choice of antibiotic is determined by the bacteriology of GABHS, clinical efficacy, patient adherence to treatment regimen, adverse effects, and cost. It is not recommended to initiate antibiotics while awaiting throat culture results in children. However, if an antibiotic is started it must be discontinued if the culture is negative.

Penicillin remains the antibiotic of choice for GABHS pharyngitis. GABHS has never shown resistance to penicillin or cephalosporins. Amoxicillin[1] can replace penicillin for treatment. (Liquid amoxicillin has a better taste than liquid penicillin.) In the penicillin-allergic patient, a first-generation cephalosporin or macrolide may be substituted. In some areas of the United States up to 8% of GABHS is resistant to macrolides and less than 1% is resistant to clindamycin (Cleocin). Antibiotics should be given for 10 days to eradicate GABHS from the pharynx. At this time, short-course (≤ 5 days) treatment cannot be recommended, except with azithromycin (Zithromax).

No clear evidence supports antibiotic treatment for group C or group G streptococcal pharyngitis. Treatment might shorten the course of infection. Treatment options are identical to those for GABHS pharyngitis.

Treatment Regimens

- Oral penicillin: PenicillinVK (Veetids)[1]: 40 mg/kg/day (up to adult dose of 1000 mg/day) in divided doses two or three times daily for 10 days.
- Amoxicillin[1]: 50 mg/kg/day (up to adult dose of 1000 mg/day) twice daily for 10 days; the FDA has approved amoxicillin ER tab (Moxatag) for patients older than 12 years at 775 mg once a day.
- Penicillin G benzathine (Bicillin-LA): Patients weighing less than 27 kg, 600,000 units IM; patients weighing 27 kg or more, 1.2 million units IM once. Penicillin G is used for patients who are unlikely to complete a full 10-day course of oral medication and for those with a personal or family history of rheumatic fever.
- First-generation oral cephalosporin: Cephalexin (Keflex) 25 to 50 mg/kg/day (up to adult dose of 1000 mg/day) twice daily for 10 days. This regimen should be used if the patient is allergic to penicillin; shorter courses are not FDA approved.
- Macrolides should be used if the patient is allergic to penicillin: Erythromycin 20 to 40 mg/kg/day (up to adult dose of 1000 mg/kg/day) in three or four doses for 10 days. Azithromycin (patients older than 6 months): Day 1: 10 mg/kg once (up to adult dose of 500 mg); days 2 to 5: 5 mg/kg once daily (up to adult dose of 250 mg/day). The dose of azithromycin is not established in infants younger than 6 months.

Tetracycline, sulfonamides, and older fluroquinalones are not recommended because of high rates of resistance. All patients should be considered infectious until they have completed 24 hours of antibiotic therapy.

Monitoring

In general, follow-up throat cultures or RADT for patients successfully treated for GABHS pharyngitis (i.e., test for cure) are not necessary. An additional RADT or throat culture is required if symptoms do not abate, symptoms recur, or the patient had previous rheumatic fever.

Patients who have repeated symptomatic episodes of GABHS have either recurrent new infections or are carriers of GABHS, with repeated superimposed viral infections.

---

[1]Not FDA approved for this indication.

GABHS carriers have positive cultures for GABHS without clinical symptoms. Approximately 20% of school-aged children are carriers. GABHS carrier status is suspected if the clinical picture is of viral pharyngitis but the patient has positive RADT or cultures both when symptomatic and when asymptomatic. Carriers do not respond to antibiotics and have no serologic response to ASO and anti-DNA B. These patients do not need to be identified or treated. These patients do not develop rheumatic fever and are not important in the spread of GABHS to others.

Patients with repeated GABHS pharyngitis have a clinical picture of recurrent bacterial pharyngitis. They respond to antibiotics and have negative RADT and culture when they are asymptomatic. They have a serologic response to ASO and anti-DNA B. Prophylactic antibiotics are not recommended for these patients. Tonsillectomy may be considered when infection attack rates do not decrease over time and no other explanation of recurrent infection can be found. Meta-analyses have found inconclusive evidence of benefit from tonsillectomy compared to nonsurgical treatment.

Patients with GABHS pharyngitis who remain symptomatic and continue to have positive cultures should receive a second course of antibiotics, with either the same antimicrobial agent or intramuscular penicillin. If a patient experiences repeated infections and there is concern that the GABHS infection is being spread among close contacts, all close and family contacts should be cultured, and only those who are positive should be treated. Family pets are not reservoirs and do not spread disease.

Mass screening should be considered in outbreaks of GABHS in a closed or semiclosed community or in outbreaks of acute rheumatic fever or poststreptococcal glomerulonephritis.

Non-GABHS pharyngitis (i.e., group C or G β-hemolytic streptococcus) is not associated with rheumatic fever, and no evidence supports treatment or follow-up culture.

Complications

The complications of GABHS pharyngitis can be classified as suppurative and nonsuppurative.

Suppurative complications occur when the infection spreads to cause conditions such as lateral pharyngeal abscess, cervical lymphandenitis, sinusitis, otitis media, retropharyngeal abscess, Lemierre's syndrome, and mastoiditis. Appropriate treatment of GABHS with antibiotics decreases these complications.

Nonsuppurative complications include acute rheumatic fever, acute poststreptococcal glomerulonephritis, and poststreptococcal reactive arthritis. Acute rheumatic fever occurs 2 to 3 weeks after GABHS pharyngitis. It is not seen after GABHS skin infections. Starting antibiotics within 9 days of symptoms can prevent acute rheumatic fever. Acute poststreptococcal glomerulonephritis can occur 10 days after pharyngeal infection and 21 days after skin infection. Antibiotics do not alter the attack rate. Poststreptococcal reactive arthritis is similar to other reactive arthritis, and the attack rate is not altered by antibiotics.

Potential complications from treatment of GABHS pharyngitis include anaphylactic reaction to antibiotics and antibiotic resistance.

References

ESCMID Sore Throat Guideline Group, Pelucchi C, Grigoryan L, et al: Guideline for the management of acute sore throat, *Clin Microbiol Infect* 18(Suppl 1):1–28, 2012. http://www.ncbi.nlm.nih.gov/pubmed/22432746.

Kociolek L, Shulman S: In the clinic pharyngitis, *Ann Intern Med* 157, 2012. ITC3-1–ITC3-16, Downloaded from http://annals.org.

Sadeghirad B, Siemieniuk RA, Brignardello-Petersen R, et al: Cortiosteroids for treatment of sore throat: Systematic Review & meta-analysis of randomized trials, *BMJ* 358, 2017. j3887/doi:10.1136/bmj.j3887.

Shulman ST, Bisno AL, Clegg HW, et al: Clinical practice guideline for the diagnosis and management of group A streptococcal pharyngitis: 2012 update by the Infectious Diseases Society of America, *Clin Infect Dis* 55:e86–e102, 2012.

PRURITUS

Method of
Hassan Bencheqroun, MD

CURRENT DIAGNOSIS

- A careful history and physical examination will reveal a clear exposure, a sick contact, a recent travel, or clues to a systemic disease.
- Antihistamines are effective in treating histamine-mediated pruritus, but they are less effective in mechanisms involving serotonin, leukotrienes, etc.
- Initial testing in the absence of improvement with nonpharmacologic methods or antihistamine should include complete blood counts, thyroid-stimulating hormone, renal and liver panel, human immunodeficiency virus (HIV) test, and chest radiograph.
- Chronic pruritus may precede a systemic illness, especially in older adults. Hodgkin lymphoma is the malignant disease most strongly associated with pruritus and occurs in up to 30% of patients diagnosed with pruritus.

CURRENT THERAPY

- Acute and localized pruritus may resolve with nonpharmacologic methods, such as skin hydration with hypoallergenic, alcohol-free, and fragrance-free moisturizing creams; decreasing the length of showers and baths as well as the temperature of the water; identifying material that may irritate the skin either in jewelry or clothing items; and avoiding scratching.
- Wound care of scratch lesions includes any cellulitic portions.
- First-line pharmacologic treatments may include the use of antihistamine and antipruritic creams. Antipruritic agents may be used as second-line treatments.
- In the absence of improvement, the management of chronic pruritus should be directed at the underlying cause, or targets on the pruritic cascade-from blockade of intracellular and intercellular signaling pathways in the skin to the modulation of neurotransmission.

Pruritus is defined as an unpleasant sensory perception that causes the desire to scratch. While it shares similarities with pain, the neurophysiology of pruritus is distinct: pain causes withdrawal, whereas pruritus induces the reflex of reaching out and scratching.

Classification

Pruritus can be distinguished as acute or chronic, with the latter defined by the International Forum for the Study of Itch (IFSI) as lasting for 6 or more weeks.

Despite many classifications over the years, there is no uniform, clinically based classification of pruritic diseases to assist in the diagnosis and management of patients with pruritus. The classification chosen for this chapter focuses on clinical signs and distinguishes between the disease with and without primary or secondary skin lesions.

1. Group 1: Pruritus of primary diseased, inflamed skin
2. Group 2: Pruritus of primary nondiseased, noninflamed skin
3. Group 3: Pruritus with chronic secondary scratch lesions

Pathophysiology

The sensation of pruritus stems from a number of different causes. It is generally transmitted through slow-conducting unmyelinated C fibers and free pruriceptive cutaneous nerve endings located superficially in the skin, which appear to be more sensitive to pruritogenic substances than pain receptors. Histamine, neuropeptide substance P, interleukin 31 (mostly in atopic dermatitis), serotonin (a key component in several diseases), bradykinin, mast cell tryptase, and other unknown mediators (e.g., in uremic pruritus, cholestatic pruritus) may be involved in the genesis of pruritus. Impulses are transmitted from the dorsal root ganglion to the spinothalamic tract. Pruritus then generates a spinal reflex response, the scratch, which is as innate as a deep tendon reflex. Other pathogenic mechanisms include neuropathic (e.g., herpes zoster), acute traumatic stress (following burns and skin grafts), chronic puritis increasingly seen in the elderly including paraneoplastic, and immune-mediated (atopic dermatitis). Lastly, opioids are known to modulate the sensation of pruritus, both peripherally and centrally.

Clinical Manifestations

Pruritus is among the most common symptoms in dermatology. While often overlooked, it is in fact rated by patients as the most quality-of-life–altering symptom of the underlying disease. Other associated symptoms depend on the etiology and may include urticarial skin lesions, dry skin, jaundice, and thyroid-related symptoms. Left untreated, itch and its associated scratching increase the risk of chronic skin changes and secondary infection.

Differential Diagnosis

The patient's workup further places him or her in one of the following categories:

1. Primary diseased, inflamed skin
   - *Inflammatory:* Atopic and contact dermatitis, psoriasis, dry skin, drug reactions
   - *Infectious:* Mycotic, bacterial and viral infections, folliculitis, scabies, pediculosis, arthropod reactions, and insect bites
   - *Autoimmune*: Bullous dermatoses, especially dermatitis herpetiformis, bullous pemphigoid, and dermatomyositis
   - *Dermatoses of pregnancy*
   - *Neoplasms:* Cutaneous T-cell-lymphoma (especially erythrodermic variants), cutaneous B-cell lymphoma, leukemic infiltrates of the skin
2. Primary nondiseased, noninflamed skin
   - Endocrine and metabolic diseases: Chronic renal failure, liver diseases/cholestasis, hyperthyroidism, malabsorption, perimenopausal pruritus
   - Infectious diseases: HIV infection, helminthosis, parasitosis
   - Hematologic and lymphoproliferative diseases, iron deficiency, polycythaemia vera, Hodgkin and non-Hodgkin lymphoma
   - Visceral neoplasms of the cervix, prostate, or colon, carcinoid syndrome
   - Pregnancy: Pruritus gravidarum with and without cholestasis
   - Drug-induced pruritus: Opioids, ACE-inhibitors, amiodarone, hydrochlorothiazide, estrogens, simvastatin, hydroxyethyl starch, allopurinol
3. Pruritus with chronic secondary scratch lesions (The underlying origin may be a systemic disease or a skin disease.)
   - Neurogenic origin (without neuronal damage), such as hepatic itch
   - Neuropathic diseases (neuronal damage causes itch)
   - Multiple sclerosis, neoplasms, abscesses, cerebral or spinal infarcts, brachioradial pruritus, postherpetic neuralgia, vulvodynia, small fiber neuropathy
   - Somatoform pruritus (e.g., obsessive-compulsive disorders)

Therapy

- Basic measures to lessen drying of skin: Limit bathing to short, cool showers with soap applied only to oily skin areas. A mild moisturizing cream is preferably applied immediately after bathing to lock in moisture. The patient's home should be humidified, especially during dry, cold winter months. Avoid contact irritants, such as wool, fiberglass, and detergents.

- Topical corticosteroids, oral melatonin[7], and clonidine (Catapres)[1] showed some efficacy in reducing nocturnal itching or improving sleep quality in nocturnal pruritus.
- Many topical and systemic medications are available, but must be chosen according to existing comorbidities, possible interactions and side effects, and patient's compliance. Ultraviolet therapy may be administered in certain cases.
- Nonspecific therapy: A wheal and flare response is a marker of histamine-induced pruritus in patients with urticaria or an allergic dermatitis. These patients benefit from long-acting antihistamines. Concurrent H1 and H2 blockers increase therapeutic effectiveness. Also exercises focused on learning to disengage patient's attention away from pruritus or pain in chronic pruritis improves the symptoms.
- Specific antipruritic therapies target several points in the pruritic cascade—from blockade of intracellular and intercellular signaling pathways in the skin to the modulation of neurotransmission.
  - Nemolizumab[5], an anti-IL-31 A receptor monoclonal antibody, was shown in a Phase II trial to induce a decrease of pruritus intensity in active treatment group when compared to placebo in atopic dermatitis patients.
  - Neurokinin 1 receptor antagonists such as aprepitant (Emend)[1] showed potential activity in chronic pruritus. Novel derivates with longer half-life time, such as serlopitant[5] or tradipitant[5], are currently investigated in clinical trials.
- Future treatments also include bile acid transport inhibitors, phosphodiesterase-4 inhibitors, and nerve ion channels modulators.
- Treatment specific: Itching gradually recedes as the primary systemic condition improves.

Complications

Pruritus is accompanied by intense scratching. Skin may thicken, displaying lichen simplex chronicus: a localized skin thickening often appearing over the posterior neck, extremities, scrotum, vulva, anus, and buttocks. In prurigo nodularis, a variant of lichen simplex chronicus, some nodules develop over areas within easy scratching reach, such as the extensor arms and legs. Impetigo may result from superinfected excoriations in patients with atopic dermatitis.

References

Cho YL, Liu HN, Huang TP, Tarng DC: Uremic pruritus: roles of parathyroid hormone and substance P, *J Am Acad Dermatol* 36:538–543, 1997.

Duval A, Dubertret L: Aprepitant as an antipruritic agent? *The New England Journal of Medicine* 361(14):1415–1416, 2009.

Ganesh E, Maxwell LG: Pathophysiology and management of opioid-induced pruritus, *Drugs* 67:2323–2333, 2007.

Ikoma A, Rukwied R, Ständer S, et al: Neurophysiology of pruritus: interaction of itch and pain, *Arch Dermatol* 139:1475–1478, 2003.

Kwa KAA, Pijpe A, Rashaan ZM, Tuinebreijer WE, Breederveld RS, Van Loey NEE: Course and predictors of pruritus following burns: a multilevel analysis, *Acta Derm Venereol* 98:636–640, 2018.

Krajnik M, Zylicz Z: Understanding pruritus in systemic disease, *J Pain Symptom Manage* 21:151–168, 2001.

McEwen MW, Fite EM, Yosipovitch G, Patel T: Drugs on the horizon for chronic pruritus, *Dermatol Clin* 36(3):335–344, 2018 Jul.

Reamy B: A diagnostic approach to pruritus, *Am Fam Physician* 84:195–202, 2011.

Reich A, Misery L, Takamori K: Pruritus: From the bench to the bedside, *Biomed Res Int* 2018:5742753, 2018 May 22.

Ruzicka T, Hanifin JM, Furue M, et al: Anti-interleukin-31 receptor A antibody for atopic dermatitis, *The New England Journal of Medicine* 376(9):826–835, 2017.

Ständer S, Siepmann D, Herrgott I, Sunderkötter C, Luger TA: Targeting the neurokinin receptor 1 with aprepitant: a novel antipruritic strategy, *PLoS ONE* 5(6), Article ID e10968.

Ständer S, Weisshaar E, Mettang T, et al: Clinical classification of itch: a position paper of the International Forum for the Study of Itch, *Acta Derm Venereol* 87:291–294, 2007.

Zirwas MJ, Seraly MP: Pruritus of unknown origin: a retrospective study, *J Am Acad Dermatol* 45:892–896, 2001.

[1]Not FDA approved for this indication.
[5]Investigational drug in the United States.
[7]Available as a dietary supplement.

RHINITIS

Method of
Masayoshi Takashima, MD; and Omar G. Ahmed, MD

Introduction

Rhinitis is defined as inflammation of the nasal mucous membranes. Despite the definition of rhinitis, there are both inflammatory and noninflammatory forms of rhinitis. Rhinitis presents as one or more of the symptoms of nasal congestion, sneezing, itching, rhinorrhea, and/or postnasal drainage. It can be divided into allergic rhinitis (AR) and nonallergic rhinitis (NAR). Often patients will have a mixed rhinitis, which has components of both allergic and nonallergic disease. AR is nasal inflammation that is mediated by immunoglobulin (Ig)E to environmental allergens. NAR is defined by non–IgE-mediated perennial symptoms. NAR shares symptoms with AR but is only distinguishable by negative allergy tests. NAR includes a broad group of diseases including vasomotor rhinitis, gustatory rhinitis, NAR with eosinophilia syndrome (NARES), occupational rhinitis, hormonal rhinitis, drug-induced rhinitis, atrophic rhinitis, and infectious rhinitis.

Most research still classifies AR according to its seasonality or its perennial nature. Seasonal AR is commonly caused by pollen allergens; perennial AR is mainly caused by dust mites and animal dander. AR can be further classified as mild or moderate/severe. Mild rhinitis is rhinitis that does not impair work, school, daily functioning, or sleep. Moderate to severe rhinitis interferes with activities of daily living, quality of life, and/or sleep. Episodic AR occurs with sporadic inhalant aeroallergen exposure not typically encountered by the patient's usual indoor and outdoor environments. Both AR and NAR can also be classified based on symptom frequency, intermittent (<4 days/week or <4 consecutive weeks/year) versus persistent (>4 days/week and >4 consecutive weeks/year).

Local allergic rhinitis (LAR) is a newly defined entity found in nonatopic patients. LAR is characterized by local inflammatory reactions including local eosinophils and localized IgE in response to aeroallergens. LAR does not show significant skin-prick testing reactions, and patients have negative systemic IgE reactions to aeroallergens.

Rhinitis may be viewed by some as a trivial disease, but it places a significant financial burden on society. The estimated direct and indirect costs to society of rhinitis were around $11.58 billion in 2002. There is a significant loss of work and school days and decreased productivity and school performance. It is estimated at least 20% to 33% decrease in productivity when patients with AR have an exacerbation of their symptoms. Patients also report significant decreased quality of life related to their rhinitis symptoms including disturbed sleep, daytime somnolence, fatigue, irritability, depression, impairment of physical and social functioning, impairment of attention and memory, and learning deficits. Appropriate recognition, diagnosis, and treatment can help alleviate these economic and societal costs.

Epidemiology/Risk Factors

The National Health and Nutrition Survey (NHANES II and III) suggests that the overall prevalence of IgE sensitivity might be increasing. Of the patients evaluated for rhinitis in the United States, 43% (58 million people) have allergic disease, 23% (19 million people) have nonallergic disease, and 34% (26 million people) have mixed rhinitis. It is estimated the prevalence of physician-diagnosed AR is up to 20% of the population and 17% to 52% for NAR. Seventy percent of allergic patients develop the disease in childhood (20 years and younger) as opposed to NAR patients, 70% of whom develop disease in adulthood. Approximately two-thirds of NAR patients have vasomotor rhinitis, and one-third have NARES. NAR has a female predominance.

Pathophysiology
Allergic
Allergic rhinitis is the result of an IgE-mediated, type I hypersensitivity allergic reaction in response to an inhaled allergen.

Allergens are proteins derived from airborne particulate matter, including dust mite feces, pollens, animal dander, and cockroach particles. Antigen presenting cells (APCs) engulf allergens, break them down, and then present these peptides to T cells (THO). These cells differentiate into the TH2 subtype and generate cytokines that regulate B lymphocytes and sequester inflammatory cells (including eosinophils). B lymphocytes produce IgE, which attach to mast cells and basophils and render them sensitized. When mast cells and basophils are exposed to the specific allergen, they degranulate and release a host of inflammatory mediators including histamine and prostaglandin. Histamine stimulates histamine type I (H1) receptors on nerve endings that cause pruritus, sneezing, and increased secretions, which constitute the early phase response of AR (minutes to 1 hour).

Eosinophils produce interleukin (IL)-5, which acts to promote activation and survival of other eosinophils. Eosinophils also produce toxic products, which damages the mucosal cells and causes nasal congestion. This damage occurs several hours after allergen exposure and constitutes the late phase.

Nonallergic Rhinitis

The nasal mucosa has two major functions: One is trapping inhaled particles through mucus production and the second is humidifying inhaled air through a complex vascular system. The mucus glands and the vascular system are regulated by the parasympathetic and the adrenergic nervous systems. Sensory nerves are stimulated by irritants in the nose through the use of a sensory receptor called a nociceptor. The nociceptive signal generates a neural reflex in the central nervous system (CNS) controlling sympathetic and parasympathetic tone in the nasal mucosa. Parasympathetic stimulation results in mucus production. Sympathetic stimulation causes vasoconstriction, which empties venous cavities. Lack of sympathetic tone causes venous engorgement and nasal congestion.

Symptomatic NAR is an exaggeration of a normal defensive mechanism. Inflammation in the nose causes an upregulation of this neural activity, resulting in the exaggerated response (also known as neural hyperresponsiveness). Hyperresponsive parasympathetic efferent nerves trigger glandular activation in the nasal mucosa, leading to vasodilation and mucus production. Excessive mucus production anteriorly causes rhinorrhea and posteriorly causes postnasal drip. This hyperresponsiveness can be due to structural or functional components of the nasal mucosa altered through genetic or pathologic factors. NAR is often associated with hyperreactivity of the nasal mucosa but the exact mechanisms is often different based on the specific type of NAR. Broadly speaking, NAR is defined as rhinitis independent of an IgE-mediated mechanism.

Infectious Rhinitis

Most infectious causes of rhinitis occur as a viral upper respiratory infection. Viruses may account for more than 95% of acute rhinitis infections, but it can be difficult to distinguish viral from bacterial infections. Viral rhinitis infections often cause nasal mucosal edema, impairment of the ciliary movement, and often obstruction of the sinonasal cavities. Duration of symptoms greater than 7 to 10 days is used clinically to distinguish viral from bacterial rhinitis/rhinosinusitis.

Clinical History

The best diagnostic tool in the evaluation of rhinitis is the clinical history. Information regarding previous evaluation and treatment should be elicited. A positive family history of rhinitis points toward allergic disease. The history of symptoms should include questions regarding congestion; sneezing; rhinorrhea; sore throat; dry throat; cough; itchy, red, or tearing eyes; voice changes; sinus symptoms of drainage; pressure or pain; snoring; ear pain or loss of hearing; and smelling difficulty.

When gathering the details of each symptom, evaluate the onset (such as those in childhood), frequency (episodic vs. persistent), pattern (seasonality), characteristics of secretions, triggers,

severity (to include quality of life evaluation), and associated geographic location or environment (home vs. work). Once a trigger is identified, history needs to be gathered even further to evaluate the possibility of modifying the exposure.

Physical Examination

As with any disease process, the physical examination provides clues into the diagnosis (Table 1). Although the physical examination in rhinitis patients should focus on the nasal mucosa, other body areas should be examined to rule out other processes. For example, the tympanic membranes should be examined for mobility, retraction, erythema, and Eustachian tube dysfunction. Examination of the eyes in AR might show conjunctival edema, erythema, and/or cobblestoning with excessive lacrimation.

TABLE 1	Clinical Manifestations of Rhinitis
TYPE OF RHINITIS	**CLINICAL FINDINGS**
Allergic rhinitis	• Symptoms of palatal itching, nasal itching, ocular symptoms, or sneezing • Allergic shiners, allergic salute, bluish boggy turbinates, mucosal stranding
Vasomotor rhinitis	• Predominantly intermittent nasal obstruction and rhinorrhea • Symptoms triggered by temperature, exercise, and environmental stimuli (odors, smoke, and dust).
NARES	• More intense symptoms, paroxysms of flares including sneezing, watery rhinorrhea, nasal itching, congestion, and hyposmia • Eosinophils on a nasal smear, but lack other allergic evidence by skin-prick testing
Gustatory rhinitis	• Nasal congestion and rhinorrhea associated with ingestion of foods and, sometimes, alcoholic beverages
Atrophic rhinitis	• Nasal crusting, dryness, and fetor due to glandular cell atrophy • Patients may have abnormally wide nasal cavities with associated squamous metaplasia
Occupational rhinitis	• Symptoms of nasal congestion and rhinorrhea triggered by an occupational exposure • Symptoms improve when away from occupation • Common substances leading to symptoms include irritating chemicals, grain dust, ozone, laboratory animal antigens, and wood
Hormonal rhinitis	• Symptoms of nasal congestion and rhinorrhea associated with pregnancy and/or menstrual cycle • Resolves 2 weeks postdelivery
Drug-induced rhinitis	• Symptoms of rhinorrhea and congestion caused by certain medications including ACE inhibitors, phosphodiesterase-5 selective inhibitors, alpha-receptor antagonists, and phentolamine
Rhinitis Medicamentosa	• Symptoms of severe rebound nasal congestion caused by prolonged and repetitive use of topical nasal decongestants
Infectious rhinitis	• Symptoms of acute-onset nasal congestion and rhinorrhea most often caused by virus. Bacterial overgrowth from virus-induced inflammation can lead to bacterial rhinosinusitis

ACE, Angiotensin-converting enzyme; *NARES,* nonallergic rhinitis with eosinophilia syndrome.

Patients with AR may also have darkening of the skin of the lower eyelids, which is also called "allergic shiners."

A nasal examination is essential for the diagnosis of rhinitis. Otolaryngologists will often use nasal endoscopy to evaluate the sinonasal cavity, but it is not necessary to diagnose different forms of rhinitis. Allergic and nonallergic nasal mucosa often will have a similar appearance with boggy, enlarged, and erythematous inferior turbinates. Bluish turbinates with allergic stranding are more common in AR. Evidence of excessive watery-clear mucus and postnasal drainage are also common findings to rhinitis. Other examination findings, which can occur in conjunction with rhinitis, are nasal polyps, sinusitis, septal deviation, septal perforation, and crusting. Looking for elongated facies, mouth breathing, and a high arch in the palate may provide a clue to the severity of the nasal obstruction in children. The tonsils and adenoids should be examined for enlargement. Posterior nasal drainage and cobblestoning in the oropharynx are common findings in rhinitis patients.

The skin examination provides useful information in the patient with AR. Atopic dermatitis or urticaria may be findings associated with allergic disease. The skin should be evaluated for dermatographism because these patients will not be able to be evaluated for allergic disease using skin-prick testing.

Diagnosis

The diagnosis of AR, NAR, and infectious rhinitis is based largely on history and physical examination. Other diagnostic testing can be performed to aid in providing a more definitive diagnosis or to rule out other causes.

AR is confirmed by IgE reactivity to environmental allergen sensitivity through skin-prick testing. When skin-prick testing is difficult to interpret or if it is not feasible, serum–allergen-specific IgE testing can be used. Nasal smears looking for eosinophils are not recommended for routine use in the diagnosis of AR. Other testing available for evaluation of rhinitis includes nasal endoscopy and radiologic imaging. Nasal endoscopy is reserved for those with atypical symptoms or an inadequate response to treatment. Radiologic imaging, such as computed tomography (CT) and magnetic resonance imaging (MRI), is used to evaluate anatomic structure and for evidence of concomitant rhinosinusitis. If a provider suspects a cerebrospinal fluid (CSF) leak, the rhinorrhea can be evaluated for beta transferrin protein, which is present only in CSF.

Differential Diagnosis

The differential for chronic rhinitis symptoms includes AR, NAR and the many subtypes described earlier, and mixed rhinitis. Many different pathologic conditions can present similarly to rhinitis including chronic sinusitis with and without nasal polyps; ciliary dyskinesia syndrome; anatomic abnormalities such as deviated septum or septal perforation; sinonasal tumors; nasal turbinate hypertrophy; cerebrospinal fluid rhinorrhea; pharyngonasal reflux; systemic disorders such as vasculitis, sarcoidosis, and autoimmune disorders; aspirin intolerance, and other medication side effects.

Treatment
Overall
Current guidelines in treatment of rhinitis do not take cost into consideration. However, the individual treatment goals should be based on factors such as age, route of administration preference (i.e., nasal vs. oral), severity, seasonality, side effects, cost, benefit to comorbid conditions, and onset of action. For example, onset of action is an important consideration for an individual who has more episodic symptoms. Also, individual patients respond differently to treatment regimens within a given group.

Avoidance
Due to the lack of high-quality evidence, implementation of avoidance measures is largely based on panel recommendations. In addition, the ubiquitous nature of allergens may limit the effectiveness of the avoidance measures. For dust mites, encasing pillows and bedding in dust mite–resistant materials may be beneficial. Pollen is seasonal and can be minimized by keeping the windows closed, using air conditioning, and limiting outdoor exposure. Using particulate filters in the home can also assist in reducing overall allergen load of pollens and dust. Avoiding basements and lowering household humidity may reduce the amount of mold exposure patients receive. Pet avoidance can only be reached by ridding the house of the pet altogether. Other, less effective measures include limiting exposure of the pet to the house and/or bedroom.

Oral Medications
Oral Antihistamine
Oral antihistamines block H1 receptors, thereby reducing nasal and palatal itching, rhinorrhea, sneezing, conjunctivitis, and urticaria. They are recommended in the treatment of AR. However, nasal congestion is not treated well with oral antihistamines. First-generation oral antihistamines are poorly selective for H1 receptors. The sedative effects of these antihistamines result from crossing the blood–brain barrier; they have been linked to industrial accidents and contribute to loss of function at work and school. Given there is no evidence of increased efficacy over second-generation antihistamines, it is not recommended to use these medications. Second-generation H1 antagonists (e.g., cetirizine [Zyrtec, generic], levocetirizine [Xyzal, generic], fexofenadine [Allegra, generic], loratadine [Claritin, generic], desloratadine [Clarinex, generic]) have excellent evidence for therapeutic efficacy and are considered first line in the treatment of AR. They particularly help the systemic symptoms associated with AR. These medications may have some role in the treatment of NAR because of their anticholinergic properties, but consideration must be given to these systemic properties, including dry mucous membranes, blurry vision, constipation, tachycardia, and urinary retention. A combination of intranasal corticosteroid treatment with oral antihistamines may be effective for sneezing and rhinorrhea in NARES.

Leukotriene Receptor Antagonists
Currently leukotriene receptor antagonists (LTRAs) are not recommended as first-line treatment for AR and are only recommended if other first-line treatments have failed. These medications were originally found to have benefits in the treatment of asthma and thus are prescribed for concomitant asthma and AR. Montelukast (Singulair, generic) is the only US Food and Drug Administration (FDA) approved form of LTRA that is clinically efficacious in perennial and seasonal AR and asthma. Montelukast is approved for children 6 months and older and has a pregnancy category B rating. However, because of the potential rare neuropsychiatric side effects including sleep disturbances, depression, anxiety, aggression, psychotic reactions, and suicidal behavior this class of medications are used as second line. Currently LTRAs have no role in the treatment of NAR.

Oral Decongestants
Oral decongestants such as pseudoephedrine reduce nasal congestion and can temporarily relieve symptoms. They can cause significant side effects including insomnia, anorexia, irritability, palpitations, and elevation in blood pressure. They are not routinely used for the treatment for AR and NAR but can help temporarily alleviate symptoms of nasal congestion in severe disease.

Systemic Corticosteroids
Systemic corticosteroids are only recommended for the treatment of severe or intractable AR. A short 5-to 7-day course is recommended in severe cases to help decrease inflammation and improve symptoms. A prolonged course greater than 3 weeks can lead to serious side effects including adrenal suppression. They have no role in the treatment of NAR.

Intranasal Medications

Intranasal Corticosteroid. Intranasal corticosteroids (INCs) are first-line treatment for moderate to severe AR and most NAR conditions. They penetrate the nasal mucosa with the result of decreased neutrophil chemotaxis, decreased eosinophil chemotaxis, reduced mast cell mediator release, and reduced basophil mediator release. Fluticasone (Flonase, generic) and beclomethasone (Beconase AQ) are the only two topical INCs approved by the FDA for NAR. In general, this class of medications are well tolerated with minimal systemic side effects.

INC side effects include irritation, bleeding, and perforation of the nasal septum; rarely, local candidiasis is seen with INC use. No single INC preparation is more efficacious than, or has any relevant difference from, any other. INC has negligible hypothalamic-pituitary-adrenal axis suppression, and systemic burden is clinically insignificant.

Intranasal Antihistamine. Azelastine (Astepro, generic) and olapatadine (Patanase, generic) are nasal sprays approved by the FDA for AR and NAR. Azelastine, considered a first-line treatment for AR, is available in 0.1% and 0.15% formulations and is thought to improve symptoms because of its antiinflammatory properties. This medication has been shown to diminish eosinophil activation and adhesion molecule expression and suppresses generation of inflammatory cytokines. Azelastine may also reduce neurogenic excitation from olfactory stimuli. These medications have a faster onset of action than INCs and are as effective in the treatment of nasal symptoms. They are more effective and have a faster onset of action than oral antihistamines for the treatment of nasal symptoms associated with AR. Intranasal antihistamine (INA) does not produce a significant amount of sedation, but side effects include headache, epistaxis, bitter taste, and nasal irritation.

Combination Intranasal Antihistamine and Intranasal Corticosteroids. The combined use of INCs and intranasal topical antihistamines is considered to be an effective treatment for both AR and NAR. It is more effective than either medication alone. The combination of the two medications can be given separately or through a combined spray with azelastine (137 mcg) and fluticasone propionate (50 mcg) called Dymista. It is currently recommended to use combination INAs and INCs for moderate to severe AR or NAR[1] that is resistant to monotherapy. The combination therapy is more effective in relieving total nasal symptom score including nasal congestion and obstruction than either drug alone.

Intranasal Anticholinergic. Ipratropium bromide (Atrovent) is the only FDA approved intranasal anticholinergic that inhibits parasympathetic function in the nasal mucosa. The parasympathetic blockade reduces the output of secretions from seromucous glands in the nose. It is mainly used in the treatment of anterior watery rhinorrhea but has a very limited role in reducing postnasal drip, nasal congestion, or sneezing. This medication is especially helpful in gustatory rhinitis and vasomotor rhinitis where there is a specific trigger for the onset of rhinorrhea. Patients can take this medication prophylactically prior to exposure of the known trigger or irritant to help control symptoms.

Nasal Cromolyn. Cromolyn (NasalCrom, generic) is a mast cell stabilizer and inhibits the release of mast cell mediators that promote IgE-mediated AR. It should be given prophylactically prior to allergen exposure in order to reduce symptoms of AR from episodic allergen exposure. It has a favorable safety profile and is considered if first-line treatments are not effective. Cromolyn has very limited usefulness for NAR conditions.

Nasal Saline. Using nasal saline to irrigate the nasal cavities helps remove mucus, enhance ciliary movement, remove allergic and irritant particles, and moisturize the dry nasal passages. There are multiple delivery methods including nose spray, bottle, pump, irrigation, or nebulizer. However, the delivery method, volume, and isotonic or hypertonic use has not been established for the treatment of AR. There is evidence that saline irrigation for AR may reduce patient-reported disease severity compared with no saline irrigation at 3 months of treatment.

Topical Decongestants

Topical decongestants reduce congestion but have no effect on itching, sneezing, or rhinorrhea. Oxymetazoline (Afrin, generic), a common topical decongestant, causes nasal vasoconstriction and can be used as a rescue medication for severe nasal congestion symptoms. There is risk for rebound congestion with prolonged use greater than 2 to 3 days and is not routinely recommended for the treatment of AR and NAR.

Surgery and Procedures for Allergic and Nonallergic Rhinitis

The role of surgery in the treatment and management of both AR and NAR is to improve symptoms that occur as a result of the disease processes rather than treat the underlying disease. Patients with symptoms of nasal obstruction and congestion will get improvement with septoplasty (if deviated and causing obstruction) and turbinate reduction. There are multiple methods to reduce the inferior turbinate, which include minimally invasive radiofrequency ablations to partial resection of the turbinate. Recently there is evidence that reduction of enlarged nasal septal swell body and nasal vestibular swell bodies can improve symptoms of nasal congestion.

Traditionally, patients with vasomotor rhinitis can also be treated with endoscopic Vidian or posterior nasal neurectomy, which improves rhinorrhea and nasal obstruction in 90% of patients. There are risks involved in this surgery including dry eye and cheek and palate numbness, which usually resolve within 6 months of the procedure. This surgery has fallen out of favor to newer in-office techniques including cryoablation and radiofrequency ablation of the posterior nasal nerve (Clarifix and Rhinaer). These procedures can be done under local anesthesia and have shown to significantly improve total nasal symptom score including nasal congestion and rhinorrhea. They are FDA approved for the treatment of chronic rhinitis and vasomotor rhinitis.

Anti-IgE

Omalizumab (Xolair) is a monoclonal antibody available for the treatment of poorly controlled asthma, but it might have a role in the treatment of AR.[1] Omalizumab binds to IgE, hindering its relationship with inflammatory cells. Omalizumab only binds to circulating IgE and not bound IgE. Due to its high cost, reports of anaphylaxis, and its injectable-only formulation, omalizumab has a limited role in AR treatment.

Immunotherapy

Allergen extract immunotherapy has been used in the treatment of respiratory allergic disease since 1911, and its efficacy has been documented since the 1970s. The amount of allergen in each immunotherapy dose is slowly increased with each dose until a maintenance phase is reached. Immunotherapy is an effective treatment for AR and is the only treatment proven to alter the course of allergic disease. Debate exists regarding which form of immunotherapy is superior (subcutaneous vs. sublingual). Contraindications to immunotherapy include beta blocker use, due to complications in treating anaphylaxis, and uncontrolled underlying diseases, such as uncontrolled asthma.

Subcutaneous immunotherapy uses the injectable form of allergen extract. Adequate treatment usually consists of a 3- to 5-year course of immunotherapy. Subcutaneous immunotherapy is indicated in those patients for whom medications and avoidance measures are inadequate, as well as those with only a few

---

[1]Not FDA approved for this indication.

[1]Not FDA approved for this indication.

relevant allergens. The inherent risk of subcutaneous immunotherapy is systemic anaphylaxis; therefore it is dosed in the physician's office. The rate of local reactions in subcutaneous immunotherapy is 0.6% to 58% and systemic reactions is 0.06% to 0.9%. Subcutaneous immunotherapy is covered by most insurance plans.

Studies for local-route immunotherapy (noninjected), many of which were carried out in Europe, have only been undertaken in adults. Local routes of immunotherapy include sublingual, local nasal, oral, and bronchial.

Sublingual immunotherapy was approved by the FDA in April 2014. The risk profile is low and therefore can be dosed at home. The rate of local reactions with sublingual immunotherapy is 0.2% to 97% and systemic reactions is 0.056%. Multiple large meta-analyses have found noninferiority when comparing sublingual to subcutaneous immunotherapy. Some medical allergy providers use subcutaneous extracts (aqueous) as sublingual therapy, but this is an off-label use.

Monitoring

The provider should consider stepping down treatment when the patient's symptoms have been controlled. The Total Nasal Symptom Score (TNSS) is a subjective assessment of the patient's specific symptoms, including rhinorrhea, nasal congestion, sneezing, and pruritus, and can be used to assess effectiveness of medications. The Rhinoconjunctivitis Quality of Life Questionnaire can also be used. Consideration for referral to an allergist might be extended to patients who have had a prolonged course, secondary infections, polyps, or other comorbid conditions including chronic sinusitis and asthma, or if immunotherapy is a consideration.

References

Brozek J, Bousquet J, Baena-Cagnani C, et al: Allergic rhinitis and its impact on asthma (ARIA) guidelines: 2010 revision, *J Allergy Clin Immunol* 126:466–476, 2010.

Chaaban M, Corey J: Pharmacotherapy of rhinitis and rhinosinusitis, *Facial Plast Surg Clin North Am* 20:61–71, 2012.

Cox L, Compalati E, Canonica W: Will sublingual immunotherapy become an approved treatment method in the United States? *Curr Allergy Asthma Rep* 11:4–6, 2011.

Dykewicz M: Management of rhinitis: guidelines, evidence basis, and systematic clinical approach for what we do, *Immunol Allergy Clin North Am* 31:619–634, 2011.

Dykewicz MS, Wallace DV, Amrol DJ, et al: Rhinitis 2020: a practice parameter update, *J Allergy Clin Immunol* 146(4):721–767, 2020, https://doi.org/10.1016/j.jaci.2020.07.007. Epub 2020 Jul 22. Review.

Greiner A, Meltzer E: Overview of the treatment of allergic rhinitis and nonallergic rhinopathy, *Proc Am Thorac Soc* 8:121–131, 2011.

Hellings PW, Klimek L, Cingi C, et al: Non-allergic rhinitis: position paper of the European Academy of Allergy and Clinical Immunology, 72:1657–1665, 2017.

Meltzer EO, LaForce C, Ratner P, et al: MP29-02 (a novel intranasal formulation of azelastine hydrochloride and fluticasone propionate) in the treatment of seasonal allergic rhinitis: a randomized, double-blind, placebo-controlled trial of efficacy and safety, 33:324–332, 2012.

Rondon C, Campo P, Galindo L, et al: Prevalence and clinic relevance of local allergic rhinitis, *Allergy* 67:1282–1288, 2012, https://doi.org/10.1111/all.12002.

Seidman MD, Schwartz SR, Bonner JR, et al: Clinical practice guideline: allergic rhinitis, *Otolaryngol Head Neck Surg* 152(1 Suppl):S1–S43, 2015.

Settipane R, Charnock D: Epidemiology of rhinitis: allergic and nonallergic, *Clin Allergy Immunol* 19:23–34, 2007.

Sin B, Togias A: Pathophysiology of allergic and nonallergic rhinitis, *Proc Am Thorac Soc* 8:106–114, 2011.

van Cauwenberge P, Bachert C, Passalacqua G, et al: Consensus statement on the treatment of allergic rhinitis. European Academy of Allergology and Clinical Immunology, *Allergy* 55:116–134, 2000.

Wallace D, Dykewicz M: The diagnosis and management of rhinitis: an updated practice parameter, *J Allergy Clin Immunol* 122:S1–S84, 2008. Young-Yuen.

Wu A: Immunotherapy: vaccines for allergic disease, *J Thorac Dis* 4:198–202, 2012.

Yan CH, Hwang PH: Surgical management of nonallergic rhinitis, *Otolaryngol Clin North Am* 51(5):945–955, 2018.

SPINE PAIN

Method of
David Borenstein, MD; and Federico Balagué, MD

CURRENT DIAGNOSIS

- Most spine pain is mechanical in origin in 95% or more of patients.
- Symptoms of mechanical acute spine pain resolve in most patients in 1 to 8 weeks.
- Most patients with spine pain do not require laboratory tests or radiographs to achieve resolution of their symptom of spine pain.

CURRENT THERAPY

- Localized neck or low back pain
  - Encouragement to remain active out of bed
  - Patient education about the natural history to improvement
  - Reassurance about the incidence of resolution
  - Effective oral drug therapy: nonsteroidal antiinflammatory drugs (NSAIDs), analgesics, muscle relaxants
  - Physical therapy with exercise program
- Radicular pain
  - Encouragement to remain active out of bed
  - Patient education about the potential for improvement
  - Efficacy of oral drug therapy: NSAIDs, analgesics, muscle relaxants, corticosteroids, antiseizure medication, epidural corticosteroid injections
  - Physical therapy: Mackenzie exercises for disk herniation
  - Surgical decompression for cauda equina, progressive motor weakness, or intractable pain

Spine pain is a common symptom that is diagnosed and treated by a wide variety of healthcare professionals. The interest in this medical problem is not limited to its incidence as a patient problem but also stems from the likelihood of spine pain being experienced by the treating physician as well. The good news about spine pain is that the vast majority of patients (about 90%) improve over 2 months with minimal intervention, but relapses are frequent. The bad news is that the smaller number of patients who develop chronic spine pain use more than the majority of health resources expended on this expensive medical problem. The goal of therapy is to relieve spine pain while it is acute so that chronic pain does not develop.

The axial skeleton may be divided into cervical, thoracic, lumbar, sacral, and coccygeal locations. The lumbar and cervical areas are the most mobile and at greatest risk for damage. These two areas will be the primary subjects of this article.

Epidemiology

Spine pain is the most common musculoskeletal complaint worldwide and produces direct and indirect costs of hundreds of billions of dollars each year in the United States. More than 80% of the world's population at some time during their lives will have an episode of low back pain. An estimated 20% of the US population has back pain every year. Neck pain occurs at a variable rate ranging from 0.055/1000 person-years (disk herniation with radiculopathy) to 213/1000 person-years (self-reported neck pain). Thoracic spine pain is relatively rare compared with the incidence of pain in the other two locations in the axial skeleton.

Persons of all ages develop spine pain. Younger people are at risk for developmental problems (idiopathic scoliosis, spondylolysis, spondylolisthesis), and older patients develop disorders associated with degeneration of spinal structures (osteoarthritis, spinal stenosis).

Risk Factors

Psychosocial factors are stronger predictors of incident low back pain than mechanical factors in adolescent populations. In adults, psychosocial difficulties are risk factors for chronicity more strongly related to outcome than any clinical or mechanical variables. Previous episodes of spine pain are strong predictors of future ones.

Studies of cohorts of twins have shown that nonspecific low back pain is more than 60% genetically determined, and work and leisure-time physical activities play a minor role. Other environmental factors, such as smoking and obesity, have not been shown to be a predictor of the development of spine pain on a consistent basis.

Pathophysiology

Most of the structures of the axial skeleton receive sensory input. The presence of anatomic alterations in these structures is not sufficient to predict the presence of pain. In general, spine pain is referred to as nonspecific because no definite pain generator can be identified. The nociceptive inputs generated by musculoskeletal structures are referred to as *somatic pain.*

In the first few decades of life, muscular sprains and strains of the paraspinous muscles in the lumbar and cervical regions are the most likely source of spinal pain. These muscular injuries occur when lifting in a position that places stress on paraspinous structures. Often the spine is in an awkward position and is mechanically disadvantaged. The subsequent muscle injury results in reflexive muscular contraction that can recruit muscles in the same myotome. Tonic contraction approximates the damaged components of the muscle but results in relative anoxia that causes the production of anaerobic metabolites that stimulate nociceptors. The number of recruited muscles may be extensive, manifested by severe spinal stiffness and limitation of motion. Most of these soft-tissue injuries to the muscle heal spontaneously without any long-term structural alterations.

Simultaneously, as people age, intervertebral disks become flatter as the nucleus pulposus loses its absorbency and the annulus fibrosus fissures and degenerates. The process results in the loss of disk integrity. Degeneration of normal biomechanical and biochemical disk properties results. Biomechanical insufficiency inevitably results in a transfer of stresses posterior to the facet joints and ligaments that are ill suited to assume compressive, tensile, and shear loads. Osteophytes form in response to these abnormal pressures, compromising the space for the neural elements. Disk degeneration itself might not be a painful process until alterations in facet joint alignment result in the onset of articular pain.

Spondylolysis is a developmental abnormality associated with a stress fracture in the growth plate of the pars interarticularis. This abnormality may be discovered as a radiographic abnormality in an asymptomatic patient. An increased risk of low back pain occurs with spondylolisthesis, the abnormality associated with instability of spinal elements in the setting of spondylolysis.

Pain generation in the axial skeleton may be somatic or neuropathic in origin. The joints, ligaments, muscles, fascia, blood vessels, and disks can be the source of localized somatic spine pain. Somatic pain, when it does radiate, tends to be less focused in distribution and exacerbated by specific positions of the spine.

Neuropathic or radicular pain is the sensation generated by damage of neural elements. Intervertebral disk herniation with compression of spinal nerve roots causes neural inflammation resulting in neuropathic and radicular pain. Radicular pain follows the path of the corresponding spinal nerve root. In addition to pain, sensory deficits and muscle weakness can occur, depending on the intensity of the nerve compression. In the setting of chronic low back pain, the role of the central nervous system in mediating persistent symptoms has been highlighted increasingly in the medical literature.

Prevention

Since the turn of the century, epidemiologic studies in adolescents have reported nonspecific spine pain at an incidence similar to that in adult populations. This finding suggests that primary prevention must be given at a very early age to have any chance of efficacy.

Among papers reporting on primary prevention, only exercise has shown effectiveness, with effect sizes ranging from 0.39 to 0.69. Other techniques, such as stress management, shoe inserts, back supports, education, and reduced lifting, were found ineffective. Some evidence in favor of occupational interventions (exercise with or without educational component) has been recently reported.

Clinical Manifestations

The most common symptoms of spinal disorders are regional pain and decreased range of motion associated in a minority of patients with radiating pain. For the majority of patients, pain has mechanical characteristics: Its intensity increases with physical activity, movements, or some postures and decreases with rest. However, it has been demonstrated that nocturnal pain is not uncommon in the absence of serious, specific spinal disorders. The precise topography of pain is often difficult for the patient to describe, and its interpretation is difficult owing to the overlap of the cutaneous projections between adjacent spinal levels and the similarities between dermatomes, myotomes, and sclerotomes.

Diagnosis

The diagnosis of spine pain is based upon the patient's history and physical examination. The history and physical examination should include a description of the pain that is as detailed as possible (e.g., past episodes, precise location, beginning of symptoms, factors increasing or decreasing pain intensity, radiating pain, neurologic symptoms, systemic symptoms), patient's medical history (e.g., past spinal surgery, neoplasia, corticosteroid treatments), and a limited physical examination focused on the posture of the spine, range of motion, muscle contraction, pain on palpation or percussion, and a brief neurologic examination.

Besides the high rate of false-positive results and financial costs, imaging studies have a negative effect on a patient's quality of life. Therefore unless there is a clear-cut surgical indication or a suspicion of an underlying life-threatening disorder, no imaging studies should be ordered on the first encounter for a patient with acute nonspecific low back or neck pain. Similarly, laboratory testing is not required unless a patient presents with clinical symptoms that suggest a systemic illness (e.g., fever, weight loss).

Differential Diagnosis

A number of guidelines are available in the literature to help a clinician in the diagnosis and treatment of patients with spine pain. The purpose of these approaches is to differentiate the vast majority of patients with mechanical disorders who will improve with noninvasive therapy without the need for radiographic or laboratory investigation from the small minority with a specific cause of spinal pain.

Traditionally, red flags have been used to identify patients with a systemic disorder causing spine pain. The red flags have included questions regarding prior history of cancer, weight loss, prolonged morning stiffness, bladder dysfunction, and bowel dysfunction. The presence of these findings suggests a diagnosis of malignancy, infection, spondyloarthropathy, or cauda equina syndrome, respectively. A study has reported that red-flag disorders occur so infrequently and have so many false-positive findings as not to be helpful in the primary care setting at the initial

TABLE 1 Mechanical Low Back Pain

FEATURE	MUSCLE STRAIN	HERNIATED NUCLEUS PULPOSUS	OSTEOARTHRITIS	SPINAL STENOSIS	SPONDYLOLISTHESIS	SCOLIOSIS
Age (year)	20–40	30–50	> 50	> 60	20	30
Pain Pattern						
Location	Back (unilateral)	Back/leg (unilateral)	Back (unilateral)	Leg (bilateral)	Back	Back
Onset	Acute	Acute (previous episodes)	Insidious	Insidious	Insidious	Insidious
Standing	↑	↓	↑	↑	↑	↑
Sitting	↓	↑	↓	↓	↓	↓
Bending	↑	↑	↓	↓	↑	↑
Straight leg	−	+	−	+ (stress)	−	−
Plain radiograph*	−	−	+	+	+	+

↑, Increased; ↓, decreased; +, present; −, absent.
*Possibility of seeing the abnormality, not a recommendation to get radiographs.
Reprinted with permission from Mechanical low back pain. In Borenstein DG, Wiesel SW, Boden SD (eds): Low back and neck pain, 3rd ed., Philadelphia, Saunders, 2004.

visit. The one exception was spine pain associated with osteoporotic vertebral compression fractures.

Despite the findings of this one report, clinicians need to be mindful of patients who would be harmed to a significant degree by delayed therapy. The disorders that require expeditious evaluation and treatment are intraabdominal vascular disorders with tearing pain and hemodynamic instability (expanding aortic aneurysm); cauda equina syndrome with bilateral sciatica; saddle anesthesia; bladder or bowel incontinence (lumbar space-occupying compressive lesions); and cervical myelopathy with balance difficulties, autonomic dysfunction, and hyperreflexia with spasticity and Babinski's sign (cervical space-occupying compressive lesions). These disorders require expeditious vessel repair or decompression surgery.

The differential diagnosis of mechanical low back pain (Table 1) and mechanical neck pain (Table 2) includes disorders ranging from muscle strain and herniated disk to scoliosis and whiplash injuries. The age of patients, pain pattern with exacerbating and mitigating factors, tension signs, and findings of plain radiographs can help differentiate among these common causes of spine pain.

Nonspecific is a term used commonly to describe the pain associated with mechanical disorders. On occasion, physicians have confused the use of "nonspecific" as meaning an absence of pathology causing pain associated with mechanical disorders. The "nonspecific" designation refers to the inability to identify the specific pain-generating anatomic structure, not the absence of somatic pain.

Therapy

Many mechanical disorders of the spine are self-limited in duration, with a vast majority of patients improving gradually over time (Box 1). This progression to "natural healing" makes placebo look efficacious in many clinical trials investigating therapies for spine pain. This situation results in evidence-based reviews of spine pain therapies revealing very few categories that have a clinically significant impact on improvement. Nonetheless, physicians need to make therapeutic choices for their patients despite this relative paucity of evidence. Therapy for spine pain includes controlled physical activity, nonsteroidal antiinflammatory drugs (NSAIDs), skeletal muscle relaxants, local and epidural corticosteroid injections, and long-term pain therapy. Surgical intervention is reserved for patients who have surgically correctable abnormalities and who have cauda equina syndrome, increasing motor weakness, spasticity, or intractable pain.

The treatment of an individual patient has to be tailored based on the patient's expectations and preferences. Goals of the treatment should be clearly defined, and the patient should be informed about the expected benefits and side effects of the treatment at the first encounter. A short trial limited to a few days may be a good start.

Self-management with education of the patient about maintaining physical activities as tolerated has been encouraged for neck and low back pain. Information on nonpharmacologic pain-management strategies and daily life activities may be provided by healthcare providers, but patients adhere more to the former than to the latter.

Exercises are slightly effective for pain and function in patients with chronic low back pain. No specific form of exercise is clearly better than others. Simply walking has shown an efficacy similar to exercising.

The use of manipulative physical techniques in the care of patients with spine pain remains controversial. The absence of clear-cut distinctions between manipulative techniques with or without thrust adds to the confusion when one analyzes the efficacy of manual therapy treatments. Overall there is some clinical trial evidence in favor of spinal manipulation for acute low back pain.

NSAIDs have short-term efficacy for both acute and chronic low back pain; however, the effect sizes are not very large. The efficacy of these drugs for patients with radicular pain has not been evaluated well enough to make general recommendations. No single class of NSAIDs has superiority to another. Cyclooxygenase 2 (COX-2) inhibitors have a better gastrointestinal (GI) safety profile but no greater efficacy. A patient's response cannot be predicted, and a trial-and-error approach is often necessary.

Opiates have not demonstrated any favorable influence in the outcome of low back pain patients. Side effects are quite common and the risk of addiction is real. When these kinds of drugs are effective, the improvement is more important in pain intensity than in terms of function. Muscle relaxants do have some efficacy for acute and chronic low back pain, but the effect size is limited. Long-term use of muscle relaxants can effect cognitive function due to their strong anticholinergic effects.

Antidepressants are not generally prescribed owing to an inconsistent improvement of patients. For patients with chronic low back pain and depression, an optimized antidepressant treatment shows a better effect on depression than on pain and functional capacity. Duloxetine (Cymbalta), a serotonin and norepinephrine reuptake inhibitor, is approved by the US Food and Drug Administration for the indication of chronic low back pain.

Evidence is lacking to support the prescription of systemic corticosteroids. However, corticosteroids have the advantage of not being toxic to the kidneys. Oral corticosteroids may be considered in patients with radicular pain from a herniated disk or spinal stenosis where epidural injections are relatively contraindicated (chronic warfarin therapy).

FEATURE	NECK STRAIN	HERNIATED NUCLEUS PULPOSUS	OSTEOARTHRITIS	MYELOPATHY	WHIPLASH
Age (year)	20–40	30–50	> 50	> 60	30–40
Pain Pattern					
Location	Neck	Neck/arm	Neck	Arm/leg	Neck
Onset	Acute	Acute	Insidious	Insidious	Acute
Flexion	+	+	–	–	+
Extension	–	+/–	+	+	+
Plain radiograph*	–	–	+	+	–

TABLE 2 Mechanical Neck Pain

+, Present; –, absent.

*Possibility of seeing the abnormality, not a recommendation to get radiographs.

Reprinted with permission from Mechanical neck pain. In Borenstein DG, Wiesel SW, Boden SD (eds): Low back and neck pain, 3rd ed., Philadelphia, Saunders, 2004.

BOX 1 Management of Low Back Pain

Acute (3–6 Weeks)
First consultation: gather information on core outcome domains.
Rule out pain of nonspinal origin.
Rule out specific causes (red flags).
No routine imaging.
Inform and reassure the patient. Advise to stay active and continue daily activities, if possible, including work.
Prescribe analgesia, if necessary. First choice: acetaminophen; second choice: NSAIDs.
Consider adding muscle relaxants (short course) or referring for spinal manipulation.
Avoid overmedicalizing, especially in patients with favorable outcome.
Be aware of yellow flags: inappropriate attitudes and beliefs about back pain, inappropriate pain behavior, emotional problems.
Subacute (6–12 Weeks) Reassessment
Bear in mind minimum clinically important difference of core outcome tools.
Consider patients' expectations.
Consider yellow flags if outcome is not favorable.
Reassess regularly by valid outcome tools to evaluate response to treatment.
Focus on function.
Give priority to active treatments.
Consider multidisciplinary program in occupational setting for workers with subacute low back pain and sick leave (>4–8 weeks).

Chronic (3–12 Weeks)
Repeat thorough clinical examination.
In cases of low impairment and disability, simple evidence-based therapies (e.g., exercises, medication, brief interventions) might be sufficient.
In cases of more-severe disability or chronicity, give priority to multidisciplinary approaches (biopsychosocial).

NSAID, Nonsteroidal antiinflammatory drug.
From Balagué F, Mannion AF, Pellisé F, Cedraschi C: Clinical update: Low back pain. *Lancet* 369(9563):726–728, 2007.

Some patients will have persistent neuropathic pain despite surgical decompression or as a result of postsurgical fibrosis. Opioid therapy is ineffective in many patients with chronic neuropathic pain. Antiseizure medicines, such as gabapentin (Neurontin)[1] and pregabalin (Lyrica), have efficacy in peripheral neuropathic pain. These same medicines are prescribed in patients with chronic neuropathic radicular pain with the hope that the mechanisms that work with peripheral neuropathy will also work for spine pain patients. Although the evidence of benefit for nonperipheral neuropathy pain has been limited. Other medicines including antidepressants (duloxetine [Cymbalta],[1] tricyclic antidepressants) have been tried when other drugs have been ineffective.

Epidural, selective nerve root, or facet joint injections have not shown adequate efficacy to be recommended on a regular basis. However, a limited number (two or three) of spinal injections may be attempted for patients with radicular pain who do not improve with oral medication.

Spinal surgery is indicated for disk herniation with radicular compromise, cervical or lumbar spinal stenosis with myelopathy or neurogenic claudication, and unstable spondylolisthesis. Controversy remains, however, concerning the relative benefit of surgical versus medical therapy for radiculopathy. Diskectomy significantly shortens (by about 8 weeks) the acute phase of pain associated with radiculopathy. However, studies with longer follow-up periods have never shown a clear difference between conservative and surgical therapies. Some studies have shown that intensive, multidisciplinary, conservative programs can be compared with surgical fusion procedures for patients with spinal instability.

For the most chronically disabled spine pain patients only, intensive multidisciplinary programs including, among others, physical reconditioning and cognitive-behavioral methods, have shown effectiveness.

Monitoring

From the standpoint of monitoring the efficacy of the treatment, five main dimensions have been recommended to evaluate the outcome of patients with spine pain. The intensity of pain is relevant but so is the perceived functional capacity, generic health status, work disability, and satisfaction with treatment. Many tools are available for the evaluation of each specific dimension. The clinician who decides to start using any specific tool needs to know, among other information, the minimal clinically meaningful changes for each tool, because differences that may be statistically significant when comparing two groups of patients may be irrelevant at the individual patient level. For example, in terms of intensity of pain, the threshold usually accepted is 3.5 to 4.7 and 2.5 to 4.5 out of 10 for patients with acute and chronic pain, respectively.

Precisely evaluating several domains with specific tools is rather time consuming. However, for busy clinicians, there are brief instruments (core set of measures) with roughly seven or eight questions that include all the previously mentioned dimensions and that have been properly validated. One example is the Core Outcome Measure Index (COMI).

[1]Not FDA approved for this indication.

Complications

The clinician should inform the patient about the possible side effects of therapies as they are initiated. At subsequent visits, specific questions regarding the potential side effects are asked. For example, the presence of hypertension, peripheral edema, and hepatic and renal dysfunction need to be evaluated in patients who are taking chronic NSAID therapy.

In addition, a majority of NSAIDs have potential GI toxicity including mild mucosal irritation, ulcers, and perforations. Hematologic and neurologic toxicity are quite variable depending on the prescribed drug. Cardiovascular toxicity may clearly be an issue, particularly for long-term treatments. The benefit of persistent use of NSAIDs for patients with chronic spine pain needs to be weighed against the increased risk of toxicities.

Besides the risks of addiction or death, the use of opiates induces constipation and urinary retention that may be a serious problem for some patients. These drugs can also produce drowsiness, headache, nausea, or vomiting.

Antidepressants also produce drowsiness and anticholinergic symptoms during the first couple of weeks of use. These drugs have specific side effects including tachycardia, weight gain, or sexual problems.

References

Balague F, Mannion AF, Pellise F, Cedraschi C: Seminar on nonspecific low back pain, *Lancet* 379(9814):482–491, 2012.

Borenstein D: Mechanical low back pain—a rheumatologist's view, *Nat Rev Rheumatol* 9:643–653, 2013.

Briggs AM, Smith AJ, Straker LM, Bragge P: Thoracic spine pain in the general population: prevalence, incidence and associated factors in children, adolescents and adults. a systematic review, *BMC Musculoskelet Disord* 10:77, 2009.

Chou R, Baisden J, Carragee EJ, et al: Surgery for low back pain: a review of the evidence for an American Pain Society Clinical Practice Guideline, *Spine* 34(10):1094–1109, 2009.

Chou R, Deyo R, Friedly J, et al: Nonpharmacoogic therapies for low back pain: a systematic review for an American College of Physicians Clinical Practice Guideline, *Ann Intern Med* 166:493–505, 2017.

Chou R, Deyo R, Firedly J, et al: Systematoic pharmacologic therapies for low back pain: a systematic review for an American College of Physicians Clinical Practice Guideline, *Ann Intern Med* 166:480–492, 2017.

Cohen SP: Epidemiology, diagnosis and treatment of neck pain, *Mayo Clin Proc* 90:284–299, 2015.

Coombs DM, Machado GC, Richards B, et al: Clinical course of patients with low back pain following an emergency department presentation: a systematic review, *Emerg Med J* 2020. https://doi.org/10.1136/emermed-2019-20929.

Deyo RA, Mirza SK, Turner JA, Martin BI: Overtreating chronic back pain: time to back off? *J Am Board Fam Med* 22(1):62–68, 2009.

Deyo RA, Mirza SK: Herniated lumbar intervertebral disk, *N Engl J Med* 374:1763–1772, 2016.

Deyo RA, Von Korff M, Duhrkoop D: Opioids for low back pain, *BMJ* 350:g6380, 2015. https://doi.org/10.1136/bmj.g6380.

Enomoto H, Fujikoshi S, Funa J, et al: Assessment of direct analgesic effect of duloxetine for chronic low back pain: post hoc path analysis of double-blind, placebo-controlled studies, *J Pain Res* 10:1357–1368, 2017.

Friedly JL, Comstock BA, Turner JA, et al: A randomized trial of epidural glucocorticoid injections for spinal stenosis, *N Engl J Med* 371:11–21, 2014.

Fritz JM, Lane E, McFadden M, et al: Physical therapy referral from primary care for acute back pain with sciatica: a randomized controlled trial, *Ann Intern Med* 174:8–17, 2021.

Hooten WM, Cohen SP: Evaluation and treatment of low back pain: a clnically focused review for primary care specialists, *Mayo Clin Proc* 90:1699–1718, 2015.

Karran EL, McAuley JH, Traeger AC, et al: Can screening instruments accurately determine poor outcome risk in adults with recent onset low back pain? A systematic review and meta-analysis, *BMC Med* 15(1):13, 2017. Erratum reported in BMC Med. 2017 Feb 17;15(1):44.

Maher C, Underwood M, Buchbinder R: Non-specific low back pain, *Lancet* 389(10070):736–747, 2017.

Qaseem A, Wilt TJ, McLean RM, et al: Noninvasive treatments for acute, subacute, and chronic low back pain: a clinical practice guideline from the American College of Physicians, *Ann Intern Med* 166:514–530, 2017.

Rubinstein SM, de Zoete A, van Middelkoop M, et al: Benefits and harms of spinal manipulative therapy for the treatment of chronic low back pain: systematic review and meta-analysis of randomised controlled trials, *BMJ* 364:l689, 2019. https://doi.org/10.1136/bmjl689.

Sowah D, Boyko R, Antle D, et al: Occupational interventions for the prevention of back pain: overview of systematic reviews, *J Safety Res* 66:39–59, 2018.

Steffens D, Maher CG, Pereira, et al: Prevention of low back pain: a systematic review and meta-analysis, *JAMA Intern Med* 176:199–2087, 2016.

Theodore N: Degenerative cervical spondylosis, *N Engl J Med* 383:159–168, 2020.

Tsiang JT, Kinzy TG, Thompson N, et al: Sensitivity and specificity of patient-entered red flags for lower back pain, *Spine J* 19(2):293–300, 2019.

Vanti C, Andreatta S, Borghi S, et al: The effectiveness of walking versus exercise on pain and function in chronic low back pain: a systematic review and meta-analysis of randomized trials, *Disabil Rehabil* 41(6):622–632, 2019.

TINNITUS

Method of
Kenneth S. Yew, MD, MPH

CURRENT DIAGNOSIS

- Tinnitus is most commonly associated with hearing loss or exposure to loud noise.
- In addition to history and examination, most patients will benefit from an audiogram.
- Unilateral or pulsatile tinnitus, focal neurologic or otologic findings, and tinnitus with vertigo warrant imaging and further evaluation.
- Patients should be evaluated for distress from tinnitus, insomnia, depression, and anxiety.

CURRENT THERAPY

- Although no cure exists for tinnitus, education and support at initial diagnosis will help to alleviate fears, dispel misconceptions, and guide expectations of treatment.
- Hearing amplification for patients with significant hearing loss can frequently resolve tinnitus.
- Cognitive behavioral therapy (CBT)—either online or in person—can relieve distress in patients with chronic tinnitus.
- Tinnitus distress should be monitored and comorbid insomnia, depression, and anxiety treated.

Definition and Epidemiology

Tinnitus is defined as a perceived sound without an external cause. It can be classified in several ways. By a traditional method of classification, the most common type of tinnitus is subjective, defined as tinnitus without a corresponding sound on auscultation. Objective tinnitus on the other hand, can be heard by the examiner as well as the patient. The 2014 American Academy of Otolaryngology–Head and Neck Surgery Foundation (AAO-HNSF) tinnitus guideline classifies tinnitus as primary or idiopathic if, after investigation, no cause other than the presence of sensorineural hearing loss (SNHL) can be determined and secondary if it is "associated with a specific underlying cause (other than SNHL) or an identifiable organic condition." Both the traditional and AAO-HNSF classifications see tinnitus from the perspective of the examiner or investigator. Another common classification is dual, based on whether the patient has nonpulsatile or pulsatile tinnitus. Tinnitus that can be modulated by movement of the head, neck, jaw, or a limb is considered to have a somatosensory component, which is detectable in up to 83% of patients with tinnitus.

Epidemiologic studies of tinnitus have assessed different age groups, definitions, and durations. Tinnitus is estimated to affect 10% to 19% of adults and to be more common with age, peaking in the sixth and seventh decades to as high as 34.4%. A minority of patients report being bothered by their tinnitus, ranging from 6% to 20%, or about 1% overall. Men have a higher prevalence than women in most studies. Pulsatile tinnitus represents less than 10% of all presentations. Prevalence for childhood tinnitus is often similar to that for adults, but some studies show a much higher prevalence. Tinnitus is often not self-reported by the pediatric population.

Risk Factors and Etiologies

The most common causes of subjective tinnitus are SNHL and occupational or leisure-time noise exposure. Other etiologies of subjective tinnitus include the following:

1. Otologic—Conductive hearing loss, cholesteatoma, Meniere disease, vestibular schwannoma (VS), traumatic cerumen removal
2. Somatic—Temporomandibular joint (TMJ) dysfunction, head or neck injury
3. Ototoxic drugs—Anti-inflammatory agents (aspirin, nonsteroidals), antimalarials (quinine, chloroquine), antimicrobials (aminoglycosides, macrolides, tetracyclines, other), antineoplastic agents, loop diuretics, local anesthetics, and other
4. Tobacco—Current or prior smoking
5. Genetic—Moderate genetic component noted in chronic tinnitus
6. Infectious
7. Metabolic/cardiovascular—Associations with hyperlipidemia, hypertension, diabetes mellitus, thyroid disease, obesity and vitamin B12 deficiency observed in epidemiologic studies
8. Neurologic—Multiple sclerosis, vestibular migraine, tension headache, type I Chiari malformation, spontaneous intracranial hypotension, and brain-stem stroke
9. Psychiatric—Stress. Most studies have found an association between chronic tinnitus and depression/anxiety symptoms. More severe tinnitus is associated with a greater likelihood of depression and/or anxiety. Neither depression nor anxiety has been demonstrated to cause tinnitus. (Data partially adapted from Yew, 2014.)

The most common causes of pulsatile tinnitus include vascular stenosis due to atherosclerosis or fibromuscular dysplasia, idiopathic intracranial hypertension, and venous malformations. Other causes include the following:

1. Arterial—Dural arteriovenous fistula, glomus tumors, arteriovenous malformation, tortuosity or aneurysm, hypertension
2. Venous—Sigmoid sinus dehiscence or diverticulum, venous hum
3. Otologic—Superior canal dehiscence, patulous eustachian tube, otosclerosis
4. Myoclonus—Stapedius, tensor tympani or palatal muscles
5. Hyperdynamic states or increased bone vascularity—pregnancy, anemia, thyrotoxicosis, Paget disease, bone invading tumors or hemangiomas
6. Somatosensory

Pathophysiology

Tinnitus is thought to arise from an intricate interaction between peripheral and central mechanisms. Although the inciting event for tinnitus may be hearing loss or cochlear damage, the actual generation and maintenance of tinnitus occurs centrally, involving both auditory and nonauditory pathways. Decreased input from the peripheral auditory system alters the excitatory/inhibitory balance within the central auditory processing system. This, in turn, may cause signal hyperactivity and increased synchrony between neural centers as the brain tries to maintain its pre–hearing loss state, a process called "homeostatic plasticity." These processes may account for a phenomenon called *central gain*, in which the central auditory system becomes hypersensitive. Human and animal studies suggest a role for the brain's emotional/cognitive areas—including the temporal, parietal, sensorimotor and limbic cortices—in the pathogenesis of tinnitus. Limbic nonauditory and auditory pathway interactions have been found in tinnitus patients using multiple functional imaging modalities, but not all investigators have confirmed differences between patients with and without tinnitus. Frontostriatal circuits appear to be critical in the development and maintenance of both tinnitus and chronic pain, consistent with the view that tinnitus, phantom limb pain, and central pain sensitization may share common pathways. The perception of tinnitus also seems to reside in somatic memory. The medial geniculate body in the thalamus is posited as the site of connection between sound perception, the auditory cortex, and the limbic system. A number of theoretical models of tinnitus psychopathology exist, but as yet none has been found to account for all findings in patients with tinnitus.

Prevention

Hearing conservation, careful use of ototoxic drugs, and smoking cessation should help to prevent tinnitus. Maintaining a healthy weight and engaging in regular physical activity should reduce tinnitus by preventing obesity and the development of metabolic risk factors. Industrial hearing conservation programs are well established; however, leisure time noise exposure is now associated with more hearing loss than occupational exposure. The use of hearing protection while firing weapons and using power tools should be encouraged. Personal listening devices (PLDs) represent the greatest current risk to hearing. A recent systematic review of studies examining short- and long-term hearing effects in PLD users found evidence of significantly poorer hearing thresholds in long-term PLD users compared with nonusers. Keeping volume settings to no more than 60% or 70% of maximum should comply with current World Health Organization guidelines to limit leisure noise to less than 70 dB for continuous exposure and less than 85 dB for up to 2 hours/days, respectively.

Clinical Manifestations

Patients report an abrupt or insidious onset of a sound in one or both ears that is continuous or intermittent. The sound may be a ringing, buzzing, roaring, or clicking; it may be high or low pitched. The tinnitus may have a pulsatile quality. Its severity and persistence may vary from transient and mild to chronic and severe. If sought carefully, the pitch or loudness of the tinnitus may be modulated by moving the head, neck, or jaw. Headache or recent head or neck injury can precede certain causes of tinnitus. Other otologic symptoms include preexisting hearing loss, hearing loss or ear fullness during tinnitus, vertigo, noise annoyance, or ear pain. How bothersome tinnitus is to patients varies by its severity and the presence of coexisting depression or anxiety symptoms.

Diagnosis

The evaluation of patients presenting with tinnitus in a primary care setting includes a thorough history and focused examination. Most patients need an audiogram and some will require imaging or standardized tinnitus impact investigations.

History

Description—Onset, pitch, quality, unilateral/bilateral, loudness, continuous/intermittent, pulsatile/nonpulsatile

Associated symptoms—Hearing loss, vertigo, otalgia, ear fullness, hyperacusis, headache, neck or TMJ pain, visual disturbance, gait problem, weakness, or paresthesia

Provocative/palliative factors—Stress; change in tinnitus with head, neck, or jaw movement

Past history—Prior tinnitus, hearing loss, occupational/leisure noise exposure, recent head, neck, or ear injury; bruxism; current or recent medications; medical history, tobacco use

Family history—Chronic tinnitus, Meniere disease or otosclerosis

Impact—Degree of tinnitus distress, insomnia, or lifestyle interference

Examination

General—Blood pressure, body mass index

Head—Masticatory muscle or TMJ tenderness; tinnitus changed by head, face, or jaw movement or contraction

Eye—Nystagmus if vertigo history and papilledema if headache history

Ear—Cerumen impaction, otorrhea, cholesteatoma, retrotympanic mass*

Neck—Neck mass, tenderness

Neurologic—Cranial nerves; neurologic exam if neurologic symptoms, headache, vertigo, or pulsatile tinnitus

Psychologic—Screen for depression and anxiety if mood symptoms or bothersome tinnitus

---

* If a retrotympanic mass suspected, the patient should be referred for a microscopic otologic exam prior to imaging.

TABLE 1	Imaging for Patients with Tinnitus	
PRESENTATION OF TINNITUS	**IMAGING CHOICE**	**COMMENT**
Uncomplicated, bilateral, and nonpulsatile	None	Hearing loss symmetric if present. No other indications for imaging, such as stroke/TIA symptoms, acute vestibular syndrome, focal neurologic exam, or retrotympanic mass.
Bilateral and nonpulsatile with asymmetric hearing loss by audiogram or unilateral and nonpulsatile	MRI of head and IAC	Vestibular Schwannoma risk ~2%.
Synchronous and pulsatile	MRI/MRA of head and IAC	If negative and there is concern for dAVF, consider 4D-CTA if available or DSA. Add MRV if concern for venous etiologies or IIH.
Synchronous pulsatile with suspicion of retrotympanic mass by microscopic examination or temporal bone disease	CTA of head and IAC with temporal bone reconstruction	
Nonsynchronous, pulsatile	MRI or CT of head	

CT, Computed tomography; *4D-CTA*, dynamic computed tomographic angiography; *dAVF*, dural arteriovenous fistula; *DSA*, digital subtraction angiography; *IAC*, internal auditory canal; *IIH*, idiopathic intracranial hypertension; *MRA*, magnetic resonance angiography; *MRI*, magnetic resonance imaging; *MRV*, magnetic resonance venography; *TIA*, transient ischemic attack.

For pulsatile tinnitus—
1. Palpate pulse—ask patient to tap out the tinnitus frequency.
2. Not pulse synchronous—consider patulous eustachian tube or myoclonic etiologies.
3. Pulse synchronous—auscultate for bruits over mastoid, preauricular area, temple, orbits, carotids, and for cardiac murmurs.
    a. To evaluate for venous etiology—apply light pressure to the ipsilateral jugular. Decreased loudness of bruit or tinnitus supports a venous etiology.
    b. To evaluate for arterial or arteriovenous etiology—apply pressure to the ipsilateral carotid. Decreased loudness of bruit or tinnitus supports an arterial or arteriovenous etiology. Use caution in elderly patients.

Although SNHL is the most common etiology for tinnitus, it is important to evaluate for other etiologies during the initial evaluation. Brief intermittent nonpulsatile tinnitus without associated headache, neurologic symptoms, hearing loss, or vertigo may be observed without further evaluation. Recent loud noise exposure, use of an ototoxic medication, or head/neck trauma can inform the diagnosis and guide both therapy and prognosis. Headache should prompt a careful search for findings suggestive of vestibular migraine, idiopathic intracranial hypertension, or spontaneous intracranial hypotension. Unilateral tinnitus with vertiginous symptoms with or without hearing loss suggests vestibular migraine, Meniere disease, or VS. An abrupt onset is more often seen in somatosensory tinnitus, migraine, Meniere disease, and brain-stem stroke or transient ischemic attack.

Tinnitus with a somatosensory component is suggested if the patient is able to change the tinnitus by movement or muscle contraction, especially if he or she has had a recent head or neck injury, coincident onset of musculoskeletal pain and tinnitus, bruxism, or TMJ pain.

An audiogram should be obtained for patients with unilateral tinnitus, suspicion of hearing loss or tinnitus lasting over 6 months, and is an option for patients with tinnitus of less than 6 months. A criterion for asymmetric hearing loss to optimize sensitivity for VS is an average 10 dB difference over the frequencies 1 to 8 kHz.

No reviewed guideline recommends laboratory testing to evaluate patients with tinnitus. Laboratory investigation in patients presenting with tinnitus can be guided by clinical suspicion and existing preventive services screening guidelines.

Table 1 lists imaging options for patients with tinnitus. Specialty consultation is helpful to evaluate the myriad causes of pulsatile tinnitus. Magnetic resonance imaging may be uncomfortable for patients with tinnitus with noise sensitivity. In such cases, contrast-enhanced computed tomography is an alternative.

Patients with tinnitus should be asked about how bothered they are by their tinnitus. If bothersome tinnitus is endorsed, then it is helpful to learn how the tinnitus is interfering with the patient's sleep, work, concentration, mood, and quality of life. This understanding will guide subsequent education, support, evaluation, and therapy. Validated questionnaires to assess tinnitus impact and monitor therapeutic response include the Tinnitus Handicap Inventory (THI), screening THI (THI-S) and Tinnitus Functional Index (TFI). The National Institute for Health and Care Excellence (NICE) tinnitus guideline highlights the TFI as it assesses global tinnitus impact, hearing acuity, sleep, anxiety, and depression. The TFI is available at https://apps.ohsu.edu/research/tech-portal/technology/view/1004796.

Differential Diagnosis

Brief spontaneous tinnitus, also called "transient ear noise," is a benign, fleeting, high-pitched, unilateral sound of unknown cause sometimes accompanied by a sensation of hearing loss. The tonal quality of tinnitus must be distinguished from the voices or music heard in an auditory or musical hallucination. Musical hallucinations can be experienced by people with SNHL or more rarely as a manifestation of epilepsy.

Treatment

Goals for treating patients with tinnitus are to help them understand that tinnitus is common, normally benign, and can improve over time; if it is chronic, therapies exist to help such patients live well with it. Table 2 lists evidence-based tinnitus therapies. Observation with support and education after negative diagnostic workup can be sufficient if tinnitus is not bothersome. In a recent observational study of patients with intrusive tinnitus, the provision of a standardized bundle of tinnitus information to all patients was associated with a nearly a fourfold drop in patients who requested further formal treatment for their tinnitus. Patient interview studies document that tinnitus support and education is beneficial at every stage of care. However, as many as 82.6% patients with tinnitus surveyed worldwide felt that their tinnitus was managed "not very effectively" or "not at all." As there is still no cure for tinnitus, part of this dissatisfaction may stem from their expectations of therapy. When US audiologists and their patients were asked about treatment goals, audiologists endorsed reduced tinnitus awareness, stress, and anxiety, whereas their patients wanted reduced tinnitus loudness or its elimination. Accurate, supportive education about tinnitus and its treatment is essential to help patients develop informed expectations. Table 3 lists selected patient education resources for tinnitus.

Aside from hearing amplification and CBT, no other therapy has proven effectiveness for tinnitus. Sound therapy to help distract from

TABLE 2 — Treatment for Patients with Chronic Tinnitus

TREATMENT	COMMENT
Support and education—in addition to providing printed or online materials, provide teaching at time of evaluation.	Help patients understand what tinnitus is and that it is typically benign. Explain that tinnitus is a result of not a cause for hearing loss. Reassure that it may persist but can improve over time. Discuss the potential for medications to cause or worsen tinnitus. Discuss prevention of tinnitus. Discuss no cures at present but management helpful to relieve distress. Review beneficial treatments and treatments unlikely to benefit.
Amplification.	Offer if hearing loss is affecting communication and consider for hearing loss without communication difficulties. Do not offer without documented hearing loss.
Sound therapy—via an in-ear or wearable device, environmental sound, smartphone, etc.	Option to offer but there is limited current evidence of efficacy.
Medications.	Avoid. Currently there is no evidence for efficacy of any medication to improve tinnitus. Medication may help with insomnia, depression, or anxiety if present.
Psychological therapies.	CBT is the most effective therapy for reducing tinnitus distress and severity. The NICE guideline suggests a stepped approach beginning with online CBT, then group therapy, then individual CBT.
Combination therapies—Tinnitus retraining therapy with amplification, with or without sound therapy.	Current evidence does not support additional efficacy of this widely practiced approach beyond usual care.
Neuromodulation—Repetitive transcranial magnetic stimulation (rTMS), transcranial direct current stimulation (tDCS), transcutaneous vagal nerve stimulation (tVNS), acoustic neuromodulation therapy and others.	Experimental. Insufficient evidence of efficacy from short-term small studies.
Other therapies—Acupuncture, herbal, vitamins, minerals and other dietary supplements.	Ineffective or inconclusive.
Treatments for somatosensory tinnitus.	Some evidence for oromyofascial therapy, dental occlusal splints, physical therapy, and relaxation training.

CBT, Cognitive behavioral therapy; NICE, National Institute for Health and Care Excellence.
Data from NICE, AAO-HNSF and European tinnitus guidelines.

TABLE 3 — Education Resources for Patients

SPONSORING ORGANIZATION	INTERNET ADDRESS
American Tinnitus Association—Podcasts, tinnitus education and support	https://www.ata.org Tinnitus Patient Navigator: https://www.ata.org/managing-your-tinnitus/tinnitus-patient-navigator
British Tinnitus Association (BTA)—A wealth of information and support for people with tinnitus	https://www.tinnitus.org.uk
"Take on Tinnitus"—Free, self-paced, brief modules from the BTA designed to help patients get information "quickly and easily"	www.takeontinnitus.co.uk
Excellent tinnitus information booklets from UK-based Action on Hearing Loss	https://www.actiononhearingloss.org.uk/how-we-help/information-and-resources/publications/tinnitus/
Tinnitus information from the Hearing Health Foundation	https://hearinghealthfoundation.org/what-is-tinnitus
How to Manage Your Tinnitus: A Step-by-Step Workbook, 3rd edition Handbook produced by the US Veterans Administration incorporating sound therapy and cognitive behavioral therapy	http://www.ncrar.research.va .gov/Education/Documents/TinnitusDocuments/HowTo MangageYourTinnitus.pdf
Hyperacusis Network—Extensive support and education about hyperacusis and tinnitus	http://www.hyperacusis.net
World Health Organization—"Make Listening Safe" brochures in multiple languages	https://www.who.int/pbd/deafness/activities/MLS/en/

or mask tinnitus may be helpful for individual patients, but evidence of its overall efficacy is limited. Tinnitus Retraining Therapy (TRT) classically combines sound-enrichment therapy and directive counseling. It can be combined with amplification. Although its individual components may be beneficial, combined TRT has not proven superior in reducing tinnitus distress compared with usual care.

Many medications as well as mineral and herbal supplements have been studied for the treatment of tinnitus, but none have proven beneficial. Available studies of acupuncture for tinnitus treatment are limited by methodologic flaws, precluding its recommendation as an effective tinnitus therapy. A variety of neuromodulation techniques to treat tinnitus have been studied; however, the studies have been small and relatively brief, with heterogeneous results. Patients with a somatosensory component to their tinnitus may experience relief from physical or dental splint therapies.

CBT targets thoughts and emotions to affect behavior. Drawing attention to inaccurate thoughts and thought patterns aided by a skilled therapist can help patients develop a more beneficial response to their tinnitus. Other cognitive-based approaches that have been studied for tinnitus include mindfulness-based CBT (MBCT) and acceptance and commitment therapy (ACT). All of these therapies have been shown to decrease the severity and distress of tinnitus but have not improved quality of life or mitigated tinnitus annoyance or loudness, depression, anxiety, or sleep. The one exception is ACT, which, compared with control patients, was found to decrease tinnitus-associated depression. Limited access to CBT therapists is an issue for many patients. Online CBT and ACT effectively reduces tinnitus severity and distress, although in-person therapy tends to have a larger effect.

Monitoring

Response to therapy can be assessed by clinical impression or a validated instrument like the TFI. As tinnitus can be associated with depression, use of a depression screening instrument such as the PHQ-9 and inquiring about suicidal ideation is recommended, especially for patients with at least moderately distressing tinnitus. If distress from tinnitus is not improving or worsens, review the completeness of the workup and discuss with the patient a referral for CBT or tinnitus specialty evaluation. Fortunately, although the severity of tinnitus may fluctuate, over time it tends not to worsen and may improve.

Complications

Carefully monitoring the level of a patient's distress from tinnitus, diagnosing treatable etiologies, and recognizing and treating comorbid conditions such as depression, insomnia, and anxiety will help to avoid most complications. It is unknown if tinnitus is a risk factor for future dementia in a person with SNHL or if screening for dementia in this setting will improve outcome.

References

Tinnitus: assessment and management (NG155). National Institute for Health and Care Excellence; March 11, 2020. Available at https://www.nice.org.uk/guidance/ng155. [Accessed 4/1/20].

Cima RFF, Mazurek B, Haider H, et al: A multidisciplinary European guideline for tinnitus: diagnostics, assessment, and treatment, *HNO* 67(Suppl 1):10–42, 2019.

Haider HF, Bojic T, Ribeiro SF, et al: Pathophysiology of subjective tinnitus: triggers and maintenance, *Front Neurosci* 12:866, 2018. Available at https://www.ncbi.nlm.nih.gov/pmc/articles/PMC6277522/pdf/fnins-12-00866.pdf. [Accessed 4 May 2020].

Hassaan A, Trinidade A: The tinnitus patient information pack: usefulness in intrusive tinnitus, *Int J Health Care Qual Assur* 32(2):360–365, 2019.

McCormack A, Edmondson-Jones M, Somerset S, et al: A systematic review of the reporting of tinnitus prevalence and severity, *Hear Res* 337:70–79, 2016.

McFerran DJ, Stockdale D, Holme R, et al: Why is there no cure for tinnitus?, *Front Neurosci* 13:802, 2019. Available at https://www.ncbi.nlm.nih.gov/pmc/articles/PMC6691100/pdf/fnins-13-00802.pdf. [Accessed 24 April 2020].

Pegge SAH, Steens SCA, Kunst HPM, et al: Pulsatile tinnitus: differential diagnosis and radiological work-up, *Curr Radiol Rep* 5(1):5, 2017. Available at https://www.ncbi.nlm.nih.gov/pmc/articles/PMC5263210/pdf/40134_2017_Article_199.pdf. [Accessed 21 March 2020].

Rosing SN, Schmidt JH, Wedderkopp N, et al: Prevalence of tinnitus and hyperacusis in children and adolescents: a systematic review, *BMJ Open* 6(6):e010596, 2016. Available at https://www.ncbi.nlm.nih.gov/pmc/articles/PMC4893873/pdf/bmjopen-2015-010596.pdf. [Accessed 18 March 2020].

Scherer RW, Formby C, Group TRTTR: Effect of tinnitus retraining therapy vs standard of care on tinnitus-related quality of life: a randomized clinical trial, *JAMA Otolaryngol Head Neck Surg* 145(7):597–608, 2019.

Trevis KJ, McLachlan NM, Wilson SJ: A systematic review and meta-analysis of psychological functioning in chronic tinnitus, *Clin Psychol Rev* 60:62–86, 2018.

Tunkel DE, Bauer CA, Sun GH, et al: Clinical practice guideline: tinnitus, *Otolaryngol Head Neck Surg* 151(2 Suppl):S1–S40, 2014.

Yew KS: Diagnostic approach to patients with tinnitus, *Am Fam Physician* 89(2):106–113, 2014.

You S, Kong TH, Han W: The effects of short-term and long-term hearing changes on music exposure: a systematic review and meta-analysis, *Int J Environ Res Public Health* 17(6):2091, 2020. Available at: https://www.mdpi.com/1660-4601/17/6/2091/htm. [Accessed 25 April 2020].

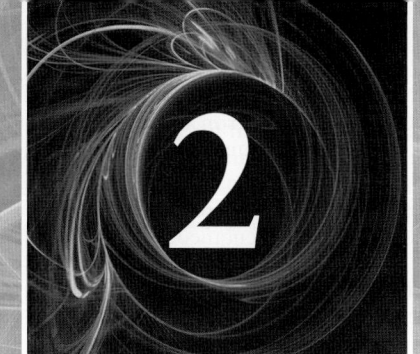

2 Allergy

ALLERGIC REACTIONS TO INSECT STINGS

Method of
James M. Quinn, MD

CURRENT DIAGNOSIS

Classify reaction based upon clinical manifestations
- Local reactions
  - Uncomplicated "usual" local reaction—mild redness, pain, and swelling limited to area of sting
  - Large local reaction—redness, pain, and swelling extending beyond area of sting
- Systemic reactions
  - Cutaneous only—flushing, urticaria, angioedema (excluding tongue, throat, larynx)
  - Anaphylaxis (cutaneous symptoms and/or respiratory symptoms, gastrointestinal symptoms, cardiovascular symptoms, uterine cramping, etc.)

CURRENT THERAPY

- Local reactions
  - Uncomplicated local reaction
    - H1 antihistamines, analgesics, cold compress
    - Discuss avoidance measures
  - Large local reaction
    - H1 antihistamines, analgesics, cold compress, avoidance measures
    - Discuss avoidance measures
    - Further evaluation, testing, epinephrine autoinjectors optional
- Systemic reactions
  - Cutaneous only
    - Based upon clinical situation and prior history
    - H1 antihistamines, epinephrine in some circumstances
    - Discuss avoidance measures
    - Further evaluation, testing, epinephrine autoinjectors optional
  - Anaphylaxis
    - Epinephrine intramuscularly
    - Consider adjunctive therapy—antihistamines, bronchodilators, intravenous fluids, vasopressors, oxygen, other supportive measures.
    - Provide epinephrine autoinjectors
    - Discuss avoidance measures
    - Consider further evaluation, testing, consideration of immunotherapy

Pathophysiology

The pathophysiology of insect sting reactions varies based upon the classification. Uncomplicated local reactions are due to direct toxic effects of the venoms. Venom components include enzymes, vasoactive amines, peptides, and other contents that directly lead to local cell death, tissue destruction, vasodilatation, altered hemostasis, and inflammation.

Fire ant stings initially follow the pattern of the uncomplicated local reactions described. Fire ant venom is unique in containing highly basic pH piperidine alkaloids. Piperidine alkaloids lead to local tissue necrosis and a pathognomonic sterile pseudopustule at the center of an otherwise uncomplicated local reaction.

Large local reactions result from an immunologic response rather than simply direct toxic effects. The reaction is a broader and more sustained immunologic late-phase response to specific antigens in the venom. It is often (up to 80% of cases) associated with and possibly mediated by venom-specific immunoglobulin E (IgE).

Systemic reactions are characterized by signs and symptoms occurring distantly from the sting site. Onset is generally rapid and can include cutaneous, respiratory, cardiovascular, gastrointestinal, and/or other symptoms. Systemic reactions are the result of mast cell degranulation from venom specific-IgE binding. Mast cells release a wide array of vasoactive amines, prostaglandins, leukotrienes, platelet activating factor, and other cytokines. These lead to vasodilatation, capillary leak, edema, bronchospasm, etc.

There are clinical situations when patients should be suspected of having an underlying mast cell disorder as a pathophysiologic contributor. These include very severe anaphylaxis, hypotension, severe anaphylaxis without cutaneous symptoms, and patients without detectable IgE.

Prevention

Prevention focuses on avoidance of stings. General strategies that may be effective include using professional exterminators for known nests with periodic reinspections; wearing fully closed-toe shoes or sandals outdoors (include socks for fire ant prevention); use of caution when or avoidance of eating or drinking outdoors, especially drinking from closed or opaque containers or straws; vigilance in wooded areas, around flowering plants, and garbage; and wearing shoes, socks, long pants, long sleeves, and hats when gardening or performing other "at-risk" outdoor activity. If the history of the sting or diagnostic testing identifies the suspected insect, teach patients about the habits and nesting of the specific insect.

Stinging insects are the Hymenoptera order and include the Apidae (bee) family of honeybees and bumblebees; the Vespidae (wasp) family of hornets, yellow jackets, and paper wasps; and the Formicidae (ant) family of the imported fire ant. Honeybees and bumblebees are generally not aggressive. They feed on nectar from flowering plants and will sting only in self-defense such as stepping barefoot on a bee in a field or with an accidental close encounter. Bees will also sting after a direct threat to their nests. Bees nests can be found in commercial hives, tree hollows, old logs, or, less commonly, in the walls of buildings. Africanized honeybees, found primarily in the southern third of the United States, differ only in that they are far more aggressive in defense of their hives. Massive and persistent retaliation can result simply from the vibration of lawn equipment several yards from their hive. The stingers of bees are barbed and often result in retention of the stinger and venom sac at the sting site. A retained stinger can occur, although less commonly, with wasps.

Yellow jackets are scavengers, seeking food wherever available—at picnics, around garbage containers, in soda cans, etc. They are highly aggressive and may sting even if unprovoked. Their nests are found underground, in rotted wood, or in wall spaces. In many areas of the country, yellow jackets are the most common cause of stings.

Hornets and paper wasps generally are not aggressive and do not sting unless defending their nests. Paper wasp nests are classically thin, paper-like honeycomb structures found under the eaves of homes, windowsills, and railings. Hornet nests are typically grayish paper mâché structures hanging from tree limbs. There are several species of hornets and wasps that have black and yellow coloring that can make them difficult to distinguish from yellow jackets and bees, making simple visual identification unreliable.

Imported fire ants are extremely aggressive, especially in defense of their nest. Fire ants are endemic to the southern United States. Fire ant nests are built underground and generally capped by a mound of overlying loose soil. Individual ants can sting multiple times and the disturbed mound easily spills out hundreds to thousands of workers prepared to sting in defense of the nest.

Clinical Manifestations

Classification of insect sting reactions based upon the clinical manifestations is important to the diagnostic and therapeutic approach. Most insect sting reactions can be classified as local or systemic. Local reactions are further subdivided as uncomplicated local reactions or as large local reactions. Systemic reactions can be further subdivided as cutaneous only or as anaphylaxis.

Uncomplicated local reactions are the expected usual reaction and are characterized by mild redness, pain, itching, and swelling limited to the area of sting generally not larger than 5 to 10 cm. These local reactions begin immediately after the sting and generally resolve over several hours but may linger up to 48 hours. Uncommonly, the pain, burning, or itch of an isolated fire ant sting goes unnoticed, but the sterile pseudopustule appears within 24 hours of the sting.

Large local reactions occur in approximately 5% to 15% of insect stings. These reactions are generally defined as larger than 10 cm or a patient's palm and can progress, involving an entire limb. Large local reactions generally begin within 6 to 12 hours, peak within 24 to 48 hours, and resolve within 3 to 10 days. Large local reactions commonly recur with repeat stings.

Systemic reactions occur in approximately 1% to 7% of stings. Systemic cutaneous-only reactions are limited to flushing, urticaria, and angioedema (excluding the airway—tongue, throat, larynx). Most systemic reactions in children are cutaneous only, whereas most systemic reactions in adults are anaphylactic.

Systemic anaphylaxis occurs in 1% to 3% of stings. Anaphylaxis is defined as the acute onset (minutes to several hours) of symptoms after a sting and include two or more of the following organ systems: cutaneous (pruritus, flushing, urticaria, angioedema), respiratory (shortness of breath, chest tightness, cough, stridor, wheezing), cardiovascular (light headedness, syncope, tachycardia, hypotension), or gastrointestinal (abdominal pain, nausea, vomiting, diarrhea). In addition, anaphylaxis can be defined as the acute onset of hypotension after exposure to a known allergen for the patient.

Toxic reactions can occur due to large numbers of stings (>20 to 50 flying Hymenoptera stings in an adult). Toxic signs and symptoms are often delayed and can include myalgia, fevers/chills, headache, rhabdomyolysis, renal failure, hemolysis, diffuse intravascular coagulation, acute respiratory distress syndrome, and death. The lethal dose for a 60-kg adult has been estimated at more than 1100 honeybee stings.

There are also unusual and rare reactions of unknown pathophysiology that include glomerulonephritis, Guillain-Barré syndrome, seizures, and serum sickness.

Diagnosis

Categorizing the type of reaction is essential for risk assessment, diagnostic evaluation, and treatment planning. History of the event, signs and symptoms, and response to therapy are important and will allow the reaction to be accurately categorized as uncomplicated local, large local, systemic cutaneous-only, or systemic anaphylaxis.

Patients experiencing uncomplicated local reactions are not at increased risk of anaphylaxis and do not require additional diagnostic evaluation.

Patients experiencing large local reactions generally do not require additional diagnostic evaluation because they have a small relative risk of future anaphylaxis. Despite the common occurrence of venom specific IgE, only 4% to 10% of patients with a history of large local reactions go on to develop a systemic reaction, and only less than 5% go on to develop anaphylaxis after repeat stings.

Patients with systemic cutaneous-only reactions generally do not require additional diagnostic evaluation because they also have a small relative risk of future anaphylaxis. Only 10% to 15% of children with systemic cutaneous-only reactions have recurrent cutaneous-only reactions and less than 3% go on to have anaphylaxis. For adults with cutaneous-only reactions, there is a less than 3% to 5% risk of progression to anaphylaxis after resting.

There may be special situations when patients with large local or systemic cutaneous-only reactions are at increased risk and would benefit from referral to consider additional diagnostic testing, epinephrine autoinjectors, and possible immunotherapy. Special situations include frequent stings, high-risk medical conditions, at-risk medications (β-blockers, angiotensin-converting enzyme [ACE] inhibitors), impaired quality of life, and/or imported fire ant stings. Data regarding future risk of repeat fire ant stings are not robust, and multiple sting attack rates are high. In these patients, the decision regarding evaluation and therapy is based on a risk-benefit discussion with the patient.

Patients with systemic anaphylaxis after stings should undergo referral for further diagnostic testing. Patients with systemic reactions to stings have a 25% to 75% chance of another systemic reaction with the highest rates of recurrence seen with more severe reactions. Systemic anaphylaxis to insect stings can be fatal. Insect stings account for up to 20% of all fatalities due to anaphylaxis and estimates are that 40 (and likely more) patients die annually from insect sting anaphylaxis in the United States.

Additional diagnostic testing may commonly include prick and intradermal skin testing, serologic assessment of specific IgE, and serum tryptase.

Therapy and Monitoring

Uncomplicated local reaction should be cleaned, and any retained stinger carefully removed. Symptomatic therapy with antihistamines, analgesics, and cold compresses can be administered. Patients should also be given advice regarding avoidance measures to prevent future stings. In the case of fire ant stings, the pseudopustule is sterile and bacteriostatic; it should not be unroofed or opened.

Large local reactions should be approached similarly to uncomplicated local reactions with symptomatic therapy. For patients with frequent painful and/or debilitating large local reactions, the unstudied method of a short burst of oral corticosteroids for 3 to 7 days is sometimes used. Efficacy with immunotherapy for large local reactions has been demonstrated in early trials, but further study is needed. Unneeded antibiotic therapy for cellulitis should be avoided. Cellulitis is unlikely at 24 to 48 hours when patients commonly present. Later presentations of large local reactions can make distinguishing cellulitis more difficult. However, after 48 hours, many large, local reactions are plateauing or improving while infection would be expected to worsen. In addition, presence of fever would suggest infection.

Systemic cutaneous-only reactions (flushing, urticaria, angioedema not involving the airway) may require a more nuanced approach. Because of the low risk of developing additional symptoms, patients with a history of prior cutaneous-only reactions can be appropriately treated with antihistamines and close observation if they present again with cutaneous-only reactions. On the other hand, patients with a history of anaphylaxis who may initially present with cutaneous-only symptoms should immediately be treated with injectable epinephrine because of the significant risk that additional symptoms will develop.

Those patients with large local reactions or systemic cutaneous-only reactions and in whom special situations exist may be given epinephrine autoinjectors, recommended to wear medical identification information, and referred to an allergist/immunologist for consideration of further evaluation.

Systemic anaphylaxis to insect stings should be treated acutely in the same way as anaphylaxis from any cause. The drug of choice, epinephrine 1 mg/mL (1:1000), should be injected intramuscularly preferentially in the lateral thigh with 0.3 to 0.5 mg in adults and 0.01 mg/kg up to 0.3 mg in children without delay. Transport to a fully capable emergency medical facility should be undertaken as soon as practicable. As available, adjunctive therapies with antihistamines, bronchodilators, intravenous fluids, vasopressors, oxygen, and other supportive measures can be considered after the administration of epinephrine based on the clinical scenario. These adjunctive therapies should not be used as a substitute for possible repeat doses of epinephrine if additional epinephrine is available and indicated. Epinephrine administration should not be delayed because delayed use of epinephrine has been associated with fatal reactions in humans. In addition, animal models demonstrate that advanced anaphylaxis can become refractory to epinephrine. Patients with a rapid and complete response to initial therapy should generally be observed for 3 to 6 hours. Prolonged observation or admission should be considered for patients with severe, prolonged, or refractory symptoms.

After acute treatment but before discharge, patients should be given an epinephrine autoinjector (Auvi-Q, EpiPen) and instructed in the proper technique for use. Patients should be instructed in basic avoidance strategies to prevent future stings and offered medical identification information. Patients should understand the significant risk of recurrence and the need to follow up for additional testing and consideration for immunotherapy. If additional evaluation identifies specific IgE to the stinging insect, immunotherapy can be offered. Immunotherapy to stinging insects is quite effective in reducing the risk of a systemic reaction while on immunotherapy and provides longer lasting risk reduction for many years after completing 3 to 5 years of immunotherapy.

References

Freeman TM: Hypersensitivity to hymenoptera stings, *N Engl J Med* 351:1978–1984, 2004.

Golden DBK: Large local reactions to insect stings, *J Allergy Clin Immunol* 3:331–334, 2015.

Golden DBK, Demain J, Freeman TM, et al: Stinging insect hypersensitivity: a practice parameter update 2016, *Ann Allergy Asthma Immunol* 118:28–54, 2017.

Jacobson RS: Entomological aspects of insect sting allergy. In Freeman TM, Tracy JM, editors: *Stinging Insect Allergy*, Switzerland, 2017, Springer, pp 17–42.

Rueff F, Przybilla M, Bilo MB, et al: Predictors of severe systemic anaphylactic reactions in patients with hymenoptera venom allergy: importance of baseline serum tryptase, *J Allergy Clin Immunol* 124:1047–1054, 2009.

Sampson HA, Munoz-Furlong A, Campbell RL, et al: Second symposium on the definition and management of anaphylaxis: summary report, *J Allergy Clin Immunol* 117:391–397, 2006.

Tracy JM, Demain JG, Quinn JM, et al: The natural history of the exposure to the imported fire ant (solenopsis invicta), *J Allergy Clin Immunol* 95:824–828, 1995.

ANAPHYLAXIS

Method of
Justin Greiwe, MD; and Jonathan A. Bernstein, MD

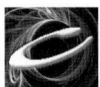

CURRENT DIAGNOSIS

- There is no universal agreement on the definition of anaphylaxis or the criteria for diagnosis.
- A comprehensive clinical history of the events surrounding the reaction provides the most valuable data along with a detailed review of current medications, recently ingested foods and/or drugs, insect stings, and physical activities before or after the event.
- While anaphylaxis remains primarily a clinical diagnosis, measurement of selected biomarkers (most commonly serum tryptase) has been used in research and clinical settings to assist in confirming this reaction.
- Cutaneous or serum-specific immunologic testing should only be performed to confirm or exclude a suspected agent under the supervision of an allergy specialist trained to interpret the meaning of the test results. Random testing to a large panel of foods or other allergens without a specific history has low diagnostic utility.

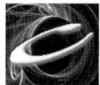

CURRENT THERAPY

- Prompt administration of intramuscular epinephrine is the gold-standard first-line medication for the treatment of anaphylaxis. Delay in treatment with epinephrine has been associated with increased morbidity and mortality.
- Patients with severe reactions can have massive fluid shifts that can occur rapidly due to increased vascular permeability which require aggressive fluid resuscitation.
- Additional treatments are considered supportive and include the addition of H1 and H2 antihistamines for itching, urticaria, and gastrointestinal complaints; albuterol for bronchospasm; oxygen; and placing the patient in the Trendelenburg position.
- Corticosteroids are not useful for the acute treatment of anaphylaxis since these medications take 4 to 6 hours to reach maximum effectiveness and there is a lack compelling evidence that corticosteroids reduce anaphylaxis severity or prevent biphasic reactions.

Introduction

Anaphylaxis is an acute, potentially life-threatening multisystem reaction caused by the sudden systemic release of preformed mediators from mast cells and basophils which include histamine, tryptase, chymase, heparin, histamine-releasing factor, and platelet-activating factor (PAF). Cellular activation also stimulates the production of lipid-derived newly formed mediators, such as prostaglandins and cysteinyl leukotrienes. These reactions are frequently, but not always, mediated by an immunologic mechanism involving two or more organs and/or are associated with hypotension or upper respiratory compromise. Other clinical manifestations include flushing, pruritus, urticaria, angioedema, shortness of breath, wheezing, nausea, vomiting, and diarrhea. Risk of death is mainly from cardiovascular collapse or asphyxiation caused by laryngeal edema. Drugs (nonsteroidal antiinflammatory drugs [NSAIDs]/antibiotics), foods, and Hymenoptera venom stings are the most common triggers; however any agent capable of inciting a sudden, systemic degranulation of mast cells can lead to anaphylaxis.

Various organizations have attempted to clarify the definition of anaphylaxis but with no consensus agreement. Experts from

TABLE 1 Comorbidities and Risk Factors for the Development of Anaphylaxis

Age: infants are at risk because manifestations might not be detected; teenagers are at risk because of "risky behavior"; elderly are at risk because of medical comorbidities and increased use of medications such as β-blockers leading to more severe cardiovascular symptoms at presentation

Gender: anaphylaxis is more common overall in females

Drugs: medications may impact severity of symptoms and response to treatment (see Table 2)

Comorbid Conditions: asthma, other respiratory diseases (e.g., chronic obstructive pulmonary disease, interstitial lung disease), cardiovascular disease, mast cell disorder (e.g., systemic mastocytosis)

Route of Administration: oral antigens are less likely to trigger anaphylaxis than parenteral antigens

Geography: prescription rates for self-injectable epinephrine devices are greater in northern than in southern states; living in a rural environment may affect incidence

Atopy: risk factor for anaphylactic and anaphylactoid reactions in general

Exposure History: the longer the interval since previous antigen exposure, the less likely a reaction will occur; previous anaphylactic reaction

Other Factors: active infections (e.g., upper respiratory tract infection, fever), physical exertion, premenstrual status, delayed administration of epinephrine, substance abuse (impairs judgement and can diminish recognition of symptoms), mental illness not well controlled

TABLE 2 Concurrent Medications That May Impact Severity of Symptoms and Response to Treatment

Possibly put patient at risk for more serious, treatment resistant anaphylaxis*

- β-adrenergic blockers
- α-adrenergic blockers
- Angiotensin-converting enzyme (ACE) inhibitors
- Angiotensin II receptor blockers
- Some tricyclic antidepressants (e.g., amitriptyline)
- Monoamine oxidase inhibitors

Potentially affect recognition of anaphylaxis

- Sedatives, hypnotics, antidepressants, ethanol, recreational drugs

Exacerbate anaphylaxis symptoms by causing nonimmunologic mast cell activation

- Ethanol, opiates, nonsteroidal anti-inflammatory drugs

Evidence of impact for most of these medications are still controversial/debatable, and expert opinion continues to shift with regard to the safety of these medications in anaphylaxis, especially with regard to concurrent use during aeroallergen and venom immunotherapy. A recent systematic review and meta-analysis of studies that assess the influence of β-blockers and ACE inhibitors on anaphylaxis suggest that the quality of evidence showing that the use of these medications increases the severity of anaphylaxis is low owing to differences in the control of confounders arising from the concomitant presence of cardiovascular diseases

the National Institute of Allergy and Infectious Disease (NIAID) and Food Allergy and Anaphylaxis Network (FAAN) met in 2005 and published diagnostic criteria for anaphylaxis. Controversy arose shortly thereafter with the World Allergy Organization (WAO) claiming that the published definition of anaphylaxis might exclude patients with clinical manifestations expressed by a single system only. Subsequent criteria published by Sampson et al. attempted to address this concern by adding single system caveats. Regardless of the continuing debate, the NIAID/FAAN criteria has been validated in real-world emergency room settings, establishing an accurate diagnosis of anaphylaxis with a sensitivity of 95% and a specificity of 71%.

Epidemiology

The prevalence of anaphylaxis in industrialized countries is estimated to range between 1.6% to 5.1%; however, rates seem to be increasing. In one study the majority (80.2%) of anaphylaxis cases were triggered by food, principally peanut and tree nut, indicating that increased rates of anaphylaxis might coincide with increasing rates of food allergy worldwide. Given increased prevalence rates, accurate recognition and management of anaphylactic episodes is of the utmost importance as a delay in treatment can lead to increased morbidity and mortality. In this regard, several consensus guidelines, including the American, European, and WAO guidelines, have been published to simplify this task.

Risk Factors

Anaphylactic reactions are becoming increasingly more common with an estimated 1500 fatalities/year caused by anaphylaxis in the United States. Comorbidities and concurrent medications may impact the severity of symptoms and response to treatment in patients experiencing anaphylaxis. Risk factors for the development of anaphylaxis and medications that may impact severity of symptoms and response to treatment are reviewed in Tables 1 and 2. Risk factors for fatal reactions include adolescence, a history of a previous anaphylactic reaction, allergy to peanut or tree nuts, history of asthma, absence of cutaneous symptoms, and delayed administration of epinephrine.

Pathophysiology

Most anaphylactic reactions are mediated by immunoglobulin E (IgE); however, not all episodes can be attributed to this mechanism. The WAO uses the term "immunologic anaphylaxis" to describe IgE-mediated, IgG-mediated, and immune complex/complement-mediated reactions. "Nonimmunologic anaphylaxis" (previously referred to as anaphylactoid reactions) is caused by agents or events that induce sudden degranulation of mast cells or basophils without the involvement of immunoglobulins like IgE.

Prevention

Avoidance of the confirmed trigger is the best way to prevent recurrence of anaphylaxis. For foods, this means educating patients about reading food labels, informing family and friends about these reactions, and being vigilant about avoiding the food(s) when eating in public establishments. Other triggers are more difficult to avoid such as venomous stinging insects or not possible in the case of idiopathic anaphylaxis (IA). In rare instances, an infection may require treatment with an antibiotic known to cause anaphylaxis in a patient. If there are no equally efficacious alternatives (i.e., penicillin for syphilis), an allergist/immunologist may perform skin testing to penicillin major and if available, minor determinants to confirm the allergy, and if positive, perform penicillin desensitization. This procedure involves relatively rapid administration of increasing amounts of the antibiotic under carefully controlled conditions by trained personnel with emergency therapy readily available until the target dose is reached. Thus desensitization results in tolerance which allows the allergic patient to take the medication without a reaction. Immunologic changes associated with immunotherapy are complicated, but the goal is to induce immune tolerance. The mechanism for inducing tolerance for different antigens is still poorly elucidated but is believed to occur by increasing regulatory T cells resulting in increased production of inhibitory cytokines like interleukin (IL)-10, transforming growth factor β (TGF-β), or both. IL-10 and TGF-β encourage the shift of antibody production from IgE toward the noninflammatory isotypes IgG4 and IgA, respectively. IL-10 is also involved in the reduction of proinflammatory cytokine release from mast cells, eosinophils, and T cells, as well as elicitation of tolerance in T cells by means of selective inhibition of the CD28 costimulatory pathway which effectively reduces lymphoproliferative responses to allergens. There also seems to be a shift in the immune response from a Th2 to a Th1 cytokine profile later in the immunotherapy course possibly mediated by the increased production of IL-12.

Long-term preventive measures include venom immunotherapy for Hymenoptera stinging insects (honey bee, wasp, yellow jacket, yellow hornet, white faced hornet) and food immunotherapy (oral, sublingual) for IgE-mediated food allergies. It is essential to recognize and manage poorly controlled comorbid conditions such as asthma and other respiratory diseases, cardiovascular disease, mastocytosis, and mast cell activation syndrome that may increase the risk for anaphylaxis. Administration of certain medications such as β-blockers and possibly angiotensin-converting enzyme (ACE) inhibitors (see Table 2) are associated with a greater risk for severe anaphylaxis by interfering with the therapeutic response to epinephrine and should be avoided if possible. This is especially true for the administration of therapeutics that place the patient at increased risk for anaphylaxis such as allergen immunotherapy (i.e., subcutaneous, sublingual, and venom immunotherapy).

Clinical Manifestations

Anaphylaxis is an acute multiorgan system reaction that generally begins within seconds to minutes but can be delayed occurring anywhere from 1 to 24 hours later after exposure to a trigger. The most common organ system involved is the skin or mucous membranes with >90% of patients presenting with some combination of pruritus, urticaria, and/or angioedema and erythema. Anaphylaxis, by nature, is unpredictable and heterogeneous in its presentation so it may be mild and resolve spontaneously or it may be severe and progress to significant respiratory or cardiovascular compromise. To help classify the severity of anaphylactic reactions, the WAO developed a universal 5-stage grading system. It was intended to more accurately assess when epinephrine should be administered during subcutaneous immunotherapy (SCIT), but has since been used to better classify all forms of systemic reactions. Each grade is based on the organ system involved defined as cutaneous, conjunctival, upper respiratory, lower respiratory, gastrointestinal, cardiovascular, or other, and the severity is based on clinical judgement (Table 3).

Anaphylaxis can present as a uniphasic response, biphasic response, or as being refractory to treatment, all of which need to be considered and recognized by the clinician evaluating these patients. Biphasic anaphylaxis is defined as a potentially life-threatening recurrence of symptoms after the resolution of the initial immediate anaphylactic episode without re-exposure to the causative agent. The delayed portion of the biphasic reaction typically occurs within 12 hours but has been reported to occur up to 72 hours after resolution of initial symptoms. Biphasic reactions have been reported to develop in up to 21% of anaphylactic episodes (all ages) and in up to 15% of children. Biphasic reactions seem to be associated with the severity of the initial anaphylactic episode. Rarely, the onset of anaphylaxis will be delayed beginning hours rather than minutes after exposure to the causative agent. This is especially true for red meat allergy, also called mammalian meat allergy or α-gal allergy. This condition is characterized by development of an IgE antibody directed against a mammalian oligosaccharide epitope, galactose-α-1,3-galactose ("α-gal") after a lone star tick bite which contains the α-gal protein. Patients typically do not develop symptoms until several hours (4 to 6 hours or even longer) after eating red meat.

Diagnosis

There is no universal agreement on the definition of anaphylaxis or the criteria for diagnosis. Table 4 summarizes the NIAID/FAAN criteria established in 2005 which continues to be generally accepted today.

While anaphylaxis remains primarily a clinical diagnosis, measurement of selected biomarkers has been used in research and clinical settings to assist in confirming this reaction. Plasma histamine, platelet activating factor, and serum tryptase can be obtained in certain situations; however, there are specific

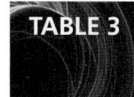

| **TABLE 3** | World Allergy Organization Subcutaneous Immunotherapy Systemic Reaction Grading System |

Grade 1:
Symptom(s)/sign(s) of 1 organ system present
Cutaneous: generalized pruritus, urticaria, flushing, or sensation of heat or warmth
or
Angioedema (not laryngeal, tongue or uvular)
or
Upper respiratory: rhinitis (e.g., sneezing, rhinorrhea, nasal pruritus, and/or nasal congestion)
or
Throat-clearing (itchy throat)
or
Cough perceived to originate in the upper airway, not the lung, larynx, or trachea
or
Conjunctival: erythema, pruritus, or tearing
Other: nausea, metallic taste, or headache

Grade 2:
Symptom(s)/sign(s) of more than 1 organ system present
or
Lower respiratory: asthma: cough, wheezing, shortness of breath (e.g., less than 40% PEF or FEV1 drop, responding to an inhaled bronchodilator)
or
Gastrointestinal: abdominal cramps, vomiting, or diarrhea
or
Other: uterine cramps

Grade 3:
Lower respiratory: asthma (e.g., 40% PEF or FEV1 drop NOT responding to an inhaled bronchodilator)
or
Upper respiratory: laryngeal, uvula, or tongue edema with or without stridor

Grade 4:
Lower or upper respiratory: respiratory failure with or loss of consciousness
or
Cardiovascular: hypotension with or without loss of consciousness

Grade 5: Death

FEV1, forced expiratory volume in one second; *PEF*, peak expiratory flow.

collection timeframes that need to be strictly adhered to for the result to be valid. Serum tryptase is the most commonly used biomarker to distinguish anaphylaxis from other conditions with a similar presentation (i.e., carcinoid syndrome, vasovagal reactions, seizures). Acute elevation of serum tryptase secondary to mast cell degranulation can occur through an IgE-mediated mechanism (i.e., venom and drug allergy) or direct degranulation of mast cells through a non-IgE mediated mechanism (i.e., NSAIDs or opiates). Tryptase can rise in serum or plasma as early as 15 minutes after clinical onset of anaphylaxis and should be collected between 30 minutes and 2 hours after symptom-onset if possible. Samples collected before or after this window are less accurate due to diminished sensitivity. Previous studies have questioned the sensitivity of serum tryptase in food-induced reactions; however a recent prospective study suggests that serum tryptase is a valuable tool in food allergic reactions as well and correlates with symptom severity. There is still debate on how serum tryptase can be used effectively in diagnosing anaphylaxis or mast cell activation with different studies quoting different cutoff values. Data on cutoffs specifically for food allergy are even harder to come by (Table 5).

According to this study comparing peak tryptase reaction levels at 2 hours with baseline is essential in correct interpretation, and a rise in tryptase of 30% above baseline is associated with a food allergic reaction. It is important to note that a normal serum tryptase level does not exclude anaphylaxis as the diagnosis.

TABLE 4	Clinical Criteria for Diagnosing Anaphylaxis

Anaphylaxis is highly likely when any one of the following three criteria are fulfilled:

1. Acute onset of an illness (minutes to several hours) with involvement of the skin, mucosal tissue, or both (e.g., generalized hives, pruritus or flushing, swollen lips-tongue-uvula)

   AND AT LEAST ONE OF THE FOLLOWING
   - a. Respiratory compromise (e.g., dyspnea, wheeze-bronchospasm, stridor, reduced PEF, hypoxemia)
   - b. Reduced BP or associated symptoms of end-organ dysfunction (e.g., hypotonia [collapse], syncope, incontinence)

2. Two or more of the following that occur rapidly after exposure to a likely allergen for that patient (minutes to several hours):
   - a. Involvement of the skin-mucosal tissue (e.g., generalized hives, itch-flush, swollen lips-tongue-uvula)
   - b. Respiratory compromise (e.g., dyspnea, wheeze-bronchospasm, stridor, reduced PEF, hypoxemia)
   - c. Reduced BP or associated symptoms (e.g., hypotonia [collapse], syncope, incontinence)
   - d. Persistent gastrointestinal symptoms (e.g., crampy abdominal pain, vomiting)

3. Reduced BP after exposure to known allergen for that patient (minutes to several hours):
   - a. Infants and children: low systolic BP (age specific) or greater than 30% decrease in systolic BP*
   - b. Adults: systolic BP of less than 90 mm Hg or greater than 30% decrease from that person's baseline

*Low systolic blood pressure for children is defined as less than 70 mm Hg from 1 month to 1 year, less than (70 mm Hg + [2 × age]) from 1 to 10 years, and less than 90 mm Hg from 11 to 17 years.
PEF, Peak expiratory flow; *BP*, blood pressure.

A comprehensive clinical history of the events surrounding the reaction provides the most valuable data along with a detailed review of current medications, recently ingested foods and/or drugs, insect stings, and physical activities before or after the event. This approach oftentimes uncovers the appropriate trigger; however, in many cases no clear trigger can be identified. More accurate diagnostic testing can be utilized in some cases when the patient or clinician suspects a specific antigen as the triggering agent. Cutaneous or serum specific immunologic testing should only be performed to confirm or exclude a suspected agent under the supervision of an allergy specialist trained to interpret the meaning of the test results. Random testing to a large panel of foods or other allergens (i.e., venoms) without a specific history has a low diagnostic utility and can result in more questions rather than answers given the high rate of false positive reactions reported, especially for foods. If diagnostic skin testing is performed, it should be delayed for at least 3 to 4 weeks after the event to obtain an accurate test result in order to allow for recovery of skin mast cells. In certain cases there may be no validated cutaneous or in vitro test to detect the potential for an IgE-mediated reaction. In these circumstances, a graded challenge or provocation test can safely be carried out under the supervision of an experienced allergist in a setting that is fully equipped to respond to any potential medical emergency including anaphylaxis. Unlike desensitization, graded challenges do not work by modifying the allergic response to the agent. Therefore patients who tolerate a graded challenge is an indication that they are not allergic to the specific agent administered.

Differential Diagnosis

Anaphylaxis can sometimes be difficult to recognize because it can mimic other conditions and is variable in its presentation. Common conditions that mimic anaphylaxis are included in Table 6.

Therapy (or Treatment)

Prompt administration of intramuscular epinephrine is the gold-standard first-line medication for the treatment of anaphylaxis. Delay in treatment with epinephrine has been associated with increased morbidity and mortality. Epinephrine autoinjectors (EAI [Auvi-Q (kaléo, Richmond, VA), EpiPen Jr, EpiPen (Mylan Inc, Canonsberg, PA)]) are commercially available in three different concentrations in the United States: 0.1 mg (7.5 to 14 kg body weight), 0.15 mg (15 to 30 kg), and 0.3 mg (>30 kg). Epinephrine can be administered intramuscularly (preferred) or subcutaneously every 5 to 15 minutes but can be given more frequently if deemed appropriate. The recommended adult dose of 1:1000 (1 mg/mL) epinephrine is 0.2 to 0.5 mg (mL), whereas the pediatric dose is 0.01 mg/kg (0.01 mL/kg/dose of 1 mg/mL solution), with a maximum dose of 0.3 mg. If not administered through an autoinjector, the epinephrine dose should be drawn up using a 1 mL syringe and injected intramuscularly into the mid-outer thigh. A higher dose (e.g., 0.5 mL) within the recommended dose range should be considered in patients with severe anaphylaxis.

Patients with severe reactions can have massive fluid shifts that can occur rapidly due to increased vascular permeability which require aggressive fluid resuscitation. Additional treatments are considered supportive and include the addition of H1 and H2 antihistamines for itching, urticaria, and gastrointestinal complaints; albuterol for bronchospasm; oxygen; and placing the patient in the Trendelenburg position. Corticosteroids are not useful for the acute treatment of anaphylaxis since these medications take 4 to 6 hours to reach maximum effectiveness. Despite this, corticosteroids are often used in the emergency treatment of anaphylaxis under the assumption that these medications may be beneficial in preventing biphasic reactions. A comprehensive literature review of 31 studies recently reported that biphasic reactions were more likely to occur in moderate to severe anaphylaxis or when anaphylaxis was not treated with timely epinephrine. Due to the potential adverse effects of corticosteroids and lack of compelling evidence demonstrating an effective role in reducing anaphylaxis severity or preventing biphasic anaphylaxis, the authors do not advocate their routine use for treatment of anaphylaxis. The appropriate observation period after an anaphylactic event often depends on the severity and duration of the initial reaction as well as the patient's response to treatment, previous reaction history, associated comorbidities, and access to medical care. Patients with moderate to severe anaphylaxis should be observed for a minimum of 4 to 8 hours; however, milder presentations can be observed for a shorter time period. All patients with a history of anaphylaxis should be given a prescription for an EAI along with instructions for self-administration and an allergy action plan specific to their trigger.

Monitoring

The main tenants of anaphylaxis management and prevention are simple in theory but difficult in practice. Complete avoidance of the triggering agent provides protection from future episodes however, accidental exposures can occur, especially for food induced anaphylaxis. Other conditions like IA occur randomly with no known triggers making avoidance impossible. While episodes of IA tend to decline in frequency over time, patients experiencing more frequent attacks often benefit from daily prophylactic treatment with H1 and/or H2 antihistamines, leukotriene receptor antagonist (LTRA), and oral prednisone as needed. In refractory cases omalizumab (Xolair) has been shown to be effective as well[1].

Carrying an EAI at all times provides patients with quick access to life-saving treatment; however, adherence has historically been poor. The predicament of poor adherence to medical treatment is a well-recognized problem; however in anaphylaxis the consequences of nonadherence can be fatal. One study from 2008 demonstrated that 48% of children prescribed an EAI did not have the device available at school, and of those with the medication on site, 78% of the autoinjectors were kept in the nurse's office or by another administrator not in close proximity to the child. Real-world data from a 2018 survey also demonstrated a poor level of adherence in patients and caregivers to anaphylaxis treatment

---

[1] Not FDA approved for this indication.

TABLE 5	Proposed Optimal Cutoffs for Tryptase Elevations Signifying Mast Cell Activation or Anaphylaxis	
AUTHOR	**CRITERIA FOR TRYPTASE INCREASE**	**CRITERIA IDENTIFY**
Phadia AB, 2008	Values above 11.4 ng/mL (upper 95th percentile)	Raised tryptase
Valent et al., 2012	20% plus 2 ng/mL over baseline level	Mast cell activation
Enrique et al., 1999	Levels >8.23 ng/mL	Anaphylaxis
Brown et al., 2009	Increase of 2 µg/L	Anaphylaxis
Egner et al, 2016	Threshold increment of 20%	Mast cell mediator release
Wongkaewpothong et al., 2014	Delta tryptase 0.8 µg/L	Anaphylaxis

TABLE 6	Differential Diagnosis of Anaphylaxis
SYSTEM	**DIFFERENTIAL DIAGNOSIS**
Cutaneous	acute generalized urticaria, acute angioedema, ACE inhibitor angioedema, hereditary/ acquired angioedema, carcinoid syndrome, postmenopause, Red man syndrome
Cardiac	vasovagal syncope, myocardial infarction, arrhythmia, shock
Respiratory	asthma or COPD exacerbation, vocal cord dysfunction syndrome, laryngospasm, pulmonary embolism, inhaled foreign body (infants/toddlers)
Psychological	panic attacks or acute anxiety, Munchausen syndrome
Other	mastocytosis and mast cell activation syndrome, pheochromocytoma, capillary leak syndrome, scombroid fish ingestion, hypoadrenergic or hyperadrenergic paroxysmal orthostatic tachycardia (POTS), hereditary alpha tryptasemia

ACE, Angiotensin-converting enzyme; COPD, chronic obstructive pulmonary disorder.

guidelines which recommend carrying more than one EAI at all times. Most (82%) did not carry two EAIs at all times, mainly due to keeping one EAI in another location; 84% respondents said they kept at least one EAI at home; however, few patients and caregivers kept more than one. More than half of the respondents (64%) said they received counseling with an emphasis on always having one EAI and keeping another in a different location, but only 27% reported counseling that emphasized always having two EAIs available. It is important to recognize that a second epinephrine dose may be required in 16% to 36% of patients; therefore a more concerted effort should be made by physicians to properly educate patients and caregivers on the importance of following standard treatment guidelines. According to a 2018 study, only 26% of milk-allergic children in the U.S. had a current EAI prescription, the lowest reported rate among the top nine food allergies.

While poor patient adherence deserves some of the blame, evidence suggests that prescribers are equally responsible for this omission. Among 208 patients identified with anaphylaxis, 64.4% were seen in the emergency department and discharged home, but only 36.6% were prescribed an EAI, and only 31.3% were referred to an allergy specialist for further evaluation. Another retrospective cross-sectional descriptive study of patients 21 years old or younger who received care for anaphylaxis reported that EAIs were prescribed to only 63%, and referral to an allergist was recommended to only 33%. Both of these studies suggest that emergency department physicians may be missing an important opportunity to empower patients with the ability to self-administer treatment for a recurrent episode and to prevent future anaphylactic reactions by not referring patients for

specialized follow-up care. Finally, a comprehensive analysis of 10,184 anaphylaxis incidents using the European anaphylaxis register revealed that in the early 2000s 27.1% of patients with anaphylaxis treated by a health professional received epinephrine while only 14.7% of lay or self-treated cases were treated with an EAI. Progress was tracked over the next decade and epinephrine administration from a health professional almost doubled to 30.6% in 2015–2017 but no significant change was found in the lay emergency respondents group.

Failing to follow published guidelines for the treatment of anaphylaxis is another barrier to timely and appropriate treatment. Oftentimes antihistamines are used as first-line agents in the treatment of an anaphylactic reaction and is the most common reason providers report for not using epinephrine, leaving patients at increased risk for life-threatening sequelae. It should be reiterated that antihistamines have no effect on arresting true anaphylactic reactions and should only be used for symptomatic relief of associated pruritus and urticaria.

Reasons for patients and caregivers not to carry or use their EAIs or to delay administration are multifaceted and complex. Teenagers and young adults are at highest risk of fatal anaphylaxis-related reactions due to delayed epinephrine injection. Cost can be a difficult barrier for patients to overcome either related to having no insurance, high insurance co-pays, and/or deductibles. The cost of the best-known autoinjector, EpiPen, made headline news in recent years when pricing rose to more than $600/2-pak by 2016. Bad press followed by public outcry led the manufacturer to produce a generic version for half the cost. Potential barriers for not carrying an EAI are summarized in Table 7.

Since many patients who have been prescribed an EAI do not routinely carry one, and emergency rooms fail to prescribe them, it is essential that life-saving EAIs be readily available in community spaces and public venues. To improve access to life-saving treatment, there is an increasing effort to distribute nonspecific EAIs to public locations including schools, parks, pools, airports, public venues, and shopping malls. In 2013, President Obama signed the "School Access to Emergency Epinephrine Act," which encouraged, but did not require, all states to adopt stock epinephrine regulations for schools. Several drug companies like Mylan Specialty (EpiPen4Schools) and Kaléo ("Q Your School") are providing free stock EAIs for schools to help improve access to epinephrine in the event a person experiences anaphylaxis in an academic setting. According to a recent EpiPen4Schools survey sponsored by Mylan Specialty, in each academic year, one in every six U.S. schools will have a student or staff member experience anaphylaxis. About 1140 episodes of anaphylaxis occurred across 6574 U.S. schools with most (89.5%) incidents involving students. More reactions were seen in high school students, who tend to be at higher risk, and food was the trigger for a majority (60%) of the reactions. Other triggers include environmental, medication, and insect stings or bites; however, 22% of severe reactions were from unknown triggers. EAIs (both stock and personal) were used to treat 77% of anaphylactic events reported. Overall this survey revealed that not only are anaphylactic events a relatively common occurrence in schools, but also that the risk extends beyond those with diagnosed allergies. A quarter of the

TABLE 7	Reasons for Patients and Caregivers Not to Carry or Use Their Epinephrine Autoinjectors or to Delay Administration

- Never prescribed
- Cost
- Inconvenience
- Lack of perception of need of the medication
  - many do not use device for years so may not think it is essential or forget how to use it properly
- Poor knowledge of appropriate use
- Lack of familiarity with different brands of autoinjectors
- Mistakenly believe EAI might be available for emergency use in many public spaces
- History of mild allergic reaction
  - might think they are not at risk for a potentially fatal reaction
- Emotional/behavioral
  - embarrassment, feeling different
- Having been OK after a past reaction without treatment
- Wait for antihistamine to work
- Rely on other medications
- Don't want to go to the emergency department
- Needle phobia

EAI, Epinephrine autoinjectors.

individuals who experienced anaphylaxis in a school setting had no known allergies. The previously stated data tend to further support the need for stock EAIs in schools, and training for staff on when and how to use them.

With increased availability of epinephrine in public settings there needs to be a focus on increased educational initiatives for the people administering life-saving treatment. Just having epinephrine available does not improve outcomes during an anaphylactic event. Healthcare professionals, first responders, and the general public need to be able to recognize classic anaphylactic symptoms and know how to properly initiate treatment. Unfortunately, when these groups are surveyed, anaphylaxis is still underrecognized and undertreated (Table 8).

Recent anaphylaxis guidelines published in the 2020 Practice Parameter Update answered five PICO questions using GRADE methodology. The first question addressed the risk of developing a biphasic reaction related to anaphylaxis and what is an appropriate observation time in the ED to monitor for a biphasic reaction. The recommendation was to take the severity of the initial anaphylaxis reaction and/or the use of one or more doses of epinephrine into account in determining the risk for a biphasic reaction and to have an extended observation period in patients considered high risk for a biphasic reaction. The second question addressed the treatment of an anaphylaxis reaction with antihistamines and glucocorticoids to prevent a biphasic reaction and recommended against this approach as epinephrine is considered more effective in this regard. The third and fourth questions asked whether patients with a history of chemotherapeutic or radiocontrast reactions should be treated with antihistamines and glucocorticoids to prevent subsequent reactions. With respect to chemotherapeutic agents this treatment was recommended; however, for radiocontrast reactions it was not, as evidence suggests using a low or iso-osmolar agent is sufficient for preventing a subsequent reaction. Finally the fifth question asked whether pretreatment with antihistamines and glucocorticoids should be used for patients undergoing rush allergen immunotherapy and the recommendation was in favor of this approach. It is important to emphasize that all of these recommendations were conditional, and the rating of evidence was very low, emphasizing the need for well designed studies to investigate best practices for the management of anaphylaxis. In general, good clinical practice requires consideration of risk versus benefit of treatment and should take into account patient preference when appropriate.

TABLE 8	Are Healthcare Professionals and First Responders Able to Appropriately Recognize and Treat Anaphylaxis?

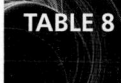

SURVEY	RESULTS
1114 pediatric emergency medicine physicians	• 93.5% correctly identified epinephrine as the treatment of choice for anaphylaxis • 66.9% used the intramuscular (IM) route of administration • 37.4% admitted affected patients for observation • Many discharge patients home after an abbreviated period
468 pediatricians (41%) responded to the survey	• 70% agreed that the clinical scenario was consistent with anaphylaxis • 72% chose to administer epinephrine • 56% of respondents agreed with both the diagnosis of anaphylaxis and treating with epinephrine • 70% did not recognize that a 30-min observation period after anaphylaxis was too short
7822 physicians, allied health, medical students, and other health professionals	• 80% of responders correctly identified the case of anaphylaxis with prominent skin and respiratory symptoms • 55% correctly recognized the case without skin symptoms as anaphylaxis • 23% of responders correctly selected risk factors for anaphylaxis

3537 paramedics	• 98.9% correctly recognized a case of classic anaphylaxis
	• 2.9% correctly identified the atypical presentation
	• 46.2% identified epinephrine as the initial drug of choice
	• 38.9% chose the IM route of administration
	  • 60.5% identified the deltoid as the preferred location
	  • 11.6% correctly identified the thigh
	• ~98% were confident they could recognize and manage anaphylaxis
	  • 39.5% carry EAIs on response vehicles
	• 95.4% were confident they could use an EAI
	  • 36.2% stated that there were contraindications to epinephrine administration in anaphylactic shock

EAI, Epinephrine autoinjectors.

Management of Complications

In general, anaphylactic reactions resolve without any major complications. Even though the prevalence rates of anaphylaxis seem to be increasing, fatal outcomes are rare, making up less than 1% of total mortality risk. In older patients, cardiovascular complications like atrial fibrillation and myocardial infarction can arise during anaphylaxis, but these events are also infrequent.

COVID-19 Vaccines and Anaphylaxis

In December 2020, the US Food and Drug Administration (FDA) issued emergency use authorizations for two mRNA-based vaccines for the prevention of coronavirus disease 2019 (COVID-19) caused by severe acute respiratory syndrome coronavirus 2 (SARS-CoV-2): Pfizer-BioNTech and Moderna. A third vaccine (Janssen) was approved in late February 2021. As with all vaccines, there is a low but recognizable risk of anaphylaxis. Given the circumstances with which these vaccinations were released, the safety and efficacy of these novel products have been under intense scrutiny since their implementation. Soon after vaccination programs were started, cases of anaphylaxis following administration of the Moderna and Pfizer-BioNTech vaccines began to be reported. Early accounts in the U.S., gathered through

01/18/2021, demonstrated fairly low risks of anaphylaxis for both vaccines: 4.7 cases/million for the Pfizer-BioNTech vaccine and 2.5 cases/million for the Moderna vaccine. Continued safety monitoring of mRNA COVID-19 vaccines have confirmed that anaphylaxis following vaccination is a rare event. Therefore the CDC only recognizes two situations where the vaccines would be contraindicated:

1. Severe allergic reaction (e.g., anaphylaxis) after a previous dose or to a component of the COVID-19 vaccine
2. Immediate allergic reaction of any severity to a previous dose or known (diagnosed) allergy to a component of the vaccine.

Although rates of anaphylaxis to the first available mRNA COVID-19 vaccines were low, locations administering these vaccines are required to adhere to CDC guidelines, including screening recipients for contraindications and precautions, having necessary supplies and staff members available to manage anaphylaxis, implementing recommended postvaccination observation periods, and immediately treating suspected anaphylaxis with intramuscular epinephrine injection.

Conclusion

Anaphylaxis is a common medical condition affecting both adult and pediatric populations and its incidence and prevalence continue to increase. Prompt recognition and treatment with epinephrine administered in a timely manner remains the mainstay of treatment for anaphylaxis. Preventive measures including patient education, immunotherapy when appropriate, antigen avoidance, and optimal management of comorbid conditions is important in preventing recurrences. There is a concerning lack of knowledge and preparedness for management of anaphylaxis at all care levels that needs to be better addressed.

Readings

Brown SGA, Blackman KE, Heddle RJ: Can serum mast cell tryptase help diagnose anaphylaxis? *Emerg Med Australas* 16:120–124, 2004.
Campbell RL, Kelso JM: Anaphylaxis: Acute diagnosis. Walls RM, ed. UpToDate. Waltham, MA: UpToDate Inc. http://www.uptodate.com (Accessed on December 04, 2018.)
CDC COVID-19 Response Team; Food and Drug Administration: Allergic reactions including anaphylaxis after receipt of the first dose of Moderna COVID-19 vaccine—United States, December 21, 2020-January 10, 2021, *MMWR Morb Mortal Wkly Rep* 70(4):125–129, 2021.
Centers for Disease Control and Prevention: Interim clinical considerations for use of COVID-19 vaccines currently authorized in the United States. Updated March 5, 2021. Accessed March 8, 2021. https://www.cdc.gov/vaccines/covid-19/info-by-product/clinical-considerations.html#:~:text=CDC%20considers%20a%20history%20of,of%20the%20COVID%2D19%20vaccine.
Centers for Disease Control and Prevention: Checklist of best practices for vaccination clinics held at satellite, temporary, or off-site locations. Updated August 18, 2020. https://www.cdc.gov/flu/business/hosting-vaccination-clinic.htm. Accessed 8 March 2021.
Commins SP, Jerath MR, Cox K, et al: Delayed anaphylaxis to alpha-gal, an oligosaccharide in mammalian meat, *Allergol Int* 65:16, 2016.
Dua S, Dowey J, Foley L: Diagnostic value of tryptase in food allergic reactions: a prospective study of 160 adult peanut challenges, *J Allergy Clin Immunol Pract* 6(5):1692–1698, 2018 Sep - Oct.
Egner W, Sargur R, Shrimpton A, et al: 17-year experience in perioperative anaphylaxis 1998-2015: harmonizing optimal detection of mast cell mediator release, *Clin Exp Allergy* 46:1465–1473, 2016.
Enrique E, García-Ortega P, Sotorra O, Gaig P, Richart C: Usefulness of UniCAP-Tryptase fluoroimmunoassay in the diagnosis of anaphylaxis, *Allergy* 54:602–606, 1999.
Grabenhenrich LB, Dölle S, Ruëff F, et al: Epinephrine in severe allergic reactions: the European anaphylaxis register, *J Allergy Clin Immunol Pract* 6(6):1898–1906, 2018 Nov - Dec.
Grossman SL, Baumann BM, Garcia Peña BM, et al: Anaphylaxis knowledge and practice preferences of pediatric emergency medicine physicians: a national survey, *J Pediatr* 163(3):841–846, 2013.
Jacobsen RC, Toy S, Bonham AJ, et al: Anaphylaxis knowledge among paramedics: results of a national survey, *Prehosp Emerg Care* 16(4):527–534, 2012.
Krugman SD, Chiaramonte DR, Matsui EC: Diagnosis and management of food-induced anaphylaxis: a national survey of pediatricians, *Pediatrics* 118(3):e554–e560, 2006.
Lee S, Bellolio MF, Hess EP, et al: Time of onset and predictors of biphasic anaphylactic reactions: a systematic review and meta-analysis, *J Allergy Clin Immunol Pract* 3:408, 2015.
Lieberman P, Nicklas RA, Randolph C, et al: Anaphylaxis--a practice parameter update 2015, *Ann Allergy Asthma Immunol* 115:341, 2015.
Phadia AB: *ImmunoCAP Tryptase. Directions for Use*, Uppsala, Sweden: Phadia AB; 2008.

Shaker MS, Wallace DV, Golden DB, et al: Anaphylaxis - a 2020 Practice Parameter Update, Systematic Review and GRADE Analysis, *J Allergy Clin Immunol* 145(4):1082–1123, 2020.
Shimabukuro TT, Cole M, Su JR: Reports of anaphylaxis after receipt of mRNA COVID-19 vaccines in the US—December 14, 2020-January 18, 2021, *JAMA*. Published online February 12, 2021.
Shimabukuro T, Nair N: Allergic reactions including anaphylaxis after receipt of the first dose of Pfizer-BioNTech COVID-19 vaccine, *JAMA*. Published online January 21, 2021.
Simons FE, Frew AJ, Ansotegui IJ, et al: Risk assessment in anaphylaxis: current and future approaches, *J Allergy Clin Immunol* 120(suppl 1):S2–S24, 2007.
Tejedor-Alonso MA, Farias-Aquino E, Pérez-Fernández E, et al: Relationship between anaphylaxis and use of beta-blockers and angiotensin-converting enzyme inhibitors: a systematic review and meta-analysis of observational studies, *J Allergy Clin Immunol Pract* 7(3):879–897, 2019 Mar.
Turner PJ, Jerschow E, Umasunthar T: Fatal anaphylaxis: mortality rate and risk factors, *J Allergy Clin Immunol Pract* 5(5):1169–1178, 2017.
Valent P, Akin C, Arock M, et al: Definitions, criteria and global classification of mast cell disorders with special reference to mast cell activation syndromes: a consensus proposal, *Int Arch Allergy Immunol* 157:215–225, 2012.
Wang J, Young MC, Nowak-Wegrzyn A: International survey of knowledge of food-induced anaphylaxis, *Pediatr Allergy Immunol* 25(7):644–650, 2014.

DRUG HYPERSENSITIVITY REACTIONS

Method of
Miriam Chan, PharmD; Ann M. Aring, MD; and Kristen Rundell, MS, MD

CURRENT DIAGNOSIS

- Detailed history should include past medical history; current diagnosis; previous and current medication use, including over-the-counter drugs and herbals as well as other nonprescribed medications; duration of the medication use; any similar reactions in the past.
- Physical examination should include vitals, temperature, and skin examination for rash.
- Laboratory testing should be conducted based on symptoms that may include complete blood count (CBC) with differential, eosinophils, sedimentation rate, liver enzymes, international normalized ratio (INR), C-reactive protein (CRP), and diagnostic skin biopsy or testing.

CURRENT THERAPY

- For life-threatening anaphylaxis reaction, start basic life support using pneumonic ACB (airway, compression, breathing) and give epinephrine immediately.
- Discontinue the offending drug if medically possible. Try drug substitution if warranted.
- An alternative option is to reduce the dose or frequency of the drug.
- Start symptomatic treatment based on the type of reaction and the offending medication.
- Some reactions may respond to treatment with antihistamines, H_2 blockers, or steroids.

Epidemiology

Drug hypersensitivity reactions are one of the many different types of adverse drug reactions (ADRs). ADRs are common, yet the more severe reactions have been estimated to cause 3% to 6% of hospital admissions. More than 100,000 deaths annually are caused by serious ADRs, making these reactions one of the leading causes of death in the United States. Early detection of all ADRs can potentially improve patient outcomes and lower health care costs.

TABLE 1   Classification of Drug Hypersensitivity Reactions

TYPE	MECHANISM	CLINICAL FEATURES	TIMING OF REACTIONS	EXAMPLES
Type 1 (IgE mediated)	Drug-IgE complex binds to mast cells	Urticaria, angioedema, bronchospasm, pruritus, GI symptoms, anaphylaxis	Immediate (minutes to hours after drug exposure, depending on the route of administration)	β-lactam antibiotic
Type II (cytotoxic)	Specific IgG or IgM antibodies directed at drug-hapten–coated cells	Hemolytic anemia, neutropenia, thrombocytopenia	Variable	Penicillin (hemolytic anemia), heparin (thrombocytopenia)
Type III (immune complex)	Antigen-antibody complexes	Serum sickness, vasculitis, drug fever	1–3 weeks after drug exposure	Penicillin (serum sickness), sulfonamides (vasculitis), azathioprine (drug fever)
Type IV (delayed, cell mediated)	Activation and expansion of drug-specific T cell	Prominent skin findings: Contact dermatitis, morbilliform eruptions	2–7 days after exposure	Topical antihistamine, penicillin, sulfonamides

Classifications

An ADR is a broad term that refers to any predictable or unpredictable reaction to a medication. A predictable (type A) reaction is dose dependent and is related to the known pharmacologic properties of the drug. Predictable reactions account for about 80% of all ADRs. An example of a type A reaction is gastritis that results from taking nonsteroidal antiinflammatory drugs (NSAIDs). The remaining 20% of ADRs are caused by unpredictable (type B) reactions. Type B reactions occur in susceptible individuals. These are hypersensitivity reactions that are different from the pharmacologic actions of the drug; they are results of interactions between the drug and the individual human immune system. Type B reactions can be further divided into drug intolerance, drug idiosyncrasy, drug allergy (immunologically mediated), and pseudoallergic reactions (anaphylactoid reactions). This chapter will focus on these type B drug hypersensitivity reactions.

Pathophysiology

Several mechanisms may play a role in the underlying etiology of immunologic drug reactions. The Gell and Coombs classification system was the original system to describe four predominant immune mechanisms. These four reaction types are listed as type I reactions (IgE medicated), type II reactions (cytotoxic), type III reactions (immune complex), and type IV reactions (delayed, cell mediated). Table 1 provides a detailed description of this classification. Type I and IV reactions are more common than type II and III reactions. Most drugs cause one type of reaction, whereas certain drugs, such as penicillin, can induce all four types of reactions.

The Gell and Coombs classification has recently been revised to reflect the functional heterogeneity of T cells. Under the new system, type IV reactions are further subclassified into four categories: IVa (macrophage activation), IVb (eosinophils), IVc (CD4⁺ or CD8⁺ T cells), and IVd (neutrophils). Nevertheless, many common hypersensitivity reactions cannot be classified in this system because of the lack of knowledge of their immune mechanism or a mixed mechanism.

A new concept of drug interaction with immune receptors has recently been developed by Pichler and colleagues. It is called the *p-i concept* (pharmacologic interaction with immune receptors). In this concept, a drug binds noncovalently to a T-cell receptor and stimulates an immune response, which can cause inflammatory reactions of different types. The stimulation of the T cell is enhanced by the additional interaction with the major histocompatibility complex molecule. This is direct stimulation of memory and effector T cells, and no sensitization is required. The skin has a high concentration of effector memory T cells, which can be rapidly stimulated by antigen penetration. The skin also possesses a dense network of dendritic cells that act as antigen-presenting cells and increase hypersensitivity reactions. As a

result, clinical symptoms by p-i drugs may appear more rapidly. Some severe reactions—such as Stevens-Johnson syndrome (SJS), toxic epidermal necrolysis (TEN), the drug rash with eosinophilia and systemic symptoms (DRESS) syndrome, or hypersensitivity syndrome—are believed to be p-i related. Examples are abacavir (Ziagen) hypersensitivity syndrome and SJS/TEN from carbamazepine (Tegretol).

Risk Factors for Hypersensitivity Drug Reactions

The chemical structure and molecular weight of the drug may help predict the type of hypersensitivity reaction. Larger drugs with greater structural complexity are more likely to be immunogenic. However, drugs with small molecular weight (< 1000 Da) can elicit hypersensitivity reactions by coupling with carrier proteins to form hapten-carrier complexes. Other drug-related factors include the dose, route of administration, duration of treatment, repetitive exposure to the drug, and concurrent illness. Topical and intravenous drug administrations are more likely to cause hypersensitivity reactions than are oral medications.

Patient risk factors include age, female gender, HIV infection or immunocompromised, atopy, specific genetic polymorphisms, previous drug hypersensitivity reactions, and inherent predisposition to react to multiple unrelated drugs.

Clinical Manifestations

Drug hypersensitivity reactions can manifest in a great variety of clinical symptoms and diseases. While some reactions are mild and often unnoticed, others, such as anaphylaxis, can be severe and even fatal. Dermatologic symptoms are the most common physical manifestation of allergic drug reactions. Drug hypersensitivity reactions can also affect various internal organs, causing diseases such as hepatitis, nephritis, and pneumonitis. The noncutaneous physical findings are generally nonspecific and may not be helpful and even delay the diagnosis and management decisions.

Dermatologic Symptoms

The most common allergic drug reactions affect the skin and can cause a variety of different exanthems. The most common skin reaction is the classic "drug rash," which is a morbilliform eruption originating on the trunk. Other dermatologic symptoms include urticaria, angioedema, acne, bullous eruptions, fixed drug eruptions, erythema multiforme, lupus erythematosus, photosensitivity, psoriasis, purpura, vasculitis, and pruritus. The most severe forms of cutaneous drug reactions are Stevens-Johnson syndrome (SJS), toxic epidermal necrolysis (TEN), and drug rash with eosinophilia and systemic symptoms (DRESS) syndrome.

Stevens-Johnson Syndrome

SJS is a systemic disorder that has cutaneous manifestations. SJS was previously thought to be synonymous with erythema multiforme major. There are now criteria that separate the two disorders. In contrast to erythema multiforme, the target lesions associated with SJS have only two rings. The inner ring may have urticaria, pustules, or necrotic lesions surrounded by macular erythema. It is a T-cell–mediated toxic reaction to the basement membrane of the epidermal cells. There is massive and widespread apoptosis, for which there are several associated cytokines. The recent theories suggest that there are two pathways, one that consists of granule-medicated exocytosis (perforin and granzyme B), and one that consists of Fas-Fas ligand interaction associated apoptosis for the keratinocytes. More recent data suggest that granulysin, which is a cationic cytolytic protein released by T lymphocytes, may play a role as well.

Interestingly, HLA genotype may predispose patients to SJS or TEN. Those patients with the HLA-B1502 found among the Han Chinese population may be associated with increased risk for developing SJS/TEN and use of carbamazepine.

SJS and TEN are on the same continuum. The definition of epidermal detachment and desquamation of epidermal cells is less than 10% of the body surface area for SJS and more than 30% for TEN. There is an overlapping diagnosis of SJS/TEN for the 10% to 30% category. To help differentiate from other ADRs, there is often a prodromal period in which a patient may have a cough and a fever. The lesions may occur up to 4 weeks after exposure to the drug. In addition, the lesions may be limited to the trunk; however, they more commonly involve the palmar surface of the hands and the dorsum of the feet, as well as the mucous membranes.

The most common drug classes associated with SJS and TENs are sulfonamides, cephalosporins, imidazole agents, and oxicam derivatives. Drugs such as carbamazepine, phenytoin (Dilantin), valproic acid (Depakote), lamotrigine (Lamictal), allopurinol (Zyloprim), nevirapine (Viramune), peramivir (Rapivab), and quinolones have been reported to cause SJS/TEN. In a retrospective chart review of 64 patients who had a diagnosis of SJS/TEN, Miliszewski et al. identified allopurinol as the single most common offending agent (20% of cases). According to the US Food and Drug Administration (FDA) Safety Alerts in 2013, acetaminophen has been associated with SJS, TEN, and acute generalized exanthematous pustulosis (AGEP). The evidence supporting causality primarily comes from a small number of cases reported in the medical literature.

The treatment is immediate cessation of the culprit drug and symptomatic treatment. Glucocorticoids are controversial and depend on the course and extent of the disease.

Toxic Epidermal Necrolysis

As previously stated, TEN is the cell-mediated disorder that involves more than 30% of the body surface. This is the more-severe form of the ADR: the mortality rates may be as high as 50%, mostly from sepsis. Patients are usually admitted to the burn unit for electrolyte and infection management. Glucocorticoids are contraindicated. There have been mixed results using IV immunoglobulin (IVIG)[1] in these patients. The IVIG is believed to inhibit the Fas-Fas ligand, which is the underlying mechanism for the basement membrane separation.

Drug Rash with Eosinophilia and Systemic Symptoms

DRESS syndrome or drug-induced hypersensitivity syndrome (DIHS) is a rare, life-threatening drug-induced reaction with a mortality rate of 10%. Therefore it is important to recognize the signs and symptoms early to initiate treatment. Most patients will have fever, lymphadenopathy (75%), eosinophilia, and an erythematous morbilliform rash on the face and body in addition to liver and multiorgan damage. The symptoms can occur 2 to 6 weeks after the drug administration. There are many drugs that can cause DRESS syndrome such as allopurinol, sulfonamides, and psychotropic medications. Based on literature review, DRESS syndrome is increasingly being recognized by psychiatrists. Carbamazepine is the most frequently reported etiology; however,

DRESS syndrome is also seen with lamotrigine, phenytoin, valproate, and phenobarbital. The treatment is drug withdrawal, systemic corticosteroids, topical treatment for lesions, and supportive care, often in the ICU or burn unit.

Acute Generalized Exanthematous Pustulosis

Acute generalized exanthematous pustulosis (AGEP) is a rare ADR that presents as a fever and small nonfollicular pustules on a widespread erythematous background. AGEP may closely mimic pustular psoriasis clinically. The presence of acanthuses and papillomatosis and a personal or family history of psoriasis favor a diagnosis of pustular psoriasis. Exposure to medication, especially antibiotics with a short latency from the initiation of the drug, favors AGEP. The eruption usually occurs within 24 hours of the initiation of the drug, and healing occurs quickly after the discontinuation of the drug. Lesions heal within 2 weeks of discontinuation without scarring. The exact mechanism of drug-specific T lymphocytes is unknown, yet IL-3 and IL-8 may be the trigger for neutrophil-activating cytokines in the skin.

Acute Interstitial Nephritis

Acute interstitial nephritis (AIN) is an important cause of acute kidney injury (AKI). More than two thirds of AIN cases are caused by drug hypersensitivity reactions. Drugs most commonly associated with AIN include antibiotics (particularly β-lactam, fluoroquinolones, and rifampicin), NSAIDs, proton pump inhibitors, phenytoin, allopurinol, and 5-aminosalicylates.

The clinical presentation of drug-induced AIN is highly variable and depends on the class of drug involved. Patients with AIN may be asymptomatic with elevation in creatinine or blood urea nitrogen or abnormal urinary sediment. When present, symptoms are nonspecific. The "classic" triad of fever, rash, and eosinophilia is present in less than 5% to 10% of patients. Each individual component of the triad also occurs at various rates.

A diagnosis of AIN should be considered in any patients with unexplained AKI, clinical manifestations of a hypersensitivity reaction, and a history of exposure to any drug associated with AIN. A definitive diagnosis of AIN is established by kidney biopsy. AIN is characterized by interstitial inflammation, tubulitis, edema, and, in some cases, eventual interstitial fibrosis. The precise disease mechanism is unclear, but the presence of T lymphocytes in the inflammatory infiltrate suggests a type IV hypersensitivity response.

Early recognition is crucial as patients can ultimately develop chronic kidney disease. The mainstay of therapy is timely discontinuation of the causative agent. If AIN persists, corticosteroids may be used to improve kidney function. However, available data on corticosteroids are inconclusive, and randomized controlled trials are needed to confirm the benefits of corticosteroids in the treatment of AIN.

Evaluation

Because the history is essential for determining whether a patient is experiencing a drug hypersensitivity reaction, it is important to review all medications and the timeline of exposure. This includes any over-the-counter medications, herbal supplements, or occasional-use medications. Occasional-use medications may include NSAIDs, acetaminophen, cold medications, and so forth. It is important to establish a temporal relationship to the onset of the medication and the initiation of the symptoms. Oftentimes, the medication may have been discontinued before the appearance of the first symptom, so a review of medications from several weeks before the symptoms is also important. In addition, because the host immune response plays a role in some of the IgE-mediated reactions, it is important to review any immunocompromising chronic or acute illnesses or states that the patient may have or is currently experiencing. This includes HIV, chronic obstructive pulmonary disease (COPD), asthma, chemotherapy, and pregnancy. For some ADRs, HLA type may be important. A patient's known genetic predisposition needs to be taken into account as well. A thorough history will also need to include any organ system or symptom that may be related to the suspected ADR.

---

[1]Not FDA approved for this indication.

A physical examination should augment and help to establish the working diagnosis of the type of ADR and the potentially offending drug. This should include vital signs of temperature, respiratory, and hydration status. The skin examination is important, as are appropriate evaluation and documentation of the type of lesion or lesions present. An examination of the oral mucosa and the conjunctiva of the eye should be done. Any lymphadenopathy, petechiae, or pallor should be noted.

Laboratory testing may be obtained to confirm or rule out a diagnosis. This may include a chest x-ray, CBC with differential, possible skin biopsy, liver function testing, creatinine, and electrolyte testing. A sedimentation rate and CRP testing may also be useful. Although additional autoimmune or antibody testing may be done, caution is suggested. There may not be a high yield on these tests, and they can be quite costly for patients.

Management

Anaphylaxis

Anaphylaxis can be a fatal drug hypersensitivity reaction because of its rapid onset. It is often underrecognized and undertreated because it can mimic other conditions and is variable in its presentation. However, respiratory compromise and cardiovascular collapse are of greatest concern, because they are the most common causes of death. Urticaria and angioedema are the most common manifestations but may be delayed or absent. The more quickly anaphylaxis occurs after exposure to the offending agent, the more likely the reaction is to be severe and potentially life threatening.

Most anaphylaxis episodes are IgE-mediated reactions resulting in a sudden mast cell and basophil degranulation. This sudden release of mediators affects the cutaneous, pulmonary, cardiac, GI, vascular, and neurologic systems. Medications are a common trigger of anaphylaxis in adults. Most cases of IgE-mediated drug anaphylaxis in the United States are due to penicillins and cephalosporins. Antibiotics are also the most common cause of perioperative anaphylaxis because skin eruptions may be missed in patients who are draped during surgery. Some anaphylaxis reactions involve other immunologic mechanisms. Administration of blood products (e.g., IVIG, animal antiserum) can cause an anaphylactoid reaction due, at least in part, to complement activation. Activation of the complement cascade can cause mast cell/basophil degranulation. Anaphylaxis episodes can also occur independently of any immunologic mechanism. Certain drugs, such as opioids, dextrans, and protamine, can cause a direct release of histamine and other mediators from mast cells and basophils. Finally, there are acute systemic reactions without any obvious triggers or mechanisms (idiopathic anaphylaxis).

Anaphylaxis is a clinical diagnosis with a short window of treatment time available. Therefore laboratory testing is limited and may not be of much value. Initially, the patient will describe flushing, pruritus, and a sense of impending doom. Some patients will have dyspnea, dizziness, syncope, or GI symptoms of diarrhea and abdominal cramping. Most patients will have cutaneous symptoms of flushing, urticaria, or angioedema. Some patients will progress to respiratory or cardiovascular complications.

The goal of therapy should be early recognition and treatment with epinephrine to prevent a progression to life-threatening respiratory or cardiovascular failure. The immediate intervention should include stopping the offending drug if possible, epinephrine injection, basic life support, high-flow oxygen, cardiac monitoring, and IV access. Epinephrine is the drug of choice for anaphylaxis. The therapeutic actions of epinephrine include α-1-adrenergic vasoconstrictor effects (decreases mucosal edema, thereby relieving upper airway obstruction, and increases blood pressure to prevent shock), β-1 adrenergic effects (increases rate and force of cardiac contractions), and β-2 effects (increases bronchodilation and decreases the release of mediators of inflammation from mast cells/basophils). Delayed epinephrine administration has been associated with fatalities. Intramuscular epinephrine in the thigh results in high-plasma concentrations and is preferred in the setting of anaphylaxis. The recommended dose of epinephrine is 0.3 mg (1 mg/mL) IM every 5 minutes. Typically, only one or two additional doses are needed. Patients in shock should receive epinephrine by slow IV infusion at 2 to 10 mcg/min with the rate titrated according to response and the presence of continuous hemodynamic monitoring. Patients taking beta-blockers may be resistant to treatment with epinephrine. In this case, glucagon[1] 1 to 5 mg IV over 5 minutes should be administered because its cardiac effects are not mediated through beta-receptors.

Adjunctive therapies for the treatment of anaphylaxis include antihistamines and corticosteroids. Consider an inhaled beta-agonist if wheezing. Diphenhydramine (Benadryl), an H_1 antihistamine, may be given intravenously at the dose of 25 to 50 mg. If an H_2 blocker is considered, give ranitidine (Zantac)[1] 50 mg/20 mL as an IV infusion over 5 minutes. Use of both diphenhydramine and ranitidine is superior to diphenhydramine alone. Corticosteroids are used to prevent a potential late-phase reaction that may occur in up to 23% of adults with anaphylaxis. There is no proven best dose or route of steroid therapy. The most common dosage is prednisone 20 to 60 mg daily for 3 to 5 days.

Angioedema

Angioedema is characterized by a deep dermal, subcutaneous, mucosal swelling. Many patients present with both urticaria and angioedema. Angioedema can progress rapidly from a mild swelling of the oral mucosal to a life-threatening laryngeal edema. With this rapid sequence of events, the most important part of treatment is obtaining and maintaining a patent airway. Epinephrine 0.3 mg IM every 10 minutes should be administered to patients who present with anaphylaxis, respiratory distress, or severe laryngeal edema. Once the airway is patent, the patient should be treated with H_1 antihistamines, H_2 blockers, and steroids. The milder cases may be treated similarly to other allergic reactions. H_1 antihistamines such as diphenhydramine and hydroxyzine (Atarax) are effective in relieving pruritus but can cause significant sedation. Therefore second-generation H_1 antihistamines[1] (loratadine [Claritin], cetirizine [Zyrtec], desloratadine [Clarinex], fexofenadine [Allegra]) are often chosen for outpatient therapy. Doxepin (Sinequan),[1] a tricyclic antidepressant with potent H_1 and H_2 blocker activities, can be used as an alternative to H_1 antihistamines. However, it should not be used as first-line treatment for acute urticaria and angioedema because of its significant side effects of severe sedation, dry mouth, and weight gain. Corticosteroids are used in patients who are not responsive to antihistamines. For most patients, a short course of oral prednisone is adequate.

In drug-induced angioedema, the offending drug should be stopped and avoided. Further trial of the medication is not recommended, because the patient will respond more quickly and with more severe symptoms on reintroduction. The patient should be counseled, and epinephrine 0.3 mg in an auto-injectable device (EpiPen, Auvi-Q, Adrenaclick) may be prescribed in case of recurrence in the future.

Specific Drugs

Almost all drugs can cause a drug hypersensitivity reaction. However, certain drugs are more frequently associated with specific types of reactions. Some of the more commonly used drugs are discussed here in more detail.

Antibiotics

Penicillin

Penicillin allergy is the most well-known drug allergy and also the most costly ADR. Although most drugs usually have type I and type IV reactions, penicillin may cause all four types of allergic drug reactions. The rate of penicillin-induced anaphylaxis after intravenous administration is approximately 1 to 2 per 10,000 treated patients.

---

[1] Not FDA approved for this indication.

Only about 10% of patients who report a penicillin drug allergy actually have a true immunologic response. The other 90% are actually able to tolerate penicillin or a cephalosporin. Patients with a penicillin allergy label are more likely to be treated with broad-spectrum or second-line antibiotics. Inappropriate use of antibiotics is linked to increased antibiotic resistance and adverse health outcomes. There is an increasing focus on penicillin allergy delabeling as an integral part of antimicrobial stewardship. Algorithms are available to clarify a patient's allergy status and expedite the evaluation for true penicillin allergy. Trubiano et al. recently developed a clinical decision tool, PEN-FAST, to aid risk stratification of patients with penicillin allergy and facilitate appropriate delabeling and prescribing strategies.

Penicillin skin testing is the best method for diagnosing an IgE-mediated penicillin allergy. A commercially available product, PRE-PEN, contains benzylpenicilloyl polylysine (PPL), which is a major antigenic determinant of penicillin. Minor determinants are metabolic derivatives of penicillin that may also produce an immune response. The current recommendations for penicillin skin testing are to administer both the major determinant (PPL) and the minor determinants (penicillin G). These two tests identify approximately 90% to 97% of the currently allergic patients. Patients with a history of penicillin allergy but negative skin testing to PPL and the minor determinants rarely experience allergic reactions on reexposure. If they should occur, the reactions are mild and self-limiting.

In general, patients who report symptoms consistent with an immediate or type I reaction or are skin-test positive to penicillin should not receive penicillin. Desensitization should be considered if penicillin is the treatment of choice for an infection and no acceptable nonpenicillin alternatives are available. Patients should be desensitized in a hospital setting. Desensitization involves administering incremental doses of oral penicillin every 15 minutes for a total of 4 to 12 hours, after which time the first dose of penicillin is given. For intravenous desensitization, three drug concentrations of penicillin are infused in 12 steps. Penicillin desensitization protocols are available in the review article by Castells et al. Desensitization is temporary and only lasts for two dosing intervals of the drug before the desensitization needs to be repeated.

Penicillin and Cephalosporin Cross-Reactivity

The rate of cross-reactivity between penicillin and cephalosporins has been historically cited to be as high as 10%. Recent data suggest that the rate may be much lower. The degree of cross-reactivity is highest between penicillins and first-generation cephalosporins, which have identical R-group side chains. In this case amoxicillin would be cross-reactive with cefadroxil (Duricef) and cefprozil (Cefzil), whereas ampicillin would be with cefaclor and cephalexin. Because of the differences in the chemical structures, second- and third-generation cephalosporins (cefdinir [Omnicef], cefuroxime [Ceftin], cefpodoxime [Vantin], and ceftriaxone [Rocephin]) are unlikely to be associated with cross-reactivity with penicillin. According to the latest guidelines for acute otitis media from the American Academy of Pediatrics and American Academy of Family Physicians, alternative initial antibiotics in patients with penicillin allergy include cefdinir, cefuroxime, cefpodoxime, or ceftriaxone.

Patients with penicillin allergy who have a negative skin-test result to penicillin (major and minor determinants) may safely receive cephalosporins. Cephalosporin treatment of patients with penicillin allergy who did not have a severe or recent penicillin reaction history shows a reaction rate of 0.1%. Use cephalosporin with caution in patients who report an immediate or accelerated penicillin allergy or those with a positive skin test to penicillin.

Sulfonamides (Sulfa Drugs)

Beside penicillins, sulfonamide antibiotics are the second most common cause of drug-induced allergic reactions. They commonly cause a delayed maculopapular/morbilliform eruption. Acute urticarial reactions (IgE mediated) to sulfamethoxazole

(SMX) or trimethoprim (TMP) are relatively infrequent; the incidence of skin rash resulting from SMX-TMP (Bactrim) in healthy subjects is estimated to be 3%. Sulfonamides are also the most common cause of SJS and TEN.

Patients with HIV have the greatest risk of sulfonamide-induced allergic reactions. The typical reaction to SMX-TMP in patients with HIV is a generalized maculopapular eruption that occurs during the second week of treatment and is usually accompanied by pruritus and fever. Because SMX-TMP is the drug of choice for a number of HIV-associated infections such as *Pneumocystis carinii* pneumonia and spontaneous bacterial peritonitis, several methods of desensitization have been devised to administer SMX-TMP to patients with HIV with a history of allergic reaction to the drug.

There are three classes of sulfonamides based on chemical structure: sulfonylarylamines (including sulfa antibiotics), nonsulfonylarylamines, and sulfonamide-moiety-containing drugs. A sulfonylarylamine has a sulfonamide moiety directly attached to a benzene ring with an amine (–NH₂) moiety at the N4 position. A nonsulfonylarylamine also has a sulfonamide moiety attached to a benzene ring, but it does not have an amine group at the N4 position. A sulfonamide-moiety–containing drug has a sulfonamide group that is not connected to a benzene ring. Table 2 presents a list of sulfonamide-containing drugs based on their chemical structure.

The N4 amine is critical for the development of delayed reactions to sulfa antibiotics. Given the important chemical differences between drugs containing sulfa antibiotics and sulfa in nonantibiotics, the risk of cross-reactivity is extremely unlikely. A retrospective cohort study by Strom and colleagues showed that approximately 90% of patients with sulfa antibiotic allergy did not have a reaction to a sulfonamide nonantibiotic. Patients with allergic reactions to sulfa antibiotics are also more likely to

TABLE 2	Classification of Sulfonamides Based on Chemical Structure

Drug

Sulfonylarylamines

Antibiotics:	*Antiinflammatory:*
Sulfadiazine	Sulfasalazine (Azulfidine)
Sulfamethoxazole	Protease Inhibitors:
Sulfisoxazole	Darunavir (Prezista)
Sulfapyridine	Fosamprenavir (Lexiva)

Nonsulfonylarylamines

Carbonic Anhydrase Inhibitors:	*Sulfonylureas:*
Acetazolamide (Diamox)	Chlorpropamide
Brinzolamide (Azopt)	Glimepiride (Amaryl)
Dorzolamide (Trusopt)	Glipizide (Glucotrol)
Methazolamide (Neptazane)	Glyburide (Diabeta)
Cyclooxygenase 2 (COX-2) Inhibitors:	Tolbutamide
Celecoxib (Celebrex)	Tolazamide (Tolinase)
Loop Diuretics:	Other Agents:
Bumetanide (Bumex)	Mafenide (Sulfamylon)
Furosemide (Lasix)	Probenecid
Torsemide (Demadex)	Tamsulosin (Flomax)
Thiazides Diuretics:	Tipranavir (Aptivus)
Chlorothiazide (Diuril)	
Chlorthalidone	
Hydrochlorothiazide	
Indapamide (Lozol)	
Metolazone (Zaroxolyn)	

Sulfonamide-Moiety-Containing Drugs

5-HT Agonists:	*Other Agents:*
Naratriptan (Amerge)	Ibutilide (Corvert)
Sumatriptan (Imitrex)	Simeprevir (Olysio)
	Sotalol (Betapace)
	Topiramate (Topamax)
	Zonisamide (Zonegran)

experience allergic reactions to the other types of sulfonamides, but this is not because of cross-sensitivity. There is no reliable skin test to rule out or confirm sulfa allergy. Some experts recommend avoiding all classes of sulfonamides in patients with serious reactions such as SJS, TEN, or anaphylaxis to any one sulfonamide.

Most diuretics are sulfonamide derivatives. The only diuretics that are not in this group are the potassium-sparing diuretics (triamterene [Dyrenium], spironolactone [Aldactone], amiloride [Midamor]) and ethacrynic acid (Edecrin). Dapsone is a sulfone that is chemically unrelated to sulfonamides. *It should also be noted that sulfates, sulfur, and sulfites are chemically unrelated to sulfonamides and do not cross-react.*

Angiotensin-Converting Enzyme Inhibitors

Angiotensin-converting enzyme inhibitors (ACEIs) have two major adverse effects: cough and angioedema. The cough is typically dry and nonproductive. The incidence of ACEI-induced cough has been reported to be 5% to 35%. Cough occurs more commonly in women, African-Americans, and Asians. The onset of cough ranges from within hours of the first dose to months after the initiation of therapy. The diagnosis is confirmed by the resolution of cough, usually within 1 to 4 weeks after discontinuation of the ACEI; however, the cough can linger for up to 3 months. The cause for ACEI-induced cough is unclear but might be related to bradykinin, substance P, or another mechanism. Angiotensin II receptor blockers (ARBs) are not associated with an increased incidence of cough and can be used as an alternative to ACEIs. Because the cough may persist for several months after stopping the ACEI, starting the ARB is not a contraindication at this time, yet the cough may persist through the initiation of the new drug.

The incidence of angioedema with ACEIs is approximately 0.1% to 0.7%. With the widespread use of ACEIs, angioedema has become a growing problem. ACEI-induced angioedema is more common in patients who are over age 65, black, or female. Angioedema frequently involves swelling of the face or upper airway and can be life threatening or fatal. It can occur within days, months, or even years after the start of treatment. However, nearly 60% of cases occur within the first week of therapy. ACEIs cause angioedema by direct interference with the degradation of bradykinin, thereby increasing bradykinin levels and leading to increased vascular permeability, inflammation, and activation of nociceptors. Bradykinin is also a prominent mediator in hereditary angioedema. Therefore ACEIs are contraindicated in patients with hereditary angioedema.

ARBs directly inhibit the angiotensin receptor and do not interfere with bradykinin degradation. Theoretically, they can be relatively safe alternatives for patients with a previous history of ACEI-associated angioedema. However, some reports of ARB-induced angioedema have recently been published. The mechanism of how ARBs cause angioedema is unclear. A meta-analysis suggests that for patients who developed angioedema when taking an ACEI, the risk of persistent angioedema when subsequently switched to an ARB is less than 10%. Therefore ARBs may be an alternative only for patients with a high therapeutic need for angiotensin inhibition. ARB treatment should be started with observation. Patients should be educated on the signs of angioedema and provided with proper emergency instructions on how to proceed if angioedema should occur.

The direct renin inhibitor aliskiren (Tekturna) does not alter local or circulating bradykinin and is believed to be an alternative in patients with ACEI- and ARB-related angioedema. However, cases of angioedema have been reported with aliskiren. As with ARBs, renin inhibitors should be used with caution in patients who previously experienced angioedema to ACEIs.

Aspirin and NSAIDs

Aspirin (ASA) and NSAIDs can cause several types of hypersensitivity reactions. The four most-common types of reactions are based on the drug pathways. Aspirin-exacerbated respiratory disease (AERD) is a serious reaction induced by ASA and NSAIDs in patients with asthma and chronic rhinosinusitis. AERD does not fit precisely into a specific type of ADR and is often referred to as a type of pseudoallergic reaction. AERD affects up to 20% of adults with asthma. It is more common in women. The usual age of onset is around 30 years. The pathophysiology of AERD is related to aberrant arachidonic acid metabolism. Patients with AERD also have increased respiratory tract expression of cysteinyl leukotriene 1 receptor and heightened responsiveness to inhaled leukotriene E_4. Administration of aspirin or an NSAID to these patients leads to inhibition of cyclooxygenase 1 (COX-1), resulting in a decrease in prostaglandin E_2 levels. Prostaglandin E_2 normally inhibits 5-lipooxygenase. As a result of decreased prostaglandin E_2 levels, arachidonic acid is preferentially metabolized in the 5-lipooxygenase pathway, leading to increased production of cysteinyl leukotrienes.

Patients with AERD typically have both rhinoconjunctivitis and bronchospasm within minutes of ingestion of a dose of ASA or NSAID. The bronchospasm can be severe and result in respiratory failure, which may require intubation and mechanical ventilation. Management of patients with AERD involves treatment of the patient's asthma and chronic rhinosinusitis and avoidance of aspirin and NSAIDs. Desensitization is available in cases when the patient has a specific therapeutic need for regular ASA or NSAID therapy. Selective COX-2 inhibitors very rarely cause reactions in patients with AERD and can be taken safely.

The second type of ASA and NSAID hypersensitivity reaction is an exacerbation of urticaria or angioedema in patients with chronic idiopathic urticaria. Approximately 20% to 40% of patients with chronic urticaria may have this drug-induced reaction. The mechanism of this reaction is related to COX-1 inhibition. The exacerbating effects are usually dose dependent. All drugs that inhibit COX-1 cross-react to cause this reaction. Selective COX-2 inhibitors are generally considered safe to take in patients with chronic idiopathic urticaria.

The third type of hypersensitivity reaction is an anaphylactic or immediate urticarial reaction or angioedema appearing soon after the intake of a specific NSAID. Other NSAIDs from other groups or even an NSAID from the same group with a slightly different chemical structure is tolerated by the patient. An IgE-mediated mechanism is implicated only in some instances. The diagnosis is made mainly by exclusion. Further research is needed in this topic.

The fourth type of hypersensitivity reaction is urticaria or angioedema caused by ASA or any NSAID that inhibits COX-1 in patients without chronic urticaria. These reactions may be either drug specific or cross-reactive to other NSAIDs. Rarely, patients may have combined respiratory and cutaneous reactions that cannot be classified into one of the four reaction types described.

Corticosteroids

Corticosteroids are the most frequently used drugs for the treatment of allergic conditions, yet they can also induce hypersensitivity reactions. Most hypersensitivity reactions to steroids can be classified into type I (immediate, IgE-mediated) and type IV (delayed, cell-mediated) mechanisms. Type I reactions are characterized by the presence of urticaria and anaphylaxis. Type IV reactions can be presented as maculopapular exanthema and delayed urticaria.

Allergic contact dermatitis (type IV reaction) caused by topical administration of steroids is the most common type of allergic reaction induced by this class of drugs, occurring at the rate of 3% to 6%. Usually this is seen as a failure to improve or a worsening of an existing dermatitis that is being treated with topical steroid. Keep in mind that the reaction can also be due to other constituents of the creams, such as neomycin or cetostearyl alcohol. The diagnosis can be done using patch testing, which detects more than 90% of allergic patients. The topical steroids most frequently involved are nonfluorinated, such as hydrocortisone and budesonide.

Inhaled and intranasal steroids can induce both local and systemic reactions. Local reactions include contact dermatitis, pruritus, nasal congestion, erythema, and dry cough and are quite often irritant in nature. Systemic reactions include eczematous lesions, particularly on the face, exanthema, and urticaria. The most frequently involved steroid is budesonide. The actual mechanism of this reaction is not clear, but it may be a T-cell–mediated reaction.

Hypersensitivity reactions to systemically administered steroids seldom occur. Most of the data come from case reports. Both immediate and delayed reactions have been described, ranging from urticaria to sudden cardiovascular collapse and death. Most immediate reactions are caused by intravenous methylprednisolone and hydrocortisone. In a few cases, the reactions can be induced by salts, such as succinate, or rarely by certain diluents such as carboxymethylcellulose or metabisulfite. Nonimmediate reactions are mainly mild, such as delayed urticaria or maculopapular exanthema. The drug involved most often is betamethasone.

Cross-reactivity between steroids is difficult to assess. Based on corticosteroid patch test results and their chemical structure, Coopman and colleagues divided the steroids into four groups: A (hydrocortisone type), B (triamcinolone acetonide type), C (betamethasone type), and D (hydrocortisone-17-butyrate type). Group D can be subdivided into D1 and D2 depending on the presence or absence of a C16 methyl substitution and/or halogenations on the C9 of the B ring. Table 3 provides the listing of the four groups. High cross-reactivity exists between corticosteroids in each group, as well as between group D2 and groups A and B, with group D1 exhibiting quite low cross-reactivity with the other groups.

Local Anesthetics
The most common immunologic reaction to local anesthetic is allergic contact dermatitis (type IV). IgE-mediated reactions (type I) to local anesthetics are very rare. Most adverse reactions are due to nonallergic factors such as vasovagal response, anxiety, dysrhythmias, and toxic reactions resulting from inadvertent IV epinephrine effects.

Any patient who presents with a history of an allergic reaction to local anesthetics should be carefully evaluated. Skin testing and graded challenge can be performed in patients who present with a history suggestive of a possible IgE-mediated allergic reaction to these drugs. A local anesthetic that does not contain epinephrine or other additives, such as parabens or sulfites, is preferred in this situation.

It is necessary to identify the type of local anesthetics to be used. Local anesthetics are classified as esters or amides based on their chemical structure. Drugs in the esters group include benzocaine (Americaine, Dermoplast, Lanacane, Hurricaine), chloroprocaine, cocaine, procaine (Novocaine), proparacaine (Alcaine, Opthaine), and tetracaine (Tetcaine). Most allergic reactions reported in the literature have been caused by agents in the esters group, which are derivatives of para-aminobenzoic acid (PABA), a known allergen. Cross-reactivity occurs among members of the ester group, but the esters do not cross-react with the amides. Agents in the amides group include bupivacaine (Marcaine), lidocaine, mepivacaine (Polocaine), prilocaine (Citanest), and ropivacaine (Naropin). Amide local anesthetics generally do not cross-react with other amides or with the esters.

Radiocontrast Media
There are two types of radiocontrast media (RCM): ionic high osmolality and nonionic low osmolality. Both of these agents contain iodine. The nonionic RCMs are much more widely used today than the ionic agents.

Allergic reactions to RCM are common and can range from mild to life threatening. Anaphylactoid reactions and severe life-threatening reactions occur in 1% to 3% and 0.22% of patients who receive ionic RCM, respectively. Less than 0.5% and 0.04% of patients who receive nonionic agents have anaphylactoid reactions and severe reactions, respectively. The fatality rate is approximately 1 to 2 per 100,000 procedures, and it is similar for both ionic and nonionic agents. RCM reactions are typically not mediated by IgE antibodies. RCM acts directly on mast cells and basophils, resulting in the release of histamine and other systemic mediators, which cause the anaphylactoid reactions. Patients at greater risk for more serious anaphylactoid reactions include females; those with asthma, heart disease, and a history of previous anaphylactoid reaction to RCM; and those taking beta-blockers. People who have seafood allergy are not at increased risk for reactions to RCM compared with the general population. The pathogenesis of anaphylactoid reactions is also not related to iodine.

Management of patients with previous RCM reactions include the use of a nonionic, low-osmolality agent and a pretreatment regimen. One common regimen consists of prednisone (50 mg PO at 13, 7, and 1 hour before the procedure), diphenhydramine (50 mg at 1 hour before the procedure), and a histamine H$_2$-receptor antagonist (1 hour before the procedure). This will significantly reduce the risk for anaphylactoid reaction with reexposure to RCM.

Delayed reactions to RCM occur 1 hour to 1 week after RCM administration. Approximately 2% of patients have delayed reactions to RCM. These reactions are generally mild, self-limited cutaneous eruptions. The mechanism is usually T-cell mediated. Rarely, more serious and life-threatening delayed reactions such as SJS, TEN, and DRESS syndrome have been reported.

Chlorhexidine
Chlorhexidine gluconate is an antiseptic agent. It is commonly available in OTC products as a skin and wound disinfectant (e.g., Betasept, Hibiclens). Hypersensitivity reactions to chlorhexidine include contact dermatitis, pruritus, urticaria, dyspnea, and anaphylaxis. Prescription chlorhexidine gluconate mouthwashes and

TABLE 3	Coopman Classification of Cross-Reactivity in Corticosteroids	
GROUP	**TYPE**	**DRUGS**
A	Hydrocortisone	Hydrocortisone (acetate, succinate, phosphate) Methylprednisolone (acetate, succinate, phosphate) Prednisolone, prednisolone acetate Tixocortol pivalate*
B	Triamcinolone acetonide	Amcinonide (Cyclocort) Budesonide (Pulmicort, Rhinocort, Entocort) Desonide (Desonate, DesOwen) Flunisolide Fluocinolone acetonide (Synalar) Fluocinolone Halcinonide (Halog) Triamcinolone Triamcinolone acetonide (Kenalog)
C	Betamethasone	Betamethasone (Celestone) Desoxymethasone Dexamethasone Paramethasone* Fluocortolone*
D1	Hydrocortisone-17-butyrate	Beclomethasone dipropionate (QVAR) Betamethasone valerate Betamethasone dipropionate Clobethasone 17-butyrate* Clobetasol 17-propyonate (Clobex)
D2	Hydrocortisone-17-butyrate	Fluticasone (Flonase) Mometasone Prednicarbate (Dermatop) Hydrocortisone 17-butyrate (Locoid) Hydrocortisone 17-propionate* Methylprednisolone aceponate*

*Not available in the United States.
From Torres and Canto (2010).

oral chips used for gum disease contain a warning about the rare but serious allergic reactions in their labels. According to a recent FDA Drug Safety Communication, the number of reports of serious allergic reactions to chlorhexidine-containing products has increased over the last several years. As a result, an anaphylaxis warning is now added to the OTC product labels under Drug Facts.

Several case reports have suggested that some patients with prior exposure to chlorhexidine and patients with chlorhexidine-induced contact dermatitis may be susceptible to anaphylaxis caused by chlorhexidine sensitization. Since chlorhexidine is the standard skin disinfectant used before surgery or invasive procedures, the exposure to the agent becomes more widespread. Even though severe anaphylaxis to chlorhexidine has been estimated to be rare, the actual rate may be higher than reported. Such reports remind clinicians to be vigilant about chlorhexidine as a hidden allergen, especially in surgical patients.

Herbal Supplements

There is a perception that herbal supplements are "natural" and therefore safe. In fact, severe allergic reactions including asthma and anaphylaxis have been well documented in patients using bee pollen products and echinacea. Echinacea is an herb belonging to a group of flowering plants known as Asteraceae. Asteraceae-derived pollens are an important cause of hay fever and asthma. Asteraceae may cause contact allergic dermatitis. Cross-reactivity exists between members of the Asteraceae family, such as ragweed, dandelion, daisy, chamomile, echinacea, feverfew, and milk thistle.

A lack of quality control has been a major concern in the herbal supplement industry. Chinese herbal products may be adulterated with synthetic medications not listed on the label. Contaminated supplements may be a potential risk for systemic contact dermatitis in nickel- and mercury-allergic patients. Because of the widespread use of herbal supplements and the underreporting of adverse events to herbs, all patients should be questioned about the use of herbal supplements when being evaluated for hypersensitivity reactions.

Conclusion

Drug hypersensitivity reactions are common; fortunately, severe and often fatal reactions are not. It is important for the clinician to have a working knowledge of common drug-induced hypersensitive reactions as well as the ability to identify and document common dermatologic findings. With that background knowledge, a thorough history and physical examination should enable the clinician to diagnose the majority of these types of reactions. A timely and appropriate management plan can then be implemented. As always, it is important to educate patients regarding their drug hypersensitivity history and the potential for future reactions.

References

American Academy of Pediatrics: Clinical practice guideline: The diagnosis and management of acute otitis media, *Pediatrics* 131:e964–e969, 2013.
Bommersbach TJ, Lapid MI, Leung JG, et al: Management of psychotropic drug-induced DRESS syndrome: A systematic review, *Mayo Clin Proc* 91(6):787–801, 2016.
Castells M, Khan DA, Phillips EJ: Penicillin allergy, *N Engl J Med* 381:2338–2351, 2019.
CDC: Sexually transmitted disease treatment guidelines 2015, *MMWR* 64(3):149–151, 2015.
Fernando SL: Acute generalized exanthematous pustulosis, *Australas J Dermatol* 53:87–92, 2012.
Harr T, French L: Toxic epidermal necrolysis and Stevens-Johnson syndrome, *Orphanet J Rare Dis* 5:39, 2010. Available at http://www.ojrd.com/content/5/1/39.
Haymore BR, Yoon J, Mikita CP, et al: Risk of angioedema with angiotensin receptor blockers in patients with prior angioedema associated with angiotensin-converting enzyme inhibitors: A meta-analysis, *Ann Allergy Asthma Immunol* 101:495–499, 2008.
Husain Z, Reddy BY, Schwartz RA: DRESS syndrome, part I. Clinical perspectives, *J Am Acad Dermatol* 68:693.e1–693.e14, 2013.
Inomata N: Recent advances in drug-induced angioedema, *Allergol Int* 61:545–557, 2012.

Joint Task Force on Practice Parameters, AAAAI, ACAAI: Drug allergy: An updated practice parameter, *Ann Allergy Asthma Immunol* 105:259–273, 2010.
Khan DA, Solensky R: Drug allergy, *J Allergy Clin Immunol* 125:S126–S137, 2010.
Lieberman P, Nicklas RA, Opperheimer J, et al: The diagnosis and management of anaphylaxis practice parameter: 2010 update, *J Allergy Clin Immunol* 126:477–480, 2010.
Miliszewski MA, Kirchhof MG, Sikora S, et al: Stevens-Johnson syndrome and toxic epidermal necrolysis: An analysis of triggers and implications for improving prevention, *Am J Med* 129(11):1221–1225, 2016.
Moka E, Argyra E, Siafaka I, Vadalouca A: Chlorhexidine: Hypersensitivity and anaphylactic reactions in the perioperative setting, *J Anaesthesiol Clin Pharmacol* 31(2):145–148, 2015.
Murata J, Abe R: Soluble Fas ligand: Is it a critical mediator of toxic epidermal necrolysis and Stevens-Johnson syndrome? *J Invest Dermatol* 127:744–745, 2007.
Perazella MA, Markowitz GS: Drug-induced acute interstitial nephritis, *Nat Rev Nephrol* 6(8):461–470, 2010.
Philips JF, Yates AB, Deshazo RD: Approach to patients with suspected hypersensitivity to local anesthetics, *Am J Med Sci* 334:190–196, 2007.
Pichler WJ: Consequences of drug binding to immune receptors: Immune stimulation following pharmacological interaction with immune receptors (T-cell receptor for antigen or human leukocyte antigen) with altered peptide-human leukocyte antigen or peptide, *Dermatol Sin* 31:181–190, 2013.
Ponka D: Approach to managing patients with sulfa allergy. Use of antibiotic and nonantibiotic sulfonamides, *Can Fam Physician* 52:1434–1438, 2006.
Sharma P, Nagarajan V: Can an ARB be given to patients who have had angioedema on an ACE inhibitor? *Cleve Clin J Med* 80:755–757, 2013.
Torres MJ, Canto G: Hypersensitivity reactions to corticosteroids, *Curr Opin Allergy Clin Immunol* 10:273–279, 2010.
Trubiano JA, Vogrin S, Chua KY, et al: Development and validation of a penicillin allergy clinical decision rule, *JAMA Intern Med* 180(5):745–752, 2020.

SERUM SICKNESS

Method of
Amy Robertson, PharmD; and Amanda Rhyne, MD

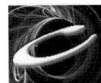

CURRENT DIAGNOSIS

- Identified by: fever, rash, joint pain (in combination or isolated)
- 7–14 days after exposure to offending agent
- Most frequently in the adult female population
- There are no disease defining labs, although complement tests may be elevated

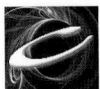

CURRENT THERAPY

- Identify and discontinue offending agent
- Symptomatic relief with analgesics and antihistamines, as needed
- Those with severe disease may be treated with oral or intravenous corticosteroids for 10–14 days
- If symptoms reappear after discontinuation of corticosteroid, reinitiate with a slow taper

Pathophysiology

Serum sickness is classified as a type III delayed immune-complex–mediated hypersensitivity reaction. It was first noted by Von Pirquet in the early 1900s after administration of equine antisera. The mechanism consists of exposure to an antigen (often a large protein) that leads to formation of an antigen-antibody complex. The immune complex load becomes too high to be appropriately excreted from the body, causing deposition in joints, tissues, and vascular endothelium. It also leads to activation of the complement pathway, which prompts mast cell and basophil degranulation with vasoactive amine release. The deposition of immune complexes and release of inflammatory mediators (histamine, serotonin) leads to the common symptoms of urticarial rash, joint pain, and fever.

Serum sickness–like reaction is not as well defined as true serum sickness. It is postulated that a non-protein drug binds to a serum protein to make a complete antigen. The newly formed antigen goes on to become an antigen-antibody complex. These complexes mimic the inflammatory cascade and symptomatic response of a true serum sickness reaction.

Epidemiology

Serum sickness is most common in the adult female population. A systematic review involving 33 cases of rituximab (Rituxan)-induced serum sickness (RISS) showed 76.7% female predominance with a mean age of 39.1 years. The majority of cases occurred in patients with an autoimmune condition, specifically immune thrombocytopenic purpura and Sjogren. Due to a lack of clear diagnostic tools and varying symptoms that can closely mimic a flare of an underlying rheumatologic illness, these reactions are often poorly documented or not identified. A study of Australian snake antivenom showed that the incidence of serum sickness was 29% ($N = 32/109$). Further research will need to be done to determine current incidence with the increasing treatment of rheumatologic disorders with immunologic medications.

Risk Factors

Risk factors for serum sickness include parenteral and cutaneous administration of chemicals, especially those with large molecular weights (e.g., proteins, serum). Heterologous (animal-derived) proteins, in particular, are associated with a high risk for a delayed immune response. Historically, equine-derived antisera and antitoxins were common causes and now includes murine and chimeric monoclonal antibodies such as rituximab (Rituxan) and infliximab (Remicade). Fewer adverse events have been reported with adalimumab (Humira), a humanized monoclonal antibody. Additional risk factors include administration of large doses, repeated dosing, and longer administration times. Patients with autoimmune disorders, circulating histamine-releasing factors, and atopy are also at an increased risk.

Serum sickness–like reactions are associated with a wider variety of molecules, including non-protein medications (e.g., antibiotics), vaccines, allergy extracts, hormones, and enzymes. See Table 1 for a list of agents commonly associated with serum sickness and serum sickness–like reactions.

Clinical Manifestations

Common manifestations of serum sickness include fever, pruritic rash (not involving mucosal membranes), and arthralgia of the metacarpophalangeal joints, knees, wrists, ankles, and shoulders. The timing of these symptoms occurs 7 to 14 days after exposure to the offending agent and can happen more promptly if there has been previous exposure. Urticaria has been reported as the most prominent symptom, present in 90% of cases. In a study of 33 cases of RISS: 78.8% presented with fever, 72.7% with arthralgia, and 69.7% with rash. The triad of fever, rash, and arthralgia were present in 48.5% of the cases. There are many less prominent manifestations of serum sickness, including headache, gastrointestinal (GI) bloating, cramps, diarrhea, and nephropathy.

Diagnosis

Recommended workup includes complete blood count (CBC), erythrocyte sedimentation rate (ESR), C-reactive protein (CRP), urinalysis (UA), and comprehensive metabolic panel (CMP). Although lab work can help to differentiate from other causes, diagnosis is made clinically. Attempts have been made to link serum sickness to elevated levels of rheumatoid factor, complement, and antibody levels without success.

Differential Diagnosis

The differential diagnoses for serum sickness include: serum sickness–like reaction, other hypersensitivity reactions, viral illness, rheumatologic disease, tick-borne disease, reactive arthritis, Stevens-Johnson syndrome, rheumatic fever, and lupus.

TABLE 1	Medications Associated With Serum Sickness and Serum Sickness–Like Reactions

Serum Sickness

Heterologous (animal-derived) proteins:
- Antivenom for snake bites: Crotalidae polyvalent immune fab, North and South American snake antivenom (CroFab)
- Chimeric (murine/human) monoclonal antibodies: rituximab (Rituxan), infliximab (Remicade)
- Equine serum heptavalent botulism antitoxin
- Equine-derived antivenom for spider bites
- Equine-derived diphtheria antitoxin
- Murine monoclonal antibodies
- Polyclonal antibodies: equine or rabbit anti-thymocyte globulin (Atgam, Thymoglobulin)

Homologous (human-derived) proteins:
- Anti-D (Rho[D]) immune globulin (RhoGAM)
- Humanized monoclonal antibodies: adalimumab (Humira), omalizumab (Xolair), natalizumab (Tysabri), alemtuzumab (Lemtrada)
- Intravenous immune globulin (Carimune NF, Gamunex-C)

Serum Sickness–like Reactions
- Allopurinol (Zyloprim)
- Antimicrobials
  - Cephalosporins (especially cefaclor [Ceclor])
  - Ciprofloxacin (Cipro)
  - Griseofulvin (Gris-PEG)
  - Isoniazid (Nydrazid, INH)
  - Minocycline (Minocin)
  - Penicillins (Pen-Vee K)
  - Streptomycin (Agri-mycin-17, Agrept)
  - Sulfonamides
- Barbiturates
- Bupropion (Wellbutrin)
- Captopril (Capoten)
- Hydantoins
- Hydralazine (Apresoline)
- Iodides
- Methyldopa (Aldomet)
- Phenytoin (Dilantin)
- Procainamide (Pronestyl, Procan-SR, Procanbid)
- Quinidine (Cardioquine)
- Thiouracils (e.g., methimazole [Tapazole])

Treatment

Treatment of serum sickness and serum sickness–like reactions are similar. Discontinuation and avoidance of the offending agent is recommended and usually leads to spontaneous resolution within several weeks. Due to the self-limiting nature and generally mild presentation, treatment is symptom driven. Low-grade fever and/or arthralgias can be treated with analgesics (e.g., acetaminophen [Tylenol]) or nonsteroidal anti-inflammatory drugs. Antihistamines and corticosteroids are commonly used, but there are limited data to support their efficacy. Antihistamines may be used to treat urticarial symptoms. Those with more severe disease (e.g., temperature >38.5°C, severe arthralgias, extensive rashes) can be treated with a short course of corticosteroids (e.g., prednisone [Deltasone] 40 to 60 mg by mouth daily). Generally oral corticosteroids are sufficient, but intravenous agents may be appropriate for some patients (e.g., methylprednisolone [Solu-Medrol] 1 to 2 mg/kg in one or two divided doses intravenously). A systematic review revealed intravenous methylprednisolone (Solu-Medrol) as the most common treatment of RISS. Other treatment options identified were intravenous betamethasone (Celestone Soluspan), intravenous hydrocortisone (Solu-Cortef), oral prednisone (Deltasone), and oral prednisolone (Millipred). This study demonstrated a mean treatment duration of 9 days with complete resolution of symptoms in all cases. Some studies recommend tapering corticosteroids over 2 weeks to avoid rebound symptoms. There are currently no evidence-based guidelines available to guide dosing or duration of therapy.

Plasmapheresis or plasma exchange is another treatment option used to eliminate immune complexes. One study reports the use of plasmapheresis in five patients post–renal transplant who experienced anti-thymocyte globulin-induced serum sickness with no improvement after administration of oral prednisone (Deltasone) 1 mg/kg/d or intravenous prednisolone (Millipred) 2 mg/kg/d. This treatment method is generally reserved for refractory cases that do not respond to corticosteroid therapy due to limited evidence of its safety and efficacy.

References

de Silva HA, Ryan NM, de Silva HJ: Adverse reactions to snake antivenom, and their prevention and treatment, *Br J Clin Pharmacol* 81(3):446–452, 2015.

Erffmeyer JE: Serum sickness, *Ann Allergy* 56:105–109, 1986.

Karmacharya P, Poudel DR, Pathak R, et al: Rituximab-induced serum sickness: a systematic review, *Semin Arthritis Rheum* 45:334–340, 2015.

Lawley TJ, Bielory L, Gascon P, et al: A prospective clinical and immunologic analysis of patients with serum sickness, *N Engl J Med* 311:1407–1413, 1984.

Lin RY: Serum sickness syndrome, *Am Fam Physician* 33(1):157–162, 1986.

Lundquist AL, Chari RS, Wood JH, et al: Serum sickness following rabbit antithymocyte-globulin induction in a liver transplant recipient: case report and literature review, *Liver Transpl* 13:647–650, 2007.

Naguwa SM, Nelson BL: Human serum sickness, *Clin Rev Allergy* 3:117–126, 1985.

Ryan NM, Kearney RT, Brown S, et al: Incidence of serum sickness after the administration of Australian snake antivenom (ASP-22), *Clin Toxicol* 54(1):27–33, 2016.

Solensky R, Khan DA, et al: Drug allergy: an updated practice parameter, *Ann Allergy Clin Immunol* 105:259–273, 2010.

Tatum AJ, Ditto AM, Patterson R: Severe serum sickness-like reaction to oral penicillin drugs: three case reports, *Ann Allergy Asthma Immunol* 86:330–334, 2011.

Tanriover B, Chuang P, Fishbach B, et al: Polyclonal antibody-induced serum sickness in renal transplant recipients: treatment with therapeutic plasma exchange, *Transplantation* 80:279–281, 2005.

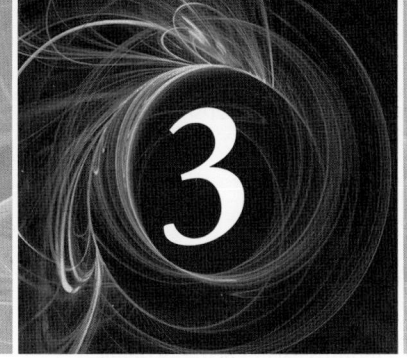

Cardiovascular System

ACUTE MYOCARDIAL INFARCTION

Method of
Kuang-Yuh Chyu, MD, PhD; and Prediman K. Shah, MD, MACC

CURRENT DIAGNOSIS

- Patients are encouraged to seek medical evaluation as soon as possible when chest pain or angina-equivalent symptoms occur.
- Early presentation leads to early recognition, diagnosis, and treatment of acute myocardial infarction.
- The diagnosis of acute myocardial infarction relies on detailed history, ECG changes consistent with myocardial ischemia, and elevation of serum biomarkers.
- Although echocardiogram is not essential to diagnose acute myocardial infarction, it is useful in diagnosing complications from acute myocardial infarction and guiding management.

CURRENT THERAPY

- Timely reperfusion of occluded coronary artery is essential in managing ST-elevation myocardial infarction (STEMI).
- Early reperfusion therapy (PCI or CABG) in non–STEMI (NSTEMI) patients with high-risk features such as congestive heart failure, dynamic ECG changes, arrhythmia, and refractory angina is beneficial.
- Medical therapy and lifestyle modification strategies are important to reduce long-term atherosclerotic cardiovascular events.

Coronary heart disease (CHD) results from atherosclerotic coronary artery disease (CAD), and its acute manifestation is acute coronary syndrome (ACS). Based on the presenting symptoms, characteristic ECG changes, and cardiac biomarkers, ACS can be further subdivided into unstable angina (USA), non–ST-elevation myocardial infarction (NSTEMI), or ST-elevation myocardial infarction (STEMI). Most patients with ACS have similar underlying pathophysiology: atherosclerotic plaque formation leading to narrowing of coronary arteries with plaque rupture or erosion and superimposed thrombus formation resulting in an acute presentation. A small portion of ACS cases can be due to conditions such as coronary artery spasm, spontaneous coronary artery dissection, coronary embolization, or cocaine use. Stress-induced acute cardiomyopathy, without angiographic signs of severely occlusive disease, can closely simulate atherothrombotic STEMI.

Although the three ACS entities share similar pathophysiology, their presentations vary widely. The initial recognition, diagnostic testing, and management strategies for these entities are similar and applicable to all patients with ACS. Diagnostically, patients with STEMI as a whole reflect a more homogeneous group of patients compared with patients with USA or NSTEMI, and patients with STEMI carry the highest risk regarding acute morbidity and mortality. The major difference in managing these three groups of patients lies in the decision for and timing of acute reperfusion of occluded culprit coronary arteries.

In the past three decades, there has been a steady decline in the incidence of STEMI and significant improvement in the outcomes of patients with STEMI with the introduction of early coronary reperfusion strategies; improved adjunctive pharmacologic therapies; adoption of guideline-directed treatments such as lipid lowering, blood pressure control, and diabetes mellitus control; and cigarette smoking cessation to effectively modify risk factors. Currently, the in-hospital mortality of STEMI has reached as low as 7%.

Diagnosis
Electrocardiogram
ECG is the most important diagnostic test to detect STEMI because clinical features, physical examination, and CAD risk factor profile only have modest sensitivity and specificity in diagnosing STEMI. Current guidelines define ST elevation at the J point in at least two continuous leads of 2 mm or greater in men or 1.5 mm or greater in women in leads V2 to V3 and/or 1 mm or greater in other contiguous chest leads or the limb leads in the absence of left ventricular (LV) hypertrophy or left bundle branch block (LBBB). Other ECG abnormalities such as paced rhythm, drug or electrolyte (hyperkalemia) effects, or Brugada syndrome also reduce the sensitivity and specificity of STEMI ECG interpretation.

Some patients present with ECG changes, although not with typical ST elevation, indicating equivalent clinical risk to STEMI, and should be treated as having a true STEMI. These STEMI-equivalent ECG patterns include (1) isolated ST depression in two or more precordial leads (V1 to V4), indicating true posterior wall myocardial infarction (MI); (2) ST depression in multiple leads with ST elevation in aVR, indicating left main or triple-vessel CAD; (3) Wellen's sign with symmetrical deep T-wave inversions in anterior precordial leads; (4) hyperacute T wave; and (5) de Winter sign showing ST depression and peaked T waves in the precordial leads. Occasionally, patients with left circumflex artery occlusion can present with a normal or near-normal ECG.

Serum Biomarkers
Serum biomarkers of myocardial necrosis such as cardiac-specific troponins T and I are complementary to diagnosing STEMI. In clinical practice, STEMI is often diagnosed with ECG alone before the laboratory result of biomarkers is available. The troponin level typically rises 4 to 6 hours after the onset of symptoms and peaks within 12 to 24 hours if reperfusion therapy succeeds in reperfusing the occluded coronary artery and patients present early in the course of STEMI; its level tends to peak after 24 hours if reperfusion therapy fails or in patients who receive no reperfusion therapy. After STEMI, successfully reperfused or not, the troponin level remains elevated for 7 to 10 days. For patients suspected of having recurrent ACS within a week after the index STEMI, given the troponin level remains elevated, creatine kinase (CK) and the MB isoform of CK (CK-MB) levels can be used as biomarkers to establish additional myocardial necrosis from a recurrent event because CK and CK-MB levels usually return to normal 48 to 72 hours after the initial index event.

Imaging

STEMI is commonly accompanied with wall motion abnormalities on echocardiogram, but echocardiogram is not essential to diagnose STEMI. Echocardiogram is extremely useful in managing patients with STEMI, especially when they present with acute complications from STEMI such as acute congestive heart failure, acute mitral regurgitation, free wall or ventricular septal rupture, pericardial effusion, cardiogenic shock, or LV thrombus.

Management of STEMI

The principal concept of managing STEMI is "time is muscle"; hence, it is important for patients to recognize symptoms for early presentation and for the medical community to administer suitable reperfusion therapy in a timely manner.

Prehospital Phase

Current guidelines recommend that patients with STEMI receive reperfusion therapy as soon as possible but within 12 hours of symptom onset to achieve optimal myocardial salvage to reduce mortality and morbidity. In daily clinical practice, a substantial number of patients still present late and miss the golden window of reperfusion. Common reasons for late presentation include (1) patients' lack of knowledge to recognize symptoms, (2) patients' inertia to seek medical care, (3) patients' lack of access to medical care, and (4) atypical symptoms that mislead patients or medical care providers to consider noncardiac problems.

Patients with suspicious myocardial ischemic symptoms are encouraged to call emergency medical services (EMS) immediately for help; this has the following benefits: (1) Patients can receive early treatment, (2) patients can receive immediate resuscitation should STEMI complications such as cardiac arrest occur en route to the hospital, and (3) an early prehospital ECG and communication with a hospital capable of percutaneous coronary intervention (PCI) by EMS significantly reduce reperfusion time and improve outcome. A recent Lifeline STEMI Accelerator Study reported only 55% of STEMI patients were transported via EMS. Improving this requires public education to enhance recognition of symptoms, implementation of an efficient EMS system, and infrastructures with standardized treatment algorithms for STEMI.

Initial management by EMS usually includes pain relief by morphine, administration of nitroglycerin,[1] oxygen, and nonenteric-coated aspirin (162–325 mg) unless contraindicated. The role of routine oxygen supplementation to patients with STEMI has been questioned. A recent randomized clinical trial (Air Versus Oxygen in Myocardial Infarction [AVOID] trial) suggests that supplemental oxygen therapy (8 L/min via face mask) in patients with STEMI without hypoxia (oxygen saturation >94%) may increase early myocardial injury and is associated with larger myocardial infarction size at 6 months.

Once STEMI is identified by a prehospital ECG performed by EMS, an assessment of candidacy for and availability of reperfusion therapy is an important next step of management to ensure immediate reperfusion and administration of its adjunctive therapy to maintain culprit coronary artery patency, limit infarct size and adverse LV remodeling, and improve outcome. To achieve the best outcome from reperfusion therapy, patients with STEMI should receive suitable reperfusion therapy within 12 hours of symptom onset—the earlier the better. Current reperfusion therapy options for STEMI include primary PCI (PPCI) or fibrinolysis. PPCI is the treatment of choice for STEMI because it confers a beneficial reduction in mortality and recurrent ischemia compared with fibrinolysis. Hence, current guidelines recommend EMS to transport patients to a PCI-capable hospital and PPCI as the preferred method of reperfusion therapy with a system goal of less than 90 minutes from first medical contact (FMC) to device time. It has been estimated that for STEMI patients with cardiogenic shock, but without out-of-hospital cardiac arrest, every 10-minute treatment delay between 60 to 180 minutes from the

---

[1]Not FDA approved for this indication

BOX 1   Contraindications and Cautions for Fibrinolytic Therapy in STEMI*

Absolute Contraindications
- Any prior ICH
- Known structural cerebral vascular lesion (e.g., arteriovenous malformation)
- Known malignant intracranial neoplasm (primary or metastatic)
- Ischemic stroke within 3 months except acute ischemic stroke within 4.5 h
- Suspected aortic dissection
- Active bleeding or bleeding diathesis (excluding menses)
- Significant closed-head or facial trauma within 3 months
- Intracranial or intraspinal surgery within 2 months
- Severe uncontrolled hypertension (unresponsive to emergency therapy)
- For streptokinase, prior treatment within the previous 6 months

Relative Contraindications
- History of chronic, severe, poorly controlled hypertension
- Significant hypertension on presentation (SBP >180 mm Hg or DBP >110 mm Hg)
- History of prior ischemic stroke >3 months
- Dementia
- Known intracranial pathology not covered in absolute contraindications
- Traumatic or prolonged CPR (>10 min)
- Major surgery (<3 weeks)
- Recent (within 2–4 weeks) internal bleeding
- Noncompressible vascular punctures
- Pregnancy
- Active peptic ulcer
- Oral anticoagulant therapy

CPR, Cardiopulmonary resuscitation; *DBP*, diastolic blood pressure; *ICH*, intracranial hemorrhage; *SBP*, systole blood pressure; *STEMI*, ST-elevation myocardial infarction.
*Viewed as advisory for clinical decision making and may not be all-inclusive or definitive.

first medical contact lead to 3.3 additional deaths per 100 PCI treated patients (FITT-STEMI trial).

Not every hospital is PCI capable. If a patient is sent to or arrives at a non-PCI-capable hospital, guidelines recommend transferring that patient to a PCI-capable hospital for PPCI with a system goal of less than 120 minutes from FMC to device time. If there is an anticipated delay of FMC to device time of 120 minutes or more, a fibrinolytic agent can be given within 30 minutes of hospital arrival if the patient has no contraindications for fibrinolysis (Box 1). Prehospital fibrinolysis, administered by EMS with physician supervision, has been shown to be feasible and safe, with a shortened reperfusion time and reduced mortality. Such strategy, however, is not used in the United States.

In real-world clinical practice, sometimes it is not possible to achieve strict time goals because of uncertainty of the initial diagnosis, necessity to treat concomitant comorbidities or complications, patient preference or consent issues, and local factors delaying transport. Therefore emphasis should be to deliver reperfusion therapy to eligible patients as rapidly as possible.

In-Hospital Reperfusion Strategy
Primary Percutaneous Coronary Intervention
PPCI performed in a high-volume hospital by experienced operators achieves a higher patency rate of infarct-related artery (IRA) and lower rate of recurrent ischemia, reinfarction, hemorrhagic stroke, and death compared with fibrinolysis. In particular, PPCI has the greatest benefit in high-risk patients such as those with cardiogenic shock. Hence, PPCI is the preferred method of

TABLE 1 Comparison of Fibrinolytic Agents

	ALTEPLASE (t-PA) (ACTIVASE)	RETEPLASE (r-PA) (RETAVASE)	TENECTEPLASE (TNK-tPA) (TNKASE)
Dose	Up to 100 mg in 90 min (weight based)	10 U + 10 U IV boluses given 30 min apart	30–50 mg based on weight
Bolus administration	No	Yes	Yes
Antigenic	No	No	No
Allergic reaction	No	No	No
Fibrin specificity	++	++	++++
90 min TIMI 2 or 3 patency rate (%)	73–84	84	85
TIMI 3 flow (%)	54	60	63

TIMI, Thrombolysis in Myocardial Infarction.
Modified from 2013 ACCF/AHA guideline for the management of ST-elevation myocardial infarction. *J Am Coll Cardiol* 2013;61:e78-140.

reperfusion whenever possible with the system goal of 90 to 120 minutes.

The reperfusion technique used in PPCI has evolved greatly in the past few decades, from balloon angioplasty, bare-metal stent (BMS), and drug-eluting stent (DES) to bioresorbable vascular scaffolds (BVSs). Compared with balloon angioplasty, BMS used in PPCI confers reduced risk for subsequent target-vessel revascularization but does not reduce the mortality rate. Compared with BMS, DES used in PPCI decreases the restenosis rate and need for reintervention without reduction in reinfarction and death. BVS is a new stent technology, with a hope of better restoration of vasomotion, less lumen loss, and reduction of target lesion revascularization in the stented vessels compared with metallic DES. However, polymer-based ABSORB BVS failed to demonstrate such benefits; instead it caused a concerning hazard of device thrombosis. A newer generation of metallic BVS (Magmaris, Biotronik) also increased late lumen loss and target lesion revascularization in STEMI patients compared with sirolimus-eluting stent in a recently published MAGSTEMI trial.

Fibrinolysis
The currently available intravenous fibrinolytic agents are tenecteplase (TNKase), reteplase (Retavase), and alteplase (Activase) (Table 1). A fibrinolytic agent should be administered to eligible patients without contraindication within 30 minutes of arrival at the emergency department. It is important to evaluate the risk/benefit ratio for each individual patient before administering fibrinolytic therapy because it carries a small but fatal risk of hemorrhage stroke (about 1%). The ideal patient to receive a fibrinolytic agent would be with symptom onset within 1 to 2 hours, low bleeding risk, and age younger than 65 years.

Although fibrinolysis achieves a reasonable patency rate of IRA (see Table 1), a substantial portion of patients fail to achieve successful reperfusion as defined by the following clinical criteria: (1) resolution of chest pain, (2) reduction of >50% of the initial ST-segment elevation pattern on follow-up ECG 60 to 90 minutes after initiation of fibrinolysis, and (3) occurrence of reperfusion arrhythmia (accelerated idioventricular rhythm [AIVR]). If fibrinolysis does not achieve resolution of ST elevation by at least 50% in the worst lead at 60 to 90 minutes, rescue PCI (transfer to PCI-capable hospital if necessary) should be strongly considered.

Percutaneous Intervention After Fibrinolysis
Approximately 40% of STEMI patients who receive fibrinolysis fail to achieve successful reperfusion and require emergent rescue PCI. Other indications for rescue PCI include severe heart failure, cardiogenic shock, persistent chest pain, or electrical instability. Hence, these patients should be transferred to a PCI-capable hospital immediately if fibrinolysis has been administered in a non-PCI capable hospital.

Otherwise, stable patients after successful fibrinolysis can undergo coronary angiography with an intent to revascularize as soon as logistically feasible, ideally between 3 and 24 hours after fibrinolysis (so-called *pharmaco-invasive strategy*). In patients older than 75 years, if a pharmaco-invasive strategy is chosen as the reperfusion strategy, a fibrinolytic agent at half dose (such as the half dose of tenecteplase used in the STREAM trial) should be used to reduce bleeding risks because patients will receive concomitant antiplatelets and anticoagulants for PCI. A recent EARLY-MYO trial confirmed the efficacy of a pharmaco-invasive strategy using half dose alteplase followed by PCI within 3 to 24 hours was noninferior to primary PCI in 30-day rates of total death, reinfarction, heart failure, or major bleeding but with a higher rate of minor bleeding. Very early PCI after successful fibrinolysis (<2–3 hours) is not recommended.

Facilitated Percutaneous Intervention
This strategy refers to a full dose or partial dose of fibrinolysis plus a glycoprotein (GP) IIb/IIIa antagonist or antithrombotic followed by immediate PCI if there is no evidence of reperfusion failure. Current guidelines do not recommend this strategy owing to potential harms such as an increase in ischemic events, bleeding, and mortality.

Patients with STEMI and Multivessel Coronary Artery Disease
About 40% to 65% of patients with STEMI undergoing PPCI for culprit IRA have multivessel CAD. Significant multivessel CAD, if left unrevascularized, is associated with a worse clinical prognosis. For patients with STEMI with cardiogenic shock, conventional paradigm deemed it reasonable to perform multivessel PPCI (or emergency coronary artery bypass grafting [CABG] in selected patients) to achieve as complete a revascularization as possible. However, a recent CULPRIT-SHOCK trial showed that initial revascularization of the culprit vessel only by PCI in patients with acute MI and multivessel ACD with cardiogenic shock resulted in a lower 30-day risk of death or renal-replacement therapy compared with a strategy of immediate multivessel PCI.

For stable patients, randomized clinical trials have demonstrated the feasibility of performing multivessel PPCI in acute settings. This approach has the following advantages: complete revascularization leading to improved LV function and prognosis, decreased vascular complications from repeated procedures, and reduced length of stay and medical costs. However, the procedure will be longer with potentially higher radiation exposure, higher risk for contrast nephropathy owing to a higher contrast load, risk of compromising viable myocardium supplied by the nonculprit coronary artery owing to procedure complications, and unnecessary stenting to the nonculprit artery without objective evidence of ischemia. Many guidelines published by the professional cardiology societies in North America and Europe

Acute Myocardial Infarction

support multivessel PCI, either at the time of PCI to the STEMI culprit vessel or as a staged procedure in selected hemodynamically stable patients. A recent COMPLETE trial further confirmed the efficacy of reducing new myocardial infarction or ischemia-driven revascularization in the complete revascularization group than in the culprit lesion PCI group but without mortality benefit. Interventional cardiologists should integrate clinical data, characteristics of lesions and procedures, clinical risks, and complications from procedures to determine the best timing and strategy to achieve the optimal benefit.

Patients With STEMI Older Than 75 Years of Age

Patients older than 75 years are usually underrepresented in STEMI clinical trials; however, revascularization with PCI still confers beneficial clinical outcomes compared with no revascularization despite age, frailty, and comorbidities. Hence PCI as a revascularization strategy for STEMI in the elderly is encouraged whenever patients' conditions allow. In the United States, the utilization of PCI for patients with STEMI older than 70 years has increased from 11% in 1998 to 35.7% in 2013 based on data from the National Inpatient Sample Database. When taking care of this group of patients, cardiologists need to pay particular attention to minimize bleeding complication (such as using radial access), monitoring patients' nonverbal responses as many patients have difficulty communicating with caregivers effectively, and identifying and treating comorbid conditions early as many elderly patients lack functional reserves in many organ systems and are prone to adverse effects of drug interactions.

Patients With STEMI Who Present Later Than 12 Hours After Symptom Onset

Patients with STEMI who present between 12 hours and 2 days after symptom onset without unstable symptoms or signs are no longer eligible for fibrinolysis but are still eligible for PPCI to salvage myocardium, which confers the benefit of reduced infarct size compared with conventional therapy guided by a predischarge symptom-limited exercise test or unplanned PCI guided by clinical instability as demonstrated in the Beyond 12 Hours Reperfusion Alternative Evaluation (BRAVE-2) trial. For patients with STEMI who present more than 48 hours after symptom onset without clinical instability, a strategy of symptom-limited stress test first or coronary angiography first to delineate high-risk features of coronary anatomy is reasonable with an intent to revascularize high-risk coronary anatomy. If patients are clinically stable without high-risk coronary anatomy noted by angiography and present between 3 and 28 days after symptom onset, PCI to open the occluded IRA does not confer a clinical benefit in reducing mortality, congestive heart failure, or nonfatal myocardial infarction compared with medical therapy as demonstrated in the Occluded Artery Trial (OAT). Irrespective of time of presentation, patients with STEMI who present with hemodynamic or electrical instability should undergo coronary angiography with an intent to revascularize the jeopardized myocardium as soon as possible.

Figure 1 summarizes current pathways of managing patients with STEMI based on their time of presentation, their clinical status, and availability of reperfusion therapy.

Adjunct Therapy
Antiplatelet Therapy
Aspirin

Unless contraindicated, 162 to 325 mg of aspirin should be administered as a loading dose immediately followed by at least 81 to 325 mg daily in all patients with STEMI, with 81 mg being the preferred maintenance dose. Patients with a history of aspirin allergy can be given clopidogrel (Plavix) instead.

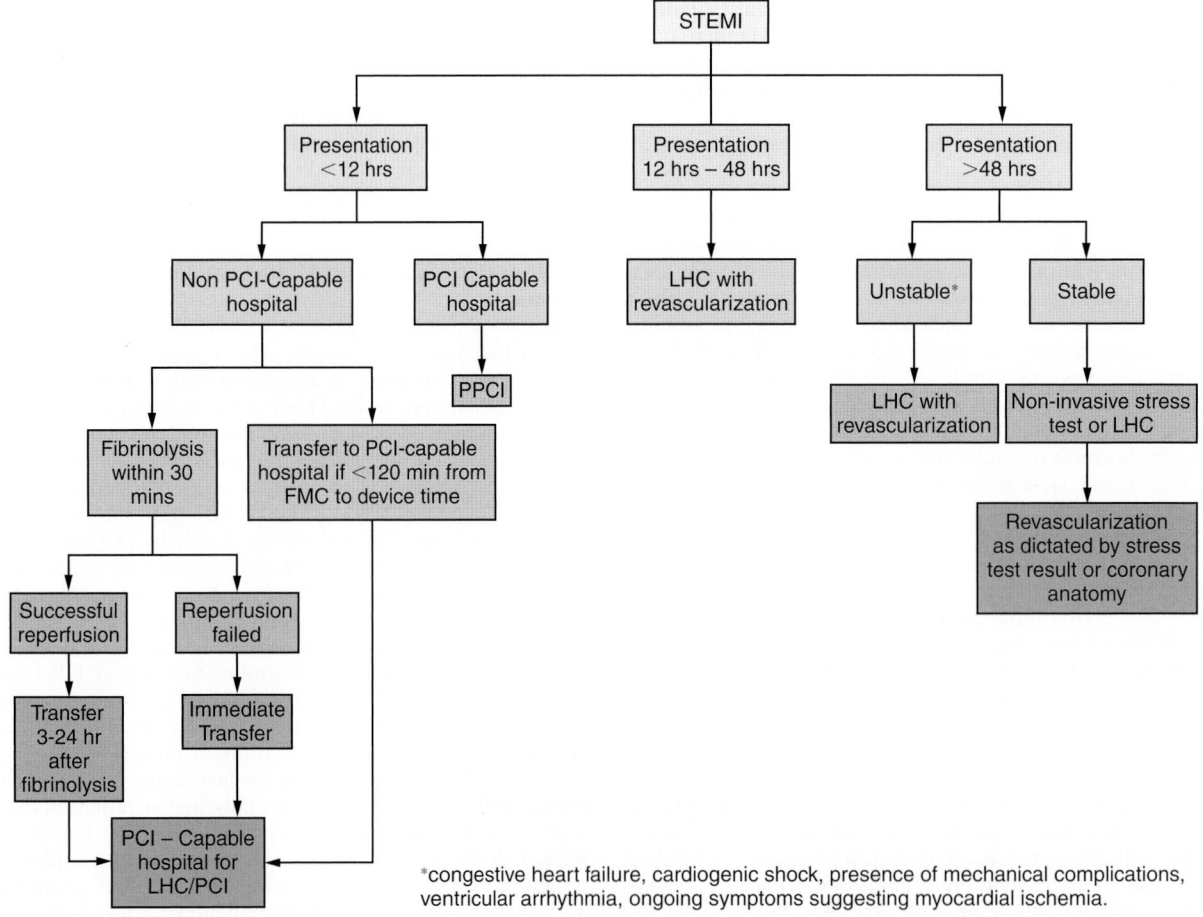

*congestive heart failure, cardiogenic shock, presence of mechanical complications, ventricular arrhythmia, ongoing symptoms suggesting myocardial ischemia.

Figure 1 Pathways of managing ST-elevation myocardial infarction *(STEMI)*. *FMC,* First medical contact; *LHC,* Left heart catheterization; *PCI,* percutaneous intervention; *PPCI,* primary percutaneous coronary intervention.

P2Y$_{12}$ Receptor Inhibitors

Clopidogrel is a second-generation thienopyridine and irreversibly blocks the platelet P2Y$_{12}$ receptor to inhibit platelet activation and aggregation. Current guidelines support the use of clopidogrel during fibrinolysis or PPCI. For patients undergoing fibrinolytic therapy, a loading dose of 300 mg followed by a maintenance dose of 75 mg daily has been recommended for patients younger than 75 years. For patients older than 75 years, only the maintenance dose of 75 mg should be given. Prasugrel (Effient) and ticagrelor (Brilinta) have not been studied and, hence, are not recommended in the setting of fibrinolysis as reperfusion therapy. For patients undergoing PPCI, depending on whether they are receiving a fibrinolytic agent and the timing of subsequent PCI, a different dosing regimen of clopidogrel may be recommended (Figure 2).

Prasugrel is a third-generation thienopyridine P2Y$_{12}$ receptor inhibitor. It is metabolized to its active form more quickly than clopidogrel and hence confers a more potent effect. In a subset of patients with STEMI in the TRITON-TIMI 38 trial, prasugrel was more efficacious in preventing composite endpoints of cardiovascular (CV) death, myocardial infarction, and stroke compared with clopidogrel, but it had a higher major bleeding rate. Prasugrel is also contraindicated in patients older than 75 years, with body weight less than 60 kg, or with prior history of stroke or transient ischemic attack.

Ticagrelor is a direct reversible P2Y$_{12}$ receptor inhibitor with a more potent, faster-acting property compared with clopidogrel or prasugrel. In the pivotal Platelet Inhibition and Patient Outcomes (PLATO) trial, ticagrelor lowered composite CV death, myocardial infarction, and stroke compared with clopidogrel but with an increase in nonprocedure-related bleeding.

Biotransformation of clopidogrel into active metabolites requires CYP2C19, whereas prasugrel mainly relies on CYP3A4 and CYP2B6 and, to a lesser extent, CYP2C19 to form active metabolites. Ticagrelor is an active P2Y$_{12}$ inhibitor and its metabolite via CYP3A4 carries equal antiplatelet potency. About 30% of the US population carries 1 or 2 CYP2C19 loss of function alleles, rendering them less responsive to the antiplatelet effect of clopidogrel. Hence genotyping CYP2C19 polymorphism could potentially affect the selection of P2Y$_{12}$ receptor inhibitor. In STEMI populations, a recent study demonstrated that genotype-guided strategy, that is, patients without loss of function of CYP2C19 were treated with clopidogrel whereas patients with loss of function received ticagrelor or prasugrel, is not inferior to a standard treatment with ticagrelor or prasugrel in the control group with respect to thrombotic events at 12 months. However, genotype-guided strategy was associated with lower risk of bleeding.

Clopidogrel, prasugrel, and ticagrelor require several hours to achieve maximal platelet inhibition. Additionally, in the setting of STEMI, the bioavailability of these oral agents may be hampered by clinical factors such as nausea, vomiting, and cardiogenic shock, leading to poor gastrointestinal (GI) absorption and leaving patients not adequately protected by platelet inhibition during immediate PPCI. Cangrelor (Kengreal) is a fast-acting, reversible adenosine diphosphate (ADP) receptor inhibitor that is administered intravenously to achieve P2Y$_{12}$ inhibition within 2 minutes. Its plasma half-life is 3 to 6 minutes, and platelet function returns to normal within 60 minutes after discontinuation of infusion. The US Food and Drug Administration (FDA) has approved cangrelor to be used as an adjunct therapy during PCI to reduce repeat coronary revascularization and stent thrombosis in patients who have not been pretreated with an oral P2Y$_{12}$ inhibitor and are not receiving a GP IIb/IIIa receptor antagonist. How to transition from cangrelor to an oral P2Y$_{12}$ inhibitor after PCI depends on which oral P2Y$_{12}$ inhibitor a patient is being

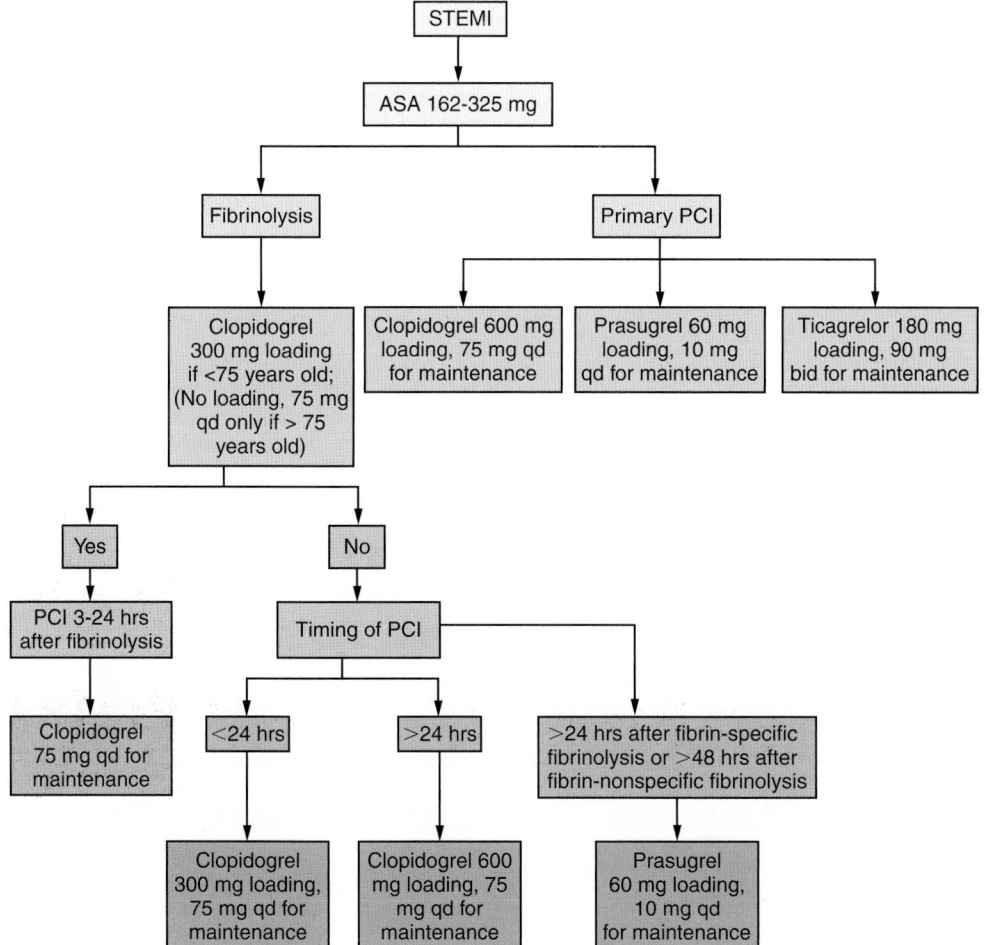

Figure 2 Oral regimen of different P2Y$_{12}$ receptor inhibitors based on reperfusion strategies. *PCI*, Percutaneous intervention. Modified from 2013 ACCF/AHA STEMI guideline.

transitioned to. Based on the CHAMPION PHOENIX trial, to transition to clopidogrel, 600 mg clopidogrel loading is necessary immediately after discontinuation of cangrelor infusion. Based on pharmacodynamic data, prasugrel 60 mg should be administered immediately after stopping cangrelor infusion, whereas ticagrelor 180 mg can be given anytime during cangrelor infusion or immediately after infusion ends.

Use and Duration of Antiplatelet Therapy

For STEMI patients, current guidelines recommend to give aspirin and one of the potent $P2Y_{12}$ inhibitors (ticagrelor or prasugrel) prior to primary PCI. When potent $P2Y_{12}$ inhibitors are not available or contraindicated, clopidogrel can be given instead.

For NSTEMI patients, it is recommended against to routinely administer $P2Y_{12}$ inhibitors in patients in whom coronary artery anatomy is not known and an early invasive management is planned. This recommendation is based on the aggregated results from several clinical trials and registries including ACCOAST, ISAR-REACT 5, DUBIUS, ARIAM-Andalucia registry, and SCAAR. Once coronary anatomy is defined and PCI deemed necessary, $P2Y_{12}$ inhibitor can be administered. This approach has the benefit of reducing unnecessary bleeding risk in patients whose NSTEMI diagnosis is disproved by coronary angiogram, reducing the wait-time for patients with suitable coronary anatomy for bypass surgery.

Current guidelines recommend 12 months of dual antiplatelet therapy (DAPT) in patients with ACS (STEMI or NSTEMI) after stent implantation. Duration of DAPT can be shortened to 6 months followed by discontinuation of $P2Y_{12}$ inhibitor if bleeding risk is high (such as PRECISE DAPT score >25). Recent trials suggest even shorter duration of dual antiplatelet therapy (3 months) followed by monotherapy (aspirin or $P2Y_{12}$ inhibitor) may be considered in patients with high bleeding risk. Continuation of DAPT beyond 12 months is reasonable in patients who tolerate DAPT, do not have bleeding complications, and are not at high bleeding risk (prior bleeding on DAPT, coagulopathy, or oral anticoagulant use).

The use and duration of DAPT becomes more complicated in patients taking oral anticoagulation therapy for a variety of reasons. Guidelines and consensus documents from North America recommend the default approach of administering triple therapy (DAPT + anticoagulation) during PCI procedure and in hospital for up to 1 week followed by clopidogrel and oral anticoagulant for 12 months. If patients are with high risk for ischemic event, the default approach is modified to use triple therapy (ASA + clopidogrel or ticagrelor + oral anticoagulant) for 1 month and discontinue ASA afterward. If patients are with high bleeding risk, default approach is modified to use clopidogrel for only 6 months. A direct oral anticoagulant (DOAC) is preferred to vitamin K antagonist as oral anticoagulant unless clinical condition prohibits the use of DOAC. Oral anticoagulant alone can be used after 12 months of treatment with additional single antiplatelet agent based on individual clinical circumstance. Other strategies including use of radial artery approach as vascular access, use of proton pump inhibitors, avoidance of GP IIb/IIIa inhibitors unless for periprocedural complications, and avoidance of nonsteroidal antiinflammatory drug (NSAID) should also be utilized.

Glycoprotein IIb/IIIa Receptor Antagonists

GP IIb/IIIa receptor antagonists include abciximab (ReoPro, a chimeric monoclonal antibody), eptifibatide (Integrilin, a synthetic peptidic inhibitor), and tirofiban (Aggrastat, a nonpeptidic inhibitor). The benefit of intravenous GP IIb/IIIa receptor antagonists in patients with STEMI was largely established before the era of oral DAPT. With current use of DAPT, contemporary trials fail to show benefit with upstream administration of GP IIb/IIIa receptor antagonists before PPCI with either unfractionated heparin (UFH)[1] or bivalirudin (Angiomax). Current US and European guidelines recommend using GP IIb/IIIa receptor antagonists for bailout situations after a large thrombus burden, no reflow or slow flow, or inadequate $P2Y_{12}$ receptor antagonist loading during PCI.

Anticoagulants

UFH,[1] low-molecular-weight heparin with enoxaparin (Lovenox) as prototype, fondaparinux (Arixtra),[1] and bivalirudin (Angiomax) are widely used in reperfusion therapy to limit thrombus propagation, reduce reocclusion and reinfarction, and improve vessel patency unless contraindicated. The choice of individual agent and its dose and duration of use depends on the choice of reperfusion therapy, concomitant use of other antiplatelet agents, and renal function (Table 2).

Given that PPCI is the preferred method of reperfusion and occurs early after presentation, and given physicians' familiarity with UFH, intravenous UFH is the preferred anticoagulant agent for PPCI. In patients with high bleeding risk, bivalirudin with DAPT is a reasonable alternative to UFH (whether the patient was pretreated with UFH) when avoidance of GP IIb/IIIa receptor antagonists is desired during PPCI.

For patients with STEMI who receive fibrinolysis as initial reperfusion therapy, UFH, enoxaparin, and fondaparinux[1] all receive a class I recommendation based on ACC/AHA guidelines. UFH is preferred since a pharmaco-invasive strategy is common or for patients who may need rescue PCI. Bivalirudin may be used after fibrinolysis in patients who develop heparin-induced thrombocytopenia and require continued anticoagulation.

Guideline-Directed Medical Therapy
Beta Blocker

Beta-blocker therapy decreases myocardial oxygen demand and improves myocardial remodeling with the benefits of reducing angina, infarct size, and mortality. Current guidelines recommend initiating oral beta blockers in the first 24 hours in patients with STEMI who are without contraindications such as congestive heart failure, evidence of a low output state, increased risk for cardiogenic shock, heart block, or reactive airway disease. If not given in the first 24 hours owing to contraindications, physicians need to reevaluate patients to determine their subsequent eligibility. Oral beta blockers should be continued for 3 years after MI as recommended by the ACC/AHA secondary prevention guideline, and longer if there are other indications (such as systolic LV dysfunction). Commonly used beta-blocker regimens are (1) metoprolol tartrate (Lopressor) 25 to 50 mg every 6 to 12 hours orally, transitioned over the next 2 to 3 days to twice-daily dosing of metoprolol tartrate or to daily metoprolol succinate (Toprol XL), and then titrated to a daily dose of 200 mg as tolerated, and (2) carvedilol (Coreg)[1] 6.25 mg twice daily, titrated to 25 mg twice daily as tolerated.

Current guidelines recommend intravenous beta blocker only for patients with refractory hypertension or ongoing ischemia without contraindications. Several small randomized clinical trials have suggested that early use of intravenous metoprolol tartrate in selected patients with STEMI with Killip class I to II and no atrioventricular (AV) block before PPCI may reduce infarct size with a higher LV ejection fraction (LVEF) or reduce the incidence of malignant arrhythmia in the acute phase without an excess of adverse events.

Angiotensin-Converting Enzyme Inhibitors or Angiotensin II Receptor Blockers

Angiotensin-converting enzyme inhibitors (ACEIs) and angiotensin II receptor blockers (ARBs) reduce afterload and decrease myocardial remodeling. Either ACEIs or ARBs should be started within 24 hours if there are no contraindications such as worsening renal function, advanced kidney disease, bilateral renal artery stenosis, hyperkalemia, or hypotension. These agents have the largest benefit in patients with anterior STEMI, congestive heart failure, or LVEF less than 40%. ACEIs may be given

---

[1]Not FDA approved for this indication

[1]Not FDA approved for this indication.

| TABLE 2 | Dosage of Anticoagulants in Reperfusion Therapy for STEMI |

	REPERFUSION THERAPY	
	FIBRINOLYSIS	**PRIMARY PCI**
Unfractionated heparin[1]	• IV bolus of 60 U/kg (maximum 4000 U) followed by an infusion of 12 U/kg/h (maximum 1000 U) initially, adjusted to maintain aPTT at 1.5–2.0 times control (approximately 50–70 s) for 48 h or until revascularization	• With GPI planned, 50–70 U/kg IV bolus, to achieve ACT 200–250 s • Without GPI planned, 70–100 U/kg IV bolus to achieve ACT 250–300 s with HemoTec or 300–350 s with Hemochron
Low-molecular-weight heparin (enoxaparin [Lovenox])	• If age <75 years: 30-mg IV bolus, followed in 15 min by 1 mg/kg subcutaneously every 12 h (maximum 100 mg for the first 2 doses) • If age ≥75 years: no bolus, 0.75 mg/kg subcutaneously every 12 h (maximum 75 mg for the first 2 doses) • Regardless of age, if CrCl <30 mL/min: 1 mg/kg subcutaneously every 24 h • Duration: for the index hospitalization, up to 8 days or until revascularization	No information
Bivalirudin (Angiomax)	No information	• With or without prior heparin: 0.75 mg/kg bolus, 1.75 mg/kg/h infusion to the end of PCI. Additional bolus of 0.3 mg/kg if needed. • Reduce infusion to 1 mg/kg/h if estimated CrCl <30 mL/min • Prefer over heparin and GPI in high-risk cases of bleeding
Fondaparinux (Arixtra)[1]	• Initial dose 2.5 mg IV, then 2.5 mg subcutaneously daily starting the following day, for the index hospitalization up to 8 days or until revascularization • Contraindicated if CrCl <30 mL/min	Not recommended as sole anticoagulant

[1]Not FDA approved for this indication.
ACT, Activated clotting time; *aPTT,* activated partial thromboplastin time; *CrCl,* creatinine clearance; *GPI,* glycoprotein IIb/IIIa inhibitors; *PCI,* percutaneous intervention; *STEMI,* ST-elevation myocardial infarction.
Modified from 2013 ACCF/AHA guideline for the management of ST-elevation myocardial infarction. *J Am Coll Cardial* 2013;61:e78-140.

routinely to all patients without contraindication, whereas ARBs are an alternative for patients intolerant to ACEIs. There is no additional benefit, only more harm if ACEIs and ARBs are given concomitantly.

Commonly used ACEI regimens are (1) captopril 6.25 to 12.5 mg three times per day to start, titrated to 25 to 50 mg three times per day as tolerated; (2) lisinopril (Prinivil) 2.5 to 5 mg/day to start, titrated to 10 mg/day or higher as tolerated; (3) ramipril (Altace) 2.5 mg twice daily to start, titrated to 5 mg twice daily as tolerated; and (4) trandolapril (Mavik) test dose 0.5 mg, titrated up to 4 mg daily as tolerated. A commonly used ARB regimen is valsartan (Diovan) 20 mg twice daily to start, titrated to 160 mg twice daily as tolerated.

HMG CoA Reductase Inhibitors (Statins)

Treatment with statins after ACS lowers the risk of CV mortality, recurrent MI, stroke, and the need for coronary revascularization. Without contraindications, all patients should receive high-intensity statins as early as possible to improve compliance. Although current guidelines do not endorse a specific low-density lipoprotein (LDL) level as a treatment goal, it is recommended to obtain a fasting lipid panel within 24 hours of presentation. A commonly used high-intensity statin regimen is atorvastatin (Lipitor)[1] 40 to 80 mg or rosuvastatin (Crestor)[1] 20 to 40 mg daily as tolerated. Statins need to be used cautiously with drugs metabolized via CYP3A4 and fibrates, with frequent monitoring for myopathy and hepatic toxicity. Statin use needs to be combined with diet and therapeutic lifestyle therapies. In patients who cannot achieve LDL-cholesterol level <70 mg/dL on adequate statin treatment, addition of PCSK9 antibody such as alirocumab (Praluent) or evolocumab (Reptha) to statin can further reduce LDL cholesterol level and risk of recurrent cardiovascular events.

Aldosterone Antagonists

Eplerenone (Inspra) improves myocardial remodeling and may reduce all-cause and CV mortality and rehospitalization. The 2013 ACC/AHA STEMI guideline recommends starting this medication 3 to 14 days after STEMI in eligible patients (creatinine ≤2.5 mg/dL in men and ≤2.0 mg/dL in women, potassium ≤5.0 mEq/L) with heart failure, with LVEF less than 35% to 40%, and already on adequate doses of beta blockers and ACEIs or ARBs. However, earlier administration (<7 days) is preferable to achieve mortality and rehospitalization benefits as suggested by a post hoc analysis of the Eplerenone Post-Acute Myocardial Infarction Heart Failure Efficacy and Survival Study (EPHESUS) trial.

Implantable Cardioverter-Defibrillator

Patients who develop ventricular tachycardia (VT) or fibrillation more than 48 hours after STEMI have the highest risk of sudden cardiac death (SCD) and, hence, are eligible for an implantable cardioverter-defibrillator (ICD) as a secondary prevention measure for SCD. For primary prevention, multiple trials have established the efficacy of prevention of SCD by ICD implantation in patients with LVEF less than 35% and New York Heart Association (NYHA) class II or III symptoms (or LVEF <30% with NYHA class I symptoms) despite optimal medical therapy 40 days after index STEMI and expectation of at least 1-year survival.

Other Medical Therapy

Morphine

Morphine is a time-honored medication used to reduce pain and anxiety, especially in patients with pulmonary edema during acute presentation of STEMI. However, analysis of results from several clinical trials and a large meta-analysis involving more than 69,000 ACS patients suggest that a morphine/P2Y$_{12}$ inhibitor interaction exists, which could lead to adverse clinical consequences. Several pharmacokinetic studies in healthy volunteers

[1]Not FDA approved for this indication.

have shown that intravenous morphine administration can reduce the level of active metabolites of clopidogrel and delay the maximal inhibition of platelet aggregation. A similar effect of morphine on ticagrelor was also reported. Given the current trend of using oral $P2Y_{12}$ receptor inhibitors before PPCI for STEMI, careful selection of patients and judicious administration of morphine with $P2Y_{12}$ receptor inhibitors deserves careful consideration.

Nitrate

Nitroglycerin reduces LV preload, increases coronary blood flow, and relieves chest pain symptoms. However, it plays no role in decreasing myocardial injury from coronary artery occlusion in STEMI. Its use in STEMI is mostly for congestive heart failure, hypertension, or rare cases of coronary spasm. It is contraindicated in patients with hypotension (systolic blood pressure [SBP] <90 mm Hg or SBP >30 mm Hg below baseline), right ventricular infarction from right coronary artery occlusion, or use of phosphodiesterase-5 inhibitors within 24 to 48 hours.

Complications of STEMI
Cardiogenic Shock

Cardiogenic shock is defined as an SBP less than 90 mm Hg for longer than 1 hour that is (1) not responsive to fluid administration alone, (2) secondary to cardiac dysfunction, or (3) associated with signs of hypoperfusion or cardiac index less than 2.2 L/min/m^2 and pulmonary capillary wedge pressure greater than 18 mm Hg. It occurs in fewer than 10% of STEMI patients (2.4% in 1986 GISSI-1 trial; 6.5% in Germany ALKK-PCI registry as reported in 2013).

Almost 75% to 80% of cases of cardiogenic shock are due to severe LV systolic dysfunction; right ventricular infarction, mechanical complications from ventricular septal rupture, acute mitral regurgitation, and free wall rupture leading to tamponade account for the rest. Other uncommon causes of noncardiogenic shock after STEMI are bleeding, systemic inflammatory response syndrome, infection, bowel ischemia, or iatrogenic (such as due to medication).

Cardiogenic shock due to mechanical complications after STEMI occurs in a bimodal fashion, with most cases occurring within 24 hours. Risk factors for mechanical complication include female gender, old age, and late or no reperfusion in the infarcted territory. An early echocardiogram is extremely helpful to delineate the etiology of cardiogenic shock to guide subsequent definitive treatment. Cardiogenic shock carries a high in-hospital mortality, approaching 50%, and is higher in patients older than 75 years. These high-mortality patients require immediate stabilization to prevent end-stage organ damage followed by emergency coronary angiography and revascularization (Box 2).

Electrical Complications
Ventricular Arrhythmia

Lethal ventricular arrhythmia, VT or ventricular fibrillation (VF), is the most common cause of out-of-hospital cardiac arrest in STEMI. For hospitalized patients, VT/VF occurs in fewer than 10% of cases in the era of reperfusion therapy, and most cases occur within 48 hours of presentation. VT/VF is often associated with congestive heart failure, cardiogenic shock, or failed reperfusion of an occluded coronary artery. Hence, correction of electrolyte and acid-base disturbance, adequate reperfusion to reduce myocardial ischemia, and treatment of heart failure or shock are important preventive measures. Early administration of beta blockers within 24 hours to patients without contraindications reduces the incidence of VF. If VT/VF occurs, treatment includes immediate defibrillation or cardioversion and an antiarrhythmic agent such as amiodarone (Cordarone). Isolated premature ventricular contractions, nonsustained VT without hemodynamic instability, and AIVR do not generally require specific treatment.

BOX 2 | Management Measures for Cardiogenic Shock

Immediate Stabilization of Patients to Prevent End-Stage Organ Damage

Maintain adequate mean arterial blood pressure with norepinephrine (Levophed), dopamine, or dobutamine with intraarterial pressure monitoring; norepinephrine preferred over dopamine for less arrhythmogenic effect

Hemodynamic monitoring with Swan-Ganz catheter to guide inotrope or fluid management

Selective use of mechanical circulatory support* if patient cannot be stabilized by previous measures

Early echocardiography to define etiology of cardiogenic shock

Early mechanical ventilation

Management of hemodynamically significant arrhythmia

Fibrinolysis in STEMI if delay to PCI >2 h

Early Coronary Angiography and Revascularization

Early transfer to regional tertiary care hospital for revascularization

Prophylactic IABP placement before transfer

PCI often the treatment of choice

CABG (with correction of mechanical complications if present) in cardiogenic shock if feasible

---

*IABP is more readily available; limited experience with other LV assist devices such as Impella and TandemHeart device.

CABG, Coronary artery bypass grafting; *IABP*, intraaortic balloon pump; *LV*, left ventricular; *PCI*, percutaneous intervention; *STEMI*, ST-elevation myocardial infarction.

Supraventricular Arrhythmia

Common supraventricular arrhythmias after STEMI include atrial fibrillation, atrial flutter, and sinus tachycardia. They are usually the consequence of or triggered by congestive heart failure, atrial infarction, pericarditis, hypoxia, or other underlying systemic problems (such as chronic obstructive pulmonary disease, bleeding, anemia, or infection). Treatment is directed to the underlying causes. For atrial fibrillation/flutter, physicians should pay special attention to anticoagulation use given the frequent concomitant use of DAPT and antithrombotics and the rate versus rhythm control strategy.

Bradycardia and Heart Block

Sinus bradycardia may occur after inferior STEMI. Because it is generally mediated through increased vagal tone, close monitoring usually suffices. High-grade AV block (second or third degree) can occur after inferior or anterior STEMI, with a worse prognosis after anterior STEMI owing to a greater degree of myocardial injury. High-grade AV block after inferior STEMI usually is transient and with a narrow complex escape rhythm, which subsides within 2 weeks. Occasionally, temporary pacemaker placement may be necessary if bradycardia causes hemodynamic instability. High-grade AV block from anterior STEMI usually requires placement of a prophylactic temporary pacing system because it is commonly associated with hemodynamic instability.

References

Bainey KR, Armstrong PW: Transatlantic comparison of ST-segment elevation myocardial infarction guidelines: insights from the United States and Europe, *J Am Coll Cardiol* 67(2):216–219, 2016.

Bates ER, Tamis-Holland JE, Bittl JA: PCI strategies in patients with ST-segment elevation myocardial infarction and multivessel coronary artery disease, *J Am Coll Cardiol* 68(10):1066–1081, 2016.

Capodanno D, Huber K, Mehran R, et al: Management of antithrombotic therapy in atrial fibrillation patients undergoing PCI: JACC state-of-the-art review, *J Am Coll Cardiol* 74(1):83–99, 2019.

Cassese S, Byrne RA, Ndrepepa G: Everolimus-eluting bioresorbable vascular scaffolds versus everolimus-eluting metallic stents: a meta-analysis of randomized controlled trials, *Lancet* 387(1018):537–544, 2016.

Chandrasekhar J, Mehran R: The ideal anticoagulation strategy in ST-elevation myocardial infarction, *Prog Cardiovasc Dis* 58:247–259, 2015.

Claassens DMF, Vos GJA, Bergmeijer TO: A genotype-guided strategy for oral P2Y12 inhibitors in primary PCI, *N Engl J Med* 381(17):1621–1631, 2019.

Damluji AA, Forman DE, van Diepen S: Older adults in the cardiac intensive care unit: factoring geriatric syndromes in the management, prognosis, and process of care. A scientific statement from the American Heart Association, *Circulation* 141:e6–e32, 2020.

Di Pasquale G, Filippini E, Pavesi PC: Complete versus culprit-only revascularization in ST-elevation myocardial infarction and multivessel disease, *Intern Emerg Med* 11(4):499–506, 2016.

Duarte GS, Nunes-Ferreira A, Rodrigues FB: Morphine in acute coronary syndrome: systematic review and meta-analysis, *BMJ Open* 9:e025232, 2019.

Elbadawi A, Elgendy IY, Ha LD: National trends and outcomes of percutaneous coronary intervention in patients > 70 years of age with acute coronary syndrome (from the National Inpatient Sample Database), *Am J Cardiol* 123(1):25–32, 2019.

Ellis SG, Kereiakes DJ, Metzger DC: Everolimus-eluting bioresorbable scaffolds for coronary artery disease, *N Engl J Med* 373(20):1905–1915, 2015.

Frampton F, Devries JT, Welch TD: Modern management of ST-segment elevation myocardial infarction, *Curr Probl Cardiol* 45(3):100393, 2020.

Guedeney P, Collet JP: Diagnosis and management of acute coronary syndrome: what is new and why? Insight from the 2020 European society of cardiology guidelines, *J Clin Med* 9(11):3474, 2020.

Hochman JS, Lamas GA, Buller CE: Coronary intervention for persistent occlusion after myocardial infarction, *N Engl J Med* 355:2395–2407, 2006.

Ibanez B, Macaya C, SÆnchez-Brunete V: Effect of early metoprolol on infarct size in ST-segment-elevation myocardial infarction patients undergoing primary percutaneous coronary intervention: the Effect of Metoprolol in Cardioprotection during an Acute Myocardial Infarction (METOCARD-CNIC) trial, *Circulation* 128(14):1495–1503, 2013.

Kragholm K, Lu D, Chiswell K: Improvement in care and outcomes for emergency medical service-transported patients with ST-elevation myocardial infarction (STEMI) with and without prehospital cardiac arrest: a mission:lifeline STEMI accelerator study, *J Am Heart Assoc* 6:e005717, 2017.

Kubica J, Kubica A, Jilma B: Impact of morphine on antiplatelet effects of oral P2Y12 receptor inhibitors, *Int J Cardiol* 215:201–208, 2016.

Mehta SR, Wood DA, Storey RF: Complete revascularization with multivessel PCI for myocardial infarction, *N Engl J Med* 381(15):1411–1421, 2019.

Pu J, Ding S, Ge H: Efficacy and safety of a pharmaco-invasive strategy with half-dose alteplase versus primary angioplasty in ST-segment-elevation myocardial infarction: EARLY-MYO trial (early routine catheterization after alteplase fibrinolysis versus primary PCI in acute ST-segment-elevation myocardial infarction), *Circulation* 136:1462–1473, 2017.

Qamar A, Bhatt DL: Current status of data on cangrelor, *Pharmacol Ther* 159:102–109, 2016.

Roolvink V, IbÆæez B, Ottervanger JP: Early intravenous beta-blockers in patients with ST-segment elevation myocardial infarction before primary percutaneous coronary intervention, *J Am Coll Cardiol* 67(23):2705–2715, 2016.

Sabate M, Alfonso F, Cequier A: Magnesium-based resorbable scaffold versus permanent metallic sirolimus-eluting stent in patients with ST segment elevation myocardial infarction: the MAGSTEMI randomized clinical trial, *Circulation* 140(23):1904–1916, 2019.

Scholz KH, Maier SKG, Maier LS, et al: Impact of treatment delay on mortality in ST-segment elevation myocardial infarction (STEMI) patients presenting with and without haemodynamic instability: results from the German prospective, multicentre FITT-STEMI trial, *Eur Heart J* 39(13):1065–1074, 2018.

Schomig A, Mehilli J, Antoniucci D: Mechanical reperfusion in patients with acute myocardial infarction presenting more than 12 hours from symptom onset: a randomized controlled trial, *J Am Med Assoc* 293(23):2865–2872, 2005.

Schwartz GG, Steg PG, Szarek M, et al: Alirocumab and cardiovascular outcomes after acute coronary syndrome, *N Engl J Med* 379(22):2097–2107, 2018.

Serruys PW, Chevalier B, Sotomi Y: Comparison of an everolimus-eluting bioresorbable scaffold with an everolimus-eluting metallic stent for the treatment of coronary artery stenosis (ABSORB II): a 3 year, randomised, controlled, single-blind, multicentre clinical trial, *Lancet* 388(10059):2479–2491, 2016.

Shah RU, Henry TD, Rutten-Ramos S: Increasing percutaneous coronary interventions for ST-segment elevation myocardial infarction in the United States: progress and opportunity, *JACC Cardiovasc Interv* 8:139–146, 2015.

Thiele H, Akin I, Sandri M: PCI strategies in patients with acute myocardial infarction and cardiogenic shock, *N Engl J Med* 377(25):2419–2432, 2017.

Yerasi C, Case BC, Forrestal BJ, et al: Optimizing monotherapy selection, aspirin versus P2Y12 inhibitors, following percutaneous coronary intervention, *Am J Cardiol* 135:154–165, 2020.

ANGINA PECTORIS

Method of
Kenneth Tobin, DO; and Kim Eagle, MD

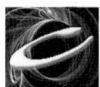

CURRENT DIAGNOSIS

- The clinical diagnosis of angina depends largely on the accurate assessment of a patient's risk factor profile for coronary artery disease and the typicality of the symptom complex.
- The most common symptom of angina pectoris is left-sided chest pain or pressure, with or without associated radiation of pain or pressure to the jaw or left arm, occurring with exertion and relieved with rest or sublingual nitroglycerin.
- Women may present with atypical symptoms such as sharp, nonexertional chest pain, generalized fatigue, shortness of breath, or right-sided chest pain.
- Basic screening tests (e.g., 12-lead electrocardiogram, laboratory data, chest radiograph) are normal in most cases.
- For an initial diagnosis, appropriate noninvasive testing or coronary angiography, or both, is important to define the amount of ischemic myocardium and an overall treatment plan.
- Even when invasive procedures are clinically indicated, aggressive medical therapy with high-dose statins, attainment of appropriate blood pressure levels, smoking cessation, and use of antiplatelet therapy is of paramount importance.
- Patients who have clinical evidence of unstable angina and laboratory evidence of myocardial ischemia most often benefit from early invasive treatment strategies.

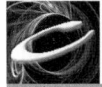

CURRENT THERAPY

Stable Angina Pectoris
- Treatment includes β-blockers, nitrates, and calcium channel blockers for symptom control.
- Consider the addition of ranolazine (Ranexa) if symptoms are not adequately controlled.

Aggressive Cholesterol Treatment Based on the American College of Cardiology (ACC)-American Hearth Association (AHA) Blood Cholesterol Guidelines
- Blood pressure management
- Antiplatelet therapy
- Lifestyle modifications:
  - Smoking cessation
  - Exercise prescription
  - Mediterranean, plant-based diet
  - Depression assessment

Unstable Angina
- With positive biomarkers for myocardial ischemia, consider coronary angiography.
- With negative biomarkers for myocardial ischemia, consider noninvasive assessment once symptoms are controlled.
- With a substantial ischemic burden identified, consider coronary angiography.
- With no or minimal ischemia identified, consider increasing medical therapy.
- With persistent symptoms, consider other treatment modalities.

Angina pectoris is defined as cardiac-induced pain that is a direct result of a mismatch between myocardial oxygen supply and demand. The initial presentation of ischemic heart disease is chronic stable angina in approximately 50% of patients; it is estimated that 16.5 million Americans are being diagnosed with this condition. Ischemic heart disease is the leading cause of death in the United States.

Stable angina refers to predictable chest discomfort during various levels of exertional activity that is predictably resolved with rest or administration of sublingual nitroglycerin (Nitrostat). Unstable angina is an acute ischemic event; this diagnosis includes patients with new-onset cardiac chest pain, angina at rest, post-myocardial infarction angina, or an accelerating pattern of previously stable angina. The terms unstable angina and non–Q wave myocardial infarction are often used interchangeably and should be further defined on the basis of myocardial necrosis as measured by serum biomarkers.

The clinical sensation of angina pectoris is caused by stimulation of chemosensitive and mechanosensitive receptors of unmyelinated nerve cells found within cardiac muscle fibers and around the coronary vessels. This stimulation cascade is thought to occur when lactate, serotonin, bradykinin, histamine, reactive oxygen species, and adenosine are released into the coronary circulation during periods of lactic acidosis. Nerve stimulation via the sympathetic ganglia occurs most commonly between the seventh cervical and fourth thoracic portions of the spinal cord. This explains from an anatomic standpoint why the most commonly recognized pain patterns for angina pectoris involve discomfort in the chest, neck, jaw, and left arm.

The most common cause of angina pectoris is coronary atherosclerosis. As plaque is initially deposited within a coronary vessel, there may be no significant internal luminal compromise during the early positive remodeling phase. However, at the point at which this compensatory mechanism fails, internal luminal compromise ensues. As long as the coronary artery segment distal to the stenosis retains the ability to vasodilate in response to increasing blood flow demands, coronary homeostasis is maintained. Once the critical threshold is passed, the blood supply cannot accommodate this demand, and angina may occur. The four major factors that determine myocardial oxygen demand are heart rate, systolic blood pressure, myocardial wall tension, and myocardial contractility.

Clinical Features

For patients with documented coronary artery disease (CAD) who have predictable episodes of classic symptoms, the diagnosis of angina pectoris is straightforward. Most patients are aware of the levels of exertion that typically induce angina symptoms. Most describe a pain or heaviness across their middle chest that may or may not radiate to the jaw or left arm. Some patients deny chest pain symptoms altogether and instead complain of exertional dyspnea or diaphoresis. Environmental situations such as cold exposure, emotional stress, or heavy meals can induce angina. The Canadian Cardiovascular Society and the New York Heart Association classification systems are used to define angina severity. Both systems use a I through IV scale, with mild angina (class I) referring to episodes that occur with extreme exertion and severe angina (class IV) to episodes that occur with minimal or no exertion. These classification systems are useful for risk stratification and for assessing medical therapy efficacy.

There are clear gender differences in the clinical presentations of angina. Pleuritic, musculoskeletal-type pain, nonexertional pain, and nocturnal pains have been reported as anginal equivalents in women. Fatigue is one of the most common presenting symptoms for CAD in women. The key to the diagnosis in men and women lies in a thorough history, which should always include the quality, location, provoking activities, and duration of pain and factors that relieve the pain. Based on a detailed clinical history, the many diagnoses that can masquerade as angina may be eliminated (Table 1).

Diagnostic Testing

A baseline electrocardiogram (ECG) is often one of the initial tests obtained in a patient with the complaint of chest pain. A normal tracing does not exclude the diagnosis of ischemic heart disease. More than 50% of patients with diagnosed angina have

TABLE 1	Differential Diagnosis of Chest Pain
Cardiac ischemia
Angina
Myocardial infarction
Vasospastic angina
Pericarditis
Aortic dissection (new-onset chest pain and new aortic insufficiency noted on auscultation is an aortic dissection until proven otherwise)
Pulmonary embolism
Esophageal spasm
Gastroesophageal reflux disease
Musculoskeletal pain
Biliary colic
Acute pneumonia

a normal ECG at rest. The baseline ECG may, however, show evidence of pathologic Q waves or left ventricular hypertrophy, either of which increases the statistical probability of significant CAD. Baseline laboratory data should include a fasting lipid panel to help define the patient's risk factor profile.

Stress testing is an appropriate screening tool for the initial diagnosis of CAD, risk stratification after acute ischemic syndrome, and assessment of treatment efficacy. Whenever feasible, it is more advantageous to obtain an exercise stress test rather than a pharmacologically based study. The additional prognostic data obtained through exercise include blood pressure response, heart rate response, heart rate recovery, metabolic equivalent level attained, and ECG assessment of the ST segment. There are several validated exercise protocols that provide additional risk stratification measures to the test results.

The predictive value of exercise treadmill stress testing ranges from 40% for single-vessel disease to 90% for three-vessel disease. A baseline left bundle branch block, paced rhythm, poorly controlled atrial arrhythmia, or left ventricular hypertrophy with secondary ischemic changes often renders the test inconclusive when assessing for ischemic changes. However, if stress testing is being performed for attainment of hemodynamic responses and achievable metabolic equivalent levels, these baseline ECG abnormalities may be overlooked.

Stress test accuracy is markedly improved by the addition of an imaging modality such as echocardiography or nuclear perfusion scanning. The sensitivity and specificity of stress echocardiography and stress nuclear imaging are 85% to 90%. Stress echocardiography is believed to be more specific, and stress nuclear imaging is thought to be more sensitive. A stress echocardiogram also allows assessment of left ventricular systolic function and valvular function and prediction of right ventricular pressure. In deciding on which stress test to perform, one should rely on the expertise of the testing facility and the individual patient's circumstance.

Risk Factor Management
Hypertension
Hypertension is a commonly occurring, well-established, major cardiovascular risk factor. Initial treatment of hypertension in patients with ischemic heart disease should always include lifestyle management. Appropriate weight loss with a goal of achieving a body mass index <25 kg/m^2 can improve hypertension control. A reduction in dietary salt intake can also have positive effects on a patient's blood pressure. Following a heart healthy diet and increased physical activity with a structured exercise program are also very important.

Discord has resulted from the publication of several recent hypertension guidelines by various medical societies, as well as the 2014 Evidence-Based Guideline for the Management of High Blood Pressure in Adults Report from the Panel Members Appointed to the Eighth Joint National Committee. It has been shown that cardiovascular risk progressively increases at blood pressures greater than 115/75 mm Hg. A meta-analysis of 61 prospective observational trials of hypertension involving 1 million adults with no known vascular disease at baseline revealed several interesting findings. Patient outcomes were related per decade of age to the usual blood pressure at the start of that decade. For example, from ages 40 to 69 years, for each increase in 20 mm Hg systolic blood pressure, a twofold increase in cardiovascular death rate occurred. These findings were much more pronounced in patients who were between 80 and 89 years old than in the youngest cohort, 40 to 49 years old. Although the relative risk was much higher in the younger group, the absolute risk was greatest among the octogenarians. These increased cardiovascular risks were not confined to subjects with blood pressures greater than 140/90 mm Hg; rather, there was a threshold of risk shown all the way down to 115/75 mm Hg. Even small reductions in blood pressure can have a significant positive impact on cardiovascular disease. Blood pressure reductions of 4 mm Hg systolic and 3 mm Hg diastolic were shown to reduce cardiovascular events by 15% in a cohort of 20,888 patients.

The Heart Outcomes Prevention Evaluation study asked the question whether all patients with atherosclerosis, regardless of blood pressure, should be treated with an angiotensin-converting enzyme inhibitor. Although many subsequent editorials implied that all patients with CAD could benefit from this therapy, a closer look at the data suggests a different interpretation. The mean blood pressure was 139/79 mm Hg, suggesting that a significant portion of the 9297 participants had a baseline blood pressure higher than this value. Compared with placebo, the treatment group had a 22% reduction in the primary outcome composite of myocardial infarction, stroke, or cardiovascular death. A small substudy using 24-hour ambulatory blood pressure monitoring showed blood pressure differences of 11 mm Hg systolic and 4 mm Hg diastolic in the treatment group compared with the placebo group, which may explain the cardiovascular event reductions reported.

The Systolic Blood Pressure Intervention Trial (SPRINT) studied cardiovascular outcomes in patients with increased cardiovascular risk (excluding diabetes) and randomized the more than 9000 participants to either intensive blood pressure control of <120 mm Hg or a standard blood pressure goal of <140 mm Hg. The trial was halted early because of the significant benefits seen in the intensive blood pressure arm. The intensive group had a 25% relative risk reduction for the primary composite endpoint compared to the standard care group. The blood pressure goal for treatment of hypertension in patients at high cardiovascular risk should be <130/80 mm Hg. High cardiovascular risk is defined as a history of clinical cardiovascular (CV) disease (established coronary artery disease, heart failure, or stroke), or an estimated 10-year atherosclerosis CV disease of ≥10%. (One must be careful with aggressive diastolic blood pressure management, as some studies have shown a J-shaped curve relationship between diastolic blood pressures and coronary events.)

Hyperlipidemia

Dyslipidemia is an important risk factor for atherosclerotic cardiovascular disease, and the lowering of low density lipoprotein (LDL)-cholesterol has been shown to correlate with reductions in cardiovascular disease event rates. Previously published cholesterol treatment guidelines recommended achieving less than 70 mg/dL LDL-cholesterol levels in CAD patients. The current guidelines published by the ACC-AHA depart from these specific values, and instead recommend using high-intensity 3-hydroxy-3-methylglutaryl coenzyme reductase inhibitors (statins) to reduce the LDL-cholesterol levels by more than 50%. These agents have been shown to be well tolerated and have

positive nonlipid pleiotropic effects, as well as the ability to dramatically lower LDL levels.

Observational evidence suggests that regardless of how cholesterol is lowered, a reduction in atherosclerotic cardiovascular disease will result. However, to achieve meaningful reductions in cardiovascular mortality, the recommended choice for lowering LDL-cholesterol levels among the currently available pharmacology are the statins. These agents have been studied exclusively using fixed-dose combinations and not dose-titrated to achieve various LDL-C levels; therefore currently available data do not support specific LDL target goals.

The Cholesterol Treatment Trialists' meta-analysis, including 90,056 subjects from 14 trials, showed a 12% reduction in all-cause mortality per 38.6 mg/dL (1 mmol/L) reduction in LDL-cholesterol, with a 19% reduction in coronary mortality, a 24% reduction in need for revascularization, a 17% reduction in stroke incidence, and a 21% reduction in any major vascular event during a mean follow-up period of 5 years. These benefits were observed in different age groups, across genders, at different baseline cholesterol levels, and equally among those with and without prior CAD and cardiovascular risk factors.

The Heart Protection Study showed that in patients with established CAD, other atherosclerotic vascular disease, or diabetes, statin therapy reduced cardiovascular events regardless of the baseline LDL-cholesterol level. The trial, which enrolled 20,536 patients aged 40 to 80 years, showed a 24% reduction in major cardiovascular events, a 25% reduction in stroke, and a 13% reduction in overall mortality with statin therapy.

Patients with a recent acute ischemic syndrome were enrolled in the Pravastatin or Atorvastatin Evaluation and Infection Therapy trial, known as Thrombolysis in Myocardial Infarction 22, which compared 80 mg atorvastatin (Lipitor) with 40 mg of pravastatin (Pravachol). The atorvastatin group achieved a median LDL level of 62 mg/dL, compared with 96 mg/dL in the pravastatin group. The relative risk reduction for this reduced LDL level was 16%. A substudy looking at the LDL-cholesterol levels achieved with atorvastatin showed that those subjects achieving a level of 40 to 60 mg/dL had a 22% reduction in events, compared with those achieving a level of 80 to 100 mg/dL. Therefore, it appears that high-dose statin therapy and aggressive LDL-lowering in this patient population lead to reduced cardiovascular events.

The Treating to New Targets trial was the first to compare a more intensely treated group with a less intensely treated group using the same agent. The design of this 10,000-patient study eliminated concerns that outcome differences were induced by dissimilar statin preparations. The mean LDL level achieved was 101 mg/dL with 10 mg atorvastatin, and 77 mg/dL with the 80 mg dose. This LDL reduction was associated with a relative risk reduction of 27% for the primary endpoint of the first major cardiovascular event.

There is an increased risk of myopathy and rhabdomyolysis in patients taking 80 mg simvastatin (Zocor), according to the Study of the Effectiveness of Additional Reductions in Cholesterol and Homocysteine (SEARCH). The US Food and Drug Administration (FDA) has subsequently restricted high-dose simvastatin to patients who have been on this dose for longer than 12 months without evidence of myopathy, and the agency has recommended that new patients should not be started on this particular dose.

To effectively achieve a greater than 50% LDL-cholesterol reduction in CAD patients utilizing currently available pharmacologic agents, the most recent treatment guidelines suggest either atorvastatin 40 to 80 mg or rosuvastatin (Crestor) 20 to 40 mg. In other patient populations that require moderate-intensity statin therapy, there are several statin choices. Because there is no currently available evidence to suggest that nonstatin lipid-altering agents effectively reduce cardiovascular mortality, these medications should not be routinely prescribed.

It is apparent from both primary and secondary prevention lipid trials that achieving lower LDL levels reduces cardiovascular event rates. Because there is no high-quality clinical evidence to support achieving specific LDL levels in patients with diagnosed

CAD, high-dose statin therapy should be the mainstay of pharmacologically based therapy, if tolerated.

Although statins are the standard pharmacologic approach for primary and secondary prevention of atherosclerotic cardiovascular disease, as many as 20% of patients may be intolerant. The numbers may be even higher if medication adherence is included. For secondary prevention in patients whose cholesterol levels are not adequately achieved on a statin or other cholesterol-lowering medication, a proprotein convertase subtilisin kexin type 9 (PCSK9) inhibitor is an FDA-approved option. PCSK9 inhibitors can also be considered for those with familial hypercholesterolemia and can be prescribed with or without a statin. The FOURIER Cardiovascular Outcomes trial studied more than 27,000 patients with stable atherosclerotic cardiovascular disease and showed that evolocumab (Repatha) reduced the primary endpoint of atherosclerotic events by 15%, without significant safety differences between treatment groups. Subgroup analyses suggested that greater benefits were seen in patients with longer exposure to evolocumab, recent acute coronary syndrome, multiple myocardial infarctions, multivessel coronary artery disease, peripheral arterial disease, as well as the subgroup who achieved very low low-density lipoprotein-cholesterol levels of below 0.3 mmol/L (10 mg/dL).

Omega-3 Fatty Acids

Omega-3 polyunsaturated fatty acids (PUFAs) are a well known part of a heart healthy diet, and are also an effective treatment for patients with elevated triglyceride levels. The Reduce-it trial studied a prescription strength omega-3 PUFA in well-controlled statin-treated patients with elevated triglycerides and either documented coronary artery disease, diabetes mellitus, or other cardiovascular risk factors. Seventy percent of the 8179 patients enrolled had a previous diagnosis of ischemic heart disease.

Patients were randomly assigned to receive 2 g of icosapent ethyl twice daily or placebo. The primary end point included cardiovascular death, nonfatal myocardial infarction, nonfatal stroke, coronary revascularization, or unstable angina. Patients treated with icosapent ethyl had a 25% risk reduction in cardiovascular events, and a 20% reduction in death due to cardiovascular causes.

This preparation of omega PUFA, icosapent ethyl (Vascepa), is pure eicosapentaenoic acid (EPA) which differs from agents used in other similar trials that contain both EPA and docosahexaenoic acid (DHA). This may explain the strongly positive outcomes that have not been shown in other similar trials.

Metabolic Syndrome

The combined presence of insulin resistance, hypertension, dyslipidemia, and abdominal obesity define metabolic syndrome. There is debate about whether this is a true syndrome or simply a clustering of cardiovascular risk factors in a particular individual. The key concept is that the concomitant presence of these particular cardiovascular risk factors markedly increases a patient's chances of developing diabetes mellitus and coronary atherosclerosis. The approach to treatment for this syndrome is no different from that for the individual components. Recognition of the components is key to the treatment of this disorder.

Smoking

Cigarette smoking is probably the most important of the identified modifiable cardiovascular risk factors. The incidence of CAD is two to four times higher in smokers than in nonsmokers. The pathophysiologic process that leads to atherosclerosis from smoking stems from induced platelet dysfunction, endothelial dysfunction, smooth muscle cell proliferation, and attenuated high-density lipoprotein cholesterol levels. Smoking cessation must be sought for every CAD patient.

Diet

Lifestyle changes for patients with CAD must incorporate healthy eating habits. The Mediterranean diet has been shown to positively affect cardiovascular disease, and conversely, a diet high in saturated fats has been shown to negatively influence multiple cardiac risk factors. Patients should be encouraged to incorporate high proportions of fruits and vegetables into their diet, along with olive oil and regular servings of fish coupled with a reduced amount of red meats and excess sugar.

Other Lifestyle Changes

Exercise should be encouraged in patients with stable angina, once all appropriate invasive and noninvasive tests have been completed and a stable medical regimen has been established.

Increasing a patient's aerobic capacity can lower the body's oxygen requirement for a given workload, which can lead to increased exercise tolerance and reduced anginal symptoms. Aerobic exercise can improve endothelial function and positively affect baroreflex sensitivity and heart rate variability in patients with CAD.

Endorphins released during exercise are thought to be mood enhancers, as well as effective muscle relaxants. Exercise itself improves sleep patterns. Cortisol levels are reduced with regular exercise, which may attenuate the body's sensation of stress and anxiety. For these reasons, appropriate exercise programs for patients with stable angina have far-reaching positive benefits. Exercise guidelines for CAD patients have been published and should be reviewed before patients begin aggressive secondary prevention efforts.

Major depression affects approximately 25% of people recovering from a myocardial infarction, and another 40% suffer from mild depression. In any given year, one of every three long-term acute ischemic syndrome survivors will develop depression. The Heart and Soul Study examined 1017 patients with stable CAD over a period of 4.8 years. Patients identified with depression were twice as likely to experience recurrent cardiovascular events. Physical inactivity was associated with a 44% greater rate of cardiovascular events. Patients with symptoms of depression were less likely to follow dietary, exercise, and medication recommendations.

Approach to Treatment
Medical Therapy

Medications used to treat angina pectoris and typical dosages are listed in Table 2.

Nitrates

Nitrates provide an exogenous source of nitric oxide, which serves to relax smooth muscle and inhibit platelet aggregation. Nitrates exert their antianginal effect by reducing myocardial oxygen demand through coronary and systemic vasodilation. Nitrates are strong venodilators, and in higher doses they can also induce arterial dilation. Reducing the preload through venodilation reduces myocardial oxygen demand. Coronary artery dilatation of stenotic vessels and intracoronary collaterals directly increases myocardial oxygen delivery. Through these mechanisms, nitrates have been shown to prevent recurrent episodes of angina and to increase exercise tolerance.

There are several nitrate preparations; they differ mainly in route of administration, onset of action, and effective half-life. Nitrate tolerance can occur with long-term use of any nitrate preparation and can be avoided by providing a 10- to 12-hour nitrate-free interval. Nitrates should be used with caution in patients with a diagnosis of hypertrophic obstructive cardiomyopathy.

β-Blockers

β-Blockers competitively inhibit catecholamines from binding to β-receptors. Over time, β-blocker therapy leads to an increase in β-receptor density. Because of receptor upregulation, acute β-blocker withdrawal may lead to a transient supersensitivity to catecholamines and subsequent angina or even myocardial infarction. There are three classes of β-receptors. Some β-blockers are receptor specific, and some exert an effect over all three receptors. However, at higher doses, even β-selective agents have cross-reactivity for all β-receptors. β-Blockers reduce myocardial

TABLE 2	Medications Used for the Treatment of Angina Pectoris

NAME	DOSAGE
β-Blockers	
Atenolol (Tenormin)	25–200 mg PO qd
Metoprolol tartrate (Lopressor)	25–200 mg bid
Metoprolol succinate (Toprol XL)	25–200 mg qd
Carvedilol (Coreg)[1]	6.25–25 mg PO bid
Carvedilol phosphate (Coreg CR)[1]	20–80 mg PO qd
Propranolol (Inderal)	80–320 mg/d, divided bid or tid
Propranolol (Inderal LA)	80–160 mg PO qd
Labetalol (Trandate, Normodyne)[1]	200–800 mg bid
Nitrates	
Isosorbide dinitrate (Isordil)	10–40 mg PO bid or tid
Isosorbide mononitrate (Imdur)	30–240 mg PO qd
Nitroglycerin (Nitrostat)	0.4 mg SL q5min
Nitroglycerin transdermal (Nitro-Dur)	0.2–0.8 mg/h 12–14 h patch
Calcium Channel Blockers	
Dihydropyridines	
Amlodipine (Norvasc)	2.5–10 mg PO qd
Felodipine (Plendil)[1]	2.5–10 mg PO qd
Nifedipine (Procardia XL)	30–90 mg PO qd
Nondihydropyridines	
Verapamil (Calan)	80–120 mg PO tid
Verapamil (Calan SR)	120–480 mg PO qd
Diltiazem (Cardizem)	360 mg/d PO, divided tid or qid
Diltiazem (Cardizem LA)	180–360 mg PO qd
Other	
Ranolazine (Ranexa)	500 mg twice daily and increase to 1000 mg twice daily as needed, based on clinical symptoms

[1]Not FDA approved for this indication.

oxygen demand through a negative inotropic effect, a chronotropic effect, and a reduction in left ventricular wall stress.

Several cardioselective β-blockers, including atenolol (Tenormin) and metoprolol (Lopressor), have been shown to be effective antianginals that are fairly well tolerated in patients with underlying bronchospastic disease. Dosing is important for β-blocker efficacy. A study comparing atenolol with placebo showed that all doses from 25 through 200 mg/day were effective in reducing angina, but only the two highest doses led to an increase in exercise tolerance. Certain β-blockers have intrinsic sympathomimetic activity, including pindolol (Visken)[1] and acebutolol (Sectral).[1] Although they may be effective in reducing angina, they should be used with caution in patients with a prior history of myocardial infarction and in those with left ventricular dysfunction, because they may not reduce heart rate or blood pressure at rest.

[1]Not FDA approved for this indication.

When β-blockers are used to treat angina, a goal resting heart rate should be between 55 and 60 beats/min. Caution should be used in patients with resting bradycardia and in those with known reactive airway disease. Atenolol is renally excreted and should be used with caution in the elderly and in those with known renal dysfunction.

Calcium Channel Blockers
Calcium channel blockers are classified as either dihydropyridines or nondihydropyridines. The former group includes amlodipine (Norvasc), felodipine (Plendil)[1], nifedipine (Procardia), and nicardipine (Cardene); the latter includes diltiazem (Cardizem) and verapamil (Calan). There are differences among the two subclasses in terms of chronotropic, dromotropic, and inotropic effects.

Calcium channel blockers positively alter myocardial oxygen supply and demand, mainly through direct arterial vasodilation. The nondihydropyridines also exhibit negative chronotropic and inotropic effects, thus further lowering myocardial oxygen demands.

One of the early quick-release preparations of a dihydropyridine calcium channel blocker, nifedipine, was reported to potentially induce myocardial infarction when used to treat angina. This was most likely due to a rapid drop in afterload leading to reflex adrenergic activation. Sustained-release preparations of nifedipine (Procardia XL), as well as the other dihydropyridines, have been proven safe and effective in patients with cardiovascular disease. Although amlodipine and felodipine are tolerated in patients with left ventricular systolic dysfunction, other calcium channel blockers should be avoided in this patient subset.

Ranolazine (Ranexa)
Ranolazine (Ranexa) is a new and unique antianginal drug approved for the treatment of stable angina. It is a sustained-release preparation that has been approved for patients who remain symptomatic while on standard angina pharmacotherapy. Its mechanism of action may be through reduction of fatty acid oxidation or effects on sodium shifts and intracellular calcium levels. QT prolongation has been reported, but a significant increase in arrhythmias has not been seen. Side effects include dizziness, constipation, and nausea. Dosing is 500 or 1000 mg twice daily, and the major route of metabolism is the cytochrome P 450 system. Ranolazine should be used cautiously in patients who are taking other pharmacologic agents that have the potential to prolong the QT interval, and in patients with liver cirrhosis.

Ivabradine (Corlanor)[1]
Heart rate has a profound effect on diastolic perfusion time and subsequent myocardial oxygen supply. Ninety percent of coronary blood flow occurs in diastole. Therefore, an elevated heart rate may result in myocardial ischemia and angina. Ivabradine (Corlanor) selectively reduces heart rate without affecting inotropic function or coronary vasomotor tone. Ivabradine does not affect central aortic pressure or ventricular repolarization.

Ivabradine is a selective and specific inhibitor of the cardiac pacemaker current (If) that controls the spontaneous diastolic depolarization in the sinus node and regulates heart rate. It is metabolized by both the liver and the gut by oxidation through the cytochrome P450 3A4 (CYP3A4). Although ivabradine has a low affinity for CYP3A4, potent inhibitors and inducers of CYP3A4 may affect its plasma levels. Although nondihydropyridine calcium channel blockers should not be co-administered, other first-line coronary artery disease medications such as β-blockers, renin-angiotensin-aldosterone system inhibitors, aspirin, and HMG-CoA reductase inhibitors can be safely combined. Starting dosage is 5 mg twice daily in patients <75 years old, and 2.5 mg twice daily for patients ≥75 years old. No dosage adjustments are necessary in patients with renal impairment or creatinine clearance >15 mL/min. In patients with moderate hepatic

[1]Not FDA approved for this indication.

impairment, caution is advised, and ivabradine is contraindicated in patients with severe liver impairment. The maintenance dose is ≤7.5 mg twice daily, with up titration possible after 4 weeks if initial dose is well tolerated, symptoms persist, and heart rate is >60 bpm. Ivabradine is contraindicated in patients with a pre-treatment resting heart rate <70 bpm.

Heart rate reduction triggered by ivabradine appears to be greatest in those patients with highest pre-treatment baseline heart rates. Borer et al. showed that ivabradine improved exercise stress testing variables in a dose-dependent fashion. In this study, ivabradine improved time to 1 mm ST-segment depression as compared to placebo ($P = .016$). In a pooled analysis of 5 randomized, double blind, parallel-group studies of patients with stable angina, ivabradine ≥5 mg/day (maximum dose 7.5 mg/day) resulted in a 14.5% heart rate reduction, a −59.4% change in the number of angina attacks per week, and a −53.7% change in the consumption of nitrates.

There is mounting clinical evidence that ivabradine improves angina symptoms and quality of life (QOL) regardless of age, gender, and pre-treatment angina class. It also appears to improve prognosis and reduce hospitalizations in angina patients with left ventricular systolic dysfunction.

Medication Combinations

Many patients with chronic stable angina require more than one antianginal medication to control their symptoms. Current guidelines recommend β-blockers or calcium channel blockers as initial therapy unless otherwise contraindicated, with the addition of nitrates as symptoms dictate. Further medications may be added and individualized to each patient based on their degree of angina and overall clinical response.

However, it is important to recognize medication side effects when deciding which agents to combine. β-Blockers block the atrioventricular (AV) node and exert a portion of their effectiveness through this mechanism. The nondihydropyridine calcium channel blockers also have AV-nodal blocking properties and therefore should be used cautiously with β-blockers, especially in patients with preexisting conduction system disease. The dihydropyridine agents do not have AV-nodal blocking effects and may be a safer choice when used in combination with β-blockers. Nitrates do not have a side-effect profile that raises concerns when they are used with β-blockers or with calcium channel blockers.

Antiplatelet Therapy

The common etiology leading to an acute ischemic syndrome is a platelet-rich clot occurring at the site of a significant coronary artery stenosis, often after a plaque rupture. Antiplatelet medications have been shown to consistently decrease morbidity and mortality in a wide array of cardiovascular disease patients. A meta-analysis suggested that for patients with stable cardiovascular disease, low-dose aspirin therapy (50 to 100 mg daily) is as effective as higher doses (>300 mg). In this patient population, aspirin therapy resulted in a 26% reduction in myocardial infarction; the number of patients needed to treat to prevent a myocardial infarction was 83.

The Antiplatelet Trialists' Collaboration study demonstrated a reduction in myocardial infarction, stroke, and death in high-risk cardiovascular patients treated with antiplatelet therapy. Consensus guidelines recommend indefinite oral aspirin for the secondary prevention of cardiovascular events in all angina patients.

Clopidogrel (Plavix)[1] is an effective alternative to aspirin for the treatment of stable cardiovascular disease in those patients with a true aspirin allergy. However, there are no compelling data to indicate that clopidogrel (or newer agents, such as prasugrel [Effient][1] and ticagrelor [Brilinta][1]) are superior to aspirin in this particular patient population. In patients with unstable angina, dual antiplatelet therapy with aspirin and clopidogrel is recommended.

---

[1] Not FDA approved for this indication.

Oral Anticoagulation

The use of vitamin K antagonists to reduce cardiac events in patients with stable ischemic heart disease has been shown to be beneficial, with results tempered by the cost of a substantial increased risk of bleeding. With the advent of newer antithrombotic agents, also referred to as direct oral anticoagulants (DOACs), there has been renewed interest in further modulating the coagulation cascade to positively affect clinical outcomes.

The recent Rivaroxaban for the Prevention of Major Cardiovascular Events in Coronary or Peripheral Artery Disease (COMPASS) study evaluated the use of a factor Xa inhibitor, rivaroxaban (Xarelto), with or without aspirin vs. aspirin monotherapy in patients with stable atherosclerotic vascular disease. Rivaroxaban (Xarelto) dosing was 5 mg twice daily as monotherapy, 2.5 mg twice daily (referred to as a vascular dose) with 100 mg ASA, or 100mg ASA.

Although the primary combined endpoint revealed positive results in the rivaroxaban plus aspirin group, this was at the cost of a significant increase in overall bleeding events. If these events are separated into fatal or critical organ bleeding only, the findings favor a vascular dose of rivaroxaban plus aspirin for treatment of stable atherosclerotic vascular disease patients. Unfortunately, these results are equivocal when all bleeding events are taken into consideration. Moreover, the positive findings of this trial are driven mainly by a reduction in ischemic stroke and not myocardial infarction (49% RRR for ischemic stroke and 14% RRR for myocardial infarction). Although atrial fibrillation and/or prior use of systemic anticoagulation were exclusion criteria, certainly the percentage of this patient population with subclinical atrial fibrillation cannot be discounted.

Therefore, at this time there is no convincing evidence that adding antithrombotic therapy to aspirin or antithrombotic monotherapy should replace goal directed medical therapy of appropriate antiplatelet medications.

Invasive Assessment

The decision to pursue an invasive treatment approach differs significantly in patients with chronic stable angina and in those with acute coronary syndromes. Within both groups, accurate risk stratification is the key consideration in choosing who will benefit from coronary angiography and subsequent percutaneous coronary intervention. An invasive strategy in unstable angina patients has been shown to reduce recurrent acute coronary syndrome events consistently in many trials. A routine invasive strategy is recommended for patients with non-ST-segment acute ischemic syndromes who have refractory ischemia, elevated cardiac biomarkers suggesting myocardial necrosis, or new ST-segment depression on ECG monitoring.

In patients with unstable angina, there are significant gender differences in outcomes related to the use of invasive therapy. Both men and women with elevated biomarkers from myocardial necrosis have comparable reductions in rates of death, myocardial infarction, and rehospitalization with invasive treatment strategies. However, in the absence of positive biomarkers, women appear to have potentially negative outcomes with an invasive approach. The current American College of Cardiology and American Heart Association guidelines recommend a conservative approach in such women.

Patients diagnosed with stable angina comprise a vast array of clinical presentations. The two most heated debates in this arena concern the initial choice of medical therapy versus an invasive approach, and when to cross over from a medical treatment plan to an invasive one. The Atorvastatin Versus Revascularization Treatment (AVERT) trial studied the effects of intensive lipid-lowering therapy on ischemic events in a relatively low-risk population of patients with single- or two-vessel disease compared with percutaneous transluminal coronary angioplasty. AVERT randomized 341 patients to medical therapy plus atorvastatin 80 mg or to angioplasty followed by usual medical care (which included the option of statin therapy at the choice of the treating physician). The medical treatment group experienced a 36%

reduction in the composite endpoint of ischemic events compared with the angioplasty group. This difference was due primarily to repeated angioplasty, coronary artery bypass grafting, or hospitalization for worsening angina. The primary outcome of this trial from a practical standpoint was that high-dose statin therapy was safe in this patient population and did not increase cardiovascular events, compared with an angioplasty-based treatment plan.

One of the keys in interpreting the available data is recognizing that by the time many of these trials are published, the percutaneous treatment choices are often outdated. Early trials used mainly balloon angioplasty; later trials used early-generation bare metal stents. Equally as important is to determine what the background medical treatment plans were for any particular trial on this subject. Often, lipid therapy was not aggressive, hypertension management was not confirmed to be adequate, and intravenous glycoprotein IIb/IIIa antagonists were either not available or not used as a standard protocol when indicated.

The Clinical Outcomes Utilizing Revascularization and Aggressive Drug Evaluation (COURAGE) trial was designed to address the potential advantages of current medical therapy over a percutaneous approach in patients with demonstrable ischemia but stable CAD. Of the 35,000 patients screened, only 2287 met the study inclusion criteria. All participants of the COURAGE trial underwent a coronary angiography, and patients with high-risk anatomic findings such as severe left main coronary artery stenosis were excluded. The biggest difference in this trial compared with previous studies was that strict guideline-based medical therapy was followed in both groups. In the entire cohort, 85% of subjects were taking a β-blocker, 93% were taking a statin, and 85% were taking aspirin. The final interpretation of the COURAGE trial results was not that medical therapy is superior for all patients with CAD, but that in selected cohorts, aggressive medical therapy is an appropriate first step in the treatment of ischemic heart disease.

It is well accepted that a coronary artery lesion ≥70% is clinically significant. Historically, the interventional cardiologist has relied on visually estimating this value during coronary angiography to determine when a percutaneous intervention is appropriate. However, physiology-guided revascularization has become an established practice in the management of patients with coronary artery disease. Both instantaneous wave free ration (iFR) and fractional flow reserve (FFR) are well-studied techniques that allow assessment of the pressure differences across a coronary artery stenosis.

iFR isolates a specific period in diastole where pressure and flow are linearly related, which is referred to as the wave-free period. During this time, competing forces (waves) that affect period diverge; an iFR value below 0.9 suggests flow restriction (normal value is 1.0). iFR is measured at rest, without the need for pharmacologic vasodilators or stressors.

FFR utilizes a guidewire that is passed through a coronary lesion and allows for measurement of both blood flow and pressure. After direct administration of the hyperemic agent adenosine (Adenocard)[1], the pressure difference across a stenosis is determined. An FFR of ≤0.80 is considered clinically significant.

Physiologic assessment of obstructive coronary artery disease adds clarity to the visual angiogram interpretation, thereby leading to more appropriate coronary interventions.

The ORBITA trial was a 200-patient placebo-controlled randomized trial assessing the efficacy of percutaneous coronary intervention (PCI) compared with a placebo sham procedure for the relief of angina in patients with severe (>70%) single-vessel coronary artery disease. Patients were randomized in a 1:1 fashion, and all patients had assessment of their coronary lesion by both FFR and iFR. All patients were assessed by cardiopulmonary exercise testing, symptom questionnaires, and dobutamine stress echocardiography before and six weeks after the procedure.

Compared with placebo, PCI reduced ischemia as assessed by stress echocardiography. However, there was no difference in the primary endpoint of exercise time between the two arms, or statistically significant differences between the two groups with respect to angina frequency. Changes in the Duke treadmill score and exercise time were both numerically higher in the PCI arm, which poses the question of small sample size effects on these outcomes.

Within the spectrum of stable ischemic heart disease, a portion of patients have coronary arteries that have chronic total occlusions (CTO). Some of these ischemic heart disease patients may suffer from coronary reserve insufficiency and develop recurrent angina.

Since a CTO lesion cannot contribute to collateral blood flow, development of further CAD is often poorly tolerated. CTO lesions are encountered in clinical practice at a frequency of 16%–18%, but only intervened upon in 5%–10% of cases. We suspect this discrepancy in prevalence and treatment is based on the combination of a high rate of technical difficulty coupled with the uncertainty of clinical benefit.

Unfortunately, successful treatment of CTO lesions does not appear to benefit all patients with chronic ischemic heart disease. Patients with underlying diabetes have a reduction in major adverse cardiac events (MACE) when compared to standard medical therapy. This same finding, however, is not seen in non diabetic patients with CTO lesions.

Novel Therapies
External Counterpulsation
External counterpulsation is a noninvasive method of increasing coronary blood flow through diastolic augmentation. Large blood pressure cuffs are placed on both legs and thighs and are inflated to a pressure of 300 mm Hg in early diastole (triggered by the patient's ECG), promoting venous return to the heart. The mechanism is unclear but may be related to enhanced endothelial function, improved myocardial perfusion, and possibly placebo effect. Several small studies have suggested a clinical reduction in angina episodes, but no positive mortality benefit has yet been published. A meta-analysis that included 13 observational studies and followed 949 patients with stable angina. Using the CCS classification scheme, there was at least a one-class improvement in 86% of the study population. Contraindications to this treatment include certain aortic valvular diseases, aortic aneurysm, and peripheral vascular disease.

Spinal Cord Stimulation
For patients whose angina is refractory to medical therapy and who are not candidates for revascularization, spinal cord stimulation may be considered. Little intermediate or long-term data are available, but many short-term studies suggest reduced angina episodes. Placement of the device and subsequent stimulation at the C7-T1 level suggests that the mechanism of action is reduced pain sensation.

Acupuncture
Acupuncture has been shown to be of benefit for the relief of both acute and chronic pain in various medical conditions. With respect to patients with documented CAD and symptomatic angina, there are only limited data currently available to recommend this modality.

A recently published randomized trial of treating chronic stable angina patients with acupuncture as an adjunct to standard medical therapy was undertaken in China. It was a small study of 398 relatively healthy angina patients. Those with prior myocardial infarction or a history of congestive heart failure were excluded. Patients were randomized to the following groups; disease-affected meridian (DAM), nonaffected meridian (NAM), sham acupuncture group, and a wait-list group. Treatment was 3 times per week for 4 weeks; each session was for 30 minutes. The greatest reduction of angina episodes occurred in the DAM group as compared to each of the other 3 groups.

---

[1] Not FDA approved for this indication.

This is the largest published clinical trial showing evidence that adding acupuncture to goal-directed medical therapy reduces angina frequency. There were some study limitations that are worth mentioning that may soften the results. Namely, the operators were not blinded to their treatment plans, angina episodes were reduced in the sham and wait-list groups (suggesting a strong placebo-associated effect), and the study population was small.

Other Causes of Angina
Syndrome X
The cardiac syndrome X refers to patients who have normal or near-normal epicardial coronary arteries and episodic chest pain. This disorder is much more common in women and is often seen in patients younger than 50 years of age. The chest pain episodes may last longer than 30 minutes and may have a variable response to sublingual nitrates. Patients with syndrome X often describe typical stress-induced angina. Risk factors include hypertension, diabetes, and hyperlipidemia. Female patients are typically postmenopausal and frequently have stress-induced symptoms and ischemia on stress imaging. They often respond to standard angina medications and typically have a better prognosis than patients with significant epicardial plaque.

Vasospastic or Prinzmetal Angina
The classic definition of Prinzmetal angina is chest pain with documented ST-segment elevation during symptoms or during exercise in the face of angiographically normal or near-normal coronary arteries. Over the years, the definition has expanded to include patients who have classic angina symptoms commonly relieved with nitrates or calcium channel blockers and minimal or no CAD. It has been shown that patients with nonobstructive CAD may be prone to focal artery spasm at the stenosis site; therefore, the previous requirement of normal coronary arteries is not an absolute necessity. Other disease states (e.g., Raynaud phenomenon) can increase a patient's development of coronary artery spasm, as can illicit drug usage (e.g., cocaine). Vasospasm is more common in active smokers. β-Blockers should be used cautiously in these patients because they may exacerbate coronary spasm. Patients with angiographically documented intramyocardial bridging may be prone to focal coronary spasm and subsequent angina pectoris.

Newer Imaging Techniques
Calcium Scoring
Coronary artery calcium scoring is a well-studied imaging modality used to assess a patient's pretest probability of CAD. With respect to evaluation for angina, one must remember that electron-beam computed tomographic (CT) scanning does not offer physiologic data and therefore does not allow determination of myocardial ischemia. This study is most useful in the workup of a low-risk patient with an atypical chest pain syndrome. If such a patient has an elevated calcium score, other studies may be reasonable and further assessment of the patient's cholesterol values should be performed.

Computed Tomographic Coronary Angiography
CT coronary angiography is a noninvasive way to image the coronary arteries. Similar to electron-beam CT, it does not provide physiologic data regarding coronary artery perfusion, but it does provide anatomic information such as the presence and percentage of coronary artery stenosis. Although selected patients with stable or unstable angina may be considered candidates for CT angiography, its main utility is to evaluate patients for chest pain who are otherwise at low risk and have a low pretest probability. Because of the volume of intravenous contrast required by CT angiography, the risk of contrast nephropathy must be considered when contemplating this study.

Summary
The approach to the patient with angina should be based on a global assessment and intensive treatment of all identified cardiovascular risk factors. It is recommended that all patients receive the appropriate dose of statin and antiplatelet therapy. Noninvasive testing is helpful for an initial diagnosis and to guide the decision for a more invasive approach. Familiarity and adherence to current treatment guidelines is of paramount importance. There are important gender differences that should not be overlooked in the clinical presentation of angina and in the approach to optimal therapy.

References
Allan BS, Krumholz HM, SM reviewing The SPRINT Research Group: N Engl J Med 2015 Nov 9 Chobanian AV, N Engl J Med, 2015 Nov 9.

Anderson JL, Adams CD, Antman EM: ACC/AHA 2007 guidelines for the management of patients with unstable angina/non-ST-elevation myocardial infarction: A report of the American College of Cardiology/American Heart Association Task Force on Practice Guidelines, J Am Coll Cardiol 5067:e1–e157, 2007.

Antithrombotic Trialists Collaboration: Collaborative meta-analysis of randomized trials of antiplatelet therapy for prevention of death, myocardial infarction, and stroke in high risk patients, BMJ 324:71–86, 2002.

Berger J, Brown D, Becker R: Low-dose aspirin in patients with stable cardiovascular disease: A meta-analysis, Am J Med 121:43–49, 2008.

Bhatt DL, Steg PG, Miller M, et al: Cardiovascular risk reduction with icosapent ethyl for hypertriglyceridemia. N Engl J Med 380:11–22, 2019.

Blood Pressure Lowering Treatment Trialists Collaboration: Effects of different blood pressure lowering regimens on major cardiovascular events: Results of prospectively-designed overviews of randomized trials, Lancet 362:1527–1545, 2003.

Boden WE, O'Rourke RA, Teo KK: Optimal medical therapy with or without PCI for stable coronary disease, N Engl J Med 35:1503–1516, 2007.

Borer JS, Fox K, Jaillon P: Antianginal and antischemic effects of Ivrabadine, a novel I(f) inhibitor, in stable angina:a randomized, double-blind, multicentered, placebo-controlled trial, Circulation 107:817–823, 2003.

Cholesterol Treatment Trialists' Collaborators: Efficacy and safety of cholesterol-lowering treatment: Prospective meta-analysis of data from 90,056 participants in 14 trials of statins, Lancet 366:1267–1278, 2005.

De Bruyne B, Fearon WF, Pijls NH: Fractional flow reserve-guided PCI for stable coronary artery disease, N Engl J Med 371:1208–1217, 2014.

Eikelboom JW, Connolly SJ, Bosch J, et al: COMPASS Investigators. Rivaroxaban with or without aspirin in stable cardiovascular disease, N Engl J Med 377:1319–1330, 2017.

Fefer P, Knudtson ML, Cheema AN, et al: Current perspectives on coronary chronic total occlusions: the Canadian multicenter chronic total occlusions registry, J Am Coll Cardiol 59:991–997, 2012.

Fihn SD, Gardin JM, Abrams J: 2012 ACCF/AHA/ACP/AATS/PCNA/SCAI/STS guideline for the diagnosis and management of patients with stable ischemic heart disease: A report of the American College of Cardiology Foundation/American Heart Association Task Force on Practice Guidelines, and the American College of Physicians, American Association for Thoracic Surgery, Preventive Cardiovascular Nurses Association, Society for Cardiovascular Angiography and Interventions, and Society of Thoracic Surgeons, J Am Coll Cardiol 60:e44–e164, 2012.

Gibbons RJ, Abrams J, Chatterjee K, et al: ACC/AHA 2007 guideline update for the management of patients with chronic stable angina: A report of the American College of Cardiology/American Heart Association Task Force on Practice Guidelines (Committee to Update the 2002 Guidelines for the Management of Patients with Chronic Stable Angina) Reston, VA, American College of Cardiology, American Heart Association Available at: www.acc.org/qualityandscience/cl inical/guidelines/stable/stable_clean.pdf (accessed August 20, 2014).

Grundy SM, Cleeman JI, Merz NB: Implications of recent clinical trials for the National Cholesterol Education Program Adult Treatment Panel III guidelines, Circulation 110:227–239, 2004.

Heart Outcomes Prevention Evaluation Study Investigators: Effects of an angiotensin-converting-enzyme inhibitor, ramipril, on cardiovascular events in high-risk patients, N Engl J Med 342:145–153, 2000.

James PA, Oparil S, Carter BL: 2014 evidence-based guideline for the management of high blood pressure in adults: Report from the panel members appointed to the eighth Joint National Committee (JNC 8), JAMA 311:507–520, 2014.

Mehta SR, Cannon CP, Fox KA: Routine vs selective invasive strategies in patients with acute coronary syndromes: A collaborative meta-analysis of randomized trials, JAMA 293:2908–2917, 2005.

Messerli FH, Mancia G, Conti CR: Dogma disrupted: Can aggressively lowering blood pressure in hypertensive patients with coronary artery disease be dangerous? Ann Intern Med 144:884–893, 2006.

Montalescot G, Sechtem U, Achenbach S: Editor's choice: 2013 ESC guidelines on the management of stable coronary artery disease: The Task Force on the management of stable coronary artery disease of the European Society of Cardiology, Eur Heart J 34:2949–3003, 2013.

Petraco R, Al-Lamee R, Gotberg M: Real-time use of instantaneous wave-free ratio: results of the ADVISE in-practice: an international, multicenter evaluation of instantaneous wave-free ratio in clinical practice, Am Heart J 168:739–748, 2014.

Ray K, Cannon C: Optimal goal for statin therapy use in coronary artery disease, Curr Opin Cardiol 20:525–529, 2005.

Sabatine MS, Giugliano RP, Keech AC: Evolocumab and clinical outcomes in patients with cardiovascular disease, N Engl J Med 376:1713–1722, 2017.

SEARCH Collaborative Group: Intensive lowering of LDL cholesterol with 80mg versus 20mg simvastatin daily in 12,064 survivors of myocardial infarction: A double-blind randomised trial, Lancet 376:1658–1669, 2010.

Stone G, Teirstein P, Rubenstein R: A prospective, multicenter, randomized trial of percutaneous transmyocardial laser revascularization in patients with noncanalizable chronic total occlusions, *J Am Coll Cardiol* 39:1581–1587, 2002.

Stone NJ, Robinson J, Lichtenstein AH, et al: 2013 ACC/AHA guideline on the treatment of blood cholesterol to reduce atherosclerotic cardiovascular risk in adults: A report of the American College of Cardiology/American Heart Association Task Force on Practice Guidelines, Circulation.

Tendera M, Borer JS, Tardif JC: Efficacy of I(f) inhibition with Ivabradine in different subpopulations with stable angina pectoris, *Cardiology* 114:116–125, 2009.

Weber MA, Schiffrin EL, White WB: Clinical practice guidelines for the management of hypertension in the community, *J Clin Hypertens* 16:14–26, 2014.

Wenger NK: *Cardiac Rehabilitation: A Guide to Practice in the 21st Century*, New York, 1999, Marcel Dekker.

Whooley MA, Jonge P, Vittinghoff E: Depressive symptoms, health behaviors, and risk of cardiovascular events in patients with coronary heart disease, *JAMA* 300:2379–2388, 2008.

Acupuncture as Adjunctive Therapy for Chronic Stable Angina: A Randomized Clinical Trial.

Zhao L, Li D, Zheng H: *JAMA Intern Med*, 2019 Jul 29.

2017 ACC/AHA/AAPA/ABC/ACPM/AGS/APhA/ASH/ASPC/NMA/PCNA Guideline for the Prevention, Detection, Evaluation, and Management of High Blood Pressure in Adults: A Report of the American College of Cardiology/American Heart Association Task Force on Clinical Practice Guidelines.

Zhu Y, Meng S, Chen M, et al: Long-term prognosis of chronic total occlusion treated by successful percutaneous coronary intervention in patients with or without diabetes mellitus: a systematic review and meta-analysis, *Cardiovasc Diabetol* 20:29, 2021.

AORTIC DISEASE: ANEURYSM AND DISSECTION

Method of
David G. Neschis, MD

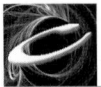

CURRENT DIAGNOSIS

- Because the majority of patients with abdominal aortic aneurysms are asymptomatic, the majority of abdominal aortic aneurysms are detected on imaging studies performed for other indications.
- Patients older than 50 years who present with abdominal or back pain of unclear etiology should be considered for evaluation of possible abdominal aortic aneurysm.
- Asymptomatic men older than 65 years who have ever smoked are eligible for abdominal aortic aneurysm screening.
- All patients older than 60 years who have a strong family history of abdominal aortic aneurysms should be considered for screening.
- Patients presenting with sudden onset of chest or back pain without clear etiology should be evaluated for dissection.
- Dissection can mimic numerous other conditions.

CURRENT THERAPY

Indications for Repair of Aneurysm
- Fusiform abdominal aortic aneurysms greater than 5.5 cm in maximum diameter
- Most saccular aneurysms and pseudoaneurysms
- Thoracic and thoracoabdominal aortic aneurysms of greater than 6 cm in maximal diameter
- Aneurysms that are symptomatic or are rapidly enlarging

Indications for Repair of Aortic Dissection
- Dissections involving the ascending aorta
- Dissections involving only the descending aorta are usually managed medically unless complicated by the following: unrelenting pain, end organ ischemia, or significant aneurysmal degeneration to greater than 6 cm in maximal diameter

Abdominal Aortic Aneurysms

Epidemiology
A ruptured abdominal aortic aneurysm is a devastating event leading to approximately 15,000 deaths per year, and it is the 13th leading cause of death in the United States. It is the 10th leading cause of death in men. Once rupture occurs, there is an 85% chance of death overall and approximately 50% mortality in the patients who make it to the hospital alive. Clearly, the goal is to identify this life-threatening lesion and repair prior to rupture. Abdominal aortic aneurysms are approximately four times more prevalent in men than in women. The overall incidence in persons older than 60 years is approximately 3% to 4%, with incidence as high as 10% to 12% in an elderly hypertensive population.

Risk Factors
Men are approximately 4 times more likely than women to develop an abdominal aortic aneurysm. Clearly, older persons, particularly those older than 60 years, are at higher risk. Tobacco use is probably the strongest preventable risk factor, with tobacco users being approximately eight times more likely to be affected than nonsmokers. Hypertension is present in approximately 40% of patients with abdominal aortic aneurysms. Family history also plays a significant role. In fact, men who have first-degree female relatives who had aneurysms are approximately 18 times more likely than the general population to develop an abdominal aortic aneurysm. There is also a strong correlation between abdominal aortic aneurysms and other peripheral artery aneurysms. Patients with bilateral popliteal artery aneurysms have an approximately 50% to 60% risk of having an abdominal aortic aneurysm.

Pathophysiology
An aneurysm is a dilatation of a blood vessel that could occur in any blood vessel in the body, even in the veins. Most commonly it is defined as a dilatation of approximately 1.5 to 2 times at that diameter of the adjacent normal vessel.

The definition of a pseudoaneurysm is often misunderstood. The attempt to describe a pseudoaneurysm in terms of the number of layers of the artery wall involved does nothing to help resolve this confusion. A pseudoaneurysm is a walled-off defect in the artery wall. A circular shell of adventitial and surrounding connective tissue contains the blood, preventing free hemorrhage. However, there remains continued flow out and back into the arterial lumen, resulting in a classic to-and-fro pattern on duplex ultrasound. The most common cause of a pseudoaneurysm is iatrogenic, from needle puncture, but it also can be caused by trauma or focal rupture of the artery at the site of an atherosclerotic ulcer.

The etiology of true aneurysms is not clear, although in the past these have been attributed to atherosclerosis. However, it is well known that the majority of patients with abdominal aortic aneurysms do not have associated significant occlusive disease. Biochemical studies have demonstrated decreased quantities of elastin and collagen in the walls of aneurysmal aortas. It is believed that a family of enzymes known as matrix metalloproteinase (MMP), particularly those that have collagenase and elastase activity, are likely involved in development of arterial aneurysms. The propensity for growth and rupture is based on Laplace's law, $T = PR$, where T represents wall tension (or in other words the propensity to rupture), P is the transmitted pressure, and R is the radius. This explains why patients with hypertension and those with larger aneurysms are at higher risk for aortic rupture.

Prevention
Currently the most effective means to prevent aneurysm rupture is early detection and elective repair. Avoidance of smoking and aggressive control of blood pressure would likely be helpful in preventing aneurysmal development and growth. Patients with known abdominal aortic aneurysms that are relatively small and at low risk for rupture are generally serially followed with imaging studies over time. These patients are advised to avoid straining (e.g., heavy lifting), avoid smoking, and keep their blood pressure well controlled.

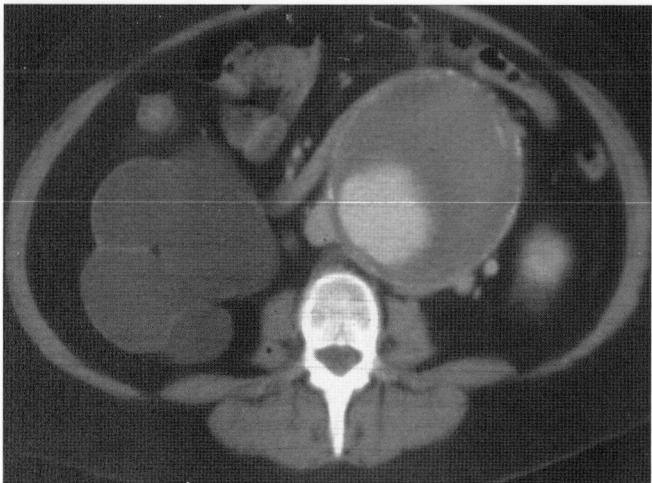

Figure 1 Large abdominal aortic aneurysm. Notice how the majority of this aneurysm is filled with laminated thrombus. The flow lumen is only mildly dilated, and this aneurysm could be missed on angiography alone.

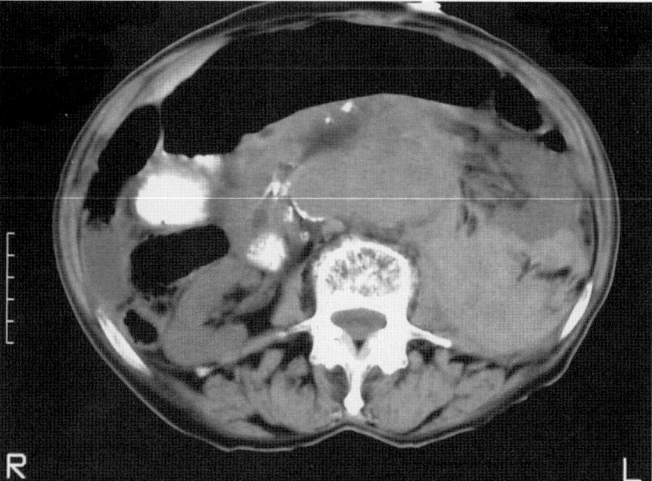

Figure 2 Classic image of a ruptured abdominal aortic aneurysm, which in this case can be seen even without the use of intravascular contrast. Note the lack of symmetry and obliteration of tissue planes in the retroperitoneum on the left.

Investigation is ongoing in efforts to develop a medication that may be helpful in slowing the growth of abdominal aortic aneurysms. It has been known since 1985 that tetracycline antibiotics have activity against MMPs. There had been several animal studies and at least one small human study suggesting that doxycycline (Vibramycin)[1] may be effective at slowing the growth of abdominal aortic aneurysms. Currently, larger human studies are ongoing. At this point, there are no formal recommendations regarding the use of doxycycline for the purpose of slowing aneurysmal growth.

Clinical Manifestations

Approximately 75% of abdominal aortic aneurysms are asymptomatic and discovered incidentally. Unfortunately, physical examination is an unreliable method for detecting aneurysms or determining aneurysm size. In heavier patients it may be simply impossible to adequately palpate the aorta. The majority of aneurysms are incidental findings identified on imaging studies performed for other reasons. Occasionally, an aneurysm is first detected upon operation for another condition.

Unfortunately, when an aneurysm becomes symptomatic, this is usually a sign of impending rupture. Symptoms related to abdominal aortic aneurysms can include abdominal or back pain. The classic triad of findings in the setting of abdominal aortic aneurysm rupture includes abdominal pain, hypotension, and a pulsatile abdominal mass. This triad, however, occurs in only approximately 20% of the patients. Often a high index of suspicion needs to be maintained.

The episode of hypotension associated with aneurysm rupture may be manifested as an episode of syncope or near-syncope before the patient arrives at the hospital. It is quite possible for the patient to have a contained rupture of the abdominal aorta and appear quite stable with a normal blood pressure in the emergency department. Although uncommon, a primary fistula between the aneurysm and gastrointestinal tract can occur and manifest as gastrointestinal bleeding.

Diagnosis

Several imaging modalities are available that can accurately diagnose and measure abdominal aortic aneurysms. Real-time B-mode ultrasound scanning has the advantage of being almost universally available, relatively inexpensive, and essentially risk free. The major disadvantage, however, is that it is technician dependent. Computed tomography (CT) scans can provide a very accurate representation of the aorta in a very short study time (Figures 1 and 2). The use of iodinated contrast is not necessary

[1] Not FDA approved for this indication.

to obtain a gross size measurement of the aorta. The contrast, however, helps delineate the flow lumen more clearly, and it is quite valuable in planning repair. Disadvantages include the use of ionizing radiation and the use of iodinated contrast material. MRI is also accurate in determining the size of the aneurysm; however, study times are longer, equipment is less widely available, and the expense is considerable. Angiography, while excellent for evaluating the status of important aortic branches and for evaluating occlusive disease, is not an accurate study for the purpose of determining maximal diameter of the aneurysm. Often aneurysms are filled with laminated thrombus, and the flow lumen, which was seen on aortography, is not representative of the true aneurysm size.

Treatment

The decision on when to intervene in an abdominal aortic aneurysm is based on a careful analysis of the patient's risk for rupture versus the risk of operative repair. Historically, open repair can be performed with less than 5% in-hospital mortality. Based on historical studies it was estimated that the risk of rupture for an approximately 5-cm aneurysm was about 1% per year, which increased dramatically to 6.6% for aneurysms between 6 and 7 cm. It has been fairly well established for years that aneurysms larger than 5.5 cm are generally recommended for repair and those less than 4 cm are generally observed over time. There remains a gray area for moderate aneurysms in the 4- to 5.5-cm category.

Two large prospective randomized trials were developed to answer this question. These include the United Kingdom Small Aneurysm Trial and the Department of Veterans Affairs Aneurysm Detection and Management (ADAM) trial. Both these studies randomized patients with moderately sized aneurysms to observation versus open repair. Results of both trials were fairly similar. The rupture rate for aneurysms under observation was 0.5% to 1% per year, and neither trial showed a difference in long-term survival. Both studies concluded that it was relatively safe to observe patients with aneurysms less than 5.5 cm in diameter, particularly in men who would be compliant with the follow-up regimen. The diameter of the aneurysm, however, should not be the only data point used for a decision on whether to repair.

Women seem to have a higher rupture rate for a particular aneurysm diameter than men, perhaps because they are starting with smaller aortas to begin with. Patients with COPD may be at higher risk for rupture as well. Saccular or eccentric-shaped aneurysms may also have a higher propensity to rupture and should not be subject to diameter recommendations for fusiform aneurysms (Figures 3 and 4). Additionally, rapidly growing

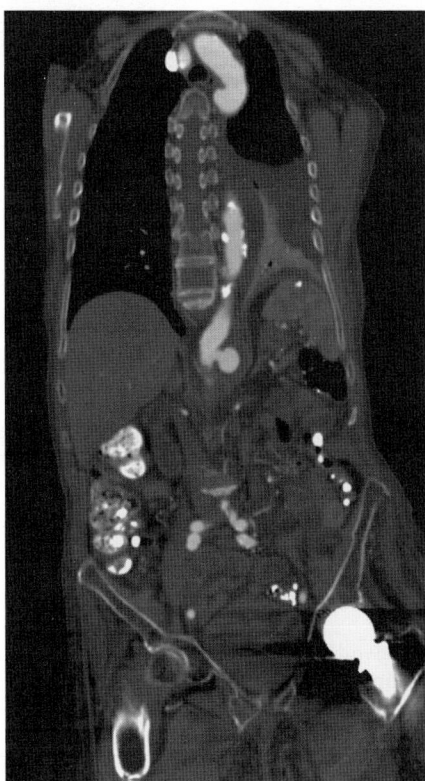
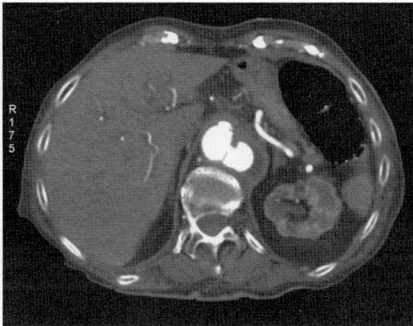
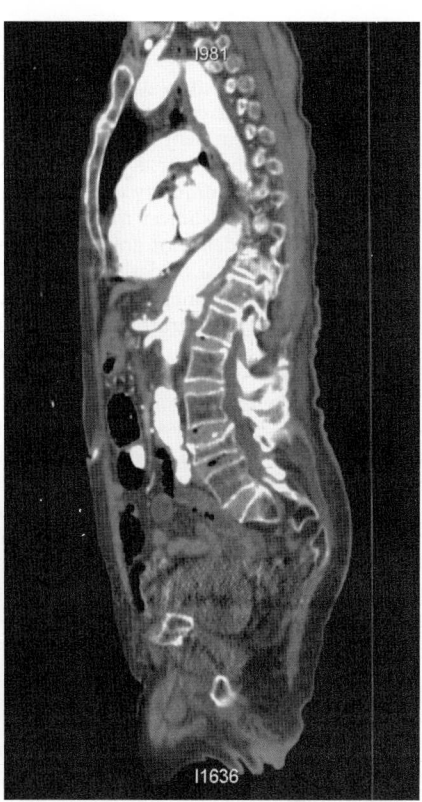

Figure 3 Axial CT slice and reconstructed images of a saccular abdominal aortic aneurysm. This lesion could also be described as a pseudoaneurysm. For these, treatment is recommended because it is thought that the risk of rupture is higher than for a similarly sized fusiform abdominal aortic aneurysm.

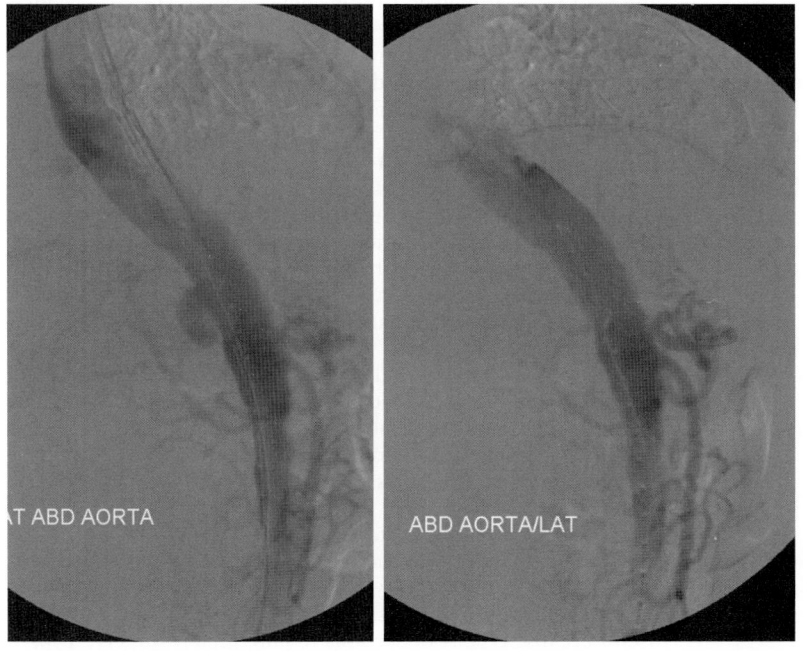

Figure 4 Angiogram of patient in Figure 3, demonstrating aneurysm before and after deployment of an endograft, which successfully excluded the lesion from the circulation.

aneurysms—growing at a rate faster than approximately 0.5 cm per year—should be considered for repair.

Once it has been determined that repair is indicated, a number of options are available. Traditional open repair involves a relatively large abdominal incision, cross clamping of the aorta, and replacement of the aneurysmal segment with a graft of polyethylene terephthalate (Dacron) or polytetrafluoroethylene (PTFE; Teflon). Often the iliac arteries are involved, and in these cases a bifurcated graft is placed. Open repair is quite durable and very effective at preventing aneurysm-related deaths. Long-term complications are rare, and patients following open repair generally enjoy 95% freedom from issues related to the repair over

the course of their lifetime. Disadvantages, however, include the large incision and an approximate 1-week hospital stay. Recovery to a relatively normal level of function occasionally takes months. In the past, many patients were deemed too old or frail to be expected to undergo open surgery.

Endograft repair has revolutionized the practice of vascular surgery. Using small incisions placed at the groin and performing the procedure under fluoroscopic guidance, devices can now be advanced into the aorta from the femoral artery. Using angiography as a guide, the graft typically is deployed below the renal arteries and effectively excludes the aneurysm from the circulation. Advantages include small incisions and very short hospital stays. Patients are typically discharged on the first or second day after aneurysm repair. Recovery to normal activity is also quite rapid, taking approximately 1 to 2 weeks. Use of this modality has allowed treatment of older and frailer patients who previously were denied treatment due to concerns of operative risk.

Endograft repair, however, is clearly not without its disadvantages. Currently, the durability of endograft repair is unknown, and these patients are subject to frequent serial imaging. Also, there is a higher incidence of graft-related complications, which can occur in up to 35% of patients. These include the development of leaks of blood into the aneurysm sac outside the graft device, issues related to graft failure and migration, and graft limb thrombosis. These grafts are also quite expensive.

Two major prospective randomized trials studying traditional open versus endograft repair are often cited. These include the United Kingdom–based EVAR-1 trial (first Endovascular Aneurysm Repair trail) and the Dutch-based DREAM trial (Diabetes REduction Assessment with ramipril and rosiglitazone Medication trial). Both studies randomized patients who were believed to be good risks for open repair to endograft versus traditional open repair. The results of both of these studies were relatively similar in that both studies demonstrated a clear early survival benefit for patients in the endograft group. However, this came at a cost of an increased incidence of graft-related complications in the endograft group and a higher cost for the endograft group. Additionally, at 2 to 4 years, there was no clear difference in long-term survival in either group.

Ultimately, the decision about whether to proceed with open or endograft repair is a decision between surgeon and patient based on the patient's aortic anatomy, overall health, and the patient's and physician's preference. It would appear, however, that older and frail patients with good anatomy should be strongly considered for endograft repair.

Monitoring

Patients with abdominal aortic aneurysms should be evaluated for the presence of femoral and popliteal aneurysms (particularly in men) and for thoracic aortic aneurysms. After open repair, a follow-up CT scan with contrast should be considered approximately 5 years out to evaluate for the integrity of the graft (i.e., pseudoaneurysms), as well as development of new aneurysms. Patients who have undergone endograft repair require more-intensive monitoring. Typical regimens include a contrast-enhanced CT scan approximately 2 weeks after repair, then 6 months after repair, and then based on the perceived stability of the graft, approximately yearly thereafter. Some centers have used duplex ultrasonography for evaluating patients after endograft repair in efforts to reduce the amount of ionizing radiation the patients receive. However, it should be remembered that duplex ultrasound is highly technician dependent, and follow-up of patients with endograft repairs using only duplex ultrasound should be performed in experienced centers.

Thoracic Aortic Aneurysms

Thoracic aortic aneurysms (TAAs) are limited to the chest cavity. Although they are less common than infrarenal abdominal aortic aneurysms, they share similar risk factors. The male-to-female ratio incidence of the TAA is approximately 1:1.

In the past, the threshold for repair was at a diameter greater than 6 cm. This threshold was chosen due to the higher operative risks associated with repair of the thoracic aorta. Now with the availability of endograft, patients with good anatomy are generally recommended for repair at a diameter similar to those for the infrarenal aorta.

Open repair involves performing a thoracotomy and cross-clamping the aorta. Repair in this location is often performed with the addition of extracorporeal bypass to maintain perfusion to the viscera and spinal cord drain performance of the repair. Although the risk of paraplegia in the treatment of infrarenal aortic is exceedingly low, the risk of paraplegia from a repair of an isolated TAA is approximately 6%. Endograft devices for repair

TABLE 1 Dissection: The Great Mimic

TERRITORY INVOLVED OR AFFECTED BY DISSECTION	MIMICS
Rupture into pericardial sac	Cardiac tamponade
Dissection through aortic valve	Acute aortic insufficiency
Dissection occluding coronary arteries	Myocardial infarction
Involvement of cerebral vessels	Stroke
Involvement of subclavian arteries	Upper extremity ischemia (cold arm)
Dissection running down descending thoracic aorta	Severe back pain and paralysis
Mesenteric artery obstruction	Mesenteric ischemia
Renal artery obstruction	Oliguria and acute renal failure
Iliac artery occlusion	Lower extremity ischemia (cold leg)

of TAA are now widely available and have reduced the incidence of paraplegia to approximately 3%.

Thoracoabdominal Aortic Aneurysms

By definition, thoracoabdominal aortic aneurysms require entrance to both the thoracic and abdominal cavity to perform repair. These lesions are usually true aneurysms of the aorta and should not be confused with dissection. Repair of thoracoabdominal aortic aneurysms is quite complex and carries risks of death and paraplegia as high as 20% in some settings. These procedures are generally performed at larger institutions with considerable experience with this condition. Unfortunately, endograft devices for the repair of thoracoabdominal aortic aneurysms are limited to a handful of centers in the United States.

Thoracic Aortic Dissection

Thoracic aortic dissection is the most common aortic emergency, even more common than ruptured abdominal aortic aneurysm. This potentially fatal condition is rare in patients younger than 50 years and is approximately two times more common in men than women. Patients at risk include patients with a history of connective tissue disorders and patients with severe, poorly controlled hypertension.

An aortic dissection occurs when there is loss of integrity of the intima and blood dissects into the media. Once in the media, there is a natural plane through which dissection is quite easy.

Although there are various classification systems for aortic dissection, the Stanford classification is perhaps the most widely used and the most useful. In this classification, any dissection that involves the ascending aorta, whether it involves the ascending aorta alone or both the ascending and descending thoracoabdominal aorta, are classified as type A. Dissections that do not involve the ascending aorta are classified as type B. This classification is useful because type A dissections require urgent surgery. Type B dissections are typically managed medically unless they are associated with complications such as unremitting pain, aneurysmal expansion, and end-organ ischemia. By convention, aortic dissections that are evaluated within 14 days after the onset of symptoms are considered acute, and those evaluated beyond 14 days are considered chronic.

Helical CAT scanners with the use of contrast are excellent at defining the location and extent of aortic dissection. However, being alert to the potential for this diagnosis requires a high index of suspicion. Aortic dissection can mimic a variety of common conditions based on the extent of the dissection and the aortic branches involved (Table 1). Uncomplicated type B dissections are typically managed medically. This is usually performed in an intensive care setting with the use of intravenous medications to control contractility and, if necessary, hypertension.

In the past, due to the friability of dissected aortic tissue, the results of operative repair for type B dissections have been particularly poor. Currently, endograft repair with the purpose of excluding the entry point of dissection and reestablishing flow to the true lumen is gaining popularity in the treatment of complex dissection. This at times may be supplemented by stenting of affected aortic side branches and fenestration to establish a connection between the true and false lumen to restore perfusion to certain organs. Once the acute phase has passed and medically treated patients are under good hypertensive control, these patients are then converted to an oral medication regimen and transferred out of the intensive care setting. Patients need to be followed up with serial CT imaging after discharge to evaluate for aneurysmal degeneration of the false lumen. This evaluation should occur every 6 months until the patient is stable and then yearly thereafter.

In cases where the total aortic diameter grows to greater than 6 cm, repair for the purpose of preventing rupture is indicated, although this is often technically more complicated than treating a fusiform aneurysm in the absence of a previous dissection. Patients should strictly adhere to their blood pressure medication regimen for life.

References

Blankensteijn JD, de Jong SE, Prinssen M, et al: Two-year outcomes after conventional or endovascular repair of abdominal aortic aneurysms, *N Engl J Med* 352(23):2398–2405, 2005.

Crawford ES, Crawford JL, Safi HJ, et al: Thoracoabdominal aortic aneurysms: Preoperative and intraoperative factors determining immediate and long-term results of operations in 605 patients, *J Vasc Surg* 3(3):389–404, 1986.

Daily PO, Trueblood HW, Stinson EB, et al: Management of acute aortic dissections, *Ann Thorac Surg* 10(3):237–247, 1970.

EVAR Trial Participants: Endovascular aneurysm repair versus open repair in patients with abdominal aortic aneurysm (EVAR trial 1): Randomised controlled trial, *Lancet* 365(9478):2179–2186, 2005.

EVAR Trial Participants: Endovascular aneurysm repair and outcome in patients unfit for open repair of abdominal aortic aneurysm (EVAR trial 2): Randomised controlled trial, *Lancet* 365(9478):2187–2192, 2005.

Lederle FA, Wilson SE, Johnson GR, et al: Immediate repair compared with surveillance of small abdominal aortic aneurysms, *N Engl J Med* 346(19):1437–1444, 2002.

Lee ES, Pickett E, Hedayati N, et al: Implementation of an aortic screening program in clinical practice: Implications for the Screen For Abdominal Aortic Aneurysms Very Efficiently (SAAAVE) Act, *J Vasc Surg* 49(5):1107–1111, 2009.

Nevitt MP, Ballard DJ, Hallett Jr : Prognosis of abdominal aortic aneurysms. A population-based study, *N Engl J Med* 321(15):1009–1014, 1989.

Nienaber CA, Rousseau H, Eggebrecht H, et al: Randomized comparison of strategies for type B aortic dissection: The INvestigation of STEnt Grafts in Aortic Dissection (INSTEAD) trial, *Circulation* 120(25):2519–2528, 2009.

Rentschler M, Baxter BT: Pharmacological approaches to prevent abdominal aortic aneurysm enlargement and rupture, *Ann N Y Acad Sci* 1085:39–46, 2006.

ATRIAL FIBRILLATION

Method of
Lin Yee Chen, MBBS, MS; and Samuel C. Dudley Jr., MD, PhD

CURRENT DIAGNOSIS

- History taking and physical examination for atrial fibrillation (AF) should focus on determining symptom severity (to decide on treatment strategy), risk of thromboembolic stroke, and associated cardiovascular risk factors.
- Symptoms include palpitations, chest discomfort, shortness of breath, and reduced exercise capacity. Some patients have no symptoms.
- Investigations include a 12-lead electrocardiogram (ECG) for confirmation; transthoracic echocardiogram to evaluate left atrial size, left ventricular ejection fraction, and rule out valvular abnormalities; and blood tests for thyroid, renal, and hepatic function.

CURRENT THERAPY

- Rate control: Achieve average ventricular rate of less than 110 beats/min by using atrioventricular node (AVN) blockers or catheter ablation of AVN
- Rhythm control: Prevent AF recurrence by using antiarrhythmic drugs or catheter ablation (pulmonary vein isolation)
- Stroke prophylaxis: Risk stratification and stroke prevention by oral anticoagulation or left atrial appendage closure
- Risk-factor management or lifestyle modification: Prevent AF by weight management, intensive blood pressure lowering, and exercise training

Epidemiology

AF is the most common sustained arrhythmia in the adult general population. Globally, the estimated number of individuals with AF in 2010 was 33.5 million. Between 1990 and 2010, the global estimated age-adjusted prevalence rate of AF increased from 569.5 to 596.2 per 100,000 men and from 359.9 to 373.1 per 100,000 women. This increase in prevalence was accompanied by a substantial increase in health burden: disability-adjusted life-years increased by 18.8% in men and 18.9% in women from 1990 to 2010. Finally, the lifetime risk for development of AF in adults at age 40 is 1 in 4.

Risk Factors and Pathophysiology

Table 1 shows the known risk factors of AF; many of these are also risk factors for atherosclerotic disease. Traditional cardiovascular risk factors such as diabetes, hypertension, and obesity can lead to AF via the following pathway: cardiovascular risk factors

TABLE 1	Risk Factors of Atrial Fibrillation
Cardiovascular risk factors	
Older age	
Male sex	
Diabetes mellitus	
Overweight and obesity	
Hypertension	
Chronic kidney disease	
Structural heart disease	
Valvular heart disease	
Cardiomyopathy (dilated, restrictive, and hypertrophic)	
Congenital heart disease	
Coronary heart disease	
Left ventricular diastolic dysfunction	
Left atrial enlargement	
Family history	
Genetics (polygenic and monogenic inheritance)	
Inflammation	
Low serum magnesium	
Heavy alcohol consumption	
Poor cardiorespiratory fitness	
Low physical activity	
Premature atrial contractions or supraventricular ectopy	

TABLE 2 | Pharmacologic Agents for Rate Control

DRUG	INTRAVENOUS ADMINISTRATION	USUAL ORAL MAINTENANCE DOSE	MAJOR SIDE EFFECTS
β Blockers			
Metoprolol (Lopressor)[1]	2.5–5 mg IV bolus; up to 3 doses	100–200 mg (long acting) daily	Bradycardia, hypotension, heart block, asthma, heart failure
Atenolol (Tenormin)[1]	N/A	25–100 mg qd	
Esmolol (Brevibloc)	50–200 µg/kg/min IV	N/A	
Propranolol (Inderal)	1–3 mg IV	10–40 mg tid	
Carvedilol (Coreg)[1]	N/A	3.125–25 mg bid	
Nondihydropyridine Calcium Channel Antagonists			
Verapamil (Calan)	5–10 mg bolus	80 mg tid or up to 360 mg (long acting) daily	Hypotension, heart block, heart failure
Diltiazem (Cardizem)	0.25–0.35 mg/kg	60 mg tid or up to 360 mg (long acting) daily	
Digitalis Glycosides			
Digoxin (Lanoxin)	0.25–0.5 mg	0.125–0.25 mg qd	Digitalis toxicity, bradycardia, heart block

[1]Not FDA approved for this indication.
IV, Intravenous.

→ left ventricular diastolic dysfunction → structural and functional alterations in the atria (enlargement, impaired function, fibrosis, etc.) → AF. The aforementioned pathway creates the substrate for AF; premature atrial contractions and supraventricular ectopic beats are the trigger for AF. Other pathophysiologic pathways include inflammation and increased oxidative stress, leading to electrical remodeling and, consequently, AF.

Clinical Manifestations
Common symptoms of AF include palpitations, irregular heartbeat sensation, lightheadedness, dyspnea, chest discomfort, and fatigue. Some patients may have no symptoms at rest but report poor stamina or easy fatigability with physical activity. Other patients, particularly among the elderly, may be asymptomatic.

Diagnosis
The absence of distinct P waves with irregularly irregular RR interval on the ECG are the sine qua non for diagnosing AF. Rhythm documentation can be obtained via the standard 12-lead ECG, Holter monitors that can record up to 48 hours, leadless patch monitors that can record up to 2 weeks, or implantable loop recorders. Newer wearable technologies that can diagnose AF include smartwatches and smartphones with specialized apps.

Paroxysmal AF is defined as AF that terminates spontaneously typically in less than 24 hours and in all cases in less than 7 days. AF that continues for more than 7 days and requires cardioversion for conversion to sinus rhythm is termed persistent AF. Long-standing persistent AF is AF that has been continuous for more than 1 year. Permanent AF exists when both patient and physician have decided not to pursue further attempts to maintain sinus rhythm.

Differential Diagnosis
These include other supraventricular arrhythmias such as atrial tachycardia, atrial flutter, long runs of premature atrial contractions, and multifocal atrial tachycardia.

Treatment
Rate Control
The goal of rate control is to prevent excessive ventricular rate response. This is a reasonable treatment strategy given data from

randomized controlled trials (RCTs) that did not show any difference in cardiovascular outcomes between rate-control and rhythm-control strategy.

The AFFIRM (Atrial Fibrillation Follow-up Investigation of Rhythm Management) trial found no difference in mortality or stroke rates between patients assigned to rhythm-control and ventricular rate-control strategies. Similarly, the RACE (Rate Control versus Electrical Cardioversion for Persistent Atrial Fibrillation) trial found that rate control was not inferior to rhythm control for prevention of death.

The RACE II study showed that lenient ventricular rate control targeting a heart rate of lower than 110 beats/min was not inferior to stricter rate control of less than 80 beats/min. Lenient rate control is more convenient and requires fewer outpatient visits and fewer medications.

Other than pharmacologic agents (Table 2), catheter ablation of the AVN is effective in controlling ventricular rate in patients with AF. AVN ablation is indicated if patients fail to achieve adequate ventricular rate control despite maximum doses of AVN blockers.

Rhythm Control
Although AF is associated with an increased risk of stroke and mortality, current evidence indicates that there is no difference in the rates of these cardiovascular outcomes between rhythm- and rate-control strategies. In the CABANA (Catheter Ablation vs Antiarrhythmic Drug Therapy for Atrial Fibrillation) trial, based on intention-to-treat analysis, there was no significant difference between catheter ablation and drug therapy with respect to a primary composite outcome of death, disabling stroke, serious bleeding, or cardiac arrest. However, in selected younger patients with paroxysmal AF, rhythm control may be a better approach. Additionally, catheter ablation to maintain sinus rhythm in selected patients with symptomatic AF and heart failure with reduced left ventricular ejection fraction may reduce mortality rate and hospitalization for heart failure. Finally, in patients who continue to have symptoms despite an adequately controlled ventricular rate, rhythm control is an appropriate next step.

Rhythm control can be achieved by the use of antiarrhythmic drugs (Table 3) or catheter ablation. In patients with paroxysmal and persistent AF who have failed at least one antiarrhythmic

TABLE 3	Pharmacologic Agents for Rhythm Control	
DRUG	**USUAL ORAL MAINTENANCE DOSE**	**MAJOR SIDE EFFECTS**
Flecainide (Tambocor)	50–200 mg bid	Hypotension, atrial flutter with high ventricular rate
Propafenone (Rythmol)	150–300 mg tid	
Propafenone Extended Release (Rythmol SR)	225–425 mg bid	
Sotalol (Betapace)	80–160 mg bid	Bradycardia, hypotension, QT prolongation, torsades de pointes
Dofetilide (Tikosyn)	125–500 µg bid	QT prolongation, torsades de pointes
Amiodarone (Pacerone)[1]	100–200 mg qd	Hypotension, bradycardia, QT prolongation
Dronedarone (Multaq)	400 mg bid	QT prolongation

[1]Not FDA approved for atrial fibrillation.

TABLE 4	CHA_2DS_2-VASc Score	
RISK FACTOR	**SCORE**
Congestive heart failure, LV dysfunction	1
Hypertension	1
Age ≥75 years	2
Diabetes mellitus	1
Stroke, TIA, or thromboembolism	2
Vascular disease (MI, PAD, complex aortic plaque)	1
Age 65–74 years	1
Sex category: female	1

MI, Myocardial infarction; *LV*, left ventricular; *PAD*, peripheral arterial disease; *TIA*, transient ischemic attack.

TABLE 5	Non–Vitamin K Oral Anticoagulants	
DRUG	**USUAL DOSE**	**COMMENTS**
Direct Thrombin Inhibitor		
Dabigatran (Pradaxa)	150 mg bid	Reversal agent (Idarucizumab [Praxbind]) FDA approved; interacts with P-glycoprotein inhibitors and inducers
Factor Xa Inhibitor		
Apixaban (Eliquis)	5 mg bid	Interacts with P-glycoprotein and CYP3A4 inhibitors and inducers
Edoxaban (Savaysa)	60 mg qd	Avoid if CrCl >95 mL/min due to increased rate of stroke
Rivaroxaban (Xarelto)	20 mg qd	Interacts with P-glycoprotein and CYP3A4 inhibitors and inducers; should be taken with evening meal

drug, catheter ablation by pulmonary vein isolation is indicated to maintain sinus rhythm. In persistent AF, the STAR AF II (Substrate and Trigger Ablation for Reduction of Atrial Fibrillation Trial Part II) showed that performing additional linear ablation or ablation targeting complex fractionated electrograms does not improve rhythm control compared with pulmonary vein isolation alone. The optimal approach to ablate persistent AF remains to be defined.

Stroke Prophylaxis
Stroke prevention is a two-stage process: determination of thromboembolic stroke risk and selection of prevention strategy. The most commonly used risk-stratification scheme for stroke prevention is the CHA_2DS_2-VASc score (https://www.mdcalc.com/cha2ds2-vasc-score-atrial-fibrillation-stroke-risk) (Table 4). Oral anticoagulation is recommended for CHA_2DS_2-VASc score of 2 or greater in men or 3 or greater in women. Aspirin should not be used for stroke prevention in AF.[1]

Oral Anticoagulants
These include vitamin K antagonists (warfarin [Coumadin]) and non–vitamin K oral anticoagulants or novel or direct oral anticoagulants (DOAC) (Table 5). Compared with warfarin, DOACs are as effective in preventing thromboembolic stroke in AF. The risk of intracranial hemorrhage from the use of DOACs is 33% to 60% less than that with warfarin. Other advantages of DOACs over warfarin include the facts that there are fewer interactions

[1] Not FDA-approved for this indication.

with food and there is no need for monitoring the international normalized ratio.

Left Atrial Appendage Closure
The Watchman device is approved by the US Food and Drug Administration (FDA) for stroke prevention in AF patients with a contraindication to long-term oral anticoagulation and who are at risk of thromboembolic stroke. Patients, however, must be able to take oral anticoagulants for at least 6 weeks after implantation of the device.

Risk Factor Management and Lifestyle Modification
Recent compelling evidence underscores the importance of a fourth pillar of AF management: risk-factor and lifestyle modifications.

Weight Loss
An RCT has shown that weight reduction with intensive risk-factor management results in a reduction of AF symptom burden and severity and reversal of cardiac remodeling.

Intensive Blood Pressure Lowering
Blood pressure lowering targeting a systolic blood pressure of 120 mm Hg is associated with lower incidence of AF compared with 140 mm Hg.

Exercise Training

A small RCT showed that, compared with nonexercise control patients, high-intensity interval training reduced AF burden and improved atrial contractile function. This time-efficient form of exercise can potentially overcome the lack-of-time problem—an oft-quoted reason for poor compliance with regular aerobic exercise.

Complications

Other than thromboembolic stroke, heart failure, and death, AF is also associated with greater cognitive decline and risk of dementia. More recently, AF has been reported to be associated with a higher risk of sudden cardiac death in the general population. Apart from stroke prevention and rate and rhythm control to prevent heart failure, we currently lack effective prevention strategies for dementia and sudden cardiac death.

Special Considerations
Subclinical Atrial Fibrillation

Subclinical AF is commonly detected from interrogation of cardiac implantable electronic devices. Whether subclinical AF poses the same health risks as clinical AF is the subject of much debate and active investigation.

Atrial Fibrillation Burden

A corollary to the problem of subclinical AF is that of AF burden—the amount of AF that a patient has. Studies based on cardiac implantable electronic devices suggest that a higher AF burden is associated with a higher risk of thromboembolic stroke, but it is unclear whether the risk increases continuously or whether a threshold exists.

References

Abed HS, Wittert GA, Leong DP, et al: Effect of weight reduction and cardiometabolic risk factor management on symptom burden and severity in patients with atrial fibrillation a randomized clinical trial, *JAMA* 310:2050–2060, 2013.

Chen LY, Bigger JT, Hickey KT, et al: Effect of intensive blood pressure lowering on incident atrial fibrillation and p-wave indices in the ACCORD Blood Pressure Trial, *Am J Hypertens* 29:1276–1282, 2016.

Chen LY, Norby FL, Gottesman RF, et al: Association of atrial fibrillation with cognitive decline and dementia over 20 years: the ARIC-NCS (Atherosclerosis Risk in Communities Neurocognitive Study), *J Am Heart Assoc* 7(6).

Chen LY, Sotoodehnia N, Bůžková P, et al: Atrial fibrillation and the risk of sudden cardiac death: the Atherosclerosis Risk in Communities (ARIC) Study and Cardiovascular Health Study (CHS), *JAMA Intern Med* 173:29–35, 2013.

Chugh SS, Havmoeller R, Narayanan K, et al: Worldwide epidemiology of atrial fibrillation: a Global Burden of Disease 2010 Study, *Circulation* 129:837–847, 2014.

January CT, Wann LS, Calkins H, et al: 2019 AHA/ACC/HRS focused update of the 2014 AHA/ACC/HRS guideline for the management of patients with atrial fibrillation: a report of the American College of Cardiology/American Heart Association Task Force on Clinical Practice Guidelines and the Heart Rhythm Society, *Circulation*, 2019. https://doi.org/10.1161/CIR.0000000000000665.

Lloyd-Jones DM, Wang TJ, Leip EP, et al: Lifetime risk for development of atrial fibrillation—The Framingham Heart Study, *Circulation* 110:1042–1046, 2004.

Malmo V, Nes BM, Amundsen BH, et al: Aerobic interval training reduces the burden of atrial fibrillation in the short term a randomized trial, *Circulation* 133:466–473, 2016.

Marrouche NF, Brachmann J, Andresen D, et al: Catheter ablation for atrial fibrillation with heart failure, *N Engl J Med* 378:417–427, 2018.

Okin PM, Hille DA, Larstorp ACK, et al: Effect of lower on-treatment systolic blood pressure on the risk of atrial fibrillation in hypertensive patients, *Hypertension* 66:368–373, 2015.

Packer DL, Mark DB, Robb RA, et al: Effect of catheter ablation vs antiarrhythmic drug therapy on mortality, stroke, bleeding, and cardiac arrest among patients with atrial fibrillation: the cabana randomized clinical trial, *JAMA* 321:1261–1274, 2019.

Van Gelder IC, Groenveld HF, Crijns HJGM, et al: Lenient versus strict rate control in patients with atrial fibrillation, *N Engl J Med* 362:1363–1373, 2010.

Van Gelder IC, Hagens VE, Bosker HA, et al: A comparison of rate control and rhythm control in patients with recurrent persistent atrial fibrillation, *N Engl J Med* 347:1834–1840, 2002.

Verma A, Jiang CY, Betts TR, et al: Approaches to catheter ablation for persistent atrial fibrillation, *N Engl J Med* 372:1812–1822, 2015.

Wyse DG, Waldo AL, DiMarco JP, et al: A comparison of rate control and rhythm control in patients with atrial fibrillation, *N Engl J Med* 347:1825–1833, 2002.

CONGENITAL HEART DISEASE

Method of
Richard A. Lange, MD, MBA; and Joaquin E. Cigarroa, MD

CURRENT DIAGNOSIS

- Examine blood pressures in arms and legs, pulse oximetry, mucous membranes and nail beds, respiratory rate, and peripheral pulses.
- In addition to listening over the precordium for heart sounds and murmurs, palpate for thrills and evidence of right or left chamber enlargement.
- Ancillary testing should include chest radiography, electrocardiography, and echocardiography.
- Consult a cardiologist if the physical examination or ancillary tests suggest congenital heart disease.

CURRENT THERAPY

- All congenital heart disease patients should have long-term follow-up for possible complications.
- Endocarditis prophylaxis is recommended for subjects with:
  - Unrepaired cyanotic congenital heart disease
  - Recently repaired congenital heart disease (<6 months after surgical or percutaneous repair)
  - Repaired congenital heart disease with residual defects
- Closure of defects with large left-to-right shunts (i.e., atrial septal defect, ventricular septal defect, atrioventricular canal, or patent ductus arteriosus) is recommended unless pulmonary vascular obstructive disease is far advanced.
- Patients with bicuspid aortic valves should be monitored for aortic root dilation.
- Pregnancy should be avoided in women with cyanotic congenital heart disease because of high maternal and fetal morbidity and mortality rates.

Congenital heart disease affects 0.4% to 0.9% of live births. Nowadays, most survive to adulthood because of improved diagnosis and treatment. Congenital cardiac defects can be categorized according to the presence or absence of cyanosis (due to right-to-left shunting) and the amount of pulmonary blood flow (Box 1).

Acyanotic Conditions
Atrial Septal Defect

Atrial septal defect (ASD) occurs in female patients two to three times as often as in male patients. Although most result from spontaneous genetic mutations, some are inherited.

The physiological consequences of ASD result from the shunting of blood from one atrium to the other; the direction and magnitude of shunting are determined by the size of the defect and the relative compliances of the ventricles. A small defect (<0.5 cm in diameter) is associated with a small shunt and no hemodynamic sequelae, whereas a sizable defect (>2 cm in diameter) usually is associated with a large shunt and substantial hemodynamic consequences. In most patients with ASD, the right ventricle is more compliant than the left; as a result, left atrial blood is shunted to the right atrium, causing increased pulmonary blood flow and dilation of the atria, right ventricle, and pulmonary arteries (Figure 1). Eventually, if the right ventricle fails or its compliance declines, the magnitude of left-to-right shunting diminishes.

In a patient with a large ASD, a right ventricular or pulmonary arterial impulse may be palpable, and wide, fixed splitting of the second heart sound is present. A systolic ejection murmur, audible in the second left intercostal space, is caused by increased blood flow across the pulmonic valve; flow across the ASD itself does not produce a murmur.

Because ASDs initially produce no symptoms or striking physical examination findings, they are often undetected for years. Small defects with minimal left-to-right shunting cause no symptoms or hemodynamic abnormalities, so they do not require closure. Even patients with moderate or large ASDs (characterized by a ratio of pulmonary to systemic blood flow of 1.5 or more) often have no symptoms until the third or fourth decade of life. Over the years, the increased blood volume flowing through the right heart chambers usually causes right ventricular dilation and failure. Obstructive pulmonary vascular disease (Eisenmenger syndrome) occurs uncommonly in adults with ASD.

The symptomatic patient with an ASD typically reports fatigue or dyspnea on exertion. Alternatively, the development of supraventricular tachyarrhythmias, right heart failure, paradoxical embolism, or recurrent pulmonary infections might prompt the patient to seek medical attention. Although an occasional patient with an unrepaired ASD survives to an advanced age, those with

sizable shunts often die of right ventricular failure or arrhythmias in their 30s or 40s.

Echocardiography can reveal atrial and right ventricular dilation and identify the ASD's location. The sensitivity of echocardiography may be enhanced by injecting microbubbles in solution into a peripheral vein, after which the movement of some of them across the defect into the left atrium can be visualized.

An ASD with a pulmonary-to-systemic flow ratio of 1.5 or more should be closed (surgically or percutaneously) to prevent worsening right ventricular dysfunction. Prophylaxis against infective endocarditis is not recommended for patients with ASD (repaired or unrepaired) unless a concomitant valvular abnormality is present.

Ventricular Septal Defect

Ventricular septal defect (VSD) is the most common congenital cardiac abnormality, with similar incidence in boys and girls. Approximately 25% to 40% of them close spontaneously by 2 years of age.

The physiological consequences of a VSD are determined by the size of the defect and the relative resistances in the systemic and pulmonary vascular beds. A small defect causes little or no functional disturbance, because pulmonary blood flow is only minimally increased. In contrast, a large defect causes substantial left-to-right shunting, because systemic vascular resistance exceeds pulmonary vascular resistance (Figure 2). Over time, however, the pulmonary vascular resistance usually increases, and the magnitude of left-to-right shunting declines. Eventually, the pulmonary vascular resistance equals or exceeds the systemic resistance; the shunting of blood from left to right ceases; and right-to-left shunting begins (e.g., Eisenmenger physiology).

A small, muscular VSD can produce a high-frequency systolic ejection murmur that terminates before the end of systole (when the defect is occluded by contracting heart muscle). With a moderate or large VSD and substantial left-to-right shunting, a holosystolic murmur, loudest at the left sternal border, is audible and is usually accompanied by a palpable thrill. If pulmonary hypertension develops, the holosystolic murmur and thrill diminish in magnitude and eventually disappear as flow through the defect decreases.

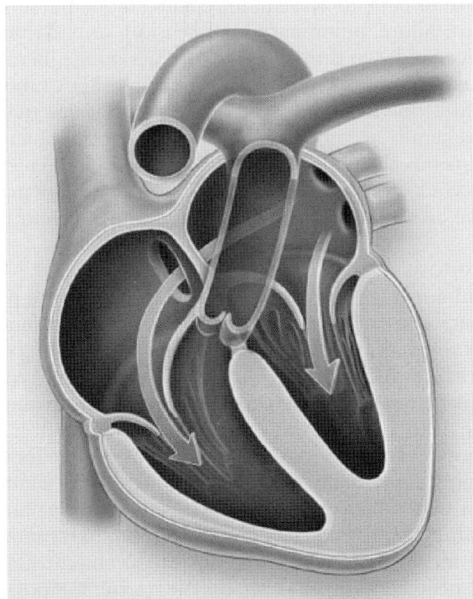

Figure 1 Atrial septal defect. Blood from the pulmonary veins enters the left atrium, after which some of it crosses the atrial septal defect into the right atrium and ventricle *(longer arrow)*. Thus left-to-right shunting occurs. (Reprinted with permission from Brickner ME, Hillis LD, Lange RA: Congenital heart disease in adults. First of two parts. N Engl J Med 2000;342:256–263.)

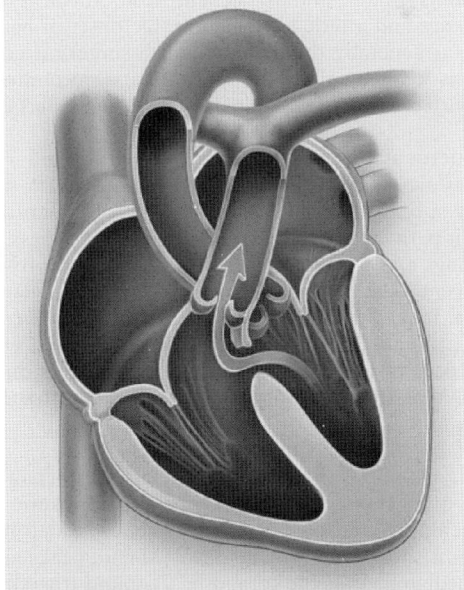

Figure 2 Ventricular septal defect. When the left ventricle contracts, it ejects some blood into the aorta and some across the ventricular septal defect into the right ventricle and pulmonary artery *(arrow)*, resulting in left-to-right shunting. (Reprinted with permission from Brickner ME, Hillis LD, Lange RA: Congenital heart disease in adults. First of two parts. N Engl J Med 2000;342:256–263.)

Echocardiography is usually performed to confirm the presence and location of the VSD and to delineate the magnitude and direction of shunting. With catheterization, one can determine the magnitude of shunting and the pulmonary vascular resistance.

The natural history of VSD depends on the size of the defect and the pulmonary vascular resistance. Adults with small defects and normal pulmonary arterial pressure are generally asymptomatic, and pulmonary vascular disease is unlikely to develop. In contrast, patients with large defects who survive to adulthood usually have left ventricular failure or pulmonary hypertension (or both) with associated right ventricular failure.

Closure of VSDs (surgically or percutaneously) is recommended if the pulmonary vascular obstructive disease is not severe. Prophylaxis against infective endocarditis is recommended for patients with unrepaired VSD and those with a residual shunt despite surgical or percutaneous closure.

Atrioventricular Canal Defect

The endocardial cushions normally fuse to form the tricuspid and mitral valves, as well as the atrial and ventricular septa. Atrioventricular (AV) canal defects are caused by incomplete fusion of the endocardial cushions during embryonic development. They are the most common congenital cardiac abnormality in patients with Down syndrome. Such cushion defects include a spectrum of abnormalities, ranging from ASD with a cleft anterior mitral valve leaflet to a common AV canal defect in which a single AV valve in association with a large ASD and VSD is present.

A common AV canal defect permits substantial left-to-right shunting at both the atrial and ventricular levels, which leads to excessive pulmonary blood flow and resultant pulmonary congestion within months of birth. Eventually, the excessive pulmonary blood flow leads to irreversible pulmonary vascular obstruction (e.g., Eisenmenger physiology).

In the patient with an AV canal defect and left-to-right intracardiac shunting, the physical examination reveals a loud holosystolic murmur audible throughout the precordium. As pulmonary vascular resistance increases, the holosystolic murmur diminishes in intensity and duration, eventually disappearing as flow through the defect decreases.

AV canal defects require surgical repair if the magnitude of pulmonary vascular obstructive disease is not prohibitive. Although such patients might initially benefit from medical treatment with diuretics and afterload reduction, the onset of heart failure symptoms is generally the point at which surgery is considered. Prophylaxis against infective endocarditis is recommended for patients with repaired and unrepaired AV canal defects.

Patent Ductus Arteriosus

The ductus arteriosus connects the descending aorta (just distal to the left subclavian artery) and the left pulmonary artery. In the fetus, it permits pulmonary arterial blood to bypass the unexpanded lungs and to enter the descending aorta for oxygenation in the placenta. Although it normally closes spontaneously soon after birth, it fails to do so in some infants, so that continuous flow from the aorta to the pulmonary artery (i.e., left-to-right shunting) occurs (Figure 3). The incidence of patent ductus arteriosus (PDA) is increased in pregnancies complicated by persistent perinatal hypoxemia or maternal rubella infection as well as among infants born prematurely or at high altitude.

A patient with PDA and a moderate or large shunt has bounding peripheral arterial pulses and a widened pulse pressure. A continuous "machinery" murmur, audible in the second left intercostal space, begins shortly after the first heart sound, peaks in intensity at or immediately after the second heart sound (thereby obscuring it), and diminishes in intensity during diastole. If pulmonary vascular obstruction and hypertension develop, the murmur decreases in duration and intensity and eventually disappears.

With echocardiography, the PDA can usually be visualized, and Doppler studies demonstrate continuous flow in the pulmonary trunk. Catheterization and angiography allow one to quantify the

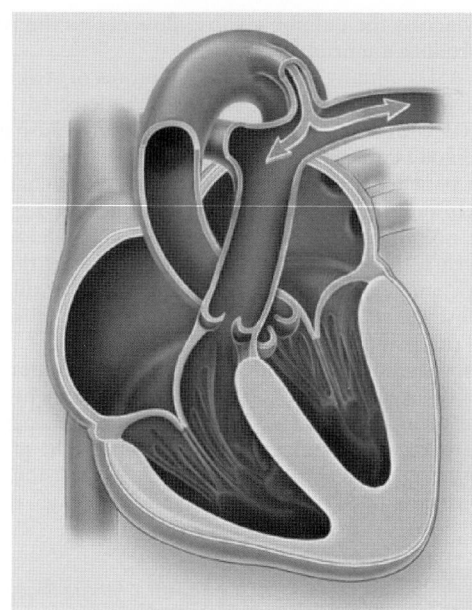

Figure 3 Patent ductus arteriosus. Some of the blood from the aorta crosses the ductus arteriosus into the pulmonary artery (arrows), with resultant left-to-right shunting. (Reprinted with permission from Brickner ME, Hillis LD, Lange RA: Congenital heart disease in adults. First of two parts. N Engl J Med 2000;342:256–263.)

magnitude of shunting and the pulmonary vascular resistance and to visualize the PDA.

The subject with a small PDA has no symptoms attributable to it and a normal life expectancy. However, it is associated with an elevated risk of infective endarteritis. A PDA of moderate size might cause no symptoms during infancy; during childhood or adulthood, fatigue, dyspnea, or palpitations can appear. Additionally, the PDA can become aneurysmal and calcified, with subsequent rupture. Larger shunts can precipitate left ventricular failure. Eventually, pulmonary vascular obstruction can develop; when the pulmonary vascular resistance equals or exceeds the systemic vascular resistance, the direction of shunting reverses.

One third of patients with an unrepaired moderate or large PDA die of heart failure, pulmonary hypertension, or endarteritis by 40 years of age, and two thirds die by 60 years of age. Because of the risk of endarteritis associated with unrepaired PDA (about 0.45% annually after the second decade of life) and the safety of surgical ligation (generally accomplished without cardiopulmonary bypass) or percutaneous closure, even a small PDA should be ligated surgically or occluded percutaneously. Once severe pulmonary vascular obstructive disease develops, ligation or closure is contraindicated.

Aortic Stenosis

A bicuspid aortic valve is found in 2% to 3% of the population and is four times more common in males than in females. The bicuspid valve has a single fused commissure and an eccentrically oriented orifice. Although the deformed valve is not typically stenotic at birth, it is subjected to abnormal hemodynamic stress, which can lead to leaflet thickening and calcification. In many patients, an abnormality of the ascending aortic media is present, predisposing the patient to aortic root dilation. Twenty percent of patients with a bicuspid aortic valve have an associated cardiovascular abnormality, such as PDA or aortic coarctation.

In patients with severe aortic stenosis (AS), the carotid upstroke is usually delayed and diminished. The aortic component of the second heart sound is diminished or absent. A systolic crescendo–decrescendo murmur is audible over the aortic area and often radiates to the neck. As the magnitude of AS worsens, the murmur peaks progressively later in systole.

In most patients, echocardiography with Doppler flow permits an assessment of the severity of AS and of left ventricular systolic

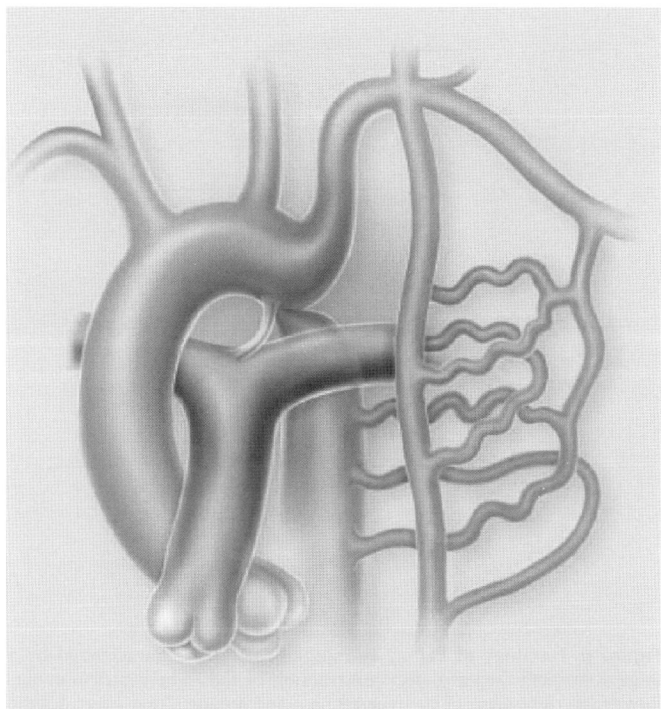

Figure 4 Coarctation of the aorta. Coarctation causes obstruction to blood flow in the descending thoracic aorta; the lower body is perfused by collateral vessels from the axillary and internal thoracic arteries through the intercostal arteries. (Reprinted with permission from Brickner ME, Hillis LD, Lange RA: Congenital heart disease in adults. First of two parts. N Engl J Med 2000;342:256–263.)

function. Cardiac catheterization is performed to assess the severity of AS and to determine if concomitant coronary artery disease is present.

The symptoms of AS are angina pectoris, syncope or near syncope, and those of heart failure (dyspnea). Asymptomatic adults with AS have a normal life expectancy. Once symptoms appear, survival is limited. The median survival is 5 years once angina develops, 3 years once syncope occurs, and 2 years once symptoms of heart failure appear. Therefore patients with symptomatic AS should undergo valve replacement.

Pulmonic Stenosis

Pulmonic stenosis (PS) is the second most common congenital cardiac malformation (after VSD). Although typically an isolated abnormality, it can occur in association with VSD.

The patient with PS is usually asymptomatic, and the condition is identified by auscultation of a loud systolic murmur. When it is severe, dyspnea on exertion or fatigue can occur; less often, patients have retrosternal chest pain or syncope with exertion. Eventually, right ventricular failure can develop, with resultant peripheral edema and abdominal swelling.

In patients with moderate or severe PS, the second heart sound is widely split, with its pulmonic component soft and delayed. A crescendo-decrescendo systolic murmur that increases in intensity with inspiration is audible along the left sternal border. If the valve is pliable, an ejection click often precedes the murmur. On echocardiography, right ventricular hypertrophy is evident; the severity of PS can usually be assessed with measurement of Doppler flow.

Adults with mild PS are usually asymptomatic and do not require a corrective procedure. In contrast, patients with moderate or severe PS should undergo percutaneous balloon dilation.

Aortic Coarctation

Aortic coarctation typically consists of a diaphragm-like ridge extending into the aortic lumen just distal to the left subclavian artery (Figure 4), resulting in an elevated arterial pressure in both arms. Less commonly, the coarctation is located immediately proximal to the left subclavian artery, in which case a difference in arterial pressure is noted between the arms. Extensive collateral arterial circulation to the lower body through the internal thoracic, intercostal, subclavian, and scapular arteries often develops in patients with aortic coarctation. Aortic coarctation, which is two to five times as common in males as in females, can occur in conjunction with gonadal dysgenesis (e.g., Turner's syndrome), bicuspid aortic valve, VSD, or PDA.

On physical examination, the arterial pressure is higher in the arms than in the legs, and the femoral arterial pulses are weak and delayed. A harsh systolic ejection murmur may be audible along the left sternal border and in the back, particularly over the coarctation. A systolic murmur, caused by flow through collateral vessels, may be heard in the back.

On chest radiography, increased collateral flow through the intercostal arteries causes notching of the posterior third through eighth ribs. The coarctation may be visible as an indentation of the aorta, and one may see prestenotic and poststenotic aortic dilation, producing the "reversed E" or "3" sign. Computed tomography, magnetic resonance imaging, and contrast aortography provide precise anatomic delineation of the coarctation's location and length.

Most adults with aortic coarctation are asymptomatic. When symptoms are present, they are usually those of hypertension: headache, epistaxis, dizziness, and palpitations. Complications of aortic coarctation include hypertension, left ventricular failure, aortic dissection, premature coronary artery disease, infective endocarditis, and cerebrovascular accidents (due to rupture of an intracerebral aneurysm). Two thirds of patients older than 40 years who have uncorrected aortic coarctation have symptoms of heart failure. Three fourths die by the age of 50 years and 90% by the age of 60 years.

Surgical repair or intraluminal stenting should be considered for patients with a transcoarctation pressure gradient greater than 30 mm Hg, with the choice of procedure influenced by the age of the patient, anatomic considerations of the coarctation, and the presence of concomitant cardiac abnormalities. Persistent hypertension is common despite surgical or percutaneous intervention, and recurrent coarctation or aneurysm formation at the repair site may occur.

Cyanotic Conditions
Ebstein's Anomaly

With Ebstein's anomaly, the tricuspid valve's septal leaflet and often its posterior leaflet are displaced into the right ventricle, and the anterior leaflet is usually malformed and abnormally attached or adherent to the right ventricular free wall. As a result, a portion of the right ventricle is atrialized, in that it is located on the atrial side of the tricuspid valve, and the remaining functional right ventricle is small (Figure 5). The tricuspid valve is usually regurgitant, but it may be stenotic. Eighty percent of patients with Ebstein's anomaly have an interatrial communication (ASD or patent foramen ovale) through which right-to-left shunting of blood can occur.

The severity of the hemodynamic derangements in patients with Ebstein's anomaly depends on the magnitude of displacement and the functional status of the tricuspid valve leaflets. On the one extreme, patients with mild apical displacement of the tricuspid valve leaflets have normal valvular function; on the other extreme, those with severe leaflet displacement or abnormal anterior leaflet attachment, with resultant valvular dysfunction, have an elevated right atrial pressure and right-to-left shunting if an interatrial communication is present.

The clinical presentation of subjects with Ebstein's anomaly ranges from severe right heart failure in the neonate to the absence of symptoms in the adult in whom it is discovered incidentally. Older children with Ebstein's anomaly often come to medical attention because of an incidental murmur, whereas adolescents and adults may be identified because of a supraventricular arrhythmia.

On physical examination, the severity of cyanosis depends on the magnitude of right-to-left shunting. The first and second heart sounds are both widely split, and a third or fourth heart sound is often present, resulting in triple or even quadruple heart sounds. A systolic murmur caused by tricuspid regurgitation is usually present at the left lower sternal border.

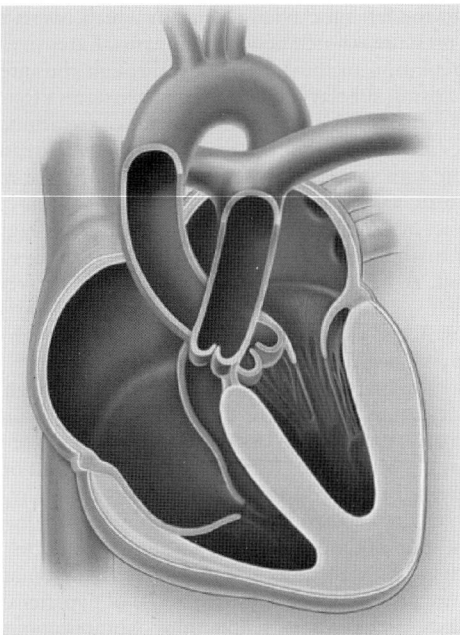

Figure 5 Ebstein's anomaly. With Ebstein's anomaly, the tricuspid valve is displaced apically, a portion of the right ventricle is atrialized (i.e., located on the atrial side of the tricuspid valve), and the functional right ventricle is small. (Reprinted with permission from Brickner ME, Hillis LD, Lange RA: Congenital heart disease in adults. Second of two parts. N Engl J Med 2000;342:334–342.)

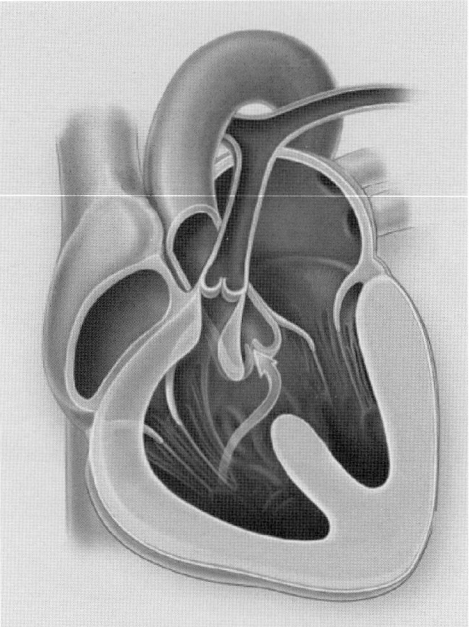

Figure 6 Tetralogy of Fallot. Tetralogy of Fallot is characterized by a large ventricular septal defect, obstruction of the right ventricular outflow tract, right ventricular hypertrophy, and an aorta that overrides the left and right ventricles. With right ventricular outflow tract obstruction, blood is shunted through the ventricular septal defect from right to left *(arrow)*. (Reprinted with permission from Brickner ME, Hillis LD, Lange RA: Congenital heart disease in adults. Second of two parts. N Engl J Med 2000;342:334–342.)

Echocardiography is used to assess the presence and magnitude of right atrial dilation, anatomic displacement and distortion of the tricuspid valve leaflets, and the severity of tricuspid regurgitation or stenosis.

Prophylaxis against infective endocarditis is recommended. Patients with symptomatic right heart failure should receive diuretics. Tricuspid valve repair or replacement in conjunction with closure of the interatrial communication is recommended for older patients with severe symptoms despite medical therapy and those with less severe symptoms who have cardiac enlargement.

Tetralogy of Fallot

Tetralogy of Fallot is characterized by a large VSD, an aorta that overrides both ventricles, obstruction to right ventricular outflow (subvalvular, valvular, supravalvular, or in the pulmonary arterial branches), and right ventricular hypertrophy (Figure 6).

Most patients with tetralogy of Fallot have substantial right-to-left shunting through the large VSD because of increased resistance to flow in the right ventricular outflow tract; the magnitude of right ventricular outflow tract obstruction determines the magnitude of shunting. Because the resistance to flow across the right ventricular outflow tract is relatively fixed, changes in systemic vascular resistance affect the magnitude of right-to-left shunting: A decrease in systemic vascular resistance increases right-to-left shunting, whereas an increase in systemic resistance decreases it.

Patients with tetralogy of Fallot typically have cyanosis from birth or beginning in the first year of life. In childhood, they might have sudden hypoxic spells, characterized by tachypnea and hyperpnea, followed by worsening cyanosis and, in some cases, loss of consciousness, seizures, cerebrovascular accidents, and even death. Such spells do not occur in adolescents or adults. Without surgical intervention, most patients die in childhood.

On physical examination, patients with tetralogy of Fallot have cyanosis and digital clubbing. A right ventricular lift or tap is palpable. The second heart sound is single, because its pulmonic component is inaudible. A systolic ejection murmur, audible along the left sternal border, is caused by the obstruction to right ventricular outflow. The intensity and duration of the murmur are inversely related to the severity of right ventricular outflow

obstruction; a soft, short murmur suggests that severe obstruction is present.

Laboratory examination reveals arterial oxygen desaturation and compensatory erythrocytosis. Echocardiography can be used to establish the diagnosis and to assess the location and severity of right ventricular outflow tract obstruction.

Complete surgical repair (closure of the VSD and relief of right ventricular outflow tract obstruction) is recommended to relieve symptoms and to improve survival; it should be performed when patients are very young. Those with tetralogy of Fallot (repaired or unrepaired) are at risk for endocarditis and therefore should receive antibiotic prophylaxis before dental or elective surgical procedures.

Patients with repaired tetralogy of Fallot require careful follow-up, because they can subsequently develop atrial or ventricular arrhythmias, pulmonic regurgitation, right ventricular dysfunction, or recurrent obstruction of the right ventricular outflow tract.

Eisenmenger Syndrome

With substantial left-to-right shunting, the pulmonary vasculature is exposed to increased blood flow under increased pressure, often resulting in pulmonary vascular obstructive disease. As the pulmonary vascular resistance approaches or exceeds systemic resistance, the shunt is reversed (right-to-left shunting develops), and cyanosis appears (Figure 7).

Most patients with Eisenmenger syndrome have impaired exercise tolerance and exertional dyspnea. Palpitations are common and most often result from atrial fibrillation or flutter. As erythrocytosis (due to arterial desaturation) develops, symptoms of hyperviscosity (visual disturbances, fatigue, headache, dizziness, and paresthesias) can appear. Patients with Eisenmenger syndrome can experience hemoptysis, bleeding complications, cerebrovascular accidents, brain abscess, syncope, and sudden death.

Eisenmenger syndrome patients typically have digital clubbing and cyanosis, a right parasternal heave (due to right ventricular hypertrophy), and a prominent pulmonic component of the second heart sound. The murmur caused by a VSD, PDA, or ASD disappears when Eisenmenger syndrome develops.

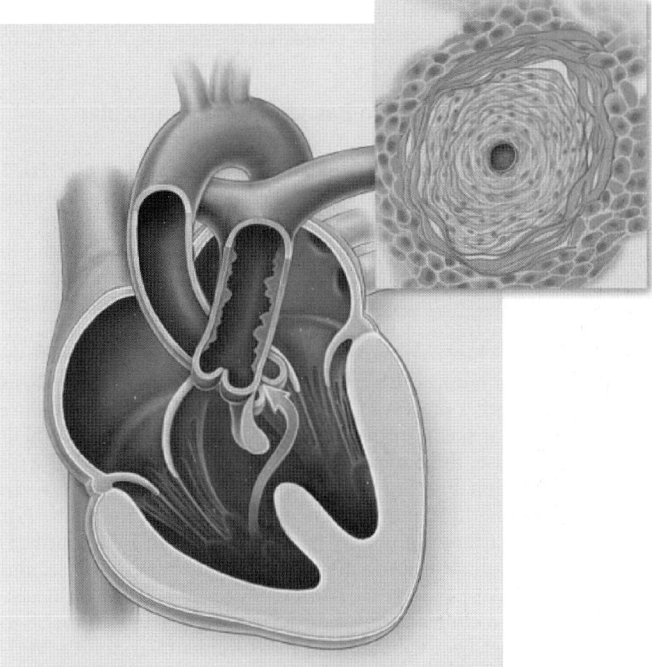

Figure 7 Eisenmenger syndrome. In response to substantial left-to-right shunting, morphologic alterations occur in the small pulmonary arteries and arterioles *(inset)*, leading to pulmonary hypertension and the resultant reversal of the intracardiac shunt *(arrow)*. In the small pulmonary arteries and arterioles, medial hypertrophy, intimal cellular proliferation, and fibrosis lead to narrowing or closure of the vessel lumina. With sustained pulmonary hypertension, extensive atherosclerosis and calcification often develop in the large pulmonary arteries. (Reprinted with permission from Brickner ME, Hillis LD, Lange RA: Congenital heart disease in adults. Second of two parts. N Engl J Med 2000;342:334–42.)

The chest x-ray reveals normal heart size, prominent central pulmonary arteries, and diminished vascular markings (pruning) of the peripheral vessels. On transthoracic echocardiography, evidence of right ventricular pressure overload and pulmonary hypertension is present. The underlying cardiac defect can usually be visualized, although shunting across the defect may be difficult to demonstrate by Doppler because of the low jet velocity.

Even though patients with Eisenmenger syndrome have severe pulmonary hypertension, they have a favorable long-term survival: 80% at 10 years after diagnosis, 77% at 15 years, and 42% at 25 years. Death is usually sudden, presumably caused by arrhythmias, but some patients die of heart failure, hemoptysis, brain abscess, or stroke.

Phlebotomy with isovolumic replacement should be performed in patients with moderate or severe symptoms of hyperviscosity; it should not be performed in asymptomatic or mildly symptomatic patients regardless of the hematocrit. Repeated phlebotomy can result in iron deficiency, which can worsen the symptoms of hyperviscosity, because iron-deficient erythrocytes are less deformable than iron-replete ones. Anticoagulants and antiplatelet agents should be avoided, because they exacerbate the hemorrhagic diathesis.

Patients with Eisenmenger syndrome should avoid intravascular volume depletion, high altitude, and the use of systemic vasodilators. Because of high maternal and fetal morbidity and mortality, pregnancy should be avoided. Patients with Eisenmenger syndrome who are undergoing noncardiac surgery require meticulous management of anesthesia, with attention to maintenance of systemic vascular resistance, minimization of blood loss and intravascular volume depletion, and prevention of iatrogenic paradoxical embolism. In preparation for noncardiac surgery, prophylactic phlebotomy (usually of 1 to 2 units of blood, with isovolumic replacement) is recommended for patients with a hematocrit greater than 65% to reduce the likelihood of perioperative hemorrhagic and thrombotic complications.

Lung transplantation with repair of the cardiac defect or combined heart–lung transplantation are options for patients with Eisenmenger syndrome who are deemed to have a poor prognosis (as reflected by the presence of syncope, refractory right heart failure, a high New York Heart Association [NYHA] functional class, or severe hypoxemia). Because of the somewhat limited success of transplantation and the reasonably good survival among patients treated medically, careful selection of patients for transplantation is imperative. Although pulmonary vasodilators improve exercise capacity, they have not been proved to improve survival.

References

Bhatt AB, Foster E, Kuehl K, et al: on behalf of the American Heart Association Council on Clinical Cardiology: Congenital heart disease in the older adult: a scientific statement from the American Heart Association, *Circulation* 131:1884–1931, 2015.

Brickner ME, Hillis LD, Lange RA: Congenital heart disease in adults. First of two parts, *N Engl J Med* 342:256–263, 2000.

Brickner ME, Hillis LD, Lange RA: Congenital heart disease in adults. Second of two parts, *N Engl J Med* 342:334–342, 2000.

Lange RA, Hillis LD, Vongpatanasin WP, Brickner ME: The Eisenmenger syndrome in adults, *Ann Int Med* 128:745–755, 1998.

Neidenbach R, Niwa K, Oto O, et al: Improving medical care and prevention in adults with congenital heart disease—reflections on a global problem—part II: infective endocarditis, pulmonary hypertension, pulmonary arterial hypertension and aortopathy, *Cardiovasc Diagn Ther* 8(6):716–724, 2018.

Stout KK, Daniels CJ, Aboulhosn JA, et al: 2018 AHA/ACC guideline for the management of adults with congenital heart disease: executive summary: a report of the American College of Cardiology/American Heart Association Task Force on Clinical Practice Guidelines, *Circulation* 139:e637–e697, 2019.

CONGESTIVE HEART FAILURE

Method of
Alex Schevchuck, MD, MS; and Mark E. Garcia, MD

CURRENT DIAGNOSIS

- Recognize clinical symptoms and signs of congestive heart failure (HF).
- Determine left ventricular ejection fraction (EF) using imaging modalities.
- Identify the potential etiologies.
- Evaluate hemodynamic status.

CURRENT THERAPY

- Current therapies differ for heart failure with preserved (HFpEF) and reduced EF (HFrEF).
- Angiotensin converting enzyme inhibitors (ACEIs), angiotensin-receptor blockers (ARBs), angiotensin receptor-neprilysin inhibitor (ARNI), and mineralocorticoid receptor antagonists (MRAs) play a pivotal role in reducing morbidity and mortality in patients with HFrEF.
- Diuretics are useful in both HFrEF and HFpEF patients to treat congestion and fluid volume removal. A patient with decompensated heart failure may need intravenous diuretic treatment for decongestion caused by intestinal edema and malabsorption of oral diuretics. High-dose IV diuretic is important for treatment of decompensated HF.
- There are limited treatment options for HFpEF. The mainstay of therapy in HFpEF is using diuretics to relieve congestion and treatment of coexisting diseases.
- In advanced heart failure, identification of high-risk features and early referral for consultation with an advanced heart failure specialist are important.

Heart Failure Definition

The definition of heart failure has been variable in part caused by a wide spectrum of etiologies and pathologic processes resulting in this disease.

Heart failure is a clinical syndrome that includes a variety of signs and symptoms of systemic and/or pulmonic congestion from cardiac dysfunction. Specifically, systolic insufficiency and/or elevated ventricular filling pressures result in decreased perfusion and congestion. The symptoms of heart failure commonly include shortness of breath with exertion or at rest, fatigue, limited exercise capacity, and edema. Figure 1 shows the new proposed universal definition of heart failure.

Heart failure can sometimes be confused for a cardiomyopathy and/or a low EF. A cardiomyopathy is a disease state of the myocardium, such as ischemic heart disease or hypertrophic cardiomyopathy. This may lead to the heart failure syndrome but is not necessarily needed to develop heart failure. Thus these terms are not synonymous or interchangeable. Likewise, a low EF does not automatically imply the diagnosis of heart failure in absence of the clinical syndrome.

There are four stages of clinical development and progression of heart failure (Table 1).

Epidemiology

Based on 2013 to 2016 NHANES data, there were 6.2 million adults with congestive heart failure in the United States, and this number has increased from 5.7 million from 2009 to 2012. This represented about 2% of the U.S. population. Projections now show that by the year 2030, the prevalence of HF may increase to nearly 3%, or >8 million adults. The prevalence of HF increases with age, approaching >12% of the population in the age group of 80 and older.

In the ARIC study, the incidence of HF in subjects ≥55 years-old was 1 million cases in 2014 and was slightly higher among women comparatively to men and among African Americans comparatively to whites.

The lifetime risk of developing heart failure is 20% to 45% in subjects ≥45 years of age. HF mortality depends on the type of heart failure, demographics, and history of hospitalizations. Although HF survival has improved with the development of contemporary therapies, 1-year mortality remains substantial,

nearing 30%. The overall cost of HF care was ~30 billion dollars in 2012. By 2030, the cost is projected to increase by 127%, to nearly 70 billion a year.

Heart Failure Classification Based on Left Ventricular Ejection Fraction (LVEF)

HF classification based on LVEF has been updated in the 2021 Universal Definition of Heart Failure document and is summarized in Table 2.

EF-based classification further implies prognostic and therapeutic differences. Thus patients with EF ≤40 benefit from specific treatments for heart failure with a reduced LVEF. HF with a mildly reduced ejection fraction has been a controversial topic and generally represents heterogeneous phenotypes that may benefit from treatments for a reduced EF and also may have a worse prognosis than patients with a preserved EF. If a patient has had heart failure with low EF that has improved to ≥40% as a result of treatment or a natural cause, the patient is subcategorized into the "HF with preserved Ejection Fraction, improved" class. Clinicians have to keep in mind the limitations of the LV assessment methods. For example, echocardiography may have variability in EF quantification based on a quantification method, reader experience/style, and image quality. An EF decrease from 41% to 39% may not necessarily represent a clinical change or deterioration from HFmrEF to HFrEF but rather be attributed to a measurement variability. Verification tests, such as cardiac magnetic resonance imaging (MRI) or multiple-gated acquisition (MUGA) scan, may be used to validate if the change is true before major therapeutic changes are made.

Functional Capacity

New York Heart Association (NYHA) Functional Class is commonly accepted classification of functional capacity in symptomatic and advanced (stages C and D) heart failure patients. Functional class has prognostic and therapeutic implications. Four NYHA functional classes (FC) are listed in Table 3.

NYFA functional class should be assessed at the time of heart failure diagnosis and then reassessed during subsequent encounters to track progress of heart failure treatment and for monitoring of disease progression.

Left Ventricular Physiology and Hemodynamic Profile

Left ventricular performance depends on three major components: preload, afterload, and contractility. The preload is the maximum amount of myocardial stretch prior to onset of ventricular systole. A clinically accepted measure of preload is the left ventricular end-diastolic pressure (LVEDP), which can be measured directly using cardiac catheterization techniques or indirectly using transthoracic echocardiography. The relationship between cardiac output (CO) and preload is described by Frank-Starling mechanism (Figure 2, Panel A). CO will continue to increase in response to increasing preload, until the LV stretch reaches the point when actin and

Figure 1 Universal definition of heart failure. BNP: Brain natriuretic peptide

TABLE 1	Stages of Development and Progression of HF			
Stage	**A** AT RISK FOR HF	**B** PRE-HF	**C** HF	**D** ADVANCED HF
Symptoms	No prior or current symptoms of HF	No prior or current symptoms of HF	Prior or current symptoms of HF	Severe symptoms of congestion, dyspnea at rest, recurrent hospitalization despite GDMT
Clinical features	Presence of HTN, CVD, DM, obesity, exposure to cardiotoxins, family history of familial cardiomyopathy	Presence of one of the following: Structural heart disease Abnormal cardiac function Elevated BNP or troponin level in case of cardiotoxins	Symptoms are caused by structural or functional heart abnormality (i.e., systolic dysfunction or elevated filling pressures)	Requires advanced therapies (VAD, transplant) or palliative care

CVD, cardiovascular disease; DM, diabetes mellitus; HTN, hypertension; GDMT: guideline-directed medical therapy; VAD: ventricular assist-device.

myosin fibers lose interlink. Any further increase in preload past this point will result in decrease in CO.

Afterload, on the other hand, has a hyperbolic relationship with the stroke volume (see Figure 2, Panel B). Any reduction in afterload results in an increase in CO and vice versa.

The contractility is a highly debated term in the myocardial physiology world and sometimes is referred to as *inotropy*. This generally implies an intrinsic force or an intensity of a myocardial contraction that is affected by positive and negative inotropic agents. Many conditions that affect the myocardium may also adversely affect the contractility.

The preload-CO relationship determines four hemodynamic profiles (Table 4).

Neurohormone and Sympathetic Nervous System Activation

Heart failure leads to a decreased cardiac output, and in this disease state multiple detrimental physiologic pathways are activated. This includes the renin-angiotensin-aldosterone system (RAAS) and the sympathetic nervous system (SNS). The RAAS is activated in this low perfusion state where the kidney senses the decreased perfusion pressure stimulating the release of renin. Renin is responsible for activating angiotensin-I, which is then further activated to its more potent form angiotensin-II by the angiotensin converting enzyme. Angiotensin-II binds to the AT1 receptor and this process triggers multiple cardiovascular and renal effects including vasoconstriction, triggering of sodium and water absorption in the renal tubules, stimulating aldosterone release, and several direct detrimental myocardium effects including hypertrophy and fibrosis.

Activation of the sympathetic nervous system during heart failure is a complex pathway that is associated with increased catecholamine levels and increased sympathetic tone. Activation of the SNS initially can be considered beneficial in early HF because this has a wide range of effects including increased heart rate and cardiac contractility, but long-term activation has significant detrimental effects leading to further cardiac remodeling and arrhythmias.

Activation of these systems directly contributes to cardiac remodeling and worsening of HF. These pathways allow for multiple different therapeutic interventions that have been proven to improve survival, decrease hospitalizations, decrease symptoms, and potentially improve cardiac function.

Diagnosis

Clinical diagnostic criteria for HF are listed in Box 1. For establishing a definite diagnosis of heart failure in this study, two major or one major and two minor criteria have to be present concurrently.

Echocardiography plays a key role in diagnosis of heart failure. Transthoracic echo (TTE) provides information about the left and right ventricular systolic function, chamber sizes, structural disease such as ventricular hypertrophy, valve structure and function, relaxation function, presence of the intracardiac shunts, and ventricular filling pressures and pulmonary artery pressure. TEE may be helpful to clarify details on cardiac structure, such as anatomy of shunts or mechanism of valve dysfunction.

Cardiac CT may provide information on cardiac and vascular structure. Cardiac MRI is excellent at the evaluation of cardiac structure, function and chamber size, as well as assessing and

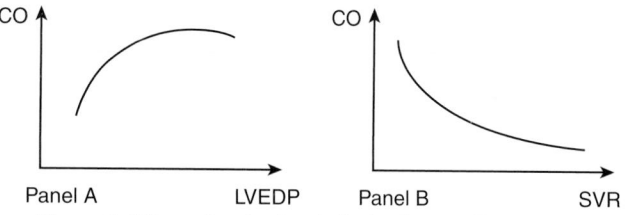

Figure 2 Effects of preload and afterload on cardiac output.

TABLE 2	Classification of Heart Failure Based on LVEF	
HF CLASS ACCORDING TO LVEF (MUST HAVE SIGNS AND SYMPTOMS)	**ACRONYM**	**LVEF, %**
HF with reduced Ejection Fraction	HFrEF	≤40
HF with mildly reduced Ejection Fraction	HFmrEF	41–49
HF with preserved Ejection Fraction	HFpEF	≥50
HF with preserved Ejection Fraction, improved	HFpEF, improved	Prior <40, now ≥40

TABLE 4	Heart Failure Hemodynamic Profiles	
	NORMAL LVEDP	**ELEVATED LVEDP**
Normal CO	A "warm and dry"	B "warm and wet"
Decreased CO	L "lethal, cold, and dry"	C "cold and wet"

TABLE 3	NYHA Functional Classification
NYHA FC	**FUNCTIONAL CAPACITY**
I	No limitations. Can perform high level of activity without symptoms (for example, running, cycling, weightlifting).
II	Slight limitations. Tolerate lower or moderate level activities well, may have limitations with higher level activities (for example, regular walking causes no symptoms, but a run may cause shortness of breath).
III	Significant limitations. Symptoms with low-level activities such as with daily activities such as walking, household chores, etc.
IV	Symptoms at rest, dyspnea with any physical activity.

BOX 1 — Clinical Criteria for CHF Diagnosis

Major Criteria
- Paroxysmal nocturnal dyspnea or orthopnea
- Neck-vein distention
- Rales
- Cardiomegaly
- Acute pulmonary edema
- S_3 gallop
- Increased venous pressure (≥16 cm of water)
- Circulation time ≥25 sec
- Hepatojugular reflux

Minor Criteria
- Ankle edema
- Night cough
- Dyspnea on exertion
- Hepatomegaly
- Pleural effusion
- Vital capacity ↓ 1/3 from maximum.
- Tachycardia (rate of ≥120/min)

Major or Minor Criterion
- Weight loss ≥4.5 kg in 5 days in response to treatment

diagnosing myocardial disease, such as tumors, fibrosis, thrombi, and inflammatory and infiltrative processes.

Nuclear radiology offers a MUGA scan that is considered a superior EF evaluation method and a myocardial perfusion viability testing, which is an important tool for evaluation of ischemic heart disease.

Left heart catheterization (a percutaneous catheter placement into the left ventricle) allows for a direct measurement of the LVEDP but is rarely performed as a standalone test because of associated risks. This is generally reserved for cases involving other percutaneous cardiac procedures, such as a coronary angiogram. A right heart catheterization (sometimes referred to as a Swan-Ganz catheter or pulmonary artery [PA] catheter) offers a lower complication risk profile and is our favorite method of invasive hemodynamic assessment.

A 12-lead electrocardiography (ECG) is an important test for HF patients. It may diagnose cardiac arrhythmias or ischemic disease, or can be suggestive of other myocardial diseases (i.e., amyloid) providing a clue to the etiology of HF.

Laboratory and Diagnostic Tests

In the newly decompensated HF patient, several laboratory tests should be obtained including serum creatinine, blood urea nitrogen, serum electrolytes, complete blood counts, urinalysis, liver function tests, thyroid stimulating hormone, and fasting lipid panel. In patients with a new HF diagnosis, it is reasonable to screen for hemochromatosis and HIV and to obtain diagnostic tests if there is a clinic concern for systemic disease such as rheumatologic diseases, amyloidosis, or pheochromocytoma.

Natriuretic peptide biomarkers include B-type natriuretic peptide (BNP) and N-terminal pro-B-type natriuretic peptide (NT-proBNP). Natriuretic peptides are released from the heart tissues when stretching (increased intracardiac volume and/or pressure). Circulating natriuretic peptides have a vasodilation and natriuretic response. BNP is the biologically active form and is inactivated by the enzyme neprilysin. Inhibition of the neprilysin enzyme is a target for sacubitril-valsartan. Natriuretic peptide levels can be useful in the ambulatory setting when the evaluation of dyspnea is unclear, assisting with the diagnosis of new onset HF, and in the emergency setting when normal natriuretic peptide levels can help rule out HF. There is no role of serial natriuretic testing in the hospitalized or ambulatory setting but it can be useful when assessing changes in symptoms and upon hospital discharge because the level can help in establishing disease severity and be a predictor of worse outcomes.

Troponin levels can be elevated in decompensated HF. Troponin elevations in HF are not diagnostic to HF but provide information on prognosis in HF and should be obtained on hospital admission.

Therapy for HFrEF
Diuretics (High Dose IV Diuretic Is Important)
Loop diuretics are the mainstay of therapy to relieve congestion in HFrEF and HFpEF. In hospitalized patients already on loop diuretic therapy, the IV dose should exceed the outpatient oral dose and should be given as intermittent boluses or infusion. Consider dosing the IV loop diuretic at 2.5 times the home oral dose. If resistant to initial IV loop diuretic dose, then consider doubling the initial dose. If resistance to IV diuretic continues then consider adding a thiazide diuretic. We prefer IV chlorothiazide, 500 mg × 1, 30 minutes before infusion of a loop diuretic. IV or PO metolazone (2.5–5 mg × 1) or HCTZ 25 mg PO × 1 can also be used. Chronic oral loop diuretics should be adjusted to maintain euvolemia.

Renin-Angiotensin-Aldosterone System Inhibitors
Angiotensin-Converting Enzyme Inhibitor (ACEI)
In patients with HFrEF, ACEIs are indicated and can reduce morbidity and mortality. ACEIs are now considered a class effect in HFrEF. ACEI block the conversion of angiotensin-I to angiotensin-II, thus avoiding vasoconstriction and other direct myocardial detrimental effects of angiotensin.

Angiotensin Receptor Blocker (ARB)
In similar fashion to ACEIs, ARBs are indicated in HFrEF to reduce morbidity and mortality. ARBs block angiotensin II from binding to the AT1 receptor and avoid the vasoconstriction and other direct myocardial detrimental effects of angiotensin.

Angiotensin Receptor–Neprilysin Inhibitor (ARNI)
ARNI is a combination drug with ARB effect and added neprilysin inhibition (Sacubitril/Valsartan [Entresto]). Neprilysin is an enzyme responsible for the degradation of BNP, and by inhibiting neprilysin circulating BNP is available for further vasodilation and natriuretic effects. ARNI provided further morbidity and mortality benefit compared with ACEI. When possible, patients should be transitioned from an ACEI or ARB to an ANRI. If already on an ACEI, then an ARNI should not be taken within 36 hours of the ACEI to avoid drug interactions. ARNI can cause hypotension, renal insufficiency, and angioedema.

Aldosterone Antagonists
Aldosterone antagonists include spironolactone (Aldactone) or eplerenone (Inspra).[1] They can further reduce morbidity and mortality in HFrEF when added to a background of ACEI/ARB/ANRI and beta blocker. In HFpEF, aldosterone antagonist can be considered to decrease hospitalization. But be aware of the risk of hyperkalemia.

Sympathetic Nervous System
There are three appropriate beta blockers for HFrEF that reduce morbidity and mortality. These include metoprolol succinate (Toprol XL), carvedilol (Coreg), and bisoprolol (Zebeta).[1] When initiating a beta blocker for HFrEF, the patient should have resolution of congestive symptoms and typically will already be on ACEI/ARB/ARNI. Beta blockers are contraindicated in cardiogenic shock.

Hydralazine and Isosorbide Dinitrate Combination
Hydralazine in combination with isosorbide dinitrate is a vasodilator. Hydralazine-isosorbide dinitrate (ISDN) combination (BiDil) or hydralazine and isosorbide dinitrate as a separate combination is indicated for patients self-described as African American and with persistent significant symptoms (NHYA III-IV) while on a background of maximal tolerated ACEI/ARB/ARNI, beta blocker, and aldosterone antagonist. Hydralazine-isosorbide dinitrate combination can also beneficial in those patients that cannot tolerate an ACEI/ARB/ARNI but not as a replacement for those that are able to tolerate.

Sodium-Glucose Cotransporter-2 Inhibitors (SGLT2 Inhibitors)
SGLT2 inhibitors are a newer therapy that is an adjunctive therapy to the existing guideline-directed medical therapy (GDMT). SGLT2 inhibitors can be considered in HFrEF patients with or without diabetes and are associated with reduced cardiovascular events.

Ivabradine
Lower heart rates in HFrEF are associated with better outcomes. Ivabradine (Corlanor, Lancora) is an adjunctive medication to the existing GDMT and can further reduce heart rate. Ivabradine can be considered in HFrEF (LVEF ≤35%) for those in sinus rhythm and on maximal tolerated beta blocker dose when the resting heart rate ≥70 beats per minute.

Digoxin
Digoxin (Lanoxin) can be added as an adjunctive medication in HFrEF and is associated with reduced hospitalizations. Digoxin should be used with caution in the elderly and those with renal dysfunction.

Treatment strategies for acute decompensated heart failure based on hemodynamic profile are described in Table 5. Treatment pathways for HFrEF stage C are shown on Figure 3.

---

[1]Not FDA approved for this indication.

Device Therapies

Medicine therapy is the cornerstone of HF treatment, but there are several other therapeutic options that need to be incorporated to further improve survival and decrease symptoms in patients that have demonstrated a lack of response to initial management and through intensification of that therapy. For patients with HFrEF, device therapy including implantable cardioverter-defibrillator (ICD) and cardiac resynchronization therapy (CRT) are proven modalities that further improve survival, and referral to an electrophysiologist and/or heart failure specialist is indicated. ICD can help prevent sudden cardiac death (SCD) in patients with ischemic or nonischemic cardiomyopathies at least 40 days post-MI with LVEF of ≤35% and NYHA II or III symptoms on GDMT or NYHA I with LVEF ≤30%. CRT is indicated in patients with an LVEF of ≤35% and LBBB with persistent symptoms. Transcatheter mitral valve repair (TMVR) using MitraClip™ (Abbott, IL, USA) is another device option in HF patients that decreases mitral regurgitation severity in secondary mitral regurgitation and improves survival in persistent HF.

Therapy for HFpEF

HFpEF is a complex heterogeneous disease where the mortality and morbidity parallel that of HFrEF. Drug therapies have

TABLE 5	Acute Decompensated HF Therapies Based on the Hemodynamic Profile	
	NORMAL LVEDP	**ELEVATED LVEDP**
Normal CO	A "warm and dry" GDMT	B "warm and wet" IV diuretic GDMT
Decreased CO	L "lethal, cold, and dry" Cardiac replacement therapy (circulatory assist devices, cardiac transplant) Palliative care	C "cold and wet" IV inotropes IV diuretics

GDMT, Guideline-Directed Medical Therapy.

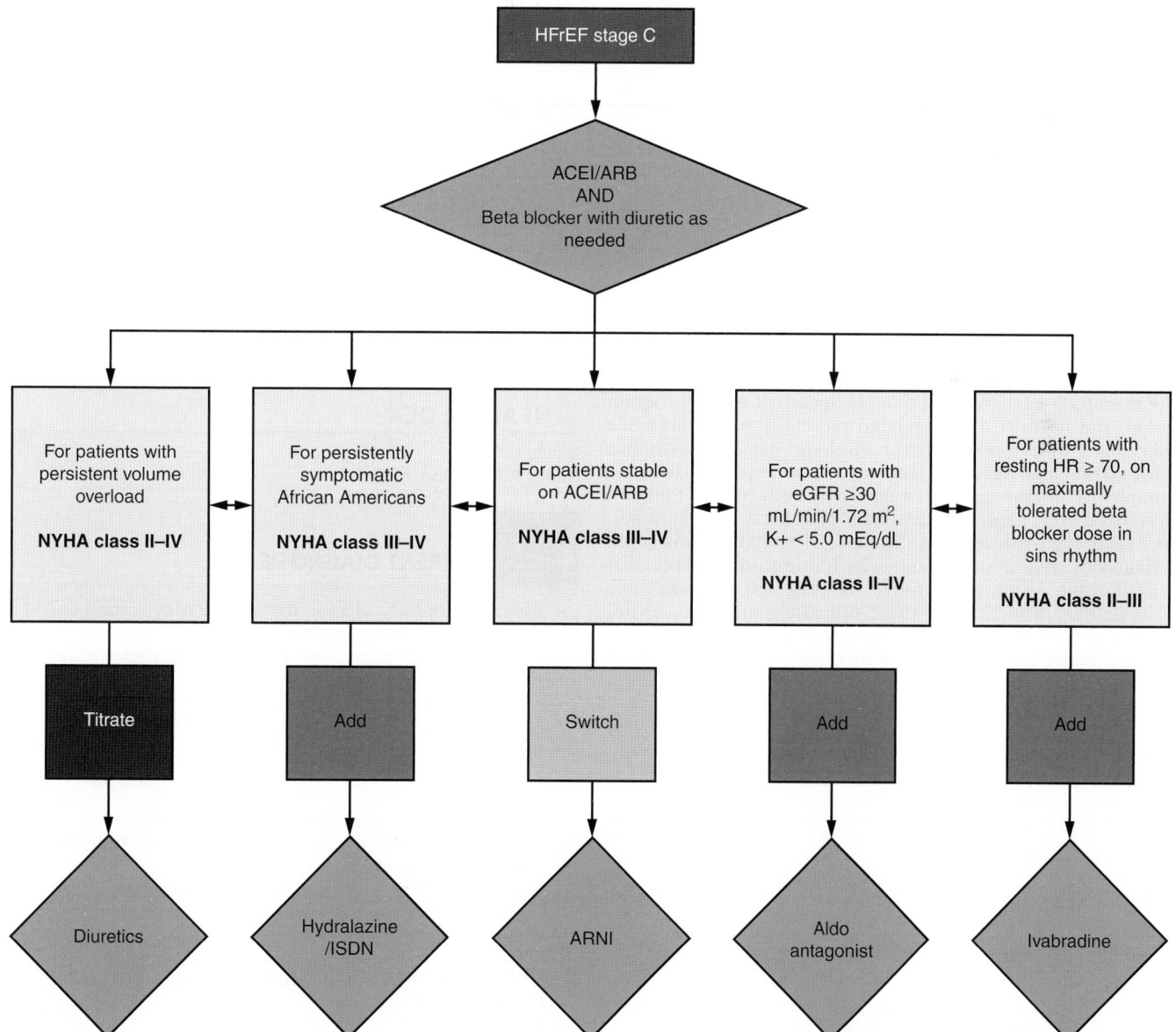

Figure 3 GDMT treatment algorithm for HFrEF stage C. Adapted from 2017 ACC Expert Consensus Decision Pathway for Optimization of Heart Failure Treatment: Answers to 10 Pivotal Issues About Heart Failure With Reduced Ejection Fraction: A Report of the American College of Cardiology Task Force on Expert Consensus Decision Pathways.

TABLE 6	I-NEED-HELP: Identifying Patients Needing Referral to an HF Specialist or an Advanced Therapy
I	Intravenous inotropes
N	New York Heart Association (NYHA) class IIIB/IV or persistently elevated Natriuretic peptides
E	End organ dysfunction
E	EF ≤35%
D	Defibrillator shocks
H	Hospitalizations ≥2
E	Edema despite escalating diuretics
L	Low systolic blood pressure (≤90), tachycardia
P	Prognostic medications; Progressive intolerance or down-titration of guideline-directed medical therapy

From Maddox, Thomas. M., et al. 2021 "Update to the 2017 ACC Expert Consensus Decision Pathway for Optimization of Heart Failure Treatment: Answers to 10 Pivotal Issues About Heart Failure With Reduced Ejection Fraction." Journal of the American College of Cardiology 77.6 (2021): 772-810.

fallen short in being able to significantly impact this disease. A few medical therapies can have impact on this disease including diuretics, which are the mainstay of therapy in relieving congestion; aldosterone antagonists have potential benefit by decreasing hospitalizations, and exercise training can be used to improve symptoms. Treatment of coexisting diseases that drive HFpEF are equally important in the management. This includes addressing coexisting systemic diseases including hypertension, diabetes, obesity, sleep apnea, ischemic heart disease, and chronic kidney disease.

Advanced Heart Failure

Stage D HF or advanced HF are those patients with symptoms at rest or with minimal exertion, recurrent hospitalizations, or refractory symptoms despite appropriate medical therapy. An important key factor in HF management is early identification of high-risk patients for consideration of advanced HF therapies. Early referral to a HF specialist or HF program is key and needs to be considered especially when there is a new onset of HF with unclear etiology, needing assistance with GDMT management, comorbid conditions that increase complexity of management, a persistent reduced LV function despite GDMT, needing referrals for possible device therapies, or having high-risk features (Table 6). These situations could potentially have a significant benefit from an HF specialist consultation. Using the acronym I NEED HELP (see Table 6) is helpful in identifying those potentially needing consideration for referral to an HF specialist for advanced therapies including transplant and mechanical circulatory support (MCS).

References

Borlaug B: Evaluation and management of heart failure with preserved ejection fraction, *Nat Rev Cardiol* 17(9):559–573, 2020.

Bozkurt B, et al: Universal definition and classification of heart failure: a report of the heart failure Society of America, heart failure association of the European Society of Cardiology, Japanese heart failure Society and Writing Committee of the universal definition of heart failure, *J Card Fail*, 2021.

Felker GM, et al: Diuretic therapy for patients with heart failure, *J Am Coll Cardiol* 75(10):1178–1195, 2020.

Maddox TM, et al: 2021 "Update to the 2017 ACC Expert Consensus Decision pathway for Optimization of heart failure treatment: answers to 10 pivotal Issues about heart failure with reduced ejection fraction," *J Am Coll Cardiol* 77(6):772–810, 2021.

McKee PA, et al: The natural history of congestive heart failure: the Framingham study, *N Engl J Med* 285(26):1441–1446, 1971.

Ponikowski P, et al: 2016 ESC Guidelines for the diagnosis and treatment of acute and chronic heart failure: the Task Force for the diagnosis and treatment of acute and chronic heart failure of the European Society of Cardiology (ESC) Developed with the special contribution of the Heart Failure Association (HFA) of the ESC, *Eur Heart J* 37(27):2129–2200, 2016.

Tsutsui H, et al: JCS 2017/JHFS 2017 guideline on diagnosis and treatment of acute and chronic heart failure—Digest version, *Circ J* 83(10):2084–2184, 2019.

Virani SS, et al: Heart disease and stroke statistics—2020 update: a report from the American Heart Association, *Circulation* 141(9):e139–e596, 2020.

Yancy CW, et al: 2013 ACCF/AHA guideline for the management of heart failure: executive summary: a report of the American College of Cardiology Foundation/American Heart Association Task Force on practice guidelines, *Circulation* 128(16):1810–1852, 2013.

Yancy CW, et al: 2017 ACC/AHA/HFSA focused update of the 2013 ACCF/AHA guideline for the management of heart failure: a report of the American College of Cardiology/American heart association Task force on clinical practice guidelines and the heart failure Society of America, *J Am Coll Cardiol* 70(6):776–803, 2017.

HEART BLOCK

Method of
Kelley P. Anderson, MD

CURRENT DIAGNOSIS

- Assess risk for heart block in the absence of symptoms or heart block on electrocardiogram (ECG).
  - Review cardiac or systemic disorders associated with cardiac conduction disease (CCD), ECG pattern, family history, maternal antibodies, cardiac interventions, and surgery.
- Evaluate documented asystole or bradycardia due to heart block.
  - Classify heart block: transient, recurrent, progressive, permanent.
  - Grade signs and symptoms: none, mild, severe.
- Evaluate signs or symptoms of possible transient heart block with no documentation.
  - Establish temporal pattern: recent versus remote onset, solitary versus recurrent, daily, weekly, monthly, yearly.
  - Grade signs and symptoms: none, mild, severe.
  - Document rhythm during symptoms: telemetry monitoring, Holter monitor, external loop recorder, implantable recorder.

- Methods of heart rate support:
  - Immediate: intravenous catecholamines, atropine, or aminophylline[1]; transcutaneous pacing
  - Short term: transvenous temporary pacing
  - Long term: permanent pacemakers
- Pacemaker configuration:
  - Number of leads: 1, 2, 3, 4
  - Lead locations: right atrial appendage, Bachman's bundle, right ventricular apex, outflow tract, left ventricle, coronary sinus
  - Programming to minimize ventricular pacing: manufacturer dependent

[1]Not FDA approved for this indication.

TABLE 1	Mechanisms of Conduction Disturbances (Examples)

- Prolonged refractory period (vagal activity, drugs, ischemia)
- Sarcolemmal ion gradient disturbances (hyperkalemia, hypokalemia)
- Sodium channel dysfunction (SCN5A mutations, sodium channel blocking drugs such as lidocaine, procainamide, flecainide [Tambocor], amiodarone [Cordarone], and imipramine [Tofranil])
- Calcium channel dysfunction (verapamil [Isoptin], diltiazem [Cardizem], mutations)
- Energy deprivation (ischemia, cyanide)
- Cell dysfunction (inflammation, barotrauma, thermal injury)
- Cell death (apoptosis, ischemic necrosis, inflammatory necrosis, surgical trauma, ablation)
- Congenital structural defects (endocardial cushion defects)
- Gap junction disturbances (fibrosis, edema, inflammation, genetic defects)
- Genetic defects (SCN5A and NKX2.5 mutations)

Heart block refers to block or delay of electrical propagation between the atria and ventricles. It is a form of cardiac conduction disease (CCD), which applies more generally to disorders of electrical impulse formation or propagation anywhere along the cardiac conduction system from the sinus node to the ventricular myocardium. Heart block or CCD may present as a syndrome, as an electrocardiographic (ECG) pattern, or as a mechanism of serious signs and symptoms such as sudden death or syncope. Pacemaker therapy is an effective treatment, but it is associated with significant short- and long-term complications. This underscores the importance of recognizing preventable and reversible causes of heart block for accurate targeting of permanent pacing. Risk stratification of patients with heart block, assessment of the benefits and risks of the therapeutic options, and patient education and guidance are largely in the domain of heart rhythm specialists. However, heart block may be encountered unexpectedly in any patient during any clinical encounter. Furthermore, some patients may require evaluation in the absence of known cardiac disease because of increased risk of CCD, or increased risk of CCD in family members or future children. A basic understanding of heart block may be useful to initiate emergency treatment and to recognize patients who warrant further evaluation or specialist referral.

Epidemiology

The prevalence and incidence of heart block are difficult to establish because they are strongly dependent on the demographic and clinical characteristics of the population sample. The prevalence is higher among the elderly and those with cardiovascular disease. First-degree heart block, defined as prolongation of the PR interval >200 ms on ECG, occurs in the population setting with prevalence of 0.7% to 2% in the young and up to 14% in the elderly. Higher degrees of heart block can be expected to be less common but similarly associated with age and underlying cardiovascular disease. In a study of the Framingham population, the prevalence of first-degree heart block was 1.6% and was associated with an incidence of pacemaker implantation of 59 per 10,000 person-years in persons with a PR interval >200 ms compared to 6 per 10,000 person-years in persons with a PR interval <200 ms. Approximately 36% of the pacemakers were for high-grade atrioventricular (AV) block.

Risk Factors

Patients with genetic or acquired CCD and patients subject to trauma or surgical procedures that can damage the conduction system are at increased risk for developing symptomatic advanced heart block. In the Framingham population, subjects with first-degree AV block had an increased risk of mortality, atrial fibrillation, and pacemaker implantation. However, the vast majority with risk factors never develop symptomatic heart block and have not been shown to benefit from intense monitoring or prophylactic pacemaker placement. The few possible exceptions are discussed below.

Pathophysiology

The function of the cardiac conduction system is to initiate and coordinate cardiac contraction to circulate blood according to physiological needs. Electrical activation is initiated by pacemaker cells of the sinus node regulated by the autonomic nervous system. Unlike conduction in common electrical circuits in which electrons flow along a conductor according to the voltage gradient, electrical activity in cardiac cells propagates from segment to segment of the cell membrane in cardiac myocytes (myocardial cells) and in specialized cardiac conduction cells. Energy-requiring ion pumps maintain an electrochemical gradient across the insulating cell membrane. Electrical activity opens voltage-sensitive ion channels causing regenerative electrical activity as ions shift along their electrochemical gradient. Electrical activity in a single cell excites several adjacent cells via gap junctions. This cascade effect makes it possible for a single cell impulse to spread rapidly throughout the myocardium to enhance synchronous contraction. This also provides a safety mechanism in that each myocardial cell can be activated by many electrical paths. In addition, specialized conduction cells exhibit automaticity (impulse formation). Although normally latent because normal activation inhibits spontaneous discharge, when the normal impulse is blocked, discharges from these subsidiary physiological pacemakers provide vital heart rate support.

Block of electrical activation can occur due to failure of any step in the process, for example, lack of metabolic energy, electrolyte imbalance, inflammatory disruption of the membrane, block of ion channels by drugs, or interference with gap junction function due to infiltration of fibrous tissue (Table 1). Because of the extensive redundancy and interconnectivity and because of the capacity to compensate for injury by electrical and anatomic remodeling, there may be extensive damage before signs or symptoms of heart block occur. Regions of the heart where there are fewer alternative paths for electrical activation, such as proximal portions of the His-Purkinje system where all conducting fibers are confined to a relatively small area, are more vulnerable to complete block. Subsidiary pacemakers sometimes fail to provide adequate rate support when heart block occurs because of pre-existing injury. If the patient survives an episode of heart block, there is a possibility for recovery due to remodeling. However, remodeling can be maladaptive and result in an adverse long-term outcome by further conduction system damage, by left ventricular dysfunction, and by bradycardia-induced ventricular tachyarrhythmias (VTAs). The mechanisms of bradycardia-induced VTAs are not known, but bradyarrhythmias precipitate torsades de pointes, a specific form of VTA, in the presence of drugs that block potassium channels, electrolyte disturbances, certain genetic abnormalities of ion channel function, heart failure, and

TABLE 2 Etiologies of Heart Block

- Frequently permanent or progressive (examples)
  - Alcohol septal ablation (acute, delayed)
  - Cardiomyopathies (hypertrophic, idiopathic, mitochondrial)
  - Catheter ablation (atrioventricular nodal reentry, accessory atrioventricular connections)
  - Congenital heart block (neonatal lupus)
  - Congenital heart disease (endocardial cushion defects)
  - Genetic disorders (SCN5A sodium channel mutations, gap junction gene mutations, fatty acid oxidation disorders, PRKAG2 mutations, LMNA gene mutations)
  - Hypertension
  - Idiopathic fibrosis and calcification (Lev's disease, Lenegre's disease)
  - Infectious disorders—destructive (endocarditis)
  - Infiltrative disorders (amyloidosis)
  - Myocardial infarction
  - Neuromyopathic disorders (myotonic dystrophy, Erb's dystrophy, peroneal muscular atrophy)
  - Noninfectious inflammatory disorders (HLA-B27–associated disorder, sarcoidosis)
  - Tumors (mesothelioma, metastatic cancer)
  - Valvular heart disease
- Frequently transient or reversible (examples)
  - Blunt trauma (baseball)
  - Cardiac surgery (valve replacement)
  - Cardiac transplant rejection
  - Central nervous system
  - Drugs (antiarrhythmics, digoxin [Lanoxin], edrophonium [Enlon])
  - Electrolyte disturbances (hyperkalemia)
  - Metabolic disturbances (hypothermia, hypothyroidism)
  - Increased vagal activity
  - Infectious disorders—nondestructive (Lyme disease)
  - Myocardial ischemia
  - Myocarditis (Chagas disease, giant cell myocarditis)
  - Rheumatic fever

myocardial hypertrophy. A comprehensive list of drugs that may account for bradyarrhythmia-related ventricular arrhythmias is available at www.torsades.org.

Although there are many potential causes of heart block, the pathophysiology is not known for the vast majority of cases because there are no tests that allow detailed structural or functional examination in patients. By the time of death, morphologic examination may reveal only nonspecific changes such as fibrosis. Instead, most etiologies are inferred by history of recent or past exposures (e.g., trauma or radiation), concomitant disorders (e.g., muscular dystrophy, cardiac sarcoidosis), abnormal test results (e.g., Lyme disease) or family history (e.g., SCN5A sodium channel mutations) (Table 2). Because most etiologies cannot be verified, the clinician must remain open to alternative explanations and accept the likelihood of multiple contributors.

Some patients, usually young, otherwise healthy individuals, present with prolonged asystole due to heart block but have no other detectable abnormalities and have excellent outcomes in the absence of intervention beyond counseling. This suggests that autonomic influences alone can cause prolonged heart block and suppression of subsidiary pacemakers. It is not known whether such responses result from an abnormality or an exaggerated normal reflex. However, the identification of such patients is important because most can be managed without pacemakers.

Prevention

Prevention of heart block is a challenge for the future. Some instances can be prevented by treatment of inflammatory disorders that cause heart block, such as Lyme disease or cardiac sarcoid. Other individuals who should be identified are those with conditions that place them, their relatives, or their unborn children at risk for heart block. This includes patients and family members with genetic disorders associated with heart block. Genetic testing and counseling may be appropriate in some patients with a family history of CCD. Neonatal lupus syndrome is a rare disorder with a high mortality rate and risk of permanent complete heart block in survivors. This occurs in pregnant women with anti-Ro/SSA or anti-La/SSB antibodies. Some such women have autoimmune disorders such as systemic lupus erythematosus and Sjögren's syndrome, but many are symptom free. Members of this group may benefit from counseling and anticipatory evaluation and treatment of offspring. Although controversial, fetal monitoring of pregnant women with anti-Ro/SSA and/or anti-La/SSB antibodies and treatment of those with signs of fetal conduction system involvement have been recommended. It should be recognized that with current methods the vast majority of heart block events cannot be predicted or prevented, and the vast majority of persons with risk factors never develop symptomatic heart block.

Clinical Manifestations

Most of the symptoms experienced by patients with heart block are common and nonspecific, including syncope, lightheadedness, fatigue, and dyspnea. Asystole or profound bradycardia may cause syncope, death, or other manifestations of hypoperfusion. Rarely, first-degree AV block results in significant symptoms (e.g., fatigue, palpitations, chest fullness), probably due to atrial contraction against a partially closed mitral valve.

Diagnosis

Because various arrhythmias and other cardiac and noncardiac disorders may be responsible for similar symptoms, it is important to identify the cause. An ECG recording of asystole or bradycardia due to heart block at the time of symptoms strongly suggests a causal relationship, but this is usually difficult to accomplish because the symptoms are often transient and infrequent. Absence of arrhythmias at the time of symptoms is also helpful in excluding heart block as the cause. Asymptomatic heart block is not infrequent. Cardiac conduction disturbances are classified by the pattern of ECG complexes. A normal 12-lead ECG lessens the probability of conduction disturbances due to structural changes but it does not eliminate the possibility of transient third-degree block due to reversible functional effects such as intense vagal activity or ischemia. Significant disease of the His bundle may be electrocardiographically silent, but more often concomitant distal disease is evident in the form of fascicular or bundle branch block or a nonspecific intraventricular conduction delay. In a patient with syncope, the presence of bifascicular block raises the possibility of transient third-degree block as the mechanism and of progression to permanent complete block. Most patients with conduction disorders are not symptomatic and do not progress to complete block. However, the combination of right bundle branch block (RBBB) and left posterior fascicle block has a greater tendency to progress to complete block than the more common RBBB and left anterior fascicle block. Nevertheless, conduction disturbances of the His-Purkinje system should not be assumed to be responsible for syncope or cardiac arrest because they are relatively common in patients with cardiovascular disorders that cause syncope or cardiac arrest due to other mechanisms. Conduction disturbances can cause dyssynchronous contraction and result in adverse remodeling. In addition, they can mask or mimic the ECG signs of myocardial infarction. Alternating bundle branch block refers to a changing ECG pattern in which both RBBB and left bundle branch block are observed or when the bifascicular block pattern switches between the anterior and posterior fascicle involvement. This pattern is considered a harbinger of complete block and warrants continuous monitoring and evaluation for permanent pacemaker implantation.

Differential Diagnosis

The challenge in second- and transient third-degree AV block is distinguishing between block in the AV node, which is often functional and reversible, and infranodal block, which often progresses to permanent complete heart block. ECG clues that block is in the AV node include normal QRS duration (<100 ms), type I

(Wenckebach) pattern, PR prolongation before blocked impulses and PR shortening after pauses, occurrence during enhanced vagal activity (e.g., sleep), narrow QRS escape complexes, and no factors favoring infranodal block. ECG clues for infranodal block include prolonged QRS duration (≥120 ms), type II pattern, and escape QRS complexes broader than intrinsic complexes. Type II second degree AV block is almost always due to block in the His-Purkinje system. Other second-degree AV block ECG patterns have poor sensitivity and specificity for site of block.

Unsustained polymorphic ventricular tachycardia is an ominous sign in any context and may result from a variety of cardiac, metabolic, and autonomic abnormalities. However, in the presence of heart block it suggests that heart rate support may be necessary to prevent sustained VTA. QT prolongation and post-pause U-wave accentuation should be sought as other harbingers of bradycardia-related VTA.

The importance and value of ECG documentation of heart block cannot be overemphasized. ECGs are subject to artifact and may be misleading when standards for acquisition and analysis are not followed. Multiple tracings of suspicious events should be obtained in multiple leads when possible. A 12-lead simultaneous rhythm recording mode is available on most modern ECG machines and should be used when continuous recordings are obtained to document arrhythmias.

Clinicians encounter heart block in three general contexts. For the patient with documented heart block, the clinician selects therapy based, in part, on whether the arrhythmia is permanent or likely to recur. There are currently no tests that provide direct information about the pathologic state of the AV conduction system. Instead, these outcomes must be inferred from functional assessment, that is, from the ECG or electrophysiological testing. Other indirect sources such as coronary angiography, magnetic resonance imaging, nuclear imaging, and myocardial biopsy, as well as a large number of specific laboratory tests, are often helpful for identifying disorders that may be causative or associated with heart block and that may affect the choice of treatment.

Another common context is the patient with symptoms for whom the objective is to verify or exclude heart block as the mechanism by correlating the cardiac rhythm with symptoms. Real-time monitoring (e.g., in-patient telemetry) is used for patients who might require immediate access to drugs or pacing devices to prevent or terminate asystole or bradycardia-dependent VTA. Holter monitoring is useful for patients who have very frequent events (at least 1 every 24 hours), and they are useful for capturing asymptomatic rhythm disturbances. External recorders are applied for a month or longer and are very helpful to associate rhythm abnormalities with symptoms and to rule out a rhythm disorder as the cause of symptoms in patients with at least one event per month. Patients with infrequent events may be candidates for implantable loop recorders, which monitor for greater than a year. Modern monitors will provide a permanent record of arrhythmias on activation by the patient or by a detection algorithm.

Electrophysiological studies allow precise measurements of AV node and His-Purkinje system function and can provide definitive information regarding the site of block if the conduction disturbance occurs during the study. Additional tests have been developed that "stress" the AV conduction system, including rapid atrial and ventricular pacing and administration of drugs such as procainamide and disopyramide (Norpace). The provocation of heart block is assumed to indicate a propensity for spontaneous AV block. Unfortunately, the sensitivity is low and a negative test does not imply a low risk of future episodes. Electrophysiological studies have the additional advantage of providing immediate test results, as well as providing the results of programmed stimulation for provocation of supraventricular and VTAs, which may be included in the differential diagnosis.

Therapy

The object of the evaluation and management for heart block is to prevent death and morbidity by (1) heart rate support in patients with poorly tolerated bradycardia; (2) monitoring and standby heart rate support in patients at high risk for asystole or severe bradycardia; (3) identifying and treating reversible causes of heart block; (4) identifying patients at high risk for sudden death, syncope, or recurrent symptoms; and (5) selecting and implanting the appropriate rate support system as soon as safety permits.

Advanced cardiac life-support guidelines apply to the patient who is unresponsive or severely compromised by heart block. However, heart block is rarely the primary problem. Therefore evaluation and treatment of other disorders should continue while efforts to obtain the appropriate heart rate are underway.

The initial evaluation should include a detailed history and physical examination and review of current and previous ECGs and rhythm strips to determine whether heart block is present or occurred in the past and whether there were symptoms or other evidence of hemodynamic compromise. Basic laboratory tests (electrolytes, metabolic panel, cardiac biomarkers, thyroid function, blood count, and coagulation studies) and basic imaging (chest x-ray and echocardiography) are usually appropriate. The patient should then be stratified for the appropriate level of care: (1) the unstable patient who requires ongoing evaluation and treatment in an intensive care setting, (2) the stable patient at high risk for asystole or complications who needs temporary transvenous pacing or other invasive procedures, (3) the patient at moderate risk who requires continuous monitoring and standby noninvasive heart rate support measures, (4) the patient at low risk who requires rapid but not immediate access to heart rate support measures that hospital monitoring provides, and (5) the patient at low risk who can be evaluated and managed as an outpatient. Additional testing and procedures may be necessary to determine the etiology of heart block and to determine whether there is a significant risk of future adverse events.

Determination of the need for long-term heart rate support, as well as other issues that may affect implantable device selection (e.g., risk for VTAs), should be accomplished as soon as possible because the risk of complications and anxiety associated with temporary heart rate support measures increases over time. Major societies have developed guidelines for implantable rhythm management devices (http://www.cardiosource.org/Science-And-Quality/Practice-Guidelines-and-Quality-Standards.aspx; http://www.escardio.org/guidelines-surveys/esc-guidelines/Pages/GuidelinesList.aspx). The reasons for the selected therapy, including the rationale for any deviation from established guidelines, should be documented and provided to the patient. This will reduce future confusion or misunderstanding about the original rationale for implantation that can affect management of patients with device complications, recalls (safety alerts), and those with a compelling need for device upgrade or explantation.

Patients with acute coronary syndromes require special consideration. The incidence of heart block in patients with myocardial infarction based on creatine phosphokinase as the marker of necrosis is approximately 10%. Although the incidence is probably lower using more sensitive markers such as troponin, heart block is still likely to be associated with increased in-hospital mortality due to larger infarct size. Tachycardia and high blood pressure increase myocardial oxygen consumption. Therefore overcorrection of heart rate and blood pressure should be avoided and ischemia should be relieved by reperfusion as soon as possible. Studies in the prethrombolytic era did not demonstrate a benefit in mortality with prophylactic temporary transvenous pacing, and complications were frequent. The risks of transvenous insertion may be higher in patients requiring administration of thrombolytics and other anticoagulants. Catheter-based revascularization methods should be given strong consideration because of established effectiveness, the possible avoidance of thrombolytic drugs, and because transvenous temporary pacing, if needed, is readily and safely accomplished during the procedure. Suggestions for standby temporary pacing (Table 3) should take into consideration the risks of transvenous pacing based on

TABLE 3 Suggestions for Temporary Pacing in Acute Myocardial Infarction

- Transvenous pacing
  - Asystole or poorly tolerated bradycardia unresponsive to atropine or aminophylline
  - Persistent third-degree AV block
  - Alternating RBBB and LBBB, or RBBB and alternating LAFB and LPFB
  - Bifascicular block, new
  - Second-degree AV block (any type) and QRS >110 ms
  - Any indication listed below at time of cardiac catheterization if performed
- Standby transcutaneous pacing
  - Any indication listed above until transvenous pacing system inserted
  - Transient asystole or poorly tolerated bradycardia
  - Bifascicular block, uncertain time of onset, or old
  - Second-degree AV block (any type) and QRS <110 ms
  - New first-degree AV block

Abbreviations: AV = atrioventricular; LAFB, LPFB=left anterior, left posterior fascicle block; LBBB, RBBB=left, right bundle branch block.

local circumstances (experience, fluoroscopic guidance, insertion site, use of anticoagulants, etc.). Most conduction disturbances associated with myocardial ischemia or infarction resolve quickly but can persist for days or weeks. The need for permanent pacemaker implantation as a consequence of myocardial infarction is rare, and prophylactic pacemaker implantation in high-risk subsets has not been shown to reduce mortality. Guidelines for temporary and permanent pacing in acute myocardial infarction have been published (http://www.cardiosource.org/Science-And-Quality/Practice-Guidelines-and-Quality-Standards.aspx; http://www.escardio.org/guidelines-surveys/esc-guidelines/Pages/GuidelinesList.aspx).

Selection of the correct therapeutic approach balances the risks and benefits of therapy against the risks of heart block for both immediate and long-term management. Catecholamines (dobutamine, dopamine, epinephrine, isoproterenol [Isuprel]) are useful for emergency, temporary, and standby heart rate support. The standby mode is accomplished by a prepared infusion at the bedside. To avoid underdoses or overdoses at the time of sudden symptomatic heart block, the optimal dose can be established in advance by test doses starting at low infusion rates. Atropine (0.5 mg every 3–5 minutes, with a maximum dose of 0.04 mg/kg or total of 3 mg) may be useful for treatment or pretreatment of patients who develop heart block at the level of the AV node in the context of elevated vagal tone (e.g., in association with nausea or endotracheal tube suction). Atropine should be avoided in patients with infranodal AV block because prolonged asystole sometimes occurs due to more frequent His-Purkinje system depolarization from increased sinus rate. Vagal activity inhibits sympathetic activity; therefore, reduction of vagal tone by atropine disinhibits sympathetic activity and may account for the unpredictable effects of atropine on heart rate. Elevations in heart rate after atropine can persist for hours and cannot be readily reversed. Aminophylline[1] (2.5–6.3 mg/kg IV) is reported to reverse heart block resistant to atropine and epinephrine by antagonizing adenosine. Stimulation of β-adrenergic receptors increases sinus node and subsidiary pacemaker rates, AV node and His-Purkinje system conduction velocities, and myocardial contractility. The effective refractory period shortens in most tissue but this effect varies with dose and specific tissue type. Dobutamine[1] (2–40 μg/kg/min) is a useful β-receptor agonist because it increases cardiac output and lowers filling pressures without excessive rise or fall of blood pressure. Dopamine[1] (2–20 μg/kg/

min IV) stimulates β1-adrenergic receptors and increases heart rate by enhancing impulse formation and conduction, as well as myocardial contractility. At higher doses (10–20 μg/kg/min) dopamine causes vasoconstriction by α1-receptor stimulation. Isoproterenol (0.02–0.06 mg IV bolus, 0.5–10.0 μg/min IV infusion) stimulates β1- and β2-adrenergic receptors and enhances vasodilation more than the other catecholamines. This can result in unwanted hypotension in some circumstances but it is also less likely to cause a reflex increase in vagal tone than drugs that cause vasoconstriction. Epinephrine (1 mg IV boluses for cardiac arrest, 0.2–1 mg subcutaneously, 0.5–10 μg/min IV) stimulates both α- and β-adrenergic receptors. It is recommended for asystolic cardiac arrest in part because it increases myocardial and cerebral flow. However, the increase of systemic vascular resistance may be detrimental by augmenting metabolic acidosis and decreasing cardiac performance in patients with poor left ventricular function. The suggested dose ranges are broad because the response to β-adrenergic stimulants such as improved AV conduction varies widely and may be affected by β-adrenergic receptor down-regulation in patients with chronic elevations in sympathetic activity such as patients with long-standing heart failure.

Temporary pacing includes primarily transcutaneous and transvenous approaches. Transthoracic, transesophageal, and transgastric approaches are rarely used. Transcutaneous pacing provides noninvasive heart rate support, as well as immediate access to countershock, but it is often so painful that most patients require sedation. For these reasons its principal uses are for short-term pacing during cardiopulmonary resuscitation and standby pacing in patients at risk for bradyarrhythmias. Capture is not achieved in some patients. Therefore users should be ready to continue mechanical cardiopulmonary support and seek alternative methods. If used in standby applications, ventricular capture should be verified in advance. Capture is often difficult to ascertain because transcutaneous stimuli cause large deflections on the ECG, and pectoral muscle stimulation can be confused with a pulse. Capture should be verified by careful ECG analysis at subthreshold and suprathreshold stimulus amplitudes and confirmed by appropriately timed femoral artery pulses, Korotkoff sounds, or arterial pressure waveforms.

Transvenous insertion of an electrode catheter is the method of choice for most patients who require temporary pacing. This approach is reliable and safe when performed by competent staff with strict aseptic technique, fluoroscopic guidance, and appropriate catheters. Small studies suggest that long-term (>5 days) temporary pacing can be accomplished with active-fixation permanent pacemaker leads attached to an external pulse generator (not approved by the US Food and Drug Administration [FDA]). Tunneling the lead may enhance stability and reduce the risk of infection.

Monitoring

Patients with high-grade or symptomatic heart block require close monitoring until the process is reversed by treatment or a pacemaker is implanted. All patients who receive pacemakers require lifelong follow-up by a trained team of physicians, nurses, and ancillary personnel using standard procedures guided by practice guidelines and manufacturer recommendations.

Complications

Catecholamines used to increase heart rate may precipitate tachyarrhythmias by electrophysiological effects mediated by adrenergic receptors or by myocardial ischemia, and they may worsen hemodynamic status. The adverse effects of catecholamines increase with duration of exposure. Ischemia and receptor-mediated electrophysiologic effects occur immediately after administration; changes in gene expression of ion channels begin as early as several hours; and long-term changes such as myocardial hypertrophy, apoptosis, and fibrosis occur

[1] Not FDA approved for this indication.

within 24 hours and may progress over much longer periods. This suggests that the duration and dose of catecholamine infusions should be minimized. Complications of temporary transvenous pacing include inadequate pacing or sensing thresholds, vascular complications, pneumothorax, myocardial perforation, infection, and dislodgment. Permanent pacemakers are highly effective, safe, and cost-effective with few contraindications. Although the complications are rarely life threatening, they should be carefully considered and acknowledged. Septicemia or endocarditis has been reported in 0.5% of patients. In patients with pacemaker-related endocarditis, the in-hospital mortality rate is reported to be over 7% with a 20-month mortality rate over 25%. The rate of significant complications has been reported to be 3.5%. About 10% of pacemakers will become infected or develop some other type of failure that may require extraction. In a recent series the rate of major complications associated with extraction was 1.4%. There is a long-term continuous risk of infection, thrombosis, and erosion. In young persons there is a periodic need to replace generators and leads. Abandoned leads block venous access and extractions are associated with significant risks. Perhaps of greater consequence is the constant inconvenience of lifelong follow-up, electromagnetic interference, and false alarms from electronic surveillance devices, as well as exclusion from important procedures, such as magnetic resonance imaging of the thorax. Conventional pacing, that is, from the right ventricular apex, is now known to be detrimental and may cause adverse ventricular remodeling, atrial fibrillation, heart failure, and premature death. Although it has been shown that patients with reduced left ventricular function are at greater risk for adverse effects, it is not known how to identify other patients at risk. Strategies for reducing the adverse effects of conventional pacing are under study, and recommendations are evolving. Because the decision for pacemaker implantation includes selection of lead configuration, lead locations, and pacing mode, patient guidance and education are complex.

Conclusions

Heart block remains a challenge because the cellular mechanisms responsible are poorly understood, prediction of symptomatic heart block (who and when) is unreliable, treatments that restore normal conduction do not exist for most conditions, and pacemaker therapy can have significant long-term adverse consequences. Fortunately, current devices and leads are much more reliable than in the past, and remote monitoring has enhanced early detection of problems and has substantially reduced the inconvenience of device monitoring. The newest generation of devices will allow many patients with pacemakers to safely undergo magnetic resonance imaging. Ongoing clinical trials will provide guidance in pacemaker configurations and programming that will minimize adverse effects. In the future, achievements in molecular biology will elucidate mechanisms and produce treatments that will relegate artificial pacemakers to museum pieces.

References

Ackerman MJ, Priori SG, Willems S, et al: HRS/EHRA expert consensus statement on the state of genetic testing for the channelopathies and cardiomyopathies, *Europace* 13:1077, 2011.

Carvalheiras G, Faria R, Braga J, et al: Fetal outcome in autoimmune diseases, *Autoimmun Rev* 11:A520, 2012.

Cheng S, Keyes MJ, Larson MG, et al: Long-term outcomes in individuals with prolonged PR interval or first-degree atrioventricular block, *JAMA* 301:2571, 2009.

Epstein AE, DiMarco JP, Ellenbogen KA, et al: ACC/AHA/HRS 2008 guidelines for device-based therapy of cardiac rhythm abnormalities, *J Am Coll Cardiol* 51:e1, 2008.

Hazinski MF, Samson R, Schexnayder S: *Handbook of emergency cardiovascular care for healthcare providers*, Dallas, TX, 2010, American Heart Association.

Smits JPP, Velkkamp MW, Wilde AAM: Mechanisms of inherited cardiac conduction disease, *Europace* 7:122, 2005.

Vardas PE, Auriccho A, Blanc JJ, et al: Guidelines for cardiac pacing and cardiac resynchronization therapy, *Eur Heart J* 28:2256, 2007.

HYPERTENSION

Method of
Timothy P. Graham, MD

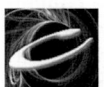

CURRENT DIAGNOSIS

- Identification of individuals with hypertension is the first step.
- Screening should begin at 18 years of age for the general population.
- Adults with risk factors should be screened annually beginning at 40 years of age.
- Stage I hypertension is established at blood pressures of 140 mm Hg systolic and 90 mm Hg diastolic.
- Stage 2 hypertension is established at blood pressures of 160 mm Hg systolic and 100 mm Hg diastolic.
- Secondary causes of hypertension should be explored and identified to optimize treatment.

CURRENT THERAPY

- Initial interventions, regardless of stage, should include lifestyle modifications, including diet and exercise.
- Optimal pharmacologic therapy should be tailored to take into account age, race, and the presence or absence of chronic kidney disease.
- For individuals 60 years of age or older, consider initiation of pharmacotherapy when systolic blood pressure is 150 mm Hg and diastolic blood pressure is 90 mm Hg.
- For individuals younger than 60 years of age but at least 18 years of age, pharmacotherapy should be initiated when systolic blood pressure is 140 mm Hg and diastolic blood pressure is 90 mm Hg.
- First-line agents for nonblack individuals should include thiazide-type diuretics, calcium channel blockers, angiotensin-converting enzyme inhibitors, or angiotensin receptor blockers.
- First-line agents for black individuals should include thiazide-type diuretics or calcium channel blockers.
- Individuals with chronic kidney disease should have therapy that includes angiotensin-converting enzyme inhibitors or angiotensin receptor blockers.

Epidemiology

Hypertension is one of the most common conditions encountered in primary care offices. The AHA/ACC definition of hypertension affects 45% of adults in the United States, which represents approximately 108 million people (cdc.gov). The most commonly affected individuals are black adults, making up 44% of the total.

In the pediatric population the prevalence of hypertension in the United States is between 1% and 5%, with obese children having the highest prevalence at 11%.

Risk Factors

Diet and Sodium Intake

Diet is a clear target for nonpharmacologic management of hypertension. Diets that are high in sodium and fat can put individuals at risk for suboptimal blood pressure control. Limiting sodium to less than 2400 mg per day confers some health benefit to individuals at risk for hypertension. Limiting even further to 1500 mg or less is more ideal and results in a significant improvement in both systolic and diastolic blood pressure typically. Additionally, putting limits on the consumption of sweets, red meat, and soda, as well as other sugar-sweetened beverages, can help weight reduction and overall health.

Sedentary Lifestyle and Obesity

Lack of physical activity is another important risk factor contributing to poor overall health and obesity. Current recommendations endorse engaging in at least 150 minutes of moderate-intensity activity per week. If patients are unable or unwilling to commit to that level of physical activity, then encouraging any physical activity is prudent, as it will convey at least some health benefit. Participation in physical activity results in absolute reduction in chronic comorbidities including hypertension, stroke, heart disease, diabetes, and metabolic syndrome. Resultant weight loss also results in significant improvement in blood pressure. It is noted that a weight loss of 22 pounds has the potential to reduce systolic blood pressure by 5 to 20 mm Hg.

For children and adolescents, elevated body mass index is the greatest risk factor for the development of hypertension.

Alcohol Intake

Although moderate alcohol intake is thought to actually reduce cardiovascular risk, heavier consumption is a risk factor for hypertension. Limiting alcohol intake to no more than two drinks per day (with "drink" defined as 12 oz. of beer, 5 oz. of wine, or 1 oz. of liquor) for men and no more than one drink per day for women (or lightweight men) is beneficial for overall health.

Smoking

Along with the myriad other reasons that smoking is not a good choice (cancer risk, chronic obstructive pulmonary disease, stroke, coronary artery disease, etc.), it is also a risk factor for hypertension. This is believed to be at least in part due to a resultant increase in sympathetic nervous system activity, which leads to an increase in myocardial oxygen demand. Additionally, smoking is the leading modifiable cause of death in the United States.

Sleep Apnea

Obstructive sleep apnea is a well-known secondary cause of and independent risk factor for hypertension. Statistically, at least half of individuals with sleep apnea also have hypertension.

Age

Age is a nonmodifiable risk factor for cardiovascular disease. Risk is higher in men 55 years of age or older and women 65 years of age or older.

Gender

Gender is another nonmodifiable risk factor. Men are at greater risk for hypertension prior to age 45. After age 45 and until age 64, the risk for men and women is approximately equivalent. At 65 years of age or older, women have a higher hypertensive risk than men.

Race

Black individuals have a higher risk of hypertension than non-black individuals. Statistics from 2015 demonstrated that in the general population aged 18 and older, approximately 34% of black individuals had hypertension, compared to approximately 24% of white individuals. Native Americans had a slightly higher risk than white individuals at 28%, and Asians had the lowest prevalence at approximately 20%. Hispanic/Latino individuals had a slightly lower prevalence than white individuals at 23%.

Family History

Family history is another nonmodifiable risk factor for cardiovascular disease. Individuals with family history of premature cardiovascular disease (men younger than 45 years of age and women younger than 55 years of age) are at increased risk themselves.

Pathophysiology

The pathophysiology of hypertension is a matter of debate. Essential hypertension, which is defined as hypertension without a clear secondary cause, makes up the majority of cases. Two primary mechanisms have been proposed for essential hypertension: neurogenic and renogenic (or nephrogenic). The neurogenic model suggests that hypertension is the result of a chronic increase in sympathetic nervous system activity. This is in contrast to the renogenic model, which attributes blood pressure increase to renal origins either through decreased renal blood flow or through renal parenchymal disease.

Prevention

Prevention of hypertension involves optimization of modifiable risk factors. Maintaining a healthy body weight, avoiding smoking, and moderating alcohol use are all key factors in minimizing risk. Additionally, engaging in regular, moderate-intensity cardiovascular exercise and eating a healthy diet without excessive sodium or fat can help significantly reduce cardiovascular risk and optimize health. These risk factors were discussed in detail in the preceding section.

Clinical Manifestations

Hypertension may have very few symptoms or none at all. If symptoms are present, they can include headaches, visual changes, dizziness, nausea, or chest pain. Oftentimes, however, there are no symptoms, and individuals can function for years without being diagnosed.

Diagnosis
Screening

As noted previously, hypertension is oftentimes an asymptomatic condition. As such, screening plays a critical role in early detection to minimize the end-organ damage that could result from untreated, long-standing hypertension. The U.S. Preventative Services Task Force (USPSTF) recommends screening for hypertension in adults who are 18 years or older (grade A recommendation). Adults 40 years and older and those with increased risk of hypertension should be screened annually. A review of the existing evidence demonstrated minimal harm in screening and a significant resultant benefit in the form of a reduction in cardiovascular events. Adults 18 to 39 years of age with no additional risk factors should be screened every 3 to 5 years. Recommended screening techniques include measurement of blood pressure in the office setting with either a manual or automatic cuff and ambulatory or home blood pressure measurement. Office measurement should be done with the patient seated and after at least 5 minutes of the patient arriving in the room. Home measurement may be beneficial after the initial screening for confirmation purposes.

For children and adolescents, the USPSTF indicates that the current evidence is insufficient to assess the risk versus benefit of screening in asymptomatic individuals (grade I evidence). The predictive value of childhood hypertension for adult hypertension is modest, with a risk for false-positive readings.

Clinical Diagnosis

Hypertension is classified in two stages based on degree of elevation. In stage 1 hypertension, systolic blood pressure is greater than or equal to 140 mm Hg to 159 mm Hg and diastolic blood pressure is greater than or equal to 90 mm Hg to 99 mm Hg. Stage 2 hypertension is reached when systolic blood pressure is 160 mm Hg or greater and diastolic blood pressure is 100 mm Hg or greater. This classification is important as the approach to treatment differs for each category, as will be discussed later.

Primary (Essential) Hypertension

Primary hypertension encompasses persistent blood pressure elevation without a discernable cause (idiopathic or of unknown cause). The majority of cases of hypertension will have no discernable cause and fall into this category.

Secondary Hypertension

Secondary hypertension is persistent blood pressure elevation that is the result of some other underlying cause. About 10% of all cases of hypertension will fall into this category. If another cause can be identified, in many cases it may be correctable.

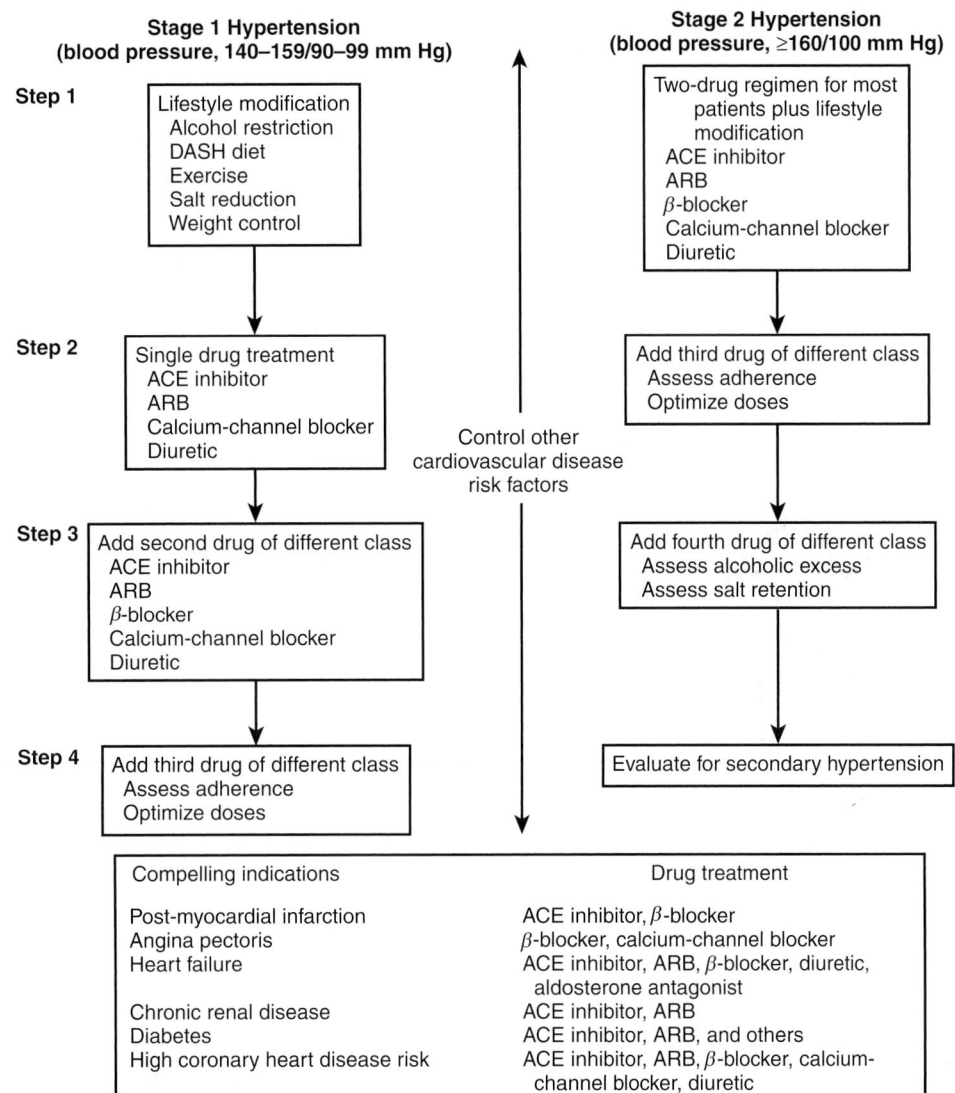

Figure 1 Algorithm for management of hypertension. *Abbreviations*: ACE = angiotensin-converting enzyme; ARB = angiotensin receptor blocker; DASH = dietary approaches to stop hypertension. (Reprinted with permission from Chobanian AV. Shattuck Lecture. The hypertension paradox— More uncontrolled disease despite improved therapy. *N Engl J Med* 2009;361:878–887.)

Looking for Secondary Causes

Identifying these underlying causes can be a challenge. Using a systematic method of investigating potential etiologies can simplify this process and improve the chances of identifying a source that with treatment can improve outcomes. One such approach is the *ABCDE* mnemonic. The A in this mnemonic stands for *accuracy* (making sure the reading is correct—such as checking the cuff for appropriate sizing and measurement technique—and repeating readings that are obtained on automatic cuffs manually), *apnea* (considering the presence of obstructive sleep apnea, which is a known contributor to difficult-to-control hypertension), and *aldosteronism* (investigating for the presence of primary hyperaldosteronism through urinary potassium excretion and an elevation in plasma aldosterone level to plasma renin activity). B stands for *bruits* (looking for renovascular sources of hypertension/renal artery stenosis, which would often present with renal bruits upon auscultation) and *bad kidneys* (hypertension resulting from renal parenchymal disease). C stands for *catecholamines* (elevation that can contribute to "white coat" hypertension, as well as overproduction with pheochromocytoma or associated with other conditions such as obstructive sleep apnea and acute stress reactions), *coarctation* (of the aorta), and *Cushing syndrome* (with mineralocorticoid effects of excess glucocorticoids in this setting). D represents both *drugs* (including nonsteroidal anti-inflammatory drugs, decongestants, estrogens, and immunosuppressive agents, as well as nicotine and alcohol) and *diet* (particularly

excess sodium intake). The final letter in the mnemonic, E, stands for *erythropoietin* (high endogenous levels—such as in chronic obstructive pulmonary disease—or exogenous levels) and *endocrine disorders* (hypothyroidism or hyperparathyroidism). Utilizing a methodical and organized approach to considering potential causes of hypertension can assist with maximizing the chances of optimally controlling blood pressure.

Differential Diagnosis

The differential diagnosis for hypertension coincides with the array of potential secondary causes that were noted earlier (see Looking for Secondary Causes section). It is important to rule out potentially treatable secondary causes in the initial phases of hypertension management.

Treatment Approaches

Approaching treatment of a patient with hypertension can be challenging. Many factors need to be considered when making these decisions, including reflection on patient age, race, gender, and comorbidities. Each of these factors can influence what the optimal treatment strategy might be. Figure 1 provides a stepwise strategy to blood pressure management.

Initial treatment should always include lifestyle modification as discussed previously, and this modification needs to be continued throughout the remainder of any management strategies.

TABLE 1	Effect of Lifestyle and Diet Modifications on Systolic Blood Pressure		
MODIFICATION	**AMOUNT**	**REDUCTION IN SBP (MM HG)**	
Dietary sodium restriction	< 30–50 mmol/d	2–8	
Moderation of daily alcohol intake	150–200 mL	2–4	
Increased physical activity	30 min 3 × per wk	4–9	
Reduction in body weight	10 kg or 22 lb	5–10	
Adoption of DASH eating plan (high potassium)		8–14	

Abbreviations: DASH = dietary approaches to stop hypertension; SBP = systolic blood pressure.

JNC-8 Guidelines

In 2014, the Eighth Joint National Committee (JNC 8) released recommendations regarding the treatment of hypertension. These guidelines were a divergence from the prior JNC 7 recommendations, effectively loosening the goals and the levels at which treatment is initiated. The following is a summary of the eight treatment recommendations from JNC 8. (Please note that the strength of recommendation that is referenced corresponds to the following: grade A—strong recommendation based on evidence; grade B—moderate recommendation based on evidence; grade C—weak recommendation with moderate certainty of a small benefit; grade D—recommendation against; grade E—expert opinion with insufficient or conflicting evidence; grade N—no recommendation for or against).

Recommendation 1

Individuals aged 60 years or older in the general population should have pharmacologic treatment initiated at a systolic blood pressure level of 150 mm Hg or a diastolic blood pressure of 90 mm Hg with treatment goals of less than 150 mm Hg systolic and less than 90 mm Hg diastolic. (Strength of recommendation: grade A.)

An additional aspect of this recommendation is that if the pharmacologic treatment results in adequate blood pressure reduction and there is no adverse effect on quality of life or patient health, then the treatment can be continued without alteration. (Strength of recommendation: grade E.)

Recommendation 2

Individuals younger than 60 years in the general population should have pharmacologic treatment initiated at a diastolic blood pressure of 90 mm Hg with a treatment goal of less than 90 mm Hg. (Strength of recommendation: grade A for ages 30–59 years, grade E for ages 18–29 years.)

Recommendation 3

Individuals younger than 60 years in the general population should have pharmacologic treatment initiated at a systolic blood pressure of 140 mm Hg with a treatment goal of less than 140 mm Hg. (Strength of recommendation: grade E.)

Recommendation 4

Individuals aged 18 years or older with chronic kidney disease should have pharmacologic treatment initiated at a systolic blood pressure of 140 mm Hg or a diastolic blood pressure of 90 mm Hg with a treatment goal of less than 140 mm Hg systolic and less than 90 mm Hg diastolic. (Strength of recommendation: grade E.)

Recommendation 5

Individuals older than 18 years with diabetes should have pharmacologic treatment initiated at a systolic blood pressure of 140 mm Hg or a diastolic blood pressure of 90 mm Hg with a treatment goal of less than 140 mm Hg systolic and less than 90 mm Hg diastolic. (Strength of recommendation: grade E.)

Recommendation 6

The treatment of nonblack individuals in the general population (including those with diabetes) who require pharmacologic treatment should include thiazide-type diuretics, calcium channel blockers, angiotensin-converting enzyme inhibitors, or angiotensin receptor blockers. (Strength of recommendation: grade B.)

Recommendation 7

The treatment of black individuals (including those with diabetes) should include thiazide-type diuretics or calcium channel blockers. (Strength of recommendation: grade B for general population, grade C for patients with diabetes.)

Recommendation 8

The treatment of individuals older than 18 years with chronic kidney disease should include, either as initial or add-on treatment, angiotensin-converting enzyme inhibitors or angiotensin receptor blockers to improve renal outcomes. (Strength of recommendation: grade B.)

Recommendation 9

The goal of hypertension treatment is to reach and maintain blood pressure goals consistent with the previous recommendations. If goals are not reached within a month of starting pharmacologic treatment, the dose of the initial agent should be increased or a second agent from recommendation 6 should be added. Blood pressure should continue to be assessed until the goal blood pressure is achieved. If blood pressure goals are not achieved with two agents, a third agent should be added.
- Angiotensin-converting enzyme inhibitors (ACEIs) and angiotensin receptor blockers (ARBs) should not be used together.
- If necessary, other classes of agents can be used if more than three agents are required or if there are contraindications to the agents in recommendation 6.
- Referral to a hypertension specialist should be considered for patients whose blood pressure goals cannot be met with the previous strategies or who are more complicated. Strength of recommendation: grade E.

ACC/AHA 2017 Hypertension Guidelines

In late 2017, the American College of Cardiology and the American Heart Association released an updated Hypertension Guideline. This guideline provided a different approach to hypertension management, particularly around blood pressure goals. Hypertension stages have tighter cut points than under the JNC-8 Guidelines. Under the ACC/AHA Guidelines, normal blood pressure is defined as less than 120/80. Blood pressure is considered elevated when systolic blood pressure is in the 120–129 mm Hg range and when diastolic remains under 80 mm Hg. Stage 1 hypertension is defined as systolic blood pressure between 130 and 139 mm Hg and a diastolic blood pressure between 80 and 90 mm Hg. Stage 2 hypertension is defined as blood pressures that are greater than 140/90. This classification is a deviation from the set points within the JNC-8 recommendations.

Nonpharmacologic

For stage I hypertension (140–159/90–99 mm Hg), the first treatment step is to aggressively modify lifestyle. This includes targeting both diet and exercise. These nonpharmacologic strategies should continue even if pharmacologic treatment is found to be necessary. The relative effects of lifestyle modification on blood pressure reduction are noted in Table 1. ACC/AHA Guidelines also recommend lifestyle changes as initial intervention for individuals with stage 1 hypertension without other cardiovascular risk factors and with a ASCVD risk of less than 10%; however, as noted above, the definition of stage 1 hypertension is at a lower blood pressure level (130-139/80-90 mm Hg.)

Diet

Dietary modifications include salt restriction to a level of less than 2400 mg per day but ideally less than 1500 mg per day. Suggested dietary interventions also include the use of the DASH (dietary approaches to stop hypertension) framework. This nutritional framework includes recommendations such as increased consumption of fruits and vegetables, preferential use of complex carbohydrates, and consumption of low-fat dairy products. The DASH diet emphasizes the intake of whole grains, fish, poultry, legumes, nuts, and nontropical vegetable oils. This diet also endorses decreasing higher-fat foods.

Exercise

Current exercise recommendations suggest that engaging in a minimum of 150 minutes of moderate-intensity exercise on a weekly basis confers the greatest health benefits. Exercise at this level of intensity reduces the risk of multiple chronic conditions including cardiovascular disease and type 2 diabetes, as well as overall all-cause mortality.

Other Lifestyle Modifications

In addition to diet and exercise, other lifestyle interventions can optimize health. Smoking cessation is an important modifiable risk factor and is the single leading cause of preventable death in the United States. Smoking increases the risk of cardiovascular morbidity and mortality, including myocardial infarction.

Alcohol consumption is another important lifestyle modification that can have a significant impact on overall health. The effects of alcohol consumption, unlike smoking, depend on quantity. It has been shown that at moderate levels of consumption, alcohol can actually decrease blood pressure (defined as no more than two drinks per day for males and no more than one drink per day for females). However, when consumed in greater quantity, alcohol can increase blood pressure, contributing to hypertension. It is emphasized that alcohol consumption should not be promoted in nondrinkers simply for the purpose of decreasing blood pressure.

Stress reduction is another lifestyle change that can have effects on blood pressure control. The mechanism of this reduction is not clear, but it is hypothesized that it may be related to decreasing autonomic nervous system output. Studies suggest that activities such as transcendental meditation can lead to modest blood pressure reduction. As such, inclusion of these activities in patient treatment plans may provide additional nonpharmacologic options.

Patients frequently ask about the utility of dietary supplements or other natural alternatives for blood pressure management. There is some evidence for select supplements in the management of hypertension, although such effects appear to be small. Examples of natural substances that may convey a small benefit include garlic and cocoa. Evidence is lacking for other agents including vitamin C, coenzyme Q10, omega-3 fatty acids, and magnesium.

Pharmacologic

In cases where hypertension is more significant or nonpharmacologic methods have failed to adequately reduce blood pressure, initiation of medications is indicated (Table 2). The selection of an agent or agents is based on a number of factors including race and comorbidities. As noted earlier, JNC 8 provides a stepwise, evidence-based approach to blood pressure management including recommended cut points where pharmacologic intervention is appropriate.

One of the points of emphasis of JNC 8 is that the point of intervention for individuals age 60 years or older is higher than those younger than that age. One should also balance the side effects or risks of medications with the benefits of intervention in this age group. The cut points for individuals with chronic kidney disease and diabetes do not differ from the general population. The choice of agent according to JNC 8 does not differ based on the presence or absence of diabetes, but does differ based on race (see recommendations 6 and 7 earlier). Individuals with chronic kidney disease also should have an ACEI or an ARB included in their treatment regimen (either as a lone agent or an add-on). In practice, decisions will need to be tailored to individual patient needs and also should consider other factors including whether or not the patient is a reproductive-age female (as ACEIs and ARBs are contraindicated in pregnancy). This is where our role as family physicians becomes increasingly important—embracing our ability to look at the whole patient when making treatment decisions.

ACC/AHA recommends the initiation of pharmacologic therapy in adults with high cardiovascular risk or preexisting cardiovascular disease and stage 1 or greater hypertension. Patients with both diabetes and hypertension are also assumed to fall into the high-risk category. Again, the defined level of blood pressure classified as stage 1 hypertension under ACC/AHA (130–139/80–90 mmHg) is lower than the JNC8 criteria as noted above. ACC/AHA also emphasizes the need to balance comorbidities as well as preferences, life expectancy, and clinical judgment when making decisions regarding antihypertensive initiation and titration in older individuals (65 or older).

A recent trial (Hygia Chronotherapy Trial) published in 2019 investigated whether timing of antihypertensive medication administration affected blood pressure control and overall outcomes. The study demonstrated that for patients on one or more antihypertensive medications, administration of at least one agent at bedtime rather than upon awakening resulted in better ambulatory blood pressure readings as well as an overall decrease in cardiovascular disease-related events. The results of this study are strongly suggestive that prioritizing bedtime dosing of antihypertensive agents for hypertensive patients leads to greater net benefit.

Monitoring

Clinical practice guidelines vary in their recommendations regarding optimal monitoring. It is clear that monitoring in the early stage or during periods of treatment change should be more frequent than during times of stability, somewhere between monthly and every 6 weeks. Once the patient is stabilized, periodic monitoring can occur either every 3 to 6 months for everyone or in a more risk-stratified manner, with lower-risk patients being seen every 6 months and higher-risk patients every 3 months.

JNC 8 recommendations, as previously discussed, suggest that patients with hypertension be monitored on at least a monthly basis until goal blood pressure is achieved, with any necessary adjustments being made at these visits.

Complications

Hypertension is often referred to as "the silent killer." This menacing name refers to the fact that this condition often presents without any discernable symptoms, which at times can make treatment compliance challenging. One of the greatest concerns with uncontrolled hypertension is the risk of end-organ damage, which is far-reaching.

Uncontrolled hypertension can lead to serious complications including myocardial infarction, stroke, peripheral artery disease, retinopathy, and renal failure. Given that hypertension is at the same time the most common condition we treat as primary care physicians, the opportunities to circumvent these sources of morbidity and mortality present themselves on a daily basis.

TABLE 2 Antihypertensive Classes

Diuretics

GENERIC	BRAND NAME	CLASSIFICATION	MECHANISM OF ACTION	DOSING
Chlorthalidone	Thalitone	Thiazide	Inhibits sodium and chloride reabsorption in distal tubules	25 mg by mouth once daily. May increase to maximum of 100 mg once daily.
Hydrochlorothiazide	Microzide	Thiazide	Inhibits sodium and chloride reabsorption in distal tubules	25 mg by mouth once daily to maximum of 50 mg in single or divided doses.
Metolazone	Zaroxolyn	Thiazide	Inhibits sodium and chloride reabsorption in distal tubules	5–20 mg by mouth once daily.
Triamterene/ hydrochlorothiazide	Dyazide	Potassium-sparing/ thiazide	Inhibits sodium reabsorption in the distal tubules	1–2 capsules by mouth once daily (37.5/25 mg capsules).
Furosemide	Lasix	Loop	Inhibits sodium and chloride reabsorption in the ascending loop of Henle	40 mg twice daily by mouth initially.
Torsemide	Demadex	Loop	Inhibits sodium and chloride reabsorption in the ascending loop of Henle	5 mg once daily by mouth initially. May increase to 10 mg once daily.

Angiotensin-Converting Enzyme (ACE) Inhibitors

Mechanism of action: Suppress the renin-angiotensin-aldosterone system

GENERIC	BRAND NAME	CLASSIFICATION	SPECIAL NOTE	DOSING
Fosinopril	Monopril	ACE inhibitor	Only ACE excreted by both renal and hepatic routes	5 mg by mouth daily initially. May be increased to 40 mg daily.
Captopril	Capoten	ACE inhibitor		Take 1 hour before meals. 25 mg two to three times daily by mouth. May increase to 50 mg two to three times daily by mouth. Maximum 450 mg per day.
Ramipril	Altace	ACE inhibitor		2.5 mg once daily by mouth. May increase to maximum of 20 mg once daily by mouth.
Enalapril	Vasotec	ACE inhibitor		5 mg daily by mouth initially. Typical dose range is 10–40 mg by mouth daily (may be divided doses).
Lisinopril	Prinivil, Zestril	ACE inhibitor		10 mg by mouth daily initial dose. Usual dose range 10–40 mg daily. Doses above 40 mg are not shown to have greater effect.
Quinapril	Accupril	ACE inhibitor		10–20 mg daily by mouth initial dose.

Angiotensin II Receptor Blockers (ARBs)

Mechanism of action: Block binding of angiotensin II to angiotensin I receptors with a resultant inhibition of angiotensin II–mediated vasoconstriction, sodium retention, and release of aldosterone

GENERIC	BRAND NAME	CLASSIFICATION	SPECIAL NOTE	DOSING
Losartan	Cozaar	ARB		50 mg daily by mouth initial dose (25 mg initial dose if also on diuretics). Titrate to a maximum of 100 mg daily.
Valsartan	Diovan	ARB	Adding a diuretic has greater effect than dose increases over 80 mg daily.	80–160 mg daily by mouth initial dose. May titrate to a maximum dose of 320 mg daily.
Olmesartan	Benicar	ARB		20 mg daily by mouth initial dose. May be titrated to 40 mg daily.
Eprosartan	Teveten	ARB		600 mg daily by mouth initial dose. May increase to 800 mg daily maximum dose. Usual range 400–800 mg daily.
Azilsartan	Edarbi	ARB		80 mg once daily by mouth. If on diuretics start at 40 mg once daily.

Beta-Blockers

GENERIC	BRAND NAME	CLASSIFICATION	MECHANISM OF ACTION	DOSING
Atenolol	Tenormin	Beta-1 selective		50 mg once daily by mouth. May increase to maximum of 100 mg once daily

Continued

TABLE 2 Antihypertensive Classes—cont'd

GENERIC	BRAND NAME	CLASSIFICATION	MECHANISM OF ACTION	DOSING
Metoprolol	Lopressor, Toprol XL	Beta-1 selective		Immediate-release formulations: 50–100 mg in single or divided doses. Maximum 450 mg per day.
				Extended-release formulations: 25–100 mg daily in a single dose. Maximum 400 mg per day.
Propranolol	Inderal LA, InnoPran XL	Beta-1 noncardioselective		Immediate-release formulations: 40 mg by mouth twice daily initial dose. Typical dosing 120–240 mg daily. Maximum 640 mg daily. Extended-release formulations: 80 mg once daily initial dose.
				Extended-release formulations: 80 mg once daily initial dose.
Bisoprolol	Zebeta	Beta-1 selective	More beta-1 specific than other beta-blockers	5 mg by mouth once daily initial dose (2.5 mg if patient has bronchospastic disease—i.e., asthma, chronic obstructive pulmonary disease). May titrate to a maximum of 20 mg per day.
Timolol		Beta-1 noncardioselective	CAUTION: Avoid abrupt discontinuation as may exacerbate ischemic heart disease.	10 mg twice daily by mouth initially. May titrate to a maximum of 60 mg per day in divided doses.
Labetalol	Trandate	Alpha and beta antagonist		100 mg twice daily by mouth (initial dose). May titrate in 2–3 days by 100 mg twice-daily increments. Maximum dose 2400 mg per day.

Calcium Channel Blockers

GENERIC	BRAND NAME	CLASSIFICATION	MECHANISM OF ACTION	DOSING
Nifedipine, extended release	Adalat CC, Procardia XL	Dihydropyridine	Binds to L-type calcium channels in sinoatrial (SA) and atrioventricular (AV) node, as well as myocardium and vasculature	30–60 mg by mouth once daily. Maximum 120 mg daily.
Diltiazem, extended release	Cardizem CD, Cardizem LA, Cartia XT, Dilacor XR	Nondihydropyridine	Binds to L-type calcium channels in SA and AV node (primarily), as well as myocardium and vasculature	180–240 mg by mouth per day initially. May titrate after 14 days. Maintenance dosing typically 180–420 mg daily. Maximum dose 480 mg per day.
Verapamil	Calan, Calan SR	Nondihydropyridine	Binds to L-type calcium channels in SA and AV node, as well as myocardium and vasculature	80 mg by mouth every 8 hours initially. Usual dose range: 240–480 mg per day.
Amlodipine	Norvasc	Dihydropyridine	Binds to L-type calcium channels in smooth muscle (vasculature)	5 mg by mouth daily (initially). May increase by 2.5 mg every 1–2 weeks. Maximum 10 mg per day.
Felodipine	Plendil	Dihydropyridine	Binds to L-type calcium channels in smooth muscle (vasculature)	2.5–5 mg by mouth once daily initially. May increase to a maximum of 20 mg by mouth once daily.*

Aldosterone Antagonists

GENERIC	BRAND NAME	CLASSIFICATION	MECHANISM OF ACTION	DOSING
Spironolactone	Aldactone	Selective aldosterone antagonist	Competes with aldosterone receptor sites. Reduces sodium reabsorption	25–100 mg by mouth once daily or divided twice daily (if being used for more than 2 weeks).
Eplerenone	Inspra	Selective aldosterone antagonist	Competes with aldosterone receptor sites. Reduces sodium reabsorption	50 mg by mouth once daily initially. May increase to twice daily if needed. (May cause hyperkalemia if doses exceed 100 mg per day.)

TABLE 2 Antihypertensive Classes—cont'd

Alpha-2 Agonists

Mechanism of action: Stimulate presynaptic aldosterone receptors, decreasing sympathetic nervous activity

GENERIC	BRAND NAME	CLASSIFICATION	MECHANISM OF ACTION	DOSING
Clonidine	Catapres, Catapres-TTS	Centrally acting alpha-2 agonist	Stimulation of alpha-2 adrenoreceptors, reducing sympathetic nervous system output	0.1 mg every 12 hours by mouth. Maximum 2.4 mg per 24 hours. (Usual dose range 0.1–0.2 mg every 12 hours.) If using transdermal formulation, 0.1 mg patch applied once every 7 days. May increase by 0.1 mg to maximum of 0.3 mg per week.
Methyldopa		Centrally acting alpha-2 agonist	Directly affects peripheral sympathetic nerves through stimulation of central alpha-adrenergic receptors	250 mg by mouth every 8–12 hours initially then can increase every 2 days. (Maximum 3 g per day.) Typical maintenance dose is 250–1000 mg by mouth divided every 6–12 hours.

Alpha Blockers

Mechanism of action: Selectively block postsynaptic alpha-1 adrenergic receptors

GENERIC	BRAND NAME	CLASSIFICATION	MECHANISM OF ACTION	DOSING
Prazosin	Minipress	Alpha-1 blocker	Competitive antagonist, reduces vascular resistance	1 mg by mouth every 8–12 hours (initial). Maintenance dose typically 6–15 mg divided every 6–8 hours. Typical maximum 20 mg per day in divided doses (although may increase to 40 mg per day in divided doses in some patients).
Terazosin	Hytrin		Selective competitive inhibitor, decreases vascular resistance	1 mg by mouth at bedtime (initial). Typical maintenance 1–5 mg daily or in divided dose every 12 hours. Maximum 20 mg per day.
Doxazosin	Cardura		Selective postsynaptic alpha-1 receptor inhibitor, vasodilation	1 mg once daily initially, titrate to maximum of 16 mg/day.

*Exceeds dosage recommended by the manufacturer.
Adapted from Medscape. Hypertension Medication. Available at: http://www.emedicine.medscape.com/article/241381-medication. Accessed May 5, 2017.

III Cardiovascular System

130

References

Al-Ansary L, et al: A systematic review of recent clinical practice guidelines on the diagnosis, assessment and management of hypertension, *PLOS One* 8(1):1–18, 2013.

Bie P, Evans R: Normotension, hypertension and body fluid regulation: brain and kidney, *Acta Physio* 219:288–304, 2017.

Carey, et al: Prevention, detection, evaluation, and management of high blood pressure in adults: synopsis of the 2017 American College of Cardiology/American Heart Association Hypertension Guideline, *Ann Intern Med* 168(5):351–358, 2018.

Chobanian AV: Guidelines for the management of hypertension, *Med Clin N Am* 101:219–227, 2017.

Garjon J, et al: First-line combination therapy versus firstline monotherapy for primary hypertension (review), *Cochrane Database Syst Rev* 1:CD10316, 2017.

Hermida RC, Crespo JJ, Domínguez-Sardiña M, et al; Hygia Project Investigators: Bedtime hypertension treatment improves cardiovascular risk reduction: the Hygia Chronotherapy Trial, *Eur Heart J* 2019 Oct 22:ehz754. Online ahead of print.

James P, Oparil S, Carter BL, et al: Evidence-based guideline for the management of high blood pressure in adults: report from the panel members appointed to the Eight Joint National Committee (JNC 8h), *JAMA* 311(5):507–520, 2014.

Kallioinen A, Hill A, Horswill MS, et al: Sources of inaccuracy in the measurement of adult patients' resting blood pressure in clinical settings: a systematic review, *J Hypertension* 35:421–441, 2017.

Langan R, Jones K: Common questions about the initial management of hypertension, *Am Fam Physician* 91(3):172–176, 2015.

Leeman L, et al: Hypertensive disorders of pregnancy, *Am Fam Physician* 93(2):121–127, 2016.

Mann S: Redefining beta-blocker use in hypertension: selecting the right beta-blocker and the right patient, *J Am Soc Hypertens* 1–12, 2016.

Onusko E: Diagnosing secondary hypertension, *Am Fam Physician* 67(1):67–74, 2003.

Oza R, Garcellano M: Nonpharmacologic management of hypertension: what works? *Am Fam Physician* 91(11):772–776, 2015.

Quyen N: Screening for high blood pressure in adults, *Am Fam Physician* 93(6):511–512, 2016.

Sexton S: Screening for high blood pressure in adults: recommendation statement, *Am Fam Physician* 93(4):300–302, 2016.

Sexton S: Screening for primary hypertension in children and adolescents: recommendation statement, *Am Fam Physician* 91(4), 2015. A–D.

Springer K: Chlorthalidone vs. hydrochlorothiazide for treatment of hypertension, *Am Fam Physician* 92(11):1015–1016, 2015.

Medscape: Hypertension. Available at: http://emedicine.medscape.com/article/241381. [accessed May 9, 2017].

HYPERTROPHIC CARDIOMYOPATHY

Method of
Sandeep Sangodkar, DO

CURRENT DIAGNOSIS

- Echocardiography is a mainstay of clinical diagnosis.
- Cardiac magnetic resonance imaging (MRI) can provide important prognostic information.
- Left ventricular outflow tract pressure and flow measurements have a classic dynamic pattern.
- Left ventricular wall thickness of at least 15 mm.

CURRENT THERAPY

Asymptomatic Disease
- Periodic follow-up to assess symptoms and risk for sudden cardiac death.
- Important to counsel patients regarding potential genetic transmission.
- Patients with concurrent atrial fibrillation should be anticoagulated.

Symptomatic Disease
- β-Blockade or calcium channel blockers are drugs of choice.
- Implantable defibrillator is indicated if the patient has risk factors for sudden cardiac death.
- Surgical myectomy may be undertaken in patients who do not respond to pharmacologic therapy.
- Alcohol ablation may be used in patients who are not candidates for surgery.

Definition
Many names, terms, and acronyms (more than 80) have been used to describe hypertrophic cardiomyopathy (HCM). Common names such as *idiopathic hypertrophic*, *subaortic stenosis*, and *hypertrophic obstructive cardiomyopathy*, popular in the literature in the 1960s and 1970s, imply that left ventricular outflow tract (LVOT) obstruction is a required component of the disease, whereas one-third of patients have no obstruction at rest or exertion. The term *HCM*, first used in 1979, encompasses both the obstructive and nonobstructive hemodynamic variants of this disease and is now considered the formal name.

Epidemiology
Although once thought of as a rare entity, HCM is now recognized as a common inherited cardiovascular disease. Epidemiologic studies from various parts of the world report a similar prevalence, thought of as 1 in 200 to 1 in 500 people, which occurs equally among sexes and ethnic groups. This may, in fact, be underreported because many people with HCM are not clinically diagnosed and achieve normal life expectancy without any HCM-related complications.

Risk Factors
HCM is caused by mutations in genes coding for thin and thick filament proteins of the sarcomere. These mutations are inherited in an autosomal dominant pattern with variable penetrance and expression. At least 11 genes have been identified as responsible for causing HCM, with 70% of successfully genotyped patients found to have mutations in the two most-common genes: β-myosin heavy chain and myosin binding protein C. More than 1500 individual gene variants have been identified, which complicates predicting prognosis for individual patients.

Clinical Manifestations
HCM is seen from pediatric to geriatric populations. A classic description of a murmur suggestive of HCM is a harsh crescendo-decrescendo systolic ejection murmur that increases in intensity with Valsalva or standing from a squatting position. Most patients with HCM are asymptomatic or only mildly symptomatic, with the most common presenting complaints being dyspnea or chest pain. The most worrisome manifestation is sudden cardiac death owing to ventricular tachyarrhythmia, seen more commonly in younger symptom-free patients. Systolic anterior motion of the mitral valve can cause significant mitral regurgitation. Heart failure with preserved ejection fraction is another manifestation of HCM; however, systolic dysfunction can be present owing to myocardial scarring. In addition, atrial fibrillation is associated with an increased risk of thromboembolism in patients with HCM and anticoagulation must be considered. Most patients with HCM have normal life expectancy without a need for major intervention.

Pathogenesis
The pathophysiology of HCM stems from multiple abnormalities, including LVOT obstruction, diastolic dysfunction, mitral regurgitation, myocardial ischemia, and arrhythmias. The peak LV outflow gradient is an important factor in determining treatment options. The obstruction was originally thought to be caused by a hypertrophied basal septum that caused ventricular outflow obstruction during systolic contraction. More recently, it is thought mitral valve systolic anterior motion and mitral-septal contact caused by venturi forces on the mitral leaflets and displacement into the outflow tract cause obstruction of LVOT. The increased LV systolic pressure in turn results in elevated diastolic pressures, mitral regurgitation, and, ultimately, decreased cardiac output.

Diagnosis
Clinically, HCM is defined as maximal end diastolic LV wall thickness of at least 15 mm based on echocardiography or cardiac MRI. Patients should have a comprehensive physical and three-generation family history as part of their initial evaluation. A distinction between HCM and physiologic LV hypertrophy from athletic conditioning must be recognized because the athletic hearts may demonstrate enlargement of the cardiac chambers and thickened septum. The likelihood of clinically significant HCM is determined by identification of sarcomere mutations, marked LV thickness (more than 25 mm), and LVOT obstruction with systolic anterior motion and mitral-septal contact. Provocative testing (exercise or pharmacologic) may elucidate the diagnosis of HCM in symptomatic patients presenting with a normal LVOT gradient at rest. Measurement of outflow gradients by echocardiography and invasive pressures by cardiac catheterization show a characteristic dynamic pattern that can be enhanced by loading conditions.

Imaging
The mainstay of imaging has been held by echocardiography. Transthoracic echocardiography is recommended in the initial evaluation of all patients with suspected HCM and family members of those diagnosed with HCM. Transesophageal echocardiography is used for diagnosis and intraprocedural guidance of surgical myectomy and alcohol septal ablation.

In recent years, cardiac magnetic resonance imaging (MRI; CMR) has proven to be an increasingly useful modality in the diagnosis and treatment of HCM. Contrast-enhanced CMR allows imaging of presumed myocardial fibrosis. Late gadolinium enhancement (LGE) is commonly seen in HCM; an extensive percentage of left ventricular mass involvement is associated with higher risk of sudden cardiac death. Consequently, an absence of LGE is associated with a lower risk of sudden cardiac death and can often provide reassurance.

TABLE 1 Pharmacologic Management of Patients With Obstructive HCM

		INITIAL DOSE	TITRATE TO MAX DOSE
Symptoms Attributable to LV Outflow Tract Obstruction			
Non-Vasodilating Beta Blockers	Metoprolol	50 mg/day	400 mg/day
	Atenolol	25 mg/day	100 mg/day
	Propranolol	60 mg/day	240 mg/day
Beta Blocker Ineffective or Not Tolerated			
Nondihydropyridine Calcium Channel Blockers	Verapamil	120 mg/day	480 mg/day
	Diltiazem	120 mg/day	360 mg/day
Severe Symptoms Despite Beta Blocker or Nondihydropyridine CCB			
	Disopyramide	200 mg BID	300 mg BID

Treatment

Asymptomatic Disease

Given that a large subset of HCM patients are symptom free and will achieve normal life expectancy, it is important to educate patients about the disease process, screen family members, and advise them to avoid strenuous activity. Coronary artery disease has an impact on survival, and thus aggressive modification of risk factors contributing to atherosclerosis (diabetes, hyperlipidemia, and obesity) is recommended. Low-intensity aerobic exercise is reasonable to allow the patient to maintain fitness. Adequate hydration and avoidance of situations leading to vasodilation are encouraged to minimize exacerbation of an existing LVOT obstruction.

Septal reduction therapy is not indicated in a symptom-free patient with any degree of obstruction.

Symptomatic Disease

Pharmacologic Management

β-Blockade is the mainstay of treatment owing to negative inotropic and negative chronotropic effect. Verapamil (Calan)[1] or diltiazem (Cardizem)[1] are reasonable alternatives to β-blockade. Disopyramide (Norpace)[1] may be added if symptomatic despite these medications (Table 1). An important role in management is to discontinue medications that promote outflow tract obstruction via vasodilatory effects such as dihydropyridine calcium channel blocking agents, angiotensin converting enzyme inhibitors, and angiotensin receptor blockers. Low-dose diuretics may provide symptomatic relief; however, high-dose diuretics should be avoided. Digitalis is potentially harmful in patients without atrial fibrillation. Phenylephrine (Neo-Synephrine)[1] is useful when treating acute hypotension in these patients.

For the treatment of atrial fibrillation in HCM, it is recommended to keep a low threshold for initiating prophylactic anticoagulation with a direct-acting oral anticoagulant or vitamin K antagonist caused by a higher risk of thromboembolic stroke.

[1]Not FDA approved for this indication.

Invasive Therapies

The major septal reduction therapies are surgical myectomy and alcohol ablation. These should be performed by experienced operators at comprehensive centers in patients with refractory symptoms.

Surgical septal myectomy is considered the most appropriate therapy for eligible patients unresponsive to optimal medical therapy. The most common procedure is a Morrow procedure in which a rectangular trough is created in the basal septum below the aortic valve, which abolishes or reduces the LVOT gradient. Eligible patients include those with severe dyspnea, chest pain, or exertional syncope despite maximal medical therapy. Hemodynamic considerations that determine eligibility consist of an LVOT gradient of at least 50 mm Hg associated with septal hypertrophy and mitral valve systolic anterior motion. Studies have shown that surgical myectomy can reverse heart failure symptoms owing to the fact it permanently removes LVOT obstruction and can reduce mitral regurgitation.

Alcohol septal ablation can benefit adult patients with HCM and LVOT obstruction. This percutaneous procedure involves injection of ethanol into a major septal perforator coronary artery, with the intent of inducing infarction of the basal septal wall near the anterior leaflet contact point. The effectiveness of alcohol septal ablation is not clear in patients with more than 30 mm of septal hypertrophy, and it should not be performed in patients with disease (coronary artery disease, mitral valve repair) that would need surgical correction regardless. Other downsides of septal ablation include an increased risk of complete heart block requiring pacemaker implantation and an undefined risk of arrhythmogenicity owing to scar tissue.

Role of Implantable Devices

Determining which patients with HCM should receive an implantable cardiac defibrillator (ICD) is challenging given the unpredictability of the disease. ICDs are the only treatment to have proven to decrease mortality given their ability to reliably abort life-threating arrhythmias. All patients with HCM need comprehensive sudden cardiac death risk stratification, with strong consideration for ICD implantation in those with personal history of ventricular fibrillation, sustained ventricular tachycardia, family history of sudden cardiac death, unexplained syncope, abnormal exercise blood pressure response, LGE >15% of LV mass, massive left ventricular hypertrophy (LVH) (>30 mm), or documented nonsustained ventricular tachycardia on Holter monitor. Device-related complications and issues such as inappropriate shocks and multiple generator changes for patients receiving a device at a young age must also be weighed when considering implantation of ICD. Risk scores can be helpful in the processes of shared decision making.

Participation in Sports

HCM has been reported as one of the most common causes of sudden death among competitive athletes; however, SCD is overall a rare event in young people. In the United States, there have been cardiovascular screening initiatives, including history and physical in addition to 12 lead electrocardiograms (ECGs), with limited success. The American College of Cardiology and American Heart Association do not currently recommend a national mandatory cardiovascular screening program.

It is reasonable for most HCM patients to engage in low-intensity competitive sports (golf, bowling) and recreational sporting activities. Participation in competitive sports is a modifiable risk factor, and it is recommended that HCM patients avoid participation in intense competitive sports regardless of age, sex, LVOT obstruction, prior septal reduction, or ICD. In addition, ICD placement should not be implanted for the sole purpose of participating in competitive athletics. For most HCM patients, mild-moderate intensity recreational exercise is beneficial for cardiovascular fitness and overall health.

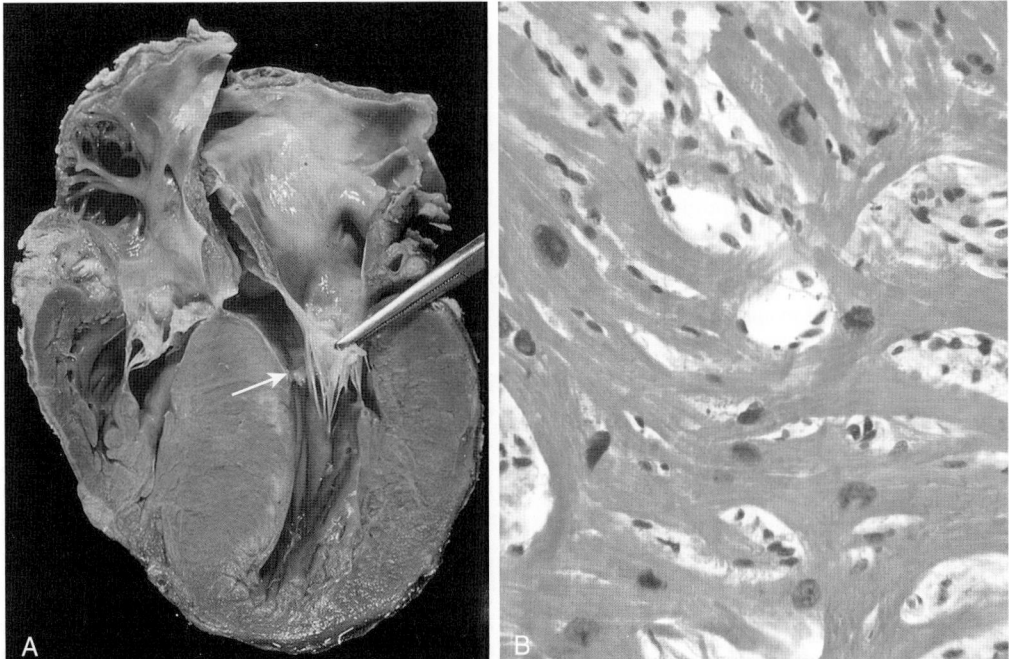

Figure 1 A, Gross anatomy section of heart demonstrating septal hypertrophy and LVOT obstruction. B, Microscopic section demonstrating myocyte hypertrophy and disarray.

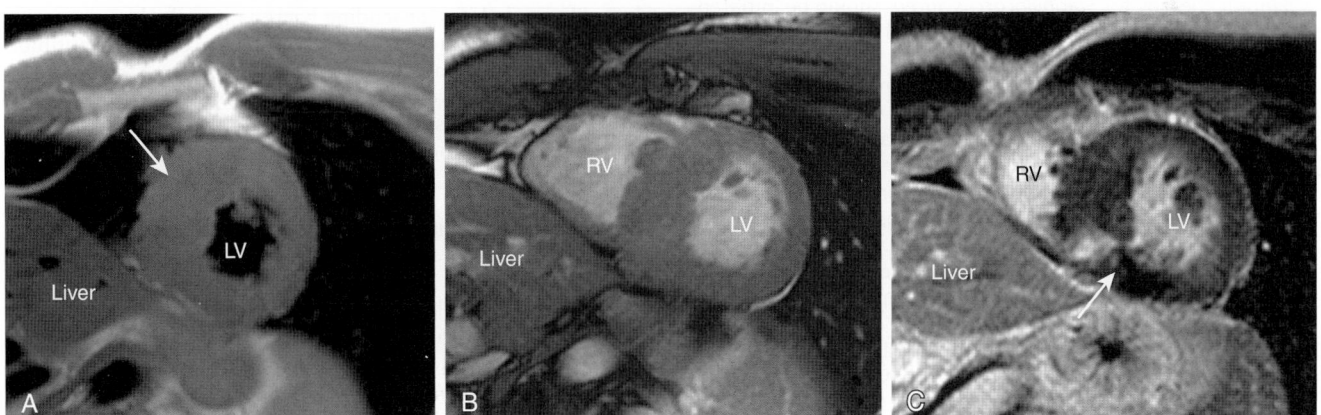

Figure 2 Cardiac MRI demonstrating septal hypertrophy (A,B) and late gadolinium enhancement (C).

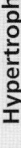
Monitoring

The unpredictability of HCM disease makes regular surveillance a necessity. Patient age has been seen as a predictor of HCM-related events, with sudden death events more common in young patients. With a family history of sudden cardiac death, periodic screening by transthoracic echocardiography (every 12–18 months) is recommended in children by the age of 12 (or younger if the child has signs of early puberty) or if there are plans for intense sports competition. Repeat transthoracic echocardiography is recommended for any change in clinical status or new cardiovascular event. As recognition of the genetic basis of this disease has improved over time, genetic screening and counseling of all first-degree family members of patients with HCM are now recommended.

Future Research

The perception of HCM has evolved from a rare and deadly condition to a more common and treatable disease. Effective use of ICDs for primary prevention and advances in surgical treatment of obstruction now allow most HCM patients to achieve normal life expectancy. Although significant progress has been made in elucidating the etiology and pathophysiology of HCM, there is much room for advancement. In addition, the relationship between genetics and environmental influences, as well as the management of family members of genotype positive–phenotype negative patients, is still unclear. Although rapid genetic testing to identify those at risk has become more widespread, further understanding of pathogenic mutations is required. Furthermore, advancement in technology will hopefully lead to therapies that can specifically target these pathways.

References

Cannan CR, Reeder GS, Bailey KR: Natural history of hypertrophic cardiomyopathy. A population based study, 1976 through 1990, *Circulation* 92:2488–2495, 1995.

Elliott PM, Anastasakis A, Borger MA: ESC Guidelines on diagnosis and management of hypertrophic cardiomyopathy, *Eur Heart J* 35:2733–2799, 2014.

Gersh BJ, Maron BJ, Bonow RO: 2011 ACCF/AHA guideline for the diagnosis and treatment of hypertrophic cardiomyopathy, *Circulation* 124:e783–e831, 2011.

Marian AJ: Recent advances in genetics and treatment of hypertrophic cardiomyopathy, *Future Cardiol* 1:341–353, 2005.

Marian AJ: Genetic determinants of cardiac hypertrophy, *Curr Opin Cardiol* 23:199–205, 2008.

Maron B, Ommen S, Semsarian C, et al: State of the art review: hypertrophic cardiomyopathy, *JACC* 64(1).

Maron BJ: Hypertrophic cardiomyopathy: a systematic review, *J Am Med Assoc* 287:1308–1320, 2002.

Robinson AK: Imaging in hypertrophic cardiomyopathy, *JACC* 24, 2018.

Ommen S, Mital S, et al: 2020 AHA/ACC guideline for the diagnosis and treatment of patients with hypertrophic cardiomyopathy, *JACC* 76(25).

INFECTIVE ENDOCARDITIS

Samuel Mathis, MD; and Oyetokunbo Ibidapo-Obe, MD

CURRENT DIAGNOSIS

- Infective endocarditis (IE) should be a diagnostic consideration in patients with fever and heart murmur.
- Healthcare related infections account for 25% to 30% of newly diagnosed cases.
- Positive blood cultures are present in approximately 90% of cases. Multiple sets should be obtained prior to initiating antibiotic therapy to improve diagnostic yield.
- Transesophageal echocardiography has the highest sensitivity and specificity in native heart evaluations while alternative imaging techniques can be used in patients with implanted heart valves.
- Complications of disease include heart failure, valvular incompetence, and structural defects such as abscess, perforation, and fistulas.

CURRENT THERAPY

- Empiric therapy for *Staphylococcus aureus* should be initiated after blood cultures have been drawn and before the results are available.
- Antibiotic choice is complex and dependent on culture results and sensitivities of organisms identified.
- Best practices propose a multidisciplinary approach to care for patients with IE and should include specialties such as cardiology, infectious disease/microbiology, and cardiothoracic surgery in cases of complicated IE or if prosthetic valves or a cardiac device is present.
- Neurology or neurosurgery consults should be accessible as up to 30% of patients will experience symptomatic neurologic events during their disease.
- Increasing numbers of patients with IE will require surgical intervention due to complications from disease such as heart failure, embolism, intracardiac abscess, or failure to control infection.
- Outpatient parenteral antibiotic therapy can be considered in a subset of patients based on their culture results and with close follow-up.

Definition

Infective endocarditis (IE) is a microbial infection of the valves or endocardium of the heart.

Epidemiology and Risk Factors

IE remains a rare disease in Western countries with incidence varying by geographic location, predisposing risk factors, and preexisting conditions.

IE has an annual incidence of 3 to 10/100,000 of the North American population with a mortality of about 30% at 30 days and 40% at 1 year.

Over the years, the epidemiology of IE has shifted with a steady increase in healthcare-associated IE accounting for about 25% to 30% of newly reported cases.

Risk factors include advancing age, prosthetic heart valves, congenital heart disease, intracardiac devices, intravenous/parenteral drug use, indwelling venous access lines, diabetes mellitus, or immunosuppression to name a few.

Developing worlds have rheumatic heart disease as a leading risk factor for IE.

Infection with *Staphylococcus aureus* is presently the most prevalent cause of IE accounting for ~26% and overtaking the Strep group, next is *Streptococcus viridans* group at ~19%, other Streptococci at 17.5% and Enterococci at 10.55. The above listed bacteria jointly account for 80% to 90% of all cases of endocarditis.

Pathophysiology

IE occurs as a result of endothelial damage, which invariably exposes the basement membrane on the valve causing a structural abnormality that allows bacteria present in the bloodstream to colonize the initially sterile vegetation (nonbacterial thrombotic endocarditis).

Bacterial involvement and growth enlarge the vegetation, impede blood flow, and cause inflammation with multiple systemic symptoms/signs.

Progressive valve dysfunction can quickly lead to heart failure, and bacterial colonization of the vegetation causes septic emboli into the bloodstream, causing sepsis, and can lead to a metastatic septic site outside of initial vegetation area on the valve.

Prevention

The mainstay of prevention of IE is antimicrobial therapy prior to procedures, which may cause IE. This has been and remains a topic of debate and varies by geographic location worldwide.

The efficacy of antimicrobial therapy as a prophylaxis depends greatly on multiple factors, which include patient's medical conditions in terms of being high risk for IE, the procedure being done, the probability of sending bacteria into the bloodstream as a result of the said procedure, and the evidence backing antibiotic prophylaxis in the patient scenario.

The guidelines have remained dynamic based on review of published literature, most of which seems to favor less use of antibiotics and better patient selection for prophylaxis if needed. See current guidelines in Box 1.

Clinical Manifestations and Diagnosis

The diagnosis of IE is based on findings of bacteremia from an organism associated with IE along with evidence of endocardial involvement. This allows for highly variable presentations of disease. Due to this variability, it is important to perform a detailed history and physical examination to help lead to the diagnosis. Blood cultures should be obtained as discussed below prior to initiating antibacterial therapy to ensure appropriate management of the causative organism. This is especially important in the setting of predisposing conditions or risk factors for IE, including recent invasive procedures, history of structural heart disease, or injection drug use. Because of the insidious nature of the disease process, many patients will present with symptoms within 2 weeks of the inciting event or infection.

The most common presentation includes fever in up to 90% of patients, though it may not be present in immunocompromised patients or those who have received previous antibiotic therapy. This can be seen in postoperative patients after valve replacement or intracardiac devices. Night sweats, fatigue, weight loss, and appetite changes are other nonspecific signs that can indicate an infection and will be present in up to half of patients with IE.

A new or changing regurgitant murmur will also be present on physical examination along with evidence of endocardial involvement. The presentation of such involvement can range from tachycardia and hypotension to embolization of the vegetations causing embolic symptoms. Approximately 25% of patients with IE will present with evidence of embolization. If left untreated, symptoms of heart failure, valvular dysfunction, and destruction of cardiac structures can occur. Other physical exam findings of IE include petechia, splinter hemorrhages, Janeway lesions, Osler nodes, and Roth spots. As these findings can occur in other conditions and have low incidence in proven cases of IE, their diagnostic use is limited.

Differential Diagnosis

There are several conditions that can mimic the symptoms of IE. Consideration of systemic lupus erythematosus, acute rheumatic fever, atrial myxoma, vasculitis, and renal cell carcinoma should be on the differential. Care must be taken to not confuse the complications of IE as the causative etiology for hospitalization. One study found that up to 50% of patients with IE were initially diagnosed with complications of their disease (pneumonia, CNS infection, septic arthritis, heart failure, stroke) before correctly identifying the causative agent. Misdiagnosis was found to significantly increase the risk of comorbidity and in hospital mortality in these patients.

Laboratory Evaluation and Blood Cultures

Blood cultures are one of the major diagnostic criteria used to diagnose IE. They are of utmost importance due to their use in the treatment of IE by identifying the microorganisms involved as well as their antibiotic sensitivities. The continuous bacteremia present in IE means that fever need not be present before ordering blood cultures. In up to 90% of cases, the etiologic agent is identified in the first two blood cultures. It is recommended that three sets of blood cultures be obtained at least 1 hour apart from separate venipunctures for the most sensitive findings (98% of cases successfully identified). Each vial should have at least 10 mL of blood to increase the chances of obtaining an appropriate amount. Alternatively, two sets of three bottles each (two aerobic, one anaerobic—six bottles total) can be drawn if timing of antibiotic therapy is a concern. Unfortunately, the most common cause of negative culture IE is due to prior administration of antibiotic therapy. This results in prolonged, broad coverage antibiotic therapy and increased uncertainty of the diagnosis.

Other lab findings that may be present in IE but are not specific for the disease include a normocytic, normochromic anemia, thrombocytopenia, leukocytosis, and elevations in erythrocyte sedimentation rate (ERS), C-reactive protein, and procalcitonin.

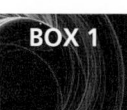

BOX 1 — Antibiotic Regimens for High-Risk Patients and Dental Procedures[1] (Taken 30–60 Minutes Prior to Procedure)

Oral: Amoxicillin 2 g (child 50 mg/kg) PO 30–60 minutes before procedure
Penicillin Allergy: Cephalexin 2 g (child 50 mg/kg) PO 30–60 minutes before procedure or clindamycin 600 mg (child 20 mg/kg)
or azithromycin or clarithromycin 500 mg (child 15 mg/kg)
Unable to tolerate oral: Ampicillin 2 g IM/IV (child 50 mg/kg)
Unable to tolerate oral and PCN allergy: Cefazolin or ceftriaxone 1 g IM/IV (child 50 mg/kg) or clindamycin 600 mg IM/IV (child 20 mg/kg)
Patients that would benefit from antibiotics due to high risk:
- Acquired valvular heart disease with stenosis or regurgitation
- Valve replacement
- Structural congenital heart disease
- Previous endocarditis
- Hypertrophic cardiomyopathy
   Dental procedures to consider antibiotic prophylaxis:
- Manipulation of the gingival or periapical region of the teeth
- Perforation of oral mucosa
- Extractions

All these regimens are not approved by the FDA for this indication.
Adapted from Bonow RO, Carabello BA, Kanu C, et al: ACC/AHA 2006 guidelines for the management of patients with valvular heart disease: A report of the American College of Cardiology/American Heart Association Task Force on Practice Guidelines (writing committee to revise the 1998 Guidelines for the Management of Patients with Valvular Heart Disease): Developed in collaboration with the Society of Cardiovascular Anesthesiologists: Endorsed by the Society for Cardiovascular Angiography and Interventions and the Society of Thoracic Surgeons. *Circulation* 114(5):e84–e231, 2006.

Imaging

Cardiac imaging should be considered if there is a strong clinical suspicion of IE. The inclusion of cardiac imaging of IE has increased the sensitivity of diagnosis (see modified Duke Criteria [Box 2]). Transthoracic echocardiogram (TTE) should be performed if there is clinical suspicion for IE. The echocardiogram should be specifically looking for any oscillating intracardiac mass on the valve or supporting structure which would indicate vegetations. It can also be used to detect abscesses, dehiscence of prostatic valve, or newly identified valvular regurgitations. The sensitivity of detecting vegetations on native valves is approximately 70% with TTE. This is increased to a sensitivity and specificity around 90% if transesophageal echocardiogram (TEE) is used instead. Due to this increased sensitivity, TEE should be used in high-risk patients with a negative TTE. Transesophageal echocardiogram should also be considered in patients with prosthetic valves, those

BOX 2 — Modified Duke Criteria for Infective Endocarditis

Definite Infective Endocarditis:
- Two major
or
- One major and three minor
or
- Five minor

Possible Infective Endocarditis:
- One major and one minor
or
- Three minor

Major Criteria
Positive blood cultures:
- Typical microorganisms consistent with IE from two separate blood culture: viridans group streptococci, *Streptococcus bovis* group, HACED group, *Staphylococcus aureus*; community acquired enterocci with abscess of primary focus
or
- Microorganisms consistent with IE from persistently positive blood cultures: at least two positive blood cultures drawn more than 12 hours apart; all of three or a majority of positive blood cultures in more than four drawn; or single positive blood culture for *Coxiella burnetii* or phage IgG antibody titer >1:800

Evidence of endocardial involvement:
- Echocardiogram positive for IE showing vegetation, abscess, psuedoaneurysm, intracardiac fistula, valvular perforation or aneurysm, new partial dehiscence of prosthetic valve
- Abnormal activity around site of a prosthetic valve detected by PET/CT assuming >3 months after surgery or radiolabeled leukocyte-SPECT/CT
- Definite paravalvular lesions by cardiac CT

Minor Criteria
- Predisposition: predisposing heart condition or injection drug use
- Fever, temperature >38°C
- Vascular phenomena (including those detected by imaging alone): arterial emboli, septic pulmonary infarcts, myotic aneurysm, intracranial hemorrhage, conjunctival hemorrhage, and Janeway lesions
- Immunologic phenomena: glomerulonephritis, Osler's nodes, Roth's spots, and rheumatoid factor
- Microbiological evidence: positive blood cultures not meeting major criteria above or serologic evidence of infection with organism consistent with IE

CT, Computed tomography; *HACEK, Haemophilus* spp, *Aggregatibacter* spp, *Cardiobacterium* hominis, *Eikenella* corrodens, *Kingella* spp; *IE,* infective endocarditis; *IgG,* immunoglobulin G; *PET,* positron emission tomography; *SPECT,* single-photon emission computed tomography.

with *S. aureus* bacteremia, and when IE-related complications have occurred such as heart block, cardiac abscess, embolism, or new/worsening murmurs.

Due to the increased number of patients with prosthetic valves or intracardiac devices, TTE and TEE may prove to be unhelpful due to the artifact from these devices. In these cases, additional imaging with F-labeled fluoro-2-deoxyglucose positron emission tomography/computed tomography (F-FDG-PET/CT) or single-proton emission computed tomography-CT (SPECT-CT) should be considered to assess for inflammation around the prosthetic or intracardiac device. These studies have been found to have a sensitivity of 93% in cases of prosthetic valve endocarditis. They have significantly lower sensitivity in cases of native heart disease (22% sensitivity). Thoracic CT scans have significant value in determining presence of perivalvular abscesses, aneurysms, or pseudoaneurysms.

Cerebral magnetic resonance imaging (MRI) should be considered in patients with evidence of embolic neurologic complications as most of these lesions are ischemic in origin.

Treatment

Treatment should be multidisciplinary and involve cardiology, cardiac surgeon, infectious disease, or microbiology. This approach improves outcomes by optimizing appropriate antibiotic regiments and assessments for surgical interventions. Initiating appropriate antibiotic therapy can improve in-hospital survival by 70% to 80%. Recommended antibiotic regimens against common organisms causing IE are listed in Table 1. These should be adjusted based on the organism and susceptibilities.

Patient with IE will require a prolonged duration of intravenous (IV) antibiotic treatment for up to 6 weeks. This is in order to ensure that all bacteria located in the vegetations are

TABLE 1 Antimicrobial Regimens Against Typical Infective Endocarditis Organisms

ORGANISM	SUSCEPTIBILITY	REGIMENT	DOSAGE	DURATION (WEEK)
Native Valve				
Streptococcus viridans, *Streptococcus bovis*	Penicillin	Penicillin G	12–18 MU IV per 24 h continuously or in four to six equally divided doses	4
		or ceftriaxone[1]	2 g IV or IM per 24 h	4
		or vancomycin	30 mg/kg IV per 24 h in two divided doses. Max: 2 g/24 h	4
	Penicillin-relative resistance	Penicillin G	24 MU IV per 24 h continuously or in four to six equally divided doses	4
		or ceftriaxone[1]	2 g IV/IM per 24 h 4	4
		plus gentamicin[1]	3 mg/kg IV/IM per 24 h in one dose	2
		or vancomycin	30 mg/kg IV per 24 h in two divided doses (limit 2 g/24 h)	4
Enterococcus spp	Penicillin	Ampicillin	12 g IV per 24 h in six divided doses	4–6
		or penicillin G[1]	18–30 MU IV per 24 h continuously or in six equally divided doses	4–6
		Plus	gentamicin 3 mg/kg IV or IM per 24 h in three divided doses	2
		or ampicillin	12 g IV per 24 h in six divided doses	6
		plus ceftriaxone[1]	2 g IV every 12 h	6
	Penicillin Resistant	Vancomycin	30 mg/kg IV per 24 h in two divided doses (limit 2 g/24 h)	
Staphylococcus spp	Oxacillin	Nafcillin[1] or oxacillin[1]	12 g IV per 24 h in four to six divided doses	6
		or cefazolin	100 mg/kg IV/IM per 24 h in three equally divided doses	6
			6 g IV per 24 h in three divided doses	6
	Oxacillin resistant	Vancomycin plus gentamicin	30 mg/kg IV per 24 h in two divided doses (goal: 1 h peak concentration 30–45 µg/mL and trough 10–15 µg/mL)	6
Prosthetic Valve				
Staphylococcus spp.	Oxacillin-susceptible	Nafcillin[1] or oxacillin[1]	12 g IV per 24 h in four to six divided doses	6
		plus gentamicin	3 mg/kg IV or IM per 24 h in three divided doses	2
		plus rifampin[1]	900 mg IV or PO per 24 h in three divided doses	6
	Oxacillin-resistant	Vancomycin	30 mg/kg IV per 24 h in two divided doses. Goal: 1 h peak concentration 30–45 µg/mL and trough 10–15 µg/mL	6
		plus gentamicin	3 mg/kg IV or IM per 24 h in three divided doses	2
		plus rifampin[1]	900 mg IV or PO per 24 h in three divided doses	6

[1]Not FDA approved for this indication.

Adapted from Bonow RO, Carabello BA, Kanu C, et al: ACC/AHA 2006 guidelines for the management of patients with valvular heart disease: A report of the American College of Cardiology/American Heart Association Task Force on Practice Guidelines (writing committee to revise the 1998 Guidelines for the Management of Patients with Valvular Heart Disease): Developed in collaboration with the Society of Cardiovascular Anesthesiologists: Endorsed by the Society for Cardiovascular Angiography and Interventions and the Society of Thoracic Surgeons. *Circulation* 114(5):e84–e231, 2006.

completely eradicated. Blood cultures should be repeated every 24 to 48 hours until resolution of bacteremia is confirmed. If surgery is required, a 4- to 6-week course of antibiotics is still recommended to reduce recurrence of IE.

In addition to IV antibiotic therapy, many patients will also be placed on parenteral therapies. In certain cases, patients may be eligible for transition to oral antibiotic to complete the duration of therapy. The criteria for step down therapy are patients who have no indication for surgery, have completed an initial course of IV antibiotics with no bacteremia, have no concerns for absorption of oral therapy in the gastrointestinal tract, have no psychological or socioeconomic concerns that would cause IV therapy to be preferred for adherence, and the organism is susceptible to the prescribed oral regiment. Oral therapy is preferred over IV due to the decreased potential for harm.

Due to increasing microorganism resistance, parenteral therapy typically consists of a beta-lactam and aminoglycoside. They should be taken close together to increase the bactericidal effect. Care should be maintained with close observation of renal function.

Complications and Surgical Indications

Infective endocarditis carries a high in-hospital mortality of up to 30% due to the development of potential complications either prior or during effective treatment. Heart failure or pulmonary edema is common, occurring in up to half of patients with IE, and is the most common indication for urgent surgery. Destruction of the valvular tissues creates significant regurgitation leading to volume overload. Conversely, severe vegetations can cause significant stenosis and lead to the same outcome. In rare cases, this can lead to cardiogenic shock, which is an immediate indication for surgery (within 24 hours). For those with symptoms of heart failure and worsening hemodynamic response, surgery should be considered within 7 days of identification. Patients with heart failure will typically require surgical intervention as medical therapy alone is insufficient at repairing the damage caused by the infection. It is important to note here that valvular or other surgical interventions for IE may be performed in the acute or active phase of infection as delay can significantly increase the mortality.

Other complications include failure to quickly eradicate infection. This can be due to inability or delays in identifying the causative organism or for severe infections. Severe localized infections can cause paravalvular or aortic root abscesses. These abscess formations usually complicate 30% to 40% of IE cases due to their contiguous spread along the tissue planes. Other risk factors for abscess formation include prosthetic valves or difficult-to-treat organisms such as fungi or multidrug-resistant organisms. For this reason, all IE cases associated with prosthetic valves should have surgical consideration. These cases are typically identified by persistently positive blood cultures despite appropriate antibiotic regiments. Abscesses are identified via TEE or the aforementioned imaging studies in patients with prosthetic valves. Due to the abscess formation and deep infection, surgical debridement or valve replacement is almost always required. Surgical evaluation and debridement is the gold standard of abscess identification.

The third major complication of IE relates to septic emboli from valvular vegetations. While one-third of patients with IE will have signs and symptoms of embolization, another one-third can be found to have silent emboli. Neurologic embolization is the most frequent site (40%), followed by lungs (20%), spleen (20%), peripheral arteries (~15%), and kidneys (10%). Embolization most often occurs prior to the initiation of antibiotic therapy and the risk of embolization is reduced by approximately 65% after 2 weeks of antibiotic therapy. Risk factors include vegetations greater than 10 mm in size and infections associated with *S. aureus* and *Streptococcus bovis*. These embolic events can further complicate treatment by causing metastatic infection sites. Embolic events are an independent risk factor for in-hospital death in IE and as such require surgical evaluation if the vegetations meet certain criteria. Surgery is indicated in valvular vegetations greater than 10 mm with embolic event while on antibiotics, in vegetations greater than 30 mm, and in those with vegetations greater than 10 mm with severe valvular (native and prosthetic) disease who are low operative risk.

Conclusion

Infective endocarditis continues to maintain a relatively high mortality rate even with the advances in both surgical and antibiotic treatment. Prompt diagnosis and targeted antimicrobial therapy are vital to improving outcomes in patients with IE. Surgical evaluation and treatment should be considered relatively early in the disease course. Even with high rates of surgical intervention, in-hospital mortality continues to remain between 15% and 20% in native valves and up to 25% in prosthetic valves. Complications associated with disease progression (heart failure, uncontrolled infections, embolic events) also increase the mortality risk. Therefore a multidisciplinary team should be involved in patients identified with IE to provide best possible outcomes. Additionally, close follow-up after hospitalization should be conducted as up to 30% of patients with IE may require surgery in the first 12 months after diagnosis.

References

Baddour LM, Wilson WR, Bayer AS, et al: On behalf of the American Heart Association Committee on rheumatic fever, endocarditis, and kawasaki disease of the council on cardiovascular disease in the young, council on clinical cardiology, council on cardiovascular surgery and anesthesia, and stroke council. Infective endocarditis in adults: diagnosis, antimicrobial therapy, and management of complications: a scientific statement for healthcare professionals from the American Heart Association, *Circulation* 132:1435–1486, 2015.

Cahill TJ, et al: Challenges in infective endocarditis, *J Am Coll Cardiol* 69(3):325–344, 2017.

Cahill TJ, Harrison JL, Jewell P, et al: Antibiotic prophylaxis for infective endocarditis: a systematic review and meta-analysis, *Heart* 103:937–944, 2017.

Chu VH, Cabell CH, Benjamin Jr DK, et al: Early predictors of in-hospital death in infective endocarditis, *Circulation* 109(14):1745–1749, 2004.

Fowler Jr VG, Miro JM, Hoen B, et al: Staphylococcus aureus endocarditis: a consequence of medical progress, *J Am Med Assoc* 293(24):3012–3021, 2005.

Gaca JG, Sheng S, Daneshmand MA, et al: Outcomes for endocarditis surgery in North America: a simplified risk scoring system, *J Thorac Cardiovasc Surg* 141:98–106, 2011.

Habib G, Lancellotti P, Antunes MJ, et al: 2015 ESC guidelines for the management of infective endocarditis: the Task Force for the Management of Infective Endocarditis of the European Society of Cardiology (ESC). Endorsed by: European Association for Cardio-Thoracic Surgery (EACTS), the European Association of Nuclear Medicine (EANM), *Eur Heart J* 36(44):3075–3128, 2015.

Kang DH, Kim YJ, Kim SH, et al: Early surgery versus conventional treatment for infective endocarditis, *N Engl J Med* 366:2466–2473, 2012.

Kiefer T, Park L, Tribouilloy C, et al: Association between valvular surgery and mortality among patients with infective endocarditis complicated by heart failure, *J Am Med Assoc* 306:2239–2247, 2011.

Li JS, Sexton DJ, Nettles R, et al: Proposed modifications to the Duke criteria for the diagnosis of infective endocarditis, *Clin Infect Dis* 30(4):633–638, 2000.

Liesman RM, Pritt BS, Maleszewski JJ, Patel R: Laboratory diagnosis of infective endocarditis, *J Clin Microbiol* 55:2599–2608, 2017.

Naderi HR, Sheybani F, Erfani SS: Errors in diagnosis of infective endocarditis, *Epidemiol Infect* 146:394–400, 2018.

Nishimura RA, Otto CM, Bonow RO, et al: 2014 AHA/ ACC guideline for the management of patients with valvular heart disease: a report of the American College of Cardiology/American Heart Association Task Force on Practice Guidelines, *J Am Coll Cardiol* 63:e57–e185, 2014.

Rajani R, Klein JL: Infective endocarditis: a contemporary update, *Clin Med (Lond)* 20(1):31–35, 2020.

Spellberg B, et al: Evaluation of a paradigm shift from intravenous antibiotics to oral step-down therapy for the treatment of infective endocarditis: a narrative review, *JAMA Intern Med*, 2020.

Task Force on the Prevention: Diagnosis, and Treatment of Infective Endocarditis of the European Society of Cardiology; European Society of Clinical Microbiology and Infectious Diseases; International Society of Chemotherapy for Infection and Cancer; ESC Committee for Practice Guidelines: Guidelines on the prevention, diagnosis, and treatment of infective endocarditis (new version 2009): the Task Force on the prevention, diagnosis, and treatment of infective endocarditis of the European Society of Cardiology (ESC), *Eur Heart J* 30(19):2369–2413, 2009.

Thornhill MH, Dayer M, Lockhart PB, Prendergast B: Antibiotic prophylaxis of infective endocarditis, *Curr Infect Dis Rep* 19(2):9, 2017.

MITRAL VALVE PROLAPSE

Method of
Kurt M. Jacobson, MD; Peter S. Rahko, MD; and Shenil Shah, MD

CURRENT DIAGNOSIS

- A midsystolic click with or without a middle- to late-peaking crescendo systolic murmur is the classic auscultatory finding of mitral valve prolapse (MVP).
- Key examination maneuvers can help differentiate MVP from other valvular heart diseases.
- Diagnostic echocardiographic findings of MVP are systolic billowing of the mitral valve leaflets 2 mm above the annulus into the left atrium.
- The presence of significant myxomatous thickening of the valve leaflets (>5 mm) is significant for prognosis.

CURRENT THERAPY

- Patients with physical findings of mitral valve prolapse (MVP) should have an echocardiogram to confirm the diagnosis, determine the severity of prolapse, determine the amount of myxomatous thickening, document the severity (if present) of mitral regurgitation, and determine left ventricular size and function.
- Uncomplicated MVP without significant mitral regurgitation can be evaluated clinically every 3 to 5 years.
- Complicated MVP (associated with significant mitral regurgitation, left ventricular structural changes, pulmonary hypertension, atrial fibrillation, or stroke) should be observed closely with serial clinical evaluation and echocardiography.
- Surgery may be required for complicated MVP associated with severe mitral regurgitation. Repair rather than replacement is the procedure of choice and should be performed at surgical centers experienced with mitral valve repair.
- Recommendations for surgery are the same for MVP as for other forms of chronic severe mitral regurgitation.
- Percutaneous intervention with the MitraClip (Abbott Vascular) is an option in symptomatic patients with moderate to severe or severe mitral regurgitation, prohibitive surgical risk, and acceptable anatomy.

Mitral valve prolapse (MVP) has been known by many names, including floppy valve syndrome, Barlow's syndrome, click/murmur syndrome, myxomatous mitral valve disease, and billowing mitral cusp syndrome. MVP is a common cardiac valvular abnormality characterized by redundant, floppy mitral valve leaflets; it is often detected initially by characteristic nonejection clicks or a middle- to late-peaking crescendo systolic murmur on physical examination.

Prevalence

MVP is the most common congenital cause of mitral regurgitation (MR) in adults and the most common indication for mitral valve surgery in the United States today. Previously, it was one of the most overdiagnosed conditions within cardiology, with suggested prevalence rates ranging from 5% to 15%. With the use of current diagnostic standards, rates are much lower; the overestimation was a consequence of diverse and nonuniformly accepted two-dimensional echocardiographic diagnostic criteria. Freed and colleagues, using the Framingham study population and applying consistent and more stringent echocardiographic diagnostic criteria, demonstrated a much lower prevalence of MVP (approximately 2.4%). The incidence appeared to be similar among men

and women. Gender differences do exist, however. Women tend to have a more benign course, whereas men tend to have more advanced myxomatous disease resulting in a greater chance of more severe MR.

Classification

Primary MVP is characterized by idiopathic myxomatous change of the mitral valve leaflets or the chordal structures or both. Secondary MVP is present when underlying conditions such as Marfan's syndrome, Ehlers-Danlos syndrome, osteogenesis imperfecta, or other collagen vascular disorders are evident. Certain congenital cardiac abnormalities, including Ebstein anomaly, aortic coarctation, hypertrophic cardiomyopathy, and ostium secundum atrial septal defects, are also associated with MVP. Familial variants with an autosomal dominant pattern of inheritance have been identified, and work to identify the genes involved is under way. The reported prevalence of MVP in first-degree relatives is between 30% and 50%.

Pathology

Macroscopic and microscopic changes can involve both the anterior and posterior leaflets as well as the chordal structures of the leaflet apparatus. Macroscopically, the surface area of the leaflet is increased, providing the accentuated, billowing appearance of the valve leaflets. Additional notable changes are thickening of the individual leaflets, increased leaflet length, thinning and stretching of the chordae, and increased circumference of the mitral valve annulus. At the microscopic level (Figure 1), normal mitral valves have three well-defined layers, each containing cells and a characteristic composition and configuration of the extracellular matrix: the fibrosa, composed predominantly of collagen fibers densely packed and arranged parallel to the free edge of the leaflet; the centrally located spongiosa, composed of loosely arranged collagen and proteoglycans; and the atrialis, composed of elastic fibers. In myxomatous mitral valves, the spongiosa layer is expanded by loose, amorphous extracellular matrix that has more proteoglycans but less collagen and more fragmented elastic fibers. What collagen is present appears to be disorganized and fragmented, giving the appearance of a haphazard layering of the spongiosa. It is this thickening that produces the classic macroscopic appearance of the myxomatous valve on two-dimensional echocardiography.

Clinical Presentation

Most patients with MVP are asymptomatic and will remain so, testifying to the often benign nature of this disease. Previously, various nonspecific symptoms, including fatigue, dyspnea, palpitations, postural orthostasis, anxiety, and panic attacks, were described as an MVP syndrome when present in association with the characteristic nonejection systolic click or middle- to late-peaking crescendo systolic murmur. Other symptoms, including chest discomfort, near-syncope, and syncope, have also been described by patients with MVP. However, in a community-based study, the prevalence of various clinical complaints including chest pain, dyspnea, and syncope was no higher in patients with MVP than in those without evidence of MVP, making such findings nonspecific. In a controlled study that compared symptomatic MVP patients with first-degree relatives with and without echocardiographic evidence of MVP, there also was no association of MVP with atypical chest pain, dyspnea, panic attacks, or anxiety. There was, however, a significant association of MVP with physical findings of systolic clicks, systolic murmurs, thoracic bony abnormalities, low body weight, and low blood pressure. Congestive heart failure, atrial fibrillation, stroke or transient ischemic attack, hypertension, diabetes, and hypercholesterolemia are no more likely in patients with MVP than in those without MVP. However, previous retrospective studies suggested a higher incidence of cerebral embolic events, infectious endocarditis, severe MR, and need for mitral valve replacement in patients with classic (complicated) versus nonclassic MVP. Symptoms of poor cardiac reserve, such as reduced exercise tolerance, dyspnea on exertion, and fatigue, may reflect the presence of significant MR and warrant clinical concern.

Diagnosis

Symptoms are not predictive of the presence or absence of MVP. Certain physical and auscultatory characteristics on examination do support the diagnosis of MVP. Patients with MVP more often have a lower body mass index, have a lower waist-to-hip ratio, and are taller. Findings of scoliosis, pectus excavatum, and hyperextensibility are also prevalent among patients with MVP. The classic auscultatory findings include a midsystolic click and a middle- to late-peaking crescendo systolic murmur heard best at the apex. The auscultatory findings are best elicited with the diaphragm of the stethoscope, and they change in relation to the first and second heart sounds (S_1 and S_2) in response to changes in left ventricular (LV) volume. Therefore the patient should be examined in several positions: supine (including lateral decubitus), sitting, standing, and, if possible, squatting. Changes in LV filling and volume affect the degree of prolapse.

The most important and most specific finding on auscultation is the presence of a nonejection midsystolic click or clicks caused by snapping of the valve apparatus as parts of the valve leaflets billow into the atrium during systole. Although these clicks can be heard over the entire precordium, they are best heard at the apex. The click can be misinterpreted as a split S_1, a true S_1 with an S_4, or a true S_1 with an early ejection click from a bicuspid valve. It can be differentiated from an ejection click heard in bicuspid aortic valves by its timing relative to the beginning of the carotid upstroke. Ejection clicks occur as the aortic valve opens and therefore precede the carotid upstroke, whereas the nonejection clicks of MVP occur afterward. Clicks from atrial septal aneurysms are uncommon but can be difficult to distinguish from those of MVP. Ejection clicks and clicks from atrial septal aneurysms are not altered by changes in loading characteristics, allowing them to be differentiated from clicks of MVP. Often, but not always, a middle- to late-peaking crescendo systolic murmur can be appreciated by itself or after a click. The murmur terminates with closure of the aortic valve (A2). This represents MR, and, in general, the duration of the murmur correlates with the severity of the MR. The earlier in systole the murmur is detected, the more severe the MR. Eventually, with more severe MR, the murmur becomes holosystolic. MVP manifestations on examination vary, and they may not always be reproducible, even in the same patient.

Certain maneuvers can aid in more accurately diagnosing MVP on examination (Figure 2). MVP is very sensitive to LV filling, and subtle changes in auscultatory findings elicited by careful examination maneuvers can be instrumental in separating MVP from other valvular abnormalities. Generally, measures that decrease LV volume or increase contractility produce earlier and more prominent systolic prolapse of the mitral leaflets, causing the systolic click and murmur to move closer to S_1. For example, in the transition from squatting to standing, LV volume is reduced, and the onset of the click and murmur is moved closer to S_1. Conversely, anything that increases LV volume, such as leg-raising, squatting, or slowing the heart rate (increased diastolic filling), delays the onset of the click or murmur and usually diminishes its duration and intensity.

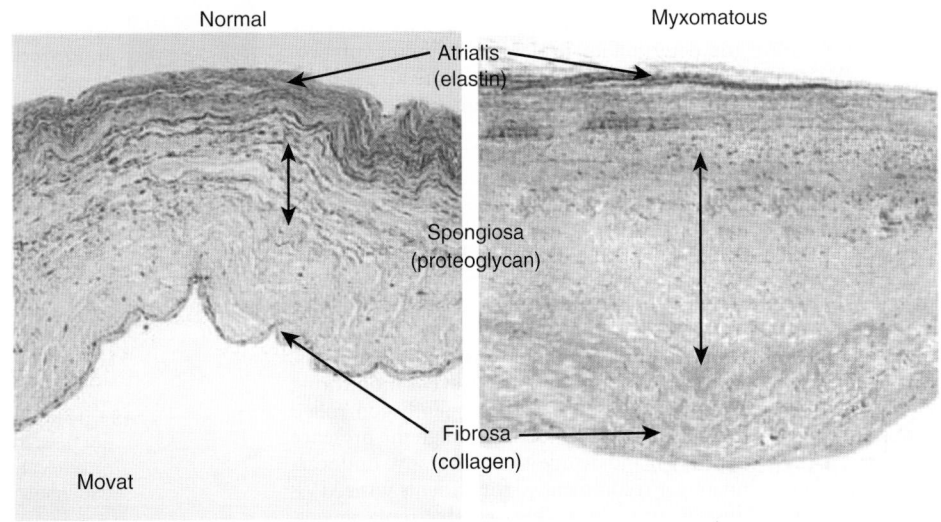

Figure 1 Morphologic features of normal mitral valves *(left)* and valves with myxomatous degeneration *(right)*. Myxomatous valves have an abnormal layered architecture: loose collagen in fibrosa, expanded spongiosa strongly positive for proteoglycans, and disrupted elastin in atrialis *(top)*. Movat pentachrome stain (collagen stains yellow, proteoglycans blue-green, and elastin black). Modified from Rabkin E, Aikawa M, Stone JR, et al: Activated interstitial myofibroblasts express catabolic enzymes and mediate matrix remodeling in myxomatous heart valves. *Circulation* 2001;104:2525.)

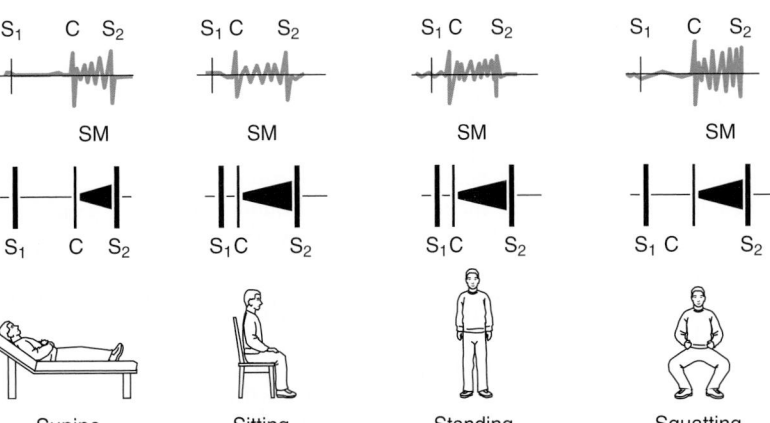

Figure 2 Auscultative findings with changes in position in patients with mitral valve prolapse (MVP). *Abbreviations*: C = click of MVP; S_1, mitral valve closure; S_2, aortic valve closure. Modified from Devereux RB, Perloff JK, Reichek N, et al: Mitral valve prolapse. *Circulation* 1976;54[1]:3–14.)

Use of Echocardiography

Two-dimensional echocardiography has proved to be the most accurate noninvasive tool for the diagnosis, assessment, and follow-up of clinically suspected MVP. In fact, physical signs of MVP in an asymptomatic patient are an American College of Cardiology/American Heart Association (ACC/AHA) class I indication for use of echocardiography to make the diagnosis of MVP and assess the severity of MR, leaflet morphology, and ventricular size and function. Once the diagnosis is made, follow-up is determined by the severity of MVP. Routine echocardiographic follow-up of asymptomatic patients with MVP is not recommended unless there are significant findings of MR or LV structural changes. Frequency of follow-up in patients with prolapse and MR is determined by the severity of MR and should be at least annual in patients with severe MR.

Diagnostic criteria for MVP on two-dimensional echocardiography are:
- Billowing of one or both mitral valve leaflets or their prolapse superiorly across the mitral annular plane in the parasternal long-axis view by greater than 2 mm during systole
- The degree of thickening of the leaflets

Combined leaflet prolapse of greater than 2 mm and leaflet thickness greater than 5 mm are supportive of classic MVP, whereas prolapse in the absence of increased thickness is considered nonclassic MVP. In addition to more often being associated with the auscultative findings of the click and murmur, the classic form is more commonly associated with increased risk of endocarditis, stroke, progressive MR, and need for mitral valve repair or replacement.

Because the mitral apparatus is saddle-shaped, certain echocardiographic views are more specific than others for determining leaflet prolapse. Most practitioners agree that the parasternal long-axis and apical two-chamber or apical long-axis views are the most accurate for determining prolapse. A finding of prolapse as determined on other views, particularly the apical four-chamber view, is much less specific and frequently leads to a false-positive diagnosis.

Medical Management

Most patients with MVP remain asymptomatic and require no additional management aside from careful observation over time. It is appropriate to provide reassurance that uncomplicated (nonclassic) MVP is a non–life-threatening condition and is unlikely to affect longevity. Periodic clinical evaluation every 3 to 5 years is reasonable. Patients who develop palpitations, lightheadedness, dizziness, or syncope should undergo Holter or event monitoring for detection of arrhythmias. Palpitations are frequently controlled with β-blockers or calcium channel blockers, although the presence of specific arrhythmias may mandate additional therapy. Endocarditis prophylaxis is no longer recommended for patients with MVP unless they have a history of endocarditis or valve replacement. Prophylaxis is recommended for patients who have undergone repair if prosthetic material was used (e.g., in ring repairs). Aspirin or warfarin (Coumadin) therapy may be recommended for certain symptomatic patients with neurologic events who have atrial fibrillation, significant MR, hypertension, or heart failure (Table 1).

Patients with classic (complicated) MVP deserve regular clinical follow-up, particularly if MR is present. These patients are more likely to develop moderate or severe MR over time. Patients with mild to moderate MR and normal LV function should be clinically evaluated at least annually and should undergo echocardiography every second or third year if stable. Patients with severe MR should have an annual echocardiogram and closer clinical follow-up. Those who have severe MR and develop symptoms or impaired LV systolic function require cardiac catheterization and evaluation for mitral valve surgery. Often the valve can be repaired rather than replaced, with a low operative mortality rate and excellent short- and long-term results when performed at experienced centers. Preservation of the native valve allows for lower risks of thrombosis and endocarditis than does prosthetic valve replacement.

Surgical Management

MVP is the most common cause of adult MR requiring mitral valve surgery. Symptoms of heart failure, severity of MR, presence or absence of atrial fibrillation, LV systolic function, LV end-diastolic and end-systolic volumes, and pulmonary artery pressure (at rest and with exercise) influence the decision to recommend mitral valve surgery. Indications for surgery in patients with MVP and MR mirror those with other forms of nonischemic severe MR. Patient outcomes after mitral valve repair are typically very good, and the surgical risk is lower than for many other forms of cardiac surgery, including mitral valve replacement.

Based on a Cleveland Clinic review of 1072 patients who underwent primary isolated mitral valve repair for MR due to myxomatous disease, the in-hospital mortality rate was 0.3%. The Mayo Clinic reviewed 1173 patients who underwent mitral valve repair for MVP from 1980 to 1999, observing mortality rates of 0.7%, 11.3%, and 29.4% at 30 days, 5 years, and 10 years, respectively.

Because of the remarkably low mortality rates associated with MVP repair, some experts advocate earlier rather than later repair of MVP in asymptomatic patients with severe MR and no evidence of LV dysfunction, pulmonary hypertension, or atrial fibrillation. AHA/ACC recommendations for surgery in patients with chronic primary mitral valve regurgitation are shown in Table 2.

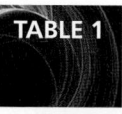

TABLE 1	ACC/AHA Recommendations for Oral Anticoagulation in Patients With Mitral Valve Prolapse
CLASS	**RECOMMENDATION**
I	ASA therapy (75–325 mg/d) for cerebral TIAs
	Warfarin (Coumadin) therapy for patients ≥65 years in atrial fibrillation with hypertension, MR, or history of congestive heart failure
	ASA therapy (75–325 mg/d) for patients <65 years in atrial fibrillation with no history of MR, hypertension, or congestive heart failure
	Warfarin therapy after stroke for patients with MR, atrial fibrillation, or left atrial thrombus
IIa	ASA therapy is reasonable in patients after stroke who do not have MR, atrial fibrillation, left atrial thrombus, or echocardiographic evidence of thickening ≥5 mm or redundancy of leaflets
	Warfarin therapy is reasonable after stroke for patients without MR, atrial fibrillation, or left atrial thrombus who have echocardiographic evidence of thickening ≥5 mm or redundancy of leaflets
	Warfarin therapy is reasonable for TIAs that occur despite ASA therapy
	ASA therapy (75–325 mg/d) can be beneficial for patients with a history of stroke who have contraindications to anticoagulants
IIb	ASA therapy (75–325 mg/d) may be considered for patients in sinus rhythm with echocardiographic evidence of complicated MVP

Abbreviations: ACC/AHA = American College of Cardiology/American Heart Association; ASA = aspirin; MR = mitral regurgitation; TIA = transient ischemic attack.

Adapted from Bonow RO, Carabello BA, Chatterjee K, et al: 2008 Focused update incorporated into the ACC/AHA 2006 guidelines for the management of patients with valvular heart disease. *Circulation* 118(15):e523–661, 2008.

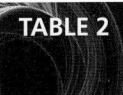

TABLE 2 ACC/AHA Recommendations for Surgery in Patients With Chronic Primary Mitral Valve Regurgitation

CLASS	RECOMMENDATION
I	Mitral valve (MV) surgery is recommended for symptomatic patients with chronic severe primary MR (stage D) and left ventricular ejection fraction (LVEF) >30%
	MV surgery is recommended for asymptomatic patients with chronic severe primary MR and left ventricular (LV) dysfunction (LVEF 30%-60% and/or left ventricular end-systolic dimension [LVESD] ≥40mm, stage C2)
	MV repair is recommended in preference to mitral valve replacement (MVR) when surgical treatment is indicated for patients with chronic severe primary MR limited to the posterior leaflet
	MV repair is recommended in preference to MVR when surgical treatment is indicated for patients with chronic severe primary MR involving the anterior leaflet or both leaflets when a successful and durable repair can be accomplished
	Concomitant MV repair or replacement is indicated in patients with chronic severe primary MR undergoing cardiac surgery for other indications
IIa	MV repair is reasonable in asymptomatic patients with chronic severe primary MR (stage C1) with preserved LV function (LVEF >60% and LVESD <40mm) in whom the likelihood of a successful and durable repair without residual MR is >95% with an expected mortality rate of <1% when performed at a Heart Valve Center of Excellence
	MV repair is reasonable for asymptomatic patients with chronic severe primary MR (stage C1) and preserved LV function (LVEF >60% and LVESD <40mm) in whom there is a high likelihood of a successful and durable repair with 1) new onset of atrial fibrillation or 2) resting pulmonary hypertension (pulmonary artery systolic arterial pressure >50mm Hg)
	MV repair is reasonable for asymptomatic patients with chronic severe primary MR (stage C1) and preserved LV function (LVEF >60% and LVESD <40mm) with progressive increase in LV size or decrease in ejection fraction on serial imaging studies
	Concomitant MV repair is reasonable in patients with chronic moderate primary MR (stage B) undergoing cardiac surgery for other indications
IIb	MV surgery may be considered in symptomatic patients with chronic severe primary MR and LVEF less than or equal to 30% (stage D)
	MV repair may be considered in patients with rheumatic mitral valve disease when surgical treatment is indicated if a durable and successful repair is likely or if the reliability of long-term anticoagulation management is questionable
	Transcatheter MV repair may be considered for severely symptomatic patients (New York Heart Association class III/IV) with chronic severe primary MR (stage D) who have a reasonable life expectancy but a prohibitive surgical risk because of severe comorbidities and remain symptomatic despite optimal goal directed medical therapy for heart failure
III Harm	MVR should not be performed for treatment of isolated severe primary MR limited to less than one half of the posterior leaflet unless MV repair has been attempted and was unsuccessful

Adapted from 2017 AHA/ACC focused update of the 2014 ACC/AHA guidelines for the management of patients with valvular heart disease. *Circulation* 135(25); e1159–e1195, 2017.

Percutaneous Management

In 2013 the FDA approved the MitraClip (Abbott Vascular) for patients with symptomatic degenerative MR who are deemed high risk for mitral valve surgery. The MitraClip technology is based on the Alfieri edge-to-edge repair in which the middle segments of the anterior and posterior leaflet are sutured together to create a double-orifice. It is approved for use in patients with New York Heart Association Class III or IV heart failure despite medical therapy, chronic moderate to severe or severe primary MR, favorable anatomy typically involving the middle segments of the anterior and posterior leaflets, reasonable life expectancy, and prohibitive surgical risk. This approval is based on the results of the Endovascular Valve Edge-to-Edge Repair Study (EVEREST II), which randomized 279 patients to either percutaneous repair or conventional surgery for repair or replacement of the mitral valve with a primary endpoint of freedom from death, from surgery for mitral valve dysfunction, and from grade 3+ or 4+ MR at 12 months. The rates of the combined primary endpoints were 55% in the percutaneous group and 73% in the surgery group (p=0.007). Rates of death (6% and 6%, respectively) and 3+ or 4+ MR (21% and 20%, respectively) were similar in each group. Major adverse events occurred in 15% of patients in the percutaneous repair group versus 48% in the surgery group at 30 days (p<0.001). Although the MitraClip was less effective at reducing MR, it was approved on the bases of its superior safety and similar clinical outcomes.

References

2008 Focused update incorporated into the ACC/AHA 2006 guidelines for the management of patients with valvular heart disease: a report of the American College of Cardiology/American Heart Association Task Force on Practice Guidelines (Writing Committee to Revise the 1998 Guidelines for the Management of Patients With Valvular Heart Disease): endorsed by the Society of Cardiovascular Anesthesiologists, Society for Cardiovascular Angiography and Interventions, and Society of Thoracic Surgeons, *Circulation* 118(15):e523–e661, 2008.

Devereux RB, Kramer-Fox R, Brown WT, et al: Relation between clinical features of the mitral prolapse syndrome and echocardiographically documented mitral valve prolapse, *J Am Coll Cardiol* 8:763–772, 1986.

Feldman T, Foster E, Glower DD, et al: Percutaneous repair or surgery for mitral regurgitation, *N Engl J Med* 364(15):1395–1406, 2011.

Flack JM, Kvasnicka JH, Gardin JM, et al: Anthropometric and physiologic correlates of mitral valve prolapse in a biethnic cohort of young adults: the CARDIA study, *Am Heart J* 138:486, 1999.

Freed LA, Benjamin EJ, Levy D, et al: Mitral valve prolapse in the general population: the benign nature of echocardiographic features in the Framingham Heart Study, *J Am Coll Cardiol* 40:1298–1304, 2002.

Freed LA, Levy D, Levine RA, et al: Prevalence and clinical outcome of mitral-valve prolapse, *N Engl J Med* 341:1–7, 1999.

Gillinov AM, Cosgrove DM, Blackstone EH, et al: Durability of mitral valve repair for degenerative disease, *J Thorac Cardiovasc Surg* 116(5):734–743, 1998.

Levy D, Savage D: Prevalence and clinical features of mitral valve prolapse, *Am Heart J* 113:1281–1290, 1987.

Marks AR, Choong CY, Sanfilippo AJ, et al: Identification of high-risk and low-risk subgroups of patients with mitral-valve prolapse, *N Engl J Med* 320:1031–1036, 1989.

Rabkin E, Aikawa M, Stone JR, et al: Activated interstitial myofibroblasts express catabolic enzymes and mediate matrix remodeling in myxomatous heart valves, *Circulation* 104:2525–2532, 2001.

Savage DD, Devereux RB, Garrison RJ, et al: Mitral valve prolapse in the general population: 2. Clinical features: The Framingham Study, *Am Heart J* 106:577–581, 1983.

Savage DD, Garrison RJ, Devereux RB, et al: Mitral valve prolapse in the general population: 1. Epidemiologic features: The Framingham Study, *Am Heart J* 106:571–576, 1983.

Suri RM, Schaff HV, Dearani JA, et al: Survival advantage and improved durability of mitral repair for leaflet prolapse subsets in the current era, *Ann Thorac Surg* 82(3):819–826, 2006.

PERICARDITIS

Method of
Amir Azarbal, MD; and Martin M. LeWinter, MD

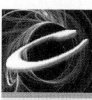

CURRENT DIAGNOSIS

- Acute pericarditis is an inflammatory syndrome thought to be caused by a viral infection in most cases. It is diagnosed when 2 of the following are present: (1) typical anterior pleuritic chest pain, (2) pericardial friction rub, (3) electrocardiography (ECG) changes (widespread ST segment elevation or PR depression, and (4) new or worsening pericardial effusion.
- Leukocytosis and an elevated high-sensitivity C-reactive protein or erythrocyte sedimentation rate (ESR) are present in most cases.
- Echocardiography is routinely used to detect pericardial effusion. Cardiac magnetic resonance imaging or computed tomography can be used to support the diagnosis.

CURRENT THERAPY

- Limitation of physical activity and high-dose aspirin[1] or other nonsteroidal antiinflammatory drugs such as ibuprofen (Advil)[1] plus colchicine[1] is the treatment of choice for idiopathic (presumed viral) pericarditis.
- Corticosteroids with gradual taper can be added for recurrences.
- Antiinflammatory drugs such as azathioprine (Imuran),[1] anakinra (Kineret),[1] and human intravenous immunoglobulin (Gammagard)[1] have been used in difficult cases of recurrent pericarditis
- Pericardiectomy is reserved for refractory cases and constrictive pericarditis.

[1]Not FDA approved for this indication.

Anatomy and Functions of the Pericardium

The pericardium consists of 2 layers. A visceral monolayer comprised of mesothelial cells is adherent to the epicardium and reflects over the origin of the great vessels, where it is continuous with the inner layer of the parietal pericardium. The latter is approximately 2 mm thick and comprised mainly of collagen and elastin. The pericardial sac is the space between visceral and parietal layers and normally contains up to 50 mL of serous fluid. The pericardium has several functions, including (1) acting as a barrier to infections, (2) providing a mechanism whereby hydrostatic pressure is exerted on the surface of the heart when gravitational or inertial forces are altered, (3) participating in neuro-humoral responses, and (4) limiting short-term distention and displacement of the heart, facilitating interactions between the cardiac chambers and modulating pressure-volume relationships and cardiac output.

Acute Pericarditis

The main inflammatory pericardial syndromes include acute and recurrent pericarditis and constrictive and effusive-constrictive pericarditis. These can be isolated to the pericardium or be a component of a systemic disease.

Acute pericarditis is the most common pericardial syndrome and is responsible for approximately 5% of emergency room visits for chest pain and 2% of patients presenting with ST elevations on ECG. An in-hospital mortality rate of approximately 1% has been reported. Acute pericarditis is more common in males. Recurrence occurs in 15% to 20% of patients within 18 months

after a first episode. Acute pericarditis can also involve the myocardium and cause myopericarditis, with elevated cardiac injury biomarkers (e.g., troponin I).

Etiology

Almost any disease that affects the pericardium can cause acute pericarditis. Acute pericarditis can also cause pericardial effusion; the incidence is highly dependent on etiology. Infectious etiologies are considered to be responsible for the majority of cases. In developed countries 80% to 90% of cases are idiopathic, that is, no specific cause is detected on routine evaluation. These cases are assumed to be viral in etiology. Bacterial and rarely fungal infections account for a small percentage of cases in the developed world. However, *Mycobacterium tuberculosis* is the most common cause of pericarditis in developing countries. Very rarely, parasitic diseases such as echinococcus and toxoplasma species can cause acute pericarditis.

Autoimmune diseases are another common cause of acute pericarditis. These include systemic autoimmune diseases such as lupus erythematosus (SLE), rheumatoid arthritis, Sjögren syndrome, and scleroderma, as well as vasculitic diseases such as eosinophilic granulomatosis with polyangiitis or allergic granulomatosis (previously named *Churg-Strauss syndrome*), Takayasu disease, and Behçet syndrome. Other autoimmune disorders associated with acute pericarditis are sarcoidosis, familial Mediterranean fever, and inflammatory bowel disease.

Malignancies affecting the pericardium also cause acute pericarditis. Almost all neoplastic pericarditis is caused by secondary metastases from extracardiac tumors, especially lung and breast cancer.

Pericarditis can occur after myocardial infarction (MI), both early (i.e., 2 to 4 days after MI) and late (Dressler syndrome, ≍1 week to 2 months after MI), and after heart surgery. The incidence of post-MI pericarditis has markedly declined because of reperfusion therapy. Trauma such as penetrating and nonpenetrating thoracic injury, esophageal perforation, and procedural complications of cardiac procedures (coronary stenting, pacemaker lead insertion, radiofrequency ablation) are all reported. Although these can cause acute cardiac tamponade, acute pericarditis occurs as a late complication within 1 to 2 weeks to as late as 3 months after the initial event. These causes are collectively termed *post-cardiac injury syndromes* and are believed to have an autoinflammatory basis. Acute pericarditis has also been reported as an immune-mediated response to various drugs.

Presentation

The diagnosis of acute pericarditis is made if two of the following are present: (1) typical anterior chest pain, (2) pericardial friction rub, (3) typical ECG changes (widespread ST segment elevation or PR depression, and (4) new or worsening pericardial effusion. In cases with typical chest pain but no other criteria, additional findings that can establish the diagnosis are elevated cardiac injury biomarkers and evidence of pericardial inflammation or thickening based on advanced imaging modalities (cardiac magnetic resonance imaging [cMRI], computed tomography [CT]). An elevation of either high-sensitivity C reactive protein (hsCRP) or the erythrocyte sedimentation (ESR) rate is supportive but not diagnostic.

Chest pain is the most common symptom of acute pericarditis, present in >90% of cases. The pain is typically sharp, located under the sternum or over the left anterior chest, and almost always pleuritic. The trapezius ridge is a classic radiation. The pain is worst supine and improved by sitting forward. Approximately one-third of patients have a pericardial friction rub (a scratchy or squeaking sound at the left sternal border) because of contact between the layers of the pericardium. The friction rub ordinarily has 3 components. Typical ECG changes include ST elevation in all leads except AVR and sometimes V1, as well as PR segment depression. Over time, these changes either simply disappear or go through a phase of ST segment normalization and T-wave inversion before disappearing. Both the friction rub and ECG changes are often evanescent. In cases where it is difficult to establish a diagnosis, repeated auscultation and ECGs can be rewarding. A pericardial effusion has been reported in as many as two-thirds of patients with acute pericarditis. The great majority are small. Sinus tachycardia and low-grade fever are also common. If cardiac tamponade is present, elevated jugular venous pressure, muffled heart sounds, hypotension, and pulsus paradoxus are seen. Other diagnoses that can be confused with acute pericarditis include acute MI, pleuritis, pulmonary embolism, costochondritis, and herpes zoster before appearance of vesicles.

Features accompanying acute pericarditis that indicate an elevated risk (mainly for development of cardiac tamponade) include fever >38.5°C, subacute onset of symptoms, moderate to large pericardial effusion, lack of response to aspirin or nonsteroidal antiinflammatory drugs (NSAIDs), immunosuppression, white blood cell count >13,000/mm³, anticoagulant therapy, and suspicion of a non-idiopathic/viral cause such as cancer, SLE, or bacterial infection.

Diagnostic Evaluation

Routine evaluation is directed toward identifying patients with or at elevated risk for cardiac tamponade or patients with a non-idiopathic/viral cause. In addition to a careful history, physical examination, and ECG, routine evaluation should include a chest radiograph, CBC, hs-CRP, routine blood chemistries, and an echocardiogram. Echocardiography should be performed in all patients to detect pericardial effusion, which can be hemodynamically significant despite a normal radiographic cardiac silhouette, and to assess cardiac function in cases with myopericarditis. In the vast majority of cases myopericarditis has no long-term prognostic significance.

Clinical Laboratory Data

Leukocytosis and elevated hs-CRP or ESR are present in most cases. The hs-CRP in particular is increased in about 75% of cases and usually normalizes within 1 to 2 weeks. Failure of normalization within this time frame is associated with higher rates of recurrence. In patients with concomitant myocarditis, markers of cardiac injury such as troponin-I are elevated.

ECG

As discussed earlier, typical ECG changes considered to be hallmarks of acute pericarditis include widespread ST segment elevations or PR segment depression (Figure 1). ECG changes are dynamic, and about 60% of patients have the following evolution over time: stage I (PR depression, ST segment elevation), stage II (ST normalization), stage III (T-wave inversion after ST segment normalization), and stage IV (ST-T normalization). These evolutionary changes have no known prognostic significance.

Imaging

The chest radiograph is normal in acute pericarditis unless a moderate- to large-size pericardial effusion or associated pulmonary pathology is present. The echocardiogram is usually normal except for the common presence of small pericardial effusions (Figure 2). In cases with associated myopericarditis, the left ventricular ejection fraction is almost always normal.

Cardiac MRI or CT typically shows pericardial thickening and enhanced gadolinium uptake (Figure 3). Advanced imaging modalities can be used to support the diagnosis of pericarditis in difficult cases.

Treatment

Treatment of common pericardial syndromes is summarized in Table 1. Reliable patients without high-risk features need not be hospitalized. For treatment of an initial episode of acute idiopathic pericarditis, avoidance of physical activity greater than walking at a normal pace is recommended until symptoms resolve and CRP has normalized. Athletes should refrain from competitive

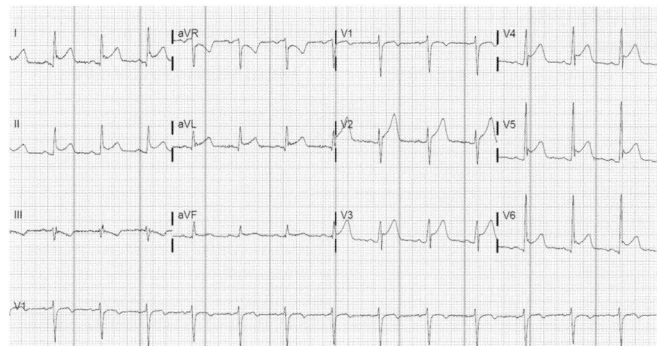

Figure 1 Electrocardiogram demonstrating typical changes of acute pericarditis. Note the widespread ST segment elevations with concomitant PR segment depression.

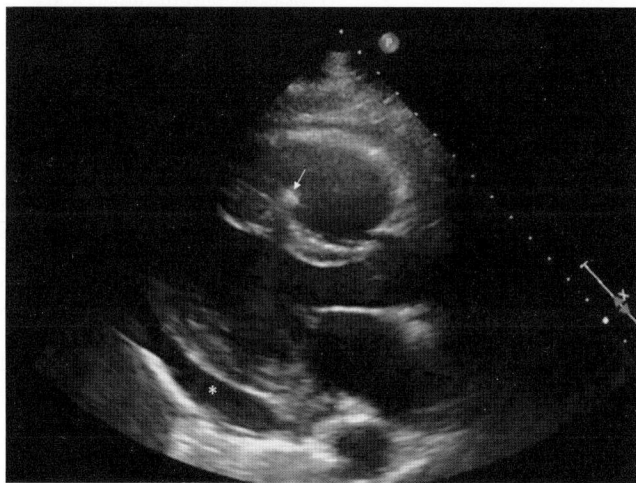

Figure 2 Parasternal long-axis view of a transthoracic echocardiogram performed in a patient with acute pericarditis showing small to moderate-sized pericardial effusion (asterisk). Also note a pacemaker lead in the right ventricle (arrow) and associated acoustic shadowing artifact.

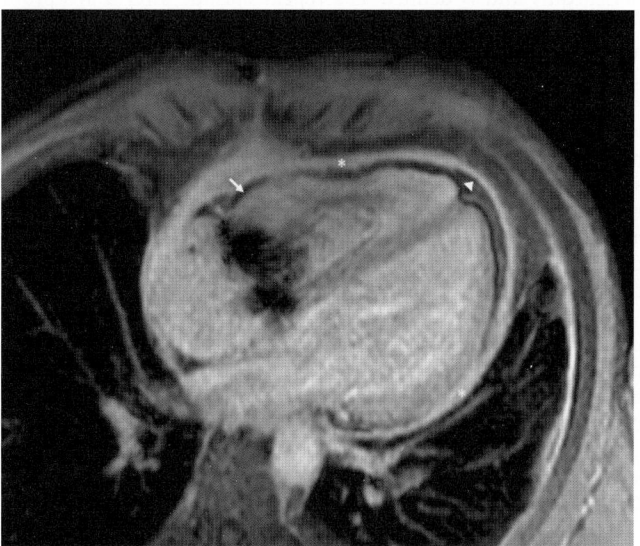

Figure 3 Cardiac MRI image in a patient with acute pericarditis after intravenous gadolinium administration. Note late gadolinium enhancement of the pericardium along with pericardial thickening indicating inflammation (asterisk). Other findings are pericardial fat (arrowhead) and trivial pericardial effusion (arrow).

TABLE 1	Treatment Summary of Common Pericardial Syndromes	
PERICARDIAL SYNDROME	**TREATMENT OVERVIEW**	**SPECIFIC CONSIDERATIONS**
Acute pericarditis	Physical activity restriction *and* NSAIDs *plus* Colchicine[1]	Restriction of physical activity until resolution of symptoms NSAIDs until symptoms resolve and CRP normalizes Colchicine for 2 to 3 months See text for pregnancy and lactation considerations
Recurrent pericarditis	Acute pericarditis treatment *plus* Corticosteroids (in refractory cases) *or* Immunosuppressive therapy (for multiple recurrences) *or* Pericardiectomy (last resort)	Restriction of physical activity until resolution of symptoms NSAIDs until symptoms resolve and CRP normalizes for 1 to 2 weeks with subsequent taper Colchicine[1] for at least 6 months For multiple recurrences, low to moderate doses of corticosteroids until resolution of symptoms and normalization of CRP followed by slow taper Immunosuppressants (anakinra [Kineret],[1] azathioprine [Imuran],[1] intravenous immunoglobulin[1]) for multiple recurrences Pericardiectomy in refractory cases (last resort)
Constrictive pericarditis	Treatment of underlying condition (ie, tuberculosis, inflammation) *or* Pericardiectomy (if chronic and refractory)	In cases of pericardial inflammation, an empiric antiinflammatory regimen may reverse the disease process and obviate the need for pericardiectomy.

[1]Not FDA approved for this indication.

sports activities for at least 3 months. NSAIDs plus colchicine[1] is a first-line pharmacologic treatment. We recommend ibuprofen (Advil)[1] 600 to 800 mg by mouth 3 times daily or aspirin[1] 2 to 4 g by mouth daily in divided doses and colchicine[1] 0.6 mg twice daily (0.6 mg once daily for patients <70 kg) until symptoms resolve and CRP normalizes. The NSAID should then be tapered over 1 to 2 weeks and colchicine continued for 3 months from onset of symptoms. All patients should receive a proton pump inhibitor while receiving NSAIDs.

In pregnancy ibuprofen, aspirin >100 mg/day by mouth, and colchicine are contraindicated after 20 weeks' gestation. Corticosteroids are preferred in this circumstance. In addition, colchicine is contraindicated during lactation.

In patients in whom a specific cause for acute pericarditis other than idiopathic/viral has been identified, the treatment should be directed at that cause. Thus, in patients with autoimmune diseases, corticosteroids may be more appropriate as the initial treatment.

Recurrent Pericarditis

Recurrent pericarditis is the most common complication of acute pericarditis and is defined as a repeat episode after a symptom-free interval of at least 4 to 6 weeks. The recurrence rate after an initial episode of acute pericarditis is approximately 15% to 20% and may increase to as much as 50% after a first recurrent episode. Patients with recurrent pericarditis can be severely incapacitated. Certain rare conditions such as familial Mediterranean fever, tumor necrosis factor receptor–associated periodic syndrome, and other periodic fever syndromes are often characterized by bouts of recurrent pericarditis. Inadequate treatment of a first episode (e.g., inadequate drug doses, too short a treatment duration or too rapid discontinuation, or tapering of medications) can be responsible for recurrences

Recurrent pericarditis after an initial bout of idiopathic/viral pericarditis is currently considered to be an autoinflammatory process (as opposed to an autoimmune disease such as SLE). It is hypothesized that, after an initial viral infection, immune system cross-reaction between viral particles and host tissue occurs. A similar mechanism is believed to be operative in the periodic fever syndromes. Of course, pericarditis due to other, specific causes can also recur.

The most feared complication of recurrent pericarditis is constrictive pericarditis. The incidence is high (≤30%) in cases of bacterial pericarditis and low to moderate (<5%) in systemic inflammatory diseases and cancer. In patients with recurrences

after an initial bout of viral/idiopathic pericarditis, symptoms almost always eventually resolve, and progression to constrictive pericarditis is very rare (<1%).

The diagnosis of a recurrence is based on the same criteria as for an initial episode (i.e., history, friction rub, ECG findings, and a new or worsening pericardial effusion). Elevated hs-CRP, ESR, and white blood cell count remain useful for monitoring disease activity and response to treatment. More advanced imaging modalities such as CT or cMRI are rarely required to diagnose a recurrence but are useful if there is a concern about development of constriction.

In general, for patients with a recurrence after an index episode of idiopathic/viral pericarditis we recommend that treatment be the same as for the initial episode (i.e., restriction of physical activity, NSAID, and colchicine[1]) until complete resolution of symptoms and normalization of hs-CRP. Some patients are able to manage recurrences by initiating treatment at the very first sign of symptoms. If the response is prompt, the recurrence is converted to a minor illness.

Use of corticosteroids for treatment of recurrent pericarditis should be reserved for cases where the above-mentioned measures have failed, especially if recurrences are frequent and severe and do not respond well to NSAIDs. Unusual patients with an initial episode who do not respond to first-line therapy are also candidates. Corticosteroids usually provide rapid relief of symptoms, and almost all patients respond favorably initially. However, corticosteroids appear to increase the chance of further recurrences, especially when high initial doses are used with rapid tapering. High doses also have a much higher incidence of adverse effects. If a decision is made to use corticosteroids, we recommend low to moderate doses (e.g., prednisone[1] 0.25 to 0.5 mg/kg/day or equivalent) usually for about 4 to 8 weeks, followed by gradual tapering (assuming symptom resolution and normalization of hs-CRP) in conjunction with colchicine. NSAIDs may also be included or added later as corticosteroids are tapered. Colchicine should ordinarily be continued for 6 months. During tapering, recurrences typically occur with doses <10 to 15 mg/day dose of prednisone or equivalent. Patients symptom free at this threshold should be treated with smaller subsequent dose decrements at intervals of 2 to 6 weeks. If possible, recurrences occurring during tapering should be treated with NSAID optimization rather than increasing corticosteroids. To prevent side effects of long-term corticosteroid use, specifically bone loss, consideration should be given to supplementary calcium and vitamin D. Bisphosphonates are recommended in all men ≥50 years and postmenopausal women in whom long-term treatment with corticosteroids at a dose of 5.0 to 7.5 mg/day of prednisone or equivalent is required.

[1]Not FDA approved for this indication.

In patients with multiple recurrences (≥3 episodes) despite the aforementioned strategies, alternative drugs have been suggested based on case reports, case series, and small randomized trials. These include azathioprine (Imuran),[1] methotrexate (Trexall),[1] and intravenous human immunoglobulin.[1] Recently, the interleukin (IL)-1β antagonist anakinra (Kineret)[1] (1 to 2 mg/kg/day up to 100 mg subcutaneously for several months) has shown considerable promise; other IL-1β antagonists are in development. Finally, as a last resort for refractory cases of recurrent pericarditis, pericardiectomy may be effective.

Constrictive Pericarditis

Etiology
Constrictive pericarditis is a consequence of chronic forms of pericarditis, especially bacterial (20% to 30%), immune-mediated, and neoplastic (2% to 5%) disease. Some cases are idiopathic. Other causes include cardiac injury syndromes, postradiation, uremia, and sarcoidosis. Before the availability of effective antimicrobial therapy, tuberculous pericarditis was the most important cause, but this is now rare in the developed world. In the third world, tuberculosis remains an important cause of pericardial disease in general and constrictive pericarditis in particular, often in association with HIV/AIDs. It is very rare (<1%) for idiopathic/viral pericarditis to result in constrictive pericarditis.

When tuberculosis was the major cause of constrictive pericarditis, cases typically presented as a very chronic disease with the features described below. Heavy pericardial calcification was a classic feature. In contemporary practice, most cases of constrictive pericarditis occur in conjunction with the syndrome of effusive-constrictive pericarditis, where pericardial effusion and constriction coexist in varying combinations.

Presentation and Physical Findings
Patients with constrictive pericarditis present with signs and symptoms of right heart failure, with small cardiac volumes and preserved ejection fraction (EF). (In extreme cases EF may be reduced due to severely impaired filling.) Symptoms include fatigue, peripheral edema, dyspnea, hepatomegaly, pleural effusions, and ascites. On physical examination, the venous pressure is markedly elevated, with an M- or W-shaped waveform caused by rapid atrial pressure descents. There is a paradoxical rise in venous pressure with inspiration (Kussmaul's sign), consistent with impaired filling of the right ventricle. A paradoxical pulse is present in as many as one-third of patients. Auscultation may reveal a pericardial knock, an early diastolic, medium-frequency sound (occurring slightly earlier than a usual third heart sound) that reflects abrupt cessation of rapid filling of the ventricles caused by the constricting pericardium. Atrial fibrillation is very common.

By definition, patients with effusive-constrictive pericarditis have pericardial effusions of variable size, which often contain adhesions and fibrous strands and are sometimes large enough to cause cardiac tamponade. In these cases, the diagnosis of constriction is often made after pericardiocentesis, when right heart filling pressures remain elevated and typical hemodynamic features become apparent.

Diagnostic Tests
The ECG often reveals nonspecific repolarization abnormalities, but there are no specific findings. In effusive-constrictive pericarditis, low-voltage and electrical alternans may be apparent if there is a large effusion. The chest X-ray film may reveal pericardial calcification, but its incidence is now low. Pleural effusions are common.

Major echocardiographic-Doppler findings include small cardiac chambers, a septal "bounce" because of exaggerated septal motion related to increased ventricular interdependence, increased mitral and tricuspid respiratory flow variation, and pericardial thickening and calcification. Interdependence is explained on the basis of a fixed intrapericardial volume, as a result of which when the volume of one ventricle changes (e.g., during respiration), the volume of the other must change reciprocally.

Cardiac catheterization reveals rapid atrial pressure descents, equalization of left- and right-sided filling pressures, increased respiratory variation in LV and RV systolic pressure (also due to ventricular interdependence) and a characteristic "dip and plateau" or "square root" sign evident in the ventricular diastolic pressure.

Cardiac CT and MRI are the best methods for imaging the pericardium. These demonstrate variable increases in pericardial thickness and calcification if present, although rare cases without increased thickness have been reported. Pericardial calcifications can be especially well visualized by cardiac CT and increased ventricular interdependence can be appreciated on real-time cine MR images. Modern cases of constrictive and effusive-constrictive pericarditis often have prominent pericardial inflammation, best imaged by gadolinium uptake during cMRI.

Treatment
Medical management of constrictive pericarditis is symptomatic and supportive, primarily consisting of diuretics to manage signs of right heart failure. It is important to avoid drugs that slow the heart rate, as these patients are critically dependent on heart rate to maintain cardiac output. Ultimately, these patients become refractory to diuretics.

Pericardiectomy has been considered the most definitive treatment for constrictive pericarditis. However, these are often difficult surgeries with high morbidity and mortality rates and delayed benefit. A number of patients are deemed too debilitated for surgery. Postradiation constriction has been considered a specific contraindication. Before pericardiectomy is undertaken, consideration should be given to a trial of an antiinflammatory regimen, especially in idiopathic cases, cases due to systemic inflammatory diseases, and cases due to post-cardiac injury syndromes. High-intensity gadolinium uptake on cardiac MRI in association with pericardial thickening is a signal that such a regimen may be successful, and apparent cures have been reported. Patients with evidence of intense inflammation often have a subacute course and belong in the subset with effusive-constrictive pericarditis. There have been no formal trials of specific antiinflammatory regimens. We favor a course of intermediate-dose prednisone[1] followed by a gradual taper similar to that recommended for recurrent pericarditis, along with colchicine[1] for at least 6 months. In cases of effusive-constrictive pericarditis presenting with cardiac tamponade, a few days of higher-dose prednisone initially may be reasonable. If an antiinflammatory regimen is to be attempted, we recommend committing to at least 2 to 3 months of prednisone treatment before tapering is begun. Reimaging the pericardium to ensure that inflammation has resolved before tapering is helpful.

References
Adler Y, Charron P, Imazio M: 2015 ESC Guidelines for the diagnosis and management of pericardial diseases. Task Force for the Diagnosis and Management of Pericardial Diseases of the European Society of Cardiology (ESC), *G Ital Cardiol (Rome)* 16:702–738, 2015.

Azarbal A, LeWinter MM: Pericardial effusion, *Cardiol Clin* 35:515–524, 2017.

Cantarini L, Lucherini OM, Brucato A: Clues to detect tumor necrosis factor receptor-associated periodic syndrome (TRAPS) among patients with idiopathic recurrent acute pericarditis: results of a multicentre study, *Clin Res Cardiol* 101:525–531, 2012.

Hoit BD: Anatomy and physiology of the pericardium, *Cardiol Clin* 35:481–490, 2017.

Imazio M, Battaglia A, Gaido L, Gaita F: Recurrent pericarditis, *Rev Med Interne* 38:307–311, 2017.

Imazio M, Brucato A, Cemin R: A randomized trial of colchicine for acute pericarditis, *N Engl J Med* 369:1522–1528, 2013.

Imazio M, Brucato A, Cumetti D: Corticosteroids for recurrent pericarditis: high versus low doses: a nonrandomized observation, *Circulation* 118:667–671, 2008.

Imazio M, Gaita F, LeWinter M: Evaluation and treatment of pericarditis: a systematic review, *JAMA* 314:1498–1506, 2015.

Kyto V, Sipila J, Rautava P: Clinical profile and influences on outcomes in patients hospitalized for acute pericarditis, *Circulation* 130:1601–1606, 2014.

LeWinter MM: Clinical practice: acute pericarditis, *N Engl J Med* 371:2410–2416, 2014.

PERIPHERAL ARTERY DISEASE

Method of
Tracie C. Collins, MD, MPH, MHCDS

CURRENT DIAGNOSIS

- Leg pain, fatigue, weakness, or numbness with walking
- Ankle-brachial index is a common initial diagnostic approach.

CURRENT THERAPY

- Risk factor control (e.g., tobacco cessation, lipid lowering therapy) is key.
- Cilostazol improves walking distance.
- Exercise rehabilitation is an important first approach in patients without severe peripheral artery disease (PAD).

Overview

Epidemiology and Risk Factors

Peripheral artery disease (PAD) is a prevalent disease affecting 20% to 30% of patients ≥50 years of age, or up to 12 million Americans. The annual age-specific incidence of PAD is 61 per 10,000 men and 54 per 10,000 women aged 65 to 74 years. The most common anatomic sites for PAD are the abdominal aorta and arteries of the lower extremities. The most common etiology of PAD is atherosclerosis, with risk factors that include age 65 years and older, smoking, diabetes mellitus, hypertension, and dyslipidemia.

Pathophysiology

PAD is atherosclerotic plaque build-up sufficient to cause a reduction of blood flow in the abdominal aorta and/or arteries of the lower extremities. The reduced blood flow can lead to exertional leg symptoms. Inflow disease is defined as blockages involving the aortoiliac and femoropopliteal arteries. Outflow disease involves the infrapopliteal (below-the-knee) arteries.

Prevention and Screening Recommendations

Prevention of PAD includes control of atherosclerotic risk factors. The US Preventive Services Task Force on PAD Screening concluded that there is no direct evidence and limited indirect evidence on the benefits of screening for PAD using the ankle-brachial index (ABI) in asymptomatic patients. Furthermore, based on available studies, there is low sensitivity and no evidence of benefit toward health outcomes with screening for asymptomatic PAD.

Clinical Manifestations

Persons with PAD may present without exertional leg symptoms (asymptomatic disease) or with symptoms of leg pain, fatigue, weakness, or numbness with walking (symptomatic disease). Symptomatic disease is categorized as atypical leg pain (pain in legs that is not classic intermittent claudication), classic intermittent claudication (exertional calf pain that resolves within 10 minutes of rest), or critical limb ischemia (ischemic rest pain, ulcers, or gangrene).

Diagnosis

The resting ABI—ratio of systolic blood pressure in the ankle to systolic blood pressure in the arm—is a commonly used, initial diagnostic test for PAD. The ABI examination is conducted by placing a patient in the supine position for 5 minutes with blood pressure cuffs placed just above each brachial artery and at each ankle. A hand-held Doppler is used to measure systolic blood pressures in both brachial arteries and in both ankles (i.e.,

the dorsalis pedis and posterior tibial arteries). The resting ABI is calculated based on the ratio of the ankle and arm pressures, based on the higher pressure for each ankle and the higher of the arm pressures. In patients with exertional leg symptoms and normal or borderline resting ABI results, exercise treadmill ABI testing is important to objectively measure functional limitations attributable to leg symptoms and PAD. The toe-brachial index provides additional diagnostic information for patients with evidence of arterial stiffness (ABI >1.40). Studies that provide more anatomic detail for patients with PAD who are being considered for invasive intervention include duplex ultrasonography, computed tomography angiography (CTA), or magnetic resonance angiography (MRA).

Ankle-Brachial Index

If the highest systolic blood pressure measured at the posterior tibialis artery is 160 and the highest systolic blood pressure measured on the upper arm is 130, then the ABI is normal at 1.23 (ankle: 160/brachial: 130 = 1.23) (Table 1).

Differential Diagnosis

The differential diagnosis for PAD includes spinal stenosis, venous claudication, popliteal artery entrapment syndrome, nerve root compression, or arthritis (Table 2). Additional history including a patient's age, approach to relieve symptoms, and/or joint involvement can help further delineate the diagnosis. PAD can certainly coexist with other chronic conditions.

Treatment

Risk Factor Control

Control of atherosclerotic risk factors is a key component to reducing systemic ischemic events in persons with PAD (Figure 1). Among persons with PAD, disease severity increases fourfold with heavy smoking and twofold with diabetes mellitus. Current guidelines for PAD management include smoking cessation, blood pressure <130/80 mm Hg (per the current American College of Cardiology/American Heart Association [ACC/AHA] guidelines), and glycosylated hemoglobin A1c level of <7%. Furthermore, all patients with PAD should have their serum low-density lipoprotein cholesterol (LDL-C) reduced to <1.8 mmol/L (<70 mg/dL).

Tobacco Cessation

Smoking cessation in patients with PAD reduces the progression of disease including the severity of claudication, occurrence of rest pain, likelihood of amputation, need for revascularization, and failure of arterial bypass grafts.

A highly successful option for smoking cessation is pharmacotherapy. Varenicline (Chantix) is efficacious for smoking cessation at a dose of 1 mg twice per day for 12 weeks. Varenicline is associated with nausea that may resolve with continued use. Use of varenicline may be associated with an increased risk of cardiovascular adverse events. In 2018 in a population-based study conducted in Canada, varenicline use was associated with a 34% higher risk for cardiovascular events in the risk compared with control interval. These findings included persons without a history of cardiovascular disease.

TABLE 1	Ankle-Brachial Index	
ABI	**RISK OF ARTERIAL DISEASE**	**REFER TO VASCULAR SPECIALIST**
≥1.0	Normal	None
0.91–0.99	Borderline	None
0.7–0.90	Some arterial disease	Treat risk factors
0.5–0.69	Moderate arterial disease	Refer
<0.5	Severe arterial disease	Refer

TABLE 2 Differential Diagnosis for Symptomatic PAD

CONDITION	LOCATION	CHARACTERISTIC	EFFECT OF EXERCISE	EFFECT OF REST	OTHER CHARACTERISTICS
Venous claudication	Entire leg, worse in calf	Tight, bursting pain	After walking	Slowly subsides	History of iliofemoral deep vein thrombosis; edema; signs of venous stasis
Popliteal artery entrapment syndrome	Calf muscles	Tight, tearing pain	After moderate to vigorous exercise (jogging)	Subsides slowly	Typically heavy muscular athletes
Spinal stenosis	Often bilateral buttocks, posterior leg	Pain and weakness	May mimic claudication	Variable relief but can take a long time to recover	Worse with standing and extending spine
Nerve root compression	Radiates down leg	Sharp lancinating pain	Induced by sitting, standing, or walking	Often present at rest	History of back problems; worse with sitting; relief when supine or sitting
Arthritis (hip, foot, or ankle)	Lateral hip, thigh, foot arch, ankle	Aching discomfort	After variable degree of exercise	Not quickly relieved	Symptoms variable; may be related to activity or present at rest

Limb improvement
• Reduce pain
• Improve walking distance
• Reduce limb loss

Cardiovascular risk reduction
• Reduce systemic ischemic events

Figure 1 Overall goals for management of peripheral artery disease.

Glycemic Control

Approaches to achieving glucose control include diet, exercise, and medications. Prior clinical trials have demonstrated the value of blood glucose control to prevent micro- but not macrovascular complications (e.g., progression of PAD). Certain minority populations are at higher risk for adverse limb outcomes compared with non-Hispanic Whites. One such outcome is lower extremity amputation. In the Strong Heart Study—an observational cohort study of cardiovascular disease and its risk factors in 13 American Indian communities—and among 1874 individuals without a lower extremity amputation at baseline, 4.4% experienced amputation within 8 years. Longer duration of diabetes mellitus and higher levels of glycosylated hemoglobin were risk factors for this adverse outcome.

Less is known of the benefit of glucose control to reduce adverse limb events in persons with PAD. However, in one retrospective cohort study involving more than 790 veterans with PAD, glucose control in African Americans was associated with a 67% reduced risk for a major limb event (i.e., lower extremity bypass surgery or lower extremity amputation). Thus there is some evidence that supports aggressive blood glucose lowering to prevent macrovascular complications in PAD.

Caution must be taken with the use of certain drugs for patients with diabetes. Specifically, the use of the sodium-glucose cotransporter-2 (SGLT-2) inhibitor, canagliflozin (Invokana), has been associated with an increased risk for lower extremity amputations, largely toe or metatarsal level, as based on results from two trials of patients with diabetes. Furthermore, in a retrospective cohort study involving 40,000 new users of SGLT-2 inhibitors, users of the SGLT-2 inhibitor were significantly more likely to undergo amputations compared with users of older antidiabetes drugs.

Antiplatelet Therapy

By reducing platelet aggregation, antiplatelet therapy reduces the risk of myocardial infarction and ischemic cerebrovascular accidents. Because of the high burden of coexisting coronary artery disease (CAD) and cerebrovascular disease in patients with PAD, antiplatelet therapy is an important part of pharmacologic therapy for this disease. In addition, aside from their systemic benefits, antiplatelet agents may reduce poor limb outcomes (i.e., reduced risk for peripheral arterial surgery and an improvement in vascular graft patency). The most common antiplatelet therapies for PAD include aspirin[1] (75–325 mg daily) and clopidogrel ([Plavix] 75 mg daily); clopidogrel is an oral P2Y12 inhibitor. Aspirin (ASA) is recommended for patients with asymptomatic PAD with stable cardiovascular disease and without contraindications or a greater risk to harm ratio (e.g., 70 years or older). Clopidogrel or ticagrelor (Brilinta)[1] (also a $P2Y_{12}$ inhibitor) monotherapy is an option for patients with symptomatic PAD without clinically manifest CAD or cerebrovascular disease. Clopidogrel is more effective than ASA to prevent a major cardiovascular event (MACE) in patients with symptomatic PAD without clinical evidence of CAD or cerebrovascular disease. Ticagrelor (90 mg twice daily) is an acceptable alternative for patients who are poor metabolizers of clopidogrel. For patients with symptomatic PAD and stable cardiovascular disease, ASA (or clopidogrel, if ASA is contraindicated) should be used to prevent MACE. For patients taking ASA who are at high risk of cardiac and ischemic limb events and 1 year out from a myocardial infarction, the addition of ticagrelor can be considered to prevent MACE or a major adverse limb event (MALE—defined as acute limb ischemia or major amputation). For patients at high risk for ischemic limb events (prior acute limb ischemia or more severe PAD as defined by an ABI <0.60), vorapaxar (Zontivity 2.08 mg daily), a protease-activated receptor-1 antagonist that inhibits thrombin-induced platelet aggregation, can be added to a regimen of ASA or clopidogrel.

Lipid Lowering Therapy

In patients with PAD and dyslipidemia, statin therapy reduces the incidence of mortality, cardiovascular events, and stroke. High-intensity statin therapy is a guideline recommended therapy for patients with PAD, per the American Heart Association. Based on results from the Heart Protection Study (HPS), there was a 13% to 27% reduction in total mortality, vascular mortality, coronary artery events, or carotid artery events during 5 years of follow-up among 6748 patients with PAD who were randomized to 40 mg of simvastatin (Zocor) therapy. These findings were independent of the coexistence of CAD at the time of randomization.

A newer treatment for lipid lowering that can be added after maximizing statin therapy is the proprotein convertase subtilisin/

---

[1]Not FDA approved for this indication.

kexin type 9 (PCSK9) inhibitor evolocumab (Repatha 140 mg every 2 weeks or 420 mg once monthly), which reduced cardiovascular events in patients with PAD. In the Further Cardiovascular Outcomes Research with PCSK9 Inhibition in Subjects with Elevated Risk (FOURIER) trial, 27,564 patients with atherosclerotic disease on statin therapy were randomized to evolocumab versus placebo and followed for a median of 2.2 years. Evolocumab significantly reduced the composite primary endpoint of cardiovascular death, myocardial infarction, stroke, hospital admission for unstable angina, or coronary revascularization in patients with PAD (hazard ratio [HR] 0.79; 95% confidence interval [CI], 0.66 to 0.94; $P = .0098$).

Statin use is also associated with a reduction in adverse limb outcomes. In the Reduction of Atherothrombosis for Continued Health (REACH) registry, statin therapy was associated with a reduction in the combined endpoint of worsening claudication, new critical limb ischemia, lower extremity revascularization, or amputation.

In the FOURIER trial, evolocumab reduced the risk of major adverse limb events (acute limb ischemia, major amputation, or urgent peripheral revascularization for ischemia) in patients with and without PAD.

Hypertension Therapy
Control of blood pressure (<130/80) is another crucial target to reduce the risk for cardiovascular morbidity and mortality in persons with PAD. The management of hypertension in patients with PAD includes lifestyle modifications and drug therapy. Thiazide diuretics are first-line agents. Angiotensin-converting enzyme inhibitors or angiotensin receptor blockers should be used in patients with renal disease or in those with chronic heart failure. Calcium channel blockers can be added for difficult-to-control hypertension. In the Heart Outcomes Protection Evaluation Study (HOPE), ramipril (Altace) at 10 mg daily significantly reduced cardiovascular events in persons with symptomatic and asymptomatic PAD; most of these patients had increased blood pressure. In the ONTARGET (Ongoing Telmisartan Alone and in Combination with Ramipril Global Endpoint Trial), telmisartan (Micardis), an angiotensin receptor blocker, was noninferior to ramipril for the composite outcome of cardiovascular death, myocardial infarction, stroke, and hospitalization for congestive heart failure. Although there has been concern with the risk for worsening of leg symptoms in persons with PAD who are prescribed β-blockers, this concern has not been validated.

Cilostazol
Cilostazol (Pletal), a phosphodiesterase type-3 with antiplatelet and vasodilator properties, is efficacious for treatment of *symptomatic* PAD (intermittent claudication). Cilostazol inhibits platelet aggregation, inhibits vascular smooth muscle proliferation, and causes vasodilatation. Cilostazol improves both pain-free and maximal treadmill walking distance. In a study involving 54 outpatient vascular clinics and 698 patients, cilostazol improved mean maximal walking distance by 54% at 6 months. Additionally, cilostazol reduces restenosis after superficial femoral artery stenting with self-expandable nitinol stents. The recommended dose is 100 mg twice daily (reduce to 50 mg twice daily for patients concomitantly taking CYP2C19 or CYP3A4 drugs).

Although several physiologic benefits of cilostazol are recognized, its mechanism of action in improving symptoms of intermittent claudication is unknown. As a phosphodiesterase type-3 inhibitor, cilostazol is in the same class of agents as milrinone (Primacor). In patients with heart failure, milrinone is associated with increased mortality. Although cilostazol has fewer cardiac inotropic effects, it has equivalent vasodilating and platelet-inhibiting effects as milrinone and is contraindicated in patients with PAD and heart failure. Cilostazol may offer some benefit toward improving lipid profiles. Rizzo and colleagues reported that cilostazol lowers plasma triglyceride levels and increases high-density lipoprotein cholesterol concentrations.

Exercise Rehabilitation and Revascularization
Walking therapy reduces walking impairment (i.e., walking distance, speed, and/or stair climbing). The exact mechanisms by which walking therapy improves lower limb function in PAD are not clear. One possible mechanism is an improvement in lower limb blood flow and walking economy (i.e., achieving gait stability without compromising walking velocity).

Walking therapy is an excellent yet underutilized component of care for persons with mild to moderately severe symptomatic PAD. Supervised treadmill walking (conducted within a clinical setting with supervision by a trained clinician) improves walking distance in patients with symptomatic PAD. Improvement is initially evident at 12 weeks, with significantly greater improvement at 24 weeks. In a typical regimen, the exercise physiologist coaches the patient to walk until there is moderate pain, to rest, and then to resume walking when pain subsides; this cycle of intermittent walking is continued for a total of 50 minutes. Short-term improvement in maximal distance with supervised treadmill walking can exceed 150%. As of May 2017, the Centers for Medicare and Medicaid has approved coverage for 36 sessions over 12 weeks of supervised exercise therapy for patients with symptomatic PAD who are referred to a cardiac rehab laboratory (hospital or outpatient) by a physician; the cost is $55 per session with a 20% copayment, which may be covered by supplemental insurance. An additional 36 sessions may also be covered without a requirement for completion of all sessions within 12 weeks; the Current Procedural Terminology (CPT) is 93668 (under Peripheral Arterial Disease Rehabilitation).

An alternative to supervised walking is a home-based walking program (community-based walking therapy). Gardner and colleagues completed a walking intervention trial that compared home-based walking to supervised walking in patients with PAD. One hundred nineteen patients were randomized and 92 completed the study. At 12 weeks, patients randomized to either home-based or supervised walking improved both their onset to pain ($P < .001$) and peak walking times ($P < .01$). A change in daily average cadence—walking rate as captured in steps per minute—was significantly greater in the home-based walking group ($P < .05$) compared with the supervised walking or usual care groups. Improvements in walking speed were also noted with a trial in which 145 participants with diabetes mellitus and PAD were randomized to a 6-month home-based walking intervention or attention control. Participants randomized to the home-based walking intervention significantly improved their walking speed ($P < .05$) and a quality of life subscale score ($P < .05$). A key challenge to the use of home-based walking is patient adherence to such therapy. Adherence to walking is impacted by several factors including patient knowledge of disease, access to environmentally safe sites, and motivation. A psychosocial mediator for behavior change, self-efficacy, was shown to positively impact home-based walking for persons with diabetes mellitus and PAD.

A multicenter trial comparing no walking to low-intensity to high-intensity walking showed the most benefit for the high-intensity group. In fact, there was no difference in the 6-minute walk distance between no walking and low-intensity walking. The main difference in the high-intensity group was that subjects walked fast enough to trigger ischemic symptoms. If medically supervised or walking at home, patients should be encouraged to walk fast enough to cause symptoms and then resume walking after symptoms resolve with rest.

Vascular Interventions
Aside from noninvasive management, patients with intermittent claudication are often referred from their primary care clinicians (e.g., internists and family medicine physicians) to vascular interventionists for consideration for lower limb revascularization. Many of these patients could be managed with exercise therapy. In patients with symptomatic PAD who have failed maximal medical therapy and exercise programs, or whose

symptoms are advanced or deteriorating, lower extremity revascularization (either surgical or, more commonly, endovascular) represents treatment options. Both strategies have demonstrated an improvement in walking performance and relief of symptoms of limb-threatening ischemia.

Similar to supervised exercise therapy, endovascular intervention improves functional outcomes in patients with PAD. The Claudication: Exercise versus Endoluminal Revascularization (CLEVER) trial randomized 111 patients with aortoiliac arterial occlusive disease to one of three treatments: optimal medical care (OMC), OMC plus supervised exercise, and OMC plus stent revascularization. The primary outcome was change in peak walking time at 6 months. Secondary outcomes included free-living step activity and quality of life. For the primary outcome, participants randomized to supervised exercise therapy and OMC experienced the greatest mean change in peak walking time 5.8 (SD 4.6) minutes. Participants randomized to stent revascularization had a mean change of 3.7 (SD 4.9) minutes and those randomized to OMC had a mean change of 1.2 (SD 2.6) minutes in peak walking time. There were statistically significant differences between the supervised exercise group compared with the OMC and stent revascularization, $P < .001$ and 0.04, respectively. Interestingly, both treatment groups experienced an improvement in quality of life, but persons randomized to stent revascularization versus supervised exercise therapy experienced the greatest improvement.

In an industry-sponsored study, 6564 patients who had received a revascularizing procedure were randomized to aspirin or the direct oral anticoagulant, rivaroxaban (Xarelto) 2.5 mg twice daily plus aspirin. The aspirin and rivaroxaban group had a significant reduction of limb ischemia, major amputation for vascular causes, myocardial infarction, ischemic stroke, or death from cardiovascular causes than aspirin alone. However, the bleeding complications were higher.

Monitoring

Over 5 years, up to 80% of patients with intermittent claudication remain stable and up to 20% worsen, based on data largely involving non-Hispanic Whites. Risk factors for disease progression are comparable to those risk factors that increase the risk for PAD. Follow-up should occur at least annually and more frequently, per the severity of PAD.

References

Bonaca MP, Nault P, Giugliano RP: Low-density lipoprotein cholesterol lowering with evolocumab and outcomes in patients with peripheral artery disease: insights from the FOURIER Trial (Further Cardiovascular Outcomes Research with PCSK9 Inhibition in Subjects with Elevated Risk), *Circulation* 137(4):338–350, 2018.

Bonaca MP, et al: Rivaroxaban in peripheral artery disease after revascularization, *N Engl J Med* 382(21):1994–2004, 2020.

Collins T, Petersen N, Suarez-Almazor M: The prevalence of peripheral arterial disease in a racially diverse population, *Arch Intern Med* 163:1469–1474, 2003.

Collins TC: PAD: medical treatment and risk reduction strategies. In Slovut D, Dean S, Jaff M, editors: *Comprehensive review in vascular and endovascular medicine*, 2012.

Gershon AS, Campitelli MA, Hawken S: Cardiovascular and neuropsychiatric events after varenicline use for smoking cessation, *Am J Respir Crit Care Med* 197(7):913–922, 2018.

Guirguis-Blake JM, Evans CV, Redmond N: Screening for peripheral artery disease using the ankle-brachial index: updated evidence report and systematic review for the US Preventive Services Task Force, *J Am Med Assoc* 320(2):184–196, 2018.

Hess CN, Hiatt WR: Antithrombotic therapy for peripheral artery disease in 2018, *J Am Med Assoc* 319(22):2329–2330, 2018.

McDermott MM, Spring B, Tian L, et al: Effect of low-intensity vs high-intensity home-based walking exercise on walk distance in patients with peripheral artery disease: the LITE randomized clinical trial, *J Am Med Assoc* 325(13):1266–1276, 2021. https://doi.org/10.1001/jama.2021.2536.

Norgren L, Hiatt WR, Dormandy JA: Inter-society consensus for the management of peripheral arterial disease (TASC II), *J Vasc Surg* 45(Suppl S):S5–S67, 2007.

Olin JW, White CJ, Armstrong EJ: Peripheral artery disease: evolving role of exercise, medical therapy, and endovascular options, *J Am Coll Cardiol* 67(11):1338–1357, 2016.

Ostergren J, Sleight P, Dagenais G: Impact of ramipril in patients with evidence of clinical or subclinical peripheral arterial disease, *Eur Heart J* 25(1):17–24, 2004.

PREMATURE BEATS

Method of
Randell Wexler, MD, MPH

CURRENT DIAGNOSIS

- The cause of a premature beat may be either atrial (premature atrial contractions or PAC) or ventricular (premature ventricular contractions or PVC) in origin.
- PACs are most often benign but are associated with increased risk of atrial fibrillation.
- PVCs may be benign, but underlying structural heart disease is not uncommon and must be ruled out with echocardiography.
- PACs and PVCs are most commonly diagnosed by EKG although Holter or event monitoring may be required.
- A heavier PVC burden is associated with increased development of cardiomyopathy and cardiovascular morbidity and mortality.

CURRENT THERAPY

- PACs are treated if their presence causes the patient symptoms and interferes with daily life.
- Beta blockers are most often used for the treatment of symptomatic PACs.
- In patients with underlying structural heart disease, the treatment of PVCs is directed at the underlying cardiac condition.
- Antiarrhythmics show no benefit in treatment of PVCs in patients with cardiomyopathy and should not be used to suppress their presence post myocardial infarction.
- Patients with a PVC burden of > 15% should see an EPS specialist for evaluation and treatment, as there is an increased risk of a significant cardiac arrhythmia.

It is not uncommon for a patient to present to a primary care physician with the complaint of their "heart pounding," "skipping beats," or having "palpitations." Though often the only symptom, patients may also complain of concomitant dizziness, lightheadedness, or frank syncope. The patient may be young or old, have underlying structural heart disease (or not), or risk factors for heart disease such as hypertension. A patient with such a history may be experiencing one of a number of cardiac arrhythmias, although it is not uncommon to find no underlying etiology at all.

Normal electrical propagation in the heart begins with the spontaneous electrical discharge at the sinoatrial node, which is then propagated along the right atrial wall to the atrioventricular node and from there to the ventricles via the His-Purkinje System. Disruption anywhere along this pathway may lead to an arrhythmia, which is defined as a rhythm that is not sinus and is accompanied by an abnormal electrical conduction.

If an arrhythmia is present, it is classified by its anatomic location of origin. Common atrial arrhythmias include atrial fibrillation/flutter, paroxysmal supraventricular tachycardia, and premature atrial contractions (PACs). Ventricular arrhythmias are often designated as premature ventricular contractions (PVCs), ventricular tachycardia, and ventricular fibrillation. Other arrhythmias that are often seen include bradycardia, tachycardia, and first-, second-, and third-degree heart block (complex morphology is normal). Age may offer clues as to etiology. As one ages, paroxysmal supraventricular tachycardia and atrial fibrillation/flutter are more likely. This chapter will review arrhythmias commonly referred to as premature beats: PACs, and PVCs.

Premature Atrial Contractions
Epidemiology and Risk Factors

PACs are common and are found in both the general population as well as in those with underlying cardiac disease. Research has established that PACs exist in up to 99% of those over the age of 50 with increasing frequency with each decade of life. It has long been believed that atrial ectopy, especially in a patient with no underlying heart disease, is benign and more of a nuisance than a risk. However, it is now understood that PACs do present an increased risk for atrial fibrillation or ischemic stroke, and although most often benign, are not entirely so.

Underlying structural heart disease (such as mitral valve disease or left ventricular dysfunction) is significantly correlated to the risk of developing PACs. Additional risk factors associated with PACs include: 1) height (potentially due to the relationship between body size and left atrial measurements); 2) those with higher levels of B natriuretic peptide (BNP); as well as 3) those with abnormalities of high-density lipoprotein (HDL) lipid metabolism in which a lower HDL is associated with increased risk of PACs. This inverse relationship has also been reported between PACs and physical activity. The difficulty in determining the clinical significance of PACs is owing to their frequent presence in the population at large.

Pathophysiology

The true etiology of PACs is not well researched and therefore not well understood. Investigation has suggested that normally functioning sino-atrial (SA) and atrio-ventricular (AV) nodes can be impacted by stimuli arising from outside of the atria. It has been proposed that this stimuli leads to reversible nodal remodeling. As a result it has been hypothesized that PACs may occur due to an adversely impacted SA or AV node subsequent to such remodeling. Others have postulated that mechanisms such as reentry and abnormal automaticity initiate PAC transmission but the actual cause is not known.

An electrocardiogram (EKG) provides an electrical account of heart function. Electrical impulses begin in the sinus node and then travel through Bachmann's bundle (the sole specialized atrial conduction system) subsequently diffusing over the atria. The P wave represents atrial electrical activity. A normal P wave as seen on the EKG is smooth and never peaked or sharp. The leads best used to review the P wave are leads II and V1.

A patient may have a left atrial abnormality (LAA), right atrial abnormality (RAA), or both. An LAA abnormality results in prolonged atrial activation times, because left atrial activation is later than right atrial activation. Such abnormalities may result in "notched" P waves because of the spatial separation of the left and right atrial peaks. When a patient has a RAA, the P wave tends to have increased amplitude due to the summation of the two peaks. Whenever possible, P wave abnormalities should be labeled left or right in nature.

A PAC will typically be seen on EKG as an abnormal P wave followed by a normal QRS complex. Morphologically, the P wave will be different than a normal (sinus) P wave. If the site of the PAC origin is near the AV node, it will be inverted, whereas if it is more distal, it will be upright. Should the PAC reach the SA node, the resulting finding on the EKG will be a longer interval between sinus beats, but it is not compensatory in nature. PACs may occur singularly or at regular intervals (every other beat is termed bigeminy) or in a group (two sequential PACs are termed a couplet). In addition, a PAC may be blocked (buried in a T wave) or conducted aberrantly (an atypical electrical configuration).

Prevention and Clinical Manifestations

The majority of PACs are idiopathic unless there is underlying heart disease. Potential non-cardiac causes include tobacco use, alcohol consumption, substance abuse, and coffee. Reducing and/or eliminating these substances can be helpful in preventing symptoms. Additionally, certain medications, supplements, or substances of abuse may cause PACs, and therefore in any patient presenting with the complaint of extra beats, a thorough review of all medications, supplements, and elicit substance use should be undertaken.

Although the vast majority of patients who are found to have PACs incidentally will not experience symptoms, patients presenting with the complaint of PACs may state that they feel that their heart is racing, skipping beats, or fluttering, or that they are experiencing palpitations. Though not common, some patients may experience dizziness.

PACs are now known to be precursors to atrial fibrillation or ischemic stroke. Thus the previous belief that atrial ectopy is benign and more of a nuisance has been shown to be incorrect. In fact, some studies suggest that a single PAC on EKG not only predicts atrial fibrillation but may also be a predictor of fatal outcome.

Diagnosis and Differential Diagnosis

The diagnosis of PACs is often made on EKG, especially if the patient is symptomatic at the time of testing. If the EKG does not demonstrate an etiology, a 24-hour Holter monitor or 30-day event monitor may also be considered. The diagnoses of a PAC can be made if the P wave has a morphology that is different from and occurs earlier in the cardiac cycle than that of a sinus P wave. Many patients experience palpitations in which the EKG evaluation suggests no underlying etiology. Therefore, in addition to electrocardiography, patients with PACs should have baseline labs drawn to include a thyroid stimulating hormone, complete blood count, magnesium and phosphate, and electrolytes. If drug use is a possible etiology, a toxicology screen can be useful.

Differential diagnosis includes other cardiac arrhythmias such as PVCs, atrial fibrillation, atrial flutter, and paroxysmal supraventricular tachycardia. Underlying disorders that may be the cause include underlying anxiety or thyroid and other metabolic disorder, as well as substance abuse.

Treatment and Monitoring

Echocardiography is helpful in determining if the patient has underlying structural heart disease requiring further evaluation and intervention. If the patient has no underlying structural heart disease, then no treatment is necessary, especially if the individual is asymptomatic and the PACs are found incidentally. If the patient does have symptomatic PACs to a degree that they interfere with the patient's quality of life, interventions include the use of beta blockers, and if they fail, a trial type IA, type IC, or type III antiarrhythmic agents may be considered. If the problem is electrophysiological in nature, catheter ablation or pulmonary vein isolation may be helpful. Elimination of tobacco, alcohol, and caffeine should be recommended.

If the patient has underlying structural heart disease, then treatment is directed at the underlying disorder. Frequent PACs can be associated with an increase in cardiovascular mortality. Patients with PACs should be educated as to the association of atrial fibrillation or stroke with instructions to notify their physician or seek attention immediately should symptoms occur. In case reports, normalization of left ventricular function has been reported following ablation.

Premature Ventricular Contractions
Epidemiology and Risk Factors

Premature ventricular contractions (PVCs) are a common cardiac finding, with upward of 40% to 75% of apparently healthy people being affected. As with PACs, they tend to increase with age. Underlying cardiovascular disease, especially ischemic heart disease increases one's risk for PVCs. As such, evaluation should be focused on excluding structural heart disease. It should be noted that PVCs are also common in those with inherited channelopathies, so a good family history is also important. PVCs are also common in well-conditioned athlete's due to autonomic tone. Although this may be a normal compensatory mechanism, structural heart disease still needs to be eliminated. PVCs associated with exercise portend increased cardiac mortality.

Pathophysiology

After propagation through the atria, the electrical impulse activates the AV node that serves as the sole pathway for electrical transmission between the atria and the ventricles. The terminal portion of the AV junction becomes the bundle of His that propagates the electrical impulse to the bundle branches, which further divide into smaller subdivisions eventually connecting to the Purkinje fibers. From the Purkinje fibers, the electrical impulse diffuses synchronously across the ventricles.

PVCs arise from ectopic foci in the ventricle and occur earlier in the cardiac cycle than expected for a sinus beat. They may be generated by increased automaticity, reentry, or triggered activity. Monomorphic PVCs suggest a triggering component whereas polymorphic PVCs tend to suggest an underlying cardiomyopathy. If the patient has no structural heart disease, the focus is likely to be the right ventricular outflow tract, whereas if the patient has structural heart disease, the left ventricle is most likely to be the site of origin.

PVCs are not preceded by a P wave and demonstrate a prolonged QRS (> 120 ms) with a compensatory pause (as opposed to a non-compensatory pause found with PACs). Conflicting ST and T wave changes are also often seen. ST depression and T-wave inversion tends to occur in R-wave dominant leads, whereas ST elevation and an upright T wave occur in S-wave dominated leads. PVCs may be unifocal or multifocal and their morphology may at times resemble right or left bundle branch blocks. If the PVC occurs with every other beat, it is termed bigeminy (or trigemini if every third, etc.), or if the PVC is paired with another PVC, it is called a couplet. One may also see an R on T phenomenon whereby the PVC occurs at or near the T wave of the previous QRS complex resulting in the R wave of the PVC blending with the T wave of the preceding beat.

Patients with frequent PVCs will often develop subsequent cardiomyopathy, though the etiology is unknown. There is an increased risk in developing cardiomyopathy the longer one is exposed to PVCs. It is suspected this may be due to a less efficient heartbeat with suboptimal cardiac output similar to bradycardia. Risk factors for progression to cardiomyopathy have been inconsistently identified but likely include increasing age, high body mass index, and male gender.

Prevention and Clinical Manifestations

Patients with symptoms caused by PVCs often present with palpitations, dizziness, chest pain, syncope, dyspnea, orthopnea, decreased exercise tolerance, and fatigue. If a patient has a cough of unknown etiology, they should be evaluated for PVCs, as PVCs are noted to produce cough as the only symptom. PVCs have also been associated with dysphagia, especially when intermittent, as well as paroxysmal choking or vomiting. As such, PVCs should be considered if a gastroenterological evaluation is normal, or if symptoms persist despite treatment for an underlying gastrointestinal disorder.

PVCs are associated with a multitude of pathologic cardiac processes including heart failure, myocardial ischemia, left ventricular hypertrophy, idiopathic ventricular tachycardia, and right ventricular dysplasia. Non-cardiac diseases with which PVCs are associated include obstructive sleep apnea, chronic obstructive pulmonary disease, and pulmonary hypertension. On exam patients may present with an irregular pulse or canon A wave. PVCs may also be associated with pulmonary or thyroid disease, the consumption of alcohol, caffeine, and the use of beta agonists. Cocaine, amphetamines, or other illicit drugs may precipitate symptoms as well. Syncope is uncommon with PVCs but, if present, represents a red flag for the presence of malignant arrhythmias.

PVCs are found on 40% to 75% of holter monitor evaluations and 1% of EKGs. They are defined as frequent if they are seen on an EKG, or are present at a rate of more than 30 an hour on event monitoring. In this instance there is a significantly increased cardiovascular risk as well as mortality. In the athlete, sinus bradycardia is common due to enhanced conditioning. This results in a lengthening of the RR interval and is thought to promote the occurrence of PVCs in this population.

The most important prognostic indicator for PVCs is the presence or absence of structural heart disease. Multifocal PVCs are considered to be risk factors for adverse cardiovascular events.

Potential contributors that are amenable to treatment include electrolyte abnormalities, hypoxia, drugs (including prescription as well as illegal), increased adrenergic drive, or ischemia.

Diagnosis and Differential Diagnosis

A 12-lead EKG is the initial test of choice. Echocardiography is necessary in individuals in which structural heart disease is suspected, or if PVC frequency is high (one or more PVCs on EKG, or more than 30 an hour on event monitoring). This is based on the understanding that the likelihood of underlying structural heart disease increases with PVC burden. In addition, if ischemia is suspected or if PVCs are triggered/evident on exertion, cardiovascular exercise stress testing is recommended. Polymorphic PVCs are more commonly seen in those with underlying cardiomyopathy.

Differential diagnosis includes ventricular arrhythmias such as ventricular tachycardia and ventricular fibrillation. Cardiac conditions include left ventricular hypertrophy in the setting of hypertension, myocarditis, acute coronary syndrome, heart failure, congenital heart disease, and hypertrophic cardiomyopathy.

Treatment and Monitoring

PVCs have been demonstrated to be an independent risk factor for cardiovascular mortality in heart failure and are associated with ejection fraction and wall motion abnormalities as well. Patients with a family history of frequent PVCs should be evaluated for inherited channelopathies such as catecholamine urgent polymorphic ventricular tachycardia. In patients with PVCs but without underlying coronary artery disease or structural heart disease, the clinical course is generally benign. It should be recalled, however, that patients with a history of PVCs can develop coronary artery disease or underlying structural heart disease, so periodic reevaluation of cardiac status is warranted.

Treatment for those with symptomatic PVCs may include beta blockers or non-dihydropyridine calcium channel blockers, but treatment is not necessary in asymptomatic patients. Use of antiarrhythmic medication to treat PVCs has not been shown to benefit patients with cardiomyopathy. In addition, treatment is not indicated following myocardial infarction to suppress PVCs that may be present. If the patient has a large PVC burden, considered to be greater than 15%, referral to an EPS specialist for consultation and possible radiofrequency ablation should be considered. If the patient has PVC-induced cardiomyopathy, catheter ablation may be considered, especially if the PVCs are monomorphic. There are no randomized controlled trials of radiofrequency ablation and antiarrhtymic drug therapy, but retrospective studies suggest decreased PVC burden in those with radiofrequency ablation.

Premature Junctional Contractions

PJCs are less common than either PACs or PVCs and are rarely seen in the setting of a normal heart. These beats arise from the atrioventricular junction. On EKG they are seen as an aberrant beat with underlying sinus rhythm. The P wave may be absent, inverted, or occur following the associated QRS complex that is morphologically normal. Causes include electrolyte and thyroid abnormalities, underlying lung or cardiac disease, or the use of excessive amounts of caffeine, nicotine, or alcohol. Medication toxicity may also be a cause, with digitalis toxicity being the classic example. If patients are asymptomatic, no treatment is required, though structural heart disease needs to be ruled out. In addition, the patient should be observed over time, as PJCs may be a harbinger of progression to a more serious arrhythmia. In the symptomatic patient, treatment is directed at the underlying cause. Supplemental oxygen may be of benefit.

References

2019 HRS/EHRA/APHRS/LAHRS: expert consensus statement on catheter ablation of ventricular arrhythmias: executive summary, *J Interv Card Electrophysiol*, 2020.

Al-Khatib SM, et al: 2017 AHA/ACC/HRS Guideline for Management of Patients With Ventricular Arrhythmias and the Prevention of Sudden Cardiac Death: A Report of the American College of Cardiology/American Heart Association Task Force on Clinical Practice Guidelines and the Heart Rhythm Society: Developed in Collaboration With the Heart Failure Society of America, *Circulation*. DOI: https://doi.org/10.1161/CIR.0000000000000549. October 30, 2017.

Cohen D, et al: Premature atrial contractions in the general population: frequency and risk factors, *Circulation*, 2012. https://doi.org/10.1161/CirculationAHA.112.112300.

Hancock EW, et al: AHA/ACCF/HRS Recommendations for the Standardization and Interpretation of the Electrocardiogram Part V: Electrocardiogram Changes Associated With Cardiac Chamber Hypertrophy: A Scientific Statement From the American Heart Association Electrocardiography and Arrhythmias Committee, Council on Clinical Cardiology; the American College of Cardiology Foundation; and the Heart Rhythm Society: Endorsed by the International Society for Computerized Electrocardiology, *Circulation* 119:e251–261. https://doi.org/10.1161/CirculationAHA.108.191097.

Giles K, Green MS: Workup and management of patients with frequent premature ventricular contractions, *Candain Journal of Cardiology* 29:1512–1515, 2013.

Lai E, Chung EH: Management of arrhythmias in athletes: atrial fibrillation, premature ventricular contractions, and ventricular tachycardia, *Curr Treat Options Cardio Med* 19:86, 2017. https://doi.org/10.1007/s11936-017-0583-x.

LaPlante L, Benzaquen BS: A review of the potential pathogencity and management of frequent premature ventricular contractions, *PACE* 39:723–730, 2016.

Lin CY, et al: Prognostic significance of premature atrial complexes burden in prediction of long-term outcome, *J Am Heart Assoc*, 2015:4e002192. https://doi.org/10.1161/JAHA.115.002192.

Marcus GM, Dewland TA: Premature atrial contractions. A wolf in sheep's clothing? *JACC* 66:242–244, 2015.

Mazella AJ, Kouri A, O'Quinn MP, Royal SH, Syed FF: Improvement in left ventricular ejection fraction after radiofrequency catheter ablation of premature atrial contractions in a 23-year-old man, *Heart Rhythm Case Rep* 5(10):524–527, 2019.

Nguen KT, et al: Ectopy on a single 12-lead ECG, incident cardiac myopathy, and death in the community, *J Am Heart Assoc* 6, 2017:e006028. https://doi.org/10.1161/JAHA.117.006028.

Stroobandt RX, Barold SS, Sinnave AF: *ECG from basics to essentials: step by step*, Wiley Publishers, 2016.

Sugumar H, Prabhu S, Voskoboinik A, Kistler PM: Arrhythmia induced cardiomyopathy, *J Arrhythm* 34(4):376–383, 2018.

TACHYCARDIAS

Method of
Alex Schevchuck, MD, MS; and Paul Andre, MD

CURRENT DIAGNOSIS

- Tachycardia is defined as cardiac rhythm with heart rate >100 bpm.
- 12-lead ECG and hemodynamic assessment are essential in each patient with tachycardia.
- Sustained arrhythmia is an arrhythmia that lasts for more than 30 seconds.
- Narrow complex rhythm (QRS ≤120 ms) favors supraventricular origin, whereas wide complex (QRS >120 ms) could be either supraventricular (with aberrant conduction) or ventricular.
- Every patient with tachyarrhythmia should be promptly assessed for hemodynamic instability and presence of symptoms (palpitations, angina, shortness of breath, lightheadedness, presyncope, syncope, volume overload).

CURRENT TREATMENT

- Vagal maneuvers may be useful for diagnosis and treatment of tachyarrhythmia.
- Direct-current (DC) cardioversion should be considered early if hemodynamic instability is present.
- If uncertain whether arrhythmia is ventricular tachycardia (VT) or supraventricular tachycardia (SVT), VT should be presumed and treated.
- Hemodynamic instability implies medical emergency, and culprit tachyarrhythmia should be treated immediately.
- A subspecialty consultation should be considered for each patient with tachyarrhythmia and high-risk features, such as syncope or family history of sudden cardiac death for diagnostic evaluation, treatment recommendations, and risk stratification.

Definition

Tachycardia is defined as a heart rate greater than 100 beats per min (bpm). This can be a normal response by the heart to the stress on the body (such as sinus tachycardia with exercise or sepsis) or a primary cardiac pathologic condition, such as atrioventricular nodal reentry tachycardia (AVNRT) or ventricular tachycardia (VT). Tachycardia present in the setting of an abnormal cardiac rhythm is defined as tachyarrhythmia.

Classification

Tachycardias classify into two major categories: wide complex (QRS duration >120 ms) or narrow-complex (QRS duration ≤120 ms). This classification is key, as wide-complex tachycardias are usually caused by an arrhythmia arising from the ventricles, such as monomorphic or polymorphic ventricular tachycardia, which are associated with considerable morbidity and mortality. On the other hand, narrow-complex tachycardias reflect ventricular activation by a competent conduction system below the atrioventricular (AV) node, indicating a source of the arrhythmia above the AV node or within the AV node or bundle of His, and are rarely life threatening.

When the tachyarrhythmia originates in the atria or within the conduction system in the AV node, it is described as a supraventricular tachycardia (SVT).

Wide-complex tachycardias include VT, supraventricular tachycardias with aberrant conduction (i.e., presence of a bundle branch block), and some types of pathway-mediated reciprocating tachycardias discussed separately.

Epidemiology

Based on the Marshfield Epidemiological Study Area (MESA) data, the incidence of SVT in the general population is 35/100,000 person-years and the prevalence is 2.25 per 1000 persons. The mean age of onset in the study was 37 years old, and the most likely presenting location was the emergency room.

Prevalence of ventricular arrhythmias is higher in men than in women, increases with age, and is strongly linked to the presence of cardiovascular disease. Fifteen percent to 16% of patients with VT have coronary atherosclerosis; and 8% to 9% have hypertension, valvular disease, or nonischemic cardiomyopathy. Only 2% to 3% of patients with VT do not have cardiovascular disease. Five percent to 10% of patients with acute MI demonstrate VT/VF, most of which occurs during the first 48 hours of hospital admission.

Pathophysiology

There are two major mechanisms of supraventricular tachycardias: automaticity and reentry.

Automaticity involves occurrence of one or multiple ectopic foci of depolarization that are located above or within the AV node. Examples of such tachycardias include focal and multifocal atrial tachycardia and junctional tachycardia.

Reentry mechanism uses a formation of an electrical circuit that may involve the AV node or accessory pathways. These tachyarrhythmias include atrial flutter, AVNRT, and AV-nodal reciprocating tachycardias (AVRT).

Ventricular tachycardias use three major mechanisms: automaticity, triggered activity, and reentry.

Automatic VTs occur from an ectopic focus of depolarization and may originate from either ventricular myocytes or Purkinje fibers. Triggered activity includes early afterdepolarization and delayed afterdepolarization. Early depolarizations occur during the repolarization phase of the membrane, usually in a setting of acquired action potential prolongation (long QT) and serves as a trigger for polymorphic VT or torsades de pointes (Figure 8). Delayed afterdepolarizations occur after a complete cell repolarization and serve as VT triggers in digoxin toxicity, right ventricular outflow tract VT, and catecholaminergic polymorphic VT. Reentry-type VT occurs when an electrical circuit forms around either an anatomic barrier (scar, artificial material in postoperative patients) or an area of a functional block. This mechanism usually results in monomorphic ventricular tachycardia.

Clinical Presentation
Clinical manifestation of tachyarrhythmias may include palpitations or fluttering sensation in the chest and neck, and signs of decreased perfusion, such as hypotension, dizziness, lightheadedness, syncope, hot flushes, altered mentation, and shock. Ventricular tachyarrhythmias in particular may result in acute loss of circulation and sudden cardiac death (SCD). Effects of tachycardia on cardiac output mostly owe to shortened diastole that affects ventricular filling and decreasing preload leading to decreased cardiac output. VTs, in turn, also result in atrioventricular and intraventricular dyssynchrony that may additionally affect cardiac stroke volume and output.

Diagnosis
In the acute setting, prompt and accurate diagnosis of the type of tachycardia is paramount. Every patient with suspected tachyarrhythmia should have a 12-lead electrocardiogram (ECG). Because many tachyarrhythmias may cause hemodynamic compromise, an expedited hemodynamic assessment should be performed (vital signs, oxygen saturation, presence of shock that may manifest as altered mentation or evidence of organ system dysfunction). An unstable patient should be treated emergently with an appropriate antiarrhythmic strategy defined by Advanced Cardiac Life Support (ACLS) algorithms.

History plays an important role in diagnosis of tachycardias. Nature and onset of symptoms, frequency of episodes and possible triggers or predisposing conditions, as well as alleviating factors, should be identified. Past medical history may be helpful in differentiation of different types of tachycardia, such as presence of ischemia or a structural heart disease that may favor VT. History of syncope, specifically if suggesting cardiogenic etiology, may help identify high-risk patients. Family history of arrhythmias or sudden cardiac death may yield important information regarding familial arrhythmias, such as Wolff-Parkinson-White (WPW) or long-QT interval syndromes.

If the patient has an implanted cardiac device, such as permanent pacemaker or a defibrillator, the device interrogation is diagnostic in most cases, especially if an AV system is present that is capable of tracking both atrial and ventricular electrical activity.

Differential Diagnosis for Narrow Complex Tachycardias
Twelve-lead ECG is the first step in differentiating between different types of narrow-complex tachycardia. Analysis of QRS regularity, axis, atrial activity, baseline and relationships between atrial and ventricular activations, and presence of delta-wave (Figure 4) or preexcitation should be performed.

Identification of atrial activity is key in differentiating between subtypes of SVT. When identification of atrial activity is difficult (as during rapid ventricular rate), vagal maneuvers, carotid sinus pressure, or administration of IV adenosine (Adenocard)[1] may assist in diagnosis or potentially terminate the arrhythmia.

Irregular tachyarrhythmia with no identifiable pattern or P waves is diagnostic of atrial fibrillation with rapid ventricular response. Variable baseline that resembles a sawtooth pattern is suggestive of atrial flutter. AV-nodal reentry usually results in a retrograde P wave that may be hidden within QRS complex or follows QRS immediately (short R-P tachycardia). Atrial tachycardia will have one or more P wave morphologies with 1:1 relationship; however, P wave morphology and axis will be different from sinus P waves. Comparison to prior ECG in sinus rhythm may be particularly helpful in this scenario.

An electrophysiology study is the gold-standard diagnostic approach if the mechanism of tachycardia is unclear from the surface ECG.

Differential Diagnosis for Wide Complex Tachycardias
Because SVT with aberrancy and some types of AVRT may result in wide QRS complex, differentiation of such arrhythmia from VT may be challenging even for experts. Orthodromic arrhythmia suggests the electrical impulse travels straight down the normal pathway, and antidromic arrhythmia suggests that the impulse travels in the opposite direction.

Atrial activity is typically not affected by the VT (unless retrograde conduction is present), leading to AV disassociation, when P waves have no relationship to the QRS complexes. This may help differentiate VT from SVT with aberrancy. Fusion and capture beats are other hallmarks of monomorphic VT. Fusion beats occur when atrial activity can conduct through the AV node down the His-Purkinje system and "fuse" with ventricular activity. The resulting QRS complex is a hybrid of the sinus rhythm narrow QRS complex and the widened VT QRS complex. Capture beats occur when atrial activity conducts down the His-Purkinje system and creates a narrow QRS complex, followed by ongoing VT. These findings are very specific for VT, but their absence does not rule it out.

Multiple algorithms have been proposed to assist in differentiating SVT from VT. We will discuss the Brugada algorithm that has excellent sensitivity and specificity (0.978 and 0.965, respectively) for diagnosis of VT. If the answer to any of the following questions is yes, subsequent steps are not necessary and the rhythm is VT (Figure 1).

Specific Tachycardias and Their Treatment
Sinus Tachycardia
Sinus tachycardia is a common narrow-complex tachycardia. It can represent a normal response to stress or a disease process (Table 1). Sinus tachycardia on a 12-lead ECG presents with ventricular rate >100 bpm and sinus P waves that are positive in leads I, II, and III, negative in aVR, and biphasic in lead V_1 with a normal PR interval (120–200 ms). Compared with an ECG in normal sinus rhythm, the P wave axis and morphology should be unchanged. A syndrome of inappropriate sinus tachycardia is a diagnosis of exclusion, when average heart rate exceeds 90 bpm over a 24-hour period and no physiologic or medical cause can be identified.

Atrioventricular-Nodal Reentry Tachycardia
AV-nodal reentry tachycardia results from activation of a dual-pathway conduit (slow and fast) that includes the AV node. This is the most common type of SVT, with a slightly higher prevalence in women. AVNRT manifests as a regular, usually rapid tachycardia with heart rates that may exceed 250 bpm. The patient will usually experience palpitations and symptoms of decreased perfusion, such as lightheadedness, dizziness, hypotension, flushing, and so forth. Syncope is rare but may occur with very rapid heart rates or in subjects with dehydration or underlying heart disease. A distinguishing symptom of AVNRT is neck palpitations. The mechanism of that is the simultaneous atrial and ventricular

---

[1]Not FDA approved for this indication.

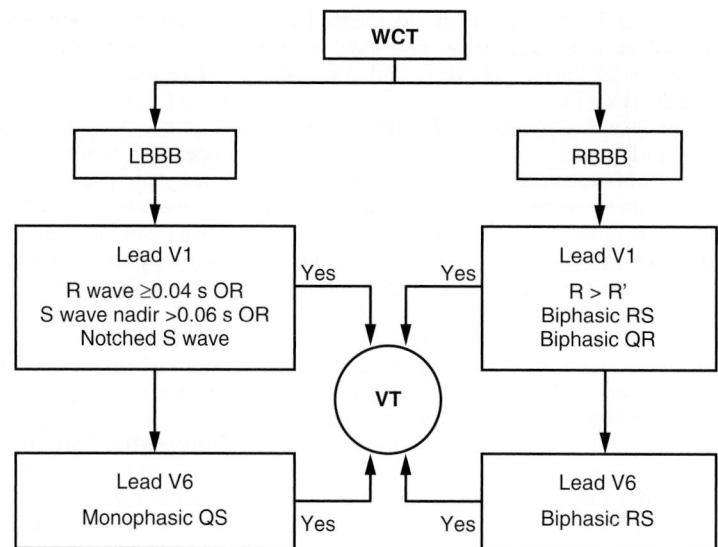

Figure 1 Brugada algorithm for differentiating supraventricular tachycardia from ventricular tachycardia. LBBB, Left bundle branch block; RBBB, right bundle branch block; WCT, wide complex tachycardia.

The algorithm questions (left side):

1. Is RS complex present in the precordial leads?
2. Is the longest R-S interval from the onset of the R wave to the deepest part of the S wave greater than 100 ms?
3. Is there AV-dissociation?
4. If none of the above, proceed with morphologic QRS criteria shown on the right

TABLE 1	Common Causes of Sinus Tachycardia	
PHYSIOLOGIC CAUSES	**PATHOLOGIC CONDITIONS**	**MEDICATIONS AND SUBSTANCES**
Exercise	Fever	Caffeine
Stress (fight or flight response)	Substance withdrawal	Nicotine
Anxiety	Hyperthyroidism	Atropine
Emotions	Pulmonary embolism	Dobutamine
Pain	Sepsis	Dopamine
	Dehydration	Pseudoephedrine
	Chronic anemia or acute blood loss	Theophylline
	Pheochromocytoma	Cocaine
	Heart failure	Methamphetamine

systole because of excitation origin located within the AV node, which is located between the atria and ventricles. This results in right atrial contraction against the closed tricuspid valve, forcing blood back into the jugular system that is subjectively perceived as palpitations in the neck. Diagnosis of AVNRT is based on a surface electrocardiogram that will classically demonstrate a rapid narrow complex tachycardia with P waves occurring within the QRS complex; therefore they are not immediately discoverable but may cause subtle deflection at the terminal portion of the QRS or immediately after the QRS (short R-P tachycardia, Figure 2). Electrophysiology study yields definitive diagnosis by demonstration of a dual-pathway physiology.

In the acute setting, as soon as AVNRT is suspected, termination of the arrhythmia should be attempted. Vagal maneuvers, such as Valsalva, carotid massage, or application of a cold wet towel to the patient's face may be helpful. Adenosine (Adenocard) has been reported to be effective in greater than 95% of patients with AVNRT. If the type of tachyarrhythmia is uncertain, adenosine may also help make a diagnosis by blocking AV conduction and causing ventricular pause that will unmask the underlying atrial activity, and may reveal arrhythmias, such as atrial tachycardia or atrial flutter. It is important to remember that adenosine has a very short half-life and should be administered as a very rapid IV injection followed by a 20 mL fluid bolus. ACLS recommends the initial dose of 6 mg followed by 12 mg if no response. The 12 mg dose can be repeated one more time. Patients taking theophylline (adenosine antagonist) may require a higher initial dose (12 mg), whereas patients with a heart transplant or on carbamazepine (Tegretol) should be given a lower initial dose (3 mg). A 12-lead ECG recording should be performed in a continuous mode while performing this intervention for more accurate rhythm identification. If these measures are ineffective to

terminate the arrhythmia, a brief assessment of hemodynamic status must be made. If patient is hemodynamically unstable, a DC cardioversion should be performed, whereas in a stable patient further treatment may include IV beta blockers, IV verapamil (Calan), or IV diltiazem (Cardizem) (Table 2). IV amiodarone (Pacerone)[1] is recommended as the next line of treatment if all prior measures are ineffective or not feasible. In a stable patient who is not responding to medications, a DC cardioversion should still be performed to restore the sinus rhythm.

Follow-up management of AVNRT should include a specialty consultation for consideration of slow pathway radiofrequency or cryo catheter ablation. The patient may be started on a maintenance oral beta blocker or a nondihydropyridine calcium channel blocker, such as diltiazem or verapamil. An antiarrhythmic medication, such as flecainide (Tambocor), may also be used to control occurrences of tachyarrhythmia; however, ischemic and structural heart disease has to be ruled out before these agents can be used because of their proarrhythmic effects with these conditions.

Pathway-Mediated Tachycardias (Orthodromic AVRT, Antidromic AVRT, WPW Syndrome)

Atrioventricular structures (AV valves and annuli) serve as an insulator, and normally there is no electrical communication between atrial and ventricular myocardium outside the normal conduction system. An accessory pathway is defined as an abnormal extranodal electrical communication between atrial and ventricular myocardium. A pathway that causes ventricular preexcitation pattern on a surface ECG (P-R interval <0.12 and presence of a delta-wave) is called a *manifest pathway*. A pathway that is not detectable on a surface ECG is called *concealed*. Accessory pathways can be located anywhere around AV annuli and may be capable of anterograde,

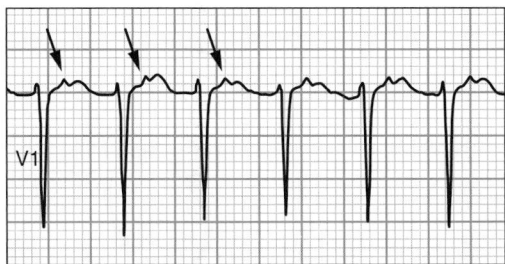

Figure 2 AV-nodal reentry (short R-P) tachycardia. Retrograde P waves are seen (arrows).

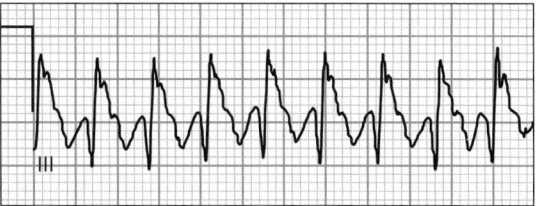

Figure 3 Antidromic reciprocating tachycardia. Wide QRS morphology results from ventricular activation via the accessory pathway. P wave is preceding the QRS complex (long R-P).

TABLE 2	Doses of Common AV Blocking Agents Used in Acute Setting for SVT Treatment
AGENT	**DOSE**
IV Metoprolol (Lopressor)[1]	2.5–5 mg over 2 min, up to 3 doses
IV Diltiazem (Cardizem)	First dose: 0.25 mg/kg over 2 min, average adult dose, 20 mg; second dose (if first dose is ineffective and tolerated): 0.35 mg/kg in 15–30 min over 2 min, average adult dose is 25 mg
IV Verapamil (Calan)	First dose: 0.075–0.15 mg/kg over 2 min; second dose (if first dose is ineffective and tolerated): 10 mg in 15–30 min over 2 min

[1]Not FDA approved for this indication.

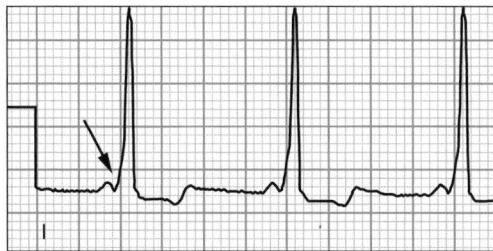

Figure 4 Manifest accessory pathway in a patient with Wolff-Parkinson-White syndrome. A short PR interval and delta-wave (arrow).

retrograde, or bidirectional conduction. They are responsible for two types of reentry tachycardias: *ORT* that uses the normal conduction system for anterograde conduction and the accessory pathway for retrograde conduction and *ART* that uses the accessory pathway for anterograde conduction and AV node for retrograde conduction.

ORT is the most common type of pathway-mediated SVT and accounts for more than 90% of AVRT cases. Because ORT uses the normal conduction system for ventricular activation, it will demonstrate a normal, narrow QRS morphology, whereas ART leads to direct ventricular activation from pathway-conducting anterograde, which results in a wide-complex QRS morphology (Figure 3).

A WPW syndrome is a bundle of a manifest accessory pathway on a surface ECG in sinus rhythm (preexcitation pattern, Figure 4) and presence of supraventricular tachyarrhythmias.

If a patient with an accessory pathway capable of rapid anterograde conduction develops atrial fibrillation, it may result in a very rapid ventricular response rate and sudden cardiac death. AV blocking agents, such as beta blockers, or calcium channel blockers (CCBs), are contraindicated for treatment of atrial fibrillation in WPW patients, as they suppress the AV node (that competes with accessory pathway for atrioventricular conduction and serves as a rate-control "gate keeper") and further facilitates the conduction down the pathway, increasing the ventricular rate. Instead, procainamide (Pronestyl)[1] should be used to suppress voltage-gated sodium channels of the accessory pathway.

Acute management of AVRT should include assessment of the 12-lead ECG for presence of preexcitation. If no preexcitation is present (ORT), the management is similar to AVNRT, as discussed previously. If preexcitation is detected (ART, WPW), AV blocking agents should be avoided or used with caution. DC cardioversion should be considered early, regardless of hemodynamic status.

For ongoing management, all patients with AVRT should undergo a subspecialty consultation for consideration of a catheter ablation procedure. Patients with a manifest accessory (e.g., WPW) pathway should also undergo risk stratification for sudden cardiac death as soon as diagnosis is made.

Atrial Tachycardias

Atrial tachycardias can be focal or multifocal. Focal atrial tachycardia is usually regular and is characterized by the presence of distinct uniform P waves on the surface ECG. Morphology of these P waves differs from those in sinus rhythm. Multifocal atrial tachycardia will contain three or more different P wave morphologies and is associated with structural heart disease, pulmonary disease, and pulmonary hypertension.

Treatment of atrial tachycardias may be challenging, with limited utility for antiarrhythmic medications and cardioversion that is often ineffective. AV-nodal blockers and ablation procedures have the most established role in treatment of these conditions.

Junctional Tachycardia

Junctional tachycardia is a rapid narrow QRS complex tachyarrhythmia with rates up to 220 bpm that originates within the AV junction and may be regular or irregular. It is more commonly seen in pediatric populations and occurs rarely in adults. In the acute setting, IV beta blockers, nondihydropyridine CCBs, or procainamide[1] can be used. For chronic suppression, oral beta-blockers, verapamil[1], diltiazem[1], or antiarrhythmic drugs may be effective.

Atrial Flutter

Atrial flutter, also known as *macroreentrant atrial tachycardia*, is a reentry arrhythmia that propagates around the tricuspid valve annulus. It most commonly involves the cavotricuspid isthmus (isthmus-dependent) and may be typical, when the signal travels up the intraatrial septum and down the lateral right atrial wall in a counterclockwise fashion around the annulus when observed from the RV apex (Figure 5, panel A), or reverse typical, or clockwise, traveling down the septum and up the atrial wall (see Figure 5, panel B).

Flutter that does not involve the cavotricuspid isthmus is called *atypical*, or *isthmus independent*.

Macroreentrant arrhythmias create a characteristic pattern on the ECG that resembles the "sawtooth" appearance of the electrical baseline, best seen in the inferior leads (Figure 6).

Counterclockwise activation creates positive deflection in lead V_1 (signal travels up the septum toward the lead) and negative deflection in the inferior leads, whereas clockwise demonstrates

[1]Not FDA approved for this indication.

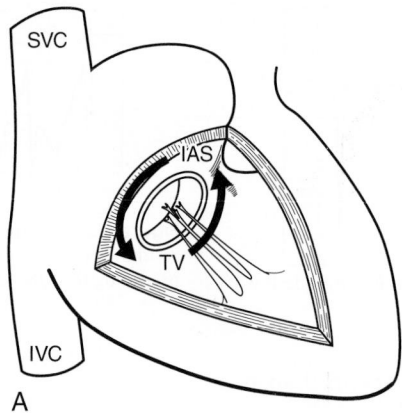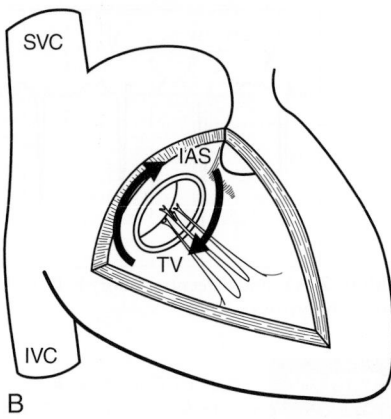

Figure 5 (Panel A) Direction of a typical, counterclockwise activation in atrial flutter. (Panel B) Direction of a reverse typical, clockwise activation in atrial flutter. IAS, Intraatrial septum; IVC, inferior vena cava; SVC, superior vena cava; TV, tricuspid valve.

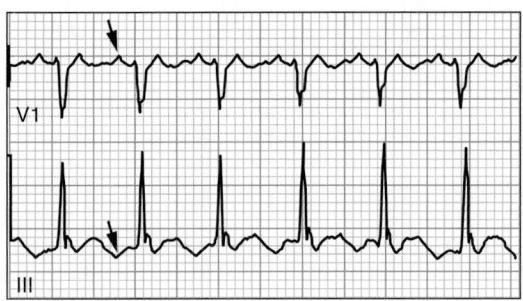

Figure 6 Macroreentrant atrial tachycardia: typical atrial flutter with 2:1 AV-nodal conduction. A variable baseline is seen that resembles a saw-tooth pattern. Positive deflections in lead V_1 and negative in lead III (arrows) indicate counterclockwise signal propagation around the tricuspid annulus.

the opposite. Because the reentrant circle uses a fairly consistent anatomic path, the cycle length of reentry is around 220 ms, resulting in an atrial waveform rate around 300 bpm. The AV node will attempt to block the portion of atrial activations, resulting in slower ventricular rates. Two-to-one conduction commonly results in a ventricular rate around 150 bpm, whereas variable conduction may lead to an irregular ventricular response, which, however, usually follows identifiable patterns with R-R intervals multiple to the flutter cycle length, or 220 ms (440 ms, 660 ms, etc.). If the tricuspid annulus is dilated or the patient is receiving an antiarrhythmic medication that slows myocardial conduction (for example, flecainide), it may increase the flutter cycle length, decreasing the flutter rate. This may have an important negative implication. Usually, AV node is able to block fast flutter, decreasing the ventricular response to 2:1. However, when the flutter rate is decreased, it allows the AV node to conduct in 1:1 fashion, leading to very rapid ventricular responses that may result in syncope and ventricular fibrillation. If flecainide is chosen as an antiarrhythmic therapy to control atrial flutter, it is important to always use it in a combination with an AV blocking agent to avoid 1:1 conduction in case of a relapse.

Medical treatment of atrial flutter may be challenging because of weaker ventricular rate responses to AV blocking agents that result in notorious difficulty with the rate-control strategy. One-to-one response should be treated as a medical emergency with a prompt DC cardioversion. For typical flutter, an EP consultation for a radiofrequency catheter ablation procedure should always be considered because of a high success rate and relative simplicity of the procedure. Atypical flutter ablations, however, may be more technically challenging with lower success rates.

Ventricular Tachycardias

Ventricular tachycardia is defined as a cardiac arrhythmia of three or greater beats at a rate of >100 bpm that originates in the ventricles. Sustained VT, just as SVT, is a VT that sustains for >30 seconds. Nonsustained VT terminates spontaneously within 30 seconds after onset.

VT that manifests with uniform beat-to-beat QRS morphology is called *monomorphic* (Figure 7). This type of morphology is more likely to represent structural or functional electrical reentry as the leading mechanism. A common substrate for such arrhythmia is a myocardial scar resulting from chronic ischemic or structural heart disease.

Polymorphic ventricular tachycardia is characterized by the presence of multiform QRS complexes and likely represents unstable myocyte membranes. Such arrhythmia may be seen in multiple conditions, including long-QT syndromes (congenital and acquired). QT should always be assessed as soon as sinus rhythm is restored. When QT prolongation is detected, a reversible cause, such as medication effect or electrolyte abnormality, should be considered and treated. If no cause can be identified, a congenital condition may be suspected.

If polymorphic VT occurs without QT prolongation, acute myocardial ischemia should be considered and promptly evaluated and treated.

Torsades de pointes represents a subtype of polymorphic VT that is usually associated with long-QT syndromes and demonstrates a characteristic ECG pattern with rotating QRS axis appearance (Figure 8).

Of all the arrhythmias seen in clinical practice, ventricular tachycardias are of most concern to practitioners because of the high morbidity and mortality associated with these disorders. Although both subtypes require emergent medical attention, polymorphic VT poses particular danger because of the often rapid deterioration of hemodynamics, loss of circulation, and death. Sustained polymorphic VT should be treated immediately with an unsynchronized DC cardioversion.

The approach to monomorphic VT starts with assessment of hemodynamic stability. Faster ventricular rates (>150 bpm) and underlying structural heart disease may be associated with more rapid hemodynamic decline. ACLS algorithms for specific types of VT must be implemented. Each patient with ventricular tachycardia should undergo a prompt specialty consultation and risk stratification for sudden cardiac death.

Artifact

All providers should be aware of telemetry and ECG artifacts that may masquerade as ventricular arrhythmias. If multilead recording is available, all leads should be examined. If sinus rhythm can be found in one or more leads, that indicates the recording is an artifact (Figure 9).

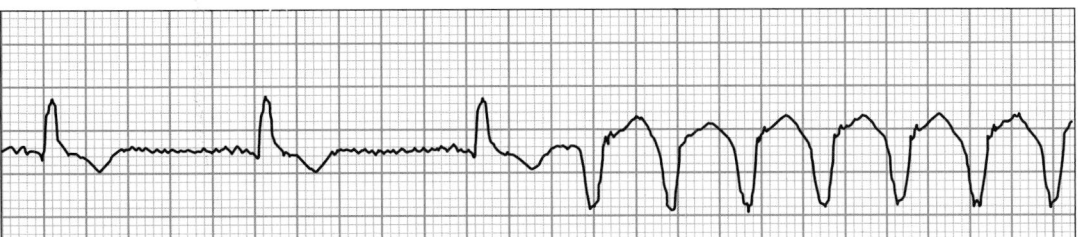

Figure 7 Onset of monomorphic ventricular tachycardia.

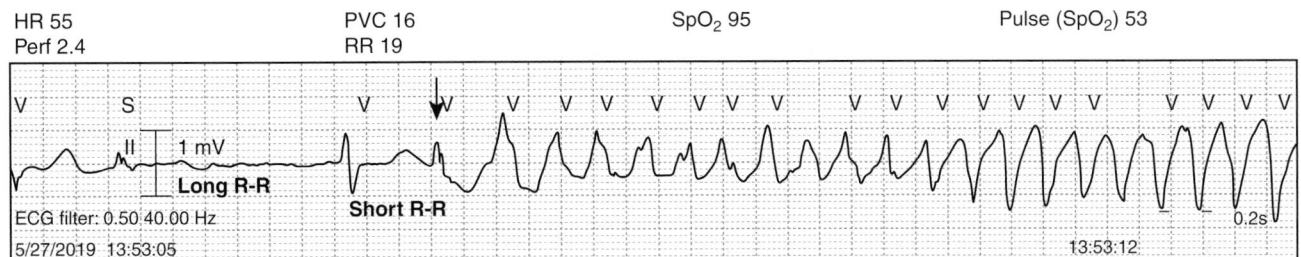

Figure 8 Polymorphic ventricular tachycardia: a premature ventricular complex (PVC, arrow), occurring during relative refractory period ("R on T" phenomenon) triggers the arrhythmia. The QT interval duration in the current R-R cycle is determined by the duration of preceding R-R cycle. A PVC that triggers VT occurs during a prolonged QT interval after a long previous R-R cycle and creates a distinctive "long-short R-R" ECG pattern.

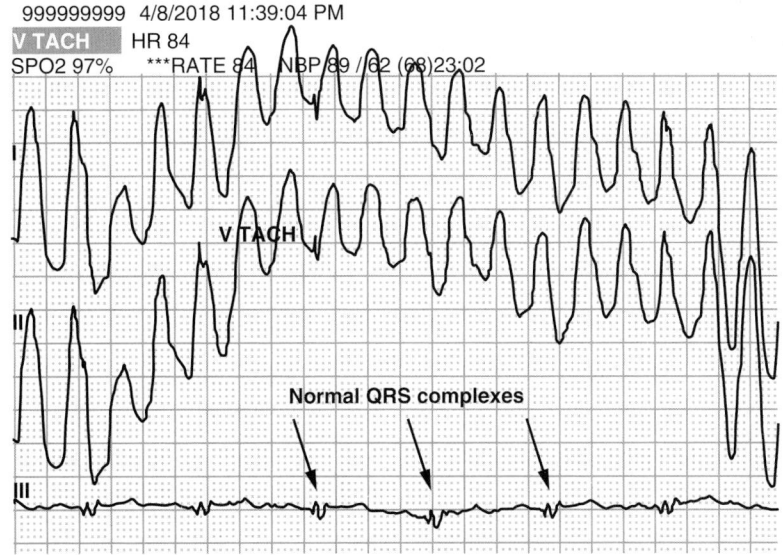

Figure 9 Artifact masquerading as ventricular tachycardia. A diagnosis of wide-complex tachycardia is dismissed by presence of sinus rhythm in lead III.

References

Al-Khatib SM, Stevenson WG: *AHA/ACC/HRS Guideline for management of patients with ventricular arrhythmias and the prevention of sudden cardiac death,* 2017.

Aronow WS, Ahn C, Mercando AD, Epstein S, Kronzon I: Prevalence and association of ventricular tachycardia and complex ventricular arrhythmias with new coronary events in older men and women with and without cardiovascular disease, *J Gerontol A Biol Sci Med Sci* 57(3):M178–M180, 2002.

Brady WJ, Mattu A, Tabas J, Ferguson JD: The differential diagnosis of wide QRS complex tachycardia, *Am J Emerg Med* 35(10):1525–1529, 2017.

Brugada P, Brugada J, Mont L, Smeets JLRM, Andries EW: A new approach to the differential diagnosis of a regular tachycardia with a wide QRS complex, *Circulation* 83(5):1649–1659, 1991.

Low PA, Sandroni P: Postural tachycardia syndrome (POTS). Primer on the autonomic nervous system, 2012, Academic Press, pp 517–519.

Meiltz A, Weber R, Halimi F: Permanent form of junctional reciprocating tachycardia in adults: peculiar features and results of radiofrequency catheter ablation, *Europace* 8(1):21–28, 2006.

Orejarena LA, Vidaillet H, DeStefano F: Paroxysmal supraventricular tachycardia in the general population, *J Am Coll Cardiol* 31(1):150–157, 1998.

Page RL: 2015 ACC/AHA/HRS guideline for the management of adult patients with supraventricular tachycardia: a report of the American College of Cardiology/American Heart Association task force on clinical practice guidelines and the Heart Rhythm Society, *J Am Coll Cardiol* 67(13), 2016.

VALVULAR HEART DISEASE

Method of
Carlos E. Sanchez, MD; Steven J. Yakubov, MD; and Arash Arshi, MD

CURRENT DIAGNOSIS

- The diagnosis of severe aortic valve stenosis is based on an integration of clinical symptoms and hemodynamic echocardiographic criteria.
- Classic symptoms of severe aortic stenosis include fatigue, dyspnea on exertion, angina, near syncope or syncope, and congestive heart failure.
- Chronic mitral regurgitation tends to be a slowly progressive disease and symptoms may not be apparent.
- Cardiac imaging, especially echocardiography, is crucial to the management of patients with valvular heart disease.
- Diagnostic echocardiographic findings of severe aortic stenosis are peak aortic valve velocity of greater than or equal to 4 m/s, transaortic mean gradient of greater than or equal to 40 mm Hg, and aortic valve area less than or equal to 1 cm² or aortic valve area index of less than or equal to 0.6 cm²/m².
- Echocardiography should be performed to determine the etiology of and characterize the severity of mitral regurgitation.
- Left ventricular size and function should be assessed in patients with mitral regurgitation.

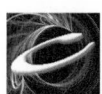

CURRENT THERAPY

- Medical therapy has not been shown to change hemodynamic progression or clinical outcomes in patients with aortic stenosis.
- Reevaluation for early symptoms and transthoracic echocardiography should be performed every 6–12 months in asymptomatic patients with severe aortic stenosis and normal left ventricular systolic function.
- Transcatheter aortic valve replacement is currently approved in patients with severe symptomatic aortic stenosis with any level of surgical risk.
- The etiology of mitral regurgitation dictates its treatment.
- Primary (degenerative) mitral regurgitation typically requires surgical repair or replacement.
- The management of secondary (functional) mitral regurgitation requires treatment of the underlying cardiomyopathy.
- Mitral transcatheter edge-to-edge repair with MitraClip (Abbott Laboratories, Abbott Park, IL) is currently indicated in secondary mitral regurgitation patients with left ventricular dysfunction who remain symptomatic despite guideline-directed medical therapy.
- The decision-making process in the management of patients with severe aortic stenosis or severe mitral regurgitation is best achieved by a multidisciplinary heart valve team and should include a systematic risk assessment of the patient's comorbidities and estimation of the 30-day cardiac surgical mortality using the Society of Thoracic Surgeons' Predicted Risk of Mortality (STS-PROM) score.

Aortic Stenosis

Aortic stenosis (AS) is the most common form of adult valvular heart disease, becoming more prevalent in the aging population. It is estimated that more than 4% of the U.S. population over age 75 have AS. Aortic valve stenosis is the most common cause of left ventricular (LV) outflow tract obstruction, while less common causes of obstruction may also occur above (supravalvular) or below (subvalvular) the level of the aortic valve and will not be discussed in this chapter.

Etiology

There are three main causes of valvular AS: congenital in origin (which is usually a bicuspid aortic valve), rheumatic valve disease, and degenerative calcification of a normal aortic valve. Congenitally affected aortic valves may be unicuspid or bicuspid and may become stenotic during childhood. In the majority of cases, a congenital bicuspid valve will develop significant calcific stenosis later in life, usually presenting after the fifth decade.

Rheumatic AS is an important cause of aortic valve disease worldwide; however, with the decline of rheumatic fever in developed countries, it is now a rare cause of AS in the United States. Rheumatic valve disease is characterized by commissural fusion, fibrosis, and calcification. Rheumatic AS is also commonly associated with rheumatic involvement of the mitral valve.

Degenerative or calcific AS is now the most common cause of AS in adults in North America. It has been associated with the same risk factors as vascular atherosclerosis including age, smoking, hypertension, diabetes, and hyperlipidemia. Histopathologic data suggest that calcific aortic valve disease is a chronic inflammatory process with lipid deposition and active leaflet calcification leading to restriction of the cusps.

Pathophysiology

In adults with AS, the gradual obstruction of the LV outflow produces a systolic pressure gradient between the left ventricle and aorta. The average time interval of disease progression from nonobstructive valve thickening (aortic sclerosis) to severe AS is 8 years. However, only 16% of individuals with aortic sclerosis will develop any grade of valve obstruction. The average rate of hemodynamic progression once moderate AS is present is an increase in aortic jet velocity of 0.3 m/s per year and mean pressure gradient of 7 mm Hg per year with a decrease in aortic valve area of 0.1 cm²/year. LV response to chronic pressure overload ultimately leads to concentric wall hypertrophy. This compensatory mechanism helps maintain normal LV contractile function to counteract the gradual increase in afterload at the expense of decreased LV compliance and delayed relaxation resulting in diastolic dysfunction.

Clinical Presentation

The cardinal symptoms of severe AS are angina, syncope, and congestive heart failure. Because symptoms in severe AS may not occur until late in the disease process, usually in the sixth to ninth decades of life, clinicians should obtain a careful history of symptoms during the patient's initial assessment. Particular attention must be directed at early symptoms of fatigue or decreased exercise tolerance as elderly patients may minimize and attribute these symptoms to aging.

Dyspnea on exertion occurs once the pulmonary capillary pressure increases as a result of excessive elevation in LV end-diastolic pressure in a poorly compliant ventricle. Symptoms of angina pectoris in severe AS may occur in a similar manner as in coronary artery disease, with symptoms precipitated by exertion and relieved by rest even in the absence of obstructive epicardial coronary artery disease. Syncope may result from the inability of the heart to increase cardiac output from the stenotic valve in the setting of transient vasodilatation during physical activity, resulting in decreased cerebral perfusion. Other causes of syncope may also be attributable to arrhythmias, either advanced forms of atrioventricular blocks from calcification impinging on the conduction system or tachyarrhythmias causing a sudden decline in cardiac output such as in atrial fibrillation.

Diagnosis and Management

Diagnosis of AS is usually suspected after a systolic ejection murmur is heard during cardiac auscultation. The classic physical findings in patients with severe AS are a loud, late-peaking

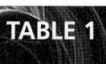

TABLE 1 Echocardiographic Stages of Aortic Valve Stenosis and Frequency of Echocardiograms in Asymptomatic Patients With Aortic Stenosis and Normal Left Ventricular Ejection Fraction

	MAXIMUM AORTIC VELOCITY	MEAN PRESSURE GRADIENT	AORTIC VALVE AREA	TTE FOLLOW-UP IN ASYMPTOMATIC PATIENTS
Mild aortic stenosis	2.0–2.9 m/s	<20 mm Hg	>1.5 cm^2	Every 3–5 years
Moderate aortic stenosis	3.0–3.9 m/s	20–30 mm Hg	1.0–1.5 cm^2	Every 1–2 years
Severe aortic stenosis	≥4.0 m/s	≥40 mm Hg	≤1.0 cm^2	Every 6–12 months
Very severe aortic stenosis	≥5 m/s	≥60 mm Hg	≤1.0 cm^2	

TTE, Transthoracic echocardiogram.

systolic murmur at the base of the heart radiating to the carotid arteries with a delayed and diminished carotid upstroke (*pulsus parvus et tardus*). The latter physical finding may be masked in elderly patients with stiff, inelastic arterial walls. Distinctively, a normally split-second heart sound is the only reliable physical finding to help exclude the diagnosis of severe AS.

A transthoracic echocardiogram (TTE) is recommended as the initial diagnostic test in the evaluation of patients with aortic valve stenosis to determine hemodynamic severity, LV size and function, and prognosis, and to evaluate timing of valve intervention. Echocardiographic valve hemodynamics define the severity of AS (Table 1). Severe AS is characterized by a peak aortic valve velocity of 4 m/s or higher, transaortic mean gradient of 40 mm Hg or higher, and aortic valve area of less than or equal to 1 cm^2 or aortic valve area index of less than or equal to 0.6 cm^2/m^2. In severe symptomatic patients with low-flow, low-gradient severe AS and abnormal LV function (<50%), a dobutamine stress echocardiogram can be used to differentiate between true severe AS and pseudo-severe AS. Low-flow, low-gradient true severe AS is characterized by a severely calcified valve with aortic valve area less than or equal to 1 cm^2 and peak aortic valve velocity less than 4 m/s that increases to 4 m/s or higher with low-dose dobutamine administration. Conversely, in pseudo-severe AS the aortic valve area increases to more than 1 cm^2 and flow normalizes during dobutamine stress echocardiogram.

Patients with asymptomatic AS require frequent monitoring owing to the progressive nature of the disease. The frequency of echocardiograms in asymptomatic patients with AS and normal LV systolic function should be performed every 6 to 12 months for reevaluation in severe AS, every 1 to 2 years for moderate AS, and every 3 to 5 years for mild AS (see Table 1). In seemingly asymptomatic patients with severe AS, exercise testing is safe and helpful to expose symptoms, arrhythmias, or abnormal blood pressure response, defined as an exercise-associated decrease of greater than or equal to 10 mm Hg in systolic blood pressure. Exercise testing should not be performed in symptomatic patients.

Treatment

Indication for intervention in patients with severe AS is dependent on the presence or absence of symptoms, the severity of AS, and LV function. Routine aortic valve replacement in asymptomatic AS is currently not recommended. Importantly, event-free survival at 2 years in asymptomatic patients with severe AS (jet velocity ≥ 4.0 m/s) is 30% to 50%, and as low as 21% in those with very severe AS (jet velocity ≥ 5.0 m/s). Close clinical follow-up to evaluate for early-onset AS symptoms and education regarding the disease course should be performed routinely. Intervention should be considered among asymptomatic patients with very severe AS (V_{max} ≥ 5.0 m/s), serum B-type natriuretic peptide (BNP) >3 times normal, or progression of V_{max} ≥ 0.3 m/s per year.

Medical therapy has not been shown to change hemodynamic progression or clinical outcomes in patients with AS. Clinical data have failed to support the use of statins specifically for the prevention of progression of AS. However, all patients with concomitant coronary artery disease or hypercholesterolemia should be treated per established guidelines. Likewise, concurrent hypertension in

patients with severe AS is common and should receive appropriate treatment per standard guidelines starting at a low dose and slowly titrating upward with frequent blood pressure monitoring. Although indicated in the treatment of acute heart failure, diuretics should be used with caution to avoid volume depletion, which may result in marked reduction in cardiac output.

Invasive Treatment

Transcatheter aortic valve replacement (TAVR) has expanded rapidly as an alternative to surgical aortic valve replacement (SAVR) since its approval in 2011, with approximately 50,000 patients treated annually in the United States alone since 2017. It is currently approved for use in patients with severe symptomatic AS with any level of surgical risk. Recent published clinical trials in low–surgical-risk candidates showed that the risk of death or disabling stroke and new onset atrial fibrillation was lower among the TAVR treated patients compared to SAVR. Additionally, rehospitalization and hospital length of stay was shorter with TAVR.

Recommendations and timing of intervention for aortic valve stenosis by either SAVR or TAVR are summarized in Table 2. Once the patient with AS is considered to meet an indication for aortic valve replacement, an important component when choosing between SAVR and TAVR is the underlying risk assessment for SAVR. In the United States, the Society of Thoracic Surgeons' Predicted Risk of Mortality (STS-PROM) risk score calculator is the initial step in predicting 30-day mortality for SAVR, with three categories: low risk defined as less than 4%, intermediate risk defined as 4% to 8%, and high risk defined as greater than 8% STS mortality risk. This risk calculator, however, does not include certain comorbid conditions that would also increase the surgical mortality risk such as frailty, porcelain aorta, liver cirrhosis, severe pulmonary hypertension, chest wall abnormalities, and hostile mediastinum. If three or more major organ systems are compromised, with severe frailty, or the morbidity and mortality risk is greater than 50%, the patient is considered prohibitive risk for SAVR. In patients with severe AS and a life expectancy less than 1 year, TAVR or SAVR is considered futile despite successful procedure and it is appropriate to avoid any intervention for severe AS. Hence the risk assessment is a combination of the STS-PROM score, frailty, disability, and major cardiovascular and noncardiovascular comorbidities.

The final treatment decision should be individualized with a risk-benefit assessment by a multidisciplinary heart team (including structural interventional cardiologists, imaging specialists, cardiovascular surgeons, and nursing professionals). The heart team assesses potential procedural outcomes based on the patient's individual procedural risk, anatomic considerations, comorbidities, life expectancy, and potential quality-of-life improvement with SAVR or TAVR. The importance of a collaborative and multidisciplinary heart team approach to the evaluation and management of patients with complex AS has been endorsed by professional guidelines to maximize appropriate outcomes.

Once the patient is considered to be a suitable candidate for TAVR, the evaluation of all patients undergoing the procedure

TABLE 2	American College of Cardiology/American Heart Association Recommendations for Timing of Intervention in Patients With Aortic Stenosis

COR	RECOMMENDATION
I	• AVR is recommended for symptomatic patients with severe high-gradient AS who have symptoms by history or on exercise testing • AVR is recommended for asymptomatic patients with severe AS and LVEF <50% • AVR is indicated for patients with severe AS when undergoing other cardiac surgery • For symptomatic patients with severe AS who are >80 years of age or for younger patients with a life expectancy <10 years and no anatomic contraindication to transfemoral TAVR, transfemoral TAVR is recommended in preference to SAVR. • In symptomatic patients with low-flow, low-gradient severe AS with reduced LVEF, AVR is recommended. • In symptomatic patients with low-flow, low-gradient severe AS with normal LVEF (Stage D3), AVR is recommended if AS is the most likely cause of symptoms.
IIa	• AVR is reasonable for asymptomatic patients with very severe AS (aortic velocity ≥ 5.0 m/s) and low surgical risk • AVR is reasonable in asymptomatic patients with severe AS and decreased exercise tolerance or an exercise fall in systolic BP equal to or greater than 10 mm Hg from baseline to peak exercise • In apparently asymptomatic patients with severe AS and low surgical risk, AVR is reasonable when the serum B-type natriuretic peptide (BNP) level is >3 times the normal level • AVR is reasonable in symptomatic patients with low-flow/low-gradient severe AS with reduced LVEF with a low-dose dobutamine stress study that shows an aortic velocity ≥4.0 m/s (or mean pressure gradient ≥40 mm Hg) with a valve area of 1.0 cm² at any dobutamine dose • AVR is reasonable for patients with moderate AS (aortic velocity 3.0–3.9 m/s) who are undergoing other cardiac surgery
IIb	• AVR may be considered for asymptomatic patients with severe AS and rapid disease progression and low surgical risk • In asymptomatic patients with severe high-gradient AS and a progressive decrease in LVEF on at least 3 serial imaging studies to <60%, AVR may be considered.

AS, Aortic stenosis; *AVR,* aortic valve replacement by either surgical or transcatheter approach; *BP,* blood pressure; *COR,* class of recommendation; *LVEF,* left ventricular ejection fraction.
Modified from Otto CM, Nishimura RA, Bonow RO, et al: 2020 ACC/AHA guideline for the management of patients with valvular heart disease: a report of the American College of Cardiology/American Heart Association Joint Committee on Clinical Practice Guidelines. *J Am Coll Cardiol.* 2021;77:e25–197.

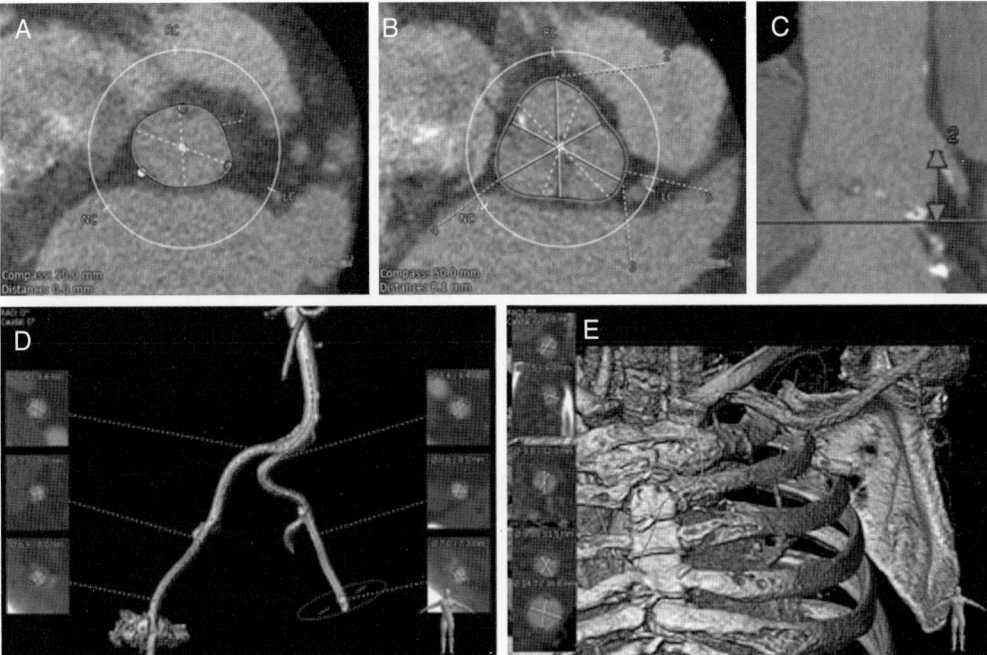

Figure 1 Multidetector computed tomography measurements of the aortic valve complex and peripheral vascular assessment. (A) Aortic annulus perimeter, area, and diameter measurement. (B) The maximum sinus of Valsalva diameters. (C) Height of the left coronary artery from the annular base. (D) Reconstructed view of the iliofemoral anatomy. (E) Left subclavian view with measurement obtained (*left* of image).

should include (1) coronary angiography to determine the presence of coronary artery disease; and (2) computed tomography of the chest, abdomen, and pelvis to determine preferred vascular access or contraindications to it and aortic annulus dimension for prosthesis sizing (Figure 1).

The currently available TAVR valves approved by the United States Food and Drug Administration (FDA) include the balloon-expandable Edwards Sapien XT and Sapien 3 (Edwards Lifesciences, Irvine, CA), and self-expandable Medtronic Evolut R and Evolut PRO systems (Medtronic, Minneapolic, MN). The choice of valve mostly depends on anatomic considerations and operator preference and experience.

A series of major procedural cardiovascular complications have been described after TAVR, including paravalvular aortic regurgitation, ischemic strokes, conduction disturbances, cardiac perforation, coronary occlusion, and vascular access complications. With the advancement of valve technology and increase in operator experience, the frequency of procedural complications has reduced since the arrival of TAVR procedures. Cerebral embolic protection has become increasingly common, but its role remains unclear in terms of reducing clinically significant strokes. Preprocedure planning by an expert heart team is essential to recognizing and preventing expected complications during and after transcatheter valve implantation.

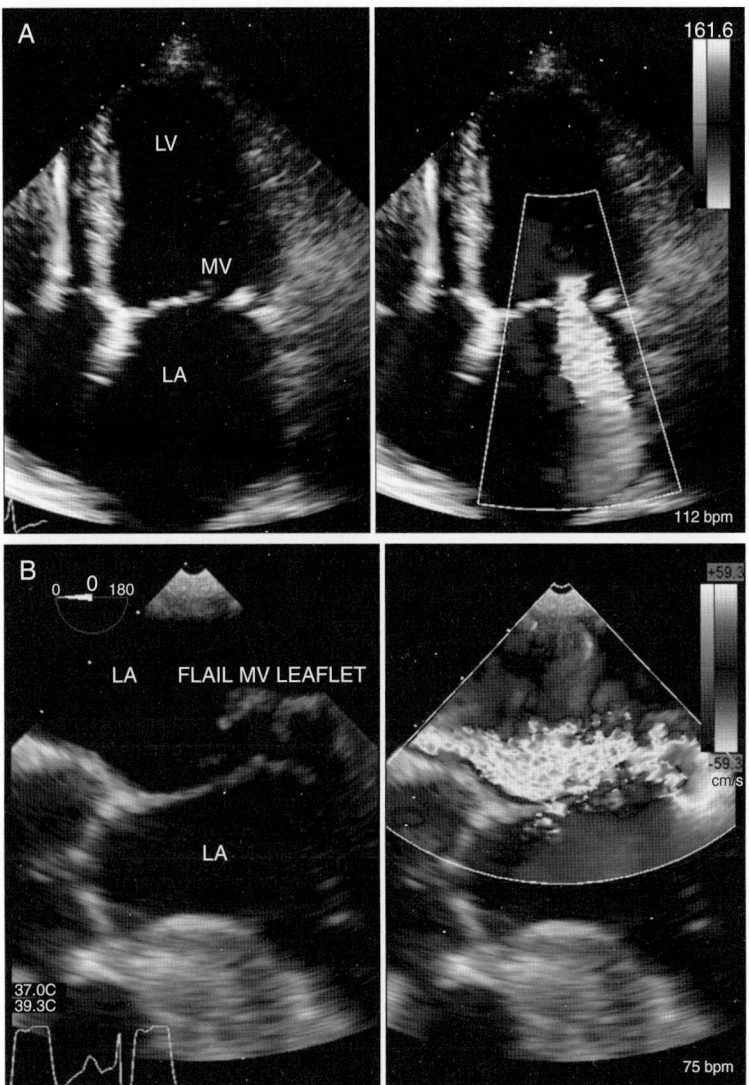

Figure 2 (A) Transthoracic echocardiogram of a patient with a dilated cardiomyopathy with annular dilation resulting in incomplete coaptation of the mitral valve leaflets and severe functional (secondary) mitral regurgitation. The regurgitant jet is central. (B) Transesophageal echocardiogram reveals a markedly myxomatous mitral valve with a large flail segment of the posterior leaflet resulting in severe degenerative (primary) mitral regurgitation. This jet is extremely eccentric. *LA*, Left atrium; *LV*, left ventricle; *MV*, mitral valve.

Currently the optimal antithrombotic regimen following TAVR is daily clopidogrel (Plavix)[1] 75 mg and aspirin[1] 75 to 100 mg for 3 to 6 months followed by daily aspirin alone for life. If there is an indication for chronic anticoagulation, it should follow current guidelines' recommendations for each individual condition (e.g., atrial fibrillation, deep venous thrombosis). The safety of antiplatelet therapy use in conjunction with oral anticoagulation should be individualized based on the patient's bleeding risk.

Mitral Regurgitation

Mitral regurgitation (MR) is a common valvular disease, and pathology in any of the structures of the mitral valve apparatus may lead to dysfunction of the valve. The base of the leaflets of the mitral valve are attached to the annulus, and the leaflets themselves are attached to the papillary muscles of the left ventricle by the chordae tendineae. The mitral valve is an integral part of both the left atrium and left ventricle, and disorders of these structures affect mitral valve function; likewise, disorders of the mitral valve lead to abnormalities of the left atrium and left ventricle.

Etiology

MR can be divided into primary (degenerative) MR and secondary (functional) MR (Figure 2). Primary MR refers to pathology of the mitral valve leaflets and chordae tendineae that results in valve dysfunction. The most common etiology is mitral valve prolapse, where the underlying pathology is myxomatous mitral valve degeneration that results in redundant leaflets, causing prolapse of the leaflets. A myxomatous mitral valve is also prone to rupture of the chordae tendineae, leading to a flail leaflet or segment of a leaflet. Other common etiologies of MR include rheumatic heart disease and endocarditis. Mitral annular calcification may cause mild to moderate MR, but severe regurgitation is uncommon.

In contrast, in secondary MR, the mitral valve itself has a relatively normal structure. Instead, the pathology is an abnormality of the left ventricle. This most commonly occurs after myocardial infarction, with focal wall motion abnormalities and displacement of the papillary muscle causing tethering of the chordae and leaflets, along with dilatation of the mitral valve annulus, resulting in incomplete coaptation of the mitral valve leaflets during systole. Secondary MR may also occur in a dilated cardiomyopathy.

Clinical Manifestations

The clinical presentation of MR is extremely variable and depends largely on the severity of the regurgitation and its acuity. MR

---

[1]Not FDA approved for this indication.

tends to be asymptomatic when mild to moderate, but severe MR frequently results in symptoms. Acute MR occurring from papillary muscle rupture complicating an acute myocardial infarction leads to rapid hemodynamic collapse and carries a high risk of mortality. These patients experience pulmonary edema due to the acute volume overload of the left ventricle and left atrium. In contrast, chronic severe MR may have a relatively indolent course, with some patients reporting few symptoms. While chronic MR typically manifests as congestive heart failure, with exertional dyspnea, orthopnea, and lower extremity edema as the hallmark symptoms, owing to the insidious nature of the disease, patients may not always recognize their symptoms. A detailed history with a specific focus on symptoms of congestive heart failure in addition to fatigue and effort intolerance must be elicited. Atrial fibrillation is a common complication of MR and is associated with worse outcomes.

Diagnosis

Physical examination classically may reveal a soft S1 and a holosystolic murmur at the apex that radiates to the left sternal border or to the axilla. However, the intensity of the murmur does not correlate to the severity of disease, nor does the absence of a murmur reliably rule out severe MR. Physical examination is important to assess the patient's volume status, with pulmonary rales and lower extremity edema suggesting congestive heart failure, and an irregularly irregular rhythm indicative of atrial fibrillation.

Cardiac imaging, in particular echocardiography, is crucial in the evaluation of suspected MR. Transthoracic echocardiography can reveal abnormalities of the mitral valve and provide important information on LV size and function and estimation of pulmonary arterial pressure. Given the orientation of the mitral valve and the limits of transthoracic echocardiography, the severity of MR can be grossly underestimated, particularly if the regurgitant jet is eccentric. Transesophageal echocardiography, especially with the availability of three-dimensional imaging, provides higher-quality images of the mitral valve and allows more precise evaluation of the severity and etiology of MR, and has become the gold-standard test in the evaluation of patients with clinically significant MR. Echocardiography with color Doppler can be used to provide a visual estimate of the severity of regurgitation. The presence of reversal of flow into the pulmonary veins during systole suggests severe regurgitation. Quantitative analysis can also be performed to determine the volume of regurgitation and the orifice of the regurgitant jet. There is currently no single echocardiographic parameter to define severe MR, but integration of multiple qualitative and quantitative measurements is recommended. Accurate assessment of LV dimensions and function is important in patients with chronic severe MR. Methods of determining the LV ejection fraction include visual estimation and volumetric analysis. Owing to the volume of blood exiting the left ventricle through both the mitral and aortic valves during systole, the ejection fraction will be increased. In the presence of severe MR, a normal LV ejection fraction approaches 70%, and LV dysfunction is deemed anything less than 60%. Even what would otherwise be considered a mildly reduced ejection fraction may indicate significant myocardial dysfunction in the presence of MR. Left atrial enlargement as a rule is found in chronic severe MR, and its absence should lead to reconsideration of the diagnosis. Exercise echocardiography can play an important role in patients with MR, especially in those with severe MR who report few symptoms, as it is an objective means to assess functional capacity and can also be used to assess changes in pulmonary pressures with exercise. In patients who have mild MR at rest but severe exertional symptoms, exercise echocardiography can identify ischemic MR with concomitant regional wall motion abnormalities.

Cardiac catheterization is performed in many patients with suspected severe MR. Right heart catheterization with measurement of right atrial, right ventricular, pulmonary arterial, and pulmonary capillary wedge pressures and cardiac outputs can help determine volume status and assess for pulmonary hypertension. Attention should be paid to the pulmonary capillary wedge

	PRIMARY (DEGENERATIVE)	SECONDARY (FUNCTIONAL)
TABLE 3 Paradigm for Management of Mitral Regurgitation Based on Etiology and Surgical Risk		
Low surgical risk	Surgical repair or replacement	CHF therapy TEER or surgery in selected patients
High surgical risk	Percutaneous repair in selected patients	CHF therapy ± TEER with MitraClip

CHF, Congestive heart failure. *TEER*, transcatheter edge-to-edge repair.

waveform, with large "v" waves, corresponding to ventricular systole, suggestive of severe MR. Left heart catheterization with selective coronary angiography is recommended to identify concomitant obstructive coronary artery disease. Left ventriculography using contrast is commonly performed, and the presence of contrast in the left atrium suggests MR. However, the clinical utility of left ventriculography is limited with the ready availability of echocardiography. The visual estimation of MR by contrast ventriculography is subjective, and the etiology of valve pathology is unable to be defined precisely. Furthermore, in a patient with congestive heart failure, the contrast load may result in acute decompensation.

Magnetic resonance imaging (MRI) is not currently a routinely used test in the evaluation of severe MR but may provide more reproducible quantification of the regurgitant volume and fraction and more accurate measurements of LV size and function. Given the importance of defining the severity of the MR and abnormalities of LV function in the management of MR, MRI may eventually have a central role in the evaluation of patients and is strongly recommended when echocardiographic data is not satisfactory.

Management and Treatment

The etiology of MR dictates its treatment (Table 3). Primary (degenerative) MR is a mechanical problem of the valve or its apparatus and requires a mechanical solution such as a surgical or percutaneous repair or replacement. Secondary (functional) MR is a problem of the left ventricle and treatment of the underlying ventricular pathology is indicated. Transcatheter edge-to-edge repair with MitraClip (Abbott Laboratories, Abbott Park, IL) in secondary MR is currently indicated in patients with LV dysfunction who remain symptomatic despite guideline-directed medical therapy.

In patients with acute severe MR, the role of medical therapy is to stabilize the patient until surgery. Afterload reduction is the initial treatment strategy, which allows for greater flow through the aortic valve, thereby increasing cardiac output while diminishing the MR. Afterload reduction may be accomplished with intravenous vasodilators such as sodium nitroprusside (Nitropress)[1] or with an intraaortic balloon pump if the clinical situation requires. The role of medical therapy for chronic severe degenerative MR is less clear, especially in asymptomatic patients with normal LV function. Symptomatic patients with a reduced ejection fraction (<60%) may be treated with heart failure therapy such as angiotensin-converting enzyme (ACE) inhibitors or angiotensin receptor blockers (ARBs), beta-adrenergic blockers, or aldosterone antagonists, in addition to loop diuretics for symptomatic relief while awaiting surgery. Ultimately most patients with severe primary MR will be referred to surgery (Table 4), and valve repair is preferable to replacement provided the anatomy is amenable to repair. If valve replacement is necessary, options include mechanical and bioprosthetic valves. Mechanical valves provide superior hemodynamic results and durability but are prone to thrombus formation and therefore require lifelong anticoagulation with warfarin (Coumadin). If after consultation with a cardiac surgeon the patient is deemed to be at prohibitive risk

---

[1]Not FDA approved for this indication.

TABLE 4	Indications for Intervention in Severe Primary (Degenerative) Mitral Regurgitation

SYMPTOMATIC

Recommended if LVEF >30%

May be considered if LVEF ≤30%

TEER may be considered if severely symptomatic with reasonable life expectancy but prohibitive surgical risk

ASYMPTOMATIC

Recommended if LV dysfunction (LVEF 30%–60% or LVESD <40 mm)

Reasonable if preserved LV function (LVEF >60% and LVESD >40 mm) if >95% chance of successful repair with <1% mortality risk

Reasonable if preserved LV function with new-onset atrial fibrillation or PASP >50 mm Hg if high likelihood of successful repair

LV, Left ventricular; *LVEF*, left ventricular ejection fraction; *LVESD*, left ventricular end-systolic dimension; *PASP*, pulmonary arterial systolic pressure; *TEER*, transcatheter edge-to-edge repair.

for surgery, transcatheter edge-to-edge repair with the MitraClip device is a reasonable alternative. This procedure is performed under general anesthesia with fluoroscopic and transesophageal echocardiographic guidance, and from the femoral vein via transseptal access, a clip is delivered to the regurgitant orifice of the mitral valve, grasping the anterior and posterior leaflets, thereby improving leaflet coaptation.

For patients with secondary MR, the target for treatment is the left ventricle. Medical therapy for the underlying cardiomyopathy is recommended, with administration of ACE inhibitors or ARBs ± neprilysin inhibitors, aldosterone antagonists, and beta-blockers. If indicated, these patients may require cardiac resynchronization therapy. With medical and device therapy, LV remodeling and function may improve, with reduction in the degree of MR. If severe MR persists despite maximally tolerated medical therapy, percutaneous mitral valve repair with the MitraClip device is the only interventional therapy currently approved that significantly reduces mortality and heart failure rehospitalizations at 2 years while improving heart failure symptoms. In patients with ischemic cardiomyopathy secondary to obstructive coronary artery disease with severe secondary MR, surgical revascularization and concomitant mitral valve repair is frequently performed if the surgical risk is not prohibitive.

MR can progress over time, as the volume overload can lead to LV dilation and worsening mitral leaflet coaptation. As the disease process may be slow and without sudden worsening of symptoms, patients will require close follow-up. Mild MR can be followed by serial transthoracic echocardiography every 3 to 5 years, and moderate MR every 1 to 2 years. In patients with asymptomatic severe MR who do not undergo surgery, transthoracic echocardiography should be performed at least annually, with special attention to LV dimensions and function.

References

Cosmi JE, Kort S, Tunick PA, et al: The risk of the development of aortic stenosis in patients with "benign" aortic valve thickening, *Arch Intern Med* 162:2345–2347, 2002.

Dal-Bianco JP, Khandheira BK, Mookadam F, et al: Management of asymptomatic severe aortic stenosis, *J Am Coll Cardiol* 52:1279–1292, 2008.

Feldman T, Foster E, Glower DD, et al: Percutaneous repair or surgery for mitral regurgitation, *N Engl J Med* 364:1395–1406, 2011.

Freeman RV, Otto CM: Spectrum of calcific aortic valve disease: pathogenesis, disease progression, and treatment strategies, *Circulation* 111:3316–3326, 2005.

Kapadia SR, Kodali S, Makkar R, et al: Protection against cerebral embolism during transcatheter aortic valve replacement, *J Am Coll Cardiol* 69:367–377, 2017.

Ling LH, Enriquez-Sarano M, Seward JB, et al: Early surgery in patients with mitral regurgitation due to flail leaflets: a long-term outcome study, *Circulation* 96:1819–1825, 1997.

Mack MJ, Leon MB, Thourani VH, et al: Transcatheter aortic-valve replacement with balloon expandable valve in low-risk patients, *N Engl J Med*, 2019. https://doi.org/10.1056/NEJMoa1814052.

Nkomo VT, Gardin JM, Skelton TN, et al: Burden of valvular heart diseases: a population-based study, *Lancet* 368:1005–1011, 2006.

Otto CM, Nishimura RA, Bonow RO, et al: 2020 ACC/AHA guideline for the management of patients with valvular heart disease: a report of the American College of Cardiology/American Heart Association Joint Committee on Clinical Practice Guidelines, *J Am Coll Cardiol* 77:e25–e197, 2021.

Otto CM, Kumbhani DJ, Alexander KP, et al: 2017 ACC Expert Consensus Decision Pathway for Transcatheter Aortic Valve Replacement in the Management of Adults with Aortic Stenosis, *J Am Coll of Cardiol* 69(10):1313–1346, 2017. https://doi.org/10.1016/j.jacc.2016.12.006.

Peltier M, Trojette F, Enriquez-Sarano M, et al: Relation between cardiovascular risk factors and nonrheumatic severe calcific aortic stenosis among patients with a three-cuspid aortic valve, *Am J Cardiol* 91:97–99, 2003.

Popma JJ, Deeb GM, Yakubov SJ, et al: Transcatheter aortic valve replacement with a self-expanding valve in low-risk patients, *N Engl J Med*, 2019. https://doi.org/10.1056/NEJMoa1816885.

Stone GW, Lindenfeld J, Abraham WT, et al: Transcatheter mitral-valve repair in patients with heart failure, *N Engl J Med* 379:2307–2318, 2018.

Wu AH, Aaronson KD, Bolling SF, et al: Impact of mitral valve annuloplasty on mortality risk in patients with mitral regurgitation and left ventricular systolic dysfunction, *J Am Coll Cardiol* 45:381–387, 2005.

Zilberszac R, Gabriel H, Schemper M, et al: Asymptomatic severe aortic stenosis in the elderly, *J Am Coll Cardiol Img* 10:43–50, 2017.

VENOUS THROMBOSIS

Method of
Andrea T. Obi, MD; and Thomas W. Wakefield, MD

CURRENT DIAGNOSIS

- Although clinical assessment and D-dimer levels are useful to rule out thrombosis, there is no combination of clinical findings and biomarker testing at this time that can rule in the diagnosis.
- Duplex ultrasound imaging is the gold standard for the diagnosis of deep venous thrombosis (DVT).
- Spiral computed tomography (CT) scanning, especially higher-resolution multidetector-row CT imaging, is preferred as the initial imaging test to establish the diagnosis of pulmonary embolism.

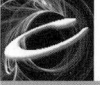

CURRENT THERAPY

- Initial preventative therapy includes anticoagulation, compression garments, and ambulation.
- The new direct oral anticoagulants (DOACs) are favored over warfarin for acute venous thromboembolism (VTE) treatment and no cancer. Rivaroxaban (Xarelto) and apixaban (Eliquis) are administered as monotherapy whereas dabigatran (Pradaxa) and edoxaban (Savaysa) require a low-molecular-weight heparin (LMWH) bridge. No bridge is needed with rivaroxaban or apixaban.
- When warfarin, dabigatran or edoxaban are used, LMWH should be administered for at least 5 days at the onset of therapy. If warfarin is used, it should be therapeutic (international normalized ratio 2.0–3.0) for 2 consecutive days before stopping LMWH.
- The duration of anticoagulation depends on a number of factors, including the presence of risk factors for thrombosis, the type of thrombosis (unprovoked or provoked), the number of times thrombosis has occurred, and risk factors for bleeding.
- Reduced-dose DOACs lessen VTE recurrences more than placebo or aspirin for long-term treatment after initial anticoagulant therapy is complete.
- Significant iliofemoral DVT may be treated with aggressive pharmacomechanical thrombolysis if a trial of anticoagulation fails to improve moderate to severe symptoms and the patient is ambulatory, has no contraindications to thrombolysis, and places a strong value on reducing the severity of postthrombotic syndrome (PTS) while accepting the inherent bleeding risk. Pulmonary embolism causing hemodynamic deterioration or right heart strain should be treated with thrombolysis.

Epidemiology

Venous thromboembolism (VTE) includes deep venous thrombosis (DVT) and pulmonary embolism (PE). VTE affects up to 900,000 patients per year and results in up to 300,000 deaths per year. The incidence has remained constant and may be increasing since the 1980s and increases with age. The annual VTE rate among persons of European ancestry ranges from 104 to 183 per 100,000 person years. Overall VTE incidence may be higher in Black populations and lower in Asians and Asian- and Native Americans. The increasing prevalence of obesity, cancer, and surgery account in part for the persistent VTE incidence. Treatment of an acute VTE appears to be associated with incremental direct medical costs of $12,000 to $15,000 (2014 US dollars) with subsequent complications to increase cumulative costs up to $18,000 to $23,000 per incident case. Sequelae from VTE including recurrent VTE, post-thrombotic syndrome (PTS), ulcers, and varicosities increase the incident cost by an average of 75%. The annual incident cost to the US healthcare system is $7 to $10 billion dollars each year.

Risk Factors

Risk factors for VTE include acquired and genetic factors. Acquired factors include increasing age, malignancy, surgery, immobilization, trauma, oral contraceptives and hormone replacement therapy, pregnancy and the puerperium, neurologic disease, cardiac disease, obesity, sepsis, pneumonia, and inflammatory bowel disease. Genetic factors include antithrombin deficiency, protein C deficiency and protein S deficiency, factor V Leiden, prothrombin 20210A, blood group non-O, abnormalities in fibrinogen and plasminogen, elevated levels of clotting factors (e.g., factors XI, IX, VII, VIII, X, and II), and elevation in plasminogen activator inhibitor-1. When a patient presents with an unprovoked VTE, family history of thrombosis, recurrent thrombosis, or thrombosis in unusual locations, a workup for hypercoagulability, including testing for the conditions noted in the previous sentence, may be indicated, although even in these situations testing is controversial. Routine testing for hypercoagulable states in the setting of a provoked DVT is generally not indicated. Hematologic diseases associated with VTE include heparin-induced thrombocytopenia and thrombosis syndrome, disseminated intravascular coagulation, antiphospholipid antibody syndrome, myeloproliferative disorders, thrombotic thrombocytopenic purpura, and hemolytic uremic syndrome. There are a number of risk prediction scores that have been advanced, the most widely used being the Caprini risk score (https://www.mdcalc.com/caprini-score-venous-thromboembolism-2005).

Pathophysiology

Although Virchow's triad of stasis, vein injury, and hypercoagulability has defined the events that predispose to VTE formation since the mid-19th century, the understanding today of events that occur at the level of the vein wall and thrombus, including the inflammatory response on thrombogenesis, thrombus resolution, and the subsequent changes to the vein wall and venous valves, is increasingly becoming apparent and may direct therapy in the future. COVID-19 has also been associated with the development of VTE. Infection with COVID-19 induces overlapping pathways that link the inflammatory response to the coagulation response. The overwhelming inflammatory response in patients with COVID-19 infection leads to a hypercoagulable state, microthrombosis, large vessel thrombosis, and ultimately can lead to death. The endothelium in multiple organs, especially the lungs, appears to play a significant role in the process going from reversible dysfunction to irreversible endothelial dysfunction. In the ICU in COVID-19 critically ill patients, the rate of VTE has most recently been reported between 25% and 30%.

Diagnosis

Deep Venous Thrombosis

The diagnosis of DVT can be ruled out with a clinical scoring system known as the Wells score (https://www.mdcalc.com/wells-criteria-dvt) and a negative D-dimer. Wells has classified patients into a scoring system that emphasizes physical presentation, and the most common physical finding is edema. Characteristics that score points in the Wells system include active cancer, paralysis or paresis, recent plaster/cast immobilization of the lower extremity, being recently bedridden for 3 days or more, localized tenderness along the distribution of the deep venous system, swelling of the entire leg, calf swelling that is at least 3 cm larger on the involved side than on the noninvolved side, pitting edema in the symptomatic leg, collateral superficial veins (nonvaricose), and a history of previous DVT. With extensive proximal iliofemoral DVT there may be significant swelling, cyanosis, and dilated superficial collateral veins. The negative predictive value of a low- or intermediate-risk patient as stratified by Wells score and a negative D-dimer is near 100%. The incidence of DVT over the next 3 months in this patient cohort is 0.0% to 0.6%, suggesting that additional testing is unlikely to improve outcomes.

Duplex ultrasound imaging is the gold standard for ruling in the diagnosis of DVT. Duplex imaging includes both a B-mode image and Doppler flow pattern. Duplex imaging demonstrates sensitivity and specificity rates greater than 95%. According to the grade criteria for the strength of medical evidence, duplex ultrasound is given a 1B level of evidence, depending on the pretest probability for DVT. Even at the level of the calf, duplex imaging is an acceptable technique in symptomatic patients. Duplex imaging is painless, requires no contrast, can be repeated, and is safe during pregnancy. Duplex imaging also identifies other causes of a patient's symptoms. Other tests available for making the diagnosis include magnetic resonance imaging (MRI) (especially good for assessing central pelvic vein and inferior vena cava [IVC] thrombosis) and spiral computed tomography (CT) scanning (especially with chest imaging during examination for PE).

A single complete negative lower extremity duplex scan is accurate enough to withhold anticoagulation with minimal long-term adverse thromboembolic complications. This requires that all venous segments of the leg have been imaged and evaluated. If the duplex scan is indeterminate owing to technical issues or to edema, treatment may be based on factors such as biomarkers, with the duplex repeated in 24 to 72 hours. Combining clinical characteristics with a high-sensitivity D-dimer assay can decrease the number of duplex scans performed in the low-risk patient. Although clinical characteristics and D-dimer levels are useful to rule out thrombosis, the converse is not true, and there is no combination of biomarkers and clinical presentation that can rule in the diagnosis. Work is ongoing to establish new biomarkers based on the inflammatory response to DVT. We have data suggesting that a combination of soluble P-selectin and the Wells score can rule in the diagnosis of DVT, whereas D-dimer plus Wells is still the best combination to rule out the diagnosis of DVT.

Conditions that may be confused with DVT include lymphedema, muscle strain, muscle contusion, and systemic problems such as cardiac, renal, or hepatic abnormalities. These systemic problems usually lead to bilateral edema.

Rarely, massive iliofemoral DVT can result in phlegmasia alba dolens (white swollen leg) or phlegmasia cerulean dolens (blue swollen leg). If phlegmasia is not aggressively treated, it can lead to venous gangrene when the arterial inflow becomes obstructed owing to venous hypertension. Alternatively, arterial emboli or spasm can occur and contribute to the pathophysiology. Venous gangrene is often associated with underlying malignancy and is always preceded by phlegmasia cerulea dolens. Venous gangrene is associated with significant rates of amputation and PE and with mortality.

Pulmonary Embolism

The diagnosis of PE historically has involved ventilation-perfusion scanning and pulmonary angiography. However, the most current techniques include spiral CT scanning and MRI, along with assessments of pretest probability and high-sensitivity D-dimer measurements. Age-adjusted D-dimer measurements may increase the diagnostic usefulness of these measurements.

INITIAL MANAGEMENT		DECISION POINT	
PRIMARY TREATMENT (3–6 MONTHS)		**SECONDARY PREVENTION**	
CASE	**INITIAL MANAGEMENT**	**PRIMARY TREATMENT**	**SECONDARY PREVENTION**
Provoked DVT of right leg following a prolonged car ride in an otherwise healthy 61-year-old man	Apixaban 10 mg BID for 7 days or rivaroxaban 15 mg daily for 21 days	Apixaban 5 mg BID for 3 months or rivaroxaban 20 mg daily for 3 months	None
PE in 79-year-old man with prostate cancer	Apixaban 10 mg bid for 7 days	Apixaban 5 mg bid	Apixaban 5 mg BID
Pulmonary emboli in a 48-year-old with ESRD	Intravenous heparin	Vitamin K antagonist (Warfarin)	None (secondary to bleeding risk with ESRD)
Unprovoked DVT in a 50-year-old male with factor V Leiden	Apixaban 10 mg BID for 7 days or rivaroxaban 15 mg daily for 21 days	Apixaban 5 mg BID for 3 months or rivaroxaban 20 mg daily for minimum of 3–6 months	Apixaban 2.5 mg BID, rivaroxaban 10 mg daily or low-dose aspirin

BID, Twice daily; *DVT*, deep venous thrombosis; *ESRD*, end-stage renal disease.

CT scanning demonstrates excellent specificity and sensitivity. Emboli down to the subsegmental level can be identified. The sensitivity for isolated chest CT imaging is increased when clinical analysis is added and when adding lower extremity imaging to the chest scan, although with the introduction of higher resolution multidetector-row CT imaging, the need for lower extremity imaging combined with CT is being questioned. Useful alternate techniques when there are contraindications to CT imaging include MRI and ventilation-perfusion imaging.

In low-risk individuals, a score of 0 on the PE Rule-out Criteria (https://www.mdcalc.com/perc-rule-pulmonary-embolism) gives confidence that further testing (D-dimer and CT) is not necessary. The PE Rule-out Criteria include (1) pulse oximetry of 94% or less, (2) heart rate of 100 beats/min or greater, (3) age of 50 years or older, (4) unilateral leg swelling, (5) hemoptysis, (6) recent trauma or surgery, (7) previous PE or DVT, and (8) exogenous estrogen use.

Axillary and Subclavian Vein Thrombosis

Thrombosis of the axillary and subclavian veins accounts for less than 5% of all cases of DVT. However, it may be associated with PE in up to 10% to 15% of cases and can be the source of significant disability. Upper extremity DVT may be primary (approximately 20%), such as from thoracic outlet syndrome, effort thrombosis, or idiopathic, or secondary (approximately 80%), such as from catheter-related, cancer-associated, surgery-related, or mediastinal tumors. Primary axillary and subclavian vein thrombosis results from obstruction of the axillary vein in the thoracic outlet from compression by the subclavius muscle and the costoclavicular space, the Paget-Schrötter syndrome, noted especially in muscular athletes. Patients with axillary and subclavian vein thrombosis present with arm pain, edema, and cyanosis. Superficial venous distention may be apparent over the arm, forearm, shoulder, and anterior chest wall.

Upper extremity venous duplex ultrasound scanning is used to make the diagnosis of axillary and subclavian vein thrombosis. A secondary DVT (such as related to a central venous catheter or other risk factor) is treated with anticoagulation alone, with the same recommendation regarding anticoagulant type, dose, and duration. If Paget-Schrötter syndrome is suspected, thrombolysis and phlebography are considered as next interventions. If phlebography is performed, it is important that the patient undergo positional phlebography with the arm abducted to 120 degrees to confirm extrinsic subclavian vein compression at the thoracic outlet once the vein has been cleared of thrombus. Because a cervical rib may be the cause of such obstruction, chest x-ray should be obtained to exclude its presence (although its incidence is quite low). Ultimately, decompression of the thoracic outlet with first rib resection (and cervical rib, if present), is necessary to prevent recurrent DVT.

Treatment
Standard Therapy for Venous Thromboembolism

The traditional treatment of VTE is systemic anticoagulation, which reduces the risk of PE, extension of thrombosis, and thrombus recurrence. Because the recurrence rate for VTE is higher if anticoagulation is not therapeutic in the first 24 hours, immediate anticoagulation should be undertaken. For PE, this usually means anticoagulation followed by testing. For DVT, because duplex imaging is rapidly obtained, usually testing precedes anticoagulation. Recurrent DVT can still occur in up to one-third of patients over an 8-year period, even with appropriate anticoagulant therapy.

The first line of therapy in the modern-day treatment of VTE is DOACs. Currently four DOACs are approved by the US Food and Drug Administration (FDA) for the treatment of DVT and one for prophylaxis of VTE. These include rivaroxaban (Xarelto) and apixaban (Eliquis) as oral monotherapy (both require a loading dose period followed by a lower dose) and dabigatran (Pradaxa) and edoxaban (Savaysa), which require a LMWH bridge, and betrixaban (Bevyxxa) for prophylaxis. Alternatively, LMWH or unfractionated heparin is given for 5 days, during which time oral anticoagulation with vitamin K antagonists (warfarin) is begun and LMWH is discontinued as soon as anticoagulation is therapeutic. With warfarin, it is recommended that the international normalized ratio be therapeutic for 2 consecutive days before stopping heparin or LMWH.

The new oral anticoagulants are favored over warfarin (grade 2B) for acute VTE and no cancer. Dabigatran targets activated factor II (factor IIa), whereas rivaroxaban, apixaban, and edoxaban target activated factor X (factor Xa). Dabigatran etexilate is FDA approved for stroke and systemic embolization prevention in patients with nonvalvular atrial fibrillation and for treatment and reduction of DVT and PE in patients who have been treated with a parenteral anticoagulant for 5 to 10 days.

Rivaroxaban is FDA approved for VTE prophylaxis in patients undergoing hip or knee replacements, for stroke and systemic embolization prevention in patients with nonvalvular atrial fibrillation, and for VTE treatment. Apixaban is currently FDA approved for the prevention of complications of nonvalvular atrial fibrillation, for prophylaxis of DVT after hip or knee replacement surgery, for the treatment of DVT/PE, and for the reduction in risk of recurrence of DVT/PE. Edoxaban has been approved for prevention of stroke and non–CNS systemic embolism in patients with nonvalvular atrial fibrillation and for treating DVT and PE in patients who have been treated with a parenteral anticoagulant for 5 to 10 days. Betrixaban is indicated for the prophylaxis of VTE in adult patients hospitalized for an acute medical illness who are at risk for thromboembolic complications due to restricted mobility and other risk factors.

When an anticoagulant bridge is required, LMWH is the standard for initial treatment. LMWH is preferred because it is administered subcutaneously, it requires no monitoring (except in certain circumstances such as renal insufficiency or morbid obesity), and it is associated with a lower bleeding potential. Additionally, LMWH demonstrates less direct thrombin inhibition, more factor Xa inhibition, and antiinflammatory properties. Compared with standard unfractionated heparin, LMWH has significantly improved bioavailability, less endothelial cell binding and protein binding, and an improved pharmacokinetic profile. The half-life of LMWH is dose independent. LMWH is administered in a weight-based fashion.

Warfarin (Coumadin), when used, should be started after heparinization is therapeutic to prevent warfarin-induced skin necrosis. For standard unfractionated heparin, this requires a therapeutic activated partial thromboplastin time (aPTT); for LMWH, warfarin is administered after an appropriate weight-based dose of LMWH is administered and allowed to circulate. Warfarin causes inhibition of protein C and S before factors II, IX, and X, leading to paradoxical hypercoagulability at the initiation of therapy. The goal for warfarin dosing is an international normalized ratio between 2.0 and 3.0.

Fondaparinux (Arixtra) is also approved for the treatment of VTE. It is a synthetic pentasaccharide that has an antithrombin sequence identical to heparin and targets factor Xa. Fondaparinux has been additionally approved for thrombosis prophylaxis in patients with total hip replacement, total knee replacement, and hip fracture; in extended prophylaxis in patients with hip fracture; and in patients undergoing abdominal surgery. It is administered subcutaneously and has a 17-hour half-life. Dosage is based on body weight. It exhibits no endothelial or protein binding and does not produce thrombocytopenia. However, no antidote is readily available. For the treatment of VTE, fondaparinux was found equal to LMWH for DVT, and for PE, it was found equal to standard heparin.

Although LMWH has been the historic standard of care for treating cancer-associated VTE, the DOACS edoxaban[1] and rivaroxaban[1] have been found effective but with a higher risk of bleeding than LMWH. A recent study found that apixaban[1] at therapeutic dose was noninferior to the LMWH dalteparin (Fragmin) with no increased risk of major bleeding for treatment of cancer-associated VTE.

With significant thrombotic complications with COVID-19, there are many studies ongoing evaluating anticoagulant treatment in these patients, to treat not only diagnosed macrothrombosis but also microthrombosis with the intent to improve mortality. Several guidelines from national and international organizations recommend prophylactic dose anticoagulation in ward (non-ICU) patients with COVID-19, and prophylactic and/or intermediate dose anticoagulation in ICU patients with COVID-19. Additionally, some guidelines suggest postdischarge anticoagulation for COVID-19 patients. This is a rapidly moving area and recommendations will change as more data is accumulated.

Duration of Treatment

The recommended duration of anticoagulation after a first episode of provoked VTE is 3 months for both proximal (grade 1B evidence) and distal thrombi (if symptomatic, grade 2C evidence) (Table 1). After a second episode of VTE, the usual recommendation is prolonged oral anticoagulation indefinitely (grade 1B), unless the patient is at high bleeding risk (two or more risk factors, grade 2B) or the patient is very young at the time of presentation. VTE recurrence is increased with homozygous factor V Leiden and prothrombin 20210A mutation, protein C or protein S deficiency, antithrombin deficiency, antiphospholipid antibodies, and cancer until resolved. Long-term oral anticoagulation is usually recommended in these situations. However, heterozygous factor V Leiden and prothrombin 20210A do not carry the same risk as their homozygous counterparts, and the length of oral anticoagulation is shortened for these conditions.

---

[1] Not FDA approved for this indication.

Regarding unprovoked DVT, in those with a low bleeding risk, the recommended length of treatment is extended therapy for more than 3 months (grade 2B evidence), provided the patient is at low or moderate risk of bleeding. Patients at high risk of bleeding should be treated for 3 months (grade 1B) and reevaluated. Additional tools that can aid in the decision making to continue or discontinue anticoagulation include thrombosis risk factors, residual thrombus burden, and coagulation system activation. The HERDOO2 score (https://www.mdcalc.com/herdoo2-rule-discontinuing-anticoagulation-unprovoked-vte) has been suggested as a way for identifying women at low risk of recurrent VTE for whom anticoagulation can be stopped. In addition, there is growing evidence that in certain circumstances, such as active cancer, the use of LMWH is superior to LMWH converted to warfarin for long-term treatment, for at least the first 3 to 6 months (grade 2C evidence). There is now evidence that rivaroxaban and apixaban may be as effective as LMWH in cancer patients, with the convenience of an oral medication. However, due to a slightly increased risk of GI bleeding, DOACs should be restricted to those patients with a non-GI malignancy and low bleeding risk.

Extended therapy is now recommended with low-dose DOACs when the risk-benefit relationship favors continued treatment. Extended rivaroxaban showed a significant decrease in recurrent VTE without a significant increase in major bleeding compared with aspirin for an additional 6 to 12 months of therapy after initial therapy. Apixaban as extended treatment of VTE has also been found to provide long-term protection against recurrent VTE. After initial treatment, an additional 12 months of apixaban therapy has been compared with placebo. There was a significant decrease in the rate of VTE without an increase in bleeding risk. In patients who cannot continue on DOACs after initial therapy for VTE and who do not have a contraindication, aspirin should be administered to prevent recurrent thrombosis. Bridging has been a complicated issue when patients on chronic anticoagulation with vitamin K antagonists (with long 5–7 days' half-lives) must undergo an operative procedure and the anticoagulation must be stopped and restarted. However, in low- to moderate-risk patients, bridging is associated with no decrease in thrombotic events but with a higher bleeding risk. In fact, bridging is only indicated currently in those patients with atrial fibrillation and a recent stroke, atrial fibrillation and a high CHADS$_2$ score (5–6), a recent VTE within the past 3 months, and mechanical cardiac valves, especially mitral valves. The availability of DOACs, with short half-lives, has dramatically decreased the need for LMWH-based bridging. In most circumstances, DOACs need to be held only for 1 day for minor procedures and 2 days for major procedures and can be started back as soon as it is felt safe from the surgical or procedural perspective.

Complications

Bleeding is the most common complication of anticoagulation. Risk factors for bleeding while on anticoagulation include age >65, previous bleeding, cancer, renal or liver failure, thrombocytopenia, previous stroke, diabetes, anemia, concurrent antiplatelet therapy, poor anticoagulant control, recent surgery, frequent falls, alcohol abuse, and nonsteroidal antiinflammatory drug use. Presence of zero risk factors (low risk) confers an absolute risk of major bleeding of 0.8% per year. Patients with one risk factor have a risk of 1.6% per year, and those with two or more have a 6.5% risk or higher per year. With standard heparin, bleeding occurs over the first 5 days in approximately 10% of patients. Warfarin is associated with a major bleeding rate of 1% to 2% per year. Even with the new DOACS, bleeding (major plus minor) may occur in 5% to 10% of cases, although the risk of intracerebral bleeding appears to be less than with warfarin. A recent real-world study of non-valvular atrial fibrillation patients suggested that rates of bleeding may be different between DOACs, with ranges between 11% and 16%. Problems specific to the DOACs include the difficulty to reliably reverse their anticoagulant effects and the difficulty with laboratory monitoring. A monoclonal antibody idarucizumab (Praxbind) for the reversal of dabigatran and a recombinant modified human Factor Xa protein andexanet alfa (Andexxa) for the reversal of Factor Xa inhibitors have been FDA approved; however, expense may limit their use. Aripazine (a Factor Xa inhibitor) is under development.

Heparin-induced thrombocytopenia (HIT) occurs in 0.6% to 30% of patients. Although historically morbidity and mortality rates have been high, it has been found that early diagnosis and appropriate treatment have decreased these rates. HIT usually begins 3 to 14 days after unfractionated heparin is begun, although it can occur earlier if the patient has been exposed to heparin in the past. A heparin-dependent antibody binds to platelets, activates them with the release of procoagulant microparticles, leading to an increase in thrombocytopenia, and results in both arterial and venous thrombosis. Both bovine and porcine unfractionated heparin and LMWH have been associated with HIT, although the incidence and severity of the thrombosis is less with LMWH. Even small exposures to heparin, such as heparin coating on indwelling catheters, can cause the syndrome. The diagnosis should be suspected with a 50% or greater drop in platelet count, when the platelet count falls below 100,000/μL, or when thrombosis occurs during heparin or LMWH therapy. The enzyme-linked immunosorbent assay detects the antiheparin antibody in the plasma. This test is highly sensitive but poorly specific. The serotonin release assay is used as a confirmatory test that is more specific but less sensitive than the enzyme-linked immunosorbent assay test.

When the diagnosis is made, heparin must be discontinued. Oral anticoagulation should not be given until an adequate alternative anticoagulant has been established and until the platelet count has normalized. Because LMWHs demonstrate high cross-reactivity with standard heparin antibodies, they cannot be substituted for standard heparin in patients with HIT. Agents that have been FDA approved as alternatives include the direct thrombin inhibitor argatroban. Fondaparinux (Arixtra)[1] has also been found effective for treatment of HIT in most cases, but it is not FDA approved for this indication.

Nonpharmacologic Treatments

The symptoms of swelling and leg fatigue can be controlled after DVT by the use of compression stockings. Additionally, walking with good compression does not increase the risk of PE, whereas it significantly decreases the incidence and severity of the PTS. A recent multicenter randomized trial has suggested that stockings do not prevent development of PTS after a first proximal DVT, and for that reason, the most recent ACCP guidelines suggest not using compression stockings to prevent PTS (grade 2B evidence). It must be remembered that the use of strong compression and early ambulation after DVT treatment can significantly reduce the symptoms of pain and swelling resulting from the DVT, even if the development of PTS is not prevented, and a new study suggests that certain surrogate markers for PTS may be lessened by the application of immediate compression, and it also reduced residual vein obstruction, which correlated with PTS.

Aggressive Therapies for Venous Thromboembolism

The goals of DVT treatment are to prevent extension or recurrence of DVT, prevent PE, and minimize the late sequela of thrombosis, namely chronic venous insufficiency. Standard anticoagulants accomplish the first two goals but not the third goal. The PTS (venous insufficiency related to venous thrombosis) occurs in up to 30% to 50% of patients after DVT and in an even higher percentage of patients with iliofemoral level DVT. It has been hypothesized that reopening the vein will alleviate venous hypertension or prevent PTS. This is known as the "open vein hypothesis." The following evidence suggests more aggressive therapies for extensive thrombosis are indicated: experimentally, prolonged contact of the thrombus with the vein wall increases damage. The thrombus initiates an inflammatory response in the

vein wall that can lead to vein wall fibrosis and valvular dysfunction. The longer a thrombus is in contact with a vein valve, the more chance that valve will no longer function.

Venous thrombectomy has proved superior to anticoagulation over 6 months to 10 years as measured by venous patency and prevention of venous reflux. Catheter-directed thrombolysis has been used in many nonrandomized studies and, in small, randomized trials, was more effective than standard therapy. Quality of life was improved with thrombus removal, and results appear to be optimized further by combining catheter-directed thrombolysis with mechanical devices. These devices include but are not limited to the Angiojet rheolytic catheter, the EKOS ultrasound accelerated catheter, and new larger bore extraction devices (Penumbra and angiovac). With these devices, thrombolysis is hastened, the amount of thrombolytic agent is decreased, and bleeding is thus decreased. Additionally, the use of venous stents for iliac venous obstruction has been shown to decrease the incidence of PTS, decrease chronic venous insufficiency, and improve disease-specific quality of life at 1, 6, and 24 months after the treatment.

To more fully elucidate the role of aggressive therapy in proximal iliofemoral venous thrombosis, the ATTRACT trial randomized 692 patients with acute proximal DVT to either anticoagulation alone or anticoagulation plus pharmacomechanical thrombolysis. This study found that more aggressive therapy did not decrease the incidence of PTS but did result in more major bleeding. The severity of the PTS was lessened by the pharmacomechanical thrombolysis, suggesting that more aggressive therapy should be offered to patients with significant iliofemoral venous thrombosis, who do not respond appropriately to a course of anticoagulation. This result also suggests that other factors need to be addressed to prevent PTS in addition to opening up the thrombosed vein.

For PE, evidence exists that thrombolysis is indicated when there is hemodynamic compromise from the embolism. It is controversial whether thrombolysis should be used in situations in which there is no hemodynamic compromise, but there is evidence of right heart dysfunction or there are positive biomarkers. For PE, PE response teams (PERTs) have become common, and they allow for a multidisciplinary group of providers to treat PE in a rapid and coordinated fashion. These teams include (for example) noninvasive clinicians, emergency physicians, clinical pharmacists, endovascular proceduralists, and cardiac, thoracic, and/or vascular surgeons. The efficacy of these teams for treatment of PE is an area of active investigation.

Inferior Vena Cava Filters

Traditional indications for the use of IVC filters include failure of anticoagulation, a contraindication to anticoagulation, or a complication of anticoagulation. Protection from PE is greater than 95% using cone-shaped, wire-based permanent filters in the IVC. With the success of these filters, indications have expanded to the presence of free-floating thrombus tails, prophylactic use when the risk for anticoagulation is excessive, when the risk of PE is thought to be high, and to allow the use of perioperative epidural anesthesia. IVC filters are not recommended as first-line therapy in patients who are treated with anticoagulants.

IVC filters can be either permanent or retrievable. If a retrievable filter is left, then it becomes a permanent filter; the long-term fate of these filters has yet to be defined adequately in the literature. Thus great efforts need to be made to remove retrievable IVC filters when the risk period is over. Most filters are placed in the infrarenal location in the IVC. However, they may be placed in the suprarenal position or in the superior vena cava.

Indications for suprarenal placement include high-lying thrombi, pregnancy or women of childbearing age, or previous device failure filled with thrombus. Although some have suggested that sepsis is a contraindication to the use of filters, sepsis has not been found to be a contraindication because the trapped material can be sterilized with intravenous antibiotics. Filters may be inserted under x-ray guidance or using ultrasound techniques, either external ultrasound or intravascular ultrasound.

---

[1] Not FDA approved for this indication.

References

Ahmed Z, Hassan S, Salzman GA: Novel oral anticoagulants for venous thromboembolism with special emphasis on risk of hemorrhagic complications and reversal agents, *Curr Drug Ther* 11:3–20, 2016.

Amin EE, Bistervels IM, Meijer K: Reduced incidence of vein occlusion and postthrombotic syndrome after immediate compression for deep vein thrombosis, *Blood* 132:2298–2304, 2018.

Bruinstroop E, Klok FA, Van De Ree MA: Elevated D-dimer levels predict recurrence in patients with idiopathic venous thromboembolism: a meta-analysis, *J Thromb Haemost* 7:611–618, 2009.

Elsharawy M, Elzayat E: Early results of thrombolysis vs. anticoagulation in iliofemoral venous thrombosis. A randomised clinical trial, *Eur J Vasc Endovasc Surg* 24(3):209–214, 2002.

Freund Y, Cachanado M, Aubry A: Effect of the pulmonary embolism rule-out criteria on subsequent thromboembolic events among low-risk emergency department patients: the PROPER Randomized Clinical Trial, *J Am Med Assoc* 319(6):559–566, 2018.

Gross PL, Weitz JI: New anticoagulants for treatment of venous thromboembolism, *Arterioscler Thromb Vasc Biol* 28:380–386, 2008.

Grosse SD, Nelson RE, Nyarko KA, Richardson LC, Raskob GE: The economic burden of incident venous thromboembolism in the United States: a review of estimated attributable healthcare costs, *Thromb Res* 137:3–10, 2016.

Guyatt GH, Akl EA, Crother M: Executive summary: antithrombotic therapy and prevention of thrombosis: American College of Chest Physicians' evidence based clinical practice guidelines, ed 9, *Chest* 141:7S–47S, 2012.

Heit JA, Spencer FA, White RH: The epidemiology of venous thromboembolism, *J Thromb Thrombolysis* 41:3–14, 2016.

Heit JA, Ashrani AA, Crusan DJ, McBane RD, Petterson TM, Bailey KR: Reasons for the persistent incidence of venous thromboembolism, *Thromb Haemost* 117:390–400, 2017.

Hull RD, Pineo GF, Brant R: Home therapy of venous thrombosis with long-term LMWH versus usual care: patient satisfaction and post-thrombotic syndrome, *Am J Med* 122:762–769, 2009.

Kahn SR, Shapiro S, Wells PS: Compression stockings to prevent post-thrombotic syndrome: a randomized placebo controlled trial, *Lancet* 383:880–888, 2014.

Kahn SR, Julian JA, Kearon C: Quality of life after pharmacomechanical catheter-directed thrombolysis for proximal deep venous thrombosis, *J Vasc Surg Venous Lymphat Disord* 8:8–23, 2020.

Kearon C, Akl EA, Comerota AJ: Antithombotic therapy and VTE disease. Antithombotic therapy and prevention of thrombosis: American College of Chest Physicians Evidence-Based Clinical Practice Guidelines, ed 9, *Chest* 141(Suppl):e419S–e494S, 2012.

Kearon C, Aki EA, Ornelas J: Antithrombotic therapy for VTE disease: chest guideline and Expert Panel Report, *Chest* 149:315–352, 2016.

Knepper J, Horne D, Obi A, Wakefield TW: A systematic update on the state of novel anticoagulants and a primer on reversal and bridging, *J Vasc Surg Venous Lymphat Disord* 1:418–426, 2013. 26.

Kucher N: Deep-vein thrombosis of the upper extremity, *N Engl J Med* 364:861–869, 2011.

Merli G, Spyropoulos AC, Caprini JA: Use of emerging oral anticoagulants in clinical practice: translating results from clinical trials to orthopedic and general surgical patient populations, *Ann Surg* 250:219–228, 2009.

Morillo R, Jimenez D, Aibar MA: DVT management and outcome trends, 2001 to 2014, *Chest* 150:374–383, 2016.

Mismetti P, Laporte S, Pellerin O: Effect of a retrievable inferior vena cava filter plus anticoagulation vs anticoagulation alone on risk of recurrent pulmonary embolism: a randomized clinical trial, *J Am Med Assoc* 313:1627–1635, 2015.

Neglen P, Hollis KC, Olivier J: Stenting of the venous outflow in chronic venous disease: long-term stent-related outcome, clinical, and hemodynamic result, *J Vasc Surg* 46:979–990, 2007.

Palareti G, Cosmi B, Legnani C: D-dimer testing to determine the duration of anticoagulation therapy, *N Engl J Med* 355:1780–1789, 2006.

Piazza G, Campia U, Hurwitz S, et al: Registry of arterial and venous thromboembolic complications in patients with COVID-19, *J Am Coll Cardiol* 76(18):2060–2072, 2020.

Righini M, Ebadi HR, Gal GL: Diagnosis of acute pulmonary embolism, *J Thromb Haemost* 15:1251–1261, 2017.

Schulman S: Advances in the management of venous thromboembolism, *Best Pract Res Clin Haematol* 25:361–377, 2012.

Schulman S, Kearon C, Kakkar AK: Dabigatran versus warfarin in the treatment of acute venous thromboembolism, *N Engl J Med* 361(24):2342–2352, 2009.

Stein PD, Fowler SE, Goodman LR: Multidetector computed tomography for acute pulmonary embolism, *N Engl J Med* 354(22):2317–2327, 2006.

Tepper PG, Mardekian J, Masseria C, et al. PloS One 13(11)e0205989. https://doi.org/10.1371/journal.pone.0205989.

Turpie AG, Bauer KA, Eriksson BI: Fondaparinux vs. enoxaparin for the prevention of venous thromboembolism in major orthopedic surgery: a meta-analysis of 4 randomized double-blind studies, *Arch Intern Med* 162(16):1833–1840, 2002.

Vedantham S, Goldhaber SZ, Julian JA: Pharmacomechanical catheter-directed thrombolysis for deep-vein thrombosis, *N Engl J Med* 377:2240–2252, 2017.

Weitz JI, Jaffer IH, Fredenburgh JC: Recent advances in the treatment of venous thromboembolism in the era of the direct oral anticoagulants, *F1000Res* 6:985, 2017.

Wells PS, Anderson DR, Rodger M: Evaluation of D-dimer in the diagnosis of suspected deep-vein thrombosis, *N Engl J Med* 349(13):1227–1235, 2003.

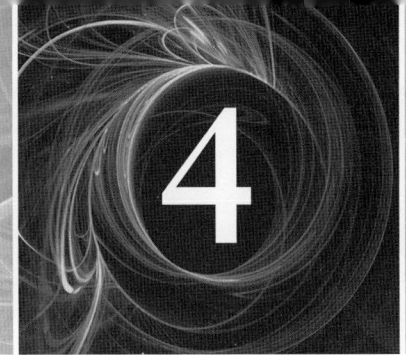

Digestive System

ACUTE AND CHRONIC PANCREATITIS

Method of
George Van Buren II, MD; and William E. Fisher, MD

CURRENT DIAGNOSIS

- Acute pancreatitis is usually caused by gallstones, and chronic pancreatitis is usually caused by alcohol abuse.
- Other less-common causes of acute and chronic pancreatitis are considered only when gallstones and alcohol are definitively ruled out.
- Pancreatic cancer and chronic pancreatitis can sometimes be difficult to distinguish.

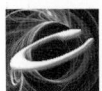

CURRENT THERAPY

- There has been a recent trend toward conservative medical therapy for acute and chronic pancreatitis, reserving surgery for select patients.
- In acute pancreatitis, try to avoid necrosectomy except in the setting of infected necrosis with organ failure.
- Asymptomatic pseudocysts can generally be observed.
- Persistent symptomatic pseudocysts can often be addressed endoscopically.
- Medical therapy for chronic pancreatitis includes pain management, nutrition, diabetes control, and cessation of drinking alcohol and smoking.
- Surgical treatment for chronic pancreatitis currently favors strict patient selection and consideration of various surgical techniques.

Acute Pancreatitis

Acute pancreatitis is an inflammatory disease of the pancreas that is associated with little or no fibrosis of the gland. It can be initiated by several factors including gallstones, alcohol, trauma, and infections, and in some cases it is hereditary (Box 1). Very often, patients with acute pancreatitis develop additional complications such as sepsis, shock, and respiratory and renal failure, resulting in considerable morbidity and mortality.

Epidemiology

The annual incidence of acute pancreatitis is probably about 50 cases per 100,000 population in the United States. Approximately 3000 of these cases are severe enough to lead to death. Studies worldwide have shown a rising but variable incidence of acute pancreatitis, including large increases in incidence in pediatric populations.

Risk Factors

Biliary tract stone disease accounts for 70% to 80% of the cases of acute pancreatitis. Alcoholism accounts for another 10%, and the remaining 10% to 20% is accounted for either by idiopathic disease or by a variety of iatrogenic and miscellaneous causes including trauma, endoscopy, surgery, drugs, heredity, infection, and toxins. Medications appear to cause less than 5% of all cases of acute pancreatitis. The drugs most strongly associated with the disorder are azathioprine (Imuran), 6-mercaptopurine (Purinethol), didanosine (Videx), valproic acid (Depakote), angiotensin-converting–enzyme inhibitors, and mesalamine (Asacol). It is difficult to determine whether the drug is responsible. Tobacco use has also been heavily linked to pancreatitis. Meta-analysis has shown cigarette smoking to be associated with acute pancreatitis development in a dose-response manner.

Pathophysiology

Pancreatitis begins with the activation of digestive zymogens inside acinar cells, which cause acinar cell injury. Digestive zymogens are co-localized with lysosomal hydrolase, and cathepsin-B catalyzed trypsinogen activation occurs, resulting in acinar cell injury and necrosis. This triggers acinar cell inflammatory events with the secretion of inflammatory mediators. Studies suggest that the ultimate severity of the resulting pancreatitis may be determined by the events that occur subsequent to acinar cell injury. These include inflammatory cell recruitment and activation, as well as generation and release of cytokines, reactive oxygen species, and other chemical mediators of inflammation, ultimately leading to ischemia and necrosis. Early mortality in severe acute pancreatitis is caused by a systemic inflammatory response syndrome with multiorgan failure. If the patient survives this critical early period, a septic complication caused by translocated bacteria, mostly gram-negative microbes from the intestine, leads to infected pancreatic necrosis. Late deaths are caused by infected necrosis, leading to septic shock and multiorgan failure.

Prevention

Gallstones are present in about 15% to 20% of patients older than 60 years, but only a fraction become symptomatic. Although gallstone pancreatitis can rarely be the first symptom of gallstones, most patients have symptoms of cholecystitis before developing pancreatitis. Thus it is important to make early and prompt referral of patients with symptomatic cholelithiasis for laparoscopic cholecystectomy to prevent life-threatening complications such as acute pancreatitis.

Clinical Manifestations

All episodes of acute pancreatitis begin with severe pain, generally following a substantial meal. The pain is usually epigastric, but it can occur anywhere in the abdomen or lower chest. It has been described as penetrating through to the back, and it may be relieved by the patient's leaning forward. It precedes the onset of nausea and vomiting, with retching often continuing after the stomach has emptied. Vomiting does not relieve the pain, which is more intense in necrotizing than in edematous pancreatitis.

On examination the patient may show tachycardia, tachypnea, hypotension, and hyperthermia. The temperature is usually only mildly elevated in uncomplicated pancreatitis. Voluntary and involuntary guarding can be seen over the epigastric region. The bowel sounds are decreased or absent. There are usually no

Alcoholism
Hereditary
Hypertriglyceridemia
Trauma (including iatrogenic: ERCP or surgery)
Drugs: azathioprine (Imuran), furosemide, mercaptopurine
    (Purinethol), opiates, pentamidine (Pentam), steroids,
    sulfasalazine (Azulfidine), sulindac (Clinoril), tetracycline,
    trimethoprim-sulfamethoxazole (Bactrim), valproic acid
    (Depakote)
Tumor
Infection (parasitic and viral)
Idiopathic

ERCP, Endoscopic retrograde cholangiopancreatography.

palpable masses. The abdomen may be distended with intraperitoneal fluid. There may be pleural effusion, particularly on the left side. With increasing severity of disease, the intravascular fluid loss may become life-threatening as a result of sequestration of edematous fluid in the retroperitoneum. Hemoconcentration then results in an elevated hematocrit. However, there also may be bleeding into the retroperitoneum or the peritoneal cavity. In some patients (about 1%), the blood from necrotizing pancreatitis can dissect through the soft tissues and manifest as a bluish discoloration around the umbilicus (Cullen sign) or in the flanks (Grey Turner sign). The severe fluid loss can lead to prerenal azotemia, with elevated blood urea nitrogen and creatinine levels. There also may be hyperglycemia, hypoalbuminemia, and hypocalcemia sufficient in some cases to produce tetany.

Diagnosis

The definition of acute pancreatitis is based on the fulfillment of two out of three of the following criteria: clinical (upper abdominal pain), laboratory (serum amylase or lipase >3× upper limit of normal) and/or imaging (computed tomographic [CT], magnetic resonance imaging [MRI], ultrasonography) criteria. Although serum amylase is often elevated in acute pancreatitis, there is no significant correlation between the magnitude of serum amylase elevation and severity of pancreatitis. Other pancreatic enzymes also have been evaluated to improve the diagnostic accuracy of serum measurements. Specificity of these markers ranges from 77% to 96%, the highest being for lipase. Measurements of many digestive enzymes have methodologic limitations and cannot be easily adapted for quantitation in emergency laboratory studies. Because serum levels of lipase remain elevated for a longer time than total or pancreatic amylase, it is the serum indicator of highest probability of the disease.

Abdominal ultrasound examination is the best way to confirm the presence of gallstones in suspected biliary pancreatitis. It also can detect extrapancreatic ductal dilations and reveal pancreatic edema, swelling, and peripancreatic fluid collections. However, in about 20% of patients, the ultrasound examination does not provide satisfactory results because of the presence of bowel gas, which can obscure sonographic imaging of the pancreas.

A CT scan of the pancreas is more commonly used to diagnose pancreatitis. CT scanning is used to distinguish milder (nonnecrotic) forms of the disease from more severe necrotizing or infected pancreatitis, in patients whose clinical presentation raises the suspicion of advanced disease (Figures 1 and 2). Pancreatic protocol CT scan of the abdomen and pelvis is recommended when not limited by renal insufficiency: a tri-phasic thin, multislice CT scan with an arterial, venous, and delayed phase in conjunction with sagittal and coronal views; no oral contrast, instead drink 1000 cc water to opacify the stomach. The scan assesses the degree of pancreatic necrosis, peripancreatic fluid collections, and the surrounding vascular structures. This tri-phasic scan can also help to detect underlying mass lesions.

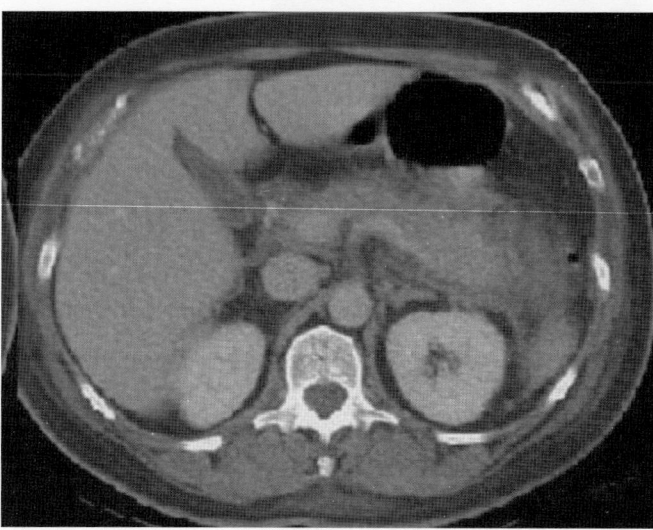

Figure 1 Computed tomographic scan confirming acute edematous pancreatitis.

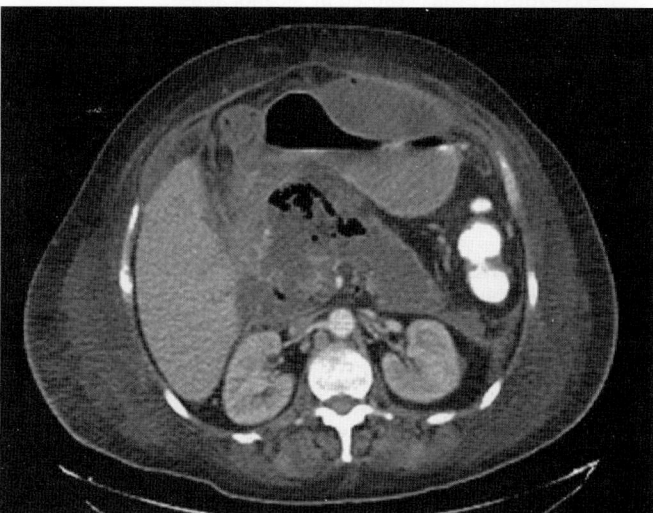

Figure 2 Computed tomographic scan confirming acute necrotizing, emphysematous pancreatitis.

Magnetic resonance cholangiopancreatography (MRCP) is also of value to assess the pancreatic duct and biliary tree. This can often reveal pancreatic ductal disruption.

Differential Diagnosis

The clinical diagnosis of pancreatitis is one of exclusion. Hyperamylasemia can also occur as a result of conditions not involving pancreatitis. The other upper abdominal conditions that can be confused with acute pancreatitis include perforated peptic ulcer and acute cholecystitis, and occasionally a gangrenous small bowel obstruction. Because these conditions often have a fatal outcome without surgery, urgent intervention is indicated in the small number of cases in which doubt persists. A tumor should be considered in a nonalcoholic patient with acute pancreatitis who has no demonstrable biliary tract disease. Approximately 1% to 2% of patients with acute pancreatitis have pancreatic carcinoma, and an episode of acute pancreatitis can be the first clinical manifestation of a periampullary tumor.

Treatment

The severity of acute pancreatitis covers a broad spectrum of illness, ranging from the mild and self-limiting to the life-threatening necrotizing variety. Some cases are so mild they can be treated in an outpatient setting. However, most cases require hospitalization for observation and diagnostic study. A conservative approach

infected pancreatic necrosis or lower mortality. Data from these well-designed trials refute prior data from less-rigorous studies suggesting prophylactic antibiotics were useful. Additional studies are required, but there is increasing concern that the prolonged use of potent antibiotics might result in an increased prevalence of fungal infections and possibly increased mortality. Currently, antibiotic therapy should be reserved for treatment of specific infections such as positive blood, sputum, and urine cultures or percutaneous or operative cultures of necrotic tissue.

Randomized clinical trials have also shown a benefit from early nasojejunal feeding compared to total parenteral nutrition. Gastric decompression with a nasogastric tube is selectively used in patients with severe ileus and vomiting but is not necessary in a majority of cases. A debate remains regarding the optimal nutritional management in the majority of pancreatitis patients. There has been a trend toward oral enteric feeding in the less severe cases.

In biliary pancreatitis, the gallbladder must eventually be removed or recurrent acute pancreatitis will occur in 30% to 60% of cases. The timing of the cholecystectomy depends on the severity of the pancreatitis. Usually laparoscopic cholecystectomy is performed during the index admission as soon as the attack of acute pancreatitis has resolved. In more severe cases, the cholecystectomy is delayed and often combined with interventions for late complications of acute pancreatitis. In cases with severe comorbidity, endoscopic sphincterotomy has been considered as an alternative to cholecystectomy. However, if the patient has a postinflammatory fluid collection, bacteria can be introduced during endoscopic retrograde cholangiopancreatography (ERCP), and sphincterotomy should be delayed.

Currently, there is no role for routine early laparotomy and necrosectomy or resection in the setting of acute necrotizing pancreatitis. If the necrotic pancreas becomes infected and the patient fails to respond to conservative treatment, then necrosectomy may be warranted. Patients with infected necrosis are rarely managed conservatively without eventual surgical intervention. However, even in the setting of infected necrosis, there has been consideration for antibiotic therapy until the acute inflammatory response has subsided, if possible, with the view that surgery that is deferred for several weeks is more easily accomplished with one intervention. Patients who suffer from infected necrosis without having clinical signs of sepsis or other systemic complications might not need immediate surgical necrosectomy.

A nonsurgical alternative for the treatment of infected necrosis is percutaneous catheter drainage. This is considered a temporary measure to allow stabilization of the patient so that a safer surgical necrosectomy can be done at a later time. Multiple large drains are required, and patients frequently undergo repeat CT and revision of the drains. Current recommendations are to postpone surgery for as long as possible, usually beyond the second or third week of the disease or later, when necrotic tissue can be easily distinguished from viable pancreas and débridement without major blood loss can be performed. When surgery is performed, tissue-preserving digital necrosectomy is the usual technique rather than a classic surgical resection of the pancreas (Figure 3).

Necrosectomy can be performed by an open anterior approach with closed lavage or with leaving the abdomen open and packing. The packing is replaced at intervals of 24 to 72 hours. Sometimes a left lateral retroperitoneal approach is helpful. Newer approaches are the video-assisted retroperitoneal débridement (VARD). This procedure is a combination of percutaneous drainage and the open lateral retroperitoneal approach. An anterior laparoscopic approach has also been described and mimics the open anterior approach using laparoscopic ports. Surgical necrosectomy is indicated in patients with sepsis caused by infected necrosis and in selected patients with extended sterile necrosis causing severe systemic organ dysfunction and sepsis without a septic focus.

In some cases, the acute inflammatory process can lead to erosion into retroperitoneal vessels, and acute hemorrhage occurs. This acute emergent complication is best managed with immediate

has been advocated in the treatment of acute pancreatitis (Box 2). Severity is assessed with imaging results and clinical parameters and is quantitated with scores such as Ranson criteria (Box 3), the Atlanta classification, and the APACHE II (Acute Physiology and Chronic Health Evaluation) score. Severe acute pancreatitis is defined by associated organ dysfunction. The Atlanta classification is based on an international consensus conference held in Atlanta in 1992 and has been updated. APACHE II was designed to measure the severity of disease for adult patients admitted to intensive care units. Though not specific to pancreatitis, APACHE II can be used in an effort to differentiate patients with mild and severe acute pancreatitis. APACHE II scores of 8 points or more correlate with a mortality rate of 11% to 18%.

Upon confirmation of the diagnosis, patients with severe disease should be transferred to the intensive care unit for observation and maximum support. Adequate fluid resuscitation optimizing organ perfusion and oxygenation is essential. The use of prophylactic intravenous antibiotics in the initial stages of severe acute pancreatitis is not proved to be useful. Two randomized, controlled studies failed to show any benefit from antibiotics. Prophylactic antibiotics did not decrease the incidence of

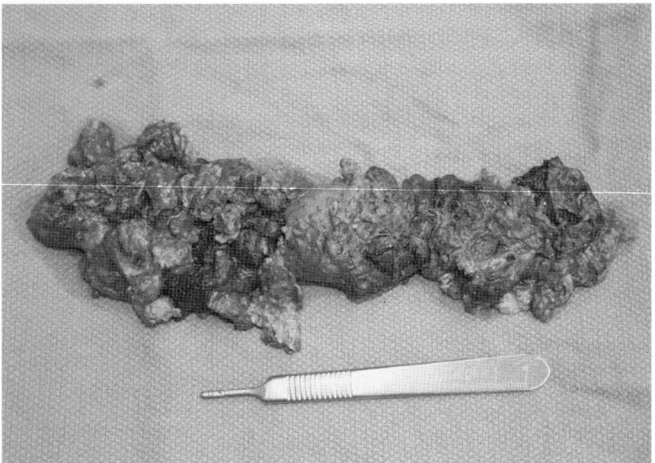

Figure 3 Necrotic material débrided from the retroperitoneum in a case of acute necrotizing pancreatitis.

angiography to determine the exact site of bleeding and can often be treated with embolization rather than surgery (Figure 4).

Although previously frowned upon, there has been a move toward enteric drainage of all necrotic collections (even when infected) when technically feasible. This can be initiated through either an endoscopic or surgical approach.

Monitoring
Despite a conservative operative approach, endocrine and exocrine insufficiency develop in as many as half of the patients and are determined by the extent of pancreatic necrosis. Therefore patients must be monitored with blood glucose measurements, stabilization of body weight, and proper nutrition.

Complications
The most common complication after successful management of acute pancreatitis is a pseudocyst. The term "pseudocyst" is currently used to broadly categorize most pancreatic and peripancreatic fluid collections (including walled-off pancreatic necrosis [WOPN] and acute peripancreatic fluid collection). The Acute Pancreatitis Classification Working Group recently proposed a revised Atlanta classification that refers to collections within 4 weeks of symptom onset as either acute peripancreatic fluid collections (APFC) or postnecrotic pancreatic fluid collections (PNPFC), depending upon the absence or presence of pancreatic/peripancreatic necrosis, respectively. After 4 weeks of the onset of symptoms, persistent collections with discrete walls are referred to as pseudocyst or WOPN, again depending upon the absence or presence of necrosis, respectively. In addition, these collections are further classified as sterile or infected and the term "pancreatic abscess" has been abolished.

The management of pseudocysts has followed a minimally invasive trend. Most pseudocysts resolve spontaneously, even beyond 6 weeks, so asymptomatic pseudocysts are usually observed (70% of pseudocysts will resolve without intervention). Endoscopic cystogastrostomy is the approach of choice for symptomatic fluid-predominant pseudocysts when there is minimal necrosis. If there is significant necrotic debris or a solid-predominant pseudocyst, surgical drainage with laparoscopic cystogastrostomy is preferred (Figure 5). This can also be performed with the traditional open technique. Cystojejunostomy (laparoscopic or open) is used in cases in which the site of the pseudocyst precludes drainage into the posterior aspect of the stomach.

Chronic Pancreatitis
Chronic pancreatitis is a chronic fibro-inflammatory disease of the pancreas characterized by irreversible morphologic changes that typically are associated with pain or permanent loss of function, or both.

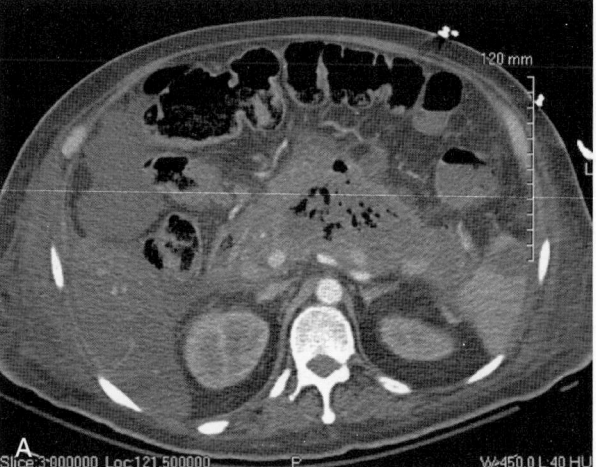

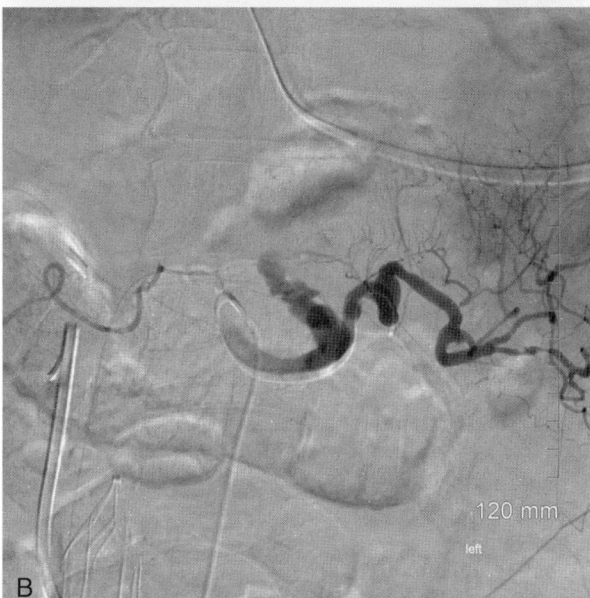

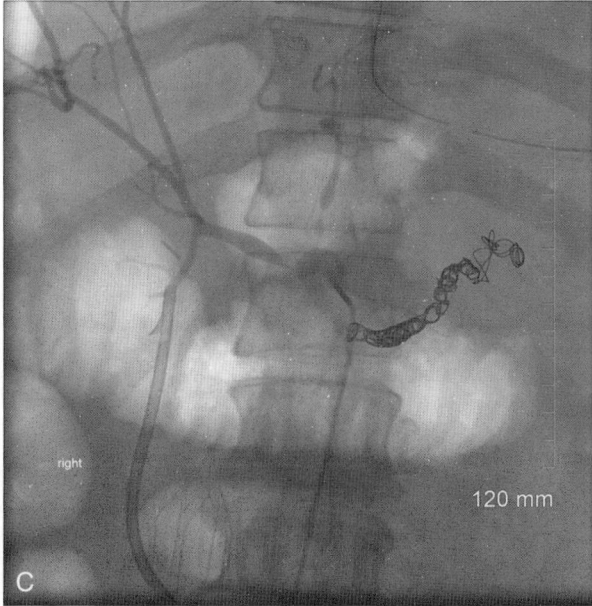

Figure 4 Acute necrotizing pancreatitis. (A) Erosion into the splenic artery as seen on computed tomography. (B) Erosion into the splenic artery as seen on angiogram. (C) This complication of acute pancreatitis is best treated with angiographic embolization.

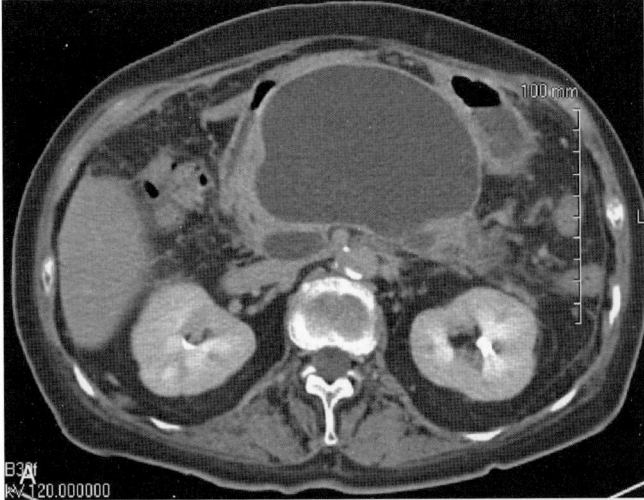

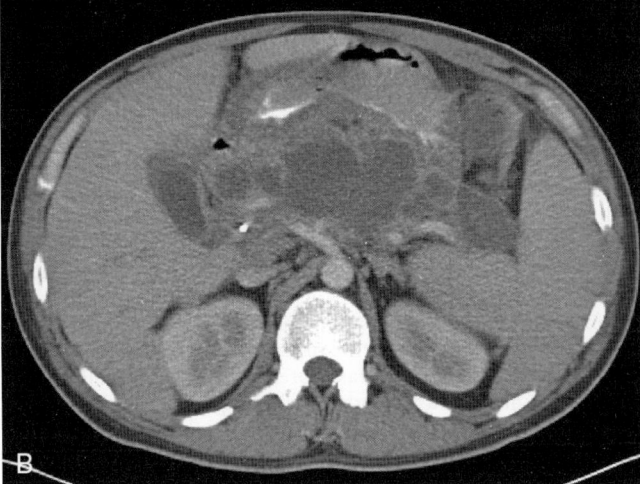

Figure 5 Computed tomographic scan showing fluid-predominant (A) and solid-predominant (B) pseudocysts. The former can be treated with endoscopic cystogastrostomy, and the latter is best treated with laparoscopic cystogastrostomy.

Epidemiology

Population studies suggest a prevalence of chronic pancreatitis that ranges from 5 to 27 persons per 100,000 population, with considerable geographic variation. Autopsy data are difficult to interpret because a number of changes associated with chronic pancreatitis, such as fibrosis, duct ectasia, and acinar atrophy, are also present in asymptomatic elderly patients. Differences in diagnostic criteria, regional nutrition, alcohol consumption, and medical access account for variations in the frequency of the diagnosis, but the overall incidence of the disease has risen progressively since the 1960s. Chronic pancreatitis in the United States currently results in more than 120,000 outpatient visits and more than 50,000 hospitalizations per year.

Risk Factors

Alcohol consumption and alcohol abuse are associated with chronic pancreatitis in up to 70% of cases. Other major causes include tropical (nutritional) and idiopathic disease, as well as hereditary causes. There is a linear relationship between exposure to alcohol and the development of chronic pancreatitis. The incidence is highest in heavy drinkers (15 drinks/day or 150 g/d). Prolonged alcohol use (four to five drinks daily over a period of more than 5 years) is required for alcohol-associated pancreatitis; the overall lifetime risk of pancreatitis among heavy drinkers is 2% to 5%. The duration of alcohol consumption is definitely associated with the development of pancreatic disease. The onset of disease typically occurs between ages 35 and 40 years, after 16

to 20 years of heavy alcohol consumption. Recurrent episodes of acute pancreatitis are typically followed by chronic symptoms after 4 or 5 years. In most cases, chronic pancreatitis has already developed and the acute clinical presentation represents a flare superimposed on chronic pancreatitis.

Tobacco use has also been heavily linked to pancreatitis. Meta-analysis has shown that both ever and current smokers had higher risks of developing pancreatitis compared with never smokers. This causative relationship was verified by the reduced or eliminated risk after smoking cessation. In comparison with current smokers, the risk of pancreatitis decreased for those who were former smokers.

Pathophysiology

Multiple episodes (or a prolonged course) of pancreatic injury ultimately leading to chronic disease is widely accepted as the pathophysiologic sequence. Abundant data indicate that acute pancreatitis may progress to recurrent acute pancreatitis and then to chronic pancreatitis in a disease continuum. Most investigators believe that alcohol metabolites such as acetaldehyde, combined with oxidant injury, result in local parenchymal injury that is preferentially targeted to the pancreas in predisposed persons. Repeated or severe episodes of toxin-induced injury activate a cascade of cytokines, which in turn induces pancreatic stellate cells to produce collagen and cause fibrosis.

The most common form of chronic pancreatitis is the calcifying type, characterized by the development of intraductal stones; the predominant causative agent is alcohol. Progressive functional impairment can develop from the dilated main pancreatic duct. Furthermore inflammatory enlargement of the pancreatic head may cause local complications such as stenosis of the pancreatic or bile duct, duodenal obstruction, or compression of retropancreatic vessels.

The pain caused by chronic pancreatitis is thought to be due to increased pressure in the pancreatic ducts and tissue, "parenchymal hypertension" from pancreatic ductal obstruction. Neural and perineural inflammation is also thought to be important in pathogenesis of pain in chronic pancreatitis. Neuropeptides released from enteric and afferent neurons and their functional interactions with inflammatory cells might play a key role.

Prevention

Because alcohol is the cause of most cases of chronic pancreatitis, cessation of alcohol consumption is recommended to prevent progression to chronic pancreatitis. Unfortunately, the majority of patients are not able to recover from alcoholism, and relapse is common.

Clinical Manifestations

Symptoms of chronic pancreatitis may be identical to those of acute pancreatitis, typically midepigastric pain penetrating through to the back. Patients with chronic pancreatic pain typically flex their abdomen and either sit or lie with their hips flexed, or lie on their side in a fetal position. Unlike ureteral stone pain or biliary colic, the pain causes the patient to be still. Nausea or vomiting can accompany the pain, but anorexia is the most common associated symptom. Patients with continuous pain can have a complication of chronic pancreatitis, such as an inflammatory mass, a cyst, or even pancreatic cancer. Other patients have intermittent attacks of pain with symptoms similar to those of mild to moderate acute pancreatitis. The pain sometimes is severe and lasts for many hours or several days.

As chronic pancreatitis progresses, endocrine and exocrine insufficiency begin to appear. Patients describe a bulky, foul-smelling, loose (but not watery) stool that may be pale and float on the surface of toilet water. Patients often describe a greasy or oily appearance to the stool or describe an "oil slick" on the water's surface. In severe steatorrhea, an orange, oily stool is often reported. As exocrine deficiency increases, symptoms of steatorrhea are often accompanied by weight loss. Patients might describe a good appetite despite weight loss, or they might have

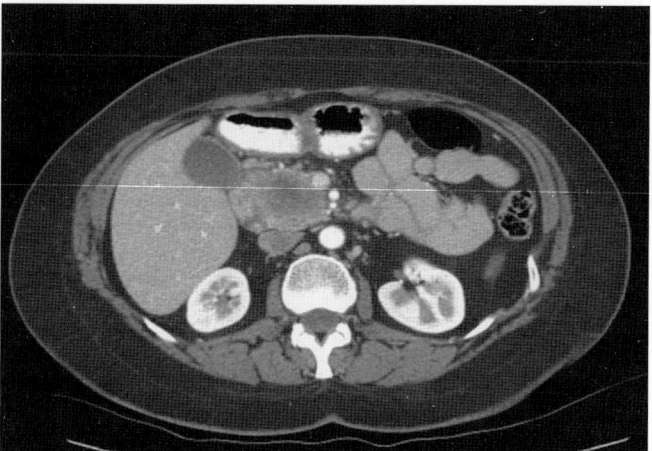

Figure 6 Computed tomographic scan of a patient with autoimmune pancreatitis and an inflammatory mass in the head of the pancreas. Preoperative diagnosis is not always possible, but surgery should be avoided because this disease often responds to steroid therapy.

diminished food intake due to abdominal pain. The combination of decreased food intake and malabsorption of nutrients usually results in chronic weight loss. As a result, many patients with severe chronic pancreatitis are below ideal body weight. Usually islet cells are spared early in the disease process despite being surrounded by fibrosis, but eventually the insulin-secreting beta cells are also destroyed, gradually leading to diabetes.

Diagnosis

The diagnosis of chronic pancreatitis depends on the clinical presentation, a limited number of indirect measurements that correlate with pancreatic function, and selected imaging studies. Diagnosis is usually simple in the late stages of the disease because of the presence of structural and functional alterations of the pancreas. Early in the disease, the diagnosis is more difficult. Various classification systems have been developed. The Cambridge classification uses imaging tests such as ERCP, CT, and ultrasound to grade severity. The Mayo Clinic system is based on functional as well as imaging results. Tests of pancreatic function include the secretin-cerulein test, Lundh test, fecal excretion of pancreatic enzymes, and quantitation of fecal fat.

Chronic pancreatitis can be classified as calcifying (lithogenic), obstructive, inflammatory, autoimmune, tropical (nutritional), hereditary, or idiopathic. Autoimmune and hereditary pancreatitis have recently been better understood and diagnosed more than before. Autoimmune pancreatitis is associated with fibrosis, a mononuclear cell (lymphocyte, plasma cell, or eosinophil) infiltrate, and an increased titer of one or more autoantibodies. It is usually associated with autoimmune diseases such as Sjögren syndrome. Increased levels of serum β-globulin or immunoglobulin (Ig)G_4 are often present, however autoimmune pancreatitis can present without these markers. This disease can be mistaken for chronic pancreatitis, with an inflammatory mass in the head of the pancreas suspicious for pancreatic cancer (Figure 6). Diagnosis is important because steroid therapy is uniformly successful in ameliorating the disease, including any associated bile duct compression.

Hereditary pancreatitis first occurs in adolescence with abdominal pain; patients develop progressive pancreatic dysfunction, and the risk of cancer is greatly increased. The disease follows an autosomal dominant pattern of inheritance with 80% penetrance and variable expression. Recent mutational analysis has revealed a missense mutation resulting in an Arg to His substitution at position 117 of the cationic trypsinogen gene, or *PRSS1*, one of the primary sites for proteolysis of trypsin. This mutation prevents trypsin from being inactivated by itself or other proteases, and it results in persistent and uncontrolled proteolytic activity and autodestruction within the pancreas. Similarly, *PSTI*, also known as *SPINK1*, has been found to have a role in hereditary pancreatitis and some cases of sporadic chronic pancreatitis. *SPINK1* specifically inhibits trypsin action by competitively blocking the active site of the enzyme.

It is likely that many of the "idiopathic" forms of chronic pancreatitis, as well as some patients with the more common forms of the disease, will be found to have a genetic linkage or predisposition.

Differential Diagnosis

There are several clinical conditions from which chronic pancreatitis needs to be distinguished. Other causes of upper abdominal pain, such as peptic ulcer disease, biliary tract disease, mesenteric vascular disease, or malignancy must be excluded. The major difficulty in the differential diagnosis of chronic pancreatitis is distinguishing it from pancreatic ductal adenocarcinoma. Chronic pancreatitis can closely mimic pancreatic cancer, both clinically and morphologically. In addition, chronic pancreatitis is a risk factor for the development of pancreatic cancer. Although in pancreatic resection specimens this problem may be finally resolved, distinguishing these two diseases preoperatively in small (needle) biopsy specimens is a formidable challenge for the pathologist. Therefore especially in the setting of an inflammatory mass in the head of the pancreas, consideration of pancreatic cancer and surgical referral is important. Workup of these patients should include a pancreatic protocol CT scan, an MRCP, and an endoscopic ultrasound to evaluate the parenchyma and the ducts of the pancreas.

Treatment

Therapy for chronic pancreatitis is aimed at managing associated digestive dysfunction and relieving pain (Box 4). It is important to first address malabsorption, weight loss, and diabetes. When pancreatic exocrine capacity falls below 10% of normal, diarrhea and steatorrhea develop. Lipase deficiency tends to manifest itself before trypsin deficiency, so the presence of steatorrhea may be the first functional sign of pancreatic insufficiency. As pancreatic exocrine function deteriorates further, the secretion of bicarbonate into the duodenum is reduced, which causes duodenal acidification and further impairs nutrient absorption. Frank diabetes is seen initially in about 20% of patients with chronic pancreatitis, and impaired glucose metabolism can be detected in up to 70% of patients.

The medical treatment of chronic or recurrent pain in chronic pancreatitis requires the use of analgesics, a cessation of alcohol use, oral enzyme therapy, and endoscopic stent therapy. Administration of pancreatic enzyme (e.g., Pancrease MT, Pancrelipase, Creon) serves to reverse the effects of pancreatic exocrine insufficiency and might also reduce or alleviate the pain[1] experienced by patients. Interventional procedures to block visceral afferent nerve conduction or to treat obstructions of the main pancreatic duct are also an adjunct to medical treatment. It has been taught that the pain of chronic pancreatitis decreases with increasing duration of the disease, the so-called burn-out phase, where endocrine and exocrine insufficiency occurs and the pain decreases.

---

[1]Not FDA approved for this indication

BOX 4 | Treatment of Chronic Pancreatitis

Pancreatic enzyme replacement
Proper nutrition and vitamin supplementation
Blood sugar control
Long-acting narcotic analgesics at lowest effective doses
Cessation of alcohol and tobacco
Endotherapy (pancreatic duct stenting and removal of stones)
Parenchymal preserving surgery (Frey, Beger) in carefully
    selected patients

However, recent studies have called this concept into question, demonstrating continued pain in patients with chronic pancreatitis despite long-standing disease and pancreatic insufficiency. Cessation of alcohol abuse, if possible, causes the pain to stop in about half of the patients.

Pain relief usually requires the use of narcotics, but these should be titrated to achieve pain relief with the lowest effective dose. Opioid addiction is common, and the use of long-acting analgesics by transdermal patch together with oral agents for pain exacerbations slightly reduces the sedative effects of high-dose oral narcotics. Celiac plexus neurolysis has been an effective form of analgesic treatment in patients with pancreatic carcinoma. However, its use in chronic pancreatitis has been disappointing, with about half of the patients deriving a benefit that lasts 6 months or less.

Pancreatic duct stenting is used for treatment of proximal pancreatic duct stenosis, decompression of a pancreatic duct leak, and drainage of pancreatic pseudocysts that can be catheterized through the main pancreatic duct. Pancreatic duct stones can also be removed endoscopically. Stent therapy in chronic pancreatitis definitely plays a role and can help select patients for successful operative therapy. However, the duration of success with stent therapy for chronic pancreatitis is probably less than with surgical therapy.

There has been significant debate over the years regarding the role and type of surgical therapy in chronic pancreatitis. Progressive functional pancreatic impairment can be delayed by surgical decompression of the dilated main pancreatic duct. Furthermore, inflammatory enlargement of the pancreatic head may cause local complications that require further treatment, such as stenosis of the pancreatic or bile duct, duodenal obstruction, or compression of retropancreatic vessels. Surgery may be superior to conservative or endoscopic treatment in terms of pain relief and preservation of pancreatic function and quality of life. Major pancreatic resections for chronic pancreatitis have a significant complication rate, both early and late. Patients with large duct disease who can have nutrition restored, are working, are not drinking alcohol, and have a supportive family structure fare better with surgical therapies. Failure to carefully select patients for either drainage or resection procedures leads to disappointing results. The surgical management of pancreatic duct stones and stenosis has been shown to be superior to endoscopic treatment in randomized clinical trials. Beger introduced the duodenum-preserving pancreatic head resection (DPPHR) in the early 1980s. Later in the decade, Frey and Smith described the local resection of the pancreatic head with longitudinal pancreaticojejunostomy, which included excavation of the pancreatic head including the ductal structures in continuity with a long ductotomy of the dorsal duct. This operation is basically a hybrid of the Beger and Puestow (Partington-Rochelle modification) procedures and is more popular in the United States (Figures 7 and 8).

Previous randomized prospective studies have compared the Whipple, Beger, and Frey procedures for chronic pancreatitis. Patients who had a Beger procedure had a shorter hospital stay, greater weight gain, less postoperative diabetes, and less exocrine dysfunction than standard Whipple patients over a 3- to 5-year follow-up. Pain control was similar between the two procedures. In a study comparing the pylorus-preserving Whipple to the Frey procedure, there was a lower postoperative complication rate associated with the Frey procedure (19%) compared to the pylorus-preserving Whipple group (53%), and the global quality-of-life scores were better (71% vs. 43%, respectively). Both operations were equally effective in controlling pain over a 2-year follow-up. Operation times, intraoperative blood loss, and transfusion requirements have been shown to be decreased with the Frey and Beger procedures compared to the Whipple procedure. In long-term (>8 years) follow-up, there was no difference between the Beger and Frey procedures in pain relief, pancreatic insufficiency, quality of life, and late mortality. Compared to the Whipple procedure, the Beger and Frey procedures may produce a lower incidence of immediate complications and diabetes but no significant differences in pain relief. Although

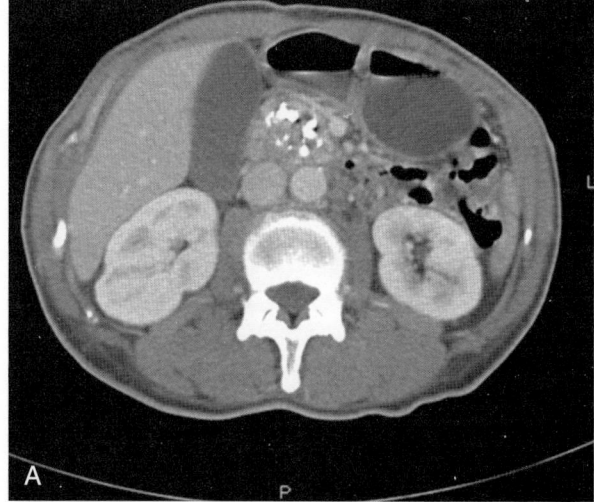

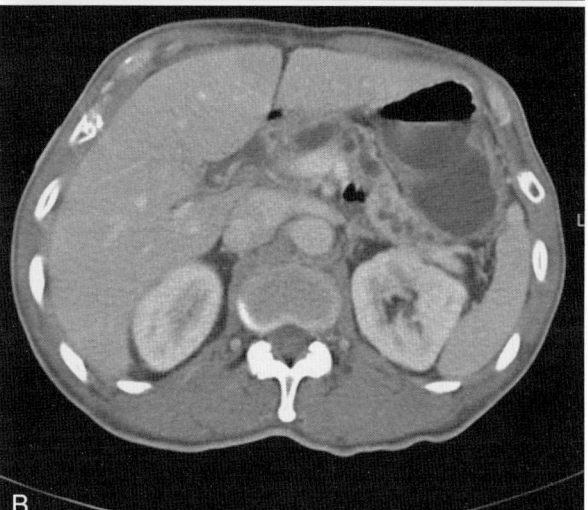

Figure 7 Computed tomographic scan of a patient with chronic calcific pancreatitis and a massively dilated pancreatic duct. (A) Axial view with calcified pancreatic head. (B) Axial view with dilated pancreatic duct.

these limited pancreatic procedures have a lower initial rate of endocrine dysfunction, the long-term risk of diabetes is more related to the progression of the underlying disease than to the effects of operation.

Recent multicenter randomized, controlled, double-blinded, trial compared DPPHR to partial pancreatoduodenectomy with a primary endpoint of quality of life within 24 months after surgery. The results showed that DPPHR was not superior to partial pancreatoduodenectomy in terms of the primary endpoint, long-term postoperative quality of life. With both resection and drainage procedures offering viable options for treatment, patient selection becomes critical in assuring there is clinical improvement postoperatively.

Recent refinements in the methods of harvesting and preserving pancreatic islets, and standardization of the methods by which islets are infused into the portal venous circuit for intrahepatic engraftment, have improved the success and rekindled interest in islet autotransplantation for chronic pancreatitis. The ability to recover a sufficient quantity of islets from a sclerotic gland depends on the degree of disease present, so the selection of patients as candidates for autologous islet transplantation is important. As success with autotransplantation increases, patients with nonobstructive, sclerotic pancreatitis may be considered for resection and islet autotransplantation earlier in their course, because end-stage fibrosis bodes poorly for transplant success. Patient selection and surgeon experience play a very large role in the outcomes of autotransplantation.

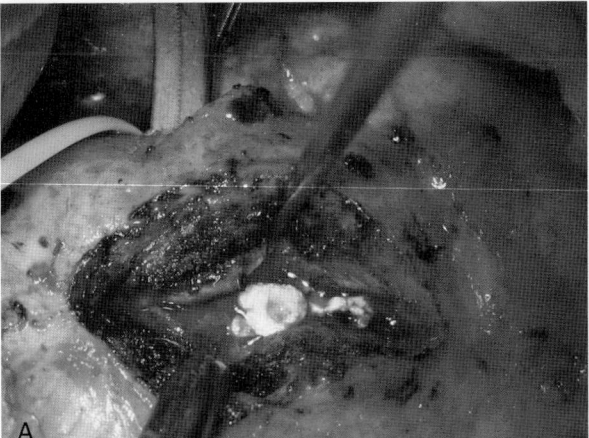

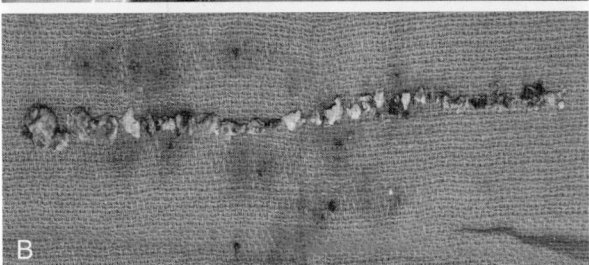

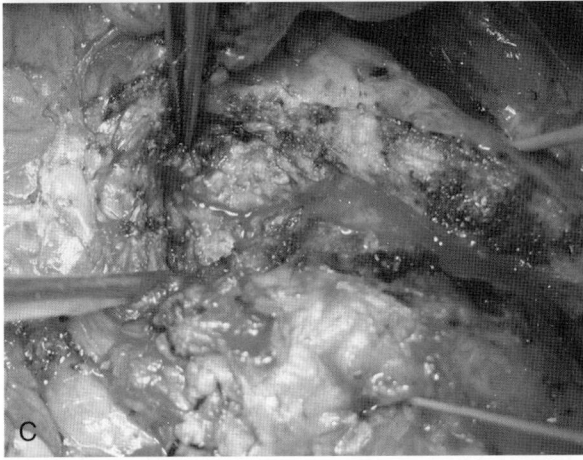

Figure 8 (A) The pancreatic duct is opened to reveal a preoperatively placed pancreatic duct stent. (B) The residual stones removed from the pancreatic duct. (C) In the Frey procedure, the head of the pancreas is cored out in addition to a longitudinal pancreatic ductotomy. The pancreas is drained with a Roux-en-Y limb of jejunum.

Monitoring

Chronic pancreatitis is of course a chronic disease, so continued monitoring and maintenance therapy is essential after an acute exacerbation of chronic pancreatitis. Pain control, proper nutrition, and alcohol and smoking cessation must be maintained as an outpatient. The clinician must also be looking for the development of common complications. An annual physical exam and CT or MRI should be considered in this population to assess for the progression of disease.

Complications

Pseudocysts in the setting of chronic pancreatitis are less likely to resolve without intervention. Often, the pancreatic duct and bile duct are compressed, and the compression might need to be addressed at the same time as the pseudocyst. A trend toward minimally invasive management remains appropriate, with endoscopic drainage preferred over laparoscopic cystogastrostomy unless additional procedures are required. Resection of a pseudocyst is sometimes indicated for cysts located in the pancreatic tail, or when a midpancreatic duct disruption has resulted in a distally located pseudocyst. Distal pancreatectomy for removal of a pseudocyst, with or without splenectomy, can be a challenging procedure in the setting of prior pancreatitis. An internal drainage procedure of the communicating duct, or of the pseudocyst itself, should be considered when distal resection is being contemplated.

Pancreatic ascites results from a disrupted pancreatic duct with extravasation of pancreatic fluid that does not become sequestered as a pseudocyst but drains freely into the peritoneal cavity. Occasionally, the pancreatic fluid tracks superiorly into the thorax, causing a pancreatic pleural effusion. Both complications are seen more often in patients with chronic pancreatitis, rather than after acute pancreatitis. Paracentesis or thoracentesis reveals noninfected fluid with a protein level greater than 25 g/L and a markedly elevated amylase level. Paracentesis is critical to differentiate pancreatic from hepatic ascites.

ERCP is most helpful to delineate the location of the pancreatic duct leak and to elucidate the underlying pancreatic ductal anatomy. Pancreatic duct stenting may be considered at the time of ERCP. Paracentesis and antisecretory therapy with the somatostatin analogue octreotide acetate, together with bowel rest and parenteral nutrition, is successful in more than half of patients. Reapposition of serosal surfaces to facilitate closure of the leak is considered a part of therapy, and this is accomplished by complete paracentesis. For pleural effusions, a period of chest tube drainage can facilitate closure of the internal fistula. Surgical therapy is reserved for those who fail to respond to medical treatment.

References

Acute Pancreatitis Classification Working Group: Revision of the Atlanta Classification of Acute Pancreatitis. Available at: http://www.pancreasclub.com/resources/AtlantaClassification.pdf. [accessed 25.08.14].

Beger HG, Matsuno S, Cameron JL: *Diseases of the pancreas: Current surgical therapy*, Berlin, 2008, Springer-Verlag.

Beger HG, Warshaw AL, Buchler MW, et al: *The pancreas: An integrated textbook of basic science, medicine, and surgery*, ed 2nd, Malden, MA, 2008, Blackwell Publishing.

Cunha EF, Rocha Mde S, Pereira FP, et al: Walled-off pancreatic necrosis and other current concepts in the radiological assessment of acute pancreatitis, *Radiol Bras* 47(3):165–175, 2014.

Dellinger EP, Tellado JM, Soto NE, et al: Early antibiotic treatment for severe acute necrotizing pancreatitis: a randomized, double-blind, placebo-controlled study, *Ann Surg* 245:674–683, 2007.

Diener MK, Hüttner FJ, Kieser M, et al: Partial pancreatoduodenectomy versus duodenum-preserving pancreatic head resection in chronic pancreatitis: the multicentre, randomised, controlled, double-blind ChroPac trial, *Lancet* 390(10099):1027–1037, 2017 Sep 9. https://doi.org/10.1016/S0140-6736(17)31960-8.

Fisher WE, Anderson DK, Bell RH, et al: Pancreas. In Brunicardi FC, Andersen DK, Billiar TR, et al: *Schwartz's principles of surgery*, ed 9th, New York, 2010, McGraw-Hill, pp 1167–1243.

Forsmark CE, Vege SS, Wilcox CM: Acute Pancreatitis, *N Engl J Med* 375(20):1972–1981, 2016 Nov 17.

Impact of smoking on the risk of pancreatitis: a systematic review and meta-analysis.

Isenmann R, Runzi M, Kron M, et al: Prophylactic antibiotic treatment in patients with predicted severe acute pancreatitis: a placebo-controlled, double-blind trial, *Gastroenterology* 126:997–1004, 2004.

Working Group IAP/APA Acute Pancreatitis Guidelines: IAP/**APA** evidence-based **guidelines** for the management of acute **pancreatitis**, *Pancreatology* 13(4 Suppl 2):e1–15, 2013 Jul-Aug. https://doi.org/10.1016/j.pan.2013.07.063.

Ye X, Lu G, Huai J, Ding J: *PLoS One* 10(4):e0124075, 2015 Apr 16, https://doi.org/10.1371/journal.pone.0124075. eCollection 2015.

Zaheer A, Singh VK, Qureshi RO, Fishman EK: The revised Atlanta classification for acute pancreatitis: updates in imaging terminology and guidelines, *Abdom Imaging* 38(1):125–136, 2013.

ACUTE DIARRHEA

Method of
Tate de Leon, MD

CURRENT DIAGNOSIS

History
- Onset, duration, and frequency of diarrhea
- Related symptoms (fever, abdominal pain, nausea, emesis, bloody stool)
- Current medications, including recent antibiotic use
- Recent sick contacts or hospitalizations
- Recent foreign travel
- Exposure to contaminated water source or undercooked meats and seafood
- Immune status

Physical Examination
- Hydration status
- Abdominal examination

Laboratory Testing
- Acute secretory diarrhea: normally not necessary
- Acute bloody diarrhea: complete blood count, stool culture, consider ova and parasite testing and *Clostridium difficile* evaluation

CURRENT THERAPY

- Symptomatic therapy
- Rehydration: enteral versus parenteral
- Antibiotics (depending on duration, severity, and other risk factors)
  - Emperic therapy
    - Adults
      - Fluoroquinolones
        - Ciprofloxacin (Cipro) 500 mg PO twice daily for 3–7 days
        - Levofloxacin (Levaquin)[1] 500 mg PO four times daily for 3–5 days
    - Children
      - Azithromycin (Zithromax)[1] 5–12 mg/kg PO four times daily for 3–5 days
  - *C difficile*
    - Metronidazole (Flagyl)[1] 500 mg PO every 8 hours for 10–14 days
    - Vancomycin (Vancocin) 125 mg PO every 6 hours for 10 days
- Antidiarrheal medications (if no contraindications such as fever or hematochezia)
  - Loperamide (Imodium) Initial 4 mg PO followed by 2 mg PO with each loose stool. Max 16 mg per day
- Probiotics[2]

[1]Not FDA approved for this indication.
[2]Not available in the United States.

Acute diarrhea in the United States is one of the most common diagnoses in general practice. Acute diarrhea can have a functional definition of a greater number of loose stools from normal lasting less than 14 days. If the episode lasts more than 14 days, it is called persistent diarrhea. If the episode lasts for more than 30 days, it is deemed chronic diarrhea. These episodes may be accompanied by nausea, vomiting, abdominal cramping, other systemic symptoms, and malnutrition. The majority of acute diarrhea cases are self-limited and do not need medical intervention.

Most often, these cases are caused by infectious agents such as viruses, bacteria, or parasites. Infection is often spread through contaminated food or drinking water or from person-to-person. Pathogens that cause diarrhea are usually transmitted through a fecal–oral route. The main risk factor for this transmission is poor hand hygiene. Other risk factors include improper food preparation, inadequate food refrigeration, and exposure to contaminated water.

Thorough investigation of a patient with acute diarrhea should include a detailed history, physical examination, and laboratory testing when indicated (Boxes 1 and 2). Acute diarrhea can be classified into two subtypes: secretory diarrhea and inflammatory diarrhea. Determining the subtype of the diarrhea is useful for suggesting the etiology and therefore the management of the diarrhea.

Secretory diarrhea is an electrolyte absorption impairment that leads to profuse, watery diarrhea that contains little or no blood or leukocytes. These episodes can last from a few hours to days. The main concern is dehydration and weight loss if oral intake is not continued. Clinical signs of severe dehydration include lethargy or unconsciousness, dry or sunken eyes, dry mouth, decreased skin turgor, and a history of poor or absent fluid intake.

Inflammatory diarrhea is bloody, usually has leukocytes, and produces less volume. The most common causes are *Salmonella*, *Campylobacter*, *Shigella*, *Escherichia coli* O157:H7, and *Entamoeba hystolytica*. The main concerns related to inflammatory diarrhea are intestinal damage, sepsis, and malnutrition. Stool cultures and evaluation for ova and parasites are recommended.

Preventive measures can help reduce the spread of infectious agents. Proper hand hygiene with soap and water, especially after exposure to feces or individuals with acute diarrhea, can help

| BOX 1 | Clinical History of Acute Infectious Diarrhea |

- Description of diarrhea
  - Duration
  - Frequency
  - Presence of blood, pus, in stool
  - Symptoms of fever, tenesmus, dehydration
  - Weight loss
- Other gastrointestinal symptoms
  - Anorexia
  - Cramping
  - Emesis
  - Nausea
- Previous episodes with similar symptoms
- Recent antibiotic exposure
- Other medication exposure
  - Anticholinergics
  - Antimotility agents
  - Aspirin (ASA)
  - Proton pump inhibitors
- Recent dietary history
  - Shellfish
  - Undercooked meat (chicken)
  - Unsanitary water
  - Animal or reptile contacts
- Travel history
  - Travel to endemic or epidemic areas
- Sexual history
- Vaccination history
- Contact with institutions, e.g., hospitals, nursing homes, day care facilities
- Employment history
- Immune status
  - Presence of HIV
  - Presence of other congenital or acquired immunodeficiencies

BOX 2	Physical Examination for Acute Infectious Diarrhea

- Vital signs
- Blood pressure (look for postural changes)
- Heart rate (look for postural changes)
- Respiratory rate
- Temperature
- Weight changes (particularly useful to assess effects of rehydration)
- Cardiovascular examination
  - Volume status
- Respiratory examination
- Rule out hyperventilation (compensatory respiratory alkalosis for metabolic acidosis resulting from dehydration and loss of bicarbonate)
- Abdominal examination
- Focal tenderness
- Guarding
- Hepatosplenomegaly
- Consider rectal examination (look for bloody stool)
- Decreased skin turgor
- Lymphadenopathy
- Rashes

limit the spread of infection. Barrier precautions are an effective adjunct when dealing with the possibility of exposure to feces in a hospital setting. For children, vaccinations have been shown to be effective in reducing rotavirus infections. Furthermore, it is imperative to separate diaper-changing areas from food-preparation areas. Proper sanitization with a bleach-based cleaner is recommended. Proper food handling and storage, along with water purification, are important means to help prevent the spread of infectious agents. Probiotics[2] are finding a home in the prevention and treatment of diarrhea. Initial studies have suggested that probiotics are useful in reducing antibiotic-associated diarrhea. Currently, more studies are needed to confirm their usefulness. Prophylactic antibiotics are usually only reserved for possible exposure to traveler's diarrhea.

Epidemiology

Worldwide, acute diarrhea still accounts for significant morbidity and mortality. The very young, the very old, and the immunocompromised populations are the most adversely affected. Acute infectious diarrhea is more prevalent in developing countries and among travelers to developing countries. Diarrhea is the second leading cause of death worldwide in children under 5 years of age. The World Health Organization estimates that globally, there are over 1.7 billion cases of acute diarrhea each year and attributes 760,000 deaths to it annually. The majority of these deaths are in children who are younger than age 5 and live in developing countries. In the United States, foodborne infectious diarrhea accounts for approximately 325,000 hospitalizations and 5000 deaths each year.

Etiology and Treatment

The precise cause of acute diarrhea is usually not found. Causes can be both infectious and noninfectious. Noninfectious causes can include medications, food allergies, and other gastrointestinal diseases. In general, clinical investigation of acute infectious diarrhea is more useful in identifying consequences of diarrhea, such as dehydration, than it is in revealing the precise etiology. Most cases of diarrhea are likely viral, as indicated by negative stool culture results in most studies. Severe cases of diarrhea tend to be a result of bacterial infection. The most common pathogens for bacteria-induced diarrhea is discussed below. To date, the optimal strategy for obtaining stool cultures has not been ascertained. It is thus reasonable to treat the patient symptomatically

for several days before obtaining a stool culture for mild to moderate cases because most cases of diarrhea are self-limited. The clinician should take into consideration individual comorbidities, immune status, the presence of severe or bloody diarrhea, underlying inflammatory bowel disease, and occupation (food handlers, day care employment, etc.) as possible indications for stool evaluation.

Bacteria

Campylobacter

Campylobacter is a common cause of diarrhea in the United States. The pathogen is often spread by consumption of undercooked meat and poultry. Symptoms may present 2 to 5 days after exposure and last up to 1 week. The patient presents with diarrhea (possibly bloody), abdominal pain, nausea, vomiting, and fever. Stool cultures are needed for a definitive diagnosis. Prevention includes thoroughly cooking all meat products, good hand and utensil hygiene before preparing foods, and avoiding unpasteurized milk. The treatment for severe *Campylobacter* diarrhea includes azithromycin (Zithromax)[1] and ciprofloxacin (Cipro), although resistance to fluoroquinolones is growing. Antimicrobial susceptibility testing is required for specific resistance. Positive stool cultures should be reported to the local health department. *Campylobacter* infections have been linked to both rheumatoid arthritis and also Guillain-Barré syndrome.

Clostridium difficile

C difficile is the organism of antibiotic-associated colitis. Antibiotics disrupt the normal flora of the GI tract, which in turn provides a window of opportunity for *C difficile* to produce toxins and flourish. The most frequent antibiotics implicated are clindamycin (Cleocin), fluoroquinolones, and beta-lactam antibiotics. *C difficile* is treated with oral metronidazole[1] (Flagyl 500 mg PO every 8 hours for 10–14 days) and vancomycin (Vancocin 125 mg PO every 6 hours for 10 days). The diagnosis is confirmed with either polymerase chain reaction (PCR), enzyme immunoassay, or anaerobic culture. Endoscopy and biopsy can also be obtained if there is a high clinical suspicion for *C difficile* with negative laboratory results or if the patient did not respond to antibiotic treatment.

E coli

E coli are a large and versatile group of pathogens that can cause widespread disease and affect multiple organ systems. *E coli* is a part of the normal flora of both human and animal digestive tract. Certain *E coli* strains can cause acute diarrhea. Pathogenic strains include enterotoxigeneic *E coli* (ETEC), enteropathogenic *E coli*, enteroinvasive *E coli*, diffusely adherent *E coli*, and enterohemorrhagic *E coli* (EHEC may also be referred as Shiga toxin-producing *E coli* or verocytotoxin-producing *E coli*). The two most common and notorious strains are ETEC and EHEC. ETEC is a major cause of traveler's diarrhea and diarrhea in children of developing countries. EHEC has led to high-profile outbreaks of diarrhea as a result of contaminated meats.

ETEC is a type of *E coli* that produces toxins that stimulate the intestines to secrete excessive fluid, thus producing diarrhea. ETEC produces two different toxins: heat-stable toxin and heat-labile toxin. Both types of toxins produce similar illnesses. Contaminated food and water is the usual source of infection. Although stool culture is needed for definitive diagnosis, ETEC infections are usually diagnosed on history and clinical symptoms. Symptoms usually appear after 1 to 2 days after exposure and may last from 5 to 7 days. Most cases of ETEC diarrhea are treated symptomatically with adequate rehydration alone. Oral rehydration salts may be used and purchased over the counter to help address electrolyte losses. Both bismuth compounds (e.g., Pepto-Bismol) and antimotility agents (e.g. loperamide [Imodium]) can help reduce severity of symptoms; they both may prolong the time the body takes to clear the toxin. Antibiotics are reserved for moderate to severe disease. The most common effective antibiotics

---

[2]Not available in the United States.

[1]Not FDA approved for this indication.

include fluoroquinolones. Antibiotics can shorten the duration of symptoms but are usually not required.

EHEC is a strain of *E coli* that produces a Shiga toxin. The toxin acts on vascular endothelium of small vessels of multiple organ systems. The toxin causes the breakdown and hemorrhage of the endothelium. When the toxin affects the vascular endothelium of the digestive tract, it causes bloody diarrhea. The pathogen often invades the kidney and lungs. Sequelae of EHEC infection include hemorrhagic diarrhea, hemolytic uremic syndrome, and thrombotic thrombocytopenic purpura. *E coli* O157 is the most common strain of EHEC. The infection is spread via the oral–fecal route, which includes consumption of contaminated food, unpasteurized milk and cheeses, and unsanitary water. Good hand hygiene is imperative. Symptoms usually appear 3 to 4 days after exposure and may last as long as 10 days. Positive stool cultures should be reported to the local health department. Supportive treatment, including rehydration, is the cornerstone of treatment. Antibiotics are contraindicated because of evidence of increased Shiga toxin release and thus increased risk of hemolytic uremic syndrome.

Salmonella

Salmonella is the most common foodborne cause of diarrhea in the United States. It is associated with ingestion of infected poultry, eggs, and milk products. *Salmonella* can also be transmitted from pets, especially reptiles. Stool cultures are required for definitive diagnosis. Fluoroquinolones remain the antibiotic of choice, although sensitivities will guide antibiotic usage.

Shigella

Shigella is the pathogen that causes dysentery and is a major cause of morbidity in developing countries. Dysentery usually presents as high fever, abdominal cramping, and bloody diarrhea. Positive stool cultures usually warrant treatment with fluoroquinolones.

Vibrio

Vibrio cholera is endemic to developing countries. Symptoms usually present 1 to 3 days after exposure. Symptoms usually include profuse watery diarrhea (rice-water stools), abdominal cramping, and vomiting. Fever is infrequent. Rehydration with appropriate electrolyte replacement is paramount. Antibiotics can be an adjunct to rehydration and include fluoroquinolones and tetracycline at 500 mg PO every 8 hours for 3 days.

Yersinia

Yersinia enterocolitica infections are less common. Symptoms include diarrhea, fever, abdominal pain, and vomiting. Stool cultures are needed to confirm the diagnosis.

Viruses

Viral pathogens are likely responsible for the majority of gastroenteritis in the United States. Given the transient nature and characteristic symptoms, the specificity of the exact virus is not usually obtained. The most common viral etiologies tend to be adenovirus, rotavirus, norovirus, and astrovirus. Rotavirus tends to affect infants and children from 3 to 36 months of age, resulting in a spectrum of disease from asymptomatic shedding to severe gastroenteritis. Vaccination has played an important role in decreasing the cases of rotavirus infections.

Norovirus (i.e., Norwalk virus) is responsible for many high-profile outbreaks in daycare centers, cruise ships, and hospitals. Norovirus can be easily transmitted from person to person, from contact of contaminated surfaces, or from exposure to contaminated food or water. Symptoms present 1 to 3 days after exposure. Symptoms include fever, explosive vomiting, and diarrhea. PCR testing can confirm the diagnosis but is not usually necessary unless there seems to be an outbreak.

Parasite

Entamoeba histolytica, *Cryptosporidium*, *Giardia*, and *Cyclospora* spp. are the most common parasitic or protozoal infections that cause diarrhea. Protozoa infections are even less common. It is usually not cost-effective to evaluate for ova and parasites unless there are specific indications, such as a history of immunocompromise, exposure to daycare centers, or history of exposure to contaminated water. Multiple stool samples are needed if there are concerns of parasite infection resulting from possible intermittent shedding. *E histolytica* can cause amoebic dysentery and lead to bloody diarrhea. Microscopy, antigen testing, and serology are all possible tests for diagnosis. Parasitic infections are usually treated with metronidazole (Flagyl), tinidazole (Tindamax 2g PO four times daily for 1–3 days) or albendazole[1] (Albenza 400 mg PO four times daily for 5 days).

Traveler's Diarrhea

Traveler's diarrhea is common to individuals from developed countries traveling to developing countries. Episodes can be caused by bacteria, viruses, and parasites. The most common pathogen is *E coli* (ETEC). Travelers should choose their food and water sources carefully. Water purification and avoiding foods prepared with contaminated water is useful. Prolonged or other symptoms such as fever or bloody stool should be further investigated.

Treatment

Fluid and electrolyte replacement are the most important therapies for acute diarrhea. The route of administration depends on the severity of the dehydration. For mild cases of diarrhea in a normally healthy individual, adequate oral intake of juices, soups, and electrolyte-infused water can be sufficient. For severe dehydration, IV fluids or oral rehydration therapy with isotonic electrolyte solutions may be needed. Oral hydration is preferred over IV fluids if possible. IV fluids are more expensive and less practical than oral rehydration. The World Health Organization has a lower-osmolarity oral rehydration solution (ORS), which is very effective in reducing stool volume and the need for switching to IV therapy in children. A number of effective ORSs are also available over the counter, including Pedialyte and Rehydralyte. IV fluids, including normal saline and lactated Ringers solution, are indicated in severe dehydration or in patients who cannot tolerate oral fluid intake.

Antimicrobial agents have a secondary role in treatment of acute diarrhea. Given the fact that most cases of diarrhea are mild, self-limited, and caused by nonbacterial pathogens, antibiotics should be used sparingly. Antibiotic treatment should be used in invasive bacterial infections, traveler's diarrhea, or in patients with immunosuppression. Empirical antibiotics can be appropriate as described above for *Campylobacter* or *C difficile* infections.

Antidiarrheal medications can be useful to help alleviate symptoms in patients with no other contraindications, such as fever or bloody diarrhea. Loperamide (Imodium initial 4 mg PO followed by 2 mg PO with each loose stool, maximum 16 mg per day) decreases intestinal peristalsis and facilitates intestinal absorption. Bismuth (Pepto-Bismol) is less effective. Bismuth produces both antisecretory and antimicrobial effects in the gastrointestinal tract.

---

[1]Not FDA approved for this indication.

References

Centers for Disease Control and Prevention: Division of Foodborne, Waterborne, and Environmental Diseases (DFWED). Available at: http://www.cdc.gov/ncezid/dfwed/a-z.html. Updated April 2013.

Fontaine O, Griffin P, Henao O, et al: Diarrhea, Acute. In Heymann DL, editor: *Control of Communicable Diseases Manual*, ed 19th, Washington, DC, 2008, American Public Health Association, pp 179–194.

Guerrant RL, Van Gilder T, Steiner TS, et al: Practice guidelines for the management of infectious diarrhea, *Clin Infect Dis* 32:331–351, 2001.

Singh SK: Diarrhea. In Andreoli TE, Benjamin IJ, Griggs RC, Wing EJ, editors: *Cecil Essentials of Medicine*, ed 8th, Philadelphia, PA, 2010, Saunders, pp 396–400.

Theilman NM, Guerrant RL: Clinical practice. Acute infectious diarrhea, *N Engl J Med* 350:38–47, 2004.

World Health Organization: Diarrheal disease. Available at: http://www.who.int/mediacentre/factsheets/fs330/en/ Updated May 2017.

BLEEDING ESOPHAGEAL VARICES

Method of
Cecilio M. Azar, MD; and Ala I. Sharara, MD

CURRENT DIAGNOSIS

- Endoscopic screening for esophageal varices is recommended in patients with liver cirrhosis.
- Noninvasive predictors of the presence of large varices, such as splenomegaly and thrombocytopenia, have limited accuracy.
- A combination of clinical and endoscopic findings including the Child-Pugh class, size of varices, and the presence of red wale markings correlates with the risk of first bleeding in patients with cirrhosis.
- Measurement of hepatic venous pressure gradient may be the best indicator of risk and severity of bleeding in patients with varices. It is an invasive test and is not widely available or used routinely in practice.

CURRENT THERAPY

- Nonselective β-blockers and endoscopic band ligation are both effective first-line therapy in the primary prophylaxis of esophageal varices.
- The management of acute variceal hemorrhage consists of prompt resuscitation and correction of coagulation abnormalities, followed by endoscopic and pharmacologic therapy with vasoactive agents. Antibiotic prophylaxis is given to decrease the risk of infection and of rebleeding. Transjugular intrahepatic portosystemic shunt (TIPS) is reserved for refractory, uncontrolled, acute variceal bleeding.
- Strategies for secondary prophylaxis of variceal bleeding include endoscopic band ligation, pharmacologic therapy with nonselective β-blockers with or without nitrates, TIPS, and surgical shunts.
- Comparative cost-effectiveness of secondary prophylaxis strategies is unknown but should take into consideration the cost of failed therapy (e.g., rebleeding, shunt revision) and that of treatment related-complications (e.g., encephalopathy, esophageal stricture).

Epidemiology

Bleeding of esophageal varices is a major complication of portal hypertension, usually in the setting of liver cirrhosis, accounting for 10% to 30% of all cases of upper gastrointestinal hemorrhage. More than any other cause of gastrointestinal bleeding, this complication results in considerable morbidity and mortality, prolonged hospitalization, and increased affiliated costs. Variceal bleeding develops in 25% to 35% of patients with cirrhosis and accounts for up to 90% of upper gastrointestinal bleeding episodes in these patients. About 10% to 30% of these episodes are fatal, and as many as 70% of survivors rebleed following an index variceal hemorrhage. Following such events, the 1-year survival is 34% to 80%, being inversely related to the severity of the underlying liver disease.

Treatment of patients with esophageal varices includes preventing the initial bleeding episode (primary prophylaxis), controlling active variceal hemorrhage, and preventing recurrent bleeding after a first episode (secondary prophylaxis). Data on the optimal management of gastric varices are much more limited, and this topic is not covered in this article.

Pathophysiology

Chronic liver disease leading to cirrhosis is the most common cause of portal hypertension. The level of increased resistance to flow varies with the level of circulatory breach and can be divided into prehepatic, hepatic or sinusoidal, and posthepatic. In cirrhosis, several organ systems are involved in the pathophysiology of portal hypertension. At the splanchnic vascular bed level there is marked vasodilatation and increase in angiogenesis, leading to increase in portal blood flow and formation of collateral circulation, such as gastroesophageal varices, along with decrease in response to vasoconstrictors. At the systemic circulation level, there is an increase in cardiac output, decrease in vascular resistance, and hypervolemia. This hyperkinetic syndrome leads to an effective hypovolemia, with a resultant increase in vasoactive factors to maintain a normal arterial blood pressure.

Varices represent portosystemic collaterals derived from dilatation of preexisting embryonic vascular channels, such as those between the coronary and short gastric veins and the intercostal, esophageal, and azygous veins. In the distal esophagus, over an area extending 2 to 5 cm from the gastroesophageal junction, veins are found more superficially in the lamina propria rather than the submucosa. This results in reduced support from surrounding tissues owing to the predominant intraluminal location of these varices and might explain the predilection for bleeding at this site. The opening and dilation of portosystemic collaterals appears to depend on a threshold portal pressure gradient (measured as hepatic venous pressure gradient [HVPG]) of 12 mm Hg, below which varices do not form. This pressure gradient is necessary but not sufficient for the development of gastroesophageal varices.

Diagnosis

The current consensus states that every patient with liver cirrhosis should undergo an upper endoscopy to detect gastroesophageal varices. The main aim behind screening for gastroesophageal varices is to identify patients requiring prophylactic treatment or further surveillance. Esophageal varices are present in 52% of screened patients and are more prevalent in more advanced disease (43% for Child–Pugh class A versus 72% in Child–Pugh class B or C). On the other hand, gastric varices are present in up to 33% of patients with portal hypertension, with progression rates for both esophageal and gastric varices from small, medium, to large varices of 10% to 15% per year. Several invasive and noninvasive procedures help in detecting portal hypertension and can, with variable accuracy, predict the presence of gastroesophageal varices. Unfortunately, none are sensitive enough to replace endoscopy. A recent meta-analysis showed that transient elastography may be a useful screening tool for the detection of significant liver fibrosis and associated portal hypertension, but it is not useful at predicting the presence or size of esophageal varices. Smaller trials have evaluated the usefulness of spleen and liver MR elastography in assessing portal hypertension and varices, but this modality has not yet found its way into clinical practice. The combination of an elastography value below 20 kPa together and a platelet count above 150,000 nearly excludes the presence of esophageal varices requiring treatment. Endoscopic videocapsule is a new modality introduced for visualizing the esophagus; it allows correct identification of varices in 80% of cases but can have poor accuracy in identifying the presence of hypertensive gastropathy and gastric varices.

Not all esophageal varices bleed; hemorrhage occurs in only 30% to 35% of patients with cirrhosis. Variceal rupture is directly related to physical factors such as the radius, thickness, and elastic properties of the vessel in addition to intravariceal and intraluminal pressure and tension. Endoscopic findings that predict a higher risk of bleeding include larger size of varices and the presence of endoscopic red signs (described as red wale markings) on the variceal wall, indicating dilated intraepithelial and subepithelial superficial veins. A combination of clinical and endoscopic findings, including the Child-Pugh class, size of varices, and the presence or absence of red wale markings, was found to correlate highly with the risk of first bleeding in patients with cirrhosis. Hemodynamic parameters examined as predictors of bleeding include HVPG, azygous blood flow, and direct measurement of intravariceal pressure.

TABLE 1 | Summary of Therapy for Esophageal Varices

	FIRST-LINE THERAPY	COMMENTS	ALTERNATIVE THERAPY	COMMENTS
Primary prophylaxis*		In advanced cirrhosis, the best therapy is unclear (probably band ligation) Transplantation should be considered for these patients		The effectiveness of combined β-blockers and band ligation is unknown Neither TIPS nor sclerotherapy is recommended for primary prophylaxis
Active variceal bleeding	Somatostatin,[2] octreotide (Sandostatin),[1] vapreotide (Sanvar),[5] or terlipressin (Glypressin)[2]	Vasoconstrictors should be continued for ≥2 days after endoscopic therapy Band ligation is superior to endoscopic sclerotherapy	Balloon tamponade or SEMS (self-expandable metal stent) TIPS	Tamponade is indicated primarily as a temporizing measure if first-line treatment fails TIPS is reserved for refractory or recurrent early bleeding but should also be considered when basal HVPG >20 mm Hg
	plus Endoscopic therapy	Antibiotic prophylaxis should be initiated	Shunt surgery	Surgery is reserved for patients with compensated liver disease in whom TIPS fails or is not technically feasible
Secondary prophylaxis	β-Blockers ± nitrates *or* Band ligation	The combination of band ligation and β-blockers ± nitrates may be more effective than either alone Nitrates alone are not recommended Patients with advanced liver disease are often intolerant of β-blockers	TIPS Shunt surgery	TIPS is best used after failure of first-line therapy or as a bridge to transplantation in patients with advanced liver disease Shunt surgery is reserved for selected patients with compensated cirrhosis in whom TIPS fails or is not feasible

Abbreviations: HVPG = hepatic venous pressure gradient; TIPS = transjugular intrahepatic portosystemic shunt.
[1]Not FDA approved for this indication.
[2]Not available in the United States.
[5]Investigational drug in the United States.
*Upon documentation of varices, variceal hemorrhage occurs in 25%–30% of patients by 2 years. β-Blockers reduce the risk to 15%–18%, and combination β-blockers plus nitrates reduce the risk to 7.5%–10%.

HVPG, calculated by the gradient of wedged and free hepatic vein pressure (normal value, 5 mm Hg), is used most often and provides reliable measurement of portal pressure in patients with cirrhosis. The extent of elevation of HVPG may be the best indicator of risk of bleeding, severity of bleeding, and survival. A rise in pressure in a patient with known varices increases the risk of bleeding, and the extent of portal pressure elevation has an inverse relationship to prognosis after hemorrhage has occurred. In general, however, a linear relationship between the degree of portal hypertension and the risk of variceal hemorrhage or formation of varices does not exist, so this technique cannot be used routinely to identify individual patients at high risk for bleeding.

Treatment
Primary Prophylaxis
The natural evolution of gastroesophageal varices without treatment is characterized by an increase in size from small to large varices, which eventually rupture and bleed. The progression rate ranges from 5% to 30% per year. The incidence of bleeding from small esophageal varices is estimated to be 4% per year, and it is as high as 15% per year for medium to large varices. In a randomized, controlled trial, the nonselective β-blocker timolol (Blocadren)[1] failed to reduce the development of varices or variceal bleeding in patients without varices. Adverse events were more common in the timolol group. Therefore, it is not recommended to start β-blockers in patients who do not yet have esophageal varices.

Based on prospective studies of cirrhotic patients with varices identified at endoscopy and of untreated groups in randomized controlled trials, the risk of bleeding from esophageal varices has been estimated at 25% to 35% at 1 year. Therapy for primary prophylaxis against variceal bleeding (prevention of a first variceal bleeding) is summarized in Table 1.

Pharmacologic Therapy
The general objective of pharmacologic therapy for variceal bleeding is to reduce portal pressure and consequently intravariceal pressure. Drugs that reduce portocollateral venous flow (vasoconstrictors) or intrahepatic vascular resistance (vasodilators) have been used and include β-blockers, nitrates, β_2-adrenergic blockers, spironolactone (Aldactone),pentoxifylline (Trental),[1] molsidomine (Corvaton),[2] and simvastatin (Zocor).[1] Because varices do not bleed at an HVPG less than 12 mm Hg, reduction to this level is ideal, but substantial reductions in HVPG (i.e., by >20%) are also clinically meaningful.

β-Blockers exert their beneficial effect on portal venous pressure by diminishing splanchnic blood flow and consequently gastroesophageal collateral and azygous blood flow. The effectiveness of β-blockers for primary prophylaxis against variceal bleeding has been demonstrated in several controlled trials. Meta-analyses have revealed a 40% to 50% reduction in bleeding and a trend toward improved survival. The estimated overall response rate is 49%, with bleeding rates of 6% in responders and 32% in nonresponders, with a number needed to treat (NNT) of 10.

The nonselective β-blockers, such as propranolol (Inderal)[1] and nadolol (Corgard),[1] are preferred because of the dual benefit of β_1- and β_2-receptor blockade. In the absence of HVPG determination, β-blockers are titrated to achieve a reduction in resting heart rate to 55 beats/min or 25% of baseline. Propranolol is generally given

[1] Not FDA approved for this indication.

[1] Not FDA approved for this indication.
[2] Not available in the United States.

as a long-acting preparation and titrated to a maximum dose of 320 mg/day. Nadolol is initiated at 80 mg daily up to a maximum daily dose of 240 mg. Carvedilol (Coreg)[1] is initiated at 6.25 mg daily and increased if tolerated to 12.5 mg/day. Carvedilol is superior to propranolol at reducing portal hypertension although available data do not allow a satisfactory comparison of adverse events. The portal pressure–reducing effects of β-blockers are not predictable; the resultant reduction in heart rate or the measurement of drug blood levels are not good indicators of response to therapy. For example, portal venous pressure is reduced in about 60% to 70% of patients who receive propranolol therapy, but only 10% to 30% of these patients show a substantial response (i.e., >20% reduction). Additionally, approximately 20% to 25% of patients have no measurable decline in portal pressure despite increasing dosage of propranolol. Non-selective beta-blockers (NSBB) are effective in preventing first and recurrent variceal hemorrhage both in patients with and without ascites. NSBB-induced reduction in portal pressure is associated with lowering the progression of cirrhosis and even death.

Refractory ascites and spontaneous bacterial peritonitis (SBP) are not absolute contraindications to NSBB as previously thought. However, high-dose NSBB (with resultant decrease in mean arterial pressure) should be used with caution because it can be associated with deleterious outcomes. Hence, careful dosing is necessary in these patients with dose reduction/discontinuation for systolic blood pressure <90 mm Hg.

In addition to β-blockers, a number of vasodilators have been investigated in patients with portal hypertension and in animal models of portal hypertension, most notably isosorbide mononitrate (Imdur).[1] Of note, there is increasing evidence that the use of β-blockers can be deleterious in patients with decompensated liver cirrhosis, refractory ascites, and severe circulatory dysfunction (systolic blood pressure 90 mm Hg, serum sodium <30 meq/fL, or hepatorenal syndrome). The exact mechanism of action of nitrates is unclear but is thought to be mediated primarily by reducing intrahepatic resistance and possibly by splanchnic arterial vasoconstriction induced in response to venous pooling and vasodilation in other regional vascular beds. Monotherapy with nitrates is ineffective in primary prophylaxis and can have detrimental effects, particularly in cirrhotic patients with ascites, and should not be used.

The addition of isosorbide mononitrate to β-blockers, however, has been shown to result in an enhanced reduction in portal pressure in humans. In a randomized, controlled trial involving 42 patients with cirrhosis and esophageal varices, a reduction of greater than 20% in HVPG was documented in only 10% in the propranolol group compared to 50% in the combination therapy group. In patients with Child-Pugh class A and B cirrhosis, the addition of isosorbide mononitrate to nadolol has been shown, in a randomized trial, to result in a greater than 50% additional reduction in variceal bleeding rate when compared with nadolol monotherapy (12% versus 29%). However, a large subsequent double-blind, placebo-controlled study failed to confirm these results. Based on the existing evidence, the combination of β-blockers and isosorbide is not recommended in primary prophylaxis.

Endoscopic Therapy

Endoscopic therapies play a prominent role in treatment of esophageal varices. Endoscopic band ligation (EBL) is the endoscopic procedure of choice in the management of esophageal varices. As of 2010, 16 randomized, controlled trials have compared EBL to β-blockers in the primary prevention of variceal bleeding. These studies suffered from significant heterogeneity, and a large number were published in abstract form. Two meta-analyses of these trials showed a slight advantage of EBL over β-blockers in terms of primary prevention of variceal bleeding, but there were no differences in mortality. A recent Cochrane database systematic review found a beneficial effect of band ligation compared to β-blockers in primary prevention of upper gastrointestinal bleeding in adult patients with esophageal varices. Again, there was no difference in mortality.

β-Blockers are cheaper and much easier to administer but are associated with issues of noncompliance and a higher incidence of adverse events (e.g., hypotension, impotence, insomnia) than EBL. However, most of these side effects are easy to manage and none require hospitalization or result in direct mortality. On the other hand, adverse events related to EBL, such as bleeding from band-related ulcers, albeit infrequent, are more significant, often requiring hospitalization and blood transfusion, and may rarely be associated with death.

According to the Baveno consensus conference, nonselective β-blockers should be considered as a first choice for preventing first variceal bleeding in high-risk patients who have not bled, and EBL should be provided for patients with contraindications or intolerance to β-blockers. The recent guidelines by the American College of Gastroenterology (ACG) and American Association for the Study of Liver Diseases (AASLD) recommend using β-blockers in low-risk patients who have medium to large varices but suggest both EBL and β-blockers for high-risk patients as first-line therapy. The optimal primary prophylaxis in patients with decompensated cirrhosis remains unclear and is arguably expedited liver transplantation. The combination of pharmacologic plus endoscopic therapy has been investigated in such patients with conflicting results. In one study, EBL plus β-blockers offered no benefit in terms of prevention of first bleeding when compared to EBL alone. In a more recent study, combination therapy significantly reduced the occurrence of the first episode of variceal bleeding and improved bleeding-related survival in a group of cirrhotic patients with high-risk esophageal varices awaiting liver transplantation.

Management of Acute Variceal Hemorrhage

Variceal hemorrhage is usually an acute clinical event characterized by rapid gastrointestinal blood loss manifesting as hematemesis (which can be massive), with or without melena or hematochezia. Hemodynamic instability (tachycardia, hypotension) is common. Although variceal bleeding is common in patients with cirrhosis presenting with acute upper gastrointestinal hemorrhage, other causes of bleeding, such as ulcer disease, must be considered. Urgent initiation of empiric pharmacologic therapy with vasoactive agents is indicated in situations where variceal hemorrhage is likely. Subsequently, direct endoscopic examination is critical to establish an accurate diagnosis and to provide the rationale for immediate and subsequent therapies. The immediate steps in the management of acute variceal bleeding include: volume resuscitation, prevention of complications, ensuring hemostasis, and initiating measures to prevent early and delayed rebleeding.

Using a MELD-based analysis, the overall 6-week mortality is estimated at 16% (5%–20%), with mortality rates worsening with more advanced disease. Recurrence rates are up to 60% within 1 to 2 years if untreated, and mortality rates as high as 33%.

Patients with variceal hemorrhage and ascites are at increased risk for bacterial infections, particularly spontaneous bacterial peritonitis. This risk appears to be increased in the setting of uncontrolled hemorrhage or as a result of transient bacteremia following endoscopic sclerotherapy or variceal ligation. Short-term systemic antibiotics (e.g., third-generation cephalosporins or fluoroquinolones for 4–10 days) have been shown to decrease the risk of bacterial infections and to reduce rebleeding as well as mortality in cirrhotic patients with gastrointestinal bleeding.

A restrictive transfusion strategy should be used, aiming for a hemoglobin of 7 to 8 gm/dL to avoid volume overexpansion and perpetuation of bleeding. The role of platelet transfusion or fresh frozen plasma administration has not been assessed appropriately. The routine administration of fresh frozen plasma in patients with active variceal bleeding may in fact be detrimental because of the resultant volume expansion and should be discouraged. Hypofibrinogenemia should be treated with cryoprecipitate aiming for levels >100 mg/dL. The use of recombinant activated coagulation factor VII (rFVIIa [Novoseven]),[1] which corrects

---

[1]Not FDA approved for this indication.

prothrombin time in cirrhotic patients, has been assessed in two randomized, controlled trials. The first trial showed, in a post hoc analysis, that rFVIIa administration might significantly improve the results of conventional therapy in patients with moderate and advanced liver failure (Child-Pugh B and C) without increasing the incidence of adverse events. A more recent trial tested rVIIa in patients with active bleeding at endoscopy and with a Child-Pugh score 8 points or higher. This trial failed to show a benefit of rVIIa in terms of decreasing the risk of 5-day failure, but it did show improved 6-week mortality. In a small prospective study involving cirrhotic patients with acute variceal bleeding and new portal vein thrombosis identified by positive intra-thrombus enhancement on contrast ultrasonography, the use of low molecular weight heparin after hemostasis is achieved by band ligation was shown to be safe, well tolerated, and effective, with complete recanalization of the portal vein within 2 to 11 days and no recurrence of bleeding.

Pharmacologic Therapy

Pharmacologic therapy can be administered early, requires no special technical expertise, and is thus a desirable first-line option for managing acute variceal hemorrhage. Drugs that reduce portocollateral venous flow (vasoconstrictors) or intrahepatic vascular resistance (vasodilators) or both have been used to achieve this effect. Vasoconstrictors work by decreasing splanchnic arterial flow, and vasodilators are used in combination with vasoconstrictors to reduce their systemic side effects, but they can also exert an added beneficial effect on intrahepatic resistance (see Table 1).

Vasopressin and Terlipressin. Vasopressin (Pitressin)[1] is a nonselective vasoconstricting agent that causes a reduction of splanchnic blood flow and thereby a reduced portal pressure. Vasopressin, which is associated with severe vascular complications, has been largely replaced by other vasoconstrictors such as its synthetic analogue, triglycyl-lysine vasopressin (terlipressin [Glypressin]).[2] Terlipressin has fewer side effects and a longer biological half-life, allowing its use as a bolus intravenous injection (2 mg every 4 hours for the initial 24 hours, then 1 mg every 4 hours for the next 24–48 hours). Terlipressin has been shown in numerous placebo-controlled trials to control bleeding in about 80% of cases and is the only pharmacologic therapy proven, as of 2010, to reduce mortality from acute variceal hemorrhage. In patients with esophageal variceal bleeding, a 24-hour course of terlipressin was shown to be as effective as a 72-hour course when used as adjunct therapy to successful variceal band ligation. Terlipressin is not currently available in the United States.

Somatostatin, Octreotide, and Vapreotide. Somatostatin,[2] a naturally occurring peptide, and its analogues, octreotide (Sandostatin)[1] and vapreotide (Sanvar),[1] stop variceal hemorrhage in up to 80% of patients and are generally considered equivalent to vasopressin (Pitressin), terlipressin[2] (Glypressin), and endoscopic therapy for the control of acute variceal bleeding. Their precise mechanism of action is unclear but might result from an effect on the release of vasoactive peptides or from reduction of postprandial hyperemia. Somatostatin is used as a continuous intravenous infusion of 250 µg/hour following a 250-µg bolus injection. Octreotide is used as a continuous infusion of 50 µg/hour and does not require a bolus injection. Side effects are minor, including hyperglycemia and mild abdominal cramps. The addition of octreotide or vapreotide to endoscopic sclerotherapy or banding improves control of bleeding and reduces transfusion requirements, with no change in overall mortality. A continuous infusion of octreotide or vapreotide is therefore recommended for 2 to 5 days following emergency endoscopic therapy.

Endoscopy

Endoscopic sclerotherapy stops variceal hemorrhage in 80% to 90% of cases. Its drawbacks include a significant risk of local complications including ulceration, bleeding, stricture, and perforation. Rare systemic complications have been reported including bacteremia with endocarditis, formation of splenic or brain abscesses, and

portal vein thrombosis. Randomized trials in patients with acute variceal bleeding have shown that EBL is essentially equivalent to endoscopic sclerotherapy in achieving initial hemostasis with lesser complications. These include superficial ulcerations, transient chest discomfort, and, rarely, stricture formation. Erythromycin infusion before endoscopy[1] in patients with acute variceal bleeding has been shown to significantly improve endoscopic visibility and to shorten the duration of the procedure.

Balloon Tamponade/SEMS

The use of the Sengstaken-Blakemore or Minnesota tube for hemostasis of variceal bleeding is based on the principle of the application of direct pressure on the bleeding varix by an inflatable—esophageal or gastric—balloon fitted on a rubber nasogastric tube. When properly applied, balloon tamponade is successful in achieving immediate hemostasis in almost all cases. However, early rebleeding following balloon decompression is high. Complications of balloon tamponade include esophageal perforation or rupture, aspiration, and asphyxiation from upper airway obstruction. Balloon tamponade or use of SEMS is generally not recommended and should largely be reserved for rescue of cases of hemorrhage uncontrolled by pharmacologic and endoscopic methods and as a temporary bridge to more definitive therapy. Self-expandable metal stents (SEMS) have recently been shown to be effective in controlling severe bleeding.

Transjugular Intrahepatic Portosystemic Shunt

Treatment with a transjugular intrahepatic portosystemic shunt (TIPS) consists of the vascular placement of an expandable metal stent across a tract created between a hepatic vein and a major intrahepatic branch of the portal system. TIPS can be successfully performed in 90% to 100% of patients, resulting in hemodynamic changes similar to a partially decompressive side-to-side portocaval shunt while avoiding the morbidity and mortality associated with a major surgical procedure. According to the American Association for the Study of Liver Diseases (AASLD) Practice Guidelines, the indications for TIPS are: (1) as rescue therapy for acute variceal hemorrhage refractory to medical and endoscopic intervention; (2) recurrent variceal hemorrhage despite medical and endoscopic treatment; and (3) an emerging indication is early TIPS within 24 to 72 hours of acute variceal hemorrhage in a select patients (e.g., those with basal HVPG >20 mm Hg). The left gastric vein is frequently embolized (embolotherapy) during TIPS creation. TIPS has been shown to be effective in treating refractory, uncontrolled, acute variceal bleeding. Patients with advanced liver disease and multiorgan failure at the time of TIPS have a 30-day mortality that approaches 100%.

Surgery

Surgery is generally considered in the setting of continued hemorrhage or recurrent early rebleeding—uncontrolled by repeated endoscopic or continued pharmacologic therapy—and when TIPS is not available or is not technically feasible. Surgical options include portosystemic shunting or esophageal staple transection alone or with esophagogastric devascularization and splenectomy (Sugiura procedure). Devascularization procedures may be useful in patients who cannot receive a shunt because of splanchnic venous thrombosis. Regardless of the choice of surgical technique, morbidity is high and the 30-day mortality for emergency surgery approaches 80% in some series. Understandably, rescue liver transplantation is not a practical option in patients with uncontrolled variceal hemorrhage.

Secondary Prophylaxis

Variceal hemorrhage recurs in approximately two thirds of patients, most commonly within the first 6 weeks after the initial episode. Patients with advanced liver disease (MELD [model for end-stage liver disease] score ≥18) have an increased risk of early rebleeding and death. Early rebleeding (within the first 5 days) is

---

[2]Not available in the United States.

[1]Not FDA approved for this indication.

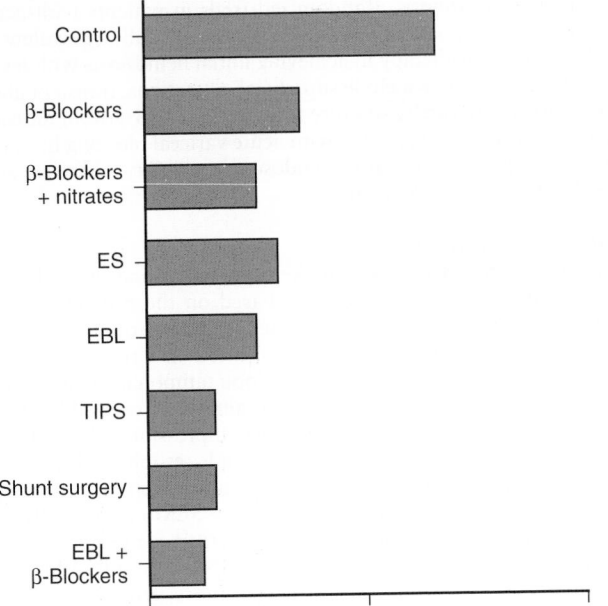

Figure 1 Relative effectiveness of available therapies for preventing recurrent variceal bleeding. The estimates shown are based on the cumulative data available in the literature for recurrent bleeding at 1 year. *Abbreviations:* EBL = endoscopic band ligation; ES = endoscopic sclerotherapy; TIPS = transjugular intrahepatic portosystemic shunt.

reduced by the adjuvant use of octreotide[1] or vapreotide[5]—and possibly terlipressin[2] and somatostatin[2]—after initial endoscopic or pharmacologic control of hemorrhage.

The severity of portal hypertension correlates closely with the severity and risk of rebleeding as well as actuarial probability of survival following an index episode. In a cohort of patients presenting with variceal hemorrhage, those with an initial HVPG greater than 20 mm Hg had a 1-year mortality of 64% compared to 20% for patients with lesser elevations in portal pressure. Given the high risk of recurrent hemorrhage and its associated morbidity and mortality, strategies aimed at prevention should be rapidly instituted following the index episode. The choice of preventive therapy should, therefore, take into consideration the efficacy of therapy, the side effects of the selected treatment, the patient's expected survival, and overall cost. Preventive strategies include pharmacologic, endoscopic, and surgical methods and are listed in Table 1. Relative effectiveness of these strategies is shown in Figure 1.

Pharmacologic Therapy

Reducing the portal pressure by more than 20% from the baseline value pharmacologically results in a reduction in the cumulative probability of recurrent bleeding from 28% at 1 year, 39% at 2 years, and 66% at 3 years to 4%, 9%, and 9%, respectively. Although adjustment of medical therapy based on portal pressure measurement would be ideal, HVPG determination might not be readily available, and treatment must be adjusted using empiric clinical parameters. Several randomized, controlled trials, including a meta-analysis, have demonstrated that β-blockers prevent rebleeding and prolong survival. The addition of isosorbide mononitrate[1] to β-blockers appears to enhance the protective effect of β-blockers alone for preventing recurrent variceal bleeding but offers no survival advantage and reduces the tolerability of therapy. A recent randomized controlled trial showed that carvedilol[1] is as effective as the combination of nadolol (Corgard)[1] plus isorsorbide-5 mononitrate in the prevention of gastroesophageal variceal rebleeding, with fewer severe adverse

events and similar survival. Compared with either sclerotherapy or endoscopic band ligation, combination medical therapy is superior in reducing the risk of recurrent bleeding in patients with esophageal variceal hemorrhage, primarily in patients with Child-Pugh class A and B cirrhosis. Notably, in patients who show a significant hemodynamic response to therapy (defined as a reduction in the hepatic venous pressure gradient to <12 mm Hg or >20% of the baseline value), the risk of recurrent bleeding and of death is significantly reduced.

Endoscopy

Endoscopic therapy has been established over the past decade as a therapeutic cornerstone for preventing esophageal variceal rebleeding. Gastric varices, however, are not effectively treated by sclerotherapy or ligation. Patients with recurrent gastric variceal hemorrhage are best treated by *N*-butyl-2-cyanoacrylate injection[1] or by nonendoscopic means such as TIPS. On the other hand, EBL is highly effective at obliterating esophageal varices and is considered the endoscopic therapy of choice for secondary prophylaxis.

Combination modality approaches, usually including an endoscopic and pharmacologic treatment, are pathophysiologically attractive and may be more effective than single therapy. Two randomized, controlled trials have shown that adding β-blockers to EBL reduces the risk of rebleeding and variceal recurrence, suggesting that if EBL is used, it should be used in association with β-blockers. One randomized, controlled trial has evaluated whether EBL could improve the efficacy of the combined administration of nadolol[1] plus isosorbide.[1] In this study, adding band ligation to nadolol plus isosorbide was shown to be superior to nadolol plus isosorbide alone in preventing variceal rebleeding, but there were no significant differences in mortality. The combination of the best endoscopic treatment (EBL) and the best pharmacologic treatment (β-blockers plus isosorbide) may be the best choice in preventing rebleeding but needs further studies for confirmation. Statins improve liver generation of NO and hepatic endothelial dysfunction in experimental models of cirrhosis and may also reduce liver fibrosis. Randomized placebo-controlled trials found that simvastatin[1] decreased HVPG and improved liver perfusion and had an additive effect in patients treated with NSBB, and showed survival benefit in patients with early stages of cirrhosis and variceal bleeding.

Transjugular Intrahepatic Portosystemic Shunt

Transjugular shunting is more effective than endoscopic therapy for preventing variceal rebleeding but offers no survival benefit. The cumulative risk of rebleeding following TIPS placement is 8% to 18% at 1 year. The trade-off, however, is that TIPS is associated with a higher incidence of clinically significant hepatic encephalopathy (new or worsened portosystemic encephalopathy was noted in about 25% of patients after TIPS). Advanced liver disease is the main determinant of poor outcome following TIPS. Consequently, in patients with advanced liver disease, TIPS is best used as a bridge to liver transplantation.

TIPS, using bare stents, has been compared with surgical shunts in two studies (8 mm portocaval H-graft shunt in one and distal splenorenal shunt in the second). Although the first study showed a significantly lower rebleeding rate in the surgical group, the second and larger trial did not find any differences in rebleeding rates, hepatic encephalopathy, or mortality, but it found a significantly higher reintervention rate in the TIPS group. However, the obstruction and reintervention rates are markedly decreased with the recent use of polytetrafluoroethylene (PTFE)-covered stents. According to these data, TIPS using PTFE-covered stents represents the best rescue therapy for failures of medical and endoscopic treatment. In addition to TIPS, balloon-occluded retrograde transvenous obliteration (BRTO) is reserved primarily for prevention of recurrent bleeding, and has recently been included in the AASLD practice guidelines. Typically, it is utilized in patients who are at high risk for TIPS, such as those with elevated MELD (>18), right-sided heart failure, or hepatic encephalopathy.

---

[1]Not FDA approved for this indication.
[2]Not available in the United States.
[5]Investigational drug in the United State.

---

[1]Not FDA approved for this indication.

Surgery

Portosystemic shunt surgery is the most effective means by which to reduce portal pressure. Although effective at eradicating varices and preventing rebleeding, nonselective portocaval shunts are associated with a significant incidence of hepatic encephalopathy, portal vein thrombosis, and occasionally liver failure. Commonly used shunts include the distal splenorenal shunt and the low-diameter (mesocaval or portocaval) interposition shunt. Rates of recurrent bleeding are on the order of 10%, with the highest risk of bleeding occurring in the first month after surgery. Devascularization procedures (i.e., esophageal transection and gastroesophageal devascularization) are usually considered in patients who cannot receive shunts because of splanchnic venous thrombosis and should be performed only by experienced surgeons. Surgical therapy has been largely supplanted by TIPS.

Cost-Effectiveness of Available Therapies

Data examining the cost of variceal bleeding and the cost-effectiveness of commonly used therapies are limited. The treatment cost of an episode of variceal bleeding has been estimated at $15,000 to $40,000. The cost-effectiveness of diagnostic methods used to guide therapy is unclear. For example, HVPG determination, which can accurately predict pharmacologic response to therapy, is an attractive, although invasive, adjunct in the management of patients with variceal bleeding, but its cost-effectiveness remains in question. Further, screening endoscopy for detecting large varices, while recommended, has not been demonstrated to be cost-effective.

There are areas in which management is controversial and not standardized. For example, given the right expertise, secondary prophylaxis with surgical shunts or TIPS may be more effective than medical or endoscopic therapy in Child-Pugh class A patients. On the other hand, patients with advanced cirrhosis are often intolerant of β-blockers—let alone in combination with nitrates—and therefore the use of combination therapy remains controversial in such patients. Arguably, the preferred treatment for such patients is TIPS as a bridge to early liver transplantation.

Therefore, when choosing a specific treatment plan, the clinician must take into consideration the direct costs of health care utilization, as well as the efficacy and morbidity of therapy. The treatment chosen should be tailored to fit the patient's clinical condition while also taking into account the possibility that the patient's liver disease can progress and thus necessitate transplantation. The cost-effectiveness of various treatment modalities should factor in the cost of failed therapy (e.g., rebleeding, shunt revision) and that of treatment-related complications (e.g., encephalopathy, esophageal stricture).

Summary

Esophageal variceal hemorrhage is a common and devastating complication of portal hypertension and is a leading cause of morbidity and mortality in patients with cirrhosis. Because the clinical outcomes are poor once variceal bleeding has occurred, primary prophylaxis with β-blockers or EBL should be considered in high-risk patients. The treatment of acute variceal hemorrhage is aimed at judicious volume resuscitation and ensuring hemostasis with pharmacologic agents and endoscopic techniques as well as prevention of complications, such as infections by the use of prophylactic antibiotics. Both NSBB and EVL are effective therapeutic options for primary prophylaxis for bleeding. NSBB have additional beneficial effects on the natural course of the disease. EVL is the treatment of choice for patients with contraindication or who are intolerant to NSBB. In patients with small size varices, NSBB is the first-line treatment option. In patients with advanced decompensated cirrhosis (arterial hypotension, hyponatremia, renal dysfunction), NSBB should be used with caution and EVL may be an alternative.

A high risk of rebleeding after an index episode mandates the institution of preventive strategies. Wedge pressure-guided medical therapy may be the preferred mode of secondary prophylaxis in patients with Child Pugh class A or B cirrhosis, but is invasive and not widely available. Patients at high risk for rebleeding, including those with decompensated or advanced liver disease, should be considered for TIPS followed by liver transplantation when applicable. Treatment with a combination of methods is pathophysiologically attractive, but the choice of therapy should ultimately be tailored to fit the patient's clinical condition, risk factors, and prognosis, taking into account issues of risk-to-benefit ratio, compliance, and cost.

References

Abraldes JG, Villanueva C, Aracil C, et al: Addition of simvastatin to standard therapy for the prevention of variceal rebleeding does not reduce rebleeding but increases survival in patients with cirrhosis, *Gastroenterology* 2016 Jan 13. Epub ahead of print.

Azam Z, Hamid S, Jafri W, et al: Short course adjuvant terlipressin in acute variceal bleeding: a randomized double blind dummy controlled trial, *J Hepatol* 56:819–824, 2012.

Bambha K, Kim WR, Pedersen R, et al: Predictors of early rebleeding and mortality after acute variceal haemorrhage in patients with cirrhosis, *Gut* 57:814–820, 2008.

de Franchis R, Baveno VIF: Expanding consensus in portal hypertension: report of the Baveno VI Consensus Workshop: stratifying risk and individualizing care for portal hypertension, *J Hepatol* 63(3):743–752, 2015.

Feu F, Garcia-Pagan JC, Bosch J, et al: Relation between portal pressure response to pharmacotherapy and risk of recurrent variceal haemorrhage in patients with cirrhosis, *Lancet* 346:1056–1059, 1995.

Garcia Pagan JC, De Gottardi A, Bosch J: Review article: the modern management of portal hypertension—primary and secondary prophylaxis of variceal bleeding in cirrhotic patients, *Aliment Pharmacol Ther* 28:178–186, 2008.

Garcia-Pagan JC, Feu F, Bosch J, Rodes J: Propranolol compared with propranolol plus isosorbide-5-mononitrate for portal hypertension in cirrhosis. A randomized controlled study, *Ann Intern Med* 114:869–873, 1991.

Garcia-Tsao G, Abraldes JG, Berzigotti A, Bosch J: Portal hypertensive bleeding in cirrhosis: Risk stratification, diagnosis, and management: 2016 practice guidance by the American Association for the study of liver diseases, *Hepatology* 65(01):310–335, 2017.

Gluud LL, Krag A: Banding ligation versus beta-blockers for primary prevention in oesophageal varices in adults, *Cochrane Database Syst Rev* 8:CD004544, 2012.

Laine L, Cook D: Endoscopic ligation compared with sclerotherapy for treatment of esophageal variceal bleeding. A meta-analysis, *Ann Intern Med* 123:280–287, 1995.

Lo GH, Chen WC, Wang HM, Yu HC: Randomized, controlled trial of carvedilol versus nadolol plus isosorbide mononitrate for the prevention of variceal rebleeding, *J Gastroenterol Hepatol* 27(11):1681–1687, 2012.

Mandorfer M, Bota S, Schwabl P, et al: Nonselective β-blockers increase risk for hepatorenal syndrome and death in patients with cirrhosis and spontaneous bacterial peritonitis, *Gastroenterology* 146:1680–1690, 2014.

Maruyama H, Takahashi M, Shimada T, Yokosuka O: Emergency anticoagulation treatment for cirrhosis patients with portal vein thrombosis and acute variceal bleeding, *Scand J Gastroenterol* 47:686–691, 2012.

Merkel C, Marin R, Sacerdoti D, et al: Long-term results of a clinical trial of nadolol with or without isosorbide mononitrate for primary prophylaxis of variceal bleeding in cirrhosis, *Hepatology* 31:324–329, 2000.

Moitinho E, Escorsell A, Bandi JC, et al: Prognostic value of early measurements of portal pressure in acute variceal bleeding, *Gastroenterology* 117:626–631, 1999.

North Italian Endoscopic Club for the Study and Treatment of Esophageal Varices: Prediction of the first variceal hemorrhage in patients with cirrhosis of the liver and esophageal varices: A prospective multicenter study, *N Engl J Med* 319:983–989, 1988.

Northup PG, Caldwell SH: Coagulation in liver disease: A guide for the clinician, *Clin Gastroenterol Hepatol* 11:1064–1074, 2013.

Polio J, Groszmann RJ: Hemodynamic factors involved in the development and rupture of esophageal varices: a pathophysiologic approach to treatment, *Semin Liver Dis* 6:318–331, 1986.

Poynard T, Cales P, Pasta L, et al: β-Adrenergic-antagonist drugs in the prevention of gastrointestinal bleeding in patients with cirrhosis and esophageal varices. An analysis of data and prognostic factors in 589 patients from four randomized clinical trials. Franco-Italian Multicenter Study Group, *N Engl J Med* 324:1532–1538, 1991.

Sersté T, Melot C, Francoz C, et al: Deleterious effects of beta-blockers on survival in patients with cirrhosis and refractory ascites, *Hepatology* 52:1017–1022, 2010.

Sharara AI, Rockey DC: Gastroesophageal variceal hemorrhage, *N Engl J Med* 345:669–681, 2001.

Shi KQ, Fan YC, Pan ZZ, et al: Transient elastography: a meta-analysis of diagnostic accuracy in evaluation of portal hypertension in chronic liver disease, *Liver Int* 33:62–71, 2013.

Sinagra E, Perricone G, D'Amico M: Tiné F, D'Amico G, Systematic review with meta-analysis: the haemodynamic effects of carvedilol compared with propranolol for portal hypertension in cirrhosis. *Aliment Pharmacol Ther* 39:557–568, 2014.

Villanueva C, Minana J, Ortiz J, et al: Endoscopic ligation compared with combined treatment with nadolol and isosorbide mononitrate to prevent recurrent variceal bleeding, *N Engl J Med* 345:647–655, 2001.

CALCULOUS BILIARY DISEASE

Method of
Zachary L. Smith, DO; and Mick S. Meiselman, MD

CURRENT DIAGNOSIS

- True biliary colic is characterized by the abrupt onset and cessation of severe mid-epigastric or, less commonly, right upper quadrant pain.
- Pain commonly starts 1 to 2 hours after eating and can be localized or radiate to the back, right shoulder, or chest.
- The onset of biliary colic commonly occurs during sleep.
- Nausea and vomiting commonly follow the onset of pain.
- Elevations of total and conjugated bilirubin, ALP, and GGT with modest elevations in AST and ALT support a suspected diagnosis of choledocholithiasis.
- A normal serum biochemistry profile has a negative predictive value of 97% for ruling out choledocholithiasis.
- Transabdominal ultrasonography is a useful and cost-effective test for diagnosing cholelithiasis; however, it has significantly lower utility for choledocholithiasis.
- For intermediate-risk patients with suspected choledocholithiasis, examination of the common bile duct with magnetic resonance cholangiopancreatography (MRCP) or endoscopic ultrasonography (EUS) is warranted.

CURRENT THERAPY

- The treatment of choice for symptomatic cholelithiasis is laparoscopic cholecystectomy. Elective laparoscopic cholecystectomy should only be performed for true biliary colic. Vague symptoms such as bloating, dyspepsia, and atypical abdominal pain are not commonly related to gallstone disease and thus are not an indication for gallbladder removal.
- Laparoscopic cholecystectomy should generally take place within 72 hours of presentation for acute cholecystitis in appropriate surgical candidates.
- Laparoscopic cholecystectomy is recommended in pregnant patients with symptomatic cholelithiasis and acute cholecystitis. This is best done by experienced surgeons in the second or early third trimesters.
- Patients who should undergo preoperative ERCP for choledocholithiasis include those with high risk stratification and those deemed intermediate risk in whom a common bile duct stone is identified on MRCP or endoscopic ultrasonography.

Cholelithiasis

Epidemiology

Gallstone disease is common in Western populations, affecting 10% to 15% of adults. It is estimated that 6.3 million men and 14.2 million women in the United States have gallstones. Although the vast majority of patients remain asymptomatic throughout their lifetime, roughly one third develop symptoms or complications.

Pathophysiology

Gallstones can be categorized based on their composition. Of patients with gallstone disease in the Western world, 80% to 90% have cholesterol stones or cholesterol-predominant stones (mixed stones). Pigment gallstones account for the remaining 5% to 10%. Patients with hemolytic disorders are prone to pigment stone formation, and therefore the correspondence with disorders such as sickle cell anemia, hereditary spherocytosis, and Gilbert's syndrome is high.

Risk Factors

Risk factors for gallstone disease include female sex, age greater than 40 years, white, Latin American, and Native American descent, family history, obesity, rapid weight loss, starvation, total parenteral nutrition, bariatric surgery, diabetes mellitus, and hypertriglyceridemia.

Clinical Manifestations

The typical symptomatic presentation of gallstone disease is biliary colic. This is described as severe pain located in the mid-epigastrium or, less commonly, the right upper quadrant, that begins and ceases abruptly. The pain is typically constant, occurring 1 to 2 hours after a meal, and can either be localized or radiate to the back or right shoulder. Often the onset of pain occurs during sleep. Nausea and vomiting commonly accompany biliary pain, and, as with most surgical entities, pain typically precedes the onset of these symptoms. Biliary colic can also manifest as chest pain and is occasionally mistaken for cardiac angina. Prolonged episodes of pain localized to the right upper quadrant often herald cholecystitis rather than biliary colic. A clinical history containing the cardinal features of biliary colic carries a high diagnostic accuracy.

Diagnosis

Transabdominal ultrasonography is the preferred initial imaging test for cholelithiasis. The sensitivity for detecting the presence of gallstones within the gallbladder lumen on ultrasonography is 97%.

Biliary Sludge

Biliary sludge is often diagnosed on transabdominal ultrasonography. It appears as low-amplitude nonshadowing echoes that layer in dependent portions of the gallbladder. The clinical course of biliary sludge varies from patient to patient. Some patients remain symptom free, and others develop overt biliary colic. A fraction of patients demonstrate resolution of biliary sludge on repeat imaging. Symptomatic biliary sludge should be treated the same as cholelithiasis. Similarly, patients with asymptomatic biliary sludge should be managed expectantly.

Treatment

In patients with symptomatic cholelithiasis, treatment should be aimed at acute pain control and prevention of recurrent episodes. In patients without contraindications, cholecystectomy is the preferred choice for treatment of symptomatic uncomplicated cholelithiasis. This is preferably done via laparoscopy, which offers lower rates of complications and postoperative pain along with better cosmetic results when compared with open cholecystectomy.

Because of the high incidence of cholelithiasis, true biliary colic should be identified before a decision is made to proceed with laparoscopic cholecystectomy. Vague symptoms such as bloating or atypical abdominal pain are not typical of gallstone disease and thus often persist after surgery. In cases of asymptomatic uncomplicated cholelithiasis, elective cholecystectomy is not recommended unless the patient is diabetic or is undergoing an operation such as gastric bypass surgery, after which there is an increased risk of gallstone formation.

There is a very limited role for medical management of gallstone disease. Nonoperative management of symptomatic cholelithiasis involves bile dissolution with ursodeoxycholic acid (Actigall). The use of medical therapy is limited based on poor efficacy and high rates of recurrence and thus should be reserved only rarely for nonsurgical candidates.

Analgesia is an important adjunct in the treatment of symptomatic cholelithiasis. In patients with severe symptoms requiring narcotic pain medication, meperidine (Demerol) is preferred over morphine because it has less effect on the sphincter of Oddi. Nonsteroidal antiinflammatory drugs (NSAIDs) are another mainstay of therapy. Parenterally administered ketorolac (Toradol) is perhaps the most commonly used agent for biliary colic in the acute care setting. Studies have shown that NSAIDs are beneficial in the management of pain due to gallstones, and at least one study has suggested that early administration of NSAIDs might decrease the progression to acute cholecystitis.

Complications
Complications that can potentially arise from cholelithiasis include acute cholecystitis, cholangitis, pancreatitis, obstructive jaundice, and, rarely, gallstone ileus.

Choledocholithiasis
Choledocholithiasis often manifests concomitantly with symptomatic gallstone disease and is a finding in 5% to 10% of patients undergoing laparoscopic cholecystectomy for symptomatic cholelithiasis. The workup for suspected choledocholithiasis combines history, physical examination, laboratory data, and various imaging modalities. If the clinical history and physical examination are suggestive, the clinician should obtain serum liver biochemistry tests including alanine aminotransferase (ALT), aspartate aminotransferase (AST), total and fractionated bilirubin, alkaline phosphatase (ALP), and γ-glutamyl transpetidase (GGT).

The typical pattern of serum biochemistry is one of cholestasis. A conjugated hyperbilirubinemia along with high levels of GGT and ALP are seen often in the setting of modest elevation to the transaminases. ALP is usually elevated out of proportion to the transaminases; however, extreme levels of AST and ALT have been described. Transaminase levels greater than 1000 U/L, although rare in gallstone disease, should not dissuade the clinician from a diagnosis of choledocholithiasis. Serum biochemistries provide the most utility in ruling out common bile duct stones. A normal biochemical profile has a negative predictive value of 97%. Clinical predictors for assessing the likelihood of choledocholithiasis in patients with symptomatic cholelithiasis are listed in Box 1.

Diagnosis
A variety of modalities are available for diagnosing choledocholithiasis. Perhaps the least expensive and most widely available test is transabdominal ultrasound. Although the sensitivity for cholelithiasis is quite high with transabdominal ultrasound, identifying stones in the common bile duct (Figure 1) is more difficult. Prospective studies have reported sensitivities ranging from 22% to 55% for detecting common bile duct stones; however, in our clinical experience the sensitivity is much lower. Other indirect indicators of choledocholithiasis such as common bile duct dilation (77%–88% sensitivity) can provide additional diagnostic clues. Based on the high false-negative rates for common bile duct stones and dilation, a negative transabdominal ultrasound scan cannot rule out choledocholithiasis. CT scanning has a higher sensitivity for choledocholithiasis than transabdominal ultrasound. Levels of radiation and cost have limited its use as a first-line diagnostic tool.

Three nonsurgical modalities offer true visualization of the common bile duct with comparable sensitivities: Magnetic resonance cholangiopancreatography (MRCP), endoscopic retrograde cholangiopancreatography (ERCP), and endoscopic ultrasonography (EUS). MRCP has a diagnostic sensitivity of 85% to 92% for detecting choledocholithiasis, and, although it is useful for helping determine which intermediate-risk patients would benefit from preoperative ERCP, small and distal common bile duct stones are often missed.

EUS and ERCP are both minimally invasive techniques useful in the diagnosis and management of choledocholithiasis. Owing to the proximity of the extrahepatic bile duct to the proximal duodenum, EUS provides high sensitivity (89%–94%) for detecting common bile duct stones and is especially useful for detecting stones less than 5 mm in diameter. ERCP provides similar diagnostic sensitivity; however, ERCP offers therapeutic capability. Because of the reasonably high risk of complications including pancreatitis (1.3%–15.1%), infection (0.6%–5.0%), gastrointestinal hemorrhage (0.3%–2.0%), and perforation (0.1%–1.1%), ERCP as an initial modality should be reserved for patients who have a high pretest probability for choledocholithiasis and particularly for those with complications such as acute cholangitis or severe pancreatitis.

Research has evaluated the use of ultrasound-guided ERCP with the goal of avoiding unnecessary bile duct cannulation, and reserving its use for therapeutic purposes only. A systematic review from 2009 showed that compared with ERCP alone, the use of EUS avoided unnecessary ERCP in 67.1% of patients in whom no common bile duct stone was identified. As more gastroenterologists become trained in this modality, EUS-guided ERCP might prove to be the preferred diagnostic modality in intermediate-risk patients for the diagnosis and initial therapy of choledocholithiasis.

Treatment
Patients with choledocholithiasis should be treated to avoid recurrent symptoms and development of complications. Stones can be extracted from the common bile duct via ERCP or laparoscopic cholecystectomy with bile duct exploration. Studies have shown similar efficacies without significant differences in morbidity or mortality; however, clinical expertise varies widely with the laparoscopic approach. Ultimately, cholecystectomy should be performed to prevent recurrence in surgical candidates. In patients undergoing laparoscopic cholecystectomy for suspected choledocholithiasis, perioperative management differs based on the risk stratification of the patient (see Box 1). High-risk patients should

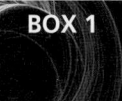

BOX 1 Strategy to Assign Risk of Choledocholithiasis in Patients with Symptomatic Cholelithiasis, Based on Clinical Predictors

Predictors of Choledocholithiasis
High Risk
1. Common bile duct stone on ultrasound, CT scan or MRI
2. Total bilirubin >4 mg/dl *and* dilated common bile duct
3. Ascending cholangitis

Intermediate Risk
1. Other abnormal liver chemistry (e.g. total bilirubin 1-8-3.9 mg/dl, elevated AST, ALT, alkaline phosphatase)
2. Age >55 years
3. Dilated common bile duct on imaging

Low Risk
None of the above are present

From ASGE Standards of Practice Committee Buxbaum JL, Abbas SM, Sultan S, et al. ASGE guideline on the role of endoscopy in the evaluation and management of choledocholithiasis. Gastrointest Endosc. 2019;89(6):1075–1105.e15.

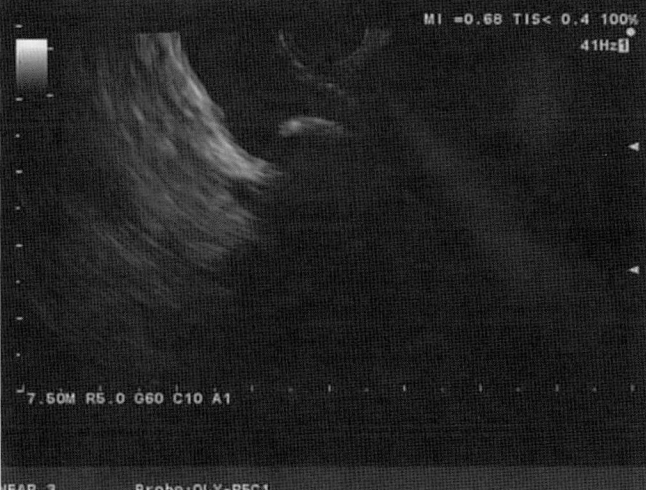

Figure 1 A large gallstone in the common bile duct (CBD) with dilatation of the CBD proximally. The endoscopic ultrasound probe is visualized in the top of the image, and a large cone-shaped shadow is cast distal to the gallstone.

proceed directly to ERCP before surgery for attempted stone extraction. In intermediate-risk patients, a preoperative MRCP or EUS should be performed, and, if the results are positive, the patient should undergo ERCP as a prelude to surgery. For suspected choledocholithiasis in low-risk patients, surgery should be performed without further imaging of the common bile duct.

Complications

The two most common adverse complications of choledocholithiasis are gallstone pancreatitis and acute cholangitis. Gallstone pancreatitis develops in 3% to 7% of patients with gallstones and is the most common cause of acute pancreatitis in the United States. The diagnosis and management of acute pancreatitis is discussed in a separate chapter.

Acute cholangitis is caused by obstruction and stasis of the biliary tract with complicating bacterial infection. The syndrome is characterized by fever, jaundice, and abdominal pain, also known as Charcot's triad. Patients who develop hypotension and changes in mental status (Reynold's pentad) have a poorer prognosis. Elderly patients often do not demonstrate the classic signs of acute cholangitis, but they can develop a delayed-sepsis–like syndrome, of which hypotension is the most pronounced feature. High biliary pressures promote the translocation of bacteria from the portal circulation into the biliary tree. The most common bacterial organism seen in acute cholangitis is *Escherichia coli* (25%–50%), followed by *Klebsiella*, *Enterobacter*, and *Enterococcus* species.

Treatment for acute cholangitis should focus on antimicrobial therapy and biliary drainage. Empiric antibiotic regimens should provide adequate activity against gram-negative and anaerobic organisms. Common regimens include monotherapy with ampicillin and sulbactam (Unasyn) or pipercillin and tazobactam (Zosyn) or combination therapy with a fluoroquinolone plus metronidazole (Flagyl).

Patients without hypotension or mental status changes commonly show initial improvement after empiric antibiotics are administered, and thus biliary drainage can be done nonurgently. In patients demonstrating signs of sepsis or severe infection, emergency biliary drainage via ERCP is warranted. Patients who are not candidates for ERCP may undergo percutaneous transhepatic biliary drainage as an alternative.

Acute Cholecystitis

Acute cholecystitis is a syndrome defined by right upper quadrant pain, fever, and leukocytosis in the setting of gallbladder inflammation. Nausea and vomiting often occur as concurrent symptoms. Patients commonly have a positive Murphy's sign on physical examination, which is defined as abrupt cessation of inspiration on deep palpation of the gallbladder fossa, just beneath the liver edge. Approximately 95% of patients with acute cholecystitis have gallstones. In these instances, cholecystitis is thought to be precipitated by obstruction of the cystic duct and by local irritation of the gallbladder wall. Local inflammation is followed by release of pro-inflammatory prostaglandins. Superimposed bacterial infection might or might not complicate acute cholecystitis. As with cholangitis, the main bacteria responsible for infections during acute cholecystitis are *E. coli* and *Klebsiella*, *Enterobacter*, and *Enterococcus* species.

Diagnosis

The diagnosis of acute cholecystitis can often be made on physical examination alone. The most common laboratory finding in acute cholecystitis is leukocytosis. Mild elevations in AST and ALT can also be seen. Elevations of bilirubin and ALP are typical of biliary obstruction and are not commonly seen in acute cholecystitis. These abnormalities, if present, should raise suspicion for other conditions such as choledocholithiasis, cholangitis, or Mirizzi's syndrome. Mirizzi's syndrome is a rare cause of obstructive jaundice characterized by an impacted cystic duct stone that causes mass effect and compression of the common bile duct or common hepatic duct.

The initial imaging study of choice for acute cholecystitis is transabdominal ultrasound. Findings suggestive of cholecystitis include cholelithiasis, pericholecystic fluid (Figure 2), and a sonographic Murphy's sign (Figure 3). Thickening of the gallbladder wall supports a diagnosis of acute cholecystitis, but it is a nonspecific finding. Transabdominal ultrasound has a sensitivity of 88% for diagnosing acute cholecystitis. Hepatobiliary cholescintigraphy (HIDA scan) (Figure 4) is recommended if the suspicion of cholecystitis remains after a negative transabdominal ultrasound. MRCP and CT scan are typically not necessary for the diagnosis, although CT scan can be useful if complications from cholecystitis such as perforation are suspected.

Treatment

The treatment for acute cholecystitis involves supportive care, analgesia, antibiotics, and either surgery or percutaneous gallbladder drainage. If treatment is delayed or inadequate, numerous potential complications can result. These include emphysematous or gangrenous cholecystitis and gallbladder perforation. All patients with acute cholecystitis should be admitted to the hospital and given supportive care including intravenous fluids. NSAIDs and opioid analgesics are typically used for pain control.

Although bacterial etiologies complicate less than half of all episodes, empiric antibiotics are commonly administered to patients with acute cholecystitis. Appropriate antibiotic regimens are the same as those used in the setting of acute cholangitis (see the discussion of complications of choledocholithiasis).

In patients who are adequate surgical candidates, cholecystectomy should be performed within 72 hours of initial presentation. Numerous prospective trials and a Cochrane Database review have evaluated early versus delayed (6–12 weeks) cholecystectomy. There is overwhelming consensus that early surgery carries no increase in complications or perioperative morbidity and is associated with shorter hospital stays. Furthermore, early laparoscopic cholecystectomy eliminates the risk of recurrent episodes of acute cholecystitis.

Acute Acalculous Cholesystitis

An estimated 5% to 10% of cases of acute cholecystitis develop without the presence of gallstones. Acute acalculous cholecystitis is often seen in the setting of serious medical illness, complicated surgery, severe blunt trauma, and burn injuries. Other conditions such as diabetes mellitus, vasculitis, AIDS, and congestive heart failure have also been implicated as risk factors. Acute acalculous cholecystitis carries major risks of gangrene (50%) and

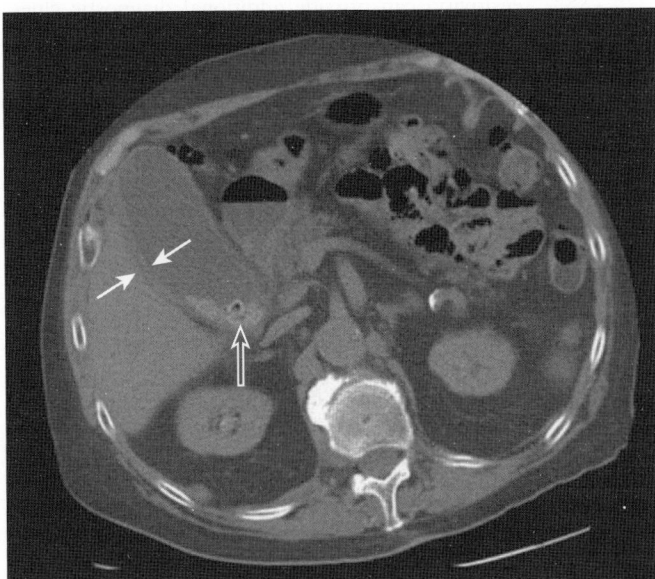

Figure 2 Computed tomography (CT) scan demonstrating acute cholecystitis. The *outline arrow* indicates gallstones within the gallbladder lumen. The two *solid arrows* highlight mural thickening of the gallbladder wall and small amounts of pericholecystic fluid. Image courtesy of Richard M. Gore, MD, Department of Radiology, NorthShore University Health System, Evanston, IL.

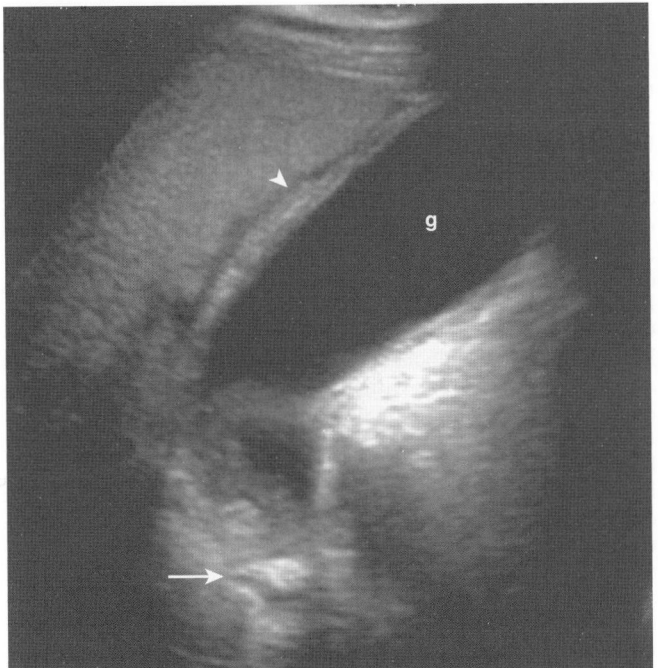

Figure 3 Acute cholecystits: ultrasound. Gallbladder *(g)* is distended, with mural thickening *(arrowhead)* and a stone in the gallbladder neck *(arrow)*. Positive sonographic Murphy sign was present.

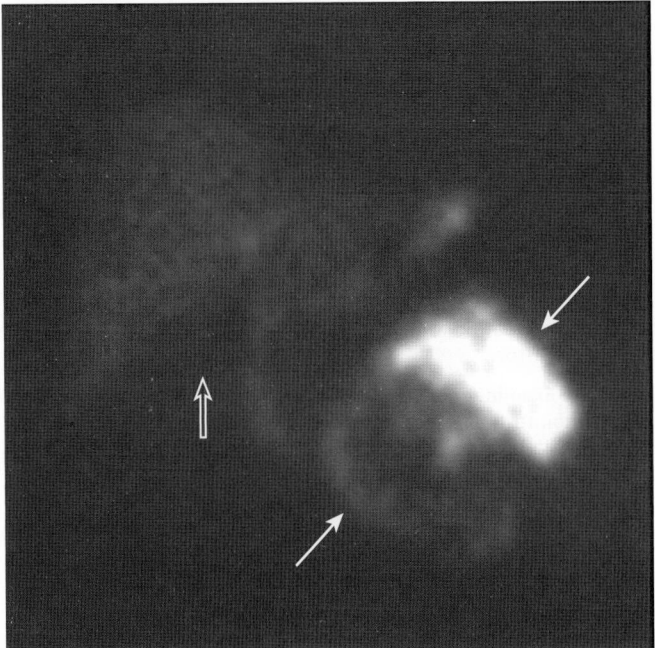

Figure 4 Hepatobiliary iminodiacetic acid (HIDA) scan demonstrating acute cholecystitis. There is nonfilling of the gallbladder *(outline arrow)*, with isotope noted in the stomach and duodenum *(solid arrows)*. Image courtesy of Richard M. Gore, MD, Department of Radiology, North-Shore University Health System, Evanston, IL.

perforation (10%), and mortality ranges from 30% to 50%. Numerous organisms have been associated with acute acalculous cholecystitis, including bacterial, viral, fungal, and parasitic infections.

The diagnosis is difficult. Patients are often critically ill and unable to elicit their symptoms. Transabdominal ultrasound is the best modality to evaluate acute acalculous cholecystitis in the critically ill patient owing to its availability, cost, and ease of performance. Hepatobiliary iminodiacetic acid (HIDA) and computed tomography (CT) scanning can have a role in difficult-to-diagnose acute acalculous cholecystitis and should be considered if ultrasound is nondiagnostic. Whereas false-positive test results can occur, a normal HIDA scan has a high negative predictive value in evaluating acute acalculous cholecystitis.

Because of the high rate of gangrene and perforation, early cholecystectomy should be performed in patients who are surgical candidates. In patients too ill to undergo surgery, biliary drainage with percutaneous cholecystostomy should be considered.

Gangrenous Cholecystitis, Emphysematous Cholecystitis, and Gallbladder Perforation

Gangrenous cholecystitis is most often seen in elderly patients and diabetics along with patients who delay seeking medical treatment for their symptoms. It is the most common complication of acute cholecystitis and carries a high mortality. Emphysematous cholecystitis is caused by gas-forming bacteria that infect the gallbladder. *E coli* and *Clostridium* species are most commonly implicated. Gas in the gallbladder may be seen on imaging, particularly CT or magnetic resonance imaging (MRI). Patients with gangrenous or emphysematous cholecystitis are at an elevated risk for gallbladder perforation. Early empiric antibiotics and cholecystectomy are crucial in the management of these complications to minimize mortality and prevent perforation of the gallbladder, a condition that carries a mortality rate of 42% to 60%.

Gallbladder Disease in Pregnancy

Pregnancy is a major risk factor for cholesterol gallstone formation. Because of anatomic changes secondary to the gravid uterus, biliary colic can be difficult to delineate from other causes of abdominal pain. Pregnant patients often have gallstones on transabdominal ultrasound, and thus a detailed history and physical examination are needed to diagnose a patient's abdominal pain as biliary. Patients with other symptoms including bloating or dyspepsia should be evaluated for other etiologies.

In pregnant patients with recurrent symptomatic cholelithiasis, laparoscopic cholecystectomy remains the treatment of choice. The second and early third trimesters are the best times to perform cholecystectomy owing to ease and lower rates of complications. Nonsurgical management of gallstones is limited in pregnancy. NSAIDs are generally avoided late in pregnancy owing to the risk of premature closure of the ductus arteriosis, especially after 30 to 32 weeks of gestation.

After appendicitis, acute cholecystitis is the second most common nonobstetric surgical emergency during pregnancy. As with nonpregnant patients, pregnant women with acute cholecystitis should be treated with cholecystectomy in addition to medical management. Early surgery for pregnant patients with acute cholecystitis has been found to decrease relapse rates and hospital readmissions. No differences in maternal or fetal morbidity and mortality have been found in patients treated conservatively versus surgically for acute cholecystitis during pregnancy.

References

Abboud PA, Malet PF, Berlin JA, et al: Predictors of common bile duct stones prior to cholecystectomy: A metaanalysis, *Gastrointest Endosc* 44:450–455, 1996.

Akriviadis EA, Hatzigavriel M, Kapnias D, et al: Treatment of biliary colic with diclofenac: a randomized, double-blind, placebo-controlled study, *Gastroenterology* 113:225–231, 1997.

ASGE Standards of Practice Committee, Buxbaum JL, Abbas fehmi SM, Sultan S, et al: ASGE guideline on the role of endoscopy in the evaluation and management of choledocholithiasis, *Gastrointest Endosc* 89(6):1075–1105.e15, 2019.

Barie PS, Eachempati SR: Acute acalculous cholecystitis, *Gastroenterol Clin North Am* 39:344–357, 2010.

Dhupar R, Smaldone GM, Hamad GG: Is there a benefit to delaying cholecystectomy for symptomatic gallbladder disease during pregnancy? *Surg Endosc* 24:108–112, 2010.

Everhart JE, Khare M, Hill M, Maurer KR: Prevalence and ethnic differences in gallbladder disease in the United States, *Gastroenterology* 117:632–639, 1999.

Freitas ML, Bell RL, Duffy AJ: Choledocholithiasis: Evolving standards for diagnosis and management, *World J Gastroenterol* 12:3162–3167, 2006.

Gore RM, Thakrar KH, Newmark GM, et al: Gallbladder imaging, *Gastroenterol Clin North Am* 39:265–267, 2010.

Gurusamy KS, Samraj K: Early versus late laparoscopic cholecystectomy for acute cholecystitis, *Cochrane Database Syst Rev* 18: CD005440.

Papi C, Catarci M, Ambrosio D, et al: Timing of cholecystectomy for acute calculous cholecystitis: A meta-analysis, *Am J Gastroenterol* 9:147–155, 2004.

CHRONIC DIARRHEA

Method of
André de Leon, MD

CURRENT DIAGNOSIS

History
- Duration, frequency, and timing
- Presence of fever/blood
- Food/medication intake
- Travel history

Physical Examination
- Gastrointestinal examination
- Hydration status
- Digital rectal examination
- Other systems: endocrine, ophthalmologic, skin

Testing
- Fecal occult blood testing
- Stool for ova/parasites, *Clostridium difficile* and other bacteria
- Stool antigen for cryptosporidium, giardia
- Fecal electrolytes (Na, K, Osm)
- Fecal leukocytes
- Erythrocyte sedimentation rate (ESR)
- Complete blood count (CBC)
- Other: iron panel (celiac sprue), TSH (hyperthyroidism), liver function tests (LFTs)
- Colonoscopy with biopsy

CURRENT THERAPY

- Supportive care and rehydration, if necessary
- Trial of discontinuation of possible offending medication/food (lactose, gluten, sorbitol)
- Dietary modification with increased fiber intake (dietary or supplementation)
- Specific therapy as directed by culture and susceptibilities or biopsy
- Empiric therapy trial with antibiotics
- Empiric trial of probiotics[1] (limited evidence of efficacy in healthy adults with chronic diarrhea)

[1]Not FDA approved for this indication.

Chronic diarrhea has traditionally been defined based on consistency, volume, and frequency of stools. However, recent studies have found that there is considerable variability in definition when using these markers. Therefore the American Gastroenterological Association has released a consensus statement suggesting that chronic diarrhea should be defined as a decrease in fecal consistency lasting for 4 or more weeks.

Epidemiology

Chronic diarrhea is a common cause of mortality in developing countries as well as the second leading cause of overall mortality in children 1 to 59 months old. The prevalence in the general population in developed nations and economic impact of chronic diarrhea has not been well established. This could be related to the variable nature of the studies that have been performed with regard to definition, population characteristics, and overall study design. The American Gastroenterological Association Burden of Illness study estimates that the direct costs of chronic diarrhea are $524 million per year and indirect costs are at least $136 million

per year. A meta-analysis of current studies suggest that chronic diarrhea can affect anywhere from 1%–5% of the population.

Classification Based on Etiology

Elucidating the exact cause of chronic diarrhea can be very challenging, as there are several hundred conditions that can be related. Consideration of comorbid symptoms and epidemiologic clues can help in constructing a differential diagnosis. Chronic diarrhea can be evaluated based on two etiologies: functional and organic. The functional chronic diarrhea category includes conditions when abdominal pain accompanies the diarrhea (e.g., irritable bowel syndrome) and when abdominal pain is absent. Organic disorders are conditions that are associated with physiologic, structural, or biochemical abnormalities. Organic disorders are more likely in adults with alarm features such as gastrointestinal (GI) bleeding, fevers, or significant weight loss.

Functional Disorders

Functional diarrhea is characterized by chronic or recurrent diarrhea not explained by structural or biochemical abnormalities. Causes may include physiologic factors (small bowel bacterial overgrowth), psychological factors (stress and anxiety), and dietary factors (carbohydrate malabsorption). Patients with functional diarrhea should not meet criteria for irritable bowel syndrome (IBS) as based on the Rome IV criteria. Patients with functional diarrhea may have abdominal pain and/or bloating, but unlike IBS, these are not predominant symptoms.

Functional Disorders: Irritable Bowel Syndrome

Multiple investigations have shown conflicting data, and no abnormality has been found to be specific for this disorder. The traditional focus has been on alterations in gastrointestinal motility and on visceral hypersensitivity; however, more recent studies have considered the role of inflammation, alterations in fecal flora, and bacterial overgrowth as possible causes. The role of food sensitivity is also being considered as a possible cause. The Rome criteria help to provide a framework for the diagnosis of IBS and emphasize pain. When these criteria are not met, then other etiologies should be considered and evaluated. The Rome criteria emphasize chronic abdominal pain that is relieved by defecation and associated with a change in stool frequency or consistency. Psychological stress also appears to correlate to the diagnosis of IBS. Patients with IBS can experience altered bowel habits with a predominance of diarrhea vs. constipation or alternating between the two (mixed type). IBS can also be postinfectious, following recovery from *Clostridrium difficile* and other bacterial infections.

Organic Disorders

Organic disorders leading to chronic diarrhea are conditions that are associated with structural, physiologic, or biochemical abnormalities. Alarm features such as gastrointestinal (GI) bleeding, fever, significant weight loss, occurrence after 50 years of age, and positive family history of colorectal cancer or inflammatory bowel disease (IBD) are more likely in organic disorders.

Organic Disorders: Fatty/Malabsorptive

Malabsorptive diarrhea is, as the name implies, secondary to impaired absorption along the gut. This can be due to structural abnormalities (gastric bypass, short bowel syndrome, celiac sprue, pancreatic insufficiency), structural abnormalities related to vascular compromise (mesenteric ischemia), or lack of enzymes that aid in digestion (e.g., lactose intolerance). Impaired absorption can also occur secondary to infections such as *Tropheryma whipplei* (Whipple's Disease), *Giardia*, small bowel bacterial overgrowth, and tropical sprue. Medications such as aminoglycoside antibiotics, orlistat (Xenical, Alli), thyroid supplementation, acarbose (Precose), and ticlopidine (Ticlid) can also cause malabsorptive diarrhea.

Organic Disorders: Inflammatory

Inflammation leading to diarrhea is often due to autoimmune, infectious, or neoplastic processes or radiation exposure.

Autoimmune processes are felt to play a large role in inflammatory bowel disease (IBD), which often manifests as Crohn disease or ulcerative colitis. Microscopic colitis may also have laboratory findings suggesting an underlying autoimmune disorder. Infections such as *Clostridium difficile, Mycobacterium tuberculosis, Yersinia, Campylobacter, Giardia, Cryptospordium, Amebae, Strongyloidedes*, cytomegalovirus, and herpes simplex virus can lead to a diarrhea with associated inflammation of the bowel. Colon cancer (villous adenocarcinoma) and lymphoma can also cause inflammatory diarrhea.

Organic Disorders: Postcholecystectomy

In the absence of a gallbladder, bile acids drain directly and more continuously into the small bowel. This increase may overcome the terminal portion of the ileum's absorptive capacity. The increased bile acids then are allowed to reach the colon, leading to diarrhea (cholerheic diarrhea).

Clinical Manifestations

History. Thorough investigation of a patient complaining of ongoing diarrhea-like features should always include a detailed medical history. A clear understanding of the patient's symptoms is vital: not all complaints may truly be defined as diarrhea but may rather be symptoms related to an interplay between fecal incontinence and stool impaction. A detailed history of travel, food intake, and medication use is essential. This can help direct the early workup and diagnostic testing. Stool frequency, volume, consistency, and timing can aid in categorization; however, they are no longer what define the condition, as noted previously. If considering the diagnosis of irritable bowel syndrome (IBS), use of the Rome IV criteria will be beneficial.

Physical Examination. The physical examination is very important to the workup and diagnosis of chronic diarrhea. Ophthalmologic findings such as episcleritis or exophthalmia can be related to IBD; skin findings such as dermatitis herpetiformis can be related to celiac sprue (seen in 15%–25% of patients with celiac disease). Prominent lymphadenopathy and weight loss can be suggestive of possible infection or malignancy. A thorough abdominal examination should include the evaluation of bowel sounds (hypermotility), skin for scars (surgical cause of diarrhea), tenderness (infection/inflammation), and masses (neoplasia) and should be followed by a digital rectal examination with fecal occult blood testing. Anoscopy can also be used to detect for ulcerations or fecal impaction, given that seepage around impacted stools can create a picture similar to diarrhea.

Testing for Diagnosis

Serum testing for chronic diarrhea should include a complete blood count (CBC), serum electrolytes, liver function tests, serum albumin, thyroid-stimulating hormone, and erythrocyte sedimentation rate. An iron panel should be performed if indicated based on the results of the CBC. Serum anti-tissue transglutaminase antibody testing may be helpful if symptoms are suggestive of celiac sprue. Stool evaluation may include fecal occult blood testing, fecal leukocytes, stool ova and parasites, stool culture (including *Salmonella*, *Shigella*, and *Campylobacter*), and stool antigen for *Giardia*. Stool testing for *Cryptosporidium* should be considered, especially in the immunocompromised. Stool pH and electrolytes may be helpful, especially when the patient is lactose intolerant. Stool testing for *C. difficile* should be performed if the patient has recently used antibiotics or been hospitalized. If medication abuse is suspected as a possible cause, a stool laxative screen (i.e., stool phenolphthalein test) may be warranted. Diagnostic testing may include a colonoscopy with biopsy.

Treatment

The exact cause of chronic diarrhea can prove elusive, and treatment trials may be warranted. Specific treatment

TABLE 1	Medications Commonly Associated with Diarrhea

Antiarrhythmic medications

- Digoxin
- Quinidine

Antibiotic medications

- Aminoglycosides
- Macrolides

Antihypertensive medications

- ACE inhibitors
- Beta blockers

Antiinflammatory medications

- 5-aminosalicylates
- Nonsteroidal antiinflammatory drugs (NSAIDs)

Antiretroviral medications (many)

Chemotherapuetic medications (many)

Dermatologic medications

- Isotretinoin (occasionally causes diarrhea)

Endocrine medications

- Alpha-glucosidase inhibitors (cause diarrhea in ≥20% of patients)
- Biguanides (cause diarrhea in ≥20% of patients)
- Thyroid hormones

Gastrointestinal medications

- Acid-reducing medications
  - H$_2$-receptor blocker
  - Proton pump inhibitors
- Antacid medications (magnesium containing)

Parasympathetic nervous system medication

- Cholinergic agonists

Psychiatric medications

- Selective serotonin reuptake inhibitors

Respiratory medications

- Xanthine derivative (Theophylline)

Data from Schiller LR, Sellin JH. Sleisenger and Fordtran's Gastrointestinal and Liver Disease: Pathophysiology/Diagnosis/Management. 9th Edition, Philadelphia, 2010, Elsevier; and Soriano M, Vaziri H. Clinical Gastroenterology, Diarrhea: Diagnostic and Therapeutic Advances, New York, 2010, Humana Press, Springer.

depends on the specific diagnosis. If there is concern about possible bacterial or protozoa infection, an empiric trial of vancomycin (Vancocin), ciprofloxacin (Cipro), or metronidazole (Flagyl) may be warranted. If there is concern for possible medication (Table 1) or food relation to diarrhea, a trial of discontinuation of offending substance/food may be reasonable. The effectiveness of probiotics[7] looks favorable; however, large intervention studies and epidemiologic investigations of long-term probiotic effects on healthy adults are largely missing. At this time, probiotics have been found efficacious in treatment of acute diarrhea, prevention of antibiotic-associated diarrhea, and prevention of traveler's diarrhea. Dietary modification continues to be an important starting point for treatment, with increased intake in bulk-forming agents such as fiber. Treatment of specific disorders such as Crohn's disease and ulcerative colitis are discussed in other chapters.

---

[7]Available as dietary supplement.

References

De Vrese M, Marteau PR: Probiotics and prebiotics: Effects on diarrhea, *J Nutr* 137:803S–811S, 2007.

Dellon ES, Ringel Y: Treatment of functional diarrhea, *Curr Treat Options Gastroenterol* 9(4):331–341, 2006.

Everhart JE, editor: *Digestive Disease in the United States: Epidemiology and impact*, Washington, DC, 1994, National Institutes of Health. (NIH Publication No. 94-1447).

Everhart JE, Ruhl CE: Burden of digestive diseases in the United States part II: lower gasteroentestinal diseases, *Gasteroenterology* 136(3):741–754. Epub 2009.

Fine KD, Schiller LR: AGA technical review on the evaluation and management of chronic diarrhea, *Gastroenterology* 116:1464–1486, 1999.

Juckett G, Trivedi R: Evaluation of chronic diarrhea, *Am Fam Physician* 84:1119–1126, 2011.

Peery AF, et al: Burden of Gastrointestinal Disease in the United States: 2012 Update, *Gastroenterology* V143(Issue 5):1179–1187, 2012, e3.

Rodrigo L: Celiac disease, *World J Gastroenterol* 12:6585–6593, 2006.

Schiller LR, et al: Chronic Diarrhea: Diagnosis and Management, *Clinical Gastroenterology and Hepatology* V15(Issue 2):182–193, 2017, e3.

Soriano M, Vaziri H: *Clinical Gastroenterology, Diarrhea: Diagnostic and Therapeutic Advances*, New York, 2010, Humana Press, Springer.

Thomas PD, Forbes A, Green J, et al: Guidelines for the investigation of chronic diarrhea, 2nd edition, *Gut* 52(Suppl. 5):v1–v15, 2003.

Whitehead WE, Borrud L, Goode PS, et al: Fecal incontinence in U.S. adults: Epidemiology and risk factor, *Gastroenterology* 137:512–517, 2009, e2.

World Health Organization. Children: Reducing mortality, Fact Sheet #178, Available at http://www.who.int/mediacentre/factsheets/fs178/en/ (accessed October 17, 2013).

CIRRHOSIS

Method of
Andres F. Carrion, MD; and Paul Martin, MD

The term *cirrhosis* is a neologism derived from the Greek *kirrhós*, which describes the yellowish discoloration of the liver during advanced stages of chronic liver disease, and the suffix *osis*, which denotes a specific condition in medical terminology. Morphologically, cirrhosis reflects the consequences of chronic hepatic necroinflammatory activity with an incomplete and disorganized repair process that results in regenerative nodules and extensive fibrosis replacing normal hepatic parenchyma with disturbance of normal hepatic physiology. Cirrhosis can result from any etiology of chronic liver disease (Table 1). Activation of hepatic stellate cells into myofibroblasts and matrix deposition are key steps in the pathogenesis of cirrhosis.

Epidemiology

The prevalence of cirrhosis varies significantly in different regions of the world and is directly influenced by the epidemiology of individual chronic liver diseases that lead to progressive hepatic fibrosis. The estimated global prevalence of cirrhosis is 4.5% to 9.5%; however, this estimate likely underestimates the real magnitude of disease burden, as a sizable proportion of asymptomatic individuals remain undiagnosed. Similarly, it is difficult to obtain accurate estimates of mortality related to cirrhosis, but countries in Central and South America and Southern Europe exhibit the highest mortality rates, particularly in males. Epidemiologic trends of cirrhosis have changed considerably over time in many countries, underscoring variations in the incidence and prevalence of specific etiologies of chronic liver disease. For instance, widespread immunization against hepatitis B virus (HBV) has markedly reduced its incidence, prevalence, and associated liver disease including cirrhosis. Alcohol consumption has varied strikingly across different regions of the globe over the past several decades. A steady decline in mortality due to cirrhosis has occurred in some European countries (mainly Mediterranean) as alcohol use has diminished. A similar trend has also been noted in North America; however, hospitalizations for acute alcoholic hepatitis have increased over the recent past in the United States. In contrast, a significant increase in mortality related to cirrhosis has been noted in some Eastern European countries with increased alcohol consumption. In addition, eradication of hepatitis C virus (HCV) is associated with a reduction in hepatic dysfunction, liver-related and all-cause mortality, and complications of cirrhosis such as hepatocellular carcinoma (HCC) and portal hypertension. The impact of highly effective direct-acting antiviral agents against HCV

TABLE 1	Etiologies of Cirrhosis
ETIOLOGY	**EXAMPLES**
Infectious	Hepatitis B Hepatitis C Hepatitis D
Autoimmune and cholestasis	Autoimmune hepatitis Biliary atresia Primary biliary cholangitis Primary sclerosing cholangitis Secondary biliary cirrhosis Secondary sclerosing cholangitis
Toxins	Alcohol Arsenic Drugs
Metabolic	Nonalcoholic steatohepatitis Alpha-1 antitrypsin deficiency Hemochromatosis Wilson disease Glycogen storage diseases Lysosomal storage diseases Galactosemia
Vascular	Cardiac cirrhosis Budd-Chiari syndrome Sinusoidal obstruction syndrome
Granulomatous	Sarcoidosis Tuberculosis Syphilis
Cryptogenic	Unrecognized metabolic-associated fatty liver disease, infections, or drugs

on the epidemiology of cirrhosis and its complications has resulted in a decline in liver transplant listings for HCV. In contrast, the growing prevalence of metabolic-associated fatty liver disease (MAFLD), previously known as nonalcoholic fatty liver disease, is reflected in its current prominence as a cause of cirrhosis. MAFLD is anticipated to become the single most frequent cause of chronic liver disease and cirrhosis in the mid to second half of this century.

Clinical Findings

In the absence of hepatic decompensation, the overwhelming majority of individuals with cirrhosis are asymptomatic and may only exhibit subtle clinical findings. Clues to the presence of cirrhosis can include elevated serum aminotransferases and/or bilirubin, decreased albumin, and prolongation of the prothrombin time. Approximately 10% to 17% of individuals with unexplained elevation of aminotransferases have unrecognized cirrhosis. Thrombocytopenia in the absence of a primary hematologic explanation is another clue to the presence of cirrhosis and primarily reflects hypersplenism due to portal hypertension but also diminished production of thrombopoietin, a platelet growth and development factor synthesized by the liver. A platelet count below $160 \times 10/\mu L$ provides the highest diagnostic accuracy for cirrhosis among routine blood tests (sensitivity 74%, specificity 88%, positive likelihood ratio 6.3, negative likelihood ratio 0.29). Thrombocytopenia is also a component of noninvasive scoring systems that predict fibrosis, such as the AST (aspartate aminotransferase) to Platelet Ratio Index (APRI) and Fibrosis-4 (FIB-4).

Physical examination may reveal somewhat diminished liver span by percussion and a firm liver edge on palpation. Splenomegaly is suggested by dullness to percussion in the left upper abdominal quadrant or a palpable spleen tip. Cutaneous signs of cirrhosis include palmar erythema, spider nevi, facial telangiectasia, decreased chest and/or axillary hair, inversion of the normal male pubic hair pattern, Terry nails ("ground glass" appearance of nails with absent lunula), and Muehrcke nails (paired, white, transverse bands separated by normal color). Nail clubbing may also be present in individuals with cirrhosis, particularly in those with hepatopulmonary syndrome. Dupuytren contracture is relatively

TABLE 2 Stages of Cirrhosis Based on Clinical Complications and 1-Year Outcome Probabilities

CIRRHOSIS	D'AMICO STAGE	COMPLICATIONS	PROBABILITY OF ADVANCING TO NEXT STAGE	1-YEAR MORTALITY
Compensated	Stage 1	(−) varices (−) ascites	7%	1%
	Stage 2	(+) varices (−) ascites	6.6%	3.4%
Decompensated	Stage 3	(+) ascites (+) varices	7.6%	20%
	Stage 4	(+) variceal hemorrhage (+) ascites	–	57%

From D'Amico G, Garcia-Tsao G, Pagliaro L: Natural history and prognostic indicators of survival in cirrhosis: A systematic review of 118 studies. *J Hepatol* 44:217–231, 2006.

TABLE 3 Child-Turcotte-Pugh Classification

CLINICAL AND LABORATORY CRITERIA	POINTS		
	1	2	3
Albumin (g/dL)	>3.5	2.8–3.5	<2.8
Ascites	None	Mild to moderate (diuretic responsive)	Severe (diuretic refractory)
Bilirubin (mg/dL)	<2	2–3	>3
Encephalopathy	None	Mild to moderate (grade 1 or 2)	Severe (grade 3 or 4)
Prothrombin time Prolongation in seconds International normalized ratio	<4 <1.7	4–6 1.7–2.3	>6 >2.3

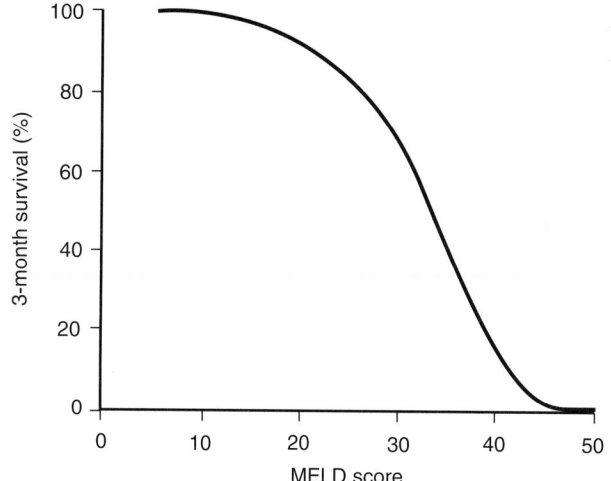

Figure 1 Relationship between Model for End-Stage Liver Disease (MELD) score and survival at 3 months. From Carrion AF, Martin P. In: *Sleisenger and Fordtran's Gastrointestinal and Liver Disease*, 11th ed., Chapter 97, page 1538. Elsevier; 2021.

common in alcohol-related cirrhosis but its pathogenesis is not well understood. Palmar erythema due to altered sex hormone metabolism is more evident on the thenar and hypothenar eminences and typically spares the central portion of the palm. Hypogonadism in both sexes and gynecomastia and testicular atrophy in males can be detected, reflecting altered sex hormone metabolism (increased production of androstenedione, enhanced aromatization to estrone, and increased conversion to estradiol). The catabolic effects of advanced cirrhosis often result in marked sarcopenia, which adversely affects quality of life and survival and is also associated with poorer outcomes after liver transplantation.

Various noninvasive methods for evaluation of liver fibrosis are now widely used in clinical practice for staging of hepatic fibrosis and diagnosis of cirrhosis. These include vibration-controlled transient elastography (Fibroscan), acoustic radiation force impulse (ARFI), shear wave and point quantification elastography, and magnetic resonance elastography.

Natural History of Cirrhosis and Prognostic Models

Cirrhosis may be broadly categorized into two distinct clinical phases, regardless of the etiology: compensated and decompensated. Compensated cirrhosis implies the absence of index complications such as jaundice, ascites, hepatic encephalopathy, or gastroesophageal variceal hemorrhage. In contrast, hepatic decompensation indicates an advanced phase of the disease, which is rapidly progressive and characterized by development of one or more complications and diminished hepatocellular function with prolongation of the prothrombin time and hypoalbuminemia. Characterizing cirrhosis as compensated or decompensated is simple and reproducible and offers useful prognostic information for clinical practice (Table 2).

More precise prognostic models such as the Child Turcotte Pugh (Table 3) and the Model for End-Stage Liver Disease (MELD) are also widely used, the latter being considered the most accurate predictor of short-term mortality for individuals with cirrhosis and serving as the basis for the current organ allocation system in liver transplantation in the United States and elsewhere (calculator available at https://optn.transplant-.hrsa.gov/resources/allocation-calculators/meld-calculator/). The most recent modification of the MELD score resulted in inclusion of the serum sodium into the formula: MELD-Na. Incorporation of the serum sodium in the MELD formula increases its prognostic accuracy in patients with relatively low scores and hyponatremia.

The specific etiology of cirrhosis may help determine its prognosis. For instance, persistent viremia in individuals with chronic HBV or HCV infection is implicated in the development of decompensated cirrhosis. Effective antiviral therapy can abort progression of chronic viral hepatitis to cirrhosis and decompensation.

Although cirrhosis per se is not an indication for liver transplantation, it is important to identify individuals with cirrhosis who should be considered for liver transplantation. Development of an index complication of cirrhosis such as gastroesophageal variceal hemorrhage, ascites, or hepatic encephalopathy is an indication to refer a patient for liver transplantation and initiate pretransplant evaluation. The MELD score provides objective and reproducible prognostication of short-term survival without liver transplantation (Figure 1), and data from a seminal study showed that liver transplantation is associated with improved survival in individuals with MELD scores greater than 17.

TABLE 4 Recommendations for Primary Prophylaxis Against Esophageal Variceal Hemorrhage

SIZE OF VARICES	RISK OF HEMORRHAGE	SURVEILLANCE INTERVAL	PRIMARY PROPHYLAXIS
No varices	CTP class A	EGD every 2 years if ongoing liver injury (i.e., obesity or alcohol abuse) or every 3 years if liver injury is quiescent (i.e., viral eradication or alcohol abstinence)	None
	CTP class B/C	EGD yearly	None
Small esophageal varices	CTP class A	EGD yearly if ongoing liver injury (i.e., obesity or alcohol abuse) or every 2 years if liver injury is quiescent (i.e., viral eradication or alcohol abstinence)	BB may be used
	CTP class B/C	EGD yearly; if BB are used, repeat EGD unnecessary	BB recommended
Large esophageal varices	CTP class A/B/C	If BB are used, repeat EGD unnecessary; if no BB, repeat EGD for EVL every 2–8 weeks until variceal eradication, then once in 3–6 months, and regularly every 6–12 months	Either BB or EVL recommended

BB, Beta blocker; *CTP*, Child-Turcotte-Pugh; *EGD*, esophagogastroduodenoscopy; *EVL*, endoscopic variceal ligation. Child-Turcotte-Pugh class obtained by adding points for each variable.
Class A: 5 to 6 points (compensated cirrhosis); class B: 7 to 9 points (decompensated cirrhosis); class C: 10 to 15 points (decompensated cirrhosis)

Major Complications of Cirrhosis

Portal Hypertension

Although portal hypertension can be inferred by clues such as splenomegaly with thrombocytopenia in a patient with cirrhosis, it is defined by a hepatic venous pressure gradient (HVPG) greater than 5 mm Hg. This gradient is calculated by subtracting the measured free hepatic vein pressure from the wedged hepatic venous pressure (a measurement that reflects portal venous pressure by using the same hemodynamic principle as the wedged pulmonary capillary pressure to assess left atrial pressure). Clinically significant portal hypertension typically occurs when the HVPG is 10 mm Hg or greater, at which threshold gastroesophageal varices and ascites occur. Unfortunately, accurate noninvasive measurement of portal pressure is not available, limiting its use in routine clinical practice as it requires passage of a transjugular catheter.

Increased intrahepatic resistance to portal venous flow aggravated by increased splanchnic blood flow in cirrhosis leads to portal hypertension. In addition to cirrhosis, which is the most common cause of portal hypertension in Western countries (hepatic schistosomiasis is the leading cause in areas where this infection is common), other disorders may result in pre- or posthepatic portal hypertension. Portal vein thrombosis is a common cause of prehepatic portal hypertension. Cardiomyopathy, constrictive pericarditis, Budd-Chiari syndrome, and inferior vena cava webs may result in posthepatic portal hypertension. Ascites and gastroesophageal variceal hemorrhage are the two most common complications of portal hypertension in cirrhosis. Less common but clinically significant complications include portal hypertensive gastropathy, hepatic hydrothorax, hepatopulmonary syndrome, portopulmonary hypertension, and hepatorenal syndrome.

Gastroesophageal Variceal Hemorrhage

Portal hypertension leads to formation of multiple portosystemic collaterals, including gastroesophageal varices. Formation of gastroesophageal varices typically occurs when the HVPG is 10 mm Hg or greater, with the risk for variceal hemorrhage increasing once HVPG is greater than 12 mm Hg. Gastroesophageal varices are present in approximately 50% of patients with cirrhosis and are more common in patients with hepatic decompensation (Child-Turcotte-Pugh class C). Variceal hemorrhage is the most dramatic complication of cirrhosis and occurs at a rate of 5% to 15% per year. Risk factors for variceal hemorrhage include larger variceal size, more advanced hepatic decompensation, and presence of vascular "red wale" signs during endoscopic evaluation. Esophageal varices are classified according to their size as small (≤5 mm) or large (>5 mm).

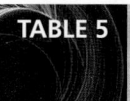

TABLE 5 Classification of Gastroesophageal and Gastric Varices and Recommendations for Primary Prophylaxis

TYPE OF VARICES	CHARACTERISTICS	PRIMARY PROPHYLAXIS
Gastroesophageal varices type 1 (GOV1)	Extension of esophageal varices along the lesser curvature into the gastric cardia	Similar to esophageal varices
Gastroesophageal varices type 2 (GOV2)	Extension of the esophageal varices along the greater curvature into the gastric fundus	BB can be used, although data not as strong as for esophageal varices
Isolated gastric varices type 1 (IGV1)	Gastric varices localized in the fundus	If high risk, consider BB or cyanoacrylate injection
Isolated gastric varices type 2 (IGV2)	Gastric varices localized in the antrum	No data, consider BB if high risk

BB, Beta blocker.

Screening for gastroesophageal varices with esophagogastroduodenoscopy (EGD) is recommended when cirrhosis is suspected. Management strategies for patients with esophageal varices that have not previously bled (primary prophylaxis) are summarized in Table 4.

Management of esophageal varices that have previously bled (secondary prophylaxis) includes a combination of a nonselective beta blocker with endoscopic variceal ligation (EVL). The dose of the nonselective beta blocker should be titrated to the maximal tolerated dose (resting heart rate of 55–60 beats/min or 25% decrease from baseline) and EVL should be repeated frequently (every 2 weeks or so) until complete variceal obliteration. Recurrence of esophageal varices may occur following EVL; thus surveillance EGD is recommended: first EGD performed 3 to 6 months after variceal obliteration and then at 6- to 12-month intervals.

Gastric varices are classified according to relationship with esophageal varices and location (Table 5).

Acute variceal hemorrhage occurs at a yearly rate of 5% to 15% and is associated with high mortality (at least 20% at

6 weeks). Adequate resuscitation is crucial in acute variceal hemorrhage with some additional precautions. Patients with variceal hemorrhage are at high risk for aspiration, and endotracheal intubation for airway protection should be performed prior to endoscopy. Overly aggressive expansion of blood volume should be avoided as it may result in increased portal venous pressure. A target hemoglobin level of between 7 and 9 g/dL is appropriate. Current guidelines recommend against correcting the international normalized ratio (INR) by use of fresh frozen plasma or recombinant factor VIIa, as this has not shown a clear benefit in individuals with acute variceal hemorrhage. There are no data to support or recommend against transfusion of platelets in this clinical scenario. Prophylactic broad-spectrum antibiotics (i.e., intravenous ceftriaxone [Rocephin][1]) reduce bacterial infections, risk of rebleeding, and mortality. Administration of vasoactive drugs such as octreotide (Sandostatin)[1] or terlipressin (Lucassin)[5] results in increased rates of initial endoscopic control of bleeding, reduced 7-day mortality, and lower transfusion requirements. EGD is recommended within 12 hours and EVL is the endoscopic treatment of choice for management of esophageal varices. Balloon tamponade (i.e., Sengstaken Blakemore, Minnesota, or Linton-Nachlas tubes) or esophageal stenting are effective rescue therapies when variceal hemorrhage cannot be controlled with standard endoscopic therapy. The role of transjugular intrahepatic portosystemic shunt (TIPS) has expanded from a salvage intervention for individuals with recurrent variceal hemorrhage following EVL to an early "preemptive" intervention in carefully selected individuals at high risk for treatment failure (Child-Turcotte-Pugh class B or C but with MELD scores ≤13) following EVL, in which case it appears to be superior to beta blocker plus EVL. Patients who survive an episode of variceal hemorrhage should receive secondary prophylaxis with a combination of a nonselective beta blocker and repeated EVL until complete obliteration of the varices is achieved. Cyanoacrylate injection, TIPS, or balloon occluded transvenous obliteration (BRTO) are the treatments of choice for management of gastric variceal hemorrhage.

Ascites

Ascites denotes pathologic accumulation of fluid in the peritoneal cavity (>25 mL) and is the most common complication of cirrhosis. Portal hypertension is required for development of cirrhotic ascites, as individuals with HVPG less than 12 mm Hg do not develop this complication. Importantly, sinusoidal hypertension appears to be a requirement for development of ascites, as prehepatic portal hypertension does not invariably result in development of this complication. Other relevant mechanisms include splanchnic vasodilatation and its consequences such as humorally mediated sodium retention and diminished free-water excretion by the kidneys, hypoproteinemia and reduced oncotic pressure, and disruption of normal lymphatic drainage in the liver due to extensive fibrosis.

Ascites can be demonstrated by physical examination when its volume is greater than 1500 mL, although ultrasonography can detect as little as 100 mL. Clinical signs include flank dullness on percussion, shifting dullness, and, if the amount of ascites present is large, demonstration of a fluid wave. A diagnostic paracentesis is mandatory in the following settings: new-onset ascites, change in clinical status including hospitalization of a patient with previously diagnosed ascites, and suggestion of spontaneous bacterial peritonitis (SBP). The following tests on the fluid are indicated: leukocyte count with differential (purple or lavender top tube with ethylenediaminetetraacetic acid [EDTA]), culture (on two blood culture bottles inoculated at the bedside), total protein, and albumin (red top tube). The appearance of the ascitic fluid may yield important clinical clues (Table 6). The serum-to-ascites albumin gradient (SAAG), obtained by subtracting the ascitic fluid albumin value from the serum albumin value, helps make a distinction between transudative and exudative ascites. A gradient of 1.1 g/dL or greater confirms portal hypertension as the etiology of ascites,

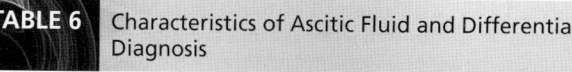

TABLE 6	Characteristics of Ascitic Fluid and Differential Diagnosis	
FLUID APPEARANCE	**DIFFERENTIAL DIAGNOSIS**	**BIOCHEMICAL HINTS ON FLUID ANALYSIS**
Clear	Uncomplicated transudative ascites due to cirrhosis	WBC <500 cells/μL, PMN <250 cells/μL, SAAG ≥1.1
Turbid/cloudy	Infection	PMN ≥250 cells/μL
Bloody	Traumatic paracentesis, hemoperitoneum	RBC >10,000 cells/μL
Milky	Chylous ascites due to obstruction or trauma of lymphatic vessels or thoracic duct	Triglycerides >200 md/dL

PMN, Polymorphonuclear cells; *SAAG,* serum-to-ascites albumin gradient; *WBC,* white blood cell.

whereas a value less than 1.1 g/dL suggests etiologies other than portal hypertension. The absolute number of polymorphonuclear (PMN) cells in the ascitic fluid is an important clue to SBP.

Cirrhotic ascites is unlikely to resolve without specific therapeutic intervention. Management of ascites is centered on sodium restriction rather than free-water restriction; total dietary intake of sodium should be less than 2000 mg (88 mmol) per day and compliance with this intervention can be documented by monitoring urinary sodium concentrations. A sodium-to-potassium concentration ratio of greater than 1 on a random urine sample correlates well with a 24-hour sodium excretion greater than 78 mmol/day and implies compliance with sodium restriction. Nevertheless, dietary restriction of sodium is efficacious in only 10% of patients, and enhanced natriuresis is typically needed to provide adequate control of ascites. Combining diuretics that work at different sites of the nephron is more effective than using a single agent. Aldosterone is upregulated in cirrhosis owing to diminished effective arterial blood volume and consequential increased renin and angiotensin activity, resulting in enhanced renal sodium and free water retention. Spironolactone (Aldactone) competitively inhibits aldosterone-dependent sodium–potassium exchange in the distal convoluted renal tubule and the collecting ducts. The recommended initial dose of spironolactone for patients with ascites due to portal hypertension is 100 mg orally daily. Administration of a loop-acting diuretic such as furosemide (Lasix)[1] is recommended in addition to spironolactone, as it potentiates natriuresis. The recommended initial dose for furosemide is 40 mg orally daily. Further increases in doses of diuretics should be made maintaining this 100:40 ratio to a maximum dose of 400 mg orally daily of spironolactone and 160 mg orally daily of furosemide, as it prevents hypo- or hyperkalemia. Renal function and electrolytes must be monitored regularly, particularly after dose modifications. Tender gynecomastia is an unpleasant side effect of spironolactone, and some patients may need to discontinue it, in which case amiloride (Midamor)[1] (10–20 mg orally daily) can be used. Two outcomes may occur in patients with ascites that is not adequately controlled with diuretics: (1) refractory ascites to maximum diuretic doses and sodium restriction, which typically recurs rapidly following large-volume paracenteses (LVP) and (2) inability to increase diuretic doses owing to symptomatic hypotension or deterioration in renal function as evidenced by increasing serum creatinine levels.

[1]Not FDA approved for this indication.
[5]Investigational drug in the United States.

[1]Not FDA approved for this indication.

Repeated LVP with removal of more than 5 L of ascitic fluid per session is a safe and effective intervention to treat refractory ascites; however, mortality within 6 months is 20% once this develops, reflecting the severity of the underlying liver disease, and thus patients should be referred for evaluation for liver transplantation. Continued dietary restriction of sodium is necessary to avoid overly frequent LVP, and continuation of diuretics should be assessed on a case-by-case basis, taking into consideration potential benefits and adverse reactions. Expansion of plasma volume for patients undergoing LVP is endorsed by current guidelines and supported by data demonstrating reduced postparacentesis circulatory dysfunction and improved survival. Plasma volume should be expanded with albumin at a dose of 6 to 8 g/L of ascitic fluid removed during or immediately after LVP.

Insertion of TIPS corrects portal hypertension and offers an attractive alternative for amelioration of refractory ascites in selected patients. TIPS is a minimally invasive technique in which an endovascular stent is used to create an intrahepatic portocaval shunt and has replaced surgical shunts. Transplant-free survival is superior with TIPS compared with repeated LVP. Assessment of systolic and diastolic heart functions is recommended prior to TIPS as significant hemodynamic changes occur following the creation of the portosystemic shunt that can result in post-TIPS heart failure in individuals with underlying systolic or diastolic dysfunction.

The MELD score is a prognostic model that was initially developed to assess risk of death following TIPS placement, and data demonstrate that patients with a MELD score greater than 18 are at high risk of death; thus TIPS should be avoided in this population. TIPS results in hepatic encephalopathy in a high proportion of patients, but pharmacologic therapy typically provides adequate treatment for this complication.

Spontaneous Bacterial Peritonitis

Cirrhosis and portal hypertension are associated with abnormal intestinal permeability leading to bacterial translocation resulting in SBP. The most commonly isolated microorganisms responsible for SBP are *Escherichia coli* (43%), *Klebsiella pneumoniae* (11%), *Streptococcus pneumoniae* (9%), other streptococcal species (19%), *Enterobacteriaceae* (4%), *Staphylococcus* (3%), and miscellaneous organisms depending on the region of the world (10%). A small-volume diagnostic paracentesis (30–60 mL) rather than LVP (which can increase the risk of hepatorenal syndrome in the setting of SBP) is mandatory for diagnosis of SBP and should be performed prior to administration of antibiotic therapy. Aerobic and anaerobic blood culture bottles should be inoculated at the bedside to avoid contamination and to increase diagnostic yield. Diagnosis of SBP is supported by the presence of 250 PMN/μL or more in the ascitic fluid without an obvious source of infection. Based on the PMN count and the microbiologic analysis of the ascitic fluid, four clinical scenarios summarized in Table 7 may be encountered.

Treatment of SBP is centered on administration of broad-spectrum empiric antibiotics with bactericidal activity against the likely infecting bacteria. Third-generation cephalosporins such as cefotaxime (Claforan) 2 g intravenously every 8 hours or ceftriaxone (Rocephin) 2 g intravenously daily offer appropriate antimicrobial coverage and are initial agents of choice for treatment of SBP. For patients allergic to beta-lactams, alternatives include fluoroquinolones such as levofloxacin (Levaquin),[1] although this agent exhibits less penetration into the ascitic fluid compared with a third-generation cephalosporin.

Current guidelines do not recommend routinely performing a follow-up paracentesis in patients with a typical initial presentation of SBP and when antibiotic therapy results in rapid clinical improvement. Repeat paracentesis, however, may be indicated to document sterility of ascitic fluid and reduction in the PMN count in patients with a slow or absent response to antibiotic therapy or in those with atypical microorganisms on initial culture results.

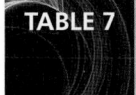

TABLE 7 Spontaneous Bacterial Peritonitis and Associated Conditions Based on Characteristics of the Ascitic Fluid

CLINICAL ENTITY	POLYMOR-PHONUCLEAR CELL COUNT	CULTURE RESULTS	ANTIBIOTICS RECOMMENDED
Spontaneous bacterial peritonitis	≥250 cells/μL	Positive, single organism	Yes
Culture-negative neutrocytic ascites	≥250 cells/μL	Negative	Yes
Monomicrobial nonneutrocytic bacterascites	<250 cells/μL	Positive, single organism	Yes
Polymicrobial bacterascites	<250 cells/μL	Positive, multiple organisms	Yes

Plasma volume expansion with albumin is an important adjunct to antibiotic therapy in patients with SBP, as it decreases the incidence of acute kidney injury and reduces mortality. The physiologic effects of intravenous infusion of albumin include increased oncotic pressure with consequential expansion of the effective arterial blood volume, as well as its ability to bind a wide range of endogenous and exogenous ligands including bacterial lipopolysaccharides, reactive oxygen species, nitric oxide and other nitrogen reactive species, and prostaglandins, thus modulating the inflammatory response. Current guidelines recommend a selective approach for administration of intravenous albumin to patients with SBP. Specifically, this therapy should be reserved for high-risk individuals such as those with serum creatinine greater than 1 mg/dL, blood urea nitrogen greater than 30 mL/dL, or total serum bilirubin greater than 4 mg/dL. The recommended dosage of albumin is 1.5 g/kg of body weight within 6 hours of establishing the diagnosis of SBP and a second dose of 1 g/kg on day 3.

Following an episode of SBP, recurrence occurs in 69% of individuals within 1 year; thus secondary prophylaxis is indicated, and current guidelines recommend long-term use of norfloxacin (Noroxin)[1] 400 mg orally twice daily or trimethoprim/sulfamethoxazole (Bactrim DS)[1] one double-strength tablet orally daily. Risk factors for recurrent SBP include ascitic fluid total protein concentration less than 1 g/dL and gastroesophageal variceal hemorrhage. Recommended antibiotic prophylaxis for patients hospitalized with gastroesophageal variceal hemorrhage include ceftriaxone[1] 1 g intravenously daily; once the patient is able to tolerate oral antibiotics, this may be changed to trimethoprim/sulfamethoxazole[1] one double-strength tablet orally daily, ciprofloxacin (Cipro)[1] 500 mg orally daily, or norfloxacin[1] 400 mg orally twice daily for a total of 7 days of antibiotic therapy. Importantly, some data suggest an increased risk for SBP in patients with cirrhosis and ascites taking proton pump inhibitors; thus unnecessary use of these agents should be avoided. The exact mechanism by which acid suppression increases the risk of SBP in cirrhosis is unclear, but intestinal bacterial overgrowth, increased intestinal permeability, and altered intestinal immune response may play important roles.

Hepatorenal Syndrome

The ominous significance of impaired renal function as a predictor of mortality in patients with cirrhosis is reflected by inclusion of the serum creatinine level in the MELD score. Renal dysfunction is commonly encountered in patients with cirrhosis, particularly in those with hepatic decompensation. Some studies reported acute kidney injury (AKI) in approximately 20% of

---

[1]Not FDA approved for this indication.

hospitalized patients with cirrhosis. The differential diagnosis of AKI in patients with cirrhosis is broad and includes common etiologies such as acute tubular necrosis and nephrotoxicity, but specific glomerulopathies associated with HBV and HCV must be considered (i.e., membranous and membranoproliferative glomerulonephritides). In addition, nonalcoholic steatohepatitis is characterized by a high prevalence of type 2 diabetes mellitus and systemic hypertension; thus patients are at increased risk for diabetic and hypertensive nephropathies. Hepatorenal syndrome (HRS) is one of several potential causes of AKI that occurs in patients with cirrhosis and portal hypertension but has also been recognized in patients with acute liver failure. Importantly, HRS is a diagnosis of exclusion, and other etiologies of AKI should be considered. The pathophysiology of HRS includes splanchnic vasodilatation causing a decline in renal perfusion with consequent reductions in the glomerular filtration rate and renal excretion of sodium (typically <10 mEq/L).

There are two distinct types of HRS depending on the acuity and severity of renal dysfunction. HRS-AKI, previously known as type I HRS, is characterized by rapid deterioration of renal function with at least a twofold increase in serum creatinine to a level greater than 2.5 mg/dL and is often precipitated by SBP, acute alcoholic hepatitis, or gastrointestinal hemorrhage. Criteria for diagnosis of HRS-AKI includes: (1) cirrhosis with ascites; (2) diagnosis of AKI according to the International Club of Ascites (ICA)-AKI criteria (increase in serum creatinine by ≥0.3 mg/dL within 48 hours, or increase in serum creatinine to ≥1.5 times baseline within 7 days); (3) absence of shock; (4) no sustained improvement of renal function (serum creatinine <1.5 mg/dL) following at least 2 days of diuretic withdrawal and volume expansion with albumin at 1 g/kg/day up to 100 g/day; (5) no current or recent exposure to nephrotoxic agents; and (6) absence of parenchymal renal disease as defined by proteinuria <0.5 g/day, no microhematuria (<50 red cells/high-power field), and normal renal ultrasonography. HRS-chronic kidney disease (CKD), previously referred to as type II HRS, is more indolent and is associated with less severe renal impairment, typically resulting in ascites resistant to diuretics. Prognosis also differs significantly for both types of HRS, with the median survival in the absence of liver transplantation being 2 weeks for HRS-AKI and 6 months for HRS-CKD.

Discontinuation of all diuretics and nephrotoxic agents is critical in patients with HRS. Plasma volume expansion with administration of intravenous albumin[1] at a dose of 1 g/kg of body weight (up to a maximum of 100 g/day) to increase renal perfusion is recommended. HRS is characterized by absent or minimal proteinuria (<500 mg/day) and normal urine sediment reflecting the lack of intrinsic renal disease. Renal ultrasonography is also recommended as it provides good assessment for chronic parenchymal changes that may suggest the presence of a chronic underlying renal disease and accurately rules out obstructive nephropathy.

Patients with HRS require either improvement in hepatic function or liver transplantation for renal function to recover. Pharmacotherapy can be used as a bridge to liver transplantation. Based on the pathophysiology of HRS-AKI, vasoconstriction with alpha-adrenergic agonists (i.e., midodrine [ProAmatine][1] or norepinephrine [Levophed][1]) or vasopressin analogs (i.e., terlipressin [Lucassin][5]) is the therapy of choice along with plasma volume expansion achieved with intravenous albumin infusion. The use of norepinephrine is reserved for critically ill patients with HRS-AKI. Terlipressin is not licensed for use in the United States. The combination of the somatostatin analog octreotide[1] along with oral midodrine and intravenous albumin infusion appears to have beneficial effects based on results from small clinical trials and is currently recommended in the United States for noncritically ill patients with HRS-AKI. Data from a meta-analysis support the efficacy of vasoconstrictor therapy (terlipressin, octreotide + midodrine, or norepinephrine) in combination with intravenous albumin in reducing short-term mortality in patients with type I HRS.

---

[1]Not FDA approved for this indication.
[5]Investigational drug in the United States.

TABLE 8 West Haven Criteria for Grading Hepatic Encephalopathy

GRADE	LEVEL OF CONSCIOUSNESS	INTELLECT AND BEHAVIOR	NEUROLOGIC FINDINGS
0	Normal	Normal	Normal examination, abnormal neuropsychiatric testing
1	Mild lack of awareness	Shortened attention span	Impaired addition or subtraction, mild asterixis
2	Lethargy	Mild–moderate disorientation, inappropriate behavior	Severe asterixis, slurred speech
3	Somnolence but arousable	Severe disorientation, inexplicable behavior	Clonus, hyperreflexia, muscular rigidity
4	Coma	Coma	Decerebrate posture

The largest randomized clinical trial to date evaluating terlipressin in combination with albumin versus placebo plus albumin showed no difference in reversal of HRS-AKI, but the terlipressin group had greater improvement in renal function. Renal replacement therapy may be needed for patients with HRS not responding to pharmacologic therapy awaiting liver transplantation; however, mortality is exceedingly high and hypotensive episodes commonly occur during hemodialysis. Following liver transplantation, renal function improves in approximately 60% of patients with HRS.

Hepatic Encephalopathy

Hepatic encephalopathy (HE) is a clinical syndrome of reversible neuropsychiatric impairment of varying severity. There is continuing controversy about its exact pathogenesis, but gut-derived toxins, including ammonia, are clearly implicated. Features of HE may be subclinical (covert) or clinically evident (overt) and include a wide range of neuropsychiatric signs and symptoms. The prevalence of HE varies depending on the clinical subtype and the severity of liver disease, with cumulative prevalence rates of up to 80% for covert HE and 30% to 40% for overt HE in patients with cirrhosis. Although the West Haven criteria are widely used for grading the severity of HE (Table 8), current guidelines recommend using three additional axes to classify HE based on the etiology, time course, and presence or absence of a precipitating factor (Table 9).

Covert HE is considered preclinical and encompasses minimal HE (features of HE that are only diagnosed by specialized neuropsychiatric testing) and grade 1 HE as per West Haven criteria. In contrast, overt HE is characterized by clinical findings of HE ranging from subtle changes in orientation and presence of asterixis to hepatic coma (grades 2–4 per West Haven criteria).

Specialized testing is necessary to establish a diagnosis of covert HE. The psychometric HE score is regarded as the gold standard, but additional assessments include the number connection test, computerized tests such as the inhibitory control test, the cognitive drug research battery, and electroencephalogram. These tests, however, are not applicable in routine clinical practice and usually require consultation with a specialist. A smartphone application that evaluates psychomotor speed and cognitive alertness has been developed and validated as a point-of-care screening tool for covert HE: EncephalApp Stroop.

The diagnosis of overt HE is clinical and supported by the presence of a wide spectrum of global neurologic deficits. Severe HE, grades 3 and 4 West Haven criteria, should prompt attention to airway protection, and endotracheal intubation ought to be considered.

TYPE OF HEPATIC ENCEPHALOPATHY	GRADE		TIME COURSE	SPONTANEOUS/PRECIPITATED
A (acute liver failure)	MHE	Covert	Episodic (one episode in 6 months)	Spontaneous: no precipitating factor discovered
B (portosystemic bypass)	1	Covert	Recurrent (more than one episode in 6 months)	
	2	Overt	Persistent (no return to normal baseline)	Precipitated by one or more specific factors
C (cirrhosis)	3	Overt		
	4	Overt		

From Patidar KR, Bajaj JS: Covert and overt hepatic encephalopathy: diagnosis and management. *Clin Gastroenterol Hepatol* 13:2048–2061, 2015.

There are no laboratory markers that can be accurately used to diagnose overt HE. Blood ammonia levels lack sensitivity and specificity and correlate poorly with the severity of encephalopathy. Furthermore, a normal ammonia level does not preclude the presence of HE, and venous ammonia levels are influenced by several other factors including phlebotomy technique and handling of the blood specimen. Efforts must be directed at identifying potential precipitating factors for HE, such as compliance with treatment of HE, new medications, gastrointestinal bleeding, AKI, electrolyte imbalances, and infections.

Management of covert and overt HE is centered on the use of nonabsorbable disaccharides and antibiotics. Lactulose (Enulose) is the most widely used nonabsorbable disaccharide. Although the exact mechanism responsible for its therapeutic efficacy is still unclear, this agent is degraded by colonic microbiota to short-chain organic acids, resulting in acidification of the intestinal lumen and increased conversion of absorbable ammonia to nonabsorbable ammonium. The starting dosage for lactulose depends on the acuity and severity of HE but must be titrated to achieve two to four soft bowel movements per day. For patients who cannot tolerate oral administration (i.e., high risk for aspiration or coma), lactulose can be administered as an enema (300 mL of lactulose solution 10 g/15 mL in 700 mL of saline or water). The cathartic effects of nonabsorbable disaccharides may result in profuse diarrhea, dehydration, and hypernatremia. Rifaximin (Xifaxan) is a broad-spectrum antibiotic with activity against gram-positive, gram-negative, and anaerobic enteric bacteria that can be used in addition to lactulose for prevention of recurrent episodes of HE. Data from clinical trials show marked reductions in HE-related hospitalization and significant improvements in health-related quality of life in patients treated with a combination of lactulose and rifaximin without an increased rate of adverse events.

The efficacy and safety of other pharmacologic therapies such as probiotics,[7] branched-chain amino acids[7], L-ornithine L-aspartate (LOLA),[7] ammonia scavengers, and other laxatives (i.e., polyethylene glycol [MiraLax][1]) need to be further confirmed by clinical trials. Because of concerns about oto- and nephrotoxicity, neomycin is no longer used.

Creation of a portosystemic shunt (now usually with TIPS) for management of complications of portal hypertension is associated with a 13% to 36% incidence of overt HE. Careful patient selection prior to insertion of TIPS and medical therapy with nonabsorbable disaccharides with or without additional rifaximin remain standard therapy; however, despite compliance, approximately 3% to 7% of patients have recurrent or persistent overt HE post-TIPS. For these patients, endovascular techniques aimed at decreasing the size of the shunt should be considered.

Liver transplantation offers definitive therapy for patients with end-stage liver disease, resulting in restoration of hepatic synthetic function and resolution of complications associated with portal hypertension. However, residual cognitive impairments may persist following liver transplantation, adversely impacting health-related quality of life.

Hepatocellular Carcinoma

Hepatocellular carcinoma (HCC) is the most common primary hepatic malignancy in adults, currently representing the fifth most common cancer and the second leading cause of cancer-related death worldwide. The epidemiology of HCC varies significantly by region and ethnicity. The majority of patients with HCC in Western populations (95%) have underlying cirrhosis (predominantly due to chronic HCV infection, alcohol-related liver disease, and nonalcoholic steatohepatitis), thus limiting applicability of surgical resection (see later) as curative therapy. In contrast, only 60% of patients with HCC in Eastern populations have cirrhosis, largely reflecting the high prevalence of chronic HBV infection and its oncogenic potential. Regions of the world with intermediate to high incidence of this malignancy (more than 3 cases per 100,000 persons per year) include Asia, sub-Saharan Africa, and Western Europe. North and South America have been typically considered low-incidence regions; however, over the past two decades there has been a steady increase in the incidence of HCC, particularly in the United States.

Current guidelines endorse implementation of surveillance strategies for early diagnosis of HCC in individuals at risk for this malignancy and recommend the use of ultrasonography every 6 months as the primary surveillance modality. Populations at risk for HCC that benefit from surveillance include individuals with cirrhosis of any etiology, Asian males with chronic HBV over age 40, Asian females with chronic HBV over age 50, patients with chronic HBV and family history of HCC, African/North American Black populations with chronic HBV, and individuals with stage 4 primary biliary cholangitis.

HCC can be accurately diagnosed without the need for liver biopsy by contrast-enhanced multiphase cross-sectional imaging modalities such as computed tomography (CT) or magnetic resonance imaging (MRI) based on specific patterns of contrast enhancement of the tumor in relation to the hepatic parenchyma. Key diagnostic characteristics for HCC on CT or MRI are contrast enhancement of the tumor during the early arterial phase and "washout" of contrast from the tumor during the portal venous and delayed phases. Additional features include presence of a capsule and interval growth of the lesion when previous imaging studies are used for comparison. Biopsy of the tumor carries a small risk for tumor seeding in the biopsy-needle tract (approximately 3%) and is rarely required to diagnose HCC owing to high accuracy of CT and MRI. The use of serum alpha-fetoprotein (AFP) has been controversial for routine surveillance owing to its low sensitivity and poor specificity; however, data from a recent meta-analysis suggest that addition of AFP to ultrasound increases the sensitivity of HCC detection. If not previously available, once a focal liver lesion is identified on imaging studies, AFP should be obtained as an additional diagnostic tool. AFP levels greater than 200 ng/mL are highly specific for HCC, and longitudinal follow-up of serum levels permits evaluation of response to therapeutic

---

[1]Not FDA approved for this indication.
[7]Available as a dietary supplement.

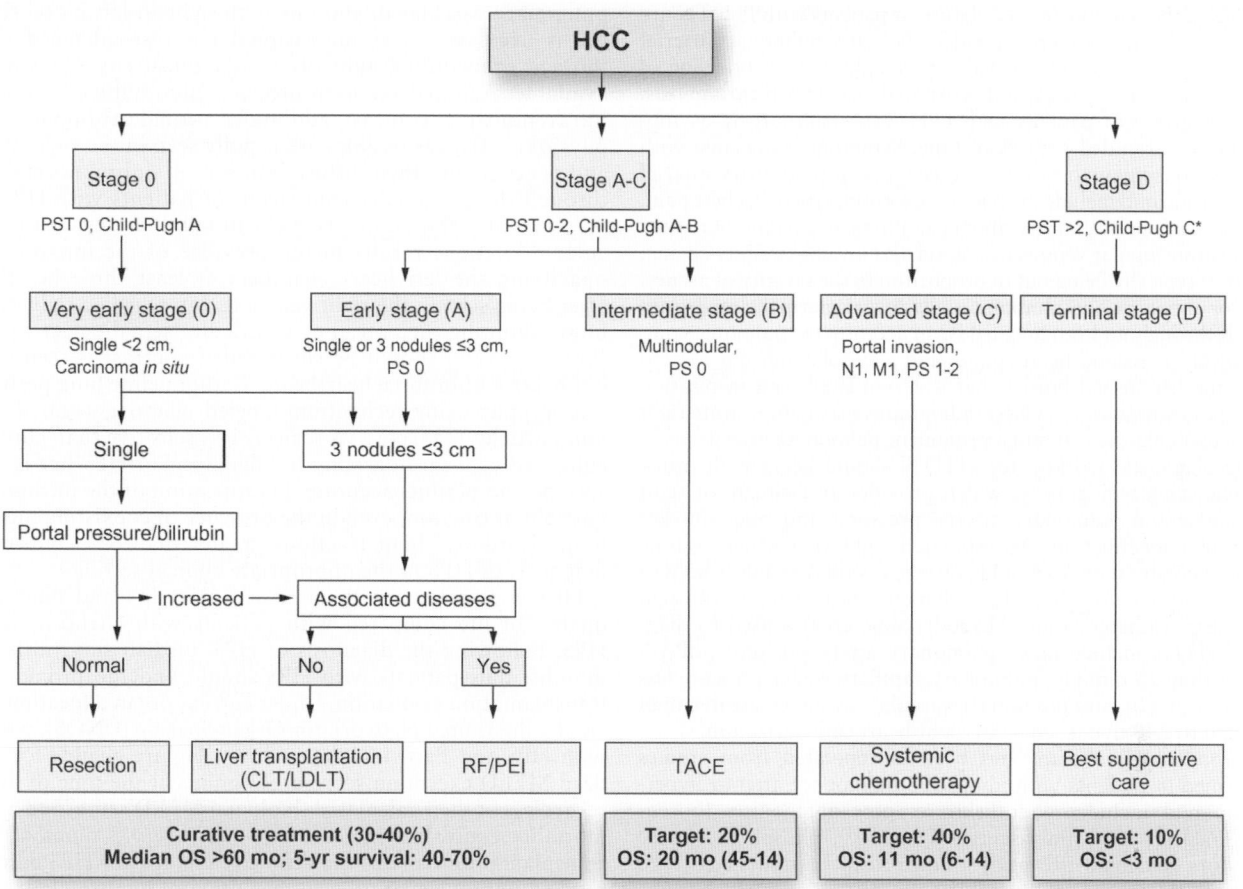

Figure 2 Barcelona Clinic Liver Cancer (BCLC) staging system for hepatocellular carcinoma (HCC). *CLT*, Cadaveric liver transplantation; *LDL*, living donor liver transplantation; *OS*, overall survival; *PEI*, percutaneous ethanol injection; *PST*, performance status; *RF*, radiofrequency ablation; *TACE*, transarterial chemoembolization. From EASL–EORTC Clinical Practice Guidelines: Management of hepatocellular carcinoma, *J Hepatol* 56(4):908–943, 2012.

interventions. Additional serologic markers for HCC include the L3 isoform of AFP (AFP-L3) and des-gamma carboxy prothrombin (DCP); however, further validation of these tests for surveillance of individuals at risk for HCC is still required.

The Barcelona Clinic Liver Cancer (BCLC) staging system can be used to categorize patients with HCC and to assist with therapeutic decisions (Figure 2). Surgical resection of HCC is reserved for patients with a single lesion and no evidence of cirrhosis or portal hypertension. Locoregional therapies include radiofrequency ablation, percutaneous ethanol injection, transarterial chemoembolization, radioembolization, and microwave ablation. These modalities are typically used for patients with early and intermediate stages (BCLC stages A and B, respectively). Liver transplantation is an effective treatment for patients with cirrhosis and HCC within the so-called Milan criteria: a single lesion up to 5 cm or no more than three lesions with the largest one being less than 3 cm, and in the absence of portal venous invasion or metastatic disease. Liver transplantation for HCC within these limits results in long-term survival equivalent to that seen in patients with cirrhosis but no HCC. Under the current organ allocation policy in the United States, patients with HCC within Milan criteria are listed for liver transplantation with their biologic MELD score (calculated by the MELD formula and without exception points) for 6 months, after which time they automatically accrue MELD exception points and the score increases to 28, with 10% increments thereafter every 3 months until the maximum score of 34 is reached. MELD exception points are granted to patients with HCC 2 cm or greater in an effort to balance risk of death that is not adequately represented by the degree of hepatic dysfunction. For patients with HCC listed for liver transplantation, the use of locoregional therapies is recommended to prevent

tumor progression that may result in dropout from the waiting list. Furthermore, active surveillance is recommended to evaluate for tumor recurrence or progression, development of new lesions, and metastatic disease while awaiting liver transplantation.

The number of systemic treatments licensed for use in patients with HCC has expanded significantly in recent years, with multiple options now available for first- and second-line therapy. First-line agents include sorafenib (Nexavar), nivolumab (Opdivo) plus pembrolizumab (Keytruda), lenvatinib (Lenvima), and bevacizumab (Avastin) plus atezolizumab (Tecentriq), cabozantinib (Cabometyx), and ramucirumab (Cyramza). Second-line therapies include nivolumab (Opdivo) either as monotherapy or in combination with ipilimumab (Yervoy), pembrolizumab (Keytruda), regorafenib (Stivarga), cabozantinib (Cabometyx), and ramucirumab (Cyramza). Adverse reactions, tolerability, and potential benefits must be carefully weighed and individualized according to overall health and performance status, as well as severity of hepatic dysfunction. The survival benefit of these agents is modest.

Portopulmonary Hypertension

Pulmonary artery hypertension in a patient with established portal hypertension is indicative of portopulmonary hypertension (PPHTN), but other etiologies of pulmonary hypertension must be excluded prior to establishing this diagnosis. The prevalence of PPHTN varies depending on the severity of liver disease and has been reported in 0.7% of patients with cirrhosis but can be as high as 12.5% in patients undergoing evaluation for liver transplantation.

The exact pathophysiology of PPHTN remains enigmatic, but increased exposure to humoral vasoconstrictors in the pulmonary vasculature due to portosystemic shunting and hyperdynamic circulation is among the most widely accepted hypotheses. Histologic findings in the pulmonary vasculature of patients with PPHTN are indistinguishable from those found in idiopathic pulmonary arterial hypertension and include medial hypertrophy with remodeling of the pulmonary artery walls and occasional in situ microthrombosis.

The majority of patients with PPHTN remain largely asymptomatic for extended periods of time. Symptoms associated with PPHTN are similar to those of other types of pulmonary arterial hypertension and include dyspnea on exertion, syncope, chest pain, fatigue, hemoptysis, and orthopnea. Physical examination may demonstrate jugular venous distention and lower extremity edema, the latter typically being out of proportion to the severity of ascites. Cardiopulmonary auscultation usually reveals normal clear breath sounds throughout both lung fields, an accentuated pulmonic component of the second heart sound, and a systolic murmur located along the left sternal border that is accentuated with inspiration (tricuspid regurgitation). Chest radiographs may demonstrate right ventricular enlargement and a prominent pulmonary artery.

The diagnostic workup for PPHTN should begin with transthoracic echocardiography, which provides an estimate of right ventricular and pulmonary arterial pressures and rules out left ventricular dysfunction. An estimated right ventricular systolic pressure greater than 50 mm Hg is typically used as a threshold to obtain more accurate direct hemodynamic measurements through right heart catheterization. Hemodynamic criteria used to diagnose PPHTN include mean pulmonary artery pressure (mPAP) greater than 25 mm Hg, pulmonary capillary wedge pressure less than 15 mm Hg, and pulmonary vascular resistance greater than or equal to 240 dyn .s. cm−5 by right heart catheterization.

Pharmacologic therapy has been extrapolated from studies performed in patients with idiopathic pulmonary arterial hypertension and includes endothelin receptor antagonists (bosentan [Tracleer][1] and ambrisentan [Letairis][1]), phosphodiesterase inhibitors (sildenafil [Revatio][1]), and prostacyclin analogs (epoprostenol [Flolan][1] and iloprost [Ventavis][1]).

Survival in PPHTN correlates with the severity of right ventricular dysfunction, and the safety and efficacy of liver transplantation are reliant on the severity of pulmonary arterial hypertension. Liver transplantation may be offered to selected patients with PPHTN but is typically contraindicated in those with mPAP greater than 35 mm Hg despite medical management, particularly if right ventricular dysfunction is present, due to considerable perioperative mortality.

Hepatopulmonary Syndrome

Hepatopulmonary syndrome (HPS) is characterized by hypoxemia due to intrapulmonary vascular dilatations with right-to-left shunting in the setting of cirrhosis and portal hypertension. Although intrapulmonary vasodilatation is encountered in over 50% of patients with cirrhosis undergoing evaluation for liver transplantation, only 15% to 30% have hypoxemia and true HPS. The most widely accepted pathophysiologic mechanism responsible for HPS is increased pulmonary synthesis of nitric oxide. Similar to PPHTN, the majority of patients with HPS are largely asymptomatic.

Clinical manifestations include dyspnea of insidious onset and two characteristic clinical findings: platypnea and orthodeoxia (worsening dyspnea and hypoxemia in upright posture, respectively). Other, more obvious but nonspecific clinical findings include spider angiomata, digital clubbing, and cyanosis. Screening for HPS relies on point-of-care oximetry indicating peripheral arterial oxygen saturation (SpO_2) less than 96% at rest and at sea level. Hypoxemia must be confirmed by arterial blood gas analysis demonstrating an arterial partial pressure of oxygen (Pao_2) less than 70 mm Hg and a widened alveolar–arterial oxygen gradient greater than or equal to 15 mm Hg (≥20 mm Hg for patients 65 years of age or older). Importantly, blood for arterial gas analysis should be obtained with the patient sitting upright, at rest, and breathing ambient air. After establishing a diagnosis of hypoxemia, documentation of

pulmonary vascular dilatations with right-to-left blood shunting is necessary. Two-dimensional contrast-enhanced transthoracic echocardiography offers high sensitivity and is widely available. Agitated saline to produce microbubbles is injected intravenously as contrast, and under normal cardiopulmonary physiology the gas bubbles are rapidly seen in the right atrium and ventricle but then diffuse into alveoli during normal flow through the pulmonary capillaries. In patients with HPS, the presence of intrapulmonary right-to-left shunting due to vascular dilatations results in the presence of the microbubbles opacifying the left heart chambers at least three heartbeats after being seen in the right ventricle. Intracardiac right-to-left blood shunting (i.e., atrial or ventricular septal defects, patent foramen ovale) should be suspected if contrast is seen in the left heart within three heartbeats. Radionuclide lung perfusion scintigraphy using technetium-labeled macroaggregated albumin particles (^{99m}Tc-MAA scan) is less sensitive than contrast-enhanced echocardiography for diagnosis of HPS but is more specific and permits accurate quantification of the intrapulmonary shunt fraction, even in the presence of coexisting intrinsic lung disorders. Shunt fractions greater than 6% confirm the diagnosis of HPS in the appropriate clinical setting.

HPS is associated with increased mortality and diminished quality of life compared with patients with cirrhosis but no HPS. Following the diagnosis of HPS, median survival is 10.6 months; thus patients with HPS should undergo prompt liver transplantation evaluation. Under current organ allocation policies by the United Network for Organ Sharing (UNOS), patients with HPS and Pao_2 less than 60 mm Hg are eligible for standard MELD exception score of 22 points at the time of listing, regardless of their calculated (biologic) MELD score, and a 10% mortality equivalent increase in points every 3 months. Liver transplantation remains the definitive therapy for HPS based on marked improvement or even resolution of hypoxemia in more than 85% of transplant recipients; however, clinically meaningful changes may be slow and take up to 1 year following transplantation.

Hepatic Hydrothorax

Hepatic hydrothorax is a transudative process leading to accumulation of more than 500 mL of fluid in the pleural space in patients with cirrhosis and portal hypertension in the absence of primary cardiopulmonary disease. Hepatic hydrothorax is thought to result from passage of ascitic fluid from the peritoneal cavity into the pleural spaces (typically on the right in up to 85% of patients) via subcentimeter defects and/or microscopic fenestrations in the tendinous portion of the diaphragm and is facilitated by negative intrathoracic pressure generated during inspiration. Clinical features include dyspnea, nonproductive cough, pleuritic chest pain, and even hypoxemia and hypotension in cases of tension hydrothorax. Fluid analysis demonstrates similar chemical characteristics than ascites: high serum–to–pleural fluid albumin gradient (>1.1 g/dL) and low total protein concentration (<2.5 g/dL).

Management of noninfected hepatic hydrothorax follows the same principles as those for ascites: sodium restriction, diuretics, repeated thoracenteses, and placement of TIPS for refractory cases. Importantly, indwelling pleural catheters should be avoided because of the high risk for complications including severe infections that may jeopardize possible liver transplant candidacy in the future.

In patients with fevers and worsening pleuritic chest pain, spontaneous bacterial empyema (SBEM) must be excluded. Similar to the diagnostic criteria for SBP, a diagnosis of SBEM is established by a PMN count greater than 250 cells/μL and a positive bacterial culture in the absence of a parapneumonic effusion. In cases in which bacterial cultures are negative, a PMN count threshold of greater than 500 cells/μL should be used to diagnose SBEM. Microorganisms responsible for this infection are also similar to those responsible for SBP; thus third-generation cephalosporins remain the antibacterial agents of choice for empiric therapy.

[1]Not FDA approved for this indication.

Liver Transplantation

Liver transplantation is effective in salvaging patients with acute liver failure (ALF) and decompensated cirrhosis, as well as selected patients with HCC (see earlier), with excellent short- and long-term outcomes. Survival after 1 and 5 years following liver transplantation is approximately 80% to 90% and 60% to 75%, respectively. Cirrhosis per se is not an indication to initiate evaluation for liver transplantation, as it is not associated with survival benefit in patients with low MELD scores. Consequently, patients should be referred for liver transplantation evaluation when the MELD score is 15 or higher or when an index complication of cirrhosis such as ascites or variceal hemorrhage occurs. Organ allocation in the United States and many other countries is based on disease severity as reflected by the MELD score for patients 12 years of age or older and the Pediatric End-Stage Liver Disease (PELD) score for patients younger than 12 years of age (includes international normalized ratio, bilirubin, albumin, and growth failure). The most recent modification of the MELD score now includes serum sodium in the mathematical equation (MELD-Na), as hyponatremia is an independent predictor of mortality in patients with cirrhosis. Some etiologies of cirrhosis result in diminished survival that is not accurately predicted by the MELD score or are associated with extremely poor quality of life; thus MELD exceptions exist. Standardized MELD exception criteria are summarized in Table 10. For patients with complications related to liver disease and associated increased morbidity and mortality not adequately reflected by the MELD score and not qualifying for standard MELD exceptions, additional points may be petitioned by the transplant center to the regional review board on a case-by-case basis with no guarantee that they will be granted. Some examples of conditions that may receive additional MELD points include recurrent bacterial cholangitis in patients with primary sclerosing cholangitis, intractable and debilitating pruritus in patients with primary biliary cholangitis, ascites refractory to maximum-tolerated doses of diuretics, HE refractory to medical therapy, and recurrent variceal hemorrhage despite adequate therapy.

Contraindications to liver transplantation continually evolve over time. Relative contraindications are usually associated with suboptimal outcomes following liver transplantation and vary widely across different transplant centers. Absolute contraindications imply that a successful outcome following liver transplantation is unlikely; thus it should not be pursued (Table 11).

ALF is an uncommon but important indication for liver transplantation owing to the high mortality associated with this condition. Although a significant proportion of patients with ALF may have spontaneous recovery, its clinical course is usually unpredictable and early referral for liver transplantation is recommended, regardless of the etiology. Patients with ALF have the highest priority for organ allocation if they meet specific criteria for UNOS status 1A (Table 12).

Evaluation for liver transplantation is a multidisciplinary process carried out over multiple encounters aimed to unveil additional medical, surgical, behavioral, social, and economic issues that may affect liver transplantation candidacy and/or outcomes. Once the patient's candidacy is deemed appropriate, formal listing occurs with UNOS. Blood type (ABO) is the major determinant for organ compatibility, and appropriate size (based on body weight) must be taken into consideration.

Living-donor liver transplantation was developed as an alternative owing to ongoing shortage of deceased-donor organs; however, living donation carries important risks for the donor that must be carefully taken into consideration. The advantages and disadvantages of living-donor liver transplantation are summarized in Table 13.

Additional approaches to try to expand donor organ supply include donation after cardiac death, using grafts from hepatitis B

TABLE 10 — Medical Conditions That Qualify for Standard MELD Exception Points

CONDITIONS	REMARKS
Hepatocellular carcinoma	T2 lesions (at least 2 cm in diameter) within Milan criteria
Hepatopulmonary syndrome	PaO_2 <60 mm Hg on ambient air
Portopulmonary hypertension	Mean pulmonary arterial pressure <35 mm Hg with treatment
Familial amyloid polyneuropathy	Confirmed by DNA analysis and histology
Primary hyperoxaluria	Need simultaneous liver–kidney transplant
Cystic fibrosis	Forced expiratory volume in 1 s (FEV_1) <40%
Hilar cholangiocarcinoma	Stage I or II, liver transplantation center must have a UNOS-approved protocol
Hepatic artery thrombosis	Within 14 days of liver transplantation, not meeting criteria for status 1A

MELD, Model for End-Stage Liver Disease; *UNOS*, United Network for Organ Sharing.

TABLE 11 — Absolute Contraindications to Liver Transplantation

CONTRAINDICATIONS TO LIVER TRANSPLANTATION

Uncontrolled sepsis

Acquired immunodeficiency syndrome

Active alcohol or substance abuse

Advanced cardiac or pulmonary disease

Intrahepatic cholangiocarcinoma

Hepatic hemangiosarcoma

Hepatocellular carcinoma with metastasis

Extrahepatic malignancy

Anatomic abnormalities that preclude liver transplantation

Lack of social support

Persistent nonadherence to medical care

TABLE 12 — Criteria for Status 1A Designation in Patients With Acute Liver Failure

Age >18 years

Life expectancy <7 days without liver transplantation

Onset of encephalopathy within 8 weeks of first symptom of liver disease

Absence of preexisting liver disease

Admission to intensive care unit, and one of the following:
• Ventilator dependence
• Requirement of renal replacement therapy
• International normalized ratio >2

Fulminant Wilson disease

Primary graft nonfunction

Hepatic artery thrombosis

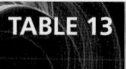

TABLE 13	Advantages and Disadvantages of Living-Donor Liver Transplantation

ADVANTAGES	DISADVANTAGES
Thorough donor screening process	Only offered in selected liver transplantation centers
Elective timing of liver transplantation permitting optimization of therapies	Donor morbidity and mortality
Diminished wait time with consequent reduction in dropout from the waiting list	Higher risk for biliary complications in the donor and recipient
Minimal cold ischemia time	

core antibody–positive and hepatitis C–positive donors, and splitting a graft for use in adult and pediatric recipients.

Adequate long-term immunosuppression prevents graft rejection and is currently centered on the use of calcineurin inhibitors (tacrolimus [Prograf] primarily, and less often cyclosporine [Neoral]) with or without concomitant antimetabolite agents such as mycophenolic acid (Myfortic) or its prodrug mycophenolate mofetil (CellCept). Additional agents include inhibitors of the mammalian target of rapamycin (mTOR) such as sirolimus (Rapamune)[1] and everolimus (Zortress).

Long-term care of liver transplant recipients should not by any means focus exclusively on graft function and prevention of rejection, but rather be comprehensive and aimed at maintaining an overall good state of health by instituting preventive health strategies and monitoring for other complications that may ensue, such as diabetes mellitus, hypertension, dyslipidemia, renal dysfunction, obesity, and alcohol relapse, among many others.

---

[1]Not FDA approved for this indication.

References

Ahluwalia V, Wade JB, White MB, et al: Liver transplantation significantly improves global functioning and cerebral processing, *Liver Transplant* 22:1379–1390, 2016.

Angeli P, Volpin R, Gerunda G, et al: Reversal of type 1 hepatorenal syndrome with the administration of midodrine and octreotide, *Hepatology* 29:1690–1697, 1999.

Arguedas MR, Singh H, Faulk DK, et al: Utility of pulse oximetry screening for hepatopulmonary syndrome, *Clin Gastroenterol Hepatol* 5:749–754, 2007.

Arroyo V, Garcia-Martinez R, Salvatella X: Human serum albumin, systemic inflammation, and cirrhosis, *J Hepatol* 61:396–407, 2014.

Bajaj JS, Heuman DM, Sterling RK, et al: Validation of EncephalApp, smartphone-based Stroop test, for the diagnosis of covert hepatic encephalopathy, *Clin Gastroenterol Hepatol* 13:1828–1835, 2015. e1.

Bass NM, Mullen KD, Sanyal A, et al: Rifaximin treatment in hepatic encephalopathy, *N Engl J Med* 362:1071–1081, 2010.

Bernardi M, Caraceni P, Navickis RJ, et al: Albumin infusion in patients undergoing large-volume paracentesis: a meta-analysis of randomized trials, *Hepatology* 55:1172–1181, 2012.

Blachier M, Leleu H, Peck-Radosavljevic M, et al: The burden of liver disease in Europe: a review of available epidemiological data, *J Hepatol* 58:593–608, 2013.

Bureau C, Thabut D, Oberti F, et al: Transjugular intrahepatic portosystemic shunts with covered stents increase transplant-free survival of patients with cirrhosis and recurrent ascites, *Gastroenterology* 152:157–163, 2017.

D'Amico G, Garcia-Tsao G, Pagliaro L: Natural history and prognostic indicators of survival in cirrhosis: a systematic review of 118 studies, *J Hepatol* 44:217–231, 2006.

Dasarathy S, Merli M: Sarcopenia from mechanism to diagnosis and treatment in liver disease, *J Hepatol* 65:1232–1244, 2016.

Escorsell À, Pavel O, Cárdenas A, et al: Esophageal balloon tamponade versus esophageal stent in controlling acute refractory variceal bleeding: a multicenter randomized, controlled trial, *Hepatology* 63:1957–1967, 2016.

Flemming JA, Kim WR, Brosgart CL, et al: Reduction in liver transplant wait-listing in the era of direct-acting antiviral therapy, *Hepatology* 65(3):804–812, 2017.

Garcia-Pagan JC, Caca K, Bureau C, et al: Early use of TIPS in patients with cirrhosis and variceal bleeding, *N Engl J Med* 362:2370–2379, 2010.

Garcia-Pagan JC, Barrufet M, Cardenas A, et al: Management of gastric varices, *Clin Gastroenterol Hepatol* 12:919–928, 2014. e1; quiz e51–2.

Garcia-Tsao G, Sanyal AJ, Grace ND, Carey W: Practice Guidelines Committee of the American Association for the study of liver D, practice Parameters Committee of the American College of G. Prevention and management of gastroesophageal varices and variceal hemorrhage in cirrhosis, *Hepatology* 46:922–938, 2007.

Garcia-Tsao G, Abraldes JG, Berzigotti A, Bosch J: Portal hypertensive bleeding in cirrhosis: risk stratification, diagnosis, and management: 2016 practice guidance by the American association for the study of liver diseases, *Hepatology* 65:310–335, 2017.

Ge PS, Runyon BA: Serum ammonia level for the evaluation of hepatic encephalopathy, *J Am Med Assoc* 312:643–644, 2014.

Gines P, Fernandez-Esparrach G, Arroyo V, et al: Pathogenesis of ascites in cirrhosis, *Semin Liver Dis* 17:175–189, 1997.

Gluud LL, Christensen K, Christensen E, et al: Systematic review of randomized trials on vasoconstrictor drugs for hepatorenal syndrome, *Hepatology* 51:576–584, 2010.

Goel GA, Deshpande A, Lopez R, et al: Increased rate of spontaneous bacterial peritonitis among cirrhotic patients receiving pharmacologic acid suppression, *Clin Gastroenterol Hepatol* 10:422–427, 2012.

Grace JA, Angus PW: Hepatopulmonary syndrome: update on recent advances in pathophysiology, investigation, and treatment, *J Gastroenterol Hepatol* 28:213–219, 2013.

Kristina Tzartzeva K, Obi J, Rich NE, et al: Surveillance imaging and alpha fetoprotein for early detection of hepatocellular carcinoma in patients with cirrhosis: a meta-analysis, *Gastroenterology* Feb 16, Epub ahead of print.

Krowka MJ, Plevak DJ, Findlay JY, et al: Pulmonary hemodynamics and perioperative cardiopulmonary-related mortality in patients with portopulmonary hypertension undergoing liver transplantation, *Liver Transplant* 6:443–450, 2000.

Kurokawa T, Zheng YW, Ohkohchi N: Novel functions of platelets in the liver, *J Gastroenterol Hepatol* 31:745–751, 2016.

Lim YS, Kim WR: The global impact of hepatic fibrosis and end-stage liver disease, *Clin Liver Dis* 12:733–736, 2008.

Lin ZH, Xin YN, Dong QJ, et al: Performance of the aspartate aminotransferase-to-platelet ratio index for the staging of hepatitis C-related fibrosis: an updated meta-analysis, *Hepatology* 53:726–736, 2011.

Llovet JM, Ricci S, Mazzaferro V, et al: Sorafenib in advanced hepatocellular carcinoma, *N Engl J Med* 359:378–390, 2008.

Marik PE, Wood K, Starzl TE: The course of type 1 hepato-renal syndrome post liver transplantation, *Nephrol Dial Transplant* 21:478–482, 2006.

Mazzaferro V, Regalia E, Doci R, et al: Liver transplantation for the treatment of small hepatocellular carcinomas in patients with cirrhosis, *N Engl J Med* 334:693–699, 1996.

Merion RM, Schaubel DE, Dykstra DM, et al: The survival benefit of liver transplantation, *Am J Transplant* 5:307–313, 2005.

Mullen KD, Sanyal AJ, Bass NM, et al: Rifaximin is safe and well tolerated for long-term maintenance of remission from overt hepatic encephalopathy, *Clin Gastroenterol Hepatol* 12:1390–1397, 2014. e2.

Ohlsson B, Nilsson J, Stenram U, et al: Percutaneous fine-needle aspiration cytology in the diagnosis and management of liver tumours, *Br J Surg* 89:757–762, 2002.

Patidar KR: Bajaj JS: covert and overt hepatic encephalopathy: diagnosis and management, *Clin Gastroenterol Hepatol* 13:2048–2061, 2015.

Pereira K, Carrion AF, Martin P, et al: Current diagnosis and management of posttransjugular intrahepatic portosystemic shunt refractory hepatic encephalopathy, *Liver Int* 35:2487–2494, 2015.

Runyon BA, Committee APG: Management of adult patients with ascites due to cirrhosis: an update, *Hepatology* 49:2087–2107, 2009.

Runyon BA, Squier S, Borzio M: Translocation of gut bacteria in rats with cirrhosis to mesenteric lymph nodes partially explains the pathogenesis of spontaneous bacterial peritonitis, *J Hepatol* 21:792–796, 1994.

Saab S, Hernandez JC, Chi AC, et al: Oral antibiotic prophylaxis reduces spontaneous bacterial peritonitis occurrence and improves short-term survival in cirrhosis: a meta-analysis, *Am J Gastroenterol* 104:993–1001, 2009; quiz 2.

Salerno F, Merli M, Riggio O, et al: Randomized controlled study of TIPS versus paracentesis plus albumin in cirrhosis with severe ascites, *Hepatology* 40:629–635, 2004.

Sort P, Navasa M, Arroyo V, et al: Effect of intravenous albumin on renal impairment and mortality in patients with cirrhosis and spontaneous bacterial peritonitis, *N Engl J Med* 341:403–409, 1999.

Udell JA, Wang CS, Tinmouth J, et al: Does this patient with liver disease have cirrhosis? *J Am Med Assoc* 307:832–842, 2012.

Vallet-Pichard A, Mallet V, Nalpas B, et al: FIB-4: an inexpensive and accurate marker of fibrosis in HCV infection. Comparison with liver biopsy and fibrotest, *Hepatology* 46:32–36, 2007.

Villanueva C, Colomo A, Bosch A, et al: Transfusion strategies for acute upper gastrointestinal bleeding, *N Engl J Med* 368:11–21, 2013.

Wang FS, Fan JG, Zhang Z, et al: The global burden of liver disease: the major impact of China, *Hepatology* 60:2099–2108, 2014.

Wells M, Chande N, Adams P, et al: Meta-analysis: vasoactive medications for the management of acute variceal bleeds, *Aliment Pharmacol Ther* 35:1267–1278, 2012.

Williams Jr JW, Simel DL: The rational clinical examination. Does this patient have ascites? How to divine fluid in the abdomen, *J Am Med Assoc* 267:2645–2648, 1992.

Zaiac MN, Walker A: Nail abnormalities associated with systemic pathologies, *Clin Dermatol* 31:627–649, 2013.

DIVERTICULA OF THE ALIMENTARY TRACT

Aaron D. Sinclair, MD

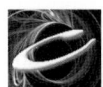

CURRENT DIAGNOSIS

- Endoscopy or barium swallow study may be used in the evaluation of most upper alimentary tract diverticula.
- Symptomatic small intestinal diverticula are difficult to diagnose and require a high index of suspicion and radiographic examination (nuclear medicine scans, capsule endoscopy, or computed tomography scans).
- Diverticulitis of the colon is most accurately identified and the treatment planned with computed tomography of the abdomen and pelvis.
- Diverticulitis of the colon that is slow to resolve may require additional imaging or direct visualization with endoscopy to identify an alternative diagnosis.

CURRENT THERAPY

- Most asymptomatic diverticula are identified incidentally and may require only monitoring.
- Surgical management of symptomatic diverticula may require surgical resection.
- Early in the disease process, uncomplicated diverticulitis of the colon may be managed on an outpatient basis with a conservative no-intervention approach or oral antibiotics.
- Complicated diverticulitis of the colon should be managed in conjunction with a surgeon and in the hospital with intravenous antibiotics.

A diverticulum is an abnormal saccular protrusion from the wall of the alimentary tract. Diverticula may be classified as either true or false. The wall of the alimentary tract is composed of submucosal, mucosal, and muscular layers. A false diverticulum is a protrusion of the submucosa and mucosa through a defect in the muscular wall of the alimentary tract. A true diverticulum is a protrusion of all layers of the alimentary tract wall. Many diverticula are asymptomatic and require no treatment. Some diverticula cause symptoms depending on their anatomic location or associated pathophysiologic complications (e.g., obstruction, infection, inflammation, or bleeding). This chapter categorizes alimentary canal diverticula by their location.

Esophagus

Zenker Diverticulum

Zenker diverticulum is a false diverticulum that develops in the upper posterior esophagus in an area known as Killian triangle, located between the inferior pharyngeal constrictors and the cricopharyngeal muscles. Zenker diverticulum typically presents after age 60 and has a male predominance for reasons that are unclear. It affects only 2 per 100,000 patients per year. Although it can be asymptomatic for years before the development of symptomatology, patients may experience dysphagia, aspiration, and regurgitation of undigested food. The exact cause is unclear, but proposed mechanisms suggest a dysfunction in coordinated swallowing muscle movement and increased intraluminal pressure in the esophagus. There may be an additive component of long-term upper esophageal sphincter irritation from acid reflux.

Diagnosis is primarily made through barium swallow, although small diverticula may be missed (Figure 1). Although endoscopic direct visualization is possible, caution should be exercised owing to the risk of perforation. Small asymptomatic diverticula can be monitored. Zenker diverticulum that are less than 2 cm but symptomatic should be evaluated for possible surgical repair. Zenker diverticulum greater than 2 cm in size, regardless of symptomatology, should be surgically evaluated and repair considered. Methods for closure include endoscopic (flexible and rigid) diverticulostomy and myotomy or traditional surgical resection. Although most patients (>90%) demonstrate symptom improvement, recurrence rates can be as high as 35%. Surgery is associated with much higher morbidity and mortality than endoscopic approaches. Emerging technologies have used different techniques (harmonic scalpel, stapler, etc.) during endoscopic repair. Morbidity and mortality are largely operator dependent.

Traction Diverticulum

Traction diverticula are the only true diverticula of the esophagus. Traction diverticula are rare. Their size tends to stay less than 2 cm. Owing to the proposed mechanism of formation, traction diverticula are isolated to the middle third of the esophagus. It is not fully clear how traction diverticula form. One proposed mechanism is related to a precedent pulmonary infection, most commonly tuberculosis or histoplasmosis, with resultant mediastinal lymph node formation. After the active infection subsides, resultant fibrosis and scarring between the tissues surrounding the mediastinal lymph nodes and esophagus occur. Initially, a small diverticulum develops from this fibrosis, which produces "traction" or a lack of mobility. Diverticular progression results when age-related changes from the dysfunction of coordinated swallowing muscle movement and increased intraluminal pressure in the esophagus develop. Surgical management is rarely needed unless these diverticula become symptomatic or complications, such as fistulas, occur.

Epiphrenic Diverticulum

Epiphrenic diverticula are false diverticula of the distal esophagus affecting only 0.015% of the general population. They are thought to arise secondary to mucosal injury from gastroesophageal reflux and muscle dysmotility. They occur within 10 cm of the gastroesophageal junction, and symptoms include dysphagia, spasmodic chest pain, and gastroesophageal reflux. There does not appear to be a correlation with between diverticular size and symptomatology. With progression of diverticular size, obstruction can become a potential complication. Diagnostic measures start with barium swallow and may be followed with additional tests, including endoscopy, 24-hour pH probe, and esophageal manometry.

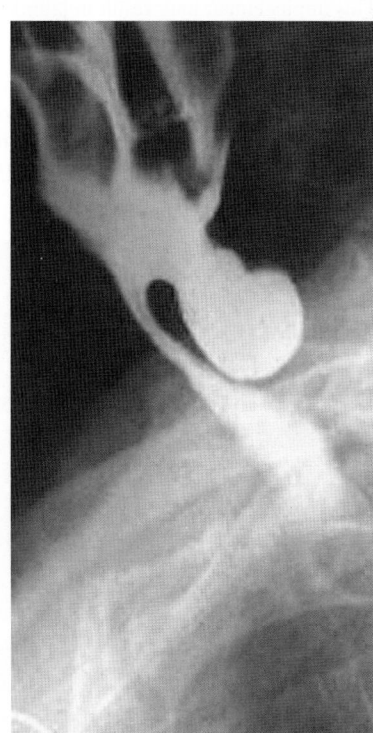

Figure 1 Zenker diverticulum. (Image courtesy Gastrolab—The Gastrointestinal Site. http://www.gastrolab.net [Accessed August 25, 2014].)

Management depends on patient symptoms and size of the diverticulum. If small (<5 cm) and asymptomatic, routine clinical and endoscopic surveillance is permissible. However, any symptomatology necessitates surgical evaluation and repair. Surgical options include open resection and laparoscopy. Partial fundoplication may be indicated, depending on the severity of gastroesophageal reflux present as indicated by ancillary testing of a 24-hour pH probe. Less invasive endoscopic myotomy procedures, successfully used to treat Zenker diverticulum, are judiciously being used to treat epiphrenic diverticulum.

Stomach

Gastric Diverticula

Gastric diverticula are rare, with an endoscopic incidence of 0.01%. Gastric diverticulum may be either true or false in nature. True gastric diverticulae (70% to 75%) are typically congenital and situated along the dorsal wall of the fundus within 2 to 3 cm of the gastroesophageal junction. False diverticulae, which are less common and typically acquired, are located around the antrum of the stomach. Most are asymptomatic and small (<3 cm). Symptoms may include epigastric pain, dyspepsia, and emesis. Rarely, ulcerations, perforations, or bleeding can occur. Diagnosis involves endoscopy, barium swallow, or contrast-aided computed tomography (CT) scan. If symptomatic, typical treatment includes a proton pump inhibitor and monitoring for symptom improvement. Continued symptoms should prompt endoscopic evaluation with biopsies of suspicious lesions with raised or irregular borders. Gastric cancers have been reported in and around gastric diverticulum. Persistent symptoms may necessitate gastrectomy of the diverticulum, especially if concerns about cancer exist.

Small Intestine

Duodenal Diverticula

Diverticula located in the duodenum are relatively common, affecting up to 22% of the general population (Figure 2). Duodenal diverticula may be either true or false diverticula. The most common location is the second portion of the duodenum. Although usually asymptomatic, ulcerative bleeding, perforation, or intermittent obstruction, particularly after eating, may occur. The size and position of the diverticula may lead to complications such as obstruction of the sphincter of Oddi and/or impingement of hepatobiliary tree drainage. This impingement may result in jaundice, right upper quadrant pain, or infection signs/symptoms similar to cholecystitis.

Duodenal diverticula may be identified on barium swallow, contrast-enhanced CT, magnetic resonance imaging, or endoscopy. Duodenal diverticula found incidentally do not require treatment. If symptoms arise, endoscopic evaluation and surgical resection should be considered. However, intervention should be considered with caution owing to a high risk (30%) of complications, in particular fistula formation and mortality.

Jejunal and Ileal Diverticula

Jejunal and ileal diverticula occur throughout the length of the small intestine in 1% to 2% of the population. There does not appear to be any statistically significant relationship with morbidity or mortality of these types of diverticula with respect to location, gender, size, number, and so forth. These false diverticula are located predominantly where the blood vessels penetrate the muscular wall of the mesenteric side of the bowel. Most are noted incidentally on radiographic studies, but some manifest with symptoms secondary to bleeding, obstruction, or infection. These symptoms are believed to be due to bacterial overgrowth that may occur within the cavity of the diverticulum. Diagnosis can be made with capsule endoscopy or a small bowel barium contrast follow-through study, although some may be noted on CT with intravenous and oral contrast. Advanced endoscopic procedures such as push enteroscopy and double balloon endoscopy can be used to further evaluate symptomatic diverticula.

Asymptomatic jejunal and ileal diverticula should not be resected. Bacterial overgrowth symptoms may respond to antibiotic treatment and intestinal promotility drug therapy. If diverticulitis is seen radiographically, intravenous antibiotics and bowel rest should be initiated. Surgical intervention with small bowel resection is indicated if symptomatic diverticula persist despite conservative management.

Meckel Diverticulum

Meckel diverticulum is a true diverticulum—a congenital anomaly that occurs owing to incomplete closure of the vitelline duct. This duct typically obliterates during the ninth week of gestational age. Owing to the embryologic origin of the diverticulum, it is almost always located within 2 feet of the ileocecal valve. Meckel diverticulum has a prevalence of 1% to 2% of the population, with a 2:1 male predominance. Approximately 2% of all existing Meckel diverticula will become symptomatic. Symptomatic diverticula most commonly cause nausea, vomiting, and abdominal pain. The sign most commonly associated with Meckel diverticulum is intussusception. This occurs owing to residual fibrous attachments to the umbilicus causing a lead point for the proximal bowel to involute onto the distal bowel. It most commonly presents with bloody mucoid stools, abdominal pain, and vomiting in children younger than 6 years of age, most commonly within the first 2 years of life. However, other symptoms may occur if ectopic tissue exists in the diverticulum. Gastric ectopic tissue may cause abdominal pain and bloody stools from ulceration of the underlying ileal tissue. Duodenal and pancreatic tissues have been identified in Meckel diverticulum but are very rare and do not typically cause symptoms.

Diagnosis in adults requires a high level of suspicion and is aided by the use of a technetium 99m (^{99m}Tc) scan to identify ectopic gastric mucosa in those patients with bleeding and symptoms of ulceration. For children with obstructive signs or symptoms, the diagnosis may be aided by ultrasound and/or computed tomographic scans. Plain film radiographs of the abdomen have low sensitivity and specificity for the diagnosis of intussusception. The sensitivity of the Meckel scan for the pediatric population is 85% to 97% but is much lower in the adult population at 62%. The choice of imaging procedure is dictated by the experience of the radiologic personnel performing the procedure.

Symptomatic Meckel diverticulum should be surgically resected. Up to 90% of intussusception secondary to Meckel diverticulum may be reduced using diagnostic ultrasonography with saline or pneumatic enema. Treatment of Meckel diverticulum largely depends on age and symptomatology because operating on asymptomatic Meckel diverticulum has been shown to have a fivefold increase in complications, such as postoperative bowel obstruction, leaks, ileus, and infection. Many experts have advocated that incidental, asymptomatic Meckel diverticulum should not be resected. Some experts advocate for selective

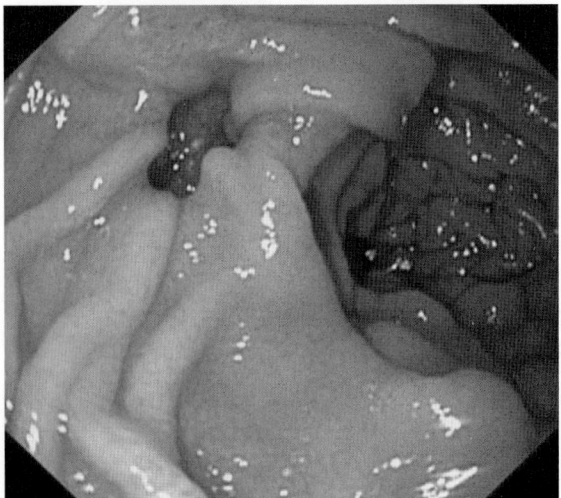

Figure 2 Duodenal diverticulum. (Image courtesy Gastrolab—The Gastrointestinal Site. http://www.gastrolab.net [Accessed August 25, 2014].)

surgical resection of asymptomatic patients with an incidentally noted Meckel diverticulum for the following: healthy young children, healthy adults younger than 50 years of age with palpable abnormalities suggestive of heterotrophic tissue, size longer than 2 cm, or a broad base wider than 2 cm.

Colon

Diverticulosis

The colon is where most diverticula occur in the alimentary tract. Owing to this predominance, this condition is commonly termed *diverticulosis* or *diverticular disease*. Diverticulum of the colon is of the false type. The incidence increases with age. The incidence of left-sided diverticulosis approaches 5% at age 40 and increases to greater than 60% at age 80. Diverticulosis is most commonly located in the sigmoid colon.

The exact pathogenesis of diverticulosis is unclear. The proposed mechanism of colonic diverticular formation places an emphasis on intraluminal pressure buildup. The pressure across the colonic wall increases as the radius of the wall decreases. Accordingly, the radius is the smallest in the sigmoid colon and thus the most likely location of diverticulosis. Normally, pressure is constant throughout the colon. However, as diverticular disease develops, abnormal pressure segmentations occur, resulting in pressure gradient changes in the colon. With increased pressure, the integrity of collagen and elastin in the wall muscle changes, the circular muscles thicken, colonic segments shorten, and the lumen narrows, leading to propagation of the disease. Several risk factors have been associated with the development of diverticular disease: smoking, lack of physical activity, and obesity. By increasing the amount of dietary fiber, it is theorized that the resultant bulking of the stools may decrease the pressure in the colon lumen and prevent diverticular disease progression. Yet, mixed results have been noted on studies of fiber intake and diverticular development and progression of disease. There is no associated risk with the ingestion of caffeine, alcohol, popcorn, seeds, or nuts and the development of diverticulosis, diverticular bleeding, or diverticulitis.

Colonic Diverticular Bleeding

Diverticula tend to develop where an arteriole penetrates the circular muscle layer of the colon. This results in vessels arching over the dome of the diverticulum. This leaves fragile vessels in a vulnerable position of a relatively thin mucosal layer prone to trauma and resultant diverticular bleeding. Bleeding typically manifests as hematochezia—a darkish to bright red bleeding that is typically characterized as brisk and acute in nature. Diverticulosis is attributed to 30% to 50% of all hematochezia. Fifteen percent of patients will experience at least one episode of bleeding in their lifetime, with a recurrent bleeding risk of up to 38%.

Most patients presenting with diverticular bleeding are asymptomatic, but some may experience bloating or cramping.

Selection of the diagnostic modality depends largely on the degree of bleeding and the cardiovascular stability of the patient. Endoscopy is the preferred treatment modality for stable patients owing to its potential for diagnosis and treatment options. Up to 80% of diverticular bleeding can be isolated with direct endoscopic visualization (Figure 3).

Endoscopic failure to identify or control diverticular bleeding may occur in the patient with massive or intermittent bleeding. Depending on the patient's cardiovascular stability and degree of bleeding, the typical evaluative progression if the site of bleeding is not identified is endoscopy, followed by tagged red blood cell scan, and then angiography. Hemodynamically unstable patients may have a high complication risk from the bowel preparation, sedation, or the procedure. Radionuclide imaging can be considered in unstable patients, nondiagnostic endoscopy, or bleeding recurrence. Radionuclide imaging requires that bleeding be active (at least 0.05 to 0.1 mL/min) to accurately isolate the location of the diverticulum. Radionuclide imaging using ^{99m}Tc sulfur colloid (shorter half-life, thus used for acute bleeding) or ^{99m}Tc pertechnetate (longer half-life more useful for intermittent bleeding)-labeled autologous red blood cells can be used to isolate the location of obscure gastrointestinal bleeding. However, numerous studies have produced highly variable sensitivities (26% to 91%). Many advocate for radionuclide imaging to be used as an ancillary test for directing more definitive treatments such as surgery or angiography-directed therapies. Angiography can be used if bleeding is active (at least 0.5 mL/min) and can isolate the bleeding location with a diagnostic yield of 40% to 78%. Angiography can be combined with embolization and/or vasopressin infusion to achieve hemostasis; however, complications may occur, including bowel infarction, rebleeding, and contrast-induced nephrotoxicity.

Diverticulitis

Diverticulosis is largely asymptomatic. Only approximately 4% will develop inflammation and infection known as diverticulitis. The disease severity and complications occur along a spectrum. The proposed mechanism of diverticulitis may be a blocked diverticulum or increased intraluminal pressure inducing. Subsequent vascular compromise and microperforation may occur, leading to localized infection and inflammation. These microperforations are usually sequestered and may lead to small localized abscess formation. This process is generally referred to as uncomplicated diverticulitis. Complicated diverticulitis is classified when a localized abscess or infection infiltrates into adjacent organs or viscera causing macroperforations, fistulas, obstructions, or enlarged abscesses.

The clinical presentation often begins with mild left lower abdominal pain, fever, and leukocytosis. Patients who seek care

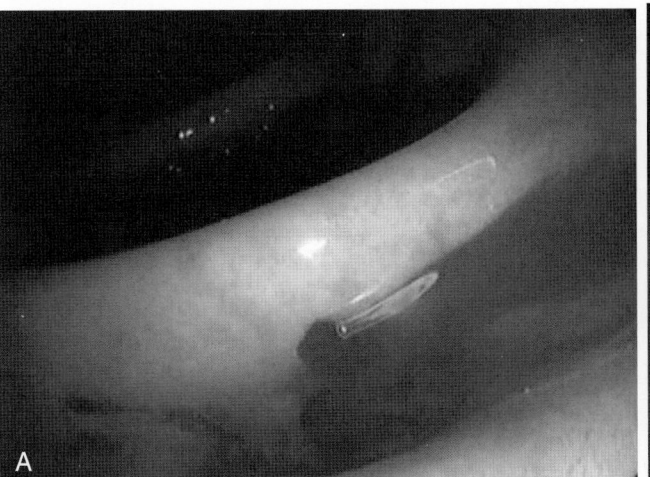 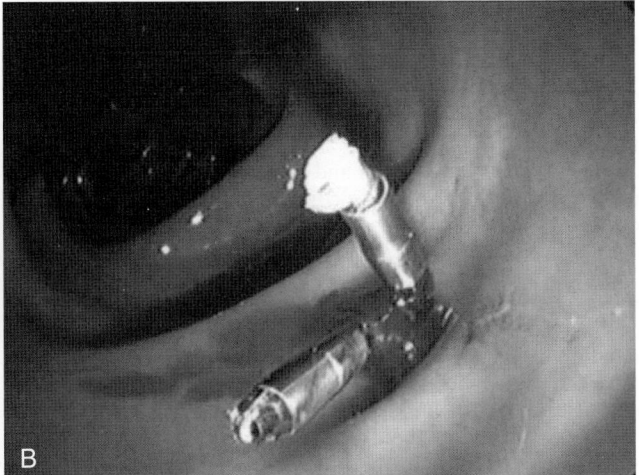

Figure 3 Colonoscopy in a patient with hematochezia from the source isolated to a diverticulum (A) and hemostasis noted after placement of two hemoclips (B). (Courtesy Janak Shah. From Feldman M. *Sleisenger and Fordtran's Gastrointestinal and Liver Disease*. 9th ed. Philadelphia: Elsevier; Figure 117.8.)

TABLE 1 Antibiotic Therapy for Diverticulitis	
OPTIONAL REGIMENS	**DOSAGE (ADULT)**
Uncomplicated Diverticulitis	
Outpatient (10–14 days)	
Ciprofloxacin (Cipro) and Metronidazole (Flagyl)	500 mg PO bid 500 mg PO tid
Amoxicillin-clavulanate (Augmentin)[1]	875 mg PO bid
Moxifloxacin (Avelox)	400 mg PO daily
Complicated Diverticulitis ***Inpatient Transitioning to Outpatient (10–14 Days Total)***	
Piperacillin-tazobactam (Zosyn)[1]	3.375–4.5 g IV every 6 h
Imipenem-cilastatin (Primaxin)	500 mg IV every 6 h
Levofloxacin (Levaquin)[1] and Metronidazole	500 mg IV every 24 h 500 mg IV every 8 h
Ceftriaxone (Rocephin) and Metronidazole	1 g IV every 24 h 500 mg IV every 8 h

[1]Not FDA approved for this indication.
Clindamycin (Cleocin) may be substituted in metronidazole intolerance/allergy.
    Antibiotics continued in complicated diverticulitis cases until negative cultures,
    clinical improvement, or sensitivities obtained on any surgical specimens.
bid, Twice a day; *tid*, three times a day.
Modified from Jacobs DO. Clinical practice: diverticulitis. *N Engl J Med.*
    2007;357:2057–2066.

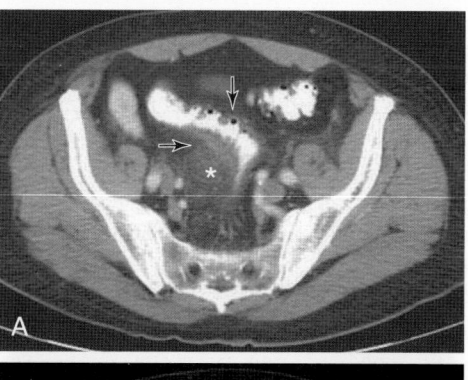

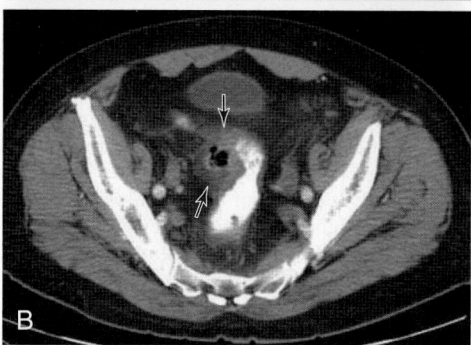

Figure 4 Diverticulitis. (A) Computed tomography (CT) image demonstrates thickened wall of the sigmoid colon *(arrows)* with stranding in the adjacent fat *(*)* indicative of diverticulitis. Fat stranding refers to abnormally increased attenuation of fat from edema and engorgement of lymphatics. (B) CT image slightly more caudal demonstrates an air-filled abscess cavity *(arrows)* with adjacent thickened sigmoid colon wall. (From McNally PR. GI/Liver Secrets Plus, 4th ed. Noninvasive Gastrointestinal Imaging: *Ultrasound, Computed Tomography, Magnetic Resonance Imaging.* Philadelphia: Mosby Elsevier; 2010, Figure 70–16.)

later in the disease process may present with sepsis or diffuse peritonitis. Initial diagnosis should be accomplished with history, physical examination, radiographic imaging, and laboratory evaluation. Abdominal radiography has limited utility but may reveal severe complications of diverticulitis such as bowel perforation or bowel obstruction. Ultrasonography and magnetic resonance imaging can be used with high levels of sensitivity and specificity in centers with demonstrated expertise. Ultrasonography has sensitivities and specificities of 92% and 90% for the detection of diverticulitis, respectively. With sensitivities and specificities of 94% and 99%, respectively, CT appears to be the imaging test of choice. This is especially true, as an alternative diagnosis was more likely to be identified with CT than with ultrasonography (50% to 100% vs. 33% to 78%). Those patients with a past medical history of diverticulitis may be empirically treated without imaging, although imaging may be needed if no clinical improvement is noted within 48 hours.

Recent data indicate no added benefit with antimicrobial therapy; thus select patients with uncomplicated diverticulitis may be treated without antibiotics and close clinical follow-up. Until further studies are done, many experts recommend that traditional treatment should include supportive care, liquid diet, and antibiotics for uncomplicated diverticulitis. Outpatient management is reasonable if the diagnosis is made early in the disease process. Uncomplicated diverticulitis responds to medical therapy in most cases. Complicated diverticulitis occurs in 25% of all diverticulitis diagnoses, requiring a surgical evaluation and intervention. Optional antibiotic regimens for gram-negative coverage and anaerobic coverage are listed in Table 1. Inpatient management is recommended with any high-risk comorbid conditions, immunosuppression, high-grade fever, leukocytosis, inability to tolerate oral fluids, and/or for elderly patients. Patient improvement should be seen within 48 hours. Those who do not improve should undergo additional evaluation such as repeat imaging or endoscopy. This is done to evaluate for underlying pathology such as cancer or inflammatory bowel disease, which would change the management strategy.

Follow-up scanning should also be considered for cases of slow-resolving diverticulitis. In the past, up to 10% of CT scans in which diverticulitis was the primary diagnosis, cancer could not be fully excluded. As CT scanner resolution has improved, newer studies have demonstrated only a small number of underlying cancers or indeterminate findings. A colonoscopy should be performed to evaluate the extent of diverticular disease and to rule out other comorbid pathology in all patients. Colonoscopy is typically recommended 6 weeks after diverticulitis symptoms have resolved, if one has not been done within the last year. Introduction of stool softeners and a high-fiber diet should begin immediately and continued indefinitely for all patients to help decrease the intraluminal pressure within the colon.

Diverticulitis that is complicated with abscess formation should be evaluated by a surgeon or radiologist for percutaneous drainage using CT or ultrasonography (Figure 4). Depending on location, aspiration or drainage tubes may be used to facilitate drainage. A general recommendation exists for consideration of drainage, preferably with interventional radiology localization, for any abscess measuring greater than 3 to 4 cm.

New research to prevent recurrent diverticulitis with medical management is emerging. Rifaximin (Xifaxan)[1] may help prevent recurrent episodes of diverticulitis. Probiotics[7] have not been shown to prevent recurrence. Fiber may be used as a beneficial supplement for the prevention of recurrent diverticulitis. Debate exists regarding elective segmental colectomy for patients who have experienced recurrent episodes of diverticulitis. Current recommendations suggest surgical consultation with discussion of the benefits and risks of surgery compared with the risks of recurrent diverticulitis. This discussion should take into account the diverticulitis frequency and severity, the impact on the patient's lifestyle, and the patient's other comorbid conditions. This consultation should at a minimum occur after the fourth recurrence of diverticulitis in patients older than age 50. There is insufficient evidence to advise a patient who has experienced fewer than four recurrent cases of diverticulitis or who is younger than age 50 on the benefit of a segmental colectomy.

[1]Not FDA approved for this indication.
[7]Available as a dietary supplement.

References

Choi JJ, Ogunjemilusi O, Divino CM: Diagnosis and management of diverticula in the jejunum and ileum, *Am Surg* 79(1):108–110, 2013.

Delavux M: Diverticular disease of the colon in Europe: Epidemiology, impact on citizen health and prevention, *Aliment Pharmacol Ther* 18(Suppl 3):71–74, 2003.

Fry RD, Mahmoud NN, Maron DJ, et al: Colon and rectum. In Townsend Jr CM, Beauchamp D, editors: *Sabiston Textbook of Surgery*, 19th ed, Philadelphia, 2012, Saunders, pp 1309–1314.

Greene CL, McFadden PM, Oh DS, et al: Long-term outcome of the treatment of Zenker's diverticulum, *Ann Thorac Surg* 100:975–978, 2015.

Ishaq S, Sultan H, Siau K, et al: New and emerging techniques for endoscopic treatment of Zenker's Diverticulum: State-of-the-art review, *Digestive Endoscopy* 30:449–460, 2018.

Jacobs DO: Clinical practice, Diverticulitis, *N Engl J Med* 357:2057–2066, 2007.

Janes SE, Meagher A, Frizelle FA: Management of diverticulitis, *BMJ* 332:271–275, 2006.

Kilic A, Schuchert MJ, Awais O, et al: Surgical management of epiphrenic diverticula in the minimally invasive era, *JSLS* 13:160–164, 2009.

Lameris W, van Randen A, Bipat S: Graded compression ultrasonography and computed tomography in acute colonic diverticulitis: Meta-analysis of test accuracy, *Eur Radiol* 18:2498–2511, 2008.

Lin S, Suhocki PV, Ludwig KA, et al: Gastrointestinal bleeding in adult patients with Meckel's diverticulum: The role of technetium 99m pertechnetate scan, *South Med J* 95:1338, 2002.

Maish MS: Esophagus. In Townsend Jr CM, Beauchamp D, editors: *Sabiston Textbook of Surgery*, 19th ed, Philadelphia, 2012, Saunders, pp 1023–1025.

Martinez-Cecilia D, Arjona-Sanchez A, Gomez-Alvarez M, et al: Conservative management of perforated duodenal diverticulum: A case report and review of the literature, *World J Gastroenterol* 14:1949–1951, 2008.

Mohan P, Ananthavadivelu M, Venkataraman J: Gastric diverticulum, *CMAJ* 182:E226, 2010.

Morris AM, Rogenbogen SE, Hardiman KM, et al: Sigmoid diverticulitis: A systematic review, *JAMA* 311:287–297, 2014.

Mulder CJ, Costamagna G, Sakai P: Zenker's diverticulum: Treatment using a flexible endoscope, *Endoscopy* 33:991–997, 2001.

Oukachbi N, Brouzes S: Management of complicated duodenal diverticula, *J Visceral Surg* 150:173–179, 2013.

Park JJ, Wolff BG, Tollefson MK, et al: Meckel diverticulum: The Mayo Clinic experience with 1476 patients (1950–2002), *Ann Surg* 241:529–533, 2005.

Sartelli M, Catena F, Ansaloni L, et al: WSES Guidelines for the management of acute left sided colonic diverticulitis in the emergency setting, *World J Emerg Surg* 11:37, 2016.

Shabanzadeh DM, Wille-Jørgensen P: Antibiotics for uncomplicated diverticulitis, Nov 14, *Cochrane Database Syst Rev* 11, 2012. https://doi.org/10.1002/14651858.

Shah J, Patel K, Sunkara T, et al: Gastric Diverticulum: A Comprehensive Review, *Inflamm Intest Dis* 3:161–166, 2018.

Shahedi K, Fuller G, Bolus R, et al: Long-term risk of acute diverticulitis among patients with incidental diverticulosis found during colonoscopy, *Clin Gastroenterol Hepatol* 11(12):1609–1613, 2013.

Sinha CK, Pallewatte A, Easty Met al, et al: Meckel's scan in children: A review of 183 cases referred to two paediatric surgery specialist centres over 18 years, *Pediatr Surg Int* 29:511–517, 2013.

Strate LL: Lower GI, bleeding: Epidemiology and diagnosis, *Gastroenterol Clin North Am* 34:643–664, 2005.

Verdonck J, Morton RP: Systematic review on treatment of Zenker's diverticulum, *Eur Arch Otorhnolaryngol* 272:3095–3107, 2015.

Weizman AV, Nguyen GC: Diverticular disease: epidemiology and management, *Can J Gastroenterol* 25:385–389, 2011.

Young-Fadok TM: Diverticulitis, *N Engl J Med* 379, 2018. 1635-164.

Zani A, Eaton S, Rees CM: Incidentally detected Meckel diverticulum: To resect or not to resect? *Ann Surg* 247:276–281, 2008.

DYSPHAGIA AND ESOPHAGEAL OBSTRUCTION

Method of
Chrisopher Vélez, MD; John E. Pandolfino, MD; Kumar Krishnan, MD

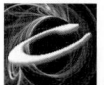

CURRENT DIAGNOSIS

- The evaluation of dysphagia begins with a careful history, though additional diagnostic testing is often required.
- Oropharyngeal dysphagia is best initially evaluated with a video fluoroscopoic examination, whereas esophageal dysphagia is best evaluated with endoscopy.
- Esophageal dysphagia with negative endoscopy and biopsy should be evaluated next with esophageal physiological testing (esophageal manometry or endoscopic functional lumen imaging probe EndoFLIP).

CURRENT THERAPY

- Underlying neuromuscular conditions such as amyotrophic lateral sclerosis, myasthenia gravis, or Guillain-Barré syndrome should be treated accordingly.
- Endoscopic therapy with dilation (often multiple) is the mainstay of treating fibrotic esophageal strictures regardless of etiology.
- Achalasia can be treated surgically or with dilation, which are equally effective. Minimally invasive endoscopic therapy for achalasia is now a well established alternative treatment approach.

Dysphagia is a symptom generated by the perceived sensation of difficulty or inability to swallow. It ranges in severity from mild difficulty with no associated clinical sequelae, to a complete inability to swallow with aspiration and severe malnutrition. Dysphagia can coexist with and must be distinguished from odynophagia, which is pain when swallowing, with associated swallowing aversion. The etiology of dysphagia is protean and includes two main categories, mechanical obstruction and motor dysfunction.

Epidemiology

Dysphagia is a common condition. In studies of outpatients, 22.6% of patients have reported dysphagia at least several times per month. Only half of these patients had discussed their symptoms with their physician. Elderly patients and women were more likely to note symptoms of dysphagia.

Pathophysiology

Effective swallowing and transfer of food bolus into the stomach requires multiple steps. These steps can be broadly placed into two phases: the oropharyngeal phase and the esophageal phase. The oropharyngeal phase of swallowing ultimately transforms the hypopharynx from a respiratory organ to a digestive organ. It requires five main coordinated steps to occur: (1) elevation of the soft palate and closure of the nasopharynx, (2) relaxation of the upper esophageal sphincter (UES), (3) traction opening of the UES, (4) closure of the laryngeal vestibule and, hence, airway protection, and (5) propulsion of the food bolus by the tongue and pharyngeal constrictors. This process is a carefully coordinated neuromuscular phenomenon with both autonomic and volitional components.

The esophageal phase of swallowing begins when a food bolus passes through the UES. During swallowing, the rapidity of bolus transit into the stomach is accomplished primarily by gravity. Esophageal peristalsis is a secondary contributor that functions to strip the bolus and clear the esophagus. Primary peristalsis is associated with oropharyngeal swallowing and propagates down through the predominantly striated muscle of the esophagus via a sequential activation pattern originating from the brainstem. This propagation then involves the esophageal smooth muscle where it also engages the intrinsic enteric nervous system to promote peristalsis through a similar but distinct mechanism. Secondary peristalsis is stimulated by distention of the proximal esophagus and will generate a propagating peristaltic contraction similar to primary peristalsis without a swallow-induced trigger. The strength, propagation velocity, and order of peristaltic contractions can be altered, with perturbations potentially leading to motor abnormalities associated with dysphagia.

Diagnosis

Dysphagia is never a normal symptom and always requires additional investigation. The first step in the diagnostic evaluation of dysphagia begins with a careful history to distinguish true dysphagia from other associated conditions such as odynophagia and globus sensation. Odynophagia can coexist with dysphagia;

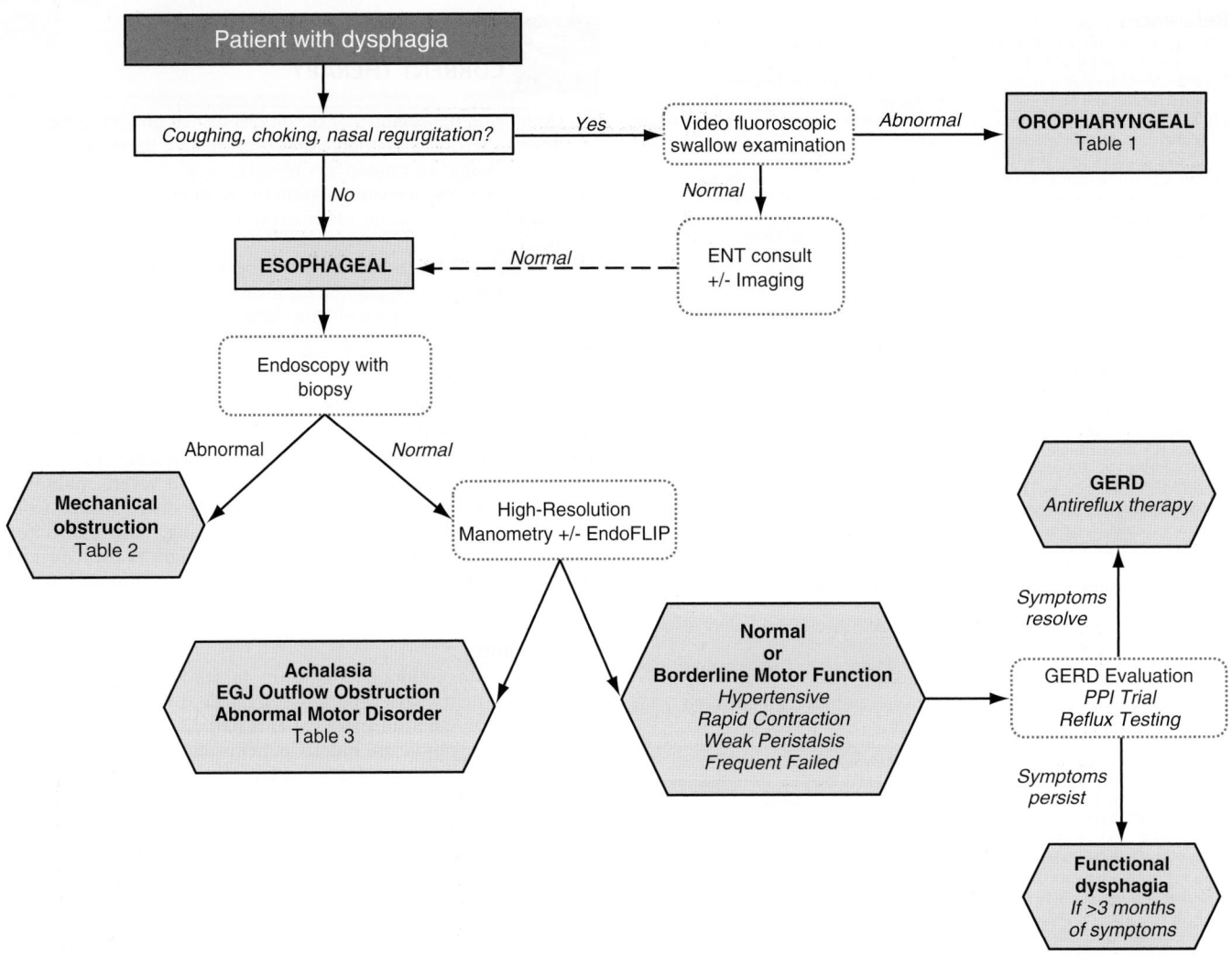

Figure 1 The workup of dysphagia and esophageal obstruction. The first step in the workup of dysphagia focuses on distinguishing oropharyngeal from esophageal dysphagia, which can be done with a history and careful assessment of swallowing during liquid swallows. The workup once this distinction is made is very different. Oropharyngeal dysphagia is typically evaluated by speech pathology and otolaryngology (ENT) based on the results of a video fluoroscopic swallow evaluation. Esophageal dysphagia is evaluated primarily with endoscopy because biopsies and interventions are often required. The primary indication for manometry is to rule out a major motor disorder in patients with a negative endoscopy. Alternatively, the functional lumen imaging probe (FLIP) can be utilized at the time of endoscopy to assess for a primary motor disorder. If a major motor abnormality is not seen on manometry or FLIP, a diagnosis of functional dysphagia should be considered; however, underlying GERD must also be addressed.

however, the predominant symptom is pain during swallowing. Globus is a sensation of a lump in the throat. It is likely a pharyngeal hypersensitivity that may coexist with other esophageal diseases or occur alone as a functional disorder. Unlike dysphagia, the symptoms in globus persist between swallows and may actually improve during the swallow.

After the above conditions have been ruled out, the next step focuses on distinguishing oropharyngeal dysphagia from esophageal dysphagia. Asking patients if their difficulty swallowing is "above-the-gulp" can differentiate oropharyngeal dysphagia. Unfortunately, patients have a difficult time communicating their symptoms because localization of the point of perceived obstruction is hampered by poor discriminant capacity and may be masked by compensatory mechanisms. Localization of dysphagia to the throat or sternal notch is unreliable because the point of obstruction may be further down in the body. However, localization in the midchest or below is more reliable that the obstruction is esophageal in origin.

As a result, the most useful and underused test for distinguishing oropharyngeal and esophageal dysphagia focuses on observing the patient swallow sips of water in the office. Often this allows the distinction between oropharyngeal and esophageal dysphagia to become apparent. Patients with oropharyngeal dysphagia will have difficulty almost immediately after initiating

a swallow, such as coughing, choking, and nasal regurgitation. Patients who can initiate a swallow without difficulty, but note symptoms soon after the swallow, are likely to have esophageal dysphagia. Furthermore, this exercise may be able to elicit associated odynophagia or regurgitation.

Physical examination plays a minor role in evaluating dysphagia outside of assessing the patient's baseline status to rule out malnutrition and dehydration because this will determine whether an expedited evaluation is required. A careful assessment of the oropharynx and a careful neck examination may unmask a mass lesion (i.e. of the thyroid), and a neurologic examination should be performed if oropharyngeal dysphagia is suspected. Additionally, a skin examination and assessment of the oropharyngeal mucosa may be helpful in assessing for potential dermatologic diseases that are associated with esophageal dysphagia. Regardless of findings, most patients will ultimately be referred for diagnostic testing, and this is dependent on the anatomic zone of interest—oropharyngeal versus esophageal (Figure 1).

Diagnostic Testing
Oropharyngeal Dysphagia
Once a distinction is made that the patient is experiencing oropharyngeal dysphagia, the next step in the evaluation should be referral for a video fluoroscopic swallowing examination, also

known as a modified barium study. Standard upper endoscopy is of limited value given the general inability to evaluate lesions in the hypopharynx and the upper esophageal sphincter. Video fluoroscopic swallow examinations have the added benefit of providing functional information in addition to anatomic information. They differ from a standard fluoroscopic examination (i.e., esophogram) by offering the patient various radiopaque food items of different consistency and are often performed by a speech pathologist. They can evaluate delay in initiation of pharyngeal swallowing, aspiration of solids and liquids, retrograde flow of ingested bolus, and residual pharyngeal contents.

If there is a suspicion for a malignancy or mechanical obstruction, a referral to otolaryngology is required. Direct laryngoscopy is used to evaluate for anatomic lesions in the nasopharynx and hypopharynx. In addition to anatomic abnormalities, function can be assessed by having the patient drink liquids with the nasal endoscope positioned in the hypopharynx. Oropharyngeal pooling of liquid indicates ineffective hypopharyngeal clearance and can suggest a high aspiration risk. Cross-sectional imaging is often an adjunct to the functional assessment of videoscopic imaging or direct laryngoscopy when an obstruction is noted without a clear lesion noted on direct examination.

Esophageal Dysphagia

If oropharyngeal dysphagia is excluded on history, the evaluation of dysphagia should proceed to upper endoscopy to rule out a mechanical obstruction. Although an esophogram can be used to assess for obstruction, most patients will eventually require endoscopy to obtain biopsies to rule out malignancy or eosinophilic esophagitis. Additionally, endoscopy has the added benefit of being therapeutic in some circumstances, and thus it is more cost-effective to begin the evaluation with endoscopy. If the endoscopy is negative, the next step is to evaluate for an underlying esophageal motor disorder. This is traditionally done by performing esophageal manometry. Recently, a novel method of assessing esophageal motor function has been developed. The functional lumen imaging probe (FLIP) is a catheter that can be placed at the time of endoscopy. Using a variety of sensors positioned along the length of the probe, it measures diameter and pressure along the esophagus. This information can be used to evaluate for contractility of the esophageal body and esophageal distensibility at the EGJ, thus providing a comprehensive assessment of esophageal motility that is complementary to esophageal manometry and can help resolve borderline cases of motility abnormality prior to the recommendation of potentially invasive surgical or endoscopic therapy. If these studies are negative, a careful evaluation for the presence of gastroesophageal reflux disease (GERD) should be performed and if suspected, the patient may benefit from ambulatory reflux testing or an empiric trial of proton pump inhibitors. Patients with no evidence of obstruction, abnormal esophageal motor function, or evidence of GERD may be classified as having functional dysphagia and they benefit from the use of neuromodulation (with agents used to treat functional gastrointestinal disorders such as tricyclic antidepressants) to improve sensory function.

Oropharyngeal Dysphagia
Differential Diagnosis

The etiology of oropharyngeal dysphagia can be broadly separated based on neuromuscular causes and anatomic causes (Table 1). The most common neurologic cause is cerebrovascular accident (CVA), with an incidence reported between 20% and 80%. CVAs involving the cerebrum, cerebellum, and brainstem can each lead to swallow dysfunction. Cerebral CVA can lead to impairment in mastication and the oral phase of swallowing and can interrupt normal pharyngeal peristalsis. CVA involving the brainstem can lead to disruption of the sensory afferents in the pharynx that help trigger pharyngeal swallow, and can also lead to motor dysfunction of laryngeal elevation, glottic closure, and cricopharyngeal relaxation/opening. Tumors in these areas can also produce similar effects. While difficulty swallowing liquids can be associated

| TABLE 1 | Oropharyngeal Dysphagia |

Iatrogenic

- Medication side effects (chemotherapy, neuroleptics, etc.)
- Postsurgical muscular or neurogenic
- Radiation
- Corrosive (pill injury, intentional)

Infectious

- Diphtheria
- Botulism
- Lyme disease
- Syphilis
- Mucositis (herpes, cytomegalovirus, candida, etc.)

Metabolic

- Amyloidosis
- Cushing's syndrome
- Thyrotoxicosis
- Wilson's disease

Myopathic

- Connective tissue disease (overlap syndrome)
- Dermatomyositis
- Myasthenia gravis
- Myotonic dystrophy
- Oculopharyngeal dystrophy
- Polymyositis
- Sarcoidosis
- Paraneoplastic syndromes

Neurologic

- Brainstem tumors
- Head trauma
- Stroke
- Cerebral palsy
- Guillain-Barré syndrome
- Huntington's disease
- Multiple sclerosis
- Polio
- Postpolio syndrome
- Tardive dyskinesia
- Metabolic encephalopathies
- Amyotrophic lateral sclerosis
- Parkinson's disease
- Dementia

Structural

- Cricopharyngeal bar
- Zenker's diverticulum
- Cervical webs
- Oropharyngeal tumors
- Osteophytes and skeletal abnormalities
- Congenital abnormalities (cleft palate, diverticula, pouches, etc.)

with oropharyngeal dysphagia, distinguishing between liquid versus solid food dysphagia is not a reliable way to differentiate this type of dysphagia from esophageal dysphagia.

A variety of neuromuscular disease can lead to bulbar symptoms, which manifest as dysphagia. This includes myasthenia gravis, amyotrophic lateral sclerosis (ALS), and Guillain-Barré syndrome (GBS). Clinicians need to be able to identify systemic manifestations of these conditions because dysphagia can often be the first manifestation of neuromuscular disorders.

The most common structural abnormalities of the hypopharynx associated with dysphagia are hypopharyngeal diverticula and cricopharyngeal bars. Acquired hypopharyngeal diverticula are most common in men after age 60 and typically present with symptoms of dysphagia, halitosis, post-swallow regurgitation, or even aspiration of material from the pharyngeal pouch. Hypopharyngeal diverticula are the result of a restrictive myopathy associated with diminished compliance of the cricopharyngeus muscle. The treatment of hypopharyngeal diverticula is cricopharyngeal myotomy with or without a diverticulectomy. Good or excellent results can be expected in 80% to 100% of Zenker's patients treated by transcervical myotomy combined with diverticulectomy or diverticulopexy. Small diverticula may spontaneously disappear following myotomy.

Other anatomic causes associated with oropharyngeal dysphagia that should be considered are cervical osteophytes and head and neck cancers. Cervical osteophytes are associated with cervical spine arthritis and may be confused with a cricopharygeal bar because the dysphagia is structural and localized to the area of the upper esophageal sphincter. It is easily differentiated on contrast studies because the cervical osteophyte can be seen impinging on the upper sphincter. Additionally, head and neck lesions of the larynx, tonsil, tongue, oral cavity, vocal cord, and nasopharynx may also impair bolus transit into the esophagus. Rapid weight loss in a patient with oropharyngeal dysphagia warrants further evaluation for malignancy; however, it is often difficult to distinguish weight loss resulting from malignancy from weight loss secondary to dysphagia. Constitutional symptoms (night sweats, fever, etc.) associated with oropharyngeal dysphagia should raise the suspicion for lymphoma.

Management

The management of oropharyngeal dysphagia is dependent on the underlying cause. Neuromuscular conditions such as stroke may respond to speech therapy and rehabilitation. Systemic neuromuscular dysfunction from conditions such as myasthenia gravis, GBS, or ALS will require treatment of the underlying condition. Patients who cannot safely take oral nutrition may need a temporary enteral feeding tube until swallow function is intact.

Management of dysphagia in patients with head and neck cancers requires a multidisciplinary approach and treatment of the underlying malignancy. Some patients are able to take adequate nutrition with dietary modification (soft or full liquid diet) while undergoing therapy. Patients who are losing weight, are dehydrated, or are unable to meet nutritional requirement by dietary modification alone may require enteral nutrition in the form of a gastrostomy tube. Although endoscopic gastrostomy tube placement is typically safe, and routinely performed in patients with head and neck cancer, there are reports of seeding the gastrostomy tube tract with malignant cells from the pharynx. In such circumstances, a direct gastrostomy tube placed by a radiologist may be preferable.

Esophageal Dysphagia

Esophageal dysphagia can be easily separated into mechanical causes and motor abnormalities after upper endoscopy is performed. Mechanical causes can be further separated into malignant and benign causes of dysphagia, and motor disorders can be conceptualized as primary motor abnormalities versus borderline motor abnormalities. Patients who have symptoms in the context of a normal endoscopy (negative biopsies for eosinophilic esophagitis) and no evidence of a primary motor disorder may also have underlying GERD or functional dysphagia (see Figure 1).

Differential Diagnosis: Mechanical Obstruction (Table 2)
Stricture

Fibrotic esophageal strictures are common and can be caused by erosive esophagitis (peptic stricture), radiation therapy, surgical anastomosis, eosinophilic esophagitis, and desquamating lesions (pemphigus, lichen planus, etc.). Peptic strictures are common and are the result of long-standing erosive esophagitis. They typically occur in the distal esophagus. Such patients often have underlying physiologic derangements that favor aggressive reflux (weak lower esophageal sphincter, hiatal hernia, poor esophageal clearance). Postsurgical anastomotic strictures are an unfortunate consequence of surgical therapy for esophageal disease, but these lesions are often amenable to endoscopic therapy.

TABLE 2 Esophageal Dysphagia (Mechanical)
Mucosal disease
GERD (peptic stricture)
Esophageal rings
Esophageal cancer
Caustic injury (e.g., lye ingestion, pill esophagitis, sclerotherapy)
Radiation injury
Infectious esophagitis
Eosinophilic esophagitis
Anastomotic stricture
Submucosal disease
Gastrointestinal stromal tumor
Sarcoidosis
Invasive carcinoma (primary or secondary)
Mediastinal disease
Tumors (lymph nodes, lung cancer)
Infection (histoplasmosis, tuberculosis)
Vascular compression
Dysphagia lusoria
Dysphagia aortica

Eosinophilic Esophagitis

Eosinophilic esophagitis (EoE) requires some focused discussion because its prevalence in patients presenting with dysphagia is increasing. EoE is a condition characterized by marked eosinophilic infiltrate within the esophageal epithelium. This infiltrate results in characteristic endoscopic findings of esophageal rings, furrows, exudate, and eventually stricture formation. The most common symptom in patients with EoE is dysphagia, which often leads to food bolus impaction. Patients are typically young Caucasians and there is a clear male predominance. Atopic conditions are more prevalent in patients with EoE. Patients should initially be treated with proton pump inhibitor (PPI) therapy because there is an overlap between GERD and EoE. Patients with persistent eosinophilia on PPI therapy can be treated by swallowing inhaled formulations of steroids (fluticasone [Flovent],[1] budesonide [Pulmicort][1]) or a food elimination diet (avoid: soy, nuts, wheat, eggs, dairy, seafood) to reduce the inflammatory component of the disease. Additional therapy with dilation will be required in many patients because histologic improvement does not always result in regression of fibrotic strictures. The esophageal body is more prone to fracture in EoE, and deep mucosal tears are often associated with dilation therapy; thus these lesions may require a more gradual and careful dilation protocol.

Rings/Webs

Esophageal webs can exist along the length of the esophagus and lead to dysphagia. The classic triad of proximal esophageal web, iron deficiency anemia, and dysphagia is Plummer-Vinson syndrome. The etiology of this condition is not entirely known; however, it is thought that iron deficiency leads to a decrease in iron-dependent oxidative enzymes, which results in degradation of esophageal tissue, resulting in web formation. Interestingly, iron supplementation alone may result in resolution of symptoms. Whereas Plummer-Vinson syndrome is a rare condition, esophageal webs are relatively common and should prompt an evaluation for caustic pill injury if localized to the transition zone along the aortic impression or distal esophagus. Medications that can be associated with pill esophagitis include NSAIDs, tetracycline, iron, bisphosphonates, potassium, and quinidine.

Malignancy

Dysphagia is often the presenting symptom in a patient with esophageal cancer. There are two subtypes of mucosal cancer in the esophagus, squamous cell and adenocarcinoma. In general,

---

[1]Not FDA approved for this indication.

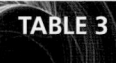 **TABLE 3**	Esophageal Dysphagia (Abnormal Motor Function)

Achalasia
EGJ outflow obstruction
Absent peristalsis
Spasm
Jackhammer

esophageal cancer has a male predominance and is slightly more prevalent among African Americans. The racial disparity is largely due to squamous cell carcinoma, which has noted a sharp decline since the 1960s. Adenocarcinoma tends to be a disease of white men (SEER database). Squamous cell carcinoma typically occurs in the mid esophagus, whereas adenocarcinoma is localized to the distal esophagus where it is associated with intestinal metaplasia (Barrett's esophagus).

Management for Esophageal Obstruction

Endoscopic dilation therapy is the most common therapeutic intervention for patients with nonmalignant mechanical dysphagia. This can be done with a single, large-diameter dilating balloon or semirigid bougie over a guide wire. There has not been any convincing data to demonstrate superiority of balloon dilators over bougie dilators. In cases of membranous webs or Schatzki rings, the goal of endoscopic therapy is to tear the lesion with a single, large-diameter dilation. In the case of a Schatzki ring, postdilation PPI therapy is associated with decreased recurrence rates.

When treating fibrotic strictures (peptic, anastomotic, radiation, EoE), the goal should be gradual stretching of the stricture. The choice of initial dilation size is based on an estimate of the diameter of the stricture. The extent to which a stricture can be dilated is expressed by the endoscopic axiom of the "rule of threes." This refers to the approach whereby the diameter of the stricture is approximated, and no more than three subsequent dilations are performed at 1-mm intervals once resistance is noted. Although there is no controlled trial for support, this approach is used to minimize the most serious risks of dilation therapy, perforation, and bleeding.

In patients with refractory strictures despite dilation therapy, several therapies have been attempted with variable efficacy. Temporary self-expanding stents have been placed to maintain lumen patency. When placed across a stricture, stents serve two purposes. First, they relieve symptoms of dysphagia by maintaining a patent lumen. In addition, the self-expanding nature of the stent provides ongoing radial force, which gradually stretches the lumen. The main disadvantage of stents is their tendency to migrate.

An alternative endoscopic approach is incisional therapy with an electrocautery knife. This is used to make incisions in the mucosa and fibrotic submucosa. This approach has been best studied in the setting of refractory anastomotic strictures; however, no head-to-head comparisons have been made between incisional therapy and other modalities.

Treatment of malignant etiologies for dysphagia will ultimately depend on the tumor type and extent of disease. Benign tumors and early-stage lesions can be treated with endoscopic resection or surgery. Endoscopic therapy using stents is also an important component of the treatment of malignancy and may be used during the treatment phase of malignant disorders or as a palliative technique for later-stage disease.

Differential Diagnosis: Motility Disorders (Table 3)

Esophageal motor disorders are defined based on patterns of contractile vigor, propagation, and the presence of deglutitive relaxation. The most common classification scheme is the "Chicago classification," at the time this chapter was written currently in its fourth version. This scheme takes advantage of advanced high-resolution manometry with modifications based on refining disorders into clinically relevant phenotypes compared to earlier classification iterations.

Achalasia

The diagnosis of achalasia is made by esophageal manometry and requires two main manometric criteria: (1) inability of the lower esophageal sphincter to relax and (2) absence of peristalsis. Recently achalasia has been subdivided into three different phenotypes using high-resolution manometry, which are associated with varying clinical outcomes. Patients typically describe both solid and liquid dysphagia. Other common symptoms are regurgitation (especially nocturnal), chest pain, and aspiration. Weight loss and malnutrition may be dominant symptoms as the disease progresses. Given that there is no treatment to reverse absent peristalsis, the treatment is focused on improving esophagogastric junction (EGJ) opening by disrupting the poorly relaxing lower esophageal sphincter. Currently, three modalities exist to treat achalasia: (1) pneumatic dilation with rigid balloons ranging in size from 3 to 4 cm; (2) surgical myotomy paired with or without a fundoplication; (3) per-oral endoscopic myotomy or POEM. It appears that the three treatment approaches are associated with good outcomes with surgery having a more durable single intervention success rate, pneumatic dilation typically requiring multiple sessions and POEM combining the benefit of one treatment session with a non-surgical approach. Botulinum toxin type A (Botox)[1] injected into the lower esophageal sphincter has been shown to reduce EGJ pressure and improve symptoms; however, this treatment only provides temporary relief and should only be reserved for poor surgical candidates or patients unwilling to undergo surgery, dilation, or endoscopic myotomy. Occasionally, esophageal dilatation may progress to a point where EGJ-directed treatment is not adequate and esophagectomy must be performed to prevent severe complications, such as aspiration and severe malnutrition. At times, dysphagia can recur after EGJ-directed therapy; EndoFLIP can help identify patients requiring re-treatment.

Esophagogastric Junction Outflow Obstruction

This pattern of motor disturbance is associated with preserved peristalsis and evidence of high pressures through the EGJ during swallowing. This may be an achalasia variant or could be associated with a subtle obstruction at the distal esophagus not evident on endoscopy. Thus recognition of this pattern should prompt an evaluation for an infiltrating tumor or other potential etiology of obstruction. Treatment is focused on the underlying cause of the obstruction. If distensibility is normal on EndoFLIP, then watchful waiting is appropriate.

Absent Peristalsis

Absent peristalsis is defined as complete absence of contractile activity on all swallows in the context of a normal or low EGJ relaxation pressure. This pattern was previously categorized as scleroderma esophagus if it was found in the context of a hypotensive lower esophageal sphincter; however, this has been abandoned because this pattern may be found in patients with severe GERD without scleroderma. Treatment is focused on aggressive antireflux therapy and lifestyle modifications to reduce dysphagia and caustic injury to the esophagus.

Distal Esophageal Spasm

Distal esophageal spasm is a rare primary motor disorder that can provoke dysphagia and is associated with premature contraction of the esophageal body. Treatment for this disorder is extremely

---

[1]Not available in the United States.

difficult and focuses on medical management with smooth muscle relaxants, such as calcium channel blockers,[1] nitrates,[1] and 5-phosphodiesterase inhibitors.[1]

Jackhammer

Jackhammer esophagus is an extreme form of nutcracker esophagus associated with contractile vigor not encountered in asymptomatic controls or under normal conditions. Previous definitions for hypertensive esophagus had a significant overlap with data from cohorts of asymptomatic controls, and thus the clinical significance of these disorders was unclear. This pattern is associated with dysphagia and chest pain and is typically treated similar to distal esophageal spasm. This motor pattern can also be seen with distal esophageal obstruction, and this should be considered in the differential diagnosis because it would alter management to focus on the obstruction.

Borderline Motor Abnormalities

Borderline motor abnormalities are those associated with ineffective esophageal motility and mild abnormalities of peristaltic propagation (rapid contraction) or hypertensive contraction. These disorders are not considered to be primary motor disorders, and secondary cause for symptoms, such as GERD and visceral sensitivity, should be considered and treated.

Monitoring

Patients with dysphagia or esophageal obstruction should be monitored for three important complications:

- Evidence of aspiration and nocturnal regurgitation because these can be associated with severe complications, such as chemical pneumonitis and aspiration pneumonia.
- Malnutrition and dehydration because this may prompt more aggressive therapy or consideration of non-oral feeding methods.
- Progressive symptoms because this could lead to progression of the disease and early therapy may avoid the above complications.

Acknowledgment

This work was supported by R01 DK079902 (JEP) from the U.S. National Institutes of Health.

---

[1]Not available in the United States.

References

Bredenoord AJ, Fox M, Kahrilas PJ, et al: Chicago classification criteria of esophageal motility disorders defined in high resolution esophageal pressure topography, *Neurogastroenterol Motil* 24(Suppl. 1):57–65, 2012.

Cook IJ, Kahrilas PJ: AGA technical review on management of oropharyngeal dysphagia, *Gastroenterology* 116:455–478, 1999.

Drossman DA: The functional gastrointestinal disorders and the Rome III process, *Gastroenterology* 130:1377–1390, 2006.

Egan JV, Baron TH, Adler DG, et al: Esophageal dilation, *Gastrointest Endosc* 63:755–760, 2006.

Francis DL, Katzka DA: Achalasia: update on the disease and its treatment, *Gastroenterology* 139:369–374, 2010.

Liacouras CA, Furuta GT, Hirano I, et al: Eosinophilic esophagitis: updated consensus recommendations for children and adults, *J Allergy Clin Immunol* 128:3–20, 2011, e26; quiz 21–2.

Pandolfino JE, Kahrilas PJ: AGA technical review on the clinical use of esophageal manometry, *Gastroenterology* 128:209–224, 2005.

Pandolfino JE, Kwiatek MA, Nealis T, et al: Achalasia: a new clinically relevant classification by high-resolution manometry, *Gastroenterology* 135:1526–1533, 2008.

Spechler SJ: AGA technical review on treatment of patients with dysphagia caused by benign disorders of the distal esophagus, *Gastroenterology* 117:233–254, 1999.

Wilkins T, Gillies RA, Thomas AM, et al: The prevalence of dysphagia in primary care patients: a HamesNet Research Network study, *J Am Board Fam Med* 20:144–150, 2007.

GASTRITIS AND PEPTIC ULCER DISEASE

Method of
Kyle Vincent, MD

CURRENT DIAGNOSIS

- Diagnosis of gastritis and peptic ulcer disease (PUD) is based on history of dyspepsia and elimination of other conditions.
- *Helicobacter pylori (H. pylori)* and nonsteroidal anti-inflammatory drugs (NSAIDs) are the most common cause of ulcer disease. Hypersecretory conditions such as Zollinger-Ellison syndrome are rare.
- If testing for *H. pylori* is indicated (test and treat strategy), IgG antibody, urea breath test, and fecal antigen test are available.
- Young patients with no "warning signs" can usually be managed on an outpatient basis without immediate endoscopy.
- Patients older than 55 with bleeding, anemia, loss of more than 10% of body weight, dysphagia, odynophagia, early satiety, history of previous malignancy, lymphadenopathy, abdominal mass, or a previously documented ulcer should undergo upper endoscopy promptly.

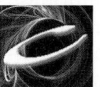

CURRENT TREATMENT

- The two principal strategies are empiric treatment or test and treat.
- In areas with an *H. pylori* infection rate of less than 10% a 4–8 week course of proton-pump inhibitors (PPIs) given empirically is appropriate.
- In patients who fail empiric PPI treatment or in areas with an *H. pylori* infection rate of greater than 10%, a test and treat strategy should be employed. A verified noninvasive *H. pylori* test should be used.
- First-line treatment of *H. pylori* consists of a PPI, clarithromycin (Biaxin), and amoxicillin (Amoxil) all taken twice a day for 14 days.
- Test of cure should be undertaken in any patient treated for *H. pylori*.
- NSAIDs should be discontinued or standard dose PPI for ulcer prophylaxis used to treat any dyspepsia.

Epidemiology

An estimated four million Americans have active gastric ulcers with 350,000 new cases diagnosed each year. The lifetime prevalence of this condition is around 10%. The incidence was previously higher in men but is currently equal in men and women. Familial clustering is now believed to result from transmission of *Helicobacter pylori (H. pylori)* from person to person or a genetic predisposition to infection with *H. pylori* rather than a genetic predisposition to gastric ulcers.

Risk Factors

Most gastric and duodenal ulcers can be attributed to *H. pylori*, NSAID use, severe physiologic stress, or hypersecretory conditions. In America, 10% of young adults harbor *H. pylori* infections, and this incidence increases with age. Lower socioeconomic status and recent immigration from areas with high rates of infection also increase the incidence of *H. pylori* infection. Hypersecretory conditions such as Zollinger-Ellison syndrome are rare, estimated to be responsible for only 0.1% of all ulcers. These conditions should not be routinely considered except in refractory or recurrent cases or in patients who have multiple ulcers.

Pathophysiology

The low pH of gastric acid is required to kill ingested bacteria and to promote proteolysis and activation of pepsin. Postprandial gastric acid production is stimulated by expression of gastrin from G cells and is inhibited in a negative feedback loop by somatostatin from antral D cells. Contrary to previous beliefs, peptic ulcer disease is not simply due to excessive acid production. Almost all patients with gastric ulcer have normal acid production and only one-third of patients with duodenal ulcer have evidence of increased acid production. The protective mechanisms of the mucosa play an important role in maintaining mucosal integrity.

The gastric and duodenal mucosa forms a gelatinous layer that is impermeable to gastric acid and pepsin. Mucosal blood flow as well as the production of mucus and bicarbonate secretion are largely regulated by E type prostaglandins (PGE). Anything that can disrupt the balance between acid production and the protective barrier has the potential to cause loss of mucosal integrity and tissue exposure to gastric acid and pepsin with subsequent inflammation and potential ulceration.

Two major mechanisms contribute to gastritis and/or ulcer formation. H. pylori is a gram-negative curved rod that produces ammonia to control the surrounding pH. Ammonia is toxic to epithelial cells, causing gastritis or duodenitis and damaging mucosal integrity. Many patients with gastritis also have a marked decrease in the number of somatostatin secreting antral D cells, leading to diminished feedback to control acid secretion during gastrin stimulation.

Prevention

The United States Preventative Task Force does not currently recommend routine screening for H. pylori in asymptomatic individuals. Prevention is based on avoidance or minimization of risk factors. Long-term NSAID use should be avoided. Prophylactic antisecretory medication should be considered when prolonged NSAID use is necessary. Proton pump inhibitors (PPIs) have better protective efficacy than histamine receptor antagonists (H2RAs) when prolonged NSAID use is necessary. Patients with a previous history of ulcer disease who use steroids or are older than 65 years of age should strongly be considered for prophylaxis with an antisecretory medication. Because of the high risk of gastric ulceration, prophylaxis is recommended for patients experiencing severe physiologic stress such as mechanical ventilation for longer than 48 hours, hypoperfusion, high dose corticosteroids, and large surface area burns (>35% total body surface). Histamine receptor antagonists such as famotidine (Pepcid),[1] cimetidine (Tagamet),[1] and ranitidine (Zantac)[1] or PPIs are recommended. No agent has shown to be clearly superior for prophylaxis in patients on steroids or undergoing physiologic stress.

No immunization against H. pylori is currently available but early stage animal trials are in progress.

Clinical Manifestations

Dyspepsia is defined by the American College of Gastroenterology as chronic or recurrent pain or discomfort centered in the upper abdomen. Discomfort is defined as a subjective negative feeling that is not painful. Discomfort can incorporate a variety of symptoms including early satiety or upper abdominal fullness. A thorough history alone is usually sufficient to establish the diagnosis and to differentiate gastritis and peptic ulcers from other common conditions, though gastritis and peptic ulcer disease are difficult to differentiate from each other. Patients with peptic ulcer disease tend to have symptoms more pronounced with food intake. A patient with a duodenal ulcer usually reports increased pain 2-3 hours after a meal; conversely, a patient with a gastric ulcer tends to have pain precipitated or exacerbated by food intake. However,

these classical findings are not reliable diagnostic indicators. Physical examination is important to rule out serious complications from peptic ulcer disease. Patient with a rigid abdomen, rebound tenderness, or guarding should be evaluated with imaging and by a surgeon to rule out perforation. The most common physical finding in peptic ulcer disease is tenderness in the epigastrium.

Differential Diagnosis

The differential diagnosis for gastritis and peptic ulcer disease is broad given its nonspecific nature, but can be narrowed down fairly quickly by a good initial history. The differential diagnosis includes gastroesophageal reflux disease (GERD), cardiac disease, gastric cancer, pancreatitis, pancreatic neoplasm, biliary disease including cholelithiasis or cholecystitis, delayed gastric emptying, or bowel ischemia. Patients presenting with a predominant complaint of heartburn or abdominal pain with heartburn more than once per week should be considered to have GERD until proven otherwise. Any symptoms associated with dyspnea or chest pressure should raise concern for a cardiac etiology. Biliary pain often radiates to the right shoulder and is associated with fatty or greasy foods. Patients with pancreatitis usually describe a severe boring type pain in the epigastrium. They may also get relief from leaning forward.

Diagnosis

While most dyspepsia symptoms can be treated on a nonurgent basis, specific "warning signs" should prompt referral or performance of upper endoscopy. These include age 55 or older, bleeding, anemia, loss of more than 10% of body weight, dysphagia, odynophagia, early satiety, history of previous malignancy, lymphadenopathy, abdominal mass, or a previously documented ulcer.

H. pylori testing is a cornerstone of managing dyspepsia. However, most other laboratory studies are usually not helpful in establishing the diagnosis in uncomplicated peptic ulcer disease or gastritis but may be helpful in eliminating other conditions in the differential diagnosis.

Noninvasive Testing

Antibody Test—Serum IgG antibodies are typically present at 21 days after the onset of H. pylori infection but can persist long after active infection. Antibody testing has a sensitivity of 85% and specificity of 79%. The positive predictive value is greatly influenced by the prevalence of the organism in the community and therefore it is less useful in areas with lower rates of H. pylori infection. The excellent negative predictive value makes IgG testing a good screening test. However, given that the IgG antibodies can persist for up to a year or longer after infection, it is not as helpful in the acute phase.

Urea Breath Test—This test identifies infection through urease activity. The patient ingests urea labeled with either ^{13}C or ^{14}C. In the presence of H. pylori, urease activity produces labeled CO_2 that is expired and can be collected and measured. Sensitivities and specificities of this test exceed 95%. It maintains a strong positive and negative predictive value despite the prevalence of H. pylori, but the test is not universally available.

Fecal Antigen Test—This assay uses either polyclonal or monoclonal antibodies to identify H. pylori antigens in the stool. The sensitivity and specificity exceed 90% in most studies. Like the breath test, it is unaffected by prevalence, however, both tests are affected by previous exposure to bismuth, antibiotics, and PPIs.

Treatment

The treatment of dyspepsia was revolutionized in the 1990s following the discovery of the role of H. pylori in pathogenesis. For patients who present with dyspepsia but no "warning signs," two separate and approximately equivalent treatment strategies are recommended. The "test and treat" option recommends using a validated noninvasive test for H. pylori and treatment of positive

---

[1]Not FDA approved for this indication.

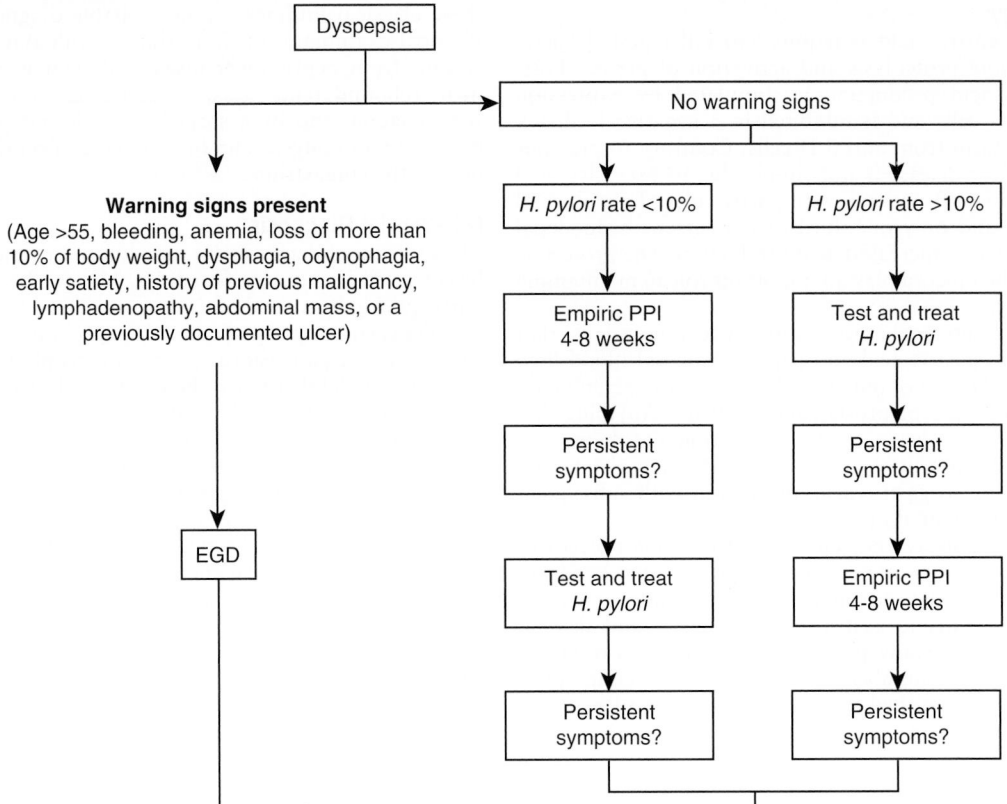

Figure 1 The treatment of dyspepsia.

tests. The "empiric" acid suppression option recommends treating with a PPI for 4-8 weeks without testing for *H. pylori*. The test and treat strategy is recommended for populations where the *H. pylori* infection rate is higher than 10%, in patients with active or past PUD, low-grade gastric mucosa-associated lymphoid tissue (MALT) lymphoma, or history of endoscopic resection of early gastric cancer. As the US prevalence varies from 10% to 40% in different communities, either strategy may be appropriate. The test and treat strategy is more appropriate for most urban areas and in communities with a high immigrant population or known high rates of *H. pylori* infection. In populations with low *H. pylori* prevalence, such as high socioeconomic areas, empiric acid suppression is an appropriate first strategy, followed by *H. pylori* testing in those patients who have continued symptoms (Figure 1).

The recommendations for eradication of *H. pylori* were updated by the American College of Gastroenterology in 2017. Previous regimens had focused on specific PPI medications. This has been replaced with a general recommendation for standard or double dose PPI of choice. There are two key considerations for selection for initial treatment: (1) Is there a penicillin allergy? and (2) Has there been any previous macrolide exposure for any reason? Current first-line treatment is the so-called triple therapy with standard or double dose PPI, clarithromycin (Biaxin), and amoxicillin (Amoxil) for 14 days. This regimen has an eradication rate of 70% to 85%. Studies show no statistical difference between 7- and 10-day treatment regimens; however, there were trends toward higher eradication rates with the longer regimen. In addition, these studies have not been duplicated in the U.S. population where 7-day regimens have shown efficacy rates below 80%. Therefore, regimens less than 10 days are not recommended and 14-day treatment should be considered. In patients who are penicillin allergic, metronidazole (Flagyl)[1] may be substituted for amoxicillin, but resistance rates for metronidazole are more than double those for amoxicillin. Second-line

therapy for those with previous macrolide exposure or penicillin allergy is the so-called quadruple therapy. This consists of standard dose PPI, bismuth subcitrate,[2] tetracycline (Sumycin),[1] and metronidazole (Flagyl).[1] Bismuth subcitrate, metronidazole, and tetracycline are available as a combination product, Pylera, which is approved to use with omeprazole for the treatment of patients with *H. pylori* infection and duodenal ulcer disease. There are multiple other regimens with similar eradication rates in European studies that have not been well validated in North America. Nonetheless, they are recommended by the American College of Gastroenterology and can be used for patients who are having difficulty with intolerance to the more common regimens. They are listed in Table 1.

Monitoring

The recommendations for routine testing for eradication of *H. pylori* were updated in 2017. Although strong evidence is lacking, expert consensus supports testing for eradication in most cases. There is clear benefit in testing patients who have persistent symptoms despite the test and treat strategy, any patient with an *H. pylori*–associated ulcer, any patient who has had a resection of any early gastric cancer, or those with an *H. pylori*–associated MALT lymphoma. In these patients, testing should be done no sooner than 4 weeks after the completion of eradication treatment. Patients requiring follow-up endoscopy, such as for an ulcer or MALT lymphoma, should undergo endoscopic testing for eradication. Patients who are not undergoing endoscopy can be tested for eradication with fecal antigen or urea breath testing. The serum antibody test is unreliable for follow-up as it can remain positive for quite some time after successful treatment.

The most common causes of treatment failure are poor compliance with the medications and antibiotic resistance by the organism. Patients should be counseled on the side effects of their regimen and the importance of compliance. About 10% of

---

[1]Not FDA approved for this indication.

[2]Not available in the United States.

TABLE 1 *H. pylori* Regimens

REGIMEN	ANTIBIOTIC			ANTACID	DURATION
Clarithromycin Triple Therapy	Clarithromycin (Biaxin) 500 mg BID	Amoxicillin (Amoxil) 1 g BID[a]		PPI (Standard or double dose)	14 days[b]
Bismuth Quadruple Therapy[c]	Tetracycline (Sumycin)[1] 500 mg QID	Metronidazole (Flagyl)[1] 500 mg QID	Bismuth subcitrate[2] or subsalicylate (Pepto-Bismol) 300 mg QID	PPI (Standard dose)	10-14 days[b]
Concomitant[c]	Clarithromycin (Biaxin) 500 mg BID	Amoxicillin (Amoxil) 1 g BID	Metronidazole (Flagyl)[1] 500 mg BID	PPI (Standard dose)	10-14 days[b]
Sequential[c]	Amoxicillin (Amoxil) 1 g BID and PPI (Standard dose)	Clarithromycin (Biaxin) 500 mg BID and metronidazole (Flagyl) 500 mg BID and PPI (Standard dose)			5-7 days
Hybrid[c]	Amoxicillin (Amoxil) 1 g BID and PPI (Standard dose)	Amoxicillin (Amoxil) 1 g BID, PPI (Standard dose), clarithromycin (Biaxin) 500 mg BID, and metronidazole (Flagyl)[1] 500 mg BID			5-7 days
Levofloxacin triple[c]	Amoxicillin (Amoxil) 1 g BID	Levofloxacin (Levaquin)[1] 500 mg daily		PPI (Standard dose)	10-14 days[b]
Levofloxacin sequential[c]	Amoxicillin (Amoxil) 1 g BID and PPI (Standard dose)	Amoxicillin (Amoxil) 1 g BID, PPI (Standard dose), levofloxacin 500 mg daily, and metronidazole (Flagyl) 500 mg BID		PPI (Standard or double dose)	5-7 days
LOAD[c]	Levofloxacin (Levaquin) 250 mg daily	Doxycycline (Vibramycin)[1] 100 mg daily	Nitazoxanide (Alinia)[1] 500 mg BID	PPI (Double dose)	7-10 days

[a]In patients with penicillin allergy, metronidazole (Flagyl) 500 mg TID can be substituted, although not FDA approved.
[b]14-day courses should be considered secondary to increased eradication rates.
[c]Not FDA approved for this treatment regimen.
[1]Not FDA approved for this indication.
[2]Not available in the United States.

patients report headaches and diarrhea with PPI use. Clarithromycin (Biaxin) can cause diarrhea, gastrointestinal upset, and altered taste. Similar effects can be seen with amoxicillin and metronidazole. Metronidazole also has disulfiram-like effects if taken with alcohol. Bacterial resistance is relatively rare, with multicenter U.S. data showing resistance rates to be 37% for metronidazole, 10% for clarithromycin, 3.9% for both antibiotics, and 1.4% for amoxicillin. For patients with persistent *H. pylori* infections, a new regimen should be attempted that does not include previously used antibiotics.

Patients who continue to have dyspepsia after successful eradication of *H. pylori* or who have persistent symptoms after a negative test and acid suppression should be considered for upper endoscopy.

Complications

Peptic ulcer disease can have severe complications, almost always requiring hospital admission. The most significant complications are gastric bleeding, perforation, or outlet obstruction.

Gastrointestinal bleeding is the most common cause of death in patients with peptic ulcer disease. Most cases of massive hemorrhage are due to erosion of a posterior ulcer into the gastroduodenal artery. Although the most common site of such hemorrhage is proximal to the ligament of Trietz, profuse bleeding can result in bright red blood from the rectum.

Approximately 5% of peptic ulcers cause perforation. This usually occurs anteriorly through the duodenum or lesser curve of the stomach. These patients often present in extremis with fever, tachycardia, dehydration, and abdominal findings of rigidity and rebound due to chemical peritonitis. Free air is commonly present under the diaphragm. Perforation is almost always requires surgical management.

Gastric outlet obstruction can occur acutely due to inflammation from peptic ulcer disease or more chronically secondary to inflammation and healing that lead to scarring and fibrosis of the duodenum. These patients can present with severe hypochloremic hypokalemic alkalosis due to the loss of hydrogen, potassium, and chloride from gastric secretions. Electrolyte derangements must be corrected prior to any attempted surgery. Initial treatment with balloon dilation can be attempted, especially in cases with newly diagnosed *H. pylori*. If the patient is negative for *H. pylori* or has successfully eradicated the organism, the long-term outcomes of dilation do not compare well to surgery.

References

Chey WD, Leontiadis GI, Howden CW, et al: ACG Clinical Guideline: Treatment of Helicobacter pylori infection, *AM J Gastroenterol* 112:112–238, 2017.

Chey WD, Wong BC: The Practice Parameters Committee of the American College of Gastroenterology: American College of Gastroenterology guideline on the management of *Helicobacter pylori* infection, *AM J Gastroenterol* 102:1808–1825, 2007.

Helicobacter pylori and peptic ulcer disease: FDA approved drug regimens. Available at. http://www.cdc.gov/ulcer/keytocure.htm. (accessed 30 December 2013).

Mercer DW, Robinson EK: Stomach. In *Sabiston Textbook of Surgery*, ed 18, Philadelphia, 2008, Saunders, pp 1223–1277.

Nordenstedt H, Graham DY, Kramer JR, et al: *Helicobacter pylori*—Negative gastritis prevalence and risk factors, *AM J Gastroenterol* 108:65–71, 2013.

Surgical critical care evidence based-medicine guidelines: Stress ulcer prophylaxis. Available at. http://www.surgicalcriticalcare.net/Guidelines/stress%20ulcer%20prophylaxis%202011.pdf. (accessed 15 December 2013).

Talley NJ, Vakil NB: The Practice Parameters Committee of the American College of Gastroenterology: Guideline for the management of dyspepsia, *AM J Gastroenterol* 100:2324–2337, 2005.

GASTROESOPHAGEAL REFLUX DISEASE (GERD)

Method of
Mustafa Abdul-Hussein, MD, MSCR; and Donald O. Castell, MD

Gastroesophageal reflux disease (GERD) is a motility disorder of the lower esophageal sphincter (LES). The definition of this disease has evolved over time, reflecting better understanding of the roles that transient LES relaxations and acid/pepsin contact with esophageal mucosa play, as well as the ability to identify these events. The diagnosis of GERD has changed from identification of a hiatal hernia, to identification of erosive esophagitis, to the currently accepted patient-centered definition: any symptom or injury to esophageal mucosa resulting from reflux of gastric contents into the esophagus. GERD should not be confused with physiologic gastroesophageal reflux, which is not associated with symptoms or esophageal mucosal injury.

The prevalence of GERD is difficult to ascertain, although several studies have indicated it to be as high as 50% of adults in Western countries, with 10% to 18% experiencing heartburn on a daily basis. Studies using health care utilization data may underestimate the prevalence because of self-treatment by individuals in the community, whereas population surveys may overestimate it because of inaccurate assessment of symptoms and absence of objective data. Regardless of the real number, the management of this disease costs more than $10 billion annually in the United States. GERD has been called a disease of white males, although recent data suggest increasing prevalence in Asia and Pacific regions.

Pathophysiology

GERD is a motility disorder of the LES characterized by inappropriate or transient relaxations that allow gastric contents to reflux into the esophagus. The LES is a tonically contracted ring of smooth muscle fibers innervated by the vagus nerve. Vagal stimulation during swallowing produces physiologic LES relaxation and is a likely source for transient LES relaxations. Gastroesophageal reflux occurs most frequently during postprandial periods, at a rate of six reflux episodes per hour, but averages two episodes per hour over the entire day. Increasing frequency of reflux in the postprandial period results from gastric distention after a meal and stimulation of tension receptors in the proximal stomach leading to transient LES relaxations (Box 1). A chronically hypotensive LES is not a major mechanism for GERD in most patients but can be seen in cases of severe erosive esophagitis.

Reflux of acidic gastric contents can lead to injury of the esophageal mucosa, including inflammation, ulceration, stricturing, Barrett's metaplasia, and adenocarcinoma. Peristaltic clearance, tissue resistance, and salivary bicarbonate make up host defense mechanisms that work by clearing reflux and neutralizing the acid residue on the mucosa. Erosive esophagitis or strictures result in the most severe form of GERD, which includes nocturnal reflux with longer acid contact times, decreased salivary production, and lower frequency of swallowing during sleep.

Complications

Acid reflux can lead to significant morbidity if it is not recognized and treated appropriately. Habitual contact of acid and activated pepsin with the stratified squamous epithelium, along with impaired defense mechanisms, results in tissue injury (Box 2). The end result of this process can be ulceration, fibrosis with stricture formation, Barrett's esophagus, or adenocarcinoma. These complications can produce alarm symptoms (Box 3). Patients presenting with alarm symptoms should undergo immediate diagnostic evaluation with an esophagogastroduodenoscopy (EGD).

Erosive Esophagitis

The endoscopic finding of erosive esophagitis is seen in fewer than 50% of patients with heartburn. The severity is stratified according to the Los Angeles Classification of Esophagitis. Treatment with a proton pump inhibitor (PPI) for 4 to 12 weeks heals erosive esophagitis in 78% to 95% of cases. The healing effect of antisecretory therapy, and particularly PPIs, demonstrates the important role of acid reflux in causing tissue injury. The recurrence rates for erosive esophagitis are high after discontinuation of PPI maintenance therapy (75%–92%), necessitating continuation of gastric acid suppression.

Strictures

Most strictures caused by GERD are peptic in origin and are located at the squamocolumnar junction. Patients with GERD and strictures, compared to those without strictures, are more likely to have a hypotensive LES, abnormal peristalsis, and prolonged acid clearance time. Stricture formation decreases the

---

BOX 1 Factors That Modulate Transient Lower Esophageal Sphincter Relaxation

Stimulants
- Gastric distention
- Pharyngeal intubation
- Upright orientation
- Foods (fatty foods, caffeine, alcohol)
- Tobacco

Inhibitors
- Recumbency
- Lateral decubitus (left side)
- Anesthesia
- Sleep

BOX 2 Esophageal Tissue Defense Mechanisms

Preepithelial
- Mucous layer
- Unstirred water layer
- Surface bicarbonate concentration

Epithelial Structures
- Cell membranes
- Intercellular junctional complexes (tight junctions, glycoconjugates/lipid)

Cellular
Epithelial transport (Na^+/H^+ exchanger, Na^+-dependent Cl^-/HCO_3^- exchanger)
- Intracellular and extracellular buffers
- Cell restitution
- Cell replication

Postepithelial
- Blood flow
- Tissue acid-base status

BOX 3 Alarm Symptoms of Gastroesophageal Reflux Disease

Presence of any of the following symptoms requires immediate evaluation:
- Dysphagia
- Odynophagia
- Weight loss
- Spontaneous resolution of GERD symptoms
- Iron deficiency anemia
- Gastrointestinal bleeding

luminal diameter, resulting in solid food dysphagia. Dysphagia in these patients is often a combination of decreased luminal diameter and dysmotility of the distal esophageal body with low-amplitude peristalsis. Patients with GERD who develop dysphagia should have immediate barium radiography and an endoscopic evaluation.

Barrett's Esophagus

Barrett's esophagus (BE) is a premalignant condition that may evolve into esophageal adenocarcinoma. The histologic abnormality involves intestinal-like metaplasia of the stratified squamous epithelium. Epidemiologic studies show Barrett's to be more common among Caucasians, males, and the elderly (mean age, 60 years). The relative risk of esophageal adenocarcinoma (EAC) in BE patients was thought to be 30- to 125-fold with an incidence of 0.5% per patient year; however, recent population studies have shown a lower incidence of 0.12% to 0.13%. Despite the prevalent use of PPIs in the treatment of GERD, the incidence of adenocarcinoma has been increasing. Current guidelines encourage endoscopic surveillance for patients with Barrett's esophagus, yet there are sparse data showing the cost-effectiveness or mortality benefit of this strategy.

Adenocarcinoma

Approximately 50% of esophageal cancers are adenocarcinomas. Since the 1970s, the incidence has been rising for reasons that are still unknown. GERD is a risk factor for esophageal adenocarcinoma, and the risk increases with the duration and severity of GERD symptoms. There is a suggestion that cagA strains of *Helicobacter pylori* are protective against development of Barrett's esophagus and adenocarcinoma. The declining incidence of *H. pylori* may be a possible explanation for the rising incidence of adenocarcinoma.

Diagnosis

GERD is largely a clinical diagnosis under the current definition (i.e., any symptom or tissue injury resulting from reflux of gastric contents into the esophagus). Patients with the typical symptoms of heartburn and regurgitation most often associated with meals have a high pretest probability of having GERD. A well-obtained history and symptom questionnaire are usually sufficient to form a presumptive diagnosis and are more cost-effective than ambulatory reflux testing or EGD. An empiric trial of PPI therapy that leads to a significant reduction or resolution of symptoms likely confirms the diagnosis.

The pathophysiology of GERD is much more complex than previously thought. It involves more than acid reflux, because nonacid reflux with a pH greater than 4 can be a common source of symptoms. This entity is unmasked when PPI therapy is found to control gastric acid secretion and impedance-pH testing identifies a temporal relationship between symptoms and episodes of nonacid reflux.

Direct-to-consumer marketing and the availability of over-the-counter PPI medications (e.g., Prilosec OTC) have led to self-treatment of GERD-type symptoms and a consequent change in the type of patients seeking medical care for their symptoms. Patients with typical GERD symptoms that do not completely respond to therapy with PPIs, including over-the-counter and prescription PPIs, warrant a more detailed evaluation of their symptoms. A separate population requiring earlier diagnostic evaluation includes patients with exclusively atypical GERD symptoms such as cough, hoarseness, throat clearing, asthma attacks, and chest pain. Less commonly, patients presenting with signs or symptoms of tissue injury, such as solid food dysphagia, should also be more rigorously tested for GERD (Box 4).

Patients who have symptoms associated with GERD, whether typical or atypical, are frequently treated empirically with PPI therapy. With a lack of discrimination regarding symptom types, this population is very heterogeneous and comprises patients with symptoms that are truly associated with GERD, not at all associated with GERD, and a combination of both. The pretest

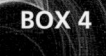

BOX 4 Clinical Spectrum of Gastroesophageal Reflux Disease–Related Symptoms and Tissue Injury

Esophageal
Symptomatic Syndromes
- Typical reflux syndrome
- Reflux chest pain syndrome

Syndromes With Tissue Injury
- Reflux esophagitis
- Reflux stricture
- Barrett's esophagus
- Adenocarcinoma

Extraesophageal
Established Association
- Reflux cough
- Reflux laryngitis
- Reflux dental erosions

Proposed Association
- Sinusitis
- Reflux asthma
- Pulmonary fibrosis
- Pharyngitis
- Recurrent otitis media

probability of GERD in this group is diluted, and nonresponders to empiric therapy are numerous. Partial responders and nonresponders to PPI therapy should undergo ambulatory reflux testing using combined multichannel intraluminal impedance (MII)-pH or standard pH. MII-pH catheters measure both esophageal pH changes and impedance changes that occur as an ion-rich refluxate passes a pair of ring electrodes, resulting in a drop in the resistance to a low-voltage current between the electrodes. The change in impedance can detect gastroesophageal reflux regardless of the acid content and can distinguish reflux types as liquid, gas, or mixed.

The goals of ambulatory reflux testing are to determine whether the esophageal acid contact time is abnormal, whether there are an abnormal number of reflux episodes, and whether a relationship between reflux and symptoms exists. The advantage of combined MII-pH is its ability to identify both acid and nonacid reflux, so that testing can be done while the patient is on acid-suppression therapy and the artifact of acidic food or beverage ingestion is eliminated; pH-only testing is affected by both of these conditions. The major disadvantage is that MII-pH testing is less available than conventional pH testing.

EGD is specific for detecting reflux-related tissue injury but is not sensitive, because fewer than 50% of patients with GERD-related heartburn have endoscopic findings of reflux. If erosive esophagitis or Barrett's esophagus is found on endoscopy, aggressive antisecretory therapy with a PPI is warranted.

A barium esophagram is unlikely to add useful diagnostic information in patients with GERD symptoms without dysphagia. It is a useful tool in distinguishing obstructive from nonobstructive dysphagia and may even be more sensitive than EGD in detecting causes of obstructive dysphagia. Achalasia is often mistaken for GERD during the onset of symptoms, and early use of esophagography may help make this diagnosis.

Management

GERD is predominantly a postprandial event involving transient LES relaxations. The primary focus in management of this disease is to eliminate or improve symptoms and prevent tissue injury. In most patients with recurrent GERD symptoms, this can be accomplished by controlling gastric acid secretion with antisecretory therapy. PPIs are the most effective pharmacologic therapy for improving symptoms and preventing tissue injury from acid reflux. Individuals with only occasional heartburn may successfully treat symptoms with a combination of lifestyle modifications and over-the-counter antacids, histamine 2 receptor antagonists, or a PPI.

Patients presenting with typical symptoms and a history consistent with GERD should be given a trial of PPI once daily for at least 4 weeks. A validated GERD symptom assessment questionnaire such as the Reflux Disease Questionnaire should be used as an initial screening tool, because symptom response is the primary outcome measure, and subsequent questionnaire responses are useful in comparison with the initial responses for measuring treatment efficacy. If symptoms have not responded or have responded only partially after this trial, then the dosing or frequency of the PPI should be increased over another 4-week period. If the response is still unsatisfactory, diagnostic testing with ambulatory combined MII-pH or pH-only monitoring is indicated.

PPIs are an effective maintenance therapy for most patients with GERD and may be stepped down or used on demand, but GERD is a chronic condition with a high recurrence rate of symptoms without some form of maintenance therapy. This creates a large population of patients on antisecretory therapy for a disease with a low mortality rate, which raises the question of drug safety. There are insufficient data available that would warrant a recommendation against long-term PPI therapy. Clinical judgment in specific patient populations should be used to determine the optimal PPI regimen.

At present, pharmacologic reflux reduction therapy consists solely of the use of baclofen (Lioresal),[1] which has been shown to reduce transient LES relaxations and associated gastroesophageal reflux. The drawback of this medication is its unwanted side effects, which include somnolence and dizziness, limiting its tolerability and clinical utility as a stand-alone therapy.

Antireflux surgery is another alternative that is effective in limiting GERD symptoms in patients with a positive reflux-symptom relationship. Candidates for surgery include younger patients who do not want to continue chronic PPI therapy and patients with symptomatic nonacid reflux. Today, most antireflux surgery is performed laparoscopically with a 360-degree Nissen fundoplication. The associated mortality rate is small (0.5%–1%), and this approach is preferred to open laparotomy. Traditional predictors for surgical success have included the presence of typical symptoms (heartburn and regurgitation), symptom response to a trial of PPIs, and an abnormal ambulatory pH study. These criteria exclude the important group of patients with atypical symptoms or symptoms related to nonacid reflux. However, such patients should be considered candidates for antireflux surgery if a positive reflux–symptom relationship can be demonstrated.

In recent years, several endoscopic therapeutic procedures have been developed for treatment of GERD. Among these procedures, transoral incisionless fundoplication (TIF) and Stretta are well studied and viable options. Stretta is the delivery of radiofrequency energy to the gastro-esophageal junction (GEJ). Stretta efficacy lays in increasing thickness of LES, decreasing compliance of GEJ without fibrosis, and decreased transient lower esophageal sphincter relaxations. Randomized trials showed improvement in GERD symptoms compared to sham procedure, though follow-up periods in these trials were only 6–12 months. A meta-analysis of 18 studies and 1441 patients concluded that Stretta is safe, well tolerated, effective in GERD symptom relief, and significantly reduces acid exposure to the esophagus, though it did not consistently normalize pH. In a recent meta analysis of 28 studies of 2468 patients with mean follow-up time of 25.4 months, Stretta improved quality-of-life scores and heartburn scores. However, 49% of the patients were still using PPIs at follow-up.

Patients with alarm symptoms and those who are partial responders to PPI therapy should also undergo EGD to aid in determining the cause of the symptoms, such as obstructive dysphagia from peptic strictures, adenocarcinoma, and bleeding esophageal ulcers (which can cause anemia). EGD findings that suggest GERD are a result of acid reflux. However, the incidence of these findings has declined with the use of PPIs.

Nonerosive reflux disease is increasingly common as more patients are converted from acid refluxers to nonacid refluxers with PPI therapy. By definition, these patients have no findings on endoscopy to suggest ongoing GERD. Absence of endoscopic findings does not exclude GERD, however, because tissue injury can occur at the microscopic as well as the macroscopic level. Patients with either erosive esophagitis or nonerosive reflux disease have dilated intercellular spaces on electron microscopy.

As previously discussed, patients with GERD may develop Barrett's esophagus. The metaplastic transformation from normal stratified squamous epithelium to an intestinal-type, columnar-lined epithelium creates a premalignant lesion with a 0.5% per year risk of progression to adenocarcinoma. Screening for Barrett's esophagus remains controversial. There is no evidence that screening results in a mortality benefit due to early detection of esophageal adenocarcinoma. Screening of all patients with GERD for Barrett's esophagus is clearly not cost-effective, but it is reasonable to target the highest-risk populations, such as Caucasian men older than 50 years of age with chronic reflux symptoms. Current American College of Gastroenterology guidelines recommend surveillance endoscopy in patients with known Barrett's esophagus at intervals determined by the degree of dysplasia. Because there have been no long-term, controlled studies, it is a grade C recommendation.

References

Bonino J, Sharma P: Barrett's esophagus, *Curr Opin Gastroenterol* 21:461–465, 2005.

Castell DO, Richter JE: *The Esophagus*, ed 4, Philadelphia, 2003, Lippincott Williams & Wilkins.

Corley DA, Katz P, Wo JM, et al: Improvement of gastroesophageal reflux symptoms after radiofrequency energy: a randomized, sham-controlled trial, *Gastroenterology*. 125:668–676, 2003.

Fass R, Cahn F, Scotti DJ, et al: Systematic review and meta-analysis of controlled and prospective cohort efficacy studies of endoscopic radiofrequency for treatment of gastroesophageal reflux disease, *Surg Endosc* 31(12):4865–4882.

Frye J, Vaezi M: Extraesophageal GERD, *Gastroenterol Clin North Am* 37:845–858, 2008.

Hila A, Agrawal A, Castell D: Combined multichannel intraluminal impedance and pH esophageal testing compared to pH alone for diagnosing both acid and weakly acidic gastroesophageal reflux, *Clin Gastroenterol and Hepatol* 5:172–177, 2007.

Hvid-Jensen F, Funch-Jensen P, et al: Incidence of adenocarcinoma among patients with Barrett's esophagus, *NEJM* 365:1375–1383, 2011.

Katz PO, Gerson LB, Vela MF: Guidelines for the diagnosis and management of gastroesophageal reflux disease, *Am J Gastroenterol* 108:308–328, 2013.

Mainie I, Tutuian R, Agrawal A, et al: Combined multichannel intraluminal impedance-pH monitoring to select patients with persistent gastro-oesophageal reflux for laparoscopic Nissen fundoplication, *Br J Surg* 93:1483–1487, 2006.

Mainie I, Tutuian R, Castell D: Comparison between the combined analysis and the DeMeester score to predict response to PPI therapy, *J Clin Gastroenterol* 40:602–605, 2006.

Mainie I, Tutuian R, Shay S, et al: Acid and non-acid reflux in patients with persistent symptoms despite acid suppressive therapy: a multicentre study using combined ambulatory impedance-pH monitoring, *Gut* 55:1398–1402, 2006.

Perry KA, Banerjee A, Melvin WS: Radiofrequency energy delivery to the lower esophageal sphincter reduces esophageal acid exposure and improves GERD symptoms: a systematic review and meta-analysis, *Surg Laparosc Endosc Percutan Tech.* 22:283–288, 2012.

Savarino E, Zentilin P, Tutuian R, et al: The role of nonacid reflux in NERD: lessons learned from impedance-pH monitoring in 150 patients off therapy, *Am J Gastroenterol* 103:2685–2693, 2008.

Vakil N: Review article: test and treat or treat and test in reflux disease, *Aliment Pharmacol Ther* 17(Suppl. 2):57–59, 2003.

Vakil N, Van Zanten SV, Kahrilas P, et al: The Montreal definition and classification of gastroesophageal reflux disease: a global evidence-based consensus, *Am J Gastroenterol* 101:1900–1920, 2006.

Verbeek RE, Siersema PD, et al: Surveillance and follow-up strategies in patients with high-grade dysplasia in Barrett's esophagus: a Dutch population-based study, *Am J Gastroenterol* 107:534–542, 2012.

Wang KK, Sampliner RE: Updated guidelines 2008 for the diagnosis, surveillance and therapy of Barrett's esophagus, *Am J Gastroenterol* 103:788–797, 2008.

[1]Not FDA approved for this indication.

HEMORRHOIDS, ANAL FISSURE, AND ANORECTAL ABSCESS AND FISTULA

Method of
Mary R. Kwaan, MD, MPH

CURRENT DIAGNOSIS

- While most anorectal complaints are caused by a benign process, it is important to be mindful that the etiology can be a malignancy or other serious medical condition, such as anorectal Crohn disease.
- A thorough, focused history is often the most helpful diagnostic tool for patients with anorectal complaints.
- In patients where no etiology for bleeding is found or where there has been a change in bowel movements, a further diagnostic work-up should be performed.
- Pain is the predominant symptom with anal fissure, thrombosed external hemorrhoids, and anorectal abscess but is not prominently featured with internal hemorrhoids.

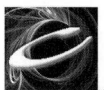

CURRENT THERAPY

- External thrombosed hemorrhoids are treated with evacuation in their early development (<72 h) but with expectant, supportive management only in their subacute phase.
- Most internal hemorrhoids can be treated with outpatient treatments, including measures to normalize bowel movements and hemorrhoidal banding or injection therapy.
- Anal fissures are treated conservatively with medical therapy but require operative therapy in a minority of cases.
- Anal fistula repair techniques have variable success rates and may require multiple procedures to treat effectively.

A number of conditions cause anorectal symptoms, but the majority of patients present with a complaint of "hemorrhoids." Most anorectal conditions can be diagnosed with a focused history and physical examination. Treatment is aimed at the relief of symptoms, education of the patient, and prevention of further symptoms. Although most anorectal complaints are caused by a benign process, it is important for clinicians to be mindful that in some cases the etiology can be a malignancy or other serious medical conditions, such as anorectal Crohn disease.

History

A thorough, focused history is often the most helpful diagnostic tool for patients with anorectal complaints. Clinicians should inquire about pain, itching, discharge, extra tissue or a lump, and bleeding. It is particularly important to understand the patient's bowel habits with respect to constipation or diarrhea as well as any change in defecatory habits. Other relevant history items include previous anorectal procedures and related medical conditions such as Crohn disease, malignancy, sexually transmitted diseases, or immunosuppression.

Pain is an important symptom to elicit from patients. In most cases, pain is the predominant symptom with anal fissure, thrombosed external hemorrhoids, and anorectal abscess. Although discomfort from internal hemorrhoids can cause aching, burning, or itching in the setting of tissue prolapse, internal hemorrhoid disease is most often painless. In contrast, external hemorrhoids that are acutely thrombosed cause pain that is acute in onset, severe, and constant. Fissure pain is often described as a tearing sensation or the feeling of "razor blades" during bowel movements that can continue for more than an hour following defecation. Patients with anal fissures might also express a fear of having bowel movements because of pain. Anorectal abscess is

often associated with pain, and patients can also present with an acute lump and occasionally a fever. Anal fistula typically is not associated with much pain, rather patients describe irritation or itching, and the most common symptom is drainage.

Anal discharge and difficulty with anorectal hygiene are also common complaints. The discharge associated with prolapsing internal hemorrhoids might contain mucus or small amounts of stool. In contrast, an anorectal fistula or abscess can spontaneously drain with associated purulent and blood-tinged output.

When a patient has bleeding, specific details to inquire about include color (bright red versus dark blood), amount, frequency, and length of time. When no etiology for bleeding is found, a flexible sigmoidoscopy or colonoscopy should be performed to evaluate for a proximal source. Even if patients are found to have some hemorrhoids, endoscopic evaluation should be strongly considered in patients over 40–50 years old. Although uncommon, the incidence of colorectal malignancy has increased this age group. Furthermore, patients 45 and older should initiate colorectal cancer screening regardless of symptoms. Stool based screening modalities identify blood in the stool. Therefore patients with anal bleeding should be encouraged to proceed with colonoscopy for screening.

Diagnosis

Although the prone jack-knife position allows the greatest exposure, the left lateral decubitus position with the knees up is preferred by patients and usually allows adequate exposure for the anorectal examination. It is critically important to have adequate lighting with a headlight as well as appropriate instrumentation to perform the anoscopy. An adjunctive test that can also be helpful in patients where mucosal (hemorrhoidal) or full-thickness rectal prolapse is suspected is to have patients bear down on the commode and then to examine externally.

The perianal skin is the skin immediately surrounding the anal verge (Figure 1). Perianal inspection includes careful examination of the surrounding skin for excoriation, an external draining orifice in the case of an anorectal fistula, lichenified skin with chronic irritation, other dermatitis, and the presence of perianal lesions. A low-lying anal fistula can be palpated as a fibrotic tract that heads from the external draining site to the anus. The anal verge is the entrance to the anal canal and is defined by the intersphincteric groove. There is frequently a clear demarcation between hair-bearing and nonhair-bearing skin in this location. Careful separation of the anoderm can help to visualize an anal fissure located at the anal verge and extending into the anal canal.

A digital rectal examination is helpful for assessing resting and squeeze anorectal tone, palpating the prostate in men, assessing for rectocele in women, detecting any palpable anorectal lesions, and evaluating for tenderness within the anal canal or at the level

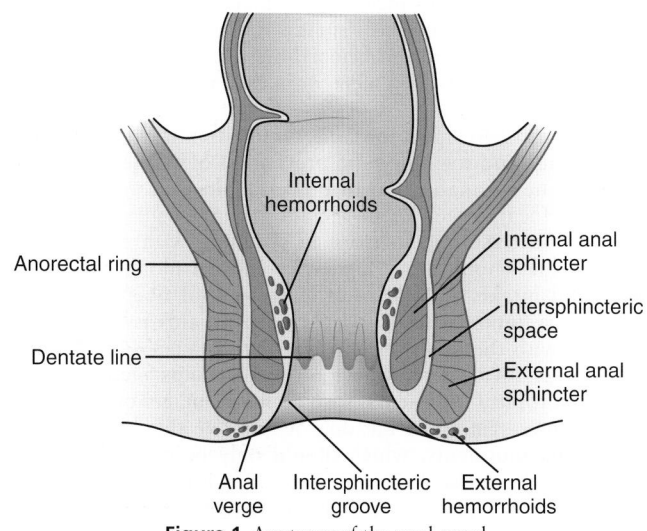

Figure 1 Anatomy of the anal canal.

TABLE 1	Staging of Hemorrhoidal Disease
GRADE	DESCRIPTION
I	Protrude only inside the lumen; seen only with the anoscope
II	Protrude during defecation; reduce spontaneously
III	Protrude during defecation; require manual reduction
IV	Permanently prolapsed and irreducible

of the levator ani muscles at the anorectal ring. Internal hemorrhoids, however, are not usually palpable as they readily compress with digital pressure and are not associated with fibrosis. Anoscopy is used to visually examine the anal canal, which is between 4 and 5 cm in length starting at the anal verge and extending to the top of the anorectal ring (top of external sphincter and levator ani muscles). Within the anal canal is the dentate line, which acts as a landmark anatomically and is located approximately 2 cm from the anal verge. The dentate line represents the transition from squamous epithelial lining of the anus to the columnar epithelial lining of the rectum. Sensation above the dentate line is mediated by autonomic fibers and results in a relative lack of sensation in comparison to the highly sensitive, somatically innervated tissue below the dentate line. The dentate line is also the location of the crypt anal glands from which anorectal abscesses and fistulas originate.

Hemorrhoids

Hemorrhoids are the anal vascular cushions that are present as normal structures in everyone. In the case of internal hemorrhoids, these cushions are arteriovenous channels that have overlying mucosa, submucosal smooth muscle, and supportive fibroelastic connective tissue. It is believed that internal hemorrhoids function by aiding with fine control of fecal continence of liquids and gases. Internal hemorrhoids enlarge and become symptomatic as fixation by submucosal smooth muscle and connective tissue becomes disrupted and loosens. This results in a sliding or prolapsing of the anal canal lining and further engorgement of the internal hemorrhoid tissues. Common exacerbating factors include constipation, diarrhea, aging, and increased abdominal pressure that can occur with chronic straining, pregnancy, heavy lifting, and decreased venous return. Internal hemorrhoids are not palpable on digital rectal examination and instead must be observed on anoscopy. Internal hemorrhoids are typically staged on a scale from I to IV based upon the extent of prolapse (Table 1).

Internal hemorrhoids, when symptomatic, most commonly present with painless bright red bleeding or prolapsing tissue (Figure 2). Patients describe bleeding with or after bowel movements. Other symptoms include itching and leakage of mucus in the setting of tissue prolapse. Pain is rarely a prominent symptom except in the case of mixed hemorrhoid disease, when there is a thrombosed external component, or in the case of grade IV incarcerated hemorrhoids.

The central principles for conservative treatment of internal hemorrhoids and for long-term prevention of worsening symptoms are the normalization of bowel habits and avoidance of straining. Ideal bowel habits include having regular, soft, and formed stool resulting in minimal straining with elimination. An ideal diet should have high fiber content along with sufficient fluid intake. A total of at least 30 g of fiber per day is generally recommended. For most patients, this is most easily achieved with the addition of a fiber supplement such as psyllium. Other medical treatment of hemorrhoids includes local anesthetic topical ointments, such as lidocaine gel or ointment, which relieve symptoms but do not improve the hemorrhoids, and steroid ointments, which should only be prescribed for a defined short course for symptoms of itching and irritation. Topical hydrocortisone can thin and atrophy the overlying tissue if used regularly.

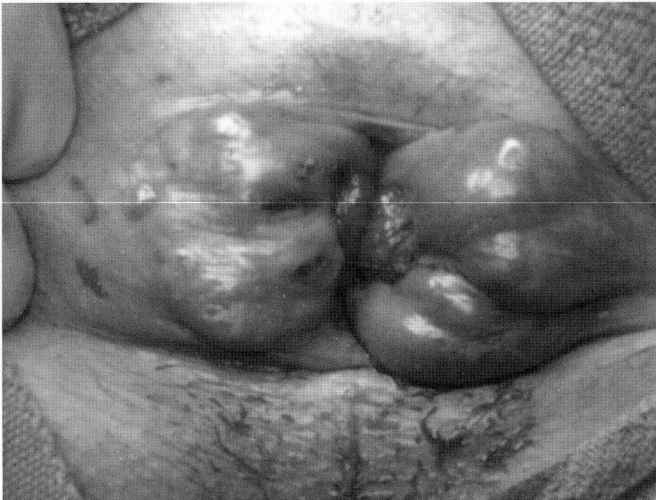

Figure 2 Prolapsing (grade III) hemorrhoids, with a prominent external component on the right and two sites of recent bleeding seen on the left.

Internal hemorrhoids might benefit from further treatment in the setting of persistent prolapse or bleeding. Injection sclerotherapy works through shrinking and scarring the internal hemorrhoid by injecting a sclerosing agent (most commonly 5% phenol in oil[1] or sodium morrhuate[1]). Alternatively, infrared coagulation may be administered at the apex of the hemorrhoid. Both procedures have moderate effectiveness but are considered less effective than rubber-band ligation, which is widely used in the office setting, with good results.

Rubber-band ligation, an office procedure, requires the use of a rubber-band ligator (either suction type or ligator with clamp) and is performed by placing a rubber band around excess hemorrhoidal tissue at the apex of the hemorrhoid. Rubber-band ligation works by strangulating and cutting off blood flow to the hemorrhoid and by creating a scar that helps to fix tissue into place. The band must be placed well above the dentate line to prevent pain. Most patients experience a sensation of pressure with the procedure. Rarely, this procedure can cause significant pain, bleeding, or a vasovagal reaction. In general, only one or two band applications are performed in the same setting to prevent excessive pain or a vasovagal reaction.

Surgical treatment for hemorrhoidal disease should be considered in patients with grade III or IV internal hemorrhoids. Grade IV hemorrhoids, especially associated with dusky prolapsed rectal mucosa, urinary retention, or significant pain should be evaluated urgently by a surgeon, as necrotic tissue requires operative debridement. Surgery is also a consideration in cases where office procedures and conservative treatment have been ineffective or when internal hemorrhoids are circumferential. In the United States, most hemorrhoidectomies continue to be performed using a closed technique, where the hemorrhoid is excised and the defect sutured closed. More recently, stapled hemorrhoidectomy (sometimes called hemorrhoidopexy) has been introduced. The stapled technique appears to work best in cases where patients have more circumferential disease and is performed by excising the rectal mucosa and disrupting blood flow, thereby shrinking hemorrhoidal tissue and lifting the prolapsing tissue into the anal canal. Although stapled hemorrhoidectomy has been demonstrated to be effective and on average less painful, it does not address external hemorrhoids, costs significantly more, and has been associated with rare but severe complications, including pelvic sepsis, rectal perforation, and rectovaginal fistula.

External hemorrhoids are generally painless, except in the case of thrombosis, and normally appear as more prominent external perianal tissue or painless skin tags. Thrombosed external

[1] Not FDA approved for this indication.

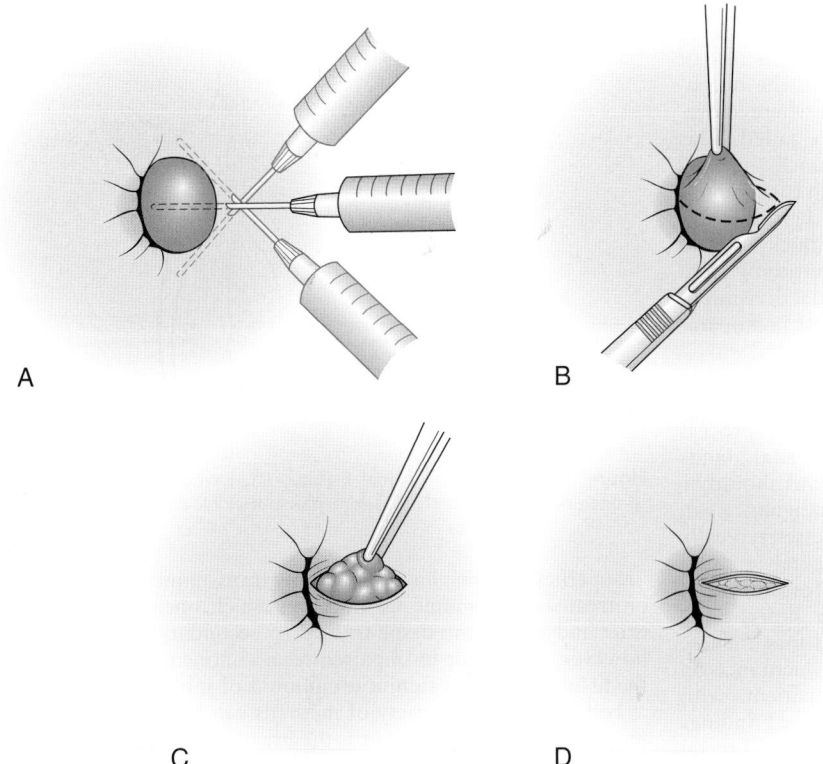

Figure 3 Incision and evacuation of an external thrombosed hemorrhoid. (A) A local anesthetic is injected into the subcutaneous surrounding tissue and at the base of the hemorrhoid. (B) The skin over the hemorrhoid is lifted and a small elliptical excision of skin is made. (C) The thrombotic clot is evacuated. Additional dissection is sometimes needed in the subcutaneous tissue to extract the clot. (D) The appearance of the evacuated area. The incision is left open and the skin heals by secondary intention.

hemorrhoids, in contrast, are associated with severe pain and a prominent external lump but not with bleeding or fever. On examination, an external thrombosed hemorrhoid appears as a prominent, blue, and firm perianal lump. Patients who present within 72 hours of the onset of symptoms benefit from an excision of the hemorrhoid rather than evacuation of the thrombosed clot (Figure 3). In contrast, patients who present after 72 hours should be treated expectantly with conservative supportive care, including sitz baths, normalization of bowel habits with fiber or stool softener, and pain management. The natural history in these cases is for the thrombosed clot to gradually be reabsorbed within several weeks. In many cases, a residual skin tag is noted by the patient and can interfere with anal hygiene.

Anal Fissure

An anal fissure is a tear in the anoderm extending proximally into the anal canal and initially resulting from a traumatic bowel movement. Fissures typically occur in the setting of constipation or frequent bowel movements. Although most fissures resulting from trauma to the anorectal region will heal, some patients have prolonged symptoms, causing them to seek medical attention. The pathophysiology of anal fissures is still not completely understood but is related to local ischemia caused by hypertonia of the internal sphincter. Most anal fissures are located at the posterior midline; some also occur at the anterior midline (Figure 4). Lateral fissures are rare and can be associated with anal malignancy, anorectal Crohn disease, HIV, syphilis, or tuberculosis. In these cases, a biopsy should be strongly considered to confirm the diagnosis.

Patients who present with anal fissure most often have a tearing pain that is associated with bowel movements and that continues after defecation and bright red bleeding with bowel movements. Physical examination demonstrates a tear in the anoderm with exposed internal sphincter upon separation of the anus. Chronic cases also demonstrate a sentinel tag overlying the distal aspect of the fissure.

Conservative treatment for acute anal fissures includes the normalization of bowel habits to minimize recurrent trauma to the anoderm and sitz baths for comfort. In cases in which the fissure is chronic or unresponsive to conservative treatment, topical therapy to relax the internal sphincter (i.e., a "chemical sphincterotomy")

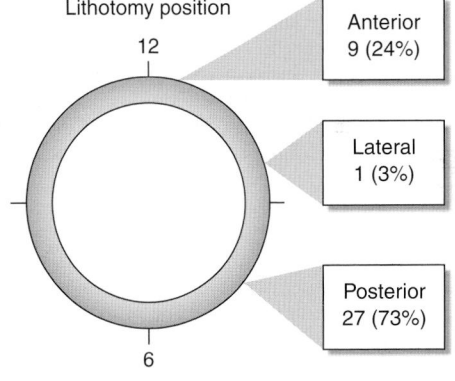

Figure 4 Distribution of the location of anal fissures.

is prescribed. Classically, nitroglycerin ointment (0.2%[1],[6] to 0.4% [Rectiv]) has been used but is associated with headaches and lightheadedness. Diltiazem ointment (2%)[1],[6] is a commonly used alternative without associated side effects. Either ointment can be applied topically two to three times per day for approximately 8 weeks. Application before bowel movements works best to help with pain on defecation. Reported healing rates are similar and range from 40% to 100%. An alternative agent that can be used for chemical sphincterotomy is botulinum toxin A (Botox)[1], which can be injected in the office or operating room with a single application into the internal sphincter. Although botulinum toxin A appears to be as effective as topical therapy, it is significantly more expensive.

[1] Not FDA approved for this indication.
[6] May be compounded by pharmacists.

Surgical lateral internal sphincterotomy is the most effective treatment for resolution of anal pain associated with fissures and to expedite healing but is associated with a small risk of fecal incontinence. This procedure is performed in the outpatient setting and should be considered in cases where more-conservative dietary and medical treatments have failed. This procedure can be performed with an open approach (incising mucosa and exposing muscle) or a closed approach (using landmarks and then dividing muscle by feel) and can be full thickness (entire internal sphincter) or tailored (partial thickness and length). Most surgeons perform a tailored sphincterotomy from the level of the top of the fissure distally, with partial division of the internal sphincter muscle to decrease the risk of postoperative fecal incontinence.

Anorectal Abscess and Fistula

Anorectal abscess is most commonly a self-limited process thought to result from obstruction and infection of anal glands located in the crypts along the dentate line. Clinicians should be aware that perianal Crohn disease, trauma, and malignancy can cause anorectal abscess or fistula. Anorectal abscesses typically manifest with acute pain in the perianal area, acutely painful defecation, an indurated painful area, or fever. Most anorectal abscesses manifest with pain and swelling either superficially at the anal verge or deeper within the ischiorectal fossa. These patients have obvious tenderness, induration, or fluctuance on external and/or digital examination. In contrast, patients with intersphincteric abscesses have severe pain but minimal findings on external examination and are only suspected on digital rectal examination.

The mainstay of therapy is surgical drainage. Superficial abscesses can be drained using local anesthesia, but more-extensive infections typically require general anesthesia. When the abscess is fluctuant and appears easily accessible, an incision and drainage with a local anesthetic can be considered in a motivated patient. Important principles in draining an anorectal abscess include keeping the patient comfortable, using aspiration with a large-bore (14- or 16-gauge) needle to help in the event of difficult localization, using a cruciate incision to ensure adequate drainage, and keeping the incision near the anus to keep any potential fistula tract as short as possible. After the abscess is drained, the area is allowed to heal by secondary intention. Patients are given analgesics and encouraged to take sitz baths. When the abscess is large and extensive, sometimes drainage tubes, débridement, or additional dressing changes are required.

In most patients, drainage of the anorectal abscess is sufficient. However, in one-third of patients, these do not heal and form a fistula with the external opening beyond the anal verge and the internal opening within an infected crypt gland at the dentate line. A recent, small randomized trial suggested that 7 to 10 days of antibiotics after abscess drainage could decrease the risk of fistula formation. Patients developing a fistula can have what appears to be a nearly healed wound but continue to intermittently drain purulent material from the external opening, and some patients continue to have signs and symptoms of infection. The tract of the fistula is most often predicted with Goodsall rule. Goodsall rule states that an anterior fistula follows a radial tract to the internal opening, typically at the anterior midline. In contrast, a posterior fistula follows a curvilinear path to the internal opening at the posterior midline. Anorectal fistulas are defined by their anatomy and path relative to the sphincter muscles and are classified typically as superficial, intersphincteric, transsphincteric, suprasphincteric, and extrasphincteric, as classically described by Parks (Figure 5). In most cases, patients can proceed directly to the operating room for initial definition of the anatomy and placement of a seton (a length of suture or other material that is looped through the fistula), which helps to allow drainage of infection within the tract, prevents recurrent infection, and allows the fistula to mature. Recurrent and complex fistulas may be better defined anatomically with the use of magnetic resonance imaging or endorectal ultrasound.

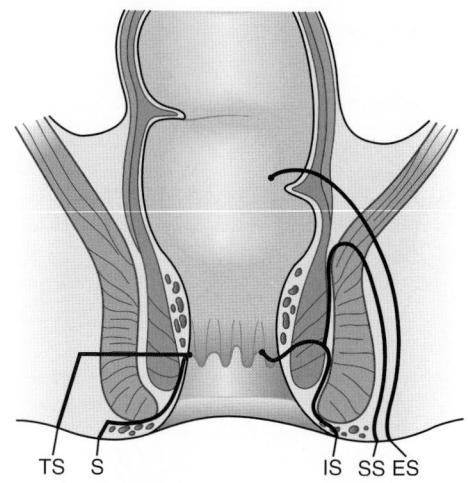

Figure 5 Classification of anal fistulas. *ES*, Extrasphincteric; *IS*, intersphincteric; *S*, superficial; *SS*, suprasphincteric; *TS*, transsphincteric.

Superficial, intersphincteric, or low transsphincteric fistulas can be treated with simple fistulotomy, which opens up the fistula tract and allows the tissue to heal by secondary intention. This, however, can result in impaired fecal continence, particularly if the fistula involves a significant amount of sphincter muscle.

Following this, a variety of methods can be used to repair the fistula. One classic technique is the use of a cutting seton, where a taut seton is progressively tightened over several weeks or months to form a scar in place of the fistula and muscle. A cutting seton may be painful, and the scar is associated with impaired continence in some cases. Fibrin glue and fistula plugs have been proposed as a method to repair a fistula, but the recurrence rate with long-term follow-up is high (>85%). Endorectal advancement flaps are the most well-established method to repair an anal fistula. With this technique, the internal orifice is closed, and healthy tissue is brought down over the internal fistula opening to allow the area to heal. This procedure can be technically difficult: failure most commonly results from ischemia of the flap, and repeat flap procedures are often not anatomically feasible owing to scarring and fibrosis. Success rates have been reported between 50% and 80%.

The ligation of intersphincteric fistula tract (LIFT) has been investigated for transsphincteric and suprasphincteric fistulas and shows modest success with the benefit of avoiding any sphincter division. In this procedure, the fistula tract is ligated and partially excised through an intersphincteric approach. Although long-term results are still unknown, reports are favorable (on the order of 60% to 80%) for the short-term success of this technique.

References

Bleier JI, Moloo H, Goldberg SM: Ligation of the intersphincteric fistula tract: An effective new technique for complex fistulas, *Dis Colon Rectum* 53:43–46, 2008.

Davis BR, Lee-Kong SA, Migaly J, Feingold DL, Steele SR: The American Society of Colon and Rectal Surgeons Clinical Practice Guidelines for the Management of Hemorrhoids, *Dis Colon Rectum* 61:284–292, 2018.

Ghahramani L, Minaie MR, Arasteh P, et al: Antibiotic therapy for prevention of fistula in ano after incision and dreainage of simple perianal abscess: A randomized single blind clinical trial, *Surgery* 162:1017–1025, 2017.

Hong KD, Kang S, Kalaskar S, Wexner SD: Ligation of intersphincteric fistula to treat anal fistula: a systematic review and meta-analysis, *Tech Coloproctol* 18:685–691, 2014.

Jayaraman S, Colquhoun PH, Malthaner RA: Stapled versus conventional surgery for hemorrhoids, *Cochrane Database Syst Rev* 4:CD005393, 2006.

Nelson R: Nonsurgical therapy for anal fissure, *Cochrane Database Syst Rev* 4:CD003431, 2006.

Nelson RL: Operative procedures for fissure in ano, *Cochrane Database Syst Rev* 1:CD002199, 2010.

Parks AG, Gordon PH, Hardcastle JD: A classification of fistula-in-ano, *Br J Surg* 63:1–12, 1976.

Shanmugam V, Thaha MA, Rabindranath KS, et al: Rubber band ligation versus excisional haemorrhoidectomy for haemorrhoids, *Cochrane Database Syst Rev* 3:CD005034, 2005.

HEPATITIS A, B, D, AND E

Method of
Varun Takyar, MD; and Marc G. Ghany, MD, MHSc

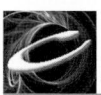

CURRENT DIAGNOSIS

Hepatitis A

- Typical prodromal symptoms are nonspecific (i.e., fever, anorexia, nausea, vomiting, diarrhea, abdominal pain, and weight loss). In about half of patients, prodromal symptoms are followed by icterus (i.e., jaundice, pruritus, and dark urine) lasting 2 weeks.
- Serum aminotransferase levels increase to 10–20 times the upper limit of normal during the prodromal phase. Total serum bilirubin rises but rarely exceeds 10 mg/dL during the icteric phase. Biochemical recovery usually occurs within 3 months.
- Acute hepatitis A virus (HAV) infection is diagnosed by the presence of anti-HAV immunoglobulin M (IgM). Anti-HAV IgG appears in the convalescent phase and remains detectable for life. Anti-HAV IgG positivity with the absence of anti-HAV IgM antibodies reflects past exposure or vaccination. The antibody test for HAV usually includes total antibodies (IgM and IgG); thus, diagnosis of acute hepatitis A requires specific anti-HAV IgM testing.

Hepatitis B

- Acute hepatitis B virus (HBV) infection may be asymptomatic or present with nonspecific symptoms of anorexia, nausea, and fever with development of icterus, pruritus, right upper quadrant pain, or, rarely, acute liver failure. Globally, it is a major cause of chronic hepatitis.
- Serum alanine aminotransferase (ALT) levels peak with the onset of symptoms.
- Suspected acute HBV infection is diagnosed by the detection of hepatitis B surface antigen (HBsAg), hepatitis B e-antigen (HBeAg), IgM antibody to hepatitis B core antigen (anti-HBc), and HBV DNA in serum in the appropriate clinical setting. Anti-HBc IgM is detected during acute HBV infection and may be detected during reactivation of chronic HBV infection.
- Chronic infection is defined as the persistence of serum HBsAg for greater than 6 months. If HBsAg is present, serum HBeAg, antibody to hepatitis B e-antigen (anti-HBe), HBV DNA, and serum ALT are used to determine the four phases of chronic infection (immune tolerant, HBeAg-positive immune active, HBeAg-negative immune active, and inactive carrier).

CURRENT THERAPY

Hepatitis A

- Treatment is predominately supportive. Avoid hepatotoxic medications and drugs metabolized by the liver. Acute liver failure with encephalopathy and impaired synthetic function occurs rarely and is more common in patients older than 50 years of age and/or those who have coexisting chronic HBV or hepatitis C virus (HCV) infections.
- Prevention includes administration of the inactivated or attenuated vaccine for children at age 1 year or older and for at-risk populations (e.g., intravenous drug users, travelers to regions with high or intermediate HAV rates, men who have sex with men, patients with chronic liver disease or clotting factor disorders).

- Preexposure passive immunization with pooled human anti-HAV immunoglobulin may be used for those at high or intermediate risk of HAV exposure.
- Postexposure passive immunization with pooled human anti-HAV immunoglobulin may be used for close personal contacts of an individual with laboratory-confirmed HAV infection, staff and attendees of childcare centers if one or more children and/or staff are diagnosed with HAV infection, and food handlers during a common-source exposure. Concurrent immunization with inactivated or attenuated vaccines for these at-risk contacts is also warranted.

Hepatitis B

- Acute HBV infection in an adult generally only requires supportive care due to high rates of spontaneous recovery. For people with evidence of acute liver failure, prompt institution of antiviral therapy with a potent nucleos(t)ide analog and referral to a transplant center is recommended. Peginterferon alfa-2a (Pegasys)[1] is contraindicated in persons with acute liver failure.
- Treatment goals of chronic hepatitis B are sustained suppression of HBV DNA to prevent the development of cirrhosis, hepatocellular carcinoma, and liver-related mortality. Cure of chronic HBV infection is currently not possible. Treatment recommendations for chronic HBV differ depending on the phase of infection but are generally indicated for immune active HBeAg-positive subjects with confirmed HBV DNA greater than 2000 to 20,000 IU/mL and serum ALT two or more times the upper limit of normal, and for immune active HBeAg-negative patients with HBV DNA greater than or equal to 2000 IU/mL with serum ALT two or more times the upper limit of normal and patients with liver biopsy–proven moderate to severe inflammation and/or moderate fibrosis. Treatment decisions outside these parameters should be individualized based on the risk for complications (e.g., older age [>40 years], family history of cirrhosis or hepatocellular carcinoma, presence of cirrhosis) and the risk of therapy (e.g., chronic kidney disease, previous treatment history). Four agents are considered first line—peginterferon alfa-2a (Pegasys), entecavir (Baraclude), tenofovir (Viread), and tenofovir alafenamide (Vemlidy)—based on their safety, effectiveness, and low rates of antiviral resistance. Peginterferon is generally recommended for those who prefer a finite course of treatment and who have clinical and laboratory features predictive of a response to peginterferon (high ALT, low HBV DNA, young age, female gender, and HBV genotype A or B). Peginterferon is contraindicated in persons with decompensated cirrhosis, autoimmune illnesses, or active psychiatric illness. Nucleos(t)ide analogs are more potent inhibitors of HBV DNA replication, generally better tolerated than peginterferon, and usually administered long term. The ideal endpoint of treatment is loss of HBsAg, though it is rarely observed with any therapy.
- Prevention includes completion of a two-three-dose HBV vaccination series for all children by 18 months of age with the first dose administered within 24 hours of birth. Infants whose mothers are HBsAg positive or whose HBsAg status is unknown should receive the last dose by 6 months of age.
- Hepatitis B immune globulin (HyperHEP B) and HBV vaccination are recommended at birth for infants whose mothers are HBsAg positive. In mothers with viral loads greater than 200,000 IU/mL, antiviral therapy with tenofovir (Viread), telbivudine (Tyzeka), or lamivudine (Epivir HBV) in the third trimester of pregnancy (gestation weeks 28 to 32) can be considered.

[1]Not FDA approved for this indication.

TABLE 1 | Hepatitis A, B, D, and E Characteristics

	HEPATITIS A	HEPATITIS B	HEPATITIS D	HEPATITIS E
Classification	Picornavirus, ssRNA(+)	Hepadnavirus, dsDNA	Deltavirus, ssRNA(−)	Hepevirus, ssRNA(+)
Source	Stool	Blood	Blood	Stool
Transmission	Enteric	Percutaneous/permucosal	Percutaneous/permucosal	Enteric
Acute infections (per 1000/year) in United States	125–200	140–320	6–13	Unknown
Epidemics	Yes	No	No	Yes
Incubation period range (weeks)	15–45 days	30–180 days	30–180 days	15–60 days
Risk of chronic hepatitis	No	Yes	Yes	Yes
Risk of HCC	No	Yes	Yes	No
Acute liver failure	0.10%	0.1%–1%	5%–20%	1%–2%#
Prevention	Pre-/post-exposure immunization	Pre-/post-exposure immunization	Pre-/post-exposure immunization	Pre-exposure immunization*

*Not available in United States.
#Higher in pregnancy at 5% to 20%.
HCC, Hepatocellular carcinoma.

Five viruses, hepatitis A through E, account for the majority of cases of acute and chronic viral hepatitis. Chronic hepatitis is arbitrarily defined as the persistence of elevated serum aminotransferase levels for 6 months or more. Complications of chronic hepatitis (predominantly cirrhosis and hepatocellular carcinoma) account for the majority of morbidity and mortality due to viral hepatitis. Effective vaccines are available for the prevention of hepatitis A, B, and D infections. In addition, safe and effective therapy is available for treatment of chronic hepatitis B and C. Therefore, it is important to screen individuals who are at high risk for chronic viral hepatitis to provide them access to care, reduce complications, and offer counseling to prevent transmission of infection.

Hepatitis A Virus
Introduction
HAV is a positive-sense, single-stranded RNA virus of the *Hepatovirus* genus belonging to the Picornaviridae family. Its genome encodes four structural and seven nonstructural proteins. Four genotypes have been identified, but there is only one serotype. Therefore, exposure to one HAV genotype confers immunity to all genotypes.

Natural History
HAV is a cause of acute hepatitis and acute liver failure but not chronic hepatitis (Table 1). In approximately 5% of cases, a prolonged cholestasis lasting more than 3 months may occur, and in approximately 10% of patients, a relapsing hepatitis has been observed up to 6 months after the acute illness with recrudescence of symptoms and flare of hepatitis. Cases of relapsing hepatitis continue to remain infectious with fecal shedding of the virus. These atypical presentations of acute hepatitis A should not be mistaken for evolution to chronic hepatitis, as resolution is the rule. Recovery of HAV is associated with development of lifelong immunity.

HAV replication occurs in hepatocytes, and the virus is shed into the intestine via the biliary system. Viral levels peak during the asymptomatic period, and virus shedding continues until around 2 weeks into the icteric phase. HAV is detectable in the blood, but levels are 1000-fold higher in the feces. Children may shed the virus longer than adults.

The incubation period usually lasts 14 to 28 days. This is followed by the onset of symptoms. The presence and severity of symptoms are variable and age related. Generally, more than 70% of adult patients have a symptomatic illness compared with only 10% of children younger than the age of 10 years. Typical symptoms are nonspecific and include fever, anorexia, nausea, vomiting, diarrhea, abdominal pain, and weight loss. This prodromal phase is followed by an icteric phase in 40% to 70% of patients with jaundice, pruritus, and dark urine. Physical examination findings are usually unremarkable, but hepatomegaly may be observed. Extrahepatic manifestations are uncommon and may include an evanescent rash and arthralgias.

Laboratory studies during the prodromal phase reveal elevated serum aminotransferase levels greater than 10 to 20 times the upper limit of normal. During the icteric phase, total serum bilirubin rises but generally does not exceed 10 mg/dL. In most patients, jaundice lasts 2 weeks and a complete clinical and biochemical recovery can be expected in 2 to 3 months.

Epidemiology
Hepatitis A occurs throughout the world (Figure 1), either sporadically or in epidemics. The prevalence of HAV correlates with the level of sanitation and hygiene of a region. In developing countries, more than 90% of children are infected before the age of 10. In developed countries, including the United States, infection rates are low. Lack of exposure at a young age leads to higher susceptibility in certain high-risk adults, including travelers to endemic areas, injection drug users, and men who have sex with men.

In the United States, HAV infection rates have declined by 95% since the introduction of the mandatory childhood vaccination in 1995. The overall incidence rate in 2016 was 0.6% per 100,000 persons due to outbreaks related to imported foods, homeless persons, and persons who use injection drugs, representing a 44% increase in cases between 2015 and 2016. HAV is spread primarily by the fecal–oral route through the ingestion of contaminated food or water. Humans are the only known reservoir of the virus.

Diagnosis
Serologic testing for antibody to HAV can confirm the diagnosis of acute infection, past exposure, and immunity to the virus. Acute HAV infection is diagnosed by the presence of anti-HAV IgM. Anti-HAV IgG appears in the convalescent phase of infection and remains detectable for life. Past exposure or vaccination confers immunity and is reflected by anti-HAV IgG positivity with the absence of anti-HAV IgM antibodies. The antibody test for HAV usually includes total antibodies (IgM and IgG). Thus, to diagnose acute hepatitis A, it is important to order anti-HAV IgM.

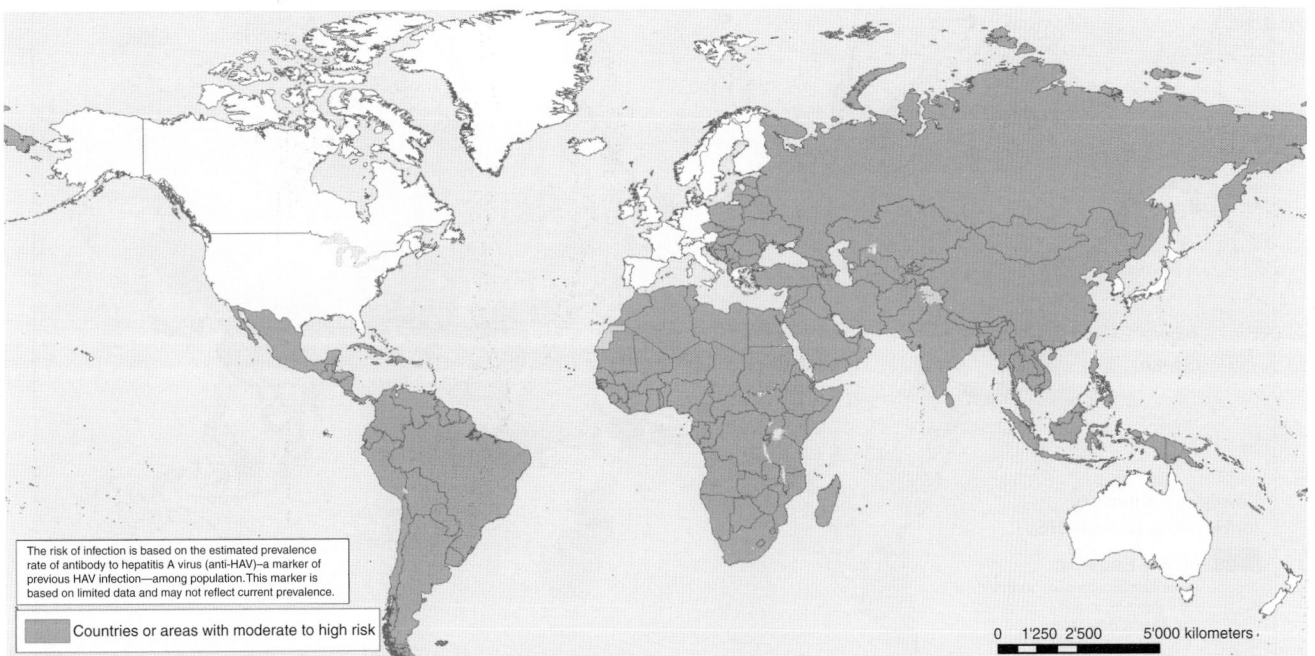

Figure 1 Global prevalence of hepatitis A and infection risk. Hepatitis A has a worldwide prevalence. Prevalence is related to the regional income, sanitation, and hygiene. High-income areas (e.g., North America, Western Europe, Australia, New Zealand, Japan, the Republic of Korea, and Singapore) have low levels of hepatitis A virus (HAV) endemicity and subsequently a high proportion of susceptible adults. Low-income regions (sub-Saharan Africa and parts of South Asia) have high endemicity levels and very few susceptible adolescents and adults. Middle-income regions have a mix of intermediate and low endemicity levels.

The risk of infection is based on the estimated prevalence rate of antibody to hepatitis A virus (anti-HAV)–a marker of previous HAV infection—among population. This marker is based on limited data and may not reflect current prevalence.

Countries or areas with moderate to high risk

0   1'250 2'500   5'000 kilometers

Treatment

Given the self-limiting nature of acute hepatitis A, treatment is predominately supportive. Caution should be taken when using hepatotoxic medications or medications metabolized predominately in the liver. Rarely, acute liver failure with encephalopathy and impaired synthetic function can occur. The patients at highest risk for this complication are generally older than 50 years of age and may have coexisting chronic HBV or HCV infections. Individuals presenting with acute liver failure are more appropriately managed at a liver transplant center.

Prevention

Both inactivated and attenuated vaccines have been licensed against HAV. Inactivated vaccines include HAVRIX (GlaxoSmithKline), VAQTA (Merck), TWINRIX (a combined hepatitis A and B vaccine from GlaxoSmithKline), AVAXIM (Sanofi Pasteur)[2], EPAXAL (Crucell)[2], and HEALIVE (Sinovac)[2]. The only live attenuated vaccine is BIOVAC-A (Pukang)[2]. The World Health Organization (WHO) recommends routine childhood vaccination for HAV in areas with intermediate infection rates. In the United States, the Advisory Committee on Immunization Practices recommends that all children at age 1 year be vaccinated. Other at-risk populations for whom vaccination is recommended include intravenous drug users, travelers to regions with high or intermediate HAV rates, men who have sex with men, persons in close contact with new adoptees from countries of high or intermediate hepatitis A endemicity, and patients with chronic liver disease or clotting factor disorders.

Passive immunization with immunoglobulin may also be used for preexposure protection among individuals who are at high or intermediate risk of HAV exposure. Pooled human anti-HAV immunoglobulins (GamaSTAN [IGIM]) decrease the HAV infection risk by 90% for up to 3 months. Passive immunization is also recommended for postexposure protection in cases of close personal contact with an individual with laboratory-confirmed HAV infection, staff and attendees of childcare centers if one or more children and/or staff are diagnosed with HAV infection, or food handlers during a common-source exposure. Concurrent immunization for HAV in these at-risk contacts is also warranted.

Hepatitis E
Introduction

Hepatitis E virus (HEV) is a nonenveloped, single-stranded, positive-sense RNA virus of approximately 7300 bases in length and the sole member of the Hepeviridae family. Its genome contains three overlapping open reading frames. ORF1 encodes four nonstructural proteins, ORF2 encodes the capsid protein, and ORF3 encodes a protein of unknown function. Four genotypes are known to infect humans, but similar to HAV, only one serotype exists, and infection with one strain confers immunity to all others. HEV is likely a zoonosis with multiple nonhuman vectors.

Natural History

HEV is a cause of acute hepatitis and acute liver failure (see Table 1). It can cause chronic hepatitis in immunocompromised individuals. The majority of acute HEV infections are asymptomatic or minimally symptomatic. The incubation period is between 15 and 60 days, and if symptoms arise, they generally consist of anorexia, nausea, vomiting, diarrhea, and abdominal pain. Acute HEV infection rarely causes jaundice, and most symptoms resolve within 6 weeks from onset. A notable exception to the generally favorable outcome is an increased risk of acute liver failure among pregnant women during the second and third trimesters in endemic regions. This leads to a high maternal mortality rate of 15% to 25% and worse maternofetal outcomes in third-trimester infections. Acute HEV infection may also be associated with a lymphocytic destructive cholangitis.

Chronic HEV infection is defined as the presence of HEV RNA in the serum or stool for more than 6 months. It is uncommon and has been observed in solid-organ transplant recipients, HIV-positive subjects, and other immunocompromised hosts. Chronic HEV infection has only been reported with HEV genotype 3 infections. It is unknown if other HEV genotypes can cause chronic HEV infection. Development of cirrhosis has been described as a consequence of chronic infection.

[2]Not available in the United States.

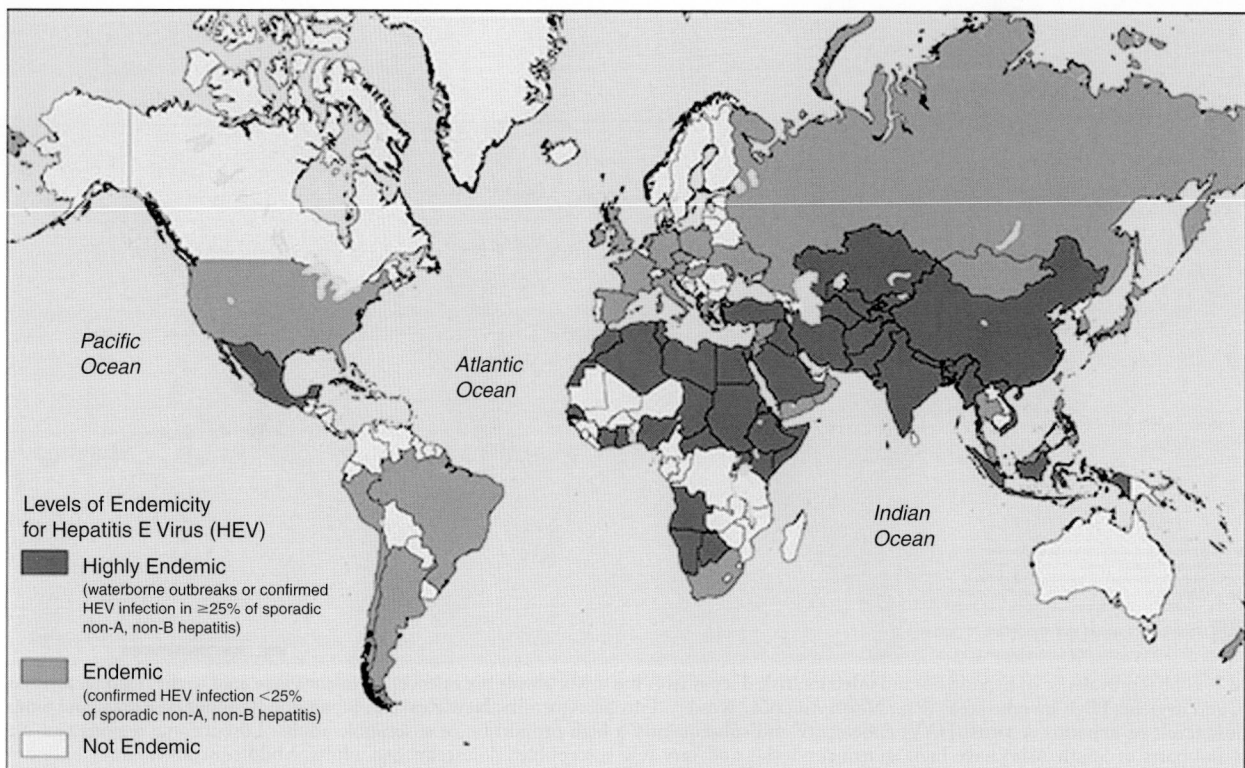

Figure 2 Global prevalence of hepatitis E virus. Hepatitis E is found worldwide. High endemic areas, defined by greater than or equal to 25% prevalence of sporadic non-A, non-B hepatitis, include parts of Central America and Mexico, Africa, the Middle East, and most of Asia. Endemic areas, defined as less than 25% prevalence of sporadic non-A, non-B hepatitis, include the United States, Europe, Russia, and parts of South America. Remaining regions are regarded as nonendemic.

Epidemiology

HEV is found worldwide and can be divided into three distinct geographical patterns: highly endemic, endemic, and nonendemic (sporadic) (Figure 2). Large waterborne epidemics in highly endemic regions are due to infection with HEV genotypes 1 and 2 in Central America, Africa, and Asia. Sporadic cases of HEV in developed countries (Europe, North America, and Far East Asia) are due to HEV genotypes 3 and 4. The reservoir for autochthonous HEV is unknown but thought to be domestic swine. Sporadic cases may occur in travelers to endemic areas. Interestingly, males are more affected than females in sporadic infections, but this gender bias is not observed during epidemics. HEV is spread by the fecal–oral route, usually through ingestion of contaminated water.

Diagnosis

There are no commercially licensed tests for HEV detection in the United States. Testing is limited to research laboratories and can be obtained through the Centers for Disease Control and Prevention.

The diagnosis of acute HEV is made by detection of anti-HEV IgM in serum or HEV RNA in stool or serum. Anti-HEV IgG has limited utility in diagnosis of HEV infections and may be a serologic marker for past infection. In immunocompromised patients, antibody testing can be falsely negative, making HEV RNA the more reliable marker of acute and chronic infection. Chronic HEV is diagnosed when HEV RNA is present in sera or stool for more than 6 months in suspected cases.

Treatment

Since most acute HEV infections are mild, the treatment is generally supportive. Patients who develop acute liver failure should be managed at a liver transplant center. The initial approach to management of chronic HEV infection in posttransplant recipients is to reduce the level of immunosuppression. If this is unsuccessful, then off-label use of antiviral therapy with peginterferon

(Pegasys)[1] or ribavirin (Rebetol)[1] may be considered. In immunocompromised individuals, therapy with peginterferon[1] or ribavirin[1] may be considered.

Prevention

Prevention of hepatitis E relies principally on good sanitation and the availability of clean drinking water. Prevention of transmission in travelers to endemic areas includes avoidance of tap water and consumption of street foods, raw vegetables, or raw or undercooked meats such as pork and seafood. A commercially available vaccine for HEV, HECOLIN[2] (Xiamen Innovax Biotech), has been available in China since 2012.

Hepatitis B

Introduction

HBV is a partially double-stranded DNA virus of approximately 3200 bases belonging to the Hepadnaviridae family. HBV consists of an outer lipid shell that surrounds a nucleocapsid consisting of the viral DNA and the polymerase. HBV has four overlapping reading frames (core, surface, polymerase, and x), which encode for seven viral proteins. HBsAg is the marker of infection and HBeAg is a marker of high viral replication and infectivity. The virus is classified into 10 major genotypes (A through J) that have a distinct geographical distribution. Four major serotypes have been described. Humans and old world primates (e.g., chimpanzees) are the only known hosts.

Natural History

Hepatitis B virus is a cause of acute hepatitis and acute liver failure (see Table 1). Globally, it is a major cause of chronic hepatitis. Infection with HBV is notable for a long incubation period ranging from 1 to 6 months. The majority (two-thirds) of persons

---

[1]Not FDA-approved for this indication.
[2]Not available in the United States.

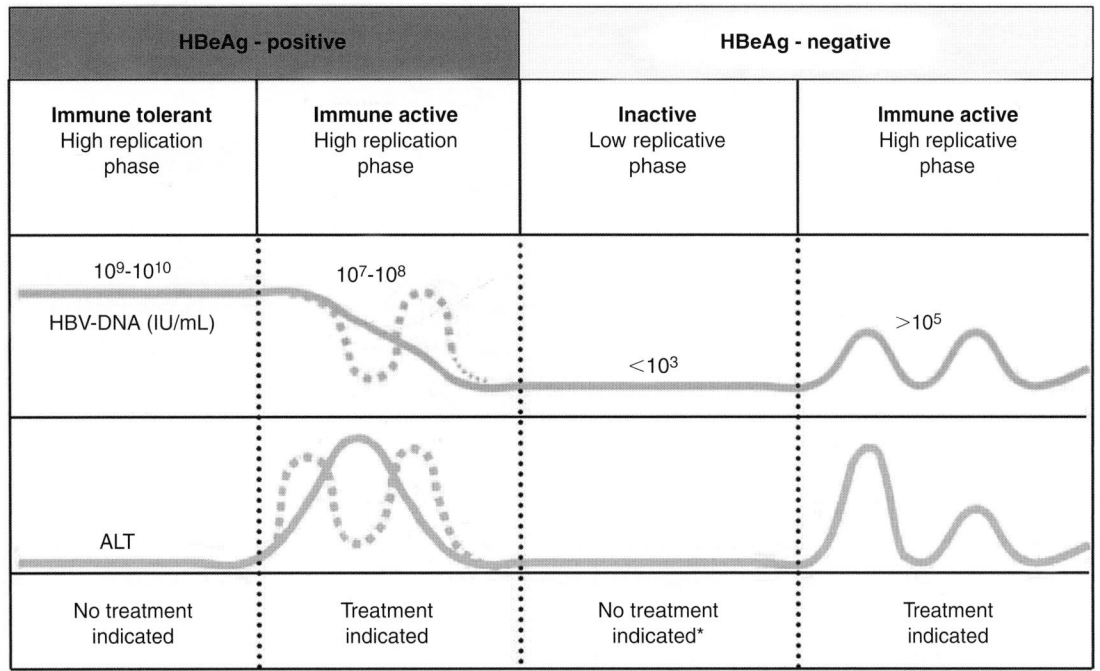

HBeAg - positive		**HBeAg - negative**	
Immune tolerant High replication phase	**Immune active** High replication phase	**Inactive** Low replicative phase	**Immune active** High replicative phase
10^9-10^{10} HBV-DNA (IU/mL)	10^7-10^8	$<10^3$	$>10^5$
ALT			
No treatment indicated	Treatment indicated	No treatment indicated*	Treatment indicated

Figure 3 Phases of chronic hepatitis B virus (HBV) infection. Chronic hepatitis B can be viewed in phases defined by HBeAg status and serum HBV DNA and ALT levels. The initial phase is the immune-tolerant phase, characterized by HBeAg positivity, high HBV DNA level ($>10^7$ IU/mL), and persistently normal ALT levels. This is seen only in persons who acquire the infection at birth or infancy and that persists for two to three decades of life. The next phase is the immune-active phase, defined by continued HBeAg positivity, high HBV viral load ($>10^5$ IU/mL), and elevated ALT levels. The next phase is characterized by loss of HBeAg and development of anti-HBe and heralds a transition from a phase of high viral replication to one of low replication. The viral load is typically less than 10^3 IU/mL and serum ALT is normal. This phase is termed the inactive carrier phase. A proportion of individuals develop raised HBV DNA and ALT levels after HBeAg seroconversion. These persons are said to have transitioned to the immune-escape or HBeAg-negative immune-active phase.

with acute HBV infection are asymptomatic, one-third have an icteric presentation, and less than 1% present with acute liver failure. Symptoms of acute HBV are nonspecific and include anorexia, nausea, pruritus, and right upper quadrant pain. Symptoms usually resolve in 1 to 3 months. Serum ALT levels peak with the onset of symptoms. The outcome of acute hepatitis B is strongly influenced by age at exposure. Resolution of acute infection occurs in 95% of persons exposed as adults, but chronic infection ensues in more than 90% of persons exposed as infants.

The natural history of chronic HBV infection depends on a complex interplay between the virus and the host immune response. Chronic HBV infection is often viewed in four phases (immune tolerant, HBeAg-positive immune active, HBeAg-negative immune active, and inactive carrier) based on HBeAg status and serum HBV DNA and ALT levels (Figure 3). This classification is useful for providing advice on prognosis and need for treatment. Approximately 25% to 40% of persons with chronic infection will be at risk for development of cirrhosis. The 5-year cumulative incidence of cirrhosis in untreated chronic HBV infection is 8% to 20%. Once cirrhosis develops, the 5-year cumulative incidence of decompensated liver disease (ascites, variceal hemorrhage, hepatic encephalopathy) is approximately 20%, and the annual risk of hepatocellular carcinoma is 2% to 5%. Persons who have resolved chronic infection (cleared HBsAg) should be counseled of the risk for viral reactivation with use of chemotherapy or other immunosuppressive therapies.

Epidemiology
An estimated 2 billion people worldwide have evidence of past HBV infection, and of these an estimated 257 million have chronic HBV infection. The prevalence of HBV infection is declining worldwide owing to the availability of an effective vaccine and implementation of successful vaccination programs. The prevalence of HBsAg, the serologic marker of chronic infection, is highest in sub-Saharan Africa and Central Asia (≥8%) (Figure 4) and lowest (<2%) in Western Europe, Australia, Canada, and the United States (except

Alaska) (see Figure 4). HBV is transmitted vertically, sexually, or through percutaneous routes and is more infectious than human immunodeficiency virus or hepatitis C virus. Individuals considered at high risk for acquiring HBV infection should be screened for chronic hepatitis B by testing for HBsAg (Table 2).

Diagnosis
A number of serologic markers (viral antigens and antibodies to the viral antigens) and nucleic acid testing are available to diagnose acute and chronic HBV infection. Cases of suspected acute HBV infection are diagnosed by the detection of HBsAg, HBeAg, IgM anti-HBc, and HBV DNA in serum in the appropriate clinical setting. Although anti-HBc IgM is detected during acute HBV infection, it is not specific for acute hepatitis B and may be seen during reactivation of chronic HBV infection.

Chronic infection is defined as persistence of HBsAg for greater than 6 months in serum. If HBsAg is present, it is advised to check HBeAg, anti-HBe, HBV DNA, and serum ALT to determine the phase of infection.

Treatment
Acute HBV infection in an adult is associated with a high rate of spontaneous recovery, and antiviral treatment is rarely required. Supportive care is advised. For persons with evidence of acute liver failure, prompt institution of antiviral therapy with a potent nucleos(t)ide analog and referral to a transplant center is recommended. Peginterferon alfa-2a (Pegasys)[1] is contraindicated in persons with acute liver failure.

The goals of treatment of chronic HBV are sustained suppression of HBV DNA to prevent the development of cirrhosis, hepatocellular carcinoma, and liver-related mortality. Cure of chronic HBV infection is currently not possible because of persistence of covalently closed circular DNA within the hepatocyte nucleus. Recommendations differ among regional guidelines, but treatment

---

[1]Not FDA approved for this indication.

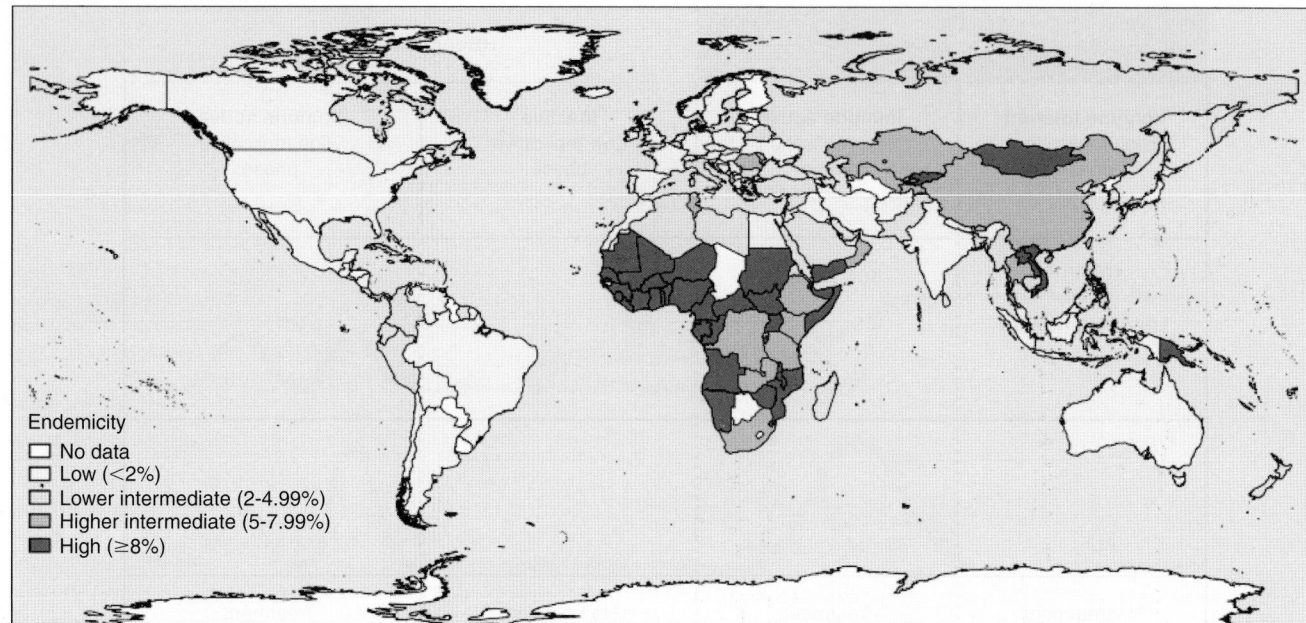

Figure 4 Global prevalence of chronic hepatitis B virus (HBV). Hepatitis B is found worldwide with varying geographical prevalence. High-prevalence areas defined as a prevalence of HBsAg greater than or equal to 8% include West sub-Saharan Africa and Mongolia. Regions of high intermediate prevalence, defined as HBsAg prevalence of 5% to 7%, include China, Southeast Asia, and the remainder of sub-Saharan Africa. Regions of low to intermediate prevalence, defined as HBsAg prevalence of 2% to 4%, include the Mediterranean region, India, the Middle East, Australia, and Japan. Regions with low prevalence, defined as HBsAg prevalence of less than or equal to 2%, include North America and Western Europe. Overall, the prevalence of HBV is declining worldwide.

Endemicity
☐ No data
☐ Low (<2%)
☐ Lower intermediate (2-4.99%)
☐ Higher intermediate (5-7.99%)
■ High (≥8%)

TABLE 2	Centers for Disease Control and Prevention Guidelines for Hepatitis B Virus (HBV) Screening

Populations recommended or required for routine testing for chronic HBV infections

Persons born in regions of high and intermediate HBV endemicity (HBsAg prevalence >2%)

US-born persons not vaccinated as infants whose parents were born in regions with high HBV endemicity (>8%)

Injection drug users

Men who have sex with men

Persons with elevated alanine aminotransferase/aspartate aminotransferase of unknown etiology

Donors of blood, plasma, organs, tissues, or semen

Hemodialysis patients

All pregnant women

Persons needing immunosuppressive therapy

Infants born to HBsAg-positive mothers

Household, needle-sharing, or sex contacts of persons known to be HBsAg positive

HIV-positive persons

Persons who are the sources of blood or body fluids for exposures the might require postexposure prophylaxis (e.g., needlestick, sexual assault)

HBsAg, Hepatitis B surface antigen.
Modified from Centers for Disease Control and Prevention. Recommendations for Identification and Public Health Management of Persons with Chronic Hepatitis B Virus Infection.

is generally indicated for HBeAg-positive subjects with confirmed HBV DNA greater than 2000 to 20,000 IU/mL and serum ALT two or more times the upper limit of normal, and for HBeAg-negative patients with HBV DNA greater than or equal to 2000 IU/ mL with serum ALT two or more times the upper limit of normal and/or liver biopsy–proven moderate to severe inflammation and/ or moderate fibrosis. The decision to treat persons outside these parameters should be individualized based on their risk for complications and risk of therapy. Eight agents are approved for the treatment of chronic HBV infection: two interferon preparations, interferon alfa-2b (Intron A) and peginterferon alfa-2a (Pegasys), and six nucleos(t)ide analogs: lamivudine (Epivir HBV), adefovir (Hepsera), entecavir (Baraclude), telbivudine (Tyzeka), tenofovir disoproxil fumarate (Viread), and tenofovir alafenamide (Vemlidy). Four agents are considered first line—peginterferon, entecavir, tenofovir, and tenofovir alafenamide—based on their safety, effectiveness, and low rates of antiviral resistance. Peginterferon is generally recommended in persons who would prefer a finite course of treatment and who have clinical and laboratory features predictive of a response to peginterferon (high ALT, low HBV DNA, young age, female gender, and HBV genotype A or B). Peginterferon is contraindicated in persons with decompensated cirrhosis, autoimmune illnesses, or active psychiatric illness. Nucleos(t)ide analogs are more potent inhibitors of HBV DNA replication and generally better tolerated than peginterferon. They are usually administered long term. The ideal endpoint of treatment is HBsAg loss, but this is rarely observed with any therapy (<10% with interferon and after 5 years of therapy with nucleos(t)ide analogs).

Prevention

Vaccination is the primary method of prevention. An effective vaccine against HBV has been available since 1981. In the United States, the Advisory Committee on Immunization Practices has recommended that all children complete the series of three vaccinations by 18 months of age with the first dose administered within 24 hours of birth. Infants whose mothers are HBsAg positive or whose HBsAg status is unknown should receive the last dose by 6 months of age. Hepatitis B immune globulin (HyperHEP B) and HBV vaccination is recommended at birth for infants whose mothers are HBsAg positive to prevent maternal–infant transmission of HBV. In mothers with viral loads greater than 200,000 IU/mL, antiviral therapy with tenofovir, telbivudine (Tyzeka), or lamivudine (Epivir HBV) in the third trimester of pregnancy (gestation weeks 28 to 32) can be considered.

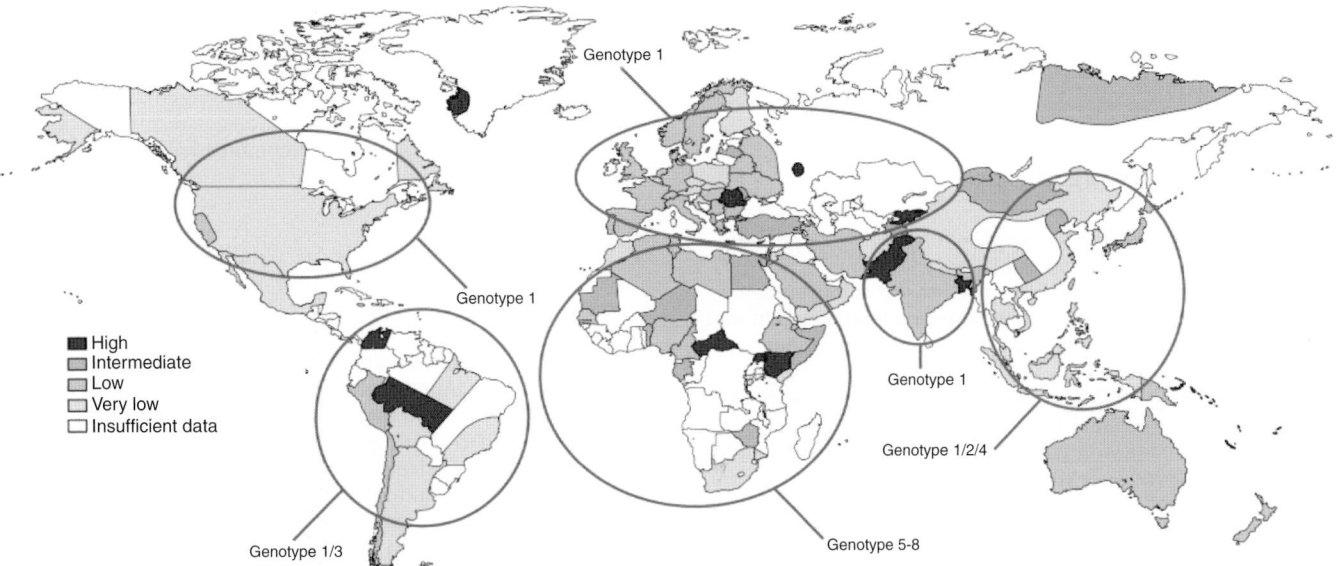

Figure 5 Global prevalence of hepatitis D virus. Hepatitis D is found globally, but its prevalence varies among geographic regions. The highest prevalence is observed in Central Africa, Central Asia, and the Amazon. Intermediate-prevalence regions include West Africa and Eastern Europe. Low-prevalence regions include North America, most of Western Europe, and Australia.

Postexposure prophylaxis is recommended for anyone who is exposed to HBV and is considered susceptible to HBV infection and consists of hepatitis B vaccination and/or hepatitis B immune globulin depending on the HBsAg status of the exposure source.

Hepatitis D

Introduction

Hepatitis D virus (HDV) is a viroid that is dependent on HBV for its lifecycle. The genome consists of a negative-sense, single-stranded circular RNA virus of approximately 1600 bases. The virus has an outer lipoprotein envelope HBsAg derived from HBV and is attached to a single structural protein, the HDV antigen (HDAg). There are eight known genotypes. Immunity to HBV prevents HDV infection.

Natural History

Hepatitis D virus is a cause of acute hepatitis, acute liver failure, and chronic hepatitis (see Table 1). Hepatitis D virus infection can occur either simultaneously with HBV (referred to as coinfection) or as an infection in a patient with chronic HBV infection (referred to as superinfection). The outcome of HBV/HDV coinfection depends on the course of acute hepatitis B infection and is generally self-limiting with a low risk of chronicity (~5%). In contrast, HDV superinfection of a chronic HBV carrier results in chronic HDV infection in more than 90% of cases. Acute liver failure is observed more commonly with coinfection than with superinfection. Chronic HDV infection has a variable course, from an asymptomatic carrier to cirrhosis and decompensated liver disease. In general, HDV infection is associated with more rapid progression to cirrhosis and decompensated liver disease and a higher rate of hepatocellular carcinoma as compared with HBV monoinfection.

Epidemiology

In developed countries, the prevalence of HDV has declined as a consequence of widespread vaccination against hepatitis B. Chronic HDV infection is predominately seen in intravenous drug users or hemophiliacs requiring frequent transfusions. HDV is prevalent in the Amazon basin, Africa, the Mediterranean basin, Central Asia, Mongolia, and Russia (Figure 5). HDV genotype 1 can be found worldwide, but all other genotypes are restricted to specific geographic areas.

HDV is spread by the same routes as HBV infection and is efficiently transmitted by parenteral and sexual exposure. In contrast to HBV, vertical transmission is not a common mode of transmission. Transmission cannot occur in the absence of HBsAg.

Diagnosis

Testing for hepatitis D should be considered in persons presenting with acute hepatitis B who have additional risk factors for HDV, including patients with a history of injection drug use, persons from endemic regions who present with a severe or protracted hepatitis, patients with chronic hepatitis B who develop an acute hepatitis of undetermined origin, and persons with HBsAg-positive chronic hepatitis B from endemic regions. Total anti-HDV (IgM and IgG) and anti-HDV IgM are the only commercially available assays in the United States. Initial testing for HDV should be with total anti-HDV. Chronic infection should be confirmed by a reverse transcriptase polymerase chain reaction assay for HDV RNA.

Treatment

The goals of treatment are long-term suppression of both HDV and HBV to prevent the development of cirrhosis, hepatocellular carcinoma, and liver-related death. There is no effective treatment for HDV. Interferon alfa (Intron A)[1] has been used for treatment of HDV. The most effective dose and duration of treatment have not been established. Peginterferon alfa-2a (Pegasys)[1] administered for 48 to 72 weeks results in sustained HDV RNA suppression after 6 months off therapy in 17% to 43% of patients. Liver transplantation with the use of hepatitis B immune globulin[1] is an option for patients with decompensated liver disease. Novel agents blocking viral entry and posttranslational prenylation are currently being investigated in clinical studies.

Financial Disclosure

The authors are employees of the US government and have no financial conflicts of interest to disclose.

Acknowledgments

This work is supported by the Intramural Research Program of the National Institute of Diabetes and Digestive and Kidney Diseases, National Institutes of Health.

References

Hoofnagle JH, Nelson KE, Purcell RH: Hepatitis E, *N Engl J Med* 367(13):1237–1244, 2012.

Hughes SA, Wedemeyer H, Harrison PM: Hepatitis delta virus, *Lancet* 378(9785):73–85, 2011.

Matheny SC, Kingery JE: Hepatitis A, *Am Fam Physician* 86(11):1027–1034, 2012.

Trépo C, Chan HL, Lok A: Hepatitis B virus infection, *Lancet* 384(9959):2053–2063, 2014.

[1]Not FDA approved for this indication.

HEPATITIS C

Method of
Arthur Y. Kim, MD

CURRENT DIAGNOSIS

- Hepatitis C virus (HCV) is a common infection in the United States, with major morbidity and mortality.
- The incidence of HCV is rising, linked to the opioid epidemic.
- Given the asymptomatic presentation and long period before complications, screening is warranted: one-time routine opt-out testing for adults age 18–79 is recommended, as is periodic repeat testing for increased risk, especially in people who inject drugs (Table 1).
- Diagnosis is made with two-stage testing: initial screening for anti-HCV antibodies followed by HCV RNA testing to confirm the presence of virus.

CURRENT THERAPY

- Novel therapeutic approaches that are safe and highly effective have revolutionized the care of HCV.
- The goal of therapy is cure of virus, which prevents liver-related complications and further transmission.
- Regimens of combination antivirals typically given for 8–12 weeks can cure over 95% of those living with HCV infection.

The diagnosis, management, and therapeutic approaches for patients living with HCV have been dramatically transformed in recent years. Most people (over 95%) living with HCV infection can be cured after 8 to 12 weeks of safe oral regimens involving combined antiviral agents. The availability of novel therapies enhances the effectiveness of screening patients for HCV infection who may otherwise be unaware of infection owing to its asymptomatic presentation.

Virology, Pathogenesis, and Natural History

HCV is a single-strand RNA virus whose genome encodes several viral proteins, including nonstructural proteins (NS3/4A, termed protease; NS5A and NS5B, termed polymerase) that may each be specifically targeted by medications. There are seven known families of virus, commonly known as genotypes 1 through 7, many with subtypes (e.g., genotype 1a or 1b).

After acute infection in the majority of individuals, the virus establishes a chronic lifelong infection characterized by high levels of viremia easily detected in plasma; in a minority, the virus is spontaneously cleared. In the latter scenario, HCV is permanently eradicated, as the polymerase is an RNA-RNA polymerase and there is no DNA intermediate to establish latency in the host. Those who achieve clearance of virus, whether spontaneously or via treatment, are susceptible to reinfection if exposed again.

Both the acute and chronic phases of HCV infection are largely asymptomatic. A minority of those with acute infection may present with nonspecific symptoms such as abdominal pain and malaise, with less than 10% presenting with jaundice. Rarely, those with chronic infection may experience extrahepatic manifestations of HCV infection, such as cryoglobulinemic vasculitis, proteinuria or glomerulonephritis, or lymphoma. Otherwise, alanine transaminase (ALT) levels may be persistently or intermittently elevated but may also be within normal range in up to 20% of infected individuals; thus, ALT is considered an imperfect screening test for HCV.

After establishment of chronic HCV infection, fibrosis occurs at a variable rate and may progress to cirrhosis in about 15%

to 20% over a 20-year period. Fibrosis may be accelerated by other liver insults, such as alcohol use, nonalcoholic steatohepatitis, and coinfection with HIV or hepatitis B virus (HBV). Those with HCV-related cirrhosis may experience significant morbidity and mortality from various complications; screening for varices and hepatocellular carcinoma is recommended (see chapter on cirrhosis).

Epidemiology

HCV is estimated to infect at least 70 million people worldwide. In the United States, it is the leading bloodborne pathogen and infects over 3 million Americans. The highest-risk groups are those born between 1945 and 1965 (so-called baby boomers), people who inject drugs, and HIV-positive men who have sex with men. In the United States, the incidence reached a peak in the 1970s and 1980s and then steeply declined; in the past decade there has been a resurgence of new incident cases linked to a widespread opioid epidemic.

Owing to the high number of infections that occurred decades ago, a large number of Americans within the baby-boomer cohort are now at risk for unidentified long-standing HCV infection, cirrhosis, and death; at present the mortality related to HCV exceeds that related to all other notifiable infectious diseases in the United States. HCV-related cirrhosis remains a leading indication for liver transplantation.

Risk Factors

HCV is most efficiently transmitted via exposure to contaminated blood or its components. In the United States, injection drug use (IDU) is the most common mode of transmission. Nosocomial exposure to contaminated blood or blood products and poorly sterilized or reused contaminated medical equipment remains an important risk, especially if strict universal precautions are not instituted. Mother-to-child transmission is not efficient, as only about 5% of children born to HCV-infected women are infected, with higher rates if HIV/HCV coinfection is present. Sexual transmission is considered very rare in the context of heterosexual relationships but does occur at higher rates in men who have sex with men, particularly with HIV and/or practices that result in exposures to blood.

Diagnosis

Two tests are used for the diagnosis of HCV infection: testing for anti-HCV antibodies and measuring HCV RNA. The suggested algorithm is initial serologic testing to assess exposure, followed by HCV RNA testing to determine current or cleared infection. Currently available anti-HCV testing is highly sensitive (>99%) but may be falsely negative in the earliest stages of infection (typically the first 4 to 12 weeks) or in the setting of immunosuppression (such as dialysis or HIV if CD4 cell counts are below 200/mm³). HCV RNA testing may be utilized to confirm current HCV RNA infection after an initial positive anti-HCV test or in settings when anti-HCV may be falsely negative. There are two types of HCV RNA tests: qualitative HCV RNA tests, which do not quantify the level of viral replication, and quantitative HCV RNA tests. Quantitative testing has improved in recent years and exhibits sensitivity similar to that of qualitative testing; therefore it is preferred in most situations.

Those with confirmed current HCV infection (positive HCV RNA) should also be tested for HIV and HBV (the latter typically by hepatitis B surface antigen [HBsAg]). Follow-up evaluation includes the HCV genotype, which defines therapeutic options. Discovery of advanced fibrosis or cirrhosis may affect the specifics of recommended antiviral regimens but also has prognostic implications. The likelihood of cirrhosis is dependent on various factors, including advancing patient age, duration of infection, and cofactors such as significant alcohol use or HIV. Noninvasive assessment with serologic testing (such as Fibrosure) or with novel imaging technologies (such as transient elastography) has largely replaced liver biopsies.

TABLE 1	Recommendations for One-Time Screening

All adults aged 18–79 years without prior ascertainment of risk

Risk factor–based screening

Risk behaviors

- Injection drug use (current or ever, including those who injected only once)

- Intranasal drug use

Risk exposures

- Persons on long-term hemodialysis (ever)

- Persons with percutaneous/parenteral exposures in an unregulated setting

- Health care, emergency medical, and public safety workers after needlesticks, sharps, or mucosal exposures to HCV-infected blood

- Children born to HCV-infected women

- Prior recipients of transfusions or organ transplants, including

  - Persons who were notified that they received blood from a donor who later tested positive for HCV infection

  - Persons who received a transfusion of blood or blood components or underwent an organ transplant before July 1992

  - Persons who received clotting factor concentrates produced before 1987

- Persons who were ever incarcerated

Other considerations

- HIV infection

- Sexually active persons about to start preexposure prophylaxis for HIV

- Unexplained chronic liver disease and/or chronic hepatitis, including elevated alanine aminotransferase levels

- Solid-organ donors (deceased and living)

- Pregnant women

HCV, Hepatitis C virus.
Modified from http://hcvguidelines.org.

Prevention

Prevention of HCV infection should be targeted to the highest-risk groups. For people who inject drugs, clean injecting equipment—including needles, syringes, and other components of drug preparation—is paramount. Risk reduction should also be achieved after viral clearance to prevent reinfection.

Prevention of fibrosis progression includes minimization or abstinence from regular alcohol use, avoidance of fatty liver, and avoidance of primary infection with or control of coexisting viruses (HIV or HBV). For individuals who are not immune, vaccination against hepatitis A virus and HBV is recommended. Patients with coexisting substance use disorder should be referred for appropriate care.

Therapy

Antiviral treatments for hepatitis C have been revolutionized with combination regimens of direct-acting antivirals (DAAs). These new drugs are used in combination with the goal to eradicate HCV. Cure is known as a sustained virologic response (SVR), defined as a negative HCV RNA test 12 or more weeks after cessation of therapy. This definition represents a durable cure in the absence of reinfection. Benefits of SVR include a significant reduction in future liver-related events, especially for those with advanced fibrosis or cirrhosis. Additional benefits include abrogation of further HCV transmission, amelioration of extrahepatic manifestations (if present), and improvement in quality of life. Virtually all patients with current HCV infection are candidates for therapy.

Agents may be classified by the viral protein they target. The following are NS3/4A protease inhibitors: simeprevir, paritaprevir (which requires pharmacologic boosting with ritonavir), glecaprevir, and grazoprevir. NS5A inhibitors include daclatasvir, elbasvir, ledipasvir, ombitasvir, and pibrentasvir; the NS5A nonnucleoside inhibitor dasabuvir; and the NS5B nucleotide polymerase inhibitor sofosbuvir. Simeprevir (Olysio), daclatasvir (Daklinza), and sofosbuvir (Sovaldi) were developed as single agents, but the majority are parts of combination regimens, as described in Table 2. The Infectious Diseases Society of America (IDSA) and American Association for the Study of Liver Diseases (AASLD) maintain guidelines for providers at http://www.hcvguidelines.org, which provides updates with approval of novel agents and as new data become available.

One major consideration in choosing a regimen is the genotype of the virus, although certain regimens such as glecaprevir/pibrentasvir (Mavyret) and sofosbuvir/velpatasvir (Epclusa) are able to treat all genotypes (termed pangenotypic). Other potential influences include presence of cirrhosis, the potential for concomitant drug interactions (including those with HIV coinfection on antiretrovirals), prior treatment experience, and adherence to therapy. Certain regimens such asglecaprevir/pibrentasvir (Mavyret) have been tested for those with advanced renal impairment. Insurance formulary preferences may also dictate the choice. One regimen in particular, elbasvir/grazoprevir (Zepatier), requires testing of genotype 1a virus for resistance-associated substitutions (RASs) associated with decreased response; if these are present, the duration should be increased and ribavirin (Ribasphere) added. In general, almost all patient groups can be offered a regimen with a rate of SVR at or above 95%.

These combinations have favorable safety profiles, with phase III trials reporting very low discontinuation rates. The most common side effects of these regimens are headache and fatigue. At times, ribavirin may be added to the regimen, particularly in the cases of relapse after previous treatment and/or cirrhosis (especially if the patient is decompensated or was previously decompensated).

Drug-drug interactions are also potentially problematic. Sofosbuvir-containing regimens should not be coadministered with amiodarone (Cordarone) owing to reports of symptomatic bradycardia with poor outcomes. Medications may significantly decrease the absorption of HCV antivirals, especially rifampin (Rifadin), carbamazepine (Tegretol), oxcarbazepine (Trileptal), and St. John's wort.[7] For the combinations of ledipasvir/sofosbuvir (Harvoni) and sofosbuvir/velpatasvir (Epclusa), care must be taken if they are coadministered with medications that decrease gastric pH. The involvement of clinical pharmacists may be very useful, along with resources such as the website maintained at the University of Liverpool: http://hep-druginteractions.org.

Monitoring

Compared with previous regimens that were associated with more side effects and complications, current treatments are far more tolerable. Clinical visits or phone calls to monitor for side effects and to promote adherence are often performed monthly during treatment. A negative HCV RNA at approximately week 4 into therapy confirms adherence. Certain regimens may require more intensive monitoring in the presence of cirrhosis, as cases of decompensation have been reported. Those with active HBV replication who are untreated are at risk for reactivation of this virus once HCV is suppressed, with rare cases of liver failure reported; cotreatment of both viruses or very close monitoring is recommended for this subgroup. At this time there are no data for the use of these agents in pregnancy or during breastfeeding.

---

[7]Available as dietary supplement.

TABLE 2 First-Line Combination Antiviral Regimens for Chronic Hepatitis C as of December 2019, Genotypes 1 to 4

GENOTYPE	COMBINATION	USE OF RIBAVIRIN (RBV)	DURATION (WEEKS)	NOTES
1	Elbasvir 50 mg/grazoprevir 100 mg FDC (Zepatier) qd	Add RBV and extend to 16 weeks if baseline NS5A RASs present (genotype 1a only)	12–16	Safe in advanced chronic kidney disease; not recommended in decompensated cirrhosis
	Glecaprevir 300 mg/ pibrentasvir 120 mg FDC (Mavyret) qd	Not proven	8–16	8 weeks for treatment naive; 12–16 weeks for certain treatment-experienced patients
	Ledipasvir 90 mg/sofosbuvir 400 mg FDC (Harvoni) qd	Add RBV if both interferon-experienced and cirrhosis (12 weeks)	8–24	Antacids reduce absorption; 8 weeks consideration only for naive patients with F0-2 and HCV RNA less than 6M IU/mL
	Sofosbuvir 400 mg/velpatasvir 100 mg FDC (Epclusa) qd	Consider in select circumstances	12–24	Antacids reduce absorption
2	Glecaprevir 300 mg/ pibrentasvir 120 mg FDC (Mavyret) qd	Not proven	8–12	8 weeks for treatment naive; 12 weeks for certain treatment-experienced patients
	Sofosbuvir/velpatasvir FDC (Epclusa) qd	Consider in select circumstances	12	Antacids reduce absorption
3	Glecaprevir 300 mg/ pibrentasvir 120 mg FDC (Mavyret) qd	Not proven	8–16	8 weeks for treatment naive (unless cirrhosis + Y93H mutation); 12–16 weeks for certain treatment-experienced patients
	Sofosbuvir/velpatasvir FDC (Epclusa) qd	Consider in select circumstances	12–24	Antacids reduce absorption
4	Elbasvir/grazoprevir (Zepatier) qd	Consider adding RBV for cirrhosis, prior nonresponder	12–16	
	Ledipasvir/sofosbuvir FDC (Harvoni) qd	Consider for previous SOF failure	12	
	Glecaprevir 300 mg/ pibrentasvir 120 mg FDC (Mavyret) qd	Not proven	8–16	8 weeks for treatment naive; 12–16 weeks for certain treatment-experienced patients
	Sofosbuvir/velpatasvir FDC (Epclusa) qd	Consider in select circumstances	12	Antacids reduce absorption

Daclatasvir may need dose adjustments with certain medications that interact with cytochrome P450.
FDC, Fixed-dose combination; *NS5A*, nonstructural protein 5A; *RASs*, resistance-associated substitutions; *RBV*, ribavirin; *SOF*, sofosbuvir.

References

AASLD/IDSA HCV Guidance Panel: Hepatitis C Guidance 2018 Update: AASLD-IDSA Recommendations for Testing, Managing, and Treating Hepatitis C Virus Infection, *Clin Infect Dis* 67(10):1477–1492, 2018.

Edlin BR, Eckhardt BJ, Shu MA, et al: Toward a more accurate estimate of the prevalence of hepatitis C in the United States, *Hepatology* 62(5):1353–1363, 2015.

Kim A: Hepatitis C virus, *Ann Intern Med* 165(5):ITC33–ITC48, 2016.

Ly KN, Hughes EM, Jiles RB, Holmberg SD: Rising mortality associated with hepatitis C virus in the United States, 2003- 2013, *Clin Infect Dis* 62(10):1287–1288, 2016.

Suryaprasad AG, White JZ, Xu F, et al: Emerging epidemic of hepatitis C virus infections among young nonurban persons who inject drugs in the United States, 2006-2012, *Clin Infect Dis* 59(10):1411–1419, 2014. 2006-2012.

INFLAMMATORY BOWEL DISEASE

Method of
Mona Rezapour, MD, MHS; Danny Avalos, MD; and Oriana M. Damas, MD*,†

Introduction and Epidemiology

Inflammatory bowel disease (IBD) is a chronic relapsing inflammatory disorder of the gastrointestinal (GI) tract that includes Crohn disease (CD) and ulcerative colitis (UC). A subset of patients with IBD have indeterminate colitis (IC), a classification that is determined when clinical features and diagnostic tests do not fit specifically into either CD or UC.

In the United States, about 3 million people have a diagnosis of IBD. Recent epidemiologic studies indicate that although the incidence of IBD in Westernized countries has stabilized, disease burden is expected to continue to rise as the annual prevalence steadily increases. The demographics of the IBD population in the US are also changing. Traditionally a disease that afflicted mainly European whites and the Ashkenazi Jewish population, IBD is now increasingly common among African Americans and Hispanic Americans.

The majority of IBD cases are sporadic. However, a little less than 20% of cases report having a relative with IBD, and this is particularly higher in patients with CD. There is also a higher IBD concordance in patients with CD compared to UC, wherein 2% to 14% of patients with CD report a family history of CD. Previous studies report that first-degree relatives of individuals with IBD have a lifetime risk of developing CD of 5% to 8% and of developing UC of 1.6% to 5.2%. With two affected parents, the risk of developing IBD in offspring increases to as high as 33%. These findings clearly support the influence of underlying genetic susceptibility in IBD development.

There are now more than 200 IBD susceptibility genetic loci associated with IBD risk, with substantial overlap seen between

* The authors disclose no relevant conflicts of interest.
† Funding for Oriana M. Damas was supported by: NIH N3U54MD010722-03S1.

UC and CD. Genome-wide association studies and meta-analyses, thereafter, provide fundamental insights into IBD pathogenesis. Implicated loci are enriched in genes involved in host-microbial interactions and are shared with other complex, immune-mediated diseases. Despite the discovery of these genetic underpinnings, established IBD loci actually explain only a fraction of the variance in disease risk and even less so of disease phenotype. This suggests that other factors, including environmental exposures, likely make larger contributions to pathogenesis and phenotype.

Clinical Features

IBD onset occurs primarily at a young age, between the second and fourth decade of life, although some studies suggest a bimodal distribution with another peak observed in the sixth and seventh decade of life. IBD can be difficult to diagnose because there is no single biomarker that can diagnose IBD. IBD diagnosis is made by a combination of clinical, serologic, radiographic, endoscopic, surgical, and histologic features. Adding further to the complexity is the fact that sometimes symptoms are vague. For example, fatigue, fever, chills, weight loss, failure to thrive in children, and development of extra-intestinal manifestations (EIMs) can at times precede luminal GI symptoms. When IBD is suspected and diarrhea is present, it is imperative that the patient's stool is examined for infectious causes because these can mimic IBD on radiographic imaging and endoscopically. Table 1 describes in detail differences in clinical presentation as well as differences in disease location between UC and CD.

Natural History

Most patients with CD and UC have a chronic, relapsing course. In CD, the natural history of intestinal inflammation can ultimately lead to the development of intestinal complications such as strictures, fistulas, and abscesses (Figure 1). This is particularly true if patients do not receive appropriate timely medical treatment. In many cases, these complications result in need for procedures (such as perianal abscess drainage or seton placements) and surgeries. Similarly, patients with untreated UC may also end up with complications including spontaneous colon perforation

or megacolon, in which case a total colectomy is curative. UC patients with longstanding disease are also at risk for colon cancer. Recent studies suggest that progression of disease of both CD and UC is preventable by timely administration of biologic therapy, which can modify the disease course.

Diagnosis

History and Physical

The diagnosis of IBD first starts with a careful clinical assessment, including a detailed history and a thorough physical exam that includes a perianal exam to look for the presence of perianal disease. A family history of IBD in the setting of GI symptoms should also raise clinical suspicion. Based on the clinical exam, the provider can then order a set of diagnostic tests to confirm the diagnosis

Laboratory Testing

It is important to order stool studies if diarrhea is present, to exclude enteric infections, as well as other causes of diarrhea (e.g., pancreatic insufficiency). A stool test to measure inflammation, such as stool fecal calprotectin or lactoferrin, is a noninvasive marker to detect the presence of enteric (mainly colonic) inflammation. These tests are useful for diagnosis and for monitoring of clinical disease activity.

Laboratory results, including presence of iron deficiency anemia, elevated C-reactive protein, and erythrocyte sedimentation rate (ESR), can clue into the diagnosis, although on their own, they are insufficient to definitely diagnose IBD. IBD-associated antibodies, including antisaccharomyces cerevisiae antibodies (ASCA IgG and IgA), perinuclear antinuclear cytoplasmic antibody (pANCA), antiflagellin (CBir1), antiouter membrane porin C (anti-OmpC), and antipseudomonas fluorescens-associated sequence I2 (anti-I2), can be measured in the blood and can aid in the diagnosis of IBD.

However, it is important to keep in mind that these antibodies can also be present in patients without IBD who have a family history of IBD. In prior studies, serologic markers such as pANCAs detect 40% to 80% of UC patients and the ASCA detect

| TABLE 1 | Clinical Presentation and Differences in Location of Disease Between Ulcerative Colitis and Crohn Disease |

CLINICAL FEATURES	ULCERATIVE COLITIS	CROHN DISEASE
Bloody diarrhea	++	±
Passage of mucus	++	±
Urgency to have a bowel movement	++	++
Tenesmus	++	±
Abdominal pain	++ (mainly left lower quadrant)	++ (can be diffuse or commonly right lower quadrant)
Weight loss	++	++
Fevers (important to exclude infection)	++	++
Fatigue and exhaustion	++	++
Presence of extra-intestinal manifestations	++	++ (especially in Crohn colitis)
Depression	++	++
Disease Location		
Small bowel involvement	– (never)	± (can be present)
Upper-gastrointestinal tract (proximal to ligament of Treitz)	– (never)	± (can be present)
Fistula presence (enteric, perianal, or entero-vaginal/vesicular or enterocutaneous)	– (never)	± (can be present)
Colonic disease	++ (always)	± (can be present)

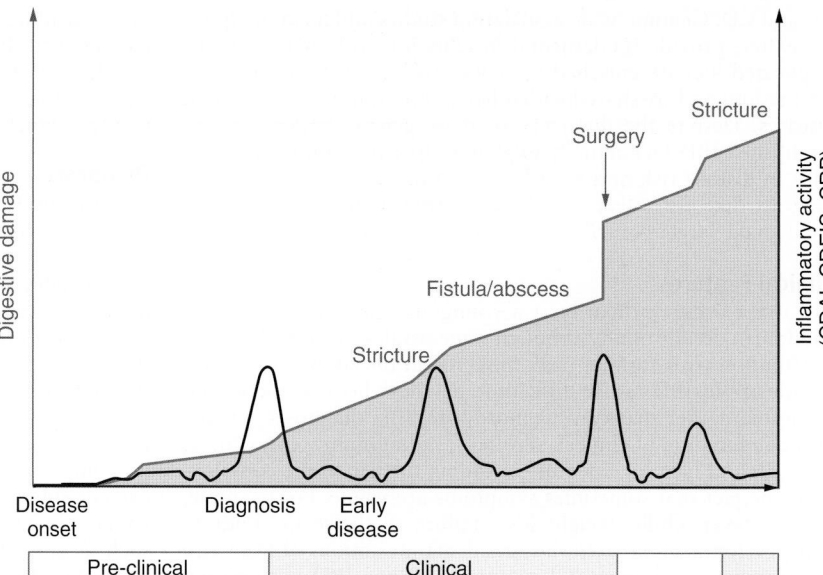

Figure 1 The natural history of Crohn disease if left untreated, (Adapted from Pariente, B, Cosnes J, Danese S, et al. Development of the Crohn's disease digestive damage score, the Lemann score. *Inflamm Bowel Dis* 17(6):1415-1422, 2011.)

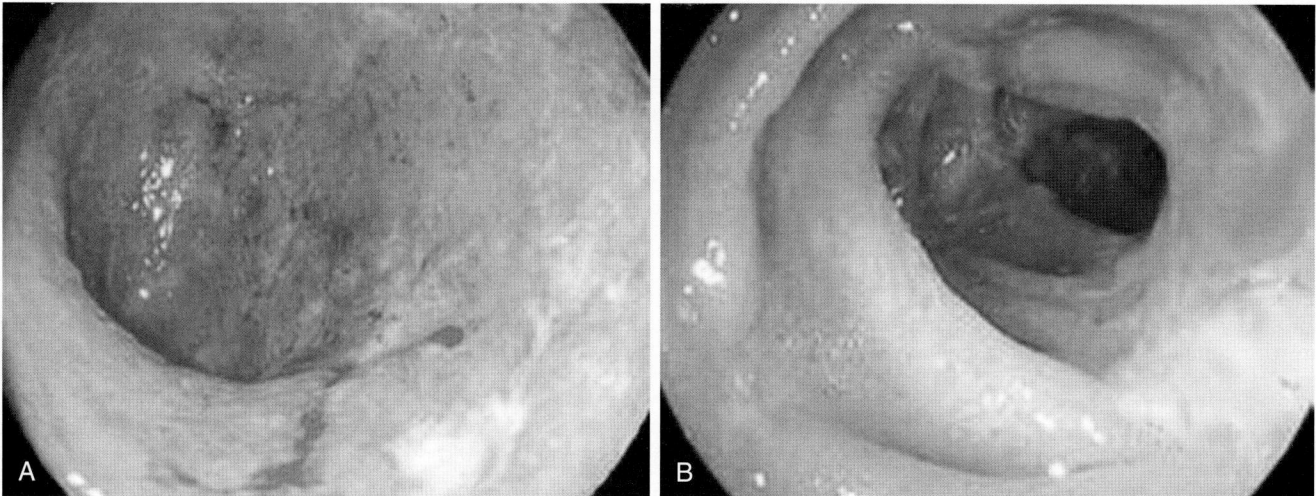

Figure 2 Endoscopic images of ulcerative colitis (UC) and Crohn disease (CD). (A) UC with luminal bleeding, loss of vascular pattern, and ulcerations. (B) CD with large deep ulcerations and edema in the terminal ileum.

about 68% of CD patients. CD patients can also carry pANCA, as seen in approximately 40% of patients who have Crohn colitis. Therefore, although helpful when positive as they can raise clinical suspicion for either CD or UC on their own, serologic markers are insufficient to diagnose IBD.

Imaging

CT and MRI provide information about the presence of inflammation in the small bowel and can be very useful in the diagnosis of IBD when there is clinical suspicion but no evidence of inflammation on ileocolonoscopy. CT or MR enterography (MRE) provide high contrast resolution that can help define mural and extra-mural complications. MREs are particularly helpful in defining the presence of disease activity in CD and in distinguishing between inflammatory and more complicated CD (such as fistulizing and/or stenotic disease). Pelvic imaging also helps identify the presence of perianal CD such as perianal/perirectal fistulas. An MRI is preferred over CT in patients younger than 17 years of age to prevent long-term exposure to radiation.

Endoscopy and Histology

Colonoscopy with ileal intubation is considered the gold standard for diagnosis of IBD. The endoscopic location and appearance can

also help distinguish between CD and UC. Endoscopic hallmarks of CD include patchy areas of inflammation with surrounding normal intervening mucosa, inflammation characterized by edema, nodularity, and ulcerations causing a cobblestone appearance (Figure 2). Endoscopic findings of UC include ulceration, friability, and loss of vascularity starting in the distal rectum and extending proximally in a continuous pattern (see Figure 2). An isolated cecal patch of inflammation can be observed in UC patients with otherwise more distal disease and this should be not be confused as a skip pattern seen in CD. Furthermore, the finding of mild ileal inflammation known as "backwash ileitis" is sometimes seen in UC patients with ileocecal valve inflammation and in the primary sclerosing cholangitis (PSC) patient. Small bowel capsule endoscopy is also helpful in visualizing the small bowel mucosa in patients with a high index of suspicion for small intestinal CD.

Histologic changes seen in CD and UC are distinct from those seen in acute infection and include mucosal separation, distortion and branching of crypts, presence of chronic inflammatory cells in the lamina propria, increase in number of lymphocytes and plasma cells in the crypt bases, and paneth cell metaplasia. In addition, the classical finding of granulomas is only seen in a minority of CD patients and although helpful, is not pathognomonic as they can also be seen in UC.

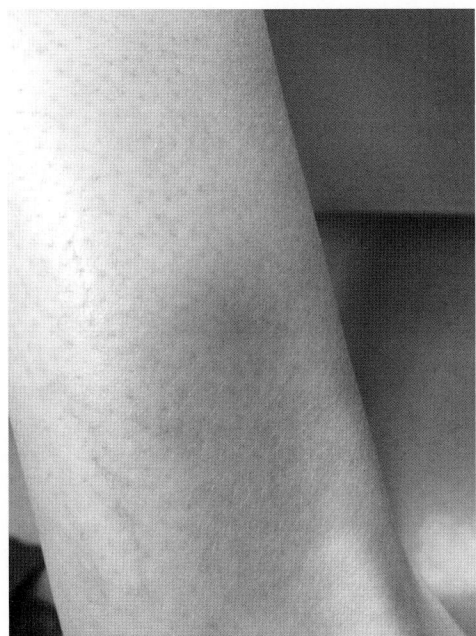

Figure 3 Picture of a patient with erythema nodosum, characterized by red/purple, painful lumps present most commonly in the lower extremities. Erythema nodosum is seen more in Crohn disease and its presence parallels active gut inflammation.

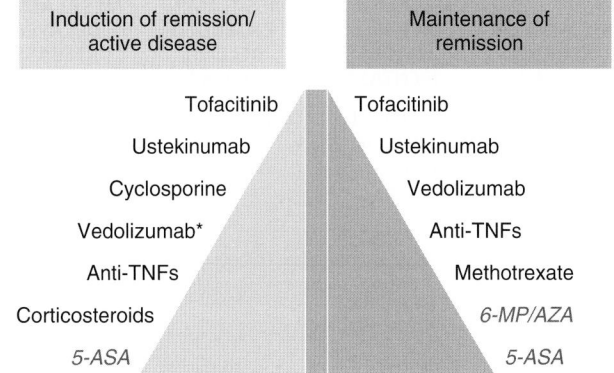

Therapeutic pyramid for IBD

Induction of remission/ active disease	Maintenance of remission
Tofacitinib	Tofacitinib
Ustekinumab	Ustekinumab
Cyclosporine	Vedolizumab
Vedolizumab*	Anti-TNFs
Anti-TNFs	Methotrexate
Corticosteroids	6-MP/AZA
5-ASA	5-ASA

Gray drugs are used in mild disease.

Figure 4 Therapeutic algorithm. Patients with milder disease benefit from 5-aminosalicylates *(5-ASA)* therapies as inductive and maintenance therapies. Other therapies are for moderate-severe disease. *Vedolizumab can be used as inductive therapy, although onset of action can take weeks. *6-MP/AZA*, 6-mercaptopurine and azathioprine.

Extraintestinal Manifestations

EIMs occur in 21% to 36% of IBD patients. Arthropathy is the most common EIM. Some EIMs are associated with disease activity and others are independent of disease activity. EIMs that parallel disease activity include aphthous ulcers and peripheral, dermatologic (erythema nodosum, Figure 3), and ophthalmologic (episcleritis and scleritis) arthropathies. EIMs that do not correlate with luminal inflammation include axial arthropathy (ankylosing spondylitis), hepatobiliary (PSC), and some dermatologic manifestations (such as pyoderma gangrenosum). Although not an EIM, by strict definition, IBD can also result in other extraluminal disease complications including thromboembolic disease and osteoporosis.

Management of Disease

In IBD, we classify therapy as induction therapy, which controls the inflammation quickly, and as maintenance therapy, which sustains control of inflammation. Figure 4 illustrates currently available inductive and maintenance therapies for IBD. The specific therapy is determined by several disease characteristics including disease location, extent of disease, and disease severity. The goal of therapy is control of inflammation, prevention of complications, and improvement in quality of life. These therapies include corticosteroids, 5-aminosalicylates (5-ASA), immunomodulators, and biologics. Therapeutic drug monitoring (TDM) of biologics is also an important component of therapy. TDM involves checking drug levels and the presence of antibodies to achieve a biologic-specific therapeutic target. TDM as a proactive or a reactive strategy is a topic of ongoing debate and beyond the scope of this chapter.

Medical Therapy

Corticosteroids

Corticosteroids, in particular prednisone, are used in both UC and CD mainly to manage disease flares. In UC, it can also be used for induction of remission in those intolerant to 5-ASAs or those who have failed to respond to 5-ASA treatment. The dose commonly used is 40 mg/day until clinical improvement and then a taper of 5 to 10 mg weekly until 20 mg, at which time a slower taper of 2.5 mg weekly is followed. Methylprednisolone (Solu-Medrol) is an intravenous medication often used in severe disease

flares in hospitalized patients in doses from 40 to 60 mg/day. Controlled-release budesonide in the ileum (Entocort EC) and controlled-release budesonide in the colon (UCERIS) also serve as effective short-term corticosteroids with fewer side effects as compared to conventional oral corticosteroids due to their high liver first-pass metabolism and low systemic bioavailability. What limits the use of corticosteroids is their substantial side effect profile that includes psychiatric disturbances, hyperglycemia, impaired wound healing, metabolic bone disease, and ophthalmologic disease. Importantly, steroids, while a convenient oral medication often interpreted as less harmful than biologics, are actually associated with a higher risk of infection than anti-TNFs and do not reliably cause mucosal healing. Steroids are also not effective for maintenance of remission, as they do not alter the natural history of the disease in the same way that biologics can.

Aminosalicylates

Aminosalicylates are compounds that contain 5-ASAs that exert a topical antiinflammatory effect on the intestinal lining. In UC, both oral and rectal formulations can be used for induction and maintenance of remission in mild-moderate disease. Their effect in CD as induction and maintenance therapy is debatable because they do not have an effect on transmural inflammation and they work mostly in the colon. See Table 2 for specific 5-ASA therapies and their location of action in the colon and/or small bowel. Patients should have yearly renal function and urine analysis testing given the rare but known side effect of acute interstitial nephritis associated with 5-ASA products.

Cytokine Inhibitors

TNF-α-antagonists (Anti-TNFs)

TNF-α-antagonists include infliximab (IFX [Remicade]), adalimumab (ADA [Humira]), certolizumab pegol (CZP [Cimzia]), and golimumab (GOL [Simponi]). They are indicated in moderately to severely active disease and most of them are effective in both UC and CD, although CZP and GOL have only demonstrated clinical efficacy in CD and UC, respectively. There is now evidence that earlier initiation of biologic therapy is more effective for induction of remission, prevention of disease complications, and reduction of steroid use. Early aggressive therapy is also associated with a higher likelihood of achieving mucosal healing, which is associated with the best clinical outcomes. Combination therapy with anti-TNF agents and immunomodulators was shown in the SONIC study to be more effective than monotherapy with anti-TNF or with immunomodulators alone in treatment-naïve patients. This finding we later learned is mainly

MEDICATION (BRAND NAME)	MESALAMINE CONTROLLED-RELEASE (PENTASA)	MESALAMINE EXTENDED RELEASE (APRISO)	MESALAMINE DELAYED RELEASE (LIALDA)	MESALAMINE DELAYED RELEASE (ASACOL HD)	SULFASALAZINE (AZULFIDINE)	OLSALAZINE (DIPENTUM)	BALSALAZIDE (COLAZAL)
Dosages	*Induction:* 1 g PO 4 times daily	*Maintenance:* 1.5 g PO daily	*Induction:* 4.8 g PO daily *Maintenance:* 2.4 g PO daily	*Induction:* 1.6 g PO 3 times daily	*Induction:* 1 g PO 4 times daily *Maintenance:* 1 g PO twice daily	*Induction*[1]: 1.5–3 g daily *Maintenance:* 500 mg PO twice daily	*Induction:* 2.25 g PO 3 times daily *Maintenance*[1]: 3–6 g PO daily
Location of release	Stomach, Jejunum, Ileum, Colon	Ileum, Colon	Ileum, Colon	Ileum, Colon	Colon	Colon	Colon
Delivery system	Controlled release gradually throughout the GI tract and not pH-dependent	Delayed release and pH-dependent	Delayed release and pH-dependent	Delayed release and pH-dependent	5-ASA linked to Sulfapyridine	Two 5-ASAs joined with one azo bond	One 5-ASA linked to an inert unabsorbed carrier molecule
Drug Monitoring	UA + renal function testing annually	UA + renal function testing annually	UA + renal function testing annually	UA + renal function testing annually	UA + renal function testing annually	UA + renal function testing annually	UA + renal function testing annually

[1]Not FDA approved for this indication.
5-ASAs, 5-Aminosalicylates; *GI*, gastrointestinal; *UA*, urinalysis.

due to the immunogenicity of anti-TNF agents, wherein introduction of immunomodulators as combination therapy reduces the frequency of antidrug antibody formation in the dual therapy group and promotes higher drug levels. Gastroenterologists starting anti-TNFs ultimately decide the need for dual therapy based on disease severity, but better algorithms for predicting who will do better on which regimen are needed.

TNF-blockers are contraindicated in patients with moderate-to-severe congestive heart failure (New York Heart Association functional class III/IV) and in patients with existing demyelinating diseases. Additionally, relative caution is advised for individuals with a prior lymphoma, known malignancies, a prior history of melanoma, and patients with a family history of demyelinating diseases. Patients should be cautioned about an increased risk of opportunistic infections, lymphoproliferative disorders, and melanoma development in patients who start anti-TNFs. However, mounting evidence suggests that the risk of lymphoproliferative disorders is actually mostly secondary to patients previously exposed to thiopurines. Recent studies show that the risk of non-Hodgkin lymphoma (NHL) is increased fourfold in IBD patients treated with thiopurines. Anti-TNF medications are also associated with an increased risk of NHL of about sixfold (6.1 per 10,000 patient-years); however, all these patients had been treated with immunomodulators previously. This is comparable to the expected rate of NHL in the general population of 1.9 per 10,000 patient-years.

Interleukin-12 and Interleukin-23 Inhibitors

Ustekinumab (Stelara) blocks both interleukin (IL)-12 and IL-23 by binding to the p40 subunit of IL-12 and IL-23, inhibiting their interaction with the IL-12 and IL-23 cell receptor binding complexes. Ustekinumab was found effective for induction of remission and as maintenance therapy for moderate to severe CD in the UNITI trials that incorporated close to 1300 CD patients. Ustekinumab is also now increasingly considered as a first-line therapy for moderate to severe CD due to its rapid onset of action, desirable safety profile, and improved efficacy when used as a first-line agent. Importantly, long-term tolerability and safety trials in both psoriasis and CD have so far reported a favorable safety profile for ustekinumab, including no serious opportunistic infections, injection-site reactions,

anaphylaxis, serum sickness-like reaction, or increased rate of malignancies. On post hoc analysis of patients in the UNITI pivotal trials, there was a 1.5-fold increase in inducing fistula response in patients with perianal fistulizing CD. Lastly, the phase 3 UNIFI trial showed that a single IV dose of ustekinumab can induce clinical remission at week 8 in patients with moderate to severe UC who have previously failed conventional or biologic therapy.

Immunomodulators

Calcineurin Inhibitors

Cyclosporine (Neoral, Sandimmune) is effective as salvage therapy in patients with severe steroid-refractory UC and was as effective as IFX in preventing colectomy in this cohort of inpatients. Cyclosporine is not effective in CD. Unfortunately, its safety profile and adverse effects limit its use. These side effects include diarrhea, nausea, vomiting, headache, tremors, hypertension, hepatotoxicity, nephrotoxicity, and neurotoxicity. Cyclosporine can be used in severe or fulminant, steroid-refractory UC, although long-term remission is only improved with the addition of either thiopurines or IFX. It can also be used in severe, steroid-refractory UC patients who have previously failed IFX therapy or have a low albumin level (particularly because low albumin is associated with high clearance of IFX), or as an inpatient bridge to vedolizumab.

Thiopurines

Thiopurines are used in both CD and UC, as either monotherapy or as adjunctive therapy to TNF-blockers. Thiopurines include azathioprine (Imuran)[1], mercaptopurine (6-MP [Purinethol])[1], and thioguanine (6-TG [Tabloid])[1]. Azathioprine is a pro-drug that is metabolized to 6-MP. The metabolic pathway of thiopurines involves three enzymes that convert 6-MP to its two by-products, 6-methylmercaptopurine (6-MMP), 6-thiouric acid, or 6-thioguanine nucleotide (6-TGN). 6-TGN is the therapeutic, targeted pathway. Thiopurine methyltransferase (TPMT) enzyme activity is tested prior to initiation of therapy to determine whether patients can obtain the drug at all and to determine the dosage. Once the drug is initiated, metabolite levels of 6-TGN

[1]Not FDA approved for this indication

and of 6-MMP are checked to assess for appropriate treatment efficacy. 6-TGN levels greater than 235 are associated with therapeutic efficacy. In addition, one study showed that 6-TGN levels greater or equal to 125 were sufficient to incur a higher level of anti-TNF in combination therapy. 6-TGN at levels above 400 can lead to myelosuppression and 6-MMP levels above 5700 can lead to hepatotoxicity. For these reasons, patients on thiopurines require more frequent blood monitoring than patients on biologics. Patients should have a hepatic function panel and a CBC checked every 4 months once steady drug dosages and drug levels have been achieved.

Methotrexate

Methotrexate[1] is used in the treatment of CD. It is a folic acid analogue that inhibits dihydrofolate reductase and subsequent folate-dependent synthetic reactions, which suppress inflammation. In CD, intramuscular methotrexate (dose 15 to 25 mg/week) is effective in the maintenance of remission. Oral methotrexate (12.5 to 15 mg/week) is not superior to placebo for maintenance of remission. In addition, methotrexate can be used as adjunctive therapy with anti-TNFs to reduce anti-TNF immunogenicity. Methotrexate is not effective in the treatment of patients with UC. The adverse effects of methotrexate include myelosuppression, alopecia, nausea, vomiting, diarrhea, hepatotoxicity, nephropathy, and neuropathy. Patients should be counseled about alcohol abstinence and contraceptive use.

Agents Targeting Leukocyte Trafficking

Leukocyte trafficking agents are now available for the treatment of severely active UC and CD. Natalizumab (Tysabri), a nonselective anti-α4 integrin antibody, interferes with the systemic trafficking of leukocytes to both vascular cell adhesion molecule-1 and mucosal addressin cell adhesion molecule-1 (MAdCAM-1). It was first approved for use in CD in 2007 when it was shown to have efficacy for induction and maintenance of remission in active CD. However, the risk of progressive multifocal leukoencephalopathy (PML) caused by JC virus has greatly limited its use in practice. Vedolizumab (Entyvio), approved in 2014, is a selective α4β7 integrin inhibitor that binds specifically to peripheral blood lymphocytes and inhibits its adhesion to a gut specific receptor, MAdCAM-1. Therefore it is a gut-specific leukocyte trafficking agent with no cases of PML reported with its use and with an overall very low systemic toxicity. Vedolizumab has a lower side effect profile, including a lower risk of systemic infections and no reported risk of lymphoproliferative disorders. It is a safer drug to use in conjunction with other immunosuppressants, for example, in patients with transplants who are already immunosuppressed. However, its slower onset of action limits its use in the acute, more urgent, setting.

Small Molecules

Agents Targeting Janus Kinase Family

Tofacitinib (Xeljanz) is the first small molecule approved for the induction and maintenance of remission of moderately to severely active UC. Tofacitinib is an oral, small molecule Janus kinase (JAK) inhibitor that preferentially inhibits *JAK3* and *JAK1*. JAK-STAT pathways regulate signaling of several immune-related mediators including type I interferon and interferon-δ. Inadvertent *JAK1* inhibition by tofacitinib results in higher rate of serious infections including herpes zoster. In addition, in psoriasis and rheumatoid arthritis patients, tofacitinib is associated with an increase in lipid levels, although the significance of this increase in causing cardiovascular events is not seen. Because of the high risk of shingles in patients taking tofacitinib, it is recommended that all patients starting tofacitinib receive the inactivated form of the herpes zoster vaccine, Shingrix, prior to starting therapy.

Pregnancy in Inflammatory Bowel Disease

Pregnancy is possible in patients with IBD. Women with IBD are more likely to have voluntary childlessness due to concerns with heritability of their IBD, risks of congenital abnormalities, and medication side effects and teratogenicity. It is important for patients and providers to know that there is no reduction in fecundity or fertility in women with IBD. This is true in most women with IBD, unless they have previously undergone pelvic surgery, such as in the setting of an ileoanal pouch anastomosis (IPAA) surgery. In this case, reduced rates of fecundity are possible but can be overcome by in vitro fertilization. Women with IBD should undergo disease activity evaluation prior to conception because active disease is the most important determining factor for a healthy, uneventful pregnancy. Patients with active disease during pregnancy are at risk for complications including premature births, low birth weight, babies born too small for gestational age, and of having cesarean deliveries.

In pregnant IBD patients, oral and rectal 5-ASAs, thiopurines, and most biologics should be continued throughout pregnancy to maintain long-term control of inflammation, which is the most influential determinant of a healthy pregnancy. However, medications such as methotrexate, cyclosporine, and allopurinol (Zyloprim)[1] are contraindicated during pregnancy and should be discontinued. Methotrexate should be discontinued in women and men planning to conceive, ideally 3 months prior to conception. Although mesalamines are considered one of the safest drugs during pregnancy, due to a few animal studies, women taking dibutyl phthalate (DBP)-containing 5-ASA (Asacol-HD) should switch to a non-DBP-containing formulation due to potential teratogenicity.

Anti-TNFs can be safely used during pregnancy. It is generally recommended to hold the last dose of an anti-TNF, due to increased placental transfer in the third trimester. That said, many GI providers may choose to continue the therapy based on presence of active inflammation and/or a historically difficult to control IBD. Certolizumab is the only anti-TNF with no placental transfer during pregnancy and can, therefore, be continued without reservations throughout the third trimester.

Several large registries have found that anti-TNFs and thiopurines have an adequate safety profile for the newborn. Studies looking at postnatal outcomes find that babies born of mothers on anti-TNF monotherapy have no increased infection risk during the first year of life. However, a small increased risk of immediate postnatal infections was seen in babies born of mothers on dual therapy with anti-TNF and immunomodulators.

Other biologics, when used as monotherapy, show similar safety profiles. Recent trials show that there are no increased safety risks to babies born of mothers treated with vedolizumab during pregnancy. Similarly, data on ustekinumab during pregnancy, largely derived from the rheumatology literature, appear to demonstrate an adequate safety profile. However, the verdict is still out on tofacitinib. So far, observed outcomes of congenital malformations (seen in 1% of patients) and spontaneous abortions (seen in 10.8% of patients) reported in tofacitinib studies mirror the background risks seen in the general population. Nevertheless, due to limited data on tofacitinib during pregnancy, no definitive conclusions or recommendations can be made regarding its use in pregnancy.

Preventive Care in Inflammatory Bowel Disease

IBD is a chronic medical condition associated with an increased risk of complications from influenza, pneumococcal pneumonia, and an increased prevalence of several cancers, including skin cancer. Despite several studies demonstrating this, IBD patients receive less preventive healthcare than other patients with chronic medical conditions. In the following we highlight important health maintenance screening measures for an IBD population. Several checklist resources are available for easy implementation into clinical practice (Figure 5).

Vaccinations

Administration of live vaccines, when deemed appropriate, should be administered to IBD patients off immunosuppression

Vaccine-Preventable Illnesses	Which Patients	How Often
Influenza (inactive)	All	Annually
Pneumococcal PCV13	If on/planning immunosuppression	Once[1]
Pneumococcal PPSV23	If on/planning immunosuppression	At baseline, repeat in 5 years
Tdap	All	Every 10 years
HPV	All aged 18-26	Once (3 doses within 6 mos.)
Meningococcal meningitis	All adult patients at risk of meningitis	Once
Hepatitis A	If non-immune	Once (2 doses within 6 mos.)
Hepatitis B	If non-immune	Once (3 doses within 6 mos.)
MMR (live vaccine)	If non-immune[2]	Once (1-2 doses)
Varicella (live vaccine)	If non-immune[2]	Once (1-2 doses within 6 mos.)
Zoster (live vaccine)	All aged > 50 years[3]	Once

Cancer Prevention	Which Patients	How Often
Cervical PAP smear	All on systemic immunosuppression[4]	Annual
Skin screen	All on systemic immunosuppression[4]	Annual
Colonoscopy	All with extensive disease for >8 years	Every 1-3 years

Other Screenings	Which Patients	How Often
DEXA Scan	High risk; women with low BMI, post-menopausal, chronic steroid exposure	At least 2 years apart
PPD or IGRA	Prior to anti-TNF or anti-IL-12/23	Once
Smoking status	All	Annual
Depression check	All	Annual

The evidence base for this checklist varies from "insufficient to assess benefits" to "moderate net benefits."

Developed by the CCFA Professional Education Committee Sub-Group: Alan Moss MD, Francis Farraye MD, MSc, Glenn Gordon MD, Raluca Vrabie MD • Approved by Committee Chairs: Samir Shah MD, Millie Long MD • V2_January_2017

1. Recommended timing of serial pneumococcal vaccination with both PPSV23 and PCV13 available in ACIP recommendation

2. Patients treated with systemic immunosuppressive therapy (steroids, thiopurines, anti-TNFs) should not receive live (attenuated) vaccines (e.g. measles, mumps, rubella, nasal influenza, varicella, and yellow fever)

3. Patients receiving anti-TNFs, anti-IL-12/23, or >20 mg prednisone should NOT be given the live zoster vaccine. Vaccine can be administered if on methotrexate < 0.4 mg/kg/week,6-mercaptopurine < 1.5 mg/kg/day or azathioprine <3 mg/kg/day

4. "Systemic immunopsuppression" currently includes azathioprine, mercaptopurine, methotrexate, anti-TNFs, anti-IL-12/23

ADDITIONAL INFORMATION
• ACG
• ACIP
• ACOG
• AGA
• National Cancer Institute
• National Osteoporosis Foundation
• PHQ-9 Depression Survey
• US Preventive Services Task Force (USPSTF) Osteoporosis
• USPSTF Tobacco

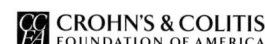

CROHN'S & COLITIS FOUNDATION OF AMERICA

Figure 5 Health maintenance checklist. At the time of this print, the inactivated form of the shingles vaccine was not available. This guideline mentions the zoster vaccine, which has now fallen out of favor in our immunosuppressed population. Adapted from the Crohn's and Colitis Foundation (website: http://www.crohnscolitisfoundation.org/science-and-professionals/programs-materials/health-maintenance-checklist.pdf).

or in patients on low dose immunosuppression. Ideally, these vaccines should be given 4 weeks or less prior to onset of immunosuppression and should be avoided within 2 weeks of initiation of immunosuppression, although vaccinations should never hold off need for urgent treatment of IBD. Low-level immunosuppression includes individuals who have received steroids at a low dose (≤ 20 mg/day) and for a short period of time (<2 weeks), or individuals taking the following medications at low doses: methotrexate ≤0.4 mg/kg/week, azathioprine ≤3.0 mg/kg/day or 6-mercaptopurine ≤1.5 mg/kg/day. Live vaccines such as the measles, mumps, and rubella vaccine (MMR), the yellow fever vaccine, and the live herpes zoster vaccine (Zostavax) are contraindicated in individuals already on immunosuppressive therapy. Fortunately, there is now an inactivated, recombinant herpes zoster vaccine (Shingrix) that is available to patients over the age of 50 and to those anticipating immunosuppression.

IBD patients should receive all age-appropriate vaccinations. Additionally, all IBD patients, irrespective of immunosuppressant medications, should receive the inactivated influenza vaccine annually and the pneumococcal vaccine (PCV13 and PPSV23). The human papilloma virus (HPV) vaccine can also be administered to patients on chronic immunosuppression from age 27 years to 45 years due to recent FDA approval extending the age group.

Cervical Cancer Screening

Women with IBD on immunosuppressive therapy are at an increased risk of cervical high-grade dysplasia and cancer. Therefore both the American College of Gastroenterology (ACG) and the European Crohn's and Colitis Organization recommend that women with IBD on immunosuppressive therapy should have annual cervical cancer screening.

Melanoma and Nonmelanoma Skin Cancer Screening

IBD increases the risk of melanoma independent of medications. Anti-TNF therapies have also been linked to an increased risk of melanoma. Nonmelanoma squamous cell skin cancer (NMSC) is associated with both current and past use of chronic immunosuppression, specifically thiopurines. In the CESAME study, the hazard ratios for NMSC in IBD who received thiopurines was 5.9 for ongoing treatment and 3.9 for past exposure. Taken altogether, it is, therefore, prudent that all IBD patients undergo evaluation by a dermatologist. Patients on anti-TNFs and on thiopurines should undergo yearly dermatologic examinations.

Depression and Anxiety Screening

IBD patients have an increased prevalence of depression and anxiety disorders, irrespective of their disease severity. In a recent systematic review, about 19% of patients with IBD developed anxiety and 21.2% developed depression. Therefore several recent guidelines now recommend screening patients with IBD for depression and anxiety. Depression and anxiety can be assessed by the Hospital Anxiety and Depression Scale, the Beck Depression inventory (BDI), the Spielberger Anxiety inventory, and the Perceived Stress Questionnaire.

Osteoporosis Screening

The pathogenesis of bone loss in IBD is multifactorial, due to steroid treatment, systemic effects of chronic inflammation, calcium and vitamin D deficiencies, and malnutrition. That said, not all IBD patients need to be screened for osteoporosis. IBD patients should be screened if they report a history of steroids for at least 3 months in a dose of greater than 7.5 mg/day or if they have any non-IBD established risk factors for osteoporosis, such as decreased body mass index, dietary deficiency of vitamin D and calcium, and previous fracture history.

Smoking Cessation Counseling in Inflammatory Bowel Disease Patients

Cigarette smoking is the strongest environmental factor impacting onset and disease course of CD. Cigarettes are associated with an increased need for steroids, development of postsurgical neo-TI strictures, and development of arthropathy. By corollary, smoking is also associated with an increased risk of colon cancer. In UC, cigarette smoking can ameliorate disease inflammation and smoking cessation can result in UC onset and/or flare-up. However, the global adverse effects of cigarette smoking are above any potential therapeutic benefit to smoking in UC.

Colon Cancer Screening and Surveillance

UC patients and CD patients with colitis are at an increased risk for colorectal cancer (CRC). The risk factors for developing CRC are similar in UC and CD and include duration, severity and extent of disease, PSC, and a family history of CRC. This risk is usually seen 8 to 10 years after the diagnosis of pancolitis. Patients with less involvement of the colon, specifically with less than a third of the colon involved, can start screening for colon cancer later, after 15 years of disease. Once screening starts, surveillance should take place every 1 to 2 years as recommended by several task force guidelines. Patients with PSC, however, need to undergo an annual surveillance colonoscopy, irrespective of duration of disease, due to their high risk of colon cancer.

Conclusion

IBD is a chronic, complex disease associated with high morbidity if untreated. In this chapter, we discuss new therapies available that can significantly alter the natural history of disease and improve quality of life. Primary care doctors, at the forefront of care, should be well acquainted with the diagnostic workup of IBD as well as with pertinent preventive health measures that are specific to an immunosuppressed population. We expect that future studies will deliver more patient-specific care models that improve delivery of healthcare, response to treatment, and ultimately IBD outcomes.

References

Beigel F, Steinborn A, Schnitzler F, et al: Risk of malignancies in patients with inflammatory bowel disease treated with thiopurines or anti-TNF alpha antibodies, *Pharmacoepidemiol Drug Saf* 23:735-744, 2014.

D'Haens G, Baert F, van Assche G, et al: Early combined immunosuppression or conventional management in patients with newly diagnosed Crohn's disease: an open randomised trial, *Lancet* 371:660–667, 2008.

Drugs for inflammatory bowel disease, *Med Lett Drugs Ther* 60:107-114, 2018.

Farraye FA, Melmed GY, Lichtenstein GR, et al: ACG clinical guideline: Preventive care in inflammatory bowel disease, *Am J Gastroenterol* 112:241–258, 2017.

Laine L, Kaltenbach T, Barkun A, et al: SCENIC international consensus statement on surveillance and management of dysplasia in inflammatory bowel disease, *Gastrointest Endosc* 81:489–501; e26, 2015.

Lichtenstein GR, Abreu MT, Cohen R, et al: American Gastroenterological Association Institute technical review on corticosteroids, immunomodulators, and infliximab in inflammatory bowel disease, *Gastroenterology* 130:940–987, 2006.

Lichtenstein GR, Loftus EV, Isaacs KL, et al: ACG clinical guideline: Management of Crohn's disease in adults, *Am J Gastroenterol* 113:481–517, 2018.

Luu M, Benzenine E, Doret M, et al: Continuous anti-TNF alpha use throughout pregnancy: possible complications for the mother but not for the fetus. A retrospective cohort on the French National Health Insurance Database (EVASION), *Am J Gastroenterol* 113:1669–1677, 2018.

Mahadevan U, Robinson C, Bernasko N, et al: Inflammatory bowel disease in pregnancy clinical care pathway: A report from the American Gastroenterological Association IBD Parenthood Project Working Group, *Gastroenterology*, 2019.

Rubin DT, Ananthakrishnan AN, Siegel CA, et al: ACG clinical guidelines: ulcerative colitis in adults, *Am J Gastroenterol* 114:384–413, 2019.

INTESTINAL PARASITES

Method of
Tarvinder Gilotra, MD

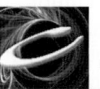

CURRENT DIAGNOSIS

Signs and Symptoms
- Watery diarrhea—Most protozoal infections: *Giardia, Blastocystis, Dientamoeba, Cryptosporidium, Cyclospora, Cystoisospora, Microsporidia*
- Dysentery—Most commonly *Entamoeba histolytica*; less commonly *Balantidium coli, Trichuris trichiura* (whipworm)
- Eosinophilia—Throughout chronic infection: *Strongyloides,* schistosomiasis, *Cystoisospora*; usually only in early infection: Ascaris, hookworm, whipworm
- Prolonged or severe diarrhea in HIV infection—Spore-forming protozoal infections: *Cryptosporidium, Cyclospora, Cystoisospora, Microsporidia*
- Visible worms passed in stool—*Ascaris, Taeniasis, Diphyllobothrium*

Diagnosis of Parasitic Infections
- Stool antigen assay: *Entamoeba histolytica, Giardia, Cryptosporidium*
- Serology:* Strongyloides, schistosomiasis
- Stool microscopy for ova and parasites: All intestinal parasites. Sensitivity is increased with repeat examinations if necessary. Concentration, preservation, and staining improve diagnosis of certain pathogens.
- Molecular tests: Traditional polymerase chain reaction (PCR), both nested and multiplexed, the real-time PCR, and newer gene amplification technologies including loop-mediated isothermal amplification (LAMP) and Luminex-based assays are gaining popularity in detecting some parasitic infections, especially in low-parasite load specimens.
- Proteomics: Mass spectrometry technique. Surface-enhanced laser desorption ionization time of flight mass (SELDI-TOF) that is based on matrix-assisted laser desorption ionization time-of-flight mass (MALDI-TOF) has been used in identifying biomarkers associated with some parasitic diseases such as African trypanosomiasis, Chagas disease, cysticercosis, and fascioliasis.

Note: Key features of intestinal parasitic infection may overlap with other conditions, including nonparasitic infections and extra intestinal parasites.

---

*Optimal method of diagnosis in returned travelers and immigrants from endemic to nonendemic areas. Does not distinguish between active and resolved infections.

Intestinal parasites are a diverse group of pathogens with local and global significance. Immigration, international adoption, travel, and the frequency of HIV/AIDS and other immune-compromising conditions (e.g., malignancy, organ transplantation) have all contributed to a need for ongoing or increased awareness of parasitic infections in the United States. Persons who reside in chronic care facilities, children in daycare, and persons whose sexual practices increase the likelihood of fecal–oral contact are also at risk for acquiring intestinal parasitic infection.

Globally, intestinal parasites are responsible for an enormous burden of disease. Although these pathogens are rarely fatal, ongoing exposure to intestinal parasites among persons in endemic areas exacerbates malnutrition, carries multiple morbidities, and causes stunting of growth and development in children, all of which have far-reaching consequences.

Patients who present with diarrheal illness (especially prolonged or travel-associated), unexplained eosinophilia, or expulsion of worms should be evaluated for intestinal parasites. In such cases, a careful history should focus on the patient's country of origin, detailed travel and recreational activities, dietary habits and new or unusual food exposures, occupation, sexual history, sick contacts, and risks for or known immunodeficiency. Some specialists advocate obtaining a complete blood count with differential to assess eosinophil count in all international adoptees and immigrants from areas where parasitic infections are common. If eosinophilia is present, antibody testing for schistosomiasis and strongyloidiasis—two chronic parasitic infections with potentially serious consequences—should be performed, and appropriate therapy should be administered if infection is discovered. For key features of common intestinal parasitic infections, see the Current Diagnosis box.

Diagnosis of intestinal parasites has improved recently with the advent of quick, simple, and accurate stool antigen tests for some major pathogens, such as *Entamoeba, Giardia,* and *Cryptosporidium* species. However, the fecal examination for ova and parasites is still the mainstay of diagnosis in many cases. Whenever possible, stool specimens should be sent to a laboratory with clinical expertise in parasitology, where wet preparation, concentration, or staining can identify most pathogens. Evaluation of fresh specimens and repeated examinations improve diagnostic sensitivity. Key diagnostic points are summarized in the Current Diagnosis box.

This review focuses on basic understanding, recognition, diagnosis, and treatment of common intestinal parasites in the United States and throughout the world. Within each section, parasites are listed in order of relative clinical significance.

Protozoa: Amoebae, Flagellates, Ciliates
Entamoeba histolytica
Entamoeba histolytica, the cause of amoebic dysentery and amoebic liver abscess, is a worldwide pathogen of major clinical significance. Approximately 10% of the world's population and up to 60% of children in highly endemic areas show serologic evidence of infection, and *E. histolytica* is estimated to cause 100,000 deaths per year globally. In the United States infection is almost exclusively found among returned travelers, immigrants from endemic areas (especially Mexico and Central and South America), men who have sex with men (MSM), and institutionalized persons. *Entamoeba dispar, Entamoeba bangladeshi,* and *Entamoeba moshkovskii* are morphologically indistinguishable from *E. histolytica.* Although these species are usually considered nonpathological species, there have been increasing reports of *E. moshkovskii* infections associated with gastrointestinal symptoms in humans in endemic areas. Other *Entamoeba,* including *Entamoeba hartmanni, Entamoeba coli, Entamoeba polecki,* and others, can be individually identified on microscopy. Again, these organisms are of uncertain pathogenicity and generally considered as commensal organisms, however, *E. polecki, Dientamoeba fragilis,* and *Iodamopeba bütschlii* have occasionally been associated with diarrheal illness.

E. histolytica exists in two forms, the hardy cyst (infective form) characterized by four nuclei, and the trophozoite (responsible for invasive disease), which has a single nucleus and survives poorly outside the human body. *E. histolytica* infection is acquired by ingestion of cysts in contaminated water or food or by sexual transmission through fecal–oral contact. Acquisition of the parasite can result in asymptomatic infection (most common), diarrheal illness, or extraintestinal infection, the latter most commonly manifest as amoebic liver abscess. An appropriately robust layer of colonic mucin may be protective against symptomatic infection, whereas trophozoite attachment to the intestinal epithelium results in penetration of the organism into the submucosal layer, where extensive tissue destruction can take place in the form of apoptosis and lysis of cells, hence the name "histolytica."

Symptoms of classic amoebic dysentery usually begin insidiously over 1 to 3 weeks after infection. Diarrhea is almost universal and typically consists of numerous small-volume stools that can contain mucus or frank blood, or both. Stools are almost always heme positive if not grossly bloody. Abdominal pain and tenesmus are common; fever is present in approximately 30% of cases. Some patients have a chronic course characterized by

weight loss, intermittent loose stools, and abdominal pain. Rare presentations of amoebic dysentery include amebomas, which can mimic malignancy, and perianal ulcerations or fistulae. Severe disease can occur in the form of fulminant colitis or toxic megacolon; the latter almost universally requires colectomy. Young age, pregnancy, corticosteroid use, malignancy, malnutrition, and alcoholism predispose to severe infection. Although persons with HIV infection or AIDS can develop invasive disease, *E. histolytica* does not appear to be a common opportunistic infection, and infection is curable in this population.

Amoebic liver abscess is the most common extraintestinal complication of *E. histolytica* that traffics to the liver via the portal venous system. Cerebral and ocular amebiasis have also been reported. Amoebic liver abscess affects children of both sexes equally, but it is up to 7 to 10 times more common in men, indicating that hormonal milieu likely plays a role. Amoebic liver abscess almost always manifests within 3 to 5 months of initial infection, but it can surface years later. Illness is characterized by fever and right upper quadrant abdominal pain that worsens over several days to weeks. Weight loss, jaundice, and cough from diaphragmatic irritation can also occur. Symptoms of dysentery usually are not present, and diarrhea is reported in less than one third of cases. Hepatomegaly and point tenderness over the liver is present in about 50% of cases. Rupture of the abscess can occur into the abdomen or pleuropulmonary space, manifesting as acute abdomen or empyema. Laboratory abnormalities include leukocytosis without eosinophilia, transaminitis, elevated alkaline phosphatase, and elevated sedimentation rate. Abscess is usually identified as a well-circumscribed hypoechoic mass on ultrasound, a low-density mass with enhancing borders on CT, and hypointense on T1 and hyperintense on T2-weighted MRI images. Chest radiograph often demonstrates elevation of the right hemidiaphragm, and pleural effusion may be present. Radionuclide uptake liver scans can help in distinguishing amoebic abscesses as "cold" compared with pyogenic abscesses that are usually "hot."

Diagnosis of intestinal *E. histolytica* infection has classically relied on stool microscopy, and this remains the only available method in most parts of the world. At least three stool specimens should be examined to improve sensitivity. Cysts visualized in stool cannot differentiate active disease from colonization, and *E. dispar, E. moshkovskii,* and *E. histolytica* species. Presence of trophozoites with ingested red blood cells (hematophagous trophozoites) on stool preparation and/or mobile amebae seen on fresh biopsy material stained with iron hematoxylin and/or Wheatley's trichrome are diagnostic of invasive intestinal amoebic disease. Contrary to the common belief, presence of hematophagous trophozoites on stool microscopy is not pathognomonic of *E histolytica,* as they can be seen with *E. dispar* infections as well.

Serology can distinguish between *E. histolytica* (makes antibodies) and *E. dispar* (does not generate antibodies) infections with good sensitivity in detecting antibodies within 5 to 7 days of infection. Positive serostatus, however, does not discriminate between acute and past infection, but negative serology is quite sensitive in endemic countries. Indirect hemagglutination serology remains the most sensitive test in nonendemic settings.

Diagnosis and species distinction of *Entamoeba* infection has improved greatly with the advent of antigen tests, now available as enzyme-linked immunosorbent assays (ELISAs), radioimmunoassay, and immunofluorescent probes. The Techlab ELISA *E. histolytica* stool antigen test is highly sensitive and specific if used on fresh stool specimens. It becomes positive with onset of symptomatic disease and resolves on treatment of infection.

Parasite DNA/RNA PCR, RT-PCR, multiplex PCR (can detect multiple pathogens), and LAMP fecal probes are highly sensitive and can differentiate *Entamoeba* species.

Aspirate of liver abscess may be necessary to distinguish from pyogenic liver abscess or when empiric therapy fails. Aspirated specimens consist mainly of necrotic hepatocytes ("anchovy paste"), and trophozoites are only seen in less than 20% of the cases. Nested multiplex PCR tests on hepatic aspirates might be useful although sensitivities range from 75% to 100%. As simultaneous colitis and amoebic liver abscess are rare, negative stool microscopy and PCR for *E. histolytica* does not preclude amoebic liver abscess. In a patient at high risk for amoebic liver abscess (e.g., young male immigrants), an adequate response to a trial of antimicrobial therapy can help confirm the diagnosis as well.

All patients who have confirmed *E. histolytica* infection and reside in nonendemic areas should be treated regardless of whether they are symptomatic because invasive disease can develop in the future. Asymptomatic cyst passers may be treated with an intraluminal agent alone, such as paromomycin or diiodohydroxyquin (iodoquinol [Yodoxin]).[2] In the United States the most readily available effective treatment for patients with amoebic colitis or liver abscess is metronidazole (Flagyl). It can be given intravenously for patients unable to tolerate oral medications. Recommended management is at least a 10-day course of the metronidazole (or tinidazole [Tindamax]) followed by an intraluminal agent (paromomycin for 7 days, diiodohydroxyquin for 20 days, or diloxanide furoate[2] for 10 days) for all cases of invasive *E. histolytica*. See Table 1 for medications and doses.

Giardiasis

Giardia duodenalis, previously known as *Giardia lamblia* or *Giardia intestinalis*, is the most commonly identified diarrheal parasitic infection in the United States, with an estimated 100,000 to 2.5 million cases per year. It is globally distributed and found in fresh water throughout mountainous regions of the United States

[2]Not available in the United States.

and Canada. The organism is a flagellated aerotolerant anaerobe that exists in a cyst and trophozoite form. Cysts can survive for several weeks in cold water. Contaminated food and water are the most common sources of infection, but the organism can also be passed by person-to-person contact. In the United States giardiasis is primarily diagnosed among international travelers, persons with recreational water exposure, institutionalized persons and children in daycare, and persons with anal–oral sexual practices.

Illness can result from ingestion of as few as 10 to 25 cysts, which transform into trophozoites in the small intestine and attach to and damage the small bowel wall. Symptomatic disease begins insidiously over approximately 2 weeks in 25% to 50% of persons who ingest *Giardia* cysts. Others become asymptomatic cyst passers (5%–15%) or have no signs of infection (35%–50%). Hallmarks of infection are watery diarrhea, bloating, flatulence, abdominal pain, and weight loss; less commonly, patients have nausea, vomiting, or low-grade fever. Steatorrhea and malabsorption, particularly secondary to *Giardia*-induced lactase deficiency, is frequently observed. Chronic *Giardia* infection should be considered in the differential diagnosis for a long-standing diarrheal illness, especially if there is history of exposure to possibly contaminated water. Patients with common variable immune deficiency, X-linked agammaglobulinemia, and immunoglobulin (Ig)A deficiency syndromes are at risk for fulminant and sometimes incurable disease, suggesting a significant role for humoral immunity in control of infection. Persons with HIV infection or AIDS usually have similar presentation as in non-HIV patients, can remain asymptomatic, and can be typically cured of infection

TABLE 1	Pharmacologic Treatment of Major Protozoan Infections			
CLINICAL SITUATION	**DRUG**	**ADULT DOSE**	**PEDIATRIC DOSE**	**COMMENTS**
Amebiasis				
Entamoeba histolytica				
Asymptomatic	Recommended: Paromomycin* *or*	25–35 mg/kg/day in 3 doses × 7 days	25–35 mg/kg/day in 3 doses × 7 days	
	Iodoquinol†,2 *or*	650 mg tid × 20 days	30–40 mg/kg/day (max 2 g) in 3 doses × 20 days	
	Diloxanide furoate‡,2	500 mg tid × 10 days	20 mg/kg/day in 3 doses × 10 days	
Mild to moderate intestinal disease	Recommended: Metronidazole *or*	500–750 mg tid × 7–10 days	35–50 mg/kg/day in 3 doses × 7–10 day	Treatment should be followed by a course of iodoquinol[2] or paromomycin in the dosage used to treat asymptomatic amebiasis.
	Tinidazole1,§	2 g once daily × 3 days	≥3 years: 50 mg/kg once daily (max 2 g) × 3 days	
Severe intestinal or extraintestinal disease	Metronidazole *or*	500–750 mg tid × 7–10 days	35–50 mg/kg/day in 3 doses × 7–10 days	Treatment should be followed by a course of iodoquinol[2] or paromomycin in the dosage used to treat asymptomatic amebiasis.
	Tinidazole§	2 g once daily × 5 days	≥3 years: 50 mg/kg once daily (max 2 g) × 5 d	
Balantidiasis				
Balantidium coli				
Symptomatic and asymptomatic disease	Recommended: Tetracycline1,‖	500 mg qid × 10 days	40 mg/kg/day (max 2 g) in 4 doses × 10 days	
	Alternatives: Metronidazole1 *or*	500–750 mg PO tid × 5 days	35–50 mg/kg/day in 3 doses × 5 days	
	Iodoquinol2,†	650 mg tid × 20 days	30–40 mg/kg/day (max 2 g) in 3 doses × 20 days	

Continued

TABLE 1 — Pharmacologic Treatment of Major Protozoan Infections—cont'd

CLINICAL SITUATION	DRUG	ADULT DOSE	PEDIATRIC DOSE	COMMENTS
Blastocystis hominis				
Symptomatic disease only				Organism's pathogenicity is uncertain.[¶]
Cryptosporidiosis				
Cryptosporidium				
Immune competent	Nitazoxanide	500 mg bid × 3 days	1–3 years: 100 mg bid × 3 days 4–11 years: 200 mg bid × 3 days ≥12 years: adult dose	FDA approved as a pediatric oral suspension for treating *Cryptosporidium* in immunocompetent children <12 years and for *Giardia*. It might also be effective for mild to moderate amebiasis. Nitazoxanide is available in 500-mg tabs and an oral suspension; it should be taken with food.
HIV-infected	No optimal therapy available			All HIV-infected patients with cryptosporidiosis should receive HAART whenever possible. Nitazoxanide,[1] paramomycin,[1] or paramomycin + azithromycin[1] may have a role in decreasing diarrhea in chronic cases of HIV-infected persons.
Cyclosporiasis				
Cyclospora cayetanensis	Recommended: TMP-SMX (Bactrim, Septra)[1] Alternative: Ciprofloxacin[1]	160 mg TMP, 800 mg SMX (1 DS tab) bid × 7–10 days 500 mg PO bid × 7 days	5 mg/kg TMP, 25 mg/kg SMX bid × 7–10 days (No recommended pediatric dose)[1]	In immunocompetent patients, usually a self-limited illness. Immunosuppressed patients might need higher doses, longer duration (TMP-SMX qid × 10 days followed by bid × 3 week) and long-term maintenance.
Dientamoebiasis				
Dientamoeba fragilis symptomatic disease only	Iodoquinol[2],[†] *or*	650 mg tid × 20 days	30–40 mg/kg/day (max 2 g) in 3 doses × 20 days	
	Paromomycin[1],[*] *or*	25–35 mg/kg/day in 3 doses × 7 days	25–35 mg/kg/day in 3 doses × 7 days	
	Metronidazole[1]	500–750 mg tid × 10 days	35–50 mg/kg/day in 3 doses × 10 days	
Giardiasis				
Giardia lamblia				
All symptomatic disease and asymptomatic carriage in nonendemic areas	Recommended:			
	Metronidazole[1] *or*	250 mg tid × 5–7 days	15 mg/kg/day in 3 doses × 5 days	
	Nitazoxanide *or*	500 mg bid × 3 days	1–3 years: 100 mg bid × 3 days 4–11 years: 200 mg bid × 3 days	
	Alternatives: Quinacrine[2],[**] *or*	100 mg tid × 5 days	6 mg/kg/d (max 300 mg/d) tid × 5 days	Albendazole[1] 400 mg daily × 5 days alone or in combination with metronidazole[1] may also be effective. Combination treatment with standard doses of metronidazole and quinacrine[2] × 3 week is effective for a small number of refractory infections. In one study, nitazoxanide was used successfully in high doses to treat a case of *Giardia* resistant to metronidazole and albendazole.

TABLE 1	Pharmacologic Treatment of Major Protozoan Infections—cont'd			
CLINICAL SITUATION	**DRUG**	**ADULT DOSE**	**PEDIATRIC DOSE**	**COMMENTS**
	Furazolidone[2] *or*	100 mg qid × 7–10 days	6 mg/kg/day in 4 doses × 10 days	
	Paromomycin[1]	25–35 mg/kg/day in 3 doses × 7 days	25–35 mg/kg/day in 3 doses × 7 days	Nonabsorbed luminal agent; may be useful for treating giardiasis in pregnancy
Cystoisosporiasis				In immunocompetent patients, usually a self-limited illness. Immunosuppressed patients might need higher doses, longer duration (TMP-SMX[1] qid × 10 days, followed by bid × 3 weeks), and long-term maintenance. For isosporiasis in sulfonamide-sensitive patients, pyrimethamine[1] 50–75 mg qd in divided doses (*plus* leucovorin[1] 10–25 mg/day) is effective.
Cystoisospora belli	Recommended: TMP-SMX[1]	160 mg TMP, 800 mg SMX bid × 7–10 days	5 mg/kg TMP, 25 mg/kg SMX bid × 7–10 days	Ciprofloxacin[1] is an alternative but may not be as effective.
Microsporidiosis				
Enterocytozoon bieneusi				
Intestinal disease	Fumagillin[+,2]	60 mg/day PO × 14 days		Oral fumagillin (Sanofi Recherche, Gentilly, France) is effective in treating *E. bieneusi* but is associated with thrombocytopenia and neutropenia. HAART can lead to microbiological and clinical response in HIV-infected patients with microsporidial diarrhea. Octreotide (Sandostatin)[1] has provided symptomatic relief in some patients with large-volume diarrhea.
	Albendazole[1]	400 mg PO bid × 21 days	15 mg/kg/day in 2 doses (max 400 mg/dose)	
Encephalitozoon intestinalis				
Diarrheal or disseminated disease	Albendazole[1]	400 mg bid × 21 days	15 mg/kg/day in 2 doses (max 400 mg/dose)	

[1]Not FDA approved for this indication.
[2]Not available in the United States.
*Should be taken with meals.
[†]Should be taken after meals.
[‡]The drug is not available commercially, but as a service it can be compounded by Panorama Compounding Pharmacy, 6744 Balboa Blvd., Van Nuys, CA 91406 (800-247-9767) or Medical Center Pharmacy, New Haven, CT (203-688-6816).
[§]A nitroimidazole similar to metronidazole, tinidazole is FDA approved and appears to be as effective and better tolerated than metronidazole. It should be taken with food to minimize gastrointestinal adverse effects. For children and patients unable to take tablets, a pharmacist may crush the tablets and mix them with cherry syrup. The syrup suspension is good for 7 days at room temperature and must be shaken before use. Ornidazole, a similar drug, is also used outside the United States. Dosing recommendations are only available for children ≥3 years of age.
[ǁ]Contraindicated in pregnant and breastfeeding women and children <8 years.
[¶]Clinical significance of these organisms is controversial; metronidazole 750 mg tid × 10 days, iodoquinol 650 mg tid × 20 days, or TMP-SMX11 double-strength tab bid × 7 days are effective. Metronidazole resistance may be common. Nitazoxanide is effective in children.
**Should be taken with liquids after a meal.
DS, Double strength; *GI*, gastrointestinal; *HAART*, highly active antiretroviral therapy; *max*, maximum; *tab*, tablet; *TMP-SMX*, trimethoprim-sulfamethoxazole.
Adapted from World Health Organization: Drugs for parasitic infections. *Med Lett Drug Ther* 8 (Suppl.), 2010.

with standard therapy. However, profound immunosuppression can be associated with more severe, atypical, disseminated, and refractory disease requiring combination therapy with quinacrine and metronidazole.

Diagnosis of giardiasis is made by examination of fresh or preserved stool or by stool antigen assays. Stool microscopy can be specific; however, it has low sensitivity because of intermittent shedding of *Giardia* cysts. Trophozoites may be directly visualized in fresh liquid stool; semiformed and preserved stool are likely to contain only cysts and should be stained with polyvinyl alcohol and/or formalin preparation. Antigen detection assays including immunochromographic assays, direct immunofluorescent assays, and ELISA assays have higher sensitivity with rapid turnaround time. Many assays are commercially available including the ImmunoCard STAT! Cryptosporidium/Giardia Rapid Assay (Meridian Bioscience, Cincinnati, Ohio) that tests for both pathogens simultaneously. Multiplex nucleic acid amplification tests (NAAT) are frequently used to detect various bacterial, viral, and parasitic pathogens as a workup for infectious diarrhea. Although it is rarely necessary, the diagnosis can sometimes be made on duodenal biopsy.

For details of treatment options, see Table 1. Tinidazole (Tindamax) and nitazoxanide (Alinia) are now the preferred agents for initial treatment of giardiasis. Metronidazole[1] is no longer the first-line therapy because of its adverse effects including metallic

[1]Not FDA approved for this indication.

taste, nausea, gastrointestinal discomfort, and headache. Patients who fail first-line therapy might have a persistent source of infection (contaminated water source, close contact with an infected person), immune deficiency predisposing to difficult eradication, or persistence of cysts. Once possible sources of reinfection have been investigated and eliminated, relapsed infections should either be retreated with a longer course of therapy (21–28 days) or treated with a different agent. Quinacrine (Atabrine)[2] is reserved for refractory cases but is contraindicated in pregnancy. Paromomycin[1] is an alternative in those with contraindications to other agents such as in pregnancy. Patients who fail more than one course of therapy should undergo immunologic workup.

Prevention of *Giardia* infection, as with other parasitic infections, involves primarily close attention to personal hygiene, hand washing, and avoidance of ingestion of fresh unfiltered water. Boiling water or use of a 0.2- to 1-μm water filter offer optimal protection against *Giardia* and other parasitic pathogens, although such filters still might not protect against *Cryptosporidium*.

Blastocystis

Blastocystis, formerly considered a yeast, has now been related to *E. histolytica* and is thought to be an anaerobic protozoan. The pleomorphic nature and karyotype diversity of this organism, its worldwide distribution, and varying diagnostic techniques have led to challenges in its identification and taxonomy. Although it has a worldwide distribution, its prevalence is higher in developing countries and is most commonly isolated in tropical regions. In temperate regions, *Blastocystis* (*B. hominis*) is detected at a high rate among MSM. It is a commensal of humans and several other animals. It appears to be transmitted via the fecal–oral route, possibly from waterborne sources. *Blastocystis* was long thought to cause only asymptomatic colonization, but there is some evidence to suggest a role in human disease, although this remains controversial. *Blastocystis* has marked morphologic variability and has been known to exist in at least four forms: vacuolated, amoeba-like, granular, and cystic, the latter of which is likely to be the infectious form. Ongoing molecular analysis has identified at least 17 subtypes of *B. hominis* (hence now referred to as *Blastocystis* spp., formerly identified as *Blastocystis hominis*) with varying degrees of pathogenicity in humans.

As suggested previously, the majority of infections appear to be entirely asymptomatic, and number of organisms does not appear to accurately predict severity of illness. Symptoms consist mainly of watery diarrhea, bloating, flatulence, abdominal cramps, urticaria, and fatigue. There are typically no pathologic findings on colonoscopy and there are no reports of invasive disease. Infection is diagnosed by stool microscopy with use of a trichrome or hematoxylin-stained preserved specimen. Fecal leukocytes are generally not found. PCR techniques have also developed with excellent sensitivity and are available worldwide. The organism is susceptible in vitro to numerous antimicrobials. Asymptomatic detection does not need treatment. Metronidazole[1] and tinidazole[1] are preferred agents for treating symptomatic disease. Trimethoprim/sulfamethoxazole (TMP-SMX, Bactrim)[1] and paromomycin[1] are alternative agents with good efficacy; details are listed in Table 1.

Dientamoeba fragilis

Dientamoeba fragilis was originally classified as an amoeba, but it is more closely related to the flagellates such as *Trichomonas vaginalis*. It is distributed globally, including in the Western nations; however, it is generally more prevalent in the areas of the world with limited public sanitation. *D. fragilis* has only recently been recognized as a clinically significant pathogen, possibly because it is difficult to visualize without specific staining techniques. Illness has commonly been found in travelers and MSM, but it can affect anyone. Some studies suggested a coinfection of *D. fragilis* with *E. vermicularis* as trophozoites were believed to survive in

E. vermicularis eggs. However, this association has not been consistently demonstrated.

Similar to most other intestinal parasites, *D. fragilis* is now known to exist in both trophozoite and cystic form, although it was only known to have trophozite phase for a long time. Despite its genetic relationship to the flagellates such as *Trichomonas*, *D. fragilis* does not have a flagellum and is immotile. Trophozoites range in size from 7 to 20 μm and can be binucleate. Cysts and precystic forms have recently been identified from human fecal specimens suggesting a fecal–oral mode of transmission.

Most patients are asymptomatic; however, numerous case reports and small series describe patients with no other organisms identified to cause their symptoms who improve significantly after treatment and documented clearance of *D. fragilis* from their stool. Illness is typically subacute to chronic, characterized by abdominal pain, watery diarrhea, anorexia, fatigue, and malaise. Unlike most other enteric parasites, *D. fragilis* is associated with marked peripheral eosinophilia and can masquerade as allergic colitis. Diagnosis can be challenging, because the trophozoites are fragile and usually missed on direct microscopy. If *D. fragilis* is suspected, stool should be preserved with polyvinyl alcohol and quickly stained with iron–hematoxylin and trichrome. PCR-based assays are very sensitive and being increasingly used for diagnosis.

Metronidazole[1] remains the drug of choice and has been efficacious in eradication of *D. fragilis* with a 10-day course. Other nitroimidazoles such as tinidazole[1] (better tolerated than metronidazole), secnidazole (Solosec),[1] and ornidazole[2] have been tested with good efficacy, but data is limited. Paromomycin[1] appears to be efficacious but is only backed up by limited data. Iodoquinol (Yodoxin)[2] has been successfully used very commonly in the past; however its availability has now declined. For full treatment information, see Table 1.

Balantidium coli

Balantidium coli is the largest protozoan that infects humans, and the only ciliate. Balantidiasis is a relatively rare cause of illness and is found primarily in rural agrarian communities in Southeast Asia, Central and South America, and Papua New Guinea. *B coli* is highly associated with animal farming, in particular, pigs and primates; humans are incidental hosts. The parasite is transmitted by direct contact with animals or on ingestion of water or food contaminated by animal excrement. Persons with malnutrition or immune deficiency are particularly susceptible to infection.

B. coli invades the intestinal mucosa from the terminal ileum to the rectum. About one half of infections are asymptomatic; the other half result in a subacute or chronic diarrheal illness with abdominal cramping, nausea, vomiting, weight loss, and occasional low-grade fever. Fewer than 5% of patients present with severe or even fulminant dysentery, and rare cases of colonic penetration with peritonitis, mesenteric lymphadenitis, or hepatic infection have been reported.

Diagnosis is made by visualization of trophozoites in fresh stool specimens or preserved and permanently stained samples. The trophozoite is relatively large (40–200 μm) and ciliated; cysts are difficult to distinguish. It displays a distinct spiraling motility that can be seen under low power. On stained sample, visualization of *B. coli*'s characteristic bean-shaped macronucleus and spiral micronucleus can help confirm the diagnosis. All patients should be treated regardless of symptoms. Tetracycline[1] (Sumycin and others) is the therapy of choice; alternative agents include metronidazole,[1] tinidazole,[1] and paromomycin[1]; see Table 1 for dosing information.

Spore-Forming Protozoa and Microsporidia
Cryptosporidium

Cryptosporidium is an intracellular pathogen with worldwide distribution that has been increasingly reported in the United States and other countries, including Nordic countries, Denmark,

Digestive System

IV

244

---

[1]Not FDA approved for this indication.
[2]Not available in the United States.

---

[1]Not FDA approved for this indication.
[2]Not available in the United States.

England, and Scotland in the last decade. Humans are most commonly infected by the recently reclassified *Cryptosporidium hominis (formerly C. parvum genotype 1)*, but *Cryptosporidium parvum (previously C. parvum genotype 2)*, primarily a bovine pathogen, also causes human disease. *Cryptosporidium* is known to be one of the important parasitic cause of diarrhea globally; however it is more frequently associated with overcrowded and poor sanitary environments. In the Unites States and other developed countries, the incidence is higher in children than in adults. *Cryptosporidium* infections have been reported as sporadic outbreaks, diarrhea and malnutrition syndrome in children from developing countries, and chronic and severe illness in immunocompromised hosts (especially with HIV infection). It is a primarily a waterborne illness and has caused multiple outbreaks in the United States secondary to recreational water exposure (e.g., swimming pools, water parks). The best-known outbreak occurred from contamination of drinking water supply in Wisconsin in 1993 that was thought to be secondary to runoff from the cattle pastures versus contaminated water from melting ice entering water treatment plants through Lake Michigan. It resulted in 403,000 documented cases of cryptosporidiosis and contributed to the deaths of dozens of persons with advanced HIV infection or malignancy.

Cryptosporidium is a coccidian spore-forming protozoa obligate intracellular parasite with a complex life cycle that matures and reproduces both asexually and sexually entirely within human hosts, thereby enabling infection to occur both from environmental sources and by direct person-to-person contact. Its oocysts, the source of infection on ingestion, are markedly hardy; they can withstand heavy chlorination, survive for months in cold water, and are small enough to occasionally evade even the smallest available water filtration systems. As few as 100 oocysts can cause infection, which results when the parasite penetrates small bowel epithelium and replicates just beneath its surface. Villous flattening and small bowel wall edema are seen on pathologic examination from infected persons.

Cryptosporidium infection can be asymptomatic or manifest as mild diarrhea to severe enteritis with or without biliary involvement. Mild illness is usually self-limited in 10 to 14 days without treatment in immunocompetent patients, although a substantial percentage of patients report a relapse of symptoms after initial improvement. It can have a protracted course with more severe symptoms in immunocompromised hosts. Fulminant and chronic infection have been frequently reported in those with HIV infection (especially those with CD4 <50), malignancy, and in malnourished children. Incubation period ranges from 3 to 28 days following the ingestion of oocysts and appears to be associated with the number of ingested oocysts. The hallmark of infection is explosive watery diarrhea, which can be so voluminous as to resemble cholera and can cause significant dehydration and electrolyte imbalance. Abdominal discomfort, nausea, vomiting, fever, malaise, and myalgia can also be present, and weight loss is common. Extraintestinal manifestations including biliary tract (cholecystitis, cholangitis, pancreatitis), and lung involvement has been reported, particularly in patients with HIV infection.

Diagnosis of *Cryptosporidium* has improved dramatically in recent years with the advent of antigen tests, which are highly sensitive and specific and can be used on a single sample of fresh stool. The ImmunoCard STAT! Cryptosporidium/Giardia Rapid Assay is useful because it can detect both pathogens. PCR is also available, has more sensitivity than direct microscopy, and can differentiate between various genotypes. When such tests are not available, stools submitted for examination should be fixed in formalin and stained for trophozoites or cysts; availability of multiple stool specimens improves the diagnostic sensitivity. Luminal fluid or biopsy specimens obtained during endoscopy can also reveal the organism.

Infection with *Cryptosporidium* is typically a self-limited illness in otherwise healthy persons, but symptoms can be improved and the course shortened with the antiparasitic nitazoxanide (Alinia).

If nitazoxanide is not available or tolerated, paromomycin[1] can be used, although it is not specifically indicated for this infection. *Cryptosporidium* remains an extremely challenging and potentially devastating infection in immunocompromised patients, especially those with HIV and a low CD4 count (counts <200 increase risk of severe illness, and counts <50 markedly increase risk). Although anticryptosporidial therapies in this population have shown very limited efficacy, restoration of immune function with HAART often affects cure. Limited data suggests a trial of nitazoxanide[1] may be reasonable in this circumstance as well. Appropriate supportive measures are also crucial in all patients with *Cryptosporidium*, including fluid and electrolyte replacement; avoiding lactose products is likely to be beneficial during the first 2 weeks after infection as the brush border regenerates. Appropriate treatment doses for nitazoxanide are listed in Table 1.

Prevention of *Cryptosporidium* infection requires a highly developed public water purification system including flocculation, sedimentation, and filtration. Use of 0.2- to 1-μm personal water filters for campers and hikers greatly reduces but does not eliminate risk of infection, whereas boiling water before drinking kills oocysts. Close attention to hygiene and avoidance of fecal–oral contact is the mainstay of prevention in the settings of institutional and community outbreaks. Patients should avoid swimming in public pools for 2 weeks after diarrhea resolution.

Cyclospora

Cyclospora cayetanensis is a coccidian with structure similar to that of *Cryptosporidium*. *C cayetanensis* is distributed worldwide, most commonly in the tropics and subtropics including Latin America (Guatemala, Peru, Mexico), the Indian subcontinent, and Southeast Asia. Outbreaks in the United States have been associated with import of contaminated produce such as raspberries and snow peas from Guatemala in 1996 and 2004, respectively. Similar outbreaks were attributed to contaminated lettuce and basil from Peru and cilantro and prepackaged salad from Mexico. It has also become increasingly recognized as a cause of infectious diarrhea in returned travelers. Unlike *Cryptosporidium*, *C cayetanensis* oocysts are shed in the stool as unsporulated oocysts (uninfected) and require few days of humid environment conditions to become sporulated infective oocysts. Hence the possibility of close person-to-person contact as a means of acquiring the infection is unlikely.

All persons are susceptible to infection, but those with HIV are at risk for more severe and prolonged disease, as seen with cryptosporidiosis and isosporiasis. Symptomatic disease appears to be most common in adults who do not have previous exposure to *Cyclospora*, such as travelers or persons who have relocated to endemic areas. Illness begins about a week after ingestion of sporulated oocysts and is characterized by watery diarrhea, abdominal cramping, bloating, anorexia, and weight loss. Low-grade fever can occur; marked fatigue is common and can last weeks or even months, and untreated infections can relapse after apparent resolution. Biliary involvement can occur in patients with HIV coinfection, as with cryptosporidiosis. Cyclosporiasis, similar to infection with other coccidians, causes damage to the small bowel epithelium, with resultant crypt flattening, edema, and inflammatory infiltrate. Lactose deficiency can remain for months after initial infection.

Diagnosis is made by stool examination. As with diagnosis of other parasitic infections, multiple stool specimens improve sensitivity. In the case of *Cyclospora*, concentration of the stool specimen also increases yield. If cyclosporiasis is suspected, specific testing should be requested because the organism exhibits unique properties. Similar to *Cryptosporidium*, organisms can be stained and visualized with Kinyoun acid-fast stain, but they are about two times the size of *Cryptosporidium* (8–10 μm in diameter). The cell wall of their oocysts also maintain its autofluorescence under ultraviolet microscopy that *Cryptosporium* does not.

---

[1]Not FDA approved for this indication.

Commonly used BioFire Film Array multiplex antigen detection test includes *C. cayetanensis*. Various conventional and real-time PCR techniques have been developed with good sensitivity. No serologic tests are available yet.

Cyclosporiasis is best treated with trimethoprim-sulfamethoxazole (Bactrim)[1]; nitazoxanide[1] and ciprofloxacin (Cipro)[1] may be effective for patients who have a sulfa allergy. Patients with HIV infection can require longer courses of treatment or chronic suppressive therapy; appropriate antiretroviral therapy is also important in the treatment of severe or relapsing infections. See Table 1 for details.

Cystoisospora

Cystoisospora belli, formerly *Isospora belli*, is a large coccidian distributed worldwide; however, infections are more frequent in tropical and subtropical areas. In United States, infections are largely identified in travelers from endemic areas and foreign-born HIV-positive patients. This is the most common parasitic cause of diarrhea in HIV-infected patients in India. Similar to *Cyclospora*, it requires a period of maturation (sporulation) outside the human body and therefore cannot be spread directly from person to person.

It appears to cause largely asymptomatic or mild infection in tropical areas to which it is endemic; the exception is among patients coinfected with HIV and particularly those with AIDS, in which it is a very common cause of chronic diarrhea in the Caribbean and Central America. Currently in wealthy countries it is found primarily in travelers returning from endemic areas. Illness is typically mild and self-limited, consisting primarily of watery diarrhea. However, some immunocompetent persons can develop a chronic sprue-like syndrome with malabsorption, and those with HIV infection or AIDS often have severe and prolonged diarrhea. *Cystoisospora* can invade to the lamina propria and can cause eosinophilia, which is different from other protozoan infections.

Diagnosis is made by observation of cysts in stool. As with *Cyclospora* and *Cryptosporidia*, they are usually not detected on routine stool ova and parasite examinations; hence acid-fast staining or ultraviolet microscopy techniques should be requested for high suspicion. Stool may also contain Charcot–Leiden crystals. No antigen detection tests are yet available. PCR tests have been developed; however, they are not widely available.

Illness is usually self-limited in immunocompetent hosts; hence antimicrobial therapy is only indicated when symptoms do not resolve spontaneously in 5 to 7 days. Symptomatic HIV-positive and other immunocompromised patients should always be treated. Trimethoprim-sulfamethoxazole (Bactrim)[1] is the treatment of choice. Ciprofloxacin (Cipro)[1] or pyrimethamine (Daraprim)[1] may be used in cases of sulfa allergy. Doses are listed in Table 1.

Microsporidia

Microsporidia are eukaryotic organisms that have been recently reclassified as fungi based on molecular genotyping. They are distributed globally, and more than 100 genera have been identified, 7 of which contain species known to be pathogenic in humans: *Encephalitozoon*, *Enterocytozoon*, *Trachipleistophora*, *Pleistophora*, *Nosema*, *Vittaforma*, and *Microsporidium*. These pathogens cause a wide variety of systemic and focal illness throughout the world.

Many immunocompetent patients in wealthy nations exhibit positive serology for certain types of microsporidial infections without a history of disease or travel. Microsporidia are most commonly associated with systemic infection in immunosuppressed persons, particularly those with HIV and a CD4 count of less than 100 or patients with organ transplants. Mode of transmission is not entirely clear, but the pathogen likely is spread both from water sources and possibly from close household contact.

Encephalitozoon intestinalis and *Enterocytozoon bieneusi* are responsible for intestinal microsporidial infections. *E. bieneusi* has been associated with self-limited diarrheal illness; *E. intestinalis* is commonly found in stool specimens throughout the developing world, but its pathogenicity is often not certain. Symptomatic infections, most often in patients coinfected with HIV, typically include a gradual onset of watery diarrhea, which may be worse in the morning and after oral intake. Significant volume and electrolyte depletion can occur, as well as fatigue, anorexia, weight loss, and malabsorption. *E. intestinalis* can disseminate and cause acute abdomen with peritonitis, cholangitis, nephritis, and keratoconjunctivitis, and *E. bieneusi* infection can result in cholangitis and nephritis as well as rhinitis, bronchitis, and wheezing. Other microsporidia are implicated in disseminated disease with a wide variety of extraintestinal manifestations including ocular, pulmonary, cerebral, renal, and muscular both in previously healthy and immunosuppressed hosts.

Diagnosis of microsporidiosis is attained by visualization of spores in stool or in tissue specimens. As suggested by their name, microsporidial spores are much smaller than those produced by spore-forming protozoal infections; most are approximately 1 μm in length and can easily be confused with bacteria or debris on slides. Special staining techniques have been described, but electron microscopy is required for species identification. PCR assays have been increasingly used for highly sensitive identification and speciation. Indirect immunofluorescence assays (IFA) are also available for *Encephalitozoon* spp. and *E. bieneusi*. Albendazole (Albenza)[1] is the treatment of choice for *E. intestinalis*. Treatment of *E. bieneusi* is more challenging. Although some response to albendazole has been reported, oral fumagillin[2] may have more efficacy. Unfortunately, it is not currently commercially available in the United States. Use of appropriate antiretroviral therapy is perhaps the most important treatment for patients with HIV infection or AIDS and chronic microsporidial infections. See Table 1 for details of treatment.

Helminths
Nematodes

Nematodes (roundworms) are cylindrical, nonsegmented organisms that are found throughout the world both as free-living species and as human and animal pathogens. Nematodes are the most common type of human parasitic infestation, found in approximately one-quarter of the world's population; often, susceptible hosts carry multiple different pathogenic nematodes. There are at least 60 species that have been shown to infect humans and 10 times that many that cause disease in other animals, but a few pathogens account for the bulk of human infections, in particular *Ascaris*, hookworm, and whipworm. These three organisms all require a period of maturation outside the human body—typically in warm, moist soil—underscoring the fact that repeated contact with fecally contaminated soil or food and water is necessary to sustain the cycle of infestation. *Strongyloides* and *Enterobius* are unique in that they can both complete their life cycle on or within human hosts and therefore can cause chronic infection and be transmitted directly by close person-to-person contact where there is the possibility of fecal–oral contamination.

Ascaris

Ascaris lumbricoides, the most common human helminthic infection, is estimated to affect 20% to 25% of the world's population. Up to 80% of community members are infected in heavily endemic areas, namely in Africa, Asia, and Central and South America. Cases of *Ascaris* infestation are also seen in rural areas in the southeastern United States. *A. lumbricoides* are white to pinkish worms that range from 10 to 40 cm in length. Transmission in humans occurs most commonly by ingestion of infectious human or pigs eggs that are oval white bodies with an adherent mucopolysaccharide capsule that clings to multiple surfaces and

---

[1]Not FDA approved for this indication.

[1]Not FDA approved for this indication.
[2]Not available in the United States.

aids in transmissibility of the parasite. Eggs are also remarkably durable, capable of surviving up to 6 years in moist soil and able to weather brief droughts and periods of freezing. Another means of transmission is by ingesting uncooked pig or chicken liver containing *A. suum* larvae.

Fecal contamination of water, food, and environmental surfaces such as doorknobs and countertops provide the means of transmission for *Ascaris,* and recurrent infection occurs as long as living conditions that predispose people to infection remain unchanged. Lack of adequate public sanitation, use of human feces as fertilizer (night soil), and frequent contact with soil or shared contaminated surfaces among close household members are risk factors for infection. Persons who move to environments with improved sanitation typically lose their infection within 2 years as all the adult worms die. Eggs excreted by an infected person must mature outside the human body for approximately 2 weeks. On ingestion by a susceptible host, mature eggs hatch in the small intestine and release larvae, which penetrate the intestinal wall and travel through the venous circulation to the lungs, where they are coughed up and swallowed. They then undergo maturation into adult worms in the intestine and produce eggs by 2 to 3 months after initial infection. The eggs are excreted in the feces and mature outside the body to continue the cycle.

Most persons with *Ascaris* infection are asymptomatic. Approximately 15% of infected people have morbidity, which is associated with young age, large burden of worms, coinfection with other intestinal parasites, and genetic predisposition. In children, infection contributes to malabsorption of protein, fat, and vitamins A and C, and treatment of heavily infected children can improve their nutritional status. *Ascaris* infection can also cause intestinal, pancreatic, or biliary obstruction as a result of worm mass or worm migration. Despite the low incidence of obstructive complications per infected person, the *Ascaris*-related acute abdomen is a significant problem on a global level given the enormous number of people infected. Some patients with intestinal *Ascaris* infection report vague abdominal complaints, such as abdominal discomfort, nausea, vomiting, or diarrhea, but these are relatively rare. Pulmonary migration of a large quantity of worms can produce Loeffler's syndrome, or eosinophilic pneumonitis.

Diagnosis is easily attained with standard saline stool preparation, and large numbers of eggs are typically seen. Larvae or worms can also sometimes be seen in sputum or stool samples. In cases of intestinal obstruction, worms may be visualized on upper gastrointestinal series, computed tomography, and even ultrasound. Multiplex PCR assays are highly sensitive at identification and quantification but are currently not routinely used. Peripheral eosinophilia with *Ascaris* infection is found only during the larval migratory phase but not at all times. Chronic eosinophilia in an at-risk person suggests another parasitic infection, often *Strongyloides.* Sputum eosinophilia and Charcot-Leyden crystals can be seen, although this is common with many parasitic eosinophilic pulmonary infections.

All persons documented to carry *Ascaris* who have migrated to nonendemic areas should be treated to prevent complications in the future; in endemic areas, adults need only be treated if they are symptomatic. Children have been shown to benefit from intermittent anthelminthic therapy in heavily affected areas of the world. For patients with intestinal obstruction, bowel rest and intravenous hydration are usually sufficient to relieve the obstruction, at which time anthelminthic therapy can be administered. In such cases, gastroenterology consultation should be obtained. In rare cases, surgical intervention is required. Treatment of pulmonary infection is controversial; however, most experts recommend steroid therapy for severe infections followed 2 to 3 weeks later (at the time full-grown worms will have migrated to the intestine) by administration of anthelminthic therapy. Strongyloides infection should be ruled out prior to corticosteroid administration as the latter can induce Strongyloides hyperinfection syndrome. The benzimidazoles (mebendazole [Vermox], albendazole [Albenza],[1]

levamisole[2]) exhibit excellent activity against *Ascaris.* Ivermectin (Stromectol)[1] and nitazoxanide[1] are suggested as reasonable alternatives. Doses and other options are listed in Table 2. Pregnant women should be treated with pyrantel pamoate (PinAway)[1] as albendazole and mebendazole carry a pregnancy class B label. Pyrantel pamoate is a depolarizing neuromuscular blocking agent that causes paralysis in helminths preventing them from invading the intestinal wall, eventually resulting in their natural expulsion for the intestinal lumen. Because no consistent teratogenic effects have been demonstrated with albendazole use in late pregnancy, the World Health Organization (WHO) has allowed the use of albendazole to treat mass infections in the second and third trimesters.

Sanitary conditions that allow for proper management of human feces are crucial in control and prevention of *Ascaris* infection; boiling water kills the eggs.

Whipworm (Trichuris)

Trichuris trichiura has become recognized in recent years as a worldwide pathogen and is frequently found as a coinfection with *A. lumbricoides* as they share a similar scope and environment conditions. Almost 90% of individuals from endemic regions are infected. Sanitary conditions that predispose to ingestion of food and water contaminated with human feces place people at risk for infection.

The adult organism is a small worm about 4 cm in length with a unique whip-like structure that allows its thin tail to become embedded in colonic crypts. Infection is acquired by ingesting *Trichuris* eggs that have undergone embryonation in the soil for 2 to 4 weeks after excretion from a previous host. Larvae emerge from eggs in the intestine and migrate into crypts, where they begin to mature. Egg production begins approximately 3 months later.

Most persons with whipworm carry few worms (approximately 20) and are asymptomatic. As with many other intestinal parasites, children are at greater risk for symptomatic infection, which can cause failure to thrive, anemia, clubbing, inflammatory colitis, and rectal prolapse. Adults with a high worm burden can also experience inflammatory colitis characterized by frequent—often bloody—diarrhea and tenesmus. Infection has been shown to result in production of tumor necrosis factor (TNF)-α by lamina propria cells in the colon, which can contribute to poor appetite and wasting that can be seen with significant infection.

Diagnosis is made by standard stool microscopy without a need to concentrate stool because large numbers of eggs are excreted. Whipworm eggs have a characteristic barrel shape with mucous (hyaline) plugs at either end. Worms can also be seen on colonoscopy, or they can be visualized grossly in cases of rectal prolapse. PCR tests are now available with improved but variable sensitivity for species identification. Peripheral eosinophilia may be seen.

Treatment of symptomatic infections can be accomplished with mebendazole (Vermox), albendazole (Albenza),[1] or ivermectin (Stromectal)[1]; see Table 2 for details.

Hookworm

Like other helminthic infections, hookworm affects a substantial portion of the world's population, particularly in rural subtropical and tropical communities where human feces are used as a component of fertilizer. Infection results primarily from parasite penetration into the skin; therefore persons with an agrarian lifestyle and significant soil contact are at greatest risk.

Two species are responsible for the majority of human hookworm: *Necator americanus* and *Ancylostoma duodenale.* *N. americanus* is smaller and a less aggressive pathogen with a longer life span than *A. duodenale.* Both parasites are found in warm climates throughout the world; *A. duodenale* exists in smaller pockets in Mediterranean countries, Iran, India, Pakistan, and the Far East, whereas *N. americanus* is widely distributed

---

[1]Not FDA approved for this indication.

---

[1]Not FDA approved for this indication.
[2]Not available in the United States.

CLINICAL SITUATION	DRUG	ADULT DOSE	PEDIATRIC DOSE	COMMENTS
Anisakiasis				
Anisaka spp. or *Pseudoterranova decipiens*	No recommended medical therapy	—	—	Successful treatment of a patient with Anisakiasis with albendazole[1] has been reported.
	Surgical or endoscopic removal of worm			
Ascariasis				
Ascaris lumbricoides	Albendazole (Albenza)[1,*] or	400 mg once	400 mg PO once	
	Mebendazole[†] (Vermox) or	100 mg bid × 3 days or 500 mg once	100 mg bid × 3 days or 500 mg once	
	Ivermectin[1,†] (Stromectol)	150–200 µg/kg once	150–200 µg/kg once	In heavy infection, therapy may be given for 3 days.
Enterobiasis (Pinworm)				
Enterobius vermicularis	Mebendazole[†] or	100 mg once, repeat in 2 weeks	100 mg once, repeat in 2 weeks	Because all family members are usually infected, treatment of the entire household is recommended.
	Albendazole[1,*] or	400 mg once, repeat in 2 weeks	400 mg once, repeat in 2 weeks	
	Pyrantel pamoate[‡]	11 mg/kg base (max 1 g) once; repeat in 2 weeks	11 mg/kg base (max 1 g) once; repeat in 2 weeks	
Hookworm				
Ancylostoma duodenale, Necator americanus	Albendazole[1,*] or	400 mg once	400 mg once	
	Mebendazole or	100 mg bid × 3 days or 500 mg once	100 mg bid × 3 days or 500 mg once	
	Pyrantel pamoate[‡,1]	11 mg/kg (max 1 g) × 3 days	11 mg/kg (max 1 g) × 3 days	
Schistosomiasis				
Schistosoma haematobium, Schistosoma mansoni	Praziquantel[§] or	40 mg/kg/day in 2 doses × 1 day	40 mg/kg/d in 2 doses × 1 day	
S. mansoni only	Oxamniquine[1, 2]	15 mg/kg once	20 mg/kg/day in 2 doses × 1 day	Praziquantel is first-line, but oxamniquine may be effective in some patients in whom praziquantel is less effective. Contraindicated in pregnancy
Schistosoma japonicum, Schistosoma mekongi	Praziquantel[§]	60 mg/kg/day in 2 or 3 doses × 1 day	60 mg/kg/day in 3 doses × 1 day	
Strongyloidiasis				
Strongyloides stercoralis	Recommended: Ivermectin[†]	200 µg/kg/day × 2 days	200 µg/kg/day × 2 days	In immunocompromised patients or in patients with disseminated disease, it may be necessary to prolong or repeat therapy or use other agents. Veterinary parenteral and enema formulations of ivermectin are used in severely ill patients unable to take oral medications.
	Alternative: Albendazole[1,*]	400 mg bid × 7 days	400 mg bid × 7 days	
Tapeworm				
Taenia solium (intestinal disease), *Taenia saginata, Diphyllobothrium latum*	Praziquantel[1] or	—	—	

Continued

CLINICAL SITUATION	DRUG	ADULT DOSE	PEDIATRIC DOSE	COMMENTS
	Niclosamide[¶, 2]	2 g once	50 mg/kg once	Available in the United States only from the manufacturer
Trichurasis (Whipworm)				
Trichuris trichiura	Recommended:			
	Mebendazole	100 mg bid × 3 days or 500 mg once	100 mg bid × 3 days or 500 mg once	
	Alternatives:			
	Albendazole[1,*] or	400 mg daily × 3 days	400 mg daily × 3 days	
	Ivermectin[†,1]	200 µg/kg daily × 3 days	200 µg/kg daily × 3 days	

[1]Not FDA approved for this indication.
[2]Not available in the United States.
*Should be taken with a fatty meal.
[†]Safety of Ivermectin in young children (<15 kg) and pregnant women not yet established. Ivermectin should be taken on an empty stomach with water.
[‡]Limited availability; can be mixed with juice or water to improve palatability.
[§]Should be taken with liquids during a meal.
[∥]Limited or no availability in the United States.
[¶]Available in the United States only from the manufacturer. Must be chewed or crushed thoroughly and swallowed with a small amount of water. Limited or no availability in the United States.
Adapted from World Health Organization: Drugs for parasitic infections. *Med Lett Drug Ther* 8 (Suppl.), 2010.

throughout impoverished rural areas of the tropics in the Americas, Asia, and Africa. *Ancylostoma ceylanicum,* a hookworm of dogs and cats, has been identified as one of the human zoonotic infections in Southeast Asia, tropical Australia, and Melanesian Pacific Islands. *Ancylostoma braziliense,* a canine intestinal pathogen, causes cutaneous larval migrans in humans because the pathogen cannot penetrate the human dermis.

Hookworms are small helminths, between 0.5 and 1 cm in length. Infection results from larval penetration of the skin on contact with contaminated soil. An intensely pruritic, erythematous, papulovesicular rash called *ground itch* can develop at the site of entry. Parasites then enter the venous or lymphatic circulation and travel to the lungs, at which point an urticarial rash with cough can develop. The larvae are swallowed and migrate to the small intestine, where they attach to the bowel wall with teeth or biting plates and take a continuous blood meal by sucking with strong esophageal muscles. As the larvae lodge in the small intestine, peripheral eosinophilia peaks, and gastrointestinal discomfort with or without diarrhea can result. Large oral ingestion of *A. duodenale* can cause Wakana syndrome, characterized by cough, shortness of breath, nausea, vomiting, and eosinophilia. The most important clinical manifestation of hookworm infection is iron-deficiency anemia, which can be mild or severe and may be accompanied by malabsorption of protein in hosts with heavy burden of disease. Infants and pregnant women can become extremely ill or even die as a result of the anemia.

Hookworm may be difficult to diagnose because light infections often do not produce enough eggs to be readily seen on stool examination; stool should therefore be concentrated if infection is suspected. Eggs do not appear in stool until approximately 2 months after dermal penetration of *N. americanus* and up to 38 weeks from cutaneous entry of *A. duodenale;* hence patients with pulmonary complaints will not yet have a positive stool examination. Multiplex PCR assays that detect *A. lumbricoides, T. trichiura,* and hookworm have higher sensitivity than direct microscopy. However, these are not as widely available yet.

Hookworm infection can be eradicated with benzimidazole antihelminthics; see Table 2 for details. Prevention of hookworm infection, as with other parasites, lies in improved sanitary conditions; wearing shoes is especially important because the majority of infections are acquired through the skin. Mass anthelminthic treatment campaigns have shown some efficacy in reducing disease in children; however, reinfection and concern for development of resistance continue to present significant challenges. Candidate vaccines are currently under investigation.

Toxocara

Human infection is most commonly from a dog ascarid, *Toxocara canis,* and rarely from the cat ascarid, *Toxocara cati.* Humans are infected with embryonated eggs shed by definite host (dogs, cats) in contaminated soil or food, and direct contact with definite hosts is usually not a classical mode of transmission. Eggs then hatch into larvae that penetrate the intestinal wall to enter the circulation and embed in various tissues leading to visceral larva migrans (lungs, liver, heart, muscle, brain) and ocular larva migrans (eyes). Visceral larva migrans (VLM) usually present as hepatitis (nodular lesions) and pneumonitis (typically with bilateral peribronchial infiltration). Pericarditis, myocarditis, Loeffler endocarditis, heart failure, cardiac tamponade, eosinophilic meningo-encephalitis, cerebral vasculitis, and myelitis have been rarely reported. Ocular larva migrans (OLM) results from granulomatous inflammatory response to embedded larva typically presenting as a whitish elevated granuloma but red eye from scleritis or uveitis. Visual impairment leading to blindness from retinal detachment are more serious complications.

ELISA IgG serology in the appropriate clinical setting is the most commonly used diagnostic modality but cannot differentiate active from past infections. Sensitivity of ELISA for OLM is lower than that for VLM. PCR testing is commercially not available yet. Definite diagnosis is established with biopsy that is rarely indicated.

Treatment of choice is albendazole (Albenza),[1] which is preferred over mebendazole (Vermox),[1] especially in neurologic disease and OLM as the latter does not cross the blood–brain barrier. Antiinflammatory corticosteroids are used as adjunctive therapy for cardiac, neurologic, and severe vision-threatening illness.

Strongyloides

Strongyloides stercoralis is a global pathogen that is estimated to affect as many as 100 million people, mostly in tropical regions of the world. In recent years, it has become more commonly recognized in the United States among immigrants as a cause of chronic eosinophilia, as well as symptomatic infection.

Strongyloides infection results when filariform larvae dwelling in fecally contaminated soil penetrate the skin or mucous membranes of a susceptible host. Larvae move to the lungs and subsequently to the trachea, where they are coughed up and swallowed. Females, about 2 cm in length, lodge in the lamina propria

[1]Not FDA approved for this indication.

of the duodenum and proximal jejunum where they begin to oviposit. Rhabditiform larvae (noninfectious form) emerge from these eggs and either transform into infectious filariform larvae (infectious form) that can repenetrate the intestinal wall (autoinfection; unique to *S. stercolaris* among other helminths) or are passed into the feces, at which point they can begin a free-living cycle and reproduce sexually or can molt directly into an infectious form ready to enter a subsequent susceptible host.

Persons infected with *Strongyloides* are typically asymptomatic. Those who have symptoms might report abdominal discomfort, diarrhea alternating with constipation, or, rarely, blood-tinged stool. Severe intestinal infections can occur and are manifest by chronic watery or mucousy diarrhea. In such cases, colonoscopy reveals excessive bowel wall thickening and copious secretions or edema (catarrhal enteritis or edematous enteritis). Parasite migration through the dermis can manifest as pathognomonic serpiginous, erythematous, and pruritic patches along the buttocks, perineum, and thighs, known as larvae currens ("running" larvae).

Strongyloides appear to attain a balanced state in their host, with similar numbers of adult worms throughout the many years of infection. During periods of host immunocompromise, in particular in patients taking corticosteroids, *Strongyloides* can enter into a state of rapid autoinfection and rampant reproduction called *hyperinfection syndrome,* which results in devastating illness. Persons with HIV infection do not seem to be at particular risk for symptomatic disease or hyperinfection, but hyperinfection has been linked to human T-lymphotropic virus (HTLV)-1 infection. *Strongyloides* has also caused hyperinfection in organ transplant patients whose donor had been infected asymptomatically with the parasite. Although it has long been thought that steroid-induced immune compromise was the major trigger for hyperinfection, growing evidence suggests that steroids themselves may be the culprit by directly inducing the accelerated life cycle in the parasite.

The hyperinfection syndrome is characterized by systemic illness with fever, cough, hypoxia, patchy or diffuse pulmonary infiltrates with alveolar microhemorrhages, and dermatitis; it can include myocarditis, hepatitis, splenic abscess, meningitis and cerebral abscess, and endocrine organ involvement. Larvae migrating out of the intestines can drag bacteria with them, resulting in gram-negative or polymicrobial sepsis. The prognosis of *Strongyloides* hyperinfection syndrome is grave even with highly effective anthelminthic treatment given the diffuse nature of this disease. However, earlier recognition and intensive supportive care can result in cure.

Diagnosis of uncomplicated *Strongyloides* infection in endemic areas can be challenging because few larvae are passed in stool, and numerous examinations may be necessary to detect them. ELISA IgG serologies to filariform larvae are highly sensitive, but positive results cannot distinguish between active and past infections. Moreover, serologies can be falsely negative in immunocompromised hosts. It is, however, the test of choice for persons who have migrated to nonendemic areas, and all persons in this setting should be treated. Ivermectin is the treatment of choice; albendazole[1] has some activity against *S. stercoralis* and can be tried as an alternative; see Table 2 for dosing. During the first days of treatment, patients can experience intense dermal pruritis as parasites die. Eosinophilia and positive ELISA can persist for months even after effective therapy.

Enterobius

Human pinworm infection, caused by the thread-like nematode *Enterobius vermicularis,* is found throughout the world and continues to be diagnosed commonly in the United States, especially in children aged 5 to 10 years. It is the most common helminthic infection in the United States and Europe. Its persistence is likely related to the fact that pinworm does not require a period of maturation outside the human body, and autoinfection or

transmission by very close contact sustains the parasite within communities. *E. vermicularis* is at maximum 1-cm long with a tapered tail and dwells in the cecum, appendix, and adjacent colon. At night, female worms travel to the anus and lay small (25–50 μm), double-walled oval eggs in the perianal skin. Within 6 hours, the eggs embryonate within their capsule and are infectious. In scratching the perianal area and subsequently bringing his or her hand to the mouth, the host ingests the embryos, which then hatch in the bowel about 2 months later and continue the cycle of infection. Embryonated eggs can also attach to bedclothes, thereby placing other household members with close contact at risk for infection. In family groups, infection is associated with close living quarters, poor hand washing, and infrequent washing of clothes and sheets. It can also be prevalent among institutionalized persons.

Infection is often asymptomatic, but it can cause perianal itching, which helps to facilitate persistent infection by encouraging frequent touching of the perianal area. Rarely, worms migrate into ectopic foci and produce painful genitourinary tract disease with granulomatous inflammation; pinworm infection rarely results in pain that mimics acute appendicitis.

Pinworm infestation is best diagnosed by the classic Scotch tape test, which involves placing and immediately removing a piece of sticky tape firmly across the perianal area early in the morning when the eggs have been deposited. The tape can then be brought into a physician's office or laboratory, where it is placed sticky-side down for microscopic examination to detect the eggs. Sensitivity can be increased by examining at least three specimens. Eggs are small (25 x 50 μm) with a characteristic "bean-shaped" appearance. It is also sometimes possible to see the white small female worms directly on the perianal region, although they are so small (8–13 mm in length) that they may easily be mistaken for residual bits of toilet paper. Although *E. vermicularis* is susceptible to standard albendazole[1] or mebendazole (see Table 2), pyrantel pamoate (Pin-Away, OTC) is most frequently used in the United States as it is cheap and effective. All household contacts should be empirically treated with the same regimen to avoid reintroducing infection from family members who may be asymptomatically carrying the parasite. Careful laundering of all bedclothes is recommended as well.

Anisakiasis

Anisakiasis is a descriptive term for human infection with parasites of two distinct genera: *Anisakis* and *Pseudoterranova.* Humans are incidental hosts for these roundworms that inhabit multiple species of fish and other marine animals (tuna, mackerel, hake, cod, sardines, and cephalopods) as intermediate hosts, and marine mammals such as whales, seals, sea lions, and walruses as final hosts. Humans acquire the parasite in its larval stage by eating undercooked or raw fish (e.g., sushi, ceviche), and therefore the condition predominates in cultures where uncooked fish is consumed. Cases are most commonly reported from Japan but are seen throughout the world in other coastal nations and among restaurateurs.

On consumption of fish with *Anisakis* larvae embedded in its musculature, humans can experience immediate symptoms in the form of itching or burning in the throat, which can provoke coughing that expels the parasite. If the parasite is swallowed, the larva attempts to embed in the gastric musculature at the pylorus. This can produce acute, short-lived epigastric abdominal pain and possibly immediate vomiting, at which point the parasite might again be ejected. If the larva does manage to penetrate gastric tissue, it dies because it is incapable of further tissue invasion in humans. An intense inflammatory response to the dead pathogen can then result, with gastric pain, nausea, and occasionally diarrhea with blood or mucus if a gastric ulcerative lesion has resulted. Eosinophilic enterocolitis, ileitis, appendicitis, and focal peritonitis and abscess formation from

[1]Not FDA approved for this indication.

[1]Not FDA approved for this indication.

penetration of larva into the peritoneum are also rarely reported. Bronchosconstriction, angioedema, and anaphylaxis have been described mimicking seafood allergy. *Pseudoterranova* appears to cause milder symptoms and less tissue invasion, and the worm might simply be vomited several days after initial ingestion and presented to a physician, often by an alarmed patient. Because the vast majority of infections are caused by a single organism, vomiting of the parasite results in a definitive cure and patients can be reassured. Diagnosis in patients with ongoing symptoms related to an embedded parasite is ultimately endoscopic. Effective cure results on endoscopic or surgical removal of the worm. Albendazole[1] as an effective therapy is reported; however, data is limited.

Trematodes
Schistosoma

Schistosomes are freshwater pathogens with areas of endemicity in Africa, South America, Southeast Asia, and parts of the Middle East. These small trematodes cause varied, often chronic infections that can carry significant morbidity, although some species cannot invade beyond the dermis in humans and result strictly in cercarial dermatitis or swimmer's itch. There are five species of schistosomes known to cause disease in humans: *Schistosoma haematobium,* found through much of Africa and parts of the Middle East; *Schistosoma mansoni,* also native to Africa and the Middle East as well as Latin America; *Schistosoma japonicum,* present in China, Southeast Asia, and the Philippines; *Schistosoma mekongi,* found only in the Mekong River basin in Laos and Cambodia; and *Schistosoma intercalatum,* endemic only in West Africa.

All persons who come in contact with schistosomes are at risk for infection, even with brief exposure to fecally contaminated freshwater in which the intermediate hosts of the pathogen (snails) reside. Frequency and degree of infection tend to be highest in children in endemic areas and then level off in the early teenage years, likely secondary to level of environmental exposure and possibly to host immunity. *S. haematobium* causes disease in the genitourinary system; the others cause intestinal, hepatic, and sometimes pulmonary diseases.

Infection is acquired rapidly on contact with freshwater (including brief swims or by repeated splashing, as can occur during river rafting), when free-living fork-tailed schistosomal larvae (cercariae) penetrate human skin and lose their tail. These schistosomulae can cause intense itching and a papulovesicular, pruritic rash at the site of penetration, swimmer's itch. Invasive schistosomulae then enter the venous bloodstream and reach the liver through portal venules, where they mature into adults. Adult worms then migrate against the portal venous flow to the mesenteric venules of the gut (*S. mansoni, S. japonicum, S. intercalatum, S. mekongi*) and vesical venous plexus (*S. hematobium*) where male and female forms mate for life. Females begin to oviposit, and the resultant inflammatory response to the eggs can cause either acute illness or chronic fibrosis and granulomatous inflammation of the tissues in which they reside.

Acute illness, called *Katayama fever,* is more common among hosts who have not been previously exposed to the organism and can be quite severe, even fatal. Katayama fever begins 3 to 8 weeks after infection, with acute onset of fever, chills, myalgias, cough, urticaria, angioedema, abdominal pain, hepatomegaly, and lymphadenopathy. Eggs might not yet be present in the stool at the time of diagnosis. Chronic schistosomiasis is a slowly progressive illness presenting chiefly with intermittent abdominal pain, diarrhea, and anorexia. Colonic ulceration with gastrointestinal bleeding and iron-deficiency anemia from huge parasitic burden has been described. Hepatosplenic schistosomiasis can be caused by granulomatous inflammation surrounding the eggs eventually leading to periportal fibrosis (Symmers' pipestem fibrosis), portal hypertension, and splenomegaly. Portal hypertension can then lead to portosystemic collateral vessel

development and deposition of eggs in the pulmonary vasculature. Granulomatous inflammation in the pulmonary tissues eventually causes endarteritis, fibrosis, pulmonary hypertension, and cor pulmonale. *S. haematobium* infection can manifest as gross or microscopic hematuria, irritative urinary symptoms, and chronic bacterial urinary tract infections; ultimately ureteral fibrosis, hydronephrosis, and granulomatous genital lesions also can ensue. Neuroschistosomiasis can cause both myelopathy and intracerebral lesions and can have varied presentation including seizures, focal deficits, encephalopathy, and rapidly progressive transverse myelitis.

Diagnosis of schistosomiasis is by observation of eggs in stool (intestinal disease), urine (urinary tract disease), or biopsy specimens, or by serum antibody testing. Concentration of stool may be necessary to detect the pathogen. The eggs of the three most common species of schistosomes can be readily identified microscopically: *S. haematobium* has an inferior spine, *S. mansoni* an inferolateral spine, and *S. japonicum* lacks a spine. Quantification of eggs is important as the parasite burden is proportional to the risk of complications and is usually reported as light (up to 100 eggs/gram), moderate (100–400 eggs/gram), and severe (>400 eggs/gram) in stool specimens. Eosinophilia is a hallmark of chronic infection and is a common cause of asymptomatic eosinophilia among immigrants from endemic regions of the world. Serology is useful particularly in returned travelers with low parasite burden; however, it can be negative in early infection as it takes 6 to 12 weeks after exposure to become positive. It is highly specific but cannot distinguish acute, chronic, or cleared infection. Antigen testing targeting specific schistosomal glycoproteins, circulating cathodic antigen (CCA, genus specific), and circulating anodic antigen (CAA, more specific to *S. mansoni*) is more sensitive than microscopy and can lead to rapid diagnosis particularly in specimens with low parasite burden. Highly sensitive PCR assays have been developed to be used on blood, stool, and urine specimens; however, these are not as widely available. Histopathology is better than microscopy particularly in ectopic manifestations but is usually not required.

All patients with schistosomiasis should be treated, and those with chronic manifestations might experience significant regression of even late-stage organ-specific disease. Treatment of choice is praziquantel (Biltricide); see Table 2 for details.

Prevention of schistosomiasis involves improving access to treated water and exploration of avenues to eliminate the intermediate snail hosts. Host immunity does appear to occur, and efforts are underway to better understand and induce such immunity in the form of a vaccine.

Cestodes
Taenia

Human tapeworm infection has long been implicated in North American oral folklore as a cause of insatiable appetite and excessive weight loss. In reality, despite their impressive size of up to 12 meters, tapeworm infection tends to be minimally symptomatic.

Taenia solium, pork tapeworm, and *Taenia saginata,* beef tapeworm, are the two most common flatworm infections of humans (humans are the only definitive hosts) worldwide and occur in any setting in which raw or undercooked meat is served and cattle and pigs have access to feed contaminated with human feces. *T. saginata* is still found in areas of North America and Europe, as well as in Central and South America and Africa; *T. solium* is common throughout Mexico, Central and South America, Africa, China, and the Indian subcontinent. Although humans are the definitive hosts for both parasites, *T. solium* is best known for its pathogenicity in the form of cysticercosis. Cysticercosis is not an intestinal parasitic infection.

Domesticated animals acquire infection on ingestion of eggs or gravid proglottids excreted by humans; the eggs mature in their musculature and develop a scolex. When humans consume infected meat, the scolex attaches in the small intestine, and the adult tapeworm develops over approximately 2 months. Adult tapeworms are made up of hundreds to thousands of gravid proglottids and can live for up to 25 years with intermittent shedding in the stool.

Symptoms tend to be mild or absent but can include nausea, abdominal pain, loose stools, anal pruritus, and occasionally weakness or increased appetite, especially in children. Serious illness rarely results when a tapeworm proglottids becomes lodged in the appendix, lodged in biliary or pancreatic ducts, or are coughed up and aspirated. Some patients come to medical attention when the worm is noted emerging from the anus or on extrusion of proglottids in the stool.

Diagnosis of taeniasis can be made on visualizing the round eggs with hooks and double wall with characteristic striations. However, the species cannot be determined unless their proglottids are examined (*T. saginatum* has 12 or more uterine branches, whereas *T. solium* has <10). Since the eggs and proglottids are shed intermittently, the sensitivity of microscopy is poor. Serum antibody and antigen tests, as well as stool PCR, have been developed for diagnosis but are not widely used in clinical practice. Eosinophilia and elevated IgE levels may be present. Single-dose praziquantel[1] (see Table 2) is curative in almost all cases, but infectious eggs can still be released in the feces for some time after worm eradication; ingestion of these could result in the subsequent development of cysticercosis, so patients should be counseled to avoid fecal–oral contact.

Proper cooking of meat is the mainstay of prevention; disposal of human waste away from animals would also be effective in interrupting the life cycle.

Diphyllobothrium

Diphyllobothrium latum (fish tapeworm) is the longest parasite known to infect humans (10–12 m). It is found in freshwater lakes in areas of the Americas, Northern Europe, Africa, China, and Japan and has a complex life cycle involving two intermediate hosts: crustaceans and small fish. Humans and other fish-eating mammals are the definitive hosts and acquire the infection on ingestion of raw fish or roe.

Eggs and proglottids are intermittently shed in human stool that embryonate in the water. Coracidiae hatch from the eggs and are ingested by small crustaceans, the first intermediate hosts. Coracidia mature into procercoid larvae in the crustaceans that are then ingested by the small freshwater fish (the second intermediate host). Procercoid larvae develop into plerocercoid larvae (sparganum) that are then passed on to the large predator fish (later intermediate host), which is then consumed by humans (definitive host). Sparganum develops into the adult worm inside the human intestine.

The mature adult tapeworm attaches within the small intestine, and hosts are usually asymptomatic. Infected persons might complain of increased appetite, nausea, or abdominal discomfort. Many patients present after the passage of portions of the tapeworm in stool, as with taeniasis. In others, diagnosis is incidental on the stool examination done for other purposes or during screening colonoscopy. As with other worms, the parasite occasionally migrates into biliary ducts or causes intestinal obstruction. Attachment of the parasite higher in the intestine competes the host for vitamin B12 absorption and can result in vitamin B12 deficiency (pernicious anemia).

Diagnosis is made either by seeing eggs with an operculum (lid-like opening) in an unconcentrated stool or by encountering the adult worm. Proglottids can be differentiated from those in taeniasis by the presence of rosette-shaped uterus. Eosinophilia is present in a minority of cases. Treatment with praziquantel[1] is curative; see Table 2. Vitamin B12 supplementation is necessary in cases of severe or symptomatic deficiency, but it will not recur once the tapeworm is eliminated. Prevention involves not ingesting undercooked fish.

---

[1]Not FDA approved for this indication.

References

Abubakar I, Aliyu SH, Hunter PR, Usman NK: Prevention and treatment of cryptosporidiosis in immunocompromised patients, *Cochrane Database Syst Rev* (1), CD004932.

Bethony J, Brooker S, Albonico M, et al: Soil-transmitted helminth infections: ascariasis, trichuriasis, and hookworm, *Lancet* 367(9521):1521–1532, 2006.

Boggild A, Yohanna S, Keystone J, Kain K: Prospective analysis of parasitic infections in Canadian travelers and immigrants, *J Travel Med* 13:138–144, 2006.

Boulware DR, Stauffer WM, Hendel-Paterson RR, et al: Maltreatment of strongyloides infection: case series and worldwide physicians-in-training survey, *Am J Med* 120:545.e1–545.e8, 2007.

Concha R, Hartington Jr W, Rogers AI: Intestinal strongyloidiasis: recognition, management, and determinants of outcome, *J Clin Gastroenterol* 39(3):203–211, 2005.

Drugs for parasitic infections, *Treat Guidel Med Lett* 11:e1–e31, 2013.

Goodgame RW: Understanding intestinal spore-forming protozoa: Cryptosporidia, microsporidia, isospora, and cyclospora, *Ann Intern Med* 124(4):429–441, 1996.

Guerrant R, Walker D, Weller P, editors: *Tropical infectious diseases: Principles, pathogens, and practice*, Philadelphia, 1999, Churchill Livingstone.

Huang DB, White AC: An updated review on Cryptosporidium and Giardia, *Gastroenterol Clin North Am* 35:291–314, 2006.

Mandell G, Bennett J, Dolin R, editors: *Mandell, Douglas and Bennett's Principles and practice of infectious diseases*, ed 5, Philadelphia, 2005, Churchill Livingstone.

Pardo J, Carranza C, Muro A, et al: Helminth-related eosinophilia in African immigrants, Gran Canaria, *Emerg Infect Dis* 12(10):1587–1589, 2006.

Stark D, Beebe N, Marriott D, et al: Dientamoebiasis: clinical importance and recent advances, *Trends Parasitol* 22(2):92–96, 2006.

IRRITABLE BOWEL SYNDROME

Method of
Arnold Wald, MD

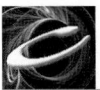

CURRENT DIAGNOSIS

- Fulfilling diagnostic criteria for irritable bowel syndrome (IBS) using Manning or Rome criteria is mandatory but not sufficient, as some organic diseases may also meet these criteria.
- Against the diagnosis of IBS is new onset in old age, a steady progressive course, frequent awakening by abdominal pain or urge to defecate, and weight loss not caused by depression.
- The diagnostic approach to patients with IBS symptoms with no "alarm signs" includes a complete blood count, stool testing for occult blood or calprotectin, C-reactive protein and colonoscopy if patient is age >50 years, has positive stool or blood test results as above, or if there is a poor response to treatment.
- After a diagnosis of IBS is established with confidence, repeated testing is counterproductive unless there is a distinct change in clinical symptoms or new alarm signs develop.

CURRENT THERAPY

- A robust patient–health care provider relationship is perhaps the most important determinant of outcome and reduced health care use in patients with IBS.
- There is significant support for the use of a low-FODMAP (fermentable oligo-, di-, and monosaccharides and polyols) diet in patients with IBS. Gluten restriction is part of this diet and will cover those patients who believe that they are gluten intolerant in the absence of celiac disease.
- Pharmacologic agents can be divided into those for IBS-C or IBS-D or in any patient with IBS to ameliorate abdominal pain. The evidence to support these agents varies in quality and strength, and none is effective in the majority of patients who have been tested.
- Cognitive behavioral therapy (CBT) can be very effective in IBS with unrelenting symptoms but may also be effective for any patient with IBS who exhibits poor stress management.

Introduction and Definitions

Irritable bowel syndrome (IBS) is a chronic functional disorder of the gastrointestinal tract characterized by chronic abdominal pain and altered bowel habits in the absence of an organic disease. In the absence of a biologic disease marker, the diagnosis has traditionally been based on a cluster of symptoms. The earliest was the so-called "Manning criteria," which was based on the presence of three or more characteristic symptoms (Table 1).

Subsequently, there have been various iterations of IBS criteria created by the Rome study groups, which are currently used for research purposes (see Table 1). When evaluating the relevant literature for IBS, it is important to note that various studies have used different criteria, which may result in variable data concerning prevalence and economic costs considerations.

From a clinical standpoint, subtypes of IBS have been defined as follows:

- **IBS with predominant constipation (IBS-C):** Patient reports that abnormal bowel movements are usually constipation (types 1 and 2 in the Bristol Stool Form Scale; BSFS; https://en.wikipedia.org/wiki/Bristol_stool_scale)
- **IBS with predominant diarrhea (IBS-D):** Patient reports that abnormal bowel movements are usually diarrhea (types 6 and 7 in the BSFS)
- **IBS with mixed bowel habits (IBS-M):** Patient reports that abnormal bowel movements are usually both constipation and diarrhea (more than one-fourth of all the abnormal bowel movements are constipation and more than one-fourth are diarrhea) using the BSFS
- **Unclassified IBS (IBS-U):** Patients who meet diagnostic criteria for IBS but cannot be accurately categorized into one of the other three subtypes

Epidemiology of IBS

Prevalence

There have been numerous surveys concerning the prevalence of IBS in the community. Most of these studies have used accepted diagnostic criteria, and some have used more than one definition within the same population. In one meta-analysis, 23 studies used the Manning criteria, 24 used Rome I criteria, 36 used Rome II criteria, and 5 used Rome III criteria. The prevalence ranged from 5% to 10% (USA, China) to 15% to 20% (Canada, Brazil, Russia). There was little or no data from Africa, Central America, and large parts of South America.

Most studies did not report the predominant stool pattern in IBS. Of the nine that included IBS-U subtypes as well, there was an even distribution, ranging from 22% to 24% mean prevalence for each of the four subgroups. In general, the pooled prevalence was higher in women than in men (14%; range 11%–16% vs. 9%; range 7.3%–10.5%), with significant heterogeneity between studies. There appeared to be no relationship between socioeconomic status in the four studies that reported it and no strong influence of age as well.

It is important to note that the meta-analysis was restricted to studies based on the general population and excluded those based on convenience samples. This makes the data more generalizable to community individuals with IBS.

Causality—a biopsychsocial conceptual model for IBS

The ability to study causality in a disorder with no biologic disease markers is fraught with difficulties. This is certainly the case with IBS as a representative of functional gastrointestinal disorders. Many hypotheses have been advanced and found wanting. The current (and in my opinion most relevant) conceptual model is the biopsychosocial construct, as shown in Figure 1.

Impact on Population Health

Although there is no mortality associated with IBS, symptoms are long lasting, and there are no curative therapies available. As a chronic illness, the economic impact of this disorder is considerable.

In a 2015 survey conducted by the American Gastroenterological Association, IBS patients reported that their symptoms interfered with work productivity on an average of 9 days per month and missed work on average of 2 days per month. Indirect costs (i.e., loss of work and reduced productivity) have been estimated to be up to $20 billion annually in the United States, with an estimated annual cost per patient of $9933 (in 2012 US dollars).

In a study of indirect costs, impairment experienced at work (presenteeism) accounted for approximately 75% of the total annual indirect costs for respondents with IBS, far in excess of absenteeism from work. Compared with control subjects, IBS respondents missed significantly more work (5.1% vs. 2.9%), experienced higher levels of presenteeism (17.9% vs. 11.3%), and had greater overall work productivity loss (20.7% vs. 13.2%) and higher daily activity impairment.

Direct Health Care Costs

It has been estimated that up to 25% of all visits to gastroenterologists in the United States were for IBS with additional others for other functional GI disorders. This accounted for 3.5 million visits to health care practitioners in 1991 and undoubtedly is much higher today. IBS patients made twice as many health care visits per year as did age-matched control subjects, and 78%

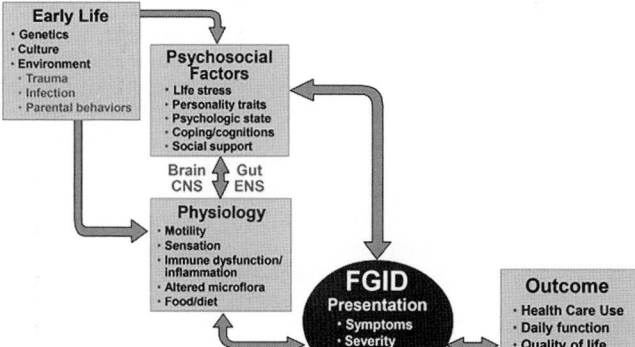

Figure 1 Predeterminants such as early life experiences, together with psychosocial factors, may interact with altered gut physiology via the brain-gut axis. This concept infers that these factors are bidirectional and mutually interactive and therefore influence both the clinical presentation of the disorder and the clinical outcomes. Among the physiological processes that may lead to GI symptoms are abnormal gut motility, visceral hypersensitivity, immune dysregulation, inflammation and barrier dysfunction, the intestinal microbiome, diet, and the brain-gut axis. No one factor alone accounts for the symptoms of IBS, and all must be considered in the management of affected patients. This becomes apparent when considering treatment approaches. *CNS*, Central nervous system; *ENS*, enteric nervous system; *FGID*, functional gastrointestinal disorder. (Reprinted with permission from Drossman DA. Functional gastrointestinal disorders: History, pathophysiology, clinical features and Rome IV. *Gastroenterology* 2016; 150:1262-79.)

TABLE 1	Criteria for IBS
Manning Criteria	**Rome IV Criteria**[*]
Looser stools with onset of pain	Recurrent abdominal pain on average at least 1 day per week in the last three months associated with two or more of the following:
More frequent bowel movements at onset of pain	
Visible distension	
Feeling of distension	Related to defecation
Mucus per rectum	
Feeling of incomplete emptying (often)	Associated with a change in stool frequency
Strict criteria > 3 of above	Associated with change in
Less strict criteria > 2 of above	form of stool (appearance)

[*]Criterion fulfilled for the last 3 months with onset of symptoms at least 6 months prior to diagnosis.

| **TABLE 2** | Diagnostic Approach to Patient With IBS Symptoms (No "Alarm Signs") |

Complete blood count
Screen for celiac disease
C-Reactive protein (inflammatory marker)
Fecal calprotectin/lactoferrin (indicators of inflammation)
Giardia (PCR or Ag)
Stool for O/P*
Colonoscopy with new onset symptoms over age 45 or positive calprotectin or lactoferrin

Rome IV (2016)

*Only if travel to high risk areas.

of the excess visits were for nongastrointestinal complaints. A subsequent analysis of this phenomenon suggests that comorbidity in IBS may be a consequence of the psychological trait for somatization, defined as the tendency to amplify the intensity and overinterpret the significance of any somatic sensation. This excess comorbidity is the primary determinant of excess health care costs associated with IBS, although it does not apply to all patients with IBS.

Recent attempts to identify factors of high users with IBS have been made, using a conceptual framework for accessing health care services, which holds that a decision to use health care is related to (1) predisposition to use services, (2) ability to use services, and (3) need for services. The important conclusion was that decisions to use health care are influenced not only by symptom-specific factors but by a variety of lifestyle and (most importantly) economic factors such as health insurance coverage.

Evaluation of Patients with Suspected IBS

The diagnosis of IBS should be made based on the clinical history, physical examination, minimal laboratory testing, and colonoscopy or other appropriate tests when clinically indicated. Fulfilling diagnostic criteria is, of course, mandatory but insufficient, because some organic diseases may also meet these criteria. The prevalence of organic disease is lowest in IBS-C and highest in IBS-D, followed by IBS-M; one of the most common considerations would be Crohn's disease. Against the diagnosis of IBS, include the new onset in old age, a steady progressive course, frequent awakening by pain or need to defecate, and weight loss not attributed to depression. Additional features that would increase concern about organic disease would include a positive family history of colorectal cancer or inflammatory bowel disease, rectal bleeding, and anemia associated with iron or vitamin B_{12} deficiency.

In the absence of "alarm signs," a consensus diagnostic approach to patients with IBS symptoms is listed in Table 2. This may vary according to clinical circumstances.

Tests of Unproven Value

A high prevalence of small intestinal bacterial overgrowth (SIBO) has been claimed by some centers, leading to the frequent utilization of either lactulose or glucose breath tests to measure hydrogen and methane in expired air. This hypothesis is based upon problematic methodology and frequently erroneous conclusions. The original studies have not been reproduced by other centers using similar and/or better techniques. This has led to the frequent use of expensive antibiotics, which can be effective in some patients with bloating and IBS, but not because these patients have SIBO. The use of lactulose breath testing should be discarded by all diagnostic centers, and glucose should be the preferred substrate but interpreted with caution. With rare exceptions, testing for food allergies

and food sensitivities should be discouraged as they have not been validated, are likely to lead to many false positive tests, and are expensive.

Lastly, after a diagnosis of IBS has been established with confidence, repeated testing is counterproductive unless there is a distinct change in clinical symptoms or new alarm signs develop. This is especially so if endoscopy procedures have already been performed.

Treatment of IBS

A validated standardized algorithm for the treatment of IBS does not exist. Treatment therefore depends on the type and severity of symptoms and the nature of associated psychosocial issues in an individual patient. A strong guiding principle is that a robust patient–health care provider relationship is an important determinant of outcome and reduction of health care use. Treatments may generally be divided into dietary and lifestyle modifications, pharmacologic agents, and behavioral therapies, all of which have been validated by randomized and controlled studies.

Dietary Modifications

Fiber supplements are widely recommended for IBS, but a meta-analysis of seven high-quality studies failed to find significant benefit, although some benefits might occur with soluble (psyllium) versus insoluble (bran) fiber in IBS-C. Unfortunately, fiber supplements may exacerbate symptoms such as abdominal bloating and discomfort.

Other dietary interventions such as gluten-free and low-FODMAP (fermentable oligo-, di-, and monosaccharides and polyols) diets have become increasingly popular. Several studies support the benefit of gluten-free diets in a subset of IBS patients in the absence of celiac disease. It remains uncertain whether the clinical benefits are a consequence of gluten withdrawal, elimination of other wheat proteins and highly fermentable short-chain fatty acids, or a placebo effect. Adding a gluten-free diet to patients who are already on a low-FODMAP diet offers no additional benefits.

There is accumulating evidence from prospective controlled studies that dietary FODMAP restriction is associated with significant symptom improvement in many patients with IBS (Table 3). It appears that restriction of both fructose and fructans is most beneficial. Significant symptom improvement was noted in IBS patients compared to several standard diets in Australia and the United States, and also a National Institute for Health and Care Excellence (NICE; England) diet.

Response to a low-FODMAP diet is usually assessed after 2 to 6 weeks. Responders are then asked to engage in a structured reintroduction of restricted foods to allow the individual to tailor his or her diet. It is optimal to involve a properly trained dietician or nutritionist oversee the care of these patients.

Pharmacologic Agents for IBS

Pharmacologic approaches to IBS may be divided into medications for IBS-C, patients with IBS-D, and for any patient with IBS in order to ameliorate abdominal pain (Table 4).

Most drugs work through different pathophysiological mechanisms. For example, for patients with IBS-C, linaclotide (Linzess), plecanatide (Trulance), and lubiprostone (Amitiza) increase intestinal chloride and water secretion to combat constipation, whereas PEG (polyethylene glycol 3350, Miralax)[1] does so through a hyperosmolar effect. For IBS-D, rifaximin (Xifaxan) is an antibiotic, loperamide (Imodium)[1] is a peripheral μ-opioid agonist, alosetron (Lotronex) works through the serotonin 3 receptor, and eluxadoline (Viberzi) has effects on all 3 opioid receptors in the gut (mu, kappa, and delta).

---

[1] Not FDA approved for this indication.

TABLE 3	Low-FODMAP Diet

AVOID OR REDUCE THESE FOODS			
FRUCTOSE	**LACTOSE**	**OLIGOS**	**POLYOLS**
Fruits: Apple, mango, pear, watermelon, juice, dried fruit	Milk: milk from cows/goats/sheep, custard, ice cream, yogurt, eggnog	Vegetables: Beets, broccoli, brussels sprouts, cabbage, fennel, garlic, onion, chicory root	Fruits: Apricot, avocado, blackberry, cherry, nectarine, peach, plum, prune, fig
Other: Asparagus, honey, high fructose corn syrup, molasses	Cheese: Soft, unripened cheese	Other: Barley, beans, chickpeas, couscous, inulin, lentils, pistachios, rye, soy milk, wheat (pasta, bread), veggie burgers	Vegetables: Cauliflower, corn, mushroom, sweet potato Sweeteners: Ending in "ol" (for example: xylitol, sorbitol), isomalt

TABLE 4	Pharmacologic Agents for IBS	
INDICATION	**DRUG**	**DOSE**
IBS-C	Linaclotide (Linzess) Plecanatide (Trulance) Lubiprostone (Amitiza) PEG-3350 (Miralax)[1] Tegaserod (Zelnorm)	72-290 µg/d[3] 3 mg/d 24 mcg bid[3] 6 mg bid
IBS-D	Rifaximin (Xifaxan) Alosetron (Lotronex)[#] Eluxadoline (Viberzi) Loperamide (Imodium)[1]	550 mg tid × 2 weeks 1 mg qd- bid 75-100 mg bid 2-16 mg/d
IBS-All	Peppermint oil[7] TCAs, i.e., Desipramine (Norpramin)[1]*	1–2 caps 20 min AC 10-100 mg/d (desipramine)

*Alternative TCAs: amitriptyline (Elavil)[1], imipramine (Tofranil)[1], nortriptyline (Pamelor)[1].

[#]Available only to physicians enrolled in the REMS Program for alosetron.

[1]Not FDA approved for this indication.

[3]Exceeds dosage recommended by the manufacturer.

[7]Available as dietary supplement.

Tricyclic agents (TCAs) presumably work via central neurochemical changes, and antispasmodics (dicyclomine [Bentyl], encapsulated oil of peppermint[7]) work largely through peripheral anticholinergic pathways. The large and diverse number of drugs are indicative of the lack of fundamental understanding of IBS. Moreover, few drugs are effective in the majority of IBS patients, and there is no more than a 10% to 15% improvement over placebo in most published studies.

The AGA guidelines used in previous chapters on IBS have been replaced by the recently published ACG guidelines, which incorporate assessment of recently introduced agents such as plecanatide (Trulance) and eluxadoline (Viberzi) and a re-assessment of tegaserod (Zelnorm), peppermint oil,[7] antispasmodics, and polyethylene glycol 3350 (PEG, MiraLax).[1]

Of the pharmacologic agents for IBS-C, linaclotide (Linzess) received a strong recommendation with high-quality evidence, lubiprostone (Amitiza) received a conditional recommendation on moderate-quality evidence, and PEG was given a conditional recommendation based on weak evidence. The first two agents showed modest benefit over placebo, whereas there are no data to support the use of PEG. For all three agents, adverse effects were relatively few, and diarrhea is perhaps the major side effect. Both linaclotide and lubiprostone are costly (as are eluxadoline and plecanatide) and may involve high out-of-pocket expenses for patients.

For IBS-D, both rifaximin (Xifaxan) and alosetron (Lotronex) received conditional recommendations based on moderate quality

[1]Not FDA approved for this indication.

evidence. The latter is approved by the FDA only for women in whom all other treatments have failed. There is a very small risk (approximately 1 case/1000 patient-years) for ischemic colitis with alosetron. Although loperamide (Imodium)[1] has very low-quality evidence to support its use, it can be very effective if used in a proactive fashion.

The case for TCAs and antispasmodics is based on low-quality evidence, but both agents can be very effective for abdominal pain and, in the case of TCAs, for reducing diarrhea in IBS patients.

Behavioral Therapy for IBS

For patients with unrelenting IBS symptoms, cognitive behavioral therapy (CBT) and gut-directed hypnosis have been found to be beneficial. Such therapies should be performed by experienced and well-trained behavioral specialists who are an integral part of the medical team that treats patients with functional GI disorders. The most robust data for efficacy is for CBT. One potential drawback is that these treatments are provider-intensive approaches, but recent studies suggest that CBT can be as effective when given in a shortened course as is the traditional method.

[7]Available as dietary supplement

References

Buono JL, Carson RT, Flores NM: Health-related quality of life, work productivity, and indirect costs among patients with irritable bowel syndrome with diarrhea, *Health Qual Life Outcomes* 15:35, 2017.

Drossman DA: Functional gastrointestinal disorders: History, pathophysiology, clinical features and Rome IV, *Gastroenterology* 150:1262–1279, 2016.

Eswaran S, Farida JP, Green J, Miller JD, Chey WD: Nutrition in the management of gastrointestinal diseases and disorders: the evidence for the low FODMAP diet, *Curr Opin Pharmacol* 37:151–157, 2017.

Gudleski GD, Satchidanand N, Dunlap LJ, Tahiliani V, Li X, Keefer L, Lackner JM, IBSOS Outcome Study Research Group: Predictors of medical and mental health care use in patients with irritable bowel syndrome in the United States, *Behav Res Ther* 88:65–75, 2017.

Lacey BL, Pimentel M, Brenner DB, et al: ACG Clinical guideline: management of irritable bowel syndrome, *Am J Gastroenterol* 116:17–44, 2021.

Lovell RM, Ford AC: Global prevalence of and risk factors for irritable bowel syndrome: a meta-analysis, *Clin Gastroenterol Hepatol* 10:712–721, 2012. e4.

Massey BT, Wald A: Small intestinal bacterial overgrowth: a guide to the use of breath testing, *Dig Dis Sci* 66:338–347, 2021.

Nellesen D, Yee K, Chawla A, Lewis BE, Carson RT: A systematic review of the economic and humanistic burden of illness in irritable bowel syndrome and chronic constipation, *J Manag Care Pharm* 19:755–764, 2013.

Radziwon CD, Lackner JM: Cognitive behavioral therapy for IBS: how useful, how often, and how does it work? *Curr Gastroenterol Rep* 19(10):49, 2017.

Rao SS, Yu S, Fedewa A: Systematic review: dietary fiber and FODMAP restricted diet in the management of constipation and IBS, *Aliment Pharm Ther* 41:1256–1270, 2015.

Skodje GI, Sarna VK, Minelle IH, et al: Fructan, rather than gluten, induces symptoms in patients with self-reported non-celiac gluten sensitivity, *Gastroenterology* 154:529–539, 2018.

Weinberg DS, Smalley W, Heidelbaugh JJ, et al: American Gastroenterological Association Institute Guideline on the Pharmacological Management of Irritable Bowel Syndrome, *Gastroenterology* 147:1146–1148, 2014.

MALABSORPTION

Method of
Lawrence R. Schiller, MD

CURRENT DIAGNOSIS

- Recognize the presence of generalized malabsorption by the combination of typical symptoms: diarrhea, greasy stools, flatulence, weight loss, fatigue, edema.
- Recognize the presence of specific malabsorption by associated symptoms and those symptoms particular to deficiency states of the malabsorbed substance: flatus, diarrhea, anemia, dermatitis, glossitis, neuropathy, paresthesias, tetany, ecchymosis.
- Documentation of generalized malabsorption is best done by stool analysis demonstrating steatorrhea and acid stools (reflecting carbohydrate malabsorption). Diagnosis depends on visualization of the small bowel by endoscopy or radiography and small bowel biopsy. Additional tests may be needed.
- Documentation of specific malabsorption is best done by demonstrating low blood levels of the malabsorbed substance or by tests designed to measure absorption of that substance. Diagnosis depends on studies designed to identify the likely diagnosis for a given situation.

CURRENT THERAPY

- Once a diagnosis is reached, therapy can be directed toward that specific problem:
  - Gluten-free diet for celiac disease
  - Antibiotics for bacterial overgrowth
  - Lactose-free diet for lactase deficiency

Every day the average human being consumes 2000–3000 kcal of food, much of it in the form of polymers or other complex molecules that must be digested and absorbed by the gut. The processes of digestion and absorption are complex and are readily disturbed by pathologic processes. More than 200 conditions have been described that can adversely affect nutrient absorption.

Strictly speaking, *maldigestion* refers to impaired hydrolysis of nutrients, usually due to lack of luminal factors, such as bile acids and pancreatic enzymes, and *malabsorption* refers to impaired mucosal transport. For clinical purposes, "malabsorption" is used to describe both processes.

Malabsorption can be generalized (panmalabsorption) or limited to a specific category of nutrients. Generalized malabsorption is usually due to maldigestion or to extensive mucosal dysfunction. Specific malabsorption occurs when a single transporter is disabled.

The causes of malabsorption can be divided into three categories: impaired luminal hydrolysis, impaired mucosal function (mucosal hydrolysis, uptake, packaging, and excretion), and impaired removal of nutrients from the mucosa (Box 1).

Diagnosis
Symptoms and Signs
Most patients with panmalabsorption have changes in their stools (Box 2). Steatorrhea (excess fat in stools) is characterized by pale color, bulkiness, greasiness, and a tendency to float (probably because of incorporated gas). Occasionally patients with malabsorption present with watery stools due to the osmotic effects of unabsorbed carbohydrates and short-chain fatty acids.

Abdominal distention and excess flatus also commonly occur due to fermentation of unabsorbed carbohydrate by colonic bacteria. This can occur not only with panmalabsorption but

---

IV Digestive System

| BOX 1 | Causes of Malabsorption or Maldigestion |

- Impaired luminal hydrolysis or solublization
  - Bile acid deficiency
  - Impaired mucosal hydrolysis, uptake, or packaging
  - Pancreatic exocrine insufficiency
  - Postgastrectomy syndrome
  - Rapid intestinal transit
  - Small bowel bacterial overgrowth
  - Zollinger-Ellison syndrome
- Brush border or metabolic disorders
  - Abetalipoproteinemia
  - Glucose-galactose malabsorption
  - Lactase deficiency
  - Sucrase-isomaltase deficiency
- Mucosal diseases
  - Amyloidosis
  - Crohn's disease
  - Celiac sprue
  - Collagenous sprue
  - Eosinophilic gastroenteritis
  - Immunoproliferative small intestinal disease (IPSID)
  - Lymphoma
  - Nongranulomatous ulcerative jejunoileitis
  - Drug-induced enteropathy (e.g., olmesartan enteropathy)
  - Radiation enteritis
  - Systemic mastocytosis
- Infectious diseases
  - AIDS enteropathy
  - *Mycobacterium avium-intracellulare*
  - Parasitic diseases
  - Small bowel bacterial overgrowth
  - Tropical sprue
  - Whipple's disease
- After intestinal resection
- Chronic mesenteric ischemia
- Impaired removal of nutrients
  - Lymphangiectasia

| BOX 2 | Symptoms and Signs of Malabsorption or Maldigestion |

- Changes in stool characteristics
  - Floating stools
  - Pale, bulky, greasy stools
  - Watery diarrhea
- Increased colonic gas production
  - Abdominal distention
  - Borborygmi, increased flatus
- Vitamin and mineral deficiencies
  - Anemia
  - Cheilosis
  - Glossitis
  - Dermatitis
  - Neuropathy
  - Night blindness
  - Osteomalacia
  - Paresthesia
  - Tetany
- Ecchymosis
- Fatigue, weakness
- Edema
- Weight loss, muscle wasting

---

also with specific malabsorption of carbohydrate (e.g., lactase deficiency).

Weight loss is typical with severe panmalabsorption, but it might not be very prominent with lesser degrees of malabsorption due to compensatory hyperphagia. Weight loss is most prominent early in the course of the illness, but body weight usually stabilizes as calorie absorption and body weight come into balance again. This is in contrast to illnesses like cancer or tuberculosis that produce continuing weight loss. If a patient with malabsorption has continuing weight loss, inflammatory bowel disease or lymphoma should be considered.

Abdominal pain is usually not present with malabsorption, although some cramping may be associated with diarrhea. Severe pain should bring chronic pancreatitis, Zollinger-Ellison syndrome, lymphoma, Crohn's disease, or mesenteric ischemia to mind.

Constitutional symptoms of fatigue and weakness commonly occur, even early in the course. In contrast, appetite is impaired only late in the course of most malabsorption states. Edema is uncommon until late in the course unless protein-losing enteropathy is present.

Vitamin and mineral deficiencies can lead to several symptoms or signs. Glossitis and cheilosis are common in patients with water-soluble vitamin deficiencies. Florid beriberi, pellagra, and scurvy are not commonly seen unless malabsorption has been particularly severe or long-lasting. Fat-soluble vitamin deficiencies also are unlikely to develop except when malabsorption has been long-standing because of substantial body stores.

Miscellaneous findings occasionally seen in patients with malabsorption can provide clues to the diagnosis. Aphthous ulcers in the mouth may be seen with celiac disease, Behçet's syndrome, or Crohn's disease. Hyperpigmentation is seen in Whipple's disease, and dermatitis herpetiformis (pruritic, blistering skin lesions) is seen in celiac disease. Scleroderma can manifest with tight skin, digital ulceration, nail changes, and Raynaud's phenomenon. Chronic sinusitis, bronchitis, and recurrent pneumonia suggest cystic fibrosis or IgA deficiency. Several systemic diseases can be associated with malabsorption syndrome (Box 3).

Tests

Routine Laboratory Tests

Routine laboratory tests (Box 4) commonly are abnormal in patients with established malabsorption syndrome. Anemia is common but not universal. Iron deficiency anemia may be the only finding in some patients with celiac disease. Microcytic anemia may be present in Whipple's disease (due to occult blood loss) and in lymphomas manifesting with malabsorption. Macrocytic anemia due to folate or vitamin B_{12} deficiency can occur in short bowel syndrome, small bowel bacterial overgrowth, or ileal disease. Lymphopenia may be present in patients with AIDS or lymphangiectasia.

Electrolyte abnormalities may be due to a combination of poor intake and excess loss in stool. Renal function usually is well maintained in malabsorption syndrome, but blood urea nitrogen may be low due to poor protein absorption, and serum creatinine concentration may be low due to depletion of muscle mass. Serum calcium levels may be low due to malabsorption, vitamin D deficiency, or intraluminal complexing of calcium by fatty acids.

Hypomagnesemia can produce hypocalcemia or hypokalemia that is resistant to intravenous repletion. Serum phosphorus, cholesterol, and triglyceride levels may be reduced due to poor intake or malabsorption. Liver tests may be abnormal due to fatty liver. Serum protein and albumin levels are well preserved in patients with malabsorption unless protein-losing enteropathy or an acute illness is present.

Prothrombin time is normal unless vitamin K malabsorption (typically associated with steatorrhea), anticoagulant therapy, antibiotic therapy, or colectomy is present.

Assays are available for several potentially malabsorbed substances, including iron, vitamin B_{12}, folate, 25-hydroxyvitamin

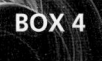

BOX 4 | Laboratory Tests for Evaluation of Malabsorption or Maldigestion

Complete Blood Count
- Hemoglobin/hematocrit
- Platelet count
- WBC differential count

Biochemistry Tests
- Blood urea nitrogen
- Potassium
- Prothrombin time
- Serum albumin
- Serum calcium
- Serum creatinine

Blood Levels of Potentially Malabsorbed Substances
- Serum iron, vitamin B_{12}, folate, 25-OH vitamin D, carotene

Fat absorption
- Qualitative fecal fat (Sudan stain)
- Quantitative fecal fat (Timed collection)

Protein Absorption and Protein-Losing Enteropathy
- α_1-Antitrypsin clearance
- Fecal nitrogen excretion

Carbohydrate Absorption
- Osmotic gap in stool water
- Quantitative excretion (anthrone)
- Stool pH <5.5
- Stool reducing substances
- D-Xylose absorption test
- Oral glucose, sucrose, and lactose tolerance tests
- Breath hydrogen tests

Vitamin B_{12} Absorption
- Serum B_{12} level

Bile Acid Malabsorption
- ^{14}C-glycocholic acid breath test
- Fecal bile acid excretion
- Serum 7α-hydroxy-4-cholesten-3-one (C4)
- ^{75}SeHCAT retention

Small Bowel Bacterial Overgrowth
- ^{14}C-glycocholic acid breath test
- ^{14}C-xylose breath test
- Glucose breath hydrogen test
- Quantitative culture of jejunal aspirate

Exocrine Pancreatic Insufficiency
- Secretin/CCK test
- Stool elastase or chymotrypsin concentration

Serologic Testing for Celiac Disease
- Anti-tissue transglutaminase antibody (IgA)
- Anti-endomysial antibody (IgA)

Abbreviations: CCK = cholecystokinin; SLE = systemic lupus erythematosus; [75] SeHCAT = selenium-75-labeled taurohomocholic acid; WBC = white blood cell.

BOX 3 | Systemic Diseases Associated with Malabsorption or Maldigestion

Endocrine Diseases
- Addison's disease
- Diabetes mellitus
- Hypoparathyroidism
- Hyperthyroidism, hypothyroidism

Collagen-Vascular and Miscellaneous Diseases
- AIDS
- Amyloidosis
- Scleroderma
- Vasculitis (systemic lupus erythematosus, polyarteritis nodosa)

D, and β-carotene. Malabsorption tends to lower blood levels, but substantial body stores of many of these can mitigate the reduction in concentration that otherwise might occur. Thus, the sensitivity and specificity of these assays for malabsorption are poor.

Tests for Malabsorption

Fat Malabsorption. The simplest test for fat malabsorption is a qualitative microscopic examination of stool using a fat-soluble stain, such as Sudan III. The finding of more than five stained droplets per high-power field is abnormal and correlates well with quantitative measurement of fecal fat excretion. The test is subject to false-positive results with some drugs and food additives, such as mineral oil, orlistat, and olestra.

A more precise estimate of fat absorption is obtained by a quantitative analysis of a timed stool collection (48 or 72 hours). During the collection, a diary of dietary intake should be maintained so that fat excretion can be assessed as a percentage of intake. Normal fat excretion is <7% of intake when stool weight is normal, but it can be twice as high due to voluminous diarrhea without indicating defective mucosal transport of fat. Thus, fat excretion must be judged against stool weight. Stool fat concentration (grams of fat per 100 grams of stool) also is of value. Pancreatic exocrine insufficiency is associated with high fecal fat concentration (>10 g/100 g stool) because, unlike hydrolyzed fat, unhydrolyzed fat does not stimulate colonic water and electrolyte secretion that would dilute fecal fat concentration.

Protein Malabsorption. Fecal nitrogen excretion can be employed as a marker of protein malabsorption, but is not often used in clinical medicine because it adds little to the evaluation. If protein-losing enteropathy is suspected, an α_1-antitrypsin clearance study can be done. In this study, fecal excretion of α_1-antitrypsin, a serum protein that is relatively resistant to hydrolysis by luminal enzymes, is divided by serum concentration of α_1-antitrypsin, and the volume of serum leaked into the lumen can be calculated. Values of more than 180 mL/day are associated with hypoalbuminemia.

Carbohydrate Malabsorption. Carbohydrate malabsorption is difficult to measure directly because fermentation of malabsorbed carbohydrate by colonic bacteria reduces the amount of intact carbohydrate that can be recovered in stool. Indirect estimates of carbohydrate malabsorption can be made by examining fecal pH (<5.5 with carbohydrate malabsorption) or fecal osmotic gap (> 100 mOsm/kg with osmotic diarrhea) based on chemical analysis of stool water. Oral carbohydrate tolerance tests may be used to evaluate absorption of sugars, such as lactose or fructose. Following an oral load of a given sugar, blood glucose levels are monitored; failure of blood glucose to increase suggests malabsorption.

Another test for carbohydrate malabsorption is the D-xylose absorption test. In this test, a 25-gram dose of D-xylose is given orally; blood xylose levels are measured 1 and 3 hours later, and urinary excretion of xylose is measured for 5 hours. Failure of blood xylose to rise above 20 mg/dL at 1 hour or above 22.5 mg/dL at 3 hours or failure of urinary excretion to exceed 5 g in 5 hours suggests malabsorption. In addition, because xylose does not require pancreatic enzymes or bile acids for absorption, an abnormal D-xylose test suggests a mucosal problem as the cause for malabsorption. The results of this test can be misleading if the patient is dehydrated or has ascites, if renal function is compromised, or if bacterial overgrowth is present in the upper small bowel.

Breath hydrogen testing is another method to assess carbohydrate absorption. If substrates such as lactose or sucrose are not absorbed in the small intestine, they pass into the colon, where bacterial fermentation produces hydrogen gas. The hydrogen is absorbed into the bloodstream and then is exhaled. The concentration of hydrogen in exhaled breath can be measured easily; a rise of more than 10 to 20 ppm after ingestion of a specific substrate is consistent with malabsorption. False-positive results can be seen in patients with small bowel bacterial overgrowth, and false-negative results can be seen in patients who lack hydrogen-producing flora or who have been on antibiotics recently.

Vitamin B$_{12}$ Malabsorption. Although the Schilling test has been used to measure Vitamin B$_{12}$ absorption, commercial testing kits are no longer available in the United States. Instead, serum B$_{12}$ levels are measured: low levels are consistent with B$_{12}$ malabsorption, but normal levels do not exclude it because B$_{12}$ is stored in the liver and can maintain serum levels for several years.

Bile Acid Malabsorption. Tests for bile acid malabsorption are not widely available in the United States. Direct measurement of bile acid excretion has been used mainly in research studies. Retention of a radioactive taurocholic acid analogue (SeHCAT, selenium-75-labeled taurohomocholic acid) is used in Europe to assess bile acid malabsorption. A breath test using ^{14}C-glycocholic acid has been used for evaluating small bowel bacterial overgrowth, but it may have application for assessing bile acid malabsorption as well. Serum 7α-hydroxy-4-cholesten-3-one (C4) reflects bile acid synthesis; higher levels reflect increased synthesis in patients with bile acid malabsorption.

Small Bowel Bacterial Overgrowth. The gold standard method used to test for small bowel bacterial overgrowth in the upper intestine is quantitative culture of jejunal fluid. The sample can be obtained during endoscopy and sent to the laboratory with instructions to quantitate the aerobic and anaerobic flora. Finding more than 10^5 bacteria per mL confirms bacterial overgrowth. Breath tests using glucose, ^{14}C-xylose, and lactulose also have been described for this purpose.

Pancreatic Exocrine Insufficiency. Tests for pancreatic exocrine insufficiency are not commonly used. The gold standard test is a secretin test. This study requires duodenal intubation, injection of secretin, and measurement of bicarbonate output. Measurement of fecal chymotrypsin or elastase activity is only moderately useful in predicting the presence of exocrine pancreatic insufficiency. For most situations, a therapeutic trial using a high dose of pancreatic enzymes with monitoring of the effect on steatorrhea is the best that can be done.

Evaluation of Suspected Malabsorption

When malabsorption is suspected because of the history, physical findings, and setting, the physician must decide if the malabsorption involves a specific nutrient or represents a generalized process (Figure 1). If the malabsorption seems to be specific, a diet and symptom diary, breath tests using the presumptively malabsorbed substrate, and stool pH to identify acid stools seen with carbohydrate malabsorption are reasonable diagnostic maneuvers.

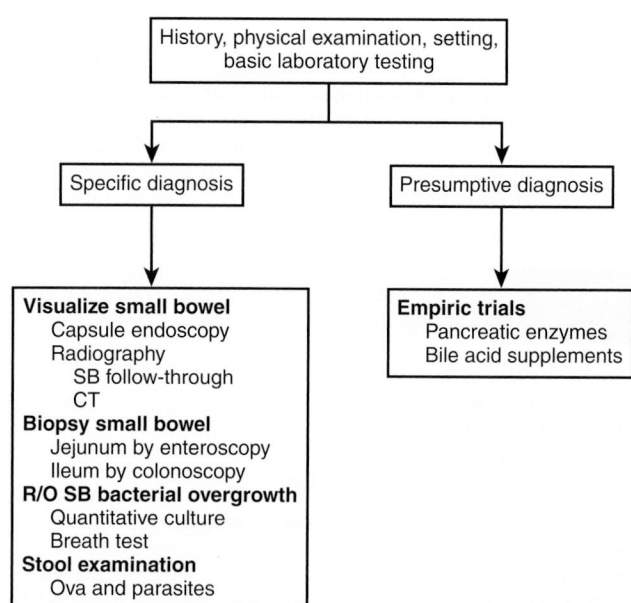

Figure 1 Flow chart for evaluation of malabsorption or maldigestion. *Abbreviations:* CT = computed tomography; R/O = rule out; SB = small bowel.

Suspected generalized malabsorption requires a more intense evaluation. Steatorrhea should be confirmed with either a qualitative fecal fat test (e.g., Sudan stain) or a quantitative stool collection for measurement of fat excretion. If steatorrhea is confirmed, the small bowel should be visualized with either capsule endoscopy or radiography (small bowel follow-through examination or computed tomography) and biopsied from above by enteroscopy and from below by colonoscopy. During enteroscopy, an aspirate of small bowel contents can be obtained for quantitative culture to look for small bowel bacterial overgrowth. An alternative method to detect small bowel bacterial overgrowth is breath testing (see earlier). Stool samples also should be examined with microscopy or immunoassay for the presence of parasites that may be associated with malabsorption.

This sequence of evaluation often leads to a specific diagnosis. When it does not, empiric trials of high-dose pancreatic enzyme replacement or low-dose bile acid supplementation can lead to a presumptive diagnosis of pancreatic exocrine insufficiency or bile acid deficiency. Hard endpoints (e.g., quantitative fat excretion) should be used to assess the effectiveness of these empiric trials.

Specific Disorders Associated With Malabsorption
Malabsorption of Specific Nutrients
Disaccharidase Deficiency
Ingested disaccharides such as lactose and sucrose and starch-digestion products such as maltotriose and α-limit dextrins must be hydrolyzed by brush border enzymes into monosaccharides for abosorption by the mucosa. If these brush border enzymes are not active or if the brush border is damaged, malabsorption of the specific carbohydrate substrate results. This can result in gaseousness or osmotic diarrhea when those substrates are ingested. This rarely occurs on a congenital basis, but it commonly occurs as an acquired disorder.

Lactase deficiency is the most common acquired disaccharidase deficiency. Infant mammals all rely on lactose as the carbohydrate source in milk, but lactase activity is shut off after weaning in most species. Most human populations lose lactase activity during adolescence as a normal part of maturation. Members of the northern European gene pool typically maintain lactase activity into adult life, but lactase activity declines gradually in many. At some point the amount of lactose ingested might exceed the ability of the remaining enzyme to hydrolyze it, resulting in lactose malabsorption and symptoms. This also can occur with acute conditions such as gastroenteritis that can disturb the mucosa and temporarily reduce lactase activity. Patients might not recognize lactose ingestion as a cause of their problem because they have not had difficulty tolerating lactose in the past. Restriction of lactose in the diet (or use of products that have predigested lactose) mitigates symptoms. Use of exogenous lactase as a tablet may only be partially effective because of incomplete hydrolysis of ingested lactose.

Transport Defects at the Brush Border
Glucose-galactose malabsorption is a rare congenital disorder resulting from an inactive hexose transporter in the brush border. Hydrolysis of lactose is intact, but transport across the apical membrane of the enterocyte fails to occur. Fructose absorption, which is mediated by a different carrier, is unaffected.

In all human beings, the ability to absorb fructose is limited by the availability of carriers in the brush border and may be overwhelmed when excess fructose is ingested. This can occur relatively easily nowadays, because high-fructose corn syrup is used frequently as a sweetener in commercial products such as soda pop. Limiting the amount of fructose ingested will reduce symptoms.

Abetalipoproteinemia is a rare condition that prevents absorption of long-chain fatty acids due to failure to form chylomicrons. Use of medium-chain triglycerides that do not require transport in chylomicrons can bypass this defect.

Pernicious anemia develops when failure to secrete intrinsic factor in the stomach prevents vitamin B_{12} absorption by the ileal mucosa. Parenteral replacement with cyanocobalamin by injection (Cyanoject) or nasal spray (Nascobal) is necessary.

Generalized Malabsorption
Celiac Disease
Celiac disease (also known as celiac sprue) is a disorder in which the mucosa of the small bowel is damaged due to activation of the mucosal immune system by ingestion of gluten, a protein component found in wheat, barley, and rye. People who have HLA-DQ2 or DQ8 are susceptible to this condition because these specific antigen-presenting proteins produce particularly strong reactions by interacting with a unique peptide digestion product of gluten. Tissue transglutaminase, an enzyme produced in the mucosa, is an important cofactor in pathogenesis by amplifying the immunogenicity of gluten peptide fragments and is the target of autoantibodies that are characteristic of this disease. The condition produces generalized malabsorption by destroying the villi of the small intestine, reducing the surface area available for absorption.

In addition to malabsorption syndrome with diarrhea and weight loss, celiac disease can produce a host of nonspecific symptoms, including abdominal pain, fatigue, muscle and joint pains, and headaches and seemingly unrelated problems such as iron deficiency anemia, abnormal liver tests, and osteoporosis. These protean manifestations mean that celiac disease must be considered in the differential diagnosis of many conditions. The clinical course is quite variable, with symptoms coming and going. Symptoms can develop during childhood and produce growth retardation or first become manifest in adulthood.

Testing for celiac disease has been simplified by the development of an assay for anti–tissue transglutaminase antibodies. This test largely supplants measurement of antigluten antibodies, although these remain of some use in evaluating adherence to a gluten-free diet. IgA antibodies are the most useful for diagnosis, but IgA deficiency is common enough that an IgA level should be measured concomitantly.

Although serologic tests have high sensitivity and specificity, the implications of adhering to a gluten-free diet are so extreme that the diagnosis of celiac disease should be confirmed whenever possible by small bowel mucosal biopsy, now obtained routinely by endoscopy. An empiric trial of a gluten-free diet may be difficult to interpret because many persons with gastrointestinal symptoms improve with dietary carbohydrate restriction. Wheat starch is particularly hard to digest; ordinarily 20% of wheat starch is not digested and absorbed by the small bowel, and enters the colon.

Treatment of celiac disease at present involves strict lifetime exclusion of gluten from the diet. This is a difficult regimen that excludes most processed foods. Assistance of a dietitian is most helpful. The prognosis with effective treatment is very good. Symptoms should respond to the diet within weeks; failure to do so should prompt an examination of compliance with the diet or reconsideration of the diagnosis. Failure to respond may be seen when lymphoma or adenocarcinoma complicate the course of celiac disease or in cases of "refractory sprue" or "collagenous sprue," which can have a different autoimmune basis from classic celiac disease and which might respond to immunosuppressive drugs such as corticosteroids or azathioprine (Imuran).[1] Persistent diarrhea may be observed in patients with celiac disease who have concomitant microscopic colitis, another condition that is linked to HLA-DQ2 and HLA-DQ8.

Olmesartan (Benicar) and perhaps other angiotensin II receptor blockers can produce enteropathies resembling celiac disease clinically, but which are not related to gluten ingestion. Diarrhea and malabsorption resolve with discontinuing the medication.

Inflammatory Diseases
Diseases that produce extensive mucosal damage by inflammation cause generalized malabsorption by reduction of mucosal surface

---

[1]Not FDA approved for this indication.

area, by promotion of small bowel bacterial overgrowth, by ileal dysfunction, or by development of enteroenteral or enterocolic fistulas. Examples include jejunoileitis due to Crohn's disease, nongranulomatous ulcerative jejunoileitis, radiation enteritis, and chronic mesenteric ischemia. With Crohn's disease, previous resection can add to the problem (see later). Therapy aimed at the underlying process can improve absorption; in some cases (e.g., radiation enteritis), no effective therapy is available for the underlying problem, and symptomatic management is all that is possible. This includes use of antidiarrheal drugs to prolong contact time between luminal contents and the small bowel mucosa, ingestion of a reduced-fat diet to reduce steatorrhea, and use of vitamin and mineral supplements to prevent deficiency states.

Infiltrative Disorders

Several conditions involve infiltration of the intestinal mucosa with cells or extracellular matrix that impede absorption or modify mucosal function by secretion of cytokines and other regulatory substances. These include eosinophilic gastroenteritis, systemic mastocytosis, immunoproliferative small intestinal disease (IPSID), lymphoma, and amyloidosis. These conditions are diagnosed by mucosal biopsy, but special stains might have to be employed to identify the infiltrating cells or matrix accurately.

Treatment of the underlying processes can improve absorption, but it is not uniformly effective. For eosinophilic gastroenteritis, a hypoallergenic (elimination) diet and corticosteroids may be useful. Mild systemic mastocytosis is treated with the mast cell-stabilizer sodium chromoglycate, H$_1$- and H$_2$-receptor antagonists, and low-dose aspirin.[1] More advanced disease might respond to interferon or cytotoxic chemotherapy. IPSID initially is treated with antibiotics, because small bowel bacterial overgrowth may be a causative factor. Once malignant change has occurred, it is treated like lymphoma with cytotoxic chemotherapy. Amyloidosis affecting the gut is not amenable to therapy and is usually fatal.

Infectious Diseases

Small Bowel Bacterial Overgrowth. Small bowel bacterial overgrowth in the jejunum can produce generalized malabsorption. It can occur whenever the mechanisms that reduce overgrowth are compromised. These situations include achlorhydria or hypochlorhydria, motility disorders of the small intestine (e.g., diabetes mellitus or scleroderma), and anatomic alterations (e.g., diverticulosis, gastrocolic fistula, or blind loops postoperatively). Fat malabsorption is attributed to bacterial deconjugation of bile acid. Bacterial toxins or free fatty acids can produce patchy mucosal damage, leading to less efficient carbohydrate and protein absorption. Bacteria also can compete with the mucosa for uptake of certain nutrients such as vitamin B$_{12}$.

Diagnosis of small bowel bacterial overgrowth can be difficult (see earlier). Treatment consists of antibiotic therapy unless a surgically correctable anatomic defect is discovered. Tetracycline is no longer uniformly effective; amoxicillin–clavulanic acid (Augmentin), cephalosporins, ciprofloxacin (Cipro), metronidazole (Flagyl), and rifaximin (Xifaxan)[1] may be employed. Therapy should be given for 1 to 2 weeks initially and then discontinued. It should be restarted when symptoms recur. If this occurs quickly, longer treatment periods should be considered. Continuous antibiotic therapy is needed rarely.

Tropical Sprue. Tropical sprue is a progressive, chronic malabsorptive condition occurring in both the indigenous population and in visitors residing in certain tropical countries for extended periods. The prevalence of tropical sprue seems to be decreasing for uncertain reasons. The disease starts as an acute diarrheal disease that becomes a persistent diarrhea associated with substantial weight loss and typically megaloblastic anemia. Villi become shortened and thickened (partial villous atrophy), but the flat mucosa of celiac disease is not usually present. Enterocytes have disrupted brush borders and can have megaloblastic changes;

the submucosa has a chronic inflammatory infiltrate. Intestinal biopsy is required for diagnosis.

Currently, tropical sprue is believed to represent a form of bacterial overgrowth with organisms that secrete enterotoxins. Most patients have evidence of excessive gram-negative bacterial colonization of the jejunum. The declining prevalence of tropical sprue may be due to improved nutrition, better sanitation, or prompt treatment of acute diarrhea with antibiotics. Treatment consists of pharmacologic doses of folic acid (folate) (5 mg daily[3]), injection of cyanocobalamin (if deficient), and antibiotic therapy for 1 to 6 months. Tetracycline 250 mg four times a day or sulfonamide is the treatment of choice. Newer antibiotics have not been tested extensively in this condition. Improvement should be noted after a few weeks. The prognosis with treatment is excellent; without treatment, tropical sprue can be fatal. Recurrence can occur.

Whipple's Disease. Whipple's disease is a rare chronic bacterial infection with multisystem involvement. The small bowel typically is heavily infiltrated with foamy macrophages containing periodic acid–Schiff (PAS)-positive material, distorting the villi. Small bowel biopsy with special stains or electron microscopy or a specific polymerase chain reaction (PCR) is diagnostic. Foamy macrophages and bacteria can be found outside the intestine in lymph nodes, spleen, liver, central nervous system, heart, and synovium. Accordingly, symptoms are protean. The bacterium has been identified as *Tropheryma whipplei*, a relative of *Acinetobacter*. It does not appear to be very contagious, and no direct person-to-person transmission has been demonstrated. Presumably, differences in host resistance allow proliferation within macrophages without clearance of the bacteria.

Whipple's disease occurs mainly in older white men, but women and all ethnic groups are susceptible. Patients can present with malabsorption syndrome or with symptoms related to the extraintestinal disease (arthritis, fever, dementia, headache, or muscle weakness). Gross or occult gastrointestinal bleeding can occur. Protein-losing enteropathy may be present.

Treatment with any of several antibiotics (penicillin, erythromycin, ampicillin, tetracycline, chloramphenicol, or trimethoprim-sulfamethoxazole [TMP-SMX]) produces excellent symptomatic responses within days to weeks, but it should be continued for months to years. Even with protracted courses, relapses are common.

Other Infections. *Mycobacterium avium–intracellulare* is another chronic bacterial infection that can cause malabsorption, particularly in patients with AIDS. Mucosal biopsy with special stains to distinguish it from Whipple's disease is essential. Antibiotic therapy can reduce the intensity of infection; clearance depends on immunologic reconstitution with antiretroviral therapy. Clarithromycin (Biaxin) and ethambutol (Myambutol) are recommended as initial therapy.

Parasitic diseases can produce malabsorption by competing for nutrients and causing mechanical occlusion of the absorptive surface and epithelial damage. Protozoa that may be associated with malabsorption include *Giardia lamblia, Cystoisospora belli, Cryptosporidium,* and *Enterocytozoon bieneusi.* Tapeworms associated with malabsorption include *Taenia saginata* (beef tapeworm), *Hymenolepis nana* (dwarf tapeworm), and *Diphyllobothrium latum* (fish tapeworm).

Giardia lamblia is a cosmopolitan parasite acquired from contaminated water or from another person by fecal-oral transmission. Cysts are relatively hardy, and ingestion of as few as 10 cysts is sufficient to establish infection. Patients with dysgammaglobulinemia (especially IgA deficiency) are likely to become infected. Diagnosis depends on finding the organism (cysts or trophozoites) in stool by microscopy (sensitivity ~50% for a single specimen), or detection of giardia antigens by immunologic testing of stool (sensitivity >90%), multiplex PCR testing (sensitivity >95%), or discovery of the organism on small bowel biopsy.

IV Digestive System

260

---

[1]Not FDA approved for this indication.

[3]Exceeds dosage recommended by the manufacturer.

Therapy consists of a single dose of tinidazole (Tindamax) (2 g), metronidazole (Flagyl)[1] (250 mg three times a day for a week), nitazoxanide (Alinia) (500 mg twice a day for three days), or quinacrine[2] (100 mg three times a day for a week).

Cystoisospora and *Cryptosporidium* spp. are coccidia, protozoa that disrupt the epithelium by intracellular invasion *(Cystoisospora)* or by attaching to the brush border, destroying microvilli *(Cryptosporidium)*. Stool examination or small bowel biopsy can identify the organism. *Cryptosporidium* can be discovered by antigen immunoassay or multiplex PCR testing on stool with excellent sensitivity. *Cystoisospora* can be treated with trimethoprim/sulfamethoxazole (TMP-SMX)[1] or furazolidone.[2] *Cryptosporidium* can be treated by nitazoxanide.

Microsporidia are intracellular organisms now believed to be most closely related to fungi and are implicated in diarrhea and malabsorption in patients with AIDS and other immunodeficiency states. Small bowel biopsy can show partial villous atrophy, and electron microscopy displays characteristic changes. Stool examination occasionally is helpful. No treatment is of proven value.

Tapeworms compete with their hosts for nutrients in the lumen. *Diphyllobothrium latum* can produce vitamin B_{12} deficiency. The others can result in more extensive nutritional deficiencies. Diagnosis is based on stool examination, and treatment depends on the particular organism identified.

Luminal Problems Causing Malabsorption

Pancreatic Exocrine Insufficiency. Pancreatic exocrine insufficiency is the most common luminal problem that results in maldigestion. Patients develop symptoms of malabsorption when pancreatic enzyme secretion is reduced by >90%. There are several clinical features that distinguish pancreatic exocrine insufficiency from mucosal disorders, such as celiac disease. When fat is not digested, it is transported through the gastrointestinal tract as intact triglyceride, which can appear as oil in the stool. In contrast, if fat is digested but not absorbed, it is in the form of fatty acids that can produce secretory diarrhea in the colon, resulting in more voluminous, even watery stools. This has two important ramifications: Fecal fat concentration is lower with mucosal disease (typically <9% by weight), and hypocalcemia due to formation of soaps (calcium plus 2 fatty acids) is seen with mucosal disease but not with pancreatic exocrine insufficiency. In addition, patients with mucosal disease tend to have more problems with water-soluble vitamin deficiencies than those with pancreatic exocrine insufficiency. In some patients with pancreatic exocrine insufficiency, carbohydrate malabsorption can produce substantial bloating, flatulence, and watery diarrhea.

Tests to document pancreatic exocrine insufficiency are not widely available or are nonspecific (see earlier), and so diagnosis usually hinges on a consistent history, demonstration of anatomic problems in the pancreas (calcification or abnormal ducts), and documentation of a response of steatorrhea to empiric treatment with a large dose of exogenous enzymes.

Bile Acid Deficiency. Bile acid deficiency is a less common cause of maldigestion, and malabsorption in this setting is limited to fat and fat-soluble vitamins. The usual setting is a patient with an extensive ileal resection (see later), but this also occurs in certain cholestatic conditions in which bile acid secretion by the liver is markedly compromised, such as advanced primary biliary cholangitis or complete extrahepatic biliary obstruction. As with pancreatic exocrine insufficiency, stools tend to have high fat concentrations (>9% by weight) when bile acid secretion is limited by hepatic or biliary disorders.

---

[1]Not FDA approved for this indication.
[2]Not available in the United States.

Zollinger-Ellison Syndrome. Zollinger-Ellison syndrome produces several abnormalities that can affect absorption. High rates of gastric acid secretion produce persistently low pH in the duodenum, which precipitates bile acid and inactivates pancreatic enzymes. In addition, excess acid can damage the absorptive cells directly.

Postoperative Malabsorption

Substantial malabsorption can result from bariatric or other gastric surgeries. Weight loss can result from inadequate intake due to early satiety or symptoms of dumping syndrome. Malabsorption can result from impaired mechanical disruption of food, mismatching of chyme delivery and enzyme secretion, rapid transit, or small bowel bacterial overgrowth due to loss of the gastric acid barrier. In addition, gastric surgery sometimes brings out latent celiac disease.

Short intestinal resections are well tolerated, but more extensive resections produce diarrhea and malabsorption of variable severity. When these symptoms are associated with weight loss or dehydrating diarrhea, short bowel syndrome is said to exist. In general, nutrient absorptive needs can be met if at least 100 cm of jejunum are preserved, but fluid absorption will be insufficient and diarrhea may be profuse. The process of intestinal adaptation permits improved absorption with time; it depends on exposure of the absorptive surface to nutrients. Absorption of specific substances, such as bile acids or vitamin B_{12}, is reduced permanently by resection of the terminal ileum.

Malabsorption in short bowel syndrome is not due solely to loss of absorptive surface area. Gastric acid hypersecretion, bile acid deficiency, rapid transit (due to loss of the ileal brake), and bacterial overgrowth may be present. These conditions are amenable to treatment and therapy with antisecretory drugs, exogenous bile acids, opiate antidiarrheals, or antibiotics can produce substantial improvement. Injection of teduglutide (Gattex), a glucagon-like peptide-2 intestinal growth factor, or growth hormone in combination with glutamine and a special diet have been approved as treatments for short bowel syndrome; they can reduce the volume of parenteral fluid or nutrients required. Results with small bowel transplantation are improving with the use of better immunosuppressive regimens, and it remains the only cure for select patients with postresection malabsorption.

Attention to nutrition is vital in any patient with malabsorption. If adequate nutrition cannot be maintained by oral intake, nutritional therapy is needed. Because of impaired bowel function, success with enteral nutrition may be impossible; parenteral nutrition may be needed. It is important to distinguish between the need for supplemental fluid and electrolytes and the need for nutrients; total parenteral nutrition is not a good choice for patients who only require fluids and electrolytes.

References

Bjørklund G, Semenova Y, Pivina L, Costea DO: Follow-up after bariatric surgery: a review, *Nutrition* 78:110831, 2020.

Diéguez-Castillo C, Jiménez-Luna C, Prados J, et al: State of the art in exocrine pancreatic Insufficiency, *Medicina (Kaunas)* 56(10):523, 2020.

Hujoel IA, Johnson DH, Lebwohl B, et al: Tropheryma whipplei infection (Whipple Disease) in the USA, *Dig Dis Sci* 64:213–223, 2019.

Hujoel IA, Murray JA: Refractory celiac disease, *Curr Gastroenterol Rep* 22(4):18, 2020.

Husby S, Murray JA, Katzka DA: AGA clinical practice update on diagnosis and monitoring of celiac disease—changing utility of serology and histologic measures: expert review, *Gastroenterology* 156:885–889, 2019.

Jansson-Knodell CL, Krajicek EJ, Savaiano DA, Shin AS: Lactose intolerance: A concise review to skim the surface, *Mayo Clin Proc* 95(7):1499–1505, 2020.

Jeejeebhoy KN, Duerksen DR: Malnutrition in gastrointestinal disorders: detection and nutritional assessment, *Gastroenterol Clin North Am* 47:1–22, 2018.

Matarese LE, Harvin G: Nutritional care for patients with intestinal failure, *Gastroenterol Clin North Am* 50(1):201–216, 2021.

Rao SSC, Bhagatwala J: Small intestinal bacterial overgrowth: Clinical features and therapeutic management, *Clin Transl Gastroenterol* 10(10):e00078, 2019.

Rubin JE, Crowe SE: Celiac disease, *Ann Intern Med* 172(1):ITC1–ITC16, 2020.

NONALCOHOLIC FATTY LIVER DISEASE

Method of
Vladimer Bakhutashvili, MD; and Adnan Said, MD, MS

CURRENT DIAGNOSIS

- Suspected in patients with steatosis noted on imaging or elevated liver enzymes (alanine aminotransferase, aspartate aminotransferase, γ-glutamyl transferase)
- Diagnosis of exclusion
  - Exclude alcohol excess by history (>21 drinks/week for men and 14 units/week for women)
  - Hepatitis C virus antibody, hepatitis B surface antigen
  - Review medications that can cause steatosis (methotrexate [Trexall], tamoxifen [Nolvadex], diltiazem [Cardizem], amiodarone [Pacerone], steroids)
  - Check serum ferritin, iron saturation (hemochromatosis)
  - Check serum ceruloplasmin and unbound copper (Wilson disease)
  - Check autoantibodies (ANA, antismooth muscle antibody) (autoimmune hepatitis)
- Liver biopsy gold standard.
  - Not essential for diagnosis
  - Useful for diagnosis of nonalcoholic steatohepatitis (NASH) and fibrosis
  - Useful in excluding other conditions (if above tests raise suspicion)
- Noninvasive serum tests (more useful for diagnosis or exclusion of advanced fibrosis and potentially in decision of whom to biopsy)
  - Nonalcoholic fatty liver disease fibrosis score
  - FIB-4 index
- Noninvasive imaging tests for diagnosis of steatosis
  - Transient elastography with controlled attenuation parameter score
  - Right upper quadrant ultrasound
  - Magnetic resonance imaging of liver with proton density fat fraction
- Noninvasive imaging tests for diagnosis of fibrosis
  - Transient elastography with FibroScan
  - Magnetic resonance elastography

CURRENT THERAPY

Lifestyle Modifications Mainstay of Therapeutic Plan
- Goal is to lose 7% to 10% of body weight gradually
- Lose no more than 1 to 2 lbs/week

Dietary Modification
- Reduce calories by 30% (500 to 1000 kcal/day)
- Reduce sugars, carbohydrates, fructose-enriched foods, and sugar sweetened beverages
- Reduce consumption of processed foods and saturated fat
- Coffee consumption (>2 cups/day, avoid adding sugar, syrups) has been shown to be beneficial

Exercise
- 150 to 200 minutes per week divided over 3 to 5 days
  - Moderate to vigorous intensity (swimming, biking, jogging, playing tennis, weights)
- Pioglitazone (Actos)[1] can be used for diabetic or nondiabetic NASH but causes weight gain and does not treat fibrosis
- Vitamin E (800 IU/day)[7] can be used for nondiabetic NASH
- Bariatric surgery can be considered if indicated for morbid obesity, complications of metabolic syndrome

---
[1]Not FDA approved for this indication.
[7]Available as a dietary supplement.

Nonalcoholic fatty liver disease

Nonalcoholic fatty liver disease (NAFLD) is defined as the presence of hepatic steatosis (hepatic fat accumulation), on imaging or liver biopsy, in the absence of secondary causes for the fat accumulation (such as excessive alcohol consumption, hepatitis C, certain medications). NAFLD is closely associated with metabolic comorbidities, including obesity, diabetes, dyslipidemia, and hypertension, and is the most common cause of chronic liver disease worldwide.

NAFLD comprises a spectrum of disease spanning from isolated steatosis (sometimes called *nonalcoholic fatty liver* or NAFL) to more advanced liver disease such as nonalcoholic steatohepatitis (NASH) (Figure 1). NASH signifies steatosis with inflammation and hepatocyte injury and has a higher likelihood of progress to cirrhosis, liver failure, and occasionally liver cancer. Besides liver disease, NAFLD is also closely associated with cardiovascular disease (CVD) and malignancy.

Epidemiology of NAFLD

The global prevalence of NAFLD is estimated at 25% according to a recent systematic review, with the highest prevalence reported in South America (31%) and the Middle East (32%) followed by Asia (27%), the United States (24%), Europe (23%), and Africa (14%). The largest datasets for these prevalence studies come from North America, Asia, and Europe, with lower numbers from the Middle East, Africa, and South America.

In the United States, the prevalence of NAFLD is highest in Hispanic Americans (22% to 45%), followed by non-Hispanic whites (15% to 33%) and blacks (13% to 24%). A significant contribution to this ethnic difference can be explained by genetic differences, particularly a single nucleotide polymorphism (SNP) in a gene (PNPLA3) that is involved in triglyceride (lipid) hydrolysis in the liver, and the ethnic prevalence that mirrors the ethnic differences in the frequency of NAFLD.

NAFLD prevalence increases with age, with a range from 22% to 30% from age 30 to a peak in the sixth decade. Very few studies report on NAFLD prevalence after age 70. Pediatric NAFLD is on the rise paralleling childhood obesity trends, but population data are scant, with estimated population prevalence of 7% to 8% in the United States. An autopsy study of 742 children (ages 2 to 19) who died of unnatural causes used liver histology as the gold standard and demonstrated a NAFLD prevalence of 9.6% adjusted for age, sex, race, and ethnicity. Pediatric obesity clinic studies have shown NAFLD prevalence of 34.2% in a meta-analysis. Differences in sex prevalence also exist, with some studies reporting the prevalence of NAFLD in men as almost double that of women.

Although the prevalence of alcohol and infectious hepatitis has remained stable, the prevalence of NAFLD has been rising in the global and US adult and pediatric population, growing in parallel with the epidemic of obesity and metabolic syndrome. From 2000 to 2015, the worldwide prevalence of NAFLD progressively increased from 20% to 27%. A recent study using data from the U.S. National Health and Nutrition Examination Survey found that NAFLD prevalence doubled between the survey periods of 1988–1994 and 2005–2008 from 5.5% to 11%.

In higher-risk populations such as patients with diabetes, the prevalence of NAFLD is higher, varying from 33% to 70%. In patients with morbid obesity attending bariatric surgery clinics, the prevalence of NAFLD has been reported at 95%.

Risk Factors for NAFLD

NAFLD is a complex disease that has genetic predispositions and is affected by various environmental factors. The degree of contribution of each of the risk factors requires further study and may vary depending on the region of the world.

NAFLD is regarded as the hepatic manifestation of the metabolic syndrome (presence of at least three of the following: abdominal obesity, hypertriglyceridemia, low high-density lipoprotein levels, hypertension, and high fasting glucose levels). Obesity (defined as waist circumference >102 cm in men or >88 cm in women or

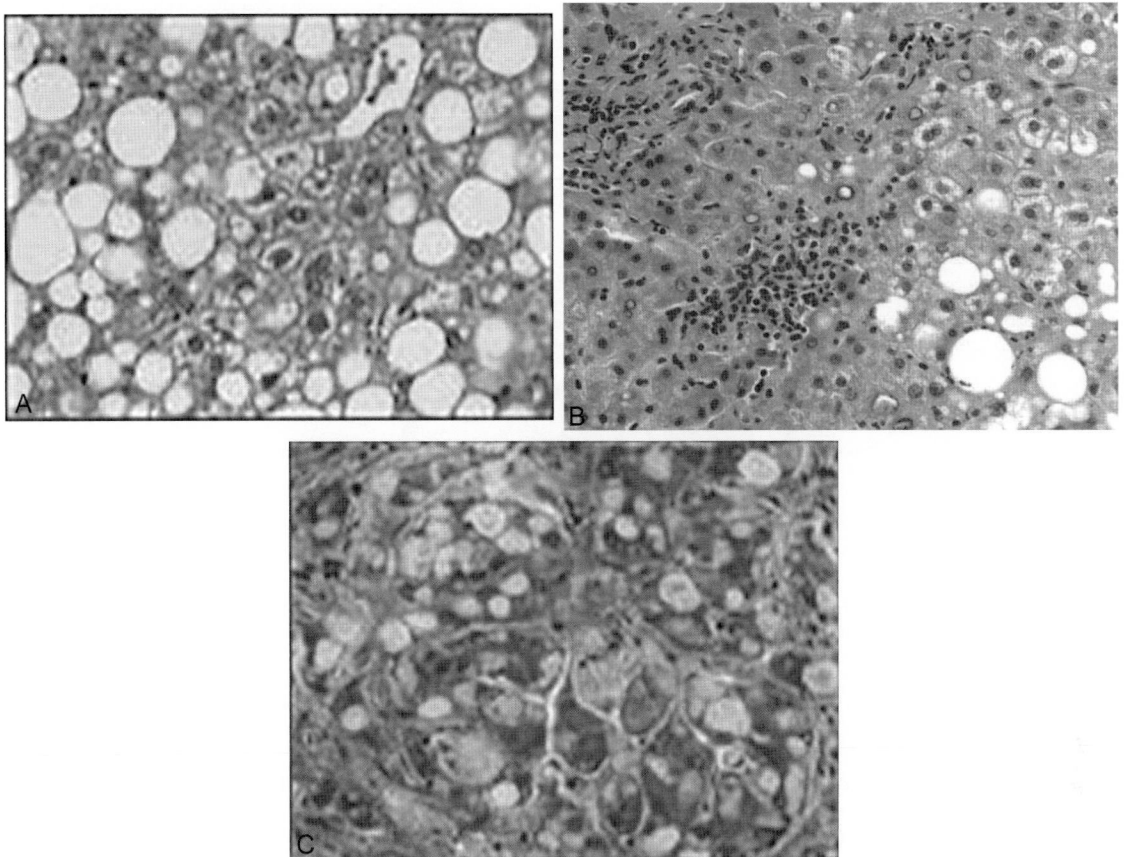

Figure 1 Histology of NAFLD. (**A**) Hepatic steatosis. Arrow points to macro-vesicular steatosis in Hepatocytes. (**B**) NASH. Arrow points to ballooned hepatocytes. Arrowhead points to lobular inflammation. (**C**) NASH with cirrhosis. Arrow points to fibrosis bands (collagen) trichrome stain.

simplified to body mass index (BMI) ≥ 30) and diabetes are two of the primary associated risk factors for NAFLD. Underpinning the rising prevalence of these associated conditions and NAFLD are societal and individual trends in unhealthy eating habits (proliferation of high-caloric processed foods and diets with a high content of sugar, corn syrup, and fat) and decreased physical activity levels. The industrialization of food production, as well as deficiencies in neighborhood planning with poor walkability and public transport system availability, are partly to blame for this epidemic. Being overweight in childhood and adolescence, especially weight gain during school years, is a significant risk factor for development of NAFLD by late childhood and adulthood.

Several genetic risk factors have been reported, with non-synonymous SNPs in two genes in particular, PNPLA3 (patatin-like phospholipase domain-containing protein 3) and TM6SF2 (transmembrane 6 superfamily member 2), being the most consistently validated. The prevalence of the PNPLA3 SNP is highest in the Hispanic population and leads to the higher prevalence of NAFLD in this population. I148M PNPLA3 genetic mutation has consistently been shown to be the most common genetic determinant of NAFLD and correlates with hepatic steatosis, as well as severity of liver disease and risk of cirrhosis and liver cancer in NAFLD.

Heavy alcohol intake and obesity have been shown to act synergistically in increasing the risk of liver disease. The effect of more moderate alcohol consumption on NAFLD is unclear currently and will require more study of cumulative lifetime alcohol consumption. There are population data suggesting that low levels of alcohol use (1 or fewer drinks per day), wine in particular, may be associated with lower risk for development of NAFLD compared with those who drink more or do not drink at all. NASH, which has a higher chance of progression to fibrosis and cirrhosis, is independently associated with diabetes, age, BMI, as well as genetic polymorphisms in PNPLA3.

Pathophysiology of NAFLD

The hallmark finding of NAFLD is accumulation of triglyceride in the cytoplasm of hepatocytes. This is caused by an imbalance between lipid buildup (fatty acid uptake and de novo lipogenesis) and removal (mitochondrial fatty acid oxidation and export as a part of very low-density lipoprotein particles). Further factors contributing to transition from a healthy liver to NAFLD include adipose tissue dysfunction, hepatic insulin resistance, dysbiosis of the gut microbiome, toxic metabolites, and genetic factors (Figure 2).

Along with storage of triglycerides, adipose tissue is involved in the secretion of hormones, cytokines, and chemokines, called *adipokines*. Overnutrition and sedentary lifestyle cause obesity and adipose tissue dysfunction, which likely plays a pivotal role in the development of insulin resistance and NAFLD. Obesity results in excess free fatty acids entering the liver through the portal circulation, which can increase lipid synthesis and gluconeogenesis. Increased levels of circulating free fatty acids also lead to peripheral insulin resistance, along with inflammation and induction of cytokine production, thereby contributing to NAFLD. In NASH, liver cell injury occurs (ballooning hepatocytes, inflammation) along with steatosis and varying degree of fibrosis.

Clinical Manifestations of NAFLD

NAFLD patients are typically symptom free until the condition progresses to cirrhosis. Early in the course of disease, it is often found incidentally on abdominal imaging including ultrasound, computed tomography (CT) or magnetic resonance imaging (MRI) (hepatic steatosis). Hepatomegaly may be the presenting symptom in some patients. Vague right upper abdominal discomfort, malaise, or fatigue can occur in patients with NASH but is very nonspecific.

The other common presentation of NAFLD is with elevation of liver enzymes, with mild to moderate elevations in aspartate aminotransferase (AST) and alanine aminotransferase (ALT).

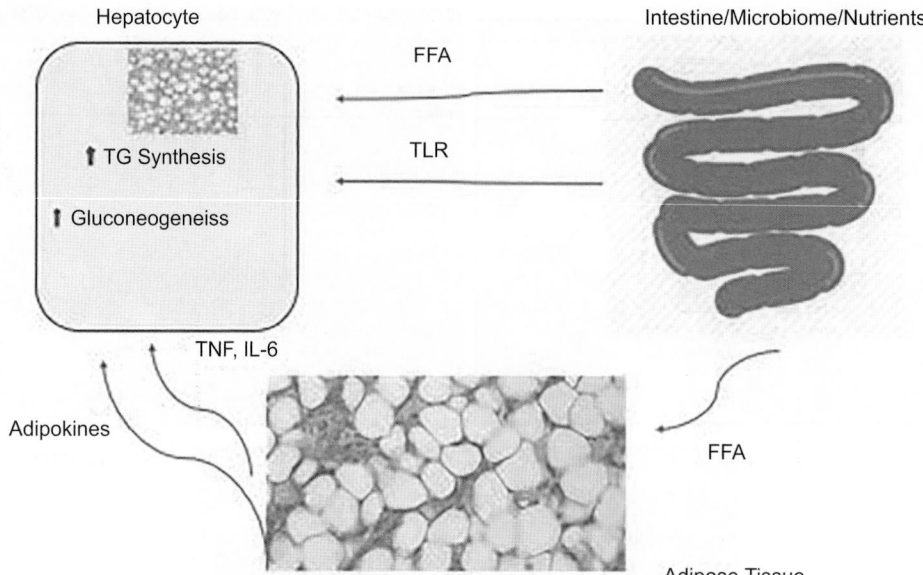

Figure 2 Pathophysiology of NAFLD. An interaction between intestine, adipose tissue and hepatocytes. *Abbreviations:* FFA = free fatty acids; TNF = tumor necrosis factor; IL = interleukin; TLR = toll-like receptor.

However, even advanced NAFLD can present with normal liver enzyme levels in up to 30% of individuals.

Patients with NAFLD frequently have comorbidities including hyperlipidemia, obesity, metabolic syndrome, hypertension, and type 2 diabetes mellitus. Associated conditions also include hypothyroidism, obstructive sleep apnea, and, less commonly, hypopituitarism, hypogonadism, polycystic ovarian syndrome, pancreaticoduodenal resection, and psoriasis among others.

In a community study of more than 7 years of follow-up from Minnesota, patients with NAFLD were shown to have excessive risk of mortality compared to population-based age- and sex-matched control subjects (SMR 1.34, 1.003-1.76). Given the commonality of risk factors for NAFLD and CVD, cardiac disease is the leading cause of death in these patients. A meta-analysis of observational studies also confirmed that the increased risk of CVD is NAFLD (odds ratio [OR] 1.64, 1.26–2.13) and in NASH as well (OR 2.58, 1.78–3.75). Obesity, diabetes, and metabolic syndrome are also risk factors for carcinogenesis, and a multitude of cancers are increased in patients with NAFLD, including liver cancer, breast cancer, kidney cancer, and colon cancer, among others. Liver disease mortality from cirrhosis and liver cancer is the third most common risk of death in these patients.

NAFLD is an increasingly common reason for decompensated cirrhosis and liver cancer. Over their lifetime 5% to 10% of patients with NAFLD progress to cirrhosis. Isolated hepatic steatosis without evidence of hepatocellular injury carries a minimal risk of progression to cirrhosis (<2%). NASH has a higher likelihood of progress to cirrhosis (5% to 12%), liver failure, and occasionally liver cancer. Patients who are older and have type 2 diabetes are at higher risk for progressing to NASH and fibrosis, and in these patients liver disease mortality predominates the clinical picture. Complications of cirrhosis, including variceal hemorrhage, ascites, hepatic encephalopathy and liver failure, can occur.

NAFLD is the second-most common cause of liver transplantation in the United States after chronic hepatitis C and is on track to becoming the most common indication by 2020. In the US general population NAFLD is already the most common reason for developing liver cancer, and the risk of developing liver cancer in patients with NAFLD related cirrhosis is 1% to 2% per year. Hepatocellular cancer (HCC) in NASH, as in most other chronic liver diseases, occurs predominantly in the setting of cirrhosis. Age, obesity, diabetes, and PNPLA3 I148M SNP are risk factors for HCC in these patients. NAFLD associated HCC is the third-most common cause of HCC in the United States, and the incidence of NAFLD-associated HCC is increasing the fastest by a 9% annual incidence rate compared with other causes of HCC.

Diagnosis of NAFLD (Figure 3)

The diagnosis of NAFLD is made by confirming the presence of hepatic steatosis on either imaging or liver biopsy, in the absence of alternative explanations for the steatosis. Diagnosing NAFLD based on elevated liver enzymes alone (without imaging or biopsy) is not recommended. Not *** are elevation of liver enzymes nonspecific, but they are also frequently normal in patients with NAFLD including in those with advanced liver disease.

Alternate causes of steatosis that must be excluded before diagnosing NAFLD include the following:

- Alcohol excess (typically defined as greater than 21 standard drinks of alcohol per week in men and greater than 14 drinks per week in women)
- Hepatitis C infection
- Medications that cause steatosis (amiodarone [Pacerone], tamoxifen [Nolvadex], methotrexate [Trexall], diltiazem [Cardizem], prednisone)
- Hemochromatosis
- Wilson disease

These conditions are easily screened for by history and serologic studies (hepatitis C virus antibody, ferritin and iron saturation, serum ceruloplasmin and copper, and serum autoantibodies).

During serologic workup in patients with suspected NAFLD, it is common to find elevated ferritin, and this is due to NAFLD itself in the majority of cases. In patients with significantly elevated ferritin and transferrin saturation, serum testing for mutations in the hemochromatosis gene (HFE) should be performed, and if there are heterozygous or homozygous mutations in this gene, then a liver biopsy should be performed for iron quantification. It is also common to find autoantibodies in NAFLD that are often elevated in autoimmune hepatitis (ANA > 1:160, Antismooth muscle antibody>1:40). These are often epiphenomena, but if the level of liver enzymes is significantly elevated (> 5 fold above normal), then a liver biopsy can be done to exclude autoimmune hepatitis.

NAFLD is usually diagnosed in one of two common scenarios: Patients with unsuspected hepatic steatosis detected on imaging done for other indications (Ultrasound or CT) or Patients with unexplained abnormal liver chemistries (liver enzymes). These patients should be assessed for associated metabolic risk factors (obesity, diabetes mellitus, or dyslipidemia).

Routine Screening for NAFLD in high-risk groups attending primary care, diabetes, or obesity clinics is not advised at this

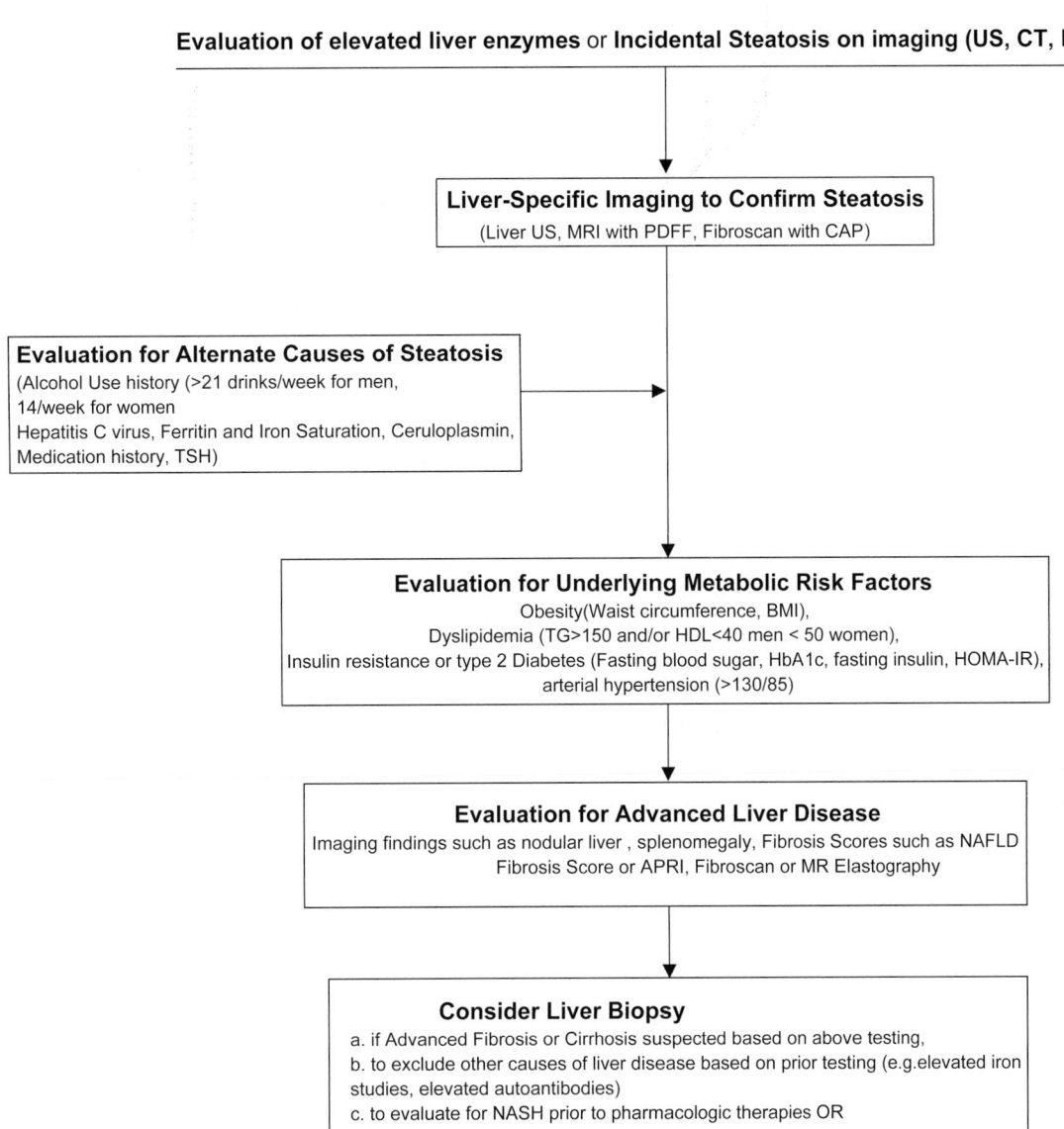

Evaluation of elevated liver enzymes or **Incidental Steatosis on imaging (US, CT, MRI)**

Liver-Specific Imaging to Confirm Steatosis
(Liver US, MRI with PDFF, Fibroscan with CAP)

Evaluation for Alternate Causes of Steatosis
(Alcohol Use history (>21 drinks/week for men,
14/week for women
Hepatitis C virus, Ferritin and Iron Saturation, Ceruloplasmin,
Medication history, TSH)

Evaluation for Underlying Metabolic Risk Factors
Obesity(Waist circumference, BMI),
Dyslipidemia (TG>150 and/or HDL<40 men < 50 women),
Insulin resistance or type 2 Diabetes (Fasting blood sugar, HbA1c, fasting insulin, HOMA-IR),
arterial hypertension (>130/85)

Evaluation for Advanced Liver Disease
Imaging findings such as nodular liver , splenomegaly, Fibrosis Scores such as NAFLD
Fibrosis Score or APRI, Fibroscan or MR Elastography

Consider Liver Biopsy
a. if Advanced Fibrosis or Cirrhosis suspected based on above testing,
b. to exclude other causes of liver disease based on prior testing (e.g.elevated iron studies, elevated autoantibodies)
c. to evaluate for NASH prior to pharmacologic therapies OR
d. to confirm steatosis if imaging equivocal

Figure 3 Diagnostic evaluation for suspected NAFLD. *Abbreviations:* US = ultrasound; PDFF = proton density fat fraction; CAP = controlled attenuation parameter; TG = triglyceride; HDL = high-density lipoprotein; HOMA-IR = homeostatic model assessment- insulin resistance; APRI = AST to platelet ratio index.

time, but there should be a high index of suspicion for NAFLD and NASH in patients with type 2 diabetes. This is primarily due to gaps in our knowledge regarding the natural history of NAFLD and treatment outcomes in NAFLD discovered by screening.

It is essential to emphasize that a diagnosis of NAFLD includes the determination of whether progressive liver disease, NASH, and fibrosis, are present to tailor treatment and monitoring. The state of comorbidities including dyslipidemia, obesity, insulin resistance, diabetes, hypothyroidism, polycystic ovary syndrome, and sleep apnea is important to evaluate at the initial evaluation to recommend specific treatment for these associated disorders.

Role of Liver Biopsy in NAFLD

Currently, the gold standard for establishing a diagnosis of NAFLD and staging fibrosis is liver biopsy. In NAFLD liver histology typically shows steatosis graded as mild (<33% of hepatocytes involved), moderate 33% to 66% or severe (>66% steatosis). Other findings seen in NASH include lobular inflammation and hepatocyte ballooning indicative of hepatocyte injury, as well as varying degrees of fibrosis from none (stage 0) to cirrhosis (stage 4).

Although liver biopsy is not essential for diagnosing hepatic steatosis, liver biopsy should be considered in patients with NAFLD who are

At increased risk of having steatohepatitis (NASH) or advanced fibrosis because no serum or radiologic marker thus far can reliably differentiate NASH from isolated steatosis. Thus patients who are older (>50), have long-standing metabolic syndrome, or have noninvasive scores that indicate advanced fibrosis (NAFLD or FIB-4 scores, or elevated liver stiffness measured by imaging techniques such as vibration-controlled transient elastography or MRE) may fall into this category.

Liver biopsy should also be considered when presence or severity of coexisting chronic liver diseases cannot be excluded without a liver biopsy. This may include patients with serum antibodies in whom coexistent autoimmune hepatitis cannot be excluded or patients with significantly elevated ferritin and iron saturation.

Despite the useful information obtained in some patients with NAFLD, liver biopsy has several limitations, including sampling error and intraobserver and interobserver variability in interpretation. It is costly and invasive and also carries risks including a mortality risk of up to 0.1% after the procedure, pain, intraperitoneal bleeding, bile leaks, and infection. As a result, it is not practical for screening millions of at-risk individuals or for frequent repeated assessments. Noninvasive approaches to diagnosis of NAFLD are thus widely used and include imaging of the liver, liver stiffness testing, and biological marker testing.

Noninvasive Testing in NAFLD
Hepatic Steatosis
Abnormal hepatic steatosis is defined by a liver fat content of ≥ 5%. The most accurate noninvasive method to quantify liver fat content is magnetic resonance spectroscopy. However, this modality requires special expertise, is time consuming to perform, and is not readily available clinically. A good alternative is MRI that uses proton density fat fraction (MRI-PDFF), which provides an accurate estimate of liver fat content, as well as spatial imaging of the liver. Conventional ultrasonography remains the most commonly used imaging modality to diagnose hepatic steatosis. It is wide availability and lower in cost than MRI, but it has limited accuracy, especially in obese individuals. It is not sensitive in detecting mild steatosis (<33%) and is also less specific than MRI with fibrosis and iron, also resulting in similar findings.

Transient elastography–based techniques are increasingly used to diagnose steatosis and estimate the degree of hepatic fibrosis. Fat and fibrosis affects shear wave propagation through tissue, and this property can be used to measure liver attenuation (steatosis) and velocity (fibrosis) using a FibroScan machine. This machine uses an ultrasonic probe placed over the skin in the right upper quadrant to produce shear waves of 50 MHz that pass through the liver. Measurements of shear wave attenuation called *controlled attenuation parameter* assess for presence and grade of hepatic steatosis. Controlled attenuation parameter has been shown to be less accurate than MRI-PDFF in diagnosing steatosis, but it is cheaper and is a point-of-care quantitative modality.

Currently there are many widely available serum-based diagnostic panels for NAFLD that use a mix of serum tests and other demographic, anthropometric measures that are combined in single measurements for diagnosis of NAFLD. Examples include fatty liver index (triglycerides, BMI, γ-glutamyl transferase, waist circumference) and NAFLD Liver Fat Score (metabolic syndrome, type 2 diabetes mellitus, fasting insulin, alanine aminotransferase, aspartate aminotransferase). These panels have been found to have sensitivities and specificities in the 70% range and show reasonable accuracy for predicting steatosis. These tests are not as accurate as imaging or biopsy tests and therefore are less often used clinically and more often used as research tools in epidemiologic research.

Assessing Fibrosis
Fibrosis is highly correlated with outcomes in liver disease and a marker of worse outcomes. Fibrosis histologically is categorized (staged) as follows on liver biopsy:
- F0: no fibrosis
- F1: portal fibrosis without septa
- F2: portal fibrosis with few septa, extending outside of portal areas
- F3: bridging fibrosis or numerous septa without cirrhosis
- F4: cirrhosis

F3 and F4 are categorized as advanced fibrosis and F0-F1 are considered none-minimal fibrosis.

Clinical decision aids such as *NAFLD fibrosis score* (https://www.mdcalc.com/nafld-non-alcoholic-fatty-liver-disease-fibrosis-score) (biomarkers evaluated: age, glucose level, BMI, platelet count, albumin, and AST/ALT ratio) or *fibrosis-4 index* (https://www.mdcalc.com/fibrosis-4-fib-4-index-liver-fibrosis((FIB-4- biomarkers measured include age, AST, platelet count, ALT) use a combination of serum and clinical variables to predict the presence of advanced fibrosis or cirrhosis. These tests are most useful in distinguishing patients who may have advanced fibrosis from those without fibrosis and thus may aid in clinical decision making including whether to perform a liver biopsy or make a referral to a liver specialist (in patients with test indicating advanced fibrosis).

Imaging-based techniques such as vibration-controlled transient elastography (FibroScan) or MRI-based elastography can be used to identify those at low or high risk for advanced fibrosis (bridging fibrosis or cirrhosis) with more accuracy than serum-based markers. The drawbacks to these methods include cost and availability (MRE) and limited utility in obesity, ascites, and acute inflammation (FibroScan). However FibroScan is increasingly available and widely used at point of care in liver clinics for fibrosis assessment.

Therapy of NAFLD (Table 1)
Treatment of NAFLD entails treatment of the liver disease, as well as of the associated metabolic syndrome (obesity, diabetes, hyperlipidemia and hypertension).

Lifestyle Modifications in NAFLD
Lifestyle modifications are integral in the treatment of NAFLD at any stage and are the principal intervention for patients with isolated steatosis and NASH without fibrosis. Patients are advised to lose ≥7% of body weight if overweight or obese (3–5% weight loss will improve steatosis, 7–10% is needed to improve histopathologic features of NASH and fibrosis).

This weight loss is best achieved gradually (losing no more than 1 to 2 lbs per week) and sustained through a combination of diet and exercise.

Basic principles of diet include reducing calories (by at least 30% or by 750–1000 kcal/day for an average US adult) and reducing consumption of simple carbohydrates and saturated fat. Reduction of sugar-sweetened beverages and of fructose-enriched food and drinks is recommended. In general, using fresh fruits and vegetable and lean meats and minimizing processed foods is recommended. Although many different diets have been studied and shown to be beneficial (Mediterranean diet), studies have also shown that any diet that follows the basic principle noted above and results in weight loss achieves the benefits of reversing NASH.

Significant alcohol use can exacerbate steatohepatitis, and limiting consumption of alcohol (≤1 drink/day for women and ≤2 drinks/day for men) is recommended.

A preponderance of epidemiologic data also shows that consumption of coffee (2 or more cups) per day is associated with reduced prevalence of NAFLD. If coffee is consumed, it should be caffeinated; addition of sweetened syrups, sugar, and large servings of milk/other calories may negate any beneficial effects.

Recommendations for physical activity include at least 150 to 200 minutes of moderate- to vigorous-intensity physical activity per week (examples are moderate jogging, weight training, sports such as tennis, swimming, or biking). For patients who do not exercise, a gradual buildup to this level is recommended. Limited data suggest that the combination of diet and exercise may be more beneficial than either in isolation.

Pharmacotherapeutics in NAFLD
Currently there are no pharmacologic agents that have an FDA indication specifically for NAFLD or NASH. There are, however, pharmacologic treatments aimed at different components of metabolic syndrome that can be used off label for NAFLD-related liver disease based on controlled trials studies and published guidelines. These agents, when used for NAFLD, should generally be limited to those with biopsy-proven NASH and fibrosis.

Pioglitazone (Actos)[1] is an insulin-sensitizing agent used in diabetes (PPAR Gamma agonist) and can be used to treat patients with and without type 2 diabetes with biopsy-proven NASH. It has been shown to improve histologic changes in NASH, including steatosis, ballooning, and inflammation but not fibrosis. For nondiabetic adults with biopsy-proven NASH, vitamin E[7] administered at a daily dose of 800 IU/day can be used as well and can cause similar histologic improvements as pioglitazone.

---

[1]Not FDA approved for this indication.
[7]Available as a dietary supplement.

TABLE 1 Therapy of NAFLD

Assessment of steatosis versus more advanced liver disease (NASH, fibrosis)

Consider pharmacotherapy or investigational agents for more advanced liver disease in addition to lifestyle modifications

Lifestyle modifications aimed at weight loss
Goals
Lose 7% to 10% of body weight
Gradual weight loss, no more than 2 lbs per week till at goal
Diet changes
Reduce calories by 30% (750–100 kcal/day), reduce simple sugars, decrease saturated fat, reduce sugar sweetened beverages and foods including fructose enriched foods
Exercise
150–200 minutes per week spaced over 5 days; moderate to vigorous intensity (e.g., jogging, playing tennis, swimming laps, biking)

Treatment of associated metabolic factors as per best practices
Diabetes
No particular agent proven beneficial as primary treatment for NAFLD although pioglitazone (Actos)[1] may benefit histologic NASH. Causes weight gain
Metformin (Glucophage)[1] no proven benefit for NASH
Insulin can cause weight gain and insulin resistance associated with NASH
Dyslipidemia
Treat per standard guidelines
Statins are safe to use if indicated (except in decompensated cirrhosis)

Pharmacotherapy for NASH
Pioglitazone[1]
Histologic benefits in diabetic and non-diabetic NASH except for fibrosis
Can cause weight gain
Vitamin E[7]
Histologic benefits in non-diabetic NASH except for fibrosis
Concerns for long term use: small risk in in all-cause mortality, increase risk of prostate cancer

Investigational trials (generally for biopsy proven NASH)

[1]Not FDA approved for this indication.
[7]Available as dietary supplement.

There are numerous pharmacologic agents in phase 1 and phase 2 trials and a few in phase 3 trials for NAFLD. Some of these agents work on glucose or lipid metabolism in the liver, whereas other are antifibrotic or antioxidant. Obeticholic acid (Ocaliva)[1] and elafibranor[5] are two compounds that show promise and are undergoing phase 3 registration trials. More safety and efficacy data are needed before they can be recommended.

Foregut bariatric surgery can be considered in otherwise eligible obese individuals with NAFLD or NASH, although it is not an established option to treat NASH specifically. Case series have shown improvement in histologic markers of NASH in patients after bariatric surgery.

Prevention of NAFLD
Prevention of NAFLD is imperative and is a societal challenge that should focus on reducing obesity and the metabolic syndrome. Early education and focus on healthy nutrition and childhood physical activity are key initiatives, as are neighborhood planning for improving access to healthy foods and healthy spaces.

Monitoring of NAFLD
Patients with NASH, especially those with significant fibrosis, are at the greatest risk for increased progression to cirrhosis and mortality. Patients with NASH and F0 or F1 fibrosis are monitored annually for liver disease progression via blood work (liver enzymes and function tests, platelet counts) and physical examinations. Evaluation of fibrosis progression in these patients through repeat liver biopsy or noninvasive testing such as FibroScan or MR elastography can be done approximately 5 years after diagnosis; however, with high interindividual variation in fibrosis progression, the timeline of testing is tailored to each individual.

For patients with more advanced fibrosis (F2 or higher) at NASH diagnosis, severity of the fibrosis governs the management. Once F3 or F4 fibrosis occurs, the risk of liver-related illness and death increases significantly, making closer follow-up appropriate.

Patients with NASH cirrhosis should be screened for gastroesophageal varices (upper endoscopy) and considered for hepatocellular carcinoma screening (guidelines from the American Association for the Study of Liver Diseases recommend ultrasound of the liver and serum alpha-fetoprotein measurements every 6 months).

[5]Investigational drug in the United States.

It must be noted that trials of these agents in NASH were generally limited to 24 months or less, and longer-term benefits are not known. Consideration to side effects must also be given; pioglitazone can cause weight gain, has been associated with osteoporosis, and has been known to exacerbate heart failure in susceptible individuals. Vitamin E has some concerns regarding increased all-cause mortality, potentially small increased risk of hemorrhagic stroke, and, in a large trial, increased risk of prostate cancer.

Patients with NAFLD are at high risk for cardiovascular morbidity and mortality, and aggressive modification of CVD risk factors should be considered in all patients with NAFLD. Statins can be used to treat dyslipidemia in patients with NAFLD, NASH, and NASH cirrhosis, but they should be avoided in patients with decompensated cirrhosis.

Currently, the following drugs are not recommended as specific treatment for NAFLD because they have shown no specific benefit for NASH: metformin (Glucophage) and GLP-1 agonists are agents that can be used for diabetes, including in patients with NAFLD; however, they have no beneficial effects specifically on NASH, although trials with GLP-1 agonists are ongoing; ursodeoxycholic acid (ursodiol [Actigall])[1] and omega-3 fatty acids[7] (can consider for hypertriglyceridemia concurrent with NAFLD) do not specifically improve NAFLD.

References

Chalasani N, Younossi Z, Lavine JE, et al: The diagnosis and management of nonalcoholic fatty liver disease: practice guidance from the American Association for the Study of Liver Diseases, *Hepatology* 67:328–357, 2018.

Diehl AM, Day C: Cause, pathogenesis, and treatment of nonalcoholic steatohepatitis, *N Engl J Med* 377(21):2063–2072, 2017.

Lindenmeyer CC, Mccullough AJ: The natural history of nonalcoholic fatty liver disease-an evolving view, *Clin Liver Dis* 22:11–21, 2018.

Loomba R: Role of imaging-based biomarkers in NAFLD: recent advances in clinical application and future research directions, *J Hepatol* 68:296–304, 2018.

Said A, Akhter A: Meta-analysis of randomized controlled trials of pharmacologic agents in non-alcoholic steatohepatitis, *Ann Hepatol* 16:538–547, 2017.

Tapper EB, Lok AS: Use of liver imaging and biopsy in clinical practice, *N Engl J Med* 377:756–768, 2017.

Tsai E, Lee TP: Diagnosis and evaluation of nonalcoholic fatty liver disease/nonalcoholic steatohepatitis, including noninvasive biomarkers and transient elastography, *Clin Liver Dis* 22:73–92, 2018.

Younossi Z, Anstee QM, Marietti M, et al: Global burden of NAFLD and NASH: trends, predictions, risk factors and prevention, *Nat Rev Gastroenterol Hepatol* 15:11–20, 2018.

Younossi ZM, Loomba R, Anstee QM, et al: Diagnostic modalities for nonalcoholic fatty liver disease (NAFLD), non-alcoholic steatohepatitis (NASH) and associated fibrosis, *Hepatology*, 2017.

PANCREATIC CANCER

Method of
Joshua S. Jolissaint, MD; and Alice C. Wei, MD, MSc

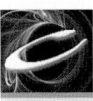

CURRENT DIAGNOSIS

- Pancreatic cancer remains highly lethal. The majority of patients present with advanced-stage disease, and 5-year survival remains below 10%.
- Patients with pancreatic cancer commonly present with jaundice, malaise, fatigue, weight loss, and abdominal pain.
- Routine screening for pancreatic cancer for patients at average risk is not recommended. For high-risk patients, screening may be considered on a case-by-case basis.
- Diagnostic workup should include a contrast-enhanced, pancreas-protocol computed tomography (CT) scan; serum carbohydrate antigen 19-9 (CA 19-9); and staging CT scans of the chest and pelvis.
- Histologic diagnosis is confirmed with endoscopic ultrasound (EUS)–guided fine-needle aspiration (FNA) or biopsy.

CURRENT THERAPY

- Surgical resection is the only available potentially curative treatment; however, only 20% of patients will have resectable disease at presentation.
- Patients with localized cancer and vascular involvement (borderline resectable [BR] or locally advanced [LA]) may be candidates for neoadjuvant therapy with chemotherapy and/or radiation. If neoadjuvant therapy is effective at stabilizing or downsizing the tumor, these patients may then be eligible for resection.
- Systemic chemotherapy is the mainstay of therapy for unresectable patients.
- Palliation of symptoms may require endoscopic or surgical management for both extrahepatic biliary obstruction and gastric outlet obstruction.

Epidemiology

In 2020 there were an estimated 57,600 new cases of pancreatic cancer in the United States. Although pancreatic cancer comprises only 3.2% of all new cancer diagnoses, it is the fourth leading cause of cancer-related death, contributing to 7.8% of cancer-associated mortality and carrying a 5-year overall survival of only <10%. Survival varies based on stage at presentation, with a 5-year survival for patients with early-stage disease of 39.4%, compared with 2.9% for those with metastatic disease. The incidence of pancreatic cancer has been relatively stable over the last decade, at approximately 12.5 cases per 10,000 person-years. Incidence increases with age, peaking between 65 and 74 years, with a median age at diagnosis of 70 years; it is higher in men than in women (14.9 vs. 11.6 per 10,000 person-years). African Americans are 12.8% to 22.8% more likely than white Americans to be diagnosed with pancreatic cancer and may have incidence rates 75% higher than patients of other races/ethnicities.

Types of Pancreatic Cancer

Cancer of the exocrine pancreas comprises 93% of pancreatic cancer cases, with pancreatic ductal adenocarcinoma (PDAC) as the most common histologic subtype. Less common subtypes include acinar cell carcinoma, adenosquamous carcinoma, and colloid carcinoma. Tumors of the endocrine pancreas, pancreatic neuroendocrine tumors (PNETs), and islet cell tumors comprise the remaining 7% of pancreatic malignancies.

Risk Factors for Pancreatic Ductal Adenocarcinoma

Multiple genetic and modifiable risk factors for PDAC have been elucidated. Smoking is the strongest risk factor and is associated with approximately one-fourth to one-third of diagnoses. Some studies have demonstrated that smoking may double an individual's risk of developing PDAC. Heavy alcohol use (three or more drinks per day) increases the risk of PDAC in a dose-dependent manner. Obesity and both types 1 and 2 diabetes mellitus are also associated with an increased risk; however, the relationship between these metabolic factors is unclear. Studies have demonstrated an increased risk of PDAC with obesity in early adulthood in addition to a greater risk associated with hyperglycemia, insulin resistance, and low levels of physical activity. Chronic pancreatitis may confer more than a seven-fold increased relative risk of PDAC, and the mechanism can be either modifiable (e.g., alcohol-related pancreatitis) or hereditary.

Approximately 10% of PDAC cases have a hereditary/genetic component (Table 1). The *BRCA1* and *BRCA2* genes encode proteins involved in DNA repair, and germline mutations in these genes are highly penetrant, significantly increasing the risk of breast and ovarian cancer in female carriers. Although the risk of PDAC among patients with *BRCA1* mutations is less well established, *BRCA2* mutations confer an approximately threefold increased relative risk. *BRCA2* mutations are seen with high frequency among both familial and sporadic PDAC cases. Other hereditary syndromes, such as Lynch syndrome or hereditary nonpolyposis colorectal cancer (HNPCC) (*MLH1, MSH2, MSH6,* or *PMS2* genes), familial adenomatous polyposis (FAP) (*APC* gene), Peutz-Jeghers syndrome (*STK11* gene), and familial atypical multiple mole melanoma (FAMMM) (*CDK2NA* gene) also confer an increased risk of PDAC. Mutations in the *ATM* gene and non-O blood groupings have also been associated with an increased risk of pancreatic cancer. In addition, having a single first-degree relative with PDAC increases a patient's risk of developing PDAC by more than four-fold; however, approximately 80% of patients with a family history of PDAC have no known predisposing genetic mutation or cause.

Lastly, 68% to 80% of hereditary pancreatitis is attributed to germline mutations in the *PRSS1* gene, which are inherited in an autosomal dominant fashion and highly penetrant (approximately 80%). Both the *SPINK1* and *CFTR* genes are also associated with familial pancreatitis. Patients who develop symptoms of pancreatitis in this setting have an increased risk of PDAC that increases with age. By the age of 75 years, patients may have a greater than 50% cumulative incidence of pancreatic cancer.

Screening

Currently there is no role for routine screening for pancreatic cancer for patients at average risk. The US Preventive Services Task Force (USPSTF) has issued a grade D rating (meaning that there is moderate or high certainty that these diagnostic methods have no benefit or that the harm outweighs the risk, thus discouraging the use of this service) for either abdominal ultrasonography, abdominal palpation, or serologic markers. For high-risk patients, those with multiple first-degree relatives with PDAC, or individuals with certain germline mutations (see "Risk Factors," earlier), screening may be considered on a case-by-case basis. Some authors have suggested the use of EUS or magnetic resonance cholangiopancreatography (MRCP), although the efficacy of these modalities as screening tools is still unknown. CA 19-9 is a serum biomarker used to track disease progression or recurrence in PDAC; however, CA 19-9 testing should not be used as a screening tool in otherwise healthy patients.

TABLE 1 Selected Genetic Syndromes With Associated Cancer Risk

SYNDROME	GENE	ESTIMATED CUMULATIVE RISK OF PANCREATIC CANCER*	ESTIMATED RISK COMPARED WITH THE GENERAL POPULATION*
Peutz-Jeghers syndrome	STKI11	11%–36% by age 65–70 years	132-fold
Familial pancreatitis	PRSS1, SPINK1, CFTR	40%–53% by age 70–75 years	26- to 87-fold
Melanoma–pancreatic cancer syndrome	CDKN2A	14% by age 70 17% by age 75 years	20- to 47-fold
Lynch syndrome	MLH1, MSH2	4% by age 70 years	9- to 11-fold
Hereditary breast-ovarian cancer syndrome	BRCA1, BRCA2	1.4%–1.5% (women) and 2.1%–4.1% (men) by age 70	2.4- to 6-fold
Familial pancreatic cancer	Unknown in most families	More than three first-degree relatives with pancreatic cancer: 7%–16% by age 70 Two first-degree relatives with pancreatic cancer: 3% by age 70	Three or more first-degree relatives with pancreatic cancer: 32-fold Two first-degree relatives with pancreatic cancer: 6.4-fold One first-degree relative with pancreatic cancer: 4.6-fold

Adapted with permission from the NCCN Clinical Practice Guidelines in Oncology (NCCN Guidelines®) for Pancreatic Adenocarcinoma V.1.2020. © National Comprehensive Cancer Network, Inc. 2020. All rights reserved. The NCCN Guidelines® and illustrations herein may not be reproduced in any form for any purpose without the express written permission of NCCN. To view the most recent and complete version of the guideline, go online to NCCN.org. The NCCN guidelines are a work in progress that may be refined as often as new significant data becomes available.
*See the associated reference for individual sources of data.

Presentation and Diagnosis

The presentation of patients with PDAC is variable. The most common presenting symptoms are jaundice and conjugated hyperbilirubinemia due to biliary tract obstruction, both of which are seen more commonly in tumors of the pancreatic head. Nonspecific complaints can include malaise, fatigue, weight loss, steatorrhea, dyspepsia, and abdominal pain radiating to the back. A new diagnosis of diabetes mellitus in patients 50 years of age or older may also indicate the presence of underlying pancreatic cancer; new-onset diabetes mellitus compared with long-standing diabetes mellitus may convey a greater than twofold increase in risk, particularly in African American and Hispanic patients.

If a diagnosis of PDAC is suspected, the initial diagnostic workup should include a contrast-enhanced dual-phase pancreas protocol CT scan and measurement of serum CA 19-9. Early multidisciplinary consultation is encouraged to optimize symptom management and establish the best treatment. Endoscopic intervention may be both diagnostic and therapeutic; if the patient presents with biliary tract obstruction, endoscopic retrograde cholangiopancreatography (ERCP) may be used to relieve jaundice and to obtain a tissue diagnosis (with ERCP and/or EUS-guided FNA and/or biopsy). Staging should be completed with cross-sectional imaging of the chest and pelvis to evaluate for distant metastases. Magnetic resonance imaging (MRI) and positron emission tomography (PET)/CT may be useful adjuncts in characterizing the tumor or ruling out metastatic disease.

Treatment

Surgical resection is the only potentially curative treatment option. However, only approximately 20% of patients with PDAC will have clearly resectable disease (i.e., without mesenteric or portovascular involvement). For this subset of patients, surgical resection is the preferred initial treatment. Tumors of the pancreatic head may be removed by pancreaticoduodenectomy (i.e., the Whipple procedure), whereas tumors of the pancreatic tail may require a distal pancreatectomy with or without splenectomy. More central or larger tumors may require a central pancreatectomy or total pancreatectomy. Patients with vascular involvement and no evidence of metastases are classified as either borderline resectable (BR) or locally advanced (LA).

The current National Comprehensive Cancer Network (NCCN) Pancreatic Adenocarcinoma guidelines recommend neoadjuvant chemotherapy with consideration of resection, depending on the patient's tolerance of chemotherapy, their fitness, and the stage of the disease. Currently accepted systemic neoadjuvant chemotherapy regimens include FOLFIRINOX-based regimens (14-day cycles of 85 mg/m² oxaliplatin [Eloxatin][1], 400 mg/m² leucovorin[1], 180 mg/m² irinotecan [Camptosar][1], and 400 mg/m² 5-fluorouracil [Adrucil] bolus followed by 2400 mg/m² infusion over 46 hours), mFOLFIRINOX (without 5-fluorouracil bolus) or gemcitabine (Gemzar) (1000 mg/m²) and N-albumin-bound (nab) paclitaxel (Abraxane) (125 mg/m²) (biweekly for 4 weeks). Some patients may benefit from chemoradiation prior to consideration of resection. The optimal duration of neoadjuvant therapy has not been established; however, most clinicians restage after 2 to 3 months of chemotherapy and reevaluate the potential for resection.

For patients who undergo upfront resection, adjuvant chemotherapy has been demonstrated to improve survival following surgery. The most active regimens include mFOLFIRINOX (85 mg/m² oxaliplatin[1], 400 mg/m² leucovorin[1], 150 mg/m² irinotecan[1], and 2400 mg/m² 5-fluorouracil infusion over 46 hours every 14 days for 12 cycles), gemcitabine plus capecitabine (Xeloda)[1] (1660 mg/m²/day on days 1 to 21 every 4 weeks), gemcitabine plus nab-paclitaxel (Abraxane), gemcitabine monotherapy, or 5-fluorouracil plus folinic acid (leucovorin) may also be offered for patients who do not tolerate other regimens due to side effects. Systemic chemotherapy dosing and recommendations for patients who do receive neoadjuvant chemotherapy are varied and dependent on clinical considerations.

Most patients will present with unresectable or metastatic disease. For these patients, FOLFIRINOX or gemcitabine plus nab-paclitaxel are the preferred regimens for those with a good performance status (European Cooperative Oncology Group [ECOG] status 0-1). For patients with ECOG performance status of 2, gemcitabine alone is recommended, whereas for patients with a performance status equal to or greater than 3, emphasis should be placed on palliation, with cancer-directed therapy administered on a case-by-case basis. Routine testing

---

[1]Not FDA-approved for this indication.

of tumor tissue for deficient mismatch repair (dMMR) or high levels of microsatellite instability (MSI-H) using immunohistochemistry (IHC), polymerase chain reaction (PCR), or next-generation sequencing (NGS) is now recommended. The programmed cell death protein 1 (PD-1) inhibitor pembrolizumab (Keytruda) has been approved as second-line therapy in patients who test positive for dMMR or MSI-H.

Managing Symptoms and Complications

Once a diagnosis of pancreatic cancer has been established, all patients should be evaluated for symptomatology, physical function, and fitness. The active treatment of symptoms and introduction of palliative care services should be considered early. Modern palliative care is not synonymous with hospice, and palliation has been shown to both improve quality of life and decrease the use of aggressive care measures at the end of life.

Pain can be a predominant symptom in patients with pancreatic cancer and may be described as a midepigastric pain radiating to the back. This can be often managed by traditional multimodal analgesia, including opioid/narcotic analgesia; however, consideration can be given to celiac plexus neurolysis or palliative radiation for refractory pain due to local tumor invasion. As described earlier, many patients will also present with **jaundice** due to extrahepatic biliary tract obstruction. Decompression can be achieved with endoscopic, surgical, or percutaneous interventions. Endoscopic stent placement is considered the first line of treatment. Although endoscopically placed stents may be associated with higher rates of readmission for in-stent occlusion or recurrent biliary obstruction, these modalities are generally associated with lower rates of adverse events than percutaneous stent placement. Current guidelines recommend placing a self-expanding metal stent (SEMS) when feasible and only after a histologic diagnosis has been made;

however, the decision as to whether to place a plastic, covered metal, or uncovered metal stent is nuanced and should be assessed by a multidisciplinary team, including a surgeon and gastroenterologist when available. For patients receiving neoadjuvant chemotherapy, fully covered SEMS are preferred as they are easily removed/exchanged. If endoscopic or percutaneous interventions are unavailable or if unresectable disease is discovered at the time of surgery, surgical biliary bypass in the form of choledochojejunostomy may be performed. This may be accompanied by a gastrojejunostomy for the treatment or prevention of **gastric outlet obstruction** (also known as a "double bypass") (Figure 1). As many as 20% of patients with PDAC of the pancreatic head will develop symptomatic gastric outlet obstruction. If not discovered intraoperatively or in patients with short prognoses or limited functional status, endoscopically placed duodenal stents can provide adequate relief of obstructive symptoms.

Pancreatic cancer is generally regarded as one of the highest risk states that predispose patients to **venous thromboembolism** (VTE), conferring a four- to sevenfold higher risk than that faced by the general population. All patients should be counseled about signs and symptoms that may indicate the presence of VTE—either deep venous thrombosis or pulmonary embolism. Current guidelines recommend the use of low molecular weight heparin (LWMH) (enoxaparin [Lovenox]) in lieu of warfarin for patients who develop a cancer-related VTE. Routine prophylactic anticoagulation has not been widely adopted due to a lack of survival benefit despite a reduction in VTE events.

Finally, patients with pancreatic cancer may develop **pancreatic exocrine insufficiency** due to pancreatic resection, tumoral destruction of the parenchyma, or blockage of the pancreatic duct. Symptoms include steatorrhea, weight loss, abdominal pain, and malnutrition due to malabsorption of fat-soluble nutrients. Pancreatic enzyme replacement may be started empirically at a dose of 25,000 to 75,000 units of pancrelipase (Creon or Zenpep) per meal with 10,000 to 25,000 units per snack (off-label dosing).

Summary

Pancreatic cancer remains a highly lethal disease. Most patients are not candidates for resection; therefore emphasis should be placed on the palliation of symptoms. However, improvements in chemotherapy over the last decade have increased both survival and rates of resectability.

References

Becker AE, Hernandez YG, Frucht H, Lucas AL: Pancreatic ductal adenocarcinoma: risk factors, screening, and early detection, *World J Gastroenterol* 20(32):11182–11198, 2014.

Heestand GM, Murphy JD, Lowy AM: Approach to patients with pancreatic cancer without detectable metastases, *J Clin Oncol* 33(16):1770–1778, 2015.

Howlader N, Noone AM, Krapcho M, editors: *SEER Cancer Statistics Review*, National Cancer Institute, 1975-2016, Bethesda, MD. (based on November 2019 SEER data submission, posted to the SEER web site, April 2020. https://seer.cancer.gov/csr/1975_2017/.

Khorana AA, Mckernin SE, Berlin J, et al: Potentially curable pancreatic adenocarcinoma: ASCO clinical practice guideline update, *J Clin Oncol* 37(23):2082–2088, 2019.

Kruse EJ: Palliation in pancreatic cancer, *Surg Clin North Am* 90(2):355–364, 2010.

Lee S, Reha JL, Tzeng CW, et al: Race does not impact pancreatic cancer treatment and survival in an equal access federal health care system, *Ann Surg Oncol* 20(13):4073–4079, 2013.

Referenced with permission from the NCCN Clinical Practice Guidelines in Oncology (NCCN Guidelines®) for Pancreatic Adenocarcinoma V.1.2020. © National Comprehensive Cancer Network, Inc. 2020. All rights reserved. Accessed March 23rd, 2020. To view the most recent and complete version of the guideline, go online to NCCN.org.

Rebours V, Lévy P, Ruszniewski P: An overview of hereditary pancreatitis, *Dig Liver Dis* 44(1):8–15, 2012.

Setiawan VW, Stram DO, Porcel J, et al: Pancreatic cancer following incident diabetes in african americans and latinos: the multiethnic cohort, *J Natl Cancer Inst* 111(1):27–33, 2019.

Sohal DPS, Kennedy EB, Khorana A, et al: Metastatic pancreatic cancer: ASCO clinical practice guideline update, *J Clin Oncol* 36(24):2545–2556, 2018.

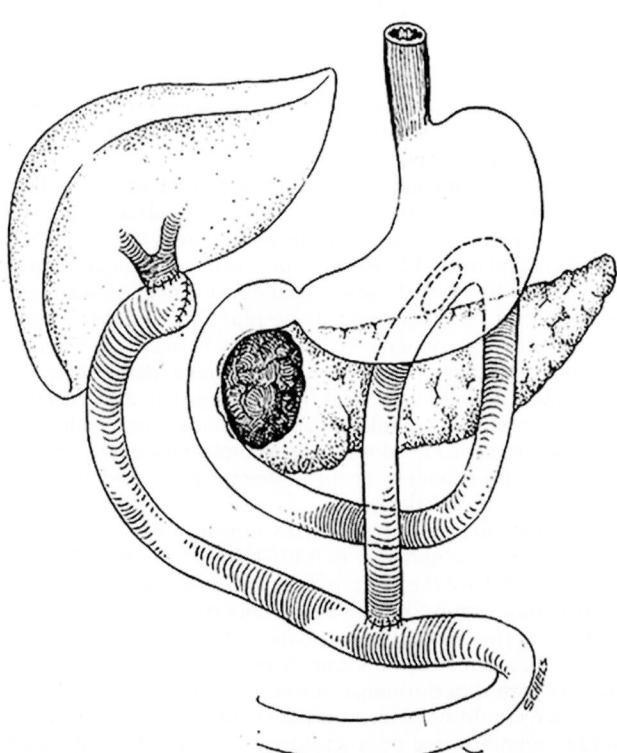

Figure 1 Double bypass showing choledochojejunostomy and gastrojejunostomy with an intact pancreatic head tumor. Reproduced with permission, Scott EN, Garcea G, Doucas H, Steward WP, Dennison AR, Berry DP: Surgical bypass vs. endoscopic stenting for pancreatic ductal adenocarcinoma, *HPB (Oxford)* 11[2]:118–124, 2009.

TUMORS OF THE COLON AND RECTUM

Method of
Pinckney J. Maxwell IV, MD; and Gerald A. Isenberg, MD

CURRENT DIAGNOSIS

- Screening of asymptomatic, average-risk patients should begin at 50 years of age.
- Colonoscopy should be performed if any screening test result is positive.
- Colonoscopy should be performed for any patient with signs or symptoms of colorectal cancer.
- Screening of high-risk patients—those with inflammatory bowel disease, familial adenomatous polyposis, or hereditary nonpolyposis colorectal cancer) and those with a significant positive family history—should begin at an earlier age and occur more frequently.

CURRENT THERAPY

- Patients with familial adenomatous polyposis or hereditary nonpolyposis colorectal cancer should undergo early, prophylactic colon resection.
- Colon tumors should be treated with segmental laparoscopic or open resection.
- Chemotherapy is offered for colon cancers with locally advanced, nodal (stage III), or metastatic (stage IV) disease.
- Rectal tumors that are small (<3 cm), involve <25% of the rectal circumference, are superficial (Tis or T1), lack nodal involvement, and have favorable pathologic characteristics should be removed by transanal techniques.
- Rectal tumors that are larger, are locally invasive, or have nodal involvement should be removed by formal open resection, with sphincter preservation if possible.
- Combination chemotherapy and radiation therapy is offered for advanced (stage II), nodal (stage III), or metastatic (stage IV) rectal cancer.
- Postoperative surveillance includes frequent office evaluations, measurements of carcinoembryonic antigen, endoscopy, and imaging.

Background, Epidemiology, and Etiology

Colorectal cancer is the third most common cancer in men and women, after prostate and lung/bronchus cancer in men and breast and lung/bronchus cancer in women. The American Cancer Society estimates that there will be 102,900 new diagnoses of colon cancer and 39,670 new diagnoses of rectal cancer in the United States in 2010. The incidence of colorectal cancer has been decreasing since the mid-1980s, with a more dramatic decrease occuring in the most recent decade. This decrease is likely related to an increase in screening with removal of precancerous polyps. The American Cancer Society expects an estimated 51,370 deaths from colorectal cancer in 2010, accounting for 9% of all cancer deaths. The mortality rate of colorectal cancer has similarly decreased since the mid-1980s, again with a sharper decline in the past decade most likely related to improved screening. Colorectal cancer is a highly treatable and frequently curable malignancy when it is detected early, highlighting the need for better screening.

The development of colorectal cancer is related to a number of factors, including age, diet, activity, environmental exposures, family history, and genetics. Ninety percent of colorectal cancers are diagnosed after the age of 50 years, and fewer than 5% of cases are diagnosed before the age of 40. The peak incidence of diagnosis is in the seventh decade of life. Dietary factors play a role in carcinogenesis. Western diets, containing high fat and low fiber, have been associated with increased rates of colorectal cancer, as has the intake of red or processed meats and alcohol. It is likely that the low-fiber Western diet slows transit time, leading to increased exposure to carcinogens. Activity level also can play a role in carcinogenesis: studies have shown an increase in cancer among those with sedentary jobs and a decreased incidence among those who exercise regularly. Exposure to cigarette smoke increases the risk of colorectal adenomas and cancers. The American Cancer Society Cancer Prevention Study II revealed that 12% of colorectal cancer deaths in the general U.S. population can be attributed to smoking. Family history and genetics also play a significant role in carcinogenesis, because approximately 10% of patients diagnosed have a first-degree relative with colorectal cancer.

Adenomatous Polyps

The progression from normal mucosa to an adenomatous polyp and then to an invasive colorectal cancer proceeds through a well-defined process over many years. Aberrant crypt foci develop into microadenomas and then into adenomatous polyps. Dysplastic cells develop within the polyp, continue to multiply, become a tumor and then break through the subepithelial barrier and invade the layers of the bowel wall, eventually spreading to pericolic tissues or to lymph nodes and distant sites. A number of genes have been implicated in carcinogenesis, including proto-oncogenes (*KRAS*, *SRC*, *MYC*), tumor-suppressor genes (*APC*, *DCC*, *TP53*, *MCC*, *DPC4*), and DNA-mismatch repair genes (*HMSH2*, *MLH1*, *PMS1*, *PMS2*, *GTBP*). Sporadic colorectal cancers develop as a result of several cumulative genetic insults involving these genes (Figure 1).

Familial Colorectal Cancer Syndromes

Familial adenomatous polyposis (FAP) is an inherited, non–sex-linked, mendelian dominant disease that accounts for approximately 1% of all colorectal cancers. The high penetrance of FAP means that there is a 50% chance of development of colorectal cancer among members of affected families. However, 20% of FAP patients have no family history, and their cases most likely represent new, spontaneous mutations. The disorder is caused by mutations in the tumor-suppressor *APC* gene, which is located on chromosome 5 (5q21–q22), or in the *MUTYH* gene, which is located on chromosome 1 (1p34.3–p32.1). FAP is characterized by the progressive development of hundreds or thousands of adenomatous polyps located throughout the entire colon. The clinical diagnosis is based on histologic confirmation of at least 100 adenomas. All patients eventually develop colorectal cancer. The adenomas typically appear by the mid-twenties, and cancers by the late thirties.

An attenuated form of FAP is recognized in which fewer adenomas (20–100) are identified. Adenomas and cancers develop somewhat later, at average ages of 44 and 56 years, respectively. FAP also exhibits extracolonic manifestations, including gastric, duodenal, and small-bowel polyps; osteomas and desmoid tumors (Gardner's syndrome); eye lesions (congenital hypertrophy of retinal pigment epithelium [CHRPE]); epidermoid cysts; and brain neoplasms (Turcot's syndrome).

Hereditary nonpolyposis colon cancer (HNPCC), also called Lynch syndrome, is an inherited, non–sex-linked, mendelian dominant disease with virtually complete penetrance. HNPCC is caused by a defect in any of a number of DNA-mismatch repair genes (*MLH1*, *MSH2*, *MSH6*, *PMS*, *PMS2*) that leads to high-level microsatellite instability (MSI-H). A number of criteria have been generated for the diagnosis of HNPCC, including the Amsterdam I and II criteria and the Bethesda guidelines (Box 1). According to the EPICOLON study, the revised Bethesda guidelines are the most discriminating set of clinical parameters for diagnosis of HNPCC.

HNPCC is subdivided into Lynch syndrome types I and II. Lynch type I refers to site-specific nonpolyposis colon cancer, and Lynch type II (formerly called familial cancer syndrome) refers to cancers that develop in the colon and related organs such as

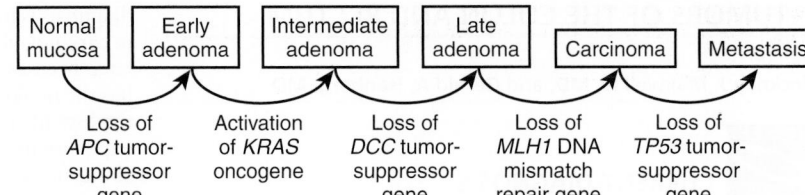

Figure 1 Sequence of progression from adenoma to carcinoma.

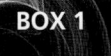

IV Digestive System

the endometrium, ovaries, stomach, pancreas, and proximal urinary tract, among others. Lynch syndrome differs from sporadic colorectal cancer in a number of important ways. It has an autosomal dominant inheritance, a predominance of proximal lesions (75% are found in the right colon), an excess of multiple primary colorectal cancers (18%), an early age at onset (average, 44 years), a significantly improved survival rate with right-sided lesions (53% at 5 years, compared with 35% for distal colorectal cancer in family members), and an increased risk for development of metachronous lesions (24%). Patients and family members of those diagnosed with HNPCC or FAP should undergo genetic testing to help improve future diagnosis and treatment options.

Inflammatory Bowel Disease

Both Crohn's disease and ulcerative colitis are associated with an increased risk of colorectal cancer; with the latter conferring approximately double the risk of the former. The duration and severity of Crohn's disease and the duration and extent (left-sided colitis versus pancolitis) of ulcerative colitis contribute to cancer risk in patients with inflammatory bowel disease. Cancer in Crohn's disease typically occurs in a stricture or bypassed segment. Neoplasia in ulcerative colitis does not follow the adenoma-carcinoma development sequence seen in sporadic colorectal cancer, and this has important screening and treatment implications.

Evaluation

Screening Average-Risk Patients

Patients with no personal history of colorectal polyps or cancers, no personal history of inflammatory bowel disease, no symptoms suspicious for colorectal cancer, no family history of colorectal polyps or cancers, and no evidence of a familial or genetic syndrome may be screened as having average risk. The two main categories of screening tests are those that detect adenomatous polyps and cancers (flexible sigmoidoscopy, colonoscopy, double-contrast barium enema, and computed tomographic [CT] colonography) and those that primarily detect cancer (fecal occult blood testing, fecal immunohistochemical testing, and stool DNA testing). The goal of screening is to reduce mortality rates by reducing the incidence of advanced disease. It seems intuitive that tests that detect polyps, the premalignant phase of colorectal cancer, would be preferred to tests that detect only cancers. However, testing for polyps and cancers is usually procedure related, whereas testing for only cancers can be conducted on stool samples alone. Screening with simple stool samples has the potential to more easily increase overall screening.

Regardless of the method used, testing in the average-risk, symptom-patient should begin at age 50 years. A total colonoscopy is required only every 10 years but involves oral bowel preparation and carries a small risk of perforation (approximately 1/1000). A flexible sigmoidoscopy is required every 5 years, in combination with annual fecal occult blood testing. Flexible sigmoidoscopy requires only enemas for preparation and carries a lower risk of perforation. Air-contrast barium enemas may be used for screening every 5 years, but they also require oral bowel preparation and are only diagnostic. CT colonography is an evolving method for screening every 5 years and offers the opportunity for more accessible screening; however, the procedure is limited in regard to identification of polyps smaller than 1 cm, also requires oral bowel prepation, and is only diagnostic. Fecal occult blood testing and fecal immunohistochemical testing are done annually. The interval for stool DNA testing is uncertain, and it tests only for a limited number of mutations. The most complete screening test, which allows removal of any precancerous lesions that are identified, remains the total colonoscopy.

Screening High-Risk Patients

High-risk patients include those with a personal history of colorectal polyps or cancers, a family history of colorectal cancer in a first-degree relative, Crohn's disease or ulcerative colitis, or a personal or family history of FAP or HNPCC. Screening in these patients has been adjusted for changes in incidence and age at onset of neoplasia (Table 1).

Symptoms and Diagnosis

Symptoms of colorectal cancer include bleeding (85%), a change in bowel habits, abdominal pain, malaise, and obstruction. Frequently, anemia is the only sign a patient exhibits. Patients with symptoms suspicious for colorectal cancer should undergo a colonoscopy. An anorectal source of bleeding should not preclude a complete colonic evaluation.

TABLE 1	Screening High-Risk Patients for Colorectal Cancer			
RISK CATEGORY	**AGE TO BEGIN**	**RECOMMENDED TEST**	**COMMENT**	
Personal history of <3 adenomas with low-grade dysplasia	5–10 y after the initial polypectomy	Colonoscopy	Examination interval should be based on other clinical factors, such as prior findings, family history, or endoscopist or patient preference.	
Personal history of 3–10 adenomas, or 1 adenoma >1 cm, or any adenoma with villous features or high-grade dysplasia	3 y after the initial polypectomy	Colonoscopy	Adenomas require compete excision. If the follow-up is normal, the next examination should be in 5 y. Presence of >10 adenomas should raise suspicion of a familial syndrome.	
Personal history of colorectal cancer	1 y after resection	Colonoscopy	Patients should undergo high-quality preoperative clearance. Follow-up after normal examinations should be extended to 3 y and then to 5 y.	
Family history of adenomas or cancer in a first-degree relative <60 y of age or in 2 first-degree relatives at any age	Age 40 y, or 10 y before the age at onset of youngest affected family member	Colonoscopy	Every 5 y	
Family history of adenomas or cancer in a first-degree relative >60 y of age or in 2 second-degree relatives with cancer	Age 40 y	Colonoscopy	Screening should be initiated at an earlier age. Intervals are based on findings or on the average-risk patient.	
FAP or suspected FAP	Age 10–12 y	Annual FS, counseling for genetic testing if showing polyps	Colectomy should be considered for positive genetic testing.	
HNPCC or risk for HNPCC	Age 20–25 y, or 10 y before the age at onset of youngest affected family member	Colonoscopy, counseling for testing	Every 1–2 y. Genetic testing should be offered to first-degree relatives of persons with a known DNA-mismatch repair gene defect or with 1 of the first 3 Bethesda criteria.	
IBD, Crohn's disease, or chronic UC	8 y after the onset of pancolitis, or 12–15 y after the onset of left-sided colitis	Colonoscopies with random four-quadrant biopsies every 10 cm for dysplasia	Screening should be offered every 1–2 y, and patients are best referred to a center with experience in the surveillance and management of IBD.	

Abbreviations: FAP = familial adenomatous polyposis; FS = flexible sigmoidoscopy; HNPCC = hereditary nonpolyposis colorectal cancer; IBD = inflammatory bowel disease.

Management

Preoperative Management

Before operative intervention is undertaken, a complete evaluation should occur, including a careful history and physical examination, routine laboratory testing, and measurement of the level of carcinoembryonic antigen. A complete evaluation of the colon is essential, including colonoscopy with biopsy, or barium enema or CT colonography if colonoscopy is incomplete. Bowel preparation is no longer indicated as a routine preoperative measure for colonic surgery.

Preoperative staging should be undertaken for colorectal cancers. CT scanning of the abdomen and pelvis are indicated to aid in evaluating the extent of localized or metastatic disease and the presence of enlarged lymph nodes. Staging of rectal cancers includes determining the distance from the anal verge, frequently with the use of a rigid proctoscope; the depth of invasion; and the presence of enlarged lymph nodes, using endorectal ultrasound or endoanal coil magnetic resonance imaging. Metastatic disease mandates neoadjuvant chemotherapy in the absence of acute symptoms of obstruction or exsanguination. Rectal cancers with evidence of local invasion into perirectal fat or adjacent structures or evidence of enlarged metastatic lymph nodes may benefit from neoadjuvant chemotherapy and irradiation. Preoperative staging allows for the application of neoadjuvant therapy in selected candidates, which can downstage and downsize tumors and can decrease rates of local recurrence in rectal cancer. Neoadjuvant therapy can also allow for sphincter-preserving procedures in patients with previously bulky or very low rectal tumors.

Surgery for Colonic Tumors

The primary therapy for tumors of the colon is operative. The basic principles of surgery for colon cancer are the following:

- Exploration: adequate visual, tactile, and potentially intraoperative hepatic ultrasound staging at the time of primary resection
- Removal of the entire cancer with enough proximal and distal bowel to encompass the possibility of submucosal lymphatic tumor spread
- Removal of the regional mesenteric pedicle, including draining lymphatics, based on the predictable lymphatic spread of the disease and the potential for regional mesenteric involvement without concurrent distant involvement
- En bloc resection of involved structures (T4 tumors)

Segmental colonic resections (right, transverse, left, or sigmoid colectomy) are undertaken based on the tumor location and blood supply with lymphatic drainage, specifically the ileocolic, middle colic, and left colic arteries. These arteries define a convenient anatomic boundary for standard colonic resection and also provide for adequate regional lymph node clearance, because the major draining lymphatics follow these blood vessels in the mesentery. Locally invasive tumors (T4) require en bloc resection of involved structures. Metastatic colonic tumors (M1) may require neoadjuvant chemotherapy before resection or palliation.

Numerous studies have verified that laparoscopic surgery is appropriate, and perhaps preferred, for colon cancer in experienced hands. The landmark Clinical Outcomes of Surgical Therapy (COST) trial in 2004 established that laparoscopic resection is equivalent to open resection for colon cancer.

Surgery for Rectal Tumors

Two approaches for rectal tumors are local excision and formal rectal resection. Local excision is the treatment of choice for a select, small group (3%–5% of all patients diagnosed with rectal cancer). Tumors amenable to transanal excision are small (<3 cm), involve less than 25% of the rectal circumference, are confined to the mucosa or submucosa (Tis or T1), lack nodal involvement by preoperative imaging, and have favorable pathologic characteristics (well or moderately differentiated with no lymphovascular invasion). Tumors in the lower or middle third of the rectum are accessible by simple transanal excision, but tumors of the upper rectum require the use of transanal endoscopic microsurgery (TEMS) techniques for resection. Local excision requires a 1-cm normal margin, but the defect usually does not require closure.

Tumors staged at T2 or greater require a formal resection, the type of which depends on the location of the tumor. Upper and middle rectal tumors can usually be managed with a low or very low anterior resection. Lower rectal tumors frequently require a proctectomy with coloanal anastomosis or an abdominoperineal resection. The goal of resection is to obtain a 5-cm distal margin, but lower tumors can be managed with a 2-cm distal margin. Very low tumors and those involving the sphincter mechanism require an abdominoperineal resection.

Rectal tumors with greater depth of rectal wall invasion (T3), evidence of fixation or local invasion (T4), or evidence of lymph nodal (N1–2) or metastatic (M1) disease mandates neoadjuvant chemoradiation therapy. Proctectomy requires a specimen-appropriate total mesorectal excision. This involves complete excision of all mesorectal tissue located behind the rectum with no carcinoma at the lateral or circumferential margins. The goal is to remove all malignant tissue, so as to reduce or eliminate the possibility of locally recurrent disease.

Locally advanced rectal tumors may preclude an effective or safe resection. Some indications for likely inoperability include extensive pelvic disease, invasion of ileofemoral vessels, extensive lymphatic involvement or significant lower extremity lymphedema, bony involvement, and life expectancy less than 3 to 6 months.

Laparoscopy is being performed for rectal malignancies in advanced centers, and studies are under way to verify the efficacy and safety of laparoscopic rectal resection in comparison with traditional open resection.

Complicated Disease

Colorectal tumors may manifest with complications such as obstruction, perforation, or significant bleeding. These presentations are generally related to more advanced disease and may preclude a complete staging workup or potential neoadjuvant therapy. Unless patients are unstable or critically ill or the tumor is unresectable, the tumor should be appropriately resected. An ostomy is usually performed, whether as an end ostomy or as a proximal loop diversion for a primary anastomosis. Colonic stenting is an attractive option for obstructing lesions as palliation or as a bridge to resection after medical stabilization and staging for potential neoadjuvant therapy.

Surgery for High-Risk Conditions

High-risk conditions for the development of colorectal malignancies include FAP, HNPCC, and chronic ulcerative colitis. Surgical management may be prophylactic or possibly therapeutic after a malignancy has been diagnosed. The mainstay of operative management in FAP and chronic ulcerative colitis is a total proctocolectomy. Reconstructive options include an ileal pouch–anal anastomosis, a continent ileostomy (Kock pouch), or an end ileostomy. A total abdominal colectomy with ileorectal anastomosis may be performed for temporary preservation of rectal function in selected cases of chronic ulcerative colitis with rectal sparing and FAP with few rectal polyps, but this requires aggressive surveillance of the remaining rectal mucosa because of the risk of malignancy. Patients with HNPCC should also undergo subtotal colectomy with ileorectal anastomosis; because of the prevalence of associated gynecological malignancies, a total hysterectomy with bilateral salpingo-oophorectomy should be offered to women as well.

Pathologic Staging and Adjuvant Therapy

Excellent pathologic sampling and review of the operative specimen provide important prognostic and therapeutic information. Current standards recommend that at least 12 lymph nodes be removed for adequate staging of colon cancer. The decision for adjuvant chemotherapy or radiation therapy or both is based on the pathologic staging. This information also provides prognostic information in terms of survival for the patient and family. A number of staging systems have been developed, but the tumor-node-metastasis (TNM) system is the one most commonly used in the United States (Table 2).

Chemotherapy is offered for patients who have colorectal cancers with locally advanced, nodal (stage III), or metastatic (stage IV) disease. The combination of chemotherapy and radiation therapy for advanced rectal cancer (stage II–IV) has decreased local recurrence and increased survival. Numerous protocols are available for treatment, with the standard of care being FOLFOX: oxaliplatin (Eloxatin), 5-fluorouracil (5-FU [Adrucil]), and leucovorin. Elderly patients and those with multiple comorbidities who may not be able to tolerate full-dose chemotherapy may be candidates for capecitabine (Xeloda) or 5-FU and leucovorin. Numerous study protocols are available at specialized centers evaluating other medications. Newer technologies continue to evolve, such as antiangiogenesis agents and immunomodulatory agents.

Metastatic Disease

Surgical therapy is also available for metastatic disease in certain situations. Metastatic liver lesions amenable to resection can be

TABLE 2	Pathologic Staging Systems for Colorectal Cancer					
PATHOLOGIC FEATURES		**STAGE**	**TNM**	**DUKES**	**ASTLER-COLLER**	**5-YR SURVIVAL (%)**
Depth of Invasion						
Lamina propria, muscularis mucosa		0	T0/Tis	A		>90
Submucosa		I	T1	A	B1	
Muscularis propria		I	T2	A	B1	
Subserosa, pericolic fat		II	T3	B	B1	70–85
Adjacent organs, perforation		II	T4	B	B2	55–65
Lymph nodal involvement						
None			N0			
1–3 nodes		III	N1	C	C1, C2	45–55
>3 nodes		III	N2	C	C1, C2	20–30
Distant metastatic disease						
Absent			M0			
Present		IV	M1	D		<5

Abbreviation: TNM = tumor-node-metastasis system.

addressed at the time of colon resection or after the patient has healed from colectomy. The lesions could be resected or treated with radiofrequency ablation, a newer technology that allows in situ destruction of liver lesions. Similarly, selected pulmonary metastases can be resected, possibly with the use of minimally invasive thoracoscopic techniques.

Surveillance

Surveillance for colon and rectal cancer is a lifelong process. Patients are seen and examined in the office every 3 months for 2 years, then every 6 months for 3 years, and then yearly for 5 years. Levels of carcinoembryonic antigen are measured at each office visit, but current literature recommends obtaining levels every 3 months for 3 years as a marker for tumor recurrence in stage II–III patients. Colonoscopy should be performed at 1 year postoperatively, assuming a high-quality preoperative study has cleared the rest of the colon. A normal colonoscopy at 1 year postoperatively would allow the next surveillance colonoscopy to be performed 3 years later. If that one is normal, subsequent examinations should be performed every 5 years. After the examination at 1 year postoperatively, the subsequent intervals should be shortened if there is evidence of HNPCC or if additional adenomas are found. As an addition to formal colonoscopies, flexible sigmoidoscopies are performed with each office visit for patients with rectal cancer. Routine imaging utilizing CT scans of the chest, abdomen, and pelvis is performed annually for 3 years in patients with colorectal cancer. Patients with increased or rising CEA levels, as noted by routine surveillance checks, or evidence of recurrent disease, as noted by history and physical examinations or routine surveillance imaging studies, can be evaluated with the use of positron emission tomography (PET), an emerging sensitive test for tumor recurrence.

References

American Cancer Society: *Cancer Facts and Figures 2013*, Atlanta, GA, 2013, American Cancer Society. Available at: http://www.cancer.org/Research/CancerFactsFigures/CancerFactsFigures/cancer-facts-figures-2013. [accessed August 25, 2014].

Beart RW, Steele Jr GD, Menck HR, et al: Management and survival of patients with adenocarcinoma of the colon and rectum: A national survey of the Commission on Cancer, *J Am Coll Surg* 181:225–236, 1995.

Bentrem DJ, Okabe S, Wong WD, et al: T1 Adenocarcinoma of the rectum: Transanal excision or radical surgery? *Ann Surg* 242:472–479, 2005.

Clinical Outcomes of Surgical Therapy Study Group: A comparison of laparoscopically assisted and open colectomy for colon cancer, *N Engl J Med* 350:2050–2059, 2004.

Desch CE, Benson 3rd AB, Somerfield MR, et al: Colorectal cancer surveillance: 2005 update of an American Society of Clinical Oncology Practice Guideline, *J Clin Oncol* 23(33):8512–8519, 2005.

Floyd ND, Saclarides TJ: Transanal endoscopic microsurgical resection of pT1 rectal tumors, *Dis Colon Rectum* 49:164–168, 2005.

Lan Y-T, Lin J-K, Li AF-Y, et al: Metachronous colorectal cancer: Necessity of post-operative colonoscopic surveillance, *Int J Colorectal Dis* 20:121–125, 2005.

Levin B, Lieberman DA, McFarland B, et al: Screening and surveillance for the early detection of colorectal cancer and adenomatous polyps, 2008: A joint guideline from the American Cancer Society, the US Multi-Society Task Force on Colorectal Cancer, and the American College of Radiology. For the American Cancer Society Colorectal Cancer Advisory Group, the US Multi-Society Task Force, and the American College of Radiology Colon Cancer Committee, *Gastroenterology* 134:1570–1595, 2008.

Maetani I, Tada T, Ukita T, et al: Self-expandable metallic stent placement as palliative treatment of obstructed colorectal carcinoma, *J Gastroenterol* 39:334–338, 2004.

Pinol V, Castells A, Andreu M, et al: Accuracy of Revised Bethesda Guidelines, microsatellite instability, and immunohistochemistry for the identification of patients with hereditary nonpolyposis colorectal cancer, *JAMA* 293:1986–1994, 2005.

Rex DK, Kahi CJ, Levin B, et al: Guidelines for colonoscopy surveillance after cancer resection: A consensus update by the American Cancer Society and the US Multi-Society Task Force on Colorectal Cancer, *Gastroenterology* 130:1865–1871, 2006.

Sauer R, Becker H, Hohenberger W, et al: for the German Rectal Cancer Study Group: Preoperative versus postoperative chemoradiotherapy for rectal cancer, *N Engl J Med* 351:1731–1740, 2004.

Stipa F, Chessin DB, Shia J, et al: A pathologic complete response of rectal cancer to preoperative combined-modality therapy results in improved oncological outcome compared with those who achieve no downstaging on the basis of preoperative endorectal ultrasonography, *Ann Surg Oncol* 13(8):1047–1053, 2006.

Winawer SJ, Zauber AG, Fletcher RH, et al: Guidelines for colonoscopy surveillance after polypectomy: A consensus update by the US Multi-Society Task Force on Colorectal Cancer and the American Cancer Society, *CA Cancer J Clin* 56:143–159, 2006.

TUMORS OF THE STOMACH

Method of
David A. Mahvi, MD; and Mark Fairweather, MD

CURRENT DIAGNOSIS

- Screening programs exist in countries with a very high incidence of gastric adenocarcinoma and can be considered elsewhere for individuals at high risk.
- Esophagogastroduodenoscopy with biopsy is the gold standard for diagnosis of stomach tumors.
- Staging workup for adenocarcinoma includes computed tomography of the chest, abdomen, and pelvis to evaluate for metastatic disease and endoscopic ultrasound to assess T-stage.

CURRENT THERAPY

Adenocarcinoma
- Treatment decisions should be made by multidisciplinary teams.
- Patients with T1a tumors and no further spread can be candidates for endoscopic or surgical resection.
- Patients with T1b tumors without nodal involvement should undergo upfront surgical resection.
- Patients with T2 or higher disease or any nodal involvement should receive perioperative chemotherapy, with the FLOT regimen being first-line (5-fluorouracil, leucovorin,[1] docetaxel [Taxotere], oxaliplatin[1]).
- Surgery consists of either a distal gastrectomy or total gastrectomy depending on tumor location and should include at least 15 lymph nodes for accurate staging.

Gastrointestinal Stromal Tumors
- All tumors greater than 2 cm should be considered for resection.
- No lymphadenectomy is required, and grossly negative margins are sufficient.
- Imatinib (Gleevec), a tyrosine kinase inhibitor, should be offered to patients after surgery with high risk of tumor recurrence (either primary tumor >5 cm or mitotic rate >5 per 50 high-powered field).

Neuroendocrine Tumors
- Type 1 and type 2 tumors can undergo endoscopic resection if less than 2 cm in size and they are not either poorly differentiated or invade beyond the submucosa.
- Surgical resection should be performed for all type 3 tumors as well as for type 1 and 2 tumors that have positive margins, recur, or have worrisome features listed above.
- Patients can develop carcinoid syndrome with liver metastases; this can be treated with somatostatin analogs, surgical cytoreduction, or liver-directed therapies.

Gastric Lymphoma
- MALT lymphomas often respond to *Helicobacter pylori* eradication.
- Other lymphomas are treated with chemotherapy, with surgery being reserved for patients with complications such as bleeding or perforation.

[1]Not FDA approved for this indication.

Gastric Adenocarcinoma

Gastric adenocarcinoma is the fourth-leading cause of cancer-related death worldwide, accounting for an estimated 768,000 deaths in 2020. Gastric cancer is the fifth-most common cancer worldwide with just over 1 million new cases annually. While the overall incidence has been downtrending due to screening in high-risk populations and the recognition of *Helicobacter pylori* as a significant risk factor, the overall crude number of cases has gradually increased due to the aging population. In the United States gastric cancer is less prevalent with the 16th highest incidence and mortality rate estimated in 2020, though with the fifth worst relative overall survival.

Classification

Historically, gastric adenocarcinomas have been divided into two main subtypes by the Lauren classification system, intestinal and diffuse. Intestinal-type gastric cancers are similar to adenocarcinomas elsewhere in the gastrointestinal tract, appearing in glandular or tubular formations. Intestinal cancers are more likely to occur in men and older patients and have a more favorable prognosis. The diffuse subtype lacks cohesive molecules, specifically E-cadherin, and will invade without gland formation.

Risk Factors

There are a number of risk factors for gastric cancer. While most cancers are sporadic, 1% to 3% are due to a genetic mutation (most commonly E-cadherin/CDH-1 mutations). Numerous dietary factors have been linked to subsequent gastric cancer development, including salty or spicy diets, processed meat, smoked fish, refined grains, and lack of adequate fruits and vegetables. Additional lifestyle factors include alcohol and cigarette use. Men are also more likely to develop the disease than women.

History of *H. pylori* infection or chronic atrophic gastritis also increase a patient's risk of developing subsequent stomach cancer. The International Agency for Research on Cancer estimates that *H. pylori* solely attributes to 36% of gastric cancers in developed countries and 47% in developing countries. Both intestinal and diffuse subtypes of gastric adenocarcinoma are associated with *H. pylori*. *H. pylori* strains with the *cagA* gene have worse prognosis. The chronic inflammation and subsequent development of atrophic gastritis can lead to intestinal metaplasia.

There has been an increasing incidence of proximal gastric cancers. Obesity and gastroesophageal reflux disease (GERD) are risk factors for more proximal lesions.

Screening

National screening programs have been established in Japan and South Korea, both of which have a relatively high incidence of gastric cancer. In Korea, screening is recommended every 2 years starting at age 40. In Japan, screening is performed every 2 to 3 years starting at age 50. Both countries have shown diagnosis at earlier cancer stages improved with utilization of their screening programs. The relative utility and cost-effectiveness of national gastric cancer screening with either upper endoscopy or upper gastrointestinal (GI) series has not been established in countries with lower relative incidence of gastric cancer. Individualized screening can be considered for those with high-risk genetic syndromes, such as CDH-1 mutation, Lynch syndrome, Peutz-Jeghers syndrome, and familial adenomatous polyposis. Screening can also be considered in patients with a strong family history of gastric cancer or previously established atrophic gastritis or intestinal metaplasia.

Clinical Manifestations

Patients with gastric adenocarcinoma often have vague symptoms that may not be present until more advanced disease is present. Epigastric abdominal pain (52%) and weight loss (62%) are the most common symptoms, but early satiety, decreased appetite, and nausea can also be present. New-onset heartburn or reflux can be a presenting symptom and warrants further workup, especially in older adults. Melena and anemia can be seen in tumors that are bleeding. A rare subset of patients may have systemic manifestations of gastric cancer. These paraneoplastic syndromes include Leser-Trelat sign, which is characterized by sudden onset

of multiple seborrheic keratoses, and acanthosis nigricans, which appears as dark pigmentation in skin folds. However, these manifestations are not specific to gastric cancer and are benign processes in the majority of patients.

Diagnosis

Esophagogastroduodenoscopy (EGD) with biopsy is the gold standard for gastric cancer diagnosis. This allows for tissue diagnosis as well as anatomic location of the primary tumor. Of note, per the American Joint Committee on Cancer (AJCC) and the Union for International Cancer Control (UICC) Tumor, Nodes, Metastases (TNM) classification, eighth edition, esophagogastric junction tumors with epicenter less than 2 cm into the proximal stomach are classified as esophageal cancers; those more than 2 cm into the stomach are staged as gastric cancers. Gastric adenocarcinomas usually appear as friable ulcerated masses endoscopically. However, it should be noted that the gastric mucosa can appear normal in linitis plastica (an aggressive form of diffuse-type adenocarcinoma), with the only endoscopic finding being poor stomach distensibility. Deep biopsies beyond the superficial mucosa must be obtained to evaluate for these lesions. Any suspicious lesion should have multiple biopsies taken to improve the diagnostic yield. For example, a single biopsy has a 70% sensitivity for diagnosis compared with 98% with seven biopsies. For this reason, six to eight biopsies are recommended for each suspicious lesion.

For lesions under 2 cm in size, endoscopic mucosal resection (EMR) or endoscopic submucosal dissection (ESD) can be considered in experienced hands, which can be both diagnostic and therapeutic depending on the pathology of the specimen. The pathology report of the biopsy should include presence of invasion, histologic subtype (intestinal or diffuse), and tumor grade. Unfortunately, in the United States the vast majority of tumors present at later stages of disease.

Staging

Once adenocarcinoma is diagnosed on endoscopic biopsy, patients should undergo computed tomography (CT) of the chest, abdomen, and pelvis to evaluate for regional and metastatic disease. Suspicious lesions in the common sites of metastatic disease such as the liver and lung should be biopsied for tissue confirmation. Ascitic fluid may be sampled by paracentesis and sent for cytologic and chemical analysis. Involvement of abdominal lymph nodes outside the standard lymphadenectomy resection (i.e., pancreatoduodenal, peripancreatic, middle colic, para-aortic) are classified as distant metastasis.

In patients without evidence of metastatic disease on CT, endoscopic ultrasound (EUS) is recommended to assess the T stage. EUS can also identify enlarged nearby lymph nodes, which can be biopsied using fine needle aspiration (FNA). If there is high clinical suspicion of metastasis but initial CT is unrevealing, integrated positron emission tomography (PET)/CT may be considered. Diagnostic staging laparoscopy may also be useful in detecting occult disease in patients with tumor invasion beyond the submucosa or in whom neoadjuvant therapy is being considered. Staging laparoscopy is superior to cross-sectional imaging for identifying peritoneal spread and allows for peritoneal fluid sampling for cytologic analysis. A complete blood count and comprehensive metabolic profile should be obtained to evaluate for anemia and electrolyte derangements.

The most recent AJCC/UICC TNM staging classifications were published in 2017. An important update in the new classification system is separate staging for patients with and without neoadjuvant therapy. Early gastric adenocarcinoma is defined as cancers that do not invade past the submucosa (T1); T1a involves the mucosa and T1b involves the submucosa. T2 tumors involve the muscularis propria, T3 penetrate to the subserosa, and T4 invade beyond the serosa (T4a) or invade adjacent structures (T4b). Regional nodal classification is N1 for 1 to 2 lymph node metastases, N2 for 3 to 6 nodes, N3a for 7 to 15, and N3b for 16 or more involved nodes. M1 stage indicates presence of metastatic disease.

Treatment

It is recommended that treatment decisions for all patients diagnosed with gastric cancer be discussed by a multidisciplinary team including medical oncology, radiation oncology, surgical oncology, gastroenterology, radiology, and pathology. Complete surgical resection of the cancer and adjacent lymph nodes offers the best opportunity for long-term survival when possible. Indicators of surgical unresectability include presence of metastatic disease, involvement of a major vascular structure such as the aorta, or encasement of the celiac axis, hepatic artery, or proximal splenic artery. It should be noted that involvement of the distal splenic artery can still represent resectable disease.

Patients with either tumor in situ (Tis) or T1a disease (tumor that does not invade past the submucosa) may be candidates for either endoscopic or surgical resection. Patients with T1b cancers (tumor that invades submucosa) should undergo upfront surgical resection. Patients with T2 or higher disease or any nodal involvement are recommended to undergo perioperative chemotherapy. Radiation therapy can be considered, especially in cases of locally advanced disease. Patients that are not candidates for curative surgical resection or with metastatic disease should be considered for palliative treatment in addition to systemic chemotherapy.

Surgery

Endoscopic resection with either EMR or ESD can be considered adequate therapy for gastric cancer less than 2 cm in size that (1) is well or moderately differentiated, (2) does not penetrate past the submucosa, and (3) does not have evidence of lymphovascular invasion.

Surgical resection typically consists of either a distal/subtotal or total gastrectomy depending on where the tumor is located. Tumors in the proximal third of the stomach typically require total gastrectomy while in the distal two-thirds a subtotal distal gastrectomy can be performed. There is no survival difference between total and distal gastrectomy for distal tumors, and the quality of life in patients has been shown to be superior with partial gastrectomy when possible oncologically. Patients undergoing surgery should be considered for a diagnostic laparoscopy to detect the possible presence of occult metastatic disease prior to committing to curative surgery. A 5 cm proximal margin should be obtained with at least a 2 cm distal margin on the duodenum. T4 tumors require en bloc resection of nearby involved organs or structures. Retrieval of at least 15 lymph nodes is necessary for accurate nodal staging.

The appropriate extent of lymphadenectomy for gastric cancer is debated. While D1 lymphadenectomy involves removal of the perigastric lymph nodes alone, D2 lymphadenectomy involves additional removal of lymph nodes around the left gastric, common hepatic, celiac, and splenic arteries. It is unclear if D2 lymphadenectomy provides an overall survival benefit, with most randomized trials not demonstrating a significant difference between D1 and D2 lymphadenectomy. However, in experienced hands, the additional D2 lymph nodes can provide improved staging information with a minimal increase in morbidity and is now what is typically performed in high-volume cancer centers. D3 lymphadenectomy (para-aortic lymph nodes), however, is associated with increased morbidity and is not presently recommended.

In cases that require reconstruction after a distal gastrectomy, options include Roux-en-Y gastrojejunostomy, Billroth I, and Billroth II. Reconstruction after total gastrectomy is performed with a Roux-en-Y esophagojejunostomy. Placement of a jejunal feeding tube should be considered at time of operation, especially if a patient is likely to receive adjuvant chemoradiation and/or their nutritional status is poor, though their use is not standardized.

Chemotherapy

The utility of chemotherapy in gastric adenocarcinoma has been established in multiple randomized trials. The first major trial (MAGIC) randomized 503 patients with resectable adenocarcinoma of the stomach, gastroesophageal junction, or lower esophagus to surgery alone versus surgery with perioperative

ECF (epirubicin [Ellence],[1] cisplatin,[1] and fluorouracil). Chemotherapy consisted of three preoperative and three postoperative cycles. Perioperative ECF resulted in improved 5-year overall survival (36% compared with 23% for patients who received surgery alone). More recently, a randomized phase II/III trial of 716 patients with resectable stage II or III gastric or gastroesophageal junction adenocarcinomas was conducted to compare perioperative ECF and perioperative FLOT (fluorouracil, leucovorin,[1] oxaliplatin,[1] and docetaxel [Taxotere]). Survival was significantly improved with FLOT, with median overall survival of 50 months compared with 35 months with ECF.

In patients who are medically fit and thereby recommended to receive perioperative chemotherapy, the FLOT regimen is recommended. Patients unable to tolerate this more aggressive chemotherapy regimen may undergo treatment with a fluoropyrimidine and oxaliplatin[1] or fluorouracil and cisplatin.[1] The ECF regimen (epirubicin,[1] cisplatin,[1] and fluorouracil) is no longer first-line therapy.

For patients who do not receive neoadjuvant therapy, treatment recommendations are guided by the pathologic tumor classification, operative margins, and extent of lymphadenectomy. Those whose final surgical pathology reveals T3, T4, or any N positive disease should be offered adjuvant chemotherapy. Those with T2N0 disease may be offered either adjuvant chemotherapy or surveillance. All patients with positive operative margins should receive adjuvant chemoradiation. Adjuvant chemotherapy is fluoropyrimidine-based. In patients who received less than a D2 lymphadenectomy, fluorouracil or capecitabine (Xeloda)[1] is recommended before and after fluoropyrimidine-based regimens. For patients that did have a D2 lymphadenectomy, oxaliplatin[1] and fluorouracil or capecitabine[1] is recommended.

Immunotherapy

There are currently ongoing preclinical and early clinical phase trials of various immunotherapy agents in the treatment of gastric adenocarcinoma. However, their use remains investigational at this time.

Radiotherapy

The benefits and indications for radiotherapy are less well established for noncardia gastric adenocarcinoma. There are currently no randomized trials comparing adjuvant chemoradiotherapy to either surgery alone or surgery and chemotherapy. Preoperative chemoradiotherapy is beneficial in patients with esophageal, gastroesophageal junction, and gastric cardia tumors as shown in the CROSS trial, but its role specifically in gastric cancer is less clear. Radiotherapy can be considered as an adjunct in multidisciplinary discussions for patients with locally advanced disease.

Palliation

The most common indications for palliative procedures in gastric cancer are gastric outlet obstruction, bleeding, and perforation. Choosing among the various palliative options with consideration of the risks and benefits specific to each patient's case as well as the patient's goals of care. For patients with an obstructing tumor, especially in the prepyloric or antral regions, surgical or endoscopic interventions may be beneficial. For a patient whose life expectancy is greater than 6 months and who is medically fit, surgical gastrojejunostomy may be preferred if technically feasible in either an open or laparoscopic fashion. If the patient is not a surgical candidate, endoscopic stent placement or endoscopic gastrojejunostomy may be considered. Finally, a venting gastrostomy tube is another alternative. However, the patient will no longer be able to eat if this is the only therapy offered, and a feeding jejunostomy tube must be considered for enteral nutrition.

Patients who present with uncontrollable bleeding may initially undergo endoscopic treatment, but this is associated with a high

---

[1]Not FDA approved for this indication.

likelihood of recurrent bleeding. Angiographic embolization or radiation therapy are potential alternatives. If these more conservative measures are unsuccessful, palliative resection should be considered. Should a patient pursue operative intervention, lymph node dissection is not required. If patients present with gastric perforation and surgery is within the patient's goals of care, urgent palliative resection may be attempted.

Monitoring

Patients successfully treated with endoscopic resection should undergo a thorough history and physical examination every 3 to 6 months after treatment for the first 1 to 2 years, then every 6 to 12 months for 3 to 5 years, followed by annual follow-up thereafter. EGD should be performed every 6 months for 1 year and then annually for up to 5 years. CT scans should be performed as clinically indicated by symptoms.

Patients with stage I disease treated by surgery should undergo a history and physical every 3 to 6 months after treatment for 1 to 2 years, then every 6 to 12 months for 3 to 5 years, followed by annual follow-up thereafter. They should have EGD and/or CT scans as clinically indicated by symptoms. These patients must additionally be monitored for nutritional deficiencies, especially involving B12 and iron.

Patients with stage II or III disease who received surgery should undergo history and physical every 3 to 6 months after treatment for 1 to 2 years, then every 6 to 12 months for 3 to 5 years, followed by annual follow-up thereafter. EGD may be performed as clinically indicated. CT of the chest/abdomen/pelvis should be performed every 6 to 12 months for the first 2 years and then annually up to 5 years. PET/CT should be considered as clinically indicated when suspicion for disease recurrence and/or metastasis is high. These patients must also be monitored for nutritional deficiencies.

Complications

In the early postoperative period, patients can develop peritonitis from an anastomotic leak or duodenal stump perforation. Bowel obstructions can also develop. It should be noted that acute afferent limb obstruction in patients that had a Billroth II reconstruction should be treated differently than other small bowel obstructions in that they typically require immediate operative intervention with either surgical revision of the gastrojejunostomy, conversion to a Roux-en-Y anastomosis, or a Braun's enteroenterostomy.

Clinically significant dumping syndrome is seen in approximately 20% of patients after distal gastrectomy. Early dumping, which occurs within an hour of eating, is associated with abdominal pain, cramping, nausea, diaphoresis, palpitations, and flushing. Late dumping occurs hours after eating and is due to hypoglycemia after the postprandial insulin peak. Most patients can be managed conservatively with small, frequent meals and avoidance of exacerbating foods. Octreotide (Sandostatin)[1] can be a useful adjunct in patients with persistent symptoms. Rarely, surgical revision to a Roux-en-Y gastrojejunostomy is required.

Gastrointestinal Stromal Tumors

Gastrointestinal stromal tumors (GISTs) are mesenchymal subepithelial neoplasms. The incidence of GIST is 7 to 15 cases per million and the most common tumor location is the stomach. GISTs account for 1% to 3% of stomach neoplasms. GISTs are thought to arise from the interstitial cells of Cajal and are identified histologically by their overexpression of CD117 (KIT). The most common presenting symptom is gastrointestinal bleeding, occurring in approximately 50% of gastric GISTs. Preoperative endoscopic biopsy is not necessary if there is a high suspicion for GIST based on endoscopic submucosal lesion appearance and it is resectable; biopsy should be performed if there is diagnostic uncertainty, if there is concern for metastatic disease, or if neoadjuvant imatinib is being considered. The prognosis for GISTs

has greatly improved after the discovery of imatinib, a receptor tyrosine kinase inhibitor that specifically targets c-KIT.

Surgery is the only curative option for patients with gastric GIST. All GISTs >2 cm should be considered for resection. Grossly negative margins are sufficient and no lymphadenectomy is required given the very low rates of lymph node metastases in these tumors. Care should be taken to preserve the tumor capsule as intraoperative rupture increases the risk of recurrence. Neoadjuvant imatinib (Gleevec) can be considered in patients with locally advanced or borderline resectable disease or in whom preoperative tumor shrinkage would potentially reduce surgical morbidity.

Imatinib is an oral medication taken at a dose of 400 mg daily. Adjuvant imatinib should be offered to patients with high risk of recurrence, specifically either primary tumor >5 cm in size and/or mitotic rate >5 per 50 high-powered field. The phase III ACOSOG Z9001 established the significant improvement in recurrence-free survival with 1 year of adjuvant therapy compared with placebo (98% vs. 83% at 1 year, $P < 0.0001$). Further, the Scandinavian Sarcoma Group XVIII phase III trial showed that 3 years of adjuvant imatinib was superior to 1 year in both recurrence-free (65.6% vs. 47.9% at 5 years) and overall survival (92.0% vs. 81.7% at 5 years). However, recurrences are not uncommon after discontinuation of imatinib, and further studies are ongoing to establish if a longer regimen may be more beneficial. For tumors resistant to imatinib, second-line therapy is sunitinib (Sutent), another tyrosine kinase inhibitor. Traditional chemotherapy and HIPEC are not standardly used now after the advent of tyrosine kinase inhibitor therapy.

Neuroendocrine Tumors

Gastric neuroendocrine tumors (gNETs) arise from enterochromaffin-like cells and were previously referred to as carcinoid tumors. The incidence of gNETs has increased 15-fold from 1973 through 2012 due to increased awareness of the disease, increased number of upper endoscopies, and possibly the increased use of PPIs. There are three distinct subtypes of gNET. Type 1 is the most common (70%–80%) and are associated with pernicious anemia and atrophic gastritis. Type 2 accounts for 5% to 10% and are associated with Zollinger-Ellison syndrome and multiple endocrine neoplasia type 1. Type 3 have normal gastrin and stomach acid levels, are solitary lesions, and are more aggressive and tend to metastasize. Neuroendocrine carcinomas are sometimes referred to as type 4 lesions and are poorly differentiated tumors that behave similar to gastric adenocarcinoma.

Upper endoscopy and biopsy are indicated for diagnosis. The mitotic rate and Ki-67 proliferation index should be measured from the specimen to allow for tumor grading. Patients with type 3 gNETs or with worrisome features (size >2 cm, high grade) should undergo multiphasic abdominal CT or MRI for staging.

Type 1 gNETs less than 1 cm can undergo endoscopic resection or surveillance. If greater than 1 cm in size, not high grade, and EUS shows no invasion beyond the submucosa, endoscopic resection can be performed. If poorly differentiated, invasion beyond the submucosa, or positive margins after endoscopic resection, surgical resection should be performed. If there is persistent or recurrent disease after surgery, an antrectomy can be considered. For type 2 tumors, gastrinoma resection or high-dose PPI should be initiated. If tumor size is under 2 cm without worrisome features on biopsy, endoscopic resection can be performed; otherwise surgical resection is recommended. Type 3 tumors, given their more aggressive behavior, should undergo anatomic surgical resection with lymphadenectomy.

If there is metastatic disease to the liver, carcinoid syndrome can occur. Surgical cytoreduction or liver-directed therapies can be offered. The most common systemic therapy utilizes somatostatin analogs (octreotide [Sandostatin] or lanreotide [Somatuline Depot]). If there is disease progression on somatostatin therapy, cytotoxic chemotherapy (i.e., etoposide [Toposar][1] with carboplatin [Paraplatin][1] or cisplatin[1]), everolimus (Afinitor), or interferon-alpha (Intron A)[1] can be given as second-line agents. Peptide

---

receptor radionuclide therapy (PRRT) delivers radiation therapy via binding of the somatostatin receptor by 177-Lu-Dotatate and may be considered in locally advanced or metastatic gNET.

Gastric Lymphomas

The stomach is the most common extranodal site of lymphoma. Gastric lymphoma accounts for approximately 3% of gastric malignancies and 10% of lymphomas. The most common presenting symptom is epigastric pain, followed by anorexia, weight loss, nausea, and bleeding. Fever and night sweats are seen in 12% of patients. Diagnosis is established by endoscopic biopsy. The two most common subtypes in the stomach are diffuse large B-cell lymphoma and marginal zone B-cell lymphoma of mucosa-associated lymphoid tissue (MALT). MALT lymphomas of the stomach often respond to *H. pylori* eradication. Patients with persistent or recurrent disease can undergo radiotherapy or chemotherapy. Surgery is only indicated in patients with complications from their disease such as significant bleeding or perforation.

---

[1]Not FDA approved for this indication.

References

Al-Batran SE, Homann N, Pauligk C, et al: Perioperative chemotherapy with fluorouracil plus leucovorin, oxaliplatin, and docetaxel versus fluorouracil or capecitabine plus cisplatin and epirubicin for locally advanced, resectable gastric or gastro-oesophageal junction adenocarcinoma (FLOT4): a randomised, phase 2/3 trial, *Lancet* 393(10184):1948–1957, 2019.

Corey B, Chen H: Neuroendocrine tumors of the stomach, *Surg Clin North Am* 97:333–343, 2017.

Cunningham D, Allum WH, Stenning SP, et al: Perioperative chemotherapy versus surgery alone for resectable gastroesophageal cancer, *N Engl J Med* 355:11–20, 2006.

DeMatteo RP, Ballman KV, Antonescu CR, et al: Placebo-controlled randomized trial of adjuvant imatinib mesylate following the resection of localized, primary gastrointestinal stromal tumor (GIST), *Lancet* 373(9669):1097–1104, 2009.

Hu Q, Zhang Y, Zhang X, Fu K: Gastric mucosa-associated lymphoid tissue lymphoma and *Helicobacter pylori* infection: a review of current diagnosis and management, *Biomark Res* 4:15, 2016.

Joensuu H, Eriksson M, Sundby Hall K, et al: One vs three years of adjuvant imatinib for operable gastrointestinal stromal tumor: a randomized trial, *JAMA* 307(12):1265–1272, 2012.

Noh SH, Park SR, Yang HK, et al: Adjuvant capecitabine plus oxaliplatin for gastric cancer after D2 gastrectomy (CLASSIC): 5-year follow-up of an open-label, randomised phase 3 trial, *Lancet Oncol* 15(12):1389–1396, 2014.

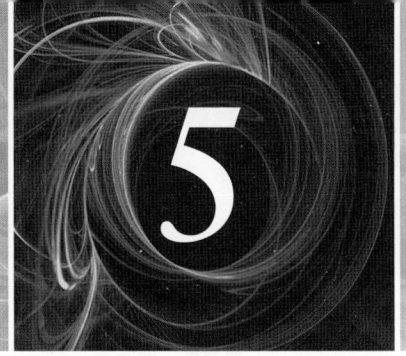

5

Endocrine and Metabolic Disorders

ACROMEGALY

Method of
Moises Mercado, MD

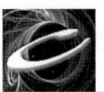

CURRENT DIAGNOSIS

Clinical
- Headaches, visual field defects
- Coarse features, increased size of hands (rings) and feet (shoes)
- Thick, oily skin, skin tags, acanthosis nigricans
- Arthralgias, osteoarthritis
- Paresthesias, carpal tunnel syndrome
- Hypertension, arrhythmia, heart failure
- Glucose intolerance, diabetes, hypertriglyceridemia
- Snoring, sleep apnea
- Risk of colon polyps or colon cancer
- Risk of thyroid cancer

Biochemical
- Glucose-suppressed growth hormone >0.4 ng/mL by ultrasensitive assays or >1 ng/mL by old radioimmunoassays
- Elevated age-adjusted insulin-like growth factor 1

Imaging
- Magnetic resonance imaging

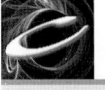

CURRENT THERAPY

- If a pituitary surgeon is available: Transsphenoidal surgery for microadenomas, intrasellar macroadenomas, and debulking or decompressing surgery in invasive macroadenomas
- Depot Somatostatin analogues (lanreotide autogel [Somatuline Depot] or octreotide LAR [Sandostatin LAR Depot]) as secondary treatment for patients failing surgery or waiting for radiotherapy effect to occur and as a primary treatment for patients with inaccessible lesions, contraindications for surgery, or preference
- Dopamine agonists: Cabergoline (DOSTINEX)[1] is effective alone or in combination with somatostatin analogues in 15% to 30% of patients
- Growth hormone receptor antagonists: Pegvisomant (Somavert) for patients resistant or intolerant to somatostatin analogues and who have tumors >5 mm from the optic chiasm
- Radiotherapy for patients resistant or intolerant to pharmacologic therapy, with clinically and biochemically active disease and a tumor remnant on MRI

[1]Not FDA approved for this indication.

Acromegaly is a disorder resulting from an excessive secretion of growth hormone (GH), with a prevalence of 40 to 60 cases per million and an annual incidence of 3 to 4 per million.

Physiology, Biochemistry, and Regulation of the GH/IGF-1 Axis

GH secretion is regulated at the hypothalamus (Figure 1). The pulsatile secretion of GH-releasing hormone (GHRH) stimulates somatotroph proliferation and GH gene transcription, whereas somatostatin, which is secreted tonically, inhibits GH synthesis. These two hypothalamic signals result in the pulsatile secretion of pituitary GH, with most pulses occurring during the night. GH is also stimulated by ghrelin, a hypothalamic and gastrointestinal orexigenic hormone that binds specific receptors in the somatotroph known as GH-secretagogue receptors. GH exerts its actions through a specific membrane receptor located predominantly in the liver and cartilage, but ubiquitously present in all tissues. One molecule of GH interacts with two molecules of GH receptor, resulting in functional dimerization and conformational changes that lead to the phosphorylation of several kinases and eventually the interaction with target genes such as the insulin-like growth factor (IGF)-1 gene.

IGF-1 is closely related to proinsulin and circulates in plasma bound to six binding proteins (IGFBPs) that are synthesized and released by the liver. IGFBP3 is the most important of these binding proteins and is also GH dependent; it forms a heterotrimeric complex composed of BP3, IGF-1, and the acid-labile subunit (ALS). IGF-1 is responsible for most of the trophic and growth-promoting effects of GH. Blood levels of IGF-1 are increased during puberty, coinciding with the acceleration of somatic growth, and decline with aging. Malnutrition, poorly controlled type 1 diabetes, hypothyroidism, and liver failure all result in diminished IGF-1 concentrations. IGF-1 is the main player in GH negative feedback regulation and it acts at both the pituitary and the hypothalamic levels. Glucose regulates GH release by increasing (hyperglycemia) or decreasing (hypoglycemia) somatostatin synthesis in the hypothalamus. Exercise and amino acids such as arginine also stimulate GH secretion.

Etiopathogenesis of Growth Hormone–Secreting Tumors

The molecular pathogenesis of pituitary tumors includes the inactivation of tumor suppressor genes, the activation of oncogenes, and the trophic effect of factors such as the hypothalamic releasing hormones. Approximately 40% of GH-producing tumors in whites harbor somatic point mutations of the α subunit stimulatory G protein coupled to the GHRH receptor (GSPα mutations). This molecular alteration causes constitutive activation of the GHRH receptor, resulting in an increased transcription of the GH gene and the promotion of somatotroph proliferation. Acromegalic patients whose tumors harbor GSPα mutations usually have a more benign clinical course and appear to be more susceptible to management with somatostatin analogues. Nonwhite acromegalic populations, including persons of Japanese, Korean, and Mexican heritage, have a much lower prevalence of GSPα mutations.

Other molecular events should be present in GSPα-negative somatotrophinomas. Menin is a protein encoded by a tumor

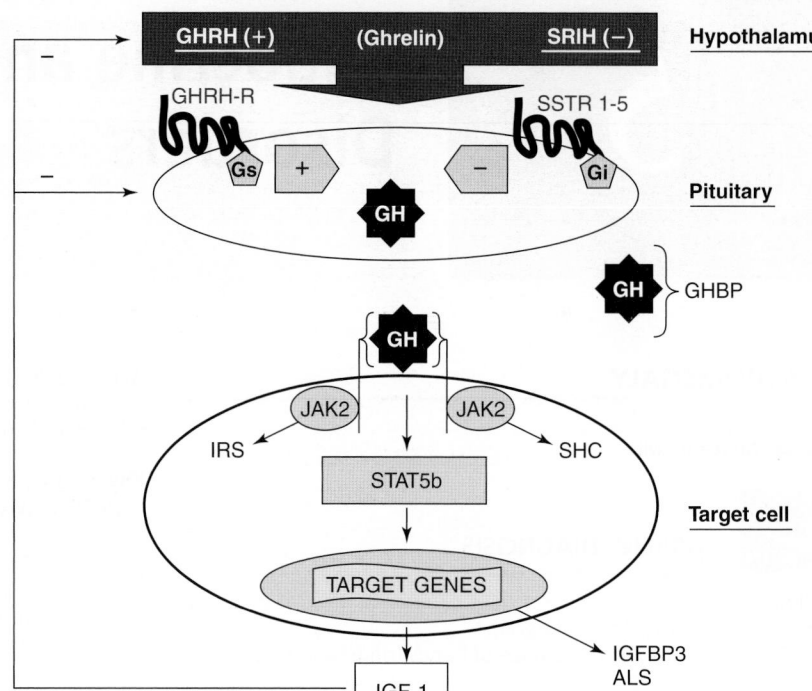

Figure 1 GH is regulated positively by GHRH and negatively by somatostatin. Fifty percent of circulating GH is bound to the GH binding protein, which represents the extracellular portion of the GH receptor. One molecule of GH dimerizes two molecules of GH receptor, and the ensuing signal transduction results in IGF-1 synthesis and secretion, which exerts negative feedback on GH secretion at the hypothalamic and pituitary levels. *Abbreviations:* ALS = acid-labile subunit; GH = growth hormone; GHRH = growth hormone–releasing hormone; IGF = insulin-like growth factor; IGFBP3 = insulin-like growth factor binding protein 3; IRS = insulin receptor S; JAK2 = Janus kinase 2; SRIH = somatostatin; SSTR = somatostatin receptor.

suppressor gene located on the short arm of chromosome 11. Inactivating mutations of menin are the molecular basis of type 1 multiple endocrine neoplasia (MEN1); however, GH-secreting tumors occurring out of this context do not have such genetic abnormalities. Inactivating mutations of other putative tumor-suppressor genes located relatively close to the menin locus have been described in several kindreds with familial acromegaly; however, they do not seem to play an important oncogenic role in the sporadic form of the disease. Other genetic alterations such as underexpression of GADD 45γ (growth arrest and DNA damage-inducible protein) and overexpression of the securing molecule PTTG (pituitary tumor transforming gene) have also been shown to be involved in the molecular pathogenesis of acromegaly. Although hereditary acromegaly is rare (less than 2% of the cases), familial somatotrophinomas account for 30% of the tumors seen in the syndrome of familial isolated pituitary adenomas. Patients with isolated familial somatotrophinomas are younger and usually have more aggressive tumors than subjects with sporadic acromegaly. Affected members do not show any molecular alterations in the MEN1 gene. However, 15% of 73 tested families harbor inactivating, germline mutations of the AIP (aryl hydrocarbon interacting protein) gene located on chromosome 11q13.3.

In more than 90% of cases, acromegaly is caused by a sporadic pituitary adenoma. In approximately 70% of these patients, these benign epithelial neoplasms are larger than 1 cm in diameter and are known as *macroadenomas*, whereas one-third of the patients harbor lesions smaller than 1 cm or *microadenomas*. One-third of the patients have tumors that cosecrete GH and prolactin (PRL) (mammosomatoroph cell adenomas). Real pituitary GH-secreting carcinomas, with documented metastasis as the irrefutable malignancy criterion, are exceedingly rare. On rare occasions, acromegaly results from GHRH-secreting neuroendocrine tumors, usually located in the lungs, thymus, or endocrine pancreas. In this scenario, the ectopically produced GHRH leads to hyperplasia of the somatotroph, with the consequent excessive production of GH. Even less common are GH-secreting tumors arising in ectopic pituitary tissue, usually located in the sphenoid sinus. A case of GH-secreting lymphoma has been reported.

Clinical Manifestations

Acromegaly develops insidiously over many years. An 8- to 10-year delay in diagnosis has been estimated from the beginning of

the first symptom. Clinical characteristics are often attributed to aging. Symptoms and signs can be divided into those resulting from the compressive effects of the pituitary tumor and those that are a consequence of the GH and IGF-1 excess.

Local Tumor Effects

Headache results from an increase in intracranial pressure and from the effects of GH itself; it is usually described as a dull pain that persists throughout the day. Occasionally, large tumors invading laterally into the cavernous sinuses give rise to cranial nerve syndromes, usually third and sixth. Visual field defects are relatively common with macroadenomas extending superiorly and compressing the optic chiasm. This usually results in different combinations of bitemporal homonymous hemianopia or quadrontopia.

Consequences of the GH/IGF-1 Excess
Skeletal Growth and Skin Changes

A GH excess developing before the pubertal closure of epiphyseal bone leads to an acceleration of linear growth, and this results in gigantism. Once the patient is in adulthood, the GH/IGF-1 excess results in acral enlargement, which is manifested by increases in ring and shoe sizes as well as enlargement of the nose, supracilliary arches, frontal bones, and mandible (Figure 2). There is thickening of soft tissues of the hands and feet; hands are fleshy and bulky and the heel pad is increased. The skin is thickened due to the deposition of glycosaminoglycans and excessive collagen production. Hyperhidrosis and seborrhea occur in 60% of patients; skin tags (previously associated with colon cancer) and acanthosis nigricans are common.

Musculoskeletal System

Generalized arthralgias are present in the majority (80%) of patients. Degenerative osteoarthritis is more common than in the general population. Paresthesias of the hands and feet and a proximal painful myopathy are often reported. Nerve entrapment syndromes such as the carpal tunnel syndrome occur in nearly half of patients.

Cardiovascular System

Arterial hypertension is found in 30% of patients, and when associated with diabetes, it contributes to the increased mortality rate of the disease. Hyperaldosteronism with low renin levels and the resulting sodium retention play an important role in the pathogenesis of

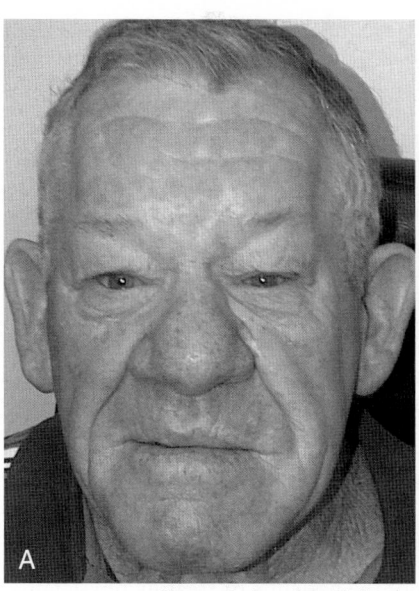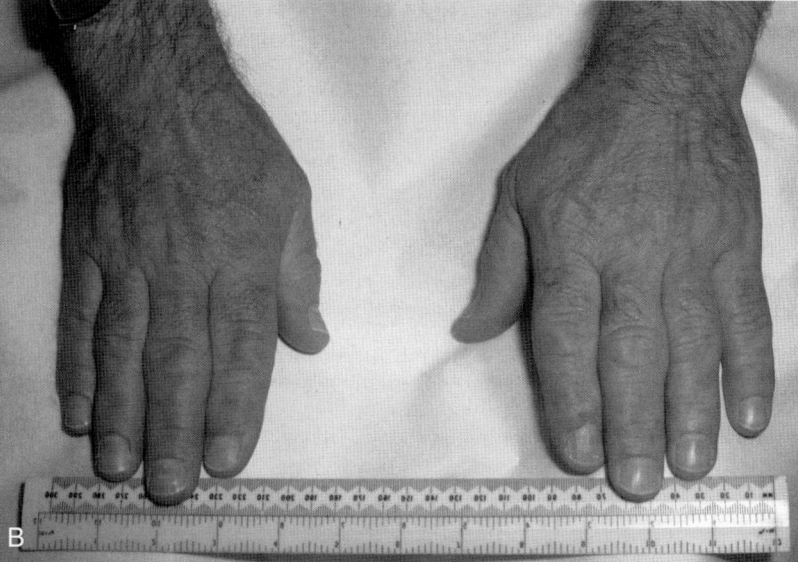

Figure 2 A and B, Skeletal growth and skin changes in acromegaly. (From Salmon JF: *Kanski's Clinical Ophthalmology,* 9th edition. Elsevier, 2020.)

hypertension, but other contributors such as an increased sympathetic tone are also present. Echocardiographic findings include left ventricular and septal hypertrophy with varying degrees of diastolic dysfunction. Symptomatic cardiac disease develops in 15% of patients and is usually due to coronary artery disease, heart failure, and arrhythmias. Although the existence of an acromegalic cardiomyopathy is still controversial, there are patients without hypertension and with angiographically normal coronaries, who develop severe congestive heart failure, in whom histologic evidence of subendocardial, subepicardial, and myocardial fibrosis and necrosis has been documented.

Respiratory Abnormalities
The majority of patients with acromegaly are affected by loud snoring. A significant fraction of these have sleep apnea (with both central and obstructive components) with significant drops in oxygen saturation, which can be complicated by arrhythmias, daytime somnolence, and chronic fatigue.

Abnormalities in Glucose Metabolism
Chronic GH hypersecretion creates a state of insulin resistance, and glucose intolerance has been reported in 30% to 50% of patients with acromegaly; the percentage with fasting hyperglycemia can be close to 30%, depending on the population. Hyperglycemia has correlated with GH concentrations in some studies and with IGF-1 levels in others. Although successful treatment of acromegaly, be it by surgical, pharmacological, or radiotherapeutical interventions, results in significant improvements in metabolic control, the prevalence of diabetes remains higher than in the general population.

Abnormalities in Lipid Metabolism
The classic lipid profile consists of diminished total cholesterol, along with elevated triglyceride concentrations. Intermediate-density lipoprotein (IDL) particles and lipoprotein(a) might also be elevated, and there is a higher percentage of the more atherogenic type II low-density lipoprotein (LDL).

Bone and Calcium Metabolism
Acromegaly is associated with hypercalciuria and hyperphosphatemia. High serum 25-hydroxyvitamin D_3 and urinary levels of hydroxyproline can be found, reflecting a state of increased bone turnover. Cortical bone mineral density is elevated, whereas trabecular bone mass is diminished.

Neoplasia
Retrospective studies suggested that colonic adenomatous polyps and adenocarcinoma were more frequent in acromegalic patients than in the general population. Prospective studies have demonstrated that the risk, albeit smaller than previously thought, is real and probably justifies screening colonoscopy in these patients. Patients with uncontrolled acromegaly have a higher risk of recurrence of premalignant polyps and a higher mortality rate from colon cancer compared with subjects with biochemically controlled disease and the general population. Recently, an increased incidence of well-differentiated thyroid carcinoma has been documented.

Associated Endocrine Abnormalities
A euthyroid goiter is often found but seldom requires specific treatment. Hypopituitarism occurs variably, depending on the size and extension of the tumor and whether the patient has undergone surgery or radiation therapy. Hypogonadotropic hypogonadism is the most common pituitary deficiency, occurring in 20% of patients. A decreased libido is a common presenting complaint in both male and female patients with acromegaly; women often have menstrual and ovulatory disturbances and men complain of impotence.

Although an elevated PRL is common, it does not always reflect cosecretion of this hormone by the somatotrophinoma, but rather an interruption of the descending dopaminergic tone by the tumor compressing the pituitary stalk. Central hypocortisolism and hypothyroidism are less common.

GH-secreting pituitary adenomas are the second, after prolactinomas, pituitary tumor occurring in the context of MEN1 (multiple parathyroid adenomas, pituitary adenoma, and pancreatic islet cell tumors). Acromegaly can also develop in patients with the McCune-Albright syndrome (polyostotic fibrous dysplasia, café au lait spots, and endocrinopathies such as sexual precocity and autonomous thyroid nodules), and occurs in the context of the Carney complex.

Mortality
Life expectancy in patients with acromegaly is decreased by about 10 to 15 years, and the standardized mortality ratio is 1.5 to 2. Most patients die of cardiovascular causes, followed by cerebrovascular events, respiratory abnormalities, and neoplastic diseases. Hormonal control has a definite impact on survival. Lowering serum GH to less than 2.5 ng/mL results in reduction of the mortality rate to levels comparable with the general population. These safe GH levels were obtained using old radioimmunoassays, and there are no equivalent studies using ultrasensitive GH assays. IGF-1 levels have not been as good as GH as independent predictors of mortality.

Other factors associated with an increased mortality include advanced age and the presence of hypertension and diabetes. Mortality rate in acromegaly can be reduced to that seen on the general population when patients are treated using a multidisciplinary approach not only aiming at controlling the GH and IGF-1 levels but also focusing on the management of comorbidities.

Biochemical Diagnosis

Due to the pulsatile nature of GH secretion, random determinations of this hormone are not useful in the diagnosis of acromegaly. The gold standard for the diagnosis is the measurement of GH after an oral glucose load of 75 g; current guidelines state that suppression to less than 0.4 ng/mL (using ultrasensitive assays) reliably excludes the diagnosis. Situations associated with decreased suppression of GH by glucose include puberty, pregnancy, use of oral contraceptives, uncontrolled diabetes, and renal and hepatic insufficiency.

IGF-1 levels reflect the integrated concentrations over 24 hours of GH and correlate well with clinical activity. Blood IGF-1 concentrations decrease with age, reflecting the parallel decline of the somatotropic axis. There is a gender difference in IGF-1 (premenopausal women have lower levels than age-matched male subjects). Other conditions that lower IGF-1 levels include malnutrition, uncontrolled diabetes, and hepatic and renal failure. Normal ranges for IGF-1 should be established in each particular center based on age. The determination of other GH-dependent peptides such as IGFBP3 and ALS has not proved to be superior to IGF-1.

Imaging

Pituitary magnetic resonance imaging (MRI) with gadolinium enhancement allows visualization of lesions as small as 2 or 3 mm in diameter. High-resolution computed tomography (CT) is a reasonable alternative, although it is much less sensitive. An ectopic source of GHRH should be suspected when the MRI is completely normal. In these rare cases, serum GHRH should be measured and the ectopic tumor should be sought, usually with high-resolution CT of the chest and abdomen.

Treatment

The decision as to what therapeutic modality should be used has to take into account medical issues (cardiopulmonary comorbidities, size, and extension of the tumor) as well as the local characteristics of the treating center. The latter refers to the availability of pituitary surgeons and radiotherapeutic technologies as well as the economic feasibility of pharmacologic therapy.

Surgery

Transsphenoidal surgery has been the traditional treatment for acromegaly and achieves biochemical cure (achievement of a post-glucose GH <1 ng/mL and normalization of IGF-1) in 80% to 90% of microadenomas. According to the latest published acromegaly consensus, biochemical cure is defined as a glucose-suppressed GH of 0.4 ng/mL as well as a normal age-adjusted IGF-1. Cure rates for macroadenomas are much lower (40%–50%), and invasive lesions have a very slight chance (<10%) of being cured by surgery. Even though surgery often fails to achieve a full biochemical cure, debulking the pituitary adenoma relieves optic chiasm compression and can result in a sufficient decrement of tumor mass (and therefore of GH production) to allow better results with either pharmacologic or radiotherapeutic regimens.

Pharmacologic Therapy

Somatostatin analogues are the most commonly used medical treatment for acromegaly. Somatostatin inhibits GH secretion and somatotroph cell growth via its interaction with five different somatostatin receptor (SSTR) subtypes. The development of long-acting somatostatin analogues such as octreotide (Sandostatin) and lanreotide (Somatuline) overcame the pharmacologic difficulties of native somatostatin (short half-life, rebound GH secretion, and need for IV administration) and resulted in a more potent inhibition of GH secretion. The most commonly used preparations are intramuscular octreotide LAR (long-acting repeatable) (Sandostatin LAR Depot) and subcutaneous lanreotide autogel (Somatuline Depot), which are administered every 4 weeks. Doses of octreotide-LAR range from 10 to 40 mg and those of lanreotide autogel from 60 to 120 mg, both administered every 4 weeks, although in specific patients the interval of injection can be increased to every 6 or even 8 weeks, thus diminishing the cost of therapy. Octreotide and lanreotide have very high affinities for SSTR-2 and to a lesser extent SSTR-5, which are precisely the most commonly expressed somatostatin receptors in GH-secreting adenomas.

When used after surgery has failed, somatostatin analogues can achieve a safe and a normal IGF-1 in 25% to 35% of patients. Primary treatment with somatostatin analogues is increasingly being used in patients with invasive tumors, when cardiopulmonary contraindications are present, and more recently as a result of the patient's or treating physician's preference. In these settings, biochemical success rates (achievement of a GH <2.5 ng/mL and normalization of IGF-1) have ranged between 30% and 80%, and more than 80% report significant relief of symptoms. More recent trials performed in unselected populations reveal that the real success rate lies between 25% and 35%. Tumor shrinkage occurs in 70% of primarily treated patients. Overall, treatment success is directly related to the abundance of SSTR-2 and SSTR-5 in the tumor. Lower pretreatment GH levels are also associated with a better response to somatostatin analogues. Side effects of somatostatin analogues, including nausea, abdominal pain, alopecia, and biliary sludge, occur in 20% of subjects. The currently recommended biochemical targets when treating patients with somatostatin analogues are the achievement of a GH of 1 ng/mL and an IGF-1 level within the normal age-adjusted range patients with somatostatin analogues is 1 ng/mL.

Pegvisomant (Somavert) is a GH mutant that prevents functional dimerization of the GH receptor, thus acting as an antagonist. Its use results in normalization of IGF-1 in more than 70% of patients, while increasing GH levels. Concern about adenoma growth due to the abolition of IGF-1 negative feedback on the tumoral somatotroph prevents its use in patients with very large lesions in close proximity to the optic chiasm. Transient elevations of liver aminotransferases can occur, although this seldom requires drug discontinuation. Pegvisomant does not compromise insulin secretion, as somatostatin analogues do. GH-receptor antagonists are expensive and should not be used as primary treatment; they are currently indicated in patients who are intolerant or have failed somatostatin analogue therapy.

Few patients respond marginally to difficult-to-tolerate large doses of bromocriptine. Newer dopamine agonists, such as cabergoline,[1] are better tolerated and achieve biochemical control in 20% to 30% of patients. Combination treatment with cabergoline and octreotide appears to be promising in cases resistant to somatostatin analogues.

Radiation Therapy

Both external-beam radiotherapy and radiosurgery are indicated in patients with persistent disease and a demonstrable tumor remnant who are either intolerant or resistant to pharmacologic treatment. Biochemical success occurs in 20% to 60% and requires many years to become apparent. Hypopituitarism, involving at least two axes, develops in more than 50% of patients within 10 years. Serious adverse effects such as brain necrosis and optic nerve damage seldom occur with the

---

[1]Not FDA approved for this indication.

currently used techniques that minimize radiation to the normal surrounding tissues. With the currently available radiation techniques, radiotherapy is an effective and safe treatment alternative. The two major drawbacks of radiotherapy are the time it takes to achieve biochemical control and the almost unavoidable induction of hypopituitarism.

Novel pharmacologic therapies are being developed, some of which will likely become useful particularly in patients who do not respond to current somatostatin analogues. These include the so-called "universal" somatostatin analogue pasireotide (Signifor LAR), which is capable of interacting not only with the SSTRs 2 and 5, but also with subtypes 1 and 3. Pasireotide seems to be slightly more effective than octreotide in achieving GH and IGF-1 targets; however, its major drawback is the worsening of hyperglycemia. Dopastatin[5] is a recently developed chimeric compound that behaves both as an analog and as a dopamine agonist; clinical trials had to be discontinued at early stages due to lack of efficacy. Oral octreotide, known as octreolin,[5] is a new preparation of octreotide acetate attached to a transient permeability enhancer, which selectively allows the translocation of the somatostatin analog through the paracellular tight junctions. Recently tested in a phase III trial its efficacy is almost equivalent as that of parenteral octreotide but it has not been approved by the FDA.

---

[5]Investigational drug in the United States.

References

Bevan JS: Clinical review: the antitumoral effects of somatostatin analog therapy in acromegaly, *J Clin Endocrinol Metab* 90:1856–1863, 2005.

Espinosa E, Ramirez C, Mercado M: The multimodal treatment of acromegaly: current status and future perspectives, *Endocr Metab Immune Disord Drug Targets* 14:169–181, 2014.

Espinosa-de-Los-Monteros AL, González B, Vargas G, et al: Clinical and biochemical characteristics of acromegalic patients with different abnormalities of glucose metabolism, *Pituitary* 14:231–235, 2011.

Espinosa de los Monteros AL, Gonzalez B, Vargas G, et al: Octreotide LAR treatment of acromegaly in "real life": long term outcome at a tertiary care center, *Pituitary* 18:290–296, 2015.

Espinosa-de-Los-Monteros AL, Sosa E, Cheng S, et al: Biochemical evaluation of disease activity after pituitary surgery in acromegaly: a critical analysis of patients who spontaneously change disease status, *Clin Endocrinol* 64:245–249, 2006.

Freda P: Current concepts in the biochemical assessment of the patient with acromegaly, *Growth Horm IGF Res* 13:171–184, 2003.

Gadelha MR, Kasuki L, Lim DST, Fleseriu M: Systemic complications of acromegaly and the impac of the current treatment landscape: an update, *Endocr Rev* 40:268–332, 2019.

Garcia Guzman B, Portocarrero Ortiz L, Dorantes Argandar A: Hereditary pituitary tumor syndromes: Genetic and clinical aspects, *Rev Invest Clin* 72:8–18, 2020.

Giustina A, Chanson P, Bronstein MD: A consensus on criteria for cure of acromegaly, *J Clin Endocrinol Metab* 95:3141–3148, 2010.

Giustina A, Chanson P, Kleinberg D, et al: Expert consensus document: a consensus on the medical treatment of acromegaly, *Nat Rev Endocrinol* 10:243–248, 2014.

Gonzalez-Virla B, Vargas-Ortega G, Martinez-Vazquez KB, Espinosa de los Monteros AL, Sosa-Eroza E, López-Felix B, Mendoza-Zubieta V, Mercado M: Efficacy and safety of fractionated conformal radiation therapy in acromegaly: A long-term follow-up study, *Endocrine* 65:386–392, 2019.

Holdaway IM, Rajasoorya RC, Gamble GD: Factors influencing mortality in acromegaly, *J Clin Endocrinol Metab* 89:667–674, 2004.

Kopchick JJ, Parkinson C, Stevens EC, Trainer PJ: Growth hormone receptor antagonists: discovery, development, and use in patients with acromegaly, *Endocr Rev* 23:623–646, 2002.

Mercado M, Abreu C, Vergara-López A, et al: Surgical and pharmacological outcomes in acromegaly: real-life data from the Mexican Acromegaly Registry, *J Clin Endocrinol Metab* 105:dga664, 2020.

Mercado M, Espinosa E, Ramirez C: Current status and future directions of pharmacological therapy for acromegaly, *Minerva Endocrinol* 41:351–365, 2016.

Mercado M, Gonzalez B, Vargas G, et al: Successful mortality reduction and of comorbidities in patients with acromegaly followed at a highly specialized multidisciplinary clinic, *J Clin Endocrinol Metab* 99:4438–4446, 2014.

Mercado M, Ramirez-Rentería C: Metabolic complications of acromegaly, *Front Horm Res* 49:20–28, 2018.

Portocarrero-Ortiz LA, Vergara-Lopez A, Vidrio-Velazquez M, et al: The Mexican Acromegaly Registry: clinical and biochemical characteristics at diagnosis and therapeutic outcomes, *J Clin Endocrinol Metab* 101:3997–4004, 2016.

ADRENOCORTICAL INSUFFICIENCY

Method of

Fabienne Langlois, MD; Elena V. Varlamov, MD; and Maria Fleseriu, MD

CURRENT DIAGNOSIS

- An initial diagnosis of adrenocortical insufficiency (AI) is based in most cases on an evaluation of morning cortisol level(s), measured at 8 AM in patients who have a normal circadian rhythm.
- A morning cortisol level less than 3 µg/dL to 5 µg/dL supports an AI diagnosis, and a value greater than 15 µg/dL effectively rules out AI.
- To confirm the diagnosis, especially in cases with intermediate cortisol values, a high-dose (250 µg) cosyntropin (Cortrosyn) stimulation test is suggested with a normal cutoff peak cortisol greater than 18 µg/dL to 20 µg/dL at 30 or 60 minutes.
- Primary AI is characterized by elevated endogenous adrenocorticotropic hormone (ACTH) levels and absence of mineralocorticoid hormones in addition to glucocorticoid (GC) deficiency; antibody screening and/or adrenal imaging is indicated.
- Secondary AI is characterized by an inappropriately normal or low endogenous ACTH level and low cortisol with preserved mineralocorticoid hormones. If an exogenous GC source/use is ruled out, pituitary hormone testing and magnetic resonance imaging (MRI) of the pituitary sella is appropriate.

CURRENT THERAPY

- Oral hydrocortisone (Cortef) is the preferred form of steroid to attain physiologic replacement. Doses are usually 15 mg to 20 mg divided into two or three daily doses, with the highest dose in the morning.
- In case of physiologic stress—such as fever, severe infection, or minor surgery—doses should be doubled or tripled (depending on the type of stress or procedure) for the duration of the event.
- In patients with primary AI, fludrocortisone (Florinef), a mineralocorticoid, should be added to the treatment regimen, with a typical dose between 0.05 mg and 0.1 mg daily.
- For adrenal crisis in patients with known AI, administer bolus hydrocortisone injection (Solu-Cortef) 100 mg followed by 50 mg to 100 mg IV every 6 hours to 8 hours or continuous infusion of 200 mg/24 h along with substantial volumes of saline.
- Patients should wear a medical alert bracelet or necklace and have frequent education regarding AI, its treatment, and the prevention of adrenal crisis.

Epidemiology

Primary adrenocortical insufficiency (AI), also known as Addison disease, has a prevalence of 100 to 140 cases per million persons. More than 90% of primary AI in the developed world is secondary to autoimmune adrenalitis, and is more common in women. Secondary AI caused by withdrawal of therapeutic glucocorticoid (GC) administration is the most prevalent; pituitary tumors and surgeries and opioid use are other common etiologies.

Risk Factors

Primary Adrenocortical Insufficiency

A personal or family history of autoimmune disease (e.g., type 1 diabetes, Hashimoto disease, vitiligo, pernicious anemia) is a risk factor for autoimmune adrenalitis. In the context of acute AI in the hospital, thrombosis and secondary adrenal hemorrhage must be ruled out and the possibility of heparin-induced thrombocytopenia (HIT) elicited if the patient is receiving parenteral anticoagulation. Miliary tuberculosis is the most frequent cause of primary AI in less economically developed countries. Infiltration in the context of malignancy is often due to a known metastatic cancer; other infiltrative diseases are rare.

Secondary Adrenocortical Insufficiency

The most common risk factor for secondary AI is prolonged use of exogenous GC. In general, patients taking more than 5 mg of prednisone or the equivalent for longer than a few weeks are at risk for secondary AI. In some patients with GC receptor hypersensitivity, even smaller doses of GC other than oral (topical, injected, or inhaled) can also suppress the hypothalamic-pituitary-adrenal axis. Immunotherapy-related hypophysitis, most often related to inhibition of cytotoxic T-lymphocyte antigen-4 (CTLA-4), but also programmed cell death protein 1 (PD-1), and/or its ligand (PD-L1) induce AI, which is rarely reversible. Chronic opioid use, especially long-acting opioids, can also suppress central ACTH and induce AI.

Patients with tumors of the hypothalamic-pituitary region or a history of treatment of such tumors with surgery and/or radiation are at significant risk. Pituitary apoplexy occurs due to hemorrhage or infarction of the pituitary tumor and causes acute secondary AI. Autoimmune lymphocytic hypophysitis is more common in women and usually occurs in the third pregnancy trimester or postpartum. Pituitary ischemia due to severe blood loss postpartum is known as Sheehan syndrome. Patients with traumatic brain injury may experience transient or permanent AI in both the acute and/or recovery phase.

Pathophysiology

Primary AI is characterized by complete destruction of the adrenal cortex, inducing deficits in all hormones: GC, mineralocorticoid, and androgens. With loss of cortisol feedback inhibition, ACTH will be markedly elevated. Secondary AI is the result of isolated low GC production; it is due a defect at the pituitary or hypothalamus level and results in low (or inappropriately normal) ACTH. Mineralocorticoid activity is maintained in secondary AI as it is controlled by the renin-angiotensin-aldosterone system.

Prevention

There is no clinically practicable strategy for preventing primary AI. Opioids and GC-associated secondary AI may be prevented through judicious use of systemic GC and opioids, with efforts made to limit administration to the lowest effective dose for the shortest possible time.

Clinical Manifestations
Primary Adrenocortical Insufficiency

The presentation of primary AI is sometimes dramatic, with a constellation of weakness, fatigue, anorexia, weight loss, nausea, abdominal pain, salt craving, and orthostatic hypotension. Symptoms start as subtle and nonspecific in some patients but may evolve rapidly in adrenal crisis, especially if a concomitant stress occurs. The skin and buccal mucosa are often hyperpigmented owing to the effect of excess ACTH on cutaneous melanocortin receptors. Hyponatremia and hyperkalemia (as a result of mineralocorticoid deficiency) are often present.

Secondary Adrenocortical Insufficiency

The presentation of secondary AI is more insidious, with weight loss, fatigue, nausea, and malaise as presenting features. This often leads to a delay in diagnosis. The production of mineralocorticoid is relatively intact in secondary AI, and as such potassium levels are usually normal. Hyponatremia may be present due to an increase in antidiuretic hormone. Hyperpigmentation is not present, reflecting normal or low ACTH levels. Other laboratory abnormalities are less common but hypoglycemia is occasionally observed, especially with concomitant growth hormone deficiency (GHD). Isolated ACTH deficiency is rare, and signs

and symptoms of other pituitary hormone abnormalities—such as hyperprolactinemia, central hypogonadism, GHD, or central hypothyroidism—may be present. Secondary AI may be masked by concomitant central hypothyroidism.

Diagnosis

Morning cortisol levels (within 2 hours of waking up) of 3 μg/dL to 5 μg/dL or less has a relatively high predictive value for AI; a morning cortisol level greater than 15 μg/dL effectively rules out AI. To confirm the diagnosis of AI, a cortisol stimulation test is performed. Insulin tolerance testing has largely been replaced by stimulation testing with synthetic cosyntropin (ACTH—Cortrosyn, Synacthen). ACTH stimulation testing of cortisol is a reliable method of evaluating adrenal reserve. However, it should not be used in cases of acute secondary AI, such as apoplexy or after recent pituitary surgery, because adrenal atrophy must have occurred for the adrenal response to cosyntropin to be blunted. In high-dose ACTH testing, a cortisol level is checked before and at 30 and 60 minutes after 250 μg of cosyntropin has been administered intravenously. A peak cortisol level greater than 18 μg/dL to 20 μg/dL at 30 or 60 minutes defines a normal response. The low-dose (1 μg) test[1] measures cortisol 20 to 30 minutes after cosyntropin administration and may be more sensitive for the diagnosis of secondary AI. However, the high-dose (250 μg cosyntropin) test remains the standard. The above-mentioned cortisol cutoffs are based on laboratory methods using polyclonal antibody immunoassays. Newer assays (liquid chromatography mass spectrometry [LC-MS/MS]) and some monoclonal antibody immunoassays) have reduced cross-reactivity with cortisol precursors and therefore result in 10% to 20% lower total cortisol levels. For example, lower stimulated cutoffs of 14 μg/dL to 17 μg/dL have been proposed. Additionally, one must consider total serum cortisol level, as this can be affected by diurnal rhythm and binding proteins, which are elevated in hyperestrogenic states and low in hypoalbuminemia. If the clinical picture is not concordant with the investigation, an endocrinology consult should be sought.

Once a diagnosis has been confirmed, a low or normal plasma ACTH level will indicate secondary AI; however, care must be taken with the methodology of the test, as some immunoassays for ACTH can give falsely low results if preanalytic precautions are not respected. An elevated ACTH level (more than twofold the upper limit of normal) typically indicates primary AI, and hyperkalemia, high plasma renin, and simultaneously low aldosterone levels will confirm associated mineralocorticoid deficiency. After the diagnosis of primary versus secondary AI has been established, an etiology should be sought (Boxes 1 and 2). Serology for antiadrenal (anti 21-hydroxylase) antibodies or evidence of other autoimmune diseases is useful in primary AI, given the very large fraction of these patients with autoimmune adrenalitis. In cases with absent antibodies, adrenal computed tomography imaging is indicated. Enlarged adrenal glands with high-density areas or calcification can suggest granulomatous disease or neoplasm. Acute hematoma or fluid collections around the adrenals during an acute adrenal crisis can indicate adrenal hemorrhage. Secondary AI is most often associated with chronic GC therapy but may be caused by a number of other diseases affecting the hypothalamic-pituitary region. If exogenous GC administration has been excluded, pituitary magnetic resonance imaging (MRI) and testing of the other pituitary axes are appropriate.

Differential Diagnosis

Presentation of AI can be subtle (especially in secondary AI), and differential diagnosis is broad and includes a number of illnesses associated with fatigue, weight loss, and malaise as well as occult malignancies, renal or hepatic dysfunction, and electrolyte disturbances. In acute AI crisis, differential diagnosis includes other systemic illnesses associated with orthostatic hypotension and electrolyte abnormalities, including dehydration and distributive and septic shock. Fever can be part of an AI crisis, but an infectious process must be ruled out as the precipitating cause.

---

[1]Not FDA approved for this indication.

BOX 1 Causes of Primary Adrenocortical Insufficiency

Autoimmune
Isolated
Autoimmune polyglandular syndromes 1 and 2

Infectious
Fungal
    Tuberculosis
    Histoplasmosis
Viral
    Human immunodeficiency virus
    Cytomegalovirus
Parasitic
Syphilis
Rarely bacterial

Bilateral Adrenal Infarction
Hemorrhage
    Anticoagulation
    Sepsis (e.g., meningococcemia)
    Trauma
Thrombosis
    Thrombophilic condition (e.g., antiphospholipid antibody syndrome)
    Heparin-induced thrombocytopenia

Neoplastic
Metastatic cancer
    Breast
    Colon
    Melanoma
    Lymphoma
Non–small cell lung cancer

Infiltrative Diseases
Hemochromatosis
Primary amyloidosis
Sarcoidosis

Bilateral Adrenalectomy
For bilateral tumors or intractable Cushing syndrome

Familial or Genetic
Classical congenital adrenal hyperplasia
Adrenoleukodystrophy
Familial glucocorticoid deficiency
Adrenocorticotropic hormone insensitivity syndromes
X-linked adrenal hypoplasia (associated with DAX-1 mutation, may be of late onset)
Triple-A or Allgrove syndrome (alacrimia, achalasia, adrenal insufficiency)

BOX 2 Etiologies of Secondary Adrenocortical Insufficiency

Iatrogenic/Medication
Chronic steroid therapy, most often oral or parenteral, but could also be inhaled, topical, or injected
Chronic opioid therapy
Immunotherapy (CTLA-4 and PD-1/PDL-1 inhibitors)
Drugs used for treatment of Cushing syndrome that can cause adrenal insufficiency
    Steroidogenesis inhibitors (ketoconazole, metyrapone, osilodrostat, mitotane, etomidate)
    Pituitary tumor directed drugs (pasireotide)
    Glucocorticoid receptor blockers (Mifepristone)

Pituitary Injury
Posttranssphenoidal or transcranial surgery
Radiation to the sella
Infarction/hemorrhage (pituitary apoplexy, Sheehan syndrome)
Traumatic brain injury

Tumors of the Sella
Pituitary adenoma
Craniopharyngioma
Meningioma
Rathke cleft cyst
Metastatic cancer

Infiltrative/Inflammatory Diseases
Sarcoidosis, tuberculosis, or other granulomatous diseases
Lymphocytic hypophysitis
Idiopathic adrenocorticotropic hormone deficiency

Congenital
Genetic mutations in transcription factors (PROP-1, PIT-1, etc.)
Midline defect
Septo-optic dysplasia

Treatment

GC replacement is recommended with oral hydrocortisone two or three times daily for primary AI and once or twice daily for secondary AI. One-half to two-thirds of the daily dose is given upon waking, and the dosage is roughly 15 mg to 20 mg/day (or 10 mg/m^2 to 12 mg/m^2 body surface area per day), typically 10 mg or 15 mg in the morning and 5 mg in the afternoon. Once-daily modified-release hydrocortisone is available in Europe and may better mimic the physiologic circadian rhythm of cortisol, but it is not yet available in the United States. Longer-acting GCs (prednisone, dexamethasone [Decadron]) may be used in patients who remain severely symptomatic in the evenings or early morning hours or who are unable to comply with a multidose hydrocortisone regimen. However, in such cases the risk of overreplacement is much higher."

Patients should be instructed to increase this dosage according to physiologic stress, as doses should be doubled or tripled for the duration of the fever or intercurrent systemic illness. Day-to-day emotional stress does not require an increment in dosing. For surgery, GC parenteral doses should be administered according to the level of surgical stress, such as 25 mg for minor stress (e.g., cataract surgery), 50 mg to 75 mg for moderate stress (e.g., cholecystectomy), and 100 mg to 150 mg daily in divided doses for major stress (e.g., heart surgery).

Patients should wear a medical alert bracelet or necklace and should be dispensed hydrocortisone or dexamethasone injection with instructions for home self-administration in case of vomiting and inability to take oral doses. If symptoms do not improve within hours after injection, patients should seek urgent medical evaluation.

Mineralocorticoid replacement is indicated in most patients with primary AI, and fludrocortisone (Florinef) is the recommended medical therapy, with a typical dose between 0.05 mg and 0.1 mg once daily.

If a patient with known AI presents in adrenal crisis, hydrocortisone (Solu-Cortef) 100 mg bolus followed by 150 mg to 250 mg/day, divided every 6 to 8 hours or as a continuous 200 mg/24 hours intravenous (IV) infusion, is an appropriate initial therapy, with the dose tapered to an appropriate oral dose as the patient's condition improves. Aggressive hydration with a saline solution will help increase the intravascular volume, and high-dose GCs have some mineralocorticoid activity; thus mineralocorticoids are not required in the treatment of acute adrenal crisis.

In critical illness, the treatment of AI should not be delayed if diagnosis cannot be established and the patient is unstable. Baseline cortisol and ACTH levels should preferably be drawn prior to the initiation of treatment and should be interpreted as a stress value (i.e., should be >18 μg/dL). If in doubt, high-dose stress GCs are administered until testing is complete and cosyntropin stimulation testing may be delayed until the patient's condition improves because hydrocortisone has to be suspended at least 24 hours before testing. The controversial entity of suboptimal cortisol response during acute stress may be associated with worse outcomes, but no consensus exists for its diagnosis and treatment. Refer to Table 1 for GC dosage recommendations.

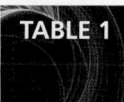

TABLE 1 Stress Dose Glucocorticoid Dosage Recommendations for Patients With Adrenal Insufficiency*,†

CLINICAL CONTEXT	MANAGEMENT
Minor surgical or medical stress (for example) Mild fever, colonoscopy, mild gastroenteritis, dental procedures	Hydrocortisone 25 mg OR twice the usual dose on days of stress
Moderate surgical or medical stress (for example) Cholecystectomy, pneumonia, severe gastroenteritis	Hydrocortisone 50–75 mg/day for 1–2 days followed by twice usual dose for 1–2 days, then resume the usual dose
Major surgical or medical stress (for example) Cardiopulmonary bypass, pancreatitis, vaginal delivery	Hydrocortisone 100–150 mg/day for 1–3 days followed by twice to thrice usual dose for 2–7 days, then resume usual dose
Adrenal crisis Critical illness (for example) Septic shock, hemodynamic instability	Hydrocortisone 100 mg bolus followed by 50–100 mg every 6–8 hours OR continuous infusion of 200 mg/24 h (or 0.18 mg/kg/day)

*For an uncomplicated course, the glucocorticoid dosage should always be individualized according to patient's clinical status.

†Patients with primary adrenal insufficiency may require slightly higher doses compared with patients with secondary adrenal insufficiency and may benefit more from additional intravenous fluids to compensate for the lack of mineralocorticoids.

The replacement of dehydroepiandrosterone (DHEA) is controversial and not recommended for all patients by present guidelines. However, a trial may be warranted in selected cases of women with primary AI and persistent symptoms, including low libido and low energy. DHEA is available only as a dietary supplement and has not been approved by the US Food and Drug Administration (FDA).

Monitoring

Patients should be interviewed and examined routinely for indicators of excess GC replacement, such as weight gain, striae, facial plethora, osteoporosis, or glucose intolerance; they should also be checked for under replacement if symptoms of AI persist. Cortisol levels and ACTH are not helpful in monitoring GC doses. Monitoring of mineralocorticoid status should include volume status, electrolytes, blood pressure, and occasionally serum renin levels. The development of hypertension, edema, or hypokalemia could mandate a dose reduction.

Complications

Adrenal crisis in patients with known AI occurs at a rate of approximately six cases per 100 patient-years. Precipitating causes of adrenal crisis are mainly gastrointestinal infection and other infections, with other stressful events (pain, surgery, severe emotional distress, and pregnancy) occurring less commonly. Iatrogenic Cushing syndrome can develop if the dose of GC replacement is supraphysiologic long-term.

Acknowledgments

The authors thank Shirley McCartney, PhD, for editorial assistance.

References

Annane D, Pastores SM, Rochwerg B, et al: Guidelines for the diagnosis and management of critical illness-related corticosteroid insufficiency (CIRCI) in critically ill patients (Part I): Society of Critical Care Medicine (SCCM) and European Society of Intensive Care Medicine (ESICM) 2017, *Crit Care Med* 45:2078–2088, 2017.

Arlt W, Allolio B: Adrenal insufficiency, *Lancet* 361:1881–1893, 2003.

Husebye ES, Pearce SH, Krone NP, Kämpe O: Adrenal insufficiency, *Lancet* 13 397(10274):613–629, 2021.

Bornstein SR, Allolio B, Arlt W, et al: Diagnosis and treatment of primary adrenal insufficiency: an Endocrine Society clinical practice guideline, *J Clin Endocrinol Metab* 101:364–389, 2016.

Charmandari E, Nicolaides NC, Chrousos GP: Adrenal insufficiency, *Lancet* 383:2152–2167, 2014.

Dillard T, Yedinak CG, Alumkal J, Fleseriu M, et al: Anti-CTLA-4 antibody therapy associated autoimmune hypophysitis: serious immune related adverse events across a spectrum of cancer subtypes, *Pituitary* 13(1):29–38, 2010.

Dorin RI, Qualls CR, Crapo LM: Diagnosis of adrenal insufficiency, *Ann Intern Med* 139:194–204, 2003.

Fleseriu M, Hashim IA, Karavitaki N, et al: Hormonal replacement in hypopituitarism in adults: an Endocrine Society clinical practice guideline, *J Clin Endocrinol Metab* 101:3888–3921, 2016.

Husebye ES, Allolio B, Arlt W, et al: Consensus statement on the diagnosis, treatment and follow-up of patients with primary adrenal insufficiency, *J Intern Med* 275:104–115, 2014.

Isidori AM, Venneri MA, Graziadio C, et al: Effect of once-daily, modified-release hydrocortisone versus standard glucocorticoid therapy on metabolism and innate immunity in patients with adrenal insufficiency (DREAM): a single-blind, randomised controlled trial, *The Lancet Diabetes & Endocrinology* 6:173–185, 2018.

Javorsky BR, Raff H, Carroll TB, Algeciras-Schimnich A, Singh RJ, Colón-Franco JM, et al: New cutoffs for the biochemical diagnosis of adrenal insufficiency after ACTH stimulation using specific cortisol assays, *Journal of the Endocrine Society*, 2021. https://doi.org/10.1210/jendso/bvab022. bvab022.

Kazlauskaite R, Evans AT, Villabona CV, et al: Corticotropin tests for hypothalamic-pituitary-adrenal insufficiency: a metaanalysis, *J Clin Endocrinol Metab* 93:4245–4253, 2008.

Rushworth RL, Torpy DJ, Falhammar H: Adrenal crisis, *N Engl J Med* 29(9):852–861, 2019. 381.

Woodcock T, Barker P, Daniel S, et al: Guidelines for the management of glucocorticoids during the peri-operative period for patients with adrenal insufficiency—guidelines from the Association of Anaesthetists, the Royal College of Physicians and the Society for Endocrinology UK, *Anaesthesia* 75(5):654–663, 2020.

CUSHING'S SYNDROME

Method of
Constantine A. Stratakis, MD, PhD

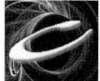

CURRENT DIAGNOSIS

- Cushing's syndrome remains one of the most challenging diagnoses in endocrine medicine.
- Cushing's disease is caused by corticotropin (ACTH)-producing pituitary adenomas (corticotropinomas) and constitutes the most common cause of endogenous Cushing's syndrome, although its prevalence varies across different age groups.
- Growth failure in children, facial plethora and rounded face, central fat deposition, supraclavicular fat accumulation, buffalo hump, purple striae, thin skin, and proximal myopathy are relatively sensitive clinical features of Cushing's syndrome.
- Ectopic ACTH syndrome occasionally has an unusual presentation of rapid onset, severe weakness, and hypokalemia without classic symptoms of Cushing's syndrome.
- A urinary free cortisol test is the most cost-effective and reliable outpatient screening test.
- A 1-mg overnight dexamethasone screening test is less useful and more expensive than the urinary free cortisol test, but it provides a good alternative for patients in whom urinary collection is impossible or unreliable.
- Midnight salivary cortisol levels greater than 3.6 nmol/L (0.13 µg/dL) have a sensitivity and specificity of approximately 95% for the diagnosis of Cushing's syndrome.
- Undetectable ACTH levels (<1 pmol/L or <5 pg/mL) indicate a primary autonomous adrenocortical disease.
- Postcontrast spoiled gradient-recalled acquisition (SPGR) magnetic resonance imaging (MRI) is superior to conventional MRI for the localization of corticotropinomas in children and adults.
- Computed tomography (CT) is used to investigate adrenal disease in patients with ACTH-independent Cushing's syndrome. Usually, conventional MRI is less useful owing to motion artifacts.

CURRENT THERAPY

Definition and Epidemiology

Cushing's syndrome remains one of the most difficult diagnoses in endocrinology. By definition, Cushing's syndrome is a multisystem disorder that develops in response to glucocorticoid excess. Iatrogenic Cushing's syndrome is common, but endogenous Cushing's syndrome is a rare condition, with an estimated incidence of 0.7 to 2.4 per million population per year. The etiology of Cushing's syndrome may be excessive adrenocorticotropic hormone (ACTH) production from the pituitary gland, ectopic ACTH secretion by nonpituitary tumors, or autonomous cortisol hypersecretion from adrenal hyperplasia or tumors (Table 1). Cushing's disease refers to the subset of Cushing's syndrome cases caused by an ACTH-producing pituitary adenoma. Cushing's disease is the most common cause of spontaneous Cushing's syndrome in almost all ages, including older children and adolescents. Approximately 20% to 30% (with the exception of very young children) of endogenous Cushing's syndrome is caused by primary adrenocortical diseases that are not ACTH-dependent. Cushing's disease and adrenocortical adenomas occur more commonly in women, with a female-to-male ratio of 3–5:1.

Pathophysiology

Cortisol inhibits the biosynthesis and secretion of corticotropin-releasing hormone (CRH) and ACTH in a negative-feedback loop that is tightly controlled. The hallmark of Cushing's syndrome is the absence of suppression of cortisol levels after low-dose dexamethasone (Decadron) administration owing to autonomous ACTH secretion by a tumor or autonomous glucocorticoid production by a primary adrenocortical disease. It is essential to understand that all diagnostic testing in Cushing's syndrome relies on the disturbance of this feedback mechanism, as revealed by dexamethasone, CRH (corticorelin ovine trifluate [Acthrel]), and all related testing.

ACTH-producing pituitary adenomas are microadenomas (<1 cm in diameter) in 80% to 90% of cases. Macroadenomas are rare and often invasive, with extension outside of the sella turcica. Chronic ACTH hypersecretion commonly leads to secondary adrenocortical hyperplasia.

Ectopic ACTH secretion is most often associated with small cell lung carcinoma, which accounts for half of the cases in adult patients with Cushing's syndrome. The ectopic ACTH syndrome

TABLE 1	Etiology of Cushing's Syndrome in Older Children, Adolescents, and Young Adults*
SYNDROME	**% OF TOTAL**
ACTH-dependent	
Cushing's disease	60–70
Ectopic ACTH syndrome	5–10
Ectopic CRH syndrome	<1
ACTH-independent	
Adrenocortical adenoma	10–15
Adrenocortical carcinoma	5
Bilateral adrenocortical disease	5–10

*In infants and younger children, the distribution is different.
Abbreviations: ACTH = adrenocorticotropic hormone; CRH = corticotropin-releasing hormone.

causes severe hypokalemia and is usually underdiagnosed in patients during advanced stages of neoplasia. Other tumors causing the syndrome are bronchial, thymic, and pancreatic carcinoids; medullary thyroid carcinoma; pheochromocytoma; or other rare neuroendocrine tumors, especially in pediatric patients.

Adrenocortical tumors are more often adenomas that are usually smaller than 5 cm. Adrenocortical carcinomas are rare but very aggressive neoplasms; they most commonly occur as large nonsecreting abdominal masses at diagnosis, and only rarely does Cushing's syndrome develop.

Up to recently, only two types of primary adrenal hyperplasias that are ACTH-independent and cause Cushing's syndrome were known: primary pigmented nodular adrenocortical disease (PPNAD) and ACTH-independent macronodular adrenocortical hyperplasia, also known as massive macronodular adrenocortical disease.

Table 2 lists no fewer than six types of bilateral adrenocortical hyperplasias. They are divided into two groups of disorders, macronodular and micronodular hyperplasias, on the basis of the size of the associated nodules. In macronodular disorders, the greatest diameter of each nodule exceeds 1 cm; in the micronodular group, nodules are less than 1 cm. Although nodules less than 1 cm can occur in macronodular disease (especially the form associated with McCune-Albright syndrome), and single large tumors may be encountered in PPNAD (especially in older patients), the size criterion has biological relevance, because we rarely see a continuum in the same subject: most patients have either macronodular or micronodular hyperplasia. We use two additional basic characteristics in this classification of bilateral adrenocortical hyperplasias: presence of tumor pigment and status (hyperplasia or atrophy) of the surrounding cortex.

Pigment in adrenocortical lesions is rarely melanin; most of the pigmentation in adrenocortical adenomas and bilateral adrenocortical hyperplasias that produce cortisol is lipofuscin. The accumulation of lipofuscin-like material results from the progressive oxidation of unsaturated fatty acids by oxygen-derived free radicals in lysosomes. Lipofuscin pigmentation appears macroscopically as light brown to occasionally dark brown or even black discoloration of the tumor or hyperplastic tissue. Lipofuscin can be seen with a light microscope, but it is better detected by electron microscopy. Massive macronodular adrenocortical disease is a bilateral disease and may be caused by abnormal hormone receptor expression or activating mutations of $G_{S}\alpha$, which lead to stimulation of steroidogenesis. About 30% to 50% of the cases may be caused by ARMC5 mutations. Another cause of ACTH-independent Cushing's syndrome is primary pigmented nodular adrenocortical disease, usually associated with a syndrome of cardiac myxomas, lentigines, and schwannomas (Carney's complex).

Clinical Manifestations

The clinical presentation of Cushing's syndrome is variable and differs in severity (Table 3). Truncal obesity is the most common

| TABLE 2 | Bilateral Adrenal Hyperplasias Causing Cushing's Syndrome | | | |

LESION	AGE GROUP	HISTOPATHOLOGY	GENETICS	GENE, LOCUS
Macronodular Hyperplasias (Multiple Nodules >1 cm Each)				
Bilateral macroadenomatous hyperplasia	Middle age	Distinct adenomas (usually 2 or 3) with internodular atrophy	MEN1, FAP, MAS, HLRCS; isolated (AD); other	Menin, *APC,GNAS*, FH, ectopic GPCRs, ARMC5, PRKACA 5
Bilateral macroadenomatous hyperplasia of childhood	Infants, very young children	Distinct adenomas (usually 2 or 3) with internodular atrophy; occasional microadenomas	MAS	*GNAS*
ACTH-independent macronodular adrenocortical hyperplasia, also known as massive macronodular adrenocortical disease	Middle age	Adenomatous hyperplasia (multiple) with internodular hyperplasia of the zona fasciculata	Isolated, AD	Ectopic GPCRs; WISP2 and Wnt-signaling; 17q22-24, other; ARMC5, PRKACA 5
Micronodular Hyperplasias (Multiple Nodules <1 cm Each)				
Isolated primary pigmented nodular adrenocortical disease	Children; young adults	Microadenomatous hyperplasia with (mostly) internodular atrophy and nodular pigment (lipofuscin)	Isolated, AD	*PRKAR1A, PDE11A; PDE8B*; 2p16; PRKACA 5 other
Carney complex–associated primary pigmented nodular adrenocortical disease	Children; young and middle aged adults	Microadenomatous hyperplasia with (mostly) internodular atrophy and (mainly nodular) pigment (lipofuscin)	CNC (AD)	*PRKAR1A*, 2p16; other
Isolated micronodular adrenocortical disease	Mostly children; young adults	Microadenomatous, with hyperplasia of the surrounding zona fasciculata and limited or absent pigment	Isolated, AD; other	*PDE11A, PDE8B*; other; 2p12-p16, other

Abbreviations: ACTH = adrenocorticotropic hormone; AD = autosomal dominant; *APC* = adenomatous polyposis coli gene; cAMP = cyclic adenosine monophosphate; CNC = Carney complex; FAP = familial adenomatous polyposis; FH = fumarate hydratase; *GNAS* = gene coding for the stimulatory subunit alpha of the G-protein (Gsα); GPCR = G-protein-coupled receptor; HLRCS = hereditary leiomyomatosis and renal cancer syndrome; MAS = McCune–Albright syndrome; MEN1 = multiple endocrine neoplasia type 1; *PDE8B* = phosphodiesterase 8B gene; *PDE11A* = phosphodiesterase 11A gene; *PRKAR1A* = protein kinase, cAMP-dependent, regulatory, type I, alpha gene; WISP2 = Wnt1-inducible signaling pathway protein 1; Wnt = wingless-type MMTV integration site family.

clinical sign and is usually the initial manifestation in most patients. Growth failure in children is the most reliable sign of Cushing's syndrome, especially when combined with continuing weight gain. Other symptoms include central fat deposition, supraclavicular fat accumulation, buffalo hump, plethora, rounded face, purple striae, thin skin, proximal muscle weakness, hypertension, impaired glucose metabolism, gonadal dysfunction, and hirsutism (see Table 3). Diabetes mellitus and hypertension also develop. Osteoporosis, mood disorders, emotional lability and cognitive deficits are commonly observed. Proximal myopathy is common, especially in older patients. Ectopic ACTH syndrome caused by small cell lung cancer can have an unusual presentation characterized by rapid onset, severe weakness, and associated hypokalemia without classic symptoms of Cushing's syndrome. In contrast, ACTH-secreting carcinoids manifest with typical clinical manifestations.

Diagnosis
Confirmation of the Diagnosis
The initial evaluation should always include a careful clinical history and physical examination. Reliable symptoms and signs of Cushing's syndrome (see Table 3) should be present in any patient who undergoes evaluation for Cushing's syndrome; patients with no reliable symptoms and signs of Cushing's syndrome should not be investigated, as this often leads to unnecessary, extensive, and expensive testing. It is essential to investigate the use of exogenous glucocorticoids and other conditions that may be associated with mild hypercortisolism, such as alcoholism, anorexia nervosa, severe depression, and morbid obesity; these are pseudo-Cushing's states and are often difficult to exclude, especially in older or chronically ill patients.

The first task in the workup of any patient is documentation of hypercortisolism. On an outpatient basis, this is typically done through the urinary free cortisol test. This is the most cost-effective and reliable outpatient screening test. We typically recommend

TABLE 3	Clinical Manifestations of Cushing's Syndrome
SIGNS AND SYMPTOMS	**INCIDENCE (%)**
Central obesity	97
Plethora	89
Moon facies	89
Decreased libido	86
Atrophic skin and easy bruising	75
Decreased linear growth	70–80
Menstrual irregularities	80
Hypertension	76
Hirsutism	56
Depression or emotional lability	67
Glucose intolerance/diabetes mellitus	70
Purple striae	60
Buffalo hump	54
Osteoporosis	50
Headache	10

collections over two or three consecutive days so that we avoid errors due to over- or undercollection that are not uncommon with single 24-hour studies. The results of the test need to be corrected for body surface area, as long as total creatinine excretion is normal. A 1-mg overnight dexamethasone test is less useful and more expensive, but it provides a good alternative for patients in whom urinary collection is impossible or unreliable. During these

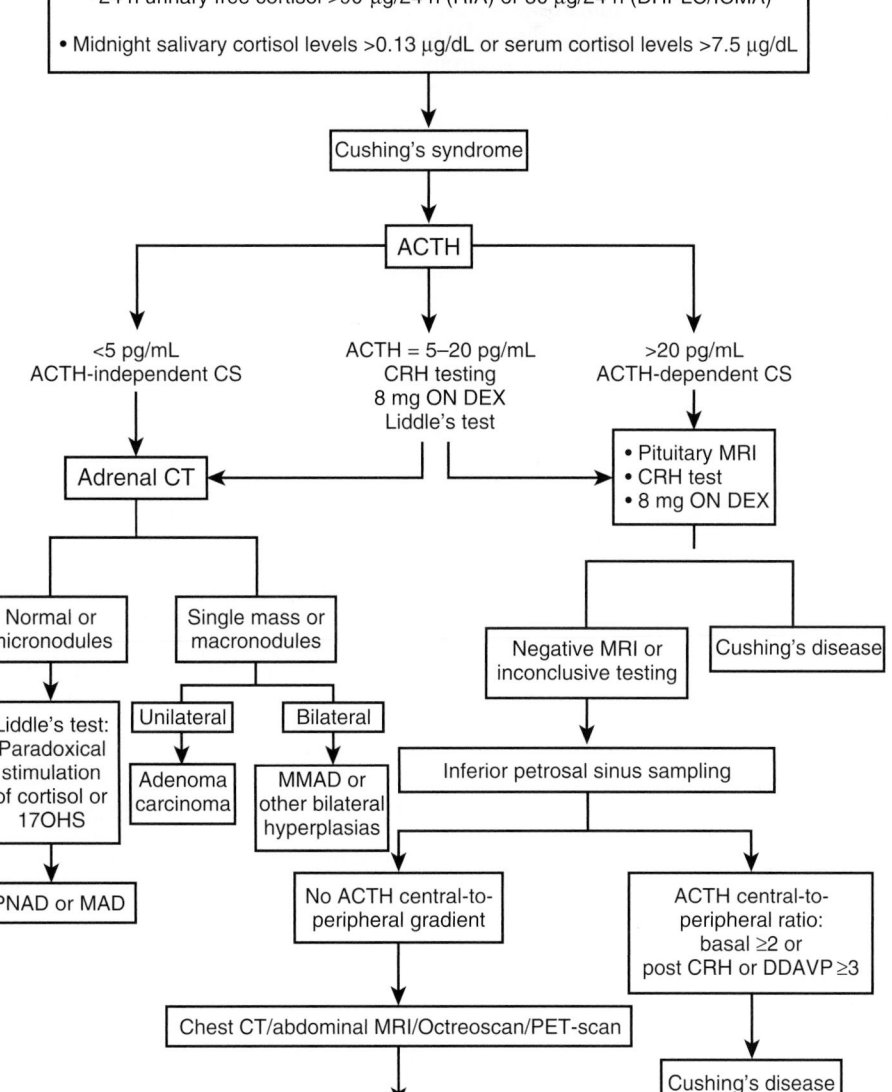

Figure 1 Algorithm for evaluating patients with Cushing's syndrome. *Abbreviations:* ACTH = adrenocorticotropic hormone; CRH = corticotropin-releasing hormone; CS = Cushing's syndrome; CT = computed tomography; DDAVP = desmopressin; DHPLC = denaturing high-performance liquid chromatography; ICMA = immunochemiluminometric assay; MAD = micronodular disease; MMAD = massive macronodular adrenocortical disease; MRI = magnetic resonance imaging; 17OHS = 17-hydroxysteroids; ON DEX = overnight dexamethasone; PET = positron emission tomography; PPNAD = primary pigmented nodular adrenocortical disease; RIA = radioimmunoassay.

screening tests for hypercortisolism, patients should avoid any activation of the hypothalamic-pituitary-adrenal axis by stress, especially physical. The baseline measurements may be repeated as needed, because cyclic hypercortisolism often precedes overt Cushing's syndrome (Figure 1).

A 24-hour urinary free cortisol excretion of greater than 250 nmol per 24 hours (90 μg/24 hours measured by radioimmunoassay) is highly specific for the diagnosis of hypercortisolism. However, pseudo-Cushing's states are often associated with abnormal levels of 24-hour urinary free cortisol. Administration of 1 mg dexamethasone (15 μg/kg for children) at 11 PM results in suppression of the hypothalamic-pituitary-adrenal axis in normal persons and a fall in plasma and urinary cortisol levels. At 8 AM, serum cortisol should be less than 50 nmol/L (1.8 μg/dL). Unfortunately, dexamethasone is primarily metabolized by the cytochrome P-450 (CYP) system; several drugs, such as phenobarbital, carbamazepine (Tegretol), and rifampicin (Rifadin), that induce the activity of CYP3A4 can lead to false-positive tests. Oral contraceptives also interfere with serum cortisol levels owing to an increase in corticosteroid-binding globulin and by increasing dexamethasone metabolism. The test can only be interpreted if the serum dexamethasone levels reach the expected range; however, this additional requirement can make the test significantly more cumbersome and expensive.

Once hypercortisolism is suspected by the urinary free cortisol or the overnight dexamethasone test, the patient may undergo testing of the cortisol diurnal rhythm. The lack of circadian rhythm of cortisol is the earliest consistent biochemical abnormality of Cushing's syndrome, even in situations of cyclic or other atypical forms of Cushing's syndrome. Serum or salivary cortisol levels at midnight may be used for this test. Normally, the level of serum cortisol begins to rise at 3 to 4 AM and reaches a peak at 7 to 8 AM, falling during the day. A sleeping midnight serum cortisol level lower than 50 nmol/L (1.8 μg/dL) excludes the diagnosis of Cushing's syndrome, whereas a midnight serum cortisol higher than 207 nmol/L (7.5 μg/dL) is highly suggestive of Cushing's syndrome. This test does require inpatient admission. Salivary cortisol levels have an excellent correlation with serum cortisol levels and offer an easy and convenient outpatient way of evaluating circadian rhythm; saliva is also stable at room temperature (for up to 7 days). Midnight salivary cortisol levels greater than 3.6 nmol/L (0.13 μg/dL) have a sensitivity and specificity of approximately 95% for the diagnosis of Cushing's syndrome (see Figure 1).

After the biochemical confirmation of hypercortisolism, the next step is to investigate the source (see Figure 1). Baseline ACTH plasma levels greater than 2 to 5 pmol/L (>20–25 pg/mL) are diagnostic of ACTH-dependent Cushing's syndrome. On the other hand, undetectable ACTH levels (<1 pmol/L or 5 pg/mL) indicate a primary autonomous adrenocortical disease. Values in between should be further investigated with dynamic testing.

High-Dose Dexamethasone Testing
Oral dexamethasone is administered as 2 mg every 6 hours for 48 hours or as a single 8 mg (120 µg/kg for children) overnight dose. Urinary and serum cortisol levels are suppressed by more than 50% in most patients with Cushing's disease.

Corticotropin-Releasing Hormone Testing
Synthetic ovine CRH (corticorelin ovine trifluate [Acthrel]), an analogue of human CRH is administered intravenously (100 µg), and plasma ACTH and cortisol levels are measured at 15-minute intervals during the next 60 minutes. Patients with Cushing's disease typically have an increase in ACTH or cortisol level of 35% and 22%, respectively. This test has a sensitivity of approximately 85% for the diagnosis of Cushing's disease, but it is often falsely positive in patients with adrenal, ACTH-independent Cushing's syndrome, who do not have a fully suppressed hypothalamic-pituitary-adrenal axis.

Inferior Petrosal Sinus Sampling
None of the noninvasive tests are 100% accurate in distinguishing pituitary (Cushing's disease) from ectopic sources of ACTH. Inferior petrosal sinus sampling (IPSS) is indicated in all cases where an ACTH-dependent source of hypercortisolism is expected but the diagnosis of Cushing's disease versus an ectopic source remains uncertain. Typically, IPSS is done when the ovine CRH and dexamethasone tests are in disagreement or when the pituitary imaging by magnetic resonance imaging (MRI) is negative. An ACTH gradient of central-to-peripheral ACTH levels of 2 or more suggests Cushing's disease. When ovine CRH, human CRH, or desmopressin (DDAVP) testing is performed during IPSS, the diagnostic accuracy of IPSS increases. After ovine CRH stimulation, a central-to-peripheral ratio of ACTH levels of 3 or more suggest the diagnosis of Cushing's disease with specificity and sensitivity greater than 95%. The test is less useful for suggesting the tumor location (right versus left side of the pituitary gland).

Imaging Studies
Pituitary Magnetic Resonance Imaging
Unfortunately, less than 50% of ACTH-producing pituitary adenomas are detectable with MRI, even with the use of contrast enhancement. Typically, we recommend against obtaining an MRI until ACTH dependency is established, because as many as 20% of the patients have an incidental pituitary microadenoma. To avoid false-negative and false-positive imaging, several centers have sought improved methods for MRI detection of ACTH-producing tumors. Our studies demonstrated that postcontrast spoiled gradient-recalled acquisition (SPGR) MRI in addition to the conventional T1-weighted spin echo was superior to conventional MRI for the diagnostic evaluation of corticotropinomas in both children and adults.

Adrenal Imaging
Computed tomography (CT) and MRI are used to investigate adrenal disease in patients with ACTH-independent Cushing's syndrome. Adrenal tumors larger than 6 cm are highly suspicious for adrenocortical carcinomas. The fat content contributes to the differentiation between benign and malignant adrenal tumors. Measurement of Hounsfield units (HU) in unenhanced CT is of great value in differentiating malignant from benign adrenal lesions. Adrenal lesions with an attenuation value of more than 10 HU in unenhanced CT or an enhancement washout of less than 50% and a delayed attenuation of more than 35 HU (on 10- to 15-min delayed enhanced CT) are suspicious for malignancy. MRI with dynamic gadolinium-enhanced and chemical shift technique is as effective as CT in distinguishing malignant from benign lesions. However, MRI is much less useful for detecting adrenal nodularity owing to motion artifacts. Thus, especially for detecting small unilateral adrenocortical adenomas or bilateral micronodular hyperplasia, we recommend a dedicated (thin-sliced) adrenal CT rather than MRI.

Ectopic Adrenocorticotropic Hormone Syndrome
High Resolution Chest-CT 7 and abdominal MRI are the recommended imaging procedures in patients with an IPSS that indicates a nonpituitary ACTH-producing source. Additionally, somatostatin receptor scintigraphy is a useful and complementary tool in the evaluation of patients with ectopic ACTH-dependent Cushing's syndrome. Recent studies have demonstrated a higher sensitivity of somatostatin receptor scintigraphy in comparison to CT or MRI for diagnosing occult ectopic tumors. Additional methods include PET-CT and FDG scans.

Treatment
Untreated chronic hypercortisolism is associated with high morbidity and mortality owing to diabetes mellitus, hypertension, cardiovascular disease, thromboembolism, and suppression of the immune system. Cushing's syndrome should be treated effectively; patients should be closely monitored to rapidly detect recurrent disease.

Treatment of Pituitary Corticotropinomas
Transsphenoidal Pituitary Surgery
The initial therapy of choice for patients with Cushing's disease is transsphenoidal surgery. This procedure is associated with low mortality and morbidity, but complications can include cerebrospinal fluid leaks, meningitis, hypopituitarism, and venous thromboembolism. The success rate for transsphenoidal surgery varies between 60% and 80%, but in experienced centers can be as high as 90% to 95%. Relapses are rare when surgery is performed in an experienced tertiary care center; it can be as high as 30% in less-experienced centers. Postoperative morning serum cortisol levels of less than 50 nmol/L (2 µg/dL) are highly predictive of remission and a low recurrence rate of less than 10% at 10 years.

After successful transsphenoidal surgery, glucocorticoid replacement therapy (hydrocortisone at 12–15 mg/m²/day; 20–30 mg daily in adults) is mandatory until the hypothalamic-pituitary-adrenal axis recovers from the chronic exposure to glucocorticoid excess; this usually takes place within a year after surgery. For recurrent disease, the choice of second-line therapy remains controversial. Repeat surgery can be successful when residual tumor is detectable on MRI imaging, but it carries a high risk of hypopituitarism. Irradiation is recommended in most cases where a tumor is not seen on MRI.

Radiotherapy
Radiotherapy has been used to suppress pituitary secretion of ACTH, but its success rate is variable (50% in some series). It can take as long as 5 years for a full effect; hypopituitarism develops in more than 70% of the patients over a period of 10 to 20 years after the therapy is completed. Stereotactic radiosurgery with gamma knife is associated with a more-rapid effect and a lower risk of hypopituitarism, but it has not been extensively studied.

Medical Treatment to Control Secretion of Adrenocorticotropic Hormone
Cushing's disease responds to the dopamine agonist cabergoline (Dostinex)[1] with a normalization of cortisol production in as many as 40% of the cases. The peroxisome proliferator-activated receptor γ (PPAR-γ) agonist rosiglitazone (Avandia)[1] was demonstrated to be effective in animal models, but it was unsuccessful in controlling ACTH oversecretion in patients with Cushing's disease. A new agent, SOM-230 (pasireotide [Signifor]), blocks both type 2 and type 5 somatostatin receptors and reduces ACTH secretion in vitro. Mifepristone (Korlym), a glucocorticoid receptor antagonist, recently became available for patients who failed surgical or irradiation therapies (see also below).

Bilateral Adrenalectomy
Bilateral adrenalectomy offers a definitive treatment that provides immediate control of hypercortisolism, but this surgery should be reserved for patients with Cushing's disease who have failed all other treatments. Bilateral adrenalectomy in active Cushing's disease often

---

[1] Not FDA approved for this indication.

TABLE 4 Medical Treatment for Hypercortisolism

MEDICATION	INITIAL DOSE	MAXIMUM DOSE	ADVERSE EFFECTS
Ketoconazole (Nizoral)[1]	100–200 mg bid/tid	1200 mg	Nausea, vomiting, abdominal pain, weakness, hypothyroidism, gynecomastia, hepatotoxicity, hypertriglyceridemia
Metyrapone (Metopirone)[1]	250 mg qid	6000 mg	Headache, alopecia, hirsutism, acne, nausea, abdominal discomfort, hypertension, weakness, leucopenia
Mitotane (Lysodren)[1]	500 mg tid	9000 mg	Nausea, vomiting, anorexia, diarrhea, ataxia, confusion, skin rash, hepatotoxicity
Aminoglutethimide (Cytadren)[2]	250 mg qid	2000 mg/d	Lethargy, nausea, anorexia, hypothyroidism, somnolence

[1]Not FDA approved for this indication.
[2]Not available in the United States.

leads to Nelson's syndrome, a condition characterized by unabated progression of a corticotropinoma (owing to the lack of negative feedback by cortisol), very high ACTH levels, and high morbidity.

Treatment of Adrenal Disease
Adrenocortical Tumors
For adrenocortical tumors, the recommended treatment is surgical. Laparoscopic adrenalectomy has become the treatment of choice for benign adrenal lesions with a diameter of less than 6 cm. In stages I to III adrenocortical carcinoma, complete tumor removal by a well-trained surgeon offers by far the best chance for cure. Surgery often needs to be extensive, with en bloc resection of invaded organs, and regularly includes lymphadenectomy. Surgery for local recurrences or metastatic disease is accepted as a valuable therapeutic option and was associated with improved survival in retrospective studies. The overall 5-year survival in different series ranged between 16% and 38%. Median survival for metastatic disease (stage IV) at the time of diagnosis is still consistently less than 12 months.

Radiotherapy has been considered ineffective for treatment of adrenocortical cancer, but it can be indicated to control localized disease not amenable to surgery.

Mitotane (o,p′-DDD [Lysodren]) is the only adrenal-specific agent available for treating adrenocortical cancer. Mitotane is indicated in metastatic adrenocortical carcinoma and can also be used as an adjuvant for tumors with a high risk of recurrence. Mitotane exerts a specific cytotoxic effect on adrenocortical cells, leading to focal degeneration of the fascicular and particularly the reticular zone. In most patients, treatment should be initiated with a dose that does not exceed 1.5 g/day; this is then rapidly increased, depending on gastrointestinal symptoms, to 5 to 6 g/day. This high-dose regimen requires measurement of mitotane blood levels 14 days after initiation of therapy. The dose is then adjusted according to the medicine's plasma concentrations (which should be greater than 14 mg/L) and tolerance of the side effects. Because mitotane treatment induces adrenal insufficiency and increases the metabolic clearance of glucocorticoids, glucocorticoid replacement is indicated, often at higher than normal doses owing to increased clearance.

Cytotoxic Chemotherapy
Cytotoxic chemotherapy includes etoposide (VePesid)[1], doxorubicin (Adriamycin)[1], and cisplatin (Platinol)[1], or streptozocin (Zanosar)[1] plus mitotane. Chemotherapy has limited efficacy for advanced adrenocortical cancer and is associated mainly with partial responses.

Bilateral Adrenal Hyperplasias
The treatment of choice for bilateral adrenal hyperplasias associated with ACTH-independent Cushing's syndrome is bilateral adrenalectomy. Patients require lifelong replacement therapy with glucocorticoids and mineralocorticoids, and they should be adequately educated about the risk of acute adrenal insufficiency.

Treatment of Ectopic Corticotropin Syndrome
The choice of treatment for ectopic ACTH syndrome depends on tumor identification, localization, and classification. The most effective treatment option is surgical resection, although this is not always possible in metastatic disease or in the case of occult tumors. Because the ectopic ACTH syndrome is usually severe and occult tumors can become evident at imaging studies only during the follow-up, medical treatment to control hypercortisolism is often necessary. Bilateral adrenalectomy may be an option to be considered when the hypercortisolism cannot be controlled by other treatment options.

Medical Adrenalectomy
Several drugs that inhibit steroid synthesis are often effective for rapidly controlling hypercortisolism in preparation for surgery, after unsuccessful transsphenoidal surgery or removal of an adrenal tumor such as extensive cancer, or while awaiting the full effect of radiotherapy in recurrent Cushing's disease (Table 4).

Most experience with inhibitors of steroidogenesis has been with metyrapone (Metopirone)[1] and ketoconazole (Nizoral)[1], two medications that appear to be more effective and better tolerated than aminoglutethimide (Cytadren)[2]. Metyrapone reduces cortisol and aldosterone production by inhibiting 11β-hydroxylation in the adrenal cortex. Ketoconazole is a broad-spectrum antifungal drug, which inhibits c17-20 desmolase, cholesterol side-chain cleavage, and 11β-hydroxylation. Ketoconazole is also associated with inhibition of testosterone biosynthesis and gynecomastia.

RU-486, or mifepristone (Korlym), is an antagonist of the progesterone and glucocorticoid receptors. Unexpectedly, the treatment of Cushing's disease with this glucocorticoid antagonist has been associated with increased ACTH secretion and consequent stimulation of cortisol production. RU-486 may be more useful in ectopic ACTH-producing tumors and in adrenal Cushing's syndrome, but its efficacy and potential side effects when administered chronically are currently unknown.

References
Allolio B, Fassnacht M: Clinical review: Adrenocortical carcinoma: clinical update, *J Clin Endocrinol Metab* 91:2027–2037, 2006.

Assie G, Libe R, Espiard S, et al: ARMC5 mutations in macronodular adrenal hyperplasia with Cushing's syndrome, *N Engl J Med* 369(22):2105–2114, 2013.

Batista D, Courkoutsakis NA, Oldfield EH, et al: Detection of adrenocorticotropin-secreting pituitary adenomas by magnetic resonance imaging in children and adolescents with Cushing disease, *J Clin Endocrinol Metab* 90:5134–5140, 2005.

Batista DL, Riar J, Keil M, Stratakis CA: Diagnostic tests for children who are referred for the investigation of Cushing syndrome, *Pediatrics* 120:e575–e586, 2007.

Bertagna X, Guignat L, Groussin L, Bertherat J: Cushing's disease, *Best Pract Res Clin Endocrinol Metab* 23:607–623, 2009.

Biller BM, Grossman AB, Stewart PM, et al: Treatment of adrenocorticotropin-dependent Cushing's syndrome: a consensus statement, *J Clin Endocrinol Metab* 93:2454–2462, 2008.

Boscaro M, Arnaldi G: Approach to the patient with possible Cushing's syndrome, *J Clin Endocrinol Metab* 94:3121–3131, 2009.

Feelders RA, Hofland LJ: Medical treatment of Cushing's disease, *J Clin Endocrinol Metab* 98(2):425–438, 2013.

Newell-Price J, Trainer P, Besser M, Grossman A: The diagnosis and differential diagnosis of Cushing's syndrome and pseudo-Cushing's states, *Endocr Rev* 19:647–672, 1998.

Terzolo M, Angeli A, Fassnacht M, et al: Adjuvant mitotane treatment for adrenocortical carcinoma, *N Engl J Med* 356:2372–2380, 2007.

---

[1]Not FDA approved for this indication.   [2]Not available in the United States.

DIABETES INSIPIDUS

Method of
Rami Mortada, MD

CURRENT DIAGNOSIS

- Diabetes insipidus (DI) is a disorder of excess urine production (i.e., "diabetes") that is dilute and tasteless (i.e., "insipidus"). DI contrasts with the concentrated and sweet urine in diabetes mellitus.
- Patients with DI present with polyuria and polydipsia; urine output is usually more than 40 mL/kg/day or more than 3 L/day.
- There are three subtypes of DI:
  - Central DI: due to relative or absolute lack of vasopressin
  - Nephrogenic DI: due to partial or total resistance to the renal antidiuretic effects of vasopressin
  - Dipsogenic DI (also called primary polydipsia): where polyuria is secondary to excessive, inappropriate fluid intake
- Initial labs should include plasma sodium and urine osmolality. Under normal physiologic conditions, the urine osmolality is less than 300 mOsm/L, but if the patient does not have sufficient fluid intake, the urine osmolality can be higher.
- The diagnosis is confirmed by examining urine output and osmolality. It can be followed by an assessment of renal response to the synthetic arginine vasopressin (AVP) analogue desmopressin (DDAVP).
- In primary polydipsia, urine concentration is normal in response to dehydration.
- In central DI, urine concentration does not increase appropriately with dehydration, but does respond to desmopressin (DDAVP). After dehydration in central DI, urine osmolality remains <300 mOsm/kg, and plasma osmolality is >290 mOsm/kg. Urine osmolality rises to >750 mOsm/kg after desmopressin.
- In nephrogenic DI, urine concentration does not increase appropriately with either dehydration or exogenous desmopressin.

CURRENT THERAPY

- The treatment goal is to control polyuria and ensure electrolyte stability.
- In Central DI:
  - The mild form might not require treatment.
  - Significant polyuria can be treated with desmopressin in divided doses: nasal spray 5 to 100 µg/day; tablets 100 to 1000 µg/day; or parenterally 0.1 to 2.0 µg/day.
  - Overtreatment can cause hyponatremia.
- In Nephrogenic DI:
  - Urine output should not be expected to normalize after DDAVP administration.
  - Correct the culprit cause (hypercalcemia or lithium [Eskalith, Lithobid] cessation).
  - Follow a low-sodium, low-protein diet, as tolerated.
  - Hydrochlorothiazide[1] 25 to 50 mg/day may be taken either alone or in combination with indomethacin (Indocin) 25 to 50 mg twice daily.
  - Symptoms may respond partly to high-dose desmopressin (e.g., 4 mcg IM twice daily).
- Primary polydipsia is treated by limiting an excessive fluid intake.

[1]Not FDA approved for this indication.

Physiology of Antidiuretic Hormone

Arginine vasopressin (AVP), also known as antidiuretic hormone (ADH), is a neurohypophysial hormone. It is a peptide hormone that promotes water retention by increasing the permeability of the kidney's collecting duct and distal convoluted tubule to water. It also increases peripheral vascular resistance, which in turn increases arterial blood pressure. In the clinical setting, the terms AVP, ADH, and vasopressin are used interchangeably.

Vasopressin is considered the main hormone involved in the regulation of water homeostasis and osmolality. The regulation and synthesis of vasopressin is under the influence of two systems: osmotic and pressure/volume status. In the case of osmoregulation, a small increase in plasma osmolality produces a parallel increase in vasopressin secretion; a small decrease in plasma osmolality causes a parallel drop in vasopressin.

Vasopressin is one among other hormones and systems that are involved in the regulation of volume and blood pressure. Other factors influence vasopressin production. For example, glucocorticoids inhibit secretion, whereas nausea and vomiting have a stimulatory effect.

Pathophysiology of Diabetes Insipidus

The kidneys exercise one of their urine-concentrating abilities by promoting water retention. If the concentration of vasopressin is decreased, polyuria occurs and diluted urine is excreted. A decrease in total body water results in an increase in the plasma osmolality. If the physiologic response is intact, thirst is stimulated, which leads to an increase in water consumption and the correction of plasma osmolarity. Therefore, unless there is a dysregulation in the thirst mechanisms or water consumption is limited due to a lack of availability (e.g., decreased level of consciousness, immobility, or physical restraints) severe dehydration does not develop.

Clinical Causes

There are three subtypes of diabetes insipidus (DI).

- DI secondary to excess water intake (primary polydipsia)

Primary polydipsia is a disorder characterized by inappropriate excess fluid intake due to a disordered thirst sensation seen mostly in patients with psychiatric illnesses. A central defect in thirst regulation plays an important role in the pathogenesis of primary polydipsia. Such patients continue drinking even if the plasma osmolality falls below normal. It is not easy to achieve or maintain a low plasma osmolality because vasopressin secretion will normally be suppressed by the fall in plasma osmolality, resulting in rapid excretion of the excess water. If vasopressin regulation is intact, primary polydipsia should not lead to clinically important disturbances in the plasma sodium concentration unless hyposmolar fluid intake overwhelms the kidneys' ability to excrete excess water. Thus the serum sodium concentration is usually normal or slightly reduced in primary polydipsia. These patients may be asymptomatic or present with complaints of polydipsia and polyuria. In rare circumstances where water intake exceeds the kidneys' ability to excrete the water load of about 500 mL/hour, symptomatic severe hyponatremia might result in severe psychosis. Psychosis from hyponatremia in primary polydipsia is most commonly seen in institutionalized patients or in individuals attempting to dilute their urine to avoid a positive urine drug test.

- DI secondary to a decrease in or absence of vasopressin secretion (central DI)

Central DI may be caused by genetic anomalies of the vasopressin gene (Table 1). Familial neurohypophyseal DI is characterized by the onset of DI with polyuria and polydipsia in childhood or early adulthood. The most common MRI finding in familial neurohypophyseal DI is the progressive disappearance of the posterior pituitary bright spot in children. The normal pituitary bright spot seen on unenhanced T_1-weighted MRI is thought to result from the T_1-shortening effect of the

TABLE 1	Central Diabetes Insipidus (DI) Etiologies
Idiopathic	Unknown etiology
Genetic	Familial neurohypophyseal DI, Wolfram's syndrome (autosomal recessive)
Mass effect	Craniopharyngiomas, primary germ cell tumors, metastatic tumors
Infiltrative diseases	Lymphoma, leukemia, sarcoidosis, amyloidosis
Autoimmune	Lymphocytic infundibuloneurohypophysitis
Trauma	Motor vehicle accident, closed head trauma
Surgical	Surgical intervention at the pituitary region

vasopressin stored in the posterior pituitary. The disappearance of the bright spot corresponds to the disappearance of vasopressin stores in the posterior pituitary. Wolfram's syndrome is a rare autosomal recessive syndrome manifested by DI, diabetes mellitus, optic atrophy, and deafness.

Central DI may be caused by mass lesions of the neurohypophysis, such as craniopharyngiomas, and primary germ cell tumors in childhood. DI can be the initial presentation. MRI often shows a thickened pituitary stalk and may show a hypothalamic mass. Metastasis to the pituitary usually is found with widespread metastatic disease and is twice as likely to involve the posterior pituitary than the anterior pituitary. DI can be associated with pituitary infiltration associated with lymphomas and leukemias.

In granulomatous disease that affects the hypothalamic-pituitary axis, there is usually clear evidence of disease elsewhere in the body. MRI shows an absence of the pituitary bright spot and widening of the hypothalamic-pituitary stalk. Lymphocytic infundibuloneurohypophysitis is a new, well-recognized cause of autoimmune DI, characterized by MRI appearance of a thickened hypothalamic-pituitary stalk and large posterior pituitary gland mimicking a pituitary tumor. Pituitary abscess is a rare cause of pituitary mass and DI. In situations where the cause is not easily diagnosed, an autoimmune process should be suspected. In some patients, the cause is idiopathic.

Central DI may be caused by surgery or trauma to the pituitary region. Vasopressin is normally secreted after any kind of surgical stress, and secretion is more pronounced after surgery to the pituitary region. Only a small percentage of patients undergoing pituitary surgery have permanent DI. A triphasic DI can occur after complete hypothalamic-pituitary stalk transection. The first phase is polyuric and appears within the first 24 hours after surgery. It is thought to be secondary to axonal shock with a resultant inability to release prefabricated vasopressin. The second phase is antidiuretic and starts on about day 6, after stalk injury. It is thought to be secondary to the unregulated release of vasopressin stores. The third phase, also polyuric, starts about day 12, after vasopressin stores have been depleted. It may result in permanent or partial DI or resolve to clinically asymptomatic disease.

The same patterns of DI that occur after pituitary surgery can be seen in patients who experience a closed head trauma. Three-quarters of traumatic induced DI are secondary to motor vehicle accidents. Trauma is usually severe and causes unconsciousness. There is a high association of anterior pituitary deficiency in association with DI induced by head trauma, so the possibility of central hypocortisolism should be considered and treated immediately. DI is reported in 50% to 90% of patients with brain death.

- DI secondary to the lack of renal response to vasopressin (nephrogenic DI)

Genetic anomalies resulting in a lack of renal response to vasopressin are caused by either a mutation in the V2 recep-

tors or a mutation of the aquaporin 2 water channels gene. The majority of the cases are X-linked recessive disorders in males. Newborns present with polyuria, vomiting, constipation, and failure to thrive. Symptoms usually occur within the first week of life.

Acquired nephrogenic DI can be caused by a kidney disease that distorts the architecture of the kidney and impairs its urine-concentrating ability (e.g., polycystic kidney disease, sickle cell disease). Decreased function of vasopressin or downregulation of aquaporin 2 channels can be caused by hypokalemia, hypercalcemia, and relief of bilateral urinary tract obstruction. Drugs such as lithium (the most common cause of drug-induced nephrogenic DI) and demeclocycline (used clinically to treat a syndrome of inappropriate ADH secretion) may cause nephrogenic DI.

Clinical Manifestations

Patients with central DI typically present with polyuria, nocturia, and polydipsia. The serum sodium concentration in untreated central DI is often in the high normal range, which provides the ongoing stimulation of thirst that replaces urinary water losses. Moderate to severe hypernatremia can develop when thirst is impaired or if there is a lack of access to free water, such as the postoperative period in patients with unrecognized DI or infants with DI. For uncertain pathophysiologic reasons, patients with central DI may develop decreased bone mineral density at the lumbar spine and femoral neck, even if treated with desmopressin.

Nephrogenic DI in its mild form can be asymptomatic. Patients with moderate to severe nephrogenic DI, as with central DI, typically present with polyuria, nocturia, and polydipsia.

Primary polydipsia is the result of an abnormal compulsion to drink water. This disorder is most often seen in middle-aged women and in patients with psychiatric illnesses. The excessive water intake initially drives the excessive urination.

Diagnosis

Polyuria must be distinguished from simple urinary frequency in the absence of excess urine volume. The initial diagnostic approach should be to confirm polyuria, defined as greater than 30 mL/kg or 3 L/day, with a urine osmolality measuring less than 300 mOsm/L. Simple metabolic causes such as hyperglycemia, uremia, and hypercalcemia should be excluded. A definitive diagnosis of DI requires testing of vasopressin production and action in response to osmolar stress. All forms of DI may be partial or complete. In primary polydipsia, the plasma sodium, blood urea nitrogen (BUN), and uric acid are relatively low. In other forms of DI, the plasma sodium and uric acid are relatively high and BUN is relatively low.

Central DI usually has an abrupt onset resulting from destruction of more than 80% of vasopressin-secreting hypothalamic neurons. The etiology of polyuria is not always evident after history and laboratory tests are completed. In that case, a water restriction test (e.g., dehydration test or water deprivation test) is completed. The water deprivation test is an indirect assessment of the AVP axis, measuring renal concentrating capacity in response to dehydration. It can be followed by assessment of the renal response to the synthetic AVP analogue desmopressin to determine whether any defect identified in urine-concentrating ability can be corrected with AVP-replacement. Office testing is acceptable unless the patient cannot be watched closely. No food or water is allowed. The patient is watched for signs of dehydration and surreptitious water drinking. Baseline measurements include weight, plasma osmolality, sodium, BUN, glucose, and urine volume and osmolality. Weight, plasma osmolality, and urine osmolality are measured hourly. The test is ended if urine osmolality has not increased to more than 300 mOsm/kg for 3 consecutive hours, plasma osmolality has reached 295 to 300 mOsm/kg, or the patient has lost 3% to 5% of body weight. All initial measurements are repeated at the end of the water restriction test. Then, 5 units of aqueous AVP (Pitressin) is administered or 2 μg of desmopressin is given subcutaneously and the plasma osmolality,

TABLE 2	Values Before and After Water Restriction			
	INITIAL PLASMA OSMOLALITY	INITIAL PLASMA SODIUM	POSTTEST URINE/PLASMA OSMOLALITY	POSTTEST URINE/PLASMA OSMOLALITY+ADH
Normal	NL	NL	>1	>1
Central DI	High (high NL)	High (high NL)	<1	>1
Nephrogenic DI	High (high NL)	High (high NL)	<1	<1
Primary polydipsia	Low (low NL)	Low (low NL)	>1	>1

TABLE 3	Treatment Options for Diabetes Insipidus
Central DI	Divide doses of two to three times per day:
	Desmopressin nasal spray 5–100 µg/day
	Desmopressin tablets 0.1–1 mg/day
	Desmopressin injection 0.1–2 µg/day
Nephrogenic DI	Low-salt, low-protein diet
	HCTZ[1] 25 mg one to two times per day
	Indomethacin[1] 25–50 mg bid
	Amiloride[1] 5–10 mg bid
Primary polydipsia	Water restriction to less than 1.5 L/day

[1]Not FDA approved for this indication.

sodium, BUN, glucose, and urine volume and osmolality are measured at 30, 60, and 120 minutes.

In primary polydipsia, urine concentration is normal in response to dehydration (Table 2).

In central DI, urine concentration does not increase appropriately with dehydration, but responds to desmopressin. Urine osmolality remains <300 mOsm/kg, accompanied by plasma osmolality >290 mOsm/kg after dehydration, and urine osmolality rising to >750 mOsm/kg after desmopressin administration.

In nephrogenic DI, urine concentration does not increase appropriately with either dehydration or exogenous desmopressin.

In practice, many results are indeterminate. If central DI is suspected, but the water deprivation test data are inconclusive, a reasonable approach is a therapeutic trial of 10 to 20 µg intranasal desmopressin per day with close monitoring of plasma sodium. If the diagnosis is confirmed, pituitary function testing and cranial MRI should follow.

Treatment

The treatment goal is to improve polyuria and polydipsia symptoms while attempting to treat the etiologic factors (Table 3). This is achieved by appropriate correction of dehydration, if present, and replacing vasopressin or augmenting its effect on the target tissue.

Mild forms of central DI may not require pharmacologic treatment. Desmopressin effectively treats polyuria and polydipsia. Desmopressin comes in different forms, and dosages usually need to be divided.

Hyponatremia from plasma dilution can be avoided by skipping treatment for a short period on a regular basis (e.g., on Sunday). No second dose of desmopressin should be given unless the patient has urine output after the first dose.

Nephrogenic DI may respond to the removal of the offending agent (e.g., lithium) or correction of the underlying electrolyte disturbance (e.g., hypercalcemia or hypokalemia). Drug-induced nephrogenic DI, however, may persist after discontinuation of the drug.

Patients should be instructed to eat a low-sodium, low-protein diet, resulting in a decrease in urine output secondary to the drop in solute excretion. If symptomatic polyuria persists, hydrochlorothiazide[1] can be started. Hydrochlorothiazide presumably acts by inducing mild hypovolemia that induces an increase in proximal sodium and water reabsorption, thereby diminishing water delivery to the vasopressin-sensitive sites in the collecting tubules and reducing the urine output. Indomethacin (Indocin[1]) is an add-on medication if there is not enough response. Given that prostaglandins antagonize the action of vasopressin, indomethacin inhibits renal prostaglandin synthesis and subsequently decreases urine output.

Amiloride (Midamor)[1] might be more effective for lithium-induced nephrogenic DI. This drug closes the sodium channels in the luminal membrane of the collecting tubule cells. These channels constitute the mechanism by which filtered lithium normally enters the collecting tubule cells and interferes with the collecting tubule response to ADH.

The approach to primary polydipsia treatment is reduction in fluid intake. Desmopressin treatment should be avoided due to the risk of hyponatremia.

Monitoring

Primary polydipsia is the most challenging of all types of DI to treat. It requires a multidisciplinary approach that frequently demands medical and psychiatric involvement.

In central DI, patients will require frequent follow-up to adjust desmopressin dosing. Once stable, patients can be seen less frequently to assess symptom control and to check plasma sodium levels to avoid overtreatment resulting in hyponatremia.

In nephrogenic DI, after the precipitating agent has been withdrawn, follow-up is needed to assess the reversibility of polyuria. If acquired nephrogenic DI becomes irreversible, patients might require prolonged pharmacological treatment. In both central and nephrogenic DI, the patient is advised to wear a medical alert bracelet stating the disease and the potential complications.

Acknowledgment

I would like to thank K. James Kallail, PhD, for his contribution to the final editing of this chapter.

[1]Not FDA approved for this indication.

References

Bockenhauer D, Bichet DG: Inherited secondary nephrogenic diabetes insipidus: Concentrating on humans, *Am J Physiol Renal Physiol* 304:F1037–F1042, 2013.

Crowley RK, Sherlock M, Agha A, et al: Clinical insights into adipsic diabetes insipidus: A large case series, *Clin Endocrinol (Oxf)* 66:475–482, 2007.

Fujiwara TM, Bichet DG: Molecular biology of hereditary diabetes insipidus, *J Am Soc Nephrol* 16:2836–2846, 2005.

Hannon MJ, Sherlock M, Thompson CJ: Pituitary dysfunction following traumatic brain injury or subarachnoid haemorrhage, *Best Pract Res Clin Endocrinol Metab* 25:783–798, 2011.

Monnens L, Jonkman A, Thomas C: Response to indomethacin and hydrochlorothiazide in nephrogenic diabetes insipidus, *Clin Sci (Lond)* 66:709–715, 1984.

Oiso Y, Robertson GL, Nørgaard JP, Juul KV: Clinical review: Treatment of neurohypophyseal diabetes insipidus, *J Clin Endocrinol Metab* 98:3958–3967, 2013.

Vande Walle J, Stockner M, Raes A, Nørgaard JP: Desmopressin 30 years in clinical use: A safety review, *Curr Drug Saf* 2:232–238, 2007.

DIABETES MELLITUS IN ADULTS

Method of
Kristine Grdinovac, MD; Candice Rose, MD, MS, RD; and David C. Robbins, MD

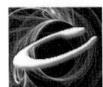

CURRENT DIAGNOSIS

- Established guidelines define diabetes as a fasting blood sugar ≥126 mg/dL or an HbA1c of ≥6.5% or a blood sugar ≥200 mg/dL 2 hours after a 75-g oral glucose load.
- Prediabetes is defined as a blood sugar of 100 to 125 mg/dL or an HbA1c between 5.7% and 6.4%.
- The diagnostic guidelines are derived from inflection points in the risk of acquiring complications at any given glucose elevation.
- People with *prediabetes* share a similar risk of cardiovascular disease (CVD) as those with diabetes. Thus, intervention with weight loss, exercise, and metformin[1] is very beneficial in this population.
- Early detection of complications can slow the progression to end-stage disease. Routine surveillance includes annual dilated eye exams, foot inspection, measurement of microalbuminuria, and measurements of blood lipids and kidney and liver function.

[1]Not FDA approved for this indication.

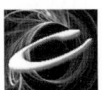

CURRENT THERAPY

- Treatment should be started early, when signs of hyperglycemia appear, including prediabetes. The risks of complications are related to the lifetime duration of hyperglycemia.
- A standard glycemic treatment goal is an HbA1c below 7%. It is justified, in a few patients, to set a higher goal when factors such as age, desire to lose weight, catastrophic risk of hypoglycemia, concurrent disease, and/or other barriers are detected.
- Because the treatment of diabetes is largely focused on prevention of atherosclerotic disease, aggressive control of blood pressure and lipids is also recommended.
- Treatment of type 2 diabetes mellitus (T2DM) is fundamentally based on diet (weight loss) and exercise with the addition of drugs (or bariatric surgery) when treatment goals are not achieved. No patient should experience uncontrolled hyperglycemia for more than 3 months without the addition of more therapy.
- Metformin is usually the first-line drug. There are now many options for additional medications that may best fit a patient's disease characteristics, financial resources, and lifestyle. Some of the newer (and more expensive) medications are weight-neutral, may promote weight loss, and have shown to reduce the risk of atherosclerotic cardiovascular disease and deterioration in renal function.
- Assessment of glucose control includes periodic measurement of HbA1c, home blood glucose monitoring, and, when appropriate, continuous glucose monitoring.
- Treatment with insulin is an option that can be introduced at any time during the course of T2DM. The goal, ideally, is to normalize the blood sugar without significant or frequent hypoglycemia.

Epidemiology

The rising prevalence of diabetes in the United States and globally has been described as an epidemic or tsunami that has the potential to overwhelm medical systems worldwide. The number of people who have been diagnosed with diabetes rose from 108 million in 1980 to about 422 million in 2014. The global prevalence has nearly doubled during the same time period, from 4.7% to 8.5%. About 34.2 million or 10.5% of Americans are known to have diabetes and a nearly equal number have the disease but are undiagnosed. The prevalence rises with age, reaching 26.8% of the population 65 years of age or older. Women have a slightly higher prevalence than men, and the disease disproportionately affects people of Hispanic and Asian descent and non-Hispanic Blacks. Not surprisingly, the proportion of people with undiagnosed diabetes is also greatest among those of color and in the lower socioeconomic strata.

The US yearly incidence of prediabetes (defined as a fasting blood sugar of 100 to 125 mg/dL or HbA1c 5.7% to 6.4%) is estimated to be approximately 35%. On average, 1 in every 10 prediabetic patients will become diabetic every year.

The risk factors for diabetes clearly include an interaction of genetic susceptibility and environmental triggers, including obesity. For example, among diabetic patients, 89% are overweight or obese. The US National Health Interview Survey has shown a striking impact of obesity on the risk of acquiring the disease. Among nearly 800,000 respondents, the lifetime risk of diabetes was approximately 7.6% among underweight men and 70.3% for those who were very obese. The effect of increasing weight on the risk of diabetes is linear, with those having a body mass index (BMI) above 30 having at least a fivefold increase in the risk of acquiring diabetes. The central or intra-abdominal accumulation of fat has also been shown to be more highly correlated with diabetes than with subcutaneous fat. Thus, individuals of the same body composition who have a predominance of central or intra-abdominal fat are much more likely to have insulin resistance, hypertension, diabetes, and dyslipidemia. Intra-abdominal fat, in contrast to subcutaneous fat, produces more free fatty acids, inflammatory cytokines, hormones associated with insulin resistance, and reduced amounts of insulin sensitizers such as adiponectin.

The widely used BMI cutoff points for overweight (25 to 30 kg/m^2) and obesity (>30 kg/m^2) are good markers for diabetic risks among non-Hispanic whites and African Americans. However, among Asians and Hispanics, diabetes incidence rises at much lower BMIs, possibly triggered by a more potent impact of central adiposity on insulin resistance and hyperglycemia. In the Diabetes Prevention Program (DPP), a BMI cutoff point of 22 kg/m^2 rather than 25 kg/m^2 was used to identify Asian participants at increased risk for diabetes. These differences should be kept in mind when counseling or treating patients of different ethnicities.

In addition to obesity, a variety of other risk factors include smoking, hypertension, hypercholesterolemia, and, most importantly, physical inactivity. Of these associated risk factors, it is clinically important to recognize that even a modest increase in physical activity and a small reduction in body weight are the only nonpharmacologic interventions prospectively shown to reduce the risk of acquiring or even occasionally reversing diabetes (as shown in the DPP).

The genetics of type 2 diabetes mellitus (T2DM) are complex and incompletely understood despite huge studies seeking the gene variations that increase risk of diabetes. Large population studies have found over 120 gene variants that account for the risk of T2DM but their contribution is small (about 3% to 10%) and, with few exceptions, any given gene variant is practically useless in assessing risk for a particular individual. Thus, while weight, waist circumference, and age are clinically useful markers of risk, genetic testing is not yet a clinical tool to predict diabetes. The predominant factors responsible for the diabetes phenotype are environmental rather than genetic. Curiously, identical monozygotic twins show a strong diabetes concordance (76%) even when the twins are raised separately from one another.

Diagnosis and Classification of Diabetes and Prediabetes

The definitions of diabetes and prediabetes are based on standardized and discrete markers of hyperglycemia. On the other hand, the complications of diabetes, most notably atherosclerosis and microvascular disease, are more or less linearly related to the exposure to hyperglycemia over time rather than appearing with any given marker of glycemia. For example, one accepted definition of diabetes is a fasting blood sugar of 126 mg/dL or higher. However, a marked increased risk of CVD is found at lower concentrations of blood glucose. Prediabetic persons, whose fasting blood sugar may range from 100 to 125 mg/dL, have nearly the same incidence of atherosclerotic heart disease as patients assigned a standardized diagnosis of diabetes.

The standard definitions of diabetes are largely based on inflection points in the risk of complications versus a given increment in glycemia. Diabetes then is defined as any of the following abnormalities:

- Hemoglobin A1c 6.5% or higher
- Fasting plasma glucose 126 mg/dL or higher
- A 2-hr glucose of 200 mg/dL or higher after a 75-g oral glucose load (oral glucose tolerance test).

It must be noted that there is some controversy over these values. Not all newly diagnosed individuals will have abnormalities in all three criteria. Furthermore, it is unsettled whether one test better predicts complications than another. Some experts insist that a patient should have at least two abnormal criteria, but this may delay justified clinical intervention and add cost and inconvenience. It is our recommendation to accept any one abnormality as a criterion for a diagnosis of diabetes and justification to begin lifestyle and possibly drug interventions.

The accepted classification of diabetes is, like the laboratory diagnosis, useful but imperfect. *The common phenotype of all types of diabetes is hyperglycemia* and a variety of more subtle abnormalities related to insulin deficiency or insulin resistance such as dyslipidemia, increased tissue oxidation, and macro- and microvascular disease, among others.

Diabetes Is Classified Into Four Categories

Type 1 Diabetes

Type 1 diabetes mellitus (T1DM) is due, in most cases, to an autoimmune destruction of the insulin-producing beta cells. About 95% of such patients have autoantibodies (glutamic acid decarboxylase-65 [GAD-65], anti-zinc transporter protein, and anti-islet cell antibodies) that mark the gradual (sometimes over many years) or rapid destruction of the beta cells. The result is a complete or near-total loss of endogenous insulin and life-sustaining dependence on insulin therapy. In general, antibody-positive persons who have all three antibodies and those with higher titers become diabetic more quickly than those with low titers of one or two antibodies.

Differentiating T1DM from T2DM can sometimes be a diagnostic challenge. *The age of onset* of T1DM peaks in the mid-teens but is not a reliable diagnostic tool because incident T1DM is seen throughout the human lifespan. Similarly, *thinness* is no longer a reliable phenotype of T1DM since so many of us are obese. *Ketoacidosis* used to be considered a hallmark of T1DM, but a subset of T2DM patients presents with ketoacidosis, recovers with treatment, and can be successfully treated with oral agents (Flatbush diabetes). The diagnosis can sometimes be even more perplexing because some new-onset T1DM patients will not require insulin for several months after presenting with ketoacidosis. This so-called honeymoon phase of diabetes usually lasts less than 6 months.

When the diagnosis is unclear, we occasionally measure C-peptide and glucose simultaneously and the GAD-65 antibody to more clearly differentiate a T1DM patient from the more common T2DM (see definition below). Those patients with very low C-peptides in the presence of elevated glucose and the positive anti-GAD-65 antibody are almost always type 1, and insulin treatment is needed from the outset.

Type 2 Diabetes

T2DM accounts for about 95% of the worldwide burden of the disease. The pathophysiology of the disease is fundamentally a simultaneous deficiency in the amount of insulin needed to overcome the insulin resistance, resulting in hyperglycemia, an event that most commonly occurs during midlife. However, the condition is increasingly manifest in childhood or early adolescence in concert with epidemic obesity and inactivity. Adolescent T2DM, now accounting for a significant proportion of diabetes in youth, appears to be a particularly aggressive form of the disease with high risk of late complications.

The cause of the hyperglycemia is complex and multifactorial. There is a progressive nonautoimmune loss of insulin production thought to be due to aging, loss of beta cells from inflammation and oxidative stress, a genetically programmed loss with age, or, for lack of a better term, pancreatic exhaustion. Resistance to insulin is also an essential aspect of the disease that may be detected long before hyperglycemia. The vast majority of patients with T2DM are obese or at least have increased amounts of central fat. Many students of T2DM argue that there are many subtypes or genotypes that share a similar clinical presentation and future classification schemes may account for those differences. About 5% of the T2DM population are thin and the cause of their noninsulin-dependent diabetes is not so clear.

Gestational Diabetes

Gestational diabetes (GDM) is typically diagnosed in the second or third trimester of pregnancy on the basis of a 50-g oral glucose tolerance test in women who were not known to be diabetic pre-pregnancy. GDM carries an increased risk of pregnancy complications (hypertension, preeclampsia, large birthweight infants) and treatment with diet, metformin[1], or insulin is commonly used. Importantly, 50% to 80% of women who had GDM will suffer from T2DM within a decade of their pregnancy.

Specific Types of Diabetes Due to Other Causes

This category may account for as much as 5% of clinical diabetes and should not be overlooked. We remind our residents to think of these "other" forms of diabetes on the first visit with every phenotypically type 2 patient. These include cystic fibrosis, glucocorticoid-induced diabetes, Cushing syndrome, hemochromatosis, certain anticancer drugs (checkpoint inhibitors, alpelisib [Piqray], etc.), and monogenic forms of diabetes. The monogenic forms of diabetes can be manifested in the first 3 months of life. Later in life an autosomal dominant form of noninsulin-dependent diabetes termed Maturity Onset Diabetes of Youth (MODY) is seen. MODY may account for a few percent of the "type 2" diabetic population and is suspected when there is onset of diabetes in the late teens or early adulthood. Genetic testing is commercially available for these polymorphisms and can identify common subtypes that are responsive to high-dose sulfonylurea medication.

Clinical Manifestations

Most patients with T2DM are discovered by elevated glucose on an incidental blood test. Population screening is generally inefficient except among those at very high risk. Otherwise, presenting symptoms include polyuria, polydipsia, nocturia, blurred vision, and/or weight loss due to catabolism. While the peak incidence of T2DM is in midlife, there is an increasing and disturbing rise in the incidence of T2DM in children and adolescents, especially those belonging to racial and ethnic minorities. This is undoubtedly correlated with childhood obesity.

Less frequently, patients can initially present with diabetic ketoacidosis (DKA) or nonketotic hyperosmolar hyperglycemic state (HHS). This typically occurs in combination with some inciting factor, such as infection, stress, or myocardial ischemia. Patients have hyperglycemia, marked dehydration, electrolyte derangements, and altered levels of consciousness and are at increased risk of death. Other common conditions that are highly

---

[1]Not FDA approved for this indication.

correlated with the development of diabetes include polycystic ovary syndrome, GDM, toxemia of pregnancy, and delivery of infants over 8 lb at birth (large for dates).

Most commonly, T2DM has an insidious onset and patients can remain asymptomatic for several years, only being diagnosed unexpectedly through routine laboratory workup. Aging, sedentariness, and obesity may tip the balance between insulin action and insulin resistance resulting in clinical hyperglycemia. At the time of diagnosis, however, asymptomatic patients may already have significant microvascular and/or macrovascular diabetic complications because there is often a long prodrome of hyperglycemia.

Without a doubt, the most common sign of insulin resistance is simply obesity (a large waist or high waist:hip ratio) or increased accumulation of central fat, a finding that occurs in 90% to 95% of T2DM patients. Other signs may include acanthosis nigricans, a velvety, hyperpigmented thickening of the skin, typically seen at the nape of the neck and within intertriginous areas such as the axilla (Figure 1). Skin tags around the base of the neck are recognized as a sign of insulin resistance. Necrobiosis lipoidica is a granulomatous skin disorder that is prevalent in up to 65% of patients. It appears as reddish-brown to yellow-brown oval-shaped plaques with central atrophy and telangiectasias that frequently ulcerate (Figure 2).

Long-Term Implications of Glycemic Control

Atherosclerotic cardiovascular disease (ASCVD), stroke and peripheral vascular disease are the major causes of morbidity and mortality in persons with diabetes. The Framingham study estimated that the relative risk of ASCVD among diabetic patients was three- to fivefold higher than in the nondiabetic cohort even when accounting for smoking, hypertension, and dyslipidemia. Diabetes itself is an independent risk factor for ASCVD, and multiple studies suggest a correlation between effective glycemic control and risk mitigation of CVD and mortality. Other risk factors for ASCVD include hypertension, dyslipidemia, tobacco use, and family history.

Treatment of hyperglycemia and associated cardiovascular (CV) risk factors has clearly been shown to be beneficial in diabetes. Several landmark trials examined the role of intensive glycemic control and ASCVD outcomes. One study, widely quoted and sometimes misinterpreted, seemed to suggest the opposite, that those assigned to very tight control experienced increased risk of death. The Action to Control Cardiovascular Risk in Diabetes (ACCORD) study evaluated the effect of tight glycemic control (HbA1c <6.0% vs. HbA1c of 7% to 7.9%) on the outcomes of nonfatal myocardial infarction (MI), nonfatal stroke, and CVD death. The trial was stopped early due to the increased mortality in the intensive therapy group. However, a subset analysis showed that patients with no history of CVD events prior to the study and baseline HbA1c less than 8% had a statistically significant reduction in CVD events. Hypoglycemia did not account for the increased deaths and the majority of the excess deaths were among those with long-term poor control and were unable to achieve tight control even when assigned to the aggressive arm of the study.

The Action in Diabetes and Vascular Disease: Preterax and Diamicron MR Controlled Evaluation (ADVANCE) trial aimed to lower HbA1c ≤6.5% in the intensive arm and measured microvascular plus macrovascular (nonfatal MI, nonfatal stroke, CVD death) outcomes. Notably, very few patients were using insulin at the start of this study, but criteria for all participants included having vascular disease or a risk factor for vascular disease. Ultimately, there was no increase in ASCVD mortality or overall mortality between the two arms. The Veteran Affairs Diabetes Trial (VADT) evaluated the value of intensive glycemic control for the primary outcomes of nonfatal MI, nonfatal stroke, CVD death, hospitalization for heart failure, and revascularization. Results of this study showed more CVD deaths in the intensive therapy group than the standard arm, although not statistically significant.

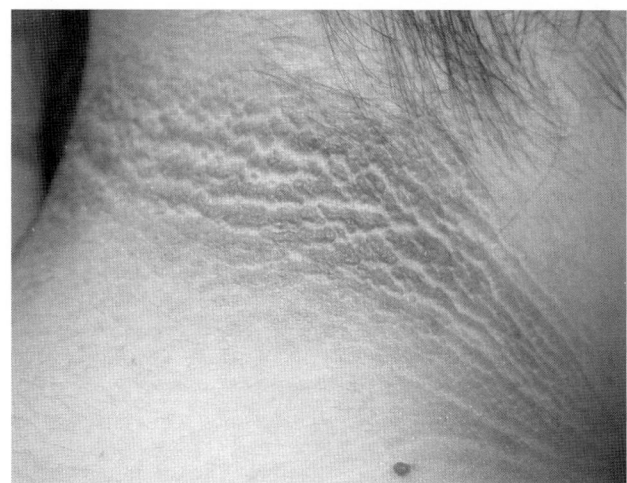

Figure 1 Acanthosis nigricans is a common exam finding of insulin resistance. It presents as a hyperpigmented, velvety, gray-to-brown thickening of the skin folds at the posterior neck and intertriginous folds. (From James WD, et al. *Andrews' Diseases of the Skin: Clinical Dermatology.* 13th ed. Elsevier; 2020.)

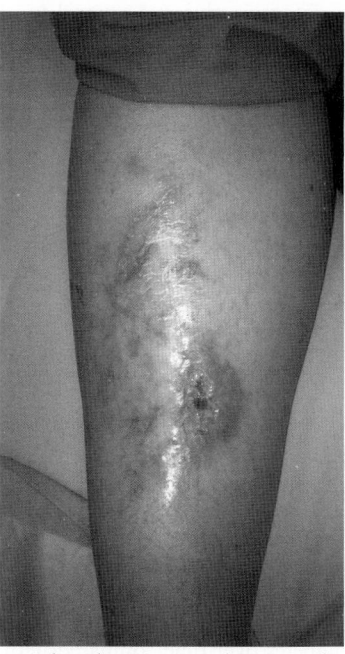

Figure 2 Necrobiosis lipoidica is a granulomatous skin disorder that is prevalent in up to 65% of patients with diabetes. It appears as reddish-brown to yellow-brown oval-shaped plaques with central atrophy and telangiectasias that frequently ulcerate.

At first glance, these studies suggest that very intensive control of diabetes may lead to increased mortality rather than improved cardiovascular outcomes. It is important to note that in all three trials, ASCVD risk factors with treated aggressively in all participants. All three studies also demonstrated more hypoglycemia in the intensive therapy groups than standard therapy groups. Hypoglycemia, however, did not explain the increased mortality in the intensively treated patients. The studies enrolled many patients who were older (mean age 60 to 66), with a long duration of diabetes (8 to 12 years) and already established CVD or known risk factors. Further subset analyses of each of these trials revealed significant benefits of intensive glycemic control for ASCVD outcomes in those patients with shorter duration of diabetes, lower initial HbA1c at entry, and/or absence of known CVD. We do not see the data from these studies as justification for not attempting tight glycemic control in most patients. *Thus, intense glycemic control may be more likely to benefit younger*

TABLE 1	Treatment Options for Overweight and Obesity in Type 2 Diabetes		
	BMI CATEGORY (kg/m²)		
Treatment (*Asian Americans in italics*)	**25.0–26.9** (*or 23.0–24.9**)	**27.0–29.9** (*or 25.0–27.4**)	**≥30.0** (*or ≥27.5**)
Diet, exercise, and behavioral therapy	Yes	Yes	Yes*
Pharmacotherapy—weight loss medications for selected patients	No	Yes	Yes*
Metabolic surgery (vertical gastroplasty or modified Roux-en-Y)	No	No	Yes*

*For obese patients with comorbidities.
BMI, Body mass index.

patients with shorter duration of diabetes in whom tight control prevents the development of future ASCVD complications.

Intensive glycemic control also reduces the risk of microvascular complications (retinopathy, nephropathy) in T2DM. As with macrovascular disease, microvascular disease may be present at the time of initial diagnosis of T2DM. Several pivotal trials demonstrated benefits of intensive versus standard blood glucose control on major microvascular outcomes in T2DM. The UK Prospective Diabetes Study (UKPDS) showed the significant impact of early, intensive glycemic control by demonstrating a 25% reduction in the development of microvascular complications in those with newly diagnosed T2DM. At the 10-year follow up, there was continued benefit in reducing microvascular risk as well as risk for MI and death from any cause, demonstrating that early, intensive control of glycemia can provide lasting positive effects on microvascular and macrovascular outcomes.

Prevention
Several large, randomized controlled trials have shown that behavior and lifestyle changes are highly effective in preventing T2DM. The strongest evidence comes from the DPP. This trial showed a reduction in incidence of T2DM among prediabetic enrollees by 58% over 3 years. The lifestyle intervention goals of the DPP were to attain and maintain a weight loss of 7% minimum and 150 minutes of physical activity per week, similar in intensity to brisk walking. Few patients actually achieved these modest goals, but the benefit was seen among most patients assigned to lifestyle changes alone. Similarly, modest reduction in weight has a significant protective effect on the progression to diabetes. The DPP study also included a metformin-only arm, and these patients also had a reduction in the incidence of diabetes (about 25%). It has been estimated that prediabetic patients following lifestyle suggestions *and* daily metformin[1] may have the lowest risk of diabetes over time compared with control groups and those receiving intensive lifestyle intervention only or daily metformin only.

General Medical Management
When caring for the typical T2DM patient, many providers face noncompliant patients with complex problems who show, over time, little progress in overcoming their disease. The treatment of diabetes is perhaps unique in medicine because it relies heavily on changes in patient lifestyle and adherence to complex regimens and imposes heavy economic burdens. The 20-minute clinic visit is unsuited for patients with multiple complaints, and after these visits providers often feel unsuccessful, frustrated with the patients, or worn out by nagging patients to adhere to their regimens.

It is important to find and practice an approach to these patients that focuses on problem solving rather than threatening, using praise for small changes, setting reasonable goals, and constantly reminding oneself that there are little victories in many patient visits that can be a source of personal reward (Table 1). In our clinic, we rely heavily on the techniques of motivational

interviewing, adapted to a short clinic visit, to help the patient identify and solve problems. In addition, we find that motivational interviewing helps the *provider* share in a sense of success, even if that change is small but in the right direction.

General Goals
The treatment of diabetes is goal driven. While there are discrete goals for average glycemia (HbA1c), blood pressure, and lipid levels, the American Diabetes Association (ADA) recognizes that the goals can be adjusted for a given patient's risks for hypoglycemia, duration of disease, presence of certain comorbidities, established vascular complications, patient preferences, and available resources and system support (Table 2).

Glycemic Goals
Assessment of glycemic control centers around HbA1c and self-monitoring blood glucose (SMBG) values. The average HbA1c correlates well with the SMBG in most instances, although certain situations, such as increased red blood cell turnover, hemoglobinopathies, or recent blood transfusions, may cause discordant results. It is also important to recognize there may be ethnic differences for HbA1c values, as studies have shown higher HbA1c values in African Americans than Caucasians with the same mean glucose. HbA1c should be measured at least quarterly in those patients who are not meeting glycemic goals or twice yearly in those patients who achieve HbA1c targets.

The ADA recommends an HbA1c target of less than 7% in most nonpregnant adults, suggesting that an even more stringent target HbA1c of less than 6.5% may be appropriate for some patients if it can be achieved without significant hypoglycemia or adverse effects. Conversely, the HbA1c goal may be loosened to less than 8% for patients who are at high risk of hypoglycemia, have limited life expectancy, have advanced complications of diabetes, or have long-standing disease. These guidelines encourage providers to individualize HbA1c goals for each patient, taking patient characteristics as well as risks and benefits into account. Similarly, the Veteran's Affairs/Department of Defense guidelines suggest shared decision-making and individualized HbA1c goals, with more aggressive HbA1c goals for patients with a long life expectancy and absent or mild microvascular complications and relaxed HbA1c goals for those with limited life expectancy and significant comorbidities.

In contrast, the American College of Physicians (ACP) recommends that clinicians target an HbA1c of 7% to 8% for most patients with T2DM, with de-escalation of pharmacologic therapy for any patients achieving an HbA1c less than 6.5%. The authors of this section do not agree with these guidelines and instead choose to follow the ADA guidelines for HbA1c targets, because HbA1c targets closer to 8% put patients at risk for developing more macrovascular and microvascular complications. While the authors do believe that HbA1c goals should be individualized and relaxed when indicated, we target A1c values of less than 7% without hypoglycemia, especially in younger patients with early diagnosis of T2DM, in an attempt to provide the greatest protection against future macrovascular and microvascular complications.

[1]Not FDA approved for this indication.

TABLE 2	Decision Factors in Selecting Glycemic Goals	
DECISION FACTORS	**HbA1c <7%**	**HbA1c >7%–8%**
Consequences of hypoglycemia	Low risk of severe hypoglycemia, patient senses hypoglycemia, has access to good support system	High risk, hypoglycemia unawareness, lives alone
Duration of diabetes	Short; tight control early in the disease promotes reduction in complications over time	There is little evidence that tight control late in the disease alters outcome
Life expectancy	Long	Short; reduction in macro- and microvascular diseases seen after years or decades of good glycemic control
Life-shortening comorbidities	Absent	Patients with life-limiting comorbidities may justifiably have glycemic goals that avoid extreme highs and lows
Well-established comorbidities such as retinopathy, nephropathy, neuropathy	Absent. However, improvement in retinopathy and delay in progression of neuropathy are recognized benefits of tight control	Many comorbidities such as end-stage renal disease, moderate-severe ischemic vascular disease, severe peripheral or autonomic nephropathy
Patient preferences	Highly motivated, strong support	Prefers less burdensome therapy, voices resistance to treatment; obstacles potentially modifiable over time
Available resources	Readily available, good health insurance, strong social network	Limited resources, including cost of medication, poor social support, etc. The provider can choose low-cost medications (human insulins, sulfonylureas, metformin) to attempt to reach glycemic goals

Home SMBG remains a mainstay for patients to evaluate and manage blood glucose levels. Patients that are on multiple daily injections (MDIs) of insulin should perform SMBG fasting, before meals, and at bedtime, which is typically three to four checks per day. For patients only on basal insulin, with or without other noninsulin agents, SMBG should be performed at least once daily, ideally fasting. It can be argued that SMBG may not provide added benefit for non-insulin treated patients, although periodic testing would still be useful to guide treatment and document hypoglycemia. Other studies have found improved glycemic control in patients without insulin therapy who still perform multiple SMBG tests per week. The ADA does not outline specific guidelines for SMBG for patients who are not on MDI.

With advances in technology, continuous glucose monitors (CGMs) are a commonly used tool to assess glucose values (Figure 3). Benefits of CGM include little to no need for SMBG, thus minimizing finger sticks, and continuous data that may alert the patient to glycemic trends and alarm for both high and low blood glucose values. Some CGMs may also be paired with insulin pumps to implement real-time data for basal insulin pump algorithms. Reports can be generated that include multiple data points not achieved with simple SMBG, such as percentage of time CGM is active, glycemic variability, and glycemic patterns over a 24-hour time frame.

A relatively new concept that is included in CGM reports is glycemic "time in range" (TIR), which accounts for the percentage of time a patient is within a desired glucose target. The TIR has a strong correlation with the HbA1c value, and it is typically reported as the "Glucose Management Indicator (GMI)" on CGM reports. In using TIR to assess control, we strive for values of 70% or higher with a coefficient of variation of less than 30%.

The most important principles in the treatment of hyperglycemia can be succinctly summarized as follows:
1. Start it early in the disease (arguably even in the prediabetic stages).
2. Don't delay additional treatment when glycemic goals are not attained. In our practice, we consider additional interventions every 3 months until the patient's glucose goals are attained.

There is strong empirical evidence supporting these principles. The Epidemiology of Diabetes Interventions and Complications (EDIC) study clearly showed that poor control early in the disease increased the prevalence of complications many years later even if tight control was implemented at some later, intermediate timepoint. This delayed risk for complications is called *metabolic memory*. Evidence from practice patterns is that patients

with poor glycemic control often stay that way for years as they promise better adherence to weight loss and exercise and negotiate with clinicians who themselves might be fearful of adding medications, especially insulin.

Monitoring
Much like driving a car without a speedometer, a diabetic patient who is unmonitored is at risk of undetected poor control and wide swings in blood sugar. There is little credible evidence that a patient can feel blood sugar highs and lows even when trained in behavioral clinical trials. Before choosing how a patient needs to be monitored, it is important to determine the frequency needed. The Diamicron MR in NIDDM Assessing Management and Improvement Control study (DINAMIC-1) randomized patients taking a sulfonylurea between no monitoring versus twice-weekly fingerstick testing groups. There was a small but significant difference in A1c between the groups (0.25%). Other studies show that the patients doing more frequent testing report a lower score on measures of quality of life while achieving comparable HbA1c levels.

Nevertheless, there are many patients who benefit from frequent monitoring. Those include patients using insulin, at risk for hypoglycemia, and perhaps a subset who insist on close monitoring as frequent reassurance that they are being properly treated. We have also observed some benefits related to self-learning. Some patients learn which foods produce high excursions in postprandial glucose and self-correct their diet over time based on these data.

Fingerstick Monitoring
The precision and accuracy of the over-the-counter (OTC) available strips are adequate to make safe clinical decisions. In general, the choice of a monitor is based on cost, insurance reimbursement, and features such as memory and the ability to upload stored results for clinical review. We find this latter feature especially useful to detect patterns of diurnal glycemia.

Continuous Glucose Monitoring
CGM offers a tremendous benefit and is extremely useful, if not necessary, in patients treated with insulin. CGM is now recommended for all patients with diabetes on multiple daily injections (MDI), continuous subcutaneous insulin infusions, and other forms of insulin therapy. Several devices are available (Freestyle Libre, Dexcom G6, Navigator, and Enlite). They are all placed on the skin. Insurance carriers often limit the use to patients treated

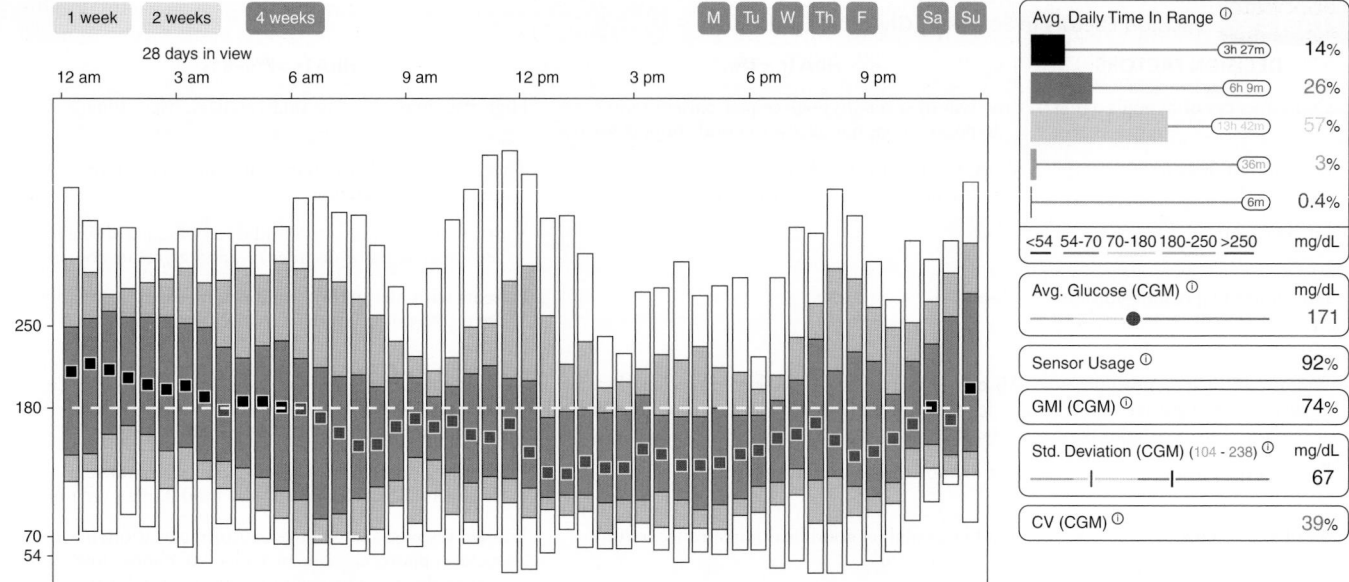

Figure 3 The report from a continuous glucose monitor contains valuable information. The time of day is along the x-axis while blood glucose is along the y-axis. On the right, average glucose, sensor usage, and time in range is documented. The clinician can see that the patient is within the glycemic goal 57% of the time, above goal 40% of the time, and hypoglycemic 3.4% of the time. The GMI is the Glucose Management Indicator, which correlates to an average A1c. In addition, the graph shows a pattern of overnight hyperglycemia (depicted by purple boxes) and daytime euglycemia with a few post-prandial low blood glucose patterns, as depicted by the green boxes and respective bars. Further information is gained by discussing daily habits and eating patterns with patients. This enables the provider to see an overall picture of glycemic control and make changes accordingly. (Photo provided by the authors, de-identified patient report.)

with at least four shots of insulin daily or insulin pumps. The most common devices are small, self-adherent to the skin, shower resistant, easy to apply, and provide continuous readings for 10 to 14 days. A few of the devices have audible low-glucose alarms, a feature useful for patients at risk for hypoglycemia without symptoms (hypoglycemic unawareness). Most do not require calibration with finger sticks and all of them can upload their data to a smartphone or independent reader, which can, in turn, be reviewed both by the patient, a family member, or clinician. "Professional" CGMs are clinic-based and can included blinded or real-time data collection for clinicians. A useful Internet site that accommodates this process with Health Insurance Portability and Accountability Act (HIPAA) compliance is Tidepool (tidepool.org). We consider the availability of continuous glucose monitoring a major advance in patient care.

Frequency of Clinical Visits

The standard frequency of visits for T2DM patients is every 3 to 6 months. We shorten that interval in patients who are in poor control as needed to prevent acute complications. The recommended interval is set, in part, on the duration needed to measure a stable change in HbA1c, which is about 3 months. Other recommendations include:

- Actions taken with each visit
  - Blood pressure (orthostatic if indicated)
  - Height, weight, vital signs
  - HbA1c if results are not available within the past 3 months
  - Skin exam
- Annual visits
  - Fundoscopic examination by eye specialist
  - Comprehensive foot exam
  - Laboratory examination to include lipid profile, liver function tests, spot urine microalbumin/creatinine
  - As indicated: electrolytes, B12, platelet count if considering fatty liver, nonalcoholic steatohepatitis (NASH), or nonalcoholic fatty liver disease (NAFLD)
- Podiatry
  - We generally refer patients to podiatry when there is evidence of reduced blood flow, infection, deformities (claw

toes, Charcot foot), heavy callouses, bunions, or neuropathy as determined by errors in sensing the 10-g fiber and loss of vibratory or position sensations. We also use these findings to order custom-fitted shoes that can prevent more serious foot disease.

- Diabetic education/nutrition
  - We find the partnership with a Certified Diabetes Care & Education Specialist (CDCES, previously known as Certified Diabetes Educator [CDE]) and/or nutritionist invaluable. Even among patients who feel fully informed, an *annual* visit can reinforce good behaviors, inform patients of new treatments, offer inroads to group and formal education, and occasionally assist in management of insulin doses depending on the regulations defining the scope of practice of diabetes educators.
- Cardiology
  - A routine referral to cardiology is not required despite the fact that the majority of T2DM patients will die of ASCVD. Cardiology visits are recommended in patients who plan on starting an intensive exercise program and those with traditional signs of ischemic heart disease (IHD). Keep in mind that diabetic patients are thought to manifest fewer symptoms of IHD and thus the threshold for referral and testing is arguably lower than for many other patients.

Early Detection of Complications

While the ultimate goal of treatment is the prevention of complications, a secondary aim is to find complications and treat them appropriately.

Hypertension

The definition of hypertension for diabetic patients varies between systolic values of less than 130 and 140 mm Hg. Currently, the ADA sets a threshold of less than 140/90 for diagnosing hypertension. We recommend three measurements in a seated patient over 15 minutes and using the average of the final two values as the recorded value. **Treatment:** angiotensin converting enzyme (ACE) and angiotensin receptor blocker (ARB) inhibitors are usually the drugs of first choice.

Retinopathy

Ophthalmoscopic examination by primary care and diabetes specialists has poor sensitivity and is not considered part of the required examination. A dilated eye exam by a qualified eye specialist is recommended in T2DM patients every year and in T1DM patients annually after 5 years of disease.

Neuropathy

Autonomic neuropathy is common among T2DM patients and is usually first detected by the loss of R-R wave variability on a long-lead electrocardiogram (ECG). Less commonly it can take the form of gastroparesis, alternating diarrhea and constipation, or orthostatic hypotension. Peripheral neuropathy can take the form of distal, symmetrical dysesthesias, hypesthesia, progressive loss of touch or vibration sensations, and heat-cold insensitivity. These patients are at risk of amputation, foot infection, and bony deformities (Charcot foot). **Treatment:** We reserve treatment for patients in whom the symptoms interfere with sleep or daily activities since drugs relieve symptoms but do not alter the course of the disease. Treatment choices for peripheral painful neuropathy include SSRIs, gabapentin (Neurontin)[1], pregabalin (Lyrica), anticonvulsants, transcutaneous electrical nerve stimulation (TENS), and, ultimately, narcotics. Gastroparesis is treated primarily on the basis of symptoms rather than studies of timed gastric emptying. Small, frequent meals and a vegetarian diet are better tolerated and there has been some success with erythromycin[1], metoclopramide (Reglan), or linaclotide (Linzess)[1] to stimulate motility.

Foot Disease

Guidelines suggest a thorough annual foot exam. We include pulses, an estimation of capillary refill, and a 10-point (5 points each foot) 10-g fiber test. Vibration sensitivity using a tuning fork is very hard to judge although it can be included in the exam, especially if using a 256 cps fork. Patients at risk should be instructed to do a daily foot exam, using a mirror to examine the plantar surface, and should promptly report early signs of infection, sores, or deformities. **Treatment:** Prevention is preferable to treatment. Custom shoes should be prescribed to patients with deformities, poor circulation, or neuropathy. Referral to podiatry is needed.

Dyslipidemia/Hyperlipidemia

Prevalence of hypercholesterolemia in diabetes is about the same as in the general population. However, at any given level of cholesterol, diabetic patients are about two to three times more likely to suffer from or die from an atherosclerotic event than nondiabetic individuals. Understandably some diabetologists consider their practice focus on glycemic control as another cardiovascular risk factor and their practice is mostly "preventive cardiology."

In contrast to relatively normal cholesterol levels, poorly controlled diabetic patients display elevated triglycerides (TG) and lowered high-density lipoproteins (HDL), and this pattern is referred to as *diabetic dyslipidemia*. The recent changes in ADA lipid treatment guidelines are now in synchrony with those of the American Heart Association (AHA) in that they focus more on risk than concentrations of blood lipids, with the exception of suggesting annual measurements of blood lipids. For patients with diabetes without preexisting CVD, the current ADA recommendations for starting pharmacological therapy are (1) an LDL cholesterol level of ≥130 mg/dL (3.35 mmol/L) and (2) a goal of less than 100 mg/dL (2.60 mmol/L) for LDL cholesterol. The AHA risk guidelines are also applied to the diabetic population. Treatment of hypertriglyceridemia is suggested with TG levels of greater than 200 to 400 mg/dL, but recognizing that the most effective treatment may be weight loss and improved glycemic control. Pharmacologic therapy is usually reserved for those with TGs greater than 400 mg/dL. Severe hypertriglyceridemia (>1000 mg/dL) carries the risk of pancreatitis and is treated with aggressive insulin management and severe caloric restriction. Markedly elevated triglycerides often plummet with fasting, and we frequently use this approach in hospitalized patients until the triglycerides are under 500 mg/dL while simultaneously treating the hyperglycemia with insulin. Statin treatment of diabetic patients is very rewarding and has a very low number needed to treat (NNT) to prevent a CV event. The Justification for the Use of Statins in Primary Prevention: An Intervention Trial Evaluating Rosuvastatin trial (JUPITER) study, for example, showed that one CV event per 5 years was prevented with every 18 patients treated with rosuvastatin. **Treatment:** Diet and drug treatment follow AHA guidelines. Diabetic dyslipidemia (low HDL, elevated TG) is responsive to improved glycemic control and weight loss. We generally reserve the use of fibrates to those in whom TGs exceed 400 mg/dL. The more potent statins (rosuvastatin [Crestor], atorvastatin [Lipitor]) are favored in patients with hypertriglyceridemia.

Depression

The prevalence of depression among diabetic patients is thought to triple that of the general population. We screen every patient on every visit with a modified Patient Health Questionnaire-9 (PHQ-9). Depression is correlated with poor diabetic control and ameliorating depression with medication or therapy is associated with an improvement in glycemic control. It has been argued that depression may be both a cause of poor control and a result of it. **Treatment:** Ideally, we prefer to combine antidepressant medications with sessions with a skilled therapist. Group diabetic visits have been shown to be helpful and efficient.

Nephropathy

Diabetes is still the most common cause of renal failure in the United States and it may be largely preventable by tight glycemic control and attainment of normal blood pressure. Screening should include a yearly spot urine test for microalbumin/creatinine. We consider any value above 30 mcg/mg creatine indicative of nephropathy even in the context of a normal glomerular filtration rate (GFR).

Treatment

The presence of microalbuminuria should trigger the prescription of an ACE or ARB inhibitor regardless of the presence of hypertension. These drugs, among others, have been shown to delay end-stage renal disease (ESRD) and slow declines in GFR. Sodium-glucose cotransporter 2 inhibitors (SGLT-2i) are also now recognized to have a benefit in stabilizing or delaying diabetic renal disease. We also carefully follow GFR and refer to nephrology when there is any rapid or otherwise unexplained rise in serum creatinine or a fall in adjusted GFR to 30 mL/min or less.

Fatty Liver Disease (NASH, NAFLD)

It is estimated that about 60% of patients with T2DM have fatty livers or NAFLD, steatosis unrelated to causes other than the metabolic disturbances of T2DM. Seventeen percent of the T2DM patients will progress to liver fibrosis, a potent risk factor for hepatocellular carcinoma (HCC). HCC is at least two to three times more prevalent among diabetic patients than the general population. NAFLD is now the leading cause of cryptogenic cirrhosis. Diagnosis of NAFLD is suspected by the presence of elevated serum transaminases, and suspicion is further raised by using one of several scoring systems (FIB4, NAFLD, or Hepcalc, a smartphone app) and ordering physiologic tests that measure loss of liver elasticity, such as the Fibroscan. We therefore include a platelet count in our routine annual labs in order to calculate the NAFLD or FIB4 and use an *indeterminate* or *likely* score as the basis for referral to hepatology. **Treatment:** Weight loss, improved metabolic control, and many diabetic medications such as pioglitazone (Actos)[1], the GLP-1 agonists, SGLT-2 inhibitors, DPP4 inhibitors, and metformin[1] may offer some benefit.

---

[1]Not FDA approved for this indication.

[1]Not FDA approved for this indication.

Hypoglycemic Unawareness

It is estimated that about 10% of deaths in T1DM are related to hypoglycemia. A small subgroup of patients loses the adrenergic response to hypoglycemia (usually a blood glucose <60 mg/dL) and are at risk for catastrophic events such as automobile accidents, neurologic decline, and trauma. Such patients must have flexible, elevated glycemic goals. Beta-blockers may contribute to the risk and alternative drugs should be considered in such patients. **Treatment:** Elsewhere in this chapter we discuss the use of glucagon (GlucaGen, Gvoke, Baqsimi) and the "rule of 15" in the treatment of various degrees of low blood sugar. These patients may derive many benefits from continuous glucose monitoring, especially with those devices that have audible alarms when the blood sugar trends down sharply. Cognitive behavioral therapy designed to teach at-risk patients to detect early clues to hypoglycemia reduces the frequency of hypoglycemic events. Some studies suggest adrenergic symptoms reappear in some patients after raising glycemic goals for a few months.

Erectile and Sexual Dysfunction

Erectile dysfunction (ED) is common among diabetic men and the clinician should not hesitate to ask if it is a problem during a visit. Surprisingly, unlike other complications, it is not clear if better glycemic control delays or prevents ED. It is also unknown if diabetic women suffer from sexual dysfunction although some claim that dryness on arousal is more common. **Treatment:** Many men respond to tadalafil (Cialis) or sildenafil (Viagra), both of which are now generic. When that fails, we refer to an experienced urologist who can consider intrapenile injections and prosthetic devices.

Lifestyle

BMI should be calculated at least annually, although it is useful to do at each visit. This can be calculated as weight in kg divided by height in meters squared (kg/m^2) or electronically in the electronic medical record (EMR) or online calculator. BMI should be classified as underweight, normal (18.5 to 24.9 kg/m^2), overweight (25 to 29.9 kg/m^2), or obese (>30 kg/m^2). In general, higher BMIs increase the risk of all-cause mortality and CVD and reduce quality of life. Weight-loss goals and intervention strategies should then be discussed (see Table 1).

Diet

A variety of eating patterns are acceptable for management of T2DM. There is no one preferred eating plan, as it should be individualized for each person. Referral to a registered dietitian nutritionist (RD/RDN) is recommended for all people with diabetes, prediabetes, and GDM to educate and help plan a diet with specific calorie and metabolic goals. People with diabetes should have medical nutrition therapy (MNT) with an RD/RDN at the time of diagnosis and as needed throughout their lives.

Reduced overall carbohydrate intake and emphasis on carbohydrates that are high in fiber and minimally processed are recommended. An eating plan emphasizing monounsaturated and polyunsaturated fats and fewer processed foods (Mediterranean-style diet) has been shown to improve glucose metabolism and lower CVD risk. In reality, a diet that is lower in calories and that the patient enjoys enough to continue can cause weight loss.

Exercise

As mentioned previously, 150 minutes per week of moderate to vigorous-intensity exercise improves insulin sensitivity, has been shown to reduce body fat, and is recommended for most patients with T1DM or T2DM. Ideally, this activity is spread over at least 3 days, with no more than 2 days in a row without exercise. Prolonged sitting has negative effects on postprandial blood glucose levels and should be avoided. People with T2DM should decrease the amount of time sitting and other sedentary behaviors. For sedentary activity lasting 30 minutes or longer, a 3-minute (minimum) break of walking, stretching, or isometric exercise is encouraged for improved glycemic control. Resistance training

should be done two to three times per week for improved strength as well as improved glycemic control. Even light activities such as housework, gardening, parking farther away, and taking the stairs all have beneficial impacts on weight and blood glucose values. If your patients do not like to "exercise," encourage an increase in normal physical activities.

Weight Loss

Treatment of obesity can delay or prevent the development of T2DM and can be very helpful in the treatment of T2DM. Behavioral therapy, including diet and physical activity, to achieve and maintain weight loss of 5% or more is recommended for patients with T2DM who are obese or overweight. Behavioral therapy should include frequent follow up with the focus on behavioral strategies, diet changes, and physical activity. For many patients a calorie deficit of 500 to 750 kcal/day will help achieve this goal. This allows for approximately 1200 to 1500 kcal/day for women and 1500 to 1800 kcal/day for men, although this depends on baseline body weight. Eating plans should be individualized for weight loss while still providing adequate protein, fat, and carbohydrates. Long-term weight maintenance programs are recommended for people who have achieved their short-term weight loss goal. These programs should include a high level of self-monitoring, including habits, food choices, and portion sizes; they should also continue to encourage a high level of physical activity (at least 200 min/week) and at least a weekly body weight check. If a body weight check is done at home, it should be done after using the bathroom first thing in the morning for consistency. Very-low-calorie diets (800 kcal/day or less) are an option for some people but should be short term (3 months) and prescribed by trained practitioners with close medical follow up. These patients still need long-term comprehensive weight maintenance counseling.

Drugs That Are Associated with Weight Loss

Medications for treatment of diabetes that are associated with modest weight loss include metformin, SGLT-2is, amylin mimetics, and alpha-glucosidase inhibitors. Glucagon-like peptide 1 (GLP-1) receptor agonists such as semaglutide (Ozempic), dulaglutide (Trulicity), liraglutide (Victoza), and exenatide (Bydureon) produce, on the average, the greatest amounts of weight loss, averaging about 1 lb per month.

Drugs That Are Weight Neutral or Cause Weight Gain

Dipeptidyl peptidase 4 inhibitors (the "gliptins") are weight neutral. Sulfonylureas, thiazolidinediones (TZDs), and insulin often cause weight gain, but the amount of weight gain is often overestimated and the benefit of glucose reduction probably counterbalances the modest weight gain associated with their use.

Drugs Used Specifically for Weight Loss

The US Food and Drug Administration (FDA) has approved a handful of medications for short-term and long-term treatment of obesity, to be used in conjunction with diet and exercise. Most of these medications have been shown to improve glycemic control in people with diabetes and delay progression to diabetes in those people at risk. Several of the GLP-1 agonists are formulated in combination with basal insulin in a pen and can be administered in a single injection.

Four medications are FDA approved for long-term weight loss in patients with BMI 27 kg/m^2 or greater with at least one obesity-associated comorbid condition (T2DM, dyslipidemia, or hypertension). These medications are orlistat (Alli, Xenical), phentermine and topiramate (Qsymia), bupropion and naltrexone (Contrave), and liraglutide (Saxenda). Phentermine (Adipex) is also approved for short-term weight loss. These medications can be helpful for patients in adhering to diet and lifestyle changes. The importance of this adherence cannot be overstated, as patients will gain back their lost weight once the medication is stopped if they have not adopted diet and lifestyle changes to continue to promote weight loss or maintenance. Providers should

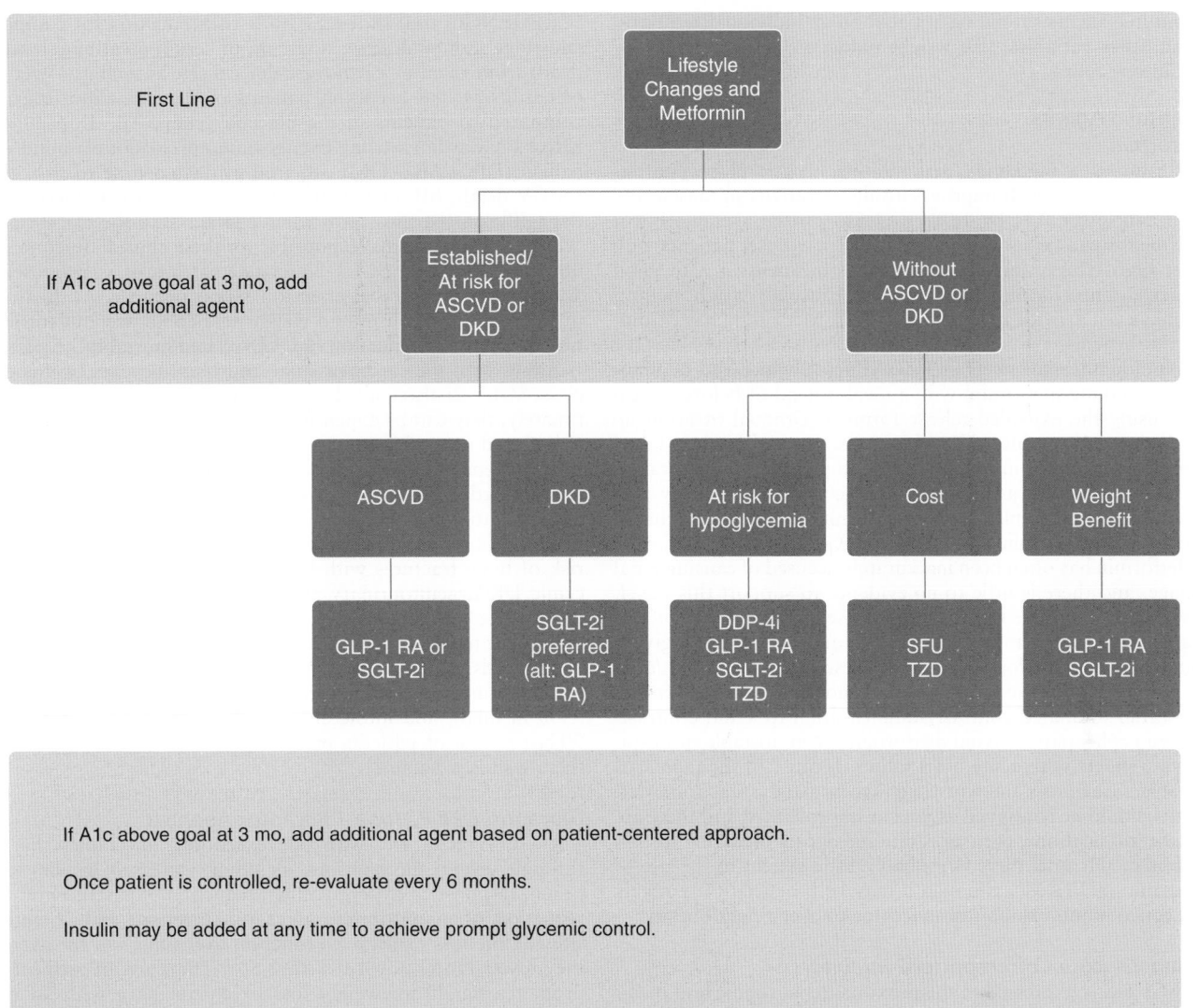

Figure 4 The choice of oral agents is based on many factors including the patient's financial resources and risk or presence of complications. In this figure, we show a decision-tree based on presence or absence of major complications. *ASCVD*, Atherosclerotic cardiovascular disease; *DPP-4i*, dipeptidyl peptidase 4 inhibitor; *DKD*, diabetic kidney disease; *Gl P-1 RA*, glucagon-like peptide 1 receptor agonists; *SGLT-2i*, sodium-glucose cotransporter 2 inhibitor; *TZD*, thiazolidinedione. (Adapted from the ADA Standards of Medical Care in Diabetes, 2020.)

be knowledgeable about the potential risks and benefits of these medications to prescribe appropriately to patients. These medications are contraindicated in women who are pregnant or trying to conceive. We urge our patients to use these in combination with a structured weight-loss program that emphasizes both short-term weight loss and maintenance.

When to Consider Bariatric Surgery

Bariatric surgery, sometimes referred to as metabolic surgery because of its weight-loss effects and treatment of T2DM, has been shown in some studies to provide better glycemic control and control of diabetes complications than medical treatment of T2DM. It should be recommended as an option to treat T2DM in patients with a BMI great than or equal to 40 kg/m² or those with BMI 30 to 39.9 kg/m² with comorbidities who have tried but not achieved weight loss with other methods. Younger age, shorter duration of diabetes, better glycemic control, and nonuse of insulin are all predictors of reversal of T2DM with bariatric surgery. Bariatric surgery has been thought of as a "last resort" but should really be considered earlier in the course of the disease. Randomized trials have shown diabetes remission rates of 30% to 60% following Roux-en-Y gastric bypass. However, over 5 to 10 years, diabetes recurrence rates are 35% to 50% but generally with improved glycemic control and less need for medications.

Pharmacologic Therapy

Along with lifestyle modifications, metformin remains the first-line agent for the treatment of T2DM because of its known effectiveness, lack of hypoglycemic effects, low cost, and relatively safe clinical profile. For patients not meeting glycemic targets with metformin alone, the ADA advises an individualized approach in selecting appropriate pharmacological therapy and escalation of treatment to achieve glycemic goals for patients with T2DM. Many agents now offer added benefits for protection against ASCVD and progression of diabetic kidney disease (DKD) as well as additional weight loss effects. A patient-centered approach should guide treatment, considering the potential for additional risk factor reduction, mitigating weight gain, hypoglycemia risk, cost, and patient preference (Figure 4). A1c should be checked every 3 months, with escalation of care if targets are not achieved. However, intensification of care, including initiation of insulin, should not be delayed in patients with markedly uncontrolled glycemia.

After metformin, providers must then consider whether patients are at risk for or have established ASCVD, heart failure, or established DKD. As such, a glucagon-like protein 1 receptor agonist (GLP-1 RA) or sodium-glucose cotransporter 2 inhibitor (SGLT-2i) should be second-line therapy. If a patient does not have high risk or established ASCVD, heart failure, or DKD, second-line agents should be initiated on an individualized basis, taking other variables, like weight reduction, hypoglycemia, or cost, into account.

Noninsulin Agents
Metformin
Metformin is a biguanide that inhibits hepatic glycogenolysis and gluconeogenesis. It improves insulin sensitivity in muscle and fat. It can lower A1c by 1.0% to 1.5% on the average, but it occasionally can be very effective even in new-onset patients with rather high HbA1c levels. Metformin is inexpensive with good efficacy and no risk of hypoglycemia. It is usually weight neutral and may even provide modest weight loss. Metformin has cardiovascular benefits.

Common adverse effects include GI upset, which can be minimized by taking metformin with a meal instead of before a meal or by using the extended release formula. Gradual titration up to full dose also reduces GI side effects, especially when taken with meals. Metformin is associated with a reduction in vitamin B12 but rarely with a deficiency. Lactic acidosis is a very rare but catastrophic complication of metformin, usually occurring in individuals with significant reduction in GFR.

Metformin has often been inaccurately accused of causing renal damage, and there is little to no evidence to support this belief. The FDA has approved metformin for use in patients with eGFR greater than 30 mL/min/1.73 m^2. The authors typically give a reduced dose of metformin for eGFR less than 60 mL/min/1.73 m^2. As metformin is renally cleared, it should be withheld for 48 hours after iodinated contrast administration to avoid contrast-induced nephropathy. Avoid metformin use in unstable or hospitalized patients with acute heart failure because of the increased risk of lactic acidosis and worsened myocardial dysfunction. Metformin should be continued as long as it is tolerated and there are no contraindications, even as additional agents including insulin are added. Of note, there is probably little benefit in the use of metformin in T1DM[1], although it may be beneficial for patients with concomitant insulin resistance due to overweight/obesity.

Sodium-Glucose Cotransporter 2 Inhibitors
The SGLT-2 is expressed in the proximal renal tubule and mediates the reabsorption of the majority of the glucose load filtered through the kidneys. SGLT-2i drugs block renal glucose reabsorption, thus promoting the excretion of glucose and sodium via glucosuria and lowering blood glucose levels in patients with T2DM. The glucose-lowering effects are independent of insulin, beta-cell function, and insulin sensitivity, thus offering an additional pathway for glucose regulation with low risk of hypoglycemia when used without insulin. These agents lower A1c by 0.5% to 1.0%. While it is appealing to use these drugs among type 1 diabetic patients, the risk of normoglycemic ketoacidosis and lack of FDA approval makes this risky, in our opinion.

Several landmark trials have demonstrated a significant benefit of the SGLT-2i for both ASCVD risk and DKD. The Cardiovascular Outcome Event Trial in Type 2 Diabetes Mellitus Patients (EMPA-REG OUTCOME) was the first pivotal trial showing reduced composite outcomes for cardiovascular death, nonfatal MI, or nonfatal stroke with the use of empagliflozin (Jardiance). There was a significant relative risk reduction in rates of CV death by 38%, all-cause mortality by 32%, and hospitalization for heart failure by 35%. As a result of this trial, empagliflozin received FDA approval for reduction of cardiovascular death in adults with T2DM and CVD. The Canagliflozin Cardiovascular Assessment Study (CANVAS) trial demonstrated reduction in cardiovascular events, but not cardiovascular death, in patients with T2DM at high risk for CVD in the canagliflozin (Invokana) group when compared to the placebo group. Subsequently, the Evaluation of the Effects of Canagliflozin on Renal and Cardiovascular Outcomes in Participants with Diabetic Nephropathy (CREDENCE) trial showed a 30% risk reduction for composite end-stage kidney disease, doubling of serum creatinine level, or death from renal or cardiovascular causes, as well as lower risk of cardiovascular events in patients of the canagliflozin group, compared to patients in the placebo group. The Dapagliflozin Effect on Cardiovascular Events randomized double-blind controlled (DECLARE-TIMI 58) trial evaluated time to first event for CV death, MI, or ischemic stroke, which was reduced in the dapagliflozin (Farxiga) arm when compared to the placebo arm. While the mechanisms responsible for these clinical outcomes are not well-described, SGLT-2i–related natriuresis is proposed to account for a favorable effect on blood pressure, while altered myocardial metabolism and weight loss could account for additional benefits to reduction in CVD-related mortality.

Along with the cardiovascular and renal benefits of this drug class, SGLT-2i also contribute to very modest weight loss. Unfortunately, they can be expensive, and there is a risk of hypoglycemia if used in combination with insulin or sulfonylureas. Because they are renally cleared, considerations for renal dose adjustment are required. There is also an FDA black-box warning for the risk of amputations with canagliflozin, a finding that has not been uniformly supported in subsequent studies. There is an increased risk of bone fractures with long-term use (canagliflozin), euglycemic DKA, genitourinary and other infections, risk of volume depletion, slight elevation of LDL cholesterol, and Fournier gangrene. The marked benefit in cardiac and renal protection of these drugs needs to be balanced against the risks of euglycemic DKA, increased urinary tract infections (UTIs) (about 10% in women, >5% in men), and intolerance due to dehydration. In balance, 90% to 95% of patients prescribed this class of drugs tolerate them well (see Table 2).

Glucagon-Like Peptide 1 Receptor Agonists
The GLP-1 RAs are, with one exception, injectables that act through several mechanisms, including increased insulin secretion in response to hyperglycemia, reduction of gastric emptying, reduction of inappropriate glucagon secretion, and potentially slowing the loss of beta-cell function over time. On the average, they lower HbA1c by 1.0% to 1.5%. This class of medications promotes significant weight loss by enhancing a sense of early satiety and has a low risk of hypoglycemia when used as monotherapy because of its glucose-dependent mechanism of action. These agents have historically been injectable, but recently a new oral GLP-1 RA (semaglutide [Rybelsus]) was approved.

Like the SGLT-2i, this class of medications has also demonstrated significant risk reductions in ASCVD and DKD. The Liraglutide Effect and Action in Diabetes: Evaluation of Cardiovascular Outcome Results (LEADER) trial included subjects at risk for CVD and found that liraglutide significantly reduced cardiovascular death, nonfatal MI, or nonfatal stroke, as well as all-cause mortality relative to placebo. Based on the LEADER data, the FDA approved liraglutide (Victoza) for the reduction of major cardiovascular events and cardiovascular deaths in adults with T2DM and CVD. Additional studies have shown benefit of GLP-1 receptor agonists in cardiovascular outcomes. The Trial to Evaluate Cardiovascular and Other Long-Term Outcomes with Semaglutide in Subjects with T2DM (SUSTAIN-6) showed statistically significant reductions in nonfatal MI, nonfatal stroke, or cardiovascular death in the semaglutide (Ozempic) group. An additional meta-analysis of seven GLP-1 RA cardiovascular outcome trials found that this drug class reduced major adverse cardiovascular events by 12%, all-cause mortality by 12%, and hospitalization for heart failure by 9%. There was also a 17% reduction in a composite of various renal outcomes.

The most common side effects of these agents include mild injection-site reactions as well as abdominal cramping, and nausea and vomiting, which are typically transient and lessened by gradual dose up-titration. There is a risk of hypoglycemia if used in combination with insulin or sulfonylureas. This class of medications has been found to increase the incidence of benign and malignant C-cell tumors in rodents and is contraindicated

---

[1]Not FDA approved for this indication.

in patients with a personal or family history of medullary thyroid carcinoma or multiple endocrine neoplasia 2A or 2B. There have also been postmarketing reports of acute pancreatitis in association with GLP-1 RAs, and they should not be initiated in patients with a history of pancreatitis. Although there are reports of increased incidence of pancreatic cancers and neuroendocrine tumors, a causal relationship has not been established and the FDA cites insufficient evidence to confirm that risk. Like the SGLT-2i, these medications may be costly, especially for patients without insurance. The drugs may be poorly tolerated in patients with gastroparesis or previous bariatric surgery. One preparation has been approved for oral use (semaglutide [Rybelsus]) but with a loss of efficacy in comparison to the injected compound.

Dipeptidyl Peptidase 4 Inhibitors
The dipeptidyl peptidase 4 (DPP-4) inhibitors work by inhibiting the degradation of incretin hormones (like GLP-1) and thus increasing the half-life to increase insulin secretion in a glucose-dependent manner and decrease glucagon secretion. They lower A1c by 0.5% to 1.0%. They are weight neutral and do not contribute to hypoglycemia if used as monotherapy. This class of medications is generally well-tolerated, but a few patients complain of upper respiratory symptoms and joint pain. There is a risk of hypoglycemia if used in combination with insulin or sulfonylureas. This class can still be used in renal failure with appropriate dose adjustments. One drug in the class, linagliptin (Tradjenta), is hepatically metabolized and no dose adjustment is needed in patients with poor renal function. Like the more potent GLP-1 RA, the DDP-4 inhibitors can be associated with pancreatitis. There is no additive benefit with a DDP-4 inhibitor with GLP-1 RA, and combination should be avoided, with preference usually for the GLP-1 RA. A dose reduction is indicated for patients with renal impairment. Of note, the ADA suggests DPP-4 inhibitors (except saxagliptin [Onglyza]) may be considered in patients with heart failure because saxagliptin may potentially exacerbate underlying myocardial dysfunction. There is a role for these agents when there is a compelling need to minimize hypoglycemia, when weight neutrality is desired, or in case of significant renal failure.

Thiazolidinediones
TZDs are insulin sensitizers that increase insulin sensitivity in muscle and fat. Pioglitazone (Actos) and rosiglitazone (Avandia) are currently available. They are potent in lowering A1c by 1.0% to 1.5%. They are not associated with hypoglycemia. Pioglitazone may reduce CVD and triglycerides. These medications may cause weight gain in the form of both volume retention and increase in fat mass. There is an FDA black-box warning against the use of these agents in congestive heart failure. They are also associated with an increased risk of bone fractures and small relative risk of bladder cancer with long-term use (pioglitazone). Pioglitazone can also raise LDL cholesterol. There is a role for these agents when patients do not want to use an injectable medication, when

cost is an issue, or when there is a need to minimize hypoglycemia. We frequently use them in the uncommon thin type 2 diabetic patient and, anecdotally, seem to have good results. Most clinicians avoid the use of TZDs in patients already taking insulin because of the risk of edema and congestive heart failure (CHF).

Secretagogues
Sulfonylureas stimulate beta-cell insulin secretion from the pancreas. They can lower HbA1c by 1.0% to 1.5%. These medications are initially effective and inexpensive. However, the authors typically do not prescribe these medications unless cost is an issue. Sulfonylureas lose their efficacy because they result in beta-cell loss over time and also cause weight gain, potentially contributing to further insulin resistance. Newer agents, such as the SGLT-2i and GLP-1 RAs, preserve islet cell function, maintain their efficacy, and have shown both cardiovascular and renal protective benefits. Sulfonylureas also have a risk of hypoglycemia and should be taken with food. Caution should be used with hepatic or renal impairment.

Other Agents
Other less used agents include amylin agonists (pramlintide [Symlin]), bile acid sequestrants (cholestyramine resin [Questran][1], colesevelam [Welchol]), and dopamine receptor agonists (bromocriptine [Cycloset]). The authors use these infrequently given their cost, modest impact on glycemia, and relative inconvenience for the patient. See Table 3 for a summary of prescribing noninsulin medications.

Insulin
Insulin is often thought of as the drug of last resort for T2DM. It has a narrow therapeutic window in that the glucose targets are near the threshold for hypoglycemia. Patients have sometimes been preconditioned with fear of insulin, having been threatened by well-intentioned providers saying, for example, "if you don't lose weight, you will need to go on insulin."

Transitioning a patient to insulin requires a fair amount of patient education, a valuable resource especially among small, isolated practices. Patients offer their own resistance seeing the cost, inconvenience, and pain. Insulin injections are sometimes seen as a mark of final deterioration in their disease and associated with catastrophic events: "My uncle lost his leg when he was put on insulin."

Arguably, insulin can be introduced at any stage of diabetes. There is some evidence that early introduction of insulin may preserve islet cell function, but long-term studies have not confirmed or rejected that concept. Conceptually, we see insulin administration as hormone replacement just as giving levothyroxine to a hypothyroid patient. We avoid using insulin as a threat, which may only increase resistance to it when it is finally needed. In practice, insulin is usually prescribed when diet and exercise, oral medications, and perhaps GLP-1 agonists have failed to achieve

[1]Not FDA approved for this indication.

TABLE 3 Noninsulin Treatment for Adults with Type 2 Diabetes: Factors to Consider for a Patient-Centered Approach

	EFFICACY	WEIGHT CHANGE	ASCVD BENEFIT	DKD BENEFIT	HYPOGLYCEMIA RISK	COST
Metformin	High	Neutral/modest loss	Benefit	Benefit	None	Low
SGLT-2i	High	Loss	Benefit	Benefit	Low	High
GLP-1 RA	High	Loss	Benefit	Benefit	Low	High
DPP-4	Low	Neutral	Neutral	Neutral	Low	High
TZD	High	Gain	Potential benefit	Neutral	None	Low
SFU	Intermediate	Gain	Neutral	Neutral	High	Low

ASCVD, Atherosclerotic cardiovascular disease; *DKD*, Diabetic kidney disease; *DPP-4*, dipeptidyl peptidase 4; *GLP-1 RA*, glucagon-like peptide 1 receptor agonist; *SFU*, sulfonylurea; *SGLT-2i*, sodium-glucose cotransporter 2 inhibitors; *TZD*, thiazolidinedione.
Adapted from the ADA Standards of Medical Care in Diabetes 2021.

treatment goals. One should not delay its use when it is needed, keeping in mind the concept of *metabolic memory* discussed earlier in this chapter; the longer the period of time patients are hyperglycemic, the more likely they are to have complications in the future.

Conceptual Approach to Insulin Administration in Type 2 Diabetes Mellitus

The primary motivation for using insulin is to achieve the treatment goal. This may go beyond reaching the desired HbA1c threshold because being an average, it does not reflect glucose variability. Evolving concepts suggest that large variations in glucose, even after meals, add to the risk of complications. Thus, TIR (percentage of time that the patient has a blood sugar of 80 to 180 mg/dL) is a concept that will likely move from the domain of the specialist to internal medicine and family practice. Whether the clinician uses a basal-bolus approach (premeal short-acting insulin with a long-acting background insulin) or combinations of regular and neutral protamine Hagedorn (NPH) insulin, the intent is to mimic the post-meal excursions in insulin and to provide a constant background of insulin action. See Table 4 for a summary of insulin preparations.

First Steps

The most common approach to initiation of insulin is to start with a single shot of basal insulin. A conservative approach is to start with 0.2 U/kg and to titrate the dose up until the patient is sleeping without hypoglycemia and waking up with acceptable blood glucose levels (typically 80 to 130 mg/dL). There are a variety of clinically tested titration protocols that allow the patient to adjust to basal insulin without further consulting the provider. These are called *treat-to-target (TTT)*. For glargine (Lantus, Basaglar) and detemir (Levemir) insulin, we suggest adding 1 unit per day to the initiating dose until the overnight and fasting targets are reached. Similarly, if the patient experiences overnight hypoglycemia, we reduce the dose by 1 unit. When prescribing ultralong insulins such as glargine 300 U/mL (Toujeo) and degludec (Tresiba), we modify the TTT by changing the dose by 2 units at 5-day intervals since the pharmacodynamic half-lives of these preparations approach 36 to 40 hours.

Next Steps

A single dose of basal insulin can achieve an HbA1c of less than 7% in at least 50% of T2DM patients. If this target is not reached, we frequently move to a dosing scheme termed *basal-plus-one*. In this case, we add short-acting insulin before the largest meal of the day. Typically, this additional dose can be estimated by dividing the basal insulin dose by one-third and adding that amount as the plus-one premeal dose. The goal of this regimen is to achieve a blood sugar of less than 180 mg/dL 2 hours after the meal. This maneuver will bring HbA1c into the target range in about half the patients who fail to be well controlled on a single dose of basal insulin.

TABLE 4 Comparison of Various Types of Insulin

TRADE NAME	GENERIC NAME	ONSET	PEAK	DURATION	COST
Rapid-acting					
Admelog	Lispro	15–30 min	30–90 min	3–5h	$$
Apidra	Glulisine	10–20 min	90–120 min	2–4 h	$$
Fiasp	Aspart + niacinamide	15–20 min	30–90 min	5 h	$$
Humalog	Lispro	10–20 min	60–180 min	3–5 h	$$
Novolog	Aspart	10–20 min	2.5–5 h	3–5 h	$$
Short-acting					
Humulin R, Novolin R	Regular human	16–30 min	4–8 h	4–12 h	$
Humulin R U500	Concentrated regular human	30 min	4–8 h	18–24 h	$$$$
Intermediate-acting					
Humulin N, Novolin N	NPH (human + protamine)	1–2 h	4–12 h	14–24 h	$
Long-acting					
Basaglar	Glargine	3–4 h	Flat	11–24 h	$$
Lantus	Glargine	3–4 h	Flat	11–24 h	$$
Levemir	Detemir	3–4 h	Flat	6–23 h	$$
Ultra-long					
Toujeo (U-300)	U300 glargine		Flat	24–36 h	$$
Tresiba (U100 and U200)	Degludec		Flat	36–42 h	$$
Combinations*					
Humulin 70/30, Novolin 70/30	NPH 70%/regular 30%	30 min	50 min–2 h and 6–10 h	18–24 h	$
Novolog Mix 70/30	NPH 70%/aspart 30%	15–30 min	50 min–2 h and 6–10 h	18–24 h	$$
Humalog Mix 75/25	NPH 75%/lispro 25%	15–30 min	50 min–2 h and 6–10 h	12–24 h	$$
Humalog Mix 50/50	NPH 50%/lispro 50%	15–30 min	2–4 h and 6–10 h	12–24 h	$$

*The fixed combination insulins generally have high inter- and intrapatient variability due to their reliance on NPH as a background or late-peaking insulin. With their use, the practitioner is trading convenience in exchange for flexible dosing. Despite these concerns, some studies have found using these combinations in T2DM produces acceptable control of glucose with slightly more hypoglycemia than multiple daily injections (separate dosing) of basal insulin + short-acting premeal insulin.
NPH, Neutral protamine Hagedorn.

Multiple Daily Injections or Basal-Bolus Therapy

MDI is used in many T2DM patients and is the standard of care in T1DM. There are a number of approaches that can be adapted for a given patient's lifestyle and motivation. A helpful statistic is that short-acting insulin in most well-controlled insulin-using patients accounts for 40% to 60% of the total daily dose (TDD).

Fixed Dose Plus Sliding Scale

In this instance the patient is prescribed a certain number of units of insulin before each meal and given a table to add insulin if the premeal glucose level is above a certain threshold. This might be acceptable in a patient who has regular meals or refuses to learn more complex premeal dose calculations. Endocrinologists frequently dislike the term "sliding scale" because it is often misused to justify giving no premeal insulin when the premeal glucose level is normal. Premeal insulin is given primarily to act on the content of the meal.

Small, Medium, Large

A conceptually simple approach is to assign three premeal doses based on the size of the meal or more specifically the amount of carbohydrate in the meal. Many patients learn to use this dosing scheme with reasonable results.

Carbohydrate Counting with a Correction Factor

This is the gold standard of calculating a premeal dose. It allows for the greatest meal flexibility but at the expense of learning to calculate the grams of carbohydrate in a meal and reliably testing the fingerstick blood glucose before the meal. In addition to working with a nutritionist, a good reference for the carbohydrate content of foods is *Calorie King*, as a paperback or free mobile phone app. Here are the steps needed to calculate carbohydrate ratio (grams of carbohydrate per unit of insulin) and the correction factor (how much insulin to take to correct for premeal hyperglycemia).

- **Estimate the total daily dose (TDD).** Typically, this is about twice the number of units used as basal insulin.
- **Estimate the carbohydrate ratio:** 500/TDD = grams of carbohydrate requiring a unit of premeal insulin
- **Estimate the correction factor:** 1600/TDD = units needed to correct premeal hyperglycemia, typically any elevation above 140 mg/dL. Patients will often remember this number as, for example, 1 extra unit for every ___ mg/dL above 130. It can also be expressed as a simple formula:
- ([blood glucose before the meal]—130)/correction factor = units needed to treat the premeal hyperglycemia

These formulas provide estimates and give the patient a starting point. Some patients find that they need different insulin dose factors at different meals. In any case, the criteria for success are that patients avoid hypoglycemia between meals and reach their glucose target before the next meal.

Other Factors Affecting Insulin Requirements

Exercise

Exercise can have a marked effect on glucose utilization and insulin sensitivity. The exercising muscle takes in glucose as needed provided that there is *some* insulin in the blood. The glucose transporter on the muscle membrane responds somewhat independently of insulin to local depletion of glucose and glycogen by accelerating glucose transport. In addition, regular exercise reduces insulin requirements both by increasing the efficiency of muscle glucose transport, improving intramuscular energy utilization, reducing insulin resistance, and increasing lean body mass/reducing body fat.

We recommend that patients reduce short-acting insulin in anticipation of exercise. Thus, for example, the premeal short-acting insulin at lunch would be reduced in anticipation of exercise before the evening meal. The amount of the reduction is variable and depends primarily on the duration and intensity of the exercise. We initially suggest decreasing the premeal insulin by one-third, but in long-duration and high-intensity exercise

premeal insulin can be reduced drastically or even eliminated in some cases. Patients need to have documented education on the impact of exercise on glycemia and to have a source of rapid-acting carbohydrate readily available to them. In the case of children or adolescents, this might mean educating coaches and teachers on the signs and treatment of hypoglycemia.

The window of vulnerability to exercise-induced hypoglycemia extends beyond the time of exercise. During post-exercise rest, muscles may continue to take up large amounts of glucose to replete glycogen stores, and hypoglycemic episodes can occur as long as 24 hours after a bout of vigorous exercise.

Sick Days

A common and unfortunate misconception held by some patients is that they don't need insulin if they don't eat. This may be true for some T2DM patients, but many will suffer uncontrolled hyperglycemia and sometimes catastrophic metabolic dysfunction when insulin is withheld for prolonged periods of time. In some patients, insulin requirements increase during illness because of the stress response. Thus, insulin-using diabetic patients should increase the frequency of blood glucose monitoring, take their basal insulin, and use short-acting insulin. Here are some guidelines:

- Check blood glucose every 4 hours.
- Check urine for ketones and report moderate or large amounts to the healthcare provider.
- If the blood glucose is under 200 mg/dL, stay hydrated with Gatorade or sugar-containing soda.
- If the blood glucose is over 200 mg/dL, drink plenty of sugar-free liquids. In patients who can tolerate a salt load, we recommend broth or soup in a cup (ramen noodle soup).
- Uncontrolled hyperglycemia, nausea and vomiting, or high ketones are indications to alert the provider as soon as possible.

Low Carb or Carbohydrate-free Meals

The popularity of paleo or keto diets confronts healthcare providers with the issue of insulin management with low carbohydrate intake. In most cases, premeal insulin can be reduced and occasionally eliminated based on postprandial blood sugar. We have occasionally observed insulin-using T2DM patients totally eliminate insulin use and return to near-normal glycemia with carefully monitored, hypocaloric ketotic diets.

Types of Insulin

Insulin preparations are categorized by their duration of action. This is referred to as the pharmacodynamics (PD) of insulin (duration of action) as opposed to pharmacokinetics (PK, circulating half-lives). The distinction between PK and PD is simply because insulin acts on membrane-bound receptors and subsequent downstream action with most insulins is much longer than the circulating half-lives (PK). All insulins sold in the United States are synthetic, derived from genetically altered yeast or bacteria. All insulins are dosed using "units," a historically interesting measure of bioactivity that was originally derived from the amount of insulin needed to reduce glucose by about 50 mg/dL in a standard laboratory rabbit. The unit now is primarily based on weight (0.0347 mg). Since the molecular weight of some synthetic insulins differs from that of human insulin, the unit is used to ensure that there is equal potency among preparations. That is, 1 unit of any given insulin preparation will be expected to have the same impact on glucose lowering. See Table 4.

The combination insulins generally have high inter- and intra-patient variability. Despite this, some studies show that twice- or thrice-daily use of these combinations produces acceptable control of glucose with slightly more hypoglycemia than basal insulin plus short premeal insulin.

- *Rapid-acting insulins.* These typically have a duration of action between 3 and 6 hours and are given right before or immediately after meals or used in insulin pumps. Fiasp, an ultrashort-acting aspart insulin, peaks a bit sooner than the short-acting analogs. Some evidence shows a modest decrease in postprandial hypoglycemia and decrease in postprandial glycemia in comparison to other short-acting analogs.

- *Short-acting insulin (human).* These are the least expensive forms of premeal insulin and are often available without prescription. The reduced cost is offset in part by inconvenience in that they should be taken 30 to 45 minutes before eating (except with premeal hypoglycemia), and they produce slightly more hypoglycemia. We consider them a good option for patients facing high drug costs.
- *Intermediate-acting insulin.* NPH is the only form of this insulin and, like regular human insulin, is much less expensive than the analog insulins. It is amorphous and thus cloudy. Before use it should be mixed by rolling the vial or pen rather than vigorously shaking the preparation. Although it can be an adequate lower-cost alternative to analog insulin, it has relatively high variability in its peak and duration of action. It is associated with slightly more frequent hypoglycemia than the newer basal and ultra-long forms of insulin. While it theoretically can be given once a day, it is usually given before breakfast and a second dose before the evening meal or bedtime. It can be used in a basal-bolus fashion with one dose at bedtime and regular insulin before each meal. The tendency of an injection of NPH to peak in the afternoon/evening makes it a logical choice in the treatment of glucocorticoid-induced hyperglycemia.[1]
- *Basal, or ultralong-acting, insulin.* These insulin preparations have a duration of action of nearly 24 hours or longer and are often the first insulin used in a treatment regimen. When cost is no object, they are usually the preferred basal preparations, with a few caveats.
  - Detemir (Levemir) has the shortest duration in the class and may not always fill the role as a once-a-day insulin. When used, we prefer to give it at night and sometimes will give it approximately every 12 hours to provide a constant background of insulin.
  - Glargine (Lantus, Basaglar, Toujeo) is an acidic insulin that cannot be mixed in the same syringe with other insulins. As such, it sometimes causes minor irritation at the injection site. The primary differences between Basaglar and Lantus, on the one hand, and Toujeo on the other, is the concentration of glargine. Toujeo is highly concentrated (300 U/mL), and this increases the duration of action by slowing its absorption from the injection site. Toujeo, then, has a more linear pharmacodynamic profile than its chemical twins and is a bit more forgiving in not requiring a precise dosing time. These insulins do not provide a post-meal peak in insulin. Thus, they may be best suited for patients who have some capacity to produce endogenous insulin to act on meal-time calories. Glargine insulin is advertised as a "flat insulin" but it develops peaks if the injected units exceed 0.3 U/kg. Thus, it is our practice to split Lantus or Basaglar into two daily shots when the required amount of insulin exceeds approximately 50 U/day. Glargine insulin is usually given at bedtime or with the evening meal, but morning dosing is successful in some patients as well.
  - Degludec (Tresiba) has the longest duration of action of the marketed insulins and has a slight benefit in that its use is associated with a bit less hypoglycemia and more flexible dosing schedules
- *Pumps.* These devices are infrequently used in general practice but it is appropriate to be comfortable with suggesting their use to the appropriate patients. Pumps are rarely helpful in patients who struggle with compliance and are in poor control. Broadly speaking, pumps fall into two classes: open-loop and semiautonomous pumps. Open-loop pumps must be programmed by the patient or provider to deliver basal doses of insulin as near-constant injections of small amounts of insulin and premeal insulin based on the calculation of the amount of insulin needed to treat premeal hyperglycemia and calorie/carbohydrate content of the meal. Closed loop pumps (semi-autonomous) are paired through Bluetooth with a continuous subcutaneous glucose monitor and are programmed to vary the amount of basal insulin to maintain a tight range of near-normal glycemia between meals. The patient is still obliged to alert the pump that it is mealtime and the patient must input the amount of anticipated carbohydrate in the meal. In practice the pumps are fairly successful at achieving near-normal glycemia with reduced variance.

Hypoglycemia

Hypoglycemia is defined as a glucose concentration of less than 70 mg/dL and is further classified into three levels. Level 1 is a glucose value less than 70 mg/dL but ≥54 mg/dL. Level 2 is a glucose value less than 54 mg/dL. Level 3 is any event with severe symptoms that require medical assistance for treatment. Hypoglycemia can present with both neurogenic (autonomic) and neuroglycopenic symptoms. Neurogenic symptoms include adrenergic responses such as tremor, palpitations, and/or anxiety, as well as cholinergic responses such diaphoresis, hunger, and paresthesias. Conversely, neuroglycopenic symptoms are those that cause an altered sensorium such as confusion, dizziness, weakness, and drowsiness but can ultimately progress to seizures or coma with severe hypoglycemia. Neuroglycopenic symptoms typically occur with glucose values less than 54 mg/dL.

Studies have suggested significant long-term risks from frequent severe hypoglycemia, including significant cognitive impairment, falls and fractures, and increased mortality. Risk factors for hypoglycemia include advanced age, African American race, longer duration of diabetes, use of sulfonylureas and/or insulin, renal impairment, dementia, alcohol ingestion, and erratic meal timing.

Hypoglycemia is also graded as mild, moderate, or severe. *Mild* is an event in which the patient feels the symptoms and treats the low level on his/her own. *Moderate* events require assistance but do not involve unconsciousness or the need for glucagon. *Severe* hypoglycemia is defined as a seizure, obtundation, need for emergency room visit, or need to call emergency medical technicians (EMTs). Many patients with well-controlled insulin-treated diabetes experience occasional mild hypoglycemia and these episodes can be acceptable provided that they are not too frequent or reach moderate-to-severe levels. Moderate and severe events should be addressed with changes in the regimen and a thorough investigation as to why the event occurred, such as skipping a meal or insulin dose error.

Clinicians should be aware that patients with poorly controlled diabetes with frequent episodes of hypoglycemia can often lose their counterregulatory responses to low blood glucose and develop hypoglycemia unawareness, in which blood glucose can drop significantly. Thus, it is important to ask patients at which glucose threshold they begin to feel symptoms of hypoglycemia. Patients can, occasionally, regain some sensitivity to hypoglycemia by relaxing blood glucose control for several weeks.

Hypoglycemia should be treated with glucose administration if the patient is alert and able to take in food by mouth. The authors educate their patients on the "Rule of 15" for treating hypoglycemia. Patients should ingest 15 g of rapid-acting carbohydrates (such as 4 oz orange juice, 4 oz regular soda, 8 oz skim milk, 3 to 4 glucose tablets, or 6 to 7 jellybeans or hard candies) every 15 minutes until finger-stick blood glucose is greater than 70 mg/dL. For prolonged hypoglycemia, we suggest a snack with complex carbohydrates, fats, and protein. It is important to always evaluate the underlying cause of hypoglycemia and adjust the treatment regimen accordingly.

For severe hypoglycemia in which the patient needs the assistance of another person or medical professional, glucagon can be administered. Glucagon is now available in intramuscular (GlucaGen), subcutaneous (GlucaGen, Gvoke), or intranasal (Baqsimi) formulations. The authors always educate patients that use of an emergency glucagon kit warrants evaluation in the emergency department after they have taken it.

---

[1]Not FDA approved for this indication.

References

American Diabetes Association Standards of Medical Care in Diabetes – 2021. *Diabetes Care* 43(Suppl 1):S1-S2, 2021.

Colberg SR, Sigal RJ, Yardley JE, et al: Physical activity/exercise and diabetes: a position statement of the American Diabetes Association, *Diabetes Care* 39(11):2065–2079, 2016.

Duckworth W, Abraira C, Moritz T, et al: VADT investigators. Glucose control and vascular complications in veterans with type 2 diabetes, *N Engl J Med* 360:129–139, 2009.

Evert AB, Dennison M, Gardner CD, et al: Nutrition therapy for adults with diabetes or prediabetes: a consensus report, *Diabetes Care* 42:731–754, 2019.

Gerstein HC, Miller ME, Genuth S, et al: ACCORD study group. Long-term effects of intensive glucose lowering on cardiovascular outcomes, *N Engl J Med* 364:818–828, 2011.

Holman RR, Paul SK, Bethel MA, et al: 10-year follow-up of intensive glucose control in type 2 diabetes, *N Engl J Med* 359:1577, 2008.

David M, Nathan DM: for the DCCT/EDIC Research Group: the diabetes control and complications trial/epidemiology of diabetes interventions and complications study at 30 years: overview, *Diabetes Care Jan* 37(1):9–16, 2014, https://doi.org/10.2337/dc13-2112.

Patel A, MacMahon S, Chalmers J, et al: ADVANCE collaborative group. intensive blood glucose control and vascular outcomes in patients with type 2 diabetes, *N Engl J Med* 358:2560–2572, 2008.

Skyler JS, Bergenstal R, Bonow RO, et al: Intensive glycemic control and the prevention of cardiovascular events: implications of the ACCORD, ADVANCE, and VA diabetes trials, *Diabetes Care* 32(1):187–192, 2009, https://doi.org/10.2337/dc08-9026.

U.S. Department of Veterans Affairs, U.S. Department of Defense: VA/DoD Clinical practice guideline for the management of type 2 diabetes mellitus in primary care, version 5.0. April 2017. Available at: https://www.healthquality.va.gov/guidelines/CD/diabetes/VADoDDMCPGFinal508.pdf. [Accessed 1 May 2020].

U.S. Preventive Services Task Force: Screening for abnormal blood glucose and type 2 diabetes mellitus: U.S preventive services task force recommendation statement, *Ann Intern Med* 163(11):861–868, 2015.

Zeitler P, Arslanian S, Fu J, et al: ISPAD clinical practice consensus guidelines 2018: type 2 diabetes mellitus in youth, *Pediatr Diabetes* 19(Suppl 27):28–46, 2018. https://doi-org.proxy.kumc.edu/10.1111/pedi.12719.

DIABETIC KETOACIDOSIS

Method of
Aidar R. Gosmanov, MD, PhD, DMSc

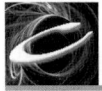

CURRENT DIAGNOSIS

- Initial evaluation includes physical examination and comprehensive metabolic panel, serum osmolality, serum ketones and β-hydroxybutyrate, complete blood count, urinalysis, urine ketones, and arterial blood gases.
- Search for precipitating causes. Omission of insulin, underlying medical illness, cardiovascular events, gastrointestinal disorders, recent surgery, stress, medications, eating disorders, psychological stress, insulin pump malfunction, and infection are potential causes; white blood cell count greater than 25,000 suggests presence of infection.
- β-Hydroxybutyrate of 3.8 mmol/L or greater in adults indicates presence of diabetic ketoacidosis (DKA), even if serum ketones are negative.
- Patients with severe chronic kidney disease (CKD) require careful evaluation of acid-base status.

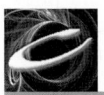

CURRENT THERAPY

- Start intravenous fluids early before insulin therapy.
- Potassium level should be more than 3.3 mEq/L before insulin therapy is initiated. Supplement potassium intravenously if needed.
- Initiate continuous insulin infusion at 0.14 U/kg/h and measure bedside glucose every 1 h to adjust the insulin infusion rate.
- Avoid hypoglycemia during the insulin infusion by initiating dextrose-containing fluids and/or reducing the insulin infusion rate until DKA is resolved.
- Transition to subcutaneous insulin only when DKA resolution is established.

Epidemiology

There were 188,965 hospital discharges for diabetic ketoacidosis (DKA) in 2014 in the United States, compared to 140,000 in 2009 and 80,000 in 1988. The in-hospital fatality rates declined consistently from 2009 to 2014 from 1.1% to 0.4%, although mortality remains high in developing countries. In 2014, the direct and indirect annual cost of DKA hospitalization was $5.1 billion.

Risk Factors

Omission of insulin is the most common precipitant of DKA. Infections, acute medical illnesses involving the cardiovascular system (myocardial infarction, stroke) and gastrointestinal tract (bleeding, pancreatitis), diseases of the endocrine axis (acromegaly and Cushing syndrome), and stress from recent surgical procedures can contribute to the development of DKA by causing dehydration, increase in insulin counterregulatory hormones, and worsening of peripheral insulin resistance. Medications such as diuretics, β-blockers, corticosteroids, second-generation antipsychotics, and anticonvulsants can affect carbohydrate metabolism and volume status and can, therefore, precipitate DKA. Other factors that can contribute to DKA include psychological problems, eating disorders, insulin pump malfunction, lower socioeconomic status, and drug abuse. It is now recognized that new-onset type 2 diabetes mellitus can manifest with DKA. These patients are obese, mostly African American or Hispanic, and extremely insulin resistant on presentation. The use of sodium-glucose cotransporter 2 (SGLT-2) inhibitors has been implicated in the development of DKA in patients with both type 1 and type 2 diabetes. Most recently, the immune checkpoint inhibitors (ICI) used in patients with advanced malignancy can cause DKA de novo in patients without a prior history of diabetes. The DKA risk is significantly more common with use of programmed cell death protein 1 inhibitors such as nivolumab (Opdivo) compared to cytotoxic T-lymphocyte associated antigen 4 inhibitors such as ipilimumab (Yervoy). Early evidence suggests that coronavirus disease 2019 (COVID-19) infection can trigger DKA in subjects without or with prior diabetes history.

Pathophysiology

Insulin deficiency, increased insulin counterregulatory hormones (cortisol, glucagon, growth hormone, and catecholamines), and peripheral insulin resistance lead to hyperglycemia, dehydration, ketosis, and electrolyte imbalance, which underlie the pathophysiology of DKA. The hyperglycemia of DKA evolves through accelerated gluconeogenesis, glycogenolysis, and decreased glucose utilization, all due to absolute insulin deficiency. Owing to increased lipolysis and decreased lipogenesis, abundant free fatty acids are converted to ketone bodies: acetoacetate and β-hydroxybutyrate (β-OHB). Hyperglycemia-induced osmotic diuresis, if not accompanied by sufficient oral fluid intake, leads to dehydration, hyperosmolarity, electrolyte loss, and subsequent decrease in glomerular filtration.

With a decline in a renal function, glycosuria diminishes, and hyperglycemia worsens. With impaired insulin action and hyperosmolar hyperglycemia, potassium uptake by skeletal muscle is markedly diminished, which, along with hyperosmolarity-mediated efflux of potassium from cells, results in intracellular potassium depletion. Potassium is lost via osmotic diuresis, causing profound total body potassium deficiency. Therefore DKA patients can present with a broad range of serum potassium concentrations. A "normal" plasma potassium concentration still indicates that potassium stores in the body are severely diminished and the institution of insulin therapy and correction of hyperglycemia will result in hypokalemia.

On average, patients with DKA have the following deficit of water and key electrolytes: water 100 mL/kg, sodium 7 to 10 mEq/kg, potassium 3 to 5 mEq/kg, and phosphorus 1 mmol/kg.

Clinical Manifestations

Polyuria, polydipsia, weight loss, vomiting, and abdominal pain usually are present in patients with DKA. Abdominal pain can be closely associated with acidosis and resolves with treatment.

TABLE 1 Laboratory Evaluation of Metabolic Causes of Acidosis

LAB VALUE	DKA	STARVATION KETOSIS	LACTIC ACIDOSIS	UREMIC ACIDOSIS	ALCOHOL KETOSIS	SALICYLATE POISONING	METHANOL OR ETHYLENE GLYCOL POISONING
pH	↓	Normal	↓	Mild ↓	↑↓	↑↓*	↓
Plasma glucose	↑	Normal	Normal	Normal	↓ or normal	Normal or ↓	Normal
Plasma ketones†	↑↑	Slight ↑	Normal	Normal	↑	Normal	Normal
Anion gap	↑	Slight ↑	↑	Slight ↑	↑	↑	↑
Osmolality	↑	Normal	Normal	↑ or normal	Normal	Normal	↑↑
Other	—	—	Lactate ↑	BUN ↑	—	Serum level +	Serum level +

*Respiratory alkalosis or metabolic acidosis.
†Acetest and Ketostix (Bayer, Leverkusen, Germany) measure acetoacetic acid only; thus, misleadingly low values may be obtained because the majority of "ketone bodies" are β-hydroxybutyrate.
BUN, Blood urea nitrogen; DKA, diabetic ketoacidosis.

Physical examination findings such as hypotension, tachycardia, poor skin turgor, and weakness support the clinical diagnosis of dehydration in DKA. Mental status changes can occur in DKA and are likely related to the degree of acidosis and hyperosmolarity. A search for symptoms of precipitating causes such as infection, vascular events, or existing drug abuse should be initiated in the emergency department. Patients with hyperglycemic crises can be hypothermic because of peripheral vasodilation and decreased utilization of metabolic substrates.

Diagnosis

Diagnostic criteria for DKA include blood glucose higher than 250 mg/dL, arterial pH 7.30 or less, bicarbonate level 18 mEq/L or less, and adjusted for albumin anion gap greater than 10 to 12. Therefore initia l laboratory evaluation should include a comprehensive metabolic panel and arterial blood gases. Positive serum and urine ketones can further support the diagnosis of DKA but are not required. In early DKA, acetoacetate concentration is low, but it is a major substrate for ketone measurement by many laboratories; therefore ketone measurement in serum by usual laboratory techniques has a high specificity but low sensitivity for the diagnosis of DKA. Conversely, β-OHB is an early and abundant ketoacid that can first signal development of DKA, but its measurement requires the use of a specific assay that is different from ketone measurement. β-OHB of 3.8 mmol/L or higher was shown to be highly sensitive and specific for DKA diagnosis.

In patients with chronic kidney disease stage 4 or 5, the diagnosis of DKA is challenging because of the presence of chronic metabolic acidosis and the possibility of mixed acid-base disorders on presentation with DKA. An anion gap greater than 20 supports the diagnosis of DKA in such patients.

Differential Diagnosis

Hyperglycemic hyperosmolar state is usually not associated with ketosis, but mixed hyperglycemic hyperosmolar state and DKA can occur. Clinical scenarios that may be accompanied by acidosis are described in Table 1. Pregnancy, starvation, and alcoholic ketoacidosis are not characterized by hyperglycemia greater than 250 mg/dL. With hypotension or a history of metformin (Glucophage) use, lactic acidosis should be suspected. Ingestion of methanol, isopropyl alcohol, and paraldehyde[2] can also alter the anion gap and/or osmolality but are not associated with hyperglycemia.

[2]Not available in the United States.

Treatment

The therapeutic goals of management include optimization of volume status, hyperglycemia and ketoacidosis, electrolyte abnormalities, and potential precipitating factors. DKA management workflow is presented in Figure 1. The efficiency of early DKA therapy can be improved by clustering key diagnostic and therapeutic steps in one protocol that is easy to understand by both nursing staff and physicians. Table 2 provides one example of such a DKA care bundle. Given the complexity of the condition management, provision of a single care bundle/order set allows the fundamentals of DKA treatment to be delivered safely and efficiently while giving the providers guidance on tackling unanticipated issues during DKA care. Special considerations should be given to patients with congestive heart failure and chronic kidney disease (CKD). These patients tend to retain fluids; therefore caution should be exercised during volume resuscitation in these patient groups.

Bicarbonate therapy is not indicated in mild and moderate forms of DKA because metabolic acidosis should correct with insulin therapy. The use of bicarbonate in severe DKA is controversial owing to a lack of prospective randomized studies. It is thought that the administration of bicarbonate actually results in peripheral hypoxemia, worsened hypokalemia, paradoxical central nervous system acidosis, cerebral edema in children and young adults, and an increase in intracellular acidosis. Because severe acidosis is associated with worse clinical outcomes and can lead to an impairment in sensorium and a deterioration of myocardial contractility, bicarbonate therapy may be indicated if the pH is 6.9 or less. Therefore the infusion of 100 mmol (2 ampoules) of bicarbonate in 400 mL of sterile water mixed with 20 mEq potassium chloride over 2 hours and repeating the infusion until the pH is greater than 7.0 can be recommended pending the results of prospective trials.

A whole-body phosphate deficit in DKA can average 1 mmol/kg. Insulin therapy during DKA will further lower serum phosphate concentration. Prospective randomized studies have failed to show any beneficial effect of phosphate replacement on the clinical outcome in DKA. However, a careful phosphate replacement is sometimes indicated in patients with serum phosphate concentration less than 1.0 mg/dL and in those with cardiac dysfunction, anemia, or respiratory depression who have a serum phosphate level between 1.0 and 2.0 mg/dL. An initial replacement strategy may include infusion of potassium phosphate at the rate of 0.1 to 0.2 mmol/kg over 6 hours, depending on the degree of phosphate deficit (1 mL potassium phosphate solution for intravenous use contains 3 mmol phosphorous and 4.4 mEq potassium). Overzealous phosphate replacement can result in hypocalcemia; therefore close monitoring of phosphorous and

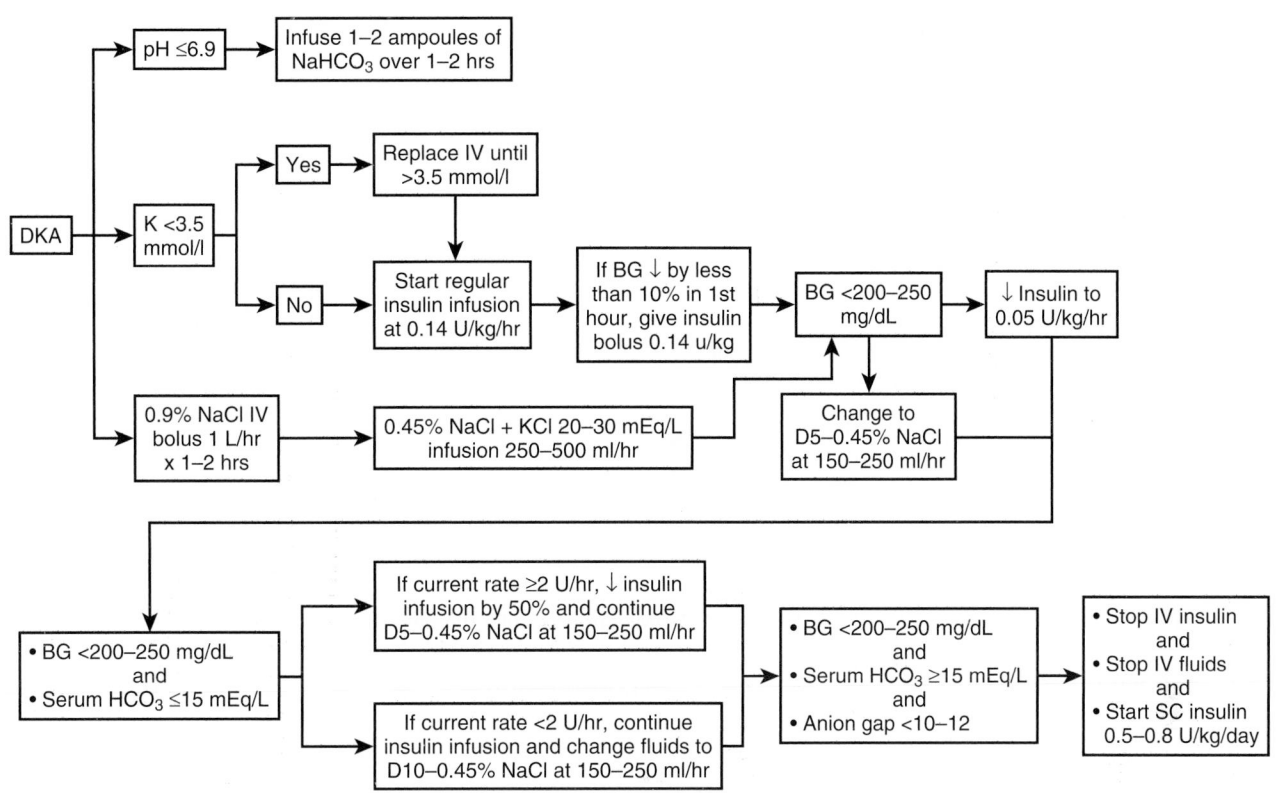

Figure 1 Diabetic ketoacidosis management protocol. *BG*, Blood glucose.

calcium levels is recommended. Patients who have renal insufficiency or hypocalcemia might need less-aggressive phosphate replacement.

When DKA is resolved, and independent of the patient's ability to tolerate oral intake, transition to subcutaneous insulin must be initiated. Patients are given intermediate neutral protamine Hagedorn (NPH) or long-acting insulin (detemir [Levemir], glargine [Lantus]) 2 hours before termination of intravenous insulin to allow sufficient time for the injected insulin to start working (Table 3). Once the patient can eat, we recommend the addition of short- or rapid-acting insulin for prandial glycemic coverage (see Table 3). This is the basal-bolus insulin regimen and provides physiologic replacement of insulin. It is common to see transition from intravenous to subcutaneous insulin using sliding-scale insulin only. This strategy as a sole approach should be discouraged because it cannot provide the necessary insulin requirement in patients recovering from hyperglycemic crisis and beta-cell failure.

If the patient used insulin prior to admission, the same dosage can be restarted in the hospital. Insulin-naïve patients require insulin at a total dose of 0.5 to 0.8 U/kg/day divided as 50% basal insulin and 50% as prandial insulin before each meal. Initially, after DKA resolution and given the possibility of fluctuating oral intake, the use of once-daily long-acting insulin such as glargine or detemir to provide basal insulin coverage is encouraged. Long-acting insulin glargine U300 (Toujeo) and insulin degludec (Tresiba), which were approved by the FDA in 2015, as well as biosimilar insulin glargine (Basaglar), which was approved in 2016, have not been studied in hospitalized patients treated for DKA and, therefore, cannot be recommended for subcutaneous administration immediately following DKA resolution. For patients who are not able to adhere to or afford multiple daily insulin injections, conversion of inpatient basal-bolus insulin regimen before discharge to split-mix insulin preparation (Humulin 70/30, Novolin 70/30, Humalog mix 75/25, Novolog mix 70/30) twice a day that contains a mixture of intermediate-acting insulin NPH and short-acting insulin formulations such as regular (Humulin R, Novolin R), aspart (Novolog), or lispro (Humalog) can be considered. Finger-stick glucose measurements before each meal and at night should be taken after discontinuation of intravenous insulin to correct for possible fluctuations in insulin needs while in the hospital.

Monitoring

Serial measurements—every 2 to 4 hours—of metabolic parameters are required to monitor therapy and then confirm the resolution of DKA. DKA is considered resolved when plasma glucose is less than 200 to 250 mg/dL, serum bicarbonate concentration is 15 mEq/L or higher, venous blood pH is greater than 7.3, and anion gap 12 or less. In general, resolution of hyperglycemia, normalization of bicarbonate level, and closure of the anion gap is sufficient to stop insulin infusion. The anion gap is calculated by subtracting the sum of Cl^- and HCO_3^+ from measured (not corrected) Na^+ concentration and can improve even before the restoration of serum bicarbonate owing to hyperchloremia from normal saline infusion. Venous pH is adequate for assessing the degree of acidosis, with consideration that it is 0.02 to 0.03 lower than arterial blood. If plasma glucose is less than 200 mg/dL but bicarbonate and pH are not normalized, insulin infusion must be continued, and dextrose-containing intravenous fluids started. The latter approach will continue to suppress ketogenesis and prevent hypoglycemia.

TABLE 2	Diabetic Ketoacidosis Order Set

Allergies: □ NKDA or □ **Other (specify):**

Baseline Labs:
□ CBC w/ Diff, CMP, Magnesium, Phosphorus, ABG, Serum Ketones, Fingerstick Blood Glucose, Hemoglobin A1c
□ Urinalysis □ Troponins q6h ×3 □ β-hydroxybutyrate □ Other (specify):

Follow-up Labs:
□ Fingerstick Blood Glucose q1h □ BMP, Magnesium, Phosphorus q2h □ VBG q____h
□ BMP, Magnesium, Phosphorus q4h □ Other (specify):

Consults: □ Endocrinology □ Diabetes Education

Nursing: □ Strict I + O

PHASE I: INITIAL MANAGEMENT

Initial Potassium Replacement for baseline potassium <3.3mmol/L
□ Potassium Chloride_____mEq IVPB (infuse at 10mEq/h)

Initial Fluid Replacement
□ 2 L bolus 0.9% NaCl at 500 mL/h OR □_____L bolus 0.9%NaCl at_____mL/h (specify)

Insulin Therapy:
Do NOT start insulin infusion until K⁺ > 3.3 mmol/L
□ Regular Human Insulin Continuous Infusion: (specify below)
□ 0.14 units/kg/h (_____units/h)
□ 0.05 units/kg/h (_____units/h) (if end-stage renal disease)

PHASE 2: USE UNTIL BLOOD GLUCOSE <250 mg/dL for the FIRST TIME during insulin therapy

BLOOD GLUCOSE (MG/DL)	INSULIN INFUSION RATE (ROUND UP TO NEAREST WHOLE NUMBER)	FLUID THERAPY
<100	See PHASE 3	
100–250	Decrease current infusion rate by half, MOVE to PHASE 3	D5 ½ NS + KCl 20 mEq/L at 200 mL/h
>250 AND: a) Glucose dropped by less than 50 mg/dL in 1 h b) Glucose dropped by 50–100 mg/dL in 1 h c) Glucose dropped by over 100 mg/dL in 1 h	a) Maintain current infusion rate and CALL MD for additional bolus (0.1 units/kg) b) Maintain current infusion rate c) Decrease current infusion rate by half	½ NS + KCl 20 mEq/L at 200 mL/h

PHASE 3: USE FOR ALL BLOOD GLUCOSE READINGS AFTER PHASE 2, or if blood glucose is <100 mg/dL at any time

BLOOD GLUCOSE (MG/DL)	INSULIN INFUSION RATE (ROUND UP TO NEAREST WHOLE NUMBER)	FLUID THERAPY
<70	1. HOLD insulin infusion and give 1 amp D50W IV 2. NOTIFY MD and check fingerstick blood glucose every 15 min until glucose >70, then every 1 h until glucose >100 3. RESTART insulin at half the previous rate when glucose >100	D5 ½ NS + KCl 20 mEq/L at 200 mL/h
70–100	1. HOLD insulin infusion and give ½ amp D50W IV 2. NOTIFY MD and recheck BG in 15 min 3. RESTART insulin at half the previous rate when glucose >100	D5 ½ NS + KCl 20 mEq/L at 200 mL/h
101–200	• If current rate ≥2 units/h, decrease rate by half • If current rate <2 units/h, continue current rate	D5 ½ NS + KCl 20 mEq/L at 200 mL/h
201–250	Maintain current infusion rate	D5 ½ NS + KCl 20 mEq/L at 200mL/h
> 250	Return to PHASE 2	

ABG, Arterial blood gas; *BMP*, basic metabolic profile; *CBC*, complete blood count; *CMP*, comprehensive metabolic panel; *IVPB*, intravenously per bag; *NKDA*, no known drug allergies; *VBG*, venous blood gas.

Complications

Hypoglycemia is the most common complication and can be prevented by the timely adjustment of insulin dosage and frequent monitoring of blood glucose levels. Hypoglycemia is defined as any blood glucose level below 70 mg/dL. If DKA is not resolved and blood glucose level is below 200 to 250 mg/dL, decreases in insulin infusion rate and/or addition of 5% or 10% dextrose to current intravenous fluids may be implemented (see Figure 1). For patients in whom DKA is resolved, strategies to manage hypoglycemia depend on whether the patient is able to eat or not. For patients who are able to drink or eat, ingestion of 15 to 20 g of carbohydrates—for example, four glucose tablets or

TABLE 3	Pharmacokinetics and Pharmacodynamics of Subcutaneous Insulin Preparations				
INSULIN	**ONSET OF ACTION**	**TIME TO PEAK**	**DURATION**	**TIMING OF DOSE**	
Regular (Humulin R, Novolin R)	30–60 min	2–3 h	8–10 h	30–45 min before meal	
Aspart (Novolog)	5–15 min	30–90 min	4–6 h	15 min before meal	
Ultra-rapid Aspart (Fiasp)	2.5 min	63 min	5–7 h	Within 0–20 min after meal start	
Glulisine (Apidra)	15 min	30–90 min	5.3 h	15 min before meal	
Lispro (Humalog)	5–15 min	30–90 min	4–6 h	15 min before meal	
NPH (Humulin N and Novolin N)	2–4 h	4–10 h	12–18 h	Twice a day	
Detemir (Levemir)	2 h	No peak	12–24 h	Once or twice a day	
Glargine (Lantus)	2 h	No peak	20–24 h	Once a day	
Glargine (Basaglar)	2 h	No peak	20–24 h	Once a day	
Glargine U-300 (Toujeo)	6 h	No peak	24–36 h	Once a day	
Degludec (Tresiba)	1 h	No peak	42 h	Once a day	

6 oz orange or apple juice or "regular" soft drink—is advised. In patients who are allowed nothing by mouth, are unable to swallow, or have an altered level of consciousness, administer 25 mL 50% dextrose IV or give 1 mg glucagon IM if no IV access is present. Blood glucose should be rechecked in 15 minutes; only if the glucose level is less than 80 mg/dL should these steps be repeated.

Non–anion-gap hyperchloremic acidosis occurs from urinary loss of ketoanions, which are needed for bicarbonate regeneration, and preferential reabsorption of chloride in proximal renal tubules secondary to intensive administration of chloride-containing fluids and low plasma bicarbonate. The acidosis usually resolves and should not affect the treatment course. Cerebral edema has been reported in young adult patients. This condition is manifested by the appearance of headache, lethargy, papillary changes, or seizures. Mortality is up to 70%. Mannitol (Osmitrol) infusion and mechanical ventilation should be used to treat this condition. Rhabdomyolysis is another possible complication resulting from hyperosmolality and hypoperfusion. Pulmonary edema can develop from excessive fluid replacement in patients with CKD or congestive heart failure.

Prevention

Discharge planning should include diabetes education, selection of an appropriate insulin regimen that the patient can understand and afford, and preparation of set of supplies for the initial insulin administration at home. Many cases of DKA can be prevented by better access to medical care, proper education, and effective communication with a healthcare provider during an intercurrent illness.

Sick-day management should be reviewed periodically with all patients. It should include specific information on when to contact the healthcare provider, blood glucose goals and the use of supplemental short- or rapid-acting insulin during illness, insulin use during fever and infection, and initiation of an easily digestible liquid diet containing carbohydrates and salt. Most importantly, the patient should be advised to never discontinue insulin and to seek professional advice early in the course of the illness. The patient or family member must be able to accurately measure and record insulin administered, blood glucose, and blood β-hydroxybutyrate with a point-of-care device when blood glucose is higher than 300 mg/dL. Recent studies demonstrated that β-OHB testing in outpatient setting is more effective than urine acetoacetate testing in preventing DKA, which may reduce the costs of care of patients with insulin-dependent diabetes. COVID-19-positive patients with diabetes outside of a hospital environment should be particularly vigilant in monitoring home blood glucose and/or β-OHB until the resolution of infection.

Because of the significant cost of repeated admissions for DKA, resources should be directed toward educating primary care providers and school personnel so that they can identify signs and symptoms of uncontrolled diabetes earlier.

References

Benoit SR, Zhang Y, Geiss LS, et al: Trends in diabetic ketoacidosis hospitalizations and in-hospital mortality--United States, 2000-2014, *MMWR Morb Mortal Wkly Rep* 67:362–365, 2018.

Cardoso L, Vicente N, Rodrigues D, et al: Controversies in the management of hyperglycaemic emergencies in adults with diabetes, *Metabolism* 68:43–54, 2017.

Desai D, Mehta D, Mathias P, et al: Health care utilization and burden of diabetic ketoacidosis in the U.S. over the past decade: a nationwide analysis, *Diabetes Care* 41:1631–1638, 2018.

Fadini GP, Bonora BM, Avogaro A: SGLT2 inhibitors and diabetic ketoacidosis: data from the FDA Adverse Event Reporting System, *Diabetologia* 60:1385–1389, 2017.

Hirsch IB: Insulin analogues, *N Engl J Med* 352:174–183, 2005.

Kamel KS, Halperin ML: Acid-base problems in diabetic ketoacidosis, *N Engl J Med* 372:546–554, 2015.

Kitabchi AE, Umpierrez GE, Miles JM, et al: Hyperglycemic crises in adult patients with diabetes, *Diabetes Care* 32:1335–1343, 2009.

Kitabchi AE, Umpierrez GE, Murphy MB, et al: Hyperglycemic crises in adult patients with diabetes: a consensus statement from the American Diabetes Association, *Diabetes Care* 29:2739–2748, 2006.

Li J, Wang X, Chen X, et al: COVID-19 infection may cause ketosis and ketoacidosis, *Diabetes Obes Metab* 22:1935–1941, 2020.

Sheikh-Ali M, Karon BS, Basu A, et al: Can serum beta-hydroxybutyrate be used to diagnose diabetic ketoacidosis? *Diabetes Care* 31:643–647, 2008.

Stamatouli AM, Quandt Z, Perdigoto AL, et al: Collateral damage: insulin-dependent diabetes induced with checkpoint inhibitors, *Diabetes* 67(8):1471–1480, 2018 Aug.

Tzamaloukas AH, Ing TS, Siamopoulos KC, et al: Pathophysiology and management of fluid and electrolyte disturbances in patients on chronic dialysis with severe hyperglycemia, *Semin Dial* 21:431–439, 2008.

Umpierrez GE, Smiley D, Kitabchi AE: Narrative review: ketosis-prone type 2 diabetes mellitus, *Ann Intern Med* 144:350–357, 2006.

Vellanki P, Umpierrez GE: Increasing hospitalizations for DKA: a need for prevention programs, *Diabetes Care* 41(9):1839–1841, 2018.

GENER AFFIRMING CARE

Method of
Molly McClain, MD, MPH, MS

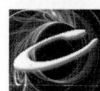

CURRENT DIAGNOSIS

- The diagnosis of gender dysphoria can be made by any clinician trained and licensed to manage behavioral health diagnoses. A team approach to care of gender expansive people, particularly youth, is optimal. Linking the expertise of primary care, endocrinology, nursing, and behavioral health is preferred though not always possible.
- Primary care is becoming the most appropriate and accessible venue to receive gender care, similar to endocrinologic diagnoses that are routinely addressed in the primary care setting, such as diabetes or thyroid anomalies.
- The diagnostic terminology has changed over time as the understanding of gender has evolved. Gender identity and expression is most accurately represented as a continuum. Diversity in gender is not a pathology. To reflect this, terms such as "transsexualism" or "gender identity disorder of children" are no longer used.
- The current diagnosis "gender dysphoria" is categorized in the Diagnostic and Statistical Manual of Mental Disorders (DSM-V). When the 11th revision of the International Statistical Classification of Diseases and Related Health Problems (ICD-11) is initiated, the diagnosis will become "gender incongruence," which will be categorized as a sexual health diagnosis. The significance of this shift is that there will no longer be a diagnostic requirement for significant distress or impairment related to one's gender.
- That gender diversity should require a diagnosis is up for debate. However, the World Health Organization included gender incongruence in the ICD-11 to ensure trans and nonbinary people's access to gender affirming care, as well as adequate health insurance coverage for these services.
- There are no current recommendations to screen for gender diversity in childhood or adolescence by primary care physicians or healthcare professionals. This may change given the increasing proportion of youth who identify as gender expansive, the long-term benefits of access to affirming care if desired, and the reticence that youth have in discussing gender identity with their families and providers.
- Box 1 defines commonly used terminology.

CURRENT THERAPY

- There is a paucity of data related to general health and long-term effects of hormone therapy or pubertal blockade for gender diverse people. The most commonly utilized guidelines from the World Professional Association of Transgender Health (WPATH), the Endocrine Society and the University of San Francisco (UCSF) Transgender Center of Excellence are based on available empirical evidence and clinician consensus.
- In addition to the above guidelines, general principles support the creation of an affirming environment for patients. Principles such as informed consent recognize that the medical provider is not a gatekeeper to desired therapies but is an advisor to the patient for their own decision making in the setting of limited empirical data.
- Trauma-informed care, or a healing-centered approach, is based on facilitating a safe environment where patient empowerment and dignity is supported, recognizing people's inherent strengths and capacities.
- Patient-centered care recognizes that everyone's gender journey is different, and there is no "full transition" that has a shared meaning. This requires the provider to follow the lead of the patient in terms of their personal gender goals, which may not include medications or surgery.
- As avoiding harm is an important ethical stance of medical professionals and use of accurate names and pronouns has been shown to dramatically reduce suicidal behavior, using correct names and pronouns are part of the care plan.
- Withholding of gender affirming treatments, or access to a physician who can, is not a neutral option given the well-documented evidence of depression, anxiety, substance use, and suicidality in the setting of lack of access to gender affirming medical therapies.

Epidemiology

The estimates of the number or percentage of those who are gender diverse are based on limited and incomplete data. The most frequently referenced estimate, using population-based probability samples, is 0.4% to 0.6% of any population. In the United States this would equate to 1 to 1.4 million adults. The dearth of data is largely related to the lack of options to select a gender other than male and female on most surveys, census data collection tools, and health system electronic medical records. In addition, the discrimination faced by gender expansive people results in reduced disclosure of gender in settings when the option to select something other than male or female is available.

Structural Determinants of Health Outcomes

The key determinant of health for gender expansive people is gender affirmation. The depth and breadth of discrimination against gender expansive people in families, education, healthcare, housing, and employment creates severe social and economic exclusion. It is this exclusion, not any biologic determinant, that leads to poorer health outcomes compared with cisgender counterparts. An observational study with nearly 28,000 trans and nonbinary respondents found that nearly 60% reported significant rejection from family because of their gender identity or harassment so severe that almost one-sixth reported leaving school in K-12 or higher education settings. Additionally, 19% were refused medical care because of their gender, and 41% reported attempting suicide (compared with 1.6% of the general population).

On the other hand, data demonstrates that gender affirmation and social/economic inclusion dramatically improves health outcomes. Use of appropriate name and pronouns have been shown to decrease suicide attempts by 56% in one study. Access to medications that suspend puberty or initiate appropriate puberty has been shown to confer lifetime protection against suicide. Even in the face of extensive institutional discrimination, family acceptance has been shown to have the most significant protective effect against homelessness, incarceration, tobacco smoking, drug and alcohol use, anxiety, depression, and suicidal behaviors.

Experts in the neurobiology of trauma describe a lack of gender affirmation as "not being seen or heard." This involves a significantly broader conceptualization of trauma than the diagnostic criteria for posttraumatic stress disorder. Many physical and behavioral health issues that gender expansive people experience stem from chronically not being seen or heard in regard to their gender. The effects of chronic trauma, or stress, on health have been well-documented. The concept of allostatic load might explain the physiologic link between discrimination and ill-health. Short bursts of stress that cause release of cortisol, adrenaline, and other hormones responsible for the "fight or flight" response is adaptive. However chronic, repeated exposures to stress and the chronic release of cortisol is similar to long-term administration of corticosteroids; no system in the human body is left unaffected. As a result, it is common for gender expansive people and anyone who has been exposed to chronic stress to experience depression, anxiety, self-harm, suicidal ideation and attempt, and substance use in addition to autoimmune issues (including mast cell activation), autonomic nervous system dysregulation (such as postural

BOX 1   Terminology

Sex: An assignment or designation made at birth (e.g., male, female, or intersex) typically on the basis of external genital anatomy. The appearance of external genital anatomy is the most common method of assigning sex at birth. Other attributes that contribute to sex include sex chromosomes, H-Y antigen, gonadal anatomy, sex hormone levels, and internal and external genitalia. Gender is not based on the appearance of external genitalia. Use of the term "assigned or designated male, female, or intersex at birth" is preferred to "female to male," "male to female," or "transgender man or woman" as these terms are limited to binary gender identities and are less precise. Use of "transgender man or woman" does not clearly indicate true gender nor the gender the individual was assigned at birth.

Gender identity: A person's concept of self as male, female, a blend of both, or neither. One's gender identity can be the same or different from sex assigned at birth. Gender identity results from a complex interaction of biologic traits, environmental factors, self-understanding, and cultural expectations.

Gender expression: The external presentation of one's gender, as expressed through one's name, clothing, behavior, social roles, hairstyle, or voice. This may or may not conform to socially defined behaviors and characteristics typically associated with being masculine or feminine.

Gender diverse/expansive: A term that is used to describe people with gender behaviors, appearances, or identities that do not align with the culturally expected norms assigned to their gender designated at birth. It can be considered an umbrella term for people who identify as transgender, genderqueer, gender fluid, gender creative, gender independent, or agender, as examples.

Transgender: A subset of gender diverse people whose gender identity does not align with their designated gender or sex at birth and is persistent, consistent, and insistent over time.

Cisgender: A term used to describe a person whose gender is congruent with the gender or sex they were assigned at birth.

Agender: A term that people may use when their identity does not align with gender at all.

Nonbinary/gender fluid: A term one might use to describe themselves if their gender does not align exclusively with male or female or if their gender identity is dynamic over time.

Gender affirmation or confirmation surgery: This term is used for both top and bottom surgeries for those interested in surgery as part of their gender journey.

Sexual orientation: This term describes an individual's attraction to other people or lack thereof. Sexual orientation and gender identity develop separately and they are not linked to each other. There are many terms that people of all genders use to describe their sexual orientation including asexual, pansexual, demisexual, bisexual, gay, straight, and aromantic, to name a few.

---

be trained on the importance of correct name and pronoun use and for all clinic employees to use their own pronouns during introductions.

At the initial visit, healthcare professionals might elicit the individual's history including the patient's gender as described by the patient, their gender journey, social support, past medical/surgical/behavioral health history, family history, whether the patient is currently engaged in behavioral health counseling, and the goals of care. Goals of care might include primary care, medical therapy for pubertal suppression or hormone therapy, and/or gender confirmation surgeries. There is no single or "correct" way that people engage in their gender journey, and it is the clinician's role to follow each individual's lead and to provide support and assistance in reaching the stated goals. It is important to use the patient's name, gender (as stated by the patient), and pronouns throughout the visit and consistently in documentation. The identification statement might read "25-year-old male (designated female at birth or DFAB, he/him) here to discuss hypertension."

The diagnosis of gender dysphoria is based on Diagnostic and Statistical Manual of Mental Disorders (DSM)-5 criteria and can be made by any clinician who has been trained and licensed to diagnose and manage behavioral health diagnoses.

The diagnosis supports the consistency (lasting 6 months or greater), and insistence and persistence of one's gender being incongruous with that designated at birth. Commonly, the description of someone's gender journey elicits elements that support the diagnosis. These elements include incongruence of one's experienced gender, their primary and/or secondary sex characteristics, desire to have their primary and secondary sex characteristics be more aligned with their experienced gender, and desire to treated by others as their experienced gender.

It is optimal for gender care to occur in the setting of team-based care consisting of primary care, endocrinology, nursing, behavioral health, and case management. However, expert consensus is consistent with the reality that this type of care is not always accessible. The Endocrine Society recommends that clinicians who diagnose and manage therapies for gender dysphoria be trained in use of the DSM and International Statistical Classification of Diseases and Related Health Problems (ICD), have the ability to determine capacity for consent, be knowledgeable in prescribing and monitoring hormone therapies, and stay abreast of the most current recommendations. Similar to other endocrinologic issues seen in primary care, referral to specialists may be warranted in specific cases but can in large part be addressed by primary care healthcare professionals.

Given the extensive discrimination experienced by gender diverse people, it is helpful for clinicians to have a healing-centered approach in all aspects of care. Healing-centered care orients the care process beyond the effects of trauma that people may have faced and brings focus toward their inherent strength and healing capacity. Creating a therapeutic alliance of safety and respect between the patient and healthcare professional is another foundation of healing-centered care. This concept can be helpful when considering physical examinations.

Many gender expansive people have experienced negative interactions with medical professionals, including inappropriate physical examinations that are incongruent with the presenting issue. To help people feel more comfortable, clinicians can consider making clear that the patient has the right to refuse anything that makes them uncomfortable and that the examination will be based only on the current needs for the visit. It is helpful to ask the patient "Is it ok with you if I listen to your heart and lungs?" and only proceed when consent has been given for each examination. There is little indication for genital examination at the initial visit unless the patient has a stated concern that would warrant it.

---

orthostatic tachycardia syndrome), chronic pain, increased rates of metabolic disorders, and increased risk of cardiovascular concerns. Recognizing the wide-ranging effects of trauma (in addition to recognition of people's resilience) can support creation of care plans that validate people's medical concerns while also attending to the likely root cause of trauma. Behavioral health providers who are skilled in the trauma-informed model, and in the many evidence-based modalities of trauma processing, can be very helpful in the care of all people with an extensive history of discrimination and social exclusion.

Evaluation

It is important to create a clinical environment that is affirming, including intake forms with gender neutral language and inclusive options for patient gender selection. All clinic staff should

Treatment
Preventive Health

While there are very few studies that have addressed preventive health in gender expansive populations, there are general principles that can help the clinician advise the patient in their choices regarding health maintenance and preventive care. If an organ is present, follow the same guidelines as for cisgender patients and use gender affirming or gender-neutral language as much as possible.

Bone health is an important consideration for people who may be status post gonadectomy and who may have had subphysiologic levels of sex hormones secondary to pubertal suppression or initiation of hormone therapy. The recommendation for all trans and nonbinary people is to start bone density screening at age 65, and for people between 50 and 64 to be considered for bone density screening if other risk factors are present.

There are mixed data on whether people on hormone therapy are at higher risk for cardiovascular disease. Therefore screening for cardiovascular disease is the same as current recommendations for all people. When calculating the atherosclerotic cardiovascular disease (ASCVD) risk score, it may be more accurate to use the patient's predominant hormonal milieu when selecting gender on the risk calculator.

There are no data that people on hormone therapy have higher rates of any type of cancer. For cancer screenings, if an individual has a particular body part or organ and meets criteria for screening based on risk factors or symptoms, the patient should be advised on risks and benefits of that screening regardless of hormone use. For breast cancer screening, if tissue is present, the patient should be advised to follow the same guidelines used for ciswomen. Cervical cancer screening is recommended for anyone with a cervix and guidelines used for ciswomen are appropriate regardless of hormone use. Cervical anatomy changes with testosterone use lead to a 10-fold higher incidence of nonsatisfactory cytology results; therefore it is advised to always perform HPV cotesting. Self-swab for HPV alone is an alternative option that can be used by people who find cotesting unacceptable.

Sexually transmitted infection screening is the same for all people as supported by the Centers for Disease Control and Prevention and the U.S. Preventive Services Task Force. Discussion of pre- and postexposure HIV prophylaxis should be considered for all who meet the criteria. Questions around sexual activity should be limited to the patient's concerns. It is helpful to ask, "What words do you use to describe your genitals?" before discussing anatomy or sexual practices. Attending to sexual health and satisfaction is an important part of whole person care. There is evidence that many people of all genders are reticent to discuss sexual health with clinicians. Inclusion of a question regarding sexual health in one's review of systems for all patients during all visits may facilitate comfort in discussing sexual health. For example, "Are you currently sexually active and do you have any questions or concerns?"

Hormone Therapy

Gender goals may include initiation of hormone therapy. The intent of hormone therapy is to express secondary sex characteristics and to feel more internally aligned with one's affirmed gender. Because gender is a spectrum and goals for hormone therapy might include masculinization, feminization, or nonbinary/gender-fluid goals, it is necessary to ask what an individual's gender and goals for therapy include. Although there is mixed evidence about the safety profile of exogenous hormones compared with endogenous hormones, it can be helpful to consider hormone therapy as initiation of an individual's true puberty and then a lifelong continuation of the hormonal milieu of their accurate gender.

Prior to initiation of hormone therapy, DSM criteria for gender dysphoria must be met and decisional capacity must be established. Any untreated psychiatric issues that affect someone's ability to make safe and informed decisions for themselves is a contraindication to initiation of hormone therapy. The provider should verify absence of hormone-sensitive malignancies and whether the patient has past or current medical issues that may increase the likelihood of side effects from the hormones. It is also imperative that the patient is informed that hormone therapy could irreversibly affect fertility yet does not protect against pregnancy or sexually transmitted illness.

Feminizing regimens consist of an antiandrogen (most commonly spironolactone [Aldactone][1] in the United States or GnRH agonist for suppression of all sex hormones) and bioidentical estradiol (Estrace, generic).[1] Prior to initiation, the medication's effects and possible side effects must be discussed. In addition to the likely effect on fertility, venous thromboembolic events (VTE) can occur while on estradiol, and the patient should have detailed information on signs and symptoms of both deep vein thrombosis and pulmonary embolism. Tobacco use increases this risk, and clinicians can work with their patients on tobacco cessation if indicated. Effects individuals might look forward to are softening of skin, thinning of body hair growth, fat redistribution, decreased muscle mass, decreased sperm production, decreased spontaneous erections, and breast development. Voice timbre is not typically affected by feminizing therapies. The most commonly used formulations are oral tablets (taken daily), patches (switched once or twice weekly), or injectables (once a week). Subcutaneous and intramuscular injections are equally effective. There is no evidence that any formulation has the capacity to cause more feminization than another as they are all the same medication. The effectiveness stems from the consistency of dosing and level of estradiol and testosterone in the serum. Prior to initiation of hormone therapy, baseline labs should be obtained to evaluate for preexisting issues (chemistry panel, hemoglobin A1c, liver function tests, lipid panel, vitamin D, complete blood count (CBC), and differential, and estradiol and testosterone levels). It is advised to start with a lower dose of antiandrogen and estradiol (50 mg spironolactone daily, and 2 mg PO, injectable at 2.5 mg once a week, or 0.05 mg/day once weekly or twice weekly transdermal patch). Per the Endocrine Society, follow-up should occur every 3 months during the first year of hormone therapy, with previsit labs (estradiol and testosterone levels and chemistry panel if on spironolactone). At each visit, doses of both medications can be adjusted based on patient preference and laboratory values. The final goal for estradiol serum level is between 100 to 200 pg per mL, and the goal for serum testosterone, if full suppression is desired, is below 50 ng per dL. Some patients may be interested in progesterone. There have not been high-quality studies performed on the effects of progesterone. Many people who advocate its use feel that it leads to mood stabilization and more rounded, though not larger, breasts. Bioidentical progesterone (Prometrium)[1] at 100 mg daily is a reasonable starting dose. People should be warned that it can decrease estradiol serum levels, so a 3-month follow-up with sex hormone levels may be helpful.

Masculinizing therapy consists of some formulation of testosterone only. The most commonly used formulations are injectable (subcutaneous is equally effective as intramuscular), topical gel (or compounded topicals), and patches. The possible side effects of testosterone must be discussed prior to initiation and include erythrocytosis and possible VTE secondary to chronic untreated erythrocytosis. Large population analyses have not shown increased risk of cardiovascular outcomes compared with cismales. Concern for metabolic effects should be considered but have not been consistently demonstrated in studies. The effects of masculinizing hormones include acne, increased body hair growth, male-pattern baldness, increased libido, clitoromegaly, vaginal atrophy, and more readily achievable fat loss and muscle gain. As with feminizing hormones, it is advised to start with a lower dose and increase based on laboratory values and patient preference. For optimized masculinization, the goal serum testosterone is between 400 and 1000 ng per dL. Prior to initiation of hormone therapy, baseline labs should be obtained to evaluate for preexisting medical problems (chemistry panel, hemoglobin A1c, liver function tests, lipid panel, vitamin D, CBC and differential, and estradiol and testosterone levels). A reasonable starting dose

---

[1]Not FDA approved for this indication.

is 30 mg injectable testosterone cypionate (Depo-Testosterone)[1] once weekly. Follow-up during the first year is every 3 months with previsit testosterone, estradiol, and hematocrit/hemoglobin levels. Dose change at these visits can be guided by patient preference and serum levels. An increase or decrease by 10 mg may be a reasonable increment at each quarterly visit.

Gender expansive goals can be achieved by lower doses of hormone therapy or "microdosing." If someone is interested in nonbinary outcomes, whether subtle feminizing or masculinizing changes are desired, all of the above instructions can be applied. However, the goal serum levels differ. For nonbinary masculinization the serum level of testosterone should be as close to 400 ng/dL as possible. This is easier to achieve with either daily topical testosterone at lower doses or low doses of injectable testosterone administered twice weekly to achieve a decreased range of peak and trough levels. If people on feminizing hormones are interested in nonbinary outcomes and/or maintenance of sexual function, the serum goal for estradiol is still between 100 and 200 pg/mL, and people can choose to use an antiandrogen to achieve the desired effect. Lower doses of spironolactone may lead to decreased feminizing effect, and the patient can balance what is most affirming to them in terms of feminization and maintenance of sexual function. As long as either estradiol or testosterone is within physiologic range, bone health is maintained.

Gender Affirming/Confirmation Surgery

As with hormone therapy, not all gender expansive people are interested in gender affirming/confirmation surgeries. The term "sex reassignment surgery" is no longer favored. For those who are interested, access to procedures improves mental health outcomes. Most guidelines suggest that people who undergo gender confirmation surgery be 18 years or older and have been on affirming hormones for at least 12 months. If patients have severe dysphoria and do not meet these criteria, clinicians can still consider supporting the medical necessity of a procedure if they feel it is indicated. "Top surgery" includes chest reduction or breast augmentation. Top surgery requires a letter from a behavioral health provider to verify the diagnosis. The patient need not be engaged in therapy long term to acquire letters for surgery. "Bottom surgery" includes hysterectomy with or without oophorectomy, orchiectomy, vaginoplasty, phalloplasty, and metoidioplasty. For any procedure that may affect fertility, two letters from behavioral health providers should be completed. The choice to undergo hysterectomy is based on patient preference. There is no evidence that hysterectomy is indicated in the setting of long-term masculinizing regimens, nor is there evidence of harms specific to people on testosterone. Those who choose to undergo hysterectomy or orchiectomy should be counseled on the need for lifelong exogenous hormones. Other procedures may include facial feminization, tracheal shave, and gluteal lift.

Insurance coverage differs by insurance carrier and state. There are some states in which the medical and surgical coverage for gender dysphoria must be supplied by insurance carriers; it is helpful for healthcare professionals to have some understanding of the legal context of the state and city they practice in for patient pursuit of surgery. It is also helpful to know what (if any) procedures are available locally and the experience that patients have with local surgeons.

Youth

Affirming care for youth includes provision of developmentally appropriate care focused on recognizing the individual's gender experience, creation of a nonjudgmental partnership with the whole family, and facilitation of discussions regarding risks and benefits of medical treatments if desired. The prevalence of youth who identify as gender diverse may be higher than that of adults. And similar to data for adults, gender expansive youth have dramatically elevated levels of depression, anxiety, disordered

eating, self-harm, substance use, suicidal ideation, and attempts compared with cisgender counterparts. Gender affirmation is the key determinant of health for gender expansive youth, as it is for adults. Data has shown that while family rejection does little to change the gender identity of youth, family acceptance has the most powerful impact on decreasing the above health outcomes. The second most impactful intervention is access to medical therapy if desired. The American Academy of Pediatrics encourages families to seek gender-informed therapy and explore legitimate fears, concerns, and confusion regarding how best to support their gender diverse or gender questioning youth. The care of youth is best provided within the context of multidisciplinary care. However, this is not always available.

Providing affirming primary care and gender care during prepubertal stages of childhood is identical to care of all children with regular well-child visits and acute care visits as needed. When youth begin to experience pubertal changes, they may experience worsening dysphoria. If desired, pubertal suppression using GnRH agonist starting at Tanner stage II or III is indicated. Pubertal suppression allows for cessation of pubertal development, which can decrease dysphoria and allow for continued clarification of gender identity. While pubertal suppression is described as reversible, the long-term effects on bone health and fertility are currently unknown and families should be informed of this. The Endocrine Society guidelines and the World Professional Association for Transgender Health (WPATH) delineate adolescent eligibility for GnRH agonist treatment that can be helpful for providers to use during evaluation of patients who desire pubertal suppression. GnRH agonists can be started if the youth has demonstrated consistent gender incongruence, has decisional capacity, and has been informed of effects and side effects and options to preserve fertility. In addition, the patient and guardians must have given consent, a pediatric endocrinologist or other clinician experienced in pubertal assessment must agree with initiation of pubertal suppression, the patient must be in Tanner stage G2/B2, and there must be no medical contraindications. It is encouraged, but not necessary, for the youth to be engaged in behavioral health support. The dosing, monitoring, and laboratory schedules for safe administration of GnRH agonists can be found in the Endocrine Society Guidelines of 2017.

The timing of pubertal induction with hormone therapy while on GnRH analogs should be based on patient and family-centered circumstances. There is no empirical evidence to support a particular age of hormone therapy initiation. The recommendation of initiation at age 16 was based on the age cut-off of certain countries regarding medical decision making and is not consistent with average age of endogenous puberty. This can make the decision of when to initiate hormone therapy more complex.

Other Considerations
Voice Training
Gender diverse individuals may want speech therapy to support their gender affirmation. Masculinizing hormones affect voice tenor permanently, but feminizing regimens do little in this regard. Some speech and language pathologists are specialized in voice feminization or masculinization practices, and for those who find this prohibitively expensive (or if this service is not available locally), there are many smartphone applications that can assist people in voice training.

Fertility Counseling, Gamete Preservation, and Contraception
While pubertal suppression and hormone therapy affect fertility, there is no data regarding the specifics with which to counsel patients and families. In terms of informed consent, it is most appropriate for people to recognize that the likelihood of having biologic children is drastically reduced, if not impossible. Patients should be counseled to seek gamete preservation if desired. If biologic children are desired, it is safest to postpone initiation of all medications until gamete preservation has been completed. At the same time, none of the medications protect against pregnancy or

---

[1]Not FDA approved for this indication.

sexually transmitted infections. Condom use is safe and effective for everyone, and for people on masculinizing hormones more acceptable forms of contraception include progesterone-only birth control pills, Nexplanon, and Mirena IUD.

Hair Removal

Hair removal from face and body may be pursued for aesthetic purposes or in preparation for surgery. It is best to suggest a hair removal specialist who provides affirming care and can offer electrolysis and laser hair removal for a tailored approach. The patient should first query their insurance carrier for possible coverage of hair removal. It is more common that insurance will cover hair removal in the setting of preoperative preparation for vaginoplasty as this is a requirement for that procedure.

Legal Considerations

Legal considerations include legal name change, change of gender and/or name on legal documents, providing letters of medical necessity for procedures, and addressing possible insurance denials of medical and/or surgical coverage. The process for legal name change, change of name and gender on birth certificates, and other state-based documents such as driver's licenses differs by state. Many states require that a medical provider write a letter demonstrating that someone meet criteria for gender dysphoria to change any legal documents, but some do not require this form of gatekeeping. Typically, if the state does require provider documentation or signatures, the format for any letter should be readily accessible and easy to create. To change federal documents, such as passports, there is a form letter that is easy to find online (https://transequality.org/know-your-rights/passports) that should be adjusted per patient and clinician as indicated, printed on letterhead, and signed in blue ink.

References

1. World Professional Association for Transgender Health. Standards of Care. Available at https://www.wpath.org/media/cms/Documents/SOC%20v7/Standards%20of%20Care%20V7%20-%202011%20WPATH.pdf?_t=1605186324. [accessed 2/24/2021].
2. Hembree WC, Cohen-Kettenis PT, Gooren L, et al: Endocrine treatment of gender-dysphoric/gender-incongruent persons: an endocrine society clinical practice guideline, *JCEM* 102:11, 2017. Available at https://academic.oup.com/jcem/article/102/11/3869/4157558. [accessed 24 February 2021].
3. USCF. Guidelines for the Primary and Gender-Affirming Care of Transgender and Gender Nonbinary People. Available at https://transcare.ucsf.edu/guidelines. [accessed 2/24/2021].
4. Rafferty J: Ensuring comprehensive care and support for transgender and gender-diverse children and adolescents, *AAP* 142:4, 2018. Available at https://pediatrics.aappublications.org/content/pediatrics/142/4/e20182162.full.pdf. [accessed 24 February 2021].
5. The Lancet. Series on Transgender Health. Available at https://www.thelancet.com/series/transgender-health. [accessed 2/24/2021].
6. National Center for Transgender Equality. U.S. Transgender Survey. Available at https://transequality.org/issues/us-trans-survey. [accessed 2/24/2021].

GOUT AND HYPERURICEMIA

Method of
Saima Chohan, MD

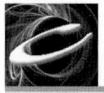

CURRENT DIAGNOSIS

- Gout is the most common inflammatory arthritis in men and is increasing in prevalence.
- A definitive diagnosis of gout requires the demonstration of monosodium urate crystals in synovial fluid or tophi.
- Gouty arthritis often begins in the joints of the lower extremity.
- Septic arthritis, rheumatoid arthritis, and calcium pyrophosphate disease (pseudogout) can mimic gout and should be ruled out.

CURRENT THERAPY

- The goals of successful gout treatment include terminating the acute attack, preventing intermittent attacks, and undertaking long-term therapy to avoid chronic arthritis.
- Indications for the chronic treatment of gout include frequent attacks, recurrent arthritis, and kidney disease.
- A serum urate level of less than 6.0 mg/dL is the goal when urate-lowering therapy is being used.
- Nonpharmacologic treatment includes lifestyle modification and dietary changes.
- The mainstay of urate-lowering therapies remains xanthine oxidase inhibition.

Epidemiology

Gout, or monosodium urate crystal deposition disease, is the most common inflammatory arthritis of men and is an increasingly common problem among postmenopausal women. It is a chronic disorder, affecting more than 5 million people in the United States and increasing in both prevalence and incidence, especially in persons older than 65 years. Gout is often accompanied by serious comorbid disorders (hypertension, cardiovascular disease, chronic kidney disease, and all of the component features of the metabolic syndrome) and is managed in primary care practice in about 90% of affected persons. Therefore identifying risk factors, optimizing diagnosis, and choosing the appropriate treatment for gout are important skills for a wide array of caregivers.

Pathophysiology and Risk Factors

Uric acid is the end product of purine metabolism in humans. Hyperuricemia, a serum urate concentration exceeding urate solubility (6.8 mg/dL), is an invariable accompaniment of gout, although serum uric acid levels might not be elevated during an acute attack. Hyperuricemia predisposes affected persons to urate crystal formation and deposition, leading to the inflammatory responses underlying the symptoms of gout. Thus treatment of gout is aimed at reducing and maintaining serum urate concentration at subsaturating levels, usually set at less than 6.0 mg/dL.

Hyperuricemia

Risk factors for hyperuricemia include obesity, hypertension, hyperlipidemia, insulin resistance, renal insufficiency, and the use of diuretics. Diets rich in certain foods are also associated with increased risk for gout. Many studies with large patient cohorts have demonstrated a relationship between hyperuricemia and hypertension, cardiovascular and peripheral vascular disease, chronic kidney disease, and diabetes mellitus. The association of hyperuricemia and metabolic syndrome has also been shown in children and adolescents. Interventional trials of asymptomatic patients with hyperuricemia and high cardiovascular risk must be performed before such treatment can be advocated.

Diagnosis

Acute gout is characterized by an abrupt onset of joint pain, erythema, and swelling, usually of one joint but less commonly of more than one. The arthritis most often occurs first in the joint of a lower extremity, especially the first metatarsophalangeal (MTP) joint at the base of the great toe. The predilection for this site is thought to be secondary to cooler acral temperature or repeated trauma and pressure on this joint.

The gold standard for the diagnosis of gout is the demonstration of monosodium urate crystals by polarized light microscopy either in joint fluid aspirated during an acute attack or between attacks or from material aspirated from suspected tophi. To aspirate the first MTP joint, the joint is first identified by palpating the space at the base of the metacarpal on the dorsal aspect while flexing and extending the toe. The needle is then inserted

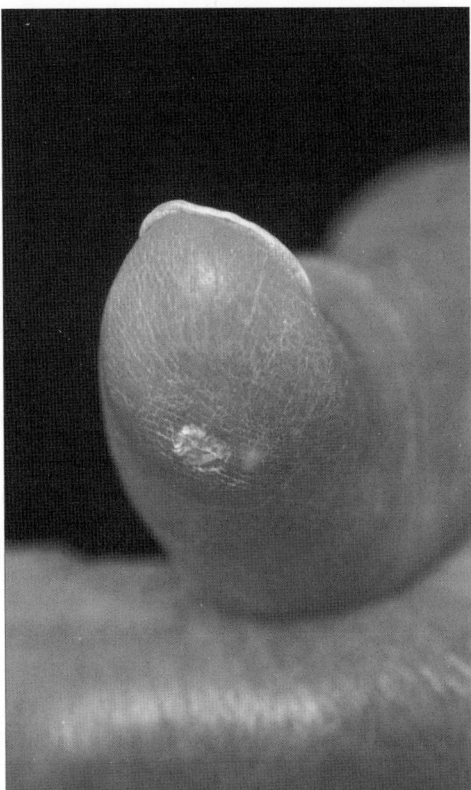

Figure 1 Intradermal urate deposit (tophus). (Reprinted with permission from Mandell BF: Gout and crystal deposition disease. In Weisman MH, Weinblatt ME, Louie JS, Van Vollenhoven R, editors: *Targeted Treatment of the Rheumatic Diseases*, Philadelphia, 2010, Saunders, pp 293–302.)

perpendicularly into the joint space to avoid the extensor hallucis tendon. Synovial fluid from affected joints should immediately be examined under polarized microscopy to confirm the diagnosis of needle-shaped crystals with negative birefringence. If polarized microscopy is unavailable, then fluid should be promptly sent in a sterile tube to an appropriate laboratory for crystal confirmation.

Unfortunately the equipment and analytical expertise necessary to make this diagnosis are not widely available to primary care physicians. As a result, the diagnosis of acute gout is commonly made on clinical grounds, using the 2015 classification criteria of the American College of Rheumatology and the European League Against Rheumatism. These diagnostic guidelines use a point system and emphasize the presence of signs of inflammation (redness, tenderness, and loss of joint function), abrupt onset, monoarticular involvement, occurrence in the first MTP joint, presence of tophi, and radiographic findings.

The initial symptoms and signs of gout often arise after many years of asymptomatic hyperuricemia. In untreated or inadequately treated patients, the course of the disease often involves acute attacks at increasing frequency, with shortening of asymptomatic periods (called intercritical gout) and, ultimately, the development of chronic joint disease (gouty arthropathy) and tophi (masses of urate crystals in a chronic inflammatory matrix) in bone, joints, skin, and even solid organs (Figure 1).

Indications for Treatment

Early in gout, patients might have attacks that are separated by years and are manageable over the course of a few days with anti-inflammatory medications and adjuncts such as joint rest and the application of ice. Over time, the attacks usually become more frequent, prolonged, and disabling, eventually requiring long-term urate-lowering treatment aimed at preventing the deposition of urate crystals and eventually abolishing acute flares and resolving tophi. Indications for urate-lowering (antihyperuricemic) therapy are listed in Box 1.

BOX 1 Indications for Urate-Lowering Therapy

- Frequent and disabling gouty attacks are often defined as two or three flares annually, although this is not evidence based; the decision to treat is based on both number of flares and the disability resulting from flares.
- Chronic gouty disease: clinically or radiographically evident joint erosions.
- Tophaceous deposits: subcutaneous or intraosseous.
- Gout with renal insufficiency.
- Recurrent kidney stones.
- Urate nephropathy.
- Urinary uric acid excretion exceeding 1100 mg/day (6.5 mmol), when determined in men younger than 25 years or in premenopausal women.

Treatment

Acute Gout

Gouty arthritis occurs suddenly, and attacks are often very painful and disabling. Patients describe an acute onset of exquisite pain, swelling, erythema, and inability to bear weight on the afflicted joint. Occasionally patients have constitutional symptoms including fever and chills, with an elevated sedimentation rate and white blood cell count. To terminate an attack, nonsteroidal antiinflammatory drugs (NSAIDs), colchicine (Colcrys), or corticosteroids can be offered. If given at full anti-inflammatory dosage, NSAIDs have a rapid onset and are quite efficacious in relieving pain and shortening the duration of an attack. The utility of this class of drugs may be limited by renal insufficiency, cardiovascular risk factors, and gastrointestinal bleeding. Although indomethacin (Indocin), sulindac (Clinoril), and naproxen (Naprosyn) are all approved by the US Food and Drug Administration (FDA) for treating acute attacks of gout, nearly every drug in this class and the selective cyclooxygenase (COX) 2 inhibitors also have considerable efficacy. High-dose salicylate therapy lowers serum uric acid by interfering in renal urate transport; low-dose aspirin[1] has the opposite effect, but it is often continued in gout patients because of its overriding importance in managing coronary artery disease.

Oral colchicine has been used to treat gout for many years as an unproven drug with no FDA dosage recommendations or prescribing information. In July 2009, however, the FDA approved Colcrys, a single-ingredient colchicine product, for the first day of treatment of acute gout attacks at a low-dose regimen of 1.2 mg followed by 0.6 mg in 1 hour (total 1.8 mg). With this regimen, colchicine can be used to abort an attack if it is taken immediately after the development of the first symptom of gout flare. Higher colchicine doses (0.6 mg every hour until symptoms improve or until gastrointestinal symptoms of diarrhea, nausea, or vomiting develop for a total of 4.8 mg over 6 hours)[3] have traditionally been recommended. A randomized placebo-controlled trial comparing the low- and high-dose regimens showed both approaches to have equivalent efficacy in pain relief at 24 hours (compared with placebo). However, adverse gastrointestinal events were significantly less common with the low-dose regimen. In subjects warranting additional flare treatment, continued use of colchicine 0.6 mg twice daily (reducing to once daily as the flare subsides) is appropriate in persons with normal renal and hepatic function. Oral colchicine is now available in generic form and in two branded versions (Colcrys, Mitigare).

Gastrointestinal symptoms are generally the first clinical signs of colchicine toxicity in patients with normal renal and hepatic function. More serious toxicities do occur and include neuromyopathy, aplastic anemia, and worsening renal and hepatic function. Patients with renal or hepatic impairment should be treated with caution; because of potentially serious drug-drug interactions, colchicine should be avoided in patients receiving cyclosporine

---

[1]Not FDA approved for this indication.

(Neoral), clarithromycin (Biaxin), verapamil (Calan), or amlodipine (Norvasc). Intravenous colchicine is not available in Europe. The FDA has stopped the marketing of unapproved injectable colchicine products in the United States and discourages the compounding of intravenous colchicine because of reports of preparation errors causing deaths.

Corticosteroids provide a safe alternative for patients with contraindications to NSAIDs or colchicine. For isolated mono-articular attacks, especially of medium or large joints, aspiration of joint fluid and intra-articular injection with triamcinolone acetonide (Kenalog) 20 to 40 mg can quickly terminate an attack. For polyarticular attacks or attacks in smaller joints, systemic corticosteroids (oral or intramuscular) may be used. Oral prednisone starting at 20 mg twice daily with a taper over 10 to 14 days is very effective. Patients can have rebound attacks if oral steroids are terminated too quickly; thus methylprednisolone (Medrol) dose packs should be avoided. If intramuscular injection is required, a single dose of triamcinolone 40 mg may be used.

There is interest in agents blocking the action of interleukin 1 (IL-1), a cytokine thought to play a major role in initiating and sustaining acute gouty inflammation. Anakinra (Kineret)[1] and canakinumab (Ilaris)[1] are potent injectable IL-1 inhibitors; studies are ongoing to assess the utility of these agents to mitigate acute attacks. In 2013 canakinumab became the first biologic agent approved for acute gout in Europe. It was approved by the European Medicines Agency for symptomatic treatment of adult patients with frequent gouty arthritis attacks in whom NSAIDs and colchicine are contraindicated, are not tolerated, or do not provide an adequate response and in whom repeated courses of corticosteroids are not appropriate. Rilonacept (Arcalyst),[1] which is also in this class, was declined approval for gout by the FDA in 2012 because of concerns about its long-term safety.

Intercritical Gout

After an attack subsides, management is directed at preventing recurrent attacks. During acute attacks of gout, normal serum urate concentration is reported in up to 40% of affected patients, and thus it is not an accurate reflection of the true urate pool. Confirmation of hyperuricemia is best achieved either before the resolution of an attack or 2 to 4 weeks after it to achieve an accurate serum urate concentration. There is a generalizable correlation between the serum urate level and the risk for a recurrent attack.

Prophylaxis of future attacks during early urate-lowering therapy can consist of colchicine at doses of 0.6 mg once or twice a day (based on renal function) or NSAIDs. If chronic NSAIDs are used, acid-reducing medications such as proton pump inhibitors or histamine-2 blockers may be used for patients at risk for gastrointestinal bleeding.

Long-Term Urate-Lowering (Antihyperuricemic) Therapy

The aim of urate-lowering therapy is to reduce and maintain serum urate at concentrations below those at which extracellular fluids are saturated with monosodium urate. In general an ultimate serum urate concentration of less than 6.0 mg/dL is advised. Urate lowering can be achieved either by increasing urinary excretion or decreasing production of urate.

Nonpharmacologic urate-lowering treatment begins with lifestyle changes. Diet and weight loss must be addressed. Obesity and weight gain are risk factors for gout, and weight loss has been shown to decrease the risk of gout. A purine-restricted diet has often been recommended to patients but is often unpalatable and impractical. Reduction in alcohol intake, namely beer and liquor, can effectively reduce urate levels. Similarly, a reduced intake of red meat and shellfish also lowers the risk of recurrent gouty attacks. Studies have shown an increased frequency of attacks in patients who consume fruit juices and soft drinks containing high-fructose corn syrup, an ingredient not found in diet drinks.

Once the decision is made to institute serum urate–lowering therapy, the duration of treatment is indefinite and must be long-term to be effective. The majority of patients with gout and tophaceous disease will continue to have attacks if therapy is discontinued; thus education is a key part of the treatment plan. Patients should be instructed that, with initiation of any urate-lowering therapy, they will be at increased risk for a flareup and thus must continue regular use of prophylactic agents as outlined earlier. At least 80% to 95% of cases of hyperuricemia and gout are attributable to impaired urate excretion, which is reflected in diminished urate clearance or fractional excretion of uric acid but not usually in low daily urine uric acid excretion. In practice, 24-hour urine collections are rarely performed. Patients are preferentially treated with xanthine oxidase inhibitors because of the easier dosing schedule and many patients have contraindications to uricosurics such as renal insufficiency and kidney stones.

Uricosurics

Relative to medications aimed at urate synthesis, uricosurics are relegated to second-line treatment of patients with elevated urate burden or tophaceous disease. The most commonly used uricosuric agent in the United States is probenecid. This is a very effective drug that concentrates and promotes urinary excretion of urate. Its utility is limited in patients with renal insufficiency, and probenecid is not recommended as first-line therapy in patients with nephrolithiasis or uric acid overexcretion. The maintenance dose of probenecid required to achieve and maintain serum urate concentration at less than 6.0 mg/dL is 0.5 to 3 g/day[3] administered in 2 or 3 daily doses. Once goal serum urate concentration has been achieved with a uricosuric agent, the risk of uric acid calculi is diminished because urinary uric acid excretion becomes normal.

Lesinurad (Zurampic) is another uricosuric agent; it is an inhibitor of renal transport proteins and was approved by the FDA in 2016. It is used at a dose of 200 mg/day in combination with a xanthine oxidase inhibitor, including allopurinol (Zyloprim) or febuxostat (Uloric). In 2017, the FDA approved a combination product of lesinurad 200 mg and allopurinol 300 mg (Duzallo), one tablet in the morning for hyperuricemia. This product is also available as a tablet containing lesinurad 200 mg and allopurinol 200 mg for patients with renal impairment. The drug has a boxed warning regarding the risk of acute renal failure.

Other drugs found to have uricosuric effects include fenofibrate (Tricor),[1] a fibric acid derivative used to treat hyperlipidemia, and the antihypertensives losartan (Cozaar)[1] and amlodipine (Norvasc).[1] These agents have mild uricosuric properties and may be useful adjuncts to urate-lowering therapy. The ingestion of skim milk has been shown to lower serum urate levels through uricosuric effects. Lower urate levels have also been seen in patients who consume coffee, but the mechanism of action is unknown.

Xanthine Oxidase Inhibitors

Allopurinol (Zyloprim) and febuxostat (Uloric) are the only FDA-approved xanthine oxidase inhibitors for the treatment of gout. Allopurinol, introduced in 1966, is approved in doses of 100 to 800 mg/day. More than 90% of patients with gout treated with urate-lowering medication in the United States are given allopurinol, but dosages of more than 300 mg/day are rarely employed and often patients do not achieve serum urate concentrations of 6.0 mg/dL or less. Appropriate use of allopurinol is limited for several reasons. There are genuine concerns about allopurinol drug interactions, gastrointestinal intolerance, rashes (ranging from mild to life threatening), and the rare but sometimes fatal hypersensitivity syndrome. Allopurinol should be avoided with the immunosuppressives azathioprine (Imuran) and 6-mercaptopurine (Purinethol) because it can increase the risk of bone marrow toxicity. That can occur because these medications are partially metabolized by xanthine oxidase. Allopurinol should not be taken with ampicillin owing to an increased risk of rash.

---

[3]Exceeds dosage recommended by the manufacturer.

[1]Not FDA approved for this indication.

Effective dosing of allopurinol is often not achieved because of compliance with published but disputed recommendations for allopurinol dose reduction in states of renal impairment. Allopurinol should be initiated at 100 mg/day in patients with creatinine clearance of 40 mL/min or greater, and it should be titrated in 100-mg increments every 2 to 4 weeks, with the endpoint of dosing determined by achievement of serum urate concentration of 6.0 mg/dL or less.

The FDA approved febuxostat (Uloric) in 2009. Unlike allopurinol, this is a nonpurine analog and selective xanthine oxidase inhibitor that is not incorporated into purine nucleotides and does not appear to affect pyrimidine metabolism. Febuxostat is primarily metabolized by oxidation and glucuronidation in the liver, with little renal excretion; this contrasts with the renal elimination of oxypurinol, the main allopurinol metabolite. The recommended starting dose of febuxostat is 40 mg/day, with an increase to 80 mg/day if serum urate concentrations do not reach goal urate levels in 2 weeks in patients with normal renal function. In Europe, higher dosages (80–120 mg/day)[3] have received approval, and studies have affirmed the efficacy and safety of dosing in this range. In the FOCUS trial, a 5-year study of efficacy and safety, febuxostat was shown to have durable maintenance of serum urate concentration at 6.0 mg/dL or less, nearly complete elimination of gouty flares, and resolution of baseline tophi in subjects. In 2019, a boxed warning was added by the FDA as studies showed that febuxostat was associated with an increased risk of cardiovascular and all-cause mortality compared with allopurinol. Although an advantage of febuxostat over allopurinol is that it can safely be taken by patients with creatinine clearance greater than 30 mL/min, we recommend allopurinol in patients with elevated cardiovascular risk.

Pegloticase

Pegloticase (pegylated porcine recombinant uricase [Krystexxa]) was granted FDA approval in 2010 for the treatment of refractory gout. Humans lack the enzyme uricase, which converts uric acid to allantoin, a more soluble purine degradation product. Replacement of this missing enzyme allows direct conversion of urate to allantoin with eventual depletion of increased body urate pools and control of disease, including resolution of tophi. Recombinant uricase therapy profoundly lowers serum urate concentration, as was demonstrated in two large trials. Pegloticase is approved at a dosage of 8 mg IV every 2 weeks.

Potential New Therapies

A number of other novel agents with new therapeutic targets for the treatment of acute and chronic gout are under investigation.

References

Becker MA, Chohan S: We can make gout management more successful now, *Curr Opin Rheumatol* 20:167–172, 2008.

Dalbeth N, Stamp L: Allopurinol dosing in renal impairment: Walking the tightrope between adequate urate lowering and adverse events, *Semin Dial* 20:391–395, 2007.

Neogi T, Jansen T, Dalbeth N et al, et al: 2015 Gout Classification Criteria: An American College of Rheumatology/European League Against Rheumatism Collaborative Initiative, *Arthr Rheum* 67:2557–2568, 2015.

Schumacher HR, Becker MA, Lloyd E, et al: Febuxostat in the treatment of gout: 5-year findings of the FOCUS efficacy and safety study, *Rheumatology* 48:188–194, 2009.

Stamp L, O'Donnell JL, Zhang M et, et al: Using allopurinol above the dose based on creatinine clearance is effective and safe in patients with chronic gout, including those with renal impairment, *Arthritis Rheum* 63:412–421, 2011.

Sundy JS, Becker MA, Baraf HS, et al: Reduction of plasma urate levels following treatment with multiple doses of pegloticase (polyethylene glycol–conjugated uricase) in patients with treatment-failure gout. Results of a phase II randomized study, *Arthritis Rheum* 58:2882–2891, 2008.

Terkeltaub R, Furst DE, Bennett K, et al: High versus low dosing of oral colchicine for early acute gout flare, *Arthritis Rheum* 62:1060–1068, 2010.

Zhu Y, Pandya BJ, Choi HK: Comorbidities of gout and hyperuricemia in the US general population: NHANES 2007-2008, *Am J Med* 125:679–687, 2012.

Macdonald TM, Ford I, Nuki G, et al: Protocol of the Febuxostat versus Allopurinol Streamlined Trial (FAST): a large prospective, randomised, open, blinded endpoint study comparing the cardiovascular safety of allopurinol and febuxostat in the management of symptomatic hyperuricaemia, *BMJ Open* 4(7):e005354, 2014. Epub 2014 Jul 10.

[3]Exceeds dosage recommended by the manufacturer.

HYPERALDOSTERONISM

Method of
Ruchi Gaba, MD; and Lawrence Chan, MD

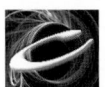

CURRENT DIAGNOSIS

- Hyperaldosteronism may be suspected in patients with severe, resistant, or early-onset hypertension and hypertensive patients with family history, hypokalemia, adrenal mass, and obstructive sleep apnea. Evaluation begins with measurement of morning plasma aldosterone concentration (PAC in ng/dL) and plasma renin activity (PRA in ng/mL/h) in a sodium- and potassium-repleted state and off of significantly interfering medications (spironolactone [Aldactone], eplerenone [Inspra], amiloride [Midamor], triamterene [Dyrenium], potassium-wasting diuretics, and licorice-derived products[7]) for at least 4 weeks.

- Elevated PRA and PAC suggest secondary hyperaldosteronism; suppressed PRA and PAC suggest conditions mimicking hyperaldosteronism; suppressed PRA but elevated PAC suggests primary hyperaldosteronism (screening positive if PAC/PRA ratio >20 to 40 and PAC >5 to 10 ng/dL).

- Positive screening of primary hyperaldosteronism should be confirmed with one of the following tests: IV saline suppression, oral salt loading, fludrocortisone (Florinef)[1] suppression, or captopril (Capoten)[1] challenge test (may skip if spontaneous hypokalemia, renin below the detection limit, and PAC >20 ng/dL).

- Once primary hyperaldosteronism is biochemically confirmed, computed tomography (CT) of the adrenal glands is recommended to exclude adrenocortical carcinoma and help subtype primary hyperaldosteronism.

- If surgical treatment is considered, adrenal vein sampling is indicated to differentiate unilateral versus bilateral lesions (may skip if the patient is <35 years with spontaneous hypokalemia, PAC >30 ng/dL, and unilateral adenoma). A cortisol-corrected aldosterone ratio from the high to the low side greater than 4:1 with cosyntropin (Cortrosyn) stimulation confirms unilateral aldosterone excess.

[1]Not FDA approved for this indication.
[7]Available as a dietary supplement.

CURRENT THERAPY

- Laparoscopic adrenalectomy is recommended for unilateral disease. Otherwise, medical treatment with a mineralocorticoid receptor antagonist (MRA; spironolactone [Aldactone] as the primary agent and eplerenone [Inspra] as an alternative) is recommended.

- Spironolactone: 12.5 to 25 mg/day titrated to a maximum dose of 400 mg/day to achieve normal blood pressure and normokalemia. Side effects include increased serum creatinine, hyperkalemia, gynecomastia, and menstrual irregularities.

- Eplerenone: 25 mg once or twice daily titrated to a maximum dose of 100 mg/day to achieve normal blood pressure and normokalemia. Side effects include increased creatinine, hyperkalemia, hypertriglyceridemia, increased liver enzymes, headache, and fatigue.

- Amiloride (Midamor)[1] or triamterene (Dyrenium)[1] (epithelial sodium channel antagonists) can be used in those who cannot tolerate MRAs or are still hypertensive/hypokalemic while on MRAs. Other antihypertensive agents are also added if necessary to control hypertension.

[1]Not FDA approved for this indication.

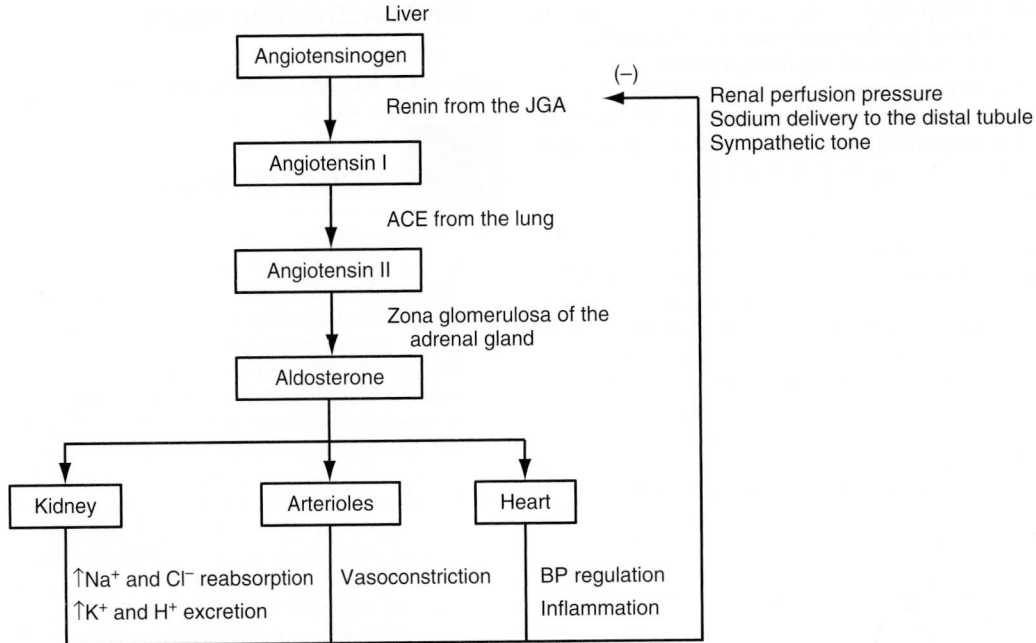

Figure 1 The renin-angiotensin-aldosterone system (RAAS). *ACE*, Angiotensin-converting enzyme; *BP*, blood pressure; *JGA*, juxtaglomerular apparatus.

Introduction

Hyperaldosteronism is a state of excessive aldosterone secretion. Primary hyperaldosteronism occurs due to autonomous hypersecretion of aldosterone relative to suppressed plasma renin, whereas secondary hyperaldosteronism occurs due to activation of the renin-angiotensin-aldosterone system (RAAS). Primary hyperaldosteronism is the most common cause of secondary hypertension, and recent reports suggest that 5% to 20% of hypertensive patients have primary hyperaldosteronism (as opposed to less than 1%, as previously reported). Secondary hyperaldosteronism includes two different categories; one is compensatory activation of the RAAS due to decreased effective circulating volume, as in congestive heart failure and liver cirrhosis; the other is overactivity of the RAAS accompanied by hypertension, as in renovascular hypertension. There are also several conditions that mimic aldosterone excess through various mechanisms that present with hypertension and other metabolic perturbations. Except for the compensatory activation of the RAAS, these conditions cause secondary hypertension with or without other metabolic consequences, such as hypokalemia and metabolic alkalosis, which bring them to medical attention. This chapter covers the current approaches to hyperaldosteronism for patients suspected of having hypertension secondary to excess aldosterone production.

Pathophysiology

Aldosterone is a steroid hormone produced by the zona glomerulosa in the adrenal gland and contributes to volume and potassium homeostasis via its action primarily on the principal cells in the collecting tubule of the kidney. The main stimuli of aldosterone secretion are angiotensin II and hyperkalemia, which increase synthesis and activity of aldosterone synthase mediated by calcium signaling. Angiotensin II releases calcium from the endoplasmic reticulum, whereas both angiotensin II and hyperkalemia depolarize membrane potential and open voltage gated calcium channels. Therefore changes in genes regulating ionic homeostasis and membrane potential can affect aldosterone secretion. Aldosterone and angiotensin II are part of the RAAS; plasma renin from the juxtaglomerular apparatus converts angiotensinogen to angiotensin I, and angiotensin-converting enzyme (ACE) converts angiotensin I to angiotensin II. Subsequently, angiotensin II stimulates secretion of aldosterone. Renin secretion is controlled by renal artery pressure, sodium delivery to the distal nephron, and sympathetic activation (via β1). Increased effective arterial circulating

volume from the action of aldosterone decreases renin secretion by negative feedback (Figure 1). Other minor factors involved in aldosterone secretion are adrenocorticotropic hormone and hyponatremia (which increase aldosterone secretion) and atrial natriuretic peptide (which decreases aldosterone secretion).

Aldosterone binds to the nuclear mineralocorticoid receptors. Activation of the mineralocorticoid receptors upregulates the basolateral Na$^+$/K$^+$ pumps and the epithelial sodium channels (ENaC), leading to increased reabsorption of Na$^+$ and Cl$^-$ and secretion of K$^+$ and H$^+$. The mineralocorticoid receptors can also be activated by other hormones with mineralocorticoid activity. Cortisol is able to bind to the mineralocorticoid receptors with similar affinity as aldosterone but normally is converted to inactive cortisone by 11β hydroxysteroid dehydrogenase 2 (11β HSD2). Mutations/inhibition of 11β HSD2 or very high cortisol levels above the capacity of 11β HSD2, as in Cushing syndrome (particularly ectopic Cushing syndrome), and glucocorticoid resistance can cause activation of the mineralocorticoid receptors. Aldosterone precursors such as deoxycorticosterone have a weak mineralocorticoid effect but can cause features of hyperaldosteronism when they are present at very high levels as in some forms of congenital adrenal hyperplasias (11β hydroxylase deficiency or 17α hydroxylase deficiency) or deoxycorticosteroid-secreting tumors. In addition, activating mutations of the ENaCs also cause increased sodium absorption and hypertension mimicking hyperaldosteronism (Liddle syndrome).

Clinical Manifestations

Primary hyperaldosteronism usually presents with normokalemic hypertension. Hypokalemia is present only in 9% to 37% of cases and may indicate more severe cases. Patients with primary hyperaldosteronism usually do not develop severe volume overload or edema because of aldosterone escape possibly related to atrial natriuretic peptide, pressure natriuresis, or decreased sodium absorption at other nephron segments. Metabolic alkalosis, mild hypernatremia (due to reset osmostat from volume expansion), and hypomagnesemia may be observed. Glomerular filtration rate and urinary albumin excretion can be elevated independent of systemic hypertension. Target organ (heart and kidney) damage and cardiovascular-related morbidity and mortality are higher in primary hyperaldosteronism than in essential hypertension with similar degrees of blood pressure (BP) elevation. Secondary hyperaldosteronism (when it is not from hypovolemia) and other conditions mimicking hyperaldosteronism can present with similar features as primary hyperaldosteronism plus specific manifestations for each disease entity. Depending on the mechanism of disease, more severe volume overload and pulmonary edema may be found (e.g., renovascular hypertension) because aldosterone escape may not work.

BOX 1   Groups Indicated for Case Detection With Relatively High Prevalence of Primary Hyperaldosteronism

- Sustained blood pressure >150/100 mm Hg on three different occasions
- Drug-resistant hypertension (>140/90 mm Hg despite three medications including a diuretic)
- Hypertension and hypokalemia (spontaneous or diuretic-induced)
- Hypertension and family history of early-onset hypertension or cerebrovascular accident at a young age (<40 years)
- Hypertension with adrenal incidentaloma
- Hypertensive first-degree relatives of primary hyperaldosteronism patients
- Hypertension with obstructive sleep apnea

Evaluation
Screening
Hyperaldosteronism may be suspected based on severe (BP >150/100 on three separate occasions) or resistant hypertension (uncontrolled BP despite use of three conventional antihypertensive agents including a diuretic, or well-controlled BP in the presence of four or more antihypertensive agents), early-onset hypertension without known risk factors, and hypertension with other features such as family history of hyperaldosteronism, early-onset hypertension, cerebrovascular accident at a young age, hypokalemia, adrenal mass, and obstructive sleep apnea. Currently there is no evidence-guided screening strategy. Some experts believe that routine screening for primary hyperaldosteronism is warranted in newly diagnosed hypertension considering its high prevalence, whereas others recommend that targeted screening is more appropriate, such as the Endocrine Society guidelines for primary hyperaldosteronism in 2016 (Box 1).

When a decision is made to screen for excessive mineralocorticoid effect, one should first examine the plasma renin and aldosterone levels; that is, plasma renin activity (PRA, ng/mL/h) and plasma aldosterone concentration (PAC, ng/dL). It is important to note that several factors can affect PRA and PAC, such as age, medications, time of day, diet (salt intake), posture, method of blood collection, level of potassium, and level of creatinine (Table 1). Diuretics (both potassium sparing and wasting) and

---

TABLE 1   Medical Factors That May Affect Aldosterone and Renin Measurement

	EFFECT ON ALDOSTERONE	EFFECT ON RENIN	EFFECT ON ALDOSTERONE–RENIN RATIO
Medications			
β-Blocker	↓	↓↓	↑
Central α₂ agonists (clonidine [Catapres], α-methyldopa [Aldomet])	↓	↓↓	↑
NSAIDs	↓	↓↓	↑
K⁺ wasting diuretics	→↑	↑↑	↓
K⁺ sparing diuretics	↑	↑↑	↓
ACE inhibitors	↓	↑↑	↓
Angiotensin II receptor blockers	↓	↑↑	↓
Dihydropyridine Ca²⁺ blockers	→↓	↑	↓
Renin inhibitors	↓	↓ plasma renin activity	↑
		↑ direct renin concentration	↓
Potassium Status			
Hypokalemia	↓	→↑	↓
Potassium loading	↑	→↓	↑
Dietary Sodium			
Sodium restricted	↑	↑↑	↓
Sodium loaded	↓	↓↓	↑
Others			
Advanced age	↓	↓↓	↑
Renal impairment	→	↓	↑
Oral contraceptives*	↑	↑ plasma renin activity	→
		↓ direct renin concentration	↑
Pregnancy	↑	↑↑	↓
Renovascular hypertension	↑	↑↑	↓
Malignant hypertension	↑	↑↑	↓

NSAIDs, Nonsteroidal antiinflammatory drugs.
*Premenopausal women have higher aldosterone level during the luteal phase and lower renin level throughout the cycle than men. False positive ARR during the luteal phase was reported when direct renin concentration was used.

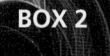

BOX 2 — Approach to Measure Plasma Renin Activity and Plasma Aldosterone Concentration

- Correct hypokalemia to 4 mmol/L.
- Liberalize sodium intake.
- Withdraw the following agents that markedly affect PRA and PAC for at least 4 weeks: spironolactone (Aldactone), eplerenone (Inspra), amiloride (Midamor), triamterene (Dyrenium), potassium-wasting diuretic, and products from licorice.[7]
- If not diagnostic and hypertension can be controlled with relatively noninterfering medications, withdraw the following agents for at least 2 weeks: β-blockers, central α_2 agonists (clonidine [Catapres], methyldopa [Aldomet]), NSAIDs, ACEIs/ARBs, renin inhibitors, and dihydropyridine calcium channel antagonists.
- If necessary, start other antihypertensive agents that have fewer effects on ARR: slow-release verapamil (Calan-SR), hydralazine (Apresoline) (with verapamil to prevent reflex tachycardia), prazosin (Minipress), doxazosin (Cardura), and terazosin (Hytrin).
- Obtain blood for PRA and PAC mid-morning after the patient has been up for at least 2 h and seated for 5–15 min.
- Establish use of estrogen products and menstrual cycles. Premenopausal females have higher ARR than men, especially during the luteal phase. False-positive ARR was reported during the luteal phase and from the use of estrogen products when direct renin concentration was used.

[7]Available as dietary supplement.

ARB, Angiotensin receptor blockers; *ARR*, aldosterone renin ratio; *NSAIDs*, nonsteroidal antiinflammatory drugs; *PAC*, plasma aldosterone concentration; *PRA*, plasma renin activity.

BOX 3 — Differential Diagnoses According to Plasma Renin Activity and Plasma Aldosterone Concentration

Causes of Primary Hyperaldosteronism: ↓ PRA and ↑ PAC (>5–10 ng/dL); ARR >20–40
- Most Common
  - Aldosterone-producing adenoma
  - Bilateral adrenal hyperplasia or idiopathic hyperaldosteronism
- Less common
  - Unilateral hyperplasia or primary adrenal hyperplasia
  - Familial hyperaldosteronism type 1 or glucocorticoid remediable aldosteronism
  - Familial hyperaldosteronism type 2
  - Aldosterone-producing adrenocortical carcinoma
  - Ectopic aldosterone-secreting tumor (ovary, kidney)
  - Multiple endocrine neoplasia type 1

Causes of Secondary Hyperaldosteronism: ↑ PRA and ↑ PAC; ARR ≈ 10
- Renovascular hypertension
- Diuretic use
- Renin-secreting tumor
- Malignant hypertension
- Coarctation of the aorta

Causes of Conditions That Mimic Mineralocorticoid Excess: ↓ PRA and ↓ PAC
- Congenital adrenal hyperplasia
- Exogenous mineralocorticoid
- Deoxycorticosterone-producing tumor
- Cushing syndrome
- 11β HSD2 deficiency
- Altered aldosterone metabolism
- Liddle syndrome
- Glucocorticoid resistance

ARR, Aldosterone-renin ratio; *PAC*, plasma aldosterone concentration; *PRA*, plasma renin activity.

mineralocorticoid antagonists can have a significant effect on PRA and PAC. Angiotensin-converting enzyme inhibitors/angiotensin receptor blockers (ACEI/ARB) and dihydropyridine calcium channel blockers can affect PRA and PAC modestly. Ideally, all medications and other factors that may affect PRA and PAC should be removed; unfortunately, it is not always practical and safe to do this because of the possibility of uncontrolled hypertension. If necessary, antihypertensive agents that affect PRA and PAC only minimally such as slow-release verapamil (Calan SR), hydralazine (Apresoline), prazosin (Minipress), doxazosin (Cardura), or terazosin (Hytrin) can be used. The Endocrine Society 2016 guidelines recommend certain caveats that optimize the chance for obtaining more easily interpretable PRA and PAC results (Box 2).

Patterns of PRA and PAC help differentiate among primary hyperaldosteronism, secondary hyperaldosteronism, and conditions mimicking hyperaldosteronism. Differential diagnoses according to different patterns of PRA and PAC are listed in Box 3. If both PRA and PAC are high, further investigation for causes of secondary hyperaldosteronism should follow. If both PRA and PAC are suppressed, further investigation for conditions that mimic hyperaldosteronism is indicated. Suppressed PRA and elevated PAC suggest primary hyperaldosteronism, and aldosterone renin ratio (ARR) should be calculated; ARR above 20 to 40 is considered screening positive for primary hyperaldosteronism. PAC greater than 15 ng/dL was recommended by some investigators to avoid false-positive ARR from very low renin level, but in many cases PAC can be less than 15 ng/dL, though this occurs more commonly in bilateral adrenal hyperplasia (BAH) than in aldosterone-producing adenoma. PAC should at least be above the level considered positive for confirmatory tests (5 to 10 ng/dL). Confirmatory tests should follow to avoid false positives. Diagnostic flow and subsequent management of hyperaldosteronism are summarized in Figure 2. Of note, there is no consensus on cutoff values for PRA, PAC, or ARR. In addition, PRA and PAC

are often obtained in a less-than-optimal condition. Therefore it is important to understand how PRA and PAC can be affected by various factors. For example, if ARR is positive while on medications that decrease PAC or increase PRA (thus decreasing ARR), ARR off this medication will be clearly positive. Screening tests should be repeated if results are inconclusive or if PA is strongly suspected but the initial screening tests are negative.

Confirmatory Tests of Primary Hyperaldosteronism
The positive screening test should be followed by one or more confirmatory tests to avoid false positives. The confirmatory tests are designed to physiologically suppress aldosterone levels that would normally occur in the absence of primary hyperaldosteronism. However, some experts believe that some aldosterone-producing lesions are not completely independent of the RAAS, and confirmatory suppression tests can give false-negative results. Other experts think that confirmatory tests are not necessary for those with obvious clinical/biochemical features. Those with spontaneous hypokalemia, renin level below the detection level plus PAC greater than 20 ng/dL may not need further confirmatory tests. Furthermore, there is no gold-standard confirmatory. Therefore factors such as cost, accessibility, feasibility, patient compliance, local expertise, and accuracy of assay should be taken into consideration in selecting confirmatory tests. The Endocrine Society guidelines in 2016 state that any of the following four confirmatory tests can be used: oral salt loading test, saline suppression test, fludrocortisone (Florinef)[1] suppression test, and captopril (Capoten)[1] challenge test (Table 2).

[1]Not FDA approved for this indication.

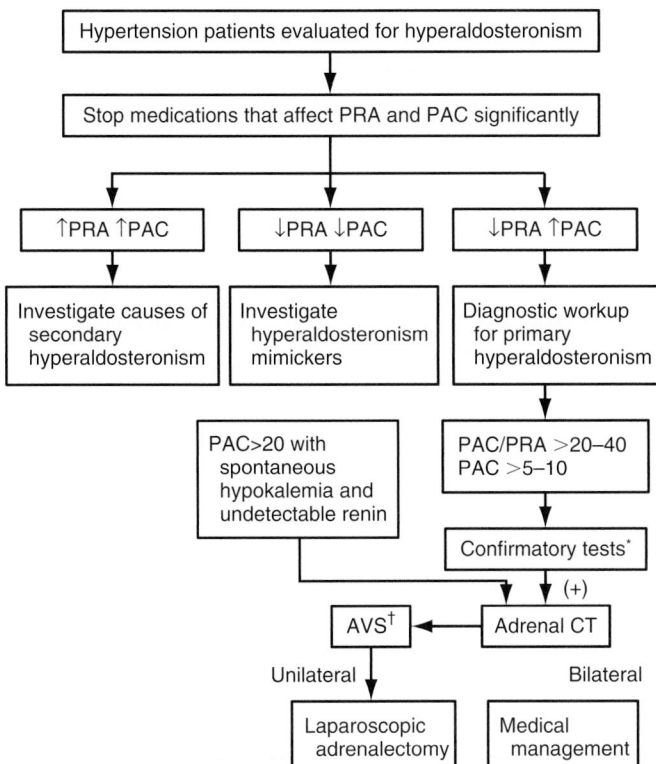

Figure 2 Evaluation of hyperaldosteronism. *AVS,* Adrenal vein sampling; *CT,* computed tomography; *PAC,* plasma aldosterone concentration in ng/dL; *PRA,* plasma renin activity in ng/mL/h. *May skip if spontaneous hypokalemia, renin level below the detection limit, and PAC >20 ng/dL. †If surgical treatment is pursued. May skip if <35 years old, spontaneous hypokalemia, PAC >30 ng/dL, and unilateral adenoma.

Figure 2 box contents:
- Hypertension patients evaluated for hyperaldosteronism
- Stop medications that affect PRA and PAC significantly
- ↑PRA ↑PAC → Investigate causes of secondary hyperaldosteronism
- ↓PRA ↓PAC → Investigate hyperaldosteronism mimickers
- ↓PRA ↑PAC → Diagnostic workup for primary hyperaldosteronism
- PAC>20 with spontaneous hypokalemia and undetectable renin
- PAC/PRA >20–40 PAC >5–10 → Confirmatory tests* → (+) → Adrenal CT → AVS†
- AVS† → Unilateral → Laparoscopic adrenalectomy; Bilateral → Medical management

Subtype Classification of Primary Hyperaldosteronism

Once primary hyperaldosteronism is biochemically confirmed, subtype classification follows to guide treatment. Lateralization of the source of excessive aldosterone production is crucial as the next step, as unilateral lesions such as aldosterone-producing adenomas (APAs) can be treated surgically; in contrast, bilateral lesions such as BAHs are treated medically. Aldosterone-producing carcinoma is rare but should be ruled out. In this regard, CT of the adrenal glands should be done first to rule out aldosterone-producing carcinoma and obtain anatomic information. However, imaging studies are usually not reliable enough to lateralize lesions. If surgical treatment is considered, adrenal vein sampling (AVS) should be performed. Most cases of primary hyperaldosteronism are sporadic; about 5% are familial, mostly via autosomal dominant inheritance. Young patients (<20 years of age) and those with family history of primary hyperaldosteronism or strokes at young age (less than 40 years) should have genetic testing for glucocorticoid remediable aldosteronism (GRA) or familial hyperaldosteronism type 1 (FH-1), which is caused by the hybrid gene of 11β hydroxylase and aldosterone synthase (increased aldosterone synthesis by adrenocorticotropic hormone). In very young patients, *KCNJ5* germline mutations, causing familial hyperaldosteronism type III, should be tested. Familial hyperaldosteronism type II is clinically indistinguishable from nonfamilial hyperaldosteronism, and can be caused by gain-of-function mutations in the *CLCN2* (chloride voltage-gated channel 2) gene. Type IV familial hyperaldosteronism generally involves patients with early onset hypertension and primary hyperaldosteronism before the age of 10. Germline mutations in the *CACNA1H* (calcium voltage-gated channel subunit alpha1H) gene occur in type IV patients who also exhibit mental retardation and developmental disorders, as well as seizures and neurological abnormalities in some patients.

Imaging

CT/MRI scans of the adrenal glands provide one of five conclusions: normal adrenal glands, unilateral macroadenomas (>1 cm), minimal unilateral adrenal limb thickening, unilateral microadenomas (≤1 cm), and bilateral macroadenomas and/or microadenomas. APAs are typically smaller than 2 cm, and BAHs exhibit either normal or nodular changes. Aldosterone-producing adrenal carcinoma are almost always larger than 4 cm in diameter and have imaging characteristics suspicious for malignancy. However, there are limitations; small APAs may be missed, hyperplasia may be misread as adenomas, and nonfunctional tumors are radiologically indistinguishable from APAs. Although several studies suggested imaging criteria for different subtypes, no study has conclusively established specific criteria that differentiate among different subtypes of primary hyperaldosteronism. In fact, CT accurately lateralizes in only about 50% to 70% of cases, and there is no evidence that MRI is superior to CT for subtype classification. Therefore AVS is required to differentiate unilateral from bilateral lesions if surgical resection is being pursued. Patients younger than 35 years with marked hyperaldosteronism with spontaneous hypokalemia and PAC greater than 30 ng/dL and solitary unilateral adenoma may not need AVS, because nonfunctioning tumors are uncommon in this young age group.

Adrenal Vein Sampling

Aldosterone levels are measured from adrenal venous blood samples (Box 4) obtained through adrenal vein cannulation to distinguish between unilateral and bilateral lesions. Unilateral lesions are associated with a marked increase in PAC on the side of the tumor (and suppressed PAC on the other side), whereas bilateral lesions have little difference between the two sides. AVS should be performed only by experienced physicians in part because recognition and successful cannulation of the right adrenal vein especially can be challenging. Complications of AVS include adrenal hemorrhage, adrenal infarction, adrenal vein perforation, and adrenal vein thrombosis, which occur only rarely (<2.5%) in the hands of a physician skilled in the procedure.

The use of cosyntropin (Cortrosyn) stimulation to minimize stress-induced fluctuation in aldosterone level is controversial, and some believe that it has no effect on AVS accuracy. If cosyntropin is not used, then AVS should be done in the morning after overnight recumbency to avoid postural aldosterone changes and reflect circadian aldosterone secretion.

In reality, different centers use different techniques, protocols, and interpretation criteria. The Endocrine Society guidelines in 2016 provide interpretation criteria with and without cosyntropin use. The first step for interpretation is to determine whether the procedure was done correctly. The adrenal vein-to-IVC cortisol ratio should be greater than 5:1 with cosyntropin given and greater than 3:1 without cosyntropin. If the ratio is significantly lower than these values, improper cannulation is implied. Next, divide the PAC values for the right and left adrenal veins by their respective cortisol values to correct the dilutional effect of the inferior phrenic vein flow into the left adrenal vein; this is termed the *cortisol-corrected aldosterone* (A/C). If cosyntropin is used, an A/C ratio of the high to the low side of greater than 4:1 indicates unilateral aldosterone hypersecretion, whereas an A/C ratio of less than 3:1 suggests bilateral aldosterone hypersecretion. These cutoffs were reported to have sensitivity of 95% and specificity of 100% for unilateral lesions. If the A/C ratio is between 3:1 and 4:1, the results of AVS should be interpreted in the context of CT, clinical findings, and other tests. Without cosyntropin, an A/C ratio of the high to the low side of greater than 2 or an A/C ratio of the high side to the periphery greater than 2.5 plus an A/C ratio of the low side to the periphery of less than 1 (suppressed contralateral aldosterone secretion) is consistent with unilateral aldosterone excess.

TABLE 2	Protocols and Interpretation of Recommended Confirmatory Tests		
	PROTOCOL	**INTERPRETATION**	**REMARKS**
Oral sodium loading test	1. Place the patient on a high-sodium diet (> 200 mmol/day) for 3 days. 2. Replace potassium to compensate for the kaliuresis induced by the high-sodium diet. 3. Collect a 24-h urine on the third day for determination of aldosterone, sodium, and creatinine; adequate if the urine sodium >200 mmol/24 h	Confirmed if the 24-h urine aldosterone is > 12 mcg (33.3 nmol) to 14 mcg (38.8 nmol). Ruled out if the 24-h urine aldosterone is <10 mcg (27.7 nmol). The test is equivocal if the value falls in between	Do not perform this test in patients with severe uncontrolled hypertension, renal failure, cardiac failure/arrhythmias, or severe hypokalemia
IV saline infusion test*	1. Place the patient supine 1 h before drawing blood for morning baseline fasting levels of renin, aldosterone, cortisol, and potassium 2. Infuse 2 L of 0.9% NaCl over 4 h, keeping the patient supine. Monitor blood pressure and heart rate 3. After 4 h, draw blood for measurement of renin, aldosterone, cortisol, and potassium	Confirmed if the PAC is >10 ng/dL (277 pmol/L). Ruled out if the PAC is <5 ng/dL (139 pmol/L). If the PAC falls between these values, the test is equivocal	Do not perform this test in patients with severe uncontrolled hypertension, renal failure, cardiac failure/arrhythmias, or severe hypokalemia
Fludrocortisone[1] suppression test	1. Give 0.1 mg fludrocortisone every 6 h for 4 days, with the potassium level checked every 6 h to be sure that it is greater than 4 mmol/L 2. Encourage a liberal sodium diet to keep urinary sodium excretion greater than 3 mmol/kg/day 3. On day 4, draw blood for an upright 7 a.m. plasma cortisol level and 10 a.m. plasma aldosterone, renin, and cortisol levels	Confirmed if the 10 a.m. PAC is >6 ng/dL, as long as PRA is <1 ng/mL/h and the plasma cortisol at 10 a.m. is less than at 7 a.m. (to exclude the ACTH effect)	The test may require hospitalization. Risks include severe hypokalemia, QT changes, worsening of left ventricular function, hypertension, and frequent phlebotomy
Captopril[1] challenge test	1. Give 25–50 mg captopril after the patient has been sitting or standing for 1 h. The patient remains seated throughout the test. 2. Draw blood for measurement of plasma renin, aldosterone, and cortisol at time 0, at 1 h, and at 2 h	Normally, captopril suppresses PAC by more than 30% from baseline. Confirmed if there is no suppression of PAC and PRA remains suppressed. The false-negative rate for this test is high because suppression occurs in more than 30% of cases. A slight decrease in aldosterone can suggest bilateral adrenal hyperplasia	

*The patient may be seated for 30 minutes before and during the infusion to improve sensitivity and PAC greater than 6 ng/dL (170 pmol/L) confirms primary hyperaldosteronism.

[1]Not FDA approved for this indication.

ACTH, Adrenocorticotropic hormone; *PAC,* plasma aldosterone concentration; *PRA,* plasma renin activity.

BOX 4	Adrenal Vein Sampling

- After both adrenal veins have been cannulated, draw baseline samples for PRA, PAC, ACTH, and cortisol from the peripheral such as cubital or iliac, right adrenal vein, and left adrenal vein.
- Inject 250 mcg of cosyntropin (Cortrosyn) after cannulation, or infuse 50 mcg cosyntropin per hour beginning 30 min before adrenal vein cannulation. This reduces stress-related fluctuations in aldosterone and cortisol values and augments the biochemical gradients. (This step is controversial.)
- Draw blood for aldosterone and cortisol levels at 5, 15, and 30 min from the peripheral site and from each adrenal vein.

ACTH, Adrenocorticotropic hormone; *PAC,* plasma aldosterone concentration; *PRA,* plasma renin activity.

Ancillary Tests

Clinical findings and other ancillary tests may help differentiate unilateral APAs from BAHs. BAHs will respond with increase in plasma aldosterone to postural stimulation, whereas APAs will not. Plasma 18-hydroxycorticosterone level tends to be higher in APAs as compared with BAHs. Iodocholesterol scintigraphy may be able to show functional correlation of anatomic abnormalities (but is not available at most centers). APA-specific tracers such as (11)C-Metomidate for positron emission tomography may be useful. Interpretation criteria of these tests are listed in Table 3. Patients with APAs tend to be younger (<40 years), predominantly female, very hypertensive with marked hypokalemia (<3 mmol/L), and tend to have a very high PAC (>25 mg/dL) compared with those with BAHs.

Treatment

Treatment of secondary hyperaldosteronism and conditions mimicking hyperaldosteronism depends on their etiology. Treatment of primary hyperaldosteronism is discussed here. The goals of treatment of primary hyperaldosteronism are (1) normalization of the serum potassium in hypokalemic patients, (2) normalization of the BP, and (3) reversal of the effects of hyperaldosteronism on the cardiovascular system. When a small group of patients were followed after treatment with adrenalectomy or mineralocorticoid receptor antagonists (MRAs), left ventricular mass was reduced (faster with adrenalectomy than MRAs), increase in carotid intima-media thickness and arterial stiffness was reversed, glomerular filtration rate and urinary albumin secretion decreased and became similar to that in essential hypertension, and excessive cardiovascular risk compared to essential hypertension

TABLE 3	Interpretation of Dynamic Testing
TEST	**FINDINGS**
Screening Test	
PAC/PRA ratio	Positive if >20–40 with PAC >5–10 ng/dL
Confirmatory Tests	
Oral sodium loading test	Positive if 24-h urine aldosterone excretion is >12–14 mcg
Saline infusion test	Positive if PAC after infusion is >10 ng/dL
Fludrocortisone[1] suppression test	Positive if upright PAC is >6 ng/dL on day 4 at 10 a.m.
Captopril[1] challenge test	Positive if PAC does not decrease by 30% and PRA remains suppressed
AVS	
With cosyntropin stimulation	A/C ratio (the high to the low side) >4:1 → unilateral aldosterone excess A/C ratio 3:1–4:1 → unclear A/C ratio <3:1 → bilateral aldosterone excess
Without cosyntropin stimulation	A/C ratio from the high to the low side >2:1 → unilateral aldosterone excess A/C ratio from the high side to the periphery >2.5 and A/C ratio from the contralateral side to the periphery <1 → unilateral aldosterone excess
If Equivocal AVS	
Postural stimulation test	PAC falls or fails to rise by 30%: consistent with APAs PAC increases by at least 33%: consistent with BAHs
Recumbent 18-hydroxycorticosterone	>100 ng/dL is consistent with APAs
NP-59 iodocholesterol scintigraphy	Unilateral early uptake (<5 days): consistent with unilateral aldosterone excess Bilateral early uptake (<5 days): consistent with bilateral aldosterone excess Negative scan does not rule out either etiology
(11)C-Metomidate positron emission tomography	Preliminary data showed (11)C-Metomidate uptake in APA

[1]Not FDA approved for this indication.

A/C ratio, Cortisol-corrected aldosterone ratio; *APA*, aldosterone-producing adenomas; *AVS*, adrenal vein sampling; *BAH*, bilateral adrenal hyperplasia; *PAC*, plasma aldosterone concentration; *PRA*, plasma renin activity.

disappeared. Cardiovascular complications were rather related to age, duration of hypertension, and smoking. In addition, there was an improvement in the quality of life at 3 months, which was sustained at 6 months. Therefore timely diagnosis and treatment is essential. For unilateral lesions, surgical resection of the affected adrenal gland is recommended mainly to obviate the need for prolonged medical treatment and side effects. For bilateral lesions, medical treatment is recommended because surgical risk outweighs benefits. BP control per se does not reduce risk of cardiovascular complications unless renin activity is restored to normal (>1 ng/mL/h), which

can be accomplished by salt restriction or increasing the dose of the MRA. MRAs are a key component of medical treatment and used as a preoperative measure or maintenance treatment (GRA should be treated with the lowest dose of glucocorticoid that can normalize BP and potassium levels rather than MRAs). A low-sodium diet (sodium <100 mEq/day = 2.3 g/day or salt 6 g/day) is also important, because left ventricular hypertrophy is associated with urine sodium excretion in primary hyperaldosteronism but not in essential hypertension. Other lifestyle changes include aerobic exercise, smoking cessation, and weight loss.

Unilateral Hypersecretion

Adrenalectomy, usually laparoscopic, is recommended. After adrenalectomy, BP improves in all patients (maximal improvement in 1 to 6 months, sometime continues to fall up to 1 year), but 30% to 60% of patients have persistent hypertension. BP and potassium level should be controlled before surgery. MRAs such as spironolactone (Aldactone) and eplerenone (Inspra)[1] can be used to control BP in patients awaiting adrenalectomy and also to prevent postoperative hypoaldosteronism. Postoperatively, normal saline is given to maintain volume status, MRAs and potassium supplements are discontinued, and antihypertensive medications may be reduced. To confirm biochemical cure, PAC and PRA should be checked shortly after the operation though renin levels might not change immediately. Risk factors for persistent hypertension after adrenalectomy include older age, duration of hypertension (>5 years), use of two or more antihypertensive agents preoperatively, BP higher than 165/100 mm Hg, low ARR preoperatively, low urine aldosterone, poor response to spironolactone preoperatively, family history of more than one first-degree relative with hypertension, and elevated serum creatinine level.

Bilateral Hypersecretion

MRAs and/or ENaC antagonists combined with other antihypertensives are used. One study showed that spironolactone had stronger antihypertensive effect than eplerenone, but there is insufficient evidence to choose one medication over another. Subtotal adrenalectomy has been tried, but only a minority of patients have responded with significant BP improvement. Unilateral adrenalectomy, however, may help selected patients by debulking aldosterone-producing tissues.

Spironolactone is the most widely used MRA. It is very effective in decreasing BP. The medication is initiated at 12.5 to 25 mg/day and can be titrated to 400 mg/day, with most patients requiring at least 200 mg/day. Potassium should be maintained at normal levels without use of potassium supplements. Use of spironolactone can be limited by side effects; antiandrogenic effects can cause gynecomastia in men and progesterone effect can cause menstrual irregularities in women. There are drug interactions to consider; spironolactone increases the half-life of digoxin (Lanoxin) and salicylates, and other NSAIDs may decrease the effectiveness of spironolactone. Serum potassium and creatinine should be closely monitored for the first 4 to 6 weeks, in particular for those with renal insufficiency or diabetes. Spironolactone is not recommended if creatinine clearance is less than 30 mL/min.

Eplerenone[1] is a competitive and selective antagonist of the aldosterone receptors. It has a lower binding affinity to androgen and progesterone receptors than spironolactone. This leads to fewer side effects. Eplerenone is 25% to 50% less potent in antagonizing the aldosterone receptors than spironolactone. Eplerenone has a short half-life and should be taken twice daily. Dosing is started at 25 mg twice daily, with a maximum dose of 100 mg/day. Again, serum potassium and creatinine should be closely monitored for the first 4 to 6 weeks in particular for those with renal insufficiency

[1]Not FDA approved for this indication.

or diabetes. Other adverse effects include hypertriglyceridemia, increased liver enzymes, headache, and fatigue. Eplerenone is contraindicated if serum potassium is greater than 5.5 mEq/L at initiation, if creatinine clearance is less than 30 mL/min, or if there is concomitant use of strong CYP3A4 inhibitors such as ketoconazole (Nizoral) and itraconazole (Sporanox).

ENaC antagonists, amiloride (Midamor)[1] and triamterene (Dyrenium)[1], can be used in patients who cannot tolerate MRAs or are still hypertensive/hypokalemic while on MRAs. Amiloride is prescribed at 10 to 20 mg/day in divided doses. Side effects include dizziness, fatigue, and impotence. Triamterene is dosed at 100 to 300 mg/day in divided doses, and its side effects are mainly dizziness and nausea. Addition of thiazide diuretics can help control BP by relieving volume overload. If BP remains uncontrolled, other antihypertensive agents such as ACEIs/ARBs or calcium channel blockers may be used.

References

Born-Frontsberg E, Reincke M, Rump LC, et al: Cardiovascular and cerebrovascular comorbidities of hypokalemic and normokalemic primary aldosteronism: results of the German Conn's registry, *J Clin Endocrinol Metab* 94:1125–1130, 2009.

Boulkroun S: Old and new genes in primary aldosteronism, *Best Pract Res Clin Endocrinol Metab* 34:101375, 2020.

Catena C, Colussi G, Lapenna R, et al: Long-term cardiac effects of adrenalectomy or mineralocorticoid antagonists in patients with primary aldosteronism, *Hypertension* 50:911–918, 2007.

Catena C, Colussi GL, Nadalini E, et al: Cardiovascular outcomes in patients with primary aldosteronism after treatment, *Arch Intern Med* 168:80–85, 2008.

Funder JW: Primary aldosteronism and cardiovascular risk, before and after treatment, *Lancet Diabetes Endocrinol* 6:5–7, 2018.

Funder JW, Carey RM, Mantero F, et al: The management of primary aldosteronism: case detection, diagnosis, and treatment: an endocrine society clinical guideline, *J Clin Endocrinol Metab* 101:1889–1916, 2016.

Gordon RD, Gomez-Sanchez CE, Hamlet SM, et al: Angiotensin-responsive aldosterone-producing adenoma masquerades as idiopathic hyperaldosteronism (IHA: adrenal hyperplasia) or low-renin essential hypertension, *J Hypertens* 5:S103–S106, 1987.

Hundemer GL, Curhan GC, Yozamp N, et al: Cardiometabolic outcomes and mortality in medically treated primary aldosteronism: a restrospective cohort study, *Lancet Diabetes Endocrinol* 6:51–59, 2018.

Kempers MJ, Lenders JW, van Outheusden L, et al: Systematic review: diagnostic procedures to differentiate unilateral from bilateral adrenal abnormality in primary aldosteronism, *Ann Intern Med* 151:329–337, 2009.

Mulatero P, Bertello C, Rossato D, et al: Roles of clinical criteria, computed tomography scan, and adrenal vein sampling in differential diagnosis of primary aldosteronism subtypes, *J Clin Endocrinol Metab* 93:1366–1371, 2008.

Parthasarathy HK, Menard J, White WB, et al: A double-blind, randomized study comparing the antihypertensive effect of eplerenone and spironolactone in patients with hypertension and evidence of primary aldosteronism, *J Hypertens* 29:980, 2011.

Pimenta E, Gordon RD, Ahmed AH, et al: Cardiac dimensions are largely determined by dietary salt in patients with primary aldosteronism: results of a case-control study, *J Clin Endocrinol Metab* 96:2813–2820, 2011.

Reincke M, Fischer E, Gerum S, et al: Observational study mortality in treated primary aldosteronism: the German Conn's registry, *Hypertension* 60:618–624, 2012.

Rossi GP: A comprehensive review of the clinical aspects of primary aldosteronism, *Nat Rev Endocrinol* 7:485–495, 2011.

Rossi GP, Barisa M, Allolio B, et al: The adrenal vein sampling international study (AVIS) for identifying the major subtypes of primary aldosteronism, *J Clin Endocrinol Metab* 97:1606–1614, 2012.

Rossi GP, Bernini G, Caliumi C, et al: A prospective study of the prevalence of primary aldosteronism in 1,125 hypertensive patients, *J Am Coll Cardiol* 48:2293–2300, 2006.

Rossi GP, Seccia TM, Pessina AC: Adrenal gland: a diagnostic algorithm—the holy grail of primary aldosteronism, *Nat Rev Endocrinol* 7:697–699, 2011.

Sawka AM, Young WF, Thompson GB, et al: Primary aldosteronism: factors associated with normalization of blood pressure after surgery, *Ann Intern Med* 135:258–261, 2001.

Sechi LA, Novello M, Lapenna R, et al: Long-term renal outcomes in patients with primary aldosteronism, *JAMA* 295:2638–2645, 2006.

Stowasser M: Update in primary aldosteronism, *J Clin Endocrinol Metab* 100:1–10, 2015.

Sukor N, Gordon RD, Ku YK, et al: Role of unilateral adrenalectomy in bilateral primary aldosteronism: a 22-year single center experience, *J Clin Endocrinol Metab* 94:2437–2445, 2009.

Zennaro MC, Boulkroun S, Fernandes-Rosa F: An update on novel mechanisms of primary aldosteronism, *J Endocrinol* 224:R63–R77, 2015.

HYPERLIPIDEMIA

Method of
Xiaoming Jia, MD; Mandeep Bajaj, MD; and Lawrence Chan, MD

CURRENT DIAGNOSIS

- Hyperlipidemia is diagnosed based on the fasting lipid profile in the context of global cardiovascular risk. The exception is when the triglyceride level is greater than 500 mg/dL because of substantial risk of pancreatitis.
- Secondary causes of hyperlipidemia, such as hypothyroidism, alcoholism, uncontrolled diabetes mellitus, kidney disorders, pregnancy, and medications, should be thoroughly investigated and treated if diagnosed.
- Possibility of familial hyperlipidemia based on the lipid profile, family history, and physical examination should be considered because cardiovascular risk can be underestimated and treatment can be challenging.

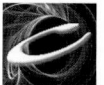

CURRENT THERAPY

- Therapy should be guided by goals of treatment based on estimated cardiovascular risk unless triglyceride level >500 mg/L, in which case lowering triglycerides to prevent acute pancreatitis is a priority.
- Low-density lipoprotein (LDL) cholesterol is a primary goal followed by non-high-density lipoprotein (HDL) cholesterol as a secondary goal. Triglycerides have also emerged as a target to further reduce residual cardiovascular risk in select patients with high cardiovascular risk.
- Therapeutic lifestyle changes should be initiated in everyone with lipid parameters above their target. Therapeutic lifestyle changes are also recommended for those with very high, high, or moderately high cardiovascular risk.
- Pharmacologic agents should be added if therapeutic lifestyle changes are not successful. Pharmacologic agents can be considered from the beginning for those with very high, high, or moderately high cardiovascular risk.
- Statin therapy is preferred if tolerated, and the intensity of therapy to use should be dictated by the degree of cardiovascular risk.
- Statins are the treatment of choice for their proven effects on cardiovascular outcomes. Other agents can be added based on response to statins and other targets such as high triglycerides.
- All other cardiovascular risk factors should be treated aggressively at the same time.

Hyperlipidemia is a condition of elevated serum lipids and lipoproteins. Hyperlipidemia is associated with an increased risk of atherosclerotic cardiovascular disease (ASCVD) and, if the triglyceride level is greater than 500 mg/dL, pancreatitis. Unless the triglyceride level is greater than 500 mg/dL, the primary goal of management of hyperlipidemia is to decrease the risk of ASCVD. ASCVD as defined by the *2018 Multisociety Guideline on the Management of Blood Cholesterol* encompasses acute coronary syndrome, history of myocardial infarction, stable or unstable angina or coronary or other arterial revascularization, stroke, transient ischemic attack, or peripheral arterial disease including aortic aneurysm, all of atherosclerotic origin. In this regard, appropriate treatment of hyperlipidemia is essential in patients with established cardiovascular disease (secondary prevention), whereas detection and treatment of hyperlipidemia are guided by the risk of ASCVD in patients without known clinical ASCVD (primary prevention).

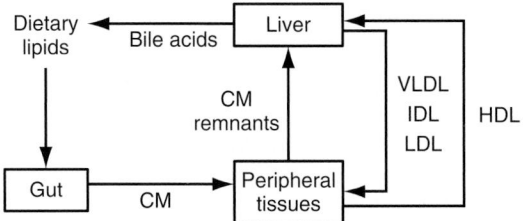

Figure 1 Overview of exogenous and endogenous pathways of lipid metabolism. *CM,* chylomicrons; *HDL,* high-density lipoproteins; *IDL,* intermediate-density lipoproteins; *LDL,* low-density lipoproteins; *VLDL,* very-low-density lipoproteins.

The prevalence of hyperlipidemia varies with the definition of hyperlipidemia and the population studied. The percentage of US adults with a total cholesterol level of 240 mg/dL or higher declined from 19% to 14% in men and from 21% to 15% in women from 1988 to 2008. This may be in part due to increased use of lipid-lowering medications, from 3.4% to 15.5%. However, major risk factors for cardiovascular disease actually have become more common: the prevalence of obesity (BMI ≥ 30 kg/m²) increased from 19.9% to 31.6% in men and from 25.2% to 34.1% in women, and the prevalence of diabetes increased from 5.5% to 11.1% in men and from 4.6% to 6.3% in women over this period. Therefore optimal treatment of hyperlipidemia to reduce cardiovascular risk is of paramount importance.

Various societies and professional organizations have published clinical guidelines for hyperlipidemia. The approach used in this chapter is mostly based on the *2013 ACC/AHA Guideline on the Treatment of Blood Cholesterol to Reduce Atherosclerotic Cardiovascular Risk in Adults: A Report of the American College of Cardiology/American Heart Association Task Force on Practice Guidelines* and the *2018 Multisociety Guideline on the Management of Blood Cholesterol.* The 2013 American College of Cardiology/American Heart Association guideline represents a substantial departure from previous guidelines in that it emphasizes the use of statins of appropriate strength according to the estimated cardiovascular risk without specific low-density lipoprotein (LDL) cholesterol targets. The 2016 European Society of Cardiology and European Atherosclerosis Society (ESC/EAS) Guidelines for the Management of Dyslipidaemias will also be integrated in the sections on Evaluation and Treatment.

Pathophysiology

Lipids have two main points of entry into the circulation: the gut (exogenous pathway) and the liver (endogenous pathway). The exogenous and endogenous pathways are interconnected by intermediate pathways (reverse cholesterol transport pathway and others). These pathways are outlined in Figure 1.

Exogenous Pathway

Lipids in food are emulsified by bile acids and then hydrolyzed into fatty acids and cholesterol by pancreatic lipases in the intestinal lumen. Inside the intestinal cells, fatty acids and cholesterol are re-esterified and then packaged with apolipoprotein (Apo) B48 into chylomicrons. Chylomicrons are secreted into the intestinal lymph and delivered to the systemic circulation. At peripheral tissues, triglycerides are hydrolyzed by lipoprotein lipase with Apo CII acting as a cofactor. Released free fatty acids are then taken up for further metabolism or storage. Chylomicron remnants are taken up by the liver via the chylomicron remnant receptors.

Endogenous Pathway

The endogenous pathway begins in the liver with the synthesis of triglyceride-rich very-low-density lipoproteins (VLDLs). Microsomal triglyceride transfer protein facilitates the transfer of lipids onto Apo B100 and stabilizes the protein for secretion as VLDLs. VLDLs, as chylomicrons, undergo lipolysis by lipoprotein lipase, releasing free fatty acids, generating smaller particles called intermediate-density lipoproteins (IDLs, also known as

TABLE 1	Classification of LDL, Total, and HDL Cholesterol and Triglycerides (mg/dL)
LDL Cholesterol (mg/dL)	
<100	Optimal
100–129	Near optimal/above optimal
130–159	Borderline high
160–189	High
≥190	Very high
Total Cholesterol (mg/dL)	
<200	Desirable
200–239	Borderline high
≥240	High
HDL Cholesterol (mg/dL)	
<40	Low
≥60	High
Triglycerides (mg/dL)	
<150	Normal
150–199	Borderline high
200–499	High
≥500	Very high

Based on the NCEP/ATPIII.
HDL, high-density lipoprotein; *LDL,* low-density lipoprotein; *NCEP/ATP III,* National Cholesterol Education Program Adult Treatment Panel III guidelines.

VLDL remnants). IDLs are either removed by the liver or further processed into cholesterol-rich LDLs. LDLs are taken up into the liver or other cells via LDL receptors, a process regulated by cellular cholesterol requirement. Macrophages in the arterial wall can also take up LDLs via the scavenger receptors and become foam cells. Foamy macrophages play a key role in the development of atherosclerosis. Recent research has further suggested that the precursors of macrophages, monocytes, can also uptake lipoprotein particles in circulation and transform into foamy monocytes, which may also play a role in atherogenesis.

Reverse Cholesterol Transport

High-density lipoproteins (HDLs) are the major lipoproteins involved in the transport of cholesterol from peripheral tissues back to the liver. HDLs are synthesized by both the hepatocytes and the enterocytes in the form of small discoidal particles containing Apo AI and phospholipids. HDLs acquire additional lipids and apolipoproteins from triglyceride-depleted chylomicrons and VLDL remnants. HDLs remove free cholesterol from tissues with the help of Apo AI and esterify it with lecithin cholesterol acyltransferase. Cholesteryl esters are then transferred to Apo B 100-containing lipoproteins (VLDLs, IDLs, and LDLs) by cholesteryl ester transfer protein (CETP). HDLs can also be taken up directly by the liver class B type I scavenger receptors (SR-BI).

Plasma Lipids and Atherosclerosis

Multiple studies have shown that total cholesterol and LDL cholesterol levels contribute to cardiovascular disease risk and that lowering of total cholesterol and LDL cholesterol levels reduces the risk. Non-HDL cholesterol (i.e., total cholesterol – HDL cholesterol = VLDL + IDL + LDL cholesterol) reflects total atherogenic lipoprotein burden and may be a better risk indicator than LDL cholesterol, especially in people with combined hyperlipidemia, diabetes, metabolic syndrome, and chronic kidney disease. Table 1 shows the classification of lipid profile.

Recent Mendelian randomization studies have suggested that triglyceride-rich lipoproteins (TRLs), including chylomicrons, VLDLs, and their remnants, also have a causal relationship with ASCVD. Therefore not only does hypertriglyceridemia represent an independent cardiovascular risk marker, it is also a significant risk factor and a target for therapy. Not surprisingly, the development of treatments targeting triglyceride pathways is an area of immense interest in the last few years. It is significant that Mendelian randomization studies suggest that HDL cholesterol does not have a causal relationship with ASCVD. Moreover, medications that increase HDL cholesterol (i.e., niacin and CETP inhibitors) have largely failed to show efficacy in ASCVD risk reduction in randomized clinical trials. Therefore, although HDL cholesterol was shown to be inversely associated with cardiovascular risk, the mechanism of the relationship between HDL cholesterol and ASCVD is not fully understood. Importantly, ASCVD cannot be viewed as a disease caused solely by a lipid disorder; rather, it is the result of a complex interplay between dyslipidemia, metabolic derangements, inflammation, and endothelial dysfunction. For instance, even mildly elevated triglycerides (>150 mg/dL) can suggest metabolic syndrome, an important risk factor for cardiovascular disease. Meanwhile, chronic systemic inflammation was shown to accelerate atherogenesis, and therapies that target inflammation have been demonstrated in clinical trials to reduce the risk for ASCVD.

Evaluation

Global Cardiovascular Risk Assessment

Risk assessment is an integral part in the evaluation of patients with hyperlipidemia. Contemporary guidelines from the United States provide detailed algorithms for risk stratification. The 2013 and 2018 cholesterol guidelines identified four subgroups of patients for whom the benefits of statin therapy outweigh the risk. Secondary prevention patients are automatically considered to be at high risk for recurrent ASCVD events and, thus, would necessitate initiation of lipid lowering therapy. In the 2018 Multisociety guideline, secondary prevention patients may be further stratified into those at very high risk, and those at not very high risk, for ASCVD, based on the presence or absence of high-risk features. The value of further delineating risk among secondary prevention patients was in part to facilitate the evidence-based use of newer nonstatin therapies (i.e., ezetimibe [Zetia][1] and PCSK9 inhibitors).

Among primary prevention patients, a history of diabetes mellitus, or significantly elevated LDL cholesterol (≥190 mg/dL or 4.9 mmol/L) signifying a likely genetic cause of hypercholesterolemia (i.e., familial hypercholesterolemia), automatically warrants initiation of lipid lowering therapy. In primary prevention patients with hyperlipidemia but without these two high-risk features, a global cardiovascular risk score can be used to further stratify a patient. Global risk scores estimate 10-year cardiovascular risk, which combines the effects of well-known risk factors, using one of several risk-calculation tools. Individual tools have been developed based on large epidemiology studies examining a limited number of available risk factors. Traditional risk factors such as age, sex, cigarette smoking, cholesterol, diabetes, and blood pressure are able to predict 80% to 90% of the cardiovascular events in people 40 years or older. However, these tools may not accurately estimate cardiovascular risk in individuals with unaccounted risk factors or those with demographics distinct from the populations used to derive the risk scores. The risk score most commonly used (and endorsed by guidelines) in the United States is the Pooled Cohort Equation (PCE). The PCE is used to estimate a 10-year risk for ASCVD for men and women aged 40 to 79 years, who are white or black race, incorporating age, sex, race, HDL and total cholesterol, diabetes, hypertension, and smoking status (http://tools.cardiosource.org/ASCVD-Risk-Estimator). The 2018 Multisociety guidelines recommend the initiation of statin therapy in patients with intermediate (≥7.5% to <20%) and high (≥20%) 10-year ASCVD risk, with consideration of statins even in select patients with borderline 10-year risk (5% to <7.5%). Of note, the risk stratification used by the European guideline is similar

to that used by the American guideline. Although patients with a history of clinical ASCVD and those with high-risk comorbidities (i.e., diabetes mellitus, significant chronic kidney disease) are also classified as higher risk, the risk assessment score used is different. The Systematic COronary Risk Evaluation (SCORE), used in the ESC/EAS Guidelines for the Management of Dyslipidemias, incorporates similar risk factors and predicts fatal cardiovascular events (www.heartscore.org).

Finally, further risk assessment for subclinical coronary atherosclerosis via the measurement of coronary calcium by computer tomography (calcium score) has also been incorporated into the most current guidelines. With the rapid advancement of cardiovascular imaging technologies, further refinement of risk assessment that incorporates calcium score or other imaging modalities will likely play a significant role in future clinical practice.

Measurement of Lipid Profiles

Lipid profiles should be measured as a part of global risk assessment, and the frequency of checkup is determined by age, sex, and risk factors for cardiovascular disease. In patients on lipid lowering therapy, a lipid panel should be performed after the initiation or dose change in therapy; it should also be performed periodically in patients on stable therapy to assess treatment efficacy and medication adherence.

A fasting lipid profile (fasting for 9 to 12 hours) is recommended to ensure the most precise lipid assessment, specifically triglycerides (subsequently LDL cholesterol if calculated using the Friedewald equation). Nonfasting lipid profile provides an accurate measurement of other lipids, including total cholesterol, HDL cholesterol, Apo B, and Apo AI. Recent studies showed that differences in triglyceride levels according to fasting time were small. Therefore lipid values from nonfasting samples should not be ignored.

LDL cholesterol can either be calculated or measured directly. The standard method used to derive LDL cholesterol from other components of the lipid panel is the Friedewald equation (LDL cholesterol = total cholesterol – HDL cholesterol – triglycerides/5). This equation should be used with appropriate caution: fasting state samples should be used; it becomes less accurate if triglycerides >200 mg/dL; it becomes invalid with triglycerides >400 mg/dL; LDL cholesterol can be underestimated at levels <70 mg/dL.

Apolipoproteins, including Apo B and Apo AI, may also be measured. The Apo B level (Apo B100) reflects the number of atherogenic lipoprotein particles. Apo B level and Apo B/Apo AI ratio are as good as traditional lipid profiles and are especially useful in certain situations such as combined hyperlipidemia, metabolic syndrome, diabetes, and chronic kidney disease. In patients with history of premature ASCVD, recurrent ASCVD events despite optimal therapy, and those with a strong family history of premature ASCVD, a measurement of lipoprotein (a) [Lp(a)] may be considered.

Other medical conditions may also affect lipid profiles. Secondary causes include hypothyroidism, nephrotic syndrome, dysgammaglobulinemia, use of progestin (especially those with androgenic activity), cholestasis, use of protease inhibitors, chronic kidney disease, uncontrolled diabetes, obesity, excessive alcohol intake, use of thiazide or β-blockers, use of corticosteroids, use of oral estrogen (not transdermal), and pregnancy. These conditions should be detected and treated, if appropriate, to improve control of hyperlipidemia.

Family history of premature cardiovascular disease and hyperlipidemia and physical findings such as xanthomas, xanthelasmas, and premature arcus cornealis may suggest familial hypercholesterolemia. As the risk for ASCVD associated with very elevated levels of atherogenic lipoproteins begins to accumulate very early in life, patients with familial hypercholesterolemia should be treated aggressively.

Treatment

Overview

Treatment is primarily aimed at lowering LDL cholesterol level, which has been shown to decrease the risk of cardiovascular disease in numerous randomized clinical trials. In clinical scenarios

[1]Not FDA approved for this indication

TABLE 2   Risk Groups and Treatment Goals (2018 Multisociety Blood Cholesterol Guideline)

	RISK CATEGORY	RECOMMENDED STATIN THERAPY TO INITIATE	NONSTATIN THERAPY
Secondary Prevention	Very high risk*	High-intensity statin (Goal LDL cholesterol reduction of ≥50%).	If LDL cholesterol ≥70 mg/dL on maximally tolerated statin then adding ezetimibe or a PCSK9 inhibitor should be considered. Ezetimibe should be tried first, given cost effectiveness.
	Not very high risk	High-intensity statin (Goal LDL cholesterol reduction of ≥50%).	If LDL cholesterol ≥70 mg/dL on maximally tolerated statin then may consider adding ezetimibe.
Primary Prevention	LDL cholesterol ≥190 mg/dL	High-intensity statin (Goal LDL cholesterol reduction of ≥50%).	If LDL cholesterol reduction of ≥50% was not achieved or if an LDL cholesterol level remains above 100 mg/dL on maximally tolerated statin, may consider ezetimibe and then a PCSK9 inhibitor if needed.
	Diabetes mellitus	Moderate-intensity statin (Goal LDL cholesterol reduction of 30% to 49%). In patients with multiple other ASCVD risk factors, high-intensity statin may be considered.	Reasonable to add ezetimibe to maximally tolerated statin therapy to reduce LDL cholesterol by ≥50%.
	High risk (10 years ASCVD risk† ≥20%)	High-intensity statin	Reasonable to add ezetimibe to maximally tolerated statin therapy to reduce LDL cholesterol by ≥50%.
	Intermediate risk (10 year ASCVD risk ≥7.5% to <20%)	If risk enhancers‡ present or if CAC score elevated, should initiate moderate intensity statin.	In patients with multiple additional ASCVD risk factors. Reasonable to add ezetimibe to maximally tolerated statin therapy to reduce LDL cholesterol by ≥50%.
	Borderline risk (10 year ASCVD risk 5% to <7.5%)	If risk enhancers present, then may consider moderate intensity statin.	
	Low risk (10 years ASCVD risk <5%)		

*Very high risk defined by a history of multiple major ASCVD events or at least 1 major ASCVD event plus multiple high-risk conditions (age ≥65 years, heterozygous familial hypercholesterolemia, history of coronary bypass surgery or percutaneous coronary intervention outside of the major ASCVD events, diabetes mellitus, hypertension, chronic kidney disease, current smoking, persistently elevated LDL cholesterol ≥100 mg/dL despite maximally tolerated statin and ezetimibe, or history of congestive heart failure).

†10 year ASCVD risk as estimated by the Pooled Cohort Equation.

‡Risk enhancers include family history of premature ASCVD, chronic kidney disease, metabolic syndrome, inflammatory disease, conditions specific to women (i.e., preeclampsia, premature menopause), ethnicity (i.e., South Asian ancestry), persistently elevated LDL cholesterol ≥160 mg/dL, persistently elevated triglycerides (≥175 mg/dL), high sensitivity C-reactive protein ≥2.0 mg/L, lipoprotein (a) >50 mg/dL or 125 nmol/L, apolipoprotein B ≥130 mg/dL, ankle-brachial index <0.9.

ASCVD, atherosclerotic cardiovascular disease; CAC, calcium; LDL, low density lipoprotein; PCSK9, proprotein convertase subtilisin/kexin type 9.

TABLE 3   LDL Cholesterol and Apo B Goals in the ESC/EAS Guideline*

	GOAL	
	LDL CHOLESTEROL (MG/DL)	APO B (MG/DL)
Very high risk: established cardiovascular disease, diabetes plus major cardiovascular risk factor(s), severe CKD (GFR <30 mL/min/1.73 m²), or 10 year fatal CVD risk ≥10%	70 or > 50% reduction if baseline 70–135	80
High risk: markedly uncontrolled risk factor(s), diabetes, moderate CKD (GFR 30–59 mL/min/1.73 m²), or 10 years fatal CVD risk 5%–10%	100 or >50% reduction if baseline 100–200	100

*10-year risk calculation using Systematic COronary Risk Evaluation (SCORE).

Apo B, apolipoprotein B; CKD, chronic kidney disease; CVD, cardiovascular disease; GFR, glomerular filtration rate; LDL, low density lipoprotein.

where the triglyceride level is >500 mg/dL, triglycerides should be lowered immediately to prevent acute pancreatitis. Every reduction of LDL cholesterol of 1 mmol/L (~40 mg/dL) is associated with ~20% reduction in cardiovascular risk. The absolute risk reduction by lowering LDL cholesterol is proportional to the global cardiovascular risk.

It should be noted that the American guidelines have shifted away from hard LDL cholesterol targets. The treatment goals and approaches according to the 2018 cholesterol guidelines are summarized in Table 2. Briefly, high-risk patients are recommended to be started on a high-intensity statin with a goal LDL cholesterol reduction of ≥50%. In high-risk patients who cannot tolerate high-intensity statins and in intermediate risk patients, a

moderate-intensity statin is recommended with a goal of LDL-C reduction of 30% to 49%. In secondary prevention patients who are determined to be at very high risk, additional validated nonstatin medications (ezetimibe and PCSK9 inhibitors) may be considered if LDL cholesterol remains ≥70 mg/dL on maximally tolerated therapy. At the time of the writing of this chapter, the Europeans, as reflected by the 2016 ESC/EAS guidelines, have maintained hard LDL cholesterol targets based on patient risk, as presented in Table 3.

As a first line, therapeutic lifestyle changes should be initiated when LDL cholesterol is above the target range. People with very high, high, or moderately high risk should also start making therapeutic lifestyle changes regardless of their LDL cholesterol level. Medications may be added at the same time as therapeutic lifestyle changes for these patients. If medications are indicated, statin is preferred because of proven efficacy that has been consistently shown in multiple clinical trials. The intensity of treatment is dictated by the patient's risk profile, ability to tolerate therapy as well as patient preference. Generally, response to treatment by a lipid panel and appropriate safety laboratory measures should be assessed 4 to 12 weeks after treatment initiation or change. Once under control, lipid panels and clinical laboratory safety profiles can be monitored every 3 to 12 months.

Therapeutic Lifestyle Changes

All patients with hyperlipidemia should be counseled on lifestyle modifications. Dietary modification to limit intake of lipids is an essential component, given that the main source of lipids is exogenous dietary fat. Saturated fatty acids and trans-unsaturated fatty acids increase LDL cholesterol, whereas dietary fibers decrease LDL cholesterol. Carbohydrates do not affect LDL cholesterol but increase triglycerides and decrease HDL cholesterol, particularly if they have a high glycemic index. Intake of fructose, a component of sucrose, increases triglycerides and decreases HDL cholesterol. Body weight reduction, increasing physical activity, and avoidance of a sedentary lifestyle have a small effect on LDL cholesterol, but they reduce triglycerides, increase HDL cholesterol, and are associated with improved cardiovascular outcome. Alcohol intake has an adverse effect on triglycerides and should be avoided.

Individual patients will need different approaches based on their cardiovascular risk and lipid profiles. Generally, total dietary fat is recommended to constitute 25% to 35% of the total

calorie intake mainly as mono- or poly-unsaturated fat, limiting saturated fat <7% and trans fat <1% of the total calorie intake. Therapeutic lifestyle changes include diets with emphasis on vegetables, fruits, whole grains, low-fat dairy products, poultry, fish, legumes, nontropical vegetable oils, and nuts as well as limited intake of sweets, sugar-sweetened beverages, and red meats; further reduction of saturated fat (<5% to 6% of the total caloric intake) and trans fat; weight reduction; and increased regular physical activity. The amount of cholesterol intake is not well correlated with LDL cholesterol level and there is no recommended limit for intake. Management of other risk factors such as smoking cessation and controlling blood pressure in hypertensive patients and blood glucose in diabetics is also very important.

Pharmacologic Agents

The currently available lipid-lowering agents can be classified based on their mechanism of action. Statins (3-hydroxy-3-methylglutaryl coenzyme A [HMG-CoA] reductase inhibitors), ezetimibe (Zetia), PCSK9 (proprotein convertase subtilisin/kexin type 9) inhibitors, and bile acid sequestrants are used primarily to reduce LDL cholesterol. Fibrates, niacin, and omega-3 fatty acid prescriptions are used primarily for the treatment of hypertriglyceridemia. These classes of agents differ with regard to degree and type of lipid lowering, and agents within the same group may differ in efficacy and side effects. Conventional dosing regimens and common adverse effects are summarized in Table 4. Expected changes in lipid profiles are shown in Table 5. The choice of drug depends on the specific lipid abnormalities, patient's tolerability to the medication, and concurrent medical conditions. In general, statins are the most effective drugs to lower cardiovascular risk and are the

---

TABLE 4 Major Drugs for Management of Hyperlipidemia

AGENT	STARTING DAILY DOSAGE	DOSAGE RANGE	MECHANISM	SIDE EFFECTS
Statins				
Lovastatin (Mevacor)	20 mg	10–80 mg	Decreased cholesterol synthesis, increased hepatic LDL receptors, decreased VLDL release	Myalgias, arthralgias, high liver enzymes, dyspepsia
Pravastatin (Pravachol)	40 mg	10–80 mg		
Simvastatin (Zocor)	20–40 mg	5–80 mg		
Fluvastatin (Lescol)	40 mg	20–80 mg		
Atorvastatin (Lipitor)	10–20 mg	10–80 mg		
Rosuvastatin (Crestor)	10 mg	5–40 mg		
Pitavastatin (Livalo)	2 mg	2–4 mg		
Cholesterol Absorption Inhibitors				
Ezetimibe (Zetia)	10 mg	10 mg	Deceased intestinal cholesterol absorption	High liver enzymes
Combination Therapies (single pill)				
Ezetimibe/Simvastatin (Vytorin)	10/20 mg	10/10–10/80 mg		
PCSK9 Inhibiting Monoclonal Antibodies (subcutaneous)				
Alirocumab (Praluent)	75 mg every 2 weeks	75–150 mg every 2 weeks	Increased hepatic LDL receptors	Injection site reactions, nasopharyngitis, upper respiratory tract infection, influenza, back pain
Evolocumab (Repatha)		140 mg every 2 weeks or 420 mg monthly		
Bile Acid Sequestrants				
Cholestyramine (Questran)	8–16 g	4–24 g	Increased bile acid excretion, increased LDL receptors	Bloating, constipation, elevated triglycerides
Colestipol (Colestid)	2 g	2–16 g		
Colesevelam (Welchol)	3.75 g	3.75 g		
Fibrates				

TABLE 4 — Major Drugs for Management of Hyperlipidemia—cont'd

AGENT	STARTING DAILY DOSAGE	DOSAGE RANGE	MECHANISM	SIDE EFFECTS
Fenofibrate (Tricor)	48–145 mg	48–145 mg	Increased LPL activity, decreased VLDL synthesis	Dyspepsia, myalgia, gallstones, high liver enzymes
Gemfibrozil (Lopid)	1200 mg	1200 mg		
Fenofibric acid (Trilipix)	45–135 mg	45–135 mg		
Niacin				
Immediate release	250 mg	250–3000 mg	Decreased VLDL synthesis	Flushing, high glucose, uric acid, high liver enzymes
Extended release (Niaspan)	500 mg	500–2000 mg		
Omega-3 Fatty Acid Prescriptions				
Icosapent ethyl (Vascepa)	4 g	4 g		Arthralgia, atrial fibrillation, lower extremity edema*
Omega-3 fatty acid ethyl esters (Lovaza)	4 g	4 g		Eructation, dyspepsia, and taste perversion

*The on-label side-effect profile of icosapent ethyl includes arthralgia. Increased rates of atrial fibrillation and lower extremity edema were reported in the REDUCE-IT trial. However, at the time of the writing of this chapter, the use of icosapent ethyl in patients meeting REDUCE-IT entry criteria would be considered off-label use.
LDL, low-density lipoprotein; *LPL*, lipoprotein lipase; *TG*, triglycerides; *VLDL*, very–low-density lipoprotein.

TABLE 5 — Metabolic Effects of Each Lipid-Lowering Drug Class

	LDL CHOLESTEROL	HDL CHOLESTEROL	TRIGLYCERIDES
Statins	↓21%–55%	↑2%–10%	↓6%–30%
Fibric acids	↓20%–25%	↑6%–18%	↓20%–35%
Niacin	↓10%–25%	↑10%–35%	↓20%–30%
Bile acid sequestrants	↓15%–25%		May ↑
Cholesterol absorption inhibitors	↓10%–18%		
PCSK9 inhibitors	↓39%–62%	↑4%–7%	↓12%–17%

Adapted from lipoprotein management in patients with cardiometabolic risk, consensus statement from the American College of Cardiology Foundation and the American Diabetes Association (ACC/ADA) (2008), and American Association of Clinical Endocrinologists' (AACE) guidelines for management of dyslipidemia and prevention of atherosclerosis (2012).

treatment of choice when medications are indicated based on the global cardiovascular risk. If the treatment goal is not achieved by statins or statins are not tolerated, other validated nonstatin therapies (ezetimibe and PCSK9 inhibitors) may be considered, followed by other agents such as bile acid sequestrants. If the primary goal is to lower triglycerides, fibrates, omega-3 fatty acids, or niacin may be more effective.

Statins

Statins are usually the first drug of choice in patients with high cholesterol levels to reduce cardiovascular risk and have been validated in multiple randomized controlled trials and their meta-analyses. Furthermore, risk reduction was apparent in a wide range of patients in both primary and secondary prevention, in men, women, smokers, patients with diabetes, as well as those with hypertension. In general, statins result in a high degree of LDL cholesterol reduction. The approximate equipotent dosages of various statins and their cholesterol-lowering effects are listed in Table 6. The 2013 and 2018 cholesterol guideline recommends moderate-or high-intensity statins (see Table 6) based on the global risk. Statins inhibit HMG-CoA reductase, the rate-limiting enzyme in cholesterol biosynthesis. By blocking cholesterol biosynthesis, statins upregulate the LDL receptor on the hepatocytes and increase clearance of IDL and LDL. In addition to their direct effects on lipid metabolism, statins have been reported to have pleiotropic effects (e.g., reduced formation of reactive oxygen species, inhibition of platelet reactivity, and decreased vasoconstriction).

Statins are usually well tolerated. Potential common side effects include myopathy, fatigue, headaches, and nonspecific gastrointestinal symptoms such as dyspepsia. Elevation of liver enzymes occurs in less than 1%. There is also a small but significant association with increase in risk of developing diabetes. Myopathy is one of the most common causes for cessation of statins. Myalgia can occur in about 10% to 20% of patients, which is much more often than reported in the clinical trials. The risk of rhabdomyolysis, however, is very low (0.1 to 0.2 per 1000 person-years). Risk for myopathy is increased in patients with advanced age, female sex, small body habitus, hypothyroidism, alcoholism, medical conditions (particularly liver or kidney disease), major surgery, excessive physical activity, history of myopathy, family history of myopathy, high-dose statins, and interacting medications or food such as grapefruit juice (>1 L/day). Simvastatin (Zocor), lovastatin (Mevacor), and atorvastatin (Lipitor) are primarily metabolized through CYP3A4, which is inhibited by protease inhibitors, cyclosporine (Neoral, Sandimmune), amiodarone (Cordarone, Pacerone), nondihydropyridine calcium channel blockers, fibrates, and other agents. Pravastatin (Pravachol) is metabolized by the kidney, not by the P450 system. Fluvastatin (Lescol) and rosuvastatin (Crestor) are primarily metabolized through CYP2C9. Pitavastatin (Livalo) is marginally metabolized by CYP2C9 and to a lesser extent by CYP2C8. Simvastatin and

TABLE 6	Equipotency and Percentage Reduction in Total Cholesterol According to the Different Types and Doses of Statins				
REDUCTION IN TOTAL CHOLESTEROL (%)	**PRAVASTATIN (PRAVACHOL), MG**	**FLUVASTATIN (LESCOL), MG**	**SIMVASTATIN (ZOCOR),* MG**	**ATORVASTATIN (LIPITOR), MG**	**ROSUVASTATIN (CRESTOR), MG**
6–15	5	10	-	-	-
15–17	10	20	5	2.5	-
22	20	40	10	5	-
27	40†	80†	20†	10†	5†
32	80†		40†	20†	10†
37		-	(80)	40‡	20‡
42	-	-	-	80‡	40‡

*See the text for the FDA warning.
†Moderate-intensity statins (reduction of low-density lipoprotein (LDL) cholesterol 30%–50%).
‡High-intensity statins (reduction of LDL cholesterol >50%).
Modified from Penning-van Beest FJA, Termorshuizen F, Goettsch WG, et al. Adherence to evidence-based statin guidelines reduces the risk of hospitalizations for acute myocardial infarction by 40%: a cohort study. *Eur Heart J.* 2007;28:154–159.

lovastatin should be avoided in patients receiving protease inhibitors. Statin dosage should be reduced in patients taking cyclosporine. Because of significant risk of myopathy and rhabdomyolysis related to high-dose simvastatin, the FDA recommends that 80 mg/day should not be used. The FDA further recommends that the dose be limited to 20 mg if the patient is also taking amiodarone, amlodipine (Norvasc), or ranolazine (Ranexa), and to 10 mg/day if taking diltiazem (Cardizem), dronedarone (Multaq), or verapamil (Calan). Addition of fibrates increases the risk of myopathy; in patients on a statin, fenofibrate (Tricor) is preferred, whereas gemfibrozil (Lopid), which has a much higher risk of rhabdomyolysis, is contraindicated. Symptoms of statin myopathy are heaviness, stiffness, cramping associated with weakness during exertion, and tendon-associated pain. Location of symptoms can be at the thighs, at the calves, or generalized. Symptoms can be very nonspecific, and differentiating statin-related myopathy from other causes is not easy. Therefore baseline symptoms, physical examination, and assessment of creatinine kinase level before the initiation of statins can be very helpful. Further decisions regarding stopping, dose reduction, or switching medications can be made based on the severity of symptoms, level of creatinine kinase elevation, and presence of rhabdomyolysis. In patients who develop myopathy while on simvastatin or atorvastatin, if the decision is to continue treatment with a statin, one option is to cautiously switch them to pravastatin, fluvastatin, or rosuvastatin, which are less prone to cause myopathy. Alternatively, lower statin dosing or less frequent dosing may be considered. For instance, rosuvastatin has a long duration of action and can be taken once every other day or weekly[1] if necessary. Theoretically, coenzyme Q10[7] may help manage statin-induced myopathy, but there is insufficient data to support its use. For patients who cannot tolerate statins, other agents should be used, starting with validated nonstatin agents.

Ezetimibe

Ezetimibe (Zetia) is the first in a new class of pharmaceutical agents that primarily targets the cholesterol transport protein Niemann-Pick C1-like 1 protein in the intestine. Ezetimibe is an efficacious and cost-effective add-on agent in people taking a statin, if the LDL cholesterol goal is not achieved or high doses of statin cannot be tolerated. Ezetimibe was shown to modestly decrease LDL cholesterol and cardiovascular events when added to simvastatin in high-risk patients in the Improved Reduction of Outcomes: Vytorin Efficacy International Trial (IMPROVE-IT) study. Moreover, ezetimibe has become a generic prescription in the United States and its safety profile is well characterized.

Elevated liver enzymes have been reported but the risk of hepatotoxicity seems to be not different from that of placebo.

PCSK9 Inhibitors

The PCSK9 (proprotein convertase subtilisin/kexin type 9) protein plays a major role in regulating the number of LDL receptors at the cell surface, including on hepatocytes. Binding of the LDL receptor by PCSK9 leads to the destruction of the LDL receptor. Therefore interference with the binding capacity of PCSK9 to LDL receptor or silencing the expression of the *PCSK9* gene allows more LDL receptors to recycle to the cell surface effecting the removal of more of the circulating plasma LDL. Over a decade ago, individuals with gain-of-function mutations of the *PCSK9* gene were found to underlie a rare form of autosomal dominant hypercholesterolemia. Subsequently, individuals with loss-of-function mutations were found to have very low LDL cholesterol levels and were protected from coronary heart disease (CHD). These discoveries led to the development of monoclonal antibodies directed against PCSK9 as a novel cholesterol-lowering agent.

Two human monoclonal antibodies against PCSK9, alirocumab (Praluent) and evolocumab (Repatha), have been approved by the FDA. Both are given by subcutaneous injection. In the Further Cardiovascular Outcomes Research With PCSK9 Inhibition in Subjects With Elevated Risk (FOURIER) trial, evolocumab was found to significantly reduce the risk for ASCVD events in patients with clinical ASCVD and LDL-C ≥70 mg/dL or a non–HDL-C level ≥100 mg/dL, who were receiving optimized lipid-lowering using high-intensity statin or at least atorvastatin 20 mg with or without ezetimibe. Similarly, in the Evaluation of Cardiovascular Outcomes After an Acute Coronary Syndrome During Treatment With Alirocumab (ODYSSEY OUTCOMES) trial, alirocumab was shown to significantly reduce the risk for ASCVD events in patients with recent acute coronary syndrome, who had a LDL-C ≥70 mg/dL, a non-HDL-C ≥100 mg/dL, or an apolipoprotein B level ≥80 mg/dL and were receiving statin therapy at a high-intensity dose or at the maximum tolerated dose. Taking into account the results, inclusion criteria, and secondary analyses from these trials, the 2018 Multisociety guidelines recommended the consideration of PCSK9 inhibitors in secondary prevention patients, especially those at very high risk, whose LDL cholesterol remains above 70 mg/dL or non-HDL cholesterol remains above 100 mg/dL on maximally tolerated statin therapy. Both alirocumab and evolocumab are also indicated for heterozygous familial hypercholesterolemia. Evolocumab is also indicated for homozygous familial hypercholesterolemia as an adjunct to other LDL-lowering therapies.

PCSK9 inhibitors are powerful LDL cholesterol lowering agents and enable reduction of LDL cholesterol by up to ~60% as a single agent or an adjunct therapy. Moreover, the absolute level of LDL cholesterol achieved may be as low as <25 mg/dL.

---

[1]Not FDA approved for this indication
[7]Available as a dietary supplement

There have been concerns regarding the potential adverse effects that may occur at such low LDL cholesterol levels, such as neurocognitive side effects. However, results from these trials and their sub-analyses have not shown a significant signal, although more long-term follow-up analysis is needed. Common side effects associated with PCSK9 inhibitors include injection site reactions, nasopharyngitis, upper respiratory tract infection, influenza, and back pain.

Currently, a significant hurdle to more widespread use of PCSK9 inhibitors is their high cost. Multiple cost-effective analyses have concluded that PCSK9 inhibitors are not yet cost effective. In 2018, the price of evolocumab was reduced by 60% by its manufacturer. Further studies will be needed to assess whether PCSK9 inhibitors are cost effective with this price reduction.

Bile Acid Sequestrants

Bile acid sequestrants have been in clinical use for many decades. These agents promote fecal excretion of bile acids. The liver responds with increased integration of cholesterol into bile acid synthesis to maintain a stable bile acid pool. The consequent decrease in cholesterol in the liver leads to upregulation of the LDL receptor and enhanced LDL clearance from the plasma. HMG-CoA synthase activity can increase, so combination therapy with statins would be synergistic, especially in patients with a suboptimal response. Available agents are cholestyramine (Questran), colestipol (Colestid), and colesevelam (Welchol). Most side effects involve the gastrointestinal tract, with constipation and bloating being the most common. These agents may interfere with the absorption of warfarin, phenobarbital, levothyroxine (Synthroid), and digoxin (Lanoxin), among other medications. Patients on multiple medications should be advised to take bile acid sequestrants 1 hour before or 4 hours after taking the other medications. These agents can also cause elevation of triglyceride level. As they are not systemically absorbed, the bile acid sequestrants may be the preferred agents when systemic absorption is to be avoided, such as during pregnancy or lactation.

Fibrates

The effect of fibrates on cardiovascular outcomes is not as favorable as with statins. However, fibrates can be useful in subsets of patients with high triglycerides and low-HDL cholesterol. Recently, the Action to Control Cardiovascular Risk in Diabetes (ACCORD) lipid trial showed that addition of fenofibrate to simvastatin in type 2 diabetic patients with cardiovascular risk factors did not improve cardiovascular outcomes, although there was a trend for better outcomes in a subgroup with triglycerides greater than 204 mg/dL and HDL cholesterol less than 34 mg/dL. Fibrates have multiple favorable metabolic effects including activation of peroxisome proliferator-activated receptor-α (contributing to the regulation of both lipid and carbohydrate metabolism), stimulation of lipoprotein lipase (increasing triglyceride hydrolysis), and downregulation of Apo CIII (improving lipoprotein remnant clearance as Apo CIII inhibits lipoprotein lipase). An enhanced VLDL-to-LDL conversion may lead to mild LDL cholesterol elevation in some patients. This effect may decrease over weeks, as the LDL receptors are upregulated. Fibrates are generally well tolerated. The most common side effect is dyspepsia. Other side effects include myopathy and hepatic enzyme elevation, particularly when fibrates are added to statins. The use of gemfibrozil (Lopid) should be avoided in patients on statin therapy due to increased risk for muscle-related adverse events. Fibrates increase the risk of gallstones, and patients on warfarin (Coumadin) may need dose adjustment. Monitoring of liver enzymes is recommended, at baseline and within 3 months and then periodically. Creatinine level can be increased through unclear mechanisms.

Niacin

Niacin or nicotinic acid effectively decreases the hepatic production of VLDL and thus, LDL cholesterol levels, and raises HDL cholesterol levels by reducing cholesterol transfer from HDL to Apo B-containing lipoproteins and HDL clearance by the liver. Niacin is also the most potent agent currently available to reduce the level of Lp(a); however, this effect on the reduction of cardiovascular events in patients with elevated Lp(a) is not known. Several trials showed the effect of niacin in preventing cardiovascular disease; however, the benefit of adding niacin to statins has not been proved. Niacin did not improve cardiovascular risk when added to simvastatin in patients with high risk for cardiovascular disease in the Atherothrombosis Intervention in Metabolic Syndrome with Low HDL/High Triglycerides: Impact on Global Health Outcomes (AIM-HIGH) study and the Heart Protection Study 2–Treatment of HDL to Reduce the Incidence of Vascular Events (HPS2-Thrive) study. There were excess adverse events and trends toward signs of harm among the niacin groups. The FDA has recently withdrawn the approval for the coadministration of niacin extended-release tablets (Niaspan) with statins. The most common side effect of niacin is flushing. This can be avoided or minimized by initiating therapy with a low dose of niacin, taking an aspirin 1 hour before niacin, avoiding hot foods or beverages at the time the niacin is taken, or switching to extended-release forms (Niaspan). Hepatotoxicity can occur at any time. Immediate-release forms are less likely to cause hepatotoxicity than sustained-release forms (Slo-Niacin). Extended-release forms can minimally elevate transaminases but significant hepatotoxicity is rare. They can, however, also cause dose-dependent reversible thrombocytopenia, which can be insidious and severe. When switching to different forms, it is recommended that one should start with low doses and titrate up to achieve desired response. Liver function tests should be monitored regularly, at baseline and every 3 months for the first year and then periodically. Other side effects include pruritus, increased uric acid levels, and hyperglycemia.

Omega-3 Fatty Acid Prescriptions

Highly purified omega-3 fatty acid preparations containing either a mixture of eicosapentaenoic acid (EPA) and docosahexaenoic acid (DHA) (Lovaza) or EPA alone (Vascepa) are effective agents used in the treatment of hypertriglyceridemia, the first FDA approved indication for these agents. Omega-3 fatty acids are polyunsaturated fatty acids (PUFA) and are essential in humans. A significant proportion of omega fatty acids is consumed in the diet. Major dietary sources of omega-3 fatty acids include nuts, vegetable oils, flax seeds, and leafy vegetables as well as fish and fish oil. EPA and DHA are the two major types of marine-derived omega-3 fatty acids. The mechanism by which omega-3 fatty acids lower triglycerides is incompletely understood.

Multiple clinical trials have been examining the efficacy of omega-3 fatty acid in improving cardiovascular outcome. Although trials using lower doses of EPA-DHA mixtures (≤1 g total daily) have shown inconsistent results, findings from recent trials assessing higher doses of pure EPA have been more favorable.

Purified EPA was first shown in the Japan Eicosapentaenoic acid (EPA) Lipid Intervention Study (JELIS) trial to significantly reduce risk for major coronary events in patients with hypercholesterolemia. Subsequently, the Reduction of Cardiovascular Events With Icosapent Ethyl–Intervention Trial (REDUCE-IT) study, a large, randomized controlled trial, assessed the efficacy and safety of purified EPA ethyl ester, icosapent ethyl (Vascepa) in secondary prevention and high-risk primary prevention patients with reasonably controlled LDL cholesterol but elevated triglycerides. The REDUCE-IT trial showed that treatment with icosapent ethyl was associated with a significant reduction in ASCVD events. In secondary analyses, icosapent ethyl has also been shown to reduce the risk for total ischemic events (first plus subsequent events). Results from REDUCE-IT suggest that in addition to LDL cholesterol lowering, high-risk patients with elevated triglycerides will likely benefit from icosapent ethyl. It is unknown whether higher doses of EPA-DHA mixtures may have similar efficacy as purified EPA; however, the relevant trial is underway. Lastly, the overall rates of adverse events were not significantly different between the treatment and control arms of REDUCE-IT. However, there were increased rates of atrial fibrillation and peripheral edema associated with patients taking icosapent ethyl observed in the trial.

References

ESC/EAS Guidelines for the management of dyslipidaemias, *Eur Heart J* 37:2999–3058, 2016.

Bhatt DL, Steg PG, Miller M, et al: Cardiovascular risk reduction with icosapent ethyl for hypertriglyceridemia, *N Engl J Med* 380(1):11–22, 2019.

Bhatt DL, Steg PG, Miller M, et al: Effects of icosapent ethyl on total ischemic events: from REDUCE-IT, *J Am Coll Cardiol*, 2019.

Brunzell JD, Davidson M, Furberg CD: Lipoprotein management in patients with cardiometabolic risk: consensus conference report from the ADA and the ACC foundation, *J Am Coll Cardiol* 51:1512–1524, 2008.

Carroll MD, Kit BK, Lacher DA, et al: Trends in lipids and lipoproteins in U.S. adults, 1988–2010, *JAMA* 308:1545–1554, 2012.

Dullaart RP: PCSK9 Inhibition to reduce cardiovascular events, *N Engl J Med* 376:1713–1722, 2017.

Eckel RH, Jakicic JM, Ard JD, et al: 2013 ACC/AHA guideline on lifestyle management to reduce cardiovascular risk: a report of the American College of Cardiology/American Heart Association task force on practice guidelines, *J Am Coll Cardiol* 63:2960–2984, 2014.

Everett BM, Smith RJ, Hiatt WR: Reducing LDL with PCSK9 inhibitors — the clinical benefit of lipid drugs, *N Eng J Med* 373:1588–1591, 2015.

Ginsberg HN, Elam MB, Lovato LC, et al: Effects of combination lipid therapy in type 2 diabetes mellitus, *N Engl J Med* 362:1563–1574, 2010.

Greenland P, Alpert JS, Beller GA, et al: 2010 ACCF/AHA guideline for assessment of cardiovascular risk in asymptomatic adults: a report of the American College of Cardiology Foundation/American Heart Association Task Force on Practice Guidelines developed in collaboration with the American Society of Echocardiography, American Society of Nuclear Cardiology, Society of Atherosclerosis Imaging and Prevention, Society for Cardiovascular Angiography and Interventions, Society of Cardiovascular Computed Tomography, and Society for Cardiovascular Magnetic Resonance, *J Am Coll Cardiol* 56:e50–e103, 2010.

Grundy SM, Cleeman JI, Merz CNB, et al: Implications of recent clinical trials for the national cholesterol education program adult treatment panel III guidelines, *Circulation* 110:227–239, 2004.

Grundy SM, Stone NJ, Bailey AL, et al: AHA/ACC/AACVPR/AAPA/ABC/ACPM/ADA/AGS/APhA/ASPC/NLA/PCNA Guideline on the Management of Blood Cholesterol: Executive Summary: a report of the American College of Cardiology/American Heart Association Task Force on Clinical Practice Guidelines, *J Am Coll Cardiol*(18)39033–39038, 2018. pii: S0735-1097.

Hlatky MA, Kazi DS: PCSK9 inhibitors: economics and policy, *J Am Coll Cardiol* 70(21):2677–2687, 2017.

Huffman MD, Capewell S, Ning H, et al: Cardiovascular health behavior and health factor changes (1988–2008) and projections to 2020: results from the National Health and Nutrition Examination Surveys (NHANES), *Circulation* 125:2595–2602, 2012.

IMPROVE-IT Investigators: Ezetimibe added to statin therapy after acute coronary syndromes, *N Eng J Med* 372:2387–2397, 2015.

Jellinger PS, Smith DA, Mehta AE, et al: American Association of Clinical Endocrinologists' guidelines for management of hyperlipidemia and prevention of atherosclerosis, *EndocrPract* 18:1–78, 2012.

Joy TR, Hegele RA: Narrative review: statin-related myopathy, *Ann Intern Med* 150:858–868, 2009.

Kazi DS, Moran AE, Coxson PG, et al: Cost-effectiveness of PCSK9 inhibitor therapy in patients with heterozygous familial hypercholesterolemia or atherosclerotic cardiovascular disease, *JAMA* 316(7):743–753, 2016.

Keaney JF, Curfman GD, Jarcho JA: A pragmatic view of the new cholesterol treatment guidelines, *N Engl J Med* 370:275–278, 2014.

Lloyd-Jones DM, Morris PB, Ballantyne CM, et al: 2017 Focused update of the 2016 ACC expert consensus decision pathway on the role of non-statin therapies for LDL-cholesterol lowering in the management of atherosclerotic cardiovascular disease risk: a report of the American Colelge of Cardiology Task Force Expert Consensus Decision Pathways, *J Am Coll Cardiol* 70:1785–1822, 2017.

Musunuru K, Kathiresan S: Surprises from genetic analyses of lipid risk factors for atherosclerosis, *Circ Res* 118(4):579–585, 2016.

O'Connell C, Horwood K, Nadamuni M: Correction of refractory thrombocytopenia and anemia following withdrawal of extended release niacin, *Am J Hematol* 91(7):E318, 2016.

Otvos JD, Collins D, Freedman DS, et al: Low-density lipoprotein and high-density lipoprotein particle subclasses predict coronary events and are favorably changed by gemfibrozil therapy in the Veterans Affairs High-Density Lipoprotein Intervention Trial, *Circulation* 113:1556–1563, 2006.

Penning-van Beest FJA, Termorshuizen F, Goettsch WG, et al: Adherence to evidence-based statin guidelines reduces the risk of hospitalizations for acute myocardial infarction by 40%: a cohort study, *Eur Heart J* 28:154–159, 2007.

Phan BAP, Dayspring TD, Toth PP: Ezetimibe therapy: mechanism of action and clinical update, *Vasc Health Risk Manag* 8:415–427, 2012.

Reiner Z, Catapano AL, De Backer G, et al: ESC/EAS guidelines for the management of dyslipidaemias: the task force for the management of dyslipidaemias of the European Society of Cardiology (ESC) and the European Atherosclerosis Society (EAS), *Eur Heart J* 32:1769–1818, 2011.

Ridker PM, Cook NR: Statins: new American guidelines for prevention of cardiovascular disease, *Lancet* 382:1762–1765, 2013.

Robinson JG, Farnier M, Krempf M, et al: Efficacy and safety of alirocumab in reducing lipids and cardiovascular events, *N Eng J Med* 372:1489–1499, 2015.

Robinson JG, Rosenson RS, Farnier M, et al: Safety of very low low-density lipoprotein cholesterol levels with alirocumab, *Journal Amn Coll Cardiol* 69(5):471–482, 2017.

Sabatine MS, Giugliano RP, Keech AC, et al: Evolocumab and clinical outcomes in patients with cardiovascular disease, *N Engl J Med* 376(18):1713–1722, 2017.

Sabatine MS, Giugliano RP, Wiviott SD, et al: Efficacy and safety of evolocumab in reducing lipids and cardiovascular events, *N Engl J Med* 372:1500–1509, 2015.

Schwartz GG, Steg PG, Szarek M, et al: Alirocumab and cardiovascular outcomes after acute coronary syndrome, *N Engl J Med* 379(22):2097–2107, 2018.

Stone NJ, Robinson J, Lichtenstein AH, et al: ACC/AHA guideline on the treatment of blood cholesterol to reduce atherosclerotic cardiovascular risk in adults: a report of the American College of Cardiology/American Heart Association task force on practice guidelines, *J Am Coll Cardiol* 63:2889–2934, 2014.

Tall AR, Rader DJ: Trials and tribulations of CETP inhibitors, *Circ Res* 122(1):106–112, 2018.

The HPS2-THRIVE Collaborative Group: Effects of extended-release niacin with laropiprant in high-risk patients, *N Eng J Med* 371:203–212, 2014.

The AIM-HIGH Investigators: Niacin in patients with low HDL cholesterol levels receiving intensive statin therapy, *N Engl J Med* 365:2255–2267, 2011.

Third report of the National Cholesterol Education Program (NCEP) expert panel on detection, evaluation, and treatment of high blood cholesterol in adults (Adult treatment panel III) final report, *Circulation* 106:3143–3421, 2002.

Tsimikas S: A test in context: lipoprotein(a): diagnosis, prognosis, controversies, and emerging therapies, *J Am Coll Cardiol* 69(6):692–711, 2017.

Wu H, Ballantyne CM: Dyslipidaemia: PCSK9 inhibitors and foamy monocytes in familial hypercholesterolaemia, *Nat Rev Cardiol* 14(7):385–386, 2017.

Xu L, Perrard XD, Perrard JL, et al: Foamy monocytes form early and contribute to nascent atherosclerosis in mice with hypercholesterolemia, *ArteriosclerThrombVasc Biol* 35:1787–1797, 2015.

Yokoyama M, Origasa H, Matsuzaki M, et al: Effects of eicosapentaenoic acid on major coronary events in hypercholesterolaemic patients (JELIS): a randomised open-label, blinded endpoint analysis, *Lancet* 369(9567):1090–1098, 2007.

HYPERPARATHYROIDISM AND HYPOPARATHYROIDISM

Method of
Claudio Marcocci, MD; and Filomena Cetani, MD

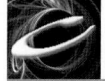

CURRENT DIAGNOSIS

Primary Hyperparathyroidism

- Third most common endocrine disorder and most common cause of hypercalcemia in the general population.
- Diagnosis based on confirmed hypercalcemia (total calcium [albumin corrected] or ionized calcium) associated with elevated or inappropriately normal serum parathyroid hormone level.
- Hypercalcemia on routine blood testing or in postmenopausal women investigated for osteoporosis is typically the first clue to the diagnosis.
- Mainly occurs as a solitary disease (90%) but may be part of hereditary syndromes.
- Genetic causes should be searched for in young patients.

Secondary Hyperparathyroidism

- Secondary hyperparathyroidism defines any condition in which the increased PTH secretion occurs as a normal physiologic response, often mediated by a decrease of serum calcium.
- Vitamin D deficiency, as a result of inadequate nutritional intake/sun exposure, malabsorption, liver diseases, or chronic renal failure, is the most common cause.
- At variance with primary hyperparathyroidism, secondary hyperparathyroidism is characterized by low or, more often, low-normal serum calcium and decreased urinary calcium excretion.

Hypoparathyroidism

- Rare disorder.
- Inadvertent removal or damage to the parathyroid gland during thyroid surgery and, much less frequently, autoimmune destruction are the most common causes.
- Diagnosis based on low serum calcium along with undetectable or inappropriately low serum parathyroid hormone level.

CURRENT THERAPY

Primary Hyperparathyroidism
- Parathyroidectomy is the only definitive therapy.
- Surgery should be considered in all cases and recommended in symptomatic patients and in those who, albeit asymptomatic, meet the surgical criteria.
- Surveillance without surgery can be considered in asymptomatic patients who do not meet the surgical criteria.
- Patients followed without surgery should be replete with vitamin D and calcium intake should not be restricted.
- Medical treatment can be considered in selected cases: antiresorptive therapy to increase bone mineral density and cinacalcet (Sensipar) to lower serum calcium.

Hypoparathyroidism
- Severe hypocalcemia is a medical emergency and treatment with intravenous calcium should be promptly instituted and maintained for 24 to 48 hours; oral therapy with calcium and active vitamin D metabolites should be started as soon as practical.
- The goal of chronic treatment is to maintain serum calcium in the low-normal range, avoiding hypocalcemic symptoms and long-term complications.
- Chronic conventional therapy is based on adequate calcium intake (calcium supplement needed in most cases) and active vitamin D metabolites.
- Recombinant full-length parathyroid hormone 1-84 (Natpara) has been approved by the U.S. Food and Drug Administration and European Medicines Agency for patients not controlled with conventional therapy.
- An individualized approach is necessary to optimize patient care. Lifelong monitoring is needed to decrease the risk of complications.

TABLE 1 Hereditary Forms of PHPT and Related Involved Gene

DISORDER	GENE	PATTERN OF INHERITANCE
Multiple endocrine neoplasia type 1	MEN1	Autosomal dominant
Multiple endocrine neoplasia type 2A	RET	Autosomal dominant
Multiple endocrine neoplasia type 4	CDKN1B	Autosomal dominant
Hyperparathyroidism–jaw tumor syndrome	CDC73	Autosomal dominant
Familial isolated hyperparathyroidism	MEN1, CDC73, CASR, GCM2, CDKN1B	Autosomal dominant
Familial hypocalciuric hypercalcemia type 1	CASR	Autosomal dominant
Familial hypocalciuric hypercalcemia type 2	GNA11	Autosomal dominant
Familial hypocalciuric hypercalcemia type 3	AP2S1	Autosomal dominant
Neonatal severe hyperparathyroidism	CASR	Autosomal recessive

Abbreviations: AP2S1 = Adaptor-related protein complex 2 sigma 1 subunit CASR = calcium-sensing receptor; CDC73 = cell division cycle 73; CDKN1B = cyclin-dependent kinase inhibitor 1B; GCM2 = glial cells missing transcription factor 2; GNA11 = G protein subunit alpha 11; MEN1 = multiple endocrine neoplasia type 1; PHPT = primary hyperparathyroidism; RET = rearranged during transfection.

Primary Hyperparathyroidism

Epidemiology
Primary hyperparathyroidism (PHPT) is currently the third most common endocrine disorder and the most frequent cause of hypercalcemia in the general population.

The disease was considered rare until the early 1970s, when its incidence in the United States rose dramatically following the introduction of serum calcium in the multichannel autoanalyzer. The incidence varies according to geographic areas and assessment measures; recent data in the United States indicate an incidence of 79.6 per 100,000 person-years in women and 35.6 per 100,000 person-years in men of all races, with the highest rate among blacks. The incidence peaks in the sixth decade of life. The prevalence ranges between 1 and 7 cases per 1000 adults. Most cases occur in women (with a female-to-male ratio of 3:1), but there is no sex difference before the age of 45 years. PHPT is rare in children and adolescents.

Pathogenesis
PHPT mainly occurs as a solitary disease (90%) but may be part of hereditary syndromes (e.g., multiple endocrine neoplasia [MEN] types 1, 2A, and 4; hyperparathyroidism–jaw tumor syndrome [HPT-JT], and familial isolated hyperparathyroidism [FIPH]) (Table 1). A single, benign adenoma is found in 80% to 85% of cases, multigland involvement in 15% to 20%, and parathyroid carcinoma in less than 1%. Multigland involvement is more common in hereditary cases, particularly MEN1. In the absence of local infiltration or metastases, the diagnosis of parathyroid carcinoma may be difficult at histology. Genetic studies (CDC73 gene mutations) and immunohistochemical studies (loss of parafibromin [the protein encoded by the CDC73 gene] expression) may help in equivocal cases. Predisposing factors are external neck irradiation in childhood and long-term lithium therapy.

PHPT is characterized by excessive parathyroid hormone (PTH) secretion from one or more parathyroid glands, due to the loss of the homeostatic control of PTH synthesis and secretion. Extracellular ionized calcium (Ca^{2+}_o) is the main regulator of PTH secretion. Ca^{2+}_o interacts with the Ca^{2+}-sensing receptor (CaSR) present on the surface of parathyroid cells; there is an inverse sigmoidal relationship between Ca^{2+}_o concentration and PTH release. In adenomas hypercalcemia is due to the loss of normal sensitivity of the parathyroid cell to the inhibitory action of Ca^{2+}_o, whereas in parathyroid hyperplasia the increased number of parathyroid cells, which have a normal sensitivity to the inhibitory action of Ca^{2+}_o, causes hypercalcemia. Serum phosphate, 1,25-dihydroxyvitamin D ($1,25(OH)_2D$), and fibroblast growth factor 23 (FGF23) are also involved in the control of PTH secretion.

Although major progress has been made in the last two decades, the molecular basis of PHPT is still unclear in the majority of cases. The clonality of most parathyroid tumors suggests a defect in the pathways that control parathyroid cell proliferation or the expression of PTH. The genes involved are listed in Table 1. Germline mutations are often found in hereditary forms. On the other hand, somatic mutations may occur in sporadic cases, even though germline mutations have also been described in apparently sporadic cases.

Clinical Presentation
In recent years the clinical presentation of PHPT in Western countries has changed from a symptomatic disease, characterized by hypercalcemia and renal (nephrolithiasis and nephrocalcinosis) and skeletal (osteitis fibrosa cystica, fragility fractures) manifestations, to one with subtle and nonspecific clinical manifestations (asymptomatic PHPT). Nephrolithiasis remains the most common classic clinical manifestation (15%–20%), and silent stones are frequently detected at ultrasound. Bone mineral density (BMD) is reduced particularly at sites rich in cortical bone (one-third distal

radius). Studies using peripheral high-resolution quantitative computed tomography (CT) has shown involvement of both cortical and trabecular sites, the latter confirmed by the trabecular bone score (TBS) at the lumbar spine. An increased rate of vertebral and nonvertebral fractures has also been documented. Nonclassical manifestations, including subtle cardiovascular abnormalities and psychological and cognitive symptoms, have also been reported.

A new variant of PHPT (normocalcemic PHPT) has recently been identified, namely patients with increased serum PTH levels in the absence of hypercalcemia (also by measurement of ionized calcium) or other causes of secondary hyperparathyroidism. This condition, called normocalcemic PHPT, has been typically recognized in persons evaluated for low BMD, in whom PTH was measured even in the absence of hypercalcemia. In some cases this new phenotype may represent an early phase of classical hypercalcemic PHPT, when PTH elevation precedes the occurrence of hypercalcemia.

Evaluation and Diagnosis

The finding of hypercalcemia on routine blood testing or in postmenopausal women investigated for osteoporosis is typically the first clue to the diagnosis of PHPT. Hypercalcemia should be confirmed in repeated testing, preferably evaluating albumin-corrected total calcium (measured total calcium in mg/dL + [0.8 × (4.0 − serum albumin in g/dL)]) or ionized calcium. The next diagnostic step is the measurement of serum PTH. An elevated (or unexpectedly normal) serum PTH in the face of hypercalcemia is virtually diagnostic of PHPT. Serum phosphate is normal or in the low-normal range in mild PHPT and low in severe cases. A low or undetectable PTH level in a hypercalcemic patient rules out the diagnosis of PHPT. The most common cause of PTH-independent hypercalcemia is malignancy, where hypercalcemia is due to the secretion by the tumor of PTH-related peptide, a molecule that shares with PTH the amino-terminal active part but does not cross-react in the PTH assay, or osteolytic lytic bone metastases. Urinary calcium should also be measured. If hypercalciuria is greater than 400 mg per day, a more extended evaluation of the stone risk profile should be performed. Urinary calcium measurement is also useful to exclude familial hypocalciuric hypercalcemia (FHH), which is suggested by the finding of the calcium-to-creatinine clearance ratio of less than 0.01.

A hereditary form of PHPT, accounting for 5% to 10% of cases, should be sought in patients younger than 30 years at diagnosis, with a family history of hypercalcemia and/or neuroendocrine tumors (see Table 1). In this setting serum calcium should be measured in first-degree relatives and genetic tests performed. Parathyroid cancer should be suspected in individuals, especially males, with marked hypercalcemia, a palpable neck mass, and serum PTH concentration 3 to 10 times the upper normal value. Some ultrasound features may raise the suspicion for cancer, such as a large (i.e., >3 cm) lobulated hypoechoic/heterogeneous parathyroid gland with irregular borders, thick capsule, suspicious vascularity, and calcifications.

Renal ultrasound should be performed in all patients, even in those with no history of nephrolithiasis, since recent studies have shown that silent kidney stones are common in patients with asymptomatic PHPT. Routine BMD testing by dual-energy x-ray absorptiometry (DXA) at the lumbar spine, hip, and distal forearm is also an essential component of the evaluation. BMD is typically low at the one-third distal radius, a site of enriched cortical bone, but a few patients may show predominant cancellous bone involvement, as documented by vertebral osteopenia or osteoporosis. The involvement of the trabecular compartment is also confirmed by the TBS at the lumbar spine. Vertebral imaging by x-ray or DXA (vertebral fracture assessment, VFA) should also be routinely performed to detect silent vertebral deformities since vertebral fracture risk is increased in asymptomatic patients.

Neck imaging (ultrasound and sestamibi scanning) has no value in the diagnosis of PHPT, but it is a useful tool for localizing the abnormal parathyroid gland in patients selected for parathyroidectomy (PTx). Sestamibi has the advantage of localizing the ectopic parathyroid gland outside the neck. The 4D computerized tomography protocol has emerged as a useful tool. Recently 18F-fluorocholine positron emission tomography (PET) has proven to be useful in the localization of hyperfunctioning parathyroid glands before surgery.

Treatment

The aim of treatment is to remove all hyperfunctioning parathyroid tissue, resolve biochemical abnormalities, improve BMD, and decrease the risk of nephrolithiasis and fractures.

Surgical Treatment

Parathyroid surgery represents the only definitive cure of PHPT. Successful PTx normalizes serum calcium and PTH, improves BMD, and decreases the risk of nephrolithiasis and fragility fractures. Patients selected for surgery should be referred to an experienced parathyroid surgeon. A focused, minimally invasive approach, guided by imaging studies associated with intraoperative monitoring of serum PTH, is the preferred surgical procedure in sporadic PHPT. In experienced hands the rate of surgical cure reaches 95% to 98% with a negligible rate of surgical complications. In hereditary cases the surgical approach (bilateral neck exploration by classical cervicotomy) may differ, since multigland involvement is common. An en bloc resection of the parathyroid lesion together with the ipsilateral thyroid lobe with clear gross margins and the adjacent structures is recommended when parathyroid carcinoma is suspected. Particular attention should be paid to avoid seeding of neoplastic parathyroid cells. Surgery should be considered for any patient with a confirmed diagnosis of PHPT and recommended in those with symptomatic disease.

Patients with mild hypercalcemia (serum calcium < 12 mg/dL [3 mmol/L]) can proceed directly to surgery. When serum calcium is higher, preoperative treatment with saline infusion eventually followed by loop diuretics, intravenous bisphosphonates, denosumab (Prolia, Xgeva)[1], or cinacalcet (Sensipar) may be considered to reduce serum calcium levels and decrease the risk of complications, particularly cardiac arrhythmias, which are associated with more severe hypercalcemia.

Surgery is also a reasonable option for patients with asymptomatic PHPT. International guidelines provide guidance to select patients who should be referred for surgery or followed without surgery. The most recent revised (2013) guidelines for surgery or monitoring are reported in Table 2. These guidelines are largely consistent with the previous ones and recommend PTx for all patients with symptomatic PHPT and asymptomatic patients who meet one or more of the indicated criteria. The new indications for surgery in asymptomatic patients include (1) the presence of silent vertebral fractures detected by x-ray, CT, magnetic resonance imaging (MRI), or vertebral fracture assessment (VFA) by DXA; and (2) a 24-hour urinary calcium excretion greater than 400 mg/dL, increased stone risk (evaluated by urinary stone risk profile), and subclinical kidney stone or nephrocalcinosis detected by x-ray, ultrasound, and CT. According to the guidelines, about 60% of patients with asymptomatic PHPT meet the criteria for surgery. As mentioned before, patients with mild PHPT may have subtle cardiovascular abnormalities and complain of psychological and cognitive symptoms. It is unclear whether and to what extent these abnormalities are reversible after successful PTx; for the time being they are not considered indications for surgery. Nonetheless, surgery could be considered in a middle-aged patient in whom asymptomatic PHPT is associated with increased cardiovascular risk (metabolic syndrome, hypertension, ischemic heart disease) if the surgical risk is low.

Randomized clinical trials have also shown that patients with sporadic asymptomatic PHPT who do not meet the surgical criteria may benefit from surgery, not only because it normalizes serum calcium and PTH, but also because it improves BMD and quality of life (QoL). On the other hand, surgery could be postponed in hereditary cases with mild hypercalcemia, because

---

[1]Not FDA approved for this indication.

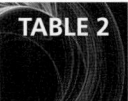

PARAMETER	GUIDELINES FOR SURGERY	GUIDELINES FOR MONITORING
Serum calcium	> 1 mg/dL (0.25 mmol/L) above the upper normal limit	Annually
Skeletal	• BMD by DXA: T-score < −2.5 at lumbar spine, femoral neck, total hip, or distal one-third radius • Vertebral fractures by x-ray, CT, MRI, or VFA	• BMD by DXA every 1–2 years at lumbar spine, total hip, or distal one-third radius • Spine x-ray of VFA when clinically indicated (e.g., back pain or height loss)

Renal	• Creatinine clearance < 60 mL/min
	• Daily urinary calcium excretion > 400 mg and increased stone risk by the urinary biochemical stone risk profile
	• Nephrolithiasis or nephrocalcinosis by x-ray, ultrasound, or CT
		• Serum creatinine annually
		• If renal stone suspected:
		  • 24-h urinary biochemical stone risk profile
		  • Renal imaging by x-ray, ultrasound, or CT

Age	< 50 years	-

Abbreviations: BMD = bone mineral density; CT = computed tomography; DXA = dual x-ray absorptiometry; MRI = magnetic resonance imaging; PHPT = primary hyperparathyroidism; VFA = vertebral fracture assessment.
Modified from Bilezikian et al. Guidelines for the management of asymptomatic primary hyperparathyroidism: Summary statement from the fourth international workshop. *J Clin Endocrinol Metab* 99:3561, 2014.

multigland disease, occasionally with asynchronous involvement of the various parathyroid glands, is not uncommon and carries an increased risk of surgical complications and recurrence/persistence of PHPT.

Therefore individual counseling addressing the benefits and risks of PTx is mandatory, and the preference of the patients should be taken into account. It is well known that parathyroid surgery, when performed by skilled neck surgeons, is safe, cost-effective, and associated with low perioperative morbidity. On the other hand, it is important to recognize that PTx, particularly if performed by inexperienced surgeons, may be associated with complications that could be invalidating and not acceptable for a patient with mild disease and a good QoL. In this regard, the choice of surgery may be reconsidered in a patient with asymptomatic PHPT in whom parathyroid surgery was initially advised or selected by the patient when preoperative imaging studies are negative. Indeed, in this setting the patient may feel uncomfortable undergoing a blind neck exploration, a surgical procedure more extensive than the minimally invasive approach and carrying the greatest risk of complications.

Nonsurgical Management
As mentioned before, many patients with PHPT do not meet the criteria for surgery. These patients, as well as those who decline surgery or have contraindications to surgery, need to be monitored.

Monitoring. Randomized clinical studies have shown stability over a short period of observation (up to 2 years) in patients with asymptomatic PHPT followed without surgery and benefits in those who underwent PTx even if they did not meet the criteria for surgery. The extension up to 5 years of one of these randomized studies has shown a more frequent occurrence of a vertebral fracture in patients belonging to the observation group than in those cured by PTx. Long-term observational studies indicate that the disease remains stable in the majority for up to 8 to 9

years, but more than one-third of patients show a progression of the disease.

Calcium intake should not be restricted, and an intake appropriate for age and sex as in the general population (preferably with food) should be recommended. Vitamin D–depleted patients should be supplemented with daily doses of 800 to 1000 IU of vitamin D; weekly or monthly doses calculated on this daily dose can also be used. A serum level of 25(OH)D greater than 20 ng/mL should be reached, and the attainment of a higher target (> 30 ng/mL) is suggested by some guidelines.

General principles for monitoring are reported in Table 2. Serum calcium and creatinine (estimated glomerular filtration rate [eGFR]) should be measured annually and BMD at the lumbar spine, total hip, and distal forearm measured every 1 to 2 years. Vertebral morphometry (by x-ray or VFA) should be performed when clinically indicated (back pain, height loss). Finally, 24-hour urinary collection for biochemical stone risk profile and renal imaging (x-ray, ultrasound, or CT) should be performed if there is a suspicion of renal stones.

Parathyroid surgery should be recommended in patients who are followed without surgery in the following instances: (1) serum calcium concentration greater than 1 mg/dL above the upper normal limit; (2) creatinine clearance less than 60 mL/min; (3) detection of nephrocalcinosis or kidney stones; (4) BMD T-score at any site less than −2.5 or the finding of a significant (greater than the least significant change as defined by the International Society for Clinical Densitometry) decrease of BMD, even if the T-score is not less than −2.5; and (5) clinical fractures or morphometric vertebral fractures, even if asymptomatic.

Medical Treatment. No medical treatment is currently available to cure PHPT. Therefore when PTx is indicated and there are no contraindications for surgery, medical treatment should not be considered a valuable alternative option. Medical treatment may be considered for patients who have contraindications to surgery or are unwilling to undergo PTx, as well as for those who have failed surgery. Treatment should be guided by the aim of therapy.

Calcimimetics. If the aim of treatment is to reduce serum calcium, the calcimimetic cinacalcet (Sensipar) can be effective. The serum calcium typically declines over a few weeks and may normalize in most patients with moderate hypercalcemia. In addition, cinacalcet increases serum phosphate and only slightly reduces PTH concentration, but has no effect on BMD. The beneficial effects are sustained over time as long as the drug is used. Adverse events are dose related: modest and transient when low doses of cinacalcet are used (up to 30 mg twice daily), but rather frequent, particularly gastrointestinal, symptoms, occasionally severe enough to require treatment withdrawal, when higher doses are employed. The use of cinacalcet has been approved by the US Food and Drug administration (FDA) for the treatment of severe hypercalcemia in patients with PHPT who are unable to undergo PTx, and by the European Medical Agency (EMA) for the reduction of hypercalcemia in patients with PHPT, for whom PTx would be indicated on the basis of serum calcium levels (as defined by relevant guidelines), but in whom surgery is not clinically appropriate or contraindicated. As clearly stated, the EMA indications leave more room for the use of cinacalcet.

Cinacalcet should not be used as an initial treatment or in patients who do not meet the approved criteria for its prescription. The long-term safety of cinacalcet has not been established. Moreover, the rather high cost is another important limit for its long-term use.

Antiresorptive Therapy. If the aim is to increase BMD, antiresorptive therapy can be considered. Alendronate (Fosamax) is the bisphosphonate that has been more extensively used and shown to be effective in reducing bone turnover markers and increasing BMD. Over a short period of time, its effectiveness in increasing BMD is comparable to that observed after successful PTx. No effect has been shown on serum calcium and PTH levels. BMD also improved in a retrospective study that included 50 elderly women treated with denodumab for 2 years.

Combined Therapy With Cinacalcet and Antiresorptive Therapy. As mentioned before, cinacalcet is effective in the control of hypercalcemia but has no effect on BMD. Conversely, bisphosphonates increase BMD, with no effect on serum calcium. Limited data indicate that combination therapy is associated with both the calcium-lowering effect of cinacalcet and the skeletal advantage of bisphosphonates. Therefore if a patient has a low BMD and serum calcium concentration appropriate for the use of cinacalcet, combined therapy could be of benefit. A recent study has shown that denosumab[1] is effective in increasing BMD and lowering bone turnover irrespective of cinacalcet treatment and might be a valid option for patients in which surgery is undesirable.

Pregnancy and Lactation

PHPT may be diagnosed during pregnancy by the finding of hypercalcemia on routine blood testing. There are some distinctive features that should be considered in the evaluation and management: (1) pregnancy is associated with hemodilution and occasionally hypoalbuminemia, and therefore it would be preferable to measure ionized calcium; (2) the hereditary form should be sought because of the young age of pregnant women; and (3) women with mild elevation of calcium should be managed conservatively, mostly by hydration—in the case of worsening of hypercalcemia PTx in the second trimester and cinacalcet[1] may be considered.

Secondary Hyperparathyroidism

Secondary hyperparathyroidism (SHPT) defines any condition in which the increased PTH secretion occurs as a normal physiologic response, often mediated by a decrease of serum calcium. Vitamin D deficiency, as a result of inadequate nutritional intake/sun exposure, malabsorption, liver diseases, or chronic renal failure, is the most common cause. Other, less common causes include vitamin D resistance (Fanconi syndrome, vitamin D receptor defects), PTH resistance (pseudohypoparathyroidism, hypomagnesemia), drugs (calcium chelators, inhibitors of bone resorption, and drugs that interfere with vitamin D metabolism [phenytoin and ketoconazole]), acute pancreatitis, and osteoblastic metastases (prostate and breast cancer).

SHPT should always be considered and ruled out before making the diagnosis of normocalcemic PHPT. At variance with PHPT, SHPT is characterized by low or, more often, low-normal serum calcium and decreased urinary calcium excretion. An elevation of serum phosphate levels can be a clue to pseudohypoparathyroidism.

A prolonged stimulation of PTH synthesis and secretion, as may occur in end-stage renal failure and severe gastrointestinal diseases, may lead to the emergence of an autonomous clone of parathyroid cells into a single gland, leading to hypercalcemia (tertiary hyperparathyroidism).

Hypoparathyrodism

Hypoparathyroidism (HypoPT) is the clinical spectrum caused by insufficient production of PTH by the parathyroid glands. The major distinguishing feature is hypocalcemia, resulting from inadequate mobilization of calcium from bone and reabsorption of calcium at the distal tubule, and decreased activity of renal 1α-hydroxylase and therefore generation of calcitriol; as a consequence, the intestinal calcium absorption will be reduced.

Epidemiology

HypoPT is a rare condition designated in both the United States and Europe as an orphan disease. The estimated prevalence is 37 and 24 per 100,000 inhabitants in the United States and Europe, respectively.

Pathogenesis

HypoPT can be congenital or acquired (Table 3).

---

[1]Not FDA approved for this indication.

TABLE 3	Classification of Hypoparathyroidism*

Congenital

- Isolated
  - Defective PTH biosynthesis (*PTH*) ^
  - Abnormal development of parathyroid glands (*GCMB, GCM2, GATA3*)
  - Autosomal dominant hypocalcemia
    - Type 1 (*CASR*)
    - Type 2 (*GNA11*)
- Associated with additional features or organ defects
  - Autoimmune
    - Isolated
    - Polyglandular syndrome type 1 (*AIRE*)
  - Di George syndrome (*TBX1*)
  - Sanjad-Sakati/Kenny-Caffey type 2 (*TBCE*)
  - Kenny-Caffey type 2 (*FAM111A*)
  - Mitochondrial DNA mutations
- Defective action of PTH
  - Pseudohypoparathyroidism
    - Type 1a (*GNAS*)
    - Type 1b (*STX16, GNAS*; in sporadic form paternal UPD)
    - Type 1c (*GNAS*)
    - Type 2 (not yet identified)

Acquired

- Destruction or removal of the parathyroid glands
  - Postoperative (neck surgery)
  - Radiation induced
  - Infiltration of the parathyroid glands (metastatic, granulomatous)
  - Deposition of heavy metals (iron, copper)
- Reversible impairment or PTH secretion or action
  - Severe magnesium deficiency
  - Hypermagnesemia (e.g., due to tocolytic therapy)
- CaSR-stimulating antibodies

*Mutated genes are indicated in parentheses.
Abbreviations: AIRE = autoimmune regulatory; CASR = calcium-sensing receptor; FAM111A = family with sequence similarity 111 member A; GATA3 = GATA-binding protein 3; GCM2 = glial cell missing homolog 2; GCMB = glial cell missing gene; GNA11 = G protein subunit alpha 11; GNAS = GNAS complex locus; PTH = parathyroid hormone; STX16 = syntaxin 16; TBCE = tubulin folding cofactor E; TBX1 = T-Box1; UPD = uniparental disomy.

Congenital HypoPT is usually hereditary and may be isolated or combined with organ defects. The autoimmune is the most common form and may be either isolated or part of the autoimmune polyglandular syndrome type 1 (APS1). The other forms are much more rare.

Acquired HypoPT is much more common than the congenital counterpart. Bilateral neck surgery for thyroid or parathyroid disorders is the most common cause. Postoperative HypoPT can be transient (caused by reversible parathyroid ischemia and resolving within a few weeks) or chronic/permanent (caused by irreversible parathyroid damage such as ischemia, electric scalpel damage, or, rarely, inadvertent removal of parathyroid glands). Its rate largely depends on the experience of the surgeon and the extent of the neck surgery.

Clinical Presentation

The clinical manifestations of HypoPT are largely related to the level of serum calcium and the speed of its fall and may range from asymptomatic cases, when hypocalcemia is mild (corrected calcium ≥ 7.0 mg/dL [1.75 mmol/L]), to a severe, life-threating condition that requires hospital admission and intensive treatment. In mild cases signs related to neuromuscular irritability, namely the Chvostek sign (twitching and/or contracture of the facial muscles produced by tapping on the facial nerve just anterior to the ear and just below the zygomatic bone) and Trousseau sign (carpal spasm evoked by inflating a sphygmomanometer cuff above systolic blood pressure for several minutes), may be present at physical examination. Moderate to severe hypocalcemia

TABLE 4 Calcium Preparation and Vitamin D Metabolites in the Management of Hypocalcemia

Calcium

AGENT	FORMULATION AND DOSE	COMMENTS
Calcium gluconate	One ampule of 10% calcium gluconate contains 93 mg; preferably diluted in 5% dextrose	Tissue necrosis may be caused by elemental calcium; preferably diluted in 5% dextrose extravasation in the adjacent subcutaneous space
Calcium salts		
Calcium carbonate	40% elemental calcium by weight: 1 g calcium carbonate contains 400 mg elemental calcium	Best absorbed with meals in an acidic environment; constipation is a common side effect
Calcium citrate	21% elemental calcium by weight, 1 g calcium citrate contains 210 mg elemental calcium	Well absorbed independent of meal and acid environment; in patients with atrophic gastritis or taking proton pump inhibitors

Vitamin D Metabolites

MEDICATION	TYPICAL DAILY DOSE	TIME TO ONSET OF ACTION	TIME TO OFFSET OF ACTION
Calcitriol [$1,25(OH)_2D$]$_3$ (Rocaltrol)	0.25–2.0 µg once or twice	1–2 days	2–3 days
Alfacalcidol* [$1\alpha(OH)D$]*	0.5–4 µg once	1–2 days	5–7 days
Dihydrotachysterol*,†	0.3–1.0 mg once	4–7 days	7–21 days
Vitamin D_2 (ergocalciferol) (Drisdol) or vitamin D_3 (cholecalciferol)‡	25,000–200,000 IU	10–14 days	14–75 days

*Not available in the United States.
†This compound is rapidly activated in the liver to 25(OH) dihydrotachysterol.
‡These compounds could be used in a setting where active vitamin D metabolites are not available and/or are too expensive.
Modified from Shoback D: Clinical practice. Hypoparathyroidism. *N Engl J Med* 2008;359:391–403, 2008.

(corrected calcium < 7.0 mg/dL [1.75 mmol/L]) is usually symptomatic, even though there is no strict relationship between the severity of symptoms and the degree of hypocalcemia. In patients with postoperative HypoPT, symptoms usually appear on the first postoperative day, but in some cases hypocalcemia may become clinically manifest even after 3 to 4 days. Classical manifestations include paresthesias, carpopedal spasm, tetany, seizures, positive Chvostek and Trousseau signs, and prolongation of the QT interval on electrocardiography. Papilledema and subcapsular cataract can be present. Pseudohypoparathyroidism is a group of genetic disorders caused by end-organ resistance to the action of PTH. Patients with the type 1a variant have a typical phenotype (Albright hereditary osteodystrophy), characterized by short stature, shortened fourth and fifth metacarpals, rounded face, and mild intellectual deficiency. Other endocrine glands, including the thyroid and the gonads, may be dysfunctional. This clinical and endocrine phenotype is also typical of patients with type 1c. Patients with type 1b have PTH resistance and in some cases partial resistance to thyroid-stimulating hormone (TSH) and mild brachydactyly. Patients with the type 2 variant have PTH resistance in the absence of the aforementioned clinical phenotype.

Evaluation and Diagnosis

The finding of low albumin-corrected serum calcium, high serum phosphate, and inappropriately low or undetectable serum PTH confirms the diagnosis of HypoPT. A recent neck surgery strongly suggests the postoperative form. A family history of hypocalcemia suggests a genetic cause. Coexistence of other autoimmune endocrinopathies (i.e., adrenal insufficiency) or candidiasis prompts consideration of APS1. Immunodeficiency and the presence of other congenital organ defects point to DiGeorge syndrome. Genetic testing may be warranted to confirm the diagnosis of this and other genetic forms. Magnesium should also be measured because magnesium deficiency impairs the secretion of PTH and its action in target tissues. Urinary calcium is usually low because of the low filtered calcium. The 24-hour calcium-to-creatinine clearance ratio is increased in patients with the activating

mutation of *CaSR*. A biochemical profile of low serum calcium and high phosphate levels, together with high serum PTH, in the absence of vitamin D deficiency, reflects the PTH-resistant state, and suggests a case of pseudohypoparathyroidism.

Treatment

The goal is to control symptoms of hypocalcemia and improve QoL while avoiding side effects and complications. The target serum calcium concentration is in the lower part of the normal range. Treatment relies on the administration of calcium (oral [dietary or supplements] or intravenous), active vitamin D metabolites, magnesium, and, where available, recombinant human PTH$_{1-84}$ (Natpara). Thiazide diuretics may help reduce hypercalciuria; a low-phosphate diet and phosphate binders may help control hypophosphatemia and lower the calcium–phosphate product.

Acute Hypoparathyroidism

Acute hypocalcemia typically follows neck surgery and may be favored by a low vitamin D status and magnesium deficiency that, when present, should be corrected before surgery. In patients with high risk (total thyroidectomy, repeated thyroid surgery), perioperative administration of calcitriol (Rocaltrol) decreases the incidence of postoperative hypocalcemia and shortens the hospital stay.

Mild Hypocalcemia. In mild hypocalcemia (corrected calcium ≥ 7.0 mg/dL [1.75 mmol/L]), oral calcium supplements (usually calcium carbonate, 1–3 grams daily in divided doses) alone or combined with active vitamin D metabolites should be administered. Calcitriol is typically initiated at an initial dose of 0.5 to 1.0 µg twice daily; equivalent doses of 1α-calcifediol[2] (1.0–2.0 µg) may also be used (see later [Chronic Hypoparathyroidism, Conventional Therapy] for more details on calcium and active vitamin D therapy) (Table 4). Serum calcium is checked weekly until optimal levels are reached.

---

[2]Not available in the United States.

Moderate to Severe Hypocalcemia. Patients with moderate to severe hypocalcemia (corrected calcium <7.0 mg/dL [1.75 mmol/L]) are usually admitted to the hospital and treated with IV calcium until an oral regimen can be started. One to two ampules of 10% calcium gluconate diluted in 50 to 100 mL of 5% dextrose should be infused over a period of 10 to 20 minutes with electrocardiographic and clinical monitoring. The calcium infusion will raise the serum calcium concentration for no more than 2 to 4 hours; thus this initial treatment should be followed by a continuous infusion (50–100 mL/h) of a solution containing 1 mg/mL of elemental calcium (11 ampules of 10% calcium gluconate added to 5% dextrose in a final volume of 1 liter). The rate should be adjusted according to corrected serum calcium level, which should be measured initially every 1 to 2 hours and subsequently every 4 to 6 hours, and maintained at the lower limit of the normal range, while the patient is asymptomatic. This calcium infusion protocol maintained for 8 to 10 hours will raise serum calcium by approximately 2 mg/dL. Oral administration of active vitamin D metabolites and calcium should be started as soon as practical. Calcitriol is typically initiated at a dose of 0.5 to 1.0 µg twice daily; oral calcium (1–3 g daily in divided doses) is also added.

If hypocalcemia is due to magnesium deficiency, the previous protocol should be applied while magnesium is being replaced by administering IV magnesium sulfate (initial dose 2 g as a 10% solution over 10–20 minutes, followed by 1 g/h in 100 mL) until a normal serum level of magnesium is reached. The only administration of magnesium will be unable to correct hypocalcemia because hypomagnesemia inhibits the secretion of PTH, and consequently the renal activation of 25OHD and induces a peripheral resistance to the action of PTH.

The rate of calcium infusion should be increased if symptoms of hypocalcemia recur. The IV infusion should be slowly tapered and discontinued when an effective regimen of oral calcium and active vitamin D is reached (up to 24–48 hours or longer) and stable desired serum calcium levels are obtained.

Chronic Hypoparathyroidism

The goal of therapy is to maintain serum calcium in the low-normal range, avoid hypocalcemic symptoms and long-term complications, and improve QoL. An individualized approach is necessary to optimize patient care. Guidelines for the management of chronic HypoPT have only recently been developed by the European Society of Endocrinology, the American Association of Clinical Endocrinologists, the American College of Endocrinology, and a panel of international experts.

Conventional Therapy. An adequate calcium intake from dietary sources (mainly dairy products) should be recommended, but calcium supplements (1–3 g daily in divided doses) are needed in almost all adult patients. Calcium carbonate is generally preferred because fewer pills per day are needed. Calcium carbonate requires an acidic gastric environment to be absorbed and should be taken with meals. Its bioavailability decreases in patients with atrophic gastritis or taking proton pump inhibitors. In these circumstances, calcium citrate, which is well absorbed independent of meal and acid environments, should be preferred. Calcium citrate might also be a preferred option for patients who complain of gastrointestinal side effects using calcium carbonate or who prefer to take calcium supplements outside mealtimes. Calcium carbonate and calcium citrate interfere with levothyroxine absorption; therefore thyroidectomized patients should be advised to take levothyroxine well apart from calcium supplements.

Prior to the availability of synthetic active vitamin D metabolites, supraphysiologic doses (25,000–200,000 IU daily) of either cholecalciferol (vitamin D_3) or ergocalciferol (vitamin D_2) were used (Table 4). Nowadays, active 1α-hydroxylated vitamin D metabolites are preferred because patients with HypoPT have impaired renal activation of 25-hydroxivitamin D. Calcitriol

(Rocaltrol) and alfacalcidol (One-Alpha)[2] have a similar time of onset, but the latter has a longer time of offset (5–7 vs. 2–3 days). Calcitriol is more potent (about 50%) than alfacalcidol when compared in terms of the calcemic effect. The daily dose of calcitriol in adults ranges between 0.25 and 2.0 µg, equal to 0.5 to 4 µg of alfacalcidol. Weight-based dosing (0.01–0.04 µg per kg peer day), eventually associated with calcium supplements (20–40 mg per kg per day) should be used in infants and young children. Adult doses should be used in older children. Another active vitamin D analog, dihydrotachysterol, is also available in some countries. Where active vitamin D metabolites are not available or too expensive, large doses of parent vitamin D can still be used, but attention should be paid to the risk of vitamin D toxicity.

A low vitamin D status is not uncommon in patients with HypoPT, and vitamin D–deficient patients treated with active vitamin D metabolites should be supplemented with vitamin D_2 or D_3, because active vitamin D metabolites do not correct hypovitaminosis D.

Active vitamin D metabolites stimulate intestinal absorption of phosphate, which may cause hyperphosphatemia and an increased calcium–phosphate product, with the risk of soft tissue calcification. In this setting the intake of phosphate-rich foods should be reduced and the daily dose of calcium supplements increased, since calcium binds phosphate.

Hypercalciuria (≥ 250 mg [6.25 mmol] in women or ≥ 300 mg [7.5 mmol] in men or > 4 mg [0.1 mmol]/kg body weight in both sexes) is a common feature in patients with chronic HypoPT, because of the lack of PTH-dependent renal tubular reabsorption of calcium. In such instances a low-sodium diet should be advised either alone or combined with the administration of a thiazide diuretic that decreases renal calcium excretion. The combination of thiazide with amiloride[1] may further lower urinary calcium excretion and decrease the risk of hypokalemia. Thiazide diuretics are not advised in autosomal dominant hypocalcemia, a condition caused by mutations of the CaSR. Magnesium deficiency, when present, should also be corrected.

Lifelong monitoring is needed in patients with chronic HypoPTH. No study has evaluated how to best monitor these patients. The target serum calcium concentration is within the low-normal range, with no symptoms of hypocalcemia. In some patients a higher serum calcium level is needed to be symptom-free. A baseline renal imaging should be obtained. The recently published guidelines of the European Society of Endocrinology suggest measuring ionized or albumin-corrected total calcium, magnesium, and creatinine (eGFR) and 24-hour urinary calcium excretion every 3 to 6 months and performing renal imaging when patients have symptoms of nephrolithiasis or increasing serum levels of creatinine. Biochemical monitoring should be performed weekly or every other week when changing the daily dose of calcium or active vitamin D metabolites or introducing a new drug. It is important to note that serum calcium may fluctuate once the therapeutic regimen has been stabilized. Several comorbidities (e.g., gastrointestinal disease, diarrhea, immobilization) and drugs (loop and thiazide diuretics, systemic glucocorticoids, proton pump inhibitors, antiresorptive drugs, cardiac glycosides, and chemotherapeutics) may interfere with calcium homeostasis, and therefore patients should be periodically asked about their occurrence or use.

Conventional therapy only partially restores calcium homeostasis, and patients with chronic HypoPT have a reduced QoL and an increased risk of comorbidities, which include nephrocalcinosis, nephrolithiasis, impaired renal function, neuropsychiatric diseases, muscle stiffness and pain, infections, and seizures. An increased rate of intracerebral calcifications and cataracts has been documented in nonsurgical HypoPT. Bone mineral content

---

[2]Not available in the United States.
[1]Not FDA approved for this indication.

is increased in patients with chronic HypoPT, but cancellous bone microarchitecture is abnormal.

Parathyroid Hormone. Until recently, HypoPT was the only major hormonal insufficiency state not treated with the missing hormone. The development of the recombinant human N-terminal 1-34 fragment ($rhPTH_{1-34}$) and the full-length 1-84 ($rhPTH_{1-84}$) molecule has stimulated several studies on its use as replacement therapy, which led to the approval by the Food and Drug Administration of $rhPTH_{1-84}$ (Natpara) for the management of chronic HypoPT.

The official recommendation is to consider $rhPTH_{1-84}$ therapy "only in patients who cannot be well-controlled on calcium and active forms of vitamin D and for whom the potential benefits are considered to outweigh the potential risk." Treatment should be started with subcutaneous administration in the thigh of 50 μg once daily, while reducing by 50% the daily dose of active vitamin D if serum calcium is greater than 7.5 mg/dL (1.875 mmol/L). Serum calcium should be monitored every 3 to 7 days and the daily dose of $rhPTH_{1-84}$ titrated every 4 weeks, aiming to reduce the daily calcium supplements to 500 mg and discontinue active vitamin D therapy while maintaining the serum calcium in the low-normal range. Afterward, serum calcium should be monitored every 3 to 6 months. Hypercalcemia has been reported in some cases, but a careful adjustment of the daily dose may decrease this risk. A "black box" in the official recommendation highlights the potential risk of osteosarcoma (studies in rats have shown that both $rhPTH_{1-34}$ and $rhPTH_{1-84}$ can cause osteosarcoma). However, there is no evidence that individuals treated with either PTH molecules are at increased risk for osteosarcoma. The safety and efficacy of $rhPTH_{1-84}$ in pediatric patients have not been established. The European Medicines Agency has approved the use of $rhPTH_{1-84}$ as an adjunctive therapy for adults with chronic hypoparathyroidism who cannot be adequately controlled with standard therapy alone.

The FDA, the European Medicines Agency, and Filomena Centani, MD, PhD have approved using $rhPTH_{1-84}$ in patient with HypoPT, and that leaves room for decision making in individual cases. The guidelines recently elaborated by a panel of international experts suggest considering the use of $rhPTH_{1-84}$ therapy, where available, in any patient with chronic HypoPT of any etiology, except in patients with autosomal dominant hypocalcemia.

Pregnancy and Lactation

There are limited data to inform treatment strategies in chronic HypoPT in pregnancy and lactation. The guidelines of the European Society of Endocrinology suggest the use of active vitamin D metabolites and oral calcium as in nonpregnant women. Frequent monitoring (every 2–3 weeks) of serum calcium, possibly ionized calcium, is recommended. No studies have addressed the use of $rhPTH_{1-84}$ therapy in pregnant women. The FDA suggests that it should be used "only if the potential benefit justifies the potential risk to the fetus."

References

Arnold A, Levine A: Molecular basis of primary hyperparathyroidism. In Bilezikan JP, et al, editor: *The Parathyroids, Basic and Clincial Concept*, London, 2015, Academic Press, pp 279–296.

Bilezikian JP, Bandeira L, Khan A, et al: Hyperparathyrodism, *Lancet* 1:168178, 2018.

Bilezikian JP, Brandi ML, Eastell R, et al: Guidelines for the management of asymptomatic primary hyperparathyroidism: summary statement from the fourth international workshop, *J Clin Endocrinol Metab* 99:3561–3569, 2014.

Bilezikian JP, Cusano NE, Khan AA, et al: Primary hyperparathyroidism, *Nat Rev Dis Primers* 2:16033, 2016.

Bilezikian JP, Khan A, Potts Jr JT, et al: Hypoparathyroidism in the adult: epidemiology, diagnosis, pathophysiology, target-organ involvement, treatment, and challenges for future research, *J Bone Miner Res* 26:2317–2337, 2011.

Bollerslev J, Rejnmark L, Marcocci C, et al: European Society of Endocrinology Clinical Guideline: treatment of chronic hypoparathyroidism in adults, *Eur J Endocrinol* 173:G1–G20, 2015.

Brandi ML, Bilezikian JP, Shoback D, et al: Management of hypoparathyroidism: summary statement and guidelines, *J Clin Endocrinol Metab* 101:2273–2283, 2016.

Cetani F, Marcocci C: Parathyroid carcinoma. In Bilezikian JP, editor: *The Parathyroids. Basic and Clincial Concepts*, London, 2015, Academic Press, pp 409–422.

Cetani F, Pardi E, Aretini P, et al: Whole exome sequencing in familial isolated primary hyperparathyroidism, *J Endocrinol Invest* 43:231–245, 2020.

Cusano NE, Silverberg SJ, Bilezikian JP: Normocalcemic primary hyperparathyroidism, *J Clin Densitom* 16:33–39, 2013.

EMA/CHMP/124164/2017 Media and Public Relations, 2017: http://www.ema.europa.eu/docs/en_GB/document_library/Press_release/2017/02/WC500222215.pdf.

Khan AA, Koch C, Van Uum SHM, et al: Standards of care for hypoparathyroidism in adults, *Eur J Endocrinol* EJE-18-0609.R1. doi:10.1530/EJE-18-0609. [Epub ahead of print], 2018.

Leere JS, Karmisholt J, Robaczyk M, et al: Denosumab and cinacalcet for primary hyperparathyroidism (DENOCINA): a randomised, double-blind, placebo-controlled, phase 3 trial, *Lancet Diabetes Endocrinol* 8:407–417, 2020.

Mannstadt M, Bilezikian JP, Thakker RV, et al: Hypoparathyroidism, *Nat Rev Dis Primers* 3:17055, 2017. http://www.ema.europa.eu/docs/en_GB/document_library/Press_release/2017/02/WC500222215.pdf.

Mannstadt M, Clarke BL, Vokes T, et al: Efficacy and safety of recombinant human parathyroid hormone (1-84) in hypoparathyroidism (REPLACE): a double-blind, placebo-controlled, randomised, phase 3 study, *Lancet Diabetes Endocrinol* 1:275–283, 2013.

Marcocci C, Bollerslev J, Khan AA, Shoback DM: Medical management of primary hyperparathyroidism: proceedings of the fourth international workshop on the management of asymptomatic primary hyperparathyroidism, *J Clin Endocrinol Metab* 99:3607–3618, 2014.

Marcocci C, Cetani F: Clinical practice, *Primary hyperparathyroidism, N Engl J Med* 365:2389–2397, 2011.

NATPARA: Shire-NPS Pharmaceuticals, Inc, 2015: [package insert]. In https://www.accessdata.fda.gov/drugsatfda_docs/label/2015/125511s000lbl.pdf.

NATPAR. https://www.ema.europa.eu/en/medicines/human/EPAR/natpar.

Rubin MR, Bilezikian JP, McMahon DJ, et al: The natural history of primary hyperparathyroidism with or without parathyroid surgery after 15 years, *J Clin Endocrinol Metab* 93:3462–3470, 2008.

Sidhu PS, Talat N, Patel P, et al: Ultrasound features of malignancy in the preoperative diagnosis of parathyroid cancer: a retrospective analysis of parathyroid tumours larger than 15 mm, *Eur Radiol* 211865-73, 2011.

Shoback D: Clinical practice. Hypoparathyroidism, *N Engl J Med* 359:391–403, 2008.

Shoback DM, Bilezikian JP, Costa AG, et al: Presentation of hypoparathyroidism: etiologies and clinical features, *J Clin Endocrinol Metab* 101:2300–2312, 2016.

Treglia G, Piccardo A, Imperiale A, et al: Diagnostic performance of choline PET for detection of hyperfunctioning parathyroid glands in hyperparathyroidism: a systematic review and meta-analysis, *Eur J Nucl Med Mol Imaging* 46:751–765, 2019.

Udelsman R, Akerstrom G, Biagini C, et al: The surgical management of asymptomatic primary hyperparathyroidism: proceedings of the fourth international workshop, *J Clin Endocrinol Metab* 99:3595–3606, 2014.

Vignali E, Viccica G, Diacinti D, et al: Morphometric vertebral fractures in postmenopausal women with primary hyperparathyroidism, *J Clin Endocrinol Metab* 94:2306–2312, 2009.

HYPERPROLACTINEMIA

Method of
Ming Li, MD, PhD; and Lawrence Chan, MD

CURRENT DIAGNOSIS

- Hyperprolactinemia is diagnosed by biochemical tests based on two-site immunoassay, which can be confounded by extreme hyperprolactinemia (hook effect) and biologically inactive macroprolactinemia.
- Hyperprolactinemia can be caused by physiological, pharmacological, or pathological conditions; careful clinical, laboratory, and radiology evaluations are required to identify its underlying cause.
- The most common causes of hyperprolactinemia include medications, prolactinoma, and other pituitary and hypothalamic/pituitary stalk diseases.
- Clinical features of hyperprolactinemia include galactorrhea, menstrual abnormalities (in women), impotence (in men), infertility, and osteoporosis.
- Patients with prolactinoma may also have local compression symptoms including headache, visual disturbance, and hypopituitarism.
- Pituitary magnetic resonance imaging (MRI) is the imaging method of choice for diagnosing prolactinoma and other sellar/parasellar lesions.

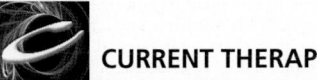

CURRENT THERAPY

- For secondary hyperprolactinemia, treatment should be directed at correcting underlying causes.
- Treatment goals for prolactinoma are relief of symptoms and the long-term effects of hyperprolactinemia, and of tumor mass effects.
- The dopamine agonists cabergoline (Dostinex) and bromocriptine (Parlodel) are effective in normalizing the prolactin level and shrinking the tumor in patients with prolactinoma.
- Surgery and radiotherapy of prolactinoma are reserved for patients resistant to or intolerant of medical therapy.
- Temozolomide (Temodar)[1] monotherapy is the first-line chemotherapy for aggressive or malignant prolactinomas after failing standard treatments.

[1]Not FDA approved for this indication.

Biochemistry and Physiology of Prolactin

Prolactin is a polypeptide hormone produced by pituitary lactotroph cells. It is also produced locally in a variety of extrapituitary tissues such as mammary glands, decidua, gonads, brain, liver, fat, pancreas, and the immune system, along with its receptors. Prolactin is highly pleiotropic in terms of its functions. Many of its actions collectively support puerperal lactation. Prolactin displays considerable sequence homology to growth hormone (GH) and placental lactogen. The prolactin and GH receptors both belong to the class I cytokine/hematopoietic receptor superfamily. Prolactin is responsible for maturation of the mammary glands during pregnancy, but it plays only a minor role for pubertal mammary development, which requires GH instead. It appears not to be an essential hormone for non-childbearing individuals. Rare patients deficient for either prolactin or its receptor are largely healthy despite difficulty with fertility and lactation.

Prolactin circulates mainly as a 23-kDa 199-aa polypeptide. Several of its cleavage products exist in blood, which may have functions unrelated to lactation; for example, one 16-kDa cleavage product of prolactin displays antiangiogenic and prothrombotic properties, and has been implicated in the development of preeclampsia and peripartum cardiomyopathy. Several forms of prolactin aggregate, known as macroprolactins, also exist in circulation at lower levels. They are formed either by covalent bonding of prolactin monomers or by their nucleating around autoimmune IgG. These macroprolactins are not biologically active in vivo and have a prolonged half-life. At times they can build up in the circulation to a level high enough to cause diagnostic difficulties.

Among the major pituitary hormones, prolactin is unique for its predominantly negative mode of regulation by the hypothalamus. It does not have a known hypothalamus-derived releasing hormone. Instead, lactotrophs are under tonic inhibition by dopamine secreted from hypothalamic neurons. Increase in prolactin output is mostly mediated by withdrawing dopaminergic control in response to environmental cues, such as physical activity, stress, and nipple stimuli (Figure 1). Under experimental and pathological conditions, several factors, including thyrotropin-releasing hormone (TRH), vasoactive intestinal peptide (VIP), oxytocin, and vasopressin, have been shown to increase prolactin secretion, but these peptides appear to play only minor and insignificant roles for the physiological regulation of prolactin.

Estrogen is the main driver of prolactin secretion during pregnancy. Stimulated by persistently elevated estrogen, lactotrophs grow in number and size. By term the pituitary gland can reach 2 to 3 times its normal size, and prolactin levels increase some 20-fold. Along with placental hormones such as estrogen, progesterone, and placental lactogen, prolactin drives the maturation of the mammary glands. Lactation starts after parturition, when estrogen withdraws from the circulation. Frequent infant suckling maintains physiological hyperprolactinemia, which is important for sustained milk production. In addition, hyperprolactinemia during this critical period provides a natural though unreliable way of contraception. This is achieved by suppression of the hypothalamus–pituitary–gonad axis. Hyperprolactinemic hypogonadism and parathyroid hormone related peptide (PTHrP) secreted from mammary epithelial cells help mobilize skeletal calcium store in support of milk production. Through its receptors in liver, intestine, fat, and pancreas prolactin also adjusts maternal nutrient metabolism for optimal milk output. In the brain, prolactin modifies parental behavior toward closer infant attendance (see Figure 1).

Pathophysiology of Hyperprolactinemia

Physiological hyperprolactinemia as occurs during pregnancy and nursing is essential for child raising through the actions of prolactin in target organs discussed above. Similar changes in these organs under the influence of persistent pathological hyperprolactinemia in the absence of pregnancy and lactation, however, are inappropriate and could lead to a variety of undesired long-term consequences.

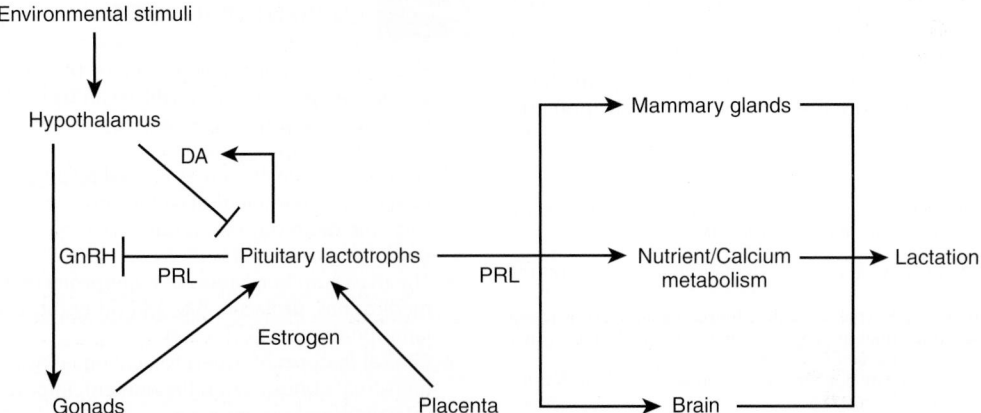

Figure 1 Physiology of prolactin and its regulation. At baseline, prolactin production and secretion are under tonic inhibition by dopamine released from hypothalamic neurons. The hypothalamus controls prolactin production by altering output of dopamine after integrating environmental stimuli and changes in hormonal homeostasis. Prolactin increases hypothalamic dopamine output, providing a negative feedback regulatory loop. Estrogen stimulates prolactin synthesis and secretion during pregnancy. Prolactin supports puerperal lactation via its action on the mammary glands, nutrient/calcium metabolism, and brain. Unlike most other anterior pituitary hormones, feedback regulation of prolactin secretion does not occur via factors produced by a peripheral endocrine target organ. Prolactin also suppresses hypothalamic-pituitary-gonadal axis by inhibiting GnRH release. *Abbreviations:* DA = dopamine; GnRH = gonadotropin releasing hormone; PRL = prolactin.

Mammary Glands

One common symptom of persistent hyperprolactinemia is galactorrhea, that is, milk production not associated with childbirth or breast-feeding. As puerperal lactation normally ends within 6 months after delivery or weaning, any milk production beyond this point is also considered galactorrhea. Since maturation of mammary glands is completed during pregnancy, galactorrhea typically happens in women between 20 to 35 years of age with previous childbirths. It also occurs in nulligravid women, postmenopausal women, and men, although less frequently.

Prolactin is a known mitogen for mammary epithelial cells, and concern has been raised regarding its potential role in the pathogenesis of breast cancer. In a large prospective study by the Women's Health Initiative (WHI), there was evidence of a significant increase in breast cancer incidence in postmenopausal women with high normal prolactin levels, which is within the highest quartile of the normal range compared with those in the lowest quartile. On the other hand, increased breast cancer risk has not been observed in patients with overt hyperprolactinemia. In fact, early parity and lactation history are strong protective factors against breast cancer. Further research is required to resolve these seemingly discrepant observations.

Female Reproductive System

Persistent hyperprolactinemia significantly diminishes the pulsatile release of gonadotropin-releasing hormone (GnRH). As GnRH neurons do not themselves express prolactin receptors, prolactin exerts its effects on their afferent neurons instead by suppression of secretion of kisspeptin, a potent secretagogue for GnRH. Prolactin receptors are also found in the gonads, and prolactin has been reported to inhibit folliculogenesis and estrogen production in the ovary directly. However, this likely has only a limited contribution to infertility and hypogonadism associated with hyperprolactinemia, for the hypothalamus-pituitary-gonad axis can be reactivated by administration of GnRH or kisspeptin, with return of ovulation and fertility in subjects with hyperprolactinemia.

Male Reproductive System

As in women, hyperprolactinemia causes secondary hypogonadism and infertility in men by suppression of GnRH pulses and a decrease in luteinizing hormone (LH) and follicle-stimulating hormone (FSH) levels. Patients often have low or low normal testosterone levels, as well as abnormal sperm counts and morphology in semen analysis. Patients usually seek medical attention for diminished libido and impotence. The central nervous system (CNS) actions of prolactin are likely partly responsible for these symptoms, as restoration of testosterone level alone is often inadequate for symptom relief, which occurs only when prolactin levels also return to normal.

Adrenal Glands

Prolactin stimulates the synthesis of androgen in the zona reticularis of the adrenal cortex. Mild elevations in serum levels of adrenal androgens, for example dehydroepiandrosterone (DHEA) and dehydroepiandrosterone sulfate (DHEA-S), are seen in approximately 50% of women with hyperprolactinemia. Symptoms of clinical hyperandrogenism such as hirsutism and acne are rare in these patients. When present, they are almost always associated with a concurrent increase in testosterone level. Elevation of adrenal androgens in hyperprolactinemia may contribute to the suppression of GnRH release in the hypothalamus and secondary hypogonadism.

Skeletal System

Premenopausal women with hyperprolactinemia have lower bone density and approximately a 4.5 times higher risk for osteoporotic fractures. Hypogonadism associated with hyperprolactinemia is the main cause of bone loss, whereas restoration of sex hormones with either hormonal replacement or correction of hyperprolactinemia improves bone density. Bone density is preserved in women with hyperprolactinemia who continue to have regular menses. Nonetheless, not all studies showed a clear correlation between the degree of bone loss and duration of amenorrhea or levels of sex hormones suggesting involvement of additional processes. For example, the levels of parathyroid hormone–related protein (PTHrP) were found to be significantly higher in patients with hyperprolactinemia, and correlated well with bone density measurements. Correction of hyperprolactinemia by dopamine agonists was shown to normalize PTHrP levels.

Etiology of Hyperprolactinemia

Any conditions that affect production or clearance of prolactin can lead to hyperprolactinemia (Table 1). Physiological hyperprolactinemia is transient and adaptive, whereas persistent

TABLE 1	Causes of Hyperprolactinemia

PHYSIOLOGICAL

Pregnancy

Lactation and breast stimulation

Neonatal period

Physical activity

Stress

Sexual intercourse

PHARMACOLOGICAL

Dopamine antagonists—antipsychotics and antiemetics

Tricyclic antidepressants

Selective serotonin reuptake inhibitors (SSRI)

Antihistamines (H2)

Verapamil (Calan)

Protease inhibitors

Dopamine synthesis inhibitors

PATHOLOGICAL

PITUITARY DISEASES

Prolactinoma

Plurihormonal adenomas

Lymphocytic hypophysitis

Empty sella syndrome

Macroadenoma with or without suprasellar extension

Idiopathic hyperprolactinemia

HYPOTHALAMIC/PITUITARY STALK DISEASES

Tumors: meningioma, craniopharyngioma, germinoma, metastasis, etc.

Granulomas

Infiltrative diseases

Irradiation

Trauma

NEUROGENIC: chest wall lesions, spinal cord lesions, herpes zoster, and epileptic seizure

PARANEOPLASTIC SYNDROME

SYSTEMIC DISEASES

End-stage renal disease

Cirrhosis

Adrenal insufficiency

Pseudocyesis

Adapted from Bronstein, 2016; Melmed et al., 2017.

hyperprolactinemia from pharmacological and pathological causes is often symptomatic with undesired long-term consequences. Pituitary adenomas over producing prolactin (prolactinomas) are the most important cause of pathological hyperprolactinemia. In addition to the elevated prolactin levels, prolactinomas also produce pathological local mass effects. Secondary hyperprolactinemia is most commonly related to disruption of dopaminergic control of lactotrophs, secondary to the use of dopamine antagonists or hypothalamic and pituitary stalk lesions.

Epidemiology and Natural History of Prolactinoma

Prolactinoma is the most common type of pituitary adenoma, contributing to approximately 40–50% of pituitary tumor cases. Prolactinomas are categorized according to size into microprolactinomas (under 1 cm) and macroprolactinomas (larger than 1 cm). Clinically these two conditions behave very differently and can be considered as separate entities. In general, macroprolactinomas tend to grow progressively and are often locally invasive; they are also generally more resistant to treatment and have a higher risk of recurrence. On the other hand, microprolactinomas rarely progress in size (~ 7% of cases) and have a good chance (~ 15% of cases) of going into remission on their own.

The prevalence of prolactinoma has been estimated to be 500 cases per million and incidence about 27 cases per million per year based on survey of asymptomatic populations. In autopsy series, however, lactotroph neoplasms staining positive for prolactin are much more common, being found in approximately 5% of the subjects. They are predominantly microadenomas. Only a small fraction of these small lactotroph neoplasms develop overt hyperprolactinemia by escaping tonic dopaminergic suppression from the hypothalamus, presumably via down-regulation of dopamine D2 receptor-mediated signaling pathway and/or bypassing the portal system for blood supply. Microprolactinomas predominantly affect women of childbearing age, with a female-to-male ratio of approximately 20:1. Macroprolactinoma, on the other hand, shows no sex predilection. Neoplastic transformation of lactotroph involves accumulation of genetic and epigenetic events. The best-understood candidate genes involved include the pituitary tumor transforming gene (PTTG) and the heparin-binding secretory transforming gene (HST). PTTG expression is positively regulated by estrogen.

Most prolactinomas occur sporadically. The vast majority of prolactinomas are benign, although they can be locally invasive. Malignant prolactinomas, as defined by the presence of extrapituitary metastases, are extremely rare. Familial cases, such as those associated with multiple endocrine neoplasia I (MEN-I) and familial isolated pituitary adenoma (FIPA), typically occur at a younger age and are more often macroprolactinomas that are locally invasive.

Clinical Manifestations

Clinical manifestations of prolactinomas fall under two categories: systemic effects of hyperprolactinemia, and local compression symptoms.

Symptoms of Hyperprolactinemia

Persistent hyperprolactinemia inappropriately recapitulates symptoms associated with normal pregnancy and nursing. In extreme cases, hyperprolactinemia has been associated with delusions of pregnancy in susceptible individuals, for example some women on psychotropic medications.

Menstrual abnormalities and infertility are the most common symptoms associated with hyperprolactinemia in women of childbearing age. These symptoms may be masked by use of oral contraceptive pills, which often delays diagnosis. The mildest cases include women presenting with infertility caused by shortened luteal phase despite preserved regular menses. As the degree of hypogonadism worsens, patients experience menstrual irregularities ranging from anovulatory cycles to oligomenorrhea and amenorrhea. Patients with amenorrhea may also experience psychological stresses and other menopausal symptoms like vaginal dryness and dyspareunia. Of note, high prolactin levels may sometimes mask vasomotor symptoms of menopausal and perimenopausal women with prolactinoma, who may develop hot flashes once they are successfully treated with dopamine agonists.

Galactorrhea occurs in up to 80% of cases of hyperprolactinemia. This will need to be differentiated from nipple discharges of other causes, especially those from breast neoplasms. Further evaluation with breast imaging and cytology is indicated when the discharge is unilateral, bloody, or associated with a breast mass. Galactorrhea is by definition milk-like in appearance, and when in doubt, Sudan Black B staining showing fat globules is confirmatory. Although considered a classic sign and symptom for hyperprolactinemia, galactorrhea per se is a poor predictor for hyperprolactinemia in the absence of additional symptoms, for it can be seen in about 10% of healthy women of childbearing age. If amenorrhea is present at the same time, the patient should be assumed to harbor a prolactinoma unless proven otherwise. The degree of galactorrhea is quite variable, from barely expressible to bothersome bra stain and copious free flow, and does not necessarily reflect the severity of hyperprolactinemia. In fact, the majority of patients with galactorrhea and normal menses have normal prolactin levels. On the other hand, in some patients with extremely high levels of prolactin, galactorrhea could be masked by severe hypogonadism.

Men with hyperprolactinemia mainly present with impotence and diminished libido, which is not always corrected with testosterone replacement. As noted in the section on pathophysiology, these symptoms are not all caused by hypogonadism but may involve the central effects of prolactin. Other symptoms and signs of hypogonadism, such as loss of body hair and muscle bulk, are less common. Infertility could also occur with decrease in sperm count and morphology, although hyperprolactinemia is only present in approximately 5% of male patients seeking treatment for infertility.

For both male and female patients, persistent hypogonadism from hyperprolactinemia leads to osteoporosis and increased risk of fracture. This could be effectively treated with either sex hormone replacement or dopamine agonists.

Mass Effects of Prolactinomas

Headache is the most common neurological symptom caused by pituitary tumors. It can occur even with microadenomas presumably caused by dural stretch. More severe headache results from larger tumors, especially those with extrasellar invasion, and occasionally from apoplexy.

Visual disturbance typically only happens with macroadenomas with suprasellar extension impinging on the optic chiasm leading to loss of visual acuity and visual field defects. The typical pattern of visual field defect is bitemporal hemianopsia, which usually starts from the upper field and progresses downward as the tumor impinges upward from below. Ophthalmoparesis typically happens in the setting of apoplexy and only rarely results from parasellar invasion of the cavernous sinus and impingement of cranial nerves III, IV, or VI.

By compressing the rest of the pituitary gland, including the stalk, prolactinoma can cause deficiencies of other anterior pituitary hormones including GH, thyroid-stimulating hormone (TSH), and adrenocorticotropic hormone (ACTH), in addition to hypogonadism from the hyperprolactinemia. The degree of the risk is proportional to tumor size.

CSF rhinorrhea occurs when a macroprolactinoma invades inferiorly into the sphenoid sinus. Other rare compressive symptoms from giant prolactinomas include epilepsy (temporal lobe involvement), exophthalmos, and hydrocephalus. Life- and vision-threatening emergencies could arise from apoplexy and CNS infection.

Laboratory Evaluation
Prolactin Assay and Pitfalls

Hyperprolactinemia is diagnosed by individual measurements of serum prolactin levels. Patients should be well rested, as physical activity stimulates prolactin secretion, but fasting is not needed.

Dynamic tests such as TRH stimulation do not appear to add to diagnostic value and are not recommended. The level of prolactin may provide valuable diagnostic clues. Secondary hyperprolactinemia rarely exceeds 150 ng/mL. On the other hand, a prolactin level of greater than 100 ng/mL is highly suggestive, and severe hyperprolactinemia of greater than 500 ng/mL is virtually diagnostic for prolactinoma. On rare occasions, secondary hyperprolactinemia can produce prolactin levels in the prolactinoma range. For example, risperidone (Risperdal)-induced hyperprolactinemia could be as high as 250 to 500 ng/mL, and patients with end-stage renal disease who are on antipsychotics or antiemetics can have prolactin levels greater than 1000 ng/mL. The size of the prolactinoma shows a rough correlation with the serum prolactin level. Patients with microprolactinomas usually have prolactin levels in the range of 50 to 300 ng/mL, whereas those with macroprolactinomas have levels of 200 to 5000 ng/mL.

Most clinical laboratories measure prolactin using a two-site immunoassay. A capture antibody first affixes prolactin in the sample to a solid matrix. Subsequently a second signal antibody is attached to the now immobilized prolactin. The signal antibody is engineered to carry either a radioisotope or a chemiluminescent enzyme to provide a readout. The assay is accurate within its designed linear range, which is typically under 10,000 ng/mL. Beyond this level both capture and signal antibodies could be saturated preventing the signal antibody to attach. As a result, signal outputs will be falsely diminished. This phenomenon, known as the hook effect, produces a falsely low reading that could lead to the misdiagnosis of a macroprolactinoma as a nonfunctioning pituitary tumor. This artifact can be circumvented by repeating the assay with a 100-fold diluted sample. Many laboratories also opt for an additional washout step to eliminate excess prolactin before adding the signal antibody, preempting the artifact.

Macroprolactinemia is another potential diagnostic pitfall masquerading as true hyperprolactinemia. Macroprolactins are biologically inactive prolactin aggregates that could accumulate in blood to a high level. Macroprolactinemia does not cause any morbidities but could contribute to analytical difficulties as the antibodies used in prolactin assays cross-react with macroprolactins. Most laboratories rely on polyethylene glycol (PEG) precipitation to determine the proportion of macroprolactins and the true concentration of monomeric prolactin. Up to 25% of monomeric prolactin can be also precipitated by PEG, potentially masking true hyperprolactinemia. Therefore patients with macroprolactinemia may still need to be further evaluated if clinical suspicion is high for true hyperprolactinemia.

Other Supporting Laboratory Tests

After confirming hyperprolactinemia, a simple chemistry panel may reveal or suggest the underlying cause such as chronic kidney disease and cirrhosis. A pregnancy test (beta human chorionic gonadotropin [βhCG] level) is essential for women of childbearing age, and hypothyroidism needs to be ruled out with a TSH assay. Both pregnancy and hypothyroidism may have presenting symptoms of sellar mass and hyperprolactinemia and therefore be mistaken for prolactinoma.

For established prolactinoma cases it is important to also assess other pituitary axes. Up to 20% of GH-secreting tumors cosecrete prolactin, and IGF-1 level is an essential screening test for these cases. If hypogonadism is suspected, levels of LH, FSH, and sex hormones (testosterone or estrogen) should be obtained. Screening for central hypothyroidism and secondary adrenal insufficiency should be done with TSH, free thyroxine (T4), and morning cortisol levels, respectively, for patients with pituitary tumors larger than 6 mm.

Neuroimaging

Pituitary imaging should be considered for all patients with unexplained significant hyperprolactinemia, especially if there are signs or symptoms of local compression. MRI with and without gadolinium contrast with dedicated pituitary protocol is the test of choice. Compared with other modalities MRI provides superior soft tissue contrast revealing the tumor's inner structure and its relationship to surrounding tissues, including cavernous sinus, pituitary stalk, and optic chiasm. Computed tomography (CT) scan still has a role for patients with metal implants or other contraindications for MRI, and is especially useful for revealing bony erosions and tissue calcification; its use is limited by suboptimal soft tissue contrast and exposure to ionizing radiation.

Visual Field Testing

A formal visual field test with a perimeter is recommended when suprasellar extension of a pituitary adenoma brings it close to the optic chiasm. Improvement or worsening in visual field often precedes imaging evidence of tumor shrinkage or expansion during treatment. Therefore visual field testing is an excellent monitoring tool for patients under treatment for macroadenoma and visual impairment.

Diagnosis

Prolactin testing is usually prompted by suggestive signs and symptoms of hyperprolactinemia such as menstrual abnormalities, infertility, and galactorrhea. A careful history, including medication use, physical examination, and routine laboratory evaluation (see preceding sections), is invaluable for uncovering secondary causes. Pituitary imaging should be performed when no other underlying causes are found especially if the levels of prolactin are higher than 100 ng/mL. A diagnostic algorithm shown in Figure 2 provides a framework for a structured and cost-effective workup of hyperprolactinemia.

Differential Diagnosis

An exhaustive list of etiologies has been provided in Table 1. A few entities deserve additional comments.

Drug-induced hyperprolactinemia is common and at times may produce serum prolactin levels matching those in patients with prolactinoma (see prior section on laboratory evaluation). A more typical range of prolactin level is 25 to 100 ng/mL for drug-induced hyperprolactinemia. It is not always possible to correlate in time the initiation of the culprit drug with the onset of symptoms, or rise of prolactin levels. The way to confirm medication-related hyperprolactinemia is to discontinue the putative offending agent(s) for three days before repeating a prolactin assay. Some medications may require a longer period of abstinence, and in such cases the level of prolactin can be retested later if the second value is reduced but still elevated. Before discontinuing psychotropic medications, one should consult with the prescribing psychiatrist to prevent worsening of the patient's mental symptoms.

Pseudoprolactinoma refers to a nonfunctioning sellar or suprasellar mass associated with hyperprolactinemia caused by stalk disruption. The prolactin level is seldom above 150 ng/mL. However, before making such a diagnosis, one must exclude hook effect with a 100-fold diluted sample. Prolactin levels are typically normalized within several days after initiation of dopamine agonists, as lactotrophs are still sensitive to dopamine, but local compressive symptoms do not improve. In contrast, patients with true macroprolactinoma experience more gradual decrease in prolactin levels after they are put on dopamine agonists, but they could expect improvement in compressive symptoms within 12 hours to days, and imaging evidence of tumor shrinkage in weeks.

Polycystic ovary syndrome (PCOS) and hyperprolactinemia are among the most common causes of menstrual irregularities and infertility, and affect women of similar ages. PCOS has also been associated with hyperprolactinemia. However, multiple studies have shown that the prevalence of hyperprolactinemia in women with PCOS is not significantly higher than that of matched populations. Although mild elevations of DHEA-S or DHEA are common in patients with hyperprolactinemia, hirsutism is rare, and when present is always associated with an increase in testosterone level, likely reflecting possible coexisting PCOS. Therefore the presence of hyperprolactinemia in patients with PCOS or hirsutism warrants additional evaluation.

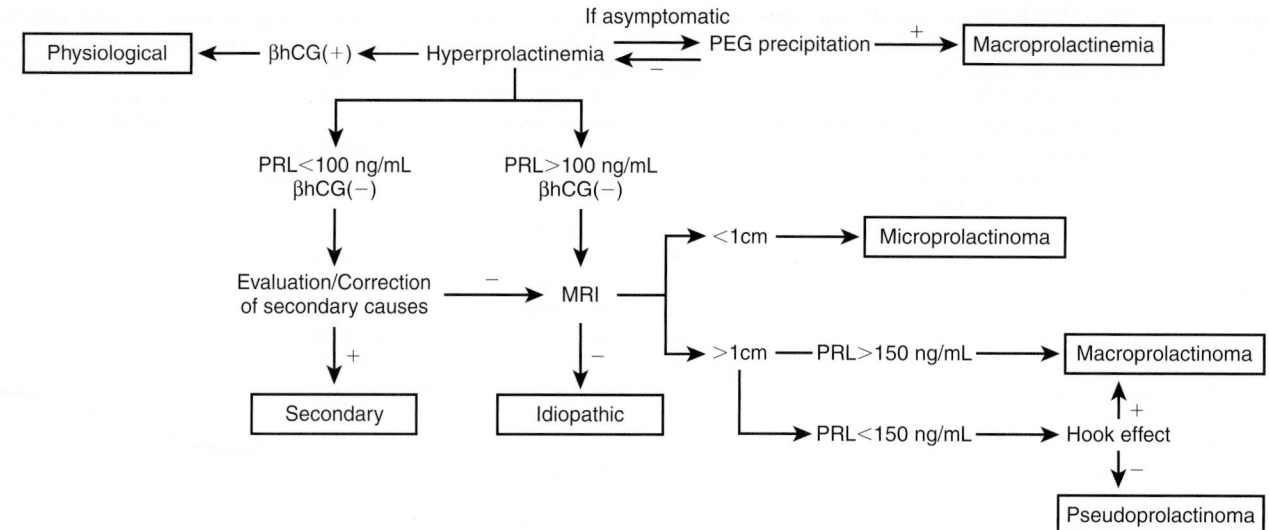

Figure 2 **Diagnostic algorithm for hyperprolactinemia.** If hyperprolactinemia occurs in the absence of relevant clinical symptoms and signs, one should rule out macroprolactinemia by PEG precipitation. When hyperprolactinemia is confirmed, pregnancy should be ruled out with a βhCG test. In the absence of pregnancy, if the PRL level is higher than 100 ng/dl, the pretest probability for a prolactinoma is high enough to justify a pituitary MRI scan, even if potential secondary causes exist. Regardless of prolactin levels, secondary causes should be carefully evaluated with medication history, physical examination, and laboratory tests such as thyroid function tests and chemistry panel, and appropriately treated. If hyperprolactinemia remains unexplained or persists despite correction of other contributing factors, a pituitary MRI is in order. Patients with negative sellar findings have idiopathic hyperprolactinemia. Patients with sellar mass may have either prolactinoma or pseudoprolactinoma. The latter is suggested by a discordant prolactin level less than 150 ng/mL for a large sellar, or a parasellar mass greater than 1 cm, after hook effect has been ruled out. *Abbreviations:* βhCG = β human chorionic gonadotropin; MRI = magnetic resonance imaging; PEG = polyethylene glycol; PRL = prolactin.

Management of Secondary Hyperprolactinemia

Treatment of secondary hyperprolactinemia should focus on correcting the underlying conditions, for example treating hypothyroidism, and resection of nonfunctioning pituitary tumors. For drug-induced hyperprolactinemia, the responsible medications should be removed or replaced with alternatives. Newer antipsychotics such as aripiprazole (Abilify) may be used in place of older agents such as risperidone (Risperdal) because they have better metabolic/hormonal profiles. For irreversible conditions such as end-stage renal disease, hyperprolactinemia can be effectively controlled with dopamine agonists. Ectopic prolactin secretion, which occurs in paraneoplastic syndrome, is a rare exception where dopamine agonists are ineffective, because extrapituitary production of prolactin is driven by alternative promoters, which do not respond to dopamine. Asymptomatic patients with modest hyperprolactinemia may not need treatment, however, and sex hormone replacement may be adequate for correcting hypogonadism if fertility is not desired.

Management of Prolactinoma

The goals for managing prolactinomas are twofold: treating symptomatic hyperprolactinemia, and relief of tumor mass effects. Treatment thus needs to be tailored to the patient's unique clinical picture and the desired outcome. Mass effects are not a concern for microprolactinomas, whereas for patients with giant prolactinomas (defined as >4 cm or >2 cm of suprasellar extension) and extreme hyperprolactinemia, normalization of prolactin levels is less likely, and treatment should focus on reversal or minimization of mass effects. The following are appropriate options in specific settings.

Observation

Active surveillance is appropriate for patients with microprolactinoma who are asymptomatic or not troubled by galactorrhea, especially if fertility is not a concern. As long as regular menses are preserved, they seem to be spared from any long-term consequences from hyperprolactinemia. Bone mineral density appears to be preserved in these patients. It is noteworthy that a significant fraction of patients may have tumor resolution during surveillance without treatment. Tumor expansion is a rare event, and serial measurements of serum prolactin level are effective for monitoring interval tumor growth. Pituitary imaging is indicated when there is significant increase in prolactin level or emergence of local compression symptoms.

Hormonal Replacement

For patients with microprolactinoma bothered only by symptoms related to hypogonadism including menstrual abnormalities, sexual dysfunction, and osteoporosis, but who no longer desire fertility, hormonal replacement is a valid alternative to dopamine agonists, especially when the latter are not tolerated or are contraindicated. This can be achieved with oral contraceptive pills in premenopausal women, or testosterone in men. This approach compares favorably to dopamine agonists in terms of cost and side effects. Patients may experience slight increases in prolactin level, but tumor progression has not been associated with use of oral contraceptive pills for up to 2 years. It would be prudent to use lower doses of estradiol (≤ 30 µg/day) and closely monitor patients for prolactin level and tumor growth.

Dopamine Agonists

Medical treatment with dopamine agonists has replaced surgery as the first-line treatment for prolactinomas, with excellent efficacy in achieving treatment goals and minimal risk. The therapeutic effects of dopamine agonists are mediated by dopamine D2 receptors in tumor cells, which inhibit prolactin synthesis and secretion, slow cell proliferation, and reduce tumor vascularity. Normalization of prolactin levels and reduction of tumor size can be expected in the majority of patients. A small fraction of prolactinomas is resistant to dopamine agonists, as defined by failure in normalizing prolactin level, reduction in tumor size by 50%, or restoration of gonadal function with standard doses. In general, microprolactinomas are more sensitive to dopamine agonists than macroprolactinomas are, and men are more likely to be drug resistant than are women. Rapid responders experience significant improvement of visual symptoms within 24–72 hours; some of them may develop complications resulting from the rapid receding of macroprolactinomas (uncorking), e.g., CSF leak, pituitary apoplexy, and optic chiasm hernia. For most patients, however, progressive reduction of tumor size occurs over the course of months to years, though some patients may never experience tumor shrinkage despite normalization of prolactin levels at the highest tolerated doses.

TABLE 2	Use of Dopamine Agonists in Hyperprolactinemia			
	ROUTE	DOSING FREQUENCY	STARTING DOSE	USUAL DOSE RANGE
Bromocriptine	PO intravaginal[1]	Twice a day	1.25 mg after dinner or before bed for 1 week, then twice a day	2.5–10 mg/day
Cabergoline	PO	Once to twice a week	0.25 mg twice a week or 0.5 mg once a week	0.5–2 mg/week

[1]Not FDA approved for this indication.

Patients with microprolactinoma may discontinue treatment upon menopause because their treatment goal has been fulfilled. Patients with macroprolactinoma, on the other hand, may require life-long treatment to prevent tumor regrowth. A meta-analysis showed that a small fraction of patients may enter long-term remission after discontinuing dopamine agonists (21% for microprolactinomas and 16% for macroprolactinomas). The odds are significantly improved if patients have been treated for at least 2 years and tumor size reduced by ≥50%. The 2011 Endocrine Society practice guidelines suggest that tapering or discontinuing dopamine agonists may be attempted in patients who have been treated for at least 2 years and experienced complete biochemical and radiographic resolution. The risk for recurrence after drug discontinuation is related to the size of adenoma at the time of the diagnosis. For tumors larger than 2 cm, especially giant prolactinomas, tapering the dopamine agonists to a lower maintenance dose for life-long treatment after achieving maximal tumor reduction would be a better strategy for these patients. Tapering or withdrawal of dopamine agonists should be followed by close surveillance of prolactin levels and pituitary MRI when prolactin level increases, especially during the first year.

Three dopamine agonists are currently used for treating hyperprolactinemia, including bromocriptine (Parlodel), cabergoline (Dostinex), and quinagolide (available only in Europe). Bromocriptine was the first dopamine agonist available, and it has the best established safety record. It is still the only dopamine agonist approved by the Food and Drug Administration (FDA) to be used in pregnancy, when indicated. Cabergoline is a more specific agonist of the D2 dopamine receptor, and is superior in many respects to bromocriptine, for example, because of dosing convenience, tolerability, and treatment efficacy. Many patients not controlled with bromocriptine may achieve normal prolactin levels after switching to cabergoline, which has become the drug of choice for cases not involving pregnancy. The safety data for cabergoline are not as extensive as those for bromocriptine. Common side effects for this class of drugs include nausea, orthostatic hypotension, fatigue, mental fogginess, and, less frequently, nasal stuffiness, Raynaud phenomenon, constipation, depression, and psychosis. Nausea is more common in patients taking bromocriptine; for these patients the intravaginal route[1] can be tried. Patients receiving higher doses of cabergoline are at risk of developing cardiac valvulopathy. This has so far been a concern for patients with Parkinson's disease, who may require much higher doses. However, the life-long exposure to high cumulative doses in patients with resistant prolactinoma is considerable, and regular echocardiogram surveillance is recommended for patients taking doses higher than 2 mg/week. Dosing regimens for bromocriptine and cabergoline are listed in Table 2. In general, patients should be started on the lowest doses and titrated upward monthly based on the serum prolactin level until treatment goals are reached.

Surgery
With the availability of the second-generation dopamine agonists, surgery is mostly reserved for the following situations: (1) patients intolerant of, or resistant to, dopamine agonists; (2) women with macroprolactinoma who are planning for conception, to forestall tumor expansion during pregnancy; (3) pituitary apoplexy

threatening neurological and visual functions if not managed urgently. Transsphenoidal tumor resection is the standard surgical approach. Perioperative mortality and morbidity are low in the hands of experienced pituitary surgeons in high-volume centers. Major surgical complications include visual loss, CNS infection, stroke, and oculomotor palsy. Craniotomy is occasionally needed for masses with extrasellar extensions that may be inaccessible by the transsphenoidal route, with higher risk for complications. Postoperatively patients need to be monitored for signs of diabetes insipidus and secondary adrenal insufficiency, which may be transient or permanent.

Radiotherapy
Radiotherapy is inadequate as a primary treatment for prolactinoma, as its efficacy is poor and latency long. It is also associated with long-term complications including permanent hypopituitarism, cerebrovascular accidents, and secondary intracranial malignancies. Currently it is reserved mostly for patients with aggressive and malignant prolactinomas failing medical/surgical treatment. Stereotactic radiosurgery is preferred over conventional fractionated radiotherapy for more convenient dosing, better efficacy, and lower rate of complications. However, radiosurgery should not be attempted for tumors in close proximity to the visual apparatus (less than 5 mm of clearance), as it is associated with an unacceptably high rate of vision loss.

Management of Prolactinoma During Pregnancy
Mild hyperprolactinemia is part of normal pregnancy, and there are concerns for the safe use of dopamine agonists in pregnant women. There is convincing evidence that as long as bromocriptine is withdrawn within a week after confirmation of pregnancy, obstetric outcome is not altered. Less robust data to date suggest that continuing bromocriptine treatment till term is also safe. Despite its longer half-life, as long as cabergoline is discontinued in early pregnancy, it also has not been found to be associated with adverse outcomes. Until there is incontrovertible evidence for the absolute safety of these dopamine agonists, however, it is prudent to discontinue these drugs as soon as pregnancy is confirmed. Given its shorter half-life and established safety record, bromocriptine is the preferred agent for fertility induction in women with hyperprolactinemia, although cabergoline would also be acceptable if bromocriptine is not tolerated. The major indication to treat prolactinomas medically during pregnancy is the concern for tumor expansion. Such risk is negligible for microprolactinomas. For patients with macroprolactinoma, however, symptomatic tumor expansion during pregnancy can occur in up to about 30% of cases. This risk can be significantly reduced if the patient has been treated with a dopamine agonist for at least a year with evidence of tumor shrinkage, or has undergone pituitary surgery or radiotherapy prior to pregnancy. Until these conditions are met, women of childbearing age with macroprolactinomas should be advised to take nonhormonal contraceptive measures. For patients who fail to achieve tumor shrinkage with dopamine agonists or cannot tolerate them, prophylactic surgery prior to pregnancy may be considered, after careful discussion with the patient on surgical risks and the possibility of permanent hypopituitarism, which further impairs fertility. The Endocrine Society practice guidelines recommend against measurement of serum prolactin levels during pregnancy. Instead the patient

[1]Not FDA approved for this indication.

should be followed clinically for any signs or symptoms of tumor expansion. MRI without gadolinium and visual field testing should be done when clinical suspicion arises. If tumor expansion is confirmed, the patient should be reinitiated on bromocriptine. Debulking surgery is reserved for patients failing or not tolerating medical treatment. Lactation usually does not cause tumor progression, and patients are encouraged to breastfeed their infants with close surveillance. They should not take either bromocriptine or cabergoline, however, as both are secreted in the milk, and are effective lactation inhibitors.

Management of Resistant and Malignant Prolactinoma

Several other treatment options are available for patients who fail the highest tolerated doses of dopamine agonists, surgery, and radiation. A small fraction of these patients have malignant prolactinoma, which is defined by extrapituitary metastasis; histopathologically, malignant prolactinomas can appear very similar to aggressive prolactinomas. An alkylating agent, temozolomide (Temodar)[1], has been successfully used in the treatment of aggressive pituitary adenoma and pituitary carcinoma. Monotherapy with temozolomide has been established as the first-line chemotherapy for these conditions, following documented tumor growth despite standard therapies. Selective estrogen receptor modulators (SERMs), including raloxifene (Evista)[1] and tamoxifen (Nolvadex)[1], have been found to be useful adjuncts that can reduce prolactin level and inhibit tumor growth.

References

Ahuja N, Moorhead S, Lloyd AJ, Cole AJ: Antipsychotic-induced hyperprolactinemia and delusion of pregnancy, *Psychosomatics* 49:163–167, 2008.

Bernard V, Young J, Chanson P, Binart N: New insights in prolactin: pathological implications, *Nat Rev Endocrinol* 11:265–275, 2015.

Bronstein MD: Disorders of prolactin secretion and prolactinomas. In Jameson JL, De Groot LJ, editors: *Endocrinology: Adult and Pediatric*, 7th ed., Philadelphia, 2016, Elsevier.

Chanson P, Maiter D: Prolactinoma. In Molmed S, editor: *The Pituitary*, 4th ed., San Diego, 2017, Elsevier.

Ciccarelli A, Daly AF, Beckers A: The epidemiology of prolactinomas, *Pituitary* 8:3–6, 2005.

Dekkers OM, Lagro J, Burman P, Jorgensen JO, Romijn JA, Pereira AM: Recurrence of hyperprolactinemia after withdrawal of dopamine agonists: systematic review and meta-analysis, *J Clin Endocrinol Metab* 95:43–51, 2010.

Filho RB, Domingues L, Naves L, et al: Polycystic ovary syndrome and hyperprolactinemia are distinct entities, *Gynecol Endocrinol* 23:267–272, 2007.

Glezer A, Bronstein MD: Prolactinomas, cabergoline, and pregnancy, *Endocrine* 47:64–69, 2014.

Grattan DR: 60 years of neuroendocrinology: the hypothalamo-prolactin axis, *J Endocrinol* 226:T101–T122, 2015.

Horseman ND, Gregerson KA: Prolactin. In Jameson JL, De Groot LJ, editors: *Endocrinology: Adult and Pediatric*, 7th ed., Philadelphia, 2016, Elsevier.

Huang W, Molitch ME: Evaluation and management of galactorrhea, *Am Fam Physician* 85:1073–1080, 2012.

Melmed S, Casanueva FF, Hoffman AR, et al: Diagnosis and treatment of hyperprolactinemia: an Endocrine Society clinical practice guideline, *J Clin Endocrinol Metab* 96:273–288, 2011.

Melmed S, Kleinberg D: Pituitary masses and tumors. In Melmed S, et al: *Williams Textbook of Endocrinology*, 13th ed., Philadelphia, 2016, Elsevier.

Miyai K, Ichihara K, Kondo K, Mori S: Asymptomatic hyperprolactinaemia and prolactinoma in the general population: mass screening by paired assays of serum prolactin, *Clin Endocrinol (Oxf)* 25:549–554, 1986.

Molitch ME: Drugs and prolactin, *Pituitary* 11:209–218, 2008.

Raverot G, Burman P, McCormack A, et al: European Society of Endocrinology Clinical Practice Guidelines for the management of aggressive pituitary tumors and carcinomas, *Eur J Endocrinol* 178:G1–G24, 2018.

Samson SL, Hamrahian AH, Ezzat S: American Association of Clinical Endocrinologists, American College of Endocrinology disease state clinical review: clinical relevance of macroprolactin in the absence or presence of true hyperprolactinemia, *Endocr Pract* 21:1427–1435, 2015.

Schlechte J, Dolan K, Sherman B, et al: The natural history of untreated hyperprolactinemia: a prospective analysis, *J Clin Endocrinol Metab* 68:412–418, 1989.

Stiegler C, Leb G, Kleinert R, et al: Plasma levels of parathyroid hormone-related peptide are elevated in hyperprolactinemia and correlated to bone density status, *J Bone Miner Res* 10:751–759, 1995.

Testa G, Vegetti W, Motta T, et al: Two-year treatment with oral contraceptives in hyperprolactinemic patients, *Contraception* 58:69–73, 1998.

Vartej P, Poiana C, Vartej I: Effects of hyperprolactinemia on osteoporotic fracture risk in premenopausal women, *Gynecol Endocrinol* 15:43–47, 2001.

HYPERTHYROIDISM

Method of
William J. Hueston, MD

CURRENT DIAGNOSIS

- Hyperthyroidism or thyrotoxicosis is most often caused by Graves' disease, toxic nodular goiter (Plummer's disease), or acute thyroiditis.
- Common symptoms in hyperthyroidism are tachycardia, elevated systolic blood pressure, tremor, and anxiety. Patients with Graves' disease also might exhibit exophthalmos. In contrast, elderly patients can present with apathetic hyperthyroidism, which can be confused with hypothyroidism.
- Hyperthyroidism should be suspected in all patients who present with atrial fibrillation, palpitations, panic disorder, or unexplained tremors.
- Thyroid storm is an acute, life-threatening condition usually occurring in patients with undiagnosed or untreated hyperthyroidism placed under physiologic stress.
- An elevated free T_4, usually with a low thyroid-stimulating hormone is the hallmark of hyperthyroidism, and anti–thyroid-stimulating hormone antibodies can help identify Graves' disease.
- Ultimately, a thyroid scan and uptake are usually necessary to differentiate the cause of hyperthyroidism.
- Subclinical hyperthyroidism is an uncommon finding of uncertain long-term clinical significance but treatment for patients over 65 with cardiac disease or osteoporosis should be considered.

CURRENT THERAPY

- In patients with Graves' disease or autonomous thyroid nodules (toxic nodular goiter), short-term treatment includes thyroid suppression medications (such as methimazole [Tapazole]) and β-blockers (such as propranolol [Inderal][1]). Long-term management with radioiodine thyroid gland ablation is often pursued once symptoms are controlled.
- Patients with acute thyroiditis might need transient β-blockade but can often be managed expectantly until symptoms abate and thyroid hormone levels normalize. A small number of patients (~10%) have persistent hypothyroidism after an episode of illness.
- Thyroid storm is a medical emergency that requires close monitoring along with an antithyroid drug, β-blockers, corticosteroids, and iodine-potassium solution (Lugol's solution).

[1] Not FDA approved for this indication.

Epidemiology

Hyperthyroidism is relatively uncommon and usually caused by three conditions: Graves' disease, toxic nodular goiter, or acute thyroiditis. Graves' disease is the most common cause of hyperthyroidism in the United States and usually affects younger patients from the teens to the 40s. Like other autoimmune diseases, women are at higher risk (seven to eight times) than men. Toxic nodular goiter accounts for 15% to 30% of hyperthyroid diagnoses. It usually occurs after age 50 years, is more common in women, and follows several decades of multinodular thyroid disease. A less-common cause is administration of amiodarone. Amiodarone is about one third iodine and can cause hyperthyroidism either through iodine-induced thyroid damage or from increased thyroxine synthesis owing to excessive iodine.

BOX 1 | Conditions Causing Hyperthyroidism

Graves' disease
Autonomous thyroid nodule (toxic nodular goiter)
Acute thyroiditis
- Hashimoto's thyroiditis
- Subacute granulomatous thyroiditis (de Quervain's thyroiditis)
- Subacute lymphocytic thyroiditis (silent or painless thyroiditis)
- Suppurative thyroiditis (bacterial infection of thyroid)
Excessive exogenous thyroid use
- Over-replacement after thyroid ablation or for hypothyroidism
- Thyroxine (Synthroid) abuse for weight loss
Iodine overconsumption
Amiodarone administration

Subclinical hyperthyroidism, defined as an abnormally low TSH but normal free thyroxine (T_4) and triiodothyronine (T_3) affects 1% to 2% of the population. This condition is most common with mild forms of hyperthyroidism but also can be observed transiently in thyroiditis. Subclinical hyperthyroidism is more common in individuals over age 70 and those with iodine-deficient diets.

Risk Factors

There are no known environmental or reversible risk factors for any of the causes of hyperthyroidism. Graves' disease is associated with a specific human leukocyte antigen (HLA) region on chromosome 6 *(CTLA 4)*.

Pathophysiology

The most common causes of hyperthyroidism are shown in Box 1.

Graves' disease is an autoimmune disorder caused by antibodies against thyroid-stimulating hormone (TSH) receptors on the thyroid gland. Graves' disease is associated with many other autoimmune diseases, including pernicious anemia, vitiligo, type 1 diabetes mellitus, autoimmune adrenal disease, Sjögren's syndrome, rheumatoid arthritis, and lupus. As with these other disorders, the etiology is unknown.

Toxic nodular goiter, also known as Plummer's disease, results from the development of autonomous thyroid adenoma. Patients who develop a toxic nodular goiter usually have a long history of many other nodules that spontaneously burn out over time, but then develop a single large nodule (usually 2.5 cm or greater) that continues to produce thyroid hormone in such large quantities that patients become hyperthyroid. No clear cause is known for the development of the nodules.

Acute thyroiditis can also produce hyperthyroidism. Several different conditions can cause thyroiditis (see Box 1). The inflammation resulting in thyroiditis is thought to be related to subacute viral infections or autoimmune reactions; suppurative thyroiditis is a rare bacterial thyroid infection, usually caused by *Staphylococcus aureus*. During the acute period of thyroid inflammation, damage to the gland leads to the release of stored thyroxine from thyroid lakes, producing hyperthyroidism. However, after the initial release of thyroid hormone from the stored lakes, damage to the gland inhibits production of new thyroxine. After the initial surge in thyroid hormone levels, thyroxine levels drop, often to levels that can result in transient hypothyroidism. Most patients return to the euthyroid state after the thyroid gland heals, but about 10% of patients with acute thyroiditis remain chronically hypothyroid.

Other, less common causes of hyperthyroidism include excessive exogenous administration of thyroid medications. This is most commonly the result of over-replacement of thyroxine (Levoxyl, Synthroid) in patients with hypothyroidism, but it may be intentional for weight loss. Because thyroxine and

triiodothyronine (T_3) are highly protein bound, over-replacement is most common if patients experience hypoproteinemia, such as in nephrotic syndrome, cirrhosis, or malnutrition.

Excessive iodine consumption, referred to as the Jod-Basedow effect, can also lead to thyrotoxicosis. The source of the iodine may include iatrogenic sources such as iodine-containing medications or radiologic contrast agents.

Several other medications, such as amiodarone (Cordarone), lithium, and interferon α (Intron A) also can cause thyrotoxicosis by causing drug-induced thyroiditis.

Prevention

There are no known strategies to prevent hyperthyroidism. For patients with hypothyroidism, annual monitoring of TSH levels is recommended to ensure that patients receive the appropriate replacement dose and not over-replacement.

Clinical Manifestations

Patients with hyperthyroidism complain of a variety of symptoms that can include anxiety, tachycardia, wide-pulse pressure hypertension, palpitations, fine tremor, weight loss, heat intolerance, and, particularly in the elderly, confusion or delirium. Patients with Graves' disease also have ophthalmopathy characterized by lid retraction and exophthalmoses that can lead to optic nerve damage. In contrast, older patients can have few of the classic signs of hyperthyroidism and instead might complain of fatigue or weakness (apathetic hyperthyroidism), unexplained delirium, weight loss, heart failure, or isolated atrial fibrillation.

Some patients have a rapid escalation of symptom severity (thyroid storm) that is life-threatening if not identified and treated promptly. These patients usually have underlying thyrotoxicosis from Graves' disease complicated by a secondary physiological stressor such as infection, surgery, or trauma. This is a medical emergency and needs immediate attention, including hospitalization with close observation.

On physical examination, patients with hyperthyroidism due to Graves' disease or thyroiditis might have a diffusely enlarged and mildly tender thyroid gland. In suppurative thyroiditis, the thyroid gland is red, hot, and very tender and accompanied by a fever and other systemic signs of severe infection. Patients with toxic nodular goiter can have palpable nodules in their thyroid gland and often have a single palpable nodule.

Diagnosis

Hyperthyroidism is diagnosed by finding an elevation in the free thyroxine (T_4) level accompanied by a low TSH level. Patients with Graves' disease often have positive anti–thyroid receptor antibody titers. Only anti-thyroglobulin receptor antibody testing is helpful because it can help differentiate Graves' disease from other causes. No other anti-thyroid tests are clinically indicated. Once the thyroid level abnormalities are found, a definitive diagnosis of the cause for the hyperthyroidism is needed to select the appropriate treatment strategy.

Other conditions can produce a depressed TSH but normal free T_4 levels. These include T_3 toxicosis and subclinical hyperthyroidism. T_3 toxicosis refers to situations where triiodothyronine (T_3) is produced in excess rather than thyroxine (T_4); this can occur in any of the conditions that can cause hyperthyroidism, as well as in surreptitious triiodothyronine (Cytomel) ingestion.

Thyroid scanning and radiolabel uptake are usually necessary to differentiate the causes of hyperthyroidism. Thyroid scanning and uptake rely on the thyroid gland to concentrate radioactive molecules, such as iodine-131 (^{131}I) or technetium. Because of the risk of thyroid storm with iodine administration, patients should be treated with antithyroid drugs for 2 to 8 weeks before a scan and the drugs should be stopped at least 4 days before the test. Patients with Graves' disease show increases in uptake and diffuse distribution of the tracer throughout the thyroid gland. Patients with toxic nodular goiter also have increased uptake, but the isotope is concentrated in a one or a few focal areas, with the remainder of the thyroid gland suppressed. In contrast, patients

TABLE 1 Treatment Strategies for Hyperthyroidism

TREATMENT	DRUG	DOSAGE
Graves' Disease and Toxic Nodular Goiter		
Thyroid hormone suppression	Methimazole Propylthiouracil	Initial: 30–40 mg/d Maintenance: 5–15 mg/d Initial: 300–400 mg/d Maintenance: 100–300 mg/d
β-Blockade	Propranolol[1] Metoprolol (Lopressor)[1]	10 mg qid 50–100 mg bid
Thyroid gland removal	Radioactive iodine ablation Thyroidectomy	
Acute Thyroiditis		
β-Blockade transiently May need thyroid replacement long term		
Thyroid Storm		
Thyroid hormone suppression	Propylthiouracil	300–400 mg/d
β-Blockade	Propranolol[1]	1 mg/min IV to max 10 mg[3]
Iodine	Lugol's solution	1–2 gtt mixed in water tid
Cardiac and fluid monitoring	Dexamethasone (Decadron)[1]	2 mg q6h

[1]Not FDA approved for this indication.
[3]Exceeds dosage recommended by the manufacturer.

with thyroiditis have decreased uptake of the radiolabel and a washed-out or mottled distribution on scanning.

Differential Diagnosis

Symptoms of hyperthyroidism also occur in patients with panic disorder and other anxiety conditions. These patients can have sinus tachycardia, tremor, and nervousness that mimic hyperthyroidism.

Treatment

Treatment depends on the cause of the hyperthyroidism (Table 1). In Graves' disease, immediate goals of treatment include reducing thyroid hormone production and blocking the peripheral effects of the excessive thyroid hormone. About 30% to 60% of patients, mostly adolescents, enter remission spontaneously, and the remission may be permanent. Remission rates are highest for those with a small goiter, no ophthalmopathy, thyroglobulin levels less than 50 µg/mL, and thyroxine levels less than 20 µg/dL. Signs of remission include a decreased ratio of T_3 to T_4, lower thyroid-stimulating thyroglobulin levels, and decreased radioactive iodine uptake on rescanning. When remissions do occur, it is usually within a year of starting antithyroid medications.

For those who do not undergo spontaneous remission, which includes most adults, consideration should be given to thyroid gland ablation to permanently treat this condition. Although the dosage can be calculated to attempt to leave patients euthyroid, permanent hypothyroidism occurs in about half of all patients treated with radioactive iodine ablation.

The initial approach to toxic nodular goiter is similar to that for symptom control, but thyroid ablation should be recommended routinely because remissions are very rare.

Thyroid gland production of hormone can be reduced rapidly with either methimazole (Tapazole) or propylthiouracil. For treatment of Graves' disease, methimazole is the preferred treatment and has the advantage of less frequent dosing, which improves compliance. Propylthiouracil is an alternative that is recommended for women in the first trimester of pregnancy and patients who cannot tolerate methimazole. However, the FDA issued a black box warning about the use of propylthiouracil in 2010 because of liver toxicity; physicians should be aware of this and use propylthiouracil only when methimazole is not suitable. With both drugs, clinicians need to be aware of drug-associated agranulocytosis, which can result in life-threatening bacterial infections. In patients on either of these medications who develop a sore throat, fever, or other signs of infection, a white blood cell count should be done immediately to ensure that they are not neuropenic. Additionally, antithyroid drugs are associated with drug-induced lupus syndromes and other forms of vasculitis.

In addition to reducing production of thyroid hormone, initial therapy for patients with Graves' disease and toxic nodular goiter should include a β-blocker to reduce the tachycardia, tremor, hypertension, and anxiety. A β-blocker that crosses the blood-brain barrier, such as propranalol (Inderal)[1] or metoprolol (Lopressor)[1], is the best choice in this situation because these also reduce the central nervous system effects such as anxiety, as well as the vascular problems caused by thyroid hormones.

Thyroid storm requires immediate attention and should be managed in the hospital setting, especially in older patients where tachycardia and hypertension can lead to cardiac instability. Prompt administration of β-blockers and propylthiouracil along with cardiac monitoring for dysrhythmias and appropriate fluid management are essential for managing this life-threatening condition. Once antithyroid drugs have been administered, iodine-potassium solution (Lugol's solution) at a dose of 1 or 2 drops three times a day should be administered, which will further reduce thyroid hormone production and reduce peripheral conversion of T_4 to T_3. Finally, corticosteroids also have been shown to rapidly reduce thyroid hormone levels in thyroid storm.

For long-term management, thyroid ablation with radioactive iodine (sodium iodide, ^{131}I) can restore patients to a permanent euthyroid state. However, radioactive iodine thyroid ablation often results in destruction of more thyroid than optimal, causing hypothyroidism. Radioactive iodine thyroid ablation is contraindicated in pregnancy. For patients in whom radioactive iodine is either contraindicated or not acceptable, thyroidectomy is an option. Thyroidectomy almost always results in permanent hypothyroidism, as well as having other risks inherent in surgery including hypoparathyroidism and recurrent laryngeal nerve damage.

In patients with hyperthyroidism associated with acute thyroiditis, symptoms often resolve by the time the evaluation is complete. In the interim, symptoms can be managed with β-blockers. β-Blocker therapy can be discontinued fairly rapidly (2 to 3 weeks) after the initial onset of symptoms.

Indications for the treatment of subclinical hyperthyroidism are less clear. Based on recommendations of the American Thyroid Association, patients with a persistently low TSH who are over age 65 or who have underlying cardiac disease or osteoporosis should be considered for treatment. The treatment strategy should be directed at the presumed cause of the condition and may include antithyroid medication for suspected Graves' Disease or thyroid ablation for toxic nodular goiter or a solitary autonomous nodule.

Monitoring

In patients on antithyroid drugs, thyroid hormone levels should be monitored frequently until they reach a stable euthyroid state. Any change in the patient's underlying health, especially changes that could alter protein levels, should prompt reevaluation. In addition, patients who have thyroid ablation need follow-up testing of TSH and free T_4 levels to ensure that sufficient thyroid tissue has been destroyed to reverse their hyperthyroidism but not make them hypothyroid. This should be done 6 to 8 weeks following ablation therapy.

[1]Not FDA approved for this indication.

Complications

Complications of hyperthyroidism include acute and chronic conditions. Acutely, the most concerning complications are cardiac dysrhythmias, especially atrial fibrillation. Chronically, excessive thyroxine is associated with cardiomyopathy and osteoporosis. In patients with ophthalmopathy, untreated Graves' disease can lead to progressive vision loss and blindness.

Hyperthyroidism in pregnancy, even when adequately treated, has been shown to be an independent risk factor for cesarean section but not for any additional pregnancy complications. Some patients with existing hyperthyroidism may experience transient increases in free T_4 levels during pregnancy that can be associated with hyperemesis gravidarum. Assessing free T_4 levels in pregnant patients who have hyperthyroidism and develop hyperemesis may be useful.

References

Cooper DS: Antithyroid drugs for the treatment of hyperthyroidism caused by Graves' disease, *Endocrinol Metab Clin North Am* 27:225–247, 1998.

Kharlip J, Cooper DS: Recent developments in hyperthyroidism, *Lancet* 373:1930–1932, 2009.

Lazarus JH: Hyperthyroidism, *Lancet* 349:339–343, 1997.

Nayak B, Hodak SP: Hyperthyroidism, *Endocrinol Metab Clin North Am* 36(3):617–656, 2007.

Zimmerman D, Lteif AN: Thyroxicosis in children, *Endocrinol Metab Clin North Am* 27:109–126, 1998.

Donangelo I, Suh SY: Subclinical hyperthyroidism: When to consider treatment, *Amer Family Phys* 95:710–716, 2017.

HYPOKALEMIA AND HYPERKALEMIA

Method of
Jie Tang, MD

CURRENT DIAGNOSIS

- The "initial approach" to the evaluation of dyskalemia is to determine if it is secondary to transcellular shifts (in vitro or in vivo) of potassium (K) or a result of a true change in total body K.
- A thorough history and physical will provide useful information regarding the causes of hypokalemia and hyperkalemia, especially in cases of low or high intake of K, and transcellular shifts.
- Key steps in the diagnostic approach to hypokalemia include assessments of urinary K excretion and acid-base status.
- Key steps in the diagnostic approach to hyperkalemia include assessments of renal function and aldosterone activity.

CURRENT THERAPY

- For both hypokalemia and hyperkalemia, it is critical to assess the underlying transcellular K shift, given the risk of rebound hyperkalemia after K repletion or hypokalemia after K restriction and removal.
- In cases of severe dyskalemia, close cardiac monitoring is needed.
- The aggressiveness of therapy for dyskalemia is directly related to the rapidity with which the condition has developed, the absolute level of serum K, and the clinical evidence of toxicity.
- In severe or symptomatic cases of hypokalemia, both intravenous and oral K repletion are often needed.
- In severe or symptomatic cases of hyperkalemia, supported by electrocardiogram (ECG) abnormalities, both immediate temporizing measures and definitive therapy for K removal are necessary.

Epidemiology

Hypokalemia is defined as a serum K level of 3.5 mmol/L or lower. It is a common electrolyte disorder encountered in clinical practice. According to one study, serum K less than 3.6 mmol/L was found in up to 20% of hospitalized patients. The majority of these patients had serum K concentrations between 3.0 and 3.5 mmol/L, but as many as 25% had values less than 3.0 mmol/L. Even mild or moderate hypokalemia increases the risks of morbidity and mortality in patients with cardiovascular disease. Hyperkalemia is defined as a serum K of 5.5 mmol/L or higher. The prevalence among hospitalized patients not yet on dialysis was reported to be about 3.3%, and among them, up to 10% had significant hyperkalemia (≥6.0 mmol/L). Hyperkalemia also carries a significantly increased risk of mortality.

Risk Factors

People most at risk for hypokalemia are those who are malnourished, with poor oral intake; those who use certain medications, such as diuretics; and those who have uncontrolled vomiting or diarrhea. People most at risk for hyperkalemia are those with reduced kidney function, those who have a history of diabetes mellitus, or those who take certain medications, such as angiotensin-converting enzyme inhibitors.

Pathophysiology

K is the most abundant cation in the human body. It regulates intracellular enzyme function and helps determine neuromuscular and cardiovascular tissue excitability. The total body store is approximately 55 mmol/kg of body weight. Over 98% of total body K is located in the intracellular fluid (primarily in muscle), and less than 2% in the extracellular fluid. A typical Western diet provides 40 to 120 mmol of K per day. Tight control of the serum K is primarily accomplished by the kidney, where approximately 95% of body K is excreted. Under normal circumstances, K losses in stool and sweat are small. In addition, the interplay of several hormonal systems (insulin, catecholamine), serum tonicity, and the internal acid-base environment contribute to the exchange of K between the extracellular fluid and intracellular fluid, which helps keep the serum K concentration tightly controlled. Hypokalemia occurs when there is a significant intracellular K shift or a reduced total body K store from poor intake, or excessive renal or extrarenal loss, whereas hyperkalemia develops when there is a significant extracellular shift, high body K load, or ineffective K elimination (aldosterone resistance/deficiency or reduced renal function).

Prevention

For patients at risk for hypokalemia, adequate dietary K intake is essential. Additional K supplements may be needed for patients taking high doses of diuretics (especially thiazide diuretics) or experiencing prolonged vomiting or diarrhea. For patients with hyperkalemia and severe kidney dysfunction, dietary K restriction is critical in maintaining body K balance. Sometimes, the empirical use of K exchange resin is needed to prevent hyperkalemia. Lastly, medications that contribute to hypokalemia or hyperkalemia should be avoided if possible.

Clinical Manifestations

Mild hypokalemia (serum K 3.0 to 3.5 mmol/L) is usually well tolerated. Moderate hypokalemia (serum K 2.5 to 3.0 mmol/L) may cause nonspecific symptoms, such as fatigue, weakness, muscle cramps, and constipation. When the serum K drops to less than 2.5 mmol/L, muscle necrosis and flaccid paralysis with eventual respiratory failure may occur. K depletion also causes supraventricular and ventricular arrhythmias, especially in patients on digitalis therapy. Although severe hypokalemia is more likely to cause complications, even minimal decreases in serum or total body K can be arrhythmogenic in patients with underlying heart disease or who are receiving digitalis therapy. Lastly, increases in systolic and diastolic blood pressures can occur in patients with hypokalemia while they are on a liberal salt diet. Overall, the

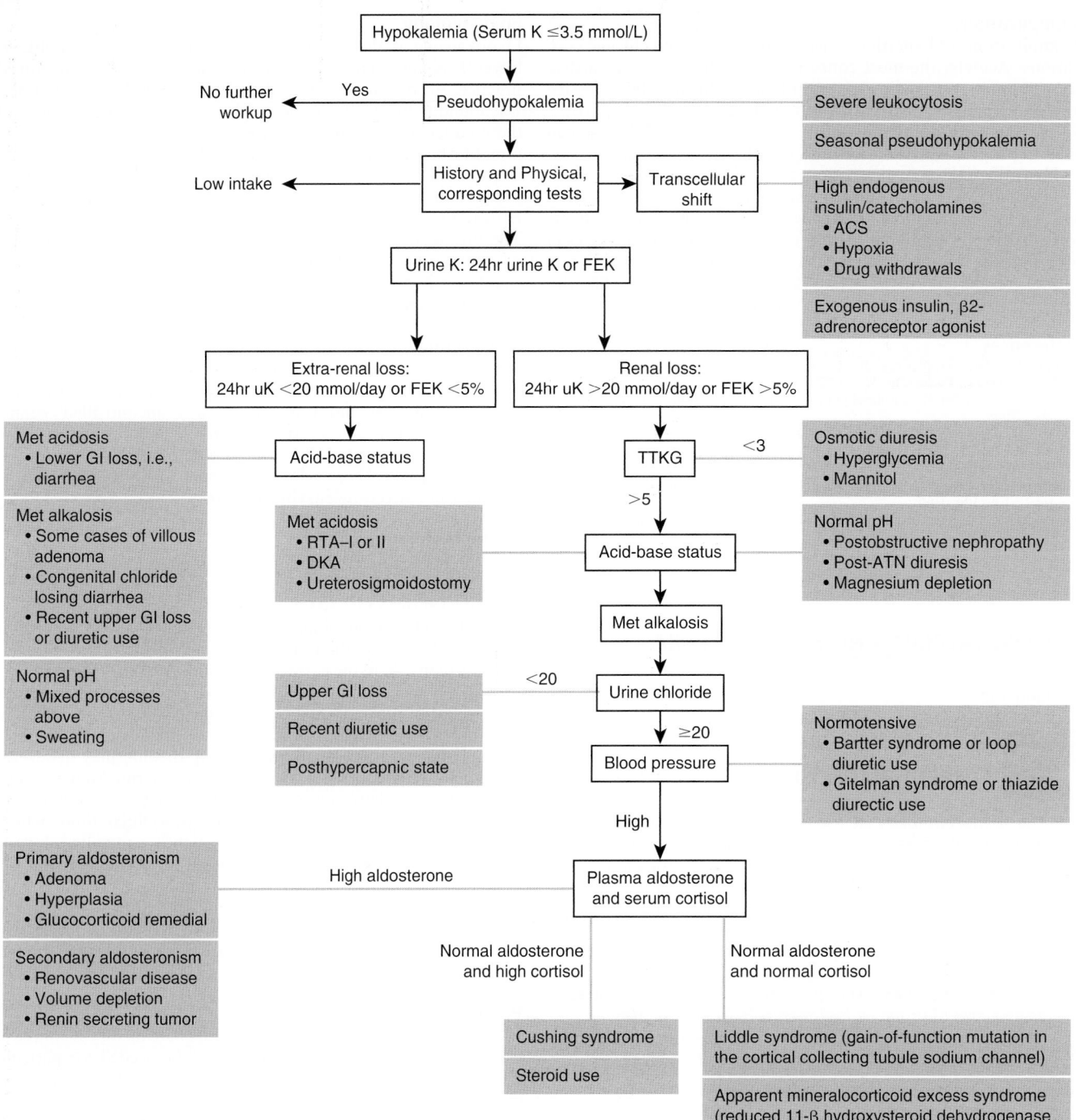

Figure 1 The diagnostic approach to hypokalemia. *ACS,* Acute coronary syndrome; *ATN,* acute tubular necrosis; *DKA,* diabetic ketoacidosis; *FEK,* fractional excretion of K; *GI,* gastrointestinal; *Met,* metabolic; *RTA,* renal tubular acidosis.

likelihood of symptoms tends to correlate with the rapidity of the decrease in serum K. As with hypokalemia, patients with hyperkalemia may present with nonspecific complaints such as fatigue and malaise. But the predominant manifestations in more severe hyperkalemia are neuromuscular and cardiac. Neuromuscular symptoms range from muscle weakness to paralysis. Cardiac arrhythmias, including asystole, ventricular tachycardia or fibrillation, and pulseless electrical activity, can also occur in severe hyperkalemia.

Diagnosis

Figures 1 and 2 illustrate the diagnostic approaches to hypokalemia and hyperkalemia. It is important to assess for pseudodyskalemia (in vitro shift of K) and dyskalemia from in vivo transcellular shift of K because neither is associated with disturbances in total body K balance. Although cellular shift of K and changes in total body K occur as isolated problems, they frequently coexist. In hypokalemia, the assessment of renal K excretion is a key step in the initial diagnostic evaluation, followed by the assessment of acid-base status. In hyperkalemia, medical history and laboratory testing can help identify altered K distribution, reduced urinary K excretion, or an excessive K load from exogenous intake or transcellular leakage. Under normal circumstances, high K intake alone is not sufficient to lead to significant hyperkalemia unless there are other risk factors present such as reduced aldosterone action or significant loss of kidney function. Measurement of the transtubular potassium gradient (TTKG) has been widely used as a diagnostic tool in both conditions. However, recent evidence

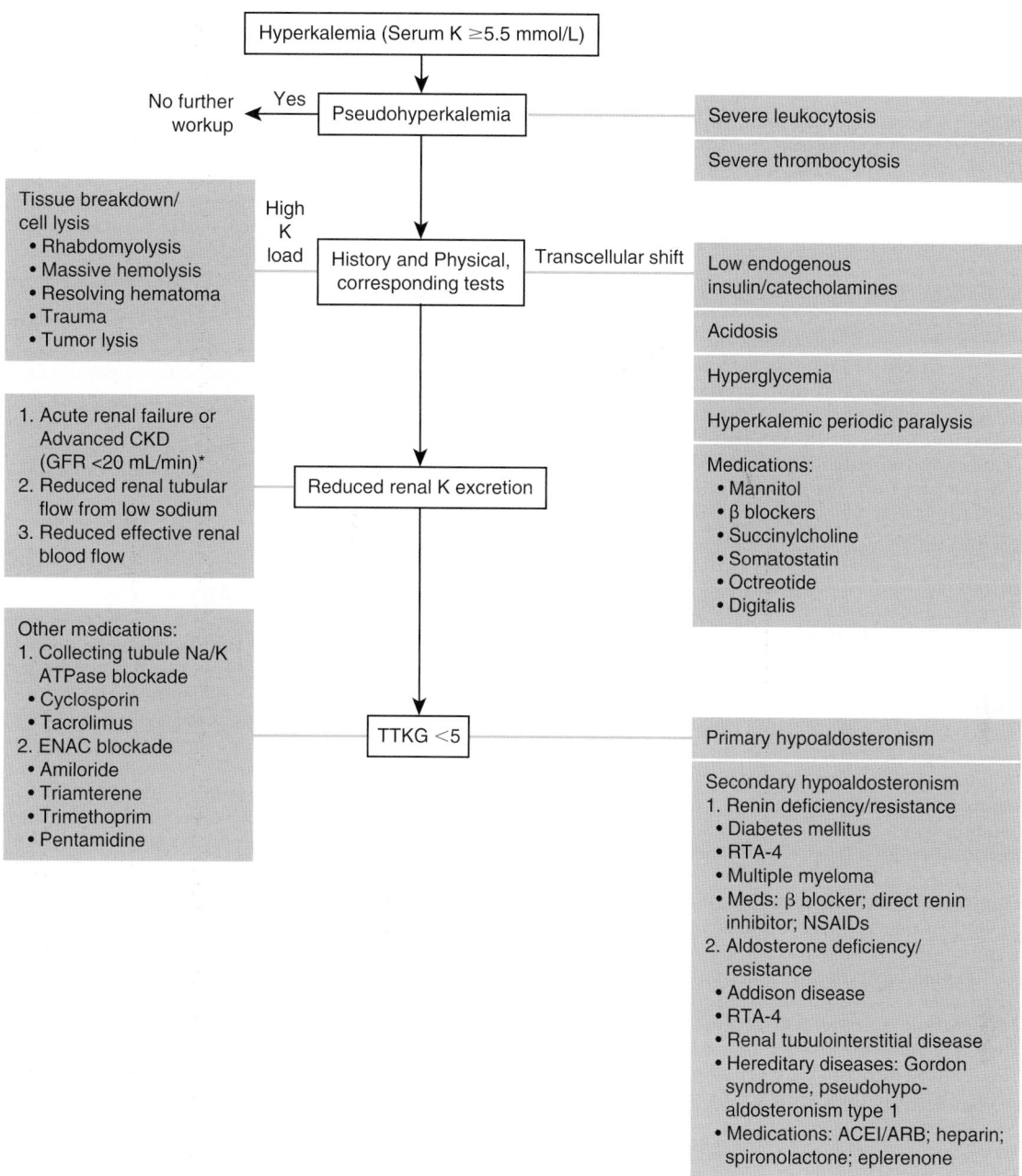

Figure 2 The diagnostic approach to hyperkalemia. *Hyperkalemia may occur with higher GFR if K load is excessive. *ACEI*, Angiotensin-converting enzyme inhibitor; *ARB*, angiotensin receptor blocker; *ENAC*, epithelial sodium channel; *GFR*, glomerular filtration rate; *NSAIDs*, nonsteroidal anti-inflammatory drugs; *RTA*, renal tubular acidosis.

suggests that the assumption inherent in the calculation of the TTKG lacks validity. That said, I still find it useful in the initial assessment.

Differential Diagnosis
Figures 1 and 2 outline a diagnostic approach, including differential diagnosis, for hyperkalemia and hypokalemia.

Therapy
The treatment of hypokalemia depends on the underlying cause, the degree of K depletion, and the risk of K depletion to the patient. In general, hypokalemia secondary to cell shift is managed by treating underlying conditions. For example, hypokalemia in the setting of catecholamine increases, as in chest pain syndromes, is managed with appropriate treatments for the pain. However, when cell-shift hypokalemia is associated with life-threatening conditions such as paresis, paralysis, or hypokalemia in the setting of myocardial infarction, the administration of K

is indicated. With K depletion, replacement therapy depends on the estimated degree of decreases in total body K. For example, decreases in total body K accompanied by a fall in serum K from 3.5 to 3.0 mmol/L are associated with a K deficit of 150 to 200 mmol. Decreases in serum K from 3 to 2 mmol/L are associated with 200- to 400-mmol additional decreases in total body K. K can be administered intravenously but in limited quantities (10 mEq/h into a peripheral vein; 15 to 20 mEq/h into a central vein). Larger K requirements can only be accomplished by oral therapy or with dialysis.

The acute management of hyperkalemia depends on the presence or absence of ECG and neuromuscular abnormalities. In the absence of symptoms or ECG abnormalities, hyperkalemia is treated conservatively—for example, by decreasing dietary K or withdrawing offending drugs. In the presence of ECG abnormalities or symptoms, the goal of therapy is to stabilize cell membranes. First-line therapy includes calcium gluconate, 10 to 30 mL IV as a 10% solution (onset of action

1 or 2 minutes). Although the mechanism remains undefined, calcium "stabilizes" the cardiac membranes. The dose can be repeated after five minutes if the ECG changes persist or recur. Other therapies include 8.4% IV sodium bicarbonate[1], 50 to 150 mEq (onset 15 to 30 minutes), and rapid-acting insulin[1] 5 to 10 units intravenously (onset 5 to 10 minutes). Insulin increases the activity of the Na-K-ATPase pump in skeletal muscle and drives K into cells. Glucose 50%, 25 g intravenously, is given simultaneously with insulin to prevent hypoglycemia. Albuterol given as 0.5 mg in D5W IV or 10–20 mg in 4 mL normal saline by nebulizer (onset 15 to 30 minutes), also activates the Na-K-ATPase and drives K into cells. K driven intracellularly generally begins to move extracellularly again after approximately 6 hours, increasing the serum K concentration. Therefore, therapy to remove K from the body should be started simultaneously. Reductions in total body K may be achieved through a K exchange resin. The primary K resin used is sodium polystyrene sulfonate (Kayexalate). One gram of this medication binds approximately 1 mEq of K and releases 1 to 2 mEq of sodium back into the circulation. This medication may be given orally (onset 2 hours) or by enema with sorbitol to induce diarrhea (onset 30 to 60 minutes).

In 2015, patiromer, a polymer that exchanges calcium for potassium in the gastrointestinal tract, was approved by the Food and Drug Administration (FDA) for the management of hyperkalemia. In 2018, sodium zirconium cyclosilicate (SZC), a novel nonabsorbed, nonpolymer zirconium silicate compound that exchanges hydrogen and sodium for potassium and ammonium was also approved by the FDA for the same indication. Both agents are well tolerated and effective. Patiromer is administered orally at an initial dose of 10 g three times a day for up to 48 hours, followed by a maintenance dose of 10 g daily (maximum daily maintenance dose 15 g/day).

If renal function is adequate, volume expansion with simultaneous diuresis can be attempted. Finally, hemodialysis is very effective in removing excess K.

The chronic management of hyperkalemia starts with dietary K restriction. Other management options include the use of diuretics, cessation or dose reduction of renin-angiotensin-aldosterone system inhibitors, and/or intermittent use of Kayexalate. Both patiromer and SZ are also well tolerated, safe, and effective in the chronic management of hyperkalemia. Just as important, they may allow the optimal use of renin-angiotensin-aldosterone system inhibitors in patients who have been previously untreated, had their dose reduced, or stopped treatment altogether.

Monitoring

Treatment for severe or symptomatic dyskalemia requires close cardiac monitoring and frequent laboratory testing to prevent overcorrection. If insulin and glucose are used in patients with hyperkalemia, blood sugars should be monitored for approximately 6 hours to identify and treat hypoglycemia from the insulin.

Complications

Complications from dyskalemia include cardiac arrhythmias, neuromuscular events, and, rarely, death. There are potential treatment-related complications if pseudodyskalemia or dyskalemia from in vivo transcellular shift is not recognized.

References

Gennari FJ: Hypokalemia, *N Engl J Med* 339:451–458, 1998.
Krishna GG, Kapoor SC: Potassium depletion exacerbates essential hypertension, *Ann Intern Med* 115:77–83, 1991.
Paice BJ, Paterson KR, Onyanga-Omara F, et al: Record linkage study of hypokalaemia in hospitalized patients, *Postgrad Med J* 62:187–191, 1986.
Stevens MS, Dunlay RW: Hyperkalemia in hospitalized patients, *Int Urol Nephrol* 32:177–180, 2000.

---

[1]Not FDA approved for this indication.

HYPONATREMIA

Method of
Beejal Shah, MD; and Susan L. Samson, MD, PhD

CURRENT DIAGNOSIS

- Perform a thorough history and physical examination with focus on the accurate assessment of volume status, neurologic symptoms and signs, current medications, and concurrent illnesses.
- Classify the hyponatremia as hypovolemic, euvolemic, or hypervolemic.
- Determine whether the hyponatremia is acute or chronic, based on the history and the clinical manifestations.
- Order key laboratory tests, including a basic metabolic panel (serum sodium, glucose, blood urea nitrogen, and creatinine), plasma osmolality, urine osmolality, and urine sodium.

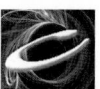

CURRENT THERAPY

- Severe and symptomatic hyponatremia should be treated with hypertonic saline (3%) at 1 to 2 mL/kg per hour. Neurologic status and serum sodium should be monitored every 2 to 4 hours. The objective is to raise sodium by 2 mEq/L per hour (or to >125 mEq/L) until deleterious neurologic symptoms improve. After this, the rate of infusion should be titrated to increase the serum sodium by 0.5 to 1.0 mEq/L per hour, with a maximum increase of 8 to 9 mEq/L over 24 hours and no more than 18 mEq/L over 48 hours, to avoid precipitating osmotic demyelination.
- As a general rule, the treatment of hyponatremia should be adjusted so that the serum sodium increases by 0.5 to 1.0 mEq/L per hour with a maximum increase of 8 to 9 mEq/L over 24 hours and no more than 18 mEq/L over 48 hours.
- Acute hyponatremia (<48 hours) may be treated more rapidly than chronic hyponatremia if dictated by neurologic findings.
- Before a diagnosis of SIADH is made, rule out adrenal insufficiency and hypothyroidism.
- Most cases of euvolemic hyponatremia are caused by the syndrome of inappropriate antidiuretic hormone (SIADH), which usually can be managed with fluid restriction, salt tablets, and vasopressin receptor antagonists ("vaptans") as indicated. Demeclocyclin is no longer used due to toxicity, expense, and the availability of vaptans.
- Discontinue thiazide diuretics in all cases of hypoosmolar hyponatremia.
- Hypovolemic and hypervolemic hyponatremia require therapy to correct the underlying cause (e.g., heart failure) and restore status to euvolemia.
- Vasopressin receptor antagonists (vaptans) are approved for short term management of euvolemic and hypovolemic hyponatremia. The same parameters apply for rate of sodium correction and monitoring as in conventional therapy.

Homeostasis maintains the concentration of sodium in the serum between 138 and 142 mEq/L (normal, 135–145 mEq/L) despite variations in water intake. Hyponatremia is defined as a serum sodium concentration of less than 135 mEq/L, although normal range values may differ slightly among laboratories, usually to a minimum normal sodium of 133 mEq/L. It is one of the most common electrolyte abnormalities found in the inpatient setting, occurring in up to 2.5% of patients, and it is a significant marker for mortality, associated with a 60-fold higher risk of death. It is not clear whether hyponatremia itself is the cause of a more adverse prognosis or whether it echoes the degree of stress caused by illness. In the outpatient setting, chronic hyponatremia is most prevalent among the elderly and nursing home residents. The approach to management of hyponatremia is highly dependent on the underlying process. Establishing the correct etiology is critical, because inappropriate treatment can worsen hyponatremia. Therapy must be administered judiciously because of the risk of severe neurologic sequelae, including central nervous system demyelination. However, with a systematic approach to the differential diagnosis of hyponatremia, the correct diagnosis can be made and therapy initiated.

Clinical Presentation
Acute hyponatremia is defined as hyponatremia of less than 48 hours in duration. Mild symptoms include headache, nausea, vomiting, confusion, and weakness, which usually occur with a sodium level of less than 129 mEq/L. More severe neurologic manifestations—seizure and coma—are seen usually below a threshold of 120 mEq/L, although there currently is no evidence-based critical sodium level above which neurologic sequelae do not occur. The neurologic manifestations of acute or recurrent symptomatic hyponatremia can be delayed, so continued monitoring is important.

In contrast, patients with chronic hyponatremia more often are asymptomatic or have blunted symptoms. In elderly patients with mild chronic hyponatremia, subtle neurocognitive manifestations can occur, with decreased balance, lowered reaction speed, memory loss, and directed gait. Mild hypoosmolar hyponatremia is not independently associated with increased morbidity and mortality. Even so, the underlying etiology needs to be determined because of the potential for other factors (e.g., new medications, dehydration, occult illness) to contribute to the development of more severe hyponatremia with its potential for neurologic injury.

Regulation of Water Balance
Approximately two thirds of total body water is contained in the intracellular fluid (ICF) and one third as extracellular fluid (ECF). Plasma osmolality is tightly regulated between 280 and 290 mOsm/kg and reflects the osmolality of the ECF. A change in plasma osmolality results in a shift of total body water between the ECF and the ICF to maintain their osmolar equivalence. Because sodium is the major osmole in the ECF, hyponatremia most often is a manifestation of decreased osmolality, so-called hypoosmolar or hypotonic hyponatremia.

Renal Handling of Water
The major osmoregulatory hormone is arginine vasopressin, also called antidiuretic hormone, which is synthesized in the paraventricular and supraoptic nuclei of the hypothalamus. It is transported along axons to the posterior pituitary, where it is processed and stored in vesicles. Vasopressin secretion is regulated by osmotic and nonosmotic stimuli. Secretion occurs with a 1% to 2% rise in osmolality (>288 mOsm/kg), as detected by receptors in the anterolateral walls of the hypothalamus adjacent to the third ventricle. Vasopressin secretion is inhibited when the plasma osmolality is lower than 280 mOsm/kg. The major nonosmotic stimulus is a decrease in effective circulating volume, which is detected by baroreceptors in the aortic arch and carotid sinuses. Although this mechanism requires a large drop (10%–15%) in blood pressure, the secretory response is more robust than for increases in osmolality. As such, acutely lowered blood pressure can override the inhibitory signal of low osmolality because of the need to maintain perfusion. Other physiologic nonosmotic stimuli include catecholamines and angiotensin II, but there is a long list of hormones and pharmacologic agents that induce or repress vasopressin secretion (Table 1).

The renal site of action of vasopressin is the V_2 receptors on the basolateral membrane of collecting duct cells in the distal nephron. The hormone-receptor interaction initiates intracellular signaling via cyclic adenosine monophosphate–dependent pathways, resulting in translocation of cytoplasmic aquaporon-2

TABLE 1	Molecules That Regulate Vasopressin Secretion	
STIMULATE VASOPRESSIN RELEASE		**INHIBIT VASOPRESSIN RELEASE**
Hormones and Neurotransmitters		
Acetylcholine (nicotinic)		Atrial natriuretic peptide
Angiotensin II		γ-Aminobutyric acid
Aspartate		Opioids (κ receptors)
Cholecystokinin		
Dopamine (D_1 and D_2)		
Glutamine		
Histamine (H_1)		
Neuropeptide Y		
Prostaglandin		
Substance P		
Vasoactive inhibitory peptide		
Pharmacologic Agents		
Adrenaline (epinephrine)		Butorphanol (Stadol)
Cyclophosphamide (Cytoxan)		Ethanol
High-dose morphine		Fluphenazine (Prolixin) Glucocorticoids
Nicotine		Haloperidol (Haldol)
Selective serotonin reuptake inhibitors		Low-dose morphine
Tricyclic antidepressants		Phenytoin (Dilantin)
Vincristine (Oncovin)		Promethazine (Phenergan)

channels to the surface of the collecting duct luminal membrane. These channels allow movement of water back into the cell for later reabsorption into the circulation. This results in a net concentration of urine and decreased plasma osmolality.

Renal Handling of Sodium
In addition to renal water handling, sodium reabsorption and excretion are important for maintenance of water homeostasis. The renin-angiotensin-aldosterone system is activated by reduced arterial perfusion pressure sensed by the juxtaglomerular apparatus of the afferent renal arteriole. Reduced arteriole effective volume (low or perceived) is sensed by the juxtaglomerular apparatus, which secretes renin, activating the renin-angiotensin system. This cascade of events ultimately stimulates aldosterone secretion, which acts at the distal nephron to cause reabsorption of filtered sodium via Na^+,K^+-adenosine triphosphatase (ATPase)–dependent sodium channels.

Central Nervous System Response to Hyponatremia/Hypoosmolality
Osmolar equivalence between the ECF and ICF is closely maintained by shifts in water between the two compartments. The major symptoms and signs of hyponatremia are neurologic in nature and are a clinical manifestation of swelling of the cells in the central nervous system, which results in cerebral edema. The most devastating consequence is herniation due to anatomic limitations on brain volume within the confines of the skull. Premenopausal women are at the highest risk for brain injury from hyponatremia.

A major compensatory mechanism in the central nervous system is the extrusion from the cells of intracellular solutes, which prevents further water influx. In the first few hours, inorganic ions (potassium, sodium, chloride) move out of the cell. After a few days of persistent hypoosmolality, the cells further compensate by extruding organic osmoles (glutamate, taurine, inositol). The clinician must be aware of this protective adaptation, because it necessitates a slower time course of correction during treatment. A rapid rise in plasma osmolality from aggressive treatment causes water to rapidly shift out of the cells, resulting in demyelination of neurons. In the past, this was termed pontine demyelinosis, but it has also been reported for extrapontine neurons and is now referred to as osmotic demyelination. The sequelae are permanent and devastating. There is clinical progression from lethargy to a change in affect, to mutism and dysarthria, and finally to spastic quadriparesis and pseudobulbar palsy.

Classification and Differential Diagnosis of Hyponatremia

Initial evaluation of hyponatremia requires a systematic and sequential approach. First, a thorough history and physical examination are required. It is important to identify any history of brain injury, stroke, mental illness, or chronic illness and the patient's current medication usage. On examination, special attention should be paid to mental status and neurologic abnormalities; manifestations of cardiac, hepatic, or renal disease; and signs of adrenal insufficiency or hypothyroidism. From the

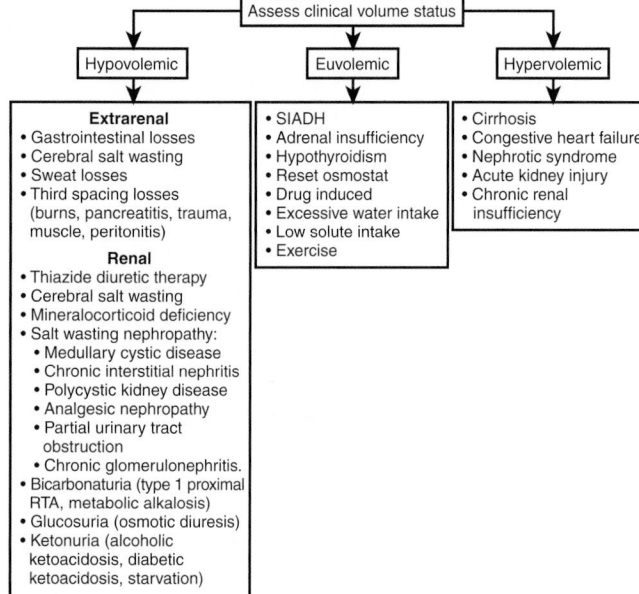

Figure 1 The differential diagnosis of hypoosmolar hyponatremia. *Abbreviations:* RTA = renal tubular acidosis; SIADH = syndrome of inappropriate antidiuretic hormone.

assessment of volume status, the hyponatremia should be classified as hypervolemic, euvolemic, or hypovolemic; each of these conditions leads in a different direction for diagnosis and treatment of the underlying cause (Figures 1 and 2). Finally, it should be determined whether the hyponatremia is acute (<48 hours) or chronic, because this can determine the time course of treatment.

For the laboratory work-up, essential basic tests are the serum sodium and potassium levels, renal function tests with blood urea nitrogen (BUN) and creatinine, and liver function tests. It is likely that these tests have already been performed, motivating the assessment of hyponatremia. After this, the plasma osmolality (P_{Osm}), urine osmolality (U_{Osm}), and urine sodium concentration are key diagnostic tests. P_{Osm} is directly measured in the laboratory and also can be calculated. Calculated osmolality is the sum of the concentrations of the known major osmoles—sodium and glucose—in the ECF and the BUN:

$$P_{Osm} = (2 \times Na) + (glucose) + (BUN)$$

The calculation is done in SI units. For sodium, mEq/L is the same as the SI unit, mmol/L; if glucose and BUN values were reported in mg/dL, they must be divided by 18 and 2.8, respectively, to convert to SI units (mmol/L). The directly measured osmolality should be within 10 to 12 mOsm/kg of the calculated value; an increased osmolar gap compared with the calculated value points toward the presence of additional osmoles in the plasma that are causing hypertonicity.

Because hyponatremia usually is a reflection of plasma osmolality, most patients also have a low P_{Osm}, and the clinician often can proceed to the differential diagnosis of hypoosmolar (or hypotonic) hyponatremia after excluding pseudohyponatremia (which usually has normal osmolality) and hyperosmolar hyponatremia. Pseudohyponatremia can occur if the plasma lipid or protein content is greatly increased in the plasma (usually to >6%–8% of volume), as in extreme hypertriglyceridemia and paraprotein disorders. These extra components decrease the aqueous portion of the plasma volume and thereby interfere with the laboratory measurement of sodium by dilutional, indirect methods such as flame photometry. Most laboratories now use direct measurement of sodium to avoid this problem.

Hyperosmolar hyponatremia can occur if there are additional osmoles present that cause water movement from the ICF into the ECF, resulting in ECF expansion and dilutional hyponatremia. Overall, the total body water and total body sodium are unchanged in this situation. An important clinical example occurs with hyperglycemia, and the reported sodium value should be corrected for high glucose by the clinician by adding 1.6 mEq/L to the measured Na for every 100 mg/dL rise in glucose above 200 mg/dL. Because glucose is included in the calculation of osmolality, there will be no significant osmolar gap.

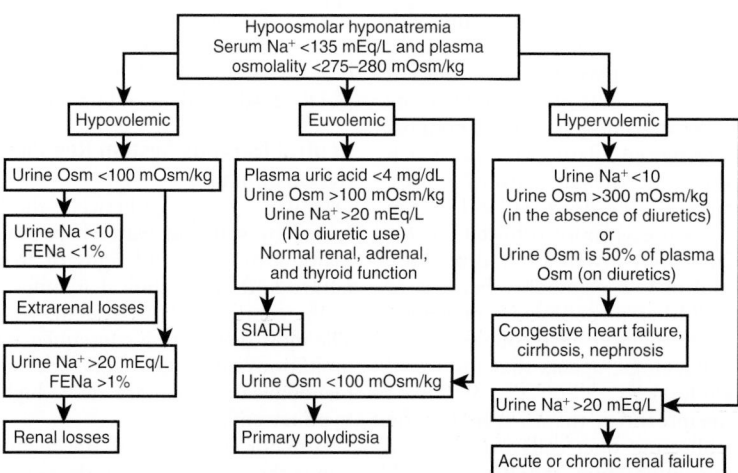

Figure 2 Laboratory findings in hypoosmolar hyponatremia. *Abbreviations:* FENa = fractional excretion of sodium; Osm = osmoles; SIADH = syndrome of inappropriate antidiuretic hormone.

Other osmotically active solutes encountered clinically are mannitol, which is used to manage increased intracranial pressure, and glycine, which is used for irrigation in urologic procedures. Mannitol and glycine are retained in the ECF and are not part of the calculated osmolality, so their presence results in an osmolar gap. High levels of alcohol or ethylene glycol also increase the osmolality, but these substances are so quickly metabolized that an osmolar gap may not be apparent by the time testing is performed.

Once pseudohyponatremia and hypertonicity have been ruled out, the diagnosis is narrowed to hypoosmolar hyponatremia. The combined physical examination and laboratory results allow classification of the patient as having hypervolemic hyponatremia with excess total body sodium, hypovolemic hyponatremia with a deficit of total body sodium, or euvolemic hyponatremia with near-normal total body sodium.

Hypovolemic Hyponatremia

The causes of hypovolemic hyponatremia can be classified as extrarenal or renal (see Figure 1). Signs of volume contraction are apparent on examination, including poor skin turgor, skin tenting (forehead), decreased or undetectable jugular venous pressure, dry mucous membranes, and orthostatic changes in blood pressure and pulse rate. If the volume status is not completely clear from the examination, laboratory values can be helpful (see Figure 2), but they need to be interpreted in the context of renal function tests. If the urine osmolality is less than maximally concentrated (<500 mOsm/kg), an infusion of 0.5 to 1 L of isotonic saline over 24 to 48 hours may help with differentiation. With hypovolemia, the sodium will begin to correct and the patient should improve clinically. Conversely, if the patient is actually euvolemic, such as with syndrome of inappropriate antidiuretic hormone (SIADH), discussed later, the serum sodium level will remain constant or decrease due to retention of free water with a concomitant increase in urinary sodium.

Extrarenal causes of hyponatremia include gastrointestinal losses and third-space losses such as in severe burns and pancreatitis. In the volume-depleted state, with intact renal function, the urine sodium is low (<10 mEq/L), reflecting a normal response by the kidney to maximally reabsorb sodium in response to volume depletion.

The renal causes of hypovolemic hyponatremia involve the inappropriate loss of sodium into the urine, and this is reflected by a urine sodium concentration of greater than 20 mEq/L.

Thiazide diuretics cause renal sodium loss, so the urine sodium is high. However, they also impair the kidney's diluting capacity, decreasing free water excretion and concentrating the urine. Only certain patients may be susceptible to hyponatremia while on thiazides. These patients may have an abnormally sensitive thirst response to the mild hypovolemia induced by the diuretics, causing increased water intake. Elderly women are the most susceptible, and hyponatremia can occur within days after initiation of thiazide therapy. Additional laboratory results reveal hypokalemia and a metabolic alkalosis. It is appropriate to stop the diuretic and restore potassium levels and volume status. Patients often have a recurrence of hyponatremia if rechallenged with thiazides. Loop diuretics, such as furosemide, are a less frequent cause of hyponatremia, which occurs only after long-term therapy.

In the absence of diuretic use, a urine sodium concentration greater than 20 mEq/L with hypovolemia is evidence for underlying renal pathology. Patients with salt-wasting nephropathy, from a number of causes (see Figure 1), usually have significant renal failure, with a creatinine value in the range of 3 to 4 mg/dL. Because of the large net sodium loss, this condition is treated with salt tablets. Renal tubular acidosis causes bicarbonaturia, which requires a compensatory excretion of urinary cations, mainly Na^+ and K^+, to maintain electroneutrality. Similarly, excretion of ketones into the urine also demands additional electrolyte losses in spite of ECF volume depletion, leading to a loss of sodium.

Cerebral salt wasting (CSW), although it could be considered an extrarenal cause, also involves the renal loss of sodium (>20 mEq/L). The biochemical presentation is very similar to that of SIADH, but the diagnosis of CSW is restricted to cases involving extreme central nervous system pathology. CSW is most commonly associated with subarachnoid hemorrhage but also has been reported with stroke, brain trauma, infection, metastases and after neurosurgery. Onset of CSW is usually within the first 10 days after the neurologic event.

CSW may be a protective mechanism against increased intracranial pressure. The proposed pathophysiologic mechanism of CSW is controversial, but one hypothesis is that the initiating event is a primary natriuresis, with renal loss of sodium, caused by the secretion of natriuretic peptides. Clinical studies have found both increased brain natriuretic peptide and increased atrial natriuretic peptide in neurosurgical patients with hyponatremia. Both hormones are vasodilators that increase the glomerular filtration rate while suppressing the renin-angiotensin system. This increases renal sodium losses, as well as water excretion, resulting in volume depletion. Vasopressin levels rise in response to low volume, so that it becomes biochemically difficult to differentiate CSW from SIADH, with a urine sodium level greater than 20 mEq/L, low uric acid, and high urine osmolality. It is helpful if CSW patients have signs of volume depletion in combination with the laboratory results. Also, the hyponatremia of CSW responds to normal saline, whereas SIADH worsens with normal saline. CSW is relatively rare in most case series, and it is important to rule out other causes for natriuresis.

Hypervolemic Hyponatremia

There are a variety of causes of hypervolemic hyponatremia (see Figure 1), all of which are a result of decreased effective circulating volume. To correct this imbalance, the ECF expands, leading to fluid retention and hyponatremia. In spite of the increased total body water and low serum sodium on testing, all of these patients have some degree of total body sodium excess. In many cases, volume overload is clinically evident from the presence of subcutaneous edema, ascites, elevated jugular venous pressure, or pulmonary edema.

In congestive heart failure (CHF), patients can develop hyponatremia with only 2 to 3 L of fluid intake per day despite normal renal function. The decreased filling pressures and cardiac output of CHF are perceived as volume depletion, detected by the baroreceptors. This stimulates vasopressin secretion, overriding the signal of low osmolality detected by the hypothalamic osmoreceptors. This lack of inhibition of vasopressin secretion is believed to be the most important contributing factor to the development of hyponatremia. In addition, decreased right atrial pressures result in inhibition of secretion of atrial natriuretic peptide, contributing to the water and sodium gain. With the low perfusion pressure, there is a decrease in the glomerular filtration rate, which is sensed by the juxtaglomerular apparatus, causing neurohumoral activation of the renin-angiotensin system and sympathetic nervous system. This leads to increased circulating levels of catecholamines, angiotensin II, and aldosterone, further stimulating tubular sodium and water reabsorption. In the absence of diuretics, the urine sodium level is very low (<10 mEq/L) in patients with CHF because of activation of the renin-angiotensin-aldosterone system and maximal tubular reabsorption of sodium. Also, there is less than maximally dilute urine (usually >300 mOsm/kg) in the absence of diuretic therapy. An elevated brain natriuretic peptide concentration helps to confirm the hypervolemia.

A similar mechanism is at work in cirrhotic patients, in whom the incidence of hyponatremia is even higher and is a strong predictor of poor outcome. In cirrhosis, low albumin results in third-spacing and decreased effective circulating volume. In addition, portal hypertension leads to splanchnic vasodilation, which also decreases the effective circulating volume. This serves to activate vasopressin secretion and the renin-angiotensin-aldosterone system.

Hyponatremia is less common in acute and chronic renal failure, but it can occur with a significant decrease in glomerular filtration rate accompanied by severe hypoalbuminemia. Interpretation of the laboratory results may be confounded by a high urine sodium concentration (>20 mEq/L) that reflects the concomitant presence of tubular dysfunction. Hyponatremia can develop in stage IV or V renal failure when fluid intake is in excess of 3 L/day.

Euvolemic Hyponatremia

Euvolemic hyponatremia is caused by impaired excretion of free water by the kidney. The differential diagnosis is more limited (see Figure 1) and the majority of cases are due to SIADH (Table 2). However, this often is a diagnosis of exclusion, and hypothyroidism and adrenal insufficiency must be ruled out clinically or biochemically in patients with euvolemic hyponatremia.

Hypothyroidism leads to reduced glomerular filtration rate and decreased flow to the distal nephron, causing maximal reabsorption of water to maintain arterial volume. Hypothyroidism has to be severe to cause hyponatremia and usually is obvious on examination. However, in the elderly population, apathetic hypothyroidism may be difficult to diagnose. Hypothyroidism can be confirmed by the presence of a high level of thyroid-stimulating hormone and a low level of free T_4 (thyroxine). Treatment involves thyroid hormone replacement and supportive care.

In primary adrenal insufficiency (Addison's disease), the concomitant aldosterone deficiency results in hyponatremia combined with hyperkalemia, prerenal azotemia, a urine sodium concentration greater than 20 mEq/L, and a urine potassium level lower than 20 mEq/L. In secondary or central adrenal insufficiency, the adrenal zona glomerulosa remains intact for the secretion of aldosterone. However, glucocorticoid deficiency still causes impaired water excretion, which can lead to dilutional hyponatremia. Vasopressin release may be stimulated by the nausea, vomiting, and orthostatic hypotension that occurs with adrenal insufficiency. Finally, corticosteroids normally inhibit vasopressin release, so their deficiency leads to enhanced vasopressin release, causing retention of free water that further contributes to the hyponatremia. The appropriate diagnostic test is a 250-μg ACTH (cosyntropin, Cortrosyn) stimulation test, although an extremely low 8 AM cortisol level (<3 μg/dL) can be diagnostic. Treatment consists of glucocorticoid replacement.

Syndrome of Inappropriate Antidiuretic Hormone

SIADH is the most common cause of euvolemic hypoosmolar hyponatremia. Edema, ascites, and orthostasis are absent, and thyroid, adrenal, and renal functions are normal. Recent diuretic use should be ruled out. The primary event is the release of vasopressin, which results in water retention. The increased intravascular volume stimulates a natriuresis, which actually is appropriate, but the resulting loss of sodium compounds the hyponatremia. There is an extensive list of causes of SIADH, usually involving pulmonary or central nervous system pathology (see Table 2). A number of medications also are known to stimulate vasopressin release or to potentiate its antidiuretic properties at the level of the kidney (see Tables 1 and 2).

The diagnosis of SIADH is suggested by a low P_{Osm} (<280 mOsm/kg) with a high U_{Osm} (>100 mOsm/kg), confirming water retention and an inappropriately concentrated urine. A spot urine sodium level will be greater than 20 mEq/L, and usually greater than 30 mEq/L. Other helpful laboratory findings include low plasma uric acid (<4 mg/dL), which has a positive predictive value of 73% to 100% for SIADH in this setting. In complicated cases confounded by use of diuretics, the fractional excretion of uric acid has a positive predictive value of 100% for SIADH when the calculated excretion is greater than 12%.

Reset osmostat can be considered a form of SIADH, but the hyponatremia is usually chronic, mild, and asymptomatic. Vasopressin release continues to be regulated, but at a lower threshold of plasma osmolality. The thirst threshold may be altered as well. Interventions to raise the sodium usually have short-lived effects, and the sodium resets at its previous value over time. Therefore, treatment is not recommended if the sodium level is stable and the patient is asymptomatic. A physiologic example of reset osmostat is seen in pregnancy, when the normal sodium range is lowered by 5 mEq/L.

TABLE 2	Causes of SIADH

CNS Disorders

Mass lesions (tumors; CNS abscess; intracranial hemorrhage or hematoma)
Stroke
CNS infections or inflammatory diseases
Spinal cord lesions
Acute psychosis
Pituitary stalk lesions
Hydrocephalus
Dementia
Guillain-Barré syndrome
Head trauma

Pulmonary Disorders

Viral/bacterial pneumonia
Positive-pressure ventilation
Bronchogenic carcinoma (small cell)
Acute respiratory failure
COPD
Tuberculosis
Aspergillosis
Pulmonary abscess

Medications/Drugs

Vasopressin analogues (desmopressin [DDAVP])
NSAIDs
Tricyclic antidepressants
Phenothiazines
Butyrophenones
SSRIs/SNRIs
Morphine
Opiates
Chlorpropamide (Diabinese)
Clofibrate (Atromid-S)[2]
Cyclophosphamide (Cytoxan)
Vincristine (Oncovin)
Nicotine
Tolbutamide (Orinase)
Barbiturates
Acetaminophen (Tylenol)
ACE inhibitors
Carbamazepine (Tegretol)
Omeprazole (Prilosec)
MDMA (Ecstasy)
Lamotrigine (Lamictal)
Sodium valproate (Depakote)
Monomaine oxidase inhibitors
Ifosfamide (Ifex)
Melphalan (Alkeran, Evomela)
Platinum agents

Other

Pain
Nausea
HIV infection/AIDS
Prolonged exercise (e.g., marathon running)
Idiopathic
Acute intermittent porphyria

[2]Not available in the United States.

Abbreviations: ACE = angiotensin-converting enzyme; AIDS = acquired immunodeficiency syndrome; CNS = central nervous system; COPD = chronic obstructive pulmonary disease; DDAVP = 1-deamino, 8-D arginine-vasopressin; MDMA = methylenedioxymethamphetamine; NSAIDs = nonsteroidal antiinflammatory drugs; SSRIs = selective serotonin reuptake inhibitors.

Other Causes of Euvolemic Hypoosmolar Hyponatremia

Primary or psychogenic polydipsia should be considered in patients presenting with hyponatremia and a history of psychiatric illness and treatment. Almost 6% to 7% of psychiatric inpatients are at risk for hyponatremia from increased water intake. The polydipsia may be related to a lowered osmolar threshold for thirst, below the threshold of suppression of vasopressin secretion. This can be further complicated by the side effect of dry mouth caused by many psychiatric medications, which compounds the increased thirst and water intake. Because the kidney is capable of excreting up to 15 to 20 L/day of dilute urine, the fact that hyponatremia develops in these patients may point toward an additional and inappropriate increase in vasopressin release or sensitivity. These patients are clinically euvolemic because of renal excretion of the excess water and have otherwise normal laboratory results except for a dilute urine (<100 mOsm/kg), which is caused by vasopressin suppression and helps differentiate primary polydipsia from SIADH. However, some patients have mildly concentrated urine (>100 mOsm/kg), in which case the psychiatric history helps with the diagnosis.

Exercise-induced hyponatremia (e.g., from marathon running) is a form of euvolemic hypoosmolar hyponatremia primarily caused by retention of water relative to fluid lost via sweating or renal excretion. Vasopressin levels are inappropriately increased during exercise-induced hyponatremia. Most importantly, it is an acute hyponatremia, developing in less than 24 hours, and should be treated accordingly.

Vasopressin levels also may be inappropriately high, secondary to pain or the use of NSAIDs, which remove prostaglandin inhibition of vasopressin release. Low solute intake combined with high fluid intake also can cause hyponatremia, as with beer potomania or a low-protein "tea and toast" diet in elderly patients. In both cases, the lack of solute in the urine does not allow retention of water in the filtrate, so the excess water is not excreted.

Hyponatremia also is common after pituitary surgery (transsphenoidal or by craniotomy) and may be a result of damage to the hypothalamic-pituitary tract that causes release of preformed vasopressin from damaged neurons. Often, hyponatremia occurs as the second phase of the classic triphasic response: transient diabetes insipidus, transient SIADH, followed by permanent diabetes insipidus. Hyponatremia can be delayed up to 1 week postoperatively, and sodium should be monitored during the second week as well. Contributions by central adrenal insufficiency and hypothyroidism also are considerations after pituitary surgery, although with these conditions there will be obvious clinical manifestations in addition to the hyponatremia.

Management

The major considerations for choosing the type and time course of treatment for hyponatremia are the duration of hyponatremia (acute or chronic) and the presence of neurologic signs and symptoms, especially severe manifestations such as altered mental status or seizure (see Table 2). Treatment options for hyponatremia include fluid restriction, saline infusion (hypertonic or isotonic), vasopressin receptor antagonists and demeclocycline (Declomycin).[1] Also, treatment of the underlying abnormality, such as CHF or salt wasting, and correction of volume status are important for hypovolemic or hypervolemic patients. Autocorrection may occur after initiation of therapy, especially in cases of hypovolemia, adrenal insufficiency, or thiazide use. Once treatment is started, the contribution of the nonosmotic stimulation of vasopressin secretion is removed, and the patient is able to raise the sodium level by 2 mEq/L per hour over 12 hours.

Acute Severe Symptomatic Hyponatremia

Acute severe hyponatremia is defined as a rapid fall in sodium in less than 48 hours to less than 120 mEq/L. Under these circumstances, most patients develop neurologic symptoms because of the rapid fluid shifts between the ECF and the ICF in the brain. If left untreated, it can result in irreversible neurologic damage and death. Because of the acute drop in sodium, initial rapid correction is acceptable and should not lead to osmotic demyelination. Treatment is aimed at raising the sodium enough to resolve the neurologic signs and symptoms. The goal is to raise the serum sodium by 1 to 2 mEq/L per hour or to greater than 125 mEq/L until symptoms resolve. Hypovolemic patients will respond to infusion of isotonic saline (normal saline 0.9%), especially if the urine sodium concentration is less than 30 mEq/L. If the neurologic findings are severe, hypertonic saline (3%) may be infused at rate of 1 to 2 mL/ kg per hour, or even up to 4 to 6 mL/kg per hour if the imbalance

is life-threatening. A loop diuretic can be combined with the saline to enhance solute-free water excretion. In exercise-induced hyponatremia, hypertonic (3%) saline is the preferred treatment to prevent cerebral edema due to water shifting into the brain along the osmotic gradient. A hypertonic (3%) saline 100 mL bolus can be given to promptly to decrease the osmotic gradient, which is promoting water entry into cells. Thereafter, in the inpatient setting, hypertonic (3%) saline infusion should be continued to promote correction of hyponatremia. Sodium levels should be monitored every 2 to 4 hours in patients undergoing hypertonic infusion. Once symptoms resolve, the rate of correction should be reduced to 0.5 to 1 mEq/hr, and the total rise in sodium should not exceed 18 mEq in 48 hours. No benefit has been observed for faster rates of correction of hyponatremia, whether acute or chronic. Useful formulas to determine the rate of infusion for fluids are provided in Figure 3. The formulas can only estimate the rate of correction, and sodium should be measured frequently.

Chronic Hyponatremia

Chronic hyponatremia is defined as a gradual fall in sodium over more than 48 hours. By this time, the brain has begun to compensate for hypoosmolality by extrusion of solutes. However, the patient is at risk of osmotic demyelination if hyponatremia is treated too aggressively. If the duration of hyponatremia is unknown, the recommendation is to assume that it is chronic. However, as with acute hyponatremia, severe neurologic symptoms and signs need to be treated with hypertonic saline until they resolve, after which the rate of correction can be slowed to 0.5 to 1 mEq/L per hour. Most cases of osmotic demyelination occur with correction rates of greater than 12 mEq/L in 24 hours, but there are cases reported with increases of 9 or 10 mEq/day. Asymptomatic hyponatremia can be treated with an infusion of isotonic saline calculated to raise the sodium by 0.5 to 1 mEq/ hour. If the patient has a dilute urine (<200 mOsm/kg), water restriction may be sufficient.

Syndrome of Inappropriate Antidiuretic Hormone

The mainstays of treatment of SIADH are fluid restriction and treatment of the underlying cause. Mild SIADH usually can be controlled with fluid restriction alone.

In most cases of SIADH, the degree of fluid restriction required can be calculated. It is dependent on three factors: the daily osmolar load, the minimum U_{Osm}, and the patient's maximum urine volume. A typical diet has a daily osmolar load of 10 mOsm/kg of body weight. For a 70-kg person, this would be 700 mOsm/day. With SIADH, the urine osmolality is held constant for that particular patient, as revealed by a spot U_{Osm}. If the U_{Osm} is 500 mOsm/ kg and the solute load is 700 mOsm, the fluid load has to be less than 700/500 or 1.4 L/day just to maintain the serum sodium level. Fluid intake above this amount will cause the sodium to decrease.

When needed, salt tablets (sodium chloride tablet 1-3 g taken once to three times daily) can help to make up for renal loss of sodium in SIADH. With symptoms and severe hyponatremia, short-term use of hypertonic saline may also be instituted to restore sodium to the ECF compartment. Loop diuretics (e.g., furosemide [Lasix]) can increase free water clearance when given with solute (e.g., hypertonic saline or salt tablets). In refractory cases, demeclocycline (300–600 mg PO twice daily)[1] can be used. Demeclocycline (Declomycin) antagonizes the actions of vasopressin by inhibiting formation of cyclic adenosine monophosphate in the collecting duct. Long-term use is limited by the side effect of photosensitivity and by nephrotoxicity in patients with underlying liver disease. Vasopressin receptor antagonists also are important adjunct treatments (see later discussion). A less commonly used treatment is urea (powder or capsules),[1,6] which causes an osmotic diuresis and increased free water excretion. Preclinical data support that urea may decrease osmotic demyelination.

Parameters for acute or chronic hyponatremia:
Do not increase serum Na by more than 9 mEq in 24 hours and 18 mEq in 48 hours

Symptomatic hyponatremia with severe neurologic symptoms (acute <48 hrs or chronic >48 hrs)
1. Correct serum Na at a rate of 1–2 mEq/l per hour (for 2 to 4 hours) until symptoms have resolved
2. Correct Na at a rate of less than 9 mEq/24 h

Acute hyponatremia symptoms
1. Correct at rate of 0.5 to 1 mEq/L per hour to a maximum of 9 mEq/24 h

Chronic hyponatremia with mild symptoms or asymptomatic
1. Correct at a rate of 0.5 mEq/L per hour with fluid restriction
2. Treat underlying etiology

Calculation of the rate of infusion of saline to correct hyponatremia
1. Change in serum sodium per liter infusate
$$(\Delta Na/L) = \frac{\text{Infusate [sodium]} - \text{Serum [sodium]}}{TBW + 1}$$
2. Amount of infusate (in L) required in 24 hours
$$L = \frac{\text{desired change in sodium } (\Delta Na) \text{ over 24 hrs}}{\Delta Na/L \text{ (from 1)}}$$
3. Rate of infusate to raise serum Na by desired amount
$$ml/hr = \frac{L \text{ (from 2)} \times 1000 \text{ mL/L}}{24 \text{ hr}}$$
4. (Simplified) Hypertonic saline infused at 1–2 mL/kg per hour

Infusate	Infusate [Na] (mmol/L)
5% sodium chloride in water	855
3% sodium chloride in water	513
Isotonic saline (0.9%)	154
Ringer's lactate solution	130
0.45% sodium chloride in water	77
0.2% sodium chloride in water	34
5% dextrose in water	0

Total Body Water (TBW) is equal to 60% of body weight in young adult men and 50% in young adult women. Older patients have less TBW. In elderly males, TBW is equal to 50% of body weight and in elderly females it is 45%.

Monitoring:
1. Monitor frequently for clinical improvement or worsening of symptoms
2. If on hypertonic saline or severely symptomatic check sodium q2–4 hrs.
3. If undergoing treatment but asymptomatic, check sodium q6–12 h.

Figure 3 Treatment of hyponatremia. *Abbreviation:* TBW = total body water.

Cerebral Salt Wasting

Management of CSW involves treatment of the underlying neurologic problem, as well as volume replacement. CSW often is difficult to differentiate biochemically from SIADH, but the rise in vasopressin in CSW is secondary to volume depletion. As a result, CSW responds to volume replacement with isotonic saline, suppressing release of vasopressin, whereas SIADH worsens with this therapy. The recommended correction rate is 0.7 to 1.0 mEq/L per hour, with a maximum of 9 mEq per 24 hours. Salt tablets may also be given to replete total body sodium. Fludrocortisone (Florinef 0.05 to 0.1 mg every 12 hours), an aldosterone receptor agonist, is a third-line treatment to encourage volume expansion and sodium retention, but the potassium concentration and blood pressure should be monitored. Fluid restriction is inappropriate for CSW and should be avoided, especially in patients with subarachnoid hemorrhage, because volume depletion can exacerbate cerebral vasospasm and cause infarction. The duration of CSW is usually 3 to 5 weeks.

Vasopressin Receptor Antagonists

Vasopressin receptor antagonists, or vaptans, are a treatment option for clinically significant euvolemic hyponatremia defined as a serum Na <125 mEq/L or if hyponatremia is symptomatic and resistant to correction with standard therapy. Vaptans also can be used for asymptomatic hypervolemic hyponatremia, but the benefit must clearly outweigh the risk, and the patient should be refractory to standard therapy. There are currently two FDA-approved vaptans, conivaptan (Vaprisol) and tolvaptan (Samsca). Conivaptan is a dual V_{1a}/V_2 arginine vasopressin receptor antagonist and tolvaptan is a selective V_2 arginine vasopressor receptor antagonist with about 29 times the affinity to the V_2 receptor compared to conivaptan. The primary action of both medications is to block the binding of vasopressin to its receptors in the distal nephron which leads to a decrease in translocation of the aquaporin-2 channels to the apical membrane of the collecting duct in the renal tubule. As a result, vaptans cause an increase in excretion of solute-free water resulting in a rise in serum sodium.

Conivaptan is an IV formulation approved for inpatient hospital use for euvolemic and hypervolemic hyponatremia. It is contraindicated for hypovolemic hyponatremia, euvolemic or hypervolemic hyponatremia with moderate to severe central nervous system (CNS) symptoms, and hypervolemic hyponatremia due to cirrhosis. Conivaptan should be used very cautiously in patients with hypervolemic hyponatremia due to heart failure because safety data are limited and efficacy has not been clearly established. Conivaptan is not recommended in those with severe renal impairment CrCl < 30 mL/min. Conivaptan is given intravenously with a bolus of 20 mg over 30 minutes in 100 mL of 5% dextrose in water (D5W) followed by a continuous infusion of 20 mg conivaptan diluted in 250 mL of D5W over 24 hours. After the initial day of treatment, conivaptan can be continued for an additional 1 to 3 days. Sodium is monitored every 2 to 4 hours and the dose may be titrated to 40 mg per 24 hours to obtain an increase in sodium of 0.5 to 1.0 mEq/L per hour. In clinical trials, the average rise in serum Na after 4 days of therapy is about 6 mEq/L. During conivaptan treatment, fluid restriction can be liberal or is not required. Close monitoring of the rate of sodium rise, neurologic status, and hemodynamic stability are required and treatment should be discontinued or resumed at a reduced dose if clinically indicated. The most common side effects of conivaptan are infusion site reactions and to a lesser degree headache, hypotension, nausea, constipation, and postural hypotension.

Tolvaptan is an oral V_2 receptor antagonist that carries the same indications for use as conivaptan. Tolvaptan should be initiated only in the hospital setting for careful monitoring of potassium and the rate of Na rise, and then can be used in the outpatient setting. The starting dose is 15 mg once daily and can be titrated to 60 mg daily after the initial 24 hours. Patients should not be on fluid restriction for the first 24 hours of tolvaptan therapy and be advised to drink based on thirst. Tolvaptan carries a risk of serious liver injury. The FDA recommends that tolvaptan should not be used for durations longer than 30 days or in any patient with underlying liver disease. Monitoring parameters are equivalent to conivaptan the drug should be stopped promptly in patients with abnormal liver tests or symptoms of hepatotoxicity. In clinical studies, the average rise in serum Na after 4 days of therapy is 4.2 mEq/L and 5.5 mEq/L after 30 days of therapy. The vaptans are a substrate and potent inhibitor of cytochrome P-450 3A4 isoenzyme (CYP3A4). Prior to initiation of therapy drug-drug interactions should be reviewed with the pharmacists and vaptans are contraindicated with other CYP3A4 inhibitors.

Summary

Hyponatremia is a common electrolyte abnormality and is usually caused by decreased plasma osmolality. Accurate assessment of volume status is a key to determining the underlying cause and choosing the correct treatment approach. The biggest risk of hyponatremia and its treatment is the possibility of severe neurologic sequelae, including fatal cerebral edema and osmotic demyelination. Therefore more aggressive initial treatment is needed in patients with neurologic manifestations (hypertonic saline), but a more conservative approach (e.g., fluid restriction) is needed for less symptomatic patients. Vasopressin antagonists are additional tools for the treatment of euvolemic or hypervolemic hyponatremia refractory to more conservative measures.

References

Androgué HJ: Consequences of inadequate management of hyponatremia, *Am J Nephrol* 25:240–249, 2005.

Cerdà-Esteve M, Cuadrado-Godia E, Chillaron JJ, et al: Cerebral salt wasting syndrome: Review, *Eur J Intern Med* 19:249–254, 2008.

Dineen R, Thompson CJ, Sherlock M: Hyponatremia presentations and management, *Clin Med (Lond)* 17:263–269, 2017.

Ellison DH, Berl T: Clinical practice: The syndrome of inappropriate antidiuresis, *N Engl J Med* 356:2064–2072, 2007.

Fenske W, Störk S, Koschker A: Value of fractional uric acid excretion in differential diagnosis of hyponatremia patients on diuretics, *J Clin Endocrinol Metab* 93:2991–2997, 2008.

Gankam Kengne F, Decauz G: Hyponatremia and the Brain, *Kidney Int Rep* 3:24–35, 2018.

Hew-Butler T, Rosner MH, et al: Statement of the Third International Exercise-Induced Hyponatremia Consensus Development Conference, *Clin J Sport Med.* 25:303–320, 2015.

Hoom EJ, Zieste R: Diagnosis and treatment of hyponatremia: Compilation of the guidelines, *J Am Soc Nephrol* 28:1340–1349, 2017.

Jovanovich AJ, Berl T: Where vaptans do and do not fit in the treatment of hyponatremia, *Kidney Int* 83:563–567, 2013.

Sterns RH, Silver AM, Hix JK: Urea for hyponatremia? *Kidney Int* 87:268–270, 2015.

⬛ HYPOPITUITARISM

Method of
Fabienne Langlois, MD; Elena V. Varlamov, MD; and Maria Fleseriu, MD

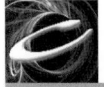

CURRENT DIAGNOSIS

- Hypopituitarism is rare and occurs most commonly due to sellar tumors and their subsequent treatment (pituitary surgery and radiation); less commonly hypopituitarism is due to infiltrative disease, cancer immunotherapy, traumatic brain injury, and congenital and other disorders.
- Heightened awareness is required, as clinical manifestations are often nonspecific and insidious, and patients can deteriorate and experience adrenal crisis if hypopituitarism is not detected and treated.
- Diagnosis is based on a combination of low baseline peripheral gland hormones (cortisol, thyroid hormone, insulin-like growth factor-1 [IGF-1], testosterone, and estrogen) and low or inappropriately normal pituitary hormones as well as complementary dynamic testing for adrenal insufficiency (AI) and growth hormone (GH) deficiency.
- Pituitary imaging should be performed when a biochemical diagnosis is confirmed or pituitary disease is suspected based on neurologic symptoms (headaches and peripheral vision loss).

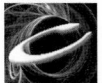

CURRENT THERAPY

- Glucocorticoid (GC) replacement is the most critical of all replacements for hypopituitarism; in such cases hydrocortisone is the preferred medication.
- Physiologic replacement of each pituitary deficiency is individualized and monitored with clinical assessment and/or laboratory measurements.
- Of note: interactions exist between different hormones, thus changes or replacement in one hormonal axis may affect other axes.

Epidemiology

Hypopituitarism results from a partial or complete pituitary hormone deficiency. Current epidemiology is not well known. A 2001 Spanish population study showed a prevalence of 45.5 cases per 100,000 and an incidence of 4.2 per 100,000 individuals per year. This estimate is likely conservative, as clinical awareness, imaging studies, and overall understanding of hypopituitarism pathophysiology have improved over the last two decades.

Pathophysiology

The pituitary gland is a small endocrine gland (~1 cm in size) located in sella turcica of the sphenoid bone at the base of the brain; its mechanism of action is closely linked to the hypothalamus and is controlled by various neurohormonal and nonhormonal inputs. The pituitary secretes hypophyseal hormones into the systemic circulation, stimulating target peripheral glands to produce specific hormones, which in turn feed back to the hypothalamic-pituitary system and maintain a highly regulated homeostasis (Figure 1).

The pituitary is composed of two functionally distinct structures that differ in embryologic development and anatomy: the adenohypophysis (anterior pituitary) and the neurohypophysis (posterior pituitary). The anterior pituitary is responsible for GH, prolactin, ACTH, TSH, LH, and FSH. The posterior pituitary stores vasopressin (or antidiuretic hormone [ADH]) and oxytocin, which are produced in the hypothalamus. Therefore any damage to the hypothalamic-pituitary unit can cause an isolated or combined hormonal deficiency (Table 1).

Different etiologies affect various hormonal patterns. In approximately 70% of cases, the anterior pituitary is affected by a locally expanding tumor, causing mass effect. The most frequent pituitary hormonal deficiency related to sellar tumors is growth hormone (GH) deficiency, followed by gonadal axis hormones (luteinizing and follicle-stimulating hormones [LH/FSH]), and thyroid-stimulating hormone (TSH) deficiencies. However, in other etiologies, the pattern of pituitary deficiency differs. For example, in immunotherapy-related hypophysitis, adrenocorticotropic hormone (ACTH) is the first and most common deficiency noted. In contrast, lymphocytic hypophysitis preferentially affects the adrenal and gonadal axes. Infiltrative diseases can also manifest as diabetes insipidus (DI) and/or anterior pituitary dysfunction. Congenital diseases may affect one or more axes and usually present in childhood; for example, an Anosmin-1 (*ANOS1*) mutation results in isolated hypogonadotropic hypogonadism (Kallmann syndrome) and failure to go through puberty, whereas a *PROP-1* mutation presents with low GH, TSH, and LH-FSH.

In severe illness, functional hypopituitarism may cause low GH, hypogonadism, and central hypothyroidism, which are transient and may recover with acute stress resolution. Traumatic brain injury may cause hypopituitarism in up to 30% to 40% of cases, most commonly as GH deficit with or without gonadal dysfunction. Many deficiencies resolve within a year. Surgery in the pituitary region can lead to one or complete pituitary hormone deficit, including transient or permanent DI.

Prevention

In most cases, hypopituitarism is not preventable. Awareness is most important for early diagnosis, as the development of hormonal deficiencies is often insidious and characterized by nonspecific symptoms such as fatigue or weight changes. Pituitary surgery should be performed by a high-volume pituitary neurosurgeon to decrease the risk of surgery-related hypopituitarism. High-dose or prolonged glucocorticoid (GC) therapy suppresses the hypothalamic-pituitary-adrenal (HPA) axis and may also alter the gonadal and thyroid axes. Prolonged opioid use can also induce hypopituitarism, especially adrenal insufficiency (AI) and hypogonadism. Limiting GCs and opioids to the lowest effective dose and for the shortest possible time allows for a reduction in the risk of HPA axis suppression.

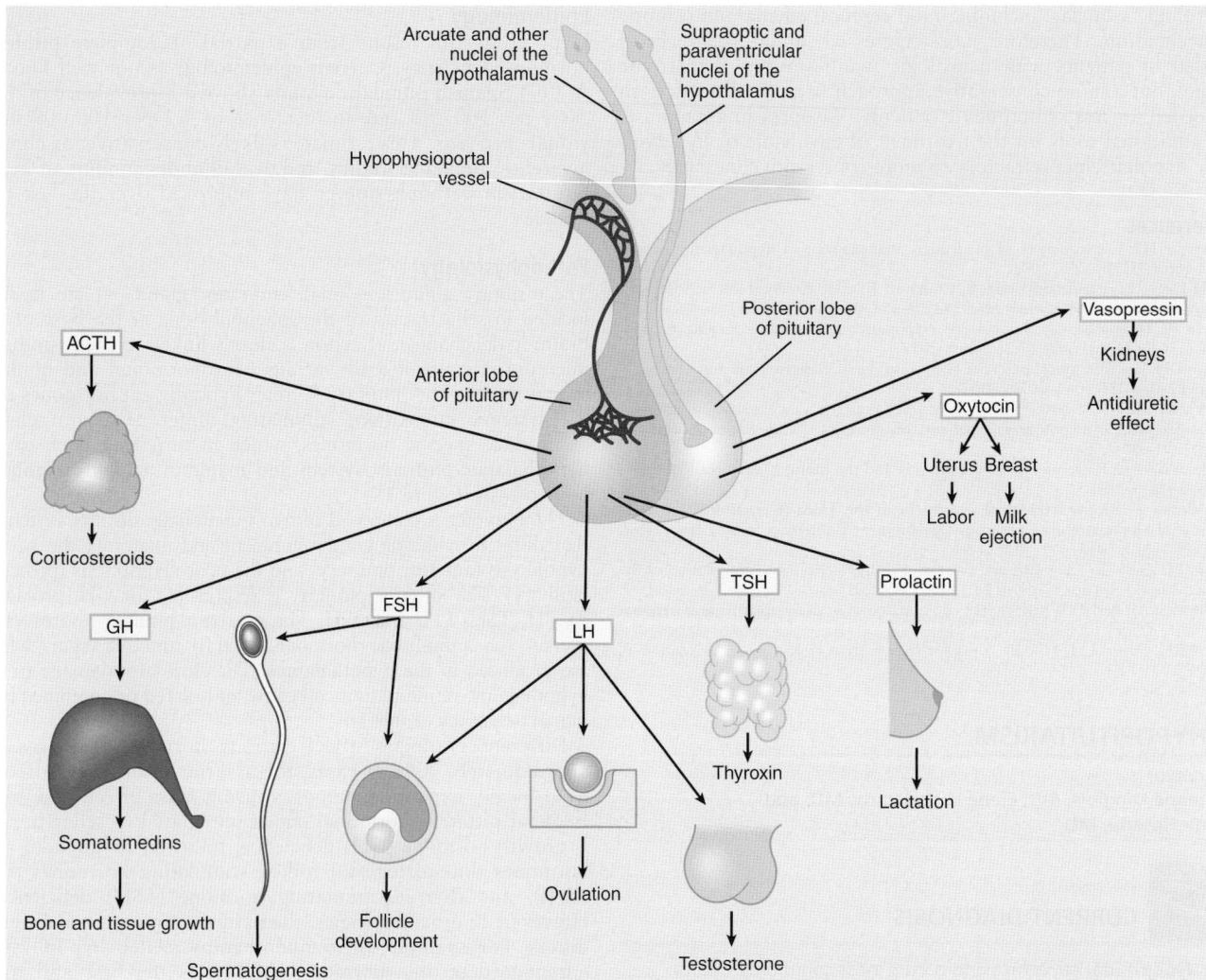

Figure 1 Relationships between hypothalamic hormones, pituitary hormones, and target organs. Numerous hormone-releasing and hormone-inhibiting factors formed in the arcuate and other hypothalamic nuclei are transported to the anterior pituitary by hypophysioportal vessels. In response to hypothalamic hormones, the anterior pituitary secretes the following: corticotropin, which evokes corticosteroid secretion by the adrenal cortex; growth hormone *(GH)*, which elicits production of insulin-like growth factors by the liver; follicle-stimulating hormone *(FSH)*, which stimulates spermatogenesis and facilitates ovarian follicle development; luteinizing hormone *(LH)*, which elicits testosterone secretion by the testes, facilitates ovarian follicle development, and induces ovulation; thyroid-stimulating hormone *(TSH)*, which stimulates thyroxin secretion by the thyroid gland; and prolactin, which induces breast tissue growth and lactation. The posterior pituitary hormones, which are formed in the supraoptic and paraventricular nuclei, are transported by nerve axons to the posterior lobe, where they are released by physiologic stimuli. Oxytocin induces the ejection of milk from the breast and stimulates uterine contractions during labor. Vasopressin increases water reabsorption by the kidneys. *ACTH,* Adrenocorticotropic hormone. From Brenner GM, Stevens CW: *Brenner and Stevens' Pharmacology,* 5th ed., pages 359–365. Elsevier; 2018.

Clinical Manifestations

Signs and symptoms of hypopituitarism vary depending on the type and severity of the pituitary hormones affected and also disease duration.

Signs and symptoms may include the following:

- ACTH deficiency—generalized fatigue, weakness, nausea, loss of appetite, failure to thrive, hypotension, hyponatremia, and hypoglycemia (note that mineralocorticoid secretion is intact; thus hyperkalemia, the hallmark of primary AI, is not present).
- TSH deficiency—fatigue, weight gain, cold intolerance, dry skin, bradycardia, and constipation.
- Gonadotropin deficiency—decreased sex drive; infertility; in women, oligo- or amenorrhea; in men, erectile dysfunction and loss of libido; gynecomastia; muscle atrophy; and decreased exercise capacity.
- GH deficiency—failure to thrive and short stature in children; some adults are symptomatic, experiencing fatigue, abdominal fat deposition, weight gain, and decreased concentration,

memory, productivity, and quality of life.
- Prolactin—inability to lactate.
- ADH deficiency—polyuria, polydipsia with excessive thirst, hypernatremia if uncompensated.

Detailed Diagnosis

The diagnosis of hypopituitarism is based on a combination of high clinical suspicion, imaging studies, and demonstration of inappropriate pituitary hormone in the setting of low levels of a target peripheral gland hormone.

In most cases, once a single pituitary hormone deficit is confirmed, other axes should be tested and pituitary magnetic resonance imaging (MRI) performed. In cases of peripheral vision deterioration with or without headaches, imaging should not be delayed.

Corticotropin (Adrenocorticotropic Hormone)

AI is confirmed when low cortisol level is measured early in the morning, before 9 a.m. An early-morning serum cortisol level greater than 15 μg/dL in a patient who is not critically ill is usually sufficient to rule out AI, and a level below 3 μg/dL to 5 μg/dL is strongly suggestive of AI. Additionally, serum cortisol testing should be repeated and interpreted in the clinical context (e.g., time of day, acute illness status) and also according to levels of cortisol binding proteins (lower in malnutrition and hypoalbuminemia and higher in hyperestrogenic states). If the serum cortisol level is between 5 μg/dL and 15 μg/dL, an ACTH stimulation test should be performed to confirm diagnosis. An ACTH stimulation test evaluates adrenal reserve that is diminished without the presence of ACTH. A standard high-dose test involves administering 250 μg of cosyntropin (Cortrosyn) and then measuring serum cortisol levels after 30 and 60 minutes. A cortisol level of higher than 18 μg/dL to 20 μg/dL at 30 or 60 minutes is considered normal. In an alternative low-dose (1 μg) test,[1] cortisol is measured 20 to 30 minutes after cosyntropin administration. This test has been suggested to be more sensitive for the diagnosis of secondary than primary AI. Nevertheless, the high-dose test is preferred. Of note, lower cortisol cutoffs (14 μg/dL to 17 μg/dL) have been proposed recently for new, more selective assays (liquid chromatography/mass spectrometry and monoclonal rather than polyclonal immunoassays), which have less cross-reactivity with cortisol precursors; however, these cutoffs need further validation. The serum ACTH level is measured concurrently with baseline cortisol to distinguish between primary and secondary AI. A low or normal ACTH level is consistent with the diagnosis of central AI, while a high ACTH level (typically greater than twice above the upper limit of normal) with primary AI (refer to AI section for further details).

Thyrotropin (Thyroid-Stimulating Hormone)

The key to a diagnosis of secondary (central) hypothyroidism is inappropriately low or normal TSH in the presence of low free T_4. Occasionally, in pituitary or hypothalamic disease, TSH is minimally elevated (usually less than 5 mU/L) and often has lower bioactivity. In contrast, in primary hypothyroidism caused by thyroid gland disorders, TSH is markedly elevated. Therefore TSH levels alone are not sufficient for diagnosis in central hypothyroidism. It is therefore important to measure paired TSH and T_4 levels.

Gonadotropins (Follicle-Stimulating Hormone and Luteinizing Hormone)

In men, central hypogonadism is diagnosed by low testosterone levels when measured between 8 a.m. and 10 a.m. in conjunction with inappropriately normal or low LH and FSH. In premenopausal women, irregular or absent periods (after exclusion of pregnancy) along with low estrogen and low or inappropriately normal gonadotrophins indicate central hypogonadism. Hyperprolactinemia, thyroid dysfunction, and hyperandrogenic states (in females) and hemachromatosis (in males), should be excluded as a cause of gonadal dysfunction. In contrast, in primary hypogonadism and in the postmenopausal state, FSH and LH are markedly elevated.

Growth Hormone

GH secretion is pulsatile, and a single low measurement of GH is not diagnostic of GH deficiency (GHD). Low age- and sex-adjusted IGF-1 in adults is suggestive of GHD; however, normal IGF-1 does not rule out GHD. Provocative testing with glucagon (GlucaGen),[1] GH-releasing hormone (GHRH), arginine (R-Gene 10), macimorelin (Macrilen), or insulin tolerance tests are recommended for the diagnosis of GHD in adults. Diagnostic cutoffs differ for different tests and for different body mass indices; therefore careful interpretation is important for accurate diagnosis. When three or more pituitary deficiencies are present along with low IGF-1 levels, confirmatory provocative testing is not required.

Vasopressin (Antidiuretic Hormone)

Hypernatremia in DI may occur due to low ADH, although it is not always present in compensated states if the patient has unlimited access to free water. When hypernatremia is suspected by polyuria and polydipsia, simultaneous measurement of serum and urine osmolality is recommended as an initial test for DI. High serum osmolality (>295 mOsmol/L) and concurrent low urine osmolality (<300 mOsmol/L) are diagnostic of DI. In subtle or unclear cases, a water deprivation test should be performed. Measurement of serum copeptin level after water deprivation, hypertonic saline, or with arginine stimulation using specific cutoffs can be helpful in diagnosis. Copeptin is derived from ADH preprohormone and is more stable than ADH; however, copeptin assays may not be available in some countries.

Differential Diagnosis

Hypopituitarism causes secondary endocrine organ failure and should be distinguished from primary failure (primary AI, primary hypothyroidism, and primary hypogonadism), where the corresponding pituitary hormone will be elevated. An ACTH stimulation test can be normal for more than 2 weeks in patients with an acute onset of central AI, such as pituitary apoplexy or after pituitary surgery, because the adrenal cortex is able to respond to stimulation for several weeks until it undergoes atrophy in the presence of low ACTH. Critical illness may result in temporary suppression of TSH, GH, and gonadotropins and does not require hormonal replacement in the acute period. Obesity can be a cause of male hypogonadotropic hypogonadism. Central DI should be distinguished from nephrogenic DI and primary polydipsia by means of a water deprivation test.

Treatment
Glucocorticoid Replacement

Oral hydrocortisone (Cortef) is the preferred GC. A typical replacement regimen is 15 mg/day to 20 mg/day as a single or divided dose (e.g., two-thirds in the morning and one-third in the early afternoon) due to its short half-life. Single doses in the morning can also be used in patients with central AI. A once-daily dual-release hydrocortisone formulation has been designed to mimic physiologic cortisol production; this is available in Europe but not in the United States. Of note, GC replacement at physiologic doses does not require treatment for bone protection or gastric ulcer prophylaxis.

Longer-acting GCs (prednisone, dexamethasone [Decadron]) may be used in patients who remain severely symptomatic in the evenings or early morning hours or who are unable to comply with a multidose hydrocortisone regimen. However, in such cases the risk of overreplacement is much higher.

Patients and families should be educated about the "sick day regimen" (i.e., to double or triple their daily dose for 3 days to 5 days according to the degree of physical stress or illness). In cases of repeated vomiting or deterioration of illness, it is recommended that patients administer injectable GC (hydrocortisone [Solu-Cortef] 100 mg IM or dexamethasone [Decadron] 4 mg IM) and seek immediate medical attention.

Minor surgical stress (e.g., cataract removal) requires additional administration of intravenous (IV) 25 mg hydrocortisone on the day of surgery only. The suggested dose for moderate stress (e.g., cholecystectomy) is 50 mg to 75 mg IV in divided doses on the day of surgery and the first postoperative day. Severe stress (e.g., coronary bypass surgery) requires 100 mg to 150 mg IV in divided doses for 2 days to 3 days with a subsequent rapid taper to the daily maintenance dose in an uncomplicated surgery (refer to the earlier section on adrenal insufficiency for further details).

Adrenal crisis and critical illness in adrenally insufficient patients are managed by administering a 100-mg IV bolus of hydrocortisone followed by 50 mg to 100 mg every 6 hours to 8 hours or continuous infusion of 200 mg/24 hours with the dose gradually decreased as the patient's condition improves. Additionally, it is recommended that patients wear a medical bracelet indicating AI risk.

---

[1]Not FDA approved for this indication.

Thyroid Deficiency

Central hypothyroidism is treated by T₄ replacement (levothyroxine [Euthyrox, Levoxyl, Synthroid]). A standard replacement dose for complete central hypothyroidism is 1.6 µg/kg/day; however, lower doses are needed in cases of partial deficiency. TSH should not be used as a marker of adequacy of replacement. Instead, one should adjust the dose to target free T₄ levels in the mid to upper half of the normal range and consider a lower target in elderly patients and in those with comorbidities in an effort to avoid over replacement.

Thyroid replacement should be administered only after corticosteroids have been replaced or adrenal function has been confirmed to be normal. Thyroid replacement in untreated AI can provoke an adrenal crisis.

Sex Hormone Deficiency

Testosterone replacement in men and estrogen (plus progesterone if the uterus is present) replacement in women is appropriate in symptomatic patients without contraindications after a discussion regarding risks and benefits. Combined oral contraceptive or hormone replacement therapy may be offered to premenopausal women. Premenopausal women not receiving estrogen replacement have an increased risk of cardiovascular disease and osteoporosis. Testosterone improves libido, sexual function, anemia, and bone density in men. Prostate, breast, and uterine cancer are contraindications to sex steroid replacement. Patients at high risk for thrombotic and cardiovascular events, including smokers, are poor candidates for hormone replacement.

Growth Hormone Deficiency

GH replacement (somatropin [Genotropin, Humatrope]) is administered as a daily injection; longer-acting formulations are in development. In GH-deficient adults, GH replacement improves body composition, has a modest effect on the maintenance of bone density, and improves quality of life. Although mortality in patients with hypopituitarism is increased, GH replacement has not been shown to improve mortality. Side effects of treatment include worsening of insulin resistance, joint pain, and peripheral edema. Although GH replacement has not been directly linked to cancer development or tumor regrowth, replacement is contraindicated in cases of active cancer.

Diabetes Insipidus

Desmopressin (DDAVP) therapy is individualized based on the patient's symptoms (severity or persistence of polyuria and polydipsia) and serum sodium levels especially during the initiation phase of therapy due to risk of hyponatremia from overcorrection. Desmopressin may be administered orally, intranasally (in some countries), or via a sublingual route; in a hospital setting it may be given via an IV or subcutaneous route. A low dose is used at initiation to avoid hyponatremia. Some patients with partial DI are only mildly symptomatic and prefer no treatment while keeping sodium levels normal with adequate water intake.

Monitoring

Patients should be periodically assessed for signs of GC over-replacement (weight gain, facial rounding, hyperglycemia, and osteoporosis) or under-replacement (nausea, fatigue, joint pain) and the GC dose adjusted accordingly.

Monitoring for thyroid, GH, gonadal deficiencies includes periodic clinical assessment and measurement of hormone levels (free T₄, IGF-1, and testosterone). Regular follow-up by an endocrinologist is warranted.

Interaction exists between the various hormone replacements. For example, thyroid replacement and GH affect GC metabolism and may cause AI in patients with low adrenal reserve.

Higher maintenance hydrocortisone doses may be required in patients who initiate GH or thyroid replacement. Oral estrogen can increase cortisol- and thyroid-binding globulins, resulting in an increase of the total cortisol and thyroxine levels and relative decrease in the bioavailable free hormone; therefore careful interpretation of test results is necessary.

Special Circumstances
Fertility and Pregnancy

New assisted reproductive techniques have led to the increased prevalence of women with hypopituitarism achieving fertility, and birth rates seem to be high in women with hypopituitarism achieving pregnancy. During pregnancy, many continuous adjustments in pituitary hormonal replacement should be considered.

Although GCs, levothyroxine, and desmopressin are safely prescribed during pregnancy, GH treatment regimens vary significantly between countries. GH is not approved for use in pregnancy, but several publications have shown that it can improve outcomes in women pursuing fertility.

In women with hypopituitarism who desire to be pregnant, close monitoring is needed, and such patients will benefit from an evaluation at a pituitary center of excellence.

Complications

Complications arise from a failure to diagnose hypopituitarism, especially in the event of an acute onset or severe illness or trauma, as untreated AI can result in cardiovascular collapse, organ failure, and death. Insufficient chronic replacement can lead to persistent symptoms and poor quality of life, whereas over replacement can result in the development of iatrogenic Cushing syndrome, iatrogenic hyperthyroidism, and other complications.

Conclusion

Early recognition and treatment of hypopituitarism is essential to reduce morbidity and mortality and improve quality of life. Care for patients with multiple pituitary deficiencies is often complex and requires expert management by an endocrinologist in conjunction with a pituitary neurosurgeon when surgical treatment for pituitary lesion is required. Although some pituitary deficiencies except adrenal and thyroid may recover or may not necessitate treatment, most patients require lifelong hormonal replacement and follow-up.

References

Brenner GM, Stevens CW: In *Brenner and Stevens'* pharmacology, ed 5, © 2018, Elsevier.

Carmichael J: Anterior pituitary failure. In Melmed S, editor: *Pituitary*, ed 4, 2007, Elsevier Inc., pp 329–364.

Fleseriu M, Hashim IA, Karavitaki N, et al: Hormonal replacement in hypopituitarism in adults: an endocrine society clinical practice guideline, *J Clin Endocrinol Metab* 101(11):3888–3921, 2016.

Higham CE, Johannsson G, Shalet SM: Hypopituitarism, *Lancet* 388(10058):2403–2415, 2016.

Honegger J, Schlaffer S, Menzel C, et al: Diagnosis of primary hypophysitis in Germany, *J Clin Endocrinol Metab* 100(10):3841–3849, 2015.

Molitch ME, Clemmons DR, Malozowski S: Evaluation and treatment of adult growth hormone deficiency: an Endocrine Society clinical practice guideline, *J Clin Endocrinol Metab* 96(6):1587–1609, 2011.

Regal M, Paramo C, Sierra SM, Garcia-Mayor RV: Prevalence and incidence of hypopituitarism in an adult Caucasian population in northwestern Spain, *Clin Endocrinol (Oxf)* 55(6):735–740, 2001.

Vila G, Fleseriu M: Fertility and pregnancy in women with hypopituitarism: a systematic literature review, *J Clin Endocrinol Metab* 105(3):e53–e65, 2020.

Javorsky BR, Raff H, Carroll TB, Algeciras-Schimnich A, Singh RJ, Colón-Franco JM, et al: New cutoffs for the biomechanical diagnosis of adrenal insufficiency after ACTH stimulation using specific cortisol assays, *J Endocr Soc*, bvab022, 2021. https://doi.org/10.1210/jendso/bvab022.

Ueland GA, Methlie P, Oksnes M, Thordarson HB, Sagen J, Kellmann R, et al: The short cosyntropin test revisited: new normal reference range LC-MS/MS, *J Clin Endocrinol Metab* 103(4):1696–1703, 2018.

HYPOTHYROIDISM

Method of
William J. Hueston, MD

CURRENT DIAGNOSIS

- Hypothyroidism is more common in women as they age.
- The signs and symptoms of hypothyroidism are nonspecific and can mimic other diseases found in the elderly, so clinicians need to have a high index of suspicion.
- The key diagnostic test is to find a low free T_4. The presence of an elevated TSH indicates primary hypothyroidism, and a low TSH indicates secondary hypothyroidism.
- There is insufficient evidence for screening for hypothyroidism in asymptomatic adults.

CURRENT THERAPY

- Thyroxine replacement with L-thyroxine (Synthroid, Levoxyl) is the treatment for hypothyroidism. Medication should be titrated to normalize the thyroid-stimulating hormone (TSH) level, which is usually achieved at an overall dose of 100 to 150 μg.
- Initial dosing for those with potential cardiac disease should be started low (25–50 μg/day) and advanced slowly every 6 to 8 weeks.
- Partial substitution of triiodothyronine (Cytomel) for thyroxine should be reserved for elderly patients with persistent neurocognitive dysfunction despite normalization of their TSH.
- Patients who have subclinical hypothyroidism with a TSH >10.0 should be considered for treatment. Patients with a TSH lower than this do not require therapy.

Epidemiology

Hypothyroidism is second only to diabetes in the prevalence of endocrine disorders in adults in the United States. Hypothyroidism occurs in up to 18/1000 population, with women outnumbering men by approximately 10:1. Rates of hypothyroidism increase dramatically with age, so that about 2% to 3% of all older women have hypothyroidism, and the prevalence is up to 5% in nursing home populations.

The prevalence of subclinical hypothyroidism, defined as an elevated TSH in the presence of normal free thyroxine (T_4) and triiodothyronine (T_3) levels increases with advancing age. Women, individuals over 65, and those from European heritage are at higher risk for subclinical hypothyroidism.

Risk Factors

Thyroid conditions are more common in patients who have a family history of thyroid disorders. In addition, hypothyroidism, as well as thyroid cancers, are more common in patients who had neck irradiation in childhood. However, most cases of hypothyroidism occur in people who have no risk factors.

Pathophysiology

Several conditions can lead to hypothyroidism (Box 1). Two categories, hypothyroidism after thyroiditis and iatrogenic hypothyroidism secondary to treatment of Graves' disease, account for the overwhelming majority of cases of hypothyroidism in the United States.

The most common non-iatrogenic condition causing hypothyroidism in the United States is Hashimoto's thyroiditis. Most idiopathic hypothyroidism also represents Hashimoto's thyroiditis that has followed an indolent course. Hashimoto's thyroiditis, also called chronic lymphocytic thyroiditis, is the most common of the inflammatory thyroid disorders and the most common cause of

goiter in the United States. The prevalence of Hashimoto's thyroiditis has been increasing dramatically since the 1960s in the United States, but the cause for this rise is unknown. In patients with acute thyroiditis, either subacute granulomatous (also known as de Quervain's) and subacute lymphocytic (also known as silent or painless), transient hypothyroidism is common after an acute attack, and 10% of these patients also develop long-term hypothyroidism.

Another common cause of hypothyroidism is a medical intervention to treat Graves' disease or thyroidectomy for chronic fibrocytic thyroiditis (Riedel's struma). Radioactive iodine ablation of the thyroid for Graves' disease often results in underproduction of thyroxine in the remaining tissue, necessitating thyroid replacement.

A third uncommon cause of hypothyroidism that should not be overlooked is secondary hypothyroidism due to hypothalamic or pituitary dysfunction. These conditions are seen primarily in patients who have received intracranial irradiation or surgical removal of a pituitary adenoma.

Finally, a variety of other conditions including infiltration of the thyroid (amyloidosis, sarcoidosis), iodine deficiency, or medications (such as amiodarone [Cordarone] or interferon) can cause hypothyroidism.

Prevention

There are no known interventions to prevent hypothyroidism. According to their 2015 analysis, the US Preventive Services Task Force found insufficient evidence to support early detection through routine screening of asymptomatic persons.

Clinical Manifestations

Individual who have hypothyroidism can present with a variety of symptoms, many of which are not specific. Consequently, clinicians must have a high index of suspicion for hypothyroidism when patients come in with any one or combination of the symptoms that could signal hypothyroidism.

Symptoms of hypothyroidism include lethargy, weight gain, hair loss, dry skin, constipation, poor concentration, trouble thinking or forgetfulness, and depression (Box 2). In older patients, hypothyroidism easily can be confused with Alzheimer's disease or other conditions that cause dementia. Patients who present with depression also should have their thyroid function assessed.

The thyroid examination in most patients with hypothyroidism is completely normal. Patients might have a painless goiter; tenderness in the thyroid is generally a sign of active inflammation consistent with acute thyroiditis. Once the thyroid inflammation has subsided, thyroid function might return to normal. Other physical findings that can occur with hypothyroidism include low blood pressure, bradycardia, nonpitting edema, generalized hair loss especially along the outer third of the eyebrows, dry skin, and

---

BOX 1   Conditions Causing Hypothyroidism

Thyroiditis
Hashimoto's thyroiditis
Subacute granulomatous thyroiditis (de Quervain's thyroiditis)
Subacute lymphocytic thyroiditis (silent or painless thyroiditis)

Iatrogenic Hypothyroidism
Radioactive iodine treatment of Graves' disease
Thyroidectomy

Secondary Hypothyroidism (Pituitary Dysfunction)
Pituitary surgery
Intercranial radiation
Congenital panhypopituitarism

Other Causes
Infiltratative diseases (sarcoidosis, amyloidosis, hemochromatosis)
Drugs (lithium, interferon, amiodarone [Cordarone])
Iodine deficiency

Common Symptoms
Lethargy
Weight gain
Constipation
Slowed mentation, forgetfulness
Depression
Hair loss
Dry skin
Neck enlargement or goiter

Physical Examination Findings
Goiter
Low blood pressure and slow pulse
Hair thinning or loss
Dry skin
Confusion
Depressed affect
Non-pitting edema

a lag in the relaxation phase of reflexes that can be assessed most easily in the ankle jerk reflexes.

Finally, there is an association between hypothyroidism and obstructive sleep apnea although it is unclear if this is a causal relationship.

Subclinical hypothyroidism usually has no, or very subtle clinical symptoms which could be explained by other conditions. The primary finding in subclinical hypothyroidism is the abnormal laboratory values. Subclinical hypothyroidism in pregnancy is associated with increases in pregnancy loss, premature rupture of membranes, and neonatal death, but limited evidence does not show a reduction in these risks with thyroid supplementation during pregnancy.

Diagnosis

The diagnosis of hypothyroidism is based on finding a low free thyroxine (T_4) level, usually with an elevation in the thyroid stimulating hormone (TSH) levels. For patients with hypothyroidism due to pituitary dysfunction, also called secondary hypothyroidism, both the free T_4 and the TSH levels are low.

One situation where clinicians need to be wary is evaluating thyroid status in patients who are severely ill. During times of acute physiological stress, patients may have mildly elevated TSH levels that suggest hypothyroidism but are, in fact, euthyroid. This condition, called euthyroid sick syndrome, does not require treatment with thyroid replacement and resolves within a few weeks of recovery, but it may be difficult to distinguish from preexisting or new-onset hypothyroidism. Clinicians need to use other clinical symptoms to try to differentiate euthyroid sick syndrome from hypothyroidism. Even though it does not require treatment, the presence of euthyroid sick syndrome in a critically ill patient is a poor prognostic sign.

In contrast to hyperthyroidism, there is no role for thyroid scans or iodine uptake testing in patients with hypothyroidism. The only exception to this is when the clinician identifies a mass on physical examination. In that situation, scanning or other imaging is essential to determine the malignancy potential of the mass.

Differential Diagnosis

The differential diagnosis for hypothyroidism is broad and depends on the primary complaints given by patients. For patients with slowed mentation, depressed affect, or confusion, clinicians should suspect depression. Patients with lethargy and a slow pulse and low blood pressure might have adrenal insufficiency. Patients with constipation need to have colonic obstruction from a mass considered as well. In the elderly, common drugs that can cause depression (such as centrally acting antihypertensive agents), bradycardia (such as β-blockers or calcium channel blockers), constipation (calcium channel blockers), hair loss, or confusion also should be considered.

In patients with pituitary failure, other pituitary hormones are likely to be deficient as well, so clinicians should look for evidence of adrenal and gonadotropic failure.

Treatment

The treatment for hypothyroidism is thyroxine replacement (Synthroid, Levoxyl). The usual dose required to achieve full replacement is between 100 μg and 150 μg, although patients who are treated with radioactive iodine and have some remaining thyroid activity might require lower doses. For patients with known heart disease or at risk for heart problems, doses should be initiated at 25 to 50 μg with increases of 25 μg every 4 to 6 weeks guided by TSH levels. Young patients who are at low risk for cardiac problems can be started at doses of 100 μg.

In choosing an agent to use for thyroid replacement, there is good evidence that generic substitutes are just as effective as brand-name drugs. A detailed study examining the metabolic effectiveness of a variety of generic drugs compared with a brand-name medication demonstrated no clinical or subclinical differences among preparations. So even though clinicians often hear that they should use a brand-name drug to maintain the stability of the replacement dose, this is not supported by the evidence.

One area of uncertainty is whether the addition of triiodothyronine (T_3, Cytomel) adds additional benefit to thyroid replacement with thyroxine. In some studies with elderly patients, subjects with continued neurocognitive dysfunction benefited from the addition of T_3 at a dose of 125 μg, with a concomitant decrease in the T_4 dose of 50 μg. However, subsequent studies of younger patients (aged 29–44 years) failed to find any benefits of partial T_3 substitution. Furthermore, studies of patients on doses of T_4 adequate to restore TSH levels to normal have been found to have normal T_3 levels. At this time, routine use of T_3 cannot be recommended; however, for selected elderly patients who have lingering confusion, depression, or slow mentation on adequate doses of T_4, a trial of T_3 partial substitution might be tried. Both the American Thyroid Association and European Thyroid Association recommend a trial of combination therapy for patients who are using single therapy with thyroxine alone who are persistently dissatisfied with their therapy.

Another situation where there is controversy is the use of thyroid replacement in patients with a mildly elevated TSH and a normal free T_4. This condition, called subacute hypothyroidism or mild hypothyroidism, is more common in white, elderly women. It has been observed that thyrotropin (TSH) levels naturally rise with age, however. In many instances these changes are simply due to aging and do not represent a pathologic process.

While some studies have shown clinical improvement in symptoms when low doses of T_4 are given to these patients, these patient populations tend to be those with preexisting thyroid disease (such as Graves' disease), and studies have had only a small number of patients. Expert panels in the US and Europe have suggested using the TSH level and the presence of anti-thyroid antibodies as guides for therapy, but that most patients with this condition will not require any therapy. Additional evidence against routine treatment is provided by a systematic review, and meta-analysis showed no improvement in quality of life or thyroid-related symptoms in patients with subclinical hypothyroidism who received levothyroxine supplementation.

When considering treatment for subacute thyroiditis, patients with a TSH under 7 generally do not require any therapy unless there are other individual patient risk factors such as existing cardiac disease or cognitive symptoms. Treatment is reasonable in those with a TSH level of 10.0 because these patients may be most symptomatic and have a progression rate of 5% to overt hypothyroidism.

When the TSH is <7, almost half of all patients will revert to normal within 2 years. Patients with a TSH <10 do not require any therapy unless there are other individual patient risk factors such as existing cardiac disease or cognitive symptoms. Treatment is reasonable in those with a TSH level of 10.0 because these patients may be most symptomatic and have a progression to overt hypothyroidism of 5%.

Monitoring

In general, once a patient receives a full replacement dose of T_4 (usually between 100 and 150 μg) and has a TSH consistently in the normal range, there is little likelihood that their thyroid requirement will change over time. Although many advocate annual retesting of TSH to ensure patients are euthyroid, there is no evidence to show this is necessary.

Some conditions do warrant closer monitoring of the TSH level. Because T_4 and T_3 are highly protein bound, any conditions where a patient's serum protein status changes should prompt additional testing. This includes conditions that lower serum protein levels, such as liver disease, nephrotic syndrome, or malnutrition, as well as those where serum proteins are increased, such as pregnancy or initiation of estrogen therapy. Because patients' dietary protein usually decreases with advancing age, older patients whose diet declines can also require monitoring and a lowering of their T_4 dose over time.

Patients with subclinical hypothyroidism also might benefit from annual retesting of their free T_4 levels. Approximately 10% of patients with subacute hypothyroidism progress to hypothyroidism within 3 years of diagnosis. Because of this, yearly testing is recommended. Also, 50% of patients with subacute hypothyroidism have positive anti-thyroid antibodies; however, routine testing for these is not recommended.

Complications

Most of the complications of hypothyroidism are associated with undertreatment or overtreatment. Patients with inadequately treated hypothyroidism are at higher risk for cardiac disease. On the other hand, over-replacement of thyroxine increases the risk of both atrial fibrillation and osteoporosis.

In addition, Hashimoto's thyroiditis is associated with other endocrine autoimmune diseases such as Addison's disease and pernicious anemia. Clinicians should be aware of these associations and not overlook new endocrine disorders that might have clinical features similar to hypothyroidism.

Finally, patients with Hashimoto's hypothyroidism also are at higher risk for the future development of lymphoma. Clinicians should educate patients about the need to have newly enlarged lymph nodes evaluated and be aggressive about evaluating symptoms or signs consistent with the development of a lymphoma.

References

Bekkering GE, Agoritsas T, Lytvyn L, et al: Thyroid hormone treatment for subclinical hypothyroidism: a clinical practice guideline, *BML* 356:I2006, 2019.
Biondi B, Cappola AR, Cooper SA: Subclinical hypothyroidism: A review, *JAMA* 322:153–160, 2019.
Bunevicius R, Kazanavicius G, Zalinkevicius R, Prange AJ: Effects of thyroxine as compared with thyroxine plus triiodothyronine in patients with hypothyroidism, *N Engl J Med* 340:424–429, 1999.
Dong BJ, Hauck WW, Gambertoglio JG, et al: Bioequivalence of generic and brand-name levothyroxine products in the treatment of hypothyroidism, *JAMA* 277:1205–1213, 1997.
Feller M, Snel M, Moutzouri E: Association of thyroid hormone therapy with quality of life and thyroid-related symptoms in patients with subclinical hypothyroidism: A systematic review and meta-analysis, *JAMA* 320:1349–1359, 2018.
Helfand M, Crapo LM: Screening for thyroid disease, *Ann Intern Med* 112:840–849, 1990.
Peeters RP: Subclinical hypothyroidism, *New Engl J Med* 376:2556–2565, 2017.
Sawin CT, Chopra D, Azizi F, et al: The aging thyroid. Increased prevalence of elevated serum thyrotropin levels in the elderly, *JAMA* 242:1386–1388, 1979.
Surks MI, Ortiz E, Daniels GH, et al: Subclinical thyroid disease: Scientific review and guidelines for diagnosis and management, *JAMA* 291(2):228–238, 2004.
U.S. Preventive Services Task Force: Screening for thyroid disease: Available at http://www.ahrq.gov/clinic/uspstf/uspsthyr.htm [accessed July 11, 2015].

OBESITY IN ADULTS

Method of
Meera Shah, MBChB, MRCP (Edin)

CURRENT DIAGNOSIS

- The diagnosis of obesity is based on the patient's body mass index (BMI), which is a ratio of weight to height. However, there are recognized limitations to using BMI alone when defining obesity.
- Waist circumference can aid the identification of patients who are not obese by BMI criteria but who are still at heightened metabolic risk.
- Certain ethnic groups, such as Asians, have a higher body fat content at a lower BMI and are therefore defined as being overweight or obese at lower BMI cutoffs.
- Diagnosing obesity early, and recognizing it as a chronic disease, allows for discussion and formulation of a plan to mitigate health risks associated with this disease.

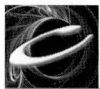

CURRENT THERAPY

- The cornerstone of any weight management program is lifestyle intervention that focuses on calorie restriction, an increase in physical activity, and behavioral modification. A multidisciplinary team approach offers the greatest benefit.
- The most effective pharmacotherapies for obesity modulate appetite regulation.
- Pharmacotherapy for obesity can be considered as an adjunct to lifestyle modification in the appropriate patient, after having a thorough discussion about benefits and associated risks.
- Weight loss procedures can be considered in patients with medically complicated obesity. This tends to be the most effective way of losing weight but is also associated with the highest risk. Therefore appropriate patient selection is key.

Obesity was recognized as a complex, chronic disease by the American Medical Association in 2013. The designation of obesity as a disease recognizes that obesity develops in response to an aberration in physiology, and its designation as a chronic disease recognizes that obesity is often present for a time period greater than a year and often requires ongoing medical attention and impairs activities of daily living.

Epidemiology

Obesity is a global phenomenon. At the current rate of growth, it is projected that by the year 2030, almost one in two adults in the United States will have a BMI of greater than 30 kg/m². With a higher prevalence of obesity comes a greater burden of obesity-associated chronic disease and comorbidities. Managing obesity is therefore a public health priority.

Obesity and Health Disparity

Obesity disproportionately affects certain racial, ethnic, and socioeconomic groups. Between 2017 and 2018, non-Hispanic Black adults (49.6%) had the highest age-adjusted prevalence of obesity, followed by Hispanic adults (44.8%), non-Hispanic White adults (42.2%) and non-Hispanic Asian adults (17.4%). Within these racial and ethnic differences, prevalence of obesity was lowest in women with college degrees compared with people with lower educational attainment, while in men there was no observable difference in obesity prevalence based on education level.

Among non-Hispanic White and Hispanic men, obesity prevalence was lower in the lowest and highest income groups compared with the middle-income group. Conversely, obesity prevalence was higher in the highest income group than in the lowest income group among non-Hispanic Black men. Among non-Hispanic White, non-Hispanic Asian, and Hispanic women, obesity prevalence was lower in the highest income group than in the middle and lowest income groups. Obesity prevalence was not affected by income in non-Hispanic Black women.

The reasons for these health disparities in adults with obesity are complex. However, there is widespread recognition of the fundamental importance of preventing childhood obesity, as children with obesity are more likely to become adults with obesity.

Diagnosis

The current definition of obesity is based on the body mass index (BMI). The BMI is defined as follows:

$$\frac{\text{Weight (kg)}}{\text{Height (m}^2)}$$

BMI is a practical measure of an individual's degree of adiposity and generally correlates well with comorbidities. However, it is well-recognized that BMI has several limitations with regard to body composition and weight distribution and may therefore be misleading if taken as the only measure of obesity, particularly at lower BMI values.

Waist circumference roughly correlates with visceral adiposity and can be an important adjunct when assessing risk associated with obesity in patients with a BMI below 35 kg/m². In adults with a BMI of 25 to 34.9 kg/m², waist circumference of greater than 102 cm (40 in.) for men and 88 cm (35 in.) for women is associated with greater risk of developing hypertension, type 2 diabetes, and coronary heart disease. Waist circumference is measured with the measuring tape situated above the iliac crest and snugged up against the skin. There is significant intraoperator variability, which limits the reproducibility and use of this metric in the longitudinal assessment of patients with obesity.

BMI cutoffs (Table 1) are applicable to the general population in the United States. Certain ethnic group such as Asians have a higher body fat content at a lower BMI and are therefore defined as being overweight or obese at lower BMI cutoffs (23–24.9 kg/m² and greater than 25 kg/m², respectively).

Assessing the Patient With Obesity in the Office

Once the patient has been diagnosed with obesity, effort then should turn toward understanding the etiology of the disease in the individual patient and assessing for comorbidities associated with obesity.

The following components in the patient's history should be elicited:
- Age of onset of weight gain
- Weight loss attempts
- Changes in dietary patterns
- History of exercise and activity in general
- A comprehensive medication history

The dietary assessment should ideally be performed by a registered dietitian.

A comprehensive medication history may identify medications that are associated with weight gain. Chief among these are psychotropic medications, antidepressants, antiepileptics, insulin secretagogues, and glucocorticoids. Progestational hormones and implants, antihistamines, and oral contraceptives may contribute to weight gain in some patients. Wherever possible, the potential for weight gain should be considered when starting patients with obesity on a new medication. If a weight-neutral alternative exists, effort should be made to switch the patient from a medication that could be contributing to weight gain as long as the underlying disease process remains adequately managed on the

TABLE 1	BMI Classification and Weight
CLASSIFICATION	**BODY MASS INDEX, kg/m²**
Underweight	≤18.5
Normal Weight	18.5–24.9
Overweight	25.0–29.9
Obesity, Class I	30.0–34.9
Obesity, Class II	35.0–39.9
Obesity, Class III	≥40

new medication. This can be difficult to achieve particularly when dealing with psychotropic medications and requires careful coordination with the patient's other prescribers.

The physical examination of the patient should focus on assessing for a pattern of weight distribution that may confer higher risk (i.e. higher waist circumference than BMI alone would confer) as well as physical findings that may elude to a secondary cause of obesity such as glucocorticoid excess, thyroid dysfunction, or dependent edema.

Comorbidities Associated With Obesity

Type 2 Diabetes

It is estimated that about 85% patients with type 2 diabetes are in the overweight or obese category.

The prevalence of diabetes has increased over the years in line with the increase in population-level obesity. The risk of developing type 2 diabetes in people with obesity increases when there is a strong family history of the disease, a prior history of gestational diabetes, or a weight distribution that is metabolically unfavorable (i.e., high waist circumference). Certain high-risk groups such as South Asians are 30% to 50% more likely to develop diabetes than their White counterparts despite having a lower BMI.

A fasting plasma glucose concentration of greater than or equal to 126 mg/dL or hemoglobin A1c of greater than or equal to 6.5% on two separate occasions can be used to make a diagnosis of type 2 diabetes.

When considering treatment for patients with type 2 diabetes and obesity, careful attention should be paid to the choice of antihyperglycemic agent. Weight-neutral options or medicines that actively promote weight loss such as GLP-1 receptor agonist or SGLT-2 inhibitors should be prioritized where possible. Conversely, patients on medications that can promote weight gain such as sulfonylureas or insulin should be counseled on alternative regimens. In patients with type 2 diabetes, weight loss of 5% to 10% is associated with hemoglobin A1c reductions of 0.6% to 1.0% and reduced need for diabetes medications.

Prevention of type 2 diabetes is possible with modest weight loss. Participants in the Diabetes Prevention program who were at high risk for developing type 2 diabetes and who were able to lose about 7% body weight through lifestyle intervention delayed development of diabetes by approximately 35%. In overweight and obese adults at risk for type 2 diabetes, average weight loss achieved with lifestyle intervention of 2.5 kg to 5.5 kg over 2 years reduces the risk of developing type 2 diabetes by 30% to 60%.

Thyroid Dysfunction

The 2021 guidelines published by European Society of Endocrinology recommends thyroid function testing in all patients with obesity, even in the absence of a clinical suspicion for hypothyroidism. The guideline is an acknowledgment of a relatively simple diagnostic test, low risk treatment, and potential for untreated hypothyroidism to adversely affect weight loss efforts. Thyroid-stimulating hormone (TSH) is the first thyroid hormone that should be measured. If this is elevated, free thyroxine (free T4) should be measured to accurately classify the disease process.

Reproductive Dysfunction

Obesity in women increases the risk for menstrual dysfunction, infertility, and adverse outcomes in pregnancy. Obesity is an independent risk factor for erectile dysfunction in men. Weight loss has been shown to improve several aspects of reproductive function in both men and women.

Cardiovascular Disease

Obesity increases the risk of coronary heart disease, heart failure, and overall cardiovascular mortality. People with obesity have a higher likelihood of developing risk factors that lead to cardiovascular disease such as hypertension and dyslipidemia.

Hypertension is a common chronic disease. Obesity has been shown to worsen hypertension; conversely there is a dose-response relationship between weight loss and improvements in blood pressure. Hence, even modest weight loss of less than 5% body weight can improve blood pressure in a clinically meaningful way.

Screening for dyslipidemia is best performed with a fasting lipid profile. Treatment guidelines for dyslipidemia are based on underlying comorbidities and calculated risk for developing atherosclerotic cardiovascular disease. Modest weight loss (less than 3 kg) leads to improvement in serum triglycerides and high-density lipoprotein (HDL) and low-density lipoprotein (LDL) cholesterol. In the presence of obesity, other modifiable risk factors such as smoking, hypertension, and sedentary lifestyle should be aggressively targeted.

Obstructive Sleep Apnea

Obstructive sleep apnea is a common but underrecognized complication of obesity. Patients with obesity who present with clinical features suspicious for sleep apnea or a neck circumference of greater than 17 inches in men or 16 inches in women should be screened for sleep apnea. Untreated sleep apnea has numerous health consequences related to the cardiorespiratory system and may also make it difficult for the patient to successfully lose weight. In addition to sleep apnea, obstructive lung disease, apnea-hypopnea syndromes, and restrictive lung disease are common complications of obesity that improve with weight loss.

Fatty Liver Disease

End-stage liver disease from nonalcoholic fatty liver disease is one of the most common reasons for liver transplantation in the world. The prevalence of nonalcoholic fatty liver disease increases as BMI increases, and up to 80% of patients with a BMI of greater than 40 kg/m^2 are estimated to have steatosis. The diagnosis of fatty liver disease is made on imaging, most commonly ultrasound. Weight loss is the first line of treatment for fatty liver disease; 5% to 10% weight loss has been shown to improve liver biochemistries and liver histology.

Mechanical Complications From Weight

Patients with overweight and obesity are at high risk of developing degenerative joint disease in weight-bearing joints. This in turn can promote further weight gain, and a vicious cycle therefore develops. A multidisciplinary approach comprising calorie restriction, behavioral therapy, physical therapy, and pain management is often necessary to achieve successful weight loss in this group of patients.

Gastroesophageal reflux is another mechanical complication from carrying excess weight, resulting from increased intraabdominal pressure from visceral adiposity. Patients who lose weight often see improvements in reflux symptoms.

Risk of Cancer

A number of malignancies are associated with obesity. In 2012 in the United States, about 28,000 new cases of cancer in men (3.5%) and 72,000 in women (9.5%) were due to overweight or obesity. The risk of developing esophageal, stomach, liver, kidney, gallbladder, pancreas, and colorectal cancers is higher in people who are overweight or obese. Endometrial carcinoma, breast cancer (in postmenopausal women), and ovarian cancer occur more commonly in women who are overweight or obese. Obesity also worsens several aspects of cancer survivorship such as quality of life, recurrence, progression, and prognosis.

Psychosocial Functioning

Patients with obesity frequently face stigma in areas such as education, employment, and healthcare, resulting in inequity and loss of opportunity. Patients with obesity often correlate their mental health and well-being with their ability to lose weight, and this can be a challenging situation to navigate. One condition that has been shown to correlate with obesity is seasonal affective disorder. Patients with this diagnosis are prone to gaining weight in the wintertime.

Treatment

Weight loss can only occur with the creation of an energy deficit in an individual. The cornerstone of any weight management program is lifestyle intervention that focuses on calorie restriction, increase in physical activity, and behavioral modification. Other modalities that can help promote weight loss include pharmacotherapy and weight loss procedures. These can be considered adjuncts to lifestyle intervention if lifestyle intervention alone does not produce the desired outcomes.

Successful management of obesity involves a multidisciplinary team working in partnership with the patient. Prior to making specific recommendations, the patient encounter should address the following:

1. Assessing the patient's readiness for change. The clinician can ask, "How prepared are you to make changes in your diet, to be more physically active, and to use behavior change strategies such as recording your weight and food intake?" A patient who is not ready to engage in changes will not be receptive to counseling on lifestyle changes.
2. Identification of barriers. Limitations to activity because of mechanical joint pain or lymphedema are relatively common and specific strategies to manage these may be necessary. Time and financial resources are also common barriers to successful weight loss. Identifying and acknowledging barriers can help build trust and forge a partnership with the patient.
3. Goal-setting. Patients are often overwhelmed by the amount of weight they need to lose. Clarifying that small but meaningful weight loss will improve health can be helpful to the patient. Aiming for 5% to 10% weight loss over 6 months is a reasonable initial goal.

Lifestyle Intervention Program

The key components of a lifestyle intervention prescription are listed in Table 2. An individualized lifestyle intervention program, based on the patient's dietary preferences, physical activity ability, and underlying motivation is most likely to result in successful weight loss.

Pharmacotherapy for Weight Loss

Appetite regulation is a complicated process that involves peripheral gut signaling, central coordination of those signals, and modulation by the environment, emotion, and behavior. Pharmacotherapy for weight loss primarily focuses on central appetite regulation and the most effective weight loss medications are appetite suppressants. Thus they act to reduce caloric intake while simultaneously often reducing cravings.

Current US Food and Drug Administration (FDA)-approved weight loss medications are indicated for individuals with a BMI ≥30 kg/m^2 or BMI ≥27 kg/m^2 with at least one obesity-associated comorbid condition who are motivated to lose weight, as an adjunct to comprehensive lifestyle intervention to help achieve targeted weight loss and health goals.

The FDA-approved weight loss medications, their dosing, and their side effect profile are listed in Table 3. All current FDA-approved weight loss medications, with the exception of weekly semaglutide, have an average reported clinical efficacy of 5% to 10% weight loss over 6 months. Because these weight loss medications are relatively similar in efficacy, choice of therapy is typically guided by the principle of minimizing medication interactions and side effects. All current FDA-approved weight loss medications are category X in pregnancy, and patients should be counseled to avoid pregnancy while taking these medications.

Phentermine (Adipex-P) is a short-acting sympathomimetic that has been approved for short-term weight loss (i.e., 12 weeks). However, phentermine is often used off-label for longer periods of time in patients who show a response to the medication in both weight loss and weight maintenance phases. Retrospective analyses of phentermine users demonstrated no increase in cardiovascular morbidity and no increase in addictive potential with phentermine use. If phentermine monotherapy is being considered as a long-term weight loss medication, the risks and benefits of this approach should be thoroughly discussed with the patient and an appropriate monitoring plan instituted.

Topiramate (Topamax) monotherapy is also used off-label to assist with weight management. Topiramate is a carbonic anhydrase inhibitor that has beneficial effects on appetite suppression and satiety. A meta-analysis on the efficacy and safety of topiramate in weight loss showed that patients on topiramate on average were able to lose an additional 5.3 kg over patients on placebo. Most common side effects with topiramate were noted to be paresthesias (tingling of the fingers), changes in taste, and psychomotor impairment.

Semaglutide (Ozempic) is a once-weekly GLP-1 receptor agonist that has been FDA approved for the treatment of obesity and for type 2 diabetes. In early 2021, a number of phase three randomized, placebo-controlled trials using semaglutide at a dose of 2.4 mg once weekly (weight loss dose) were published. The Semaglutide Treatment Effect in People with Obesity (STEP) randomized controlled trials were designed to study the weight loss effect of high-dose semaglutide in patients with and without type 2 diabetes (STEP 1, 2, and 3) and weight maintenance in patients without type 2 diabetes (STEP 4 and 5). On average, participants taking 2.4 mg semaglutide subcutaneously once weekly were able to achieve 15% weight loss compared with patients on placebo who achieved 2% to 5% weight loss. Overall, the gastrointestinal (GI)-related side effect profile was higher in the semaglutide group (nausea, constipation, diarrhea, gallbladder-related conditions), and treatment discontinuation was seen in approximately 3% of participants in that group.

Monitoring Patients on Weight Loss Medications

Patients on weight loss medications should be evaluated early and often to ensure continued efficacy of the drug and to monitor for side effects. The best predictor of overall response to a weight loss medication is weight loss achieved in the first 3 months. In general, 5% weight loss in the first 3 months is indicative of a "responder." If a patient with a previously upward weight trend is able to maintain their weight on the new medication after 3 months of use, then that patient may still be considered a responder. Patients who have had significant changes to their health, overall medication regimen, or physical activity routine may not achieve the goal of 5% weight loss over 3 months; in these situations a longer duration of follow-up might be necessary to determine whether the patient is a responder to the medication.

Except for the scenarios listed above, patients who do not achieve a 5% weight loss over 3 months have several options. If appetite suppression is inadequate per clinical history, then a higher dose of the drug or a different weight loss medication could be considered. Patients could also benefit from meeting with a dietitian to ensure that their dietary plan is adequately calorie-restricted. If a patient has significant side effects from the medication, then an alternative weight loss medication could be considered.

TABLE 2	Components of a Lifestyle Intervention Program
COMPONENT	
Diet	*Calorie restriction of 300–500 kcals/day.* Goal for most women: 1200–1500 kcals/day. Goal for most men: 1500–1800 kcals/day. There is no specific dietary macronutrient composition that promotes long-term weight loss. The best predictor of weight loss is dietary adherence; hence patients should be counseled on dietary strategies that are most likely to be sustained.
Physical activity	*Goal: ≥150 minutes a week of moderate-intensity exercise* Patients should be encouraged to increase physical activity wherever able. The first goal may be to decrease sedentary time. Patients can aim for 10 minutes of activity at a time. Self-monitoring of activity, such as using a step-counter, can be helpful. Patients with multiple comorbidities and limitations to activity may benefit from a specific physical activity prescription from a physical therapist.
Behavioral therapy	Behavioral modification is key to ensuring long-term success. Daily monitoring of food and activity can help patients make behavioral changes. Ideally, patients will also be enrolled in a structured behavioral modification curriculum supervised by a behavioral psychologist. Patients benefit from regular feedback and support of their efforts.

Adapted from Heymsfield SB, Wadden TA. Mechanisms, pathophysiology, and management of obesity. *N Engl J Med.* 2017;376(15):1492.

TABLE 3	FDA-Approved Pharmacologic Agents for Weight Loss	
NAME/TRADE NAME	**DOSING**	**COMMON SIDE EFFECTS**
Orlistat/ Xenical™	120 mg TID with meals	Bloating, abdominal cramps, diarrhea, steatorrhea
Phentermine-Topiramate ER/ Qsymia®	3.75/23 mg daily for 2 weeks, then 7.5/46 mg daily thereafter High dose therapy is 11.25–69 mg daily for 2 weeks, then 15–92 mg daily thereafter	Phentermine side effects: Constipation, dry mouth, tachycardia, insomnia, hypertension Topiramate side effects: Paresthesias, dizziness, cognitive dysfunction, kidney stones, glaucoma
Naltrexone-SR/bupropion-SR/ Contrave®	Each tablet contains 8 mg naltrexone and 90 mg bupropion. Titrate by 1 tablet a week until maximal therapeutic dose of 2 tablets twice daily	Nausea, constipation, dry mouth, headache
Liraglutide/Saxenda®	Titrate by 0.6 mg daily every week until maximal therapeutic dose of 3 mg daily subcutaneously	Nausea, abdominal discomfort, constipation, or diarrhea.
Semaglutide/Wegovy®	Start at 0.25 mg subcutaneously weekly for 4 weeks; then 0.5 mg weekly for 4 weeks; then 1 mg weekly for 4 weeks; then 1.7 mg weekly for 4 weeks; then 2.4 mg weekly	Nausea, vomiting, constipation or diarrhea, gallbladder-related symptoms

Patients should be seen every 3 to 6 months to assess their weight loss trends and monitor for side effects and the potential for new medication interactions. Patients with a clinically meaningful weight loss can also be retested for improvements in their metabolic profile (e.g., fasting glucose), as this may affect therapeutic decision making.

Weight loss typically slows down after about 6 months of therapy, sometimes referred to as a "weight plateau"; this is a physiologic adaptation to weight loss. Specifically, it is estimated that for each kilogram of lost weight, calorie expenditure decreases by about 20 to 30 kcal/day whereas appetite increases by about 100 kcal/day above the baseline level prior to weight loss. Hence, the default trend is for weight loss followed by weight regain. This is an important phenomenon to highlight with patients who can become frustrated that their efforts are not yielding results. Patients may be more willing to engage in modifications to their dietary intake or energy expenditure to overcome this when they understand how metabolic adaptation occurs with weight loss.

Procedural Interventions for Weight Loss

Endoscopic Interventions

Endoscopic weight loss procedures, such as the endoscopic sleeve gastroplasty (ESG) and endoscopic intragastric balloon are increasing in popularity because of their efficacy and noninvasive nature.

The ESG is a procedure whereby the patient's stomach capacity is endoscopically reduced, creating a gastric sleeve the size of a small banana. A systematic review and meta-analysis to evaluate the efficacy and safety of ESG in adults showed the average total body weight loss to be approximately 17%. 2.2% of patients in this cohort experienced side effects, most commonly GI-related.

Most patients included in the analysis had a BMI between 30 and 40 kg/m^2, thus this procedure may not yield similar results in patients with class III obesity (BMI greater than 40 kg/m^2). The procedure is also technically challenging and may therefore not be widely available. Patients interested in the ESG should continue to be counseled on making sustainable lifestyle changes following the procedure to ensure long-term weight maintenance.

Intragastric balloon devices are approved to treat obesity in patients with a BMI greater than 30 kg/m^2. In this procedure, a gastric balloon is endoscopically inserted and filled with saline. It remains in place for 6 months, after which it is removed following endoscopic deflation. The intragastric balloon increases satiety and decreases gastric emptying, thus promoting decreased caloric intake and ultimately weight loss. Total body weight loss at 12 months is approximately 10%; patients who lose weight with the balloon in place often see some degree of weight regain following balloon removal. Adverse effects are most commonly seen in the first week following balloon placement and consist of nausea and constipation. Balloons that are left in place for greater than 6 months run the risk of causing gastric erosion.

Cellulose and Citric Acid (Plenity®)

Plenity is an FDA-cleared, prescription-only aid for weight management. It is made from naturally derived cellulose and citric acid, forming a three-dimensional (3D) matrix in the stomach when ingested with water, and is not absorbed systemically. This product is indicated in overweight and obese adults with a BMI of 25 to 40 kg/m^2, when used in conjunction with diet and exercise.

It is currently the only FDA-approved weight loss aid that can be used in patients with a BMI as low as 25 kg/m^2. Access to Plenity is currently limited but should become broader by late 2021.

In a multicenter, double-blind, placebo-controlled 24-week study of 436 patients with a mean BMI 33 to 34 kg/m^2, patients were randomized to either 3 Gelesis100 (former name of Plenity) capsules taken with 500 mL water 20 to 30 minutes before lunch and dinner or placebo. Participants were prescribed a hypo caloric diet and asked to do 30 minutes of moderate-intensity exercise a day. Mean weight loss achieved was 6.4% in the treatment arm versus 4.4% in the placebo arm. Approximately 60%

of participants in the treatment arm achieved at least a 5% weight loss, a threshold that is considered clinically relevant. Adverse GI effects were higher in the treatment arm (38% vs. 28%), but the dropout rate was similar in both groups.

Bariatric Surgery

Bariatric (or metabolic) surgery results in significant weight loss leading to remission or resolution of several weight-related comorbidities. Compared with usual obesity care, bariatric surgery has also been shown to prolong life expectancy. Bariatric surgery is indicated in patients with a BMI greater than 40 kg/m^2 or in patients with a BMI greater than 35 kg/m^2 with associated weight-related comorbidities. There is compelling data that patients with diabetes with a BMI as low as 27 kg/m^2 may benefit from bariatric surgery, but this has not been adapted into practice.

Candidacy for bariatric surgery is determined on medical and psychological grounds. Patients interested in bariatric surgery should be motivated and ready for the significant and lifelong changes that occur after surgery. Psychological contraindications to pursuing surgery include untreated major depression or psychosis, other active psychiatric illness including chemical dependency, binge-eating disorders, and the inability to comply with nutritional requirements including lifelong vitamin supplementation.

There are several types of bariatric surgeries. Here we present the two most common, which are the laparoscopic Roux-en-Y gastric bypass (RYGB) and the laparoscopic sleeve gastrectomy (Figure 1).

Roux-en-Y Gastric Bypass

In this surgery, a small "pouch" is formed from the proximal part of the stomach, which is divided and separated from the distal part of the stomach. The pouch has a capacity of approximately 1 tbsp at the time of creation. The small intestine is divided approximately 100 cm distal to the pylorus; one end forms the anastomosis with the pouch and the other and is anastomosed at the jejunum about 75 to 100 cm distal to the pouch. These anatomic alterations result in restriction of food intake and decrease absorption capacity of the small intestine, thus leading to weight loss. The average weight loss seen after gastric bypass surgery is approximately 30% of total body weight.

Patients who undergo gastric bypass surgery often develop an aversion to high sugar content and fatty foods (i.e., calorie-dense foods). This in turn does help decrease total caloric intake. Patients can often develop lactose intolerance as well, which limits their total dairy consumption.

Guidelines for multivitamin supplementation following RYGB is outlined below (Table 4).

Complications from RYGB can be categorized as either surgical complications or nutritional complications. In the immediate postoperative period, anastomotic ulcerations and strictures may occur, requiring reintervention. Longer-term surgical complications may include the development of intestinal obstruction from internal hernias or adhesions. Overall, the mortality from bariatric surgery is less than 1%. Nutritional deficiencies after RYGB most commonly involve deficiencies of iron, vitamin D, and calcium. This is partly driven by the exclusion of the proximal duodenum, which is the major side of absorption of these specific nutrients.

Sleeve Gastrectomy

The sleeve gastrectomy is the most widely performed bariatric procedure worldwide. In this surgery, approximately 80% of the body of the stomach is removed, leaving behind a tubular structure that resembles a shirtsleeve. The average weight loss seen with the sleeve gastrectomy is approximately 15% to 25% of total body weight. The sleeve gastrectomy is the preferred bariatric procedure in patients who have a need to be consistent with absorption of specific medications, for example antirejection medications after organ transplantation.

Guidelines for multivitamin supplementation following sleeve gastrectomy is outlined below (Table 4).

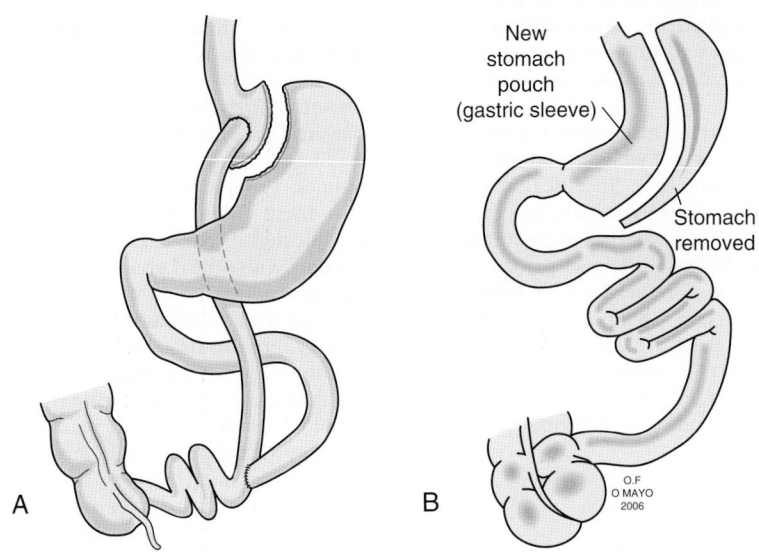

Figure 1 Techniques commonly used for the surgical treatment of obesity: (A) Roux-en-Y gastric bypass; (B) laparoscopic sleeve gastrectomy.

Postoperative complications of the sleeve gastrectomy include staple line leak or dilation of the gastric sleeve. Approximately 15% of patients who undergo sleeve gastrectomy can develop new or worsening gastroesophageal reflux symptoms. Patients who have undergone a sleeve gastrectomy often do not develop food aversion and are able to continue eating a wide variety of foods.

Monitoring After Bariatric Surgery
Nutrition
Patients who have undergone bariatric surgery should obtain annual levels of complete blood count, ferritin, 25 hydroxy vitamin D, fasting glucose, and lipid profile (if indicated). B12 levels should be checked if the patient is not taking a parenteral formulation of B12 as absorption in the altered GI anatomy can be variable. Patients who have undergone more malabsorptive procedures such as the biliopancreatic diversion/duodenal switch or very long limb RYGB may be screened for deficiencies in vitamins A, zinc, and copper.

Patients who have undergone gastric bypass surgery and other malabsorptive bariatric procedures should also have annual measurements of 24-hour urine volume, calcium, creatinine, and oxalate excretion. This is the most reliable way of ensuring adequate calcium absorption while screening for hyperoxaluria.

An annual dietitian review is strongly recommended to ensure that patients are adhering to nutritional guidelines and meeting their nutritional goals.

Physical Activity
Patients should be encouraged to pursue moderate intensity physical activity for at least 150 minutes a week (i.e., 30 minutes a day). When advising on the intensity of physical activity, patients can be guided to choose options that result in the following: "Your breathing quickens, but you're not out of breath. You develop a light sweat after about 10 minutes of activity. You can carry on a conversation, but you can't sing."

Data from the National Weight Control Registry shows that the majority of nonsurgical weight loss patients engage in a structured and consistent daily physical activity program to successfully maintain their weight.

Weight
In a recent prospective, long-term study of patients who had undergone RYGB, 93% of patients maintained at least a 10% weight loss from baseline, 70% maintained at least a 20% weight loss, and only

TABLE 4	Guidelines for Standard Multivitamin and Mineral Supplementation After Bariatric Surgery
SUPPLEMENT	**DOSING AND SUPPLY**
200% of recommended daily allowance for vitamins and minerals	Two chewable multivitamins daily Patients with renal impairment may need dose adjustment
Elemental calcium	1500–2000 mg daily with meals, in divided doses. If supplements are required, calcium citrate is better absorbed in a low acid environment such as post-gastric bypass
Vitamin D	3000–5000 units of vitamin D3 daily, total through dietary intake and supplements
B12	1000 mcg deep subcutaneous injection monthly OR 500–1000 mcg orally daily

40% maintained at least a 30% weight loss after 12 years. Weight regain is therefore a reality that tends to occur after the second postoperative year in a proportion of patients who undergo bariatric surgery. Weight regain may lead to relapse of weight-related comorbidities and can be psychologically difficult for the patient.

When a patient who has undergone bariatric surgery presents with weight regain, a number of factors should be considered. The patient's dietary habits should be evaluated by a dietitian familiar with bariatric surgery. The patient's physical activity habits should also be evaluated and assistance from a physical therapist can be considered for patients with significant limitations to exercise. Anatomic changes such as dilation of the gastrojejunal anastomosis or the presence of a gastro-gastric fistula can contribute to excess calorie intake and weight regain; these can be detected with an upper GI contrast study. The patient's medication record should be carefully evaluated to identify medications that may predispose to weight gain. Finally, a psychology evaluation may uncover behaviors that may be predisposing to weight regain, for example graze-eating, nighttime eating, or binge-eating.

Patients who experience weight regain after bariatric surgery should be offered a multidisciplinary approach to management. In addition to dietary and behavioral intervention, patients may also be candidates for antiobesity medications or procedures that revise their postbariatric surgery anatomy.

Specific Complications of Roux-en-Y Gastric Bypass

There are number of unique complications that can occur following RYGB as a result of anatomic alterations. Here, we will highlight two—nephrolithiasis and alcohol use disorder.

Nephrolithiasis

The risk for nephrolithiasis after gastric bypass surgery is moderately high, with reported prevalence rates of 7.65% to 13%. Solely gastric restrictive operations such as the gastric sleeve are not associated with higher risk for kidney stone formation beyond that attributed to obesity alone. Nephrolithiasis can present as early as the first year after surgery; as such, patients should be counseled on interventions to prevent kidney stone formation soon after surgery. Current guidelines recommend completing a 24-hour urine super saturation between 6 and 12 months after surgery. This can assess for adequacy of hydration status, calcium ingestion, oxalate excretion, and citrate excretion (low urinary citrate predisposes to kidney stone formation).

Patients with nephrolithiasis should be counseled on adequate fluid intake (1500–2000 mL of urine output per day), a low-fat diet, a low oxalate diet, and adequate dietary or supplemental calcium with meals. Hypocitraturia may be treated with potassium citrate salts. Patients with nephrolithiasis after gastric bypass may benefit from more frequent visits with a dietitian to help meet the patient's nutrition and hydration goals.

Alcohol Use Disorder

Alcohol use disorder is a rare complication that can occur in the long-term after gastric bypass. Changes in the gastrointestinal anatomy following gastric bypass surgery alter the pharmacokinetics of alcohol metabolism, leading to early and higher blood alcohol concentration peaks accompanied by a greater feeling of drunkenness. Additionally, there is decreased clearance of alcohol through the first pass mechanism. In practical terms, peak blood alcohol levels achieved after consuming about two drinks in women who have had RYGB surgery resembles that observed after consuming about four drinks in women who have not had surgery.

Large prospective observational studies show that the prevalence of alcohol use disorder after RYGB increases over time since surgery. Risk factors for developing alcohol use disorder after gastric bypass surgery include male sex, younger age, smoking, and any alcohol consumption presurgery. Although baseline alcohol consumption is a risk factor, about 20% of patients diagnosed with alcohol use disorder within 5 years of RYGB reported no alcohol consumption the year prior to surgery. Patients undergoing gastric bypass surgery should therefore be routinely screened for and counseled on the effects of alcohol use after surgery.

References

Adams TD, Davidson LE, Litwin SE, et al: Weight and Metabolic Outcomes 12 Years after Gastric Bypass, *N Engl J Med* 377(12):1143–1155, 2017.

Arnold M, Pandeya N, Byrnes G, et al: Global burden of cancer attributable to high body-mass index in 2012: a population-based study, *Lancet Oncol* 16(1):36–46, 2015.

Bhatti UH, Duffy AJ, Roberts KE, Shariff AH: Nephrolithiasis after bariatric surgery: a review of pathophysiologic mechanisms and procedural risk, *Int J Surg* 36(Pt D):618–623, 2016.

Canales BK, Hatch M: Kidney stone incidence and metabolic urinary changes after modern bariatric surgery: review of clinical studies, experimental models, and prevention strategies, *Surg Obes Relat Dis* 10(4):734–742, 2014.

Carlsson LMS, Sjoholm K, Jacobson P, et al: Life Expectancy after Bariatric Surgery in the Swedish Obese Subjects Study, *N Engl J Med* 383(16):1535–1543, 2020.

Centers for Disease C, Prevention: Prevalence of overweight and obesity among adults with diagnosed diabetes-United States, 1988-1994 and 1999-2002, *MMWR Morb Mortal Wkly Rep* 53(45):1066–1068, 2004.

Clinical Guidelines on the Identification, Evaluation, and Treatment of Overweight and Obesity in Adults-The Evidence Report. National Institutes of Health, *Obes Res* 6(Suppl 2):51S–209S, 1998.

Davies M, Faerch L, Jeppesen OK, et al: Semaglutide 2.4 mg once a week in adults with overweight or obesity, and type 2 diabetes (STEP 2): a randomised, double-blind, double-dummy, placebo-controlled, phase 3 trial, *Lancet* 397(10278):971–984, 2021.

Fabbrini E, Sullivan S, Klein S: Obesity and nonalcoholic fatty liver disease: biochemical, metabolic, and clinical implications, *Hepatology* 51(2):679–689, 2010.

Greenway FL, Aronne LJ, Raben A, et al: A Randomized, Double-Blind, Placebo-Controlled Study of Gelesis100: a Novel Nonsystemic Oral Hydrogel for Weight Loss, *Obesity (Silver Spring)* 27(2):205–216, 2019.

Hagedorn JC, Encarnacion B, Brat GA, Morton JM: Does gastric bypass alter alcohol metabolism?, *Surg Obes Relat Dis* 3(5):543–548, 2007; discussion 8.

Hales CM, Carroll MD, Fryar CD, Ogden CL: Prevalence of Obesity and Severe Obesity Among Adults: United States, 2017-2018, *NCHS Data Brief* (360)1–8, 2020.

Hedjoudje A, Abu Dayyeh BK, Cheskin LJ, et al: Efficacy and Safety of Endoscopic Sleeve Gastroplasty: a Systematic Review and Meta-Analysis, *Clin Gastroenterol Hepatol* 18(5):1043–10453 e4, 2020.

Hendricks EJ, Srisurapanont M, Schmidt SL, et al: Addiction potential of phentermine prescribed during long-term treatment of obesity, *Int J Obes (Lond)* 38(2):292–298, 2014.

Heymsfield SB, Wadden TA: Mechanisms, Pathophysiology, and Management of Obesity, *N Engl J Med* 376(15):1492, 2017.

Himpens J, Dobbeleir J, Peeters G: Long-term results of laparoscopic sleeve gastrectomy for obesity, *Ann Surg* 252(2):319–324, 2010.

Jakicic JM, Marcus BH, Lang W, Janney C: Effect of exercise on 24-month weight loss maintenance in overweight women, *Arch Intern Med* 168(14):1550–1559, 2008; discussion 9–60.

Jensen MD, Ryan DH, Apovian CM, et al: 2013 AHA/ACC/TOS guideline for the management of overweight and obesity in adults: a report of the American College of Cardiology/American Heart Association Task Force on Practice Guidelines and The Obesity Society, *J Am Coll Cardiol* 63(25 Pt B):2985–3023, 2014.

King WC, Bond DS: The importance of preoperative and postoperative physical activity counseling in bariatric surgery, *Exerc Sport Sci Rev* 41(1):26–35, 2013.

King WC, Chen JY, Courcoulas AP, et al: Alcohol and other substance use after bariatric surgery: prospective evidence from a U.S. multicenter cohort study, *Surg Obes Relat Dis* 13(8):1392–1402, 2017.

Knowler WC, Barrett-Connor E, Fowler SE, et al: Reduction in the incidence of type 2 diabetes with lifestyle intervention or metformin, *N Engl J Med* 346(6):393–403, 2002.

Kramer CK, Leitao CB, Pinto LC, Canani LH, Azevedo MJ, Gross JL: Efficacy and safety of topiramate on weight loss: a meta-analysis of randomized controlled trials, *Obes Rev* 12(5):e338–e347, 2011.

Kumar RB, Aronne LJ: Iatrogenic Obesity, *Endocrinol Metab Clin North Am* 49(2):265–273, 2020.

Lee JW, Brancati FL, Yeh HC: Trends in the prevalence of type 2 diabetes in Asians versus whites: results from the United States National Health Interview Survey, 1997-2008, *Diabetes Care* 34(2):353–357, 2011.

Lieske JC, Mehta RA, Milliner DS, Rule AD, Bergstralh EJ, Sarr MG: Kidney stones are common after bariatric surgery, *Kidney Int* 87(4):839–845, 2015.

Parrott J, Frank L, Rabena R, Craggs-Dino L, Isom KA, Greiman L: American Society for Metabolic and Bariatric Surgery Integrated Health Nutritional Guidelines for the Surgical Weight Loss Patient 2016 Update: Micronutrients, *Surg Obes Relat Dis* 13(5):727–741, 2017.

Pepino MY, Okunade AL, Eagon JC, Bartholow BD, Bucholz K, Klein S: Effect of roux-en-y gastric bypass surgery: converting 2 alcoholic drinks to 4, *JAMA Surg* 150(11):1096–1098, 2015.

Polidori D, Sanghvi A, Seeley RJ, Hall KD: How strongly does appetite counter weight loss? quantification of the feedback control of human energy intake, *Obesity (Silver Spring)* 24(11):2289–2295, 2016.

Rubino D, Abrahamsson N, Davies M, Hesse D, Greenway FL, Jensen C, et al: Effect of Continued Weekly Subcutaneous Semaglutide vs Placebo on Weight Loss Maintenance in Adults With Overweight or Obesity: The STEP 4 Randomized Clinical Trial, *J Am Med Assoc* 325(14):1414–1425, 2021.

Salminen P, Helmio M, Ovaska J, et al: Effect of laparoscopic sleeve gastrectomy vs laparoscopic roux-en-y gastric bypass on weight loss at 5 years among patients with morbid obesity: the SLEEVEPASS Randomized Clinical Trial, *J Am Med Assoc* 319(3):241–254, 2018.

Schauer PR, Bhatt DL, Kashyap SR: Bariatric surgery or intensive medical therapy for diabetes after 5 years, *N Engl J Med* 376(20):1997, 2017.

Shaker M, Tabbaa A, Albeldawi M, Alkhouri N: Liver transplantation for nonalcoholic fatty liver disease: new challenges and new opportunities, *World J Gastroenterol* 20(18):5320–5330, 2014.

Singh S, de Moura DTH, Khan A, et al: Intragastric Balloon Versus Endoscopic Sleeve Gastroplasty for the Treatment of Obesity: a Systematic Review and Meta-analysis, *Obes Surg* 30(8):3010–3029, 2020.

Sjostrom CD, Lissner L, Wedel H, Sjostrom L: Reduction in incidence of diabetes, hypertension and lipid disturbances after intentional weight loss induced by bariatric surgery: the SOS Intervention Study, *Obes Res* 7(5):477–484, 1999.

Smith MD, Patterson E, Wahed AS, et al: Thirty-day mortality after bariatric surgery: independently adjudicated causes of death in the longitudinal assessment of bariatric surgery, *Obes Surg* 21(11):1687–1692, 2011.

Sohn CH, Lam RW: Update on the biology of seasonal affective disorder, *CNS Spectr* 10(8):635–646, 2005. quiz 1-14.

Svensson PA, Anveden A, Romeo S, et al: Alcohol consumption and alcohol problems after bariatric surgery in the Swedish obese subjects study, *Obesity (Silver Spring)* 21(12):2444–2451, 2013.

Wadden TA, Bailey TS, Billings LK, et al: Effect of Subcutaneous Semaglutide vs Placebo as an Adjunct to Intensive Behavioral Therapy on Body Weight in Adults With Overweight or Obesity: the STEP 3 Randomized Clinical Trial, *J Am Med Assoc* 325(14):1403–1413, 2021.

Ward ZJ, Bleich SN, Cradock AL, et al: Projected U.S. State-Level Prevalence of Adult Obesity and Severe Obesity, *N Engl J Med* 381(25):2440–2450, 2019.

Wilding JPH, Batterham RL, Calanna S, et al: Once-Weekly Semaglutide in Adults with Overweight or Obesity, *N Engl J Med* 384(11):989, 2021.

PARENTERAL NUTRITION IN ADULTS

Method of
**Meetal Mehta, MD; Kris M. Mogensen, MS; and
Malcolm K. Robinson, MD**

CURRENT DIAGNOSIS

- Reserve parenteral nutrition (PN) for patients with intestinal dysfunction or failure.
- Reserve PN for conditions such as short-bowel syndrome, severe malabsorption, ileus or intestinal dysmotility, intractable vomiting, and severe diarrhea.
- Always reevaluate the need for PN and work toward a transition to enteral nutrition or an oral diet, if possible, to limit complications associated with PN.

CURRENT THERAPY

- Correct electrolyte abnormalities and hyperglycemia prior to the initiation of PN.
- Start with no more than 150 to 200 g dextrose on the first day of PN; start with 100 to 150 g dextrose for patients with diabetes or patients at risk for the refeeding syndrome.
- Advance PN by 100 to 150 g dextrose daily until the goal is achieved.
- Maintain blood glucose <180 mg/dL.
- Monitor electrolytes, including phosphate and magnesium, until stable; the frequency of laboratory monitoring can be decreased based on stability.
- Monitor closely for complications associated with PN: electrolyte abnormalities, hyper/hypoglycemia, PN-associated liver disease, and central line infections.

Since the inception of parenteral nutrition (PN) in the 1960s, the science of PN has matured in a number of ways. The initial excitement of being able to feed basic nutrients, vitamins, and trace elements intravenously has been tempered by the realization that indiscriminate use of PN can be harmful. Although PN can still be lifesaving, it is imperative that it be used judiciously and only as long as necessary. This chapter discusses the current use of PN in adult patients.

Indications and Contraindications

Enteral nutrition (EN) is the preferred method of nutrition support, primarily because it is associated with fewer infectious and metabolic complications. However, total PN (TPN), which is the provision of all nutrient requirements intravenously, may be indicated when feeding through the gastrointestinal (GI) tract is not possible. PN may be appropriately initiated in those who cannot receive enteral nourishment and are malnourished or at risk for developing malnourishment. Malnourishment can be defined as unintentional loss of more than 10% of usual body weight or greater than 7 to 10 days of inadequate nutrient intake. The body stores of well-nourished persons are generally sufficient to provide the essential nutrients, resist infection, promote wound healing, and support other necessary physiologic functions for this time period. In patients who are anticipated not to be able to receive adequate EN for longer than 10 days, it is not necessary to wait 10 days before initiating PN. This may include patients with short-bowel syndrome and others who are expected to have prolonged GI dysfunction.

According to the American Society for Parenteral and Enteral Nutrition (ASPEN) guidelines, EN is contraindicated in conditions such as diffuse peritonitis, intestinal obstruction, early stages of short-bowel syndrome, intractable vomiting, paralytic ileus, severe GI bleeding, and severe diarrhea and malabsorption

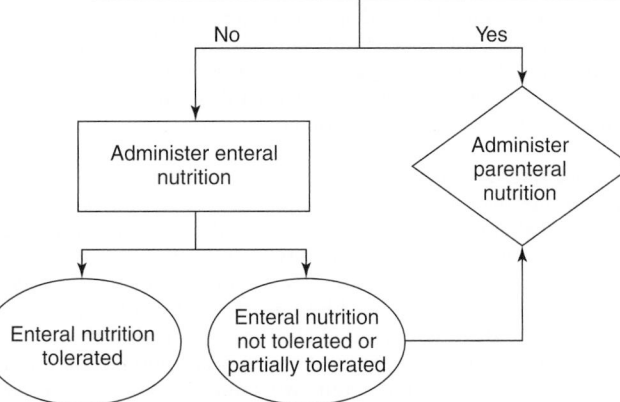

Figure 1 Determining route of feeding.

syndromes. Other relative contraindications to EN include severe pancreatitis and enterocutaneous fistulas, although depending on the clinical circumstances, EN may be indicated. PN and EN may be provided concomitantly, although in patients who are critically ill, PN should not be started until all strategies to maximize enteral feeding (such as the use of postpyloric feeding tubes and motility agents) have been attempted. PN support is unlikely to benefit a patient who will be able to take EN within 4 or 5 days after the onset of illness or who has a relatively minor injury (Figure 1).

There are four key steps to consider before initiating PN, including assessing nutritional status, determining energy needs, evaluating GI function, and estimating the length of time a patient will require PN (Box 1).

Assessment of Nutritional Status

Nutrient depletion is associated with increased morbidity and mortality, and up to 60% of hospitalized patients are estimated to have malnutrition. Therefore it is imperative to identify patients who have or are at risk for developing protein-energy malnutrition or have specific nutrient deficiencies. A patient's risk of developing malnutrition-related medical complications needs to be quantified, and it is necessary to monitor the adequacy of nutritional therapy.

Nutrition assessment begins with a thorough history and physical examination in conjunction with select laboratory tests aimed at detecting specific nutrient deficiencies in patients who are at high risk for future abnormalities. The nutrition assessment should establish whether the patient will need maintenance therapy or nutrition repletion and should assess the status of the patient's GI tract, especially if nutrition support will be required.

A thorough history includes an assessment of recent weight changes, dietary habits, GI symptoms, and changes in exercise tolerance or physical abilities that would indicate functional

BOX 1   Decision-Making Steps When Initiating Parenteral Nutrition

Assess the patient's nutritional status. Nutrition support (PN or EN) should not be initiated in well-nourished patients unless they have received a suboptimal diet for more than 7 days.

Determine whether the patient has extreme energy needs (hypermetabolism) that warrant the early use of nutrition support (PN and/or EN) within 7 days of injury or illness. These are typically critically ill patients who have suffered severe burns or trauma.

Evaluate the function of the GI tract; if it is intact and can be used safely, PN should be avoided. PN support is indicated until enteral access is established and the patient can meet nutrient needs via tube feedings.

Estimate how long the patient will require PN support. If GI function is expected to return within 5 days, there is no known benefit of initiating PN.

EN, Enteral nutrition; *GI*, gastrointestinal; *PN*, parenteral nutrition.

---

capacity deficiencies. Screening for malnutrition risk, using a validated nutrition screening tool (e.g. Mini Nutritional Assessment, Malnutrition Screening Tool, Malnutrition Universal Screening Tool, Nutritional Risk Index, Nutrition Risk Screening-2002, etc.), may identify these relevant changes. Diagnosis of malnutrition includes further history taking and a physical examination. This includes inspection for subcutaneous fat and muscle wasting, which indicate a loss of body energy and protein stores; edema and ascites, which can also indicate altered energy demands or decreased energy intake; and signs of vitamin and mineral deficits such as dermatitis, glossitis, cheilosis, neuromuscular irritability, and coarse easily pluckable hair.

Several nutritional biomarkers have traditionally been used to quickly assess nutritional status. The serum proteins prealbumin, transferrin, and retinol-binding protein have a rapid turnover rate and short half-lives and therefore may be used as indicators of recent nutritional intake. However, these proteins are affected by the metabolic responses to stress and illness, as well as other conditions, including iron status (transferrin) and renal status (retinol-binding protein, prealbumin). This can limit their usefulness in acute and chronic inflammatory states.

Prealbumin is least affected by fluctuations in hydration status and by liver and renal function compared with other plasma proteins. However, prealbumin levels drop in acute inflammatory conditions during which the liver prioritizes production of positive acute-phase reactants, decreasing negative acute-phase reactants such as prealbumin. A rise in C-reactive protein, a protein synthesized by the liver as part of the acute-phase response, indicates an active inflammatory state. Thus C-reactive protein, when measured along with prealbumin, can help differentiate a low prealbumin due to nutritional inadequacy versus low prealbumin due to an acute-phase response.

The serum albumin, another negative acute-phase reactant, has traditionally been used as an indicator of nutritional status. Although it is a good preoperative predictor of outcome for patients undergoing surgery, its sensitivity to many variables in the acute care setting make it an unreliable marker to assess nutritional status under such conditions or in the immediate postoperative period. Additionally, redistribution of albumin, increases in GI and renal losses, and alterations in tissue catabolism during inflammatory states affect its intravascular concentrations.

Notably these serum markers are affected only after weeks of starvation in noninflammatory states and do not increase with adequate nutritional support, making it a poor initial indicator of nutritional status or muscle mass. However, they may be used to indicate inflammatory status and nutritional risk, instead of nutritional status and muscle mass.

A simple and practical index of malnutrition is the degree of weight loss. Unintentional weight loss of greater than 10% within the previous 6 months indicates protein-energy malnutrition and is a good prognosticator of clinical outcome. Weight can also be compared with an ideal or desirable weight, or an index of body weight relative to height. The body mass index (BMI), reported as weight in kilograms divided by height in meters squared, is the best known such index, and can be used to detect both undernutrition and overnutrition. This index is dependent on height, and the same standards apply to both men and women. A BMI of 18.5 to 25 kg/m^2 is considered normal, 25 to 29.9 kg/m^2 is considered overweight, and greater than 30 kg/m^2 is considered obese. Patients with a normal or high BMI can still have nutrient deficiencies and therefore can be malnourished if they have recently lost a significant amount of weight. In addition, a BMI of 18 kg/m^2 or less in an adult indicates moderate malnutrition and a BMI less than 15 kg/m^2 is associated with increased morbidity.

Another practical tool for evaluating nutritional status is the subjective global assessment (SGA) that encompasses historical, symptomatic, and physical parameters. The SGA technique determines whether nutrient assimilation has been restricted because of decreased food intake, maldigestion, or malabsorption; whether any effects of malnutrition on organ function and body composition have occurred; and whether the patient's disease process influences nutrient requirements. The findings of the history and physical examination are subjectively weighted to rank patients as being well nourished, moderately malnourished, or severely malnourished and are used to predict their risk for medical complications (Box 2).

Estimating Nutritional Requirements

Historically, TPN often provided nutrients in excess of actual requirements. This was based on the assumption that patients requiring nutritional intervention were severely depleted and required aggressive repletion; hence, the misnomer "hyperalimentation." Overfeeding is associated with increased carbon dioxide production and difficulty weaning from a ventilator as well as metabolic complications, such as hyperglycemia, which can lead to increased infection, morbidity, and mortality. Thus nutritional support should be titrated to match actual metabolic requirements.

In addition, there are times when *underfeeding* calories may be necessary and beneficial. In such cases, this is referred to as "permissive" underfeeding to distinguish it from underfeeding that occurs due to the unintentional inadequate delivery of nutrients. For example, permissive underfeeding may be appropriate for some critically ill patients with obesity who are receiving adequate protein. Such permissive underfeeding for critically ill patients with obesity is now the recommendation of ASPEN and the Society of Critical Care Medicine (SCCM).

Energy Requirements

There are four components of daily energy requirement. The first is the basal metabolic rate (BMR), which is the amount of energy expended under complete rest shortly after awakening and in a fasting state (12–14 hours). BMR varies with age, sex, and body size; correlates roughly with body surface area; and is proportional to lean tissue mass. This relationship holds true even among persons of different ages and sexes. Resting metabolic rate or resting energy expenditure (REE) represents the amount of energy expended 2 hours after a meal under conditions of rest and thermal neutrality. Although it is often used synonymously with BMR, the REE is typically 10% higher.

The second component of daily energy expenditure is the thermic effect of exercise or the energy used in physical activity. The contribution of this component increases markedly during intense muscular work. However, admission to a hospital generally results in a marked decrease in physical activity. Hospital activity in ambulatory patients accounts for a 20% to 30% increase in BMR. Critically ill patients who are on a ventilator generally have low activity levels (BMR increases by only 5%–10%) because the ventilator performs the work of breathing, and they are not ambulatory.

The third component of energy expenditure is diet-induced thermogenesis, the increase in BMR that follows food intake. The digestion and metabolism of exogenous nutrients, whether delivered to the gut or vein, result in an increase in metabolic rate. The magnitude of the thermic effect of food varies depending on the amount and composition of the diet and accounts for approximately 10% of daily energy expenditure.

Finally, acute illness adds an additional stress factor to the daily energy expenditure and correlates with disease severity. For example, a patient's metabolic rate increases by 10% to 30% after a major fracture, from 20% to 60% with severe infection, and from 40% to 110% with a severe third-degree burn. In addition, fever accelerates chemical reactions, and the BMR rises approximately 10% for each degree Celsius increase in temperature. Alternatively, cooling of febrile patients produces a reduction in BMR of approximately 10% per degree Celsius.

The first step of estimating energy requirements is to estimate the BMR. This is usually accomplished using one of several predictive equations. The most commonly used method is based on the predictive equations reported by Harris and Benedict in 1919. The Harris-Benedict equations are as follows:

$$BMR\,(men) = 66.47 + 13.75(W) + 5.0(H) - 6.76(A)$$

$$BMR\,(women) = 655.1 + 9.56\,(W) + 1.85(H) - 4.68\,(A)$$

where W is weight in kg, H is height in cm, and A is age in years.

After the BMR is calculated, it is adjusted for the level of stress induced by injury or the disease process and activity level. Activity factors for hospitalized patients are 1.0 to 1.1 for intubated patients, 1.2 for patients confined to bed, and 1.3 for patients out of bed. Stress factors may vary from 1.1 for patients with minimal stress, 1.3 for patients with moderate stress, up to 2.0 for patients with severe burns. Therefore the patient's energy requirements (total energy expenditure [TEE]) are finally calculated:

$$TEE = BMR \times Activity\ factor \times Stress\ factor$$

The thermic effect of feeding is generally not included in the calculation of energy requirements for hospitalized patients.

Alternatively, some clinicians estimate energy requirements based on actual body weight, providing about 25 to 30 kilocalories (kcal)/kg administered to critically ill patients. Predicting energy expenditure in patients with obesity can be difficult because using predictive formulas with actual body weight can lead to high TEE and potentially to overfeeding. Determining energy requirements for critically ill patients with obesity is discussed later in this chapter. The Harris-Benedict equation using the average of actual and ideal weight and a stress factor of 1.3 predicts REE in acutely ill patients with obesity with a BMI of 30 to 50 kg/m^2.

Indirect calorimetry is a more precise, clinically practical, and individualized method to determine energy expenditure, particularly in patients in whom estimating requirements through predictive equations is difficult, such as those who continue to lose weight despite what appears to be an adequate caloric intake, who are critically ill, or who have rapidly changing energy needs. Indirect calorimetry measures changes in oxygen consumption and carbon dioxide production to calculate the REE. As indirect calorimetry accounts for the effects of disease state, stress, and trauma, a stress factor is not necessary in calculating energy needs. However, the measurement occurs at rest, and therefore an activity factor of 1.0 to 1.3, depending on whether the patient is intubated, bedridden, or ambulatory, must be applied.

Nutrient Requirements

The recommended daily protein allowance for most healthy persons who are not hospitalized is 0.8 g/kg, or about 60 to 70 g of protein each day. The stressed, critically ill patient generally needs a higher dose of protein in the range of 1.2 to 2.0 g/kg/day. For most patients, providing protein beyond 1.5 g/kg/day is not beneficial. In fact, providing excess protein does not enhance uptake and can lead to increased ureagenesis, which can cause renal injury in some patients.

The calorie-to-nitrogen ratio for most PN solutions is typically about 150:1, with an acceptable range of 100:1 to 180:1. Nitrogen content is used as a marker for protein, and, hence, the two terms are used interchangeably. Usually, 6.25 g of protein is equal to 1.0 g of nitrogen. The conversion factor is slightly higher (6.4) for PN solutions, such as those with higher concentrations of crystalline amino acids.

Vitamin and mineral requirements are altered in certain disease states due to increased losses, greater use, or both. Guidelines for parenteral vitamin and trace elements, developed by the Nutrition Advisory Group of the American Medical Association, were approved by the US Food and Drug Administration (FDA) in 1979 and amended in 2000 (Table 1).

Composition of Central and Peripheral Venous Solutions

Central venous access is required for providing TPN because of the hypertonicity of the formulas infused (1900 mOsm/kg). The infusion of a hypertonic solution into a peripheral vein, known as *peripheral parenteral nutrition* (PPN), can result in thrombophlebitis and venous sclerosis unless the PN is drastically diluted to lower the tonicity. To minimize the hypertonicity of PPN solutions, dextrose is limited to 5% to 10%, and amino acids are limited to 2.5% to 3.5%. Lipids are isotonic and therefore provide a significant portion of the caloric substrate of PPN formulas.

TABLE 1	Recommended Daily Doses of Parenteral Vitamins and Trace Elements

MICRONUTRIENT	PARENTERAL DOSE
Vitamins	
Vitamin A	3300 IU
Vitamin D	200 IU
Vitamin E	10 IU
Vitamin K	150 μg
Ascorbic acid (vitamin C)	200 μg
Folic acid	600 μg
Niacin	40 mg
Riboflavin (vitamin B2)	3.6 mg
Thiamine (vitamin B1)	6 mg
Pyridoxine (vitamin B6)	6 mg
Cyanocobalamin (vitamin B12)	5 μg
Pantothenic acid	15 mg
Biotin	60 μg
Trace Elements	
Zinc	2.5–5 mg
Copper	0.3–0.5 mg
Chromium	10–15 μg
Manganese	60–100 μg
Selenium	20–60 μg

Data from American Medical Association, Department of Foods and Nutrition: Multivitamin preparations for parenteral use. A statement by the Nutrition Advisory Group. *JPEN J Parenter Enteral Nutr* 3:258–62, 1979; Food and Drug Administration: Parenteral multivitamin products: Drugs for human use: Drug efficacy study implementation: Amendment. *Federal Register* 65(77):21200–21201, 2000.

Central venous solutions, which are prepared by the hospital's pharmacy, typically combine carbohydrate in the form of dextrose, protein as crystalline amino acids, and lipids. Lipid emulsions come in many forms, with differing oil sources which provide varying amounts of essential fatty acids and phytosterols. The first lipid emulsion approved for PN uses a polyunsaturated long-chain triglyceride soybean oil base. It provides adequate essential fatty acids but has inflammatory properties due to its high phytosterol and omega-6 fatty acid content, which may play a role in PN-associated liver disease. Newer lipid emulsions have been approved by the FDA that provide different types of oils including a blend of soybean, medium chain triglyceride, olive, and fish oils (SMOFlipid®, Fresenius Kabi USA, Melrose Park, IL); soybean and olive oils (Clinolipid, Baxter, Deerfield, IL); and fish oil (Omegaven®, Fresenius Kabi USA, Melrose Park, IL; currently only approved for use in children in the United States). Fish oil and mixed lipid emulsions have more favorable, antiinflammatory profiles and studies suggest that they may prevent or reverse PN associated liver disease. For this reason, these newer lipid emulsions should be considered in patients who are at risk for developing PN associated liver disease.

Vitamins, electrolytes, and trace elements are added to the formulation as needed. Typical substrate profiles of carbohydrate, protein, and lipids in central PN are shown in Table 2. A usual PN prescription administers 1 to 2 L of a solution each day. Administration of 500 mL of a 20% fat emulsion 1 day each week is sufficient to prevent essential fatty acid deficiency. Alternatively, if additional calories from lipids are needed on a daily basis, they can be administered as a separate infusion or most commonly as part of the mixture of dextrose and amino acids, a technique known as *triple mix* or *three-in-one*.

Including lipid injectable emulsion into a parenteral admixture changes the conventional nutritional solution into an emulsion. Various electrolytes and micronutrients can adversely influence emulsion stability, and therefore their concentration in three-in-one solutions is limited to prevent "cracking" of the PN solution, in which microscopic or macroscopic precipitates are formed. The higher the cation valence, the greater the destabilizing influence to the emulsifier. Therefore trivalent cations such as ferric ion (iron dextran) are more disruptive than divalent cations such as calcium or magnesium ions, which are more disruptive than monovalent cations such as sodium or potassium. No concentration of iron dextran is safe in triple-mix formulations. In-line filters prevent infusion of precipitates and are necessary for all PN solutions (including triple-mix solutions) because it is impossible to visually detect precipitates until they are grossly incompatible and unsafe for infusion.

Once the basic solution is created, electrolytes are added as needed (Table 3). Sodium or potassium salts are given as chloride or acetate depending on the patient's requirements. Normally, equal amounts of chloride and acetate are provided. However, if chloride losses from the body are increased, which can occur in patients who have nasogastric tubes, then most of the salts should be given as chloride. Similarly, more acetate should be given to patients when additional base is required because acetate generates bicarbonate when it is metabolized. Sodium bicarbonate is incompatible with PN solutions and cannot be added to the mixture. Phosphate may be given as the sodium or potassium salt. Lipid injectable emulsions contain an additional 15 mmol/L of phosphate.

Commercially available preparations of fat-soluble and water-soluble vitamins, minerals, and trace elements are added to the nutrient mix unless they are contraindicated. Adequate thiamine is essential for patients receiving PN and can be provided separately. Vitamin K is now a component of standard IV multivitamin preparations. Trace element preparations that include copper, manganese, selenium, and zinc are added to the PN solution in amounts consistent with the American Medical Association guidelines (Table 1). Manganese accumulation can be toxic, and overexposure can lead to progressive neurodegenerative damage. Manganese is usually supplied in the PN solution at a daily dose of 0.5 mg as part of a multiple trace element additive. Because manganese is primarily eliminated via biliary excretion, patients with biliary obstruction or cholestasis can accumulate potentially toxic levels of manganese. Hence, manganese should be removed from the PN of patients with hyperbilirubinemia. Higher doses, 10 to 15 mg/day, of zinc are provided to patients with excessive GI losses.

Iron is not a part of commercial additive preparations because it is incompatible with triple-mix solutions and can cause anaphylactic reactions when it is given intravenously. Patients who need this trace element should receive it orally or by injection. Iron is avoided in patients who are critically ill because hyperferremia can increase bacterial virulence, alter polymorphonuclear cell function, and increase host susceptibility to infection.

PPN is less commonly used than central PN and can be disadvantageous. Because of the low concentration of dextrose, greater volumes (typically >2 L/day) are required to provide sufficient calories, which might not be feasible in fluid-restricted patients. PPN generally does not approximate a patient's energy needs because PPN provides only 1000 to 1500 kcal/day, and a large percentage of the calories (60%) are derived from fat. High-fat infusions are undesirable because they are associated with impaired reticuloendothelial system function and are potentially immunosuppressive. There is no evidence that lipid injectable emulsions improve outcomes or significantly decrease nitrogen losses. Generally, PPN should be avoided unless it is combined with enteral feeding in patients who cannot tolerate full enteral feeding, patients who

TABLE 2	Central Versus Peripheral Parenteral Nutrition	
PROPERTY	CENTRAL NUTRITION	PERIPHERAL NUTRITION
Volume of fluid required (mL)	1500–2500	2500–3500
Duration of therapy (d)	>7–14	5–14
Route of administration	Dedicated central venous catheter	Peripheral vein or multiuse central catheter
Substrate profile	150–600 g/day dextrose	150–300 g/day dextrose (5%–10% of final concentration)
		50–100 g/day amino acid (3% of final concentration)
Osmolarity (mOsm/L)	1300–1800	600–900

TABLE 3	Electrolyte Concentrations in Parenteral Nutrition
ELECTROLYTE	RECOMMENDED PN DOSES
Potassium	1–2 mEq/kg
Sodium	1–2 mEq/kg
Phosphate	20–40 mmol
Magnesium	8–20 mEq
Calcium	10–15 mEq
Chloride	As needed*
Acetate (mEq/L)	As needed*

*Depending on acid-base balance

cannot get a central venous catheter, or patients with low body weights in whom PPN can meet at least two-thirds of estimated needs.

Administration and Venous Access

Typically, central PN solutions are administered into the superior vena cava. Access to this vein can be achieved by cannulation of the subclavian or internal jugular veins. Peripherally inserted central venous catheters (PICCs), typically inserted via an antecubital vein and advanced into the superior vena cava, are the most commonly used central venous access devices for providing PN. PICC placement offers the advantage of central venous access, while avoiding the risks associated with accessing the subclavian or jugular veins, such as hemothorax, pneumothorax, and arterial injury.

Tunneled catheters or catheters with indwelling ports should be considered for patients who will need prolonged central venous nutrition (e.g., >6 weeks). Patients who will be using their catheters solely for daily central PN and who require home IV nutrition may be best served by a tunneled catheter rather than an indwelling port. Tunneled catheters may be more easily used and cared for, which can minimize the risk of infection.

Inserting a dedicated line for infusing hypertonic solutions requires strict aseptic technique and maximal barrier protection: hat, mask, gown, and gloves must be worn. The position of the catheter tip in the superior vena cava is confirmed by chest x-ray before any concentrated solutions are administered. Once the position of the tip has been confirmed, the line should be used exclusively for administering the hypertonic nutrient solution.

Multiple-lumen central venous catheters are most commonly used. Although at least one lumen is dedicated to the infusion of the PN solutions, the other(s) may be used for monitoring, blood drawing, or medication. The rate of catheter sepsis associated with multiple-port catheters may be the same as or slightly greater than the rate associated with the use of single-port catheters.

However, multiple-port PICCs are used to infuse PN solutions for a shorter period of time, which can minimize their inherent risk. Multiple-port catheters should be carefully maintained, including dressing changes, maintaining the dedicated lumen, careful handling of the other lumens, and removing the catheter as soon as it is no longer needed.

Infusion and Patient Monitoring

It is advisable to start with 1 L of central PN and increase the volume as needed, depending on the patient's metabolic stability. Blood glucose levels should be closely monitored and maintained at <180 mg/dL, tissue perfusion should be adequate, and Po_2, Pco_2, electrolytes (especially potassium, phosphate, and magnesium) and acid-base balance should be near normal before starting or advancing to the goal solution. The solutions should be administered using a volumetric pump set at a constant rate. It is important not to modify the infusion rate during any given day to try to compensate for excess or inadequate administration of the PN solution, such as when the PN solution arrives later than expected. A cyclic schedule (10–16 hours/day) for patients requiring long-term PN can be initiated once the patient is metabolically stable. In situations when the central PN solution must be suddenly discontinued, a 10% dextrose solution may be given at the same infusion rate as was used for the PN unless the patient is severely hyperglycemic. PN solutions may be administered at one-half the infusion rate to patients who are undergoing surgical procedures because circulating glucose and electrolyte levels are easier to control.

In addition to hyperglycemia, metabolic complications include hyper- and hypophosphatemia, hyper- and hypokalemia, hyper- and hypomagnesemia, and hyper- and hypocalcemia. Thus it is important to monitor the patient's serum electrolytes closely, especially when initiating TPN. In the inpatient setting, once the patient stabilizes on the individual nutritional prescription, serum chemistries should be obtained at least twice weekly to measure chloride, CO_2, potassium, sodium, blood urea nitrogen, creatinine, calcium, and phosphate levels and once weekly for a full profile that includes liver function, magnesium, and triglyceride levels. Stable home PN patients may have less frequent chemistry monitoring, typically starting with once per week monitoring, then decreasing to twice per month and then monthly, depending on overall stability and clinical status.

Patients With Special Needs
Glucose Intolerance

Hyperglycemia is the most common metabolic complication related to PN, and glucose regulation may be especially difficult in patients who have diabetes mellitus or who develop insulin resistance in response to severe stress or infection. Control of blood glucose levels is important for all patients who receive PN because uncontrolled hyperglycemia may be associated with complications such as fluid and electrolyte disturbances and increased infection risk due to impairment of host defenses, including decreased polymorphonuclear leukocyte mobilization, chemotaxis, and phagocytic activity. Intensive insulin therapy, maintaining blood glucose concentrations between 80 and 110 mg/dL, was once considered standard practice for critically ill patients. However, more recent literature has demonstrated significant morbidity and mortality with this approach. For hospitalized patients, a target blood glucose of 140 to 180 mg/dL is recommended. Select circumstances may require more stringent blood glucose goals (110–140 mg/dL) if this can be maintained without hypoglycemic episodes.

Patients with difficult glycemic control may best be managed by continuous insulin infusion, which is safe, effective, and more timely than subcutaneous insulin therapy. Hypoglycemia that occurs during this type of infusion generally is short lived and more easily corrected than hypoglycemia resulting from subcutaneous insulin administration. A separate IV insulin infusion can be used rather than adding incremental doses of insulin to the PN bag every 24 hours in patients for whom glycemic control is difficult. Many intensive care units (ICUs) have an insulin drip infusion protocol in which there are frequent checks of serum glucose and adjustments of the insulin infusion drip (e.g., every 1–2 hours) to maintain target glucose levels. The conventional approach of using sliding scale insulin to cover high blood glucose levels may be unsafe and ineffective, and repetitive doses of subcutaneous insulin in the edematous patient can have a cumulative effect leading to prolonged hypoglycemia. In addition, adjusting insulin in the PN bag every 24 hours might not achieve the desired rapid correction of hyperglycemia deemed appropriate based on the literature, which indicates worse outcomes for those with poor glucose control.

Abrupt discontinuation of PN can lead to hypoglycemia and should be avoided. Instead, it is recommended to decrease the PN infusion rate by one-half for the last hour of infusion prior to discontinuation to prevent rebound hypoglycemia.

Pancreatitis
Most cases of pancreatitis are mild, and nutritional support is not needed. However, 10% to 20% of patients with pancreatitis develop severe disease that results in a hypermetabolic, hyperdynamic, systemic inflammatory response syndrome that creates a highly catabolic stress state. In an evidence-based report evaluating nutrition support in acute pancreatitis patients, EN delivered to the small intestine (distal to the ligament of Treitz) is preferred over PN; EN patients are less likely to suffer from multiorgan failure, systemic infections, and death.

Initiation of PN should be delayed in patients with acute pancreatitis who cannot tolerate EN even though they might eventually require PN. Providing PN within 24 hours of admission has been shown to worsen outcome, and providing PN after resuscitation and abatement of the acute inflammatory process appears to improve outcome compared with standard therapy. Consequently, if EN is not feasible, the initiation of PN should be delayed for at least 5 days after admission to the hospital, when the peak period of inflammation has abated.

Acute Kidney Injury and Chronic Kidney Disease
Acute kidney injury (AKI) is associated with severe nutritional deficits. Most patients with AKI are catabolic and have energy requirements 50% to 100% greater than resting requirements, likely the result of other coexisting conditions such as sepsis, trauma, and burns. Energy is provided to patients with AKI in sufficient quantities to minimize protein degradation, generally in the range of 20 to 30 kcal/kg/day. Lipid injectable emulsions can be used as a source of concentrated energy in patients who require a fluid restriction.

Protein loss is accelerated and protein synthesis is impaired in patients with AKI. Loss of amino acids in the dialysate and renal replacement therapies add to the protein deficit and increase individual protein needs. Approximately 10 to 12 g of amino acids are lost with each dialysis therapy, depending on the type of dialyzer membrane, blood flow rate, and dialyzer reuse procedure, and approximately 10 to 16 g/day of amino acids are lost through continuous renal replacement therapies (CRRT). The provision of protein at 1.2 g/kg/day and up to 2.5 g/kg/day is recommended for AKI patients receiving hemodialysis and CRRT, respectively.

Protein is provided with a standard solution containing both essential and nonessential amino acids. Although some data suggest essential amino acids alone may be beneficial compared with a mixture of both essential and nonessential amino acids, the efficacy of using essential amino acid solutions remains uncertain. The goal is to provide adequate protein while treating the patient aggressively with dialysis to prevent the accumulation of nitrogenous waste products.

Fluid and electrolyte balance are often impaired in patients with AKI. The amount of fluid from the PN might need to be adjusted daily, depending on the phase of AKI, whether the patient is receiving dialysis, and whether dialysis is continuous or intermittent. Serum potassium and phosphate levels typically rise in patients with AKI until dialysis is initiated, at which time levels might drop, especially with the provision of PN. Potassium, phosphate, and magnesium levels need close monitoring and adjustment to correct imbalances. Acetate salts of potassium or sodium can be administered to help correct a metabolic acidosis.

Standard doses of the water-soluble vitamins and additional folic acid (1 mg/day total) and pyridoxine (vitamin B6) (10 mg/day) might need to be added to the solution for patients who are being dialyzed because these vitamins are lost from the body in the dialysate bath. Thiamine losses are increased with CRRT and repletion (100 mg/day) must be provided for patients receiving this therapy. The dose of vitamin C might need to be restricted to 100 mg/day to prevent oxalate deposits. However, additional vitamin C (250 mg/day) should be provided to patients receiving CRRT. The supplementation of fat-soluble vitamins is usually not required, especially in patients who also are eating, because excretion of fat-soluble vitamins is reduced in renal failure. For example, serum vitamin A levels may be elevated in AKI due to enhanced hepatic release of retinol and retinol-binding protein, decreased renal catabolism, and decreased degradation of vitamin A transport protein by the kidneys. Vitamin D levels may be decreased because of impaired activation of 1,25-dihydroxycholecalciferol in the kidneys. In anuric patients, trace elements may be withheld from the PN solution; however, for prolonged PN, trace elements and fat-soluble vitamins should be monitored and replaced accordingly.

Patients with chronic kidney disease (CKD) also have nutritional deficits due to anorexia, amino acid losses into the dialysate, concurrent illness, metabolic acidosis, and endocrine disorders. However, unlike those suffering from AKI, patients with CKD have normal energy requirements. Protein intake generally is restricted in predialysis patients to 0.6 g/kg/day or 0.75 g/kg/day if the patient is malnourished. Protein is required in higher amounts in patients on dialysis, depending on the type of dialysis: 1.2 g/kg/day for hemodialysis; 1.2 to 1.5 g/kg/day for peritoneal dialysis. Predialysis patients who become acutely ill should be given protein 1.2 to 1.5 g/kg/day even if this precipitates the need for dialysis. Starvation from insufficient calories or protein in the patient with renal dysfunction increases the risk of nutritionally related complications and should be avoided in the severely ill patient regardless of the potential need for dialysis.

Intradialytic PN is the provision of IV amino acids, carbohydrates, and fat directly into the venous drip chamber of the hemodialysis unit during treatment. It is a method of providing additional calories and protein in malnourished chronic hemodialysis patients. It is associated with significant increases in body weight and serum albumin in patients with end stage renal disease. However, intradialytic PN is expensive and the benefits have not been fully elucidated. A typical solution contains about 1100 kcal and 50 g of protein, which is provided three times per week with hemodialysis. For example, in a dialysis patient who requires 2500 kcals and 70 g protein/day, intradialytic PN will provide approximately 20% of the weekly energy and approximately 30% of the weekly protein needs. Thus intradialytic PN is reserved for patients with end-stage renal disease on hemodialysis who cannot ingest sufficient nutrients by mouth and who are not candidates for nutritional support via EN or PN due to GI intolerance, venous access problems, or other reasons. Appropriate use of intradialytic PN should be limited to a very small fraction of people who are on hemodialysis.

Hepatic Dysfunction and Liver Failure

Hepatic dysfunction is associated with a variety of abnormalities including metabolic abnormalities, malabsorption, maldigestion, anorexia, and early satiety due to ascites. Dietary restrictions also can contribute to malnutrition.

Protein intake in patients with stable chronic liver disease depends on the patient's nutritional status and protein tolerance. Nutritionally depleted patients can require as much protein as 1.5 g/kg estimated dry weight. In a minority of patients who have protein-sensitive hepatic encephalopathy, protein intake might need to be decreased to 0.5 to 0.7 g/kg/day and gradually increased to 1.0 to 1.5 g/kg/day, as tolerated. These patients have deranged plasma amino acid profiles, with increased concentrations of aromatic amino acids (phenylalanine, tyrosine, and tryptophan) and methionine and decreased branched-chain amino acids (leucine, isoleucine, and valine). Randomized, controlled trials that provided parenteral or enteral formulas enriched with branched-chain amino acids have been inconsistent with regard to improvements in encephalopathy, morbidity, and mortality. These specialty products should be reserved for patients with disabling encephalopathy who do not tolerate standard proteins and have not responded to other therapies, such as lactulose or neomycin administration.

Energy requirements are difficult to predict in patients with liver failure. Whereas most patients have a normal metabolic rate, up to one-third may be hypermetabolic. Although providing 25 to 30 kcal/kg/day is a guideline for providing energy needs, basing requirements on indirect calorimetry is often recommended.

Fluid restriction due to ascites and edema often necessitates increasing the dextrose concentration in the PN so as to maintain sufficient calories in a restricted volume. Sodium is reduced in the formula because liver-failure patients excrete nearly sodium-free urine. Vitamin and mineral deficiencies often occur as a result of suboptimal nutrient intake, decreased absorption, decreased storage, and in some cases alcohol use, which decreases thiamine (vitamin B1) and folate absorption. Copper and manganese may be contraindicated because a major route of excretion for these substances is the biliary system. Zinc deficiency is common in cirrhotic patients, and supplementation of this mineral may be necessary, especially if there are excessive GI losses.

Acute Respiratory Distress Syndrome

Patients with protein-calorie malnutrition have an increased incidence of pneumonia, respiratory failure, and acute respiratory distress syndrome (ARDS). Nutritional support is indicated in patients with ARDS. Notably, underfeeding and overfeeding can be detrimental to pulmonary function.

Overfeeding calories, and particularly glucose, can lead to increased minute ventilation, increased dead space, and increased carbon dioxide production and ultimately to difficulty weaning from a ventilator. Hypercapnia from increased carbon dioxide production is the result of glucose combustion causing more carbon dioxide production and excess calories triggering lipogenesis. A healthy person increases ventilation in response to increased calories and thus avoids hypercapnia. However, patients with compromised ventilatory status might not be able to compensate with increased ventilation and can develop respiratory distress, acute respiratory failure, and difficulty weaning from mechanical ventilation. Thus the use of indirect calorimetry measurements to determine energy expenditure is imperative in patients with ARDS.

Critically Ill Patients With Obesity

Obesity is a growing problem worldwide, and management of critically ill patients with obesity poses many challenges. These patients are at risk for hyperglycemia, hyperlipidemia, and hypercapnia, all of which can be exacerbated by metabolic changes associated with critical illness. As with any critically ill patient, those with obesity will preferentially use protein and carbohydrate for energy and cannot effectively draw upon adipose tissue for energy. These patients require nutrition support to minimize loss of lean body mass.

The concept of "hypocaloric feeding" has emerged as the preferred way to feed critically ill patients with obesity. Energy delivery is restricted to approximately 60% to 70% of estimated energy requirements and protein delivery is high (typically >2 g/kg ideal body weight [IBW]). This is to avoid hyperglycemia, hyperlipidemia, and hypercapnia while providing the protein required to spare lean body mass and support recovery. Small-scale studies employing this feeding method have demonstrated that patients can achieve positive nitrogen balance. One study found decreased ICU length of stay, decreased antibiotic days, and a trend toward decreased mechanical ventilation days.

Energy and protein delivery for critically ill patients with obesity is guided by BMI. The ASPEN-SCCM guidelines recommend providing 11 to 14 kcal/kg of actual weight for patients with a BMI of 30 to 50 kg/m² or 22 to 25 kcal/kg IBW for patients with a BMI >50 kg/m². For protein delivery, ASPEN and SCCM recommend protein provision of ≥2 g/kg IBW for patients with class I and class II obesity (BMI of 30–35 kg/m² and 35–40 kg/m², respectively) and for patients with class III obesity (BMI >40 kg/m²) protein provision should be ≥2.5 g/kg IBW.

Other Conditions and Nutritional Treatments

The catabolic response to major surgery, trauma, burn, and sepsis is characterized by a net breakdown of body protein stores to provide substrates for gluconeogenesis and acute-phase protein synthesis. Adequate nutrition can attenuate whole-body catabolism but rarely, if ever, prevents or reverses the loss of lean body mass during the acute phase of injury. Several strategies to prevent the loss of lean body mass have been investigated, including growth hormone, growth factors, and conditionally essential amino acids, such as glutamine.

Growth hormone is a potent anabolic agent, and administration to humans increases the rate of wound healing, decreases rates of wound infection, and decreases the catabolism and muscle wasting of critical illness. However, a large European trial found increased morbidity and mortality in patients with prolonged critical illness who received high doses of growth hormone. Thus the use of growth hormone in patients who are in the acute phase of critical illness is not recommended.

Alternative anabolic agents such as oxandrolone (Oxandrin)[1] and testosterone[1] are being pursued to induce positive nitrogen balance and enhance wound healing in critically ill patients. These anabolic steroid hormones increase protein synthesis

---

[1]Not FDA approved for this indication.

and can reduce the rate of protein breakdown. In a study of patients with alcoholic hepatitis, administration of oxandrolone was associated with lower mortality compared with patients receiving placebo. The patients receiving oxandrolone had improvements in the severity of their liver injury and the degree of malnutrition. Several studies have demonstrated a benefit of oxandrolone use in the burn patient population. Other anabolic steroid hormones, such as methandienone[2] and nandrolone decanoate (Deca Durabolin),[2] have been shown to increase protein anabolism and nitrogen balance in hospitalized patients.

Hormone treatment should be reserved for patients with major burns and documented impaired healing, patients who have large wounds or enterocutaneous fistulae who have impaired healing, patients with muscle wasting and weakness associated with AIDS or other failure to thrive conditions and, in general, patients who have not responded to aggressive nutritional support but whose underlying disease processes are controlled. Growth factors have not been shown to decrease length of time on a respirator in ICU patients. In fact, such factors can increase ventilator time and worsen outcome.

Glutamine-supplemented PN solutions administered to trauma or critically ill patients can improve overall nitrogen balance, enhance muscle protein synthesis, improve intestinal nutrient absorption, decrease gut permeability, improve immune function, and decrease hospital stays and costs in some patient populations. A review of 14 randomized trials in surgical and critically ill patients found that glutamine supplementation was associated with reduced mortality, lower rates of infectious complications, and a decreased hospital stay. The greatest benefit was in patients receiving high-dose (>0.29 g/kg/day) parenteral glutamine.

However, a recent randomized trial of glutamine and antioxidant micronutrient supplementation in critically ill patients showed a trend toward increased 28-day mortality and significant in-hospital and 6-month mortality in patients receiving glutamine supplementation. There were limitations in this study in that baseline glutamine levels were not checked for all patients; in a subset of 66 patients with plasma glutamine levels evaluated, all had normal levels at baseline. This suggests that glutamine supplementation may not be appropriate for all critically ill patients. In addition, patients received approximately 50% of goal energy requirements and approximately 45% of goal protein delivery from glutamine. The total amount of glutamine given in this study was significantly higher than the dose of glutamine usually recommended. This raises the possibility that there is an optimal "therapeutic window" for glutamine administration: Giving too little glutamine may not be efficacious and giving too much may be toxic. Further investigation is required before a definitive recommendation can be given based on this study alone.

Patients with intestinal dysfunction requiring PN, such as those with short-bowel syndrome or mucosal damage following chemotherapy and/or radiation therapy, might benefit from glutamine-containing PN. Glutamine-containing PN might also be beneficial in patients with immunodeficiency syndromes, including AIDS, immune-system dysfunction associated with critical illness, and bone marrow transplantation; patients with severe catabolic illness, such as major burns; patients with multiple trauma; and patients with other diseases associated with a prolonged ICU stay. Glutamine-supplemented solutions should not yet be considered routine care and should not be used in patients with significant renal insufficiency or in patients with significant hepatic failure. A recent ASPEN position paper summarizes recommendations for use of both enteral and IV glutamine.

---

[2]Not available in the United States.

Common Complications and Management

Catheter Sepsis

Catheter-related bloodstream infection (CRBSI) is an infection that originates from the catheter itself and is confirmed by culture. Central line–associated bloodstream infection (CLABSI) is a bloodstream infection without another identified focus of infection in a patient with a central line in place for at least 48 hours prior to the development of infection. Central venous CRBSIs range from 3% to 20% in hospitalized patients and is the most common complication of central venous catheters. Colonization of the skin, intraluminal contamination from manipulation of the catheter hub or IV connectors, and seeding of microorganisms from the bloodstream are common sources of infection. Common organisms associated with CRBSIs include *Staphylococcus epidermidis*, *Staphylococcus aureus*, *Enterococcus* spp., *Candida albicans*, *Escherichia coli*, *Klebsiella* spp., *Pseudomonas* spp., and *Enterobacter* spp. as well as resistant strains such as methicillin-resistant *S. aureus* and vancomycin-resistant enterococci.

Management of patients with catheter infection depends on their clinical condition. In extremely ill patients with high fevers who are hypotensive or who have local signs of infection around the catheter site, the catheter should be removed, its tip cultured, and peripheral and central venous blood cultures should be obtained. In CRBSI, the organisms that grow from the catheter tip are the same those identified in the peripheral blood culture, and typically more than 10^3 organisms are grown from cultures of the catheter tip.

Specific therapy should be initiated against the primary source in patients in whom a source of infection other than the catheter tip is present. Peripheral blood cultures should be obtained. Blood cultures should not be taken from the central venous catheter port dedicated for PN because this increases the risk of contaminating the line. If the infection resolves, central venous feedings can be continued, while making sure to maintain euglycemia. If a source is not identified and the symptoms persist, the catheter should be removed and its tip should be cultured. If the culture of the catheter tip returns positive or if the index of suspicion is high, empiric antibiotic therapy is initiated and later narrowed to target the specific microorganism once culture and susceptibility data become available. If removal of the catheter is indicated and is not possible due to lack of access sites or high risk of bleeding complications, then salvage therapy (systemic antibiotics plus antibiotic lock therapy) or, as a last resort, exchange of the catheter over a guidewire with systemic antibiotics and antibiotic lock therapy may be considered, with long-term ethanol lock therapy to prevent further infections. Central venous feedings may be continued during this interval if the patient is stable. It is important to note that changing the site of catheter, rather than salvage therapy or guidewire exchange, is preferred in patients in whom infection is suspected.

Other Complications

Common complications, their etiologies, and treatments are outlined in Table 4. Prolonged administration of PN can result in altered hepatic function and can lead to liver failure. One to 2 weeks after initiating PN, transaminases may be elevated, but this often resolves without any change in the composition of PN or rate of administration. However, in patients receiving long-term PN (>20 days), prolonged elevations of alkaline phosphatase followed by elevated levels of serum transaminases can occur, even after therapy is discontinued.

Serum levels of alkaline phosphatase and bilirubin initially remain normal, but they rise in many patients who receive long-term PN. Patients who do not receive lipids in the PN solution have more frequent and severe hepatic abnormalities, most likely due to higher carbohydrate loads. Excess glucose increases insulin

TABLE 4 Possible Etiologies and Treatment of Common Complications of Central Parenteral Nutrition

PROBLEM	POSSIBLE ETIOLOGY	TREATMENT
Glucose		
Hyperglycemia, glycosuria, hyperosmolar nonketotic dehydration, or coma	Excessive dose or rate of infusion, inadequate insulin production, concomitant steroid administration, infection	Decrease the amount of glucose given, increase insulin, administer a portion of calories as fat
Diabetic ketoacidosis	Inadequate endogenous insulin production and/or inadequate insulin therapy	Give insulin Decrease glucose intake
Rebound hypoglycemia	Persistent endogenous insulin production by islet cells after long-term high-carbohydrate infusion	Give 5%–10% glucose before parenteral infusion is discontinued
Hypercarbia	Carbohydrate load exceeds the ability to increase minute ventilation and excrete excess CO_2	Limit glucose dose to 5 mg/kg/min Give greater percentage of total caloric needs as fat (up to 30%–40%)
Fat		
Hypertriglyceridemia	Rapid infusion	Decrease rate of PN infusion
	Decreased clearance	Allow clearance (~12 h) before testing blood
Essential fatty acid deficiency	Inadequate essential fatty acid administration	Administer essential fatty acids in doses of 4%–7% of total calories
Amino Acids		
Hyperchloremia metabolic acidosis	Excessive chloride content of amino acid solutions	Administer Na^+ and K^+ as acetate salts
Prerenal azotemia	Excessive amino acids with inadequate caloric supplementation	Reduce amino acids Increase the amount of glucose calories
Miscellaneous		
Hypophosphatemia	Inadequate phosphorus administration with redistribution into tissues	Give 15 mmol phosphate/1000 IV kcal Evaluate antacid and Ca^{2+} administration
Hypomagnesemia	Inadequate administration relative to increased losses (diarrhea, diuresis, medications)	Administer Mg^{2+} (15–20 mEq/1000 kcal)
Hypermagnesemia	Excessive administration; renal failure	Decrease Mg^{2+} supplementation
Hypokalemia	Inadequate K^+ intake relative to increased needs for anabolism; diuresis	Increase K^+ supplementation
Hyperkalemia	Excessive K^+ administration, especially in metabolic acidosis; renal decompensation	Reduce or stop exogenous K^+ If ECG changes are present, treat with calcium gluconate, insulin, diuretics, and/or Kayexalate
Hypocalcemia	Inadequate Ca^{2+} administration; reciprocal response to phosphorus repletion without simultaneous calcium infusion	Increase Ca^{2+} dose
Hypercalcemia	Excessive Ca^{2+} administration; excessive vitamin D administration	Decrease Ca^{2+} and/or vitamin D administration
Elevated liver transaminases or serum alkaline phosphatase and bilirubin	Enzyme induction secondary to amino acid imbalances or overfeeding	Reevaluate nutritional prescription Cycle TPN Avoid overfeeding calories Consider change to a blended lipid rather than 100% soybean oil-lipid Consider administering carnitine

PN, Parenteral nutrition; *TPN,* total parenteral nutrition.

secretion, which stimulates hepatic lipogenesis and results in hepatic fat accumulation. Fatty infiltration is the initial histopathologic change; it is readily reversible and might not be accompanied by altered liver function tests.

Longer PN therapy may be associated with cholestasis, cholelithiasis, steatosis, and steatohepatitis and can progress to active chronic hepatitis, fibrosis, and eventual cirrhosis. The management of PN-related liver dysfunction is summarized in Box 3.

Complications are minimized and nutritional therapy maximized when the care of patients who require specialized nutritional support is supervised by a nutrition support team. Ideally, the nutrition support team consists of a pharmacist, dietitian, nurse, and physician.

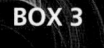 **BOX 3** Management of Parenteral Nutrition-Related Liver Dysfunction

Have the patient eat, if possible.
Avoid administering large amounts of glucose or protein calories.
Supply IV fat emulsions (up to 30% of total calories).
Consider addition of blended lipid emulsions with lower concentrations of soybean oil.
Cycle the parenteral nutrition, infusing for 10 to 12 hours/day.
Reevaluate energy needs; reduce energy delivery if liver dysfunction persists.

References

Al-Omran M, Albalawi ZH, Tashkandi MF, Al-Ansary LA: *Enteral versus parenteral nutrition in acute pancreatitis*, Cochrane Database Syst Rev, 2010. https://doi.org/10.1002/14651858.CD002837.pub2. CD002837.

A.S.P.E.N. Board of Directors: Guidelines for the use of parenteral and enteral nutrition in adult and pediatric patients: *JPEN J Parenter Enteral Nutr* 26:1SA–138SA, 2002.

A.S.P.E.N. Ayers P, Adams S, Boullata J, et al: Parenteral nutrition safety consensus recommendations, *JPEN J Parenter Enteral Nutr* 38:296–333, 2014.

Bistrian BR, McCowen KC: Nutritional and metabolic support in the adult intensive care unit: key controversies, *Crit Care Med* 34:1525–1531, 2006.

Boullata JI, Gilbert K, Sacks G, et al: A.S.P.E.N. Clinical guidelines: parenteral nutrition ordering, order review, compounding, labeling, and dispensing, *JPEN J Parenter Enteral Nutr* 38(3):334–377, 2014.

Butler SO, Btaiche IF, Alaniz C: Relationship between hyperglycemia and infection in critically ill patients, *Pharmacotherapy* 25:963–976, 2005.

Evans DC, Corkins MR, Malone A, et al: The use of visceral proteins as nutrition markers: an ASPEN position paper, *Nutr Clin Pract* 36:22–28, 2021.

Heyland DK, Dhaliwal R, Suchner U, Berger MM: Antioxidant nutrients: a systematic review of trace elements and vitamins in the critically ill patient, *Intensive Care Med* 31:327–337, 2005.

Heyland D, Muscedere J, Wischmeyer PE, et al: A randomized trial of glutamine and antioxidants in critically ill patients, *N Engl J Med* 368:1489–1497, 2013.

Li Y, Tang X, Zhang J, Wu T: Nutritional support for acute kidney injury, *Cochrane Database Syst Rev*, 2010. https://doi.org/10.002/14651858.CD005426. pub2, CD005426.

McClave SA, Chang W-K, Dhaliwal R, Heyland DK: Nutrition support in acute pancreatitis: a systematic review of the literature, *JPEN J Parenter Enteral Nutr* 30:143–156, 2006.

McClave SA, Taylor BE, Martindale RG, et al: Guidelines for the provision of nutrition support therapy in the adult critically ill patient: Society of Critical Care Medicine (SCCM) and American Society for Parenteral and Enteral Nutrition (A.S.P.E.N.), *JPEN J Parenter Enteral Nutr*. 40:159–211 40:1200, 2016. Erratum in: JPEN J Parenter Enteral Nutr 2016.

McMahon MM, Nystrom E, Braunschweig C, et al: A.S.P.E.N. Clinical guidelines: nutrition support of adult patients with hyperglycemia, *JPEN J Parenter Enteral Nutr* 37:26–36, 2013.

O'Grady NP, Alexander M, Burns LA, et al: Guidelines for the prevention of intravascular catheter-related infections, *Clin Infect Dis* 52:e162–e193, 2011. Also available at http://www.cdc.gov/hicpac/BSI/BSI-guidelines-2011.html. accessed December 5, 2013.

Vanek VW, Matarese LE, Robinson M, et al: A.S.P.E.N.Position paper: parenteral nutrition glutamine supplementation, *JPEN J Parenter Enteral Nutr* 26:479–494, 2011.

Worthington P, Balint J, Bechtold M, et al: When is parenteral nutrition appropriate? *JPEN J Parenter Enteral Nutr* 41:324–377, 2017.

PHEOCHROMOCYTOMA

Method of
Katherine I. Wolf, BS; and Karel Pacak, MD, PhD, DSc

CURRENT DIAGNOSIS

- The most common clinical sign of a pheochromocytoma/paraganglioma (PPGL) is hypertension; when combined with the triad of headache, palpitations, and diaphoresis, the diagnosis should be suspected.
- A biochemical diagnosis of PPGL should be established with elevated plasma free or urinary fractionated metanephrines and plasma methoxytyramine.
- Localize tumors with anatomic imaging (computed tomography [CT] or magnetic resonance), followed by specific functional imaging using positron emission tomography modalities.
- Following diagnosis, a thorough medical and family history should be obtained to assess for syndromic clinical presentations of PPGL. If available, all patients with confirmed PPGL should undergo genetic testing.
- If a causative mutation is identified, the patient's first-degree relatives should be appropriately tested. Positive individuals should be presymptomatically screened with plasma free or urinary fractionated metanephrines and imaging as described, if appropriate.

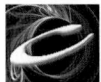

CURRENT THERAPY

- Prompt surgical excision remains the primary treatment for PPGL. If feasible, cortical sparing adrenalectomies should be attempted in patients with bilateral or hereditary PPGLs (except succinate dehydrogenase subunit B [*SDHB*]–related disease) to prevent lifelong corticosteroid supplementation.
- One to two weeks prior to the operation, regardless of biochemical activity, patients should be started on a preoperative α- followed by β-adrenoceptor blockade to avoid unopposed α-adrenoceptor stimulation leading to vasoconstriction and hypertension crisis. At minimum, a normotensive patient should be maintained on low-dose calcium channel blockers.
- After surgery, scheduled clinical follow-up is necessary, particularly in cases of underlying genetic mutations or large tumors (>5 cm), which are more likely to metastasize.
- Management of metastatic PPGL requires a multidisciplinary approach involving surgical excision alongside pharmacologic, radio-, and chemotherapies.

The 2017 World Health Organization (WHO) Classification of Tumors of Endocrine Organs defines pheochromocytoma (PHEO)* as a chromaffin cell tumor arising from the adrenal medulla. Paragangliomas (PGLs) are functionally similar tumors that arise along the extra-adrenal ganglia and are further classified as parasympathetic or sympathetic. Predominantly located in the head and neck, parasympathetic PGLs are locally invasive, rarely develop metastases, and secrete dopamine/methoxytyramine. In contrast to their parasympathetic counterparts, sympathetic PGLs are concentrated primarily in the abdomen and pelvis, with 2% found in the mediastinum and 1% in the neck. Abdominal PGLs often derive from the organ of Zuckerkandl, a collection of neural crest cells above the bifurcation of the aorta at the origin of the inferior mesenteric artery (Figure 1). Biochemically, PHEOs are characterized by the synthesis, metabolism, storage, and usually, but not always, secretion of catecholamines, metanephrines, and/or methoxytyramine.

Epidemiology

Previously, PHEOs were primarily diagnosed at autopsy. However, as the sensitivity of biochemical and imaging assays increased, the incidence of PHEO likewise swelled. A recent European analysis estimates that the age-standardized incidence rate increased from 0.29 to 0.46 from 1995 to 2015, respectively. While PHEO can occur at any age (including childhood, particularly when associated with germline genetic mutations), the average age of diagnosis is most commonly in the fifth decade. Although no consistent gender preference has been reported, in the Netherlands, a statistically significant number of PHEOs occurred in females (55%) compared to their male counterparts (45%). The PHEO to PGL ratio is approximately 0.80 to 0.20, respectively. Approximately 30% to 40% of patients with PHEO carry a germline or somatic mutation in one of the 25 known PHEO susceptibility genes (see "Genetics" below). The rate of malignancy varies from 0% to 71% depending on genetic background, with succinate dehydrogenase subunit B (*SDHB*)–related disease, the most clinically aggressive.

Genetics

While complete consensus is lacking, 30% to 40% of PHEOs are hereditary, with a significant percentage (upwards of 20%) of apparently sporadic tumors carrying somatic mutations. Identification of a genetic alteration allows for appropriate treatment algorithms and management of subsequent endocrinopathies or syndromic neoplasias in the proband and at-risk relatives as well.

---

*From this point forward, PHEO represents pheochromocytoma and paraganglioma unless otherwise specified.

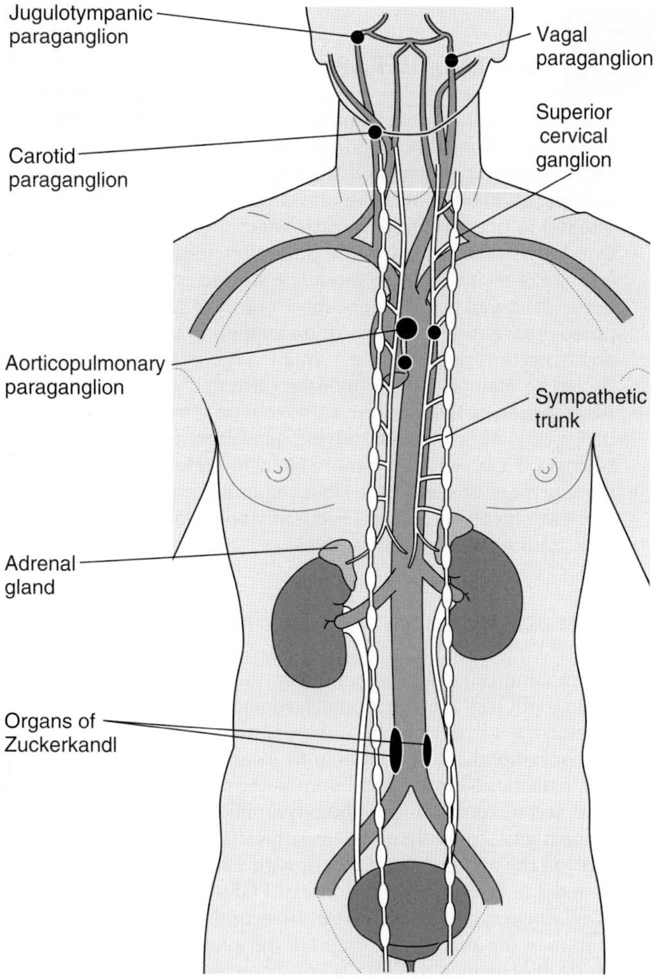
Jugulotympanic paraganglion
Vagal paraganglion
Superior cervical ganglion
Carotid paraganglion
Aorticopulmonary paraganglion
Sympathetic trunk
Adrenal gland
Organs of Zuckerkandl

Figure 1 Important anatomic distribution of chromaffin tissue composing paraganglia.

At present, at least 25 PHEO susceptibility genes have been discovered, which can broadly be categorized into major and minor contributors, with the major genes representing 85% to 90% of all hereditary tumors. Well-known hereditary genetic mutations include von Hippel-Lindau tumor suppressor (*VHL*), *RET* proto-oncogene resulting in multiple endocrine neoplasia (MEN) types 2A and 2B, neurofibromin 1 (*NF1*) tumor suppressor, and the succinate dehydrogenase (*SDHx*) subunits *SDHB* and *SDHD* genes. The minor susceptibility genes, representing 10% to 15% of hereditary tumors include *SDHA*, *SDHC*, succinate dehydrogenase assembly factor 2 (*SDHAF2*), fumarate hydratase (*FH*), Myc-associated factor X (*MAX*), hypoxia-inducible factor 2 alpha (*HIF2A*), malate dehydrogenase 2 (*MDH2*), isocitrate dehydrogenase 1 (*IDH1*), *H-RAS* and *K-RAS* proto-oncogenes, transmembrane protein 127 (*TMEM 127*), cold-shock domain containing E1 (*CSDE1*), mastermind like transcriptional coactivator 3 (*MAML3*) fusion genes, prolyl hydroxylase 1 and 2 (*PHD1/2*), iron regulatory protein 1 (*IRP1*), *MDH2*, kinesin superfamily member (*K1F1B*), dihydrolipoamide *S*-succinyltransferase (*DLST*), and DNA methyltransferase 3 alpha (*DNMT3A*). Characteristics of the most important hereditary tumor syndromes are described in Table 1.

Several well-established PHEO syndromes (Box 1) exhibit characteristic clinical features. Rare PGL-associated syndromes include Carney triad and Carney-Stratakis syndrome, which are characterized by *SDHB* and *SDHD*-related gastrointestinal stromal tumors (GISTs). The novel recently described Pacak-Zhuang syndrome consists of *HIF2A*-associated PGLs in the setting of polycythemia, duodenal somatostatinomas, and marked, permanent choroidal thickening and tortuous dilated veins in the choroid and retina. Another rare, recently described PHEO syndrome is characterized by giant cell tumors associated with a postzygotic *H3F3A* mutation.

In conjunction with the United States Endocrine Society Clinical Practice Guidelines, recent publications have emphasized genetic counseling and subsequent testing in all patients diagnosed with PHEO, regardless of suggestive family history or age at presentation. Within the United States, several commercially available PHEO gene panels screen patients for the most prevalent hereditary genetic syndromes via DNA sequencing and deletion/duplication analysis. However, broad, comprehensive genetic panels covering 10 to 12 genes are expensive and may not be covered by insurance. In patients with a confirmed PHEO, an algorithm (Figure 2) based on family history, syndromic clinical features, and biochemical phenotype can be used to tailor genetic testing and reduce the financial burden. If genetic testing is positive for hereditary PHEO, all first-degree relatives should undergo genetic evaluation. Asymptomatic carriers should undergo annual biochemical evaluation with plasma free metanephrines and whole-body magnetic resonance (MR) imaging every other year for surveillance. Genetic testing in children (Box 2) should be approached on an individual basis following discussion with parents/guardians, geneticists, and psychiatrists due to the ethical and legal ramifications. Children should only be screened if they will be offered regular surveillance.

Clinical Manifestations

As a result of episodic catecholamine secretion on - and β-adrenoceptors, the clinical manifestations of PHEO are related to hemodynamic and metabolic instability. While the majority of primary clinical indicators (Box 3) for PHEO are nonspecific, when several symptoms are taken in conjunction, the diagnosis should be considered. Classically, patients experience paroxysmal hypertension accompanied with headaches, palpitations secondary to tachyarrhythmia, and diaphoresis. However, pallor, nausea, flushing, fatigue, and psychological symptoms—including anxiety, panic attacks, and nervousness—are common. Symptoms may occur spontaneously or as a result of direct tumor manipulation, anesthesia, or ingestion of tyramine-rich foods, which trigger catecholamine release and subsequent crisis. Unfortunately, patients may not exhibit any signs or symptoms of PHEO, thereby delaying a timely diagnosis. Therefore, if biochemistry or imaging suggests PHEO, the diagnosis may not be excluded based on the patient's asymptomatic state.

Differential Diagnosis

Referred to as the "great mimic," PHEO manifests with a myriad of signs and symptoms that are easily misconstrued for more common disorders, which often prevents a timely diagnosis. Consideration should be given to conditions that also result in sympathomedullary activation, including hyperadrenergic and renovascular hypertension, panic disorders, menopausal syndrome, temporal epilepsy, and other neuroendocrine tumors that release vasoactive substances. Patients with a presumptive diagnosis of PHEO should be screened biochemically. If results are unequivocal, a normal response to the clonidine suppression test will effectively rule out PHEO.

Biochemical Evaluation

PHEOs are capable of secreting all, none, or any combination of catecholamines—epinephrine, norepinephrine, and dopamine. Plasma free metanephrines (the *O*-methylated metabolites of parent catecholamines) is the current gold-standard diagnostic criteria to detect and exclude a diagnosis of PHEO. Twenty-four-hour urinary metanephrines is a comparable alternative when plasma is not available. Definitive diagnosis is likely when biochemical evaluation is greater than two times the upper reference limit (URL) (Figure 3). To reliably interpret test results, specific conditions (Box 4) should be ensured throughout the blood draw. Additionally, there are a variety of foods and medications (Table 2) that interact either directly or indirectly with catecholamine measurement and should therefore be avoided

TABLE 1 | Characteristics of Hereditary Pheochromocytoma Syndromes and Gene Mutations

SYN-DROME	MUTA-TION	GENE	PROTEIN FUNCTION	PENETRANCE	BILATERAL	MALIG-NANT	PHEO OR PGL	PEAK AGE (Y)	BIOCHEMICAL PHENOTYPE+
MEN2	10q11.2	*RET*	Receptor tyrosine kinase	50%	50–80%	Rare	PHEO	40	ADR
VHL	3p25-26	*VHL*	VHL protein/E3 ubiquitin protein ligase	10–30%	50%	5%	PHEO	30	NA
NF-1	17q11	*NF-1*	NF-related protein	1–2%	16%	5–10%	PHEO	50	ADR
PGL1	11q23	*SDHD*	Membrane-spanning subunit; D subunit of SDH	90% if paternally transmitted†	Inconsistent Reports	5–20%#	PHEO/PGL	35–40	NA and/or DA; some biochemically silent
PGL2 SDHD5	11q12.2 Assembly factor for SDHA	*SDHAF2/*		100% if paternally transmitted		Unknown	PGL	30–40	
PGL3	1q21	SDHC	Membrane-spanning protein; C subunit of SDH	Inconsistent Reports	Inconsistent Reports	Rare	PHEO/PGL	38	NA and/or DA; some biochemically silent
PGL4	1p36	SDHB	Catalytic iron-sulfur protein; B subunit of SDH	30-50%	Rare	31–71%	PHEO/PGL	30	NA and/or DA; some biochemically silent
PGL5	5p15	SDHA	Catalytic flavoprotein; A subunit of SDH	10–13%‡	Inconsistent Reports	30-66%	PHEO/PGL	40	NA and/or DA; some biochemically silent
-	2q11.2	TMEM127	Transmembrane protein	Inconsistent Reports	33%	<5%	PHEO	43	ADR
-	14q23	MAX	bHLHLZ transcription factor	Inconsistent Reports*	67%	<25%	PHEO	32	Mixed ADR and NA+

Abbreviations: Adrenergic (*ADR*), Basic helix-loop-helix leucine zipper (*bHLHLZ*), Dopaminergic (*DA*), Multiple endocrine neoplasia (*MEN*), Noradrenergic (*NA*), Neurofibromatosis (*NF*), Paraganglioma (*PGL*), Pheochromocytoma (*PHEO*), Succinate dehydrogenase (*SDH*), von Hippel-Lindau (*VHL*)

Adrenergic: Phenotype characterized by increased levels of epinephrine or epinephrine/metanephrine. Noradrenergic: Phenotype characterized by increased levels of norepinephrine or norepinephrine/normetanephrine

†Observations at the National Institutes of Health report lower penetrance

#Excluding head and neck PGLs, where the rate of malignancy is approximately 5–10%

‡Observations at the National Institutes of Health report a much lower penetrance, almost zero percent

*Probable paternal transmission only

for 12 hours prior to collection. Patients with acute or chronic kidney disease, particularly those on dialysis, commonly have elevated plasma metanephrines (although likely less than three to four times the URL of normal). If necessary, liquid chromatography with tandem mass spectrometry is a quick and cost-effective means to detect and remove potentially interfering substances. Previously, the glucagon[1] stimulation test was utilized, but this has been abandoned due to poor sensitivity and provocation of hypertension.

Confirmatory follow-up testing is necessary in almost all cases of PHEO given the high false-positive rate. Repeat plasma or urinary metanephrines and catecholamines, or the clonidine suppression test, can be used in equivocal cases, as secondary validation or in patients in whom interfering drugs cannot be stopped. Prior to clonidine suppression testing, patients should undergo

a complete medication review with consideration to hold antihypertensives given predilection for profound hypotension in response to clonidine. Additionally, diuretics, antidepressants, and β-adrenoceptor blockers have been reported to interfere with test results and should be held when appropriate. The patient should be fasting overnight and resting comfortably supine for 20 minutes prior to baseline blood draw. Clonidine (Catapres)[1] is administered at a dose of 0.3 milligrams (mg) per 70 kg, with appropriate dose adjustments as necessary (upwards of 0.5 mg based on weight), and subsequent repeat blood draw 3 hours after administration.

With an increasing proportion of hereditary PHEO, it is important to distinguish their various catecholamine profiles, which can help guide genetic testing. In the last several years, the *O*-methylated metabolite of dopamine—methoxytyramine—has been used to confirm head and neck PGLs, which solely secrete dopamine and are therefore missed with standardized biochemical analysis. Furthermore, recent literature points to plasma

---

[1]Not FDA approved for this indication.

BOX 1 — Important Syndromic Pheochromocytoma Presentations

von Hippel-Lindau Syndrome
Type 2A
- Retinal and central nervous system hemangioblastomas
- Pheochromocytoma
- Endolymphatic sac tumors
- Epididymal cystadenomas

Type 2B
- Renal cell cysts/carcinomas
- Retinal and central nervous system hemangioblastomas
- Pancreatic cysts/neoplasms
- Pheochromocytoma
- Endolymphatic sac tumors
- Epididymal cystadenomas

Type 2C
- Pheochromocytoma

Multiple Endocrine Neoplasia
Type 2A
- Medullary thyroid carcinoma
- Pheochromocytoma
- Hyperparathyroidism
- Cutaneous lichen amyloidosis

Type 2B
- Medullary thyroid carcinoma
- Pheochromocytoma
- Marfanoid habitus

FMTC: Familial Medullary Thyroid Carcinoma
Neurofibromatosis Type 1
- Neurofibromas
- Café-au-lait macules
- Lisch nodules
- Scoliosis
- Cognitive impairment
- Pheochromocytoma

Other Pheochromocytoma Syndromes
Carney Triad
- Gastrointestinal stromal tumor
- Pulmonary chondroma
- Paraganglioma

Carney-Stratakis Syndrome
- Gastrointestinal stromal tumor
- Paraganglioma

Pacak-Zhuang Syndrome
- Paraganglioma
- Somatostatinoma
- Polycythemia
- Retinal abnormalities
- Pheochromocytoma and giant cell tumors with *H3F3A* mutations

Adapted from Lenders JW, Eisenhofer G, Mannelli M, et al: Phaechromocytoma. *Lancet* 366:665–675, 2005.

methoxytyramine as a novel biomarker for metastatic PHEO, which can be used in conjunction with large tumor size, germline genetic mutations (particularly *SDHx*), and the presence of extra-adrenal PGLs to indicate a higher likelihood of malignancy.

Localization of Pheochromocytoma

Imaging should only be pursued after clear biochemical evidence is confirmed. For optimal results, initial anatomic scans should consist of whole-body CT or MR imaging. T2-weighted MR imaging is preferred in patients in whom radiation exposure should be limited, those with a CT contrast allergy, and for the detection of skull-based lesions with the presence of known surgical clips. Ultrasound is not recommended for the localization of PHEO but may be utilized in children and during pregnancy if MR imaging is unavailable. Anatomic imaging is only sufficient for PHEO confirmation if the adrenal gland is the sole site of involvement (tumors <5 cm in size) and the metanephrine level is very high—all other patients should proceed with functional imaging, which is also useful in ruling out metastatic disease.

Currently, there are four primary nuclear imaging techniques used to confirm or detect metastatic PHEO (iodine-123 metaiodobenzyl-guanadine [^{123}I-MIBG], gallium-68 DOTA coupled somatostatin analogs [^{68}Ga-SSTa], fluorine-18-fluorodihydroxyphenylalanine [^{18}F-FDOPA], and 18-fluronine-fluorodexoyglucose [^{18}F-FDG]). Several algorithms (Figure 4) have been proposed based on tumor location, genetic predisposition, and presence of metastatic disease. While ^{18}F-FDG was previously preferred for comprehensive localization of metastatic disease, recent systematic reviews have reported the superiority of ^{68}Ga-SSTa in apparently sporadic and *SDHx*-related PHEO. However, for other inherited PHEO (*NFI, VHL, RET, MAX*), ^{18}F-FDOPA is the preferred positron emission tomography (PET) radiopharmaceutical. Given the relatively novel status of ^{68}Ga-SSTa and ^{18}F-FDOPA, these modalities may not be available at a particular institution. In this case, physicians should proceed with traditional ^{18}F-FDG. The use of ^{123}I-MIBG scintigraphy should be limited to patients with known metastatic PHEO in the evaluation and eligibility for targeted radionuclide therapy.

Treatment

The preferred, localized treatment for PHEO is surgical resection. Even in patients with metastatic disease or where complete excision is not feasible, debulking procedures are favorable to reduce hormonal secretion and prevent anatomic complications. To ensure patient safety throughout the perioperative period, a multidisciplinary team should include a medical internist/endocrinologist, anesthesiologist, and surgeon, preferably in an experienced center (see "Perioperative Management" for details). For metastatic, systemic treatment options, see "Metastatic Pheochromocytoma."

Preoperative Medical Preparation

Surgical resection bears high perioperative risks and complications, which can be mitigated with an appropriate - and β-adrenoceptor blockade. Over the past decade, multiple case series have called into question the necessity of such medical management. However, the United States Endocrine Society Clinical Practices guideline continues to recommend an α-adrenoceptor blockade to ensure the protection of patients, secondary to prolonged circulating catecholamines. While patients are most at risk for a catecholamine and subsequent hypertensive crisis during induction of anesthesia and direct tumor manipulation, daily psychological and physical stressors are just as likely to result in a sudden release of catecholamines. Therefore, it is imperative patients be adequately blocked even without a surgical plan.

At minimum, blood pressure should be treated preoperatively for 7–14 days barring extenuating circumstances (Figure 5). The most commonly used nonselective α-adrenoceptor blocker is phenoxybenzamine (Dibenzyline). However, this medication may be expensive, poorly covered by insurance, and is associated with nasal congestion, fatigue, and ejaculatory dysfunction—which may be rate limiting for patients. Selective α1-adrenoceptor blockers include doxazosin (Cardura), prazosin (Minipress), and terazosin (Hytrin). Selective adrenoceptor blockers have a shorter duration of action and are more likely to result in first-dose orthostatic hypotension, while the long-acting phenoxybenzamine is associated with postoperative hypotension. In low-risk, normotensive patients, calcium channel blockers and metyrosine (Demser) can be utilized if available within the institution.

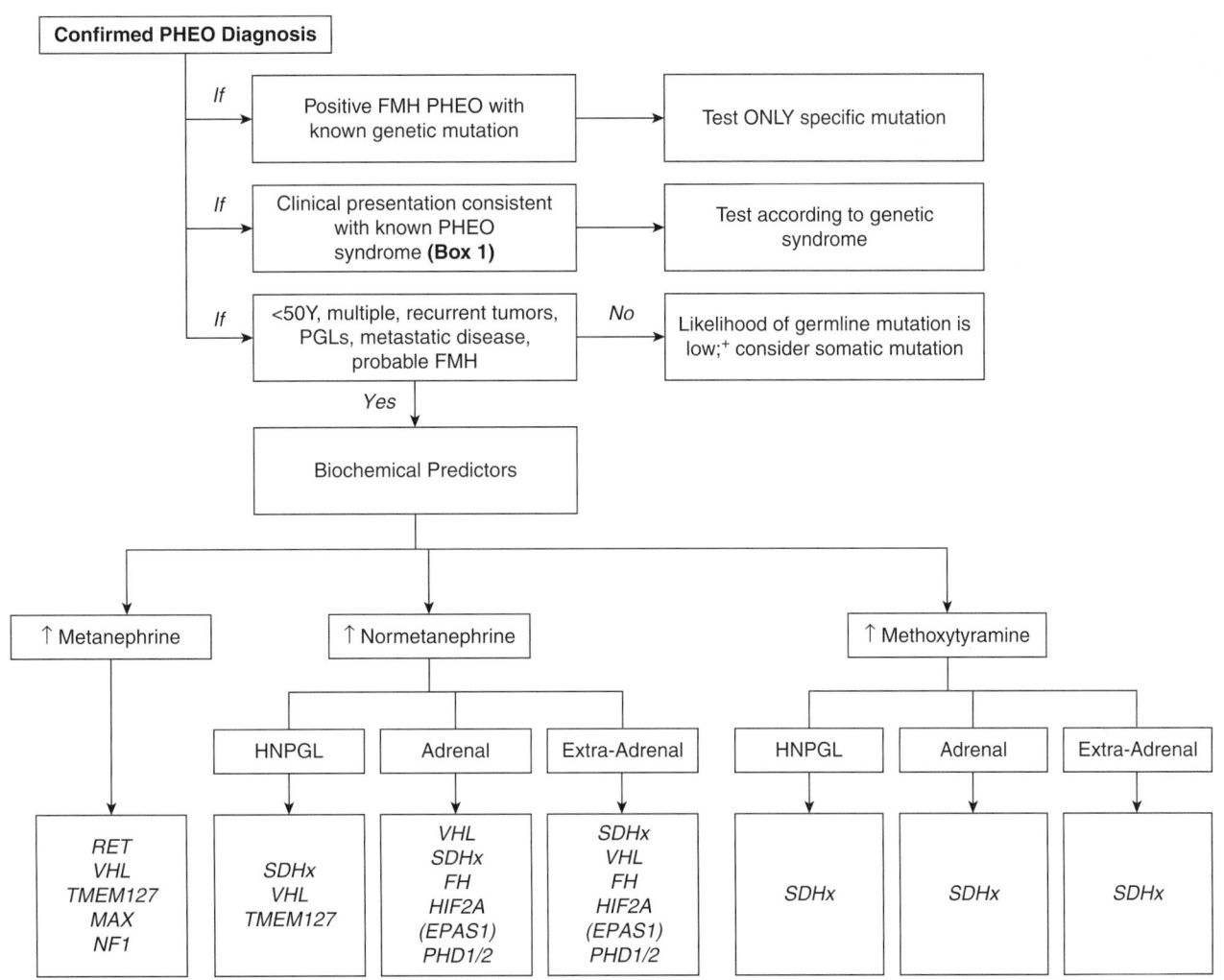

Figure 2 Targeted algorithm for genetic analysis in patients with confirmed pheochromocytoma. If both normetanephrine and methoxytyramine are elevated, follow the algorithm for methoxytyramine. If both normetanephrine and metanephrine are elevated, follow the algorithm for metanephrine. *SDHAF2* mutation screening should be considered in patients who suffer exclusively from head and neck paragangliomas and who have familial antecedents, multiple tumors, or a very young age of onset and in whom *SDHB/C/D* gene mutations are negative. Only the most common genes are listed. *FMH*, Family medical history. (Adapted from Karasek D, Shah U, Frysak Z, et al: An update on the genetics of pheochromocytoma. *J Hum Hypertens* 27[3]:141–147, 2013.)

Considerations for Pediatric Genetic Testing

- Parent/Guardian should meet with geneticist and/or psychiatrist in the absence of the child to discuss implications for genetic testing and subsequent screening recommendations if positive.
- Parent/Guardian should be given adequate time to reflect on their consultation and develop a plan to discuss why the child is undergoing the testing and the implications of the results.
- Medical providers should work with the family to avoid testing or revealing results close to or falling on birthdays, religious holidays, or important school activities, as this may negatively impact the memory of these events.
- If possible, avoid simultaneously testing multiple siblings given the potential impact of discordant results.
- If positive, genetic counselors should emphasize the importance of "at risk" vs. "being ill" and provide all parties with the appropriate space to express their immediate reactions, ask questions, and process their emotions.

Adapted from Lahlou-Laforet K, Consoli SM, Jeunemaitre X, et al: Presymptomatic genetic testing in minors at risk of paraganglioma and pheochromocytoma: our experience of oncogenetic multidisciplinary consultation. *Horm Metab Res* 44:354–358, 2012.

If tachycardia ensues, cardioselective β1-adrenoceptor blockers, such as atenolol (Tenormin) or metoprolol (Lopressor), can be initiated 2 to 3 days after α-adrenoceptor administration. β-Adrenoceptor blockers *cannot* be given prior to initiation of an α-adrenoceptor blocker as unopposed antagonism can result in severe hypertensive crisis. In patients with persistent tachyarrhythmia, ivabradine (Corlanor) can be used; however, it is not approved by the FDA for this indication.

Perioperative Management

As stated previously, an appropriate preoperative blockade is a necessity to ensure 24 hours of systolic blood pressure less than 140 mm Hg prior to surgery. Orthostatic hypotension is tolerated, but not below 80/45 mm Hg. Operative approach should be decided on an individual basis by the surgeon. When appropriate and feasible, small, nonmetastatic PHEOs and retroperitoneal PGLs should be surgically excised with a minimally invasive technique. Locoregional invasion is difficult to assess preoperatively; therefore, suspected cases should initially be explored by laparoscopy with conversion to an open procedure in the face of critical adhesions. In non-*SDHB*-related bilateral PHEO, an adrenocortical sparing procedure is recommended to avoid permanent glucocorticoid deficiency.

Intraoperatively, direct communication between the surgeon and anesthesiologist—particularly during tumor manipulation

BOX 3 Clinical Indications to Screen for Pheochromocytoma

- Patients with a known pheochromocytoma susceptibility gene mutation or a positive family history.
- Patients with triad of headaches, sweating, and tachycardia (regardless of blood pressure).
- Patients with recent onset of uncontrolled hypertension on greater than three to four standard oral therapies.
- Patients with previous history of hypertension, tachycardia, or arrhythmia following anesthesia, surgery, or ingestion of medications known to precipitate symptoms of pheochromocytoma.
- Patients with an incidental adrenal mass.

and excision—is imperative to minimize hemodynamic fluctuations secondary to massive catecholamine release. Careful and continued monitoring of postoperative hemodynamic stability is crucial. Common complications include hypertension, hypotension, arrhythmias, adrenocortical insufficiency, and hypoglycemia. Within the immediate (first 24 hours) postoperative period, transient hypertension is likely attributable to pain, volume overload, or autonomic instability, which should be treated symptomatically. However, persistent hypertension should be concerning for incomplete tumor resection, metastatic disease, excess fluid administration, or underlying essential hypertension. Recommended first-line management is with short-acting, easily titratable agents, such as nicardipine (Cardene) or labetalol (Trandate). Attempts to repeat plasma/urinary metanephrine levels to assess for residual disease burden should be delayed for five to seven days following surgery to ensure resolution of operative catecholamine spikes. In a postoperative hypotensive (SBP <90 mm Hg) patient,

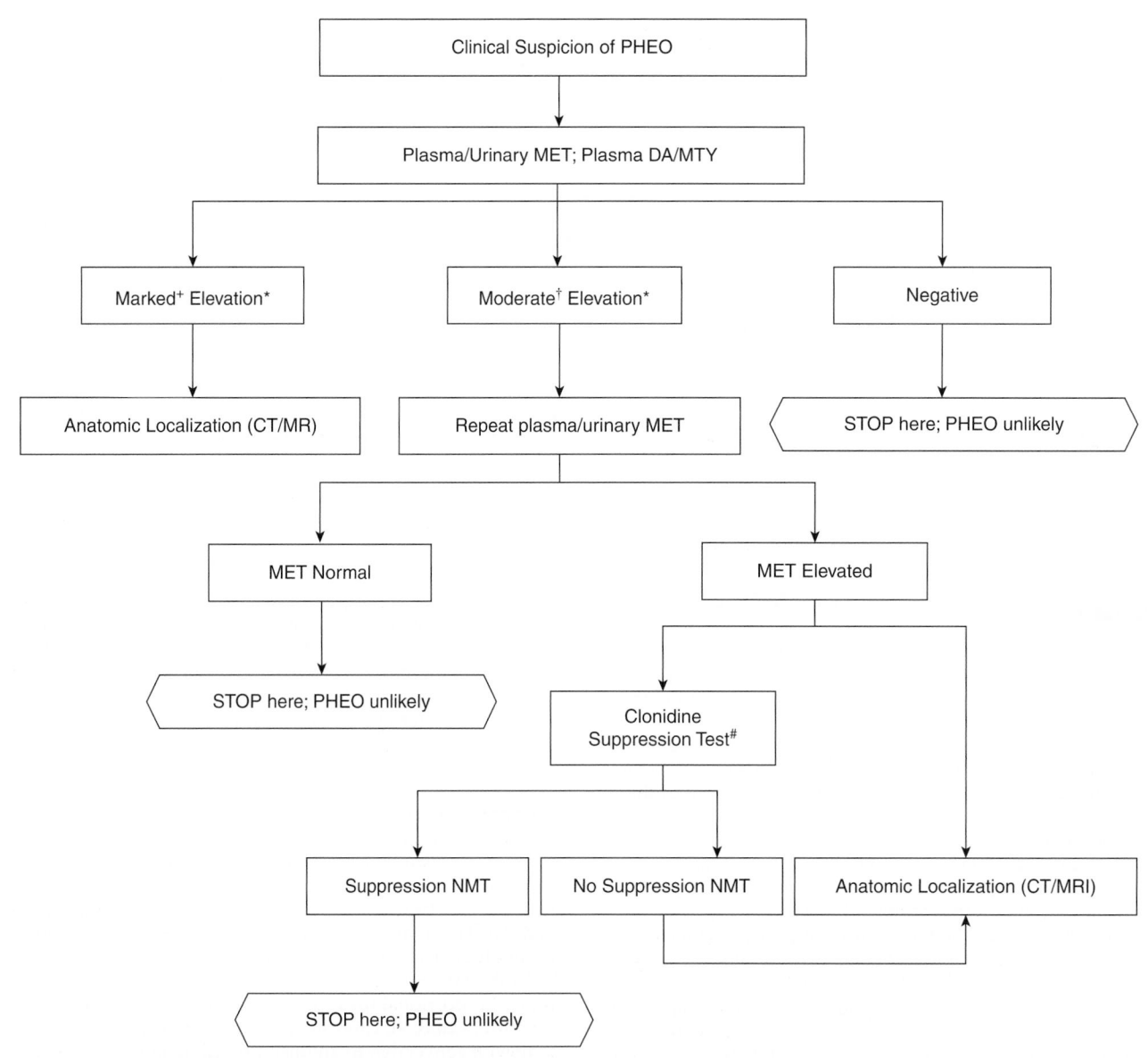

†Marked: greater than 2x the URL of normal
†Moderate; less than 2x the URL of normal
*First rule out any drug-related false elevation of MET/MTY (see Table 2) or renal failure
#If suspicion for PHEO is low or interfering drugs cannot be held

Figure 3 Algorithm for biochemical diagnosis of pheochromocytoma.

hemorrhage should be excluded before deliberating a differential. Alternative etiologies include prolonged -adrenoceptor blockade action, abrupt cessation of serum catecholamines, chronically low circulating plasma volume, or blood loss. The primary treatment modality is fluid resuscitation or blood transfusion, if needed. Vasopressors should be used sparingly, especially when metyrosine or long-acting β-adrenoceptor blockers were used preoperatively.

Postoperative tachyarrhythmias (>100 beats/min) are likely due to continued catecholamine secretion or the use of intraoperative inotropes, while bradyarrhythmias (<60 beats/min) are due to a variety of concerns. For persistent abnormal rhythms, expert evaluation is recommended. If adrenal insufficiency is expected postoperatively, patients should receive 50 to 100 mg hydrocortisone (Cortef) prior to induction, followed by 25 to 50 mg every 8 hours thereafter. Barring any postoperative complications, transition to an oral steroid regimen 24 to 48 hours after surgery (glucocorticoid and mineralocorticoid) and provide appropriate education on adrenal crisis, emergency bracelets, and dosage adjustments in times of sickness. In the absence of catecholamine excess, upregulated liver glycogenolysis and inhibition of insulin secretion may cease, leading to postoperative hypoglycemia. Importantly, the classic signs and symptoms may be masked in the immediate postoperative period and should be routinely monitored for the first 24 hours following surgery.

Hypertensive Crisis

The most dangerous PHEO-related complication, a hypertensive crisis, can manifest with a severe headache, visual disturbances, myocardial infarction, congestive heart failure, or a cerebrovascular accident. Immediate treatment with repetitive 5-mg intravenous boluses of phentolamine (Regitine)—a short-acting, reversible, nonselective α-adrenoceptor agonist—should be repeated every 2 minutes until hypertension is adequately controlled (or initiate a continuous infusion). If unavailable, continuous infusions of sodium nitroprusside (Nitropress), labetalol (Trandate), or nicardipine (Cardene) are alternative options, with appropriate dose de-escalation upon the resolution of hypertension and subsequent symptoms related to the crisis.

Metastatic Pheochromocytoma

According to the 2017 WHO report, metastatic PHEO is only established by the presence of chromaffin cells where they are normally absent. PHEO metastasizes via a hematogenous or lymphatic route with the bones, lymph nodes, liver, and lungs being the most common sites of disease progression. Recent data suggest that almost half of patients with metastatic PHEO present within 1 year of initial diagnosis, while greater than 70% of patients will develop metastatic disease within 5 years of their primary diagnosis. At the time of primary tumor resection, over 75% of metastatic PHEO patients have a tumor larger than 5 centimeters (cm), with one study reporting a median tumor diameter of 7.0 cm. From a genetic perspective, around half of all patients with metastatic disease do not express a germline mutation and are apparently sporadic; however, of the remaining 50%, anywhere from 10% to 42% have been associated with SDHB-related disease. Biochemically, markedly elevated norepinephrine and/or dopamine methoxytyramine are

TABLE 2	Diet and Medication-Induced* Interference of Fractionated Plasma Metanephrines		
		NE	NMT
Diet			
Tomatoes, beans, coffee, cheese, wine, fermented foods		↑	↑
Medications			
Acetaminophen‡		↑	-
TCA		↑↑	↑↑
SNRI#		↑↑	↑↑
MAOi##		↑	↑
Phenoxybenzamine		↑	↑
Sympathomimetics+		↑↑	↑↑
Labetalol		↑	↑
Cocaine		↑↑	↑↑
β-Adrenoceptor Blocker		↑	↑
Methyldopa/Carbidopa		↑	↑
Buspirone		↑↑	↑↑

*All increases are relative and depend on drug dose, duration of treatment, and quantity of food.
‡Drug interference is not seen with mass spectrometry-based assays. Elevated NE is related to contamination during high-performance liquid chromatography.
#Reported cases of SSRIs potentially leading to elevated norepinephrine level.
##Also elevated MN and MTY.
+Pseudoephedrine, nicotine, amphetamines.
↑Moderate elevation.
↑↑Marked elevation.
MAOi, Monoamine oxidase inhibitor; NE, norepinephrine; NMT, normetanephrine; SSRI, selective serotonin reuptake inhibitor; SNRI, serotonin norepinephrine reuptake inhibitor; TCA, tricyclic antidepressants.

associated with the presence of metastases, especially in patients with SDHx-related disease, and can be utilized to monitor disease progression. Current publications indicate that the 5-year overall survival ranges from 62% to 85%, while the median overall survival varied between 6 and 24 years. Location and type of tumor also indicate a higher likelihood of malignancy, with extra-adrenal PGLs the most worrisome for metastatic disease. Meanwhile, head and neck PGLs were associated with improved prognosis and very rarely reported cases of rapidly progressive disease.

Management of metastatic PHEO (Figure 6) requires a multidisciplinary approach, consisting of targeted pharmacology, radiotherapy, chemotherapy, and surgery. Surgical debulking procedures continue to be the mainstay of palliative treatment. Delaying any procedures is positively correlated with rapidly progressive metastatic disease and should be avoided whenever possible. Chemotherapy with cyclophosphamide (Cytoxan)[1], vincristine (Oncovin)[1], and dacarbazine (DTIC-Dome)[1], CVD, is the primary therapeutic modality in patients with rapidly progressive (within 3 to 6 months) PHEO. While only 30% of the metastatic PHEO population exhibits clinical benefit, the reported advantages in SDHB-related disease is as high as 80%. Temozolomide (TMZ [Temodar])[1] is the only other chemotherapeutic agent with significant experience in PHEO patients.

For patients with slow to moderate progression, eligibility for targeted radiolabeled therapy should be considered with ^{131}I-MIBG and peptide receptor radionuclide therapy (PRRT) if they have avid disease on ^{123}I-MIBG and ^{68}Ga-SSA, respectively. Currently, lutetium-177 DOTATATE (Lutathera) is not approved by the FDA for metastatic PHEO in the United States;

---

[1] Not FDA approved for this indication.

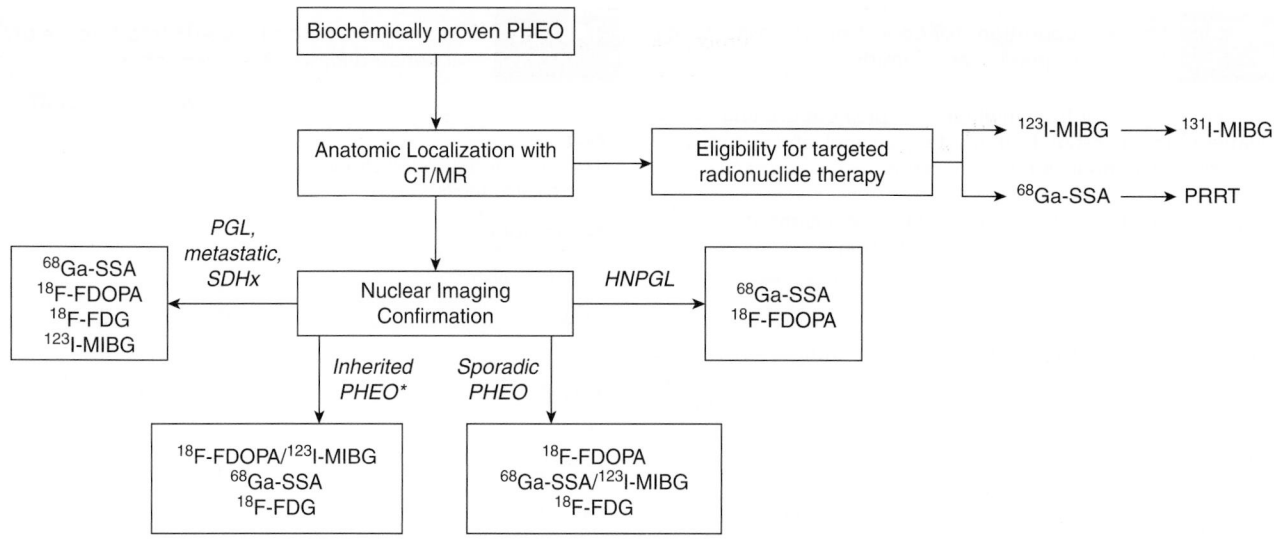

Figure 4 Imaging algorithm for pheochromocytoma localization. (Adopted from Taieb D, Hicks RJ, Hindie E, et al.: European Association of Nuclear Medicine Practice Guidelines/Society of Nuclear Medicine and Molecular Imaging Procedure Standard 2019 for Radionuclide Imaging of Pheochromocytoma and Paraganglioma. *Eur J Nucl Med Mol Imaging* 46(10):2112–2137, 2019; and Taieb D, Jha A, Treglia G, et al: Molecular imaging and radionuclide therapy of pheochromocytoma and paraganglioma in the era of genomic characterization of disease subgroups. *Endocr Relat Cancer.* 26[11]:R627–R6, 2019.)

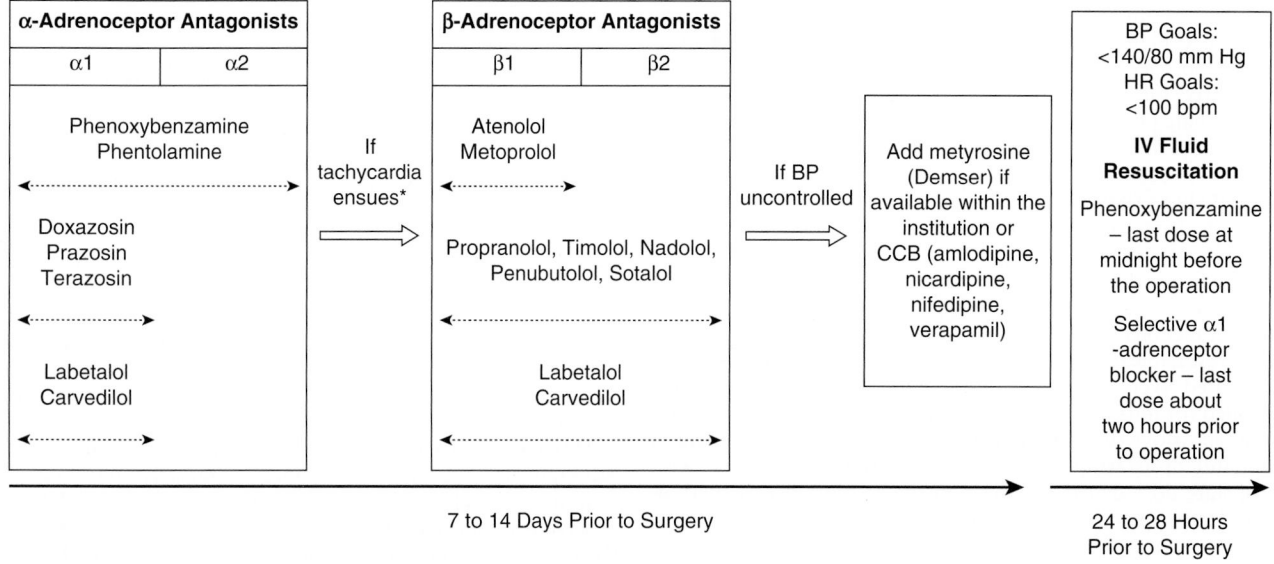

Figure 5 Preferred preoperative treatment regimen for pheochromocytoma. (Adapted from Wolf KI, Santos JRU, Pacak K: Why take the risk? We only live once: The dangers associated with neglecting a preoperative alpha adrenoceptor blockade in pheochromocytoma patients. *Endocr Pract.* 25[1]:106–108, 2019.)

however, international reports have shown success in neuroendocrine tumors, and clinical trials are ongoing.

There are several up-and-coming novel therapeutic agents that will hopefully be approved for treatment of metastatic PHEO after further validation, including HIF-2α, mTOR, and P13K inhibitors, as well as immunotherapy.

Prognosis and Monitoring

The long-term survival of patients after surgical excision of a benign, solitary PHEO is the same as age-adjusted normal subjects.

A longitudinal follow-up study determined that recurrences are more likely in patients with extra-adrenal PGLs and those with germline mutations. Following treatment, 25% of patients continue to have well-controlled hypertension on oral medications. Periodic, lifelong biochemical and/or imaging surveillance is required for all patients, but especially for those with an underlying hereditary disorder. Frequency of follow-up depends on the surgical pathology, presentation at diagnosis, and biochemical profile. Patients with metastatic disease should have routine, scheduled observation with a specialist to ensure proper care.

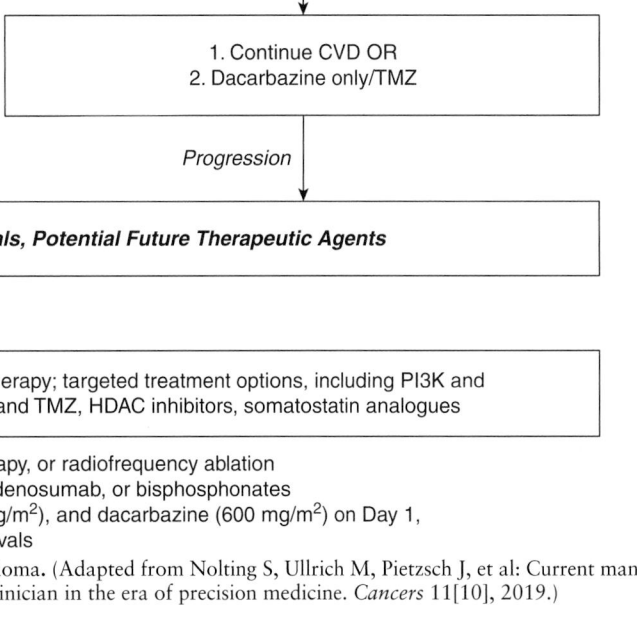

Pheochromocytoma

*Arterial embolization, chemoembolization, selective radiotherapy, or radiofrequency ablation

+ Consider conventional radiotherapy, cyberknife procedures, denosumab, or bisphosphonates

#Averbuch: cyclophosphamide (750 mg/m²), vincristine (1.4 mg/m²), and dacarbazine (600 mg/m²) on Day 1, followed by dacarbazine (600 mg/m²) on Day 2 at 21-day intervals

Figure 6 Treatment algorithm for metastatic pheochromocytoma/paraganglioma. (Adapted from Nolting S, Ullrich M, Pietzsch J, et al: Current management of pheochromocytoma/paraganglioma: A guide for the practicing clinician in the era of precision medicine. *Cancers* 11[10], 2019.)

References

Alrezk R, Suarez A, Tena I, Pacak K: Update of pheochromocytoma syndromes: genetics, biochemical evaluation, and imaging, *Front Endocrinol* 27(9):515, 2018.

Berends AMA, Buitenwerf E, de Krijger RR, et al: Incidence of pheochromocytoma and sympathetic paraganglioma in the Netherlands: a nationwide study and systematic review, *Eur J Intern Med* 51:68–73, 2018.

Bjorklund P, Pacak K, Crona J: Precision medicine in pheochromocytoma and paraganglioma: current and future concepts, *J Intern Med* 280(6):559–573, 2016.

Crona J, Lamarca A, Ghosal S, et al: Genotype-phenotype correlations in pheochromocytoma and paraganglioma: a systematic review and individual patient meta-analysis, *Endocr Related Cancer* 26(5):539–550, 2019.

Darr R, Kuhn M, Bode C, et al: Accuracy of recommended sampling and assay methods for the determination of plasma-free and urinary fractionated metanephrines in the diagnosis of pheochromocytoma and paraganglioma: a systematic review, *Endocrine* 56(3):495–503, 2017.

Dmitriev PM, Wang H, Rosenblum JS, et al: Vascular changes in the retina and choroid of patients with epas1 gain-of-function mutation syndrome, *JAMA Opthalmol*, 2019. Epub ahead of print.

Eisenhofer G, Goldstein DS, Walther MM, et al: Biochemical diagnosis of pheochromocytoma: how to distinguish true from false-positive test results, *J Clin Endocrinol Metab* 88(6):2656–2666, 2003.

Eisenhofer G, Lenders JW, Siegert G, et al: Plasma methoxytyramine: a novel biomarker of metastatic pheochromocytoma and paraganglioma in relation to established risk factors of tumour size, location and SDHB mutation status, *Eur J Cancer* 48(11):1739–1749, 2012.

Else T, Marvin ML, Everett JN, et al: The clinical phenotype of SDHC-associated hereditary paraganglioma syndrome (PGL3), *J Clin Endocrinol Metab* 99(8):E1482–E1486, 2014.

Gupta G, Pacak K: Precision medicine: an update on genotype/biochemical phenotype relationships in pheochromocytoma/paraganglioma patients, *Endoc Pract* 23(6):690–704, 2017.

Hamidi O, Young Jr WR, Iniguez-Ariza NM, et al: Malignant pheochromocytoma and paraganglioma: 272 patients over 55 years, *J Clin Endocrinol Metab* 102(9):3296–3305, 2017.

Hescot S, Curras-Freixas M, Deutschbein T, et al: Prognosis of malignant pheochromocytoma and paraganglioma (MAPP-Prono Study): a european network for the study of adrenal tumors retrospective study, *J Clin Endocrinol Metab* 104(6):2367–2374, 2019.

Jha A, de Luna K, Balili Ca, et al: Clinical, diagnostic, and treatment characteristics of *SDHA-related* metastatic pheochromocytoma and paraganglioma, *Front Oncol* 22(9):53, 2019.

Jochmanova I, Pacak K: Genomic landscape of pheochromocytoma and paraganglioma, *Trends Cancer* 4(1):6–9, 2018.

Jochmanova I, Wolf KI, King KS, et al: SDHB-related pheochromocytoma and paraganglioma penetrance and genotype-phenotype correlations, *J Cancer Res Clin Oncol* 143(8):1421–1435, 2017.

Karasek D, Shah U, Frysak Z, et al: An update on the genetics of pheochromocytoma, *J Hum Hypertens* 27(3):141–147, 2012. 2013.

Lahlou-Laforet K, Consoli SM, Jeunemaitre X, et al: Presymptomatic genetic testing in minors at risk of paraganglioma and pheochromocytoma: our experience of oncogenetic multidisciplinary consultation, *Horm Metab Res* 44:354–358, 2012.

Lenders JW, Duh QY, Eisenhofer G, et al: Pheochromocytoma and paraganglioma: an endocrine society clinical practice guideline, *J Clin Endocrinol Metab* 99(6):1915–1942, 2014.

Lenders JW, Eisenhofer G, Mannelli M, Pacak K: Phaeochromocytoma, *Lancet* 366(9486):665–675, 2005.

Mamilla D, Araque KA, Brofferio A, et al: Postoperative management in patients with pheochromocytoma and paraganglioma, *Cancers* 11(7), 2019.

Muth A, Crona J, Gimm O, et al: Genetic testing and surveillance guidelines in hereditary pheochromocytoma and paraganglioma, *J Intern Med* 285(2):187–204, 2019.

Neumann HP, Bausch B, McWhinney SR, et al: Germ-line mutations in nonsyndromic pheochromocytoma, *N Engl J Med* 346(19):1459–1466, 2002.

Nolting S, Ullrich M, Pierzsch J, et al: Current management of pheochromocytoma/paraganglioma: a guide for the practicing clinician in the era of precision medicine, *Cancers* 11(10), 2019.

Pacak K: Preoperative management of the pheochromocytoma patient, *J Clin Endocrinol Metab* 92(11):4069–4079, 2007.

Pacak K, Eisenhofer G, Carrasquillo JA, et al: Diagnostic localization of pheochromocytoma: the coming of age of positron emission tomography, *Ann N Y Acad Sci* 970:170–176, 2002.

Rao D, Peitzsch M, Prejbisz A, et al: Plasma methoxytyramine: clinical utility with metanephrines for diagnosis of pheochromocytoma and paraganglioma, *Eur J Endocrinol* 177(2):103–113, 2017.

Taieb D, Hicks RJ, Hindie E, et al: European association of nuclear medicine practice guideline/society of nuclear medicine and molecular imaging procedure standard 2019 for radionuclide imaging of pheochromocytoma and paraganglioma, *Eur J Nucl Mol Imaging* 46(10):2112–2137, 2019.

Taieb D, Jha A, Treglia G, Pacak K: Molecular imaging and radionuclide therapy of pheochromocytoma and paraganglioma in the era of genomic characterization of disease subgroups, *Endocr Related Cancer* 26(11):R627–R652, 2019.

Tella S, Jha A, Taieb D, et al. A Comprehensive Review of Evaluation and Management of Cardiac Paragangliomas. *Heart*. Submitted, in publication.

Toledo RA, Qin Y, Cheng ZM, et al: Recurrent mutations of chromatin-remodeling genes and kinase receptors in pheochromocytomas and paragangliomas, *Clin Cancer Res* 22(9):2301–2310, 2016.

van Hulsteijn LT, Dekkers OM, Hes FL, et al: Risk of malignant paraganglioma in SDHB-mutation and SDHD-mutation carriers: a systematic review and meta-analysis, *J Med Genet* 49(12):768–776, 2012.

Wolf KI, Santos JRU, Pacak K: Why take the risk? We only live once: the dangers associated with neglecting a pre-operative alpha adrenoceptor blockade in pheochromocytoma patients, *Endocr Pract* 25(1):106–108, 2019.

THYROID CANCER

Method of
Michael Holyoak, MD; and Rudruidee Karnchanasorn, MD

CURRENT DIAGNOSIS

- Most thyroid cancer will present as incidentally discovered thyroid nodules.
- The vast majority of thyroid nodules are benign and risk of malignancy can be reliably estimated based on sonographic features.
- Thyroid function should always be assessed if a nodule is discovered. If thyroid stimulating hormone (TSH) is low, a thyroid uptake and scan should be obtained.
- The American Thyroid Association (ATA) and the American College of Radiology's (ACR's) Thyroid Imaging Reporting and Data System (TIRADS) uses ultrasound features to determine risk of malignancy and the need for fine needle aspiration (FNA).
- Approximately 90%–95% of thyroid nodules are benign and can be monitored with serial ultrasound. FNA is only indicated for nodules equal to or greater than 1 cm.
- Benign nodules can be monitored with ultrasound at intervals based on their risk of malignancy.
- The vast majority of thyroid cancer is classified as differentiated thyroid cancer (DTC). Medullary thyroid cancer (MTC) is less common and somewhat more aggressive. Anaplastic thyroid cancer (ATC) is a rare and very aggressive thyroid cancer that typically presents at a more advanced stage.

CURRENT THERAPY

- Although thyroid cancer is relatively common, it is responsible for a very small portion of cancer-related mortality.
- Some experts have expressed concern about potentially unnecessary morbidity associated with overtreatment of very low risk DTCs, particularly micropapillary carcinoma.
- Most patients with thyroid cancer should be managed surgically. Smaller, lower-risk differentiated cancers can be treated with lobectomy. Larger or higher-risk tumors should be treated with total thyroidectomy and compartment neck dissections based on the presence of lymphadenopathy.
- Radioactive iodine (RAI) should be utilized based on the ATA risk stratification.
- Patients with DTC should be monitored longitudinally using serum thyroglobulin (Tg) levels and serial ultrasound.
- TSH suppression is indicated for many patients postoperatively, initially based on their ATA risk and later on their response to therapy.
- Patients with MTC should undergo surgery and be monitored with serial carcinoembryonic antigen (CEA) and calcitonin levels in addition to imaging studies.
- Patients with ATC typically require aggressive surgery, often including tracheostomy and management by a multidisciplinary team.

Epidemiology

Thyroid nodules are highly prevalent. Data show that approximately 5% to 10% of patients will have palpable nodules and approximately 34% of patients will have nodules detectable by ultrasound. The prevalence of nodules increases significantly with age, and they are three to four times more common in women. Only a small portion of thyroid nodules are malignant, about 5% to 15%. In 2015, it was estimated that at least 62,000 cases of thyroid cancer were diagnosed in the United States, making it the most common form of endocrine cancer. The incidence of thyroid cancer has been increasing steadily for the past several decades. This is likely attributable to the increased utilization and sensitivity of diagnostic imaging. It is important to note that the climbing thyroid cancer incidence has not been accompanied by an increase in thyroid cancer deaths. Low-risk differentiated thyroid cancers (DTCs) such as micropapillary carcinomas are responsible for a large proportion of newly diagnosed thyroid cancers. There is significant concern that many individuals with low-risk DTCs may receive treatment associated with unnecessary risk and morbidity. Papillary thyroid carcinomas (PTCs) are particularly slow-growing cancers. In one study involving patients with low-risk DTCs who were monitored without surgery, only 10% were found to have disease progression at a median follow-up interval of 6 years.

Risk Factors

The majority of thyroid cancer cannot be attributed to specific risk factors. Nutritional factors including iodine intake have been associated with an increased risk of thyroid nodularity. Childhood exposure to ionizing radiation is one particularly well-documented risk factor for thyroid cancer. In a large retrospective study, individuals treated with radiation for Hodgkin disease, were 27 times more likely to have thyroid nodules than those treated without radiation. An elevated thyroid stimulating hormone (TSH) level in the setting of thyroid nodularity has been associated with an increased risk of thyroid cancer. Cigarette smoking has actually been negatively correlated with risk of thyroid cancer.

Pathophysiology

DTCs are derived from follicular cells and are responsible for more than 95% of cases of thyroid cancer (Table 1). DTC includes PTC and follicular thyroid carcinoma (FTC) as well as the follicular

TABLE 1	Overview of Thyroid Tumor Subtypes				
SUBTYPE	**ORIGIN CELL TYPE**	**% OF THYROID CANCER**	**5-YEAR SURVIVAL**	**COMMON MUTATIONS**
PTC	Follicular	~80%	~99%	*BRAF, TKR*
FTC	Follicular	~15%	~98%	*RAS, PAX8-PPARG*
NIFTP	Follicular	0.4%–2.6%	N/A	*RAS*
PDTC	Follicular	~1%	~62%	*RAS, P53*
MTC	Parafollicular/C-cell	~3%	~90%	*RET*
ATC	Follicular	~1%	~7%	*BRAF, TERT, P53*

ATC, Anaplastic thyroid cancer; *MTC*, medullary thyroid cancer; *NIFTP*, neoplasm with papillary-like nuclear features; *PDTC*, poorly differentiated thyroid carcinomas.

variants including Hurthle cell cancer. Another related variant of thyroid tumor termed noninvasive follicular thyroid neoplasm with papillary-like nuclear features (NIFTP) has an exceptionally low recurrence rate of less than 1% at 15 years. NIFTP is best described as a benign tumor and does not require completion thyroidectomy or radioactive iodine (RAI). PTC metastasizes via the lymphatic system, typically to cervical lymph nodes. FTC and its variants classically spread hematogenously, which contributes to a less favorable prognosis. The *BRAF* mutation is the most frequently encountered mutation in non-medullary thyroid cancer (MTC) and is present in 50% to 70% of patients with PTC. *TERT* mutations are frequently present in high-risk forms of PTC. Mutations in the *RAS* family of oncogenes are also commonly present in FTC.

Poorly differentiated thyroid carcinomas (PDTC) are high-risk cancers that classically spread hematogenously to lung and bone. These cancers are also derived from follicular cells.

MTC originates from parafollicular or calcitonin-producing C cells. Mutations of the *RET* proto-oncogene are thought to be responsible for the majority of cases. *RET* mutations are classically inherited in an autosomal dominant pattern; however, they can occur sporadically. All patients diagnosed with MTC should be screened for *RET* mutations. If such testing is positive, first-degree relatives should be screened as well. Specific *RET* mutations result in specific phenotypes with varying risks of MTC. Knowledge of the specific *RET* mutation guides the need and timing of prophylactic thyroidectomy; this is of particular importance in the pediatric setting. MTC is part of the classic presentation of patients with multiple endocrine neoplasia type 2 (MEN 2), which also includes a risk of pheochromocytoma and parathyroid adenomas.

Anaplastic thyroid cancer (ATC) is an uncommon (<1%) but aggressive form of cancer. Despite its rarity, ATC is responsible for as much as 50% of thyroid cancer–related mortality. Patients usually present with advanced disease, commonly with symptoms of hoarseness or dysphasia due to local invasion. Approximately 50% of ATCs arise from a known DTC, with the hypothesis of dedifferentiation changes from preexisting DTC to aggressive ATC.

Clinical Manifestations

Most patients with thyroid cancer, particularly with DTCs, present asymptomatically with incidentally discovered thyroid nodularity on imaging. More aggressive forms of thyroid cancer, including poorly differentiated cancers and ATC, can present with symptoms related to regional invasion, including dysphasia, hoarseness-related recurrent laryngeal nerve injury, and tracheal compression.

Diagnosis

All patients suspected of having thyroid nodules should undergo ultrasound and measurement of serum their TSH levels. A TSH below normal should prompt a scintigraphic evaluation with thyroid uptake and scan to assess for functioning or "hot" nodules. Fine needle aspiration (FNA) is not generally indicated for hyperfunctioning nodules due to a low likelihood of malignancy. Thyroid scintigraphy is not needed when serum TSH is normal or elevated. Serum calcitonin measurement used as a screening test for MTC remains controversial due to its low specificity.

Ultrasound is a critical step in evaluating thyroid nodules. It is not only safe and cost effective but also reliably determines risk of malignancy and therefore need for FNA. Suspicious sonographic features of nodules associated with increased risk of malignancy include hypoechogenicity (darker than normal thyroid parenchyma), microcalcifications that are taller than wide on transverse view, and irregular or infiltrative nodule margins. Ultrasound of the central and lateral neck compartments is critical to screen for suspicious lymphadenopathy, which can influence the surgical approach. The American Thyroid Association (ATA) recommends FNA utilizing a risk stratification system based on size and sonographic patterns. FNA is recommended for nodules equal to or greater than 1 cm with intermediate (10% to 20% malignancy risk) or high suspicion patterns (>70% to 90% risk), 1.5 cm for low suspicion (5% to 10% risk) and 2 cm for very low suspicion (<3%). Purely cystic nodules are benign and do not need FNA.

The Thyroid Imaging Reporting and Data System (TIRADS) is another validated clinical tool produced by the American College of Radiology (ACR). It uses a points system based on sonographic features to stratify nodules into one of five TIRADS categories: TR1, benign; TR2, not suspicious; TR3, mildly suspicious; TR4, moderately suspicious; and TR5, highly suspicious, with malignancy risks of 0.3%, 1.5%, 4.8%, 9.1%, and 35%, respectively. TR1 and TR2 nodules do not require FNA. FNA is indicated for TR3 nodules starting at 2.5 cm, TR4 at 1.5 cm, and TR5 at 1 cm. Nodules less than 1 cm are too small for FNA based on both the ATA and ACR-TIRADS owing to the slow-growing nature of micropapillary thyroid cancer. Other considerations governing the need for FNA include specific risk factors of thyroid cancer or syndromes associated with thyroid cancer, such as MEN, Cowden syndrome, familial adenomatous polyposis, and Carney complex. In addition, fluorodeoxyglucose-avid nodules are associated with a malignancy rate of about 35%. However, the recommended FNA size of these nodules remains at least 1 cm or greater.

The 2017 Bethesda system has been the standard method of cytology diagnosis of thyroid nodules, consisting of six categories. Category I, nondiagnostic (ND) or unsatisfactory, represents a 5% to 10% malignancy risk; in such cases repeat FNA is required unless the lesion is mostly cystic or ultrasound features of very low suspicion. Category II, benign, represents approximately 70% of specimens and a less than 3% risk of malignancy. Both category III, atypia of undetermined significance/follicular lesion of undetermined significance (AUS/FLUS), and category IV, follicular neoplasm or suspicious for follicular neoplasm (FN/SFN), are associated with a slightly higher malignancy risk, 10% to 30% in AUS/FLUS and 25% to 40% in FN/SFN. The management of both categories III and IV is not straightforward, and various molecular assessments can be utilized to help with decision making. Currently available molecular tests—including the Afirma GSC, RNA seq panel, and ThyroSeq3 112-gene panel—have high sensitivity and specificity, functioning as rule-out and rule-in tests to decrease the number of unnecessary thyroid surgeries. Category V (suspicious for malignancy [SFN]) and category VI (malignant), carry high rates of malignancy (60% to 75% and 97% to 99%, respectively) and should prompt referral for operative management.

Nodules that do not meet the initial threshold for cytologic assessment require continued sonographic surveillance, the recommended interval of which ranges from 6 to 24 months based on sonographic features. FNA should be performed if there is a 50% increase in the tumor volume calculated with three-dimensional measurement or once nodules reach the threshold size. A nodule with two negative biopsies should be considered benign.

Therapy

Papillary thyroid microcarcinoma (PTMC) is defined as a small PTC equal to or less than 10 mm in size. PTMCs generally grow very slowly and carry an excellent prognosis. Although many individuals are asymptomatic and do not require treatment, an increased rate of detection has likely resulted in overtreatment. It has been shown that PTMCs in young patients are more likely to progress more than those in elderly patients. Active surveillance for most PTMCs has been shown to be safe, and FNA is not recommended for thyroid nodules smaller than 1 cm. Active surveillance should not be considered in the presence of high-risk features such as nodal metastasis or distant metastasis, vocal cord paralysis due to invasion of the recurrent laryngeal nerve, high-grade malignancy on cytology, or in the case of PTMCs attached to the trachea or located along the path of the recurrent laryngeal nerve. Ultrasound-guided percutaneous ethanol ablation (UPEA) by experienced specialists has been shown to be a safe and well-tolerated definitive minimally invasive alternative for PTMC patients who do not wish to have surgery and are uncomfortable with active surveillance, although UPEA is currently available at only a limited number of centers.

Treatment of thyroid cancer is mainly based on individualized risk stratification, accounting for both mortality based on TNM (tumor, node, and metastases) staging, the risk of disease recurrence, and the persistence of structural disease.

Although DTC carries a very low risk of mortality as compared with other cancers, the TNM staging system remains an accurate predictor of mortality. Recent changes to the system recommend that patients younger than 55 years of age at the time of diagnosis receive only stage 1 (no distant metastases) or stage II (distant metastases present) classification. Ten-year disease-specific survival rates for stages I to IV were 99.5%, 94.7%, 94.1%, and 67.6%, respectively.

In addition to TNM staging, an individualized risk stratification outlined by the ATA 2015 guidelines is an important milestone for the assessment of risk of thyroid cancer recurrence and persistence of structural disease. The ATA system utilizes variables such as histology, extent of the first surgery, and postoperative thyroglobulin (Tg) to guide initial postoperative therapy and treatment in follow-up. Patients with tumor sizes less than 4 cm without clinical lymph node metastases or micrometastases measuring less than 2 mm in five or fewer lymph nodes can be classified as ATA low risk. Intermediate-risk disease is defined as DTC with minimal extrathyroidal extension or aggressive histology. High-risk disease includes patients with gross extension, distant metastases, any lymph node metastases greater than 3 cm, as well as FTC with greater than 4 foci of vascular invasion. In contrast, minimally invasive FTC is considered low risk.

The ATA recommends either total thyroidectomy or lobectomy for low-risk patients with DTC. The decision to proceed with total thyroidectomy or lobectomy primarily depends on tumor size and patient preference. Low-risk patients are not routinely treated with RAI.

Use of RAI is based on individualized risk stratification accounting for extent of tumor, histology type, age, and presence of distant metastases. Radioiodine is typically delayed several months after surgery to allow for complete recovery and assessment of the biochemical response with Tg. Serum Tg reaches its nadir approximately 4 to 6 weeks postoperatively, and measurement at this point is perhaps the most accurate method of appraising the quality of surgery and probability of cure.

RAI remnant ablation uses a low dose of radioiodine-131 (131-I), around 30 mCi, to destroy any residual thyroid tissue postoperatively. Remnant ablation thus facilitates the interpretation of subsequent serum Tg levels and follow-up RAI whole-body scans to detect any residual or recurrence disease or metastatic foci. Remnant ablation is not routinely recommended in ATA low-risk DTC patients.

Adjuvant treatment utilizes a higher dose of 131-I (75 to 150 mCi) postoperatively to destroy microscopic thyroid cancer and/or suspected residual disease to potentially decrease recurrence and mortality. RAI adjuvant treatment should be considered in ATA intermediate-risk DTC patients.

Primary treatment with RAI uses 100 to 200 mCi of 131-I to destroy known locoregional and/or distant metastasis with a goal of cure, reduced recurrence and mortality, and/or palliation among high-risk DTC patients.

Serum TSH should be elevated prior to proceeding with RAI, as TSH potentiates RAI uptake by iodine-avid tissues including normal thyroid tissue and most thyroid cancers. This has historically been accomplished by withdrawing thyroid hormone replacement for approximately 2 weeks until TSH increases to 30 or more. During this time patients should be instructed to consume a low-iodine diet. The use of recombinant human TSH (Thyrogen) is also a safe and effective alternative to thyroid hormone withdrawal in the detection of recurrent/residual thyroid cancer and facilitation of RAI ablation.

Localized treatments with external beam radiation are sometimes needed for gross residual disease or bone metastases. Surgery may be necessary when bone metastases threaten a limb's function.

Systemic treatments for advanced DTC and MTC include tyrosine kinase inhibitors (TKIs). These agents are reserved for patients with progressive or unresectable disease or tumor that is threatening vital structures. TKI-associated adverse effects are common and include hypertension, hand-foot skin reactions, diarrhea, rash, fatigue, and weight loss. The dose of TKI often needs to be titrated based on tolerability.

Most patients with MTC have advanced disease at the time of diagnosis, leading to an unfavorable prognosis. Cure is much more probable if all disease is intrathyroidal at the time of diagnosis. Early identification and complete surgical resection are ideal for the definite treatment of MTC. Calcitonin is a specific serum marker and its doubling time is the most important prognostic factor for survival and disease progression. Serum carcinoembryonic antigen (CEA) is usually elevated in advanced cases and is often used as a tumor marker in conjunction with calcitonin. The risk of recurrence is low when postoperative calcitonin is undetectable. Patients with low but detectable calcitonin level less than 150 pg/mL likely have persistent or recurrent disease confined to neck lymph nodes and can be followed every 6 to 12 months with physical examination, neck ultrasound, and serial measurement of calcitonin and CEA. If postoperative calcitonin is greater than 150 pg or has a rapid doubling time, additional imaging studies are required to evaluate for distant metastases. If there is concern for disease progression, systemic therapy with vandetanib (Caprelsa) or cabozantinib (Cometriq) should be considered. Before starting this, the possibility of using a local treatment should be evaluated to delay systemic therapy, along with a multidisciplinary team approach.

Patients with ATC usually present with a rapidly enlarging neck mass that can cause compressive neck symptoms and invasion of the adjacent recurrent laryngeal nerve, leading to dysphonia, or compression of the trachea, causing airway obstruction. Ultrasound remains the primary imaging study for ATC, but additional studies including computed tomography (CT) with contrast of neck, abdomen, and pelvis; positron emission tomography CT (PET-CT) if available, and brain magnetic resonance imaging (MRI) can be used. Due to the risk of acute airway compromise, an expeditious diagnosis and management plan by a multidisciplinary team is crucial. Ideally a care team would include a pathologist, head and neck surgeon, medical oncologist, radiation oncologist, and endocrinologist. A palliative care physician should also be involved, given ATC's extremely poor prognosis. Patients with ATC and their families should take part in an in-depth discussion about the natural history of the disease, goals of treatment, treatment toxicities, and expected outcomes. Most untreated patients will die of asphyxiation; therefore treatment addressing the primary neck disease, even with a goal of only palliation, is a priority. Hospice care could be the best option for patients who do not wish to pursue aggressive therapy. Tracheostomy to prevent airway obstruction as a part of palliative care is controversial but may be appropriate for patients with impending airway compromise. In contrast, patients with limited disease should initially be treated with surgery followed by chemoradiotherapy (intensity-modulated radiotherapy [IMRT] plus taxane-based chemotherapy) as a standard of care when feasible, unless hospice is alternatively elected. Patients with widely metastatic or stage IVC disease should instead be treated with palliative systemic therapy or best supportive care.

Recent studies have indicated improvements in overall survival in early multimodality therapy, especially with recent advancements in systemic therapy including targeted and immunotherapies such as the *BRAF* inhibitor dabrafenib (Tafinlar) and the *MEK* inhibitor trametinib (Mekinist), anti-PD1 monoclonal antibody spartalizumab,[5] and newer agents such as the peroxisome proliferator-activated receptor (PPAR)-γ agonist efatutazone,[5] and mammalian target of rapamycin (mTOR) inhibitors, which seem to provide a more efficacious treatment in advanced ATC.

Monitoring

Regardless of the initial risk assessment, patients with DTC should be monitored longitudinally and classified as having either an excellent, indeterminate, or incomplete response, both biochemically and structurally, to therapy. An excellent response (1% to 4% recurrence rate) is defined as no clinical, biochemical, or structural evidence of disease. Serum Tg should be less than 0.2 ng/mL with a suppressed TSH, or less than 1 ng/mL if TSH is stimulated. Patients with an indeterminate response (15% to 20% recurrence rate) will have nonspecific biochemical or structural findings. A biochemical incomplete response (20% recurrence rate) reflects abnormally elevated Tg or Tg antibody levels (Serum Tg >1 ng/mL basal or >10 ng/mL if TSH is stimulated or increasing Tg antibodies) in the absence of disease. A structural incomplete response (50% to 85% recurrence rate) includes persistent or newly identified locoregional or distant metastasis with or without abnormal Tg or Tg antibodies.

TSH suppression therapy (TST) requires supraphysiologic doses of exogenous thyroid hormone, with the goal of lowering serum TSH. TSH has trophic effects on thyroid tissue, and a subnormal serum TSH may minimize tumor growth and reduce the risk of progression of advanced thyroid cancer. Aggressive TST is not recommended for low-risk patients but may improve survival outcome for those at high risk. Serum TSH levels that were consistently maintained in the subnormal to normal ranges have led to better outcomes in patients at all stages of disease compared with subjects whose serum TSH levels were in the normal to elevated ranges.

Management of Complications

Immediate surgical complications following thyroidectomy are adversely correlated with low-volume surgeons. High-volume surgeons are also associated with an increased risk of postoperative complications; however, this is likely attributable to overall greater case complexity. Potential complications include injury of the recurrent laryngeal nerve leading to temporary or permanent hoarseness, airway difficulty due to bilateral vocal cord paralysis, and need for tracheostomy. Total thyroidectomy can lead to transient or permanent hypoparathyroidism with resultant hypocalcemia. Adequate preoperative vitamin D replacement can help to maintain normocalcemia. Postoperatively the parathyroid hormone (PTH) level should be checked; calcitriol (Rocaltrol) may be needed in addition to calcium supplementation if the PTH level is low or undetectable. Serial calcium levels should be obtained following discharge.

---

[5]Investigational drug in the United States.

Long-term TST can result in adverse outcomes such as osteoporosis, fracture, and cardiovascular disease, including atrial fibrillation. In general, daily levothyroxine (Levoxyl, Synthroid) doses of 1.6 to 1.8 µg/kg are the initial treatment following thyroidectomy, whereas doses of 2.0 to 2.2 µg/kg are needed to suppress the serum TSH. The dosage requirements of individual patients are highly variable and depend on multiple factors, including body mass index, the concomitant use of other medications, and patient adherence. The ATA recommends maintaining serum TSH levels between 0.5 and 2 mU/L in low-risk and intermediate-risk patients with an excellent response to treatment. Mild TSH suppression (TSH 0.1 to 0.5 mU/L) should be used for high-risk patients who have had an excellent response (negative imaging and undetectable suppressed Tg). Mild TSH suppression is also recommended in patients with a biochemically incomplete response. More significant TSH suppression (i.e., serum TSH <0.1) is recommended in patients with residual structural disease or a biochemically incomplete response if they are young or at low risk for complications from iatrogenic hyperthyroidism.

Adverse effects of RAI—including radiation thyroiditis, sialadenitis, and tumor hemorrhage or edema—occur in 10% to 30% of patients. The possibility of adverse effects is dose dependent. Long-term risk of secondary malignancies has been reported; however, the risk is considerably lower when the total dose is less than 100 mCi. Immediately after patients have been treated with RAI, an appropriate isolation protocol is required to protect household members from radiation exposure, especially women who are pregnant as well as infants. The required duration of isolation is predominantly based on RAI dose and rate of clearance.

Conclusion

Thyroid nodules are very common and are often discovered incidentally. The vast majority of nodules, approximately 90% to 95%, are benign. Thyroid sonography should be obtained for all nodules, as this reliably predicts the risk of malignancy and need for FNA. DTCs are indolent; FNA is not indicated for nodules less than 1 cm in size. Thyroid function should be assessed prior to proceeding with FNA. Patients with a TSH below normal should undergo thyroid uptake and scan to investigate for an autonomously functioning nodule or nodules. Most nodules can be monitored with ultrasound alone. Guidelines produced by either the ATA or ACR can reliably determine the need for FNA. PTC is the most common type of DTC and typically has a very favorable prognosis. Lower-risk patients with DTC can be managed with lobectomy. Patients with larger tumors (>4 cm), extrathyroidal extension, or higher-risk cytology should be treated with total thyroidectomy and central neck dissection. Lateral compartment neck dissections should be completed if there is FNA-positive disease.

Low-risk patients with DTC do not need treatment with RAI, whereas intermediate- and high- risk cases should receive RAI. All patients should be monitored longitudinally after initial therapy, both radiographically and biochemically, utilizing serum Tg. The ATA categorizes patient response as excellent, indeterminate, or incomplete. Patients should receive appropriate levels of TSH suppression, initially based on their ATA risk and subsequently on their response to therapy. TSH suppression poses multiple risks if continued long-term.

MTC should be considered of higher risk than DTC and is managed surgically. MTC is often detected later and is usually more advanced than DTC. Calcitonin and CEA levels can be monitored longitudinally. Calcitonin doubling time is a particularly important prognostic factor for following these patients.

ATC is a rare but extraordinarily aggressive and rapidly growing form of thyroid cancer. Patients should be managed by a multidisciplinary team with consideration for tracheostomy due to risk of asphyxiation in the setting of rapid tumor growth. Aggressive resection as well as prompt chemotherapy are appropriate treatment options in appropriately selected patients with less advanced disease.

References

Biondi B, Cooper DS: Thyroid hormone suppression therapy, *Endocrinol Metab Clin North Am* 48(1):227–237, 2019, https://doi.org/10.1016/j.ecl.2018.10.008.

Brito JP, Hay ID: Management of papillary thyroid microcarcinoma, *Endocrinol Metab Clin North Am* 48(1):199–213, 2019, https://doi.org/10.1016/j.ecl.2018.10.006.

Cabanillas Maria E, David G: Mcfadden, and cosimo durante. "Thyroid cancer, *The Lancet* 388(10061):2783–2795, 2016. Print.

Chintakuntlawar AV, Foote RL, Kasperbauer JL, Bible KC: Diagnosis and management of anaplastic thyroid cancer, *Endocrinol Metab Clin North Am* 48(1):269–284, 2019, https://doi.org/10.1016/j.ecl.2018.10.010.

Cho A, Chang Y, Ahn J, Shin H, Ryu S: Cigarette smoking and thyroid cancer risk: a cohort study, *British journal of cancer* 119(5):638–645, 2018, https://doi.org/10.1038/s41416-018-0224-5.

Du L, Wang Y, Sun X, Li H, Geng X, Ge M, Zhu Y: Thyroid cancer: trends in incidence, mortality and clinical-pathological patterns in Zhejiang Province, Southeast China, *BMC cancer* 18(1):291, 2018, https://doi.org/10.1186/s12885-018-4081-7.

Haugen BR, Alexander EK, Bible KC, Doherty GM, Mandel SJ, Nikiforov YE, Wartofsky L: 2015 American Thyroid Association management guidelines for adult patients with thyroid nodules and differentiated thyroid cancer: the American Thyroid Association guidelines task force on thyroid nodules and differentiated thyroid cancer, *Thyroid: official journal of the American Thyroid Association* 26(1):1–133, 2016, https://doi.org/10.1089/thy.2015.0020.

Maxwell C, Sipos JA: Clinical diagnostic evaluation of thyroid nodules, *Endocrinol Metab Clin North Am* 48(1):61–84, 2019.

Mayson SE, Haugen BR: Molecular diagnostic evaluation of thyroid nodules, *Endocrinol Metab Clin North Am* 48(1):85–97, 2019, https://doi.org/10.1016/j.ecl.2018.10.004.

Miyauchi A, Ito Y: Conservative surveillance management of low-risk papillary thyroid microcarcinoma, *Endocrinol Metab Clin North Am* 48(1):215–226, 2019, https://doi.org/10.1016/j.ecl.2018.10.007.

Nikiforov YE, et al: Nomenclature revision for encapsulated follicular variant of papillary thyroid carcinoma: a paradigm shift to reduce overtreatment of indolent tumors, *JAMA Oncol* 2(8):10–1029, 2016.

Viola D, Elisei R: Management of medullary thyroid cancer, *Endocrinol Metab Clin North Am* 48(1):285–301, 2019, https://doi.org/10.1016/j.ecl.2018.11.006.

Xing M: Genetic-guided risk assessment and management of thyroid cancer, *Endocrinol Metab Clin North Am* 48(1):109–124, 2019, https://doi.org/10.1016/j.ecl.2018.11.007.

THYROIDITIS

Method of
Leigh M. Eck, MD

CURRENT DIAGNOSIS

- Thyroiditis is a term used to describe a diverse group of disorders associated with thyroid inflammation.
- Thyroiditis can be associated with a euthyroid state, thyrotoxicosis, or hypothyroidism.
- The clinical presentation of thyroiditis will direct the evaluation with useful testing to include measurement of thyroid hormone levels, thyroid antibody testing, white blood cell count, erythrocyte sedimentation rate, thyroid scintigraphy, and thyroid ultrasound.

CURRENT THERAPY

- Abnormalities of thyroid hormone levels resulting from thyroiditis may be transient and require no or only short-term therapy.
- If symptomatic thyrotoxicosis is present, beta-blocker therapy should be initiated.
- Thyroiditis associated with persistent hypothyroidism is managed with synthetic thyroxine (T4, Levoxyl, Synthroid).
- Thyroid pain associated with subacute thyroiditis is managed with a nonsteroidal antiinflammatory drug or, if ineffective, glucocorticoid therapy.
- Acute suppurative thyroiditis requires immediate parenteral antibiotic therapy as well as surgical drainage, if indicated.

Thyroiditis is a term used to describe a diverse group of disorders characterized by inflammation of the thyroid gland (Table 1). Presentation of thyroiditis is variable depending on the etiology. The most common thyroid disorder in the United States, Hashimoto's thyroiditis, most often presents with hypothyroidism. Other forms of thyroiditis may present with thyrotoxicosis because of inflammation in the thyroid gland resulting in the release of stored hormone. Painful thyroiditis is seen with subacute, suppurative and radiation-induced thyroiditis, while other variants are most often painless.

Epidemiology

The most common cause of hypothyroidism in iodine-sufficient areas of the world is *Hashimoto's thyroiditis,* also known as *chronic autoimmune thyroiditis.* Elevated serum antithyroid peroxidase antibody concentrations are found in ~ 5% of adults and ~ 15% of older women; overt hypothyroidism is seen in up to 2% of the population. A variant of chronic autoimmune thyroiditis, *postpartum thyroiditis,* is a destructive thyroiditis induced by an autoimmune mechanism that occurs within 1 year of parturition. Postpartum thyroiditis occurs in up to 10% of women in the United States. *Silent thyroiditis* is indistinguishable from postpartum thyroiditis, with the exception of lack of temporal relationship to pregnancy. Silent thyroiditis may account for about 1% of all cases of thyrotoxicosis. Many medications are associated with an alteration in thyroid function testing; however, only a few are known to provoke an autoimmune or destructive inflammatory thyroiditis, including amiodarone (Cordarone), lithium, interferon alfa, interleukin-2, tyrosine kinase inhibitors, and checkpoint inhibitor immunotherapy. *Riedel's thyroiditis* is a progressive fibrosis of the thyroid gland with a prevalence of only 0.05% among patients with thyroid disease requiring surgery. *Subacute thyroiditis* is the most common cause of thyroid pain. It occurs in up to 5% of patients with clinical thyroid disease. *Suppurative thyroiditis,* most commonly caused by bacterial infection, is rare because of the thyroid gland's encapsulation, high iodine content, rich blood supply, and extensive lymphatic drainage. *Radiation-induced thyroiditis* occurs in approximately 1% of patients who receive radioactive iodine therapy for hyperthyroidism.

Risk Factors

Hashimoto's thyroiditis is more common in women, particularly older women. Hashimoto's thyroiditis is associated with several gene polymorphisms, suggesting a role for genetic susceptibility. Subacute thyroiditis frequently follows an upper respiratory tract infection, with its incidence highest in summer. Suppurative thyroiditis is most likely to occur in patients with preexisting thyroid disease, those with congenital anomalies such as pyriform sinus fistula, and those who are immunosuppressed.

Pathophysiology

Hashimoto's thyroiditis, postpartum thyroiditis, and silent thyroiditis all have an autoimmune basis. The antithyroid immune response begins with activation of thyroid antigen-specific helper T cells. Once helper T cells are activated, they induce B cells to secrete thyroid antibodies; thyroid antibodies most frequently measured are those

TABLE 1	Causes of Thyroiditis
Autoimmune thyroiditis: Hashimoto's thyroiditis, postpartum thyroiditis, silent thyroiditis	
Subacute thyroiditis, also known as de Quervain's thyroiditis or subacute granulomatous thyroiditis	
Suppurative thyroiditis, also known as infectious thyroiditis or pyrogenic thyroiditis	
Riedel's thyroiditis, also known as fibrous thyroiditis	
Therapy induced thyroiditis: amiodarone (Cordarone), interferon-alpha, interleukin-2, lithium, tyrosine kinase inhibitors, radioactive iodine, checkpoint inhibitor immunotherapy	

directed against thyroid peroxidase and against thyroglobulin. The mechanism for autoimmune destruction of the thyroid likely involves both cellular immunity and humoral immunity. Riedel's thyroiditis is the local involvement of the thyroid in a systemic disease, multifocal fibrosclerosis; the etiology of Riedel's thyroiditis is not known. Although a viral cause of subacute thyroiditis has been proposed, clear evidence for this proposed etiology is lacking. Suppurative thyroiditis is most often associated with a bacterial pathogen; however, fungal, mycobacterial, or parasitic infections may also be the cause. Although rare, radiation-induced thyroiditis may occur following the treatment of hyperthyroidism with radioactive iodine because of radiation-induced injury and necrosis of thyroid follicular cells and associated inflammation.

Clinical Manifestations

A symmetrical, painless goiter is frequently the initial finding in Hashimoto's thyroiditis. The usual course of Hashimoto's thyroiditis is gradual loss of thyroid function. Among patients with this disorder who have subclinical hypothyroidism, overt hypothyroidism occurs at a rate of about 5% per year. The classic presentation of postpartum thyroiditis occurs in only approximately 30% of afflicted women, with the characteristic sequence of hyperthyroidism, followed by hypothyroidism, and then recovery. Persistent hypothyroidism is seen in up to 30% of women following an episode of postpartum thyroiditis. Silent thyroiditis is marked by a similar characteristic sequence of thyroid hormone dysfunction. However, it

is not temporally associated with pregnancy; 20% will have residual hypothyroidism. *Medication-induced thyroiditis* is variable in its presentation. Amiodarone (Cordarone), rich in iodine, is associated with hypothyroidism and hyperthyroidism; type 2 amiodarone-induced thyrotoxicosis is due to a destructive thyroiditis process. Lithium is more commonly associated with hypothyroidism. Interferon-alfa and interleukin-2 can cause both permanent and transient hypothyroidism likely related to the ability of these substances to induce or exacerbate thyroid autoimmune disease. Riedel's thyroiditis presents with neck discomfort or tightness, dysphagia, hoarseness, and a diffuse goiter that is hard, fixed, and often not clearly separable from the adjacent tissues. Generally, patients are euthyroid, and their antithyroid antibody concentrations are often high. Subacute thyroiditis manifests with a prodrome of myalgias, pharyngitis, low-grade fever, and fatigue with subsequent fever and neck pain, and up to 50% of patients have symptoms of thyrotoxicosis. Patients with suppurative thyroiditis are usually acutely ill with fever, dysphagia, dysphonia, anterior neck pain with erythema, and a tender thyroid mass. Radiation-induced thyroiditis presents 5 to 10 days following radioactive iodine treatment with neck pain and tenderness. In addition, there can be a transient exacerbation of hyperthyroidism.

Diagnosis and Differential Diagnosis

The diagnostic approach to suspected thyroiditis can be focused based on an association with thyroid pain and circulating thyroid hormone status (Figure 1). Hashimoto's thyroiditis is diagnosed

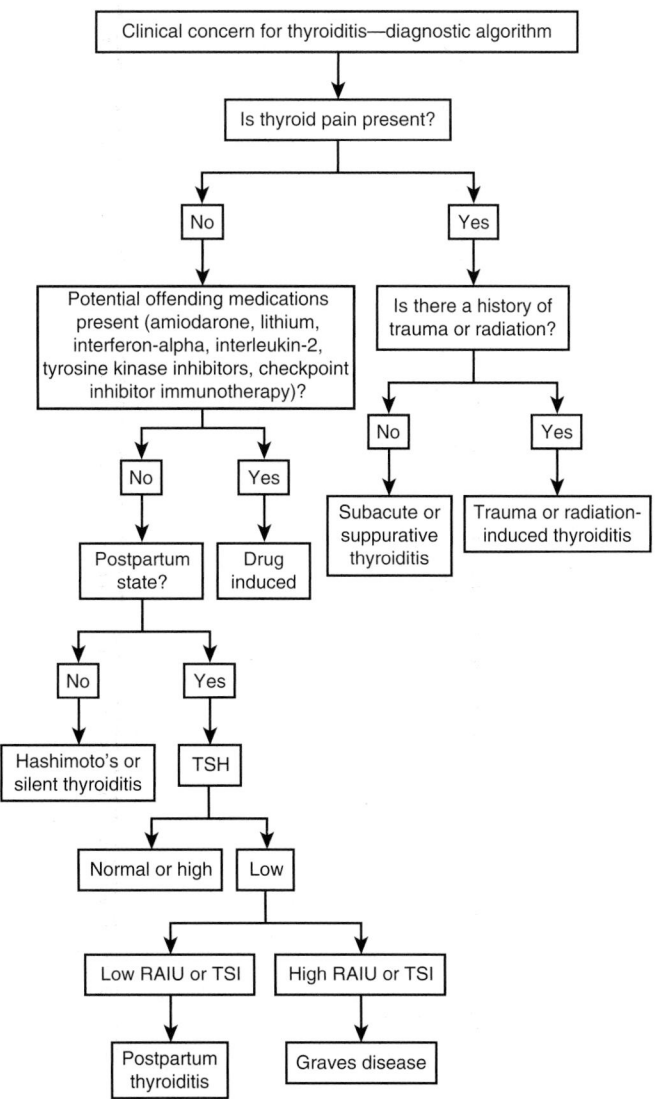

Figure 1 Clinical concern for thyroiditis—diagnostic algorithm. *Abbreviations:* RAIU = radioactive iodine uptake; TSI = thyroid-stimulating immunoglobulins.

when a goiter is found on examination with a subsequently noted elevation of thyroid antibodies or when subclinical or overt hypothyroidism is detected with associated elevated thyroid antibodies. Screening for postpartum thyroiditis with a measurement of TSH and free thyroxine should be undertaken in women presenting with symptoms of thyroid dysfunction in the postpartum period. If hyperthyroidism is present, thyroid scintigraphy (if not contraindicated, e.g., breastfeeding) or measurement of thyroid-stimulating immunoglobulins is helpful in the differentiation of postpartum thyroiditis from Graves' disease. The diagnostic approach to silent thyroiditis is similar. The laboratory hallmark of subacute thyroiditis is a markedly elevated erythrocyte sedimentation rate; the leukocyte count is normal or slightly elevated. Thyrotoxicosis may be present; if so, thyroid scintigraphy will reveal a low iodine uptake state. Thyroid antibody testing is typically normal. Thyroid ultrasound reveals a hypoechogenic gland with low to normal vascularity. Suppurative thyroiditis is typically associated with normal thyroid function. Leukocyte counts and erythrocyte sedimentation rates are elevated. Fine-needle aspiration with Gram stain and culture is the diagnostic test of choice. Radiation-induced thyroiditis should be considered if a temporal relationship to radioactive iodine treatment is present. If there is an exacerbation of hyperthyroidism immediately following radiation treatment for the same, consideration of radiation-induced thyroiditis due to the release of preformed thyroid hormone associated with destruction of follicular cells should be considered as an etiology of thyrotoxicosis in addition to the underlying disease process.

Treatment

Once overt hypothyroidism is present in the patient with Hashimoto's thyroiditis, treatment with synthetic L-thyroxine (Levoxyl, Synthroid) therapy is indicated. The average replacement dose of thyroxine in adults is approximately 1.6 mcg/kg body weight per day. Adjustment of dosage is undertaken every 6 weeks until a euthyroid status is achieved. The majority of women with postpartum thyroiditis will not need treatment during either the hyperthyroid or hypothyroid phase. If symptomatic hyperthyroidism is present, beta-blocker therapy can be used; antithyroid medications have no utility in the management of postpartum thyroiditis. Women with symptomatic hypothyroidism should be treated with synthetic thyroxine therapy; in asymptomatic women, initiation of thyroxine therapy should be considered if TSH is >10 mU/L. Management of silent thyroiditis is the same as that for postpartum thyroiditis. Symptoms associated with Riedel's thyroiditis may be relieved with prednisone; a small case series associated improvement and even resolution of the process

with tamoxifen (Nolvadex)[1] therapy. Surgery is indicated in Riedel's thyroiditis if compressive symptoms are present. The goal of therapy in subacute thyroiditis is to provide symptom relief. Nonsteroidal antiinflammatory medications are often adequate to control pain; if insufficient, glucocorticoid therapy should be initiated. Beta-blockade therapy can ameliorate symptoms of thyrotoxicosis if indicated. Suppurative thyroiditis is managed with appropriate antibiotics and drainage of any abscess; the disease may prove fatal if diagnosis and treatment are delayed. Pain associated with radiation-induced thyroiditis can be managed with nonsteroidal antiinflammatory therapy or, if ineffective, a short course of glucocorticoid therapy. Radiation-induced thyroiditis is a self-limited process and will resolve spontaneously within days to weeks.

Monitoring

In the patient with Hashimoto's thyroiditis with a euthyroid state, routine TSH testing should be undertaken given the risk of development of overt hypothyroidism at 5% per year. Any woman who has had postpartum thyroiditis should be monitored very closely for thyroid dysfunction with future pregnancies, as reoccurrence is likely. For women who have fully recovered from postpartum thyroiditis, yearly TSH measurements should be considered because of underlying chronic autoimmune thyroiditis and risk for overt hypothyroidism. Although overall recurrence rates for silent thyroiditis have not been well established, a similar monitoring plan is warranted for this variant of chronic autoimmune thyroiditis. Subacute thyroiditis recurs in only about 2% of patients. Routine monitoring following resolution of process has not been defined.

---

[1]Not FDA approved for this indication.

References

Bogazzi F, Bartalena L, Martino E: Approach to the patient with amiodarone-induced thyrotoxicosis, *J Clin Endocrinol Metab* 95:2529–2535, 2010.

Cooper DS, Ladenson PW: The thyroid gland. 2011. In Gardner DG, Shoback D, editors: *Greenspan's Basic & Clinical Endocrinology*, 9th ed., New York, 2011, McGraw-Hill, (Available at. http://accessmedicine.mhmedical.com/content.aspx?bookid¼380&Sectionid¼39744047. Accessed 23 January 2014.

De Groot L, Abalovich M, Alexander ED, et al: Management of thyroid dysfunction during pregnancy and postpartum: an Endocrine Society clinical practice guideline, *J Clin Endocrinol Metab* 97:2543–2565, 2012.

Pearce EN, Farwell AP, Braverman LE: Thyroiditis, *N Engl J Med* 348:2646–2655, 2003.

Samuels MH: Subacute, silent and postpartum thyroiditis, *Med Clin North Am* 96:223–233, 2012.

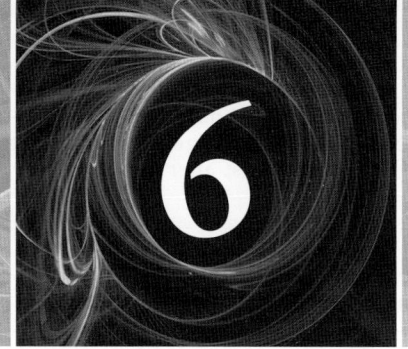

6 Hematology

ACUTE LEUKEMIA IN ADULTS

Method of
William Blum, MD

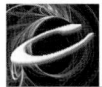

CURRENT DIAGNOSIS

- Diagnosis of acute leukemia is made based on the presence of myeloid (acute myeloid leukemia [AML]) or lymphoid (T- or B-cell acute lymphoblastic leukemia [ALL]) blasts in blood and/or bone marrow. Acute leukemia may uncommonly have an ambiguous lineage or mixed phenotype.
- Medical history taking should identify risk factors such as prior exposure to chemotherapy for other malignancies (or nonmalignant disorders), antecedent hematologic disorders, familial hematologic disorders, or other inherited genetic disorders (e.g., Down syndrome, others).
- Clinical examination should identify extramedullary sites of involvement such as meninges/central nervous system (CNS), active infection, hemorrhage, or disseminated intravascular coagulation (DIC).
- AML requires the presence of at least 20% blasts in blood or marrow except in selected subsets of disease with specific cytogenetic aberrations associated with more favorable clinical outcomes, which do not require at least 20% blasts. These favorable subsets are t(8;21)(q22;q22), inv(16)(p13q22) or t(16;16)(p13;q22), and t(15;17)(q22;q12). Testing for additional cytogenetic and molecular aberrations is critical for diagnosis, prognosis, and therapy.
- Acute promyelocytic leukemia (APL) with *PML-RARA* gene fusion, detected by genetic methods or cytogenetics showing t(15;17), is a unique entity requiring different therapy; APL has a favorable prognosis.
- ALL is subcategorized based on B- or T-lymphocyte lineage and requires at least 20% blasts in blood or marrow. Less than 20% blasts constitutes lymphoblastic lymphoma, which is treated similarly.
- For B-ALL (also in mixed phenotype acute leukemia), identification of the Philadelphia chromosome t(9;22)(q34.1;q11.2) or its *BCR-ABL1* gene fusion is essential for proper diagnosis and treatment. As with AML, testing for an established group of other specific chromosomal and molecular aberrations is standard.

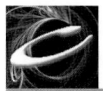

CURRENT THERAPY

- AML is typically treated with intensive initial therapy (induction) followed by repetitive cycles of intensive postremission therapy (consolidation). Induction chemotherapy most commonly consists of anthracycline plus cytarabine (Cytosar). Several acceptable postremission approaches are used; often, these are repetitive high-dose cytarabine–based regimens.
- APL is uniquely treated with all-*trans*-retinoic acid (tretinoin [Vesanoid]) and arsenic trioxide (Trisenox), instead of chemo-

therapy, although cases with high presenting white blood cell (WBC) counts may require chemotherapy for cytoreduction.
- ALL is treated with multidrug regimens for induction and postremission therapies. Postremission therapies include further intensification cycles and prolonged lower-dose maintenance therapy. CNS-directed therapy is a critical component of treatment even in patients without clear involvement. Most acute leukemias of ambiguous lineage are treated with ALL-type regimens, although clinical outcomes are poor.
- The use of pediatric ALL regimens for adolescents and young adults has improved outcomes.
- Older patients or those with medical infirmities may require less intensive treatment regimens; because of more resistant disease and also higher toxicities, such patients fare worse than younger patients.
- Because of high relapse risks, allogeneic hematopoietic stem cell transplantation (alloHCT) in first remission is an important consideration for all eligible patients with AML except those with favorable-risk disease. High-risk older patients with ALL are also offered early transplantation. All patients who relapse should be considered for transplantation if remission is again achieved.
- Several subsets of acute leukemia can be treated by new effective therapies that target specific aberrant signaling or enzymatic activities or that are directed to unique biologic targets of disease. Most important among these are the tyrosine kinase inhibitors (TKIs), which are used in treating acute leukemia (typically ALL) with *BCR-ABL1*.
- Advances in immunology have rapidly and dramatically improved the options for treatment, especially for those with relapsed B-ALL. Novel antibody constructs and genetically engineered autologous cellular products directed to eliminate B-lymphocytes can induce durable remissions in B-ALL.

Epidemiology

According to data from the National Institutes of Health, the incidence of acute myeloid leukemia (AML) in the United States is 4.2 per 100,000 per year, with an estimate of 19,940 new cases for 2020. According to the American Cancer Society, AML accounts for about 1.3% of all new cancer cases and 31% of all new leukemia cases (but 62% of leukemic deaths). AML is far more common than acute lymphoblastic leukemia (ALL) in adults. Although AML affects all age groups, the incidence increases with advancing age, presenting at a median age of 67 years. ALL is estimated to occur in 6150 cases in the United States for 2020 and has a bimodal distribution across ages, with a peak in early childhood and a second peak around the age of 70 years.

Risk Factors

Most cases of acute leukemia in adults have no established cause. Genetic predisposition, drugs, and radiation have been associated with the development of acute leukemia, particularly AML. Several rare genetic syndromes—including Down syndrome, Fanconi anemia, Bloom syndrome, neurofibromatosis type I, and ataxia telangiectasia—are associated with an increased risk for developing acute leukemia. AML with germline predisposition represents an uncommon but important subset of disease. Germline mutations associated with increased risk of developing a myeloid neoplasm include *CEBPA*, *DDX41*, *RUNX1*, *ANKRD26*, *ETV6*, and *GATA2*. Down syndrome–associated AML and ALL pose an increased risk of toxicity with standard chemotherapy and require dose adjustment (and expert management).

Anticancer drugs are the leading cause of therapy-associated AML. Alkylating agent–associated leukemias typically occur 4 to 6 years after exposure; affected individuals often have multilineage dysplasia and monosomy/aberrations in chromosomes 5 and 7. Topoisomerase II inhibitor–associated leukemias typically occur with shorter latency, 1 to 3 years after exposure; affected individuals often have AML with monocytic features and aberrations involving chromosome 11q23.

Pathophysiology

Acute leukemias are hematologic malignancies arising from hematopoietic progenitor (stem) cells in the bone marrow. Clonal immature cells accumulate in the blood, bone marrow, and occasionally in the extramedullary tissues. These malignant cells divide and proliferate, but they do not differentiate into functional cells (i.e., neutrophils, lymphocytes, or others). Patients with acute leukemia are immunocompromised and have impaired oxygen-carrying capacity (anemia) and bleeding diathesis (because of thrombocytopenia or disrupted coagulation).

Patients experience complications directly from the accumulation of abnormal immature blasts or indirectly from the reduction in functional hematopoietic cells in the marrow and blood. Leukemic involvement of the bone marrow often results in pancytopenia—patients may present with cytopenias in all hematopoietic cell lineages. Patients with acute leukemias typically have evidence of circulating leukemic blasts in the peripheral blood (sometimes with high white blood cell [WBC] counts consisting entirely of blasts), or they may have pancytopenia with no circulating blasts at all. Patients typically require transfusions of red blood cells and platelets and are at risk of life-threatening infectious complications due to neutropenia. Most patients with acute leukemia die from infection or, less frequently, hemorrhage.

Patients with morphologically similar acute leukemias may experience vastly different clinical outcomes. Increasingly, this is understood by karyotyping or genetic sequencing studies that demonstrate marked heterogeneity in the cytogenetic and mutational profiles among patients with acute leukemia. It is clear that morphology and cytochemical staining alone to establish diagnosis does little to explain the pathophysiology of these varied hematologic cancers. Genetic sequencing studies demonstrate common dysregulation of several critical cellular pathways but also a myriad of genetic differences that occur only in small (or very small/unique) subsets. In adults, most cases of AML ultimately arise against the backdrop of a limited number of mutations that accumulate with advancing age. As noted earlier, cases with a clear cause, such as germline predisposition or drug exposure, are rare. The Cancer Genome Atlas (cancergenome.nih.gov) and other databases have shown that up to 5% to 6% of healthy individuals over 70 years of age have blood cells with potentially "premalignant" mutations that are associated with clonal expansion. There appear to be a variety of "final insults" that transform these expanded clones to AML. However, how all these genetic aberrations contribute to leukemic transformation remains incompletely understood. Although the number of mutations per cell in AML is relatively small (median of 13 mutations) compared with other cancers (e.g., melanoma and non–small cell lung cancer may have several hundred mutations per cell), great heterogeneity exists in the mutations identified between individual patients with AML. The same can be said of ALL. Indeed, dramatic differences in mutations/genetic signatures have been observed between patients with childhood, adolescent, young adult, and older adult ALL, respectively.

Great heterogeneity exists not just between patients with different types of acute leukemia but within each individual patient. Each patient may have several leukemic clones and subclones with slightly different mutational profiles. The presence of genetically different clones and subclones helps to explain why a patient may achieve remission but then experience relapse with more resistant disease, since sensitive clones are eliminated by chemotherapy whereas surviving clones are more resistant to subsequent treatment. Furthermore, clones that persist after treatment may emerge with additional novel mutations.

Clinical Manifestations

Patients with any type of acute leukemia present with similar symptoms. Most have vague symptoms that are consequences of pancytopenia. Typically, the onset of illness is no more than 3 months before diagnosis unless the leukemia is associated with an antecedent hematologic disorder. Fatigue is common, as are anorexia and weight loss. Fever or infection is also common but not universal at presentation. Patients may have evidence of abnormal hemostasis (bleeding, easy bruising). Bone pain, lymphadenopathy, nonspecific cough, headache, and diaphoresis (excessive sweating) may also occur. Bone pain, typically vaguely localized to the pelvis or back, is frequent. Patients with ALL (as compared with AML) are more likely to have lymphadenopathy, splenomegaly, or extramedullary involvement at other sites, such as the testicles or CNS. However, involvement at any of these sites is not exclusive to ALL; their presence is not diagnostic of that type. Rarely, patients present with primary symptoms caused by extramedullary leukemia. Extramedullary disease in AML is known as a myeloid sarcoma (also called a *granulocytic sarcoma* or *chloroma*). This is a tumor mass consisting of myeloid blasts and is most commonly seen in the skin, lymph nodes, gastrointestinal tract, soft tissue, or testis. Patients who present with isolated myeloid sarcoma typically develop blood or marrow involvement quickly thereafter; such patients thus require systemic treatment (not solely surgical resection or local radiation). CNS involvement at initial presentation (headache, cranial nerve palsies) is uncommon. Patients with ALL, however, have an increased risk of CNS disease and should thus be given intrathecal chemotherapy as prophylaxis even without such symptoms (or detectable CNS involvement).

Severe hemorrhagic complications are relatively infrequent at presentation but are most commonly encountered in acute promyelocytic leukemia (APL). Recognition of this risk at the time of initial presentation is critical, as replacement of fibrinogen or plasma may be lifesaving. Patients with APL often present with disseminated intravascular coagulation (DIC)-associated hemorrhage and may have intracranial hemorrhage or bleeding at other sites. Appropriate therapy for APL such as all-*trans*-retinoic-acid (Tretinoin [Vesanoid]) should be initiated upon suspicion and not withheld pending genetic confirmation of the classic $t(15;17)$ rearrangement. Thrombosis is a less frequent but well-recognized feature of APL. Bleeding associated with coagulopathy may also occur in monocytic AML and with extreme degrees of leukocytosis or thrombocytopenia in other acute leukemias. Retinal hemorrhage caused by thrombocytopenia and extreme leukocytosis is detected in approximately 15% of patients.

Laboratory parameters are quite variable with any type of acute leukemia. Although many patients present with leukocytosis and high levels of circulating blasts, it is important to note that presenting with low WBC counts or even no circulating blasts is not rare. Typically, though, review of the peripheral blood smear identifies the classic blast—fine, lacy chromatin with one or more nucleoli and a high nucleus-to-cytoplasm ratio, which is characteristic of immature cells. The presence in blasts of abnormal rod-shaped granules called *Auer rods* on light microscopy indicates a diagnosis of AML.

Anemia is observed at diagnosis in nearly all patients but is not severe. Decreased erythropoiesis often results in a reduced reticulocyte (immature red blood cell) count; red blood cell survival may be shortened by accelerated destruction. Most patients also present with at least mild thrombocytopenia (below the normal lower limit value of 150,000/μL); severe thrombocytopenia (<10,000/μL) can be life threatening and requires immediate platelet transfusion.

Diagnosis

When acute leukemia is clinically suspected, in addition to morphologic and flow cytometric analyses, cytogenetic and genetic tests are mandatory to aid rapid diagnosis, assess prognosis, and inform the best approach to treatment. That said, clinical features also remain important. These include a history of antecedent hematologic disorder or prior chemotherapy, advanced age, and a strong family history of acute leukemia or related hematologic disorder (all favoring AML); all of these have an adverse prognosis. In ALL, a high WBC count at presentation (>100,000/μL for B-ALL and >30,000/μL for T-ALL) and T-cell phenotype have an adverse prognosis.

Initial assessments should evaluate cardiovascular, pulmonary, hepatic, and renal systems; patients should also be evaluated and treated for infection or DIC. Preparation for transfusion of blood or platelets requires blood type and cross-match to be determined, and human leukocyte antigen (HLA) testing is required early in the treatment course (before chemotherapy) in consideration of future allogeneic hematopoietic stem cell transplantation (alloHCT). Cytogenetic analysis typically requires bone marrow. Genetic testing (from blood or marrow) continues to evolve and is critical for successful diagnosis, prognosis, and therapy.

The diagnosis of AML is based on a finding of at least 20% myeloid blasts by histology, cytochemistry, or flow cytometry. However, this 20% threshold is not required for the diagnosis if any of the following recurrent cytogenetic abnormalities is present: $t(15;17)$, $t(8;21)$, inv(16), or $t(16;16)$. Myeloid blasts stain positive for myeloperoxidase; by flow cytometry, myeloid blasts are typically positive for CD13 and CD33. A prognostic schema developed by the European LeukemiaNet assigns prognostic risk based on cytogenetic and genetic features of disease (Table 1). Some morphologic features are associated with specific cytogenetic or molecular findings such as $t(15;17)$ and APL, or dysplastic eosinophils and inv(16) or $t(16;16)$. The expression of B-cell markers (CD19, PAX5, cytoplasmic CD79a) is not infrequent in $t(8;21)$.

The diagnosis of ALL likewise requires at least 20% lymphoid blasts. By immunohistochemical methods, lymphoid blasts stain positive for terminal deoxynucleotidyl transferase (TdT); by flow, lymphoid blasts are typically positive for CD10, CD19, CD22, and CD20 (variable) for B-ALL and CD3, CD7, CD4, and CD8 for T-ALL.

Patients may uncommonly present with acute leukemia of ambiguous lineage (undifferentiated or mixed phenotype). However, more common are AML cases that express an aberrant B- or T-cell marker (e.g., CD7 on myeloid blasts); this is called an aberrant immunophenotype. Likewise, B-ALL may aberrantly express CD13 or CD33.

Molecular testing is an important component of diagnosis. For AML, molecular testing should include assessment of FLT3 (with allelic ratio), NPM1, CEBPA (biallelic), IDH1, IDH2, RUNX1, ASXL1, and TP53. For ALL, testing is equally complex but is still evolving in terms of commercial availability for important molecular analyses. Critical to the initial assessment of ALL is testing for the BCR-ABL1 fusion by molecular methods that are widely available; tyrosine kinase inhibitors (TKIs) targeting this lesion are now an important part of treatment. Likewise, testing by interphase fluorescence in situ hybridization for the major recurrent cytogenetic abnormalities seen in ALL—including ETV6-RUNX1, TCF3-PBX1, and KMT2A rearrangements, among others—is mandatory. Although not yet widely available, testing in B-ALL for the "BCR-ABL1-like" genetic signature identifies a subset of patients with adverse prognosis but potential responsiveness to TKI therapies. BCR-ABL1-like disease as a subset has several common genetic features including disruption of B-lymphoid transcription factors including IKZF1, CRLF2, JAK2, and others. Diagnostic testing guidelines for both AML and ALL are delineated and annually updated by the National Comprehensive Cancer Network (NCCN.org).

Cytogenetic analysis should be performed on the bone marrow aspirate taken at diagnosis in any patient suspected to have acute leukemia. Prognosis is determined by the presence of structural or numeric chromosomal abnormalities and is then more fully informed by additional genetic testing. Broadly speaking, patients with AML with $t(15;17)$, known as APL as described earlier, have an excellent prognosis, with 80% to 90% cured. Patients with $t(8;21)$ or inv(16) also have a favorable prognosis. Patients with

Acute Leukemia in Adults

405

TABLE 1	2017 European LeukemiaNet Risk Stratification by Genetics for Acute Myeloid Leukemia*
RISK CATEGORY[†]	**GENETIC ABNORMALITY**
Favorable	$t(8;21)(q22;q22)$; RUNX1-RUNX1T1 inv(16)(p13.1q22) or $t(16;16)(p13.1;q22)$; CBFB-MYH11 Mutated NPM1 without FLT3-ITD or with FLT3-ITD[low‡] Biallelic mutated CEBPA
Intermediate	Mutated NPM1 and FLT3-ITD[high‡] Wild type NPM1 without FLT3-ITD or with FLT3-ITD[low‡] (w/o adverse-risk genetic lesions) $t(9;11)(p21.3;q23.3)$; MLLT3-KMT2A[§] Cytogenetic abnormalities not classified as favorable or adverse
Adverse	$t(6;9)(p23;q34.1)$; DEK-NUP214 $t(v;11q23.3)$; KMT2A rearranged $t(9;22)(q34.1;q11.2)$; BCR-ABL1 inv(3)(q21.3q26.2) or $t(3;3)(q21.3;q26.2)$; GATA2,MECOM(EVI1) –5 or del(5q); –7; –17/abn(17p) Complex karyotype,[¶¶] monosomal karyotype[¶] Wild type NPM1 and FLT3-ITD[high‡] Mutated RUNX1[**] Mutated ASXL1[**] Mutated TP53[††]

*This table excludes acute promyelocytic leukemia. Frequencies, response rates, and outcome measures should be reported by risk category and, if sufficient numbers are available, by specific genetic lesions indicated.

[†]Prognostic impact of a marker is treatment-dependent and may change with new therapies.

[‡]Low, low allelic ratio (<0.5); high, high allelic ratio (>0.5); semiquantitative assessment of FLT3-ITD allelic ratio (using DNA fragment analysis) is determined as ratio of the area under the curve (AUC) "FLT3-ITD" divided by AUC "FLT3-wild type"; recent studies indicate that acute myeloid leukemia with NPM1 mutation and FLT3-ITD low allelic ratio may also have a more favorable prognosis and patients should not routinely be assigned to allogeneic hematopoietic-cell transplantation.

[§]The presence of $t(9;11)(p21.3;q23.3)$ takes precedence over rare, concurrent adverse-risk gene mutations.

[¶¶]Three or more unrelated chromosome abnormalities in the absence of one of the World Health Organization–designated recurring translocations or inversions, i.e., $t(8;21)$, inv(16) or $t(16;16)$, $t(9;11)$, $t(v;11)(v;q23.3)$, $t(6;9)$, inv(3) or $t(3;3)$; AML with BCR-ABL1.

[¶]Defined by the presence of one single monosomy (excluding loss of X or Y) in association with at least one additional monosomy or structural chromosome abnormality (excluding core-binding factor AML).

[††]TP53 mutations are significantly associated with AML with complex and monosomal karyotype.

[**]These markers should not be used as an adverse prognostic marker if they co-occur with favorable-risk AML subtypes.

Adapted from Döhner H, Estey E, Grimwade D, et al: Diagnosis and management of AML in adults: 2017 ELN recommendations from an international expert panel, *Blood* 129:424–447, 2017.

no cytogenetic abnormalities (cytogenetically normal AML; CN-AML) have an intermediate prognosis. Patients with a complex karyotype, $t(6;9)$, inv(3), or –7 (absence of chromosome 7), respectively, have an adverse prognosis with few cures, particularly in older patients. Genetic testing provides valuable additional information, especially in CN-AML. Favorable genetic risk is observed in those with NPM1 mutations without a high allelic ratio of FLT3 internal tandem duplication (FLT3-ITD) and also in those with biallelic CEBPA mutations. Conversely, TP53 mutations (often but not exclusively observed in the setting of complex karyotype) are associated with adverse risk. Mutations in genes encoding isocitrate dehydrogenase (IDH) enzymes may contribute to prognostication but, more importantly, identify patients who are likely to respond to novel therapies that target these aberrant pathways.

Cytogenetic testing for ALL enables classification into several groups, including, for example, BCR-ABL1 fusion disease. This fusion, known cytogenetically as $t(9;22)$ and colloquially referred to as the Philadelphia (Ph) chromosome (based on the city where it was originally identified) has a poor prognosis. However, the incorporation into multiagent regimens of TKIs that target the aberrantly active kinase has improved clinical outcomes. Other important ALL subsets include *KMT2A* rearrangements at chromosome 11q23 (with various translocation partners but often chromosome 4 in B-ALL). Both *BCR-ABL1* and *KMT2A* aberrant ALLs are associated with an unfavorable prognosis. Many other subsets of ALL exist in the World Health Organization (WHO) classification. Favorable risk is seen in patients with B-ALL with *t*(12;21)(p13.2;q22.1), the *ETV6-RUNX1* fusion. T-ALL is characterized by activation mutations in *NOTCH1* (present in about 60% of cases) and deregulation of a number of transcription factors; immunophenotyping showing an early T-cell precursor (ETP) phenotype (low expression of CD1a, CD8, CD5) has been associated with an adverse prognosis.

Historically, the diagnosis and classification of acute leukemia was based on the French-American-British morphologic and cytochemical criteria, which assigned patients with AML to one of eight groups designated M0 to M7. Likewise, ALL was classified into L1, L2, and L3 groups. These categories, while still in the vernacular on the clinical wards, are practically obsolete. Diagnosis and classification are based instead on the complex morphologic, flow, cytogenetic, and molecular characterization schemas outlined by the WHO for myeloid neoplasms and acute leukemia.

Differential Diagnosis

The differential diagnosis for acute leukemia includes many bone marrow disorders that present with pancytopenia. However, the presence of excess blasts in the blood or marrow limits the diagnosis to AML, ALL, or acute leukemia of ambiguous lineage. For patients without circulating blasts in the blood, highest in the differential diagnosis of pancytopenia are other hematologic cancers with marrow infiltration or bone marrow failure syndromes such as aplastic anemia. Advanced myeloproliferative disorders with bone marrow fibrosis and myelodysplastic syndromes can also present similarly, occasionally with rare circulating blasts. Rarely, the pancytopenia caused by the displacement of hemopoietic bone marrow tissue by fibrosis, tumor, or granuloma (called myelophthisis) mimics acute leukemia (but without blasts). Examples include solid organ cancers with extensive marrow involvement and granulomatous disease such as tuberculosis. However, essentially only acute leukemia is the appropriate diagnosis in patients with high-level circulating blasts visualized on light microscopy.

Treatment of Acute Myeloid Leukemia

Treatment of the newly diagnosed adult patient with AML is usually divided into two phases: (1) induction and (2) consolidation (i.e., postremission management). The aim of induction chemotherapy is complete remission (CR), defined as fewer than 5% blasts on a bone marrow aspirate, with recovery of blood counts (absolute neutrophil count >1000/μL *and* platelet count >100,000/μL). Additional defining criteria of CR include absent circulating blasts and no detectable extramedullary disease. Achievement of CR (or failure to do so) is the best predictor of long-term clinical outcome. The definition of CR is further refined based on the detection of measurable residual disease (MRD) by cytogenetics, flow cytometry, and/or molecular testing. Marrow response *without* full blood count recovery meets lesser response definitions (often termed CR with incomplete count recovery, or CRi); patients with such responses have outcomes inferior to those with CR. Blood count recovery occurs approximately 4 weeks after the initiation of intensive induction chemotherapy. CR is achieved in 60% to 90% of younger patients (depending on molecular risk) and in approximately 2% to 60% of older patients (>60 years). Notably, for older patients this estimate is from the subset limited to those who are actually offered intensive therapy; many older patients are not treated intensively (or at all) owing to medical comorbidities. Such patients would likely fare even worse than the estimates provided if offered intensive treatment. Long-term survival estimates are approximately 60% for younger patients with favorable-risk disease (see Table 1), 40% for intermediate-risk disease, and 20% for adverse-risk disease.

Older patients do poorly in each group; indeed, there are very few long-term survivors among older patients with adverse-risk disease.

Induction and consolidation therapies are chosen based on the patient's age, overall fitness, and cytogenetic/molecular risk. Intensive induction therapy is the norm in younger patients (<60 years). In older patients, the benefit of intensive therapy is more controversial in all but those with a favorable-risk profile; novel approaches for selecting patients predicted to be responsive to treatment and new therapies remain under investigation. Notably, large datasets have demonstrated that even more infirm older patients with AML benefit from treatment as compared with only palliative care.

Standard induction therapy for AML consists of cytarabine (cytosine arabinoside, AraC; Cytosar), 100 to 200 mg/m^2 per day administered as a continuous infusion for 7 days, and daunorubicin (Cerubidine), 60 to 90 mg/m^2/day for 3 days, commonly known as the 7 + 3 schedule. Idarubicin (Idamycin; 12 mg/m^2/day) is equivalent to daunorubicin. Resistant disease is more frequent in older patients and those with prior hematologic disorders, therapy-related AML, or cytogenetic and genetic abnormalities that adversely affect clinical outcome (which are more frequent in older patients). In older patients, the long-term outcome is generally poor owing to the higher frequency of resistant disease in this group plus an increased rate of treatment-related mortality. As an alternative to intensive induction, unfit or adverse-risk older patients may instead receive lower-intensity therapy with a hypomethylating agent (such as decitabine [Dacogen][1] or azacytidine [Vidaza][1]). For patients older than 75 years or those who are not candidates for intensive therapy, the FDA recently approved venetoclax (Venclexta) in combination with hypomethylating agent therapy. A randomized trial demonstrated improved survival and higher remission rates with azacytidine in combination with venetoclax, compared to azacytidine alone. All older patients should be considered for clinical trials, but older patients in adverse-risk groups should ideally be offered investigational approaches whenever available.

Induction of first CR (CR1) is critical to long-term survival in AML. However, without further therapy, virtually all patients in CR will eventually relapse. Patients are estimated to have 10^{12} leukemic cells at diagnosis, which intensive induction chemotherapy reduces by four to five orders of magnitude. Although this reduces the disease burden by 99.9%, approximately 10^8 residual leukemic cells still remain after successful induction therapy. These residual cells may not be measurable at all or may be measurable only by sensitive techniques such as multiparameter flow cytometry or quantitative reverse transcriptase polymerase chain reaction (RT-PCR). They cannot be detected by morphology alone. Thus postremission therapy is designed to eradicate residual (typically undetectable) leukemic cells to prevent relapse and prolong survival. As for induction, the type of postremission therapy in AML is selected for each individual patient based on age, fitness, and cytogenetic/molecular risk.

Postremission treatment options include chemotherapy and/or transplantation. The choice between consolidation with chemotherapy or transplantation is complex and based on age, risk, and practical considerations. In younger patients receiving chemotherapy, postremission therapy with intermediate/high-dose cytarabine for two to four cycles is standard practice. It is clear that alloHCT is the best relapse-prevention strategy currently available for AML. However, the benefit of alloHCT in reducing relapse risk is offset somewhat by increased morbidity and mortality from complications including graft-versus-host disease. Given that relapsed AML is typically resistant to chemotherapy, alloHCT in CR1 is a favored strategy for patients at high risk for relapse. Transplantation is generally recommended for physically fit patients less than 75 years of age who do not have favorable-risk disease and have a suitable donor. Donors are typically HLA matched (related or unrelated) or, increasingly,

---

[1]Not FDA approved for this indication.

haploidentical (half-matched sibling, parent, or child). Prognostic factors help in selecting the appropriate postremission therapy in patients in CR1. Generally speaking, patients with favorable-risk AML in CR1 are treated with chemotherapy alone; patients with adverse-risk disease should proceed to alloHCT at CR1 if possible. The decision for alloHCT versus chemotherapy in CR1 for intermediate-risk patients remains in debate.

Recent years have seen FDA approvals for several targeted drugs. For AML patients with *FLT3* mutation, midostaurin (Rydapt, in combination with initial chemotherapy) and gilteritinib (Xospata, as monotherapy for relapsed AML), respectively, have improved outcomes compared to chemotherapy alone. Likewise, agents targeting mutated IDH enzymes 1 or 2 (in AML patients with *IDH1* or *IDH2* mutations) have been shown effective in both relapsed and initial therapy settings. Another non-targeted drug, CPX-351 (Vyxeos, a liposomal combination of daunorubicin [an anthracycline] and cytarabine), has demonstrated superiority to initial standard chemotherapy in patients with secondary AML or AML with myelodysplasia-related changes. All of these drugs, as well as venetoclax and many other novel agents, are currently in additional clinical trials.

APL is uniquely treated with all-*trans*-retinoic acid (tretinoin [Vesanoid]) and arsenic trioxide (Trisenox), instead of chemotherapy, although cases with high presenting WBC counts (>10,000/μL) may require chemotherapy for cytoreduction. Cases with high WBC counts are at increased risk for fatal hemorrhage and other complications. Low-risk patients (WBC <10,000/μL) have a virtually nonexistent frequency of resistant disease. Patients with APL require expert management to address complications of DIC and hemorrhage and the so-called APL syndrome (formerly known as differentiation syndrome, retinoic acid syndrome). APL syndrome is marked by a rising WBC count, fever, hypoxia, shortness of breath, and fluid accumulation; it occurs up to 3 weeks after treatment initiation. It is common, especially in presentations with higher WBCs, and requires urgent therapy consisting of steroids, diuresis, and possibly cytoreduction.

Treatment of Acute Lymphoblastic Leukemia

Standard chemotherapy treatment of ALL is of much more extended duration and regimen complexity than that of AML. However, the same general principles apply—achievement of CR1 with initial therapy is the critical first step for long-term survival. Postremission therapy in ALL is broken into different segments of various intensity, including interim maintenance, delayed intensification, and prolonged (24 months) maintenance. CNS-directed therapy (systemic chemotherapy with intrathecal chemotherapy, or cranial radiotherapy) is an important mandatory feature of ALL treatment. Generally, treatment approaches include variations on a five-drug induction combination of cyclophosphamide (Cytoxan), prednisone[1] or dexamethasone[1] (Decadron), anthracycline (doxorubicin [Adriamycin]; or daunorubicin [Cerubidine]), PEGylated asparaginase (Oncaspar), and vincristine (Oncovin). The principle of therapy is continuous exposure to multiple chemotherapy agents with nonoverlapping resistance mechanisms; all ALL regimens use alternating chemotherapy regimens given over an extended period of time. Additional agents include methotrexate, cytarabine, 6-mercaptopurine (Purinethol), and others. Examples of treatment strategies are the BFM (Berlin-Frankfurt-Munster) approach and the hyper-CVAD (hyperfractionated cyclophosphamide, vincristine, Adriamycin, Dexamethasone) regimen.

Unfortunately, although children with B-ALL have favorable long-term survival in the 80% to 90% range, adults fare far worse. Estimated long-term survival rates for adults with ALL are only 30% to 40%. Encouraging data have come from recent cooperative group studies: adolescents and young adults (age 16 to 40 years) treated with "pediatric inspired" regimens have outcomes far better than those treated with "adult" regimens. Pediatric regimens have a greater focus on less myelotoxic therapies

such as PEGylated asparaginase, vincristine, and steroids. Unfortunately, older adults (>40 years) have difficulty tolerating such approaches. The addition of nelarabine (Arranon) to first-line therapy has improved outcomes in T-ALL.

As noted previously, the identification of the Ph chromosome *t(9;22)* or the *BCR-ABL1* fusion is a very important part of the initial diagnosis of B-ALL or mixed-phenotype acute leukemia. The introduction of TKI for Ph-positive patients into multiagent induction and postremission treatment has dramatically improved outcomes and is now standard. Whether Ph-positive B-ALL should have mandatory alloHCT in CR1 is now controversial. Imatinib (Gleevec) is a standard TKI; second- or third-generation TKIs such as dasatinib (Sprycel), nilotinib (Tasigna)[1], or ponatinib (Iclusig) are also commonly used for the treatment of Ph-positive acute leukemia.

Additional advances to traditional approaches over the last 5 years include the use of CD20 monoclonal antibodies (rituximab [Rituxan][1]) for patients with B-ALL whose lymphoid blasts express this surface marker and nelarabine in T-ALL. Nelarabine is a purine analog with increased activity in T-lymphoid blasts and 30% response rates in the relapsed setting; it is being incorporated into front-line multiagent trials. AlloHCT in adult ALL is more controversial than in AML, although most trials offer alloHCT in CR1 for high-risk disease.

Immune-Based Therapies in Acute Leukemia

Beyond the use of alloHCT, recent years have seen remarkable progress in immunologic therapies for acute leukemia. The US Food and Drug Administration recently approved exciting engineered cellular therapies for relapsed malignancies of B-lymphocytes: chimeric antigen receptor (CAR) T-cells that target CD19 (in B-ALL and non-Hodgkin lymphoma). In these cases, autologous B cells are collected by apheresis from the patient, genetically engineered *ex vivo* to target CD19, then infused back into the patient to treat CD19+ malignancy (typically after some type of lymphodepleting therapy). In the process, CD19+ normal B cells are also eliminated. High response rates and long-term remissions have been reported in patients with ALL with highly refractory disease using CAR T-cell therapy; complete response rates in the range of 70% to 90% have been observed in CD19+ cancers: ALL, chronic lymphocytic leukemia, and diffuse large B-cell lymphoma (Figure 1). Challenges of CAR T-cells include issues with uncontrolled immune cell activation, killing of normal

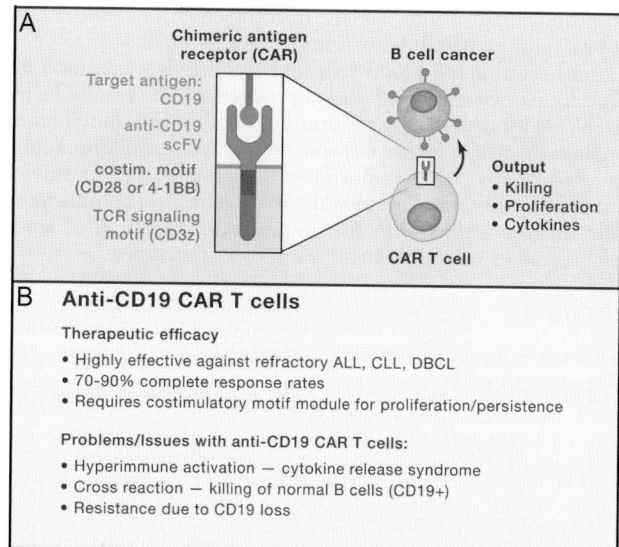

Figure 1 Chimeric antigen receptor T cells. Reprinted with permission from Lim WA, June CH: The principles of engineering immune cells to treat cancer, *Cell* 168:724–740, 2017.)

[1]Not FDA approved for this indication.

[1]Not available in the United States.

CD19+ B cells, and resistance due to loss of CD19 expression on leukemic cells (e.g., CD19-negative relapse). Whether CAR retargeting can be successfully applied to other hematologic targets beyond CD19 remains to be seen; results targeting the BCMA antigen in myeloma, CD22, and CD123 are promising.

Several novel antibodies have also recently been approved. Inotuzumab ozogamicin (Besponsa; targeting CD22 in B-ALL) and gemtuzumab ozogamicin (Mylotarg; targeting CD33 in AML) are antibody-drug conjugates that deliver the toxin calicheamicin to lymphoid or myeloid blasts, respectively. Blinatumomab (Blincyto) is a CD3-CD19 bispecific antibody. Bispecific agents targeting CD33, CD123, and CD20 are in ongoing clinical trials.

Monitoring

Measurement of residual disease is an important component of management in acute leukemia. It is not surprising that initial responsiveness to chemotherapy is a useful predictor for long-term outcome. Lack of early clearance of blasts (by days 7 to 14) has adverse prognostic value (especially in ALL). Persistence of abnormal karyotype after induction among patients in CR is also associated with poor clinical outcomes. For patients in morphologic CR, measurement of MRD is an emerging standard (ALL) and intensive research (AML) area. More sensitive methods of MRD measurement beyond light microscopy and cytogenetics are increasingly used to aid decision making. Examples of sensitive MRD assessment include immunophenotyping to detect minute populations of blasts or quantitative RT-PCR and other molecular methods to detect leukemia-associated molecular abnormalities. Particularly in B-ALL, early clearance of MRD is favorable. In ALL and in APL, MRD assessment is a very useful and reliable tool to assess prognosis, detect early relapse, and direct the initiation of additional therapy. In AML, MRD identifies high risk patients, but how to utilize that data to mitigate risk is not yet established in most cases. Specifically, quantitative measurement of mutated *NPM1* transcript levels during first remission provides important and potentially actionable information in that subset of AML.

Management of Complications

The treatment of acute leukemia involves repeated cycles of myelotoxic or immunosuppressive chemotherapy, requiring intensive supportive care. The emergence of infections with multidrug-resistant organisms is a growing concern. In addition, invasive fungal infections are associated with early death. Standard infection precautions include reverse isolation, air filtration, and prophylactic antimicrobials. Recommendations on the latter are best tailored based on institutional antibiograms.

Transfusion of red blood cells and platelets is a common and necessary part of treatment. Blood products should ideally be leukodepleted (done by the American Red Cross in the United States) to reduce the risk of febrile transfusion reaction and alloimmunization. Particularly in the multicourse induction and postremission therapies in ALL, it is clear that the management of complications while still proceeding with the on-time administration of subsequent therapies whenever possible improves outcomes.

References

Arber DA, Orazi A, Hasserjian R, et al: The 2016 revision to the World Health Organization classification of myeloid neoplasms and acute leukemia, *Blood* 127:2391–2405, 2016.

Brown AL, Churpek JE, Malcovati L, et al: Recognition of familial myeloid neoplasia in adults, *Semin Hematol* 54:60–68, 2017.

Ding L, Ley TJ, Larson DE, et al: Clonal evolution in relapsed acute myeloid leukaemia revealed by whole-genome sequencing, *Nature* 481:506–510, 2012.

Döhner H, Estey E, Grimwade D, et al: Diagnosis and management of AML in adults: 2017 ELN recommendations from an international expert panel, *Blood* 129:424–447, 2017.

Iacobucci I, Mullighan CG: Genetic basis of acute lymphoblastic leukemia, *J Clin Oncol* 35:975–983, 2017.

Lim WA, June CH: The principles of engineering immune cells to treat cancer, *Cell* 168:724–740, 2017.

Maude SL, Frey N, Shaw PA, et al: Chimeric antigen receptor T cells for sustained remissions in leukemia, *N Engl J Med* 371:1507–1517, 2014.

National Comprehensive Cancer Network (NCCN): Clinical practices guidelines in oncology, Available at NCCN.org [Accessed February 2018].

Papaemmanuil E, Gerstung M, Bullinger L, et al: Genomic classification and prognosis in acute myeloid leukemia, *N Engl J Med* 374:2209–2221, 2016.

TCGA Research Network, Ley TJ, Miller C, et al: Genomic and epigenomic landscapes of adult de novo acute myeloid leukemia, *N Engl J Med* 368:2059–2074, 2013.

Welch JS, Ley TJ, Link DC, et al: The origin and evolution of mutations in acute myeloid leukemia, *Cell* 150:264–278, 2012.

BLOOD COMPONENT THERAPY AND TRANSFUSION REACTIONS

Method of
Theresa Nester, MD

CURRENT DIAGNOSIS

- Fever greater than 1°C rise during or within 4 hours after transfusion should prompt evaluation of the patient and consideration of a transfusion reaction.
- Fever and pain are the most common manifestations of an acute hemolytic transfusion reaction.
- The point of the transfusion reaction laboratory investigation is to evaluate for hemolysis, either intravascular or extravascular. The majority of reactions are negative for hemolysis.
- The differential diagnosis of a transfusion reaction with respiratory symptoms includes febrile nonhemolytic and circulatory overload (common), allergic or anaphylactic reaction, transfusion-related acute lung injury, acute hemolytic reaction, and bacterial contamination (rare).

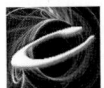

CURRENT THERAPY

- The decision to transfuse red blood cells to a patient should depend more on the clinical state of the patient than on an absolute trigger for hemoglobin or hematocrit.
- A transfusion trigger of less than 7 g/dL is recommended for hospitalized adult patients who are hemodynamically stable, including critically ill patients. A transfusion trigger of 8 g/dL is recommended for patients undergoing orthopedic or cardiac surgery, as well as those with preexisting cardiovascular disease.
- For severe autoimmune hemolytic anemia, maintenance of hemoglobin at greater than 4 g/dL in younger patients and greater than 6 g/dL in older patients or patients with cardiovascular disease is appropriate.
- Platelets are not typically indicated in thrombotic thrombocytopenic purpura, autoimmune thrombocytopenic purpura (ITP), and heparin-induced thrombocytopenia (HIT) unless the patient has significant bleeding.
- Currently available coagulation tests are not very useful for predicting bleeding in patients with end-stage liver disease. These patients establish a new equilibrium between coagulation, anticoagulation, and fibrinolysis that results in relatively less bleeding than predicted by the international normalized ratio.
- The goal during massive transfusion scenarios should be to prevent marked acidosis, hypothermia, and coagulopathy. The latter is often achieved with replacement of coagulation factors using plasma or cryoprecipitate within the first hour of the resuscitation.
- Cryoprecipitate is useful as a source of concentrated fibrinogen. In a patient who is actively bleeding and has a fibrinogen less than 100 mg/dL, cryoprecipitate is indicated.
- Fibrinogen concentrates are available for select patient populations.

Therapeutic Use of Blood Components

The community blood supply depends on two types of donors: whole blood donors and apheresis donors. Units of whole blood are centrifuged and then separated into components within a closed system. Using apheresis techniques, individual components of whole blood can be collected. Citrate is used to keep blood components from clotting.

The decision to transfuse blood to a patient should always include a consideration of the risks versus the benefits. Risks of transfusion-transmitted diseases are small with current testing standards. Transfusion reactions do occur; the most common ones are not life-threatening unless the patient cannot tolerate tachycardia or hypertension. Rarely, a patient experiences a life-threatening reaction. Thus it is important to ensure that the need for the blood component outweighs the risks. Additionally, in a bleeding patient, it is important to check coagulation parameters (platelet count, prothrombin time [PT], international normalized ratio [INR], activated partial thromboplastin time [aPTT], fibrinogen) in addition to hematocrit (Hct) to ensure that the component that will best address the bleeding is being used.

Red Blood Cells
Indications
Red blood cells should be given to increase oxygen-carrying capacity. The hemoglobin (Hb) and Hct levels alone should not be used to determine the need for transfusion; instead, the patient's clinical picture should drive the decision to transfuse. The patient's intravascular volume status, cardiopulmonary function, and baseline vital signs in the presence of anemia should all be considered. When anemia has persisted over weeks and months, large volume transfusion is often not indicated because compensatory mechanisms have had time to work.

Transfusion Triggers
The most recent clinical practice guideline from AABB (formerly known as the American Association of Blood Banks) has the following recommendations: in hospitalized adult patients who are hemodynamically stable, including critically ill patients, a transfusion threshold of 7 g/dL is acceptable. In patients undergoing orthopedic or cardiac surgery, and those with preexisting cardiovascular disease, a transfusion threshold of 8 g/dL is recommended. The recommendations do not apply to patients with acute coronary syndrome, severe thrombocytopenia, or chronic transfusion dependent anemia, because of insufficient evidence.

Dosage
One unit of packed red blood cells will increase the hemoglobin by 1 g/dL and hematocrit by 3% in the patient who is not bleeding or experiencing hemolysis (Table 1).

Autoimmune Hemolytic Anemia
Special Situation
When the autoantibody responsible for autoimmune hemolytic anemia reacts at body temperature, all red blood cell units can appear incompatible. This is because the antibody binds to an epitope common to all red blood cells, such as the band 3 protein. The clinician needs to decide when to transfuse the (apparently) incompatible units. In a patient who has never received a transfusion or been pregnant, there is little possibility of red blood cell alloantibodies in circulation, and the chance of hemolysis (beyond that being caused by the autoantibody) is low. For the patient who has received a transfusion or who has been pregnant in the past, the risk that a circulating red blood cell alloantibody is present and is being masked by the autoantibody is higher; special studies are available to reduce the risk of an alloantibody being overlooked. The transfusion trigger depends on whether the anemia is acute or chronic. For acute severe anemia, maintenance of hemoglobin at greater than 4 g/dL in younger patients and greater than 6 g/dL in older patients or patients with cardiovascular disease is appropriate.

TABLE 1 Component Therapy: Dosage and Expected Increment

COMPONENT	DOSE	EXPECTED INCREMENT	AVERAGE VOLUME
Red blood cells	1 unit	Hct 3%, Hb 1 g/dL	250 mL
Whole blood platelets	1 unit	Platelet count increased by 5000–10,000/μL	50 mL/unit (1 pool of 6 = 300 mL)
Apheresis platelet	1 unit	Platelet count increased by 20,000–60,000/μL	300 mL/unit
Plasma	10 mL/kg	Factor levels increased by 20%	300 mL/unit
Cryoprecipitate	1 unit	Fibrinogen increased by 5 mg/dL	15 mL/unit
Prepooled cryoprecipitate	1 6-unit pool	Fibrinogen increased by 45 mg/dL	120 mL/pool

Abbreviations: Hb = hemoglobin; Hct = hematocrit.

Platelets
Platelets are required as part of normal clotting. The first stage of clot formation is development of a platelet plug over the site of endothelial injury.

Indications
The indications for platelet transfusion may be divided into prevention of bleeding and treatment of bleeding in the setting of thrombocytopenia or platelet dysfunction.

Transfusion Triggers
Prevention of Bleeding. In a stable patient with normal platelet function, transfusion is appropriate if the platelet count is less than 10,000/μL. One randomized, controlled trial has shown that transfusion at platelet counts of 5000/μL to 10,000/μL prevents bleeding in the stable patient. In a stable patient with other hemostatic abnormalities (e.g., on anticoagulation), transfusion is appropriate with a platelet count less than 50,000/μL.

Before a planned invasive procedure such as open lung biopsy, transfusion is appropriate with a platelet count of <50,000/μL. For lumbar puncture, consensus guidelines suggest that a platelet count of 50,000/μL is appropriate, although there are a few large studies suggesting that counts between 20,000 and 50,000/μL may be adequate. A patient undergoing major surgery should receive platelets if the count is less than 50,000 to 100,000/μL. The transfusion should take place as close to the procedure as possible so the platelets remain in circulation while the procedure is occurring.

Treatment of Bleeding. Platelets may be transfused with a major hemorrhage (e.g., gastrointestinal or genitourinary) and a platelet count less than 30,000 to 50,000/μL. For bleeding with major surgery or trauma, transfusion is appropriate for counts less than 80,000/μL. For bleeding into critical areas (e.g., central nervous system bleeding or diffuse alveolar hemorrhage), platelets may be given for counts less than 100,000/μL.

Dosage
Dosage is determined on the basis of the baseline platelet count, desired platelet count, and estimated blood volume. For a 70-kg patient, 3×10^{11} platelets (four to six units of pooled whole blood platelets or one unit of apheresis platelets) increases platelet count by approximately 30,000 to 50,000/μL in the absence of alloimmunization or excessive consumption. For prophylactic therapy, lower dosages have been shown to be as effective as higher dosages in the prevention of bleeding.

Out of ABO Group Platelet Transfusion

Because platelets can only be stored for a maximum of 7 days following collection, and the community platelet supply is collected from volunteer donors, a platelet product that is identical to the patient's ABO type might not be available (Table 2 and Box 1). Thus it may be necessary to infuse a small volume of incompatible plasma (suspending the platelets) to the patient. There is therefore a small risk of hemolysis of the patient's red blood cells if the isoagglutinin (anti-A or anti-B) titer in the donated plasma is high. Studies of healthy blood donors indicate that these antibody titers are typically low and do not precipitate hemolysis. Transfusion services often have policies that limit the amount of incompatible plasma a patient has received with platelet transfusion. Alternatively, some centers measure the antibody titer in the donated product and give high-titer products only to patients whose red blood cells lack the corresponding ABO antigen.

Unresponsiveness to Platelet Transfusion

A number of clinical factors can result in a patient's less-than-optimal response to platelet transfusion. In addition to consumption, some of these factors include splenomegaly, fever, and antifungal therapy. Patients who have been sensitized to foreign human leukocyte antigens through prior pregnancy or transfusion can also have a poor response to platelet transfusion. Transfusion medicine consultation regarding the evaluation of refractoriness to platelet transfusion may be indicated.

Special Situations

Uremia. Patients who are dialysis dependent might have an acquired platelet defect as a result of the uremic environment. Transfusion of platelets into this environment will render the transfused platelets dysfunctional. Thus if optimal platelet function is desired, dialysis should be performed frequently. Consider performing dialysis without heparin if the patient is actively bleeding.

Purpura and Thrombocytopenia. In patients with autoimmune thrombocytopenic purpura (ITP), thrombotic thrombocytopenic purpura (TTP), or heparin-induced thrombocytopenia (HIT), platelet transfusion is not indicated unless the patient has significant bleeding. Other therapies, such as steroid administration for ITP and plasma exchange for TTP, should be initiated to address the condition.

Plasma

Plasma contains all of the coagulation proteins needed for clot formation, as well as all of the fibrinolytic proteins that prevent systemic thrombosis. There are currently several kinds of plasma, such as fresh frozen, FP24, thawed, and liquid. All contain hemostatic levels of coagulation factors as long as they are stored appropriately. The effect of plasma transfusion on the PT and INR is 4 to 6 hours, owing to the short half-life of coagulation factor VII. Thus other, longer-lasting means of restoring coagulation factors, such as vitamin K administration, should be undertaken if a more durable response is desired.

When replacing coagulation factors with plasma, it is not necessary to have 100% factor replacement as the goal. Hemostasis is typically able to occur if circulating coagulation factor levels are between 40% and 50%. It is important to understand that the relationship between the INR and the percentage factor level is a logarithmic, rather than a linear, relationship (Figure 1). Thus whether the INR is 9 or 1.8, the initial dosage of plasma should be 10 to 20 mL/kg, with recheck of the laboratory values a few minutes after infusion. The more prolonged the INR, the more significant the impact of the dose on the INR.

Transfusion Triggers

For bleeding or imminent surgery that cannot be corrected in a timely manner by vitamin K administration, use plasma to correct an INR greater than 1.8 to 2.0. The exception is patients with end-stage liver disease (see later).

Dosage

At a dosage of 10 mL/kg, each unit has an average of 300 mL (3–5 units in a 70-kg adult). This dosage should increase circulating coagulation factors by 20% immediately after infusion.

Special Situations

Liver Disease. The INR is a less useful test in patients with end-stage liver disease. The destruction of liver tissue leads to decreased production of coagulation and fibrinolytic proteins such that a new balance is established. Patients with end-stage liver disease have been shown to have normal levels of circulating thrombin and reduced levels of certain anticoagulant proteins (e.g., protein C), which could explain why they do not bleed as often as predicted with the elevation in INR. Thus the prophylactic use of plasma to correct a mildly prolonged laboratory value in the absence of bleeding is not indicated. It will lead to unnecessary plasma infusion, and the risk of volume overload and transfusion reactions outweighs the benefit in these patients.

Massive Transfusion. In trauma patients, patients with ruptured aortic aneurysms, and patients with other arterial bleeding, massive transfusion may be necessary. The basic principles of such a scenario include taking steps early into the resuscitation to

TABLE 2	ABO Compatibility*		
PATIENT'S ABO	**ANTIBODIES IN CIRCULATION**	**COMPATIBLE PACKED RED BLOOD CELLS**	**COMPATIBLE PLASMA**
O	anti-A, anti-B	O	O, A, B, AB
A	anti-B	O or A	A or AB
B	anti-A	O or B	B or AB
AB	None	O, A, B, AB	AB

*For platelet compatibility, see text.

BOX 1	Rh(D) compatibility

Rh(D) negative patients should receive Rh negative red blood cells and platelet units.*†

Rh(D) positive patients can receive Rh positive or Rh negative red blood cells and platelet units.

Rh compatibility does not apply to acellular components (plasma and cryoprecipitate).

Only 15% of blood donors are Rh negative.

* In times of shortage, it becomes necessary to preserve the Rh(D) negative red blood cell inventory for females of childbearing potential (< 50 years old).

† Platelet components contain very few red blood cells; Rho(D) immune globulin (RhoGAM) may be administered if prevention of anti-D formation is deemed appropriate. Consult with a transfusion medicine physician if further discussion is needed.

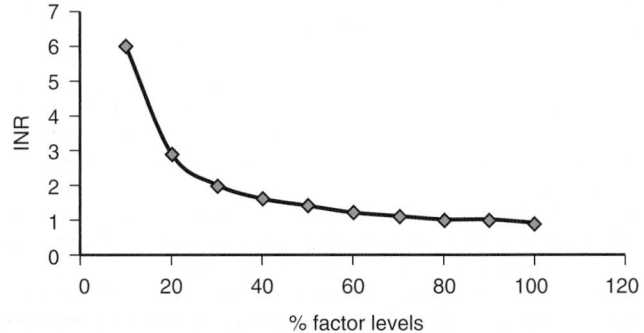

Figure 1 American Association of Blood Banks international normalized ratio (INR) compared with percentage factor levels. Reprinted with permission from Nester T, AuBuchon J: Hemotherapy decisions and their outcomes. In Roback JD (ed): AAB Technical Manual, 17th ed. Bethesda, MD, American Association of Blood Banks, 2011, p 592.

prevent the patient from becoming too cold, acidotic, or coagulopathic to reverse the situation. Some plasma (and cryoprecipitate, if the fibrinogen is very low) should be infused early into the resuscitation to help prevent coagulopathy. Red blood cells and plasma should be infused through a blood warmer, if possible.

Isolated Prolonged aPTT. Other than a deficiency in coagulation factor XI, bear in mind that the differential of an isolated prolonged aPTT includes entities that do not typically require plasma (refer to Figure 2). Hemophilia A, hemophilia B, and von Willebrand disease are no longer treated by plasma but can require factor concentrates to prevent bleeding. Systemic administration of heparin must be reversed by protamine, if fast reversal is desired. Note that plasma transfusion will not reverse the effect of heparin. One of the most common causes of a prolonged aPTT is a lupus anticoagulant; this is an antibody directed against phospholipids that typically leads to thrombosis rather than hemorrhage.

Intracranial Hemorrhage or Life-Threatening Bleeding. Reversal of anticoagulation in the setting of intracranial hemorrhage or life-threatening bleeding depends on the anticoagulant. For patients taking warfarin (Coumadin), refer to Box 2.

Prothrombin complex concentrates (PCCs) may be used to replenish factors II, VII, IX, and X rapidly. For reversal of dabigatran (Pradaxa), a direct oral anticoagulant (DOAC), idarucizumab (Praxbind) is approved by the Food and Drug Administration (FDA) as a reversal agent. KCentra is a 4-factor PCC that has been FDA approved to treat life-threatening hemorrhage in adult patients on warfarin. For reversal of apixaban (Eliquis) and rivaroxaban (Xarelto) in life-threatening bleeding, andexanet alfa (Andexxa) is available.

Cryoprecipitate

Cryoprecipitate contains fibrinogen, coagulation factors VIII and XIII, and von Willebrand factor. The most common current use is as a source of concentrated fibrinogen. It may also be used to treat hemorrhage in the rare patient with factor XIII deficiency.

Indications

Clinical scenarios that increase probability for low fibrinogen include any clinical situation where disseminated intravascular coagulation (DIC) may be present. These include obstetric bleeding, trauma involving head injury or crush injury, and sepsis. Clinical events that can lead to an isolated decrease in serum fibrinogen concentration include administration of L-asparaginase (Elspar) and surgeries that disrupt bladder or salivary gland endothelium. Fibrinogen concentrates are available for patients who will not accept cryoprecipitate.

Transfusion Triggers

Transfusion is appropriate in patients with low serum fibrinogen, typically less than 100 mg/dL. In cases of massive transfusion, a trigger of 150 mg/dL is considered practical, so that the patient becomes less coagulopathic in the time that it takes to draw and review new laboratory values. New evidence indicates that a fibrinogen level of less than 300 mg/dL predicts severe postpartum hemorrhage, as a normal postpartum fibrinogen level is in the 600 mg/dL range. Because component therapy aims to replete coagulation factors to hemostatic (rather than completely normal) levels, consensus guidelines suggest maintaining a fibrinogen level greater than 200 mg/dL during a postpartum hemorrhage.

Dosage

Dosage depends on the type of cryoprecipitate available. If the product requires resuspension in saline before pooling, then one unit (average 15 mL volume) will increase fibrinogen by 5 mg/dL. If the product has been pooled in plasma before freezing, then one unit will increase fibrinogen by 7 to 8 mg/dL; a six-unit pool will increase fibrinogen by 45 mg/dL. Check with the transfusion service laboratory regarding which product is available and the expected increment.

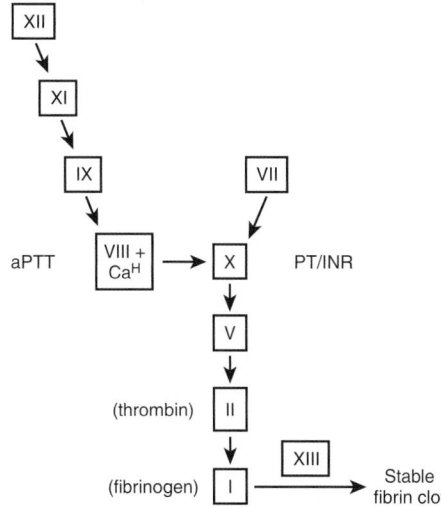

In vitro coagulation cascade (simplified)

Figure 2 Coagulation cascade.

BOX 2 Guidelines for Correction of Excessive Warfarin Anticoagulation

INR Higher than Therapeutic but <5, No Significant Bleeding
Lower anticoagulant dosage.
Temporarily discontinue drug, if necessary.

INR >5 but <9, No Significant Bleeding
Omit 1 or 2 doses, monitor INR, resume when INR is in therapeutic range.
Alternative if patient is at increased risk of hemorrhage:
• Omit 1 dose
• Give 1–2.5 mg vitamin K orally.
For rapid reversal before urgent surgery:
• Give 2–4 mg vitamin K orally.
• Give 1–2 mg at 24 hours if INR remains elevated.

INR >9, No Significant Bleeding
Omit warfarin; give 2.5–5.0 mg vitamin K orally.
Closely monitor INR; give additional vitamin K, if necessary.
Resume warfarin at lower dose when INR is within therapeutic range.

Serious Bleeding at Any Elevation of INR
Omit warfarin.
Give 10 mg vitamin K by slow IV infusion.
Supplement with plasma or prothrombin complex concentrate depending on urgency of correction.
Vitamin K infusions may be repeated every 12 hours.

Life-Threatening Hemorrhage
Omit warfarin.
Give prothrombin complex concentrate with 10 mg vitamin K by slow IV infusion.
Repeat as necessary, depending on INR.

Abbreviation: INR = international normalized ratio.
From Nester T, AuBuchon J: Hemotherapy decisions and their outcomes. In Roback JD (ed): AAB Technical Manual, 17th ed. Bethesda, MD, American Association of Blood Banks, 2011, p 571–616.

Special Situation

DIC is a state where fibrinogen is consumed at a faster rate than other circulating coagulation factors. This is because DIC is typically a thrombin-generating process (thrombin cleaves fibrinogen into fibrin for clot formation). Thus, although all coagulation factors are being consumed in DIC, timely repletion of fibrinogen by use of cryoprecipitate can result in more-timely cessation of bleeding in a patient with active DIC. The target value is fibrinogen at least 100 mg/dL. If the PT and INR are still prolonged with fibrinogen greater than 100 mg/dL, administration of plasma will replete other coagulation factors being consumed.

Transfusion Reactions

Reactions to transfusion are relatively common; life-threatening reactions are rare (Tables 3 and 4).

Because fever is a feature of both common and dangerous reactions, a transfusion reaction evaluation should be initiated with fever greater than 1°C above patient's baseline temperature at the start of the transfusion. The infusion of product should cease, at least until the laboratory results are known and the patient has responded to treatment. The main point of the laboratory investigation is to evaluate the plasma for abnormal (usually red) color in an effort to detect intravascular hemolysis as quickly as possible. If the clerical check and hemolysis direct antiglobulin tests are negative, one might consider restarting the transfusion with careful surveillance of the patient. A direct antiglobulin test is performed to detect the presence of antibody coating red blood cells in circulation; a positive result could indicate extravascular hemolysis, which is not as dangerous as intravascular hemolysis.

Most-Common Reactions
Febrile Nonhemolytic Reaction

Presentation. A febrile nonhemolytic transfusion reaction manifests as fever greater than a 1°C rise above the patient's baseline, often accompanied by rigors. Hypertension, tachypnea, and transient decrease in oxygen saturation can also occur until the symptoms are treated. Evidence of hemolysis will be absent on laboratory evaluation. These reactions can manifest during or 2 to 3 hours after the transfusion.

Pathophysiology. Cytokines produced by white blood cells present in cellular blood components (red blood cell and platelet units) are responsible for the clinical presentation. Platelets also secrete cytokines; thus leukoreduction of platelet units might not be successful in preventing the reaction.

Acute Management. Administration of an antipyretic is the routine treatment; meperidine (Demerol)[1] may be required to address severe rigors. Slow IV push of 25 mg as a first dose is recommended; an additional 25-mg dose can be given 10 to 15 minutes later if rigors persist.

[1]Not FDA approved for this indication.

TABLE 3	Transfusion Reactions	
MOST-COMMON REACTIONS	**INCIDENCE**	
Allergic reaction of mild severity	1:33 to 1:100	
Febrile nonhemolytic reaction	1:100 to 1:1000 with leukocyte reduction	
Transfusion-related circulatory overload	< 1:100	
MOST DANGEROUS REACTIONS	**INCIDENCE**	
Acute hemolytic reaction	1:38,000 to 1:70,000	
Anaphylactic reaction	1:20,000 to 1:50,000	
Transfusion-related acute lung injury	1:1200 to 1:190,000	
Bacterial contamination of red cell unit with gram-negative organisms	1:1,000,000	

TABLE 4	Transfusion Reactions with Respiratory Symptoms		
REACTION	**CLASSIC SIGNS**	**RELATIVE FREQUENCY**	**ACUTE MANAGEMENT (TRANSFUSION STOPPED IN ALL CASES)**
Febrile nonhemolytic reaction	Transient tachypnea in the presence of rigors and fever	Common	Antipyretic ± meperidine (Demerol)[1]
Circulatory overload	Hypoxia Crackles in lower lung fields Increased BP Chest radiograph consistent with volume overload	Common	Diuresis
Allergic reaction of moderate severity	Wheezes Possible perioral or periorbital edema Possible hives	Uncommon	IV antihistamines and possibly epinephrine (Adrenalin)
Allergic reaction of marked severity	Wheezes, swollen lips, tongue, uvula Stridor or other signs of airway compromise Very decreased BP	Rare	Epinephrine IV fluids and airway management Bronchodilators and glucagon (GlucaGen)[1] for patient on β-blockers
Transfusion-related acute lung injury	Tachypnea and hypoxia during or within 6 of transfusion Persisting for several hours Chest radiograph consistent with bilateral white out	Rare	Respiratory support of noncardiogenic pulmonary edema
Acute hemolytic reaction	Red urine and red serum Hypotension and diffuse oozing may be present Tachypnea (10% of patients)	Rare	Supportive (possibly ICU) care Administration of crystalloid solution Blood component therapy if DIC is present
Bacterial contamination with Gram-negative organism	Very decreased BP Fever Nausea, vomiting Possible tachypnea	Rare	Intensive care for support of Gram-negative sepsis

Abbreviations: BP = blood pressure; DIC = disseminated intravascular coagulation; ICU = intensive care unit.
[1]Not FDA approved for this indication.

Prevention with Future Transfusion. Antipyretic may be administered prior to transfusion. Ordering leukoreduced red blood cells and platelets (if the hospital inventory is not entirely composed of leukoreduced components) is also a preventive measure. For recurring reactions with platelets, volume reduction of the component can reduce the incidence.

Allergic Reaction of Mild Severity

Presentation. Urticaria or flushing occurs during a transfusion. Evidence of hemolysis is absent on laboratory evaluation.

Pathophysiology. Allergic reactions are immunoglobulin (Ig) E-mediated reactions against some allergen in the donor plasma. Because all blood components have some amount of plasma, it is possible to experience an allergic reaction with any blood product.

Acute Management. Slowing the infusion rate may be all that is required to alleviate the reaction. Antihistamine administration also addresses the symptoms.

Prevention with Future Transfusion. A reaction of this type may be a one-time event. For patients with recurrent reactions, transfusing the blood product more slowly (maximum of transfusion over 4 hours), or premedication with antihistamines will reduce the incidence.

Transfusion Associated Circulatory Overload (TACO)

Presentation. The patient has respiratory distress, typically during the transfusion, and increase in blood pressure unless cardiac decompensation occurs. Tachycardia, tachypnea, and decrease in oxygen saturation are often present. Jugular venous distension may be seen. Radiographic findings include pleural effusions, perihilar edema, and increased vascular pedicle width.

Pathophysiology. The reaction results in cardiogenic pulmonary edema.

Acute Management. Diuretic should be administered. Supplemental oxygen may be required temporarily to improve oxygen saturation.

Prevention with Future Transfusion. Slowing the infusion rate with a maximum time of transfusion over 4 hours can prevent the reaction. Diuretic administration may be necessary in patients with poor heart function.

Most-Dangerous Reactions

Acute Hemolytic Transfusion Reaction (AHTR)

Presentation. The most common signs include fever with or without rigors and pain. The more commonly reported sites of pain include flank, back, chest, or abdomen. Nausea and vomiting and dyspnea can also occur. In more severe presentations, hemodynamic instability is present, accompanied by oozing from line sites or petechial hemorrhage if DIC is occurring. Red or cola-colored urine is another manifestation of an acute hemolytic transfusion reaction and represents overwhelming of the renal capacity to recirculate free heme.

Pathophysiology. Red blood cells have proteins and carbohydrates on the cell surface that are antigenic. These epitopes are categorized into blood groups based on structure and sharing of a parent protein. A patient who lacks particular epitopes can develop antibodies through pregnancy or transfusion. Such red blood cell alloantibodies then lyse transfused red blood cells that possess the cognate antigen. When time allows for pretransfusion testing, the antibodies are identified, and antigen-negative units are provided. The ABO blood group system is unusual in that almost all patients older than 4 months have naturally occurring antibodies to the A and B antigens that they did not inherit. These antibodies are capable of activating complement and causing intravascular lysis when bound to their cognate antigen. Thus it is of utmost importance to avoid transfusing red blood cells against the ABO antibody in circulation. Refer to the ABO compatibility table (see Table 1).

Acute Management. Management is largely supportive. The end result of intravascular hemolysis and activation of the complement cascade can be shock, uncontrolled bleeding secondary to DIC, and renal failure. Therefore prompt infusion of intravenous crystalloid solutions are indicated to maintain blood pressure and renal perfusion. The goal for urine flow rate should be more than 1 mL/kg per hour. Coagulation laboratory values should be obtained to determine whether DIC is present; if so, component therapy to reverse the DIC is indicated. If the reaction is severe, intensive care is appropriate, because cardiac monitoring and mechanical ventilation may be necessary to support the patient.

Prevention with Future Transfusion. An acute hemolytic reaction is one of the most feared complications of transfusion. It is also often one of the most preventable. Great care should be given to the pretransfusion blood sample draw, comparing the label to the patient's unique identifiers, and labeling the tube at the patient's bedside as soon as the blood is in the tube. Just before transfusion, the unit label attached to the blood product should be compared with the patient's armband to ensure that the product is intended for this particular patient. To prevent intravascular hemolysis from antibodies directed against non-ABO antigens, pretransfusion testing (antibody screen or crossmatch) should be done in advance of the need for red cell transfusion for any patient whose clinical situation indicates a likelihood of needing blood. The exception is a patient who is hemodynamically unstable because of acute red blood cell loss, where uncrossmatched red blood cells are indicated. If the patient's identity is known, a call to the hospital transfusion service in this situation is warranted; explain that the patient needs uncrossmatched red blood cells and ask if there are transfusion records that indicate a need for antigen-negative units.

Allergic Reaction of Marked Severity (Anaphylaxis)

Presentation. Significant drop in blood pressure occurs, typically early into the transfusion. Wheezes, difficulty breathing, and stridor may be present. Tongue or facial edema and hives may be observed.

Pathophysiology. Anaphylaxis is an IgE-mediated reaction against an allergen in the donor plasma. In a patient with absolute IgA deficiency, naturally occurring anti-IgA can precipitate this reaction on binding IgA in the plasma. Anti-haptoglobin antibodies can also induce a severe reaction.

Acute Management. Airway and blood pressure support should be provided with the patient recumbent and the lower extremities elevated. The treatment of choice is epinephrine (Adrenalin) 1 mg/mL, also labeled as 1:1000 or 0.1%, using an adult dosage of 0.3 to 0.5 mg per single dose, typically administered intramuscularly to the mid-quadriceps area. If symptoms persist, the dose may be repeated every 5 to 15 minutes for a maximum of three times, unless palpitations, tremors, or extreme anxiousness occurs. Supplemental oxygen should be administered and the airway maintained. Intravenous fluid administration is also recommended. Bronchodilators such as albuterol can be given as adjunctive treatment for bronchospasm that does not appear to respond to epinephrine. For patients on β-blockers, the addition of intravenous glucagon[1] (GlucaGen) 1 to 5 mg administered over 5 minutes, followed by infusion of 5 to 15 µg/minute, may be required. The addition of glucocorticoids can help prevent the biphasic reaction that occurs in some patients.

Prevention with Future Transfusion. Slow administration with careful observation of any transfusion is required. Premedication with intravenous antihistamines is appropriate. Steroids may be administered, although their effectiveness has not been confirmed through controlled trials. Epinephrine should be available at the bedside. For severe allergic reactions, a discussion with the transfusion service physician regarding washed components is appropriate.

---

[1]Not FDA approved for this indication.

Transfusion-Related Acute Lung Injury

Presentation. The signs of transfusion-related acute lung injury (TRALI) are difficulty breathing, tachypnea, and hypoxia during or within 6 hours of a transfusion of any blood component. Ideally, signs of underlying lung disease or circulatory overload are absent. Chest radiograph may show diffuse bilateral opacities (white-out). Diuretic administration does not result in improvement. The hypoxemia can progress to the point that the patient requires mechanical ventilation, and thus the patient should be closely monitored while the reaction is occurring.

Pathophysiology. The factors that result in TRALI are not entirely known. In a portion of cases, antibodies against white blood cell antigens are present in donor plasma. These antibodies are believed to bind the cognate antigens on the patient's white blood cells, leading to degranulation and a capillary leak syndrome involving the lungs. Other theories regarding the pathophysiology of TRALI exist. One such theory implicates biologically active substances such as lipids and cytokines in the stored blood products. These substances are believed to prime the patient's granulocytes and activate pulmonary endothelium, setting the stage for an additional trigger to cause acute lung injury. Regardless of the cause of TRALI, the end result is an increase in pulmonary vascular permeability and noncardiogenic pulmonary edema. The estimated mortality rate from TRALI is 5% to 8%.

Acute Management. Management consists of supportive care, with particular regard to respiratory support. With adequate supportive care, the process most often reverses over 48 to 96 hours.

Prevention with Future Transfusion. Marked respiratory compromise is occasionally due to white blood cell antibodies in the patient, which bind cognate antigens in the donated red blood cells or platelet unit ("reverse TRALI"). In these cases, leukoreduction of cellular blood products may reduce the severity of subsequent transfusions, although solid evidence to support this is lacking. For TRALI caused by white blood cell antibodies in the donated product, there are no preventive measures for the clinician to take. The majority of US blood suppliers provide plasma from only male donors, in an effort to reduce the incidence of TRALI caused by multiparous women with white blood cell antibodies.

Bacterial Contamination of a Blood Component

Presentation. The most-common presentation includes fever and rigors, nausea and vomiting, and possible onset of moderate hypotension during or after a platelet transfusion. Rarely, presentation includes signs of overt septic shock, including marked hypotension, typically early into the transfusion of a red blood cell or platelet component. Bacterial contamination of plasma or cryoprecipitate is extremely rare.

Pathophysiology. The most-common organisms to contaminate a platelet product are gram-positive organisms such as *Staphylococcus epidermidis*. These organisms are thought to be introduced into the collection bag via a skin plug that results from phlebotomy using a large-gauge needle when sterilization of the phlebotomy site has been ineffective.

The most common organisms to contaminate a red blood cell unit are gram-negative, endotoxin-producing organisms such as *Yersinia enterocolitica*. This organism is introduced into the blood product as a result of asymptomatic bacteremia in the donor, from sources such as the gastrointestinal tract. The donor-screening questionnaire and vital sign assessment at the time of donation help to make collection from such a donor a very rare event. Transfusion of a bacterially contaminated red blood cell unit is most often a fatal event. It is important to remember that platelets can also be contaminated by the same gram-negative, endotoxin-producing organisms; in this case, signs of septic shock may be manifest.

Acute Management. Blood cultures from the patient should be drawn, and then prompt intravenous antibiotic administration should begin. Supportive care including inotropic agents and close nursing attention may be required.

Prevention with Future Transfusion. Bacterial contamination is associated with a donor product, and thus preventive measures for the patient do not apply. Blood suppliers perform bacterial detection tests on platelet components, and transfusion services have strict policies related to visual inspection of all blood products before they are issued to a patient-care area. However, these measures are not completely effective. The FDA recently approved pathogen inactivation technology for platelets, which may further lower the risk.

Other Reactions

Delayed Hemolytic Transfusion Reaction

Presentation. The main finding with a delayed hemolytic transfusion reaction is usually an unexplained decrease in hematocrit within 2 to 7 days after transfusion. The patient often remains symptom free unless the decline in hemoglobin is poorly tolerated. Jaundice can occur, and laboratory values consistent with hemolysis may be positive (elevated indirect bilirubin, elevated lactate dehydrogenase, decreased haptoglobin). Rarely, signs of intravascular hemolysis can occur.

Pathophysiology. The most common source of this reaction is a red blood cell alloantibody that the patient developed with prior transfusion or pregnancy; the antibody titer wanes over time such that pretransfusion testing does not detect the antibody. A unit of red blood cells positive for the cognate antigen is then transfused, and within a few days the patient's memory B cell response produces the antibody again. Transfused cells are then cleared, most often by an extravascular mechanism.

Acute Management. Most transfusion services have a policy to notify the clinician that a serologic delayed hemolytic transfusion reaction is present on testing a new plasma sample from the patient. If the patient's hematocrit has declined, it may be useful to determine a clinical correlation by obtaining the laboratory values just described. This is of particular importance when the distinction between hemolysis and bleeding will lead to different management strategies for the patient. Although extravascular clearance of hemoglobin is fairly well tolerated by the kidneys, the conservative approach is to increase renal perfusion with intravenous crystalloid solutions if possible.

Prevention with Future Transfusion. For a patient who routinely receives care through one hospital system, the transfusion service will keep a record of the red blood cell alloantibody and provide antigen-negative cells for transfusion. The prevention, then, is to plan ahead for transfusion when possible, so that fully compatible units can be provided. Uncrossmatched red blood cells may be positive for the cognate antigen.

Allergic Reaction of Moderate Severity

Presentation. The patient has labile blood pressure, either hyper- or hypotension, accompanied by at least one of the following: throat scratchiness, respiratory wheezes, or perioral or periorbital edema. Hives may be present. Gastrointestinal symptoms such as crampy abdominal pain may also be present.

Pathophysiology. This is an IgE-mediated reaction against an allergen in the plasma of the donated product.

Acute Management. Treatment is administration of intravenous antihistamines. If the respiratory component does not resolve, consider epinephrine administration and treat similarly to anaphylaxis (see previous section).

Prevention with Future Transfusion. Slower infusion of blood products can reduce further episodes of this type of reaction. If the patient is atopic, intravenous antihistamines may be administered as a premedication. If the patient requires chronic transfusion and experiences this type of reaction on a repeated basis, discussion with the transfusion service regarding washed components may be warranted.

Hypotensive Transfusion Reaction

Presentation. The patient has isolated hypotension (drop in systolic BP greater than 30 but less than 80 mm Hg) that responds quickly to cessation of the transfusion. The reaction classically occurs within the first 15 minutes of infusion of the blood product.

Pathophysiology. Pathophysiology is unclear. Some research indicates that the patient may have slower ability to metabolize bradykinin compared to other individuals.

Acute Management. Stop the transfusion.

Prevention with Future Transfusion. Prevention is unclear. In the author's experience, rate of infusion has a role. Slower infusion may help to prevent this type of reaction.

Transfusion Associated Dyspnea

Presentation. Mild respiratory distress that occurs within 24 hours of cessation of transfusion.

Pathophysiology. Pathophysiology is unclear.

Acute Management and Prevention with future transfusion. Management is supportive and prevention is unclear.

References

Abdel-Wahab OI, Healy B, Dzik WH: Effect of fresh-frozen plasma transfusion on prothrombin time and bleeding in patients with mild coagulation abnormalities, *Transfusion* 46:1279–1285, 2006.

Carson JL, Guyatt G, Heddle NM, et al: Clinical practice guidelines from the AABB: Red cell transfusion thresholds and storage, *JAMA* 316(19):2025–2035, 2016.

Carson JL, Stanworth SJ, Alexander JH, et al: Clinical trials evaluating red blood cell transfusion thresholds: An updated systematic review and with additional focus on patients with cardiovascular disease, *Am Heart J* 200:96–101, 2018.

Cuker A, Burnett A, Triller D: Reversal of direct oral anticoagulants: Guidance from the anticoagulation forum, *Am J Hematol* 94(6):697–709, 2019.

Cushman M, Lim W, Zakai NA: *2011 Clinical Practice Guide on Anticoagulant Dosing and Management of Anticoagulant-Associated Bleeding Complications in Adults*, Washington, DC, 2014, American Society of Hematology.

Kaufman RM, et al: Platelet transfusion: A clinical practice guideline from the AABB, *Ann Internal Med* 162(3):205–213, 2015.

Lisman T, Porte RJ: Rebalanced hemostasis in patients with liver disease: Evidence and clinical consequences, *Blood* 116:878–885, 2010.

Nester T, Jain S, Poisson J: *Hemotherapy decisions and their outcomes. AABB Technical Manual*, 18th ed, Bethesda, MD, 2014, AABB Press.

Savage WJ, Hod EA: Noninfectious complications of blood transfusion. In Fung MK, editor: *AABB Technical Manual*, ed 19th, Bethesda, MD, 2017, American Association of Blood Banks, pp 569–599.

Tummula R, et al: Specific antidotes against direct oral anticoagulants: a comprehensive review of clinical trials, *Int J Cardiol* 214:292–298, 2016.

CHRONIC LEUKEMIAS

Method of
Jatin Rana, MD; and Daniel Isaac, DO

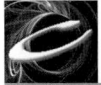

CURRENT DIAGNOSIS

Chronic Myelogenous Leukemia
- Clinical symptoms
  - Constitutional symptoms
  - Splenomegaly (abdominal discomfort, early satiety)
- Laboratory parameters
  - Elevated white blood cell count, ~100,000/μL, with differential consisting of various stages of granulocyte maturation from myeloblasts to mature neutrophils
  - Absolute basophilia
- Genetic parameters
  - Presence of *bcr-abl1* by cytogenetics, fluorescence *in situ* hybridization, or reverse transcriptase-polymerase chain reaction

Chronic Lymphocytic Leukemia
- Clinical symptoms
  - B symptoms (fevers, night sweats, weight loss)
  - Lymphadenopathy and/or organomegaly
  - Recurrent infections
- Laboratory parameters
  - Absolute lymphocytosis
  - Anemia
  - Thrombocytopenia
- Immunophenotypic analysis by flow cytometry
  - Monoclonal population of light-chain restricted mature B cells that express CD19, CD20(dim) and CD23 and co-expressing CD5

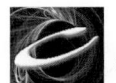

CURRENT THERAPY

Chronic Myelogenous Leukemia: Chronic Phase
- Front-line therapy
  - Imatinib mesylate (Gleevec) 400 mg daily
  - Dasatinib (Sprycel)
  - Nilotinib (Tasigna)
  - Bosutinib (Bosulif)
- Second-line therapy
  - Imatinib mesylate (Gleevec) 800 mg daily
  - Dasatinib (Sprycel)
  - Nilotinib (Tasigna)
  - Bosutinib (Bosulif)
  - Ponatinib (Iclusig)
  - Omacetaxine mepesuccinate (Synribo)
- High risk for failure
  - Allogeneic stem cell transplantation

Chronic Lymphocytic Leukemia
- Chemotherapy
  - Fludarabine (Fludara)
  - Cyclophosphamide (Cytoxan)
  - Chlorambucil (Leukeran)
  - Bendamustine (Treanda)
- Immunotherapy (monoclonal antibodies)
  - Rituximab (Rituxan)
  - Ofatumumab (Arzerra)
  - Obinutuzumab (Gazyva)
  - Alemtuzumab (Campath)
- Targeted therapy
  - Idelalisib (Zydelig)
  - Duvalisib (Copiktra)
  - Ibrutinib (Imbruvica)
  - Venetoclax (Venclexta)
  - Acalabrutinib (Calquence)

Chronic Myelogenous Leukemia

Chronic myelogenous leukemia (CML) is a myeloproliferative disorder with malignant clonal expansion and pathogenic leukemogenesis. It is defined by a translocation of chromosomes 9 and 22—the Philadelphia (Ph) chromosome—with the resultant formation of a fusion gene product *bcr-abl* (Figure 1). In 2001, the management of the disease changed dramatically with the approval and clinical use of imatinib mesylate (Gleevec), the first tyrosine kinase inhibitor (TKI) targeting the BCR-ABL1 oncoprotein.

Epidemiology and Risk Factors

The worldwide incidence of CML is 1 to 2 cases per 100,000 adults. In the United States, the disorder accounts for approximately 11% to 15% of all new adult cases of leukemia annually. CML is predominately a disorder of adults with the median age at diagnosis of 55 to 60 years. The disease has a slight predominance to males, with a male-to-female ratio of 1.4 to 1.0. The number of patients living with CML is expected to continually increase due to the successful management of the disorder with TKI therapy. Other than prior radiation exposure, little is known regarding potential risk factors. No specific genetic or familial predisposition to the pathogenesis of CML has been identified.

Pathogenesis

The reciprocal translocation between chromosomes 9 and 22 giving rise to the Ph chromosome is key to the pathogenesis of CML. There is an exchange of genetic material with a portion of the Abelson murine leukemia *(abl1)* gene on the long arm of chromosome 9 relocating next to the breakpoint cluster region *(bcr)* on the long arm of chromosome 22. The presence of the newly formed Ph chromosome (t9;22)(q34;q11.2) is a characteristic

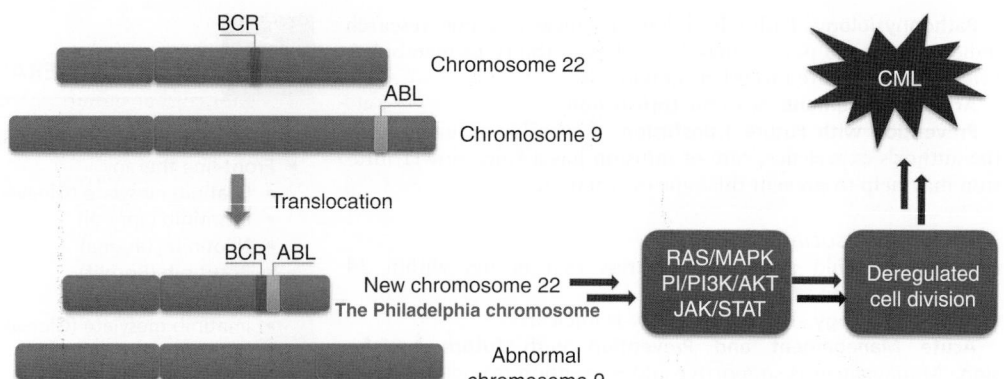

Figure 1 Schematic of the formation of Philadelphia chromosome (the new chromosome 22) and its physiological consequences. (From Chen, et al. *Protein Kinase Inhibitors as Sensitizing Agents for Chemotherapy*, Fig. 2.1. Elsevier, 2019.)

rearrangement seen in approximately 95% of CML cases. This leads to the creation of a hybrid oncogene *bcr-abl1*, which in turn translates into a BCR-ABL1 protein. There are three distinct breakpoint regions in the *BCR* gene each associated with a unique disease phenotype. The transcript from the most common breakpoint region (major breakpoint cluster region [M-BCR]) is translated into the p210BCR-ABL1 oncoprotein with the molecular consequence of constitutive tyrosine kinase activity. This leads to activation of signal-transduction proteins and upregulation of several key signaling pathways (RAS, JAK/STAT, and PI-3-kinase) with consequential alterations in cellular proliferation, differentiation, adhesion and survival.

The clinical course of CML can be divided into three distinct phases of the disorder: the chronic phase, in which the vast majority (90% to 95%) of patients are diagnosed, or the more aggressive accelerated and blast phases. The malignant clone acquires additional mutations with time with subsequent progression to the advanced phases of CML. The aberrations most commonly seen at the chromosomal level include trisomy 8, amplification of t(9,22), abnormalities in chromosome 17, trisomy 19, trisomy 21, and monosomy 7, which if present at diagnosis may have a negative prognostic impact on survival. Changes at the molecular level (e.g., *bcr-abl1* kinase domain mutations) are associated with clinical resistance to TKI therapy.

Clinical and Laboratory Characteristics

The malignant disorder of hematopoietic stem cells produces marked myeloid hyperplasia in the bone marrow and resultant uncontrolled proliferation of myeloid cells, erythroid cells and platelets in the peripheral blood. Up to 50% of CML patients in the United States are asymptomatic at diagnosis and have abnormalities only noted on routine physical examination or with the presence of abnormalities on a complete blood count (CBC). Clinical manifestations seen at presentation include fatigue, weight loss, splenomegaly leading to abdominal fullness and early satiety, malaise, and acute gouty arthritis. Laboratory findings include a markedly elevated white blood cell count (~100,000/μL) with a differential consisting of various stages of granulocyte maturation from myeloblasts to mature neutrophils. There is presence of absolute basophilia and often associated absolute eosinophilia. The findings of an elevated platelet count and anemia can be seen at presentation in approximately 20% to 30% and 50% of patients, respectively. High levels of lactate dehydrogenase (LDH) and uric acid can be seen due to increase cellular turnover associated with the disorder.

Without therapy, a patient in the chronic phase of CML will eventually progress to the more aggressive phases in 3 to 5 years. A consensus is lacking on the definition of accelerated phase; however, common features include an increase in the number of peripheral blood myeloblasts and basophils, development of low platelet counts, or discovery of additional clonal cytogenetic abnormalities. The definition of blast phase by the International Bone Marrow Transplant Registry (IBMTR) uses criteria of at least 30% blasts in the peripheral blood or bone marrow, or the presence of

extramedullary infiltrates of the clonal leukemic cells. The blast phase of CML presents clinically like acute leukemia (30% having a lymphoid morphology, 60% as acute myeloblastic leukemia, and the remainder as megakaryocytic or undifferentiated) with worsening constitutional symptoms, anemia and bleeding tendencies.

Diagnosis

Clinical suspicion of a CML diagnosis is made from a patient presenting with the typical laboratory abnormalities with or without any physical manifestations (see the Current Diagnosis box). Examination of a peripheral blood smear reveals increased neutrophils and immature circulating myeloid cells, increased basophils and eosinophils, normal to increased number of platelets, and possible normocytic anemia. Obtaining a bone marrow examination with aspirate is essential in the initial workup of a CML patient to appropriately stage the disorder and in assessing for the presence of the Ph chromosome by cytogenetics. The routine cytogenetic study is valuable to evaluate for clonal evolution denoted by the presence of additional karyotypic changes, which may poorly impact prognosis. Utilizing fluorescence *in situ* hybridization (FISH) or reverse transcriptase-polymerase chain reaction (RT-PCR) amplification studies for the detection of the *bcr-abl1* hybrid gene or its transcripts is important both as a baseline confirmatory test for CML and its continued monitoring. FISH analysis has the ability to detect the *bcr-abl1* molecular anomaly using specific probes targeting the chimeric oncogene among interphase nuclei in the peripheral blood. Qualitative RT-PCR can reveal the presence of bcr-abl1 transcripts, whereas continued monitoring of CML patients for the amount of residual disease can be assessed by obtaining quantitative RT-PCR levels. The techniques involving FISH analysis and RT-PCR have both demonstrated high concordance in simultaneous sampling of peripheral blood and bone marrow specimens.

Differential Diagnosis

At presentation, CML can be routinely differentiated from leukemoid reactions, which typically have lower white blood cell counts, absence of basophilia, and presence of Döhle's bodies and toxic vacuolation of granulocytes. Temporary extreme neutrophilia and associated left shift can be present after corticosteroid use. The detection of *bcr-abl1* can aid in differentiating CML from other myeloproliferative disorders (essential thrombocytosis, polycythemia vera), chronic neutrophilia leukemia, chronic myelomonocytic leukemia, chronic eosinophilia leukemia, chronic basophilic leukemia, or myelodysplastic syndromes. Rarely, patients can have *bcr-abl1* negative or atypical CML, in which additional mutations (*CSF3R, KRAS/NRAS, SETBP1*) may be present and are associated with a poor outcome.

Prognosis

The introduction of imatinib mesylate and additional TKIs in the 2000s has changed a dismal prognosis of CML into a manageable chronic disorder with a near normal lifespan. Prior to the current TKI-based era, the median survival for patients with CML was 5 to 7 years. Oral chemotherapeutics (hydroxyurea [Hydrea] and busulfan [Busulfex, Myleran]) and injectable interferon alfa (interferon alfa-2b [Intron A][1] and peginterferon alfa-2a [Pegasys][1]) were important in achieving hematologic remissions, reducing thrombotic complications, and increasing median survival. Allogeneic stem cell transplantation (allo-SCT) remains a vital option for patients with advanced phases of CML or following failure of multiple TKIs.

CML prognostic scoring systems (Sokal, Euro) have traditionally used basic hematologic data, spleen size, and age to stratify patients into risk groups. Compared to the prior conventional cytotoxic-based scoring systems (Sokal), the new EUTOS Long Term Survival (ELTS) score takes into consideration the current TKI treatment era and age does not hold such a negative impact in the scoring.

The mainstay of managing CML is the continuation of long-term TKI therapy to maintain a remission and has resulted in most patients achieving a normal life expectancy. More recently there has been a greater acceptance to the concept of TKI therapy discontinuation in carefully chosen patients, for example, chronic phase patients with a minimum TKI therapy duration of 3 years and sustained deep molecular remission of at least 1 year. In such patients, there is an emphasis on more frequent molecular testing and monitoring for adverse events associated with discontinuation (TKI withdrawal syndrome). The recent success of maintaining prolonged treatment-free remission (TFR) is promising. Importantly, in those that have lost a major molecular response (MMR), nearly all patients were able to regain their response with resumption of TKI treatment.

Monitoring Response to Tyrosine Kinase Inhibitor Therapy

First-line TKI use in CML is aimed at achieving a maximal reduction of leukemia burden with the goal of obtaining a complete cytogenetic response within 12 months of therapy initiation. Peripheral CBCs with differential are frequently ordered until a complete hematologic response is achieved. Quantitative RT-PCR (international scale, IS) is followed every 3 months to assess for residual *bcr-abl1* transcripts relative to *abl1* transcripts, and the degree of molecular response. Cytogenetics and FISH analysis can be helpful in patients with atypical translocations and atypical *bcr-abl1* transcripts, and in those with additional chromosome abnormalities. Milestones of hematologic, cytogenetic, and molecular response to therapy and monitoring recommendations are summarized in Tables 1 and 2. Testing for *bcr-abl1* kinase mutations is recommended in patients who fail to achieve a timely optimal response or display resistance/loss of response to a first-line TKI. Salvage therapy consists of alternative TKI use or consideration of allo-SCT for advanced phases of CML.

Treatment

There are currently four tyrosine-kinase inhibitors approved for front-line CML: imatinib (Gleevec), dasatinib (Sprycel), nilotinib (Tasigna), and bosutinib (Bosulif). Each of these TKI therapeutic agents are acceptable options for a patient with newly diagnosed chronic phase CML. The decision of which TKI to choose is dependent on a variety of factors including patient comorbidities, drug toxicity profile, cost, and disease characteristics.

In 2001, the development of imatinib mesylate (Gleevec) changed the treatment landscape for patients with CML. The first generation TKI was established as the standard of care for front-line patients with chronic phase CML following the International Randomized Study of Interferon Alpha Versus STI571 (IRIS). A total of 1106 patients with chronic phase CML were randomized to receive imatinib (400 mg daily) versus interferon alfa (Intron-A)[1] (5 million units/m^2 daily) plus low-dose cytarabine (Cytosar) (20 mg/m^2 daily for 10 days per month). At 18 months, the imatinib arm was found to have superior outcomes including tolerability, hematologic responses, complete cytogenetic response (76.2% vs. 14.5%, $P < .001$), and freedom from progression to advanced phase (accelerated or blast) CML (96.7% vs. 91.5%, $P < .001$). Long-term outcomes revealed that the imatinib assigned group had an overall survival rate of 83.3%, a cumulative complete cytogenetic response rate of 83%, and a 10-year MMR rate of 93%. Due to the high crossover rate from the interferon alfa plus cytarabine arm, no comparative survival benefit was seen with the use of the TKI.

The suggested starting dose of imatinib is 400 mg once daily taken with a meal. Higher doses (600 mg daily or 800 mg daily) are associated with increased toxicity without proven overall survival benefit. Although well tolerated by most patients, common side effects include superficial edema, muscle cramps, abdominal pain, nausea, rash, and diarrhea. Patients should be routinely assessed for low blood counts (cytopenias), and those with liver or kidney impairment may require closer monitoring and dose adjustments. Since its introduction, the cost of brand-name imatinib has risen from $30,000 per year to an annual price of $140,000, illustrating the financial toxicity associated with potential long-term TKI based therapy for CML. Since 2015, the availability of generic imatinib has reduced the annual cost in the United States, albeit the price remains higher compared to other regions of the world.

Second generation TKIs approved for frontline chronic phase CML include dasatinib (Sprycel), nilotinib (Tasigna), and bosutinib (Bosulif). Compared to the use of imatinib, these agents have demonstrated faster and deeper responses, and less disease progression to the advanced accelerated and blast phases. Thus,

[1]Not FDA approved for this indication.

[1]Not FDA approved for this indication.

| TABLE 1 | Milestones for Treating Chronic Myelogenous Leukemia Expressed as BCR-ABL1 on the International Scale |

	OPTIMAL	WARNING	FAILURE
Baseline	NA	High-risk ACA, high-risk ELTS score	NA
3 months	≤10%	>10%	>10% if confirmed within 1–3 months
6 months	≤1%	>1%–10%	>10%
12 months	≤0.1%	>0.1%–1%	>1%
Any time	≤0.1%	>0.1%–1%, loss of ≤0.1% (MMR)*	>1%, resistance mutations, high-risk ACA

*Loss of MMR (BCR-ABL1 >0.1%) indicates failure after TFR.
For patients aiming at treatment-free remission, the optimal response (at any time) is BCR-ABL1 ≤0.01% (MR^4). A change of treatment may be considered if MMR is not reached by 36–48 months.
ACA, Additional chromosome abnormalities in Ph+ cells; *ELTS,* EUTOS long term survival score; *MMR,* major molecular response; *NA,* not applicable.
From Hochhaus A, Baccarani M, et al. European LeukemiaNet 2020 recommendations for treating chronic myeloid leukemia. *Leukemia.* 2020;34:966–984.

TABLE 2	European LeukemiaNet Definitions and Monitoring Recommendations		
	HEMATOLOGIC RESPONSE	**CYTOGENIC RESPONSE**	**MOLECULAR RESPONSE**
Definitions			
	Complete: Platelet count <450 × 10⁹/L WBC count <10 × 10⁹/L Differential without immature granulocytes and with <5% basophils Nonpalpable spleen	Complete: Ph+ 0% Partial: Ph+ <35% Minor: Ph+ 36–65% None: Ph+ >95%	Complete: transcript nonquantifiable and nondetectable Major: ≤0.10
Monitoring			
	Check every 2 wk until complete response achieved and confirmed, then every 3 mo unless otherwise required	Check at 3 and 6 mo, then every 6 mo until complete response achieved and confirmed; thereafter every 12 mo if molecular monitoring cannot be ensured; check always for occurrence of treatment failure or unexplained cytopenia	Check every 3 mo until major response is achieved; conduct mutation analysis in case of failure, suboptimal response, or increase in transcript level

Ph, Philadelphia chromosome; *WBC,* white blood cell.

Used with permission from Baccarani M, Saglio G, Goldman J, et al: Evolving concepts in the management of chronic myeloid leukemia: Recommendations from an expert panel on behalf of the European LeukemiaNet. *Blood* 108:1809–1820, 2006; Baccarani M, Cortes J, Pane F, et al: Chronic myeloid leukemia: an update of concepts and management recommendations of European LeukemiaNet. *J Clin Oncol* 27:6041–6051, 2009.

second generation TKIs may be the preferred choice for chronic phase CML patients with high-risk disease.

The phase III ENESTnd trial evaluated the efficacy and safety of nilotinib versus imatinib in 846 newly diagnosed chronic phase CML patients. Patients in the nilotinib (300 mg twice daily) arm were shown to have improved cumulative rates of MMR (77.7% vs. 62.5%, P < .0001) compared to imatinib 400 mg daily, with no difference in 10-year progression free survival (86.2% vs. 87.2%). There are increased rates of ischemic heart disease, ischemic cardiovascular events and peripheral artery disease among those treated with nilotinib, especially at a higher dose (400 mg twice daily). Additional adverse events associated with nilotinib therapy include elevation in blood glucose levels, headaches, rash, QTc prolongation, pancreatitis, and increased liver enzyme levels.

The DASISON was a randomized trial of 519 patients with frontline chronic phase CML assigned to dasatinib (100 mg daily) or imatinib (400 mg daily). Treatment with the second generation TKI demonstrated earlier and more robust MMR rates at 3 months (84% vs. 64%, P < .0001) and deeper molecular response with 4.5-log reduction of *bcr-abl1* transcripts (<0.0032 IS, MR4.5) (42% vs. 33%). Dasatinib therapy is associated with less nausea, rash, and muscle aches. Patients should be monitored for potential low blood counts and the development of pleural effusions. We await longer follow-up for a recent trial, which has shown effective activity of lower dose dasatinib (50 mg daily) with a more acceptable safety profile.

In the BFORE randomized trial, the bosutinib (400 mg daily) arm achieved significantly higher MMR rates (47% vs. 37%, P = .02) and complete cytogenetic response rates (77% vs. 66%, P = .007) at 12 months compared to imatinib (400 mg daily) therapy. There were similar rates of 2-year survival with both drugs. Patients taking the second generation TKI are more likely to experience gastrointestinal adverse effects (diarrhea, liver enzyme elevation), which may necessitate dose reductions and temporary holding of the medication.

The preference of using a second generation TKI as the initial treatment of chronic phase CML should be performed in the context of the available data, understanding the unique side effect profile of each drug, assessing cost-effectiveness of long-term treatment, and appropriate patient selection. The ability to achieve response milestones faster and with a deeper response (MR4.5 rates) displays the potential of using second generation TKIs for patients in whom eventual TKI discontinuation would be considered. The lack of overall survival benefit of these agents compared to imatinib seen in clinical trials could be secondary to effective salvage therapy.

Continuation of long-term therapy with TKIs can be difficult for the patient and provides additional challenges to the treating physician. Routine monitoring for and managing TKI-associated toxicities is as vital as regular assessment of disease response. Despite many short- and long-term toxicities from TKIs graded as mild, they have resulted in poorer quality-of-life patient reported scores and often can lead to treatment nonadherence. Newly prescribed medications should also be assessed for potential drug-drug interactions with the TKI, which may require dose adjustments.

Other Therapeutic Options

Patients on frontline TKI that fail to meet treatment response milestones, display intolerance to the medication, or have progression/relapse should be assessed for treatment adherence and evaluated for possible drug interaction impacting TKI metabolism. Bone marrow examination should be performed to ensure the patient has not progressed to an advanced phase of the disease. Often acquisition of novel point mutations in *bcr-abl1* leads to treatment resistance. Determining the type of mutation guides the appropriate switching to an alternative TKI. Most of the mutations displaying resistance to imatinib therapy can be overcome by the use of a second generation TKIs. These have the ability to once again achieve high rates of response, especially when compared to increased doses of imatinib (400 mg twice daily). The T315I mutation is a unique alteration, which confers resistance to all available second generation TKI. Ponatinib (Iclusig), a third generation TKI, is effective in heavily pretreated CML patients and is the only approved TKI with activity displayed against the T315I mutation. However, the drug at the approved dose (45 mg daily) is associated with considerable risk of vascular occlusive disease, thrombotic events, heart failure, and hepatotoxicity. Ongoing studies in patients with acquired T315I mutations are evaluating efficacy and tolerability with lower ponatinib dosing (15 or 30 mg daily) as well as the use of additional novel third-generation TKIs.

As the only curative option for patients with CML, an evaluation for allo-SCT candidacy is appropriate if optimal response is not achieved after two or more TKIs due to resistance, drug intolerance, or inadequate response to ponatinib for those harboring the T315I mutation. Patients with accelerated phase CML are treated initially with TKI therapy (second or third generation preferred) and early consideration of allo-SCT based on a lack of optimal response. Blast phase CML requires a more aggressive combined approach using the newer generation TKIs and intensive chemotherapy, followed by immediate allo-SCT in responders. For the advanced phases of the disease TKI therapy is typically administered at a higher starting dose: imatinib 600 mg daily for accelerated phase and 800 mg daily for blast phase, dasatinib 140 mg daily, nilotinib 400 mg twice daily, bosutinib 500 or 600 mg daily, and ponatinib 45 mg daily. In 2012, omacetaxine mepesuccinate (Synribo) subcutaneous injection was approved for patients with resistance or intolerance to two or more prior TKIs. The drug joins a list of potential palliative options including hydroxyurea, hypomethylating agents, cytarabine, and busulfan. Unfortunately, survival in end-phase CML is measured in months.

Chronic Lymphocytic Leukemia

Chronic lymphocytic leukemia (CLL) is a chronic, mature B-cell neoplasm and is the most common type of leukemia in Western countries. CLL is a heterogeneous disease and not all patients require treatment at the time of diagnosis, as randomized trials have failed to demonstrate a survival advantage with early treatment strategies. Molecular profiling and whole exome sequencing have led to improved understanding of the pathogenesis of CLL and significant improvements in our therapeutic approach. Historically, therapy for CLL included alkylating agents, purine analogues, and CD20 directed monoclonal antibodies. However, over the past several years the treatment approach to CLL has rapidly evolved with the advent of targeted agents such as Bruton tyrosine kinase (BTK) inhibitors, B cell leukemia/lymphoma 2 (BCL2) inhibitors, and phosphoinositide 3-kinase (PI3K) inhibitors. The development of such agents has led to significant improvement in outcomes for these patients including those with high-risk genomic aberrations that had historically been resistant to standard chemotherapies.

Epidemiology and Risk Factors

CLL accounts for approximately 30% of all leukemias in the United States. It is a disease of older adults with a median age at diagnosis of 70 years. CLL occurs more commonly in men than women with a male to female ratio of approximately 1.7:1. The incidence of CLL also varies by race with a higher incidence being seen in Caucasians. Furthermore, the incidence of CLL in Asian countries is quite low. While the exact reasons racial disparities exist are not clear, it appears that genetic factors are the most likely explanation. CLL does appear to be seen at a higher frequency among those with a first-degree family member with CLL. There are no clearly identified environmental or occupational risk factors. Most cases of CLL are preceded by development of monoclonal B-cell lymphocytosis (MBL). However, despite the presence of MBL only a small portion of patients will progress to CLL at a rate of 1% to 2% per year.

Pathogenesis

CLL is a disease of clonal B-cell lymphocytes arrested in B-cell differentiation. The pathogenesis of CLL is complex and many steps in the developmental pathway have yet to be elucidated. Nevertheless, the development of CLL appears to follow a two-step process in which one first develops MBL due to an unknown event (i.e., gene mutation, epigenetic changes, cytogenetic abnormalities, antigenic stimulation) resulting in proliferation of a clone of B-cells. A second event or "hit" occurs (i.e., further cytogenetic changes) leading to accumulation of the malignant clone and subsequent progression to CLL. Malignant cells accumulate due to their inability to undergo apoptosis. This is thought to be mediated by overexpression of anti-apoptotic proteins such as BCL2. The exact cell of origin likely differs between cases specifically related to the mutational status of the immunoglobulin variable region genes. FISH detects chromosomal abnormalities in 70% to 80% of patients with CLL and certain genetic abnormalities are clearly associated with disease prognosis (see the following). Furthermore, it appears that karyotypic abnormalities are acquired throughout the disease course and such clonal evolution has been associated with progressive disease.

Clinical Manifestations

The clinical manifestations of CLL vary widely with most patients displaying no clinical symptoms and diagnosis made by routine blood counts showing lymphocytosis. Persistent lymphadenopathy is another common presenting symptom and is present in up to 90% of patients. The spleen is the most commonly enlarged lymphoid organ and splenomegaly is detected in up to 50% of patients. Splenomegaly can lead to a variety of clinical symptoms including abdominal discomfort or early satiety contributing to poor oral intake and weight loss. Up to 10% of patients may present with "B" symptoms such as unintentional weight loss (10% or more of body weight within previous 6 months), fevers not associated with infection, drenching night sweats, and/or profound fatigue. Importantly, patients with CLL are immunocompromised and can present with recurrent infections. Autoimmune complications of CLL should be considered including hemolytic anemia, immune thrombocytopenia, and pure red cell aplasia, to name a few. Anemia and thrombocytopenia are findings consistent with advanced disease.

Diagnosis

A diagnosis of CLL is suspected when one presents with lymphocytosis with an absolute lymphocyte count greater than 5000/μL. Subsequent peripheral blood flow cytometry demonstrates immunophenotypic evidence of a monoclonal B-cell population that co-expresses the T-cell antigen CD5 and B-cell surface antigens CD19, CD20 (usually low/dim expression) and CD23 (Table 3). Typically, there is a low level of surface membrane immunoglobulin (most often IgM) along with a single immunoglobulin light chain, kappa or lambda, which confirms the clonal nature. The presence of a monoclonal B-cell population with the same immunophenotypic profile but with an absolute lymphocyte count less than 5000/μL is termed MBL. Bone marrow aspirate and biopsy are not required for the diagnosis of CLL but may be helpful in certain circumstances.

Differential Diagnosis

Peripheral lymphocytosis can occur in viral or other infectious processes and immunophenotyping by peripheral flow cytometry is helpful to distinguish between reactive and malignant causes and allows one to establish the diagnosis of CLL. Caution must be taken to differentiate from other low-grade B-cell malignancies (see Table 3). Importantly, one must distinguish mantel cell lymphoma from CLL. As CLL expresses CD23, MCL is typically CD23 negative and is characterized by strong expression of cyclin D1. A lymph node biopsy should be pursued when immunophenotyping of the peripheral blood fails to yield a diagnosis.

Prognosis

While most patients with CLL are diagnosed with early stage disease, the prognosis and clinical course is highly heterogeneous. Historically, risk stratification using the Rai or Binet clinical staging systems have been the mainstay of predicting prognosis in clinical practice (Tables 4 and 5). Over the past several years, our understanding of the molecular biology and underlying genetic aberrations in CLL have led to complementary prognostic variables to predict survival, which are widely used in clinical practice today. FISH testing to identify cytogenetic aberrations prior to treatment has allowed for more robust risk stratification. Specifically, deletion of 13q and trisomy 12 are favorable prognostic abnormalities, whereas deletion 17p and deletion 11q are higher risk abnormalities. Deletion 17p and/or aberrations in TP53 predict an aggressive disease course and refractoriness to conventional chemoimmunotherapy regimens. The mutational status of immunoglobulin heavy chain variable genes (IGHV) is also associated with survival. Unmutated *IGHV* genes have a more aggressive clinical course and shorter survival compared to those with mutated *IGHV* genes. Other prognostic factors have also been identified such as lymphocyte doubling time, Beta-2 microglobulin levels, expression of CD38 by flow-cytometry, and ZAP-70 expression in addition to clinical factors (i.e., age, sex, performance status). The CLL-IPI score has been validated by several groups and uses five independent prognostic factors: TP53 deletion and/or mutation, *IGHV* mutational status, serum

TABLE 3 Differential Diagnosis of Chronic Lymphocytic Leukemia by Immunophenotype

DISEASE	CD5	CD10	CD20	CD23	SURFACE IMMUNOGLOBULIN	OTHER
Chronic lymphocytic leukemia	+	–	+ (dim)	+	+ (dim)	
B-cell prolymphocytic leukemia	±	–	+	±	+ (bright)	
Mantle cell lymphoma	+	–	+	–	+ (bright)	t(11;14)
Hairy cell leukemia	–	–	+	–	+	CD11c, CD103, CD123 positive
Lymphoplasmacytic lymphoma	– (rarely +)	–	+	±	+	Most have monoclonal IgM paraprotein. Associated with MYD88 mutations.
Splenic marginal zone lymphoma	±	–	+	±	+ (bright)	

TABLE 4 Rai Staging System for CLL

RISK	STAGE	CLINICAL DESCRIPTION
Low	0	Lymphocytosis
Intermediate	I	Lymphocytosis + lymphadenopathy
	II	Lymphocytosis + hepatomegaly or splenomegaly (± lymphadenopathy)
High	III	Lymphocytosis + anemia (Hb <11 g/dL)
	IV	Lymphocytosis + thrombocytopenia (<100,000/μL)

TABLE 5 Binet Staging System for Chronic Lymphocytic Leukemia

STAGE	CLINICAL DESCRIPTION
A	Two or less lymphoid areas enlarged
B	Three or more lymphoid areas enlarged
C	Anemia (<10 g/dL) or thrombocytopenia (<100,000/μL)

B2-microglobulin concentration, clinical stage and age. This has identified four distinct prognostic subgroups with 5-year overall survival rates ranging from 93% in the low-risk group to 23% in the very high-risk group. More recently, the International Prognostic Score for Early-stage CLL (IPS-E) scoring system has been developed to predict time to first treatment in early stage, asymptomatic patients. This system identified three covariates independently correlated with time to first treatment including unmutated *IGHV* genes, absolute lymphocyte count greater than 1500/μL and the presence of palpable lymphadenopathy. However, it should be noted that none of these prognostic scoring systems have yet to affect the decision of when to initiate therapy.

Treatment

Not all patients with CLL require treatment at the time of diagnosis. CLL-directed treatment is indicated for those with active disease as defined by the International Workshop on Chronic Lymphocytic Leukemia Treatment (i.e., progressive marrow failure, symptomatic splenomegaly, bulky lymphadenopathy, rapid lymphocyte doubling time and/or constitutional symptoms). Therapy for patients with active disease has rapidly evolved over the past several years. It is important to note, however, that patients with advanced CLL are not cured with conventional therapy and thus, treatment is directed at alleviating symptoms,

improving quality of life and prolonging survival. With the incorporation of monoclonal antibodies into standard therapy with purine analogues, we began to see significant improvements in patient outcomes with prolonged remissions in some patients. Additionally, the development of BTK and BCL2 inhibitors has yielded a significant advancement in the treatment of advanced stage CLL leading to deep remissions, prolonged progression-free survival, and improved overall survival. Importantly, such therapies have yielded marked improvement in outcomes in patients with high-risk disease who historically do not respond or relapse soon after conventional chemoimmunotherapy. Nevertheless, CLL remains an incurable disease, short of allo-SCT.

First-Line Therapy

The choice of front-line therapy in CLL should be made based on patient characteristics and patient preferences/goals, as well as tumor characteristics. Typically, the preferred initial therapy depends on genetic risk stratification and the patient's ability to tolerate therapy. Genetic risk stratification is typically based on *IGHV* mutational status and the presence of 17p deletion or *TP53* mutation. Patients with *IGHV*-unmutated disease with or without 17p deletion or *TP53* mutations are typically treated with targeted agents such as BTK inhibitors or BCL2 inhibitors with or without monoclonal antibodies. For those with IGHV-mutated disease without 17p deletions or TP53 mutations, conventional chemoimmunotherapy and targeted therapy remain treatment options with no single agreed upon standard treatment.

First-line therapy with fludarabine (Fludara), cyclophosphamide (Cytoxan), and rituximab (Rituxan) (FCR) has historically been the most commonly used chemoimmunotherapy combination. The addition of rituximab (Rituxan) to fludarabine and cyclophosphamide represented significant progress in the treatment of CLL with an overall response rate approaching 95% and a complete response rate of 70%. FCR remains an acceptable initial treatment option for younger patients with active disease, specifically those with IGHV-mutated disease who do not harbor 17p deletions or *TP53* mutations. For patients who are elderly

(>65 years) or those who cannot tolerate FCR, the combination of bendamustine (Treanda) and rituximab (Rituxan) (BR) offers similar efficacy with improved tolerability compared with FCR. Again, BR is a reasonable front-line therapy for those with *IGHV*-mutated disease without a 17p deletion or *TP53* mutation only.

BTK inhibitors such as ibrutinib (Imbruvica) and acalabrutinib (Calquence) and the BCL2 inhibitor venetoclax (Venclexta) are highly effective therapies that have been shown to improve progression-free survival and overall survival. In patients with high-risk disease (17p deletion and/or *TP53* mutations or *IGHV* unmutated) treatment with targeted agents are preferred given improved outcomes demonstrated in multiple clinical trials. In those with standard risk disease (*IGHV* mutated without 17p deletion or *TP53* mutations) chemoimmunotherapy and targeted agents appear to be similar in efficacy and the choice of which to use must be individualized. There are no trials directly comparing targeted agents and the choice of which agent to use must be based on patient preferences and comorbidities. Options include single agent ibrutinib (Imbruvica) (with or without rituximab [Rituxan] for younger patients), the combination of venetoclax plus obinutuzumab (Gazyva) or acalabrutinib. While the combination of ibrutinib plus venetoclax has shown promise in early studies, this is not yet recommended in routine clinical practice.

Other Therapeutic Options
Treatment of relapsed disease in those who achieve at least a partial remission to front-line therapy requires assessment of time to progression from prior therapy. Early relapse is considered for those who experience disease progression at a shorter interval than the median expected for that treatment (i.e., within 5 to 6 years of targeted therapy and 2 to 3 years of FCR). Targeted therapy with *BTK* inhibitors or *BCL2* inhibitors is preferred treatment at the time of relapse with the choice of therapy depending on numerous factors including patient preferences, comorbidities, and front-line therapy received. Additionally, PI3K inhibitors idelalisib (Zydelig) plus rituximab and duvelisib (Copiktra) have gained the US Food and Drug Administration (FDA) approval for patients with relapsed CLL after one or two prior lines of therapy, respectively.

Hematopoietic stem cell transplantation remains the only curative therapy for CLL; however, the ideal timing is not clear and data are limited in nature. Perhaps, more important is the associated considerable treatment-related morbidity and mortality. Chimeric antigen receptor (CAR)-T cell therapy has been investigated in patients with relapsed or refractory CLL and has shown promising activity in early phase studies with complete response rates in the largest series of ~28%. Further work is needed to better define the role of CAR-T therapy in patients with relapsed CLL. Patients with relapsed CLL should be encouraged to participate in ongoing clinical trials.

Complications
The most common complications that occur in patients with CLL are related to intrinsic immune dysfunction. Specifically, patients with CLL have abnormal immune responses and thus are at a high risk for infectious complications. Infections are the major cause of mortality in patients with CLL and patients with recurrent major bacterial infections should be considered for intravenous immunoglobulin therapy (IVIg) (Gammagard S/D). Anemia can be related to direct bone marrow infiltration or hypersplenism. In such circumstances, CLL-directed therapy results in improvement in anemia. Additionally, autoimmune hemolytic anemia and pure red cell aplasia can also occur. Similarly, thrombocytopenia may be related to autoimmune destruction, hypersplenism, or disease burden. CLL transformation to aggressive B-cell lymphomas (most commonly diffuse large B-cell lymphoma), called Richter's transformation, is seen in 5% to 10% of patients. Patients with CLL have a higher risk of secondary malignancies, both hematologic and solid tumors. A retrospective review of the Surveillance, Epidemiology and End Results (SEER) program showed that ~11% of patients with CLL developed a secondary solid tumor. Thus, appropriate screening must be undertaken in this population.

References
Condoluci A, Bergamo T, Langereins P, et al: International prognostic score for asymptomatic early-stage chronic lymphocytic leukemia, *Blood*, 2020. https://doi.org/10.1182/blood.2019003453.
Faderl S, et al: The Biology of Chronic Myeloid Leukemia, *N Engl J Med* 341:164–172, 1999.
Hallek M, Shanafelt T, Eichhorst B: Chronic lymphocytic leukemia, *Lancet* 391(10129):14–20, 2018.
Hochhaus A, Baccarani M, et al: European LeukemiaNet 2020 recommendations for treating chronic myeloid leukemia, *Leukemia* 34:966–984, 2020.
Jabbour E, Kantarjian H: Chronic myeloid leukemia: 2020 update on diagnosis, therapy and monitoring, *Am J Hematol* 95:691–709, 2020.
Rawstron AC, Bennett FL, O'Connor SJ, et al: Monoclonal B-cell lymphocytosis and chronic lymphocytic leukemia, *N Engl J Med* 359:575–583, 2008.
Siegel RL, Miller KD, Jemal A: Cancer statistics, 2020, *CA Cancer J Clin* 70(1):7, 2020.

DISSEMINATED INTRAVASCULAR COAGULATION

Method of
Kenneth Byrd, DO

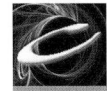

CURRENT DIAGNOSIS

- Disseminated intravascular coagulation (DIC) is an abnormal activation of the coagulation system that is caused by predisposing conditions such as sepsis, malignancy, and trauma.
- Clinical manifestations include organ injury due to microvascular thrombosis and less commonly macrovascular thrombosis. DIC can alternatively present with severe bleeding.
- Laboratory findings include thrombocytopenia, elevated D-dimer, elevated international normalized ratio (INR) and partial thromboplastin time (PTT), and sometimes decreased fibrinogen.
- The International Society on Thrombosis and Haemostasis (ISTH) scoring system predicts overt DIC if score ≥5.

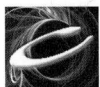

CURRENT TREATMENT

- Aggressive and prompt treatment of the underlying condition causing DIC is paramount.
- If the patient is bleeding or undergoing a procedure, aggressive transfusion support with platelets and fresh frozen plasma (FFP) or cryoprecipitate is often advised.
- Unless the patient is bleeding or undergoing a procedure, FFP or cryoprecipitate is usually not indicated, and platelets are only transfused if less than 20×10⁹/L. The major exception is acute promyelocytic leukemia (APL).
- Prophylactic low-molecular-weight heparin (LMWH) is often indicated in DIC.
- Therapeutic heparin/LMWH is rarely indicated in DIC unless there is clear evidence of a severe prothrombotic state.
- No other treatments are routinely used for DIC, including antithrombin, activated protein C, antifibrinolytics, and thrombomodulin. However, the role of these agents continues to be evaluated.

Introduction
Disseminated intravascular coagulation (DIC) is a complex and often life-threatening manifestation of an acquired disease process. This process is initiated by a strong procoagulant cascade that leads to microthrombi throughout the vasculature. A risk of hemorrhage often follows due to a depletion of platelets, consumption of coagulation factors, and accelerated plasmin formation.

Epidemiology

DIC has been reported in approximately 10% to 20% of critical care admissions. It is an independent predictor of mortality and the risk of death in a patient with sepsis is doubled when accompanied by DIC. Mortality rates vary based on the scoring system used but can be as high as 46%. The mortality rate appears to correlate with the severity of laboratory abnormalities at diagnosis.

Pathophysiology

DIC is primarily a coagulation dysfunction due to excessive procoagulant activity. The overactivation is multifactorial but is mainly due to the generation of excessive thrombin, which is mediated by the extrinsic pathway involving tissue factor and factor VIIa. Thrombin excess leads to increased platelet aggregation and thrombotic occlusion of small and midsize vessels with fibrin. Vascular occlusion leads to the derangement of oxygen supply and tissue demand, which can compromise multiple organs. This effect is compounded by defects in inhibitors of coagulation along with fibrinolytic suppression. Antithrombin activity is diminished due to increased consumption, degradation, and impaired synthesis. Likewise, protein C, tissue factor-pathway inhibitor (TFPI), and thrombomodulin activity are decreased in part due to excess inflammatory cytokines. Fibrinolytic suppression occurs in many instances of DIC due to an increase in plasminogen activator inhibitor-1 (PAI-1), which is the principal inhibitor of the fibrinolytic system.

The excessive activation of the coagulation pathway predictably leads to the depletion of platelets and clotting factors. However, the cause of bleeding in DIC is multifactorial, including consumption of clotting factors, thrombocytopenia, platelet dysfunction, endothelial damage, and excess fibrin degradation products (FDPs) that cause feedback anticoagulant effect.

Clinical Manifestations

The manifestations of DIC are often obscured by the underlying causative etiology. Many times, the diagnosis of DIC is solely laboratory based without any clear clinical manifestations. At other times, DIC may be overtly symptomatic. Recently, it has been suggested that DIC could be divided into clinical subtypes that include asymptomatic, bleeding, and organ failure types. The presentation depends on whether there is a predominance of thrombosis from excessive thrombin activation or bleeding from consumptive coagulopathy.

Overall, the incidence of major bleeding in DIC is 5% to 12%. DIC that presents with acute bleeding is most commonly seen in acute leukemia, obstetric disorders, and trauma. Typical hemorrhagic features of DIC include bleeding from venipuncture sites or indwelling catheters, generalized ecchymosis that develops spontaneously or with minimal trauma, bleeding from mucous membranes, unexpected and major bleeding from around drain sites or tracheostomies, and concealed hemorrhage in serous cavities such as retroperitoneal hemorrhage.

Thrombotic organ failure type of DIC is most commonly seen with sepsis. The incidence of organ involvement secondary to thrombosis is 10% to 40%. This occurs due to thromboses in small and midsize vessels. Many organs can be involved, but it is most commonly seen in the kidneys, lungs, liver, and brain. This can manifest as respiratory distress syndrome, acute kidney injury, confusion, and seizures. The skin can also be involved and present as purpura fulminans or acral ischemia. Macrovascular thrombosis such as venous thromboembolism may present as a later manifestation. COVID-19 frequently presents with a DIC-like coagulopathy. Unlike classic acute DIC, fibrinogen is often elevated and there is excessive thrombotic risk.

Diagnosis

Making the diagnosis of DIC starts with identifying an underlying associated disease state. Table 1 lists the known risk factors for DIC. Once this is established, the diagnosis entails a combination of laboratory values along with an analysis of the clinical

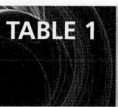

TABLE 1	Risk Factors for Disseminated Intravascular Coagulation (Incidence of Disseminated Intravascular Coagulation Per Etiology)

- Sepsis (35%)
  - Most commonly bacterial
- Severe trauma (up to 50%)
  - Most commonly brain injury or burns
- Malignancy
  - Metastatic cancer (up to 20%)
  - Acute leukemia (15%)
  - Acute promyelocytic leukemia (90%)
  - COVID-19
- Obstetrical
  - Placental abruption
  - Amniotic fluid embolism
  - Postpartum hemorrhage
  - Acute fatty liver of pregnancy
- Vascular malformations
  - Kasabach-Merritt syndrome
  - Large aortic aneurysms
  - Other large vascular malformations
- Severe immunologic reaction
  - Acute hemolytic transfusion reaction
  - Anaphylaxis
- Heat stroke
- Postcardiopulmonary resuscitation

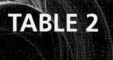

TABLE 2	International Society on Thrombosis and Haemostasis Scoring System

Platelet count × 10⁹/L
- ≥100 = 0
- <100 = 1
- <50 = 2

Fibrin marker levels (D-dimer, fibrin degradation products)
- No increase = 0
- Moderate increase (>ULN but <5× ULN) = 2
- Strong increase (≥5× ULN) = 3

Prothrombin time
- <3 s (*INR <1.3) = 0
- ≥3 but <6 s (*INR 1.3–1.5) = 1
- ≥6 s (*INR ≥1.6) = 2

Fibrinogen
- >100 mg/dL = 0
- ≤100 mg/dL = 1

*Assuming the International Survey Index value of the thromboplastin reagents used is close to 1
- A score of ≥5 points is compatible with overt DIC
- The scoring system is only appropriate in patients with an underlying disorder that can be associated with DIC
- If the score if <5 and DIC is still suspected, then consider repeating labs in 1–2 days

DIC, Disseminated intravascular coagulation; *ULN*, upper limits of normal.

presentation. The difficulty with diagnosing DIC is that there is no gold standard and no pathognomonic test. There have been several scoring systems developed for DIC to assist in standardizing the diagnosis. The most commonly utilized is the International Society on Thrombosis and Haemostasis (ISTH) scoring system, which was originally devised in 2001 and has been subsequently validated. The scoring system is outlined in Table 2. A score of ≥5 suggests overt DIC. A score of < 5 indicates a lack of DIC or nonovert DIC (i.e., subtle and compensated hemostatic dysfunction). The ISTH scoring system has a sensitivity of 93% and a specificity of 98%. Most other available scoring systems are more sensitive but less specific for DIC. Importantly, if DIC is suspected but not confirmed, then labs should be repeated to assess trends.

The decreased platelet count in DIC is due to excessive thrombin activation and is almost always less than 100 × 10⁹/L and often

TABLE 3	Differential Diagnosis of Disseminated Intravascular Coagulation		
DISEASE	**SIMILARITIES**	**DIFFERENCES**	**COMMENTS**
Liver disease	Low plt; prolonged PT/PTT; low fibrinogen; increased FDP (DIC > Liver disease)	No schistocytes in liver disease; worsening labs in DIC and more stable in liver disease	Factor VIII not very helpful for differentiation. Normal or elevated in liver disease (not synthesized in liver). However, as an acute phase reactant, often normal or elevated in DIC
Thrombotic microangiopathy (TMA)	Low plt; increased FDP (DIC > TMA); decreased ADAMTS13 (TMA lower than DIC)	MAHA in TMA; normal PT/PTT and fibrinogen in TMA; numerous schistocytes common in TMA, but not DIC	Extremely low plt with normal PT/PTT is common in TMA but unusual in DIC; TMA includes TTP, HUS, secondary TMAs
Heparin-induced thrombocytopenia (HIT)	Low plt, increased FDP	Normal PT/PTT in HIT; low fibrinogen unusual in HIT	Plt <20 × 10⁹/L is uncommon in HIT
Catastrophic antiphospholipid syndrome (CAPS)	Low plt; increased FDP; PTT elevation (false elevation of PTT commonly due to LA)	Normal PT in CAPS; lab diagnosis of APLS in CAPS	Normal plt often seen in CAPS and severe thrombocytopenia is rare; microvascular thromboses in both; macrovascular thrombosis is a more common initial presentation of CAPS than DIC
Hemophagocytic lymphohistiocytosis (HLH)	Low plt; prolonged PT/PTT; low fibrinogen; increased FDP	HLH with very high ferritin, TGs, organomegaly, and often hemophagocytosis	

APLS, Antiphospholipid antibody syndrome; *DIC*, disseminated intravascular coagulation; *FDP*, fibrin degradation products; *LA*, lupus anticoagulant; *MAHA*, microangiopathic hemolytic anemia; *plt*, platelet count; *PT*, prothrombin time; *PTT*, partial thromboplastin time; *TG*, triglycerides; *TTP*, thrombotic thrombocytopenic purpura.

trending down. A normal platelet count without a downward trend would essentially rule out DIC. The INR and PTT are often elevated due to consumption of coagulation factors but can be normal in up to 50% of cases. The vast majority of DIC is also marked by an increase in fibrin-related markers due to increased fibrinolysis. Traditionally, FDPs were used but have largely been replaced by D-dimer. Fibrinogen is traditionally decreased in DIC but is often normal as it frequently surpasses compensated consumption only later in the clinic course. It can also be falsely normal or even elevated as it is an acute phase reactant. It is only rarely severely diminished. A fibrinogen level of <100 mg/dL is seen in <50% of DIC and usually reflects the late, severe, consumptive stage of DIC.

Thromboelastography (TEG) and rotational thromboelastometry (ROTEM) testing have been evaluated to assess overall coagulation, including platelet function, and clot dissolving potential. TEG has demonstrated good correlation with clinically important organ dysfunction and survival, although its advantage over usual coagulation assays has not yet been confirmed. The role of these two modalities in DIC is still unclear.

DIC often presents with a small population of schistocytes. If the red blood cell population is > 10% schistocytes, then an alternative diagnosis is more likely (i.e., TMA). Of note, a low ADAMTS13 can be seen in DIC but is usually >30%. There is also frequently a reduction in antithrombin and protein C. These tests are not done routinely and are likely not as sensitive as the ISTH scoring system. Finally, factor VIII can be low in DIC due to consumption, but it can also be elevated at times as it is an acute phase reactant.

The differential diagnosis of DIC is explained in Table 3.

Therapy

The foundation of treatment for DIC is to treat the underlying disorder. If the underlying disorder is reversed, then DIC typically resolves.

During active DIC there may be a need for transfusion support. It is important to note that the following transfusion recommendations are mostly based on low-quality evidence, including expert opinion. In the presence of bleeding, platelet transfusions should be given to keep platelet count greater than 30 to 50 × 10⁹/L. Similarly, in the setting of invasive procedures, platelets

should be maintained greater than 20 to 50 × 10⁹/L, depending on the risk of the procedure. Importantly, in the absence of bleeding or procedure, platelets should be transfused only if platelet count is less than 20 × 10⁹/L (a range of 10 to 30 × 10⁹/L has been proposed by various sources). The exception to this threshold would be acute promyelocytic leukemia (APL), in which platelets should be maintained greater than 30 to 50 × 10⁹/L even in the absence of bleeding (less commonly some suggest a 20 × 10⁹/L threshold).

A similar approach to the replacement of factors is indicated. If the patient is bleeding or undergoing a high risk procedure and fibrinogen is less than 150 mg/dL or PT/PTT is greater than 1.5 upper limits of normal (ULN), then fresh frozen plasma (FFP) or cryoprecipitate is recommended. Keep in mind that FFP contains all factors of the soluble coagulation system, while cryoprecipitate contains a concentrated subset of plasma factors including fibrinogen, factor VIII, von Willebrand factor, and factor XIII. The choice between FFP and cryoprecipitate is made on a case-by-case basis and can often be influenced by fluid status. The recommended dose of FFP is 15 to 30 mL/kg and cryoprecipitate is 5 to 10 units. A less frequently used option is 2 g of fibrinogen concentrate. Factor replacement is not indicated in the absence of bleeding or procedure. An exception to this threshold is APL, in which factor replacement could be considered if fibrinogen is less than 100 to 150 mg/dL, even in the absence of bleeding.

In addition to transfusion support and treatment of the underlying etiology, heparin[1] can be considered in a few circumstances. Most importantly, guidelines recommend prophylactic heparin or low-molecular-weight heparin (LMWH)[1] in the absence of bleeding as long as platelet count is greater than 20 to 30 × 10⁹/L, INR greater than 1.5, and fibrinogen greater than 100 mg/dL. This is especially vital in prothrombotic DIC (i.e., sepsis, solid tumor malignancy). An exception to the general use of LMWH prophylaxis is in hyperfibrinolytic DIC (i.e., APL and prostate cancer), in which more caution is advised with heparin use. Therapeutic heparin is uncommonly advised in DIC, but it can be considered in prothrombotic DIC, as evidenced by thromboembolism, purpura fulminans, or acral ischemia. As heparin can partially

---

[1]Not FDA approved for this indication.

inhibit activation of the coagulation, it would make sense that it could help offset DIC. In small studies, heparin has shown beneficial effects on coagulation parameters. However, improvement in clinically important outcomes in DIC has not been clearly demonstrated.

Other therapies that have been studied in the treatment of DIC include antithrombin concentrate (AT [Thrombate III]),[1] activated protein C (APC), recombinant thrombomodulin, and antifibrinolytics. Currently, these agents are rarely, if ever, indicated for use. AT and APC have been extensively studied in the setting of sepsis. One of the issues in assessing the benefit of AT and APC is that many clinical trials assess the general sepsis population and do not limit analysis to those specifically with DIC. For AT, there has been no significant reduction in mortality in these studies. However, there is a suggestion that there may be significant benefit in the subset of patients with severe sepsis and DIC. This requires prospective validation. APC has also shown promise at times, including improvement in mortality in an early randomized controlled trial (RCT). However, subsequent studies showed an increased risk of serious bleeding and lack of survival benefit. Therefore, the FDA advised to stop using APC for DIC in 2011.

Caution is advised with the use of antifibrinolytics in DIC. Since the excessive fibrin deposition appears in part to be due to insufficient fibrinolysis, further inhibition of the fibrinolytic system would clearly not be appropriate. This is especially the case in sepsis, but there are a few exceptions to this. Antifibrinolytics can be considered in hyperfibrinolytic DIC (i.e., APL or prostate cancer) only in the setting of life-threatening bleeding. The other exception is in acute trauma. A large RCT showed that early use of antifibrinolytics in trauma was beneficial. However, once the acute phase has passed, further thrombin generation eventually predominates, and the balance is tipped toward thrombosis.

Recombinant soluble thrombomodulin continues to be actively evaluated and shows some potential. While efficacy outcomes have been heterogeneous, a 2020 meta-analysis suggested a 28-day mortality benefit of recombinant thrombomodulin[5] in patients with sepsis and coagulopathy. Results of ongoing studies are pending.

Finally, it is worth mentioning that a Cochrane review evaluated recombinant factor VIIa (NovoSeven)[1] and concluded that it does not have proven efficacy in DIC and that there is an increased risk of arterial thrombotic events. Its use is not advised.

<hr/>

[1]Not FDA approved for this indication
[5]Investigational drug in the United States.

References

Asakura H, Ogawa H: COVID-19-associated coagulopathy and disseminated intravascular coagulation, *Int J Hematol* 113(1):45–57, 2021.

Bakhtiari K, Meijers JC, de Jonge E, Levi M: Prospective validation of the International Society of Thrombosis and Haemostasis scoring system for disseminated intravascular coagulation, *Crit Care Med* 32(12):2416–2421, 2004.

Bernard GR, Vincent JL, Laterre PF, et al: Efficacy and safety of recombinant human activated protein C for severe sepsis, *N Engl J Med* 344(10):699–709, 2001.

Gando S, Levi M, Toh CH: Disseminated intravascular coagulation, *Nat Rev Dis Primers* 2:16037, 2016.

Levi M: Pathogenesis and diagnosis of disseminated intravascular coagulation, *Int J Lab Hematol* 40:15–20, 2018.

Levi M, Scully M: How I treat disseminated intravascular coagulation, *Blood* 131(8):845–854, 2018.

Sanz MA, Grimwade D, Tallman MS, et al: Management of acute promyelocytic leukemia: recommendations from an expert panel on behalf of the European Leukemianet, *Blood* 113(9):1875–1891, 2009.

Squizzato A, Hunt BJ, Kinasewitz GT, et al: Supportive management strategies for disseminated intravascular coagulation, *ThrombHaemost* 116(05):896–904, 2016.

Valeriani E, Squizzato A, Gallo A, et al: Efficacy and safety of recombinant human soluble thrombomodulin in patients with sepsis-associated coagulopathy: A systematic review and meta-analysis, *J Thromb Haemost* 18(7):1618–1625, 2020.

Wada H, Thachil J, Di Nisio M, et al: Guidance for diagnosis and treatment of disseminated intravascular coagulation from harmonization of the recommendations from three guidelines, *J ThrombHaemost* 11(4):761–767, 2013.

Warren BL, Eid A, Singer P, et al: High-dose antithrombin III in severe sepsis: a randomized controlled trial, *JAMA* 286(15):1869–1878, 2001.

HEMOCHROMATOSIS

Method of
Paul C. Adams, MD

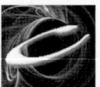

CURRENT DIAGNOSIS

- Consider the diagnosis in patients with Northern European ancestry.
- Initial testing is transferrin saturation or unsaturated iron binding capacity and serum ferritin.
- Secondary testing is the C282Y genetic test.
- More than 90% of typical hemochromatosis patients are homozygotes for the C282Y mutation.
- If genetic testing is not typical, reassess the diagnosis and consider secondary iron overload related to cirrhosis, alcoholism, viral hepatitis, or an iron-loading anemia.
- A number of other hemochromatosis genetic mutations are relevant to only a minority of patients.
- Not all patients need a liver biopsy.
- Siblings are at highest risk in a family study.

CURRENT THERAPY

- Iron overload from hemochromatosis is treated by the weekly removal of 500 mL of blood until the serum ferritin is in the low-normal range of approximately 50 µg/L.
- Some but not all patients require maintenance therapy with three to four phlebotomies per year. In some countries, this can be a voluntary blood donation.
- Excess alcohol, high doses of vitamin C, and iron supplementation should be avoided, but strict dietary restrictions are not recommended.
- Siblings and children of patients should be tested for hemochromatosis with transferrin saturation, ferritin, and genetic testing.

Hemochromatosis is the most common genetic disease in populations of European ancestry. The diagnosis can be elusive because of the nonspecific nature of the symptoms. With the discovery of the hemochromatosis gene (*HFE*) in 1996 came new insights into the pathogenesis of the disease and new diagnostic strategies.

A fundamental issue that arose after the discovery of the *HFE* gene is whether the disease hemochromatosis should be defined strictly on phenotypic criteria such as the degree of iron overload (i.e., transferrin saturation, ferritin, liver biopsy, hepatic iron concentration, iron removed by venesection therapy), or whether the condition should be defined as a familial disease in Europeans most commonly associated with the C282Y mutation of the *HFE* gene and varying degrees of iron overload. Because the genetic test has been increasingly used as a diagnostic tool, most studies now use a combination of phenotypic and genotypic criteria for the diagnosis of hemochromatosis.

Clinical Features

Although hemochromatosis is often classified as a liver disease, it should be emphasized that it is a systemic genetic disease with multisystem involvement. The liver is central in both diagnosis and prognosis. Hepatomegaly remains one of the more common physical signs in hemochromatosis, but it is not always present in the young, asymptomatic homozygote. In a study of 717 homozygotes from Australia, 8% of men and 1.7% of women had cirrhosis of the liver at the time of diagnosis. The prevalence of cirrhosis in asymptomatic or screened patients is much lower. It is likely that there are factors other than iron overload that contribute to cirrhosis in hemochromatosis. These can include the effects of alcohol or comodifying genes. The effect of iron depletion therapy is usually stabilization of the liver disease, and fibrosis improves with repeat liver biopsy after iron depletion. This may account for the relatively small number of C282Y homozygotes that require liver transplantation. The other common clinical manifestations are arthralgias, pigmentation, congestive heart failure, impotence, and fatigue. Several large population studies failed to demonstrate an increase in diabetes compared with a control population. A population-based study estimated that only 28% of male and 1% of female C282Y homozygotes will develop symptoms of iron overload. A larger population-based screening study (UK Biobank) identified 2,890 C282Y homozygotes in 451,243 participants and found that male hemochromatosis patients had an odds ratio of 4.30 for liver disease and 10.5 for hepatocellular carcinoma. Women were much less affected.

Diagnosis

A paradox of genetic hemochromatosis is that the disease is underdiagnosed in the general population and overdiagnosed in patients with secondary iron overload.

Preliminary population studies using genetic testing demonstrate a prevalence of homozygotes of approximately 1:227 among whites. The fact that many physicians consider hemochromatosis to be rare implies either a lack of penetrance of the gene (nonexpressing homozygote) or a large number of patients who remain undiagnosed in the community.

Transferrin Saturation

Previous studies had suggested that transferrin saturation would be a good screening test and diagnostic test for hemochromatosis.

The sensitivity of transferrin saturation in population-screening studies designed to detect C282Y homozygotes (genotypic case definition) was only approximately 75%, and transferrin saturation can be in the normal range in young female homozygotes. A large biologic variation in transferrin saturation within an individual patient has also been reported.

Serum Ferritin

The relationship between serum ferritin and total body iron stores was clearly established by strong correlations with hepatic iron concentration and the amount of iron removed by venesection. However, ferritin can be elevated secondary to chronic inflammation and histiocytic neoplasms. A major diagnostic dilemma in the past was whether the serum ferritin concentration was related to hemochromatosis or to another underlying liver disease, such as alcoholic liver disease, chronic viral hepatitis, or nonalcoholic steatohepatitis. It is likely that most of these difficult cases can now be resolved by genetic testing.

MR Imaging

Liver MR imaging continues to advance and is ideally performed in centers with special expertise. Liver iron concentration, fat concentration, tumor detection, and fibrosis score from MR elastrography can be provided with this noninvasive tool.

Liver Biopsy

Liver biopsy was previously the gold-standard diagnostic test for hemochromatosis; however, it has shifted from a major diagnostic tool to a method of estimating prognosis and concomitant disease. The need for liver biopsy seems less clear now in the young, asymptomatic C282Y homozygote in whom there is a low clinical suspicion of cirrhosis based on history, physical examination, and liver biochemistry. A large study conducted in France and Canada suggested that C282Y homozygotes with a serum ferritin concentration of less than 1000 µg/L, a normal aspartate transaminase (AST) concentration, and no hepatomegaly have a very low risk of cirrhosis. C282Y homozygotes with a ferritin level greater than 1000 µg/L, an elevated AST, and a platelet count of less than 200,000/mm^3 have an 80% chance of having cirrhosis. Hepatic elastography is another noninvasive tool to assess liver fibrosis in hemochromatosis.

Patients with cirrhosis have a 5.5-fold relative risk of death compared with noncirrhotic hemochromatosis patients. Cirrhotic patients are also at increased risk of hepatocellular carcinoma. Liver biopsy is considered in typical C282Y homozygotes with liver dysfunction and in potentially iron-overloaded patients without the typical C282Y mutation. Simple C282Y heterozygotes, compound heterozygotes (C282Y/H63D), H63D homozygotes, and patients with other risk factors (e.g., alcohol abuse, chronic viral hepatitis) who have moderate to severe iron overload (ferritin > 1000 µg/L) may be considered for liver biopsy.

Since the introduction of genetic testing, hepatic iron concentration and hepatic iron index have become less useful in the diagnosis of hemochromatosis.

Genetic Testing

A major advance stemming from the discovery of the hemochromatosis gene is the use of a diagnostic genetic test. Most studies report that more than 90% of typical hemochromatosis patients were homozygotes for the C282Y mutation. A second minor mutation, H63D, was also described in the original report. Compound heterozygotes (C282Y/H63D) and, less commonly, H63D homozygotes, resemble C282Y homozygotes with mild to moderate iron overload. Genetic mutations involving ferroportin, hemojuvelin, transferrin receptor 2, ceruloplasmin, and hepcidin are associated with iron overload. It is likely that, as more mutations are found, they will be relevant to only a minority of patients. Commercial tests are rarely available for these rare genetic mutations.

Some patients with clinical pictures indistinguishable from genetic hemochromatosis are negative for the C282Y mutation. Most of these cases appear to be isolated, although a few cases of familial iron overload with negative C282Y testing have been reported. A negative C282Y test should alert the physician to question the diagnosis of genetic hemochromatosis and to reconsider secondary iron overload related to cirrhosis, alcoholism, viral hepatitis, or an iron-loading anemia. If no other risk factors are found, the patient should begin phlebotomy treatment, similar to any other hemochromatosis patient.

The interpretation of the genetic test in several settings is shown in Box 1. Genetic discrimination is a concern, given the widespread use of genetic testing, but discrimination has been rarely reported in screening studies. In the case of hemochromatosis, the advantages of early diagnosis of a treatable disease outweigh the disadvantages of genetic discrimination.

Family Studies

Once the proband case is identified and confirmed with the genetic test for the C282Y mutation, family testing is imperative. Siblings have approximately one in four chance of carrying the gene and should be screened with the genetic test (C282Y and H63D mutation), transferrin saturation, and serum ferritin. A cost-effective strategy now possible with genetic testing is to test the spouse for the C282Y mutation to assess the risk in the children. If the spouse is not a C282Y heterozygote or homozygote, the children will be obligate heterozygotes, assuming paternity and excluding another gene or mutation causing hemochromatosis. This strategy is particularly advantageous if the children are geographically separated or in different health care systems.

Treatment

The treatment of hemochromatosis continues to use the medieval therapy of periodic bleeding. Blood is removed, with the patient in the reclining position over 15 to 30 minutes. Initial treatment consists of the weekly removal of 500 mL of blood. A hemoglobin test is done before each phlebotomy. If the hemoglobin concentration has decreased to less than 10 g/dL, the phlebotomy schedule is modified to 500 mL every 2 weeks. Phlebotomies are continued until the serum ferritin concentration is approximately 50 µg/L. Serum ferritin levels are drawn monthly in patients with significant iron overload and increased to weekly as the ferritin decreases to < 200 µg/L. The concomitant administration of a

BOX 1 | Interpretation of Genetic Testing for Hemochromatosis

"C282Y Homozygote"

This is the classic genetic pattern seen in more than 90% of typical cases. Expression of disease ranges from no evidence of iron overload to massive iron overload with organ dysfunction. Siblings have a one in four chance of being affected and should have genetic testing. For children to be affected, the other parent must be at least a heterozygote. If iron studies are normal, false-positive genetic testing or a nonexpressing homozygotic state should be considered

"C282Y/H63D Compound Heterozygote"

This patient carries two copies of the minor mutation. Most patients with this genetic pattern have normal iron studies. A small percentage have mild to moderate iron overload. Severe iron overload is usually seen in the setting of another concomitant risk factor (e.g., alcoholism, viral hepatitis)

"C282Y Heterozygote"

This patient carries one copy of the major mutation. This pattern is seen in approximately 10% of the white population and is usually associated with normal iron studies. In rare cases, the results of iron studies are high, in the range expected in a homozygote rather than a heterozygote. These patients may carry an unknown hemochromatosis mutation, and liver biopsy is helpful to determine the need for phlebotomy therapy

"H63D Homozygote"

Most patients with this genotype will have normal iron studies. A small percentage have mild to moderate iron overload. Severe iron overload is usually seen in the setting of another concomitant risk factor (e.g., alcoholism, viral hepatitis)

"H63D Heterozygote"

This patient carries one copy of the minor mutation. This pattern is seen in approximately 20% of the white population and is usually associated with normal iron studies. This pattern is so common in the general population that the presence of iron overload can be related to another risk factor. Liver biopsy is required to determine the cause of the iron overload and the need for treatment in these cases

"No HFE Mutations"

If iron overload is present without any mutations in the hemochromatosis gene (HFE), a careful history for other risk factors must be reviewed, and liver biopsy can be useful to determine the cause of the iron overload and the need for treatment. Most of these are isolated, nonfamilial cases. There are cases described involving genetic mutations in ferroportin, hemojuvelin, transferrin receptor 2, ceruloplasmin, and hepcidin genes. Genetic tests for these mutations are not widely available

---

salt-containing sport beverage (e.g., Gatorade) is a simple method of maintaining plasma volume during the phlebotomy.

Maintenance phlebotomies after iron depletion, consisting of three to four phlebotomies per year, are performed in most patients, although the rate of iron reaccumulation is highly variable. Maintenance therapy is initiated when the serum ferritin rises from 50 µg/L to > 300 µg/L. The transferrin saturation remains elevated in many treated patients and does not normalize unless the patient becomes iron deficient. In some countries, patients with mild iron abnormalities are encouraged to become voluntary blood donors. Iron depletion has been demonstrated to improve fibrosis and reduce the risk of hepatocellular carcinoma.

Chelation therapy[1] is not recommended for hemochromatosis. Patients are advised to avoid oral iron therapy and alcohol abuse, but there are no dietary restrictions. Patient support groups have been concerned by the practice of iron fortification of foods, but much of this iron is in an inexpensive form with poor bioavailability.

Hemochromatosis is a common and often underdiagnosed disease. Early diagnosis and treatment result in an excellent long-term prognosis. The development of a diagnostic genetic test has improved the feasibility of the goal of prevention of morbidity and mortality from hemochromatosis.

---

[1]Not FDA approved for this indication.

References

Adams PC, Reboussin DM, Barton JC, et al: Hemochromatosis and iron overload screening (HEIRS) study: Screening in a racially diverse of primary care population, N Engl J Med 352:1769–1778, 2005a.

Adams PC: Hemochromatosis case definition: Out of focus, Nat Clin Pract Gastroenterol Hepatol 3:178–179, 2006.

Adams PC, Barton JC: How I treat hemochromatosis, Blood 116:317–325, 2010.

Allen KJ, Gurrin LC, Constantine CC, et al: Iron-overload-related disease in HFE hereditary hemochromatosis, N Engl J Med 358:221–230, 2008.

Atkins JL, Pilling LC, Masoli J, et al: Association of hemochromatosis HFE p.C282Y homozygosity with hepatic malignancy, JAMA 324:2048–2057, 2020.

Bacon BR, Adams PC, Kowdley K, et al: Diagnosis and management of hemochromatosis: AASLD practice guidelines, Hepatology 54:328–343, 2011.

Bardou-Jacquet E, Morandeau E, Anderson G, et al: Regression of fibrosis stage with treatment reduces long-term risk of liver cancer in patients with hemochromatosis caused by mutation in HFE, Gastroenterol Hepatol 18:1851–1857, 2020.

Beaton M, Guyader D, Deugnier Y, et al: Non-invasive prediction of cirrhosis in C282Y-linked hemochromatosis, Hepatology 36:673–678, 2002.

Brissot P, Pietrangelo A, Adams PC, de Graaf B, McLaren C: Loreal O, Haemochromatosis Nature Reviews Disease Primers, 4:18016, 2018, https://doi.org/10.1038/nrdp.2018.16.

Falize L, Guillygomarch A, Perrin M, et al: Reversibility of hepatic fibrosis in treated hemochromatosis: A study of 36 cases, Hepatology 44:472–477, 2006.

Gordeuk V, Lovato L, Vitolins M, et al: Relationship between dietary iron intake and serum ferritin concentration in HFE homozygotes, Can J Gastroenterol 26:345–349, 2012.

Ong SY, Gurrin LC, Dolling L, et al: Reduction of body iron in HFE-related haemochromatosis and moderate iron overload: a multicentre, participant-blinded, randomised controlled trial. Lancet Haematol 4:e607-e614, 2017.

Pilling LC, Tamosaukaite J, Jones G, et al: Common conditions associated with hereditary haemochromatosis genetic variants: cohort study in UK Biobank, BMJ 364:k5222, 2019, https://doi.org/10.1136/bmj.k5222.

HEMOLYTIC ANEMIAS

Method of
Thomas G. DeLoughery, MD

CURRENT DIAGNOSES

- Suspect hemolysis when anemia is accompanied by signs of red cell breakdown—high low-density lipoprotein and indirect bilirubin with a low haptoglobin.
- The reticulocyte count is often high.
- A positive direct antibody test confirms the diagnosis of autoimmune hemolytic anemia in the presence of hemolysis.
- In patient with non-immune hemolysis, specific testing is required to make the diagnosis.

At the most basic level, hemolytic anemias are caused by red blood cell destruction. This destruction can be due to factors either intrinsic or extrinsic to the red blood cell. The pace of the hemolysis can vary from being only detectible by laboratory abnormalities to fulminant acute severe anemia. A useful way to think about hemolytic anemias is to divide them into hereditary disorders and acquired disorders (Table 1). Defects in any part of the red blood cell lead to inherited disorders, whereas acquired disorders are caused by immune-related processes and other etiologies extrinsic to the red blood cell.

Pathophysiology

Congenital

The major components of the red blood cell are the membrane, hemoglobin, and enzymes; therefore the three major classes of hereditary hemolytic anemias are due to defects in any of these three red blood cell components.

Hereditary spherocytosis is the most common hemolytic anemia caused by membrane defects. This condition is caused by mutations in the proteins that make up the red blood cell skeleton, which leads to an unstable membrane. The red blood cells in hereditary spherocytosis initially have a normal biconcave disc structure, but after repeated passage through the spleen, they gradually lose portions of the membrane and become more spherical as they age (a process known as *splenic conditioning*). These spherocytes are less deformable and because of that are ultimately trapped and destroyed in the spleen. Less common anemias due to membrane defects are hereditary elliptocytosis and pyropoikilocytosis. In elliptocytosis the skeletal defects are not as profound, so the clinical presentation is usually milder. Most patients with pyropoikilocytosis are homozygous for mutations that cause elliptocytosis and have very unstable red blood cell membranes; often fragments of red blood cells are seen in the circulation.

The most common red blood cell enzyme defect is glucose-6-phosphate dehydrogenase (G6PD) deficiency. An adequate supply of reduced glutathione (GSH) is necessary to protect the erythrocyte from oxidative damage. G6PD catalyzes the conversion of glucose-6-phosphate to 6-phosphogluconate, in the process reducing NADP to NADPH. NADPH is necessary for the conversion of glutathione (GSSG) to reduced GSH. The erythrocyte does not have any other source of NADPH and so is dependent solely on this pathway for reducing power. When G6PD is deficient, this leads to decreased NADPH, which leads to decreased GSH. When the red blood cell undergoes oxidative stress, this lack of reducing power results in damage of red blood cell proteins, especially hemoglobin. These damaged proteins can aggregate, causing membrane damage and red blood cell destruction as the crystalized proteins are removed by the spleen.

Pyruvate kinase deficiency is a hemolytic anemia caused by an enzymatic defect in the glycolytic pathway. Pyruvate kinase catalyzes conversion of phosphoenolpyruvate to pyruvate, generating ATP in the same reaction. Deficiency of pyruvate kinase results in decreased levels of erythrocyte ATP. Lack of ATP results in a leaky cell membrane and loss of water and potassium. This leads to cellular dehydration and rigid, nondeformable cells, which are susceptible to destruction within the spleen.

By far the most common hereditary hemolytic hemoglobin defect is sickle cell anemia. The abnormal hemoglobin protein forms long polymers that disrupt red blood cell integrity. There are also very rare defects in hemoglobin that can cause unstable molecules that can crystallize and lead to hemolysis—most often due to splenic removal of damaged proteins.

Acquired

Autoimmune hemolytic anemias (AIHA) can be mediated by either anti-red blood cell immunoglobulin G (IgG) or immunoglobulin M (IgM) antibodies. In IgG-mediated disease, the antibody binds to red blood cell membrane proteins. The antibody-coated red blood cells are then phagocytized by macrophages found primarily in the spleen, leading to hemolysis.

In IgM-mediated hemolysis ("cold agglutinin disease"), the antibody binds to the red blood cell most often in the periphery of the body. The "cold" appellation comes from the fact that the antibody binds more strongly when below body temperature. Most commonly, complement is fixed only through C3, and then the C3-coated red blood cells are taken up by the macrophages. In rare patients the IgM can fix complement rapidly, leading to intravascular hemolysis by formation of the end product of complement the membrane attack complex.

Rare patients can develop immune hemolysis induced by medication. There have been three mechanisms proposed for drug AIHA. The hapten mechanism is most often associated with the use of high-dose penicillin. High doses of penicillin lead to drug incorporation into the red blood cell membrane by binding to proteins. Another mechanism is the formation of an immune complex of drug, antibody, and red blood cell membrane, which leads to hemolysis. Finally, patients taking certain drugs such as methyldopa will develop a positive direct antibody (DAT) after 6 months of therapy and hemolysis, which is indistinguishable from warm antibody AIHA.

In paroxysmal nocturnal hemoglobinuria (PNH), red blood cells lack the regulatory membrane proteins that inhibit activated complement proteins. These proteins include membrane inhibitor of reactive lysis (CD59) and decay-accelerating factor (CD55). The molecular defect in PNH is a mutation of the phosphatidyl inositol glycan complementation group A gene located on the X-chromosome. This enzyme is required for synthesis of glycosyl phosphatidylinositol (GPI)–linked proteins. Cells derived from the PNH stem cells are deficient in all proteins that are linked to the membrane by a GPI-molecule, including those that inactivate complement. Normally there is baseline activation of complement; it is believed that one of the functions of red blood cells is inactivation of these active complement proteins. When activated complement binds PNH red blood cells instead of being destroyed, the resulting membrane attack complex leads to lysis of the red blood cell.

Microangiopathic hemolytic anemias (MAHA) result from destruction of circulating red cells. Although MAHA is commonly associated with thrombotic microangiopathies such as thrombotic thrombocytopenia purpura (TTP) and hemolytic uremic syndrome (HUS), there are many other possible associated disease states. For example, patients with malignant hypertension can have very severe hemolysis due to increased shearing of red blood cells traversing damaged glomeruli. There may also be associated thrombocytopenia, which can lead to concern that TTP may be present. Hemolysis associated with malignant hypertension resolves rapidly with control of the blood pressure. Scleroderma renal crisis is often accompanied by a MAHA due to both severe hypertension and renal damage.

TABLE 1	Hemolytic Anemia: Classification of Common Causes

Congenital

Membrane Defects

Hereditary Spherocytosis
Hereditary Elliptocytosis
Hereditary Pyropoikilocytosis

Enzymatic Defects

G-6-PD Deficiency
Pyruvate Kinase Deficiency

Hemoglobin Defects

Sickle Cell Disease
Unstable Hemoglobins

Acquired

Autoimmune

Warm Antibody IgG
Cold Antibody IgM
Drug-Induced
Paroxysmal Nocturnal Hemoglobinuria

Mechanical

Microangiopathic
Toxins
Parasites

Cardiac valvular disease can lead to a MAHA. This is seen most commonly after mitral valve repair if there is a small defect at the site where the valve ring is sewn in. Ventricular contraction leads to a small resurgent jet, which results in a high-shear situation in the jet and red blood cell destruction. In some cases, this can result in severe hemolysis and a transfusion-dependent anemia.

Ventricular assist devices (VAD) to support heart failure patients can also lead to hemolysis. This is blood flowing through the device being subjected to high shear rates. Most patients have low levels of hemolysis, but with VAD thrombosis there is an abrupt increase in hemolysis due to higher shear forces; a rising LDH is an indication to look for VAD thrombosis.

Along with MAHA, there are several other syndromes that may cause mechanical damage to the red blood cells. Clostridium infections can lead to hemolysis by direct damage to red blood cell membranes. The bacteria secrete an alpha-toxin that has phospholipase activity and leads to the red blood cell membrane literally dissolving—which causes the hemoglobin to leak out of the cells. In some cases this can be so severe that the measured hemoglobin may equal the hematocrit. Empty red blood cell "ghosts" may be seen on the smear.

Wilson's disease may cause episodes of hemolysis along with the neurologic and hepatic disease. This is caused by large amounts of hepatic copper entering the circulation and inducing an oxidative hemolysis. The smear can show spherocytes and "bite cell." The hemolysis is often transient because it is related to high levels of copper in the serum.

Spur cell anemia is a hemolytic process seen in patients with end-stage liver disease. The lipid metabolism alterations induced by severe liver disease lead to cholesterol crystal formation in the red cell membrane. These crystals are removed by the spleen and can lead to both hemolysis and deformed red cells—"spur cells."

Prevention

There are a few supportive steps in patients with hemolysis. Although most food is supplemented with folate, high red cell turn over can increase the need for this vitamin. Patients with hemolysis are often supplemented with folic acid 1 mg daily.[1]

A key preventive measure for those with G6PD deficiency is avoiding agents that can lead to oxidative stress of red cells. The most complete list of medications found at https://www.g6pd.org/ and common medications are listed in Table 2. Some rarer red blood cell enzymatic or hemoglobin defects are also sensitive to oxidative stress, so these medications should be avoided in those disease also.

Clinical Manifestations
Inherited

The severity of congenital hemolytic anemia varies tremendously. Some children are very symptomatic right after birth, whereas older patients may only present with mild anemia and subtle laboratory findings. A common presentation is a burst of hemolysis with oxidative or other stressors. Hereditary hemolytic anemias are often more severe right after birth, and severity may decrease with age. Patients with congenital anemia can present with extrahematologic problems. Given that the serum bilirubin is increased and more bilirubin is excreted in the bile, they may present with pigmented gallstones. Patients can present with gallbladder disease in their teens or twenties, and this should raise the suspicion of hemolytic anemia. These patients may be more prone to skin ulcers around the ankle, which may not heal well.

Classically patients with congenital hemolytic anemias can develop three types of crises. The first is the "hemolytic crisis." When patients develop fevers or encounter other stresses, the rate of hemolysis may increase, and any inflammation can suppress erythropoiesis, leading to severe anemia. The second type of crisis is the "megaloblastic crisis" where patients become folic acid deficient because of the high folate demand associated with

TABLE 2	Drugs That May Precipitate a Hemolytic Crisis With G6PD Deficiency
Acetanilide (Antifebrin)[4]	
Dapsone	
Furazolidone[2]	
Isobutyl Nitrate[4]	
Methylene Blue	
Nalidixic acid[2]	
Naphthalene	
Nitrofurantoin (Macrobid)	
Pamaquine[2]	
Phenazopyridine (Pyridium)	
Phenylhydrazine	
Primaquine	
Quinolones	
Sulfacetamide	
Sulfamethoxazole	
Sulfanilamide	
Sulfapyridine	

[2]Not available in the United States.
[4]Not yet approved for use in the United States.

increased red blood cell production. With mass supplementation of folate in the food supply, this incidence has fallen. The final crisis is the "aplastic crisis" where red blood cell production is temporarily compromised and the reticulocyte count plummets. This is most commonly found with infections with parvovirus B-19. The infection clears in most patients within 1 week, but patients often require transfusion support during this time.

Hereditary spherocytosis is most prevalent in northern European populations and occurs with a frequency of approximately 1 in 5000. Most cases (75%) show an autosomal dominant pattern of inheritance. The remainder is due to autosomal recessive inheritance and new mutations. Common clinical features of hereditary spherocytosis include anemia, jaundice, reticulocytosis, splenomegaly, and microspherocytes. Anemia later in life is variable and usually mild. Complications include hemolytic crises, leg ulcers, and gallstones.

With hereditary elliptocytosis, most patients are symptom free, and the frequent finding of elliptocytes on the blood smear is of no clinical consequence. However, approximately 10% to 15% of patients have significant hemolysis and may develop anemia. Mild hereditary elliptocytosis is inherited in an autosomal dominant fashion. The incidence is higher in African and Asian populations because of its beneficial impact on malarial infection. Patients with pyropoikilocytosis have severe hemolysis.

G6PD deficiency is the most common enzyme defect in humans and affects an estimated 600 million people worldwide. G6PD deficiency is transmitted as an X-linked recessive condition. Hundreds of G6PD variants have been identified. Enzymatic activity varies from normal with no clinical consequences to severe deficiency resulting in chronic hemolysis and shortened red blood cell life span, even in the absence of stressors. The two most common variants are the G6PD A variant, which has moderate enzyme deficiency (10%-15% activity), and the G6PD Mediterranean mutation, which has almost no detectable enzyme activity. Despite this, patients with G6PD Mediterranean have a nearly normal erythrocyte life span except under conditions of metabolic or oxidative stress.

The classic presentation of hemolysis with G6PD deficiency is with oxidant stress. For example, certain medications such as

[1]Not FDA approved for this indication.

sulfonamides can lead to increased oxidative stress. Patients with G6PD deficiency cannot generate enough reducing power to overcome this stress, which leads to oxidative damage to proteins, especially hemoglobin. The patient presents with fulminant hemolysis that can lead to a severe anemia. Because of membrane damage, the blood smear can show spherocytes and "bite cells"—red blood cells with defects caused by splenic conditioning. Treatment is removing the offending agent and is otherwise supportive. A unique presentation is "favism." After patient eats fava beans, an overwhelming hemolysis develops. This can be idiosyncratic and occur even in patients who have safely eaten the beans in the past.

Pyruvate kinase deficiency is inherited as an autosomal recessive condition. Anemia is variable and may range from a presentation in early infancy requiring transfusions to fully compensated hemolysis presenting with jaundice alone. Many patients have moderate anemia, jaundice, and splenomegaly. Patients with this disorder are also susceptible to the crises identified above. Splenectomy may be helpful in severe cases, but response is variable.

Acquired

AIHA patients who have IgG as the offending antibody are said to have warm antibody AIHA. The name warm comes from the fact that the antibody reacts best at body temperature. The incidence varies by series but is about 1 in 100,000 patients per year, and women are affected more often than men.

Warm AIHA can complicate several diseases. Lupus patients can develop warm AIHA as part of their disease complex. Of malignances, that with the strongest association with AIHA is chronic lymphocytic leukemia (CLL). Series show that 5% to 10% of patients with CLL will have warm AIHA. The disease can appear concurrently with CLL or may develop during the course of the disease.

A rare but important variant of warm AIHA is Evan's syndrome. This is the combination of AIHA and immune thrombocytopenia. One to three percent of AIHA is the Evan's variant. The immune thrombocytopenia can precede, occur concurrently, or develop after the AIHA. The diagnosis of Evan's syndrome should raise the concern of underlying disorders. In pediatric and young adult patients, immunodeficiencies such as autoimmune lymphoproliferative disease needs to be considered. In older patients, Evan's syndrome is often associated with T-cell lymphomas.

In rare patients with warm AIHA, IgA or IgM antibodies are implicated. Patients with IgM AIHA often have a severe course with a fatal outcome. Patients' plasma may show spontaneous hemolysis and agglutination. The DAT may not be strongly positive or show C3 reactivity. The clinical clues are C3 reactivity with no cold agglutinins and severe hemolysis, sometimes with intravascular hemolysis.

In cold agglutinin disease, in addition to hemolysis, patients often note symptoms related to agglutination of red blood cells in the peripheral circulation. For example, acrocyanosis will be noted in cold weather. Rare patients will have abdominal pain when eating cold food due to ischemia related to agglutination of red blood cells in the viscera. Some patients with cold agglutinins can have an exacerbation of their hemolysis with cold exposure.

In young patients, cold AIHA is often post-infectious (such as from viral and mycoplasma infections), and the course is self-limited. The hemolysis usually starts 2 to 3 weeks after the illness and will last for 4 to 6 weeks. In older patients, the etiology in more than 90% of cases is a B-cell lymphoproliferative disorder, usually with monoclonal kappa B-cells. The most commonly seen are marginal zone lymphoma, small lymphocytic lymphoma, and lymphoplasmacytic lymphoma.

A unique cold AIHA is paroxysmal cold hemoglobinuria (PCH). This AIHA is most often post-viral affecting children; in the past it complicated any stage of syphilis. The antibody is IgG directed against the P antigen on the RBC. Binding is best in the "cold," but then complement is activated at body temperature. Because this antibody can fix complement, hemolysis can be rapid and severe, leading to extreme anemia.

Drug-induced AIHA is a rare drug reaction with a lower incidence than drug-related immune thrombocytopenia. The rate of severe drug-related AIHA is estimated at 1 in 1 million, but less severe cases may be missed. Most patients will have positive DAT without signs of hemolysis, although rare patients will have relentless hemolysis resulting in death. With hapten-related AIHA, very few patients will have hemolysis, and in those cases the hemolysis will resolve a few days after discontinuation of the offending drug. With immune complex disease, most often the patient will only have a positive DAT, but rare patients on exposure or reexposure will have life-threatening hemolysis. The onset of this hemolysis is rapid, with signs of acute illness and intravascular hemolysis. The classic associated drug is quinine, but many other drugs have been implicated.

A virulent form of immune complex hemolysis is associated with both disseminated intravascular coagulation and brisk hemolysis. Patients who receive certain second- and third-generation cephalosporins (especially cefotetan [Cefotan] and ceftriaxone [Rocephin]) have developed this syndrome. The clinical symptoms start 7 to 10 days after receiving the drug—often the patient has only received the antibiotic for surgical prophylaxis. Warm DAT hemolysis with an acute hematocrit drop, hypotension, and disseminated intravascular coagulation develop. The patients are often believed to have sepsis and are then often reexposed to the cephalosporin, resulting in worsening of the clinical status. The outcome is often fatal because of massive hemolysis and thrombosis.

Hemolysis caused by methyldopa is indistinguishable from warm AIHA, which is consistent with the notion that methyldopa induces an autoimmune hemolytic anemia. The hemolysis often resolves rapidly after stopping the methyldopa, although the Coombs test result may remain positive for months. This type of drug-induced hemolytic anemia has been reported with levodopa, procainamide (Pronestyl), and chlorpromazine (Thorazine).

In MAHA, the course of the presentation is dictated by the underlying cause. In valvular hemolysis, the onset of hemolysis is soon after the cardiac procedure and may require transfusion support. With VAD hemolysis, most patients have only mild hemolysis, but with pump thrombosis, the hemolysis can be severe. Patients with spur cell anemia have findings of severe liver disease—high INRs and bilirubin (mean of 9.5 mg/dL). Spur cell hemolysis is associated with an ominous prognosis and average survival of a few months.

PNH is characterized by episodes of hemolysis and a propensity for thrombosis and pancytopenia. Often patients can have PNH for years before the diagnosis is made. The hemolysis can range from being well compensated to transfusion dependence. Patients with PNH often have severe thrombophilia; the leading cause of morbidity and death (before the release of effective therapy) has been thrombosis. The cause of the hypercoagulable state is unknown, but complement-activated platelets have been implicated.

Diagnosis

There are two steps in the diagnosis of hemolytic anemia—first determining the presence of hemolysis, and then finding the cause. Hemolysis is demonstrated by evidence of both red blood cell breakdown as well as the compensatory increase in red blood cell production this stimulates. When red blood cells undergo hemolysis, their contents, mostly hemoglobin and the enzyme LDH, are released. Hemoglobin is by haptoglobin, and the heme moiety is broken down, first to bilirubin and then to urobilinogen, which is excreted in the urine.

The following tests are performed to investigate hemolysis:

LDH: Lactate dehydrogenase is an enzyme found in high concentration in the red blood cell; hemolysis releases this enzyme into the plasma. Most patients with hemolysis will have an elevated LDH level, making this a sensitive test. However, many other processes, including liver disease, pneumonia, and more, will also increase the serum LDH.

Serum bilirubin: Heme is broken down to produce bilirubin. Initially unconjugated, the bilirubin is delivered to the liver where it is conjugated and excreted into the bile. In hemolysis the unconjugated ("indirect bilirubin") is increased as opposed to liver disease, where the conjugated ("direct bilirubin") is increased. If a patient has coexisting liver disease with an elevated direct bilirubin, this test is not reliable.

Serum haptoglobin: Haptoglobin binds free serum hemoglobin and is taken up by the liver. Haptoglobin usually falls to very low levels in hemolysis. It's important to remember that haptoglobin is also an acute-phase reactant that can rise with systemic disease or inflammation. However, patients with advanced liver disease will have low haptoglobin due to a lack of synthesis, and up to 2% of the population may congenitally lack haptoglobin.

Hemoglobinemia: If the hemolysis is very rapid, the amount of free hemoglobin that is released will overwhelm haptoglobin and lead to the presence of free hemoglobin in the plasma. This can be crudely quantified by examining the plasma. Even minute amounts of free hemoglobin will turn the plasma pink. In fulminant hemolysis, the serum will be cola colored.

Urine hemosiderin: When hemoglobin is excreted by the kidney, the iron is deposited in the tubules. When the tubule cells are sloughed off, they will appear in the urine. The urine can be stained for iron, and, if positive, this is another sign of hemolysis. This is a later sign because it takes a week for enough iron-laden tubule cells to be excreted in detectable quantities.

Mean corpuscular volume (MCV): The MCV may be larger in hemolysis for several reasons. The size of reticulocytes is larger than normal red blood cells, so a brisk reticulocytosis will have a higher MCV. In cold agglutinin disease, the aggregation of red blood cells will falsely increase the MCV. Finally, hemolysis can lead to folate deficiency and a rise in MCV.

Reticulocyte count: With hemolysis the breakdown of red blood cells is accompanied by an increase in the reticulocyte count as marrow tries to compensate. The reticulocyte percentage needs to be adjusted for the hematocrit—a correct value of above 1.5% is considered raised. Recently, automated complete blood count machines have taken advantage of the fact that reticulocytes will absorb certain stains, and these machines can directly measure the reticulocyte count via flow cytometry.

This results in an "absolute" reticulocyte count. This does not have to be corrected for hematocrit, and levels about 90,000/μL are consider elevated. However, the reticulocyte count can also be increased in blood loss or in patients who have other causes of anemia (such as treated iron deficiency). In addition, as many of 25% of patients with AIHA will never have elevated reticulocyte counts for reasons such as nutritional deficiency, autoimmune destruction of red blood cell precursors, or lack of erythropoietin.

The blood smear provides vital information (Table 3). The finding of abnormal red blood cell shapes can be a clue to autoimmune hemolysis or red blood cell membrane defects. For example, spherocytes are seen in autoimmune hemolytic anemia, heredity spherocytosis, Wilson's disease, clostridial sepsis, and severe burns. Schistocytes are a sign of microangiopathic hemolytic anemia and should prompt concerns for such disease processes as thrombotic thrombocytopenia purpura, vavular hemolysis, VAD, march hemoglobinuria, among many examples.

In hereditary spherocytosis, the blood smear suggests the diagnosis. Confirmation is by demonstrating an increased osmotic fragility, although direct genetic screening for the molecular defects is becoming more common. The blood smear is also critical for diagnosing hereditary elliptocytosis and hereditary pyropoikilocytosis, although there is an increasing role for genetic diagnosis. Patients with hereditary pyropoikilocytosis are usually homozygous or compound heterozygous for one of the mutations causing mild hereditary elliptocytosis.

Diagnosis of G6PD deficiency is made by measuring enzyme activity. This is best done after the hemolytic episode is over, because reticulocytes have higher G6PD levels and can lead to falsely normal enzyme activity levels.

AIHA demonstrate either IgG or complement on the red blood cell. This is done by the "direct antibody" or "Coombs test." IgG bound to red blood cells will not agglutinate them. However, if IgM that is directed against IgG or C3 is added, the red blood cells will agglutinate, proving that there is IgG or C3 on the red blood cell membrane. The finding of a positive DAT in the setting of a hemolytic anemia is diagnostic of AIHA.

TABLE 3	Typical Blood Smear Findings in Hemolysis
Bite Cells	
Oxidative Hemolytic Anemia Such as G6PD Deficiency	
Elliptocytes	
Heredity Elliptocytosis Schistocytes Thrombotic Thrombocytopenic Purpura, Valvular Hemolysis,	
Spherocytes:	
Hereditary Spherocytosis, Autoimmune Hemolytic Anemia, Wilson's Disease, Burns	
Spur Cells:	
Severe Liver Disease	

There are several pitfalls to the DAT. One is that a positive DAT can be found in 1 in 1000 patients in the normal population and up to several percent of ailing patients, especially those with elevated gamma globulin such as patients with liver disease or HIV. Administration of IVIG can also create a false-positive DAT. Conversely, patients can have AIHA with a negative DAT. Some patients have a low amount of IgG binding the red blood cell, which is below the detection limit of the DAT reagents. Other patients can have IgA or "warm" IgM as the cause of the AIHA. Specialty laboratories can test for these possibilities. The diagnosis of DAT-negative AIHA should be made with caution, and other causes of hemolysis-like hereditary spherocytosis or PNH should be excluded.

The DAT in patients with cold AIHA will show cells coated with C3. The blood smear will often show agglutination of the blood, and if the blood cools before being analyzed, the agglutination will interfere with the analysis. Titers of cold agglutinin can range from 1 in 1000 to 1 in > 1 million. The autoantibodies are most often directed against the I/i antigen system, with 90% against I. The I specificity is typical with primary cold agglutinin disease and also following mycoplasma infection. The i-specific antigen is most typical of Epstein-Barr and cytomegalovirus infections.

In PCH the DAT is often weakly positive but can be negative. The diagnostic test is the Donath-Landsteiner test. This complex test is performed by incubating samples in three temperature ranges: one at 0°C to 4°C, one set at 37°C, and one incubated first at 0°C to 4°C and then 37°C. The diagnosis of PCH is made if only the third tube shows hemolysis.

For many patients, the first clue to drug-associated AIHA is the finding of a positive DAT in a patient taking a suspect drug (Table 4). Specialty laboratories such as Wisconsin Blood Center or the L.A. Red Cross can perform in vitro studies of drug interactions that can produce a certain diagnosis.

For PNH, the diagnosis had been based on an in vitro demonstration of increased sensitivity of red blood cells to complement lysis. Currently, flow cytometry is performed to examine cells for the absence of GPI-anchored proteins (CD55 or CD59 on red cells, other GPI-anchored proteins on white blood cells). In patients with microangiopathy the smear will show abundant schistocytes with a marked elevated LDH.

Therapy

Splenectomy is curative for most cases of hereditary spherocytosis but is reserved for patients with severe symptoms. For patients with hereditary pyropoikilocytosis, splenectomy can also be useful.

Most patients with G6PD deficiency require no special management beyond the avoidance of provocative medications and food. Highly symptomatic patients with pyruvate kinase deficiency may respond to splenectomy, and in clinical trials a small molecule agent that can increase enzyme activity.

Initial management of warm AIHA is prednisone starting at 1 mg/kg daily. It can take up to 3 weeks to see a response. Once the hematocrit is > 30%, the prednisone is slowly tapered. Eighty

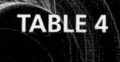

TABLE 4	Drugs Implicated in Autoimmune Hemolytic Anemia

Most Common

Cefotetan (Cefotan)
Ceftriaxone (Rocephin)
Piperacillin (Pipracil)
Fludarabine (Fludara)

Other Implicated Drugs

Acetaminophen
Amphotericin B
Beta-lactams (any)
Carboplatin (Paraplatin)
Cephalosporins (any)
Chlorpromazine (Thorazine)
Chlorpropamide (Diabinese)
Cimetidine (Tagamet)
Ciprofloxacin (Cipro)
Diclofenac (Voltaren)
Doxycycline
Enalapril (Vasotec)
Erythromycin
Isoniazid
Levodopa
Melphalan (Alkeran)
Methyldopa
Nonsteroidal Antiinflammatory Agents
Omeprazole (Prilosec)
Oxaliplatin (Eloxatin)
Probenecid
Procainamide
Quinidine
Quinine
Rifampin
Sulfa drugs
Teniposide (Vumon)
Tetracycline
Thiazides
Thiopental (Pentothal)
Tolbutamide (Orinase)
Tricyclic Antidepressants

[1]Not FDA approved for this indication.

percent of patients will respond to steroids, but the steroids can be fully tapered off in only 30%. For patients who can be maintained on 10 mg or less of steroids daily, this maybe the most reasonable long-term therapy.

Current data show that adding rituximab (Rituxan)[1] to steroids for warm AIHA will improve overall response and should be considered early in most patients. These responses appear to be durable, and for relapses, repeating treatment is effective. It is important to remember that, for most patients, the response to rituximab is a gradual one over months; one should not expect a rapid response. Most studies have used the "traditional" 375 mg/m² dosing weekly for 4 weeks, and another option is 1000 mg repeated once 14 days apart.

Splenectomy is now reserved for patients with warm AIHA who do not respond to steroids or rituximab. Reported response rates in the literature range from 50% to 80%, with 50% to 60% remaining in remission. Timing of the procedure is a balance between allowing time for the steroids to work and the risk of toxicity of steroids. A patient who is at low risk for surgery and has either refractory disease or an inability to be weaned from high doses of steroids should have splenectomy considered early.

For patients who do not respond to either splenectomy or rituximab, the therapy is less certain. Although intravenous immune globulin is a standard therapy for immune thrombocytopenia, response rates are low in warm AIHA. Numerous therapies have been reported in small series, but there is no clear approach. Options include the following:

- Azathioprine (Imuran)[1] 75-150 mg/day
- Cyclophosphamide (Cytoxan)[1] 1000 mg monthly bolus IV
- Mycophenolate (CellCept)[1] 500-1000 mg bid
- Cyclosporine (Neoral)[1] 5 mg/kg daily divided in two doses
- Danazol (Danocrine)[1] 200 mg tid

Our approach has been to use mycophenolate for patients who require high doses of steroids or need transfusions. Patients needing lower doses of steroids may be good candidates for danazol to help wean them off steroids.

The sparse literature on Evan's syndrome suggests it can be more refractory to standard therapy, with response rates to splenectomy being in the 50% range. In patients with lymphoma, antineoplastic therapy is crucial. Data are accumulating for patients with autoimmune lymphoproliferative disease: mycophenolate or sirolimus (Rapamune)[1] starting at 2 mg/m² may be effective for splenectomy or rituximab failures.

The importance of diagnosing cold AIHA and differentiating it from warm AIHA is the fact that standard therapy for warm disease steroids is ineffective. Because C3-coated red blood cells are taken up through the reticulo-endothelial system, especially in the liver, as well as the spleen, splenectomy is an ineffective therapy.

Simple measures to help with cold AIHA should be used. Patients should be kept in a warm environment and should try to avoid the cold. If transfusions are needed, they should be infused via blood warmers to prevent hemolysis. In rare patients with severe hemolysis, plasma exchange can be considered. Given the culprit antibody is IgM—mostly intravascular—use of plasma exchange can slow the hemolysis to give time for other therapies to take effect.

Therapy of cold AIHA remains difficult. Currently the drug of choice is rituximab.[1] Response can be seen in 45% to 75% of patients but is almost always a partial response; retreatment is often necessary. As with other autoimmune hematologic diseases, there can be a delay in response. There are data to support adding bendamustine (Treanda)[1] 90 mg/m² to rituximab. The response rates are higher, but so are the complications of therapy. Although more toxic, this combination can be considered in patients with aggressive disease. Soon to be approved is sutimlimab[5], which is a monoclonal antibody that blocks complement 1s and dramatically reduces hemolysis.

For most patients with drug-induced AIHA, stopping the offending drug is sufficient. It is doubtful that steroids or other autoimmune-directed therapy is effective. For patients with the DIC-hemolysis syndrome, there are anecdotes that plasma exchange may be helpful. Therapy for patients with positive DAT without signs of hemolysis is uncertain. If the drug is essential, then the patient can be observed. If the patient has hemolysis, the drug needs to be discontinued and the patient observed for signs of end-stage organ damage.

Transfusions can be very difficult in AIHA. The presence of the autoantibody can interfere with typing of the blood and almost always interferes with the cross-match, because this final step consists of mixing the patient's serum with donor red blood cells. In most patients with AIHA the autoantibodies will react with any donor cells, rendering a negative cross-match impossible. Without the cross-match the concern is that underlying alloantibodies can be missed, which can lead to transfusion reactions.

Some of these concerns may be allayed by remembering that patients who have never been transfused or pregnant will rarely have alloantibodies. Second, a patient who has undergone transfusion in the remote past may have an amnestic antibody response but not an immediate hemolytic reaction.

When a patient is first suspected of having AIHA, a generous sample of blood should be given to the transfusion service. This will allow for adequate testing of the sample. Second, many centers will test the blood not only for blood groups ABO and D but will also perform full Rh typing and check for Kidd, Duffy, and Kell status. This can allow transfusion of phenotypically matched blood to lessen the risk of alloantibody formation.

One difficult issue is timing of transfusion. Clinicians are often hesitant to transfuse patients with AIHA due to fear of reactions. But in frail patients with severe anemia—especially elderly

[5]Investigational drug in the United States

patients or those with heart disease—transfusion can be lifesaving. Because in some cases it can take hours to screen for alloantibodies, it is often preferable to transfuse patients with severe anemia while carefully observing for reactions.

The treatment for PNH is the complement inhibitor eculizumab (Soliris), a humanized monoclonal antibody that targets complement protein C5, thereby preventing assembly of the terminal complement complex during complement activation. In studies, treatment with eculizumab has been shown to reduce hemolysis, as well as improve anemia, fatigue, and quality of life in patients with PNH. In addition, eculizumab has demonstrated efficacy in reducing thrombosis. Just approved is ravulizumab (Ultomiris), another anti-C5 monoclonal antibody that needs infusion only every 8 weeks instead of every 2 weeks (eculizumab).

Management of Complications

The most concerning complication of splenectomy is overwhelming post-splenectomy infection. In adults, the spleen appears to play a minimal role in immunity except for defense from certain encapsulated organisms. Patients will often present with disseminated intravascular coagulation and will rapidly progress to purpura fulminans. Approximately 40% to 50% of patients will die of sepsis even when detected early. The overall lifetime risk may be as high as 1 in 500. The organism most commonly found in these cases is *Streptococcus pneumoniae*, which is reported in more than 50% of cases. *Neisseria meningitidis* and *Haemophilus influenzae* have also been implicated in many cases.

Patients who have undergone splenectomy need to be warned about the risk of overwhelming post-splenectomy infection and instructed to report to the emergency department immediately if they develop a fever greater than 101° or shaking chills. Once in the emergency department, blood cultures should be rapidly obtained and the patient started on antibiotic coverage with agents that cover encapsulated organisms. Patients who are planning to have or are being considered for a splenectomy should be vaccinated for pneumococcal, meningococcal, and H influenza infections. If patients are planning to be treated with rituximab first, they should also be vaccinated because after receiving rituximab, they will not be able to mount an immune response.

The major side effects of rituximab are infusion reactions—often worse with the first dose. These can be controlled with antihistamines, steroids, and, for severe rigors, meperidine (Demerol).[1] Rare patients can develop neutropenia (about 1 in 500) that appears to be autoimmune in nature. Infections appear to be only minimally increased with the use of rituximab. One group at higher risk are patients who are chronic carriers of hepatitis B. These patients may have reactivation of the virus that can be fatal in some cases; patients being considered for rituximab need to be screened for hepatitis B. Progressive multifocal leukoencephalopathy is a very rare risk that is more common in cancer patients and heavily immunosuppressed patients. The overall risk is unknown but is less than 1 in 50,000.

Eculizumab and ravulizumab are well tolerated, except for a risk of meningococcal infection estimated at 1 in 500 risk. All patients receiving this agent should be vaccinated and need to report to the emergency department with any sign of infection.

---

[1]Not FDA approved for this indication.

References

Berentsen S: Cold agglutinin disease, *Hematology Am Soc Hematol Educ Program* 2016:226–231, 2016.

Brodsky RA: Warm autoimmune hemolytic anemia, *N Engl J Med* 15; 381(7):647–654, 2019.

Cappellini MD, Fiorelli G: Glucose-6-phosphate dehydrogenase deficiency, *Lancet* 371(9606):64–74, 2008.

Go RS, Winters JL, Kay NE: How I treat autoimmune hemolytic anemia, *Blood* 129:2971–2979, 2017.

Haley K: Congenital hemolytic anemia, *Med Clin North Am* 101:361–374, 2017.

Hill A, DeZern AE, Kinoshita T, Brodsky RA: Paroxysmal nocturnal haemoglobinuria, *Nat Rev Dis Primers* 3:17028, 2017.

Liebman HA, Weitz IC: Autoimmune Hemolytic Anemia, *Med Clin North Am* 101:351–359, 2017.

HEMOPHILIA AND RELATED CONDITIONS

Method of
Meera Chitlur, MD; Bulent Ozgonenel, MD; and Roshni Kulkarni, MD

CURRENT DIAGNOSIS

- The hemophilias and von Willebrand disease (VWD) account for 80% to 85% of inherited bleeding disorders. Hemophilia A and B are X-linked, whereas VWD and rare bleeding disorders (RBDs) are autosomal disorders.
- The diagnosis of hemophilia and other inherited bleeding disorders should be confirmed by specific laboratory assays because screening tests such as prothrombin time (PT) and activated partial thromboplastin time (aPTT) may be normal. Plasma levels of deficient factor determine clinical severity and management.
- Major complications associated with hemophilia are inhibitor development, hemarthrosis, and intracranial hemorrhage. Hemarthrosis is the most common and debilitating complication, and central nervous system (CNS) bleeding is the most common cause of mortality in hemophilia. Mucosal bleeding and menorrhagia are the most common manifestations of VWD. Bleeding manifestations of RBDs are mild, although homozygotes can present with severe disease.
- Newborns have normal levels of factor VIII; therefore, the diagnosis of hemophilia A can be established at birth. Vacuum delivery should be avoided to prevent head bleeds.
- Women and adolescents with menorrhagia and no underlying pathology should be investigated for a bleeding disorder.

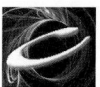

CURRENT THERAPY

- Currently there is a paradigm shift in the treatment of hemophilia. In addition to the traditional plasma-derived and recombinant concentrates, the new extended half-life recombinant products have reduced the treatment burden by reducing the frequency of intravenous injections. Novel, subcutaneously administered, nonfactor replacement therapy with prolonged hemostatic efficiency has been a game changer for patients both with and without inhibitors. Gene therapy is on the horizon, offering a promise of cure. Even for von Willebrand disease (VWD) and rare bleeding disorders (RBDs) such as deficiencies of factors VII, XI, XIII, X, fibrinogen, replacement factor concentrates are currently available. Early and effective treatment and prophylaxis can prevent bleeding episodes, including repeated hemarthrosis and joint destruction in persons with hemophilia. Patients should be tested annually for the presence of inhibitors. Cryoprecipitate is not recommended for the treatment of hemophilia because of concerns regarding transmission of bloodborne pathogens.
- For mild and moderate hemophilia A and VWD, the use of desmopressin (DDAVP) coupled with antifibrinolytics can obviate the use of concentrates. Continued vigilance should be implemented for inhibitory antibodies and new and emerging bloodborne pathogens.
- All patients with inherited bleeding disorders should be immunized against hepatitis A and B and followed in close collaboration with the local hemophilia treatment center (HTC) (https://www.cdc.gov/ncbddd/hemophilia/htc.html). The National Hemophilia Foundation's (https://www.hemophilia.org) Medical and Scientific Advisory Committee (MASAC) guidelines for updated recommendations and product choice should be followed.

Hemophilia A and Hemophilia B

Hemophilia is an X-linked congenital bleeding disorder caused by a deficiency of factor VIII (hemophilia A) or factor IX (hemophilia

B). Hemophilia A is the most common severe bleeding disorder and affects 1 in 5000 males in the United States; hemophilia B occurs in 1 in 30,000 males.

Pathophysiology

The *factor VIII* gene is one of the largest genes and spans 186 kb of genomic DNA at Xq28. Intron 22 of the *factor VIII* gene is particularly large and is therefore susceptible to inversion mutations. Inversions of this intron account for 50% of all severe hemophilia A cases, and inversions of other introns, deletions, point mutations, and insertions account for the remainder.

Hepatic and reticuloendothelial cells are presumed sites of factor VIII synthesis. Factor VIII is synthesized as a single chain polypeptide with three A domains (A1, A2, and A3), a large central B domain, and two C domains (Figure 1). The binding sites for von Willebrand factor (VWF), thrombin, and factor Xa are on the C2 domain, and factor IXa binding sites are on the A2 and A3 domains. The B domain can be deleted without any consequences. VWF protects factor VIII from proteolytic degradation in the plasma and concentrates it at the site of injury.

The *factor IX* gene is 34 kb long and located at Xq26. It is a vitamin K–dependent serine protease composed of 415 amino acids. It is synthesized in the liver and its plasma concentration is approximately 50 times that of factor VIII. Gene deletions and point mutations result in hemophilia B.

Role of Factors VIII and IX in Coagulation

Factor VIII circulates bound to VWF. It is a cofactor for factor IX and is essential for factor X activation. In the classic coagulation cascade, activation of the intrinsic or extrinsic pathway of coagulation results in sufficient thrombin generation. The fact that bleeding still occurs in hemophilia despite an intact extrinsic pathway has led to the revised cell-based model of coagulation.

The revised pathway incorporates all coagulation factors into a single pathway initiated by Factor VII and tissue factor. The contact factors (XI, XII, kallikrein, and high-molecular-weight [HMW] kininogen) are not essential but serve as a backup. Following injury, encrypted tissue factor is exposed and forms a complex with F VIIa. The tissue factor–factor VIIa complex activates factor IX to IXa (which moves to the platelet surface) and factor X to Xa. This generates small amounts of thrombin that activates platelets, converts platelet factor V to Va and factor XI to XIa, and releases factor VIII from VWF and activates it. The factor XIa activates plasma factor IX to IXa on the platelet surface, which together with factor VIIIa forms the tenase complex (factor VIIIa/IXa) that converts large amounts of factor X to Xa. Factor Xa

forms a prothrombinase complex with FVa and converts large amounts of prothrombin to thrombin, called *thrombin burst*. This results in the conversion of sufficient fibrinogen to fibrin to form a stable clot. In hemophilia, lack of factor VIII or IX produces a profound abnormality. Factor Xa generated by FVIIa and tissue factor is insufficient because this pathway is inhibited by tissue factor pathway inhibitor (TFPI) as part of a negative feedback, and factors VIII and IX, which are required for amplifying the production of Xa, are absent. The primary platelet plug formation and initiation phases of coagulation are normal. Any clot that is formed (from the initiation phase) is friable and porous.

Clinical Features

The diagnosis of hemophilia is often made following a bleeding episode or because of a family history; however, 50% of cases have no family history. Based on the plasma levels of factor VIII or IX (normal levels are 50%–150%) that correlate with severity and predict bleeding risk, hemophilia is classified as mild (>5%), moderate (1%–5%), and severe (<1%) (Table 1). Approximately 65% of persons with hemophilia have severe disease, 15% have moderate disease, and 20% have mild disease. Most cases of severe disease manifest by 4 years of age; moderate or mild disease is diagnosed later and often following bleeding secondary to trauma or surgery.

Hemophilia can be diagnosed in the first trimester, using chorionic villus sampling and gene analysis. In the second trimester, fetal blood sampling can be performed. Prenatal diagnosis to determine fetal gender can aid in the management of pregnancy and delivery.

The hallmark of severe hemophilia is hemarthrosis, or bleeding into the joint, that can occur spontaneously or with minimal trauma. The immediate effects of a joint bleed are excruciating pain, swelling, warmth, and muscle spasms, and the long-term effect of recurrent hemarthrosis is the hemophilic arthropathy, which is characterized by synovial thickening and chronic inflammation. Repeated hemorrhage results in a target joint. Knees, elbows, ankles, hips, and shoulders are commonly affected. Disuse atrophy of surrounding muscles leads to further joint instability. Limitation of joint range of motion due to hemarthrosis often correlates positively with older age, non-White race, and increased body mass index, and it adversely affects quality of life.

Muscle hematomas, another characteristic site of bleeding, can lead to compartment syndrome, with eventual fibrosis and peripheral nerve damage. Iliopsoas bleeds manifest with pain and flexion deformity. Gastrointestinal bleeding and hematuria occur less often.

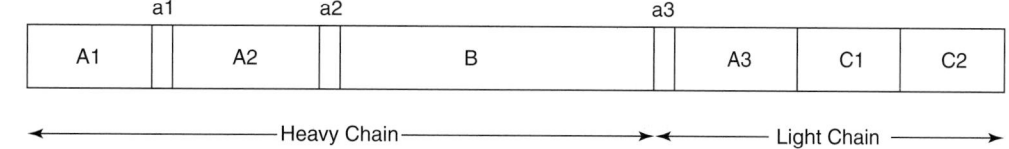

Figure 1 Factor VIII protein structure.

TABLE 1	Hemophilia Severity and Clinical Manifestations		
CHARACTERISTICS	**SEVERE (50%–70%)**	**MODERATE (10%)**	**MILD (30%–40%)**
Factor VIII or IX activity (normal 50%–150%)	<1%	1%–5%	>5%
Age of diagnosis	Birth to 2 years	Childhood or adolescence	Adolescence or adult
Bleeding patterns	2–4/month	4–6/year	Rare
Clinical manifestations	Hemarthroses, muscle, central nervous system, gastrointestinal bleeding, hematuria	Bleeding into joints or muscle following minor trauma, surgical procedure, dental bleeding Rarely spontaneous	Surgical procedures (including dental) and major trauma

Central nervous system (CNS) hemorrhage is a rare but serious complication with a 10% recurrence rate and is the leading cause of mortality in hemophiliacs. Although most newborns with severe hemophilia experience an uneventful course following vaginal delivery, vacuum extraction is associated with an increased CNS bleeding risk. The incidence of intracranial hemorrhage in newborns with hemophilia is 1% to 4%.

Diagnosis

Hemophilia A and B are clinically indistinguishable, and specific factor assays are the only way to differentiate and confirm the diagnosis. Both should be differentiated from VWD. The prothrombin time (PT), platelet function analysis (PFA)-100, and fibrinogen activity are normal. (PFA, a platelet-function screening test, replaces bleeding time because the bleeding time has low sensitivity and specificity and is operator dependent.) The activated partial thromboplastin time (aPTT) is prolonged when the factor levels are less than 30%. Table 2 shows the characteristics and differences between the hemophilias and VWD.

Female carriers may be asymptomatic except for those with extreme lyonization resulting in low factor VIII or IX levels. It is important to note that carriers may experience bleeding episodes (such as heavy menstrual bleeding, postpartum hemorrhage, joint bleeding, etc.) even with levels of FVIII or IX in the 40% to 60% range. Factor VIII levels increase throughout pregnancy and drop to prepregnancy levels following delivery, but factor IX levels remain constant throughout pregnancy.

Treatment

The treatment for hemophilia consists of replacement therapy with intravenous factor VIII or factor IX concentrates produced by purification of donor plasma (plasma derived) (e.g., factor VIII [human]: Hemofil M, Koate; factor IX [human]: AlphaNine SD, Mononine) or in cell culture bioreactors (recombinant) (e.g., factor VIII [recombinant]: Advate, Afstyla, Kogenate FS, Nuwiq, Xyntha; factor IX [recombinant]: BeneFIX, Ixinity, Rixubis). Careful screening of donors combined with heat treatment and viral inactivation methods have made plasma-derived products safer. Plasma-derived and recombinant products appear to have equivalent clinical efficacy. Cryoprecipitate is no longer recommended because of concerns regarding pathogen safety.

Treatment administered only during bleeding symptoms is known as *episodic therapy*, and periodic administration of factor concentrates to prevent bleeding is known as *prophylactic therapy*. Response to treatment is more effective when it is administered early. Although prophylaxis prevents the development of joint disease, the high cost of factor replacement coupled with the need for venous access makes it expensive and difficult and out of reach for patients in the developing world.

The goal of treatment is to raise factor levels to approximately 30% or more for minor bleeds (hematomas or joint bleeds) and 100% for major bleeds (CNS or surgery). Administering 1 U/kg of factor concentrate raises plasma factor VIII levels by 2% and factor IX levels by 1.5% (except with the recombinant factor IX product, where it increases by 0.8%). The half-life of factor VIII is 8 to 12 hours, and that of factor IX is up to 24 hours with standard factor products.

Factor concentrates can also be given by continuous infusion (3–4 U/kg/h). The bolus dose varies from 25 to 50 U/kg depending on the severity, site, and type of bleeding and is dosed to the available vial size because of the cost of the products. Table 3 lists the dosing schedule for various types of bleeds.

For prophylaxis, factor VIII 25 to 40 U/kg administered every other day or factor IX 25 to 40 U/kg twice weekly (because of the longer half-life of factor IX) is aimed at preventing joint disease. Prophylaxis may begin at 1 to 2 years of age and is continued lifelong. Self-infusion before any planned strenuous activity is recommended. Because of the complications of central venous catheters (infections, thrombosis, and mechanical), use of a peripheral vein is encouraged.

Extended half-life (EHL) factor products have increased the half-lives by 1.5-fold in the case of factor VIII and 2.4- to 4.8-fold in the case of factor IX products. EHL factor products have been developed with an aim to decrease the frequency of infusions and improve quality of life for patients with hemophilia, achieved through PEGylation or fusion of the factor protein to the Fc fragment of an immunoglobulin (Ig) or albumin. The first of these EHL products were approved by the US Food and Drug Administration (FDA) in 2014: factor IX (recombinant), Fc fusion protein (Alprolix) for use in patients with hemophilia B, and factor VIII (recombinant), Fc fusion protein (Eloctate) for use in patients with hemophilia A. Subsequently, PEGylated recombinant factor VIII (Adynovate, Takeda Pharmaceuticals, approved 2015) and PEGylated recombinant factor IX (Rebinyn, Novo Nordisk-approved in 2017 but not for prophylaxis) and recombinant albumin fusion Factor IX (Idelvion, CSL Behring) have been approved for use in patients with hemophilia. Recently further extension of the half-life of factor VIII was achieved by a novel fusion protein called BIVV001,[5] consisting of a single recombinant FVIII protein fused to a dimeric FC, a D'D3 domain of VWF (FVIII binding domain), and two XTEN polypeptides. The mean half-life of BIV001 was three to four times that of rFVIII (37.6 h–42.5 h vs. 9.1–13.2 h, respectively) thereby allowing weekly dosing.

Novel Therapies for the Treatment of Hemophilia

In recent years, the field of hemophilia treatment has seen dramatic changes. Treatment options that do not target replacement of the missing factor are currently being tested. Factor VIII mimetics such as the bispecific factor IXa– and factor X–directed antibody emicizumab (Hemlibra) (see later) are FDA-approved nonfactor therapy. Rebalancing agents that inhibit endogenous anticoagulants and restore coagulation include small interfering RNA (siRNA) targeting antithrombin (Fitusiran [Sanofi Pharmaceuticals]),[5] anti-TFPI antibody e.g., Concizumab [Novo Nordisk][5]), and products targeting the anticoagulant effect of activated prothrombin complex (APC) are in clinical trials. The advantages are that these rebalancing agents can be given to either hemophilia A or B patients, provide the benefits of prophylaxis, and can be given subcutaneously, thereby eliminating the need for intravenous injection. More data are needed regarding the safety and efficacy of these medications.

Gene therapy offers promise of a cure, and trials of gene therapy for both hemophilia A and B are currently in process. Two gene therapy trials for hemophilia B had shown subtherapeutic or transient expression of factor IX. In December 2011, Nathwani and colleagues reported that a single injection of factor IX–expressing adeno-associated virus (AAV) vector was effective in treating patients with hemophilia B for more than a year. Since this breakthrough, there have been more successful gene therapy trials that are currently going on for the treatment of both hemophilia A and B. The trials have incorporated modifications of promoters, transgenes and AAV serotypes, and lentiviral vectors. This has been a significant breakthrough in the treatment of hemophilia.

Complications of Treatment

One of the most serious complications of hemophilia treatment is the development of inhibitors or neutralizing antibodies (IgG) that inhibit the function of substituted factor VIII and factor IX. Five percent to 10% of all hemophiliacs and up to 30% of patients with severe hemophilia A develop inhibitors. The incidence of inhibitors in hemophilia B is lower (1%–3%). Most factor VIII inhibitors arise after a median exposure of 9 to 12 days in patients with severe hemophilia A. They can be transient or permanent and should be suspected if a patient fails to respond to an appropriate dose of clotting factor concentrate. Inhibitors can exacerbate bleeding episodes and hemophilic arthropathy.

[5]Investigational drug in the United States.

CHARACTERISTIC	HEMOPHILIA A	HEMOPHILIA B	VON WILLEBRAND DISEASE
Incidence	1:5000	1:30,000	1%–3% of US population
Abnormality	Factor VIII deficiency	Factor IX deficiency	VWF (qualitative and quantitative defect)
Inheritance	X-linked, affects males Gene at the tip of X chromosome	X-linked, affects males Gene at the tip of X chromosome	Autosomal dominant (gene: chromosome 12) Some are recessive or compound heterozygotes
Production site	Unknown, liver endothelium	Liver (vitamin K–dependent)	Megakaryocytes and endothelial cells
Function	Cofactor; forms tenase complex with factor IX and activates factor X, leading to thrombin burst that results in conversion of large amounts of fibrinogen to fibrin	Serine protease (inactive form: zymogen) activated by factor XI or VIIa; forms a tenase complex with factor VIII and activates factor X	Platelet adhesion to site of injury or damaged endothelium
			Protects factor VIII from proteolysis
Classification (normal levels 50%–150%)	Mild (>5%)	Mild (>5%)	Type 1
	Moderate (1%–5%)	Moderate (1%–5%)	Type 2 (2A, 2B, 2M, 2N)
	Severe (<1%)	Severe (<1%)	Type 3
Clinical presentation	Positive family history (30% new mutation) Hemarthroses, hematomas, hematuria, intracranial hemorrhage, gastrointestinal hemorrhage, etc.	Positive family history (30% new mutation) Milder disease, although identical hemorrhage sites as hemophilia A	Positive family history Mucocutaneous bleeding (epistaxis, menorrhagia, postdental bleeding, gastrointestinal bleeding in adults) Type 3 can manifest as hemophilia A
PFA, bleeding time	Normal	Normal	May be prolonged
PT	Normal	Normal	Normal
aPTT	Prolonged	Prolonged	Prolonged or normal
Factor VIII assay	Decreased or absent	Normal	Decreased or normal (absent type 3)
Factor IX assay	Normal	Decreased or absent	Normal
VWF:Ag	Normal	Normal	Decreased or absent (type 3)
VWF:RCo	Normal	Normal	Decreased or abnormal
VWF multimers	Normal	Normal	Abnormal in types 1, 2A, 2B; absent in type 3
Specific treatment	Recombinant factor VIII (preferred)	Recombinant factor IX	DDAVP (intranasal or intravenous) (FDA approved for type 1)
	Pathogen-safe plasma-derived concentrates	Pathogen-safe plasma-derived concentrates	VWF concentrates (pathogen-safe plasma derived or recombinant VWF)
	DDAVP for mild cases	DDAVP ineffective	
Inhibitor patients	Immune tolerance, recombinant factor VIIa, APCC	Immune tolerance, recombinant factor VIIa	Inhibitors are rare
Adjunct therapy	Antifibrinolytics	Antifibrinolytics	Hormonal therapy (oral contraceptives), antifibrinolytics

APCC, Activated prothrombin complex concentrates; *aPTT,* activated partial thromboplastin time; *DDAVP,* desmopressin; *PFA,* platelet function analyzer; *PT,* prothrombin time; *RCo,* ristocetin cofactor; *VWF,* von Willebrand factor; *VWF:Ag,* von Willebrand factor antigen.

Inhibitor levels, measured using Bethesda units (BU), are classified as high titer (>5 BU) or low titer (<5 BU). In patients with low-titer inhibitors, higher than normal doses of factor VIII or IX may be used to treat bleeding. For those with high-titer inhibitors, agents that bypass factor VIII or factor IX are used. These include recombinant activated factor VII and, in the case of hemophilia A, APC concentrates (APCCs) or recombinant porcine factor VIII (currently in prelicensure clinical trials). Immune tolerance induction, a long-term

TABLE 3 Treatment of Bleeding Episodes and Desired Plasma Levels in Hemophilias A and B

TYPE OF BLEEDING	FACTOR DOSE	DURATION OF TREATMENT	COMMENTS
Persistent or profuse epistaxis Oral mucosal bleeding (including tongue and mouth lacerations) Dental procedures Acute hemarthrosis Intramuscular hematomas Physical therapy	Single dose	1–2 days	Local pressure, antifibrinolytics, fibrin glue for local control, WoundSeal Powder for epistaxis Sedation in small children with tongue laceration
Dental procedures	Single dose	1 h before procedure	Antifibrinolytics for 7–10 days
Acute hemarthrosis, intramuscular hematomas	Single dose	1–3 days	Use lower doses if treated early. Non–weight bearing on affected joint.
Physical therapy	Single dose	Treat before PT	Consider synovectomy (surgical, radioisotope or chemical) for target joints.
Gastrointestinal bleeding	Single dose	2–3 days	May use oral antifibrinolytics
Persistent painless gross hematuria	Single dose	1–2 days	Increase PO or IV fluids with low-dose antifibrinolytics; risk of clotting in the urinary tract with factor replacement
Life-threatening bleeding such as intracranial hemorrhage, major surgery, and trauma	Double dose	10–14 days	Bolus dose followed by continuous infusion (3–4 U/kg/h); may switch to bolus before discharge

"Single dose" refers to a factor dose that aims to achieve 40% to 50% factor level and is ~20 to 25 units/kg for factor VIII products and ~50 units/kg for factor IX products.

"double dose" refers to a factor dose that aims to achieve 80% to 100% factor level and is ~40 to 50 units/kg for factor VIII products and ~80 to 100 units/kg for factor IX products.

Factor doses are dosed closest to the vial.

PT, Physical therapy.

approach designed to eradicate inhibitors, is effective in 70% to 85% of patients with severe hemophilia A; the most important predictor of success of immune tolerance induction is an inhibitor titer of less than 10 BU at the start of immune tolerance induction.

A novel treatment for hemophilia A with inhibitors is emicizumab (Hemlibra®), a chimeric humanized antibody that triggers and propagates thrombin generation by binding to both factor IX and factor X. By binding to these coagulation factors, the antibody mimics the function of factor VIII. The medication is given subcutaneously; making it a preferred drug in young children. Emicizumab showed remarkable success in preventing bleeding complications in patients with severe hemophilia A with inhibitors, and received FDA approval initially for routine prophylaxis to prevent or reduce the frequency of bleeding episodes in patients with hemophilia A with inhibitors in 2017, but this approval was extended to hemophilia A without inhibitors in 2018 following studies in noninhibitor patients. Emicizumab can be administered subcutaneously once a week, every 2 weeks, or every 4 weeks, and all these regimens have been found to be equally effective. In general, emicizumab has been well accepted by hemophilia patients, especially children and those with difficult venous access as its treatment regimen does not require intravenous dosing and the dose frequency is much easier to manage than prophylaxis with conventional factor VIII products. Emicizumab (Hemlibra) treatment is safe by itself, but thrombotic microangiopathy and thrombotic complications have been observed in hemophilia A with inhibitor individuals receiving concomitant high doses of APCC for management of breakthrough bleeds while on emicizumab (>100 U/kg of FEIBA for >24 hours). Hence it is recommended that recombinant factor VIIa (NovoSeven RT) be used as the first line of treatment for management of breakthrough bleeds in inhibitor patients on emicizumab (MASAC document #255).

Although inhibitors are rare in hemophilia B, they can result in anaphylaxis with exposure to factor IX–containing products. Immune tolerance regimens are associated with nephrotic syndrome and are successful in eradicating the inhibitor only in 40% of cases.

Another important complication of treatment is the transmission of bloodborne pathogens such as hepatitis B and C viruses and

human immunodeficiency virus (HIV). In the 1970s, lyophilized plasma factor concentrates of low purity resulted in the transmission of HIV, causing the deaths of many hemophiliacs. Currently, donor screening for pathogens coupled with viral attenuation by heat or solvent detergent technology make these products pathogen safe. However, nonenveloped viruses (parvovirus and hepatitis A) and prions can resist inactivation and can be potentially transmitted.

Patients with bleeding disorders should be encouraged to attend the comprehensive hemophilia treatment centers (HTCs), where they are seen by a multidisciplinary team of hematologists, nurses, social workers, geneticists, physical therapists, dental hygienists, nutritionists, and so on, who educate patients and address issues such as self-care, transitions, and quality of life. Patients are trained to self-infuse and calculate dosage, maintain treatment logs, and call for serious bleeding episodes. The mortality rate among patients who receive care at HTCs is lower than among those who do not: 28.1% versus 38.3%, respectively. At the HTCs, hemovigilance for bloodborne and emerging pathogens was maintained through participation in the Centers for Disease Control and Prevention (CDC) Universal Data Collection (UDC) project. The grant cycle of the UDC was completed in 2012, and a new surveillance instrument is currently in use (Community Counts) that incorporates collecting information on comorbidities and complications of bleeding disorders in this population. Routine vaccination against hepatitis A and B is recommended.

von Willebrand Disease

VWD is an inherited (autosomal dominant) bleeding disorder caused by deficiency or dysfunction of VWF, a plasma protein that mediates platelet adhesion at the site of vascular injury and prevents degradation of factor VIII. A defect in VWF results in bleeding by impairing platelet adhesion or by decreasing factor VIII.

VWF is synthesized in endothelial cells and undergoes dimerization and multimerization, forming low, intermediate, and HMW multimers. The HMW multimers are most effective in promoting platelet aggregation and adhesion. Circulating HMW multimers are cleaved by the protease ADAMTS13, which is deficient in patients with thrombotic thrombocytopenic purpura.

TABLE 4 Clinical Variants of von Willebrand Disease

TYPE	FACTOR VIII	VWF AG	RISTOCETIN COFACTOR	RIPA	MULTIMER
1	↓	↓	↓	↓ or normal	Normal
2A	↓ or normal	↓↓	↓	↓↓	Large and intermediate multimers absent
2B	↓ or normal	↓↓	↓ or normal	↓ to low dose	Large multimers absent
2M	Variably ↓	Variably ↓	↓	Variably ↓	Normal
2N	↓↓	Normal	Normal	Normal	Normal
3	↓↓↓↓	↓↓↓↓	↓↓↓↓	None	Absent
Platelet type	↓ or normal	↓ or normal	↓	↓ to low dose	Large multimers absent

Ag, Antigen; *RIPA*, ristocetin-induced platelet aggregation; *VWF*, von Willebrand factor.

VWD is the most common bleeding disorder, affecting 1% or more of the population. It occurs worldwide and affects all races. VWD is classified into three major categories: partial quantitative deficiency (type 1), qualitative deficiency (type 2), and total deficiency (type 3). There are several different variants of type 2 VWD: 2A, 2B, 2N, and 2M based on the phenotype. Approximately 75% of patients have type 1 VWD.

Clinical Presentation

Mucous membrane–type bleeding (e.g., menorrhagia, epistaxis) and excessive bruising are characteristic clinical features in VWD. Bleeding manifestations vary considerably, and in some cases the diagnosis is not suspected until excessive bleeding occurs with a surgical procedure or trauma. Although excessive menstrual bleeding may be the initial manifestation, it takes 16 years for a diagnosis of bleeding disorder. It is for this reason that the American College of Obstetrics and Gynecology recommended screening for hemostatic disorders in all adolescents and women presenting with menorrhagia and no pathology and before hysterectomy for menorrhagia. In infants or small children with type 3 (severe) VWD, excessive bruising and even joint bleeding (due to very low levels of factor VIII) can mimic hemophilia A.

Diagnosis

Laboratory evaluation for VWD requires several assays to quantitate VWF and characterize its structure and function. Many variables affect VWF assay results, including the patient's ABO blood type. Persons of blood group AB have 60% to 70% higher VWF levels than those of blood group O.

Clinical conditions and disorders with elevated VWF levels include pregnancy (third trimester), collagen vascular disorders, postoperative period, liver disease, and disseminated intravascular coagulation. Low levels are seen in hypothyroidism and the first 4 days of the menstrual cycle.

Symptoms are modified by medications like aspirin or nonsteroidal antiinflammatory drugs (NSAIDs), which can exacerbate the bleeding; oral contraceptives can decrease the bleeding in women with VWD by increasing VWF levels. VWF levels in African American women are 15% higher than in White women. Clinical symptoms and family history are important for establishing the diagnosis of VWD, and a single test is sometimes not sufficient to rule out the diagnosis.

Initial workup should include a complete blood count, aPTT, PT, fibrinogen level, or thrombin time. These tests do not rule out VWD but help rule out thrombocytopenia or factor deficiency as the cause for bleeding. The closure times on the PFA-100, which has replaced the bleeding time as a screening test in some centers, may be prolonged. The aPTT in VWD is only abnormal when factor VIII is sufficiently reduced.

Specific tests for VWD include ristocetin cofactor assay, a factor VIII activity, and VWF antigen (VWF Ag) assay. The ristocetin cofactor activity measures induced binding of VWF to platelet glycoprotein Ib and is subject to significant intra- and interlaboratory variability, making it an unreliable assay for the diagnosis. In addition, certain mutations in the A1 domain of the VWF, especially the D1472H mutation, have been found to attenuate the VWF-Ristocetin binding, leading to misdiagnosis of VWD. This has led to the development of the glycoprotein 1bM assay (direct measure of platelet-binding activity of VWF), collagen binding assay (measure of mutimeric function), and genotyping (especially for type 2 VWD, which are the new tests available to assist with the diagnosis). Multimer analysis is done by agarose gel electrophoresis using anti-VWF polyclonal antibody and is available at reference laboratories.

In type 1 VWD, the VWF is subnormal in amount, with normal multimer structure. Those with types 2A and 2B VWD lack the HMW multimers. In type 2B, the VWF has a heightened affinity for platelets, often resulting in some degree of thrombocytopenia from platelet aggregation. A useful laboratory test for type 2B is the low-dose ristocetin-induced platelet aggregation (RIPA) assay.

In type 3 (severe) VWD, the affected person has inherited a gene for type 1 VWD from each parent, resulting in very low levels (3%) of VWF (and low factor VIII, because there is no VWF to protect factor VIII from proteolytic degradation). Less commonly, a person with type 3 is doubly heterozygous. Table 4 provides a quick overview of the laboratory findings in the different variants of VWD.

Treatment

See the section on general hemostatic agents for a discussion on the use of desmopressin and antifibrinolytic agents.

For type 3 patients and in persons with type 1 VWD who do not respond adequately to desmopressin (DDAVP), an intermediate-purity plasma-derived concentrate rich in the hemostatically effective HMW multimers of VWF (such as Humate-P) should be used to treat moderately severe or severe bleeding episodes and before surgery. Prophylaxis with VWF concentrates is effective in reducing the bleeding episodes and joint disease in severe VWD. A recombinant VWF concentrate enriched with HMW multimers, Vonvendi (does not contain any factor VIII), is now available and approved for use only in adults.

As in hemophilia, antifibrinolytics are an effective adjunctive treatment for invasive dental procedures or other bleeding in the oropharyngeal cavity. These may be effective even when used alone in some VWD women with menorrhagia. For epistaxis, Nosebleed QR, a hydrophilic powder (over-the-counter [OTC] product), can help.

Special Situations
Pregnancy

VWF (and factor VIII) levels increase during the third trimester of pregnancy, and women with type 1 VWD have a decrease in bruising or other bleeding symptoms. However, those with type 2 VWD (abnormal VWF) and type 3 (no VWF) have no change in the bleeding tendency. Even in type 1 VWD, VWF levels fall following delivery, so treatment (with IV desmopressin or Humate P) may be needed.

TABLE 5 Rare Bleeding Disorders: Inheritance, Clinical Features, and Treatment

FACTOR	PREVALENCE	TYPE	INHERI-TANCE	MANIFESTATION AND DIAGNOSIS	TREATMENT	HEMOSTATIC LEVELS	HALF-LIFE
Factor I	1:1,000,000	Afibrinogenemia Dysfibrinogenemia Hypofibrinogenemia	AR AD AD	Mild bleeding CNS, umbilical, joint bleeding Recurrent miscarriage PT, aPTT, TT prolonged Low FI levels Paradoxical thrombosis	FFP 15–20 mL/kg Cryoprecipitate 1 bag/5–10 kg Fibrinogen concentrate (RiaSTAP) Treatment q3–5d	50 mg⁻¹ g/dL	2–5 days
Factor II	1:2,000,000	Type I: hypoprothrombinemia Type II: dysprothrombinemia	AR AR	Hematomas, hemarthroses, menorrhagia CNS, umbilical, postpartum hemorrhage PT abnormal	FFP, PCC 20–30 U/kg for prophylaxis or treatment	20%–30%	3–4 days
Factor V	1:1,000,000	Parahemophilia, labile factor, proaccelerin, Owren disease	AR	Mucosal bleeding, postpartum hemorrhage, CNS bleeding Platelet factor V deficiency more reflective of bleeding potential Prolonged PT, aPTT Normal TT	FFP Platelet transfusions Antiplatelet antibodies can develop with repeated platelet transfusions	15%–20%	36 h
Factor VII	1:500,000	Proconvertin or stable factor	AR	Menorrhagia; mucosal, muscle, intracranial bleeds (15%–60%); hemarthrosis Prolonged PT Normal aPTT, TT, FI, liver functions	Recombinant factor VIIa (NovoSeven), 15–30 µg/kg q 2h for major bleeds FFP, PCC 20–30 U/kg for prophylaxis or treatment Plasma-derived factor VII concentrates[2],*	15%–20%	4–6 h
Factor X	1:1,000,000		AR	Menorrhagia; umbilical, joint, mucosal, muscle, intracranial bleeding Prolonged PT, aPTT	FFP, PCCs 20–30 U/kg Pd FX (Coagadex)	15%–20%	24–48 h
Factor XI (common in Ashkenazi Jews)	1:1,000,000		AR	Posttraumatic bleeding, menorrhagia Prolonged aPTT Normal PT	Hemoleven,*,§ FFP 15–20 mL/kg Inhibitors can occur	15%–20%	
Factor XIII	1:2,000,000		AR	Intracranial, joint, umbilical bleeding Delayed wound healing Recurrent miscarriages PT, aPTT normal ↓FXIII assay	Factor XIII concentrate (Corifact) 40 IU/kg q28d to maintain trough level of 5%–20% FFP 15–20 mL/kg. Tretten, a recombinant FXIII-A subunit concentrate 3.5 units/kg/month for prophylaxis. Use in patients with FXIII A subunit deficiency Cryoprecipitate 1 bag/5–10 kg q3–4 weeks	2%–5%	11–14 days
Combined factor V and VIII	1:2,000,000			Mucosal bleeding Prolonged PT, aPTT (disproportionately)	Factor VIII concentrates and FFP	15%–20%	
Vitamin K-dependent multiple deficiencies	1:2,000,000			Umbilical stump, intracranial, postsurgical bleeding Skeletal abnormalities Hearing loss	Oral vitamin K, FFP, PCC	15%–20%	

*Available in Europe.

AD, Autosomal dominant; aPTT, activated partial thromboplastin time; AR, autosomal recessive; CNS, central nervous system; FFP, fresh frozen plasma; FI, fibrinogen; PCC, prothrombin complex concentrate; PT, prothrombin time; TT, thrombin time.

[2]Not available in the United States.

§Investigational drug in the United States.

Acquired von Willebrand Disease

Acquired VWD occurs in persons who do not have a lifelong bleeding disorder. Conditions associated with acquired VWD include underlying autoimmune disease (lymphoproliferative disorders, myeloproliferative disorders, or plasma cell dyscrasias), valvular and congenital heart disease, Wilms tumor, chronic renal failure, and hypothyroidism. The mechanism of acquired VWD is unknown. Medications such as valproic acid can also cause VWD. Removal of the underlying condition often corrects the VWF. Desmopressin, Humate P, recombinant factor VIIa, or plasma exchange may be tried, if necessary, to treat bleeding.

Rare Bleeding Disorders

The RBDs account for 3% to 5% of inherited coagulation deficiencies, other than factor VIII, factor IX, or VWF deficiencies. They are autosomal recessive and affect both sexes. The prevalence of RBDs ranges from 1:500,000 to 1:2,000,000. Bleeding manifestations are restricted to persons who are homozygotes or compound heterozygotes. RBDs are common in countries such as Iran, where consanguineous marriages are customary. Ashkenazi Jews are particularly affected by factor XI deficiency. Deficiency of factor XII is a risk factor for thrombosis but not for bleeding. Most cases of RBDs are identified by abnormal screening tests coupled with specific factor assays.

Factor concentrates (recombinant or plasma derived) are available for some of the deficiencies such as FVII, X (Coagadex [human]), XIII (Tretten [recombinant], Corifact [human]), XI (in Europe), and fibrinogen concentrate (human) (Fibryga, RiaSTAP). The advantages of concentrates are pathogen safety and small volume. The use of antifibrinolytics and fibrin glue as adjunct therapy for bleeding manifestations is encouraged. Table 5 lists the inheritance, frequency, manifestations, and treatments of the RBDs.

General Hemostatic Agents

For short-term therapy (before dental procedures and minor bleeding episodes), the synthetic vasopressin analog desmopressin acetate (DDAVP injection, Stimate Nasal Spray) is useful both in mild hemophilia A and type 1 VWD, and occasionally in type 2A VWD.[1] Some young women with menorrhagia have also benefited from its use at the onset of menses, with a second dose given after 24 hours. The mechanism of action for desmopressin is increase in plasma concentrations of factor VIII and VWF by stimulating release of the endothelial stores of VWF. The levels of both factor VIII and VWF increase by three- to fivefold within 15 to 30 minutes following infusion. A DDAVP trial to determine response is helpful in selecting patients who might benefit from such therapy. For hemostatic purposes, intravenous (IV) (0.3 µg/kg in 50 mL of normal saline infused over 15–30 minutes) or intranasal dose (150 µg) can be used. The intranasal dose is 15 times larger than that recommended for diabetes insipidus. A multidose intranasal spray formulation (Stimate nasal spray in the United States and Octostim nasal spray in Canada, 1.5 mg/1 mL) delivers 150 µg per spray. The recommended dosage is one spray for patients who weigh less than 50 kg and two sprays (one in each nostril) for those who weigh more than 50 kg. (Note that Ferring Pharmaceutical issued a voluntary recall of Stimate in July 2020 because of higher than specified doses in the sprays. Stimate is not anticipated to be released until 2023. This recall does not affect intravenous doses). The IV route, which was usually used for surgical coverage or for severe bleeding episodes requiring hospitalization, is now the only[1] available route until the intranasal medication is released again.

When necessary, repeat doses may be given at 12- to 24-hour intervals. Tachyphylaxis (diminished response to repeated doses of the medication) occurs due to depletion of endothelial VWF stores. Tachyphylaxis is less commonly seen in VWD patients than in hemophilia patients. It is important to monitor free water intake following DDAVP administration because it can cause hyponatremia and seizures.

Desmopressin can also be used in the treatment of bleeding in patients with platelet dysfunction secondary to uremia.[1] Desmopressin seems to be effective in reducing blood loss during cardiac surgery in patients who are taking antiplatelet medications.[1] Since desmopressin requires the presence of either factor VIII or VWF to be able to show its effect, it is ineffective in moderate to severe hemophilia A, type 2M VWD, type 2N VWD, and type 3 VWD (there is no VWF to be released from storage sites). Desmopressin should be used with caution in type 2B VWD[1] as it can exacerbate the thrombocytopenia. Some patients with type 2A VWD may respond to desmopressin,[1] and a desmopressin test may be needed to determine benefit. Desmopressin is ineffective in hemophilia B and other coagulation disorders.

Antifibrinolytics such as ε-aminocaproic acid (Amicar) and tranexamic acid (Cyklokapron or Lysteda)[1] are used as adjunct therapies and in mild hemophilia and can decrease the need for factor concentrates. The recommended dosage for ε-aminocaproic acid is 50 to 100 mg/kg/dose intravenously or orally every 4 to 6 hours (maximum 30 g/24 h). The recommended dosage for tranexamic acid is 10 mg/kg/dose intravenously or 25 mg/kg body weight orally, three times daily.

General Measures

Aspirin and aspirin-containing compounds should be avoided in persons with bleeding disorders because they interfere with platelet function and can exacerbate bleeding.

---

[1]Not FDA approved for this indication.

References

Aledort LM: Do hemophilia carriers bleed? Yes, *Blood* 108(1):6, 2006.

Arnold WD, Hilgartner MW: Hemophilic arthropathy. current concepts of pathogenesis and management, *J Bone Joint Surg Am* 59(3):287–305, 1977.

Bolton-Maggs PH, Pasi KJ: Haemophilias A and B, *Lancet* 361(9371):1801–1809, 2003.

d'Oiron R, O'Brien S, James AH: Women and girls with haemophilia: lessons learned, *Haemophilia* 27(Suppl 3):75–78, 2021.

Flood VH, Gill JC, Morateck PA, et al: Common VWF exon 28 polymorphisms in African Americans affecting the VWF activity assay by ristocetin cofactor, *Blood* 116(2):280–286, 2010.

Franchini M, Mannucci PM: Non-factor replacement therapy for haemophilia: a current update, *Blood Transfus* 14:1–5, 2018.

Gill JC, Wilson AD, Endres-Brooks J, Montgomery RR: Loss of the largest von Willebrand factor multimers from the plasma of patients with congenital cardiac defects, *Blood* 67(3):758–761, 1986.

Hoffman M, Monroe 3rd DM: A cell-based model of hemostasis, *Thromb Haemost* 85(6):958–965, 2001.

Miller CH, Dilley AB, Drews C, et al: Changes in von Willebrand factor and factor VIII levels during the menstrual cycle, *Thromb Haemost* 87(6):1082–1083, 2002.

Miller CH, Dilley A, Richardson L, et al: Population differences in von Willebrand factor levels affect the diagnosis of von Willebrand disease in African-American women, *Am J Hematol* 67(2):125–129, 2001.

Mulder K, Llinas A: The target joint, *Haemophilia* 10(Suppl. 4):152–156, 2004.

National Hemophilia Foundation Medical and Scientific Advisory Council (MASAC): *MASAC recommendations concerning the treatment of hemophilia and other bleeding disorders*, Available at http://www.hemophilia.org/Researchers-Healthcare-Providers/Medical-and-Scientific-Advisory-Council-MASAC/MASAC-Recommendations.

Pabinger-Fasching I: Pipe S: Innovations in coagulation: improved options for treatment of hemophilia A and B, *Thromb Res* 131(2):S1, 2013.

Pierce GF, Lillicrap D, Pipe SW, Vandendriessche T: Gene therapy, bioengineered clotting factors and novel technologies for hemophilia treatment, *J Thromb Haemost* 5(5):901–906, 2007.

Shapiro A: Development of long-acting recombinant FVIII and FIX Fc fusion proteins for the management of hemophilia, *Expert Opin Biol Ther* 13(9):1287–1297, 2013.

Soucie JM, Nuss R, Evatt B, et al: Mortality among males with hemophilia; relations with source of medical care. the hemophilia surveillance system project investigators, *Blood* 96(2):437–442, 2000.

Veldman A, Hoffman M, Ehrenforth S: New insights into the coagulation system and implications for new therapeutic options with recombinant factor VIIa, *Curr Med Chem* 10(10):797–811, 2003.

Warrier I, Ewenstein BM, Koerper MA, et al: Factor IX inhibitors and anaphylaxis in hemophilia B, *J Pediatr Hematol Oncol* 19(1):23–27, 1997.

Weyand AC, Pipe SW: New therapies for hemophilia, *Blood* 133(5):389–398, 2019.

BLOOD, 1 JULY 2006. VOLUME 108, NUMBER 1

---

[1]Not FDA approved for this indication.

HODGKIN LYMPHOMA

Method of
Anusha Vallurupalli, MBBS

CURRENT DIAGNOSIS

- Typically presents as painless cervical or mediastinal lymphadenopathy.
- "B" symptoms (fevers, drenching night sweats, and weight loss >10% of body weight) may be present.
- Tissue diagnosis is made by identifying Reed Sternberg cells on either excisional (preferable) or incisional biopsy. Fine needle aspiration (FNA) is never adequate and should be avoided.

CURRENT THERAPY

- Limited-stage disease (stages I to IIA) with favorable risk factors, termed "early favorable" can be treated with combined modality therapy, (*Adriamycin, bleomycin, vinblastine,* and *dubarbazine* [ABVD]), for 2 cycles followed by 20 Gy involved-field radiation.
- Limited-stage disease (I to IIA) with unfavorable risk factors, termed "early unfavorable," may be treated with either combined-modality therapy, 4 cycles of ABVD followed by 30 Gy involved-field radiotherapy, or with 6 cycles of ABVD alone. Decisions about therapy should be decided in a multidisciplinary setting and are usually based on patient age and sex, disease bulk, and area of involved field radiation.
- Advanced-stage disease (IIB to IV) can now be treated with either ABVD or A +AVD for 6 cycles.
- Clinical trials should always be considered for the treatment of disease at any stage, if available.

Epidemiology

There were 8500 estimated new cases of Hodgkin lymphoma (HL) in 2018 with 1050 deaths according to the SEER database. 86.6% patients who underwent treatment were surviving at 5 years between 2008 and 2014. There has been a downward trend in new cases and deaths due to HL over the last 10 years. The median age at diagnosis is 39 years and there is a bimodal age distribution with the highest risk in the age group of 20 to 34 years.

Pathology

HL is classified broadly into classical Hodgkin lymphoma (CHL) and nodular lymphocyte predominant Hodgkin lymphoma (NLPHL) based on the WHO classification system. CHL is the most common type, accounting for 95% of the cases. There are four distinctive histologic subtypes of CHL, Nodular Sclerosis (NS), Mixed Cellularity (MC), Lymphocyte Rich (LR), and Lymphocyte depleted (LD) with NS being the most common subtype.

Pathologically, CHL is characterized by the presence of definitive "Reed Sternberg" (RS) cells, which express CD30 and CD15 on their cell surface. NLPHL, on the other hand, is characterized by "popcorn cells" that express CD20 and CD45 on the cell surface.

Risk Factors

Most cases of CHL are sporadic with no clear risk factors. NS is the most common subtype in United States and developed countries. MC and LR are more common in developing countries and are associated with prior Epstein Barr Virus (EBV) infection. HIV infection is associated with a 5 to 10 times higher risk due to immune suppression and associated EBV infection. The incidence of HL in HIV patients may be increasing in the era of antiretroviral therapy. Increased risk is also seen in other acquired or congenital immunodeficiencies.

There is also increased risk of CHL in families with an index case. According to a Nordic study, there is a threefold increase over the general population risk and the risk is the highest in siblings. Familial risk varies by subtypes and is the highest in the LR subtype.

Clinical Presentation

Painless lymphadenopathy either in the neck (75%) or mediastinal lymph nodes (60%) is the most common presentation for CHL, whereas NLPHL usually presents with painless peripheral lymphadenopathy. "B" symptoms, which include fever higher than 38°C, unintentional weight loss of more than 10% of body weight over 6 months, and drenching night sweats can be present and are often considered unfavorable risk factors. Patients may present with local symptoms from bulky lymphadenopathy such as dyspnea, chest pressure or cough due to mediastinal masses, and neck discomfort and trouble swallowing from cervical lymphadenopathy. Prolonged dyspnea, cough, or chest pressure should be evaluated with appropriate imaging in a young patient when CHL is a consideration in the differential diagnosis. Pruritus can also be seen in some patients and often improves with the treatment of CHL.

Spleen involvement can be seen in 20% of cases and is considered as nodal involvement in CHL. Other extra nodal involvement (e.g., bone marrow, lungs, liver, and bone) is uncommon and is usually associated with advanced unfavorable disease and a poor prognosis. CNS involvement is extremely rare.

Initial lab testing may not show any major abnormalities in early stage and favorable risk patients. The Erythrocyte Sedimentation Rate (ESR) is prognostic in CHL and should be performed at diagnosis in all patients. Anemia, lymphopenia, leukocytosis, and hypoalbuminemia may be seen on labs in advanced and unfavorable risk patients and are a result of cytokine response.

Diagnosis

Adequate tissue sampling is essential in the diagnosis of any lymphoma and is even more indispensable in HL. CHL is characterized by background inflammatory cells, which include polyclonal reactive lymphocytes, neutrophils, and eosinophils with the actual malignant RS cells configuring only 1% to 2% of the total cellularity. As a result, diagnosis is often missed on FNA, which is considered a very insensitive diagnostic methodology. Excisional biopsy is preferable and in cases where it is not possible, multiple core needle biopsies or mediastinoscopic biopsies can be considered, based on the location.

On Haemotoxylin and eosin (H&E) staining of the biopsy, the classic presentation for CHL is a rich inflammatory background interspersed with positive CD15 and CD30 RS cells. RS cells are typically large with bilobed eosinophilic nucleoli and abundant cytoplasm. Mononuclear variants also occur. On immunohistochemistry, RS cells are usually negative for the panlymphoid marker CD45 and the B-cell marker CD20. The presence of RS cells will rule out other conditions in the differential diagnosis, including Non-Hodgkin lymphoma, autoimmune diseases, and infections. The NS subtype also presents with dense bands of fibrosis on H&E staining.

NLPHL is also characterized by atypical malignant cells amidst a polyclonal inflammatory microenvironment composed primarily of small lymphocytes in large nodular meshworks of follicular dendritic cells. The "popcorn" cells characteristic of NLPHL express CD20 and CD45, rather than CD15 an CD30, which is the major pathologic differentiating factor from CHL.

Staging and Risk Prognostication

Staging starts with a thorough history and physical exam. "B" symptoms, pruritus, fatigue, alcohol intolerance, and decrease in performance status may all be noted on the history. Careful palpation and measurements of lymph nodes and spleen as well as documentation of extra nodal involvement are important and can be followed after the initiation of treatment for a clinical response assessment.

The Ann Arbor classification is used for staging. CHL is broadly divided into four stages based on the spread of the lymphoma. Stage I disease is confined to a single lymph-node region, while Stage II is the involvement of multiple lymph-node regions on the same side of the diaphragm, Stage III has involvement of nodal regions on both sides of the diaphragm and Stage IV has

TABLE 1 Staging Hodgkin Disease

STAGE	DEFINITION
I	Confined to single lymph-node region*
II	Involvement of multiple lymph-node regions on a same side of diaphragm
III	Involvement of nodal regions on both sides of the diaphragm
IV	Extensive involvement of extranodal site(s)
Sub Classification	
A	Absence of "B" symptoms
B	Presence of "B" symptoms
Modifiers	
E	Localized focus of extranodal disease or localized extension of nodal disease into an extranodal site.
S	Splenic involvement (the spleen is considered a nodal site in Hodgkin lymphoma)
X (Cotswold modifier)	Bulky disease (>10 cm or >0.33 of the maximal intrathoracic diameter for mediastinal mass per NCCN guidelines)

*Lymph node regions include: right cervical (including cervical, supraclavicular, occipital, and preauricular lymph nodes), left cervical, right axillary, left axillary, right infraclavicular, left infraclavicular, mediastinal, hilar, periaortic, mesenteric, right pelvic, left pelvic, right inguinal femoral, and left inguinal femoral.
NCCN, National Comprehensive Cancer Network.

extensive involvement of an extranodal site or sites. Each stage is subdivided into "A" and "B" depending on the presence or absence of B symptoms. The Cotswold classification includes an "X" category for bulky disease (Table 1).

Radiographic staging is performed with CT scans in conjunction with PET scanning at diagnosis and repeated after two cycles of chemotherapy and at the end of treatment (EOT). Positron emission tomography–computed tomography (PET-CT) imaging leads to a change in staging in 10% to 30% of patients, more often upstaging. Bone marrow aspirate/biopsy is no longer required for the routine evaluation of patients with HL due to the high sensitivity of PET scan. CNS staging with lumbar puncture (LP) and MRI of the brain is only done if there is a high suspicion based on symptoms and physical examination. Routine staging laparotomy and bilateral bone marrow biopsies are no longer performed.

Laboratory evaluation includes a complete blood count with differential, complete metabolic profile, including albumin, ESR, and baseline HIV testing. Due to the routine use of anthracyclines, an echocardiogram or multigated acquisition scan (MUGA; also called equilibrium radionuclide angiogram) is necessary prior to initiation of chemotherapy to assess left ventricular ejection fraction. Pulmonary function testing is performed and a detailed tobacco smoking history should be obtained due to the use of bleomycin. A pregnancy test should be performed on all women of childbearing age prior to the initiation of therapy. Fertility counseling is recommended for age appropriate patients even though the infertility risk is low (2% to 10%) with the ABVD regimen. The risk of infertility is higher with other regimens such as bleomycin, etoposide, doxorubicin hydrochloride (Adriamycin), cyclophosphamide, vincristine (Oncovin), procarbazine, and prednisone (BEACOPP).

Regardless of the stage, CHL is highly curable and 86.6% patients were alive at 5 years following treatment. Therefore, it is highly important to diagnose and treat patients appropriately and to monitor for long-term complications in survivors. Staging and risk prognostication are essential in deciding the appropriate treatment regimen. Age greater than 50, bulky disease more than 10 cm, elevated ESR, presence of "B" symptoms, involvement of greater than three nodal groups, and bulky mediastinal

mass greater than 0.33 (maximum width of the mass/maximum intrathoracic diameter) are all unfavorable factors in limited stage disease (Stage I to II). In advanced-stage CHL, the international prognostic score is generated using seven adverse risk factors, which include male sex, age greater than 45 years, stage IV disease, serum albumin of less than 4 g per deciliter, a hemoglobin level of less than 10.5 g per deciliter, leukocytosis (a white-cell count of at least 15,000 per cubic millimeter), and lymphocytopenia (a lymphocyte count of less than 600 per cubic millimeter, a count that was less than 8% of the white-cell count, or both). The score predicted the rate of freedom from progression of disease with 42% survival in patients with a score of 5 or higher.

Treatment

Stage I to IIA constitutes limited stage disease and Stage IIB to IV constitutes advanced disease.

Limited Stage Classical Hodgkin Lymphoma

Combined modality treatment using a combination of radiotherapy (RT) and chemotherapy is the treatment of choice for early stage limited disease with favorable risk factors. Various trials over decades have established the role of combined modality treatment with RT alone or chemotherapy alone being the comparator arms.

The HD 10 trial investigated the reduction of number of cycles of doxorubicin (Adriamycin,[1] bleomycin, vinblastine, and dubarbazine [ABVD]) and the dose of involved field radiation (IFRT) in patients with no unfavorable risk factors. One thousand three hundred and seventy patients were randomized into four different groups. Early stage favorable risk factor patients who received 2 cycles of ABVD followed by 20 Gy IFRT had similar 5 year overall survival (OS) as the patients who received 4 cycles of ABVD followed by 30 Gy IFRT. ABVD for 2 cycles followed by 20 Gy IFRT is now the standard of care for Stage IA to IIA disease with favorable risk patients. Four cycles of ABVD followed by 30 Gy of IFRT or 6 cycles of ABVD is recommended for limited stage (stage I to IIA) disease with unfavorable risk factors or bulky disease. Stanford V and BEACOPP (bleomycin, etoposide [Toposar],[1] Adriamycin,[1] cyclophosphamide, vincristine [Oncovin], procarbazine [Matulane], and prednisone) regimens are considered alternate treatment options and generally yield similar excellent results with 5 year OS rates of 90% to 95%. ABVD is the most commonly used regimen due to greater tolerability and less cumulative dosage of anthracyclines.

Advanced-Stage Classical Hodgkin Lymphoma

Advanced-stage CHL (Ann Arbor stages IIB to IV) used to be a fatal disease until the development of the MOPP (mechlorethamine, vincristine [Oncovin], procarbazine, and prednisone) regimen in the 1960s. ABVD for 6 to 8 months was compared to MOPP in a randomized landmark clinical trial and ABVD was found to be equally or more effective and was associated with less toxicity. ABVD is administered on days 1 and 15 of a 28-day cycle for 6 total cycles. Modern outcomes with ABVD for advanced-stage disease produced 5-year freedom from progression and OS of 78% and 90%, respectively. Combined modality treatment with IFRT is considered in patients with bulky disease for tumor consolidation or in patients with an incomplete response to chemotherapy.

Alternative regimens include escalated BEACOPP and Stanford V. Neither of these regimens improved OS when compared to ABVD and were associated with increased treatment-related toxicity. Most recently, brentuximab vedotin (BV) (Adcetris) in combination with an Adriamycin, vinblastine, and dacarbazine (A+AVD) regimen has been approved in the United States for advanced stage CHL based on the phase III randomized ECHELON-1 study. This regimen had a 4.9 percentage-point lower combined risk of progression, death, or noncomplete response when compared with the use of subsequent anticancer therapy at 2 years in comparison to ABVD with a tolerable safety profile. The modified end point is considered a caveat for this study and long-term survival data for this study is still pending. Both

---

[1]Not FDA approved for this indication

ABVD and A+AVD are reasonable first line options in patients with Stage III and IV disease and should be chosen based on the patient's age, financial status, and preference and comorbidities. There are not enough data at this time to recommend A+AVD over ABVD. There are ongoing clinical trials evaluating the efficacy and tolerability of combination regimens with BV and checkpoint blockade (nivolumab [Opdivo]) in front line settings. As of now, ABVD is still the preferred regimen in United States with ongoing debate in regard to alternative regimens.

Relapsed/Refractory Classical Hodgkin Lymphoma

CHL carries an overall excellent prognosis and approximately 85% of patients are cured. However, approximately 15% of patients do relapse or have primary refractory disease and will require salvage treatment. Prognosis, especially in patients with refractory disease or who relapse within 12 months of treatment, has historically been poor with conventional salvage chemotherapy. However, with the advent of targeted therapy and checkpoint blockade, response rates and OS rates for this group have improved significantly. Currently, conventional salvage chemotherapy followed by autologous stem cell transplant, which offers a 50% cure rate, remains the second line option.

BV maintenance is offered starting 30 to 45 days after stem cell transplant for a total of 16 cycles, 3 weeks apart based on phase III randomized AETHERA trial data. Patients randomized to receive brentuximab consolidation had significantly improved progression-free survival of 43 months, compared with 24 months in placebo-treated patients. There are ongoing clinical trials evaluating newer agents in second-line settings and enrollment in clinical trials is preferable for these patients. Patients who relapse after autologous stem cell transplant are usually considered for allogeneic stem cell transplant after they have demonstrated a response with next line options.

BV is a monoclonal antibody that is active against CD30 bound to the microtubule toxin monomethyl auristatin E (MMAE). BV has been FDA approved for third-line treatment after a pivotal phase II study resulted in an ORR of 75% and CR of 34% compared to single agent treatment. BV is administered every 3 weeks by intravenous infusion at a dose of 1.8 mg/kg. BV is now also used in combination with Bendamustine (Bendeka)[1], which, in multiple single institutional retrospective data, showed improved response rates of around 92% compared to BV alone.

Mostly recently, immunotherapy with checkpoint blockade has been studied in CHL after identification of 9p24.1 amplification, which results in universal overexpression of programmed death-1(PD-1) ligands. Nivolumab and pembrolizumab (Keytruda), which are both PD-1 inhibitors, have been studied in phase II studies and have shown overall response rates of around 69% and 67%, respectively. Nivolumab is FDA approved for patients who have relapsed after autologous stem cell transplant and have failed BV. Pembrolizumab is approved for patients who have failed BV. Further studies are evaluating the role of combination treatments with these agents. There are also ongoing clinical trials evaluating newer treatment options such as CD30 engineered CAR T cells.

Treatment of Nodular Lymphocyte-Predominant Hodgkin Lymphoma

Nodular lymphocyte-predominant Hodgkin lymphoma (NLPHL) is typically an indolent disease and presents with early stage disease in peripheral nodal locations. Early stage patients are treated with IFRT alone with excellent response rates. Ten year OS is 95% in these patients. Advanced-stage NLPHL is relatively uncommon and can be treated with either single agent rituximab (Rituxan),[1] due to CD20 positivity on malignant cells, or combination chemotherapeutic regimens such as ABVD and RCHOP (*r*ituximab, *c*yclophosphamide, *h*ydroxydaunomycin [doxorubicin], *O*ncovin, and *p*rednisone), depending on the extent of disease and patient comorbidities.

Response Assessment

End-of-treatment (EOT) assessment is more accurate with PET-CT imaging. The Deauville score, which is a 5-point scoring system, is used to assess responses with PET scan imaging. A score of 1, 2, or 3 is considered a complete metabolic response. There is no indication for routine surveillance scans after the EOT assessment. A score of 4 or 5 is considered a suboptimal response and may require a change of treatment plan. Interim PET scanning after two cycles of ABVD therapy has prognostic significance. However, the significance of interim PET scanning with newer combination regimens has not been validated.

Complications and Long-Term Monitoring

CHL is a curable cancer. Short- and long-term complications from treatment require close monitoring, especially given the young age of presentation in most patients. Most short-term side effects are fatigue, nausea, emesis, constipation, increased risk of infections, and peripheral neuropathy. Patients need long-term cardiac monitoring due to the risk of congestive heart failure with anthracyclines and combination IFRT, and the risk of coronary artery disease with IFRT. Bleomycin can cause long-term pulmonary toxicity and patients should be monitored while on active treatment. Prompt discontinuation of bleomycin is warranted if there is any suspicion of pulmonary complications. There is a long-term risk of secondary malignancies and myelodysplastic syndrome in patients treated for HL.

Patients should undergo regular cancer screenings. Yearly complete blood count is warranted. Thyroid evaluation once a year is recommended for patients who have received neck or superior mediastinal IFRT. Mammography is recommended for women starting 8 years after IFRT to mediastinum.

References

Advani RH, Hoppe RT, Baer D, et al: Efficacy of abbreviated Stanford V chemotherapy and involved-field radiotherapy in early-stage Hodgkin lymphoma: mature results of the G4 trial, *Ann Oncol* 34:1044–1048, 2013.

Armand P, Engert A, Younes A, et al: Nivolumab for relapsed/refractory classic hodgkin lymphoma after failure of autologous hematopoietic cell transplantation: extended follow-up of the multicohort single-arm Phase II CheckMate 205 Trial, *J Clin Oncol* 36(14):1428–1439, 2018 May 10.

Canellos GP, Anderson JR, et al: Chemotherapy of advanced Hodgkin's Disease with MOPP, ABVD, or MOPP alternating with ABVD, *N Engl J Med* 327:1478–1484, 1992.

Chen RC, Chin MS, Ng AK, et al: Early-stage, lymphocyte-predominant Hodgkin's lymphoma: patient outcomes from a large, single-institution series with long follow-up, *J Clin Oncol* 28:136–141, 2010.

Cheson BD, Fisher RI, Barrington SF, et al: Recommendations for initial evaluation, staging, and response assessment of hodgkin and non-Hodgkin lymphoma: the Lugano classification, *J Clin Oncol* 32(27):3059–3067, 2014 Sep 20.

Connors JM, Jurczak W, Straus DJ, et al: Brentuximab vedotin with chemotherapy for stage III or IV Hodgkin's lymphoma, *N Engl J Med* 378:331–344, 2018.

Eichenauer DA, Fuchs M, Pluetschow A, et al: Phase 2 study of rituximab in newly diagnosed stage IA nodular lymphocyte-predominant Hodgkin lymphoma: a report from the German Hodgkin Study Group, *Blood* 118:4363–4365, 2011.

Engert A, Plutschow A, Eich HT, et al: Reduced treatment intensity in patients with early-stage Hodgkin's lymphoma, *N Engl J Med* 363:640–652, 2010.

Gallamini A, Hutchings M, Rigacci L, et al: Early interim 2-[18 F]fluoro-2-deoxy-Dglucose positron emission tomography is prognostically superior to international prognostic score in advanced-stage Hodgkin's lymphoma: a report from a joint Italian-Danish study, *J Clin Oncol* 25:3746–3752, 2007.

Hasenclever D, Diehl V: A prognostic score for advanced Hodgkin's disease. International Prognostic Factors Project on Advanced Hodgkin's Disease, *N Engl J Med* 339(21):1506–1514, 1998 Nov 19.

Jacobson CA, Abramson JS: HIV-associated Hodgkin's lymphoma: prognosis and therapy in the era of cART, *Adv Hematol* 2012:507257, 2012.

Kharazmi E, Fallah M, Pukkala E, et al: Risk of familial classical Hodgkin lymphoma by relationship, histology, age, and sex: a joint study from five Nordic countries, *Blood* 126(17):1990–1995, 2015 Oct 22.

LaCasce AS, Bociek RG, Sawas A, et al: Brentuximab vedotin plus bendamustine: a highly active first salvage regimen for relapsed or refractory Hodgkin lymphoma, *Blood* 11:815183, 2018.

Meyer RM, Gospodarowicz MK, Connors JM, et al: ABVD alone versus radiation-based therapy in limited-stage Hodgkin's lymphoma, *N Engl J Med* 366:399–408, 2012.

Moskowitz CH, Nademanee A, et al: Brentuximab vedotin as consolidation therapy after autologous stem-cell transplantation in patients with Hodgkin's lymphoma at risk of relapse or progression (AETHERA): a randomised, double-blind, placebo-controlled, phase 3 trial, *Lancet* 385(9980):1853–1862, 2015 May 9.

Moskowitz CH, Zinzani PL, Fanale MA, et al: Pembrolizumab in relapsed/refractory classical Hodgkin lymphoma: primary end point analysis of the Phase 2 Keynote-087 Study, *Blood* 128:1107, 2016.

Younes A, Gopal AK, Smith SE, et al: Results of a pivotal phase II study of brentuximab vedotin for patients with relapsed or refractory Hodgkin's lymphoma, *J Clin Oncol* 30(18):2183–2189, 2012 Jun 20.

[1]Not FDA approved for this indication

IRON DEFICIENCY ANEMIA

Method of
Susan Evans, MD

CURRENT DIAGNOSIS

- The presence of symptoms and signs depends on the degree of iron deficiency, the time course of the development of iron deficiency, and the overall physiologic state of the patient. Patients may be asymptomatic. Signs and symptoms are more likely if anemia and/or hemodynamic instability are present.
- Symptoms include fatigue, poor exercise tolerance, weakness, headache, pica, dyspnea, dizziness, vertigo, and angina pectoris.
- Signs include pallor, dry and rough skin, brittle nails, defects of the nail bed (koilonychias), atrophy of the lingual papillae, and cheilosis.
- Systolic heart murmur if anemia is present
- Neonates: delayed growth and development
- Adolescents: learning and behavior problems
- Blood loss is the most common cause of iron deficiency
- Iron deficiency is the most common cause of anemia

Laboratory Findings
- Decreased iron on bone marrow aspirate is the gold standard but is rarely used
- Low serum hemoglobin to diagnose anemia
- Low mean corpuscular hemoglobin: late finding
- Low mean corpuscular volume: late finding
- Low serum iron
- High serum iron-binding capacity
- Low percent transferrin saturation (TSAT)
- Low serum ferritin, but may be normal in the presence of inflammation

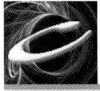

CURRENT THERAPY

Oral Replacement
- Ferrous sulfate (or another equivalent iron preparation) 325 mg (65 mg elemental iron) three times daily.
- Avoid taking with meals to increase absorption.

Parenteral Replacement
- Recommended when blood loss exceeds the ability to replace orally, in the context of malabsorption and if oral iron is not tolerated
  - Ferric carboxymaltose (Ferinject and Injectafer)
  - Ferric gluconate (Ferrlecit)
  - Ferumoxytol (Feraheme)
  - Iron sucrose (Venofer)

Unstable Patient
- If the patient is hemodynamically unstable due to anemia, consider blood transfusion

Treatment Endpoint
- Continue iron replacement for 3 months after anemia is resolved and iron replaced.

Epidemiology
Anemia affects more than one-third of the world's population, or 2 billion people. Iron deficiency continues to be the most common cause of anemia. Iron deficiency is the only micronutrient deficiency that remains a significant problem in both developing and developed countries. Iron deficiency refers to a decrease in iron stores below a normal level and can cause fatigue even without anemia. In the case of iron deficiency without anemia, iron stores are still adequate for erythropoiesis. Iron deficiency anemia is a more serious condition in which there is not enough erythroid iron available, leading to anemia. Worldwide levels of iron deficiency are estimated to be twice that of iron deficiency anemia.

Risk Factors
Risk factors for iron deficiency anemia include age, socioeconomic status, gender, diet, disease, and medical treatment. Several groups of people are at an increased risk of iron deficiency based on age or their stage in life. Infants and children ages 0 to 5 years old are at risk for iron deficiency because of their rapid rate of growth, which necessitates increased iron stores. Adolescent girls and women of child bearing age are also at risk due to iron loss through menstruation. In 2016, 32.8% of women of reproductive age were considered anemic. The 2025 Global Nutrition Targets aim to decrease the prevalence by 50%. During pregnancy, a woman's iron needs triple because of the expansion of red cell mass, the placenta, and the growth of the fetus. Worldwide, anemia affects 38% of pregnant women and is known to increase the risk of cesarean section and maternal mortality. Elderly people are also at risk for iron deficiency for a number of reasons, including inadequate diet, poor absorption due to disease or antacid medicines, or as a complication of chronic disease.

Dietary causes of iron deficiency anemia include lack of access to or preference against eating a diet including iron rich foods. While 90% of iron in the body is recycled every day, dietary iron is essential for replacing lost iron, which is mainly excreted in bile. Iron supplementation of common foods such as breads and rice in the United States decreases the risk of dietary iron deficiency. Iron is found naturally in both animal products such as meat and in plant based foods such as green leafy vegetables, sweet potatoes, and legumes. As long as they eat a healthy and well-balanced diet, vegetarians and vegans have not been shown to be at an increased risk for iron deficiency; such diets have many other health benefits.

Any illness or therapy that leads to decreased iron absorption or blood loss may cause iron deficiency. Common causes of blood loss include gastrointestinal diseases such as cancer, inflammatory bowel disease, and ulcer disease. Taking aspirin, nonsteroidal anti-inflammatory drugs (NSAIDs), or anticoagulants also increases the risk of gastrointestinal blood loss. Iron absorption is decreased in the context of celiac disease, post gastric bypass surgery, and *Helicobacter pylori* infection. Chronic diseases associated with iron deficiency include chronic kidney disease, rheumatoid arthritis, cancer, obesity, and chronic heart failure. There are also medical treatments that may cause iron deficiency such as antacid medicines, which decrease iron absorption, dialysis that causes blood loss, and erythropoietin therapy that depletes iron stores through increased erythropoiesis. Frequent phlebotomy, including repetitive blood donation or treatment for polycythemia or hemochromatosis, decrease iron stores. Rarely, there may be a genetic cause for iron deficiency anemia such as iron-refractory iron deficiency anemia.

Pathophysiology
Iron in the body can be broken down into two main types: functional iron and storage iron. Functional iron plays many essential roles in the human body. It is found in hemoglobin, which carries oxygen from the lungs to body tissues, and in muscles as myoglobin, which helps with oxygen use and storage. Iron plays a role in enzymatic reactions, DNA synthesis, mitochondrial energy generation, and cell proliferation. Storage iron is found in ferritin, hemosiderin, and transferrin. Iron homeostasis is very important to the body and is regulated through the diet, gastrointestinal absorption, and the recycling of the iron in red blood cells. Total body iron stores are about 3.5 g for men and 2.5 g for women. Approximately 20 to 25 mg of iron is needed daily for red cell production and body processes. Dietary absorption of iron is limited to about 1 to 2 mg/day; the daily requirement is

produced through the recycling of iron in used red blood cells by macrophages.

Dietary iron is found in two forms. Heme iron (Fe^{2+}) is found in animal products such as meat, poultry and seafood and is more easily absorbed than plant-based iron. Nonheme iron (Fe^{3+}) is found in plant sources such as beans and lentils, baked potatoes, dark green leafy vegetables, tofu, and cashews. Dietary iron is also found in iron fortified breakfast cereals and enriched breads. Adding foods high in vitamin C to a meal with nonheme iron can increase iron absorption. There are other foods that inhibit the absorption of iron, including polyphenols found in some vegetables, tannins found in tea, and calcium found in dairy products. Dietary iron absorption takes place almost exclusively in the duodenum and upper jejunum.

The recycling of iron from used red blood cells provides about 90% of body iron and is essential for maintaining normal iron levels in the body. Hepcidin, a peptide hormone mainly synthesized in the liver, controls the process of iron absorption and recycling. When serum iron levels are high, hepcidin levels increase in response, which leads to breakdown of the iron transporter called ferroportin. A decrease in ferroportin leaves more iron inside macrophages, enterocytes, and hepatocytes, and the serum iron level decreases. When serum iron levels drop, expression of hepcidin should decrease as well. However, inflammation and infection can cause hepcidin to increase inappropriately; this is one of the ways in which chronic disease contributes to iron deficiency.

Prevention

Prevention plays a large role in the treatment of iron deficiency anemia worldwide and includes both dietary interventions and supplementation. A food-based approach to prevention would include encouraging patients to eat more iron rich foods such as meats and dark green leafy vegetables. A list of iron rich foods is found in Table 1. Heme iron, found in animal sources, is easily absorbed; however, the absorption of nonheme iron from plant sources is affected by the foods with which they are eaten. Foods that can inhibit the absorption of iron include the tannins in tea and coffee and the calcium found in milk. It is best to eat these foods separately from iron rich foods to increase iron absorption. Certain foods increase the absorption of nonheme iron when they are eaten at the same time, including foods that contain heme (such as meat) or foods that contain vitamin C (such as fruit, orange juice, or broccoli). Encouraging iron fortified foods, which in the United States include cereals, rice, pasta, and bread, is another effective way to prevent deficiency. There are some cases when the risk of developing iron deficiency is so high that supplementation with an oral iron supplement is recommended. The World Health Organization recommends universal supplementation for low-birth-weight infants with 2 mg/kg daily from age 2 months to 23 months. They also recommend universal supplementation for pregnant women with 60 mg iron per day. While supplementation for pregnant women is common practice in the United States, the US Preventive Services Task Force states that there is insufficient evidence to show that these practices help prevent adverse maternal health and birth outcomes. According to the US Preventive Services Task Force, evidence is also insufficient to recommend screening children age 6 months to 2 years of age for iron deficiency anemia in the United States.

Clinical Manifestations

Patients with iron deficiency may be asymptomatic. The presence of symptoms and signs of iron deficiency depend on the degree of deficiency, the time course of the development of iron deficiency, and the overall physiologic state of the patient. Common symptoms of iron deficiency include fatigue, weakness, irritability, poor concentration, decreased exercise intolerance, dry mouth, headache, and restless leg syndrome. Severe iron deficiency can cause pica, a craving to eat substances such as ice, dirt, clay, or paint. Signs of iron deficiency include pallor and a systolic heart murmur if anemia is present, hair loss, atrophy of lingual papillae, and nail changes such as koilonychias.

Diagnosis

Normal hemoglobin levels depend on age, gender, pregnancy status, altitude, and smoking, but in general, an adult male is considered anemic with a hemoglobin level less than 13 g/mL and an adult female at less than 12 g/mL. However, these thresholds were first recommended by the World Health Organization in 1968 and and were not developed using current laboratory and epidemiological methods. The World Health Organization is in the process of evaluating and updating the guidelines for assessment and diagnosis of anemia. Iron deficiency may be present with or without anemia; therefore, measuring hemoglobin level is neither a sensitive nor a specific test for iron deficiency. Absolute iron deficiency occurs when the amount of total body iron is low. Functional iron deficiency occurs when there is not enough iron available to meet the demand of body tissues and processes because iron is sequestered either in macrophages or the reticuloendothelial system.

Diagnosing iron deficiency is not straightforward because serum ferritin level, which is often used as a screening test, is affected by gender, age, inflammation, infection, and chronic diseases such as liver disease and cancer. While a serum ferritin concentration less than 12 µg/L makes iron deficiency very likely, a person with inflammation or chronic disease may have iron deficiency at much higher ferritin levels. Increasing the cutoff for normal ferritin concentration to 30 µg/L has been shown to increase sensitivity for iron deficiency, and an even higher cutoff of 100 µg is recommended by some specialty societies. For this reason, utilizing more than one iron status indicator to make the diagnosis is important. A low iron level (<50 µg/dL) and an elevated total iron binding capacity (TIBC >450 µg/dL) also support the diagnosis of iron deficiency. Other supporting labs include a drop in transferrin saturation (TSAT) to less than 16% or less than 20% if inflammation or disease is present. Low mean corpuscular volume (MCV) may be another sign of iron deficiency, but this is generally a late finding, so MCV may be in the normal range. Low MCV can also be seen in thalassemia. Low mean corpuscular hemoglobin concentration (MCHC) is another late finding in iron deficiency. Decreased iron seen on bone marrow aspiration is still considered the gold standard for diagnosing iron deficiency, but it is rarely done due to both cost and patient discomfort. A new test being developed to diagnose iron deficiency measures the level of serum soluble transferrin receptors (sTfR), which increase in the context of iron deficiency and are not affected by inflammation. A drawback for the test is that the sTfR level may be elevated in those with hemolytic anemia or chronic

TABLE 1	Iron Rich Foods
IRON TYPE	**DIETARY SOURCES**
Heme Iron	Beef
	Chicken
	Fish
	Organ Meats
	Oysters
Nonheme Iron	Dark Green Leafy Vegetables
	Beans
	Lentils
	Tofu
	Baked Potato
	Cashews
	Fortified Cereals, Breads and Pasta

lymphocytic leukemia as well as in those using recombinant human erythropoietin.

Differential Diagnosis

The differential diagnosis of iron deficiency includes causes of fatigue and exercise intolerance such as hypothyroidism, electrolyte disturbances due to diuretic therapy, left ventricular dysfunction, chronic lung disease, malignancies, or liver disease.

Anemia of chronic disease can mimic iron deficiency anemia and may be found concurrently in the same patient. A low MCV on blood count can also be a sign of thalassemia.

Treatment

The goal of treatment is to replace iron so that hemoglobin levels normalize, and iron stores are replenished. Treatment of iron deficiency must take into consideration the type of patient being treated and the source and amount of iron deficit or blood loss. Patients who are severely anemic and hemodynamically unstable may be candidates for blood transfusion. For people in groups that are at high risk for iron deficiency, such as infants, toddlers, adolescents, and menstruating women, it is reasonable to start with oral supplementation with iron and only proceed with further work up if that is unsuccessful. However, in patients at low risk for iron deficiency, such as men and post-menopausal women, it is important to determine the underlying cause of iron deficiency. Blood loss is the most common cause of iron deficiency, so this work-up includes evaluation for a source of bleeding. Urinalysis and heme-occult testing are preliminary tests, and upper and lower endoscopy is needed to evaluate for gastrointestinal pathology including cancer, colitis, or celiac disease. If those tests are inconclusive, consider proceeding to video capsule endoscopy to further evaluate the small intestine. Heavy gynecologic bleeding may require further evaluation and treatment. Persistent blood noted on urinalysis would warrant referral to urology for further testing.

Oral iron supplementation continues to be the first line treatment for iron deficiency anemia. Common forms include ferrous sulfate (Feosol), ferrous gluconate (Fergon), and ferrous fumarate (Ferro-Sequels). A typical dose of ferrous sulfate is 325 mg, which is 65 mg elemental iron, three times daily. However, there is now evidence that a dose of oral iron increases serum hepcidin, which then decreases iron absorption. Based on these findings, an alternate recommendation would be to give a single dose of iron on alternate days. This dosing schedule may increase iron absorption and adherence to treatment as a simpler regimen with decreased side effects. Iron is best absorbed when taken between meals; however, this can also worsen side effects. It is best to take iron separate from acid reducing medicines and foods that inhibit iron absorption. Common side effects of oral iron include diarrhea, nausea, epigastric discomfort, and constipation. Side effects can be lessened by taking iron with food, taking smaller doses, or changing to ferrous gluconate 325 mg (35 mg elemental iron).

Parenteral iron may be indicated when oral therapy is unsuccessful due to malabsorption, when oral iron is not tolerated, or when the rate of absorption with oral supplementation is insufficient due to the rate of blood loss. New forms of parenteral iron are safer and less likely to cause hypersensitivity reactions than older high-molecular weight iron dextran. The dose of IV iron needed can be calculated with the following formula: body weight in kilograms x 2.3 x hemoglobin deficiency (target hemoglobin level—patient hemoglobin level). Add another 500 to 1000 mg iron to replace low iron stores. Parenteral iron preparations licensed for use in the United States include iron sucrose (Venofer), ferumoxytol (Feraheme), ferric carboxymaltose (Ferinject and Injectafer), and ferric gluconate (Ferrlecit). A common dose for iron sucrose is 200 mg IV over 2 to 5 minutes, which is often repeated 5 times or until the target dose of iron is reached. Ferumoxytol has a usual dose of 510 mg IV infusion over at least 15 minutes which can be repeated 3 to 5 days after the initial dose. For patients who weigh ≥50 kg, the dose of ferric carboxymaltose is 750 mg IV over 15 to 30 minutes, and this can be repeated 7 days after the first dose. Ferric gluconate is generally used for patients on dialysis, and the typical dose is 125 mg IV over 10 minutes or IV infusion over 60 minutes per dialysis session.

Monitoring

The earliest marker for successful iron replacement is an increase in the reticulocyte count, which occurs within 5 to 10 days of initiation of iron replacement. Darkening of stools after 2 or 3 days of starting oral iron replacement is a reliable marker of compliance. A hemoglobin increase of 2 g/dL is considered an appropriate response to oral iron replacement. Reaching a serum ferritin level of 100 µg/L will ensure good iron stores in nearly all patients. Once iron deficiency has been corrected, a complete blood count and labs to evaluate iron stores should be checked monthly for 3 months and then every 3 months for a year. If iron levels are not maintained, then further work up is indicated to discover the cause.

Management of Complications

If properly treated, iron deficiency has few complications in adults. Untreated iron deficiency in infants and small children can lead to cognitive development and growth deficits. Treating iron deficiency without identifying the source and cause of blood loss could result in a delay or failure to diagnose gastrointestinal malignancies or other serious clinical problems.

Plummer–Vinson syndrome is a rare clinical condition characterized by a triad of iron deficiency anemia, postcricoid esophageal webs, and dysphagia. The pathogenesis of Plummer-Vinson syndrome remains unclear, though iron and other nutritional deficiencies, genetic predisposition, and autoimmunity have all been implicated in the formation of the webs. Treatment includes the correction of iron deficiency and endoscopic dilation of the esophageal webs to relieve dysphagia.

References

Auerbach M, Adamson JW: How we diagnose and treat iron deficiency anemia, *Am J Hematol* 91(1):31–38, 2016 Jan.

Bermejo F, Garcia-Lopez S: A guide to diagnosis of iron deficiency and iron deficiency anemia in digestive diseases, *World J Gastroenterol* 15(37):4638–4643, 2009 Oct 7.

Camaschella C: Iron-deficiency anemia, *N Engl J Med* 372(19):1832–1843, 2015 May 7.

Centers for Disease Control. Recommendation to Prevent and Control Iron Deficiency in the United States. Available at https://www.cdc.gov/MMWR/preview/mmwrhtml/00051880.htm. [Accessed April 16, 2019].

Craig WJ, Mangels AR, American Dietetic Association: Position of the American Dietetic Association: vegetarian diets, *J Am Diet Assoc* 109(7):1266–1282, 2009 Jul.

Engebretsen KV, Blom-Hogestol IK, Hewitt S, et al: Anemia following Roux-en-Y gastric bypass for morbid obesity; a 5-year follow-up study, *Scand J Gastroenterol* 53(8):917–922, 2018 Aug.

Lopez A, Cacoub P, Macdougall IC, Peyrin-Biroulet L: Iron deficiency anaemia, *Lancet* 387(10021):907–916, 2016 Feb 27.

Parrott J, Frank L, Rabena R, Craggs-Dino L, Isom KA, Greiman L: American Society for Metabolic and Bariatric Surgery Integrated Health Nutritional Guidelines for the Surgical Weight Loss Patient 2016 Update: Micronutrients, *Surg Obes Relat Dis* 13(5):727–741, 2017 May.

Peyrin-Biroulet L, Williet N, Cacoub P: Guidelines on the diagnosis and treatment of iron deficiency across indications: a systematic review, *Am J Clin Nutr* 102(6):1585–1594, 2015 Dec.

Stoffel NU, Cercamondi CI, Brittenham G, et al: Iron absorption from oral iron supplements given on consecutive versus alternate days and as single morning doses versus twice–daily split dosing in iron–depleted women: two open–label, randomised controlled trials, *Lancet Haematol* 4(11):e524–33, 2017.

World Health Organization/UNICEF/UNU: Iron Deficiency Anaemia: Assessment, Prevention, and Control. A guide for Programme Managers, Geneva, Switzerland, 2001, World Health Organization. Available at https://www.who.int/nutrition/publications/en/ida_assessment_prevention_control.pdf. [Accessed 17 April 2019].

MULTIPLE MYELOMA

Method of
S. Vincent Rajkumar, MD; and Robert A. Kyle, MD

CURRENT DIAGNOSIS

- Malignant clonal plasma cell disorder
- Characterized by presence of a monoclonal immunoglobulin in the serum or urine in most patients
- Typical manifestations include anemia, osteolytic bone lesions, and renal failure
- Initial work-up should include a bone marrow aspiration and biopsy with fluorescent in situ hybridization studies to determine molecular cytogenetic typ0065
- Standard risk: trisomies (hyperdiploidy), t(11;14), and t(6;14)
- High risk: del(17p), gain 1q, t(4;14), (t14;16) or t(14;20)

CURRENT THERAPY

- Do not begin treatment until symptomatic multiple myeloma develops (CRAB: *c*alcium elevated, *r*enal failure, *a*nemia, *b*one lesions) or other myeloma defining events are present. Patients with high risk smoldering multiple myeloma are candidates for preventive therapy with lenalidomide (Revimid) or lenalidomide plus dexamethasone (Decadron)[1] (Rd)
- Decide whether an autologous stem cell transplant is feasible. If it is, one must avoid melphalan (Alkeran) therapy as initial treatment.
- Initial therapy typically consists of a triplet regimen such as lenalidomide (Revlimid), bortezomib (Velcade), and dexamethasone[1] (VRd). Alternatives are daratumumab (Darzalex), lenalidomide, and dexamethasone (DRd).
- Patients who are candidates for autologous stem cell transplantation should collect stem cells after 3 to 4 cycles of induction. After collection, patients proceed to either early transplantation, or resume initial therapy and postpone transplant until relapse. After transplant, and after initial therapy in patients who delay transplant, patients should receive maintenance therapy.
- Patients who are not stem cell transplant candidates who are treated with VRd receive about 8 to 9 cycles of triplet therapy followed by maintenance. If DRd is used as initial therapy, the triplet is continued at maintenance doses. Frail patients can be treated with the doublet regimen of Rd, in which case therapy is continued until progression if tolerated.
- Relapsed or refractory myeloma should be treated with one of the active drugs given alone or in combination. Active agents include thalidomide, lenalidomide, bortezomib, carfilzomib (Kyprolis), pomalidomide (Pomalyst), daratumumab (Darzalex), ixazomib (Ninlaro), elotuzumab (Empliciti), panobinostat (Farydak), isatuximab (Sarclisa), belantamab mafodotin (Blenrep), melphalan flufenamide (Pepaxto), selinexor (Xpovio), ide-cel (Abecma), corticosteroids, anthracyclines, and alkylators.

[1]Not FDA approved for this indication.

Multiple myeloma is characterized by the neoplastic proliferation of clonal plasma cells. It is typically associated with a monoclonal (M) protein in the serum and/or urine.

Epidemiology

In the United States, multiple myeloma constitutes 1% of all malignant diseases and slightly more than 10% of hematologic malignancies. The annual incidence is 4 to 5 per 100,000; the incidence in African Americans is twice that in whites. The apparent recent increase in rates is probably caused by increased availability and use of medical facilities and improved diagnostic techniques, particularly in the older population. The median age at diagnosis is approximately 70 years.

Risk Factors

The cause of multiple myeloma is unclear. Exposure to radiation might play a role. Persons in agricultural occupations who are exposed to pesticides, herbicides, or fungicides have an increased risk of multiple myeloma. Benzene and petroleum products, hair dyes, engine exhaust, furniture worker products, obesity, and chronic immune stimulation have also been reported as risk factors. The risk of developing multiple myeloma is higher for patients with a first-degree relative with the disease. Clusters of two or more first-degree relatives or identical twins have been recognized.

Clinical Manifestations

Weakness, fatigue, bone pain, recurrent infections, and symptoms of hypercalcemia or renal insufficiency should alert the physician to the possibility of multiple myeloma. Anemia is present in 70% of patients at the time of diagnosis. An M protein is found in the serum or urine in more than 97% of patients with multiple myeloma by immunofixation studies and the serum free light chain (FLC) assay. Lytic lesions, osteoporosis, or fractures are present at diagnosis in 80% of patients and are best detected by whole body low-dose computed tomography (CT) or positron emission tomography (PET)/CT. Magnetic resonance imaging (MRI) and PET/CT are also helpful in patients who have skeletal pain but no abnormality on radiographs or when there are other clinical concerns about the extent of the disease. Conventional radiography is less sensitive and is no longer recommended. Hypercalcemia is present in 15% of patients, and the serum creatinine value is 2 mg/dL or greater in almost 20% of patients at diagnosis.

Diagnosis

If multiple myeloma is suspected, the patient should have, in addition to a complete history and physical examination:
- Determination of values for hemoglobin, leukocytes with differential count, platelets, serum creatinine, calcium, and uric acid
- A radiographic survey of bones, including humeri and femurs using low-dose whole body CT or PET-CT.
- Serum protein electrophoresis with immunofixation
- Quantitation of immunoglobulins (Igs), serum FLC assay
- Bone marrow aspirate and biopsy
- Routine urinalysis
- Electrophoresis and immunofixation of an adequately concentrated aliquot from a 24-hour urine specimen
- Fluorescence in situ hybridization (FISH)
- Measurement of β_2-microglobulin, C-reactive protein, and lactate dehydrogenase

Box 1 lists the International Myeloma Working Group updated criteria for diagnosis of myeloma and related disorders. Metastatic carcinoma, lymphoma, leukemia, and connective tissue disorders can resemble multiple myeloma and must be considered in the differential diagnosis. Patients with multiple myeloma must be differentiated from those with monoclonal gammopathy of undetermined significance (MGUS) and smoldering (asymptomatic) multiple myeloma (SMM). Patients with MGUS and low-risk SMM may remain stable for long periods and not require treatment (see Box 1). Patients with high-risk SMM (any two or more of the following: >20% bone marrow plasma cells, >2g/dL serum M protein, >20 serum FLC ratio) should be considered for lenalidomide (Revlimid) or lenalidomide plus dexamethasone (Decadron)[1] as preventive therapy.

[1]Not FDA approved for this indication.

Monoclonal Gammopathy of Undetermined Significance
- Serum M protein <3 g/dL
- Clonal bone marrow–plasma cells <10%
- Absence of end-organ damage (CRAB) attributable to a plasma cell proliferative disorder

Smoldering Multiple Myeloma
- Serum M protein ≥3 g/dL and/or clonal bone marrow–plasma cells 10%–60%
- Absence of myeloma defining events or amyloidosis

Multiple Myeloma
- Presence of clonal bone marrow plasma cells 10% or greater or biopsy-proven plasmacytoma
- Presence of end-organ damage (CRAB) thought to be related to a plasma cell proliferative disorder or other myeloma defining event (clonal bone marrow plasma cells 60% or higher, serum free light chain ratio 100 or more provided involved free light chain level is 100 mg/L or more, more than one focal lesion on magnetic resonance imaging)

CRAB, Calcium elevated, renal failure, anemia, bone lesions; M, monoclonal.
Derived from Rajkumar SV, Dimopoulos MA, Palumbo A, et al. International Myeloma Working Group updated criteria for the diagnosis of multiple myeloma. *Lancet Oncol.* 2014;15:e538–e548.

Treatment

Patients with symptomatic multiple myeloma may be classified as having high-risk or standard-risk disease. High-risk disease is defined as the presence of del(17p), gain 1q, t(4;14), t(14;16), or t(14;20) with FISH. Detection of p53 mutations by sequencing is also considered a cytogenetic high-risk factor. The presence of two high-risk cytogenetic abnormalities is considered "double-hit" myeloma; and the presence of three high-risk abnormalities is considered triple-hit myeloma. Lactate dehydrogenase, circulating plasma cells, and β_2-microglobulin levels are additional important risk factors. Approximately 15% to 20% of patients with symptomatic multiple myeloma have high-risk disease.

Initially, patients are classified into those eligible for an autologous stem cell transplant (SCT) versus those not eligible. An autologous SCT adds approximately 1 year of survival on average when compared with patients treated with conventional-dose chemotherapy alone.

Eligibility for autologous SCT in multiple myeloma varies from country to country. In the United States, decisions are made on a patient-by-patient basis depending on the physiologic age rather than the chronologic age. In most institutions, patients older than 70 years or with serum creatinine greater than 2.5 mg/dL, Eastern Cooperative Oncology Group (ECOG) performance status of 3 or 4, or New York Heart Association (NYHA) functional status class III or IV are considered ineligible for autologous SCT. Although patients with kidney failure may have an autologous SCT, the morbidity and mortality are higher.

Initial Therapy for Transplant-Eligible Patients

The approach to treatment of newly diagnosed myeloma in patients eligible for stem cell transplantation is summarized in Figure 1A. Bortezomib (Velcade), lenalidomide (Revlimid), dexamethasone (Decadon) (VRD)[1] is the preferred standard initial therapy for multiple myeloma. In a randomized trial conducted by the Southwest Oncology Group, VRD was superior to lenalidomide plus dexamethasone (Rd) in terms of progression-free survival (PFS) and overall survival (OS). Bortezomib and dexamethasone are typically administered once weekly. In the VRD regimen lenalidomide is given at a dose of 25 mg daily on days 1 to 14 of a 21-day cycle. Bortezomib should be given using the

once-weekly schedule to reduce the risk of peripheral neuropathy. It is also preferable to administer bortezomib subcutaneously to diminish the risk of neuropathy. An alternative to VRD is daratumumab (Darzalex), lenalidomide, dexamethasone (DRD). For patients who are initiated on DRD, all three drugs are continued until progression, with daratumumab administered once-monthly after the first 6 months of therapy. The addition of daratumumab (Darzalex) to VTD (Velcade, thalidomide, dexamethasone) has shown better response rates and PFS compared with VTD, but more data on OS are needed before this approach can be recommended. Further data from randomized trials on the addition of daratumumab to the current standard of VRD is also needed. Bortezomib plus cyclophosphamide (Cytoxan) 300 mg/m² orally once weekly plus dexamethasone 40 mg once weekly (VCD) is an option for patients presenting with acute renal failure. If lenalidomide is not available, an alternative for initial therapy is bortezomib, thalidomide (Thalomid), and dexamethasone (VTD). For high-risk patients less than 65 years of age, daratumumab plus VRD can be considered as an alternative. In all regimens, it is preferable to administer dexamethasone at a dose no greater than 40 mg per week unless there is need for urgent cytoreduction as in patients with acute renal failure and cast nephropathy.

Autologous Stem Cell Transplantation

Following 3 to 4 months of induction therapy with one of the initial regimens, one must collect the stem cells in patients eligible for transplantation. The stem cells must be collected before the patient is exposed to prolonged therapy, especially melphalan (Alkeran). Granulocyte colony-stimulating factor (G-CSF, Neupogen) with or without cyclophosphamide (Cytoxan) is used for mobilizing stem cells. G-CSF plus cyclophosphamide is preferred in patients who are treated with lenalidomide plus dexamethasone induction, who are older than 65 years, or who have received such therapy for over 4 months. Plerixafor (Mozobil) may also be used for mobilization of hematopoietic stem cells. It is advisable to collect 6×10^6 CD34+ cells/kg, which is sufficient for two transplants in patients below 65 years of age.

The timing of autologous SCT takes into account the patient's wishes, and it may be done early (when the patient recovers from stem cell collection) or delayed until relapse. There is no difference in OS even at 8 years of follow up among patients who receive an autologous SCT immediately following collection of stem cells and those who receive it at first relapse. In general, we prefer an early transplant because this provides a better quality of life and time without therapy.

Melphalan 200 mg/m² is the preferred conditioning regimen for autologous SCT. Tandem transplantation is not recommended for most patients. An exception would be young patients (below 65 years of age) with high-risk multiple myeloma, in whom such an approach can be considered on a case-by-case basis.

The mortality rate with autologous SCT is approximately 1%. Unfortunately, multiple myeloma is not eradicated, and the autologous peripheral stem cells are contaminated by myeloma cells or their precursors.

Bone marrow transplantation from an identical twin donor (syngeneic) is the treatment of choice if such a donor is available. Results are superior to allogeneic transplantation.

Maintenance Therapy Following Autologous Stem Cell Transplantation

Randomized trials have tested the value of lenalidomide as maintenance therapy following stem cell transplantation. An OS benefit has been observed in a meta-analysis of three trials. This benefit appears to be mainly restricted to standard-risk patients. An increased risk of second cancers has been noted with lenalidomide maintenance and further follow-up is needed. In another randomized trial improved OS with bortezomib maintenance has been reported, but it is not clear whether the benefit is due to the maintenance therapy or differences in induction therapy between the two groups. We recommend lenalidomide maintenance for standard-risk patients following autologous SCT, and following

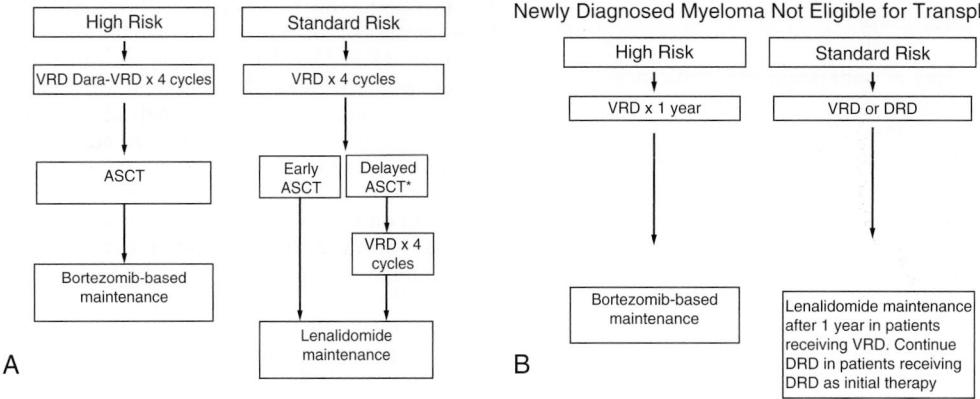

Figure 1 Approach to the treatment of newly diagnosed myeloma in patients eligible for stem cell transplantation (A) and approach to the treatment of newly diagnosed myeloma in patients not eligible for stem cell transplantation (B). *ASCT*, Autologous stem cell transplantation; *DRD*, daratumumab, lenalidomide, dexamethasone; *Dara*, daratumumab; *VRD*, bortezomib, lenalidomide, dexamethasone. Modified from Rajkumar SV. Multiple myeloma: 2020 update on diagnosis, risk-stratification, and management. *Am J Hematol.* 95(5):548–567, 2020.

approximately 12 months of initial therapy in patients not eligible for SCT and in patients who delay SCT. In high-risk patients, we recommend bortezomib-based maintenance.

Allogeneic Transplantation

Allogeneic bone marrow transplantation (myeloablative and non-myeloablative) has been tested in myeloma, but treatment-related mortality is high and graft-versus-host disease is a troublesome problem. Furthermore, only a small proportion of patients with multiple myeloma are eligible. Allogeneic transplantation is currently not recommended for routine use outside of a clinical trial. An exception to this are young patients with high-risk disease in first relapse after autologous transplantation who are willing to assume the high treatment-related mortality associated with allogeneic SCT.

Initial Therapy for Patients Who Are Ineligible for Autologous Stem Cell Transplantation

The initial therapy for patients not eligible for transplantation now resembles that of transplant-eligible patients. The current approach to treatment of newly diagnosed myeloma in patients not eligible for stem cell transplantation is summarized in Figure 1B. Currently, we prefer VRD as initial therapy. An alternative that has been recently approved for initial therapy in the United States is DRD. Other options include VCD and VTD. For frail patients, the doublet regimen of Rd can be used.

When using VRD, we continue the initial chemotherapy regimen for approximately 8 to 9 cycles followed usually by lenalidomide maintenance in standard-risk patients and bortezomib plus lenalidomide maintenance in high-risk patients.

Relapsed or Refractory Multiple Myeloma

Almost all patients with multiple myeloma who survive eventually relapse. If relapse occurs more than 6 months after treatment is discontinued, the initial chemotherapy regimen should be reinstituted. Most patients respond again, but the duration and quality of response are usually inferior to the initial response. Recently, several new drugs have been approved for the treatment of multiple myeloma including pomalidomide (Pomalyst), carfilzomib (Kyprolis), daratumumab (Darzalex), elotuzumab (Empliciti), panobinostat (Farydak), ixazomib (Ninlaro), selinexor (Xpovio), isatuximab (Sarclisa), belantamab mafodotin (Blenrep), melphalan flufenamide (Pepaxto), and idecabtagene vicleucel (ide-cel [Abecma]).

Thalidomide

Thalidomide (Thalomid) is usually instituted in a dose of 50 to 100 mg daily and, if necessary, escalated to 200 mg daily if tolerated. It is most often used in combinations such as VTD. Side effects include sedation, fatigue, constipation, rash, deep venous thrombosis (DVT), edema, bradycardia, and hypothyroidism. Virtually all patients develop a sensorimotor peripheral neuropathy. The use of thalidomide in pregnancy is contraindicated, and the System for Thalidomide Education and Prescribing Safety (STEPS) program must be followed to prevent teratogenic effects.

Bortezomib

Bortezomib (Velcade) is a proteasome inhibitor that produces a response rate of approximately 35% in patients with relapsed or refractory myeloma. It is most often used in combinations such as VRD, VCD, or VTD to maximize response rates. The most troublesome side effect is peripheral neuropathy, which can occur in 35% to 40% of patients. The neuropathy is often painful but does improve in most patients after discontinuing bortezomib. The risk of neuropathy can be greatly reduced by using bortezomib in a once-weekly subcutaneous schedule.

Lenalidomide

Lenalidomide (Revlimid) as a single-agent produces an objective response in approximately 30% of patients with relapsed or refractory multiple myeloma. The major side effects are cytopenias, and the dose needs to be modified accordingly. The combination of lenalidomide plus low-dose dexamethasone (Rd) is the backbone of several myeloma treatment regimens.

Carfilzomib

Carfilzomib (Kyprolis) is a new proteasome inhibitor approved for the therapy of patients with multiple myeloma who have received at least two prior therapies, including both an immunomodulatory agent and bortezomib, and have disease progression on or within 60 days of the completion of the last therapy. Carfilzomib needs to be administered intravenously twice weekly. In a recent randomized trial, the combination of carfilzomib, lenalidomide, and dexamethasone (KRD) was found to have superior response rate, PFS, and OS compared with Rd.

Pomalidomide

Pomalidomide (Pomalyst) is an analog of lenalidomide and thalidomide. It has shown significant clinical activity in patients who are refractory to both bortezomib and lenalidomide (dual refractory). It is approved for patients with multiple myeloma who received at least two prior therapies, including both lenalidomide and bortezomib, and have disease progression on or within 60 days of the completion of the last therapy. It is administered orally at a dose of 2 to 4 mg daily for 21 days every 28 days. The major side effects are cytopenias and fatigue.

Panobinostat

Panobinostat (Farydak) is a pan-deacetylase inhibitor that is approved for the treatment of multiple myeloma in patients who have received at least two prior therapies, including both an immunomodulatory agent and bortezomib. It is administered orally at a starting dose of 20 mg three times a week for 2 weeks every 3 weeks. It is given in combination with bortezomib and dexamethasone. It is associated with severe diarrhea in approximately 25% of patients, so use must be restricted to younger patients in good performance status who have failed other treatments but are not yet refractory to bortezomib. If the drug is used, the dose must preferably be lower than the approved label dose, and the dose of bortezomib and dexamethasone must also be reduced to a once-weekly schedule. The drug approval carries a black box warning concerning cardiac arrhythmias and severe diarrhea.

Elotuzumab

Elotuzumab (Empliciti) is a monoclonal antibody that is approved for the treatment of relapsed myeloma. It targets the signaling lymphocytic activation molecule F7 (SLAMF7). In a randomized trial of 646 patients, elotuzumab plus Rd was superior to Rd, median PFS 19.4 months versus 14.9 months, respectively ($P < .001$).

Daratumumab

Daratumumab (Darzalex) is a monoclonal antibody that is approved for the treatment of relapsed myeloma. It targets CD38, a molecule universally expressed on myeloma cells. Daratumumab has a response rate of approximately 30% in heavily pretreated patients. Two randomized trials have found improvement in PFS with the addition of daratumumab to Rd and bortezomib-dexamethasone, respectively.

Ixazomib

Ixazomib (Ninlaro) is an oral proteasome inhibitor approved for the treatment of relapsed myeloma. It is a boronic acid derivative similar to bortezomib. It is administered once weekly orally. Compared with bortezomib, it has a lower risk of peripheral neuropathy.

Selinexor

Selinexor (Xpovio) is an oral drug that acts by binding to nuclear export protein 1 (XPO1) and selectively blocking the transport of various proteins within the cell. It has been approved in combination with low dose dexamethasone for patients with relapsed or refractory multiple myeloma who have received at least 4 prior therapies, and whose disease is refractory to at least 2 proteasome inhibitors, at least 2 immunomodulatory agents, and an anti-CD38 monoclonal antibody. It is administered orally at a dose of 80 mg twice a week. However, due to toxicities, a once weekly regimen is likely more preferable.

Belantamab mafodotin

Belantamab mafodotin (Blenrep) is an antibody drug conjugate targeting B-cell maturation antigen (BCMA) that is expressed on plasma cells. Belantamab mafodotin has been approved as a single agent in patients with relapsed or refractory multiple myeloma who have received at least 4 prior therapies, including an anti-CD38 monoclonal antibody, a proteasome inhibitor, and an immunomodulatory agent. It has a response rate of approximately 30%. The main adverse effect of concern is grade 3 to 4 keratopathy, which can be seen in approximately 40% of patients, necessitating ophthalmologic evaluation prior to starting therapy and periodically during therapy.

Idecabtagene vicleucel

Idecabtagene vicleucel (ide-cel; Abecma) is a chimeric antigen receptor T cell therapy (CAR-T) targeting BCMA. It has been approved for patients with relapsed refractory myeloma after 4 or more prior therapies, including an immunomodulatory drug, a proteasome inhibitor, and an anti-CD38 antibody. Ide-cel is well tolerated, with less than 5% of patients experiencing severe cytokine release syndrome or neurological toxicity. It has a response rate of 73%, with a response duration of approximately 9 months.

Isatuximab

Isatuximab (Sarclisa) is a monoclonal antibody targeting CD38 and is an alternative to daratumumab. It has been approved in combination with pomalidomide and dexamethasone, as well as in combination with carfilzomib and dexamethasone. In certain patients, isatuximab may be significantly less expensive than daratumumab, which may be a consideration.

Melphalan flufenamide

Melphalan flufenamide (Pepaxto) is a new peptidase-potentiated alkylating agent. It has been approved for the treatment of patients with relapsed refractory myeloma who have received at least 4 prior lines of therapy and whose disease is refractory to at least one proteasome inhibitor, one immunomodulatory agent, and one CD-38 directed monoclonal antibody. More data is needed to determine the role of this agent and whether it has any advantage in response rate to conventional alkylators such as cyclophosphamide and melphalan.

Other New Drugs

New drugs that are in clinical trials include new bi-specific antibodies such as teclistamab[5] and AMG-701[5] (targeting BCMA and CD3), talquetamab[5] (targeting GPRC5D and CD3), and cevostamab[5] (targeting FcRH5 and CD3). Venetoclax (Venclexta)[1] has shown promise against t11;14 subtype of multiple myeloma. Iberdomide[5] is a new cereblon targeting agent that has also shown promise. Other BCMA directed CAR-T therapies are also showing promise, including cilta-cel[5].

Supportive Therapy
Radiotherapy

Palliative radiation in a dose of 20 to 30 Gy should be limited to patients who have disabling pain and a well-defined focal process that has not responded to chemotherapy. Analgesics in combination with chemotherapy usually can control the pain. This approach is preferred to local radiation because pain often occurs at another site, and local radiation does not benefit the patient with systemic disease. In addition, the myelosuppressive effects of radiotherapy and chemotherapy are cumulative and can restrict future therapy. Radiation is required for spinal cord compression from plasmacytoma. Postsurgical radiation after stabilization of fractures or impending fractures is rarely needed.

Hypercalcemia

Hypercalcemia must be suspected if the patient has anorexia, nausea, vomiting, polyuria, increased constipation, weakness, confusion, stupor, or coma. If it is untreated, renal insufficiency usually develops. Hydration, preferably with isotonic saline and prednisone (25 mg orally four times daily), is effective in many patients with mild to moderate hypercalcemia (calcium < 13 mg/dL). If more-severe hypercalcemia occurs, zoledronic acid (Zometa) at a dose of 4 mg intravenously over 15 minutes or pamidronate (Aredia) 90 mg given intravenously over at least 2 hours is indicated. Calcitonin (Miacalcin) may be used if rapid reduction of calcium levels is needed. Hemodialysis may be necessary for extremely severe hypercalcemia. The dosage of prednisone must be reduced and discontinued as soon as possible.

Renal Insufficiency

Approximately 20% of patients with multiple myeloma have a serum creatinine level of 2.0 mg/dL or more at diagnosis. Myeloma kidney (cast nephropathy) and hypercalcemia are the

---

[1]Not FDA approved for this indication.
[5]Investigational drug in the United States.

two major causes. Myeloma kidney is characterized by the presence of large, waxy, laminated casts in the distal and collecting tubules. Some light chains are very nephrotoxic, but no specific amino acid sequence of the nephrotoxic light chain has been identified.

Dehydration, infection, nonsteroidal antiinflammatory agents, and radiographic contrast media can contribute to acute kidney failure. Hyperuricemia or amyloid deposition can produce renal insufficiency. Nephrotic syndrome rarely occurs in multiple myeloma unless amyloidosis is present.

Maintenance of a high fluid intake producing 3 L of urine per 24 hours is important for preventing kidney failure in patients with Bence Jones proteinuria. If hyperuricemia occurs, allopurinol (Zyloprim) in doses of 300 mg daily provides effective therapy.

Acute kidney failure should be treated promptly with appropriate fluid and electrolyte replacement. Patients with kidney failure should be treated with either VCD or VTD to reduce the tumor mass as quickly as possible. A trial of plasmapheresis is reasonable in an attempt to prevent chronic dialysis. Hemodialysis and peritoneal dialysis are equally effective and are necessary for patients with symptomatic azotemia.

Anemia

Almost every patient with multiple myeloma eventually becomes anemic. Increased plasma volume from the osmotic effect of the M protein can produce hypervolemia and can spuriously lower the hemoglobin and hematocrit values. Patients with significant symptoms should be considered for red blood cell transfusion. If a transfusion is indicated, irradiated leukocyte-reduced red cells are preferred.

In patients with newly diagnosed myeloma, induction chemotherapy is often associated with a prompt improvement in hemoglobin levels, so it is better to avoid the use of erythropoietin. Erythropoietin (Epogen) should be seriously considered in relapsed patients receiving chemotherapy who have a persistent, symptomatic hemoglobin level of 10 g/dL or less.

Erythropoietin reduces the transfusion requirement and increases hemoglobin concentration in more than half of patients. Those with low serum erythropoietin values are more likely to respond. Most physicians proceed with a trial of erythropoietin 150 U/kg three times weekly or 40,000 U once a week. Darbepoetin, a long-lasting erythropoietin (Aranesp), may be given weekly or biweekly. Erythropoietin should be discontinued when the hemoglobin reaches 11 g/dL.

Skeletal Lesions

Bone lesions manifested by pain and fractures are a major problem. A skeletal radiographic survey should be repeated at 6-month intervals or sooner if pain develops. Patients should be encouraged to be as active as possible because confinement to bed increases demineralization of the skeleton. Trauma must be avoided because even mild stress can result in a fracture. Fixation of long bone fractures or impending fractures with an intramedullary rod and methyl methacrylate gives excellent results.

All patients with multiple myeloma who have lytic lesions, pathologic fractures, or severe osteopenia should receive an intravenous bisphosphonate. Pamidronate (Aredia) 90 mg intravenously over 2 hours every 4 weeks or zoledronic acid (Zometa) 4 mg intravenously over 15 minutes every 4 weeks are equally efficacious. The dosage of bisphosphonates should be reduced with renal insufficiency. Because renal insufficiency or nephrotic-range proteinuria can occur, serum creatinine and 24-hour urine protein monitoring is necessary. One should seriously consider stopping the intravenous bisphosphonate in patients who have responsive or stable disease after 2 years of therapy. In other patients, we recommend reducing the dose to once every 3 months. A randomized trial has found that

denosumab (Xgeva), a monoclonal antibody targeting RANKL, may be as effective in reducing skeletal events as zoledronic acid and may be an option for selected patients with significant renal impairment.

Bisphosphonates should be resumed upon relapse with new-onset skeletal-related events. Osteonecrosis of the jaw can occur in patients receiving bisphosphonates. Although the relationship is unclear, it is essential to obtain a complete dental evaluation and perform preventive dental treatment before beginning bisphosphonates. The patient should practice good oral hygiene during therapy. Invasive procedures (especially dental extractions) should be avoided during bisphosphonate therapy. Osteonecrosis of the jaw should be managed conservatively.

Vertebroplasty or kyphoplasty may be helpful for patients with an acute compression fracture of the spine. Both have been associated with pain relief. Results appear to be better when the procedure is performed shortly after the compression fracture. Leakage of the methyl methacrylate is a potential adverse event. A choice between vertebroplasty and kyphoplasty depends on the expertise of the physician performing the procedure.

Infections

Bacterial infections are more common in patients with myeloma than in the general population. All patients should receive pneumococcal and influenza immunizations despite their suboptimal antibody response. Substantial fever is an indication for appropriate cultures, chest radiography, and consideration of antibiotic therapy. The greatest risk for infection is during the first 3 months after chemotherapy is initiated, and prophylactic antibiotics (levofloxacin [Levaquin] or cotrimoxazole [Bactrim]) should be considered during this period. Antiviral prophylaxis (acyclovir [Zovirax] 400 mg twice daily or valacyclovir [Valtrex] 500 mg once daily) should be given to all patients receiving bortezomib because of the increased risk of herpes zoster. Intravenous immunoglobulin (IVIg, Gammagard)[1] may be helpful in selected patients who have recurrent serious infections despite the use of prophylactic antibiotics. It is inconvenient, associated with side effects, and very expensive. Consequently, few of our patients receive IVIg.

Hyperviscosity Syndrome

Symptoms of hyperviscosity can include oronasal bleeding, gastrointestinal bleeding, blurred vision, neurologic symptoms, or congestive heart failure. Most patients have symptoms when the serum viscosity measurement is more than 4 cP, but the relationship between serum viscosity and clinical manifestations is not precise. The decision to perform plasmapheresis, which promptly relieves the symptoms of hyperviscosity, should be made on clinical grounds rather than serum viscosity levels. Hyperviscosity is more common in IgA myeloma than in IgG myeloma.

Extradural Myeloma (Cord Compression)

The possibility of cord compression must be considered if weakness of the legs or difficulty in voiding or defecating occurs. The sudden onset of severe radicular pain or severe back pain with neurologic symptoms suggests compression of the spinal cord. MRI or CT of the entire spine must be performed immediately. Radiation therapy in a dose of approximately 30 Gy is beneficial in about one half of patients. Dexamethasone (Decadron)[1] should be administered in addition to radiation therapy. Surgical decompression is necessary only if the neurologic deficit does not improve.

---

[1]Not FDA approved for this indication.

Venous Thromboembolism

Patients with multiple myeloma have an increased risk of venous thromboembolism. This is due to the malignancy itself, as well as therapy with lenalidomide, thalidomide, or pomalidomide. All patients receiving lenalidomide (or thalidomide or pomalidomide) need DVT prophylaxis with aspirin[1] (81 mg or 325 mg daily) or full-dose warfarin (Coumadin)[1] or low-molecular-weight heparin.[1]

Emotional Support

All patients with multiple myeloma need substantial and continuing emotional support. The physician's approach must be positive in emphasizing the potential benefits of therapy. It is reassuring for patients to know that some survive for 10 years or more. It is vital that the physician caring for patients with multiple myeloma has the interest and capacity for dealing with incurable disease over the span of years with assurance, sympathy, and resourcefulness.

References

Anderson K, Ismaila N, Flynn PJ, et al: Role of bone-modifying agents in multiple myeloma: American Society of Clinical Oncology Clinical Practice Guideline Update, *J Clin Oncol*, 2018 Jan 17, JCO2017766402. Available at: 10.1200/JCO.2017.76.6402 [Epub ahead of print].

Attal M, Lauwers-Cances V, Marit G, et al: Lenalidomide maintenance after stem-cell transplantation for multiple myeloma, *N Engl J Med* 366:1782–1791, 2012.

Chari A, Vogl DT, Gavriatopoulou M, et al: Oral selinexor–dexamethasone for triple-class refractory multiple myeloma, *N Engl J Med* 372(381):727–738, 2019.

Dimopoulos MA, Oriol A, Nahi H, et al: Daratumumab, lenalidomide, and dexamethasone for multiple myeloma, *N Engl J Med* 375(14):1319–1331, 2016.

Durie BGM, et al: Bortezomib with lenalidomide and dexamethasone versus lenalidomide and dexamethasone alone in patients with newly diagnosed myeloma without intent for immediate autologous stem-cell transplant (SWOG S0777): a randomised, open-label, phase 3 trial, *Lancet* 389(10068):519–527, 2017.

Facon T, Kumar S, Piesner T, et al: Daratumumab plus lenalidomide and dexamethasone for untreated myeloma, *N Engl J Med* 380(22):2104–2115, 2019.

Krishnan A, Pasquini MC, Logan B, et al: Autologous haemopoietic stem-cell transplantation followed by allogeneic or autologous haemopoietic stem-cell transplantation in patients with multiple myeloma (BMT CTN 0102): a phase 3 biological assignment trial, *Lancet Oncol* 12:1195–1203, 2011.

Kyle RA, Rajkumar SV: Epidemiology of the plasma-cell disorders, *Best Pract Res Clin Haematol* 20:637–664, 2007.

Lonial S, Dimopoulos M, Palumbo A, et al: Elotuzumab therapy for relapsed or refractory multiple myeloma, *N Engl J Med* 373:621–631, 2015.

Lonial S, Lee HC, Badros A, et al: Belantamab mafodotin for relapsed or refractory multiple myeloma (DREAMM-2): a two-arm, randomised, open-label, phase 2 study, *Lancet Oncol* 21:207–221, 2020.

McCarthy PL, Owzar K, Hofmeister CC, et al: Lenalidomide after stem-cell transplantation for multiple myeloma, *N Engl J Med* 366:1770–1781, 2012.

Moreau P, Attal MA, Hulin C, et al: Bortezomib, thalidomide, and dexamethasone with or without daratumumab before and after autologous stem-cell transplantation for newly diagnosed multiple myeloma (CASSIOPEIA): a randomised, open-label, phase 3 study, *Lancet* 394(10192):29–38, 2019.

Moreau P, Masszi T, Grzasko N, et al: Oral ixazomib, lenalidomide, and dexamethasone for multiple myeloma, *N Engl J Med* 374(17):1621–1634, 2016.

Munshi NC, Anderson LD, Shah N, et al: Idecabtagene vicleucel in relapsed and refractory myeloma, *N Engl J Med* 384:705–716, 2021.

Palumbo A, Chanan-Khan A, Weisel K, et al: Daratumumab, bortezomib, and dexamethasone for multiple myeloma, *N Engl J Med* 375(8):754–766, 2016.

Raje N, Terpos E, Willenbacher W, et al: Denosumab versus zoledronic acid in bone disease treatment of newly diagnosed multiple myeloma: an international, double-blind, double-dummy, randomised, controlled, phase 3 study, *Lancet Oncol* Feb 8. pii: S1470-2045(18)30072-X. Available at: https://doi.org/10.1016/S1470-2045(18)30072-X.

Rajkumar SV, Jacobus S, Callander NS, et al: Lenalidomide plus high-dose dexamethasone versus lenalidomide plus low-dose dexamethasone as initial therapy for newly diagnosed multiple myeloma: an open-label randomised controlled trial, *Lancet Oncol* 11:29–37, 2010.

Rajkumar SV, et al: International Myeloma Working Group updated criteria for the diagnosis of multiple myeloma, *Lancet Oncol* 15:e538–e548, 2014.

San Miguel J, Weisel K, Moreau P, et al: Pomalidomide plus low-dose dexamethasone versus high-dose dexamethasone alone for patients with relapsed and refractory multiple myeloma (MM-003): a randomised, open-label, phase 3 trial, *Lancet Oncol* 14:1055–1066, 2013.

Sonneveld P, Schmidt-Wolf IGH, van der Holt B, et al: Bortezomib induction and maintenance treatment in patients with newly diagnosed multiple myeloma: results of the randomized phase III HOVON-65/ GMMG-HD4 trial, *J Clin Oncol* 30:2946–2955, 2012.

Stewart AK, et al: Carfilzomib, lenalidomide, and dexamethasone for relapsed multiple myeloma, *N Engl J Med* 372(2):142–152, 2015.

---

[1]Not FDA approved for this indication.

MYELODYSPLASTIC SYNDROMES

Method of
Jamile M. Shammo, MD

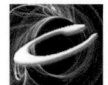

CURRENT DIAGNOSIS

- Myelodysplastic syndromes (MDSs) are diseases of the elderly.
- Chronic unexplained cytopenias should be evaluated to rule out MDS.
- Bone marrow biopsy with cytogenetic testing is necessary to make the diagnosis.
- The International Prognostic Scoring System (IPSS) and the Revised IPSS (IPSS-R) are important tools for risk stratification and choice of therapy.

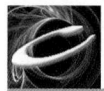

CURRENT THERAPY

- MDSs are broadly divided into two therapeutic categories per the IPSS: low-risk disease (encompassing low and intermediate-1 risk groups), and high-risk disease (encompassing intermediate-2 and high-risk groups).
- The IPSS-R defines five prognostic groups (very low, low, intermediate, high, and very high risk). Treatment options are also dependent on risk category.
- Patients with low-risk disease should receive supportive care and hematopoietic growth factors or luspatercept (Reblozyl); those with the deletion 5q abnormality should be treated with lenalidomide (Revlimid).
- Patients with high-risk disease should be treated with a hypomethylating agent and should be considered for allogeneic stem cell transplantation.

Epidemiology

The MDSs represent a group of heterogeneous clonal stem cell disorders that affect the elderly. The reported annual incidence of approximately 4.4 per 100,000 of the general US population is highest among Caucasians and non-Hispanics. The onset of an MDS before the age of 50 years is rare; the incidence rises with age such that in patients older than 70 years, the incidence exceeds 45 per 100,000 persons. Men are nearly twice as likely to be affected as women (5.8 vs. 3.3 per 100,000 per year).

Risk Factors

De novo or primary MDS refers to cases in which no prior toxic exposure can be documented. Therapy-related MDS, on the other hand, occurs in patients who have previously been treated with either chemotherapy, radiotherapy, or both. Median onset of therapy-related MDS varies with the agents used and usually occurs 2 to 5 years after initial exposure to radiation or chemotherapy.

Tobacco use and occupational exposure to solvents and agricultural chemicals have also been associated with the development of MDS. A minority of MDS cases might have evolved from an antecedent hematologic disorder such as aplastic anemia or paroxysmal nocturnal hemoglobinuria (PNH). Several rare and inherited genetic disorders—such as Fanconi anemia, dyskeratosis congenita, Diamond-Blackfan syndrome, and Shwachman-Diamond syndrome—have been associated with a higher risk of developing MDS.

Pathophysiology

A variety of pathophysiologic processes resulting in ineffective hematopoiesis and peripheral cytopenias have been described in association with MDS. These processes include excessive apoptosis of myeloid progenitors, abnormal responses to cytokines and growth factors, epigenetic aberrations resulting in gene silencing, chromosomal abnormalities, and a defective bone marrow microenvironment. Several somatic point mutations affecting multiple genes have recently been identified in up to 80% of MDS patients. However, the initiating events remain unknown.

Clinical Manifestations

Some patients with MDS are symptom free, but the majority present with peripheral blood cytopenias, of which anemia is the most common. Patients might complain of fatigue, weakness, and exercise intolerance. Those with significant neutropenia and thrombocytopenia can present with infections or bleeding. Systemic symptoms are less common; when present, however, they can herald disease progression to acute leukemia. Similarly, the presence of Sweet syndrome (acute febrile neutrophilic dermatosis) can herald transformation to acute myelogenous leukemia (AML). Organomegaly and lymphadenopathy are uncommon. Infection is the cause of death in approximately 20% to 35% of cases. Transformation to acute leukemia occurs in about 30% of all patients with MDS.

Diagnosis

The diagnosis of MDS can be challenging because its clinical and pathologic characteristics can overlap with those of other disorders such as aplastic anemia, myeloproliferative neoplasms, and acute leukemia.

A thorough history and physical examination should be performed on every patient with one or more peripheral blood cytopenias, along with basic laboratory tests such as iron studies, vitamin B12, and folate levels. However, many disorders can cause pancytopenia; therefore consideration for a hematology referral should be entertained for the evaluation of pancytopenia or persistent otherwise unexplained cytopenias, in which case a bone marrow biopsy may be necessary to identify an etiology.

The diagnosis of MDS requires an evaluation of the peripheral blood smear, a bone marrow biopsy, and aspirate to ascertain the presence of myeloid dysplasia; iron stains, which are necessary for the detection of ring sideroblasts; and cytogenetic studies to detect abnormal clones. Bone marrow dysplasia involving at least 10% of the cells of a specific myeloid lineage is the hallmark of MDS. Conventional karyotyping can detect cytogenetic abnormalities in 50% of patients with de novo MDS and in 95% of patients with therapy-related MDS. The presence of certain cytogenetic abnormalities can aid in making the diagnosis of MDS, particularly when dysplastic features are not prominent. It should be noted that the presence of +8, −Y, or del(20q) is not considered to be MDS-defining in that setting.

Next-generation sequencing (NGS) has recently allowed for the identification of point mutations in the majority of patients with MDS. These mutations involve genes encoding for splicing factors, epigenetic modifiers, and transcription factors, among others. NGS is increasingly utilized in this patient population to assist in making the diagnosis (SF3B1 in MDS-RS) or to provide important prognostic information (TP53 in del 5q MDS).

Differential Diagnosis

MDS should be distinguished from a variety of disorders including megaloblastic anemia, aplastic anemia, large granular lymphocyte leukemia, myelofibrosis, copper deficiency, autoimmune disorders, and HIV infection, which can cause anemia and dysplastic features in the bone marrow. Exposure to certain drugs and toxins can result in marrow dysplasia. These include mycophenolate mofetil (Cellcept), ganciclovir (Cytovene), lead, and excess zinc. Such changes are reversible once the offending agent has been discontinued. The diagnosis of MDS can be made by performing a bone marrow biopsy to detect dysplasia and rule out other disorders that can also cause pancytopenia. Every effort should be made to rule out other reactive causes of dysplasia prior to making a diagnosis of MDS.

Classification and Risk Stratification

Since 1982, there have been various proposals for the classification and risk stratification of MDS. The French-American-British (FAB) classification scheme was the first attempt developed to address the broad range of morphologic features and clinical outcomes in MDS. It identified five subtypes based on morphology and percentage of marrow blasts: refractory anemia (RA), refractory anemia with ringed sideroblasts (RARS), refractory anemia with excess blasts (RAEB), refractory anemia with excess blasts in transformation (RAEB-t), and chronic myelomonocytic leukemia (CMML). This classification allowed MDS to be separated into distinct subsets relative to survival and evolution to acute leukemia.

The World Health Organization (WHO) revised the FAB system to further refine MDS subsets by adding a category of refractory cytopenia with multilineage dysplasia, recognizing 5q-deletion syndrome as a separate clinical and pathologic entity, and lowering the blast percentage from 30% to 20% to diagnose AML. The WHO system was revised in 2008 and again in 2016. The most recent revision eliminated reference to RA and modified the terminology to identify six general MDS categories based on the presence of single- or multilineage dysplasia, ring sideroblasts, blast percentage, and del(5q) (Table 1).

The IPSS was introduced in 1997 to address the variability in prognosis within FAB subtypes. It predicts survival and risk of evolution to acute leukemia. The IPSS is calculated by adding scores assigned to three variables: blast cell count, cytogenetics, and number of cytopenias (Table 2). The IPSS was revised in 2012 (IPSS-R) to incorporate five cytogenetic categories and account for the depth of cytopenias in MDS (Tables 3 and 4). The IPSS and IPSS-R are widely used to predict the prognosis and clinical behavior of patients with various forms of MDS and to guide choice of therapy.

Treatment

A variety of therapeutic options exist for the treatment of MDS patients, spanning the spectrum from supportive care to allogeneic stem cell transplantation. Choice of therapy should take into account the patient's age, comorbidities, and the IPSS/IPSS-R score.

The treating physician should consider the ultimate goal of therapy and whether it is intended to cure, extend survival, or merely palliate symptoms. In the first decade of the 21st century, several novel therapeutic options for MDS emerged. Clinical trials evaluating novel agents are being conducted to help identify effective agents for patients who have relapsed or failed to respond to standard therapies.

Supportive Care

Supportive care has been the cornerstone of MDS therapy for decades; it includes red blood cell transfusion for symptomatic anemia, platelet transfusion to reduce the risk of bleeding or to treat bleeding, and use of hematopoietic growth factors such as erythropoiesis stimulating agents (ESAs) and colony-stimulating factors such as granulocyte colony-stimulating factor (G-CSF), filgrastim (Neupogen)[1], and granulocyte-macrophage colony-stimulating factor (GM-CSF) sargramostim (Leukine)[1]. The last two cytokines have limited efficacy and are not routinely recommended for the treatment of MDS-related neutropenia.

Two ESAs are currently available: a recombinant human erythropoietin (rhu-EPO; epoetin alfa [Epogen, Procrit])[1] and a supersialylated form of EPO (darbepoetin alfa [Aranesp])[1]. These are considered the standard of care for the treatment of anemia in patients with low-risk MDS. A predictive model for response to such treatment has been developed by the Nordic MDS study group to guide patient selection. In general, patients with a serum EPO level less than 500 mU/mL and low transfusion burden are likely to respond by improving their hemoglobin level and reducing their need for transfusions.

---

[1]Not FDA approved for this indication.

TABLE 1 | World Health Organization 2016 Classification of Myelodysplastic Syndromes

NAME	DYSPLASTIC LINES	CYTOPENIAS*	RING SIDEROBLASTS AS % OF MARROW	BM AND PB BLASTS	CYTOGENETICS BY CONVENTIONAL KARYOTYPE ANALYSIS
MDS with single-lineage dysplasia (MDS-SLD)	1	1 or 2	<15% <5% + *SF3B1* mutation	BM <5%, PB <1%, no Auer rods	Any unless patient fulfills all criteria for MDS with isolated del(5q)
MDS with multilineage dysplasia (MDS-MLD)	2 or 3	1–3	<15% <5% + *SF3B1* mutation	BM <5%, PB <1%, no Auer rods	Any unless patient fulfills all criteria for MDS with isolated del(5q)
MDS with ring sideroblasts (MDS-RS)					
MDS-RS with single-lineage dysplasia (MDS-RS-SLD)	1	1 or 2	≥15% ≥5% + *SF3B1* mutation	BM <5%, PB <1%, no Auer rods	Any, unless fulfills all criteria for MDS with isolated del(5q)
MDS-RS with multilineage dysplasia (MDS-RS-MLD)	2 or 3	1–3	≥15% ≥5% + *SF3B1* mutation	BM <5%, PB <1%, no Auer rods	Any, unless fulfills all criteria for MDS with isolated del(5q)
MDS with isolated del(5q)	1–3	1–2	None or any	BM <5%, PB <1%, no Auer rods	del(5q) alone with 1 additional abnormality except –7 or del(7q)
MDS with excess blasts (MDS-EB)					
MDS-EB-1	0–3	1–3	None or any	BM 5%–9% or PB 2%–4%, no Auer rods	Any
MDS-EB-2	0–3	1–3	None or any	BM 10%–19% or PB 5%–19% or Auer rods	Any
MDS, unclassifiable (MDS-U) with 1% blood blasts	1–3	1–3	None or any	BM <5%, PB = 1% (PB blasts must be recorded on at least 2 separate occasions) no Auer rods	Any
MDS with single-lineage dysplasia and pancytopenia	1	3	None or any	BM <5%, PB <1%, no Auer rods	Any
MDS based on defining cytogenetic abnormality	0	1–3	<15%	BM <5%, PB <1%, no Auer rods	MDS-defining abnormality
Refractory cytopenia of childhood	1–3	1–3	None	BM <5%, PB <2%	Any

BM, Bone marrow; *MDS*, myelodysplastic syndrome; *PB*, peripheral blood.
*Cytopenias are defined as Hgb <10 g/dL, pLT <100 x 10⁹/L, and ANC <1.8 x 10⁹/L.

TABLE 2 | International Prognostic Scoring System for Myelodysplastic Syndromes

PROGNOSTIC VARIABLE	SCORE VALUE				
	0	0.5	1.0	1.5	2.0
Marrow blasts (%)	<5	5–10	11–20	—	21–30
Karyotype*	Good	Intermediate		Poor	
Cytopenia†	0/1	2/3			

*Cytogenetics: Good = normal, –Y alone, del(5q) alone, del(20q) alone; Poor = complex (≥3 abnormalities) or chromosome 7 anomalies; Intermediate = other abnormalities. This excludes karyotypes t(8;21), inv16, and t(15;17), which are considered to be AML, not MDS.
†Cytopenias: neutrophil count <1800/μL, platelets <100,000/μL, Hb <10 g/dL.

TABLE 3	Survival and Progression by International Prognostic Scoring System Risk Category				
RISK CATEGORY	% IPSS POP.	OVERALL SCORE	MEDIAN SURVIVAL (Y) IN THE ABSENCE OF THERAPY	25% AML PROGRESSION (Y) IN THE ABSENCE OF THERAPY	
Low	33	0	5.7	9.4	
Intermediate 1	38	0.5–1.0	3.5	3.3	
Intermediate 2	22	1.5–2.0	1.2	1.1	
High	7	≥2.5	0.4	0.2	

AML, Acute myelogenous leukemia; *IPSS,* International Prognostic Scoring System.

TABLE 4	The Risk Score International Prognostic Scoring System–Revised						
PROGNOSTIC VARIABLE	0	0.5	1	1.5	2	3	4
Cytogenetics	Very good	—	Good	—	Intermediate	Poor	Very poor
Blasts BM, %	≤2	—	2%–5%	—	5%–10%	>10%	—
Hb	≥10	—	8–10	<8	—	—	—
Platelets	≥100	50–100	<50	—	—	—	—
Neutrophils	≥0.8	<0.8	–	—	—	—	—

INTERNATIONAL PROGNOSTIC SCORING SYSTEM-REVISED PROGNOSTIC RISK CATEGORIES/SCORE

RISK GROUPS	RISK SCORE
Very low	≤1.5
Low	>1.5–3
Intermediate	>3–4.5
High	>4.5–6
Very high	>6

CYTOGENETIC RISK GROUPS

PROGNOSTIC SUBGROUP	CYTOGENETIC ABERRATION	MEDIAN SURVIVAL, YEARS	MEDIAN AML—EVOLUTION 25%, YEARS
Very good	–Y, del(11q)	5.4	NR
Good	Normal, del (5q), del (12p), del (20q), double including del (5q)	4.8	9.4
Intermediate	del (7q), +8, +19, il7q, any other single or double independent clones	2.7	2.5
Poor	–7, lnv(3)/1(3q)/del(3q), doublet including –7/del(7q), complex: 3 abnormalities	1.5	1.7
Very poor	Complex: >3 abnormalities	0.7	0.7

AML, Acute myelogenous leukemia.
From Greenberg PL, Tuechler H, Schanz J, et al. Revised International Prognostic Scoring System (IPSS-R) for myelodysplastic syndromes, *Blood* 120:2454–2465, 2012.

Thrombopoietin agonists such as romiplostim (N-Plate)[1] and eltrombopag (Promacta)[1] are in clinical trials to evaluate their safety and efficacy in low-risk MDS patients with thrombocytopenia.

Immunomodulatory Drugs

The novel class of immunomodulatory drugs includes thalidomide (Thalomid)[1] and lenalidomide (Revlimid). Thalidomide was investigated initially with some success in patients with low-risk disease. However, its use was compromised because of poor tolerability. Lenalidomide has been approved for the treatment of patients with low-risk MDS who harbor deletion 5q cytogenetic abnormality because it was shown in clinical trials to result in transfusion independence in about two-thirds of such patients.

Luspatercept (Reblozyl)

A recombinant fusion protein that acts as a ligand trap for TGF-B super family has shown positive results in early phase trials in ameliorating anemia in transfusion-dependent MDS patients. The

Pivotal MEDALIST trial was a randomized, double-blind, placebo-controlled trial that evaluated the efficacy of luspatercept as defined by the proportion of patients who achieved red blood cell (RBC) transfusion independence during any consecutive 8-week period between weeks 1 and 24 of therapy and enrolled 229 transfusion-dependent patients with low-risk MDS with ring sideroblasts who were randomized at 2:1 to either luspatercept or placebo. The trial demonstrated that 37.9% of those who were randomized to luspatercept achieved the primary efficacy endpoint compared with 13.2% who received placebo (*P* <.0001). Subsequently, the drug was approved by the FDA on April 3, 2020, for the treatment of anemia in transfusion-dependent patients with MDS with ring sideroblasts (MDS-RS), and MDS-RS-T.

Hypomethylating Agents

Two parenteral hypomethylating agents are currently approved for the treatment of MDS: 5-azacitidine (Vidaza) and decitabine (Dacogen). These agents are cytosine analogues known to inhibit and deplete DNA methyltransferase, which adds a methyl group to cytosine residues in newly formed DNA, resulting in the formation of a hypomethylated DNA in vitro. The exact mechanism of action in vivo has not yet been identified. Results of randomized clinical trials comparing these agents to best supportive care in patients with MDS have demonstrated a statistically significant improvement in response rate and hematologic improvement. It has been shown for the first time that treatment with 5-azacitidine was reported to result in prolongation of survival in patients with Int-2 and high-risk disease. Both drugs have myelosuppressive properties and comparable response rates.

More recently, in 2020, an oral hypomethylating agent (Inqovi) combining decitabine and cedazuridine was approved by the FDA for MDS.

Immunosuppressive Therapy

Immunosuppressive therapy with antithymocyte globulin (Thymoglobulin)[1] or cyclosporine (Neoral)[1] or both was evaluated in several clinical trials and was shown to result in durable hematologic responses in a subset of MDS patients—specifically, younger patients with low-risk disease, hypocellular marrows, PNH clone, human leukocyte antigen (HLA)-DR 15 phenotype, and low transfusion need.

Hematopoietic Stem Cell Transplantation

Allogeneic stem cell transplantation is the only curative therapy for MDS patients; this option is feasible for a small subset: typically younger patients with good performance status and an available HLA-matched donor. Approximately 40% of patients can be cured with this modality. The recent introduction of reduced-intensity conditioning regimens and nonmyeloablative transplants has resulted in expanding the age limit for performing the procedure, thus reducing transplant-related complications and mortality. However, it has been associated with a higher risk of relapse. Because stem cell transplantation is associated with a high rate of treatment-related death—estimated at 39% at 1 year—and the development of acute and chronic graft versus host disease, such treatment is recommended only to patients with high-risk disease. Patients with low-risk MDS may be considered for transplant at disease progression.

Conclusion and Future Direction

MDS is a chronic disease characterized by features reminiscent of bone marrow failure states with a variable propensity for leukemic evolution. It is curable only by allogeneic stem cell transplantation, which is feasible in only a small subset of patients. For all others, the treatment goal is aimed at improving quality of life and prolonging survival. A variety of ongoing clinical trials are evaluating novel agents and combinations of drugs to further optimize the outcome of patients with this disease. Meanwhile, a great deal of research is focused on understanding the molecular underpinning of this heterogeneous disorder so as to enhance our understanding of its biology.

References

Arber DA, Orazi A, Hasserjian R, et al: The 2016 revision to the World Health Organization (WHO) classification of myeloid neoplasms and acute leukemia, *Blood* 127:2391–2405, 2016.

Bejar R, Stevenson K, Abdel-Wahab O, et al: Clinical effect of point mutations in myelodysplastic syndromes, *NEJM* 364:2496–2506, 2011.

Bennett JM, Catovsky D, Daniel MT, et al: Proposals for the classification of the myelodysplastic syndromes, *Br J Haematol* 51:189–199, 1982.

Brunning RD, Porwit A, Orazi A, et al: Myelodysplastic syndromes/neoplasms. In Swerdlow S, Campo E, Lee Harris N, et al: *WHO Classification of Tumors of Hematopoietic and Lymphoid Tissues*, 4th ed, Lyon, France, 2008, IARC, pp 88–103.

Cutler CS, Lee SJ, Greenberg P, et al: A decision analysis of allogeneic bone marrow transplantation for the myelodysplastic syndromes: Delayed transplantation for low-risk myelodysplasia is associated with improved outcome, *Blood* 104(2):579–585, 2004.

Fenaux P, Mufti GJ, Hellstrom-Lindberg E, et al: Efficacy of azacitidine compared with that of conventional care regimens in the treatment of higher-risk myelodysplastic syndromes: A randomized, open-label, phase III study, *Lancet Oncol* 10:223–232, 2009.

Fenaux P, Platzbecker U, Mufti GJ, et al: Luspatercept in patients with lower-risk myelodysplastic syndromes, *N Engl J Med* 382:140–151, 2020.

Godley LA, Larson RA: Therapy-related myeloid leukemia, *Semin Oncol* 35:418–429, 2008.

Greenberg PL: The smoldering myeloid leukemic states: Clinical and biologic features, *Blood* 61:1035–1044, 1983.

Greenberg PL, Cox C, LeBeau MM, et al: International scoring system for evaluating prognosis in myelodysplastic syndromes, *Blood* 89:2079–2088, 1997.

Greenberg PL, Tuechler H, Schanz J, et al: Revised International Prognostic Scoring System (IPSS-R) for myelodysplastic syndromes, *Blood* 120:2454–2465, 2012.

Hellstrom-Lindberg E, Negrin R, Stein R, et al: Erythroid response to treatment with G-CSF plus erythropoietin for the anaemia of patients with myelodysplastic syndromes: Proposal for a predictive model, *Br J Haematol* 99(2):344–351, 1997.

Kantarjian H, Issa JP, Rosenfeld CS, et al: Decitabine improves patient outcomes in myelodysplastic syndromes: Results of a phase III randomized study, *Cancer* 106(8):1794–1803, 2006.

List A, Dewald G, Bennett J, et al: Lenalidomide in the myelodysplastic syndrome with chromosome 5q deletion, *N Engl J Med* 355(14):1456–1465, 2006.

Ma X, Does M, Raza A, Mayne ST: Myelodysplastic syndromes: Incidence and survival in the United States, *Cancer* 109(8):1536–1542, 2007.

Martino R, Iacobelli S, Brand R, et al: Retrospective comparison of reduced-intensity conditioning and conventional high- dose conditioning for allogeneic hematopoietic stem cell transplantation using HLA-identical sibling donors in myelodysplastic syndromes, *Blood* 108:836–846, 2006.

Molldrem J, Leifer E, Bahceci E, et al: Antithymocyte globulin for treatment of the bone marrow failure associated with myelodysplastic syndromes, *Ann Intern Med* 137(3):156–163, 2002.

Nisse C, Lorthois C, Dorp V, et al: Exposure to occupational and environmental factors in myelodysplastic syndromes: Preliminary results of a case-control study, *Leukemia* 9:693–699, 1995.

Owen C, Barnett M, Fitzgibbon J: Familial myelodysplasia and acute myeloid leukaemia—a review, *Br J Haematol* 140:123–132, 2008.

Rollison DE, Howlader N, Smith MT, et al: Epidemiology of myelodysplastic syndromes and chronic myeloproliferative disorders in the United States, 2001–2004 using data from the NAACCR and SEER programs, *Blood* 112:45–52, 2008.

Silverman LR, Demakos EP, Peterson BL, et al: Randomized controlled trial of azacitidine in patients with the myelodysplastic syndrome: A study of the Cancer and Leukemia Group B, *J Clin Oncol* 20(10):2429–2440, 2002.

Soppi E, Nousiainen T, Seppa A, Lahtinen R: Acute febrile neutrophilic dermatosis (Sweet's syndrome) in association with myelodysplastic syndromes: A report of three cases and a review of the literature, *Br J Haematol* 73(1):43–47, 1989.

Tefferi A, Vardiman JW: Myelodysplastic syndromes, *N Engl J Med* 361(19):1872–1885, 2009.

Vardiman JW, Harris NL, Brunning RD: The World Health Organization (WHO) classification of myeloid neoplasms, *Blood* 100:2292–2302, 2002.

NON-HODGKIN LYMPHOMA

Method of
Kevin A. David, MD; and Andrew M. Evens, DO, Msc

CURRENT DIAGNOSIS

- The etiology of non-Hodgkin lymphoma (NHL) is not known, although several risk factors and conditions are associated with an increased risk of developing lymphoma, including congenital immunosuppression conditions (ataxia-telangiectasia, Wiskott-Aldrich syndrome, and X-linked lymphoproliferative syndrome), acquired immunodeficiency states (e.g., human immunodeficiency virus [HIV] and after solid organ transplantation), viruses (e.g., human T-lymphotropic virus [HTLV]-1 and hepatitis C virus [HCV]), and autoimmune disorders (e.g., Sjögren syndrome, celiac sprue, and systemic lupus erythematosus).

- Patients most commonly present clinically with enlarged, painless lymph nodes, splenomegaly, and bone marrow involvement, but they may also present with other extranodal disease sites (e.g., stomach, skin, liver, bone, brain).

- NHL has many different clinicopathologic subtypes—more than 65 types are included in the World Health Organization (WHO) classification of lymphoid neoplasms. The natural history and prognosis of these vary greatly from indolent and slow-growing types (over many years) to highly aggressive (within weeks) types.

Excisional lymph node biopsy is the gold standard procedure in establishing the precise NHL histology. Expert hematopathology review incorporating morphologic, immunophenotypic, and genetic features is essential for an accurate diagnosis.

- Indolent lymphomas are low-grade and represent slow-growing NHL that may remain stable with low tumor burden, not warranting therapy for several years. The disease is highly responsive to treatment with a variety of treatment options (remission rates exceeding 90% with combined rituximab (Rituxan)/chemotherapy), although the clinical course is characterized by repetitive relapses. Outside of early-stage disease and therapy with allogeneic stem cell transplantation, low-grade NHLs are not curable.
- Transformation of follicular lymphoma to a high-grade NHL occurs in 2% to 3% of patients each year; it is less common in other indolent subtypes. Transformation is typically heralded by an aggressive change in the patient's clinical condition.
- Diffuse large B-cell lymphoma (DLBCL), the most common aggressive NHL, is curable in all stages in a majority of patients with rituximab (Rituxan)-based chemotherapy. A variety of primary extranodal DLBCL clinical subtypes warrant specialized therapy, such as primary central nervous system (CNS) lymphoma and testicular lymphoma.
- Long-term survivors are at increased risk for second cancers. The highest relative risk of developing a secondary malignancy occurs more than 21 to 30 years after original diagnosis. Patients who received an anthracycline (e.g., doxorubicin [Adriamycin]) as part of therapy are at a long-term increased risk for cardiovascular disease.

The term *malignant lymphoma* was originally introduced by Billroth in 1871 to describe neoplasms of lymphoid tissue. Generally speaking, lymphomas are neoplasms of the immune system. Traditionally, lymphomas are divided into Hodgkin lymphoma (HL) and non-Hodgkin lymphoma (NHL).

There are many different clinicopathologic subtypes of NHL (>60). By cell of origin, the majority of NHLs are of B-cell origin (85%–90%); T-cell NHLs account for 10% to 15% of lymphomas in the United States, whereas natural killer cell or histiocytic lymphomas are rare (<1%). The NHL subtypes for lymphoid, histiocytic, and dendritic neoplasms as classified by the WHO were updated in 2016.

NHLs manifest most commonly clinically with involvement of lymph nodes, spleen, and bone marrow, but they can involve other extranodal sites (stomach, skin, liver, bone, brain, etc.). Peripheral blood involvement uncommonly occurs (leukemic phase of lymphoma). The natural history and prognosis vary greatly among the different subtypes of NHL, from indolent subtypes that are often slow-growing (i.e., therapy not warranted for years) to very aggressive and rapidly fatal types (within weeks) if not treated. Most NHL subtypes are highly treatable with initial remission rates greater than 90% using combined rituximab (Rituxan)/chemotherapy; however, indolent NHLs are generally incurable, whereas the goal of treating most aggressive NHLs is cure.

Epidemiology

Currently, NHL represents approximately 5% of all cancer diagnoses, being the seventh most common cancer in women and men. Estimates from the American Cancer Society indicate that in 2021 approximately 90,000 new cases of NHL will be diagnosed in the United States and approximately 22,000 people will die of the disease. In addition, there are approximately 900,000 people living with NHL in the United States.

Geographic Distribution

The incidence of NHL varies throughout the world, in general being more common in developed countries, with rates in the United States of more than 15 per 100,000 compared with 1.2 per 100,000 in China. In the United States the incidence rates of NHL more than doubled between 1975 and 1995, representing one of the largest increases of any cancer. The increases have been more pronounced in White populations, males, older adults, and those with NHL diagnosed at extranodal sites. Similar findings have been reported in other developed countries. The incidence rates of NHL began to stabilize in the late 1990s, although the temporal trends vary by histologic subtype, as well as by race and sex (Figure 1). Some of the increase may be related to improved diagnostic techniques and access to medical care and the increased risk of NHL attributable to human immunodeficiency virus (HIV) infection. However, additional factors are likely responsible for this unexpected increase in incidence.

Age

Overall, NHL incidence rises exponentially with increasing age. In persons older than 65 years, the incidence is 90.9 per 100,000 population compared with 7.1 per 100,000 population for persons aged 20 to 49 years. Except for high-grade lymphoblastic and Burkitt lymphomas (the most common types of NHL seen in children and young adults), the median age at presentation for most subtypes of NHL exceeds 60 years.

Race and Ethnicity

Incidence varies by race and ethnicity, with White people overall having a higher risk than Black people and Asians (incidence rates increased 50%–60% in White people compared with Black people). Most NHL subtypes are more common in White people than in Black people; however, peripheral T-cell lymphoma (PTCL), mycosis fungoides, and Sézary syndrome occur more often in Black people than in White people.

Etiology and Risk Factors
Chromosomal Translocations and Molecular Rearrangements

Nonrandom chromosomal and molecular rearrangements play an important role in the pathogenesis of many lymphomas and often correlate with histology and immunophenotype. These chromosomal changes often result in oncogenic gene products; for example, t(11;14)(q13;q32) translocation results in overexpression of *bcl-1* (cyclin D1) in mantle cell lymphoma (MCL), whereas translocation with 8q24 leads to c-*myc* overexpression in nearly all Burkitt lymphomas and in 10% to 15% of patients with diffuse large B-cell lymphoma (DLBCL). Research to discover more information regarding the prognostic and pathogenic importance of these oncogenes continues, although they are currently used primarily in clinical practice for diagnostic purposes. In addition, these genes serve as potential targets for novel therapeutics.

Environmental Factors

Environmental factors may also play a role in the development of NHL, including particular occupations (e.g., chemists, painters, mechanics, machinists) and chemicals (solvents and pesticides). Patients who receive chemotherapy or radiation therapy for any indication are also at increased risk for developing NHL as a secondary cancer as discussed later.

Viruses

Several viruses have been implicated in the pathogenesis of NHL, including Epstein-Barr virus, human T-lymphotropic virus (HTLV-1), Kaposi sarcoma–associated herpesvirus (KSHV, also known as human herpesvirus 8 [HHV-8]), and hepatitis C virus (HCV). Meta-analyses have shown 13% to 15% seroprevalence of HCV in certain geographic regions among persons with B-cell NHL. Furthermore, HCV infection is associated with the development of clonal B-cell expansions and certain subtypes of NHL, particularly in the setting of essential (type II) mixed cryoglobulinemia. HTLV-1 is a human retrovirus that establishes a latent infection through reverse transcription in activated T-helper cells. A minority (5%) of carriers will develop adult T-cell leukemia lymphoma. KSHV-like DNA sequences are often detected in primary effusion lymphomas in patients with HIV infection and in those with multicentric (plasma cell variant) Castleman disease.

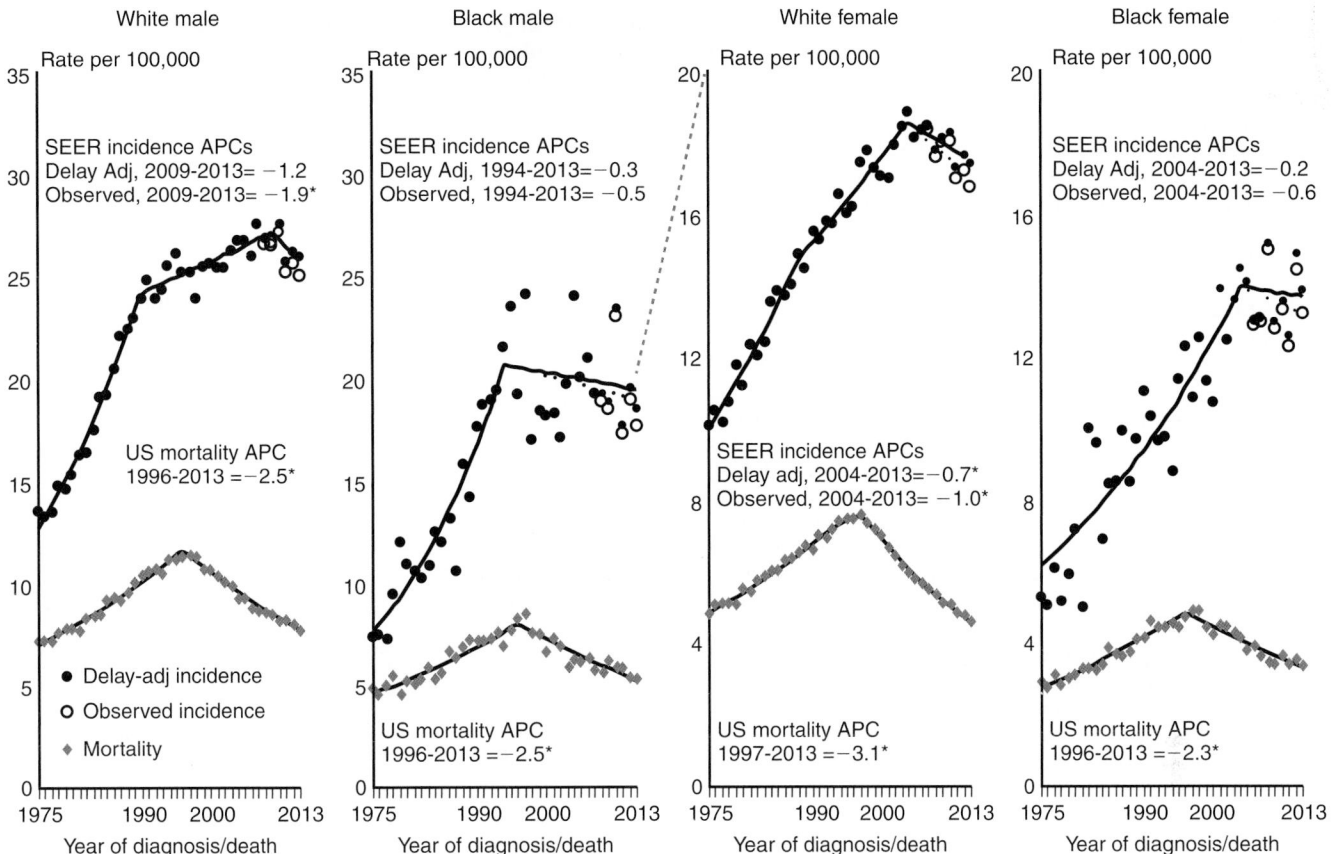

White male	Black male	White female	Black female
Rate per 100,000	Rate per 100,000	Rate per 100,000	Rate per 100,000

SEER incidence APCs
Delay Adj, 2009-2013= −1.2
Observed, 2009-2013= −1.9*

SEER incidence APCs
Delay Adj, 1994-2013=−0.3
Observed, 1994-2013= −0.5

SEER incidence APCs
Delay Adj, 2004-2013=−0.2
Observed, 2004-2013= −0.6

US mortality APC
1996-2013 =−2.5*

SEER incidence APCs
Delay adj, 2004-2013=−0.7*
Observed, 2004-2013= −1.0*

- Delay-adj incidence
○ Observed incidence
♦ Mortality

US mortality APC
1996-2013 =−2.5*

US mortality APC
1997-2013 =−3.1*

US mortality APC
1996-2013 =−2.3*

Year of diagnosis/death (×4)

Source: SEER 9 areas and US mortality files (National Center for Health Statistics, CDC).
aRates are age-adjusted to the 2000 US Std population (19 age groups - census P25-1103).
Regression lines and APCs are calculated using the joinpoint regression program version 4.3.0.0. April 2016, National cancer institute.
The APC is the annual percent change for the regression line segments. The APC shown on the graph is for the most recent trend.
*The APC is significantly different from zero P < .05.

Figure 1 Surveillance, epidemiology, and end results (SEER) observed incidence, SEER delay adjusted incidence, and US death rates for non-Hodgkin lymphoma, by race and sex.

Bacterial Infections

Gastric mucosa-associated lymphoid tissue (MALT) lymphoma is seen most often, but not exclusively, in association with *Helicobacter pylori* infection. Infection with *Borrelia burgdorferi* has been detected in approximately 35% of patients with primary cutaneous B-cell lymphoma in Scotland. Studies indicate that *Campylobacter jejuni* and immunoproliferative small intestinal disease are related. European reports have noted an association between infection with *Chlamydia psittaci* and ocular adnexal lymphoma. The infection was found to be highly specific and does not reflect a subclinical infection among the general population. Furthermore, remission of NHL to antibiotics has been reported. Attempts to confirm this association in the Western hemisphere have been unsuccessful.

Immunodeficiency

Patients with congenital conditions of immunosuppression are at increased risk of NHL. These conditions include ataxia-telangiectasia; Wiskott-Aldrich syndrome; X-linked lymphoproliferative syndrome; severe combined immunodeficiency; acquired immunodeficiency states, such as HIV infection; and iatrogenic immunosuppression. Relative risk of NHL is increased 150- to 250-fold among patients with acquired immunodeficiency syndrome (AIDS); patients usually develop high-grade NHLs, such as Burkitt lymphoma or DLBCL. The incidence of posttransplantation lymphoproliferative disorders (PTLDs) after solid organ transplantation ranges from 1% to 3% in kidney transplant recipients to 10% to 12% in heart and multiorgan transplant recipients, the latter who require more potent immunosuppressive therapy.

Autoimmunity

An increased incidence of gastrointestinal lymphomas is seen in patients with celiac (nontropical) sprue and inflammatory bowel disease, particularly Crohn disease. An aberrant clonal intraepithelial T-cell population can be found in up to 75% of patients with refractory celiac sprue before overt T-cell lymphoma develops. Sjögren disease is associated with a sixfold increased risk of NHL overall, with risk varying in part on severity of disease (5–200 times); moreover, the risk specifically of parotid marginal zone lymphoma is increased 1000-fold. In addition, systemic lupus erythematosus and rheumatoid arthritis have been associated with a slightly increased risk of B-cell lymphoma.

Genetic Susceptibility

Several studies have implicated a role for genetic variants in the risk of NHL, including genes that influence DNA integrity and methylation, genes that alter B-cell survival and growth, and genes that involve innate immunity, oxidative stress, and xenobiotic metabolism.

Signs and Symptoms

Fever, weight loss, and night sweats, referred to as B symptoms, are more common in advanced and aggressive subtype NHLs, but they may be present at all stages and in any histologic subtype.

Low-Grade or Indolent Lymphomas

Painless, slowly progressive peripheral adenopathy is the most common clinical presentation in patients with low-grade lymphomas. Patients sometimes report a history of waxing and waning adenopathy before seeking medical attention. Spontaneous regression of enlarged lymph nodes can occur, which may cause a low-grade lymphoma to be confused with an infectious condition. Primary extranodal involvement and B symptoms are uncommon at presentation; however, both are more common in advanced or end-stage disease and in particular indolent NHL subtypes (e.g., gastric MALT and nongastric extranodal MALT). Bone marrow is frequently involved, sometimes in association with cytopenias. Splenomegaly is seen in approximately 40% of patients, but the spleen is rarely the only involved site besides the specific subtype of splenic marginal zone lymphoma.

High-Grade or Aggressive Lymphomas

The clinical presentation of high-grade lymphomas is more varied. Although the majority of patients present with adenopathy, more than one-third present with extranodal involvement alone or with adenopathy, the most common sites being the gastrointestinal tract (including Waldeyer ring), skin, bone marrow, sinuses, genitourinary tract, bone, and central nervous system (CNS). B symptoms are more common, occurring in approximately 30% to 40% of patients. Lymphoblastic lymphoma often manifests with an anterior mediastinal mass, superior vena cava syndrome, and leptomeningeal disease. American patients with Burkitt lymphoma often present with a large abdominal mass and symptoms of bowel obstruction. In addition, certain histologic NHL subtypes manifest with symptoms unique to that particular lymphoma subtype; for example, angioimmunoblastic T-cell lymphoma (AITL) in addition to lymphadenopathy presents with disease features including organomegaly, skin rash, pleural effusions, arthritis, eosinophilia, and varied immunologic abnormalities such as positive Coombs test, cold agglutinins, hemolytic anemia, antinuclear antibodies, and polyclonal hypergammaglobulinemia.

Screening

No effective methods are currently available for screening patients or populations for NHL.

Diagnosis

A definitive diagnosis can be made only by biopsy of pathologic lymph nodes or tumor tissue. It is critical in most cases to perform an *excisional* lymph node resection to avoid false-negative results and inaccurate histologic classification; fine-needle aspirations or core biopsies are often insufficient for diagnostic purposes. When clinical circumstances make surgical biopsy of involved lymph nodes or extranodal sites prohibitive, a core biopsy obtained under computed tomography (CT) or ultrasonographic guidance may suffice, but it often requires the integration of histologic examination and immunophenotypic and molecular studies for accurate diagnosis. A formal review by an expert hematopathologist is mandatory. In addition to morphologic review and immunostaining of tissue, other studies such as detailed cellular immunophenotyping and genotyping for relevant oncogenes are often needed to complete the diagnosis.

In addition to a detailed history and physical examination, baseline staging studies are warranted. These consist of blood tests (complete blood count with differential, complete metabolic panel including liver function tests, and lactate dehydrogenase [LDH]); CT of chest, abdomen, and pelvis; and bone marrow biopsy and aspirate (Box 1). For aggressive NHL histologies, functional imaging is advocated (i.e., fluorodeoxyglucose [18F] positron emission tomography [FDG-PET]), as is assessment of ejection fraction in anticipation of anthracycline-based chemotherapy. Testing for history of hepatitis B virus (HBV) is recommended, especially before starting anti-CD20 antibody therapy; evidence suggests that anti-CD20 antibody therapy (e.g., rituximab [Rituxan]) increases the risk of HBV reactivation above the known rate of chemotherapy-associated reactivation. HIV serology should be obtained in patients with relevant risk factors, especially for DLBCL and Burkitt lymphoma. HTLV-1 serology is recommended in patients who present with cutaneous T-cell lymphoma lesions, especially if they have hypercalcemia.

BOX 1 | Initial Assessment and Workup for Non-Hodgkin Lymphoma

- Excisional tissue biopsy
- Detailed history and physical examination
- CBC with differential, metabolic panel (including liver function), and LDH
- CT scans (chest, abdomen, pelvis)
- Nuclear functional imaging (i.e., FDG-PET)*
- Bone marrow biopsy and aspirate
- Heart function (e.g., MUGA) if anthracycline therapy anticipated
- EGD, colonoscopy, or both†
- HIV and HBV testing (with risk factors and/or if monoclonal antibody therapy planned)
- Consider TB testing (i.e., PPD with energy panel) with history of exposure
- Assessment of CSF (when applicable or with risk factors)‡
- Consider early institution of TLS prophylaxis (e.g., intravenous fluids, allopurinol [Zyloprim])*,†,‡

CBC, Complete blood count; *CSF*, cerebrospinal fluid; *CT*, computed tomography; *EGD*, esophagogastroduodenoscopy; *FDG-PET*, fluorodeoxyglucose (18F) positron emission tomography; *HBV*, hepatitis B virus; *HIV*, human immunodeficiency virus; *LDH*, lactate dehydrogenase; *MCL*, mantle cell lymphoma; *MUGA*, multigated acquisition [scan]; *NHL*, non-Hodgkin lymphoma; *PPD*, purified protein derivative [tuberculosis test]; *TB*, tuberculosis; *TLS*, tumor lysis syndrome.
*Primarily for aggressive NHL subtypes.
†With clinical suspicion of involvement; EGD for NHL head and neck involvement (e.g., tonsil, base of tongue, nasopharynx), and consider colonoscopy for MCL (if symptomatic).
‡Consider for aggressive histologies with less than 1 extranodal site and elevated LDH and for particular unique lymphoma locations (e.g., testicular, sinus, breast, adrenal, paraspinal).

Examination of cerebrospinal fluid and consideration of intrathecal chemotherapy prophylaxis or integration of intravenous high-dose methotrexate are applicable for patients with DLBCL with bone marrow, epidural, testicular, paranasal sinus, breast, or multiple extranodal sites (especially when in conjunction with elevated LDH). Testing is mandatory for high-grade lymphoblastic lymphoma and Burkitt lymphoma and its variants and primary CNS lymphoma if there is no evidence of increased intracranial pressure. Upper gastrointestinal endoscopy or gastrointestinal series with small bowel follow-through is recommended in patients with head and neck involvement (tonsil, base of tongue, nasopharynx) and those with primary gastrointestinal disease. MCL is associated with a high incidence of occult gastrointestinal involvement. In addition, magnetic resonance imaging (MRI) of the complete craniospinal axis and ocular examination is advocated with any brain or leptomeningeal disease involvement to rule out multifocal disease.

Classification

The 1965 Rappaport Classification of malignant lymphomas was based solely on architecture and cytology. Since then, with the help of advanced cellular and genetic technologies, numerous new unique NHL entities have emerged. The WHO classification was revised in 2016, which continues to emphasize immunophenotyping, genotyping, and clinical features. Another way to group the many different lymphoma histologies is by clinical presentation and prognosis (Table 1).

Prognosis

International Prognostic Index

The International Prognostic Index (IPI) was developed as a prognostic factor model for aggressive NHLs treated with doxorubicin (Adriamycin)-containing regimens (Box 2). In the pre-rituximab (Rituxan) era, persons with no risk factors or one risk factor had a predicted 5-year overall survival (OS) rate of 73%, compared with 26% for high-risk patients with four or five risk factors.

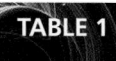

LYMPHOMA TYPE	PERCENTAGE OF ALL NON-HODGKIN LYMPHOMAS
Indolent or Low-Grade Non-Hodgkin Lymphomas	
Follicular lymphoma	20–25
Small lymphocytic lymphoma	7
MALT-type marginal zone lymphoma	7
Nodal-type marginal zone lymphoma	<2
Lymphoplasmacytic lymphoma	<2
Aggressive or High-Grade Non-Hodgkin Lymphomas	
Diffuse large B-cell lymphoma	30–35
T-cell lymphomas: peripheral or systemic (multiple subtypes)	10–12
Mantle cell lymphoma	6
Lymphoblastic lymphoma	<2
Burkitt lymphoma	<1

TABLE 1 Clinical Prognostic Classification of Adult Immunocompetent Non-Hodgkin Lymphomas

Subtypes are listed in order of most to least common.
MALT, Mucosa-associated lymphoid tissue.

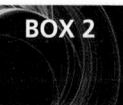

BOX 2 Enhanced International Prognostic Index Risk Factors and Associated Approximate Cure Rates for Diffuse Large B-Cell Lymphoma

Factors/Scoring
- Age, years
- >40 to ≤60: 1
- >60 to ≤75: 2
- >75: 3
- Lactate dehydrogenase (LDH), normalized
- >1 to ≤3: 1
- >3: 2
- Ann Arbor stage III–IV: 1
- Extranodal disease*: 1
- Performance status ≥2: 1
- Five-Year Progression-Free Survival Rates Based on Score at DiagnosisScore 0–1: 91%
- Score 2–3: 74%
- Score 4–5: 51%
- Score ≥6: 30%

*Disease in bone marrow, central nervous system, liver/GI tract, or lung.

In the postrituximab era, the survival rates have improved (see Box 2). A variant of the IPI is also useful in predicting outcome in patients with follicular low-grade lymphoma (FLIPI), MCL (MIPI), and most recently in Burkitt lymphoma.

Molecular Profiling

DNA microarray technology for gene expression profiling has identified distinct prognostic subgroups in many NHL subtypes including DLBCL and follicular NHL. Patients with germinal center B-like DLBCL have an improved OS compared with other molecular profiles. Studies in follicular NHL have identified gene expression signatures that also predicted survival. Interestingly, the genes that defined the prognostic signatures were not expressed in the tumor cells but were expressed by the nonmalignant tumor-infiltrating cells—primarily T cells, macrophages, and dendritic cells.

Treatment

The therapeutic approach for NHL differs for each clinicopathologic subtype. Chemotherapy remains an important modality. However, in some instances, radiation therapy or, rarely, surgical resection plays a role. Biologic approaches, including monoclonal antibodies and antibody-drug conjugates, have shown significant activity and are currently incorporated into many treatment paradigms. In addition, other novel therapeutics targeting the cell surface of lymphoma cells or varied transcription factors continue to be incorporated into treatment paradigms. Autologous and allogeneic stem cell transplantation are mostly reserved for patients with recurrent or refractory disease, although there are some subtypes in which consolidative autologous transplantation after frontline therapy is considered (e.g., MCL and PTCLs).

Indolent B-Cell Non-Hodgkin Lymphomas

Indolent lymphomas are low-grade and represent slow-growing NHLs that may be stable with low tumor burden that may not warrant therapy for several years. The disease is responsive to treatment (remission rates greater than 90% with combined rituximab/chemotherapy), although the clinical course is characterized by repetitive relapses. Outside of early-stage disease and therapy with an allogeneic stem cell transplant, low-grade NHLs are not curable. The median survival of patients with advanced-stage follicular lymphoma in the prerituximab era was 9 to 10 years, although that is currently significantly longer (≈16–18 years). Transformation to a high-grade NHL occurs in 2% to 3% of patients each year with follicular lymphoma (less common in other indolent subtypes) and is typically heralded by an aggressive change in the patient's clinical condition (e.g., B symptoms, rapidly rising LDH).

General Principles

Only a minority of patients present with early-stage disease (i.e., stage I or II). Low-dose involved field radiotherapy is a valid treatment option for these patients (especially stage I without central sites of disease), and associated 20-year disease-free survival rates are greater than 50%. Treatment for patients with advanced-stage disease ranges from observation (i.e., watchful waiting) to anti-CD20 monoclonal antibody therapy (rituximab [Rituxan] or obinutuzumab [Gazyva]) with or without chemotherapy. Treatment choice depends in part on tumor burden and the patient's individual disease characteristics and baseline functional status. Treatment with frontline anti-CD20 monoclonal antibody with chemotherapy (outpatient therapy given once every 3–4 weeks typically for 6–8 cycles) followed by 2 years of maintenance therapy with anti-CD20 monoclonal antibody for patients with high tumor burden is associated with median progression-free survival (PFS) rates of approximately 9 to 10 years.

Treatment options for relapsed indolent lymphoma include repeating rituximab with or without a different chemotherapy regimen, radioimmunotherapy, oral lenalidomide (Revlimid) immunomodulatory therapy, or stem cell transplantation. There is a small subset of follicular lymphoma patients who experience early progression to first line therapy (i.e., within 2 years), and survival rates are significantly inferior with conventional therapies. Autologous stem cell transplantation is an option for patients with relapsed disease, especially early progressors, although an improvement in OS is debated. Allogeneic stem cell transplantation is a potential curative modality for patients with relapsed or refractory disease, although patient selection is critical owing to potential morbidity and mortality related to this therapeutic option.

Special Considerations

Localized gastric MALT lymphoma cases often may be managed with therapy for *H. pylori* infection; radiation is typically reserved for failure to eradicate *H. pylori*. Patients with lymphoplasmacytic lymphoma (Waldenström macroglobulinemia) can present clinically with hyperviscosity or cryoglobulinemia, which may be managed acutely with plasmapheresis, but ultimately systemic therapy similar to that for other indolent NHLs is warranted. More recently, the Bruton tyrosine kinase (BTK) inhibitor, ibrutinib (Imbruvica), was approved by the US Food and Drug Administration (FDA) for the treatment of relapsed or refractory marginal zone lymphoma patients who require systemic therapy after at least one anti-CD20–based therapy.

Aggressive or High-Grade Non-Hodgkin Lymphomas

High-grade B- and T-cell NHLs are typically aggressive lymphomas that are fatal in weeks to a few months if not treated. However, many of these NHLs are curable with multiagent chemotherapy.

General Principles

DLBCL, the most common aggressive NHL, is curable in all stages in the majority of patients (60%–70%). A common treatment is anti-CD20 monoclonal antibody combined with anthracycline-based chemotherapy: rituximab–cyclophosphamide, doxorubicin (hydroxydaunorubicin), vincristine (Oncovin), prednisone (R-CHOP). The number of treatment cycles depends on stage of disease and response to treatment. Standard therapy for advanced-stage disease is six R-CHOP cycles, whereas patients with early-stage disease may receive three or four cycles with or without involved field radiation. There are emerging data regarding the prognostic importance of *MYC* rearrangement (from tumor testing) as a single finding and especially in conjunction with *BCL-2* and/or *BCL6* (i.e., double or triple hit) by molecular studies as well as with immunohistochemical staining. Outcomes with R-CHOP for DLBCL patients with a molecular double hit (e.g., presence of MYC and *BCL-2* rearrangements) are modest; more intensive and novel therapeutic options should be considered. Therapy for relapsed DLBCL typically includes abbreviated salvage non–cross-resistant chemotherapy followed by autologous stem cell transplantation for patients who have chemotherapy-sensitive disease, which is curative in approximately 35% to 45% of patients.

MCL is a B-cell NHL with initial high remission rates (>90%–95%), but it has more modest long-term outcomes, and it is difficult to cure. With standard chemotherapy regimens (e.g., R-CHOP), the median PFS rates are only 18 to 20 months. With more-intensive chemotherapy regimens, especially ones incorporating high-dose cytarabine as a component of induction therapy, 5-year PFS rates are near 70%. Some groups advocate induction therapy with aggressive high-dose cytarabine (Cytosar)[1]-based chemotherapy followed by consolidative autologous stem cell transplantation in first remission. As noted later, there has been the integration of several novel therapeutic agents into the treatment paradigm of MCL. Bendamustine (Bendeka, Treanda) in combination with rituximab has also become a widely used and more tolerable induction regimen, especially in older patients with MCL.

Burkitt lymphoma and related high-grade NHLs (e.g., lymphoblastic lymphomas) are often rapidly growing malignancies with a doubling time of 24 hours. Prompt initiation of therapy, including aggressive supportive care measures, is often warranted. With aggressive chemotherapy regimens, including prophylactic intrathecal chemotherapy, the majority of Burkitt patients younger than age 40 years are cured (>70%–80%). In addition, there are data showing high efficacy using lower-intensity treatment consisting of infused etoposide (Toposar),[1] doxorubicin, and cyclophosphamide with vincristine, prednisone, and rituximab (EPOCH-R), especially for patients untreated Burkitt lymphoma without CNS involvement, including HIV related.

Systemic (i.e., noncutaneous) PTCLs are mostly aggressive malignancies. They are treatable; however, cure rates are lower compared with most aggressive B-cell NHLs. Standard therapy had consisted of CHOP-based chemotherapy with or without autologous stem cell transplantation in first remission as consolidation. Recently published data from the ECHELON-2 trial combining the antibody drug conjugate, brentuximab vedotin (Adcetris), with cyclophosphamide, doxorubicin, and prednisone (CHP) chemotherapy versus standard CHOP for untreated CD30+ PTCLs was associated with significantly improved PFS and OS. This regimen (i.e., brentuximab vedotin + CHP) was subsequently FDA approved for this indication. Several additional novel targeted agents have also been FDA approved over the past several years for the treatment of T-cell NHL (see later).

Special Considerations

There are several clinical subtypes of DLBCL that present as primary extranodal manifestations such as primary testicular DLBCL and primary gastric DLBCL. If these lymphomas are localized, treatment typically consists of abbreviated cycles (3–4) of R-CHOP followed by involved field radiation. In addition, CNS prophylaxis with either intrathecal chemotherapy or agents such as intravenous high-dose methotrexate[1] is warranted for testicular DLBCL given the relatively high risk of CNS involvement or relapse.

Primary CNS lymphoma is typically DLBCL; high-dose methotrexate chemotherapy is a key component of therapy.

A long-standing therapeutic maneuver for solid organ transplant–related PTLDs has been reduction of immunosuppression, although, using this approach alone, mortality rates have ranged from 50% to 60% in most series. Evidence with use of initial rituximab-based therapy suggests significantly improved outcomes in the modern era.

The majority of AIDS-related NHLs are aggressive or high-grade types: DLBCL or Burkitt lymphoma. Similar therapy as immunocompetent NHL is often recommended. Response to therapy, including cure rate, has improved significantly with better control of opportunistic infections and highly active antiretroviral therapy (HAART).

Mycosis fungoides and Sézary syndrome are cutaneous T-cell lymphomas that initially might show eczematous lesions. It is often difficult to establish the diagnosis, but eventually the lesions develop into plaques and tumors. Lymph nodes, spleen, and visceral organs may be involved. Sézary syndrome is a variant of mycosis fungoides and shows peripheral blood involvement; patients usually have diffuse erythroderma. Skin-targeted modalities for treatment of early-stage mycosis fungoides include psoralens with ultraviolet A (PUVA) light, narrowband-ultraviolet light, skin electron-beam radiation, and topical steroids, retinoids, carmustine (BiCNU) and nitrogen mustard (Mustargen).[1] Treatment goals in advanced stages are to reduce tumor burden and to relieve symptoms. Treatment options also include monochemotherapy or polychemotherapy including CHOP, extracorporeal photopheresis, interferons, retinoids, monoclonal antibodies, recombinant toxins, histone deacetylase inhibitors, and most recently, the antibody drug conjugate brentuximab vedotin (Adcetris) and humanized antibody against CCR4, mogamulizumab (Poteligeo) (Study of KW-0761).

During therapy for aggressive/high-grade NHLs, attention should be paid to preventing tumor lysis syndrome. Measures to prevent this complication include aggressive hydration, allopurinol (Zyloprim), and frequent monitoring of electrolytes, uric acid, and creatinine. Rasburicase (Elitek), a recombinant urate oxidase enzyme, is an expensive but potent agent for treating hyperuricemia.

Novel Treatment Options and Modalities

Many new agents targeting specific molecular targets have become available for the treatment of lymphoma (Tables 2 and 3). Novel agents in lymphoma include bortezomib (Velcade) and lenalidomide (Revlimid), which are FDA approved for relapsed or refractory MCL (and lenalidomide also for relapsed follicular lymphoma),

---

[1]Not FDA approved for this indication.

---

[1]Not FDA approved for this indication.

TABLE 2 Targeted Therapeutics FDA Approved for the Treatment of B-Cell Non-Hodgkin Lymphoma[1]

BTK inhibitors	**Mechanism:** Small molecule binds Bruton tyrosine kinase (BTK) and inhibits downstream signaling pathways initiated by B-cell receptor **Notable toxicities:** atrial fibrillation, myelosuppression, rash, arthralgias, headache, bleeding, and impaired wound healing (should be held perioperatively and prior to other invasive procedures)	
	Drug Name	*Indication and Year Approved*
	Ibrutinib (Imbruvica)	Mantle cell lymphoma (2013) CLL/SLL (2014) Waldenström macroglobulinemia (2015) Marginal zone lymphoma (2017)
	Acalabrutinib (Calquence)	Mantle cell lymphoma (2017) CLL/SLL (2019)
	Zanubrutinib (Brukinsa)	Mantle cell lymphoma (2019)
Anti-CD20 monoclonal antibodies	**Mechanism:** Bind to CD20 molecule on B lymphocytes and induce a variety of responses, including antibody-mediated cytotoxicity, complement-mediated cytotoxicity, and apoptosis. **Notable toxicities:** infusion reactions, hypogammaglobulinemia, hepatitis B virus reactivation, progressive multifocal leukoencephalopathy (rare)	
	Drug Name	*Indication and Year Approved*
	Rituximab (Rituxan)	Relapsed indolent B-cell lymphomas (1997) Untreated DLBCL with CHOP (2006) CLL (2010) Follicular lymphoma maintenance (2011) Waldenström macroglobulinemia, with ibrutinib (2018)
	Obinutuzumab (Gazyva)	Untreated CLL with chlorambucil (Leukeran) (2013) Relapsed rituximab refractory follicular lymphoma with bendamustine (Bendeka) (2016) Untreated follicular lymphoma with bendamustine (2017) Untreated CLL with ibrutinib (2019)
	Ofatumumab (Arzerra)	Relapsed CLL (2016)
Anti-CD79b monoclonal antibody	**Mechanism:** Binds to CD79b molecule on B lymphocytes. Conjugated monomethyl auristatin E (MMAE) is then internalized by lymphocyte. MMAE binds tubulin, resulting in cell cycle arrest. **Notable toxicities:** neuropathy, immunosuppression, fatigue, diarrhea	
	Drug Name	*Indication and Year Approved*
	Polatuzumab vedotin (Polivy)	Relapsed DLBCL with bendamustine and rituximab (2019)
Immunomodulators	**Mechanism:** affects T-cell stimulatory pathways, angiogenesis, and cell proliferation **Notable toxicities:** myelosuppression, fatigue, rash, thrombosis (prophylactic aspirin or anticoagulants typically advised)	
	Drug Name	*Indication and Year Approved*
	Lenalidomide (Revlimid)	Relapsed mantle cell lymphoma (2013) Relapsed follicular lymphoma and marginal zone lymphoma (2019)
Anti-CD19 monoclonal antibody	**Mechanism:** monoclonal antibody that binds to CD19 antigen and mediates B-cell lysis through apoptosis and immune effector mechanisms, including antibody-dependent cellular cytotoxicity (ADCC) and antibody-dependent cellular phagocytosis **Notable toxicities:** neutropenia, fatigue, anemia, diarrhea, thrombocytopenia, cough, pyrexia, and peripheral edema	
	Drug Name	*Indication and Year Approved*
	Tafasitamab-cxix (Monjuvi) in combination with lenalidomide	Relapsed DLBCL
Phosphatidylinositol-3-kinase (PI3Kδ) inhibitors	**Mechanism:** small molecule inhibitors of PI3 kinase, resulting in inhibition of various cellular processes, such as cellular growth, proliferation, and intracellular trafficking **Notable toxicities:** pneumonitis, colitis, transaminitis, hypertension, hyperglycemia (copanlisib)	
	Drug Name	*Indication and Year Approved*
	Idealisib (Zydelig)	Relapsed CLL/SLL and follicular lymphoma (2014)
	Copanlisib (Aliqopa)	Relapsed follicular lymphoma (2017)
	Duvelisib (Copiktra)	Relapsed CLL/SLL and follicular lymphoma (2018)
PD-1 (programmed cell death-1) inhibitors	**Mechanism:** blocks PD-1 on cellular surface, facilitating T-cell–mediated immune killing **Notable toxicities:** pneumonitis, colitis, dermatitis, endocrinopathies (hypothyroidism)	
	Drug Name	*Indication and Year First Approved*
	Pembrolizumab (Keytruda)	Relapsed primary mediastinal large B-cell lymphoma (2018)

Continued

TABLE 2	Targeted Therapeutics FDA Approved for the Treatment of B-Cell Non-Hodgkin Lymphoma[1]—cont'd	
Chimeric antigen receptor (CAR) T-cell therapy	**Mechanism:** CD19-directed genetically modified autologous T cells target CD19-expressing lymphoma cells **Notable toxicities:** cytokine release syndrome (fever, hypotension, organ dysfunction), neurotoxicity (mental status changes, confusion, seizures), cytopenias	
	Drug Name	*Indication and Year Approved*
	Axicabtagene ciloleucel (Yescarta)	Relapsed DLBCL (2017) Relapsed follicular lymphoma (2021)
	Tisagenlecleucel (Kymriah) Brexucabtagene autoleucel (Tecartus)	Relapsed DLBCL (2018) Relapsed mantle cell lymphoma (2020)
	Lisocabtagene maraleucel (Breyanzi)	Relapsed DLBCL (2021)
BCL-2 inhibitors	**Mechanism:** small molecule inhibits antiapoptotic activities of protein BCL2 **Notable toxicities:** tumor lysis syndrome, myelosuppression, fever, diarrhea	
	Drug Name	*Indication and Year Approved*
	Venetoclax (Venclexta)	Relapsed CLL/SLL (2016) Untreated CLL/SLL in combination with obinutuzumab (2019)
Proteasome inhibitors	**Mechanism:** inhibits proteasomal clearance of multiple molecules, including proapoptotic molecules **Notable toxicities:** peripheral neuropathy, fatigue, diarrhea	
	Drug Name	*Indication and Year Approved*
	Bortezomib (Velcade)	Relapsed mantle cell lymphoma (2006) Untreated mantle cell lymphoma with chemotherapy (2014)
Nuclear export inhibitor	**Mechanism:** actively binds to export protein 1 (XPO1 or CRM1) inhibiting the nuclear export of tumor suppressors, growth regulators, and antiinflammatory proteins **Notable toxicities:** fatigue, nausea, diarrhea, appetite decrease, weight decrease, constipation, vomiting, pyrexia; dizziness and mental status changes; thrombocytopenia, neutropenia, anemia, and hyponatremia	
	Drug Name	*Indication and Year Approved*
	Selinexor (Xpovio)	Relapsed DLBCL
Radioimmunotherapy	**Mechanism:** monoclonal antibodies deliver targeted radiation to lymphoma cells **Notable toxicities:** cytopenias (delayed), fatigue, MDS	
	Drug Name	*Indication and Year Approved*
	Ibritumomab tiuxetan (Zevalin)	Relapsed follicular lymphoma (2002) Consolidation for follicular lymphoma after initial chemotherapy (2009)

CHOP, Cyclophosphamide, doxorubicin, Oncovin, prednisone; *CLL/SLL,* chronic lymphocytic leukemia/small lymphocytic lymphoma; *DLBCL,* diffuse large B-cell lymphoma; *MDS,* myelodysplastic syndrome.
[1]Not FDA approved for this indication.

and histone deacetylase inhibitors, which are approved for cutaneous T-cell lymphoma and peripheral T-cell NHLs as well. In addition, bortezomib is FDA approved for untreated MCL patients in combination with immunochemotherapy. Other newer agents that are FDA approved for the treatment of patients with chronic lymphocytic leukemia (CLL), including in higher-risk patient populations (e.g., p53 mutated), are idelalisib (Zydelig), an inhibitor of PI3K delta; the BTK inhibitor ibrutinib (Imbruvica), which is also FDA approved for patients with CLL and MCL; and venetoclax (Venclexta), a BH3 mimetic acting as an inhibitor of BCL2. There are several recently published and a number of ongoing clinical studies to evaluate the optimal sequence and varied combinations for patients with CLL, especially vis-à-vis harnessing frontline targeted therapeutics.

The BTK inhibitor acalabrutinib (Calquence) is FDA approved for relapsed or refractory MCL patients who have received at least one prior therapy. Two other PI3K inhibitors (i.e., copanlisib [Aliqopa] and duvelisib [Copiktra]) are approved for adult patients with relapsed or refractory follicular lymphoma. New anti-CD20 antibodies have also been approved for the treatment of CLL (e.g., obinutuzumab [Gazyva]) as well as antibody drug conjugates, which contain potent drugs that are conjugated to an antibody. These include brentuximab vedotin (Adcetris), which is FDA approved for newly diagnosed CD30-positive T-cell lymphomas and relapsed anaplastic (T-cell) large-cell lymphoma, and the anti-CD79b monoclonal antibody drug complex, polatuzumab vedotin (Polivy), that the FDA approved in combination with rituximab and bendamustine for relapsed/refractory DLBCL.

These novel therapeutic agents are mostly FDA approved for patients with relapsed or refractory disease; however, there are a multitude of ongoing studies in the frontline/untreated setting and in varied sequences and combinations.

There is also great excitement in the continued application of new immunotherapy approaches in NHL such as checkpoint inhibitors (e.g., programmed death-1 [PD-1] inhibitors) as well as chimeric antigen receptor (CAR) T-cell therapy, which involve removal of T cells from patients followed by bioengineered CARs (e.g., CD19) that facilitate T-cell expansion and antigen/tumor recognition when reinfused into the patient. Axicabtagene ciloleucel (Yescarta), tisagenlecleucel (Kymriah), and lisocabtagene maraleucel (Breyanzi) are anti-CD19 CAR T-cell therapies the FDA approved for patients with relapsed or refractory DLBCL. Overall response rates range from 50% to 72%, with complete remission rates of 32% to 51%. Furthermore, 25% to 35% of patients appear to experience longer-term disease remission. There are a multitude of other CAR T-cell and natural killer-based constructs being studies across several lymphoma subtypes.

TABLE 3	Targeted Therapeutics FDA Approved for the Treatment of T-Cell Non-Hodgkin Lymphoma	
Histone Deacetylase Inhibitors	**Mechanism:** modules acetylation of key targets, including genes involved in cancer-related cellular pathways **Notable toxicities:** QT prolongation, electrolyte abnormalities, cytopenias (especially thrombocytopenia), nausea, fatigue	
	Drug Name	*Indication and Year Approved*
	Romidepsin (Istodax)	Relapsed CTCL (2009) Relapsed PTCL (2011)
	Vorinostat (Zolinza)	Relapsed CTCL (2006)
	Belinostat (Beleodaq)	Relapsed PTCL (2014)
Anti-CD30 monoclonal antibody	**Mechanism:** Binds to CD30 molecule on T lymphocytes. Conjugated monomethyl auristatin E (MMAE) is then internalized by lymphocyte. MMAE binds tubulin, resulting in cell cycle arrest. **Notable toxicities:** peripheral neuropathy, diarrhea, cytopenias, fatigue, pancreatitis	
	Drug Name	*Indication and Year Approved*
	Brentuximab vedotin (Adcetris)	CD30-positive mycosis fungoides and cutaneous anaplastic large cell lymphoma (2017) Untreated CD30-expressing PTCL (2018)
Anti-CCR4 monoclonal antibody	**Mechanism:** binds CCR4 (CC chemokine receptor type 4) and inhibits downstream signal transduction pathways and chemokine-mediated cellular migration and T-cell proliferation **Notable toxicities:** infusion reactions, infection, rash, fever, edema, nausea, headache, cytopenias	
	Drug Name	*Indication and Year Approved*
	Mogamulizumab (Poteligeo)	Mycosis fungoides (2018) Approved outside US for adult T-cell leukemia/lymphoma
Folate antagonists	**Mechanism:** folate analog that accumulates in lymphoma cells and impairs DNA synthesis **Notable toxicities:** mucositis, myelosuppression, nausea, fatigue	
	Drug Name	*Indication and Year Approved*
	Pralatrexate (Folotyn)	Relapsed PTCL (2009)

CTCL, Cutaneous T-cell lymphoma; *PTCL*, peripheral T-cell lymphoma.

Follow-Up of Long-Term Survivors

Relapse

Among patients with aggressive lymphomas, such as DLBCL, most recurrences are seen within the first 2 years after the completion of therapy, although later relapses occur uncommonly. Physical examination and laboratory testing at 2- to 3-month intervals and follow-up CT scans at 6-month intervals for the first 2 years after diagnosis are recommended; however, there is ongoing debate regarding the impact that postsurveillance scans have on disease outcomes. Detection of recurrent disease is important in part because these patients may be candidates for potentially curative therapy (e.g., stem cell transplantation). Patients with advanced low-grade NHL are at a constant risk for relapse, as discussed before.

Secondary Malignancies

Long-term NHL survivors are at an increased risk for second cancers. In general, the risk is increased with history of radiation use, but it is also seen with chemotherapy. In a survey of 28,131 Dutch registry patients with NHL who survived 2 years or longer, significant excesses of second cancers were seen for nearly all solid tumors as well as acute myelogenous leukemia (AML) and HL. The standardized incidence ratio (SIR) for solid tumors after NHL was 1.65. The SIRs for solid tumors are increased for up to 30 years after NHL diagnosis, with the highest relative risk of developing a secondary malignancy occurring more than 21 to 30 years after original diagnosis.

Late Treatment Complications

There has been more selective use of radiation as part of therapy for NHL. Thus the risk of certain radiation-induced complications has been reduced in patients treated more recently. Nevertheless, the risk still exists. Transplant recipients are at increased risk for secondary myelodysplasia and AML, regardless of whether they received radiation. All chemotherapy agents may cause long-term morbidity; in particular, patients who received an anthracycline (e.g., doxorubicin [Adriamycin]) are at a long-term increased risk of cardiovascular disease. Among Dutch and Belgian NHL patients treated with at least six cycles of doxorubicin-based chemotherapy, cumulative incidence of cardiovascular disease was 12% at 5 years and 22% at 10 years. Risk of coronary artery disease matched that of the general population; however, risk of chronic heart failure was significantly increased (SIR, 5.4), as was stroke (SIR, 1.8). Risk factors associated with excess risk included younger age at start of NHL treatment (<55 years), preexisting hypertension, any salvage treatment, and use of radiotherapy; risk relating to radiotherapy was dose-dependent. Continued studies are needed to develop optimal secondary prevention strategies.

References

Burger JA, et al: Ibrutinib as initial therapy for patients with chronic lymphocytic leukemia, *N Engl J Med* 373(25):2425–2437, 2015.

Dunleavy K, Pittaluga S, Shovlin M, et al: Low-intensity therapy in adults with Burkitt's lymphoma, *N Engl J Med* 369(20):1915–1925, 2013.

Evens AM, Danilov AV, Jagadeesh D, et al: Burkitt lymphoma in the modern era: real world outcomes and prognostication across 30 US Cancer Centers, *Blood* 137:374–386, 2021.

Fischer K, Al-Sawaf O, Bahlo J, et al: Venetoclax and obinutuzumab in patients with CLL and coexisting conditions, *N Engl J Med* 380(23):2225–2236, 2019.

Gopal AK, Kahl BS, de Vos S, et al: PI3Kδ inhibition by idelalisib in patients with relapsed indolent lymphoma, *N Engl J Med* 370(11):1008–1018, 2014.

Hemminki K, Lenner P, Sundquist J, Bermejo JL: Risk of subsequent solid tumors after non-Hodgkin's lymphoma: effect of diagnostic age and time since diagnosis, *J Clin Oncol* 26(11):1850–1857, 2008.

Horwitz S, O'Connor OA, Pro B, et al: Brentuximab vedotin with chemotherapy for CD30-positive peripheral T-cell lymphoma (ECHELON-2): a global, double-blind, randomised, phase 3 trial, *Lancet* 393(10168):229–240, 2019.

Marcus R, Davies A, Ando K, et al: Obinutuzumab for the first-line treatment of follicular lymphoma, *N Engl J Med* 377(14):1331–1344, 2017.

Morton LM, Curtis RE, Linet MS, et al: Second malignancy risks after non-Hodgkin's lymphoma and chronic lymphocytic leukemia: differences by lymphoma subtype, *J Clin Oncol* 28:4935–4944, 2010.

Moser EC, Noordijk EM, van Leeuwen FE, et al: Long-term risk of cardiovascular disease after treatment for aggressive non-Hodgkin lymphoma, *Blood* 107:2912–2919, 2006.

Neelapu SS, Locke FL, Bartlett NL, et al: Axicabtagene ciloleucel CAR T-Cell therapy in refractory large B-Cell lymphoma, *N Engl J Med* 377(26):2531–2544, 2017.

Olszewski AJ, Jakobsen LH, Collins GP, et al: Burkitt lymphoma international prognostic Index, *J Clin Oncol*, 2021. pre-published.

Prince HM, Kim YH, Horwitz SM, et al: Brentuximab vedotin or physician's choice in CD30-positive cutaneous T-cell lymphoma (ALCANZA): an international, open-label, randomised, phase 3, multicentre trial, *Lancet* 390(10094):555–566, 2017.

Roberts AW, et al: Targeting BCL2 with Venetoclax in relapsed chronic lymphocytic leukemia, *N Engl J Med* 374(4):311–322, 2016.

Schuster SJ, Bishop MR, Tam CS: Tisagenlecleucel in adult relapsed or refractory diffuse large B-Cell lymphoma, *N Engl J Med* 380(1):45–56, 2019.

Shanafelt TD, Wang XV, Kay NE, et al: Ibrutinib-rituximab or chemoimmunotherapy for chronic lymphocytic leukemia, *N Engl J Med* 381(5):432–443, 2019.

Siegel RL, Miller KD, Fuchs HE, et al: Cancer statistics, 2021, *CA Cancer J Clin* 71(1):7–33, 2021.

Swerdlow SH, Campo E, Pileri SA, et al: The 2016 revision of the World Health Organization classification of lymphoid neoplasms, *Blood* 127(20):2375–2390, 2016.

Trappe RU, Dierickx D, Zimmermann H, et al: Response to rituximab induction is a predictive marker in B-cell post-transplant lymphoproliferative disorder and allows successful stratification into rituximab or R-CHOP consolidation in an international, prospective, multicenter phase II trial, *J Clin Oncol* 35(5):536–543, 2017.

Wang ML, Rule S, Martin P, et al: Targeting BTK with ibrutinib in relapsed or refractory mantle-cell lymphoma, *N Engl J Med* 369(6):507–516, 2013.

Woyach JA, Ruppert AS, Heerema NA, et al: Ibrutinib regimens versus chemoimmunotherapy in older patients with untreated CLL, *N Engl J Med* 379(26):2517–2528, 2018.

Zhou Z, Sehn LH, Rademaker AW, et al: An enhanced International Prognostic Index (NCCN-IPI) for patients with diffuse large B-cell lymphoma treated in the rituximab era, *Blood* 123(6):837–842, 2014.

PERNICIOUS ANEMIA/MEGALOBLASTIC ANEMIA

Method of
Anusha Vallurupalli, MBBS

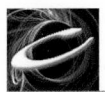

CURRENT DIAGNOSIS

- Megaloblastic anemia is defined as macrocytic anemia with large, structurally and functionally abnormal red blood cells in the bone marrow and peripheral blood and is most commonly associated with folate or B12 deficiencies.
- In adults, folate deficiency is most commonly due to inadequate dietary intake. Vitamin B12 deficiency is mainly due to cobalamin malabsorption from food due to pernicious anemia, an autoimmune disorder, and gastrointestinal malabsorption.
- Megaloblastic anemia often presents with macrocytosis and hypersegmented neutrophils on peripheral smear.

CURRENT TREATMENT

- Prompt recognition and diagnosis are essential to prevent both short-term and long-term complications.
- Recognition of the underlying etiology for megaloblastic anemia is essential for a long-term treatment plan.
- Vitamin B12 deficiency can be treated with both oral and parenteral therapy and the route and duration of treatment is usually based on underlying etiology.
- If vitamin B12 deficiency is untreated, folate repletion will correct the megaloblastic anemia but not the associated neuropathic changes that occur with B12 deficiency.
- Folate replacement is generally accomplished through the oral route.
- Preventive B12 and folate dosing is warranted in certain high risk patients.
- Both B12 and folate replacements are generally well tolerated.

Introduction

Anemia is one of the most common hematologic disorders encountered on a regular basis in various clinical settings. In 2010, the global prevalence of anemia was 32.9%; that is, more than 2.2 billion people were affected. The World Health Organization (WHO) defines anemia as a hemoglobin (Hb) count of less than 13 g/L in men, less than 12 g/L in nonpregnant women, and less than 11 g/L in pregnant women and the elderly. A Hb of less than 10 g/L in any patient should trigger an evaluation. The etiology of anemia is oftentimes multifactorial, especially in elderly patients. In elderly patients, anemia can exacerbate comorbid cardiac complications such as cardiac ischemia and congestive heart failure. Most of the causes of anemia, especially nutritional causes, can usually be treated efficiently. Therefore, the cause of anemia should be identified and treated promptly to decrease the risk of complications.

Megaloblastic anemia, in general, is defined as macrocytic anemia with large, structurally and functionally abnormal red blood cells in the bone marrow and peripheral blood. Hypersegmented neutrophils are also commonly seen on the peripheral smear. The mean corpuscular volume (MCV) is elevated. Megaloblastic anemia is most commonly associated with nutritional deficiencies, specifically B12 and folate. In most cases, diagnosis is made by blood testing.

Epidemiology

The incidence and prevalence of anemia is highly variable and depends on age, sex, ethnicity, country of origin, socioeconomic status, and multifactorial comorbid conditions.

A retrospective study of 1784 randomly selected older adults living at home found macrocytosis in 6.3% of men and 3.3% of women. Folate and B12 deficiencies are the most common causes of megaloblastic anemia. Folate and B12 nutritional deficiencies are often easily treated.

Etiology

Folate Deficiency

Deficiency of folate is the most common cause of megaloblastic anemia. Folate is abundant in green leafy vegetables and approximately 60% of dietary folate is absorbed in the small intestine. However, folate is not stored in the body for a long duration and needs to be constantly replaced. Body stores of folate only last for approximately 6 months. Other causes include malabsorption and factors affecting folate metabolism (Table 1).

Vitamin B12 Deficiency

Deficiency of vitamin B12 can occur due to insufficient capture of the vitamin B12 from dietary sources because of inadequate intake, as seen in vegetarians and vegans or in patients who are malnourished. Malabsorption, as seen in patients with pernicious anemia, atrophic gastritis, or following gastric surgery, is another major cause (Table 2).

Pernicious Anemia

Pernicious anemia is characterized by malabsorption of B12 due to a deficiency of intrinsic factor. It is often associated with other co-existing autoimmune disorders such as celiac disease, Hashimoto thyroiditis, and Sjögren syndrome. Pernicious anemia is usually diagnosed by checking for intrinsic factor antibodies in the blood or by biopsy-proven immune atrophic gastritis. Intrinsic factor neutralizing antibodies are found in the setting of atrophic immune gastritis. *Helicobacter pylori*-related atrophic gastritis is in the differential and, if there is a clinical suspicion, should be evaluated by gastric biopsy. Intrinsic factor antibodies should not be checked after parenteral B12 administration for at least 2 weeks, as it will result in a false negative result.

Clinical Manifestations

Symptoms of anemia and laboratory findings (Table 3) from folate deficiency and B12 deficiency are essentially indistinguishable.

TABLE 1	Causes of Folate Deficiency

Dietary Deficiency

Malabsorption due to abnormalities of the jejunum
- Celiac disease
- Jejunal resection
- Tropical sprue

Drug-induced malabsorption
- Sulfasalazine (Azulfidine)

Increased requirement
- Pregnancy
- Prematurity
- Chronic hemolytic anemias (sickle cell anemia and autoimmune hemolytic anemias)
- Malignant diseases
- Chronic inflammatory disease

Increased loss
- Some skin diseases
- Long-term dialysis

Acquired abnormality of folate metabolism: dihydrofolate reductase inhibitors (methotrexate and sulfamethoxazole/trimethoprim [Bactrim])

Complex or uncertain mechanism
- Ethanol abuse (some cases)
- Anticonvulsant drugs (some cases)
- Oral contraceptive drugs, glutethimide, and cycloserine

Inherited abnormalities of folate absorption and metabolism
- Hereditary folate malabsorption
- Glutamate formiminotransferase-cyclodeaminase deficiency

Adapted from Wickramasinghe SN. Diagnosis of megaloblastic anemias. *Blood Rev.* 2006;20(6):299–318.

TABLE 2	Causes of B12 Deficiency

Dietary Deficiency

Impaired release of B_{12} from food—food cobalamin malabsorption

Inadequate secretion of intrinsic factor
- Pernicious anemia
- Total or partial gastrectomy
- Congenital intrinsic factor deficiency
- Congenitally abnormal intrinsic factor

Impaired release of B_{12} from B_{12}–R binder complex
- Pancreatic insufficiency
- Zollinger-Ellison syndrome

Diversion of dietary B_{12}
- Abnormal intestinal bacterial flora—jejunal diverticula, small intestinal strictures, and stagnant intestinal loops (blind loop syndrome)
- Fish tapeworm infestation

Malabsorption due to abnormalities in the terminal ileum
- Ileal resection
- Crohn disease
- Chronic tropical sprue
- Other acquired diseases
- Imerslund-Gräsbeck syndrome (selective malabsorption with proteinuria)

Drug-induced malabsorption (amino salicylic acid, neomycin, colchicine, slow-release potassium chloride, metformin, phenformin, biguanides, and cholestyramine)

Inactivation of methyl cobalamin by nitrous oxide

Inherited abnormalities of B_{12} transport or intracellular B_{12} metabolism
- Deficiency or abnormality of transcobalamin II
- Defective methyl cobalamin synthesis (hyper homocysteinemia)
- Defective synthesis of both methyl cobalamin and adenosyl cobalamin (hyper homocysteinemia and methylmalonic acidemia)

Adapted from Wickramasinghe SN. Diagnosis of megaloblastic anemias. *Blood Rev.* 2006;20(6):299–318.

TABLE 3	Laboratory Findings in Megaloblastic Anemia

Common for both B12 and folate deficiencies:
- Macrocytosis with elevated MCV, often greater than 100
- Megaloblasts and hypersegmented neutrophils on peripheral smear
- Anemia
- Elevated homocysteine levels

Specific for B12 deficiency:
- Elevated MMA levels
- Elevated LDH, indirect bilirubin, and low haptoglobin in the setting of intravascular hemolysis, which can be seen in severe B12 deficiency.
- Positive intrinsic factor antibodies in patients with pernicious anemia.

LDH, Lactate dehydrogenase; *MCV,* mean corpuscular volume; *MMA,* methylmalonic acid.

TABLE 4	Signs and Symptoms of B12 Deficiency

Neurological Symptoms/Signs
- Dysesthesia and hypoesthesia
- Subacute combined degeneration presenting with ataxia, decreased proprioception, and vibratory sensation
- Extrapyramidal signs (e.g., dystonia, dysarthria, and rigidity)
- Abnormal deep tendon reflexes
- Ataxia or positive Romberg test

Gastrointestinal Symptoms/Signs
- Glossitis
- Abdominal pain
- Dyspepsia likely related to atrophic gastritis or *H. pylori* infection

Psychiatric Symptoms
- Depression or mood impairment
- Psychosis
- Dementia

Rare Manifestations
- Skin hyperpigmentation
- Grey hair

Anemia Symptoms
- Fatigue
- Palpitations
- Exertional dyspnea
- Chest pain
- lightheadedness

B12 deficiency can manifest without anemia and is also characterized by neuropsychiatric symptoms (Table 4). The cause of neurological symptoms is thought to be secondary to the role that vitamin B12 plays in neuronal myelination, although the exact mechanism is not known.

Diagnosis

The diagnosis of pernicious anemia is based on laboratory testing (see Table 3). Complete blood count with differential, peripheral blood smear, complete metabolic profile including total and indirect bilirubin, lactate dehydrogenase, and serum folate and B12 levels are all included in the initial diagnostic testing. Methylmalonic acid (MMA) and homocysteine levels in indeterminate situations where the B12 or folate serum levels are borderline low may be helpful. MMA levels are increased in B12 deficiency, whereas MMA levels are normal in folate deficiency. Homocysteine levels are increased in both folate and B12 deficiencies. There may be fluctuations in MMA and homocysteine levels due to underlying concurrent conditions such as renal insufficiency (increased MMA levels), methylmalonic aciduria (increased MMA levels) and hereditary homocystinemia (increased homocysteine levels), and additional bacterial overgrowth in the small intestine (increased MMA levels), in addition to other rare conditions. Intrinsic factor antibody testing should be ordered prior to initiation of parenteral B12 replacement in patients with pernicious anemia.

TABLE 5 Differential Diagnosis of Macrocytic Anemia

- Chronic alcohol abuse
- Myelodysplastic syndromes
- Hypothyroidism
- Chronic lung disease with hypoxia
- Heavy smoking
- Chronic liver disease
- Chronic hemolytic anemia
- Therapy with certain anticonvulsant drugs
- Myeloma (some cases)
- Hypoplastic and aplastic anemia
- Physiologic
- Normal neonates
- Normal pregnancy (some cases)

Adapted from Wickramasinghe SN. Diagnosis of megaloblastic anemias. *Blood Rev.* 2006;20(6):299–318.

Bone marrow aspiration and biopsy are not routinely recommended and should be reserved for cases in which there is persistent anemia despite replacement of both B12 and folate with resultant normalized levels. Patients with pernicious anemia should be evaluated for underlying gastric cancer with esophagogastroduodenoscopy. A systematic meta-analysis of 27 studies revealed a pooled gastric cancer incidence rate in patients with pernicious anemia of 0.3/100 person-years and an estimated sevenfold relative risk of gastric cancer.

Differential Diagnosis

The differential diagnosis for macrocytic anemia includes anemia related to chronic alcohol use (with or without liver disease), thyroid failure, and myelodysplastic syndromes (Table 5). Symptoms of copper deficiency can mimic B12 deficiency, can occasionally present with macrocytosis and should be ruled out with serum copper level testing if the patient does not respond to B12 supplementation.

Prevention

Providing food sources with nutrients rich in folic acid and/or B12 is best for preventing megaloblastic anemia. Therapeutic supplementation may be necessary, especially for the very old. The Institute of Medicine (United States) Standing Committee on the Scientific Evaluation of Dietary Reference Intakes has recommended fortification of cereals with multiple B vitamins, including B12. Prophylactic folate treatment should be administered to patients with increased requirements such as those with chronic hemolytic anemias and women who are pregnant. Preventive therapeutic replacement should be offered to all patients who have undergone bariatric gastric surgery or patients with compromised small intestine absorption due to various causes.

Treatment

General Principles

All patients who are identified as having B12 deficiency and/or folate deficiency should be treated. Replacement of the nutrients usually corrects the anemia. Blood transfusions are generally reserved for emergency situations such as severe symptomatic anemia and in patients with cardiac complications (i.e., chest pain, heart failure) associated with anemia. Oral replacement is generally well tolerated and is the first line treatment of choice. Parenteral replacement, especially for B12 deficiency, should be considered in patients with severe B12 deficiency who present with symptomatic anemia, severe neurologic symptoms,

pernicious anemia, as well as in patients who are at risk for malabsorption and in women who are pregnant. Replacement with oral folate in a patient with undiagnosed B12 deficiency will improve the anemia but will not reverse the neurological symptoms.

The underlying cause for B12 deficiency and/or folate deficiency should be identified and treated. The duration of therapy depends on the underlying cause of the deficiency. Lifelong replacement is recommended for patients with irreversible causes (e.g., gastric bypass surgery and pernicious anemia). Short term treatment is recommended for patients with reversible causes (e.g., drug induced, reversible causes of malabsorption, inadequate dietary intake, and alcoholism). Both B12 and folate are water soluble vitamins and do not generally cause any major adverse effects.

Treatment of B12 Deficiency

Vitamin B12 is available in oral, sublingual, intramuscular (IM), subcutaneous (SC), and intranasal formulations. Cyanocobalamin is the most available formulation in United States. The oral formulation is generally effective in patients with a reversible cause and is administered at a dosage of 1000 µg daily for at least 1 month followed by either continuation of the same dose for maintenance or the dose can be decreased to 100 to 500 µg daily in patients with mild reversible deficiencies. The parenteral formulation is preferably administered IM at a dose of 1000 µg daily for 1 week followed by 1000 µg once a week for 1 month. The maintenance dose for IM or parenteral deep SC injection is 1000 µg monthly and indefinitely, depending on the etiology. Patients are usually taught to self-administer the injections to minimize the inconvenience of travel, improve compliance, and decrease costs.

Treatment of Folate Deficiency

The replacement dose for folic acid varies between 1 and 5 mg/day. Usually, therapy is continued for at least 3 to 6 months, provided that the underlying causes of the deficiency have been corrected.

Complications and Long-Term Monitoring

Patients with undiagnosed megaloblastic anemia can develop severe anemia and cardiac comorbidities. Neuropsychiatric changes can become irreversible if the B12 deficiency is not treated promptly. Patients may also develop long-term complications from undiagnosed underlying etiologies.

There is no need for frequent monitoring of B12 and folate levels once the underlying cause of the deficiency has been identified and appropriate treatment has been started.

References

Carmel R, Agrawal YP: Failures of cobalamin assays in pernicious anemia, *N Engl J Med* 367:385–386, 2012.

Green R: Vitamin B₁₂ deficiency from the perspective of a practicing hematologist, *Blood* 129:2603–2611, 2017.

Inelmen EM, D'Alessio M, Gatto MR, et al: Descriptive analysis of the prevalence of anemia in a randomly selected sample of elderly people living at home: some results of an Italian multicentric study, *Aging (Milano)* 6:81–89, 1994.

Kassebaum NJ, Jasrasaria R, Naghavi M, et al: A systematic analysis of global anemia burden from 1990 to 2000, *Blood* 123:615–624, 2014.

Lahner E, Capasso M, et al: Incidence of cancer (other than gastric cancer) in pernicious anemia: a systematic review with meta-analysis, *Digestive and Liver Disease* 50(8):780–786, 2018.

Wazir SM: Ghobrial I: Copper deficiency, a new triad: anemia, leucopenia, and myeloneuropathy, *J Community Hosp Intern Med Perspect* 7(4):265–268, 2017 Oct.

Wang H, Li L, Qin LL, et al: Oral vitamin B12 versus intramuscular vitamin B12 for vitamin B12 deficiency, *Cochrane Database Syst Rev* 3:CD004655, 2018.

Wickramasinghe SN: Diagnosis of megaloblastic anemias, *Blood Reviews* 20(6):299–318, 2006.

PLATELET-MEDIATED BLEEDING DISORDERS

Eric H. Kraut, MD

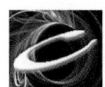

CURRENT DIAGNOSIS

- Platelet-mediated bleeding disorders commonly present with bleeding from mucosal surfaces or skin. Bleeding caused by reduced platelet counts may present with petechiae or purpura, whereas abnormalities of function are more likely to present with bleeding after injury or menstruation.
- Evaluation of platelet function used to be measured by the bleeding time. However, it is now more commonly evaluated by the platelet function analysis (PFA)-100 or platelet aggregation studies.
- Thrombocytopenia is most commonly caused by deficient production of platelets from the bone marrow, decreased platelet survival in the circulation, or sequestration of platelets by an enlarged spleen.
- Patients may bleed after trauma at platelet counts less than 50,000/μL and develop petechiae or purpura at platelet counts less than 20,000/μL, but they usually do not have severe bleeding unless platelet counts drop to less than 10,000/μL.
- The most common causes of new thrombocytopenia in the hospitalized patient are drugs or infection, whereas the usual cause of new platelet function abnormalities are medications.
- Patients in the hospital and placed on heparin should have their platelet counts monitored, and a reduction of 50% should be evaluated for heparin-induced thrombocytopenia (HIT).
- Immune thrombocytopenic purpura (ITP) usually presents in outpatients as new-onset mucocutaneous bleeding associated with only a reduced platelet count or unexplained asymptomatic isolated thrombocytopenia.
- Drugs that inhibit platelet activation and aggregation, such as aspirin, clopidogrel (Plavix), and dipyridamole (Persantine) can lead to significant bleeding, especially after surgery or procedures. This effect may last for 7 to 10 days.
- Patients presenting with a lifetime history of easy bruising and or heavy menses should have careful evaluation of their bleeding history and family history of bleeding. If positive, studies to rule out von Willebrand disease or hereditary disorders of platelet granules such as storage pool disorder should be done.

CURRENT THERAPY

- Patients with severe thrombocytopenia (platelet counts <10,000/μL) that is due to impaired production are at risk of severe bleeding and should be considered for platelet transfusions. The benefit of transfusing platelets when the platelet count reaches this level and the patient is not bleeding has been demonstrated as reducing bleeding in some patients in a recent study.
- Standard practice for platelet transfusions is to maintain platelet counts greater than 50,000/μL for patients with gastrointestinal bleeding and 75,000 to 100,000/μL for neurosurgical procedures. Platelet transfusions should be considered for certain other invasive procedures.
- Patients with immune thrombocytopenia should not receive platelet transfusions unless they are having significant bleeding because response to platelet transfusion occurs in less than 10% of patients and is short lasting.
- Patients with immune thrombocytopenic purpura (ITP) who have no bleeding and platelet counts greater than 30,000/μL can be followed without treatment because the risk of bleeding is low.

- In patients with ITP and thrombocytopenia less than 10,000/μL, initial treatment with high doses of corticosteroids in combination with intravenous immunoglobulin (IVIG; Gamunex) induces a rapid rise in platelets, usually within 24 hours.
- Current treatment for patients with ITP who fail prednisone treatment include splenectomy, rituximab (Rituxan),[1] or thrombopoietin agonists (romiplostim [Nplate] or eltrombopag [Promacta]).
- Patients with chronic renal failure can develop severe bleeding diathesis, which appears to be multifactorial including platelet dysfunction. Dialysis can reduce bleeding but not completely correct it. Other treatment that may help to include desmopressin (DDAVP),[1] tranexamic acid (Lysteda),[1] and synthetic erythropoietin (Epogen).[1]
- Patients with drug induced platelet dysfunction who may need to undergo surgery or who are bleeding may require platelet transfusions.
- Patients with inherited platelet disorders and mild bleeding can be treated with DDAVP but, if severe, may require platelet transfusions.

[1]Not FDA approved for this indication.

Platelets are small nonnucleated blood cells that are derived from bone marrow megakaryocytes. Their production is controlled by the hormone thrombopoietin produced in the liver, and they survive in the circulation for 8 to 10 days. On blood vessel injury, they form a seal or plug at the site of injury to limit bleeding. This initial event, termed *primary hemostasis*, occurs after endothelial injury when the subendothelial surface is exposed to circulating blood. Platelets are drawn to the site via von Willebrand factor (VWF), which, in combination with other proteins including fibrillar collagen, fibronectin, and laminin, leads to platelet adhesion. After platelets adhere to the vessel wall, they are activated, undergo a shape change, and release products from their granules. These platelet granule products, including adenosine diphosphate (ADP) and thromboxane A_2, further potentiate this process. Fibrinogen then binds to platelets via GPIIb/IIIa on the platelet surface causing firm platelet aggregation. The platelet secretory release reaction and aggregation recruits other platelets forming a firm hemostatic plug. Platelets also support the coagulation phase by interacting with circulating clotting factors and providing a surface for generation of thrombin. Secondary hemostasis occurs and thrombin-mediated fibrin mesh stabilizes the platelet plug.

Clinical Manifestations

The hallmark of platelet-mediated bleeding disorders is mucocutaneous bleeding such as nose bleeds, prolonged bleeding after tooth extractions, and heavy menstrual bleeding. When the platelet count drops to less than 30,000/μL, one may also see petechiae or purpuric lesions, especially on lower extremities.

Quantitative Platelet Disorders (Thrombocytopenia)

Primary hemostasis depends on an adequate number of platelets to prevent bleeding. A significant reduction in platelets or thrombocytopenia is usually defined as less than 100,000/μL. However, bleeding usually does not occur until the platelet count drops much lower. For example, spontaneous bleeding may only occur when the platelet count is less than 20,000/μL and severe life-threatening bleeding occurs only less than 10,000/μL. Thrombocytopenia can develop due to inadequate platelet production from the bone marrow, reduced platelet survival in the circulation, or sequestration of platelets in the spleen. Differentiating the cause requires evaluation of the patient's associated medical problems, physical findings, drug history, blood chemistry analysis, and possibly bone-marrow sampling.

Decreased platelet production is often the result of chemotherapeutic drugs for cancer, some antibiotics and antivirals (Table 1),

TABLE 1	Drugs Commonly Implicated as Causes of Drug-Induced Thrombocytopenia
CATEGORY	**IMPLICATED IN SEVERAL REPORTS**
Heparin	Unfractionated and low-molecular-weight heparin
Cinchona alkaloids	Quinidine, quinine
Platelet inhibitors	Abciximab (RepPro), eptifibatide (Integrilin), tirofiban (Aggrastat)
Antirheumatic agents	Gold salts
Antimicrobial agents	Linezolid (Zyvox), rifampin, sulfonamides, vancomycin
Sedatives and anticonvulsants	Valproic acid, phenytoin, carbamazepine
Histamine receptor antagonists	Cimetidine
Diuretic agents	Chlorothiazide
Analgesic agents	Acetaminophen, naproxen, diclofenac
Chemotherapy agents	Oxaliplatin (Eloxatin), fludarabine (Fludara), and others

or radiation therapy. These drugs may cause bone marrow injury, including damage to the megakaryocytes. Complete recovery may occur after stopping the offending agent. One common agent that can induce thrombocytopenia is alcohol. Thrombocytopenia associated with reduction in the white blood cell count and or red blood cell count should alert physicians to the possibility of a bone marrow disorder such as forms of leukemia or aplastic anemia. In cases where the cause is not evident, a bone marrow biopsy may be necessary to demonstrate whether there is a malignancy that may require urgent treatment.

Patients with reduced platelet production can often be observed without intervention depending on the severity of the thrombocytopenia, presence of bleeding, or the need to perform invasive procedures. Guidelines for transfusion of platelets to prevent bleeding (prophylactic transfusion) have changed in the last few years. With evidence that severe bleeding may not occur in most patients until the platelet count is less than 10,000/μL, limited platelet resources, and potential for development of alloimmunization to platelets, transfusions are not usually given unless sustained platelet counts are less than 10,000/μL. When platelets are transfused, it is appropriate to measure the response with a platelet count 1 hour post transfusion. The platelet count should rise 30,000 to 40,000/μL for the usual four-pack of platelet transfusion. Patients requiring frequent transfusions may require single-donor apheresis or human leukocyte antigen–matched platelets to obtain a good response.

Thrombocytopenia Resulting from Increased Platelet Destruction

Normally, platelets live in the circulation for 10 days, and the bone marrow replenishes them at the same rate that they are destroyed. Platelet survival may be altered by both nonimmune and immune processes. Severe infections will often lead to increased platelet destruction, and the platelet count returns to normal when the infection is adequately treated. Consumption of platelets also can occur in association with microangiopathic hemolytic anemia, as seen in disseminated intravascular coagulation (DIC) and thrombotic thrombocytopenic purpura and hemolytic uremic syndrome (TTP/HUS). It is important to review the blood smear to document fragmented red blood cells and evaluate coagulation parameters to help differentiate DIC from TTP/HUS and other causes of consumption. TTP/HUS may require specific and urgent treatment to prevent life-threatening complications.

Platelet transfusions are not usually given for TTP because there are reports of patients deteriorating after transfusions.

Immune-mediated platelet destruction is seen in response to several common drugs, including the sulfonamides and vancomycin. The characteristic pattern of immune-mediated platelet destruction is a sharp drop in the platelet count 7 to 10 days after starting the drug. The platelet count may drop to 5000/μL or less. Recognition is important because significant bleeding may occur, and the platelet count will only improve after discontinuation of the drug. Glycoprotein IIa/IIIb inhibitors, which are often used after cardiac stent placement, may cause a dramatic drop in the platelet count to as low as 1000/μL within hours of administration. This is important to recognize because this is one case where platelet transfusions may be necessary to prevent severe bleeding and it can be easily confused with other causes of low platelet counts.

Heparin-induced thrombocytopenia (HIT) is a unique drug reaction for several reasons. First, although thrombocytopenia is the initial sign of this entity, the major and feared complication is arterial and venous thromboses. It appears to affect 4% to 5% of patients exposed to unfractionated heparin and approximately 0.5% of patients exposed to low-molecular-weight heparin. Those at highest risk are female surgical patients who receive a minimum of 4 days of either type of heparin. The classic pattern is exposure to heparin at any dose with development of antibodies to heparin at day 4 and a 50% reduction in platelet count by day 6. The antibodies responsible are to the heparin–platelet factor 4 complex (IgG-PF4). A suspicious clinical pattern and a high antibody titer measured by an enzyme-linked immunosorbent assay are often diagnostic. Patients suspected of having HIT are at a high risk of thromboembolic disease within the first 24 hours of the drop in platelet count, and the heparin should be immediately stopped. However, despite the reduced platelet count, bleeding is unusual. Patients should be placed on an alternative anticoagulant, usually a direct thrombin inhibitor. The platelet count takes approximately 2 weeks to return to normal, and warfarin (Coumadin) should not be started until the platelet count returns to normal to avoid warfarin-associated necrosis. By reducing protein C and protein S, warfarin creates a temporary hypercoagulable state and places the patient at risk for warfarin-associated necrosis during the time when patients are most susceptible to thrombosis from HIT.

Immune thrombocytopenic purpura (ITP), previously termed *idiopathic thrombocytopenic purpura* affects 1 to 3 people per 100,000 but is probably the most common cause of severe isolated thrombocytopenia seen in the outpatient setting. It affects all ages, although ITP in childhood has a unique natural history. Childhood ITP is often associated with viral illness, is commonly transient, and may not need treatment. In adults, 40% of patients may have protracted or recurrent episodes of ITP, and the majority of patients need treatment. It was demonstrated in the 1950s that ITP is caused by circulating antiplatelet antibodies, and, like many autoimmune diseases, it is more common in women. When ITP presents in association with other diseases such as systemic lupus erythematosus or chronic lymphatic leukemia, or in patients with HIV, management of the underlying disease is important. The clinical presentation of ITP depends on the degree of thrombocytopenia. Mild thrombocytopenia of 20,000 to 80,000/μL is often asymptomatic, whereas platelet counts less than 20,000/μL may present with mucocutaneous bleeding and diffuse petechiae and purpura. Thrombocytopenia, an otherwise normal blood count, and peripheral blood smear without evidence of splenomegaly in a patient with no other illness helps to make a tentative diagnosis. A bone marrow biopsy is no longer considered necessary to confirm the diagnosis.

Treatment of ITP has changed over the past several years, and initial treatment after the diagnosis requires evaluation of the platelet count, whether it is increasing or decreasing, and the presence or absence of bleeding. Patients who have counts greater than 20,000/μL without bleeding and who are not in need of an invasive procedure can be observed without intervention. Patients with counts between 10,000 and 20,000/µL may be started on oral prednisone at 1 mg/kg. Patients with severe thrombocytopenia less than 10,000/µL and those who are bleeding can receive high-dose dexamethasone (Decadron) at 40 mg daily for 4 days and intravenous immunoglobulin (IVIG; Gamunex). There is usually a response to treatment within 24 hours. Although usually not helpful or required, approximately 10% of patients will have a response to platelet transfusion, and this can be considered for patients presenting with low platelet counts and bleeding. Refractory or recurrent ITP is a common problem in these patients, and recommendations for treatment include splenectomy, rituximab (Rituxan)[1], or thrombopoietin agonists. The choice of which to use depends on the patient and his or her clinical condition.

Thrombocytopenia Due to Hypersplenism
The platelet mass is distributed 70% in the circulation and 30% in the spleen. Enlargement of the spleen and/or alteration of blood flow in portal hypertension may increase platelet sequestration in the spleen and reduce the platelet count in the peripheral blood circulation. Patients' counts rarely drop to less than 20,000/µL. Thus thrombocytopenia caused by hypersplenism does not usually need any intervention. Patients with hepatitis C and cirrhosis may present with low platelet counts, and this may represent both hypersplenism and secondary immune thrombocytopenia. A trial of steroids may be used if these patients' clinical situation requires therapy.

Qualitative Platelet Function Disorders
Acquired Qualitative Platelet Function Disorders
Acquired disorders of platelet function are commonly seen, because platelets are the target of medications used to prevent arterial and cardiac stent thrombosis. Spontaneous bleeding is not common, but bleeding resulting from trauma or surgery can be a significant clinical problem. Because many patients may be on multiple antiplatelet agents or anticoagulants at the same time, the risk of bleeding needs to be recognized. Acquired qualitative disorders of platelet function may be due to drugs, hematologic diseases, or medical illnesses.

Drugs are the most common cause of acquired platelet dysfunction with differing risks of bleeding due to different targets. Aspirin causes irreversible acetylation of cyclooxygenase I (COX-1) and inhibits generation of prostaglandin A2. Although it is considered a weak antiplatelet agent with up to 25% resistance, aspirin increases the risk of bleeding in otherwise normal patients. Major bleeding was seen in up to 3.7% of patients and, when aspirin is used in combination with other antiplatelet agents or in patients with underlying bleeding disorders, the bleeding risk is higher. Clopidogrel (Plavix) is a thienopyridine prodrug, and the active metabolite irreversibly inhibits the surface receptor $P2Y_{12}$ on platelets. In clinical trials the risk of major bleeding in patients taking clopidogrel was similar to what is described with aspirin. Clopidogrel may significantly increase bleeding after surgery. GPIIb/IIIa receptor antagonists used after cardiac stent placement inhibit platelet aggregation and can induce severe thrombocytopenia.

Malignancies of the bone marrow may produce abnormally functioning platelets or alter platelet function by affecting VWF. The myeloproliferative and myelodysplastic disorders may produce platelets with reduced numbers of granules and may have associated increased risk of gastrointestinal bleeding and bleeding after invasive procedures. Acquired von Willebrand disease, an infrequent cause of abnormal bleeding, can be seen in patients with lymphoproliferative disease, multiple myeloma, and Waldenström macroglobulinemia.

Systemic illness can alter platelets and increase the bleeding risk. Acute and chronic renal failure are common causes of platelet-function abnormalities. In uremia, hemorrhagic complications include upper gastrointestinal bleeding, pericardial bleeding, and intracranial bleeding. Bleeding in renal failure is believed to be multifactorial and includes impaired release of platelet granules, decreased prostaglandin formation, VWF dysfunction, and presence of severe anemia. Effective treatment includes improvement of the anemia with erythropoietin (Epogen)[1] or DDAVP[1] or conjugated estrogens (Premarin).[1]

Hereditary Qualitative Platelet Function Disorders
Inherited abnormalities of platelet function are infrequent disorders that give rise to bleeding of varying severity. Inherited abnormalities of platelet function are often classified according to the type of genetic defect. Bernard-Soulier syndrome (BSS) is a severe bleeding disorder with autosomal recessive inheritance characterized by thrombocytopenia, decreased platelet adhesion, reduced platelet survival, and giant platelets on blood smear. Patients with BSS have defects in the GPIb-IX-V complex leading to reduced binding to VWF. Glanzmann thrombasthenia is an autosomal recessive disorder with defects of integrin αIIbβ3, a receptor on activated platelets that normally binds platelets during aggregation. Platelet aggregation to ADP and thrombin is abnormal. Patients with BSS and Glanzmann thrombasthenia who need treatment require platelet transfusions.

Hereditary disorders of platelet secretion are common reasons patients present to clinicians for evaluation of mucocutaneous bleeding. Defects in platelet dense granules (δ storage pool disease) are suspected in patients with a negative work-up for von Willebrand disease. Diagnosis is made by platelet electron microscopy and or platelet aggregation studies. Granule deficiency associated with abnormalities of other lysosome-related organelles may lead to specific phenotypes such as Hermansky-Pudlak and Chediak-Higashi disease. Gray platelet syndrome (GPS), or alpha granule deficiency, is an autosomal recessive disorder with mild bleeding. GPS patients may also be thrombocytopenic. Treatment for bleeding or in preparation for surgery includes DDAVP[1] or platelet transfusions.

---

[1]Not FDA approved for this indication.

References
Aster RH, Curtis BR, McFarland JG, Bougie DW: Drug-induced immune thrombocytopenia: pathogenesis, diagnosis, and management, *J Thromb Haemost* 7:911–918, 2009.

Barbour T, Johnson S, Cohney S, Hughes P: Thrombotic microangiopathy and associated renal disorders, *Nephrol Dial Transplant* 27:2673–2685, 2012.

Estcourt L, Stanworth S, Doree C, et al: Prophylactic platelet transfusion in prevention of bleeding in patients with hematologic disorders and stem cell transplantation, *Cochrane Database Syst Rev* 5:CD004269, 2012. 10.1002/14651858. CD004269.pub.

Hedges SJ, Dehoney SB, Hooper JS, et al: Evidence-based treatment recommendations for uremic bleeding, *Nat Clin Pract Nephrol* 3:138–153, 2007.

Jackson S: Arterial thrombosis: insidious, unpredictable, and deadly, *Nat Med* 17:1423–1436, 2011.

Kam T, Alexander M: *Drug induced immune thrombocytopenia, J Parm Pract* 27:430–439, 2014.

Neunert C, Tenell D, Arnold DM: American Society of Hematology 2019 guidelines for immune thrombocytopenia, *Blood Adv* 10:3829–3866, 2019.

Nurden A, Nurden P: Advances in our understanding of the molecular basis of disorders of platelet function, *J Thromb Haemost Suppl* 1:76–91, 2011.

Raschke RA, Gallo T, Cunz SC, et al: Clinical effectiveness of a Bayesian algorithm for the diagnosis and management of heparin induced thrombocytopenia, *J Thromb Haemost* 15:1640–1645, 2017.

Stanworth SJ, et al: Risk of bleeding and use of platelet transfusions in patients with hematologic malignancies: recurrent event analysis, *Haematol* 100(6):740–747, 2015.

Tsantes AE, Nikolopoulos GK, Tsirigotis P, et al: Direct evidence for normalization of platelet function resulting from platelet count reduction in essential thrombocytosis, *Blood Coagul Fibrinolysis* 22:457–462, 2011.

Warkentin AE, Donadni MP, Spencer FA, et al: Bleeding risk in randomized controlled trials comparing warfarin and aspirin: a systemic review and meta-analysis, *J Thromb Haemost* 10:512–520, 2012.

Zucker ML, Hagedorn CH, Murphy CA, et al: Mechanism of thrombocytopenia in chronic hepatitis C as evaluated by the immature platelet fraction, *Int J Lab Hematol* 34:525–532, 2012.

POLYCYTHEMIA VERA

Method of
Peter R. Duggan, MD; and Sonia Cerquozzi, MD

CURRENT DIAGNOSIS

- Polycythemia vera (PV) should be considered when there is persistent elevation of hemoglobin (> 165 g/L in men and > 160 g/L in women) or hematocrit (> 49% in men and > 48% in women).
- *JAK2V617F* mutation testing and erythropoietin levels should be performed when PV is suspected.
- Bone marrow biopsy and aspiration may be necessary in some cases to confirm the diagnosis of PV and to distinguish PV from other myeloproliferative neoplasms (MPNs).
- PV is highly likely when *JAK2V617F* mutation is present and erythropoietin level is subnormal. When *JAK2V617F* mutation is seen with normal erythropoietin level, PV is possible; bone marrow biopsy is recommended to differentiate PV from other MPNs. When *JAK2V617F* is normal and erythropoietin is low, consider *JAK2* exon 12 mutational analysis or alternative diagnosis of congenital polycythemia. Wildtype *JAK2V617F* with normal or high erythropoietin level makes PV very unlikely, and patients should be investigated for secondary causes of polycythemia.
- Investigations for secondary polycythemia that may be indicated include:
  - Chest x-ray
  - Pulse oximetry
  - Arterial blood gas including carboxyhemoglobin and methemoglobin levels
  - Kidney and liver function tests
  - Abdominal imaging studies (ultrasound or computed tomography [CT] scan)
  - Oxyhemoglobin dissociation curve
  - Nocturnal polysomnography

CURRENT THERAPY

- All patients should be treated with phlebotomy and/or cytoreductive therapy to target hematocrit less than 45%.
- Low-dose aspirin[1] (acetylsalicylic acid [ASA]) should be used in *all patients* without a contraindication.
- In *high-risk* patients with PV (age ≥ 60 years and/or history of thrombosis), cytoreductive therapy should be used in combination with ASA.
- Alkylating agents should be avoided as cytoreductive therapy owing to the risk of acute leukemia.
- Conventional cardiovascular risk factors (diabetes, hypertension, hyperlipidemia) should be aggressively managed, and cigarette smoking should be discouraged.
- Thromboembolic events should be managed according to accepted management guidelines. Thromboprophylaxis should be used after surgery and in other high-risk situations.

[1]Not US Food and Drug Administration (FDA) approved for this indication.

Polycythemia vera is a clonal stem cell disorder characterized by an increase in red cell production independent of the stimulation by erythropoietin. PV is the most common of the chronic myeloproliferative neoplasms (MPNs), occurring in approximately 2 to 3 people per 100,000 annually. The median age at diagnosis is 70 years, and it is rare in patients younger than 40 years.

A mutation of the tyrosine kinase Janus kinase 2 (*JAK2*) is consistently found in PV. This sheds some light on the pathogenesis of the disease and is useful in the diagnosis of PV and other MPNs. A single acquired mutation (*V617F*) of the gene for the JH-2 domain of *JAK2* can be found in 90% to 95% of patients with PV. The JH-2 domain functions to inhibit *JAK2* activity. In normal erythropoiesis, binding of erythropoietin to its receptor lifts this inhibition and allows *JAK2* stimulation of cell division and differentiation. In mutated *JAK2*, this inhibitory function is absent, leading to constitutive activity of the tyrosine kinase. This mutation is also present in about half of patients with essential thrombocytosis and primary myelofibrosis. The small number of patients with PV who are negative for the common *JAK2V617F* mutation have another functionally similar mutation within *exon 12*.

Presentation

Many patients with PV are asymptomatic, and PV is diagnosed after the incidental finding of an elevated hemoglobin or hematocrit on routine complete blood count. Splenomegaly is present in 30% to 40% of patients. Up to half of patients experience nonspecific symptoms such as weight loss, sweating, headache, fatigue, epigastric discomfort, visual disturbances, and dizziness. Many of these symptoms are likely caused by decreased blood flow due to an increased blood viscosity from polycythemia.

Generalized pruritus is often described, often after a warm bath or shower (aquagenic pruritus). Although the cause of this is unknown, it is thought to be due to the degranulation of increased numbers of mast cells in the skin of patients, releasing histamine and other inflammatory mediators. However, the symptom responds poorly to antihistamines, and it does not always resolve with treatment of PV.

Venous and arterial thromboembolic events are a major cause of morbidity and mortality in PV. Thrombosis at presentation occurs in up to 40% of patients. Ischemic stroke, transient ischemic attack, and myocardial infarction are common, especially among elderly patients. These, along with deep venous thrombosis and pulmonary embolus, are the most common thrombotic events and often result in serious morbidity, disability, and even death. Thrombotic events that are considered unusual in the general population, such as Budd-Chiari syndrome; portal, mesenteric, and other abdominal vein thrombosis; and cerebral venous thrombosis, occur more commonly among patients with PV. The possibility of an underlying MPN should be considered when a patient presents with such an event.

PV can manifest with symptoms of peripheral vascular disease. Patients with erythromelalgia describe a painful burning sensation of the hands and feet; pallor, erythema, or cyanosis of the extremities; and sometimes cutaneous ulceration. Erythromelalgia results from microvascular thrombosis and ischemia due to platelet activation and aggregation and responds well to platelet reduction and antiplatelet agents such as aspirin (ASA).[1]

Almost all patients with PV are iron deficient at diagnosis, even before the onset of therapeutic phlebotomy. Other manifestations of PV include acute gouty arthritis, peptic ulcer disease, erosive gastritis, and hypertension.

Diagnosis and Differential Diagnosis

The 2016 World Health Organization (WHO) diagnostic criteria for PV are shown in Box 1. The *JAK2V617F* mutation is present in about 95% of cases of PV. Erythropoietin level is decreased in more than 90% and is rarely elevated. Few patients with PV carry a mutation of exon 12 (~4%) of the *JAK2* gene instead of the more common *JAK2V617F* mutation. A *JAK2* mutation can also be found in about half of patients with essential thrombocytosis and primary myelofibrosis.

Leukocytosis and thrombocytosis are present in the majority of cases of PV. Red cell mass is increased. A nuclear medicine study measuring red cell mass and plasma volume is rarely required with the availability of *JAK2* testing, but it may be useful when

[1]Not FDA approved for this indication.

VI Hematology

470

BOX 1 2016 World Health Organization Diagnostic Criteria for Polycythemia Vera

Diagnosis requires three major criteria or first two major criteria and minor criterion.*

Major Criteria
1. Hemoglobin > 165 g/L in men, 160 g/L in women,
   or
   Hematocrit > 49% in men, > 48% in women,
   or
   Other evidence of increased red cell volume†
2. Bone marrow biopsy: hypercellular for age with trilineage growth (panmyelosis)
3. Presence of *JAK2V617F* or *JAK2* exon 12 mutation

Minor Criterion
1. Subnormal serum erythropoietin level

---

*Bone marrow biopsy may not be required in sustained erythrocytosis—hemoglobin > 185 g/L (hematocrit > 55.5%) in men or > 165 g/L (hematocrit > 49.5%) in women—if major criterion 3 and minor criterion are present.
†> 25% above mean normal predicted value.

BOX 2 Differential Diagnosis of Polycythemia

Normal Red Cell Mass
Relative polycythemia
Gaisböck syndrome

Elevated Red Cell Mass
Primary Polycythemia
Polycythemia vera

Secondary Polycythemia
- Congenital EPO receptor mutations
- Chuvash polycythemia
- High-affinity hemoglobin
Appropriately elevated EPO (hypoxia driven)
- Chronic hypoxic lung disease
- Cardiac shunts or cyanotic heart disease
- Sleep apnea
- Methemoglobinemia
- High altitude
- Chronic carbon monoxide poisoning
- Cigarette smoking
- Renal artery stenosis
Inappropriately elevated EPO
- Renal cell carcinoma
- Hepatocellular carcinoma
- Hemangioblastoma
- Uterine fibroids
Other causes:
- Erythropoetin stimulating agents (ESA)
- Androgens (testosterone)
- Kidney transplant

Abbreviation: EPO = erythropoietin.

BOX 3 Thrombotic Risk in Polycythemia Vera

Low Risk
Age < 60 years and no history of thrombosis

High Risk
Age ≥ 60 years and/or history of thrombosis

---

relative polycythemia is suspected. Bone marrow biopsy and aspiration are not often needed for a diagnosis of PV but have been included as a major criterion within the revised WHO classification. Bone marrow examination can be important for diagnosing PV in the rare cases where *JAK2* is negative and to differentiate PV from other *JAK2*-positive MPNs when the distinction cannot be made based on peripheral blood counts.

Erythrocytosis can occur as a result of a number of other conditions in the absence of PV (Box 2). A careful history and physical examination with selected investigations can usually distinguish PV from secondary polycythemia and relative polycythemia (see Current Diagnosis). In relative (apparent, spurious) polycythemia, there is usually only a modest increase in the hematocrit, because of a decrease in plasma volume rather than a true increase in red cell mass. Thrombocytosis, leukocytosis, and splenomegaly should be absent. Causes include smoking, dehydration, and use of diuretics, and it is also described in middle-aged, obese, hypertensive men (Gaisböck syndrome).

Red cell mass can be elevated owing to increased stimulation of erythropoiesis by high levels of erythropoietin. Erythropoietin can be increased as an appropriate response to chronic hypoxia (sleep apnea, right-to-left cardiac shunts, chronic lung disease, high altitude, smoking, methemoglobinemia), and it can be inappropriately elevated owing to erythropoietin-secreting tumors (renal cell carcinoma, hepatocellular carcinoma, cerebellar hemangioma, uterine fibroids) or decreased kidney perfusion (renal artery stenosis). Familial causes of polycythemia include high-affinity hemoglobins, erythropoietin receptor mutations, and Chuvash polycythemia. Polycythemia occurs in 10% to 15% of patients following kidney transplantation, and this may be due to erythropoietin secretion by the native kidneys or increased sensitivity to erythropoietin. Polycythemia can be drug induced, such as with the use of performance-enhancing drugs (erythropoietin [Epogen], androgens) in athletes and testosterone replacement in men.

Prognosis

Patients with PV have a reduced life expectancy compared with the general population, with a median survival of approximately 14 years, or 24 years if younger than age 60 at diagnosis.

Despite therapy, thrombosis remains an important cause of mortality. Cardiac disease, ischemic stroke, pulmonary embolus, and other thrombotic events account for 40% of deaths among patients with PV. Nonfatal thrombosis is common, occurring in almost 4% of patients annually. Age and a history of prior thromboembolic events are independent risk factors for thrombosis and

can be used to predict a patient's risk of future events (Box 3). Low-risk patients are younger than 60 years and have no history of thrombosis. They experience new events at a rate of 2% per year. For patients older than 60 years or with a past history of thrombosis, this rate is 5% annually, but it can be as high as 11% when both risk factors are present.

The contribution of other cardiovascular risk factors (smoking, diabetes, hypertension, hyperlipidemia) to thrombotic risk in PV has been studied, with inconclusive results. However, because these are major contributors to the development of cardiovascular disease in the general population, they should also be considered when assessing risk in patients with PV. Leukocytosis (white blood cell count > 15×10^9/L) has been associated with a higher risk of arterial thrombosis.

Conversely, the risk of major hemorrhage is low, with fatal bleeding responsible for less than 5% of all deaths. However, there is considerable excess mortality from malignancy, in particular transformation to a myelodysplastic syndrome, myelofibrosis, or acute leukemia. The rate of leukemic transformation is less than 10% at 20 years. Risk factors for leukemic transformation include advanced age, leukocytosis, and abnormal karyotype. Approximately 10% of patients transform to myelofibrosis (post-PV myelofibrosis). Risk factors for post-PV myelofibrosis include leukocytosis and *JAK2V617F* allele burden of greater than 50%.

Treatment

The goals of treatment in PV are to lower the risk of thrombosis while minimizing toxicity. This is achieved by a combination of phlebotomy, aspirin,[1] and hydroxyurea (Hydrea)[1] or other cytoreductive agents. The use of these therapies can be individualized based on a patient's risk of developing future thromboembolic events. Risk stratification (Box 3) aims at identifying patients with PV at higher risk of thrombotic events who require cytoreductive therapy. Because cerebrovascular and cardiovascular disease are among the main causes of morbidity and mortality for these patients, careful attention should be paid to the management of conventional cardiovascular risk factors. Hypertension, diabetes, and hyperlipidemia should be controlled with standard measures based on current guidelines, and patients should be encouraged to stop smoking. As the hematocrit increases in PV, there is a dramatic increase in blood viscosity. Phlebotomy is the fastest, most effective way to normalize a patient's hematocrit, and it should be initiated immediately in those with newly diagnosed PV. Blood volume should be reduced as rapidly as possible. Usually, 500 mL of blood is removed every 1 or 2 days until the hematocrit is less than 45%. The frequency of phlebotomy or volume of blood removed can be decreased in elderly patients, those with cardiovascular disease, or others who do not tolerate this schedule. The optimal target in patients with PV is to maintain a hematocrit less than 45% to lower the risk of major thrombotic events and death from cardiovascular causes. Regular phlebotomy eventually results in iron deficiency, at which point most patients' phlebotomy needs decrease dramatically. Iron replacement should be avoided.

Aspirin

Previous studies did not support the routine use of aspirin to prevent thrombosis in PV. However, high doses of aspirin were used in these early studies, resulting in excess bleeding in the treatment arm. The results of a recent large randomized trial show that low-dose aspirin (100 mg/day) reduces major thrombotic events (nonfatal myocardial infarction, nonfatal stroke, pulmonary embolism, major venous thrombosis). This was accomplished without an increase in bleeding risk. Although there was a trend suggesting more minor bleeding events in those receiving aspirin, the rates of major bleeding were identical for those receiving aspirin or placebo. The benefit from aspirin was seen, even though this study included many low-risk patients without a prior history of thromboembolism. Low-dose aspirin (75–100 mg daily)[1] should be started in all patients without a contraindication to the drug (history of bleeding or intolerance). Because of the risk of bleeding from acquired von Willebrand disease that can occur with extreme thrombocytosis, aspirin should be held when platelets are more than 1500×10^9/L until the count can be lowered by cytoreduction.

Cytoreductive Therapy

Cytoreductive therapy is recommended for high-risk patients with PV (Box 3). Hydroxyurea (HU)[1] is the cytoreductive agent most commonly used to treat PV. Hydroxyurea can safely control blood counts and decreases spleen size in PV and other MPNs. Randomized data are limited, but hydroxyurea also appears to reduce thrombotic complications. A starting dosage of 15 to 20 mg/kg daily (1000–1500 mg daily) is used. Occasional phlebotomy is still required to maintain hematocrit less than 45%, but the frequency usually decreases. Myelosuppression is the main toxicity. The lowest dosage that provides therapeutic effect should be used, and excess myelosuppression should be avoided. The dosage can be titrated to ensure that the white cell count remains higher than 3.0×10^9/L, neutrophils are higher than 2.0×10^9/L, and platelets are in the normal range.

Hydroxyurea has been associated with leg ulcers and other skin changes, especially after long-term use. There is growing evidence that hydroxyurea does not contribute to the excess rates of acute leukemia seen in PV; rates are no different than in those treated with phlebotomy alone. However, transformation is clearly associated with the use of other chemotherapeutic agents such as chlorambucil (Leukeran)[1], busulfan (Myleran)[1], and pipobroman (Vercyte),[2] accounting for one-third of the deaths among patients with PV treated with these agents. The use of these agents should be avoided. Hydroxyurea resistance can occur in up to 11% of patients and is associated with increased risk of death. Both hydroxyurea resistance and intolerance are defined according to the European Leukemia Net (ELN) criteria.

Interferon-α2b (IFN-α2) (Intron A)[1] is an alternative treatment option in the setting of hydroxyurea resistance and/or intolerance and often is considered in young patients with PV. IFN-αb is available in both short-acting and controlled-release (pegylated) formulations. IFN-α is commonly administered subcutaneously with a starting dose of 3 million units daily, or pegylated IFN-α (Peg-Intron)[1] is given at 45 to 90 μg weekly. Studies have shown its efficacy in controlling blood counts in addition to achieving complete hematologic and molecular responses. The inconvenience of its administration and its side effects including mood disturbances and flulike illness make it a less desirable therapy. Controlled studies are comparing hydroxyurea with pegylated forms of IFN-α. At present, both are first-line cytoreductive treatment options with recommendations that IFN-α be used in females with childbearing potential.

JAK Inhibitors

Ruxolitinib (Jakafi), a *JAK1/2* inhibitor, was originally approved in patients with myelofibrosis, including myelofibrosis evolving from PV. There was a significant reduction in spleen size and constitutional symptoms in almost half of these patients. In the phase III RESPONSE trial, ruxolitinib illustrated its effectiveness in controlling hematocrit (< 45%), reducing spleen size (≥ 35%), and improving symptoms in patients with PV who had hydroxyurea intolerance or resistance, resulting in its approval as a second-line cytoreductive agent in PV. The most common side effects are anemia, thrombocytopenia, and atypical infection risk.

Other Treatment Issues

Hyperuricemia is common in myeloproliferative neoplasms and occasionally results in kidney stones or gout. Allopurinol (Zyloprim) 300 mg daily can be used to reduce uric acid levels in patients with these complications. For those with intractable pruritus, several agents have been used with variable success. Some patients respond to aspirin,[1] hydroxyurea[1], cimetidine (Tagamet)[1], cyproheptadine (Periactin)[1], and paroxetine (Paxil)[1] 20 mg daily. Both IFN-α[1] and ruxolitinib have been successful in the majority of cases.

Less than 60% of pregnancies occurring in patients with PV are successful. First-trimester fetal loss is the most common complication, and third-trimester fetal loss, preterm birth, and intrauterine growth restriction are also common. Phlebotomy should be used to keep the hematocrit at less than 45%. Interferon-α2b[1] is recommended for those requiring cytoreductive therapy during pregnancy; other cytoreductive agents are contraindicated owing to possible teratogenic effects. There is some evidence that the use of low-dose aspirin[1] throughout pregnancy improves live birth rate. It is recommended that prophylactic low-molecular-weight heparin (LMWH) be used for 6 weeks postpartum.

Surgery in patients with PV has a high risk of both operative bleeding and postoperative thromboembolism. Elective surgeries should be delayed until cytoreductive measures and phlebotomy can be used to achieve good control of blood counts. Aspirin should be held for 1 week before surgery to reduce the risk of hemorrhage. LMWH should be given after surgery to prevent deep venous thrombosis. Mechanical compression stockings are

---

[1]Not FDA approved for this indication.

[1]Not FDA approved for this indication.
[2]Not available in the United States.

an option for patients with bleeding that prevents the use of anti-coagulation. When thromboembolic events do occur, treatment should be according to current management guidelines. Venous thromboembolism is treated with LMWH and warfarin (Coumadin). Indefinite anticoagulation should be considered because of the high risk of recurrent events. Low-dose aspirin is indicated in those with a history of arterial events such as stroke and myocardial infarction.

References

Arber DA, Orazi A, Hasserjian R, et al: The 2016 revision to the World Health Organization classification of myeloid neoplasms and acute leukemia, *Blood* 127(20):2391–2405, 2016.

Barosi G, Birgegard G, Finazzi G, et al: A unified definition of clinical resistance and intolerance to hydroxycarbamide in polycythemia vera and primary myelofibrosis: results of a European LeukemiaNet (ELN) consensus process, *Br J Haematol* 148:961–963, 2010.

Finazzi G, Caruso V, Marchioli R, et al: for the ECLAP Investigators: Acute leukemia in polycythemia vera: an analysis of 1638 patients enrolled in a prospective observational study, *Blood* 105(7):2664–2670, 2005.

Kiladjian JJ, Cassinat B, Chevret S, et al: Pegylated interferon-alfa-2a induces complete hematologic and molecular responses with low toxicity in polycythemia vera, *Blood* 112:3065–3072, 2008.

Landolfi R, Marchioli R, Kutti J, et al: Efficacy and safety of low-dose aspirin in polycythemia vera, *N Engl J Med* 350:114–124, 2004.

Marchioli R, Finazzi G, Landolfi R, et al: Vascular and neoplastic risk in a large cohort of patients with polycythemia vera, *J Clin Oncol* 23(10):2224–2232, 2005.

Marchioli R, Finazzi G, Specchia G, et al: Cardiovascular events and intensity of treatment in polycythemia vera, *N Engl J Med* 368:22–33, 2013.

Passamonti F: How I treat polycythemia vera, *Blood* 120(2):275–284, 2012.

Passamonti F, Rumi E, Caramella M, et al: A dynamic prognostic model to predict survival in post-polycythemia vera myelofibrosis, *Blood* 111(7):3383–3387, 2008.

Quintas-Cardama A, Kantarjian H, Manshouri T, et al: Pegylated interferon alfa-2a yields high rates of hematologic and molecular response in patients with advanced essential thrombocythemia and polycythemia vera, *J Clin Oncol* 27:5418–5424, 2009.

Tefferi A, Barbui T: Polycythemia vera and essential thrombocythemia: 2015 update on diagnosis, risk-stratification and management, *Am J Hematol* 90(2):163–173, 2015.

Tefferi A, Guglielmelli P, Larson DR, et al: Long-term survival and blast transformation in molecularly annotated essential thrombocythemia, polycythemia vera, and myelofibrosis, *Blood* 124(16):2507–2513, 2014.

Tefferi A, Rumi E, Finazzi G, et al: Survival and prognosis among 1545 patients with contemporary polycythemia vera: an international study, *Leukemia* 27:1874–1881, 2013.

Vannucchi AM, Kiladjian JJ, Griesshammer M, et al: Ruxolitinib versus standard therapy for the treatment of polycythemia vera, *N Engl J Med* 372:426–435, 2015.

PORPHYRIAS

Method of
Marshall Mazepa, MD; and Gregory Vercellotti, MD

CURRENT DIAGNOSIS

- Making the diagnosis relies on, first, an awareness and index of suspicion for these rare conditions, which manifest as either unexplained abdominal pain and neurologic symptoms, photosensitive skin lesions (some blistering and some not), or both.
- Patients with inexplicable recurrent abdominal pain may request an evaluation for acute intermittent porphyria (AIP), which can be excluded with a spot urine aminolevulinic acid (ALA) and porphobilinogen (PBG) test. Urine ALA and PGB will be extremely elevated at the time of acute attack, which is the ideal time to make the diagnosis, but levels *will remain elevated* (many times the upper limit of normal) for many weeks to months afterward, which can facilitate making the diagnosis in the nonacute setting.
- Porphyria cutanea tarda (PCT), the most common form of porphyria, is typically acquired, concurrent with iron overload, hepatitis C infection, and/or smoking. It classically presents with blistering skin lesions on the backs of the hands due to sun exposure.

CURRENT THERAPY

- Patients should avoid alcohol consumption, smoking, hormone therapy, and drugs known to trigger attacks.
- Treatment of acute neurovisceral pain attacks includes outpatient oral carbohydrate loading or intravenous hemin (Panhematin) for treatment of severe attacks that require hospitalization.
- For patients with an acute hepatic porphyria (AHP) and recurrent severe neurovisceral attacks, givosiran (Givlaari), a small interfering RNA targeting aminolevulinic acid synthase-1 (ALAS-1), was recently US Food and Drug Administration (FDA) approved as a preventive therapy to reduce the frequency of attacks.
- For patients with erythropoietic protoporphyria (EPP), afamelanotide (Scenesse), an analogue of human α-melanocyte-stimulating hormone (α-MSH) that stimulates melanin production, was recently FDA approved for reduction in EPP-related photosensitivity.

The porphyrias refer to a family of metabolic disorders of heme synthesis, where symptoms occur due to abnormal accumulation of metabolites, and most are congenital. Porphyria cutanea tarda (PCT) is the exception, which is caused by the acquired inhibition of hepatic uroporphyrinogen decarboxylase (UROD), commonly associated with hepatitis C virus (HCV) infection and iron overload. The porphyrias can be classified by the organ of heme precursor overproduction and acuity—the acute and chronic hepatic porphyrias and the acute erythropoietic porphyrias. This new system of classification has largely been driven by the development of new therapies that specifically target the metabolic driver of disease in the acute hepatic porphyrias (AHPs), including the recent FDA approval of givosiran (Givlaari) for AHPs. From a more practical standpoint, we recommend considering classifying the patient's symptoms as either neurovisceral alone, neurovisceral plus dermatologic, or dermatologic alone, because the symptoms inform potential diagnoses and requisite testing.

While there are at least nine porphyrias, from a therapy perspective, three porphyrias are the most important to recognize. Acute intermittent porphyria (AIP) is likely the most common AHP. Patients with unexplained recurrent abdominal pain may request an evaluation for this disorder from their primary care doctor or consultant. PCT is likely overall the most common porphyria, and treatment with phlebotomy and avoidance of alcohol and other triggers can lead to profound relief of symptoms. Erythropoietic protoporphyria (EPP) is a very rare porphyria with dermatologic findings only, and a new FDA-approved therapy increases melanocyte melanogenesis, which is protective against ultraviolet (UV) light-associated painful skin manifestations, the first of its kind. Given that these conditions are rare, we suggest coordinating diagnosis and management with an expert. The American Porphyria Foundation (APF) website (porphyriafoundation.org) provides an important resource for patients and providers alike, including US experts in the field.

Pathophysiology and Clinical Manifestations

The heme synthetic pathway includes eight enzymes (Table 1). Heme is primarily synthesized in bone marrow (giving rise to hemoglobin in erythroblasts) and about 20% in the liver. While the pathways to synthesize heme are similar in the two organs, regulation of the two pathways differs. Aminolevulinic acid synthase-1 (ALAS-1) regulates heme synthesis in the liver and other organs; ALAS-2 regulates heme synthesis in the bone marrow. Both heme (the end product of the pathway) and glucose down-regulate ALAS-1 activity through negative feedback, observations which inform treatment. Conversely, demand for ALAS-1 activity can be

TABLE 1 Heme Synthesis Pathway

METABOLITES	ENZYME	DISEASE	PATHOLOGY
Succinyl coenzyme A (CoA) and glycine			
Delta aminolevulinic acid (ALA)	ALA synthase (ALAS-1)	X-linked protoporphyria (XLP)	Gain-of-function mutation in ALA synthase Mimics EPP <10% of erythropoietic porphyrias (EPs) Males > females
Porphobilinogen (PBG)	ALA dehydratase	ALA dehydratase deficiency porphyria (ADP)	Elevated urine ALA
Hydroxymethylbilane	Porphobilinogen deaminase	**Acute intermittent porphyria (AIP)**	Elevated urine ALA and PBG
Uroporphyrinogen III	Uroporphyrinogen synthase	Congenital erythropoietic porphyria (CEP)	Excess erythrocyte, plasma porphyrins, urinary and fecal porphyrins; hemolytic anemia
Coproporphyrinogen III	Uroporphyinogen decarboxylase (UROD)	**Porphyria cutanea tarda (PCT)**	Elevated plasma and urine uroporphyrins Normal urine ALA and PBG
Protoporphyrinogen IX	Coproporphyrinogen oxidase (CPOX)	Hereditary coproporphyria (HCP)	Elevated urine ALA and PBG Plasma and stool porphyrins to differentiate VP
Protoporphyrin IX	Protoporphyrinogen oxidase (PPOX)	Variegate porphyria (VP)	Elevated urine ALA and PBG Plasma and stool porphyrins to differentiate HCP
Heme	Ferrochelatase	**Erythropoietic protoporphyria (EPP)**	Elevated erythrocyte, plasma, stool porphyrins

increased by many inducers of cytochrome P450 because heme is central to the function of these enzymes. Hence, drugs that induce cytochrome P450 should be avoided in patients with porphyria.

Clinical manifestations of the porphyrias include neurovisceral and/or dermatologic symptoms. The term *neurovisceral* refers to unexplained generalized abdominal pain plus neurologic symptoms ranging from mild neurologic manifestations (e.g., paresthesias and weakness) to, rarely, severe manifestations, including seizures and respiratory failure. Patients commonly describe a prodrome they recognize over time. Some patients can abort severe attacks with home measures such as carbohydrate consumption, rest, and hydration. They may also recognize extreme alcohol intolerance, triggers of attacks from new medications, herbs, or supplements, and, in women, onset of symptoms after puberty and during the luteal (premenstrual) stage of their menstrual cycle when progesterone levels are highest. Women are more commonly diagnosed with AHPs than men (estimated 4:1). Due to a delay in diagnosis, many patients have had multiple nondiagnostic evaluations or surgical interventions. Hyponatremia may occur during episodes and prompt treatment should be given to avoid precipitating seizures. Dark or reddish-tinged urine may also be present during an acute episode.

The dermatologic manifestations of the porphyrias include photosensitivity and either blistering or nonblistering skin lesions on sun-exposed areas. By far the most common manifestation is PCT, which has isolated blistering skins findings, classically on the backs of hands and other sun-exposed areas. In erythropoietic porphyria, skin lesions are nonblistering, but extremely painful and have a prodrome of escalating pain with light exposure. Coordination of care and management with a dermatologist is frequently necessary for diagnosis because there are many other blistering skin lesions and causes of photosensitivity. Liver damage in the form of cholestatic hepatitis is an uncommon complication, as well as are porphyrin-containing gallstones.

Diagnosis
The diagnosis of the porphyrias relies on the presence of symptoms (neurovisceral and/or dermatologic) consistent with the diagnosis and biochemical abnormalities to confirm the diagnosis. A careful history shows painful episodes, prodrome, exacerbating, and alleviating factors, including alcohol tolerance, skin rashes or dermatologic evaluations, and neurologic manifestations (most commonly weakness). In addition to alcohol and tobacco histories, a careful review of all current and past medications and their associations with attacks should evaluated. Among the more common inducers of attacks include oral contraceptives and many anticonvulsants. An excellent resource for drug safety in the porphyrias is provided at the APF website (porphyriafoundation .org). An account of the most recent painful episode and timing from testing may also be helpful when considering testing.

The linchpin to the diagnosis of the AHPs, AIP in particular, is the spot urine ALA, porphobilinogen (PBG), and urine creatinine test (creatinine normalizes the measurement and negates the need for a 24-hour urine collection). While the likeliest time to find extreme elevations in heme metabolites will be during an attack, because testing is now done exclusively at reference laboratories, it is often impractical to base a diagnosis and treatment plan on acute testing. However, testing should be sent if the diagnosis is being considered during an episode of acute abdominal pain. In the outpatient setting, often there is confusion about the utility of testing outside of an acute episode. Because this is a congenital metabolic disorder, for most porphyrias, including AIP, a spot ALA, PBG, and urine creatinine test is sufficient to make the diagnosis. The levels of ALA and PBG outside of an acute episode will often remain high for many weeks. Hence, even without acute abdominal pain, levels greater than four to five times the upper limit of normal will make the diagnosis. Conversely, a common error in diagnosis is to measure levels of *all* porphyrins in the urine. Drugs whose metabolism induces cytochrome P450 (and hence heme synthesis), excess alcohol, and other chronic illnesses can result in relatively minor elevations in downstream porphyrins and lead to confusion about the diagnosis.

The APF website (porphyriafoundation.org) is an excellent resource for providers and patients alike. There are a limited number of reference laboratories with the proficiency to perform the diagnostic assays for these disorders, which are listed on the APF website. Most helpful to a specialist is for the patient to be given the spot urine ALA, PGB, and urine creatinine test prior to referral for evaluation of the AHPs.

TABLE 2 | Diagnosis and Treatment of Porphyrias

	SPECIFIC PORPHYRIAS	NEURO-VISCERAL	DERMATOLOGIC	TREATMENT	TREATMENT MECHANISM
Acute hepatic porphyrias	AIP (most common), ADP, HCP, VP	Yes	AIP, ADP—none VP and HCP photosensitive blistering	Hemin (Panhematin)—acute Givosiran (Givlaari)—prophylaxis	Hemin—negative feedback on ALAS-1 Givosiran—direct inhibition of transcription of ALAS-1
Chronic hepatic porphyrias	PCT	No	Photosensitive blistering	1. Phlebotomy plus 2. HCV eradication HIV treatment Alcohol and tobacco cessation	1. Iron reduction 2. Elimination/reduction of susceptibility factors
Erythropoietic porphyrias	EPP, XLP, CEP	No	Photosensitive nonblistering	Sun avoidance Afamelanotide (Scenesse)—EEP only	Prevention of blue light (410 nM) to activate pathogenic metabolites to cause dermatologic damage Afamelanotide—increase melanin to absorb light and improve sunlight tolerance

ADP, ALA dehydratase deficiency porphyria; *AIP*, Acute intermittent porphyria; *ALAS-1*, aminolevulinic acid synthase-1; *CEP*, congenital erythropoietic porphyria; *EPP*, erythropoietic protoporphyria; *HCP*, hereditary coproporphyria; *HCV*, hepatitis C virus; *PCT*, porphyria cutanea tarda; *VP*, variegate porphyria; *XLP*, X-linked protoporphyria.

For PCT, the diagnosis can be suspected by visual inspection of blistering skin lesions, aided by the evaluation of a dermatologist, including a skin biopsy and confirmation with biochemical testing. The first step in diagnosis is to measure plasma porphyrins. If elevated, then typically laboratories will reflexively fractionate the different porphyrins, which reveals elevated uroporphyrin and heptacarboxyl porphyrins. Given that blistering skin lesions are not specific to PCT, a spot urine porphyrin test should also be done concurrently. In PCT, urine ALA and PBG will be normal, in contrast to the hereditary coproporphyrias (HCPs) that have blistering skin lesions. After the diagnosis of PCT is made, evaluation for susceptibility factors that could lead to the finding of PCT (given that 80% are acquired) should also be done, including HCV and HIV infections, alcoholic liver disease, and iron overload. Genetic predisposition to iron overload due to mutations in the HFE gene (pathogenic in hereditary hemochromatosis) is frequently found.

For the very rare erythropoietic porphyrias, including EPP, a more specialized approach is needed, including evaluation by a dermatologist. EPP in particular is diagnosed by elevated protoporphyrin in red blood cells (erythrocyte protoporphyrin), plasma, and stool (normal in urine), which shares a phenotype with the very rare X-linked protoporphyria (XLP) but differs in the genetic lesion.

Given that these metabolic disorders are genetic in origin (PCT is the exception), there may be a temptation to perform genetic testing over biochemical testing to make the diagnosis. However, genetic testing should only be performed to confirm the diagnosis *after* discovery of biochemical evidence to support the diagnosis. The incomplete penetrance in these disorders has been well established so that to begin with genetic testing would likely falsely assign the diagnosis to patients whose symptoms should not be attributed to the disorder.

Management
Acute Hepatic Porphyrias
The main principle of management of all AHPs is *avoidance* of inducers of heme biosynthesis to reduce production of excess toxic metabolites that drive the clinical disease manifestations (Table 2). In AHPs, where neurovisceral and/or skin symptoms are hallmarks, patients should be counseled to avoid alcohol use, smoking, oral contraceptives (both estrogen and progestins have been associated with attacks), and physicians should carefully prescribe drugs that induce cytochrome P450. The APF website (porphyriafoundation.org) has an excellently curated and searchable drug database that should be consulted before starting any new medication. Patients should also be counseled about the risks of over-the-counter medications, herbal medicines, and supplements as potential inducers of attacks. Patients should also be counseled about environmental or situational inducers of attacks that in general would be considered metabolic stressors, such as physical or emotional stress, infection, fasting (e.g., as with fad diets), pregnancy (also a high progesterone state), and surgery. For women with attacks that are regularly triggered by menstrual cycles, ovarian suppression with gonadotropin-releasing hormone analogue can be used as a preventive measure as well.

When patients experience the prodrome of an acute attack (neurologic symptoms, tachycardia, vague abdominal pain), some are able to abort attacks by oral carbohydrate loading (at least 300 g/day). For patients who present for medical attention, in addition to withdrawal of any identifiable precipitants of the attack (new medications, supplements, or alcohol), IV dextrose (10% dextrose in 0.45% normal saline) can be used as a temporizing measure if hemin is not available or for treatment of mild attacks. Carbohydrates directly but weakly inhibit ALAS1, so hemin is preferred for treatment of attacks that require more than therapy at home.

Intravenous hemin (Panhematin) rapidly reduces plasma PBG and ALA by reducing ALAS-1 activity through negative feedback. The primary acute toxicity from this therapy is phlebitis so it is strongly recommended to deliver this therapy by a central catheter. The drug is dosed once per day for 4 consecutive days at a dose of 3 to 4 mg/kg and reconstituted in albumin for better stability. Other supportive measures for an acute attack include antiemetics and analgesics (opioids commonly required for pain control). While seizures are highly uncommon, management is quite challenging given that the most common anticonvulsants are also strong precipitants of porphyric attacks. Thus, electrolyte abnormalities and other precipitants of seizures should be carefully managed.

Some patients with frequent attacks require regular treatment with hemin or preventive hemin infusions. However, because the effect of this therapy is short lived, this can lead to iron overload and poor quality of life. Givosiran (Givlaari) was recently approved exclusively as a preventive therapy for AHPs. This novel therapy is a small interfering RNA therapy that inhibits ALAS-1, and hence is a potent inhibitor of hepatic heme synthesis. The most commonly reported toxicities in the trials included injection-site reactions, nausea, rash, and elevated transaminases. The phase 3 clinical trial found a significant reduction in attacks when this therapy was given as a once-monthly subcutaneous injection overall by about 70% over placebo and nearly half had no attacks. Hemin (see Treatment of Acute Attacks) was still effective as a rescue therapy for acute attacks.

Porphyria Cutanea Tarda

Blistering skin lesions are attributed to the presence of iron overload in addition to other predisposing factors that cause UROD deficiency. By treating iron overload with phlebotomy, plus removing or treating underlying triggers such as alcohol and tobacco use, hepatitis C (HCV) infection, or HIV infection, PCT can be effectively managed. Phlebotomy can be initiated on an every 2-weeks schedule with careful attention to the patient's hemoglobin and symptoms of anemia. While ideally iron deficiency is the target (ferritin <20), a careful balance between symptoms of PCT and symptoms of iron deficiency should be considered. In addition to phlebotomy, skin protection from sun exposure is the other important management strategy, along with supportive care of blistering lesions, including treatment of secondary bacterial infections.

If phlebotomy is poorly tolerated, then hydroxychloroquine (Plaquenil)[1] 100 mg twice weekly is another effective treatment. In a randomized trial, this therapy has been shown to reduce PCT symptoms and plasma porphyrin levels as quickly as phlebotomy (≈6 months).

Patients with HCV infection should be considered for eradication therapy and/or screened for cirrhosis and hepatocellular carcinoma. It is not known whether HCV eradication alone will cause remission in PCT, but certainly it is beneficial to reduce the patient's risk of HCV-related complications such as cirrhosis. HIV infection should be treated and smoking cessation should be pursued. Patients often avoid alcohol because they recognize its deleterious effects, but for those with alcohol use disorder, cutting back on use or abstinence is much more challenging and management should be coordinated with an addiction specialist. Similarly, tobacco cessation is strongly encouraged.

Erythropoietic Porphyrias

In treatment of erythropoietic porphyrias, where EPP is the more common of these rare diseases, trigger avoidance is the mainstay of treatment. From a young age, patients can identify the prodrome of an attack during sunlight exposure. Thus, avoidance of sunlight exposure is the primary preventive strategy. It should be noted that UV light exposure still occurs through glass. When necessary, precautions should be made and a physician letter may be necessary to allow window tinting in the patient's car. In addition, exposure from other sources of UV light such as fluorescent lights can cause photosensitivity. For any patient with EPP who is undergoing surgery, particular attention needs to be paid to avoid excess UV exposure from operating room lights. Transparent sunscreens block UV light only and are not effective for prevention of symptoms in EPP. Regular use of protective clothing and hats was the only treatment for EPP until recently. Avoidance of sunlight also frequently leads to vitamin D deficiency.

Afamelanotide (Scenesse) is a synthetic analogue of alpha-melanocyte stimulating hormone. This recently approved drug, the first drug approved for EPP, increases melanin and skin pigmentation, and hence, improves sunlight tolerability. The drug is administered, as a monthly controlled-release implant. Overall, this new therapy is well tolerated and though it improves sunlight tolerability it does not affect the underlying cause.

References

American Porphyria Foundation. https://porphyriafoundation.org/.

Bissell DM, Montgomery Bissell D, Anderson KE, Bonkovsky HL: Porphyria, *New Engl J Med* 377:862–72, 2017.

Langendonk JG, Balwani M, Anderson KE, et al: Afamelanotide for Erythropoietic Protoporphyria, *N Engl J Med* 373:48–59, 2015.

Sardh E, Harper P, Balwani M, et al: Phase 1 Trial of an RNA Interference Therapy for Acute Intermittent Porphyria, *N Engl J Med* 380:549–58, 2019.

Singal AK: Porphyria cutanea tarda: Recent update, *Mol Genet Metab* 128:271–81, 2019.

Singal AK, Kormos-Hallberg C, Lee C, et al: Low-dose hydroxychloroquine is as effective as phlebotomy in treatment of patients with porphyria cutanea tarda. *Clin Gastroenterol Hepatol* 10:1402–9, 2012.

Wang B, Rudnick S, Cengia B, Bonkovsky HL: Acute Hepatic Porphyrias: Review and Recent Progress, *Hepatol Commun* 3:193–206, 2019.

[1]Not FDA-approved for this indication.

SICKLE CELL DISEASE

Method of
Enrico M. Novelli, MD; Mark T. Gladwin, MD; and Lakshmanan Krishnamurti, MD

CURRENT DIAGNOSIS

- Sickle cell disease (SCD) is diagnosed by neonatal screening in the United States.
- Persons with congenital hemolytic anemia should be tested for SCD by hemoglobin electrophoresis regardless of their ethnic background.
- Infection with parvovirus B19 should be suspected in children presenting with acute anemia and reticulocytopenia.
- Human leukocyte antigen (HLA) class I and II testing should be performed in all patients with SCD and unaffected siblings to identify candidates for hematopoietic stem cell transplant.
- Transcranial Doppler screening for primary prevention of stroke is indicated in children with homozygous SCD.
- Acute chest syndrome is diagnosed in patients presenting with fever, hypoxemia, and a radiographic pulmonary infiltrate.
- Screening for kidney disease should be performed by obtaining a spot urine sample for microalbuminuria
- Screening for iron overload by ferritin, quantitative liver magnetic resonance imaging (MRI), cardiac MRI, or liver biopsy is indicated in all patients who have received more than 10 lifetime transfusions.
- Pulmonary hypertension screening by transthoracic echocardiogram is indicated in all patients with homozygous SCD.

CURRENT THERAPY

- All children with sickle cell disease (SCD) should receive penicillin prophylaxis.
- High fever should be treated empirically with coverage for *Streptococcus pneumoniae* pending results of blood cultures.
- Children with high transcranial Doppler velocity need to be placed on a chronic transfusion regimen to keep the hemoglobin (Hb) S less than 30%.
- Painful vasoocclusive episodes warrant prompt treatment with an individualized intravenous opiate regimen, as well as supportive care and incentive spirometry.
- Preoperative transfusion should aim at a target hemoglobin level of 10 g/dL regardless of the HbS percentage and is indicated in all patients with SCD undergoing major surgery.
- Therapy with hydroxyurea (Droxia, Siklos) is indicated in all patients at all ages with HbSS disease and HbSβ-thalassemia, and in patients with HbSC with a severe phenotype on a case-by-case basis.
- Erythropoietin-stimulating agents can be used in conjunction with hydroxyurea to prevent or ameliorate reticulocytopenia and in patients with underlying renal insufficiency.
- Iron chelation is indicated in all patients with findings of iron overload.
- Treatment of acute chest syndrome includes parenteral antibiotics to cover atypical microorganisms and transfusion, with exchange transfusion reserved for the most severe cases.
- Patients with pulmonary hypertension should receive optimal hematologic care (maximal hydroxyurea and/or chronic transfusion therapy) and specific therapy for pulmonary hypertension in severe cases, with coordination and referral to a pulmonary hypertension specialist.
- Stem cell transplantation should be offered to all patients who have a matched donor and display a severe phenotype.

Epidemiology

Sickle cell disease (SCD) affects 70,000 to 100,000 persons in the United States and millions worldwide. The hemoglobin S (HbS) mutation arose in West-Central Africa approximately 7300 years ago and then propagated to vast tropical and subtropical areas due to the selective pressure of malaria infection. It is predominantly found in persons of African, Mediterranean, Arab, or Indian ancestry. In the United States, approximately 1 in 15 African Americans harbors the HbS (sickle hemoglobin) mutation and 1 in 400 is affected by the disease. Most patients with SCD in the United States are homozygous for HbS (SS), with heterozygous HbSC being the second most common abnormality. Conversely, in Mediterranean countries, HbS/β-thalassemia is the most common SCD syndrome, and in the Arab peninsula HbSS in combination with hereditary persistence of fetal hemoglobin (HPFH) is particularly prevalent.

Pathophysiology

SCD consists of a group of inherited hemoglobinopathies characterized by a qualitatively abnormal hemoglobin molecule that affects the structure and integrity of the red blood cells (RBCs). SCD is an autosomal recessive disease due to homozygosity for HbS, characterized by a single base substitution in the β-globin gene of the hemoglobin tetramer, leading to an amino acid substitution (valine to glutamic acid), or coinheritance of HbS with other abnormal hemoglobins such as hemoglobin C, D, E, and O or β-thalassemia.

HbS is less soluble than normal hemoglobin (HbA) in the deoxygenated state and polymerizes when sickle RBCs are exposed to hypoxic conditions in the microcirculation. In the classic pathophysiologic explanation of SCD, sickled RBCs containing HbS polymers are less deformable and remain trapped in the microcirculation, causing end-organ ischemia and necrosis. Compounding this mechanism, more recent literature has emphasized the role of cellular adhesion, abnormal cytokine levels, ischemia-reperfusion injury, oxidative damage, sterile inflammation, and an abnormal endothelial milieu (Figures 1 and 2). HbS polymers also lead to deformity and fragility of the RBC membrane, with resulting intravascular and extravascular hemolysis.

Patients with SCD suffer from severe chronic hemolytic anemia and acute episodes of RBC trapping and destruction in the microvasculature (vasoocclusive episodes). Vasoocclusive episodes are the hallmark of SCD and are characterized by more intense episodic vasoocclusion, often with increasing hemolysis, and are due to exogenous or endogenous factors that acutely alter the rheologic properties of the RBCs. The main determinants of RBC sickling and vasoocclusion are hypoxemia, RBC dehydration, RBC concentration, high HbS relative to fetal hemoglobin (HbF), and blood viscosity; these can occur in a multitude of clinical settings. Most common clinical inciting events leading to vasoocclusive episodes are dehydration due to inadequate replacement of fluid losses, thermal changes, surgical stress, exposure to low oxygen tension, infections, and psychological stressors.

Epidemiologic studies indicate that the risk of vasoocclusive episodes and acute chest syndrome is related to high steady-state hemoglobin levels, leukocytosis, and low HbF levels. These findings are consistent with pathogenic mechanisms of altered red cell rheology, higher viscosity, HbS polymerization, and inflammatory cellular adhesion. Interestingly, the epidemiologic risk factors associated with chronic vascular complications such as pulmonary hypertension (PH), cutaneous leg ulceration, priapism, systemic systolic hypertension, renal failure with proteinuria, and possibly stroke are different and include a low steady-state hemoglobin level, increased hemolytic intensity, iron overload, and markers of low nitric oxide (NO) bioavailability. One hypothesis is that SCD is driven by two overlapping but different mechanisms of disease: on one hand, vasoocclusion causes vasoocclusive episodes and acute chest syndrome, and on the other hand, hemolytic anemia leads to endothelial dysfunction and chronic vasculopathy. Both are caused fundamentally by HbS polymerization.

Prevention

See "Evidence-Based Management of Sickle Cell Disease: Expert Panel Report, 2014" at http://www.nhlbi.nih.gov/health-pro/guidelines/sickle-cell-disease-guidelines for detailed, consensus guidelines on prevention and treatment.

Bacterial Infections

Before the antibiotic era, most patients with SCD succumbed to bacterial sepsis from encapsulated organisms. A landmark multicenter, randomized, double-blind, placebo-controlled clinical trial of prophylaxis with oral penicillin in children with sickle cell anemia published in 1986 showed that bacterial prophylaxis started at birth reduced by approximately 80% the incidence of infection in the penicillin group, as compared with the group given placebo. This study became the foundation for universal screening of SCD. Results of the Penicillin Prophylaxis in Sickle Cell Study II (PROPS 2) trial show that prophylaxis can be safely discontinued at age 5 years as long as there is no history of prior serious pneumococcal infection or surgical splenectomy and in the setting of appropriate comprehensive care. All children should also receive both the 13-valent pneumococcal conjugate (Prevnar 13) and 23-valent pneumococcal polysaccharide (Pneumovax) vaccines, and adults should receive Pneumovax. Vaccinations for *Haemophilus influenzae* and *Neisseria meningitidis* are also indicated.

Neurologic Events

Stroke is a devastating complication of SCD and affects predominantly children with HbSS and abnormal transcranial Doppler (TCD) results. Silent cerebral infarcts are magnetic resonance imaging (MRI)-detectable abnormalities that also carry a high risk of morbidity, including overt stroke and cognitive impairment. There is conclusive evidence that chronic transfusions are effective in the primary and secondary prevention of both overt and silent strokes in SCD. The first landmark trial (STOP) published in 1995 showed that the first stroke can be prevented by placing children with abnormal TCD on prophylactic monthly transfusions with a target HbS of less than 30%. Transfusions were later found to also have a beneficial effect on reducing the incidence of the recurrence of silent cerebral infarcts, as shown by the SIT trial. The importance of continuing transfusions for more than 30 months was underscored by the STOP 2 trial, where TCD abnormalities recurred and the incidence of silent cerebral infarctions on MRI was higher in the transfusion-halted group. The enthusiasm over the beneficial effects of transfusions was tempered by the concerns about the side effects of long-term, possibly indefinite use of this therapeutic strategy. Therefore there has been an interest in exploring whether hydroxyurea (Droxia, Siklos) could represent an alternative to transfusion in high-risk children. Specifically, the SWiTCH trial explored the hypothesis that hydroxyurea and phlebotomy could maintain an acceptable stroke recurrence rate and significantly reduce the hepatic iron burden as compared with a prophylactic chronic transfusion regimen. Unfortunately, the trial was terminated early because of a significantly higher stroke recurrence rate in the hydroxyurea arm compared with the transfusion arm, with equivalent hepatic iron burden in both groups. Thus the issue of when, if ever, it is safe to discontinue transfusions for the secondary prevention of stroke is still unknown. Conversely, as shown by the results of the TWiTCH trial, another study halted prematurely by the National Institutes of Health, hydroxyurea is not inferior to chronic transfusions in lowering TCD velocities in children at high risk but without a history of stroke, thereby suggesting that this drug may be equally effective in the primary prevention of neurologic complications.

Clinical Manifestations

Multiple genetic and epigenetic factors affect the SCD phenotype. Patients homozygous for HbS (SS) or compound heterozygous for HbS and a nonfunctional β^0-thalassemia allele tend

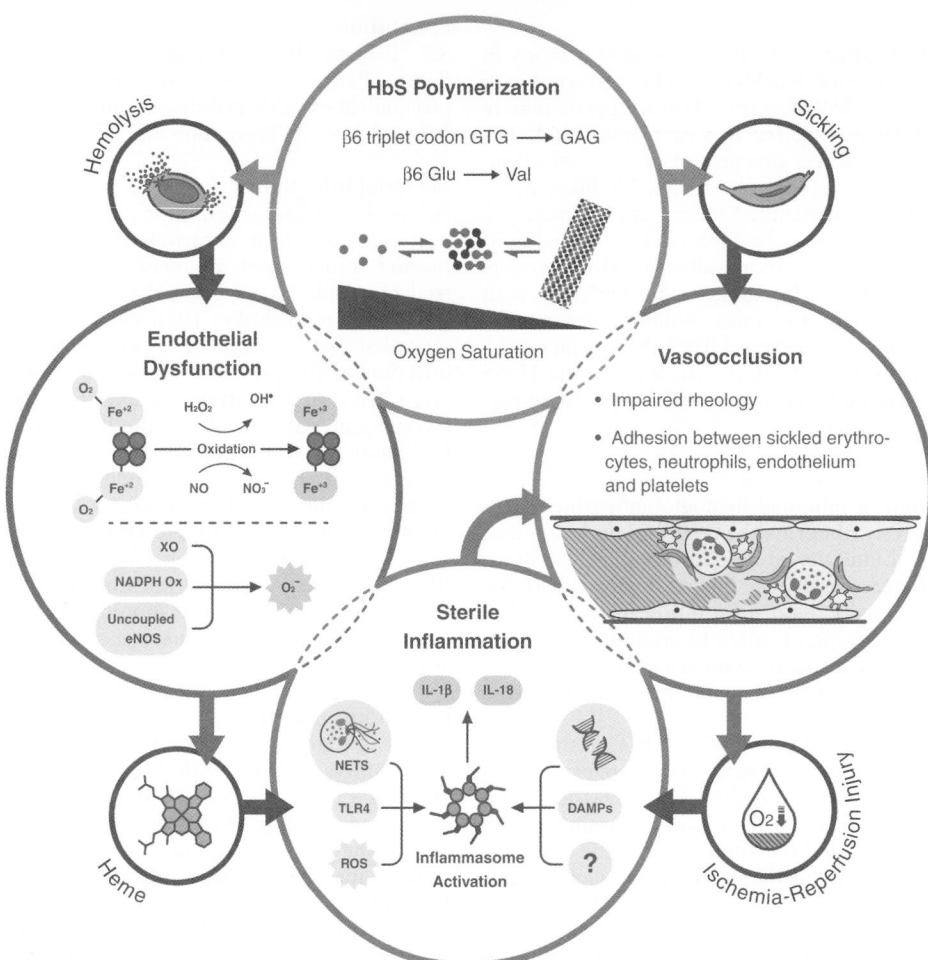

Figure 1 Molecular pathophysiology of SCD. A mutation in the β-globin gene leads to substitution of valine for glutamic acid at the 6th position in the β-globin chain. Following deoxygenation, the mutated hemoglobin (HbS) molecules polymerize to form bundles (top circle). The polymer bundles result in erythrocyte sickling (clockwise), which results in impaired rheology of the blood and aggregation of sickle erythrocytes with neutrophils, platelets and endothelial cells to promote stasis of blood flow referred to as "vaso-occlusion" (right circle). Vaso-occlusion promotes ischemia-reperfusion (I-R) injury (clockwise). Hb polymer bundles (top circle) also promote hemolysis or lysis of erythrocytes (counter-clockwise) that releases cell free Hb into the circulation. Oxygenated Hb (Fe2+) promotes endothelial dysfunction (left circle) by depleting endothelial nitric oxide (NO) reserves to form nitrate (NO3-) and methemoglobin. Alternatively, Hb can also react with H_2O_2 through the Fenton reaction to form hydroxyl free radical (OH·) and methemoglobin (Fe3+). Also, NADPH oxidase (NADPH ox), Xanthine oxidase (XO) and uncoupled endothelial NO synthase (eNOS) generate oxygen free radicals to promote endothelial dysfunction. Methemoglobin (Fe3+) degrades to release cell free heme (counter-clockwise), which is a major eDAMP. Reactive oxygen species (ROS) generation, toll-like-receptor-4 (TLR4) activation, neutrophil extracellular traps (NETs) generation, release of tissue or cell derived DAMPs, DNA and other unknown factors (?) triggered by cell free heme or I-R injury can contribute to sterile inflammation by activating inflammasome pathway in vascular and inflammatory cells to release IL-1β (bottom circle). Finally, sterile inflammation further promotes vaso-occlusion through a feed-back loop by promoting adhesiveness of neutrophils, platelets and endothelial cells. (Reproduced with permission from the Annual Review of Pathology: Mechanisms of Disease, Volume 14 © 2019 by Annual Reviews, http://www.annualreviews.org.)

to display the most severe manifestations. On the other end of the spectrum, HPFH, particularly common in Saudi Arabia, or coinheritance of β-thalassemia mitigates the phenotype. Although the net effect of high HbF levels on the phenotype of SCD is beneficial, coinheritance of one or two α-thalassemia alleles has a more complex effect. α-Thalassemia is present in approximately 30% of patients with SCD and is associated with higher hemoglobin, lower mean corpuscular volume (MCV), and decreased rate of hemolysis. These effects are protective toward stroke and leg ulcers but lead to increased rates of vasoocclusive episodes, osteonecrosis, and acute chest syndrome because of increased blood viscosity related to the higher hemoglobin level. Patients with HbSC and HbS/β+-thalassemia have an intermediate severity phenotype (Table 1). Haplotypes of polymorphic sites in the β-globin gene cluster in chromosome 11 have been associated with different disease severity and rates of complications. Other yet unidentified genetic factors predispose certain patients to develop a particularly severe hemolysis with brisk reticulocytosis and a high rate of specific complications that include leg ulcers, priapism, and PH.

Hematology

This section describes the main clinical manifestations of SCD in each organ system (Figure 3 and Table 2).

Baseline or Steady-State Hematologic Abnormalities

Chronic intravascular and extravascular hemolysis causes a chronic anemia of moderate to severe intensity in HbSS and HbS/β0-thalassemia, with a hemoglobin range of 6 to 9 g/dL. In HbSC and HbS/β+-thalassemia, the anemia may be mild or absent. The anemia of SCD is usually normocytic in HbSS, with anisocytosis and poikilocytosis and a population of small dehydrated dense cells, irreversibly sickled cells, numerous reticulocytes, and schistocytes. Reticulocytosis is common but not compensatory, and nucleated RBCs are seen in acute exacerbations of the anemia such as in splenic or hepatic sequestration. Baseline leukocytosis with neutrophilia is also common and is a poor prognostic sign associated with acute chest syndrome in adults and frequent vasoocclusive episodes in children. Preclinical studies have shown that leukocytes are not simply a marker of disease activity and acute phase but also have a direct pathogenic role in cellular adhesion

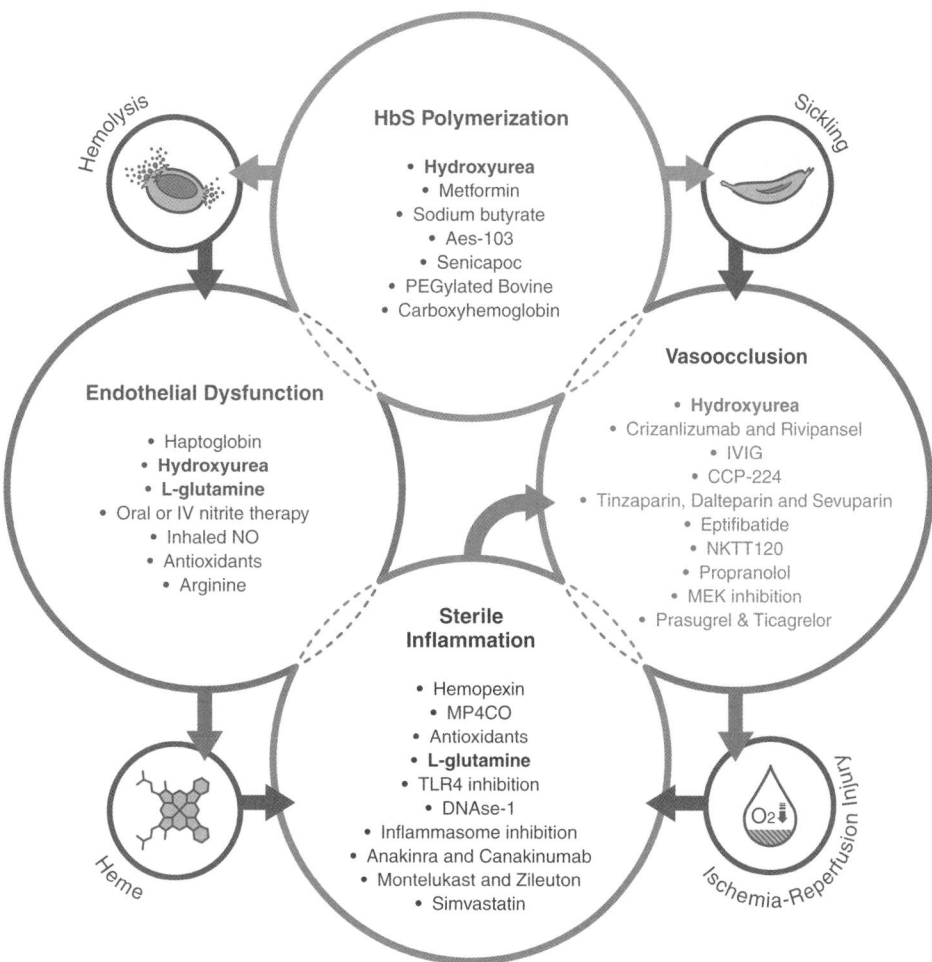

Figure 2 FDA approved and experimental therapies targeting the molecular pathobiology of sickle cell disease. The FDA approved drugs are in bold. (Reproduced with permission from the Annual Review of Pathology: Mechanisms of Disease, Volume 14 © 2019 by Annual Reviews, http://www.annualreviews.org.)

TABLE 1 Severity of the Main Sickle Cell Syndromes

GENOTYPE	CLINICAL SEVERITY	HEMOGLOBIN (G/DL)
HbSS	Usually marked	6–10
HbS-β⁰-thalassemia	Moderate to marked	6–10
HbS-β⁺-thalassemia	Mild to moderate	9–12
HbSC	Mild to moderate	10–15
HbSS-HPFH	Mild	

HbSC, Heterozygous phenotype; *HbSS*, homozygous phenotype; *HPFH*, hereditary persistence of fetal hemoglobin.

and vasoocclusion. The platelet count is commonly elevated in SCD, particularly in patients who are autosplenectomized as a result of repeated splenic infarction, and platelet activation is increased. In the subset of patients with HbSC and HbS/β⁺-thalassemia who retain a functional spleen and develop splenomegaly, features of hypersplenism may instead be observed with resulting mild pancytopenia.

Hematologic Indices During Vasoocclusive Episodes
In acute vasoocclusive episodes the total Hb decreases as a result of hemolysis (by 1.6 g/dL in acute chest syndrome). The lactate dehydrogenase (LDH), reticulocyte count, and other markers of hemolysis such as aspartate transaminase (AST) and indirect bilirubin are elevated in steady state, and in many—but not

all—patients are further increased during vasoocclusive episodes. Haptoglobin levels are chronically depressed in SCD and typically not measurable, even in steady state, in patients with HbS homozygosity. In patients with HbSC, vasoocclusive episodes may be due to increased blood viscosity and RBC sickling, and worsening hemolysis might not be readily appreciated.

Splenic sequestration crises occur mostly in childhood and are characterized by anemia disproportionate to the degree of hemolysis, reticulocytosis, and acute splenomegaly. Splenic sequestration and repeated episodes of splenic infarction eventually lead to autosplenectomy, although some patients develop splenomegaly. Splenic infarction usually manifests with left upper-quadrant pain and may be massive, involving more than 50% of the splenic tissue.

In severe vasoocclusive episodes, massive bone marrow infarction can also occur. In these instances, the peripheral blood smear reveals a leukoerythroblastic picture with immature neutrophilic forms, nucleated RBCs, and teardrop cells. Fat emboli syndrome, a life-threatening complication of vasoocclusive episodes, can then develop as bone marrow fat embolizes to peripheral capillary beds, leading to multiorgan failure.

Red Blood Cell Alloimmunization
RBC alloimmunization is a common complication of transfusional therapy in SCD and occurs in approximately 30% of patients. It is primarily due to the disparate expression of RBC antigens in African Americans as compared with the donor pool, which is mostly composed of whites. Alloimmunization complicates RBC matching and leads to delayed hemolytic transfusion reactions. Alloantigens that become undetectable by indirect Coombs test 2 months after

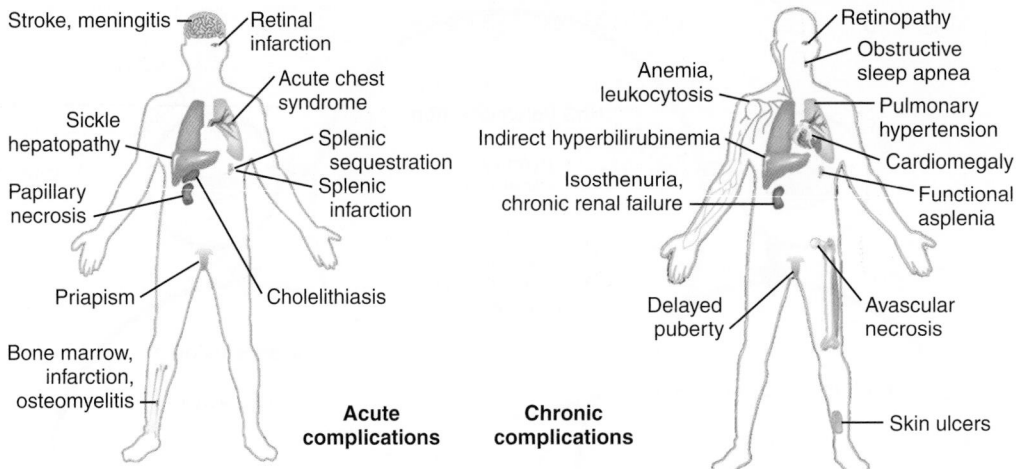

Figure 3 Acute and chronic complications of sickle cell disease.

exposure to mismatched blood have the potential to result in future false-negative cross-matching results. A subset of heavily alloimmunized patients with SCD undergoes life-threatening hemolytic reactions upon exposure to mismatched RBC units. In these hyperhemolytic crises, there is intense hemolysis of transfused and non-transfused RBCs and acute anemia. Treatment of hyperhemolytic crises is empirical and includes erythropoietin-stimulating agents (ESAs), parenteral steroids, and intravenous immunoglobulins (Gammagard).[1]

Iron Overload

Hemosiderosis is the other major complication of transfusional therapy in SCD and is characterized by iron deposition in the heart, liver, and endocrine glands, leading to organ failure and significant morbidity and mortality. It commonly occurs in patients who have received more than 10 lifetime transfusions or more than 20 packed RBC units. Liver biopsy is the "gold standard" for diagnosis, but it is an invasive and uncomfortable procedure. Hepatic and myocardial iron quantitation by MRI is supplanting liver biopsy as the preferred test to diagnose iron overload and monitor therapy with iron chelators, although when this is not available diagnosis often rests on the finding of an elevated ferritin and transferrin saturation in the appropriate clinical setting.

Hemostatic Activation and Thrombosis

Numerous studies have shown that arterial and venous thrombosis are common in SCD and include pulmonary embolism, in situ pulmonary thrombosis, and stroke. In SCD, alterations at all levels of the hemostatic system have been described: patients with SCD exhibit increased basal and stimulated platelet activation, increased markers of thrombin generation and fibrinolysis, increased tissue factor activity, and increased von Willebrand factor (vWF) antigen and thrombogenic ultralarge vWF multimers with depressed ADAMTS13 activity. Interestingly, hemostatic activation is amplified during vasoocclusive episodes, as shown by increases in multiple markers of thrombosis as compared with steady state, suggesting a link between hemolysis and thrombosis.

Neurology

Ischemic stroke is common in SCD, with the highest incidence between 2 and 5 years of age. Patients may develop overt stroke from large vessel occlusion (5% to 8% of patients with HbSS) or silent infarcts from focal ischemia detectable by MRI without symptoms of acute stroke (20% to 35% of patients with HbSS). The pathophysiology of stroke in SCD is unclear, although genetic factors and an unbalance between oxygen demand and supply have been postulated. Multiple epidemiologic studies have shown that the risk factors for ischemic stroke in adult

patients include HbSS genotype, severity of anemia, systolic hypertension, male gender, and increasing age. Patients with repeated strokes are at risk for development of anatomic abnormalities and Moyamoya pattern of vascularization, which predisposes to both ischemic and hemorrhagic stroke later in life. The highest incidence of intracerebral hemorrhages occurs in patients older than 20 years.

Both overt and silent strokes have a negative impact on IQ and cause cognitive impairment measurable by psychometric testing. Children and adults with SCD can develop cognitive impairment and subtle signs of accelerated brain aging and vascular dementia even in the absence of focal ischemia by MRI, with a low hematocrit being a predictor of neuropsychological dysfunction. These abnormalities are probably due to chronic and diffuse, as opposed to focal, cerebral anoxia and may be unmasked by psychometric testing.

Ophthalmology

Retinal abnormalities are common in SCD and are often asymptomatic until the occurrence of ophthalmologic emergencies. Retinal disease is due to arteriolar occlusion, with subsequent vascular proliferation, neovascularization, retinal hemorrhage (stage IV), and detachment (stage V). Patients with HbSC are more prone to retinal complications, possibly as a result of increased blood viscosity.

Nephrology

Renal abnormalities are common in SCD and manifest primarily as hematuria, proteinuria, and renal tubular acidosis. Hematuria is usually due to papillary necrosis and is an acute finding that requires supportive care and carries a good prognosis. Rarely, gross hematuria requires urologic consultation. Tubular functional defects include an inability to concentrate the urine (hyposthenuria) and renal tubular acidosis. Hyposthenuria often manifests with enuresis in childhood, and it is clinically relevant because it predisposes patients to an increased risk of dehydration. Renal tubular acidosis similar to type IV renal tubular acidosis is a common finding in SCD and may lead to hyperkalemia, an important consideration in patients already predisposed to hyperkalemia with intravascular hemolysis and whenever therapy with angiotensin-converting enzyme inhibitors is entertained.

Hyperphosphatemia and hyperuricemia are also often observed in SCD. Microalbuminuria may be detected in early adulthood and tends to progress to nephrotic range proteinuria. Focal segmental glomerulosclerosis is the most common glomerular abnormality and it is probably due to glomerular sickling and infarction. There are currently no approved therapies to prevent progression to end-stage renal disease, which occurs in up to 20% of patients and at a median age of 37 years. Renal replacement therapy is often needed in older adults with SCD. Serum creatinine and 24-hour creatinine clearance are not adequate for screening

---

[1]Not FDA approved for this indication.

TABLE 2 Landmark Randomized Clinical Trials in Sickle Cell Disease

YEAR OF PUBLICATION	TITLE	MAIN FINDINGS
1986	Prophylaxis with oral penicillin in children with sickle cell anemia: A randomized trial	84% reduction in incidence of infection and no deaths from pneumococcal septicemia in the penicillin group
1995	Multicenter Study of Hydroxyurea in Sickle Cell Anemia (MSH)	Reduced incidence of painful crises, ACS, and transfusion in the hydroxyurea group Survival benefit in follow-up study
1995	Preoperative Transfusion in Sickle Cell Disease Study	A conservative transfusion regimen was as effective as an aggressive regimen in preventing perioperative complications in patients with sickle cell anemia
1996	Multicenter investigation of bone marrow transplantation for sickle cell disease	HCT is safe in SCD with survival and event-free survival at 4 years of 91% and 73% and can lead to cure
1998	Stroke Prevention Trial in Sickle Cell Anemia (STOP)	Transfusion reduces the risk of a first stroke by 92% in children with sickle cell anemia who have abnormal results on transcranial Doppler ultrasonography
2005	Optimizing Primary Stroke Prevention in Sickle Cell Anemia (STOP 2)	Discontinuation of transfusion for the prevention of stroke in children with sickle cell disease results in a high rate of reversion to abnormal blood-flow velocities on Doppler studies and stroke
2009	Improving the Results of Bone Marrow Transplantation for Patients with Severe Congenital Anemias	Nine of 10 adults who received nonmyeloablative allogeneic hematopoietic stem cell transplantation for severe sickle cell disease achieved stable, mixed donor–recipient chimerism and reversal of the sickle cell phenotype, without acute or chronic GVHD.
2011	Pediatric Hydroxyurea Phase III Clinical Trial (BABY HUG)	Children ages 9–18 months randomized to receive hydroxyurea irrespective of disease severity for 2 y had decreased pain episodes, dactylitis, ACS, hospitalization, leukocyte count, and transfusion and increased hemoglobin as compared with children receiving placebo.
2014	Silent Infarct Trial (SIT)	Children with silent cerebral infarcts and normal TCD velocity who were randomized to chronic transfusion therapy had a 58% relative risk reduction in the recurrence of silent cerebral infarct or stroke as compared to those in the observation arm.
2017	Sustain Study	Crizanlizumab, a monoclonal antibody that targets P-selectin, reduced the rate of VOE to a median/year of 1.63 compared to 2.98 with placebo and increased the median time to the first and second crisis.

ACS, Acute chest syndrome; GVHD, graft-versus-host disease; HCT, hematopoietic cell transplantation; SCD, sickle cell disease; TCD, transcranial Doppler; VOE, vasooc-clusive crisis.

and monitoring of progression of kidney disease, because tubular secretion of creatinine is preserved and glomerular hyperfiltration is common in SCD, leading to a relatively low creatinine and a high glomerular filtration rate even in patients with underlying kidney impairment. Testing for microalbuminuria, plasma cystatin C levels, and hemoglobinuria may instead be used as screening tools for chronic kidney disease.

Leg Ulcers
Leg ulcers occur in 10% to 20% of patients with HbSS and have been associated with a chronically high hemolytic rate. They are usually located over the malleolar areas and are exquisitely painful, debilitating, disfiguring, and nonhealing. Vascular and plastic surgery consultations are recommended and aim at excluding local vascular problems that can complicate management of the ulcers and at providing prompt débridement and skin grafting. Although hydroxyurea is associated with development of leg ulcers in patients with myeloproliferative disorders, there is no such link with leg ulcers in SCD. Although wound healing may be impaired with hydroxyurea use, patients who develop an increase in fetal hemoglobin and have reduced sickling as a result of hydroxyurea therapy might have a net benefit in terms of tissue oxygenation and perfusion. Transfusional therapy, including exchange transfusional therapy, topical nitrates[1], and nutritional zinc[7] or L-arginine[7] supplementation, have shown benefit in anecdotal reports, but the evidence is inconclusive.

Gastroenterology
Nausea, vomiting, and dyspepsia in SCD are related to delayed gastric emptying and gastrointestinal motility disorders, autonomic neuropathy, or medical therapy. Opiates are often responsible for acute nausea and vomiting, whereas other medications such as hydroxyurea and deferasirox (Exjade) are occasionally responsible for chronic symptoms. Gastroparesis may be due to damage of the microvasculature of autonomic nerves (vasa vasorum) from repeated episodes of sickling.

The liver may be episodically affected by hepatic sequestration crises, heralded by direct hyperbilirubinemia, right upper quadrant pain from distention of the hepatic capsule, acute anemia, and reticulocytosis or by sinusoidal vasoocclusion leading to severe episodes of intrahepatic cholestasis. Supportive therapy and transfusions are indicated for hepatic vasoocclusive complications. Exchange transfusion may be the preferred modality for hepatic sequestration with the goal of preventing erythrocytosis once the pooled RBCs are released back into the circulation. Elevation of liver injury tests may be drug induced (hydroxyurea, deferasirox) but also related to hepatic sickling, particularly if it occurs during a vasoocclusive episode.

---

[1]Not FDA approved for this indication.

[7]Available as dietary supplement.

Infectious Disease

Patients homozygous for HbSS develop functional asplenia during childhood. This is due to repeated episodes of splenic infarction leading to fibrosis and autosplenectomy. As a result, children are susceptible to overwhelming bacterial sepsis from encapsulated organisms such as *Streptococcus pneumoniae, H. influenzae,* and *N. meningitidis.* High pediatric mortality from sepsis was therefore common before a landmark study published in 1986 demonstrated the benefit of penicillin prophylaxis instituted at birth. Vaccination for encapsulated organisms is also standard of care in children and adults. In spite of preventive measures, the incidence of life-threatening bacterial infections is increased in SCD, and high fever should be treated empirically as in splenectomized patients, with coverage for penicillin-resistant *S. pneumoniae* pending blood culture results. Patients with indwelling venous catheters are at risk of catheter-related bacteremia.

Viral infections with bone marrow–tropic viruses such as Epstein-Barr virus, cytomegalovirus, and predominantly parvovirus B19 place patients at risk for myelosuppression, which can further worsen chronic anemia. In children, infections with parvovirus B19 are responsible for transient red cell aplasia and severe aplastic crises, characterized by acute anemia and reticulocytopenia due to intramarrow destruction of erythroid precursors. Treatment of these episodes includes transfusion and intravenous immunoglobulins[1], besides supportive measures.

Individuals with SCD are known to be particularly vulnerable to H1N1 influenza, which has raised concerns about the outcomes

of SARS-CoV-2 infection and COVID-19 in SCD. Epidemiological data show that African Americans have been disproportionately affected during the COVID-19 pandemic, but large studies on the outcomes of COVID-19 in SCD have not yet been published.

Pulmonology

A subset of patients with vasoocclusive episodes develop acute chest syndrome, the major pulmonary complication of SCD. Acute chest syndrome is a lung injury syndrome defined by fever, pleuritic chest pain, oxygen desaturation, and multilobar radiographic infiltrates associated with severe vasoocclusive episodes, infection, and bone marrow fat embolization (Figure 4). It usually develops 2 to 3 days after hospitalization for vasoocclusive episodes and is often misdiagnosed as nosocomial pneumonia or aspiration pneumonia, particularly because it displays a predilection for the lower lobe of the lungs. Although pneumonia often accompanies acute chest syndrome, proper diagnosis is important because acute chest syndrome warrants simple or exchange transfusion in addition to antibiotic therapy and supportive measures. Common infectious pathogens identified in cases of acute chest syndrome include *Chlamydia pneumoniae, Mycoplasma pneumoniae,* and *Legionella pneumophila,* thus dictating inclusion of a macrolide in the antibiotic cocktail. Pulmonary embolism with resulting infarct is also in the differential diagnosis of acute chest syndrome and may occur concurrently in 17% of patients. If not recognized and treated promptly, acute chest syndrome leads to pulmonary failure and carries a high mortality.

Airway hyperreactivity is common in children with SCD and needs to be actively diagnosed and aggressively treated because

---

[1]Not FDA approved for this indication.

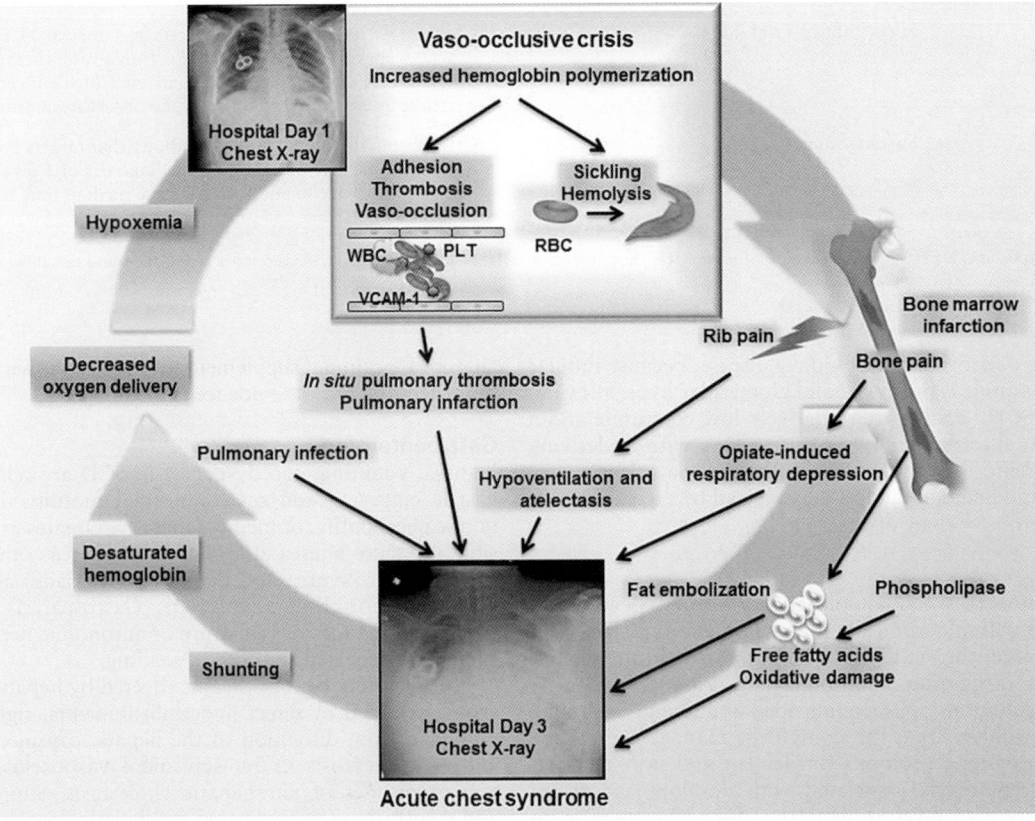

Figure 4 Vicious cycle of acute chest syndrome (ACS). Vasoocclusive crises are characterized by increased intraerythrocytic polymerization of deoxygenated hemoglobin S, leading to red blood cell sickling, cellular hyperadhesion, hemolysis, and vasoocclusion in the microvasculature. These processes are responsible for acute pain (pain crisis) and bone marrow necrosis. ACS typically occurs in a subset of patients 2 to 3 days after hospitalization for a vasoocclusive episode, and radiographically may present as new multilobar, basilar infiltrates on a chest x-ray. Fat embolization from the necrotic marrow is a recognized cause of ACS and is diagnosed by identifying lipid-laden macrophages in the bronchoalveolar lavage. However, pulmonary infection is the most common trigger of ACS and may be superimposed over existing pulmonary infarction. Hypoventilation and molecular pathogens such as reactive oxygen species from ischemia-reperfusion injury and by-products of hemolysis may also play a role in inducing or exacerbating lung injury. Finally, in situ pulmonary thrombosis has been frequently identified as a comorbid condition in patients with ACS and may be caused by endothelial and hemostatic activation. As a result of lung injury, ventilation-perfusion mismatches and shunting ensues, with subsequent hemoglobin desaturation and hypoxemia. Tissue hypoxia in turn triggers further hemoglobin S polymerization and sickling in a vicious cycle.

it is associated with worse SCD outcomes. Children with chronic respiratory symptoms should be tested for bronchial hyperresponsiveness.

Chronic complications of SCD include pulmonary fibrosis and PH. PH is an emergent complication of SCD and is associated with a high morbidity and mortality. Multiple epidemiologic studies have shown that a high baseline hemolysis rate, low hemoglobin, increasing age, a history of leg ulcers, liver dysfunction, iron overload, and kidney failure are risk factors for the development of PH. Three epidemiologic studies and a randomized clinical trial have shown that an elevated tricuspid regurgitant jet velocity (TRV) measured by Doppler echocardiography is a common occurrence in SCD with 30% of the patients having a TRV of 2.5 m/s (2 standard deviations [SDs] above the normal mean) or higher, and 10% of the patients having a TRV of 3.0 m/s (3 SDs above the normal mean) or higher. These have proven to be valuable cutoff values, as a TRV of less than 2.5 m/s, when combined with an N-terminal pro B-type natriuretic peptide (NT-proBNP) value less than 160 has a high negative predictive value for PH. A TRV of 3.0 m/s or higher confers a positive predictive value for having PH by right heart catheterization (RHC) of 60% to 75% and a relative risk for death of 10.6. Controversy exists on the significance of an intermediate TRV value of 2.5 to 2.9 m/s, because it is unclear how accurately it predicts RHC-diagnosed PH. In three subsequent studies, patients with intermediate or high TRV values had a prevalence of PH by RHC ranging from 25% to 65% depending on what specific cutoff value was used as the criteria to perform an RHC (2.5 vs. 2.8) and on whether patients with evidence of end-organ damage were included or excluded. However, it is worrisome that regardless of the prevalence of PH, patients with an intermediate TRV are as a whole at increased risk of death (relative risk 4.4). One screening approach is to consider RHC in all patients with TRV of 3.0 or higher and in patients with intermediate TRV values of 2.5 to 2.9 m/s if the NT-proBNP is greater than 160 pg/mL or the 6-minute walk is less than 333 m or there is a high clinical pretest probability of having PH (mosaic perfusion pattern on computed tomography [CT] scan, low diffusing capacity of the lung for carbon monoxide (DLCO), significant dyspnea on exertion, etc.). It is likely that intermediate TRV values will need to be combined with other measures of right ventricular function and functional capacity such as NT-proBNP, and 6-minute walk to derive a highly predictive composite biomarker of PH. All studies have been concordant on the high risk of death conferred by PH in SCD whether measured by echocardiography, NT-proBNP, or RHC. Noninvasive transthoracic Doppler echocardiography is recommended by the American Thoracic Society as a screening test in homozygous SCD due to its safety, low cost, and availability. However, the definitive diagnosis of PH requires a confirmatory RHC.

RHC studies of patients with SCD and PH reveal a hyperdynamic state similar to the hemodynamics characteristic of portopulmonary hypertension. It is increasingly clear that pulmonary pressures rise acutely in vasoocclusive episodes and even more during acute chest syndrome. This suggests that acute PH and right heart dysfunction represent a major comorbidity during acute chest syndrome, and right heart failure should be considered in patients presenting with acute chest syndrome.

Cardiology
Similar to other conditions with chronic anemia, SCD is associated with a hyperdynamic state, low peripheral vascular resistance, and normal blood pressure or hypotension. In this setting, even mild elevation of the blood pressure can indicate relative hypertension and represent a risk factor for stroke. Because there are no studies on the treatment of hypertension in SCD, general guidelines on antihypertensive therapy are applied.

Coronary artery disease is rarely observed in SCD, although many patients complain of chest pain during vasoocclusive episodes. In these instances, the usual work-up for acute coronary syndrome is recommended. It is possible that myocardial microvascular occlusions are the predominant ischemic event in SCD.

Left-sided heart disease in SCD is primarily due to diastolic dysfunction (present in approximately 13% of patients), although systolic dysfunction and mitral or aortic valvular disease (2% of patients) can also occur. The presence of diastolic dysfunction alone in SCD patients is an independent risk factor for mortality. Patients with both pulmonary vascular disease and echocardiographic evidence of diastolic dysfunction are at a particularly high risk for death (odds ratio, 12.0; 95% confidence interval [CI], 3.8 to 38.1; $P < .001$).

Cardiac dysfunction is a late complication and the major cause of death in patients with iron overload. Heart failure and conduction defects are the most common abnormalities and warrant emergent iron chelation treatment. Among the iron chelators, deferiprone (Ferriprox) appears to be particularly apt at reducing cardiac iron content. Chelators may be used in combination for cases of severe cardiac decompensation from hemosiderosis.

Methadone (Dolophine) is associated with a risk of QTc prolongation, which carries a risk of arrhythmias and sudden death, particularly in the setting of PH and iron overload. Frequent electrocardiographic (ECG) monitoring, as well as dosage reduction or discontinuation, are warranted in this group, particularly if the QTc is greater than 500 ms.

Endocrinology
Iron overload is a common cause of endocrinopathy in SCD and thalassemia, with the hypophysis, gonads, and thyroid glands being particularly affected. Patients with iron overload should therefore undergo screening for endocrine dysfunction as it is mandated in thalassemia.

However, patients with SCD are at risk for specific endocrine problems regardless of their iron status. Delayed growth and puberty are relatively common, presenting in females with delayed age of menarche by 2 to 3 years and in males with small testicular size and hypospermia. Likely pathogenic factors include increased catabolism, chronic hypoxemia, hospitalizations with prolonged immobility, ischemic insults during vasoocclusive episodes, and chronic use of opiates.

Priapism
Priapism is the most common urogenital complication in patients with the HbSS genotype. It is a sustained, painful erection in the absence of sexual stimulation from occlusion of the penile blood return. It is defined as stuttering if it lasts from minutes to less than 3 hours and as prolonged if it lasts more than 3 hours. The latter is considered a urologic emergency because of the risk of permanent fibrosis and impotence and requires a urologic consultation. Pseudoephedrine (Sudafed)[1] may lead to detumescence in nonemergency settings, whereas aspiration of the corpus cavernosum is required in the emergency setting and is performed under conscious sedation and local anesthesia. This is usually accompanied by installation of epinephrine. Other supportive measures, such as intravenous fluids and parenteral opiates, are usually indicated.

Penile shunts are used as a last resort to prevent further episodes of priapism by increasing the cavernous blood flow using native vessels or by creating an arteriovenous shunt. They invariably result in erectile dysfunction, which can be ameliorated by implantation of an inflatable penile prosthesis. There are data showing that sildenafil (Viagra)[1] therapy can prevent priapism by altering vascular smooth muscle tone through inhibition of phosphodiesterase 2 activity.

Diagnosis
The diagnosis of SCD rests on the hemoglobin electrophoresis or high-performance liquid chromatography (HPLC), which allows detection of most hemoglobin variants. In patients with microcytosis α-globin gene sequencing may reveal coinheritance of an α-thalassemia trait.

[1]Not FDA approved for this indication.

Neonatal Screening

Children with SCD have an increased susceptibility to bacteremia due to *S. pneumoniae*, which can occur as early as 4 months of age and carries a case fatality rate as high as 30%. Acute splenic sequestration crises also contribute to mortality in infancy. Diagnosis by newborn screening and immediate entry into programs of comprehensive care, including the provision of effective pneumococcal prophylaxis, can reach infants who might otherwise be lost to the healthcare system and has been demonstrated to decrease morbidity and improve survival. Currently, newborn screening and follow-up of SCD are carried out in all 50 states in the United States, as well as in most developed countries, and initiatives are under way to introduce universal newborn screening in most sub-Saharan African countries.

Late Diagnoses and Misdiagnoses

Rarely, patients who were born before the adoption of universal screening or who were lost at the time of follow-up of positive neonatal screening results are only diagnosed late in life. This occasionally occurs in patients with HbSC who might have normal hemoglobin and hematocrit and a mild disease phenotype. Alternatively, the disease may be misdiagnosed as iron deficiency in patients with HbS/β⁺-thalassemia on account of their microcytosis, which places them at risk of futile and potentially harmful prolonged trials of iron supplementation. Patients who have a low HbS level (< 40%) due to recent transfusion or who have only mildly decreased hemoglobin (HbSC or HbS/β⁺-thalassemia) may receive an erroneous diagnosis of sickle cell trait (carrier state).

Treatment

From the original description of SCD in 1910 to the 1970s, there was no efficacious therapy for SCD, and most patients died within the first 2 decades of life, with infectious complications being responsible for the majority of pediatric fatalities. Several preventive and pharmacologic milestones since then, and the realization that care has to occur in a multidisciplinary setting, have profoundly affected the natural history of the disease (Table 3). Median age at death in resource-rich countries was 42 years in male patients and 48 years in female patients with HbSS, according to data from the Cooperative Study of Sickle Cell Disease in the 1980s (a prehydroxyurea setting), thereby still lagging approximately 2 to 3 decades behind that of the general African-American population. The following sections summarize the therapeutic approach to the most important complications of SCD.

Vasoocclusive Episodes

Acute pain from vasoocclusive episodes in SCD is extremely intense, affects both children and adults, and is due to ischemia or necrosis of the vascular beds. Most patients report severe pain in the bones and joints of the extremities, as well as lower back, although acute ischemia and pain can affect unusual sites such as the mandibular area. Infants and young children may experience dactylitis, a painful swelling of the hands from bone marrow infarct in the small bones of the digits. Occasionally, adults may also experience the typical signs of inflammation, such as edema, warmth, and erythema in an affected limb, but a paucity or absence of signs is the norm. Imaging studies such as MRI, positron emission tomography (PET), and bone scan can reveal signs of acute bone marrow infarction in a painful bony area, but they are not routinely used in the work-up of a pain episode, unless osteomyelitis or septic arthritis are suspected.

Intravenous opiates are the mainstay of treatment of a pain episode. Even in opiate-naïve patients with SCD, opioid dosages often exceed those required for other indications. For instance, doses of intravenous hydromorphone (Dilaudid) of 1 to 2 mg are typical in adult patients. However, most patients, are on an oral pain regimen at home and have a history of multiple admissions for vasoocclusive episodes. In these cases, individualized care based on prior effective regimens and the patient's own perception of the intensity of pain are recommended. After an attempt at controlling the pain with three or four closely spaced opiate boluses is made, patients who are in persistent discomfort or have evidence of underlying complications triggering the vasoocclusive episode should be admitted and ideally placed on patient controlled analgesia. Nonsteroidal antiinflammatory drugs such as ketorolac (Toradol) have fallen out of favor due to their risks in patients with renal disease and their questionable efficacy. The

TABLE 3	Manifestations of Sickle Cell Disease With Key Prevention and Treatment Strategies	
MANIFESTATION	**PREVENTION**	**TREATMENT**
Pneumococcal sepsis	Penicillin, Prevnar/Pneumovax vaccination	Antibiotic therapy for penicillin-resistant *Streptococcus pneumoniae*
Splenic or liver sequestration	—	Exchange transfusion
Painful vasoocclusive episode	Hydroxyurea (Droxia), prevention of exposure to triggers	Intravenous fluids, parenteral opiates, supplemental oxygen
Acute chest syndrome	Incentive spirometry during VOE, hydroxyurea	Transfusion, broad-spectrum antibiotics with atypical coverage
Iron overload	Optimization of transfusion therapy	Iron chelation with deferasirox (Exjade) or deferoxamine (Desferal)
RBC alloimmunization	Transfusion with leukoreduced RBCs	—
CVA	Chronic transfusion in children with high transcranial Doppler velocity	Exchange transfusion and thrombolytics in selected cases
Pulmonary hypertension	Hydroxyurea?, treatment of predisposing conditions such as obstructive sleep apnea, hypoxemia, thromboembolism	Hydroxyurea, chronic transfusion therapy, specific therapy
Kidney disease	Antihypertensive therapy?, hydroxyurea?, ACE inhibitors?	ACE inhibitors?, renal replacement therapy, kidney transplant
Priapism	Hydroxyurea?	Pseudoephedrine (Sudafed)[1], aspiration of corpus cavernosum, sildenafil (Viagra)[1]
Leg ulcers	Hydroxyurea?, topical sodium nitrite?, voxelotor?	Surgical débridement, surgical grafting

ACE, Angiotensin-converting enzyme; *CVA*, cerebrovascular accident; *RBCs*, red blood cells; *TCD*, transcranial Doppler; *VOE*, vasoocclusive episode (crisis).
[1]Not FDA approved for this indication.

American Pain Society and the National Heart, Lung and Blood Institute (NHLBI) have published guidelines for the treatment of acute and chronic pain in SCD, followed by other institutions in the past decade.

Common obstacles to prompt and effective care in SCD are the health professional's fear of overdosing the patient, as well as misconceptions about addiction and pseudoaddiction. In general, healthcare professionals tend to overestimate the prevalence of opioid use disorder in SCD and tend to undertreat patients significantly, leading to patients' frustration and anger when their pain demands are not met (pseudoaddiction).

Nonpharmacologic therapies such as biofeedback, relaxation, and localized heat may be effective and should be incorporated into the management of pain episodes whenever possible. Care for vasoocclusive episodes should also include management of possible precipitating factors: dehydration and hypovolemia should be corrected with hypotonic crystalloids, and an infection work-up should be initiated in patients with fever, hypoxemia, or leukocytosis above baseline. Antiemetics and antipruritus therapy are also usually required.

Prior experiences in multiple institutions have shown that a dedicated facility for effective and rapid management of uncomplicated vasoocclusive episodes reduces hospitalizations and length of stay and facilitates integration of care—psychological, socioeconomic, and nutritional—in a multidisciplinary approach. This experience is the basis of the concept of the day hospital in SCD and relies on the need to provide prompt assessment and treatment of pain, safe dose titration to relief, monitoring of adverse effects, and adequate disposition (emergency department, inpatient admission, home) in a clinical environment familiar with SCD and the individual patient.

Chronic Pain

Chronic pain is common, and a study using pain diaries compiled by patients shows that most patients with SCD experience pain on an almost daily basis (PiSCES study). Orthopedic problems such as avascular necrosis (AVN) are common and tend to develop early in patients with HbSS disease, thus exposing patients to a lifetime of pain. There is an increasing realization that central sensitization and opiate-induced hyperalgesia also play a significant role in chronic pain in SCD. Unfortunately, there is a dearth of safe and effective strategies to manage chronic pain in SCD. At times, short-acting and long-acting opiates are required to empower the patient to manage pain at home and minimize use of the emergency department. Drugs for neuropathic pain, such as gabapentin (Neurontin)[1], may also be used in combination with opiates because neuropathic pain may develop as a result of tissue ischemia and necrosis.

Patients who have successfully transitioned from pediatric to adult care, have a good support system, and are distracted by their work or school schedules tend to cope better and require less pharmacologic support.

Because analgesic care is life-long, consultation with pain specialists is often valuable, particularly in patients for whom more-sophisticated pain regimens are needed. For instance, the mu-opioid receptor partial agonist buprenorphine (Buprenex, Butrans), opioid rotation, and methadone used as analgesic can help to reduce the total opiate requirements. Several States in the United States have approved the use of marijuana for medical purposes for several conditions including SCD. Although controlled studies on the benefits and risks of medical marijuana in SCD are lacking, studies in sickle mice and anecdotal reports hold promise. Urine toxicology screens and written "opiate agreements" are indicated in patients receiving opiates to ensure adherence with the therapy and to minimize the risk of use of illicit substances, particularly at a time of heightened surveillance for opiate abuse in the United States. The ASH guidelines published in 2020 emphasized an individualized approach in the management of chronic pain in SCD due to the lack of extensive evidence

on the benefits of opioids for chronic pain in this population. In addition, they recommended "against the initiation of chronic opiate therapy unless pain is refractory to multiple other treatment modalities" in children and adults with chronic pain from SCD. All recommendations on opioids for chronic pain were "conditional" based on very low certainty in the evidence about effects, and reflect a more guarded stance on opioids due to the deeper appreciation of the risks of chronic opioids for noncancer pain that has emerged in the past few years.

Transfusional Therapy

In SCD, the benefits of transfusion in terms of improved hemodynamics and oxygenation need to be balanced with the risks of iron overload, alloimmunization, transfusion reactions, and viral transmission of infectious agents. Leuko-reduced, sickle-negative RBCs with extended phenotypic matching for Rh Cc, Ee, and Kell, which account for 80% of detected antibodies, are required. By using extended phenotypic matching, the rate of alloimmunization decreased from 3% to 0.5% per unit, and the rate of delayed hemolytic transfusion reactions decreased by 90% in the STOP study. In previously immunized patients, a full RBC match also inclusive of matching for the Duffy, Kidd, and S antigens is recommended. Indications for transfusion include hemoglobin less than 5 g/dL or less than 6 g/dL with symptoms and any severe complication such as stroke, aplastic anemia, splenic or hepatic sequestration, or acute chest syndrome.

Prophylactic transfusions have been considered standard of care before surgery (with the exclusion of minor procedures such as intravenous port placement); the benefit of preoperative transfusions in preventing SCD-related complications in HbSS patients has also been confirmed in a small randomized clinical trial (the TAPS study). As to the type of transfusion strategy to be used, a clinical trial published in 1995 showed that a conservative prophylactic transfusion regimen to achieve a target hemoglobin of 10 g/dL and any HbS value was as effective as an aggressive regimen to achieve a hemoglobin of 10 g/dL and a target HbS value of less than 30% in preventing postsurgical complications such as acute chest syndrome.

Exchange transfusion (erythrocytapheresis with RBC exchange) is usually reserved for the most severe complications, which include acute chest syndrome with impending pulmonary failure, acute stroke and its prevention in children, multiorgan failure, and sepsis. Box 1 summarizes the main indications for simple and exchange transfusion in SCD, as well as the areas of uncertainty.

Iron Chelation

Patients who have received more than 10 transfusions or 20 units of packed RBCs should be screened for iron overload. Most authorities recommend initiation of iron chelation based on a ferritin level consistently greater than 1000 ng/mL, based on data from the thalassemia literature, although liver iron quantitation by MRI or biopsy should be obtained, when available, prior to therapy and to monitor its effectiveness. In the United States, the oral chelating agents deferasirox (Exjade) and deferiprone (Ferriprox) and the parenteral deferoxamine (Desferal) are available and should be administered until the ferritin level is less than 500 ng/mL for three consecutive measurements. Patients on iron chelation with deferasirox and deferoxamine require monitoring of hepatic, renal, auditory, and visual toxicity, and particular caution has to be exercised in the setting of renal disease, because transient, reversible increases in serum creatinine and rare instances of irreversible acute kidney injury have been reported in patients with underlying renal insufficiency. Deferiprone has been associated with agranulocytosis and neutropenia, mandating close monitoring of the absolute neutrophil count during therapy.

Erythropoietic Stimulating Agents

Although a brisk reticulocytic response is common in SCD, patients who develop renal failure or aplastic crises or who receive therapy with hydroxyurea may experience a relative or absolute reticulocytopenia (<100,000 reticulocytes/mL) and a worsening

---

[1]Not FDA approved for this indication.

BOX 1 Indications for Transfusion

No Indication
Chronic steady-state anemia
Uncomplicated painful episode
Infections
Minor surgery without general anesthesia
Aseptic necrosis of hip or shoulder
Uncomplicated pregnancy

Unclear Indication
Intractable or frequent painful episodes
Leg ulcers
Before receiving intravenous contrast dye
Complicated pregnancy
Cerebrovascular accident in adults
Chronic organ failure

Simple Transfusion
Symptomatic anemia
- High output cardiac failure
- Dyspnea
- Angina
- Central nervous system dysfunction
Sudden decrease in hemoglobin
- Aplastic crisis
- Acute splenic sequestration
Severe anemia (hemoglobin ~5 g/dL) with fatigue or dyspnea
Preparation for surgery with general anesthesia

Exchange Transfusion
Acute cerebrovascular accident
Multiple organ system failure
Acute chest syndrome
Hepatic sequestration
Retinal surgery

of their baseline anemia. In these situations, therapy with ESAs may be beneficial.

Because of bone marrow expansion in patients with HbSS, higher starting doses of erythropoietin (Epogen, (Epogen, Procrit)[1] than in patients without SCD may be considered. For darbepoetin (Aranesp)[1], a reasonable starting dose is 100 to 200 µg/weekly or every 2 weeks. ESAs can be titrated by 20% to 25% increases in dose per week in patients who do not respond adequately. Weekly monitoring of hematocrit is essential to avoid overdosage and relative erythrocytosis, which can lead to hyperviscosity and vasoocclusive episodes.

Nutritional Considerations

Malnutrition, growth retardation, and stunting with findings of low lean and fat body mass are highly prevalent in children and adolescents with SCD, due to their increased caloric demands and a hypermetabolic state. Macronutrient and micronutrient deficiencies are common, and nutritional counseling is warranted. Hypovitaminosis D and low bone mineral density are also prevalent in children and adults. Folic acid[1] is indicated at the dose of 1 mg daily as in other hemolytic diseases, particularly where folate nutritional supplementation programs are absent. Strategies aimed at decreasing iron intake and absorption should be implemented early. There is also growing interest in antioxidant nutraceuticals, particularly in light of the clinical trial showing beneficial effects with L-glutamine (Endari) in SCD; however, evidence on other substances remains limited. The small subset of patients who are overweight or obese is at risk for exacerbating or precipitating common orthopedic problems in SCD such as AVN of the femoral head and its resulting disability. These patients should also receive targeted nutritional counseling.

Hydroxyurea

Since the pediatric hematologist Janet Watson suggested in 1948 that the paucity of sickle cells in the peripheral blood of newborns was due to the presence of increased HbF, there has been interest in developing therapies to modulate the hemoglobin switch from fetal to newborn life and prolong HbF production. Several antineoplastic agents, including 5-azacytidine (Vidaza)[1] and hydroxyurea, became the focus of attention after they were found to increase HbF levels in nonhuman primates and individuals with SCD.

The landmark Multicenter Study of Hydroxyurea in Sickle Cell Disease (MSH) showed that the incidence of painful crises was reduced from a median of 4.5 per year to 2.5 per year in hydroxyurea-treated patients with SCD. The rates of acute chest syndrome and blood transfusion were also reduced significantly. A follow-up for up to 9 years of 233 of the original 299 subjects showed a 40% reduction in mortality among those who received hydroxyurea. This study led to the approval of hydroxyurea (Droxia, Siklos) as the first disease-modifying therapy in adults with SCD. More recent studies showed that hydroxyurea is safe and effective in children and adults with SCD. The recently concluded BABY HUG study showed that children 9 to 18 months with HbSS disease randomized to receive 2 years of hydroxyurea therapy, irrespective of the disease severity, had less dactylitis and fewer pain episodes, hospitalizations, and transfusions than children receiving placebo.

On the molecular and cellular levels, the benefits of hydroxyurea are mostly related to increased intracellular HbF, which prevents the formation of HbS polymers and sickling. In addition to this mechanism, some patients on hydroxyurea who do not adequately increase their HbF levels also display clinical benefits, suggesting that hydroxyurea might have other beneficial rheologic properties.

Although the MSH study only included patients with HbSS, its findings traditionally have been extrapolated to other sickle cell syndromes such as HbSC and HbS/β-thalassemia. A report from Greece, where S/β-thalassemia is highly prevalent, has confirmed that hydroxyurea similarly reduces complications and mortality in patients with HbS/β⁰-thalassemia, with a nonsignificant benefit also observed in HbS/β⁺ thalassemia. Existing guidelines also recommend hydroxyurea in patients with HbSC disease, but there is still no high-level evidence to support this practice.

Hydroxyurea has been indicated at a dosage of 15 mg/kg (7.5 mg/kg in patients with renal disease) in patients with frequent pain episodes, history of acute chest syndrome, other severe vasoocclusive episodes, or severe symptomatic anemia, although another sensible approach is to prescribe it to all patients with HbSS regardless of their phenotype. End points are less pain, increase in HbF to 15% to 20%, increased hemoglobin level to 7 to 9 g/dL in severely anemic patients, improved well-being, and acceptable myelotoxicity. The dosage can be increased by 500 mg every other day every 8 weeks to a maximum of 35 mg/kg if no toxicity is encountered. Considering the potential myelotoxicity, hepatotoxicity, and nephrotoxicity of this medication, laboratory monitoring needs to be performed every 2 weeks at the time of initiation or escalation and monthly during maintenance therapy. Laboratory studies should include a complete blood cell (CBC) count, differential and reticulocyte count, and serum chemistries. Measurements of HbF can be performed every 3 months. An elevated MCV is a marker of adherence to the therapy.

Criteria for holding hydroxyurea are listed in Figure 5. Patients need to be counseled on the teratogenic potential, as demonstrated in animal studies, as well as the risks of infertility and leukemogenesis, although a growing body of evidence shows that these risks may have been overestimated in patients with SCD.

Other side effects that can affect compliance include, but are not limited to, weight gain, alopecia, skin and nail hyperpigmentation (melanonychia), nausea and vomiting, and mucosal

[1]Not FDA approved for this indication.

[1]Not FDA approved for this indication.

Start therapy if one or more of the following conditions are present:
- frequent pain episodes
- history of acute chest syndrome
- other severe VOE
- severe symptomatic anemia

Starting dose: 15 mg/kg or 7.5 mg/kg if the patient has kidney disease

Endpoints:
- less pain
- increase in HbF to 15%–20%
- increased hemoglobin level to 7–9 g/dL
- improved well-being
- acceptable myelotoxicity

Dose escalation: increase dose by 500 mg every other day every 8 weeks if no toxicity encountered to a maximum of 35 mg/kg

Lab monitoring:
- At time of initiation or escalation: check CBC/differential/reticulocyte count every 2 weeks; serum chemistries every 2–4 weeks, percent HbF every 6–8 weeks
- During maintenance: check CBC/differential/reticulocyte count chemistries monthly, percent HbF every 3 months

Criteria to hold:
- ANC <2000
- Hb <9.0 g/dL and reticulocyte count <80,000 (alternatively start Epo)
- Platelet count <80,000
- Raising creatinine
- 2-fold elevation of AST or ALT over baseline
- 2 months prior to planned conception/pregnancy

Figure 5 Protocol for hydroxyurea treatment.

ulcerations. Because of the toxicity concerns, as well as factors intrinsic to long-term preventive therapy, hydroxyurea therapy has had low effectiveness in spite of high efficacy, with underprescribing by healthcare professionals and poor patient compliance being major obstacles to its widespread adoption.

Therapy of Pulmonary Hypertension

Because evidence-based guidelines for managing PH in patients with SCD are not available, recommendations are based upon the pulmonary arterial hypertension literature, case reports, small open-label studies, and expert opinion. For patients with mild PH (tricuspid regurgitant velocity [TRV], 2.5 to 2.9 m/s), it is important to identify and treat risk factors associated with PH such as rest, exercise or nocturnal hypoxemia, sleep apnea, pulmonary thromboembolic disease, restrictive lung disease or fibrosis, left ventricular systolic and diastolic dysfunction, severe anemia, and iron overload. These patients may benefit from aggressive SCD management, including optimization of hydroxyurea dosage and initiation of a chronic transfusion program in those who do not tolerate or respond poorly to hydroxyurea. Consultation with a pulmonologist or cardiologist experienced in PH is also recommended.

For patients with TRV 3 m/s or more, we recommend following the guidelines for TRV 2.5 to 2.9 m/s. In addition, RHC is necessary to confirm diagnosis and to directly assess left ventricular diastolic and systolic function. We would consider specific therapy with selective pulmonary vasodilator and remodeling drugs if the patient has pulmonary arterial hypertension defined by RHC and exercise limitation defined by a low 6-minute walk distance.

US Food and Drug Administration (FDA)-approved drugs for primary pulmonary arterial hypertension include the endothelin receptor antagonists (bosentan [Tracleer] and ambrisentan [Letairis]), prostaglandin-based therapy (epoprostenol [Flolan], treprostinil [Remodulin, Tyvaso, Orenitram], and iloprost [Ventavis]), the phosphodiesterase-5 inhibitors (sildenafil [Revatio]), and riociguat (Adempas), the first member of a new class of drugs, the soluble guanylate cyclase (sGC) stimulators.

No published randomized studies in the SCD population exist for any of these agents, although a multicenter placebo-controlled trial of sildenafil for PH of SCD was stopped early because of an unexpected increase in hospitalizations for vaso-occlusive crisis in the treatment group receiving sildenafil.

Anticoagulation is indicated in patients who have evidence of pulmonary thromboembolic complications and is supported by evidence of benefit in other populations with PH.

Hematopoietic Stem Cell Transplantation

Despite improvement of supportive care in SCD, life expectancy remains lower than for those not affected. In addition, quality of life for patients with SCD is usually significantly impaired. Although hydroxyurea can decrease acute complications of SCD such as vasoocclusive episodes and acute chest syndrome, no satisfactory measures exist to prevent the development of irreversible organ damage in adults. Furthermore, therapy with hydroxyurea is lifelong, and only 20% to 30% of eligible patients are prescribed or actually take the drug.

Currently, allogeneic hematopoietic stem cell transplantation (HCT) remains the only curative treatment. Indications for HCT have been empirically determined from prognostic factors derived from studies of the natural history of SCD. The most common indications for which patients with SCD have undergone HCT are a history of stroke, recurrent acute chest syndrome, or frequent vasoocclusive episodes.

Allogeneic HCT after myeloablative therapy has been performed in hundreds of pediatric and numerous adult patients with SCD. The backbone of the preparative regimens have consisted of busulfan (Busulfex)[1] 14 to 16 mg/kg and cyclophosphamide (Cytoxan)[1] 200 mg/kg. Additional immunosuppressive agents used have included antithymocyte globulin (Atgam)[1], rabbit antithymocyte globulin (Thymoglobulin)[1], antilymphocyte globulin, or total lymphoid irradiation (Figure 6). Cyclosporine A (Neoral)[1], alone or with mercaptopurine (Purinethol)[1] or methotrexate[1], has been used for posttransplant graft-versus-host disease prophylaxis.

The outcome of HCT for patients with SCD from matched siblings is excellent. Of 1000 recipients of human leukocyte antigen (HLA)-identical sibling transplants performed between 1986 and 2013 and reported to the European Blood and Marrow Transplant, Eurocord, and the Center for International Blood and Marrow Transplant Research, the 5-year event-free and overall survival were 91.4% (95% CI 89.6% to 93.3%) and 92.9% (95% CI 91.1% to 94.6%), respectively. Event-free survival was lower with increasing age at transplantation (hazard ratio [HR] 1.09; $P < .001$) and higher for transplantations performed after 2006 (HR 0.95, $P = .013$). Twenty-three patients experienced graft failure; 70 patients (7%) died, the most common cause of death being infection. Stabilization or reversal of organ damage from SCD has been documented after HCT. In patients who have stable donor engraftment, complications related to SCD resolve, and there are no further episodes of pain, stroke, or acute chest syndrome. Patients who successfully receive allografts do not experience sickle-related central nervous system complications and have evidence of stabilization of central nervous system disease by cerebral MRI. However, the impact of successful HCT on reversal of cerebral vasculopathy has been variable. Current research is focused on improving the applicability of HCT to a greater proportion of patients with SCD by the development of novel conditioning regimens minimizing myeloablation (see Figure 6), the use of novel sources of hematopoietic stem cells such as umbilical cord blood, extending HCT to adult recipients and alternate donors such as matched unrelated donors and haploidentical donors. The aim of these studies is to develop safe and effective alternatives for patients without matched sibling donors, thus increasing the applicability of curative therapy for SCD.

[1]Not FDA approved for this indication.

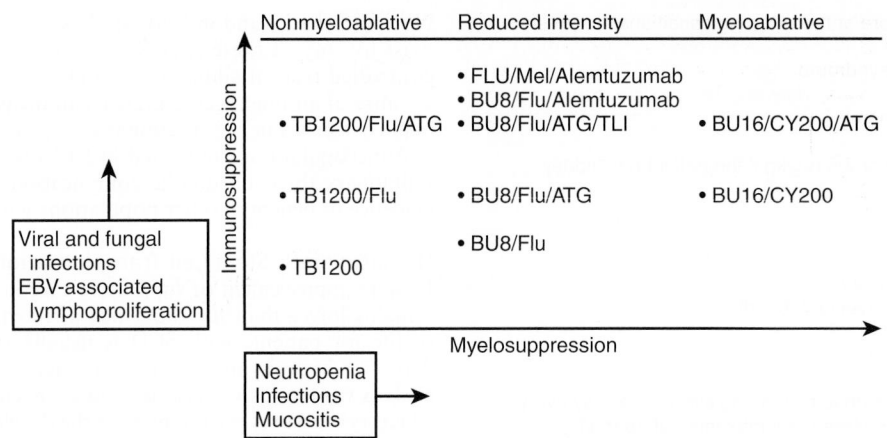

Figure 6 Spectrum of immunosuppression and myelosuppression in preparative regimens in hematopoietic stem cell transplantation (HCT) in sickle cell disease (SCD). Most preparative regimens for HCT in SCD have used a backbone of busulfan (BU) (Busulfex)[1] and cyclophosphamide (CY) (Cytoxan)[1]. Additional immunosuppressive agents include equine antithymocyte globulin (Atgam)[1] or leporine antithymocyte globulin (Thymoglobulin) (ATG)[1], antilymphocyte globulin, total lymphoid irradiation (TLI) or total body irradiation (TBI), fludarabine (Flu) (Fludara)[1], and alemtuzumab (Campath)[1]. Attempts to reduce the intensity of preparative regimens for patients with SCD have been based on one of two approaches. The first is the use of reduced-intensity conditioning regimens to produce less myeloablation. These require donor marrow infusion for hematopoietic recovery. The second is the use of nonmyeloablative regimens, which do not eradicate host hematopoiesis and allow hematopoietic recovery even without donor stem cell infusion. [1]Not FDA approved for this indication. Adapted with permission from Krishnamurti L. Hematopoietic cell transplantation: a curative option for sickle cell disease. *Pediatr Hematol Oncol.* 2007;24:569–575.

New and Experimental Therapies

The last few years have witnessed a flourishing of new therapeutic approaches for SCD. Three new drugs have received FDA approval and have been incorporated in the clinical practice across the United States, and several are in the pipeline or being reviewed in accelerated approval pathways by the FDA. Several decades of preclinical research in sickle mouse models are finally bearing fruit with pathologic pathways identified in sickle mice being harnessed for the development of molecular targeted biologicals. Finally, gene therapy is currently on the horizon with several gene therapy and gene editing approached being developed simultaneously.

Antioxidant Strategies

In 2018, pharmacologic *L*-glutamine (Endari) received FDA approval as the second disease-modifying drug in SCD. A randomized, phase III multicenter trial showed that patients in the *L*-glutamine group had significantly fewer pain crises and hospitalizations than those in the placebo group. Of note, two-thirds of the patients in both arms received concomitant hydroxyurea. Reassuringly, the drug had relatively mild side effects including nausea and fatigue. *L*-glutamine presumably acts by reducing oxidant stress in the sickle RBCs, although its effects on major disease parameters such as hemolysis are unclear.

Modulation of Cellular Adhesion

Adhesive interactions between RBCs, white blood cells, and platelets, and between cells and endothelium are implicated in the pathogenesis of vasoocclusive episodes. Recently, several compounds have been developed to target specific adhesion molecules such as E-selectin and P-selectin. This is a particularly promising area of research that has yielded two compounds in advanced phases of development. The P-selectin inhibitor crizanlizumab has shown significant reduction of the rate of crises per year and longer median time to the first crisis and second crisis when given as intravenous prophylaxis in a double-blind, randomized, phase II clinical trial. FDA approved crizanlizumab (Adakveo) for the prevention of vaso-occlusive episodes in SCD in November 2019. As in the case of *L*-glutamine, crizanlizumab can be used with and without concurrent hydroxyurea therapy. The pan-selectin inhibitor rivipansel[5] had shown promising results in a phase II

trial of treatment of vaso-occlusive episodes but failed to meet the primary end point of time to readiness for discharge and other key secondary endpoints in a phase III trial.

Modulation of Hemoglobin Oxygen Affinity

Deoxygenation of HbS leads to polymerization, sickling, and hemolysis. Thus strategies aimed at increasing the oxygen affinity of HbS may be beneficial. Clinical trials in adults and children have shown reduced hemolysis and improved hemoglobin with voxelotor, a once daily oral drug that increases the oxygen affinity of hemoglobin maintaining it in the oxygenated state and reducing polymerization and sickling. Unfortunately, these changes were not accompanied by a statistically significant reduction in vaso-occlusive episodes. Voxelotor (Oxbryta) was also approved by the FDA for the treatment of SCD in November 2019.

Modulation of Nitric Oxide

NO is an active biogas and a free radical species that mediates arterial relaxation, cellular adhesion to endothelium, hemostasis, and blood viscosity. In SCD, NO bioactivity is reduced as a result of decreased production due to endothelial perturbation and NO scavenging by cell-free hemoglobin generated during intravascular hemolysis. Dietary supplementation with *L*-arginine, a precursor of NO, and delivery of exogenous NO or NO bioactivity to the microvasculature in SCD, should promote dilatation of the terminal arterioles where obstruction to flow and tissue damage occurs, improvement of lung ventilation and perfusion is matching, decrease in pulmonary artery pressures, and inhibition of platelet aggregation and cellular adhesion. Although two recent clinical trials on *L*-arginine supplementation and inhaled NO (DeNOVO trial) for vasoocclusive episodes failed to show a clinical benefit, optimization of timing and dosing and novel strategies to target the NO pathway might lead to valuable NO therapeutics in the future.

Gene Therapy

The ultimate cure for SCD, gene therapy, is finally on the horizon. A French group first reported that a patient had been successfully treated with lentiviral-mediated insertion of an anti-sickling β-globin gene into autologous stem cells. The transduced cells were then transplanted into the patient who has since experienced long-term remission from SCD. Subsequently, in a clinical trial at the

---

[5]Investigational drug in the United States.

National Institutes of Health (NIH), several patients were treated with autologous hematopoietic stem cells transduced with a lentiviral vector that encodes for a nonsickling hemoglobin with very promising results. Other gene therapy approaches have targeted fetal hemoglobin induction and have harnessed the CRISPR-Cas9 gene editing technology.

Several hurdles need to be overcome before gene therapy will become a viable, large scale therapeutic option for SCD, including technical limitations (e.g., the need for *ex vivo* gene transduction or editing, with the potential loss of stem cell viability), toxicity concerns (e.g., the need for myeloablative chemotherapy to accommodate the auto transplant), cost considerations, and ethical concerns. It is also important to note that gene therapy approaches may not necessarily lead to a cure if they do not result in permanent and high-level suppression of HbS polymerization. Further compounding these concerns, in early 2021 a company performing clinical trials of a lentiviral gene therapy approach for SCD has halted its studies after one gene therapy recipient developed acute myeloid leukemia and another a myelodysplastic syndrome. The causes of this serious setback are currently being investigated.

Surgical Issues

Preoperative patient optimization includes prophylactic transfusion, close monitoring of pulse oximetry, adequate analgesia based on the patient's opiate tolerance, and monitoring for sickle cell–related complications.

AVN of the femoral heads, and more rarely of the humeral heads, is the most common orthopedic problem in SCD. Surgery is usually deferred until the pain and disability from AVN become intolerable and usually involves total hip or shoulder arthroplasty. This is usually a more involved procedure than in the general population on account of the altered bone anatomy in SCD. Patients with bone marrow expansion may experience thinning of the cortical bone and prosthetic instability, whereas some may suffer from the opposite problem of obliteration of the medullary shaft by sclerotic bone in response to multiple necrotic events.

Patients with SCD tend to develop pigmented gallstones and cholelithiasis. Cholecystectomy is performed in patients with SCD with cholelithiasis, right upper quadrant pain, and a positive hepatobiliary iminodiacetic acid (HIDA) scan. In SCD, the rate of intraoperative complications is higher and so is the rate of reversion from laparoscopic to open cholecystectomy.

Splenectomy has been reserved for patients with massive splenic infarction (>50% of the spleen volume); intractable, recurrent splenic pain; and splenic abscess in the setting of splenic infarction. It is important to limit splenectomy to these few specific circumstances, because overwhelming sepsis and acute PH have been reported in the postsplenectomy period in SCD.

Kidney transplantation has been successfully performed in patients with SCD on chronic renal replacement therapy, although survival at 7 years is lower than in African Americans without SCD (67% vs. 83%). This difference is mostly due to vasoocclusive complications in the transplanted kidney, possibly exacerbated by the higher hematocrit in the postoperative period from resumption of endogenous erythropoietin production and increased blood viscosity. It is therefore critical to closely monitor ESA therapy in the posttransplantation period to prevent overdosing and relative erythrocytosis. A chronic transfusion program to prevent intrarenal sickling and maximization of hydroxyurea therapy should also be entertained, although its benefits need to be balanced against the risk of HLA alloimmunization and rejection. Combined solid organ and HCT protocols are being developed to overcome these complications. Recently, lung transplantation has been successfully performed in a SCD patient with severe pulmonary arterial hypertension and pulmonary venoocclusive disease.

References

Adams RJ, Brambilla D: Discontinuing prophylactic transfusions used to prevent stroke in sickle cell disease, *N Engl J Med* 353:2769–2778, 2005.

Adams RJ, Brambilla DJ, Granger S, et al: Stroke and conversion to high risk in children screened with transcranial Doppler ultrasound during the STOP study, *Blood* 103:3689–3694, 2004.

Ataga KI, et al: Crizanlizumab for the prevention of pain crises in sickle cell disease, *N Engl J Med* 376:429–439, 2017.

Bunn HF: Pathogenesis and treatment of sickle cell disease, *N Engl J Med* 337:762–769, 1997.

Charache S, Terrin ML, Moore RD, et al: Effect of hydroxyurea on the frequency of painful crises in sickle cell anemia. Investigators of the Multicenter Study of Hydroxyurea in Sickle Cell Anemia, *N Engl J Med* 332:1317–1322, 1995.

DeBaun MR, et al: Controlled trial of transfusions for silent cerebral infarcts in sickle cell anemia, *N Engl J Med* 371(8):699–710, 2014.

Falletta JM, Woods GM, Verter JI, et al: Discontinuing penicillin prophylaxis in children with sickle cell anemia. Prophylactic Penicillin Study II, *J Pediatr* 127:685–690, 1995.

Gaston MH, Verter JI, Woods G, et al: Prophylaxis with oral penicillin in children with sickle cell anemia. A randomized trial, *N Engl J Med* 314:1593–1599, 1986.

Gladwin MT, Sachdev V: Cardiovascular abnormalities in sickle cell disease, *J Am Coll Cardiol* 59:1123–1133, 2012.

Gladwin MT, Sachdev V, Jison ML, et al: Pulmonary hypertension as a risk factor for death in patients with sickle cell disease, *N Engl J Med* 350:886–895, 2004.

Gladwin MT, Vichinsky E: Pulmonary complications of sickle cell disease, *N Engl J Med* 359:2254–2265, 2008.

Gluckman E, Cappelli B, Bernaudin F, et al: Sickle cell disease: An international survey of results of HLA-identical sibling hematopoietic stem cell transplantation, *Blood* 129(11):1548–1556, 2017.

Hoppe CC, Inati AC, Brown C, et al: Initial results from a cohort in a phase 2a study (GBT440- 007) evaluating adolescents with sickle cell disease treated with multiple doses of GBT440, a HbS polymerization inhibitor, *Blood* 130.

Howard J, Malfroy M, Llewelyn C, et al: The Transfusion Alternatives Preoperatively in Sickle Cell Disease (TAPS) study: A randomised, controlled, multicentre clinical trial, *Lancet* 381:930–938, 2013.

Hsieh MM, Fitzhugh CD, Weitzel RP, et al: Nonmyeloablative HLA-matched sibling allogeneic hematopoietic stem cell transplantation for severe sickle cell phenotype, *JAMA* 312(1):48–56, 2014.

Jeong GK, Ruchelsman DE, Jazrawi LM, Jaffe WL: Total hip arthroplasty in sickle cell hemoglobinopathies, *J Am Acad Orthop Surg* 13:208–217, 2005.

Krishnamurti L, Kharbanda S, Biernacki MA, et al: Stable long-term donor engraftment following reduced-intensity hematopoietic cell transplantation for sickle cell disease, *Biol Blood Marrow Transplant* 14:1270–1278, 2008.

Lee MT, Piomelli S, Granger S, et al: Stroke Prevention Trial in Sickle Cell Anemia (STOP): Extended follow-up and final results, *Blood* 108:847–852, 2006.

Little JA, McGowan VR, Kato GJ, et al: Combination erythropoietin-hydroxyurea therapy in sickle cell disease: Experience from the National Institutes of Health and a literature review, *Haematologica* 91:1076–1083, 2006.

Mehari A, Alam S, Tian X, et al: Hemodynamic predictors of mortality in adults with sickle cell disease, *Am J Respir Crit Care Med* 187:840–847, 2013.

Merkel KH, Ginsberg PL, Parker JC, Post MJ: Cerebrovascular disease in sickle cell anemia: A clinical, pathological and radiological correlation, *Stroke* 9:45–52, 1978.

Morris CR, Kato GJ, Poljakovic M, et al: Dysregulated arginine metabolism, hemolysis-associated pulmonary hypertension, and mortality in sickle cell disease, *JAMA* 294:81–90, 2005.

Noguchi CT, Rodgers GP, Serjeant G, Schechter AN: Levels of fetal hemoglobin necessary for treatment of sickle cell disease, *N Engl J Med* 318:96–99, 1988.

Novelli EM, Huynh C, Gladwin MT, et al: Pulmonary embolism in sickle cell disease: A case-control study, *J Thrombosis and Hemostasis* 10:760–766, 2012.

Ohene-Frempong K, Weiner SJ, Sleeper LA, et al: Cerebrovascular accidents in sickle cell disease: Rates and risk factors, *Blood* 91:288–294, 1998.

Niihara Y, et al: A phase 3 trial of l-glutamine in sickle cell disease, *N Engl J Med* 379:226–235, 2018.

Platt OS: The acute chest syndrome of sickle cell disease, *N Engl J Med* 342:1904–1907, 2000.

Platt OS, Brambilla DJ, Rosse WF, et al: Mortality in sickle cell disease. Life expectancy and risk factors for early death, *N Engl J Med* 330:1639–1644, 1994.

Platt OS, Thorington BD, Brambilla DJ, et al: Pain in sickle cell disease. Rates and risk factors, *N Engl J Med* 325:11–16, 1991.

Reiter CD, Wang X, Tanus-Santos JE, et al: Cell-free hemoglobin limits nitric oxide bioavailability in sickle-cell disease, *Nat Med* 8:1383–1389, 2002.

Ribeil J, et al: Gene therapy in a patient with sickle cell disease, *N Engl J Med* 376:848–855, 2017.

Scheinman JI: Sickle cell disease and the kidney, *Nat Clin Pract Nephrol* 5:78–88, 2009.

Smiley D, Dagogo-Jack S, Umpierrez G: Therapy insight: Metabolic and endocrine disorders in sickle cell disease, *Nat Clin Pract Endocrinol Metab* 4:102–109, 2008.

Steinberg MH: Management of sickle cell disease, *N Engl J Med* 340:1021–1030, 1999.

Steinberg MH, Barton F, Castro O, et al: Effect of hydroxyurea on mortality and morbidity in adult sickle cell anemia: Risks and benefits up to 9 years of treatment, *JAMA* 289:1645–1651, 2003.

Telen MJ, Wun T, McCavit TL, et al: Randomized phase 2 study of GMI-1070 in SCD: Reduction in time to resolution of vaso-occlusive events and decreased opioid use, *Blood* 125:2656–2664, 2015.

Vichinsky EP, Neumayr LD, Earles AN, et al: Causes and outcomes of the acute chest syndrome in sickle cell disease, *N Engl J Med* 342:1855–1865, 2000.

Vichinsky E, Hoppe CC, Ataga KI, et al: A phase 3 randomized trial of voxelotor in sickle cell disease, *N Engl J Med* 381(6):509–519, 2019.

Walters MC, Patience M, Leisenring W, et al: Bone marrow transplantation for sickle cell disease, *N Engl J Med* 335:369–376, 1996.

Walters MC, Storb R, Patience M, et al: Impact of bone marrow transplantation for symptomatic sickle cell disease: An interim report. Multicenter investigation of bone marrow transplantation for sickle cell disease, *Blood* 95:1918–1924, 2000.

Yawn BP, et al: Management of sickle cell disease: Summary of the 2014 evidence-based report by expert panel members, *JAMA* 312(10):1033–1048, 2014.

THALASSEMIA

Method of
Sarah A. Holstein, MD, PhD; and Raymond J. Hohl, MD, PhD

CURRENT DIAGNOSIS

- Complete blood count: anemia (very severe in β-thalassemia major, mild in β-thalassemia minor and α-thalassemia trait), low mean corpuscular volume, variable leukocytosis, thrombocytopenia (secondary to splenomegaly) or thrombocythemia (after splenectomy)
- Peripheral blood smear: hypochromia, microcytosis, anisocytosis, poikilocytosis, target cells, Heinz bodies, nucleated red blood cells
- Evidence of hemolytic anemia: indirect hyperbilirubinemia, elevated lactate dehydrogenase, decreased haptoglobin
- Hemoglobin electrophoresis pattern:
  - β-Thalassemia minor: elevated HbA2 ($\alpha_2\delta_2$)
  - β-Thalassemia intermedia: elevated HbA2, elevated HbF ($\alpha_2\gamma_2$), and decreased HbA ($\alpha_2\beta_2$)
  - β-Thalassemia major: absence of HbA, markedly elevated HbF, and elevated HbA2
  - α-Thalassemia trait: normal
  - Hemoglobin H disease: decreased HbA, presence of HbH (β_4) and HbBart (γ_4)
  - Hemoglobin Barts hydrops fetalis: HbBart, absence of HbA, HbA2, and HbF
- Timing of symptomatic disease:
  - β-Thalassemia minor: asymptomatic
  - β-Thalassemia intermedia: variable
  - β-Thalassemia major: within first year of life
  - α-Thalassemia trait: asymptomatic
  - Hemoglobin H disease: symptomatic at time of birth
  - Hemoglobin Barts hydrops fetalis: death during gestation

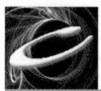

CURRENT THERAPY

- Chronic packed red blood cell transfusions for β-thalassemia major (1–3 units of packed leukoreduced erythrocytes every 3–5 weeks) with a target hemoglobin concentration of 9–10.5 g/dL; variable transfusion needs for β-thalassemia intermedia and hemoglobin H disease
- Splenectomy with antibiotic prophylaxis and vaccination
- Iron chelation: deferoxamine (Desferal), or deferasirox (Exjade); deferiprone (Ferriprox)
- Osteoporosis management: calcium with vitamin D supplementation; bisphosphonates
- Allogeneic hematopoietic cell transplantation for β-thalassemia major
- Luspatercept (Reblozy) for transfusion-dependent adults with beta-thalassemia

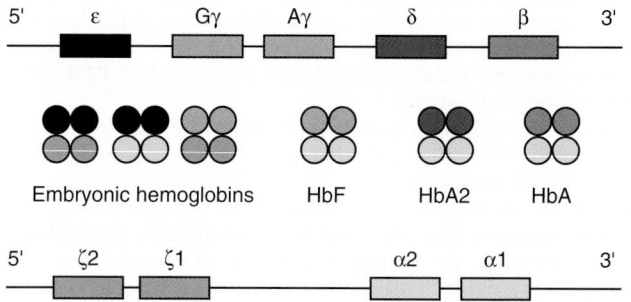

Figure 1 Representation of the β and α globin gene clusters. Also shown are the globin tetramers produced during embryonic development.

Globin Gene Arrangements

Thalassemia syndromes encompass a spectrum of hemoglobin disorders that arise from impaired production of globin chains. The genes that encode globins are located in two clusters: the β gene cluster on chromosome 11 and the α gene cluster on chromosome 16 (Figure 1). The β gene cluster includes the adult globin genes (β and δ) as well as the fetal Aγ and Gγ genes and the embryonic ε gene. The arrangement of the 5′ to 3′ sequence of these genes parallels the order of their developmental expression. Functional hemoglobin is a tetramer that includes two α and two β globin units. The α gene cluster includes two fetal/adult α genes (α1 and α2) and the embryonic ζ genes. In the embryo, three hemoglobins are found ($\zeta_2\varepsilon_2$, $\alpha_2\varepsilon_2$, and $\zeta_2\gamma_2$). Fetal hemoglobin (HbF) is composed of two α chains and two γ chains ($\alpha_2\gamma_2$). In adults, the predominant hemoglobin is hemoglobin A (HbA), consisting of two α chains and two β chains ($\alpha_2\beta_2$) (see Figure 1). Hemoglobin A2, consisting of two α chains and two δ chains ($\alpha_2\delta_2$), is a normal variant in adults and typically represents less than 3% of the total hemoglobin (see Figure 1).

In β-thalassemia, there is diminished production of β globin genes, resulting in an excess of α globin chains. Conversely, in α-thalassemia there is impaired production of α globin genes, resulting in an excess of β globin chains. This imbalance of globin production is variable, and the degree of accumulation of unpaired globin chains is directly related to the severity of the disease phenotype. The genetic basis of thalassemia is heterogeneous, and several hundred mutations have been identified. These mutations may affect any level of globin gene expression, including arrangement of the globin gene complex, gene deletion, splicing, transcription, translation, and protein stability. In general, β-thalassemia occurs as a result of mutations, whereas α-thalassemia occurs as a result of gene deletion.

It has been estimated that there are 270 million carriers of thalassemia in the world, including 80 million β-thalassemia carriers. The frequency of β-thalassemia carriers is highest in the malarial tropical and subtropical regions of Asia, the Mediterranean, and the Middle East. The term thalassemia, derived from Greek, refers to the Mediterranean Sea. This distribution is secondary to the selective advantage of heterozygotes against malaria. β-Thalassemia is subdivided into major, intermedia, and minor types (Table 1). α-Thalassemia is classified into four syndromes: α-thalassemia trait 2 (loss of one α globin gene [αα/α–];α-thalassemia trait 1, also referred to as α-thalassemia minor (loss of two α globin genes [αα/– – or α–/α–]); hemoglobin H (HbH) disease (loss of three alleles [α–/– –]); and hemoglobin Barts hydrops fetalis (loss of all four α globin loci [– –/– –]).

Pathophysiology

The clinical manifestations of thalassemia and their severity are a consequence of the relative excess of unpaired globin chains. In particular, excess α globin chains are unstable and insoluble and therefore precipitate inside the red blood cell (RBC). These

TABLE 1 Summary of Hematologic and Clinical Features of the Thalassemias

TYPE	HEMATOLOGIC FINDINGS	HEMOGLOBIN ELECTROPHORESIS PATTERN	CLINICAL FEATURES
β-Thalassemia major	Severe anemia, microcytosis, hypochromia, target cells, nucleated RBCs	Absence of HbA, markedly elevated HbF, elevated HbA2	Splenomegaly, jaundice, skeletal abnormalities, abnormal facies; transfusion dependent
β-Thalassemia intermedia	Mild to moderate anemia, microcytosis, hypochromia	Elevated HbA2, elevated HbF, decreased HbA	Splenomegaly; variable transfusion dependence
β-Thalassemia minor	Mild anemia, microcytosis, target cells	Elevated HbA2	None
Hemoglobin Barts hydrops fetalis	Severe anemia, anisopoikilocytosis, hypochromia, nucleated RBCs	HbBart; absence of HbA, HbA2, and HbF	Death during gestation; fetus with massive hepatosplenomegaly, generalized edema
Hemoglobin H disease	Moderately severe anemia, anisopoikilocytosis, microcytosis, Heinz bodies	Decreased HbA; HbH and HbBart present	Splenomegaly, jaundice; generally transfusion dependent
α-Thalassemia trait 1	Mild anemia, hypochromia, microcytosis, target cells	Normal	None
α-Thalassemia trait 2	Normal	Normal	None

Hb, Hemoglobin; *HbA*, hemoglobin A; *HbF*, fetal hemoglobin; *HbH*, hemoglobin H; *RBCs*, red blood cells.

inclusions (precipitated hemoglobin) may be visualized as Heinz bodies. The accumulation of α globin chains leads to a variety of insults to the erythrocyte, including changes in membrane deformability and increased fragility. Free β chains are more soluble than free α chains and are able to form a homotetramer (HbH). The hallmark of thalassemia is an anemia that is a consequence of both increased destruction (i.e., hemolysis) and decreased production (i.e., ineffective erythropoiesis). The bone marrow typically displays erythroid hyperplasia.

Oxidant injury is closely linked with the pathology of thalassemia. Under normal conditions, a small amount of methemoglobin (Fe^{3+}) is formed via oxidation and can then be reduced back to hemoglobin (Fe^{2+}). However, isolated globin chains can be oxidized to hemichromes, some forms of which are irreversibly oxidized. The hemichromes can then generate reactive oxygen species, which can oxidize membrane components, leading to cell injury. There is an increase in membrane rigidity in β-thalassemia, and this appears to be secondary to the binding of partially oxidized α globin chains to components of the membrane skeleton. Increased membrane rigidity in turn leads to decreased membrane deformability and increased destruction. In α-thalassemia, HbH has a left-shifted oxygen disassociation curve and therefore does not readily transport oxygen. HbH erythrocytes have increased rigidity, which is thought to be secondary to interactions between excess β globin chains and the membrane. Unlike with β-thalassemia, HbH erythrocytes have increased membrane stability. Inclusion bodies have been identified in HbH cells, and there appears to be a correlation between RBC age and solubility of HbH. As cells age, the amount of soluble HbH decreases, and the level of inclusions increases.

It has also been recognized that there is increased phagocytosis of thalassemia RBCs compared with in normal controls. The etiology is not completely understood, but it may be a consequence of reduction in surface levels of sialic acid, increase in surface immunoglobulin G binding, and changes in phosphatidylserine localization.

Despite the pronounced hemolysis and marrow erythroid hyperplasia, patients with thalassemia generally do not display the compensatory reticulocytosis that is indicative of the other basis for anemia, ineffective erythropoiesis. Accumulation of α chain aggregates is thought to lead to death of erythrocyte precursors. Furthermore, abnormal assembly of membrane proteins in erythroid precursors has been demonstrated.

Iron overload is one of the primary causes of morbidity. Even without transfusion, the long-standing anemia, however mild, leads to increased iron absorption in the gut and eventual chronic iron overload. Excessive iron deposition causes devastating damage to multiple organs, particularly affecting the heart, liver, and endocrine organs.

β-Thalassemia Major

Symptoms of β-thalassemia major are not present at birth, because HbF ($\alpha_2\gamma_2$) is present. However, as HbF levels decline over the first year, the signs and symptoms of severe hemolytic anemia begin to manifest. Affected individuals display hepatosplenomegaly from expansion of the reticuloendothelial system, as well as extramedullary hematopoiesis, pallor, growth retardation, and abnormal skeletal development. If left untreated, 80% of children with β-thalassemia major will die before the age of 5 years.

Laboratory Features

Thalassemia major is characterized by a severe microcytic anemia. Hemoglobin levels may be as low as 3 to 4 g/dL. The peripheral blood smear is markedly abnormal and is notable for hypochromia, microcytosis, anisocytosis, poikilocytosis, target cells, and tear drop cells. Routine stains show the presence of precipitated α globin chains as Heinz bodies. The reticulocyte count is often low. The white blood cell count is often high but may be artifactually elevated as a consequence of automated inclusion of high numbers of circulating nucleated RBCs. The platelet count is typically normal, but progressive hypersplenism can result in decreased platelet counts. Patients who have undergone splenectomy often have increased white blood cell and platelet counts. Iron studies reveal elevated serum iron, transferrin saturation, and ferritin. Consistent with hemolysis and ineffective erythropoiesis, indirect bilirubin and lactate dehydrogenase levels are increased, and haptoglobin levels are low.

Clinical Features

Unique to β-thalassemia major is the development of extramedullary erythropoiesis. This may be so severe that the masses of bone marrow lead to broken bones and spinal cord compression. Sites of involvement include the sinuses and the thoracic and pelvic cavities. The expansion of the erythroid bone marrow can lead to a number of skeletal changes. In particular, characteristic changes in the facial bones and skull result in frontal bossing, overgrowth of the maxillae, and malocclusion. This has sometimes been referred to as chipmunk facies. Other bones are also affected, and premature fusion of the epiphyses results in shortened limbs.

Compression fractures of the spine may occur. Even if the disease is managed appropriately with transfusions and iron chelation, patients will still suffer from osteopenia and osteoporosis. Possible mechanisms include changes secondary to hypogonadism or increased bone resorption secondary to vitamin D deficiency.

Hepatomegaly and splenomegaly, secondary to extramedullary erythropoiesis and RBC destruction, are prominent. Injury to Kupffer cells and hepatocytes from chronic overload leads to fibrosis and end-stage liver disease. Hepatic iron overload is probably caused in part by comparatively high levels of transferrin receptors. Iron overload, and perhaps other factors, increase susceptibility to viral hepatitis. Laboratory studies show indirect hyperbilirubinemia, hypergammaglobulinemia, and elevated liver markers. The chronic hemolysis leads to formation of bilirubin gallstones, although cholecystitis or cholangitis is not common. Splenic dysfunction results in immune dysfunction. The shortened erythrocyte survival time leaves patients susceptible to aplastic crisis induced by parvovirus B19 infection. Extramedullary hematopoiesis may also affect the kidneys, and patients often have large kidneys. Rapid cell turnover leads to hyperuricemia, and children may develop gouty nephropathy.

A number of endocrine abnormalities are commonly seen in β-thalassemia major, including hypogonadism, growth failure, diabetes, and hypothyroidism. These abnormalities occur even in chronically transfused patients and may be in part related to iron overload. Endocrine glands, such as liver and heart, have high levels of transferrin-receptor and therefore are more susceptible to iron overload. The typical growth pattern for a child with β-thalassemia major is relatively normal until the age of 9 to 10 years. After that time, the growth velocity slows, and the pubertal growth spurt is either absent or reduced. Although secretion of growth hormone does not appear to be altered in thalassemic patients, a reduction in peak amplitude and nocturnal levels of growth hormone has been observed. Amenorrhea is quite common, with 50% of girls presenting with primary amenorrhea. Secondary amenorrhea also develops, particularly in patients who do not receive regular chelation therapy. In males, impotence and azoospermia is common. Primary hypothyroidism typically appears during the second decade of life. The prevalence of diabetes mellitus and impaired glucose intolerance has been estimated at 4% to 20%. Unlike type 1 diabetes mellitus, diabetes associated with thalassemia is rarely complicated by diabetic ketoacidosis. The risk of diabetic retinopathy is lower, but the risk of diabetic nephropathy is higher. Patients with a high ferritin level (greater than 1800 μg/L) experience a faster progression to hypothyroidism, hypogonadism, and other endocrinopathies.

Thalassemic patients suffer from extensive cardiac abnormalities. Chronic anemia causes cardiac dilation. Although long-term transfusion can help prevent cardiac dilation, the resulting iron overload leads to cardiac hemosiderosis. Pericarditis, ventricular and supraventricular arrhythmias, and end-stage cardiomyopathy can develop. Ventricular arrhythmia is a common cause of death. Patients may also develop pulmonary hypertension. The degree of iron overload in the heart has traditionally been assessed by cardiac biopsy, but cardiac magnetic resonance imaging (MRI) is increasingly being used.

Vitamin and mineral deficiencies may occur. Folic acid deficiency may develop in patients, presumably as a consequence of increased cell turnover. Although the cause is unknown, patients with β-thalassemia major often have very low serum zinc levels. Serum levels of vitamin E and vitamin C may also be low.

Management of β-Thalassemia Major
Transfusion
The key intervention for the management of β-thalassemia major is chronic transfusion therapy. In particular, during the first decade of life, regular transfusion results in improvements in hepatosplenomegaly, skeletal abnormalities, and cardiac dilation. Patients typically require 1 to 3 units of packed RBCs every 3 to 5 weeks. The optimal target total hemoglobin level has yet to be determined. Alloimmunization does occur, and some blood centers try to leukodeplete their products, match donors by ethnicity,

and limit the donor pool for any particular patient. Although the risk of bloodborne infections is currently quite small, regular transfusion of blood products still carries a risk for infections such as human immunodeficiency virus (HIV) and hepatitis C.

Splenectomy
The general indication for splenectomy is an increase of more than 50% in the RBC transfusion requirement over the period of 1 year. Splenectomy may initially yield a decrease in the RBC transfusion requirement. It has been noted that thalassemia patients are at higher risk for infection after splenectomy than are those patients splenectomized for other reasons. The bacteria that most frequently cause infections in these patients include *Streptococcus pneumoniae, Haemophilus influenzae, Neisseria meningitidis, Klebsiella, Escherichia coli,* and *Staphylococcus aureus.* The increased susceptibility to infection compared with other splenectomized patients is thought to be a result of greater immune dysfunction secondary to iron overload. In particular, it has been reported that iron-overloaded macrophages lose the ability to kill intracellular pathogens. Antibiotic prophylaxis with penicillin, amoxicillin, or erythromycin is recommended for children up to age 16 years. In addition, patients should receive immunizations, including the pneumococcal, influenza, and *Haemophilus influenzae* vaccines.

Iron Chelation Therapy
Because of increased iron absorption and long-term transfusion therapy, iron overload develops. As noted earlier, iron overload causes damage to multiple organs. Because iron is poorly excreted, removal must be accomplished by phlebotomy (not an option in thalassemic patients) or by chelation therapy. Historically, deferoxamine (Desferal) has been the most widely used chelator. This agent may be administered subcutaneously (SQ), intramuscularly (IM), or intravenously (IV). The dosing for chronic iron overload is 1000 to 2000 mg/day (or 20 to 40 mg/kg/day) SQ or 500 to 1000 mg/day IM or 40 to 50 mg/kg/day IV. The IV-only route is indicated for patients with cardiovascular collapse. Multiple studies have shown that deferoxamine therapy improves long-term survival. In addition, intensive therapy with deferoxamine has been shown to improve cardiac function in patients with severe iron overload. However, compliance with daily injections has been a particular problem, and, unless regular therapy is given, iron will reaccumulate.

Deferiprone (Ferriprox) was the first orally active chelator to be introduced. It is given three times daily (total of 75 mg/kg/day). Studies have indicated that deferiprone may be as effective as deferoxamine in lowering iron levels. A recent Cochrane Review concluded that deferiprone is indicated in the treatment of iron overload in thalassemia major if deferoxamine therapy is contraindicated or inadequate. Agranulocytosis associated with deferiprone has been reported, and, because of this risk, the drug is currently not available in the United States except through the US Food and Drug Administration (FDA) Treatment Use Program. Deferiprone is available in Europe and Asia. There has also been interest in combined therapy with deferiprone and deferoxamine, and one study showed that the combination was more effective in removing cardiac and hepatic iron but did not further improve cardiac function.

Deferasirox (Exjade) is the first orally active agent approved for use in the United States. Its longer half-life in comparison with deferiprone allows this drug to be given once daily (total of 20 to 40 mg/kg/day). A phase III trial comparing deferasirox to deferoxamine in patients with thalassemia revealed similar decreases in liver iron concentrations. Side effects include gastrointestinal complaints (abdominal pain, nausea, vomiting, diarrhea) and skin rash. There have been postmarketing reports of acute renal failure, hepatic failure, and cytopenias. It is recommended that serum creatinine, ferritin, and alanine aminotransferase be monitored monthly during therapy. A prospective, randomized study comparing deferiprone and deferoxamine versus deferiprone and deferasirox in 96 patients with β-thalassemia major demonstrated that both regimens reduced iron overload. However, the latter regimen was found to be superior with respect to improving cardiac iron, patient compliance, and patient satisfaction.

The "gold standard" for measurement of liver iron concentration has been liver biopsy with iron measurement by atomic absorption spectrometry. More recently, there has been increasing use of MRI technology to measure liver iron levels. In general, iron content determined by MRI methodology correlates with liver iron concentration determined by biopsy. However, the precision of liver MRI measurement appears to be dependent on iron levels, liver fibrosis, and calibration. Hepatic iron concentration has also been measured using a superconducting quantum interference device (SQUID), although reported consistency has varied and widespread use of this technique has been limited by expense and complexity.

Management of Osteoporosis

Even with calcium and vitamin D supplementation, iron chelation, transfusion therapy, and hormonal therapy, bone loss continues to be a significant problem for thalassemia patients. Recently, there has been interest in the use of bisphosphonates. This class of drugs, which includes clodronate (Bonefos)[2], alendronate (Fosamax), pamidronate (Aredia), zoledronate (Zometa), and neridronate (Nerixia)[2], inhibit osteoclastic bone resorption and have found extensive use in the management of Paget disease, osteoporosis, and skeletal metastases. Small studies performed in thalassemia patients have failed to show benefit with clodronate 100 mg IM every 10 days or 300 mg IV every 3 weeks. A very small study using alendronate (Fosamax)[1] 10 mg PO daily revealed an increase in bone mineral density only at the femoral level. Conversely, in a study involving pamidronate (Aredia)[1] 30 or 60 mg IV every month, there was an increase in bone density only at the lumbar level. The most promising results have been achieved with the most potent member of the class, zoledronate. Several trials demonstrated that zoledronate (Zometa)[1] 4 mg IV every 3 or 4 months results in significant improvement in femoral and lumbar bone mineral density and reduces bony pain. The largest randomized trial involved 118 β-thalassemia patients who received calcium plus vitamin D with or without neridronate (given every 90 days). At 6 and 12 months, there was increased bone mineral density as well as decreased back pain and analgesic use in the neridronate arm. Larger, long-term trials are necessary before this agent finds widespread use in the management of thalassemia-induced osteoporosis.

Hematopoietic Cell Transplantation

Hematopoietic cell transplantation is the only curative strategy for patients with hemoglobinopathies. Patients are assigned to a risk class (Pesaro class) based on adherence to regular iron chelation therapy, presence or absence of hepatomegaly, and presence or absence of portal fibrosis. Those children with no or little hepatomegaly, no portal fibrosis, and regular iron chelation therapy (class I) have a better than 90% chance of cure, whereas those with both hepatomegaly and portal fibrosis (class III) have long-term survival rates of approximately 60% in older studies. More recent reports indicate that class III survival has improved to 90%.

The use of human leukocyte antigen (HLA)-identical sibling donors has been preferred, because the use of HLA-mismatched donors has produced inferior results and is associated with increased graft rejection, graft-versus-host disease, and infection. However, it is estimated that only one-third of patients will have a matched donor. The use of unrelated donors has been explored, and initial studies showed poorer outcomes. However, more recent data suggest that matched unrelated donors might be a viable option if a suitable sibling donor is lacking, thanks to improved donor selection and transplantation techniques. The use of partially HLA-matched unrelated cord blood has been reported, although four of nine children did not engraft.

Another emerging technique is the use of reduced-intensity conditioning regimens, although long-term success has yet to be achieved. However, no randomized controlled studies have been performed evaluating the role of transplant in thalassemia patients.

Gene Therapy

Globin gene therapy, achieved through manipulation of autologous stem cells, is an attractive alternative to allogeneic transplantation. There are three major scientific hurdles that must be overcome: design of vectors that yield therapeutic levels of globin gene expression, ability to isolate and transduce autologous stem cells, and development of transplantation conditions that will permit host repopulation. In addition, the safety of viral and nonviral transfections is an issue. Initial studies involved ex vivo transduction of autologous hematopoietic stem cells with a lentiviral vector carrying the transgene. This gene therapy has been administered intravenously or via intrabone injection following a myeloablative conditioning regimen. Many of the patients treated to date have achieved transfusion independence, and thus far no unusual toxicities have been observed. The first gene therapy to obtain regulatory approval is Zynteglo[2], which was granted conditional approval by the European Commission. Zynteglo therapy involves the ex vivo transduction of autologous CD34+ cells with the gene encoding β^{A-T87Q}-globin via a BB305 lentiviral vector. Following a myeloablative conditioning regimen with busulfan (Busulfex)[1], the transduced CD34+ cells are administered (single dose of 5.0×10^6 cells/kg). Zynteglo is currently approved only for patients with transfusion-dependent non-β^0/β^0-thalassemia who are 12 years and older. Another approach that is currently under investigation involves the use of genome editing techniques such as CRISPR.

Pharmacologic Induction of Fetal Hemoglobin

Induction of HbF expression has been proposed as a therapeutic strategy. For β-thalassemia, induced γ globin gene expression would be predicted to decrease globin chain imbalance by complexing with free α chains. Hydroxyurea (Hydrea)[1] is an antimetabolite thought to interfere with DNA synthesis. It is well established in the management of sickle cell disease, where it has been shown to increase levels of HbF. The use of hydroxyurea in β-thalassemia is much less well established. In the United States, hydroxyurea has been approved for use in sickle cell disease but not for thalassemia. Studies published elsewhere in the world have generally shown improvements in hemoglobin levels in thalassemia intermedia patients, with some patients becoming transfusion independent. A recent meta-analysis on the use of hydroxyurea in patients with transfusion dependent β-thalassemia concluded that this agent might offer some benefit but that double-blinded placebo-controlled studies are lacking.

5-Azacytidine (azacitidine [Vidaza])[1], an inhibitor of DNA methyltransferase, has been shown to induce HbF. However, concerns regarding long-term use have prevented further evaluation in thalassemia. Decitabine (Dacogen)[1], an analog of 5-azacytidine, has been shown to increase HbF levels in patients with sickle cell disease refractory to hydroxyurea. A small pilot study of low-dose decitabine in β-thalassemia intermedia patients demonstrated an increase in total hemoglobin and hemoglobin F levels. Butyrate[5], an inhibitor of histone deacetylases, is another agent capable of inducing HbF. However, butyrate and its derivatives (arginine butyrate[5], sodium isobutyramide[5], and sodium phenylbutyrate [Buphenyl][1]) have failed to show significant clinical benefit in thalassemia patients. Therefore, at this time, no agent has been approved for use in thalassemia patients. A number of hypotheses have been proposed to explain the lack of success of inducers of HbF in thalassemia: there is simply too little γ globin production to significantly affect globin chain balance; these agents decrease expression of partially active β-thalassemia genes; these agents increase expression of α-globin genes; chronic transfusions appear to reduce HbF levels; and these agents suppress erythropoiesis.

Novel Agents Targeting Ineffective Erythropoiesis

An alternative strategy that is being investigated involves the targeting of ineffective erythropoiesis. Luspatercept-aamt (Reblozyl)

---

[1]Not FDA approved for this indication.
[2]Not available in the United States.

---

[1]Not FDA approved for this indication.
[2]Not available in the United States.
[5]Investigational drug in the United States.

and sotatercept (ACE-011)[5] are activin receptor trap ligands that were developed to treat postmenopausal osteoporosis but were noted to increase Hb levels. Initial phase 2 studies with these agents in thalassemia patients revealed reductions in transfusion burden, increase in Hb, and reduction in liver iron levels. A phase 3 study comparing luspatercept plus best supportive care to placebo plus best supportive care revealed that 21.4% of patients receiving luspatercept achieved a reduction in transfusion burden compared with 4.5% in the placebo group. Luspatercept (1 mg/kg SQ every 3 weeks) is approved by the FDA for the treatment of anemia in adult patients with β-thalassemia who require regular RBC transfusions. Janus kinase 2 (JAK2) plays a key role in erythropoiesis, and there is interest in the potential use of JAK2 inhibitors in thalassemia. A phase II study with ruxolitinib (Jakafi)[1] showed a trend toward reduction in transfusions as well as a reduction in spleen size.

Antioxidants

Oxidative damage is believed to be an important cause of tissue damage, and there has been interest in the use of antioxidants in thalassemia patients. A variety of substances have been investigated, including ascorbate[1], vitamin E[1], N-acetylcysteine (Mucomyst)[1], flavonoids, and indicaxanthin[5]. A variety of antioxidant effects have been observed in vitro with these agents, but none have been shown to improve anemia in patients with thalassemia.

β-Thalassemia Intermedia

Given the underlying genetic heterogeneity, it is not surprising that the clinical manifestations of β-thalassemia intermedia are also quite varied. Some patients with more mild forms of β-thalassemia intermedia do not require long-term transfusion therapy. There is not a clear consensus about when long-term transfusion should be initiated. Factors that are considered for children include growth patterns, spleen size, and bone development. Transfusion may be necessary during infection-induced aplastic crises. In some instances, transfusions are begun in childhood to help with growth and then discontinued after puberty. Some adults gradually become more anemic and eventually require transfusion. Some authors have argued that starting transfusions early in life is advantageous, because the prevalence of alloimmunization appears to increase if transfusion is started after the first few years of life.

Splenomegaly usually develops in all patients, including those who do not require transfusion. With progression of splenomegaly and the accompanying sequestration and hemolysis, there is usually worsening of anemia, to the point at which transfusions may be required. Most patients achieve transfusion independence after splenectomy. Gallstones may develop, and a prophylactic cholecystectomy is sometimes performed at the same time as the splenectomy. As with β-thalassemia major patients, intermedia patients are at increased risk for infection and should be appropriately vaccinated.

For reasons that are not entirely clear, there is an increased risk of thromboembolic complications in intermedia patients compared with thalassemia major patients. An Italian study reported that 10% of thalassemia intermedia and 4% of thalassemia major patients experienced a thromboembolic event. Another study reported that thromboembolism occurred four times more frequently in patients with intermedia versus major disease. This report noted that venous events were more common in the thalassemia intermedia population, whereas arterial events were more common in the thalassemia major population. An even higher rate of venous thrombotic events (29%) was reported in a population of splenectomized patients with thalassemia intermedia. It has been suggested that exposed anionic phospholipids on the surface of damaged RBCs may induce a procoagulant effect. There is no consensus regarding the prophylactic use of antiplatelet agents or anticoagulants in this population.

Patients with thalassemia intermedia may develop iron overload, although it is less severe than in patients with thalassemia major. Even those that are not regularly transfused may develop a degree of iron overload, because there is increased iron absorption. Iron overload may be managed with the iron chelating agents as described earlier. Cardiac toxicity, including congestive heart failure, valvular problems, and pulmonary hypertension (leading to secondary right-sided heart failure), resulting from iron overload is not infrequent in the thalassemia intermedia population.

Bone abnormalities and osteoporosis may develop in thalassemia intermedia patients. In a North American study, the prevalence of fractures in these patients was 12%. Leg ulcers involving the medial malleolus are common and are often difficult to treat. Hypogonadism, hypothyroidism, and diabetes may occur, with frequency related to the severity of anemia and iron overload. Pseudoxanthoma elasticum, a syndrome consisting of skin lesions, angioid streaks in the retina, calcified retinal walls, and aortic valve disease, is more common in thalassemia intermedia than in thalassemia major. Currently, no effective therapy exists, although it has been reported that aluminum hydroxide (Alternagel)[1] reduces skin calcification.

β-Thalassemia Minor

Most patients with β-thalassemia minor are asymptomatic. However, they have an abnormal complete blood count that may sometimes lead to the misdiagnosis of iron deficiency. Although these patients have a microcytic anemia, it is much less severe than in patients with β-thalassemia major. In general, the hematocrit is greater than 30%. The mean corpuscular volume is typically less than 75 fL and the RBC distribution width index is normal, in contrast to iron deficiency, in which the degree of microcytosis is less and the distribution width index is usually increased. The peripheral blood smear shows the presence of target cells. Hemoglobin electrophoresis typically reveals an increase in HbA2. The normal anemia experienced during pregnancy may sometimes be exacerbated in patients with β-thalassemia minor, necessitating transfusion. Otherwise, no long-term effects of β-thalassemia minor have been described, and no interventions are required.

α-Thalassemia
Laboratory and Clinical Features

Patients with α-thalassemia trait 2 are symptom free and have normal laboratory values, including complete blood count, peripheral smear, and hemoglobin electrophoresis. Individuals with α-thalassemia trait 1 are symptom free, and the disease resembles β-thalassemia minor. The peripheral smear shows a hypochromic microcytic anemia with the presence of target cells. Hemoglobin electrophoresis is normal.

HbH disease does produce symptoms. Unlike β-thalassemia major, in which HbF production protects the fetus, individuals with HbH disease develop hemolytic anemia during gestation and are symptomatic at birth. This is because α globin production is required for HbF ($\alpha_2\gamma_2$). As with β-thalassemia major, patients with HbH disease suffer from the consequences of chronic hemolytic anemia, although the severity is somewhat less. The transfusion requirements for HbH patients resemble those for patients with β-thalassemia intermedia, with transfusion support initiated in the second and third decades of life. These patients also develop iron overload, necessitating treatment with chelation therapy.

Hydrops fetalis with hemoglobin Barts is usually fatal in utero. The utter lack of α globin chain production results in absence of HbF. Hemoglobin Barts, a homotetramer consisting of four γ globin genes, is unable to deliver oxygen to tissues. Severe tissue hypoxia develops, leading to widespread tissue ischemia. High cardiac output failure leads to massive edema (hydrops). In most cases, death occurs in the third trimester or late second trimester. There have been reports of live births after intrauterine transfusion, but survival beyond the perinatal period is exceedingly rare. Prenatal diagnosis of hemoglobin Barts hydrops fetalis may be achieved through DNA-based testing using amniocytes from amniocentesis or chorionic villi sampling. Noninvasive testing is under development, including methods that isolate circulating fetal DNA in maternal peripheral blood.

---

[1]Not FDA approved for this indication.
[5]Investigational drug in the United States.

---

[1]Not FDA approved for this indication.

Management

Patients with α-thalassemia 2 and 1 traits do not require treatment. The management of HbH disease is similar to that described for β-thalassemia.

References

Algiraigri A, Wright N, Paolucci EO, et al: Hydroxyurea for lifelong transfusion-dependent β-thalassemia: A meta-analysis, *Pediatr Hematol Oncol* 34(8): 435–448, 2017.

Bayanzay K, Khan R: Meta-analysis on effectiveness of hydroxyurea to treat transfusion-dependent beta-thalassemia, *Hematology* 20(8):469–476, 2015.

Bhardawj A, Swe KM, Sinha NK, Osunkwo I: Treatment for osteoporosis in people with β-thalassaemia, *Cochrane Database Syst Rev* 3:CD010429, 2016.

Cappellini MD, Motta I: New therapeutic targets in transfusion-dependent and – independent thalassemia, *Hematology Am Soc Hematol Educ Program*(1) 278–283, 2017.

Delvecchio M, Cavallo L: Growth and endocrine function in thalassemia major in childhood and adolescence, *J Endocrinol Invest* 33(1):61–68, 2010.

Jagannath VA, Fedorowicz Z, Al Hajeri A, et al: Hematopoietic stem cell transplantation for people with β-thalassaemia major, *Cochrane Database Syst Rev* 10:CD008708, 2014.

Porter JB, Garbowski MW: Interaction of transfusion and iron chelation in thalassemias, *Hematol Oncol Clin North Am* 32(2):247–259, 2018.

Porter J: Beyond transfusion therapy new therapies in thalassemia including drugs, alternate donor transplant, and gene therapy, *Hematology Am Soc Hematol Educ Program*(1)361–370, 2018. 2018.

Saliba AN, Harb AR, Taher AT: Iron chelation therapy in transfusion-dependent thalassemia patients: current strategies and future directions, *J Blood Med* 6:197–209, 2015.

Taher AT, Weatherall DJ, Cappellini MD: Thalassemia, *Lancet* 391(10116):155–167, 2018.

THROMBOTIC THROMBOCYTOPENIC PURPURA

Method of
Ravi Sarode, MD

CURRENT DIAGNOSIS

- A provisional diagnosis based on unexplained microangiopathic hemolytic anemia (MAHA) and thrombocytopenia in the absence of oliguric renal failure is sufficient to initiate emergent plasma exchange (PLEX) for a suspected diagnosis of autoimmune acquired thrombotic thrombocytopenic purpura (TTP).
- The final diagnosis is usually established by the documentation of a severe deficiency (<10% activity) of ADAMTS13 (*a disintegrin and metalloproteinase with thrombospondin 1 motif, 13th member of the family).
- These laboratory tests are recommended for patient evaluation:
  - Complete blood count ([CBC] shows anemia and decreased platelet count, usually <30,000/uL)
  - Peripheral blood smear (shows "schistocytes/fragmented red blood cells," a hallmark of thrombotic microangiopathy [TMA])
  - Reticulocyte count (elevated)
  - Haptoglobin (usually undetectable in TTP)
  - Lactate dehydrogenase ([LDH] usually more than twice the upper limit of normal in TTP)
  - Blood urea nitrogen, serum creatinine (determine nonoliguric renal insufficiency, serum creatinine <2.5 mg/dL)
  - Liver function tests, including direct and indirect bilirubin
  - Troponin (some patients have an ischemic cardiac injury)
  - Plasma ADAMTS13 activity: (<10% is diagnostic of TTP) and inhibitor level (usually detected in 90% of cases of acquired TTP) or ADAMTS 13 antibodies by enzyme-linked immunosorbent assays (ELISA) (almost all acquired TTP)
  - Prothrombin time, partial thromboplastin time, fibrinogen, and D-dimers (to rule out disseminated intravascular coagulopathy [DIC])
  - Direct antiglobulin test (to rule out autoimmune hemolytic anemia)
  - Urinalysis

CURRENT THERAPY

- The goal is to normalize ADAMTS 13 levels (>50%)
- Daily PLEX using plasma as a replacement fluid (1–1.5 total body plasma volume) until the platelet count is greater than 150,000/μL for 2 days. Thereafter, the frequency of PLEX may be guided more judiciously if ADAMTS13 levels are obtained once or twice a week during hospitalization.
- Caplacizumab (Cablivi, 11 mg IV loading dose followed by daily 11 mg SQ), a nanobody that interferes with the binding of von Willebrand factor (vWF) to the GPIb domain on platelets and disrupts the pathophysiology of the disease in severe presentations or refractory cases, may prevent deaths and reduce the number of PLEXs needed. Given daily until ADAMTS13 levels >20% to 30%.
- Prednisone 1 mg/kg/day tapered gradually as platelet count remains >150,000/uL
- Rituximab (Rituxan)[1] (either 100 mg fixed dose or 375 mg/m² weekly for 4 weeks) upfront as soon as the diagnosis of autoimmune TTP is confirmed (reduces length of stay, number of PLEXs, and exacerbations and relapses, and thus overall cost)
- Plasma (10–15 mL/kg) or cryoprecipitate (one dose = 10 units of pooled cryoprecipitate) infusion, if PLEX will be delayed more than 6 hours on day 1.
- ADAMTS13 testing during follow-up to detect early biologic relapse and preemptive Rituxan to avoid clinical relapse and hospitalization.
- Exacerbation or relapsing TTP
  - Rituximab (Rituxan)[1] (100 mg fixed dose or 375 mg/m²) weekly for 2 to 4 weeks
  - Cyclosporine (Neoral)[1] (2–3 mg/kg/day up to 6 months)
  - Vincristine (Oncovin)[1] (1.4 mg/m² once a week for 4 weeks)
  - Bortezomib (Velcade)[1] (1.3 mg/m² one to two cycles or 1 mg fixed dose weekly for 4 weeks)
  - Splenectomy as a last resort

[1]Not FDA approved for this indication.

Thrombotic thrombocytopenic purpura (TTP) is a rare (one to two cases per million) but life-threatening thrombotic microangiopathy (TMA) disorder characterized by the presence of microthrombi in the microcirculation of various organs, including the brain, kidneys, heart, and abdominal viscera. Microthrombi consist of platelets and von Willebrand factor (VWF), resulting in microangiopathic hemolytic anemia (MAHA) and thrombocytopenia. MAHA refers to the fragmentation of red blood cells (schistocytes) during their passage through partially occluded arterioles and capillaries by microthrombi. TTP diagnosis requires a high degree of suspicion because a delay in initiating plasma exchange (PLEX), the current standard of care, could result in a poor response or fatal outcome. In the past, diagnosis of TTP was made based on a pentad that included MAHA, thrombocytopenia, neurologic involvement, renal affection, and fever. This pentad was found in patients who had died of TTP, indicating advanced disease; therefore, one should not wait for the development of a pentad, which could delay TTP diagnosis and lead to a potentially fatal outcome. Currently, unexplained MAHA and thrombocytopenia in the absence of oliguric renal failure are sufficient to make a working diagnosis of TTP and initiate emergent PLEX. Patients may present with only severe thrombocytopenia and/or with warm autoimmune hemolytic anemia and be managed as nonresponding immune thrombocytopenia/Evan syndrome. However, after a few days, such patients may develop MAHA, establishing a TTP diagnosis. Therefore, such patients not responding to standard therapy should have high suspicion of TTP. Similarly, but rarely, a young patient may present with unexplained ischemic stroke without hematologic features and later develop hematologic features.

Pathophysiology

In congenital TTP (Upshaw-Shulman syndrome), ultralarge (UL) multimers of vWF were detected during remission but were absent during relapse. Later, a ADAMTS13 (a disintegrin and metalloproteinase with thrombospondin 1 motif, 13th member of the family), vWF-cleaving protease, was identified that was responsible for cleaving UL multimers secreted from endothelium into normal-sized vWF multimers seen in normal plasma. This cleavage occurs under high-shear-rate flow conditions in smaller blood vessels where the UL-vWF undergoes unfolding, exposing the cleavage site for ADAMTS13. ADAMTS13 is severely deficient (<10%) in patients with both congenital and acquired (autoimmune) TTP. Persistence of UL-vWF multimers in the microcirculation results in unfolding of the molecule, enabling it to bind to platelets at GPIb, thus producing platelet-vWF microthrombi in capillaries and arterioles that cause end organ ischemic damage

(Figure 1). Elevated lactate dehydrogenase (LDH) reflects not only MAHA but also tissue damage; hence very high LDH reflects more severe disease.

Classification

TTP can be divided into (1) a congenital form resulting from a genetic defect in the *ADAMTS13* gene and (2) an acquired form due to an autoantibody against the ADAMTS13 enzyme (Figure 2). Congenital TTP can present in the neonatal period, early childhood, or later in life, when it is usually associated with an inciting trigger in the form of pregnancy, severe infection, surgery, or other stress. Acquired TTP is usually idiopathic without an underlying disorder, or secondary when associated with an underlying autoimmune disorder such as systemic lupus erythematosus (SLE), human immunodeficiency virus (HIV), use of ticlopidine (Ticlid),[2] and so on. Other clinical conditions that present with MAHA and thrombocytopenia with nonsevere ADAMTS13 deficiency are grouped under the broader term TMA.

---

[2] Not available in the United States.

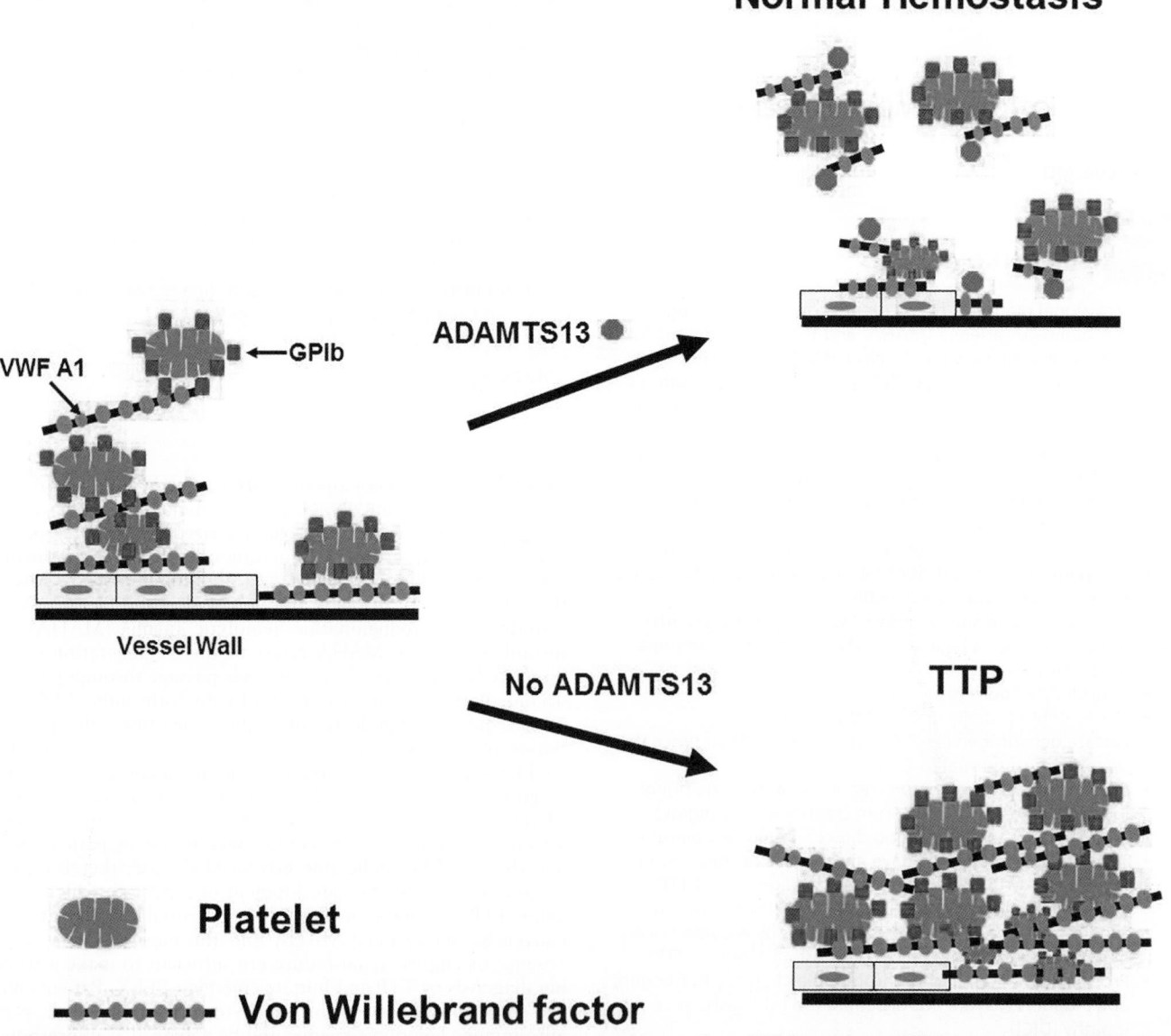

Figure 1 During normal hemostasis, *ADAMTS13* enzyme cleaves ultralarge multimers of von Willebrand factor (vWF) in normal sizes and prevents the formation of platelet-vWF aggregates under high shear rates. However, in the absence of *ADAMTS13* (a disintegrin and metalloproteinase with thrombospondin 1 motif, 13th member of the family) due congenital deficiency or autoantibodies, vWF persist as ultralarge multimers that unfold under high shear rates in small blood vessels and induce vWF-platelet microthrombi in various organs, causing ischemic damage.

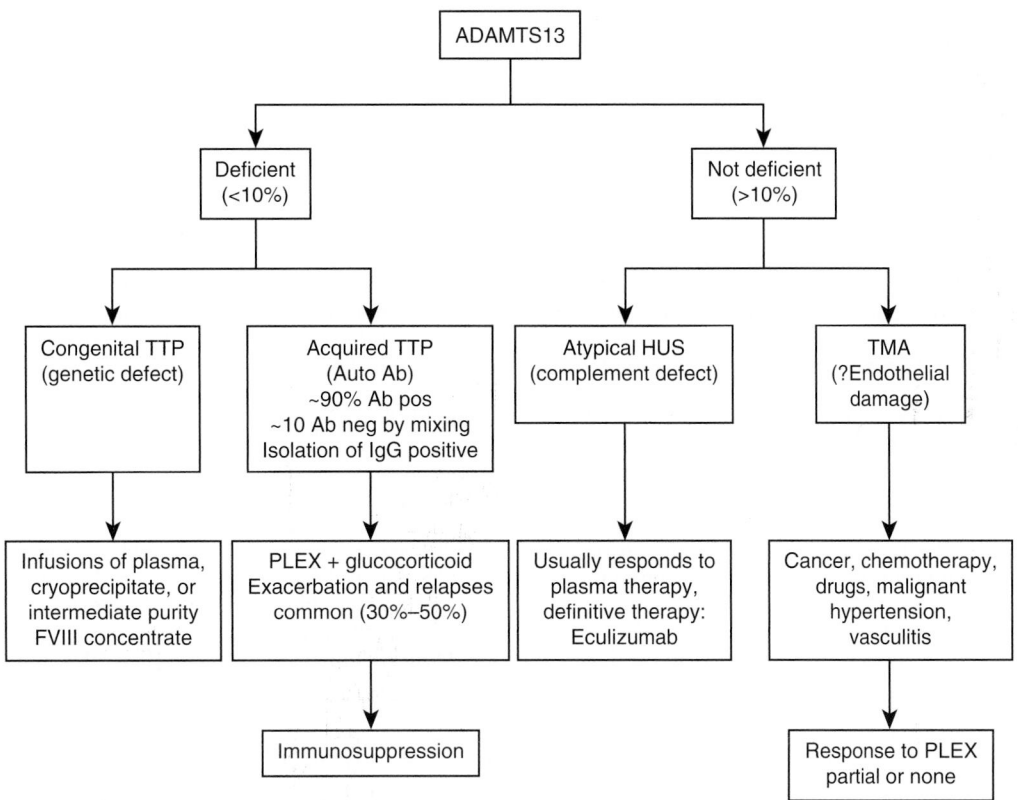

Figure 2 Classification of TTP. *Ab*, Antibody; *ADAMTS13*, a disintegrin and metalloproteinase with thrombospondin motif 1, 13th member of the family; *HUS*, hemolytic uremic syndrome; *MAHA*, microangiopathic hemolytic anemia; *PLEX*, plasma exchange; *TMA*, thrombotic microangiopathy; *TTP*, thrombotic thrombocytopenic purpura.

Clinical Presentation

Autoimmune TTP is a disease of young adults (20–50 years of age, female-to-male ratio 2:1), with the majority being African American. Most patients present in the emergency department with an acute onset of vague, anemia-like symptoms (malaise, fatigue, weakness) and thrombocytopenia (petechiae, bleeding gums). Detailed evaluation reveals that these symptoms had their onset several days before presentation. Up to 70% to 80% of patients have some neurologic features, including severe headaches, visual disturbances, focal neurologic deficits, transient ischemic attacks, memory deficits, unusual behavior, confusion, seizures, paraparesis, stupor, and coma. Mild renal insufficiency is seen in less than 50% and fever in less than 15%. Because of the generalized nature of the disease, any organ system can be affected, and ischemic insult to the heart is not uncommon.

Diagnosis

Unexplained MAHA and thrombocytopenia constitute the diagnostic features and are associated with elevated LDH, reticulocytosis, undetectable haptoglobin, elevated bilirubin, and nonoliguric renal insufficiency in some patients. A severe deficiency of ADAMTS13 (<10% activity with a detectable inhibitor in up to 90% of patients and antibodies by enzyme-linked immunosorbent assays [ELISA] in almost all) confirms the diagnosis. Because this test is usually sent to a reference laboratory, this level is unavailable in most hospitals at the time of clinical diagnosis. Therefore, based on the initial clinical and laboratory features, PLEX should be initiated emergently because a delay can increase not only morbidity but also mortality. A sample for ADAMTS13 must be drawn before initiating PLEX or plasma/cryoprecipitate infusion to avoid measuring enzyme from transfused products. ADAMTS13 is a stable enzyme; if a sample for ADAMTS13 could not be drawn before plasma therapy, a routine coagulation test sample may be used. In congenital TTP, a persistent severe deficiency of ADAMTS13 (without an inhibitor) is associated with *ADAMTS13* gene defect. However, this diagnosis is sometimes made difficult because many

patients, especially children and young adults, are often misdiagnosed as having immune thrombocytopenia or anemia of unknown origin or the hemolysis elevated liver enzymes and low platelets (HELLP) syndrome in pregnancy.

Differential Diagnosis

The differential diagnosis of TTP includes clinical conditions that present with MAHA and thrombocytopenia but without severe ADAMTS13 deficiency—that is, TMA. These conditions include hematopoietic stem cell transplantation, drug toxicities (mitomycin, clopidogrel [Plavix], cyclosporine A [Neoral], etc.), malignant hypertension (usually mild to moderate thrombocytopenia), HELLP syndrome with severe preeclampsia, mechanical cardiac devices (for example, left ventricular assist devices, intraaortic balloon pumps, and mechanical heart valves), disseminated intravascular coagulation (DIC), vasculitis, and both diarrhea-associated and atypical hemolytic uremic syndrome (HUS).

Treatment

PLEX is the standard of care therapy. Its use has reduced mortality from more than 90% to less than 20%. Ideally it should be initiated within 4 to 6 hours of suspected diagnosis. The patient's plasma (which contains autoantibody) is selectively removed during PLEX (1.0–1.5 plasma volume processed) and replaced with donor plasma containing ADAMTS13. Neurologic symptoms usually disappear within 24 to 48 hours. The platelet count is the most useful laboratory parameter in the assessment of initial response. Complete clinical response, defined as normalization of platelet count for at least 2 days with near normal LDH, is generally achieved in most patients with seven to nine daily PLEXs. Thereafter, a gradual taper—that is, PLEX every other day in the first week, twice in the next week, and once in the third week—may be performed. However, the number of PLEXs can be guided by frequent ADAMTS13 measurements to avoid unnecessary PLEXs and reduce exposure to hundreds of plasma donors, thus reducing the risk of transmitting known and unknown pathogens. Another option is to use pathogen-inactivated plasma such as Octaplas (Octapharma Plasma Centers), which is approved by the FDA for the treatment of TTP. Given the autoimmune nature of the disease, glucocorticoid therapy is often given from the beginning. Approximately 30% to 50% of patients will have an exacerbation of the disease (worsening of clinical or laboratory features after initial response) or relapses (recurrence of the disease 30 days after discontinuation of PLEX). Such patients require additional PLEXs and other immunomodulatory therapies (e.g., rituximab [Rituxan],[1] cyclosporine [Neoral],[1] vincristine [Oncovin],[1] bortezomib [Velcade],[1] or splenectomy as a last resort). Early rituximab use, within the first week, has recently been shown to reduce number of PLEXs, length of stay, and exacerbation/relapse. Preliminary data also suggest that a lower dosage of rituximab (100 mg weekly for 4 weeks) elicits a similar clinical response as a higher dosage (375 mg/m^2 weekly for 4 weeks). However, the former offers the benefits of reduced cost, lower infusion time, and fewer side effects. A dialysis-type catheter is required for PLEX and can be placed with ultrasound guidance in patients with platelet counts as low as 5000/μL. With the exception of a life-threatening bleed, platelet transfusion is contraindicated in TTP because it is a thrombotic disorder of platelet consumption and transfused platelets may worsen the condition (with the appearance of new neurologic symptoms, myocardial infarction, etc.). Most fatalities occur during the first few days of diagnosis, probably because of the severity of the disease or delay in the initiation of PLEX. If initiation of PLEX is likely to be delayed, either plasma or cryoprecipitate can be infused temporarily to supplement ADAMTS13.

Caplacizumab (Cablivi), a nanobody that binds to the A1 domain of vWF and blocks its interaction with GPIb/IX/V receptors on platelets, has recently been approved by the FDA for the treatment of TTP. A randomized clinical trial showed that caplacizumab given once as an intravenous (IV) bolus (of 11 mg) followed by daily subcutaneous injections (of 11 mg) up to 30 days post-PLEX led to normalization of the platelet count slightly faster and reduced the numbers of PLEXs, disease exacerbations, and possibly deaths but also led to more relapses compared with placebo. It seems that the use of caplacizumab can definitely benefit severe and refractory TTP and may be tailored based on frequent ADAMTS13 testing during the treatment course. Once ADAMTS13 levels are greater than 20% to 30%, caplacizumab should be discontinued to prevent a bleeding tendency due to development of acquired von Willebrand syndrome. Congenital TTP is treated with plasma infusions (10–15 mL/kg); however, cryoprecipitate

and intermediate purity Factor VIII concentrate that contain adequate ADAMTS13 have been used successfully to avoid volume overload in susceptible patients. In congenital TTP, a recombinant ADAMTS13 has recently been shown to produce very promising results in a phase I clinical trial.

Monitoring
Considering the relatively high frequency of cardiac involvement, cardiac monitoring should be performed initially. Although PLEX is an otherwise safe procedure, complications related to catheter infection and line thrombosis are not uncommon and should be identified as soon as possible to avoid exacerbation of the disease. Exacerbation of TTP is often related to an infection. There is increasing awareness of delayed long-term psychological and psychosocial effects in up to 50% patients; a careful follow-up is recommended to identify and manage these issues.

Prognosis
Although PLEX has reduced TTP mortality in the last two decades, most deaths occur within 24 to 48 hours of presentation and are due to delay in the administration of PLEX for a variety of reasons, including a delay in diagnosis or line placement or nonavailability of PLEX at the institution. After one PLEX, survival rates can increase to greater than 90%. Importantly, no clinical or laboratory parameter exists to predict outcome or relapse. Frequent ADAMTS13 monitoring is now used during follow-up to detect early biologic relapse (drop in activity <30%–50%); preemptive rituximab[1] has been used to prevent overt hematologic and clinical relapse and avoid hospitalization.

---

[1]Not FDA approved for this indication.

References
Fujimura Y, Matsumoto M, Isonishi A, et al: Natural history of Upshaw-Schulman syndrome based on ADAMTS13 gene analysis in Japan, *J Thromb Haemost* 9(Suppl 1):283–301, 2011.

Peyvandi F, Rock GA, Shumak KH, Buskard NA, et al: Comparison of plasma exchange with plasma infusion in the treatment of thrombotic thrombocytopenic purpura. Canadian Apheresis Study Group, *N Engl J Med* 325:393–397, 1991.

Sarode R, Bandarenko N, Brecher ME, et al: Thrombotic thrombocytopenic purpura: 2012 American Society for Apheresis (ASFA) consensus conference on classification, diagnosis, management, and future research, *J Clin Apher*, https://doi.org/10.1002/jca.21302.

Shah N, Rutherford C, Matevosyan K, et al: Role of ADAMTS13 in the management of thrombotic microangiopathies including thrombotic thrombocytopenic purpura (TTP), *Br J Haematol* 163:514–519, 2013.

Tsai HM: Thrombotic thrombocytopenic purpura and atypical hemolytic uremic syndrome—An update, *Hematol Oncol Clin North Am* 27:565–584, 2013.

---

[1]Not FDA approved for this indication.

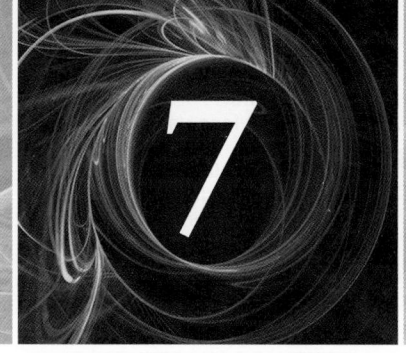

Head and Neck

DRY EYE SYNDROME

Method of
Curtis E. Margo, MD, MPH; and Lynn E. Harman, MD

CURRENT DIAGNOSIS

- Symptoms of mild to moderate dry eye are nonspecific and include ocular burning, stinging, irritation, foreign body sensation, episodic tearing, and momentary blurred vision cleared with blinking.
- Symptoms are often age-related exacerbated by fans, air conditioning, and low humidity.
- Many topical medications and contact lens use may worsen symptoms.
- Symptoms of dry mouth suggest Sjögren syndrome.
- Clinical signs of dry eyes beyond nonspecific conjunctival injection are subtle and difficult to appreciate without slit lamp magnification.
- Tear osmolarity, tear matrix metalloprotein-9 concentration, tear breakup time, Schirmer test, and grading of ocular surface dye staining are adjuvant studies used to diagnose dry eye and monitor therapy.
- Several systemic disorders can cause dry eye, including Sjögren syndrome, thyroid eye disease, sarcoidosis, and ocular cicatricial pemphigoid.
- Other ocular surface and eyelid disorders often coexist with dry eye and need to be considered in management strategies.

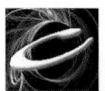

CURRENT THERAPY

- Titrated use of artificial tears based on symptoms is the mainstay of treatment for mild to moderate dry eye.
- Correction or management of exacerbating disorders such as blepharitis or lagophthalmos also need to be addressed.
- Preservative-free artificial tears are indicated for persons using more than three or four drops a day.
- A half-inch ribbon of ocular ointment/gel placed in the lower cul-de-sac will disperse in tear film, providing longer-lasting lubrication at bedtime.
- An antiinflammatory topical medication approved by the US Food and Drug Administration (FDA) for dry eye is indicated for persons whose symptoms persist despite using artificial tears or when frequency of use is burdensome.
- Escalation of therapy for persistent symptoms is individualized and may include such measures as punctal occlusion (temporary and less often permanent), autologous serum drops, oral cholinergic agonists, and rigid gas-permeable scleral lenses.

Epidemiology

Dry eye is a common age-related disorder whose epidemiologic features are incompletely characterized in part because of variable definitions and lack of a universal standard for diagnosis. In terms of pathophysiology, dry eye reflects a breakdown of homeostasis of the tear film related to a decreased or abnormal tear film or from increased tear loss through evaporation. Synonyms for symptomatic dry eye include dry eye syndrome, keratoconjunctivitis sicca, and dry eye disease. These terms imply a more definitive nosologic entity than may exist, since inadequate surface lubrication is caused by diverse, often concurrent and unrelated conditions. Population-based studies show that the prevalence of dry eye symptoms progressively rises from age 40 years onward, usually from single percentile proportions to the high teens. Further epidemiologic generalizations can be misleading because of the heterogenous nature of dry eye and common confounding conditions that also result in inadequate surface lubrication.

Risk Factors

Increasing age is a common factor associated with dry eye. Dry eyes are also caused by systemic disease, many of which are age related. Estimates are that roughly 10% of patients with severe dry eyes have Sjögren syndrome, an autoimmune disorder of exocrine glands. Other systemic conditions that may result or exacerbate dry eyes are thyroid eye disease, Parkinson disease (attributed to reduced blink), acquired immunodeficiency syndrome (AIDS), graft-versus-host disease, and atopy. Any condition that reduces the integrity of the ocular surface—such as Stevens-Johnson syndrome, alkali or acid burns, or ocular cicatricial pemphigoid—can result in dry eyes (Figure 1).

The association of dry eye with chronic blepharitis (itself a multifaceted disorder) confounds the discussion of risk factors because the conditions are closely linked. Dry eye, for example, is reported in roughly half of patients with staphylococcal blepharitis. Dry eye is also found in a substantial proportion of persons with seborrheic blepharitis, meibomian gland dysfunction (MGD), and ocular rosacea. Symptoms of dry eye and chronic blepharitis overlap, and each condition exacerbates the other. The evaluation and management of dry eye must take into consideration the close association it has with the major forms of chronic blepharitis: staphylococcal, seborrheic, and MGD.

Pathophysiology

Proper lubrication of the eye depends on the interactions of surface epithelium, tear film production and composition, normal eyelid anatomy, and blink reflex. The classic three-layer precorneal tear film consists of a thin outer oil coat that inhibits evaporation, a middle aqueous compartment, and an inner mucinous layer that acts as surfactant; however, this scheme is probably an oversimplification. Conceptually, it is useful in understanding different paths leading to an inadequate tear film. The integrity of the precorneal tear film can be lost by a deficiency in one or more of its components. A variety of factors may contribute to these deficiencies. The superficial lipid layer, which reduces ambient evaporation, for example, is produced by sebaceous glands of the lid. Disorders that interfere with normal sebaceous gland function (estrogen replacement therapy, blepharitis, MGD, etc.) can adversely affect tear evaporation (see Figure 1).

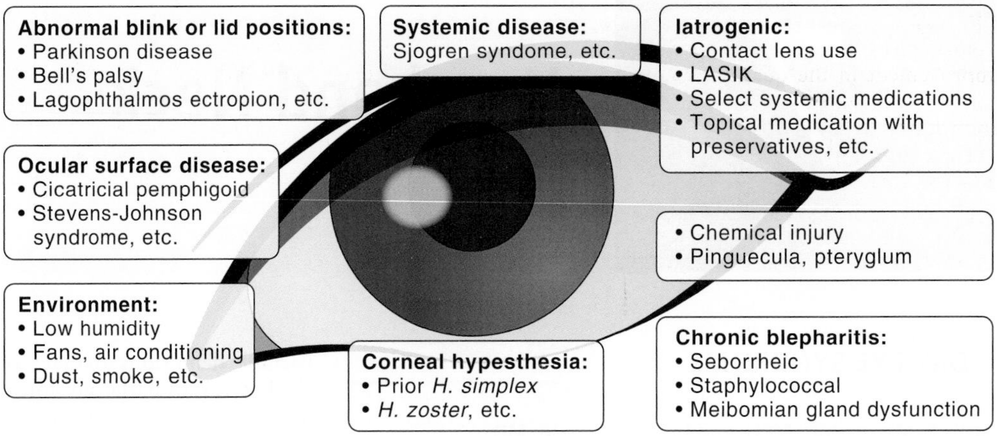

Abnormal blink or lid positions:
• Parkinson disease
• Bell's palsy
• Lagophthalmos ectropion, etc.

Ocular surface disease:
• Cicatricial pemphigoid
• Stevens-Johnson syndrome, etc.

Environment:
• Low humidity
• Fans, air conditioning
• Dust, smoke, etc.

Systemic disease:
Sjogren syndrome, etc.

Iatrogenic:
• Contact lens use
• LASIK
• Select systemic medications
• Topical medication with preservatives, etc.

• Chemical injury
• Pinguecula, pteryglum

Corneal hypesthesia:
• Prior *H. simplex*
• *H. zoster*, etc.

Chronic blepharitis:
• Seborrheic
• Staphylococcal
• Meibomian gland dysfunction

Figure 1 Illustration showing the diverse and interrelated conditions that can result in dry eye symptoms and signs. The lists are incomplete but emphasize the importance of addressing factors that contribute to inadequate tear film beyond prescribing artificial tear substitutes.

The aqueous layer of the tear film contains electrolytes, antimicrobial proteins such as lysozyme, immunoglobulins, and various growth factors. Major and accessory lacrimal glands produce aqueous tears, a process that slowly declines with age. Primary diseases of these glands will adversely affect tear production. The classic example is Sjögren syndrome. The aqueous layer is also rich in a mucinous glycocalyx, which comes from goblet cells. These macromolecules are chemically attracted to epithelium-bound mucins and enhance surface interface contact. Loss of goblet cells due to various diseases such as Stevens-Johnson syndrome or injury from a chemical burn will result in poor surface wetting.

Healthy eyelids and a normal blink reflex disperse tears over the ocular surface. Any disease or injury that affects eyelid margins or the blink reflex has the potential to adversely affect the dispersion of tears over the surface of the eye. The list of conditions that fall into this realm is extensive and ranges from Bell palsy and eyelid trauma to Parkinson disease and the reduced blink rate associated with computer use and reading.

The normal tear film also depends on normal corneal innervation. Partial loss of corneal sensation from previous infection with herpes zoster or herpes simplex or past laser-assisted in situ keratomileusis (LASIK) surgery will reduce basal tear production.

Clinical Manifestations

Early or initial symptoms of dry eye—including ocular burning, stinging, irritation, tearing, foreign body sensation, and mild mucous discharge—are nonspecific. Vision can be affected, usually transiently, and clears with blinking. Symptoms are worsened by low humidity or proximity to a fan or gusty wind. Many topical eyedrop medications and contact lenses exacerbate symptoms. Symptoms may also worsen for persons taking antihistamines, antidepressants, and antianxiety medications.

The severity of dry eye may be subdivided into mild, moderate, and severe, which serve as a guide for instituting therapy. Mild dry eye consists of ocular surface symptoms from burning and stinging to foreign body sensation. The threshold of *severe* is reached when vision becomes impaired with periodic blurring that clears with blinking. As the condition worsens, blurring becomes more frequent and of longer duration. The category of moderate dry eye falls between these reference points. Although subjective, this basic scheme is useful in initiating therapy and monitoring responses to treatment.

Diagnosis

Other than ocular injection, signs of dry eye are difficult to appreciate without the magnification of a slit lamp. The normal 1-mm inferior tear meniscus at the lid margin is reduced, the corneal surface lacks luster, and the tear film breaks up rapidly, in less than 10 seconds. These findings are more easily appreciated when fluorescein is applied to the tear film, using either a saline-moistened fluorescein strip or a drop of 1% to 2% solution. As the fluorescein becomes dilute, inferior punctate erosions of the cornea may be seen. A 1% solution of Rose Bengal, which is mildly irritating, will detect conjunctival involvement by staining cells in the interpalpebral zone. There is no universally preferred diagnostic test for dry eye. Tear osmolarity, tear production measured by Schirmer strip, and tear matrix metalloproteinase-9 assay have different sensitivities, specificities, and proficiency profiles.

The tear deficiency state is often accompanied by other disorders of the eyelid or blink or conditions of the ocular surface that confound the singular diagnosis of dry eye. Age-related lid laxity, ectropion, entropion, pinguecula, and pterygium will worsen dry eye symptoms and signs of inadequate tear film. Absence of complete eyelid closure (lagophthalmos) will contribute to dry eye through increased evaporative tear loss.

Dry eyes are also accompanied by lid margin diseases such as MGD, rosacea, and chronic blepharitis. Early signs of these disorders are difficult to detect without the slit lamp. Suspicions of ocular allergies may arise because of papillary tarsal changes (or the dominant complaint of itching). Contact lens use can also lead to symptomatic dry eye.

Secondary dry eye following injury to the surface of the eye is usually evident from past medical history. The range of ocular surface disorders giving rise to dry eye include acid or alkali burns, past LASIK surgery, ocular cicatricial pemphigoid, and Stevens-Johnson syndrome, to name a few.

Evaluation for systemic disease in patients with more severe manifestations of dry eye (and those with dry mouth) involves general medical history and examination. Laboratory studies are directed at primary and secondary Sjögren syndrome. Thyroid eye disease should be considered in persons with stare or lagophthalmos.

Differential Diagnosis

The major diagnostic challenge in evaluating dry eye is diagnosing common concurrent conditions and estimating how much they are contributing to symptomatology. Is a dry eye contributing to symptoms of chronic blepharitis or vice versa? Such clinical judgments guide therapeutic priorities. If, for example, a patient with dry eye symptoms has 3 to 4 mm of lagophthalmos, successful management will need to address abnormal lid closure. The need for tear film supplements will likely change as eyelid position is corrected. A similar scenario might exist for a patient with Bell palsy whose need for topical lubricants will change as blink and lid function improve.

Therapy

Management of dry eye can be divided into two domains: (1) improvement in the quality or amount of the tear film and (2) correction or improvement of concomitant comorbid conditions contributing to symptoms.

The algorithm for improving an inadequate tear film because of underproduction or evaporation begins by removing or minimizing harmful exposures, including topical eye drops with preservative that might disrupt a normal tear film, oral medications such as antihistamines, or environmental irritants, including smoke and dust when possible. The list of potential medications that can worsen dry eye is considerable. Since causal associations are not always evidence, a trial of withdrawal and reexposure may be indicated.

The use of over-the-counter artificial tear supplements is a starting point for essentially all forms of dry eye, although frequency of use and dose escalation vary depending on severity of symptoms. Artificial tears are mixtures of electrolytes, a water-soluble polymer, and preservative adjusted to various tonicities and pH. Commonly used polymers include polyvinyl alcohol, povidone, dextran, propylene glycol, and derivatives of methylcellulose. Although some differences in viscosity and ability to promote tear film stability exist among polymers, most are therapeutically equivalent. There is limited to no evidence of improved efficacy of artificial tear supplements that contain lipids and vitamins.

Prolonged or frequent exposure to some preservatives can adversely affect surface epithelium. Preservative-free tear substitutes are recommended when used more than three to four times a day.

Ointments/gels applied before sleep prolong the duration of topical lubrication and are particularly helpful in persons with lagophthalmos for retarding evaporation. Persons using continuous positive airway pressure also benefit from their use. Major components of these products are mineral oil ointments, lanolin, and petrolatum. When applied in a thin half-inch ribbon in the lower conjunctival cul-de-sac, they dissolve at body temperature and disperse within the tear film. Ointments and gels will inhibit absorption of topical prescription medications, so their use must be separated in time from lubricants. Ointments and gels are well suited for protecting the cornea when lid closure is incomplete (lagophthalmos, Bell palsy, etc.), but they are poorly tolerated during wakeful periods as they cause blurred vision.

When further dose escalation is undesirable, antiinflammatory therapy with topical 0.05% cyclosporine (Restasis) twice daily can be considered. Roughly two-thirds of patients with dry eye—mild, moderate, or severe—report improvement with cyclosporine; however, the benefits may not be appreciated for weeks after starting therapy. Topical cyclosporine may reduce the need for artificial tear supplements. Discontinuation after prolonged use (>1 year) may diminish the need for further supplemental artificial tears.

Another topical antiinflammatory agent, lifitegrast (Xiidra), an integrin antagonist that blocks interaction of lymphocytes with upregulated adhesion molecules in dry eye, has received FDA approval for the treatment of dry eye. Signs and symptoms of dry eye are improved using lifitegrast twice daily over 3 months, but its long-term effectiveness remains to be determined.

Topical corticosteroids have limited use in dry eye beyond short-term control of inflammation, until long-term therapies take effect.

A preservative-free water-soluble polymeric insert (Lacrisert) is an option for patients unable to apply topical drops. A small cylindric rod containing 5 mg of hydroxypropyl cellulose is placed in the lower conjunctival recess, where it dissolves over 12 to 24 hours. Some observers note that insertion of the rod each day may require greater manual dexterity than that needed to use eyedrops. The role of polyunsaturated fatty acid supplements containing omega-3 and/or omega-6 components is uncertain. Clinical studies have provided favorable but inconsistent results. Given the safety of oral supplement therapy, further investigations using outcomes that lend themselves to pooled data analysis is anticipated.

Punctal occlusion is an alternative for persons with aqueous tear deficiency not able to obtain relief with topical supplements. Occlusion of either upper or lower punctum appears to have an equivalent improvement on the height of the lower tear meniscus. Although plugs can be retained for months or years following insertion, they are prone to fall out in 30% to 50% of patients over 24 months. The largest-diameter silicone plugs should be used. They occasionally cause irritation or epiphora but can be removed should side effects develop. Plugs rarely become displaced, although this is a complication that is likely to be underreported. Relief of symptoms despite failure to retain silicone plugs for prolonged periods raises the option of permanent occlusion using thermal cautery or laser-induced burns. It would be ill advised to attempt permanent punctal closure without a trial with plugs to gauge the potential benefit.

Anecdotal experience guides the management of persons with persistent symptoms who are using maximal tolerable artificial lubricants, antiinflammatory agents, and punctal occlusion. In persons with Sjögren syndrome, symptoms of dry eye may improve with oral cholinergic agonists, although patients in studies reported greater relief in dry mouth symptoms. Pilocarpine (Salagen) 5 mg orally four times a day is associated with predictable side effects like excessive sweating. A small proportion of patients find muscarinic side effects intolerable. Pilocarpine and cevimeline (Evoxac) are both FDA approved for treatment of dry mouth of Sjögren syndrome. Their efficacy in treating dry eye in persons without Sjögren syndrome is unknown.

Autologous serum formulations applied as topical drops have shown some benefit in persons with Sjögren syndrome and graft-versus-host disease. Studies of effectiveness are limited and disadvantages include inconvenience of collection, need for sterile preparation facility, and repeated blood draws.

The long-term effectiveness of ridged gas-permeable scleral lenses and humidified goggles is not well documented, but both are options for severe dry eye. Vigilant monitoring is necessary because the potential for secondary infection is high in persons with a severely impaired tear film.

References

Cornea/External Disease Preferred Practice Pattern Panel 2017-2018: *Blepharitis Preferred Practice Pattern*, San Francisco, 2018, American Academy of Ophthalmology.

Cornea/External Disease Preferred Practice Pattern Panel 2017-2018: *Dry Eye Preferred Practice Pattern*, San Francisco, 2018, American Academy of Ophthalmology.

Downie LE, Ng SM, Lindsley KB, et al: Omega-3 and omega-6 polyunsaturated fatty acids for dry eye disease, *Cochrane Database Syst Rev* 2019(12):CDO11016, 2019.

Duncan K, Jeng BH: Medical management of blepharitis, *Curr Opin* 26:289–294, 2015.

Pan Q, Angelina A, Marrone M, et al: Autologous serum eye drops for dry eye, *Cochrane Database Syst Rev* 2:CD009327, 2017.

Perez VL, Pflugfelder SC, Zhang S, et al: Lifitegrast, a novel integrin antagonist for treatment of dry eye disease, *Ocul Surf* 14:207–2015, 2016.

Pflugfelder SC, de Paiva CS: The pathophysiology of dry eye disease, *Ophthalmology* 24:S4–S13, 2017.

Pflugfelder SC, Solomon A, Stern ME: The diagnosis and management of dry eye. A twenty-five-year review, *Cornea* 19:644–649, 2000.

Pucker AD, Ng SM, Nichols JJ: Over the counter (OTC) artificial tears drops for dry eye syndrome cochrane, *Database Syst Rev* 2:CD009729, 2016.

Schwartz LM, Woloshin S: A clear-eye view of restasis and chronic dry eye disease, *JAMA Intern Med* 178:181–182, 2018.

Su MY, Perry HD, Barsam A, et al: The effect of decreasing the dosage of cyclosporine a 0.05% on dry eye disease after 1 year of twice-daily therapy, *Cornea* 30:1098–1104, 2011.

GLAUCOMA

Method of
Albert P. Lin, MD; and Kristin Schmid Biggerstaff, MD

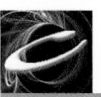

CURRENT DIAGNOSIS

Primary Open Angle Glaucoma

- Primary open angle glaucoma is an irreversible optic neuropathy typically associated with elevated intraocular pressure.
- Primary open angle glaucoma is the most common form of glaucoma, affecting over three million Americans. It is more common in African Americans (6% to 7%), Asians (2% to 3%), and Hispanics (2%) and less common in whites (1%). It is more common in older adults: 1 to 2% in 50-year-olds compared with 6% to 12% in 80-year-olds.
- Primary open angle glaucoma is diagnosed by a complete ophthalmic examination, including dilated stereoscopic optic nerve examination and formal visual field.
- Untreated primary open angle glaucoma can lead to slow irreversible loss of vision and blindness. Other common causes of slow and progressive vision loss in older adults include cataracts, macular degeneration, and diabetic retinopathy.

Acute Angle Closure Glaucoma

- Pupillary block in susceptible patients leads to block of aqueous drainage and sudden and extreme rise of intraocular pressure. Acute angle closure can damage the optic nerve, resulting in acute angle closure glaucoma.
- About 0.5% to 1.0% of US adults are at risk for acute angle closure. It is more common in Inuits and Asians and rare in African Americans. The risk of acute angle closure increases with age. It is also more common in hyperopes.
- Patients can present with blurry vision, red eye, pain, headache, nausea, or vomiting. Acute angle closure is sometimes misdiagnosed as migraines or gastrointestinal illnesses. Patients with conjunctivitis, keratitis, uveitis, and corneal abrasion can also present with the same symptoms.
- Peripheral iridotomy prevents acute angle closure in susceptible patients. High intraocular pressure can result in irreversible damage of the optic nerve within hours, making acute angle closure one of the true ophthalmic emergencies.

CURRENT THERAPY

Primary Open Angle Glaucoma

- Topical eye drops, including β-blockers, selective α_2 agonists, carbonic anhydrase inhibitors, prostaglandin analogues, and rho kinase inhibitors, can be used to reduce intraocular pressure.
- Oral carbonic anhydrase inhibitors are typically used in recalcitrant cases until surgery can be performed.
- Laser trabeculoplasty may be used as first-line or adjunct therapy.
- Glaucoma surgery, including trabeculectomy, tube shunt, and cyclodestruction, may be performed if goal intraocular pressure cannot be reached with medical therapy or in nonadherent patients.

Acute Angle Glaucoma

- All glaucoma eye drops are used to reduce intraocular pressure.
- Oral and intravenous medications are added sequentially to reduce intraocular pressure as needed.
- Laser iridotomy can be performed as prophylactic treatment or acutely to break the pupillary block if the patient is unresponsive to medical intervention.
- Emergency glaucoma incisional surgery is performed if the patient is unresponsive to all other treatments.

Glaucoma is an optic neuropathy with characteristic optic nerve head appearance: narrowing of the neuroretinal rim. The optic nerve is a collection of more than 1 million axons from the retinal ganglion cells. The anterior 1-mm portion of the optic nerve within the globe is referred to as the *optic disk* or simply the *disk*. When the disk is examined with direct or indirect ophthalmoscopy, a cup, or a physiologic empty space, is observed centrally. The remainder of the disk, which has a yellow-orange appearance, contains the axons and is referred to as the *neuroretinal rim*. The area of the cup compared to the entire disk is the cup-to-disk ratio, which is normally less than 0.4 (Figure 1A). When patients develop glaucoma, axons are lost from the neuroretinal rim and the size of the cup increases in relation to the disk. Narrowing of the neuroretinal rim and increased cup-to-disk ratio are the hallmarks of glaucomatous optic neuropathy (see Figure 1B).

Glaucoma can result in significant and irreversible loss of vision and is one of the leading causes of blindness in the United States. Early in the disease state, glaucoma is asymptomatic; it is sometimes called "the sneak thief of sight." As the disease progresses, the patient develops decreased peripheral vision and eventually loss of the central vision.

Glaucoma is typically associated with increased intraocular pressure (IOP), but it is possible to have normal-tension or low-tension glaucoma. Glaucoma treatment is focused on the reduction of IOP to prevent or slow optic nerve damage and preserve visual function.

Glaucoma is classified in many ways, and it is most useful to approach it clinically based on the status of the angle, the area between the cornea and iris where aqueous humor exits the globe through the trabecular network. We further discuss primary open angle glaucoma, the most common form of glaucoma in the United States, and the management of acute angle closure, one of the true ophthalmic emergencies.

Primary Open Angle Glaucoma

Glaucoma is one of the leading causes of blindness in older adults, especially in patients of African American descent. Vision loss from glaucoma is irreversible, and the treatment goal is to reduce IOP, slow disease progression, and preserve visual function during the patient's lifetime. Glaucoma is a slowly progressive disease, and progression to blindness often takes more than 10 years, even in untreated patients. Given its slow progression and the fact that central vision loss occurs in late disease, most patients do well with early diagnosis and treatment. Treatment is more difficult in late disease because the rate of disease progression and visual deterioration is accelerated, sometimes despite good control of IOP.

Due to the early asymptomatic nature of the disease, the patient's adherence to and persistence with treatment is often less than optimal. Studies have shown patients who obtain glaucoma information from physicians other than their ophthalmologists have a higher rate of medication adherence. Ophthalmologists have the options to use treatment modalities such as laser and surgery to obtain pressure control and decrease or eliminate the need for medication use.

The American Academy of Ophthalmology recommends asymptomatic patients older than 40 years be referred for ophthalmic evaluation once every several years for early detection of glaucoma and other chronic eye diseases. However, the US Preventive Services Task Force found insufficient evidence to recommend for or against screening for glaucoma in adults. Risks, benefits, and cost effectiveness of screening are beyond the scope of this chapter, but symptomatic patients or patients at high risk for glaucoma (African American ethnicity and family history) might benefit from ophthalmology consultation. It is possible to diagnose glaucoma by direct ophthalmoscopy, but this is not a substitute for binocular assessment of the disk through dilated pupils and formal visual field testing. If glaucoma is suspected or diagnosed, primary care visits should include inquiries regarding glaucoma medication use, medication side effects, and the time

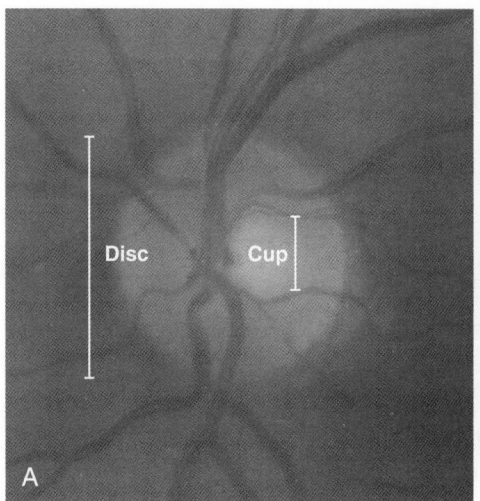
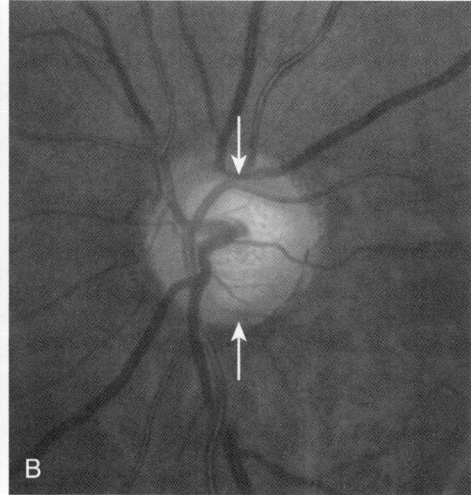

Figure 1 Disk appearance. (A) Normal disk. Cup-to-disk ratio is less than 0.4. (B) Glaucoma. Increased cup-to-disk ratio and narrow neuroretinal rim superiorly and inferiorly *(arrows)*.

			CARBONIC			
CLASS	**β-BLOCKER**	**SELECTIVE α₂ AGONIST**	**ANHYDRASE INHIBITOR**	**PROSTAGLANDIN ANALOGUE**	**RHO KINASE INHIBITOR**	**COMBINATION**
Medication	Timolol (Timoptic) Betaxolol (Betoptic) Levobunolol (Betagan)	Brimonidine (Alphagan)	Dorzolamide (Trusopt) Brinzolamide (Azopt)	Latanoprost (Xalatan) Travoprost (Travatan) Bimatoprost (Lumigan) Latanoprostene bunod (Vyzulta)	Netarsudil (Rhopressa)	Timolol/Dorzolamide (Cosopt) Timolol/Brimonidine (Combigan) Brimonidine/Brinzolamide (Simbrinza) Netarsudil/latanoprost (Rocklatan)
Dosing	qd (Timoptic), bid (Betoptic), or qd to bid (Betagan)	bid	bid	qhs	qd	bid (Cosopt, Combigan), or tid (Simbrinza), or qd (Rocklatan)
Cap color	Yellow	Purple	Orange	Teal	White	Blue (Cosopt, Combigan), or light green (Simbrinza), white (Rocklatan)
Side effects	Bradycardia, COPD, and asthma exacerbation	Allergic conjunctivitis, dry mouth, and fatigue in elderly	Stinging and bitter taste	Hyperemia, lash growth, and increased pigmentation	Hyperemia	See individual components

TABLE 1 Topical Glaucoma Medications: Carbonic Anhydrase Inhibitors

COPD, Chronic obstructive pulmonary disease.

of last eye examination. Primary care physicians can improve glaucoma outcome by promoting adherence to medication and follow-up. Glaucoma patients need to follow up with their ophthalmologists at least annually, and in severe cases every 3 months, for intraocular pressure checks.

Treatment

Topical Glaucoma Medications

Topical glaucoma medications are administered once or twice daily. Patients should look up, pull down their lower eye lid, drop the medication on the inferior conjunctival cul-de-sac, and keep their eyes closed for 5 minutes. Applying gentle pressure next to the bridge of the nose to occlude the puncta can improve absorption of the medication. Medication bottle caps are color-coded by their class, and patients can usually identify their eye drops by color. Glaucoma medications are not subject to first-pass effect through the liver and can sometimes have significant systemic side effects, especially the β-blockers. Topical glaucoma medications are described later and summarized in Table 1.

Prostaglandin Analogues. Latanoprost (Xalatan), travoprost (Travatan), and bimatoprost (Lumigan) are prostaglandin analogues and are color-coded by teal caps. They are administered once at bedtime but may be administered once at any time during the day to promote adherence. They decrease IOP by increasing uveoscleral outflow. Latanoprostene bunod (Vyzulta) is converted into latanoprost and nitric oxide inside the eye and decreases IOP by promoting aqueous outflow through both the uveoscleral and trabecular meshwork pathways. It is considered a prostaglandin analogue with an additional mechanism of action. Side effects are primarily local and include increased conjunctival hyperemia, increased lash growth, and possible irreversible increase in periocular and iris pigmentation.

β-Blockers. Timolol (Betimol, Istalol, Timoptic), levobunolol (Betagan), and betaxolol (Betoptic) are color-coded by yellow caps. They are administered once or twice daily and decrease IOP by decreasing aqueous production. Side effects include bradycardia, exacerbation of chronic obstructive pulmonary disease (COPD) and asthma, impotence, and decreased serum

TABLE 2 | Oral and Intravenous Glaucoma Medications

	ACETAZOLAMIDE (DIAMOX)	METHAZOLAMIDE (NEPTAZANE)	MANNITOL (OSMITROL)	GLYCERIN 50%[1]
Class	CAI	CAI	Hyperosmotic	Hyperosmotic
Dosage	250 or 500 mg bid	25 mg or 50 mg bid	1 g/kg in 30 min	1 g/kg once
Route	PO or IV	PO	IV	PO
Side effects	Bitter taste, indigestion, paresthesia, tinnitus, polyuria, kidney stones, hypokalemia, aplastic anemia, and sulfa allergy		Polyuria, dehydration Exacerbate CHF and diabetes (glycerin)	

CAI, Carbonic anhydrase inhibitor; *CHF*, congestive heart failure
[1]Not FDA approved for this indication.

high-density lipoprotein (HDL) cholesterol. Physicians need to be aware that a topical β-blocker is a potential cause of acute changes in cardiovascular or pulmonary status. There are several reported incidents of death following the use of topical β-blockers mostly due to exacerbation of asthma.

Selective α₂ Agonists. Brimonidine (Alphagan) and apraclonidine (Iopidine) belong to the class of selective α₂ receptor agonists, and brimonidine is more commonly prescribed; it is color-coded by purple caps. It is administered twice daily and decreases IOP by decreasing aqueous production. Allergic conjunctivitis has been reported in up to 25% of patients. Rarely, it causes dry mouth and chronic fatigue and drowsiness in the elderly.

Carbonic Anhydrase Inhibitors. Dorzolamide (Trusopt) and brinzolamide (Azopt) are color-coded by orange caps and are sulfa-based medications. They are administered twice daily and decrease IOP by decreasing aqueous production. This class of medication has minimal systemic side effects. However, some patients complain about transient stinging and a bitter taste in the mouth after administration. These side effects, if tolerable, are not indications for discontinuing therapy.

Rho Kinase Inhibitors. Netarsudil (Rhopressa) affects actin and myosin contraction and decreases IOP by increasing aqueous outflow through the trabecular meshwork. It is color coded white and administered once daily. Conjunctival hyperemia is reported in up to 50% of the patients. Ophthalmologists have also observed pinpoint conjunctival hemorrhages and corneal verticillata (lipid deposits on the corneal epithelium) because these observations are asymptomatic and generally not reported by the patients. Compared to other medications, rho kinase inhibitor has a unique mechanism of action and is considered to be an excellent adjunct medication to lower IOP when other medications are already in use.

Combined Topical Medications. Timolol and dorzolamide (Cosopt) and timolol and brimonidine (Combigan) are color-coded by blue caps. Brimonidine and brinzolamide (Simbrinza) are color-coded by a light green cap. Netarsudil and latanoprost (Rocklatan) are color-coded by white caps. Combined medications decrease exposure to preservatives and can decrease irritation and problems with dry eyes. Adherence might also be improved.

Oral Carbonic Anhydrase Inhibitors
Oral carbonic anhydrase inhibitors include acetazolamide (Diamox), 250 mg or 500 mg given twice daily, and methazolamide (Neptazane), 25 mg or 50 mg given twice daily. They are sulfa-based medications and decrease IOP by decreasing aqueous production. Oral carbonic anhydrase inhibitors are not commonly used today because effective topical medications are available. They are typically used on a short-term basis to achieve IOP control in acute or refractory cases. Side effects can include aplastic anemia, kidney stones, bitter taste, indigestion, paresthesia of the extremities, tinnitus, and polyuria. Clinicians need to consider the possibility of hypokalemia when patients take other diuretics to control blood pressure (Table 2). Acetazolamide may also be given intravenously.

Laser Trabeculoplasty
Argon or selective laser trabeculoplasty can be used to increase aqueous outflow. Laser trabeculoplasty is noninvasive and safe, and it can be performed in the office in less than 10 minutes. Compared to surgery, IOP reduction is limited, up to 25% as primary treatment, but less as an adjunct modality. It is ineffective or less effective in some patients with light trabecular meshwork pigmentation. The effect of laser decreases over time but may be repeated in the case of selective laser trabeculoplasty.

Surgery
The most commonly performed glaucoma surgeries are trabeculectomy, tube shunt, and cyclodestruction. Trabeculectomy (with or without Xen gel stent) and tube shunt are procedures that create an opening in the sclera to increase aqueous outflow. Cyclodestruction destroys the ciliary body and decreases aqueous production. The procedure can be transscleral or endoscopic; the endoscopic method is typically done at the time of cataract surgery. Alternative surgical methods such as deep sclerectomy, Trabectome, canaloplasty, iStent, Kahook dual blade, and Hydrus are performed at the time of cataract surgery to minimize the invasiveness and potential complications associated with traditional glaucoma surgery. However, these minimally invasive glaucoma surgeries (MIGS) are not as effective at lowering the IOP.

Visual Impairment and Blindness
Patients who are visually impaired (Snellen vision of <20/40) or legally blind (Snellen vision of <20/200 or visual field of <20 degrees) may have significantly decreased mobility and ability to function. Continued glaucoma treatment is still important in these patients because even maintenance of count-finger vision can allow the patients some degree of independence. Low-vision devices and services, including high-contrast video magnifiers, audiobooks, eccentric viewers, and mobility training, can allow patients maximal use of their residual vision and improve their confidence and quality of life.

Acute Angle Closure Glaucoma
Pupillary block in susceptible patients blocks aqueous drainage and leads to sudden and extreme rise of intraocular pressure. Acute angle closure can damage the optic nerve, resulting in acute angle closure glaucoma.

About 0.5% to 1.0% of US adults are at risk for acute angle closure. It is more common in Inuits and Asians and rare in African Americans. The risk of acute angle closure increases with age. It is also more common in hyperopes (farsightedness).

Mechanism of Acute Angle Closure: Pupillary Block
After aqueous is produced in the ciliary body in the posterior chamber, it travels through the pupil and exits the anterior chamber through the trabecular meshwork located between the iris and the cornea. Pupillary block occurs when the iris contacts the lens and obstructs the flow of aqueous through the pupil. Increased posterior chamber pressure displaces the iris anteriorly against the trabecular meshwork and stops aqueous outflow.

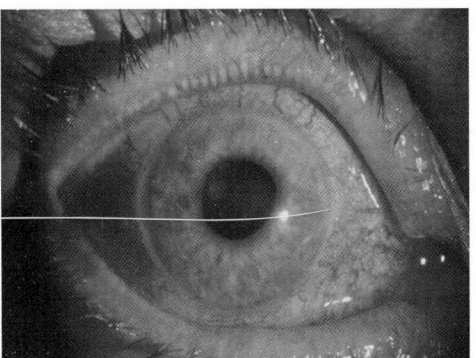

Figure 2 Acute angle closure patient with red eye and mid-dilated and nonreactive pupil.

Patients at risk for acute angle closure have narrow occludable angles. These patients have smaller eyes, allowing the lens to contact the iris to initiate papillary block. The distance between the iris and the lens is the shortest when the pupil is mid-dilated. Therefore, patients who present with acute angle closure might have a history of dim light exposure (movies) or use of medications with anticholinergic properties (antihistamines, decongestants, antispasmodics). High IOP causes iris and corneal endothelial cell dysfunction, resulting in nonreactive pupil and hazy cornea, respectively. High IOP also results in inflammation and red eye, as well as severe pain, nausea, and vomiting (Figure 2). Elevated IOP can damage the optic nerve within hours, and acute angle closure needs to be treated on an emergency basis to prevent permanent loss of vision.

Diagnosis

Patients with acute angle closure can present with blurry vision, red eye, pain, headache, nausea, or vomiting. History can include hyperopia, onset after exposure to a dim environment, or taking anticholinergic medications. Examination findings include decreased vision, conjunctival hyperemia, mid-dilated, nonreactive pupil with or without an afferent papillary defect, and increased IOP (by palpation or tonometry). Acute angle closure is sometimes misdiagnosed as migraines or gastrointestinal illness. Patients with conjunctivitis, keratitis, uveitis, and corneal abrasion can also present with the same symptoms.

Treatment

If acute angle closure is suspected, an emergent referral to ophthalmology is indicated. If an ophthalmologist is not immediately available, the goal will be to medically control the IOP as soon as possible. One drop of topical aqueous suppressant—β-blocker, selective α2 agonist, or carbonic anhydrase inhibitor—should be administered (timolol, brimonidine, and dorzolamide) (see Table 1). The maximum dose of oral or intravenous carbonic anhydrase inhibitor is given: acetazolamide 500 mg or methazolamide 50 mg (see Table 2). The patient is placed in the supine position to allow the lens and iris to fall posteriorly. The patient is reassessed in 30 minutes, and if the condition is not improved, topical drops are repeated. If there is no improvement after another 30 minutes, a hyperosmotic, oral glycerin[1] 1 g/kg or intravenous mannitol (Osmitrol) 1 g/kg over 30 minutes, is administered. Hyperosmotics may be contraindicated in patients with congestive heart failure, and glycerin can cause severe hyperglycemia in diabetic patients.

An ophthalmologist can break the pupillary block by medically lowering the IOP or by performing anterior chamber paracentesis, compression gonioscopy, laser peripheral iridotomy, and, in recalcitrant cases, emergent trabeculectomy. Once the pressure is controlled, it is important to perform an iridotomy in both eyes to prevent future episodes. Patients with patent iridotomies may safely take anticholinergic medications.

---

[1]Not FDA approved for this indication.

References

Allingham RR, Damji KF, Freedman S, et al: *Shield's Textbook of Glaucoma*, ed 5, Philadelphia, 2005, Lippincott Williams & Wilkins, pp 155–190.

American Academy of Ophthalmology: Available at: Practice guidelines. Preferred practice patterns. Primary angle closure. http://www.aao.org/preferred-practice-pattern/primary-angle-closure-ppp–october-2010, October 2010. [Accessed 10 July 2015].

American Academy of Ophthalmology: Practice guidelines. Preferred practice patterns. Primary open-angle glaucoma, September 2005. Available at: http://www.aao.org/preferred-practice-pattern/primary-openangle-glaucoma-ppp–october-2010 October 2010 [accessed July 10, 2105].

Congdon N, O'Colmain B, Klaver CC, et al: Eye Diseases Prevalence Research Group; Causes and prevalence of visual impairment among adults in the United States, *Arch Ophthalmol* 122:477–485, 2004.

Friedman DS, Wolfs RC, O'Colmain BJ, et al: Eye Diseases Prevalence Research Group: Prevalence of open-angle glaucoma among adults in the United States, *Arch Ophthalmol* 122(4):532–538, 2004.

Lin AP, Orengo-Nania S, Braun UK: PCP's role in chronic open-angle glaucoma, *Geriatrics* 64:20–28, 2009.

Nordstrom BL, Friedman DS, Mozaffari E, et al: Persistence and adherence with topical glaucoma therapy, *Am J Ophthalmol* 140:598–606, 2005.

Schwartz GF, Quigley HA: Adherence and persistence with glaucoma therapy, *Surv Ophthalmol* 54:S57–S68, 2008.

US Preventive Services Task Force: Screening for glaucoma, Available at: http://www.uspreventiveservicestaskforce.org/Page/Topic/recommendation-summary/glaucoma-screening; March, 2005 October 2013 [accessed July 10, 2015].

MÉNIÈRE'S DISEASE

Method of
Terry D. Fife, MD

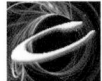

CURRENT DIAGNOSIS

- Ménière's disease is characterized by recurrent attacks of severe vertigo, nausea, and vomiting typically lasting 1 to 6 hours.
- Ménière's disease causes tinnitus on the side of the affected ear; the tinnitus can change in pitch and loudness during attacks of vertigo.
- Attacks of vertigo are associated with reduced or muffled hearing on the side of the affected ear.
- Fluctuating unilateral hearing loss and low-frequency hearing loss on the side of the affected ear is characteristic.

CURRENT THERAPY

- Initial therapy includes a sodium-restricted diet (preferably <1500 mg of sodium daily) and a diuretic agent (e.g., thiazide diuretics).
- Betahistine,[1] a medication widely used in Europe that may be obtained at compounding pharmacies in the United States, may be helpful in selected patients at a dosage 16 to 24 mg three times daily though some authors have recommended even higher dosages.
- Transtympanic infusion of gentamicin[1] or corticosteroids and endolymphatic sac surgery may be considered as minimally invasive options in patients with serviceable hearing. Gentamicin poses a moderate risk of inducing hearing loss.
- Vestibular nerve sectioning is highly effective in stopping vertigo attacks with a reasonably low risk of causing further hearing loss, but it is a more invasive procedure.
- Labyrinthectomy is highly effective in stopping vertigo attacks but causes complete hearing loss, so it is only an option for patients who have already lost all useful hearing.

Patients who have undergone procedures that cause acute loss of vestibular function often have vertigo for a while after the surgery; the vertigo improves more quickly with vestibular rehabilitative therapy.

---

[1]Not FDA approved for this indication.

Ménière's disease is a disorder of the inner ear that results in recurrent, spontaneous episodes of vertigo, hearing loss, ear fullness, and tinnitus affecting the same ear. The hearing loss often fluctuates early in Ménière's disease, but fluctuating hearing is not always present. Eventually permanent hearing loss occurs, affecting the low frequencies initially but ultimately affecting all frequencies.

Epidemiology

The reported prevalence of Ménière's disease varies from about 50 to 200 per 100,000. Females are somewhat more prone to Meniere's disease than males, with a female/male ratio of about 1.9:1.

Risk Factors

Possible risk factors for later development of Ménière's syndrome include autoimmune disorders, migraine, syphilitic otitis and viral infection of the inner ear, head trauma, and a family history of Ménière's disease.

Pathophysiology

The underlying mechanism is generally thought to be due to endolymphatic hydrops, a type of swelling of the endolymphatic compartment that ultimately leads to permanent damage of the inner ear structures. Possible reasons for this periodic swelling of the endolymph compartment include mechanical obstruction of endolymph flow or at least dysregulation of the electrochemical membrane potential between endolymph and perilymph compartments.

Endolymphatic hydrops appears to be the mechanism for a number of conditions that can lead to Ménière's syndrome. When no primary cause is identified, the idiopathic form of the syndrome is called Ménière's disease. When an underlying cause is found, it is referred to as Ménière's syndrome or secondary Ménière's or secondary endolymphatic hydrops. Secondary Ménière's syndrome can result from delayed endolymphatic hydrops in which symptoms come on years after a prior disorder or viral injury of the labyrinth, syphilitic otitis, autoimmune inner ear disease, and trauma.

Prevention

There is no known way of preventing the development of Ménière's disease because it occurs in many people with no risk factors.

Clinical Manifestations

Ménière's disease can manifest with periodic unilateral (or, less commonly, bilateral) hearing loss or isolated attacks of vertigo. Not uncommonly, Ménière's disease has both elements present at its onset, but the vertigo is usually the symptom that gets the most attention. Vertigo usually lasts 1 to 6 hours but can last as little as 30 minutes or as long as all day. Patients prone to motion sickness often report that their dizziness lasts longer because the aftereffect of vertigo lingers longer in those who are motion sensitive. Vertigo attacks in Ménière's disease are often quite severe and generally render patients unable to move around owing to the vertigo, nausea, and recurrent vomiting.

The hearing loss is usually unilateral, and patients might notice fluctuation in hearing accompanied by ear fullness and a low-pitched roaring tinnitus either before or coincident with the vertigo. If audiometry can be performed during this time, low-frequency (250–1000 Hz) hearing loss may be documented and might improve after the attack ceases. This signature fluctuating low-frequency sensorineural hearing loss is very helpful (Figure 1) when found, but getting patients with vertigo attacks in for testing while they are in the acute stage of vertigo is usually not feasible.

Occasionally, patients with Ménière's have sudden random drop attacks in which they abruptly fall without loss of consciousness. These spells, referred to as otolithic crises of Tumarkin, can lead to serious injury and should prompt aggressive treatment. The mechanism is presumed to be related to sudden mechanical deformation or sudden neural discharges related to the otolith structures of the inner ear. Because there is no specific treatment for Tumarkin crises, treatment entails the standard treatments for Ménière's disease in general.

As Ménière's disease progresses, usually over months to years, permanent low-frequency hearing loss develops that gives way to hearing loss at all frequencies. Eventually, the patient can lose all or most hearing on the affected side. Meanwhile, with each vertigo attack, some vestibular function is lost, and so as vertigo attacks continue, vestibular loss ensues, often paralleling the hearing loss. Ménière's occasionally burns out, meaning that enough vestibular function has been lost that acute hydrops no longer produces vertigo. Patients might report less severe dizziness or just a vague feeling of unsteadiness. This usually indicates advanced Ménière's, and unilateral hearing and vestibular loss should be expected.

Bilateral Ménière's disease is present at the time of initial diagnosis in about 10% of cases and by 10 years of symptoms, about 35% have bilateral involvement. Bilateral Ménière's disease has treatment implications because treating one side alone will be unlikely to stop the vertigo attacks, which could be emanating

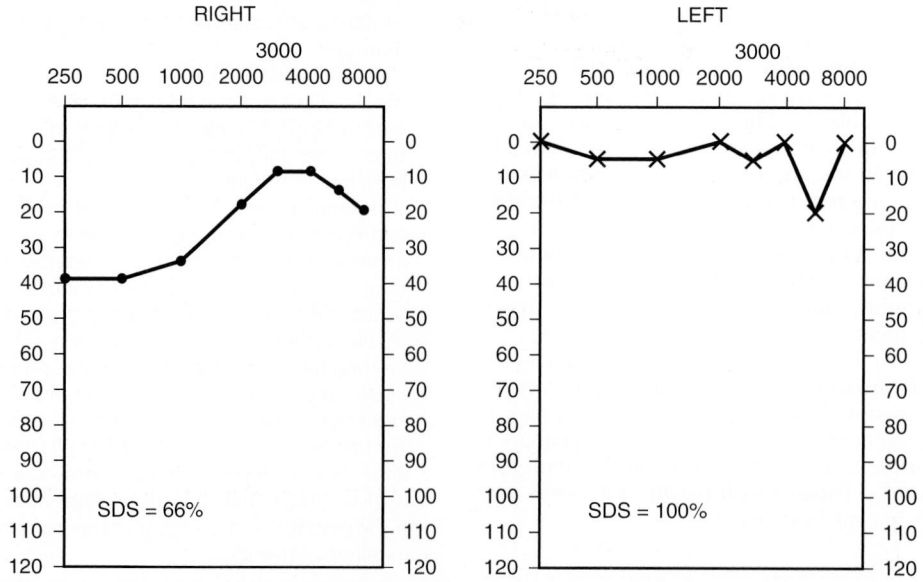

RIGHT-SIDED MÉNIÈRE'S DISEASE

Figure 1 Audiogram showing typical low-frequency hearing trough of Ménière's disease affecting the right ear.

from the untreated side. Surgical treatment of both sides is also problematic because it could leave the patient with bilateral hearing loss, vestibular loss, or both.

Diagnosis

The diagnosis of Ménière's disease is made clinically based on unilateral hearing loss, tinnitus, ear fullness, and episodic vertigo typically lasting 1 to 6 hours. The criteria for definite, probable, and possible Ménière's disease are listed in Box 1. Several recent studies using three-dimensional fluid-attenuated inversion recovery (3D-FLAIR) 24 hours after administration of bilateral intratympanic gadolinium (Gd) injection and similar techniques have demonstrated abnormalities consistent with endolymphatic hydrops. MRI at this point, however, is not yet established as useful in affirming the diagnosis of Ménière's disease.

Differential Diagnosis

Vestibular neuritis causes a single attack of vertigo, sometimes with acute hearing loss (labyrinthitis), but it can usually be distinguished from Ménière's disease because vestibular neuritis has a lifetime recurrence rate of only 2%, whereas Ménière's vertigo attacks recur multiple times and cause fluctuating and gradual decline in hearing.

When a patient reports episodic vertigo attacks in the absence of unilateral tinnitus, ear fullness, and hearing loss, one must be cautious in diagnosing Ménière's disease because vestibular migraine (basilar-type migraine) can produce a similar pattern. Diagnostic criteria have been published for vestibular migraine (Lempert, 2013).

Benign paroxysmal positional vertigo causes brief recurrent spells of spinning without hearing loss, so it is rarely confused with Ménière's disease.

Vertebrobasilar insufficiency can cause isolated vertigo, but the duration is usually only several minutes and without hearing loss, whereas Ménière's attacks last hours and are associated with unilateral auditory symptoms.

Acoustic neuroma (vestibular schwannoma) typically leads to slowly progressive unilateral sensorineural hearing loss, but vertigo is infrequently a prominent feature because patients compensate gradually as their vestibular function wanes due to compressive effects of the tumor.

Fluctuating unilateral hearing loss, ear fullness, and tinnitus can occur without vertigo and is referred to as cochlear hydrops. Such symptoms can precede the development of vertigo but may be treated as Ménière's nonetheless. Lermoyez's syndrome refers to transiently improved hearing and tinnitus during attacks of vertigo. More commonly, however, hearing declines around and during vertigo spells.

Treatment

Medical Management

Treatment of Ménière's disease is mainly aimed at preventing the vertigo attacks, but no treatments are known that reliably restore or arrest hearing loss or tinnitus. It is presumed that if attacks of vertigo, ear fullness, fluctuating hearing, and tinnitus are all stopped, hearing should stabilize, but this is still a supposition. The management of Ménière's is hierarchical, starting with a low-sodium diet and a diuretic and proceeding to more-invasive or destructive surgical procedures only when initial medical treatment fails. When a patient has very frequent vertigo attacks and is disabled, more-aggressive treatment may be considered sooner.

Dietary sodium should be restricted to 1000 to 1500 mg daily. The average person consumes about 4000 mg daily, and the maximum recommended daily intake of sodium is 2300 mg. Because more than 70% of the daily sodium comes from processed foods, this dietary restriction generally requires more than simply stopping the use of table salt, which generally accounts for only about 10% of daily sodium intake for most people.

A diuretic is usually added to the sodium restriction. The most commonly prescribed diuretic is hydrochlorothiazide 25 mg combined with triamterene 37.5 mg (Dyazide)[1] because this combination usually obviates the need for potassium supplementation. Acetazolamide (Diamox)[1] 125 to 250 mg bid or furosemide (Lasix)[1] 10 to 20 mg daily are also options. Patients with severe sulfa allergy can use low-dose ethacrynic acid (Edecrin)[1] 12.5 to 25 mg daily.

An acute attack of vertigo from Ménière's disease can be managed with vestibular suppressants such as dimenhydrinate (Dramamine)[1] 50 mg, meclizine (Antivert) 25 to 50 mg, diazepam (Valium)[1] 2 to 5 mg, or promethazine (Phenergen)[1] 12.5 to 50 mg. Scopolamine in patch form (Transderm-Scōp)[1] is too slow to be useful because it takes hours to be absorbed transdermally. Scopace (oral scopolamine) has been discontinued and is no longer being manufactured in the United States. Scopolamine tablets[1] may be available in certain compounding pharmacies. Nausea can additionally be managed with prochlorperazine (Compazine) 10 mg orally or 25 mg by suppository, with oral or sublingual ondansetron (Zofran)[1] 4 to 8 mg, or with other antiemetics. Generally, the vertigo attacks subside in several hours even without treatment.

Betahistine hydrochloride or dihydrochloride[2] may also be helpful in Ménière's, although it is not commonly used in the United States. The role of betahistine is not firmly established, although it is widely prescribed for vertigo throughout the world. Betahistine may be helpful when successful medical management with diet and diuretics has helped but is inadequate to stop attacks. Betahistine is a vasodilator, a modest H_1 histamine agonist, and a powerful H_3 histamine receptor antagonist. Its method of action in Ménière's is unknown, though it may influence perfusion of the stria vascularis to reduce pressure in the endolymphatic space. Doses of betahistine may start at 8 mg PO three times daily and may be increased to 48 mg three times daily. It is available outside the United States in the form of Serc®, Vertin®, Vertipress®, Betavert® and many other trademarks throughout the world. Betahistine may be made within the United States at compounding pharmacies with a physician prescription[1] and may also be imported from outside the United States for personal use. This is often done using an encapsulated powder form of betahistine dihydrochloride USP (from manufacturers such as

---

BOX 1   Diagnostic Criteria for Ménière's Disease

Definite Ménière's Disease
1. Two or more spontaneous attacks of vertigo, each lasting 20 minutes to 12 hours
2. Audiometrically documented low- to mid-frequency SNHL in the affected ear on at least 1 occasion before, during, or after 1 of the episodes of vertigo
3. Fluctuating aural symptoms (hearing loss, tinnitus, or ear fullness) in the affected ear
4. Other causes excluded by other tests

Probable Ménière's Disease
1. At least 2 episodes of vertigo or dizziness lasting 20 minutes to 24 hours
2. Fluctuating aural symptoms (hearing loss, tinnitus, or fullness) in the affected ear
3. Other causes excluded by other tests

Basura GJ, Adams ME, Monfared A, et al: Clinical practice guideline: Ménière's disease, *Otolaryngol Head Neck Surg* 162:415–434, 2020.

---

[1]Not FDA approved for this indication.
[2]Not available in the United States.

TABLE 1 Procedures Used in the Management of Ménière's Disease

METHOD	TECHNIQUE	ADVANTAGES	DISADVANTAGES
Procedures Intended to Spare Serviceable Hearing			
Intratympatic corticosteroids	Injection of steroid through the tympanic membrane to the middle ear to be absorbed in the inner ear	Minimally invasive, few side effects	Effectiveness unclear when compared to placebo
Intratympanic gentamicin (Garamycin)[1]	Injection of gentamicin through the tympanic membrane to the middle ear to be absorbed in the inner ear	Simple office-based procedure, low risk profile	Number of injections is unpredictable; some risk of hearing loss
Endolymphatic mastoid shunt	Placing a shunt from the endolymphatic sac to the mastoid air cells	Effective in 50%–75% of cases; low risk of hearing loss; day procedure	Vertigo can recur; effectiveness depends on surgical experience and technique
Vestibular neurectomy	Surgical sectioning of the vestibular part of cranial nerve VIII, sparing the auditory part of the nerve	Highly effective in eliminating vertigo attacks	Requires general anesthesia; risk of facial weakness, hearing loss
Procedures Expected to Eliminate Residual Hearing			
Labyrinthectomy or cochleosacculotomy	Several methods of removing all or part of the labyrinth	Highly effective in stopping vertigo attacks	Inevitable complete hearing loss

[1]Not FDA approved for this indication.

Fagron, Inc., St. Paul, MN USA) by weight in capsules with or without filler. Side effects are few, although occasionally patients report some gastrointestinal upset or mild headache. Betahistine is not histamine, and has not been found to cause or aggravate urticaria.

Oral corticosteroids are often used but rarely seem effective except in cases of bilateral Ménière's resulting from autoimmune inner ear disease (AIED). Oral corticosteroids rarely seem to be effective in typical Ménière's disease.

Ménière's attacks have been said to be triggered by caffeine, chocolate, stress, visual stimuli, and dropping barometric pressure. Such triggers should be avoided when possible, but strong associations with these triggers can also occur in migrainous vertigo. Vestibular rehabilitative therapy is not generally helpful in Ménière's because most vertigo attacks remit and the patients have few vestibular symptoms between attacks. However, when vestibular loss has occurred and the patient appears to have not compensated well for it, vestibular rehabilitation can be helpful.

Bilateral Ménière's Disease
The estimated incidence of bilateral Ménière's disease varies in the literature but is estimated to occur in about 15% of cases and bilateral involvement increases over time. The possibility of bilateral involvement weighs on the decision-making for any procedures that sacrifice hearing or vestibular function because it leaves the patient with only one functioning labyrinth.

Serviceability of Hearing
Serviceable hearing is residual hearing that can be useful to the patient by wearing hearing aids. In general, because hearing loss is permanent, one should avoid sacrificing any serviceable hearing.

Injections and Surgical Treatments
Patients who continue to have disabling vertigo despite a low-salt diet, diuretics, and possibly betahistine are considered to have failed conservative medical therapy. The next step in treatment depends on the age, health status, and residual hearing and vestibular function of the patient and also on the surgeon's opinion and experience with the various options. If spells are infrequent, symptomatic management of vertigo attacks may be the best option. Table 1 outlines some of the additional interventional options.

Intratympanic Gentamicin
Transtympanic gentamicin (Garamycin)[1] administration has become increasingly used as an effective treatment of Ménière's disease. This is partly due to the ease of administration of gentamicin and its relative safety. Gentamicin is a commonly used aminoglycoside antimicrobial agent with activity against gram-negative bacteria that also happens to be ototoxic. It damages hair cells of the labyrinth and preferentially affects hair cells of the vestibular neuroepithelium over that of the cochlea. Even so, transtympanic administration still has some risk of causing hearing loss. Gentamicin is administered by injecting a small amount (usually about 0.5 mL) of gentamicin sulfate (80 mg/2 mL) solution through the tympanic membrane into the middle ear space. To avoid rapid drainage through the eustachian tube, the injection is done with the patient supine and kept in that position for an hour or so to allow the gentamicin to absorb through the round window into the inner ear. There are many protocols, but commonly an injection is given once, and additional injections can be considered every 3 to 4 weeks until improvement in vertigo attacks is realized. Studies suggest that intratympanic gentamicin is an effective treatment for vertigo complaints in Ménière's disease but there is some risk of hearing loss.

Endolymphatic Sac Surgery
Another option for patients with residual functional hearing is endolymphatic sac shunt or decompression. This procedure eliminates vertigo in 50% to 75% of those treated. Nevertheless, its effectiveness compared with placebo has remained a point of contention based on a number of studies. It has been suggested that the procedure's effectiveness depends on the operative technique and experience of the surgeon.

Intratympanic Steroids
Sometimes, a trial of intratympanic corticosteroids may be offered (Basura, 2020), although its effectiveness in controlled trials is still not compelling. Even so, a trial of corticosteroids administered in this manner poses little risk.

[1]Not FDA approved for this indication.

Vestibular Neurectomy

The most definitive procedure for stopping vertigo attacks in Ménière's when the goal is to preserve hearing is vestibular neurectomy. This procedure involves craniotomy and severing the vestibular nerve while preserving the cochlear nerve. This procedure requires overnight hospitalization and general anesthesia, and it does pose some risk to facial nerve function and hearing on the affected side.

Labyrinthectomy

For patients who have unilateral Ménière's disease and no serviceable hearing, labyrinthectomy is a commonly used procedure. This procedure entails the removal of the membranous labyrinth and is highly effective in stopping recurrent vertigo attacks from that ear. In elderly patients or those who are poor surgical candidates, a more limited transtympanic cochleosacculotomy may be performed.

Meniett Treatment

The Meniett device is a portable, low-frequency, pressure-wave delivery system that administers a wave of pressure of about $12 \mathrm{cm} \mathrm{H}_2\mathrm{O}$ to the middle ear via a tympanostomy tube for about 0.6 seconds pulsed at 6 Hz for 5 minutes about three to five times daily. Quality randomized trials demonstrating effectiveness of this treatment are lacking, and it is recommended by a recent evidence-based guideline that this treatment should NOT be prescribed (Basura, 2020).

Monitoring

Following patients with Ménière's disease should include monitoring of the frequency and severity of vertigo spells and the fluctuation in hearing, ear fullness, and tinnitus. Periodic audiometry is probably the most sensitive measure of stabilization of the condition. Vestibular testing may be considered when changes might alter the treatment strategy. Brain imaging is only helpful in excluding other disorders, but does not yet have a role in the management of Ménière's disease.

Complications

Known complications include the progression of unilateral and occasionally bilateral hearing and vestibular function. There may also be complications associated with some of the treatments as described earlier. Owing to the unpredictability of the vertigo attacks, many patients avoid certain activities and might even develop agoraphobic features because the attacks are so severe and disruptive. In most cases, these avoidance behaviors improve if Ménière's disease can be controlled.

Conclusion

The management of Ménière's disease is still part art and part science. Treatment options are many, but patients should be reassured that, in most cases, something can be offered to help improve their vertigo and quality of life.

References

Basura GJ, Adams ME, Monfared A, et al: Clinical practice guideline: Ménière's disease, *Otolaryngol Head Neck Surg* 162:415–434, 2020.
Lempert T: Vestibular migraine, *Semin Neurol* 33:212–218, 2013.
Lopez-Escamez JA, et al: Diagnostic criteria for Ménière's disease, *J Vestib Res* 25(1):1–7, 2015.
Nevoux J, Franco-Vidal V, Bouccara D, et al: Diagnostic and therapeutic strategy in Ménière's disease. Guidelines of the French Otorhinolaryngology-Head and Neck Surgery Society (SFORL), *Eur Ann Otorhinolaryngol Head Neck Dis*, 134(6):441–444, 2017.
Pullens B, van Benthem PP: Intratympanic gentamicin for Ménière's disease or syndrome, *Cochrane Database Syst Rev*(3), 2011. https://doi.org/10.1002/1465185 8.CD008234.pub2. CD008234.
Pullens B, Verschuur HP, van Benthem PP: Surgery for Ménière's disease, *Cochrane Database Syst Rev* 28(2), 2013. CD005395.
Russo FY, Nguyen Y, De Seta D, et al: Meniett device in meniere disease: Randomized, double-blind, placebo-controlled multicenter trial, *Laryngoscope* 127:470–475, 2017.
Yaz F, Ziylan F, Smeeing DPJ, Thomeer HGXM: Intratympanic treatment in Meniere's disease, efficacy of aminoglycosides versus corticosteroids in comparison studies. A systemic review, *Otology and Neurotology* 41(1):1–10, 2020.

OTITIS EXTERNA

Method of
Kimberly Williams, MD

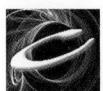

CURRENT DIAGNOSIS

- Pain, itching, or fullness of the ear
- Tenderness of tragus, pinna, or both
- Onset <48 h
- Physical examination findings of erythema, edema, ± drainage and debris

CURRENT THERAPY

- Aural toilet
- Topical antimicrobials
- Analgesic treatment

Otitis externa is an inflammation of the ear canal and can be either acute or chronic. It is often called swimmer's ear.

Epidemiology

Acute otitis externa is a common problem seen in the primary care office. The annual incidence falls between 1:100 and 1:250 with a lifetime incidence approaching 10%. Peak incidence is in children 7 to 12 years old. It does appear to have a genetic link, because it occurs more often in people with blood group type A. Chronic otitis externa affects 3% to 5% of the population.

Risk Factors

Otitis externa is more common in warmer climates with high humidity. Increased water exposure, especially from swimming, places a person at higher risk. Other risk factors include debris from dermatologic conditions such as psoriasis, trauma due to use of hearing aids and ear plugs and abrasions from cleaning of the ear canal. Cerumen helps prevent microbial growth by providing an acidic pH; when cerumen is removed in cleaning, an environment ready for microbial growth is set up.

Pathophysiology

Approximately 95% of acute otitis externa is due to bacterial infection (Figure 1). The other 5% can be attributed to fungal infections or, less commonly, herpes zoster. Fungal infection is more common in chronic otitis externa. Of the bacterial infections, 20% to 60% are due to *Pseudomonas aeruginosa*. *Staphylococcus aureus* is the next major causative organism. Gram-negative organisms account for 2% to 3% of bacterial infections.

Prevention

Prevention is aimed at avoiding water accumulation and retention in the ear canal. Using ear plugs while swimming and using a hair dryer to dry the ear canal after water exposure can be beneficial. The use of acidifying eardrops, such as acetic acid 2% (Vosol), before and after swimming can also help prevent otitis externa. Other preventive measures include stopping the removal of cerumen and avoiding trauma to the ear canal. Finally, proper treatment of dermatologic conditions such as eczema and psoriasis can help reduce debris that can be a risk factor for infection.

Clinical Manifestations

Otitis externa usually develops rapidly over 1 to 2 days. Most patients complain of a feeling of ear pain, fullness, or itching. Hearing loss may be another symptom. Key physical examination findings include tenderness on palpation of the tragus, discomfort with

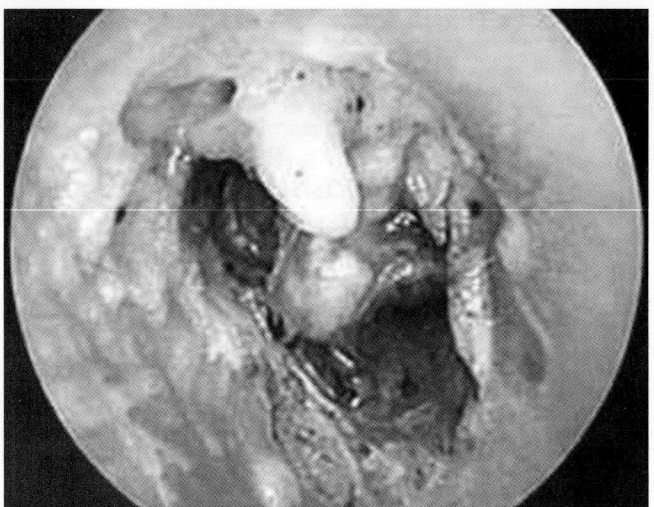

Figure 1 Acute otitis externa with the canal somewhat narrowed from edema and obstructed by desquamating epithelium, soft cerumen, and purulent discharge; this must be removed to visualize the tympanic membrane and to allow ototopical therapy to penetrate to all the superficially infected areas of the canal skin. Reprinted with permission from Osguthorpe JD, Nielsen DR. Otitis externa: review and clinical update. *Am Family Physician*. 2006;76:9.

traction on the pinna, edema of the ear canal, and erythema of the canal. Pain may be out of proportion to examination findings. Regional lymphadenitis and cellulitis of the pinna and adjacent skin can also be present.

Diagnosis

The diagnosis of otitis externa is made clinically by history and physical examination. The history should be positive for otalgia, itching, or sense of fullness. The exam should be positive for tenderness if the tragus is palpated or if the pinna is pulled up and out. If the cause is bacterial, purulent drainage is usually present. Otoscopy will show diffuse canal edema, usually present with erythema. Often there will be copious amounts of debris. Debris should be cleared to visualize the tympanic membrane. There should be good mobility of the tympanic membrane and the tympanometry curve will be normal unless there is concomitant acute otitis media.

Differential Diagnosis

Middle ear disease should be distinguished from external disease by ensuring that the tympanic membrane is normal. Acute otitis media with perforation of the tympanic membrane may result in purulent middle ear secretions into the external ear canal. Contact dermatitis of the ear canal can mimic otitis externa, and a thorough history of exposure to metals such as nickel and copper, chemicals such as new soaps, topical antibiotics, detergents, cosmetics, and other irritants should be obtained. Fungal infection of the ear canal can mimic bacterial otitis externa. Fungus tends to infect the medial portion of the ear canal and has spores and filaments that can be seen both macroscopically and microscopically. Also in the differential are carcinoma of the external auditory canal, which mimics chronic infection; herpes, which is rare and forms vesicles on the outer ear canal; and radiation therapy.

Therapy

Topical therapy is the treatment of choice in mild to moderate disease in healthy patients. The choice of topical agent is based on cost, ease of administration, and risk of side effects (Table 1). Topical aminoglycoside and fluoroquinolone antibiotics have a response rate of more than 70%. If there is a perforation of the tympanic membrane, ciprofloxacin topical solutions are preferred because of the risk of ototoxicity from aminoglycosides and neomycin. Using a topical steroid in conjunction with topical antibiotic therapy has been shown to shorten duration of ear pain. Duration of topical therapy should be 7 to 10 days. Clotrimazole 1%[1] may be used for superficial fungal infections of the ear canal.

[1]Not US Food and Drug Administration approved for this indication.

TABLE 1 Topical Otic Preparations for Treatment of Otitis Externa.

ACTIVE DRUGE	BRAND NAME	DOSING	COMMENTS
Acetic acid 2% solution with steroid	Vosol HC, Acetasol HC	q4–6h	Can sting/local irritation
Ciprofloxacin/ hydrocortisone	Cipro HC	q12h	Approved if tympanic membrane is perforated
Ciprofloxacin/ dexamethasone	Ciprodex	q12h	Approved if tympanic membrane is perforated
Neomycin, polymyxin B, hydrocortisone	Cortisporin Otic	q6h	Neomycin can cause local irritation, ototoxic potential
Ofloxacin	Floxin Otic	q24h	Can cause local irritation
Tobramycin[1]	Tobrex	q6h	Minimally irritating, ophthalmic preparation, ototoxic potential
Gentamycin[1]	Garamycin	q6h	Ophthalmic preparation, ototoxic potential

[1]Not FDA approved for this indication.

For the topical therapy to be effective, it must be delivered to the tissue of the ear canal. First, the canal must be cleared of debris. This can be done in the physician's office under direct visualization or with lavage of the ear canal using saline or hydrogen peroxide warmed to body temperature. The patient should then be instructed on the proper delivery of the eardrops. Eardrops are administered more effectively if another person delivers the drops. The patient should lie on his or her side with the affected ear up, and drops should be placed in the ear canal until it is filled. The patient should remain on his or her side for 3 to 5 minutes. If greater than 50% of the canal is edematous, a wick made of cellulose material should be placed to facilitate delivery of the drops. The wick may fall out or can be removed by either patient or clinician once the edema has resolved.

Systemic therapy should be used in patients who are immune compromised, including those with diabetes, and in patients with surrounding cellulitis. The systemic therapy chosen should be effective against pseudomonas.

Adequate pain control is another important factor in the treatment of otitis externa. Often this can be achieved with nonsteroidal antiinflammatory medications, but opioid analgesics may be necessary, especially to remove debris. Analgesics should be used early in treatment of the disease.

Monitoring

Patients should respond to therapy in 48 to 72 hours. If therapy fails, the clinician should evaluate adherence to therapy and ability of the drug to be delivered properly. Alternative diagnoses should be considered, including fungal infections, dermatitis, foreign bodies, and middle ear disease with perforation of the tympanic membrane. If the infection has spread outside of the ear canal, systemic therapy should be started.

Complications

One complication of simple otitis externa is malignant otitis externa, an invasive infection of the external auditory canal causing osteomyelitis of the temporal bone. It most commonly occurs in elderly diabetic patients or the immunocompromised. Complications include meningitis, dural sinus thrombosis, cranial abscess, and cranial nerve neuropathy including facial nerve paralysis. Diagnosis may require computed tomography and cultures. Treatment includes systemic antipseudomonal antibiotics and surgical débridement. Contact dermatitis from the topical antimicrobials prescribed for otitis externa may also complicate treatment. This is due to a delayed-type hypersensitivity reaction to one or more of the components of the topical therapy. Neomycin is the most common cause, but hypersensitivity reactions can also occur from other agents including preservatives and fragrances. The reaction is characterized by pruritus, edema, and inflammation of the skin in the auditory canal. It can spread beyond the canal to the pinna and even the skin of the neck. This is treated with topical steroids and by stopping the offending agent.

OTITIS MEDIA

Method of
Gretchen M. Irwin, MD, MBA

CURRENT DIAGNOSIS

- History of acute onset of symptoms
- Middle ear effusion
  - Bulging tympanic membrane
  - Limited mobility of tympanic membrane or air fluid level visible behind tympanic membrane
- Middle ear inflammation
  - Erythema of tympanic membrane or distinct otalgia

CURRENT THERAPY

- Watchful Waiting—appropriate for children:
  i. Greater than 2 years of age with nonsevere illness
  ii. Greater than 6 months of age with uncertain diagnosis and nonsevere illness
  iii. Greater than 2 years of age with severe illness, but uncertain diagnosis
  - Need close follow-up in 48 hours
  - Consider delayed prescription
- Antibiotics
  - First line should be amoxicillin (Amoxil) 80 to 90 mg/kg/day[3]
  - Treat 10 days if child less than 6 years of age, 5 to 7 days if greater than 6 years of age
  - Follow-up if not improving in 48 hours
- Analgesia
  - Acetaminophen (Tylenol), ibuprofen (Motrin, Advil)
  - Benzocaine in combination with antipyrine (Allergen, Auroguard), benzocaine with antipyrine and acetic acid (Auralgan)
- Antihistamines and decongestants are of no benefit
- Surgery—consider tympanostomy tubes when:
  i. First AOM episode at less than 6 months of age and child with 2 or more episodes in 6 months or 3 in 24 months
  ii. First AOM episode at more than 12 months of age and child with 3 episodes in 6 months, 5 episodes in 12 months or 7 episodes in 24 months

---
[3]Exceeds dosage recommended by the manufacturer.

Epidemiology

Acute otitis media (AOM) is a common condition of childhood, with one in four children having at least one episode of AOM by age 10. In fact, 86% of children will have at least one episode of AOM within the first year of life. Younger children are more likely to be affected, with peak incidence noted between ages 6 and 20 months likely because of the relative immaturity of the immune system and eustachian tube function. On average, 5 billion dollars are spent per year on office visits, lost productivity, and diminished parental quality of life due to AOM infections. As a result, research has focused on effective strategies both to prevent episodes of AOM and also to efficiently treat episodes that do occur.

Risk Factors

Identifying children at risk for AOM has been an important strategy to attempt to limit instances of AOM. Unfortunately, many of the risk factors associated with AOM are not modifiable, including male sex, Native American ethnicity, presence of siblings within the home, and a family history of recurrent AOM. Additional risk factors include low socioeconomic status, premature birth, attendance at out-of-home daycare, lack of breastfeeding, and history of poor maternal health during pregnancy. Limited studies have suggested that interventions such as avoiding supine feeding or bottle propping, reducing pacifier use after the first 6 months of life, and eliminating passive tobacco exposure can help to reduce incidence; however, the evidence in which these interventions demonstrate clear impact is limited. Public health programs that encourage breastfeeding and optimal maternal health during pregnancy, as well as those focused on reducing tobacco use, have perhaps the best opportunity to impact AOM incidence rates.

Not only are these identified risk factors for any episode of AOM, but children with these characteristics are also more likely to have recurrent AOM. Although many children will be affected in their lifetimes, those with recurrent disease are most at risk of complications leading to morbidity or mortality. Other risk factors specifically for recurrent AOM include an early onset of first episode and low parental education.

Pathophysiology

AOM has classically been associated with three bacteria; namely, *Streptococcus pneumoniae*, *Moraxalla catarrhalis*, and *Haemophillus influenzae*. The introduction of pneumococcal vaccines has led to a shifting in the frequency with which each pathogen causes disease. In 1999, *S. pneumoniae* was responsible for 40% to 45% of acute otitis media, while *H. influenzae* was responsible for 25% to 30%. In 2017, the bacteria were responsible for 15% to 25% and 50% to 60%, respectively. The frequency of *M. catarrhalis* infections has remained consistent at 12% to 15%.

The bacteria responsible for AOM become pathogenic in the setting of eustachian tube dysfunction. A relative obstruction of the eustachian tube develops most commonly secondary to secretions from an antecedent viral upper respiratory infection or allergies, but may result from neuromuscular conditions or abnormal anatomy. Such relative obstruction creates a negative pressure within the middle ear leading to serous effusion and secondary infection of this collection of interstitial fluid. Thus prevention of AOM is aimed at both reducing the presence of pathogenic bacteria and preventing upper respiratory infections that may create eustachian tube dysfunction.

Prevention

The successes of immunization programs in virtually eliminating childhood illnesses such as measles, polio, and varicella have led to great interest in the development of vaccines capable of eradicating the causative agents of AOM. Immunizations targeting the specific bacteria most commonly associated with AOM have had mixed success, however.

For example, although the serotypes contained in the 7-valent pneumococcal conjugate vaccine (PCV, Prevnar) are responsible for approximately 66% of pneumococcal-related AOM, only moderate effectiveness has been noted in reducing AOM incidence among vaccinated children. After the introduction of the 7-valent PCV into practice in February of 2000, AOM incidence decreased only 6% to 7% among vaccinated children. The 9-valent and 11-valent PCVs[2] have been shown to result in a risk reduction of S pneumoniae isolates in children with AOM of 17% and 34%, respectively. An increase in serotype 19A has been noted that is not covered in the 7-, 9-, or 11- valent PCVs[2] but is included in the new 13-valent PCV (Prevnar 13). The 13-valent PCV was incorporated into the recommended childhood immunization schedule in February 2010. Since 2010, there has been a steady decline in otitis media attributable to S. pneumoniae.

Similar vaccines are in development for H influenzae and M catarrhalis as causative agents of AOM. The current H influenzae b vaccine, or Hib, has had little impact on AOM, because less than 5% of episodes are caused by the type b strain of Haemophilius. Instead non-typeable H influenzae is a much more common cause of AOM.

Although the vaccines targeting specific bacteria that have been shown to cause AOM have been successful, so too has the influenza vaccine been shown to impact the course of AOM. In several studies, children who received seasonal influenza vaccine (Fluzone) were found to have fewer episodes of AOM than unvaccinated children. Furthermore, those who did have an AOM episode were found to use fewer antibiotics and have shorter duration of middle-ear effusion compared with unvaccinated counterparts.

With evidence that reducing incidence of viral influenza may reduce the occurrence of secondary AOM, several other interventions aimed at reducing viral upper respiratory infection incidence have been studied for their impact on AOM rates. The use of zinc[7] and propolis[7] as agents to prevent viral upper respiratory infections, for instance, has been shown to have mixed benefit in reducing AOM in children. In multiple studies, zinc has been well tolerated with no contraindications to use identified. Zinc as a single agent has been shown to prevent AOM only when used in children under age 5 who are also malnourished. However, when combined with propolis, zinc was shown to be effective at reducing AOM episodes for children with a history of recurrent AOM. Of note, in several trials zinc did not reduce upper respiratory infection rates; rather, rates of secondary AOM alone were decreased. Although not necessarily effective as a preventive measure for all children, zinc and propolis may be an option for children with recurrent infection.

Similarly, probiotics[7] added to infant formula have been shown to be beneficial for some children. Although breastfeeding as compared to formula supplementation has been shown to be most beneficial in preventing AOM, infant formulas supplemented with Lactobacillus rhamnosus GG and Bifidobacterium lactis Bb-12 (Enfamil Premium, Nestle Good Start) were shown to reduce incidence of AOM over the first 7 months and the first 1 year. Children who received placebo formula had an incidence of AOM of 50% in the first 7 months, whereas children who received the probiotic-supplemented formula had an incidence of only 22%.

Dietary supplementation to limit AOM is not limited to infant formulas, however. Xylitol[7], a polyol sugar alcohol found in birch plants, plums, strawberries, and raspberries, has been demonstrated in several studies to be effective at preventing both dental caries and AOM, although its dosage forms make administration difficult. Xylitol is available as a chewing gum, which raises concern as a choking hazard in young children. Similarly, in its oral syrup form, xylitol must be administered five times daily to be effective. Studies of thrice-daily dosing have not been able to demonstrate the same preventive effect as dosing five times daily despite a consistent total daily dose of 10 grams per day. Furthermore, emerging evidence suggests that xylitol must be given daily to remain effective at reducing AOM episodes, because

prophylaxis only during winter months or use only during upper respiratory tract infections is ineffective. Of note, children who have already received tympanostomy tubes receive no prevention benefit from xylitol administration. Research is ongoing to increase physician awareness of xylitol as a possible prophylactic measure because current studies suggest less than one half of US physicians are aware of xylitol and less than one fourth discuss or recommend its use to patients.

Echinacea[7] and osteopathic manipulation have also been cited as potential prophylactic treatments, particularly for children at high risk of recurrence. However, little evidence exists that either are effective. In fact, one large study demonstrated an increased risk of AOM with Echinacea use during an upper respiratory tract infection episode and no benefit to manipulation treatment. Ongoing studies are examining the use of these modalities.

Clinical Manifestations

AOM presents with a rapid onset of symptoms that may include fever, chills, ear pain, or ear pulling. In fact, ear pulling and ear rubbing have been demonstrated to be quite sensitive for the diagnosis of AOM in the setting of a history consistent with AOM and middle ear effusion. Often, symptoms may be preceded by upper respiratory symptoms such as rhinorrhea, cough, or congestion. Children who have had tympanostomy tubes placed will likely have a far different presentation, with fever and pain being quite unlikely; rather, a thin, yellow or milky discharge may be the only sign that AOM is present.

Diagnosis

The 2013 update of the guidelines of the American Academy of Pediatrics for the diagnosis and treatment of AOM acknowledged that no gold standard exists for the clinical diagnosis of AOM. History and physical examination should be consistent with rapid onset of inflammation in the middle ear. Both pneumatic otoscopy and tympanometry may be useful in the diagnosis of AOM. Tympanic membranes should be evaluated for position, mobility, color, and degree of translucency using pneumatic otoscopy to assess for presence of middle ear effusion or inflammation. Moderate to severe bulging of the tympanic membrane, new onset of otorrhea without other cause, or mild bulging of the tympanic membrane with intense erythema or ear pain should prompt diagnosis of AOM. Furthermore, tympanomtry may be useful in determining whether an effusion is present if the diagnosis is otherwise unclear.

One concern of physicians has been accurately diagnosing middle ear inflammation after a child has been vigorously crying. A study of 125 healthy children, age less than 30 months, assessed the impact of crying on tympanic membrane color by performing otoscopy both before and after administering at least two immunizations. While crying can cause a pinkening of the tympanic membrane, it should disappear when the child quiets and should be less intense than what is observed with inflammation. True middle ear inflammation results in an angry, red eardrum, not the milder, pink flush seen with vigorous crying. The presence of effusion should also help to support a diagnosis of inflammation.

Differential Diagnosis

Otitis media with effusion is often misdiagnosed as an episode of AOM. Like AOM, OME is common, with 2.2 million episodes annually representing an estimated cost of 4 billion dollars. OME can also occur with a viral upper respiratory infection and may follow or precede an episode of AOM. OME differs from AOM, however, because fluid may be present in the middle ear with OME, but there are no signs of acute infection.

Although OME is not associated with acute infection, it is nonetheless critical to diagnose, because research has demonstrated that chronic OME is associated with hearing loss and subsequent developmental delay. In fact, OME in infancy has

---

[2] Not available in the United States.

[7] Available as a dietary supplement.

TABLE 1 | Treatment Options for Acute Otitis Media

AGE OF CHILD	AOM WITH OTORRHEA		AOM WITHOUT OTORRHEA		AOM WITH SEVERE SYMPTOMS*	
	UNILATERAL	BILATERAL	UNILATERAL	BILATERAL	UNILATERAL	BILATERAL
6 months to 2 years	Antibiotics	Antibiotics	Antibiotics or observation	Antibiotics	Antibiotics	Antibiotics
>2 years	Antibiotics	Antibiotics	Antibiotics or observation	Antibiotics or observation	Antibiotics	Antibiotics

*Severe symptoms include toxic-appearing child, persistent otalgia for >48 hours, temperature >39°C in past 48 hours, or uncertain access to follow-up.

been shown to be associated with, on average, a 7-point reduction in IQ at age 7.

The cornerstone of treatment for OME is observation for 2 to 3 months to allow the effusion to clear. Avoidance of allergens and tobacco exposure that may worsen eustachian tube dysfunction is also important. Decongestants and antihistamines are not effective. If an effusion does not clear within 2 months, a single course of amoxicillin (Amoxil) or penicillin may be given.

Audiometry should be performed in all children with OME for longer than 3 months or, in the setting of language delay, learning problems or suspected hearing loss in a child with OME. If the effusion persists, or if a child has multiple episodes of OME or has hearing or learning difficulties as a result of OME, surgical intervention should be considered.

Initial surgical intervention for children with persistent OME should be myringotomy with placement of tympanostomy tubes. Tonsillectomy and myringotomy alone are not indicated for treatment of OME. However, adenoidectomy may have a role, particularly in children ages 4 to 8 years. Current recommendations include adenoidectomy only if repeat surgery for OME is needed. However, emerging evidence suggests adenoidectomy may decrease the need for surgical retreatment, reduce ongoing hearing loss, and be of benefit during initial surgery for older children.

Treatment

The treatment of AOM has been controversial in recent years. Because it is the most common childhood bacterial infection for which antibiotics are prescribed worldwide, debate continues about both the most effective regimen and appropriate time to treat AOM. On average, 2.8 billion dollars are spent per year on antibiotics for episodes of AOM, yet emerging evidence suggests that watchful waiting is appropriate for some children. Judicious use of antibiotic therapy remains key in the prevention of morbidity and mortality associated with otitis media but is not an appropriate therapy for every child. All children require analgesia of some type, as well as close, scheduled follow-up, but use of observation or antibiotic varies with severity of illness and age of the child. Treatment options are summarized in Table 1.

Treatment Options: Observation

For some children with AOM, observation has been shown to be an appropriate therapy that avoids the possible side effects of antibiotics, with low risk of complications developing from an untreated otitis media. Evidence suggests that 78% of AOM episodes will spontaneously resolve within the first few days of infection. In fact, for every 100 otherwise healthy at-risk children with AOM, 80 will improve within 3 days without antibiotic therapy. If the same 100 children were all treated with amoxicillin or ampicillin, 92 would improve, although 3 to 10 would develop a rash and 5 to 10 would develop diarrhea. Thus, in a typical family medicine practice, 16 children with AOM would need to be treated with antibiotics to prevent 1 child from experiencing ongoing otalgia, whereas 1 of every 24 children treated will experience harm related to therapy. Hence, the use of antibiotics is not without risk. Multiple studies have demonstrated that even in children as young as 2 months of age, many will improve without antibiotic therapy, and delaying antibiotics may prevent undesirable side effects without

exposing the child to undue risk. No studies have demonstrated a resurgence of either mastoiditis or meningitis with implementation of watchful waiting for AOM.

If observation is chosen as a management strategy for AOM, it is important to re-evaluate the child in 48 to 72 hours to ensure that they are improving and that a rescue antibiotic is prescribed if symptoms are not resolving. Delayed prescriptions are one strategy that has been effective at reducing antibiotic use, maintaining parental satisfaction, and improving healthcare efficiency.

Physicians are often concerned that parental satisfaction will decrease if watchful waiting for an episode of AOM is recommended. Interestingly, satisfaction has been tied to the receipt of an antibiotic prescription, though not necessarily the administration of antibiotics to the child. Declines in satisfaction are noted when parents are advised to return to care in 2 to 3 days if the child is not improving while undergoing watchful waiting. By offering a delayed prescription, the parent can avoid the difficulties associated with needing to be re-seen if the child fails to improve, and parental satisfaction is maintained even if the child never receives any medication. Parents should be educated that up to one third of children who initially are treated with observation will eventually need antibiotic therapy. Although this suggests up to two thirds of children can avoid unnecessary antibiotics, parents should be aware that many children will go on to need antibiotic therapy. Clearly, however, not every child is a candidate for observation therapy.

Treatment Options: Antibiotic Therapy

Antibiotic therapy may be associated with less duration of pain, less analgesic use, and less absence for both children and parents from school and work, respectively. The American Academy of Pediatrics and the American Academy of Family Physicians in a joint position statement have recommended that, when a decision is made to use antibiotics, amoxicillin (Amoxil) be given as a first-line agent at a dose of 80 to 90 mg/kg/day.[3] For penicillin-allergic children, cefdinir (Omnicef), cefpodoxime (Vantin), or cefuroxime (Ceftin) may be used. Although the cross-reactivity of cephalosporins and penicillins is likely lower than previously believed, if concern exists about treating a child with a cephalosporin, clindamycin (30–40mg/kg/day) may be used. Macrolide antibiotics may have limited efficacy. Ceftriaxone (Rocephin) may be used as a single dose for a child unable to tolerate oral medications.

Although amoxicillin continues to be the preferred first-line agent, 30% to 70% of S pneumoniae strains have become penicillin and macrolide resistant whereas 20% to 40% of H influenzae has beta-lacatamase–producing capabilities. Given the various resistance patterns of organisms, a child who fails to improve on amoxicillin should receive amoxicillin with clavulanate (Augmentin) or ceftriaxone as second-line therapy. Clindamycin (Cleocin) or tympanocentesis to identify a causative organism may also be considered.

Current evidence continues to suggest that a 10-day course is optimal for children younger than age 2 years. Less benefit to longer-duration therapy is noted in older children, and therefore

Otitis Media

513

---

[3]Exceeds dosage recommended by the manufacturer.

a shorter 5- to 7-day course is recommended for those older than 2 years.

If a child has a perforation of the tympanic membrane, treatment considerations may be slightly different. Oral antibiotics continue to be recommended if perforation is a result of the AOM episode; however, if a child has an episode of AOM with tympanostomy tubes in place, topical 0.3% ciprofloxacin/0.1% dexamethasone (Ciprodex Otic) should be added to oral amoxicillin. See Table 2 for antibiotic dosing recommendations.

Regardless of the decision to implement watchful waiting or antibiotic therapy, any child with AOM should be expected to improve within 48 to 72 hours. If improvement is not occurring, the child should be re-evaluated.

Treatment Options: Surgery

For some children, AOM will not be an isolated event. Instead, they will have recurrent infections and require multiple antibiotic courses throughout a year, prompting consideration of tympanostomy tube placement. Currently, referral for evaluation for tympanostomy tubes is recommended when a child has had three or more episodes of AOM within a 6-month period or more than four episodes within a 12-month period. Some have argued, however, that this recommendation should be considered within the context of the child's age at first presentation. A child who has the first episode of AOM before 6 months of age is likely to go on to have many more episodes. Ultimately, they will likely meet the criteria for myringotomy and thus may warrant a more aggressive approach from the outset. Conversely, a child who presents with a first episode of AOM as an older child is less likely to have recurrent episodes and can therefore be treated in a more conservative manner.

Using an age-stratified approach, children who experience a first episode of AOM prior to 6 months of age should receive tympanostomy tubes if they have two episodes in a 6- or 12-month time period or three episodes in 24 months. Similarly, children who have a first episode of AOM after 1 year of age should receive tympanostomy tubes only if they have three episodes within 6 months, five within 12 months, or seven within 24 months.

Referral may also occur if a child has a history of AOM associated with meningitis, facial nerve paralysis, coalescent mastoiditis, or brain abscess. Tympanostomy tubes are also often placed due to prolonged OME resulting in hearing loss and language delay. Myringotomy without tube placement may be considered for either diagnosis of an infection that has not responded to numerous antibiotics or for relief of severe otalgia.

AOM episodes will continue to occur despite tympanostomy tube placement. However, episodes will likely be less severe, of shorter duration, and less frequent. In addition to ongoing AOM episodes, tympanostomy tubes can be problematic if they become clogged. New studies in animal models suggest that applying colchicine[1] in the external ear may prevent this complication.

Treatment Options: Analgesia

Regardless of a decision to pursue watchful waiting or antibiotics, analgesics are an important component in the treatment of AOM. Multiple homeopathic interventions and home remedies including application of heat, ice, or mineral oil (Min-O-Ear)[1] have been used for pain control, although no studies exist to verify their effectiveness. Acetaminophen (Tylenol), ibuprofen (Motrin), narcotics, and tympanostomy have all been demonstrated to be effective at reducing pain. However, the side effects of altered mental status, gastrointestinal upset, and respiratory depression with narcotics, as well as the skill needed to perform tympanostomy, limit the usefulness of these interventions in primary care practice. Topical medications may help avoid the systemic

---

[1]Not FDA approved for this indication.

TABLE 2	Antibiotic Selection for Specific Patient Populations			
	ANTIBIOTIC OF CHOICE	DOSE (mg/kg/day)	ROUTE	DURATION OF THERAPY
AOM in child older than 2 years	Amoxicillin (Amoxil)	80–90[3]	PO	5–7 days
AOM in child younger than 2 years	Amoxicillin	80–90[3]	PO	10 days
AOM in child with allergy to penicillin	Cefdinir (Omnicef) Cefpodoxime (Vantin) Cefuroxime (Ceftin)	14 10 30	PO PO PO	10 days 5 days 10 days
AOM with inability to tolerate oral medications	Ceftriaxone (Rocephin)	50	IV/IM	1 day
AOM with amoxicillin failure	Amoxicillin with clavulanate (Augmentin) Ceftriaxone (Rocephin)	90 of amoxicillin and 6.4 of clavulanate[3] 50	PO IV/IM	10 days 3 days[3]
AOM with amoxicillin/ clavulanate failure	Ceftriaxone (Rocephin)	50	IV/IM	3 days[3]
AOM with ceftriaxone failure and tympanocentesis not available	Clindamycin (Cleocin)[1]	30–40[3]	PO	10 days
Perforated tympanic membrane	Amoxicillin	80–90[3]	PO	10 days
Tympanostomy tube in place	Amoxicillin and topical 0.3% ciprofloxacin/0.1% dexamethasone (Ciprodex Otic)	80–90 8 drops	PO Topical bid	10 days 7 days

[1]Not FDA approved for this indication.
[3]Exceeds dosage recommended by the manufacturer.
Abbreviation: AOM = acute otitis media.

effects of oral medication. Antipyrine and benzocaine are the only topical analgesics available in the United States. Topical benzocaine has been demonstrated to have minimal side effects and in patients older than 5 years of age may offer more relief than acetaminophen alone. Benzocaine is available in combination with antipyrine (Allergen Ear Drops, Auroguard Otic). Benzocaine is also available with antipyrine and acetic acid (Auralgan) but may be expensive. In other countries, antipyrine, also known as phenazone, is available in combination with procaine and is effective.

Antihistamines have often been prescribed, as have decongestants, in an attempt to reduce the fluid volume in the middle ear and hence provide relief. Unfortunately, use of antihistamines and decongestants has been shown to result in a fivefold to eightfold increase in the risk of side effects with no benefits, including no decreased time to cure, no prevention of surgery or complications, and no increased symptom resolution. Therefore antihistamines and decongestants have not been routinely recommended.

Conclusion

AOM continues to be one of the most costly and common childhood illnesses in developed nations throughout the world. Successful management of this condition requires much more than choosing amoxicillin at an appropriate dose and duration or appropriately timing a surgical referral. Vigilant attention to modifying risk factors when possible, promoting immunization, and limiting the spread of viral illnesses has been shown to prevent AOM instances. Furthermore, adherence to diagnostic criteria to attempt to accurately distinguish between AOM and OME, as well as implementing observation when appropriate, can significantly reduce antibiotic usage, thereby minimizing side effects for patients and opportunity to develop resistance in pathogens.

RED EYE

Lynn Fisher, MD; and John N. Dorsch, MD

CURRENT DIAGNOSIS

- Bacterial, viral, and allergic conjunctivitis can often be distinguished by the course of spread in the eye, the type of ocular discharge present, and associated symptoms.
- Subconjunctival hemorrhage can occur from trauma, increased intrathoracic pressure, anticoagulants, or idiopathically.
- Physicians should consider referring to an ophthalmologist patients with traumatic injury to the eye, loss of vision, extreme pain not explained by pathology, keratitis, suspected uveitis or glaucoma, chemical injury, or nonhealing corneal abrasion.

CURRENT THERAPY

- Do not use eye patches in patients with corneal abrasions.
- Do not use topical anesthetics for the eye outside a clinic or hospital setting because corneal toxicity can occur.
- Patients with corneal abrasions should be reexamined the following day.
- Patients with corneal abrasions from extended-wear contact lenses often become colonized with *Pseudomonas aeruginosa* and should be treated with appropriate antibiotics (quinolones).

In the primary care office, the most common causes of red eye are conjunctivitis, subconjunctival hemorrhage, and corneal abrasions due to a foreign body. Other common causes of red eye include blepharitis and hordeolum. Less common but serious causes of red eye include viral keratitis, uveitis, scleritis, and angle-closure glaucoma. Other usually less serious causes of red eye include episcleritis, pingueculum, and pterygium. All primary care physicians should have expertise in recognizing and treating the common causes of red eye and should recognize and refer patients with higher-stakes diagnoses (Boxes 1 and 2).

BOX 1 | Approach to the Patient with Red Eye

The following questions are often helpful in making the diagnosis in patients with red eyes.
- *Is one eye or are both eyes involved?* Infections, allergy, and systemic illness are more likely to cause bilateral eye involvement.
- *Does the patient have intense eye pain?* If yes, likely diagnoses include acute angle closure glaucoma, uveitis, scleritis, keratitis, foreign body, or corneal abrasion.
- *Does the patient have a foreign body sensation?* If so, consider corneal abrasion, trauma, dry eye, keratitis, and other corneal disorders.
- *Is there a discharge?* If it is very copious and purulent, consider gonococcal conjunctivitis. If it is discolored and purulent, consider bacterial conjunctivitis. Copious watery discharge is typical of viral conjunctivitis. Stringy, mucoid discharge is typical of allergic or chlamydial conjunctivitis.
- *Do the eyes itch?* If so, consider blepharitis or allergy in the differential.
- *Are the eyelids swollen?* Consider allergy or infection.
- *Do the eyelids have lumps?* Hordeolum and chalazion should be considered.
- *Do the eyes burn?* Consider blepharitis or dry eye.
- *Is the eye redness recurrent?* Consider herpes keratitis, uveitis, and allergic conjunctivitis.
- *Does the patient have photophobia?* Corneal problems (abrasions, keratitis) and uveitis should be considered.
- *Is there loss of vision?* Consider corneal ulcer, uveitis, and angle closure glaucoma.
- *Is the patient using ocular medications?* Prolonged use of neomycin and sulfa ophthalmic medications can cause sensitization and redness of the eyes.

BOX 2 | Red Eye

Common Causes
- Conjunctivitis: bacterial, viral, allergic
- Subconjunctival hemorrhage
- Corneal abrasion
- Blepharitis

Less Common Causes
Less Serious
- Episcleritis
- Pingueculum
- Pterygium

More Serious
- Viral keratitis
- Uveitis
- Scleritis
- Angle closure glaucoma

Physical Examination

Always check visual acuity in any patient with an eye complaint. Fluorescein strips (Flu-Glo, Fluorets), topical anesthetic drops, and cobalt blue light are used to examine the cornea for abrasions, keratitis, and ulceration. Cotton-tipped applicators are used to evert the upper eyelid and look for a foreign body.

Pupillary reaction is often affected by angle closure glaucoma and uveitis, but it is rarely affected by conjunctivitis, blepharitis, and corneal disorders. The pupil may be irregular in the patient with uveitis.

Patients with uveitis often have pain in the closed affected eye when a bright light is shined in the normal eye or with convergence of the eyes. This is due to consensual reflex of the pupils to light and accommodation.

Examine the conjunctiva by pulling the lower eyelid down with the examiner's finger. If the bulbar or palpebral conjunctivae are inflamed (i.e., hyperemic, edematous, discharge), conjunctivitis is present. Palpable preauricular nodes may be present with viral conjunctivitis and chlamydial conjunctivitis.

Conjunctivitis

Conjunctivitis is the most common cause of red eye encountered by primary care clinicians. Among the etiologies of conjunctivitis, viral conjunctivitis is the most common. Although patients with conjunctivitis might have some minor irritation of the eyes, they usually do not complain of pain in the eye or loss of vision. Ocular discharge is generally considered to be an important diagnostic feature of conjunctivitis (Table 1). Although much has been written about characterizing conjunctivitis by the nature of the discharge, one meta-analysis failed to find evidence of the diagnostic usefulness of clinical signs or symptoms in distinguishing bacterial conjunctivitis from viral conjunctivitis.

Viral Conjunctivitis

Viral conjunctivitis is often seen in epidemics and is most commonly caused by members of the Adenovirus family. Typically, viral conjunctivitis starts in one eye and spreads to the other eye a few days later. The conjunctivae appear red and swollen, with copious watery discharge (Figure 1). The natural course of viral conjunctivitis is self-limiting, lasting 10 to 14 days. Tender preauricular lymph nodes, when present, indicate the presence of viral or chlamydial conjunctivitis. Management should be directed at scrupulous hygiene. Patients must be informed that their infection is highly contagious. They should avoid close contact with other persons (e.g., towels, direct contact, swimming pools) for 2 weeks and wash hands or use hand sanitizer frequently to prevent the spread of their infection. Topical antibiotics have been prescribed to try to prevent bacterial superinfection, but there is no good evidence that they have any significant impact. Symptomatic treatment with cold compresses and topical vasoconstrictors may be helpful. Conjunctivitis has been reported in patients with coronavirus. If a patient has a red eye with burning and watery discharge that is also associated with fever, cough, shortness of breath, fatigue, or loss of taste/smell, coronavirus should be considered as a potential cause. Clinically significant conjunctivitis was observed in less than 4% of inpatients and 2% of outpatients with confirmed mild to moderate coronavirus from one 2020 study in a training and research hospital in Istanbul, Turkey. There is no specific treatment for conjunctivitis caused by coronavirus.

Bacterial Conjunctivitis

Bacterial conjunctivitis typically starts abruptly in one eye and spreads to the other eye in 1 to 2 days. Usually a purulent discharge is present that persists throughout the day. A variety of gram-positive and gram-negative organisms cause bacterial conjunctivitis, but the most common causes are *Staphylococcus aureus, Streptococcus pneumoniae,* and *Haemophilus pneumoniae.* Treatment of bacterial conjunctivitis is usually empiric, but conjunctival scraping for smears and cultures should be done in infants, immunocompromised patients, and patients

TABLE 1	Conjunctivitis		
TYPE	**COURSE**	**CHARACTERISTICS**	**DISCHARGE**
Bacterial	Starts in one eye, often spreads to other eye		Purulent
Allergic	Accompanies allergic rhinitis	Itchy eyes	Mucus
Viral	Usually bilateral	Very red eyes	Watery

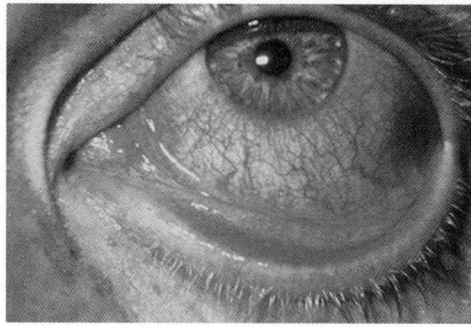

Figure 1 Viral conjunctivitis. Reproduced with permission from the University of Michigan Kellogg Eye Center, https://www.kellogg.umich.edu.

with hyperacute conjunctivitis in which *Neisseria gonorrhoeae* or *Chlamydia trachomatis* infection is suspected. Treatment of bacterial conjunctivitis (excluding gonococcal or chlamydial conjunctivitis) usually consists of a topical antibiotic used four times a day (Table 2). Topical antibiotics are usually prescribed for 5 to 7 days, and resolution of conjunctivitis is expected within that time.

Hyperacute bacterial conjunctivitis has an abrupt onset, copious purulent discharge, and rapid progression, and it is usually associated with gonococcal infection in a sexually active patient. Chemosis (edema of the conjunctivae) may be present.

Chlamydial conjunctivitis is acquired through exposure to infected secretions from the genital tract, either direct or indirect. The infection is usually unilateral (at least initially), and often there is involvement of the preauricular node on the ipsilateral side. Gonococcal and chlamydial infections are treated systemically (Box 3).

Conjunctivitis of the Newborn

Chlamydial conjunctivitis is the most common cause of infectious conjunctivitis of the newborn in the United States. Onset of conjunctivitis is 3 to 10 days after birth, but it has been reported as late as 2 months after birth. Erythromycin ointment (Ilotycin 0.5%) or tetracycline ointment[2] given shortly after delivery is effective in preventing chlamydial conjunctivitis but not systemic chlamydial infections. *Chlamydia trachomatis* infections, causing pneumonia and otitis media, can be treated either with ethylsuccinate (EryPed Drops) orally 50 mg/kg/day in four divided doses for 14 days or azithromycin (Zithromycin)[1] 20 mg/kg/day orally up to 1 g daily for 3 days. Chlamydial infections of rectal and urogenital sites can only be treated with erythromycin ethylsuccinate orally 50 mg/kg/day in four divided doses for 14 days.

Gonococcal conjunctivitis of the newborn is a hyperacute infection that occurs 2 to 4 days after birth. It can cause corneal ulceration and loss of vision. Gonococcal conjunctivitis can be prevented with silver nitrate drops[2] or erythromycin (Ilotycin) or tetracycline ointment[2] administered shortly after delivery. Silver nitrate commonly causes a self-limited chemical conjunctivitis, which can delay visual bonding of the infant to the parents in the

---

[1]Not FDA approved for this indication.
[2]Not available in the United States.

TABLE 2 Topical Antibiotics Used to Treat Bacterial Conjunctivitis

DRUG	DOSAGE
Bacitracin (Ak-Tracin, Bacticin) ointment	Apply 0.5 inch in eye q3–4 h
Ciprofloxacin (Ciloxan) 0.3% ophthalmic solution	1–2 gtt in eye q15 min × 6 h, then q30 min × 18 h, then q1 h × 1 d, then q4 h × 12 d[3]
Gatifloxacin (Zymaxid) 0.5% ophthalmic solution	1 gtt in eye q2 h up to 8 ×/d on day 1, then 1 gtt 2–4 ×/day on day 2–7
Gentamicin (Gentak, Gentasol) 0.3% ophthalmic solution or ointment	Ointment: 0.5 inch applied to eye 2–3 times per day Solution: 1–2 gtt in eye q4 h
Levofloxacin (Quixin) 0.5% ophthalmic solution	1–2 gtt in eye q2 h × 2 d while awake, then q4 h while awake × 5 d
Moxifloxacin (Vigamox) 0.5% ophthalmic solution	1 gtt in eye tid × 7 d
Neomycin/polymyxin B/ gramicidin (Neosporin) ophthalmic solution	1–2 gtt in eye q4 h × 7–10 d
Ofloxacin (Ocuflox) 0.3% ophthalmic solution	1–2 gtt in eye q2–4 h × 2 d, then 1–2 gtt in eye qid × 5 d
Polymyxin B and trimethoprim (Polytrim) ophthalmic solution	1 gtt in eye q3 h × 7–10 d
Sulfacetamide (Isopto Cetamide, Ocusulf-10, Sodium Sulamyd, Sulf-10, AK-Sulf) 10% ophthalmic solution, ointment	Ointment: 0.5-inch ribbon in eye q3–4 h and q h × 7 d Solution: 1–2 gtt in eye q2–3 h × 7–10 d
Tobramycin (AK-Tob, Tobrex) 0.3% ophthalmic solution	1–2 gtt in eye q4 h

[3]Exceeds dosage recommended by the manufacturer.

BOX 3 Treatment of Chlamydial and Gonococcal Conjunctivitis

Chlamydial Conjunctivitis
- Doxycycline (Vibramycin) 100 mg PO bid × 7 days
- Or
- Azithromycin (Zithromax) 1 g PO X 1
- Treat partners

Gonococcal Conjunctivitis
- Ceftriaxone (Rocephin 1 g IM x 1 in patients ≥150 kg, or 500 mg IM x 1 in patients <150 kg)
- Azithromycin (Zithromax) 1 g PO x 1

first few hours of life. Gonococcal conjunctivitis of the newborn is treated with Ceftriaxone (Rocephin) 25 to 50 mg/kg up to 125 mg IM/IV.

Conjunctivitis–Otitis Media Syndrome
Conjunctivitis–otitis media syndrome is a common condition in which children with otitis media also have purulent bilateral ocular discharge. It responds to treatment of otitis media; no topical treatment of conjunctivitis is required.

Methicillin-Resistant *Staphylococcus Aureus* Conjunctivitis
Increasing numbers of cases of bacterial conjunctivitis are caused by methicillin-resistant *S. aureus* (MRSA). MRSA conjunctivitis manifests as bacterial conjunctivitis resistant to conventional therapy and is treated with the same drugs used to treat MRSA

BOX 4 Patient Hygiene Measures for Conjunctivitis

- Do not wear contact lens until the conjunctivitis has cleared and resume wear with a new set. Wear and clean your contact lens as recommended by your eye doctor.
- Avoid touching the eyes and if you do, immediately wash your hands. Use a clean towel or tissue each time you wipe your face and eyes.
- Wash your hands or use hand sanitizer frequently. Always wash them before and after eating, after using bathroom, and after sneezing/coughing.
- Do not use eye makeup while an eye is infected with conjunctivitis. Replace eye makeup if the eye becomes infected and never share makeup.

in other parts of the body (Doxycycline [Vibramycin],[1] vancomycin [Vancocin], sulfamethoxazole-trimethoprim [Bactrim][1]). Cultures should be obtained when MRSA is suspected.

Allergic Conjunctivitis
Allergic conjunctivitis is an immunoglobulin E (IgE)-mediated condition characterized by bilateral eye involvement, itchy eyes, and mucoid discharge. *Seasonal* conjunctivitis is caused by exposure to common allergens (e.g., pollens, dander) and usually accompanies allergic rhinitis. *Perennial* allergic conjunctivitis is similar to seasonal allergic conjunctivitis, but the symptoms are usually less severe. Patients are usually treated with a systemic antihistamine. Ophthalmic (topical) medications include antihistamine or decongestants, mast cell inhibitors, nonsteroidal antiinflammatory drugs (NSAIDs), H_1-antagonists, and various combinations of these (Table 3). Milder cases can be treated with a decongestant-antihistamine combination for about 2 weeks. Moderate to more severe cases can require longer use of these medications or the addition of systemic antihistamines or mast cell inhibitors. Some patients require topical corticosteroids or cyclosporine (Restasis)[1] for severe allergic conjunctivitis, but these should be evaluated by an ophthalmologist because of potential complications of therapy.

Subconjunctival Hemorrhage
In subconjunctival hemorrhage, the redness of the eye is localized and sharply circumscribed, and the underlying sclera is not visible (Figure 2). Conjunctivitis is not present, and there is no discharge. There is typically no pain or visual change. Subconjunctival hemorrhage may be spontaneous, but it can also result from trauma, hypertension, bleeding disorders, or increased intrathoracic pressure (e.g., straining, coughing, retching). No treatment is necessary, but investigation may be warranted if the etiology is in question or the hemorrhage is recurrent. Referral to an ophthalmologist should be considered if the subconjunctival hemorrhage is from trauma or has not resolved within 2 to 3 weeks.

Corneal Abrasion
Corneal abrasions typically result from scratching of the corneal epithelium due to trauma, but they can also occur from extended-wear contact lenses. Patients with corneal abrasions present with pain, excessive tearing from the involved eye, photophobia, a foreign-body sensation (like having sand in the eye), and blurry vision.

Corneal abrasions are identified by staining the cornea with fluorescein and examining under cobalt blue light (Figure 3). The eye should also be examined carefully to check for foreign bodies. Topical anesthetic is administered to make the patient comfortable during the examination, but continued use can cause corneal damage.

Management of corneal abrasions consists of pain relief and prevention of infection. Pain can be relieved with topical NSAIDs

[1]Not FDA approved for this indication.

	TABLE 3	Topical Medications for Allergic Conjunctivitis		
GENERIC NAME	**BRAND NAME(S)**	**DOSING**	**MODE OF ACTION**
Azelastine 0.05% solution	Optivar	1 gtt in eye(s) bid	H_1-antagonist, mast cell inhibitor
Cromolyn 4% solution	Crolom, generic	1–2 gtt in eye(s) 4–6 times per day	Mast cell inhibitor
Emedastine 0.05% solution	Emadine	1 gtt in eye(s) qid	H_1-antagonist
Epinastine 0.05% solution	Elestat	1 gtt in eye(s) bid	H_1- and H_2-antagonist, mast cell inhibitor
Ketorolac 0.5% solution	Acular	1 gtt in eye(s) qid up to 1 week	NSAID
Diclofenac 0.1% solution[1]	Voltaren ophthalmic	1 gtt in eye(s) qid × 2 weeks	NSAID
Lodoxamide 0.1% solution	Alomide	1–2 gtt in eye(s) qid up to 3 months	Mast cell inhibitor
Loteprednol 0.2% susp.	Alrex	1 gtt in eye(s) qd	Corticosteroid
Naphazoline/pheniramine (solution)	• Naphcon-A (OTC) • Opcon-A (OTC) • Visine-A (OTC)	1–2 gtt in eye(s) qd-qid prn	Antihistamine, decongestant
Nedrocomil 2% solution	Alocril	1–2 gtt in eye(s) bid	H_1-antagonist, mast cell inhibitor
Olopatadine 0.1% solution	Patanol	1 gtt in eye(s) bid	H_1-antagonist, mast cell inhibitor
Olopatadine 0.2% solution	Pataday	1 gtt in eye(s) qd	Mast cell inhibitor

[1]Not FDA approved for this indication.
NSAID, Nonsteroidal antiinflammatory drug.

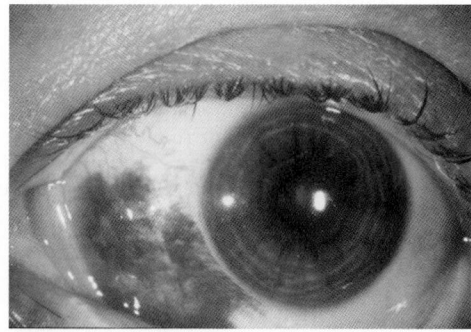

Figure 2 Subconjunctival hemorrhage. Reprinted with permission from American Academy of Ophthalmology: Managing the red eye. eye care skills for the primary care physician series. San Francisco: American Academy of Ophthalmology, 2001.

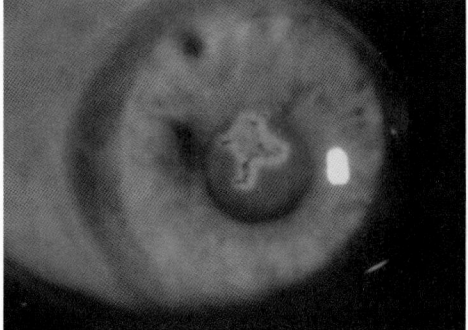

Figure 3 Corneal abrasion with fluorescein stain with cobalt blue light. Reprinted with permission from American Academy of Ophthalmology: Managing the red eye. eye care skills for the primary care physician series. San Francisco: American Academy of Ophthalmology, 2001.

such as ketorolac (Acular)[1] and diclofenac (Voltaren),[1] oral over-the-counter analgesics, and occasionally oral narcotics. Topical antibiotics are usually prescribed to prevent infection. Antibiotic ointments are lubricating and soothing to the eye, making them

a good option for traumatic corneal abrasions. Topical ophthalmic antibiotic ointments commonly used are bacitracin (Bacticin), erythromycin (Ilotycin), and gentamicin (Gentak).

In patients who have corneal abrasions from contact lens overwear, eyes are commonly colonized with *Pseudomonas aeruginosa.* These patients should be treated with topical antibiotics such as ciprofloxacin (Ciloxan) or ofloxacin (Ocuflux) solutions.

Patching of the eye, though a common practice of the past, has not shown evidence of benefit in recent studies. It was found that eye patching can actually cause harm, so this practice is no longer recommended.

Infrequently, patients have traumatic uveitis accompanying corneal abrasion. Traumatic uveitis usually causes significantly more pain than a corneal abrasion, and, if uveitis is suspected, the clinician should consider referral to an ophthalmologist.

Patients with corneal abrasions should be reexamined in 24 hours. Corneal abrasions typically should be healed or greatly improved in 24 hours. If the abrasion is not completely healed after 24 hours, the patient should be examined again in 2 or 3 days. Referral should be considered if any worsening occurs or if the abrasion does not heal within 5 days. Corneal abrasions can be prevented by using protective eyewear.

Other Causes of Red Eye
Other causes of red eye are somewhat less common.

Blepharitis
Blepharitides are inflammatory conditions of the eyelid caused by infection or obstruction of eyelid glands (Table 4). Blepharitis may be accompanied by conjunctivitis. Staphylococcal blepharitis arises from the accessory glands to the eyelashes and causes discharge from the eyelid, often associated with erythema, induration, loss of eyelashes, and crusting of the eyelid (Figure 4). This is treated with hot, moist packs to the eyes, baby shampoo scrubs (3 oz. water and 3 drops baby shampoo used on a washcloth bid), and erythromycin ointment (Ilotycin) at bedtime. Seborrheic blepharitis, a more chronic form of blepharitis, arises from the meibomian glands and causes scaling of the eyelids (Figure 5). Seborrheic blepharitis is often associated with skin disorders such as rosacea, eczema, and seborrheic dermatitis. This is treated with hot, moist packs and baby shampoo scrubs. Resistant cases are treated with oral tetracycline (Sumycin) (or one of its derivatives).

[1]Not FDA approved for this indication.

TABLE 4 Blepharitis

TYPE	SITE OF ORIGIN	CLINICAL CHARACTERISTICS	TREATMENT
Staphylococcal	Accessory glands of eyelids	Erythema and induration of eyelid; crusting; discharge; loss of eyelashes	• Warm compresses • Baby shampoo scrubs • Erythromycin ointment (Ilotycin)
Seborrheic	Meibomian glands	More chronic, scaling	1. Warm compresses 2. Baby shampoo scrubs 3. Oral tetracycline for resistant cases

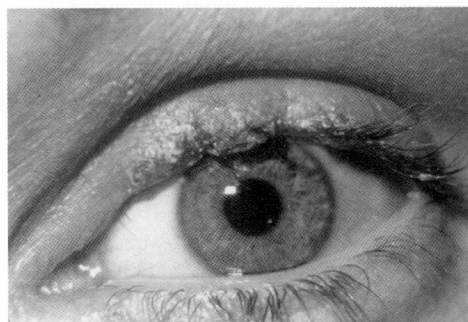

Figure 4 Staphylococcal blepharitis. Reprinted with permission from American Academy of Ophthalmology: Managing the red eye. eye care skills for the primary care physician series. San Francisco: American Academy of Ophthalmology, 2001.

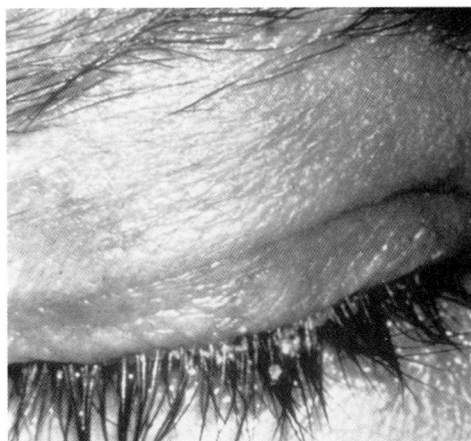

Figure 5 Seborrheic blepharitis. Reprinted with permission from American Academy of Ophthalmology: Managing the red eye. eye care skills for the primary care physician series. San Francisco: American Academy of Ophthalmology, 2001.

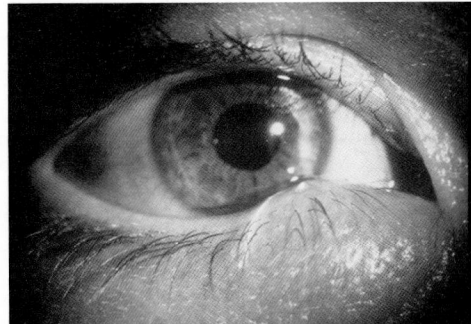

Figure 6 Hordeolum. Reprinted with permission from American Academy of Ophthalmology: Managing the red eye. eye care skills for the primary care physician series. San Francisco: American Academy of Ophthalmology, 2001.

Hordeolum (Stye)

A hordeolum is an acute, painful mass of the eyelid that is caused by inflammation of the glands (Figure 6). It does not usually cause the eye to become red as well. Warm compresses to the eyelid four times a day for 3 to 5 minutes typically causes resolution within 1 week. Because they arise from the same glands, hordeola and blepharitis commonly occur together.

Episcleritis

Episcleritis is a self-limited inflammation of the episcleral vessels and is believed to be autoimmune. It has a rapid onset and usually minimal discomfort. Redness is most often confined to a sector of the eye. Episcleritis usually resolves in 7 to 10 days. Recurrence is not uncommon. Oral NSAID drugs may be prescribed, but treatment is usually not necessary.

Scleritis

Scleritis is, fortunately, much less common than episcleritis. Patients with scleritis experience intense inflammation and deep eye pain. Scleritis is commonly associated with rheumatoid arthritis and inflammatory bowel disease. The patient should be promptly referred to an ophthalmologist if scleritis is suspected.

Acute Angle Closure Glaucoma

Acute angle closure glaucoma is characterized by acute ocular pain and is often accompanied by vomiting, blurred vision, acute photophobia, pupils unreactive to light, and circumcorneal redness (ciliary flush). Treatment of glaucoma with pilocarpine (Isopto Carpine), topical timolol (Timoptic), and acetazolamide (Diamox) should be started, and the patient should be given an urgent referral to an ophthalmologist.

Anterior Uveitis

Uveitis is the inflammation of the iris and ciliary muscle, often associated with autoimmune disease. Trauma can also cause uveitis. Signs of uveitis include ocular pain, ciliary flush, and occasionally irregularity of the pupil. Prompt referral should be arranged for a patient in whom uveitis is suspected.

In general, referral to an ophthalmologist should be considered for the following:
• Traumatic injury to the eye
• Loss of vision
• Extreme eye pain not explained by pathology
• Keratitis
• Suspected uveitis or glaucoma
• Chemical injury (especially alkali)
• Corneal abrasion not healing

References

Ackay B, Kardes E, Kiray G, et al: Evaluation of ocular symptoms in COVID-19 subjects in inpatient and outpatient settings, *International Ophthalmology* 41:1541–1548, 2021.

American Optometric Association: *Optometric clinical practice guideline: Care of the patient with anterior uveitis*, June 23, 1994. Revised March 1999. PDF available at www.aoa.org/documents/CPG-7.pdf. June 23, 1994 [accessed July 10, 2015].

Arbour JD, Brunette I, Boisjoly HM, et al: Should we patch corneal abrasions? *Arch Ophthalmol* 115(3):313–317, 1997.

Au YK, Henkind P: Pain elicited by consensual pupillary reflex: a diagnostic test for acute iritis, *Lancet* 2:1254–1255, 1981.

Avdic E, Cosgrove SE: Management and control strategies for community-associated methicillin-resistant *Staphylococcus aureus*, *Expert Opin Pharmacother* 9(9):1463–1479, 2008.

Boder F, Marchant C, et al: Bacterial etiology of conjunctivitis-otitis media syndrome, *Pediatrics* 76:26–28, 1985.

Bradford CA: *Basic Ophthalmology*San Francisco, ed 8, 2004, American Academy of Ophthalmology.

Centers for Disease Control and Prevention. Zika Virus. Symptoms, diagnosis, and treatment. Available at www.cdc.gov/zika/symptoms. Accessed Feb. 3, 2016.

Centers for Disease Control and Prevention: *Sexually Transmitted Diseases Treatment Guidelines*, 2015. Available at www.cdc.gov/std/tg2015/default.htm. Accessed May 25, 2021.

De Toledo AR, Chandler JW: Conjunctivitis of the newborn, *Infect Dis Clin North Am* 6(4):807–813, 1992.

Frith P, Gray R, MacLennan S, et al: *The Eye in Clinical Practice*, Oxford, 1994, Blackwell Scientific.

Jackson WB: Blepharitis: Current strategies for diagnosis and treatment, *Can J Ophthalmol* 43(2):170–179, 2008.

Khan J, Mack H: Management of conjunctivitis and other causes of red eye during the COVID-19 Pandemic, *AJGP* 49(10):656–661, 2020.

Kimberlin D, Brady M, Jackson M: *Red Book. Report of the Committee on Infectious Diseases*, ed 31, AAP Committee on Infectious Diseases, 2018.

Liebowitz HM: The red eye, *N Engl J Med* 343(5):345–351, 2000.

Patterson J, Fetzer D, Krall J, et al: Eye patch treatment for the pain of corneal abrasion, *South Med J* 89(2):227–229, 1996.

Prochazka AV: Diagnosis and treatment of red eye, *Primary Care Case Reviews* 4:23–31, 2001.

Rietveld RP, van Weert H, Riet G, Bindels P: Diagnostic impact of signs and symptoms in acute infectious conjunctivitis: systematic literature search, *BMJ* 327(4):789, 2003.

Tarabishy A: Jeng B: Bacterial conjunctivitis: A review for internists, *Cleve Clin J Med* 75(7):507–512, 2008.

Talbot EM: A simple test to diagnose iritis, *BMJ* 295:812–813, 1987.

Trobe JD: *The Physician's Guide to Eye Care*, ed 2, San Francisco, 2001, Foundation of the American Academy of Ophthalmology.

Wilson SA, Last A: Management of corneal abrasion, *Am Fam Physician* 70:123–130, 2004.

Wong AH, Barg SS, Leung AK: Seasonal and perennial allergic conjunctivitis, *Recent Pat Inflamm Allergy Drug Disc* 3(2):118–127, 2009.

RHINOSINUSITIS

Method of
Ann M. Aring, MD

CURRENT DIAGNOSIS

- Because inflammation of the sinuses rarely occurs without concurrent inflammation of the nasal mucosa, rhinosinusitis is a more accurate term for what is commonly called sinusitis.
- Most cases of sinusitis are caused by viral infections associated with the common cold. Viral rhinosinusitis improves in 7 to 10 days.
- Four signs and symptoms with a high likelihood ratio for acute bacterial sinusitis are double sickening, purulent rhinorrhea, erythrocyte sedimentation rate (ESR) >10mm, and purulent secretion in the nasal cavity. A combination of at least three of these four symptoms and signs has a specificity of 0.81 and sensitivity of 0.66 for acute bacterial rhinosinusitis.
- Acute rhinosinusitis lasts up to 4 weeks, subacute rhinosinusitis lasts from 4 to 12 weeks, and chronic rhinosinusitis lasts 12 weeks or longer. Recurrent acute rhinosinusitis is defined as four or more episodes per year with complete resolution between episodes.
- Radiographic imaging in a patient with acute rhinosinusitis is not recommended unless a complication or an alternative diagnosis is suspected. Computed tomography of the sinuses without contrast media is the imaging method of choice.

CURRENT THERAPY

- Mild rhinosinusitis symptoms of less than 7 days' duration can be managed with supportive care including analgesics, saline nasal irrigation, and intranasal corticosteroids.
- Antibiotic therapy is recommended for patients with sinusitis symptoms that do not improve within 7 to 10 days or that worsen at any time.
- First-line antibiotics include amoxicillin with or without clavulanate.
- Macrolides and trimethoprim sulfamethoxazole (Bactrim) are not recommended for empiric therapy owing to high rates of resistance among *Streptococcus pneumoniae* and *Haemophilus influenzae*.
- For adults allergic to penicillin, doxycycline may be used as an alternative regimen for initial empiric therapy for bacterial rhinosinusitis. According to a recent US Food and Drug Administration (FDA) safety alert, fluoroquinolones such as levofloxacin (Levaquin) and moxifloxacin (Avelox) should be reserved for patients who do not have other treatment options.
- In adults with confirmed acute rhinosinusitis, more than 70% will clinically improve after 2 weeks with or without antibiotic therapy.
- Antibiotic use increases the absolute cure rate by 5% compared with placebo at 7 to 15 days.

Epidemiology of Acute Rhinosinusitis and Predisposing Factors

Each year in the United States, rhinosinusitis affects one in seven adults and is diagnosed in 31 million patients. Rhinosinusitis is the fifth most common diagnosis for which antibiotics are prescribed. Rhinosinusitis has a higher frequency in the winter months and lower frequency in the summer and autumn months.

Predisposing Factors

Predisposing factors for acute rhinosinusitis include viral upper respiratory infections and allergic rhinitis. Anatomic malformations including polyps, deviated nasal septum, foreign bodies, and tumors can also predispose to acute rhinosinusitis.

Pathogenesis and Etiology of Rhinosinusitis

Most cases of acute rhinosinusitis are caused by viral infections associated with the common cold. The most common viruses in acute viral rhinosinusitis are rhinovirus, adenovirus, influenza virus, and parainfluenza virus. Mucosal edema occurs with the viral infection with subsequent obstruction of the sinus ostia. In addition, viral and bacterial infections impair the cilia, which help transport the mucus. The ostia obstruction and slowed mucus transport cause stagnation of secretions and lowered oxygen tension within the sinuses. This environment is an excellent culture medium for both viruses and bacteria and the infectious particles grow rapidly. The body responds with an inflammatory reaction. Polymorphonuclear leukocytes are mobilized, which results in pus formation. The most common bacteria found in acute community-acquired bacterial rhinosinusitis are *S pneumoniae*, *H influenzae*, *Staphylococcus aureus*, and *Moraxella catarrhalis*. Acute adult rhinosinusitis most commonly involves the maxillary and ethmoid sinuses. More than one of the paranasal sinuses can be affected.

Diagnosis of Acute Rhinosinusitis

Diagnosis of acute bacterial rhinosinusitis requires that symptoms persist for longer than 10 days or worsen after 5 to 7 days. Four signs and symptoms with a high likelihood ratio for acute bacterial sinusitis are double sickening, purulent rhinorrhea, ESR

TABLE 1	Signs and Symptoms of Acute Bacterial Rhinosinusitis			
SIGN/SYMPTOM	SENSITIVITY (%)	SPECIFICITY (%)	LR +	ODDS RATIO
Symptoms after upper respiratory tract infection	99	8	1.1	2.1
Facial pain on bending forward	90	22	1.2	0.9
Nasal congestion	90	14	1.0	1.1
Purulent rhinorrhea	89	42	1.5	1.6
Bilateral facial pain, pressure, or fullness	78	32	1.2	1.4
Double sickening	72	65	2.1	*
Previous sinusitis	57	38	0.9	0.4
Upper teeth pain	50	50	1.0	1.2
Unilateral facial pain, pressure, or fullness	46	73	1.7	1.9

Abbreviation: LR = Likelihood ratio.
*No data given in reference.

TABLE 2	Indications for Subspecialist Referral for Acute Bacterial Rhinosinusitis

Anatomic defects causing obstruction

Complications such as orbital involvement, altered mental status, meningitis, cavernous sinus thrombosis, intracranial abscess, Pott's puffy tumor (osteomyelitis of front bone)

Evaluation of immunotherapy for allergic rhinitis

Frequent recurrences (3–4 episodes per year)

Fungal sinusitis, granulomatous disease, or possible neoplasm

Immunocompromised host

Nosocomial infection

Severe infection with persistent fever >102°F or 39°C

Treatment failure after extended antibiotic courses

Unusual or resistant bacteria

From Aring AM, Chan MM. Current concepts in adult acute rhinosinusitis. Am Fam Physician 2016;94[2]:97–105.

>10mm, and purulent secretion in the nasal cavity. A combination of at least three of these four symptoms and signs has a specificity of 0.81 and sensitivity of 0.66 for acute bacterial rhinosinusitis. Table 1 lists the sensitivity, specificity, likelihood ratio, and odds ratio of criteria used to diagnose acute rhinosinusitis. If resistant pathogens are suspected or if the patient's immune system is compromised, bacterial culture of the secretions may be used for diagnosis and to direct therapy.

Imaging
For uncomplicated acute rhinosinusitis, radiographic imaging is not recommended. Plain sinus radiography shows air–fluid levels in patients with both viral and bacterial rhinosinusitis. Sinus computed tomography should not be used for routine evaluation of acute bacterial rhinosinusitis. However, sinus computed tomography without contrast media can be used to identify suspected complications and define anatomic abnormalities.

Differential Diagnosis
The signs and symptoms of acute bacterial rhinosinusitis and prolonged viral upper respiratory infection are similar, which can lead to overdiagnosis of acute bacterial rhinosinusitis. Other conditions that mimic bacterial rhinosinusitis are migraine headache, tension headache, trigeminal neuralgia, and temporomandibular joint disorders.

Treatment of Acute Rhinosinusitis
Symptomatic Treatment
Mild rhinosinusitis symptoms less than 7 days in duration can be managed with supportive care including analgesics, saline nasal irrigation, and intranasal corticosteroids. There are no randomized controlled trials that evaluate the effectiveness of decongestants in patients with sinusitis. Nasal saline is used to soften viscous secretions and improve mucociliary clearance. The mechanical cleansing of the nasal cavity with saline has been shown to benefit patients with rhinosinusitis. Most studies of intranasal corticosteroids are industry sponsored. A 2013 Cochrane review found that patients receiving intranasal corticosteroids were more likely to

experience symptom improvement after 15 to 21 days compared with those receiving placebo (73% vs. 66.4%; $p<.05$; number needed to treat [NNT]=15). Antihistamines should not be used for symptomatic relief of acute rhinosinusitis, except in patients with a history of allergic rhinitis.

Antibiotic Treatment
Antibiotic therapy is recommended for patients with sinusitis symptoms that do not improve within 7 to 10 days or that worsen at any time. Amoxicillin with or without clavulanate is recommended as the first-line antibiotic in adults with acute bacterial rhinosinusitis. "High-dose" amoxicillin-clavulanate (Augmentin XR) is recommended for patients with high risk of *S pneumoniae* resistance, recent antibiotic use, or treatment failure. Macrolides and trimethoprim sulfamethoxazole are not recommended for empiric therapy owing to high rates of resistance among *S pneumoniae* and *H influenzae*. Fluoroquinolones are not recommended as first-line antibiotics because they do not demonstrate benefit over beta-lactam antibiotics and are associated with a variety of adverse effects. According to a recent FDA safety alert, fluoroquinolones should be reserved for patients who do not have other treatment options.

Complications and Referral
Complications of acute bacterial rhinosinusitis are estimated to occur in 1 in 1000 cases. Patients with acute bacterial rhinosinusitis who present with visual symptoms (diplopia, decreased visual acuity, disconjugate gaze, difficulty opening the eye), severe headache, somnolence, or high fever should be evaluated with emergency computed tomography with contrast. Sinonasal cancers are uncommon in the United States, with an annual incidence of less than 1 in 100,000 patients. However, cancer should be included in the differential diagnosis. Referral to an otolaryngologist is needed if symptoms persist or progress after maximal medical therapy when computed tomography shows evidence of sinus disease. Table 2 summarizes indications for subspecialist referral in a patient with acute bacterial rhinosinusitis.

References
Aring AM, Chan MM: Current concepts in adult acute rhinosinusitis, *Am Fam Physician* 94(2):97–105, 2016.
Chow AW, Benninger MS, Brook I, et al: IDSA clinical practice guideline for acute bacterial rhinosinusitis in children and adults, *Clin Infect Dis* 54(8):e72–112, 2012. Epub 2012 Mar 20.

Cornelius RS, Martin J: Wippold, FJ 2nd, et al. ACR appropriateness criteria sinonasal disease, *J Am Coll Radiol* 10(4):241–246, 2013.

DeSutter AI, Lemiengre M, Campbell H: Antihistamines for the common cold, *Cochrane Database Syst Rev* CD009345, 2015.

Hayward G, Heneghan C, Perera R, Thompson M: Intranasal corticosteroids in management of acute sinusitis: A systematic review and meta-analysis, *Ann Fam Med* 10:241–249, 2012, https://doi.org/10.1370/afm.1338.

King D, Mitchell B, Williams CP, Spurling GKP: Saline nasal irrigation for acute upper respiratory tract infections, *Cochrane Database of Syst Rev* 4, 2015, https://doi.org/10.1002/14651858.CD006821.pub3.

Lemiengre MB, van Driel ML, Merenstein D, et al: Antibiotics for acute rhinosinusitis in adults, *Cochrane Database Syst Rev* 9:CD006089, 2018.

Lindbaek M, Hjortdahl P, Johnsen U: Use of symptoms, signs, and blood tests to diagnose acute sinus infections in primary care: Comparison with computer tomography, *Fam Med* 23:183–188, 1996.

Rosenfeld RM, Piccirillo JF, Chadrasekhar SS, et al: Clinical practice guideline (update): Adult sinusitis, *Otolaryngol Head Neck Surg* 152(2S):S1–39, 2015.

U.S. Food and Drug Administration. FDA Drug Safety Communication: FDA updates warnings for oral and injectable fluoroquinolone antibiotics due to disabling side effects. Available at http://www.fda.gov/Drugs/DrugSafety/ucm511530.htm [accessed January 28, 2017].

Zalmanovici Trestioreanu A, Yaphe J: Intranasal steroids for acute sinusitis, *Cochrane Database Syst Rev* 12, 2013.

TEMPOROMANDIBULAR DISORDERS

Method of
Jeffrey P. Okeson, DMD

Temporomandibular disorder (TMD) is a collective term that includes a number of clinical complaints involving the muscles of mastication, the temporomandibular joints (TMJs) and associated orofacial structures. Other commonly used terms are Costen's syndrome, TMJ dysfunction, and craniomandibular disorders. TMDs are a major cause of nondental pain in the orofacial region and are considered a subclassification of musculoskeletal disorders. In many TMD patients the most common complaint is not with the TMJs but rather the muscles of mastication. Therefore the terms *TMJ dysfunction* or *TMJ disorder* are actually inappropriate for many of these complaints. It is for this reason that the American Dental Association adopted the term *temporomandibular disorder*.

Signs and symptoms associated with TMDs are a common source of pain complaints in the head and orofacial structures. These complaints can be associated with general joint problems and somatization. Approximately 50% of patients suffering with TMDs do not first consult with a dentist but seek advice for the problem from a physician. The family physician should be able to appropriately diagnose many TMDs. In many instances the physician can provide valuable information and simple therapies that will reduce the patient's TMD symptoms. In other instances, it is appropriate to refer the patient to a dentist for additional evaluation and treatment.

Epidemiology

Cross-sectional population-based studies reveal that 40% to 75% of adult populations have at least one sign of TMJ dysfunction (e.g., jaw movement abnormalities, joint noise, tenderness on palpation), and approximately 33% have at least one symptom (e.g., face pain, joint pain). Many of these signs and symptoms are not troublesome for the patient, and only 3% to 7% of the population seeks any advice or care. Although in the general population women seem to have only a slightly greater incidence of TMD symptoms, women seek care for TMD more often than men at a ratio ranging from 3:1 to 9:1. For many patients TMDs are self-limiting or are associated with symptoms that fluctuate over time without evidence of progression. Even though many of these disorders are self-limiting, the health care provider can provide conservative therapies that will minimize the patient's painful experience.

Signs and Symptoms

The primary signs and symptoms associated with TMD originate from the masticatory structures and are associated with jaw function (Box 1). Pain during opening of the mouth or during chewing is common. Some persons even report difficulty speaking or singing. Patients often report pain in the preauricular areas, face, or temples. TMJ sounds are often described as clicking, popping, grating, or crepitus and can produce locking of the jaw during opening or closing. Patients commonly report painful jaw muscles, and, on occasion, they even report a sudden change in their bite coincident with the onset of the painful condition.

It is important to appreciate that pain associated with most TMDs is increased with jaw function. Because this is a condition of the musculoskeletal structures, function of these structures generally increases the pain. When a patient's pain complaint is not influenced by jaw function, other sources of orofacial pain should be suspected.

The spectrum of TMD often includes commonly associated complaints such as headache, neckache, or earache. These associated complaints are often referred pains and must be differentiated from primary pains. As a general rule, referred pains associated with TMDs are increased with any activity that provokes the TMD pain. Therefore, if the patient reports that the headache is aggravated by jaw function, it could very well represent a secondary pain related to the TMD. Likewise, if the secondary symptom is unaffected by jaw use, one should question its relationship to the TMD and suspect two separate pain conditions. Pain or dysfunction due to non-musculoskeletal causes such as otolaryngologic, neurologic, vascular, neoplastic, or infectious disease in the orofacial region is not considered a primary TMD even though musculoskeletal pain may be present. However, TMDs often coexist with other craniofacial and orofacial pain disorders.

Anatomy and Pathophysiology

The TMJ is formed by the mandibular condyle fitting into the mandibular fossa of the temporal bone. The movement of this joint is quite complex as it allows hinging movement in one plane and at the same time allows gliding movements in another plane.

Separating these two bones from direct articulation is the articular disk. The articular disk is composed of dense fibrous connective tissue devoid of any blood vessels or nerve fibers. The articular disk is attached posteriorly to a region of loose connective tissue that is highly vascularized and well innervated, known as the retrodiscal tissue. The anterior region of the disk is attached to the superior lateral pterygoid muscle.

The movement of the mandible is accomplished by four pairs of muscles called the muscles of mastication: the masseter, temporalis, medial pterygoid, and lateral pterygoid. Although not considered to be muscles of mastication, the digastric muscles also play an important role in mandibular function. The masseter, temporalis, and medial pterygoid muscles elevate the mandible and therefore provide the major forces used for chewing and other

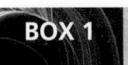

| **BOX 1** | Common Primary and Secondary Symptoms Associated with Temporomandibular Disorders |

Primary Symptoms
Facial muscle pain
Preauricular (TMJ) pain
TMJ sounds: jaw clicking, popping, catching, locking
Limited mouth opening
Increased pain associated with chewing

Secondary Symptoms
Earache
Headache
Neckache

Abbreviation: TMJ = temporomandibular joint.

jaw functions. The inferior lateral pterygoid muscles provide protrusive movement of the mandible, and the digastric muscles serve to depress the mandible (open the mouth).

When discussing the pathophysiology of TMD, one needs to consider two main categories: joint pathophysiology and muscle pathophysiology. Because etiologic considerations and treatment strategies are different for these conditions, they are presented separately.

Pathophysiology of Intracapsular TMJ Pain Disorders

Several common arthritic conditions such as rheumatoid arthritis, traumatic arthritis, hyperuricemia, and psoriatic arthritis can affect the TMJ. These conditions, however, are not nearly as common as local osteoarthritis. As with most other joints, osteoarthritis results from overloading the articular surface of the joint, thus breaking down the dense fibrocartilage articular surface and ultimately affecting the subarticular bone. In the TMJ, this overloading commonly occurs as a result of an alteration in the morphology and position of the articular disc. In the healthy TMJ, the disc maintains its position on the condyle during movement because of its morphology (i.e., the thicker anterior and posterior borders) and interarticular pressure maintained by the elevator muscles. If, however, the morphology of the disc is altered and the discal ligaments become elongated, the disk can be displaced from its normal position between the condyle and fossa. If the disc is displaced, normal opening and closing of the mouth can result in an unusual translatory movement between the condyle and the disc, which is felt as a click or pop. Disc displacements that result in joint sounds might or might not be painful. When pain is present it is believed to be related to either loading forces applied to the highly vascularized retrodiscal tissues or a general inflammatory response of the surrounding soft tissues (capsulitis or synovitis).

Pathophysiology of Masticatory Muscle Pain Disorders

The muscles of mastication are a very common source of TMD pain. Understanding the pathophysiology of muscle pain, however, is very complex and still not well understood. The simple explanation of muscle spasm does not account for most TMD muscle pain complaints. It appears that a better explanation would include a central nervous system effect on the muscle that results in an increase in peripheral nociceptive activity originating from the muscle tissue itself. This explanation more accurately accounts for the high levels of emotional stress that are commonly associated with TMD muscle pain complaints. In other words, an increase in emotional stress activates the autonomic nervous system, which in turn seems to be associated with changes in muscle nociception.

These masticatory muscle pain conditions are further complicated when one considers the unique masticatory muscle activity known as bruxism. Bruxism is the subconscious, often rhythmic, grinding or gnashing of the teeth. This type of muscle activity is considered to be parafunctional and can also occur as a simple static loading of the teeth known as clenching. This activity commonly occurs while sleeping but can also be present during the day. These parafunctional activities alone can represent a significant source of masticatory muscle pain, and certainly bruxism in the presence of central nervous system–induced muscle pain can further accentuate the patient's muscle pain complaints.

Etiology

Because TMD represents a group of disorders, any of several etiologies may be associated. Problems arising from intracapsular conditions (clicking, popping, catching, locking) may be associated with various types of trauma. Gross trauma, such as a blow to the chin, can immediately alter ligamentous structures of the joint, leading to joint sounds. Trauma can also be associated with a subtler injury such as stretching, twisting or compressing forces during eating, yawning, yelling, or prolonged mouth opening.

When the patient's chief complaint is muscle pain, etiologic factors other than trauma should be considered. Masticatory muscle

pain disorders have etiologic considerations similar to other muscle pain disorders of the neck and back. Emotional stress seems to play a significant role for many patients. This can explain why patients often report that their painful symptoms fluctuate greatly over time.

Although most TMD patients do not have a major psychiatric disorder, psychological factors can certainly enhance the pain condition. The clinician needs to consider such factors as anxiety, depression, secondary gain, somatization, and hypochondriasis. Psychosocial factors can predispose certain people to TMD and can also perpetuate TMD once symptoms have become established. A careful consideration of psychosocial factors is therefore important in the evaluation and treatment of every TMD patient.

TMDs have a few unique etiologic factors that differentiate them from other musculoskeletal disorders. One such factor is the occlusal relationship of the teeth. Traditionally it was thought that malocclusion was the primary etiologic factor responsible for TMD. Recent investigations, however, do not support this concept. Still, in certain instances occlusal instability of the teeth can contribute to a TMD. This may be true in patients with or without teeth. Poorly fitting dental prostheses can also contribute to occlusal instability. The occlusal condition should especially be suspected if the pain problem began with a change in the patient's occlusion (e.g., following a dental appointment).

History and Examination

All patients reporting pain in the orofacial structures should be screened for TMD. This can be accomplished with a brief history and physical examination. The screening questions and examination are performed to rule in or out the possibility of a TMD. If a positive response is found, a more extensive history and examination is indicated. Box 2 lists questions that should be asked during a screening assessment for TMD. Any positive response should be followed by additional clarifying questions.

Patients experiencing orofacial pain should also be briefly examined for any clinical signs associated with TMD. The clinician can easily palpate a few sites to assess tenderness or pain, as well as assess for jaw mobility. The masseter muscles can be palpated bilaterally while asking the patient to report any pain or tenderness. The same assessment should be made for the

---

BOX 2	Recommended Screening Questionnaire for Temporomandibular Disorder

All patients reporting pain in the orofacial region should be screened for TMD with a questionnaire that includes these questions. The decision to complete a comprehensive history and clinical examination depends on the number of positive responses and the apparent seriousness of the problem for the patient. A positive response to any question may be sufficient to warrant a comprehensive examination if it is of concern to the patient or viewed as clinically significant by the physician.

1. Do you have difficulty, pain, or both when opening your mouth, for instance when yawning?
2. Does your jaw get stuck or locked or go out?
3. Do you have difficulty, pain, or both when chewing, talking, or using your jaws?
4. Are you aware of noises in the jaw joints?
5. Do your jaws regularly feel stiff, tight, or tired?
6. Do you have pain in or about the ears, temples, or cheeks?
7. Do you have frequent headaches, neckaches, or toothaches?
8. Have you had a recent injury to your head, neck, or jaw?
9. Have you been aware of any recent changes in your bite?
10. Have you been previously treated for unexplained facial pain or a jaw joint problem?

Abbreviation: TMD = temporomandibular disorder.

temporal regions, as well as the preauricular (TMJ) areas. While the examiner's hands are over the preauricular areas, the patient should repeatedly open and close the mouth. The presence of joint sounds should be noted along with whether these sounds are associated with joint pain.

A simple measurement of mouth opening should be made. This can be accomplished by placing a millimeter ruler on the lower anterior teeth and asking the patient to open as wide as possible. The distance should be measured between the maxillary and mandibular anterior teeth. It is generally accepted that less than 40 mm is a restricted mouth opening.

It is also helpful to inspect the teeth for significant wear, mobility, or decay that may be related to the pain condition. The clinician should examine the buccal mucosa for ridging and the lateral aspect of the tongue for scalloping. These are often signs of clenching and bruxism. A general inspection for symmetry and alignment of the face, jaws, and dental arches may also be helpful. A summary of this screening examination is shown in Box 3.

Treatment

Most recent studies suggest that TMDs are generally self-limiting, and symptoms often fluctuate over time. Understanding this natural course does not mean these conditions should be ignored. TMD can be a very painful condition leading to a significant decrease in the patient's quality of life. Understanding the natural course of TMD does suggest, however, that therapy might not need to be very aggressive. In general, initial therapy should begin very conservatively and only escalate when therapy fails to relieve the symptoms.

When the physician identifies a patient with a TMD, he or she has two options. The physician can elect to treat the patient or refer the patient to a dentist who specializes in TMD for further evaluation and treatment. The decision to refer the patient should be based on whether the patient needs any unique care provided only in a dental office. The following are some indications for referral to a dentist:

- History of trauma to the face related to the onset of the pain condition
- The presence of significant TMJ sounds during function
- A feeling of jaw catching or locking during mouth opening
- The report of a sudden change in the occlusal contacts of the teeth
- The presence of significant occlusal instability
- Significant findings related to the teeth (e.g., tooth mobility, tooth sensitivity, tooth decay, tooth wear)
- Significant pain in the jaws or masticatory muscles upon awakening

- The presence of an orofacial pain condition that is aggravated by jaw function and has been present for more than several months

The specific therapy for a TMD varies according to the precise type of disorder identified. In other words, masticatory muscle pain is managed somewhat differently than intracapsular pain. Generally, however, the initial therapy for any type of TMD should be directed toward the relief of pain and the improvement of function. This initial conservative therapy can be divided into three general types: patient education, pharmacologic therapy, and physical therapy.

Patient Education

It is very important that patients have an appreciation for the factors that may be associated with their disorder, as well as the natural course of the disorder. Patients should be reassured and if necessary, convinced by appropriate tests, that they are not suffering from a malignancy. Properly educated patients can contribute greatly to their own treatment. For example, knowing that emotional stress is an influencing factor in many TMDs can help the patient understand the reason for daily fluctuations of pain intensity. Attention should be directed toward changing the patient's response to stress or, when possible, reducing exposure to stressful conditions. Patients with pain during chewing should be told to begin a softer diet, chew slower, and eat smaller bites. As a general rule the patient should be told "if it hurts, don't do it." Continued pain can contribute to the cycling of pain and should always be avoided. The patient should be instructed to let the jaw muscles relax, maintaining the teeth apart. This will discourage clenching activities and minimize loading of the teeth and joints.

When pain is associated with a clicking TM joint, the patient should be informed of the biomechanics of the joint. This information often allows the patient to select functional activities that are less traumatic to the joint structures. For example, some patients may report that the pain and clicking are less when they chew on a particular side of the mouth. When this occurs, they should be encouraged to continue this type of chewing.

Pharmacologic Therapy

Pharmacologic therapy can be an effective adjunct in managing symptoms associated with TMDs. Patients should be aware that medication alone will not likely solve or cure the problem. Medication, however, in conjunction with appropriate physical therapy and definitive treatment, does offer the most complete approach to many TMD problems. Mild analgesics are often helpful for many TMDs. Control of pain is not only appreciated by the patient but also reduces the likelihood of other complicating pain disorders such as muscle co-contraction, referred pain, and central sensitization.

Nonsteroidal antiinflammatory drugs (NSAIDs) are very helpful with many TMDs. Included in this category are aspirin, acetaminophen (Tylenol), and ibuprofen. Ibuprofen (Motrin, Advil, Nuprin) is often very effective in reducing musculoskeletal pains. A dosage of 600 to 800 mg three times a day for 3 to 5 days commonly reduces pain and stops the cyclic effects of the deep pain input. For patients with gastrointestinal issues, short-term use of a cyclooxygenase-2 (COX-2) inhibitor such as celecoxib (Celebrex) can also be useful.

Physical Therapy

In many patients with TMD, symptoms are relieved with very simple physical therapy methods. Simple instructions for the use of moist heat or cold can be very helpful. Surface heat can be applied by laying a hot, moist towel over the symptomatic area. A hot water bottle wrapped inside the towel will help maintain the heat. This combination should remain in place for 10 to 15 minutes, not to exceed 30 minutes. An electric heating pad may be used, but care should be taken not to leave it on the face too long. Patients should be discouraged from using the heating pad while sleeping because prolonged use is likely.

Like thermotherapy, coolant therapy can provide a simple and often effective method of reducing pain. Ice should be applied directly to the symptomatic joint or muscles and moved in a circular motion without pressure to the tissues. The patient will initially experience an uncomfortable feeling that will quickly turn into a burning sensation. Continued icing will result in a mild aching and then numbness. When numbness begins the ice should be removed. The ice should not be left on the tissues for longer than 5 minutes. After a period of warming a second cold application may be desirable.

The physician should be aware that many TMDs respond to the use of orthopedic appliances such as occlusal appliances, bite guards, and splints. These appliances are made by the dentist and are custom fabricated for each patient. Several types of appliances are available. Each is specific for the type of TMD present. The dentist should be consulted for this type of therapy.

Other Therapeutic Considerations

Sometimes TMDs become chronic and, as with other chronic pain conditions, might then be best managed by a multidisciplinary approach. If the patient reports a long history of TMD complaints, the physician should consider referring the patient to a dentist associated with a team of therapists, such as a psychologist, a physical therapist, and even a chronic pain physician. Generally, patients with chronic TMD are not managed well by the simple initial therapies discussed in this chapter. Often other factors, such as mechanical conditions within the TMJs or psychological factors, need to be addressed. The physician who attempts to manage these conditions in the private practice setting can become very frustrated with the results. It is therefore recommended that if the patient's history suggests chronicity or if initial therapy fails to reduce the patient's symptoms, referral is indicated.

References

de Leeuw RE: *Orofacial Pain: Guidelines for Assessment, Diagnosis, and Management*, ed 5, Chicago 2013, Quintessence.
Okeson JP: *Management of Temporomandibular Disorders and Occlusion*, ed 8, St. Louis, 2019, Elsevier.
Okeson JP: *Bell's Orofacial Pains*, ed 7, Chicago, 2014, Quintessence.
Scrivani SJ, Keith DA, Kaban LB: Temporomandibular disorders, *N Engl J Med* 359(25):2693–2705, 2008.

UVEITIS

Method of
Curtis E. Margo, MD, MPH; and Lynn E. Harman, MD

CURRENT DIAGNOSIS

- Uveitis is classified by anatomic location and etiology.
- Most forms of uveitis are due to infectious or immune-mediated disease.
- Drug-induced uveitis and masquerade disorders (neoplasms) must be excluded in diagnostic evaluations.
- Patients with first-time uveitis should have a medical history, physical examination, and basic laboratory studies, with the possible exception of adults who have a single episode of mild anterior uveitis that responds to therapy and who have no systemic signs or symptoms.
- Diagnostic evaluation must differentiate infectious from noninfectious uveitis.
- Patients who are immunosuppressed are at higher risk of infectious uveitis and their clinical presentations may be atypical.
- Uveitis in children is uncommon and deserves a thorough medical evaluation at initial presentation.
- Uveitis is managed optimally through a collaborative multidisciplinary approach.

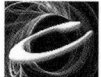

CURRENT THERAPY

- Eradication of infection is the primary objective in infectious uveitis but may require judicious use of local antiinflammatory agents to mitigate structural and functional damage to intraocular tissues.
- The goal of therapy in noninfectious uveitis is to suppress and eliminate inflammation, achieving lasting remission through the stepwise implementation of therapy.
- First-time anterior uveitis in adults with negative medical history and review of systems can be treated with topical corticosteroids and cycloplegic agents and careful clinical monitoring.
- Corticosteroids can be delivered topically, through periocular and intravitreal injection, via sustained release devices implanted in the eye, and systemically.
- Immunomodulating therapy using alkylating agents, antimetabolites, biologic response modulators, or inhibitors of T-lymphocyte signaling are indicated for uveitis not responsive to systemic corticosteroids.
- A thorough history, physical examination, and select laboratory studies are required before initiating immunomodulating therapy.

Current Diagnosis

Uveitis describes a heterogeneous group of disorders that have in common inflammation of the uveal tract (i.e., iris, ciliary body, and choroid). Symptoms are nonspecific, usually involving various combinations of blurred vision, ocular discomfort, intolerance to light, and floaters. Onset may be sudden or insidious. Children may have no symptoms. The essential signs of uveitis are the presence of inflammatory cells in the aqueous humor and/or vitreous gel. Sufficient magnification with a slit lamp is required to confidently detect these inflammatory cells and avoid confusion with suspended red blood cells or pigment epithelial cells. Although the uveal tract is the conceptual epicenter of uveal inflammation, there is spillover inflammation in the aqueous humor and vitreous gel, the two anatomic locations used to quantify the severity of inflammation and to monitor response to therapy. Grading schemes for recording the severity of anterior chamber and vitreous inflammatory cell density and protein content (flare) have been published by the Standardization of Uveitis Nomenclature (SUN) Classification Working Group.

Clinical Features and Diagnosis

The anatomic classification of intraocular inflammation into anterior, intermediate, and posterior uveitis and panuveitis guides the diagnostic workup toward the determination of etiology. When the anterior chamber is the principal site of inflammation, the terms iritis or iridocyclitis are often used. When the vitreous is the primary focus of inflammation, the term intermediate uveitis is preferred, but posterior cyclitis or vitritis are commonly used synonyms. Pars planitis falls within the category of intermediate uveitis and is characterized by a layering of inflammatory cells over the pars plana and anterior retina called a "snowbank lesion." Posterior uveitis embraces diverse conditions that are anatomically characterized by terms such as chorioretinitis, retinochoroiditis, or neuroretinitis.

Most cases of uveitis are caused by infection or immune-mediated disease. A substantial proportion of immune-mediated disease is a manifestation of systemic disease. Arriving at a diagnosis of infectious or noninfectious uveitis requires exclusion of drug-induced uveitis and so-called masquerade disorders (usually neoplasms) that mimic uveal inflammation. Most idiopathic forms of uveitis are localized immune-mediated disease whose pathogenesis is not yet understood. A number of immune-mediated uveitides have overlapping features with infectious disease. For instance, syphilis and Lyme disease have been mistaken for several of the uveal white dot syndromes (see later). Tuberculosis can resemble serpiginous choroiditis. The diagnostic evaluation for persons with noninfectious uveitis and no known systemic disorders involves a complete history, review of systems, physical examination, and select laboratory tests. The optimal use of laboratory testing in this setting is unresolved.

The anatomic categories of posterior uveitis and panuveitis have vastly expanded the number of potential diagnoses. The pattern and distribution of inflammatory lesions of the choroid, retina, and optic nerve, along with a host of other clinical findings (e.g., vascular or perivascular involvement, severity of overlying inflammation, color and shape of choroidal and retinal lesions, etc.) are critical to narrowing the differential diagnosis. The importance of pattern recognition in the diagnosis of posterior uveitis and panuveitis cannot be overstated. Toxoplasma chorioretinitis, the most common form of posterior uveitis, can usually be confidently diagnosed by clinical ophthalmoscopic appearance of a yellow-white retina with overlying vitreal inflammation adjacent to a hyperpigmented chorioretinal scar. On the other hand, the disorders belonging to the so-called white dot syndromes (acute posterior multifocal placoid pigment epitheliopathy, multifocal chorioretinitis with panuveitis, punctate inner choroidopathy, multiple evanescent white dot syndrome, and birdshot chorioretinopathy) require special studies such as fluorescein angiography and optic coherence tomography to elucidate. Most of these disorders, and a few others such as Vogt-Koyanagi-Harada disease and sympathetic ophthalmia, are clinically defined syndromes. Laboratory studies in the context of a clinically defined syndrome are used to exclude conditions that could possibly mimic their appearance.

Uveitis occurs in children substantially less often than adults. Although a majority of the same infectious and noninfectious etiologies that occur in adults also affect children, juvenile idiopathic arthritis has a relatively unique clinical presentation in young patients. All four subtypes of juvenile idiopathic arthritis are associated with anterior uveitis, but the pauciarticular category may present with anterior chamber inflammation and advanced band keratopathy with few or no symptoms. This degree of incongruity between symptoms and clinical findings on slit-lamp examination is unusual in adults.

Current Therapy

The heterogeneous nature of uveitis limits the generalizability of a universal therapeutic algorithm. When the cause of uveitis is infection, the goal of therapy is to eradicate the infectious organism while controlling inflammation during the process. For noninfectious uveitis, the goal of therapy is to suppress and eliminate inflammation and to achieve lasting remission. This is approached through the stepwise implementation of therapeutic agents, beginning with an agent that has a satisfactory safety profile and can suppress inflammation. The severity and pattern of inflammation at presentation and the perceived risk to vision and ocular integrity guide the initial selection of therapy. Timing of treatment escalation and transition to noncorticosteroid therapy are decisions based on multiple factors, including the patient's general medical health. Simultaneous therapies, particularly local and systemic antiinflammatory agents, are commonly used. Multidisciplinary management is ideally suited to combine the expertise needed to track the ocular response to treatment and to prescribe and monitor many of the systemic mediations.

Anterior Uveitis

Anterior uveitis, the most common subset of uveitis, is usually noninfectious. A minority of cases are attributed to viruses, most often herpes simplex virus (HSV), varicella zoster virus (VZV), and cytomegalovirus (CMV). Clinical manifestations of viral anterior uveitis depend on the immune status of the patient. Once appropriate diagnostic evaluation is complete and viral anterior uveitis is suspected or established for HSV or VZV, therapy with oral acyclovir (Zovirax),[1] valacyclovir (Valtrex),[1] and famciclovir (Famvir)[1] is started. Following clinical resolution of inflammation, maintenance therapy with an oral antiviral drug for HSV should be considered. Anterior uveitis due to CMV is treated with

intravenous ganciclovir (Cytovene).[1] Maintenance therapy with topical ganciclovir (Zirgan)[1] or oral valganciclovir (Valcyte)[1] should be considered. Duration of maintenance therapies for viral anterior uveitis has not been subject to rigorous study.

The vast majority of anterior uveitis is noninfectious, for which the mainstay of treatment is topical corticosteroids with cycloplegics (Table 1). There are nearly 20 different preparations of topical

TABLE 1	Topical Medications for Anterior Uveitis
DRUG NAME (TRADE NAMES)	FORMULATION	STARTING DOSE SCHEDULE*
Topical Corticosteroids		
Dexamethasone (Decadron phosphate [Maxidex])	0.1% suspension; 0.1% solution; 0.05% ointment[2]	4 times per day
Difluprednate (Durezol)	0.05% emulsion	4 times per day
Fluorometholine alcohol (Flarex, FML)	0.1 and 0.25% suspensions; 0.1% ointment	2–4 times per day; 1–3 times per day
Loteprednol etabonate (Lotemax)	0.5% suspension	4 times per day
Leteprednol etabonate (Alrex)	0.2% suspension[1]	3 times per day
Prednisolone acetate (Pred Forte, Econopred Plus; AK-Tate)	1.0% suspension	4 times per day
Prednisolone sodium phosphate (Inflamase Forte; AK-Pred)	1.0% solution	4 times per day
Prednisolone acetate (Pred Mild; Econopred)	0.12% suspension	4 times per day
Topical Cycloplegic Agents		
Atropine sulfate (Isopto atropine)	1.0%	Once or twice a day
Cyclopentolate hydrochloride (Cyclogyl)[1]	0.5% and 1.0%	Twice a day
Homatropine hydrobromide (Isopto homatropine)	2.0%–5.0%	Once or twice a day
Scopolamine hydrobromide (Isopto hyoscine)	0.25%	Once or twice a day
Tropicamide (Mydriacyl)[1]	0.5% and 1.0%	2–3 times a day
Topical Nonsteroidal Antiinflammatory Medications		
Bromfenac (BromSite; Prolensa; Xibrom)[1]	0.075%–0.09% solution	Once or twice daily
Diclofenac (Voltaren)[1]	0.1% solution	2 times per day
Flurbiprofen (Ocufen)[1]	0.03% solution	2 times per day
Ketorolac (Acular LS; Acular)[1]	0.4%–0.5%	3 times per day
Nepafenac (Ilevro; Nevanac)[1]	0.1%–0.3% suspension	1–3 times a day, based on formulation

*More frequent use of corticosteroids dictated by severity of inflammation then tapered based on clinical response.
[1]Not FDA approved for this indication.
[2]Not available in the United States.

---

[1]Not FDA approved for this indication.

[1]Not FDA approved for this indication.

corticosteroid (e.g., dexamethasone sodium phosphate 0.1% solution; prednisolone acetate 1.0% suspension [Pred Forte]) that come in suspension or solution (and some as ointment) and in different concentrations. Dose and duration of use is tailored to the clinical setting.

Topical nonsteroidal antiinflammatory agents (e.g., diclofenac 0.1% [Voltaren][1]; ketorolac 0.4% [Acular][1]; flurbiprofen 0.03% [Ocufen]) are less effective than topical corticosteroids in controlling the inflammation of anterior uveitis. Their use in combination with topical corticosteroids may be additive.[1]

Topical cycloplegics provide pain relief, and the mydriasis they produce reduces the risk of iridolenticular scarring. The selection of a long-acting (e.g., atropine sulfate 1% [Isopto Atropine] twice daily) versus short-acting cycloplegic agent (e.g., cyclopentolate hydrochloride 0.5%–1.0% [Cyclogyl] two or three times a day) is based on clinical features such as severity of inflammation, presence of synechial scarring, age of patient, ability to take topical medications, and so on. Duration of action varies from 1 to 2 weeks for topical atropine to approximately half a day for cyclopentolate.

Noninfectious anterior uveitis is commonly associated with surgical trauma and accidental blunt trauma (concussive injury). They are usually effectively managed with tapering regimens of topical corticosteroids and cycloplegics.

Oral prednisone (1 mg/kg/day) may be needed for severe or recalcitrant anterior uveitis. Strategies for therapeutic escalation beyond oral corticosteroids parallel that of intermediate or posterior uveitis.

Although topical corticosteroids and cycloplegics do not play a primary role in intermediate and posterior uveitis, they are used as adjuvant therapies for comfort and to minimize the formation of peripheral and posterior synechiae.

Intermediate Uveitis

Intermediate uveitis, characterized by inflammatory cells in vitreous, peripheral retina, and pars plana, can be associated with systemic disorders such as multiple sclerosis, sarcoidosis, syphilis, toxocariasis (in children), and Lyme disease. Vitritis is also a presenting sign of endogenous endophthalmitis and can be mimicked by primary vitreoretinal lymphoma. Once infection, drug-related uveitis, and masquerading conditions are excluded, the approach to therapy for noninfectious forms of intermediate uveitis is similar to the stepladder approach (described later) that typically begins with oral corticosteroids (Table 2). For pars planitis recalcitrant to medical therapy, options include peripheral ablation of the snowbank lesion with indirect laser photocoagulation and pars plana vitrectomy. Their effectiveness has not been rigorously tested in clinical trials.

Periocular injections of depot corticosteroids (40 mg triamcinolone acetonide [1 mL of 40 mg/mL Kenalog-40][1]) delivers medication closer to the site of inflammation and may be used as a bridge to oral steroid therapy or to reduce the dose of oral steroids. Intravitreal corticosteroid injection through the pars plana (4 mg triamcinolone acetonide suspension [0.1 mL 40 mg/mL Kenalog-40[1]; Triesence]) is often tried before moving to immune modulator therapy. The risk of endophthalmitis and the need for repeat injections are drawbacks.

Posterior Uveitis and Panuveitis

The general diagnostic approach to posterior uveitis and panuveitis begins by excluding infection and drug-induced uveitis and not overlooking the possibility of a masquerade condition. The optimal strategy for laboratory testing to identify a culpable systemic disorder responsible for noninfectious uveitis is a matter of debate. Many posterior and pan uveitides are clinically defined syndromes. For example, Behçet disease, multifocal choroiditis with panuveitis, acute posterior multifocal placoid pigment epitheliopathy, serpiginous choroiditis, punctate inner choroidopathy, multiple evanescent white dot syndrome, Vogt-Koyanagi-Harada disease, and sympathetic ophthalmia are diagnoses based on clinical findings (e.g., ophthalmoscopy,

fluorescein angiography, optical coherence tomography, etc.). These syndromes have no confirmatory laboratory tests, other than several with strong human leukocyte antigen (HLA) haplotype associations (e.g., Behçet disease [HLA-B51] and birdshot chorioretinpathy [HLS-A29]).

Management of inflammation associated with noninfectious posterior uveitis requires systemic medications. Most clinicians initiate oral corticosteroids, understanding that high-dose long-term use is associated with serious and predictable side effects. The risk of systemic side effects may be reduced with judicious use of periocular or intravitreal corticosteroid injections, but those routes of administration also have their own potential adverse effects and complications. These range from elevated intraocular pressure and glaucoma to infectious endophthalmitis. A sustained-release corticosteroid implant is another option. Corticosteroids are embedded to either a biodegradable or nonbiodegradable vehicle to achieve sustained release. The implants are injected into the vitreous or surgically fixed to the sclera. Dexamethasone (Ozurdex, 0.7 mg) has a delivery span of 6 months, and fluocinolone acetonide (Iluvien 0.19 mg[1]; Retisert 0.59 mg; Yutiq 0.18 mg) 18 to 36 months.

The optimal time to transition to noncorticosteroid immunomodulatory therapy is not well defined. The guidelines for treatment escalation are also imprecise, relying on clinical judgment, individual patient input, and shared decision making. Immunomodulatory therapy for the treatment of uveitis falls into four drug categories: antimetabolites, inhibitors of T-lymphocyte signaling, biologic response modifiers, and alkylating agents (Table 3). Their judicious use has been shown to reduce or eliminate the need for systemic corticosteroids, improve long-term visual prognosis, and reduce ocular complications from inflammation. Meaningful clinical responses should occur within 3 months of initiating therapy. Following achieved clinical end points, drugs can be carefully tapered over 24 months. A thorough history, physical examination, and select laboratory tests and imaging studies should be completed prior to initiation of therapy.

The most commonly used antimetabolites for the treatment of noninfectious uveitis are methotrexate (Rheumatrex),[1] azathioprine (Imuran),[1] and mycophenolate mofetil (Cellcept).[1] Oral methotrexate, 7.5 to 15 mg once per week with daily folic acid[1] 1 mg, can be increased to 20 to 25 mg/week based on clinical response. Appropriately adjusted intravenous dose can be tried for persons with gastrointestinal intolerance. Intravitreal injection of 400 µg/0.1 mL has been used for refractory inflammation. Oral azathioprine is begun at 1 mg/kg/day. Depending on clinical response, it can be incrementally increased to 2.5 mg/kg/day. Mycophenolate mofetil is started at 1 to 2 g orally per day in divided doses up to 3 g/day. The manifold side effects of antimetabolites necessitate close clinical monitoring.

Most experience in treating noninfectious uveitis with inhibitors of T-lymphocyte signaling, or calcineurin inhibitors, is with cyclosporine (Sandimmune).[1] Given 2.5 to 5 mg/kg/day in divided doses, cyclosporine can cause nephrotoxicity, bone marrow suppression, and hypertension.

Alkylating agents used to treat noninfectious uveitis include cyclophosphamide (Cytoxan)[1] and chlorambucil (Leukeran).[1] These immunomodulating drugs are titrated to keep white blood cell counts in the range of 3000 to 4500 cells per cubic millimeter. Chlorambucil is started at 0.15 mg/kg/day and cyclophosphamide at 1 to 3 mg/kg/day. Regular monitoring for bone marrow suppression and opportunistic infection is needed for both drugs. Risks of hemorrhagic cystitis with cyclophosphamide may be reduced by consuming generous amounts of water daily.

Biologic response modifiers, or "biologics," have expanded the therapeutic arsenal for treating advanced and severe noninfectious uveitis. This family of medications consists of antibodies directed against key cytokines in the immune response pathway. Most experience in treating noninfectious uveitis has been with tumor necrosis factor-α (TNF-α) inhibitors (infliximab [Remicade][1] and

---

[1]Not FDA approved for this indication.

[1]Not FDA approved for this indication.

TABLE 2	Treatment of Infectious Uveitis		
DIAGNOSIS	**INFECTIOUS ORGANISM(S)**	**TREATMENT**	**COMMENT**
Acute retinal necrosis	Herpes zoster virus (HZV) Herpes simplex virus (HSV) I and II	Acyclovir (Zovirax)[1] 13 mg/kg/dose divided every 8 h IV for 7 days, followed by 800 mg PO 5 times/day for 3–4 months or Famciclovir (Famvir)[1] 500 mg PO q8h or Valacyclovir (Valtrex)[1] 1000–2000 mg PO q8h for induction Ganciclovir (Cytovene)[1] 500 mg IV q12h; maintenance: (duration varies with response) Valganciclovir (Valcyte)[1] 900 mg PO BID for 3 weeks then 450 mg PO BID Ganciclovir[1] 1000 mg PO TID	Adjuvant intravitreal injection options: Ganciclovir (200–2000 µg/0.1 mL)[6] Foscarnet (Foscavir)1 (1.2–2.4 mg/0.1 mL)[6]; Possible role for prednisone (0.5–2.0 mg/kg/day po for up to 6–8 weeks)
Anterior uveitis, viral	HSV	Valacyclovir[1] 1000 mg PO TID Acyclovir[1] 400 mg PO × 5/day 4 weeks Famciclovir 250 mg PO TID	Topical corticosteroids and cycloplegic recommended. Alternative options include an intravitreal ganciclovir (2 mg/0.05 mL).[6] After active infection eradicated, consider maintenance therapy for HSV and CMV
	HZV	Valacyclovir[1] 1 g PO TID Acyclovir[1] 800 mg PO × 5/day 5–6 weeks Famciclovir[1] 500 mg PO TID 5–6 weeks	
	Cytomegalovirus (CMV)	Ganciclovir[1] 5 mg/kg IV BID 2–3 weeks Valganciclovir[1] 900 mg PO BID × 6 weeks, then 450 mg PO BID × 6 weeks	Gancyclovir gel 0.15% 5/day (optional)
Cat-scratch disease	*Bartonella henselae*	Doxycycline (Vibramycin)[1] 100 mg PO BID 2 to 4 weeks	Children: antibiotic selection based on age, dental maturity.
Cytomegalovirus retinitis	Cytomegalovirus	Ganciclovir 5 mg/kg/day IV BID for 2–3 weeks followed by maintenance 5 mg/kg/day PO Cidofovir (Vistide)[1] 5 mg/kg/week IV for 2 weeks then 5 mg/kg every 2 weeks Valganciclovir 900 mg BID PO, then PO qd for maintenance. Foscarnet 90 mg/kg IV BID × 2 wks; maintenance 90–120 mg/kg IV daily	Immune reconstitution targets cause of immune compromise.
Diffuse unilateral subacute neuroretinitis (DUSN)	Possible larva of *Baylisascaris procyonis*, *Toxocara canis*	Photocoagulation of intraretinal nematode	Destruction of intraretinal larva may preserve vision.
Lyme disease	*Borrelia burgdorferi*	Doxycycline[1] 100 mg PO BID × 21 days (adults) Amoxicillin[1] 500 mg PO BID (adult); 50 mg/kg PO in divided doses × 14–21 days (children)	Alternative: cefuroxime axetil (Ceftin) 500 mg PO BID × 14–21 days (adult); 30 mg/kg/day PO (children)
Metastatic endophthalmitis (endogenous)	Numerous bloodborne bacteria and fungi	Sepsis treatment protocol; antibiotic selections based on cultures and sensitivities	Role and timing of intravitreal antibiotics and of vitrectomy less well defined
Onchocerciasis	*Onchocerca volvulus*	Ivermectin (Stromectol) 150 µg/kg single oral dose; repeat at 6 months for the lifespan of adult worm	Corticosteroids to control ocular inflammation; route of administration depends of site of inflammation
Syphilis	*Treponema pallidum*	Aqueous penicillin G 18–24 million units, IV qd divided doses for 10–14 days	Ocular syphilis is considered a subset of neurosyphilis
Toxocariasis	*Toxocara canis* or *Toxocara catis*	Prednisone 1 mg/kg/day PO; timing of antihelminthic therapy unresolved.	Laser ablation and vitrectomy depending on stage of disease. Intraocular larval death incites considerable inflammation
Toxoplasmosis	*Toxoplasma gondii*	Pyrimethamine (Daraprim): loading dose 50–100 mg PO; treatment dose 25–50 mg/day PO; and sulfadiazine: loading dose 2–4 g PO; treatment dose 1.0 g PO QID, and prednisone (0.5–1.0 mg/kg/day PO) Trimethoprim-sulfamethoxazole (Bactrim DS)[1] 160 mg/80 mg PO BID, plus above regimen of prednisone	Modify doses if pregnant or immune compromised. Some recommend adding clindamycin or azithromycin.
Tuberculosis	*Mycobacterium tuberculosis*	Follow recomendations for first line therapy for active tuberculosis on CDC website	

BID, Twice a day; *IV*, intravenous; *PO*, by mouth; *TID*, three times a day.

[1]Not FDA approved for this indication.

[6]May be compounded by pharmacists.

TABLE 3 Immune Modulator Therapy for Uveitis

GENERIC (TRADE) NAME	DOSE (ROUTE)*	COMMENT/INDICATIONS†
Alkylating Agents		
Chlorambucil (Leukeran)[1]	0.15 mg/kg/day (oral)	Behçet disease; juvenile idiopathic arthritis; pars planitis; sympathetic ophthalmia
Cyclophosphamide (Cytoxan)[1]	1 mg/kg/day (oral)	Sclerouveitis; sympathetic ophthalmia
Antimetabolites		
Azathioprine (Imuran)[1]	1–1.5 mg/kg/day (oral) can increase to 2.5 mg/kg/day	Severe anterior uveitis; panuveitis, juvenile idiopathic arthritis; pars planitis, sarcoidosis; sympathetic uveitis; Vogt-Koyanagi-Harada disease (VKH)
Methotrexate (Otrexup, Rasuvo, Rheumatrex, Trexall)[1]	7.5–15 mg/week (oral)	Anterior, intermediate, and posterior uveitis; juvenile idiopathic arthritis; sympathetic uveitis
Mycophenolate mofetil (Cellcept)[1]; Mycophenolate sodium (Myfortic)[1]	Mofetil: 1 g (oral) divided dose/day; Sodium: 360 mg (oral)/day	Anterior, intermediate, and posterior uveitis
Calcinernin Inhibitors		
Cyclosporine (Gengraf, Neoral, Sandimmune)[1]	2.5–5 mg/kg/day (oral) divided dose	Often given with prednisone 10–20 mg/day; Behçet disease; birdshot chorioretinopathy; pan uveitis; posterior uveitis; sarcoidosis; sclerouveitis; sympathetic uveitis; VKH
Tacrolimus (Prograf, Astagraf XL, Envasus XR)[1]	0.15–0.3 mg/kg/day (oral)	Behçet disease; birdshot chorioretinopathy; posterior uveitis
Biologic Response Modifier Tumor Necrosis Factor (TNF)-α Inhibitor		
Adalimumab (Humira)	40 mg every other week subcutaneous injection	Anterior, intermediate and posterior uveitis; juvenile idiopathic arthritis; sarcoidosis
Infliximab (Remicade)[1]	3 mg/kg/day (intravenous) weeks 0, 2, and 6	Behçet disease; anterior uveitis; juvenile idiopathic arthritis; sarcoidosis
Certolizumab pegol (Cimzia)[1]	400 mg subcutaneous induction 1–3 doses; 200 mg every 2 weeks	Refractory uveitis
Golimumab (Simponi)[1]	50 mg subcutaneous every 4 weeks	Juvenile idiopathic arthritis; Behçet disease
Biologic Response Modifier Interluekin-1 Inhibitor		
Anakinra (Kineret)[1]	100 mg subcutaneous daily	Behçet disease
Canakinumab (Ilaris)[1]	150–300 mg subcutaneous every 4–8 weeks	Behçet disease; juvenile idiopathic arthritis
Biologic Response Modifier Anti-Interleukin 6 Receptor		
Tocilizumab (Actemra)[1]	4–8 mg/kg (intravenous) every 2– 4 weeks	Juvenile idiopathic arthritis; Behçet disease; persistent macular edema
Biologic Response Modifier Anti-Cd20		
Rituximab (Rituxan)[1]	375 mg/m² intravenous weekly, modify accordingly	Refractory uveitis; juvenile idiopathic arthritis; refractory VKH;

*Therapeutic doses and schedules in clinical trials have differed in loading doses and maintenance doses. Cited doses reflect lower ranges.
†Refers to reported success at controlling or eliminating inflammation as a single or as a steroid-sparing agent. Strength of recommendations will vary by level of evidence.
[1]Not FDA approved for this indication.

adalimumab [Humira]). Although other biologics have been used to treat advanced or severe noninfectious uveitis, their equivalence or superiority to the drugs already mentioned are under study. Etanercept (Embrel)[1] may increase the risk of anterior uveitis in persons with ankylosing spondylitis.

Infliximab (Remicade) is given intravenously beginning with two loading doses of 3 to 5 mg/kg each given 2 weeks apart. Injections are then continued at 4-week intervals. Based on clinical response, dose can be gradually increased to 10 mg/kg. Side effects include infection from activation of latent tuberculosis or hepatitis, drug-induced autoimmune disease, and demyelinating disease. There is also a small risk of increased overall cancer mortality compared with a nonimmunosuppressed population of patients. Adalimumab (Humira) is given subcutaneously starting at 40 mg/kg every 2 weeks. Children are started at a reduced dose. Its adverse risk profile is similar to that of infliximab.

Other biologics used to treat noninfectious uveitis such as anti-CD20 monoclonal antibody (Rituximab [Rituxan][1]) have less established positions in the stepwise implementation of therapy. Interferon alfa-2a (Roferon-A),[1] known for its antiviral and antineoplastic effects, has been used to treat Behçet disease with persistent macular edema. It is given as a subcutaneous injection of 3 to 9 million international units daily for a week then tapered over 3 to 6 months. Interferon alfa-2a is associated with flu-like symptoms and depression, which may limit patient acceptance.

Complications of Uveitis

Chronic uveitis gives rise to a variety of ocular complications such as secondary glaucoma; macular edema; corneal dysfunction; neovascularization of the iris, angle, and retina; retinal tears and detachments; cyclitic membrane formation; and uveal effusion, as well as other conditions. These ocular complications are typically approached by controlling or eliminating ocular inflammation and managing the structural/functional problems according to standards guidelines.

Disease-Specific Recommendations

Strength of recommendations for disease-specific noncorticosteroid immunomodulatory therapy is constrained by the relative lack of prospective clinical trials, drug-to-drug comparison trials, studies that have included patients with diverse forms of uveitis, and the small size of studies. Given these limitations, the strength of recommendations is tempered by a level of evidence for most drugs of 2B or lower on the Oxford Centre for Evidence-Based Medicine level of evidence scale. Mycophenolate preparations,[1] azathioprine,[1] methotrexate,[1] cyclophosphamide,[1] cyclosporine,[1] sirolimus (Rapamune),[1] infliximab,[1] adalimumab, and etanercept[1] have demonstrated varying degrees of success in controlling inflammation, improving visual outcome, and reducing corticosteroid use in severe anterior, intermediate, and posterior uveitis and in panuveitis. Control of inflammation and improved visual acuity in Vogt-Koyanagi-Harada disease have been achieved with systemic methotrexate,[1] azathioprine,[1] mycophenolate preparations,[1] infliximab,[1] adalimumab,[1] and interferon alfa-2a.[1] The uveitis of Beçhet disease, juvenile idiopathic arthritis, pars planitis, and sympathetic ophthalmia responds to chlorambucil.[1] Mycophenolate preparations[1] have had success in various forms of anterior, intermediate, and posterior uveitis. The inflammation of Beçhet disease has been controlled with azathioprine,[1] infliximab,[1] adalimumab,[1] rituximab,[1] and interferon alfa-2a.[1] Sarcoid uveitis has responded to infliximab,[1] and adalimumab.[1] The systemic disease of juvenile idiopathic arthritis has been successfully managed with methotrexate, cyclosporine,[1] mycophenolate mofetil,[1] azathioprine,[1] and TNF-α inhibitors adalimumab and infliximab.[1] Therapeutic vitrectomy and/or laser ablation has been used in different forms of noninfectious uveitis, but evidence of long-term effectiveness is sparse.

Systemic Drug Use in Pregnancy and in Children

Because the teratogenic potential of many immunosuppressive drugs is incompletely understood, it may be prudent to discuss contraception when they are administered to women. The largely unknown teratogenic effects of immunosuppressive agents in men should also be considered. Although prednisone is well tolerated during pregnancy, its use should be carefully comanaged with an obstetrician.

The effects of immunosuppressive drugs are less well studied in children than in adults. Children on immunosuppressive agents should not receive live virus vaccine for 3 months after immunosuppressive use has ended. This would include high-dose corticosteroids. The impact of immunosuppressive drugs and systemic corticosteroids on growth and their collateral effects on social development are not inconsequential. Osteoporosis, adrenal suppression, and heightened susceptibility to infections related to cell-mediated immunity are among the side effects that require monitoring in children. Calcium supplements and vitamin D may be beneficial in some circumstances.

---

[1]Not FDA approved for this indication.

References

Dick AD, Rosenbaum JT, Al-Dhibi HA, et al: Guidance on noncorticosteroid systemic immunomodulatory therapy in noninfectious uveitis. Fundamentals of Care for UveitiS (FOCUS) Initiative, *Ophthalmology* 125:757–773, 2018.

Foster CS, Kothari S, Anesi SD, et al: The Ocular Immunology and Uveitis Foundation preferred practice patterns of uveitis management, *Surv Ophthalmol* 61:1–17, 2016.

Jabs DA, Nussenblatt RB, Rosenbaum JT: Standardization of Uveitis Nomenclature (SUN) Work Group. standardization of uveitis nomenclature for reporting clinical data. results of the first international workshop, *Am J Ophthalmol* 140:509–516, 2005.

Jap A, Soon-Phaik C: Viral anterior uveitis. diagnosis and management, *Focal Points* 34(5):1–18, 2016. Available at https://store.aao.org/clinical-education/product-line/focal-points.html.

Levy-Clarke G, Jabs DA, Read RW, et al: Expert panel recommendations for the use of anti-tumor necrosis factor biologic agents in patients with ocular inflammatory disorders, *Ophthalmology* 121:785–796, 2014. e783.

London NJS, Garg SJ, Moorthy MS, et al: Drug-induced uveitis, *Focal Points* 33(5):1–10, 2015. Available at https://store.aao.org/clinical-education/product-line/focal-points.html.

Lower CY, Lima BR: Pediatric uveitis, *Focal Points* 32(3):1–11, 2014. Available at https://store.aao.org/clinical-education/product-line/focal-points.html.

Schwartzman S: Advancements in the management of uveitis, *Best Prac Res Clin Rheumatol* 30:304–316, 2016.

Wakefield D, McCluskey P, Wildner G, et al: Inflammatory eye disease: pretreatment assessment of patients prior to commencing immunosuppressive and biologic therapy: recommendations from an expert committee, *Autoimmun Rev* 16:213–222, 2017.

Yeh S, Suhler ER, Moorly RS, et al: Biologic response modifiers in uveitis, *Focal Points* 30(3):1–16, 2012. Available at https://store.aao.org/clinical-education/product-line/focal-points.html.

VISION REHABILITATION

Method of
August Colenbrander, MD; and Donald C. Fletcher, MD

CURRENT DIAGNOSIS

- The need for vision rehabilitation needs to be considered whenever patients indicate that they have difficulty performing visual tasks.
- Sometimes, however, patients do not recognize the visual causes of their complaints, therefore:
  - Vision rehabilitation needs to be considered whenever visual acuity is reported as 20/50 or less.
  - Vision rehabilitation also needs to be considered for all patients with reported visual disorders, such as visual field deficits or contrast vision deficits, who have not received this service yet,

CURRENT THERAPY

- Simple cases of reduced visual acuity can be addressed with a variety of magnifying devices, ranging from stronger glasses to electronic devices.
- Improved task lighting can often be helpful.
- Orientation and mobility training can be indicated for patients with visual field loss, even if their visual acuity is still adequate.
- As for any other specialized service, referral to a dedicated low vision service may be indicated.

Vision rehabilitation refers to the multidisciplinary effort of assisting those with various degrees of vision loss in coping with the *consequences* of that loss. To describe vision rehabilitation, the nature of vision itself must be understood. Vision is the major source of information about our environment. The eyes alone contribute as much information to the brain as all other organs combined. It is not surprising therefore that many people fear loss of vision almost as much as loss of life.

Most people will state that "we see with our eyes." On closer examination, this is not true. An isolated eyeball cannot produce any vision; our brain, however, can produce exquisite visual imagery in our dreams, without any input from the eyes.

The ultimate goal of vision is to facilitate interaction with the environment, not just to read letters on a letter chart. To achieve this goal, the visual process goes through three distinct stages. Each stage comes with its own specific problems.

- First is the *optical stage*, where the refractive media of the eye deliver an image to the retina. Familiar problems in this area include refractive errors and cataracts.

- Second is the *receptor stage*, where the optical image is translated into neural impulses. Age-related macular degeneration (AMD) is a significant problem of the receptor stage, which is becoming increasingly common as the population ages.
- Third are various stages of *neural processing*, initially in the inner retina (glaucoma), then in the visual cortex, and finally in higher cortical centers, where the visual input gives rise to visual perception and to visually guided behaviors, actions, and interactions.

The most common visual problems vary for different ages. Today, brain-damage-related vision problems (cerebral visual impairment [CVI]) are the single most prevalent cause of visual impairment in *infants and young children.* Given that vision is so important for normal development, vision loss in infants constitutes a developmental emergency and should be detected and addressed as early as possible. When a child does not smile back at the mother, the mother may be inclined to leave the baby in its crib, instead of holding him or her to provide extra tactile stimulation to compensate for missing visual stimulation.

At *school age* and later, visual health is critical because reading becomes important for academic development. For *adults,* vision is important for maintaining independence in activities of daily living (ADL) and development of vocational skills. For *seniors,* vision loss may exacerbate other age-related dysfunctions. Studies of the elderly have shown correlations between visual impairment and depression, falls, and reduced longevity. In all of these instances, early detection and early intervention are essential; the primary care physician plays a crucial role in this respect.

Four Aspects of Vision Loss
Vision is a complex phenomenon.

A convenient framework for discussing the various impacts of vision loss is to consider four aspects of visual functioning (Figure 1). At a basic level, we may consider how various external causes may result in *structural changes* to the eyes and the visual pathways. For this aspect, the focus is on the tissue; an ocular pathologist is needed to describe the pathologic condition. However, structural changes alone do not determine how well the eyes actually function. Clinicians need to measure various *organ functions,* such as visual acuity, visual field, and contrast sensitivity.

Yet even knowing how the eyes function does not tell us how the person functions. In other words, the *abilities* of the person to perform tasks, such as reading, mobility, face recognition, and ADL, must be considered. Occupational therapists (OTs) and other rehabilitation professionals work with patients to teach them how residual vision can be used most effectively. OTs also assess the person in a societal context. For example, do the visual

changes have an impact on the person's *participation* in society, on his or her ability to perform necessary tasks, and on general satisfaction with one's quality of life? It is clear that to cover all aspects of vision rehabilitation, a team approach is necessary and that the patient must be part of that team.

A single ADL may cover several of the above aspects. When reading, the aspect of minimum print size falls under organ function (retinal resolution). Reading speed (words/minute) and reading endurance (hours/day) define abilities of the person; reading endurance may be poor, even if reading acuity is adequate. Reading enjoyment, finally, falls under the aspect of quality of life.

It is helpful to draw a line between the organ side of Figure 1 on the left and the person side on the right. On the left side of the diagram, we discuss *visual functions,* which describe how each eye functions. On the right side, we speak of *functional vision,* which describes how the person functions in vision-related activities. Medical specialists are well versed in dealing with the left side of the diagram. Yet the ultimate goal of all interventions is to improve the patient's quality of life. It is the function of vision rehabilitation to make sure that "eye" doctors become "people" doctors by extending their interest to the right side of the diagram as well.

Comprehensive Vision Rehabilitation
Considering all of these aspects, comprehensive vision rehabilitation involves much more than the patient's performance on a letter chart and requires teamwork by different professionals who specialize in different aspects of vision loss. All vision loss starts with some medical condition, so primary care physicians are well positioned to coordinate team activities. Primary care physicians need to be aware of what other team members can contribute and should know where to locate vision rehabilitation resources and to make appropriate referrals.

Figure 2 illustrates that comprehensive vision rehabilitation involves much more than the traditional optical low vision care offered in the past, and is still relevant today.

Low vision is a term used to describe individuals whose vision (with appropriate optical correction) is less than normal (low) but who are not blind (vision). Unfortunately, many people in this category do not yet receive the services they need. Such services should include adequate refractive, medical, and surgical care as well as rehabilitative care. The latter may include vision enhancement, vision substitution, and vision assistance as well as the honing of coping skills.

Vision enhancement, which is the traditional focus of low vision care, is primarily oriented at improving residual visual

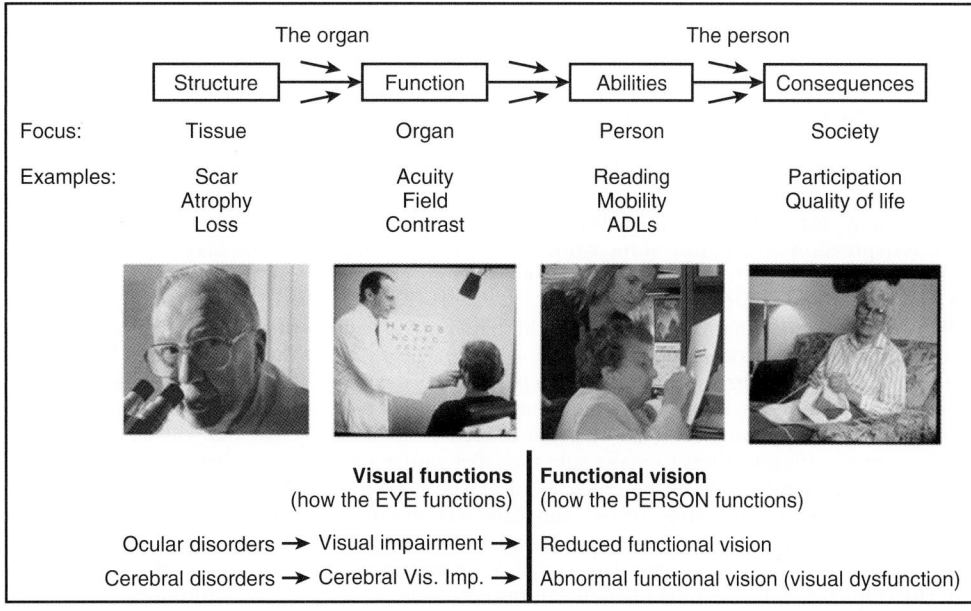

Figure 1 Aspects of vision loss.

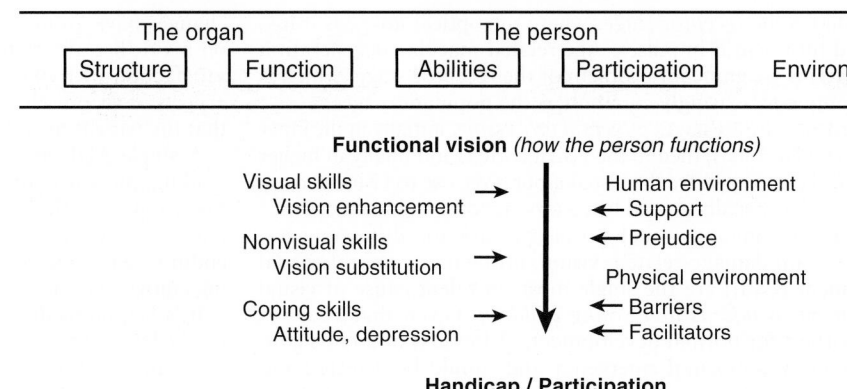

| Structure | Function | Abilities | Participation | Environment |

Functional vision (how the person functions)

Visual skills
  Vision enhancement →   Human environment
                              ← Support
Nonvisual skills   ← Prejudice
  Vision substitution →
                            Physical environment
Coping skills   →   ← Barriers
  Attitude, depression   ← Facilitators

Handicap / Participation

Figure 2 Comprehensive vision rehabilitation.

function through visual aids, including a wide range of magnification devices. Additionally, enhancement of contrast, illumination, and filters need to be explored.

Low vision is distinct from blindness (i.e., no vision). For blindness, the emphasis of rehabilitation is entirely on vision substitution. Patients with severe or profound low vision may combine the use of low vision rehabilitation skills with some blindness rehabilitation skills.

Vision substitution expands the options for rehabilitation by optimizing the use of other senses. This can range from using simple tactile markings to sense the position of a stove dial to devices such as talking books, a long cane for travel, and braille for reading. Vision enhancement and vision substitution are not mutually exclusive. A patient may use a magnifier to read price tags and may prefer talking books for recreational reading. A patient with retinitis pigmentosa, which causes reduced night vision, may have normal mobility in the daytime and need a cane at night. Digital audio books may have braille labels.

Vision assistance. A special form of vision substitution involves using the eyes of others. Family members, caregivers, and office personnel should be familiar with *sighted guide* techniques to effectively assist visually impaired patients with minimal embarrassment. *Guide dogs* are also a possibility. Using a guide dog requires training of the patient as well as of the dog so that they can work as a team. Dog users must also demonstrate mastery of long cane travel skills.

Coping skills. How different patients will accept visual aids may differ greatly. It is important to recognize that vision loss often causes a reactive depression. On the one hand, a depressed patient will be less receptive to rehabilitative suggestions. On the other hand, demonstration of rehabilitative success can be a powerful tool to lift a reactive depression and to motivate the patient for further success. It has been shown that the teaching of general problem-solving skills may improve the effectiveness of vision rehabilitation.

Many professionals may be involved in vision rehabilitation. Technicians may prescribe various magnifiers, rehabilitation workers may teach daily living skills, and psychologists may address depression. Acceptance of the work of these professionals will be improved if the trusted primary care physician is credited with making the referrals.

Beyond the factors that directly involve the patient, the environment must also be considered.

The *human environment* is important. As patients go through the stages of adaptation, a supportive home environment is essential. As patients are counseled, it is important to include spouses, children, or significant others to make sure that they understand the condition, know what can be expected, and know how to support the patient. Answering family and caregiver questions directly is often better than leaving this to the patient, who initially may not have absorbed everything that was said. An overprotective environment, which deprives patients of opportunities to do things for themselves, can be as detrimental as an overdemanding one that puts too much emphasis on the patient's shortcomings. The same holds true for the work or school environment and for social groups.

Initially, patients often feel isolated and believe that they are the only ones experiencing these problems. *Peer support groups* can be helpful; in these groups, patients can experience how others are dealing with similar problems.

Finally, the *physical environment* needs to be considered. An uncluttered environment, where things have a defined, fixed place is helpful because it reduces the need for searching. Good general illumination and task lighting often help, because at higher illumination levels retinal cells that are damaged but not dead can still contribute to vision. Good contrast is important: Do not serve milk in a white Styrofoam cup; mark the edges of steps and stairs. The triangles and circles on men's and women's bathrooms are designed to be visible for those with very low vision; braille labels in elevators are useful for people who are totally blind.

How Blind Is Blind?

The most common visual function test is the letter chart, developed by Snellen in 1862. That test determines how large a letter, or other symbol, must be to be recognized by the patient. That size is then compared with the size recognized by a standard observer. If the magnification requirement is 2×, visual acuity is said to be 1/2; if it is 5×, visual acuity is said to be 1/5, etc. That fraction can be recorded in different ways; in the United States, it is customary to use 20 as the numerator (1/2 = 20/40, 1/5 = 20/100); in the British Commonwealth, 6 is used as the numerator (6/12, 6/30); in Europe, decimal fractions are common (0.5, 0.2).

Those calculations are simple; unfortunately, the terminology used to describe various ranges of vision loss is confusing. Figure 3 shows progressively degraded pictures with examples of the terminology used to describe different degrees of visual impairment. The visual acuity level represented by each picture can be determined from the number of lines that are readable on the low vision letter chart.

The first picture shows the visual acuity level that is labeled as "low vision" by the World Health Organization (WHO). Although the bottom lines of the letter chart cannot be read, the appearance of the room is near normal. The next picture shows what the US Social Security Administration considers "statutory blindness" for its programs. Although reading regular print is not possible without magnification devices, it is clear that this is far from actual blindness. Other US programs use a different definition for "legal blindness," and the WHO does not consider a person "blind" until he or she has reached the status of the last picture. At that level, reading even the special letter chart is not possible, but one can still navigate the room. Even this level of visual impairment does not constitute actual blindness.

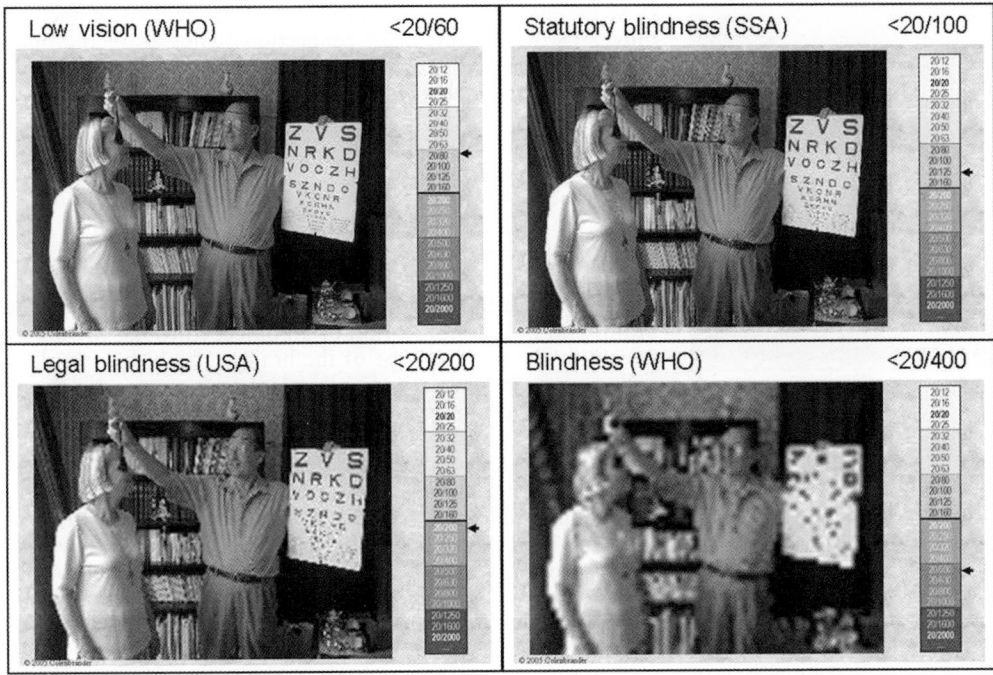

Figure 3 Ranges of vision loss.

The widespread use of the word "blindness" is unfortunate because it cannot be used with modifiers. One is either blind or sighted; one cannot be "a little bit blind." This black-and-white thinking has hampered the acceptance of vision rehabilitation. Terms such as *vision loss* or *visual impairment* are preferred because they can be used with modifiers, including mild, moderate, severe, profound, and total vision loss. Although "legal blindness" and "severe vision loss" (ICD-9-CM) have the same definition, there is a big difference between telling a patient "you *are* legally blind" and "you *have* a severe visual impairment." The first statement might be followed by "I am sorry, there is nothing more we can do for your eyes"; the second statement leads to the question, "What can we do to help you cope with this problem?"

Vision Rehabilitation Techniques and Devices

Having considered the general outlines of vision rehabilitation, some details of rehabilitative interventions can be discussed. Primary care physicians should know what vision rehabilitation techniques are available so that they can make appropriate referrals.

Optical Problems

The most commonly encountered visual problems are those involving the optical system of the eye.

Refractive errors are the easiest visual problems to deal with. Refractive errors can be corrected with glasses or contact lenses, and for those who hate glasses, by refractive surgery. Even if there are other causes of vision loss, determining the best refractive correction is still important.

Uncorrected refractive error accounts for about half of all visual impairment worldwide. In developed countries, the question may be why people do not avail themselves of the solutions that are available. In developing countries, availability and accessibility of eye care and of the means for correcting refractive errors often do not exist. Providing these services is a matter of infrastructure, not of individual healthcare.

Opacities disrupt visual image formation. Cataracts are the most familiar opacity; they can be removed by surgery. Other opacities of a temporary or permanent nature may occur in the cornea, in the anterior chamber, or in the vitreous cavity. Corneal and conjunctival infections may cause corneal scarring, as is the case in trachoma, a condition that does not exist in the developed world anymore but is still a major cause of vision loss worldwide.

Letter chart acuity is a good way to measure optical problems. It should be understood, however, that letter chart acuity only measures the function of the retinal area where the letter read is projected. Even for a patient with 20/200 acuity, this area is less than 1 degree in diameter. For optical problems this does not matter because foveal defocus predicts equal defocus in all other areas of the retina. For retinal problems, however, visual acuity alone is not sufficient to characterize the visual status.

Magnification is the primary way to compensate for reduced acuity. One way to provide magnification is to bring print closer to the eye. For older adults, this requires reading glasses with extra power. Alternatively, large print may be helpful. Larger print on medicine labels, as required in several states, can reduce medication errors by older adults, who often take several medications. Handheld magnifiers are another option; today, many have built-in LED illumination to provide more light. Video-magnifiers with a table-mounted large screen are ideal for prolonged reading; they can also enhance contrast and brightness, while some devices can even read the text out loud. Tablets, smartphone apps, and dedicated devices can provide similar advantages in a portable form. Today, these electronic means of magnification are increasingly popular because they can provide not only magnification but also contrast enhancement. They also have a larger field of view and allow a more comfortable reading distance with binocular viewing.

Retinal Problems

While primitive forms of cataract surgery have existed for centuries, the study of retinal disorders has only been possible since the invention of the ophthalmoscope in 1851. The ability to effectively treat some retinal disorders is even more recent. Important retinal disorders include the following.

Age-related macular degeneration (AMD) is the most frequent diagnosis encountered in low vision rehabilitation services in the Western world. Because the condition is age-related, its frequency will increase in the future as our population ages. This has caused profound changes in the nature of low vision care. Until the mid-20th century, most low vision care was provided by special education teachers serving young students in schools for the blind. Today, the majority of low vision patients are seniors. This has resulted in a significant influx of OTs into the field with skills in addressing multiple geriatric impairments. Yet the needs of seniors to be served still outstrip the available services.

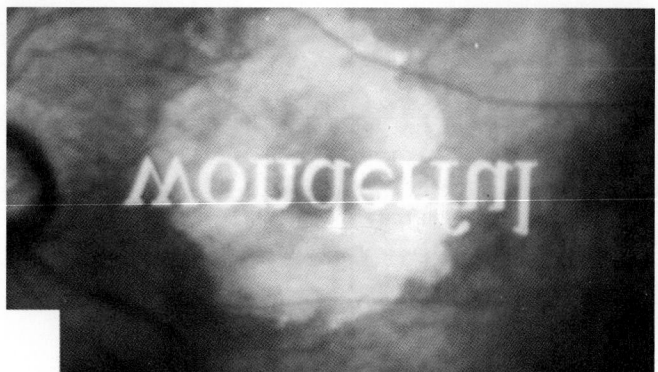

Figure 4 Ring scotoma.

Given that macular degeneration affects central vision and the ability to read, most patients will ultimately seek rehabilitation help. However, if only one eye is affected, AMD may go unnoticed. The patient may only complain when the second eye starts to deteriorate; at that point, the damage in the first eye may be beyond repair. Therefore, it is useful to ask patients to periodically cover each eye to see whether there is any vision difference between the eyes. If there is, this is a reason for referral.

Glaucoma is another age-related condition. It causes loss of peripheral vision and affects central vision only in the late stages. Glaucoma often goes undetected because patients are not spontaneously aware of visual field loss, as little as they are spontaneously aware of an increased blood pressure. Therefore, glaucoma must be sought out, primarily by measuring the intraocular pressure.

Diabetic retinopathy is not limited to seniors. As the incidence of diabetes is rising worldwide, so is the incidence of diabetic retinopathy. Even if treated adequately, it will cause scattered blind spots throughout the visual field.

There are many other hereditary and nonhereditary retinal conditions that may cause vision loss, but they occur in smaller numbers. They all require the help of vision rehabilitation professionals to help patients cope effectively.

Scotomata. Whatever the cause, retinal conditions will generally cause localized blind spots (scotomata). Therefore, when retinal damage is suspected, visual acuity alone is no longer a sufficient descriptor of visual impairment because the retinal area where the letter chart symbol is projected does not predict anything about other retinal areas. In addition to letter chart acuity, the condition of the visual field and the presence of blind spots (scotomata) must be considered (Figure 4).

Figure 4 shows a retinal image, where a word is projected across a ring scotoma that leaves only a small central island of vision. This patient will be able to recognize the central letter but will not be able to read the word. Clinicians must be careful when providing such patients with magnification because too much magnification will mean that fewer letters fit into the central area. This example also makes it clear that when retinal involvement is suspected, a reading test may be more informative than a letter chart test, given that reading requires a larger retinal area.

Neural Processing Problems
As stated earlier, the most important stages of the visual process take place after the retinal receptors have translated the optical image into neural impulses.

The first transformations take place in the *inner retina*. Here, the input from 100 M receptors in each eye is preprocessed and compressed for transmission through 1 M nerve fibers in each optic nerve. The optic nerve fibers do not simply transmit a pixel-by-pixel image, as does a digital camera. Different retinal ganglion cells probably transmit different aspects of the image, such as edges, movement, color, brightness, and so on. These separate "movies" are transmitted in parallel. At a later stage of neural processing, these different aspects of the image are merged again to contribute to a single visual perception.

At the first synaptic station in the lateral geniculate nucleus, only 20% of the incoming connections come from the optic nerves; the other 80% come from other cortical centers and probably contribute to filtering based on attention and other factors.

In the visual cortex, the visual information is analyzed for shapes and contours. In higher cortical centers, the visual information is further processed. Here, the flow of information is no longer strictly visual because it is combined with information from other senses. This results in identification and recognition of objects through comparison to stored concepts (through the ventral stream to the temporal lobe of the brain) and in spatial location of an object (through the dorsal stream to the parietal lobe of the brain), which then result in voluntary or involuntary visually guided action.

Our knowledge of these processes is still relatively new. It has been greatly helped by new modalities for neural and retinal imaging. Today, neural processing problems are increasingly recognized in all age groups.

In young children, CVI is now recognized as the most frequent cause of visual perceptual problems. CVI is often caused by perinatal ischemia, which may cause cortical as well as subcortical changes (periventricular leukomalacia). Because this ischemia is not localized, impairments are often not limited to the visual system. Schools for the blind have increasingly developed into schools for children with multiple disabilities.

In contact sports, the results of repeated subclinical injuries are now recognized.

In veterans, traumatic brain injuries may cause problems that may be hard to define. Often visual interpretation and decision making are impaired; oculomotor system problems are often found. Traffic accidents may cause similar damage.

In older adults, strokes may cause more localized problems and agnosias for specific tasks. In all of these cases, the term *visual impairment* may be used when visual acuity and/or visual field are impaired. The term *visual dysfunction* may be more appropriate when the visual input from the eyes to the brain is normal but the processing of this information in the brain is not.

Patient-Centered Functional Priorities
Vision problems affect all aspects of a patient's life. It is no longer sufficient for clinicians to determine that nothing more can be done about the *causes* of vision loss, because much more can be done about the *consequences* of vision impairment.

To determine the range of services that may be appropriate for an individual with vision impairment, the American Academy of Ophthalmology recommends consideration of the following functional priority areas:

- Reading—for many patients, this is their foremost concern.
- ADL—even though reading may be the most prominent complaint, most people spend the larger part of their day performing vision-dependent activities other than reading for self-care and home management.
- Safety—Patients with visual field loss must be made explicitly aware of this loss and the problems it may cause in navigating the environment. Are they at risk for falls? How do they cross the street? Do they drive?
- Community participation—can the individual still participate in community events, including religious gatherings?
- Physical, cognitive, and psychosocial well-being—because many patients with vision loss are older, this is an important aspect that should not be overlooked. If cognitive problems exist, it may affect the recommendations to be made.

Based on these considerations, patient-centered priorities can be set and specific rehabilitation goals formulated that reflect the patient's needs and desires. The primary care physician can then make appropriate referrals for rehabilitation.

References

American Academy of Ophthalmology: The Academy's Initiative in Vision Rehabilitation. Available at www.aao.org/low-vision-and-vision-rehab Verified 2021-03-28.

Bourne RA, et al: Magnitude, temporal trends, and projections of the global prevalence of blindness and distance and near vision impairment: a systematic review and meta-analysis, et al. *Lancet Glob Health* 5(9):e888–e897, 2017.

Colenbrander A: Measuring vision and vision loss. In Tasman W, Jaeger EA, editors: *Duane's Ophthalmology*, Vol. 5. Philadelphia, 2013, Lippincott Williams & Wilkins.

Colenbrander A: Towards the development of a classification of vision-related functioning—a potential framework. In Dutton GH, Bax M, editors: *Visual Impairment in Children Due to Damage to the Brain*, London, 2010, Mac Keith Press.

Fletcher DC, Schuchard RA: Preferred retinal loci relationship to macular scotomas in a low-vision population, *Ophthalmology* 104:632–638, 1997.

Fletcher DC, Schuchard RA, Watson G: Relative locations of macular scotomas near the PRL: effect on low vision reading, *J Rehabil Res Dev* 36:356–364, 1999.

Schoessow KA: Shifting from compensation to participation: a model for occupational therapy in low vision, *Br J Occup Ther* 73:160–169, 2010.

Additional Website Sources

The AFB website (www.AFB.org) has information for all age groups, including a section on aging.

The MDsupport website (www.MDsupport.org) specializes in support and documentation for AMD patients and care givers.

The Lighthouse Guild International in New York (www.lighthouseguild.org) offers extensive resources for all forms of vision loss.

These websites contain links to many more websites with additional information and often can provide information about local resources.

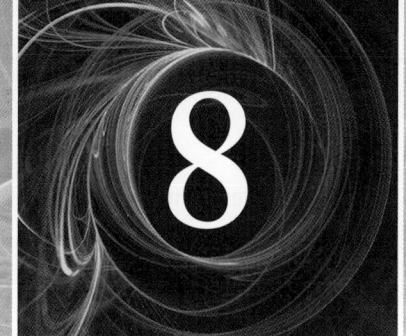

8 Infectious Diseases

AMEBIASIS

Method of
Koji Watanabe, MD, PhD

CURRENT DIAGNOSIS (SEE ALSO BOX 1)

- Amebiasis is transmitted by the ingestion of fecally contaminated water or food and by high-risk sexual behaviors (men who have sex with men [MSM] or oral–anal sexual contact).
- Although self-limiting mild to moderate colitis is the most common disease presentation, various severe illnesses (liver abscess, peritonitis, pleurisy, and pericarditis) can also occur.
- Diagnostic value of microscopic stool or abscess ova and parasite examination (O&P) is low. Antigen detection in stool shows high sensitivity for severely diarrheal and/or dysentery cases (amebic colitis), but shows relatively low sensitivity for mild colitis or asymptomatic cases. Serology shows high sensitivity but cannot distinguish current infection from past infection, and it is ideally used in conjunction with fecal antigen detection or polymerase chain reaction (PCR).

CURRENT THERAPY (SEE ALSO BOX 2)

- Infected individuals who are asymptomatic should be treated with a luminal agent (e.g., paromomycin), because they can be a source of new infection and can develop invasive amebiasis after long-term asymptomatic infection.
- Mild to severe colitis and extraintestinal disease require initial treatment with a tissue-active agent (e.g., metronidazole) followed by a luminal agent.
- Reinfection can occur frequently in endemic settings. The clinician should discuss methods to prevent re-exposure to *Entamoeba histolytica* with treated patients.

Epidemiology and Risk Factors for Acquisition

Amebiasis is transmitted by oral ingestion of the transmissible cyst form of *Entamoeba histolytica* in human stools. Transmission occurs by the ingestion of fecally contaminated food and water, mainly in developing countries. It also transmits directly from human to human by sexual contact or in institutions for the cognitively impaired. Food- or water-borne infection occurs in settings of poor sanitation. It is estimated to be the second most common cause of parasite infection–related mortality worldwide, accounting for 40,000 to 70,000 deaths annually. In developed countries, people who travel to or immigrate from developing countries are at higher risk for this parasitic disease. In the United States, amebiasis is the second most common cause of diarrhea in returning travelers. However, over the last two decades amebic infection has been increasingly reported as a sexually transmitted infection in East Asian developed countries and Australia. In one report from Taiwan, men who have sex with men (MSM) and people engaging in oral–anal sex were more likely to be seropositive for *E. histolytica*. While older studies from the United States have shown that amebiasis in MSM was due to nonpathogenic *Entamoeba dispar*, more recently MSM was shown to be an independent risk factor for amebiasis-related mortality. Also, *E. histolytica* infection has been reported as a common comorbidity among HIV-infected MSM or as a sexually transmitted infection in developed European countries. It is important for primary care physicians to take detailed histories of sexual behavior as well as travel whenever amebiasis is suspected.

Pathophysiology and Susceptible Host Factors to Invasive Diseases

E. histolytica has two different forms: the tissue-invasive "trophozoite form" and the infectious "cyst form," which is responsible for transmission. Cysts are notable for environmental stability, demonstrating considerable resistance to chlorination and desiccation, with several outbreaks resulting from the contamination of drinking water. Once cysts are ingested, excystation occurs at the terminal ileum or large intestine, forming motile trophozoites. Trophozoites bind to the mucous layer and the underlying intestinal epithelial cells via a parasite Gal/GalNAc lectin. Blockade of activity of the Gal/Gal lectin prevents contact-dependent cytolysis. Moreover, it has been shown that antilectin IgA in stool or breast milk has a protective effect against future acquisition of amebic infection in cohort studies. These results indicate that the Gal/GalNAc lectin plays a crucial role in amebic infection.

Host factors are also important for susceptibility to amebiasis. Amebiasis is more common in malnourished children, and the nutritional hormone leptin is protective, with a single nucleotide mutation of leptin receptor being the predominant genetic factor controlling amebiasis susceptibility in Bangladeshi children. Amebic liver abscess (ALA) is 10 times more common in men than in women and is uncommon in children. Also, the very young or old, malnourished people, pregnant women, and patients using corticosteroids are at increased risk of severe amebiasis.

Clinical Manifestations and Complications of Amebiasis

Asymptomatic self-limiting infection is the most common disease form of amebiasis. Up to 80% to 90% of people exposed to cysts have no or mild symptoms and clear the infection spontaneously. However, asymptomatic infection persists for a long time in some individuals who are reported as asymptomatic cyst passers or as fecal occult blood–positive, which is incidentally diagnosed by colonoscopy. These asymptomatically infected individuals can be a source of a new infection in the community. Also, some develop symptomatic invasive diseases after long-term latent infection.

Symptomatic intestinal amebiasis (amebic colitis) generally has a subacute onset. Usually it takes 1 to 3 weeks from disease onset to make a diagnosis. Abdominal symptoms range from mild diarrhea to severe dysentery with abdominal pain, diarrhea, and bloody stools. Weight loss and fever are common but not universal symptoms. Intestinal fistula or perforation of the large intestine, resulting in peritonitis, is a rare but life-threatening complication of intestinal amebiasis. Toxic megacolon also can be caused by amebiasis. Amebic colitis sometimes mimics acute appendicitis. In this situation, appendectomy without amebicidal treatment may result in severe postoperative complications, such as abdominal sepsis, gastrointestinal fistula, or hemorrhage. Periodic acid–Schiff (PAS) stain, or ideally, immunoperoxidase with anti-E. histolytica antibodies, in addition to routine hematoxylin and eosin (H&E) stain can help to identify the parasite by the histopathology. Thus, intestinal amebiasis sometimes presents as severe and complicated clinical illnesses.

E. histolytica infection also may have extraintestinal dissemination. Liver abscess is the most common form of extraintestinal amebiasis. Patients usually present with 1 to 2 weeks of fever with or without right upper quadrant abdominal pain. Other common symptoms may include cough, sweating, malaise, weight loss, anorexia, and hiccough. Two-thirds of patients lack intestinal symptoms. Physical examination reveals hepatomegaly and tenderness over the liver in approximately half of cases. Complications can occur by direct invasion of trophozoites or the indirect effect of inflammation. Up to 10% of patients with ALA have accompanying thoracic amebiasis (pleuritic and pleural effusion). Pericarditis is the next most common form of extraintestinal amebiasis; it may result from rupture of a liver abscess in the left lobe or through extension of pleural amebiasis. Cerebral amebic abscesses are a rare form of extraintestinal amebiasis; they usually accompany other metastatic lesions, such as liver abscesses and thoracic amebiasis.

Thus, amebiasis can have various clinical presentations. The diagnosis can be very difficult to make in severe cases and in atypical clinical presentations because of secondary bacterial infection at the site of amebic invasion.

Diagnosis

Sensitivity of each diagnostic test is shown in Box 1. Although microscopic stool ova and parasite examination (O&P) is frequently used in many countries including the United States, it has low sensitivity. Identification of trophozoites by microscope in aspirated fluid from amebic abscess is more challenging because trophozoites are present only at the edge of the abscess. Moreover, microscopic examination cannot distinguish pathogenic E. histolytica from nonpathogenic E. dispar or Entamoeba moshkovskii by shape.

Currently, the combination of antigen detection in stool and/ or sera and serologic testing is the best diagnostic pathway. Antigen detection in feces by the TechLab E. histolytica II enzyme-linked immunosorbent assay (ELISA) is rapid to perform (<2 hours) and can distinguish E. histolytica from E. dispar and E. moshkovskii. These antigen tests have highly sensitive diagnostic value for amebic colitis, that is, Bristol stool scale 6 or 7 (60% to 95%), whereas sensitivity is relatively low for asymptomatic carrier, that is, Bristol stool scale 5 or lower (20% to 50%). In one report, when used on patients' sera, ELISA showed high sensitivity in ALA cases but only before metronidazole treatment began. Real-time polymerase chain reaction (PCR) in stool is superior in sensitivity to stool antigen detection, but is still technically complex for diagnostic use in clinical settings. Serologic tests are sensitive (approximately 90% during the convalescent phase) and noninvasive diagnostic tools for amebiasis. Antibodies are detectable in 70% or more of patients within 5 to 7 days of acute infection and persist for years after treatment. Therefore, a negative serologic result is helpful for exclusion of disease, whereas a positive result cannot distinguish between present and previous infection.

Histopathologic examination using biopsy or resected samples is sometimes useful for the diagnosis of intestinal amebiasis. As mentioned, PAS stain in addition to H&E can increase sensitivity in detection of Entamoeba. However, identification of Entamoeba in biopsy specimens is often challenging. About half of cases with gross ulcerative lesions in the large intestine, in which E. histolytica was proven by PCR, had a negative result on histopathology.

Therapy

Recommended treatment regimens are shown in Box 2. Therapy for invasive infection differs from therapy for noninvasive

---

BOX 1 Sensitivity of Tests for Diagnosis of Amebiasis.*

Test	Colitis	Liver Abscess
Microscopy (stool)	25%–60%	10%–40%
Stool antigen detection (e.g., E. histolytica II enzyme-linked immunosorbent assay (ELISA)	80%	40%
Serum antigen detection	65%	>95%
Microscopy (abscess fluid)	N/A	<20%
Real time polymerase chain reaction	>95%	>95%
Serologic testing (indirect hemagglutination)		
Acute	70%	70%–80%
Convalescent	>90%	>90%
Histopathology by biopsy	45%	N/A

*Before the initiation of therapy.
Modified from Mandell G, Bennett JE, Dolin R, et al. *Mandell, Douglas, and Bennett's Principles and Practice of Infectious Diseases.* 7th ed. Philadelphia: Elsevier Saunders; 2009.

BOX 2 Treatment Recommendations for Amebiasis in Adults.

Asymptomatically Infected Individuals
Paromomycin (Humatin) 30 mg/kg/d PO tid × 5–10 days
or
Iodoquinol (Yodoxin)[2] 650 mg PO tid × 20 days

Mild to Severe Intestinal and Extraintestinal Disease
Metronidazole (Flagyl)* 750 mg PO tid × 10 days
or
Tinidazole (Tindamax) 2 g PO once daily × 5 days
Followed by
Paromomycin[1] 30 mg/kg/d PO tid × 5–10 days
or
Iodoquinol 650 mg PO tid × 20 days

*Use of intravenous form of metronidazole (500mg q8h) is limited to patients who cannot take oral medications.
[1]Not FDA approved for this indication.
[2]Not available in the United States
Modified from Mandell G, Bennett JE, Dolin R, Blaser MJ. *Mandell, Douglas, and Bennett's Principles and Practice of Infectious Diseases.* 7th ed. Philadelphia: Elsevier Saunders; 2009.

---

infection. Noninvasive infections (treatment for asymptomatically infected individuals) require treatment with luminal-active agents: paromomycin (Humatin) is currently recommended because of its high potency in asymptomatic cyst passers. Recently, it is increasingly reported that macroscopically visible colonic ulcers by E. histolytica are unexpectedly diagnosed from asymptomatic individuals. Treatment for asymptomatic patients with colonic ulcers is currently undetermined; however, tissue-active agents are commonly administered prior to luminal-active agents in reported cases. Future proof of concept study is warranted for appropriate treatment regimen for such cases.

For symptomatic patients, tissue-active agents should be administered before luminal-active agents. Most patients with mild to moderate colitis and uncomplicated liver abscess respond to treatment with tissue-active agents, such as metronidazole (Flagyl) and tinidazole (Tindamax). Tinidazole has the advantage of less frequent dosing than metronidazole. Treatment with tissue-active agents should be followed by luminal-active agents because parasites persist in the intestine in up to 40% to 60% of patients who receive tissue-active agents. Broad-spectrum antibiotics and/ or surgical treatment should be added to tissue-active agents in patients with fulminant colitis in which perforation and peritonitis or bacteremia are suspected. Therapeutic needle aspiration or catheter drainage is not routinely required for uncomplicated liver abscesses. Those interventions in addition to medical treatment are recommended if there is clinical deterioration or lack of response to initial medical treatment, or if alternative diagnoses need to be excluded. Also, some reports suggest that clinicians should consider those interventions for patients with a high risk of abscess rupture, as defined by a cavity with a diameter of more than 5 cm or by the presence of lesions in the left lobe, although these criteria were not conclusive in case-control studies.

Symptoms (diarrhea, dysentery, fever, pain, and tenderness) and laboratory markers (white blood cell counts, red blood cell counts, and C-reactive protein) rapidly improve after effective treatment even in patients with extraintestinal lesions. In contrast, radiologic findings, such as abscess size, often remain unchanged for months after completion of treatment.

Monitoring After Treatment and Disease Prevention

Although routine monitoring after treating amebiasis is not recommended, it is well known that reinfection frequently occurs in endemic situations, including both water- or food-borne infections and sexually transmitted infections. In developed countries, in order to prevent reinfection, it is important for the primary physician to inform patients of behaviors that will place them at risk for acquisition of the cyst and how to avoid them, such as avoiding nonsterilized water or food in developing countries, unsafe homosexual contact, and oral–anal sexual contact. In developing countries, more than 1 billion people still have no access to safe food and water, resulting in the urgent need for an effective vaccine. Induction of acquired mucosal immunity is the current goal for vaccine development. Although there is currently no vaccine in human clinical trials, a vaccine containing the naïve or recombinant Gal/GalNAc lectin of *E. histolytica* has strong immunogenicity and protective effect against amebic colitis and liver abscess in animal models. Continuous effort will be needed to develop an effective vaccine to save the lives of affected people in endemic areas.

References

Barwick RS, Uzicanin A, Lareau S, et al: Outbreak of amebiasis in Tbilisi, Republic of Georgia 1998, *Am J Trop Med Hyg* 67:623–631, 2002.

Blessmann J, Tannich E: Treatment of asymptomatic intestinal *Entamoeba histolytica* infection, *N Engl J Med* 347:184, 2002.

Chavez-Tapia NC, Hernandez-Calleros J, Tellez-Avila FI, et al: Image-guided percutaneous procedure plus metronidazole versus metronidazole alone for uncomplicated amoebic liver abscess, *Cochrane Database Syst Rev* CD004886, 2009.

Duggal P, Guo X, Haque R, et al: A mutation in the leptin receptor is associated with *Entamoeba histolytica* infection in children, *J Clin Invest* 121:1191–1198, 2011.

Gunther J, Shafir S, Bristow B, et al: Short report: amebiasis-related mortality among United States residents, 1990–2007, *Am J Trop Med Hyg* 85:1038–1040, 2011.

Haque R, Mollah NU, Ali IK, et al: Diagnosis of amebic liver abscess and intestinal infection with the TechLab *Entamoeba histolytica* II antigen detection and antibody tests, *J Clin Microbiol* 38:3235–3239, 2000.

Hung CC, Chang SY, Ji DD: Entamoeba histolytica infection in men who have sex with men, *Lancet Infect Dis* 12:729–736, 2012.

Hung CC, Wu PY, Chang SY, et al: Amebiasis among persons who sought voluntary counseling and testing for human immunodeficiency virus infection: a case-control study, *Am J Trop Med Hyg* 84:65–69, 2011.

Kobayashi T, Watanabe K, Yano H, et al: Underestimated Amoebic appendicitis among hiv-1-infected individuals in Japan, *J Clin Microbiol* 55:313–320, 2016.

Korpe PS, Liu Y, Siddique A, et al: Breast milk parasite-specific antibodies and protection from amebiasis and cryptosporidiosis in Bangladeshi infants: a prospective cohort study, *Clin Infect Dis* 56:988–992, 2013.

Leder K, Weller PF: Intestinal and extraintestinal *Entamoeba histolytica* amebiasis. UpToDate. Available at: http://www.uptodate.com/contents/search. [Accessed 22 April 2019].

Petri Jr WA, Haque R: *Entamoeba* species, including amebic colitis and liver abscess. In Bennett JE, Dolin R, Blaser MJ, editors: *Mandell, Douglas, and Bennett's principles and practice of infectious diseases*, ed 8th, Philadelphia, 2015, Elsevier Saunders, pp 3047–3058.

Saidin S, Othman N, Noordin R: Update on laboratory diagnosis of amoebiasis, *Eur J Clin Microbiol Infect Dis* 38:15–38, 2019.

Yanagawa Y, Shimogawara R, Endo T, et al: Utility of the rapid antigen detection test E. histolytica quik chek for the diagnosis of *Entamoeba histolytica* infection in nonendemic situations, *J Clin Microbiol* 58:e01991-20, 2020.

ANTHRAX

Method of
Shingo Chihara, MD

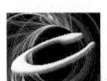

CURRENT DIAGNOSIS

Cutaneous Anthrax
- Incubation period of 1 to 7 days from exposure to cattle
- Painless or pruritic lesion progresses to ulcer and eschar
- Significant swelling
- Gram stain and culture of lesion

Gastrointestinal
- Incubation period of 1 to 6 days after consumption of raw or undercooked meat
- Nonspecific symptoms followed by abdominal pain, ascites
- Diarrhea uncommon
- Obtain blood culture and ascitic fluid for culture and Gram stain

Inhalational
- Incubation period of 1 to 7 days (up to 43 days)
- Biphasic: fever, malaise, myalgia followed by dyspnea
- Widened mediastinum seen on chest x-ray and computed tomography (CT) of chest
- Blood cultures turn positive in most

Injection
- Injection drug use
- Significant swelling seen; eschar rare

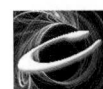

CURRENT THERAPY

Systemic Anthrax With Possible/Confirmed Meningitis
- Ciprofloxacin (Cipro) 400 mg IV every 8 hours or levofloxacin (Levaquin) 750 mg IV every 24 hours or moxifloxacin (Avelox)[1] 400 mg IV every 24 hours
  plus
- Meropenem (Merrem)[1] 2 g IV every 8 hours or imipenem/cilastatin (Primaxin)[1] 1 g IV every 6 hours or doripenem (Doribax)[1] 500 mg IV every 8 hours
- If penicillin-susceptible strains, then penicillin G 4 million units IV every 4 hours or ampicillin[1] 3 g IV every 6 hours could be an alternative to carbapenems
  plus
- Linezolid (Zyvox)[1] 600 mg IV every 12 hours or clindamycin (Cleocin) 900 mg IV every 8 hours or rifampin (Rifadin) 600 mg IV every 12 hours or chloramphenicol 1 g every 6 to 8 hours

Systemic Anthrax When Meningitis Has Been Excluded
- Ciprofloxacin 400 mg IV every 8 hours or levofloxacin 750 mg IV every 24 hours or moxifloxacin[1] 400 mg IV every 24 hours
  or
- Meropenem[1] 2 g IV every 8 hours or imipenem/cilastatin[1] 1 g IV every 6 hours or doripenem[1] 500 mg IV every 8 hours
  or
- Vancomycin (Vancocin)[1] 60 mg/kg/day IV divided every 8 hours (goal trough 15–20 µg/mL)
  or
- If penicillin-susceptible strains, then penicillin G 4 million units IV every 4 hours or ampicillin[1] 3 g IV every 6 hours
  plus
- Clindamycin[1] 900 mg IV every 8 hours or linezolid[1] 600 mg IV every 12 hours
  or

Anthrax has been described for centuries and the name is derived from Greek for "burnt coal" owing to eschar formation from cutaneous anthrax. Anthrax is rarely seen in developed countries, including the United States, but it is important to be aware of this condition because of its potential as a bioterrorism agent. When anthrax is suspected, the clinician needs to contact the local or state health department immediately. Anthrax has historical significance because it was the agent used in Koch's postulate during the 19th century when Koch proved that *Bacillus anthracis* is responsible for anthrax in cattle.

Background

B. anthracis is the bacterium responsible for anthrax. It forms spores that can survive in soil for years. It is hyperendemic in the Middle East and in sub-Saharan Africa. Systemic anthrax is primarily a disease of grazing animals. In naturally-acquired anthrax, humans are accidentally infected from exposure to the animal or its products.

Epidemiology

Since the mid-20th century, there has been a precipitous decline in anthrax owing to animal and human vaccines, improvement in factory hygiene, sterilization procedures for imported animal products, and increased use of alternatives to animal hides or hair. Cutaneous anthrax comprises over 95% of naturally-acquired human anthrax and there are an estimated 2000 cases annually. Between 1900 and 2001 there were 18 cases of inhalational anthrax in the United States, of which 16 were fatal. Over the last decade, there have been several cases of inhalational and cutaneous anthrax related to African drum makers. In late 2001, there were 22 cases of anthrax in the United States from spores delivered in the mail, of which five were fatal. In 1979, accidental release of dried anthrax spores from a biologic weapons facility in Sverdlovsk in the former Soviet Union resulted in 68 deaths from inhalation anthrax.

Pathophysiology

B. anthracis is a gram-positive, encapsulated, spore forming, nonmotile, nonhemolytic, nonmotile rod-shaped bacterium. Infection with anthrax requires three components: the edema factor, the lethal factor, and protective antigen. The edema factor combines with protective antigen and becomes edema toxin, which causes edema and impairment of the immune system. The lethal factor combines with protective antigen and becomes lethal toxin, which causes lysis of macrophages. For cutaneous anthrax, these exotoxins result in extensive edema and tissue necrosis locally. In inhalation anthrax, spores that reach the alveoli or alveolar ducts are phagocytized by the alveolar macrophage and transported to the mediastinal lymph nodes where they replicate and cause hemorrhagic mediastinitis. With gastrointestinal tract infection, *B. anthracis* is transported from the gastrointestinal tract to mesenteric lymph nodes where they multiply and cause mesenteric lymphadenitis, ascites, and sepsis.

Clinical Manifestations

There are four distinct clinical presentations: cutaneous, inhalation, gastrointestinal tract, and injection anthrax, depending on the site of entry. Meningitis is a devastating complication that could occur with any of the four infections.

Cutaneous Anthrax

Cutaneous anthrax is the most common form and seen in developing countries as a result of contact with infected animals or animal products such as wool, hair, or hides. Spores invade through either skin abrasions or hair follicles. Subsequently, they germinate and multiply. The incubation period is commonly 5 to 7 days with range of 1 to 19 days. The lesions appear in exposed areas such as head, neck, forearms, and hands and begin as a small, painless papule. They are pruritic at times and form blisters. Subsequently, they evolve into painless necrotic ulcers with a black, depressed eschar with extensive edema and lymphadenopathy.

Inhalation Anthrax

Inhalation anthrax occurs when spores are aerosolized while working with contaminated animal products or when they are released intentionally in bioterrorism. The incubation period is 1 to 7 days but could be as long as 43 days. The course of disease is usually biphasic. Initially, nonspecific symptoms such as fever, malaise, and myalgia are present, resembling influenza. These symptoms last for several days before the bacteremic phase starts. The manifestations include rapidly, fulminant progressive respiratory symptoms such as severe dyspnea, as well as hypoxemia and shock. Once in this phase, the patient dies within a few days despite support in the intensive care unit. Therefore it is important to suspect anthrax in the prodromal phase, which is difficult owing to its rarity and lack of specific symptoms. Widening of the mediastinum on a chest x-ray may be helpful in establishing the diagnosis. This finding was seen in 7 out of 10 cases of inhalation anthrax from 2001. Hilar abnormalities, pulmonary infiltrates, or consolidation and pleural effusion may be seen.

Gastrointestinal Tract Anthrax

Gastrointestinal tract anthrax occurs after ingestion of raw or undercooked meat from an animal infected with anthrax. Gastrointestinal infection is relatively common and has been reported from mouth to ascending colon. The incubation period is 1 to 6 days. Initially, nonspecific symptoms such as asthenia, headache, low-grade fever, facial flushing and conjunctival injection occur. They are followed by abdominal pain, abdominal distention from ascites, nausea, and vomiting. Diarrhea occurs less frequently. As the disease progresses, abdominal pain becomes severe and findings of hypotension and intravascular depletion are seen. When the infection occurs in the oropharynx, necrotic ulcers with pseudomembranes cause pain and edema.

Injection Anthrax

An outbreak of injection anthrax was described in 2009. It was reported in Scotland among injection heroin users. Among the 47 confirmed cases, typical eschar formation seen in cutaneous anthrax was not seen in all but one case. Prominent edema was seen in most patients and some developed compartment syndrome.

Meningitis

Meningitis is a complication seen with all forms of anthrax. About half of patients with inhalation anthrax develop hemorrhagic meningitis. Symptoms such as altered mental status, seizures, cranial nerve palsies, and myoclonus may be seen. When anthrax is suspected, lumbar puncture should be done on presentation unless there are contraindications.

Diagnosis

When diagnosis of anthrax is suspected, the provider must notify the local department of health and the clinical microbiology laboratory. There has been reported transmission of anthrax to laboratory personnel handling *B. anthracis* and specimen handling in biosafety level 3 facilities is recommended. Because the genus *Bacillus* is part of the normal skin flora, it is crucial for the microbiology laboratory to distinguish *B. anthracis* from other non-*anthracis* species of *Bacillus*. Conventional culture and staining are used for distinction. *B. anthracis* is nonmotile and nonhemolytic and those characteristics are used to distinguish it from non-*anthracis* species of *Bacillus*. Most microbiology laboratories have the ability to make a presumptive identification of an organism, and the identification is confirmed by a reference laboratory.

Specimen Collection

When collecting clinical specimens for suspected anthrax, proper personal protective equipment such as disposable gloves, disposable aprons, and boots, should be used. When there is any potential of aerosolization of spores, then face shields and respirators are recommended. Hand washing with soap and water will reduce the endospore contamination of the skin, but alcohol handrubs are not effective against these endospores. For cutaneous anthrax, the edge of the eschar should be lifted, and two specimens of vesicular fluid should be collected by rotating a swab. One swab will be used for culture and Gram stain while the other would be used for polymerase chain reaction (PCR). Punch biopsy of the cutaneous lesion is an alternative. When inhalational anthrax is suspected, blood cultures must be obtained prior to use of antibiotics. If pleural fluid is present, then thoracentesis should be performed for Gram stain, culture, and PCR. For alimentary tract anthrax, blood cultures must be obtained. If there are oral lesions, then specimens could be collected with swabs similar to a cutaneous lesion. If ascites is present, then paracentesis should be performed for Gram stain, culture and PCR. For meningitis, cerebrospinal fluid (CSF) should be collected for culture, Gram stain and PCR.

There are unique findings observed in routine laboratories with systemic anthrax. Marked hemoconcentration may be seen in the complete blood count, and the initial white blood cell count is frequently within normal limits. In chemistry, decreased sodium, increased blood urea nitrogen, mild transaminitis and hypoalbuminemia are seen. Inflammatory markers such as erythrocyte sedimentation rate and C-reactive protein are elevated in most cases except in cases of injection anthrax, when C-reactive protein is low.

Treatment

Supportive Care

Hospitalization is required for all patients with systemic infections. Only uncomplicated cutaneous anthrax could be treated on an outpatient basis. Close monitoring is warranted because the patient status may deteriorate rapidly. Hemodynamic support should be given, including fluids, vasopressors, blood products, and invasive hemodynamic monitoring. Mechanical ventilation may be needed because of respiratory distress, airway protection for altered mental status, or for airway edema. Adjunctive corticosteroids may be indicated in four situations: patients with history of endocrine or corticosteroid therapy; edema of head or neck; anthrax meningitis; or

vasopressor-resistant shock. Pleural fluid and ascites should be drained aggressively. Surgery is indicated in certain situations. Surgery for cutaneous anthrax has led to dissemination and poor outcome. Therefore, in cutaneous anthrax, indication for surgery is limited to tracheotomy for airway obstruction and surgery for compartment syndrome. In gastrointestinal anthrax, surgery might be considered for complications such as bowel ischemia or infarct and perforation. In injection anthrax, removal of necrotic nidus would help reduce the toxin and spore reservoir.

Antimicrobial Treatment for Systemic Disease with Possible Meningitis

At least three intravenous antibiotics with good penetration to the central nervous system are recommended. At least one drug should have bactericidal activity, and at least one drug should inhibit protein synthesis. These should be continued for at least 2 weeks or until clinically stable, whichever is longer. The fluoroquinolone class is bactericidal, has good penetration to the central nervous system, and has no reported resistance by *B. anthracis*. Intravenous ciprofloxacin (Cipro) is the primary bactericidal component in the treatment of systemic disease. Levofloxacin (Levaquin) and moxifloxacin (Avelox)[1] are considered to be alternatives. The carbapenem class has good central nervous system penetration, and meropenem (Merrem)[1] is the preferred second antibiotic in treatment of systemic disease with possible meningitis. Imipenem/cilastatin (Primaxin)[1] and doripenem (Doribax)[1] are considered alternatives. Penicillin G or ampicillin[1] could be used in place of carbapenems when the isolate is known to have a minimum inhibitory concentration (MIC) of less than 0.125 μg/mL. As for protein synthesis inhibitor, linezolid (Zyvox)[1] is preferred because it provides good central nervous system penetration. If there is contraindication to linezolid use such as drug–drug interaction or myelosuppression, then clindamycin (Cleocin)[1] is the alternative. When both linezolid and clindamycin cannot be used, rifampin (Rifadin)[1] could be used for synergistic effect in combination with the bactericidal drugs. Chloramphenicol is another antibiotic that is a protein synthesis inhibitor. It could be used if linezolid, clindamycin, and rifampin are unavailable. Doxycycline (Vibramycin) is an inhibitor of protein synthesis but does not adequately penetrate the central nervous system. Therefore doxycycline should not be used when meningitis is not ruled out. If the patient had been exposed to aerosolized spores, then the patient should be transitioned to oral antibiotics after completion of initial intravenous combination therapy to prevent relapse from spores.

Antimicrobial Treatment for Systemic Disease when Meningitis is Ruled Out

At least two antimicrobial agents are recommended for systemic anthrax without meningitis. At least one should be bactericidal and at least one should be a protein synthesis inhibitor. This combination should be administered intravenously for at least 2 weeks or until clinically stable, whichever is longer. For penicillin-susceptible strains, penicillin G is considered equivalent to ciprofloxacin. Vancomycin (Vancocin)[1] is an acceptable alternative bactericidal agent. Clindamycin[1] and linezolid[1] are equivalent first choices for protein synthesis inhibitors. Doxycycline is an alternative agent. If the patient had been exposed to aerosolized spores, then the patient should be transitioned to oral antibiotics after completion of initial intravenous combination therapy to prevent relapse from spores.

Treatment for Cutaneous Anthrax without Systemic Involvement

A single oral antibiotic is adequate to treat cutaneous anthrax without systemic involvement. Fluoroquinolones and doxycycline are considered first-line agents. Clindamycin[1] is a second-line agent when first-line agents are unavailable or

---

[1]Not FDA approved for this indication.

contraindicated. Penicillin or amoxicillin[1] may be used if the isolate is found to be sensitive in vitro. It is important to give an adequate dose because resistance may develop when underdosed.

Antitoxins
There are three antitoxins in the Centers for Disease Control and Prevention (CDC) Strategic National stockpile: raxibacumab, obiltoxaximab, and anthrax immune globulin intravenous (AIGIV). These agents are not readily available to the public. They inhibit binding of protective antigen to the anthrax toxin receptor and translocation of lethal factor and edema factor into cells. There are human and animal data from the pre-antibiotic era that suggest that there is lower mortality in those who received the antitoxin in cutaneous anthrax compared with those who did not. Whether this agent should be given for systemic anthrax is controversial owing to lack of data. Because the mortality rate with systemic anthrax is high whereas the complication of antitoxin treatment is low, the potential benefit from antitoxins outweighs the potential risk from the antitoxins in systemic anthrax. This agent should be given in addition to appropriate antibiotics when systemic anthrax is suspected.

Pregnancy
Overall management is similar to that in the nonpregnant patient. In pregnancy, ciprofloxacin is preferred over doxycycline for both treatment and prevention. Newer fluoroquinolones such as levofloxacin and moxifloxacin[1] are not preferred because embryo toxicity has been observed in animal studies. This was not seen with ciprofloxacin. Transplacental transmission of anthrax is known to occur. Ciprofloxacin, levofloxacin, meropenem,[1] ampicillin,[1] penicillin, clindamycin,[1] and rifampin[1] are known to have adequate concentration in the placenta and at least one agent should be used with treatment.

Prognosis
Uncomplicated cutaneous anthrax has a mortality rate of less than 2% with treatment. Injection anthrax has a mortality rate of 28%, and gastrointestinal anthrax has a mortality rate of 40%. Inhalational anthrax has mortality of 45% despite antibiotics and modern intensive care. Meningitis from anthrax is almost always fatal.

Prevention
Postexposure prophylaxis should be started as soon as possible after exposure. Sixty days of antibiotics for immediate protection and a three-dose series of Anthrax Vaccine Adsorbed (AVA, BioThrax) for long-term protection are recommended by the United States Advisory Committee on Immunization Practices. Ciprofloxacin and doxycycline are recommended as first-line antibiotic therapy for postexposure prophylaxis and are FDA-approved for this indication. Alternative agents include levofloxacin, moxifloxacin, amoxicillin, or penicillin VK (if sensitive); and clindamycin. AVA should be administered at diagnosis and at 2 and 4 weeks. AVA is not FDA-approved for postexposure prophylaxis.

---

[1]Not FDA approved for this indication.

References
Anthrax. Available at http://www.cdc.gov/anthrax/ [accessed 31.01.15].
Hendricks KA, Wright ME, Shadomy SV, et al: Centers for disease control and prevention expert panel meetings on prevention and treatment of anthrax in adults, *Emerg Infect Dis* 20, 2014. https://doi.org/10.3201/eid2002.130687.
Knox D, Murray G, Millar M, et al: Subcutaneous anthrax in three intravenous drug users, *J Bone Joint Surg* 93:414–417, 2011.
Logan NA, Hoffmaster AR, Shadomy SV, Stauffer KE: In Versalovic J, editor: *Manual of clinical microbiology*, 10th ed., Washington DC, 2011, ASM Press, pp 381–402.
Meaney-Delman D, Zotti ME, Creanga AA, et al: Special considerations for prophylaxis for and treatment of anthrax in pregnant and postpartum women, *Emerg Infect Dis* 20, 2014. https://doi.org/10.3201/eid2002.130611.
Ruoff KL, Clarridge J, Bernard K: In Garcia LS, editor: *Clinical microbiology procedures handbook*, ed 3rd, Washington DC, 2010, ASM Press. 3.18.1.
Singh K: Laboratory-acquired infections, *Clin Infect Dis* 49:142–147, 2009.

BABESIOSIS

Method of
Cheston B. Cunha, MD; and Burke A. Cunha, MD

CURRENT DIAGNOSIS

- Suspect babesiosis in patients from Ixodes tick-endemic areas who present with a malaria-like illness (MLI) with fever, chills, headache, fatigue, and malaise.
- Clinically, babesiosis usually presents as an acute febrile illness with high fevers (>102 °F), relative bradycardia, and shaking chills accompanied by fatigue and myalgias.
- Myalgias may suggest an influenza-like illness (ILI).
- Severe headaches may suggest an alternate diagnosis, e.g., meningitis.
- Some patients with babesiosis may be short of breath and may go on to develop acute respiratory distress syndrome (ARDS).
- Consider babesiosis for unexplained fevers following blood transfusion.
- In prolonged fevers that meet the definition of fever of unknown origin (FUO), consider babesiosis in patients from endemic areas.
- With babesiosis, there are usually no localizing signs except for splenomegaly. Importantly, no rash is present. If rash is present, consider an alternate diagnosis.
- In babesiosis, nonspecific laboratory test results, considered together, are helpful in excluding or narrowing diagnostic possibilities.
- Common nonspecific laboratory findings of babesiosis include a normal/slightly decreased white blood cell count, relative lymphopenia, atypical lymphocytes, thrombocytopenia, elevated total bilirubin, and high lactate dehydrogenase levels. Sera are mildly elevated.
- The erythrocyte sedimentation rate is usually highly elevated (>90 mm/h) as are serum ferritin levels.
- Definitive babesiosis diagnosis is by peripheral blood smears (thick and thin); thick smears are best for the detection of babesia and thin smears are best to assess the degree of parasitemia.
- In normal hosts, the degree of parasitemia is usually low (1%–5%), but high in compromised hosts (>10%). Severe babesiosis may occur in asplenic individuals (Howell-Jolly bodies reflect the degree of splenic dysfunction), the immunosuppressed, the elderly, and those with coinfections, e.g., ehrlichiosis, Lyme disease.
- If present, babesiosis is diagnosed by peripheral stained blood smears demonstrating the characteristic (but uncommon) "Maltese cross" in tetrads (four merozoites).
- In nonmalarious areas, babesiosis may be diagnosed by demonstrating intraerythrocytic ring forms on the peripheral smear.
- Babesiosis, like malaria, has intracellular ring forms, but babesiosis, unlike malaria, has no intracellular pigment (hemozoin).
- Alternatively, *Babesia microti* serology in the Northeastern United States is diagnostic if IgM titers are highly elevated (>1:64).
- Polymerase chain reaction to detect Babesia is more sensitive than blood smear review. It is particularly useful in patients with a low level of parasitemia.

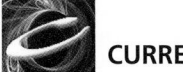

CURRENT THERAPY

TABLE 1	Babesiosis	
PREFERRED THERAPY	**ALTERNATE THERAPY**
Azithromycin (Zithromax)[1] 500 mg PO×1, then 250 mg PO q24h×7 days **plus** Atovaquone suspension (Mepron)[1] 750 mg PO q12h×7 days	Clindamycin (Cleocin)[1] 600 mg PO q8h×7 days **plus** Quinine[1] 650 mg PO q8h×7 days

From Cunha BA, editor. Antibiotic Essentials. 12th ed. Sudbury, MA: Jones & Bartlett; 2013, p. 253–268.
[1]Not FDA approved for this indication.

Epidemiology

Babesiosis is a tick-borne zoonosis that clinically presents as a malaria-like illness (MLI). There are many *Babesia* species, but only five are pathogenic in humans. The geographic distribution of babesiosis mimics that of hard-bodied *Ixodes dammini* (*I. scapularis*) ticks and their vertebrate hosts, e.g., dogs, cats, cattle, and rodents. The primary reservoir for babesiosis in the Northeastern United States is the white-footed mouse (*I. dammini* nymphs) and the white-tailed deer (*I. dammini* adults). Sporadic cases of babesiosis also occur in states with the tick vector/vertebrate hosts. Babesiosis may also be acquired by blood/blood product transfusions.

Clinical Features

In the Northeastern United States, babesiosis is usually *B. microti* and clinically manifests as an MLI. Babesiosis may be asymptomatic (IgG seropositive) or a mild, self-limited influenza-like illness (ILI). The incubation period for naturally acquired babesiosis is 1 to 6 weeks and 6 to 9 weeks for transfusion-acquired babesiosis. Clinical presentations in normal hosts are subacute with fever, fatigue, headache, malaise, and anorexia often mimicking Epstein-Barr virus infectious mononucleosis (with false-positive Monospot test results). Babesiosis presenting in patients with prolonged fevers of unknown origins (FUOs) and anorexia/weight loss may mimic a lymphoreticular malignancy. Presentation may be acute in those with impaired splenic function, those on immunosuppressives, or the elderly. Babesiosis may be viewed clinically as the "malaria of Long Island/Nantucket" as it presents with many malarial features, e.g., fever, chills, headache, sweats, myalgias. Excluding epidemiologic considerations, babesiosis differs in geographic distribution from malaria. Clinically, babesiosis differs from malaria in two important aspects. The clinical hallmarks of malaria are acute onset, intermittent fevers, and the classic "malaria paroxysm." Babesia reproduce by asynchronous asexual budding, which is clinically manifest as constant/nonintermittent fever. With malaria, fevers are intermittent with fever periodicity related to the *Plasmodium* species. Only *P. falciparum* has no fever periodicity and like babesiosis has no hepatic phase. Malaria and babesiosis both have extraerythrocytic ring forms, but babesiosis has two distinct morphologic features: extracellular merozoites (tetrads), known as "Maltese crosses," and no extraerythrocytic pigment, which malaria does have.

Unless the liver or spleen is enlarged, the physical features in babesiosis are limited to the fever. The fever curve of babesiosis is remittent without periodicity; fever is between 102 °F and 105 °F and accompanied by relative bradycardia. Rash is not a feature. When babesiosis is suspected, the presence of a rash is either indicative of coinfection, e.g., Lyme disease, or an alternative cause, e.g., viral or drug exanthem. Babesiosis should not be in the differential diagnosis of Rocky Mountain spotted fever with rash on the wrists/ankles. Babesiosis may clinically resemble ehrlichiosis. Peripheral blood smears are the best way to differentiate babesiosis from ehrlichiosis. Nonspecific laboratory abnormalities in babesiosis include normal/decreased white blood cell (WBC) count (leukopenia). Relative lymphopenia is usually present. Atypical lymphocytes are frequently present in the peripheral smear. Thrombocytopenia is a constant finding. The erythrocyte sedimentation rate (ESR) is highly elevated (usually >90 mm/h and often >100 mm/h) as is C-reactive protein (CRP). Since the pathophysiology of babesiosis is that of an acute hemolytic anemia, like malaria, intravascular hemolysis in babesiosis is manifested by increased lactate dehydrogenase (LDH)/total bilirubin. Increased LDH and total bilirubin are the most sensitive indicators of the degree of intravascular hemolysis in babesiosis. The hemoglobin/hematocrit is decreased later in more severe cases. Ferritin levels are highly elevated and prolonged (higher/longer) than would occur with acute-phase ferritin elevations. Since babesiosis impairs T cell function, as in malaria, serum protein electrophoresis often shows polyclonal gammopathy reflecting compensatory B cell hyperactivity. Serum transaminases are mildly elevated, but alkaline phosphatase is unelevated. Cold agglutinins are not a feature of babesiosis. In patients with decreased/absent splenic function, Howell-Jolly bodies are present in the peripheral smear. The number of Howell-Jolly bodies present is inversely proportional to the degree of splenic dysfunction.

Diagnosis of babesiosis is microscopic or serologic. Like malaria, babesiosis may be diagnosed on Giemsa stained blood smears. If malaria is not a diagnostic consideration (geographic distribution, blood transfusion), the presence of intraerythrocytic ring forms is diagnostic. Less common, but more specific, are pathognomonic tetrads (Maltese crosses) of babesiosis in peripheral smears. Also, unlike malaria, there is no extraerythrocytic pigment in babesiosis. Alternatively, elevated IgM *Babesia* species titers are diagnostic.

Therapy

The preferred therapy of babesiosis consists of 7 days combination therapy of azithromycin (Zithromax)[1] plus atovaquone (Mepron).[1] Alternatively, clindamycin (Cleocin)[1] plus quinine[1] for 7 days may be used (Table 1).

Treatment failure may occur in those with impaired T cell function, e.g., patients with HIV or with decreased splenic function. In such cases, exchange transfusion may be lifesaving.

[1]Not FDA approved for this indication.

References

Bonoan JT, Johnson DH, Cunha BA: Life-threatening babesiosis in an asplenic patient treated with exchange transfusion, azithromycin and atovaquone, *Heart Lung* 27:424–428, 1998.

Cunha BA, Raza M, Schmidt A: Highly elevated serum ferritin levels are a diagnostic marker in babesiosis, *Clin Infect Dis* 60:827–829, 2015.

Cunha BA, Mickail N, Laguerre M: Babesiosis mimicking Epstein Barr Virus (EBV) infectious mononucleosis: another cause of false positive Monospot test, *J Infect* 62:531–532, 2012.

Cunha BA, Cohen YZ, McDermott B: Fever of unknown origin (FUO) due to babesiosis in an immunocompetent host, *Heart Lung* 37:481–484, 2008.

Cunha BA, Nausheen S, Szalsa D: Pulmonary complications of Babesiosis: case report and literature review, *Eur J Clin Microbiol Infect Dis* 26:505–508, 2007.

Cunha BA, Crean J, Rosenbaum G: Lipid abnormalities in babesiosis, *Am J Med* 15:758–759, 2000.

Cunha CB: Infectious diseases differential diagnosis. In Cunha BA, editor: *Antibiotic Essentials*, ed 12th, Sudbury, MA, 2013, Jones & Bartlett, pp 474–506.

Hildebrandt A, Gray JS, Hunfeld KP: Human babesiosis in Europe: what clinicians need to know, *Infection* 41:1057–1072, 2013.

Kim N, Rosenbaum GS, Cunha BA: Relative bradycardia and lymphopenia in patients with babesiosis, *Clin Infect Dis* 26:1218–1219, 1998.

Krause PJ, Daily J, Telford SR, et al: Shared features in the pathology of babesiosis and malaria, *Trends Parasitol* 23:605–610, 2007.

Larkin JM: Ticks and tick-related illness, *Med Health RI* 91:209–211, 2008.

Leiby DA: Transfusion-transmitted Babesia spp: bull's-eye on Babesia microti, *Clin Microbiol Rev* 24:14–28, 2011.

Merch K, Holmaas G, Frolander PS, et al: Severe human Babesia divergens infection in Norway, *Int J Infect Dis* 23:37–38, 2014.

Nathavitharana RR, Mitty JA: Diseases from North America: focus on tick-borne infections, *Clin Med* 15:74–77, 2015.

Panduranga V, Kumar A: Severe babesiosis presenting as acute respiratory distress syndrome in an immunocompetent patient, *Conn Med* 78:289–291, 2014.

Rosenbaum GS, Johnson DH, Cunha BA: Atypical lymphocytosis in babesiosis, *Clin Infect Dis* 20:203–204, 1995.

Sharon KP, Krause PJ: Babesiosis. In Cunha BA, editor: *Tickborne infectious diseases diagnosis and management*, New York, 2007, Information Healthcare, pp 111–120.

Usmani-Brown S, Halperin JJ, Krause PJ: Neurological manifestations of human babesiosis, *Handb Clin Neurol* 114:199–203, 2013.

Wudhikarn K, Perry EH, Kemperman M, et al: Transfusion-transmitted babesiosis in an immunocompromised patient: a case report and review, *Am J Med* 124:800–805, 2011.

BACTERIAL MENINGITIS

Method of
Martha L. Muller, MD, MPH

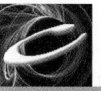

CURRENT DIAGNOSIS

Patient age often determines clinical presentation:
- Neonates-nonspecific symptoms
- Classic features: fever, headache, neck stiffness, altered mental status
- Cerebrospinal fluid (CSF) evaluation
- Elevated opening pressure
- Elevated white blood cell count
- Decreased glucose: CSF to blood glucose ratio <0.60
- Elevated protein

CURRENT THERAPY

Neonates <2 mo
- Most common organisms: *S. agalactiae* (GBS), *E. coli*, or other gram-negative enteric organism, occasional *L. monocytogenes*
- Empiric therapy: Ampicillin, cefotaxime or ceftriaxone (should be discussed with an infectious diseases pharmacist to determine risk factors for use)

Infants and Children >2 mo
- Most common organisms: *S. pneumoniae, N. meningitidis, H. influenzae* type B
- Empiric therapy: Ceftriaxone and vancomycin (used for potential penicillin-resistant *S. pneumoniae*)

Adults
- Most common organisms: *S. pneumoniae, N. meningitidis*
- Empiric therapy: Ceftriaxone and vancomycin

Adults >50 years of age
- Most common organisms: *S. pneumonia, N. meningitidis, L. monocytogenes*
- Empiric therapy: Ceftriaxone, vancomycin, and ampicillin

Bacterial meningitis is a serious, life-threatening infection of the central nervous system. This inflammation of the meninges and subarachnoid space, including the cerebrospinal fluid (CSF), may potentially affect the brain cortex and parenchyma. Bacterial meningitis can occur via several pathophysiologic mechanisms (Table 1). In the neonatal period, most of the offending organisms have colonized mucosal surfaces after contact and aspiration of maternal intestinal and genital tract secretions during the delivery process. The most common mechanism noted outside of the neonatal period involves nasopharyngeal colonization, penetration of the nasopharyngeal mucous membrane barrier with entrance to the interstitial space, and entrance into the capillary bloodstream with subsequent delivery to the meninges or choroid plexus. Once organisms penetrate the CSF an advantage in their favor exists. In a usual physiologic state, there is essentially an absence of capsule-specific immunoglobulins, complement factors, polymorphonuclear lymphocytes and other plasma cells within the CSF. Available host defenses are apparently ineffectual against encapsulated organisms. Inflammation of the meninges results in vasospasm, potential arterial thrombosis, and cerebral vein occlusions. Additionally, bacterial and neutrophil-associated inflammatory products may traverse the pial barrier, potentially resulting in neuronal necrosis or compress cranial nerves.

The majority of bacterial meningitis cases occur sporadically. Worldwide bacterial meningitis is linked with significant morbidity and mortality, evidenced by approximately 16 million reported cases in 2013, associated with 1.6 million years lived with disability annually. An incidence of 0.8 per 100,000 in the United States has been reported, with a noted decrease of 64% from 1997 to 2014. Although dependent on many factors, including etiologic agent, age, risk factors, etc., case fatality rates for bacterial meningitis have been reported between 17% to 40%.

A disease formally dominated by *H. influenzae* in infants has now transitioned to one caused by *S. pneumoniae*, largely affecting elderly patients. On the whole, *S. pneumoniae* meningitis causes meningitis in children <5 years of age and in the elderly, greater than 65 years of age. Contrastingly, *N. meningitidis* tends to cause meningitis in older children and young adults.

Many intrinsic and extrinsic factors increase the risk for developing bacterial meningitis and impact the potential offending bacteria (see Table 1). Additionally, general factors such as poor living conditions and crowded day-care centers influence the potential development of bacterial meningitis.

Diagnosis

The clinical presentation of bacterial meningitis is greatly influenced by patient age. Neonates and infants generally present with nonspecific signs and symptoms, including poor feeding, respiratory distress, fussiness, general weakness, and irritability. Although not universal, fever and seizures may also be present in <40% and 15% to 34% of babies with bacterial meningitis, respectively. Similarly, hypothermia may be a presenting symptom. In general, patients with bacterial meningitis beyond the neonatal period present with more classic symptoms, including fever, neck stiffness, photophobia, significant headache, nausea,

TABLE 1	Pathophysiologic Mechanisms Associated With the Development of Bacterial Meningitis
MECHANISM	**EXAMPLES**
Hematologic	Nasopharyngeal colonization with penetration
Traumatic	Skull fractures
Iatrogenic	Cochlear implantation; ventriculoperitoneal shunt placement
Congenital	Dermal sinus
Contiguous infection	Sinuses; middle ear

and vomiting. Those patients with associated systemic compromise have higher potential for poor disease outcome.

Physical examination findings are also associated with age, generally displaying more characteristic findings with increasing age. Meningeal irritation may be demonstrated by neck stiffness, the Brudzinski sign (hips and knees reflexively flex when the neck is flexed), and Kernig's sign (flexion of the thigh with the hip and knee at 90-degree angles results in pain knee extension). A high degree of suspicion for bacterial meningitis in the appropriate clinical setting should be maintained despite physical examination findings as they are not always indicative of the disease. An adult prospective study demonstrated that the classic signs of meningeal irritation demonstrated sensitivity of only 5% to 30%. Elderly patients >65 years of age may present without typical symptoms. Additionally, patients with bacterial meningitis in this population may frequently present with nonspecific confusion. These elderly patients may also not uncommonly have nuchal rigidity not associated with bacterial meningitis.

In general, lumbar puncture should be sought without delay, with few contraindications to suggest otherwise. Indications for obtaining neuroimaging prior to conducting a lumbar puncture include the presence of focal neurologic findings in children and immunocompromised condition, previous history of central nervous system disease, new onset seizure, and focal neurologic findings in adults. CSF examination is crucial to the diagnosis of bacterial meningitis. CSF obtained for suspected bacterial meningitis should routinely be evaluated for cell count (red blood cells; white blood cells with differential as appropriate), glucose, protein, gram stain, and culture (Table 1). CSF culture serves as the gold standard for diagnosis, with reported positivity in 50% to 90% of patients. CSF should be evaluated as soon as possible after obtaining it as white blood cells deteriorate within 30 minutes and elevated white blood cell counts have the potential to metabolize CSF glucose. In general, characteristic CSF findings include elevated white blood cells, low glucose, and elevated protein values (Table 2). It is important to note that the CSF white blood cell count may infrequently be normal, especially very early in the course of illness. Blood cultures should also be obtained for patients with concerns for bacterial meningitis, with reported positivity in 50% to 80% of cases.

The receipt of antibiotics prior to CSF evaluation may lend to decreased organism recovery via culture. Effective antibiotic therapy can result in sterile cultures within 2 hours for *N. meningitidis* and begin the sterilization process within 4 hours for *S. pneumoniae*. Although CSF glucose and protein values in children may rarely be affected (in general, irregular values tend to

persist for many days despite appropriate therapy), a diagnosis of bacterial meningitis may often still be made based on the CSF analyses in the setting of antibiotic pretreatment. Polymerase chain reaction (PCR) is a promising tool in the arsenal for diagnosis of bacterial meningitis, especially in the setting of antibiotic pretreatment. Thirty percent to 50% of culture-negative CSF cultures have been found to positive when tested via PCR. A prospective study from Sweden reviewing CSF from repeat lumbar puncture demonstrated PCR positivity in 89% of samples taken on days 1 to 3, 70% of samples taken on days 4 to 6, and in 33% of samples taken on days 7 to 10. In contrast, all CSF cultures taken from the same samples were negative. Its utilization rising, PCR sensitivity has been reported as 61% to 100%, 88% to 94%, and 72% to 92% for *S. pneumoniae*, *N. meningitidis*, and *H. influenzae*, respectively. Additionally, false-negative PCR results are rare, occurring in approximately 5% of cases. Latex agglutination and coagglutination techniques, best for detection of bacteria that are actively proliferating and shedding polysaccharide, are infrequently used for the diagnosis of bacterial meningitis.

Complications of bacterial meningitis may occur anytime during the course of the illness and include circulatory collapse, disseminated intravascular coagulation, gangrenous digits, focal neurologic findings, seizures, and subdural effusions.

The differential diagnosis of bacterial meningitis in infants and young children includes otitis media, pharyngitis, pneumonia, retropharyngeal abscess, and lymphadenopathy. Additional diagnoses include brain abscess, tuberculous meningitis, aseptic meningitis, meningitis caused by atypical organisms, and sinusitis.

Antibiotic Management

Underscored by an almost 100% mortality noted for untreated bacterial meningitis, prompt, appropriate antibiotic administration is paramount, generally increasing the chances of survival. This is particularly notable for infants and children where case fatality rates are decreased to <10% and <5% for meningococcal meningitis in the setting of appropriate therapy.

Empiric antibiotic therapy should be chosen based on a variety of factors, including most likely bacterial etiology (local antibiograms and resistance patterns should be considered) (Tables 3 and 4), ability to penetrate the blood-brain barrier and achieve adequate CSF levels, and bactericidal mechanism of action. Beta-lactam antibiotics are frequently used to treat bacterial meningitis and generally effective against the most commonly associated bacteria. CSF concentrations of these antibiotics, even in the setting of minimal meningeal inflammation, are generally adequate for the minimal inhibitory concentrations for susceptible bacteria. Bacterial resistance patterns also greatly influence empiric antibiotic therapy. Worldwide, penicillin resistance in *S. pneumoniae* has impacted recommendations to use vancomycin as part of the empiric antibiotic regimen. Antibiotics should be provided at maximal clinically indicated doses parenterally (Table 5). Antibiotic therapy should not be delayed by the need to obtain neuroimaging. Once a specific organism is isolated, antibiotic therapy should be tailored to treat that organism, completing an appropriate duration of therapy (Table 6).

Adjunctive Therapy

With a goal of decreasing inflammation leading to neuronal death and brain damage, dexamethasone (Decadron)[1] administration is the cornerstone of adjunctive therapy for bacterial meningitis. Data from studies evaluating the effect of steroids on outcomes of infants and children with bacterial meningitis have demonstrated improved meningeal inflammatory indices and decreased audiologic and neurologic sequelae compared with those receiving placebo; this benefit is most notable for *H. influenzae* meningitis. The data for dexamethasone use to treat *S. pneumoniae* meningitis in children are less vigorous. Additionally, animal models

TABLE 2	Anticipated Cerebrospinal Fluid (CSF) Findings in Bacterial Meningitis

CSF PARAMETER	TYPICAL FINDINGS
White Blood Cell Count	>1000 cells/mm³ (may be affected by immunosuppression, neutropenia, atypical pathogens)
Glucose	<40 mg/dL (CSF to blood glucose ratio <0.60)
Total Protein	>100 mg/dL (increased above normal values for age)
Gram Stain	Positivity depends on bacterial burden. Stains positive 97% of the time when cultures grow >10⁵ CFU Specific yield of 70%–90% for *S. pneumoniae* Specific yield of 30%–90% for *N. meningitidis* Sensitivity low for *L. monocytogenes* as few organisms are generally present in CSF
CSF Opening Pressure	>200 mm/CSF (may be >300 mm/CSF. Continued elevation for first 24–48 hours before decrease)

Bacterial Meningitis

---

[1]Not FDA approved for this indication.

TABLE 3 Empiric Antibiotic Therapy Based on Contributing Factors*

CONTRIBUTING FACTOR	POTENTIAL ORGANISMS	ANTIBIOTIC THERAPY
Age		
<1 month	*S. agalactiae*, *E. coli* (gram-negative enteric organisms), *L. monocytogenes*	Ampicillin and cefotaxime or ceftriaxone (discuss use in this population with pharmacist)
1–2 years	*S. pneumoniae*, *N. meningitidis*, *H. influenzae* type B, *S. agalactiae*, *E. coli*	Ceftriaxone or cefotaxime, and vancomycin
2–50 years	*S. pneumoniae*, *N. meningitidis*	Ceftriaxone or cefotaxime and vancomycin
>50 years	*S. pneumoniae*, *N. meningitidis*, *L. monocytogenes*	Ceftriaxone or cefotaxime, ampicillin and vancomycin
Head Trauma		
Penetrating trauma	*S. aureus*, coagulase negative *Staphylococci*, aerobic gram-negative organisms (including *P. aeruginosa*)	Vancomycin with either cefepime[1] or meropenem
Neurosurgery	*S. aureus*, coagulase negative *Staphylococci*, aerobic gram-negative organisms (including *P. aeruginosa*)	Vancomycin with either cefepime[1] or meropenem
CNS Shunt Placement	*S. aureus*, coagulase negative *Staphylococci*, aerobic gram-negative organisms (including *P. aeruginosa*)	Vancomycin with either cefepime[1] or meropenem

*This table was adapted from the Infectious Diseases Society of America Practice Guidelines for Bacterial Meningitis.
[1]Not FDA approved for this indication.

TABLE 4 Special Patient Characteristics Associated With Specific Organisms

BACTERIA	PATIENT CHARACTERISTICS
S. pneumoniae	Immunocompromised status
N. meningitidis	Complement deficiencies; asplenia; smoking; antibody deficiency
H. influenzae type B	American Indian children; Alaska Native children
L. monocytogenes	Immunocompromised status
S. aureus	Neurosurgical procedures; shunt device placement; trauma; underlying disease (i.e., diabetes mellitus, human) immunodeficiency virus, cardiovascular disease; intravenous drug use

of bacterial meningitis demonstrated decreased vancomycin concentrations and penetration rates in the CSF for those animals receiving dexamethasone. This is important given the potential need to use vancomycin in the treatment of penicillin-resistant *S. pneumoniae* bacterial meningitis.

The American Academy of Pediatrics Committee on Infectious Diseases does endorse the use of dexamethasone for *H. influenzae* type B meningitis. However, the Committee does not make a recommendation for routine dexamethasone use in *S. pneumoniae* meningitis. They do provide a consideration of its use in children >6 weeks of age after risks and benefits have been reviewed. There is inadequate data to make a recommendation for dexamethasone use during the neonatal period. The data available demonstrating decreased unfavorable outcomes in adults when using dexamethasone have prompted the Infectious Diseases Society of America to routinely recommend dexamethasone for adults with suspected or proven pneumococcal meningitis. When given, dexamethasone should be provided at a dose of 0.15 mg/kg every 6 hours for 2 to 4 days. It should be given 10 to 20 minutes before or concurrent with the first dose of antibiotic therapy.

Vaccination Prevention

Between 1990 and 2013, global mortality caused by *S. pneumoniae*, *N. meningitis*, and *H. influenza* type B decreased by 29%, 25%, and 45%, respectively. Conjugate vaccination strategies have played an important role in improving that landscape. The introduction of *H. influenzae* type B and *S. pneumoniae* conjugate vaccines during the 1990s and 2000s contributed to reports of a decrease in bacterial meningitis, in both vaccinated and nonvaccinated populations. The introduction of conjugated *H. influenzae* type B vaccination programs provided a significant contribution to reducing bacterial meningitis, wherein bacterial meningitis caused by this organism has decreased by almost 100%. Interestingly, initiation of the 7-valent pneumococcal conjugate vaccine (Prevnar 7) in the United States was accompanied by a noted decrease in meningitis caused by vaccine serotypes, initially in children followed by a decrease in adults. However, a concurrent increase in nonvaccine serotypes was noted in response. Likewise, the introduction of the 13-valent pneumococcal conjugate vaccine (Prevnar 13) has also been met with an increased prevalence of nonvaccine serotypes causing bacterial meningitis. Despite the concerns regarding serotype replacement, receipt of several pneumococcal conjugate vaccines in the United States led to a 66% and 33% reduction in rates of pneumococcal meningitis for children <2 years of age and adults >65 years of age, respectively. Vaccination against *N. meningitidis* has also resulted in a decrease in bacterial meningitis demonstrating a rate decrease from 13.5 per 100,000 in 1968 to 1985 to 5.2 per 100,000 in 1989 to 2011.

Immunization against *H. influenzae* type B, *S. pneumoniae*, and *N. meningitidis* have been incorporated into the routine childhood vaccination schedule in the United States. The Advisory Committee on Immunization Practices provides specific vaccine recommendations.

Outcomes/Sequelae

The consideration of patient outcomes is multifactorial, including patient age, time to antibiotic administration especially as it relates to symptom onset, host factors such as immune response to infection, and time to CSF sterilization. In general, the greatest morbidity and mortality are seen at the extremes of ages (i.e., neonates and the elderly). Mortality associated with bacterial meningitis has been 20% to 25% for numerous decades. Pneumococcal meningitis is associated with the highest case fatality rates, reported as 20% to 37% in high-income countries and as high as 51% in low-income countries. This is in contrast to case fatality rates reported as 3% to 10% worldwide for meningococcal meningitis.

TABLE 5	Antibiotics Commonly Used to Treat Bacterial Meningitis	
ANTIBIOTIC	**ADULT DOSING**	**PEDIATRIC DOSING**
Ampicillin	2 grams every 4 hours	300–400 mg/kg/day divided every 4–6 hours; maximum daily dose: 12 g/day
Cefotaxime*	2 grams every 4–6 hours	225–300 mg/kg/day divided every 6–8 hours
Ceftriaxone	2 grams every 12 hours	50 mg/kg/dose every 12 hours
Cefepime	2 grams every 8 hours	50 mg/kg/dose every 8 hours
Meropenem	2 grams every 8 hours	40 mg/kg/dose every 8 hours
Vancomycin+	15–20 mg/kg/dose every 8–12 hours	15 mg/kg/dose every 6 hours

*There is currently not a reliable method by which to obtain this drug in the United States.
+Appropriate loading and level monitoring should be performed by an infectious diseases pharmacist.
1Not FDA approved for this indication.

TABLE 6	Duration of Antibiotic Therapy for Uncomplicated Infections Caused by Specific Organisms
PATHOGEN	**DURATION OF THERAPY**
S. agalactiae (GBS)	14 days
E. coli (gram-negative enteric organisms)	21 days
L. monocytogenes	21 days
S. pneumoniae	10–14 days
N. meningitidis	7 days
H. influenzae type B	7–10 days

Neurologic difficulties have been reported in 20% to 30% of bacterial meningitis events. Similarly, longstanding neuropsychological sequelae have been reported in as many as 50% of those who survive bacterial meningitis. Compared with their well siblings who did not have bacterial meningitis, infants and children with bacterial meningitis are more likely to experience seizures, hearing loss, cognitive disturbances, and behavioral concerns. Similarly, there have been reports of disturbed executive functioning, memory, and intelligence in adults who have recovered from bacterial meningitis.

Seizures, hearing loss, and cognitive impairment are the most commonly reported disabilities after a diagnosis of bacterial meningitis. Seizures complicate bacterial meningitis and have an individual link to increased morbidity. It is important to note that this differs from febrile seizures, with a multicenter study reporting less than 1% of their population with complex febrile seizures having bacterial meningitis. Longstanding neuropsychological sequelae have been reported in as many as 50% of those who survive bacterial meningitis. Hearing loss is a common complication of bacterial meningitis. It has the potential to be transient or permanent and is often associated with *S. pneumoniae* meningitis. Sustained hearing loss is generally sensorineural, with incidence reported as 14% for mild hearing loss and 5% for severe hearing loss. The hearing loss typically occurs during the initial days of the infection and can be transient or permanent, underscoring the need for formal hearing evaluation to occur in all patients diagnosed with bacterial meningitis.

References

American Academy of Pediatrics RedBook report of the Committee on infectious diseases 2018-2021, 31st Edition.
Brouwe MC, van de Beek D: Epidemiology of community-acquired bacterial meningitis, *Curr Opin Infect Dis* 31:78–84, 2018.
Costerus JM, et al: Community-acquired bacterial meningitis, *Curr Opin Infect Dis* 30:135–141, 2017.
Davis LE: Acute bacterial meningitis, *Continuum (Minneap Minn)* 24:1264–1283, 2018.
Figueiredo AHA, et al: Acute community-acquired bacterial meningitis, *Neurol Clin* 809–820, 2018.
Kim KS: Acute bacterial meningitis in infants and children, *Lancet Infect Dis* 10:32–42, 2010.
Lexicomp Online: *Pediatric and neonatal Lexi-Drugs online*, Hudson, Ohio, 2021, UpToDate, Inc.
Lexicomp Online: *Adult Lexi-Drugs online*, Hudson, Ohio, 2021, UpToDate, Inc.
Liechti FD, et al: Bacterial meningitis: insights into pathogenesis and evaluation of new treatment options: a perspective from experimental studies, *Future Microbiol* 10:1195–2213, 2015.
McGill F, et al: Acute bacterial meningitis in adults, *Lancet* 388:3036–3047, 2016.
Obaro S: Updating the diagnosis of bacterial meningitis, *Lancet Infect Dis* 19:1160–1161, 2019.
Oordts-Speets AM, et al: Global etiology of bacterial meningitis: a systematic review and meta-analysis, *PloS One* 13:e0198772, 2018, https://doi.org/10.1371/journal.pone.0198772.
Posadas E, et al: Pediatric bacterial meningitis: an update on early identification and management, *EB Medicine* 15:1–20, 2018.
Saez-Llorens X, McCracken Jr GH: Bacterial meningitis in children, *Lancet* 361:2139–2148, 2003.
Tunkel AR, et al: Practice guidelines for the management of bacterial meningitis, *CID* 39:1267–1284, 2004.
van de Beek D, et al: Community-acquired bacterial meningitis, *Nat Rev Dis Primers* 2:1–20, 2016.

BRUCELLOSIS

Method of
Xinghong Yang, PhD

CURRENT DIAGNOSIS

- The diagnosis of brucellosis relies on the serologic reaction of antibodies to *Brucella's* lipopolysaccharide (LPS) located on the cell surface of smooth *Brucella melitensis, Brucella abortus,* and *Brucella suis*.
- Although the rough species, *Brucella canis,* does not have an intact LPS layer, its detection requires the antigens specifically prepared from *B. canis*.
- Rose Bengal test is regularly used to diagnose infection with smooth *Brucella* spp.
- When patients with brucellosis symptoms test negative by Rose Bengal test, the microagglutination test and 2-mercaptoethanol rapid slide agglutination test are used to determine whether the patient is infected with rough *Brucella* spp.

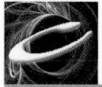

CURRENT THERAPY

- Three aspects of therapy are critical when using antibiotics to treat brucellosis:
  - The antibiotics must be able to penetrate macrophages to take effect because *Brucella* spp. are intracellular pathogens and normally reside within professional and nonprofessional phagocytes.
  - Multiple antibiotics are typically used to minimize relapses commonly seen when only a single antibiotic is used.
  - In complicated cases, in addition to antibiotic treatment, surgical intervention may be required to remove infected tissues.

Brucellosis is an ancient disease recorded by the Romans more than 2000 years ago. Since *Brucella* was identified as the cause of brucellosis in sick soldiers in 1887 by Sir David Bruce, brucellosis has been defined as an emerging disease. *Brucella* is a zoonotic bacterial pathogen, causing approximately 500,000 new cases annually worldwide. Although rarely fatal (<5% mortality rate), it causes an undulating fever leading to a dramatic decrease in the quality of life. Its incubation time can vary between 1 and 8 weeks, and often infection is asymptomatic; however, serious complications can lead to disability or death. Because no human vaccine is available, antibiotic therapy is the only option for treatment.

A total of ten *Brucella* species have been identified to date (Table 1). Four of these—*Brucella melitensis*, *Brucella abortus*, *Brucella suis*, and *Brucella canis*—commonly cause human brucellosis, and their genomes have been sequenced.

Epidemiology

Wildlife and domesticated animals can serve as natural reservoirs for *Brucella* spp. Humans acquire brucellae by exposure to contaminated foods or aerosols or by direct contact. Often contaminated or unpasteurized animal products, such as milk, soft cheese, and butter are consumed, causing oral exposure. *Brucella* spp. can spread via contaminated aerosols or by aerosolization of contaminated animal by-products, resulting in lung infection. *Brucella* can also infect by direct contact of skin cuts or abrasions with sick animals or their products and enter into the blood or lymphatic system and, regardless of route, produce infection,

causing a bacteremia. Among the three routes, food ingestion and aerosol inhalation can result in brucellosis. Aerosolized brucellae can be used as a bioweapon because the dosage required for infecting 50% of the population is as little as 1885 colony-forming units (CFUs).

Currently, brucellosis is endemic to Latin America, Africa, the Mediterranean rim, the Middle East, and Central Asia. To prevent human infection, animal immunization campaigns were adopted by many countries, including the United States and the former Soviet Union. The campaigns successfully curbed animal infection and consequently reduced human infection in these areas. When the programs were stopped, the incidence of brucellosis rapidly increased. Thus maintenance of animal immunization programs is essential for protecting humans from infection.

Although transmission of brucellae among humans occurs rarely, several cases have been reported. It may be disseminated via sexual contact, milking, and organ transplantation. *B. melitensis* is the most commonly isolated species from brucellosis patients, followed in descending order by *B. abortus*, *B. suis*, and *B. canis*. *B. melitensis* and *B. abortus* can cause acute brucellosis and display the most severe symptoms, which can lead to complications. *B. suis* can cause extended duration of illness and results in suppurating lesions in infected tissues. Patients with *B. canis* infections display mild to moderate illness and rarely develop complications.

Risk Factors

The susceptible population includes those who live or travel in the endemic areas, particularly veterinarians, microbiologists, and those who work with or process livestock. The current animal vaccines are all infectious to human, and consequently veterinarians who administer these vaccines are at high risk for being infected. Microbiologists or laboratory workers also can acquire brucellosis through close contact, and indeed laboratory outbreaks are frequently reported. Thus *Brucella* is also considered an occupational disease or a laboratory-acquired disease.

Pathophysiology

Brucella can be phagocytized by nonprofessional and professional phagocytic cells to establish an intracellular replication niche. Once inside host cells, brucellae stay in early-formed phagosomes, where they prevent phagosomes from fusing with late-formed endosomes and lysosomes and survive intracellularly. Antibiotics must be able to penetrate the host cell membrane to kill brucellae or inhibit their growth.

Brucella uses numerous mechanisms to evade detection by the immune system. Unlike LPS from other gram-negative bacteria, *Brucella* LPS does not trigger an inflammatory response or activate the alternative complement system, so it helps brucellae avoid recognition. *Brucella*'s LPS endows brucellae with a phenotype highly resistant to cationic bactericidal peptides. The intracellular brucellae do not cause cell death in macrophages or apoptosis in respiratory epithelial cells. Thus the LPS reduces the chances of exposure to the immune system, which aids brucellae survival and meanwhile diminishes the stimulation of the host immune system. *Brucella* inhibits the macrophage response to interferon-γ (IFN-γ), a critical cytokine for stimulating innate and adaptive immunity. Additionally, to maintain vigorous intracellular survival and replication, brucellae equip their outer membranes with phosphatidylcholine and synthesize cyclic β-1,2-glucans to preclude fusion between phagosome and lysosome.

Diagnosis

Accurate diagnosis of brucellosis is always a challenge because brucellosis exhibits symptoms similar to numerous other febrile illnesses (Table 2). In many patients, the symptoms are mild and moderate; thus in a number of cases the diagnosis might not be even considered.

Isolation of brucellae from blood, bone marrow, urine, cerebrospinal fluid, or joint aspirate serves as the gold standard for diagnosing brucellosis. However, under many circumstances, brucellae cannot be cultured from patients' samples. The rate of

TABLE 1	*Brucella* Species, Preferred Animal Hosts, and Human Infection Potential	
SPECIES	**HOST ANIMALS OR RESERVOIR**	**HUMAN INFECTION?***
B. melitensis	Goats, sheep, camels	Yes
B. abortus	Cows, bison, camels, yaks	Yes
B. suis	Pigs, wild hares, caribou, reindeer, wild rodents	Yes
B. canis	Dogs	Yes
B. cetaceae	Seals, harbor porpoises	Yes
B. inopinata	Unknown	Yes
B. microti	Common voles, red foxes, soil	Unknown
B. neotomae	Rodents	No
B. ovis	Sheep	No
B. pinnipedialis	Minke whales, dolphins	No

*"Yes" and "no" mean *Brucella* spp. are able or unable to infect humans, respectively; "unknown" indicates that it is not confirmed whether *Brucella* spp. are able to infect humans.

blood culture positivity ranges from 16% to 90%. Hence, other indices are used to identify brucellosis. Testing for antibodies against *Brucella* is commonly used. *Brucella* agglutination titer of 1:160 is considered a clear diagnostic index as long as the patient presents signs and symptoms of the disease. Recommended tests are the Rose Bengal test, the serum agglutination test alone or with 2-mercaptoethanol or dithiothreitol reduction, Coombs' antiglobulin, the complement-fixation test, and the enzyme-linked immunosorbent assay (ELISA). The results of a combination of tests such as the serum agglutination test and Coombs' antiglobulin can be used to assess the stage of evolution of the disease at the time of diagnosis. In the blood sample, infection may also be associated with low levels of red and white blood cells, low platelets, and elevated liver function. A biopsy of body tissues can also assist in making the diagnosis because patients can experience bone marrow hypoplasia or liver fibrosis and cirrhosis.

Depending on the patient's symptoms and severity of the illness, an investigation may be undertaken. Examinations may include computed tomography (CT) scan or magnetic resonance imaging (MRI) to identify signs of inflammation or abscesses in the brain or other tissues. Electrocardiogram (ECG) may be performed to investigate heart infection or damage, and x-rays can show bone and joint deformations.

Differential Diagnosis

Because human brucellosis mimics the symptoms of many other diseases, disease complications vary from patient to patient, and the latency time between exposure and the occurrence of symptoms is irregular and relatively long, making the differential diagnosis tedious and difficult. Therefore, before diagnosis, answers to three questions can help narrow the focus to brucellosis:

- Did the patient have direct contact with large or small ruminants, their carcasses, or their products?
- Did the patient consume unpasteurized dairy products?
- Does the patient live in or travel to areas where brucellae are endemic in humans or epidemic in animals?

In spite of the difficulties in diagnosing brucellosis, some clinical features can still be used to distinguish brucellosis from other infectious diseases. If left untreated, fever of brucellosis displays an undulating pattern. In about 50% of patients, the fever of brucellosis is associated with musculoskeletal symptoms; however, these symptoms are rarely observed in typhoid and malaria fevers.

In patients with hepatosplenomegaly or lymphadenopathy, the differential diagnosis includes glandular fever–like illnesses, such as cytomegalovirus (CMV) infection, Epstein-Barr virus (EBV) infection, HIV infection, toxoplasmosis, and tuberculosis (TB). CMV patients can develop antibodies to the virus. Also, in the active infection phase, CMV can be detected from the blood, saliva, urine, or other body tissues. These indices can be used to differentiate CMV infection from the brucellosis. EBV patients have an elevated white blood cell count, an increased total number of lymphocytes, and greater than 10% atypical lymphocytes, but brucellosis patients usually show a decrease in the white blood cell count.

HIV infection can induce antibodies against HIV, and virologic tests can detect HIV antigens or RNA. HIV infection can be further confirmed by a supplemental antibody test, such as Western blot and indirect immunofluorescence assay. Brucellosis patients' sera do not display any reaction in these tests. For toxoplasmosis patients, serum immunoglobulin (Ig)G and IgM titers can be used to detect whether the patient is infected by *Toxoplasma*.

For TB patients, a skin test or a special TB blood test can be used for diagnosis, and other tests such as chest x-ray and a sample of sputum coughed up from deep in the lungs may be used for confirmation. In patients with osteomyelitis or septic arthritis, the most important alternative diagnosis is TB.

In patients with acute epididymoorchitis, the differential diagnosis includes mumps and surgical problems, such as torsion. For mumps patients, buccal swab specimens are collected for viral detection via culturing virus in cell lines or using real-time polymerase chain reaction (RT-PCR) to detect mumps viral RNA. For testicular torsion in men, an ultrasound examination of the spermatic cord can provide valuable information regarding whether the patient requires emergency surgery.

Treatment

To date, the only option for treating brucellosis is by means of antibiotics. However, in cases of complications, such as heart brucellosis and spinal brucellosis, antibiotic treatment in combination with surgical intervention may be needed. Antibiotics commonly used are doxycycline (Vibramycin), rifampin (Rifadin),[1] streptomycin, cotrimoxazole (TMP-SMX [Bactrim]),[1] and gentamicin (Garamycin)[1] (Table 3). Regimens of a combination of 2 or 3 antibiotics are recommended to reduce the unacceptably high relapse rates with monotherapy. Antibiotic regimens vary and depend on the patient's age, the severity of the disease, pregnancy, cost of the medicine, and availability of the medicine.

Doxycycline combined with rifampin[1] for a full 6-week course is a commonly used therapy recommended by the World Health Organization. It is considered the most effective regimen, particularly when combined with an aminoglycoside. In patients with spondylitis or sacroiliitis, doxycycline plus streptomycin is an

TABLE 2	Symptom Pattern of Human Brucellosis	
SYMPTOMS	**PERCENT***
Fever	93
Chills	82
Sweats	87
Aches	91
Lack of energy	95
Joint and back pain	86
Arthritis	40
Spinal tenderness	48
Headache	81
Loss of appetite	78
Weight loss	65
Constipation	47
Abdominal pain	45
Diarrhea	7
Cough	24
Testicular pain, epididymoorchitis	21†
Rash	14
Sleep disturbance	37
Ill appearance	25
Pallor	22
Lymphadenopathy	32
Splenomegaly	25
Hepatomegaly	19
Jaundice	1
Central nervous system disorder	4
Cardiac murmur	3
Pneumonia	1

Data from Corbel MJ: Brucellosis in humans and animals. Geneva, World Health Organization, 2006.
*Percentage based on 500 patients.
†Percentage based on 290 male patients.

---

[1]Not FDA approved for this indication.

TABLE 3 Treatment for Brucellosis

MEDICATION	ADULT DOSAGE	DOSAGE ADJUSTMENT				ADVERSE EFFECTS
		PEDIATRIC DOSAGE	RENAL FAILURE	HEPATIC INSUFFICIENCY		
Doxycycline (Vibramycin)	100 mg PO q12h	2.2–4.4 mg/kg[3] PO div q12h (>8 y)	No change	No change		Dizziness, headache, photosensitivity, nausea, diarrhea, hemolytic anemia, hepatotoxicity
Rifampin (Rifadin)[1]	600–900 mg PO qd	20 mg/kg PO qd (do not exceed 600 mg qd)	No change	Moderate: caution Severe: avoid		Heartburn, epigastric distress, anorexia, nausea, flatulence, cramps, liver dysfunction, jaundice
Streptomycin	15 mg/kg IM q24h or 1 g IM qd × 2–3 wk	20–40 mg/kg IM qd (do not exceed 1 g/d)	Necessary	No change		Nausea, vomiting, vertigo, face paresthesias, rash, fever, urticaria, angioedema, eosinophilia
Trimethoprim-sulfamethoxazole (TMP-SMX) (Bactrim)[1]	1 DS tab PO q12h (160 mg TMP/800 mg SMX)	8–12 mg/kg TMP PO given in divided doses q12h	Necessary Avoid use in CrCl <15 mL/min	No change		Nausea, vomiting, anorexia, rash, urticaria
Gentamicin (Garamycin)[1]	2 mg/kg[3] IM/IV q8h or 5 mg/kg IM/IV q24h[1] or 240 mg q24h	2.5 mg/kg q8–12h IM/IV	Necessary	No change		Nephrotoxicity, dizziness, vertigo, tinnitus, hearing loss, numbness, skin tingling, muscle twitching, convulsions

Abbreviations: CrCl = creatinine clearance; DS = double strength.
[1]Not FDA approved for this indication.
[3]Exceeds dosage recommended by the manufacturer.

effective combination. For pediatric patients older than 8 years, doxycycline plus gentamicin[1] is the recommended therapy. For children younger than 8 years, trimethoprim-sulfamethoxazole (TMP-SMX) therapy for 3 weeks followed by a 5-day course of gentamicin[1] is most effective. TMP-SMX[1] is also effective in treating pregnant women, either as a single agent or in combination with rifampin[1] or gentamicin[1] (see Table 3).

Once brucellosis is diagnosed, immediate therapy is critical because it can alleviate symptoms and also prevent the development of complications. Nevertheless, even when treatment is executed according to the doctor's prescription, rates of relapse can still reach up to 5% to 10%. Depending on the severity or complications of the illness and the treatment time applied, the recovery time can last from several weeks to several months.

Monitoring

After antibiotic therapy is initiated, patients are periodically monitored by doctors to evaluate whether the therapeutic regimen is effective and whether relapse occurs. Because relapse is indicated by the recurrence of a positive blood culture result during the post-therapy period or signs and symptoms of brucellosis infection, routine examination of the patient includes serum culture for *Brucella* organism and assessment for brucellosis symptoms after the treatment phase. In addition to monitoring brucellosis symptoms, both doctors and patients should monitor any adverse effects of medication. For instance, adverse reactions to TMP-SMX occur in 50% to 100% of patients with AIDS compared with about 14% of patients without AIDS. Up to 57% of AIDS patients treated with TMP-SMX[1] require a change in therapy owing to the adverse effects.

Generally, brucellosis patients should be followed up clinically for up to 2 years to detect relapse. Patients should be monitored for regaining of body weight. IgG antibody should be checked by serum agglutination test for levels that remain in the diagnostic range for more than 2 years. Complement fixation titers should fall to normal within 1 year of treatment. Relapse should respond to a prolonged course of the same therapy originally used.

Complications

Brucellae are transported into the lymphatic system and can replicate in spleen, liver, kidney, breast tissue, and joints to cause both localized and systemic infections. Infection of the reproductive system can cause fetal abortion. Owing to the low virulence, low toxicity, and multiple mechanisms to protect them from the immune system, brucellae can survive and reproduce in nearly any tissues or organs. At 1 year after infection, the disease can develop into chronic brucellosis that can further cause one or multiple complications in one organ or the whole body.

There are seven major types of complications from *Brucella* infection.

- Endocarditis: Brucellae can infect the heart's inner lining, which can destroy the heart valves and, if left untreated, will lead to death of the patient.
- Meningitis and encephalitis: Brucellae can infect the central nervous system to cause an inflammation of the brain, the membranes surrounding the brain, and the spinal cord. This is fatal if the patient is not treated in time.
- Arthritis: Osteoarthritis caused by *Brucella* infection is typically associated with pain, stiffness, and swelling of the joints, such as the knees, hips, ankles, wrists, spine, shoulder, elbow, sternoclavicular, and small joints. Spondylitis caused by brucellae is characterized by joint inflammation between the vertebrae bones of the spine or between the spine and pelvis. Spondylitis is difficult to treat and can cause lasting damage. These osteoarticular complications are the clinical forms most commonly observed.
- Epididymitis and epididymoorchitis: Brucellae can infect the epididymis to cause swelling and pain of the testicle.
- Cutaneous complications: Brucellae can infect skin to cause lesions, rashes, nodules, erythema nodosum, papules, petechiae, and purpura.
- Respiratory complications: Inhalation of brucellae can result in lung infection, which can lead to pneumonia, bronchopneumonia, pleural effusion with a predominance of monocytic or lymphocytic infiltrates, and paroxysmal dry cough.
- Hematologic complications: Aspartate aminotransferase (AST) or alanine aminotransferase (ALT) levels can be elevated and are associated with pain in the right upper quadrant or jaundice.

Complications are common in brucellosis patients. Young patients tend to have cutaneous, hematologic, and respiratory complications. Adult patients tend toward osteoarticular and cardiac complications. Middle-aged patients tend to develop genitourinary, neurologic, and gastrointestinal complications.

Prevention

Maintaining hygienic habits is very important for avoiding *Brucella* infection. These include consuming only pasteurized milk and cheese. Meat must be cooked thoroughly before consumption. In these regards, education is beneficial for preventing infection by this pathogen. People who handle animals or animal products should wear personal protective equipment, including glasses, rubber gloves, and clothing to protect skin and eyes from exposure or direct contact. Laboratory workers should use a Biosafety Level 3 (BSL-3) facility to handle the *Brucella* organisms and work according to the laboratory's standard operating procedures. Animal immunization programs must be maintained all over the world to cut off the transmission chain from livestock to humans. In addition, primary care physicians should be familiar with the clinical and laboratory findings of brucellosis symptoms and complications.

References

Centers for Disease Control and Prevention: *Sexually Transmitted Diseases Treatment Guidelines, 2010: Epididymitis*, 2012. Available at http://www.cdc.gov/std/treatment/2010/epididymitis.htm (accessed 07.09.15).

Corbel MJ: *Brucellosis in humans and animals*, Geneva, 2006, World Health Organization.

Dokuzoguz B, Nurcan Baykam N: Brucellosis. In Bope ET, Kellerman RD, Rakel RE, editors: *Conn's Current Therapy 2011*, Philadelphia, 2011, Saunders, pp 74–78.

Gür A, Geyik MF, Dikici B, et al: Complications of brucellosis in different age groups: A study of 283 cases in southeastern Anatolia of Turkey, *Yonsei Med J* 44:33–44, 2003.

Harrison's Practice. Answers on Demand. Brucellosis, 2012, Available at. http://www.harrisonspractice.com. (Accessed 8.11.16).

Joint WHO/FAO Expert Committee on Brucellosis: Sixth report, *World Health Organ Tech Rep Ser* 740:1–132, 1986.

Mayo Clinic. Brucellosis: Complications, 2012. Available at. http://www.mayoclinic.com/health/brucellosis/DS00837/DSECTION=complications. 2012 [accessed 07.09.15].

Pappas G, Akritidis N, Bosilkovski M, et al: Brucellosis, *N Engl J Med* 352:2325–2336, 2005.

Pappas G, Bosilkovski M, Akritidis N, et al: Brucellosis and the respiratory system, *Clin Infect Dis* 37:e95–399, 2003.

Skalsky K, Yahav D, Bishara J, et al: Treatment of human brucellosis: Systematic review and meta-analysis of randomised controlled trials, *BMJ* 336:701–704, 2008.

Yang X, Skyberg JA, Cao L, et al: Progress in Brucella vaccine development, *Front Biol* 8:60–77, 2013, https://doi.org/10.1007/s11515-012-1196-0.

CLOSTRIDIOIDES DIFFICILE COLITIS

Method of
Jeffery D. Semel, MD

CURRENT DIAGNOSIS

- *Clostridium difficile* (renamed *Clostridioides difficile*) infection is diagnosed by a combination of clinical and laboratory-findings.
- Diagnosis requires a positive test for the presence of *C. difficile* toxins.
- GDH, or glutamate dehydrogenase, produced by *C. difficile*, can be detected in stool. However, it is not specific and can be produced by non-toxigenic *C. difficile*.
- Enzyme immunoassay testing for toxin A and or B has a variable sensitivity and specificity and a turnaround time of about 24 hours and correlates well with disease activity.
- Polymerase chain reaction testing has a high sensitivity and specificity and a turnaround time of less than 4 hours; correlates less with disease activity, thus identifying patients with colonization as well as active infection. Increasingly, combination testing is being employed to imrove diagnostic accuracy.
- Laboratory testing for *C. difficile* toxins should only be performed on patients with ≥3 unformed stools per 24 hours, who are not on laxatives and is not useful as a test of cure.
- Pathologic findings can help to confirm diagnosis.

CURRENT THERAPY

- If possible, the clinician should first consider discontinuing concurrent antibacterial therapy.
- Treatment should be initiated only after a positive test result for *C. difficile* toxin unless the patient is at high risk for *C. difficile* infection or is severely ill, in which case empirical therapy is justified.
- Treatment recommendations depend on the severity of the disease and whether the patient has a first-time diagnosis or recurrence.
- Clinical parameters that guide treatment include increasing age, leukocytosis, elevation of serum creatinine, and presence of hypotension, shock, ileus, or megacolon.
- Oral vancomycin (Vancocin) or fidaxomicin (Dificid), are preferred for initial therapy. Metronidazole (Flagyl)[1] oral, can be used for non-severe disease if these are not available.
- Intravenous metronidazole and or rectal vancomycin (enema)[1],[6] can be added for severe disease.
- FMT (fecal microbiota therapy) is a safe and effective option for recurrent disease, and has shown promise in studies of severe or fulminant *C. difficile* infection.
- Antimicrobial stewardship programs are a safe and cost-effective method of reducing the burden of *C. difficile* infections.

[1]Not FDA approved for this indication.
[6]May be compounded by pharmacists.

Pseudomembranous colitis is an inflammatory disease of the colon that is almost always associated with the toxin-producing bacteria *Clostridioides difficile*. In very rare cases, other organisms can be responsible. In this article I discuss *C. difficile* as an important cause of pseudomembranous colitis.

Epidemiology and Risk Factors

C. difficile is the most common infectious cause of health care–associated diarrhea. Studies in US hospitals showed that mortality rates related to *C. difficile* infection nearly quadrupled from 1999 through 2004. An active population and laboratory based study done by the US Centers for Disease Control and Prevention in 2011 suggested that 453,000 new cases occur in the United States annually; with a 30-day mortality rate of 6.4%. Higher rates of infection were found in whites, females, and those >65 years of age. A Canadian study in 2011 prospectively followed 5422 hospitalized patients and showed that 7.4% had asymptomatic colonization only (60% of these were positive at the time of admission); 2.8% developed *C. difficile* infection during hospitalization. Another study by the CDC found decreased hospital-associated infection rates in US hospitals between 2011 and 2015 but no change in the rate of *C. difficile* infections. Colonization of asymptomatic hospitalized patients with *C. difficile* ranges from 0%–22% and is higher in residents of long-term care facilities.

Additional risk factors for the development of *C. difficile* infection include antimicrobial or chemotherapeutic drug exposure, severe underlying illness, prior hospitalization (acute or long-term care), use of feeding tubes, recent gastrointestinal surgery, and gastric acid suppression. Exposure to antibiotics has been shown to lead to an alteration in the type and quantity of bacterial species found in the normal human intestinal microbiome. Most antibiotics have been associated with *C. difficile* infection. Increased antimicrobial duration and dosage appear to be associated with higher risk of *C. difficile* infection.

Epidemic strains have been described by pulsed-field gel electrophoresis (NAP1,4,7,11 etc.) that are associated with decreased regulatory gene function and increased toxin production. The risk and severity of infection are increased after exposure to the NAP1 strains. Failure of standard first-line therapy for *C. difficile* infection may increase to 10% to 35% during infection with NAP strains.

C. difficile infection occurs rarely without prior antibiotic exposure. Healthy peripartum women, children, and postsurgical patients rarely have *C. difficile* infection develop after a single dose of an antibiotic. Newborns have a higher rate of colonization but generally a low rate of *C. difficile* infection.

Infection is costly. It is estimated that each episode costs the US health care system $3,427–$16,307 per episode or $1.2 billion–$5.9 billion per year.

Microbiology and Pathophysiology

C. difficile is a gram-positive, spore-forming, anaerobic rod. *C. difficile* can exist as either a spore or vegetative form. The vegetative form is highly oxygen sensitive; slight exposure can kill the bacteria. The spore form is highly heat-stable and can survive harsh conditions such as the high acidity of the stomach. Spores have been shown to resist many commercial disinfectants. *C. difficile* reproduces in intestinal crypts and releases exotoxins A and B, leading to severe inflammation. Toxin A (enterotoxin) attracts neutrophils and monocytes, and toxin B (cytotoxin) degrades colonic epithelial cells. Most strains of *C. difficile* produce both toxin A and B; however, toxin production, and thus detection may fluctuate during infection. Toxins disrupt cell membranes and cause shallow ulcerations on the intestine mucosal surface. Ulcer formation leads to the release of proteins, mucus, and inflammation manifesting as a pseudomembrane. A pseudomembrane is virtually pathognomonic for *C. difficile* infection.

Transmission occurs via the fecal–oral route, person to person, or via fomites. Following exposure to antibiotics, the normal gut flora is altered ("dysbiosis"), allowing *C. difficile* to become more dominant. Exposure to *C. difficile* spores may result in no acquisition, asymptomatic colonization, mild diarrhea, or infection. Evidence showing colonization occurring during hospitalization as opposed to prior to hospitalization poses an increased risk for *C. difficile* infection, suggests that colonization in some patients induces immunity, and that more virulent strains are present in the hospital.

In addition, the host immune response to spore exposure is important in determining the clinical outcome. Approximately 60% of people have detectable levels of antibodies to toxin A and B. It is likely that prior exposure to *C. difficile* spores or related clostridial species and subsequent colonization stimulates antibody production and immunity. *C. difficile* has been found to be capable of creating a biofilm in vitro, which may impair the antibacterial activity of antibiotics such as metronidazole (Flagyl). Various studies are attempting to define the role of active or passive immunotherapy, including vaccination with nontoxigenic *C. difficile*, to prevent *C. difficile* infection.

Clinical Features

C. difficile infection is diagnosed by a combination of clinical and laboratory findings. Diarrhea is defined as the passage of three or more unformed stools in a 24-hour period. Symptoms include fever, diarrhea, and cramplike abdominal pain. Patients can have nausea, vomiting, or hematochezia. In severe cases, abdominal tenderness and distention are present. Signs of septic shock can develop. The extent of leukocytosis frequently correlates with disease severity. Plain abdominal radiographs might show distended loops of bowel, ileus, or, in severe cases, toxic megacolon. Computed tomography (CT) image findings include colonic wall thickening and dilatation, mesenteric edema, and, rarely, perforation. Endoscopy can reveal pseudomembranes. However, sigmoidoscopy or colonoscopy may be complicated by perforation in severely ill patients and should be performed with caution.

Differential Diagnosis

The differential diagnosis includes bacterial causes such as *Shigella*, *Salmonella*, or *Campylobacter* species, protozoan infections such as *Entamoeba histolytica* or *Strongyloides stercoralis* (immunosuppressed patients), inflammatory disorders such as ulcerative colitis or Crohn's disease, drug toxicity (e.g., chemotherapeutic agents), and vascular disorders such as ischemic bowel disease.

Diagnosis

Various tests have been developed for the diagnosis of *C. difficile* infection. Glutamate dehydrogenase (GDH) is a protein produced by *C. difficile* and can be detected in stool. It is very sensitive for *C. difficile* but can be produced by non-toxigenic *C. difficile* and thus is non-specific.

Enzyme immunoassays (EIA) for toxin A and or B detect toxin production. The sensitivity is 63%–94% and specificity is 75%–100%. GDH and toxin assays correlate well with clinical disease activity, but may not detect the presence of small amounts of toxin.

Molecular tests such as polymerase chain reaction (PCR) can be performed in less than 4 hours. The sensitivity is approximately 93% and specificity is 97%. These tests target toxin genes and do not always correlate with clinical disease. Since the introduction of PCR, the number of cases diagnosed has increased further (though some may represent colonization). Thus positive *C. difficile* testing must be correlated with clinical disease activity to determine if treatment is indicated. Increasingly, authors have recommended two-step testing using PCR, or, GDH/toxin EIA, followed by PCR when GDH/toxin EIA are discordant.

Treatment

If possible, the clinician should first consider discontinuing concurrent antibacterial therapy, unless there is a compelling clinical indication to continue. Antimotility agents should be avoided because decreased gut motility can increase the potential for tissue toxin exposure and toxic megacolon. Treatment for *C. difficile* infection should be initiated only after a positive *C. difficile* test result unless the patient is at high risk for *C. difficile* infection or is severely ill, in which case empirical therapy is reasonable even with negative test results.

Antibacterials used to treat *C. difficile* infection can be administered orally, intravenously, or rectally. Oral therapies are preferred. Oral vancomycin (Vancocin) is not absorbed in the gastrointestinal tract and is eliminated in the feces. Fidaxomicin (Dificid), a macrocyclic antibiotic, has been shown to have equal efficacy to vancomycin but with a potentially lower rate of *C. difficile* recurrence. Fidaxomicin is approved for patients 18 years or older. Oral metronidazole (Flagyl), a nitroimidazole antibiotic, is eliminated primarily in the urine, although 6% to 15% is eliminated in the feces, and may be less active as inflammation subsides.

The Society for Healthcare Epidemiology of America (SHEA) and the Infectious Diseases Society of America (IDSA) published treatment guidelines in 2018. Recommendations for the treatment of *C. difficile* infection depend on the severity of the disease. Clinical parameters that correlate with severity include increasing age, leukocytosis, and elevation of the serum creatinine.

For all patients with a first episode of *C. difficile* infection vancomycin 125 mg four times daily or fidaxomicin 200 mg twice daily, by mouth (PO) for 10 days is recommended. If these drugs are not available, metronidazole (Flagyl)[1] 500 mg three times daily by mouth can be used but should be avoided if the disease is severe.

A white blood cell count of at least 15,000 cells/μL or a serum creatinine at least 1.5 times the premorbid level suggests the possibility of severe infection.

Patients with an initial episode that is complicated by hypotension, shock, ileus, or megacolon should be treated with vancomycin 500 mg PO 4 times per day, plus metronidazole 500 mg IV[1] every 8 hours. If the patient has a complete ileus, the clinician may consider adding a rectal instillation of vancomycin[1,6] 500 mg every 6 hours. It is recommended that trained personnel administer the enema to decrease the chances of rectal perforation.

---

[1]Not FDA approved for this indication.
[6]May be compounded by pharmacists.

Monitoring

The response to therapy should be monitored clinically. Reversal of hemodynamic instability, decreasing stool frequency, and a declining white blood cell count are objective measures of response. Stool tests for *C. difficile* toxin are not valuable for monitoring disease elimination, because these tests can remain positive after improvement.

Complications and Recurrence

Another challenging problem in *C. difficile* infection is recurrence. Recurrence is defined as another episode that occurs within eight weeks following resolution of the initial episode. Recurrence occurs in approximately 20% to 30% of cases. Continued use of antibacterials (other than treating agents), increased age, female sex, use of proton pump inhibitors or corticosteroids, living in a nursing home, longer hospitalization, severe underlying disease, and inadequate antitoxin antibody response are risk factors for relapse. Even though treatment failure and relapse are common, resistance to metronidazole or vancomycin is uncommon.

For an initial recurrence, a tapered, pulsed dose regimen of vancomycin is often employed. This consists of vancomycin 125 mg PO 4 times per day for 2 weeks, followed by 125 mg PO 2 times per day for 1 week, followed by vancomycin 125 mg PO once daily for 1 week, followed by 125 mg PO once every 2 to 3 days for 2 to 8 weeks.

Fidaxomicin may be considered as an alternative to vancomycin for an initial recurrence.

Another option for recurrent *C. difficile* infection is fecal reconstitution or fecal microbiota therapy (FMT). The goal is to reverse dysbiosis and restore normal colonic flora. Healthy donor stool is infused via colonoscopy, intraduodenal, or by frozen capsule. Numerous studies have shown the efficacy of FMT, although the exact place, timing and mode of installation continue to be under evaluation. A second FMT installation may improve efficiency. Donor stool must be screened for infectious agents prior to installation. Additional promising options for prevention of recurrences include the addition of monoclonal antibodies directed against *C. difficile* and the oral administration of non toxigenic *C. difficile* strains. A monoclonal antibody directed at *C. difficile* toxin B, bezlotoxumab (Zinplava), is available for the prevention of recurrence in patients at high risk. Additionally, should antibiotic therapy be required in a high risk patient, prophylaxis with vancomycin appears to be beneficial in reducing the risk of *C. difficile* colitis.

Probiotics[7] are live organisms that seek to restore the normal gastrointestinal microflora. Most studies have used *Lactobacillus* species or *Saccharomyces boulardii* in an effort to prevent, or treat *C. difficile* infection. A recent Cochrane analysis has shown that the use of probiotics during antimicrobial administration may decrease the subsequent development of *C. difficile* colitis. The optimal probiotic formula, dosing, and side effect profile remains to be determined. Probiotics have not shown benefit during active infection. Occasional cases of fungemia or bacteremia have been reported in immunocompromised patients and those with central venous catheters treated with probiotics. Probiotics should be avoided in these patients.

Recently, Fischer et al. have reported promising results using fecal microbiota transplant with oral vancomycin in the treatment of severe or fulminant *C. difficile* colitis as a possible option to avoid surgery in critically ill patients. Total colectomy is often considered as a last measure for patients who remain critically ill despite standard therapy. The exact indications for surgery are not clear, although refractory shock, signs of peritonitis, megacolon, and multiorgan failure are most often cited. As expected, the mortality rate after total colectomy is high, ranging from 35% to 80%. Neal and colleagues reported that in a series of 42 patients, performance of a diverting loop ileostomy and intraoperative colonic lavage with polyethylene glycol, followed by postoperative antegrade vancomycin flushes, resulted in 19% mortality and 93% colon preservation.

Prevention

Given the current difficulties in controlling the spread of *C. difficile*, prevention is critical. *C. difficile* spores resist desiccation and can survive in the hospital environment for months. Environmental contamination is highest in and around the rooms of patients with *C. difficile* infection. The risk of hospital-associated *C. difficile* has been found to be increased for patients occupying the bed of a previous patient who received antibiotics. Items that have been found to harbor *C. difficile* spores include clothing, blood pressure cuffs, telephones, toilets, doorknobs, oral and rectal thermometers, and other medical equipment. In addition, the hands of health care workers have been found to be a vehicle of transmission.

Current recommendations for prevention of transmission of *C. difficile* include the following. Careful hand hygiene with soap and water is essential. Programs to monitor the compliance and technique of hand hygiene are recommended. Alcohol-based hand rubs, which are widely used, have been shown to be less effective at removing spores than conventional hand washing. Thus alcohol-based hand rubs should not be used for *C. difficile* isolation when *C. difficile* outbreaks are present. Barrier precautions with gowns and gloves should be used. Programs to ensure adequate and effective cleaning of health care facilities after use are recommended. Disposable electronic thermometers are recommended. Antimicrobial stewardship programs aimed at promoting the judicious use of antibacterial therapy have been found to be effective in reducing *C. difficile* infection rates and are encouraged.

References

Agrawal M, Aroniadis OC, Brandt LJ, et al: The long-term efficacy and safety of fecal microbiota transplant for recurrent, severe, and complicated *Clostridium difficile* infection in 146 elderly individuals, *J Clin Gastroenterol* 50(5):403–407, 2016.

Feazel L, Malhotra A, Perencevich E, et al: Effect of antibiotic stewardship programmes on Clostridium difficile incidence: a systematic review and meta-analysis, *J Antimicrob Chemother.* 69:1748–1754, 2014.

Fischer M, Sipe B, Cheng Y, et al: Fecal microbiota transplant in severe and severe-complicated *Clostridium difficile*: A promising treatment approach, *Gut Microbes* 8(3):289–302, 2017.

Goldenberg JZ, Yap C, Lytvyn L, et al: Probiotics for the prevention of Clostridium difficile-associated diarrhea in adults and children, *Cochrane Database Syst Rev* 12:CD006095, 2017.

Hsu J, Abad C, Dinh M, et al: Prevention of endemic healthcare-associated *Clostridium difficile* infection: reviewing the evidence, *Am J Gastroenterol* 105:2327–2339, 2010.

Jiang ZD, Ajami NJ, Petrosino JF, et al: Randomised clinical trial: faecal microbiota transplantation for recurrent Clostridum difficile infection - fresh, or frozen, or lyophilised microbiota from a small pool of healthy donors delivered by colonoscopy, *Aliment Pharmacol Ther* 45(7):899–908, 2017.

Johnson SW, Brown SV, Priest DH: Effectiveness of oral vancomycin for prevention of healthcare facility-onset *Clostridioides difficile* infection in targeted patients during systemic antibiotic exposure, *Clin Infect Dis* 27:ciz966, 2019, https://doi.org/10.1093/cid/ciz966. {epub ahead of print}.

Kyne L, Warny M, Qamar A, et al: Asymptomatic carriage of *Clostridium difficile* and serum levels of IGG antibody against toxin A, *N Engl J Med* 342:390–397, 2000.

Kwon JH, Olsen MA, Dubberke ER: The morbidity, mortality, and costs associated with Clostridium difficile infection, *Infect Dis Clin N Am* 29:123–134, 2015.

Ma GK, Brensinger CM, Wu Q, et al: Increasing incidence of multiply recurrent *Clostridium difficile* infection in the United States: A cohort study, *Ann Intern Med* 167:152–158, 2017.

Magill SS, O'Leary SJ, Janelle DL, et al: Changes in prevalence of health - care associated infections in U.S. hospitals, *N Engl J Med* 379:1732–1744, 2018.

McDonald LC, Gerding DN, Johnson S, et al: Practice Guidelines for Clostridium difficile Infection in Adults and Children: 2017, *Clin Infect Dis* 66:987–994, 2018.

Neal M, Alverdy JC, Hall DE, et al: Diverting loop ileostomy and colonic lavage: An alternative to total abdominal colectomy for treatment of severe, complicated *Clostridium difficile* associated disease, *Ann Surg* 254:423–427, 2011.

Oksi J, Aalto A, Sailla P, et al: Real-world efficacy of bezlotoxumab for prevention of recurrent *Clostridium difficile* infection: a retrospective study of 46 patients in five university hospitals in Finland, *Eur J Clin Microbiol Infect Dis* 38:1947–1952, 2019.

Shim JK, Johnson S, Samore MH, et al: Primary symptomless colonisation by *Clostridium difficile* and decreased risk of subsequent diarrhea, *Lancet* 351:633, 1998.

---

[7]Available as a dietary supplement.

CAT SCRATCH DISEASE

Method of
Ronen Ben-Ami, MD

CURRENT DIAGNOSIS

- The combination of a compatible clinical syndrome of regional lymphadenopathy with a primary inoculation lesion and cat contact is highly suggestive of cat scratch disease.
- Results of *Bartonella henselae* serology are helpful in confirming the diagnosis; however, up to 20% of patients remain seronegative throughout their disease.
- Detection of *B. henselae* DNA by polymerase chain reaction from pus obtained by needle aspiration or lymph node biopsy is a highly sensitive diagnostic modality and may be particularly useful in seronegative patients.

CURRENT THERAPY

- Typical cat scratch disease is a self-limited disease; therefore, systemic antimicrobials are not routinely indicated in immunocompetent patients with uncomplicated cat scratch disease.
- Indications for antimicrobial therapy include an immunocompromised host, endocarditis, retinitis, and other atypical syndromes.
- Treatment may also be considered for patients who have typical cat scratch disease along with extensive or bulky lymphadenopathy and are highly symptomatic.
- Suppurative lymph nodes should be drained by large-bore needle aspiration.

Cat scratch disease is a worldwide zoonotic infection caused by *Bartonella henselae*, an intracellular, pleomorphic, gram-negative bacillus. Other *Bartonella* species have rarely been implicated. The disease typically manifests as benign regional lymphadenopathy, but atypical disease can involve almost any organ system and is associated with significant morbidity.

Epidemiology

B. henselae infection is widespread among domestic cats and other felids worldwide, and serologic studies indicate a higher prevalence in warm, humid climates. Transmission among cats occurs via an arthropod vector, the cat flea *Ctenocephalides felis*. *B. henselae* bacteremia is detected at higher rates in feral than in domesticated cats and in kittens as compared to adult cats, explaining the higher infectivity of these animals. Cats infected with *B. henselae* are asymptomatic. Transmission to humans occurs via a scratch, bite, or lick; contamination of cat scratches by flea feces may enhance *Bartonella* transmission.

Cat scratch disease has been estimated to occur in the United States at a rate approaching 10 per 100,000 population. There is some seasonality, with incidences peaking between September and January. Although traditionally considered a disease of childhood, epidemiologic surveys have found a similar incidence of cat scratch disease in adults, and 6% of those patients are aged 60 years or older. Cat contact is the most important risk factor: Almost all patients are cat owners or were otherwise exposed to cats, and about half can recall a recent bite or scratch, most commonly by a kitten.

Clinical Manifestations

Cat scratch disease is divided into two clinical syndromes. Typical cat scratch disease is a subacute, self-limited regional lymphadenopathy and constitutes 80% to 90% of cases. Atypical cat scratch disease encompasses Parinaud oculoglandular syndrome and other clinical entities with systemic extranodal involvement. Bacillary angiomatosis and bacillary peliosis are manifestations of *B. henselae* infection in immunocompromised persons and are not discussed here.

Typical Cat Scratch Disease

A primary skin lesion, usually a papule or pustule, appears at the site of inoculation 3 to 10 days after cat contact and persists for 1 to 3 weeks. Regional lymphadenopathy develops within 1 to 7 weeks and resolves spontaneously after 2 to 4 months. The primary lesion is still present in about two thirds of patients when they present for evaluation of lymphadenopathy. The most commonly involved lymph nodes are, in descending order of frequency, axillary and epitrochlear nodes, head and neck nodes, and femoral and inguinal nodes. One third of patients develop lymphadenopathy at multiple sites. Lymph nodes are often painful and red; suppuration occurs in 10% of nodes. Mild constitutional symptoms, including low-grade fever and malaise, are noted in about half the cases. Rash, night sweats, anorexia, and weight loss are uncommon. Infection results in lifelong immunity.

Atypical Cat Scratch Disease

Parinaud oculoglandular syndrome, the most common form of atypical cat scratch disease, is a specific type of regional lymphadenopathy that occurs following conjunctival inoculation of *B. henselae*. The syndrome includes granulomatous conjunctivitis and preauricular lymphadenopathy. Endocarditis and encephalitis represent severe forms of *B. henselae* infection and are more common in elderly patients. Encephalitis manifests with various degrees of altered mental status, agitation, headache, and seizures. Cerebrospinal fluid lymphocytic pleocytosis occurs in only one third of cases, and brain-imaging studies usually fail to show any abnormalities. Neuroretinitis manifests as sudden unilateral loss of visual acuity. The diagnosis is suspected based on typical findings on fundoscopic examination: papilledema and macular exudates in a starlike configuration. However, these findings are not pathognomonic of cat scratch disease. Other infrequent manifestations are self-limited granulomatous hepatitis and splenitis and osteoarticular disease. Prolonged fever of unknown origin is a rare manifestation. Patients present with relapsing fever, weight loss, and night sweats, often with organ involvement, specifically hepatosplenic lesions, abdominal or mediastinal lymphadenopathy, and ocular disease.

Diagnosis

A compatible clinical syndrome in a person with a positive history of cat exposure suggests cat scratch disease. The diagnosis is most commonly confirmed with specific serologic assays. Immunofluorescence and enzyme immunoassays are comparably sensitive, although cross-reactivity can occur with other organisms such as *Chlamydia* species, *Coxiella burnetii*, and non-*henselae Bartonella* species. A single elevated titer of immunoglobulin (Ig)M or IgG in the acute phase or a fourfold increase of IgG in convalescent serum supports the diagnosis.

Biopsy and histopathologic examination of lymph nodes are usually only performed when malignancy is suspected. Necrotizing granulomas are typically observed. The pleomorphic gram-negative bacilli are best visualized with the Warthin-Starry stain;

TABLE 1	Antibiotic Treatment Regimens for Cat Scratch Disease		
CLINICAL SYNDROME	FIRST CHOICE	SECOND CHOICE	COMMENTS
Typical cat scratch disease	Not indicated*	Azithromycin (Zithromax)[1] 500 mg PO on day 1, then 250 mg PO × 4 days	Drain suppurative nodes using large-bore aspiration
Endocarditis	Gentamicin (Garamycin)[1] 1 mg/kg IV q8h × >14 days plus doxycycline (Vibramycin) 100 mg IV/PO bid × 6 wk	Doxycycline 100 mg PO bid plus rifampicin (Rifadin)[1] 300 mg PO bid × 6 wk	Some experts recommend extending oral doxycycline treatment × 3–6 mo Surgical valve excision may be required
Neuroretinitis	Doxycycline 100 mg PO bid plus rifampicin[1] 300 mg PO bid × 4–6 wk	NA	Spontaneous resolution is the rule; the utility of treatment remains unproven
Other atypical cat scratch disease	As for neuroretinitis	NA	Treatment duration should be individualized

*Treatment may be considered for patients with bulky or extensive lymphadenopathy and for immunocompromised patients.
[1]Not FDA approved for this indication.
NA, Not available.

however, the sensitivity of this method is too low to be clinically useful. Similarly, culture lacks sensitivity and requires prolonged incubation, making it impractical for routine use.

Polymerase chain reaction assays for the detection of *B. henselae* in pus aspirated from suppurative lymph nodes or primary skin lesions is highly sensitive and specific, and it can be performed with a rapid turnaround time. However, these assays are not widely available in most clinical microbiology laboratories.

Differential Diagnosis

Cat scratch disease should be differentiated from other infectious and noninfectious causes of regional lymphadenopathy. Importantly, lymphoma and solid tumors with metastases to lymph nodes may be confused with cat scratch disease. Malignancy should be suspected in patients who have marked constitutional symptoms, who are seronegative, or whose lymphadenopathy fails to resolve spontaneously after more than 6 months. Unlike cat scratch disease, pyogenic lymphadenitis manifests with rapid progression, high-grade fever, and a septic-appearing patient. Mycobacterial infection, syphilis, bubonic plague, tularemia, histoplasmosis, and sporotrichosis should be considered based on the presence of specific risk factors and endemic exposures. *Bartonella* endocarditis must be differentiated from other causes of culture-negative endocarditis, specifically Q fever and brucellosis.

Treatment

Because of the self-limiting course of typical cat scratch disease, patients usually only require observation and reassurance of its benign nature. The goals of therapy are alleviation of symptoms in patients with bulky lymphadenopathy and drainage of suppurating lymph nodes to prevent spontaneous formation of chronic sinus tracts. If drug treatment is initiated, azithromycin (Zithromax)[1] is the agent of choice based on a small randomized placebo-controlled study that showed more-rapid resolution of lymphadenopathy in the azithromycin arm as determined by ultrasound. Suppurative nodes should be drained by large-bore needle aspiration. Incisional drainage is best avoided because it can promote sinus tract formation.

Atypical cat scratch disease syndromes usually require treatment, but there are scant data to support specific regimens and treatment duration is not well defined. For patients with endocarditis, treatment with an aminoglycoside for at least 14 days is associated with a higher likelihood of recovery and survival. Uncontrolled data suggest that, for patients with neuroretinitis, treatment with antibiotics and corticosteroids is associated with better visual outcomes than treatment with antibiotics alone (Table 1).

Prevention

Flea control in domestic cats can reduce the likelihood of *Bartonella* bacteremia and transmission to humans. Bites and scratches should be promptly rinsed. HIV-infected patients and other immunocompromised persons should be cautioned about the risks of cat exposure because they are susceptible to disseminated visceral *B. henselae* infection, as well as other zoonotic infections such as toxoplasmosis.

References

Ben-Ami R, Ephros M, Avidor B, et al: Cat-scratch disease in elderly patients, *Clin Infect Dis* 41:969–974, 2005.
Giladi M, Kletter Y, Avidor B, et al: Enzyme immunoassay for the diagnosis of cat-scratch disease defined by polymerase chain reaction, *Clin Infect Dis* 33:1852–1858, 2001.
Habot-Wilner Z, Trivizki O, Goldstein M, et al: Cat-scratch disease: ocular manifestations and treatment outcome, *Acta Ophthalmol* 96(4):e524–e532, 2018.
Hansmann Y, DeMartino S, Piemont Y, et al: Diagnosis of cat scratch disease with detection of *Bartonella henselae* by PCR: A study of patients with lymph node enlargement, *J Clin Microbiol* 43:3800–3806, 2005.
Jackson LA, Perkins BA, Wenger JD: Cat scratch disease in the United States: An analysis of three national databases, *Am J Public Health* 83:1707–1711, 1993.
Jacobs RF, Schutze GE: *Bartonella henselae* as a cause of prolonged fever and fever of unknown origin in children, *Clin Infect Dis* 26:80–84, 1998.
Raoult D, Fournier PE, Vandenesch F, et al: Outcome and treatment of *Bartonella* endocarditis, *Arch Intern Med* 163:226–230, 2003.
Rolain JM, Brouqui P, Koehler JE, et al: Recommendations for treatment of human infections caused by *Bartonella* species, *Antimicrob Agents Chemother* 48:1921–1933, 2004.
Zangwill KM, Hamilton DH, Perkins BA, et al: Cat scratch disease in Connecticut. Epidemiology, risk factors, and evaluation of a new diagnostic test, *N Engl J Med* 329:8–13, 1993.

[1]Not FDA-approved for this indication.

CHIKUNGUNYA

Method of
Scott Kellermann, MD, MPH; and Rick D. Kellerman, MD

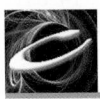

CURRENT DIAGNOSIS

- Clinically, chikungunya is a diagnosis of exclusion, particularly when laboratory testing is not available. Accurate diagnosis depends on the patient's clinical symptoms and the epidemiology of endemic disease.
- Acute symptoms include incapacitating relapsing bilateral symmetrical polyarthralgia accompanied by high fever, headache, backache, and fatigue. Some may have a pruritic maculopapular rash at onset.
- Chronic symptoms include episodic incapacitating symmetrical polyarthralgia. Many have long-term asthenia and depression.
- Virus isolation provides definitive diagnosis.
- Immunoglobulin M antibody levels peak 3 to 5 weeks after the onset of illness and persist for approximately 2 months.
- Immunoglobulin M antibody levels peak 3 to 5 weeks after the onset of illness and persist for approximately 2 months.
- Paired acute-phase and convalescent-phase antibody sampling may be required for diagnosis.

CURRENT THERAPY

- Medical treatment is primarily supportive.

The word "chikungunya" is a derivation of the Kimakonde (a Mozambique dialect) word "kungunyala" meaning "to become desiccated or contorted." In the Democratic Republic of the Congo, it is called "buka-buka," translated as "broken-broken," reflecting the incapacitating arthralgias that are common manifestations of Chikungunya fever.

Epidemiology

Chikungunya, first diagnosed in Tanganyika in 1952, is found in a large percentage of countries in Africa, Asia, and Southeast Asia and is prevalent in India. Chikungunya virus often causes large outbreaks with high attack rates, affecting one-third to three-quarters of the population. Dense human populations and lack of herd immunity likely contribute to the explosive nature of chikungunya epidemics in many regions. In India during 2006, more than 1,250,000 cases of chikungunya were reported, with *Aedes aegypti* implicated as the vector. In late 2013, the first locally acquired cases were reported on Caribbean islands. By the end of 2017, more than 2.6 million suspected cases had been reported in the Americas. From 2010 through 2013, 110 cases of chikungunya were reported among US travelers. Following the outbreak in the Americas, there were >4,000 cases reported in US travelers from 2014 to 2017, 13 of which were locally acquired in the continental United States in 2020, there were 22 cases reported from 10 states, all from returning travelers. There were no reported cases from US territories. All reported cases occurred in travelers returning from affected areas. No locally transmitted cases have been reported from U.S. states.

A 2014 study, undertaken by the Puerto Rico Department of Health and the CDC, demonstrated that chikungunya cases are underreported in Puerto Rico. In passive surveillance of 250 participants, 70 (28%) tested positive for past or current chikungunya virus infection. However, only two of 25 participants (8%) with chikungunya infection who sought care had been reported to health authorities.

It is believed that chikungunya virus originated in Africa and migrated to Asia 200 years ago. Evidence derived from molecular genetics suggests it evolved around 1700; the first recorded outbreak of this disease was probably in 1779.

Interestingly, some medical historians believe that a pandemic of chikungunya occurred in the western hemisphere in the 1800s but was diagnosed as dengue fever. The 21st-century researchers who have examined the accounts of this pandemic now speculate that it was caused by chikungunya because the cases exhibited severe joint arthritis, which is more indicative of chikungunya than dengue. The virus then disappeared from the Americas until it reemerged during the last decade. Chikungunya epidemics appear suddenly and unpredictably and proceed explosively.

Risk Factors

Individuals at the highest risk of contracting chikungunya and suffering from more-severe symptoms are those who have chronic arthritis, underlying chronic medical conditions, those over the age of 65 years, and pregnant women. Travelers who spend extended periods of time in endemic areas are at greater risk. These include missionaries, humanitarian aid workers, and those who frequently work outdoors.

Pathophysiology

Chikungunya is an arthropod transmitted disease caused by a single-stranded RNA arbovirus. As with dengue fever and yellow fever, chikungunya cycles from mosquito to human to mosquito. The mosquito *Aedes aegypti* is the usual vector for transmission of chikungunya. *Aedes albopictus*, the Asian tiger mosquito, is also a vector. Both species are found in the southeastern United States and limited parts of the southwest. The *Aedes albopictus* species survives further north into the Mid-Atlantic states and into the lower Midwest. The risk of person-to-mosquito transmission is highest during the viremic first week of illness. Human and non-human primates are the main amplifying reservoirs for the virus. Transmission is possible through a needle stick, the handing of blood, and through aerosol laboratory exposure. No transfusion-related cases have been identified. The intrapartum period is the most critical for vertical transmission of chikungunya. Rates up to 48.3% have been observed in neonates born from mothers with active viremia during labor. Neonatal infections can result in fever, poor feeding, maculopapular rash, limb edema, and meningoencephalitis. There are no reported cases transmitted by breastfeeding. Previous infection will convey permanent immunity.

Prevention

Currently, no vaccine or preventive drug is available. Several candidate vaccines are in various stages of development. The best preventive measures are wearing permethrin-treated, bite-proof long sleeves and trousers and using a mosquito repellant such as 30% DEET, 20% oil of lemon eucalyptus, or 30% picaridin. Screening windows and doors has only a limited effect, because most contacts between the *Aedes* mosquitoes and humans occur outside.

Standing water, a breeding ground for mosquitoes, should be drained. *Aedes aegypti* breeding sites are associated with human habitation and are seemingly innocuous (i.e., flower vases, water storage vessels and birdbaths). Customary blood handling procedures are recommended.

If a Chikungunya epidemic were to occur in the United States, the standard public health measures of avoidance and mosquito control would be major lines of defense. To prevent local spread, the patient diagnosed with chikungunya should use mosquito repellant for 1 week after onset of fever.

Clinical Manifestations

Chikungunya virus infection should be considered in patients with acute onset of fever and polyarthralgia, especially in travelers who have recently returned from areas with endemic chikungunya. The incubation period of the chikungunya virus ranges from 1 to 12 days, most typically 3 to 7 days. Seventy two percent to 97% of those infected develop symptoms. Clinical onset is abrupt. The hallmarks of chikungunya are erratic, relapsing, and incapacitating polyarthralgia accompanied by high fever, backache, headache, and fatigue. Polyarthralgia is reported in 87% to 98% of cases and represents the most characteristic symptom. The joint pain is mostly polyarticular, bilateral, and symmetrical and occurs mainly in peripheral joints (wrists, ankles, and phalanges) and some large joints (shoulders, elbows and knees). Joint swelling is less frequent, occurring in 25% to 42% of cases. Typically, the fever lasts for 2 days and then will defervesce abruptly. Headache and an extreme degree of prostration may persist for a variable period, usually about 5 to 7 days. Symptoms typically resolve in 7 to 10 days. Rare symptoms include uveitis, retinitis, myocarditis, hepatitis, nephritis, hemorrhage, and neurologic problems such as myelitis, meningoencephalitis, Guillain-Barré syndrome, and cranial nerve palsies.

In 40% to 50% of cases, skin involvement is present consisting of a pruritic maculopapular rash, predominantly on the thorax, localized petechia, and facial edema. Though rarely affected, children may exhibit a bullous rash with pronounced sloughing. The case fatality ratio is approximately 1 per 1000, with most deaths occurring in newborns, the elderly, and the infirm.

Diagnosis

The instructions for serum diagnostic testing are found on the Centers for Disease Control and Prevention's website (http://www.cdc.gov/chikungunya/hc/diagnostic.html). The virus may be cultured within the first 3 days of illness. Virus isolation provides the most definitive diagnosis but requires 1 to 2 weeks for completion and must be processed in a biosafety level 3 laboratory. Chikungunya viral RNA may be identifiable by RT-PCR during the first 8 days of illness. Chikungunya virus antibodies usually develop by the end of the first week of illness. IgM antibody levels peak 3 to 5 weeks after the onset of illness and persist for approximately 2 months. In some cases, paired acute-phase and convalescent-phase antibody sampling may be required for accurate diagnosis. False-positive results may occur due to infection from closely related viruses.

A complete blood count may show lymphopenia and thrombocytopenia. Liver enzymes may elevate, and the serum creatinine might also increase. There are no pathognomonic radiologic findings, and biologic markers of inflammation are normal or modestly elevated.

In many parts of the world, chikungunya is a clinical diagnosis of exclusion, particularly when laboratory testing is not readily available. The probability of accurate clinical diagnosis depends on the epidemiology of endemic diseases and the patient's clinical symptoms.

Differential Diagnosis

The differential diagnosis for chikungunya includes influenza, malaria, rickettsia, and a multitude of viruses, especially dengue fever. Dengue and chikungunya viruses are transmitted by the same mosquitoes, may have similar clinical features, and can occasionally coinfect the same individual. Clinically differentiating chikungunya from dengue may be difficult; however, in chikungunya the onset of fever is typically more abrupt and shorter lived, with severe arthralgia, rash, and lymphopenia more prevalent, whereas infection with dengue is more likely to present with neutropenia, thrombocytopenia, hemorrhage, shock, and death.

Seasonally, chikungunya is more likely to be seen in the summer months when *Aedes* mosquitos proliferate.

Treatment

Medical treatment is primarily supportive. The use of antiviral agents is unproven. Acetaminophen is recommended and, once dengue has been excluded, nonsteroidal antiinflammatory agents and corticosteroids can be useful for the treatment of joint pain. During the first week of the illness, those infected with chikungunya should be protected from further mosquito exposure to reduce the risk of local transmission.

Monitoring

Chikungunya is a nationally notifiable disease. Cases should be immediately reported to state or local health department officials to facilitate diagnosis and mitigate the risk of local transmission.

Complications

Over the 3 years after the 2006 La Reunion outbreak, 60% of patients experienced continued symptoms of arthralgia, typically episodic, symmetrical (90%), highly incapacitating (77%), and polyarthralgias (70%). Local swelling, asthenia, and depression were common long-term complaints. Age >35 years and the presence of joint pain 4 months after the disease onset were risk factors for long-term arthralgia. Chikungunya is one of the agents researched as a potential biologic weapon.

References

Centers for Disease Control and Prevention: Chikungunya: atypical and severe disease manifestations. http://www.cdc.gov/chikungunya/pdfs/Chikungunya-atypical-severe-disease_Healthcare-provider-factsheet-10-07-2014.pdf.

Centers for Disease Control and Prevention: Chikungunya virus. http://www.cdc.gov/chikungunya/. Accessed May 25, 2019.

Centers for Disease Control and Prevention: Chikungunya virus in the United States, https://www.cdc.gov/chikungunya/geo/united-states-2020.html.

Centers for Disease Control and Prevention: Infectious Diseases Related to Travel chikungunya. https://wwwnc.cdc.gov/travel/yellowbook/2020/travel-related-infectious-diseases/chikungunya.

Cerny T, Schwarz M, Schwarz U: The range of neurological complications in Chikungunya fever, *Neurocrit Care* 27:447–457, 2017.

Couderc T, Khandoudi N, Grandadam M: Prophylaxis and therapy for Chikungunya virus infection, *J Infect Dis* 200:516–523, 2009.

Escobar M, Nieto S, Barona J: Pregnant women hospitalized with chikungunya virus infection, Colombia, 2015, *Emerging Infectious Diseases* 23(11), 2017.

Gerardin P, Barau G, Michault A: Multidisciplinary prospective study of mother-to-child chikungunya virus infections on the island of La Reunion. https://journals.plos.org/plosmedicine/article/file?id=10.1371/journal.pmed.0050060&type=printable.

Mohan A, Kiran DHN, Manohar IC, Kumar DP: Epidemiology, clinical manifestations, and diagnosis of chikungunya fever: lessons learned from the re-emerging epidemic, *Indian J Dermatol* 55:54–63, 2010.

Morens DM, Fauci AS: Perspective: Chikungunya at the door—Déjà vu all over again? *N Engl J Med* 371:885–887, 2014.

Morrison TE: Reemergence of Chikungunya virus, *J Virol* 88:11644–11647, 2014.

Pialoux G, Gaüzère B-A, Jauréguiberry S, Strobel M: Chikungunya, an epidemic arbovirus, *Lancet Infect Dis* 7:319–327, 2007.

Ramful D, Carbonnier M, Pasquet M: Mother-to-child transmission of Chikungunya virus infection, *Pediatr Infect Dis J* 26:811–815, 2007.

Schilte C, Staikovsky F, Couderc T: Chikungunya virus-associated long-term arthralgia: a 36-month prospective longitudinal study, *PLoS Negl Trop Dis* 7(3):e2137, 2013.

Schwameis M, Buchtele N, Wadowski PP: Chikungunya vaccines in development, *Hum Vaccin Immunother* 12:716–731, 2016.

Sharp TM, Roth NM, Torres J, Chikungunya, et al: cases identified through passive surveillance and household investigations–Puerto Rico, May 5-August 12, *MMWR* 63(48):1121–1128, 2014.

Staples JE, Fischer M: Perspective: Chikungunya virus in the Americas—what a vectorborne pathogen can do, *N Engl J Med* 371:887–889, 2014.

Taksandel A, Vilhekar KY: Neonatal Chikungunya infection, *J Prevent Infect Control* 1:8, 2015.

Thiberville SD, Moyen N, Dupuis-Maguiraga L: Chikungunya fever: epidemiology, clinical syndrome, pathogenesis and therapy, *Antiviral Res*, 99. 2013, pp 345–370.

World Health Organization. Chikungunya. https://www.who.int/en/news-room/fact-sheets/detail/chikungunya. 15 September, 2020.

CHOLERA

Method of
Mark Pietroni, MD, MBA

Cholera affects about 3 million people per year and kills approximately 100,000. It can kill within hours of the onset of symptoms, and even today the impact of an outbreak of cholera can be catastrophic in locations in which the water and sanitation infrastructure is weak, especially in crisis or war situations. The 21st century has already seen large-scale cholera epidemics in Haiti, Zimbabwe, Pakistan and Yemen, as well as many smaller outbreaks in countries and areas in which cholera is endemic. When cholera is untreated, mortality can be as high as 60% to 70%, but even in epidemics, with appropriate management and well-run diarrhea treatment centers, mortality can be reduced to well below 1%.

Oral rehydration therapy (ORT) is now the mainstay of treatment (Table 1). Developed in the 1960s in Dhaka, Bangladesh, ORT was used to great effect during the Bangladesh Liberation War of 1971. Cholera broke out in the refugee camps outside Calcutta, and the medical services ran out of intravenous fluid. ORT was not accepted as routine therapy by the medical profession at that time. The courageous decision to treat people with ORT saved thousands of lives and convinced the world of the effectiveness of ORT in the management of cholera.

Pathophysiology

Cholera is caused by a gram-negative, comma-shaped bacterium called *Vibrio cholerae*. Clinical disease is caused by two serogroups: *V. cholerae* O1 (which has two biotypes: classical and El Tor) and *V. cholerae* O139. Humans are the only known natural host, and asymptomatic human carriage is rare. *V. cholerae* is rapidly killed by boiling water, but it can lie dormant for months in blue-green algae, crustaceans, and copepods in brackish water, especially in estuaries. The Ganges delta provides an ideal habitat and is believed to be the place cholera first emerged.

Human infection is caused by ingestion of contaminated food or drink or from poor hand hygiene in epidemic situations. Relative or absolute achlorhydria facilitates passage through the stomach. Proliferation occurs in the small intestine, where a number of toxins are released. This results in massive secretion of isotonic fluid into the gut. The fluid passes out of the anus full of vibrios to perpetuate the cycle of transmission. Killing the host does not appear to interrupt this cycle!

The cholera toxin is secreted only by the O1 and O139 serogroups. It has two subunits: A (active) and B (binding). Subunit B binds to receptors in the small intestine and subunit A activates adenylate cyclase. This causes the active secretion of a number of ions into the gut, which drags water by osmosis and also blocks the reabsorption of sodium from the gut. The net result is a massive loss of water, sodium chloride, and bicarbonate. This cannot be replaced by drinking a sodium solution because sodium reabsorption is blocked. However, the addition of glucose to a solution of sodium activates a sodium–glucose co-transporter; sodium is absorbed and water follows by osmosis. This is the basis of oral rehydration therapy for diarrhea today.

Clinical Presentation and Diagnosis

Cholera manifests as an acute watery diarrhea without blood in the stool or (usually) abdominal cramps. The majority of cases are clinically indistinguishable from other causes of watery diarrhea. About 10%-20% will develop dehydration but most require only oral rehydration fluid as treatment. However, some will progress to classic or severe cholera.

The classic picture is of the rapid onset of profuse watery diarrhea (rice-water stool) and vomiting, which is painless and can result in circulatory collapse within hours without effective treatment. The history is usually less than 24 hours, although it may be longer if the patient is taking oral rehydration solution. Abdominal cramps can occur. Fever is absent. Patients usually remain alert, but severe electrolyte abnormalities such as hypoglycemia and hyponatremia can cause a reduced level of consciousness or convulsions, especially in children. Acidosis is often severe and results in tachypnea, which is commonly misdiagnosed as pneumonia. Patients should be reassessed for the presence or absence of pneumonia 1 to 2 hours after adequate rehydration. The diagnosis of cholera can be confirmed by the presence of rapidly motile vibrios detected by dark-field microscopy or by stool or rectal swab culture. However, the classic history, appearance of the stool, and rapid presentation mean that the diagnosis is usually clinical.

Treatment

A clinical syndrome of acute watery diarrhea (three or more watery stools in the last 24 hours) of short duration (24–48 hours) with or without vomiting associated with dehydration in anyone older than 2 years in an endemic or epidemic situation should be treated as cholera. Children younger than 2 years may be managed in the same way, but other diagnoses such as rotavirus should be considered. The mainstay of management (whatever the causative organism) is appropriate early rehydration,

TABLE 1	Composition (mEq/L) of Common Solutions Used for Rehydration						
SOLUTION	**NA⁺**	**K⁺**	**CL⁻**	**HCO₃⁻**	**CITRATE**	**CA²⁺**	**GLUCOSE OR CARBOHYDRATE**
Intravenous Solution							
Normal saline	154	—	154	—	—	—	—
Ringer's lactate	130	4	109	28	—	3	—
Ringer's lactate + D$_5$	130	4	109	28	—	3	278
Cholera saline (Dhaka solution)	133	13	98	48	—	—	140
Oral Solution							
Standard ORS	90	20	80	—	10	—	111
Hypo-osmolar ORS	75	20	65	—	10	—	75
ReSoMal*	45	40	76	—	7	—	125

Abbreviations: D$_5$ = 5% dextrose; ORS = oral rehydration solution; ReSoMal = reduced osmolarity ORS for malnourished children.
Reprinted with permission from Harris JB, Pietroni M: Approach to the child with acute diarrhea in developing countries. UpToDate. Available at http://www.uptodate.com/contents/approach-to-the-child-with-acute-diarrhea-in-developing-countries (accessed August 11, 2016).
*Also contains Mg 6 mmol/L, Zn 300 μmol/L, Cu 45 μmol/L.

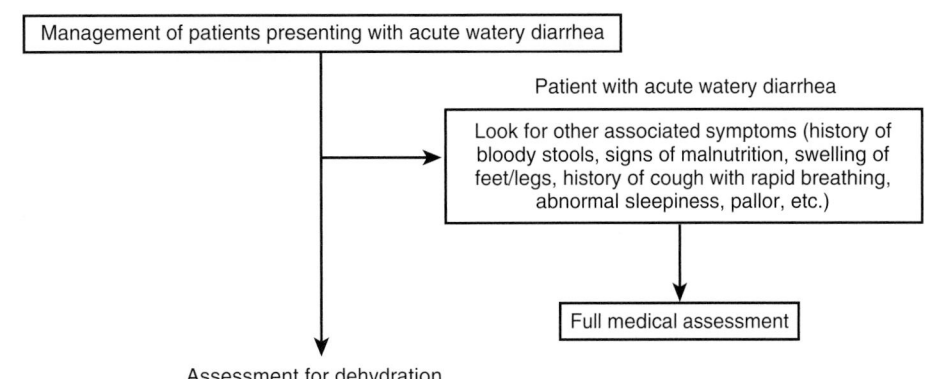

Assess	Condition	Normal	Irritable/less active*	Lethargic/comatose*
	Eyes	Normal	Sunken	Sunken
	Tongue	Normal	Dry	Dry
	Thirst	Normal	Thirsty (drinks eagerly)	Unable to drink*
	Skin pinch	Normal	Goes back slowly*	Goes back very slowly*
	Radial pulse	Normal	Reduced*	Uncountable or absent*
Diagnosis		No sign of dehydration	If at least 2 signs, including one (*) sign, are present, diagnose *some dehydration*	If some dehydration plus one of the (*) signs are present, diagnose *severe dehydration*
Management		A	B	C

A. No sign of dehydration—ORS
- 50 mL ORS per kg body weight *plus* ongoing losses
- Send patient home with 4 packets of ORS
- Continue feeding, including breast milk for infants and young children

B. Some dehydration—ORS
- 80 mL ORS per kg body weight over 4–6 hours plus ongoing losses
- Observe patient for 6–12 hours
- Continue feeding, including breastmilk for infants and young children
- Reassess patient and dehydration status hourly.
- In case of frequent vomiting (>3 times in 1 hour): Treat with IV fluid

C. Severe dehydration—Start IV fluid immediately (100 mL/kg)

IV solution containing sodium, potassium, chloride and bicarbonate (e.g., Ringer's Lactate)

Children <1 year or malnourished
30 mL/kg in first 1 hour
70 mL/kg in next 5 hours

Adults and children >1 year
30 mL/kg in first 1/2 hour
70 mL/kg in next 2 1/2 hours

- Encourage the patient to take ORS as soon as he/she is able to drink
- Antibiotic, if needed, after rehydration
- Zinc[1] 20 mg/day for 10 days in children 6 months to 5 years old, 10 mg/day for 10 days in children under 6 months

Figure 1 Quick identification of cholera cases can be made using a standard case definition. During an outbreak, cholera should be suspected in any patient who is older than 2 years, is attending a health facility, and has a history of acute watery diarrhea (passage of at least three stools in the last 24 hours) of a short duration (less than 24 hours), with or without vomiting, and with signs of dehydration. (Flow chart modified from International Centre for Diarrhoeal Disease Research, Bangladesh (ICDDR,B) internal treatment protocol.) *Abbreviation:* ORS = oral rehydration solution.

and time should not be wasted worrying about investigations or which antibiotic to use (Figure 1).

The initial assessment should be brief but must:
- Confirm the diagnosis of acute watery diarrhea
- Assess the level of dehydration
- Assess the presence or absence of malnutrition
- Recognize any other comorbidities

Accurate assessment and rapid, appropriate treatment of dehydration is critical to the management of cholera. A simple scoring system based on five clinical signs is sufficient and can accurately predict patients with 5% to 10% (some) dehydration and greater than 10% (severe) dehydration. Common mistakes include overreliance on individual clinical signs and giving too little intravenous fluid during the initial phase and too much during the recovery phase. Patients with less than 5% (no) dehydration and

5% to 10% (some) dehydration can be managed with oral rehydration alone (Box 1) unless there is a reduced level of consciousness or inability to take fluids by mouth. Those with 5% to 10% (some) dehydration must be reassessed every 1 to 2 hours to make sure that hydration is improving.

Patients with severe dehydration require an immediate intravenous fluid bolus of 100 mL/kg given over 3 hours with one third in the first 30 minutes (double the duration in children who are younger than 1 year or have malnutrition). If possible, the intravenous fluid should contain sodium, potassium, and bicarbonate—Ringer's lactate or cholera saline—but normal saline with 5 to 10 mmol/L of potassium may also be used. Oral rehydration should start at the same time. Once the intravenous fluid bolus has finished, further intravenous fluids are usually not required.

BOX 1 Fluids for Patients without Signs of Dehydration

Acceptable
Oral rehydration solution (optimal for both repletion and maintenance)
Salted drinks (salted rice water or salted yogurt drink)
Broth or soup (salted vegetable or meat soup)
Water
Rice water
Coconut water (unsweetened)
Weak tea (unsweetened)
Fresh fruit juice (unsweetened)

Unacceptable
Carbonated beverages
Sweetened juices
Coffee
Medicinal teas or infusions

Fluids containing salt should be encouraged. Unacceptable fluids include carbonated beverages and sweetened juices; the sugar in these fluids may worsen diarrhea. Coffee and medicinal teas or infusions are also unacceptable since they can have diuretic and purgative effects.

Reprinted with permission from Harris JB, Pietroni M: Approach to the child with acute diarrhea in developing countries. UpToDate. Available at http://www.uptodate.com/contents/approach-to-the-child-with-acute-diarrhea-in-developing-countries (accessed August 11, 2016).

BOX 2 Antibiotics in Cholera

Antibiotics should be given to all patients with severe dehydration. Choice of antibiotic depends on local sensitivity pattern. If ciprofloxacin is used a 3-day course is now needed due to rising MICs.

First-Line Drug (If Susceptibility Report Is Not Available)
Adults
Azithromycin (Zithromax)[1] 1 g (500 mg × 2) PO as a single dose after correcting severe dehydration

Children
Azithromycin[1] 20 mg/kg PO as a single dose after correction of dehydration and cessation of vomiting (if any)

Second-Line Drug (Not Recommended for Children < 5 Years or Pregnant Women)
Adults
Ciprofloxacin (Cipro)[1] 1 g (500 mg × 2) PO for 3 days after correction of severe dehydration

Children
Ciprofloxacin[1] 20 mg/kg PO for 3 days after correction of dehydration and cessation of vomiting (if any)

Third-Line Drugs
Doxycycline (Vibramycin) 300 mg as a single dose after food (not in children or pregnant women)

[1]Not FDA approved for this indication.

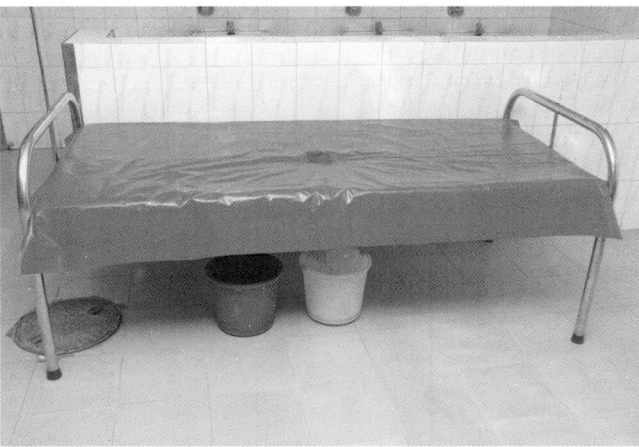

Figure 2 Cholera cot.

Patients are best managed using a cholera cot, especially in an epidemic situation. The cholera cot is a bed (or sometimes a chair) covered with a nonabsorbent sheet with a hole that allows the passage of stool and urine directly to a bucket under the bed (Figure 2). The sheets and bucket should be replaced three times a day and between patients. They may be washed, sterilized, and reused. Patients do not need to use a toilet (which can be several times an hour), linen is not soiled, and body fluids are prevented from running on the floor. This system enables adequate infection control to be maintained with limited resources.

After an initial assessment has been made and fluids started, a fuller clinical assessment can take place. Patients with significant comorbidities can require individually tailored treatment plans.

Antibiotics reduce the length of stay and fluid requirement in patients with severe dehydration due to cholera (Box 2). A single dose is sufficient, but this should be repeated if the dose is vomited back. The choice of antibiotic should be guided by local sensitivities where these are available. If not, a single dose of azithromycin (Zithromax)[1] 1 g in adults and 20 mg/day for 10 days in children 6 months to 5 years old, 10 mg/day for 10 days in children under 6 months. All children between 6 months and 5 years of age should receive zinc[1] 20 mg/day for 10 days because this reduces subsequent mortality and further episodes of diarrhea.

Recovery from cholera is rapid, and mortality is extremely low if the dehydration is treated appropriately. The Cholera Hospital run by the International Centre for Diarrhoeal Disease Research, Bangladesh (ICDDR,B), in Dhaka treats around 120,000 patients a year. The average length of stay is 16 hours, and the mortality rate is zero.

Prevention

Because the transmission of cholera is feco-oral, cholera can be prevented by good hand hygiene and by providing safe drinking water and appropriate sanitation. Standard food and hygiene precautions should be followed by people travelling in endemic areas (e.g., eat only boiled or fried foods; drink only boiled or bottled water). The FDA recently approved a single-dose live oral cholera vaccine, called Vaxchora in the United States. Vaxchora is indicated for adults 18–64 years old who are traveling to an area of active cholera. Two other oral inactivated cholera vaccines, Dukoral and ShanChol, are not available in the United States. These two cholera vaccines provide around 60% to 80% efficacy for 6 months. They are not recommended for the occasional traveler or tourist but may be given to people working in high-risk situations, such as aid workers in a cholera outbreak. The World Health Organization recommends the use of oral cholera vaccine in endemic areas as part of disease control programmes and maintains a global cholera vaccine stockpile for use in epidemic situations.

References

Ali M, Nelson AR, Lopez AL, Sack D: Updated global burden of cholera in endemic countries. *PLoS Negl Trop Dis* 9(6):e0003832, 2015. https://doi.org/10.1371/journal.pntd.0003832.

Alam NH, Ashraf H: Treatment of infectious diarrhea in children, *Paediatr Drugs* 5:151–165, 2003.

Harris JB, Pietroni MAC: Approach to the child with acute diarrhea in resource limited countries. In: UpToDate, Calderwood, S.B. & Bloom, A. (Eds), UpToDate, Waltham, MA, 2017.

Pietroni MAC: Case management of cholera, *Vaccine* 38(1):A105–A109, 2020.

Roy SK, Tomkins AM, Akramuzzaman SM, et al: Randomised controlled trial of zinc supplementation in malnourished Bangladeshi children with acute diarrhea, *Arch Dis Child* 77:196–200, 1997.

Saha D, Karim MM, Khan WA, et al: Single-dose azithromycin for the treatment of cholera in adults, *N Engl J Med* 354:2452–2462, 2006.

UNICEF Cholera Toolkit www.unicef.org/cholera_toolkit/ especially Chapter 8: Case management and infection control in health facilities and treatment sites pp 110–135. Accessed 10/3/2018.

[1]Not FDA approved for this indication.

COVID-19

Method of
Lucius M. Lampton, MD

CURRENT DIAGNOSIS

- Coronavirus disease 2019 (COVID-19; the illness caused by SARS-CoV-2) presents with a broad spectrum of multisystem clinical manifestations, including fever, dry cough, dyspnea, fatigue, sore throat, gastrointestinal symptoms, headache, chills, myalgias, anosmia, and ageusia.
- Transmission of SARS-CoV-2 most commonly occurs via respiratory droplets from face-to-face contact and by surface contamination.
- Diagnosis is based on detection of SARS-CoV-2 by viral testing of a respiratory sample, usually a nasopharyngeal swab. A serologic test can detect antibodies from past infection or vaccination.
- Other factors critical for diagnosis and treatment include exposure history, computed tomography (CT) findings, laboratory tests, and clinical manifestations of SARS-CoV-2 infection.

CURRENT THERAPY

- Since there are few proven therapies for this novel coronavirus, prevention and protection via utilization of a SARS-CoV-2 vaccine is paramount and offers the possibility of containing COVID-19 worldwide.
- Other pragmatic recommendations focus on prevention of person-to-person transmission and infection control, which are accomplished by social distancing, hand washing, source control measures, screening, quarantine, contact tracing, and personal protective equipment (PPE) for healthcare workers.
- Initial treatment is symptomatic, and patients with mild disease usually recover at home with rest and hydration.
- Patients with moderate or severe disease may require hospitalization and intensive care.
- The utilization of monoclonal antibody therapy, dexamethasone, oxygen supplementation, and remdesivir should be considered in appropriate settings; however, the provision of supportive care and respiratory support for infected patients remains the keystone of treatment in more severe cases.
- Older adults and individuals with severe underlying medical conditions are at higher risk for morbidity and mortality from COVID-19.

Epidemiology

A novel coronavirus, severe acute respiratory syndrome coronavirus 2 (SARS-CoV-2), was first recognized in December 2019 as the etiologic agent of a serious respiratory illness soon designated coronavirus disease 2019 (COVID-19). This potentially fatal disease possesses extraordinary global public health significance with enormous human casualties and a tragic worldwide economic impact. Since COVID-19 was first reported in Wuhan, the capital of Hubei, China, COVID-19 has reached a pandemic level, spreading over the world and multiplying more hurriedly than any infectious disease of recent memory with more than 218 million confirmed cases and more than 4,528,900 deaths, according to the latest figures (September 1, 2021) from the World Health Organization (WHO). The outbreak has spread to 219 countries beyond China, and in the United States, there have been more than 39 million confirmed cases and more than 641,937 deaths.

This new, highly contagious coronavirus causes a respiratory illness with such symptoms as fever, cough, shortness of breath, and, in some cases, a deadly acute respiratory syndrome, which can lead to pneumonia, respiratory failure, or septic shock. Infected persons have shown a range of symptoms from mild to severe illness and death. Symptoms may appear in as few as a couple of days to as long as 14 days after exposure. Genetic analysis of the virus indicates that it originated in bats, although it is still unclear whether it jumped directly from bats or an intermediary host existed. It appears similar to other zoonotic coronaviruses, like SARS-CoV, which emerged in 2002. Although there is a near-consensus view that the causative agent of COVID-19 has a natural zoonotic origin, several of its characteristics are not easily explained by this hypothesis and suggest the possibility of an alternate hypothesis of a laboratory leak origin. There remains much to be learned about the possible source and evolutionary path of this emerging disease.

In many countries, healthcare facilities have been stressed by a surge in cases, especially patients requiring ventilatory support and intensive care. In order to slow the disease spread and allow more time for public health and hospitals to become better prepared, public health efforts have focused on flattening the epidemic curve with recommendations for physical distancing (referred to by some as social distancing) in order to minimize person-to-person transmission. Closure of schools and workplaces has occurred, as well as cancellation of public events and services such as public transport. Classic public health strategies, including quarantine, have also been implemented as effective countermeasures. However, limited data exist on the comparative effectiveness of these varied policy interventions. The brisk emergence of this devastating pandemic caused by a previously unknown pathogen underscores the perpetual challenges facing modern public health of emerging infectious diseases and the necessity of sustained preparedness.

The availability of safe and effective SARS-CoV-2 vaccines asserts the possibility of controlling COVID-19 both in the United States and worldwide. However, the emergence of several new variants of the original virus have been recognized that appear to cause significant changes in the way the pathogen behaves, including alterations to its transmissibility. Reports from around the world reveal that the new variants are penetrating populations previously thought immune from vaccination or past infection, indicating the need for booster vaccinations.

Risk Factors

Exposure history to individuals with COVID-19 is the essential risk factor. Individuals who have had close contact with a known positive patient or who have traveled to an area with high community transmission should be screened if they are symptomatic. Employment as a healthcare worker engaged in the direct care of patients is also a risk factor. Individuals at higher risk of morbidity and mortality if infected are adults over the age of 65 years, especially those in long-term care facilities and those with chronic illnesses such as hypertension, diabetes, obesity, chronic kidney disease, chronic obstructive pulmonary disease (COPD), asthma, immunocompromised conditions, pregnancy, heart failure, and sickle cell disease. Studies have also revealed that a disproportionate percentage of COVID-19 hospitalizations and deaths occurs in minority and lower-income populations. Children seem to be relatively unaffected by COVID-19, although rare cases of severe disease, including death, have been reported.

Pathophysiology

Coronaviruses (CoVs) are enveloped, positive sense single-stranded RNA viruses, which are characterized by club-like glycoprotein spikes on their surface that mediate receptor binding and cell entry during infection. These spikes on the envelope give coronaviruses a crown-like appearance under an electron microscope, which is the source of its name, *coronam* being the Latin term for crown. They are the largest group of viruses belonging to the *Nidovirales* order, which includes *Coronaviridae*,

Arteriviridae, Mesoniviridae, and *Roniviridae* families. The *Coronavirinae* comprise one of two subfamilies in the *Coronaviridae* family. Coronaviruses possess an unusually large RNA genome and cause a wide spectrum of multisystem diseases in birds and mammals ranging from upper respiratory infections in chickens to enteritis in pigs and cows to potentially fatal human respiratory disease. To date, only seven human coronaviruses have been identified. Several cause common colds and self-limiting upper respiratory infection. However, at least three have caused widespread deadly outbreaks, including the highly pathogenic severe acute respiratory syndrome coronavirus (SARS-CoV), Middle Eastern respiratory syndrome coronavirus (MERS-CoV), and most recently SARS-CoV-2.

Genomic analyses indicate that SARS-CoV-2 probably originated and evolved from a strain found in bats. Most researchers suggest that there probably was an amplifying mammalian host, intermediate between bats and humans. However, it is not certain whether an intermediary exists, as the original strain's mutation could have directly jumped from bats to humans. Although animal-to-human transmission was first presumed, the main exposure mechanism appears to be human-to-human transmission, with symptomatic individuals the most frequent source of spread, although pre- and asymptomatic individuals may also contribute to this spread. The transmission is believed to occur through respiratory droplets spread by coughing, sneezing, or talking, although aerosol transmission in closed spaces is also possible. Studies also reveal that SARS-CoV-2 can contaminate objects and surfaces for hours and days. One study found the virus on plastic and stainless steel for up to 2 to 3 days, on cardboard for up to 1 day, and copper up to 4 hours. SARS-CoV-2 has been found on a variety of surfaces, from floors to trash receptacles to computer mouses. SARS-CoV-2 RNA has also been detected in blood and stool, although fecal-oral transmission has not been documented, which suggests that the presence of viral RNA does not necessarily predict that the virus is also viable and infectious.

Like other coronaviruses, SARS-CoV-2 is sensitive to ultraviolet rays and heat, although the inactivation temperature must be further studied. These viruses can be effectively inactivated by lipid solvents including ether, ethanol, chlorine-containing disinfectants, and peroxyacetic acid.

Prevention

Vaccination is the most effective way to prevent SARS-CoV-2 infection. Although there over 100 COVID-19 vaccines in various stages of development across the world, three vaccines were authorized for emergency use by the US Food and Drug Administration (FDA) and have been used extensively in the United States: Comirnaty/Pfizer-BioNTech, Moderna, and Johnson & Johnson's Janssen.

The Pfizer-BioNTech COVID-19 vaccine, which is marketed as Comirnaty, was the first FDA-approved vaccine for the prevention of COVID-19 disease in individuals 16 years of age and older. This mRNA vaccine also continues to be available under emergency use authorization (EUA), including for individuals 12 through 15 years of age and for the administration of a third dose in certain immunocompromised individuals. The vaccine consists of two shots given 3 weeks (21 days) apart, with full vaccination occurring 2 weeks after the second shot. Although it is recommended to obtain the second shot as advised, the second shot may be given up to 6 weeks (42 days) after the first dose, if necessary.

Moderna COVID-19 vaccine, also an mRNA vaccine, is authorized for emergency use in individuals 18 years of age and older. The vaccine consists of two shots given 4 weeks (28 days) apart, with full vaccination achieved 2 weeks after the second shot. (As with the Pfizer vaccine, the second shot may be given up to 6 weeks after the first dose, if necessary.)

The Centers for Disease Control and Prevention (CDC) has recommended that certain immunocompromised individuals receive a third dose of either mRNA COVID-19 vaccines at least 28 days after the completion of the initial vaccine series. Also, third or

booster doses of the mRNA vaccines may start for other patients at 6 months from the last dose. With the mRNA COVID-19 vaccinations, mild side effects are common within 7 days of getting vaccinated, and there has been a rare association recognized with myocarditis, especially in young adult and adolescent males.

The third vaccine authorized, Johnson & Johnson's Janssen (J&J/Janssen) COVID-19 vaccine, is a viral vector vaccine and allowed for use in individuals 18 years of age and older. This vaccine consists of one shot, with full vaccination occurring 2 weeks after the shot. Mild side effects were common within 7 days of getting vaccinated, and there did emerge a plausible causal relationship between the vaccine and thrombosis and thrombocytopenia syndrome (TTS).

Thus far, these three vaccines appear to provide strong protection against COVID-19 and its new variants, although the duration of protection is uncertain and breakthrough cases have been reported. Booster development specific to new variants is ongoing.

Currently, there is no known agent that can be administered to prevent infection before exposure to SARS-CoV-2 as preexposure prophylaxis (PrEP). Clinical trials are investigating several possible agents, including ivermectin, emtricitabine plus tenofovir alafenamide or tenofovir disoproxil fumarate, hydroxychloroquine, monoclonal antibodies, and supplements such as zinc, vitamin C, and vitamin D.

A postexposure prophylaxis (PEP) authorized by the FDA for emergency use is the anti-SARS-CoV-2 monoclonal antibodies casirivimab plus imdevimab. This combination may be utilized either as a subcutaneous injection or an intravenous infusion for PEP for people with a high-risk exposure who are at risk for progression to severe COVID-19 if infected with SARS-CoV-2 and who were not fully vaccinated or who are vaccinated but are not expected to mount an adequate immune response. There are a number of other agents (hyperimmune gammaglobulin, ivermectin, convalescent plasma, interferons, tenofovir with or without emtricitabine, and vitamin D) currently being investigated for PEP. Hydroxychloroquine has also been studied for PEP in several trials with no evidence of efficacy.

Other preventive strategies should focus on isolation of patients and rigid infection control, which includes appropriate measures to provide clinical care for infected patients. Transmission of SARS-CoV-2 is believed to occur usually through respiratory droplets spread from an infectious person to others within 6 feet. Airborne transmission of small droplets to persons more than 6 feet away can occur less commonly. Also, in rare instances, an individual just passing through a room that was previously occupied by an infected individual may become infected. For the general public, the primary preventive action is physical distancing (maintaining 6 feet between people) and isolation in order to minimize transmission. Other general recommendations include avoidance of close contact with individuals suffering from acute respiratory infections; washing hands frequently, especially after any contact with infected individuals and their environment; individuals with acute airway infections or symptoms should keep their distance from others and follow cough and hand hygiene; high-risk or immunocompromised individuals should avoid public gatherings; and the utilization of strict hygiene measures in clinical settings to prevent and control infections. One of the most important strategies is frequent hand washing and the use of portable hand sanitizers, as well as avoiding contact with one's face after interacting in an environment that might have contamination.

Studies indicate that the combination of isolation and contract tracing with physical distancing can effectively reduce disease transmission in communities. A variety of public health interventions have been implemented worldwide during the pandemic to reduce transmission. Among the more effective associated with reduced rates of transmission are the use of home quarantine after infection, the restriction of mass gatherings, travel restrictions, and social distancing. Studies assert that risk of resurgence follows when these interventions are lifted. A key priority is identifying optimal protective measures, which result in the least economic and societal disruption while adequately controlling transmission and infection.

Source control is an important prevention strategy and refers to use of cloth face coverings or face masks to cover an individual's mouth and nose to prevent spread of respiratory secretions when talking, sneezing, or coughing. Due of the potential for asymptomatic and presymptomatic spread, source control measures appear to be an effective prevention tool.

Medical providers should utilize infection prevention and control (IPC) practices during the COVID-19 pandemic, along with standard protocols, in providing routine healthcare delivery to patients. These practices should apply to care for all patients, not just those with suspected or confirmed SARS-CoV-2 infection. Telehealth strategies offer a resource for high-quality medical care with the reduction of possible SARS-CoV-2 transmission. When providing in-person clinical care, points of entry into the facility should be limited and monitored. Patients should be advised to reschedule their appointments if they have symptoms of COVID-19, and triage protocols should be developed to determine whether an in-person appointment is necessary or if the patient can be managed from home. If a symptomatic patient must come in for a visit, advise triage personnel that they and the patient must take appropriate preventive protocol interacting with the patient. Patients who do not have symptoms of COVID-19 should be advised to utilize a face mask to come inside the facility. Also, clinic staff should screen and triage everyone entering the facility for signs and symptoms of SARS-CoV-2 infection, as well as establishing policy to be sure all adhere to source control measures, physical distancing, and hand hygiene practices while in the healthcare facility. These screening stations should be outside the facility to screen patients, staff, and visitors before they enter. Supplies for respiratory hygiene should be provided for patients and staff, including alcohol-based hand sanitizers with 60% to 95% alcohol, tissues, and no-touch receptacles. If a patient must be examined who might have COVID-19, they should not wait among other patients and should be evaluated in a separate, well-ventilated space following protective protocols. Considering the level of local transmission, facilities should explore designating a separate area at the facility or nearby where patients with COVID-19 symptoms can be evaluated. Healthcare staff should wear a face mask at all times while they are within the facility, including break rooms and any space where they might interact with coworkers. As well, medical staff should remove their work respirator or face mask, perform hand hygiene, and replace their face covering at the end of their shift when leaving a facility.

Filtering facepiece respirators (FFR), which include N95 respirators, are half facepiece respirators used in healthcare that filter out particles and are critical tools to prevent viral transmission. The masks are commonly referred to as an N95 and should be fitted for each wearer. This "fit testing" is typically done at the workplace. Healthcare workers caring for COVID-19 infected patients should at all times use strict contact and airborne precautions, which include such required PPE as an N95 mask, eye protection, gowns, and gloves in order to prevent viral transmission.

It is unclear whether COVID-19 infection and recovery imparts partial or complete immunity, and if immunity is achieved, it is unknown for how long it lasts. As well, it is also unclear whether serologic testing can be utilized to provide guidance when patients can safely end isolation or return to work. The presence of antibodies may not confer immunity because not all antibodies produced in response to infection are neutralizing. Whether second infections with SARS-CoV-2 can occur remains unknown, but these have been reported. Whether presence of antibody changes susceptibility to subsequent infection or how long antibody protection lasts are unknown.

Clinical Manifestations

COVID-19 patients can manifest a wide variety of symptoms, with pulmonary inflammation its main pathologic manifestation.

The estimated incubation period for COVID-19 is up to 14 days from exposure, with a median incubation time of 4 to 5 days. The spectrum of illness can range from asymptomatic infection to severe pneumonia with acute respiratory distress syndrome (ARDS) and death. Patients usually report fever; dry cough; shortness of breath; gastrointestinal symptoms such as abdominal pain, diarrhea, anorexia, and vomiting; myalgias; headaches; dizziness; anosmia; dysgeusia; sore throat; fatigue; and chills. Mild pneumonia can occur, but in more severe cases tachypnea, dyspnea, and significant pneumonia can be seen, which can develop into a critical stage with respiratory failure, septic shock, and multiorgan failure. Older adult patients occasionally present with delirium or altered mental status. Adults with severe disease usually present during the second week of illness, a period that coincides with declining viral loads but increasing markers of inflammation, which suggests that host tissue damage is mediated by hyperinflammatory and maladaptive immune responses.

As is found in many other viral infections, there appears to be a two-phase immune response in COVID-19. The first is the body's response directly to the viral infection. This is followed by a second, reactive stage infection, which precipitates a cytokine release syndrome, a consequence of the host's reaction to the infection and the resulting cytokine activation cascade, which causes autoimmune-induced damage to lung, vascular endothelium, gastric mucosa, and other structures. This is mediated by non–T leukocytes and is found to be associated with lymphocytopenia, elevated ferritin levels, a decreasing platelet count, and elevated erythrocyte sedimentation rate. This cytokine storm and its extensive tissue damage and dysfunctional coagulation are felt to be a result of interleukin 6 (IL-6) overexpression.

Thrombotic aberration in COVID-19 patients is common and appears to contribute to organ failure and death. Platelet hyperreactivity, which is recognized in COVID-19, also contributes to morbidity through increased platelet–platelet and platelet–leukocyte interactions. Hemostatic alterations that mimic disseminated intravascular coagulopathy associated with sepsis often present with severe COVID-19 illness, with elevated risk of thrombosis rather than bleeding.

Most children with COVID-19 present either without symptoms or with symptoms milder than in adults. Symptoms resemble routine acute chest infections, with pyrexia, dry cough, sore throat, sneezing, myalgia, and lethargy. Less commonly, wheezing, diarrhea, and vomiting have also been noted. An uncommon disorder, multisystem inflammatory syndrome in children has also been associated with SARS-CoV-2, resulting in severe illness in previously healthy children and adolescents.

Diagnosis

The diagnosis of COVID-19 is established by a suggestive clinical history including exposure history and clinical manifestations of SARS-CoV-2 infection, as well as detection by a nucleic acid amplification test (NAAT) of SARS-CoV-2 RNA in an upper respiratory sample (i.e., a nasopharyngeal, nasal, or oropharyngeal specimen). Lower respiratory tract specimens have a higher viral load and are recommended for intubated or mechanically ventilated patients with clinical signs and symptoms of COVID-19. This molecular or antigen test, which detects viral RNA, is the reference standard for the screening of COVID-19 and should be used to diagnose acute SARS-CoV-2 infection. Other diagnostic tests are available, including antigen-based diagnostic tests that detect viral antigens and serologic tests that detect anti-SARS-CoV-2 immunoglobulins. If the initial viral test results are positive for SARS-CoV-2, the patient should be considered to have COVID-19, regardless of whether other findings are also present. Because of false-negative test result rates of SARS-CoV-2 viral testing, other data such as imaging and laboratory tests are often helpful in making a presumptive diagnosis.

Since pulmonary inflammation is the major pathologic manifestation of COVID-19, chest radiography should be an initial imaging study. A plain chest radiograph (CXR) in COVID-19 may reveal peribronchial thickening (which is typical in viral infections), pneumonia, nonspecific findings, or even negative findings. A chest computed tomography (CT) scan is usually more helpful in providing a definitive diagnosis. Multiple studies reveal that COVID-19 pneumonia is more likely to have a peripheral distribution, ground-glass opacity (GGO), fine reticular opacity, bilateral consolidations, and vascular thickening. These studies also reveal that COVID-19 is less likely to have a central plus peripheral distribution, pleural effusion, and lymphadenopathy. However, differentiating radiographic findings of COVID-19 pneumonia, influenza virus pneumonia, and other viral pneumonias in clinical practice remains difficult.

Despite its diagnostic benefits, a chest CT is not recommended as a first-line screening test for those with suspected COVID-19 infection. As well, a chest CT should be used sparingly and reserved for hospitalized patients with clinical indications for CT. If a patient medically declines, a chest CT may be indicated to better assess pulmonary status and disease progression. In the first 2 weeks after symptoms onset, there can be a rapid evolution of CT abnormalities, after which these findings recede gradually.

Laboratory testing also plays a role in initial evaluation and diagnosis of COVID-19, especially in the workup of hospitalized patients. Multiple abnormalities are often seen in positive patients and can assist in assessing whether a patient is improving or declining. Among typical abnormal results are elevations in serum C-reactive protein, lactate dehydrogenase, ferritin, procalcitonin, creatine kinase, alanine aminotransferase, and aspartate aminotransferase. Many patients also present with a low albumin. Lymphocytopenia, which is associated with an elevated risk of ICU care and acute kidney injury, is the most common hematologic abnormality seen, although leukopenia and leukocytosis are also common. A modest prolongation of prothrombin times, a mild thrombocytopenia, and elevated D-dimer values often are seen, which has also been associated with higher rates of ARDS and mortality. However, some of these laboratory findings are nonspecific, being common in pneumonia in general, and their clinical utility remains uncertain.

Differential Diagnosis

In its initial stages, COVID-19 appears clinically like many other viral and bacterial respiratory illnesses, presenting with a broad range of nonspecific and varied signs and symptoms. These other illnesses not only need to be considered in the differential diagnosis but also may occur simultaneously with COVID-19 infection.

Viral infections in the differential diagnosis include influenza, parainfluenza, coronavirus, adenovirus, respiratory syncytial virus, infectious mononucleosis, acute HIV, human rhinovirus/enterovirus, and human metapneumovirus. Bacterial pneumonias, which should be considered in the differential diagnosis, include *Streptococcus pneumoniae*, *Haemophilus influenza*, *Chlamydia pneumoniae*, and *Moraxella catarrhalis*. Atypical pneumonias in the differential include *Legionella pneumophila* and *Mycoplasma pneumoniae*. In immunocompromised hosts, *Pneumocystis jirovecii* should be considered. If patients have returned from international travel, such illnesses as dengue and malaria should be considered.

In addition to these infectious illnesses, the differential may include noninfectious disorders such as pulmonary embolism, COPD exacerbation, asthma, pulmonary edema, vasculitis, cor pulmonale, pneumonitis, ARDS, acute coronary syndrome, CHF, valvular disease, cancer, or acute chest syndrome in sickle cell disease.

Treatment

The pathogenesis of COVID-19 is propelled by two main processes and possesses two major phases. Early in the clinical course, the replication of SARS-CoV-2 launches the disease. Later in the clinical course, the disease's driver becomes a dysregulated inflammatory and immune reaction to SARS-CoV-2, which results in profound tissue injury. Understanding this biphasic disease evolution, pragmatic therapies should directly target SARS-CoV-2 early in the disease course and focus on immunosuppressive and antiinflammatory strategies in its later stages. Although multiple therapeutic agents have been proposed and are being evaluated for the treatment of COVID-19, few have yet been proven efficacious. With limited high-quality data to support specific protocols, current management is focused on reducing viral spread and providing supportive care and respiratory support for infected patients. Initial treatment is symptomatic. Patients who present with mild symptoms, such as a fever, cough, or myalgias, can be treated at home with antipyretics, analgesics, or antitussives, with oral hydration encouraged. Infected patients should be encouraged to isolate themselves as much as possible away from others within their homes. Any shared common areas within the house should be disinfected frequently and a mask worn if any interaction with others occurs. Oxygen therapy via nasal cannula is an early and essential step in addressing evolving respiratory impairment and can be arranged at home. Monitoring of oxygen saturations is also recommended if dyspnea is an issue. Telemedicine can effectively be utilized to monitor infected patients.

The therapeutic use of anti-SARS-CoV-2 monoclonal antibodies (mAb) should be considered early in the course of the illness in nonhospitalized patients at high risk for progression to severe COVID-19. REGEN-COV (casirivimab and imdevimab, administered together) and sotrovimab are authorized for the treatment of mild-to-moderate COVID-19 in adults and pediatric patients (12 years of age and older weighing at least 40 kg) with positive results of viral testing and who are at high risk for progression to severe disease. Casirivimab/imdevimab and sotrovimab are recombinant human immunoglobulin (Ig)G1 mAb that target the surface spike glycoprotein that mediates viral entry into host cells. Casirivimab plus imdevimab may be given by either intravenous infusion or subcutaneous injection, and sotrovimab is given intravenously. Early evidence suggests that mAb treatment can reduce the viral load of SARS-Cov-2, which results in milder infection with less hospitalization and death. Treatment using mAb should be initiated as soon as possible after a patient receives a positive viral test and within 10 days of symptom onset.

Most patients with COVID-19 require hospitalization when they begin to experience respiratory distress, chest discomfort, altered mental status, somnolence, or cyanosis. Patients can sometimes decline precipitously from normal breathing to respiratory arrest, which is felt to be precipitated by an excessive and hyperactive inflammatory response. Although aerosol-generating procedures, such as high-flow oxygen and noninvasive positive-pressure ventilation, are high risk for healthcare providers, they can be utilized with strict isolation precautions. Nebulized medications can also be considered in patients with acute bronchospasm with preexisting asthma or COPD. Otherwise, these agents have not proven to be effective and come with a high level of risk to providers. Use of a hydrofluoroalkane (HFA) is a safer option for providers and can also be considered. Respiratory failure refractory to oxygen therapy may require noninvasive and invasive mechanical ventilation, which would require intensive care. Heated high-flow nasal canula oxygen has been administered. Prone positioning, which is a higher positive end-expiratory pressure strategy, has also been utilized to facilitate oxygenation. The intubation threshold in COVID-19-related respiratory distress is uncertain and controversial, largely due to many patients experiencing normal breathing work with critical but well-tolerated hypoxemia. Whether earlier or later intubation is better for patient survival is unclear. Standard updated best practice guidelines for supportive management of acute hypoxemic respiratory failure and ARDS should be followed. The use of a conservative fluid management strategy for COVID-19 patients is also strongly advised.

Although most hospitalized COVID-19 patients are treated with broad-spectrum antibiotics, observational studies suggest a low incidence of bacterial or fungal coinfection and that it may be prudent to withhold antibacterial drugs in the majority of patients unless and until they present with radiologic or laboratory findings compatible with coinfection or unless they are immunocompromised or critically ill.

The use of systemic corticosteroids for viral pneumonia and ARDS is recommended, with studies suggesting that they may modulate inflammation-mediated lung injury and reduce fatal progression of respiratory failure. The Randomized Evaluation of COVID-19 Therapy (RECOVERY) trial demonstrated that 6 mg daily of dexamethasone for up to 10 days (given orally or intravenously) reduced 28-day all-cause mortality by one-third among critically ill COVID-19 patients. It should be noted that there was no benefit found among patients with shorter symptom duration and no supplemental oxygen requirement. Systemic corticosteroids when used in combination with antivirals and immunomodulators such as baricitinib or tocilizumab have also demonstrated clinical benefit in subsets of COVID-19 hospitalized patients.

Although the incidence of venous thromboembolism in COVID-19 patients is not well established, thromboembolic prophylaxis with subcutaneous low molecular weight heparin is recommended for all hospitalized adults with COVID-19. Microvascular thrombosis is theorized to be a part of hypoxemic respiratory failure in many COVID-19 patients. Whether critically ill COVID-19 patients should receive therapeutic-intensity anticoagulation without venous thromboembolism is unknown; however multiple trials are ongoing to assess whether certain patients would benefit from therapeutic dosing. Postdischarge thromboprophylaxis should also be considered for hospitalized COVID-19 patients due to increased risk for embolic events after discharge.

Multiple antiviral therapies are being studied. Preliminary results from a large, randomized trial suggest that a 10-day course of intravenous remdesivir (an inhibitor of RNA polymerase with in vitro activity against multiple RNA viruses, including Ebola) was superior to placebo in the treatment of hospitalized patients with COVID-19 who had evidence of lower respiratory tract involvement and required supplemental oxygen therapy. Despite the effectiveness of the drug, high mortality persists and future strategies propose utilizing antiviral agents in combination with other therapeutic approaches to maximize patient outcomes. Several other antiviral agents such as favipiravir and oseltamivir have also been proposed for the treatment of COVID-19 patients.

Among the more controversial investigational therapies for COVID-19 are chloroquine and hydroxychloroquine, antimalarial agents that have demonstrated antiviral activity and immunomodulatory effects. Hundreds of clinical trials are ongoing; however due to multiple safety issues, most notably QT prolongation and cardiac complications, current research does not support the off-label use of chloroquine/hydroxychloroquine. It has also been suggested that azithromycin and other macrolides have therapeutic benefits on viral infections and that there exists a synergistic effect via the combination of hydroxychloroquine or chloroquine and azithromycin. Evidence of efficacy of this combination or of azithromycin alone is lacking. A potential risk of QT prolongation induced by the association of the two drugs has also not yet been established but should be considered. Ongoing randomized clinical trials should provide more guidance in the future. Lopinavir/ritonavir and other HIV protease inhibitors are also being studied, but their clinical benefit has not been demonstrated.

Ivermectin, a widely used and generally well-tolerated antiparasitic drug, has shown broad-spectrum activity in vitro against many viruses and has been shown to inhibit the replication of SARS-CoV-2 in cell cultures. Several ongoing clinical trials are evaluating the use of ivermectin for the treatment of COVID-19.

Statins, H2 receptor blockers, angiotensin-converting enzyme (ACE) inhibitors, and angiotensin receptor blockers (ARBs) have all been hypothesized to play a beneficial role in the treatment and prevention of SARS-CoV-2 infection. Insufficient evidence exists on their benefits; thus they are not recommended for treatment of COVID-19. As well, news agencies promoted reports that nonsteroidal antiinflammatory drugs (NSAIDs) might worsen COVID-19 outcome. The FDA has stated that there is no evidence linking NSAIDs with worsening COVID-19 outcome and that patients should continue to use NSAIDs as directed.

Some clinicians encourage the use of vitamin and mineral supplements, such as zinc sulfate, vitamin C, and vitamin D, to treat respiratory viral infections and COVID-19. Multiple ongoing studies are evaluating the use of these supplements for both the prevention and treatment of SARS-CoV-2 infection. However, due to the lack of clinical evidence, most guidelines do not endorse the use of any of these supplements above the recommended dietary allowance for the treatment of COVID-19.

The use of convalescent plasma containing neutralizing antibody donated by people who have recovered from COVID-19 has been reported to show improvement in some patients. Hightiter convalescent plasma, which may help suppress the virus and modify the inflammatory response, has been authorized for emergency use for the treatment of certain hospitalized COVID-19 patients. Other promising alternative therapies being studied include the use of convalescent plasma-derived hyperimmune globulin and mesenchymal stem cells.

Complications

The majority of those infected with COVID-19 will be asymptomatic or experience only mild disease with total recovery. However, patients with underlying illnesses are at high risk for potential complications, including intubation and death. Long-term complications have the potential to be wide-ranging, since research now underscores that coronavirus is a multisystem disease that causes damage not only to the lungs but also to the heart, kidneys, liver, pancreas, brain, neurologic system, gastrointestinal tract, and skin. The hospital mortality from COVID-19 is approximately 15% to 20% but rises up to 40% among patients with more severe disease requiring ICU admission. However, there is much variation across communities and the globe regarding thresholds for hospitalization and differences in outcome. Hospital mortality impacts age groups differently, with mortality less than 5% among patients under age 40 years to 35% for patients aged 70 to 79 years to greater than 60% for patients aged 80 to 89 years. It is postulated that actual mortality figures from COVID-19 are higher than what is reported because not all people who died during the pandemic were tested for the illness.

After improvement and recovery from the initial illness, a patient should be advised to isolate for a minimum of 7 days after the first onset of symptoms and for at least 3 days after resolution of fever and improvement in respiratory symptoms. A test-based strategy is not recommended by the CDC to determine when transmission-based precautions can be discontinued. Additional local guidance regarding the duration of isolation should also be consulted.

Researchers and clinicians have focused most intensely on the acute phase of COVID-19, but the persistence of a diverse range of symptoms has been reported, suggesting continued monitoring of patients after discharge for sequelae is prudent. Some patients appear to suffer a postviral syndrome, lasting several months and sometimes longer. This phenomenon has become known as "long COVID" and presents with a wide range of physical and mental symptoms, including dyspnea, cough, chest pain, fatigue, muscle and joint pain, altered smell, altered taste, headaches, and diarrhea. Other common symptoms frequently seen are cognitive impairment, memory loss, sleep disorders, and anxiety. Individuals with long COVID often report impaired quality of life, with increased issues with mental health and employment. Multidisciplinary care involving the long-term monitoring of symptoms may be necessary in order to identify and address ongoing complications, which may require extended physical rehabilitation, mental health treatment, and social services support.

Although most children and adolescents with SARS-CoV-2 infection have only mild cases of COVID-19, clinicians have recognized an uncommon new childhood hyperinflammatory disorder during the pandemic. Appearing 2 to 4 weeks after SARS-CoV-2 infection in previously healthy pediatric patients, this disorder has been termed multisystem inflammatory syndrome in children (MIS-C) and presents with cardiovascular shock, fever, and hyperinflammation. Mucocutaneous manifestations similar to those of Kawasaki disease have been described, as well as other features including toxic shock syndrome, acute abdominal conditions, encephalopathy, elevated inflammatory markers, and multisystem involvement. Early reports suggest that the syndrome chiefly affects adolescents and children above age 5 years and may disproportionately impact racial and ethnic minorities. Critical illness can lead to intensive care in some patients, with prominent cardiac involvement and coronary-artery aneurysms reported. Most patients have recovered after treatment with a broad range of immunomodulatory agents and intensive care support. Most patients have been treated in a manner following Kawasaki disease or other inflammatory disorders, thus specific therapy for MIS-C still needs to be established.

Conclusions

Much remains unknown in our understanding of the transmission, infection, and management of this novel coronavirus (SARS-CoV-2). Several medical organizations, including the Infectious Diseases Society of America, the World Health Organization, and the National Institutes of Health, have developed interim guidelines that have been modified as more information becomes available during this rapidly evolving pandemic. Most of these guidelines emphasize that there are few proven treatments for COVID-19, that few randomized clinical trials have been published to guide effective management, and that further randomized trials are needed. The foundation of prevention of COVID-19 is vaccination, and the most effective current therapy centers on the early use of neutralizing mAb. This unprecedented pandemic requires therapeutic flexibility and a continuous reshaping of treatment protocols based on available scientific evidence for best patient outcomes.

References

Aiyegbusi OL, Hughes SE, Turner G, et al: Symptoms, complications and management of long COVID: a review, *J R Soc Med*, 2021 Jul 15. 1410768211032850.

Coronavirus (COVID-19) at Centers for Disease Control and Prevention. Available at: https://www.cdc.gov/coronavirus/2019-nCoV/index.html. Accessed on August 21, 2021.

del Rio C, Malani PN, Omer SB. Confronting the Delta variant of SARS-CoV-2, Summer 2021. JAMA. Published online August 18, 2021.

Feldstein LR, Tenforde MW, Friedman KG, et al: Characteristics and outcomes of US children and adolescents with multisystem inflammatory syndrome in children (MIS-C) compared with severe acute COVID-19, *J Am Med Assoc* 325(11):1074–1087, 2021.

Infectious Diseases Society of America. Infectious Diseases Society of America guidelines on the treatment and management of patients with COVID-19. April 11, 2020, with updates to 6/25/21. https://www.idsociety.org/practice-guideline/covid-19-guideline-treatment-and-management/. Accessed August 17, 2021.

Johns Hopkins Coronavirus Resource Center. COVID-19 Dashboard by the Center for Systems Science and Engineering (CSSE) at Johns Hopkins University. https://coronavirus.jhu.edu/map.htm. Accessed August 23, 2021.

Marovich M, Mascola JR, Cohen MS: Monoclonal antibodies for prevention and treatment of COVID-19, *J Am Med Assoc* 324(2):131–132, 2020.

McCullough PA, Kelly RJ, Ruocco G, et al: Pathophysiological basis and rationale for early outpatient treatment of SARS-CoV-2 (COVID-19) infection, *Am J Med* 134(1):16–22, 2021 Jan.

National Institutes of Health. Coronavirus disease 2019 (COVID-19) treatment guidelines. https://www.covid19treatmentguidelines.nih.gov/. Accessed August 21, 2021.

RECOVERY Collaborative Group: Azithromycin in patients admitted to hospital with COVID-19 (RECOVERY): a randomised, controlled, open-label, platform trial, *Lancet* 397(10274):605–612, 2021 Feb 13.

RECOVERY Collaborative Group, Horby P, Lim WS, et al: Dexamethasone in hospitalized patients with Covid-19, *N Engl J Med* 384(8):693–704, 2021 Feb 25.

Rosenberg ES, Holtgrave DR, Dorabawila V, et al. New COVID-19 cases and hospitalizations among adults, by vaccination status — New York, May 3–July 25, 2021. MMWR Morb Mortal Wkly Rep. ePub: August 18, 2021.

Segreto R, Deigin Y, McCairn K, et al: Should we discount the laboratory origin of COVID-19? [published online ahead of print, 2021 Mar 25], *Environ Chem Lett* 1–15, 2021.

Tenforde MW, Self WH, Naioti EA, et al. Sustained effectiveness of Pfizer-BioNTech and Moderna vaccines against COVID-19 associated hospitalizations among adults — United States, March–July 2021. MMWR Morb Mortal Wkly Rep. ePub: August 18, 2021.

Weinreich DM, Sivapalasingam S, Norton T, et al: Trial investigators. REGN-COV2, a neutralizing antibody cocktail, in outpatients with Covid-19, *N Engl J Med* 384(3):238–251, 2021 Jan 21.

World Health Organization. Therapeutics and COVID-19: living guideline. Available at: https://www.who.int/publications/i/item/WHO-2019-nCoV-therapeutics-2021. Accessed on August 22, 2021.

EBOLA VIRUS DISEASE

Method of
Uma Malhotra, MD

CURRENT DIAGNOSIS

- Detection of viral RNA in the blood by reverse transcriptase-polymerase chain reaction (RT-PCR) beginning 3 days after the onset of symptoms.
- Repeat testing may be necessary for patients with illness duration shorter than 3 days.
- Details on specimen collection and handling can be found on the Centers for Disease Control and Prevention (CDC), and World Health Organization (WHO) websites.

CURRENT THERAPY

- Intensive fluid management to correct volume losses and electrolyte abnormalities.
- Aggressive use of antiemetics, antidiarrheals, and rehydration solutions.
- Respiratory and hemodynamic support.
- Blood products for management of coagulopathy.
- Evaluate and treat any concomitant infections.
- There are no approved antiviral therapies. However, monoclonal antibody therapies, REGN-EB3 (Inmazeb) and mAb114 (Ebanga), improve survival in patients with disease due to the *Zaire* species.
- Strict infection control measures, with contact and droplet precautions, must be used.
- Personnel trained in the correct use of personal protective equipment (PPE) should care for the patients.
- The rVSV-ZEBOV Ebola vaccine (Ervebo), a replication-competent, live attenuated vaccine is now approved by the Food and Drug Administration (FDA) for the prevention of disease caused by *Zaire ebolavirus* in adults aged ≥18 years at high risk for occupation exposure. A second vaccine, Ad26.ZEBOV/MVA-BN-Filo,[5] given in two doses, has been found to be safe and immunogenic when given to at-risk populations in regions where there is no active disease transmission and is expected to provide longer protection.

---

[5]Investigational drug in the United States.

Filoviridae, derived from the Latin word "filum," meaning threadlike, is a family of viruses with a filamentous structure that can cause severe hemorrhagic fever and fulminant septic shock. Filoviruses have been divided into two genera: Ebola-like viruses with six species—*Zaire, Sudan, Tai Forest, Bundibugyo, Reston,* and *Bombali*; and Marburg-like viruses with a single species—*Marburg*, which has caused outbreaks in Central Africa. Using paleoviruses (genomic fossils) found in mammals, we can extrapolate that the viruses probably diverged several thousand years ago, and that the family itself is at least tens of millions of years old.

Epidemiology

Of the six Ebola virus species only four—*Zaire, Sudan, Tai Forest,* and *Bundibugyo*—cause disease in humans. Since its first recognition in 1976, *Zaire ebolavirus* has caused multiple outbreaks in Central Africa. It is the causative agent of the 2014 West African epidemic, with an initial estimated case fatality rate as high as 70%, although as the epidemic evolved, lower fatality rates in the range of 30% to 40% were observed.

The 2014 epidemic began in Guinea, when a 2-year-old child became infected in late 2013, and *Zaire ebolavirus* subsequently spread to Liberia, Sierra Leone, Nigeria, Senegal, and Mali. The epidemic resulted in over 28,000 cases and 11,000 deaths, with more than 800 infections occurring in health care workers. Outbreaks due to the Zaire species continue to occur in the Democratic Republic of the Congo (DRC). *Sudan* virus has been associated with a case-fatality rate of approximately 50% in four epidemics, which occurred in Sudan and Uganda between 1970 and 2004. *Tai Forest* virus has been identified as the cause of illness in one person following exposure during a necropsy on a chimpanzee found dead in the Tai Forest. *Bundibugyo* virus, most closely related to the Ivory Coast species, emerged in Uganda in 2007, causing an outbreak with a case fatality rate of approximately 30%. *Reston* virus, discovered after an outbreak of lethal infection in macaques imported into the United States in 1989, is maintained in animal reservoirs in the Philippines. *Bombali* virus RNA has been found in African bats.

Risk Factors/Transmission

Outbreaks generally begin when an individual becomes infected through contact with the tissue or body fluids of an infected animal. The virus then spreads to others who come into contact with the infected individual's blood, skin, or other body fluids. Prior to the 2014 epidemic in West Africa, outbreaks occurred in remote regions with low population density and were controlled within short periods. However, this epidemic showed that movement of infected individuals facilitates the extensive and rapid spread of the virus.

Transmission occurs most commonly through direct contact of broken skin or mucous membranes with virus-containing body fluids from an infected person, the most infectious being blood, feces, and vomit. During the early phase of illness, the level of virus in the blood is typically quite low, but then increases rapidly to very high levels in advanced stages of the illness, when patients become highly infectious. In fact, corpses of persons who die from Ebola are highly infectious, and ritual washing of bodies at funerals has played a significant role in the spread of infection. The virus has also been detected in urine, semen, saliva, breast milk, tears, and sweat, and can persist in some of these fluids much longer than in blood. Ebola virus may also be transmitted though contact with contaminated surfaces where the virus can remain infectious from hours to days.

Transmission to health care workers may occur when appropriate PPE is not used, especially when caring for severely ill patients in advanced stages of illness. During the 2014 outbreak in West Africa, a large number of health care workers became infected. In Sierra Leone, the incidence of confirmed cases at the peak of the epidemic was about 100-fold higher in health care workers than in the general population. Several factors have contributed to the high rates of infections among health providers, including failure to recognize infection among patients and corpses, limited availability and training in the use of appropriate PPE, and inadequate management of contaminated waste and burial of corpses. Although there is no evidence of respiratory transmission, the virus is highly infectious when released in laboratory experiments as a small-particle aerosol, and therefore health care workers may be at risk if exposed to aerosols generated during procedures.

Human infection can occur through contact with infected wild animals during hunting, butchering, and preparing meat, with several episodes having occurred following contact with infected gorillas or chimpanzees. To prevent infection, food products should be properly cooked to inactivate the virus, and basic hygiene measures should be followed. Direct transmission of virus infection from bats to wild primates or humans has not been proven, although Ebola RNA sequences and antibodies have been detected in bats in Central Africa. Bats likely form a major reservoir.

Pathophysiology

Ebolavirus is a negative-sense, single-stranded RNA virus resembling rhabdoviruses and paramyxoviruses in its genome organization and replication mechanisms. The tubular virions contain the nucleocapsid surrounded by an outer envelope, which is derived from the host cell membrane and studded with viral glycoprotein spikes. The virions attach to host cell receptors through the spikes and are then endocytosed into vesicles. Initially, productive infection occurs primarily in dendritic cells, monocytes, and macrophages, resulting in impaired interferon production and release of proinflammatory cytokines, which have secondary effects on innate and adaptive immune responses, inflammation, and vascular integrity. Neutrophils are activated, with resultant degranulation, and lymphocytes undergo apoptosis. The virus then spreads to regional lymph nodes, resulting in further rounds of replication, followed by dissemination to the liver, spleen, thymus, and other lymphoid tissues.

When the virus infects cells, it hijacks the cell and forces it to become a virus-producing factory, churning out new copies of the virus, which results in a loss of cellular function and eventual cell death by apoptosis. As the disease progresses, there is extensive tissue necrosis accompanied by a systemic inflammatory response induced by the release of various cytokines, chemokines, and proinflammatory mediators, as well as a severe coagulopathy triggered by the release of tissue factors. This systemic inflammatory response may contribute to gastrointestinal dysfunction, and ultimately there is a multisystem failure caused by the damage to vascular and coagulation systems.

Clinical Manifestations and Laboratory Findings

Patients with Ebola virus disease (EVD) typically have an abrupt onset of symptoms 5 to 10 days after exposure, with a range of 2 to 21 days. The first phase of the illness is characterized by high fever, chills, headaches, myalgia, and malaise. The second phase is marked by gastrointestinal symptoms, which develop by day 3 to 5, and includes watery diarrhea, nausea, vomiting, and abdominal pain. Patients may also develop chest pain, hiccups, shortness of breath, conjunctival injection, and rash. The rash is usually diffuse erythematous, maculopapular, involving the face, neck, trunk, and arms. Respiratory symptoms such as cough are rare. Common neurologic symptoms include delirium, manifested by confusion, slowed cognition, or agitation, and less frequently, seizures.

The final phase, beginning in the second week, is marked by either progression to shock and death or gradual recovery. Fatal disease is characterized by development of multisystem failure usually as a consequence of massive fluid losses that lead to shock, loss of consciousness, and renal failure. Major bleeding, typically hemorrhage from the gastrointestinal tract, is infrequent and seen in less than 5% during the terminal phase of illness. Patients who survive begin to improve during the second week of illness, with a prolonged convalescence marked by weakness, fatigue, myalgias, headache, and memory loss. About half of the survivors are plagued by chronic debilitating joint pain and a quarter experience eye problems. The virus can persist in the eye for months, leading to uveitis, cataracts, and sometimes blindness. The prevalence of uveitis, unlike other causes, continues to increase until at least two years after symptom onset, with about 33% of the patients affected by that point.

During acute illness patients typically develop leukopenia, lymphopenia, thrombocytopenia, serum transaminase elevations, and proteinuria. They may develop renal insufficiency and electrolyte disturbances as a result of the gastrointestinal losses. Severe cases develop coagulation abnormalities with prolonged prothrombin and partial thromboplastin times, and elevated fibrin degradation products, consistent with disseminated intravascular coagulation.

Diagnosis

The approach to evaluating patients depends on whether or not appropriate signs and symptoms are evident, and if an exposure occurred within 21 days prior to the onset of symptoms. Infection control precautions must be used for all symptomatic patients with an identifiable risk for EVD. All symptomatic patients should be isolated in a single room with a private bathroom, and implementation of contact and droplet precautions. Only essential personnel who are well trained in the use of PPE should interact with the patient. Phlebotomy and laboratory testing should be limited to essential tests. Both the CDC and the WHO have provided detailed recommendations for approach to the evaluation of persons who may have been exposed to the virus.

Rapid diagnostic tests are the most commonly used tests for diagnosis. Viral RNA is generally detectable by RT-PCR in the blood 3 days after the onset of symptoms. Repeat testing may be necessary for patients with illness duration shorter than 3 days. A negative RT-PCR test greater than or equal to 72 hours after the onset of symptoms rules out EVD. Details on specimen collection and handling can be found on the CDC website. For clinicians outside the United States, the WHO has issued guidance for the collection and shipment of specimens from patients with suspected disease.

Rapid immunoassays that detect virus antigen have also been developed. However, the tests are associated with both false positives and false negatives. Therefore they must be verified using RT-PCR test. The rapid immunoassays are mostly useful to make a provisional diagnosis in the appropriate clinical setting when RT-PCR is not readily available.

Differential Diagnosis

Acute onset of febrile illness in a person who lives or has recently been in West or Central Africa may be caused by a variety of local infectious diseases, which must be considered in the differential diagnosis. **Malaria** may have similar findings and might occur concurrently. Examination of blood smears and rapid antigen tests are typically used to diagnose malaria. **Typhoid** is characterized by fever and abdominal pain, and diagnosed by blood cultures.

Patients with **Lassa fever** may develop a severe clinical syndrome resembling EVD and progress to fatal shock. The illness is restricted to West Africa, where it is transmitted through exposure to the aerosolized excretions of rodents, and diagnosed by RT-PCR testing and/or serology. Clinical manifestations of **Marburg virus disease** are similar to EVD, and cases have been identified in Central Africa. The diagnosis is made by RT-PCR. Patients with **influenza** may have a similar initial presentation, but respiratory signs and symptoms are prominent.

Therapy

Good supportive care can significantly improve the chances of recovery from EVD. Mortality rates have been as low as 18% among those cared for in the US and Europe, receiving careful fluid and electrolyte management, nutritional support, and critical care. Large volumes of intravenous fluids and electrolytes are often needed to correct dehydration and electrolyte abnormalities resulting from gastrointestinal losses. Supportive care is required for complications such as shock, hypoxia, hemorrhage, and multiorgan failure. Patients may develop secondary bacterial infections, which may require concurrent management with antimicrobials. Infection prevention and control measures are critical; all bodily fluids and tissues must be considered potentially infectious. The illness is associated with high rates of pregnancy-associated hemorrhage and fetal death. The Centers for Disease Control and Prevention and the American College of Obstetrics and Gynecology have issued recommendations for the care of pregnant women with EVD. However, there are no definitive data to recommend cesarean section versus vaginal delivery or the preferred timing for delivery. According to WHO guidelines from 2020, labor should not be induced. Additionally, procedures such as cesarean delivery, episiotomy, and vacuum extraction should only be performed for maternal indications, with the overall goal of reducing maternal morbidity and mortality.

No FDA-approved antiviral drugs or therapeutic vaccines are available, although several are currently in various stages of testing. Several monoclonal antibodies (mAbs) have been evaluated in animal studies and in clinical trials. Two products, mAb114 (ansuvimab-zykl, Ebanga) and REGEN-EB3 (atoltivimab/maftivimab/odesivimab, Inmazeb) were approved for use by the US Food and Drug Administration (FDA) in 2020, and recommended for use by the WHO during the recent 2021 outbreak in the DRC. The first, mAb114, was isolated from a survivor of EVD and shown to protect 100 percent of macaques from lethal infection when administered up to five days after virus challenge. The second, REGN-EB3, contains three mAbs (atoltivimab, maftivimab, odesivimab) that target the virus surface glycoprotein, providing potent virus neutralization. In rhesus macaques, a single infusion prevented death, even when administered after the onset of illness. The antibodies showed modest reductions in overall mortality in the range 14.6%–17.8% when compared to ZMapp, a three mAb combo, that had previously shown a small reduction in mortality compared to placebo (22% versus 37%). Clinicians may contact the CDC's Emergency Operations Center for additional information on use of experimental therapeutics for treatment of EVD.

Long-Term Follow-up

The WHO suggests close follow-up of patients after hospital discharge for the first year. A suggested schedule is first follow-up 2 weeks after discharge, then monthly for 6 months, and then every three 3 months to complete 1 year. Survivors with ocular findings require follow-up to assess for cataracts. Semen testing should be done at follow-up visits until negative for Ebola virus RNA. If semen testing is unavailable, then WHO recommends that men practice safe sex for 12 months from onset of illness.

If patients develop fever, then they should be assessed for relapse, while also being evaluated for other causes of infection. Development of uveitis and meningitis may suggest relapse. Spinal fluid analysis should be done when meningitis is suspected, even if the blood tests are negative for Ebola virus RNA.

Prevention

Two vaccines have shown promise in the prevention of EVD. The recombinant vesicular stomatitis virus-Zaire Ebola vaccine (rVSV-ZEBOV) has been found to have an efficacy of 97.5% when given as part of a ring vaccination strategy, where contacts of infected people are vaccinated, as are any subsequent contacts of those people. In November 2019, the WHO specified that the vaccine met standards for implementation in the prevention of EVD. The greatest role for the vaccine may be in disease prevention when given promptly post-exposure. The FDA approved rVSV-ZEBOV (Ervebo) on December 19, 2019. In the US, the vaccine is recommended for pre-exposure prophylaxis in adults at risk for occupation exposure to the *Zaire* virus species.

A second vaccine, Ad26.ZEBOV/MVA-BN-Filo[5], was introduced in the DRC in November 2019 in response to the ongoing Ebola epidemic. Given in two doses, 56 days apart. this prime-boost vaccine has been found to be safe and immunogenic. In contrast to the rVSV-ZEBOV vaccine, which is being employed in a ring vaccination strategy for health care workers in the outbreak area, the Ad26.ZEBOV/MVA-BN-Filo vaccine will be given to at-risk populations in regions where there is no active disease transmission and is expected to provide longer protection.

Recommendations for travelers to an area affected by an Ebola outbreak or those residing in such an area are as follows:
- Practice careful hand hygiene and avoid contact with an infected person's blood or body fluids, including personal items that may have come in contact with blood and body fluids.

---

[5]Investigational drug in the United States.

- Avoid unprotected contact with the body of a deceased person who was infected with EVD.
- Avoid contact with bats and nonhuman primates, including blood, bodily fluids, and tissues from these animals.
- Monitor health for 21 days after return from an Ebola endemic region, and seek medical care immediately if any symptoms develop.

Health care workers at risk for exposure to Ebola must wear PPE and notify appropriate health officials at their institutions if they have unprotected contact with the blood or bodily fluids of a person infected with EVD. Finally institutions must have proper infection control and sterilization measures in place for handling of biohazardous materials. Clinicians may contact the CDC for additional information on use of experimental therapeutics and vaccines for prophylaxis following a high-risk occupational exposure to Ebola virus.

Monitoring

Local authorities may have specific regulations for management of asymptomatic individuals with Ebola virus exposure. This includes self-monitoring versus direct observation by a health official, and the need for quarantine. In general, asymptomatic persons who have had an exposure should be monitored for 21 days after the last known exposure, and should immediately report the development of fever or other clinical manifestations suggestive of EVD to the health authorities.

References

Bah EI, Lamah MC, Fletcher T, et al: Clinical presentation of patients with Ebola virus disease in Conakry, Guinea, *N Engl J Med* 372:40–47, 2015.
Chertow DS, Kleine C, Edwards JK, et al: Ebola virus disease in West Africa—clinical manifestations and management, *N Engl J Med* 371:2054–2057, 2014.
Lamontagne F, Fowler RA, Adhikari NK, et al: Evidence-based guidelines for supportive care of patients with Ebola virus disease, *Lancet* 391(10121):700, 2018.
Mulangu S, Dodd LE, Davey Jr RT, et al: A randomized, controlled trial of Ebola virus disease therapeutics, *N Engl J Med* 381:2293, 2019.
PREVAIL III Study Group, Sneller MC, Reilly C, Badio M, Bishop RJ, et al: A longitudinal study of Ebola sequelae in Liberia, *N Engl J Med* 380(10):924, 2019.
United States Centers for Disease Control and Prevention (CDC). Ebola (Ebola virus disease). Available at http://www.cdc.gov/vhf/ebola/.
WHO Ebola Response Team: Ebola virus disease in West Africa—the first 9 months of the epidemic and forward projections, *N Engl J Med* 371:1481–1495, 2014.
World Health Organization (WHO). Ebola. Available at https://www.who.int/health-topics/ebola/.

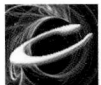

FOODBORNE ILLNESSES

Method of
Anita Devi K. Ravindran, MD; and Viswanathan K. Neelakantan, MD

CURRENT DIAGNOSIS

- Infective foodborne illnesses are innumerable and are caused by various microorganisms. Some microorganisms are established agents, several others are emerging pathogens, and the pathogenicity of the remainder is still under speculation.
- Classification of these illnesses is best done according to their incubation periods, the symptoms they produce, or both.
- Nausea and vomiting predominate in illnesses with short incubation periods caused by preformed toxins, whereas diarrhea predominates in those with long incubation periods caused by toxins produced in the intestine.
- Undercooked charcuterie, meat, poultry, and seafood account for a majority of foodborne illness, but dairy products, salads, pastries, fruits, and vegetables can also cause illness.
- Contaminated water acts as a vehicle in almost all instances.

CURRENT THERAPY

- The majority of infective foodborne illnesses with symptoms confined to the gastrointestinal tract, although apparently alarming, are self-limiting and need only supportive measures including replacement of water and electrolytes.
- Antimicrobial agents are indicated only in certain patients, including those with systemic illnesses, extremes of age, immunocompromised and malnourished states, and severe life-threatening illness.
- Antitoxin is useful in botulism poisoning.
- Vaccines are available against *Vibrio cholerae*, *Salmonella typhi*, hepatitis A virus, and rotavirus, but their effectiveness and cost-effectiveness are debatable.

The Centers for Disease Control and Prevention (CDC) estimates that each year roughly one in six Americans (about 48 million people) gets sick from foodborne illnesses; 128,000 are hospitalized, and 3000 die. These figures are higher in developing nations, and many cases are not brought to light because they occur in remote villages. The 2011 estimates provide the most accurate picture of infective foodborne illnesses, of which bacteria, viruses, and parasites account for the majority. Processing of ready-to-eat foods increases the risk of acquiring foodborne illness because of increased food handling, leading to introduction and growth of pathogens. Increased international travel and migration have also resulted in a greater risk because travelers are at high risk for developing foodborne gastroenteritis caused by pathogens to which they have not been exposed at home.

Classification of Foodborne Illnesses

Agents causing foodborne diseases may be classified in several ways. The most common scheme is a taxonomic combined with a classification based on mode of action (Tables 1 to 3).

Bacteria

Aeromonas Species

Species of *Aeromonas* are ubiquitous and autochthonous in aquatic environments, more so after the tsunami that followed the Indonesian earthquake in December 2004. These aeromonads share many biochemical characteristics with members of the Enterobacteriaceae. The mesophilic species *Aeromonas caviae*, *Aeromonas hydrophila*, and *Aeromonas veronii* are principally associated with gastroenteritis; *A. caviae* particularly infects children younger than 3 years.

Transmission is documented as occurring from a contaminated piped water source, as seen in community-based outbreaks, especially among children. The probability of occurrence of *Aeromonas* infection increased significantly when the mean seasonal temperature exceeded 14°C (57°F), and this was exacerbated where the mean free chlorine concentration fell below 0.1 mg/L.

Aeromonas species are potential food-poisoning agents. *A. hydrophila* is psychrotrophic and has been associated with spoilage of refrigerated animal products including chicken, beef, pork, lamb, fish, oysters, crab, and milk.

The incubation period for *Aeromonas*-associated traveler's diarrhea is 1 to 2 days. It usually causes a sporadic illness. Usually a mild to moderate but self-limiting diarrhea occurs, but it can be severe enough in children to require hospitalization. *Aeromonas* gastroenteritis can occur as a nondescript enteritis, as a more-severe form accompanied by bloody stools, as the etiologic agent of a subacute or chronic intestinal syndrome, as an extremely rare cause of cholera-like disease, or in association with episodic traveler's diarrhea. By far the most common presentation of *Aeromonas* gastroenteritis is watery enteritis. The most serious complication resulting from *Aeromonas* gastroenteritis is hemolytic uremic syndrome.

TABLE 1	Classification of Foodborne Illnesses
SIGNS AND SYMPTOMS OR MECHANISM	**PATHOGENS**
Based on Symptoms and Duration of Onset	
Nausea and vomiting within 6 h	*Staphylococcus aureus, Bacillus cereus*
Abdominal cramps and diarrhea within 8–16 h	*Clostridium perfringens, Bacillus cereus*
Fever, abdominal cramps, and diarrhea within 16–48 h	*Salmonella, Shigella, Vibrio parahemolyticus,* enteroinvasive *Escherichia coli, Campylobacter jejuni*
Abdominal cramps and watery diarrhea within 16–72 h	Enterotoxigenic *E. coli, Vibrio cholerae* O1, O139 Bengal, *Vibrio parahemolyticus,* NAG (nonagglutinable) vibrios, *Norovirus*
Fever and abdominal cramps within 16–48 h	*Yersinia enterocolitica*
Bloody diarrhea without fever within 72–120 h	Enterohemorrhagic *E. coli* O157:H7
Nausea, vomiting, diarrhea, and paralysis within 18–36 h	*Clostridium botulinum*
Based on Pathogenesis	
Food intoxications resulting from the ingestion of preformed bacterial toxins	*Staphylococcus aureus, Bacillus cereus, Clostridium botulinum, Clostridium perfringens*
Food intoxications caused by noninvasive bacteria that secrete toxins while adhering to the intestinal wall	Enterotoxigenic *E. coli, Vibrio cholerae, Campylobacter jejuni*
Food intoxications that follow an intracellular invasion of intestinal epithelial cells	*Shigella, Salmonella*
Diseases caused by bacteria that enter the bloodstream via the intestinal tract	*Salmonella typhi, Listeria monocytogenes*
Based on Toxin Production	
The organisms responsible produce two major types of toxins, or they may be invasive, with no toxin production.	
Secretory toxins are enterotoxins produced by microbes that colonize the intestines in large numbers by attaching to the mucosal epithelial cells without invasion of mucosa, and, hence, there is no fever or other systemic symptoms as a result of lack of inflammatory response. Massive quantities of fluid and electrolytes are lost into the large bowel as its reabsorbing capacity is exceeded by the hypersecretion of isotonic fluid produced by the enterotoxins.	*Vibrio cholerae,* enterotoxigenic *E. coli, Shigella dysenteriae, Salmonella typhimurium*
Cytotoxins are those that destroy the epithelial cells of the mucosa.	*Shigella dysenteriae* elaborating Shiga toxin, causing destructive colitis, enterohemorrhagic *E. coli,* producing a similar toxin causing hemorrhagic colitis and hemolytic uremic syndrome (HUS), and *Vibrio parahemolyticus*) *Clostridium perfringens,* which produces a secretory enterotoxin, also has a cytotoxic action.
Secretory toxins, cytotoxins, and/or neurotoxins that are preformed are ingested directly in food.	*Bacillus cereus, Staphylococcus aureus, Clostridium botulinum*
Certain invasive microbes produce systemic symptoms such as fever, headache, and myalgia, in addition to gastrointestinal symptoms.	Salmonellosis typhoid fever, shigellosis, and brucellosis

Pathogenesis

Mesophilic *Aeromonas* spp. can express a range of virulence factors, including attachment mechanisms and production of a number of toxins. Toxins include aerolysin (a pore-forming cytolysin that attaches to cell membrane, leading to leakage of cytoplasmic contents) and a cytotonic enterotoxin with activity similar to that of cholera toxin. Strains of *A. hydrophila* produce lectins and adhesins, which enable adherence to epithelial surfaces and gut mucosa.

Laboratory Diagnosis

Samples are best transported using Cary-Blair medium. *Aeromonas* forms a bull's-eye–like colony on the selective medium cefsulodin irgasan novobiocin (CIN) agar owing to fermentation of D-mannitol. Ampicillin blood agar has an advantage over CIN agar in that hemolytic colonies can readily be tested for oxidase. *Aeromonas* species produce hemolysis on sheep blood agar.

Treatment

In *Aeromonas* infections, ciprofloxacin (Cipro)[1] 500 mg PO or 400 mg IV twice daily is the antimicrobial treatment of choice. Piperacillin-tazobactam (Zosyn)[1] 4.5 g IV three times daily or ceftazidime (Fortaz)[1] 2 g IV daily may be added in severe infections. The organism is also susceptible to aminoglycosides and carbapenems. Resistance is now becoming a problem because *Aeromonas* can produce β-lactamases and carbapenemases. Therefore it is preferable to initiate therapy with a fluoroquinolone when the organism is isolated.

Bacillus cereus

Bacillus cereus is found abundantly in the environment and vegetation. It is known to produce two forms of food poisoning, emetic and diarrheal. The emetic (short-incubation) type of illness is associated with contaminated fried rice that is not refrigerated.

---

[1]Not FDA approved for this indication.

TABLE 2 Common Organisms Implicated in Infective Foodborne Illness

ETIOLOGIC AGENT	USUAL INCUBA-TION PERIOD	SYMPTOMS	DURATION OF SYMPTOMS	COMMON VEHICLES
Upper Gastrointestinal Tract Symptoms (Nausea, Vomiting) Occur First or Predominate				
Staphylococcus aureus (preformed toxin)	1–6 h	Sudden onset of severe nausea and vomiting Abdominal cramps, diarrhea, and fever may be present	24–48 h	Unrefrigerated or improperly refrigerated meat, potato and egg salads, cream pastries
Bacillus cereus (preformed toxin)	1–6 h	Sudden onset of severe nausea and vomiting Diarrhea may be present	24 h	Improperly refrigerated cooked or fried rice, meat
Lower Gastrointestinal Tract Symptoms (Abdominal Cramps, Diarrhea) Occur First or Predominate				
Bacillus cereus (diarrheal toxin)	10–16 h	Abdominal cramps, watery diarrhea, nausea	24–48 h	Meat, stew, gravy, vanilla sauce
Clostridium perfringens (toxin)	8–16 h	Watery diarrhea, nausea, abdominal cramps; fever is rare	24–48 h	Meat, poultry, gravy, dried or precooked foods, time- and/or temperature-abused food
Vibrio cholerae	2 h to 5 d	Rice-water purging diarrhea leading to dehydration, shock, acidosis, renal failure, abdominal pain Cholera sicca is a severe form; patient dies before diarrhea is manifest; ileus and abdominal bloating result	2–7 d	Sewage-contaminated water Seafood: fish, shellfish, crabs, oysters, clams Contaminated rice, millet gruel, vegetables
Vibrio parahaemolyticus	12–24 h	Watery diarrhea, abdominal cramps, nausea, vomiting Neurologic symptoms can occur, as with *Clostridium botulinum* and *Trichinella spiralis*	2–5 d	Raw or undercooked seafood
Shigella	1–4 d	Abdominal cramps, fever, diarrhea Stool might contain blood and mucus	4–7 d	Food or water contaminated with fecal matter Ready-to-eat food touched by infected food worker
Salmonella (not *typhi*)	1–3 d	Diarrhea, fever, abdominal cramps, vomiting	4–7 d	Contaminated eggs, unpasteurized milk or juice, cheese, contaminated raw fruits and vegetables
Enterotoxigenic *Escherichia coli*	1–3 d	Watery diarrhea, abdominal cramps, some vomiting	3–7 d (or longer)	Food or water contaminated with human feces
Shiga toxin–producing *E. coli*, including *E. coli* O157:H7	2–6 d	Severe diarrhea that is often bloody; abdominal pain and vomiting Usually little or no fever	5–10 d	Undercooked beef, especially hamburger, unpasteurized milk and juice, raw fruit and vegetables (e.g., sprouts), salami (rarely), contaminated water
Campylobacter jejuni	2–5 d	Diarrhea, cramps, fever, vomiting Diarrhea may be bloody	2–10 d	Raw and undercooked poultry, unpasteurized milk, contaminated milk
Vibrio vulnificus	1–7 d	Vomiting, diarrhea, abdominal pain Fever, bleeding within the skin, ulcers requiring surgical removal Can be fatal to people with liver disease or weakened immune systems	2–8 d	Undercooked or raw seafood, especially oysters
Yersinia enterocolitica	3–7 d	Appendicitis-like symptoms: diarrhea, vomiting, fever, abdominal pain	Can remit and relapse over weeks to 1 mo	Drinking water, food contaminated with human fecal matter
Cyclospora	7–10 d	Diarrhea (usually watery), loss of appetite, weight loss, stomach cramps, nausea, vomiting, fatigue	Can remit and relapse over weeks to 1 mo	Fresh herbs and produce (e.g., raspberries, basil, lettuce)
Giardia lamblia (beaver fever)	7–10 d	Diarrhea (acute or chronic), stomach cramps, flatulence, weight loss, malabsorption, developmental delay	Days to weeks	Drinking water, food contaminated with human fecal matter

Continued

ETIOLOGIC AGENT	USUAL INCUBA- TION PERIOD	SYMPTOMS	DURATION OF SYMPTOMS	COMMON VEHICLES
Entamoeba histolytica	1–4 wk	Intestinal: diarrhea, fever, abdominal pain, dysentery, colitis, bowel perforation, ameboma Extraintestinal amebiasis: liver abscess with anchovy-sauce pus, spread to viscera, lungs, and brain	Days to weeks	Drinking water Food contaminated with human fecal matter
Both Upper and Lower Gastrointestinal Tract Symptoms				
Rotavirus	18–36 h	Acute onset of fever and vomiting followed 12–24 h later by frequent watery stools	3–7 d	Contaminated drinking water, food, fomites
Norovirus and other caliciviruses	12–48 h	Nausea, vomiting, cramping, diarrhea, fever, myalgia, some headache Diarrhea is more prevalent in adults; vomiting is more prevalent in children	12–60 h	Food (including shellfish) or water contaminated with human fecal matter Ready-to-eat food touched by an infected food worker
Generalized Symptoms				
Listeria monocytogenes	9–48 h or GI symptoms; 2–6 wk for invasive disease	Fever, muscle aches, nausea or diarrhea Pregnant women can have mild flulike illness, and infection can lead to premature delivery or stillbirth Elderly and immunocompromised patients can have bacteremia or meningitis	Variable	Fresh soft cheese, unpasteurized milk, ready-to-eat deli meat, hot dogs
Balatidium coli	4–5 d	Mostly asymptomatic Chronic diarrhea, occasional dysentery, nausea, foul breath, colitis, abdominal pain, weight loss, deep intestinal ulcerations, possible perforation of the intestine, pneumonia-like illness	Variable	Water contaminated with pig feces
Salmonella typhi	8–14 d	Fever, anorexia, lethargy, malaise, headache, rose spots, constipation or diarrhea, hepatosplenomegaly	4–6 wk	Contaminated water; contaminated food, mainly via food handlers; shellfish from polluted water
Ascoris lumbricoides	4–16 d	Nausea, abdominal pain, intestinal obstruction, malnutrition, Loeffler's syndrome (cough, pneumonitis, eosinophilia), biliary colic, colangitis, pancreatitis, appendicitis	Variable (chronic)	Soil-contaminated raw food, food handlers, water
Trichinella spiralis	1–2 wk	Asymptomatic or chronic diarrhea, abdominal pain Allergy leading to rash, periorbital edema, vasculitis, intramural thrombi Weakness of jaw, biceps, diaphragm, intercostals Eosinophilia, subconjunctival, splinter hemorrhages Muscle penetration: myalgia, orbital pain, diplopia Chronic phase: neurologic symptoms	Variable Acute phase: 1–3 wk	Raw or undercooked meat of pig, horse, wild boar, bush pig, warthog, bear
Infective cysticerci of *Taenia solium* (pork tape worm)	2 months on average	Seizures, vasculitis, focal neurologic deficits, intracranial hypertension, hydrocephalus, mental changes, encephalitis and Brun's syndrome (intermittent obstruction of cerebral aqueduct), myosists, vasculitis	Highly variable	Undercooked charcuterie (pork), contaminated raw vegetables, salads, water
Hepatitis A	15–50 d	Diarrhea, dark urine, jaundice, flulike symptoms, fever, headache, nausea, aversion to food, vomiting, abdominal pain; distaste for cigarettes	Variable: 2 wk to 3 mo	Food (including shellfish) or water contaminated with human fecal matter Inadequately cooked clams, oysters, mussels, cockles Contaminated lettuce, slush beverages, frozen strawberries and salad items Ready-to-eat foods touched by an infected food worker

TABLE 2 — Common Organisms Implicated in Infective Foodborne Illness—cont'd

ETIOLOGIC AGENT	USUAL INCUBA-TION PERIOD	SYMPTOMS	DURATION OF SYMPTOMS	COMMON VEHICLES
Brucella species	1–8 wk	Flulike illness; undulating fever, malaise, arthralgia, anorexia, hepatosplenomegaly, pleurisy, nausea, vomiting, diarrhea, new onset of increased desire to sleep after lunch	Variable	Unpasteurized dairy products, undercooked meat, bone marrow Contact with laboratory cultures and tissue samples Accidental injection of live brucellosis vaccine
Hepatitis E	3–8 wk	Prodrome: anorexia, nausea, vomiting, arthralgia, myalgia, weight loss, dehydration, abdominal pain Icteric phase: jaundice, pruritus, light-colored stool Urticaria, diarrhea, malaise	Variable (several weeks)	Fecally contaminated drinking water and food Raw and undercooked shellfish incriminated in sporadic outbreaks Possibly zoonotic spread
Microsporidium: *Encephalitozoon,* *Pleistophora,* *Nosema,* *Vittaforma,* *Trachipleistophora,* *Brachiola,* *Microsporidium,* *Enterocytozoon*	Unknown	Watery or bloody or unspecified diarrhea, abdominal discomfort, cramps, flatulence, weight loss, loss of appetite, wasting syndrome, subfebrile temperatures Extraintestinal: pneumonitis, myositis, keratoconjunctivitis, seizures, nephritis, cholangiopathy	Variable; self-limiting (1–2 wk) in immunocompetent patients	Contaminated water, food, or inhalation

Abbreviation: GI=gastrointestinal.

TABLE 3 — Rare and Emerging Infections

ETIOLOGIC AGENT	USUAL INCUBA-TION PERIOD	SYMPTOMS	DURATION OF SYMPTOMS	COMMON VEHICLES
Bacillus subtilis	10 min to 14 h (average, 2.5 h)	Vomiting, diarrhea, abdominal cramps, nausea, headache, flushing, sweating	1.5–8 h	Sausage rolls, meat pasties, turkey stuffing, chicken stuffing, pizza, whole-grain bread, steak pie, pork sandwiches
Cyanobacteria: *Microcystic aeuroginosa,* *Anabaena circinalis,* *Anabaena flosaquae,* *Aphanizomenon flosaquae,* *Cylindrospermopsis racibarskii*	3–6 h	Diarrhea, vomiting, allergic reactions, breathing difficulty, dizziness, tingling and numbness, liver and kidney toxicity	8–16 h	Drinking water from untreated surface sources, inhaling aerosols from jet-skis and boats, consuming dietary supplements contaminated by microcystin
Anisakis	Few hours to days	Gastric: abdominal pain, nausea, vomiting Allergic: urticaria, anaphylaxis Intestinal: ileus, perforation, peritonitis, stenosis	2 wk	Raw, lightly pickled, or salted marine fish: Mackerel, squid, horse mackerel, salmon, bonito Squid, cuttlefish Sushi, sashimi
Astrovirus	1–4 d	Watery diarrhea (especially in children), vomiting, fever, anorexia, abdominal pain	3–4 d	Sewage-polluted water and food
Pleisomonas shigelloides	5 d	Diarrhea with blood and mucus, abdominal pain, headache, nausea, chills, fever, vomiting	1–7 d	Contaminated water used for drinking or rinsing foods to be eaten raw Contaminated raw shellfish, salted fish, crabs, oysters
Cyclospora	7 d	Frequent watery diarrhea, weight loss, abdominal pain, bloating, flatulence, vomiting, nausea, low-grade fever, fatigue, malabsorption, cholecystitis	1–4 wk Relapse is common	Fecally contaminated fresh raspberries, snow peas, mesclun

Continued

	TABLE 3	Rare and Emerging Infections—cont'd			
ETIOLOGIC AGENT	USUAL INCUBA-TION PERIOD	SYMPTOMS	DURATION OF SYMPTOMS	COMMON VEHICLES
Iosospora belli	8–11 d	Diarrhea, steatorrhea, headache, fever, malaise, abdominal pain, vomiting, dehydration, weight loss Mesenteric lymph node, liver, spleen involvement	Variable; runs a chronic course in immunocompromised patients	Contaminated food and water
Edwardisella tarda	Not defined	Nausea, vomiting, diarrhea, dysentery, colitis, wound infections, septicemia	Variable: 1–2 wk or longer	Fecal contamination of food, water, raw fish
Citrobacter species	Not defined	Diarrhea, hemolytic uremic syndrome, thrombocytopenic purpura		Meat and milk Parsley (in green butter) from organic gardens using pig manure
Arizona	Not defined	Diarrhea		Cream pie, chocolate eclairs, custard, eggs, chicken, turkey
Achromobacter xylosoxidans	Not defined	Abdominal pain, diarrhea, headache, vomiting		Raw milk, spoiled canned food, contaminated well water

The organism is present in uncooked rice, and the spores survive boiling. The illness is usually self-limiting, with recovery in a day. It is mediated by a heat-stable, preformed enterotoxin resembling that of *Staphylococcus aureus*. The first major outbreak of *Bacillus cereus* food poisoning was in 1971 in England. The diarrheal (long-incubation) type of illness is produced by a heat-labile diarrheal enterotoxin formed in the intestine, which activates adenylate cyclase, causing intestinal fluid secretion, similar to *Escherichia coli* LT toxin and the toxin of *Clostridium perfringens*.

Pathogenesis
During the slow cooling of cooked rice, spores germinate and vegetative bacteria multiply; then they sporulate again. Sporulation is also associated with toxin production. The toxin is heat stable and can easily withstand the temperatures used to cook fried rice.

Laboratory Diagnosis
The disease is diagnosed by the isolation of *B. cereus* from the incriminated food (emetic type) or from stool and food (diarrheal type). Isolation from stools alone is not sufficient because gastrointestinal colonization with *B. cereus* occurs in many persons.

Treatment
B. cereus food poisoning may be symptomatically managed with replacement of fluids and electrolytes. Antimicrobials have no role in treatment. *B. cereus* is also known to produce a variety of ocular and systemic infections such as meningitis, osteomyelitis, pneumonia, and endocarditis. These are usually not foodborne, and it is in this situation that vancomycin (Vancocin)[1] becomes the drug of choice, with clindamycin (Cleocin)[1] and carbapenems being the alternative drugs, both being used along with aminoglycosides for synergistic action.

Campylobacter jejuni
Campylobacter jejuni are harbored in the reproductive and alimentary tracts of some animals. Other than gastrointestinal symptoms, the patient has malaise and headache. The organism may be shed in the patient's stool for up to 2 months. Bacteremia is observed in a small minority of cases. The disease is usually self-limiting. Guillain-Barré syndrome and Reiter's syndrome are recognized sequelae.

Pathogenesis
As few as 500 organisms can cause enteritis. The organism is invasive but generally less so than *Shigella*. *Campylobacter* produces adenylate cyclase–activating toxins resembling *E. coli* LT and cholera toxin.

Laboratory Diagnosis
The feces may be inoculated in enrichment medium or on selective media such as Campy-BAP or Skirrow's medium.

Treatment
Indications for antibiotic therapy in *C. jejuni* infections are prolonged fever, severe diarrhea, dysentery, and persistent symptoms for more than a week. Therapy of *Campylobacter* infection with ciprofloxacin (Cipro 500 mg orally twice daily for 7 days) early in the course of the illness shortens its duration. Unfortunately, this has led to the emergence of fluoroquinolone-resistant *Campylobacter* infections. Erythromycin eradicates carriage of susceptible *C. jejuni* and might shorten the duration of illness if given early in the disease. Erythromycin (Ery-Tab)[1] 250 mg PO four times daily is the drug of choice in *Campylobacter* enteritis. Azithromycin (Zithromax)[1] is also useful and has the advantage of shorter duration of therapy.

Gentamicin (Garamycin), carbapenems, amoxicillin-clavulanate (Augmentin),[1] and chloramphenicol[1] are useful in systemic infections. The usual duration of treatment is 2 weeks. The therapy is prolonged in immunocompromised persons and in patients with endovascular infections.

Clostridium botulinum
Clostridum botulinum is widely distributed in soil, in sediments of lakes and ponds, and in decaying vegetation. *C. botulinum* elaborates the most potent toxin known in humans. When the toxin is ingested, paralysis occurs, often requiring prolonged artificial ventilation. Common signs and symptoms include vomiting, thirst, dry mouth, constipation, ocular palsies, dysphagia, dysarthria, bulbar paralysis, and death due to respiratory paralysis. Coma or delirium occurs in some. Infants present with lethargy, poor feeding, loss of head control, and sometimes sudden infant death syndrome (SIDS).

The incriminated foods are corn syrup, home-canned or bottled meat, fruits, fish, vegetables, herb-infused oils, and

---

[1]Not FDA approved for this indication.

cheese sauce. Infant botulism is associated with consumption of honey; honey should not be given to infants younger than 1 year.

Pathogenesis
Not all strains of *C. botulinum* produce botulinum toxin. Toxigenic types of the organism, designated A, B, C1, D, E, F, and G, produce immunologically distinct forms of botulinum toxin. Lysogenic phages encode toxin C and D serotypes.

Foodborne botulism is not an infection but an intoxication because it results from the ingestion of foods that contain the preformed clostridial toxin. If contaminated food has been insufficiently heated or canned improperly, the spores can germinate and produce botulinum toxin. The toxin is released only after cell lysis and death. The toxin resists digestion and is absorbed by the upper gastrointestinal tract and enters the blood. The toxin blocks release of acetylcholine by binding to receptors at synapses and neuromuscular junctions and causes flaccid paralysis.

Laboratory Diagnosis
Spoilage of food or swelling of cans or presence of bubbles inside the can indicate growth of *C. botulinum*. Food is homogenized in broth and inoculated in Robertson cooked meat medium and blood agar or egg-yolk agar, which is incubated anaerobically for 3 to 5 days at 37°C. The toxin can be demonstrated by injecting the extract of food or culture into mice or guinea pigs intraperitoneally.

Treatment
Hospitalization in an intensive care unit with immediate administration of botulinum antitoxin is vital in the management of botulism. The antitoxin neutralizes only toxin molecules unbound to nerve endings and does not reverse the paralysis. It should be given within 24 hours after the diagnosis is made. Penicillin is the antimicrobial of choice. Intubation and mechanical ventilation are needed for respiratory failure. If swallowing difficulty persists, intravenous fluids or alimentation should be given through a nasogastric tube.

Clostridium perfringens
C. perfringens is heat resistant and elaborates two toxins that can induce specific pathology in the human intestinal tract. It is the third leading cause of foodborne illnesses in United States, after norovirus and *B. cereus*. It is present abundantly in the environment, vegetation, sewage, and animal feces.

Human diseases caused by this organism are the more common *C. perfringens* type A food poisoning and the less common, but more serious, *C. perfringens* type C food poisoning producing necrotic enteritis. Necrotic enteritis is characterized by vomiting, severe abdominal pain, and bloody diarrhea. The incubation period is 2 to 5 days. Progression to necrosis of the jejunum and death occur.

Pathogenesis
Spores in food can survive cooking and then germinate when the food is improperly stored. When these vegetative cells form endospores in the intestine, they release enterotoxins. Food poisoning is mainly caused by type A strains, which produce alpha and theta toxins. The toxins result in excessive fluid accumulation in the intestinal lumen.

Laboratory Diagnosis
Because the bacterium is present normally in intestines, isolation from feces might not be sufficient to implicate it as the cause of the illness. Similarly, isolation from food, except in large numbers ($>10^9$/g), might not be significant. The homogenized food is diluted and plated on selective medium, as well as Robertson cooked meat medium, and subjected to anaerobic incubation. The isolated bacteria must be shown to produce enterotoxin.

Treatment
Food poisoning due to *Clostridium perfringens* is managed conservatively with hydration and replacement of electrolytes. *C. perfringens* is susceptible to benzylpenicillin (penicillin G), which may be useful in managing severe infections (1 mU IV every 4 hours). Vancomycin,[1] clindamycin,[1] cefoxitin (Mefoxin), and metronidazole (Flagyl) are alternatives. *C. perfringens* type C toxoid vaccine[2] (two doses, 4 months apart) is preventive in pigbel.

Cronobacter sakazakii
Cronobacter sakazakii causes neonatal meningitis or necrotizing enterocolitis and bacteremia, which results in an alarming mortality rate. Surviving patients sometimes develop ventriculitis and cerebral abscess. *C. sakazakii* has been isolated from infant formulas.

Enterobacter species are generally resistant to the cephalosporins, except cefepime (Maxipime),[1] but are responsive to carbenicillin (Geocillin),[1] piperacillin (Pipracil),[1] ticarcillin (Ticar),[1] amikacin (Amikin),[1] and tigecycline (Tygacil).[1]

Enterohemorrhagic Escherichia coli
Many serogroups of *E. coli*, including O4, O26, O45, O91, O111, O145, and O157, are pathogenic, but the most common pathogenic serotype is O157:H7. Cattle are the main sources of infection; most cases are associated with the consumption of undercooked beef burgers and similar foods from restaurants and delicatessens. The latest outbreak of *E. coli* O157:H7 during the fall of 2019 and 2020 was linked to leafy greens (romaine salad greens).

Pathogenesis
Enterohemorrhagic *E. coli* (EHEC) strains can produce one or more types of cytotoxins, which are collectively referred to as Shiga-like toxins because they are antigenically and functionally similar to Shiga toxin produced by *Shigella dysenteriae*. (Shiga-like toxins were previously known as verotoxins.) The toxins provoke cell secretion and kill colonic epithelial cells, causing hemorrhagic colitis and hemolytic-uremic syndrome (HUS), leading occasionally to disseminated intravascular coagulation (DIC). A fibrin layer forms in the glomerular capillary bed, and acute renal failure occurs due to DIC. These are most likely to occur in children, elderly patients, and pregnant women. The young recover fully, but at times dialysis is warranted.

Laboratory Diagnosis
Laboratory diagnosis is performed by culturing the feces on McConkey's agar or sorbitol McConkey's agar. Strains can then be identified by serotyping using specific antisera. Shiga-like toxins can be detected by enzyme-linked immunosorbent assay (ELISA), and genes coding for them can be detected by DNA hybridization techniques.

Treatment
Hydration with electrolyte replacement is the mainstay of treatment in *E. coli* O157:H7 infection, and patients should be monitored closely and constantly for the development of HUS, which requires management in an intensive care setting with blood transfusion and dialysis. Although dysentery is self-limiting, the use of rifaximin (Xifaxan), a nonabsorbable agent, is recommended in those who are increasingly susceptible to infections. In the absence of dysentery, early institution of drugs like ciprofloxacin (Cipro) or azithromycin (Zithromax),[1] especially in traveler's diarrhea, decreases the duration of illness.

Enterotoxigenic Escherichia Coli
Enterotoxigenic *E. coli* (ETEC) is now ubiquitous in nature. Wild animals and cattle act as reservoirs of the organism. *E. coli* is carried normally in the intestine of humans and animals. Some

---

[1]Not FDA approved for this indication.
[2]Not available in the United States.

specific serotypes harbor plasmids that code for toxin production. This bacterium is responsible for a majority of traveler's diarrhea. The disease is self-limiting and resolves in a few days.

Pathogenesis
The bacteria colonize the gastrointestinal tract by means of fimbriae, attaching to specific receptors on enterocytes of the proximal small intestine. Enterotoxins produced by ETEC include the LT (heat-labile) toxin and the ST (heat-stable) toxins. LTs are similar to cholera toxin in structure and mode of action, consisting of A and B subunits. The B (binding) subunit of LTs binds to specific ganglioside receptors (GM1) on the epithelial cells of the small intestine and facilitates the entry of the A (activating) subunit, which activates adenylate cyclase. Stimulation of adenylate cyclase causes an increased production of cyclic adenosine monophosphate (cAMP), which leads to hypersecretion of water and electrolytes into the lumen and inhibition of sodium reabsorption.

Laboratory Diagnosis
The sample of feces is cultured on McConkey's agar. The ETEC stains are indistinguishable from the resident E. coli by biochemical tests. These strains are differentiated from nontoxigenic E. coli present in the bowel by a variety of in vitro immunochemical, tissue culture, or DNA hybridization tests designed to detect either the toxins or the genes that encode for these toxins. With the availability of a gene probe method, foods can be analyzed directly for the presence of ETEC in about 3 days. LTs can be detected by ligated rabbit ileal loop test and by observing morphologic changes in Chinese hamster ovary cells and Y1 adrenal cells. ELISA, immunodiffusion, and coagglutination are also used in diagnosis.

Listeria monocytogenes
Listeria monocytogenes is quite hardy and resists the deleterious effects of freezing, drying, and heat remarkably well for a bacterium that does not form spores. It is capable of growing at 3°C and multiplies in refrigerated foods. The latest implicated food in a February 2021 outbreak is queso fresco cheese.

Pathogenesis
L. monocytogenes invades the gastrointestinal epithelium. Once the bacterium enters the host's monocytes, macrophages, or neutrophils, it is bloodborne and can grow. Its presence in phagocytes also permits access to the brain and transplacental migration to the fetus in pregnant women. Granulomatosis infantisepticum is a feature of listeriosis. The pathogenesis of L. monocytogenes centers on its ability to survive and multiply in phagocytic host cells.

Laboratory Diagnosis
The diagnosis of listeriosis is most commonly made by isolation of L. monocytogenes from a normally sterile site. β-Hemolytic colonies, which test negative for catalase, hydrolyze hippurate, and have a positive cAMP reaction, form on blood agar. Serologic testing is not useful in diagnosing acute invasive disease, but it can be useful in detecting asymptomatic disease and gastroenteritis in an outbreak or in other epidemiologic investigations. Stool testing is not commercially available.

Treatment
Ampicillin[1] (2g IV every 4 hours) is the drug of choice in Listeria monocytogenes infections. Aminoglycosides are added for synergistic effect. Trimethoprim-sulfamethoxazole (TMP-SMX)[1] (Bactrim, 20 mg of trimethoprim/day IV every 6 hours) is an alternative for patients allergic to penicillin. Ampicillin and TMP-SMX may be used in combination. Vancomycin (Vancocin),[1] linezolid (Zyvox),[1] carbapenems, macrolides, and tetracyclines are also

effective. Cephalosporins are ineffective in the treatment of listeriosis and should not be used. The duration of therapy is highly variable depending on the clinical situation and is 14 days for bacteremia, 21 days for meningitis, 42 days for endocarditis, and 56 days for neurologic infections. Patients whose disease is promptly diagnosed and treated recover fully, but permanent neurologic sequelae are common in patients with cerebral illnesses. Consuming only pasteurized dairy products and fully cooked meats, meticulously cleaning utensils, and thoroughly washing fresh vegetables before cooking will prevent foodborne listerial infections. Pregnant women and others at risk should avoid soft cheeses and thoroughly reheated ready-to-serve and charcuterie foods.

Nontyphoidal Salmonellosis
Nontyphoidal salmonellosis consists of several causative organisms classified under the family Enterobacteriaceae; one such organism is Salmonella enteritidis. It does not occur normally in humans, but several animals act as reservoirs.

The diarrhea may be watery, with greenish, foul-smelling stools. This may be preceded by headache and chills. Other findings include prostration, muscle weakness, and moderate fever. In August 2020, a multi-state outbreak of Salmonella enteritidis was linked to peaches packed or supplied by Prima Wawona packing company. An outbreak of Salmonella stanley infection was linked to wood ear mushrooms (dried mushrooms, also called kikurage/dried black fungus) imported to to the U.S. Yet another non-typhoidal Salmonella infection reported in July 2020 was caused by Salmonella newport. The likely source was identified as potentially contaminated red onions. A food-borne illness recently reported from Mexico was caused by Salmonella poona and linked to consumption of cucumbers.

Pathogenesis
The organism penetrates and passes through the epithelial cells lining the terminal ileum. Multiplication of bacteria in lamina propria produces inflammatory mediators, recruits neutrophils, and triggers inflammation. Release of lipopolysaccharides and prostaglandins causes fever and also loss of water and electrolytes into the lumen of the intestine, resulting in diarrhea.

Laboratory Diagnosis
Culture in selenite F broth and then subculture on deoxycholate citrate agar isolates the organisms. Plates are incubated at 37°C overnight, and growth is identified by biochemical and slide agglutination tests.

Treatment
The antibiotics recommended for gastroenteritis due to nontyphoidal salmonellosis are ciprofloxacin (Cipro)[1] 500 mg PO twice daily, and ceftriaxone (Rocephin) 2 g IV daily, for 3 to 7 days. Amoxicillin (Amoxil)[1] and TMP-SMX[1] are also effective. Therapy is prolonged in bacteremia, endocarditis, or meningitis.

Shigella Species
Shigella species belong to the family Enterobacteriaceae. Bacillary dysentery is caused by Shigella flexneri, Shigella boydii, Shigella dysenteriae, and Shigella sonnei. S. flexneri is most common in developing countries where hygiene is poor and clean drinking water is unavailable; S. sonnei is most common in developed countries. The watery diarrhea that is present initially becomes bloody after a day or two owing to spread of infection from the ileum to the colon. The illness is caused by exotoxin acting in the small bowel.

Extraintestinal manifestations are recognized, including HUS, Reiter's syndrome, meningitis, Ekiri syndrome (reported in Japanese children and consisting of a triad of encephalopathy due to cerebral edema, bizarre posturing, and fatty degeneration of liver), vaginitis, lung infections, and keratoconjunctivitis. Toxic megacolon, pneumatosis coli, perforation, and rectal prolapse are recognized complications.

Tossed salads, chicken, and shellfish are the commonly incriminated foods. Person-to-person spread by anal intercourse or oral

---
[1]Not FDA approved for this indication.

sex also occurs. Prepared food acts as a vehicle of transmission. Spread of infection is also linked to flies.

Children are at high risk during the weaning period, and increasing age is associated with decreased prevalence and severity. Children in daycare centers, persons in custodial institutions, migrant workers, and travelers to developing countries are also at high risk.

Pathogenesis

The virulence factor is a smooth lipopolysaccharide cell wall antigen, which is responsible for the invasive features, and the Shiga toxin, which is both cytotoxic and neurotoxic. Shigellae survive the gastric acidity and invade and multiply within the colonic epithelial cells, causing cell death and mucosal ulcers, and spread laterally to involve adjacent cells but rarely invade the bloodstream.

Laboratory Diagnosis

Shigellosis can be correctly diagnosed in most patients on the basis of fresh blood in stool. Neutrophils in fecal smears strongly suggest infection. Any clinical diagnosis should be confirmed by cultivation of the etiologic agent from stools. Cary-Blair medium is the transport medium of choice, and MacConkey agar or deoxycholate citrate agar (DCA) as well as a highly selective medium such as xylose-lysin deoxycholate (XLD), Hektoen enteric (HE), or Salmonella-Shigella (SS) agar are also used.

Treatment

Ciprofloxacin (Cipro, 500 mg PO twice daily for 3 days) is the antibiotic of choice for shigellosis. Alternative agents are pivmecillinam (Selexid),[2] ceftriaxone (Rocephin),[1] and azithromycin (Zithromax).[1]

Staphylococcus aureus

A notable incident of staphylococcal food poisoning occurred in February 1975 when 196 of 344 passengers and one flight attendant aboard a jet from Tokyo to Copenhagen via Anchorage contacted a gastrointestinal illness characterized by nausea, vomiting, and abdominal cramps. The flight attendant and 142 passengers were hospitalized. Symptoms developed shortly after a ham and omelet breakfast had been served. S. aureus was incriminated as the offending agent and ham as the vehicle of the outbreak. The source was traced to a cook with pustules on his fingers.

S. aureus is ubiquitous in the environment. Only strains that produce enterotoxin cause food poisoning. Food is usually contaminated by infected food handlers.

Pathogenesis

If food is stored for some time at room temperature, the organism can multiply in the food and produce enterotoxin. Most food poisonings are caused by enterotoxin A, and the isolates commonly belong to phage type III. These are heat stable, and ingestion of as little as 23 μg of enterotoxin can induce symptoms. The toxin acts on the receptors in the gut, and sensory stimulus is carried to the vomiting center in the brain by vagus and sympathetic nerves.

Because the ingested food contains preformed toxin, the incubation period is very short. In severe illness, profound hypotension occurs. Death is known to occur at extremes of age and in the malnourished.

Laboratory Diagnosis

The presence of a large number of S. aureus in food can indicate poor handling or sanitation; however, it is not sufficient evidence to incriminate the food as the cause of food poisoning.

Staphylococcal food poisoning can be diagnosed if staphylococci are isolated in large numbers from the food and their toxins are demonstrated in the food or if the isolated S. aureus is shown to produce enterotoxins. Dilutions of food may be plated on Baird-Parker agar or mannitol salt agar. Enterotoxin may be detected and identified by gel diffusion.

Treatment

Therapy is mainly supportive. Antibiotics have no role in the treatment because they are not antitoxins. Intravenous fluids and electrolyte replacement are imperative in the severely dehydrated patient.

Yersinia Species

The Yersinia species that cause food poisoning are commonly Yersinia enterocolitica and rarely Yersinia pseudotuberculosis. Pigs and other wild or domestic animals are the hosts, and humans are usually infected by the oral route. Serogroups that predominate in human illness are O:3, O:5, O:8, and O:9.

Yersiniosis is common in children and occurs most often in winter. Y. enterocolitica is associated with terminal ileitis and Y. pseudotuberculosis with mesenteric adenitis, but both organisms can cause mesenteric adenitis and symptoms that cause a clinical picture resembling appendicitis, resulting in surgical removal of a normal appendix. Rarer strains of Y. enterocolitica are likely to cause systemic infections, especially in patients with diabetes or in iron overload states. In Japan, a form of vasculitis, called Izumi fever, occurs, and in Russia a scarlet fever–like illness has been reported.

Pathogenesis

Yersinia organisms can survive and grow during refrigerated storage. Strains that cause human yersiniosis carry a plasmid that is associated with a number of virulence traits. Ingested bacteria adhere and invade M cells or epithelial cells.

Laboratory Diagnosis

Suspect food is homogenized in phosphate-buffered saline and inoculated into selenite F broth and held at 4°C for 6 weeks. The broth is subcultured at weekly intervals on deoxycholate citrate (DCA) or Yersinia-selective agar plates. This is termed cold-enrichment technique.

Treatment

Antibiotics are not recommended for gastroenteritis caused by Yersinia enterocolitica and the less-common Yersinia pseudotuberculosis, but bacteremia and extraintestinal infections require treatment with ciprofloxacin[1] (500 mg PO or 400 mg IV twice daily for 2 weeks). Third-generation cephalosporins (cefotaxime[1] [Claforan]), amoxicillin[1] (Amoxil), TMP-SMX[1] (Bactrim), amoxicillin-clavulanate[1] (Augmentin), carbapenems, and gentamicin (Garamycin) are also effective agents in therapy.

Viruses

Noroviruses

Noroviruses (formerly called Norwalk or Norwalk-like viruses and small round structured viruses [SRSV]) and sapoviruses belong to the family Caliciviridae and are the most common cause of gastroenteritis. They account for about 90% of epidemic nonbacterial outbreaks of gastroenteritis around the world. Norovirus infection often affects people during the winter months and is therefore sometimes called winter vomiting disease; however, people may be affected at any time of the year. After a norovirus infection, immunity lasts only for 14 weeks and is incomplete. Persons with blood group O are more susceptible to infection, whereas those with groups B and AB are partially protected. Norovirus infection outbreaks more commonly occur in closed or semiclosed communities, such as prisons, dormitories, cruise ships, schools, long-term care facilities, and overnight camps—places where infection can spread rapidly from human to human or through tainted food and surfaces. Infection outbreaks can also result from food handled by an infected person.

Outbreaks have often been linked to consumption of cold foods, including salads, sandwiches, and bakery products. Salad

[1]Not FDA approved for this indication.
[2]Not available in the United States.

[1]Not FDA approved for this indication.

dressing, cake icing, and oysters from contaminated waters have also been implicated in gastroenteritis outbreaks. Weight loss, lethargy, low-grade fever, headache, and (rarely) ageusia occur. Vomiting is more likely with infections caused by norovirus than sapovirus.

Pathogenesis

Norovirus strains that infect humans are found in genogroups I, II, and IV. GII.4 strains are more commonly associated with person-to-person transmission, and GI strains are identified more commonly in shellfish-associated outbreaks.

Noroviruses were shown to differentially bind to histo-blood group antigens, and the binding pattern correlates with susceptibility to infection and illness. A number of enzymes are important in the synthesis of histo-blood group antigens, including fucosyl transferase-2 (FUT-2, secretor enzyme), FUT-3 (Lewis enzyme), and the A and B enzymes. The glycan produced by FUT-2 H type 1, serves as a viral receptor for noroviruses.

Laboratory Diagnosis

The virus can be recovered from the infected person's stool and vomitus during illness for about 2 weeks. Electron microscopy and reverse-transcriptase polymerase chain reaction (RT-PCR) antigen-detection assays are performed on stool samples. Serologic assays are not available for clinical use. However, infection can be diagnosed by identifying a fourfold or greater increase in antibody titer between acute and convalescent sera using norovirus virus-like particles as antigen.

Treatment

There is no specific treatment for norovirus infection. Hydration is generally adequate for most patients. In developing countries, oral rehydration therapy is the treatment of choice. Effective hand washing, careful food processing, and education of food handlers along with chlorination of water are important preventive measures. A vaccine for norovirus is in clinical trials.

Rotavirus

Among the seven rotavirus species (A to G), rotavirus A, B, and C can cause disease in humans. Rotavirus A is the most common and is the major cause of waterborne outbreaks in humans. Infections are referred to as infantile diarrhea, winter diarrhea, or acute viral gastroenteritis. Children 6 months to 2 years of age, premature infants, the elderly, and the immunocompromised are particularly prone to more-severe symptoms caused by infection with group A rotavirus. Rotavirus can survive in water for days to weeks, depending on water quality and temperature. Waterborne outbreaks are most common, followed by spread by fomites. Rotaviruses infect intestinal enterocytes; diarrhea may be caused by malabsorption secondary to the destruction of enterocytes, villus ischemia and activation of the enteric nervous system, and intestinal secretion stimulated by the action of rotavirus nonstructural protein 4 (NSP4), a novel enterotoxin and secretory agonist with pleiotropic properties.

Outbreaks caused by group B rotavirus, also called adult diarrhea rotavirus, have also been reported in the elderly and adults. Such infections are rare and usually subclinical. Group C rotavirus has been associated with rare and sporadic cases of diarrhea in children in many countries. Subclinical infection to severe gastroenteritis leading to life-threatening dehydration can occur. The illness has an abrupt onset, with vomiting often preceding the onset of diarrhea. Up to one third of patients have fever of about 39°C. The stools are characteristically watery and only occasionally contain red or white cells. Symptoms generally resolve in a week.

Respiratory and neurologic features in children have been reported. Rotavirus infection has been associated with other clinical conditions including sudden infant death syndrome (SIDS), necrotizing enterocolitis, Kawasaki's disease, and type 1 diabetes.

Laboratory Diagnosis

Electron microscopy, direct antigen detection assays (ELISA, immunochromatography, latex agglutination), and nucleic acid detection (e.g., RT-PCR, polyacrylamide gel electrophoresis [PAGE]), are used mainly in epidemiologic studies during outbreaks.

Treatment

Dehydration due to group A rotavirus infection is treated with early institution of oral and intravenous fluids. The role of probiotics,[7] bismuth subsalicylate (Pepto Bismol),[1] inhibitors of enkephalinase, and nitazoxanide (Alinia)[1] are not clearly defined. Antimicrobials and antimotility agents should be avoided. A marked fall in deaths from childhood diarrhea following introduction of rotavirus vaccines (Rotarix, RotaTeq) has been reported from various parts of the world, and surveillance information has not revealed an association of any serious adverse reactions with the vaccine.

Other Pathogens

Cryptosporidium

Transmission of *Cryptosporidium* is usually by the fecal-oral route, often through food and water contaminated with livestock mammal feces. Persons most likely to be infected by *Cryptosporidium parvum* are infants and young children in daycare centers; those whose drinking water is unfiltered and untreated; those involved in farming practices such as lambing, calving, and muckspreading; people engaging in anal sexual practices; patients in a hospital setting (from other infected patients or health care workers); veterinarians; and travelers.

Pathogenesis

Cryptosporidium spp. are believed to be noninvasive. Malabsorption resulting from the intestinal damage caused by prolonged protozoal infection can be fatal. Although host cells are damaged in cryptosporidiosis, the means by which the organism causes damage is not known. Mechanical destruction and the effects of toxins, enzymes, or immune-mediated mechanisms, working alone or together, may be instrumental. In the immunocompromised, the illness is much more debilitating, with cholera-like diarrhea.

Laboratory Diagnosis

Traditionally, cryptosporidiosis is diagnosed by microscopic observation of developmental stages of the organism in an intestinal biopsy specimen. Oocysts can be recovered from stool samples by formalin-concentration techniques, staining with a modified Ziehl-Neelsen acid-fast stain. Serologic tests (ELISA, immunofluorescence antibody, PCR) are of added value.

Treatment

Nitazoxanide (Alinia, 500 mg PO twice daily for 3 days) is recommended with antiretrovirals for HIV-positive patients. Fluid replacement and antidiarrheal agents are also given.

Trichinosis

Trichinosis is due to *Trichinella spiralis* infection, commonly as a result of consuming improperly cooked pork. Recent outbreaks in North America have been attributed to consumption of bear meat rather than pork. The parasite lodges in the extraocular muscles, deltoid, biceps, intercostals, diaphragm, tongue, or masseter and produces severe weakness with pain, fever, and cough along with splinter hemorrhages and eosinophilia.

Moderate *T. spiralis* infection is treated with mebendazole (Vermox 200–400 mg PO three times daily for 3 days) or albendazole[1] (Albenza 400 mg PO twice daily for 7–14 days). For severe infections, prednisone is added in a dose of 1 mg/kg/day for 5 days.

---

[1]Not FDA approved for this indication.
[7]Available as dietary supplement.

TYPE OF POISONING	TOXINS	SOURCES OF TOXINS	PRIMARY VECTOR	ACTION TARGET
PSP	Saxitoxins and gonyautoxins	*Alexandrium* spp., *Gymnodinium* spp., *Pyrodinium* spp.	Shellfish	Voltage-gated sodium channel 1
NSP	Brevetoxins	*Kerenia brevis, Chatonella marina, C. antiqua, Fibrocapsa japonica, Heterosigma akashiwo*	Shellfish	Voltage-gated sodium channel 5
	Yessotoxins	*Protoceratium reticulatum, Lingulodinium polyedrum Gonyaulax spinifera*	Shellfish	Voltage-gated calcium/sodium channel?
CFP	Ciguatoxins	*Gambierdiscus toxicus*	Coral reef fish	Voltage-gated sodium channel 5
CFP	Maitotoxins	*Gambierdiscus toxicus*	Coral reef fish	Voltage-gated calcium channel
AZP	Azaspiracids	*Protoperidinium crassipes*	Shellfish	Voltage-gated calcium channel
Palytoxin poisoning	Palytoxins	*Ostrepsis siamensis*	Shellfish	Na₊K₊ATPase

Neurocysticercosis

Neurocysticercosis is caused by *Taenia saginata* infection, commonly as a result of consuming improperly cooked pork or contaminated raw vegetables and water. The parasite lodges in the central nervous system and skeletal muscle and presents as intracranial calcifications and ring-enhancing lesions on radioimaging studies. Other than leukocytosis, eosinophilia, and raised erythrocyte sedimentation rate, antibodies to species-specific antigens of *T. solium* can be detected by immunosorbent assay and complement fixation-tests. Treatment is aimed at controlling seizures and relief of hydrocephalus. Albendazole (15 mg/kg/day for 8–28 days) or praziquantel (50–100 mg/kg/day in three divided doses for a month) are given for parenchymal cysticerci with glucocorticoids to suppress the inflammatory response around the dying parasites. Surgery may be required to reduce intracranial pressure.

Dinoflagellate toxins

Dinoflagellates, a very large and diverse group of eukaryotic algae in the marine ecosystem, are the major group producing toxins that impact humans. Dinoflagellate toxins are structurally and functionally diverse, and many present unique biological activities. Five major seafood poisoning syndromes caused by toxins have been identified from the dinoflagellates (Table 4): paralytic shellfish poisoning (PSP), neurotoxic shellfish poisoning (NSP), amnesic shellfish poisoning (ASP), diarrheic shellfish poisoning (DSP) and ciguatera fish poisoning (CFP). Symptoms include allergic manifestations, neurologic including paresthesia of the extremities, headache, ataxia, vertigo, cranial nerve palsies, and paralysis of respiratory muscles as well as gastrointestinal. Symptomatic treatment and antihistamines are the mainstay of treatment.

Tetrodotoxin poisoning

It is a neurotoxin concentrated in the skin and viscera of puffer fish, and other fishes of the order Tetraodontiformes and in some amphibian, octopus, and shellfish species. Human poisonings occur when the flesh or organs of the fish are improperly prepared and eaten. Tetrodotoxin acts by blocking the conduction of nerve impulses along nerve fibers and axons and interferes with the transmission of signals from nerves to muscles. Onset of symptoms usually is 30–40 minutes but may be as short as 10 minutes; it includes lethargy, paraesthesia, emesis, ataxia, weakness, and dysphagia; ascending paralysis occurs in severe cases with high mortality (1-2 mg is lethal). Management is symptomatic.

Group B Sreptococcus (GBS)

GBS bacteria is found in 15%–30% of adult human intestines and urinary tract. Rarely implicated in infections of skin, joints, heart and brain, a recent outbreak of food-borne illness caused by the Type III GBS ST283 strain was reported in Singapore during the period of January–July 2015. It is the largest of its kind and first association to food-borne transmission of GBS to people via consumption of "yusheng-style" raw fresh water fish. The primary case presented with giddiness and suffered bouts of vomiting and diarrhea. Further studies are ongoing to establish the link between increase in cases of Group B streptococcus (GBS) infection to consumption of raw fish. Treatment is symptomatic.

Newer Trends in Foodborne Illness

New or unusual pathogens and food hazards are identified in course of investigating outbreaks. In 2011, a novel outbreak of sprout-associated illness caused by a strain of *Escherichia coli* O104:H4 was reported from Germany and France. This enteroaggregative and Shiga toxin-producing strain caused severe illness leading to HUS and death. In 2008, an outbreak following consumption of chicken caused by *Arcobacter butzleri* (found in poultry) was reported from Wisconsin. The calcivirus Sapovirus is emerging as the likely cause of oyster-associated foodborne outbreaks in Japan. New and unsuspected food vehicles are also being identified that had not been previously recognized as problematic (Box 1).

Changing patterns of disease presentation have seen important foodborne challenges emerging. Chagas disease is emerging as a foodborne infection linked to fresh, unpasteurized acai and guava juice. Infected triatomid insects present in fruits are implicated. Outbreaks of Nipah virus encephalitis in Bangladesh and India have been linked to drinking of palm sap, toddy, and well water contaminated with urine of feeding giant fruit bats, the vector of Nipah virus.

More syndromes and other systemic disease presentations are being linked to foodborne infection. The feco-oral transmission of pathogens leading to other systemic manifestation include Campylobacter sp. (Guillain-Barre syndrome, irritable bowel syndrome), Toxoplasma gondii (behavior changes and neuropsychiatric manifestations) and Salmonella choleraesuis (aortitis). Foodborne outbreak of Group G streptococci (GGS) pharyngitis in a school dormitory in Japan (2016) presented with sore throat and fever in a majority; implicated food was a broccoli salad.

BOX 1 New Food Vehicles Identified in Outbreaks

Bagged spinach
Carrot juice
Peanut butter
Broccoli powder on a snack food
Dry dog food
Frozen potpies
Canned chilli sauce
Hot peppers
White and black pepper
Raw cookie dough (likely the flour)
Hazelnuts
Fenugreek sprouts
Papayas
Pine nuts
Raw scrapped tuna

Reprinted from Braden C, Tauxe R: Emerging trends in foodborne diseases, *Inf Dis Clinics N Am* 27:517-533, 2013.

BOX 2 Miscellaneous Organisms Implicated in Foodborne and Waterborne Illnesses

Adenovirus 40, 41
Bacillus anthracis
Bacillus mycoides
Burkholderia cepacia
Burkholderia pseudomallei
Clostridium bifermentans
Corynebacterium diphtheriae
Coxiella burnetii
Dientamoeba fragilis
Enterococcus faecalis, E. faecium
Erysipelothrix rhusiopathiae
Francicella tularensis
Klebsiella spp.
Leptospira spp.
Mycobacterium bovis
Parvovirus B
Pediococcus
Pestivirus
Picobirnavirus
Proteus spp.
Pseudomonas aeruginosa
Pseudomonas cocovenanans
Reovirus
Streptobacillus moniliformis
Taenia solium, T. saginata
Torovirus
Toxoplasma gondii

Miscellaneous

Many other organisms are implicated in foodborne and waterborne illnesses (Box 2). Some are discussed elsewhere in this book. Amebiasis, brucellosis, cholera, hepatitis A and E, giardiasis, typhoid fever, and other foodborne intestinal nematodes and cestodes are covered in the infectious diseases section of this text and are not covered in this section.

References

Baker AC, Goddard VJ, Davy J, et al: The identification of a diagnostic marker to detect freshwater cyanophages of filamentous cyanobacteria, *Appl Environ Microbiol* 72:5713–5719, 2003.
Braden CR, Tauxe RV: Emerging trends in foodborne diseases, *Infect Dis Clin North Am* 27(3):517–533, 2013

Centers for Disease Control and Prevention: *A–Z index for foodborne illness*, 2012. http://www.cdc.gov/foodsafety/diseases/. 2012 [accessed August 11, 2016].
Centers for Disease Control and Prevention: *CDC Estimates of Foodborne Illness in the United States*, 2012. Available at: http://www.cdc.gov/foodborneburden/PDFs/FACTSHEET_A_FINDINGS.pdf. 2012 [accessed August 11, 2016].
Centers for Disease Control and Prevention. The National Institute for Occupational Safety and Health (NIOSH) Emergency Response Safety and Health Database; Category Index: Biotoxins, http://www.cdc.gov/niosh/ershdb/emergencyresponsecard_29750019.html. August 11, 2016.
Centers for Disease Control and Prevention: Tetrodotoxin Poisoning Associated with Eating Puffer Fish Transported from Japan — California, 1996, *Morb Mortal Wkly Rep* 45(19), 1996.
Gamarra RM. Food poisoning- Clinical presentation. Drugs and Diseases, Medscape. updated June 26, 2015, http://emedicine.medscape.com/article/175569-clinical#b5. [Accessed August 11, 2016].
Hajmeer MN, Fung DYC: Other bacteria. In Riemann H, Cliver DO, editors: *Foodborne Infections and Intoxications*, 3rd ed, New York, 2006, Academic Press, pp 341–363.
Hale TL, Keusch GT: Shigella, 1996: In Baron S, editor: *Medical Microbiology*, 4th ed, Galveston, 1996, TX: University of Texas Medical Branch at Galveston. PMID: 21413252 (PubMed). Available at: http://www.ncbi.nlm.nih.gov/books/NBK7627 (accessed August 11, 2016).
Hedberg CW, Osterholm MT: Outbreaks of food-borne and waterborne viral gastroenteritis, *Clin Microbio Rev* 6:199–210, 1993.
Janda JM, Abbott SL: The genus Aeromonas: Taxonomy, pathogenicity, and infection, *Clin Microbiol Rev* 23:35–73, 2010.
Juranek DD: Cryptosporidiosis: Sources of infection and guidelines for prevention, *Clin Infect Dis* 21:S57–61, 1995.
Ministry of Health, Singapore, National Environment Agency, Agri-food & Veterinary Authority of Singapore 24 July 2015. Update on Investigation into Group B Streptococcus Cases, https://www.moh.gov.sg/content/moh_web/home/pressRoom/pressRoomItemRelease/2015/update-on-investigation-into-group-b-streptococcus-cases.html. [Accessed August 11, 2016].
Nataro JP, Kaper JB: Diarrheagenic Escherichia coli, *Clin Microbiol Rev* 11:142–201, 1998.
Niyogi SK: Shigellosis, *J Microbiol* 43:133–143, 2005.
Ortega YR, Sanchez R: Update on Cyclospora cayetanensis, a food-borne and waterborne parasite, *Clin Microbiol Rev* 23:218–234, 2010.
Parashar UD, Bresee JS, Gentsch JR, Glass RI: Synopsis: Rotavirus, *Emerg Infect Dis* 4:561–570, 1998.
Sodha SV, Griffin PM, Hughes JM: Foodborne disease. In Mandell GL, Bennett JE, Dolin R, editors: *Principles and Practice of Infectious Diseases*, 7th ed, Philadelphia, 2009, Churchill Livingstone, pp 1413–1427.
University of Maryland: *Chemical Ecology: Tetrodotoxin- Mode of action*, 2001. http://www.life.umd.edu/grad/mlfsc/zctsim/ionchannel.html.
Wang D-Z: Neurotoxins from Marine Dinoflagellates: A Brief Review, *Marine Drugs* 6(2):349–371, 2008, https://doi.org/10.3390/md20080016.
Yamaguchi T, Kawahara R, et al: Foodborne outbreak of group G streptococcal pharyngitis in a school dormitory in Osaka, Japan, *J Clin Microbiol* 56(5):e01884–17, 2018. https://doi.org/10.1128/JCM.01884-17.

GIARDIASIS

Method of
Rodney D. Adam, MD

CURRENT DIAGNOSIS

- Giardiasis is the most common intestinal protozoan infection worldwide.
- Most cases result from exposure to contaminated drinking or recreational water.
- The clinical manifestations range from asymptomatic to chronic diarrhea with malabsorption and weight loss.
- The diagnosis can be established by stool microscopy or by immunoassays of fecal specimens.
- Occasionally, the trophozoites can be found in duodenal specimens when fecal assays are negative.
- Serologic testing plays no role in the diagnosis.
- Irritable bowel symptoms are very common after successful treatment of giardiasis.

Giardia lamblia is the most common parasitic cause of diarrhea. It is found globally with manifestations that range from asymptomatic to chronic diarrhea with weight loss and malnutrition. Infection occurs when cysts are ingested, most commonly from contaminated water or more direct fecal oral transmission. Less commonly, infections are acquired from food or from zoonotic sources. The cysts excyst in the small intestine and replicate as trophozoites, which cause the disease associated with the organism. The diagnosis is made by the microscopic detection of cysts or trophozoites from fecal samples or by immunoassays of fecal samples. The treatment of choice for symptomatic patients is tinidazole (Tindamax) or metronidazole (Flagyl),[1] while treatment of asymptomatic people depends on the circumstances. Irritable bowel syndrome is common after symptomatic infection, so patients with persistent symptoms should only be treated when persistent infection is documented.

Background

Giardia lamblia (syn. *Giardia intestinalis, Giardia duodenalis*) was initially described by Leeuwenhoek in the 17th century while doing a microscopic examination of his own diarrheal feces. However, *G. lamblia* was not widely accepted as a human pathogen until the 1960s, when a number of outbreaks were reported in travelers to endemic areas. The presumed source of infection in these cases was contaminated drinking water. Subsequently, *Giardia* has become the most commonly identified parasitic cause of diarrhea, and, along with *Cryptosporidium* species, is among the most commonly identified parasitic causes of water-borne diarrheal disease.

Organism

Giardia species are members of the diplomonad (two bodies) group of flagellated protozoans. The life cycle consists of the environmentally resistant cyst, which infects its host on ingestion. It is oval in shape, is about 8 μm × 12 μm in size and contains four nuclei. It excysts into pear-shaped trophozoites in the proximal small intestine that are about 10 to 12 μm by 5 × 7 μm in size. Two symmetrically placed nuclei are in the body of the trophozoites and four pairs of flagella aid with motility. A ventral concave disk uses primarily mechanical means to attach to the intestinal wall of the host. While still in the small intestine, some of the trophozoites then encyst into the cyst form, which is passed in the feces to continue the cycle of infection. The *Giardia* species are all parasitic and were initially assigned to species on the basis of host of origin. However, in 1952, they were divided into three species (*Giardia agilis*,

[1]Not FDA approved for this indication.

amphibians; *Giardia muris*, rodents; *G. duodenalis* [*G. lamblia*], mammals and birds) that could easily be distinguished on the basis of morphologic appearance of the trophozoites. Subsequently, the *G. lamblia* morphologic group has been divided into additional species based on differences that can be seen at the ultrastructural or molecular level. Of the organisms that remain assigned to *G. lamblia*, all are found in mammals but are divided into eight genotypes or assemblages (A through H) on the basis of molecular differences with varying host specificities. Only genotypes A and B have been found in humans. It is likely that at least some of these eight genotypes will eventually be assigned to separate species.

Epidemiology

Giardiasis is the most commonly diagnosed human protozoan infection and is one of the most commonly identified forms of gastroenteritis. Most cases occur from ingestion of contaminated water or by human-to-human transmission through the fecal–oral route. Thus the epidemiology of human infections can be understood by examining these mechanisms of transmission. In the United States most cases are sporadic and occur more often in the summer, probably reflecting infection from recreational water exposure. Infections were more commonly reported in children from ages 1 to 9 years, especially those younger than 4 years of age. In general, the incidence is higher in the northern states, perhaps because cysts survive longer in cool, moist environments.

Direct human-to-human transmission by the fecal oral route also occurs, leading to the higher prevalence found in children in daycare centers. The occasional reports of food-borne transmission most likely occurred because of food being contaminated by infected food handlers.

The greater incidence in children could reflect an increased use of recreational water facilities, daycare exposure, or increased susceptibility to symptomatic disease. The epidemiology of giardiasis in the United States is similar to that found in other developed countries located in temperate regions. However, in developing regions with inadequate availability of purified water, the epidemiology is very different. For example, in a shantytown near Lima, Peru, children were almost universally infected by the age of 2 years, and when treated, they were rapidly reinfected, but there were no symptoms that could clearly be correlated with their infections. Perhaps an outbreak at a ski resort town in the United States can explain these different epidemiologic patterns. In this water-borne outbreak, tourists were disproportionately affected despite drinking from the same water source as the local residents. The conclusion was that the local residents had repeatedly been exposed to water contaminated by *Giardia* cysts and were less susceptible to symptomatic disease.

The degree of zoonotic transmission of giardiasis remains controversial. Human acquisition of infection from dogs or cats has not been well documented, and usually the *Giardia* genotypes found in cats or dogs are distinct from those found in humans (A and B), even in regions where both are endemic. However, genotypes A and B have sometimes been identified in dogs or other animals, so the question is not totally resolved. On the other hand, beavers have been implicated as a source of contaminated water leading to human infections.

Risk Factors

People with hypogammaglobulinemia, and possibly those with IgA deficiency, are at increased risk for prolonged giardiasis. In animal models, deficiency in cell-mediated immunity (CMI) has been associated with increased risk, but in humans the increased risk has not been associated with defects in CMI.

Pathogenesis

Infection is initiated by the ingestion of as few as 10 cysts. After passage through the acidic environment of the stomach, each cyst excysts into two trophozoites in the proximal small intestine. However, gastric acidity is not required, and people with achlorhydria or who are treated with suppressors of gastric acid remain vulnerable to giardiasis. The trophozoites replicate in the proximal small intestine, where they attach to the intestinal mucosa by their ventral disks. The attachment appears to occur by mechanical means facilitated by the suction generated by the ventral disk and the four pairs of flagella as they provide motility. Although the trophozoites attach to the intestinal wall and leave imprints after separating from the wall, there is no well-documented evidence of invasion, either of the intestinal wall or at extraintestinal sites. Toxins have not been identified as causes of diarrhea. However, cysteine proteases, which are also involved in encystation, may be important contributors to the symptoms. The host parasite interaction leads to enterocyte apoptosis and epithelial barrier disruption. The host immune response is mediated through a TH17 response that includes IgA production. An inadequate immune response results in persistence of organisms and an excessive response may be responsibility for the prolonged diarrhea and malabsorption that is commonly found in symptomatic people. Irritable bowel syndrome as well as chronic fatigue are common after giardiasis with a rate over 30% in a large Norwegian outbreak in 2004. The trophozoites are coated with a cysteine-rich protein encoded by one of a family of related genes, and expression can be switched from one to another, perhaps contributing to the chronicity of the infection.

Prevention

The strategies for prevention should be determined by the most prevalent risk factors in specific situations. For travelers to endemic regions, the major risk is from the ingestion of contaminated water. Therefore drinking water should be purified by boiling for 1 minute or by filtration through a pore size of <1 μm. Halogenization with iodine or chlorine requires a prolonged contact time (hours) to inactivate cysts and is not recommended. In daycare centers and for food handlers, the best preventive measure is effective hand washing. In addition, children or workers who are infected should be treated.

Clinical Features

Most people with giardiasis are symptom-free, but the percentages range from rates of diarrhea no higher than background among children in some highly endemic regions to attack rates of nearly 100% in visitors to endemic regions. Symptomatic patients typically present for evaluation only after several days or even weeks of illness because of the subacute onset. The symptoms of giardiasis typically develop after an incubation period of 1 to 2 weeks and consist of diarrhea that is characterized by loose, foul-smelling stools and abdominal discomfort described as cramping or bloating (Table 1). Fatigue is very common, but fever is unusual and, when present, is mild and occurs only within the first few days. Malabsorption and weight loss are often present. The majority of cases resolve within several weeks, but occasionally the symptoms will last for months in the absence of treatment. The prolonged symptoms are often due to postinfectious irritable bowel syndrome and/or chronic fatigue, especially if not accompanied by weight loss. Relapse is relatively uncommon after effective treatment.

Diagnosis

The gold standard of diagnosis has been the microscopic evaluation of three separate fecal samples, including concentrated specimens for cysts or, less commonly, trophozoites. The identification of trophozoites is typically associated with symptomatic infection, but cysts may be found in symptom-free persons. Because of the challenges in obtaining three fecal specimens

TABLE 1	Symptoms of Giardiasis*
SYMPTOM	**AVERAGE (%)**
Diarrhea	95
Abdominal cramps	70
Weakness or malaise	70
Nausea	60
Weight loss	50
Anorexia (decreased appetite)	50
Abdominal distention (bloating/distension)	50
Flatulence	50
Vomiting	30
Fever	20

From Adam RD. Giardiasis. *Hunter's Tropical Medicine and Emerging Infectious Diseases,* Eds: Magill AJ, Ryan ET, Hill DR, Solomon T. Elsevier, 2019.
*The table includes the approximate frequency of the signs and symptoms reported in six studies of symptomatic giardiasis, but it is important to note that there is substantial variability of symptoms among studies.

and the interobserver variability in skill at identifying *Giardia* cysts, antigen detection tests have come into widespread use. The enzyme immunoassays are more commonly used and have high degrees of sensitivity and specificity. A direct fluorescent assay is slightly more sensitive than the enzyme immunoassays and can also detect *Cryptosporidium* species, but it requires the availability of fluorescent microscopy. Polymerase chain reaction (PCR) tests have also been described and are more sensitive but more expensive and not widely available. Some patients have negative workups of stool samples, but *Giardia* trophozoites can be detected in duodenal contents with the string test. The patient swallows a capsule on a string, which is left in situ for 4 hours to overnight. The string is then removed and examined microscopically for trophozoites. Alternatively, endoscopy with sampling of duodenal contents and duodenal biopsy can be used. Endoscopy has the added advantage of being able to detect other possible diagnoses, such as celiac disease or tropical sprue.

Differential Diagnosis

The diagnosis of giardiasis should be suspected in patients presenting with prolonged (>5–7 days) diarrhea without blood in the stools and no fever. In patients presenting relatively early in the course of illness, the major considerations in the differential diagnosis are other infectious etiologies of diarrhea, particularly *Campylobacter jejuni, Salmonella, Cryptosporidium,* and *Cyclospora cayetanensis.* Thus patients presenting with compatible symptoms should have stool samples submitted for culture and for microscopic examination for ova and parasites (O and P). Watery diarrhea is uncommon, and bloody stools are not seen with giardiasis; thus these findings should prompt the search for other etiologies.

For patients presenting with more prolonged symptoms, a number of noninfectious illnesses should be added to the differential diagnosis. Irritable bowel syndrome and lactose intolerance are among the more common etiologies and should be considered in patients presenting with diarrhea but no weight loss. Gluten enteropathy, tropical sprue, and, rarely, Whipple's disease are among the noninfectious etiologies of diarrhea accompanied by weight loss.

Treatment

Patients with symptomatic giardiasis should be treated. The criteria for treatment of patients with asymptomatic giardiasis are not

	DOSE				
DRUG	**ADULT**	**PEDIATRIC***	**FREQUENCY**	**DURATION**	**EFFICACY (%)**
Metronidazole[1] (Flagyl)	250 mg	5 mg/kg	tid	5–7 days	90–100
Tinidazole (Tindamax)	2 g	50 mg/kg	Single dose	Single dose	90–100
Quinacrine[2] (Atabrine)	100 mg	2 mg/kg	tid	5–7 days	80–100
Furazolidone[2] (Furoxone)	100 mg	1.5 mg/kg	qid	10 days	80–94
Paromomycin[1] (Humatin)	500 mg	8–10 mg/kg	tid	10 days	55–90
Albendazole[1] (Albenza)	400 mg qd	15 mg/kg	Daily	5 days	90–100
Nitazoxanide (Alinia)	500 mg bid	7.5 mg/kg	bid	3 days	70–80

*The adult dose is the maximum pediatric dose.
[1]Not FDA approved for this indication.
[2]Not available in the United States.

well defined, but in general, patients in regions with low prevalence or linked with outbreaks should be treated. On the other hand, in settings where the prevalence is high and recurrence rates are high, there is probably no value to treating asymptomatic infection.

The most commonly used agents for treatment of giardiasis are the nitroimidazoles. Metronidazole (Flagyl),[1] tinidazole (Tindamax), and secnidazole (Solosec)[1] are available in the United States, while orinidazole (Tiberal)[2] is available in other countries (Table 2). These agents are completely absorbed from the gastrointestinal tract and are inactivated primarily by hepatic metabolism. Metronidazole has been available in the United States for decades and has generally been considered the drug of choice for treatment of giardiasis in most situations. More recently, tinidazole has become available and is the only agent available in the United States with a high degree of efficacy when given as a single dose. A meta-analysis of 60 randomized clinical trials for treatment of giardiasis concluded that tinidazole was more effective than metronidazole or albendazole. Metronidazole is mutagenic in bacterial assays and showed some carcinogenic activity in an animal model. However, carcinogenicity in humans has not been documented. Serious adverse reactions to the nitroimidazoles are rare, but nausea and a metallic taste are common and may decrease the compliance of patients with metronidazole. The problem with noncompliance can be addressed by the use of tinidazole or the other agents that can be given as a single dose.

Albendazole (Albenza)[1] is a tubulin inhibitor that was introduced as a broad-spectrum antihelminthic, but it also has good activity against *Giardia* trophozoites. It is generally well tolerated and in areas with endemic helminth infections has the added advantage of antihelminthic activity.

The first trimester of pregnancy poses a special problem because none of the agents have been adequately studied or approved for use during this time. Paromomycin (Humatin)[1] is a nonabsorbed aminoglycoside and is expected to be safe during pregnancy. Therefore it is usually the preferred choice in that setting; however, it is somewhat less effective than other agents. Specialty consultation should be considered for treatment of patients in their first trimester. Metronidazole is used extensively during the second and third trimesters for other indications; thus it can be considered the drug of choice for those patients.[1] Albendazole is known to be teratogenic and should be avoided during pregnancy.

[1]Not FDA approved for this indication.
[2]Not available in the United States.

Nitazoxanide (Alinia) has been approved in the United States for treatment of giardiasis (and cryptosporidiosis) and is very well tolerated. However, the somewhat lower efficacy compared with nitroimidazoles and albendazole, along with the requirement for twice daily dosing, limits its role.

Treatment failures are not uncommon but may or may not be due to true drug resistance because in vitro cultures are not routinely performed, and in vitro testing is not standardized. When treatment failure occurs, the patient may respond to the same or an alternative drug. Treatment-refractory cases have been treated successfully with a combination of metronidazole[1] plus quinacrine[2] or albendazole.[1] The most common reason for persistence of symptoms after treatment is due to postgiardiasis irritable bowel syndrome, which can occur in over 30% of patients. Thus it is important to reevaluate stool specimens from patients with symptoms that persist after therapy.

Diet
Lactose intolerance is quite common while patients have giardiasis and potentially for months thereafter, so lactose ingestion should be moderated or eliminated as needed.

[1]Not FDA approved for this indication.

References

Adam RD. *Giardia duodenalis;* Biology and Pathogenesis, *Clinical Microbiology Reviews,* 2021.

Coffey CM, Collier SA, Gleason ME, Yoder JS, Kirk MD, Richardson AM, Fullerton KE, Benedict KM: Evolving epidemiology of reported giardiasis cases in the United States, 1995–2016, *Clinical Infectious Diseases* 72:764–770, 2020.

Cooper MA, Sterling CR, Gilman RH, Cama V, Ortega Y, Adam RD: Molecular analysis of household transmission of *Giardia lamblia* in a region of high endemicity in Peru, *J Inf Dis* 202:1713–1721, 2010.

Hanevik K, Dizdar V, Langeland N, Hausken T: Development of functional gastrointestinal disorders after giardia lamblia infection, *BMC Gastroenterology* 9:27, 2009.

Lengerich EJ, Addiss DG, Juranek DD: Severe giardiasis in the United States, *Clin Infect Dis* 18:760–763, 1994.

Morrison HG, McArthur AG, Gillin FD, Aley SB, Adam RD, Olsen GJ, Best AA, Cande WZ, Chen F, Cipriano MJ, et al: Genomic minimalism in the early diverging intestinal parasite, *Giardia lamblia Science* 317:1921–1926, 2007.

Ordonez-Mena JM, McCarthy ND, Fanshawe TR: Comparative efficacy of drugs for treating giardiasis: a systematic update of the literature and network meta-analysis of randomized clinical trials, *Journal of Antimicrobial Chemotherapy* 73:596–606, 2018.

Singer SM, Fink MY, Angelova VV: Recent insights into innate and adaptive immune responses to *Giardia, Advances in Parasitology* 106:171–208, 2019.

HUMAN IMMUNODEFICIENCY VIRUS: TREATMENT AND PREVENTION

Method of
Allison K. Cormier, MD; Tyler K. Liebenstein, PharmD; and Ryan P. Westergaard, MD, PhD, MPH

CURRENT DIAGNOSIS

- National guidelines recommend universal screening for human immunodeficiency virus (HIV) infection for all adult and adolescent patients in all healthcare settings after notification that testing will be done, unless the patient specifically declines testing (opt-out testing). Patients with behavioral risk factors, sexually transmitted diseases, or tuberculosis should be screened annually.
- Revised HIV testing algorithms reflect the increased sensitivity of newer diagnostic assays during early infection, such as fourth-generation HIV-1/2 antigen/antibody combination immunoassays.
- Acute HIV infection is recognized as a variable syndrome including fever, pharyngitis, rash, and arthralgias. As many as half of patients may be asymptomatic during seroconversion and early infection.

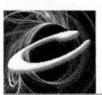

CURRENT THERAPY

- Combination antiretroviral therapy (ART) should be offered to all patients with HIV infection, regardless of CD4+ cell count.
- Initial ART regimens preferred for most patients include a combination of two nucleoside analogue reverse transcriptase inhibitors (NRTIs) and an integrase strand transfer inhibitor (INSTI), which are often co-formulated into single-tablet preparations that can be administered once daily.
- While ART decisions are often made by providers with specialized training, all providers who care for people living with HIV should be aware of the risk of antiretroviral drug interactions, particularly interactions involving the pharmacokinetic enhancing agents ritonavir (Norvir) and cobicistat (Tybost).
- Since 2014, co-formulated emtricitabine-tenofovir disoproxil fumarate (Truvada) has been approved for daily oral administration for preexposure prophylaxis (PrEP) as an HIV prevention strategy for people at elevated risk of HIV transmission. In 2019, emtricitabine-tenofovir alafenamide (Descovy) was also approved for PrEP in men who have sex with men (MSM) and transgender women.

Introduction

Remarkable advances in therapeutics, leading to the development of ART, have transformed HIV infection from an almost universally fatal illness to a chronic disease that can be managed over decades with an enlarging repertoire of treatment options. Further developments in ART have also provided opportunities for preventing HIV infection in high-risk individuals. This chapter provides an overview of the current understanding of HIV pathogenesis, epidemiology, and reviews guidelines for the initial evaluation and long-term management of HIV infection in adult patients.

Pathophysiology

HIV is an enveloped, single-stranded RNA virus belonging to the family Retroviridae. It was recognized as the causative agent of AIDS within 3 years after the initial description of the syndrome in 1981, and ongoing characterization of its molecular biology has

provided the identification of multiple targets for drug development. Two types of human immunodeficiency viruses exist: HIV-1 and HIV-2. HIV-1 has worldwide distribution, accounts for most infections outside western Africa, and is the focus of this chapter.

HIV-2 infection is endemic in West Africa and has limited spread outside this area. It should be considered in infections in patients of West African origin or those who have had sexual contact or shared needles with people of West African origin. HIV-2 generally has a longer asymptomatic stage, lower plasma HIV-2 viral loads, and overall lower mortality rate. Approximately 25% to 30% of patients with HIV-2 who do not receive ART will have HIV-2 RNA levels below the rate of detection and some will also have clinical progression and CD4 cell count decline. HIV-2 can progress to AIDS over time. HIV-1 and HIV-2 coinfection may occur and should be a consideration in patients from high prevalence HIV-2 areas. Patients diagnosed with HIV-2 infection should be managed by an HIV specialist.

Genetic heterogeneity of HIV-1 is reflected in categorization of the virus into three groups (M, O, and N) and several subtypes (B, C, D, AE, and CRF01_AE), some of which have overlapping geographic distribution around the world. Subtype C is prevalent in southern and eastern Africa, China, India, South Asia, and Brazil and accounts for 50% of HIV subtypes, whereas subtype B, the most common subtype in the United States, accounts for 12%.

The HIV viral genome is encoded in single-stranded RNA, packaged in core protein structures, and surrounded by a lipid bilayer envelope that is derived from the cell membrane of the host cell as the virus buds from the cell surface after replication. This outer viral membrane contains HIV-specific glycoproteins, including gp120 and gp41, which facilitate attachment and entry into host cells through interaction with the cell surface receptor, CD4, and coreceptors CCR5 and CXCR4. CD4+ helper T lymphocytes are the predominant host cell affected by HIV; this molecular tropism explains the immune system destruction manifested in chronic HIV infection and provides the rationale for clinical staging of HIV infection using CD4+ T-cell counts. After host cell entry, the key enzyme responsible for viral replication is reverse transcriptase, an RNA-dependent DNA polymerase that is packaged within the virion core. This enzyme facilitates conversion of the HIV genome into a double-stranded DNA intermediate molecule. The second key enzymatic step is integration of this intermediate nucleic acid product into the host genome, which is facilitated by the viral protein integrase. Protein synthesis with packaging of new viral particles ensues, utilizing an HIV-specific protease. The integrase inhibitor class of drugs acts by blocking this step of integration.

Natural History

Within 1 to 4 weeks after the initial HIV infection, seroconversion may be accompanied by a nonspecific, self-limited illness, often referred to as acute retroviral syndrome. This illness has variable manifestations but may include fever, malaise, myalgias, arthralgias, generalized lymphadenopathy, pharyngitis, and rash. The associated rash may be maculopapular, urticarial, or roseola-like. An illness resembling acute infectious mononucleosis syndrome, similar to that caused by Epstein-Barr virus or cytomegalovirus (CMV), and aseptic meningitis has been described. Diagnosis of acute HIV infection requires a high index of suspicion, which does not commonly occur unless the patient reports a recent history of a high-risk exposure.

During the acute phase of infection, high levels of viremia are present (often exceeding 10 million copies/mL) as HIV becomes widely disseminated throughout the body and the host defenses begin to counteract circulating virus through cell-mediated and humoral (antibody-mediated) immune mechanisms. Antibodies against HIV usually become detectable 2 to 4 months after infection. The initial, high-level viremia plateaus and then begins a decline as neutralizing antibodies are established. Ongoing replication is partially controlled by the immune response, resulting in a steady-state level of viremia. This virologic level differs from patient to patient and is one of the determinants of the rate of disease progression. A small number of HIV-infected persons are able to control viral replication to levels below the limit of detection, and they tend to have a more benign course of disease. In these patients, designated "elite suppressors" by researchers, HIV replication continues to occur, and HIV RNA can be isolated from latently infected cells by means of specialized laboratory techniques.

After the establishment of HIV infection and seroconversion, a period of asymptomatic infection ensues, during which patients are free of evidence of immune suppression and opportunistic infections (OIs) are uncommon. This phase of clinical latency lasts a median of 8 to 10 years, based on observational studies from the pre-ART era. Ongoing viral replication leads to gradual decline in CD4 counts.

The symptomatic stage of HIV infection can begin at any time after infection, but clinical manifestations become more likely as the CD4 count falls farther below the normal range of 800 to 1200 cells/mm^3. For example, *Pneumocystis jirovecii* (formerly *Pneumocystis carinii*) pneumonia (PJP) usually occurs in patients with a CD4 count of less than 200 cells/mm^3 or a percentage less than 10%. CMV retinitis occurs almost exclusively in patients with a CD4 count of less than 50 cells/mm^3 or a percentage less than 5%. Mucocutaneous candidiasis (oral thrush), herpes zoster, HIV-associated nephropathy, peripheral neuropathy, tuberculosis, and community-acquired bacterial pneumonia occur with increased frequency at earlier stages of infection and are less reliably predicted by CD4+ cell measurement.

Diagnosis

The current recommended testing algorithm incorporates fourth-generation antigen/antibody combination HIV-1/2 immunoassay with a confirmatory HIV-1/HIV-2 antibody differentiation immunoassay. The fourth-generation assay detects both HIV-1 and HIV-2 antibodies and HIV p24 antigen. It has increased sensitivity due to its ability to diagnose acute/early infection, because HIV p24 antigen is detected before seroconversion has occurred. If the fourth-generation combination assay is positive, the HIV-1 and HIV-2 antibody differentiation immunoassay both confirms the positive result and determines if the patient is infected with HIV-1 or HIV-2. If the fourth-generation assay is positive but the confirmatory antibody differentiation immunoassay is indeterminate or negative, a plasma HIV RNA level should be obtained.

In facilities where fourth-generation testing is not available, a two-step approach is utilized via enzyme-linked immunosorbent assay (ELISA) to detect HIV antibodies with subsequent confirmation using HIV-1/HIV-2 differentiation assay. ELISA detects HIV IgM and IgG antibodies as early as 3 weeks after virus exposure. This modality has excellent sensitivity and specificity for diagnosing chronic HIV infection; however, diagnosis may be missed in patients with early HIV infection who have not yet had seroconversion. If concern exists for acute/early HIV infection, plasma HIV RNA can be assessed.

False-negative and false-positive tests occur rarely. False-negative screening tests can occur with ELISA-only testing during acute/early HIV infection. This occurs less often using the fourth-generation antigen/antibody assay, which is more sensitive in detecting early HIV infection by identifying the p24 antigen. False-positive screening test results can occur for several non-HIV reasons, including cross-reaction from alloantibodies in pregnant females, autoantibodies from autoimmune diseases or malignancy, and the influenza vaccine. False-positive results in both screening and confirmatory testing are particularly uncommon.

Indeterminate test results occur when the initial screening test is positive and subsequent confirmatory testing is indeterminate or negative. In the event of a positive fourth-generation antigen/antibody test and negative HIV differentiation assay, the detection of p24 antigen would yield a positive result but the differentiation assay would be negative, as no antibody is present. In all patients with indeterminate test results, a plasma HIV RNA should be obtained, as viremia is present prior to antibody seroconversion. A detectable plasma HIV RNA level is diagnostic of HIV infection. If HIV RNA is negative, the patient should be reassured that HIV infection is unlikely. A repeat screening test can be repeated after 3 months for further reassurance. If the patient had a recent high-risk exposure, another plasma HIV RNA can be performed in 1 to 2 weeks. All patients with indeterminate testing should be counseled to avoid activities with potential to transmit HIV to others until evaluation is completed.

Consent

HIV screening should be voluntary and pursued only after discussion with the patient regarding testing. In the United States, written consent is no longer obligatory in any state, but individual states may have policies regarding documentation of the consent process and related counseling. Confidentiality, access to post-testing counseling, and services to support prompt linkage to HIV care for patients with positive results are important resources in HIV testing settings.

Screening

Early detection of HIV infection and subsequent initiation of ART can dramatically reduce morbidity and mortality of affected patients. A relatively normal life span is possible in patients in the United States who are diagnosed early in their infection and successfully treated. Such early treatment also can reduce the transmission of HIV. One-time testing is recommended for patients without high-risk factors for HIV exposure in patients 13 to 75 years of age. Pregnant women should be screened for HIV early in their pregnancy, even if they have been screened during prior pregnancies.

In patients with elevated risk of HIV exposure, more frequent testing is recommended. Men who have sex with other men, along with patients who have sex with sexual partners who have HIV or with persons of unknown serostatus may benefit from HIV screening at least every 6 months. This is especially important in patients aged 13 to 24 years, because this demographic group has experienced the highest rate of new infections in recent years. Other high-risk groups include patients who use injection drugs and sex workers.

Approach to the Patient with HIV Infection

HIV patient care is an ever-changing field, with routinely updated professional guidelines and new medications. The quality of care received by patients with HIV has been shown to correlate with the healthcare provider's experience and comfort in treating these patients. Referral to an HIV specialist is recommended for new HIV diagnoses, complications of HIV or antiretroviral drugs, and for treatment failure.

All patients with HIV should have a comprehensive history, physical examination, and laboratory evaluation when establishing care. This baseline evaluation can help establish and define the patient's goals and plan of care. In a patient who has already established treatment with ART and presents for initial evaluation with a new healthcare provider, it is important to document the complete antiretroviral history and drug resistance testing results, if available.

Patients with HIV are often faced with many medical, psychiatric, and social issues. These are best addressed through a patient-centered, multidisciplinary approach. In patients with a new diagnosis of HIV, it is important to counsel them regarding HIV infection and assess their understanding of the disease and its transmission. They should also be assessed for readiness to initiate ART, potential high-risk behaviors, mental illness, substance abuse, social support, medical comorbidities, and/or economic factors, because these are potential issues that may impair adherence to ART.

Antiretroviral Therapy

There are currently six major classes of antiretroviral medications used to treat patients with HIV. Although dozens of such medications are available, only a small selection of agents is currently preferred as initial treatment regimens (Table 1). For most patients, ART includes a combination of two NRTIs plus a third medication from a different class, although two-drug regimens are preferred for some patients.

When to Initiate Antiretroviral Therapy

Combination ART first became available in the mid-1990s and provided life-saving therapy for millions of patients suffering from HIV and AIDS. While the early ART regimens were effective

GENERIC NAME (TRADE NAME) AND RECOMMENDED ADULT DOSING	SINGLE TABLET REGIMEN?	IMPORTANT POINTS
INSTI + 2 NRTIs		
Bictegravir/emtricitabine/tenofovir alafenamide (Biktarvy) 50/200/25 mg—1 tablet by mouth once daily	Yes	Bictegravir has been shown to raise serum creatinine from baseline by a median 0.1 mg/dL due to inhibition of creatinine secretion, not a true reduction in GFR
Dolutegravir/abacavir/lamivudine (Triumeq) 50/600/300 mg—1 tablet by mouth once daily	Yes	Dolutegravir has been shown to raise serum creatinine from baseline by a mean of 0.15 mg/dL due to inhibition of creatinine secretion, not a true reduction in GFR Dolutegravir has a drug interaction with metformin (maximum daily metformin dose is 1000 mg) Must be confirmed HLA-B*5701 negative before starting to avoid abacavir hypersensitivity reaction
Dolutegravir (Tivicay) 50 mg—1 tablet by mouth once daily **PLUS** Tenofovir alafenamide/emtricitabine (Descovy) 25/200 mg—1 tablet by mouth once daily OR Tenofovir disoproxil fumarate/emtricitabine (Truvada) 300/200 mg—1 tablet by mouth once daily	No	Dolutegravir has been shown to raise serum creatinine from baseline by a mean of 0.15 mg/dL due to inhibition of creatinine secretion, not a true reduction in GFR Dolutegravir has a drug interaction with metformin (maximum daily metformin dose is 1000 mg) Descovy generally preferred over Truvada due to fewer bone and kidney toxicities
Raltegravir (Isentress HD) 600 mg—2 tablets by mouth once daily OR Raltegravir (Isentress) 400 mg—1 tablet by mouth twice daily **PLUS** Tenofovir alafenamide/emtricitabine (Descovy) 25/200 mg—1 tablet by mouth once daily OR Tenofovir disoproxil fumarate/emtricitabine (Truvada) 300/200 mg—1 tablet by mouth once daily	No	Isentress HD generally preferred over Isentress due to once daily dosing Descovy generally preferred over Truvada due to fewer bone and kidney toxicities
INSTI + 1 NRTI		
Dolutegravir/lamivudine (Dovato) 50/300 mg—1 tablet by mouth once daily	Yes	This two-drug regimen should not be used in those with HIV RNA >500,000 copies/mL, HBV coinfection, or in whom ART is to be started before the results of HIV genotypic resistance testing for reverse transcriptase or HBV testing are available Dolutegravir has been shown to raise serum creatinine from baseline by a mean of 0.15 mg/dL due to inhibition of creatinine secretion, not a true reduction in GFR Dolutegravir has a drug interaction with metformin (maximum daily metformin dose is 1000 mg)

*Biktarvy [package insert]. Foster City, CA: Gilead Sciences, Inc.; 2021.
bTivicay [package insert]. Research Triangle Park, NC: ViiV Healthcare; 2020.
ART, Antiretroviral therapy; *GFR,* glomerular filtration rate; *HBV,* hepatitis B virus; *HIV,* human immunodeficiency virus; *HLA,* human leukocyte antigen; *INSTI,* integrase strand transfer inhibitor; *NRTIs,* nucleoside analogue reverse transcriptase inhibitors.
Adapted from: Panel on Antiretroviral Guidelines for Adults and Adolescents. Guidelines for the Use of Antiretroviral Agents in Adults and Adolescents with HIV. Department of Health and Human Services. Available at https://clinicalinfo.hiv.gov/sites/default/files/guidelines/documents/AdultandAdolescentGL.pdf. Section accessed March 9, 2021 [Table 6a].

in helping patients with AIDS recover, they were also associated with many toxicities and side effects. In 2006, the US Department of Health and Human Services, the International AIDS Society–USA, and the British HIV Society recommended CD4 counts of 200 cells/mm³ as the threshold for initiating ART treatment in asymptomatic patients. More recently, the paradigm has shifted toward earlier initiation of ART based on accumulating evidence for the beneficial effects of treatment initiation earlier in the course of infection. Antiretroviral therapies have advanced significantly since their conception, consisting of multiple drug classes, fewer toxicities, less pill burden, and overall improved tolerance. Failure to suppress viral loads on these medications is more likely to be due to therapy nonadherence than medication failure.

HIV patients are now achieving normal life spans, and non-AIDS-defining illnesses are becoming more prominent. Cardiovascular, renal, and hepatic disease complications are lower in patients who started ART at higher CD4 thresholds (>350 cells/mm³). Earlier initiation of ART is also associated with reduced risk of transmission and improved immune restoration.

Current Recommendations for Antiretroviral Therapy

ART should be offered to all patients with HIV infection, regardless of CD4 count. The goal of ART is to prevent morbidity, mortality, and transmission associated with HIV. This is accomplished by maximally inhibiting HIV replication to achieve an undetectable HIV viral load. Based on guidelines from the US Department of Health and Human Services, INSTI-based regimens are currently the first-line recommendation as initial therapy for most patients with HIV based on high rates of virologic suppression and tolerability demonstrated in large clinical trials. Nonnucleoside reverse transcriptase (NNRTI) and protease inhibitor (PI)-based regimens are recommended in certain clinical situations (Table 2). Monotherapy with any antiretroviral drug is not recommended due to increased risk of drug resistance and therapy failure.

TABLE 2	Recommended Initial Regimens in Certain Clinical Situations

GENERIC NAME (TRADE NAME) AND RECOMMENDED ADULT DOSING	SINGLE TABLET REGIMEN?	IMPORTANT POINTS
INSTI + 2 NRTIs		
Elvitegravir/cobicistat/tenofovir alafenamide/emtricitabine (Genvoya) 150/150/10/200 mg—1 tablet by mouth once daily OR Elvitegravir/cobicistat/tenofovir disoproxil fumarate/ emtricitabine (Stribild) 150/150/300/200 mg—1 tablet by mouth once daily	Yes	Genvoya generally preferred over Stribild due to fewer bone and kidney toxicities Drug interactions with other medications are prevalent with both products due to cobicistat, a CYP3A4 inhibitor
NNRTI + 2 NRTIs		
Rilpivirine/tenofovir alafenamide/emtricitabine (Odefsey) 25/25/200 mg—1 tablet by mouth once daily OR Rilpivirine/tenofovir disoproxil fumarate/emtricitabine (Complera) 25/300/200 mg – 1 tablet by mouth once daily	Yes	Rilpivirine should only be used if HIV RNA <100,000 copies/mL and CD4 >200 cells/mm^3 Odefsey generally preferred over Complera due to fewer bone and kidney toxicities PPIs contraindicated with rilpivirine. H2 blockers may be used once daily, but must be spaced 12 h apart from rilpivirine. Should be taken with food
Doravirine/tenofovir disoproxil fumarate/lamivudine (Delstrigo) 100/300/300 mg—1 tablet by mouth once daily OR Doravirine (Pifeltro) 100 mg—1 tablet by mouth once daily PLUS Tenofovir alafenamide/emtricitabine (Descovy) 25/200 mg—1 tablet by mouth once daily	Yes, for Delstrigo	May be taken with or without food Doravirine does not have any restrictions with acid-suppressive medications
Efavirenz/tenofovir disoproxil fumarate/emtricitabine (Atripla) 600/300/200 mg—1 tablet by mouth once daily	Yes	High rates of neuropsychiatric adverse effects (e.g., vivid dreams, depression, suicidal ideation)
PK-enhanced PI + 2 NRTIs		
Darunavir/cobicistat/emtricitabine/tenofovir alafenamide (Symtuza) 800/150/200/10 mg—1 tablet by mouth once daily OR Darunavir/cobicistat (Prezcobix) 800/150 mg—1 tablet by mouth once daily OR Darunavir (Prezista) 800 mg —1 tablet by mouth once daily + Ritonavir (Norvir) 100 mg—1 tablet by mouth once daily PLUS Tenofovir alafenamide/emtricitabine (Descovy) 25/200 mg—1 tablet by mouth once daily OR Tenofovir disoproxil fumarate/emtricitabine (Truvada) 300/200 mg—1 tablet by mouth once daily OR Abacavir/lamivudine (Epzicom) 600/300 mg—1 tablet by mouth once daily	Yes, for Symtuza	Prezcobix generally preferred over the combination of Prezista and Norvir due to single tablet and potentially fewer GI side effects and drug interactions Drug interactions with other medications are prevalent with both cobicistat and ritonavir due to CYP3A4 inhibition. Ritonavir also inhibits and induces several other CYP enzymes. Careful attention should be given to manage drug interactions. Descovy generally preferred over Truvada due to fewer bone and kidney toxicities If using Epzicom, must be confirmed HLA-B*5701 negative before starting to avoid abacavir hypersensitivity reaction
Atazanavir/cobicistat (Evotaz) 300/150 mg—1 tablet by mouth once daily OR Atazanavir (Reyataz) 300 mg—1 tablet by mouth once daily + Ritonavir (Norvir) 100 mg—1 tablet by mouth once daily PLUS Tenofovir alafenamide/emtricitabine (Descovy) 25/200 mg—1 tablet by mouth once daily OR Tenofovir disoproxil fumarate/emtricitabine (Truvada) 300/200mg—1 tablet by mouth once daily	No	Darunavir-containing regimens generally preferred over atazanavir-containing regimens Atazanavir is known to increase serum bilirubin. This generally does not require further workup if patient is asymptomatic Evotaz generally preferred over the combination of Reyataz and Norvir due to single tablet and potentially fewer GI side effects and drug interactions Drug interactions with other medications are prevalent with both cobicistat and ritonavir due to CYP3A4 inhibition. Ritonavir also inhibits and induces several other CYP enzymes. Careful attention should be given to manage drug interactions. Descovy generally preferred over Truvada due to fewer bone and kidney toxicities

CYP3A4, Cytochrome P450 3A4; GI, gastrointestinal; H2, histamine H2 receptor; HIV, human immunodeficiency virus; HLA, human leukocyte antigen; INSTI, Integrase strand transfer inhibitor; NNRTI, non-nucleoside reverse transcriptase inhibitor; NRTI, nucleoside reverse transcriptase inhibitor; PI, protease inhibitor; PPI, proton pump inhibitor.

Adapted from: Panel on Antiretroviral Guidelines for Adults and Adolescents. Guidelines for the Use of Antiretroviral Agents in Adults and Adolescents with HIV. Department of Health and Human Services. Available at https://clinicalinfo.hiv.gov/sites/default/files/guidelines/documents/AdultandAdolescentGL.pdf. Section accessed March 9, 2021 [Table 6a].

Selection of an Antiretroviral Regimen

ART regimens should be individualized based on a regimen's side effect profile, pill burden, potential drug interactions, virologic efficacy, cost, and resistance test results. Before starting ART in any patient with HIV, the following factors must be considered:

- Pretreatment HIV RNA level
- Pretreatment CD4 count
- HIV genotypic drug resistance testing results
- HLA-B*5701 status (if planning to use abacavir-based ART regimen)
- A patient's individual preference
- Anticipated medication adherence

Other factors that are important to consider when choosing an initial regimen include the patient's medical comorbidities (cardiovascular, renal, psychiatric disease), pregnancy or the potential to become pregnant, and coinfections with tuberculosis, hepatitis C virus, and hepatitis B virus (HBV).

The currently recommended ART for most patients includes two NRTIs, abacavir/lamivudine (ABC/3TC [Epzicom]) or either tenofovir alafenamide/emtricitabine (TAF/FTC [Descovy]) or tenofovir disoproxil fumarate/emtricitabine (TDF/FTC [Truvada]), plus an INSTI. INSTI-based regimens are well tolerated, have convenient dosing, and provide excellent virologic suppression. Regimens including NNRTI or PK-enhanced PIs remain effective, but are now only recommended in certain clinical scenarios.

The NRTI combinations of ABC/3TC, TAF/FTC, and TDF/FTC are available as fixed-dose combination tablets. The 3TC and FTC components have few adverse effects. The main differences between these combinations involve ABC, TAF, and TDF. The advantages of TAF and TDF include activity against HBV, and HLA-B*5701 testing is not required prior to use. TDF has some association with lower lipid levels when compared to TAF, but also may cause decline in renal function and reduced bone mineral density. TAF is associated with less bone and kidney toxicity and its use is preferred in patients with underlying bone and kidney disease or those at risk for these conditions. The advantage of ABC is that it has less bone mineral loss and less nephrotoxicity than TDF and does not require dose adjustment in patients with renal insufficiency. Potential drawbacks to ABC include an observed association with cardiovascular events in some studies and a hypersensitivity syndrome, necessitating screening for HLA-B*5701 prior to treatment initiation.

Once the combination NRTI backbone has been chosen, a third drug from another class must be added to the regimen. Current recommendations for most patients favor the INSTI class due to its high efficacy, fewer side effects, and no significant CYP3A4-associated drug interactions.

Darunavir (DRV [Prezista])–based regimens may still be preferred in certain patients with difficulty maintaining medication adherence, and a high genetic barrier to resistance is favored or in a situation when ART should be initiated prior to receipt of resistance test results. Darunavir boosted with ritonavir (Norvir) (DRV/r) has a low rate of transmitted PI resistance, high genetic barrier to resistance, and a low rate of treatment-emergent resistance. Dolutegravir (DTG [Tivicay]) or a Bictegravir-containing regimen (BIC/FTC/TAF [Biktarvy]) is also a consideration for patients in whom it is necessary to initiate ART prior to resistance testing results due to its high barrier of resistance.

NNRTI-based regimens include efavirenz (EFV [Sustiva]), rilpivirine (RPV [Edurant]), or doravirine (DOR [Pifeltro]) and may be appropriate choices in certain patients with good medication adherence. These medications have a low genetic barrier to resistance. EFV has minimal PK interactions with rifamycins, which makes it an excellent option in patients who require treatment for tuberculosis. EFV has a high rate of central nervous system–related side effects, which lowers its overall tolerability for some patients. RPV has fewer side effects than EFV, but its virologic efficacy is reduced in patients with high baseline HIV RNA and low CD4 counts. RPV also requires acid for absorption; it is contraindicated with proton pump inhibitors and must be spaced 12 hours apart from histamine 2 receptor antagonists.

More recently, two large, randomized controlled trials showed that a two-drug regimen of DTG plus lamivudine (DTG/3TC [Dovato]) was noninferior to DTG plus TDF/FTC. This is another potential initial regimen for most people with HIV except for patients with pre-treatment HIV RNA greater than 500,000 copies/mL, who are known to have active HBV coinfection, or who will initiate ART before results of HIV genotype testing for reverse transcriptase or HBV testing are available.

In 2021, the first complete long-acting injectable ARV regimen, cabotegravir and rilpivirine (Cabenuva®), was approved as an option to replace the current ARV regimen in adults with HIV. Once-monthly cabotegravir and rilpivirine intramuscular (IM) injections can be used as an optimization strategy for people with HIV currently on oral ART with documented viral suppression (HIV-1 RNA less than 50 copies per mL) for at least 3 months. Candidates for cabotegravir and rilpivirine long-acting injections should have no baseline resistance to either medication, have no prior virologic failures, should not have hepatitis B virus (HBV) infection (unless also receiving an oral HBV active regimen), should not be pregnant or planning to become pregnant, and should not be receiving medications with significant drug interactions with cabotegravir and rilpivirine. Before initiation of the IM injection, patients should receive oral cabotegravir (Vocabria) and oral rilpivirine (Edurant) for approximately one month as an oral lead-in period to assess tolerance to these drugs. Cabotegravir and rilpivirine injections should be administered by healthcare providers as gluteal IM injections. Administration variances of +/–7 days are allowed. The product is refrigerated and should be brought to room temperature prior to administration. Unopened vials may remain at room temperature for up to 6 hours. Medication drawn into a syringe may remain in the syringe for up to 2 hours.

Monitoring Response to Antiretroviral Therapy

HIV disease progression and response to ART can be monitored via CD4 T lymphocyte (CD4) cell count and HIV RNA (viral load). CD4 count should be measured prior to initiation of ART and provides information regarding the patient's immune function and risk of OI. Recommendations for monitoring viral load and CD4 count are shown in Table 3.

CD4 counts can be highly variable, and significant change is only considered with 30% difference in absolute count or an increase or decrease in CD4 percentage by 3 percentage points. CD4 cell recovery is most rapid in the first 3 months after initiating ART, later followed by more gradual increases. For most patients on ART, adequate response is considered as an increase in CD4 count in the range of 50 to 150 cells/mm^3 during the first year of treatment. Subsequent increases may average 50 to 100 cells/mm^3 per year until a steady-state level is reached. Peripheral blood CD4 cell counts in most HIV patients will continue to increase over a decade as long as viral suppression is maintained. Most individuals will eventually recover CD4 counts within the normal range (>500 cells/mm^3). For approximately 15% to 20% of patients, especially those who initiate ART at very low CD4 counts (<200 cells/mm^3), low CD4 counts may persist, which is associated with increased morbidity and mortality. These patients should be evaluated for reversible causes of CD4 cell lymphopenia, including offending medications, untreated coinfections, and underlying malignancy. In patients with appropriate virologic suppression, the addition of more antiretroviral agents or transitioning to a different ART regimen has not been demonstrated to improve CD4 cell recovery.

CD4 counts should be repeated 3 months after ART initiation to monitor immune reconstitution and can be monitored in many patients at 3- to 6-month intervals for the first 2 years of ART. In virally suppressed patients with consistent CD4 counts between 300 and 500 cells/mm^3 for at least 2 years, CD4 can be checked annually. While ART is recommended for all patients with HIV, patients who remain untreated should have CD4 counts monitored every 3 to 6 months to assess the need for OI prophylaxis.

Viral load functions as a marker for ART response and should be monitored at initiation of therapy and regularly thereafter.

CLINICAL SCENARIO	VIRAL LOAD MONITORING	CD4 COUNT MONITORING
Before initiating ART	At entry into care If ART initiation is deferred, repeat before initiating ART. In patients not initiating ART, repeat testing is optional.	At entry into care If ART is deferred, every 3–6 months
After initiating ART	Preferably within 2–4 weeks (and no later than 8 weeks) after initiation of ART; thereafter, every 4–8 weeks until viral load is suppressed.	3 months after initiation of ART
After modifying ART because of drug toxicities or for regimen simplification in a patient with viral suppression	4–8 weeks after modification of ART to confirm effectiveness of new regimen	Monitor according to prior CD4 count and duration on ART, as outlined below.
After modifying ART because of virologic failure	Preferably within 2–4 weeks (and no later than 8 weeks) after modification; thereafter, every 4–8 weeks until viral load is suppressed. If viral suppression is not possible, repeat viral load every 3 months or more frequently if indicated.	Every 3–6 months
During the first 2 years of ART	Every 3–4 months	Every 3–6 months
After 2 years of ART (VL consistently suppressed, CD4 consistently 300–500 cells/mm^3) After 2 years of ART (VL consistently suppressed, CD4 consistently >500 cells/mm^3)	Can extend to every 6 months for patients with consistent viral suppression for greater than or equal to 2 years.	Every 12 months Optional
While on ART with detectable viremia (VL repeatedly >200 copies/mL)	Every 3 months or more frequently if clinically indicated	Every 3–6 months
Change in clinical status	Every 3 months	Perform CD4 count and repeat as clinically indicated

ART, Antiretroviral therapy.
Adapted from: Panel on Antiretroviral Guidelines for Adults and Adolescents. *Guidelines for the Use of Antiretroviral Agents in Adults and Adolescents Living with HIV.* Department of Health and Human Services. Available at https://clinicalinfo.hiv.gov/sites/default/files/guidelines/documents/AdultandAdolescentGL.pdf. Section accessed March 9, 2021 [Table 4].

Pre-treatment viral load can also provide useful information regarding selection of an initial ART. Commercially available HIV-1 RNA assays do not detect HIV-2 viral load. Decreases in viral load following ART initiation are associated with a reduction in risk of disease progression to AIDS or death. Optimal viral suppression is defined as a viral load persistently below the level of detection. Low-level viremia refers to a patient with confirmed detectable HIV RNA less than 200 copies/mL. This may be detected using real-time polymerase chain reaction (PCR) assays and may be predictive of developing viral rebound. Viral rebound, or virologic failure, is considered to occur when a patient with confirmed virologic suppression has HIV RNA greater than or equal to 1000 copies/mL. If virologic suppression occurs and the patient is found to have a single isolated detectable HIV RNA level with return to virologic suppression in subsequent tests, this is referred to as a virologic blip. This is not usually associated with virologic failure, and does not require a change in ART. Acute illness, stress, and recent immunizations are a few potential causes of virologic blips. A repeat viral load can be rechecked in 3 months to confirm return to appropriate viral suppression.

If a patient has a very high HIV viral load at the time of ART initiation, it may take several weeks for a measurable virologic response to occur. Certain ART regimens may also have slower rates of virologic suppression than others. A patient who has received ART for at least 24 weeks and has not yet had documented virologic suppression should be evaluated for antiretroviral drug resistance.

The use of ART to prevent HIV transmission is called treatment as prevention (TasP), also known as Undetectable = Untransmittable (U = U). Maintaining HIV RNA levels less than 200 copies/mL with ART prevents HIV transmission to sexual partners. Patients who start ART should use another form of prevention with sexual partners for at least the first 6 months of treatment and until an HIV RNA level less than 200 copies/mL has been achieved. Patients who have HIV and who rely on ART for prevention require high ART adherence because transmission is possible during periods of poor compliance or treatment interruption.

Treatment Failure

Patients who are receiving ART and who do not achieve HIV RNA levels below the lower limit of detection or who are shown to have sustained virologic rebound are at risk for developing resistance mutations to their current ART regimen, especially at HIV RNA levels greater than 500 copies/mL. Virologic failure has a strong association with suboptimal medication adherence and drug intolerance/toxicity leading to self-discontinuation of ART.

Some factors that may increase the risk of ART nonadherence include active substance use, neurocognitive impairment, and mental health disorders. Unstable housing and other socioeconomic and psychosocial factors can make ART adherence particularly difficult. The patient's inability to afford the medication may lead to intermittent adherence or nonadherence. Some patients will stop taking ART due to adverse effects of their regimen. Others may not be able to adhere to a high pill burden or frequency of dosing.

Less common causes of treatment failure include existing or newly developed drug resistance. Patients with HIV-2 or HIV-1/HIV-2 coinfection can have innate resistance to certain ART regimens. Others may have adverse drug–drug interactions with other medications, suboptimal virologic potency, or error in their medication prescription.

If a patient is experiencing virologic failure, it is important to determine the cause because there is potential for choosing a subsequent therapy regimen that promotes better adherence. Management of a patient who is experiencing treatment failure is often complex; consultation with an HIV specialist can prove beneficial.

Drug Resistance and Resistance Testing

Two types of resistance assays exist to assess viral strains and direct treatment strategies: genotypic and phenotypic. These assays provide useful information in regard to resistance to NRTIs, NNRTIs, PIs, and INSTIs. In some settings, INSTI resistance tests can be ordered separately. In patients with newly diagnosed HIV infection, resistance testing can guide therapy selection to optimize virologic response. Genotypic assays detect drug resistance mutations by sequencing reverse transcriptase, protease, and integrase genes. Interpreting these test results requires knowledge of the mutations selected by different antivirals and the potential for cross-resistance to other drugs. Clinical trials have shown that consultation with HIV specialists regarding drug resistance interpretation improves virologic outcomes.

Adverse Drug Reactions and Drug-Drug Interactions

Adverse drug reactions to ART are common, especially when first initiating therapy. Generally, reactions such as nausea, fatigue, and headache often resolve within 1 to 2 weeks of starting ART. Severe or persistent adverse drug reactions should prompt consideration of change to a different agent. Each ART drug class has different characteristic adverse drug reactions. Additionally, each individual ART agent carries its own characteristic adverse drug reactions (Table 4). As drug therapies have evolved and new medications discovered, preferred agents have been updated to avoid those that have tended to cause more frequent and severe adverse effects. For example, older agents in the NRTI class (e.g., stavudine [Zerit] and didanosine [Videx]) were commonly associated with hepatic steatosis, lipodystrophy, and insulin resistance. Newer generation NRTIs, which have much lower rates of these serious adverse effects, have largely supplanted the use of these older drugs.

All providers who care for patients who receive ART should be aware of the possibility of antiretroviral drug–drug interactions. The use of the pharmacokinetic enhancing agents ritonavir (Norvir) and cobicistat (Tybost) in many combination ART regimens can pose serious risks to patients who receive other drugs metabolized through the cytochrome P450 pathway, including numerous anti-coagulant drugs and synthetic glucocorticoids. When prescribing or altering one or more drugs in an ART regimen, the potential for drug interactions must be explored. It is critical to carefully review the patient's other medications for potential interactions. If multiple drugs with similar or conflicting metabolic pathways are prescribed, healthcare providers should carefully monitor for appropriate therapeutic efficacy and concentration-related toxicities.

Viral Hepatitis Coinfection

Approximately 5% to 10% of patients with HIV in the United States have coinfection with chronic HBV. Disease progression to cirrhosis, end-stage liver disease, and hepatocellular carcinoma is more rapid in these patients. Some antiretroviral toxicities and complications may be attributed to flares of HBV after initiation or discontinuation of ART.

FTC, 3TC, TDF, and TAF[1] are approved for treatment of HIV and are also active against HBV. Discontinuation of these drugs can potentially cause significant hepatic damage due to reactivation of HBV. The anti-HBV drug entecavir (Baraclude) has activity against HIV[1]. When entecavir is used to treat HBV in patients with HBV/HIV coinfection who are not taking ART, the drug can select for M184V mutation, resulting in HIV resistance to 3TC and FTC. When 3TC is the only active drug used to treat HBV in coinfected patients, 3TC resistance develops in approximately 40% to 90% of patients after 2 to 4 years on 3TC monotherapy.

Before ART is initiated, all patients who test positive for HBV surface antigen (HBsAg) should also be tested for HBV DNA using a quantitative assay. This test should be repeated every 3 to 6 months to ensure effective HBV suppression. In patients with HBV/HIV coinfection, immune reconstitution following initiation of treatment for HIV, HBV, or both can be associated with elevated transaminases.

Complications

Diagnosis and Management of Opportunistic Infections

The widespread availability and use of ART have significantly reduced OI-related mortality in persons with HIV infection. OIs continue to cause considerable morbidity and mortality, however, due to the increasing number of undiagnosed cases of HIV and patients with known HIV infection but who are not on ART or unable to maintain adherence to ART.

Pneumocystis pneumonia (PJP) is an infection caused by a ubiquitous fungus, *P. jirovecii*. Most cases occur in patients with an advanced compromised immune system (CD4 count <100 cells/mm^3). The most common manifestations are dyspnea, fever, non-productive cough, and chest discomfort. Onset of symptoms

[1]Not FDA-approved for this indication.

TABLE 4	Monitoring Recommendations for Antiretroviral Toxicity of Selected Drugs	
DRUG	**TOXICITY**	**MONITORING**
NRTIs		
Abacavir (Ziagen)	Liver Abacavir hypersensitivity syndrome	LFTs Screening for HLA-B*5701 (should be confirmed negative prior to abacavir initiation) Symptoms of abacavir hypersensitivity may include fever, rash, nausea, vomiting, diarrhea, abdominal pain, malaise, fatigue, or respiratory symptoms such as sore throat, cough, or shortness of breath
Emtricitabine (Emtriva)	Minimal toxicity Liver Hyperpigmentation/skin discoloration	Serum creatinine LFTs Hepatitis B (prior to initiation of therapy) Severe acute exacerbation of hepatitis may occur in patients with HBV/HIV coinfection who discontinue emtricitabine. In patients where discontinuation of tenofovir is necessary, ensure an agent active against HBV is administered.
Lamivudine (Epivir)	Minimal toxicity Liver	Serum creatinine LFTs Hepatitis B (prior to initiation of therapy) Severe acute exacerbation of hepatitis may occur in patients with HBV/HIV coinfection who discontinue lamivudine. In patients where discontinuation of tenofovir is necessary, ensure an agent active against HBV is administered.

VIII Infectious Diseases

590

DRUG	TOXICITY	MONITORING
Tenofovir (disoproxil fumarate [Viread], alafenamide [Vemlidy])	Renal toxicity (tubulopathy) Decreases in bone mineral density Liver	Serum creatinine Urine glucose and protein (prior to initiation and as clinically indicated during therapy) Serum phosphorus (in patients with chronic kidney disease) Bone mineral density testing (if history of bone fracture or risk factors for bone loss) LFTs Hepatitis B (prior to initiation of therapy) Tenofovir alafenamide (Vemlidy) is associated with lower rates of bone and kidney toxicity compared to tenofovir disoproxil fumarate Severe acute exacerbation of hepatitis may occur in patients with HBV/HIV coinfection who discontinue tenofovir. In patients where discontinuation of tenofovir is necessary, ensure an agent active against HBV is administered.
NNRTIs		
Efavirenz (Sustiva)	Rash Neuropsychiatric symptoms Hyperlipidemia Hepatotoxicity QT interval prolongation	LFTs Lipid panel (prior to therapy periodically during) Signs and symptoms of neuropsychiatric effects (e.g., vivid dreams, depression, suicidal ideation)
Rilpivirine (Edurant)	Rash Depression, insomnia, headache Hepatotoxicity QT interval prolongation	LFTs Lipid panel
Doravirine (Pifeltro)	Nausea Dizziness Abnormal dreams	None specific
PIs		
All	GI intolerance, nausea, vomiting, diarrhea Hyperglycemia Insulin resistance Hepatotoxicity Fat maldistribution Hyperlipidemia	Serum glucose LFTs (at baseline and as clinically indicated thereafter)
Atazanavir (Reyataz)	Indirect hyperbilirubinemia	Bilirubin
Darunavir (Prezista)	Skin rash	Darunavir contains a sulfonamide moiety; Stevens-Johnson syndrome, toxic epidermal necrolysis, acute generalized exanthematous pustulosis, and erythema have been reported. Risk of cross-reactivity between darunavir and sulfonamide medications is very low. However, use caution in patients with severe sulfonamide allergies.
INSTIS		
All	INSTIs typically well tolerated for most patients GI intolerance Insomnia Headache Depression and suicidal ideation (rare, usually in patients with pre-existing psychiatric conditions) CPK elevation, muscle weakness, and rhabdomyolysis (primarily reported with raltegravir [Isentress]) Possible association with weight gain	LFTs Serum creatinine (dolutegravir [Tivicay] and bictegravir) CPK (if signs of muscle toxicity)

CPK, Creatinine phosphokinase; *GI,* gastrointestinal; *HBV,* hepatitis B virus; *HIV,* human immunodeficiency virus; *HLA,* human leukocyte antigen; *INSTI,* integrase strand transfer inhibitor; *LFT,* liver function test; *NRTI,* nucleoside reverse transcriptase inhibitor; *NNRTI,* non-nucleoside reverse transcriptase inhibitor; *PI,* protease inhibitor. Table is not all inclusive.

Adapted from: Panel on Antiretroviral Guidelines for Adults and Adolescents. Guidelines for the Use of Antiretroviral Agents in Adults and Adolescents with HIV. Department of Health and Human Services. Available at https://clinicalinfo.hiv.gov/sites/default/files/guidelines/documents/AdultandAdolescentGL.pdf. Section accessed March 9, 2021 [Appendix B, tables 3–6].

is usually subacute and progressive over days to weeks. Mild cases may present with normal pulmonary physical examination findings at rest but develop dyspnea, tachycardia, and rales with exertion. Hypoxemia is often present to varying severity. Laboratory findings are consistent with lactate dehydrogenase levels greater than 500 mg/dL and elevated serum 1,3 β-d-glucan. Chest radiography may show diffuse, bilateral, ground-glass interstitial infiltrates, but chest radiography can appear unremarkable in patients with early disease. In patients with normal chest plain films, computed tomography (CT) of the chest can show underlying abnormalities consistent with PJP. HIV-infected patients, including pregnant women and those on ART, should receive PJP chemoprophylaxis if they have CD4 counts less than 200 cells/mm^3. Patients who receive pyrimethamine (Daraprim)–sulfadiazine for treatment or suppression of toxoplasmosis do not require additional prophylaxis for PJP. Trimethoprim-sulfamethoxazole (TMP-SMX [Bactrim]) is the first-line prophylactic agent at one double-strength tablet daily (which also confers prophylaxis against toxoplasmosis[1]) or three times weekly. In those who cannot tolerate TMP-SMX, alternative prophylactic options include dapsone[1], dapsone plus pyrimethamine[1] plus leucovorin[1], aerosolized pentamidine (Nebupent), and atovaquone (Mepron).

Toxoplasma gondii is a protozoan infection and is associated with reactivation of latent tissue cysts. Patients at greatest risk have CD4 counts less than 50 cells/μL. Clinical disease is rare in patients with CD4 counts greater than 200 cells/μL. In patients with AIDS, the typical presentation of infection is focal encephalitis, including headache, confusion, focal motor weakness, and fever. In the absence of treatment, disease progression may lead to seizures, coma, and death. CT and MRI of the brain may show multiple contrast-enhancing lesions within the gray matter of the cortex or basal ganglia, often with associated edema. HIV-infected patients with toxoplasma encephalitis are usually seropositive for toxoplasma IgG antibodies. Definitive diagnosis requires the combination of clinical presentation, identification of one or more mass lesions via CT or MRI, and detection of the organism in a sample, with brain biopsy being the most preferred method. Therapy of choice includes pyrimethamine plus sulfadiazine plus leucovorin[1].

Disseminated *Mycobacterium avium* complex (MAC) disease typically occurs in patients with CD4 counts less than 50 cells/mm^3. Other factors associated with increased susceptibility to MAC disease include HIV RNA levels greater than 100,000 copies/mL, previous OIs, and previous colonization of the respiratory or gastrointestinal tract with MAC. In HIV-infected patients with AIDS who are not on ART, MAC disease usually presents as a disseminated, multiorgan infection. Symptoms may be minimal at first but may include fever, night sweats, weight loss, diarrhea, fatigue, and nonspecific abdominal pain. Laboratory abnormalities may include anemia out of proportion for that expected from HIV alone and an increase in liver alkaline phosphatase. Physical exam or imaging may note nonspecific hepatomegaly, lymphadenopathy, and/or splenomegaly. Diagnosis is based on a combination of clinical symptoms and the isolation of MAC from cultures obtained from blood, lymph nodes, bone marrow, or other sterile sites. Initial treatment should consist of at least two antimycobacterial medications in an effort to prevent the development of resistance. Infectious disease specialists should be consulted regarding treatment. MAC isolates should be tested for susceptibility to clarithromycin (Biaxin) and azithromycin (Zithromax).

Cryptococcus neoformans meningitis occurs more commonly in patients with CD4 counts less than 100 cells/μL. It can present as a subacute or acute meningoencephalitis associated with fever, headache, and malaise. Classic meningeal symptoms may be absent. Disseminated disease is usually present when diagnosed in a patient with HIV infection and can involve virtually any organ. Diagnosis of meningitis via cerebral spinal fluid (CSF) often demonstrates elevated opening pressure, elevated protein, low-to-normal glucose, and lymphocytic pleocytosis. Numerous yeast forms may be visualized on Gram stain or India ink preparations of CSF. CSF cryptococcal antigen (CrAg) is often positive. Serum CrAg may be positive in both meningeal and nonmeningeal involving infections and its presence can be detected weeks to months prior to the onset of symptoms. A positive serum CrAg should proceed to lumbar puncture to rule out meningeal disease. Treatment of cryptococcosis occurs in three stages: induction, consolidation, and maintenance therapy.

CMV disease can cause disseminated and localized end-organ damage in HIV-infected patients with suppressed immune states with CD4 counts less than 50 cells/mm^3. Clinical disease is usually the result of reactivation of latent infection. Risk factors include not receiving or failing to respond to ART, previous OIs, high level of CMV viremia, and high HIV viral load (>100,000 copies/mL). Retinitis is the most common clinical manifestation of CMV end-organ disease and is often unilateral but can progress to bilateral if therapy or immune recovery are not pursued. Retinitis may present with floaters, scotomata, or peripheral visual field defects. Colitis is another manifestation of CMV disease and may be associated with weight loss, abdominal pain, significant diarrhea, and malaise. Hemorrhage and bowel perforation can be life threatening. CMV viremia can be measured via PCR and is usually present in end-organ disease.

Mucocutaneous candidiasis of the oropharynx and esophagus occurs commonly in HIV-infected patients and is often an indication of underlying immune suppression (CD4 count <200 cells/mm^3). Oropharyngeal candidiasis is usually painless and affects the oropharyngeal mucosa and tongue surface. Esophageal candidiasis may be associated with retrosternal discomfort and odynophagia. Oropharyngeal candidiasis is usually diagnosed clinically. Diagnosis of esophageal candidiasis is made based on symptoms, response to therapy, or visualization of mucosal lesions on examination.

Many treatment guidelines recommend initiating ART within 2 weeks for most diagnosed OI. In patients with cryptococcal meningitis and possible tuberculous meningitis, ART should be deferred due to the risks of serious immune reconstitution syndrome outweighing the benefits of ART. In patients with AIDS-associated OI for which no effective therapy exists (e.g., progressive multifocal leukoencephalopathy [PML], cryptosporidiosis, and microsporidiosis), improvement in immune function with ART can potentially improve disease outcomes.

Neurologic

Both central nervous system disease and peripheral nerve abnormalities are common in advanced AIDS. HIV infection can directly cause distal sensory neuropathy, which may manifest as dysesthesia or hypersensitivity, decreased reflexes, and chronic neuropathic pain. Inflammatory demyelinating polyneuropathy (e.g., Guillain-Barré syndrome) has known associations with some enteric pathogens and causes ascending motor weakness, typically without sensory involvement. CMV infection may cause polyradiculopathy, transverse myelitis, and encephalitis/ventriculitis in patients with CD4 counts lower than 50 cells/mm^3. CMV end-organ disease, including retinitis (a vision-threatening condition), requires prompt diagnosis and initiation of appropriate anti-CMV therapy.

Focal central nervous system lesions can arise from infectious and malignant conditions. Cerebral toxoplasmosis usually occurs in patients with prior exposure to *T. gondii* who develop reactivation disease when the CD4 count is lower than 100 cells/mm^3. The main differential diagnosis for one or several enhancing brain lesions includes toxoplasmosis and primary central nervous system lymphoma (PCNSL). PCNSL is associated with Epstein-Barr virus, and detection of nucleic acid for Epstein-Barr virus in cerebrospinal fluid carries a high specificity for this condition in the proper radiographic context. PML, a rare and potentially devastating demyelinating condition, is caused by reactivation of JC virus and can manifest as focal neurologic deficit, seizures, or cognitive dysfunction. *C. neoformans* is a common cause of meningitis in AIDS patients and may manifest with central nervous system mass lesions, pulmonary disease, or gastrointestinal disease. Worldwide, tuberculosis accounts for a large proportion of HIV-associated meningitis; less commonly, it can manifest as single or multiple focal lesions (tuberculomas). Neurosyphilis

---

[1]Not FDA approved for this indication.

should be considered in patients with unexplained neurologic disease and sexual risk factors.

Respiratory Complications

Respiratory illnesses are among the most common causes of morbidity in HIV-infected patients. Community-acquired bacterial pneumonia occurs at a significantly higher rate in HIV-infected compared with HIV-noninfected patients, regardless of CD4 count, and is one of the most common reasons for hospitalization. *P. jirovecii* (formerly *P. carinii*) pneumonia (PCP) manifests with fever, cough, and dyspnea. Findings on physical examination and chest radiography can be variable, making the diagnosis difficult in the absence of high clinical suspicion. Elevated lactate dehydrogenase and oxygen desaturation with ambulation can be diagnostic clues. More than 90% of cases occur among patients with CD4 counts lower than 200 cells/mm³. The diagnosis is established by visualization of organisms in induced sputum (sensitivity, 50% to 90%) or in bronchoalveolar lavage specimens (sensitivity, 90% to 99%), most commonly with the use of immunofluorescent staining.

The risk of reactivation of latent TB is increased 100-fold in patients with HIV infection. Patients with HIV infection who are latently infected have a 10% annual risk of developing symptomatic tuberculosis, compared with a 10% lifetime risk among the general population. The risk of reactivation increases with decreasing CD4 count, and patients with counts lower than 350 cells/mm³ are more likely to have atypical radiographic presentations, including middle- and lower-lobe infiltrates without cavitation. Patients with low CD4 counts are more likely to have extrapulmonary tuberculosis. Diagnostic approaches to tuberculosis in patients with HIV infection are similar to those in patients without HIV infection. Tuberculin skin testing can be used to diagnose latent tuberculosis infection, although the recommended cutoff for a positive test is 5 mm of induration. Treatment of coinfection with *Mycobacterium tuberculosis* and HIV requires consultation with experienced clinicians and pharmacists because of extensive drug–drug interactions among antiretroviral drugs and rifamycins.

Gastrointestinal Complications

Oropharyngeal candidiasis (thrush) commonly manifests as white plaques on the tongue, palate, or buccal mucosa that are painless and are easily scraped off. Although thrush is typically uncomplicated and easily treatable with topical preparations such as nystatin (Mycostatin) and clotrimazole (Mycelex troche), in the proper clinical setting it can alert the clinician to the presence of esophageal candidiasis. Esophageal involvement should be suspected in patients with dysphagia and odynophagia; retrosternal chest pain may also be present. Thrush is usually present but is not required for the diagnosis, which is often made on clinical grounds rather than being confirmed with endoscopy. Patients with esophageal candidiasis typically respond after several days of treatment, and 7 to 14 days of antifungal therapy is usually sufficient. For cases not responsive to empiric treatment for candidiasis, referral for endoscopy should be considered. Esophagitis caused by CMV or herpes simplex virus requires a histopathologic diagnosis.

Acute diarrhea, defined as three or more loose or watery stools per day for 3 to 10 days, is common among patients with HIV infection, and more than 1000 different enteric pathogens have been described. Data from a large cohort indicate that the most common pathogens isolated are *Clostridium difficile*, *Shigella* spp., *Campylobacter jejuni*, *Salmonella* spp., *Staphylococcus aureus*, and MAC. Culture of the stool can yield a microbiologic diagnosis in many cases, particularly for acute diarrheal illnesses caused by *Campylobacter*, *Yersinia*, *Salmonella*, and *Shigella* species. Infection with *C. difficile*, the most common bacterial enteric pathogen in the United States for both HIV-infected and HIV-uninfected persons, is diagnosed in most settings by detection of cytotoxin in the stool by enzyme immunoassay (EIA) or PCR, although the more laborious tissue culture is considered the gold standard. Enteric viruses are present in 15% to 30% of HIV-infected persons with acute diarrhea. Definitive diagnosis is not feasible in most clinical laboratories; viral enteritis should be suspected in the setting of community outbreaks because of the high transmissibility of viral pathogens. Treatment is supportive with fluid resuscitation and antimotility agents.

Chronic diarrhea (duration 30 days) was a common manifestation of advanced-stage AIDS in the pre-HAART era. Most pathogens that cause acute gastroenteritis can also cause chronic symptoms. Pathogens that should be suspected in cases of chronic watery diarrhea include protozoa such as *Cryptosporidium parvum*, *Isospora belli*, and *Microsporidia* spp. These entities are self-limited in the absence of severe immunosuppression. In advanced HIV infection, pathogen-specific antimicrobial therapy is infrequently effective, and symptoms commonly do not improve without immune reconstitution in response to ART. *Giardia lamblia* causes watery diarrhea, abdominal bloating, and occasionally malabsorption syndrome, and can occur at any CD4 count. CMV infection can affect any segment of the gastrointestinal tract and is a common cause of chronic diarrhea. Diagnosis of gastrointestinal CMV disease is difficult without biopsy. Detection of CMV viremia with PCR does not correlate well with presence of CMV disease in HIV-infected patients, and CMV can be undetectable in serum in patients with extensive gastrointestinal disease.

Other Conditions

ART has dramatically increased the survival of individuals living with HIV, and the HIV elderly population is expanding. There are few clinical trials or studies systematically focused on this cohort. Older adults with HIV may develop comorbidities that can complicate their HIV management. ART-related CD4 cell recovery in older patients has been observed to be slower and to be of lower magnitude than in younger patients. Hepatic and renal functions decrease as the body ages and may lead to impaired drug elimination and increased drug exposure in older patients.

Immune Reconstitution Inflammatory Syndrome

Immune reconstitution inflammatory syndrome (IRIS) is a collection of inflammatory disorders often associated with paradoxical worsening of preexisting infectious diseases after initiation of ART. IRIS is usually accompanied by an increase in CD4 count and can occur at any CD4 count. It usually occurs in the first 4 to 8 weeks after initiation of ART. Clinical features are often associated with the type and location of the preexisting OI and can be localized or systemic. Patients should continue on ART and should receive treatment for the underlying OI as quickly as possible. If the patient's presentation involves paradoxical worsening of a previously diagnosed OI that is already receiving treatment, OI therapy should also be continued. Disseminated MAC accounts for up to one-third of the cases of IRIS in the United States. Other important causes of IRIS are tuberculosis, CMV infection, viral hepatitis, and candida infections.

Management of Human Immunodeficiency Virus in Pregnancy and Women of Childbearing Potential

Human Immunodeficiency Virus in Pregnant Women

Every pregnant woman with HIV should be given ART regardless of her immunologic or virologic status in order to improve her health and prevent transmission of HIV to the fetus. Increased perinatal transmission risk exists in pregnant women who experience early HIV infection and high-level viremia. Pregnant women with newly diagnosed HIV infection should start ART as soon as possible to prevent perinatal HIV transmission. The goal of ART is to achieve and sustain viral suppression throughout the pregnancy. Resistance testing should be performed prior to initiating ART, but therapy may be started before receiving resistance testing results. ART regimen can be modified at a later date once resistance testing results are available.

In 2019, the U.S. Department of Health and Human Services announced that data on neural tube defects (NTDs) in infants born to women who received DTG (Tivicay) around the time of conception showed lower prevalence of NTDs than initially reported (0.3%); however, the rate is still higher than the rate reported for infants born to individuals who received ART that did not contain DTG (0.1%). Current recommendations concerning DTG use include discussing the benefits and risks of NTDs with persons of childbearing potential to allow the patient to make an informed decision about care. DTG may be used as an alternative ART in women of childbearing potential who are trying to conceive and those who are sexually active and not using contraception. For individuals who are using effective contraception, DTG is a recommended option.

In a patient already taking a regimen containing EFV [Sustiva] who presents for prenatal care during the first trimester and has virologic suppression, EFV can be continued. The risk of fetal NTDs is limited to the first 5 to 6 weeks of pregnancy, and pregnancy is often not recognized before weeks 4 to 6. Unnecessary changes to a patient's ART regimen during pregnancy may result in loss of viral suppression with increased risk of perinatal transmission.

In a pregnant patient with an HIV RNA viral load greater than or equal to 1000 copies/mL (or viral load is unknown) near delivery, IV infusion of zidovudine (Retrovir) during labor is recommended regardless of the patient's antepartum ART regimen or resistance profile. Maternal ART should be continued following delivery. Following delivery, the patient should continue to follow up with their HIV care provider as recommended for non-pregnant adults.

Maternal adherence to ART reduces but does not completely eliminate the risk of transmission of HIV in breast milk. Post-natal HIV transmission can occur despite maternal ART adherence, and patients should be counseled to avoid breastfeeding. There have also been reports of mother-to-child transmission of HIV via mothers pre-masticating food and feeding it to their infants.

Preexposure Prophylaxis of Human Immunodeficiency Virus Infection

Globally, up to 2 million new HIV infections occur per year. It is estimated that up to 50,000 new HIV infections occur annually in the United States. The highest incidence of new HIV infections occur in men having sex with other men, especially among young African American males. For uninfected patients with a high risk of HIV acquisition, PrEP is an evidence-based method for preventing infections in those at risk. Since 2012, tenofovir disoproxil fumarate-emtricitabine (TDF-FTC [Truvada]) has been approved for PrEP and is at least 90% effective in reducing risk of HIV transmission. In 2019, TAF-FTC (Descovy) was also approved for PrEP, although only for selected patients; it is not currently approved for use in patients who have receptive vaginal sex. Efficacy is dependent on medication adherence.

Daily oral PrEP is recommended as one HIV prevention option for people who are sexually active with men, adult heterosexually active men and women who are at increased risk of acquiring HIV infection, and adult injection drug users at increased risk of acquiring HIV infection (Table 5). PrEP therapy should be discussed with heterosexually active women and men with sexual partners known to have HIV infection to prevent virus transmission during conception and pregnancy.

Prior to initiating PrEP, it is important to obtain a detailed sexual and drug use history to identify patients likely to benefit from PrEP. Pertinent information includes frequency of condom use, penile-anal or penile-vaginal sex, number of sex partners, HIV serostatus of sex partner(s), drug use during sex, and history of sexually transmitted infections (STIs). It is important to determine sexual practices with a patient's main sexual partner, casual partners, and whether they have any anonymous partners. A drug history over the prior 6 months should be obtained and include injection drug use and sharing of needles. The 2017 PrEP guidelines published by the US Public Health Service recommend the following questions to initiate these discussions with patients regarding their behaviors in the previous 6 months:
- Have you had sex with men, women, or both?
- (If men or both sexes) How many men/women have you had sex with?
- How many times did you have vaginal sex when neither you nor your partner wore a condom?
- How many times did you have receptive anal sex (you were the bottom) with a man who was not wearing a condom?
- How many of your male sex partners were HIV positive?
- (If any positive) With these HIV-positive male partners, how many times did you have insertive anal sex (you were on top)/vaginal sex without wearing a condom?
- Have you used methamphetamines (such as crystal meth or speed)?

TABLE 5	Preexposure Prophylaxis		
	MEN WHO HAVE SEX WITH MEN	**HETEROSEXUAL WOMEN AND MEN**	**INJECTION DRUG USERS**
Detecting substantial risk of acquiring HIV infection	HIV-positive sexual partner Recent bacterial STI High number of sex partners History of inconsistent or no condom use Commercial sex work	HIV-positive sexual partner Recent bacterial STI High number of sex partners History of inconsistent or no condom use Commercial sex work In high-prevalence area or network	HIV-positive injection partner Sharing injection equipment
Clinical eligibility	Documented negative HIV test result before prescribing PrEP No signs/symptoms of acute HIV infection Normal renal function; no contraindicated medications Documented hepatitis B infection and vaccination status		
Prescription	Daily, continuing, oral doses of FTC/TDF (Truvada), ≤90-day supply		
Other services	Follow-up visits at least every 3 months to provide the following: HIV test, medication adherence counseling, behavioral risk reduction support, side effect assessment, STI symptom assessment At 3 months and every 6 months thereafter, assess renal function Every 3–6 months, test for bacterial STIs		
	Do oral/rectal STI testing	For women, assess pregnancy intent Pregnancy test every 3 months	Access to clean syringes/needles and drug treatment services

HIV, Human immunodeficiency virus; *PrEP,* preexposure prophylaxis; *STI,* Sexually transmitted infection.
Preexposure Prophylaxis for the Prevention of HIV Infection In the Unites States—2017 Clinical Practice Guideline. US Public Health Service. Available at https://www.cdc.gov/hiv/guidelines/preventing.html. Accessed March 9, 2021 [Table 1].

- Do you have a history of STIs?

Patients screened for PrEP must be screened for common bacterial STIs, including serologic testing for syphilis and nucleic acid amplification tests for gonorrhea and chlamydia. This includes swabs of the oropharynx in patients who participate in oral sex and anal swabs for recipients of anal intercourse. Screening for trichomonas and bacterial vaginosis are not required prior to initiating PrEP because they lack strong correlation with HIV coinfection.

Plasma HIV testing with fourth-generation antigen/antibody test should be obtained to confirm that the patient does not have undiagnosed HIV infection. Additional HIV RNA testing should be performed in patients with signs or symptoms of acute HIV infection in the last 4 weeks, those with indeterminate antigen/antibody test results, and patients with high-risk HIV exposure in the preceding 4 weeks.

TDF-FTC (tenofovir disoproxil fumarate/emtricitabine [Truvada]) is generally tolerated well by most patients; however, screening for persons at increased risk of adverse effects should be performed prior to PrEP initiation. TDF is associated with acute and chronic kidney disease in HIV-infected patients. Its safety in patients without HIV and eGFR less than 60 mL/min/1.73 m^2 has not been documented. Serum creatinine should be measured as PrEP is not recommended for patients with estimated glomerular filtration rate less than 60 mL/min/1.73 m^2. In patients without reduced kidney function but who have risk factors for developing renal disease, urinalysis to document baseline proteinuria can be obtained for monitoring purposes. A different formulation of tenofovir, TAF (tenofovir alafenamide fumarate [Vemlidy])[1], has less association with renal and bone toxicity compared to TDF. In the United States, once-daily TAF-FTC (tenofovir alafenamide/emtricitabine [Descovy]) can be prescribed for PrEP in high-risk MSM and transgender women, particularly those who have bone or renal contraindications to TDF.

Screening for undiagnosed hepatitis B infection should be performed via hepatitis B surface antigen, hepatitis B core antibody, and hepatitis B surface antibody. If the patient's serology shows nonimmunity, vaccination against HBV should be pursued, as individuals engaging in high-risk sexual and drug-use behaviors have an increased risk of HBV infection. If the patient's serology reveals chronic HBV, it must be determined whether the patient requires HBV treatment. TDF and TAF are first-line treatment choices for chronic HBV and can be used for PrEP and treatment of chronic HBV. In those with chronic HBV who do not require HBV treatment, there is a low risk of HBV flare if TDF or TAF is discontinued.

TDF is also associated with decreased bone density; therefore, patients considering PrEP should be screened for osteoporosis risk factors. The greatest amount of bone loss has been associated with the first 6 months of treatment. In patients with known osteopenia or osteoporosis, the risk of acquiring HIV versus further bone loss must be considered. If PrEP is pursued in these patients, a baseline dual-energy x-ray absorptiometry (DXA) scan should be obtained prior to PrEP initiation if a recent test is not available. Repeat DXA testing on TDF therapy should be considered on a case-by-case basis given that no guidelines for monitoring have been defined. Due to lower rates of bone and renal toxicity, TAF should be considered over TDF in patients with significant risk for bone-related complications.

Females with childbearing potential should be screened for pregnancy. TDF and FTC are felt to be safe in pregnancy (category B), although some concerns have been raised regarding fetal bone development with TDF use. In patients who are pregnant, the risk of acquiring HIV must be considered against the risk of using antiretroviral medication during pregnancy. Limited data are available regarding PrEP efficacy during pregnancy. TAF has not been assigned a pregnancy category due to lack of data.

Initiating Preexposure Prophylaxis
The combination tablet of TDF-FTC (Truvada) or TAF-FTC (Descovy) should be taken once daily for a duration of as long as the infection risk continues. It should be dispensed as a 90-day supply and renewed at each 3-month clinic follow-up. Condom use is encouraged while using PrEP. For patients who are not willing to use condoms consistently, CDC recommends condom use to prevent acquisition of HIV (and other STIs) for the first 7 days after starting PrEP if engaging in receptive anal sex and 21 days if engaging in receptive vaginal sex. Common side effects of once-daily TDF-FTC and TAF-FTC include nausea and vomiting. These symptoms usually improve and resolve within the first 4 weeks of use.

Some patients who only have discrete periods of high-risk HIV exposure may not wish to take PrEP at all times. In this situation, PrEP should be initiated at least 1 week prior to high-risk sexual activity for male patients and 3 weeks for female patients. After the period of high-risk behavior ends, PrEP should be continued for at least 1 month. These recommendations are based on pharmacokinetic data and not clinical trials.

Preexposure Prophylaxis Monitoring and Follow-Up
Patients on PrEP should have routine follow-up with their prescribing medical provider. The first follow-up should occur 1 month after initiating PreP and every 3 months thereafter. More frequent follow-up should occur for patients with exposures or symptoms of STIs or medication side effects.

Every 3 months, patients should be screened for HIV infection with fourth-generation antigen/antibody testing, screened for symptoms of acute HIV infection, pregnancy testing, screened for STIs appropriate for recent sexual behaviors, assessed for medication adherence as well as sexual and drug use behaviors. Serum creatinine should be monitored after the first 3 months of PrEP and can be monitored at least every 3 months thereafter in patients with risk factors for kidney disease and every 6 months for patients without kidney disease. Appropriate counseling should be provided to encourage medication adherence and reduce high-risk sexual and drug use behaviors.

Postexposure Prophylaxis of Human Immunodeficiency Virus Infection
The most effective means to prevent HIV infection include preventing exposure to the virus. In the event that an isolated occupational, sexual, or injection drug-related exposure occurs, postexposure prophylaxis can be a second line of defense against HIV acquisition.

Occupational Exposure
Healthcare personnel include all paid and unpaid persons working in a healthcare setting with potential for exposure to infectious materials such as bodily fluids, contaminated medical supplies, or environmental surfaces. In the occupational setting, prevention of exposures to blood and bodily fluids from infected sources is the key to preventing occupationally acquired HIV infection. The overall risk of becoming infected with HIV after inadvertent exposure to body fluids from an HIV-infected patient is low. It is estimated that the average risk for HIV transmission following percutaneous exposure to HIV-infected blood is 0.3% and after mucous membrane exposure is 0.09%. The average risk of HIV transmission following nonintact skin exposure has not been defined; however, it is estimated to be lower than mucous membrane exposure. Healthcare personnel at the highest risk are those who received an accidental inoculation containing blood from a known HIV-infected source.

---

[1]Not FDA-approved for this indication.

Initial Laboratory Evaluation

All patients initiating post-exposure prophylaxis (PEP) after potential HIV exposure should be tested for HIV antigens and antibodies at baseline prior to PEP initiation. If baseline HIV testing indicates existing HIV infection, PEP should not be initiated. Repeat HIV testing should be performed at 4 to 6 weeks and 3 months following the exposure to determine if HIV infection has occurred. Administration of PEP should not be delayed while awaiting the results of HIV testing and can be discontinued if the source patient is found to not have HIV infection. PEP is most effective when taken as soon as possible following exposure.

Initiating Preexposure Prophylaxis/Choosing Appropriate Preexposure Prophylaxis Therapy

PEP is most effective when initiated as soon as possible following the exposure incident. If PEP is delayed, the effectiveness of therapy may be significantly reduced if initiated 72 hours or more following exposure. Initiating therapy after 72 hours might still be considered if the exposure is proven to be of an extremely high risk of transmission.

The current recommendation for PEP therapy is FTC plus TDF (which can be dispensed as a fixed-dose combination tablet [Truvada]) plus raltegravir (RAL [Isentress]) or DTG [Tivicay] for 4 weeks. Overall, this regimen has acceptable tolerability, convenient dosing, and minimal drug interactions. In patients with significant underlying renal disease, an acceptable PEP alternative is zidovudine plus lamivudine (Combivir)[1] in addition to RAL or DTG.

PEP regimens include three (occasionally more) antiretroviral medications. Due to the potential for medication-related side effects, it is important to choose a PEP regimen with a lower toxicity profile to improve patient tolerance and encourage completion of PEP therapy.

HIV PEP should be offered to pregnant or breastfeeding healthcare providers based on the same criteria as any other provider with a similar exposure. Risk of HIV transmission from mother to child during acute HIV infection is increased during pregnancy and breastfeeding.

Additional resources regarding PEP are available (e.g., PEPline at http://www.nccc.ucsf.edu/about_nccc/pepline; (888)-448-4911).

References

Baeten JM, Donnell D, Ndase P, et al: Antiretroviral prophylaxis for HIV prevention in heterosexual men and women, *N Engl J Med* 367(5):399–410, 2012.

Centers for Disease Control and Prevention. *HIV Surveillance Report: Estimated HIV Incidence and Prevalence in the United States 2010–2015*, vol 23. Atlanta, GA: CDC; 2016.

Centers for Disease Control and Prevention: *HIV Surveillance Report: Diagnoses of HIV Infection in the United States and Dependent Areas*, vol 28. Atlanta, GA: CDC; 2016.

Dominguez KL, Smith DK, Thomas V, et al: Updated guidelines for antiretroviral postexposure prophylaxis after sexual, injection drug use, or other nonoccupational exposure to HIV-United States, centers for disease control and prevention, U.S. Department of Health and Human Services, 2016.

Global UNAIDS: *AIDS Update*, 2016. http://www.unaids.org/sites/default/fil es/media_asset/global-AIDS-update-2016_en.pdf.

Grant RM, Lama JR, Anderson PL, et al: Preexposure chemoprophylaxis for HIV prevention in men who have sex with men, *N Engl J Med* 363(27):2587–2599, 2010.

Kaplan JE: Guidelines for The Prevention and Treatment of Opportunistic Infections in Hiv-Infected Adults and Adolescents, 2013.

Kuhar DT, Henderson DK, Struble KA, et al: Updated US Public Health Service guidelines for the management of occupational exposures to human immuno- deficiency virus and recommendations for postexposure prophylaxis, *Infect Control Hosp Epidemiol* 34(9), 2013.

US Public Health Service. Preexposure prophylaxis for the prevention of HIV infection in the United States—2019.

---

[1]Not FDA approved for this indication.

INFECTIOUS MONONUCLEOSIS

Method of
Ben Z. Katz, MD

CURRENT DIAGNOSIS

- The classic triad of acute infectious mononucleosis consists of fever, lymphadenopathy, and pharyngitis.
- The diagnosis of infectious mononucleosis is usually based on the clinical picture, the presence of at least 10% atypical lymphocytes in the peripheral blood, and positive heterophil serology (monospot test).

CURRENT THERAPY

- In most patients, infectious mononucleosis is self-limited and requires only symptomatic treatment.
- Steroids and antiviral therapy have no place in the therapy of uncomplicated acute infectious mononucleosis in healthy persons.

Epidemiology and Risk Factors

One must distinguish between the epidemiology of Epstein-Barr virus (EBV) infection and that of infectious mononucleosis (IM), the most common symptomatic manifestation of primary EBV infection. Almost all adults have been infected with EBV. The symptomatology of primary EBV infection varies with the infected person's age at the time, with younger children usually having inapparent or mild infections. In developing countries and in lower socioeconomic groups in industrialized nations, up to 90% of children acquire primary EBV infection by 6 years of age, and IM frequently never develops. In contrast, in higher socioeconomic groups, only 40% to 50% of adolescents have previously experienced EBV infection. From 10% to 20% of susceptible adolescents and adults contract EBV every year thereafter, with IM developing in about half of these patients.

Pathophysiology

Saliva is the main vehicle for transmission of EBV, a double-stranded DNA herpesvirus. Transmission usually requires direct and prolonged contact with infected oropharyngeal secretions, with salivary exchange being the main mode of transmission. The infection begins with viral replication in oropharyngeal epithelial cells and then spreads to local B lymphocytes, which then disseminate throughout the reticuloendothelial system and induce vigorous T- and NK-cell responses and neutralizing antibodies. The atypical lymphocytes that are produced are mainly suppressor T cells directed against EBV-infected B cells.

It is thought that most of the clinical manifestations of IM are due to these T- and NK-cell responses, which might explain why young children, whose immune responses are incompletely developed, are often asymptomatic with primary EBV infection. It is also possible that viral load determines symptomatology, and, because young adults likely spread more virus via salivary exchange than toddlers, young adults are more likely to be symptomatic. All EBV-seropositive persons shed virus intermittently throughout their lives. EBV may rarely be spread via blood transfusion or transplantation.

Clinical Manifestations

IM is usually an acute, self-limited, benign lymphoproliferative disease. EBV is responsible for nearly all heterophil-positive and most heterophil-negative cases. Other causes of heterophil-negative mononucleosis include cytomegalovirus, toxoplasmosis, hepatitis A and B, adenovirus, HIV, rubella, and human herpesvirus 6.

The classic triad of IM consists of fever, lymphadenopathy, and pharyngitis. Other typical findings include lymphocytosis with atypical lymphocytes and the presence of heterophil antibodies. After a 4- to 6-week incubation period, the illness begins with a 3- to 5-day prodrome of malaise, headache, and fatigue, typically followed in about half of the cases by onset of the triad. Additional symptoms can include anorexia, nausea, vomiting, periorbital or facial edema, and generalized lymphadenopathy, which is usually symmetrical. Splenomegaly occurs by the second or third week of illness in about half of all cases; rarely, splenic rupture can occur, which very rarely may be fatal. Hepatomegaly occurs in 10% to 15%, with hepatitis occurring in about 5% of cases. Up to 20% of patients have a rash that may be erythematous, maculopapular, morbilliform, scarlatiniform, or urticarial, especially if ampicillin or one of its derivatives has been given. Other symptoms can include arthritis and jaundice.

IM is a self-limited disease in nearly all patients. Median illness duration is 16 days.

Diagnosis

The diagnosis is usually based on the clinical picture, atypical lymphocytosis, and positive heterophil serology. Most adolescents and young adults with IM have most or all of these features, as well as an elevated white blood cell count with a relative lymphocytosis. Atypical lymphocytes generally represent more than 9% to 10% of the white blood cell count. Many infected persons also have mild thrombocytopenia and elevated hepatocellular enzymes. Heterophil antibody positivity is usually measured as a positive monospot test. If IM is suspected and heterophil antibodies are negative, specific titers for EBV, including viral capsid antigen (VCA) IgM and IgG, early antigen (EA), and Epstein–Barr nuclear antigen (EBNA), should be obtained, as well as serologic testing for cytomegalovirus (CMV) and toxoplasmosis. Acute EBV infection is characterized by the presence of IgM and IgG VCA antibodies and EA antibodies and the absence of EBNA antibodies.

Differential Diagnosis

If liver chemistry values are markedly elevated and antibodies against EBV, CMV, and toxoplasmosis are unrevealing, serology for hepatitis A, B, and C should be measured. If risk factors are present, HIV antibodies should be checked. A throat culture is indicated in patients with pharyngitis or tonsillitis because the tonsillitis of acute IM can be indistinguishable from that of group A streptococcal pharyngitis.

Treatment

In most patients, IM is self-limited and requires only symptomatic treatment, including bed rest, acetaminophen (Tylenol, 10–15 mg/kg every 4–6 hours), aspirin (10–15 mg/kg every 4–6 hours), or nonsteroidal antiinflammatory agents such as ibuprofen (Advil, 5–10 mg/kg every 6–8 hours). Saline gargles can be useful in treating a sore throat. In severe cases, meperidine (Demerol, 1–1.5 mg/kg every 3–4 hours) may be required.

Although a short, tapering course of corticosteroid therapy (e.g., a Medrol Dosepak[1]) is often prescribed, there is little evidence for its clinical efficacy, and caution is warranted. Infection is ultimately self-limited in nearly all cases, and rare reports of neurologic or septicemic complications after steroid use have appeared. Long-term immune responses following steroid use appear to be normal. Corticosteroid therapy should, however, be considered for the treatment of severe cases of IM associated with hemolysis, respiratory embarrassment, or thrombocytopenic purpura. The use of corticosteroids in atypical or antibody-negative cases is inappropriate because the diagnosis of lymphoma can then be confounded.

Parenteral administration of acyclovir[1] (Zovirax, 10–20 mg/kg IV every 8 hours) to patients with acute IM secondary to EBV reduces the level of oropharyngeal viral replication; however, replication returns to the previously high levels after cessation of treatment, little or no reduction is seen in the number of EBV-infected B cells in the peripheral circulation, and the drug has little or no effect on the clinical course. Acyclovir administered in high doses orally (20 mg/kg, maximum dose of 800 mg qid for 5

days) is also ineffective. Antiviral therapy is therefore not recommended for acute IM in a normal host.

In immunosuppressed or severely ill patients, however, specific therapy has a role in many cases. For example, etoposide (VePesid)[1], a drug that reduces macrophage activation, is often used in cases of infection-associated hemophagocytic syndrome. In posttransplant lymphoproliferative disorders, first-line therapy is often a reduction in immunosuppression; other options include rituximab[1] (Rituxan, 375 mg/m^2 IV weekly for 4 weeks). Oral leukoplakia in patients with AIDS responds to oral acyclovir[1] (20 mg/kg, maximum dose of 800 mg qid for 20 days), whereas a tapering course of steroids (as recommended earlier) may be used for lymphocytic interstitial pneumonitis (see below).

Monitoring

Quarantine is not indicated. Ampicillin and related drugs should be avoided when treating secondary bacterial complications because of their association with rash in persons with IM. Contact sports should be avoided as long as splenomegaly is still evident because of the rare possibility of splenic rupture, which usually occurs within 3 weeks of onset of IM but has been reported as late as 7 weeks into the illness.

Complications

Complications of acute IM can be neurologic (seizures, cranial nerve palsies, aseptic meningitis, encephalitis, optic neuritis, transverse myelitis, infectious polyneuritis [Guillain-Barré syndrome], psychosis, Alice in Wonderland syndrome, or acute cerebellar ataxia), hematologic (hemolytic or aplastic anemia, thrombocytopenic purpura, agranulocytosis, or agammaglobulinemia), cardiac (pericarditis or myocarditis), pulmonary (cough or atypical pneumonia), renal (glomerulonephritis, acute kidney failure, or acute interstitial nephritis), or ophthalmologic (conjunctivitis) in nature. In about 10% of adolescents and young adults, fatigue can persist for 6 months or longer, and many of these patients meet the criteria for chronic fatigue syndrome. Young adults with more severe acute IM and certain predisposing symptoms and laboratory findings are more likely to meet criteria for chronic fatigue syndrome 6 months later.

Rare patients have very high titers of EBV antibodies, and a chronic active EBV infection associated with unusual clinical manifestations such as uveitis or lymphoma can occur. EBV is also associated with lymphoproliferative disorders in persons with underlying abnormal immune systems. These include X-linked lymphoproliferative syndrome, in which affected males usually die of acute EBV infection, and the related infection-associated hemophagocytic syndrome, which is most commonly (about 75% of the time) triggered by EBV and seems to be due to an overly exuberant macrophage response to EBV-infected lymphocytes. Transplant recipients can acquire EBV-associated lymphoproliferative disease that can range from an asymptomatic infection to fatal IM or lymphoma. Finally, although not seen much anymore due to combination antiretroviral therapy, patients with AIDS are susceptible to several serious complications of EBV infection, including lymphocytic interstitial pneumonitis, oral leukoplakia, leiomyosarcoma, and lymphoma.

References

Candy B, Hotopf M: Steroids for symptom control in infectious mononucleosis, *Cochrane Database Syst Rev*(3)CD004402, 2006.

Cohen JI, Jaffe ES, Dale JK, et al: Characterization and treatment of chronic active Epstein–Barr virus disease: A 28-year experience in the United States, *Blood* 117:5835–5849, 2011.

Jason LA, Cotler J, Islam MF, Sunnquist M, Katz BZ. Risks for developing ME/CFS in college students following infectious mononucleosis: a prospective cohort study. *Clin Infect Dis* 2021; (in press).

Katz BZ: Commentary on "Steroids for symptom control in infectious mononucleosis (Review)" by B Candy and M Hotopf, *Evid Based Child Health* 7:447–449, 2012.

Katz BZ, Reuter C, Lupovitch Y, Gleason Y, McClellan D, Cotler J, Jason LA: A validated scale for assessing the severity of acute infectious mononucleosis, *J Pediatr* 209:130–133, 2019.

Odumade OA, Hogquist KA, Balfour Jr HH: Progress and problems in understanding and managing primary Epstein- Barr virus infections, *Clin Microbiol Rev* 24(1):193–209, 2011.

Rouphael N, Talati NJ, Vaughan C, et al: Infections associated with haemophagocytic syndrome, *Lancet Infect Dis* 7:814–822, 2007.

Soltys K, Green M: Posttransplant lymphoproliferative disease, *Pediatr Infect Dis J* 24:1107–1108, 2005.

[1]Not FDA approved for this indication.

INFLUENZA

Method of
Jeffrey A. Linder, MD, MPH

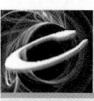

CURRENT DIAGNOSIS

- Influenza should be considered in any patient with respiratory symptoms between October and May in North America.
- The single most important piece of information when considering a diagnosis of influenza is the community prevalence of influenza.
- During influenza outbreaks, sudden onset of fever and cough has a positive predictive value of about 85%.
- Rapid testing should be done with molecular tests (e.g., reverse transcriptase polymerase chain reaction [RT-PCR]), which have a high sensitivity and specificity.

CURRENT THERAPY

- The influenza vaccine is the best means of preventing influenza. The inactivated influenza vaccine is recommended for all persons age 6 months and older.
- Influenza vaccination should be prioritized for essential workers and people at high-risk for influenza or COVID-19 complications.
- The antivirals zanamivir (Relenza) and oseltamivir (Tamiflu) can be used for prophylaxis of influenza in unimmunized patients, in close contacts of infected patients, and during institutional outbreaks of influenza.
- Early antiviral treatment should not be delayed and should be used for patients who are hospitalized; have severe, complicated, or progressive illness; or are at higher risk for complications.
- Antivirals may be prescribed within 48 hours of symptom onset for outpatients not at higher risk for influenza complications.

Influenza is a highly contagious viral infection that should be considered in any patient with respiratory symptoms between October and May in North America. Influenza infects 5% to 20% of the population of the United States in a typical year, sickens 3% to 11% of Americans, and is responsible for up to 431,000 hospitalizations and 51,000 deaths per year. Influenza can range in severity from mild illness to life-threatening disease. Those at highest risk of hospitalization, death, or complications from influenza are children younger than 2 years old, adults older than 65 years, people of any age who have underlying medical conditions or immune compromise, and pregnant women.

Information about influenza changes rapidly. Emergence of severe acute respiratory syndrome coronavirus 2 (SARS-CoV-2) and associated coronavirus disease 2019 (COVID-19) has complicated influenza diagnosis and management. To care optimally for patients with influenza-like illness during the influenza season, clinicians need to keep abreast of updated recommendations and the current prevalence of influenza and COVID-19 in their community. The influenza vaccine remains the best means of reducing the incidence, severity, and complications from influenza, but antiviral medications and symptomatic treatments have an important role in the prevention and treatment of influenza (Box 1).

Microbiology

There are two types of influenza viruses, A and B. Influenza A is separated into subtypes based on two surface antigens: hemagglutinin (H) and neuraminidase (N). The predominant circulating strains of influenza in recent decades have been influenza A (H1N1), influenza A (H3N2), and influenza B. Influenza

A (H3N2) subtypes generally cause more severe influenza and are associated with higher mortality than other types. Influenza viruses undergo slight genetic changes from year to year, termed *antigenic drift*. Major changes in surface glycoproteins are termed *antigenic shift* and can result in severe pandemic influenza in a nonimmune population, which happened with an antigenically novel influenza A (H1N1) virus in 2009. Because of antigenic drift, and because immunity to a given type or subtype of influenza provides limited cross-immunity to other types and subtypes, the influenza vaccine needs to be reformulated and administered most years.

Patients contract influenza by being exposed to large-sized respiratory droplets from an infected person or contact with surfaces harboring influenza virus. Influenza has a latency of 1 to 4 days before the onset of symptoms. Adults are infectious from the day before symptom onset through approximately day 7 of illness, but immunosuppressed adults and children shed the virus for longer periods. Symptoms generally last from 7 to 14 days.

Beyond the emergence of SARS-CoV-2 in 2019, several other novel, highly pathogenic respiratory viruses—avian influenza A (H5N1), avian influenza A (H7N9), and Middle East respiratory syndrome coronavirus (MERS-CoV)—have case-fatality rates ranging from 34% to 53%. Collectively there have been more than 5000 human cases. These pathogens, if they acquire the ability to be highly transmissible between humans, have the potential to cause pandemic respiratory disease.

Prevention

Influenza vaccination is between 20% and 90% effective in preventing influenza or complications of influenza. Influenza vaccination is highly cost-effective and can even be cost-saving in high-risk groups. Influenza vaccination is less effective in younger children, in adults older than 65 years, in adults with comorbid conditions, and when there is a poor match between the influenza vaccine and circulating influenza. The Centers for Disease Control and Prevention (CDC) Advisory Committee on Immunization Practices puts out annual recommendations and supplementary updates on the prevention and treatment of influenza (www.cdc.gov/flu). The Advisory Committee on Immunization Practices recommends vaccinating all persons 6 months of age and older.

At present, there are four commonly administered, recommended types of influenza vaccine: trivalent inactivated influenza vaccine (IIV3), quadrivalent inactivated influenza vaccine (IIV4), quadrivalent recombinant influenza vaccine (RIV4), and quadrivalent live attenuated influenza vaccine (LAIV4). The IIV4 (Afluria Quadrivalent, Fluarix Quadrivalent, Flucelvax Quadrivalent, FluLaval Quadrivalent, Fluzone Quadrivalent), IIV3 (Afluria),[2] adjuvant IV3 (Fluad), and RIV4 (Flublok Quadrivalent) vaccines are administered as an intramuscular injection. Inactivated influenza vaccines in the United States will be available in IIV4 formulation only.

Different products are approved for administration in different lower age limits. A high-dose IIV4 (Fluzone High-Dose Quadrivalent), an adjuvanted IIV3 (Fluad), and an adjuvanted IIV4 (Fluad Quadrivalent) are available for patients aged 65 years or older, who are less likely to respond immunologically to standard inactivated influenza vaccine (IIV). The main adverse effect of the IIV is soreness at the injection site. Patients often report a mild immune response of fever, malaise, myalgia, and headache that can last for 1 to 2 days, but rates of most of these symptoms are no different from those in patients who receive placebo injection.

Allergic reactions to egg proteins or other vaccine components (e.g., antibiotics and inactivating compounds) include hives, angioedema, asthma, and anaphylaxis. For patients with egg allergy who have only hives, any otherwise appropriate IIV or RIV can be administered. For patients with more severe reactions to egg or who received treatment for an allergic reaction can also receive any recommended IIV or RIV in an inpatient or outpatient medical setting and observed for at least 15 minutes by a clinician able to recognize and manage severe allergic reactions. The recombinant influenza vaccine (RIV4; FluBlok Quadrivalent) and cell culture derived quadrivalent (ccIIV4; Flucelvax) are considered egg free. Patients who have had severe allergic reaction to influenza vaccine should not receive the vaccine.

Vaccination should be deferred in patients with confirmed or suspected COVID-19 or with any acute febrile illness, but patients with more moderate illness can be vaccinated. Guillain-Barré syndrome was associated with the 1976 swine flu vaccine, but there is no consistent evidence that modern influenza vaccines are associated with Guillain-Barré syndrome.

The LAIV4 (FluMist Quadrivalent) is administered as a nasal spray and is approved for patients ages 2 to 49 years. The LAIV4 is contraindicated in children aged 2 to 4 years with recurrent wheezing or asthma; children who are receiving aspirin or aspirin-containing products; patients with comorbid conditions or immunosuppression; pregnant women; family members or close contacts of severely immunosuppressed patients, who require a protected environment (e.g., hematopoietic stem cell transplant recipients); cerebrospinal leak or cochlear implants; and receipt of oseltamivir (Tamiflu) or zanamivir (Relenza) in the previous 48 hours, peramivir (Rapivab) in the previous 5 days, or baloxavir (Xofluza) in the previous 17 days. The LAIV4 should not be administered to those with severe nasal congestion. Adverse effects of the LAIV4 include runny nose, nasal congestion, headache, sore throat, chills, and tiredness, although these are only slightly more common than in patients receiving placebo. Those receiving the LAIV4 should avoid contact with severely immunosuppressed persons for 7 days.

Patients should be vaccinated in the fall when the seasonal vaccine becomes available, even as early as August. In the event of vaccine shortages, higher-risk patients should receive priority (see Box 1). Patients should continue to be vaccinated until February and beyond because in the majority of recent influenza seasons the peak has been February or later. Children 6 months to 8 years of age who have not been previously immunized against influenza should be given two doses separated by at least 4 weeks.

BOX 1 Influenza Vaccine Recommendations.

- All persons aged ≥6 months should be vaccinated annually
- Vaccination efforts should prioritize essential workers and people at higher risk of influenza and COVID-19 complications:
  - Age 6 months to 5 years
  - Age ≥50 years
  - Chronic pulmonary (including asthma), cardiovascular (except hypertension), renal, hepatic, neurologic, hematologic, or metabolic (including diabetes mellitus) disorders
  - Immunosuppressed
  - Pregnant during the influenza season
  - Age 6 months to 18 years old receiving long-term aspirin therapy and who therefore might be at risk for Reye syndrome
  - Residents of nursing homes and other long-term care facilities
  - American Indians/Alaska Natives
  - Morbidly obese (body mass index ≥40)
- Vaccination efforts should also prioritize those likely to transmit influenza to higher risk people:
  - Healthcare personnel
  - Household contacts and caregivers of children aged <5 years and adults aged ≥50 years, with particular emphasis on vaccinating contacts of children aged <6 months
  - Household contacts and caregivers of persons with medical conditions that put them at higher risk for severe complications from influenza

---

Evaluation

Community Prevalence of Influenza

In caring for a patient with suspected influenza, the single most important piece of data is the community prevalence of influenza among patients with influenza-like illness. This ranges from near 0% during summer months to approximately 30% during a typical influenza seasonal peak. The prevalence may be higher during a particularly severe outbreak. In the United States clinicians can check the local prevalence of influenza and COVID-19 among patients with influenza-like illness through the CDC (www.cdc.gov/flu) and their state department of public health.

History and Physical Examination

Beyond the local prevalence of influenza, the diagnosis of influenza rests on the patient's history. All methods of diagnosing influenza—symptom complexes, clinician judgment, and testing—generally are highly specific but have poor sensitivity. Thus it is important to consider a diagnosis of influenza in any patient with respiratory symptoms during influenza season. Influenza is classically described as the very sudden onset of fever, headache, sore throat, myalgias, cough, and nasal symptoms. Children can also have otitis media, nausea, and vomiting. In differentiating influenza from nonspecific upper respiratory tract infections, it is most useful to consider the circulating prevalence of influenza, the abruptness of onset, and the severity of symptoms. Although COVID-19 and influenza symptoms overlap, COVID-19 may be more likely to include more profound shortness of breath, loss of taste or smell, nausea, vomiting, or diarrhea.

Certain symptom complexes have been shown in trials of antiviral treatment to strongly suggest influenza. For example, in an area with circulating influenza, prior to the emergence of SARS-CoV-2, the acute onset of cough and fever can have a positive predictive value as high as 85%. Other studies have shown that clinician judgment performed as well as or better than hard-and-fast symptom complexes or rapid testing.

The physical examination in influenza primarily serves to identify the severity of influenza, complications, and worsening of underlying medical conditions. Clinicians should record vital signs and perform examinations of the ears, nose, sinuses, throat, neck, lungs, and heart for all patients suspected of having influenza.

Testing

Testing may not be required to make a diagnosis of clinical influenza, but can help differentiate influenza from other respiratory viruses. Treatment for patients at high risk for influenza complications should not wait for test results. Testing may also help inform antiviral use, antibiotic prescribing, site-of-care decisions, and infection control measures. Specimens (nasopharyngeal swab, nasal swab, nasal wash, or nasal aspirate, depending on the particular test) should ideally be collected within 3 to 4 days of symptom onset.

Molecular assays such as reverse transcriptase polymerase chain reaction (RT-PCR) testing are highly sensitive (90% to 95%) and specific. Some can produce results in 15 to 45 minutes, and some can differentiate influenza types and subtypes. RT-PCR should be considered for hospitalized patients, institutional outbreaks, or other situations when clinicians are concerned about false-negative rapid test results. Other nucleic acid amplification tests, which can differentiate influenza from other respiratory pathogens, are becoming more available. The CDC recommends that all hospitalized patients with suspected influenza be tested with a high-sensitivity, high-specificity molecular assay.

Rapid influenza diagnostic tests (RIDTs) are much less sensitive (50% to 70%) and somewhat less specific (90%) than molecular tests. Negative results do not exclude the possibility of influenza, especially if the circulating prevalence of influenza is high (>30%). Some RIDTs can distinguish influenza A from influenza B and can provide a point-of-care result in less than 15 minutes.

In the event of a high prevalence of influenza or a high risk of complications from influenza, empiric antiviral treatment is indicated. Testing may be particularly helpful for hospitalized patients to rule out a need for antibiotics, but antiinfluenza treatment should not be withheld solely on the basis of a negative test result. Chest radiography, cultures, and blood tests are not routinely indicated, but they should be obtained for patients with suspected pneumonia or to identify other suspected complications.

Complications

Complications of influenza include primary complications, suppurative complications, and worsening of comorbid conditions. Primary complications of influenza include viral pneumonia, which is a feared complication and is likely a main cause of death in pandemic influenza. Other, less common primary complications of influenza include myositis and rhabdomyolysis, Reye syndrome, myocarditis, pericarditis, toxic shock syndrome, and central nervous system disease (e.g., encephalitis, transverse myelitis, and aseptic meningitis). Children can have a severe course with influenza, including signs and symptoms of sepsis along with febrile seizures. Suppurative complications of influenza include bacterial pneumonia, otitis media, and sinusitis. Influenza can cause worsening of comorbid conditions such as asthma, chronic obstructive pulmonary disease, congestive heart failure, and chronic kidney disease.

Chemoprophylaxis

Antiviral medications can be used to prevent influenza in patients who did not receive the influenza vaccine, cannot receive the influenza vaccine, received the vaccine in the prior 2 weeks (before reliable immunity develops), or in the event of poor matching between vaccine and circulating influenza strains (Table 1). Chemoprophylaxis should also be considered for close contacts of patients with confirmed influenza or for patients with immune deficiency who are unlikely to respond to the influenza vaccine but who are at high risk for having complications from influenza (see Box 1).

Amantadine (Symmetrel) and rimantadine (Flumadine) are not recommended for chemoprophylaxis or treatment because of a high prevalence of resistant influenza A strains. The neuraminidase inhibitors oseltamivir (Tamiflu), and zanamivir (Relenza) are approximately 80% effective in preventing influenza in household contacts of persons with influenza, and more than 90% effective in preventing influenza in institutional settings. Chemoprophylaxis should be taken for 7 days after last known exposure. For hospital or long-term care facility outbreaks, chemoprophylaxis should be taken and for a minimum of 2 weeks or until 1 week after the end of the outbreak. For patients allergic to or unable to respond to the vaccine, chemoprophylaxis should be used for the duration of circulating influenza. The IIV can be given to patients receiving chemoprophylaxis. The LAIV should not be given from 2 days before to 14 days after taking an antiviral medication. Patients who receive the LAIV in this window should be revaccinated at a later date.

TABLE 1 Antiviral Agents for the Treatment and Prophylaxis of Influenza.

ANTIVIRAL AGENT	TREATMENT*		PROPHYLAXIS†		COMMENTS
	CHILDREN	ADULTS	CHILDREN	ADULTS	
Oseltamivir (Tamiflu)	Any age‡ Dose for 5 days bid: <1 year: 3 mg/kg per dose; ≤15 kg: 30 mg; 16–23 kg: 45 mg; 24–40 kg: 60 mg; >40 kg: 75 mg	75 mg PO bid for 5 days	3 months to 1 year: 3 mg/kg/day‡ Dose qd: ≤15 kg: 30 mg; 16–23 kg: 45 mg; 24–40 kg: 60 mg; >40 kg: 75 mg	75 mg PO qd	For patients with creatinine clearance < 30 mL/min, oseltamivir adult dosing should be reduced to 30 mg qd for treatment and to 30 mg qod for prophylaxis
Zanamivir (Relenza)	Approved for children ≥7 years; 10 mg (2 inhalations) bid for 5 days	10 mg (2 inhalations) bid for 5 days	Approved for children ≥5 years; 10 mg (2 inhalations) qd	10 mg (2 inhalations) qd	Avoid in patients with chronic lung disease (e.g., asthma, chronic obstructive pulmonary disease)
Peramivir (Rapivab)	2–12 years: One 12-mg/kg dose, up to 600 mg maximum IV over minimum 15 min	≥13 years: One 600-mg IV dose over a minimum of 15 min	NA	NA	For patients with creatinine clearance 30–49 mL/min, the dose should be reduced to 200 mg; For patients with creatinine clearance 10–29 mL/min, the dose should be reduced to 100 mg
Baloxavir (Xofluza)	≥12 years and older weighing at least 40 kg: one 40-mg dose	40 to <80 kg: one 40-mg dose; ≥80 kg: one 80-mg dose	≥12 years of age following contact with an individual who has influenza. Dose: <80 kg: 1 40 mg tablet ≥80 kg: 1 80 mg tablet	NA	For patients within 2 days of illness onset. Avoid in pregnant women or breastfeeding mothers

*Suspected or confirmed influenza among persons with severe influenza or for persons at higher risk for influenza complications up to 5 days after symptom onset. For outpatients not at higher risk for influenza complications, treatment should be started within 48 hours of symptom onset.

†Prophylaxis should be given for 7 days after last known exposure and for institutional outbreaks for at least 2 weeks or until 1 week after the end of the outbreak.

‡Oseltamivir is approved by the US Food and Drug Administration for treatment in children 14 days and older and prophylaxis in children 1 year and older. Treatment in children <14 days old and prophylaxis in children <1 year old is recommended by the Centers for Disease Control and Prevention and the American Academy of Pediatrics.

IV, Intravenous; NA, not approved; PO, per os (orally).

Adapted from Centers for Disease Control and Prevention. Influenza Antiviral Medications: Summary for Clinicians. Available at http://www.cdc.gov/flu/professionals/antivirals/ (accessed June 14, 2021).

Treatment

The influenza vaccine is the best means of reducing influenza-related morbidity and mortality, but its limitations include production problems, low vaccination rates, and variable effectiveness. Given these limitations, there is an important role in management for influenza-specific antiviral medications (see Table 1). Antiviral medications reduce the duration of influenza symptoms by approximately 1 day, reduce complications requiring antibiotics by 30% to 50%, might decrease hospitalizations, decrease mortality among hospitalized patients, and are cost-effective. Early antiviral treatment, which should not wait for test results, starting up to 5 days after symptom onset can reduce complications for patients who are hospitalized; have severe, complicated, or progressive illness; or are at higher risk for complications (see Box 1). For outpatients not at higher risk for complications, antiviral treatment must be started within 48 hours of symptom onset.

Oseltamivir (Tamiflu) is taken as a capsule or oral suspension. The dose of oseltamivir should be reduced in patients with renal disease. Adverse effects of oseltamivir include nausea, vomiting, and perhaps behavioral changes. Oseltamivir, oral or enterically administered, is the drug of choice for hospitalized patients and those with severe illness. Zanamivir (Relenza) is taken as an oral inhaled powder and is not recommended for patients with underlying lung or heart disease. Adverse effects of zanamivir include worsening of underlying lung disease and allergic reactions. Amantadine and rimantadine are not recommended because of a high prevalence of resistant influenza A strains.

Peramivir (Rapivab), an intravenous neuraminidase inhibitor, was approved in the United State in December 2014 for patients within 48 hours of symptom onset. Peramivir has been associated with diarrhea, rashes including Stevens-Johnson syndrome, and neuropsychiatric changes.

Baloxavir (Xofluza), a cap-dependent endonuclease inhibitor, is active against both influenza A and B. Baloxavir has been associated with diarrhea. It has the advantage of requiring only one dose.

Antibiotics are generally not necessary, but they should be prescribed to treat suppurative complications of influenza. Antitussives such as guaifenesin with codeine (Robitussin AC) help coughing patients to sleep at night. β-Agonists, such as albuterol (Proventil)[1], can help patients with cough, especially if there is wheezing on examination. Analgesics and antipyretics such as acetaminophen (Tylenol) and ibuprofen (Motrin) reduce fever and generally help patients to feel better. Patients should be encouraged to rest and drink plenty of fluids.

Patients with suspected influenza should minimize contact with others to avoid spreading the infection. Use of face masks and hand hygiene can reduce the transmission of influenza.

---

[1]Not FDA approved for this indication.

References

Centers for Disease Control and Prevention: Influenza (Flu): information for health professionals, http://www.cdc.gov/flu/professionals/index.htm. Accessed 3 July 2020.

Ebell MH, Afonso AM, Gonzales R, et al: Development and validation of a clinical decision rule for the diagnosis of influenza, *J Am Board Fam Med* 25:55–62, 2012.

Falsey AR, Murata Y, Walsh EE: Impact of rapid diagnosis on management of adults hospitalized with influenza, *Arch Intern Med* 167:354–360, 2007.

Grohskopf LA, Alyanak E, Broder KR, et al: Prevention and control of seasonal influenza with vaccines: Recommendations of the Advisory Committee on Immunization Practices — United States, 2020–21 Influenza Season, *MMWR Recomm Rep* 69(No. RR-8):1–24, 2020.

Tokars JI, Olsen SJ, Reed C: Seasonal incidence of symptomatic influenza in the United States, *Clin Infect Dis* 66:1511–1518, 2018.

LEISHMANIASIS

Method of
Luigi Gradoni, PhD

CURRENT DIAGNOSIS

- Infected tissues must be sampled for microscopy demonstration of *Leishmania* organisms in Giemsa-stained impression smears or cultures. Polymerase chain reaction (PCR) detection of *Leishmania* DNA increases diagnostic sensitivity.
- Different tissue samplings are performed depending on the clinical form of leishmaniasis: For visceral leishmaniasis, aspirate or biopsy specimens are obtained from spleen, bone marrow, the liver, or enlarged lymph nodes. For cutaneous and mucocutaneous leishmaniasis, the material is obtained by skin lesion scraping or biopsy.
- Serology is useful when the diagnosis of visceral leishmaniasis proves difficult with other methods.

CURRENT THERAPY

- The therapy of leishmaniasis relies on a limited number of drugs, most of which are old and relatively toxic. Systemic drug administration requires hospitalization and monitoring of the patient.
- The pentavalent antimony (Sb) drugs sodium stibogluconate (Pentostam)[10] and meglumine antimoniate (Glucantime)[2] are equivalent and used in all clinical forms of leishmaniasis. Dosage is Sb 20 mg/kg/day IM for 21 to 28 days. In cases of uncomplicated cutaneous leishmaniasis, use intralesional administration intermittently over 20 to 30 days.
- Liposomal amphotericin B (Ambisome) is the gold standard for treating visceral leishmaniasis. Dosage: Total dose of 18 to 21 mg/kg IV using one of the following schedules: 3 mg/kg/day on days 1 to 5 and 10; 3 mg/kg on days 1 to 5, day 14, and day 21; 10 mg/kg/day for 2 days.
- Amphotericin B desoxycholate (Fungizone) is used in visceral leishmaniasis[1] and mucocutaneous leishmaniasis. Dosage is 0.5 mg/kg IV every other day for 14 days.
- Other parenteral drugs: Pentamidine isethionate (Pentam 300)[1] is used to treat some forms of New World cutaneous leishmaniasis; dosage is 2 mg/kg IM every other day for 7 days. Paromomycin (aminosidine) sulfate[2] is used for Indian visceral leishmaniasis; dosage is 11 mg/kg/day IM for 21 days.
- Miltefosine (Impavido)[5] is recommended for visceral leishmaniasis therapy in India and Ethiopia and for cutaneous leishmaniasis therapy in Colombia and Bolivia. Dosage is 2.5 mg/kg/day (not exceeding 100 mg/day) PO for 28 days.

[1]Not FDA approved for this indication.
[2]Not available in the United States.
[5]Investigational drug in the United States.
[10]Available in the United States from the Centers for Disease Control and Prevention.

Epidemiology

Leishmaniases are diseases caused by members of the genus *Leishmania*, protozoan parasites infecting numerous mammal species, including humans. The flagellated forms (promastigotes) are transmitted by the bite of phlebotomine sand flies and multiply as aflagellated forms (amastigotes) within cells of the mononuclear phagocyte system. The diseases range over the intertropical zones of America and Africa and extend into temperate regions of Latin America, Southern Europe, and Asia. About 20 named *Leishmania* species and subspecies are pathogenic for humans, and 30 sand fly species are proven vectors. Each parasite species circulates in natural foci of infection where susceptible phlebotomines and mammals coexist. The epidemiology and clinical manifestations of the diseases are largely diverse, being usually grouped into two main entities: zoonotic leishmaniases, where domestic or wild animal reservoirs are involved in the transmission cycle and humans play a role of accidental host, and anthroponotic leishmaniases, where humans are the sole reservoir and source of the vector's infection.

Visceral leishmaniasis (VL) is caused by *Leishmania donovani* in the Indian subcontinent and East Africa (anthroponotic entity) and by *L. infantum (L. chagasi)* in the Mediterranan basin, parts of Central Asia, and Latin America (a zoonotic entity with domestic dogs acting as the main reservoir host). Several species of *Leishmania* cause cutaneous leishmaniasis (CL) or mucocutaneous (MCL) leishmaniasis. The most common are *L. major* (rural zoonotic entity) and *L. tropica* (urban anthroponotic entity) in the Old World and *L. mexicana, L. braziliensis, L. amazonensis, L. panamensis, L. guyanensis,* and *L. peruviana* (sylvatic zoonotic entities) in the New World.

Globally, 80 Old World and 21 New World countries are endemic for human leishmaniasis, with an estimated yearly incidence of 0.7 million to 1.2 million cases of CL forms and 0.2 million to 0.4 million cases of VL forms. Overall estimated prevalence is 12 million people with a disability-adjusted life years burden of 860,000 for men and 1.2 million for women. The disease affects the poorest people in the poorest countries: 72 are developing countries, of which 13 are among the least developed. The incidence is not uniformly distributed in endemic areas: 90% of CL cases are found in only seven countries (Afghanistan, Algeria, Brazil, Iran, Peru, Saudi Arabia, and Syria), whereas 90% of VL cases occur in rural and suburban areas of five countries (Bangladesh, India, Nepal, Sudan, and Brazil). These figures, however, must be regarded as underestimates; currently, it appears that the global incidence of human leishmaniases is higher than before, owing to environmental and human behavioral factors contributing to the changing landscape of these diseases.

Risk Factors

Risk factors for leishmaniasis are primarily associated with geographically and temporally defined human exposure to phlebotomine vectors. In the Old World, colonization and urbanization of desert areas have been identified as the major risk factor for outbreaks of zoonotic CL. Tourists and military personnel are often exposed to *L. major* or *L. tropica* infections in rural or urban endemic settings of North African and Middle Eastern countries. In the New World, the colonization of the primary forest associated with activities of deforestation, road building, mining, and tourism is responsible for the domestication of sylvatic cycles of CL and MCL agents. Increase in density and geographic range of phlebotomine vectors resulting from climate changes, together with the increased mobility of infected pet dogs, has been identified as a cause of northward spreading of zoonotic VL in Europe.

Individual risk factors play a major role in VL disease. Most of the *L. donovani* and *L. infantum* infections are asymptomatic or subclinical in well-nourished immunocompetent persons. Malnourished persons, infants younger than 2 years, and severely immunosuppressed adults are at high risk for acute VL when exposed to infection. Before the era of HAART (highly active antiretroviral therapy), the AIDS epidemics in southern Europe caused more than 2000 HIV and VL co-infection cases among men aged 39 years on average. Other conditions have been reported that influence the clinical outcome of VL, such as immunosuppressive therapies after organ transplantation, corticosteroid and anti–tumor necrosis factor α (TNF-α) treatments for immunologic disorders, hematologic neoplasia, and chronic conditions of hepatic cirrhosis. However, most acute VL episodes in adults remain unexplained. Other factors associated with impaired immune response to *Leishmania* (e.g., genetic factors) are probably involved.

Pathophysiology

Ingestion of metacyclic promastigotes inoculated by the vector in the skin is mediated by several types of receptors found in resident macrophages, monocytes, neutrophils, and dendritic cells. *Leishmania* lipophosphoglycan, the most abundant surface glycoconjugate, is the main factor of virulence. Once in the cell phagolysosome, amastigotes survive from hydrolase activity through pH acidification while selectively inhibiting production of reactive oxygen species. Multiplication of parasites, infection of new cells, and dissemination to tissues are contrasted by the host's inflammatory and specific immune responses. Even in most susceptible natural mammal hosts, most infections are efficiently controlled, giving rise to asymptomatic latent infections. Leishmaniases have typical immunologic polarity: Cure or control are associated with robust cellular immune responses driven by production of interleukin (IL) 12, whereas acute or chronic diseases are characterized by the absence of such responses and the presence of high levels of nonprotective serum antibodies, a condition often associated with high levels of IL-10 production. In spite of this polarity, analysis of cytokine patterns in tissues reveals a less-polar situation, as both T_H1 and T_H2 cytokines were found to be secreted in specimens from tissues infected with CL, MCL, and VL.

Prevention

There are no human vaccines available for the immune protection against leishmaniasis. Promising data on safety and immunogenicity have been provided for the only *Leishmania* candidate vaccine under development, consisting of the recombinant polyprotein antigen LEISH-F1 with MPL-SE as adjuvant. Preventive measures are thus limited to the individual protection from sand fly bites or to community protection through reservoir control. Individual protection is through the use of repellents or insecticide-impregnated nets. Reservoir control measures are largely diverse, depending on the epidemiologic entity of leishmaniasis. Examples related to zoonotic entities with synanthropic reservoir hosts are the destruction of rodent populations around human dwellings (e.g., to control zoonotic CL due to *L. major*) and the fight against canine infections through the mass use of topical insecticides or drug treatments (e.g., to control zoonotic VL due to *L. infantum*). Early diagnosis and treatment of human cases is the main control measure against anthroponotic entities of VL (*L. donovani*) and CL (*L. tropica*).

Clinical Manifestations
Visceral Disease

VL, also known as kala-azar, results from the multiplication of *Leishmania* in the phagocytes of the reticuloendothelial system. In endemic settings, the ratio of incident asymptomatic infections to incident clinical cases varies from 4:1 to 50:1 depending on the epidemiologic type (anthroponotic VL is normally more virulent) and the poverty of the affected country. Classic VL manifests as pallor, fever, and hard splenomegaly; hepatomegaly is less common. Laboratory findings document pancytopenia and hypergammaglobulinemia. The clinical incubation period ranges from 3 weeks (exceptional) to more than 2 years, but 4 to 6 months is average. Patients report a history of fever resistant to antibiotics; on physical examination, the spleen is typically appreciated 5 to 15 cm below the left costal margin. Symptomatic VL is 100% fatal when left untreated.

Cutaneous Disease

CL results from multiplication of *Leishmania* in the phagocytes of the skin. In the classic course of the disease, lesions appear first as papules, advance slowly to nodules or ulcers, and then spontaneously heal with scarring over months to years. The clinical incubation period ranges from 1 week (exceptional) to several months; lesions caused by *L. major* and *L. mexicana* tend to evolve and resolve quickly, whereas those caused by *L. braziliensis, L. tropica,* and dermotropic strains of *L. infantum* can have longer periods of incubation and spontaneous healing.

Mucosal Disease

MCL results from parasitic metastasis in the nasal mucosal that eventually extends to the oropharynx and larynx. It can develop from CL lesions caused by *L. braziliensis* and *L. panamensis.* Typically, MCL evolves slowly (3 years on average) and does not heal spontaneously.

Diagnosis

The standard diagnosis method for all forms of leishmaniasis is still the microscopy demonstration of *Leishmania* organisms in Giemsa-stained impression smears or cultures from samples of infected tissues. In general, sensitivity increases when both staining and culture are performed. Polymerase chain reaction (PCR) detection of *Leishmania* DNA on samples further increases the diagnostic sensitivity and also might allow species identification by target DNA sequencing or restriction fragment length polymorphism analysis.

Different tissue samplings must be performed depending on the clinical form of leishmaniasis. For VL, aspirate or biopsy specimens are obtained from the spleen, bone marrow, the liver, or enlarged lymph nodes. Higher diagnostic yields are obtained with spleen aspirates (more than 98%), although bone marrow aspirates (80% to 98% of yield) are usually preferred. For CL and MCL, material is obtained by scraping tissue juice from a nodular lesion or from the edge of an ulcer or by taking punch biopsies of inflamed tissue. Diagnostic yields of about 80% are obtained with impression smears and cultures during the first half of the natural course of the lesion. After that, standard parasitologic diagnosis becomes more difficult and PCR remains the only reliable method.

Serology is useful when the diagnosis of VL proves difficult with other methods. Commercially available dipstick tests using recombinant antigen K39 can be used in decisions for or against treatment. Negative serology results are common in CL and MCL, as well as in VL when patients are severely immunosuppressed.

Differential Diagnosis
Visceral Disease

The differential diagnosis depends on the local disease pattern associated with endemic areas. In many of them it includes chronic malaria, disseminated histoplasmosis, hepatosplenic schistosomiasis, typhoid fever, brucellosis, tuberculosis, endocarditis, relapsing fever, and African trypanosomiasis. Other cosmopolitan diseases include syphilis, lymphomas, chronic myeloid leukemia, sarcoidosis, malignant histiocytosis, and liver cirrhosis.

Cutaneous Disease

A typical history of CL—an inflammatory, slowly developing, and painless skin lesion associated with recent exposure to sand fly bites—can strongly support a clinical diagnosis of disease. However, there is an extensive differential diagnosis, which includes acute or chronic forms of CL. For the former, insect bites, furuncular myiasis, and bacterial tropical ulcers are the most common; for the latter, keloid, lupus vulgaris, discoid lupus erythematosus, and sarcoidosis.

Treatment

The therapy of leishmaniasis relies on a limited number of drugs, most of which are old and relatively toxic compounds. Systemic drug administration requires hospitalizing and monitoring the patient.

Pentavalent Antimonials

Organic salts of pentavalent antimony (Sb) are still the mainstay therapy for all clinical forms of leishmaniasis. Two preparations are available that are equal in efficacy and toxicity when used in equivalent Sb doses: sodium stibogluconate (Pentostam),[10] available in English-speaking countries, and meglumine antimoniate (Glucantime),[2] available in Southern Europe and Latin America.

The recommended dosage of Sb is 20 mg/kg/day for 21 to 28 days, given intramuscularly or intravenously. Treatment should be prolonged for 40 to 60 days in areas with documented Sb-resistant VL (e.g., in Bihar State, India). The drugs can be administered intralesionally in cases of uncomplicated CL, intermittently over 20 to 30 days. Systemic toxicity caused by the antimonials relates to the total dose administered and includes anorexia, pancreatitis, and changes on electrocardiography (e.g., prolongation of the QT interval), which can precede dangerous arrhythmias.

Amphotericin B Drugs

Liposomal amphotericin B (Ambisome) is the current gold standard for VL treatment, being highly effective and nontoxic. However, the high cost of the drug precludes its use in developing countries where leishmaniasis is endemic. Liposomal amphotericin B is given intravenously at the total dose of 18 to 21 mg/kg, with various treatment schedules similarly effective: 3 mg/kg/day on days 1 to 5 and 10; 3 mg/kg on days 1 to 5, 14, and 21; or 10 mg/kg/day for 2 days.

Amphotericin B desoxycholate (Fungizone) is a relatively toxic compound used in Sb-resistant VL[1] and MCL, administered intravenously at the low dosage of 0.5 mg/kg every other day for 14 days. Doses in excess of 1 mg/kg/day commonly result in severe infusion-related side effects (fever, chills, and bone pain) and delayed side effects (toxic renal effects).

Other Parenteral Drugs

Other parenteral drugs include old second-line drugs whose use is limited. Pentamidine isethionate (Pentam 300)[1] is a toxic compound used to treat some forms of New World CL resistant to Sb therapy and is given intramuscularly at the low dose of 2 mg/kg every other day for 7 days. Treatment in excess of this dosage can result in common side effects such as myalgias, nausea, headache, and hypoglycemia. Paromomycin (aminosidine) sulfate injection[2] (manufactured by Gland Pharma, India, on behalf of Institute of One World Health) is an old aminoglycoside that is being reevaluated as a first-line drug for Indian VL. It is given intramuscularly at the dose of 11 mg base per kg per day for 21 days. Elevation of alanine aminotranferease (ALT) and aspartate aminotransferase (AST) liver enzymes is usually seen during therapy.

Miltefosine, the First Oral Drug for Leishmaniasis

Miltefosine (Impavido)[5] is a hexadecylphosphocholine originally developed as an anticancer agent. It is the first recognized oral treatment for leishmaniasis and is available in Germany and India. So far, it is recommended for VL therapy in India and Ethiopia and for CL therapy in Colombia and Bolivia. The drug is administered at 2.5 mg/kg/day (not exceeding 100 mg/day) for 28 days. Miltefosine administration does not require the patient to be hospitalized for monitoring. Mild gastrointestinal toxicity may be common. The drug is contraindicated in pregnancy.

Monitoring

In VL patients, fever recedes by day 3 to 5 of treatment, and well-being returns by the first week. Hematologic indices start to improve during the second week. Hemoglobin, serum albumin, and body weight are the most useful indicators of progress. The spleen tends to normalize 1 to 2 months after the end of therapy, although it can take up to 1 year to regress completely. Parasitologic assessment of cure is not normally necessary. Relapses can occur after apparent clinical cure from 2 to 8 months after treatment has been discontinued.

In CL patients, clinical response to drugs is rapid, but complete reepithelialization of lesions is observed in only one third of patients by the end of 3- to 4-week treatment courses.

---

[2]Not available in the United States.
[10]Available in the United States from the Centers for Disease Control and Prevention.

---

[1]Not FDA approved for this indication.
[2]Not available in the United States.
[5]Investigational drug in the United States.

References

Alvar J, Aparicio P, Aseffa A, et al: The relationship between leishmaniasis and AIDS: The second 10 years, *Clin Microbiol Rev* 21:334–359, 2008.

Alvar J, Vélez ID, Bern C: Leishmaniasis worldwide and global estimates of its incidence, *PLoS One* 7:e35671, 2012.

Aronson N, Herwaldt BL, Libman L, et al: Diagnosis and treatment of leishmaniasis: clinical practice guidelines by the Infectious Diseases Society of America (IDSA) and the American Society of Tropical Medicine and Hygiene (ASTMH), *Clin Infect Dis* 63:e202–e264, 2016.

Berman JJ: Treatment of leishmaniasis with miltefosine: 2008 status, *Expert Opin Drug Metab Toxicol* 4:1209–1216, 2008.

Bern C, Adler-Moore J, Berenguer J, et al: Liposomal amphotericin B for the treatment of visceral leishmaniasis, *Clin Infect Dis* 43:917–924, 2006.

Bhattacharya SK, Sinha PK, Sundar S, et al: Phase 4 trial of miltefosine for the treatment of Indian visceral leishmaniasis, *J Infect Dis* 196:591–668, 2007.

Chappuis F, Sundar S, Hailu A, et al: Visceral leishmaniasis: what are the needs for diagnosis, treatment and control? *Nat Rev Microbiol* 5:873–882, 2007.

González U, Pinart M, Rengifo-Pardo M, et al: Interventions for cutaneous and mucocutaneous leishmaniasis, *Cochrane Database Syst Rev*(2), 2009, CD004834.

Gradoni L, Soteriadou K, Louzir H, et al: Drug regimens for visceral leishmaniasis in Mediterranean countries, *Trop Med Int Health* 13:1272, 2008.

Gramiccia M, Gradoni L: The current status of zoonotic leishmaniases and approaches to disease control, *Int J Parasitol* 35:1169–1180, 2005.

Sundar S, Agrawal N, Arora R, et al: Short-course paromomycin treatment of visceral leishmaniasis in India: 14-day vs 21-day treatment, *Clin Infect Dis* 49:914–918, 2009.

LEPROSY

Method of
Carolina Talhari, MD, PhD; Maria Lucia Penna, MD, PhD; and Gerson O. Penna, MD, PhD

CURRENT DIAGNOSIS

- Contact of susceptible person with untreated leprosy cases; travel to or residence in a leprosy-endemic country
- Skin lesion(s) with altered sensation
- Thickened or enlarged peripheral nerve, with sensory loss and/or weakness in the muscles supplied by the nerve
- Presence of acid-fast bacilli in a slit skin smear
- Skin biopsy with the presence of acid-fast bacilli or typical lesions, thereby aiding disease classification

CURRENT THERAPY

Paucibacillary leprosy (6 months)
Adult (50–70 kg)
- Dapsone: 100 mg daily
- Rifampin (Rifadin)[1]: 600 mg once a month under supervision
- Clofazimine (Lamprene): 50 mg daily and 300 mg once a month under supervision

Child (under 10 years)
- Dapsone: 1 mg/kg daily
- Rifampin[1]: 10/kg mg once a month under supervision
- Clofazimine: 1 mg/kg/day

Multibacillary leprosy (12 months)
Adult (50–70 kg)
- Dapsone: 100 mg daily
- Rifampin (Rifadin)[1]: 600 mg once a month under supervision
- Clofazimine (Lamprene): 50 mg daily and 300 mg once a month under supervision

Child (under 10 years)
- Dapsone: 1 mg/kg daily
- Rifampin: 10/kg mg once a month under supervision
- Clofazimine: 1 mg/kg/day

[1]Not FDA approved for this indication.

Epidemiology

Leprosy is a chronic disease caused by *Mycobacterium leprae* that affects skin and nerves, often resulting in physical disabilities. The disease has been found around the world, showing that transmission occurs regardless of climate.

Disease transmission has ceased in nearly all developed nations, most likely because of better nutrition and socioeconomic development. Currently, new autochthonous cases are found in all tropical countries, with India and Brazil having the highest number of cases annually. Some insular countries located in the Pacific and Indian Oceans have the highest rates of new case detection, indicating a high risk of transmission.

In the Gulf region of the United States, mostly in the states of Louisiana and Texas, native cases are still diagnosed. There are armadillos (*Dasypus novemcinctus*) in the area that have been infected with strains of *M. leprae* found also in autochthonous human cases. This suggests that leprosy might be a regional zoonosis, even though *M. leprae* was introduced into the Americas by Europeans and Africans. There are also records of *M. leprae* infection in armadillos in Central and South America. Furthermore, cases in African chimpanzees raise the possibility that these animals could be helping to maintain leprosy transmission in Africa.

The mechanisms of leprosy transmission are not well known because there is no easy way to diagnose infection. It is presumed that in endemic areas, infection is much more frequent than actual disease onset. The incubation period can vary from a few months to more than 10 years, with an average of 2 to 5 years for paucibacillary (PB) and 5 to 10 years for multibacillary (MB).

It is known that MB cases excrete large numbers of viable bacilli through nasal mucus, suggesting that transmission may be by respiratory route, and, in fact, this is believed to be the main source of transmission. Because *M. leprae* can be eliminated from ulcerated skin lesions, breast milk, urine, and feces, and remains viable in the environment for many days, especially in humid climates, it is possible to theorize the existence of many different forms of transmission. The role of insects as vectors of bacilli is arguable.

Leprosy cases are not uniformly distributed in a community but tend to form clusters within different geographic regions, villages, or groups of domiciles. In most countries, cases are more common among men, and the 15- to 29-year-old age group tends to present the highest risk of disease. In areas where transmission is declining, the incidence tends to be higher among the elderly, affecting those who lived during a period with a higher risk of infection.

Until recently, *M. leprae* was the only agent responsible for leprosy until, in 2008, a new species called *Mycobacterium lepromatosis* sp. was described in Mexico as responsible for a diffuse form of the disease associated with increased morbidity and mortality. However, the clinical significance of this new entity, both in magnitude and in distribution, as well as particularities of the immune response to this pathogen, are not well known.

Risk Factors

In endemic areas, the main risk factors are a history of household contact with leprosy cases and low socioeconomic standing. It is estimated that home contacts of MB patients show a 5 to 10 times increased risk of becoming ill; PB case contacts present a 2 to 3 times increased risk, compared with a group with no history of home exposure. In general, the increased risk between contacts reflects the proximity of these individuals, inside the house, with the potential source of infection. Also important is the sharing of other factors by household members, such as genetic markers, behavior, diet, intercurrent infections, and contextual aspects related to socioeconomic and environmental conditions.

An important fact in leprosy is that, even when living for a long time and in the same house with an untreated MB patient, most people do not get sick. It is estimated that 90% of the population have natural defenses against *M. leprae*. Today, there is evidence that susceptibility and resistance to *M. leprae* are genetically determined. The low frequency of genetically determined susceptibility may be the cause of the wide difference between infection and disease that is believed to exist.

Recent studies confirmed the association between risk of incident leprosy and socioeconomic factors as demonstrated by the Norwegian study almost a century ago.

Prevention

Vaccination with bacille Calmette-Guerin (BCG)[1] reduces the risk of leprosy, with studies showing a variable efficacy of 20% to 80%. The revaccination of household contacts also provides protection, especially against the MB forms of the disease.

Chemoprophylaxis of contacts or high-risk groups with a single dose of rifampin (Rifadin)[1] has been shown to be effective for a period of 2 years. However, although the chemoprophylaxis trials reported a benefit, the relatively short duration of protection indicates functional limitations.

Combined strategies, including the integration of rapid diagnostic tests to facilitate the detection of early or asymptomatic leprosy cases, as well as both chemoprophylaxis and immunization, is suggested as an active control strategy with a great potential of reducing the incidence of leprosy.

Improving socioeconomic conditions in the general population in endemic areas is also a very effective strategy for disease control. This can be seen when comparing the current epidemiologic situation in the Hawaiian Islands with Micronesia or the Marshall Islands, where leprosy continues with a high incidence rate.

Pathophysiology

M. leprae is an intercellular microorganism with a particular tropism for skin and peripheral nerve cells. It cannot be cultivated in vitro, but can be inoculated in mouse footpads and armadillos, although growth is quite slow. Active *M. leprae* infection is characterized by a wide clinical range, varying from a disease in which few bacilli are present in the body to one in which a high bacterial load is found in skin lesions.

Upon entering the organism, *M. leprae*, through its PAMPS (molecular patterns associated with pathogens), is recognized by pattern recognition receptors (PRRs) expressed in antigen-presenting cells (APCs), mainly dendritic cells (DCs), macrophages, monocytes, fibroblasts, and Schwann cells. Thus the innate immune response of the host is initiated, in which the bacilli can be eliminated with a local inflammatory response, avoiding the disease, or, when this does not occur, the innate immunity can, according to the pattern of cytokines produced by APCs, regulate the response of host adaptive immunity.

In the adaptive immunity, the bacilli multiply within macrophages, enter the lymph stream and bloodstream, reach the regional lymph nodes, and from there move on to the organs of the mononuclear phagocyte system. The mycobacterial antigens are then processed and presented by APCs that can be Langerhans cells, DCs, or others from the monocyte-macrophage system that induce the hapten-protein conjugates to link the HLA-DR class II molecules to the CD4 þ lymphocytes. In those individuals where there is stimulation of the T-helper 1 cell response, these lymphocytes will produce interferon (IFN)-gamma cytokines, tumor necrosis factor (TNF-α), interleukin-2 (IL-2), IL-17, IL1-β, and IL-12 that will promote the differentiation of macrophages in epithelioid cells that will undergo a fusion process resulting in giant cells. This inflammatory response will be sufficient to reduce *M. leprae* in the tuberculoid form of leprosy. In the presence of massive tissue infiltration by CD4 T lymphocytes, large production of these cytokines occurs along with the chemokine CXCL-10, leading to edema and tissue inflammation of the leprosy type 1 reaction. The production of TNF-α and IFN-γ by Schwann cells will lead to neural damage, which is also more significant in the type 1 reaction.

On the other hand, in the presence of stimulation of the TH2 subpopulation of T lymphocytes (TLs), these will produce the cytokines IL-4, IL-5, IL-6, IL-13, TNF-α, and IL-10 and TGF-β, these two produced by regulatory T lymphocytes (T-reg). The

TGF-β, IL-4, and IL-10 are suppressors of macrophage activation, leading to an insufficient immune cell response to combat the level of *M. leprae* proliferation within the macrophages. This characterizes the more infectious forms of the disease at the lepromatous end of the spectrum. The cytokines IL-4, IL-5, IL-6, and IL-13 activate plasma cells and B lymphocytes, which together with complement activation, will form the immunocomplexes that will trigger leprosy type 2 reactions.

Clinical Manifestations

Due to the complexity of the parasite-host relation and the variable efficacy of the host's cellular immune response, the clinical manifestations of the disease cross a wide spectrum. This can vary from an isolated nerve lesion or a single skin patch to a systemic disease with the presence of nodules or tubercles, generally on the face. The disease can affect several organs beyond skin and nerves, including eyes, testicles, and kidneys.

Ridley and Jopling, in 1966, proposed a case classification system that takes into consideration clinical, bacteriologic, histopathologic, and immunologic parameters: tuberculoid (TL), borderline-tuberculoid (BTL), borderline-borderline (BBL), borderline-lepromatous (BLL), and lepromatous (LL). Indeterminate leprosy (IL) can be considered the first clinical manifestation of the disease. It can be cured spontaneously or evolve into one of the other clinical forms.

Indeterminate Leprosy

This is characterized by one or more hypochromic macules with imprecise borders and reduced thermal sensitivity, although pain and tactile sensation may be preserved (Figure 1). These may occur as areas of sensory disturbance with no alteration in skin color, sweat glands, or hair growth. Any alteration in nerve function is preliminary and, therefore, there are no physical disabilities described with this classification. Bacilloscopic readings are negative.

Tuberculoid Leprosy

This type is characterized by erythematous or hypochromic skin lesions with clear, raised borders (Figure 2). These are limited in number with an asymmetrical distribution and altered thermal sensation. Pain and tactile sensation may also be altered. Reduced perspiration and restricted partial or full alopecia may also be seen. Nerves can be affected intensively but this usually only happens to a few. Slit skin smear results are negative.

Among children, TL lesions may have the appearance of nodules or tubercles, generally only one on the face, named nodular benign leprosy of childhood. Although these lesions tend to regress spontaneously, treatment should continue as per standard ethical practice.

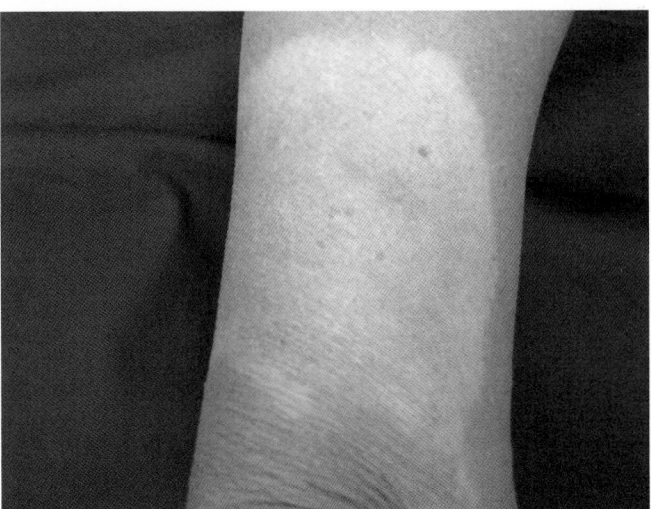

Figure 1 Indeterminate leprosy.

---

[1]Not FDA approved for this indication.

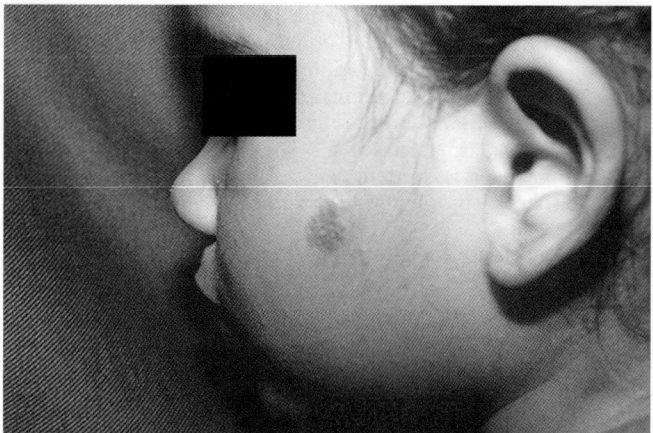
Figure 2 Tuberculoid leprosy in child.

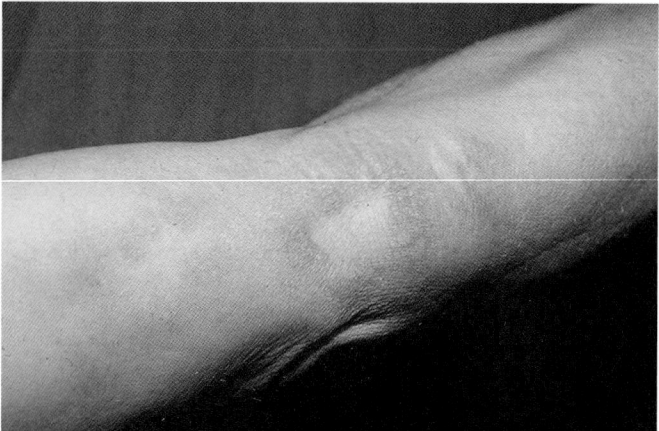
Figure 4 Borderline-borderline leprosy.

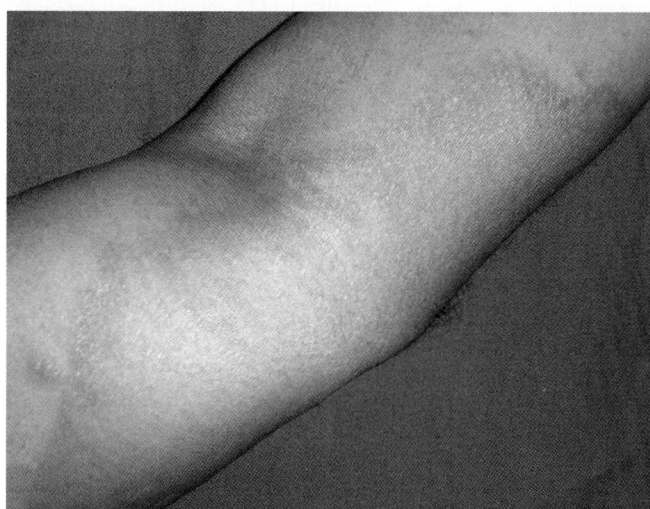
Figure 3 Borderline-tuberculoid leprosy.

Borderline-Tuberculoid Leprosy
This form is characterized by lesions similar to those seen at the TL end of the spectrum, although more numerous. In general, there are more than five lesions with a diameter of 10 cm or more, less clearly defined borders, and containing possible satellite lesions (Figure 3). These lesions tend to be more symmetrical and several nerves may be affected. However, most patients with this disease type will still have a negative bacilloscopy.

Borderline-Borderline Leprosy
This is a relatively rare variation, given that it commonly evolves quickly toward the lepromatous pole, often spurred on by reaction episodes. There are usually many foveal lesions (infiltrated plaques with expanding outer borders and well-defined inner borders with apparently normal skin in the middle) (Figure 4). Generally, nerves are intensively affected, and skin smears are almost always positive.

Borderline-Lepromatous (Virchowian) Leprosy
A wide number of lesions are present with a range of possible clinical manifestations (infiltrations, papules, plaques, foveae, and nodules) that are common to the lepromatous form. However, with this type there is a tendency to see some delimitation between the lesions and areas of healthy skin. Bacilloscopy is positive with a high bacterial load.

Lepromatous (Virchowian) Leprosy
This form has the highest bacterial burden of human bacterial infections. Extensive lesions tend to be symmetrical, erythematous, infiltrated, and without clear delineation from normal skin areas. Simple lesions evolve to become papules, tubercles, and

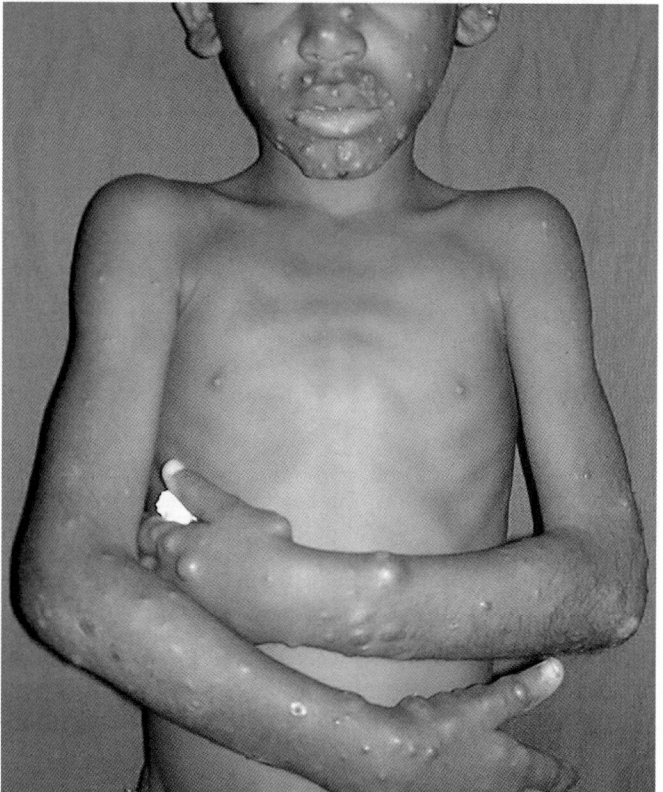
Figure 5 Lepromatous (Virchowian) leprosy.

nodules that can eventually ulcerate and that are especially full of bacilli (Figure 5). There is diffuse infiltration of the face, with auricular appendages affected in the vast majority of cases and bilateral madarosis also common. Hands and feet may also be infiltrated or showing signs of xerodermia.

LL is a systemic disease that can affect, when patients are not treated properly and opportunely, the liver, spleen, adrenal glands, lymph nodes, eyes, and nose. Nasal obstruction can be present with little or no response to vasoconstrictors. Often the nasal cavities will be affected, and the oropharynges will be full of nasal secretion highly abundant in bacilli. Subsequent nasal dryness can lead to secondary ulceration and infection with possible perforation and destruction of the nasal septum, resulting in what is commonly referred to as saddle nose. With olfactory bulb dysfunction, anosmia will often be the outcome.

Lesions to the palate, lips, gum, and uvula can further compromise the pharynx, nasopharynx, and tonsils. The eyes may show erythema, dryness, dacryocystitis, lagophthalmos, and/or diminished sensation in the cornea. Likewise, iritis and iridocyclitis

TABLE 1	Main Differential Diagnosis by Leprosy Forms	
INDETERMINATE LEPROSY	**TUBERCULOID AND BORDERLINE-TUBERCULOID LEPROSY**	**BORDERLINE-BORDERLINE, BORDERLINE-LEPROMATOUS, AND LEPROMATOUS LEPROSY**
Eczematidis (Pityriasis alba)	Seborrheic dermatitis	Erythema nodosum
Seborrheic dermatitis	Dermatofitosis	Diffuse (anergic) cutaneous leishmaniasis
Localized scleroderma (morphea)	Granuloma annulare	Cutaneous and mucosal leishmaniasis
Residual hypochromia and achromia	Cutaneous leishmaniasis	Systemic lupus erythematous and other rheumatologic diseases
Pityriasis versicolor	Discoid lupus erythematous	Neurofibromatosis (von Recklinghausen disease)
Vitiligo	Pityriasis rosea Gibert	Pityriasis rosea Gibert
Hypochromic nevus	Psoriasis	Congenital syphilis, secondary syphilis, tertiary syphilis
	Sarcoidosis	Cutaneous lymphoma (Mycosis fungoides)
	Secondary syphilis	
	Cutaneous tuberculosis	

may be present, so proper intervention is necessary to ensure prevention of early onset of blindness.

The testes may also be directly affected by bacilli, as witnessed by atrophy of the testicular parenchyma and diffuse fibrosis with eventual sterility and alteration of sexual function. When secondary amyloidosis is present, renal insufficiency may result.

Variations of Lepromatous Leprosy
Histoid Lepromatous Leprosy (or Wade's Lepromatous)
This form of leprosy is rare. Nodular lesions are present, well defined, and of varying sizes. These may be round or oval with a reddish or pink color. These lesions contain a large number of bacilli and are normally associated with sulfone resistance. Histiocytes with a spongy appearance are present under histologic analysis.

Diffuse Lepromatous Leprosy
Described by Lucio, Alvarado, and Latapi, this is a diffuse form of LL, also called "beautiful" leprosy because this form confers a pinkish and healthy appearance to the skin. It is more frequently seen in Mexico and is characterized by the diffuse infiltration of the skin, altered sensation that starts in the hands and feet, loss of eyebrows, and telangiectasias in the face and torso. Recently a mycobacterium was isolated in cases of diffuse lepromatous leprosy (DLL) with Lucio phenomenon, whose DNA cannot be amplified using usual *M. leprae* primers. As a result, a new species has been proposed under the name *M. lepromatosis*, but many specialists do not yet accept that this is a separate microorganism.

Pure Neural Leprosy
This type presents only nerve lesions without any cutaneous patches. The most common nerves affected are the ulnar, tibial, and fibular. The radial, median, facial, trigeminal, and auricular nerves, among others, may also be damaged.

Neuropathic pain is often present spontaneously or when the nerve is palpated, either with or without thickening of the nerve. This can evolve to sensory loss, paresthesia, or muscular atrophy in the corresponding area, in addition to autonomic dysfunction and nerve abscess.

Leprosy Diagnosis
The patient is examined to locate any possible skin lesions with diminished sensation and/or areas of sensory alteration that may be due to compromised peripheral nerves. Lighting must be adequate, and it is important to observe the entire body surface moving from head to toe. Where there are possible signs of disease, thermal, pain, and tactile sensation testing should be done, also looking for areas of alopecia and/or anhidrosis. It must be noted if there is any type of physical disability.

Bacilloscopy consists of the collection and examination of skin smears taken from a suspected lesion, both earlobes, and

both elbows, and helps to classify a patient as PB with a negative examination result or MB when positive.

The bacilloscopic results will generally be negative in the IL, TL, and BTL, which are considered the PB group. Similarly, they tend to be positive in LL, BLL, and BBL, which are MB group.

Ideally, the bacilloscopic reading should be expressed quantitatively as a bacteriologic index (BI) so that it is possible to monitor the patient's progress during treatment. In patients with positive bacilloscopy at the time of diagnosis, it is recommended to repeat it at the end of therapy. Smear microscopy is important for differential diagnoses between reactions and relapse.

The histologic examination of a skin biopsy also helps to provide a more precise disease classification and can help confirm diagnosis in cases that are bacilloscopy negative. In IL, there is a nonspecific inflammatory infiltrate, consisting of lymphocytes and sometimes histiocytes, around superficial and deep vessels, affecting the cutaneous appendages, especially the neural fillets. The TL and BTL forms are characterized histologically by the presence of granulomas-histiocytes, which differentiate into epithelioid cells, giant cells, and lymphocytes, located around vessels, cutaneous appendages, and nervous fillets. Bacillus research is almost always negative. In BLL and LL forms, the inflammatory infiltrate is characterized by the predominance of foamy or vacuolated histiocytes, with large numbers of bacilli, isolated or grouped in structures called globias.

In regions with limited access to laboratory resources, clinical diagnosis is sufficient to warrant the beginning of the standard leprosy treatment regimen, keeping in mind that this is the only dermatologic disease with altered sensation in lesions. The World Health Organization (WHO) suggests the classification of cases as either PB or MB based on the number of skin lesions, with MB cases having five or more such patches.

Available serologic testing does not show sufficient accuracy for disease diagnosis or infection. A recent meta-analysis using a fixed model to estimate or for the association of phenolic glycolipid (PGL)-1 positivity and clinical leprosy demonstrated that PGL-1 appears not to be a useful test in the decision of which contacts should receive chemoprophylaxis.

Real-time polymerase chain reaction is available for leprosy and can act as a means of confirmation for diagnosis of PB cases.

Differential Diagnosis
Differential diagnoses of leprosy include a variety of dermatologic conditions, given the wide range of clinical manifestations in leprosy. The sensory loss symptomatic of leprosy can also be difficult to determine in children and in other diseases that produce changes in the normal skin characteristics (Table 1).

Treatment
Leprosy treatment, like tuberculosis treatment, must deal with bacillar resistance and persistence. Single-drug therapy selects

drug-resistant bacilli and should be avoided. Therapy duration has, as a target, the reduction of the number of persistent bacilli that could lead to relapses.

Standard multidrug therapy (MDT) with dapsone, rifampin (Rifadin),[1] and clofazimine (Lamprene) for 12 months for MB cases and 6-month MDT with dapsone and rifampin for PB cases has dramatically changed the prognosis for leprosy patients. However, the evidence is rather weak on the efficacy of this drug regimen, especially regarding the necessary length of time for treatment, both in terms of the proportion of relapse cases and other outcomes, such as physical disability. The use of rifampin once a month was determined for financial reasons, and there is no study comparing this schedule with daily use. For this reason, research on new drugs and treatment regimens continues.

Shorter regimens were used but had shown high relapse rates: daily doses of rifampin[1] and ofloxacin (Floxin)[1] for 4 weeks; single-dose course of rifampin, ofloxacin, and minocycline (Minocin)[1] for single-lesion patients.

Fluoroquinolones (pefloxacin,[2] ofloxacin, and moxifloxacin [Avelox][1]), macrolides (clarithromycin [Biaxin][1]), and tetracycline (minocycline) are effective against *M. leprae*. Only rifampin, its derivative rifapentine (Priftin),[1] and moxifloxacin are bactericidal drugs; all others are bacteriostatic.

In cases of intolerance or resistance to dapsone, this can be removed from the drug regimen, and for PB patients, clofazimine is used instead. For MB patients, in these cases, minocycline or ofloxacin can be used instead of dapsone, without alteration in treatment duration. Where similar intolerance or resistance is related to rifampin, this should be substituted with a daily dose of 400 mg of ofloxacin. This alternate course lasts 6 months for cases and 24 months for MB.

For those who cannot take either dapsone or rifampin, PB patients can be treated with ofloxacin (400 mg/day) or minocycline (100 mg/day), and clofazimine (50 mg/day) in self-administered doses for 6 months. Similarly, MB patients can use ofloxacin plus minocycline plus clofazimine during the first 6 months of treatment (intensive phase), followed by 18 months with daily doses of ofloxacin or minocycline and clofazimine (maintenance phase).

Perspectives on the Use of a Uniform Treatment for All Forms, Regardless of Clinical or Laboratory Classification

Despite the success of MDT, the complexity for the operationalization of the scheme throughout the health system, the prolonged treatment time, and the difficulty of patient adherence reinforce the need for shorter regimens that can be easily implemented in primary care. Since 2002, the WHO recommended clinical studies to investigate the viability of a uniform treatment (U-MDT) for all leprosy cases, regardless of classification, with 6 months' duration.

The first randomized and controlled study on U-MDT, "Estudo independente para determinar efetividade do esquema Uniforme de MDT de seis doses (U-MDT) em pacientes de hanseníase, (U-MDT-CT- BR)," was performed in Brazil and evaluated the efficacy of daily intake of dapsone plus clofazimine and monthly rifampicin for 6 months for both PB and MB leprosy patients, regardless of classification criteria. Between 2012 and 2018, 14 scientific articles were published from U-MDT-CT-BR; these showed that the reduction in the duration of treatment did not increase relapse rates, reaction frequency, or neural damage. The Brazilian study also demonstrated no statistical differences in BI decline, between regular MDT and U-MDT. Moreover, the same study showed that U-MDT reduced *M. leprae*-specific antibodies during and after treatment.

Together with the results from three previous studies performed in China, India, and Bangladesh, U-MDT-CT-BR support the premise that U-MDT is an acceptable option to be adopted in endemic countries to treat leprosy patients in the field worldwide. These studies led WHO to recommend the addition of clofazimine to the PB treatment in 2019.

A recent study showed the existence of a high susceptibility genetic profile among leprosy patients predisposing to disease recurrence. The authors showed that recurrence or reinfection is not related to time of treatment but rather to individual genetic susceptibility. Additionally, a population-based study for the search for *M. leprae* resistance reported the emergence and transmission of resistant strains in a former leprosy colony located in the Brazilian Amazon. Taken together, these studies demonstrated the need to save the unnecessary use of these drugs and strongly support the decision to adopt the shorter uniform treatment for leprosy.

Dapsone and rifampin resistance have been reported. Although reports of clofazimine-resistant isolates of *M. leprae* are rare, multidrug-resistant leprosy reports are increasing and should be regularly monitored.

Leprosy Reactions and Control

Over the course of this chronic disease, around 30% of the patients develop acute inflammatory episodes called leprosy reactions. These reactions can occur before diagnosis, as well as during or after MDT treatment. They are commonly grouped into (1) type 1 (reversal) reactions (T1Rs) resulting from vigorous cell-mediated immune response and (2) type 2 reactions (T2Rs), the clinical manifestation of which is frequently erythematous nodosum leprosum (ENL) that comes about mainly from immunocomplex deposits. In patients with BBL and BLL, it is possible to have both reaction types simultaneously. There is also Lucio phenomenon, which is an immune system response with important clinical manifestations. Its physiopathology is not well understood, with abundant infection of *M. leprae* in endothelium, which can lead to thrombosis in the most superficial vases from immunocomplex deposits with hemorrhaging and cutaneous infarction.

In the literature, a robust positive association has been demonstrated between bacterial load and the frequency of leprosy reactions. A reaction can be set off by various factors, such as pregnancy, childbirth, vaccinations, puberty, intercurrent infections, stress (physical, psychological, or surgical), use of potassium iodate/iodide (SSKI), and immune reconstruction inflammatory syndrome (IRIS) linked to antiretroviral and/or immune-based therapies.

Those patients who experience leprosy reactions during MDT treatment should continue taking their regimen without modification while also beginning a specific and concurrent treatment for the appropriate reaction type.

Type 1 Reaction or Reversal Reaction

Clinically speaking, lesions become more erythematous and infiltrated, and those with previously diminished sensation can become more sensitive to touch. Desquamation may occur and some lesions may even ulcerate. New lesions can erupt along with edema in the hands, feet, and face, as well general systemic symptoms. These reactions can last for years in some patients. It is important to begin an immediate intervention, given that neuritis is the most common, serious, and potentially disabling clinical manifestation of T1R.

The drug of choice for T1R treatment is prednisone (or prednisolone [Millipred]) with a dosage of 1 to 2 mg/kg/day for at least 12 weeks, at which point it can be tapered off until discontinuing medication around the 24th week.

Alternative drugs in type 1 reaction:

Azathioprine (Imuran)[1]: 1 to 2 mg/kg/day, until reaction control.
Cyclosporine (Neoral, Sandimmune)[1]: 5 to 8 mg/kg/day, until reaction control.
Clofazimine: 300 mg to 30 days/200 mg to 30 days/100 mg to 30 days.

---

[1]Not FDA approved for this indication.
[2]Not available in the United States.

---

[1]Not FDA approved for this indication.

Type 2 Reaction

This occurs in MB patients, and ENL is the most frequent clinical manifestation of T2Rs. Other variations of T2R are polymorphic erythema and vasculitis.

Clinically, ENL is a systemic condition with the eruption of painful and often symmetrical erythematous nodules on the arms and legs. When deeper, these nodules are more easily palpated than the more visible ones but will often ulcerate. Neuritis is frequent, although it is less aggressive than seen in T1Rs. The systemic impact can produce edema, myalgia, fever, malaise, asthenia, weight loss, cephalalgia, iritis, episcleritis, iridocyclitis, glaucoma, epistaxis, arthralgia, and orchiepididymitis with testicular atrophy, glomerulonephritis, chronic renal insufficiency, hepatosplenomegaly, and amyloidosis.

The most common medication used for ENL is thalidomide (Thalomid) in variable dosage, from 100 to 400 mg/day, depending on the severity of the reaction. The distribution of thalidomide is restricted in some countries due to its teratogenic effects. For this reason, it should be given under strict supervision with proper medical, ethical, and legal measures in place.

For ENL associated with neuritis, iritis, orchitis, and/or hand-foot reactions, or in women of childbearing age, a course of corticosteroids should be given (prednisone at 1–2 mg/kg/day).

In chronic cases and those that are nonresponsive to treatment, it is possible to administer clofazimine along with steroids at the initial dosage of 100 mg three times per day for a maximum of 12 weeks. This should be reduced to 100 mg twice daily for another 12 weeks and finally 100 mg/day for 12 to 24 weeks. Cyclosporine (Neoral, Sandimmune)[1] may also offer some benefit to the patient with serious ENL, as can the association of azathioprine (Imuran),[1] methotrexate,[1] and corticosteroids.

Alternative drugs in type 2 reaction:

Azathioprine[1]: 1 to 2 mg/kg/day, until reaction control.
Cyclosporine[1]: 5 to 8 mg/kg/day, until reaction control.
Methotrexate[1]: 15 mg (IM/SC or PO)/week, until reaction control.
Pentoxifylline: (Trental)[1] 1200 mg/day, until reaction control.
Clofazimine: 300 mg to 30 days/200 mg to 30 days/100 mg to 30 days.

Lucio Phenomenon

Lucio phenomenon can occur in forms of LL. The skin lesions can be discrete and limited in number, pinkish or cyanotic, often very painful, and potentially necrotizing and ulcerative. This condition can lead to death. Treatment is based on a course of corticosteroid therapy appropriate for each patient.

Differential Diagnosis Between Relapse and Reaction

Relapse rates are very low whereas reactions are quite frequent, even after completing treatment. Table 2 shows the main differences between reaction type 1 and type 2 relapse. Recently *M. leprae* whole genome sequencing technique was used to discriminate between cases of relapse and reinfection.

Complications

Leprosy complications are the result of permanent nerve damage.

Lesions to the large nerve trunks, such as the ulnar, median, and tibial, cause motor and sensory loss leading to disabilities such as claw hand and footdrop.

The absence of sensation in the hands, soles of the feet, and cornea leaves these areas predisposed to common wounds and pressure ulcers. This reality demands that patients take specific care to avoid ulcers and detect them as soon as possible to prevent secondary infection. In addition, corneal ulcers can result in blindness.

Acknowledgment

We thank Dr. Anna Maria Salles for the patient pictures.

---

[1]Not FDA approved for this indication.

TABLE 2 Differences Between Reaction Type 1 and Relapse	
REVERSAL REACTION	**RELAPSE**
Generally occurs during course of multidrug therapy or within 6 months of treatment completion	Occurs at least 2 years after treatment completion
Sudden and unexpected onset	Slow and insidious onset
Can be accompanied by fever and malaise	In general, no systemic symptoms present
Old lesions become erythematous, shiny, and infiltrated	Old lesions may present erythematous edges
In general, many new lesions	Few new lesions
There may be ulceration of the reaction lesions	Ulceration may occur on arms and legs in addition to the lesions
Regression with desquamation	No desquamation present
Can quickly affect several nerve trunks, with presence of pain, sensory alteration, and decreased motor function	May affect a single nerve and functional alterations often take place very slowly
Excellent response to corticosteroid therapy	Does not respond well to corticosteroid therapy
Bacteriologic index stable or falls	Bacteriologic index rises

References

Andrade KVF, Nery JS, Penna MLF, Penna GO, Pereira SM: Effect of Brazil's Conditional Cash Transfer Programme on the new case detection rate of leprosy in children under 15 years old, *Lepr Rev* 89:13–24, 2018 https://doi.org/10.1016/S1473-3099(19)30624-3.

Andrade KVF, Nery JS, Pescarini JM, et al: Geographic and socioeconomic factors associated with leprosy treatment default: an analysis from the 100 Million Brazilian Cohort, *PloS Negl Trop Dis* 13(9):e0007714, 2019.

Becx-Bleumink M: Relapses among leprosy patients treated with multidrug therapy: experience in the leprosy control program of the All Africa Leprosy and Rehabilitation Training Center (ALERT) in Ethiopia; practical difficulties with diagnosting relapses; operational procedures and criteria for diagnosing relapses, *Int J Lepr Other Mycobact Dis* 60:421–435, 1992.

Butlin CR, Pahan D, Maug AKJ, et al: Outcome of 6 months MBMDT in MB patients in Bangladesh—preliminary results, *Lepr Rev* 87:171–182, 2016.

Cruz RCDS, Bührer-Sékula S, Penna GO, et al: Clinical trial for uniform multidrug therapy for leprosy patients in Brazil (U-MDT/CT-BR): adverse effects approach, *An Bras Dermatol* 93:377–384, 2018.

Cambau E, Perani E, Guillemin I, Jamet P, Ji B: Multidrug-resistance to dapsone, rifampicin, and ofloxacin in M leprae, *Lancet* 349:103–104, 1997.

Cruz RCDS, Bührer-Sékula S, Penna MLF, Penna GO, Talhari S: Leprosy: current situation, clinical and laboratory aspects, treatment history and perspective of the uniform multidrug therapy for all patients, *An Bras Dermatol* 92(6):761–773, 2017.

da Silva Rocha A, Cunha Dos Santos AA, Pignataro P, et al: Genotyping of Mycobacterium leprae from Brazilian leprosy patients suggests the occurrence of reinfection or of bacterial population shift during disease relapse, *J Med Microbiol* 60:1441–1446, 2011.

Ferreira IP, Bührer-Sékula S, De Oliveira MR, et al: Patient profile and treatment satisfaction of Brazilian leprosy patients in a clinical trial of uniform six-month multidrug therapy (U-MDT/CT-BR), *Lepr Rev* 85(4):267–274, 2014.

Fine PE: Leprosy: the epidemiology of a slow bacterium, *Epidemiol Rev* 4:161–188, 1982.

Gelber RH, Grosset J: The chemotherapy of leprosy: an interpretive history, *Lepr Rev* 83:221–240, 2012.

Gillis TP, Scollard DM, Lockwood DN: What is the evidence that the putative Mycobacterium lepromatosis species causes diffuse lepromatous leprosy? *Lepr Rev* 82:205–209, 2011.

Gonçalves H de S, Pontes MA, Bührer-Sékula S, et al: Brazilian clinical trial of uniform multidrug therapy for leprosy patients: the correlation between clinical disease types and adverse effect, *Mem Inst Oswaldo Cruz* 107(Suppl 1):74–78, 2012.

Guerra JG, Penna GO, Castro LCM: Eritema Nodoso Hansênico: atualização clínica e terapêutica, Erythema Nodosum Leprosum: clinical and therapeutic update, *An Bras Dermatol* 77:389–407, 2002.

Han XY, Sizer KC, Velarde-Félix JS, et al: The leprosy agents Mycobacterium lepromatosis and Mycobacterium leprae in Mexico, *Int J Dermatol* 51:952–959, 2012.

Hungria EM, Bührer-Sékula S, Oliveira RM, et al: Mycobacterium leprae-specic antibodies in multibacillary leprosy patients decrease during and after treatment with either the regular 12 doses multidrug therapy (MDT) or the uniform 6 doses MDT, *Front Immunol* 9:915, 2018.

Hungria EM, Bührer-Sékula S, de Oliveira RM, et al: Leprosy reactions: the predictive value of Mycobacterium leprae-specific serology evaluated in a Brazilian cohort of leprosy patients (U-MDT/CT-BR), *PLoS Negl Trop Dis* 11(2):e0005396, 2017.

Hungria EM, Oliveira RM, Penna GO, et al: Can baseline ML Flow test results predict leprosy reactions? An investigation in a cohort of patients enrolled in the uniform multidrug therapy clinical trial for leprosy patients in Brazil, *Infect Dis Poverty* 5(1):110–120, 2016.

International Federation of Anti-Leprosy Associations: Available at http://www.ilep.org.uk/about-ilep/. [Accessed July 9, 2015].

Kroger A, Pannikar V, Htoon MT, et al: International open trial of uniform multidrug therapy regimen for 6 months for all types of leprosy patients: rationale, design and preliminary results, *Trop Med Int Health* 13:594–602, 2008.

Lie H: Why is leprosy decreasing in Norway? *Trans R Soc Trop Med Hyg* 22(4):357–366, 1929.

Lockwood DN, Shetty V, Penna GO: Hazards of setting targets to eliminate disease: lessons from the leprosy elimination campaign, *BMJ* 348:1136, 2014.

Maeda S, Matsuoka M, Nakata N, Kai M, Maeda Y, et al: Multidrug resistant M leprae from patients with leprosy, *Antimicrob Agents Chemother* 45:3635–3639, 2001.

Matsuoka M, Kashiwabara Y, Namisato Y: A M leprae isolate resistant to dapsone, rifampicin, ofloxacin, and sparfloxacin, *Int J Lepr* 68:452–455, 2000.

Matsuoka M, Kahiwabara Y, Liangfen Z, Goto M, Kitajima S: A second case of multidrug-resistant Mycobacterium leprae isolated from a Japanese patient with relapsed lepromatous leprosy, *Int J Lepr* 71(3):240–243, 2003.

Moura RS, Penna GO, Cardoso LP, et al: Description of leprosy classification at baseline among patients enrolled at the uniform multidrug therapy clinical trial for leprosy patients in Brazil, *Am J Trop Med Hyg* 92(6):1280–1284, 2015.

Moura RS, Penna GO, Fujiwara T, et al: Evaluation of a rapid serological test for leprosy classification using human serum albumin as the antigen carrier, *J Immunol Methods* 412:35–41, 2014.

Nery JS, Ramond A, Pescarini JM, et al: Socioeconomic determinants of leprosy new case detection in the 100 Million Brazilian Cohort: a population-based linkage study, *Lancet Glob Health* 7(9):e1226–e1236, 2019.

Nery JS, Pereira SM, Rasella D, et al: Effect of the Brazilian conditional cash transfer and primary health care programs on the new case detection rate of leprosy, *PLoS Negl Trop Dis* 8:e3357–e3360, 2014.

Norman G, Joseph G, Ebenezer G, et al: Secondary rifampin resistance following multi-drug therapy – a case report, *Int J Lepr Other Mycobact Dis* 71(1):18–21, 2003.

Opromolla DVA, Costa HC, Oliveira PRD: Resistência medicamentosa múltipla secundária na hanseníase, *Hansen Int* 18(1,2):11–16, 1993.

Pedrosa VL, Dias LC, Galban E, et al: Leprosy among schoolchildren in the Amazon region: a cross-sectional study of active search and possible source of infection by contact tracing, *PLoS Negl Trop Dis* 12:e0006261, 2018.

Penna GO, Bührer-Sékula S, Kerr LRS, et al: Uniform multidrug therapy for leprosy patients in Brazil (U-MDT/CT-BR): results of an open label, randomized and controlled clinical trial, among multibacillary patients, *PLoS Negl Trop Dis* 11:e0005725, 2017.

Penna GO, Pontes MA, Cruz R, et al: A clinical trial for uniform multidrug therapy for leprosy patients in Brazil: rationale and design, *Mem Inst Oswaldo Cruz* 107(Suppl 1):22–27, 2012.

Penna ML, Bührer-Sékula S, Pontes MA, et al: Primary results of clinical trial for uniform multidrug therapy for leprosy patients in Brazil (U-MDT/CT-BR): reactions frequency in multibacillary patients, *Lepr Rev* 83(3):308–319, 2012.

Penna ML, Bührer-Sékula S, Pontes MA, et al: Results from the clinical trial of uniform multidrug therapy for leprosy patients in Brazil (U-MDT/CT-BR): decrease in bacteriological index, *Lepr Rev* 85(4):262–266, 2014.

Penna ML, Penna GO: Leprosy frequency in the world, 1999–2010, *Mem Inst Oswaldo Cruz* 107(Suppl 1):3–12, 2012.

Penna ML, Penna GO, Iglesias PC, et al: Anti-PGL-1 positivity as a risk marker for the development of leprosy among contacts of leprosy cases: systematic review and metaanalysis, *PLoS Negl Trop Dis* 10:e0004703, 2016.

Pescarini JM, Strina A, Nery JS, et al: Socioeconomic risk markers of leprosy in high-burden countries: a systematic review and meta-analysis, *PLoS Negl Trop Dis* 12(7):e0006622, 2018.

Rosa PS, D'Espindula HRS, Melo ACL, et al: Emergence and transmission of drug/multidrug-resistant Mycobacterium leprae in a former leprosy colony in the Brazilian Amazon, *Clin Infect Dis* ciz570, 2019.

Santos SD, Penna GO, Costa MCN, et al: Leprosy in children and adolescents under 15 years old in an urban center in Brazil, *Mem Inst Oswaldo Cruz* 111:359–364, 2016.

Shen J, Yan L, Yu M, et al: Six years' follow-up of multibacillary leprosy patients treated with uniform multi-drug therapy in China, *Int J Dermatol* 54:315–318, 2015.

Shetty VP, et al: Primary resistance to single and multiple drugs in Leprosy—a mouse foot pad study, *Lepr Rev* 67, 1996.

Stefani MMA, Avanzi C, Bührer-Sékula S, et al: Whole genome sequencing distinguishes between relapse and reinfection in recurrent leprosy cases, *PLoS Negl Trop Dis* 11(6):e0005598, 2017.

Talhari C, Mira MT, Massone C, et al: Leprosy and HIV coinfection: a clinical, pathological, immunological, and therapeutic study of a cohort from a Brazilian referral center for infectious diseases, *J Infect Dis* 202:345–354, 2010.

Talhari C, Talhari S, Penna GO: Clinical aspects of leprosy, *Clin Dermatol* 33:26–37, 2015.

Talhari S, Gontijo B, Vale ECS, Marques SA: Editorial—new perspectives for the treatment of Hansen's disease, *An Bras Dermatol* 92(6):760, 2017.

Talhari S, Neves RG, Penna GO, Oliveira MLWR: In *Hanseníase*, 4th ed, Manaus, 2006, Gráfica Tropical.

Truman RW, Singh P, Sharma R, et al: Probable zoonotic leprosy in the southern United States, *N Engl J Med* 364:1626–1633, 2011.

Uaska Sartori PV, Penna GO, Bührer-Sékula S, et al: Human genetic susceptibility of leprosy recurrence, *Sci Rep* 10:1284, 2020.

Van Brakel W, Cross H, Declercq E, et al: Review of leprosy research evidence (2002–2009) and implications for current policy and practice, *Lepr Rev* 81:228–275, 2010.

Van Veen NH, Lockwood DN, Van Brakel WH, et al: *Interventions for erythema nodosum leprosum (Review)*, *Cochrane Collaboration*, John Wiley & Sons, p 53, 2012.

Vieira MCA, Nery JS, Paixão ES, Andrade KVF, Penna GO, Teixeira MG: Leprosy in children under 15 years of age in Brazil: a systematic review of the literature, *PLoS Negl Trop Dis* 12(10):e0006788, 2018.

WHO Expert Committee on Leprosy. World Health Organ Tech Rep Ser., 968:1–61, 2012.

WHO: In *Global leprosy strategy 2016–2020: Accelerating towards a leprosy-Free world*, WHO, 2016.

LYME DISEASE AND POST-TREATMENT LYME DISEASE SYNDROME

Method of
Carlos R. Oliveira, MD, PhD; and Eugene D. Shapiro, MD

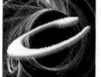

CURRENT DIAGNOSIS

- Lyme disease, caused by the spirochete *Borrelia burgdorferi*, is the most common vector-borne infection in both the United States and Europe.
- Early localized Lyme disease is a clinical diagnosis that is based on the presence of a single erythema migrans rash. The rash presents as an expanding circular macule that is often uniformly erythematous but occasionally can have central clearing that gives it the appearance of a target lesion. Erythema migrans usually appears 7 to 14 days after a tick bite (although the bite often is not recognized). If untreated, it persists for about 3 to 4 weeks.
- Early disseminated Lyme disease can present as multiple erythema migrans, cranial nerve palsy, lymphocytic meningitis, radiculomyelitis (Bannwarth syndrome), or carditis.
- Arthritis is the primary manifestation of late Lyme disease. Typically it is an oligoarthritis that most often involves a single knee.
- Patients with no objective signs but only nonspecific symptoms (e.g., arthralgia, myalgia, fatigue, or perceived cognitive difficulties) are highly unlikely to have active Lyme disease as the cause regardless of the result of antibody tests.
- Antibody test results for Lyme disease are usually negative in patients with erythema migrans (single or multiple); therefore testing for antibody generally is only indicated for patients with non-cutaneous manifestations of Lyme disease.
- The IgG antibody test has good sensitivity for patients with Lyme disease ≥4 weeks after initial infection.
- Tests for antibodies to *B burgdorferi* should use a two-tier procedure, first with a sensitive quantitative test, usually either a whole-cell or C-6 peptide enzyme-linked immunosorbent assay (ELISA); if that result is either positive or equivocal, a more specific test, the Western immunoblot, is done to confirm a positive test result. The presence of antibodies against at least either 2 (for IgM) or 5 (for IgG) proteins of *B burgdorferi* is required for the immunoblot result to be considered positive.
- In patients with symptoms present for 4-6 weeks or longer, Lyme disease should not be diagnosed based on a positive IgM antibody result alone.
- Sensitivity of PCR assays of both blood and CSF are poor because concentrations of *B burgdorferi* in these fluids are low.
- Once serum antibodies to *B burgdorferi* develop, both IgG and IgM antibodies may persist for decades despite adequate treatment; therefore elevated concentrations of antibodies in serum do not necessarily indicate active infection.

CURRENT THERAPY

- An oral course of doxycycline (Vibramycin)[1] for 10 days or of amoxicillin (Amoxil)[1] or cefuroxime axetil (Ceftin) for 14 days is highly effective for treating early localized Lyme disease.
- A 14-day course of the same antimicrobials also is highly effective in treating multiple erythema migrans and other manifestations of early disseminated Lyme disease, although patients with Lyme meningitis or complete atrioventricular block should be treated either parenterally with ceftriaxone (Rocephin)[1] or cefotaxime (Claforan)[1] or, in some instances, orally with doxycycline.[1]
- A 28-day course of an oral regimen is recommended for the treatment of Lyme arthritis.
- Doxycycline (Vibramycin) is contraindicated in women who are pregnant or are breastfeeding.
- The most effective preventive measure is avoidance of tick-infested areas. If exposure is unavoidable, visual inspection and prompt removal of embedded ticks, use of tick repellents with N, N-diethyl-3-methylbenzamide (DEET), and use of protective clothing have all been found to be modestly effective.
- An infected tick generally must be attached for 36 to 72 hours or longer for there to be a substantial risk of transmission of B burgdorferi. If a tick that has been embedded for at least 36 hours is removed, a single dose of doxycycline (Vibramycin) 8.8 mg/kg, maximum 200 mg,[1] given within 72 hours of removing the engorged tick, can be effective in preventing Lyme disease.
- Multiple or prolonged courses of antibiotics have not been shown to be effective and are not recommended for patients with only chronic, subjective symptoms after completing appropriate antibiotic treatment for Lyme disease.

[1]Not FDA approved for this indication.

Epidemiology and Ecology

Lyme arthritis was first described in 1977 when an unusual cluster of children with arthritis in Lyme, Connecticut, was reported. Soon after, Willy Burgdorfer identified the causative bacterial agent, a spirochete that was later named *Borrelia burgdorferi*, in *Ixodes scapularis*, the deer tick. Lyme disease, the most common vector-borne illness in both the United States and Europe, is transmitted by hard-bodied ticks of the *Ixodes* genus. In the United States, *Ixodes scapularis* (in the East and upper Midwest) and *Ixodes pacificus*, the Western black-legged tick (on the Pacific coast), can be vectors of Lyme disease. More than 90% of all cases in the United States occur in nine states: Connecticut, Maryland, Massachusetts, Minnesota, New Jersey, New York, Pennsylvania, Rhode Island, and Wisconsin. In Europe and in Asia, *Ixodes ricinus* (the sheep tick) and *Ixodes perscultatus* (the tiaga tick) can transmit *B burgdorferi*. *Ixodes* ticks feed once in each of the three stages of their 2-year life cycle: larva, nymph, and adult. There are a number of genomospecies of *Borrelia burgdorferi* sensu lato that cause Lyme disease. In the United States, Lyme disease is almost exclusively caused by *B burgdorferi* sensu stricto, whereas in Europe and in Asia, *Borrelia afzelii* and *Borrelia garinii*, in addition to *B burgdorferi* sensu stricto, are the major causes of Lyme disease.

Lyme disease is a zoonosis. The primary reservoir for *B burgdorferi* are small mammals, such as mice and chipmunks, although birds and other mammals, such as foxes and coyotes, can also serve as reservoirs of the organism. Deer are not a competent reservoir for *B burgdorferi*, but they are important for supporting the life cycle of the deer tick. Ticks are uninfected when they hatch. They can become infected after they feed on an infected animal. The bacteria live in the midgut of the tick, which must remain attached to a host for 36 to 48 hours or longer for the spirochete to travel to the salivary glands so it can be injected into the host. Although ticks may become infected at any stage of the life cycle, nymphs are more likely to transmit the organism. This is because their small size (<2 mm) makes them more difficult to detect than adult ticks and because the organism can be transmitted more rapidly from an infected nymph than from an infected adult tick. Consequently, nymphal ticks are less likely than are adult ticks to be removed before the organism can be transmitted. The most important risk factor for Lyme disease is exposure to ticks in an area in which the disease is endemic. Most cases of Lyme disease occur in the spring and summer, which correlates with peak activity of nymphal ticks and with frequent outdoor activity of humans.

Pathophysiology

The pathogenesis of Lyme disease is predominantly driven by the host immune response to the spirochete. During the first stage of infection, after transfer of the organism to the skin, inflammation ensues that leads to an erythematous lesion at the site of inoculation. The spirochete does not produce toxins; however, it can disseminate via the bloodstream or through the lymph vessels. After dissemination, the spirochete can adhere to distal tissues, and an immune-mediated inflammatory reaction at these sites leads to the characteristic clinical manifestations of Lyme disease.

Prevention

No vaccine is currently available to prevent Lyme disease in humans. The most effective preventive measure is avoidance of tick-infested areas. Tick repellents that contain N, N-diethyl-3-methylbenzamide (DEET) and the use of protective clothing (long sleeves and pants) have been found to be modestly effective at preventing Lyme disease. If exposure is unavoidable, frequent visual inspection with prompt removal of ticks is recommended. In endemic areas, if a nymphal or adult *Ixodes* tick is removed that is partially engorged (has been attached for at least 36 hours), a single dose of doxycycline (Vibramycin)[1] administered within 72 hours of removing the tick can be effective in preventing Lyme disease.

Clinical Manifestations

The clinical manifestations of Lyme disease can be divided into three stages: early localized disease, early disseminated disease, and late disease. About two-thirds of patients with Lyme disease in the United States have early localized disease, which is characterized by a single erythema migrans (EM) rash at the site of the tick bite (although the tick bite is recognized in only a minority of cases). The rash starts as an erythematous macule or papule and then expands as an annular macule that is often uniformly erythematous (about two-thirds of cases of EM), although it can have central clearing that gives it the appearance of a classic target lesion. EM usually appears 7 to 14 days (range 3–30 days) after the tick bite and, if untreated, may expand to an average of 15 cm in diameter before resolving after 2 to 4 weeks or longer. The rash may be asymptomatic or it may be accompanied by systemic symptoms such as fever, malaise, headache, stiff neck, myalgia, or arthralgia.

The second most common manifestation of Lyme disease is multiple EM, which accounts for 15% to 23% of the reported cases in the United States. Multiple EM, a manifestation of early disseminated Lyme disease, occurs when the spirochete disseminates via the bloodstream and presents as multiple erythematous round or ovoid macules that are usually smaller than most single EM lesions and are often accompanied by fever and other systemic symptoms. Other manifestations of early disseminated Lyme disease include cranial nerve palsy (especially facial palsy), lymphocytic meningitis, radiculomyelitis, and carditis. Cranial nerve palsies, especially facial nerve palsy, occur more commonly in children and account for approximately 3% to 5% of all cases of Lyme disease. In most cases, facial nerve palsy resolves within 4 to 8 weeks usually leaving minor, if any, obvious residua.

[1]Not FDA approved for this indication.

Lyme meningitis occurs less frequently (1% to 2% of cases) and typically has a subacute presentation similar to, though often of longer duration, than that of enteroviral meningitis. There is a mononuclear pleocytosis in cerebrospinal fluid. Increased intracranial pressure with papilledema is not uncommon. Neurologic involvement in Lyme disease is more common in Europe and in Asia, presumably because local strains of the bacteria are more neurotropic. Carditis, which is found in fewer than 1% of cases, typically causes various degrees of heart block, which usually is asymptomatic and may be detected only with an electrocardiogram, but may manifest as syncope, dyspnea, or dizziness due to complete heart block. Sudden death due to Lyme carditis has been reported but is very rare.

Arthritis is the main manifestation of late Lyme disease, and in North America accounts for approximately 6% to 8% of reported cases. Lyme arthritis typically is an oligoarthritis that involves a single knee about 90% of the time. Symptoms of arthritis develop 2 to 6 months after the tick bite and present with objective signs of inflammation of the joint. Arthritis typically resolves 2 to 6 weeks after appropriate treatment, although it may persist or recur in 10% to 20% of treated patients.

In Europe and in Asia, uncommon manifestations of Lyme disease include borrelial lymphocytoma, a painless nodule commonly located on the ear, breast, or scrotum; and acrodermatitis chronica atrophicans, a chronic fibrosing skin lesion typically found on the extensor surfaces of the extremities.

Diagnosis

Early localized Lyme disease is a clinical diagnosis based on a history of potential exposure to ticks in an endemic area and the presence of the characteristic EM rash. Antibodies to the organism typically appear 3 to 4 weeks after the initial infection. Consequently, serologic tests are not indicated in patients with EM because most will not have detectable antibodies. Although more patients with multiple erythema migrans may be seropositive at the time of presentation, a majority will still be seronegative early on. Moreover, detectable antibodies may never develop in patients who are treated early in their courses. In patients with extracutaneous manifestations of Lyme disease, serologic testing is useful in making a diagnosis. Tests for antibodies to *B burgdorferi* should use a two-tier procedure, in which a sensitive quantitative test, usually an enzyme-linked immunosorbent assay (ELISA) against either "whole cell" or C6 peptide antigens of the bacteria, is performed. If the result of the quantitative test is either positive or equivocal, a Western immunoblot is done to confirm the specificity of the result. As with most infections, once they develop, elevated concentrations of both IgM and IgG antibodies may persist for decades in symptom-free patients who have been cured of Lyme disease. A positive test result is evidence of prior exposure to the organism and is not evidence of active infection. In addition, false-positive antibody test results are common, especially in patients with a low prior probability of Lyme disease, such as those with chronic nonspecific symptoms such as arthralgia, myalgia, or fatigue, who do not have concomitant objective findings associated with Lyme disease. False-positive IgM test results are especially common. A diagnosis of Lyme disease should rarely be based on a positive IgM test result alone, especially in patients who have had symptoms for a month or longer.

Polymerase chain reaction (PCR) assays can detect the organism in skin biopsies, CSF, blood, or synovial fluid. However, because concentrations of the organism are low in both the blood and the CSF, sensitivity of PCR assays of these fluids is poor. Because the rash is so characteristic and because virtually all patients with Lyme arthritis will have a positive result for IgG antibodies to *B burgdorferi*, such assays rarely are needed to make a diagnosis. The organism can be cultured using special media, but sensitivity generally is poor, and it takes weeks for the organism to grow.

Differential Diagnosis

The differential diagnosis of Lyme disease depends on the clinical stage of the illness. Single EM may be confused with ringworm, cellulitis, nummular eczema, granuloma annulare or insect bites. Southern tick–associated rash illness (STARI) manifests in a rash identical to EM. However, it occurs at the site of a bite from the lone star tick (*Amblyomma americanum*) and is most common in the south-central United States. The cause of STARI is unknown, but, unlike with Lyme disease, it is not associated with significant extracutaneous manifestations. Multiple EM may look very similar to erythema multiforme. Lymphocytic meningitis occurs with numerous viral infections, most commonly enterovirus. There are many other causes of carditis, including a number of viruses, as well as rheumatologic diseases such as lupus and rheumatic fever. There is substantial variation in how Lyme arthritis presents. Most often it is a subacute arthritis that may mimic rheumatoid arthritis or other more chronic arthritides, with <50,000 white blood cells/mL in the synovial fluid. However, it can present acutely and may mimic acute bacterial arthritis (like that due to *Staphylococcus aureus*), with >100,000 white blood cells/mL in synovial fluid.

Relapse Versus Reinfection

Resistance of *B burgdorferi* to recommended antimicrobials has not been reported. First-line antimicrobial therapy for Lyme disease is highly efficacious, and bacteriologic treatment failures are very rare. In a study of patients with two or more episodes of EM that occurred years apart, it was shown that the episodes were caused by different strains of bacteria, indicating that reinfection, rather than persistence of the original organism, was the cause of repeated episodes of EM. Reinfection rarely occurs in patients with late Lyme disease, indicating that most such patients are immune. On the other hand, patients with early Lyme disease who are treated may become reinfected from a new tick bite, presumably because the organism was killed before a protective immune response could occur. Persistent or recurrent arthritis does occur in 10% to 20% of patients with Lyme arthritis. So-called antibiotic-refractory arthritis occurs when frank arthritis persists despite two or more courses of antimicrobial treatment. This may be due to either an autoimmune process or slow clearance of antigens of dead organisms. There is no evidence that the cause is failure of the antibiotic to kill the organisms.

Post-Treatment Lyme Disease Syndrome and "Chronic" Lyme Disease

A small minority of patients with Lyme disease who have completed appropriate treatment may continue to have nonspecific symptoms, such as fatigue, arthralgia, myalgia, or perceived cognitive difficulties, for weeks or months after completing treatment. These have been termed *post-treatment Lyme disease symptoms* and, if they persist for 6 months or longer and are disabling, they are referred to as *post-treatment Lyme disease syndrome* (PTLDS). It is not clear whether the frequency or the nature of these symptoms in patients with PTLDS is greater than that among the general population. In addition, several placebo-controlled, randomized clinical trials of prolonged courses (6 weeks or longer) of intensive antimicrobial treatment (e.g., with ceftriaxone) in patients with PTLDS have found there was virtually no benefit and substantial risk of adverse side effects of this treatment. Consequently, the Infectious Diseases Society of America, the American Academy of Pediatrics, the American Academy of Neurology, the American College of Rheumatology, and expert professional societies from many European countries do not recommend prolonged treatment with antimicrobials in patients with PTLDS. These patients are distinguished from patients with so-called "chronic" Lyme disease, who have complaints similar to those with PTLDS but who do not have evidence of ever having had Lyme disease. Of course, prolonged antimicrobial treatment is not indicated for these patients, who might better be described as having medically unexplained symptoms. Patients with either PTLDS or "chronic Lyme disease" are best managed by focusing on alleviating symptoms rather than with additional courses of antibiotic therapy. This is because long-term treatment with antibiotics has not been shown to provide benefit and is associated with substantial risks. Managing these patients can be challenging. Ideally, management decisions should

TABLE 1	Antimicrobials Recommended to Treat Lyme Disease		
MANIFESTATION	**FIRST-LINE AGENTS**	**ALTERNATIVE AGENTS**	**DURATION**
Single or multiple erythema migrans, cranial nerve palsy, carditis that is asymptomatic or for which the patient is not hospitalized	Doxycycline (Vibramycin)[1] 4.4 mg/kg/day in 2 divided doses (maximum 100 mg/dose)	Azithromycin (Zithromax)[1] 10 mg/kg/day in 1 dose (maximum 500 mg/dose)	14 days; for single EM, 10-days of doxycycline or 7–10 days of azithromycin is effective
	Amoxicillin (Amoxil)[1] 50 mg/kg per day in 3 divided doses (maximum 500 mg/dose)	Clarithromycin (Biaxin)[1] 7.5 mg/kg in 2 divided doses (maximum 500 mg/dose)	
	Cefuroxime axetil (Ceftin) 30 mg/kg PO in 2 divided doses (maximum 500 mg/dose)	Erythromyciin (E.E.S.)[1] 12.5 mg/kg in 4 divided doses (maximum 500 mg/dose)	
Severe carditis, meningitis,* radiculomyelitis	Ceftriaxone (Rocephin)[1] 50–75 mg/kg IV in 1 dose (maximum 2 g/dose)	Cefotaxime (Claforan)[1] 150–200 mg/kg/day IV in 3 divided doses (maximum 2 g/dose) Penicillin G (Pfizerpen)[1] 200,000-400,000 U/kg/day in 6 divided doses (maximum 4 million U/dose)	14 days; for severe carditis and for meningitis, an oral agent may be used to complete a course of treatment after substantial clinical improvement
Lyme arthritis[†]	Same oral agents used for EM	Same oral agents used EM	28 days

[1]Not FDA approved for this indication.

*Some experts treat Lyme meningitis with doxycycline (Vibramycin)[1], administered orally, 4.4 mg/kg/day in 2 divided doses (maximum 100 mg/dose), for 14 days.

[†]Patients with persistent or recurrent arthritis 4 weeks after completing treatment may receive either a second 4-week course of treatment orally or 2 weeks of treatment with a parenterally administered antimicrobial listed above.

be directed by a clinician who can both form a long-term therapeutic relationship with the patient, and who has substantial experience managing medically unexplained symptoms. Clinicians need to be aware that while there is no scientific evidence to support the existence of "chronic" Lyme disease, many of these patients are suffering, and thus, are vulnerable to those who would offer inappropriate and potentially harmful therapies.

Chemoprophylaxis

A single dose of doxycycline (Vibramycin; 8.8 mg/kg, maximum 200 mg)[1] taken within 72 hours of a deer tick bite was effective in preventing Lyme disease. However, because the risk of Lyme disease after a recognized tick bite is low, prophylaxis generally is not recommended routinely, but only for those at higher risk, such as someone in an endemic area who removes an engorged nymphal stage deer tick.

Treatment

Antimicrobial treatment of Lyme disease is highly effective and complications are rare (Table 1). The recommendations for treatment are summarized in the table. Antimicrobials that are highly effective and are considered first-line agents to treat Lyme disease orally include doxycycline (Vibramycin)[1], amoxicillin (Amoxil)[1] and cefuroxime axetil (Ceftin). Amoxicillin (Amoxil) is the preferred agent for women who are either pregnant or breastfeeding. Because the risk of staining of teeth is low, use of doxycycline for ≤21 days of treatment in children <8 years of age is now considered acceptable. Doxycycline (Vibramycin) is the preferred oral agent due to its good activity against other tick-borne illnesses such as human granulocytic anaplasmosis. Although macrolides such as azithromycin (Zithromax),[1] clarithromycin (Biaxin),[1] and erythromycin (EES)[1] are effective for treating early Lyme disease, they may not be as effective as the first-line agents. When parenteral treatment is indicated, ceftriaxone (Rocephin)[1] is the preferred agent because of once-a-day dosing. Alternative antimicrobials such as cefotaxime (Claforan)[1] and penicillin G (Pfizerpen-G)[1] also are highly effective, although penicillin G is rarely used because of frequent dosing due to its short half-life.

For patients with single EM, a 10-day course of doxycycline or a 14-day course of either amoxicillin or cefuroxime is recommended. For multiple EM, cranial nerve palsy (without apparent meningitis) or carditis that is asymptomatic and for which the patient is not hospitalized, a 14-day course of an oral antimicrobial is recommended. For complicated carditis (complete heart block) and for meningitis, a 14-day course of a parental agent is recommended, althought there is evidence that 14 days of doxycycline orally may be adequate for treating meningitis. Some experts complete a course of initial parenteral treatment with oral therapy after the patient has improved clinically. Patients with Lyme meningitis should be carefully evaluated for increased intracranial pressure which, if present, should be managed appropriately. There is no evidence that steroids are beneficial for patients with facial palsy due to Lyme disease. For treatment of Lyme arthritis, a 28-day course of an oral antimicrobial is recommended. Nonsteroidal antiinflammatory drugs may be effective for treating the pain and inflammation associated with Lyme arthritis.

References

Centers for Disease Control. Lyme disease: *Data and statistics*. Available at https://www.cdc.gov/lyme/stats/index.html [Accessed April 10,2018].

Feder HM Jr, Johnson BJB, O'Connell S, et al: A critical appraisal of "chronic lyme disease." *N Engl J Med* 357:1422–1430, 2007.

Hatcher S, Arroll B: Assessment and management of medically unexplained symptoms, *BMJ* 336:1124–1128, 2008.

Klempner MS, Hu LT, Evans J, et al: Two controlled trials of antibiotic treatment in patients with persistent symptoms and a history of Lyme disease, *N Engl J Med* 345:85–92, 2001.

Lantos PM: Chronic Lyme disease: the controversies and the science, *Expert Rev Anti Infect Ther* 9:787–797, 2011.

Lantos PM, Rumbaugh J, Bockenstedt LK, Falck-Ytter YT, et al: Clinical practice guidelines by the Infectious Diseases Society of America (IDSA), American Academy of Neurology (AAN), and American College of Rheumatology (ACR): 2020 guidelines for the prevention, diagnosis and treatment of Lyme disease, *Clin Infect Dis* J.23;72(1):1–8, 2021.

Ljøstad U, Skogvoll E, Eikeland R, et al: Oral doxycycline versus intravenous ceftriaxone for European Lyme neuroborreliosis: a multicentre, non-inferiority, double-blind, randomised trial, *Lancet Neurol* 7:690–695, 2008.

Nadelman RB, Nowakowski J, Fish D, et al: Tick bite study group: prophylaxis with a single-dose doxycycline for the prevention of Lyme disease after an Ixodes scapularis tick bite, *N Engl J Med* 345:79–84, 2001.

Shapiro ED: Clinical practice: Lyme disease, *N Engl J Med* 370:1724–1731, 2014.

Steere AC, Strle F, Wormser GP, et al: Lyme borreliosis, *Nat Rev Dis Primers* 2:1–18, 2016.

[1]Not FDA approved for this indication.

MALARIA

Nestor Sosa, MD; and José Antonio Suárez, MD

CURRENT DIAGNOSIS

- Malaria is endemic in tropical and subtropical areas of Africa, Asia, Oceania, and Central and South America.
- Suspect malaria in returning travelers and recently arrived immigrants from an endemic region with fever, accompanied by headaches, chills, malaise and body aches.
- The microscopic examination of Giemsa-stained thin and thick peripheral blood smears is the standard diagnostic method for malaria.
- Rapid diagnostic antigen detection and polymerase chain reaction (PCR) testing can be used for initial diagnosis, but species confirmation and level of parasitemia require microscopy.

CURRENT THERAPY

- Treatment selection should be based on *Plasmodium* species involved, geographic area where the infection was acquired, presence of resistance to antimalarial drugs, and disease severity.
- Intravenous (IV) artesunate (available from Centers for Disease Control and Prevention [CDC])[5] is the recommended therapy for severe malaria. Alternative treatments are artemether-lumefantrine (Coartem)[1], atovaquone-proguanil (Malarone)[1] or quinine (Qualaquin)[1] plus doxycycline[1] or clindamycin[1].
- Uncomplicated malaria caused by chloroquine-sensitive *Plasmodium* species can be treated with chloroquine or hydroxychloroquine (Plaquenil). Radical cure of *Plasmodium vivax* and *Plasmodium ovale*[1] requires subsequent therapy with primaquine or tafenoquine (Krintafel).
- Artemisinin combination therapies (i.e., artemether-lumefantrine [Coartem]) are the primary regimens for uncomplicated malaria caused by chloroquine-resistant *P. falciparum* or *P. vivax*[1].

[5]Investigational drug in the United States.
[1]Not FDA approved for this indication.

Introduction

Malaria is an important parasitic disease caused by protozoa of the genus *Plasmodium (Phylum Apicomplexa)* and transmitted primarily by the bite of female *Anopheles* mosquitoes.

Malaria remains a formidable health problem, especially in sub-Saharan Africa, and other tropical regions in Southeast Asia, Oceania, and Latin America. The World Health Organization (WHO) estimates that in 2018, there were 228 million new cases of malaria and 405,000 deaths worldwide. Two thirds of all deaths occur in children under 5 years of age. The economic losses from the disease, only in Africa, are estimated to reach US$12 billion per year.

In recent years, a significant investment has been made in malaria control and elimination efforts. According to the 2019 WHO World Malaria Report, an estimated US$ 2.7 billion was invested by governments of malaria-endemic countries and international partners in 2018. The incidence rate of malaria declined globally between 2010 and 2018 from 71 to 57 cases per 1000 population at risk; the number of countries with zero or less than 100 indigenous cases have also increased in the same period of time. These advances in malaria control can be explained by the use of long-lasting insecticidal nets, indoor residual spraying programs, rapid diagnostic testing, and access to artemisinin combination therapy (ACT).

Epidemiology

Most cases of malaria occur in Africa, but cases are reported in other tropical and subtropical regions of Southeast Asia (the Greater Mekong Region), Oceania, India, and Central and South America (Figure 1).

Five different species of *Plasmodia* have been associated with the disease: four human malaria parasites, *P. falciparum*, *P. vivax*, *P. ovale*, and *P. malariae*, and one simian plasmodia of macaques monkeys, *P. knowlesi*, which affects humans in Borneo and Peninsular Malaysia.

P. falciparum is responsible for the great majority of cases overall, is the most prevalent in sub-Saharan Africa, and it is associated more frequently with the most severe and fatal forms of the disease. *P. vivax* is the most prevalent species in Southeast Asia and Central and South America; *P. ovale* circulates with a very low incidence in Africa, Asia and Oceania; and *P. malariae* is rare but has been reported worldwide.

The infection is transmitted primarily from person to person, via the bite of the female mosquito of the genus *Anopheles*. More than 30 different species of *Anopheles* have been associated with malaria transmission worldwide. Environmental factors, like relative humidity, elevation, and temperature, influence the transmission of malaria in the endemic areas. Highest transmission occurs during the wet or rainy season. Other less common modes of transmission are mother to child (congenital malaria), blood transfusions, needle sharing, and via solid organ transplants.

Most cases in nonendemic areas are reported in travelers and immigrants arriving from areas with local malaria transmission. Rarely, infected mosquitos can be accidentally transported in airplanes and cause cases in and around airport terminals in nonendemic regions, the so-called "airport malaria." In the United States, the CDC report about 2000 imported malaria cases every year and it is a nationally reportable disease. Travelers to sub-Saharan Africa have the greatest risk of acquiring the disease. Sixty-seven percent of the cases reported in the United States in 2015 were caused by *P. falciparum*, 12% by *P. vivax*, 4% by *P. ovale*, 3% by *P. malariae*, and less than 1% by more than one species.

One of the greatest challenges for the prevention and treatment of malaria has been the development of drug resistance, especially among *P. falciparum*, but also reported with *P. vivax*. The patterns and geographical distribution of drug-resistant parasites is complex. Resistance to malaria medication continues to be an essential consideration when selecting drugs for treatment and chemoprophylaxis.

Since the 1970s, chloroquine resistance in *P. falciparum* has been confirmed in every continent where malaria is endemic, sparing only Mexico, Central America west of the Panama Canal, Haiti, the Dominican Republic, and a few Middle Eastern countries. High-grade chloroquine resistance in *P. vivax* has been reported in Papua New Guinea, the Solomon Islands, India, Myanmar, and Indonesia.

The emergence of resistance of *P. falciparum* to mefloquine (Lariam) has been documented in Myanmar (Burma), Lao People's Democratic Republic (Laos), Thailand, Cambodia, China, and Vietnam. Resistance to sulfadoxine/pyrimethamine (Fansidar)[2] and atovaquone/proguanil (Malarone) has also been reported. The resistance to these drugs has made ACT the treatment of choice for most cases of *P. falciparum* malaria. Unfortunately, there have been recent reports of clinical failures and resistance to artemisinin derivatives from the five countries of Greater Mekong Subregions: Cambodia, Laos, Myanmar, Thailand, and Vietnam.

[2]Not available in the United States.

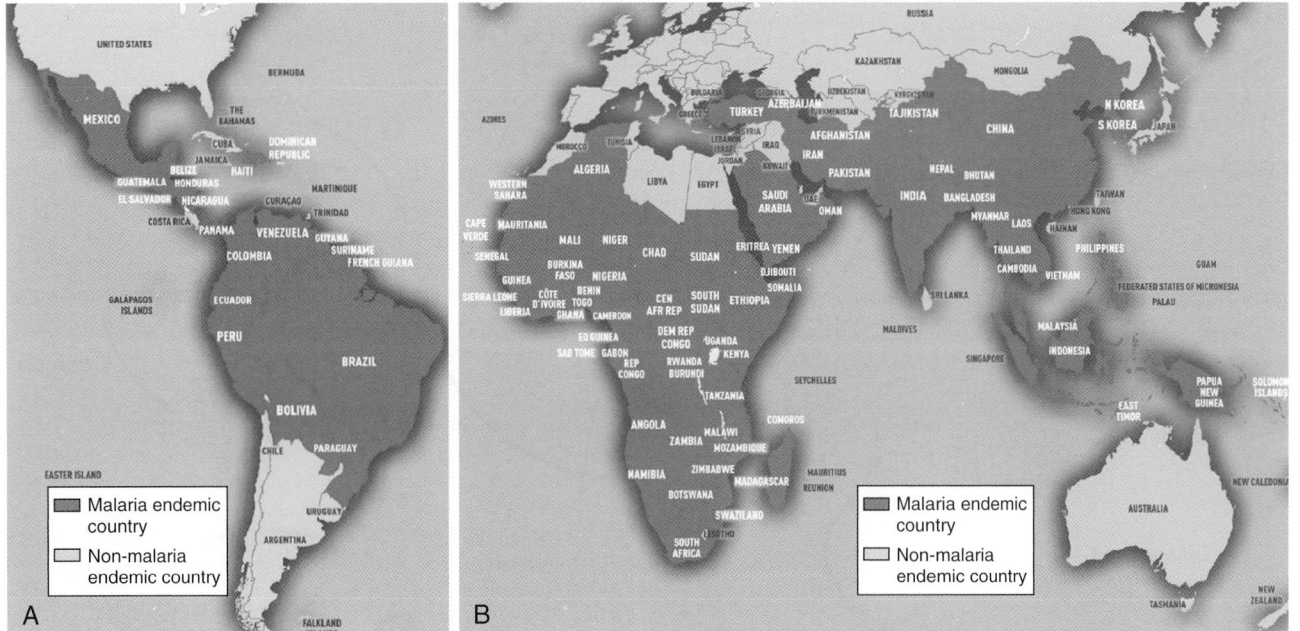

Figure 1 Malaria-endemic countries in the (A) Western and (B) Eastern Hemispheres. Transmission occurs across most of Africa, Central and South America, and Southern and Southeast Asia, as well as parts of the Caribbean, Eastern Europe, and the South Pacific. Countries are shaded completely even if the area of endemicity is only in a small area of the country. (Adapted from Centers for Disease Control and Prevention: *CDC Health Information for International Travel 2016*, New York, 2016, Oxford University Press. Public Domain.)

Parasite Life Cycle

The life cycle of the different species of *Plasmodia* are similar (Figure 2). The sexual cycle occurs in the mosquito, and repeated asexual cycles in the human host. The human infection starts when between 10 and 100 sporozoites—present in the salivary glands of the female *Anopheles* mosquito—enter the human host when the insect takes a blood meal. These sporozoites migrate from the dermis, invade the hepatocytes, and differentiate into hepatic schizonts that produce merozoites that later are liberated and invade circulating erythrocytes. *P. vivax* and *P. ovale* preferentially invade younger erythrocytes (reticulocytes); *P. falciparum* invades all types of erythrocytes.

Differences in the duration of these exo-erythrocytic cycles explain the variations in the incubation period of the different species of malaria. *P. knowlesi* incubation period is from 9 to 12 days and *P. falciparum* is often 9 to 14 days, while *P. vivax* ranges from 12 to 17 days and *P. ovale* from 16 to 18 days. *P. malariae* is the most variable with ranges from 18 to 40 or more days.

The erythrocytic cycles of invasion and growth take approximately 24 hours in *P. knowlesi*; 48 hours in *P. falciparum*, *P. ovale* and *P. vivax*; and 72 hours in *P. malariae*. These differences explain the periodicity of the fever paroxysm seen with the different parasites.

Once in the red blood cells, the merozoites develop into ring forms, and mature into trophozoites and schizonts and finally merozoites that rupture the cells and invade other erythrocytes, repeating and amplifying this erythrocytic asexual phase.

Some of the trophozoites in the red cells mature into gametocytes—the form that, when taken up by the mosquitoes, start the sexual cycle. The sexual cycle takes approximately 1 to 2 weeks within the mosquito. The gametocytes cross-fertilize in the mosquito midgut and become diploid zygotes that form an ookinete and finally close to 1000 sporozoites that migrate to the salivary glands and can infect another human host.

In *P. vivax* and *P. ovale* infection, parasites may remain latent in the liver as hypnozoites and reactivate after months, or even years, causing relapses of the disease.

Malaria Immunity

Acquired immunity to malaria is not sterilizing, but it protects against symptomatic and severe disease. It increases with age, number of episodes of the infection, and time spent living in the endemic area.

Several genetic polymorphisms seem to confer resistance to severe *P. falciparum* infection. Its relative increased prevalence in areas that are endemic for malaria demonstrates the natural selection forces of this disease over the human genome. Hemoglobin gene alterations like sickle cell disorders, thalassemia, hemoglobin C, hemoglobin E, and hemoglobin F, and blood cell enzyme deficiencies like glucose-6-phospate dehydrogenase and certain blood group antigens (Duffy negative and ABO type O), have been associated with relative protection to infection or severe malaria.

Malaria is uncommon in neonates. The presence of fetal hemoglobin (hemoglobin F) and maternal antibodies may, in part, explain this observation.

Clinical Manifestations

The incubation period ranges from 9 to 40 days and it is influenced by the specific parasite species involved, the immune status of the host, the administration of chemoprophylaxis, and the infecting dose of sporozoites.

After a vague prodromal period of 2 to 3 days, malaria classically manifests as an acute febrile illness with episodes of paroxysms characterized by chills (classically described as "teeth chattering, bed shaking chills"), rigor, high temperature (T ≥40°C) and profuse sweating, usually followed by fatigue and sleep. Other common symptoms include headache, weakness, insomnia, arthralgia, myalgia, and, less frequently, diarrhea, abdominal pain, or respiratory symptoms.

Individuals with prior immunity and children may present only with fever and headache; infants and very young children may present with irritability and a decrease in food intake.

The malaria paroxysms may recur every 24 *(P. knowlesi)*, 48 (tertian fever in *P. vivax* and *P. falciparum*), or 72 hours (quartan fever in *P. malariae*). In primary infections, this periodicity may take several days to become apparent. The patient may be relatively asymptomatic between these paroxysms.

On physical exam the patients may exhibit pallor, hepatosplenomegaly and, in severe cases, jaundice, altered mental status, and convulsions. Rash, pulmonary manifestation and lymphadenopathy are rare.

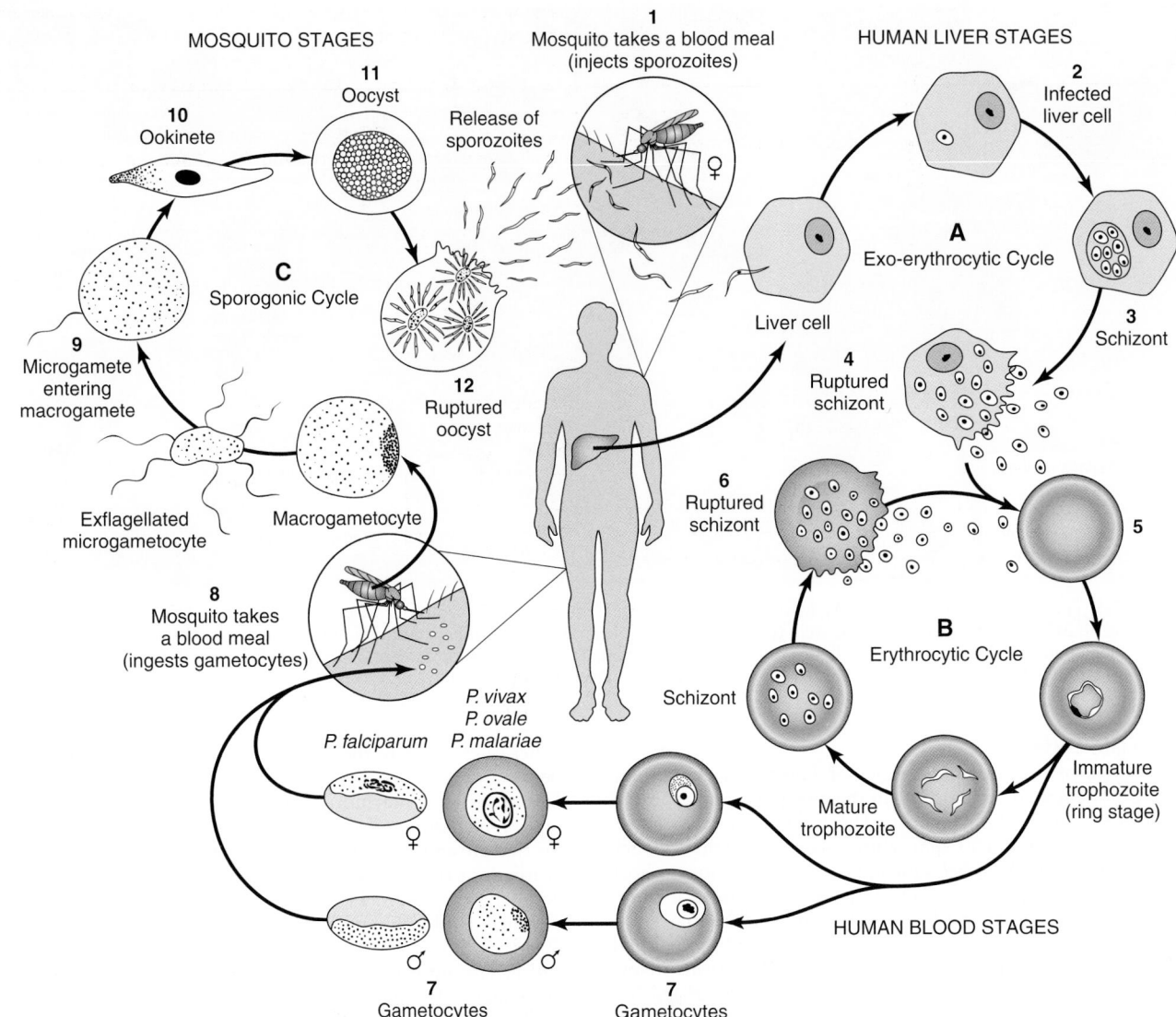

Figure 2 The malaria parasite life cycle involves two hosts. During a blood meal, a malaria-infected female *Anopheles* mosquito inoculates sporozoites into the human host (1). Sporozoites infect liver cells (2) and mature into schizonts (3), which rupture and release merozoites (4). (In *Plasmodium vivax* and *Plasmodium ovale*, a dormant stage [hypnozoites] can persist in the liver and cause relapses by invading the bloodstream weeks to years later.) After initial replication in the liver via exoerythrocytic cycle or tissue schizogony (A), the parasites undergo asexual multiplication in erythrocytes via erythrocytic cycle or blood schizogony (B). Merozoites infect red blood cells (5). The ring stage trophozoites mature into schizonts, which rupture, releasing merozoites (6). Some parasites differentiate into sexual erythrocytic stages (gametocytes) (7). Blood stage parasites are responsible for the clinical manifestations of the disease. The gametocytes—male (microgametocytes) and female (macrogametocytes)—are ingested by an *Anopheles* mosquito during a blood meal (8). The parasites' multiplication in the mosquito is known as the sporogonic cycle (C). While in the mosquito's stomach, the microgametes penetrate the macrogametes, generating zygotes (9). The zygotes in turn become motile and elongated (ookinetes) (10), and invade the midgut wall of the mosquito, where they develop into oocysts (11). The oocysts grow, rupture, and release sporozoites (12), which make their way to the mosquito's salivary glands. Inoculation of the sporozoites (1) into a new human host perpetuates the malaria life cycle.

Severe or Complicated Malaria

Nonimmune individuals such as children or travelers to endemic areas or pregnant females may develop more severe manifestations of malaria. Complicated malaria, more commonly associated with *P. falciparum* infection, has been recently reported with *P. knowlesi* and *P. vivax*. The most important clinical and laboratory findings of complicated malaria are listed in Table 1. In parasitemic patients, the presence of any of the clinical or laboratory features of severe malaria represents a medical emergency, and hospitalization, admission into critical care units, and rapid initiation of specific treatment are important. Even in patients with less severe disease, because of the ability of *P. falciparum* infection to progress in just a few hours to severe and life-threatening complications, it is advisable to hospitalize all nonimmune individuals during their initial period of treatment.

The clinical presentation of complicated malaria may be different in children and adults. Cerebral malaria (see later) is more common in children; multiorgan system involvement is more frequent in adults. Important clues in the physical exam are prostration, deep breathing, a decreased level of consciousness, slow capillary filling, signs of congestive heart failure, hepatosplenomegaly, pallor, and decreased urine output. Mortality rates of complicated or severe malaria range between 15% and 22% in adults, and between 8.5% and 10.9% in children.

Cerebral Malaria

Parasite sequestration in the cerebral microvasculature is associated with a variable and potentially lethal constellation of symptoms that include a decreased level of consciousness, coma, generalized seizures and/or focal neurologic deficits. Histopathologic findings frequently exhibit the presence of sequestered parasites, ring hemorrhages, perivascular leukocyte infiltrates, and immune-histochemical evidence of endothelial activation. In children with cerebral malaria, intracranial pressure is usually increased. Among those who survive, neurologic recovery can be rapid and complete, but sequelae have been reported in

TABLE 1 — Features of Complicated or Severe Malaria

FINDING	DESCRIPTION
Cerebral malaria	Diminished consciousness, Blantyre Coma Score of ≤2 in children, Glasgow Coma Scale <9 in adults or seizures
Respiratory distress/pulmonary edema	Radiographic evidence, hypoxemia
Hyperparasitemia	>2% or >100,000/μL in low transmission settings; or >5% or >250,00 in high transmission settings
Severe anemia	<5g Hgb or <15% hematocrit
Hypoglycemia	<2.2 mmol/L or 40 mg/dL
Jaundice/icterus	Clinically evident
Renal failure	Creatinine >265 mmol/L
Hemoglobinuria	
Metabolic acidosis or hyperlactatemia	HCO$_3$ <15 mmol/L or lactate >5 mmol/L
Shock	SBP <70 mm Hg in adults; SBP <50 mm Hg in children
Abnormal spontaneous bleeding	

HCO3, Bicarbonate; *SBP*, systolic blood pressure.

up to 15% of children with cerebral malaria. In patients with malaria that present with neurologic manifestations, it is important to exclude other conditions like meningitis, hypoglycemia, and other causes of encephalopathy. Fundoscopic examination may be useful, revealing retinal hemorrhages and white exudates suggestive of malarial retinopathy.

Respiratory Failure/Respiratory Distress Syndrome

Noncardiogenic pulmonary edema is a complication of severe *P. falciparum* malaria, seen more frequently in adults than children. Sequestration of infected erythrocyte in the lungs is thought to be associated with the production of cytokines, increased vascular permeability, pulmonary edema, dyspnea, hypoxia and progression to acute lung injury, and respiratory distress syndrome. Patients may become hypoxemic and require mechanical ventilation.

Acute Kidney Injury

Although mild proteinuria and oliguria can be present in uncomplicated malaria, acute renal failure—secondary to decreased renal perfusion, intravascular hemolysis, hemoglobinuria, acute tubular necrosis, and anuria—is a complication of severe malaria. Renal replacement therapy and general support through the critical period is associated with complete recovery of renal function in the majority of patients.

Malaria During Pregnancy

Malaria during pregnancy, especially in nonimmune primigravidas, is associated with increased morbidity and mortality. The relative immunosuppression of pregnancy and parasite accumulation in the placenta related to its affinity with abundant chondroitin sulfate A (CSA) seem to be contributing factors for this phenomenon. Complications such as premature delivery, intrauterine growth retardation, low neonatal birth weight, increased newborn mortality, and maternal hypoglycemia and pulmonary edema have been reported. Placental malaria during subsequent pregnancies tends to be less severe than in the first pregnancy due to the development of immunity to CSA-binding parasites.

Non-Falciparum Malaria

P. vivax and *P. ovale* are usually not associated with severe disease, but acute lung injury and splenic rupture may occur. Severe cases of *P. vivax* have been reported in Papua New Guinea and Indonesia, with complications like severe anemia, cerebral malaria and respiratory distress. Relapses of *P. vivax* and *P. ovale* due to reactivation of the hypnozoites months or years after the initial infection is another characteristic of these two *Plasmodium*.

P. malariae, the etiology of quartan fever, is associated with very low parasitemia, chronic indolent infection, but nephrotic syndrome has been reported in young children in endemic areas.

In *P. knowlesi*, clinical presentation is similar to uncomplicated *P. falciparum* malaria, but approximately 10% of the cases may present with daily fever spikes, hyperparasitemia, metabolic acidosis, hepatic and renal dysfunction, respiratory distress, severe anemia and refractory hypotension.

Laboratory Diagnosis

The microscopic examination of Giemsa-stained thin and thick peripheral blood smears is the standard diagnostic method for malaria. Thick smears concentrate red cell layers by lysing the erythrocytes and are used to screen a relatively large amount of blood. Thin smears are used to determine the *Plasmodium* species based on the morphology and characteristics of the circulating forms.

P. falciparum infections are characterized by the presence of thin ring forms, frequently positioned at the red cell membrane, multiple infected cells, banana-shaped gametocytes, and the absence of trophozoites and schizonts that are sequestered in the microvasculature. The smears of *P. vivax* and *P. ovale* have thicker rings, ameboid trophozoites, schizonts and round gametocytes. Erythrocyte enlargement and Schüffner dots are common in *P. vivax* and *P. ovale* but absent in other malaria species. *P. malariae* has characteristic band forms and *P. knowlesi* rings are similar to *P. falciparum*, but its mature forms and gametocytes are indistinguishable from *P. malariae*.

In addition to direct microscopy, other diagnostic methods, such as rapid diagnostic antigen detection (RDT), PCR, and serology are used in different settings.

RDTs are increasingly useful, especially in situations where microscopy is not immediately available. RDTs are immunochromatographic tests that detect *Plasmodium* antigens, like *P. falciparum* histidine-rich protein 2 (PfHRP2) or pan-malarial *Plasmodium* aldolase (PMA). Some of these tests are specific for *P. falciparum* or *P. vivax*, whereas others detect antigens common to several *Plasmodium*.

The reported sensitivies and specificity of most RDTs are high, frequently around 95% and 99%, respectively. In patients with low parasitemia (less than 100 parasites/μL), the sensitivity decreases.

Even when RDTs are positive, direct microscopy is indicated to confirm the diagnosis to the species level (based on morphology) and to estimate the level of parasitemia. Most RDTs are not useful to evaluate treatment response because they may remain positive for several weeks after successful treatment.

PCR detects segments of the parasite DNA using amplification. It is very specific and may be useful in very low parasitemia, but it is not yet readily available in most clinical settings where malaria patients are diagnosed.

Serologic tests, like indirect fluorescent antibody (IFA), are not useful for routine diagnosis of acute cases of malaria. Antibody positivity may take several days or weeks to develop. Serology is useful to screen blood donors in transfusion-related cases, as part of the evaluation of tropical splenomegaly syndrome (TSS) to detect infection when parasitemia is below the level of detection for microscopy or RDTs, and for the testing of treated and cured malaria patients.

Other nonspecific clinical laboratory abnormalities frequently detected in patients with malaria are anemia, with decreased hemoglobin and hematocrit, increased lactic dehydrogenase (LDH) levels, and decreased haptoglobin levels. The anemia is normocytic normochromic, but microcytosis is not infrequent—especially in patients with iron deficiency or thalassemia. The white cell count may be increased, decreased or normal. Platelet

TABLE 2 Antimalarial Drugs: Activity and Side Effects

DRUG (TRADE NAME)	ACTIVITY	INDICATION	SIDE EFFECTS	COMMENTS
Chloroquine (Aralen) Hydroxychloroquine (Plaquenil)	Blood schizonts (all *Plasmodia*) and gametocytes (*P. ovale, malariae, vivax, knowlesi*)	Treatment of choice for chloroquine susceptible *Plasmodium*	GI symptoms, headache, dizziness, insomnia, visual changes, ototoxicity, retinopathy, and peripheral neuropathy	Safe in children and pregnant patients
Atovaquone/Proguanil (Malarone)	Blood and tissue schizonts	Chemoprophylaxis and treatment of uncomplicated malaria outside endemic areas (in combination with artesunate[1] or primaquine[1])*	Headache, cough, and GI upset, dizziness, mucosal ulcerations, increased LFTs	Safe in children >5 kg of body weight Contraindicated in severe renal dysfunction
Artemisinin Derivatives**: artemether, artesunate, dihydroartemisin	Blood schizonts and gametocytes	Treatment of choice for uncomplicated and severe *P. falciparum* malaria[1] in endemic areas	GI symptoms, dizziness, headache, neutropenia, elevated LFTs	Contraindicated in the first trimester of pregnancy
Quinine sulfate (Qualaquin) and Quinidine gluconate***	Blood schizonts of all *Plasmodium* species, gametocytes of *P. vivax, P. ovale,* and *P. malariae*	Uncomplicated or severe malaria when ACTs are not available or cannot be used (early pregnancy)[1]	Tinnitus, hearing impairment or loss, nausea, headache, dizziness, dysphoria, visual changes, QT prolongation, angina, hypotension, vertigo, vomiting, diarrhea, hypoglycemia	Can be used in the first trimester of pregnancy
Tetracyclines: Doxycycline (Vibramycin), tetracycline	Blood schizonts of all *Plasmodium* species	Chemoprophylaxis of *P. falciparum*. Treatment of chloroquine-resistant *P. falciparum* and *P. vivax*[1] in combination with quinine	GI symptoms, dry mouth, stomatitis, photodermatitis, *Candida vaginitis*, anal pruritus	Contraindicated in children <8 years and pregnant patients
Clindamycin (Cleocin)	Blood schizonts of all *Plasmodium* species	Severe[1] or uncomplicated malaria[1] in combination with artemisinin derivatives or quinine	GI symptoms (including *Clostridium difficile* colitis), rash	Not to be used as monotherapy
Mefloquine (Lariam)	Blood schizonts of all *Plasmodium* species	Chemoprophylaxis of all *Plasmodium* species.[1] Treatment of *P. falciparum* malarias part of ACTs	GI symptoms, neuropsychiatric symptoms like anxiety, irritability, paranoia, depression, hallucinations and depression	Violent behavior reported with prolonged use Safe during pregnancy
Primaquine sulfate	Exo-erythrocytic forms (hypnozoites), gametocytes	Chemoprophylaxis *P. vivax* endemic areas[1] Treatment of *P. vivax* and *P. ovale* hypnozoites[1] (prevention of relapses or radical cure)	GI symptoms, severe hemolytic anemia in G6PD-deficient patients	Level of G6PD should be checked before primaquine use

*Not recommended in endemic areas due to resistance to atovaquone.

**Used in combination with other agents, artemisinin-based combination therapy (ACT) is considered the treatment of choice for *P. falciparum* malaria in endemic areas. (Available ACT: artemether + lumefantrine (Coartem) (only FDA-approved treatment), artesunate + amodiaquine (Coarsucam)[2], artesunate + mefloquine (Artequin)[2], artesunate + sulfadoxine-pyrimethamine (Arsuamoon[2]/Fansidar[2]), and dihydroartemisinin + piperaquine (Eurartesim)[2]

***Quinidine gluconate IV formulation is the only FDA approved treatment for severe malaria in the United States, but it is no longer available. Cardiac monitoring is recommended during treatment with this drug.

G6PD, Glucose 6 phosphate dehydrogenase; *GI*, gastrointestinal; *LFTs* liver function tests.

[1] Not FDA approved for this indication.

[2] Not available in the United States.

counts may be decreased or normal. Mild hyponatremia may be present secondary to inappropriate secretion of antidiuretic hormone, vomiting or urinary losses.

In severe cases of malaria, hyperbilirubinemia, metabolic (lactic) acidosis, increased creatinine, albuminuria and hemoglobinuria may be present. Hypoglycemia may occur in patients with malaria. Contributing factors to hypoglycemia are impaired hepatic neoglucogenesis, decreased oral intake, and increased glucose consumption due to the hypermetabolic state and hyperinsulinemia—secondary to drugs like quinine or quinidine.

In African children with malaria, secondary bacterial infection, including bacteremia, is not uncommon.

Antimalarial Drugs

There are multiple drugs used in the treatment and prevention of malaria. Their indication depends on the species involved, availability of the medication, presence of drug resistance and severity of the disease. Some of the drugs have activity against the

erythrocytic phase or asexual forms and are referred to as blood schizonticides. Other antimalarial substances kill tissue or exo-erythrocytic parasites in the liver and are called tissue schizonticides. Tissue schizonticides prevent disease relapses in patients with *P. vivax* and *P. malariae*. Finally, other drugs demonstrate activity against gametocytes and decrease disease transmission, preventing the sexual stage in the mosquito. See Table 2 for the name, activity and side effects of the most commonly used antimalarial drugs.

Chloroquine (Aralen) and hydroxychloroquine (Plaquenil) are two of the oldest antimalarial drugs. They are considered blood schizonticides and also have gametocidal activity. They can be used in the prevention and treatment of all *Plasmodium* species in the absence of drug resistance, and are considered the treatment of choice for *P. vivax, P. malariae, P. ovale,* and *P. knowlesi*. Unfortunately, chloroquine resistance in *P. falciparum* is widespread and these drugs are no longer recommended for prevention or treatment, except in limited areas of Central America, the Caribbean, and the Middle East.

The combination of atovaquone/proguanil (Malarone) demonstrates activity against both tissue and blood schizonts and is frequently used in malaria prophylaxis, or as part of multidrug regimens with primaquine[1] or artesunate[5] for the treatment of uncomplicated chloroquine-resistant malaria in returning travelers outside endemic areas. The emergence of resistance to the atovaquone component limits its use in endemic areas.

Artemisinin derivatives, like artemether, artesunate[5], and dihydroartemisinin[2], have activity against blood schizonts and gametocytes. These substances are originally derived from the Chinese medicinal plant quinghaosu (Artemisia annua) and are frequently used in combination with other drugs. The available combinations are artemether + lumefantrine (Coartem, FDA approved), artesunate + amiodaquine (Coarsucam)[2], artesunate + mefloquine (Artequin)[2], dihydroartemisinin + piperaquine (Eurartesim)[2] or artesunate (Arsuamoon)[2] + sulfadoxina + pyrimethamine (Fansidar)[2] and are collectively referred to as artemisinin combination therapy (ACT).

ACT is considered the first-line treatment of uncomplicated *P. falciparum* malaria in endemic areas. The recent emergence of *P. falciparum* resistant to ACT in Southeast Asia is compromising the efficacy of these two drug combinations. A recent study demonstrated improved efficacy of three-drug regimen (dihydroartemisinin + piperaquine + mefloquine) in areas with artemisinin resistance. Artemisinin derivatives can be used in children and pregnant woman but are contraindicated during the first trimester of pregnancy. Oral monotherapy with artemisinin derivatives is strongly discouraged to prevent the development of resistance.

Quinine sulfate (Qualaquin), one of the oldest antimalarial drugs, derived from the bark of the Cinchona tree (*Cinchona calisaya*), demonstrates activity against blood schizonts and gametocytes of *P. vivax*, *P. ovale*, and *P. malariae*. It is used in combination with other drugs in severe malaria[1] and for uncomplicated chloroquine-resistant malaria species during pregnancy. Quinine has a narrow therapeutic index, and can produce cardiac conduction disturbances (e.g., QT prolongation, angina) and lead to cardiac arrest. Hyperinsulinemic hypoglycemia has been observed in children, elderly patients and pregnant women. IV preparations of quinine dihydrochloride and the antiarrhythmic quinidine gluconate had been used as antimalarial drugs but are no longer available in the United States.

The antibiotics, tetracycline and doxycycline (Vibramycin), display activity against blood schizonts; the latter is frequently used in travelers as prophylaxis for chloroquine and mefloquine resistant *P. falciparum* malaria. Tetracyclines can be employed in combination with quinine for the treatment of uncomplicated *P. falciparum* malaria and chloroquine-resistant *P. vivax*[1]. These antibiotics should not be used as monotherapy against malaria, and are contraindicated during pregnancy and for children younger than 8 years.

Clindamycin (Cleocin) is another antibiotic that acts as a blood schizonticide for all *Plasmodium* species. It is effective in combination with quinine for the treatment of uncomplicated *P. falciparum* malaria, and chloroquine resistant *P. vivax* when tetracyclines are contraindicated[1].

Mefloquine (Lariam) is an antimalarial structurally related to quinine. It has a long half-life and has activity against blood schizonts of all *Plasmodium* species. It is used in prophylaxis of malaria but can be used as an alternative treatment of uncomplicated *P. falciparum* malaria, and in combination with primaquine[1] (tissue schizonticide) in cases of chloroquine-resistant *P. vivax* infection. It is generally well tolerated, but central nervous system and psychiatric side effects, like anxiety, depression, paranoia, hallucinations, and violent behavior, have been reported.

Primaquine is active against tissue or exoerythrocytic forms and gametocytes of malaria parasites. It is indicated in the radical cure of *P. vivax* and *P. ovale*[1] eliminating the hypnozoites and preventing relapses of the disease. Primaquine can be used for prophylaxis in travelers to areas when greater than 90% of the cases of malaria are caused by *P. vivax*[1]. In patients with glucose-6-phosphate dehydrogenase (G6PD) deficiency, primaquine administration may cause acute hemolytic anemia. The activity of the G6PD enzyme should be measured before its usage. Primaquine is also contraindicated during pregnancy and breastfeeding, unless the infant has been tested for G6PD deficiency.

Tafenoquine (Arakoda, Krintafel), an FDC-approved antimalarial drug related to primaquine, is recommended for prophylaxis of all *Plasmodium* species (Arakoda), and as a radical cure of *P. vivax* infection combined with chloroquine only (Krintafel). Like primaquine, tafenoquine should not be used in people with G6PD deficiency, during pregnancy or while breastfeeding.

Lumefantrine is an antimalarial drug used in combination with artemether (as Coartem) in the treatment of uncomplicated *P. falciparum* malaria. It is active against erythrocytic stages of all *Plasmodium* species. Possible serious adverse effects reported with this combination include QT prolongation, bullous eruption, urticaria, splenomegaly hepatomegaly, hypersensitivity reaction, and angioedema. Artemether-lumefantrine (Coartem) is assigned a pregnancy category C by the US Food and Drug Administration (FDA) and its use during pregnancy should only be considered when the benefits outweigh the risks.

For the specific adult and pediatric dosing, clinical indication, treatment duration, and primary and alternative antimalarial regimens, see Table 3.

Treatment of Uncomplicated Malaria

The CDC provides advice to healthcare providers on the diagnosis and treatment of malaria and can be reached through the CDC Malaria Hotline (770) 488-7788 (or, toll free: [855] 856-4713) Monday–Friday, 9 am to 5 pm EST. Off-hours, weekends, and federal holidays, call (770) 488-7100 and ask to have the malaria clinician on-call paged.

For *P. falciparum* or species not identified acquired in areas with chloroquine resistance, there are four regimens: Artemether-lumefantrine (Coartem) is the preferred regimen; alternatives are atovaquone-proguanil (Malarone), quinine plus either doxycycline[1], tetracycline[1], or clindamycin[1], and the fourth regimen is mefloquine (Lariam). For cases of *P. falciparum* acquired in areas without chloroquine resistance, either chloroquine or hydroxychloroquine can be used. Alternatively, the same drugs used for chloroquine-resistant *P. falciparum* can be used.

Chloroquine or hydroxychloroquine can be used for most cases of malaria caused by *P. ovale* and *P. vivax*, *P. malariae*, and *P. knowlesi*. If these drugs are not available, artemether-lumefantrine (Coartem)[1], atovaquone-proguanil (Malarone)[1], mefloquine (Lariam)[1], or quinine[1] plus either doxycycline[1], tetracycline[1], or clindamycin[1] can be used. These regimens can be used for infections where chloroquine-resistant *P. vivax* has been reported (Papua New Guinea, Indonesia, Burma, and certain areas of Central and South America).

To eradicate *P. vivax* and *P. ovale* hypnozoites, patients should also be treated with either tafenoquine (Krintafel)[1] or primaquine phosphate[1]. Tafenoquine can be used in patients 16 years of age or older and is given as a single dose. If primaquine phosphate is used, CDC recommends a dose of 30 mg (base) by mouth daily for 14 days. Due to reduced efficacy of primaquine in patients over 70 kg, the total dose of primaquine should be adjusted in these patients to 6 mg/kg. This total dose should be given in daily doses of 30 mg for the number of days needed to complete the total dose. As mentioned before, quantitative G6PD enzyme activity should be measured before the use of primaquine or tafenoquine.

Treatment of Severe Malaria

Patients with severe malaria should be treated promptly. IV artesunate[5] is the treatment of choice regardless of the species involved. Clinicians caring for patients with suspected severe malaria should call CDC to obtain IV artesunate, as part of an

---

[1] Not FDA approved for this indication.
[2] Not available in the United States.
[5] Investigational drug in the United States.

---

[1] Not FDA approved for this indication.
[5] Investigational drug in the United States.

TABLE 3 Antimalarial Regimens and Dosing by Clinical Diagnosis and Resistance

CLINICAL DIAGNOSIS/PLASMODIUM SPECIES/DRUG SUSCEPTIBILITY	DRUG/PRESENTATION	PEDIATRIC DOSE#	ADULT DOSE
Primary Regimens			
Uncomplicated malaria/*P. falciparum*/chloroquine-sensitive or uncomplicated malaria/*P. malariae* or *P. knowlesi*	Chloroquine phosphate 1 tab = 500 mg (salt) (300 mg of base)	10 mg base/kg PO then 5 mg base /kg PO at 6, 24, 48 h. Total 25 mg base/kg	1 g salt (600 mg base) PO, then 500 mg in 6 h, then 500 mg daily × 2 days. Total dose 2500 mg
	Hydroxychloroquine 1 tab = 200 mg (salt) (155 mg of base)		800 mg salt (620 mg base) PO, then 400 mg daily × 2 days. Total dose 2000 mg
Primary Regimens			
Uncomplicated malaria/*P. falciparum* or species not identified Chloroquine resistance or unknown resistance	Artemether/lumefantrine (Coartem)* 1 tab = 20 mg/120 mg	The patient should receive the initial dose, followed by the second dose 8 h later, then 1 dose bid for the following 2 days. 5–<15 kg: 1 tablet per dose 15–<25 kg: 2 tablets per dose 25–<35 kg: 3 tablets per dose ≥35 kg: 4 tablets per dose	4 tabs PO in a single dose, then 4 tabs after 8 h, then 4 tabs every 12 h × 2 days
	Atovaquone/proguanil (Malarone)** Adult tab = 250 mg/100 mg Ped tab = 62.5 mg/25 mg	5–<8 kg: 2 peds tabs PO qd × 3 days 8–<10 kg: 3 peds tabs PO qd × 3 days 10–<20 kg: 1 adult tab PO qd × 3 days 20–<30 kg: 2 adult tabs PO qd × 3 days 30–<40 kg: 3 adult tabs PO qd × 3 days ≥0 kg: 4 adult tabs PO qd × 3 days	4 adult tabs PO in a single dose daily × 3 days
	Quinine sulfate (Qualaquine) 1 tab = 324 mg plus one of the following: doxycycline[1] 100 mg,*** tetracycline[1] 250 mg,*** or clindamycin[1] 450 mg	**Quinine sulfate:** 10 mg/kg PO tid × 3 days (7 days if SE Asia) + **Clindamycin:** 20 mg/kg/day divided tid × 7 days for children under 8 years of age or **Doxycycline:** 2.2 mg/kg/bid × 7 days or **Tetracycline:** 25 mg/kg/day PO divided qid × 7 days	**Quinine sulfate:** 648 mg PO tid × 3 days (7 days if SE Asia) + **Doxycycline:** 100 mg PO bid × 7 days or **Tetracycline:** 250 mg PO qid × 7 days or **Clindamycin:** 20 mg/kg/day PO divided tid × 7 days
	Alternative Regimens		
	Mefloquine**** 1 tab = 250 mg	15 mg salt/kg (13.7 mg base) PO as initial dose, then 10 mg salt/kg (9.1 mg base/kg) PO given 6–12 h after initial dose Total dose: 25 mg salt/kg	750 mg (684 mg base) PO as initial dose, then 500 mg PO × 1 dose 6–12 h later.^ Total 1250 mg
Primary Regimens			
Uncomplicated malaria/*P. vivax* or *P. ovale* chloroquine sensitive	Chloroquine phosphate or hydroxychloroquine plus either primaquine[1] phosphate 1 tab = 15 mg (base) or tafenoquine[1] (Arakoda): 1 tab = 100 mg (Krintafel): 1 tab = 150 mg	**Chloroquine phosphate or hydroxychloroquine** same as above **Primaquine phosphate:** 0.5 mg/kg base PO qd × 14 days or **Tafenoquine succinate:** 300 mg PO × 1 dose (children ≥16 years old)	**Chloroquine** phosphate: same as above **Primaquine phosphate:** 30 mg base = 2 tab PO qd × 14 days or **Tafenoquine succinate:***** 300 mg PO × 1 dose
Primary Regimens			
Uncomplicated malaria/*P. vivax* In case of suspected chloroquine-resistant *P. vivax*	1. Artemether-lumefantrine (Coartem)[1] plus either primaquine phosphate or tafenoquine	**Artemether-lumefantrine:** see doses above **Primaquine phosphate:** see doses above **Tafenoquine:** see doses above	**Artemether-lumefantrine:** see doses above**Primaquine phosphate:** see doses above **Tafenoquine:** see doses above
	2. Atovaquone-proguanil (Malarone)[1] plus either primaquine phosphate or tafenoquine	**Atovaquone-proguanil:** see doses above **Primaquine phosphate or Tafenoquine:** see doses above	**Atovaquone-proguanil:** see doses above **Primaquine phosphate or Tafenoquine:** see doses above
	3. Quinine sulfate[1] plus either doxycycline[1] or tetracycline[1] plus either primaquine phosphate or tafenoquine	**Quinine sulfate:** see doses above for 3 days **Doxycycline or Tetracycline:** see doses above **Clindamycin:** see doses above **Primaquine phosphate:** see doses above **Tafenoquine** can be used instead of primaquine in children ≥16 years: 300 mg PO × 1 dose	**Quinine sulfate:** see doses above for 3 days **Doxycycline or Tetracycline:** see doses above **Clindamycin:** see doses above **Primaquine phosphate or Tafenoquine:** see doses above
	4. Mefloquine plus either primaquine phosphate or tafenoquine	**Mefloquine:** see doses above **Primaquine phosphate:** see doses above **Tafenoquine** can be used instead of primaquine in children ≥16 years: 300 mg PO × 1 dose	**Mefloquine:** see doses above **Primaquine phosphate or Tafenoquine:** see doses above

CLINICAL DIAGNOSIS/PLASMODIUM SPECIES/DRUG SUSCEPTIBILITY	DRUG/PRESENTATION	PEDIATRIC DOSE[#]	ADULT DOSE
Severe malaria	1. Artesunate IV[5]110 mg/vial follow with a complete oral course of one of: artemether/lumefantrine[1] atovaquane/proguanil[1] quinine[1] plus doxycycline[1]	**Artesunate:** <20 kg 3.0 mg/kg IV at 0, 12, 24 h. Continue q24h if unable to take oral medication **Atovaquane/proguanil** × 3 days (see doses above) **Artemether/lumefantrine** × 3 days (see doses above) **Quinine sulfate:** × 3 days (7 days if SE Asia) plus **Doxycycline:** 2.2 mg/kg q12h × 7 days	**Artesunate:** 2.4 mg/kg IV at 0, 12, 24 h. Continue q24h if unable to take oral medication **Atovaquane/proguanil** × 3 days (see doses above) **Artemether/lumefantrine** × 3 days (see doses above) **Quinine sulfate:** × 3 days (7 days if SE Asia) plus **Doxycycline:** 100 mg q12h × 7 days

*Artemether-lumefantrine: Take with food. Drug of choice in second/third trimester of pregnancy. Recommended by experts in the first trimester but not yet in the official guidelines.

**Atovaquone-proguanil: Take with food; repeat dose if patient vomits within 30 minutes; Not recommended in pregnancy.

***Doxycycline and tetracycline: Not recommended during pregnancy or in children less than 8 years old. Avoid concomitant intake of divalent cations and antacids. American Academy of Pediatrics now permits less than 21 days for any acute infection for children of all ages.

****Mefloquine: Not effective against strains of *P. falciparum* from SE Asia.

*****Tafenoquine succinate: if G6PD normal.

[#]Pediatric dose should not be higher than adult dose.

[1]Not FDA approved for this indication.

[5]Investigational drug in the United States.

[^]This is an off-label dose.

expanded-use investigational new drug (IND) protocol (see CDC contact information earlier). Oral therapies should be started while waiting for IV artesunate to arrive. The preferred antimalarial for interim oral treatment is artemether-lumefantrine (Coartem)[1] because of its fast onset of action. Other oral options include atovaquone-proguanil (Malarone)[1], quinine[1] plus doxycycline (Vibramycin)[1], and mefloquine (Lariam)[1]. Patients on treatment for severe malaria should have one set of blood smears (thick and thin) performed every 12 to 24 hours until a negative result (no *Plasmodium* parasites are detected) is reported.

After the course of IV artesunate is completed, if parasite density is ≤1% (assessed on a blood smear collected 4 hours after the last dose of IV artesunate), and the patient can tolerate oral treatment, a full treatment course with a follow-up regimen must be administered (see Table 3).

Antimalarial Drugs in Pregnancy

Monitoring the safety of antimalarial drugs and understanding their pharmacokinetics is particularly important in pregnancy—with the altered maternal physiology and the risks to the developing fetus. The scheme will depend on drug susceptibility, the region where infection was acquired, gestational age, severity of the disease, and drug category.

For infections with chloroquine-sensitive *P. falciparum*, *P. vivax*, *P. ovale*, and *P. knowlesi*, chloroquine or hydroxychloroquine can be used during pregnancy. If resistance to chloroquine is suspected, quinine sulfate[1] + clindamycin[1] or mefloquine[1] can be used for treatment during the first trimester of pregnancy. Artemether-lumefantrine (Coartem)[1] is the treatment of choice during the second and third trimesters of pregnancy in chloroquine-resistant malaria infections.

Primaquine and tafenoquine should not be given during pregnancy. Pregnant patients with *P. vivax* and *P. ovale* infections should receive chloroquine prophylaxis[1] (300 mg [base] PO once a week) for the duration of the pregnancy to prevent relapses. After delivery, patients with normal G6PD activity should be treated with primaquine or tafenoquine or continue with chloroquine prophylaxis for a total of 1 year. For women who are breastfeeding, infants should be tested for G6PD deficiency and, if found to have normal activity, oral primaquine can be given to the mother. Tafenoquine is not recommended during breastfeeding.

---

[1]Not FDA approved for this indication

Treatment of Pediatric Patients

The majority of cases and deaths, especially in sub-Saharan Africa, occur in young children. Prompt diagnosis and therapy initiation is key to prevent complications, like cerebral malaria in young children. Treatment regimens recommended are essentially the same as in adults, with few differences. Weight-based dose adjustments are necessary and pediatric doses should not exceed those given to adults. Tetracycline and doxycycline should be avoided in children younger than 8 years. Tafenoquine is not indicated in those younger than 16 years of age. For complete details on dosing and treatment duration in pediatric patients, see Table 3.

Prevention of Malaria

Prevention of malaria includes both chemoprophylaxis and measures taken to reduce the number of mosquito bites. Malaria vaccines are still experimental or in early pilot implementation phases. They have been studied primarily in children in endemic areas and are not universally recommended.

Travelers to endemic areas can reduce mosquito bites by using N,N-diethyl-meta-toluamide (DEET 10% to 50%) or 7% picaridin-containing insect repellents on exposed skin (applied after sunscreen), wearing permethrin-treated clothing, wearing clothes and footwear that cover as much skin as possible, sleeping under permethrin-treated bed nets, staying in housing with air-conditioning and well-screened areas cleared of mosquitoes, and refraining from outdoor activity during peak *Anopheles* biting hours (from dusk to dawn).

Recommendations for chemoprophylaxis based on the country being visited can be found on the CDC's website at, https://www.cdc.gov/malaria/travelers/country_table/a.html

Several considerations have to be taken into account for the chemoprophylaxis in travelers to malarial areas. An individualized risk benefit assessment should be conducted for every traveler, considering not only the region or country to be visited but also the itinerary and duration, specific cities or rural areas, types of accommodations, season (rainy or dry), and type of travel (adventure or business).

It is important to consider that no chemoprophylactic regimen is 100% effective, and other measures to decrease mosquito bites, as described previously, should be considered. If a person develops malaria while taking chemoprophylaxis, that particular drug should not be used as part of the treatment regimen.

The recommended regimens according to the *Plasmodium* species and its pattern of resistance are detailed in Table 4.

TABLE 4	Chemoprophylaxis of Malaria		
LOCAL RESISTANCE PATTERN	**DRUG**	**PEDIATRIC DOSE**	**ADULT DOSE**

Primary Regimens

LOCAL RESISTANCE PATTERN	DRUG	PEDIATRIC DOSE	ADULT DOSE
Chloroquine sensitive *Plasmodium falciparum*	1. Chloroquine phosphate 1 tab = 500 mg (salt) (300 mg of base)	8.3 mg/kg (5 mg/kg of base) PO 1×/week up to 300 mg (base) max dose. Starting 1–2 weeks before travel, during travel and 4 weeks post-travel	500 mg (300 mg base) PO per week. Starting 1–2 weeks before travel, during travel and 4 weeks post-travel
	2. Atovaquone/ proguanil (Malarone)*1 adult tab = 250/100 mg 1 ped tab = 62.5/25 mg	5–8 kg ½ peds tab 9–10 kg ¾ peds tab 11–20 kg 1 peds tab 21–30 kg 2 peds tab 31–40 Kg 3 peds tab >40 kg 1 adult tab per day with food. One day prior to, during and 7 days post travel	One adult tab (250/100 mg) per day with food. One day prior to, during and 7 days post travel

Alternative Regimens

LOCAL RESISTANCE PATTERN	DRUG	PEDIATRIC DOSE	ADULT DOSE
	1. Tafenoquine** (Arakoda) ≥16 years only 1 tab = 100 mg		Prior to malaria-endemic area (loading regimen): 200 mg once daily × 3 days (starting 3 days before travel) In endemic area (maintenance regimen) 200 mg once weekly (starting 7 days after last loading regimen dose) Post travel: 200 mg one-time dose (7 days after last maintenance dose)
	2. Doxycycline 1 tab = 100 mg***	8–12 years: 2.2 mg/kg once/day up to 100 mg/day. 1–2 days before, during and for 4 weeks post-travel	100 mg PO qd. 1–2 days pre-travel, during and 4 weeks post travel
	3. Mefloquine 1 tab = 250 mg****	Weekly dose by weight in kg 5–<10 kg: 31.25 mg (1/8 tablet) 10–<20 kg: 62.5 mg (1/4 tablet) 20–<30 kg: 125 mg (1/2 tablet) 30–45 kg: 187.5 mg (3/4 tablet) >45 kg: 250 mg (1 tablet) Start 1–2 weeks before travel and continue 4 weeks after leaving endemic area.	250 mg (228 mg base) 1 tab PO once per week, 1–2 weeks before, during and 4 weeks after travel
Nonchloroquine resistant *Plasmodium vivax*	Primaquine phosphate1 1 tab = 15 mg (base)	0.5 mg/kg base (0.8 mg/kg salt) up to adult dose 30 mg base (52.6 mg salt) daily Start 1–2 days prior, during, and 7 days after travel	30 mg base PO daily in non-pregnant, G6PD-normal travelers Start 1–2 days prior, during, and 7 days after travel

Primary Regimens

LOCAL RESISTANCE PATTERN	DRUG	PEDIATRIC DOSE	ADULT DOSE
Chloroquine resistant *Plasmodium falciparum*	1. Atovaquone/ proguanil* 1 adult tab = 250/100 mg 1 ped tab = 62.5/25 mg	5–8 kg ½ peds tab 9–10 kg ¾ peds tab 11–20 kg 1 peds tab 21–30 kg 2 peds tab 31–40 kg 3 peds tab >40 kg 1 adult tab Daily with food 1–2 days prior to, during and for 7 days post travel in endemic area	1 adult tab/day with food 1–2 days prior to, during and for 7 days post travel in endemic area

Alternative Regimens

LOCAL RESISTANCE PATTERN	DRUG	PEDIATRIC DOSE	ADULT DOSE
	1. Tafenoquine (Arakoda) 1 tab = 100 mg**	Not approved for malaria prophylaxis in <18 years of age	Prior to malaria-endemic area (loading regimen): 200 mg once daily × 3 days (starting 3 days before travel) In endemic area (maintenance regimen) 200 mg once weekly (starting 7 days after last loading regimen dose) Post travel: 200 mg one-time dose (7 days after last maintenance dose)
	2. Doxycycline 1 tab = 100 mg***	8–12 years: 2.2 mg/kg once/day up to 100 mg/day 1–2 days before, during and for 4 weeks post-travel	100 mg PO qd. 1–2 days pre-travel, during and 4 weeks post travel
	3. Mefloquine 1 tab = 250 mg****	Weekly dose by weight in kg <9 kg 5 mg/kg 15–19 kg ¼ adult dose 20–30 kg ½ adult dose 31–45 kg ¾ adult dose >45 kg adult dose	250 mg (228 mg base) 1 tab PO once per week, 2–3 weeks before, during and 4 weeks after travel

*Atovaquone-proguanil: preferred for short trips due to increase adherence.

**Tafenoquine: must have G6PD activity greater than 70% normal on a quantitative test. Preferred for longer trips due to few adverse effects.

***Doxycycline: the American Academy of Pediatrics now recommends that doxycycline can safely be administered for short durations (≤21 days) regardless of patient age; this does not apply to malaria prophylaxis due to required duration of dosing.

****Mefloquine: start 3 weeks ahead, if feasible, to assess for intolerance. This is the current best option for pregnancy.

1Not FDA approved for this indication.

References

Ansong D, Seydel K, Taylor T: Malaria. In Ryan E, Hill D, Solomon T, et al, editors: *Hunter's Tropical Medicine and Emerging Infectious Diseases, 2020,* 10th ed, Syracuse, 2020, Elsevier, pp 734–754.

Centers for Disease Control and Prevention: Malaria and travelers for U.S. residents. Available at: https://www.cdc.gov/malaria/travelers/index.html. Accessed 17 April 2020.

Centers for Disease Control and Prevention: Malaria treatment (United States). Available at: https://www.cdc.gov/malaria/diagnosis_treatment/treatment.html. Accessed 17 April 2020.

Fairhurst R, Wellems T: Malaria (*Plasmodium* species). In Bennett J, Dolin R, Blaser M, editors: *Mandell, Douglas and Bennett's Principles and Practice of Infectious Diseases, 2019,* 9th ed, Philadelphia, 2019, Elsevier, pp 3299–3320.

RTS, S Clinical Trials Partnership: Efficacy and safety of RTS, S/AS01 malaria vaccine with or without a booster dose in infants and children in Africa: final results of a phase 3, individually randomized, controlled trial, *Lancet* 386:31–45, 2015.

Van Der Pluijm R., Tripura R., Hoglund R., et al. Triple artemisinin-based combination therapies versus artemisinin-based combination therapies for uncomplicated *Plasmodium falciparum* malaria: a multicenter, open label, randomized clinical trial. www.thelancet.com Published online March 11, 2020. Available at: https://doi.org/10.1016/S0140-6736(20)30552-3.

World Health Organization: Malaria. Available at: https://www.who.int/malaria/en/. Accessed 17 April 2020.

World Health Organization: World malaria report 2019. Available at: https://www.who.int/news-room/feature-stories/detail/world-malaria-report-2019. Accessed 17 April 2020.

MEASLES (RUBEOLA)

Method of
Jane A. Weida, MS, MD

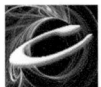

CURRENT DIAGNOSIS

- Measles is a highly contagious viral illness with a prodrome of high fever, cough, conjunctivitis, and coryza.
- A pathognomonic enanthem (Koplik spots—small white lesions) may appear on buccal mucosa.
- The incubation period is about 10 days to the onset of fever; the typical rash appears after about 14 days.
- Measles produces a red maculopapular rash beginning on the face and then becoming generalized.
- Patients usually have a history of exposure, particularly of travel to an endemic area or of contact with carriers or non-immunized individuals.

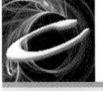

CURRENT THERAPY

- No specific antiviral therapy is available
- Adequate hydration
- Bed rest
- Antipyretics
- Antibiotics if needed for bacterial complications

Epidemiology

Before measles vaccines were introduced, measles caused millions of deaths worldwide each year. In the decade before the first measles vaccine was licensed in 1963, there were about 549,000 measles cases and 495 deaths annually in the United States. It is estimated that the actual incidence was much higher, possibly 3 to 4 million.

Measles was declared to have been eliminated from the United States in 2000, but outbreaks have occurred since then. There were no measles cases reported in the United States during 2021, as of March 5, 2021. In 2020 there were 13 cases in the United States. Conversely, in 2019 there were 1282 cases of measles in 31 states, the largest outbreak since 1992. The majority of these cases involved people who had not been vaccinated.

Most measles cases are due to either travel to endemic areas or exposure to carriers or persons who had not been immunized. Travelers with measles continue to bring the disease to the United States. Measles can spread when it reaches an area where groups of people are unvaccinated, including areas where immunity dips below 95%.

Measles continues to be a major problem in many regions of the world. Due to increased worldwide measles vaccination, reported cases and estimated measles deaths have dropped, but the numbers have increased in recent years. Since 2000, measles deaths worldwide have decreased 62%, and it is estimated that measles vaccination has prevented 25.5 million deaths.

Risk Factors

Being unvaccinated is the largest risk factor for measles in the United States. Infants who have lost maternal immunity but are too young to be immunized are at higher risk, as are individuals with vitamin A deficiency. Travel to international areas where measles is more common or where there is an outbreak also increases the risk of contracting the disease. If measles is suspected in a patient, a careful travel history should be obtained.

Pathophysiology

Measles is caused by an RNA respiratory virus of the family *Paramyxoviridae* and genus *Morbillivirus.* It is one of the most highly contagious of the communicable diseases. The virus spreads from person to person via respiratory droplets from coughing or sneezing or via direct contact. Patients are usually contagious from about 4 days before to about 4 days after the rash appears. The fact that the disease is contagious before the onset of symptoms makes quarantining particularly difficult. The incubation period is generally 10 days before the prodrome and 14 days before the onset of the rash, but it may vary from 6 to 21 days.

The virus triggers an aggressive immune response. This leads to a suppression of the immune response to other pathogens, which makes the individual susceptible to secondary infections. This immune suppression can last for a few weeks to a few months, but in some cases it may last for 2 to 3 years.

Once a measles infection has cleared, the affected person gains lifelong immunity provided that they remain immunocompetent. Infants are protected by maternal antibodies for about 1 month in the case of an immunized mother and for about 4 months in the case of a mother who had a prior measles infection.

Prevention

The best way to prevent measles is with measles vaccination. The Centers for Disease Control and Prevention (CDC) recommends measles-mumps-rubella (MMR) vaccination at ages 12 to 15 months, with the second dose at 4 to 6 years of age. Two doses are more than 99% effective. Students at post–high school institutions who are not immune to measles should have two doses of MMR vaccine at least 28 days apart. Adults born during or after 1957 who do not have evidence of immunity should receive at least one dose of MMR vaccine. The vaccine should not be given to pregnant women or immunocompromised individuals.

International travelers should be protected against measles. Infants 6 to 11 months of age who are traveling should receive one dose of MMR vaccine. Children 12 months of age and older should have documentation of two doses of MMR vaccine at least 28 days apart. Teenagers and adults born during or after 1957 without evidence of immunity should have two documented doses of MMR vaccine.

Despite the importance of measles prevention, some parents refuse to vaccinate their children. A study published in the United Kingdom in 1998 claimed to find a link between autism and MMR vaccine. The study was later proven to be erroneous and fraudulent. Subsequent studies have consistently shown that there is no link between vaccines and autism. It is vital for clinicians to educate parents about the importance—which cannot be overstated—of MMR vaccination.

Clinical Signs and Symptoms

Measles generally presents with a prodrome that includes high fever, malaise, anorexia, conjunctivitis, coryza, and nonproductive cough. Fever may reach over 40°C. Conjunctivitis may include redness, swelling, photophobia, and discharge. Koplik spots, which are small white spots surrounded by a red ring, appearing on the buccal mucosa, are pathognomonic but are not always present.

The measles rash is erythematous and maculopapular. It usually appears first on the face and behind the ears and then spreads to the trunk and extremities. The rash lasts 3 to 7 days. Recovery begins soon after the rash appears.

Diagnosis

Measles is usually diagnosed clinically, based on the presenting signs, vaccination history, and travel exposure history. Clinical diagnosis can be difficult when the incidence of measles is low. The World Health Organization clinical case definition for measles is a person with fever and maculopapular rash and at least one of the symptoms of cough, coryza, or conjunctivitis.

Laboratory findings include leukopenia unless there is a secondary bacterial infection, as well as thrombocytopenia and proteinuria. The most commonly used serologic test is virus-specific immunoglobulin M (IgM) in serum or oral fluid. IgM antibodies may not be detectable until 4 or more days after the rash appears. Viral cultures may be obtained, although measles is technically difficult to culture. Nasopharyngeal swabs may also be obtained for detection of virus by polymerase chain reaction (PCR).

Measles is a reportable illness in the United States; therefore, suspected cases should be reported to the local health department without delay. The CDC recommends that serologic and viral specimens be collected in suspected cases of measles; clinicians can contact their local laboratories to find out which specimens to collect.

Differential Diagnosis

During the prodromal stage, measles can easily be mistaken for other upper viral respiratory illnesses. Although Koplik spots are pathognomonic, they are easy to overlook. Once the rash has appeared, measles can still be mistaken for other illnesses, including erythema infectiosum, infectious mononucleosis, enterovirus, Kawasaki disease, chikungunya, Rocky Mountain spotted fever, rubella, and scarlet fever.

Treatment

No specific antiviral treatment is available for measles. Treatment is supportive, including rest, adequate fluids, and antipyretics. Patients should be kept at bed rest until they are afebrile. Prompt recognition and treatment of secondary bacterial infections is essential. The World Health Organization recommends the administration of vitamin A[1] to all those with measles. The CDC recommends treatment with vitamin A of children with severe cases of measles, such as those who are hospitalized. It is given immediately when the disease is diagnosed and then repeated the following day. In the United States, vitamin A is not routinely given for milder cases of measles.

Monitoring

Most measles patients do not need hospitalization. For those who do, both standard and respiratory precautions should be initiated. Respiratory precautions should continue for 4 days after onset of rash for healthy children and for the duration of the illness for immunocompromised patients.

For those who have been exposed to measles and are not immune, MMR should be administered within 72 hours of exposure or Ig (GamaSTAN) administered within 6 days of exposure.

[1]Not FDA approved for this indication.

Complications

Complications of measles can occur in up to 40% of patients; complications are highest in the very young, the very old, and those who are malnourished. Often the complications affect the respiratory tract, with pneumonia being the leading cause of death associated with measles. Pneumonia may be caused by a secondary bacterial or viral infection or by the measles virus itself. Otitis media is another common complication. Gastrointestinal complications include diarrhea and stomatitis. Measles keratoconjunctivitis is a common complication, especially in children with vitamin A deficiency.

Rarely, measles can cause severe central nervous system (CNS) complications. About 1 in 1000 cases of measles results in post-measles encephalomyelitis, leading to fever, seizures, and neurologic abnormalities. Measles causes about 1 to 2 deaths per 1000 due to respiratory or neurologic complications. Subacute sclerosing panencephalitis is a rare delayed neurologic complication of measles, occurring in about 1 in 10,000 to 100,000 patients. This fatal complication causes seizures and progressive intellectual and behavioral deterioration about 7 to 10 years following a measles infection.

References

Bester J: Measles and measles vaccination a review, *JAMA Pediatr* 170(12):1209–1215, 2016.

Clark E, Shandera WX: Viral & rickettsial infections: measles. In Papadakis MA, McPhee SJ, editors: *Current medical diagnosis and treatment 2021*, 60 ed, McGraw Hill Education, pp 1418–1421, 2021.

Centers for Disease Control and Prevention. Measles Cases and Outbreaks. Available at: https://www.cdc.gov/measles/cases-outbreaks.html

Centers for Disease Control and Prevention: Measles Elimination. Available at: https://www.cdc.gov/measles/elimination.html.

Centers for Disease Control and Prevention: Measles for Healthcare Providers. Available at: https://www.cdc.gov/measles/hcp/index.html.

Centers for Disease Control and Prevention: Progress Toward Regional Measles Elimination — Worldwide, 2000-2019. Available https://www.cdc.gov/mmwr/volumes/68/wr/mm6848a1.htm.

Measles, Kimberlin DW, Brady MT, Jackson MA, Long SS, Itasca IL: In *Red Book: 2018 Report of the Committee on Infectious Diseases*, 31 ed, American Academy of Pediatrics, 2018, pp 537–550.

Moss W: Measles, *Lancet* 390:2490–2502, 2017.

METHICILLIN-RESISTANT *STAPHYLOCOCCUS AUREUS*

Method of
Elissa Rennert-May, MD, MSc; and John M. Conly, MD

CURRENT DIAGNOSIS

- Healthcare-associated methicillin-resistant *Staphylococcus aureus* (HA-MRSA) is endemic in many hospital settings. The strains are polyclonal, resistant to many non–β-lactam antimicrobials, and typically cause pneumonia, line-related infection, surgical site infection, bacteremia, and infrequently skin and soft tissue infections.

- Strains of community-associated MRSA (CA-MRSA) have risen exponentially over the past two decades. The strains are clonal, sensitive to many non–β-lactam antimicrobials, harbour multiple virulence factors, and typically cause pyogenic skin and soft tissue infections and occasionally severe necrotizing pneumonia, fasciitis, and multifocal osteomyelitis.

- HA-MRSA infections typically affect patients with multiple co-morbidities in the healthcare setting, but CA-MRSA typically affects previously healthy persons.

- It can be difficult to differentiate infectious syndromes due to β-hemolytic streptococci versus CA-MRSA.

CURRENT THERAPY

- Methicillin-resistant *Staphylococcus aureus* (MRSA) strains harbor resistance to the β-lactam antimicrobials, including oxacillin, dicloxacillin, cloxacillin[2], nafcillin, methicillin[1], and first-, second-, and third-generation cephalosporins.
- Healthcare-associated MRSA (HA-MRSA) strains are typically resistant to macrolides, clindamycin (Cleocin), aminoglycosides, and quinolones (with the exception of delafloxacin [Baxdela]) and are variably resistant to tetracycline and trimethoprim-sulfamethoxazole (Bactrim). They are sensitive to vancomycin (Vancocin) and the lipoglycopeptides, fusidic acid[2], rifampin (Rifadin)[1], the oxazolidinones linezolid (Zyvox) and tedizolid (Sivextro), daptomycin (Cubicin), ceftaroline (Teflaro), and ceftobiprole (Zevtera)[2].
- Community-associated MRSA (CA-MRSA) strains are resistant to macrolides and quinolones (with the exception of delafloxacin [Baxdela]) but usually are sensitive to aminoglycosides such as gentamicin (Garamycin), clindamycin, (Cleocin) and trimethoprim-sulfamethoxazole (Bactrim)[1], in addition to vancomycin (Vancocin), the lipoglycopeptides, fusidic acid[2], rifampin (Rifadin)[1], the oxazolidinones linezolid (Zyvox) and tedizolid (Sivextro), daptomycin (Cubicin), ceftaroline (Teflaro), and ceftobiprole (Zevtera)[2].
- Empiric antimicrobial therapy should be guided by the clinical presentation, and when full sensitivities are available, the antimicrobials may be tailored accordingly.

[1]Not FDA approved for this indication.
[2]Not available in the United States.

Epidemiology

Staphylococcus aureus is one of the most frequently encountered bacteria causing human infections and may be considered as either methicillin-sensitive *S. aureus* (MSSA) or methicillin-resistant *S. aureus* (MRSA). MRSA was first described in 1961 and is resistant not only to the traditional antistaphylococcal β-lactam antibiotics (methicillin[2] , nafcillin, oxacillin, cloxacillin[2], and dicloxacillin) but also other important β-lactam antibiotics, including the first- to fourth-generation cephalosporins and the carbapenem family, thus eliminating an important class of antibiotics from the clinician's armamentarium. The only β-lactams that have activity against MRSA are the advanced-generation cephalosporin agents ceftaroline (Teflaro) and ceftobiprole (Zevtera)[2].

MRSA strains acquired in the hospital or other healthcare settings have traditionally been referred to as healthcare-associated MRSA (HA-MRSA), whereas community-associated MRSA (CA-MRSA) has referred to isolates acquired in the community setting and in the absence of traditional hospital or healthcare exposures for at least 1 year (overnight stays in an acute care or long-term care facility, surgery, dialysis, or presence of a central venous catheter). The term *community-onset HA-MRSA* has been used to describe the occurrence of MRSA infection in the setting of the presence of a healthcare exposure within the past year. MRSA has been recognized as a healthcare-associated pathogen since the 1970s and became endemic in hospitals in many countries, including the United States, United Kingdom, and many European countries, with exceptions being Denmark, the Netherlands, Scandinavia, and Canada. For several decades, MRSA was typically considered a hospital pathogen. Novel and virulent MRSA strains arising in the community and not associated with any traditional healthcare exposure risks were first encountered in the late 1990s in the United States, Australia, and some European countries and have since risen explosively on a global basis to become the predominant clone of *S. aureus* associated with community infections. Methicillin resistance among community

isolates of *S. aureus* has been reported to be as high as 75% in some US communities. More recently livestock-associated MRSA (LA-MRSA) has been reported on a global basis, and transmission of these strains from swine, cattle, and horses has been implicated as a source of human infections, particularly in farmers, abattoir workers, and veterinarians.

Specific genetic and molecular distinctions initially distinguished the HA- and CA-MRSA strains (Table 1) and have been used to characterize MRSA strains as likely of community versus healthcare origin. The HA-MRSA strains were found to harbor large staphylococcal cassette chromosome (SCC*mec*) types known as SCC*mec* types I, II, or III; to have multidrug resistance to non–β-lactam antimicrobials; to have the absence of specific virulence characteristics such as carriage of the Panton-Valentine Leukocidin *(PVL)* gene; and to have varying multilocus sequence types (ST5, ST239, ST 247, ST250). On the other hand, the CA-MRSA strains have been found to harbor SCC*mec* types IV, V, and more recently VI to XIII have been described; to have paucidrug resistance to non–β-lactam antimicrobials; to have the presence of specific virulence characteristics such as carriage of the *PVL* gene, and to have multilocus sequence types ST1, ST8, and ST80. LA-MRSA strains often are nontypeable or harbor SCC*mec* V, have high rates of tetracycline resistance, carry multiple virulence factors, and are most often multilocus sequence types ST398 or ST9. However, over the past few years, healthcare-associated strains have moved into the community and likewise community strains have spread rapidly within hospitals, and the original distinctions between CA-MRSA and HA-MRSA from an epidemiologic perspective have become increasingly blurred. The point of transmission of MRSA is not always possible to identify with certainty, making the classification of CA and HA strains increasingly imprecise.

Risk Factors

The risk factors for HA-MRSA may be viewed from the perspective of the healthcare environment and patient-specific risk factors. A major risk factor for acquiring HA-MRSA is exposure to a healthcare setting and particularly in hospital or other institutional settings where the prevalence of carriage of MRSA among patients is high. Additional risk factors in the healthcare environment include poor hand hygiene practices among hospital employees, contaminated bedside equipment and surfaces, overcrowding, and reduced healthcare worker-to-patient ratios. Patient risk factors (see Table 1) include aging, multiple comorbidities, receipt of antibiotics within the preceding 3 months, prolonged duration of hospital stay, admission to a long-term care facility or hospital in the previous year, invasive procedures, and the presence of indwelling catheters or other devices. Initial risk groups for CA-MRSA were injection drug users, homeless populations, incarcerated persons, and indigenous peoples. The Centers for Disease Control and Prevention have suggested the five Cs (Figure 1 and Table 2) as contributing factors implicated in the transmission among these groups. The initial risk groups have expanded (Table 3) to include men who have sex with men (MSM), athletes (especially those involved in team and contact sports), military personnel, those with a prior history of abscesses, individuals with chronic skin disorders, individuals with recent antibiotic receipt, underserved urban populations, individuals who have contact with colonized pets or livestock, and veterinary workers. In the drug-using and underserved urban populations, prevalence and social networking studies have identified hospices, shooting galleries, and crack houses as key sites in which CA-MRSA transmission may occur. Recent outbreaks have been reported in hospital nurseries, daycare settings, nursing home workers, schools, and college dormitories. Sexual transmission has been reported, but it may reflect close skin-to-skin genital contact rather than a true sexually transmitted pathogen. CA-MRSA has now become endemic in the general population in many communities, and the elderly and the very young seem to have a predilection for infection, especially if other risk factors are present. Risk groups for LA-MRSA include farmers, their family members and farm hands who are engaged in livestock production (especially swine and cattle), abattoir workers, veterinarians, and

[2]Not available in the United States.

TABLE 1 General Features Differentiating HA- and CA-MRSA*

CHARACTERISTIC	HA-MRSA	CA-MRSA
Drug resistance to non–β-lactams	Multiresistance	Pauciresistance
Pathogenicity islands	Few	Multiple
Age predilection	Older	Younger
Comorbidities	Multiple	None
Traditional risk factors	Healthcare contact, prolonged hospital stay, poor hand hygiene, contaminated equipment, invasive procedures, medical devices, recent antibiotic use	Crowded community environment, lack of cleanliness, loss of skin integrity, intravenous drug user, homelessness, incarceration, aboriginal, HIV+, contact sports, athletes, military, chronic skin disorder, veterinary worker

*Features are generalizations only given the appearance of community strains replacing traditional hospital strains in the health care setting and the appearance of typical HA strains in the community setting.
CA, Community-associated; *HA*, healthcare-associated; *HIV*, human immunodeficiency virus; *MRSA*, methicillin-resistant *Staphylococcus aureus*.

The "5 Cs" for Transmission of CA-MRSA

- **C**rowding
- **C**ontact with skin
- **C**ompromised skin
- **C**ontaminated personal care items
- **C**leanliness lack

Figure 1 The five Cs implicated in transmission of community-associated methicillin-resistant *S. aureus*. Adapted from the US Centers for Disease Control and Prevention.

veterinary assistants. Recent transmission of strains of LA-MRSA has been reported in the hospital setting as well.

Pathophysiology

The resistance to the antistaphylococcal β-lactam antibiotics in MRSA strains is imparted by the presence of an altered configuration for a specific penicillin-binding protein (PBP) known as PBP2a in the cell wall of staphylococci. Normally the PBPs would act as a site for the attachment of the active moieties of the β-lactam agent, which then would inhibit further cell wall assembly. The alteration in the configuration of PBP2a occurs as the result of the presence of the SCC*mec* gene in *S. aureus*, which confers resistance to the β-lactam antibiotics. The origins of the *mec* gene and its insertion into the SCC*mec* element are not known with certainty. Once the MRSA strains acquired resistance to the antistaphylococcal β-lactam antibiotics in the healthcare setting, it is not difficult to appreciate how it emerged as a predominant pathogen in the hospital setting over the years, with increasing acuity of illness in the patient populations and increased use of broad-spectrum antimicrobials.

The appearance and rapid spread of CA-MRSA with the clinical impression of more virulent and lethal infections than what had been seen with traditional HA-MRSA strains may be explained by several factors. The SCC*mec* IV genetic element is very widely distributed among *S. aureus* isolates, which may explain its appearance in multiple settings globally, and these strains appear to have more rapid growth rates than typical HA-MRSA strains, larger numbers of virulence factors, pathogenicity islands, and higher levels of expression of the virulence factors produced. Recently α-type phenol-soluble modulins were described in strains of CA-MRSA, which are produced at very high levels and are potent lysins of neutrophils. High levels of α-toxin production by these strains, which act as pore-forming toxins for multiple cell types, may also contribute to their virulence. The vast majority of CA-MRSA strains also produce the genes for PVL and it functions as a dermonecrotic factor in skin lesions, a potent cell lysin in high concentrations, and a potent inflammatory mediator in lower concentrations. However, there is controversy about the role of PVL as a single predominant virulence factor, because strains of CA-MRSA that have this gene knocked out have demonstrated no difference in pathogenicity in both vertebrate and invertebrate animal models and in human settings when the PVL is not present.

Prevention

Controlling the spread of HA-, CA-, or LA-MRSA from an infected or colonized person to others in the hospital, family, or community is a key goal of prevention. In the hospital setting, strict adherence to hand hygiene, application of barrier precautions (gloves, gowns, and private rooms) for patients colonized or infected with MRSA, environmental and equipment cleaning, and antimicrobial stewardship are the key preventive strategies. Active surveillance cultures to identify colonized patients and decolonization may be effective in selected settings, but its general application is controversial. In the community setting, practicing hygienic measures including good personal hygiene, consistent hand hygiene, ensuring all draining skin and soft tissue lesions have adequate dressings, not sharing potentially contaminated personal articles, and keeping the household environment hygienic are important. Public health organizations may also contribute to the prevention of CA-MRSA by instituting education programs targeting healthcare providers and individuals in high-risk groups in the community, and by promoting appropriate antimicrobial use. In sports settings, in addition to the basic hygienic measures mentioned previously, avoidance of sharing of towels and other personal items, showering after every practice or tournament, cleaning of communal showering and bathing areas, and cleaning or laundering of equipment after each use are also important.

Clinical Manifestations

The specific clinical infections associated with MRSA parallel those associated with MSSA. Almost any body site, organ, or appendage may be affected by infections due to *S. aureus*, but there are specific predilections associated with HA- and CA-MRSA. In the hospital or other healthcare setting, the most commonly encountered sites of infection include pneumonia, line-related infection, surgical site infection, bacteremia, and less often skin and soft tissue infections. In the community setting, the most common sites (>80%) are skin and soft tissue infections (furuncles, cellulitis, and soft tissue abscesses) and less commonly severely invasive infections such as necrotizing pneumonia, necrotizing fasciitis,

TABLE 2 Risk Factor Associations Reported for CA-MRSA Infections

RISK CATEGORIES	FACTOR	DETAILS FROM REPORTS
High-risk populations	Younger and older age	Age distribution in CA-MRSA younger than HA-MRSA High rate of CA-MRSA in children under 2 years CA-MRSA more common in children compared to adults Outbreaks in hospital nurseries Outbreaks in nursing homes with elderly residents
	Indigenous populations: Native or Aboriginal or African American	Aboriginal communities in midwestern United States, Canada, and Australia Alaskan natives More common in African Americans
	Athletes (predominantly contact sports)	Outbreaks on football teams Outbreaks on wrestling team Other competitive sports
	Injection (intravenous) drug users (IVDUs)	San Francisco IVDUs Canadian report of USA300 strain outbreak
	Men who have sex with men (MSM)	CA-MRSA described in HIV+ population of MSM
	HIV+ individuals	Risk associated with overlapping social networks, intravenous drug use, hemodialysis, and CD4 counts <200 reported as independent risks
	Military personnel	3% of US Army soldiers colonized
	Inmates of correctional facilities	Reports of outbreaks in US prisons Two outbreaks (total 10 inmates) in Canada
	Students in elementary schools and college dormitories	Reports of outbreaks in schools and college dormitories
Previous positive MRSA cultures	MRSA carriage Past MRSA infection	Colonized soldiers more likely to get CA-MRSA disease Prior abscess risk factor for CA-MRSA
Medical history	Chronic skin disorder	Dermatologic condition most common underlying medical disorder for CA-MRSA infection Classroom contact of index CA-MRSA case had chronic dermatitis
	Recurrent or recent antibiotic use	Antibiotic use associated with CA-MRSA infection in rural Alaska
Environmental	Homelessness and living in shelters Overcrowding Contact with colonized pet Veterinary workers and family members	Medically underserved populations at higher risk of CA-MRSA Reports of USA300 strain outbreak involving individuals living in shelters or homeless Close contact implicated in jail outbreaks Neonatal intensive care unit transmission Family dog source of recurrent infection Veterinarians working with horses and livestock Family members of animal care workers Small animal veterinarians Swine farmers

CA, Community-associated; *HA*, healthcare-associated; *HIV*, human immunodeficiency virus; *MRSA*, methicillin-resistant *Staphylococcus aureus*.
Adapted from Barton-Forbes M, Hawkes M, Moore D, et al. Guidelines for the prevention and management of community associated methicillin resistant *Staphylococcus aureus* (CA-MRSA): a perspective for Canadian Health Care Practitioners. *Can J Infect Dis Med Microbiol*. 2006;17(suppl C):1B–24B.

627

multifocal osteomyelitis/septic arthritis, epidural abscess, pelvic septic thrombophlebitis, and bacteremia with toxic shock syndrome. The skin and soft tissue infections often affect young previously healthy patients and are characteristically very painful and pyogenic with an initial black eschar that patients presume was a "spider bite" as the initiating process.

Diagnosis

The diagnosis of MRSA infections is based on the clinical presentation and the isolation of the causative organism from purulent discharge, sputum, or urine, or from specimens obtained from normally sterile body fluids (joint fluid, abscess or tissue aspirates, and blood). The organism appears on Gram stain as a gram-positive organism in clusters and is usually seen in association with neutrophils and may be either intracellular or extracellular. The organism is very hardy and grows readily on typical media in the microbiology laboratory within 24 to 48 hours. Some laboratories are using rapid agglutination tests to detect the PBP2a protein or polymerase chain reaction (PCR)-based techniques to provide same-day or next-day identification. In settings where no cultures have been obtained or in the setting of toxic shock syndrome where cultures are often negative, the diagnosis may be difficult and only suspected based on a typical clinical presentation.

Treatment

MRSA strains harbor resistance to the β-lactam antimicrobials, including oxacillin, dicloxacillin, cloxacillin[2], nafcillin, methicillin[2], and first-, second-, and third-generation cephalosporins. The newer advanced-generation cephalosporin antimicrobials ceftaroline (Teflaro) and ceftobiprole (Zevtera)[2] have activity against MRSA strains. The majority of HA-MRSA strains are resistant to macrolides, clindamycin (Cleocin), aminoglycosides, and quinolones (with the exception of delafloxacin [Baxdela]) and are variably resistant to tetracycline and trimethoprim-sulfamethoxazole (Bactrim)[1], depending on local epidemiologic patterns. They are sensitive to vancomycin (Vancocin) and the lipoglycopeptides such as dalbavancin (Dalvance), telavancin

[2] Not available in the United States

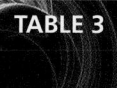

| TABLE 3 | Principles of Empiric Treatment of Minor Skin and Soft Tissue Infections (Folliculitis, Furuncles, Small Abscesses Without Cellulitis, Impetigo, Secondarily Infected Lesions Such as Eczema, Ulcers, or Wounds) Where the Etiology Is Unknown But May Include MRSA as a Possibility |

Recommendations

One or more of the following measures may be employed:
- Local therapy using hot soaks, elevation, and dressings as appropriate
- Incision and drainage of furuncles or small abscesses without antimicrobial therapy
- Topical 2% mupirocin ointment (Bactroban) or fusidic acid[2] for impetigo and secondarily infected lesions if local strains are likely sensitive
- Topical antiseptics may be considered
- Antimicrobial therapy is recommended in addition to local measures if one or more of the following is present: multiple sites of infection, evidence of progression, clinical evidence of systemic symptoms and signs, presence of comorbidities, extremes of age, immunosuppression, septic phlebitis, or difficult site for incision and drainage.
- In follow-up, routine screening for colonization of the nares or other body sites is not recommended.

[2]Not available in the United States.
MRSA, Methicillin-resistant *Staphylococcus aureus*.

| TABLE 4 | Principles of Empiric Treatment of Non–Life-Threatening Skin and Soft Tissue Infections Other Than Minor Skin Infections Where the Etiology Is Unknown But May Include MRSA as a Possibility |

Recommendations
- Antibiotic choice should be based on the severity of illness at presentation, clinical judgment, and regional susceptibility patterns of strains
- Empiric therapy for CA-MRSA and β-hemolytic streptococci is recommended*

*The IDSA guideline suggests to differentiate purulent and nonpurulent cellulitis and reserve empiric therapy for β-hemolytic streptococci only in nonpurulent cellulitis but acknowledges it is an area of controversy. The UK and Canadian guidelines explicitly recommend coverage for β-hemolytic streptococci and do not differentiate cellulitis into different types.
CA, Community-associated; *IDSA*, Infectious Diseases Society of America; *MRSA*, methicillin-resistant *Staphylococcus aureus*.

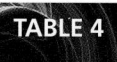
| TABLE 5 | Principles of Empiric Treatment of Life-Threatening Infections Where the Etiology Is Unknown But May Include MRSA as a Possibility |

Recommendations
- Include MRSA coverage, regardless of prevalence rates of CA-MRSA in the community
- Include an agent effective against MSSA until susceptibility results become available

CA, Community-associated; *MRSA*, methicillin-resistant *Staphylococcus aureus*; *MSSA*, methicillin-sensitive *Staphylococcus aureus*.

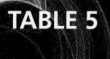

(Vibativ), and oritavancin (Orbactiv) and usually sensitive to fusidic acid[2], rifampin (Rifadin)[1], the oxazolidinones linezolid (Zyvox) and tedizolid (Sivextro), and daptomycin (Cubicin). For hospitalized patients where *S. aureus* is considered a possible etiology of any major infectious syndrome, it should be considered as methicillin-resistant until proven otherwise. Empiric choices of vancomycin or lipoglycopeptides such as dalbavancin (Dalvance), telavancin (Vibativ) or oritavancin (Orbitactiv), linezolid (Zyvox) or tedizolid (Sivextro), daptomycin (Cubicin) or advanced-generation cephalosproins such as ceftaroline (Teflaro) or ceftobiprole (Zevtera)[2] should be considered as appropriate to the presenting syndrome. CA-MRSA strains are resistant to macrolides and often quinolones (with the exception of delafloxacin [Baxdela]) but usually are sensitive to aminoglycosides such as gentamicin (Garamycin), clindamycin, and trimethoprim-sulfamethoxazole (Bactrim)[1],but the resistance patterns vary depending on local resistance patterns. In addition, these strains are sensitive to vancomycin (Vancocin) and the lipoglycopeptides, fusidic acid[2], rifampin (Rifadin)[1], linezolid (Zyvox), daptomycin (Cubicin), ceftaroline (Teflaro), and ceftobiprole (Zevtera)[2]. LA-MRSA strains are almost always resistant to tetracyclines; often resistant to quinolones, macrolides, and clindamycin, and variably resistant to aminoglycosides and trimethoprim-sulfamethoxazole.

In addition, these strains are sensitive to vancomycin (Vancocin) and the lipoglycopeptides, fusidic acid[2], rifampin (Rifadin)[1], the oxazolidinones linezolid (Zyvox) and tedizolid (Sivextro), daptomycin (Cubicin), ceftaroline (Teflaro) and ceftobiprole (Zevtera)[2]. Treatment guidelines for MRSA with a focus on the ambulatory setting have been published in Canada, the United Kingdom, and the United States, and provide both empiric choices for common infectious presentations of unknown etiology and definitive treatment once an etiology of MRSA is known. The treatment options for both empiric and definitive use where MRSA is considered or proven are presented in Tables 3 through 6 and represent a constellation of the various guidelines that have been published. A recent randomized controlled trial assessed the efficacy of combination therapy in patients with MRSA bacteremia (vancomycin or daptomycin with flucloxacillin[2]). They found that the number of patients with persistent bacteremia after 5 days was lower in the combination arm. However, due to increased nephrotoxicity in the combination arm the trial was stopped early. Further studies are required to determine the role and benefit of combination therapy for MRSA infections.

[2] Not available in the United States.

TABLE 6   Guidelines for the Management of MRSA Infections

CLINICAL DISEASE	KEY FEATURES	MANAGEMENT PRINCIPLES	ANTIMICROBIAL CHOICES AND COMMENTS*
Skin and Soft Tissue Infection (SSTI)			
Localized lesion	Infected scratches and minor wounds Insect bites Furuncles Small abscesses Absence of systemic illness	Culture selectively[†] No antibiotic therapy recommended *Exceptions: multiple sites of infection, evidence of progression, systemic symptoms and signs, presence of comorbidities, extremes of age, immunosuppression, septic phlebitis, or difficult site for incision and drainage: antimicrobial therapy is recommended in addition to local measures* Cover draining lesions Emphasize personal hygiene Close follow-up Return if worsening	Generally not indicated, although some evidence exists for treatment with clindamycin PO or trimethoprim-sulfamethoxazole (Bactrim)[1] PO, in conjunction with incision and drainage for small simple abscesses Topical antibacterial (e.g., mupirocin [Bactroban] or fusidic ointment[2]) therapy may be considered Systemic antimicrobial therapy indicated if one or more of the following: multiple sites of infection, evidence of progression, systemic symptoms and signs, presence of comorbidities, extremes of age, immunosuppression, septic phlebitis, or difficult site for incision and drainage
Cellulitis (not extensive) or multiple abscesses with minimal or no associated systemic features for oral treatment consideration	Classic features of rubor, dolor, calor, and swelling suggesting cellulitis with or without associated drainage or exudate	Culture site (if purulent or drainage) Drainage of abscess or needle aspiration Oral therapy in older child and adult Appropriate infection control measures Imaging for extent and complications as appropriate Close follow-up Return if worsening	*Empiric:* Include coverage for β-hemolytic streptococci[¶] Clindamycin (Cleocin) 300–450 mg tid-qid PO for adults and 30–40 mg/kg/day[3] ÷ q6–8h PO for children TMP-SMX (Bactrim)[1] 1–2 DS tab bid PO for adults and 8–12 mg/kg/day (of TMP) ÷ q12h PO for children PLUS coverage for β-hemolytic streptococci (e.g., amoxicillin, cephalexin [Keflex]) Doxycycline (Vibramycin) 100 mg bid PO for adults and 4.4 mg/kg/day mg/kg/day ÷ q12h PO for children** PLUS coverage for β-hemolytic streptococci (e.g., amoxicillin, cephalexin) Delafloxacin (Baxdela) 450 mg bid PO for adults *Comment:* Recently became the first fluoroquinolone approved by the FDA for MRSA SSTI Linezolid (Zyvox) 600 mg bid PO for adults and 30 mg/kg/day ÷ q8h PO for children, not to exceed 600 mg/dose; for children older than 12 years of age 600 mg bid PO *Comment:* Linezolid is more expensive than the other options and may not always be readily available depending on the setting *Comment:* If parenteral therapy considered, see choices for severe SSTI Tedizolid (Sivextro) 200 mg PO/IV once daily for 6 days; safety and efficacy have not been established for children *Proven MRSA:* As above, based on sensitivity testing If parenteral therapy necessary, see choices for SSTI with systemic features
Cellulitis (severe or rapidly spreading or extensive) or complicated SSTI (deep soft tissue infection, surgical or traumatic wound infection, large or multiple abscesses, or infected ulcers and burns) and/or associated systemic features for parenteral treatment consideration	Classic features of rubor, dolor, calor, and swelling suggesting cellulitis with or without associated drainage or exudate with systemic features of fever, chills, malaise, prostration	Culture (blood if febrile, site if purulent) Hospitalize as appropriate Drainage of abscess or needle aspiration Parenteral therapy Imaging for extent and complications as appropriate Appropriate infection control measures Consultation as indicated	*Empiric:* Include coverage for β-hemolytic streptococci[¶] Vancomycin (Vancocin) 15–20 mg/kg/dose q8–12h IV for adults and 40–60[3] mg/kg/day ÷ q6h IV for children *Proven MRSA:* Based on sensitivity testing Vancomycin 15–20 mg/kg/dose q8–12h IV for adults and 40–60[3] mg/kg/day ÷ q6h IV for children Clindamycin 600–900 mg q8h IV/IM for adults and 30–40 mg/kg/day[3] ÷ q6–8h IV for children Linezolid 600 mg q12h PO/IV for adults and 30 mg/kg/day ÷ q8h PO/IV for children, not to exceed 600 mg/dose; for children older than 12 years of age 600 mg bid PO/IV Tedizolid (Sivextro) 200 mg PO/IV once daily for 6 days; safety and efficacy have not been established for children Ceftaroline (Teflaro) 600 mg IV q12h for adults; safety and efficacy have not been established for children Daptomycin (Cubicin) 4 mg/kg/dose once daily IV for adults and under investigation in children Dalbavancin (Dalvance) 1000 mg IV followed by 500 mg IV 1 week later for adults; safety and efficacy not established in children Telavancin (Vibativ) 10 mg/kg/dose IV once daily Oritavancin (Orbactiv), given as a single 1200 mg 3-hour infusion; not approved for children Delafloxacin (Baxdela) 300 mg bid IV *Comment:* Linezolid, tedizolid, daptomycin, ceftaroline, ceftobiprole,[2] dalbavancin, oritavancin and telavancin are more expensive than the other options and may not always be readily available depending on the setting

Continued

| TABLE 6 | Guidelines for the Management of MRSA Infections—cont'd |

CLINICAL DISEASE	KEY FEATURES	MANAGEMENT PRINCIPLES	ANTIMICROBIAL CHOICES AND COMMENTS*
Necrotizing fasciitis (NF)	Clinically indistinguishable from group A streptococcus NF disease Extreme toxicity High complication rate	Cultures (blood, tissue) Imaging for extent and complications Surgical débridement Consultation as indicated Parenteral therapy Infection control measures	*Empiric:* Include coverage for β-hemolytic streptococci Vancomycin 15–20 mg/kg/dose q8–12h IV for adults and 40–60[3] mg/kg/day ÷ q6h IV for children Clindamycin 600–900 mg q8h IV/IM for adults and 30–40 mg/kg/day[3] ÷ q6–8h IV for children *Proven MRSA:* Based on sensitivity testing Vancomycin 15–20 mg/kg/dose q8–12h IV for adults and 40–60[3] mg/kg/day ÷ q6h IV for children Clindamycin 600–900 mg q8h IV/IM for adults and 30–40 mg/kg/day[3] ÷ q6–8h IV for children Linezolid 600 mg q12h PO/IV for adults and 30 mg/kg/day ÷ q8h PO/IV for children, not to exceed 600 mg/dose; for children older than 12 years of age 600 mg bid PO/IV TMP/SMX[1] 8–12 mg/kg/day (of TMP) ÷ q8–12h IV for adults and 8–12 mg/kg/day (of TMP) ÷ q6h IV for children *Comments:* Adjuncts such as IVIG (Gamunex)[1] may be considered in severe cases with septic shock Few data available for the use of TMP-SMX in this indication

Musculoskeletal Infection (MSI)

CLINICAL DISEASE	KEY FEATURES	MANAGEMENT PRINCIPLES	ANTIMICROBIAL CHOICES AND COMMENTS*
Osteomyelitis/septic arthritis	Preceding trauma Tendency for multifocal involvement Disease in adjacent muscle not uncommon Progression to chronic osteomyelitis possible May be complicated by deep venous thrombosis	Cultures (blood, bone, and tissue) Imaging for extent and complications Involve surgical team (early débridement and drainage) Consultation as indicated Parenteral therapy Consider combination therapy for severe cases or if slow to respond Infection control measures Look for other infected sites (imaging)	*Empiric:* Vancomycin 15–20 mg/kg/dose q8–12h IV for adults and 40–60[3] mg/kg/day ÷ q6h IV for children Clindamycin 600–900 mg q8h IV/IM for adults and 30–40 mg/kg/day[3] ÷ q6–8h IV for children Linezolid[1] 600 mg q12h PO/IV for adults and 30 mg/kg/day ÷ q8h PO/IV for children, not to exceed 600 mg/dose; for children older than 12 years of age 600 mg bid PO/IV Daptomycin[1] 6 mg/kg/dose once daily IV for adults and 6–10 mg/kg once daily for children TMP/SMX[1] 8–12 mg/kg/day (of TMP) ÷ q8–12h IV for adults and 8–12 mg/kg/day (of TMP) ÷ q6h IV for children *Comments:* Linezolid and daptomycin are more expensive than the other options and may not always be readily available depending on the setting Few data available for the use of TMP-SMX in these indications for children *Proven MRSA:* As above, based on sensitivity testing Addition of rifampin (Rifadin)[1] may be considered for osteomyelitis
Pyomyositis	May be extensive Tendency for multifocal involvement	Cultures (blood, tissue) Imaging for extent and complications Surgical drainage Consultation as indicated Parenteral therapy Infection control measures	

Respiratory Tract Infection (RTI)

CLINICAL DISEASE	KEY FEATURES	MANAGEMENT PRINCIPLES	ANTIMICROBIAL CHOICES AND COMMENTS*
Pneumonia	Influenza-like prodrome, hemoptysis, fever, shock, leukopenia, pneumatoceles, multifocal abscesses, consolidation, frequent empyema, respiratory failure, and high mortality	Cultures (blood, pleural fluid, sputum) Imaging for extent and complications Consultation as indicated Intensive care unit as appropriate Infection control measures Combination parenteral therapy Chest tube drainage for empyema	*Empiric:* Vancomycin 15–20 mg/kg/dose q8–12h IV for adults and 40–60[3] mg/kg/day ÷ q6h IV for children Linezolid 600 mg q12h PO/IV for adults and 30 mg/kg/day ÷ q8h PO/IV for children, not to exceed 600 mg/dose; for children older than 12 years of age 600 mg bid PO/IV Clindamycin 600–900 mg q8h IV/IM for adults and 30–40 mg/kg/day[3] ÷ q6–8h IV for children TMP/SMX[1] 8–12 mg/kg/day (of TMP) ÷ q8–12h IV for adults and 8–12 mg/kg/day (of TMP) ÷ q6h IV for children Telavancin (Vibativ) 10 mg/kg/dose IV once daily for adults for hospital or ventilator acquired pneumonia Ceftaroline (Teflaro) 600 mg IV q12h for adults with community-acquired pneumonia; safety and efficacy have not been established for children Ceftobiprole (Zevtera)[2] 500 mg IV q8h for adults with community-acquired and hospital-acquired pneumonia; safety and efficacy have not been established for children *Comment:* Daptomycin not indicated because it is inactivated by lung surfactant *Proven MRSA:* As above, based on sensitivity testing

TABLE 6 Guidelines for the Management of MRSA Infections—cont'd

CLINICAL DISEASE	KEY FEATURES	MANAGEMENT PRINCIPLES	ANTIMICROBIAL CHOICES AND COMMENTS*
Other			
Sepsis syndrome Bacteremia Native valve endocarditis	Shock Multiple-organ failure May have purpura fulminans Associated SSTI, MSI, and RTI May be complicated by Waterhouse-Friedrichsen syndrome High mortality	Blood cultures Culture any pus or fluid collection Look for primary or secondary focus Imaging for identification of source including echocardiography Consultation as indicated ICU care Imaging: look for occult abscesses, bone infection, or endocarditis Involve surgery and other specialists as needed Infection control measures Parenteral, multidrug therapy Prolonged therapy for endovascular source infections	*Empiric:* Vancomycin 15–20 mg/kg/dose q8–12h IV for adults and 40–60[3] mg/kg/day ÷ q6h IV for children Daptomycin 6 mg/kg/dose once daily IV for adults and 4–10[3] mg/kg/dose once daily for children[1] *Comments:* Doses of daptomycin of up to 10 mg/kg/dose[3] once daily have been used in adults in this indication Some recommendations have included linezolid in this setting at the doses described above *Proven MRSA:* As above, based on sensitivity testing. *Comment:* New IDSA guidelines for the treatment of *S. aureus* bacteremia are in progress

*Choice of antimicrobial therapy depends on local susceptibility patterns.

†Patients with risk factors, as a part of an outbreak investigation, patients with slowly responding or recurrent lesions.

¶The IDSA guideline suggests to differentiate purulent and nonpurulent cellulitis and reserve empiric therapy for β-hemolytic streptococci only in nonpurulent cellulitis but acknowledges it is an area of controversy. The UK and Canadian guidelines explicitly recommend empiric coverage for β-hemolytic streptococci and do not differentiate cellulitis into different types. A recent randomized controlled trial in the United States found no significant difference in efficacy between clindamycin and trimethoprim-sulfamethoxazole when used for treatment of uncomplicated skin and soft tissue infections, which were thought to be secondary to either β-hemolytic streptococci or *S. aureus*. Another recent placebo-controlled trial in the United States found that clindamycin or trimethoprim-sulfamethoxazole in conjunction with incision and drainage improved outcomes in patients with simple small abscesses (<5 cm) compared with incision and drainage alone.

[1]Not FDA approved for this indication. Dosing has varied in published reports and specific dosing guidelines are not available.

[2]Not available in the United States.

[3]Exceeds dosage recommended by the manufacturer.

**Not recommended for pediatric patients younger than 8 years of age or in pregnancy.

ICU, Intensive care unit; *IDSA*, Infectious Diseases Society of America; *IVIG*, intravenous immunoglobulin; *MRSA*, methicillin-resistant *Staphylococcus aureus*; *TMP-SMX*, trimethoprim-sulfamethoxazole.

References

Barton-Forbes M, Hawkes M, Moore D, et al: Guidelines for the prevention and management of community associated methicillin resistant *Staphylococcus aureus* (CA-MRSA): a perspective for Canadian Health Care Practitioners, *Can J Infect Dis Med Microbiol* 17(Suppl. C):1B–24B, 2006.

Chambers HF, Deleo FR: Waves of resistance: *Staphylococcus aureus* in the antibiotic era, *Nat Rev Microbiol* 7:629–641, 2009. https://doi.org/10.1038/nrmicro2200.

Daum RS, Miller LG, Immergluck L: A placebo-controlled trial of antibiotics for smaller skin abscesses, *N Engl J Med* 376(26):2545–2555, 2017.

David MZ, Daum RS: Community-associated methicillin resistant *Staphylococcus aureus*: epidemiology and clinical consequences of an emerging epidemic, *Clin Microbiol Rev* 23:616–687, 2010. https://doi.org/10.1128/CMR.00081-09.

Fluit AC: Livestock-associated *Staphylococcus aureus*, *Clin Microbiol Infect* 18:735–744, 2012. https://doi.org/10.1111/j.1469-0691.2012.03846.x.

Geriak M, Haddad F, Khulood R, et al: Clinical data on daptomycin plus ceftaroline versus standard of care monotherapy in the treatment of methicillin-resistant *Staphylococcus aureus* bacteremia, *Antimicrob Agents Chemother*, 2019. https://doi.org/10.1128/AAC.02483-18.

Gorwitz RJ, Jernigan DB, Powers JH, et al: *Strategies for clinical management of MRSA in the community: summary of an experts' meeting convened by the Centers for Disease Control and Prevention, 2006:* 2006. Available at www.cdc.gov/%20ncidod/dhqp/pdf/ar/CAMRSA_ExpMtgStrategies.pdf (accessed 02.01.2013).

Gould FK, Brindle R, Chadwick PR, et al: Guidelines (2008) for the prophylaxis and treatment of methicillin resistant *Staphylococcus aureus* (MRSA) infections in the United Kingdom, *J Antimicrob Chemother* 63:849–861, 2009. https://doi.org/10.1093/jac/dkp065.

Kaplan SL, Hulten KG, Gonzalez BE, et al: Three-year surveillance of community-acquired *Staphylococcus aureus* infections in children, *Clin Infect Dis* 40:1785–1791, 2005.

Klevens RM, Morrison MA, Nadle J, et al: Invasive methicillin resistant *Staphylococcus aureus* infections in the United States, *JAMA* 298:1763–1771, 2007.

Kock R, Becker K, Cookson B, et al: Methicillin resistant *Staphylococcus aureus* (MRSA): burden of disease and control challenges in Europe, *Euro Surveill* 15:19688, 2010.

Lakhundi S, Zhang K: Methicillin-resistant *Staphylococcus aureus*: molecular characterization, evolution, and epidemiology, *Clin Microbiol Rev* 31, 2018. e00020-18. https://doi.org/10.1128/CMR.00020-18.

Liu C, Bayer A, Cosgrove SE, et al: Clinical practice guidelines by the Infectious Diseases Society of America for the treatment of methicillin resistant *Staphylococcus aureus* infections in adults and children: executive summary, *Clin Infect Dis* 52:285–292, 2011. https://doi.org/10.1093/cid/cir034.

Miller LG, Daum RS, Creech CB, et al: Clindamycin versus trimethoprim-sulfamethoxazole for uncomplicated skin infections, *N Engl J Med* 372(12):1093–1103, 2015.

Muto CA, Jernigan JA, Ostrowsky BE, et al: SHEA guideline for preventing nosocomial transmission of multidrug-resistant strains of *Staphylococcus aureus* and enterococcus, *Infect Control Hosp Epidemiol* 24:362–386, 2003.

Nathwani D, Morgan M, Masterton RG, et al: Guidelines for UK practice for the diagnosis and management of methicillin resistant *Staphylococcus aureus* (MRSA) infections presenting in the community, *J Antimicrob Chemother* 61:976–994, 2008. https://doi.org/10.1093/jac/dkn096.

Tong SYC, Lye DC, Yahav D, et al: Effect of vancomycin or daptomycin with vs without an antistaphylococcal β-lactam on mortality, bacteremia, relapse, or treatment failure in patients with MRSA bacteremia: a randomized clinical trial, *JAMA* 323(6):527–537, 2020.

MUMPS

Method of
Kristen Rundell, MS, MD

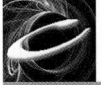

CURRENT DIAGNOSIS

- Parotitis (swelling of the parotid salivary glands): unilateral or bilateral
- Fever
- Headache
- Malaise
- Myalgias
- Anorexia
- Increased serum amylase

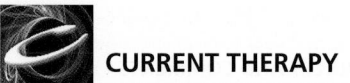

CURRENT THERAPY

- Supportive care
- Warm or cold packs on the parotid
- Analgesics and/or antipyretics (such as acetaminophen [Tylenol] or ibuprofen [Motrin])
- IV fluids or hospitalization for cases of pancreatitis, meningitis, or severe orchitis

Epidemiology

Mumps is an extremely contagious, self-limiting virus that had disease rates of 99% until the vaccine was introduced in 1967. Since 2006, there have been several outbreaks, in the United States, these usually present in young people and those who are not vaccinated, and have increased transmissibility on college campuses, in close knit communities and large social gatherings. For the United States and Finland, mumps is almost eradicated. For the rest of the world, mumps is still endemic as a result of a vaccination rate of only 61%.

Pathophysiology

Mumps is a single-stranded RNA virus and a member of the *Paramyxovirus* genus. It is transmitted through respiratory secretions, saliva, and contact with contaminated fomites.

Prevention

With the high rate of transmission and no antiviral therapy, prevention for mumps relies on community immunity as a result of high vaccine rates. There are two formulations of the mumps vaccine currently available in the United States: the measles-mumps-rubella vaccine (MMR) and the measles-mumps-rubella-varicella vaccine (MMRV, ProQuad). The dosing schedule for children calls for the first dose at age greater than 12 months to 15 months, and the second dose for children greater than 4 years to 6 years of age. For infants aged 6 through 11 months who are traveling internationally, a single MMR vaccine is recommended. These children should be revaccinated with 2 doses of MMR vaccine with the first dose at ages 12 months to 15 months and the second dose at ages 4 years to 6 years. During an epidemic, a single dose for adults born before 1957 is recommended and may be required by some health care professionals. The first dose gives approximately 80% immunity. Persons receiving both doses may still get the mumps virus if there is outbreak or if they travel to an endemic area. To avoid exposure or contraction of the disease during travel, it is suggested that travelers wash hands frequently and use alcohol-based sanitizers to decrease the contraction or spread of disease.

The vaccine is contraindicated for patients who are pregnant or planning to conceive in the 28 days after vaccination. Vaccine administration is also contraindicated for those who have a severe anaphylactic reaction to the vaccine or one of the components, and those individuals who are severely immunocompromised.

Clinical Manifestations

The incubation period for the mumps virus is 16 to 18 days. At the onset of the illness, patients may develop acute viral infection symptoms of fever, headache, and malaise. The parotitis, swelling of the parotid gland, is the diagnostic hallmark of the mumps virus. This is caused by the infection and inflammation of the parotid ductal epithelium. The swelling may last up to 10 days. Close to 30% of persons may not have this symptom and may be only mildly symptomatic.

Diagnosis

Diagnosis is made by the history and the constellation of symptoms and physical findings. It is difficult to use IgM to determine active infection, because the response may be short in duration, delayed, or even absent. PCR testing is available and requires early sampling.

Differential Diagnosis

Viral infections such as parainfluenza (also in the paramyxovirus genus) coxsackievirus, influenza A, Epstein-Barr, adenovirus, HIV, and cytomegalovirus may present with similar symptoms as mumps. There are also noninfectious etiologies of parotitis, which include salivary stones or tumors, sarcoid, Sjögren's syndrome, and thiazide diuretics.

Therapy (or Treatment)

Treatment for mumps virus is largely supportive. For complicated cases of pancreatitis, meningitis, encephalitis, and orchitis, patient may need to be hospitalized for additional care. The additional care usually includes fever reduction, analgesia, fluid resuscitation, and treatment of secondary bacterial infections.

Monitoring

For persons with active mumps, it is suggested that they be isolated from school or work for 5 days after the onset of symptoms. Shedding of virus usually occurs 4 days prior to the onset of symptoms. For this reason, it is difficult to slow down outbreaks of the disease. The last outbreak in the United States was in 2010.

Complications

Complications from mumps are rare. In children, pancreatitis and hearing loss are the sensorineural complications most often diagnosed. For adolescents and adults the complications are more common and usually more severe. These include aseptic meningitis; orchitis in males, which rarely leads to sterility; oophoritis in females; pancreatitis; and arthritis. Even more uncommon are Guillain–Barré/ascending polyradiculitis, transverse myelitis, facial palsy, interstitial nephritis, and myocardial involvement.

Mumps in pregnancy has been associated with increased fetal loss. There are no known teratogenic effects.

References

American Academy of Pediatrics: Mumps. In Pickering LK, Baker CJ, Kimberlin DW, Long SS, editors: *Red Book: 2009 Report of the committee on Infectious Diseases*, ed 28, Elk Gove Village IL, 2009, American Academy of Pediatrics, pp 468–472.

Centers for Disease Control and Prevention (CDC): Exposure to mumps during air travel—United States, April 2006, *MMWR Morb Mortal Wkly Rep* 55(401), 2006.

Centers for Disease Prevention and Control Website 5/1/2021.

Dayan GH, Rubin S: Mumps outbreaks in vaccinated population: are available mumps vaccines effective enough to prevent an outbreak? *Clin Infect Dis* 47:1458, 2008.

Kleiman MB: Mumps virus. In Lenette EH, editor: *Laboratory Diagnosis of Viral Infections*, ed 2, New York, 1992, Marcel Dekker. p. 549.

Kutty PK, Barskey AE, Gallagher KM: *Mumps. Infectious diseases related to travel*, CDC Yellowbook, 2012(chapter 3).

Wharton M, Cochi SLK, William S: Measles, mumps and rubella vaccines, *Infect Dis Clin North Am* 4:47, 1990. www.cdc.gov/travel/yellowbook.

MYALGIC ENCEPHALOMYELITIS/CHRONIC FATIGUE SYNDROME

Method of
Stephen J. Gluckman, MD

Myalgic encephalomyelitis/chronic fatigue syndrome (ME/CFS) is an often-misunderstood syndrome that should not be confused with malingering, hypochondriasis, or just fatigue. Patients with ME/CFS are truly suffering from their often-disabling symptoms. It is impossible to successfully treat a patient with ME/CFS unless the clinician believes the patient is genuinely symptomatic. ME/CFS also should not be confused with the isolated symptoms of fatigue. Fatigue is a common patient complaint, whereas ME/CFS has a much lower prevalence.

Definition

ME/CFS is not a new disease; the syndrome has been described since at least the mid-1700s. However, since that time it has been mistakenly ascribed to a number of incorrect pathologic and infectious causes. In the past it has been called febricula, neurasthenia, effort syndrome, Da Costa syndrome, chronic brucellosis, chronic Lyme disease, chronic Epstein-Barr syndrome, total allergy syndrome, chronic candidiasis, and multiple chemical sensitivity syndrome. More recently it has been falsely attributed to infection with xenotropic murine leukemia virus–related virus (XMRV) and related retroviruses, such as murine leukemia virus (MLV). None of these possible causes has proved to be correct.

In 1988, in an attempt to be descriptive rather than to attribute an incorrect etiology to the disease, the term *chronic fatigue syndrome* was coined. Therefore, the name is relatively new but the syndrome is not. The disease is chronic and fatigue is a cardinal feature, but it is more than being chronically tired. This working case definition was published by the Centers for Disease Control and Prevention and then modified in 1992 by the National Institute of Allergy and Infectious Diseases. In March 2015 the Institute of Medicine (IOM; now the National Academy of Medicine [NAM]) issued an extensive and thorough review of the topic. As a result of this review they proposed a name change to systemic exertion intolerance disease (SEID). This comprehensive report has three major themes: (1) ME/CFS has acquired a great deal of negative connotation with associated misunderstanding and prejudice. The name change to SEID is an attempt to disconnect this disease from past misunderstandings. However, this name change has not caught on. (2) The criteria for diagnosis were greatly simplified, with emphasis on the major features (Box 1). (3) By using the term "disease" and by supplying ample reference support in the document, the IOM unequivocally underscores the very real nature of this malady. The IOM report is by far the most thorough examination of the topic and it unequivocally supports the validity of this disease.

One note of caution: This case definition is an epidemiologic and research tool and not a strict clinical tool. It is useful for studying the disease. However, some patients do not completely fit this definition. ME/CFS can nonetheless be diagnosed by a knowledgeable clinician who is willing to consider this diagnosis.

Because some immune abnormalities are often seen in these patients, some people have called this "chronic fatigue and immune dysregulation syndrome." The immune abnormalities seen in ME/CFS patients are mild and differ from patient to patient. Most significantly, these patients are not immunosuppressed or at risk for opportunistic infections.

It has been noted that many of the symptoms of fibromyalgia overlap with ME/CFS, and some clinicians consider fibromyalgia and ME/CFS to be different aspects of the same disease because both often include pain and fatigue. These different names for the same syndrome can be confusing to patients and clinicians, and when managing patients with ME/CFS it is important to explain this to them.

Epidemiology

Although chronic fatigue is an extremely common symptom, ME/CFS is not. The former has been noted to have a prevalence of 10% to 25% in a number of studies. However, the point prevalence of ME/CFS has been estimated to be in the range of 0.1%. ME/CFS is overrepresented in young and middle-aged women, but it has been described in both men and women and in all age groups.

Pathophysiology

The cause of ME/CFS is unknown. Much effort has gone into trying to discern an infectious, endocrine, immune, or psychiatric cause, but to date none has been proven. Studies have shown a link between ME/CFS and the presence of certain genes that mediate immune and stress responses. The findings suggest that difficulty managing stress may be linked to the development of ME/CFS. They also suggest that there may not be a single cause of ME/CFS but that there may be a number of stress-related triggers (physical or emotional) in those with a genetic predisposition. This is consistent with the typical course, in which a previously healthy person develops an acute illness that resolves but initiates ME/CFS.

Clinical Features and Diagnosis

Although there is, as yet, no diagnostic test, the history, physical examination, and laboratory testing are generally very characteristic and allow a clinician to confidently make the diagnosis. The typical story is one of a previously highly functioning person who develops an acute illness or other stressor. The acute problem resolves; however, from that time on, symptoms of ME/CFS are triggered. Despite often-profound symptoms, physical examination is persistently normal, as is laboratory testing. Symptoms are exacerbated by physical activity. The pre-ME/CFS medical history of the patient is not one of multiple medical problems. Affected patients are typically high functioning persons who are "struck down" with this disease. Features to emphasize in addition to the case definition noted in Box 1 are included in Box 2.

In a patient with a typical history and examination, laboratory testing should be limited (Box 3). Testing for diseases with

---

BOX 1	Criteria for CFS/SEID

Diagnosis requires that the patient have the following three symptoms:

- A substantial reduction or impairment in the ability to engage in pre-illness levels of occupational, educational, social, or personal activities that persists for more than 6 months and is accompanied by fatigue, which is often profound, is of new or definite onset (not lifelong), is not the result of ongoing excessive exertion, and is not substantially alleviated by rest
- Postexertional malaise
- Unrefreshing sleep

    At least one of the two following manifestations is also required:

- Cognitive impairment
- Orthostatic intolerance

CFS, Chronic fatigue syndrome; *SEID,* systemic exertion intolerance disease.

BOX 2	Frequent Features of Chronic Fatigue Syndrome

- Sudden onset of fatigue after a relatively common illness or other stressor
- Previously active and healthy person
- Symptoms very sensitive to exacerbation by physical activity
- Normal physical examination and laboratory testing
- Altered sleep
- "Foggy" thought processes
- Lack of progression to organ failure or any significant objective organ abnormality
- Joint and muscle aching without physical evidence of inflammation
- Feverish feeling (sustained elevated temperatures [>37.4°C] should prompt a search for an alternative diagnosis because the chronic fatigue syndrome patient is not truly febrile)
- Diffuse aching that is not well localized to joints or muscles, but without erythema, effusion, or limitation of motion
- Muscles that are easily fatigued (however, strength is normal, as are biopsies and electromyograms)
- Occasional mild cervical and/or axillary lymphadenitis (painful lymph nodes [lymphadenia] are a common complaint, but this is not a true lymphadenopathy)

a low pretest likelihood runs the serious risk of false-positive results. This can result in further testing, diagnostic confusion, and unnecessary treatments. Specifically, the signs and symptoms of ME/CFS are not those of systemic lupus, Lyme disease, cytomegalovirus, bartonellosis, ehrlichiosis, or babesiosis, among others. Serologic testing for these diagnoses is not helpful and can be harmful if the presence of antibodies results in the initiation of unwarranted medications. The presence of antibodies does not mean active disease. The analogy that patients can relate to is to remind them that they likely have antibodies to chickenpox but that they clearly do not have active chickenpox. For similar reasons, neuroimaging without objective clinical findings is not indicated. Although abnormalities can be found, they are nonspecific and of no clinical utility. Tilt-table testing seems to be abnormal in many patients with ME/CFS; however, testing is expensive and uncomfortable, and abnormal results do not alter the management. Of course, if history, physical examination, and initial laboratory testing do reveal abnormalities, further laboratory evaluation should be undertaken to elucidate the cause of the aberration(s).

Treatment

There is no established cure for ME/CFS, but patients should be counseled that a number of things can be done to manage this often-disabling illness (Box 4). These can be divided into things the clinician should do and things the patient should do.

Things the Clinician Should Do

To successfully manage ME/CFS, a clinician must believe that the patient is truly symptomatic. Patients with ME/CFS are not malingering. Because they often appear well and have consistently normal objective testing, they often become very defensive about their limitations. They are sensitive to the validity of their symptoms. Not only are they suffering, but also they are blamed for it. Many patients with ME/CFS are partially or totally disabled. Their outward healthy appearance belies the internal sense of ill health. It is common for relatives and colleagues to believe they are malingering. A vicious cycle of frustration, anger, and depression commonly ensues.

As part of establishing the validity of the diagnosis, a clinician should review the history of ME/CFS, emphasizing that this is not a new disease but was originally described centuries ago.

For successful management, a clinician should give the patient enough time, specifically inquire about other diagnoses the patient is concerned about, and explain why they are not correct. The clinician should see the patient at regular intervals.

Make sure that the patient has reasonable expectations. Most patients with ME/CFS have not had previous chronic illnesses or significant prolonged limitations. It is often necessary to review the information about ME/CFS with the patient's family and to emphasize that this disabling illness is not volitional.

Although it is generally wise to avoid a discussion about whether the origin of ME/CFS is psychiatric or organic, depression is an expected consequence of any chronic illness. Depression has specific treatments, and it should be aggressively diagnosed and treated. The patient should be told that successful management of depression will help him or her cope with ME/CFS.

If a sleep disturbance exists, it also should be aggressively managed, if necessary, by a sleep specialist. Sleep deprivation makes other symptoms more difficult to deal with.

Chronic pain is very enervating. If pain is prominent, that also should be aggressively managed, often by a pain specialist.

It is important for the clinician to be cautious about ascribing all of a patient's symptoms to ME/CFS. Such patients are, of course, not protected from getting additional, unrelated illnesses. Each symptom should be considered on its own before defaulting it to ME/CFS.

Complementary therapies must be discussed or the patient might get the impression that the clinician is not comfortable in considering them; this can partially undermine the clinician–patient relationship. Although all are of unproved benefit and often undetermined risk, "complementary" therapies that are not dangerous, such as acupuncture, or expensive are reasonable to consider.

Things the Patient Should Do

Of the 350 studies that have looked at treatment options for ME/CFS, only cognitive behavioral therapy and graded exercise therapy have been shown to be of possible benefit. In cognitive behavioral therapy, the patient undergoes a series of 1-hour sessions designed to alter beliefs and behaviors that might delay recovery. Although exercise can exacerbate symptoms, deconditioning will also do so. Limiting activity can worsen weakness and depression. The risk of exacerbating symptoms can be reduced by cautiously setting less-ambitious activity/exercise goals. Because many patients with ME/CFS were particularly active before the onset of their illness and are impatient to get their former lives back, they often need strict guidelines to try to prevent overdoing exercise while at the same time getting a clear prescription to exercise. The exercise prescription should be individualized based on the degree of impairment, but it is wise to initially set goals on the low side to avoid exacerbating symptoms.

As part of the management of ME/CFS, patients, their families, and, when appropriate, their employers need to reframe their expectations. ME/CFS patients have a chronic, disabling illness. Families and others need to understand that patients cannot do all that they were able to do before the onset of ME/CFS and that patients cannot "will" the disease away any more than they could will away a more visible disability.

Things That Should Not Be Done
There are many suggested remedies for ME/CFS. Most are either unstudied or disproved. In particular, treatments that are expensive or potentially harmful should be avoided. There is no role for antimicrobial therapy. There is no role for antiviral therapy, including treatment for retroviruses. There is no role for intravenous immunoglobulin, corticosteroids, special diets, or vitamin treatments.

Prognosis
The likelihood for complete recovery from ME/CFS is only fair. The disease tends to wax and wane over time, but in only a minority of patients does it completely resolve. If sustained improvement occurs, it is generally over several years. Several features have been associated with a poorer prognosis, including age older than 38 years, more than eight symptoms, duration longer than 1.5 years, less than 16 years of formal education, a history of a dysthymic disorder, and a sustained belief that the disease is due to a physical cause.

Monitoring
Despite the lack of very effective treatment, many patients benefit from regular monitoring of their condition. Knowing they have scheduled visits minimizes the number of crises and emergency visits and allows the patient to reconnect with a validating physician. Follow-up on a quarterly basis is a reasonable interval.

References
Bouquet J, Gardy JL, Brown S, et al: RNA-seq analysis of gene expression, viral pathogen, and B-cell/T-cell receptor signatures in complex chronic disease, *Clin Infect Dis* 64:476, 2017.
Clark MR, Katon W, Russo J, et al: Chronic fatigue: risk factors for symptom persistence in a 212-year follow-up study, *Am J Med* 98:187–195, 1995.
Fulcher KY: White PD: randomised controlled trial of graded exercise in patients with the chronic fatigue syndrome, *BMJ* 314:1647–1652, 1997.
Goertzel BN, Pennachin C, de Souza Coelho L, et al: Combinations of single nucleotide polymorphisms in neuroendocrine effector and receptor genes predict chronic fatigue syndrome, *Pharmacogenomics* 7:475–483, 2006.
Goldenberg DL, Simms RW, Geiger A, et al: High frequency of fibromyalgia in patients with chronic fatigue seen in a primary care practice, *Arthritis Rheum* 33:381–387, 1990.
Green CR, Cowan P, Elk R, et al: National Institutes of Health pathways to prevention workshop: advancing the research on myalgic encephalomyelitis/chronic fatigue syndrome, *Ann Intern Med* 162:860, 2015.
Haney E, Smith ME, McDonagh M, et al: Diagnostic methods for myalgic encephalomyelitis/chronic fatigue syndrome: a systematic review for a National Institutes of Health Pathways to Prevention Workshop, *Ann Intern Med* 162:834, 2015.
IOM (Institute of Medicine): *Beyond Myalgic encephalomyelitis/chronic fatigue syndrome: redefining an illness*, Washington, DC, 2015, The National Academies Press. https://www.ncbi.nlm.nih.gov/25695122.
Lightfoot Jr RW, Luft BJ, Rahn DW, et al: Empiric parenteral antibiotic treatment of patients with fibromyalgia and fatigue and a positive serologic result for Lyme disease. A cost-effectiveness analysis, *Ann Intern Med* 119:503–509, 1993.
Schwartz RB, Garada BM, Komaroff AL, et al: Detection of intracranial abnormalities in patients with chronic fatigue syndrome: comparison of MR imaging and SPECT, *Am J Roentgenol* 162:935–941, 1994.
Wessely S, Chalder T, Hirsch S, et al: The prevalence and morbidity of chronic fatigue and chronic fatigue syndrome: a prospective primary care study, *Am J Public Health* 87:1449–1455, 1997.
White PD, Goldsmith KA, Johnson AL, et al: Comparison of adaptive pacing therapy, cognitive behaviour therapy, graded exercise therapy, and specialist medical care for chronic fatigue syndrome (PACE): a randomised trial, *Lancet* 377:823–836, 2011.

NECROTIZING SKIN AND SOFT-TISSUE INFECTIONS

Method of
Kalyanakrishnan Ramakrishnan, MD

CURRENT DIAGNOSIS

- Physical examination of the affected area may detect:
  - Exquisite pain and tenderness out of proportion to local signs of infection.
  - Cutaneous anesthesia, firm woody subcutaneous tissue, edema, and tenderness extending outside involved skin margins, hemorrhage or bullae of the overlying skin, and soft tissue crepitus.
  - Laboratory Risk Indicator for Necrotizing Fasciitis (LRINEC) score is useful in diagnosing necrotizing fasciitis. Imaging (computed tomography [CT] or magnetic resonance imaging [MRI] in adults; ultrasonography [US] in children) is usually confirmatory. Imaging should not delay surgery if indicated based on suspicion.

CURRENT TREATMENT

- Empiric high-dose intravenous polymicrobial antibiotics and surgical debridement remain the cornerstones of initial management of necrotizing skin and soft-tissue infections. Organism-specific antibiotics are continued until resolution of infection and debridement complete (usually 7–14 days).

Epidemiology
Necrotizing skin and soft tissue infections are rare with an estimated annual incidence of 1000 cases in the United States. These infections may be polymicrobial or monomicrobial. Polymicrobial infections are more common (70%–80%) and generally caused by synergistic activity of aerobes and anaerobes originating from the bowel or genitourinary tracts. They are more prevalent among older and immunocompromised patients, individuals with significant comorbidities, and those with underlying abdominal pathology. These infections typically involve the trunk and perineal regions, and follow penetrating abdominal injuries or surgery, genital or perianal sepsis, or decubitus ulcers. They have a more indolent course and thus are easier to diagnose. Monomicrobial infections (20%–30%) frequently follow minor trauma and are usually caused by group A streptococcus (GAS), occasionally by methicillin-resistant *Staphylococcus aureus* (MRSA), or by clostridia. They are more aggressive, involve the extremities and occur more often in younger healthy individuals. Type 3 infections follow exposure to contaminated fresh or warm seawater or ingestion of raw seafood; organisms responsible include *Aeromonas hydrophila*, *Vibrio vulnificus*, *Mycobacterium marinum*, *Pasteurella multocida*, *Haemophilus* and *Klebsiella* species. Type 4 (fungal) infections generally follow burns or major trauma. Both types 3 and 4 infections are rare, progress rapidly, and have a high mortality rate, especially in immune-suppressed patients.

Risk Factors
Cardiopulmonary disease, debility, diabetes mellitus, hepatorenal disease, immunocompromised states, obesity, arteriovenous/lymphatic insufficiency, and senescence all increase risk of skin and soft tissue infections by reducing tissue vascularity and oxygenation, increasing fluid stasis and risk of trauma, and decreasing ability to counter infections. Diabetes mellitus and hepatic

cirrhosis favor polymicrobial infections due to staphylococcus and streptococcus species, anerobes, and gram-negative bacilli. Neutropenia, intravenous drug use, and hot tub exposure promote pseudomonas infection. Human and animal bites cause infections with oral flora, staphylococci, *Pasteurella multocida*, and anerobes. Poor sanitation and soil contamination propagate clostridial infections. Postoperative infections typically follow wound contamination with microorganisms from the patient during surgery.

Pathophysiology

Necrotizing skin and soft tissue infections advance rapidly, breaking down and traversing anatomic barriers, initiating extensive destruction of the subcutaneous tissue, fascia, and muscle and damaging the neurovascular bundle, thrombosing the subcutaneous vessels, and causing overlying skin necrosis. Most infections follow a rift in the protective cutaneous barrier due to trauma or increased tissue tension. Necrotizing fasciitis may also result from blunt injuries (bruise, muscle strain) and, occasionally vascular or lymphatic spread from a distant focus of infection. Various toxins expressed by the organisms (GAS and clostridia) display local and systemic effects (platelet aggregation and thrombosis, decreasing phagocytosis, neutrophil function and vascular tone, myocardial inhibition) triggering the systemic inflammatory response syndrome (SIRS) and multiple organ failure.

Prevention

Preserving cutaneous integrity prevents infection. Abrasions and lacerations should be washed with antibacterial solutions, foreign bodies should be removed, and dead/devitalized tissue excised to minimize infection risk. Preoperative skin cleansing with chlorhexidine/alcohol (Hibiclens) or povidone iodine diminishes rates of superficial and deep incisional infections. Intranasal 2% mupirocin ointment (Bactroban) twice daily with chlorhexidine total body wash daily for 5 days in nasal carriers of MRSA reduces hospital-acquired deep surgical–site infections, as does administering antibiotics (aminopenicillins, a second- or third-generation cephalosporin) 60 minutes before incision, sterile surgical technique, minimal tissue handling, and minimally invasive surgery.

Clinical Manifestations

Features of inflammation (redness, warmth, swelling, pain) and loss of function characterize necrotizing skin and soft tissue infections. Altered mental status, anorexia, diaphoresis, fatigue, fever, hypotension, nausea, and tachycardia suggest systemic spread of infection. The extremities, trunk, or anogenital regions are usually involved. Induration denotes cutaneous involvement. Patients with necrotizing fasciitis have severe pain disproportionate to the physical findings and rapid progression of infection. Examination reveals cutaneous anesthesia, firm and woody subcutaneous tissue, edema and tenderness extending beyond involved skin, hemorrhage or bullae of the overlying skin, and crepitus (indicates soft tissue gas; seen especially with gas-forming organisms such as clostridia). Tense edema and bullae have high specificity and positive predictive value for necrotizing fasciitis. Fournier gangrene is a form of polymicrobial necrotizing soft-tissue infection involving the loose groin and genital skin, where subcutaneous vessel thrombosis causes extensive tissue loss.

Diagnosis

Diagnosis is based on a strong clinical suspicion followed by confirmatory laboratory and imaging studies (if time permits), and surgery. Leukocytosis with a marked left shift, elevated C-reactive protein, elevated serum creatinine and creatine phosphokinase (denotes muscle injury), and low serum bicarbonate (suggests acidosis) signify severe infection. The LRINEC score (https://www.mdcalc.com/lrinec-score-necrotizing-soft-tissue-infection) uses six different laboratory parameters (hemoglobin, white blood cell count, C-reactive protein, glucose, creatinine, sodium) to predict risk of necrotizing fasciitis (score ≥ 6 suggestive, ≥ 8 strongly predictive). White blood cell count (< 15,000 mm^3) and serum sodium (> 135 mmol/L) levels alone are useful in ruling out necrotizing fasciitis (99% negative predictive value). Gram stains and cultures of aspirates or tissue biopsies, and blood cultures are valuable for detecting the infecting organisms and systemic spread; contamination may yield false-positive results. Biopsy or debridement typically demonstrates swollen gray soft tissue with undermining of the overlying skin, a brownish and odorous exudate and non-contractile muscle. Imaging (plain x-rays, ultrasonography [US], computed tomography [CT], magnetic resonance imaging [MRI]) may show edema or thickening, fluid collections or free air in the soft tissues. US, CT and MRI are highly sensitive (MRI highest) in detecting deep soft tissue involvement characteristic of necrotizing fasciitis; specificity is lower. US is sufficient in children, whose tissues are thin enough to allow adequate evaluation on imaging. Imaging should not delay debridement, if considered necessary.

Therapy

Patients with necrotizing skin and soft-tissue infections typically require in-hospital management, because many have underlying unstable comorbid illnesses, systemic sepsis, severe dehydration and acidosis, muscle breakdown, and organ dysfunction. Initial resuscitation may require airway and oxygen support, large-volume rehydration, and invasive monitoring. High-dose intravenous (IV) broad-spectrum antibiotics effective against the usually infecting polymicrobial spectrum of pathogens are commenced, followed by early and aggressive debridement of all necrotic tissue. IV antibiotics are maintained until the patient is afebrile for 48 to 72 hours and tolerates oral intake, debridement is completed and culture results are available. For polymicrobial necrotizing fasciitis acceptable antimicrobial choices include vancomycin plus piperacillin/tazobactam (Zosyn), a carbapenem (meropenem [Merrem], ertapenem [Invanz] or imipenem-cilastatin [Primaxin]), or cefotaxime (Claforan) with metronidazole (Flagyl) or clindamycin (Cleocin). Streptococcal and clostridial infections are treated with penicillin G and clindamycin. Antibiotic options in methicillin-susceptible *S. aureus* infections include nafcillin oxacillin or cefazolin. Options for methicillin-resistant *S. aureus* (MRSA) infections and in penicillin-allergic patients include vancomycin, daptomycin (Cubicin), or linezolid (Zyvox). Antibiotic doses are modified in children. Recommended duration is 7 to 14 days; longer as needed. Doxycycline combined with ciprofloxacin (Cipro) treats *Vibrio vulnificus* infection. Ceftriaxone (Rocephin) or cefotaxime combined with doxycycline is useful in aeromonos infections. Doxycycline is contraindicated in children (< 8 years), as is ciprofloxacin (< 17 years), unless the infection is considered life-threatening. Fungal infections respond well to fluconazole (Diflucan), voriconazole (Vfend) or amphotericin B; the antifungals usually continued for 2 weeks after resolution of symptoms. Debridement/drainage is repeated until all diseased tissue or collections are eliminated and healing begins. Wound vacuum dressings help remove drainage and encourage formation of healing granulation tissue. The tissue defect heals by secondary intention or may require skin grafting or flap closure. Hyperbaric oxygen (3–4 daily treatments at 2–3 atmosphere pressure for 30–90 minutes each) is useful, especially in clostridium-related synergistic infections. Adding intravenous immunoglobulin[1] 0.5–2 g/kg daily for 3 days has shown some success, and is an option in critically ill hemodynamically unstable patients not responding to conventional measures, especially in those with streptococcal toxic shock syndrome. Fournier gangrene is managed along the same principles as above.

---

[1]Not FDA approved for this indication.

Monitoring

Patients in shock or with acute respiratory distress syndrome, SIRS, or multi-organ failure are best managed in an intensive care unit and often require invasive monitoring, cardiorespiratory and renal support, and occasionally, endotracheal intubation.

Complications

Significant disfigurement, limb loss, respiratory and renal failure, and mortality (14%–50%) may eventuate despite timely and appropriate treatment; the mortality influenced by age, extent of infection, degree of biochemical/acid-base imbalance, presence of comorbidities, and treatment delay.

References

Kaafarani HMA, King DR: Necrotizing skin and soft tissue infections, *Surg Clin North Am* 94:155–163, 2014.

Hakkarainen TW, Kopari NM, Pham TN, Evans HL: Necrotizing soft tissue infections: review and current concepts in treatment, systems of care and outcomes, *Curr Probl Surg* 51:344–362, 2014.

Morgan MS: Diagnosis and management of necrotizing fasciitis: a multiparametric approach, *J Hosp Infect* 75:249–257, 2010.

Stevens DL, Bisno AL, Chambers HF, et al: Practice guidelines for the diagnosis and management of skin and soft tissue infections: 2014 update by the Infectious Diseases Society of America, *Clin Infect Dis* 59:e10–e52, 2014.

Ramakrishnan K, Salinas RC, Agudelo Higuita NI: Skin and soft tissue infections, *Am Fam Physician* 92:474–483, 2015.

OSTEOMYELITIS

Method of
Wissam El Atrouni, MD, MSc; John Sojka, MD; Mitchell Birt, MD; and Kim Templeton, MD

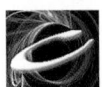

CURRENT DIAGNOSIS

- Osteomyelitis in adults typically occurs as a result of spread from adjacent soft tissues or direct inoculation of bone, such as after trauma or surgery. Hematogenous bacterial seeding leading to osteomyelitis is more common in children than in adults. When it occurs in adults, it is almost exclusively in the spine.
- Open fractures can lead to osteomyelitis due to contamination of bone at the time of injury; even small soft tissue wounds can indicate the presence of an open fracture. Due to the risk of infection, open fractures should be treated emergently.
- Infections around implanted hardware, especially joint arthroplasties or hardware in the spine, require urgent referral. These infections can occur at the time of hardware placement or later due to hematogenous seeding from distant infections. Patients with late arthroplasty infections usually demonstrate new pain in the area of a previously well-functioning joint.
- Diabetes mellitus is one of the more common chronic health conditions that increases the risk of developing osteomyelitis. Osteomyelitis in this population of patients usually occurs in the foot as a result of progressively deepening soft tissue ulcers and secondary infection. These infections are frequently polymicrobial.
- Initial evaluation of patient suspected of having osteomyelitis includes obtaining plain films. However, plain film findings are usually not specific for infection. Additional radiographic modalities, such as magnetic resonance imaging (MRI) scan and/or a variety of nuclear medicine studies, can provide additional information regarding diagnosis and extent of involvement.

CURRENT THERAPY

- In the absence of sepsis, antibiotics for patients with suspected osteomyelitis are not started until adequate cultures can be obtained, through aspiration or biopsy of the bone or during surgical debridement of the affected area.
- Antimicrobial therapy for osteomyelitis in adults typically lasts 4–6 weeks, while in children it may only be needed for 2–3 weeks, depending on the clinical picture.
- Surgical intervention for osteomyelitis of long bones is indicated for patients with chronic infections, infections adjacent to joint replacements, or to address bone abscesses. Surgery in these instances requires extensive debridement of infected and necrotic bone to remove all microabscesses and then irrigation to dilute any remaining bacterial load.
- Treatment of patients with diabetes-related foot infections and underlying osteomyelitis may require revascularization of the affected limb to decrease the need for amputation.

Introduction

Normal bone is typically highly resistant to infection. Infections in bone can arise when the host immune system is compromised or there is injury to the bone. Osteomyelitis occurs either due to hematogenous spread, extension from infections in adjacent soft tissues or joints, or as a result of direct inoculation of the bone due to trauma or surgery. Osteomyelitis can lead to devastating outcomes, including amputation or sepsis, if not addressed early, especially in patients with other health conditions.

Various classification systems have been developed to describe osteomyelitis. The Lew and Waldvogel classification described the etiology of the infection (in order of decreasing frequency: contiguous focus, vascular insufficiency, or hematogenous); however, this classification system does not guide or indicate the results from treatment. The Cierny-Mader system is based on the location (intramedullary) and extent (localized vs. diffuse) of the infection, as well as the degree of compromise of the patient. Unlike the Lew and Waldvogel classification, the Cierny-Mader (C-M) staging systems correlates with outcomes and can help guide treatment. Mandell et al. recommend considering C-M type 1 as early (intramedullary) hematogenous osteomyelitis, type 2 as early contiguous spread, and types 3 (localized) and 4 (diffuse) as more advanced disease.

Osteomyelitis can be described as acute, usually being present for 2 weeks or less, subacute, and chronic. Chronic osteomyelitis can be more challenging to eradicate due to the development of avascular areas of bone (sequestra) and surrounding bone sclerosis (involucra) that help to wall off the sequestra, making it difficult to adequately address these areas with systemic antibiotics.

Epidemiology

The incidence of osteomyelitis appears to be increasing, especially among adults. This may reflect better evaluation and diagnostic measures or the increased prevalence of comorbidities, such as diabetes mellitus, or the aging of the population, as the risk increases with age. The reported age- and sex-adjusted annual incidence has been reported to be approximately 24 cases per 100,000 person-years and is higher among men than women.

No similar increased prevalence of osteomyelitis has been identified among children or young adults. However, other demographic differences have been noted. African American children have the highest rates of hospitalization related to osteomyelitis, while the lowest rates are among children of Asian or Hispanic descent. In addition, children who live in households with low median incomes or whose care is covered by private funds or Medicaid are more likely than children from other socioeconomic backgrounds to be hospitalized with acute osteomyelitis.

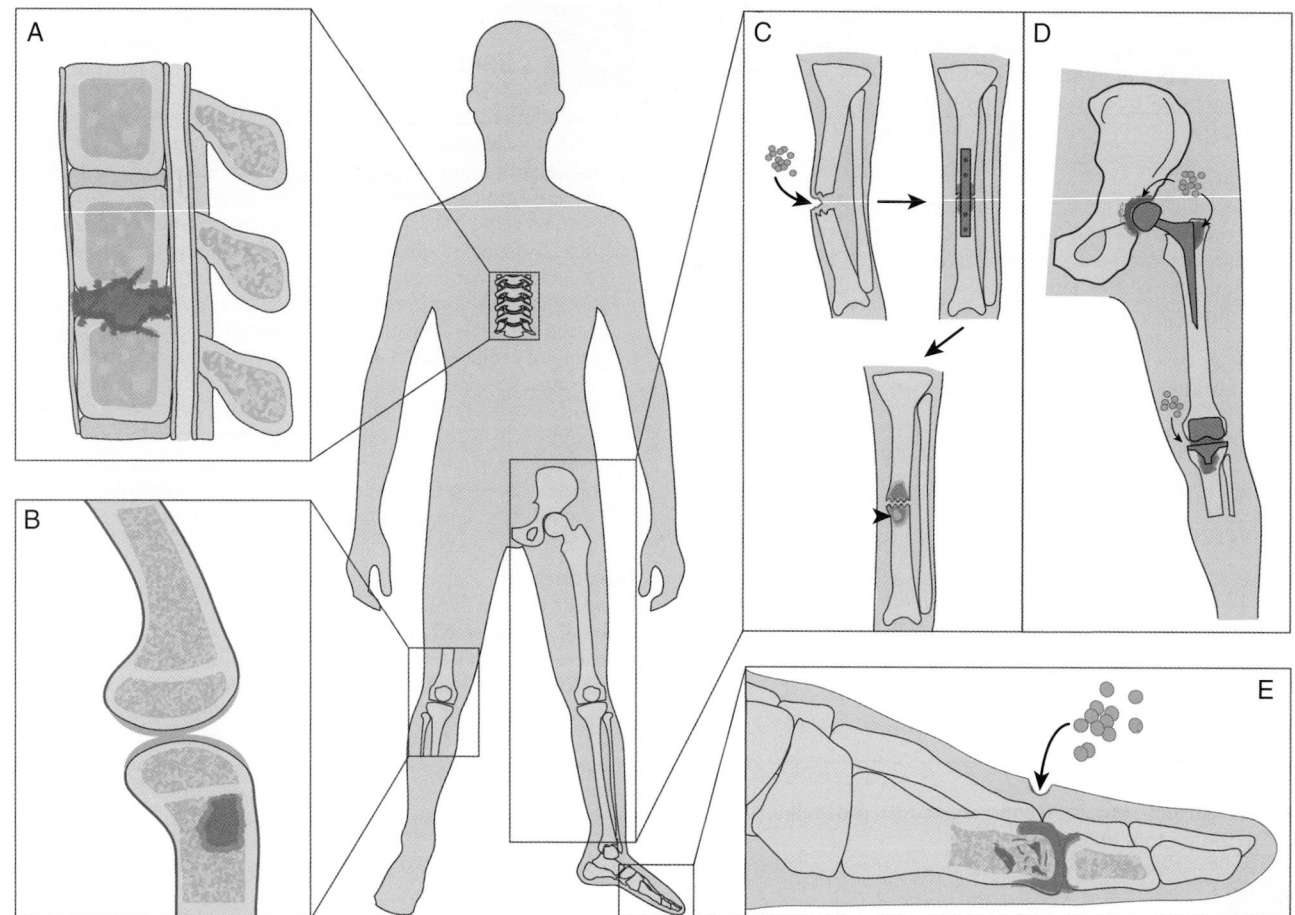

Figure 1 A diagram showing three categories of osteomyelitis. **A** and **B**, Primary hematogenous (bloodborne) spread of bacteria mainly afflicts the vertebral bodies at all ages or the metaphysis of skeletally immature patients. **C** and **D**, Contiguous bone infection is most commonly seen with direct contamination of bacteria in open fractures or joint replacement surgery with prosthetic implants. **E**, Vascular or neurologic disease associated osteomyelitis most commonly affects the lower extremity. (From Birt MC, Anderson DW, Toby WB, et al: Osteomyelitis: recent advances in pathophysiology and therapeutic strategies, *J Orthop* 14:45–52, 2017.)

Pathogenesis

Osteomyelitis can occur via hematogenous seeding, direct extension from an adjacent area of infection, or due to inoculation of the bone as a result of trauma or surgery (Figure 1). *Staphylococcus aureus*, in particular, has receptors for fibronectin, laminin, collagen, and sialoglycoproteins that are present in the bone matrix, leading to seeding of the bone and consequent inflammatory reaction. Hematogenous osteomyelitis is more common among children than among adults. In adults, hematogenous osteomyelitis is almost exclusively seen in the spine, resulting from seeding of the disc space from a distant infected site (Figure 2). This can then involve the adjacent vertebral bodies and, with time, result in epidural extension. When hematogenous osteomyelitis occurs in the long bones of children and adolescents, it is almost always in the metaphysis. It is thought that this reflects the circulation in that area, with slowing of bone flow in the terminal capillaries along the area of the physis. In young children, there is connection between the metaphyseal and epiphyseal vessels that can allow infection of the epiphysis and eventually the adjacent joint. This is much less likely to occur in adults.

Bone infections due to trauma are typically related to presence of open fractures. Open fractures usually reflect significant levels of trauma to the bone and secondary soft tissue involvement. Infections can arise in these situations due to direct contamination of the soft tissues and bone with materials from the environment, including clothing, grass, and dirt, with contained bacteria. Open fractures are graded with the system described by Gustilo and Anderson and range from small puncture wounds over the fracture site to soft tissue stripping from the bone to open fractures

with associated vascular injury. This classification system can help in determining the prognosis: patients with higher grade injuries typically have a greater incidence of subsequent infection—up to 50% among patients with concomitant vascular injury. While a small puncture wound over a fracture may seem inconsequential, these wounds usually indicate that bone was exposed at some point and was at risk for bacterial contamination. Open fractures are surgical emergencies and need immediate referral.

Bone infections can develop at sites of prior surgery, especially past surgical sites that include implantation of hardware. Many of these infections are thought to occur during the time of hardware placement. While such infections can occur at the site of any hardware, it is most common among patients who have undergone joint arthroplasty and is one of the most devastating complications of these procedures. The rate of infection after primary joint arthroplasty ranges from 0.3% to 2.4% for total hip arthroplasties (THAs) and 1.0% to 3.0% for total knee arthroplasties. Infection rates are higher among patients who undergo revision surgeries. Patients with infected arthroplasties may present in the first few weeks after surgery or may note onset of new pain in a previously well-functioning joint. The bacteria in these cases not only exist on the surface of the implant but also extend into adjacent bone and soft tissues (Figure 3). Patients with prior surgery of the spine, with or without the placement of hardware, are also at risk of developing late infections in the range of 0.2% to 9%. Suspected infections in areas of prior surgery, especially if implants are in place, require urgent referral.

Osteomyelitis is more likely to occur in patients with serious and/or chronic health conditions, including obesity, malignancy,

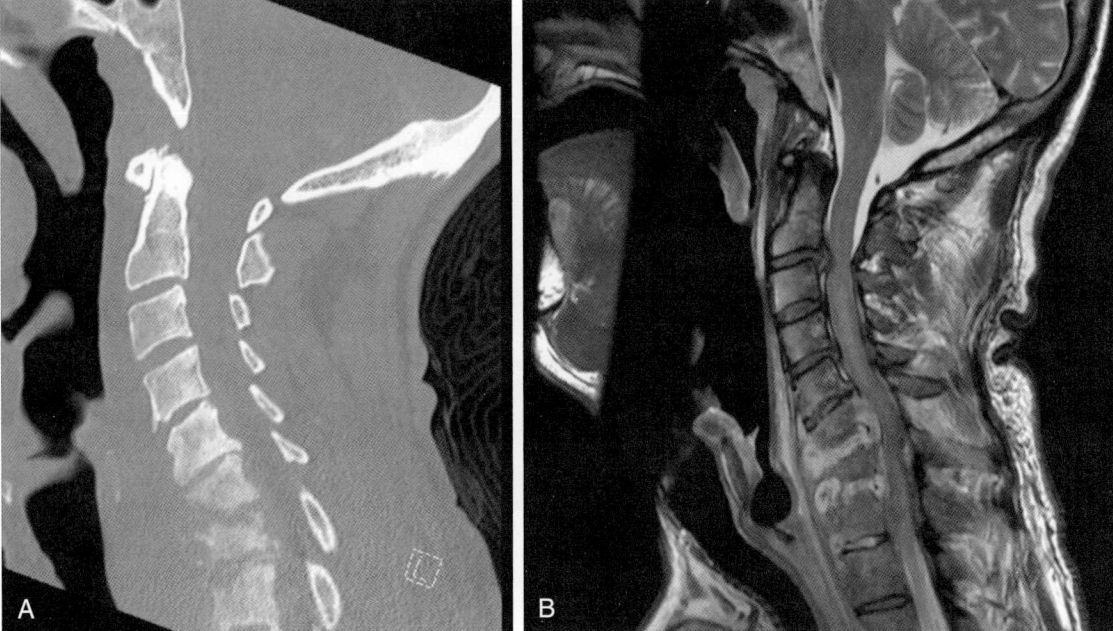

Figure 2 A, Sagittal computed tomography scan demonstrating C6-8 spondylodiskitis. Note the cortical irregularity of the vertebral end plates. There is disc space narrowing and loss of the normal cervical spine curvature. Severe cortical destruction is present due to bacterial infection of the bone and intervertebral disc. **B,** Sagittal T2 magnetic resonance imaging reveals diffuse T2 signal throughout the vertebral body and disc. Evident is loss of the normal cortical line of the endplates compared to adjacent levels and hyperintensity that extends posteriorly to the soft tissues.

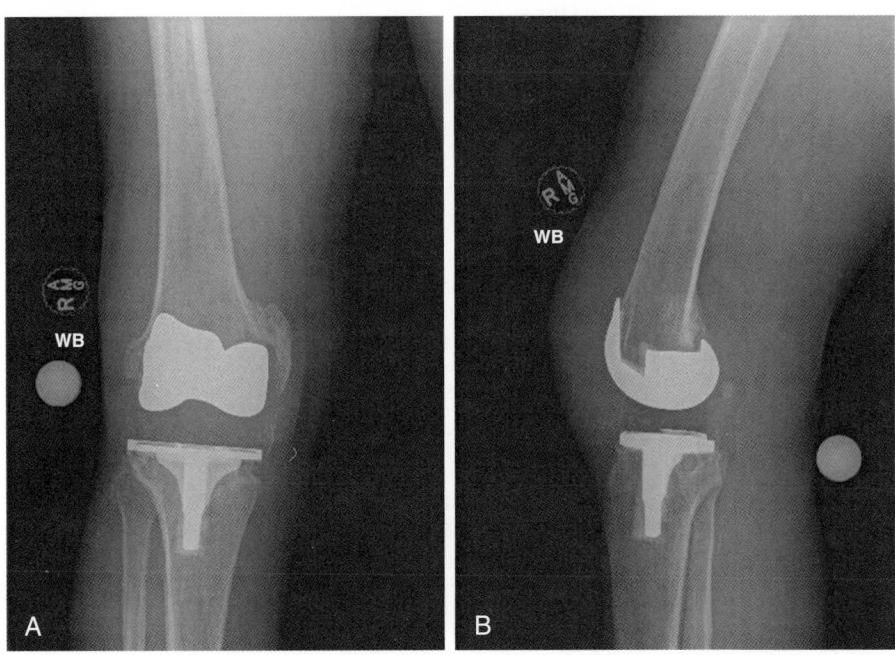

Figure 3 A, Anteroposterior radiograph of an infected total knee arthroplasty. The radiograph shows resorption of the bone, especially the femur, adjacent to the implant. **B,** Lateral radiograph of the knee demonstrating lucencies extending posterior along the femur and interface between the femur and implant.

immune compromise, substance abuse, and malnutrition. One of the most common of conditions increasing the risk for development of osteomyelitis is diabetes mellitus. An estimated 25% of diabetic patients will develop a foot ulcer at some point in their lifetime, with increased morbidity and mortality, compared to patients with diabetes without foot ulcers. Of these foot ulcers, 20% to almost 60% will harbor underlying osteomyelitis (Figure 4). Infected foot ulcers are the most common risk factor for lower extremity amputations in this population. Diabetic foot ulcers usually start as superficial breaks in the skin or ulcers, which, if they become chronic, are at risk of infection. Infections of foot ulcer in the setting of diabetes are greater among patients with peripheral neuropathy or peripheral vascular disease; these comorbidities can also lead to masking of the signs and symptoms of inflammation,

making a diagnosis of infection more challenging. Superficial infections in diabetic foot ulcers can eventually affect deeper tissues, in some patients progressing to osteomyelitis. Depth of the ulcer, especially in the presence of elevated inflammatory markers, can aid in the diagnosis of osteomyelitis. Involvement of bone can be confirmed with plain films; other imaging modalities, such as magnetic resonance imaging (MRI), white blood cell (WBC) scintigraphy, and 18F-fluorodeoxyglucose (18F) positron emission tomography (FDG-PET)/computed tomography (CT) may be useful in confirming the diagnosis but have variable reported sensitivities and specificities. Treatment of these ulcers and associated infections is multidisciplinary: in addition to administration of antibiotics for culture-confirmed infections and potential surgical debridement of involved tissue, treatment includes local

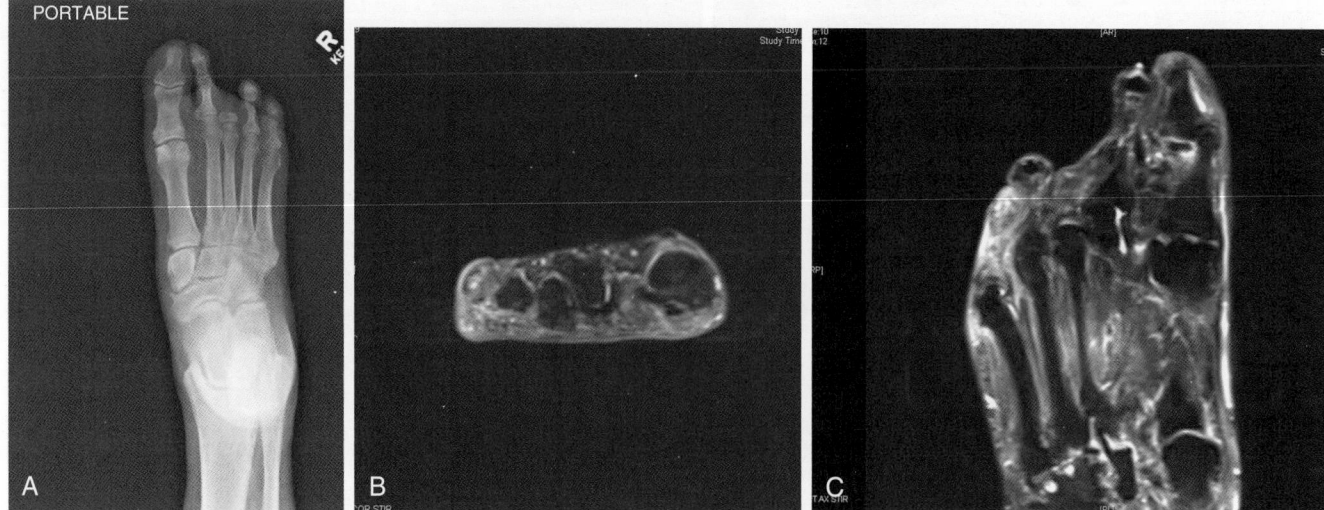

Figure 4 Osteomyelitis associated with diabetes/vascular insufficiency. **A,** Anteroposterior radiograph revealing diffuse osteopenia within the fifth toe and subtle cortical disruption along lateral aspect of the proximal phalanx. Note previous amputation of third toe. Patients with loss of protective sensation and poor vascular supply have recurrent or multiple episodes of wound infections that can extend to involve adjacent bone. **B** and **C,** Coronal and axial short tau inversion recovery (STIR) magnetic resonance images. Hyperintense STIR signal along the proximal phalanx and adjacent soft tissues of the fifth toe, consistent with infection and inflammation.

wound care (although evidence of type of wound care is mixed), evaluating and addressing, if needed or possible, peripheral vascular disease; off-loading of the involved portion of the extremity; and appropriate glycemic control.

Etiology

In children, most cases of acute hematogenous osteomyelitis are caused by a single organism, most commonly *S. aureus*. These cases typically involve the vascular metaphysis of long bones. Coagulase-negative staphylococci can also be an etiology in infants in intensive care with vascular catheters. Other gram-positive cocci include Streptococci: *Streptococcus pneumoniae* in incompletely immunized children, or young children with underlying conditions and *Streptococcus pyogenes* (group A), especially following primary varicella-zoster and *Streptococcus agalactiae* (group B) in neonates. Culture-negative cases occur frequently, and these are usually presumed to be due to *S. aureus* and treated as such. In children 6 to 36 months old, *Kingella kingae*, a gram-negative component of the oral flora, is a major pathogen that causes non-long bone osteomyelitis. *Haemophilus influenzae* type b (Hib) is a rare cause of hematogenous osteomyelitis in young children after the wide implementation of Hib vaccination. Enteric gram-negative bacilli can cause osteomyelitis in infants and children with sickle cell disease. Those with hemoglobinopathies and HIV infection are also at risk for Salmonella osteomyelitis.

In adults, hematogenous osteomyelitis primarily presents as vertebral osteomyelitis and is caused by *S. aureus* in more than half of cases in case series in developed countries. The proportion of the cases of hematogenous osteomyelitis due to methicillin-resistant *S. aureus* (MRSA) depends on local epidemiology. Other etiologic organisms include aerobic gram-negative bacilli after genitourinary instrumentation, pyogenic streptococci including group B and C/G in diabetics, viridans and anginosus-group streptococci, enterococci, *Pseudomonas aeruginosa*, coagulase-negative staphylococci in patients with indwelling venous catheters, and injection drug users. In endemic areas, *Brucella* species and *Mycobacterium tuberculosis* should be considered. Disseminated *Mycobacterium avium complex* (MAC) can involve the spine in patients with AIDS. Fungal vertebral osteomyelitis is rare but can occur in people at risk such as individuals who live in endemic areas for dimorphic fungi like *Histoplasma, Blastomyces,* and *Coccidioides*; intravenous drug users who can get *Candida* osteomyelitis; and immunocompromised hosts who can develop infections with Aspergillus.

TABLE 1	Microbiology of Osteomyelitis
Common >50%	**Rare <5%**
• *Staphylococcus aureus* (MSSA, CA-MRSA) • Coagulase-negative staphylococci	• *Salmonella* • *Mycobacterium tuberculosis* • *Brucella* • *Coxiella* • Dimorphic fungi
Occasional 25%–50%	• *Mycobacterium avium* complex
• *Streptococci* • *Enterococci* • *Pseudomonas* • *Enterobacter* • *Proteus* • *Escherichia coli* • *Serratia* • Anaerobes (*Finegoldia, Clostridium, Bacteroides*)	• Atypical mycobacteria • *Aspergillus* • *Mycoplasma* • *Tropheryma* • *Actinomyces* • *Bartonella* • *Pasteurella* • *Eikenella*

CA, Community-associated*; MRSA,* Methicillin-resistant *Staphylococcus aureus; MSSA,* Methicillin-susceptible *Staphylococcus aureus.*
Adapted from *Mandell, Douglas, and Bennett Principles and Practice of Infectious Diseases,* 9th edition, chapter 104, pages 1418–1429.

Among adults with trauma or open fractures, diabetic and vascular insufficiency foot infections are more likely to develop polymicrobial osteomyelitis with staphylococci, streptococci, enterococci, gram-negative bacilli, and anaerobes (Table 1). After animal or human bites, *Pasteurella multocida, Eikenella corrodens,* and oral anaerobic gram-positive cocci are usually identified.

Clinical Manifestations

Patients with osteomyelitis typically present with pain and tenderness in areas with or without prior injury. They may experience pain with activity but also note pain at rest and that awakens them at night. Symptoms may be acute and localized or gradual onset and nonspecific; the latter may be subtle, making clinical suspicion crucial. There may be noted warmth and erythema, especially in more superficial bones. Patients may also present with fever and other systemic signs of infection. Symptoms of pain at rest and constitutional signs may be interpreted as representing an underlying neoplasm, especially in children, in whom osteomyelitis and Ewing sarcoma often have nearly identical presentations. Patients whose bone infection has involved an adjacent native joint are reluctant to use that joint and have significant pain, even with limited attempts at range of motion. Patients with

| TABLE 2 | Medical Treatment of Osteomyelitis |

ORGANISM	FIRST CHOICE	ALTERNATIVE
MSSA	Nafcillin, oxacillin or cefazolin	Vancomycin, some add rifampin to nafcillin/oxacillin
MRSA	Vancomycin or daptomycin	Linezolid or levofloxacin + rifampin
Penicillin susceptible *Streptococci*	Penicillin G, ceftriaxone, or cefazolin	Vancomycin
Enterococci and Streptococci with Penicillin MIC >0.5	Penicillin G, ampicillin with optional gentamicin	Vancomycin with addition of gentamicin
Enterobacteriaceae	Ceftriaxone or ertapenem	Ciprofloxacin or levofloxacin
Pseudomonas aeruginosa	Cefepime, meropenem, or imipenem	Ciprofloxacin or ceftazidime

MIC, Minimum inhibitory concentration; *MRSA*, Methicillin-resistant *Staphylococcus aureus*; *MSSA*, Methicillin-susceptible *Staphylococcus aureus*.
Adapted from *Mandell, Douglas, and Bennett Principles and Practice of Infectious Diseases*, 9th edition, chapter 104, page 1418–1429.

long bone infections, especially children, are reluctant to utilize that extremity, including bearing weight, if the infection involves a lower extremity. Patients with new onset pain in the setting of implanted hardware, especially joint arthroplasties, should be assumed to have an infection until proven otherwise. Patients with vertebral osteomyelitis usually present with unremitting back pain. The diagnosis can be difficult to make, because the symptoms may seem consistent with degenerative changes in the spine and initial plain radiographs prove nondiagnostic. However, continued infections in this area can lead to epidural extension, with neurologic changes that require rapid referral.

Diagnosis/Confirmation

The clinical diagnosis of osteomyelitis is confirmed by a combination of serum studies, radiographic findings, microbiology or culture results, and pathology, if the patient undergoes surgery. Plain radiographs are an inexpensive initial study; however, their sensitivity in diagnosing osteomyelitis is limited, as the findings of bone loss and periosteal reaction can be attributed to a number of aggressive bone conditions, including neoplasms. In addition, bone loss of approximately 30% to 40% is required before being noted on plain radiographs. MRI provides additional sensitivity and specificity in diagnosis, even in early osteomyelitis, especially if obtained with and without contrast. MRI findings include reduced T1- and heightened T2-weighted bone marrow signals, representing fatty marrow replaced by inflammation. Contrast enhancement patterns can also help to differentiate infection from neoplasia. CT is an alternative to MRI if the latter is not available or the patient is unable to tolerate the examination. CT findings can include gas along fascial plains, decreased density of infected bone, soft tissue masses, and abscesses, as well identifying the course of overlying sinus tracts. Nuclear medicine imaging modalities are more expensive than other imaging options. While in some reports nuclear medicine imaging modalities have been noted to be more sensitive in identifying osteomyelitis, they are less specific, with high false-positive rates. However, they can be useful in imaging areas in which hardware is present, because such metal can significantly limit the details seen on MRI or CT. Nuclear medicine imaging modalities include three-phase Tc99m MDP scan—ideal for bones not affected by underlying conditions, gallium 67 scan (usually performed as sequential bone then gallium scan for comparison), 111-indium radiolabeled WBC scans, or Tc99m sulfur colloid bone marrow scans performed in sequence with WBC scans. These additional imaging modalities are usually used in complicated cases or cases in which the diagnosis is unclear based on other, less expensive tests.

The identification of the infecting organism is crucial to optimal medical management. In cases of presumed osteomyelitis, antibiotics should be withheld until material for culture is obtained, usually via needle aspiration of the area. If the patient requires surgical debridement, tissue can be sent for culture and for pathologic evaluation. Pathology in these instances can help to rule out neoplasia and will demonstrate acute, chronic, or acute on chronic inflammatory cells. Swab cultures of draining sinuses demonstrate poor correlation with adjacent bone cultures, except for *S. aureus*. Material obtained for culture should be sent for both aerobic and anaerobic assessment.

Treatment
Medical Treatment

Vertebral osteomyelitis without associated neurologic deficit or nerve compression, and acute hematogenous osteomyelitis in children, are usually treated with systemic antimicrobials without the need for surgical debridement. Most other osteomyelitis syndromes in adults require a combination of medical and surgical treatments to eradicate infection and restore function. A cornerstone of medical therapy for osteomyelitis is identification of the causative organisms in culture. In the absence of associated active soft tissue infection or sepsis, antimicrobials are usually held until adequate cultures are obtained either by aspiration/biopsy or during surgical debridement of the affected bone. Vancomycin (Vancocin) and beta-lactams including cephalosporins have been used extensively for the treatment of osteomyelitis (Table 2). Although most experience is with intravenous antimicrobials, some data support the use of highly orally bioavailable antibiotics like trimethoprim-sulfamethoxazole (Bactrim)[1], rifampin[1], clindamycin, and quinolones. Duration of antimicrobial treatment is generally 4 to 6 weeks based on experimental models and limited prospective studies. Parenteral antimicrobials can be continued outside the hospital using peripherally inserted central catheters (PICCs). In children with hematogenous osteomyelitis, parenteral therapy can be changed to oral when the child is afebrile and able to tolerate oral medications, and duration of therapy as short as 2 to 3 weeks has been reported to be effective.

Fracture site infections following open fractures are treated with debridement, cultures, and organism-directed antimicrobial therapy. Considering that it is common to use or retain fracture fixation devices, long-term oral antimicrobial suppression following induction treatment for 6 weeks is used until fracture healing is documented on imaging. At that point, antimicrobial suppression can be stopped.

Vertebral osteomyelitis treatment might require drainage of associated paravertebral or psoas abscesses by radiology. Duration of antimicrobial therapy might be longer than 6 weeks in patients with undrained abscesses, MRSA infections, or end-stage renal disease. Follow-up at the end of treatment includes assessment of resolution or improvement in pain and in level of inflammation markers in the erythrocyte sedimentation rate C-reactive protein (ESR, CRP) test. A 25% or more reduction in these inflammation markers at the end of treatment is associated with treatment success. Repeat MRI is not routinely recommended and is reserved for patients with failure to improve or worsening symptoms. In 1 to 2 years after successful therapy, spontaneous fusion of the affected vertebral levels usually occurs.

Diabetic foot osteomyelitis management requires evaluation of the vascular supply to the affected area and revascularization is needed in patients with peripheral arterial disease to optimize surgical outcome and minimize need for amputation. Because most of these infections are polymicrobial, use of antimicrobials with anaerobic spectrum of activity is recommended (piperacillin-tazobactam [Zosyn][1], ampicillin-sulbactam [Unasyn][1], ertapenem

Osteomyelitis

---
[1] Not FDA approved for this indication.

[Invanz][1], cephalosporins with metronidazole [Flagyl], quinolones with metronidazole or clindamycin).

Surgical Treatment

Surgery is often performed in conjunction with antibiotic treatment in cases of osteomyelitis of long bones, especially in cases of chronic osteomyelitis or in the presence of bone abscesses, typically in cases of chronic osteomyelitis or in the presence of bone abscesses, especially in the presence of implanted hardware. Surgery for osteomyelitis of the spine is usually reserved for patients whose infection does not completely respond to antibiotic treatment or who develop neurologic deficits. Surgical treatment of osteomyelitis of long bones is primarily performed with wide excisional debridement and copious irrigation. The order in which the operations are performed is very important because a large bacterial load can be pushed further into surrounding bone and soft tissues by irrigating before debridement. The adage "the solution to pollution is dilution" accurately describes the intent of copious irrigation at a site of bone infection.

Bacteria identified within bone, either causing a biologic breakdown of the structure of the bone (infection) versus bacteria on or near bone (colonization), are two distinct clinical pictures. The structure of bone is similar to that of sponge; bacteria resulting in osteomyelitis can "hide" in the caverns and nooks of cancellous bone quite readily, leading to small local abscess communities in the bone, bone marrow, and surrounding soft tissues, making it difficult to eradicate them through the host inflammatory response or with systemic antibiotics. In addition, bacteria in these areas may not be exposed to antibiotic agents, WBCs, or irrigation solutions. Therefore, they can exist and multiply until the bone reacts and begins to break down at the site of the infection. Given this analogy, it is understandable that there is the need to irrigate a site of osteomyelitis thoroughly to dilute the bacterial load and then allow antibiotics the opportunity to work to eliminate the remaining pathogens from the infected bone.

To rid the bone of infection, surgeons typically debride bone that is obviously infected and/or necrotic, while healthy bone can and will be removed up to the margin of infected bone to improve the likelihood of healing in the absence of infection. This is critical to the success of the procedure but can lead to large defects. In addition, adjacent soft tissues should be sharply debrided back to healthy, bleeding tissue. As a result, WBCs can come into the area along with antibiotic agents delivered via the healthy, small blood vessels to complete the task of eliminating the bacteria. It is important that tissue removed during these procedures is sent for culture, as well as for pathologic examination.

Debridement involving infected bone with orthopedic implants adjacent to the site can be challenging. These implants and any surrounding necrotic tissue can be colonized by bacteria, often in the form of a surrounding glycocalyx or exopolysaccharide coating that envelops the bacteria. In some patients, this can necessitate the removal of rods, plates, screws, or the components of a joint replacement, as systemic antibiotics are unable to access bacteria housed in this biofilm. Removing the implant results in removal of the glycocalyx and reduces the bacterial load but frequently necessitates subsequent reconstructive surgeries.

Often, with obvious purulent infections, several surgical procedures are required to accomplish the task of bacterial elimination. The initial bacterial load can be so great that even after significant tissue (both bone and soft tissue) has been excised and irrigated, the surgeon cannot confidently close the wound for the completion of the case. Surgical decision making may include a second or third procedure to assess the site and determine the need for further tissue removal and irrigation versus wound closure. When multiple (staged) procedures are performed, wound coverage techniques can help to continue to minimize or eliminate bacteria during the patient's hospitalization.

A vacuum-assisted closure (VAC) device is one such coverage technique. These devices apply a vacuum or negative pressure environment to the wound with an evenly applied suction level to allow for continued bacterial debridement while keeping the wound covered during the time that the patient is out of the operating room. The VAC can be applied after the excisional debridement and irrigation procedure has been completed. VACs are typically used in anticipation of a return to the operating room for a second or third procedure.

A wound VAC device is applied to the bed of the wound utilizing three key elements: (1) a sponge substrate (for even application of the suction), (2) a plastic tape to seal the wound edges, and (3) a suctioning device or pump to apply the negative pressure to the wound. Once applied, these devices can continue to promote healthy tissue growth and create a hostile environment for bacteria, thereby limiting bacterial proliferation.

Conclusion

Patient outcomes after treatment of osteomyelitis have improved over the years with development of new imaging technologies to improve diagnostic accuracy, development of new antibiotics and antibiotic delivery methods, and expanded surgical techniques. Most importantly, treatments, both medical and surgical, are based on a better understanding of the pathogenesis of this infection. However, given the continued increase in prevalence of this condition, we need additional research to better understand the contribution of various risk factors and comorbidities so that we can improve prevention efforts and continue to tailor multidisciplinary interventions.

References

Birt MC, Anderson DW, Toby EB, Wang J, Osteomyelitis: Recent advances in pathophysiology and therapeutic strategies, J of Orthopaedics 14:45–52, 2017.

Bouchoucha S, Gafsi K, Trifa M, et al: Intravenous antibiotic therapy for acute hematogenous osteomyelitis in children: a short versus long course, Arch Pediatr 20:464–469, 2013.

Chong BSW, Brereton CJ, Gordon A, Davis JS: Epidemiology, microbiological diagnosis, and clinical outcomes in pyogenic vertebral osteomyelitis: a 10-year retrospective cohort study, Open Forum Infect Dis 5(3), ofy037, 2018 Epub.

Cierny G, Mader JT, Penninck JJ: The Classic: A clinical staging system for adult osteomyelitis, CORR 414:7–24, 2003.

Crenshaw AH, ed: Campbell's Operative Orthopedics, 8th ed. edition

Dartnell J, Ramachadran M, Katchburian M: Haematogenous acute and subacute paediatric osteomyelitis: a systemic review of the literature, J Bone Joint Surg Br 94(5):584, 2012.

Euba G, Murillo O, Fernadez-Sabe N, et al: Long-term follow up trial of oral rifampin-cotrimoxazole combination versus intravenous cloxacillin in treatment of chronic staphylococcal osteomyelitis, Antimicrob Agents Chemother 53:2672–2676, 2009.

Gehrke Alijanipour P, Parvizi J: The management of an infected total knee arthroplasty, Bone Joint J 97-B(10 Suppl A):20–29, 2015.

Gustilo RB, Mendoza RM, Williams DN: Problems in management of type III (severe) open fractures: a new classification of type III open fractures, J Trauma 24:742–746, 1984.

Kim UJ, Bae JY, Kim S-E, et al: Comparison of pyogenic postoperative and native vertebral osteomyelitis, Spine J 19:880–887, 2019.

Kremers HM, Nwojo ME, Ransom JE, et al: Trends in the epidemiology of osteomyelitis: a population-based study, 1969 to 2009, JBJS(A) 97:837–845, 2015.

Lew DP, Waldvogel FA: Osteomyelitis. Lancet 364(9431):369–379, 2004.

Lew DP: Waldvogel FA: Current concepts: osteomyelitis, NEJM 336:999–1007, 1997.

Lindbloom BJ, James ER, McGarvey WC: Osteomyelitis of the foot and ankle: diagnosis, epidemiology, and treatment, Foot Ankle Clin N Am 19:569–588, 2014.

Lipsky BA, Senneville E, Abbas ZG, et al: Guidelines on the diagnosis and treatment of foot infection in persons with diabetes (IWGDF 2019 update), Diabetes Metab Res Rev 36(S1):e3280, 2020.

Mandell JC, Khurana B, Smith JT, et al: Osteomyelitis of the lower extremity: pathophysiology, imaging, and classification, with an emphasis on diabetic foot infection, Emerg Radiol 25:175–188, 2018.

Masters EA, Trombetta RP, de Mesy Bentley KL, et al: Evolving concepts in bone infection: redefining "biofilm", "acute vs. chronic osteomyelitis", "the immune proteome" and "local antibiotic therapy", Bone Res 7:20, 2019.

Okubo Y, Nochioka K, Testa M: Nationwide survey of pediatric acute osteomyelitis in the USA, J Pediatric Ortho 26:501–506, 2006.

Park KH, Cho OH, Lee JH, et al: Optimal duration of antibiotic therapy in patients with hematogenous vertebral osteomyelitis at low risk and high risk of recurrence, Clin Infect Dis 262:1262–1269, 2016.

Miller M, ed: Review of Orthopaedics, 3rd ed.

Samara E, Spyropoulou V, Tabard-Fougère A, et al: Kingella kingae and osteoarticular infections, Pediatrics 144(6), 2019, Epub.

Senneville E, Lipsky BA, Abbas ZG, et al: Diagnosis of infection in the foot in diabetes: a systematic review, Diabetes Metab Res Rev 36(S1):e3281, 2020.

Zalavras CG, Marcus RE, Levin LS, Patzakis MJ: Management of open fractures and subsequent complications, JBJS (A) 4:884–895, 2007.

PLAGUE

Method of
Nelson Iván Agudelo Higuita, MD; and Douglas A. Drevets, MD

CURRENT DIAGNOSIS

- Plague should be suspected when a person develops abrupt onset of fever, lymphadenopathy, or sepsis and there is history of a flea bite or possible exposure to an infected animal or person.
- *Yersinia pestis* is an aerobic gram-negative coccobacilli that exhibits bipolar staining with Giemsa, Wright's, and Wayson stains.
- Automated diagnostic systems may misidentify *Y. pestis* as another organism.

CURRENT THERAPY

- Timely and appropriate management is imperative for a good outcome.
- Despite their toxicities, aminoglycosides are the treatment agents of choice.
- Respiratory droplet precautions should be instituted when pneumonic plague is suspected.
- Postexposure prophylaxis is indicated for close contacts.

Historical descriptions indicate that *Yersinia pestis* probably caused Justinian's Plague (AD 541), which led into the first plague pandemic. The second plague pandemic, also known as the Black Death, began in Central Asia in 1347 and then spread to Europe, Asia, and Africa. It killed an estimated 50 million people. The current (third) plague pandemic began in China and then spread worldwide along shipping routes in 1899–1900. *Y. pestis* is a gram-negative, nonmotile, facultatively anaerobic, non-spore-forming coccobacillus that is approximately 0.5 to 0.8 μm in diameter and 1 to 3 μm in length. Genomic sequencing shows that *Y. pestis* is a recently emerged clone of *Y. pseudotuberculosis*.

Epidemiology

Plague is a zoonosis for which urban and sylvatic rodents (e.g., rats, prairie dogs, and marmots) are the most important enzootic reservoirs. Additionally, domestic cats and dogs have been linked to human disease. Human plague occurs in North and South America, Asia, and Africa. Recent outbreaks reported to the World Health Organization (WHO) have occurred in the Democratic Republic of Congo (2005, 2006), China (2009), and Peru (2010). Plague is endemic in Madagascar, and between 2004 and 2009, 30% of all human cases worldwide were reported from this country. The largest epidemic in a quarter of a century was identified August 1, 2017, and was contained November 27, 2017. A total of 2417 cases (77% pneumonic) with a 9% case fatality ratio were reported. From 2000 to 2009, a total of 21,725 cases of plague with a 7.4% fatality rate were reported worldwide. The incidence of plague in most of the world is otherwise declining. In 2018, only 5 countries reported cases of plague. In North America, most human cases occur in New Mexico, Arizona, California, Colorado, and Texas. Between 1900 and 2012, 1006 confirmed or probable cases have occurred in the U.S. with over 80% of these attributable to bubonic plague.

Modes of Transmission

Most human infections are transmitted from rodent to humans via the bite of an infected flea. Infection also can be acquired by contact with body fluids from infected animals, such as during field dressing of game or by inhalation of respiratory droplets from animals, particularly cats, or humans with pneumonic plague.

Bioterrorism Threat

Plague was used as an agent of biowarfare by the Japanese in World War II and was a focus of intensive research and development in the former Soviet Union during the Cold War. Primary pneumonic plague is the most likely form of exposure because of biowarfare or bioterrorism. Recent increases in terrorism worldwide have increased the focus of public health management groups to develop comprehensive statements regarding plague as a biological weapon.

Pathogenesis and Clinical Syndromes

Transdermal inoculation of bacilli from the bite of an infected flea ultimately leads to infection of the regional lymph nodes in which massive replication of bacteria creates the bubo (derived from the Greek *bubon* or "groin"), a swollen, erythematous, and painful lymph node in the groin, axilla, or cervical region. Bacteremia and septicemia frequently develop and lead to secondary infection of other organs including the lungs, spleen, and central nervous system. Primary pneumonic plague is a rare natural occurrence and results from the inhalation of respiratory droplets containing *Y. pestis* bacilli from another case of pneumonic plague, usually in humans or in cats. Although plague in dogs is rare, human outbreaks have been traced to sick dogs with wildlife exposure. Secondary pneumonic plague results from seeding of the lungs by blood-borne bacteria in the setting of either bubonic or septicemic plague. Septicemic plague also begins with transdermal exposure but manifests as primary bacteremia/septicemia without the bubo. Less common manifestations include meningitis, pharyngitis, and gastroenteritis.

Bubonic plague is an acute febrile lymphadenitis that develops 2 to 8 days after inoculation. Inflamed lymph nodes are usually 1 to 6 cm in diameter and painful. Abrupt onset of fever is an almost universal finding and occurs simultaneously with, or up to 24 hours before, the appearance of the bubo. Headache, malaise, and chills are frequent, along with nausea, vomiting, and diarrhea. Most patients are tachycardic, hypotensive, and appear prostrate and lethargic with episodic restlessness. Leukocytosis with a left shift is typical. Complications include pneumonia, shock, disseminated intravascular coagulation, purpuric skin lesions, acral cyanosis, and gangrene. The differential diagnosis of bubonic plague includes tularemia and Group A β-hemolytic streptococcal adenitis with bacteremia.

Symptoms of septicemic plague are similar to those caused by other gram-negative bacteria, and are very similar to those of bubonic plague except that abdominal pain is more common in septicemic plague. Septicemic plague must be differentiated from fulminating septicemia caused by other gram-negative bacteria. Primary pneumonic plague has an abrupt onset of fever and influenza-like symptoms 1 to 5 days after inhalation exposure. Symptoms include shortness of breath, cough, chest pain, and bloody sputum with rapid progression to fulminating pneumonia and respiratory failure. Patients with secondary pneumonic infection show respiratory symptoms in addition to those attributed to the bubo or sepsis. Radiographic findings include patchy bronchopneumonia, multilobar consolidations, cavitations, and alveolar hemorrhage and are not pathognomonic of *Y. pestis*. Plague pneumonia must be differentiated from severe influenza, inhalation anthrax, and overwhelming community-acquired pneumonia.

Diagnosis

Plague is diagnosed by demonstrating *Y. pestis* in blood or body fluids such as a lymph node aspirate, sputum, or cerebrospinal fluid. A tentative diagnosis of bubonic plague can be made rapidly with fluid aspirated from a bubo showing gram-negative coccobacilli with bipolar staining. It is important to remember that automated diagnostic systems might misidentify *Y. pestis*. In an outbreak in Colorado, the misidentification of *Y. pestis* as

Pseudomonas luteola delayed the recognition of the outbreak. Serology showing a fourfold rise in antibody titers to F1 antigen or a single titer of more than 1:128 is also diagnostic. Rapid tests using monoclonal antibodies to detect *Y. pestis* F1 antigen in bubo aspirates and sputum have been developed and field tested. The use of mass spectrometry as a more rapid and cost-effective diagnostic tool has also been studied.

Treatment

The aminoglycosides (gentamicin[1] and streptomycin), the fluoroquinolones (ciprofloxacin [Cipro] moxifloxacin [Avelox] and levofloxacin [Levaquin]) and doxycycline (Vibramycin) are the first-, second-, and third-line classes of antibiotics, respectively. Typical minimal inhibitory concentrations for 90% (MIC_{90}) of tested strains for the fluoroquinolones are less than 0.03 to 0.25 μg/mL compared with less than 1.0 μg/mL and less than 1.0 μg/mL to 4.0 μg/mL for gentamicin and streptomycin, respectively, and less than 1.0 μg/mL for doxycycline. Streptomycin (15 mg/kg up to 1 g intramuscularly [IM] every 12 hours) and gentamicin (5 to 7 mg/kg/day intravenously [IV]/IM in one or two doses daily) are the drugs of choice for severe infection. Standard fluoroquinolone dosing includes ciprofloxacin 400 mg IV/500 mg orally every 12 hours; levofloxacin 500–750 mg IV/orally daily; and moxifloxacin 400 mg IV/orally daily. Doxycycline is administered starting with a 200 mg loading dose followed by 100 mg IV/orally every 12 hours. Chloramphenicol (25 mg/kg IV/orally every 6 hours) can be used in select circumstances. Antibiotic therapy should be continued for a total of 10 days; some experts will extend the duration of therapy to 14 days when a bacteriostatic agent like a tetracycline is used.

Prevention and Control

Standard infection control procedures should include a disposable surgical mask, latex gloves, devices to protect mucous membranes, and good hand washing. Hospitalized patients with known or suspected pneumonic plague should be isolated under respiratory droplet precautions for at least 48 hours after appropriate antibiotics are initiated. Patients without respiratory plague can be managed under standard precautions. Postexposure prophylaxis should be given to individuals with close contact (less than 2 meters) with an infectious case or who have had a potential respiratory exposure. The recommended adult antibiotics for prophylaxis are doxycycline or ciprofloxacin in the same doses used for treatment. Postexposure prophylaxis can be given orally and should be continued for 7 days following exposure. Currently, there is no licensed plague vaccine. An encapsulated *Y. pseudotuberculosis,* strain V674pF1, is an efficient live oral vaccine against pneumonic plague in mice. Recently, flea resistance to insecticides such as DDT and Deltamethrin in Madagascar has prompted an immediate need for alternative insecticides to prevent future plague outbreaks.

References

Andrianaivoarimanana V, et al: Understanding the persistence of plague foci in Madagascar, *PLoS Negl Trop Dis.* 7(11):e2382, 2013.
Boulanger LL, Ettestad P, Fogarty JD, et al: Gentamicin and tetracyclines for the treatment of human plague: review of 75 cases in New Mexico, 1985–1999, *Clin Infect Dis* 38:663–669, 2004.
Boyer S, et al: Xenopsylla cheopis (Siphonaptera: Pulicidae) susceptibility to deltamethrin in Madagascar, *PLoS One* 9(11), 2014, e111998.
Butler T: A clinical study of bubonic plague. Observations of the 1970 Vietnam epidemic with emphasis on coagulation studies, skin histology and electrocardiograms, *Am J Med* 53:268–276, 1972.
Butler T: Plague gives surprises in the first decade of the 21st century in the United States and worldwide, *Am J Trop Med Hyg* 89(4):788–793, 2013.
CDC. Maps and Statistics. http://www.cdc.gov/plague/maps/index.html.
Cler DJ, Vernaleo JR, Lombardi LJ, et al: Plague pneumonia disease caused by Yersinia pestis, *Semin Respir Infect* 12:12–23, 1997.
Derbise A, Cerdà Marín A, et al: An encapsulated *Yersinia* pseudotuberculosis is a highly efficient vaccine against pneumonic plague, e1528 *PLoS Negl Trop Dis* 6(2), 2012. Feb.
Gage KL, Dennis DT, Orloski KA, et al: Cases of cat-associated human plague in the Western US, 1977–1998, *Clin Infect Dis* 30:893–900, 2000.
Inglesby TV, Dennis DT, Henderson DA, et al: Plague as a biological weapon: Medical and public health management. Working Group on Civilian Biodefense, *JAMA* 283:2281–2290, 2000.
Perry RD, Fetherston JD: *Yersinia pestis*—etiologic agent of plague, *Clin Microbiol Rev* 10:35–66, 1997.
Prentice MB, Rahalison L: Plague, *Lancet* 369:1196–1207, 2007.
Runfola JK, et al: Outbreak of human pneumonic plague with dog-to-human and possible human-to-human transmission, *MMWR Morb Mortal Wkly Rep* 64(16):429–434, 2015.
Wang H, et al: A dog-associated primary pneumonic plague in Qinghai Province, China, *Clin Infect Dis* 52(2):185–190, 2011.
WHO external Situation report 14 - 04 December 2017.
Wong JD, Barash JR, Sandfort RF, Janda JM: Susceptibilities of *Yersinia pestis* strains to 12 antimicrobial agents, *Antimicrob Agents Chemother* 44:1995–1996, 2000.
World Health Organization. Plague Outbreaks Situation Report.
World Health Organization: Plague around the world in 2019, *Weekly Epidemiological Record* 94(25):289–292, 2019.

POST-COVID SYNDROME

Method of
Victor S. Sierpina, MD; Justin Seashore, MD; and Sagar Kamprath, MD

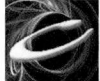

CURRENT DIAGNOSIS

- The postacute COVID syndrome is defined as symptoms extending 3 weeks to 3 months after the acute disease and long-haul COVID syndrome defined as symptoms persisting beyond 3 months.
- Predominant symptoms are new onset shortness of breath, cough, palpitations, fatigue, and brain fog. Other common symptoms include gastrointestinal (GI) disturbances, headaches, hair loss, new onset nondescript pain, depression, anxiety, and posttraumatic stress.
- Results of testing are not part of the current definition because many patients were not tested and are or were asymptomatic carriers.
- The broad spectrum of clinical manifestations of post-COVID syndrome should encourage clinicians and medical educators to include it in the differential of any of a number of new or worsening complaints.

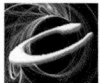

CURRENT TREATMENT

- Evidence for optimal management of long-haul COVID may be lacking at this time but is evolving with best practices being described by multiple professional bodies.
- Multidisciplinary management and rehabilitation are essential to whole person care.
- Organ and system specific care is appropriate and must be prioritized as to serious versus milder long-term problems.
- Self-management and peer support can plan important roles and must include shared decision making.
- Appropriate consultation and use of currently established practice guidelines that are disease or organ specific is foundational to optimal treatment planning.
- Quality of care principles for long-haul COVID include accessing care, reducing burden of illness, taking clinical responsibility, having continuity of care, undertaking multidisciplinary rehabilitation, evidence-based investigation and management, and conducting further research and development of appropriate and evidence-based clinical services.

Over the past year we have endured an ever-changing multimodal disease process, devastating millions of people not only as a result of severe infection but also because of mild or asymptomatic forms of the disease. Our understanding and definitions of what

---

[1]Not FDA approved for this indication.

spectrum of conditions the post-COVID syndrome (PCS) or long-haul COVID encompasses is in the stage of medical discovery. Current estimates are between 10% to 30% of COVID infected patients may be left with residual symptoms.

What we present in this chapter is a foundational program that is holistic and methodical, offering low invasive procedures and management strategies. This approach will offer post-COVID patients an improved quality of life with low risk, cost effectiveness, and common-sense healthcare approaches. The evidence base for this approach is grounded in current best practices but continues to evolve with new knowledge about the course of PCS. In parallel, we need to guide patients away from high-risk, high-cost, invasive therapies that have no proven benefit.

The role of peer support is clearly important to those with PCS who may otherwise feel isolated and misunderstood. Healthcare professionals must be cognizant of the range of real physical long-term impacts of COVID; address them with clinical discernment, understanding, and empathy; and be careful not to label all such presentations as related to stress, anxiety, depression, or other psychological epiphenomena.

Pathophysiology

COVID-19 is caused by the severe acute respiratory syndrome coronavirus 2 (SARS-COV-2) and is genetically similar to the SARS coronavirus, which was responsible for the SARS outbreak in 2002. Coronaviruses that circulate among human are usually benign and are responsible for about a quarter of all common cold illnesses with a total of seven human coronaviruses in known existence. However, it is likely that bats, a natural animal reservoir, facilitated the mutation of the virus in China in late 2019. As another spillover possibility, the escape of modified virus from a research laboratory in Wuhan is being debated. This novel coronavirus is composed of single-stranded RNA with its envelope surrounded by spike proteins resembling a crown, typically transmitted through respiratory droplets and fecal oral transmission. The incubation period is about 5 days, follow a week of worsening symptoms that may lead to hospitalization. Of those who are symptomatic, about 20% need further hospital/ICU while the rest often improve with the aid of the innate immune system, which tends to get weaker with age. Interferon (IFN) is a key component which affects the mechanism of viral infection. Higher viral loads and delayed interferon responses are seen in severe infection, and it may be likely that patients most susceptible to severe disease are those that cannot adequately mount an effective early antiviral response.

The virus attaches to cells via the ACE2 receptor, found in the tongue, nose, throat, stomach, small intestine, liver, brain, kidneys, and lungs. In the lungs it binds to type 2 alveolar cells, where it replicates. The cells subsequently send a distress signal of cytokines and down regulate the ACE2 decreasing angiotensin 1 to 9 and 1 to 7 (provasodilation and antifibrotic). Angiotensin 1 receptors are more stimulated, which leads to a proinflammatory and profibrotic stage. COVID-19 also favors disordered endothelial function, which contributes to protein accumulation in the alveolar space seen in the "cytokine storm" directly related to capillary leak and the cases of ARDS seen in advanced states of the disease. Unfortunately, this is not only limited to the lungs but predisposes the entire body system to a prothrombotic state, as seen in cases of stroke and other ischemic dysfunctions. In this inflammatory state, vascular endothelial and smooth muscle cells produce large amounts of IL-6, which stimulates the acute phase response increasing fibrinogen production favoring clot formation.

COVID-19 remains a complex disease process of the endothelium, and future therapies may focus on antiinflammatory therapies and promoting endothelial homeostasis. Obesity is one of the major risk factors for the cytokine storm as it induces a constant state of low-grade inflammation characterized by acute-phase reactants, reactive oxygen species, and proinflammatory cytokines. Moderate exercise over time, however, enhances the immune system mobilizing NK and CD8+ T cells, and overall improves immunosurveillance and lowers inflammation.

Prevention

Conventional prevention includes the well-known Centers for Disease Control and Prevention (CDC) guidelines regarding masking, social distancing, handwashing/avoidance of touching the face, various isolation, quarantine measures, and vaccination. Large droplets are the primary mode of spreading which can be greatly mitigated with widespread mask wearing in addition to adequate ventilation.

Monoclonal antibodies may also be used in acute infection because they bind to the spike proteins of the coronavirus and can reduce the viral load, theoretically reducing the severity of the illness. Currently, two monoclonal antibodies are available: bamlanivimab[5] by Eli Lilly and casirivimab with imdevimab (REGEN-COV)[5] by Regeneron. These measures may be used for COVID-19 positive individuals who are not sick enough to be admitted to the hospital but are at risk for progression to hospitalization because of medical comorbidities such as diabetes, immunosuppression, or obesity.

Rates of anxiety and depression have gone up during the pandemic, which subsequently attenuate our immune system. Managing these appropriately and promptly will be helpful to improve not only immunity but also quality of life. Spending time outside and physical activity can also help strengthen our immune system and mitigate the cabin fever of COVID-19. Breathing techniques such as resonant breathing or 4-7-8 breathing can also help increase parasympathetic tone, increase heart rate variability, and decrease stress. At least 7 hours of sleep prior to vaccination provides for a more robust antibody response from the immune system.

The recent mRNA vaccines offer hope for prevention of infection and transmission with current projections of being 94.5% effective in reducing severe disease. Additionally, as new variants occur, these newly developed vaccines continue to protect up to 100% against severe COVID 19 infection. However, it is recommended to continue wearing masking and engage in social distancing even after vaccination. Some recent reports have indicated that patients suffering with post-COVID symptoms found that getting the COVID vaccine relieved those symptoms. The exact mechanism of this is unknown and bears further study but may have to do with clearing residual virus or reducing autoimmune and inflammatory processes.

Other less proven but widely used methods include use of various supplements such as vitamin C,[1] vitamin D,[1] quercetin,[7] zinc,[1] probiotics,[7] and antiinflammatory compounds like fish oil[1] and other supplements. None of these are proven in prospective trials but are widely used, and there is some historical evidence for their utility and mechanisms of action in other coronavirus-like infections such as the common cold. An open discussion with patients regarding the limited evidence for them may be helpful while respecting patient autonomy and desire for agency in selecting self-care strategies in the presence of fear and uncertainty.

Vitamin C remains a potent antioxidant and anecdotally beneficial in several studies, though there is insufficient evidence to recommend supplementation. For prevention, one may focus on increasing consumption of foods high in vitamin C such as citrus.

Vitamin D is an important regulator of human immune function and may stimulate the innate immune response to provide front-line protection against infectious agents. On the whole, people are spending less time outside in the sunlight, which hampers the production of the active form of vitamin D. Recently it was noted the higher vitamin D levels correlated with a decreased number of COVID cases and mortality. This could be caused by low vitamin D being a marker of a sedentary lifestyle and thus is likely an overall health risk. Whether one is COVID+, taking vitamin D may be beneficial with a dose around 4000 IU daily. There

---

[5]Investigational drug in the United States.
[1]Not FDA approved for this indication.
[7]Available as dietary supplement

is also evidence vitamin K_2[1] may be helpful in the absorption of vitamin D but should be avoided for those on blood thinners.

Quercetin is a naturally occurring dietary flavonoid with antiviral properties and may disrupt the infectious mechanism of the coronavirus. It is an antioxidant found in many plant foods including capers, red onions, apples, leafy greens, dill, cilantro, fennel, berries, sweet potato, tomatoes, broccoli, and tea. Quercetin can also be purchased as a supplement and is often combined with vitamin C to increase absorption and taken up to 500 mg twice a day.

Zinc impairs replication in RNA viruses and may enhance cytotoxicity when used with a zinc ionophore such as quercetin. Long-term zinc supplementation may result in copper deficiency, and thus replacing copper is recommended.

N-acetylcysteine (NAC),[1] a glutathione precursor, at 600 mg orally twice may help improve oxidative stress and inflammatory response in patients with upper respiratory tract infections. NAC assists the liver in reducing glutathione, which in turn helps the liver in removing toxins. A case report has noted that glutathione supplementation has improved dyspnea in COVID-19 patients. These may represent a novel treatment approach in blocking NF kappa-b and attenuating the cytokine storm seen in COVID-19.

Clinical Manifestations

According to the CDC, the most reported long-term symptoms include (Box 1) the following:
- Fatigue
- Shortness of breath
- Cough
- Joint pain
- Chest pain
  Other reported long-term symptoms include the following:
- Difficulty with thinking and concentration (sometimes referred to as "brain fog")
- Depression
- Muscle pain
- Headache
- Intermittent fever
- Fast-beating or pounding heart (also known as heart palpitations)
  More serious long-term complications appear to be less common but have been reported. These have been noted to affect different organ systems in the body. These include the following:
- Cardiovascular: inflammation of the heart muscle
- Respiratory: lung function abnormalities
- Renal: acute kidney injury
- Dermatologic: rash, hair loss
- Neurologic: smell and taste problems, sleep issues, difficulty with concentration, memory problems
- Psychiatric: depression, anxiety, changes in mood

Diagnosis

In our experience, the predominant symptoms leading patients to seek help are focused on new onset shortness of breath, cough, palpitations, fatigue, and brain fog. Other common symptoms include GI disturbances, headaches, hair loss, new onset nondescript pain, depression, anxiety, and posttraumatic stress.

The postacute COVID syndrome is defined as extending 3 weeks to 3 months after the acute disease occurs and after the long-haul COVID syndrome with symptoms persisting beyond 3 months after the infection has resolved.

Results of testing are not part of the current definition as many patients were not tested and are or were asymptomatic carriers. Even antibody testing is not entirely reliable as we are unsure of the durability of IgG results postinfection.

Those with risks for long-haul COVID include any of the following, which make it two to three times more likely: persistent cough, hoarseness, headache, diarrhea, loss of appetite, and shortness of breath in the first week.

[1]Not FDA approved for this indication.

646

BOX 1

The most commonly reported long-term symptoms include the following:
- Fatigue
- Shortness of breath
- Cough
- Joint pain
- Chest pain
  Other reported long-term symptoms include the following:
- Difficulty with thinking and concentration (sometimes referred to as "brain fog")
- Depression
- Muscle pain
- Headache
- Intermittent fever
- Fast-beating or pounding heart (also known as heart palpitations)
  More serious long-term complications appear to be less common but have been reported. These have been noted to affect different organ systems in the body. These include the following:
- Cardiovascular: inflammation of the heart muscle
- Respiratory: lung function abnormalities
- Renal: acute kidney injury
- Dermatologic: rash, hair loss
- Neurologic: smell and taste problems, sleep issues, difficulty with concentration, memory problems
- Psychiatric: depression, anxiety, changes in mood

Centers for Disease Control and Prevention. Long-Term Effects of COVID-19. Available at https://www.cdc.gov/coronavirus/2019-ncov/long-term-effects.html. [accessed 3/22/21].

Persons with more than five symptoms in the first week of their illness were four times more likely to develop long-haul COVID than those with fewer symptoms. The five most predictive symptoms of long-haul COVID in the first week of illness were fatigue, headache, shortness of breath, hoarse voice, and myalgia. Long-haul COVID was also more likely to occur in women, older people, and those with obesity.

Indeed, PCS may be four syndromes or more rather than one distinct postviral entity but may include postintensive care syndrome, postviral fatigue syndrome, and long-haul COVID syndrome. Symptoms may fluctuate and present nonlinearly and nonsequentially unpredictable ways.

Such conditions have been seen in other postinfectious conditions largely because the persistence of the immune response, ongoing inflammation, and effects on blood coagulation. After the Spanish Flu of 1918, which killed an estimated 20 to 50 million people, late-occurring neurologic sequela included long-lasting brain damage in up to a million people. SARS, MERS, myalgic encephalomyelitis, and chronic fatigue syndrome are other syndromes that share overlapping symptoms to PCS.

Evidence for optimal management of long-haul COVID may be lacking at this time, but as an evolving clinical problem, it has important public health considerations as the pandemic continues and even after it abates.

Therapy

Once PCS or long-haul COVID is suspected or diagnosed, determining the patient's baseline status helps organize and systematize clinical interventions. Addressing evolving exacerbations and life-threatening manifestations must take priority. Avoidance of unproven, high-cost, invasive experimental therapies outside of clinical trials should be avoided.

An excellent summary diagram for a primary care approach to PCS is shown in General Principles of Management and is derived from a monograph by the National Center for Health and Care Excellence (NICE) (Box 2).

For clinicians, a standardized approach to patients in the initial setting is important. Functional and behavioral assessments are of great importance because the rehabilitation of patients requires management of both. Multidisciplinary teams to direct care and address newly developing symptoms should be used.

To begin evaluation of the PCS patient, initial screening with standardized questionnaires using shortness of breath scales such as the UCSD SOB scale, and activity scale assessing ADLs and iADLS should be done. Nutritional evaluation (e.g., SGA), GAD-7, PHQ9, and IES-6 are examples of behavioral assessments to evaluate anxiety, depression, and posttraumatic stress. Along with an evaluation of ongoing symptoms evaluation, these scales should be used with each visit to allow for individualized evaluations of improvement. To see an example of a comprehensive, holistic intake form from our institution as a sample and link to these tools, see Box 3.

Using a multidisciplinary rehabilitation team including physicians, rehabilitation therapists, psychologists, nutritionists, and social workers to review these screenings allows developing personalized, patient-directed care.

Shared decision making with patients is key, given the vast number of symptoms patients may be experiencing. Discussing which are most troubling and limiting to the patient is of importance in goal setting. From this baseline, establish plans to address the most severe symptoms initially and those which can be readdressed in the future.

Just as the presentation of acute COVID-19 presents with a vast range of symptoms, patients recovering from COVID show heterogeneity as well. Some have few or no residual symptoms after the acute infection, while others show sustained symptoms at higher or lesser clinical penetrance.

Pulmonary

For many, respiratory symptoms may be the predominating symptom; therefore, proper pulmonary examination is important. Pulmonary function testing, a 6-minute walk test, and chest x-ray are good starting points. Using pulmonary rehabilitation will help guide patients through this new sensation of SOB and reduce symptom burden. This aspect of rehabilitation should not be limited to patients with only abnormal pulmonary function testing. Home monitoring with pulse oximetry is recommended.

Several breathing techniques have been offered to help patients deal with breathlessness, improving diaphragmatic breathing and helping normalize lung functioning (Box 4).

The question of whether to use inhaled bronchodilators remains. A potential practice is trial with short-acting agent to be used when symptomatic. If patient notes temporary benefit and the need to use frequently, a trial of long beta agonist plus inhaled cortical steroid can be considered. COVID-19 is known to induce an inflammatory response, and this may abate symptoms. Ensure a plan to step down therapy as one would do with asthma.

As pulmonary symptoms such as cough and shortness of breath have predominated presenting concerns in PCS patients, a program at Yale called RECOVERY has been developed, which could be a model for approaching pulmonary and other systems (Figure 1).

Cardiac

Another key organ affected by COVID infection is the heart. Cardiotoxicity from the infection can cause inflammation of the heart (myocarditis), rhythm disturbances, and damage to the heart muscle (cardiomyopathy). Sudden cardiac death, heart attacks, and heart failure have all been observed, including Takotsubo heart syndrome.

Cardiac symptoms such as palpitations or increased resting heart rate can be further evaluated with long-term cardiac monitoring, such as Holter monitor. If it is unclear whether symptoms

BOX 2 | Management of Post-COVID Syndrome

These recommendations are for healthcare professionals providing care for people with ongoing symptomatic COVID-19 or post–COVID-19 syndrome in primary care and community settings or in multidisciplinary assessment and rehabilitation services.

Self-Management and Supported Self-Management
- Give advice and information on self-management to people with ongoing symptomatic COVID-19 or post–COVID-19 syndrome, starting from their initial assessment. This should include the following:
  - Ways to self-manage their symptoms, such as setting realistic goals
  - Who to contact if they are worried about their symptoms or they need support with self-management
  - Sources of advice and support, including support groups, social prescribing, online forums and apps
  - How to get support from other services, including social care, housing, and employment, and advice about financial support
  - Information about new or continuing symptoms of COVID-19 that people can share with their family, careers, and friends (see the section on common symptoms of ongoing symptomatic COVID-19 and post-COVID syndrome).
- Explain to people that it is not known whether over-the-counter vitamins and supplements are helpful, harmful, or have no effect in the treatment of new or ongoing symptoms of COVID-19.
- Support people in discussions with their employer, school, or college about returning to work or education, for example, by having a phased return. For advice on returning to work, follow national guidance, for example, NICE's guideline on workplace health: long-term sickness absence and capability to work.

Multidisciplinary Rehabilitation
- Assess people who have been referred to integrated multidisciplinary rehabilitation services to guide management. Include physical, psychological, and psychiatric aspects of rehabilitation. Ensure that any symptoms that could affect the person being able to start rehabilitation safely have been investigated first. See also the recommendation on multidisciplinary rehabilitation teams.
- Work with the person to develop a personalized rehabilitation and management plan that is recorded in a rehabilitation prescription and should include the following:
  - Areas of rehabilitation and interventions based on their assessment
  - Helping the person to decide and work toward goals
  - Symptom management for all presenting symptoms, for example, advice and education on managing breathlessness, fatigue, and brain fog
- Encourage people to keep a record of, or use a tracking app to monitor, their goals, recovery, and any changes in their symptoms (also see the section on follow-up and monitoring).

Support for Older People and Children
- Consider additional support for older people with ongoing symptomatic COVID-19 or post–COVID-19 syndrome, for example, short-term care packages, advance care planning, and support with social isolation, loneliness, and bereavement, if relevant.
- Consider referral from 4 weeks for specialist advice for children with ongoing symptomatic COVID-19 or post–COVID-19 syndrome.

COVID-19 rapid guideline: managing the long-term effects of COVID-19 (NG188) © NICE 2020. All rights reserved. Subject to Notice of rights (https://www.nice.org.uk/terms-andconditions# notice-of-rights). Pages 18, 19.

BOX 3 Online Resources for Management of Post-COVID Syndrome

UTMB Health Post COVD Recovery Clinic intake questionnaire
https://www.utmbhealth.com/postcovid-19-clinic
UCSD SOBQ
https://doi.org/10.1378/chest.113.3.619
ADL's/IADL's
https://aging.ufl.edu/files/2012/05/ADLTable.pdf
https://www.alz.org/careplanning/downloads/lawton-iadl.pdf
SGA
https://nutritioncareincanada.ca/sites/default/uploads/files/SGA%20Tool%20EN%20BKWT_2017.pdf
GAD 7
https://adaa.org/sites/default/files/GAD-7_Anxiety-updated_0.pdf
PHQ 9
https://www.apa.org/depression-guideline/patient-health-questionnaire.pdf
IES-R
https://emdrfoundation.org/toolkit/ies-scoring.pdf

BOX 4 Breathing Techniques for Post-COVID Syndrome

About 80% of the work of breathing is done by the diaphragm. After illness or general deconditioning, the breathing pattern may be altered, with reduced diaphragmatic movement and greater use of neck and shoulder accessory muscles. This results in shallow breathing, increasing fatigue, breathlessness, and higher energy expenditure. The breathing-control technique is aimed at normalizing breathing patterns and increasing the efficiency of the respiratory muscles (including the diaphragm), resulting in less energy expenditure, less airway irritation, reduced fatigue, and improvement in breathlessness. The patient should sit in a supported position and breathe in and out slowly, preferably in through the nose and out through the mouth, while relaxing the chest and shoulders and allowing the tummy to rise. They should aim for an inspiration to expiration ratio of 1:2. This technique can be used frequently throughout the day, in 5- to 10-minute bursts (or longer, if helpful).

Other breathing techniques—such as diaphragmatic breathing, slow deep-breathing, pursed lip breathing, yoga techniques, Buteyko—are used in strategies to manage patients' breathing patterns and breathlessness but require specialist advice to identify which technique best suits each patient.

Greenhalgh T, Knight M, A'Court C, Buxton M, Husain L. Management of post-acute covid-19 in primary care. BMJ. 2020;370:m3026.

are cardiac versus pulmonary driven, a cardiopulmonary exercise test and or echocardiogram can assist in delineating between the two.

The appropriate type of testing and therapy for post-COVID cardiac syndrome will need to be determined. ECG and rhythm monitoring, echocardiography, and close clinical observation with directed questions about cardiac function will be required for months, perhaps years. Cardiac biopsy may be needed, as well as special imaging such as cardiac MRI.

Special consideration to cardiac rehabilitation must be given in PCS patients and modifying or suspending rehabilitation exercises is indicated in the following:

- Saturation <88% to 93%
- Heart rate <40 beats per minute or >120 beats per minute
- Systolic blood pressure <90 mm Hg or >180 mm Hg
- Body temperature fluctuations >37.2°C
- Respiratory symptoms and fatigue that worsen during exercise and are not alleviated after rest
- Symptoms such as chest tightness or pain, difficulty in breathing, severe cough, dizziness, headache, unclear vision, palpitations, sweating, and instability

Long-term physiotherapy and cardiology consultation may be needed.

Fatigue

Prevention of deconditioning while managing the risks of overexertion can be a balancing act in the PCS patient.

Exercise rehabilitation for athletes and others requires careful titration and personalization because excessive exercise can set back progress. This has also been seen in treatment of fibromyalgia and chronic fatigue syndrome where even slowly graded exercise increases can cause worsening. Likely what we have learned from other conditions such as myalgic encephalomyelitis, chronic fatigue, and fibromyalgia syndrome may be transferrable and helpful, including some safe approaches from complementary and integrative medicine, including mind-body therapies, yoga, tai chi, acupuncture, personalized nutritional and fitness prescriptions, and carefully selected supplements, minerals, and vitamins.

A general rule of thumb for the post-COVID rehabilitation is that, if a patient feels excessively fatigued the day following exercise, the program needs to be backed down to prevent overdoing. Controlled breathing exercises, careful pacing, goal setting, low-intensity exercise, and stress reduction are all critical.

Detailed guidelines (see Stanford Guidelines in references) have been offered on returning to sports activities that can help

physicians in addressing appropriate measures, timing, and rehabilitation of multiple systems: pulmonary, cardiac, neurologic, psychological, musculoskeletal, and overall exercise rehabilitation for returning to vigorous activities. The risk for postacute COVID deconditioning is significant and needs to be considered on returning athletes to activity.

Dysautonomia

Providers should be familiar with syndromes such as chronic fatigue, postural orthostatic tachycardia syndrome, and mast cell activation syndrome. These syndromes are commonly brought up within the post–COVID-19 community.

Dysautonomia may be particularly challenging because it presents with rapid heartbeat, anxiety, numbness, dizziness, low blood pressure, and extreme fatigue. Orthostatic intolerance may be caused by viral or autoimmune damage to the autonomic system, a postural orthostatic tachycardia (POTs)–like syndrome. This condition is best managed with established measures such as patient education, maintaining volume, adjusting positional changes gradually, structured exercise including isometrics, compression garments, and in some cases pharmacologic agents to retain sodium and fluid such as fludrocortisone (Florinef),[1] midodrine (Proamatine), and others affecting adrenergic surge such as beta blockers, methyldopa,[1] and clonidine(Catapres).[1]

Neurological

Patients with COVID may suffer severe central nervous system insults resulting in strokes, severe brain inflammation (encephalomyelitis, a multiple sclerosis-like or Guillain-Barre type of demyelination), weakness, numbness, confusion, delirium, memory loss, headache, and psychosis. A complaint of enduring brain fog is common. Some of these problems occur early, others late. They may be hard to detect in intensive care unit (ICU) patients who are very sick, hypoxemic, sedated; and for whom an MRI scan can be difficult to obtain.

Full neuropsychological testing and/or neurologic consultation should be considered in cases in which cognitive changes persist post-COVID.

---

[1]Not FDA approved for this indication.

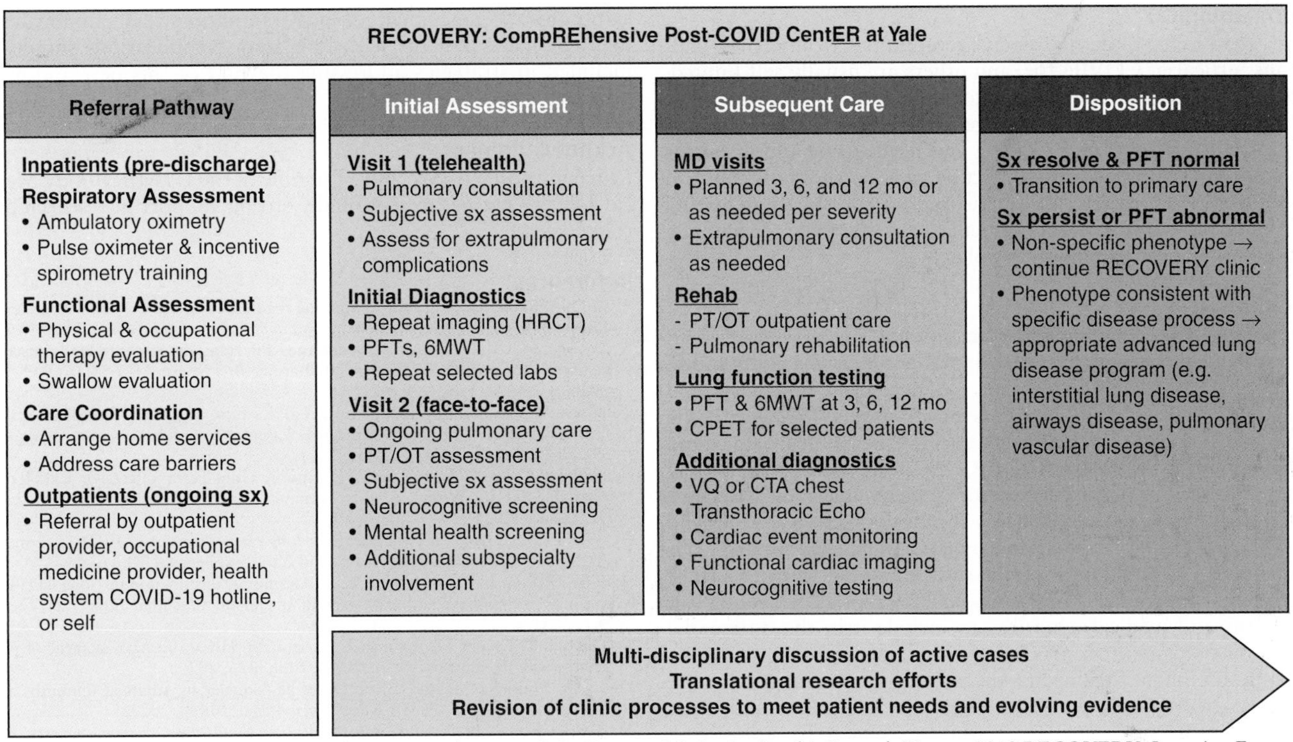

Figure 1 The RECOVERY Clinic Model. From Lutchmansingh D, Knauert M, Antin-Ozerkis D, et al. Disease 2019 RECOVERY: Learning From the Past, Looking to the Future. Chest 2021;159(3):953.

Anosmia is another neurologic symptom of COVID and can be quite debilitating, though patients often recover with time. It can lead to appetite and weight loss and depression. Therapy for persistent anosmia can include olfactory training, which includes repeated sniffing of a set of odorants to speed recovery.

Mental Health

Mental health support for many will be of importance as patients cope with the unknown. Sorting out somatic from psychosomatic problems will require clinical acumen, patience, perseverance, and continuity of care. Psychiatric consequences may be severe and related to the immune response and/or from psychological stressors such as social isolation, worries about a potentially fatal illness, concerns about infecting others, stigma of disease, impact on employment, finances, and relationships in general.

The immune response to coronaviruses induces local and systemic production of cytokines, chemokines, and other inflammatory mediators, all of which combine to worsen the burden of preexisting depression, anxiety, posttraumatic stress disorder (PTSD), and other mental health disorders, particularly in female patients.

Mental health issues may end up being one of the most serious, enduring, yet largely hidden impacts seen in the post-COVID patient, and thus management and monitoring must address this domain to maintain a holistic approach.

Therapeutic trials of holistic, integrative, and functional medicine are appropriate given low harm and potential benefit. These may include antiinflammatory diets, acupuncture, meditation, and selected supplements such as fish oil,[1] magnesium,[1] SAMe,[7] valerian,[7] B vitamins,[1] and others.

Hematological

Thrombotic sequelae and hypercoagulable states need monitoring and management and may require prolonged anticoagulation especially in those with significant deep vein thromboses or pulmonary or cardiac emboli. Many patients will need transient anticoagulation, though some may require ongoing therapy if clotting abnormalities persist.

Gastrointestinal

Diarrhea and other gastrointestinal complaints, if continuing, likely reflect viral impact on the microbiota. An antiinflammatory diet, Mediterranean-type diet, hypoallergenic elimination diet, or other personalized nutritional strategies should be considered. Optimizing nutritional support for vulnerable elderly and those with continued anosmia and dysgeusia is likewise vital. Though not yet well defined in terms of dosing and speciation, replacing microbiota with food-sourced or encapsulated prebiotics and probiotics is worth considering as a safe and potentially useful strategy in this population.

Renal

Acute kidney injury during the infectious stage may result in longer term decreases in glomerular filtration rate (GFR) and other renal parameters. This is likely to be worse in those already at risk with existing chronic kidney disease, diabetes, or hypertension. Nephrology consultation should be sought in appropriate cases.

Endocrine

Loss of control of diabetes and even diabetic ketoacidosis has been observed after resolution of acute COVID symptoms, sometimes weeks or months later. New cases of prediabetes and diabetes have been reported. COVID may also activate latent autoimmune thyroid disease, resulting in thyroiditis or thyrotoxicosis in the aftermath and resolution of respiratory disease. Risks for osteoporosis may also increase because of a multiplicity of factors such as immobilization, inflammation, steroid use, and other lifestyle or dietary factors. Weight gain and inactivity during lockdowns have contributed to these conditions as well.

Being alert to the potential for the occurrence or exacerbation of endocrinological issues will enhance our ability to respond quickly and appropriately in our management.

---

[1]Not FDA approved for this indication.
[7]Available as dietary supplement

Dermatological

The broad range of dermatologic presentations from rashes, chilblains, urticaria, COVID-toe, and others are usually self-limited, not prolonged, and treated with topical steroids, antihistamines, or oral steroids. Hair loss (telogen effluvium) is a particularly distressing problem from COVID and needs to be addressed for its emotional and cosmetic impact. It may be short-lived but, if prolonged, must be part of a holistic program of care including dermatologic consultation, particularly if there is an ongoing autoimmune or inflammatory etiology.

Monitoring

Supportive and rehabilitative care is what we have now. This includes adequate rest, nutrition, immune support, activity modification, mental stimulation, stress management, and heart and lung rehabilitation including supplemental oxygen for some. Using standard and evidence treatments for lung, heart, neurologic, and renal problems is a logical start. Given protracted and relapsing symptoms, it is important to reassure patients that most cases will recover with time and supportive, symptomatic care. Registries and post-COVID clinics are needed to track and manage these serious sequelae of COVID. Our awareness is the first line of defense. The diffuse and protean manifestations of PCS should be driving our clinicians and medical educators to include it in the differential diagnosis of many other presenting complaints.

Multidisciplinary teams are key to long-term management but are not always easily accessible. Self-care and online and other forms of support groups have sprung up widely for emotional, social support, and peer-led practical advice in managing PCS. Much of the awareness of PCS has been brought to public and professional awareness by such peer groups. Further research and support in this area will be helpful.

Quality of care principles for a long COVID include access to care, reducing burden of illness, taking clinical responsibility, continuity of care, multidisciplinary rehabilitation, evidence-based investigation and management, and further research and development of appropriate and evidence-based clinical services. Given the disproportionate impact of COVID on communities of color, additional attention must be given to social determinants of health, healthcare access, and enhanced research efforts regarding the genetic and racial differences in disease impact, both acute and long term.

Complications

We remain in the early phases of understanding of COVID-19 and its potential long-term complications. This provides many areas for clinicians and researchers to examine. As with COVID-19 infection itself, long-term complications may broadly affect multiple body systems. Addressing these symptoms starts with recognition.

One persistent neurologic complication that remains of concern is cognitive decline, which many describe as brain fog. Additional symptoms of neuropathic pain and headaches may require further evaluation by a neurologist.

Myocardial inflammation seen in some COVID-19 infections may lead to future reduced cardiac function, arrhythmias, scarring, or cardiomyopathy. The prevalence currently remains unknown but is a major concern in our younger population and athletes.

Pulmonary complications are common in hospitalized patients requiring ventilatory assistance. Our experience in post-COVID population shows that fibrotic conversion, if it occurs, is rare, but reduction in diffusion capacity may persist. This reduction is a sign of parenchymal disease and should be monitored if patients develop future reductions in lung volumes in comparison to standard population.

Hematologic complications such as thrombosis and long-term risk remain unknown and further study remains necessary. Can a patient with COVID-19 and a thrombosis be safely managed as a short-term event as a provoked clot or is there a prolonged inflammatory cascade that leaves a prolonged risk?

The behavioral health component remains of utmost importance as with so much unknown and unclear duration of symptoms. Management of posttraumatic stress, anxiety, and depression for patients with long-term complications should be included in strategies addressing the care of this new and ever-growing at-risk population.

Acknowledgment

Much gratitude to Ms. Julie Trumble of the UTMB Moody Medical Library for her exceptionally strong support in research and referencing.

References

Alwan NA: Surveillance is underestimating the burden of the COVID-19 pandemic, *Lancet* 396(10252):e24, 2020.

Barker-Davies RM, O'Sullivan O, Senaratne KPP, et al: The Stanford Hall consensus statement for post-COVID-19 rehabilitation, *Br J Sports Med* 54(16):949–959, 2020.

Calabrese M, Garofano M, Palumbo R, et al: Exercise training and cardiac rehabilitation in COVID-19 patients with cardiovascular complications: state of art, *Life (Basel)* 11(3):259, 2021.

Centers for Disease Control and Prevention. Long-Term Effects of COVID-19. Available at https://www.cdc.gov/coronavirus/2019-ncov/long-term-effects.html. [accessed 3/22/21].

COVID-19 rapid guideline: managing the long-term effects of COVID-19, London, 2020, National Institute for Health and Care Excellence (UK).

Dani M, Dirksen A, Taraborrelli P, et al: Autonomic dysfunction in "long COVID": rationale, physiology and management strategies, *Clin Med (Lond)* 21(1):e63–e67, 2021. d.

Greenhalgh T, Knight M, A'Court C, Buxton M, Husain L: Management of post-acute covid-19 in primary care, *BMJ* 370:m3026, 2020.

Logue JK, Franko NM, McCulloch DJ, et al: Sequelae in Adults at 6 months after COVID-19 infection, *JAMA Netw Open* 4(2):e210830, 2021.

Mahase E: Long covid could be four different syndromes, review suggests, *BMJ* 371:m3981, 2020.

Mendelson M, Nel J, Blumberg L, et al: Long-COVID: an evolving problem with an extensive impact, *S Afr Med J* 111(1):10–12, 2020.

Nabavi N: Long covid: How to define it and how to manage it, *BMJ* 370:m3489, 2020.

Nalbandian A, Sehgal K, Gupta A, et al. Post-acute COVID-19 syndrome. *Nat Med.* Available at https://doi.org/10.1038/s41591-021-1283-z.

NIHR Themed Review: *Living with Covid19*, 2020, pp 1–29.

PSITTACOSIS

Method of
Christopher C. McGuigan, MB, ChB, MPH

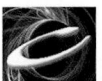

CURRENT DIAGNOSIS

- The key to successful management of psittacosis is to consider this diagnosis, particularly in cases of community-acquired pneumonia (CAP), especially given a history of bird contact.
- The typical clinical pictures are of CAP, influenza-like illness, or fever of unknown origin. Psittacosis causes 1% of incident CAP cases. Onset is usually sudden with fever, chills and a prominent headache. Consider this diagnosis in a patient with CAP unresponsive to β-lactam antibiotics.
- Investigation will typically reveal a normal or slightly elevated white blood cell count with a left shift or toxic changes, increase in C-reactive protein (CRP) or erythrocyte sedimentation rate (ESR), mildly abnormal liver function tests, hyponatremia, and mild renal impairment. Chest x-ray may be more abnormal than examination alone would predict.
- Diagnosis can be confirmed with (ideally) paired serum samples: using either the complement fixation test (widely used but unable to differentiate between *Chamydophila* species), or the microimmunofluorescence test, which is specific for individual *Chamydophila* species. Either a single high titer or a fourfold rise in titer using samples collected at least 14 days apart are interpreted as positive. More recently, real-time polymerase chain reaction (rt-PCR) tests are used to detect specific DNA. These can provide a more rapid diagnosis, as well as subspecific genotype.

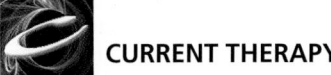

CURRENT THERAPY

- Therapy should commence when the diagnosis is suspected on clinical presentation and initial investigation.
- Tetracyclines are the drugs of choice; for example, doxycycline (Vibramycin) 100 mg bid for 10 to 14 days.
- Macrolides are suitable (but probably less effective) alternatives in those intolerant of tetracyclines (e.g., children and pregnant women).
- Notification to health authorities facilitates public health investigation and interventions to reduce transmission and control outbreaks.

Psittacosis is caused by infection with the bacterium *Chlamydophila psittaci* (formerly *Chlamydia psittaci*). It is twice as common in men than in women, and mainly affects adults typically aged 40 to 50 years. The main reservoir for psittacosis is birds, particularly psittacine birds (parrots, parakeets, budgerigars and cockatoos), but other bird species and mammals can be infected.

Risk Factors

The most common etiological factor is exposure to infected birds—especially a new, sick, or dead one—typically a pet or via occupational exposure (e.g., work as a veterinarian, zoo keeper, or poultry-worker). Most cases are sporadic, but outbreaks have occurred associated with pet shops, aviaries, and poultry-processing plants and with mowing lawns in areas with large numbers of psittacine birds. Person-to-person transmission is rare. Ingestion of poultry products is *not* a risk factor.

Pathophysiology

C psittaci infection is via the respiratory tract and is typically thought to be by inhalation of an aerosol of dried feces or other avian secretion. It then either travels via the blood to the liver and spleen (where it replicates, causing a secondary bacteremia) or directly infects respiratory epithelial cells.

Prevention

Prevention is aimed at controlling disease or colonization in susceptible host species: usually birds. This is facilitated by import restrictions including quarantine and treatment of suspected infections with tetracycline-impregnated feeds. Notification of health authorities is important for initiating public health investigations and interventions to reduce transmission and control of outbreaks.

Clinical Manifestations

The incubation period varies from 4 to 14 or more days. The typical presentation of psittacosis is of an influenza-like illness with sudden onset of fever, chills, and prominent headache, with or without rigors. A more gradual onset is also seen. A typically mild, dry cough usually starts later. There may also be diarrhea, pharyngitis, altered mental state, or shortness of breath. Chest examination is usually abnormal, but the findings are often minimal and less prominent than symptoms or x-ray findings would suggest. Pleural effusion is rare.

Patients might present with a fever of unknown origin without obvious respiratory involvement, or the disease can be misdiagnosed as meningitis because of prominent headache, sometimes with photophobia.

The white blood cell count is usually normal or slightly raised, but there is often a left shift or toxic changes. Increases in the C-reactive protein (CRP) and erythrocyte sedimentation rate (ESR) are common. Mildly abnormal liver function tests, hyponatraemia, and mild renal impairment are also common. The cerebrospinal fluid sometimes contains a few mononuclear cells but is otherwise normal. The chest x-ray usually shows more

(nonspecific) abnormality than examination findings might predict. The most common finding is lobar consolidation, but bilateral consolidation and interstitial opacities are also common.

Confirmation of diagnosis is more commonly performed using serology. The complement fixation (CF) test is widely used, but cannot differentiate between *Chlamydophila* species. A fourfold rise in titer, using samples collected at least 14 days apart, or a single titer of 1:128 or higher, is interpreted as positive, but this test is not widely available. Culture of *C psittaci* is difficult and hazardous. Polymerase chain reaction (PCR) assays have been developed, but are not yet widely available for routine clinical use.

Diagnosis

Diagnosis is facilitated by eliciting a history of recent bird contact from a patient with a compatible clinical syndrome, most commonly an influenza-like presentation, community acquired pneumonia (CAP), or a fever of unknown origin. The diagnosis should be considered in a patient with CAP and prominent headache, splenomegaly, or failure to respond to β-lactam antibiotics.

Differential Diagnosis

Differential diagnosis of an atypical CAP, includes infection with *Legionella* species, *Mycoplasma pneumoniae*, or *Chlamydophila pneumoniae*.

Treatment

When the diagnosis is suspected on clinical presentation and initial investigations, empiric therapy should be commenced. Tetracyclines are the drugs of choice, for example doxycycline (Vibramycin) 100 mg bid for 10 to 14 days. Tetracycline treatment usually leads to improvement in symptoms (including fever) within 24 to 48 hours. Macrolides are usually recommended for pregnant women, children, and other patients intolerant of tetracyclines. However, erythromycin (Erythrocin)[1] has been shown to fail in situations where a tetracycline was effective, and there are few clinical data on the efficacy of the other agents in this class. Some data suggest that quinolones may be effective. Tetracycline hydrochloride or doxycycline (4.4 mg/kg/d divided into two infusions) may be given intravenously for critically ill patients.

Monitoring

Symptomatic improvement usually occurs within 24 to 48 hours of starting a tetracycline; typically including reduction of fever.

Complications

The degree of illness varies from asymptomatic to life threatening. Given appropriate antimicrobial therapy, subsequent case-fatality is less than 1%. Elderly persons and pregnant women are susceptible to more severe illness. Neurologic consequences (e.g., meningo-encephalitis) are recognized but rare. Other less-common sequelae include hemoptysis, proteinuria, hepatosplenomegaly, and encephalitis. Cardiac manifestations include relative bradycardia and, rarely, myocarditis, culture-negative endocarditis, and pericarditis. Erythema nodosum and other skin manifestations have also been described. *C psittaci* has been demonstrated by PCR to be present in ocular adnexal lymphoma (OAL) in parts of Eurasia. Up to one half of such cases respond to antibiotic treatment. However, studies elsewhere suggest that this organism might not commonly play a role in OAL. Recovery with minimal residual deficit is normal.

References

Contini C, Seraceni S, Carradori S, et al: Identification of *Chlamydia trachomatis* in a patient with ocular lymphoma, *Am J Hematol* 84:597–599, 2009.

Grayston JT, Thom DH: The chlamydial pneumonias, *Curr Clin Top Infect Dis* 11:1–18, 1991.

Heddema ER, Beld MG, De Wever B, et al: Development of an internally controlled real-time PCR assay for detection of *Chlamydophila psittaci* in the LightCycler 2.0 system, *Clin Microbiol Infect* 12:571–575, 2006.

[1]Not FDA approved for this indication.

Hogerwerf L, DE Gier B, Baan B, Van Der Hoek W: Chlamydia psittaci (psittacosis) as a cause of community-acquired pneumonia: a systematic review and meta-analysis. [Review], *Epidemiol Infect* 145(15):3096–3105, 2017.

Hughes P, Chidley K, Cowie J: Neurological complications in psittacosis: a case report and literature review, *Respir Med* 89:637–638, 1995.

National Association of State Public Health Veterinarians. Compendium of measures to control *Chlamydophila psittaci* infection among humans (psittacosis) and pet birds (avian chlamydiosis), 2010. Available at: http://www.nasphv.org/Documents/Psittacosis.pdf [accessed July 9, 2015].

Richards M. Psittacosis, Up to date 2006; Available at http://www.uptodate.com/physicians/pulmonology_toclist.asp [accessed 31.12.12; subscription required].

Wallensten A, Fredlund H, Runehagen A: Multiple human–to–human transmission from a severe case of psittacosis, Sweden, January–February 2013, *Euro Surveill* 19(42):20937, 2014.

Williams J, Tallis G, Dalton C, et al: Community outbreak of psittacosis in a rural Australian town, *Lancet* 351:1697–1699, 1998.

Yung AP, Grayson ML: Psittacosis: a review of 135 cases, *Med J Aust* 148:228–233, 1988.

Q FEVER

Method of
Didier Raoult, MD, PhD

Q fever is a widespread zoonosis caused by *Coxiella burnetii*, a small, coccoid, strict intracellular gram-negative bacterium. It lives within the phagolysosome of its eukaryotic host cell at very low pH (4.5–4.8). It had previously been classified in the rickettsial family; however, recent phylogenic data based on study of the 16S rRNA gene sequence have shown that it belongs to *Legionellales* with the *Legionella* species and *Francisella tularensis*.

The bacterium has a sporelike life cycle, which explains its marked resistance to physicochemical agents. In cultures, *C. burnetii* exhibits a phase variation (from virulent phase I to avirulent phase II) caused by a spontaneous chromosome deletion. The avirulent form paradoxically generates high antibody levels in patients, but only patients with chronic infection have high antiphase I immunoglobulin G (IgG) and IgA antibody titers.

The reservoir of *C. burnetii* is wide, and nearly all tested mammals, birds, and ticks can be infected. Outbreaks have also been reported in association with the birth products of mammals (including ungulates and pets), raw milk, slaughterhouses, and farm work. Laboratory outbreaks have been reported. The disease is prevalent everywhere in the world but in New Zealand and South Pacific Islands, but because its clinical spectrum is wide and nonspecific, the observed incidence is directly related to physician interest in Q fever. A recent outbreak has been observed in the Netherlands.

Clinical Features

Q fever is a reportable disease in the United States. In humans, infection is symptomatic in only 50% of patients. Most symptomatic patients experience a flulike syndrome lasting 2 to 7 days and consisting of severe headaches and cough; 5% to 10% of infected patients may be sick enough to be investigated. They initially have high fever and one or several of pneumonia, hepatitis, meningoencephalitis, rash, myocarditis, and pericarditis. Routine laboratory investigation commonly shows mildly elevated transaminase levels and mild thrombocytopenia. The local strain may influence the clinical manifestations. In French Guyana, the disease is more commonly symptomatic and severe.

In special hosts such as immunocompromised patients (specifically those with splenectomy), *C. burnetii* can cause endocarditis. In pregnant women it can lead to recurrent miscarriage, low-birth-weight offspring, and prematurity. *C. burnetii* could contribute to the evolution of lymphoma.

In patients with valvular heart disease and those with arterial aneurysms or a vascular prosthesis, it can cause chronic endocarditis or vascular infection in patients in the 2 years following primary infection. The clinical picture is that of a chronic blood culture–negative endocarditis; the modified Duke criteria are of diagnostic value in such cases. It is spontaneously fatal in most cases. Recently, acute endocarditis associated with anticardiolipin antibodies was described. Criteria specifically adapted to Q fever may be used to diagnosed focalized infections. This denomination appears to be more appropriate than "chronic Q fever."

Diagnosis

Because Q fever is pleomorphic, the diagnosis is based mainly on comprehensive serum testing in patients with an unexplained infectious syndrome. Liver biopsy may be of diagnostic value, because the typical doughnut granuloma is quasispecific to acute Q fever. Valves obtained at surgery or autopsy can be used for culture, direct immunostaining, and polymerase chain reaction (PCR).

Three serologic techniques are used. Complement fixation lacks sensitivity, and one-third of patients with acute Q fever do not exhibit complement-fixing antibodies within 1 month after onset of the disease. However, a fourfold increase in antibodies to phase II antigen indicates acute Q fever, and antibody levels against phase I that are higher than 1:200 indicate persistent focalized Q fever. Indirect immunofluorescence assay is the reference method. A single titer of 1:200 for IgG antiphase II associated with a titer of 1:50 for IgM is diagnostic of acute infection. IgG antibody levels against phase I that are greater than 1:800 and IgA antibody levels greater than 1:50 are highly predictive of endocarditis or vascular infection. Enzyme-linked immunosorbent assay (ELISA) is useful for diagnosing acute infection in detecting IgM antiphase II.

PCR has recently been developed to detect *C. burnetii* DNA in the sera of patients with Q fever. Real-time PCR using multicopy gene *IS1111* is the more-sensitive technique. It is positive in the sera of patients with acute Q fever before IgG antibodies to *C. burnetii* become apparent. It is also positive in patients with untreated endocarditis. Contamination of PCR can occur, and many unconfirmed results are reported in the literature. Detection of patients at risk for endocarditis may be provided by systematic echocardiography in patients with acute Q fever specifically seeking for aortic bicuspidy and serologic follow-up at 3 and 6 months after acute infection. Antiphospholipid antibodies are relatively common during acute Q fever and predictive of endocarditis and deep vein thrombosis.

Use of a positron emission tomography (PET) scanner may help in the diagnosis of endocarditis (and may reveal mycotic aneurysms), vascular infection, and joint infection.

Treatment

To be active against Q fever, an antibiotic compound has to enter the cell, be effective at an acidic pH (where *C. burnetii* multiplies), and have activity against *C. burnetii*. No antibiotic is bactericidal, but bactericidal activity can be achieved by the addition of hydroxychloroquine (Plaquenil)[1] to doxycycline (Vibramycin).

For acute Q fever, the reference treatment is doxycycline 100 mg orally twice daily for 2 to 3 weeks. Other compounds have been reported to be effective, such as trimethoprim-sulfamethoxazole (TMP-SMX) (Bactrim)[1], Rifampin (Rifadin)[1] 300 mg twice daily, and ofloxacin (Floxin)[1] 200 mg twice daily. In the case of Q fever in pregnant women, one double-strength TMP-SMX tablet (trimethoprim 160 mg, sulfamethoxazole 800 mg)[1] twice daily until delivery prevents fetal death (Table 1). Patients with acute Q fever and high antiphospholipid antibodies may be treated with hydroxychloroquine[1] until normalization.

Persistent focalized and acute endocarditis should be treated for 18 months to 2 years, and antibody levels should be monitored. Patients with prosthetic valves may be treated for 2 years. Two protocols have been evaluated: doxycycline 200 mg daily combined with ofloxacin[1] 400 mg daily for 4 years to lifetime, and doxycycline combined with hydroxychloroquine[1] for 1.5 to 2 years in an amount to achieve a 1 ± 0.20 µg/mL plasma concentration. Doxycycline serum levels greater than 4.5 µg/mL are

---

[1] Not FDA approved for this indication.

TABLE 1 Treatment

Q FEVER	RECOMMENDED TREATMENT	ALTERNATIVE TREATMENT
Acute	Doxycycline (Vibramicyn) 100 mg PO q12h × 14 d	Ofloxacin (Floxin)[1] 200 mg PO q8h[3] × 14 d Cotrimoxazole (Bactrim)[1] 160/800 mg/PO q12h × 14 d
Acute Q fever with high antiphospholipid antibodies	Hydroxychloroquine (Plaquenil)[1] 200 mg PO q8h as long as high antiphospholipid antibodies persist	
Endocarditis	Doxycycline 100 mg PO q12h *plus* hydroxychloroquine (Plaquenil)[1] 200 mg PO q8h[3] × 18–24 mo	Doxycycline 100 mg PO q12h *plus* ofloxacin[1] 200 mg PO q8h[3] for 3 y to lifetime
Acute in a patient with a valvular lesion	Same as chronic Q fever for 12 mo	
In pregnancy	Trimethoprim/ Sulfamethoxazole (Bactrim)[1] 160/800 mg PO q12h until term	

[1]Not FDA approved for this indication.
[3]Exceeds dosage recommended by the manufacturer.

associated with a more rapidly favorable outcome. This last regimen is apparently more efficacious in terms of relapse. However, regular ophthalmologic surveillance is critical to detect the accumulation of chloroquine in the retina. Both regimens expose the patient to a major risk of photosensitization.

The combination of doxycycline and hydroxychloroquine for 1 year has demonstrated efficacy in preventing endocarditis. Patients with high-level antiphospholipid antibodies may be treated by the same treatment until normalization of the antibody level.

Prevention

Prevention depends on avoiding exposure, particularly by pregnant women and patients with valvulopathy. No vaccine is currently available outside Australia.

References

Eldin C, Melenotte C, Mediannikov O, et al: From Q fever to *Coxiella burnetii* infection: a paradigm shange, *Clin Microbiol Rev* 30:115–190, 2017.

Klee SR, et al: Highly sensitive real-time PCR for specific detection and quantification of Coxiella burnetii, *BMC Microbiol* 19:2, 2006.

Maurin M, Raoult D: Q fever, *Clin Microbiol Rev* 12:518–553, 1999.

Merhej V, Cammilleri S, Piquet P, et al: Relevance of the positron emission tomography in the diagnosis of vascular graft infection with *Coxiella burnetii*, *Comp Immunol Microbiol Infect Dis* 35(1):45–49, 2012.

Melenotte C, Epelboin L, Million M, et al: Acute Q fever endocarditis: a paradigm shift following the systematic use of transthoracic echocardiography during acute Q fever, *Clin Infect Dis* 13;69(11):1987-1995, 2019.

Million M, Bardin N, Bessis S, et al: Thrombosis and antiphospholipid antibody syndrome during acute Q fever: a cross-sectional study, *Medicine (Baltimore).* 96(29):e7578, 2017 Jul.

Million M, Roblot F, Carles D, et al: Reevaluation of the risk of fetal death and malformation after Q fever, *Clin Infect Dis* 59(2):256–260, 2014.

Million M, Thuny F, Richet H, Raoult D: Long-term outcome of Q fever endocarditis: a 26-year personal survey, *Lancet Infect Dis* 10:527–535, 2010.

Million M, Walter G, Thuny F, et al: Evolution from acute Q fever to endocarditis is associated with underlying valvulopathy and age and can be prevented by prolonged antibiotic treatment, *Clin Infect Dis* 57(6):836–844, 2013.

Raoult D: Chronic Q fever: expert opinion versus literature analysis and consensus, *J Infect* 65:102–108, 2012.

Rolain JM, Maurin M, Raoult D: Bacteriostatic and bactericidal activities of moxifloxacin against Coxiella burnetii, *Antimicrob Agents Chemother* 45:301–302, 2001.

RABIES

Method of
Alan C. Jackson, MD

CURRENT DIAGNOSIS

- A history of animal bite or exposure is often absent in rabies acquired in North America.
- Pain, paresthesias, and pruritus are early neurologic symptoms of rabies, probably reflecting infection in local sensory ganglia.
- Autonomic features are common including hypersalivation, gooseflesh, cardiac arrhythmias, and priapism.
- Hydrophobia is a highly specific feature of rabies.
- Paralytic features may be prominent, and the clinical presentation can resemble that of Guillain-Barré syndrome.
- Saliva samples for reverse transcription polymerase chain reaction (RT-PCR) and a skin biopsy should be obtained to detect rabies virus antigen to make a laboratory diagnosis of rabies.

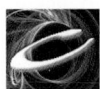

CURRENT THERAPY

- Details of an exposure determine whether postexposure rabies prophylaxis should be initiated.
- Wound cleansing is important after potential rabies exposure.
- Active immunization with a schedule of four doses of rabies vaccine (RabAvert or Imovax Rabies) at intervals is recommended. The four- dose series is a new Centers for Disease Control and Prevention (CDC) recommendation and is not yet reflected in the package insert, which calls for five doses.
- Passive immunization (if previously the patient was not immunized) consists of infiltrating human rabies immune globulin (HyperRAB, Imogam Rabies, or KamRAB) into the wound, with the remainder of the 20 IU/kg dosage given intramuscularly.

Rabies is an acute infection of the nervous system caused by rabies virus, which is a member of the family Rhabdoviridae in the genus *Lyssavirus*. Other lyssaviruses have only very rarely caused rabies in locations outside of the Americas.

Pathogenesis

Rabies virus is usually transmitted by bites from rabid animals. Transmission has rarely occurred through an aerosol route (in a laboratory accident or bat cave containing millions of bats) or by transplantation of infected organs or tissues (e.g., corneas). The virus is in the saliva of the rabid animal and is inoculated into subcutaneous tissues or muscles via a bite.

During most of the long incubation period (lasting 20–90 days or longer), the virus is close to the site of inoculation. The virus binds to the nicotinic acetylcholine receptor at the postsynaptic neuromuscular junction and travels toward the central nervous system (CNS) in peripheral nerves by retrograde fast axonal transport. There is rapid dissemination throughout the CNS by fast axonal transport. Under natural conditions, degenerative neuronal changes are not prominent, and it is thought that the rabies virus induces neuronal dysfunction by mechanisms that are not well understood. In rabies vectors, the encephalitis is associated with behavioral changes that lead to transmission by biting. After the CNS infection is established, the virus spreads by autonomic and sensory nerves to multiple organs, including the salivary glands of rabies vectors in which the virus is secreted in saliva.

Clinical Features

In North America, where the bat is the most common rabies vector for human disease, a history of an animal bite is usually absent, and there may be no known contact with animals. The incubation period is usually between 20 and 90 days, but it occasionally lasts 1 year or longer. Prodromal features are nonspecific and include malaise, headache, and fever, and patients can also have anxiety or agitation. Approximately half of patients experience pain, paresthesias, or pruritus at the site of the wound, which has often healed, and these symptoms likely reflect infection and inflammation involving local sensory ganglia. Approximately 80% of patients with rabies have encephalitic rabies; approximately 20% have paralytic rabies.

In encephalitic rabies, there are characteristic periods of generalized arousal or hyperexcitability separated by lucid periods. Autonomic dysfunction is common and includes hypersalivation, gooseflesh, cardiac arrhythmias, and priapism. Hydrophobia is the most characteristic feature of rabies and occurs in 50% to 80% of patients; contractions of the diaphragm and other inspiratory muscles occur on swallowing. This can become a conditioned reflex, and even the sight or thought of water can precipitate the muscle contractions. Hydrophobia is thought to be caused by inhibition of inspiratory neurons near the nucleus ambiguus.

In paralytic rabies, prominent muscle weakness usually begins in the bitten extremity and progresses to quadriparesis; typically there is sphincter involvement. Patients have a longer clinical course than in encephalitic rabies. Paralytic rabies is often misdiagnosed as Guillain-Barré syndrome.

Coma subsequently develops in both clinical forms. With aggressive medical therapy, a variety of medical complications develop, and multiple organ failure is common. Survival is very rare and has usually occurred in the context of incomplete postexposure rabies prophylaxis that included administration of one or more doses of rabies vaccine.

Epidemiology

Worldwide about 60,000 human deaths per year are attributed to rabies. The impact is particularly significant in terms of years of life lost because children are commonly the victims. Most human rabies cases occur through transmission from dogs in developing countries with endemic dog rabies, particularly in Asia and Africa. Travelers to endemic regions may develop rabies after they return home if they have not received effective postexposure rabies prophylaxis after an exposure. In the United States and Canada, transmission of rabies virus occurs most commonly in human cases from insect-eating bats, and often there is no known history of a bat bite or exposure to bats. A bat bite might not be recognized. The rabies virus variants responsible for most human cases are found in silver-haired bats and tricolored bats, and also in Brazilian (Mexican) free-tailed bats. These are small bats. Other rabies vectors in North American wildlife include skunks, raccoons, and foxes, but these species are rarely responsible for transmission to humans. This is likely because postexposure rabies prophylaxis is administered after recognized exposures.

Diagnosis

Most cases of rabies can be diagnosed clinically or the diagnosis will be strongly suspected, which is particularly important so that appropriate barrier nursing techniques can be initiated to prevent exposures of many health care workers. Some patients are candidates for an aggressive therapeutic approach. A serum-neutralizing titer can be useful for diagnosis in a previously unimmunized person, but a positive titer might not develop until the second week of clinical illness or later, and the result of the test might not be readily available. Detection of rabies virus antigen in a skin biopsy obtained from the nape of the neck using a fluorescent antibody technique is a useful diagnostic test. Detection of rabies virus ribonucleic acid (RNA) in saliva or in skin biopsies using RT-PCR amplification is an important recent advance for rapid rabies diagnosis. Rabies virus antigen can be detected in brain tissue obtained by brain biopsy or postmortem. Negative antemortem diagnostic laboratory tests do not exclude rabies and the tests may need to be repeated on subsequent samples.

Prevention

After a rabies exposure is recognized, rabies can be prevented with initiation of appropriate steps, including wound cleansing and active and passive immunization. After a human is bitten by a dog, cat, or ferret, the animal should be captured, confined, and observed for a period of at least 10 days; initiation of postexposure rabies prophylaxis is not necessary if the animal remains healthy. The animal should also be examined by a veterinarian prior to its release. If the animal is a stray, unwanted, shows signs of rabies, or develops signs of rabies during the observation period, the animal should be killed immediately, and its head should be transported under refrigeration for a laboratory examination. The brain should be examined via an antigen-detection method using the fluorescent antibody technique and viral isolation using cell culture or mouse inoculation.

The incubation period for animals other than dogs, cats, and ferrets is uncertain; these animals should be killed immediately after an exposure, and the head should be submitted for examination. If the result is negative, one may safely conclude that the animal's saliva did not contain rabies virus; if immunization has been initiated, it should be discontinued. If an animal escapes after an exposure, it should be considered rabid unless information from public health officials indicates this is unlikely, and rabies prophylaxis should be initiated. The physical presence of a bat might warrant postexposure prophylaxis when a person (such as a small child or sleeping adult) is unable to reliably report contact that could have resulted in a bite.

Local wound care should be given as soon as possible after all exposures, even if immunization is delayed, pending the results of an observation period. All bite wounds and scratches should be washed thoroughly with soap and water. Devitalized tissues should be débrided.

Purified chick embryo cell culture vaccine (RabAvert) and human diploid cell vaccine (Imovax Rabies) are licensed rabies vaccines in the United States and Canada. Other vaccines grown in either primary cell lines (hamster or dog kidney) or continuous cell lines (Vero cells) are also satisfactory and available in other countries. A regimen of four 1-mL doses of rabies vaccine should be given IM in the deltoid area (anterolateral aspect of the thigh is also acceptable in children). The four-dose series is a recent CDC recommendation and is an update from the five doses recommended in the current package insert. Ideally, the first dose should be given as soon as possible after exposure, but failing that, it should be given regardless of the length of a delay. Three additional doses should be given on days 3, 7, and 14. Pregnancy is not a contraindication for immunization. Live vaccines should not be given for 1 month after rabies immunization.

Local and mild systemic reactions are common. Systemic allergic reactions are uncommon, and anaphylactic reactions may be treated with epinephrine and antihistamines. Corticosteroids can interfere with the development of active immunity. Immunosuppressive medications should not be administered during postexposure therapy unless they are essential. The risk of developing rabies should be carefully considered before deciding to discontinue vaccination because of an adverse reaction. A serum-neutralizing antibody determination is necessary only after immunization of immunocompromised patients. Less-expensive vaccines derived from neural tissues are still used in some developing countries; these vaccines are associated with serious neuroparalytic complications.

Human rabies immune globulin (Imogam Rabies, HyperRAB, or KamRAB) should also be administered as passive immunization for protection before the development of immunity from the vaccine. It should be given at the same time as the first dose of vaccine and no later than 7 days after the first dose. Rabies vaccine and human rabies immune globulin should never be administered at the same site or in the same syringe. The recommended dose of human rabies immune globulin is 20 IU/kg; larger doses should not be given because they can suppress active immunity from the vaccine. After wounds are washed, they should be infiltrated with human rabies immune globulin (if anatomically feasible), and the remainder of the dose should be given IM in the gluteal area. Current updated recommendations by the World Health Organization do not recommend giving the remainder of the dose intramuscularly under certain circumstances. If the exposure involves a mucous membrane, the entire dose should be administered IM. With multiple or large wounds, the human rabies immune globulin might need to be diluted for adequate infiltration of all of the wounds. Adverse effects of human rabies immune globulin include local pain and low-grade fever.

After an exposure, a previously immunized patient should receive two 1-mL doses of rabies vaccine on days 0 and 3, but the patient should not receive human rabies immune globulin.

Management of Human Rabies

About 30 people have survived rabies, and 29 received rabies vaccine prior to the onset of their disease; there have been many recent survivors in India due to supportive critical care measures, and most have neurological sequelae (see Jackson, 2021). The possibilities for an aggressive approach were reviewed (see Jackson et al., 2003). There was one survivor in Wisconsin in 2004 who did not receive rabies vaccine. It is now doubtful whether the therapy she received played a significant role in her favorable outcome because a similar approach has failed in many cases (see Jackson, 2013), and there are concerns about its scientific rationale (see Zeiler and Jackson, 2016). Palliation is an important alternative approach and may be appropriate for many patients in whom rabies develops (see Jackson, 2021).

References

Fooks AR, Banyard AC, Horton DL, et al: Current status of rabies and prospects for elimination, *Lancet* 384:1389–1399, 2014.
Fooks AR, Jackson AC, editors: *Rabies: scientific basis of the disease and its management*, 4th ed., London, UK, 2020, Elsevier Academic Press.
Jackson AC: Therapy of human rabies. In Fooks AR, Jackson AC, editors: *Rabies: scientific basis of the disease and its management*, 4th ed., London, UK, 2020, Elsevier Academic Press, pp 547–566.
Jackson AC: Current and future approaches to the therapy of human rabies, *Antiviral Res* 99:61–67, 2013.
Jackson AC, Warrell MJ, Rupprecht CE, et al: Management of rabies in humans, *Clin Infect Dis* 36:60–63, 2003.
Jackson AC: Treatment of rabies. In: Hirsch MS, Edwards MS, Mitty J, eds. UpTo-Date. Waltham, MA: Wolters Kluwer, 2021.
Manning SE, Rupprecht CE, Fishbein D, et al: Human rabies prevention—United States, 2008: Recommendations of the Advisory Committee on Immunization Practices, *MMWR Recomm Rep* 57(RR-3):1–28, 2008.
World Health Organization: *WHO expert consultation on rabies. Third report*, WHO Technical Report Series 1012, Geneva, 2018, WHO.
Zeiler FA, Jackson AC: Critical appraisal of the Milwaukee protocol for rabies: this failed approach should be abandoned, *Can J Neurol Sci* 43:44–51, 2016.

RAT-BITE FEVER

Method of
Jatin M. Vyas, MD, PhD

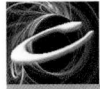

CURRENT DIAGNOSIS

- Exposure to rats is the major risk factor. Transmission can occur with simple contact with infected animals or excreta.
- A maculopapular rash and septic arthritis after initial symptoms of fever or sepsis should raise the suspicion of rat-bite fever.
- Clinicians must maintain a high index of suspicion for this diagnosis.
- Notify microbiology laboratory of clinical suspicion (slow growth, 5%–10% CO_2 microaerophilic conditions, 20% normal rabbit serum media supplementation, and avoidance of sodium polyanethol sulfonate when collecting blood cultures from the patient).

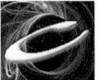

CURRENT THERAPY

Bite Site
- Clean and disinfect the bite site.
- Administer tetanus toxoid (tetanus-diphtheria toxoids, Td), if indicated.
- Postexposure rabies prophylaxis (Imovax Rabies) for animal bites should be considered in consultation with local public health authorities, though there are no reports of rat-to-human transmission of the rabies virus.

Established and Suspected Cases
- Give intravenous penicillin G at a dose of 1.2 million U/day for 5 to 7 days, followed by oral penicillin (PenVK)[1] or ampicillin (Omnipen)[1] 500 mg qid for an additional 7 days.
- For penicillin-allergic patients, consider doxycycline (Vibramycin)[1] 100 mg IV/PO twice daily or tetracycline (Achromycin)[1] 500 mg PO four times daily.
- *S. moniliformis* can be resistant to gentamicin (Garamycin),[1] tobramycin (Nebcin),[1] ciprofloxacin (Cipro),[1] and levofloxacin (Levaquin).[1]

[1]Not FDA approved for this indication.

Rat-bite fever (RBF) is a systemic, febrile disease caused by infection with *Streptobacillus moniliformis* or *Spirillum minus*. As the name implies, this infection is transmitted by a rat bite. However, the bacteria can also be transmitted by simple contact with infected rats or even through ingestion of food contaminated with rat excreta. Diagnosis can be difficult, and a high degree of suspicion is necessary to make a correct diagnosis. Recognition and early treatment are crucial, because case fatality is as high as 25% in untreated cases.

Epidemiology

S moniliformis is part of the normal respiratory flora of the rat. From 50% to 100% of healthy wild, laboratory, and pet rats harbor *S moniliformis* in the nasopharynx. *S moniliformis* is also excreted in the urine. *S minus* causes rat-bite fever mostly in Asia, but this organism is found worldwide. *S minus* has been demonstrated in rat conjunctival secretions and blood. Thus rat-bite fever can be transmitted not only from a bite but also through scratches, handling of dead rats, handling litter material, or by contamination of rat excreta.

Although the rat is the natural reservoir and major vector of the disease, *S moniliformis* has also been found in other rodents such as mice, squirrels, gerbils, and weasels. No precise data are available on the true incidence of rat-bite fever because it is not a reportable disease. It appears to be unusual in Western countries, a rarity that might reflect failed diagnosis, empiric treatment of infected bites and scratches caused by animals, or spontaneous recovery.

Risk Factors

The major risk factor is exposure to rats, either as an occupational hazard for persons such as laboratory workers, veterinarians, or pet shop employees, or for persons who have rats for pets or feed rats to snakes, especially children. Classically, homelessness and lower socioeconomic status were described as major factors, but most cases reported in the last few years have involved pet rats. Thirty percent of patients with rat-bite fever do not report any exposure to rats or other rodents. Therefore the lack of documented exposure does not exclude this diagnosis.

Pathophysiology

Very little is known about the pathophysiology of *S moniliformis* infections. Presumably, the failure of local control by dendritic cells, tissue macrophages, neutrophils, and other components of the innate immune system results in deeper infection, leading to bacteremia. Studies using histologic analysis have revealed intravascular thrombosis near the port of entry.

Prevention

The role of prophylactic antibiotics is unknown, but some authors recommend the use of oral penicillin V (PenVK)[1] after documented exposure to rats and a break in the skin. Penicillin V should be given for 3 days at a dose of 2 g per day for adults. Primary prevention should be encouraged for patients with occupational risk by using protective gloves to handle animals or cages.

Clinical Manifestations

Rat-bite fever is a systemic febrile disease. Classically, following a rat bite and a short incubation of 2 to 10 days, systemic dissemination of the organism is associated with an abrupt onset with intermittent relapsing fever, rigors, myalgias, arthralgias, headache, sore throat, malaise, and vomiting. These symptoms are followed within the first week by the development of a maculopapular rash in 75% of patients. The rash can be pustular, purpuric, or petechial, and it typically involves the extremities, in particular the palms and soles. The bite site typically heals promptly, with minimal inflammation and no significant regional lymphadenopathy.

Following the rash, approximately 50% of infected patients develop an asymmetric migrating polyarthritis, which appears to be exceedingly painful and affects large and middle-sized joints. Joint effusion appears more common in adults. Infection can occur in any tissue. Although most cases of rat-bite fever resolve spontaneously, there have been reports of complications. These include meningitis, endocarditis (including prosthetic valve endocarditis), myocarditis, pericarditis, pneumonia, brain abscess, septic arthritis, DIC (disseminated intravascular coagulation), and infarcts of the spleen and kidneys. The mortality rate in untreated cases is around 10% to 15%, and it rises to more than 50% in the rare cases with cardiac involvement.

Two closely related variants have been described. In Haverhill fever, the organism is transmitted by ingestion of contaminated food. Haverhill fever tends to occur in epidemics and also causes rashes and arthritis, but upper respiratory tract symptoms and vomiting appear more prominent. It is important to note that these patients do not provide a history of exposure to rodents. Sodoku is a rat-bite fever caused by *S minus*; it is common in Japan. The course is more subacute, arthritic symptoms are rare, and if the bite initially heals, it then ulcerates and is associated with regional lymphadenopathy and a distinctive rash. *S minus* cannot be grown using synthetic media, and thus microbiologic diagnosis rests on visualization of these organisms in infected tissues.

Diagnosis

Diagnosis is difficult and requires a high clinical index of suspicion. The initial symptoms of rat-bite fever are nonspecific, triggering a broad differential diagnosis. Additionally, the fastidious nature of this organism makes isolation from blood cultures difficult. Clinicians should ask about rodent exposure when compatible symptoms are seen in patients. Rat-bite fever should not be ruled out in the absence of bite history, because transmission can occur without a bite, and pet owners or laboratory workers can minimize the significance of the bite, especially in the absence of a local reaction.

No reliable serologic test is available, and the definitive diagnosis requires isolation of *S moniliformis* from the wound, blood, or synovial fluid in patients with septic arthritis. The microbiology laboratory should be specifically notified of any clinical suspicion to enhance the chances of recovering the pathogen.

---

[1]Not FDA approved for this indication.

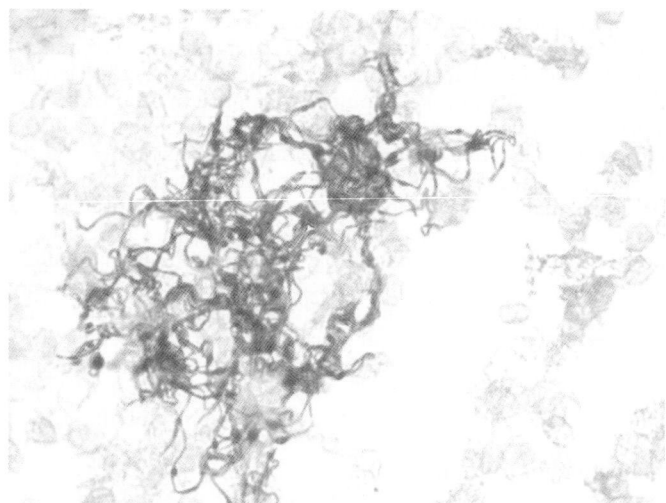

Figure 1 Gram stain of *Streptobacillus moniliformis*. Gram stain of growth from anaerobic bottle, ×100 magnification [microphotography]. Reprinted with permission from Partners' Infectious Disease Images; accessed on August 11, 2016, from http://www.idimages.org/images/detail/?imageid=373.

S moniliformis is a highly pleomorphic, nonencapsulated, nonmotile, gram-negative rod, which can stain positively on Gram stain (Figure 1). It is often dismissed as proteinaceous debris because of its numerous bulbous swellings with occasional clumping (*moniliformis*="necklace-like"). It grows slowly and requires a microaerophilic environment with 5% to 10% CO_2 or anaerobic conditions and media supplementation with 20% normal rabbit serum. Cultures can take up to 7 days to turn positive. Some experts recommend holding blood cultures for 21 days to permit sufficient time to grow this organism. *S moniliformis* is also inhibited by sodium polyanethol sulfonate, a common adjunct in most commercial blood culture media at a concentration as low as 0.0125%. *S moniliformis* has been identified using polymerase chain reaction amplification and 16S ribosomal ribonucleic acid (rRNA) sequencing, which shows great promise though it is available at reference laboratories. Fatty acid profiles obtained by gas-liquid chromatography can also be used for identification.

S minus, the other etiologic agent of rat-bite fever, is a short, thick, gram-negative, tightly coiled spiral rod that measures 0.2 to 0.5 μm and has two to six helical turns.

Differential Diagnosis

Differential diagnosis for fever, rash, and polyarthritis is broad. Malaria, typhoid fever, and neoplastic disease can cause relapsing fevers, and the presence of a rash and polyarthritis might suggest viral and rickettsial diseases including Rocky Mountain spotted fever. An asymmetric oligoarthritis suggests disseminated gonococcal and meningococcal diseases in the context of cutaneous lesions on the palms and soles. Lyme disease, leptospirosis, or secondary syphilis can have a similar clinical presentation. Finally, when classic infectious symptoms such as fever or rash are missing, any causes of polyarthritis, from crystal-induced arthropathies to rheumatoid arthritis, should be considered.

Treatment

All established cases of rat-bite fever should be treated with antibiotics because of the associated mortality and potential for complications. Intravenous penicillin G at a dose of 1.2 million units per day should be initiated as soon as the clinical diagnosis is made. Empiric therapy is necessary and should not be delayed for laboratory confirmation of this bacterial infection. The intravenous treatment should continue for 5 to 7 days. After treatment with IV penicillin and suitable clinical response, therapy should be continued with oral penicillin (PenVK)[1] or ampicillin (Omnipen)[1] at a dose of 500 mg qid for an additional 7 days. For patients allergic to penicillin, intravenous doxycycline (Vibramycin)[1] at a dose of 100 mg every 12 hours or oral tetracycline (Achromycin)[1] at a dose of 500 mg four times a day can be used.

Streptomycin[1] and cephalosporins including cefotamxine (Claforan)[1] have been reported to be potentially useful. Other antibiotics including azithromycin (Zithromax),[1] erythromycin,[1] carbapenems,[1] aztreonam (Azactam),[1] clindamycin (Cleocin),[1] vancomycin (Vancocin),[1] and nitrofurantoin (Macrodantin)[1] have shown efficacy in vitro, but they lack good clinical correlation to recommend them for routine use. Erythromycin has been associated with treatment failures. Trimethoprim-sulfamethoxazole (Bactrim),[1] polymyxin B,[1] gentamicin (Garamycin),[1] tobramycin (Nebcin),[1] ciprofloxacin (Cipro),[1] and levofloxacin (Levaquin)[1] should not be used because in vitro resistance has been demonstrated.

Typically, the bite site heals promptly. It should be cleaned and disinfected, as is typical for management of other wounds. Tetanus prophylaxis (tetanus-diphtheria toxoids, Td) administration is indicated as required by the patient's immunization record. Rabies prophylaxis (Imovax Rabies) is usually not required for rodent bite, but consultation with local public health authorities is encouraged. There are no reports of transmission of the rabies virus from rats to humans.

---

[1]Not FDA approved for this indication.

References

Abusalameh M, Mahankali-Rao P, Earl S, et al: Discitis caused by rat bite fever in a rheumatoid arthritis patient on tocilizumab-first ever case, *Rheumatology (Oxford)* 57:1118–1120, 2018.

Adam JK, et al: Notes from the field: fatal rat-bite Fever in a child - San Diego County, California, 2013, *MMWR Morb Mortal Wkly Rep* 63(50):1210–1211, 2014.

Chen PL, Lee NY, Yan JJ, et al: Prosthetic valve endocarditis caused by *Streptobacillus moniliformis*: A case of rat bite fever, *J Clin Microbiol* 45:3125–3126, 2007.

Crews JD, Palazzi DL, Starke JR: A teenager with fever, rash, and arthralgia. *Streptobacillus moniliformis* infection, *JAMA Pediatr* 168(12):1165–1166, 2014.

Elliott SP: Rat bite fever and *Streptobacillus moniliformis*, *Clin Microbiol Rev* 20:13–22, 2007.

Fenn DW, et al: An unusual tale of rat-bite fever endocarditis, *BMJ Case Rep*. 2014, 2014.

Gaastra W, Boot R, Ho HT, Lipman LJ: Rat bite fever, *Vet Microbiol* 133:211–228, 2009.

Giorgiutti S, Lefebvre N: Rat bite fever, *N Engl J Med* 381(18):1762, 2019.

Graves MH, Janda JM: Rat-bite fever (*Streptobacillus moniliformis*): A potential emerging disease, *Int J Infect Dis* 5:151–155, 2001.

Holroyd KJ, Reiner AP, Dick JD: *Streptobacillus moniliformis* polyarthritis mimicking rheumatoid arthritis: An urban case of rat bite fever, *Am J Med* 85:711–714, 1988.

King HY. Rat Bite Fever. UpToDate. http://www.uptodate.com/contents/rat-bitefever; [accessed April 21, 2018].

Lambe DW Jr, McPhedran AM, Mertz JA, Stewart P: *Streptobacillus moniliformis* isolated from a case of Haverhill fever: Biochemical characterization and inhibitory effect of sodium polyanethol sulfonate, *Am J Clin Pathol* 60:854–860, 1973.

Miura Y, Nei T, Saito R, Sato A, Sonobe K, Takahashi K: Streptobacillus moniliformis bacteremia in a rheumatoid arthritis patient without a rat bite: a case report, *BMC Res Notes* 8(1):694, 2005 Nov 19, https://doi.org/10.1186/s13104-015-1642-0.

Schachter ME, Wilcox L, Rau N, et al: Rat-bite fever, Canada, *Emerg Infect Dis* 12:1301–1302, 2006.

Stehle P, Dubuis O, So A, Dudler J: Rat bite fever without fever, *Ann Rheum Dis* 62:894–896, 2003.

Torres-Miranda D, Moshgriz M, Siegel M: Streptobacillus moniliformis mitral valve endocarditis and septic arthritis: the challenges of diagnosing rat-bite fever endocarditis, *Infect Dis Rep* 10(2):7731, 2018.

Washburn RG: Streptobacillus moniliformis (rat–bite fever). In Mandell GL, Bennett JE, Dolin R, editors: *Principles and Practice of Infectious Diseases*, vol 2, 6th ed, Philadelphia, 2005, Elsevier, pp 2708–2710.

RELAPSING FEVER

Method of
Diego Cadavid, MD

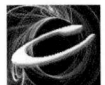

CURRENT DIAGNOSIS

- There are two forms of relapsing fever: epidemic and endemic.
- Epidemic relapsing fever is transmitted from person to person by the body louse *Pediculus humanus*.
- Endemic relapsing fever is transmitted from rodent reservoirs to humans exposed to endemic areas by soft-bodied ticks of the genus *Ornithodoros*.
- The hallmark of relapsing fever is two or more febrile episodes separated by periods of relative well-being.
- The diagnosis is confirmed by visualization of the etiologic spirochetes in thin peripheral blood smears prepared at times of febrile peaks by phase-contrast or darkfield microscopy or light microscopy after Wright or Giemsa staining.

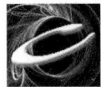

CURRENT THERAPY

- The antibiotic of choice for treatment of relapsing fever is doxycycline except in children or pregnant women. In children <8 years of age, erythromycin[1] or oral penicillin is used instead of tetracycline (Table 3).
- Relapsing fever, if severe or complicated with neuroborreliosis, requires treatment with the intravenous antibiotics ceftriaxone or penicillin G (Table 3).
- The louse-borne epidemic form is treated with a single dose, whereas the endemic tick-borne form is treated with multiple doses for at least 1 week (Table 3).
- Antibiotic treatment of relapsing fever results in the Jarisch-Herxheimer reaction (JHR) in as many as 60% of cases, more often in the epidemic than in the endemic forms. It is characterized by the sudden onset of tachycardia, hypotension, chills, rigors, diaphoresis, and high fever. To reduce the risk of JHR, antibiotics should be started between but not at times of febrile peaks.

---

[1]Not FDA approved for this indication.

657

Relapsing fever is one of several diseases caused by spirochetes. Other human spirochetal diseases are syphilis, Lyme disease, and leptospirosis. Notable features of spirochetes are wavy and helical shapes, length-to-diameter ratios of as much as 100 to 1, and flagella that lie between the inner and outer cell membranes. The spirochetes that cause relapsing fever are in the genus *Borrelia*. Other *Borrelia* species cause Lyme disease, avian spirochetosis, and epidemic bovine abortion. Table 1 shows the main *Borrelia* species of relapsing fever, their vectors, and an estimate of their geographic ranges. In the United States, relapsing fever was considered a disease endemic only in the West. However, the recent finding of relapsing fever–like *Borrelia* in ticks and dogs in the eastern United States suggests that the risk of relapsing fever may extend into the East.

Epidemiology

There are two forms of relapsing fever: epidemic transmitted to humans by the body louse *Pediculus humanus* (louse-borne relapsing fever [LBRF]) and endemic transmitted to humans by soft-bodied ticks of the genus *Ornithodoros* (tick-borne relapsing fever [TBRF]). In LBRF, itching caused by skin infestation

TABLE 1 Relapsing Fever *Borrelia* Species Pathogenic to Humans

RELAPSING FEVER	*BORRELIA* SPECIES	ARTHROPOD VECTOR	DISTRIBUTION OF DISEASE
Endemic	*Borrelia hermsii*	*Ornithodoros hermsi*	Western North America
	Borrelia turicatae	*Ornithodoros turicata*	Southwestern North America and northern Mexico
	Borrelia venezuelensis	*Ornithodoros rudis*	Central America and northern South America
	Borrelia hispanica	*Ornithodoros marocanus*	Iberian peninsula and northwestern Africa
	Borrelia crocidurae	*Ornithodoros erraticus*	North and East Africa, Middle East, southern Europe
	Borrelia duttoni	*Ornithodoros moubata*	Sub-Saharan Africa
	Borrelia persica	*Ornithodoros tholozani*	Middle East, Greece, Central Asia
	Borrelia uzbekistan	*Ornithodoros pappilipes*	Tajikistan, Uzbekistan
	Borrelia miyamotoi	Ixodes spp.	Asia, Europe, North America
Epidemic	*Borrelia recurrentis*	*Pediculus humanus*	Worldwide (recently only in East Africa including immigrants to Europe)

with lice leads to scratching, which may result in crushing of lice and release of infected hemolymph into areas of skin abrasion. Louse infestation is associated with cold weather and a lack of hygiene. Migrant workers and soldiers at war are particularly susceptible to this infection. Historically, massive outbreaks of LBRF occurred in Eurasia, Africa, and Latin America, but currently the disease is found only in Ethiopia and neighboring countries. However, immigrants can spread LBRF to other parts of the world.

The main risk factor for TBRF is exposure to endemic areas (Table 1). The risk of infection increases with outdoor activities in areas where rodents nest, like entering caves or sleeping in rustic cabins. *Ornithodoros* ticks are soft-bodied and feed for short periods of time (minutes), usually at night. They can live many years between blood meals and may transmit spirochetes to their offspring transovarially. Infection is produced by regurgitation of infected tick saliva into the skin wound during tick feeding. There are several natural vertebrate reservoirs for TBRF, but most common are rodents (deer mice, chipmunks, squirrels, and rats). In contrast, the body louse *Pediculus humanus* is a strict human parasite, living and multiplying in clothing. Hard-tick-borne relapsing fever (HTBRF) is an emerging infectious disease throughout the temperate zone caused by *Borrelia miyamotoi*. *Borrelia miyamotoi* is a spirochete closely related to the bacteria that cause TBRF. It is more distantly related to the bacteria that cause Lyme disease. First identified in 1995 in ticks from Japan, *B miyamotoi* has since been detected in two species of North American ticks, the black-legged or "deer" tick (Ixodes scapularis) and the western black-legged tick (Ixodes pacificus). These ticks are already known to transmit Lyme disease, anaplasmosis, and babesiosis.

Clinical Diagnosis

Relapsing fever should be suspected in any patient presenting with two or more episodes of high fever and constitutional symptoms spaced by periods of relative well-being. The index of suspicion increases if the patient has been exposed to endemic areas for TBRF or to countries where LBRF still occurs (Table 1). Whereas LBRF is usually associated with a single febrile relapse, TBRF usually has multiple relapses (up to 13). Only about 10% of cases of HTBRF have febrile relapses. In LBRF the second episode of fever is typically milder than the first; in TBRF the multiple febrile periods are usually of equal severity. The febrile periods last from 1 to 3 days, and the intervals between fevers last from 3 to 10 days. During the febrile periods, numerous spirochetes are circulating in the blood. This is called *spirochetemia* and is sometimes unexpectedly detected during routine blood smear examinations.

TABLE 2 Frequent Clinical Manifestations of Tick-Borne Relapsing Fever

SIGN OR SYMPTOM	FREQUENCY (%)
Headache	94
Myalgia	92
Chills	88
Nausea	76
Arthralgia	73
Vomiting	71
Abdominal pain	44
Confusion	38
Dry cough	27
Ocular pain	26
Diarrhea	25
Dizziness	25
Photophobia	25
Neck pain	24
Rash	18
Dysuria	13
Jaundice	10
Hepatomegaly	10
Splenomegaly	6

Between fevers, spirochetemia is not observed because the numbers are low. The fever pattern and recurrent spirochetemia are the consequences of antigenic variation of abundant outer membrane lipoproteins of relapsing fever *Borrelia* species that are the target for serotype-specific antibodies.

The mean latency between exposure to ticks in the endemic form or to lice in the epidemic form and onset of symptoms is 6 days (range, 3–18 days). Because *Ornithodoros* ticks feed briefly and painlessly at night, patients with TBRF may not be able to recall having been bitten by a tick. The clinical manifestations of TBRF and LBRF are similar, although some differences do exist. Table 2 lists the frequency of the most common manifestations of TBRF.

The usual initial presentation is sudden onset of chills followed by high fever, tachycardia, severe headache, vomiting, myalgia and arthralgia, and often delirium. In the early stages, a reddish rash may be seen over the trunk, arms, or legs. The fever remains high for 3 to 5 days, and then it clears abruptly. After an asymptomatic period of 7 to 10 days, the fever and other constitutional symptoms can reappear suddenly. The febrile episodes gradually become less severe, and the person eventually recovers completely. As the disease progresses, fever, jaundice, hepatosplenomegaly, cardiac arrhythmias, and cardiac failure may occur, especially with LBRF. Jaundice is more common at times of relapses. Patients with LBRF are more likely to develop petechiae on the trunk, extremities, and mucous membranes; epistaxis; and blood-tinged sputum. Rupture of the spleen may rarely occur. Multiple neurologic complications can occur as a result of disseminated intravascular coagulation in LBRF and as a result of infection of the meninges and cranial and spinal nerve roots by spirochetes in TBRF. The most common neurologic complications of TBRF are aseptic meningitis and facial palsy. Relapsing fever in pregnant women can cause abortion, premature birth, and neonatal death. Sometimes patients can have nonfebrile relapses, consisting of periods of severe headache, backache, weakness, and other constitutional symptoms without fever that occur at the time of expected relapses. Delirium may persist for weeks after the fever resolves, and, rarely, symptoms may be protracted.

Relapsing fever may be confused with many diseases that are relapsing or cause high fevers. These include typhoid fever, yellow fever, dengue, African hemorrhagic fevers, African trypanosomiasis, brucellosis, malaria, leptospirosis, rat-bite fever, intermittent cholangitis, cat-scratch disease, and echovirus 9 infection, among others. Relapsing fever *Borrelia* spp. have antigens that are cross reactive with Lyme disease *Borrelia* spp. and inasmuch as the endemic areas of relapsing fever and Lyme disease overlap to some extent, confusion between the two infections can be expected. In fact, the same species of ticks can transmit HTBRF and Lyme disease, although erythema migrans rash is rare in the former and common in the latter.

Laboratory Diagnosis

Although the pattern of recurring fever is the clue to diagnosing relapsing fever, confirmation of the diagnosis requires demonstration of spirochetes in peripheral blood taken during an episode of fever. The comparatively large number of spirochetes in the blood during relapsing fever provides the opportunity for the simplest method for laboratory diagnosis of the infection, light microscopy of Wright- or Giemsa-stained thin blood smears or darkfield or phase-contrast microscopy of a wet mount of plasma. The blood should be obtained during or just before peaks of body temperature. Between fever peaks, spirochetes often can be demonstrated by inoculation of blood or cerebrospinal fluid (CSF) into special culture medium (BSK-H with 6% rabbit serum available from Sigma) or experimental animals. Enrichment for spirochetes is achieved by using the platelet-rich fraction of plasma or the buffy coat of sedimented blood. In the United States the most common causes of relapsing fever are *Borrelia hermsii* and *Borrelia turicatae*; both grow in BSK-H medium and in young mice or rats. Whereas direct visual detection of organisms in the blood is the most common method for laboratory confirmation of relapsing fever, immunoassays for antibodies are the most common means of laboratory confirmation for Lyme disease. Although serologic assays have been developed for the agents of relapsing fever, these are not widely available and of dubious utility. The antigenic variation displayed by the relapsing fever species means there are hundreds of different "serotypes." If a different serotype or species is used for preparing the antigen, only antibodies to conserved antigens may be detected. For this reason, a standardized enzyme-linked immunosorbent assay (ELISA) with Lyme disease *Borrelia* as antigen may be the best available serologic assay for relapsing fever. ELISA for *Borrelia burgdorferi* antibodies is routinely done across the United States and Europe.

TABLE 3 Treatment Options for Tick-Borne Relapsing Fever*

Adults

Nonsevere forms

1. Doxycycline (Doryx oral), 100 mg PO bid for 1–2 wk†

2. Tetracycline (Sumycin), 500 mg PO qid for 1–2 wk

3. Erythromycin (Erythrocin),[1] 500 mg PO tid for 1–2 wk

Severe forms

1. Ceftriaxone (Rocephin),[1] 2 g IV qd for 1–2 wk

2. Penicillin G parenteral aqueous (Pfizerpen),[1] 4 million U IV q4h for 1–2 wk

Children (≤8 y)

Nonsevere forms

1. Erythromycin suspension oral (EryPed),[1] 30–50 mg/kg/d divided tid for 1–2 wk

2. Azithromycin oral suspension (Zithromax),[1] 20 mg/kg on the first day followed by 10 mg/kg/d for 4 more days

3. Penicillin V (Pen-Vee K),[1] 25–50 mg/kg/d divided qid for 1–2 wk

4. Amoxicillin (Amoxil),[1] 50 mg/kg/d divided tid for 1–2 wk

Severe forms

1. Ceftriaxone (Rocephin),[1] 75–100 mg/kg/d IV for 1–2 wk

2. Penicillin G parenteral aqueous (Pfizerpen),[1] 300,000 U/kg/d given IV in divided doses q4h for 1–2 wk

Abbreviations: IV = intravenous; PO = orally.
[1]Not FDA approved for this indication.
*The same oral agents are used for treatment of louse-borne (epidemic) relapsing fever but given as a single dose.
†In general, treatment for 1 wk is recommended in early/milder cases and for up to 2 wk for more severe cases.

If a positive result for IgM or IgG antibodies is obtained, the Western blot for antibodies to *B burgdorferi* antigens would be expected to discriminate current or past Lyme disease from relapsing fever, as well as from syphilis, another cause of false-positive Lyme disease ELISA results. Other frequent laboratory abnormalities can occur in relapsing fever but are not diagnostic. These include elevated white blood cell count with increased neutrophils, thrombocytopenia, increased serum bilirubin, proteinuria, microhematuria, prolongation of the prothrombin time (PT) and partial thromboplastin time (PTT), and elevation of fibrin degradation products.

Treatment

Relapsing fever *Borrelias* are very sensitive to several antibiotics, and antimicrobial resistance is rare. Table 3 summarizes the treatment options for adults and children younger than 8 years. Children older than 8 years can be treated with the same antibiotics as adults, but the doses should be adjusted by weight. Before antibiotics are given, the possibility of causing the Jarisch-Herxheimer reaction (JHR) should be considered (see later). The tetracycline antibiotics are most commonly used for treatment of LBRF and TBRF. The first antibiotic of choice in adults and children older than 8 years is doxycycline (Doryx). In general, shorter treatments are needed for LBRF than for TBRF. Single-dose therapy is usually recommended for LBRF. In contrast, in TBRF even multiple doses of tetracyclines for up to 10 days may fail to prevent relapses, and retreatment can be required. *B. miyamotoi* is susceptible in vitro to doxycycline, azithromycin, and ceftriaxone. Physicians have successfully treated patients infected with *B miyamotoi* with a 2 to 4-week course of doxycycline.

Alternative oral antibiotics to the tetracyclines are erythromycin (E-Mycin)[1], azithromycin (Zithromax)[1], amoxicillin (Amoxil)[1], penicillin[1], and chloramphenicol (Chloromycetin).[1] However, oral chloramphenicol is not available in the United States. Erythromycin, azithromycin, and penicillin do not appear as effective as the tetracyclines; however, they are recommended for children younger than 8 years and for pregnant women. Amoxicillin is another alternative for young children with early Lyme disease; however, it is ineffective for human granulocytic ehrlichiosis, which sometimes occurs as a co-infection with Lyme disease. *Borrelia miyamotoi* may be resistant to amoxicillin.

Although treatment with antibiotics is usually given orally, they may need to be given intravenously if severe vomiting makes swallowing impractical. If there are symptoms and signs of meningitis or encephalitis without clinical or radiologic signs of increased intracranial pressure, the CSF should be examined to rule out central nervous system (CNS) infection. The finding of elevation of CSF cells and protein demands the use of parenteral antibiotics, such as penicillin G[1] or ceftriaxone (Rocephin).[1] Optimally, antibiotic treatment should be started during afebrile periods when the spirochetemia is low. Starting therapy near the peak of a febrile period may induce JHR, in which high fever and a rise and subsequent fall in blood pressure, sometimes to dangerously low levels, may occur. Dehydration should be treated with fluids given intravenously. Severe headache can be treated with pain relievers such as codeine, and nausea or vomiting can be treated with prochlorperazine (Compazine).

Jarisch-Herxheimer Reaction

Antibiotic treatment of relapsing fever causes JHR in as many as 60% of cases. JHR is more common in LBRF than in TBRF. It can also occur in HTBRF. It is characterized by the sudden onset of tachycardia, hypotension, chills, rigors, diaphoresis, and high fever. Patients with JHR have said that they felt as if they were going to die. JHR is caused by the rapid killing of circulating spirochetes 1 to 4 hours after the first dose of antibiotic, which results in the release of large amounts of *Borrelia* lipoproteins in the circulation followed by massive release of tumor necrosis factor and other cytokines. If possible, patients with JHR should be transferred to an intensive care unit for close monitoring and treatment. Over several hours, the temperature declines and the patient feels better. Large amounts of intravenous fluids (0.9% sodium chloride solution) may be required to treat hypotension. Steroids and nonsteroidal antiinflammatory agents have no effect on the frequency or severity of the JHR. One study found that pretreatment with anti-TNF-alpha monoclonal antibody (Humira)[1] suppressed JHR after penicillin treatment for LBRF and reduced the associated increases in plasma cytokines. Death can occur as a result of JHR secondary to cardiovascular collapse in up to 5% of patients with treated LBRF and much less frequently in TBRF.

Outcome

Complete recovery occurs in 95% or more of adequately treated patients. The prognosis for untreated cases or if treatment is delayed varies. A mortality rate as high as 40% is reported in untreated epidemics of LBRF. Relapsing fever also has a high mortality rate in neonates. Some neurologic sequelae can occur in patients with TBRF complicated with neuroborreliosis.

Prevention

Prevention of TBRF involves avoidance of rodent- and tick-infested dwellings such as animal burrows, caves, and abandoned cabins. Wearing clothing that protects skin from tick access (e.g., long pants and long-sleeved shirts) is also helpful. Repellents and acaricides provide additional protection. Diethyltoluamide (DEET) repels ticks when applied to clothing or skin, but it must be used with caution. It loses its effectiveness within 1 to several hours when applied to skin and must be reapplied; it is absorbed through the skin and may cause CNS toxicity if used excessively. Picaridin (KBR 3023), which has been used as an insect repellent for years in Europe and Australia, is now available in the United States in 7% solution as Cutter Advanced Repellent (Spectrum Brands). The US Centers for Disease Control and Prevention (CDC) is recommending it as an alternative to DEET. Permethrin Insect Repellent, an acaricide, is more effective than DEET but should not be applied directly to skin. When applied to clothing, it provides good protection for 1 day or more. In LBRF, prevention can be achieved by promoting personal hygiene and by dusting undergarments and the inside of clothing with malathion[1] powder[2] or lindane[1] powder[2] when available. Widespread antibiotic use may be necessary to control epidemics of LBRF, using one or two doses of 100 mg doxycycline[1] given within 1 week of exposure.

---

[1]Not FDA approved for this indication.

[2]Not available in the United States

References

Barbour AG, Hayes SF: Biology of *Borrelia* species, *Microbiol Rev* 50:381–400, 1986.

Bryceson AD, Parry EH, Perine PL, et al: Louse-borne relapsing fever, *Q J Med* 39:129–170, 1970.

Cadavid D, Barbour AG: Neuroborreliosis during relapsing fever: Review of the clinical manifestations, pathology, and treatment of infections in humans and experimental animals, *Clin Infect Dis* 26:151–164, 1998.

Fekade D, Knox K, Hussein K, et al: Prevention of Jarisch-Herxheimer reactions by treatment with antibodies against tumor necrosis factor alpha, *N Engl J Med* 335:311–315, 1996.

Kazragis RJ, Dever LL, Jorgensen JH, Barbour AG: In vivo activities of ceftriaxone and vancomycin against *Borrelia* spp. in the mouse brain and other sites, *Antimicrob Agents Chemother* 40:2632–2636, 1996.

Melkert PW: Fatal Jarisch-Herxheimer reaction in a case of relapsing fever misdiagnosed as lobar pneumonia, *Trop Geogr Med* 39:92–93, 1987.

Southern P, Sanford J: Relapsing fever, *Medicine* 48:129–149, 1969.

Taft W, Pike J: Relapsing fever. Report of a sporadic outbreak including treatment with penicillin, *JAMA* 129:1002–1005, 1945.

RUBELLA AND CONGENITAL RUBELLA

Method of
Dee Ann Bragg, MD

CURRENT DIAGNOSIS

- Given its clinical overlap with other viral syndromes, suspected rubella infection must be confirmed with laboratory testing.
- Rubella serology or viral polymerase chain reaction (PCR) testing are available options for confirming a suspected diagnosis.

CURRENT THERAPY

- Rubella infection is largely self-limited with no specific treatment indicated.
- Infection during pregnancy should prompt further evaluation and counseling regarding risks and potential outcomes.
- Treatment of children with congenital rubella syndrome requires a multidisciplinary effort based on individual manifestations.
- Vaccination is essential in reducing the risk of rubella and congenital rubella syndrome.

---

[1]Not FDA approved for this indication.

Rubella typically presents in children and adults as a mild viral illness, but is one of the TORCH infections (toxoplasmosis, other, rubella, cytomegalovirus, herpes) known to cause congenital anomalies. Although vaccination efforts have led to the successful eradication of rubella in the United States, it remains a significant cause of morbidity and death worldwide. Its name is derived from Latin and means "little red." Initially considered a variant of measles or scarlet fever, rubella was first described as its own entity in the German medical literature in 1814. Thus it is still often referred to as "German measles" in common nomenclature.

Pathophysiology and Virology

Rubella virus, a single-stranded RNA virus and the only member of the Rubivirus genus, is part of the Togaviridae family and is the causative agent of rubella infection. There are 13 recognized genotypes of rubella, each with minor differences in nucleotide sequencing and gene expression. Rubella typically presents as a mild and self-limited illness. During pregnancy, however, it can infect the placenta and disrupt organogenesis by creating systemic inflammation and inhibiting actin assembly. Outcomes of antenatal infection are variable but can include miscarriage, fetal death, and congenital rubella syndrome (CRS).

Multiple factors are involved in the pathogenesis of CRS. Rubella infection can cause necrosis of the chorionic epithelial and endothelial cells. These cells then enter fetal circulation and can incite thrombotic or ischemic lesions in the eyes, ears, brain, and heart. The virus also appears to trigger an immune-modulated upregulation of interferon and cytokines, which can alter the normal development and differentiation of fetal cells.

Epidemiology

Although rubella is less contagious than other viruses such as influenza or measles, large epidemics are associated with significant morbidity from complications including encephalitis, fetal loss, deafness, and blindness. Norman Gregg, an Australian ophthalmologist, was the first to recognize the teratogenic potential of rubella when in 1941 he noted an unusually high incidence of congenital cataracts after an area outbreak.

Rubella was successfully eradicated from the United States in 2004 due to widespread vaccination efforts, and most sporadic cases since that time have been documented in foreign-born young adults. In endemic areas, annual springtime outbreaks are common. However, sporadic cases can occur year-round in temperate climates. Outbreaks typically affect early school–aged children, and the mean age for an infected host is 5 to 9 years. Because lifelong immunity develops after natural infection, large cyclical epidemics tend to occur every 3 to 8 years as population immunity wanes.

Humans are the only known host of rubella infection, and the virus is transmitted from person to person through respiratory droplets. After transmission, rubella virus replicates in the respiratory mucosa and cervical lymph nodes before entering systemic circulation and spreading to target organs.

Clinical Manifestations

Acquired Rubella

After an incubation period of about 14 days (range, 12–23), a variety of clinical symptoms can appear. These are generally mild, and about 50% of cases are asymptomatic. In children, a skin rash is typically the initial manifestation of rubella. The rash usually appears on the face and then progresses downward from the head to the feet. It lasts about 3 days and is characteristically maculopapular, presenting with small pink non-coalescing papules that are occasionally pruritic. Bathing or showering in hot water tends to make the rash more evident.

Adults more often have a prodromal period of low-grade fever, malaise, and adenopathy lasting 1 to 5 days before the onset of skin findings. Lymphadenopathy may begin up to a week before the rash and can last for several weeks. The postauricular nodes are particularly commonly involved, and posterior cervical or suboccipital nodes may also be affected.

Sequelae

Polyarthritis and polyarthralgia are the most common complications of rubella, particularly in adult women, in whom they are seen up to 70% of the time. They appear with such frequency that they are often considered intrinsic to the virus itself rather than complications. Joint symptoms typically present around the same time or just after the onset of the rash. They usually last 3 to 4 days but can remain for up to 1 month. The most commonly affected joints are fingers, wrists, and knees. Chronic arthritis is rarely observed.

Other complications are uncommon but can carry a high degree of morbidity and death. Hemorrhagic events are more likely in children than adults and occur in about 1 in 3000 cases. They manifest as a result of vascular damage or thrombocytopenia. Skin purpura is the most common presentation, but gastrointestinal, cerebral, or intrarenal hemorrhage can occur. Encephalitis occurs in about 1 in 6000 cases, more commonly in adults than children. Rare complications include orchitis, neuritis, progressive panencephalitis, and Guillain-Barré syndrome.

Congenital Rubella Syndrome (CRS)

CRS can present transiently with low birth weight, thrombocytopenic purpura, or hemolytic anemia. However, permanent defects are the hallmark of CRS because it classically involves a triad of cataracts, cardiac anomalies, and sensorineural deafness. Of these, hearing loss is the most common and sometimes the only complication observed. Cardiac abnormalities can include patent ductus arteriosus, ventricular septal defect, pulmonary artery hypoplasia, and coarctation of the aorta. Other ocular defects such as glaucoma, retinopathy, and microphthalmia can also occur. Additional manifestations can include microcephaly, intellectual disability, psychomotor retardation, and delayed speech.

Notably, it can take 2 to 4 years for certain neurologic, endocrine, or cardiac abnormalities associated with CRS to manifest. Diabetes mellitus, thyroid disease, autism, and progressive panencephalopathy can all occur as late effects of CRS.

The risk of CRS and its associated congenital defects is greatest when infection occurs in the first trimester. Up to 85% of infants born under these conditions are found to be affected, whereas defects are rare when infection occurs after 20 weeks' gestation.

Diagnosis

Given its nonspecific nature and similarity to other viral infections, clinical diagnosis of rubella is challenging and largely unreliable. Suspected infection should be confirmed by 1 of 3 diagnostic methods: (1) rubella immunoglobulin M (IgM) serology, (2) a demonstrated rise in rubella virus immunoglobulin G (IgG) between acute and convalescent phases, or (3) detection of rubella virus by PCR.

Among the existing options for laboratory diagnosis, rubella IgM is the most accessible and widely used. However, collection timing is important to consider. Rubella IgM will only be detectable in about 50% of cases on the day of rash appearance but will be present in nearly all cases by 7 to 10 days after the rash. It will then remain positive for 4 to 12 weeks. Importantly, serum IgM testing is most sensitive and specific in the setting of local outbreaks. False-positive results occur more frequently in sporadic cases, and in those instances, additional means of analysis should be performed to confirm diagnosis.

Rubella IgG testing can be used to diagnose acute rubella infection under two circumstances: either (1) a negative rubella IgG during acute infection followed by a positive IgG in the convalescent phase, or (2) a fourfold increase in IgG titer over 10 to 14 days. IgG avidity testing may also be useful. This measures the strength of antigen-antibody binding, which is typically weaker in acute infection and increases over time. Therefore a low avidity index would indicate a more recent infection.

Viral isolation of rubella by PCR is quite valuable for diagnostic confirmation and can be performed on samples obtained from throat or nasopharyngeal swabs. These tests are not as widely available in postvaccination settings and may need to be performed in conjunction with local health departments or national epidemiology centers.

Diagnosis of CRS in infants can similarly be confirmed by one of three methods: (1) rubella IgM detection in serum or cord blood, (2) persistence of rubella IgG >6 months of age (past the time frame of passive maternal immunity), or (3) PCR isolation of rubella virus from respiratory or urinary samples. Because both rubella virus and IgM remain positive for several months in patients with CRS, the time frame for testing is less crucial than in cases of postnatal infection.

Treatment

There is no specific treatment for rubella and, because acquired cases are generally mild and self-limiting, basic supportive care is recommended. Detection of rubella infection in pregnancies before 18 weeks' gestation should prompt further investigation including maternal-fetal medicine referral, detailed ultrasound examination, support for adverse outcomes including neonatal hospice services, and follow-up examination and screening of the newborn. Maternal infections after 18 weeks can be followed with routine ultrasound monitoring along with newborn evaluation and testing.

Prevention

Rubella Vaccine

The first rubella vaccines became available in 1969, and a number of strains have been developed since that time. Of these, the RA 27/3 vaccine has been the most enduring, and all other strains were discontinued at the time of its introduction in 1979. The RA 27/3 rubella vaccine is a live attenuated virus that is administered in conjunction with measles and mumps as MMR, or with measles, mumps, and varicella as MMRV (ProQuad). Single-antigen rubella vaccine is not available in the United States.

Vaccination against rubella is safe and effective. Adverse events such as fever and rash are mild and are generally attributable to the measles and mumps portions of the vaccines. After a single dose, more than 95% of those vaccinated have serologic confirmation of rubella immunity, with evidence of lifelong immunity in the vast majority of responders. MMR or MMRV is recommended for all children at 12 months of age, followed by a second dose between 4 and 6 years of age. The second dose is generally indicated to stimulate measles and mumps immunity in those who did not respond to the first vaccine. MMR and MMRV are contraindicated in immunosuppression, pregnancy, and in patients with a history of anaphylaxis to neomycin or other vaccine components.

Preconception Counseling and Prenatal Care

Rubella immunity, defined as serum rubella IgG of 10 IU/mL or greater, should be documented in all women attempting to conceive. MMR vaccine should be given in cases of nonimmunity, and although it is recommended at least 4 weeks before conception, inadvertent vaccination after that time is unlikely to be associated with adverse events. Rubella IgG should likewise be checked in all pregnant females as part of routine obstetric care, and MMR should be administered postpartum to nonimmune women.

Eradication and Future Goals

Despite widely available effective vaccines and evidence of sustained eradication in the Western Hemisphere, there are still approximately 100,000 cases of CRS annually worldwide. Although some African and Asian nations have introduced routine rubella vaccination, public health efforts have been inconsistent in many developing countries. Dedicated personnel and funding will likely be necessary to decrease rubella incidence and its complications on a global scale.

References

Baltimore RS, Nimkin K, Sparger K, et al: Case 4-2018: a newborn with thrombocytopenia, cataracts, and hepatosplenomegaly, *N Engl J Med* 378:564–572, 2018.

Bouthry E, Picone O, Hamdi G, et al: Rubella and pregnancy: diagnosis, management and outcomes, *Prenat Diagn* 34:1246–1253, 2014.

Centers for Disease Control and Prevention: *Epidemiology and Prevention of Vaccine-Preventable Diseases, 13th Edition.* Hamborsky J, Kroger A, Wolfe S, eds. Washington, DC: Public Health Foundation, pp 325–340, 2015.

Lambert N, Strebel P, Orenstein W, et al: *Rubella, Lancet* 385(9984):2297–2307, 2015.

Papania M, Wallace G, Rota P, et al: Elimination of endemic measles, rubella, and congenital rubella syndrome from the western hemisphere: the US experience, *JAMA Pediatr* 168:148–155, 2014.

Tipples G: Rubella diagnostic issues in Canada, *J Infect Dis* 204(Suppl 2):S659–S663, 2011.

SALMONELLOSIS

Method of
Arelis Santana, MD, MPH

CURRENT DIAGNOSIS

- Nontyphoidal Salmonellae (NTS) represent a significant cause of infectious diarrhea globally.
- Underlying comorbidities, the virulence of the pathogen, and the size of inoculum can affect the severity of the infection.
- The most common clinical manifestation of NTS is self-limited acute gastroenteritis.
- Bacteremia and invasive infections (mycotic aneurysms, aortitis, among others) should be suspected in patients with high-grade fevers and predisposing risk factors (e.g., aneurysms and atherosclerotic disease).
- Diagnosis of NTS infection is confirmed by laboratory isolation of Salmonellae from the stool, blood, or sterile body fluid.

CURRENT THERAPY

- Treatment for uncomplicated Salmonella gastroenteritis is based on supportive care with fluid and electrolyte replenishment.
- Antimicrobial therapy may be warranted for those with severe infection (severe diarrhea, high fever, need for hospitalization) or risk factors for invasive disease.
- Chronic carriage of NTS can occur in less than 1% of patients. Antimicrobial therapy may be of some utility in patients with chronic carriage; however, there is no strong evidence yet supporting its routine use.
- Adequate hand hygiene practices, appropriate food handling, and standard precautions are still the best way to avoid NTS spread.

Salmonellae was named after Dr. Daniel Elmer Salmon, a veterinary pathologist chief of the Bureau of Animal Industry, who helped with the eradication of contagious bovine pleuropneumonia in the United States. His colleague and professor, Dr. Theobald Smith, was the first to isolate *Salmonella choleraesuis* from porcine intestines in 1885. This microorganism can grow in both humans and animals, causing a broad range of clinical manifestations. Clinical presentations comprise gastroenteritis, bacteremia, endovascular infections, localized infections, and chronic carrier state. However, the most common presentation of salmonellosis is uncomplicated gastroenteritis.

Microbiology

Salmonella is a genus of gram-negative bacilli belonging to the family of Enterobacteriaceae. The genus of Salmonellae is divided into two species: *enterica and bongori. Salmonella enterica* is further divided into six different subspecies based on DNA resemblances. Subspecies are also differentiated into serotypes. Salmonellae serotypes are designated based on the immunoreactivity of cell surface structures, the O and H antigens. These serotypes are classified using the Kauffmann–White classification scheme. Salmonella has more than 2500 serotypes. However, less than 100 have been found to be pathogenic in humans.

Salmonellae species are nonspore forming, motile, facultative anaerobes that can measure 2 to 3 μm by 0.4 to 0.6 μm in size. All Salmonellae are motile utilizing a flagellum, except for *S. Gallinarum-*and *S. Pullorum.* Similar to other Enterobacteriaceae, they can produce acid on glucose fermentation. Most of the species do not ferment lactose and appear white on MacConkey agar plates, except for approximately 1% of them, which can make their identification challenging. Another important feature of identification is that most of the species, except for *S. Typhi,* produce hydrogen sulfide on sugar fermentation, which can be detected on the selective indicator plates.

Epidemiology

Nontyphoidal Salmonellae (NTS) represent a significant cause of infectious diarrhea globally. Approximately, there are 93.8 million cases of gastroenteritis Salmonella species and 155,000 deaths per year. According to the Centers for Disease Control and Prevention (CDC), there are approximately 1.35 million illnesses and 420 deaths due to NTS yearly in the United States, with an estimate of 39 cases of salmonellosis for each culture-confirmed case. The Salmonella serotypes most frequently isolated are *S. enteritidis, S. typhimurium,* and *S. newport.*

Salmonellae can inhabit the intestinal tract and can be found in the feces of humans and animals. These include but are not limited to birds (including poultry), reptiles, and amphibians. Infection can occur from the ingestion of animal food products such as undercooked meat, poultry, eggs, and dairy products, or from cross-contamination due to improperly handled food or water. Other possible sources include animal bodies contaminated with Salmonella. For example, reptiles can commonly harbor this organism. Also, areas where animals live, such as water tanks and cages, may be contaminated with these organisms and can be potential sources of infection. NTS outbreaks have also been associated with fresh produce, milk, nuts, fruits, and raw vegetables. These products can become contaminated by manure or water and then are distributed.

The emergence of antibiotic resistance in NTS has been on the rise and is currently a global concern as antibiotic treatment options are becoming limited and ineffective. Antibiotic resistance has been associated with the use of antimicrobials in animal feeds. The mechanisms of resistance described in NTS include active efflux pumps to remove antibiotics from inside the cell, hydrolytic enzyme production, mutations in target genes to evade the action of antibiotics, and decreased permeability of the outer membrane, among others.

In the United States, the National Antimicrobial Resistance Monitoring System (NARMS) monitors antibiotic resistance, including Salmonella. According to their last report in 2015, approximately 4% of NTS isolates were resistant to five or more antimicrobials, 4.7% of NTS strains were nalidixic acid resistant, 0.4% were resistant to ciprofloxacin, and 2.7% were resistant to ceftriaxone. Resistance to nalidixic acid is a good indicator of a decreased susceptibility to fluoroquinolones. In summary,

TABLE 1	Predisposing Factors for Salmonellosis
Gastrointestinal	
Achlorhydria	
Gastric surgery	
Inflammatory bowel disease	
Infections	
HIV/AIDS (decreased T-cells)	
Bartonellosis	
Malaria	
Schistosomiasis	
Immune or structural compromise	
Age (<6 months, >60 years)	
Lymphoma	
Splenectomy	
Cirrhosis with portal hypertension	
Diabetes mellitus	
Chronic uremia	
Hemolytic anemia (iron overload)	
Sickle cell (bone infarct, autosplenectomy)	
Systemic lupus	
Atheromata, aortic aneurysm	
Drugs	
H2-blockers, proton pump inhibitors	
Antibiotic administration	
Antimotility agents	
Chemotherapy	
Corticosteroids	
Transplant antirejection agents	

resistance rates to fluoroquinolones or third-generation cephalosporins in the United States are not high but warrant careful monitoring.

Pathogenesis

A combination of factors related to both the pathogen and the host affects the pathogenesis of Salmonella infection and clinical presentation. Underlying conditions and the size of inoculum can affect the severity of the infection. NTS infection commences with the ingestion of organisms in contaminated food or water and usually requires approximately 10^6 organisms to produce the disease. However, infants or persons with certain underlying predisposing factors could develop the disease with smaller inoculums. Some of these predisposing risk factors include impaired cellular immunity, achlorhydria, alteration in the intestinal flora and integrity, and the extreme of ages (Table 1). These risk factors can lead to a more severe initial infection and complications such as bacteremia and/or metastatic infection. Gastric acidity is the initial barrier to Salmonellae; therefore, underlying conditions or medications that increase the pH of the stomach can predispose a person to infection. Salmonellae invade by binding to the gastrointestinal mucosa and submucosal lymphoid systems. After the invasion of Salmonella and the translocation of bacterial proteins into the host cell cytoplasm, the intestinal mucosa secretes interleukin-8 (IL-8), a strong neutrophil chemotactic factor. This causes an extensive polymorphonuclear leukocyte infiltration in both small and large intestinal mucosa. Degranulation and release of toxic neutrophils result in damage to the intestinal mucosa, producing diarrhea.

Clinical Presentation

Gastroenteritis

The most common clinical manifestation of NTS is self-limited acute gastroenteritis. The incubation period is usually 6 to 48 hours following the exposure, but more extended incubation periods of up to 7 days have been reported. Symptoms include sudden onset of nausea and vomiting, followed by fever, constitutional symptoms, abdominal pain, and watery diarrhea. On rare occasions, bloody diarrhea can also be present. Symptoms subside within 3 to 7 days in uncomplicated gastroenteritis. In patients with predisposing factors (see Table 1), the clinical illness may be more complex, including bacteremia. Patients with inflammatory bowel disease can have serious complications like toxic megacolon that can potentially be life-threatening.

Higher inoculum of bacteria and virulence of different strains may correlate with the severity of diarrhea and the length of the disease course. The stool can contain polymorphonuclear leukocytes, or occult blood and leukocytosis can also be seen in the complete blood cell count.

Invasive Infections

Bacteremia can result as a complication from Salmonella gastroenteritis in up to 5% of the patients, and it should be suspected in patients with high-grade fevers or with predisposing risk factors. Bacteremia can lead to a variety of extraintestinal manifestations such as endocarditis, mycotic aneurysm, hepatic abscesses, or osteomyelitis. *S. choleraesuis and S. Dublin* are commonly associated with more invasive infections.

Although these are uncommon, NTS endovascular infection, including aortitis and mycotic aneurysms, should be suspected in patients with high-grade bacteremia or persistent bacteremia, or with pre-existing valvular heart disease, prosthetic vascular graft, or aortic aneurysm.

Intraabdominal infections due to NTS are also rare but can occur as hepatic and/or splenic abscesses, or cholecystitis, more commonly in patients with underlying hepatobiliary abnormalities. Other rare manifestations of invasive disease are meningitis (more common in infants 1 to 4 months old), pneumonia, and urinary tract infections. Salmonella osteomyelitis is most commonly seen with sickle cell disease, or underlying bone disease.

Diagnosis

Diagnosis of NTS infection is confirmed by laboratory isolation of Salmonellae from the stool, blood, or sterile body fluid. The definitive diagnosis of NTS gastroenteritis requires the identification in stool culture. Blood cultures should be performed whenever a patient has a prolonged or recurrent fever with NTS gastroenteritis. Endovascular infection should be suspected if there is high-grade bacteremia or persistent bacteremia. If an aortic or vascular infection is suspected, further imaging with computed tomography or magnetic resonance imaging (preferably with contrast angiographic analysis) should be performed.

Additionally, if a localized infection is diagnosed, such as an intraabdominal abscess or osteomyelitis, a body fluid drainage and culture is recommended. Salmonellosis is a nationally notifiable disease for which most states require that isolates of Salmonella be sent for serotyping to the local public health laboratory.

Treatment

NTS gastroenteritis is usually self-limited; therefore, antibiotics are routinely not recommended for an uncomplicated infection. Antibiotic therapy has been associated with prolonged bacterial shedding and potentially extending carriage.

Supportive care with fluid and electrolyte replenishment, preferably via the oral route, is the mainstay of treatment for Salmonella gastroenteritis. Patients that present with severe dehydration or profuse vomiting should initially receive intravenous fluid repletion and may require hospitalization. Antiemetics such as, but not limited to, prochlorperazine (Compazine) or promethazine (Phenergan) may be helpful for symptom control. Antimotility agents are not recommended as they can increase the risk of complications.

There are specific clinical settings where antimicrobial therapy may be warranted for those with severe disease (severe diarrhea, high fever, need for hospitalization) or risk factors for invasive disease. When antimicrobial therapy is indicated, empiric treatment is started, and it must be tailored to susceptibility data once results are available.

Fluoroquinolones are usually the agents commonly used for adults and adolescents without contraindications to such antibiotics (Table 2). Fluoroquinolones are often avoided in children due to association with the development of cartilage defects. Additionally, note that serious adverse reactions have been associated with fluoroquinolones, including tendonitis, tendon rupture, peripheral neuropathy, and QT prolongation, among others. Other antibiotic options (see Table 2) include trimethoprim-sulfamethoxazole (Bactrim)[1], amoxicillin[1], ceftriaxone (Rocephin)[1], or azithromycin (Zithromax)[1]. For patients with severe infection who cannot tolerate oral intake, intravenous fluoroquinolone or a third-generation cephalosporin such as ceftriaxone[1] is a good option. The duration of antibiotic therapy for NTS gastroenteritis in the absence of bacteremia is 3 to 7 days, depending on clinical response.

In the case of NTS bacteremia without other focal infection or immunocompromised state, 14 days of antibiotics are appropriate. Longer duration of antibiotics of 2 to 6 weeks of antibiotic therapy is recommended in patients with an immunocompromised state, including patients with advanced HIV with CD4 cell counts less than 200 cells/μL and organ transplant recipients in order to prevent a relapse of the infection.

Prolonged antibiotic therapy may be needed in patients with extraintestinal and endovascular infections, and eradication of the infection may require surgical intervention. Focal infections may require removal of the fluid collection like joint lavage in septic arthritis or abscess drainage if clinically indicated. In addition, graft or prosthetic material removal may be necessary for the eradication of the infection. The duration of the antibiotic course will depend on the infection site (see Table 2).

Chronic Carriage

Asymptomatic excretion or carriage of Salmonella can occur after NTS infection. This can last up to 5 weeks; however, more extended periods have been reported. Chronic carriage of NTS is defined as excretion of the organism for more than 12 months, identified in stool culture 1 month after illness, followed by repeat positive cultures. Less than 1% of patients develop NTS chronic carriage. Routine follow-up cultures are not recommended after an uncomplicated Salmonella gastroenteritis in immunocompetent patients after the resolution of symptoms. However, in the United States, public health departments may require one or more negative stool cultures for individuals who work in specific settings such as childcare, food preparation, or health care in order to return to work.

---

[1] Not FDA approved for this indication.

TABLE 2	Recommended Antibiotic Therapy for Nontyphoidal Salmonella Infection in Adults		
	ANTIBIOTIC	**DOSE**	**DURATION**
Severe gastroenteritis	Ceftriaxone (Rocephin)[1]	1–2 g IV daily	3–7 days (Immunosuppressed patients may require longer treatment of 2–6 weeks)
	Cefotaxime (Claforan)[1]	2 g IV Q8h	
	Amoxicillin[1]	1 g PO TID	
	Trimethoprim-sulfamethoxazole Bactrim DS[1]	160/800 mg PO BID	
	Azithromycin (Zithromax)[1]	1000 mg PO on day 1, then 500 mg PO daily	
	Ciprofloxacin (Cipro)[1]	500 mg PO BID or 400 mg IV Q12h	
Bacteremia	Ceftriaxone[1]	2 g IV daily	7–14 days (Immunosuppressed patients may require longer treatment of 2–6 weeks)
	Cefotaxime[1]	2 g IV Q8h	
	Ciprofloxacin[1]	400 mg IV Q12h	
	Trimethoprim-sulfamethoxazole[1]	8–10 mg/kg/day of TMP component IV TID	
	Ampicillin	2 g IV Q4h	
Endovascular infection*	Ceftriaxone[1]	2 g IV daily	6–8 weeks
	Cefotaxime[1]	2 g IV Q8h	
	Ciprofloxacin[1]	400 mg IV Q12h	
	Ampicillin[1]	2 g IV Q4h	
Extraintestinal focal infection**	Ceftriaxone[1]	2 g IV daily	4–6 weeks
	Ampicillin[1]	2 g IV Q4h	
	Ciprofloxacin[1]	400 mg IV Q12h or 750 mg PO BID	

*Treatment includes antibiotic regimen with surgical intervention.
**Bone and joint infection should be treated for 4–6 weeks along with surgical intervention if clinically indicated.
[1]Not FDA approved for this indication.

An antibiotic course for asymptomatic carriage has not been proved to be effective and may promote resistance; hence, it is not recommended. Antimicrobial therapy may be of some utility in patients with chronic carriage; however, there is no strong evidence yet supporting its routine use.

Prevention

Prevention of NTS infections involves personal and institutional efforts. Currently, there are no vaccines to prevent NTS infection. Adequate hand hygiene practices and standard precautions are still the best way to avoid NTS spread. Individuals with the condition should remain out of work until the symptoms of gastroenteritis and diarrhea resolve, especially individuals that work in food handling, childcare, health care, or direct contact with immunosuppressed patients. This approach will decrease the possibility of outbreaks. Cross-contamination can occur when uncooked meat or poultry is being prepared. Therefore, utensils and the cutting board used in the preparation of these should be washed to prevent other foods from contamination.

Additionally, the CDC advises that children less than 5 years old, adults older than 65 years of age, and immunosuppressed individuals should not handle or touch amphibians or reptiles. They also recommend keeping the equipment used to handle reptiles out of the kitchen. The CDC also recommends that live poultry should not be kept inside the house, particularly in areas of food preparation. Also, strict hand hygiene precautions are recommended after touching live fowl. Children under 5 years of age or immunocompromised patients should not handle live poultry.

References

Benenson S, Raveh D, Schlesinger Y, et al: The risk of vascular infection in adult patients with nontyphi Salmonella bacteremia, *Am J Med* 110:60–63, 2001.

Center for Disease Control and Prevention (CDC): *National Antimicrobial Resistance Monitoring System for Enteric Bacteria (NARMS): Human Isolates Surveillance Report for 2015 (Final Report)*, Atlanta, GA, 2018, US Department of Health and Human Services. https://www.cdc.gov/narms/pdf/2015-NARMS-Annual-Report-cleared_508.pdf. Accessed 29 April 2020.

Eaves DJ, Randall L, Gray DT, et al: Prevalence of mutations within the quinolone resistance-determining region of gyrA, gyrB, parC, and parE and association with antibiotic resistance in quinolone-resistant Salmonella enterica, *Antimicrob Agents Chemother* 48:4012–4015, 2004.

Hohmann EL: Nontyphoidal salmonellosis, *Clin Infect Dis* 32:263, 2001.

Majowicz SE, Musto J, Scallan E, et al: The global burden of nontyphoidal Salmonella gastroenteritis, *Clin Infect Dis* 50:882, 2010.

Panel on Opportunistic Infections in HIV-Infected Adults and Adolescents. Guidelines for the prevention and treatment of opportunistic infections in HIV-infected adults and adolescents: Recommendations from the Centers for Disease Control and Prevention, the National Institutes of Health, and the HIV Medicine Association of the Infectious Diseases Society of America. http://aidsinfo.nih.gov/contentfiles/lvguideline s/adult_oi.pdf. Accessed on April 28, 2020.

Pegues D, Miller S: Salmonella species. In Bennett J, Dolin R, Blaser M, Mandell, Douglas, editors: *Bennett's Principles and Practice of Infectious Diseases*, ed 8, Philadelphia, PA, 2015, Elsevier/Saunders, pp 2559–2568.

Riddle MS, DuPont HL, Connor BA: ACG clinical guideline: diagnosis, treatment, and prevention of acute diarrheal infections in adults, *Am J Gastroenterol* 111:602, 2016.

Schultz M: Theobald Smith, *Emerg Infect Dis* 14(12):1940–1942, 2008. https://doi.org/10.3201/eid1412.081188.

Tindall BJ, Grimont PA, Garrity GM, Euzéby JP: Nomenclature and taxonomy of the genus Salmonella, *Int J Syst Evol Microbiol* 55:521, 2005.

SEVERE SEPSIS

Method of
Jerome Larkin, MD; and David P. Rakel, MD

CURRENT DIAGNOSIS

Systemic Inflammatory Response Syndrome (SIRS)
- Diagnosis is based on the presence of two or more of the following:
  - Temperature >38°C or <36°C
  - Pulse >90 beats/min
  - Respirations >20 breaths/min or arterial partial pressure of carbon dioxide ($Paco_2$) <32 mm Hg
  - White blood cell count >12,000 or <4000 cells/mm³ or >10% bands

Sepsis
- Diagnosis is based on a finding of SIRS plus proven or suspected infection as the cause.

Severe Sepsis
- Diagnosis is based on a finding of sepsis plus organ dysfunction of one or more major systems (typically kidney, lung, or heart; less often, central nervous system).

Septic Shock
- Diagnosis is based on a finding of severe sepsis plus persistent hypotension despite aggressive fluid resuscitation (i.e., vasopressors are required to maintain mean arterial pressure >65 mm Hg).

Supportive Laboratory Findings
- Hyperglycemia
- Lactic acidosis
- Hyperbilirubinemia
- Acute renal failure
- Thrombocytopenia
- Coagulopathy
- Leukocytosis or leukopenia
- Elevated erythrocyte sedimentation rate or C-reactive protein

Supportive Physical Findings
- Decreased capillary refill or mottling of skin
- Mental status changes or obtundation
- Tachypnea or respiratory failure
- Tachycardia
- Anuria or oliguria
- Edema

CURRENT THERAPY

Initial 6 Hours
- Initiate fluid resuscitation with crystalloid or colloid to achieve central venous pressure of 12 mm Hg (or 15 mm Hg if intubated).
- Add dopamine (Intropin) or norepinephrine (Levophed) for persistent hypotension (mean arterial pressure <65 mm Hg).
- Obtain blood, urine, and other appropriate cultures (cerebrospinal fluid, abscess drainage, catheter tip, tissue, sputum).
- Administer empiric antimicrobial therapy.
- Perform appropriate imaging studies with urgent source control as indicated and allowed by clinical status; remove potentially infected foreign bodies.
- All interventions should be undertaken simultaneously and initiated within 1 hour after making a presumptive diagnosis of sepsis.

Subsequent Interventions
- Maintain glycemic control with a target blood glucose level of less than 150 mg/dL.
- Use unfractionated or low-molecular-weight heparin for prophylaxis against deep venous thrombosis.
- Use a histamine 2 (H_2) blocker or proton pump inhibitor for gastric ulcer prophylaxis.
- Initiate therapy with dobutamine (Dobutrex) for low cardiac output in the face of adequate filling pressures.
- Consider therapy with activated protein C (drotrecogin alfa [Xigris]) for patients with an Acute Physiology and Chronic Health Evaluation (APACHE) II score of 25 or greater.
- Consider therapy with hydrocortisone (Solu-Cortef)[1] for patients with continued hypotension despite adequate fluid resuscitation and vasopressors.
- Achieve adequate sedation.

[1]Not FDA approved for this indication.

Epidemiology

Sepsis is the tenth most common cause of death in the United States. The incidence is highest during the winter, most likely reflecting increased respiratory viral infections that precede the development of community-acquired pneumonia, which is itself a medical condition with increased risk of developing severe sepsis.

A remarkable aspect of sepsis, severe sepsis, and septic shock is the relatively small number of associated pathogens out of the more than 1000 microorganisms known to cause human disease. *Staphylococcus aureus*, streptococci, enterococci, and gram-negative rods are the most commonly isolated species. *Escherichia coli*, *Klebsiella*, *Pseudomonas*, *Serratia*, *Acinetobacter*, *Enterobacter*, *Citrobacter*, and *Neisseria meningitidis* (a gram-negative coccus) constitute the most common gram-negative pathogens. This relative paucity of etiologic bacterial pathogens has implications for empiric antimicrobial therapy. The emergence of resistant organisms, particularly methicillin-resistant *S. aureus* (MRSA) and gram-negative bacteria harboring extended-spectrum β-lactamases, increases the risk of antibiotic failure and attendant mortality. Fungal pathogens, particularly non-candidal species, continue to increase in incidence. This is most likely the result of better empiric management of gram-negative and candidal sepsis in patients with hematologic malignancies.

Although sepsis is most typically a disease of the elderly, the immune suppressed, and those with chronic medical problems, otherwise young and healthy individuals can also be stricken with no clear cause or known risk factor, such as in meningococcemia, toxic shock syndrome, and necrotizing fasciitis.

Definitions

The term *sepsis* derives from a Greek word that generally implies putrefaction. It also has a colloquial meaning, understood by most laypeople to mean a serious, potentially overwhelming infection. Historically, it has been intuitively understood by physicians to mean an infection, once localized, that has now disseminated and is life threatening. Bacteremia is implied if not always proven. Sepsis was usually fatal in the preantibiotic era, and its morbidity and mortality remain substantial.

Sepsis is a systemic inflammatory response syndrome (SIRS) with an immune activation characterized by the findings of fever with tachycardia, tachypnea, and/or leukocytosis or leukopenia. Although sensitive, this definition is so overly broad as to be rather unhelpful to an experienced clinician who would not need to resort to such terms to understand that a patient is seriously ill. Nonetheless, it provides a useful construct in beginning to arrive at a specific definition of sepsis. Both infectious and noninfectious processes—severe burns and pancreatitis being the most notable examples of the latter—can cause SIRS.

Sepsis is defined as the finding of SIRS in the presence of known or suspected invasion by a microbe into a normally sterile body site. Severe sepsis is sepsis that has become more generalized.

The cardinal finding is organ dysfunction that is unrelated to the primary site of infection. Other typical findings include hyperglycemia, thrombocytopenia, hyperbilirubinemia, acidosis, coagulopathy, edema, oliguria, hypotension, ileus, hypoxia, and poor perfusion. Heart, kidney, and respiratory failure are the most common forms of organ dysfunction. Altered sensorium is also common. Septic shock refers to the presence of hypotension with systolic blood pressure lower than 90 mm Hg or mean arterial pressure lower than 60 mm Hg despite adequate fluid resuscitation. These terms (sepsis, severe sepsis, and septic shock) are all part of a continuum, implying a progressively graver degree of illness with associated increasing mortality. No single symptom, physical finding, organ dysfunction, or laboratory abnormality serves to make or exclude the diagnosis, although isolation of a microorganism in the setting of such findings is highly suggestive. Increasing numbers of physical findings and other abnormalities correlate with an increasing likelihood of the diagnosis of sepsis.

Pathophysiology

Infection of the immunocompetent host by a microorganism typically leads to immune activation. This serves to isolate the site and source of infection. Local tissue is often damaged, but eventually the infection is cleared, and repair and regeneration occur. This process is highly regulated, with a number of different cell types and mediators involved, all in delicate balance between proinflammatory and antiinflammatory effects. The patient may have few or no symptoms, or there may be systemic evidence of infection (i.e., SIRS). Sepsis is the failure of localization such that the process becomes generalized and leads to tissue destruction remote from the site of infection. Why the immune system enters this state of dysregulation remains unknown, although an enormous amount of research over the past 4 decades has elucidated many of the pathways and mediators involved. Tumor necrosis factor, platelet-activating factor, interleukins, eicosanoids, interferons, and nitric oxide are among the biologically active molecules characterized to date. Particular microbes also contribute to this process through the elaboration of toxins (typically by gram-positive organisms) and endotoxins (gram-negative–derived lipopolysaccharide). These events lead to tissue destruction as a result of ischemic insult, direct cytotoxicity, and accelerated apoptosis. The characterization of inflammatory mediators has led to attempts to modify the immune response through the use of novel therapies such as monoclonal antibodies directed against tumor necrosis factor. To date such attempts have not met with success, and investigation continues.

Diagnosis

The diagnosis of sepsis ultimately relies on the clinical suspicion of infection in the setting of SIRS. A constellation of other supportive evidence establishes a greater or lesser likelihood of the presence of sepsis (see the Current Diagnosis box). It is rare that specific microbiologic evidence for infection is available in a manner timely enough to determine that sepsis is present or to help guide the initial, typically urgent, therapy. When it is available, it usually is a Gram stain or other type of specialized microbiology stain that confirms the presence of a potential pathogen in a site where none should be (e.g., gram-positive cocci in cerebrospinal fluid). Early therapy therefore relies on aggressive resuscitative measures and the administration of empiric antibiotics.

Treatment

Early Goal-Directed Resuscitation: The First 6 Hours

Initial treatment of sepsis should focus on correction of hemodynamic parameters, early administration of antibiotics, and source control of potential sites of infection. The 2008 guidelines from the Surviving Sepsis Campaign, an international initiative to improve sepsis outcomes, emphasized the importance of aggressive fluid resuscitation. Therapy should be implemented according to a protocol directed at achieving the following specific goals:

- Central venous pressure 8 to 12 mm Hg, or 12 to 15 mm Hg in those who are mechanically ventilated or have decreased left ventricular compliance

- Central venous or mixed venous oxygen saturation 70% or greater
- Mean arterial pressure (MAP) 65 mm Hg or greater
- Urine output 0.5 mL/kg/hr or greater

Administration of fluid boluses of 1000 mL or more of crystalloids or 300 to 500 mL of colloids over 30 minutes should begin as soon as hypoperfusion is recognized. There is no evidence that one type of fluid is superior to the other, although crystalloid is substantially cheaper. In cases of profound intravascular volume depletion, more rapid and more frequent fluid administration may be needed. Hemodynamic improvement (decreased heart rate, increased blood pressure, increased urine output) and the goal of optimizing central venous pressure should direct the need for continued infusion of fluid while avoiding the development of volume overload and pulmonary edema. Transfusion of packed red blood cells should be considered if anemia is present, with a goal of achieving a hemoglobin level of 7.0 to 9.0 g/dL. If tissue hypoperfusion or hypoxia persists (central mixed venus oxygen saturation <70%) despite achieving a central venous pressure of 12 mm Hg, therapy with dopamine (Intropin) or norepinephrine (Levophed) should be initiated with a goal of achieving a MAP of 65 mm Hg. There is no role for the use of low-dose dopamine for renal protection. An arterial line for more precise and continuous measurement of blood pressure should be inserted as soon as possible after the initiation of vasopressor therapy. Ideally, vasopressors should not be introduced to increase MAP until after the fluid deficit has been corrected. However, in cases of severe shock, vasopressor therapy may be needed early in the resuscitation effort to improve perfusion to the peripheral vascular beds. If there is no response to dopamine and norepinephrine, the patient should be treated with epinephrine (Adrenalin).[1]

Appropriate antibiotics should be administered within 1 hour after diagnosis of severe sepsis or septic shock, because mortality increases in a linear fashion with each hour of delay. All efforts should be made to obtain appropriate cultures, in particular at least two sets of blood cultures. At least one of these should be peripheral, with the second from any long-term (>48 hours) vascular device. Cultures of urine, sputum, wounds, abscesses, and cerebrospinal fluid should also be obtained as appropriate and before the administration of antibiotics, assuming that such specimens can be obtained during the first hour. Specific antibiotic choices are discussed later.

Source Control

A survey for potential sources of infection should be performed, and early resuscitation efforts should occur concomitantly. Elimination of the source of infection is critical to reversing septic shock. Conditions that require emergent intervention, such as necrotizing fasciitis, cholangitis, and intestinal infarction, should be ruled out within the first 6 hours after presentation. Potentially infected indwelling devices should be removed as soon as possible. Necrotic tissue should be débrided and abscesses drained if either condition is detected. Practitioners must consider the risks and benefits of the specific invasive procedures and the timing of such interventions for each patient individually. Every effort should be made to limit the invasiveness of necessary procedures, to avoid further stress in patients with an already hemodynamically fragile state. Imaging studies such as computed tomography of the head, chest, abdomen, and pelvis are necessary to identify or rule out potential sources of infection. An exception to the mandate to drain or débride infected collections is the presence of infected pancreatic necrosis, in which case surgical intervention should be delayed.

Other Interventions

After hemodynamic parameters have been stabilized with fluid and vasopressors, cultures have been obtained, antibiotics have been administered, and initial source control of infected foci has

---

[1]Not FDA approved for this indication.

been achieved, other interventions may be appropriate. Many of these are typical components of good critical care.

Cardiac Dysfunction. Patients who have adequate left ventricular filling pressures (as determined by a central venous pressure ≥12 mm Hg) but low cardiac output may benefit from therapy with dobutamine (Dobutrex) to increase cardiac output and improve tissue perfusion.

Corticosteroid Therapy. Activation of the hypothalamic-pituitary axis and the consequent increase in serum cortisol levels are vital aspects of the body's acute stress response to shock. Recent data suggest that critical illness–related corticosteroid insufficiency is more prevalent in septic shock than previously thought, with rates as high as 60%. Therapy with corticosteroids is indicated only for those patients who have continued hypotension in the face of adequate fluid resuscitation and vasopressor support. Hydrocortisone (Solu-Cortef)[1] should be administered intravenously 200–300 mg/day for 7 days, either divided every 6 hours or as a continuous infusion. Dexamethasone (Decadron)[1] should not be used unless hydrocortisone is not available. Because of the unclear long-term benefits and the known immunosuppressive side effects of corticosteroids, patients should be weaned from hydrocortisone as soon as vasopressors are no longer necessary. If another form of corticosteroid other than hydrocortisone is used, then fludrocortisone (Florinef)[1] at a dose of 50 mcg/day should be added for mineralocorticoid effect.

Activated Protein C. Patients who are at increased risk of death with Acute Physiology and Chronic Health Evaluation (APACHE) II scores (https://www.mdcalc.com/apache-ii-score) of 25 or higher and those with multiple organ dysfunction may benefit from infusion of activated protein C (drotrecogin alfa [Xigris]). This drug has numerous contraindications, including current active bleeding, recent (within 3 months) hemorrhagic stroke, recent (within 2 months) severe head trauma or intracranial or intraspinal surgery, trauma with a risk of life-threatening bleeding, presence of an epidural catheter, and intracranial neoplasm or mass lesion or evidence of herniation. It is not recommended for use in children. It is given as a 96-hour continuous infusion.

Glycemic Control. Maintenance of the blood glucose concentration lower than 150 mg/dL is associated with decreased mortality and length of stay in the intensive care unit. Control should be achieved with intravenous insulin, paying close attention to serum glucose levels every 1 to 2 hours until stable, with adjustments made on the basis of a validated protocol. Patients receiving intravenous insulin should simultaneously receive some form of glucose as a calorie source to minimize the risk of hypoglycemia.

Sedation and Paralytics. Sedation and treatment of pain should be aggressively managed according to validated protocols. Daily interruption of sedation allows for more accurate titration of drug and decreases the total time of mechanical ventilation. Paralytics should be avoided or used only briefly if required.

Anticoagulation. Patients should receive prophylaxis for deep venous thrombosis with either low-molecular-weight heparin or unfractionated heparin unless contraindicated by severe thrombocytopenia, recent intracranial bleeding, or coagulopathy. Those patients who cannot receive heparin should receive prophylaxis with graduated compression stockings or intermittent compression devices. Patients who are at especially high risk for deep venous thrombosis (e.g., prior history of clot, orthopaedic surgery, trauma) should receive both pharmacologic and mechanical prophylaxis. Low-molecular-weight heparin is preferred to unfractionated heparin in high-risk patients.

Ulcer Prophylaxis. Patients should receive prophylaxis with a proton pump inhibitor or a histamine 2 (H_2) blocker to prevent upper gastrointestinal bleeding.

Bicarbonate Therapy. There is no role for the administration of bicarbonate to correct acidosis or improve hemodynamic status.

---

[1]Not FDA approved for this indication.

Antibiotics

Antibiotic choices should take into account the most likely pathogens for the suspected site or process. In general, initial empiric therapy (Table 1) should be broad, with an intention to narrow therapy once a microorganism has been isolated or a more precise clinical diagnosis has been made. Such a reevaluation should take place approximately 72 hours after the initiation of therapy. Numerous studies have documented the mortality associated with initial therapy that did not include agents active against the pathogen eventually isolated. In general, drugs from the β-lactam and related classes of antibiotics should be preferred for at least a part of most empiric regimens.

Special considerations include patients with neutropenia and fever, who should always be treated with at least one agent active against *Pseudomonas*. Some debate continues regarding the use of two anti-pseudomonal drugs as part of the initial antibiotic regimen. Given the possibility of resistance on the part of this pathogen, it would seem reasonable to use two drugs initially, until *Pseudomonas* has been isolated (if present) and its susceptibilities are known, allowing coverage to be narrowed. The Surviving Sepsis Campaign guidelines advocate this approach. There is no benefit in treating with two drugs known to be active in an attempt to achieve a supposed synergy.

Patients with hematologic malignancies are at increased risk for sepsis from fungal organisms. Severe sepsis or septic shock in such patients warrants empiric treatment with an echinocandin, a broad-spectrum azole such as voriconazole (Vfend) or posaconazole (Noxafil), or amphotericin (Fungizone).

MRSA continues to increase in incidence nationally and is now common as a community-acquired pathogen. It is also to be suspected as a cause of postinfluenza bacterial pneumonia. Empiric treatment with an antibiotic active against this bacterium, such as vancomycin (Vancocin), linezolid (Zyvox), or daptomycin (Cubicin), should be strongly considered in septic patients in communities where the rate of MRSA in bloodstream infections exceeds 10%. This pathogen should always be considered in a patient with a long-term intravenous catheter, prosthetic device, or other indwelling foreign body. Although vancomycin-resistant *S. aureus* is extremely rare, caution should be taken when using daptomycin and linezolid as empiric therapy, because resistance has been reported.

Prior administration of antibiotics and the attendant risk of infection by a pathogen resistant to the previous therapy should be considered in arriving at a course of empiric therapy. A typical scenario is a patient who presents with a catheter-related bloodstream infection while taking vancomycin. One would expect a gram-negative bacterium, a fungal organism, or, potentially, a vancomycin-resistant enterococcus as the pathogen. Recent hospitalization or residence in a nursing home places patients at risk for colonization and subsequent infection with resistant gram-negative rods.

Prognosis and Limits of Care

Patients who present with severe sepsis or septic shock often have substantial prior medical morbidity, decreasing their chances of survival. The overall mortality rate remains between 20% and 40%. Patients often have expressed wishes regarding limits of care to family members or others close to them before becoming ill. It is always appropriate to discuss goals of therapy, possible and probable outcomes, and plans for further evaluation and treatment with patients (if possible) and their proxies in all instances. Decisions to proceed with or limit care should be made within the context of a patient's expressed or expected wishes and should take into account unfolding clinical data and circumstances. Time spent in this endeavor can substantially decrease the amount of futile care rendered to a patient and lead to care that more truly reflects the patient's wishes regarding life-prolonging measures. The stress and anxiety experienced by family members may also be reduced.

Substantial progress has been made in the past 3 decades in decreasing the mortality associated with severe sepsis and septic shock. Nevertheless, the mortality rate remains unacceptably high, and the overall incidence and severity of disease appear to be

TABLE 1 Empiric Antibiotic Choices for Severe Sepsis*

SOURCE	ANTIBIOTIC AND DOSE	COMMENTS
Community-acquired pneumonia	Ceftriaxone (Rocephin) 2 g q24h *plus* azithromycin (Zithromax) 500 mg q24h	Should include atypical coverage; alternative is moxifloxacin (Avelox)
Health care–associated pneumonia	Piperacillin/tazobactam (Zosyn) 4.5 g q6h *or* meropenem (Merrem)[1] 2 g q8h[3]*plus* vancomycin (Vancocin)[1] 1 g q12h	Should cover for *Pseudomonas* and other resistant gram-negative rods
Neutropenia/fever	Piperacillin/tazobactam[1] 4.5 g q6h *or* meropenem[1] 2 g q8h[3]	Consider empiric fungal coverage for prolonged neutropenia
Abdominal sepsis	Ampicillin/sulbactam (Unasyn) 3 g q6h *or* piperacillin/tazobactam 4.5 g q6h	Consider coverage for yeast, MRSA
Urosepsis	Ampicillin/sulbactam[1] 3 g q6h *or* piperacillin/tazobactam[1] 4.5 g q6h	Obtain imaging and decompression as appropriate
Foreign body/vascular catheter–related sepsis	Piperacillin/tazobactam[1] 4.5 g q6h *or* meropenem[1] 2 g q8h[3] *plus* vancomycin 1 g q12h	Vascular catheters or other foreign bodies should be removed urgently
Meningitis	Ceftriaxone 2 g q12h *plus* vancomycin[1] 750 mg q8h *plus* rifampin (Rifadin)[1] 600 mg q24h	Consider steroid therapy before or simultaneously with administration of antibiotics
Soft-tissue infection	Cefazolin (Ancef) 2 g q8h *plus* vancomycin 1 g q12h	Image for abscess with débridement as appropriate
Necrotizing fasciitis	Ampicillin/sulbactam 3 g q6h *plus* vancomycin 1 g q12h *plus* clindamycin (Cleocin) 900 mg q8h	Obtain urgent surgical consultation
Unknown	Piperacillin/tazobactam 4.5 g q6h *or* meropenem 2 g q8h[3] *plus* vancomycin 1 g q12h *plus* tobramycin (Tobrex) 7 mg/kg q24h	Obtain appropriate imaging studies, especially of abdomen, pelvis, central nervous system

[1]Not FDA approved for this indication.
[3]Exceeds dosage recommended by the manufacturer.
*In all cases, prior antimicrobial therapy, kidney and liver dysfunction, and the probable source of sepsis should be carefully considered. Always consider coverage for methicillin-resistant *Staphylococcus aureus* (MRSA) in areas where incidence in bloodstream isolates is >10%.

increasing, by as much as 1.5% annually by some estimates. The risk of death for an individual patient appears to stabilize approximately 6 months after the original illness. Many patients who do survive remain with the same risk factors (e.g., diabetes, vascular disease, prosthetic devices, immunosuppression) that contributed to their infection and therefore are at risk for recurrence. Moreover, certain organisms, such as MRSA, resistant gram-negative rods, and fungi, remain difficult to treat, and success rates are relatively low despite aggressive, timely, and prolonged therapy.

References

Bone RC: Immunologic dissonance: A continuing evolution in our understanding of the systemic inflammatory response syndrome (SIRS) and the multiple organ dysfunction syndrome (MODS), *Ann Intern Med* 125:680–687, 1996.

Delinger RP, Levy MM, Carlet JM, et al: Surviving Sepsis Campaign: Internatonal guidelines for management of severe sepsis and septic shock—2008, *Crit Care Med* 36:296–327, 2008.

Dombrovskiy VY, Martin AA, Sunderram J, Paz HL: Rapid increase in hospitalization and mortality rates for severe sepsis in the United States: A trend analysis from 1993 to 2003, *Crit Care Med* 35:1244–1250, 2007.

Ibrahim EH, Sherman G, Ward S, et al: The influence of inadequate antimicrobial treatment of bloodstream infections on patient outcomes in the ICU setting, *Chest* 118:146–155, 2000.

Jimenez MF, Marshall JC: Source control in the management of sepsis, *Intensive Care Med* 27(Suppl 1):S49–S62, 2001.

Kumar A, Roberts D, Wood KE, et al: Duration of hypotension before initiation of effective antimicrobial therapy is the critical determinant of survival in human septic shock, *Crit Care Med* 34:1589–1596, 2006.

Leibovici L, Shraga I, Drucker M, et al: The benefit of appropriate empirical antibiotic treatment in patients with bloodstream infection, *J Intern Med* 244:379–386, 1998.

Levy MM, Fink MP, Marshall JC, et al: 2001 SCCM/ESICM/ACCP/ATS/SIS International Sepsis Definitions Conference, *Intensive Care Med* 29:530–538, 2003.

Martin GS, Mannino DM, Easton S, et al: The epidemiology of sepsis in the United States from 1979 through 2000, *N Engl J Med* 348:1546–1554, 2003.

McDonald JR, Friedman ND, Stout JE, et al: Risk factors for ineffective therapy in patients with bloodstream infection, *Arch Intern Med* 165:308–313, 2005.

Miller PJ, Wenzel RP: Etiologic organisms as independent predictors of death and morbidity associated with bloodstream infection, *J Infect Dis* 156:471–477, 1987.

Sasse KC, Nauenberg E, Long A, et al: Long-term survival after intensive care unit admission with sepsis, *Crit Care Med* 23:1040–1047, 1995.

SMALLPOX

Method of
Raul Davaro, MD

CURRENT DIAGNOSIS

- Human-to-human transmission of variola virus occurs by inhalation of large, virus-containing airborne droplets of saliva from an infected person.
- Before smallpox was eradicated, the disease had a secondary household or close contact attack rate of approximately 60% among unvaccinated individuals.
- There are four main clinical forms of smallpox, each with different characteristics.
- During the smallpox era, the case-fatality rate differed for the different clinical forms, but it was approximately 30% overall in unvaccinated individuals.

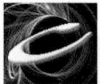

CURRENT THERAPY

- There is no proven treatment for smallpox disease in people sick with smallpox.
- Isolating patients in a negative-pressure room and insuring vaccination is the main course of therapy.

Smallpox is caused by the variola virus (VARV) and is highly infectious by the respiratory route. Susceptible persons have up to a 90% chance of contracting the disease if they are exposed to someone who is infected, and the overall fatality rate is estimated at 30% among those who have not been vaccinated. The VARV is unique among the orthopoxviruses in that it is known to be a sole human pathogen.

The World Health Organization (WHO) declared smallpox eradicated in 1980 and today is the only human disease to be eliminated by the WHO. The eradication of smallpox through vaccination has not eliminated the risk of reintroduction of the infection by the accidental or intentional release of the VARV.

This viral infection, spread by respiratory droplets, continued to have worldwide distribution at the beginning of the 20th century. Because smallpox confers immunity in the survivors of an attack, its persistence depends on the contact of nonimmune persons with infected persons in the initial 2 weeks of acquiring the infection.

The WHO designed an Intensified Eradication Program based on a ring vaccination strategy that began in 1966 and eradicated smallpox from humans in an unprecedented effort in less than 10 years. The last natural case was documented in Somalia in 1977. Routine immunization against smallpox ceased in the United States in 1972 and worldwide in 1980. It was thought that without a human reservoir, the reemergence of this infection would not occur.

Smallpox virus stocks are still available in the United States at the Centers for Disease Control and Prevention (CDC) in Atlanta, Georgia, and in Russia at the State Center for Virology and Biotechnology in Novosibirsk, Siberia. These stocks are maintained under strict biocontainment measures. In the aftermath of the terrorist attacks on September 11, 2001, and the deliberate distribution of *Bacillus anthracis* afterward, President Bush announced plans to immunize health care workers and first responders against smallpox by 2003. Although the plan fell short of its goals, 40,000 first responders and health care workers were vaccinated by the end of 2003.

The Agent

Smallpox is a single, linear, double-stranded DNA virus that belongs to the *Orthopoxvirus* genus, family Poxviridae. The poxviruses replicate in the cell cytoplasm. They are brick shaped and measure about 300 by 250 by 200 nm.

Epidemiology

The natural reservoir of smallpox is the patient suffering from the disease. Smallpox spreads from person to person through droplet nuclei or fine-particle aerosols released from the pharynx of infected persons. Smallpox can also be transmitted by fomites such as clothing and bedding. Smallpox patients are not infectious until the third day of the clinical disease, typically 1 day before the skin eruption. The secondary attack rate of smallpox is 37% to 88% among unvaccinated contacts, depending on many variables.

Clinical Presentation

Smallpox occurs as either variola major or variola minor (alastrim). Variola major had a mortality rate of 30% compared with 1% for variola minor.

After an incubation period of 10 to 14 days, the illness begins with intense prostration and high fever lasting 4 to 6 days (Figure 1). Headache, photophobia, and vomiting are noted. During the prodrome phase, most patients are bedridden. Around the fourth day, the fever breaks and the patient feels better.

The eruptive phase is signaled by an enanthem involving the buccal mucosa and pharynx and a centrifugal exanthem that begins on the face and forearms. The initial rash is macular and turns pustular in 1 to 2 days. Within 2 days, the papules evolve into vesicles that become cloudy and pustular. Most patients exhibit lesions on their soles and palms. A typical feature of variola is that the exanthem everywhere is in the same state of evolution, unlike the exanthem of chickenpox, in which lesions exhibit all stages of evolution. At the end of days 8 to 10, the skin rash crusts and dries; it takes 3 to 4 weeks from the onset of the disease for all the scabs to fall off. The period of contagiousness ends when the last scab falls off. Scarring and pitting of the skin are common sequelae.

Patients with the hemorrhagic disease develop severe prostration, high fever, abdominal pain, petechiae, and extensive cutaneous ecchymoses. In the malignant or flat form, the lesions fail to

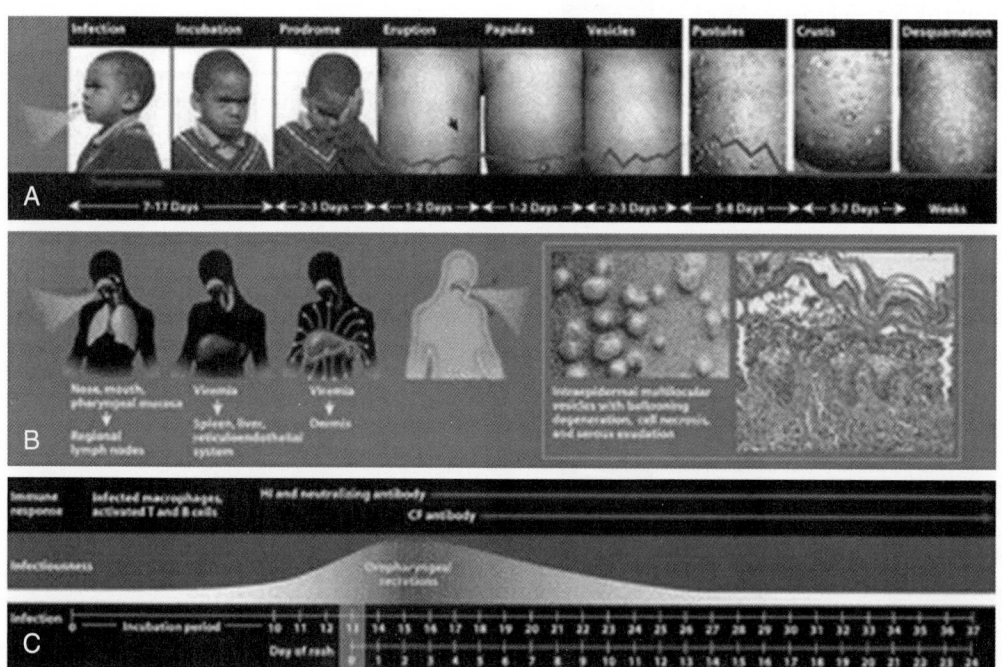

Figure 1 Clinical manifestations and pathogenesis of smallpox and the immune response. **A,** The initial phases of infection and the clinical manifestations include temperature spikes and progressive skin lesions (photographs of lesions courtesy of Dr. David Heymann, World Health Organization). **B,** The pathogenesis of the infection. The photographs on the *right* show the characteristic features of the vesicles caused by smallpox (H&E, × 90). **C,** The immune response to smallpox and the period of infectiousness. *CF,* Complement fixation; *HI,* hemagglutination inhibition. (Reprinted with permission from Breman JG, Henderson DA: Diagnosis and management of smallpox, *N Eng J Med* 346:1300–1308, 2002.)

progress to the pustular stage. In the hemorrhagic and the malignant forms, death invariably occurs within 1 week.

Complications
Bacterial infections of the skin and other organs are common. Ocular involvement may result in blindness. Encephalitis (1 in 500 cases of variola major) is a devastating complication.

Differential Diagnosis (Figure 2)
Many rashes can be confused with smallpox, especially at the outset of the eruption, when the rash is maculopapular. Herpes zoster, chickenpox, herpes simplex, impetigo, scabies, erythema multiforme, and syphilis are some of the conditions that can be confused with smallpox (Box 1). When smallpox was endemic, chickenpox was the most common condition confused with smallpox. The most useful clinical points of smallpox are the following:
- Centrifugal distribution of the lesions
- All the lesions in the same stage of development
- Progression of the rash from the face to the arms, trunk, and legs
- A severe prodrome phase that lasts 4 days
- In an epidemic, known contact with an active case

Diagnosis
The identification of a suspected case of smallpox should be treated as an international health emergency. Clinical samples may be collected from vesicular or pustular fluid, blood, tonsillar swabs, and skin biopsy and must be transported to a biosafety level 4 facility for processing and testing with real-time polymerase chain reaction (PCR) assays to detect virus DNA.

Lesions of varicella zoster virus (chickenpox, herpes zoster) demonstrate multinucleated giant cells on Tzanck smears; lesions of smallpox do not. Serology or electronic microscopy is not recommended for the diagnosis of smallpox because these modalities cannot distinguish among different orthopoxviruses.

Treatment
A suspected case of smallpox should be placed in a negative-pressure room with strict respiratory and contact isolation

---

BOX 1   Conditions That Might Be Confused with Smallpox

Maculopapular stage
Measles
Rubella
Drug eruptions
Secondary syphilis
Erythema multiforme
Scabies, insect bites
Acne
Scarlet fever

Vesicular/Pustular stage
Chickenpox
Disseminated herpes zoster
Disseminated herpes simplex virus
Drug eruptions
Contact dermatitis
Erythema multiforme (including Stevens-Johnson syndrome)
Enteroviral infections
Secondary syphilis
Acne
Generalized vaccinia
Monkeypox
Impetigo
Scabies, insect bites
Disseminated molluscum contagiosum

---

precautions. Ideally, to minimize the risk of contagion in health care personnel, patients with smallpox should be assisted by providers documented to have been immunized against this condition. Patients with smallpox require careful care of their eyes to avoid complications, and this is accomplished with daily eye rinsing. Patients must receive adequate nutrition and hydration. Skin and soft tissue infections must be treated with an antistaphylococcal β-lactam and, initially pending results of cultures, an antimicrobial with activity against methicillin-resistant *Staphylococcus aureus*. Tecovirimat (TPOXX) is an inhibitor of the orthopoxvirus VP37 envelope wrapping protein and is indicated for the treatment of human smallpox disease in adults and pediatric patients weighing at least 13 kg. The effectiveness of TPOXX for treatment of smallpox disease has not been determined in humans because adequate and well-controlled field trials have not been feasible, and inducing smallpox disease in humans to study the drug's efficacy is not ethical. TPOXX efficacy may be reduced in immunocompromised patients based on studies demonstrating reduced efficacy in immunocompromised animal models. The recommended dosage of tecovirimat in adults weighing at least 40 kg is 600 mg (three 200-mg capsules) taken twice daily orally for 14 days. No adequate and well-controlled studies in pregnant women were conducted; therefore, there are no human data to establish the presence or absence of tecovirimat-associated risk. Common adverse reactions in healthy adult subjects (≥2%) were headache, nausea, abdominal pain, and vomiting.

Vaccines and Vaccination
The current smallpox live vaccine, ACAM2000 (Sanofi Pasteur Biologics), is based on the traditional Jenner vaccine (using the related virus, vaccinia) and is administered in a single percutaneous dose. Vaccination after exposure—but before the rash is present—can abort or attenuate the clinical manifestations of the disease. This live vaccine is contraindicated for persons with severe immunosuppression, and newer-generation vaccinations have been developed for these populations. The virus begins growing at the injection site causing a localized infection or "pock" to form. A red, itchy sore spot at the site of the vaccination within 3 to 4 days is an indicator that the vaccination was successful; that is, there is "a take." A blister develops at the vaccination site and then dries up, forming a scab that falls off in the third week, leaving a small scar. If no evidence of vaccine take is apparent after 7 days, the person can be vaccinated again.

The vaccine causes local and systemic symptoms. There is an eruption at the injection site with redness and pain, systemic symptoms such as fever, and headaches. Swelling and tenderness of regional lymph nodes begin 3 to 10 days after vaccination and can last up to a month.

The Modified Vaccinia Ankara (MVA [JYNNEOS]) was compared with ACAM2000. The immune responses and attenuation of the major cutaneous reaction suggest that this MVA vaccine protected against variola infection.

Complications
The vaccine (ACAM2000) is not without risk: it is estimated that pericarditis or myocarditis may develop in 5.7 per 1000 vaccinees. In addition, eczema vaccinatum, generalized vaccinia, progressive vaccinia, and vaccinia encephalitis can also occur (Table 1). The most common complication is inadvertent autoinoculation causing self-limited satellite lesions. Generalized vaccinia results from viremia and may be life threatening in immunocompromised patients. Progressive vaccinia is characterized by necrosis at the inoculation site and distal sites such as bones and internal organs. Progressive vaccinia is often a fatal complication. Myopericarditis was observed with the use of adult vaccines in the United States in 2002 (see Table 1).

Contraindications to Vaccination
Persons who are immune compromised or who have severe eczema or who are pregnant should not receive postexposure

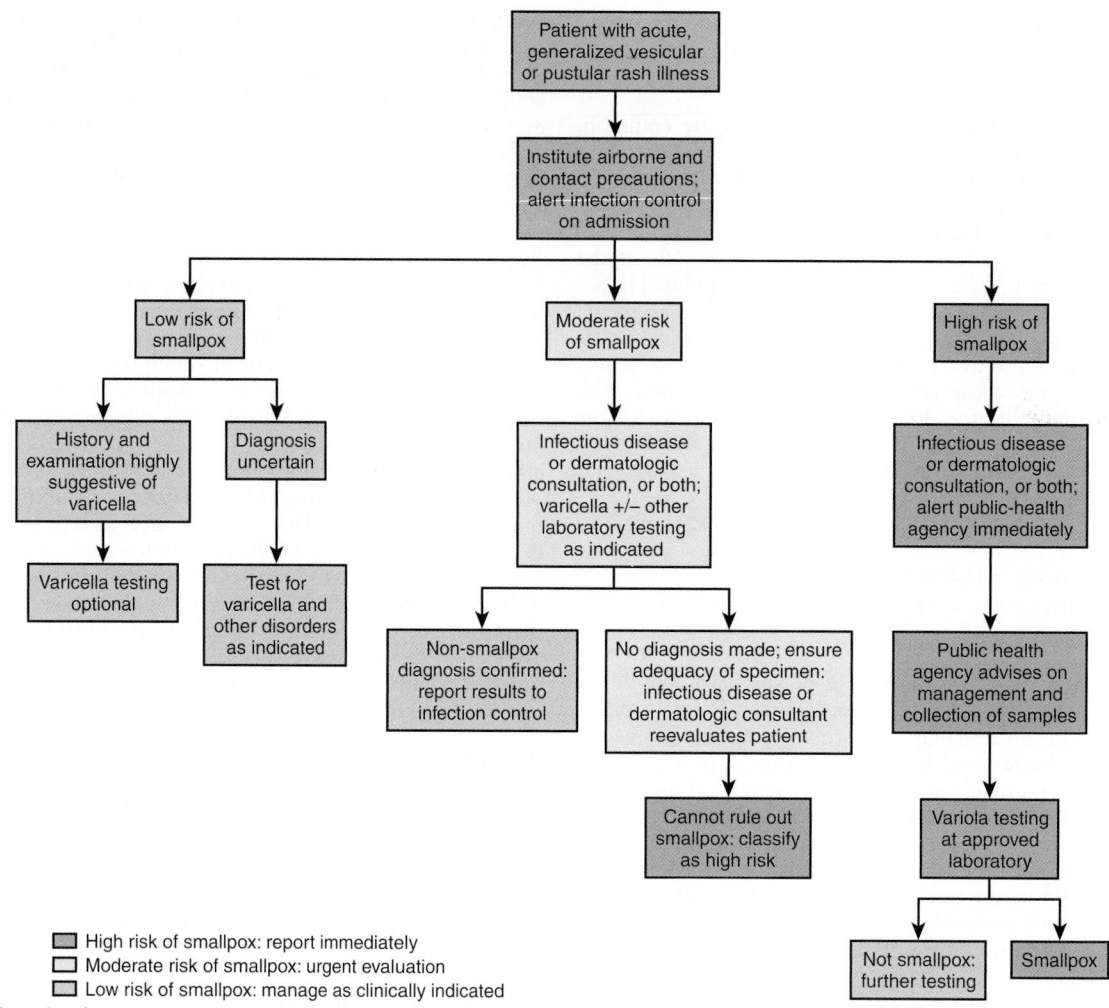

Figure 2 Algorithm for assessing patients for smallpox. (Reprinted with permission from Moore ZS, Seward JF, Lane JM: Smallpox, *Lancet* 367:425–435, 2006.)

TABLE 1	Rates of Complications from Vaccinia, According to Vaccination Status and Age[a]							
	PRIMARY VACCINATION (N = 650,000)				**REVACCINATION (N = 996,000)**			
Complications	0–4 Years	5–19 Years	> 20 Years	All Ages	1–4 Years[b]	5–19 Years	> 20 Years	All Ages
Accidental infection	564	371	606	529	198	48	25	42
Generalized vaccinia	263	140	212	242	0	10	9	9
Erythema multiforme	299	87	30	165	73	2	9	10
Eczema vaccinatum	39	35	30	39	0	2	5	3
Postvaccinal encephalitis	15	9	0	12	0	0	5	2
Progressive vaccinia	3	0	0	2	0	0	7	3
Other	222	214	6636	266	18	24	55	39

[a]Data are from a 1968 survey of 10 states. No deaths occurred.
[b]No children younger than 1 year were revaccinated.
Reprinted with permission from Breman JG, Henderson DA: Diagnosis and management of smallpox, *N Engl J Med* 346:1300–1308, 2002.

vaccination against smallpox. However, in the event of exposure to a patient with smallpox, no absolute contraindication is applicable.

Use in Warfare

Because natural smallpox has been eradicated, the only possibility of a smallpox outbreak is the deliberate release of smallpox in a population by a nation or a terrorist group to inflict casualties in a civilian population. Preemptive vaccination of first responders and ring immunization of those exposed

are the means available to avoid the massive propagation of smallpox. Smallpox stocks have been earmarked for destruction since the eradication of the disease in 1980. Yet, successive meetings of the World Health Assembly have postponed making a final recommendation while the threat of reemergence from elsewhere remains. At its last meeting in September 2018, the Advisory Committee on Variola Virus Research told WHO that live virus is still needed for the development of new antivirals, with split opinions on whether it is needed for diagnostics.

References

Adalja AA, Toner E, Inglesby TV: Clinical management of potential bioterrosism related conditions, *N Engl J Med* 372:954–962, 2015.

Behbehani A: The smallpox story: Life and death of an old disease, *Microbiol Rev* 47:455–509, 1983.

Breman JG, Henderson DA: Diagnosis and management of smallpox, *N Engl J Med* 346:1300–1308, 2002.

Bronze MS, Huycke MM, Machado LJ, et al: Viral agents as biological weapons and agents of bioterrorism, *Am J Med Sci* 323:316–325, 2002.

Centers for Disease Control and Prevention: Smallpox vaccination. Information for Health Care professionals. Available at http://www.bt.cdc.gov/agent/smallpox/vaccination/ [accessed 05.05.15].

Cleri DJ, Porwancher RB, Ricketti AJ, et al: Smallpox as a bioterrorist weapon: Myth or menace? *Infectious Dis Clin North Am* 20:329–358, 2006.

Grosenbach DW, Honeychurch K, Rose EA, et al: Oral tecovirimat for the treatment of smallpox, *N Engl J Med* 379:44–53, 2018.

Kempe HC: Variola. In Beeson PB, McDermott W, editors: *Textbook of Medicine*, ed 12, Philadelphia, 1967, WB Saunders, pp 44–46.

Lofquist J, Weimert NA, Hayney MS: Smallpox: a review of clinical disease and vaccination, *Am J Health Syst Pharm* 60:749–758, 2003.

Moore ZS, Seward JF, Lane JM: Smallpox, *Lancet* 367:425–435, 2006.

Pittman PR, Hahn M, HeeChoon S Lee, et al: Phase 3 efficacy trial of modified vaccinia ankara as a vaccine against smallpox, *N Engl J Med* 381:1897–1908, 2019.

Weiss MM, Weiss PD, Mathisen G, et al: Rethinking smallpox, *Clin Infect Dis* 29:1668–1673, 2004.

Whitley RJ: Smallpox: a potential agent of bioterrorism, *Antiviral Res* 57(7–12), 2003.

TETANUS

Method of
Dilip R. Karnad, MD

Tetanus is a potentially fatal illness caused by the neurotoxin produced by the spore-bearing anaerobic bacterium *Clostridium tetani*. As the causative organism and its spores are ubiquitous, nonimmune individuals in any part of the world may get tetanus unless they are protected by the highly effective vaccine.

Epidemiology

As a result of effective universal immunization, tetanus is rare in the developed world. Twenty to 40 cases of tetanus occur annually in the United States and 12 to 15 cases per year have been reported from the United Kingdom in the last 10 years. Although progressively declining in the developing world due to improved immunization coverage, according to WHO figures, more than 500 cases were reported in 2012 from each of these nations: Angola, Bangladesh, Congo, India, and Uganda. While tetanus may affect individuals of all ages, a significant number of cases in developed countries are elderly people who did not receive a primary immunization or lacked the booster dosage needed to maintain protective immunity. In developing countries, most cases are neonates (*tetanus neonatorum*), children who are born to nonimmunized mothers and thus lack transplacentally acquired passive immunity. Infection of the umbilical stump due to poor hygiene results in severe tetanus that has mortality in excess of 60%.

The infection is caused by the gram-positive, spore-bearing bacterium *C. tetani*, the spores of which exist in the soil, in animal feces, and even in the human gastrointestinal tract. Spores remain dormant and viable for several months and are destroyed by autoclaving at 1 atmosphere pressure at 120°C for 15 minutes. When inoculated into human or animal tissues, they transform into motile bacilli in an anaerobic environment that produce a potent exotoxin, tetanospasmin, which produces the manifestations of tetanus. It must be emphasized that tetanus is not transmitted from human to human, and patients do not require isolation.

Risk Factors

Elderly individuals are at increased risk, as they may not have received adequate immunization or may have waning immunity. Other predisposed groups include immigrants from countries with an unreliable immunization program, immunosuppressed individuals (with HIV infection or receiving immunosuppressive drugs), and intravenous drug addicts. Local factors include wounds with crushed, devitalized tissue or contaminated by dirt or rust, such as open fractures, punctures, and abscesses. However, even scratches, chronic ulcers, or tattooing may cause tetanus. In developing countries, unsafe practices related to termination of pregnancy may cause maternal tetanus; newborn babies born outside of medical facilities are at risk of neonatal tetanus.

Pathophysiology

Tetanospasmin is a highly toxic protein released by *C. tetani*. It is absorbed into the circulation and reaches the ends of motor axons all over the body, from where it is transported proximally along the axonal cytoplasm to motor nuclei in the brainstem and spinal cord at a rate of 3 to 13 mm/hour. A fragment of the toxin then binds inhibitory interneurons that produce gamma-amino butyric acid (GABA) and glycine and inactivates synaptobrevin, a protein that is essential for the release of these neurotransmitters from presynaptic vesicles.

The loss of normal inhibition at motor and autonomic neurons results in spontaneous discharge of nerve impulses as well as exaggerated responses to stimuli manifesting as tonic muscle contraction with superadded intermittent muscle spasms. As tetanospasmin reaches the motor nuclei of the shortest motor axons first, muscles innervated by motor cranial nerves are affected first, followed by trunk muscles, and finally the extremities. Autonomic overactivity results in severe tachycardia, swings in blood pressure, profuse sweating, and (rarely) ileus. An exaggerated startle-like response to stimuli with motor and autonomic components is also typical. Generalized spasms may mimic tonic seizures.

Clinical Manifestations

An attempt should be made to locate the predisposing wound, such as cuts, abrasions, burns, puncture wounds, and other skin lesions. Uncommon causes include needle-sticks in intravenous drug abusers, ulcerated malignant tumors, and chronic middle-ear infection in children (otogenic tetanus). In up to 30% of patients, no site of infection is discovered. The incubation period is the interval between the injury and the onset of symptoms and can range from a few days to a few months (usually 3–21 days). A short incubation period (<7 days) suggests the likelihood of developing severe tetanus; however, a long incubation period does not necessarily indicate a milder disease. The period of onset (the interval between the first symptom and first paroxysmal muscle spasm) is a better predictor of severity: early elective tracheal intubation and mechanical ventilation are usually required if the interval is <48 hours.

Generalized Tetanus

Initial symptoms include an inability to open the mouth (lockjaw or trismus), difficulty in chewing and swallowing, and stiffness of neck muscles. The contraction of facial muscles produces the characteristic sneering smile (*risus sardonicus*) (Figure 1). In severe cases, intermittent spasms are provoked by attempts to speak or swallow. Pooled saliva from hypersalivation and dysphagia may trigger cough and laryngeal spasms; if prolonged, these may prove fatal. Rigidity of paraspinal muscles follows, and hyperextension of the spine results in opisthotonus (Figure 2). Finally, proximal muscles of the extremity are also affected. Deep tendon reflexes are always exaggerated and ankle clonus is common. Tonic muscle spasms may affect head and neck muscles and laryngeal muscles, or may be generalized. Paroxysmal spasms occur spontaneously or in response to loud noise, bright lights, or attempts to speak or swallow. Prolonged spasms may compromise breathing.

The Ablett classification is commonly used to grade the severity of tetanus. Grade I (mild) tetanus is characterized by moderate trismus and general spasticity without spasms, dysphagia, or respiratory distress. Grade II (moderate) tetanus has severe trismus, intermittent short spasms, mild tachypnea, and dysphagia.

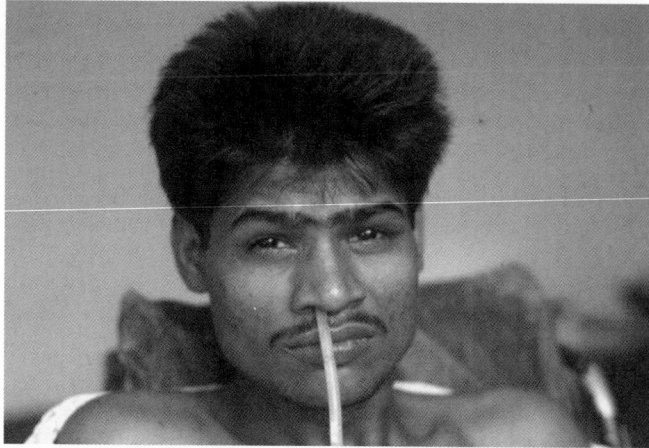

Figure 1 Typical facial expression with the sneering smile *(risus sardonicus)*, wrinkled forehead, narrow palpebral fissures, and "crow's feet" at the lateral palpebral margins from the tonic contraction of muscles of facial expression in moderate tetanus.

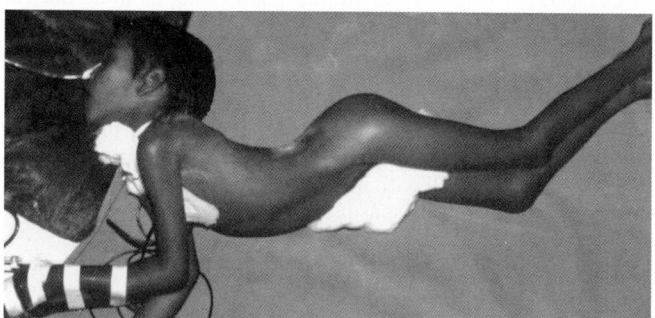

Figure 2 Spasm of paraspinal muscles, producing the hyperextended opisthotonic posture in severe tetanus.

Grade III (severe) tetanus is associated with severe rigidity, prolonged spasms, severe dysphagia, tachypnea, apneic spells, and tachycardia. The presence of additional violent autonomic disturbances with persistent or intermittent episodes of severe hypertension and tachycardia alternating with hypotension and bradycardia is classified as Grade IV (very severe) tetanus. Cardiac arrhythmias, peripheral vasoconstriction, and sudden asystole may also occur in very severe tetanus.

Despite the use of antitetanus immune globulin (HyperTET) to neutralize circulating tetanus toxin, the disease may progress for up to 2 weeks as more intraaxonal toxin continues to reach the central nervous system. Manifestations persist for another 2 to 3 weeks before gradually subsiding. During this period, an apparently stable patient is at risk of developing sudden asphyxia due to severe generalized or laryngeal spasms. Patients may develop fever, rhabodomyolysis, and hyperthermia due to excessive muscular activity.

Cephalic Tetanus
Following injuries to the head or face, in some patients, the toxin reaches the local motor nuclei earlier and produces a combination of partial paralysis and overactivity—more severely affected motor neurons stop functioning while the remaining fibers are overactive and cause muscle spasm (Figure 3).

Localized Tetanus
In this rare form of tetanus, manifestations are restricted to muscles in the region of the wound. These patients have a good prognosis.

Diagnosis
C. tetani can be isolated from the wound in <30% of cases, and microbiological and other laboratory tests do not help in

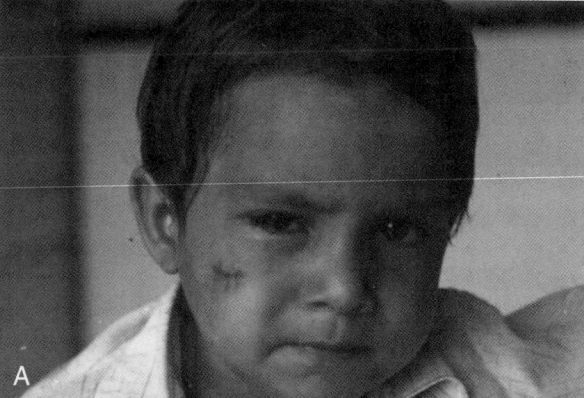

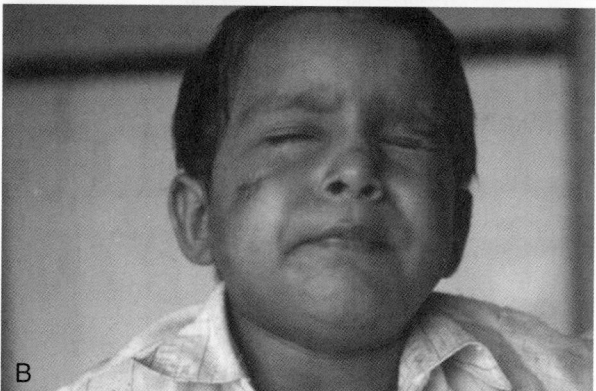

Figure 3 Cephalic tetanus: This 6-year-old child developed mild tetanus 3 weeks after a wound on his right cheek was sutured. He had cephalic tetanus characterized by partial paralysis of the right facial nerve along with overactivity of the unaffected nerve fibers. **A,** Note the overactivity of the facial muscles with a narrow palpebral and prominent nasolabial fold on the same side as the injury. On asking him to shut his eyes tight (**B**), weakness of the orbicularis oculi and other facial muscles on the right side become manifest.

confirming the diagnosis. The diagnosis is entirely clinical. In an individual with a predisposing injury, the presence of trismus, rigidity of neck, abdominal and paraspinal muscles, and severe hyperreflexia are suggestive. The spatula test is a useful bedside test: A spatula (tongue depressor) is inserted into the mouth to touch the posterior pharyngeal wall. Normally, a gag reflex is activated in an attempt to expel the spatula. In tetanus, severe spasms of the masseters results in the patient biting on the spatula, making it difficult to withdraw—a positive test. In one study, the spatula test was positive in 94% of patients with tetanus and in none without tetanus. The electromyogram shows the continuous discharge of motor units in moderate tetanus and the absence of the normal silent period.

Differential Diagnosis
While the diagnosis of tetanus is easy in severe tetanus, it may be mistaken for other conditions in its initial stages (Table 1). The spatula test is negative in other conditions causing trismus. Abdominal muscles usually relax after adequate sedation. As in spasticity due to cord compression, deep reflexes are exaggerated; however, the plantar response, which is extensor in spinal cord disorders, is always flexor with tetanus. Unlike seizures or other intracranial diseases, the patient with tetanus is always fully alert and awake.

Treatment
In patients with life-threatening spasms, prompt, adequate sedation is the first step in management. Patients must be observed in an intensive care unit because the disease may rapidly worsen. They should be nursed in a quiet, dimly lit room in order to keep

TABLE 1 Conditions that Mimic Clinical Manifestations of Tetanus

CLINICAL FEATURE	DIFFERENTIAL DIAGNOSIS
Trismus	Acute tonsillar abscess, temporomandibular joint disease, extraptramidal reaction to drugs, dental pathology
Neck stiffness	Cervical spine disease; extrapyramidal reaction to drugs such as antipsychotics, antiemetics, or metoclopramide; meningitis; subarachnoid hemorrhage
Abdominal rigidity	Acute abdomen
Dysphagia	Myasthenia gravis, acute bulbar paralysis, rabies
Muscle spasms	Seizures, spasticity due to spinal cord disease, stiff man syndrome

external stimuli to a minimum—this is difficult in modern intensive care units.

Neutralization of Toxin

Although unsupported by randomized studies, human tetanus immune globulin (HyperTET) (3000–6000 units) is administered intramuscularly to neutralize the circulating toxin. This does not bind to the toxin that has already entered neurons. There is insufficient evidence favoring intrathecal administration[1] of tetanus immune globulin over the usual intramuscular route, although one randomized study showed a shortening of the course of tetanus. Equine antiserum[2] (10,000–20,000 units) may be administered after skin testing for hypersensitivity. Though rarely used today due to the risk of anaphylaxis or serum sickness, it has the advantage of being administered intravenously.

Control of Clostridial Infection

Benzylpenicillin (Penicillin G) in a dose of 10 to 12 million units per day is given intravenously for 10 days. In one study, metronidazole (Flagyl) (500 mg every 6 hour for 10 days) was superior to procaine penicillin (Wycillin),[1] presumably because procaine and penicillin are GABA antagonists and may worsen manifestations of tetanus. However, a more recent study showed that a single intramuscular injection of 1.2 million units of benzathine penicillin (Bicillin LA)[1] was as effective as benzylpenicillin or metronidazole. Fortunately, resistance to these antibiotics has not been reported. Debridement of the infected wound and abscess drainage should be performed after spasms have been adequately controlled.

Control of Muscle Spasms

Benzodiazepines (diazepam [Valium] or lorazepam [Ativan][1]) are the preferred drugs and act by enhancing the effect of GABA on its receptor on the postsynaptic membrane, thus potentially antagonizing the effect of tetanospasmin. However, as very little GABA is released in tetanus, large doses (up to 1000 mg/day[3]) of diazepam may be required to achieve adequate sedation and muscle relaxation. Diazepam may be administered intravenously (10–30 mg in 5 mg boluses every 5 minutes)[3] or through a nasogastric tube (10–40 mg every 1 to 2 hours).[3] Barbiturates and chlorpromazine (Thorazine)[1] are alternative agents. Other sedative hypnotic agents such as midazolam (Versed)[1] and propofol (Diprivan)[1] have also been used with good effect. In mild to moderate tetanus, drug doses can be titrated to achieve moderate sedation and control rigidity and spasms without causing respiratory depression. In severe cases, however, spasms may not be controlled despite large doses,

increasing the risk of severe central nervous system (CNS) depression. In these patients, heavy sedation combined with neuromuscular blockade and mechanical ventilation is required. In about 10% of cases, benzodiazepines may produce paradoxical excitation instead of sedation; increasing doses make the patient more wakeful, agitated, and delirious, with increased spasms. Discontinuation of diazepam and the use of barbiturates and chlorpromazine may prevent the need for paralysis and mechanical ventilation. Pancuronium (Pavulon),[1] vecuronium (Norcuron),[1] and rocuronium (Zemuron)[1] are often used for neuromuscular blockade. Atracurium (Tracrium)[1] could also be used but may have unfavorable cardiovascular effects. Intravenous and intrathecal baclofen (Lioresal Intrathecal)[1] have been used in some case.

Airway Management

Tracheostomy or endotracheal intubation is required in moderate and severe tetanus to prevent respiratory failure due to laryngeal spasm and aspiration of oropharyngeal secretions. In most developing countries, elective tracheostomy is performed early in severe tetanus. In countries with superior intensive care facilities, heavy sedation, neuromuscular blockade, endotracheal intubation, and mechanical ventilation are preferred, with tracheostomy being reserved for those who need prolonged ventilation.

Control of Autonomic Disturbances

With good intensive care, mortality due to respiratory failure has been drastically reduced. Autonomic dysfunction is now the major challenge in patients with severe tetanus; it is common even in sedated and paralyzed patients. Various measures to control autonomic fluctuations include intravenous fluid loading, oral and parenteral beta-blockers, alpha-blockers, centrally acting sympatholytics such as clonidine (Catapres)[1] or dexmedetomidine (Precedex),[1] and epidural or spinal bupivacaine (Marcaine).[1] More recently, infusion of dexmedetomidine has been used by some authors. Many patients may develop sudden asystole, possibly due to sudden parasympathetic discharge, catecholamine-induced myocardial damage, or sudden loss of sympathetic drive. Consequently, the use of long-acting antiadrenergic drugs should be avoided. Increasing the level of sedation itself is also effective, to a significant extent.

The agent most frequently used for autonomic dysfunction is intravenous magnesium sulfate.[1] A randomized controlled trial in Vietnamese patients showed that magnesium sulfate did not decrease mortality, ICU stay, or the need for mechanical ventilation but did reduce the dose of sedatives and neuromuscular blocking drugs required. This study used a loading dose of 40 mg/kg over 30 minutes, followed by intravenous infusion of 2 g/hour in patients >45 kg and 1 to 5 g/hour in patients ≤45 kg. Infusion was titrated to maintain serum magnesium levels between 2 and 4 mmol/L.

Other Measures

Continuous muscle hyperactivity and spasms greatly increase caloric requirements. Most patients require nasogastric tube feeding because of trismus and dysphagia. A catabolic state similar to sepsis may develop in very severe tetanus. Consequently, patients lose up to 15% of their body weight during the illness. Good nursing care is essential to prevent pressure sores, deep vein thrombosis, stress ulcers, and aspiration pneumonia. Urinary catheterization is required in most patients as urinary retention is common and distension of the urinary bladder may provoke spasms and autonomic overactivity. All patients should be started on a primary immunization schedule against tetanus.

Complications

Respiratory failure may occur due to laryngeal obstruction, prolonged spasm of respiratory muscles, aspiration pneumonia, or

---

[1]Not FDA approved for this indication.
[2]Not available in the United States.
[3]Exceeds dosage recommended by the manufacturer.

[1]Not FDA approved for this indication.

sedative drugs. Severe spasms may result in tongue-bite, compression fractures of midthoracic vertebrae, rhabdomyolysis, myoglobinuria, and renal failure. Rarely, patients may develop acute respiratory distress syndrome (ARDS) either due to tetanus itself or as a result of secondary bacterial sepsis. Cardiac arrhythmias and sudden asystole are common in patients with autonomic dysfunction. Acute myocardial infarction may occur in elderly patients with underlying coronary artery disease due to sympathetic overactivity. Deep vein thrombosis and pressure sores are preventable complications. The overall mortality ranges from 40% to 60% in countries with inadequate health care facilities. With good intensive care, mortality as low as 10% is reported in some series. Mortality is higher in neonates, the elderly, and patients with a short incubation period and period of onset.

Prevention

Adsorbed tetanus toxoid (Tt), derived from formaldehyde-treated tetanus toxin, is extremely effective in inducing active immunity. It is available as a single-antigen preparation or in combination with diphtheria toxoid as pediatric diphtheria-tetanus toxoid (DT) or adult tetanus-diphtheria (Td), and with both diphtheria toxoid and acellular pertussis vaccine as DTaP (Infanrix, Tripedia) or Tdap (Adacel, Boostrix) (lower-case alphabets indicate lower doses of antigens). Pediatric vaccines (DT and DTaP) contain identical amounts of tetanus toxoid as adult vaccines, but three to four times as much diphtheria toxoid. The usual schedule for primary immunization in children <7 years consists of four doses of DTaP or DT at age 2, 4, 6, and 15 to 18 months. A booster dose is recommended at 4 to 6 years of age. In individuals aged 7 years or older, three doses of the adult formulation are administered; the second dose is given 4 to 8 weeks after the first, and the third dose after another 4 to 6 months. Further booster doses are needed every 10 years to maintain antibody titers above the protective level of 0.1 IU/mL.

After administration of Tt to individuals with wounds, protective titers of antibody are achieved after at least 2 weeks. Consequently, passive immunization with 250 units of human tetanus immune globulin (HyperTET) or 1500 units of equine antitetanus serum[2] administered intramuscularly is needed to confer protection during these initial few weeks. This is especially required in individuals with tetanus-prone wounds who have not received at least three doses of tetanus toxoid in the past. Previously unimmunized individuals with clean, minor, nontetanus prone wounds do not need any passive immunization, but should receive active immunization. Passive immunization is not necessary in those who have received three or more doses of the toxoid. These individuals should receive a dose of Tt (or Td) if more than 10 years have elapsed since the last booster dose and they have nontetanus prone wounds or if >5 years have elapsed after the booster dose and they have a tetanus-prone wound. In countries where neonatal tetanus is common, primary immunization of women during pregnancy has been advocated as a public health program to prevent neonatal tetanus.

References

Apte NM, Karnad DR: The spatula test: A simple bedside test to diagnose tetanus, *Am J Trop Med Hyg* 53:386–387, 1995.
Centers for Disease Control and Prevention: In Atkinson W, Wolfe S, Hamborsky J, editors: *Epidemiology and Prevention of Vaccine-Preventable Diseases*, ed 12, Washington, DC, 2011, Department of Health and Human Services, Centers for Disease Control and Prevention, pp 291–299.
Farrar JJ, Yen LM, Cook T, et al: Tetanus, *J Neurol Neurosurg Psychiatry* 69:292–301, 2000.
Gibson K, Uwineza JB, Kiviri W, Parlow J: Tetanus in developing countries: A case series and review, *Can J Anaesth* 56:307–315, 2009.
Lisboa T, Ho YL, Filho GTH, et al: Guidelines for the management of accidental tetanus in adult patients, *Rev Bras Ter Intensiva* 23:394–409, 2011.
Rodrigo C, Samarakoon L, Fernando SD, Rajapakse S: A meta-analysis of magnesium for tetanus, *Anaesthesia* 67:1370–1374, 2012.
Roper MH, Vandelaer JH, Gasse FL: Maternal and neonatal tetanus, *Lancet* 370:1947–1959, 2007.
Thwaites CL, Yen LM, Loan HT, et al: Magnesium sulphate for treatment of severe tetanus: A randomized controlled trial, *Lancet* 368:1436–1443, 2006.
Trujillo MH, Castillo A, Espana J, et al: Impact of intensive care management on the prognosis of tetanus. Analysis of 641 cases, *Chest* 92:63–65, 1987.

TICKBORNE RICKETTSIAL DISEASES (ROCKY MOUNTAIN SPOTTED FEVER AND OTHER SPOTTED FEVER GROUP RICKETTSIOSES, EHRLICHIOSES, AND ANAPLASMOSIS)

Method of
Robert Wittler, MD

CURRENT DIAGNOSIS

- Early diagnosis of Rocky Mountain spotted fever (RMSF) and other tickborne rickettsial diseases is made clinically. RMSF should be considered in the setting of fever, headache, rash, and a history of possible tick exposure. The rash is not always present and typically occurs 2 to 4 days after the onset of fever.
- Diagnostic laboratory tests for rickettsial diseases, particularly RMSF, are usually not helpful in making a timely diagnosis during the initial states of illness.
- Tickborne rickettsial diseases can be confirmed by polymerase chain reaction (PCR) during the acute stage if readily available (whole blood for ehrlichiosis and anaplasmosis and skin biopsy or whole blood for RMSF) or at later stages by subsequently demonstrating a fourfold increase between acute and convalescent (ideally 2 to 4 weeks apart) serum immunoglobulin G (IgG) indirect immunofluorescence antibody titers. PCR of whole blood for RMSF has low sensitivity, although sensitivity increases in patients with severe disease.
- Typical findings of ehrlichiosis and anaplasmosis include fever, headache, malaise, leukopenia, thrombocytopenia, and elevated serum transaminases. Rash is often not present.

CURRENT THERAPY

- Treatment of choice for all tickborne rickettsial diseases in patients of all ages (including children less than 8 years of age) is doxycycline (Vibramycin).
- The dose for doxycycline is 100 mg twice daily (intravenously [IV] or orally depending on severity of illness) for adults. For children weighing <45 kg,[1] the recommended dose is 2.2 mg/kg/dose IV or orally twice daily.
- Delay in recognition and appropriate treatment is the most important factor associated with death from RMSF. Empiric treatment within 5 days of the onset of symptoms with doxycycline is the best way to prevent morbidity and death. Treatment decisions should never be delayed while awaiting laboratory confirmation, nor should treatment be discontinued solely on the basis of a negative test result with an acute-phase specimen.
- Although optimal duration of therapy has not been well studied, a common treatment course for RMSF and ehrlichiosis is at least 3 days after the patient defervesces (typically the minimum total course is 5–7 days) or longer for severe illness. Anaplasmosis should be treated for 10 days to provide appropriate therapy for possible coinfection with *Borrelia burgdorferi*.
- Historically chloramphenicol has been recommended for the treatment of RMSF during pregnancy based on adverse effects of older tetracycline drugs (but not specifically doxycycline). Although there is limited evidence, doxycycline has not been associated with teratogenicity or maternal hepatic toxicity during pregnancy, and doxycycline has been used successfully to treat tickborne rickettsial disease in several pregnant women without adverse effects.

- Chloramphenicol is not an alternative treatment for human monocytic ehrlichiosis (HME) or HGA. Chloramphenicol treatment of RMSF has been associated with a greater risk of death compared with doxycycline treatment.
- Limited case report data suggest that rifampin[1] can be used as an alternative to doxycycline for the treatment of confirmed (RMSF ruled out) mild anaplasmosis during pregnancy or with documented tetracycline allergy.

[1]Not FDA approved for this indication.

Tickborne rickettsial diseases in humans often share clinical features but are epidemiologically and etiologically distinct. In the United States included diseases are (1) Rocky Mountain spotted fever (RMSF) caused by *Rickettsia rickettsii*; (2) other spotted fever group (SFG) rickettsioses, caused by *Rickettsia parkeri* and *Rickettsia* species 364D; (3) *Ehrlichia chaffeensis* ehrlichiosis, also called human monocytic ehrlichiosis (HME); (4) other ehrlichioses, caused by *Ehrlichia ewingii* and *Ehrlichia muris*-like agent; and (5) anaplasmosis, caused by *Anaplasma phagocytophilum*, also called human granulocytic anaplasmosis (HGA). The reported incidence of tickborne rickettsial diseases has increased in the United States. Tickborne rickettsial diseases, especially RMSF, continue to cause severe illness and death in otherwise healthy adults and children, despite the availability of effective antibiotic therapy. SFG rickettsioses (including RMSF), ehrlichioses, and anaplasmosis are nationally notifiable diseases in the United States. Providers report potential cases to state or local health departments. In 2010, the reporting category of RMSF was changed to spotted fever rickettsiosis, as serology does not readily distinguish RMSF from other SFG rickettsioses.

Epidemiology

Tickborne rickettsial pathogens are maintained in natural cycles involving domestic or wild vertebrates and ticks. The epidemiology of each disease reflects the geographic distribution and seasonal activities of the tick vectors and the natural vertebrate hosts, as well as the human activities resulting in tick exposure. Although cases have been reported in every month, most cases occur during April to September, coincident with peak levels of tick host-seeking activity.

RMSF is the rickettsiosis in the United States that is associated with the highest rates of severe and fatal outcomes. The case-fatality rate in the preantibiotic era was ~25%. Current case-fatality rates are estimated at 5% to 10%. From 2008–2012, the estimated average annual incidence from passive surveillance of SFG rickettsioses was 8.9 cases per million persons. Reported annual incidence has increased during the past two decades. The highest incidence occurs in persons aged 60 to 69 years, and the highest case-fatality rate is among children aged <10 years. Additional epidemiologic risk factors for fatal RMSF include age ≥40 years, alcohol abuse, and glucose-6-phosphate dehydrogenase deficiency. From 2008 to 2012, 63% of reported SFG rickettsiosis cases came from Arkansas, Missouri, North Carolina, Oklahoma, and Tennessee. SFG rickettsiosis has been reported from all the contiguous 48 states and the District of Columbia.

In the United States, the tick species most frequently associated with transmission of *R rickettsii* is the American dog tick, *Dermacentor variabilis*, which is found primarily in the eastern, central, and Pacific Coast regions. The Rocky Mountain wood tick, *Dermacentor andersoni*, is associated with transmission in the western United States. Larval and nymphal stages of most *Dermacentor* spp ticks usually do not bite humans. Adult *D variabilis* and *D andersoni* ticks bite humans, but the principal hosts are deer, dogs, and livestock.

The brown dog tick, *Rhipicephalus sanguineus*, which is located throughout the United States, is an important vector in parts of Arizona and along the United States–Mexico border. All stages (larvae, nymphs, and adults) of *Rh sanguineus* bite humans

and can transmit *R rickettsia*. Domestic dogs are the preferred host. On Arizona tribal lands, the warm climate and proximity of ticks to domiciles (tick-infested dogs) provide a suitable environment for *Rh sanguineus* to remain active year-round, resulting in cases of RMSF in Arizona every month of the year.

Rickettsia parkeri is transmitted by the Gulf Coast tick, *Amblyomma maculatum*. *R parkeri* rickettsiosis cases have not been documented in children, and no fatal cases have been reported. The first confirmed case of Rickettsia species 364D was in 2010 and likely transmitted by the Pacific Coast tick, *Dermacentor occidentalis*. All reported cases have been from California.

The average annual incidence of ehrlichiosis from 2008 to 2012 was 3.2 cases per million persons, with the most common cause being *E chaffeensis*. The highest incidence is in persons aged 60 to 69 years. The case fatality rate is ~3% and is highest among children aged <10 years, adults aged ≥70 years, and immunosuppressed persons. *E chaffeensis* is transmitted to humans by the lone star tick, *Amblyomma americanum*, which is the most commonly encountered tick in the southeastern United States, with a range that extends into areas of the Midwest and New England. Arkansas, Delaware, Missouri, Oklahoma, Tennessee, and Virginia have the highest reported incidence. The white-tailed deer is an important natural reservoir for *E chaffeensis*, and most cases occur during May to August.

The principal vector for *E ewingii* ehrlichiosis is also *A americanum*. Cases have primarily been reported from Missouri. No fatal cases of *E ewingii* ehrlichiosis have been reported. *Ehrlichia muris*–like agent (EML) has recently been recognized as a human pathogen. Reported cases have been from Minnesota and Wisconsin. The blacklegged tick, *Ixodes scapularis*, is an efficient vector for EML in experimental studies. EML agent DNA has been detected in *I scapularis* collected in Minnesota and Wisconsin but has not been detected in *I scapularis* from other states.

The incidence of human anaplasmosis during 2008–2012 was 6.3 cases per million persons. Incidence is highest in the northeastern and upper midwestern states, and the geographic range seems to be expanding. The case fatality rate is <1%. *I scapularis* is the vector for *Anaplasma phagocytophilum* in the northeastern and midwestern United States, whereas the western blacklegged tick, *Ixodes pacificus*, is the principal vector along the West Coast. The seasonality is bimodal, with the first peak June–July and a smaller peak in October, corresponding to the emergence of the adult stage of *I scapularis*. *I scapularis* also transits *Borrelia burgdorferi* (Lyme disease), *Babesia microti* (babesiosis), *Borrelia miyamotoi* (tickborne relapsing fever), and deer tick virus (a cause of tickborne encephalitis). Simultaneous infections with *A phagocytophilum* and *B burgdorferi* or *B microti* have occurred.

Pathophysiology

The agents causing RMSF, ehrlichiosis, and anaplasmosis are all obligate intracellular pathogens, but the target host cells they infect and subsequent pathology vary by organism.

R rickettsii is transmitted from the tick to humans via a painless bite, which often goes unrecognized. The organism resides in the salivary gland of the tick and is passed during acquisition of a blood meal. *R rickettsii* can be transmitted as early as 10 to 24 hours after tick attachment. When transmitted to a human host, *R rickettsia* localize and multiply in vascular endothelial cells, and, less commonly, underlying smooth muscle cells of small and medium vessels, resulting in vasculitis. The vasculitis is the underlying mechanism for most of the clinical features and laboratory abnormalities of RMSF. Injury to the vascular endothelium results in increased capillary permeability, microhemorrhage, and platelet consumption. Late-stage complications of pulmonary edema (acute respiratory distress syndrome) and cerebral edema are consequences of the microvascular leakage.

E chaffeensis predominantly infects monocytes and tissue macrophages and replicates in cytoplasmic vacuoles called morulae. Unlike RMSF, direct vasculitis and endothelial injury are rare in human monocytic ehrlichiosis. Frequent pathologic findings include granuloma formation, myeloid hyperplasia, and megakaryocytosis in the bone marrow. The severe pathology and multiorgan involvement in severe and fatal HME in immunocompetent patients is believed to be due to dysregulation of the host immune response that leads to tissue damage and eventually multiorgan failure. *E ewingii* has a predilection for neutrophils, and morulae can be observed in granulocytes of the blood, cerebrospinal fluid (CSF), and bone marrow.

A phagocytophilum is found predominantly in neutrophils in the peripheral blood and tissues from infected individuals. *A phagocytophilum* has the unique ability to selectively survive and multiply within cytoplasmic vacuoles (morulae) of polymorphonuclear cells by delaying their apoptosis. Infection with *A phagocytophilum* induces a systemic inflammatory response, which is believed to be the mechanism for tissue damage. Pathologic findings with human granulocytic anaplasmosis include normocellular or hypercellular bone marrow, erythrophagocytosis, hepatic apoptosis, focal splenic necrosis, and mild interstitial pneumonitis and pulmonary hemorrhage.

Clinical Manifestations

A detailed history should include information about known tick bites or activities that might be associated with tick exposure. Unrecognized tick bites are common. A history of a tick bite within 14 days of illness onset is reported in only 50% to 60% of RMSF cases and 68% of ehrlichiosis cases. Absence of a tick bite should never dissuade providers from considering tickborne rickettsial disease in the appropriate clinical context. Contact with pets, especially dogs, and a history of tick attachment or recent tick removal from pets can be useful in assessing human tick exposure.

Tickborne rickettsial diseases commonly have nonspecific clinical signs and symptoms early in the course of disease. Although there is overlap in the clinical presentations of tickborne rickettsial diseases, the frequency of certain associated signs and symptoms (e.g., rash and other cutaneous findings) and typical laboratory findings differ by pathogen and assist providers in developing a differential diagnosis, beginning appropriate antibacterial treatment, and ordering confirmatory diagnostic tests.

Symptoms of RMSF typically begin 3 to 12 days after the bite of an infected tick or 4 to 8 days after discovery of an attached tick. The incubation period is generally shorter (≤5 days) in patients who develop severe disease. Initial symptoms are often nonspecific and include the sudden onset of fever, chills, malaise, and myalgia. Clinical suspicion for RMSF should be maintained in cases of nonspecific febrile illness and sepsis of unclear cause, particularly during the spring and summer months.

The classic triad of fever, rash, and reported tick bite is present in only a minority of RMSF patients during the initial presentation to health care; therefore it is crucial not to wait for development of this triad before considering a diagnosis of RMSF and beginning treatment. A rash typically occurs 2 to 4 days after the onset of fever; however, many patients initially seek medical care before the rash. In one large series of patients with RMSF, 88% of patients had a rash, but only 49% had a rash in the first 3 days. Children more frequently have rash (97%) and develop the rash earlier. The rash typically begins as small, blanching macules on the ankles, wrists, or forearms that then spreads to the palms, soles, arms, legs, and trunk, usually sparing the face. The generalized petechial rash appears later (day 5 or 6) and is indicative of advanced disease. An inoculation eschar is rarely present with RMSF. In addition to rash, the most frequent clinical findings at any point in the illness are fever (99%), headache (91%), and myalgia (82%).

The total white blood cell count is typically normal or mildly increased with RMSF, and increased numbers of immature neutrophils are often present. Thrombocytopenia, slight elevations of AST or ALT, and hyponatremia might be present, particularly as the disease advances. Laboratory values cannot be relied on to guide early treatment decisions because they are often within or slightly deviated from normal reference values

early in the course. When CSF is obtained, a lymphocytic (less commonly neutrophilic) pleocytosis can be present, along with a moderately elevated CSF protein. CSF glucose is generally normal.

R parkeri rickettsiosis is a milder illness compared with RMSF; no severe manifestations or death has been reported. Symptoms develop a median of 5 days (range, 2–10 days) after the bite of an infected tick. The first manifestation in nearly all patients is an inoculation eschar, which generally is nonpruritic, nontender or mildly tender, and surrounded by an indurated, erythematous halo and occasionally a few petechiae. Shortly after the onset of fever (0.5–4 days later), a nonpruritic maculopapular or vesicopustular rash develops in 90% of patients. The rash primarily involves the extremities and trunk and in ~half of patients involves the palms and soles. Headache (86%) and myalgia (76%) are common. Laboratory findings include modest elevation of hepatic transaminases (78%), mild leukopenia (50%), and thrombocytopenia (40%).

Few patients with *Rickettsia* species 364D have been reported, so the full clinical spectrum has yet to be described. It does appear to be relatively mild and characterized by an eschar or ulcerative skin lesion with regional lymphadenopathy. Fever, headache, and myalgia occur, but rash has not been a notable feature.

Symptoms of *E chaffeensis* ehrlichiosis typically occur a median of 9 days (range, 5–15 days) after an infected tick bite. Fever (96%), headache (72%), malaise (77%), and myalgia (58%) are common. Abdominal pain, vomiting, and diarrhea can occur, particularly in children. Rash (maculopapular, petechial, or diffuse erythema) occurs in approximately one-third of patients and is more frequent in children. The rash occurs a median of 5 days after illness onset and can involve the palms and soles. Neurologic manifestations are present in ~20% of patients. Characteristic laboratory findings in the first week include leukopenia, thrombocytopenia, and elevated levels of hepatic transaminases. *Ehrlichia ewingii* and *Ehrlichia muris*-like agent ehrlichiosis have similar clinical and laboratory features as *E chaffeensis* ehrlichiosis, although rash and gastrointestinal symptoms are less common.

Symptoms of human granulocytic anaplasmosis typically occur 5 to 14 days after an infected tick bite. Fever (92%–100%), headache (82%), malaise (97%), and myalgia (77%) are common. Rash is present in <10% of patients, and central nervous system involvement is rare. Laboratory findings are similar to ehrlichiosis.

Diagnosis

Early diagnosis and initiation of treatment of tickborne rickettsial diseases is based on clinical and epidemiologic findings, as rapid confirmatory assays are often not available or reliable to guide treatment decisions early in the clinical course. Confirmatory diagnostic tests are serologic assays, nucleic acid detection, immunostaining of biopsy tissue, blood-smear microscopy, and culture.

Assays using paired acute and convalescent sera (ideally collected 2–4 weeks apart) are the standard for serologic confirmation. Assays are insensitive during the first week of rickettsial infection. After 7 days of illness, the sensitivity increases. Assays are highly sensitive 2 to 3 weeks after illness onset. Early therapy with doxycycline may diminish or delay the development of antibodies in RMSF.

A diagnosis of tickborne rickettsial diseases is confirmed with a ≥fourfold increase in antibody titer in patients with a clinically compatible acute illness. A single IgG antibody reciprocal titer ≥64 is supportive of, but not confirmatory for, the diagnosis. In the United States, *R rickettsia*–reactive IgG antibody reciprocal titers ≥64 can be found in 5% to 10% of the population who do not acutely have RMSF. Some laboratories also perform assays for IgM antibodies. However, because of the lower specificity of IgM compared with IgG assays, IgM titers should not be used as a stand-alone method for diagnosis.

PCR amplification of DNA from whole blood specimens collected during the acute stage of illness is particularly useful for confirming *E chaffeensis*, *A phagocytophilum*, *E ewingii*, and EML agent infections due to the tropism of those organisms for circulating cells. PCR detection of *R rickettsia* in whole blood is less sensitive, as low numbers of rickettsiae typically circulate in the blood in the absence of advanced disease. Tissue specimens such as a skin biopsy are a more useful source of SFG rickettsial DNA compared with blood samples. Doxycycline treatment decreases the sensitivity of PCR. Obtaining blood before treatment is recommended to decrease false-negative results.

Immunostaining of a skin punch biopsy is useful for diagnosing RMSF with 100% specificity and 70% sensitivity. Microscopic examination of blood smears or buffy-coat preparations during the first week of illness may reveal leukocyte morulae in patients infected with *E chaffeensis* or anaplasmosis, although it is relatively insensitive, and accuracy is dependent on having experienced microscopists. Culture is the reference standard for microbiologic diagnosis, but the agents that cause tickborne rickettsial diseases require cell culture techniques that are not widely available.

Differential Diagnosis
The differential diagnosis of fever and rash is broad, and during the early stages of illness tickborne rickettsial diseases can be indistinguishable from many viral exanthams, particularly in children. In addition to viral infections, conditions that should be considered include meningococcemia, Kawasaki disease, secondary syphilis, disseminated gonococcal infection, bacterial endocarditis, scarlet fever, leptospirosis, typhoid, drug eruptions, Stevens-Johnson syndrome, toxic shock syndrome, and thrombotic thrombocytopenic purpura.

Treatment
Doxycycline is the drug of choice for treatment of all tickborne rickettsial diseases in patients of all ages and should be initiated immediately in persons with signs and symptoms suggestive of rickettsial disease. Treatment decisions should never be delayed awaiting laboratory confirmation. Multiple studies have noted a delay in appropriate treatment of tickborne rickettsial diseases, particularly after the fifth day of illness for RMSF, to be a significant potentially preventable risk factor for severe disease, increased mortality rates, and long-term sequelae. Because of the nonspecific signs and symptoms of tickborne rickettsial diseases, concomitant empiric treatment for other conditions in the differential diagnosis should be administered (e.g., treatment with ceftriaxone for meningococcemia).

The recommended dose of doxycycline is 100 mg twice daily (IV or oral) for adults and 2.2 mg/kg twice daily (IV or oral) for children weighing <45 kg.[1] Oral therapy is appropriate for patients with early-stage disease who can be treated as outpatients. The recommended duration of therapy for RMSF and ehrlichiosis is at least 3 days after fever resolves and until evidence of clinical improvement is noted; typically, the minimum total course is 5 to 7 days. Severe or complicated disease could require a longer course. HGA should be treated for 10 days to provide appropriate therapy for possible coinfection with Lyme disease.

The use of doxycycline to treat children with suspected tickborne rickettsial disease should no longer be a subject of controversy. The American Academy of Pediatrics and CDC recommend doxycycline as the treatment of choice for children of all ages with suspected tickborne rickettsial disease. Doxycycline used at the recommended dose and duration for RMSF in children aged <8 years, even after multiple courses, has not resulted in tooth staining or enamel hypoplasia.

Chloramphenicol in the past was used as an alternative drug for treating RMSF. However, chloramphenicol has been associated with a higher risk of death compared to patients treated with a tetracycline; in vitro evidence indicates that chloramphenicol is not effective treatment for ehrlichiosis or anaplasmosis. Chloramphenicol is no longer available in the oral form in the United States, and the IV form is not readily available at all institutions.

Chloramphenicol has been recommended for the treatment of RMSF during pregnancy based on adverse effects of older tetracycline drugs (but not specifically doxycycline). Although there is limited evidence, doxycycline has not been associated with teratogenicity or maternal hepatic toxicity during pregnancy, and doxycycline has been used successfully to treat tickborne rickettsial diseases in several pregnant women without adverse effects.

Rifamycins demonstrate in vitro activity against *E chaffeensis* and *A phagocytophilum*. Case reports document favorable outcomes in small numbers of pregnant women treated with rifampin for anaplasmosis. Rifampin[1] could be an alternative for treatment of confirmed mild anaplasmosis (RMSF ruled out) during pregnancy or documented allergy to tetracycline-class drugs. Rifampin is not acceptable treatment for RMSF or potential coinfection with *B burgdorferi*.

Treatment of symptom-free persons seropositive for tickborne rickettsial disease is not recommended, regardless of past treatment, because antibodies can persist for months to years after infection.

Monitoring and Complications
Fever with tickborne rickettsial diseases typically subsides within 24 to 48 hours when treated with doxycycline in the first 4 to 5 days of illness. Lack of a clinical response within 48 hours of early treatment with doxycycline could indicate the illness is not a tickborne rickettsial disease, and alternative diagnoses or coinfection should be considered. Severely ill patients may require >48 hours of treatment before clinical improvement is noted. Patients with mild disease treated on an outpatient basis need close follow-up to ensure they are responding appropriately.

Patients with evidence of organ dysfunction, severe thrombocytopenia, mental status changes, or the need for supportive therapy should be hospitalized. Other considerations for hospitalization include the likelihood and ability to take oral medication and existing comorbid conditions, including the patient's immune status. Infection with RMSF and to a somewhat lesser extent HME are most likely to have a severe disease or death. Severe, late-stage manifestations of RMSF include meningoencephalitis, acute respiratory distress syndrome (ARDS), acute renal failure, arrhythmia, and seizures. Severe manifestations of HME include ARDS, shock-like syndromes, renal failure, hepatic failure, coagulopathies, and hemorrhagic complications.

Severe or life-threatening manifestations are less frequent with anaplasmosis than with RMSF or HME. Predictors of a more severe course of anaplasmosis include advanced age, immunosuppression, comorbid medical conditions, and delay in diagnosis and treatment. Confirmed *A phagocytophilum* coinfection has been reported in <10% of patients with Lyme disease. Response to treatment can provide clues to possible coinfection with Lyme disease or babesiosis. If the clinical response to treatment with doxycycline is delayed, coinfection or an alternate infection should be considered. Conversely, if Lyme disease is treated with a beta-lactam antibiotic in a patient with unrecognized *A phagocytophilum* infection symptoms could persist.

Prevention
The best prevention for all the tickborne rickettsial diseases is to avoid tick bites, perform regular tick checks on humans and pets, and promptly remove attached ticks. Longer periods of tick attachment increase the probability of transmission of tickborne diseases. Repellents and protective clothing can reduce the risk for tick bites. Products containing 20% to 30% N,N-Diethyl-meta-toluamide (DEET) effectively repel ticks and can be applied directly to the skin. DEET is not recommended for use on infants younger than 2 months. Permethrin-treated or -impregnated clothing can significantly reduce tick bites. Prophylactic treatment is not recommended in persons who have had recent tick bites and are well.

---

[1] Not FDA approved for this indication.

References

Biggs HM, Behravesh CB, Bradley KK, et al: Diagnosis and management of tick-borne rickettsial diseases: Rocky Mountain spotted fever and other spotted fever group rickettsioses, ehrlichioses, and anaplasmosis—United States, *MMWR Recomm Rep* 65:1–44, 2016.

Buckingham SC, Marshall GS, Schutze GE, et al: Clinical and laboratory features, hospital course, and outcome of Rocky Mountain spotted fever in children, *J Pediatr* 150:180–184, 2007.

Cross R, Ling C, Day NPJ, McGready R, Paris DH: Revisiting doxycycline in pregnancy and early childhood—time to rebuild its reputation? *Expert Opin Drug Saf* 15:367–382, 2016.

Dahlgren FS, Holman RC, Paddock CD, Callinan LS, McQuiston JH: Fatal Rocky Mountain spotted fever in the United States, 1999–2007, *Am J Trop Med Hyg* 86:713–719, 2012.

Hamburg BJ, Storch GA, Micek ST, Kollef MH: The importance of early treatment with doxycycline in human ehrlichiosis, *Medicine (Baltimore)* 87:53–60, 2008.

Helmick CG, Bernard KW, D'Angelo LJ: Rocky Mountain spotted fever: clinical, laboratory, and epidemiological features of 262 cases, *J Infect Dis* 150:480–488, 1984.

Ismail N, McBride JW: Tick-borne emerging infections: ehrlichiosis and anaplasmosis, *Clin Lab Med* 37:317–340, 2017.

Kirkland KB, Wilkinson WE, Sexton DJ: Therapeutic delay and mortality in cases of Rocky Mountain spotted fever, *Clin Infect Dis* 20:1118–1121, 1995.

Marshall GS, Stout GG, Jacobs RF, et al: Antibodies reactive to Rickettsia rickettsii among children living in the southeast and south central regions of the United States, *Arch Pediatr Adoles Med* 157:443–448, 2003.

TOXIC SHOCK SYNDROME

Method of
Alwyn Rapose, MD

CURRENT DIAGNOSIS

- Clinical diagnosis: High index of suspicion when there is a combination of fever, rash—initially erythematous followed by desquamation, hypotension, and multiorgan injury.
- There needs to be a thorough search for a focus of infection like retained foreign body or tampon, deep-seated abscess or peritonitis, necrotizing fasciitis, or postoperative wound infection.
- Blood cultures and deep tissue cultures (from the site of the suspected infection) are recommended in all cases.

CURRENT THERAPY

- Aggressive fluid resuscitation.
- Broad antibiotic coverage initially, followed by deescalation to target the organism identified in cultures.
- Intravenous immunoglobulin may help in patients who fail to respond to standard care.

Introduction

Toxic shock syndrome (TSS) is an acute illness, which as the name suggests is caused by a toxin, and the patient presents with hypotension (shock) and multiorgan involvement (syndrome). It was initially described in children with *Staphylococcus aureus* infection, but a similar syndrome is associated with *Streptococcus* infections as well as clostridial infections in children and adults. Different toxins—acting either directly or via different cytokine pathways—have been implicated in the pathogenesis of the disease. TSS carried a high mortality risk (40% to 60% in streptococcal TSS). However, early recognition and aggressive interventions have resulted in much improved outcomes in the era of modern medicine.

Historical Aspects

A review of the medical literature indicates this was first described in 1978 when J. Todd and colleagues reported a collection of seven cases in children. In the early years following its description, a majority of cases were seen in young menstruating women who used tampons, with the onset of illness within a few days of onset of their menstrual period. A large number of investigators evaluated tampons, contraceptive sponges, sanitary pads, and other medical and surgical materials and as the medical community became more familiar with this syndrome, there was a decrease in tampon-associated TSS and an increased incidence of nonmenstrual TSS associated with respiratory infections, necrotizing skin infections, deep-seated abscesses, and postoperative infections including gynecologic surgeries.

TSS is classically associated with *S. aureus* infection. The clinical features included fever, skin rash, hypotension, and multiorgan involvement with various combinations of respiratory, renal, and hepatic injury. Similar features following infection with *Streptococcus pyogenes* (*group A Streptococcus* [GAS] as well as other streptococci) resulted in a description of streptococcal toxic shock–like syndrome (TSLS). In patients with complications of medical or spontaneous abortions and infection with *Clostridium species* similar clinical features were seen along with very high mortality, and this condition was also included when describing TSS.

Pathogenesis

The *S. aureus* isolates from patients with menstruation-related TSS revealed a toxin that was first called toxic shock syndrome toxin 1 (TSST-1). Since then, however, multiple other toxins associated with *S. aureus* (enterotoxins B-F) have been described to be associated with TSS. Similarly, streptococcal exotoxins (A, B, and C)—superantigens—are potent activators of T lymphocytes and can also directly cause high fever (pyrotoxins) and shock, as well as tissue damage.

These bacterial toxins induce production of tumor necrosis factor (TNFα), interferons (IFNγ), interleukins (IL-1, IL-2), and other cytotoxins by human monocytes and lymphocytes that result in a cascade of proinflammatory cytokines (cytokine storm). These cytokines are responsible for fever, damage to vascular endothelium resulting in tissue injury, as well as the loss of intravascular volume and hypotension.

In contrast, clostridial infection is associated with direct tissue damage by secreted clostridial toxins.

Clinical Features

The surveillance case definition developed by the Centers for Disease Control and Prevention (CDC) included five clinical criteria: Fever, rash, hypotension, and involvement of three or more organ systems. The rash usually subsided with desquamation, which is the fifth clinical criterion. The patient may have prodromal symptoms like myalgia, arthralgia, and headache. Fever associated with a diffuse erythematous skin rash (sheets of erythema) involving the face trunk and extremities is rapidly followed by hypotension, decreased urine output, and features of septic shock (Figures 1 through 3). Detailed history taking and a thorough clinical examination is essential to determine the focus of infection—either menstrual tampon, retained foreign body, necrotizing infection in a closed space (fasciitis), postoperative wound infection, or, more recently described, peritonitis-associated TSS. Subtle differences between TSS and TSLS have been described. Clostridial infection following septic abortion or other gynecologic surgery is associated with severe abdominal and pelvic pain, uterine tenderness (endometritis), and a foul-smelling vaginal discharge. A delay in diagnosis and intervention results in a rapid progression of systemic involvement. A cytokine storm in the lungs can result in respiratory complications like acute respiratory distress syndrome (ARDS), and there can be acute renal injury secondary to hypotension or toxin-induced acute interstitial nephritis, shock liver, and in severe situations, altered mental status. In the recovery phase, the erythematous rash subsides with desquamation.

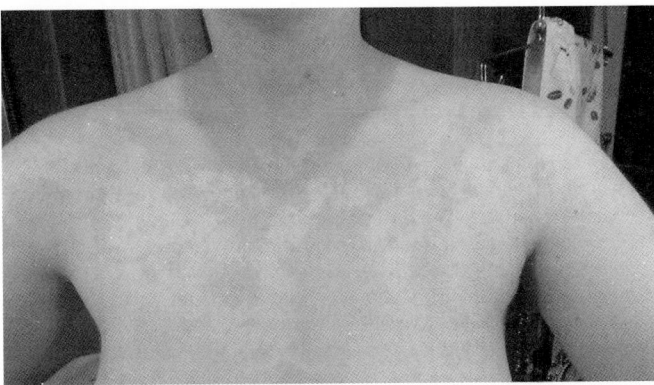

Figure 1 Diffuse erythematous rash on the trunk.

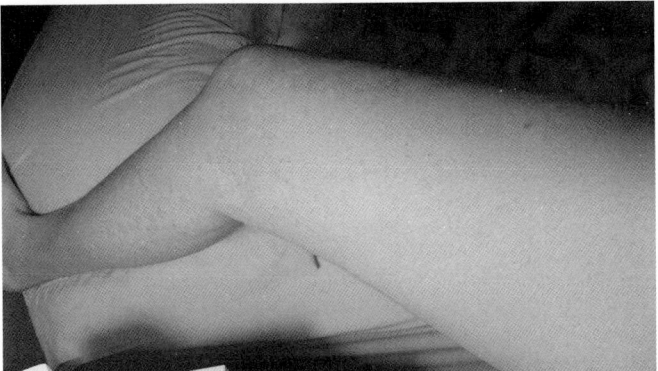

Figure 2 Diffuse erythematous rash on the lower extremity.

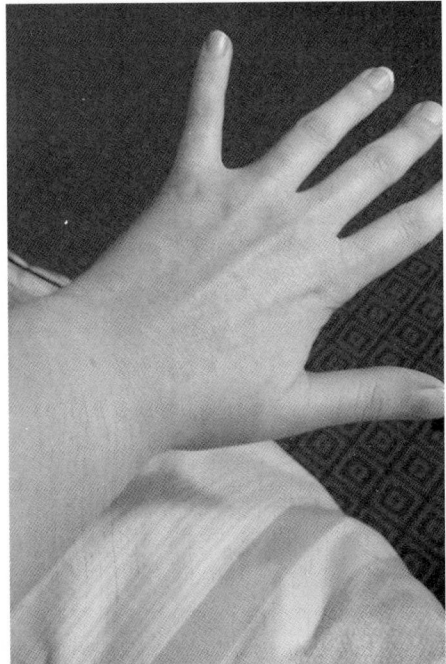

Figure 3 Diffuse erythematous rash on the upper extremity.

Management

Early diagnosis, rapid intervention with intravenous (IV) fluids, IV antibiotics as well as IV immunoglobulin (IVIG)[1] in some circumstances, along with supportive therapy like mechanical ventilation in patients with respiratory failure and dialysis for patients with severe renal injury, are key to survival in patients with TSS. Patients in circulatory shock are treated in an intensive

[1]Not FDA approved for this indication.

care unit with ionotropic agents such as norepinephrine (Levophed) and vasopressin (Pitressin) to provide pressor support. A multidisciplinary team, including intensivists, infectious disease specialists, pulmonologists, and nephrologists, is required for the management of these patients because they often develop respiratory failure and acute renal injury.

Removal of the focus of infection—be it an infected tampon, retained products of conception, surgical drainage of deep-seated abscess, aggressive debridement in patients with necrotizing fasciitis, or postoperative wound infection—is an essential component in the management of TSS.

Blood cultures should be obtained at presentation, and tissue cultures should be obtained at the time of surgery. Ascitic fluid cultures are essential in cases with suspected peritonitis.

Patients should be initially treated with aggressive IV fluid resuscitation along with antibiotic combinations that will provide broad coverage against *Staphylococcus*, *Streptococcus*, and anaerobic organisms. Vancomycin (15 to 20 mg/kg every 12 hours) along with a carbapenem (meropenem [Merrem] 1 g every 8 hours, imipenem [Primaxin] 500 mg every 6 hours, or ertapenem [Invanz] 1 g every 24 hours), or vancomycin along with piperacillin-tazobactam (Zosyn 4.5 g every 6 to 8 hours) (though there has been reported a higher risk of nephrotoxicity with this compared to the combination of vancomycin with carbapenem) is often the first choice for broad coverage. These antibiotics need dose adjustments based on a patient's renal function. In addition, antibiotics like clindamycin (600 to 900 mg every 8 hours) and linezolid (Zyvox 600 mg every 12 hours) are included because of their direct antitoxin effect (suppress toxin production and accelerate phagocytosis). These antibiotics do not need renal dose adjustments. When the patient is on vancomycin, there should be close monitoring of vancomycin troughs or vancomycin area under the curve, as well as creatinine, to optimize vancomycin dosage and reduce the risk of nephrotoxicity. If linezolid is used, vancomycin will not be required. Newer agents like ceftaroline (Teflaro 600 mg every 12 hours) also provide coverage against methicillin-resistant *S. aureus* (MRSA). The results of microbiology cultures help guide the final antibiotic choice (deescalation of antibiotics). If an infection is caused by a *Streptococcus* species, and no *S. aureus* is identified, vancomycin/ceftaroline can be discontinued and IV penicillin (12 to 24 million units per day as a continuous infusion or in six divided doses) combined with clindamycin is recommended. The duration of antibiotic therapy depends on the patient's clinical response. IVIG[1] has been used in patients who are failing standard therapy. It probably acts by providing antiinflammatory mediators and antibodies against some of the toxins and superantigens and has been shown to improve survival especially in TSLS.

New Research and Developments

Newer antibiotics recently approved for use in skin and skin structure infections, including dalbavancin (Dalvance), oritavancin (Orbactiv), delafloxacin (Baxdela), and omadacycline (Nuzyra), have great coverage against *S. aureus*, including MRSA and *Streptococcus*. However, these have not been approved for use in TSS.

There is ongoing research into the development of immunological agents (monoclonal antibodies and vaccines) that can target toxins and other superantigen-induced cytokine pathways. These nonantibiotic therapies have the potential to block the toxin-induced shock without the side effects commonly associated with antibiotic use.

[1]Not FDA approved for this indication.

References

Burnham JP, Kollef MH: Understanding toxic shock syndrome, *Intensive Care Med* 41(9):1707–1710, 2015.

Emgard J, Bergsten H, McCormick JK, et al: MAIT cells are major contributors to the cytokine response and group A streptococcal toxic shock syndrome, *Proc Natl Acad Sci USA* 116(51):25923–25931, 2019.

Jayouhey E, Bolze PA, Jamen C, et al: Similarities and differences between staphylococcal and streptococcal toxic shock syndromes in children: results from a 30-case cohort, *Front Pediatr* 6:360, 2018.

Krakauer T: FDA-approved immunosuppressants targeting staphylococcal super antigens: mechanisms and insights, *Immunotargets Ther* 6:17–29, 2017.

Krakauer T: Staphylococcal superantigens: pyrogenic toxins induced toxic shock, *Toxins (Basel)*. 11(3), 2019.

Linner A, Darenberg J, Sjolin J, et al: Clinical efficacy of poly-specific intravenous immunoglobulin therapy in patients with streptococcal toxic shock syndrome: a comparative observational study, *Clin Infect Dis* 59(6):851–857, 2014.

Reingold AL, Hargrett NT, Shands KN, et al: Toxic shock syndrome surveillance in the United States. 1980 to 1981, *Ann Intern Med* 96(6 Pt 2):875–880, 1982.

Shibl AM: Effect of antibiotics on production of enzymes and toxins by microorganisms, *Rev Infect Dis* 5(5):865–875, 1983.

Tierno Jr PM, Hanna BA: Ecology of toxic shock syndrome: amplification of toxic shock syndrome toxin 1 by materials of medical interest, *Rev Infect Dis* 11(Suppl 1):S182–S186, 1989.

Todd J, Fishaut M: Toxic-shock syndrome associated with phage-group-1 staphylococci, *Lancet* 2:1116–1118, 1978.

Wannamaker LW: Streptococcal toxins, *Rev Infect Dis*(5 Suppl 4)S723–S732, 1983.

Zumla A: Super antigens, T cells and microbes, *Clin infec Dis* 15(2):313–320, 1992.

TOXOPLASMOSIS

Method of
Carlo Contini, MD

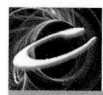

CURRENT DIAGNOSIS

- The diagnosis of *Toxoplasma gondii* infection mostly relies on serologic detection of specific IgM and IgG antibodies.
- Specific IgM antibodies with low IgG (IgG-avidity testing) are consistent with recent infection in immunocompetent persons. Positive IgG antibodies in the absence of IgM in healthy persons indicate past infection and resistance to reinfection.
- Amniocentesis and polymerase chain reaction (PCR)–based analysis on amniotic fluid (AF) [past 18 weeks' gestation] are useful to establish a certain or presumed seroconversion in pregnancy and to determine whether the infection was transmitted to the offspring.
- IgM, IgA, or both at birth indicate probable congenital infection.
- Serologic testing is not useful for the diagnosis of TE in AIDS patients, who should instead undergo computed tomography (CT) or magnetic resonance imaging (MRI), cerebrospinal fluid (CSF)–*T-gondii* DNA PCR testing, or demonstration of tachyzoites by histology.
- Serologic screening is helpful in identifying transplant patients at risk, especially seronegative recipients with seropositive donors, and can help in establishing the diagnosis by showing seroconversion. Serologic follow-up combined with PCR after allogeneic hematopoietic stem cell transplantation (HSCT) is recommended in all patients at risk for toxoplasmosis.

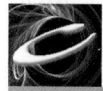

CURRENT THERAPY

- All immunocompetent patients, as well as nonpregnant women with acute toxoplasmosis presenting with lymphadenitis and fever, generally do not require specific antimicrobial treatment because the infection is self-limited and usually subclinical.
- Pyrimethamine (Daraprim) plus sulfadiazine[1] plus folinic acid (Leucovorin)[1] is the standard and preferred regimen against toxoplasmosis. It is recommended for acute *T gondii* infection in immunocompetent adults with acute illness; pregnant women who acquire the infection after 18 weeks' gestation or in whom fetal infection is documented (positive PCR-AF); and immunosuppressed patients, including AIDS patients. Patients who do not tolerate the standard regimen should be given alternative drugs such as clarithromycin (Biaxin),[1] azithromycin

(Zithromax),[1] atovaquone (Mepron),[1] and dapsone.[1]
- Trimethoprim-sulfamethoxazole (TMP-SMX, Bactrim)[1] has been shown to have efficacy similar to pyrimethamine-sulfadiazine and may be used as an alternative if patients do not have sulfa allergy and pyrimethamine is not tolerated or is not available.
- Oral spiramycin (Rovamycine)[2] is the drug most often used in the prenatal therapy of congenital toxoplasmosis (before 18 weeks of gestation) because of high concentration in placenta without crossing it and of its relative lack of toxicity compared with the teratogenic effects of pyrimethamine. Spiramycin is more efficacious when administered early after maternal seroconversion.
- TMP-SMX[1] should be given as a prophylaxis to HIV-positive patients who have CD4+ cell counts that are less than 100/mm³ and IgG *T gondii* antibodies and who are not already receiving a PCP prevention regimen, as well as to patients with active toxoplasmosis, transplant patients, and workers after accidental laboratory exposure.
- In ocular toxoplasmosis, corticosteroid therapy, if given, should be always monitored to prevent severe tissue destruction.
- Universal prophylaxis with TMP/SMX in allo pre-HCTSP patients should be implemented by all transplantation programs.

[1]Not FDA approved for this indication.
[2]Not commercially available in the United States.

Toxoplasma gondii is a ubiquitous protozoan parasite that is extremely widespread and of great medical importance, infecting all mammalian cells and responsible for human and veterinary diseases. It was initially described in Tunis by Nicolle and Manceaux (1908) in the tissues of the rodent gundi (*Ctenodactylus gundi*) and later in Brazil by the microbiologist Alfonso Splendore (1908) in the rabbit. Its identification was rapidly followed by the recognition that it was a human pathogen. In this regard, the Italian bacteriologist Castellani (1914) was probably the first to describe a *T gondii*–like parasite in smears of blood and spleen from a 14-year-old Singhalese boy who died of a disease characterized by severe anemia, fever, and splenomegaly. However, it was not until the 1960s and 1970s that the parasite was identified as a coccidian and the cat recognized as the definite host.

Toxoplasma belongs to the phylum *Apicomplexa*, which contains many other protozoan pathogens of human and veterinary importance, such as *Plasmodium* spp. (malaria), *Cryptosporidium* spp (cryptosporidiosis), and *Eimeria* spp (poultry coccidiosis).

Disease can occur through acute infection after recent contact with *T gondii* cysts or oocysts or through endogenous reactivation. Primary infection is usually subclinical, but in some patients cervical or occipital lymphadenopathy or ocular disease is present. Infection acquired during pregnancy can cause severe damage to the fetus if *Toxoplasma* crosses the placental barrier, and it causes abortion or congenital birth defects if the mother becomes infected for the first time shortly before or during pregnancy.

In patients with AIDS and others who are immunocompromised, reactivation of latent disease can cause life-threatening encephalitis. Ocular infection by *Toxoplasma* is a major cause of retinochoroiditis in several geographic areas in both immunocompetent and immunocompromised persons. Due to the heterogeneous parasitologic outcomes and limited immunological data, the role of aging in toxoplasmosis evolution remains poorly understood.

Epidemiology and Risk Factors

Toxoplasmosis is a cosmopolitan zoonotic disease that has important implications for public health because it affects one-third of the world's population. It is also a significant veterinary pathogen that can infect many species of warm-blooded animals. *T gondii* is one of the world's most successful parasites, in part because of its ability to infect and persist in most warm-blooded animals. In general, the prevalence in animals is much higher than

VIII Infectious Diseases

that in humans. In China, among the major animals monitored, pigs were the most frequently infected by *T gondii*, reaching 70% in some areas and farms. This high *T gondii* prevalence increases the risks of human infection through meat consumption, because pork is the main meat Chinese people consume. Among other meat-producing animals, sheep and chickens have also high *T gondii* infection rates, and economic losses caused by abortions and other diseases from sheep toxoplasmosis are predicted to be huge in the forthcoming decades.

In humans, the incidence of positive serology for *Toxoplasma* varies greatly around the world and is influenced by different cultures. In Colombia, approximately half of the women of childbearing age have *T gondii* antibodies, and the clinical disease in congenitally infected children is more severe than in Europe. In humans, seroprevalence of *T gondii* infection rises with age; does not vary greatly between sexes; and is lower in cold regions, hot and arid areas, and at high elevations. Prevalence rates, which range worldwide from <10% to >60%, are thought to depend on food production and harvesting practices, water treatment, environment, climate, and exposure to soil or sand. In the United States, the seroprevalence of *T gondii* appears to be declining. Seroprevalence in Europe is high, up to 54% in southern European countries; it decreases with increasing latitude to 5% and 10% in northern Sweden and Norway, respectively. As is the case of most other protozoa, the prevalence of *Toxoplasma* is higher in Africa, South America, and in developing areas of the world. In Brazil, there is a higher prevalence of *T gondii* infection among male patients (79.0%) than among female patients (63.4%), according to data obtained from a blood bank.

The sexual cycle of *T gondii* occurs in felines. The estimated seroprevalence for *T gondii* in domestic cats (*Felis catus*), worldwide, is 30% to 40%. Most feline infections occur postnatally through ingestion of infected tissue cysts or rarely oocysts, although congenital infections occur. Tens of millions of unsporulated oocysts may be released in the feces of a single cat in a day, depending on the stage of *T gondii* ingested. These sporulate in 1 to 21 days and are highly infectious to the parasite's intermediate hosts (asexual cycle), which include almost any warm-blooded animal, such as birds, humans, and sea otters.

Sporulated oocysts are very resistant to environmental conditions and to disinfectants; however, they are killed within 1 to 2 minutes by heating to 55°C to 60°C, and the risk of infection is reduced by deep-freezing meat (–12°C or lower) before cooking.

Feline infections are typically subclinical. Common symptoms of *T gondii* infection in cats can include fever, ocular inflammation, anorexia, lethargy, abdominal discomfort, and neurologic abnormalities. Occasionally, pneumonia, liver damage, and loss of vision develop. Why only some cats show symptoms is not known.

Identification of locally prevalent risk factors is critical for health education, and it is generally important for policy. The most important recognized factors influencing the risk of *T gondii* infection are having a cat or a dog, doing household work, having a lower education level, having poor hygiene habits, eating raw vegetables, and working in contact with soil.

Most people are infected inadvertently, and thus the specific route of transmission usually cannot be established. Contact with this obligate intracellular protozoan can occur through the ingestion of oocysts containing sporozoites or cysts containing bradyzoites in contaminated food or water. The major risk factors for *T gondii* exposure are directly related to exposure to cats and more specifically to cat feces, which represent the source of ingestion of sporozoites from the environment. Because cats are the primary host for *T gondii*, cats in the house or stray cats in and around the house or property are considered a primary risk factor for acquiring this parasite during pregnancy. Moreover, any job or activity that puts a pregnant woman in direct contact with soil, sand, or materials such as fruit, vegetables, or drinking water that could have been contaminated by cat feces puts her at risk for being infected. In this setting, rain and surface water can transport infectious oocysts into drinking water supplies and

irrigation waters. Coprophagous insects that can contaminate food and fertilizer also contribute to the spread of oocysts. Climate plays an indirect role in allowing better (in the case of moist and hot climate) or worse (in the case of dry and cold climate) survival of oocysts in the environment.

Consumption of undercooked meat of secondary hosts such as pigs and sheep is also a major route of transmission of the disease to humans. The ingestion of undercooked or raw meat during pregnancy is also an important risk factor, because the tissue can contain *T gondii* cysts that, unless destroyed by cooking or by food-preparation practices, could infect a pregnant woman. Heating at 60°C to 100°C for 10 minutes, freezing at either –10°C for 3 days or –20°C for 2 days, or irradiation at doses of 75 to 100 kilo rad is sufficient to kill tissue cysts. Tissue cysts are also killed by gamma irradiation at a dose of 1.0 kGy, but irradiation of meat has not been approved in the European Union (EU). Neither cooking in a microwave oven nor chilling at 5°C for 5 days is sufficient to kill tissue cysts.

The risk of infection rises also in women who taste meat when preparing meals or who eat raw or undercooked beef, lamb, or other meats, but not pork. Eating raw horsemeat imported from non-EU countries can expose consumers to high inocula of highly virulent atypical *T gondii* strains, which can cause a life-threatening primary infection or severe congenital toxoplasmosis with atypical outcome. Transmission during breast-feeding or direct human-to-human transmission other than from mother to fetus (discussed later in the chapter) has not been recorded. Drinking unpasteurized milk and consuming milk products also correlates with increased risk of infections. Although oral transmission is considered the main route of infection, it does not explain the common occurrence of toxoplasmosis in a variety of hosts, such as herbivorous animals, birds, and wild rodents. In this regard, *T gondii* infection has been discovered in particular ticks (i.e., *Haemaphysalis longicornis*) that could serve as a reservoir for secondary toxoplasmosis transmission to other common hosts, if ingested. Other routes are transplacental infection of the fetus, transfusion of white blood cells, and organ transplantation from a seropositive donor to a seronegative recipient.

It is not uncommon for health care professionals, laboratory workers, pet lovers (especially cat owners), butchers, cooks (those handling raw meat), veterinarians, and farmers to acquire acute toxoplasmosis.

Finally, an interesting hypothesis suggested that toxoplasmosis may be transmitted from infected men to noninfected women during unprotected sexual intercourse, resulting in the most dangerous form of disease, the congenital toxoplasmosis. *T gondii* tachyzoites in fact, are present in the seminal fluid and tissue of the testes of various animals including humans.

Dogs can also have a role in the transmission of toxoplasmosis as a mechanical vector by rolling in foul-smelling substances and by ingesting fecal material. Unlike in cats, *T gondii* does not replicate in the dog's gut and no cysts are shed. In areas where dogs and cats are plentiful, immunocompromised persons and pregnant women should be warned of the possibility of acquiring *T gondii* from dogs, as well as from soil contaminated by cats. People should be encouraged to wash their hands after contact with soil, dogs, or cats, as well as before eating.

Pathophysiology

Disease can occur through acute infection after recent contact with *T gondii* cysts or oocysts or through endogenous reactivation. After ingestion, the sporozoites or bradyzoites invade the intestinal epithelium and differentiate to tachyzoites, which disseminate in the blood and replicate within the new host. The parasite translocation into the blood stream may be a possible consequence of localized intestinal inflammation and enteropathy generated by the parasite, which collectively results in impaired integrity of the intestinal mucosa and gut–blood barrier. Transport of the parasite via the bloodstream can occur intracellularly within dendritic cells or monocytes or as a free tachyzoite. Certain Toxoplasma surface antigens aid in the interaction between the tachyzoite and the host cell. One is the perforin-like protein 1 (PLP-1) forming pores in the host cell membrane after binding, as well as playing a role in egress. The success of *Toxoplasma* as a widespread pathogen is due to the effortlessness with which it can be transmitted among the intermediate hosts. Once inside a host, the parasite develops powerful tools to modulate its host cell and to develop into a chronic infection, undergoing bradyzoite development that can evade the host's immune system as well as, in contrast with acute toxoplasmosis, all known antitoxoplasmic drugs.

Host protection from *T gondii* results from a complex cell-mediated immune response involving inflammatory cells, lymphocytes and macrophages, and cytokines. Inoculum size, parasite virulence (strain), genetic background, time of infection (congenital versus postnatal contamination), and sex also contribute to affect the course of infection in human beings and animal models of toxoplasmosis. In particular, the *T gondii* genotype affects its replication rate, migration, and tendency to differentiate to bradyzoites, virulence, and epidemiologic pattern of occurrence. Type II genotypes (most strains isolated from AIDS patients and newborns with congenital disease) and type III genotypes (mostly isolated from animals) are generally less virulent and more cystogenic compared with type I genotypes (also found in congenital disease). Ocular toxoplasmosis in humans is associated with type I but not type II or III genotypes.

Other than the three major Toxoplasma clonal lineages designated as types I, II and III, which are only predominant in Europe and North America (mostly type 2 strain), there are highly polymorphic strains referred to as atypical in South America and Africa, termed Africa 1, 2, and 3.

Genetic background also plays a significant role in increased susceptibility to *T gondii* in humans; HLA-DQ3 appears to be a genetic marker associated with susceptibility to development of TE in patients with AIDS. The mechanisms by which *T gondii* invades host cells and forms an intracellular niche have been extensively reviewed, and several aspects of this process are directly relevant to immunity and pathogenesis. During invasion, three successive waves of proteins are secreted from parasite organelles, (the micronemes, dense granules, and rhoptries) into the host cell. Rhoptry proteins are the major virulence factors of *T gondii* and are located in different parts of the host cells. Blocking the cell intrinsic defense mechanisms of the host lets *T gondii* invade, parasitize, and proliferate in the host successfully. These proteins can alter host cell function and inhibit the immune response directed toward the parasite.

During infection in the intermediate host, *T gondii* undergoes stage conversion between the rapidly dividing tachyzoite that is responsible for acute toxoplasmosis and the slowly replicating, encysted bradyzoite stage. This process of tachyzoite-bradyzoite interconversion is central to the pathogenesis and longevity of infection. In normal conditions, the tachyzoite stage is thwarted by the prompt and efficient interferon-γ-dependent cell-mediated immune response, which eventually kills off the majority of the disseminating tachyzoites before eventually entering the persistent form, the bradyzoite. Bradyzoites are encysted within various tissues, most notably the brain but also muscle, eye, and lung, and are infectious to another intermediate host or the cat if eaten. Cell-mediated immune mechanisms thus play a major role in the control of *T gondii* infection because the parasite is exclusively localized intracellularly.

After infection, *T gondii* evokes a powerful and persistent T-helper-1 (Th1) response (dendritic cell activated) together with neutrophils, inflammatory monocytes, and macrophages. The response is characterized by production of proinflammatory cytokines, including interleukin (IL)-12, INF-α and tumor necrosis factor (TNF)-α, which, together with other immunologic mechanisms, protect the host against rapid replication of tachyzoites and subsequent pathologic changes. The outcome of toxoplasmic infection depends on a balance between proinflammatory (IL-12, TNF-α) and downregulatory (IL-10, IL-27) cytokines that suppress parasite proliferation and control the inflammatory response, respectively.

Clinical Presentation in the Immunocompetent

Acute acquired toxoplasmosis has traditionally been considered an oligosymptomatic and self-limited infection in previously healthy patients. The typical clinical presentation of acute *T gondii* infection is a short flulike or mononucleosis-like illness that includes prolonged fever, headache, persistent enlarged but firm lymph nodes (rarely painful but initially tender) unattached to the overlying skin, and, occasionally, myalgia and gastrointestinal symptoms that rarely need treatment. Other infectious or noninfectious diseases cause similar symptoms and should always be included in the differential diagnosis: mononucleosis, cat scratch disease, tuberculosis, primary HIV infection, sarcoidosis, metastatic cancer, and lymphoma. In these cases, serologic testing is the initial and primary method of diagnosis.

Lymph node biopsy should be reserved for when *Toxoplasma* serology is uncertain and all other infectious serologic investigations are negative. Hepatomegaly and hepatitis with a moderate increase in liver enzyme levels (a 5- to 10-fold elevation) are common. Lymphocytosis and atypical lymphocytes are other laboratory hallmarks of toxoplasmosis. The spleen appears to be involved early in toxoplasmosis, but palpable splenomegaly is uncommon.

Pneumonia as well as myocarditis, polymyositis, or encephalitis are rarely described in immunocompetent hosts.

Although malaria and dengue are the most common causes of fever in travelers, toxoplasmosis should be considered in the differential diagnosis of fever, particularly in travelers with nonspecific symptoms such as fatigue, fever, headache and lymphadenopathy.

Latent toxoplasmosis is characterized by the lifelong presence of cysts of the parasite in different host tissues, including the nervous system, and by the presence of anamnestic *T gondii* immunoglobulin (Ig) G antibodies in the serum. Long considered asymptomatic, latent toxoplasmosis might increase the risk of schizophrenia and Parkinson's disease; influence human personality and behavior; impair psychomotor performance and increase the risk of suicide (suicide rates have been shown higher in countries with greater *T gondii* prevalence, regardless of national wealth or gross domestic product), traffic accidents, and the probability of the birth of male offspring. Recent studies have also hypothesized that *T gondii* is a risk factor for increasing aggressiveness as well as a murder behavior in women.

Higher rates of *T gondii* seropositivity have been reported for several psychiatric conditions affecting neurotransmitters, especially dopamine, that are implicated in the emergence of psychosis and behavioral Toxoplasma-induced abnormalities and in inducing brain inflammation by the direct stimulation of inflammatory cytokines in the central nervous system. Also, there is increasing evidence for a prominent role of immune dysregulation in psychosis and bipolar disorders. Accumulating evidence suggests that a permeabilized gut–blood barrier is present in psychiatric disorders, as demonstrated through studies of microbial translocation and microbiome sequencing that seem to indicate an actively dysbiotic environment in subsets of individuals with psychiatric disorders. RhD phenotype seems to play an important role in the strength and direction of association between latent toxoplasmosis and personality and intelligence.

Toxoplasmosis should also be regarded as an epilepsy risk factor. Epileptogenic mechanisms are probably multifactorial (direct lodgment of parasite, direct modulation of neuronal functions, abnormalities in GABA, role of calcium, etc.), etc. Recently, it was suggested that chronic latent neuroinflammation caused by the parasite may be responsible for the development of several neurodegenerative diseases manifesting with the loss of smell. Olfactory dysfunction reported in Alzheimer's disease, multiple sclerosis, and schizophrenia was frequently associated with the significantly increased serum anti-*T gondii* immunoglobulin G antibody levels.

In addition to above-mentioned manifestation, several recent studies performed in human and animal models have demonstrated that latent or acute toxoplasmosis is associated with reproductive organs disorders, infertility, sperm abnormalities, behavioral changes, and neurological disorders in pregnant women and other people.

A meta-analysis also suggested chronic toxoplasmosis as a possible risk factor for type 2 diabetes mellitus. However, more accurate studies are needed to better understand this association.

A very important aspect that has emerged in recent years concerns the possible occurrence of toxoplasmosis in patient receiving biotherapies, particularly anti-TNF-α agents for the treatment of rheumatologic diseases and other conditions that need biotechnological drugs. *Toxoplasma* serology should be performed in patients before treatment with TNF-α antagonists is initiated, and patients should be advised to avoid situations that increase risk of exposure to *Toxoplasma*.

Clinical Presentation in Immunocompromised Patients

The presence of latent bradyzoite cysts, along with the ability of bradyzoites to reconvert into the active and rapidly growing tachyzoites that can result in often fatal injury, explains the high incidence of acute toxoplasmosis often observed in immunocompromised persons. In immunocompromised hosts and in patients with AIDS, the central nervous system (CNS) is the site most typically affected by infection, and toxoplasmic encephalitis (TE) is the most common manifestation, which typically consists of single or multiple brain lesions. In individuals with AIDS and a CD4 T-cell count <100 cells/μL, the incidence of TE is 28% in seropositive patients not taking prophylaxis. Ocular and pulmonary diseases are the most common extracerebral sites of infection. For *Toxoplasma*, various mechanisms have been proposed for CNS entry, including the so-called "Trojan horse" mechanism, whereby an infected immune cell crosses the BBB, bringing the intracellular parasite with it. TE is also the third most common condition associated with AIDS in Brazil, still accounting for high mortality and morbidity rates despite free access to antiretroviral therapy (ART). However, as in transplant patients or those with malignant hemolymphopathies or solid tumors, other organs such as the lungs or eyes may be involved. Most of these cases result from reactivation of latent infection, although reinfection with a different *T gondii* strain in the transplanted organs can also occur. Although the mortality rate of pulmonary toxoplasmosis was high before the advent of ART, patients with AIDS and recipients of bone marrow transplants are also at risk for development of pulmonary toxoplasmosis, especially patients with very low CD4 cell counts. The clinical manifestations are nonspecific and are similar to those of *Pneumocystis jirovecii*.

In immunocompromised patients with suspected pulmonary toxoplasmosis, conventional staining is the most appropriate method to diagnose for experienced microbiology laboratories, whereas *T gondii*–specific PCR may be useful for laboratories with less experience in parasitology.

The predictive value of elevated blood levels of lactate dehydrogenase is of uncertain value. Patients with TE typically present with headache, confusion, altered mental status, and motor weakness. Focal neurologic deficits or seizures, weakness, sensory abnormalities, cerebellar signs, and neuropsychiatric manifestations are also common. Fever is usually, but not reliably, present. Accompanying nausea or vomiting usually indicates elevated intracranial pressure. Computed tomography (CT) scan or magnetic resonance imaging (MRI) of the brain typically shows multiple contrast-enhancing lesions, often with associated edema. These should be distinguished from other infectious or noninfectious CNS diseases in the course of AIDS.

In immunocompromised patients, the infection can disseminate rapidly and manifests with nonspecific symptoms such as fever and malaise. It can affect a number of organs, including the brain, cerebellum (an uncommon presentation), eye, liver, and lungs, as well as skeletal muscle, bone marrow, bladder, and spinal cord. Cardiac toxoplasmosis can occur during the course of multivisceral dissemination. However, in patients with AIDS, it is usually asymptomatic and found only at autopsy, typically in the setting of widely disseminated infection. Acquired toxoplasmosis with cutaneous involvement can also occur in the pediatric population, particularly in immunocompromised patients after stem cell transplantation. Early diagnosis and treatment of this life-threatening opportunistic infection may improve patient outcomes.

Toxoplasmosis of the Eye

Ocular toxoplasmosis is the major cause of visual impairment in high *T gondii* endemic regions of the United States and Europe, where it accounts for 30% to 50% of the infectious posterior uveitis. Toxoplasmosis can affect the retina and the underlying choroid, causing retinochoroiditis, the most common manifestation of ocular toxoplasmosis, which consists in an acute focal-necrotizing retinochoroiditis often adjacent to an old chorioretinal scar. Although the inner retina is the primary site of infection, vitreous, choroid, and sometimes sclera are secondarily affected. Many lesions are self-limiting and heal, forming characteristic unilateral or bilateral pigmented scars in the retina, where Toxoplasma cysts are found. Ocular lesions can recur in adolescence and adulthood, even after treatment in infancy. The severity of the disease is mainly a function of the parasite genotype and the host's immune status. Diagnosis in immunocompetent patients is based on the findings of typical ocular manifestations, including eye pain and decreased visual acuity, and may be confirmed by biologic tools applied to intraocular samples for antibody detection (local synthesis of specific antibodies), although PCR is becoming more widely available for direct identification of the parasite DNA in the vitreous and aqueous humor, especially with new methods of detection that can improve its sensitivity. When the clinical symptoms first manifest in immunocompetent patients, the intraocular inflammatory response may reduce the parasitic burden in the aqueous humor and vitreous, thus decreasing the amount of target DNA for PCR amplification. Secretory IgA antibodies in tears have been suggested as a reliable marker of acute ocular toxoplasmosis. Symptoms and signs in immunocompromised patients do not distinguish ocular toxoplasmosis from other ocular infections in HIV, including tuberculosis, *P jirovecii* pneumonia, and CMV retinitis. Toxoplasmic chorioretinitis appears as raised yellow-white, cottony lesions in a nonvascular distribution, unlike the perivascular exudates of CMV retinitis. Vitreal inflammation is usually present, in contrast to ocular toxoplasmosis in immunocompetent patients. Up to 63% of AIDS patients with Toxoplasma chorioretinitis have concurrent CNS lesions.

Maternal Infection and Congenital Toxoplasmosis

Infection with *T gondii* is particularly dangerous for pregnant women because it can lead to the transplacental passage of the parasite from the circulation of the primarily infected mother. Successful pregnancy involves an elegant equilibrium in organizing the immune system at the fetal-maternal and uteri milieu resulting in tolerance (TH2) of the fetus and defense (TH1) against the pathogenic agents. The placenta also plays an important role in trans-placental transmission, as it is a natural barrier to protection of the fetus against infectious agents and also a target tissue for parasite multiplication. In fact, the placental barrier is more efficient to inhibit the tachyzoites transmission at the beginning of gestation, but becomes more permeable at the end of pregnancy.

As tachyzoites bypass the placental blood barrier and invade the fetal organs, they propagate and compromise the embryonic developmental process.

During pregnancy, the prevalence of toxoplasmosis increases throughout the second and third quarter of gestation; simultaneously, progesterone and 17β-estradiol also increase and can aggravate or reduce parasite reproduction. Infection of the placenta is a prerequisite for congenital transmission. More than 60% of infected pregnant women do not experience any symptoms or signs, and the clinical features, when present, are the same as in other immunocompetent persons.

Currently, congenital toxoplasmosis is the second most common intrauterine infection and remains a public health problem throughout the world. The global annual incidence of congenital toxoplasmosis has been estimated to be 190,100 cases (95% credible interval, CI: 179,300–206,300). This is equivalent to a burden of 1.20 million DALYs (95% CI: 0.76–1.90). High burdens are seen in South America and in some Middle Eastern and low-income countries. The risk of transmission of *T gondii* to the fetus ranges from 0.6 to 1.7 per 1000 pregnant women.

According to Massachusetts Department of Health (United States), about 1 case of congenital toxoplasmosis occurs for every 10,000 live births. Moreover, from 4,000,000 live births each year in the United States, 400 have acquired congenital toxoplasmosis. This rate is markedly higher for other developing countries. In France, about 300 cases are reported each year to the National Reference Center. The frequency of transmission and severity of disease are inversely related.

The development of possible consequences depends on many factors, including the degree of parasitemia in the mother, the maturity of the placenta, the age of the fetus, and immunologic maturity. Early maternal infection (first trimester) can cause severe congenital toxoplasmosis and can result in death of the fetus in utero and spontaneous abortion. Clinical manifestations of congenital toxoplasmosis observed in infancy are numerous and include jaundice, rash, hepatosplenomegaly, anemia, thrombocytopenia, hydrocephalus, microcephalus, intracranial calcifications, convulsions, psychomotor and mental retardation, chorioretinitis, microphthalmia, blindness, strabismus, visual and auditory inflammatory disorders, cardiovascular abnormalities, and pains. All these signs and symptoms are included in the general workup of suspected congenital TORCH infections: *toxo*plasmosis, *other* (syphilis, varicella-zoster, parvovirus B19, HIV infection, listeriosis, hepatitis B, Zika virus), *r*ubella, *c*ytomegalovirus, and *h*erpes. The classic triad of bilateral chorioretinitis, hydrocephalus, and cerebral calcifications is exceptional.

Fetal infection at the second trimester results in milder complications, which include splenomegaly, hepatomegaly, cerebral calcifications, pneumonitis, anemia, epilepsy, thrombocytopenia-induced petechiae, rash, and retinochoroiditis. When maternal infection occurs during the third trimester, most of neonates (more than 80%) are asymptomatic; however, retinochoroiditis and neurologic deficits in newborn who may be at high risk for seizures, mental retardation, or delay in growth, as well as in early adulthood, might be developed if these newborns are not treated appropriately in early age. In multiparous women, the risk of infections has been shown twice as high as in nulliparas.

The clinical course of the disease in a child with congenital toxoplasmosis is not influenced by whether the mother showed any clinical symptoms of the disease or was entirely asymptomatic. Infants born to women infected simultaneously with HIV and *T gondii* should be evaluated for congenital toxoplasmosis, considering the increased risk of reactivation of parasitemia and disease in these mothers.

Diagnosis in the Immunocompetent

In immunocompetent persons, confirmation of acute infection can exclude other potentially more serious etiologies. In other clinical settings where *Toxoplasma* infection can result in severe sequelae, the interpretation of laboratory findings poses significant challenges. The parasite can in fact be present in acute, chronic, latent, or reactivated form. Thus, discrimination of these forms is often crucial in understanding clinical relevance. A schematic diagnostic pathway that can be followed for the diagnosis of toxoplasmosis is shown in Figure 1. Methodical serologic screening for *T gondii* IgG and IgM antibodies in adult symptomatic immunocompetent persons, in pregnant women as early in gestation as possible (preferably in first trimester), and in seronegative women each month or trimester thereafter is optimal. Such screening allows detection of seroconversion and early initiation of treatment.

The laboratory tests used most commonly for initial investigation are serologic, targeting detection of IgG, IgM, and IgA specific for *T gondii* by available commercial kit. In addition to confirming infection, these tests can aid in determining prognosis,

influence management, and assist in monitoring response to treatment. Typically, acute-phase IgM appears first about 1 to 2 weeks after infection, closely followed by IgA and IgE. Generally, IgM peaks at about 2 months. The time at which immunoglobulins can no longer be detected is highly variable depending on the test employed, usually about 6 to 9 months. In a small minority of cases IgM can persist at high levels for up to 18 months or for years, leading to an inaccurate assessment of when the exposure occurred. This circumstance can be problematic because congenital toxoplasmosis can occur if the mother was infected during her pregnancy, and it is thus important to ascertain in which trimester of pregnancy the infection occurred. IgA antibodies are considered to be a marker of acute toxoplasmosis as their kinetics are faster than those of IgM antibodies; however, they can also persist for more than a year, and their detection, together with IgM detection, strongly suggests neonatal infection. IgE serology is highly specific in pregnant women but has low sensitivity, remaining detectable for less than 4 months after infection; moreover, it is not useful in samples from newborns.

To date, an IgM test is still used by most laboratories to determine if a patient has been infected recently or in the distant past, but confirmatory testing (double sandwich or capture IgM-ELISA [enzyme-linked immunosorbent assay] kits and the immunosorbent agglutination assay [IgM-ISAGA]) should always be performed owing to the difficulties in interpreting a positive IgM test result for the relatively high incidence of false-positive results (due to the rheumatoid factor and antinuclear antibodies in some IgM-IFA tests). Thus, a positive IgM test result in a single serum sample can be interpreted as a true-positive result in the setting of a recently acquired infection, a true-positive result in the setting of an infection acquired in the distant past, or a false-positive result. IgM levels decline more rapidly than IgG antibodies, which typically reach maximal levels at about 4 months, then decline to a lower level over the next 12 to 24 months but persist for decades. Elevated IgG levels confirm if a patient has been exposed to the parasite, but they do not differentiate between a recent or past exposure, because IgG persists at a low level throughout the life of the patient. The absence of IgG antibodies in early pregnancy indicates that women are at risk for acquiring toxoplasmosis.

The most commonly used tests for the measurement of IgG antibody are the Sabin-Feldman dye test (still considered the gold standard diagnostic test; it measures primarily IgG antibodies to *T gondii*, but it requires viable *Toxoplasma* organisms), the ELISA, the IFA, and the modified direct agglutination test. Other immunological methods, including chemiluminescence assays (CLIA), enzyme-linked fluorescence assay (ELFA), and immunochromatographic test (ICT), have been developed to improve the ability of diagnosis of *T gondii* infection.

Depending on the method used, the avidity tests currently available (serum IgG avidity test and immunosorbent agglutination assays (ISAGA) are helpful primarily to rule out that a patient's infection occurred within the prior 4 to 5 months and that the fetus is not at risk for congenital toxoplasmosis. The avidity test that shows low IgG values in a recent *T gondii* infection is most important when only a single serum sample is available at the time when critical decisions must be made. A major problem with this test is that the maturation of the IgG response after a primary *Toxoplasma* infection varies considerably among patients; in fact, low-avidity results can persist for as long as 1 year, and substantial numbers of patients have borderline or equivocal results. These equivocal cases require that in addition to a more careful interpretation of all laboratory test results in conjunction with other clinical findings, other serologic methods should then be undertaken in serology reference laboratories. Recently, a growing number of studies have demonstrated the potential advantages of chimeric or synthetic peptide antigens (EC2 (containing MIC1 and MIC2 antigenic regions) and EC3 (containing M2AP, GRA3 and GRA7 antigenic regions) for the serological diagnosis of toxoplasmosis.

The employment of polymerase chain reaction (PCR) to identify *T gondii* DNA in amniotic fluid (AF) obtained by

First-level T. gondii Diagnostic Test

Detection of serum anti–T. gondii IgM and IgG in first trimester
- If IgM and IgG negative: absence of specific immunity; mother prophylaxis, monthly serologic control*
- If only IgG is detected: infection likely took place 6–12 months before or before pregnancy; immunity
- If only IgM is detected: initial phase seroconversion of false IgM positivity†
- If IgM and IgG are detected: possible recent infection; consider a more thorough workup (reference laboratory) to try to determine the time of infection in the mother‡

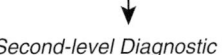

Second-level Diagnostic Test

IgG avidity assay
- If negative (high avidity): infection occurred 3–5 months before testing
- If positive (low avidity): probable recent *T. gondii* infection; repeat serology 3 weeks after the first sample; start spiramycin, ecographic surveillance
Try to establish a certain or presumed seroconversion in pregnancy and to determine whether the infection was transmitted to the product of conception.

Third-level Diagnostic Tests (further maternal and fetal assessment)

In the mother

Detection of T. gondii-specific DNA by PCR-AF at 18 weeks of gestation§
- If positive: the fetus has been infected; consider starting treatment and monthly fetal ultrasound examination to detect abnormalities; start pyrimethamine-sulfadiazine‖
- If negative: fetus unaffected; *T. gondii* has not crossed the placental barrier; continue spiramycin¶
- Parasite isolation on tissue culture: mouse inoculation**

In the newborn

Detection of serum anti-T. gondii IgM and IgA††
- If IgM and/or IgA are present at birth: probable connatal infection
- If IgM and/or IgA are not present at birth: monthly control

Western blot assay of serum IgG and IgM from mother-baby pairs‡‡
- If positive: confirmation of early postnatal diagnosis; therapy and serological control§§
- If negative: monthly control for the first 3 months

Figure 1 A schematic diagnostic pathway for the diagnosis of toxoplasmosis. *No treatment is required. †Repeat the tests weekly to detect the appearance of IgG antibodies to confirm the seroconversion. ‡Given that IgM may persist for several months, try to date the beginning of infection through education and counseling to guide the prenatal diagnosis of the patient. §PCR sensitivity is significantly higher for infections occurred between the 17th and 21st week of gestation. ‖If ecographic abnormalities, consider abortion. ¶A negative PCR cannot completely rule out congenital infection; consider follow-up through ultrasounds and continue prophylaxis with spiramycin (Rovamycine) until delivery and neonatal testing. **For confirmation of PCR results; however, they are complex, expensive, and relatively insensitive. ††Limitations because IgA antibodies may persist for several months and are not always produced. ‡‡This test is not widely used mainly because of its technical complexity and high price. §§Administer pyrimethamine (Daraprim)-sulfadiazine therapy and serologic controls after cessation of therapy and every 6 months for the first 2 years.

amniocentesis at 18 weeks and later represents a milestone in the early diagnosis of intrauterine *T gondii* infection, thereby avoiding the use of more invasive procedures on the fetus. Sensitivity and specificity of PCR may even increase when performed on AF samples obtained from the sixteenth week of pregnancy onward. The specificity and positive predictive value of PCR on AF samples is close to 100%, although different protocols influence its sensitivity and specificity. PCR is generally carried out with various gene targets, of which the most widely used is the 35-fold repetitive gene *B1*. Following it, several multicopy targeting genes including 18S rRNA-, P30-, B1-genes, 529-bp repeat fragment or the AF146527 element have been used for the detection of *T gondii* in different biologic samples. In particular, PCR with the 529-bp RE gene is 10–100 times more sensitive than the B1 gene.

Results of studies indicated that loop-mediated isothermal amplification (LAMP) and real-time-PCR using AF and CSF are more sensitive and specific methods in congenital infection and immunocompromised patients, respectively, and could be used for early diagnosis of infection and also in follow-up after treatment. Moreover, LAMP on cord blood or whole blood is highly sensitive, specific, and easy to perform, as it doesn't require expensive equipment.

However, a definitive correlation between the number of *Toxoplasma* organisms in AF and the severity of congenital infection has not yet been demonstrated. PCR should be considered for pregnant women (without a contraindication for the procedure) with positive diagnostic serology or highly suggestive of an infection because of ultrasonographic abnormalities in the fetus acquired during gestation or shortly before conception. If the PCR-AF test result is negative, the fetus should be unaffected, presumably because *T gondii* has not yet crossed the placental barrier even if it is theoretically possible that fetal infection can occur later in pregnancy from a placenta that was infected earlier in gestation. Samples obtained by cordocentesis, funipuncture, or periumbilical fetal blood sampling should not be used, because fetal risk of contamination with maternal blood is higher than with amniocentesis, and cordocentesis is less sensitive.

In the newborn, diagnosis of infection is based on detection of serum anti-*Toxoplasma* IgM and IgA antibodies that do not cross the placenta, unlike maternal IgG antibodies. Better results are obtained if the ISAGA method is used. Maternal IgG antibodies present in the newborn can reflect either past or recent infection in the mother and require serologic follow-up of the newborn for the 1st year of life until the complete disappearance of these antibodies. A negative *T gondii*–specific IgG test result at 1 year of age essentially rules out congenital toxoplasmosis. Detection of IgG in oral fluid appears to be a promising tool for monitoring infants with suspected congenital toxoplasmosis.

Detection of specific IgA antibodies appears to be more sensitive than detection of IgM antibodies for establishing infection in the newborn, because these antibodies may be present when there is no *T gondii*–specific IgM, and the converse can also occur. However, transmission of maternal IgM or IgA antibodies can occur during the birth process. Because of the relatively brief half-life of IgM and IgA, positive tests for these antibodies usually must be confirmed by repeat testing at 2 to 4 days of life in the case of IgM antibodies and at 10 days of life for IgA antibodies.

Evaluation of infants with suspected congenital toxoplasmosis should always include ophthalmologic examination, electroencephalogram, hearing test, blood tests, non-contrast CT scanning or ultrasound of the brain, and examination of CSF. Although CT scanning is the first-line diagnostic method used in the United States to detect CNS abnormalities caused by toxoplasmosis, ultrasound can be used as an alternative diagnostic method to avoid the effects of radiation in the neonatal period. Ultrasound is recommended for women with suspected or diagnosed acute infection acquired during or shortly before gestation. This technique can reveal fetal abnormalities, including hydrocephalus, brain or hepatic calcifications, splenomegaly, and ascites. Because most infants do not show signs of toxoplasmosis at birth, a negative ultrasound does not rule out the possibility of infection and might need to be followed by a CT scan for confirmation, because ultrasound results can vary depending on the examiner and technology used. Newborns thus need a thorough examination after birth and follow-up blood tests during the first year of life.

Diagnosis in the Immunocompromised

In immunocompromised persons and AIDS patients with TE, indirect serologic methods widely used in immunocompetent patients are unreliable because they fail to produce significant titers of specific antibodies. Although incidence of TE among HIV-infected persons directly correlates with the prevalence of anti–*T gondii* antibodies, the absence of IgG antibody makes a diagnosis of toxoplasmosis unlikely, but not impossible. Anti-*Toxoplasma* IgM antibodies are usually absent. CSF findings are normal or show nonspecific alterations such as lymphocytic pleocytosis and discrete CSF hyperproteinorrachia.

In clinical practice, the diagnosis of TE is presumptive and mainly based on clinical presentation, imaging, and laboratory test results. Imaging includes CT or MRI, preferably with gadolinium contrast, and shows isodense or hypodense single or multiple lesions with a mass effect, taking up the contrast dye in a ringlike or nodular manner in more than 90% of cases. However, as neither CT nor MRI can reliably distinguish CNS infections, such as toxoplasmosis, from lymphoma in HIV-1–positive patients, the use of FDG-PET has been shown to offer better sensitivity to noninvasively differentiate cerebral toxoplasmosis and other infectious diseases from primary CNS lymphoma. Laboratory results include the presence of serum-specific *T gondii* IgG antibodies. Diagnosis is also made from an objective response, on the basis of clinical and radiographic improvement, to specific anti–*T gondii* therapy in the absence of a likely alternative diagnosis. In general, the occurrence of low CD4+ T-cell count (less than 150–200/mm3) and the presence of *T gondii* IgG antibody is habitually accepted as being a good predictor of TE reactivation, although less than 6% of TE patients show negative tests. If the suspected diagnosis of toxoplasmosis is correct, clinical or radiographic improvement should become evident by more than 50% within 7 to 14 days. If symptoms persist, a brain biopsy should be performed. This should be considered in immunocompromised patients with presumed CNS toxoplasmosis with a single MRI

lesion, absence of IgG antibodies, or an unsatisfactory clinical response to specific anti–*T gondii* treatment.

Diagnosis of TE is crucial because other brain diseases—such as CNS lymphoma, bacterial abscess, progressive multifocal leukoencephalopathy, viral or fungal encephalitis, neurotuberculosis, cytomegalovirus encephalitis, and focal lesions caused by fungi (*Cryptococcus neoformans*, *Aspergillus* spp., and *Nocardia* spp.)—could share similar clinical and CT scan signs. In general, no imaging technique is completely specific. Thallium single-photon emission computed tomography (SPECT) and positron emission tomography (PET) can be useful in distinguishing toxoplasmosis or other infections from CNS lymphoma. CNS lymphoma has greater thallium uptake on SPECT and greater glucose and methionine metabolism on PET than neurotoxoplasmosis or other infections.

Definitive diagnosis of TE is made by pathologic examination of brain tissue obtained by open or stereotactic CT-guided brain biopsy, although there is morbidity and even death associated with the biopsy procedure. Tachyzoites are demonstrated on hematoxylin and eosin stains or immunoperoxidase staining, which can increase diagnostic sensitivity, or by Giemsa on cytocentrifuged CSF samples. *Toxoplasma* organisms must be distinguished from other intracellular organisms such as *Histoplasma*, *Trypanosoma cruzi*, and *Leishmania*.

Since the turn of the twenty-first century, molecular techniques have allowed significant improvement and have been shown to be an important diagnostic tool in laboratory diagnosis of TE. Their use is principally appropriate for immunocompromised patients because these techniques are not affected by the immunologic status of the host. PCR-based assays, in particular, have been shown to be rapid, sensitive, and specific enough to be used as a frontline test for detecting CSF *T gondii* DNA in most patients with CNS infection, thus avoiding invasive and expensive brain biopsy procedures. However, results usually are negative once specific anti-*Toxoplasma* therapy has been started. Moreover, parasite levels in blood and CSF may be very poor in some patients and cause difficulties in interpreting the PCR product. For this reason, a number of quantitative real-time PCRs with specific *T gondii* genome sequence have been developed in the last decade and used in patients with AIDS and CNS damage with different rates of sensitivity and specificity. In this setting, the recent sensitive and specific real-time PCR technique targeting the 529-bp repeat fragment of the *AF146527* element repeated 300 times in the genome of *T gondii* has been demonstrated to exactly quantify the parasite load, allowing correlation with clinical symptoms and impact of treatment. Moreover, the use of real-time PCR with primers targeting the genes SAG4 and MAG1 (located in the bradyzoites) and SAG1 (located in tachyzoites) has shown to be useful to identify relapses of TE in patients in whom the use of PCR with B1 gene failed to detect DNA, in AIDS patients and other immunocompromised patients especially, when prophylaxis or treatment has been started.

Diagnosis of TE in AIDS patients can also be supported by demonstration of intrathecal antibody production based on detection of oligoclonal bands in CSF with antibody-specific index (ASI) and affinity-mediated immunoblot (AMI) techniques. This approach has also been shown to discriminate TE from other opportunistic CNS infections in AIDS.

In non-AIDS–immunocompromised patients, regular PCR follow-up of allogeneic hematopoietic stem-cell transplant (allo-HSCT) patients could guide preemptive treatment and improve outcome.

Treatment

An ideal treatment for toxoplasmosis should achieve therapeutic, systemic brain and eye concentrations to be effective in the organs where the majority of disease occurs and should be active against both the acute replicating tachyzoite and latent bradyzoite stages of the parasite. However, current treatments are only capable of suppressing the rapidly dividing tachyzoyte stage of the organism. The main goal of treatment is to interrupt the replication of the parasite and prevent further damage to the organs involved. Nonpregnant immunocompetent patients with acute toxoplasmosis plus lymphadenitis generally do not require antimicrobial therapy because the infection is self-limiting and usually subclinical. Chronic lymphadenopathy accompanied by fever and marked weakness can be cured with specific therapy. Patients whose *T gondii* infection occurred during laboratory accidents or blood transfusions need specific treatment. Pregnant women must be treated to reduce the risk and severity of congenital infection. Immunocompromised patients, including patients with AIDS and transplant recipients, should always be treated with antitoxoplasmic agents. For eye disease, treatment usually includes anti-*Toxoplasma* agents plus systemic corticosteroids. The most important treatment and prophylactic regimens for the therapy of toxoplasmosis are shown in Tables 1 and 2.

The folate synthesis pathway being the best-known therapeutic target against Toxoplasma, the main enzymes targeted by pharmaceuticals are the dihydropteroate synthase and dihydrofolate reductase. Since the dihydropteroate enzyme is not found in mammalian cells, it provides a specific target against Toxoplasma. The standard pyrimethamine (Daraprim) and trimethoprim (Trimpex)[1] are the most widely used dihydrofolate reductase inhibitors. Pyrimethamine, however, is more effective then trimethoprim and is usually administered in conjunction with a dihydropteroate synthase inhibitor (sulfonamide compounds such as sulfadiazine and sulfamethoxazole).

First-line therapy for acquired toxoplasmosis in both immunocompetent and immunodeficient patients consists of the synergistic combination of pyrimethamine and sulfadiazine. Pyrimethamine plus sulfadiazine[1] plus folinic acid (Leucovorin)[1] to prevent hematologic toxicity is the preferred regimen. Azithromycin (Zithromax)[1] or atovaquone (Mepron)[1] may be used as alternate therapy in combination with pyrimethamine or sulfonamides for the treatment and prophylaxis of toxoplasmosis when first-line line therapy is contraindicated. Both compounds have been shown to be partially effective against tissue cysts in experimental studies. More recently, however, the search for new and efficient pharmacologic treatments directed against proliferating tachyzoites or the tissue cyst of Toxoplasma is under intense and frequent evaluation.

Treatment During Pregnancy

Management of maternal and fetal infection of *T gondii* varies considerably between different countries and even centers in the same country. According to the European Multicentre Study on Congenital Toxoplasmosis (EMSCOT) data, which suffer from the lack of a large-scale controlled clinical trial, treatment for the fetus should be started immediately (within 3 weeks of infection) after diagnosis of recently acquired maternal infection. This has been shown to significantly reduce sequelae and to have a beneficial effect when therapy is begun soon after birth. Later treatment has been shown to have no effect.

The macrolide antibiotic spiramycin (Rovamycine)[2] is prescribed immediately after diagnosis of maternal infection in most centers in Europe and the United States, and there has been no evidence that this drug is teratogenic. Spiramycin does not cross the placenta but is concentrated in the placenta and protects the fetus from contact with the parasite. It has been estimated to reduce the incidence of vertical transmission of *T gondii* by about 60%. It is used 1 g every 8 hours in many EU countries, especially France, and in Asia and South America and does not seem to have any fetal effects, although a small percentage of women have developed gastrointestinal side effects.

Spiramycin should be continued as prophylaxis until delivery, along with periodic ultrasound examination, because the placenta could have been infected earlier in gestation.

In the case of positive PCR-AF at or immediately after 18 weeks' gestation, or with high probability of fetal infection acquired late in the second trimester (after 18 weeks) or during the third trimester of gestation (because of ultrasound abnormalities), and in women who cannot undergo amniocentesis, the spiramycin regimen should be replaced with the drug combination of sulfadiazine[1] and pyrimethamine plus folinic acid (Leucovorin).[1] This treatment strategy varies in some U.S. and European centers. Folinic acid prevents the toxicity of pyrimethamine without activity against Toxoplasma. This combination therapy is used only after confirmed or strongly suspected fetal infection and is never administered in the first trimester of pregnancy due to its teratogenic and hematological adverse effects, in addition to symptoms of nausea in the mother.

Throughout the pregnancy, therapy with pyrimethamine in conjunction with folinic acid should be continued to prevent hematologic toxicities, along with monitoring of blood cell counts and rigorous periodic ultrasound examination. Because spiramycin does not readily cross the placenta, it is not reliable for the treatment of infection in the fetus. In the absence of clinical and laboratory signs suggestive of congenital toxoplasmosis, therapy is not indicated in infants, but it is necessary to inform the specialist and to plan, with the specialist, periodic clinical and serologic controls. In symptomatic infants, the combination of pyrimethamine plus sulfadiazine plus leucovorin is recommended. The duration of this treatment is not specifically defined, but it must be continued for up to a year, possibly alternating cycles of antifolate for 4 weeks with spiramycin cycles of equal duration.

Ocular Toxoplasmosis

In immunocompetent patients, *Toxoplasma*-related chorioretinitis is usually a self-limited infection and generally may resolve spontaneously in a period of 4 to 8 weeks. However, treatment is recommended for lesions within the vascular arcades, adjacent to the optic disk, or larger than 2 optic disk diameters to reduce the chance of vision loss. In general, pyrimethamine, sulfadiazine[1] plus folinic acid[1], and corticosteroids form the most common drug combination currently used to treat ocular toxoplasmosis. Patients may also be treated with TMP-SMX,[1] which appears to be a safe and effective substitute for pyrimethamine, sulfadiazine, and folinic acid, or with azithromycin[1] or intravitreal clindamycin (Cleocin)[1] and prednisone for 4 to 6 weeks. Pyrimethamine plus azithromycin is another drug combination that is similar to the standard treatment and can be considered an acceptable alternative treatment for sight-threatening ocular toxoplasmosis. *Toxoplasma* retinochoroiditis in immunocompromised patients requires immediate treatment. Atypical presentations also warrant treatment.

Recurrent toxoplasmic retinochoroiditis, probably related to the rupture of the dormant retinal cyst or *Toxoplasma* circulating in peripheral blood, remains a major health crisis and can be associated with severe morbidity if the disease extends to structures critical for vision, including the macula and optic disk. Severe morbidity can also occur if there is damage to the eye from inflammation or if there are complications such as retinal detachment or neovascularization. In patients with frequent recurrences, the rate of recurrent toxoplasmic retinochoroiditis can be significantly reduced by long-term intermittent treatment with TMP-SMX 160 mg/800 mg (Bactrim DS)[1], with one tablet administered three times a week as a prophylactic regimen. Intravitreal clindamycin[1] injection and possibly steroids may be an acceptable alternative to the classic treatment in ocular toxoplasmosis. It can offer the patient more convenience, a safer systemic side effect profile, greater availability, and fewer follow-up visits and hematologic evaluations. Although research has identified wide variation in practices regarding the use of corticosteroids, a recent Cochrane review did not identify evidence from randomized controlled trials for the role of corticosteroids in the management of ocular toxoplasmosis. The question of foremost importance, however, is whether they should be used as adjunct

---

[1] Not FDA approved for this indication.
[2] Not commercially available in the United States.

| TABLE 1 | Treatment Regimens for Toxoplasmosis |

PATIENTS	DRUG OF CHOICE	RECOMMENDED DOSAGE	LENGTH OF ADMINISTRATION	ADVERSE EFFECTS
Acute infection in *T gondii* seropositive pregnant patients with undocumented fetal infection	Spiramycin (Rovamycine)[2]	1000 mg PO q8h (without food)	Throughout pregnancy or until fetal infection is documented	Mild GI disturbances, possible skin eruptions
Acute infection in a pregnant patient with documented fetal infection (positive PCR-AF)	Pyrimethamine (Daraprim)* *plus*	Loading dose, 50 mg PO q12h × 2 d, then 50 mg PO daily	Throughout pregnancy; avoid before 18th wk of gestation because of high risk of teratogenesis	Pyrimethamine is a potential teratogen (kidney and heart malformation) and should be used only after the first trimester
	Sulfadiazine[1] *plus*	Loading dose 75 mg/kg PO, then 50 mg/kg q12h (max 4 g daily)	Throughout pregnancy; do not administer before 18th wk of gestation[†]	Sulfadiazine can cause crystal-induced nephropathy[‡]
	Folinic acid (Leucovorin)[1]	10–20 mg PO daily	During and for 1 wk after pyrimethamine use	Complete regimen: rash, fever and dose-dependent myelosuppression; weekly monitoring of blood cell counts
Congenital infection in the infant	Pyrimethamine *plus*	Loading dose 2 mg/kg PO daily × 2 d; then 1 mg/kg PO daily × 2–6 mo; then 1 mg/kg tiw	1 y	Same as above
	Sulfadiazine[1] *plus*	50 mg/kg PO q12h	1 y	
	Folinic acid[1]	10 mg/kg PO tiw	During and for 1 wk after pyrimethamine use	
Acute *T gondii* infection in adult immunocompetent patients and in pregnant patients infected > 6 mo before conception	Treatment not recommended or, if acutely ill: Pyrimethamine *plus*	Loading dose 200 mg PO daily in 2 divided doses, then 0.5–1 mg/kg/d (max 50 mg/d; 75 mg (if >60 kg)	4–6 wk, or 1–2 wk after resolution of symptoms	Same as above
	Sulfadiazine[1] *plus*	1000–1500 mg PO q6h	During and 1 wk after pyrimethamine use	
	Folinic acid[1]	5–20 mg PO tiw		
Chorioretinitis in immunocompetent patients	Pyrimethamine[§,1] *plus*	200 mg loading dose, then 50–75 mg PO daily	1–2 wk after resolution of symptoms	
	Sulfadiazine[§,1] *plus*	1000–1500 mg PO q6h	1–2 wk after resolution of symptoms	
	Folinic acid[1] *plus*	5–20 mg PO tiw	During and for 1 wk after pyrimethamine use	
	Prednisone	1 mg/kg daily in 2 divided doses	Until resolution of signs and symptoms	
Alternatives				
	TMP-SMX (Bactrim)[1] *or*	160–800 mg q12h	6 wk	Skin rash, fever, leukopenia, thrombocytopenia, hepatotoxicity; also available as an IV formulation
	Azithromycin (Zithromax)[1] alone or associated with pyrimethamine *or*	500 mg/d	5 wk	Not reported
	Intravitreal clindamycin (Cleocin)[1]-dexamethasone (Decadron)	One injection 1–400 mcg	Not reported	Not reported
For untreatable cases only				
	Photocoagulation	Not usually done	Not reported	Not reported

TABLE 1   Treatment Regimens for Toxoplasmosis—cont'd

PATIENTS	DRUG OF CHOICE	RECOMMENDED DOSAGE	LENGTH OF ADMINISTRATION	ADVERSE EFFECTS
Immunocompro-mised patients and patients with TE[||]	Pyrimethamine *plus*	Loading dose 200 mg PO, then 50–75 mg PO daily	At least 4–6 wk after signs and symptoms resolve	Same as above
	Folinic acid[1] *plus either*	10–20 mg PO or IV or IM daily (max 50 mg daily)		
	Sulfadiazine *or*	1000–1500 mg PO q6h	During and for 1 wk after pyrimethamine use	Rash, fever, diarrhea, hepatotoxicity
	Clindamycin[1,¶] *plus*	600 mg PO or IV q6h (max 1200 mg q6h)	At least 4–6 wk after signs and symptoms resolve	Fever, rash, diarrhea, hepatotoxicity
	Prednisone	1 mg/kg daily in 2 divided doses	Until improvement of edema or mass effect related to focal lesion	
	Alternatives TMP-SMX[1] alone *or*	5 mg/kg TMP PO or IV q12h (max 15–20 mg/kg/d)	Same as above	Same as above
	Pyrimethamine *plus* folinic acid[1] *plus one of the following:*	Same as abovepyrimethamine and folinic acid doses 500 mg PO q12h	Same as above	Same as above
	Clarithromycin (Biaxin)[1]	750 mg PO q6h	At least 4–8 wk after resolution of signs and symptoms	
	Atovaquone (Mepron)[1]	1200–1500 mg PO daily	Not reported	Atovaquone can increase LFTs and skin rash Take with a meal to enhance absorption
	Azithromycin[1]	100 mg PO daily	Not reported	
	Dapsone[1]	750 mg PO q6h	Not reported	
	Atovaquone (Mepron)[1] alone or with sulfadiazine	1000–1500 mg PO q6h	Not reported	
Acute infection in patients with *T gondii* and HIV infection**	Spiramycin[2] (as for immunocompetent pregnant women)	1,000 mg PO q8h (without food)	Throughout pregnancy or until fetal infection is documented	

[1]Not FDA approved for this indication.
[2]Not commercially available in the United States.
*Take with food to minimize gastrointestinal adverse effects.
†This might change in some European countries.
‡Should be taken on an empty stomach with adequate water.
§Take both for 3 weeks followed by 1 week off; repeat for 3 or 4 cycles.
||After initial phase of therapy, maintenance therapy must be continued as long as the patient remains immunocompromised.
¶Clindamycin can be used instead of sulfadiazine in patients intolerant to sulfonamides.
**Amniocentesis should be avoided because of the risk of transmitting HIV infection to the fetus.
Abbreviations: GI, gastrointestinal; LFT, liver function test; PCR-AF, polymerase chain reaction testing of amniotic fluid; TMP-SMX, trimethoprim-sulfamethoxazole.

therapy (that is, in addition) to antiparasitic agents. There is no evidence to support that one antibiotic regimen is superior to another, so choice needs to be informed by the safety profile. Intravitreous clindamycin with dexamethasone[1] seems to be as effective as systemic treatments. There is currently level I evidence that intermittent trimethoprim-sulfamethoxazole prevents recurrence of the disease.

Toxoplasmosis in Immunosuppressed Patients

With the advent of the ART, the natural course of HIV infection has markedly changed, and opportunistic infections including toxoplasmosis have declined and changed in presentation, outcome, and incidence. However, TE is a major cause of morbidity and mortality, especially in resource-poor settings, and it is a common neurologic complication in some countries despite the availability of ART and effective prophylaxis. The initial therapy of choice in TE patients consists of the combination of pyrimethamine, which is able to penetrate the brain parenchyma efficiently even in the absence of inflammation, plus sulfadiazine or clindamycin[1] plus folinic acid.[1]

Adjunctive corticosteroids should be administered when clinically indicated only for treatment of a mass effect associated with focal lesions or associated edema and for a short time because of their potential immunosuppressive effects. Patients receiving corticosteroids should be closely monitored for the development of other effects, including CMV retinitis and tuberculosis. Anticonvulsants should be administered to patients with a history of seizures, but should not be administered prophylactically to all patients. Drug interactions between anticonvulsants and antiretroviral agents should be carefully evaluated, and doses should be adjusted according to established guidelines. The preferred alternative regimen for patients unable to tolerate or who fail to respond to first-line therapy is pyrimethamine plus clindamycin[1] plus leucovorin.[1]

Common clindamycin toxicities include fever, rash, nausea, diarrhea (including pseudomembranous colitis or diarrhea related to *Clostridium difficile* toxin), and hepatotoxicity. Other alternative regimens shown in Table 1 are active in the treatment of TE and may be used in sulfa-intolerant patients or those who have not responded to treatment, although their relative efficacy compared with the previous regimens is unknown.

The combination of atovaquone (Mepron)[1] with either pyrimethamine or sulfadiazine has demonstrated utility for the treatment of acute TE in patients with a Karnofsky

TABLE 2	Prophylaxis Regimens for Toxoplasmosis			
PATIENTS WHO SHOULD RECEIVE PROPHYLAXIS	**DRUG OF CHOICE***	**RECOMMENDED DOSAGE**	**LENGTH OF ADMINISTRATION**	
Primary prophylaxis for immunocompromised patients, including advanced pregnant HIV-positive women (CD4+ count < 100 cells/mm³ and *T gondii* IgG positive)	First choice: TMP-SMX (Bactrim)[1]	1 DS tab 160–800 mg PO daily	For life or until immunoreconstitution has occurred[†]	
	Alternatives			
	Pyrimethamine (Daraprim)[1] *plus*	50–75 mg/wk		
	Dapsone[1] *plus*	50 mg/d		
	Folinic acid[1] *or*	25 mg/wk		
	Pyrimethamine-sulfadoxine (Fansidar)[1] *plus*	1 tab twice weekly	Same as above	
	Folinic acid[1] *or*	25 mg/wk	Same as above	
	Atovaquone (Mepron)[1]	1,500 mg PO daily	Same as above	
Secondary prophylaxis for immunocompromised patients after primary or induction treatment	Same regimen used in the acute phase: TMP-SMX[1]	Half doses of those used in the acute phase 2.5 mg/kg TMP PO or IV q12h, max 15–20 mg/kg/d	For life or until immunoreconstitution has occurred[†]	
Prophylaxis in adults receiving heart, lung, or liver transplant, especially in the case of a seropositive donor (D +) and seronegative recipient (R –)[‡]	First choice: TMP-SMX[1]	80 mg TMP/400 mg SMX (1 tab single-strength Bactrim) twice daily	For 6 wk after transplant	
	Alternative			
	Pyrimethamine[1] *plus*	50–75 mg PO daily	Same as above	
	Folinic acid[1]	5–10 mg PO daily	During and for 1 wk after pyrimethamine use	
Prophylaxis in adults receiving bone marrow and allogeneic stem cell transplants[§] Prophylaxis for accidental laboratory exposure and blood transfusions	First choice: TMP-SMX[1] *Alternatives*[¶]: Pyrimethamine[1] *plus* Clindamycin (Cleocin)[1] *plus* Folinic acid[1]	Same as above[‖] Not standardized	For more than 6 mo Not reported	
	Pyrimethamine[1] *plus* Sulfadiazine[1] *plus* Folinic acid[1]	Same as for acute infection**	2 wk	

[1]Not FDA approved for this indication.
*For side effects, see Table 1.
[†]In patients with AIDS, primary and secondary prophylaxis are generally discontinued when the patient's CD4+ cell count has returned to more than 200 cells/μL and HIV PCR peripheral blood viral load has been reasonably controlled for at least 6 months following ART.
[‡]Preemptive antiparasite treatment should be considered for all symptomatic, seropositive, immunocompromised patients in whom toxoplasmosis is suspected.
[§]There are no clear recommendation for anti–*T gondii* prophylaxis in allogeneic stem cell transplantation, because the optimal regimen has not yet been determined.
[‖]Not specifically codified.
[¶]Alternative regimen in sulfonamide-allergic patients.
**Presumptive therapy should be given with the same dosages as for acute infection and monitored serologically for several months after the exposure or until seroconversion is noted; that is, testing immediately after the exposure, weekly for at least 1 month, and at least monthly thereafter. Seroconversion can occur despite presumptive therapy. Although presumptive therapy typically prevents disease or at least substantial morbidity, it does not necessarily prevent infection.
Abbreviations: ART, highly active retroviral therapy; PCR, polymerase chain reaction; TMP-SMX, trimethoprim-sulfamethoxazole.

Performance Status Score greater than 30, which combines the ability to work, to undertake normal activities without external assistance, and to take care of personal needs. Acute therapy should be continued for at least 6 weeks, if there is clinical and radiologic improvement. This should be followed by maintenance therapy (lifelong secondary prophylaxis), usually with the same regimen that was used in the acute phase but at half doses (see Table 2).

Recent findings indicate that daily pyrimethamine-based maintenance therapy is likely more efficacious in preventing TE relapse compared with intermittent therapy. Moreover, the likelihood of relapse associated with pyrimethamine-based therapy in patients with HIV and TE decreased after the introduction of HAART to approximately 11%. Relapse may thus affect a patient's

[1]Not FDA approved for this indication.

disease severity and prognosis, increase utilization of health care resources, and result in additional health care expenditure. Currently, maintenance treatment should be continued for the life of the patient or until underlying immunosuppression has ceased (immune reconstitution resulting from ART). Adult and adolescent patients appear to be at low risk for recurrence of TE when they have successfully completed initial therapy, remain asymptomatic with respect to signs and symptoms, and have a sustained (i.e., more than 6 months) increase in their CD4+ T-lymphocyte counts to greater than 200 cells/μL on ART. AIDS patients with CD4+ T-cell counts less than 100/μL and IgG *Toxoplasma* antibody should receive primary prophylaxis for toxoplasmosis. Fortunately, the same daily regimen of one double-strength tablet of TMP/SMX (Bactrim DS) used for *Pneumocystis jirovecii* prophylaxis provides adequate primary protection against toxoplasmosis. Secondary prophylaxis for toxoplasmosis may be discontinued in the setting of effective ART and when CD4+ T-cell counts increase to more than 200/μL for 6 months.

Prophylaxis and treatment measures of disease in bone marrow transplant recipients as well as in those receiving organ transplantation are shown in Table 2. Universal prophylaxis with TMP/SMX in allo pre-hematopoietic cell transplant seropositive recipients (HCTSP) should be implemented by all transplant programs. Preemptive treatment with routine blood PCR monitoring is an option if prophylaxis cannot be used.

T *gondii* Infection During Pregnancy in HIV-Positive Women

Immunocompromised women with chronic infection do rarely transmit the parasite to the fetus, resulting in congenital infection. This includes women with AIDS, as well as those on immunosuppressive treatment. Vertical transmission occurs in up to 4% of cases, particularly when the CD4+ count is less than 100/mm³. The risk of transmission is low when the CD4+ count is greater than 200/mm³ (see Table 2).

Consideration should be given to screening all immunosuppressed women for evidence of maternal *T gondii* serologic status to establish an early diagnosis of reactivation. Seropositive women with low CD4 counts should receive TMP-SMX (Bactrim)[1] to prevent reactivation of *Toxoplasma*. Because of reports of congenital toxoplasmosis in mildly or moderately immunosuppressed women, it is recommended that immunocompromised women not infected with HIV and women who are infected with HIV and who have CD4 counts less than 200/mm³ be treated with spiramycin (Rovamycine)[2] for the duration of the pregnancy. A nonpregnant woman who has been diagnosed with an acute *T gondii* infection should be counseled to wait 6 months before attempting to become pregnant. Each case should be considered separately in consultation with an expert.

Detailed ultrasound examination of the fetus specifically evaluating for hydrocephalus, cerebral calcifications, and growth restriction should be done for HIV-1-infected women with suspected primary or symptomatic reactivation of *T gondii* during pregnancy.

Prevention

Strategies for the primary prevention of toxoplasmosis in pregnant women and in immunosuppressed patients with negative serology are shown in Box 1.

Screening

Secondary prevention by serologic monitoring of seronegative pregnant women should be closely connected with detailed primary prevention. Routine toxoplasmosis screening programs for pregnant women have been established in France, Austria, and Brazil. In France, guidelines recommend that nonimmune pregnant women be tested monthly throughout pregnancy to detect seroconversion to *Toxoplasma* infection. In the United States, routine serologic screening is not performed. In Italy, serologic screening is recommended to prevent congenital toxoplasmosis as part of the antenatal care protocol (TORCH). Serologic screening of women should begin before conception, with follow-up monthly tests during pregnancy to detect seroconversion. This is the basis for the French screening program and the Austrian Toxoplasmosis Prevention Program, which recommend routine serologic testing. Treatment is recommended if one of the tests suggests definite or probable primary maternal infection.

Vaccine

Vaccination is one of the most efficient strategies to prevent and control the spread of toxoplasmosis by immunization of humans and animals (the source of infection). To date, there is much debate about whether a human vaccine is feasible. Costs, target population, method for testing the vaccine, and risks associated with the vaccine are important factors affecting development of the vaccine. Much of the work has been focused on SAG1, a surface antigen expressed on tachyzoites, in attempts to induce protective immune response when introduced to the host with various adjuvants. SAG1 is primarily involved in adhesion, signal transduction, invasion, material transport and host immune responses. Thus, this protein may be crucial for both the diagnosis of *T gondii* infection and the ability to immunize against this parasite.

In general, a simpler route to prevent human disease would be to vaccinate animals (cats and intermediate hosts) that are responsible

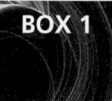

BOX 1 Strategies for the Primary Prevention of Toxoplasmosis in Pregnant Women and in Immunosuppressed Patients With Negative Serology

- Check immunity to toxoplasmosis. If the patient has no protection (absence of anti-*Toxoplasma* IgG), take direct or indirect prophylactic measures against cats, food, and water.
- Universal prophylaxis with TMP/SMX[1] in all pre-HCTSP patients should be implemented by all transplant programs. Preemptive treatment with routine blood PCR monitoring is an option if prophylaxis cannot be used.
- Avoid contact with food (including unwashed fruit or vegetables) or water potentially contaminated with cat feces. Wash before consuming.
- Avoid any job or activity that requires contact with dirt, soil, or other material potentially contaminated with cat feces (e.g., gardening or handling cat litter). Wear gloves when gardening or handling cat litter.
- Keep cats inside. Do not adopt or handle stray cats. Do not feed cats raw or undercooked meat but only canned or dried commercial food or well-cooked food. Do not obtain a new kitten or cat during pregnancy.
- Disinfect the cat litter box with near-boiling water for 5 minutes before handling.
- Wash hands thoroughly after contact with raw meat.
- Kitchen surfaces and utensils that have come in contact with raw meat should be washed.
- Avoid ingesting raw or dried meat, raw eggs, or unpasteurized milk.
- Avoid eating raw oysters, clams, or mussels.
- Protect foods from flies, cockroaches, and other insects.
- Avoid touching the eyes or face or any mucous membrane during or immediately after preparing food.
- Cook meat thoroughly. Pork, lamb, beef, veal, and poultry should be cooked until the meat reaches 80°C in the center.
- Refrain from skinning animals.
- Avoid children's sandboxes.
- Avoid contact with stray dogs (xenosmophilia); if this is not possible, wash your hands after contact.

[1]Not FDA approved for this indication.

---

[1]Not FDA approved for this indication.

for transmission to humans, as demonstrated using a live attenuated vaccine developed for the prevention of chronic infection in sheep. However, it cannot be used in humans because of the risk of reversion to a pathogenic form. Vaccine development to prevent feline oocyst shedding is ongoing, mostly involving live vaccines. More recently, *T gondii* dense granule proteins including GRA-6, a secretory vesicular organelle that produces proteins that participate in the modification of the parasitophorous vacuole, have been shown to be suitable as possible DNA vaccines for immunity against toxoplasmosis. Recombinant rhoptry effector protein 54 (ROP54) plasmid has demonstrated to provide partial protection against acute and chronic toxoplasmosis. Finally, aspartic protease 1 (Asp 1) has also shown to play an essential role in the *T gondii* lifecycle, thus being a potential vaccine candidate against toxoplasmosis.

In summary, the immune evasive nature and complex life cycle of *T gondii* has made the design of immunotherapeutics aimed at providing complete protection, a discouraging challenge. Generally, vaccine studies thus far have shown that multi-antigenic formulations confer better protection than single-subunit vaccines.

---

[1]Not FDA approved for this indication.

References

Alaa Tareq Shakir Al-Hassnawi: Toxoplasma gondii may be an advisor for aggressiveness: seroprevalence of toxoplasmosis in murderer women in Iraq, *American Journal of Biology and Life Sciences* 2(6):187–190, 2014.

Boothroyd JC: Toxoplasma gondii: 25 years and 25 major advances for the field, *Int J Parasitol* 39:935–946, 2009.

Connolly MP, Haitsma G, Hernández AV, Vidal JE: Systematic review and meta-analysis of secondary prophylaxis for prevention of HIV-related toxoplasmic encephalitis relapse using trimethoprim-sulfamethoxazole, *Pathog Glob Health*. 111(6):327–331, 2017 Sep, https://doi.org/10.1080/20477724.2017.1377974.

Contini C: Clinical and diagnostic management of toxoplasmosis in the immunocompromised patient, *Parassitologia* 50:45–50, 2008.

Contini C, Seraceni S, Cultrera R, et al: Evaluation of a real-time PCR-based assay using the lightcycler system for detection of Toxoplasma gondii bradyzoite genes in blood specimens from patients with toxoplasmic retinochoroiditis, *Int J Parasitol* 35:275–283, 2005. Epub 2005 Jan 18.

Del Grande C, Contini C, Schiavi E, et al: Bipolar disorder with psychotic features and ocular toxoplasmosis: a possible pathogenetic role of the parasite? *J Nerv Ment Dis* 205(3):192–195, 2017.

Derouin F, Pelloux H: ESCMID study group on clinical parasitology: prevention of toxoplasmosis in transplant patients, *Clin Microbiol Infect* 14:1089–1101, 2008.

Dupont CD, Christian DA, Hunter CA: Immune response and immunopathology during toxoplasmosis, *Semin Immunopathol* 34:793–813, 2012. Epub 2012 Sep 7.

Elmore SA, Jones JL, Conrad PA, et al: Toxoplasma gondii: epidemiology, feline clinical aspects, and prevention, *Trends Parasitol* 26:190–196, 2010.

Flegr J, Preiss M, Klose J: Toxoplasmosis-associated difference in intelligence and personality in men depends on their Rhesus blood group but not ABO blood group, *PLoS One* 8, 2013. e61272.

Homan W, Vercammen M, De Braekeleer J, Verschueren H: Identification of a 200- to 300-fold repetitive 529 bp DNA fragment in Toxoplasma gondii, and its use for diagnostic and quantitative PCR, *Int J Parasitol*. 30:69–75, 2000.

Jasper S, Vedula SS, John SS, et al: Corticosteroids for ocular toxoplasmosis, *Cochrane Database Syst Rev* 30(4), 2013. CD007417.

Maenz M, Schlüter D, Liesenfeld O, et al: Ocular toxoplasmosis past, present and new aspects of an old disease, *Prog Retin Eye Res* 39:77–106, 2014.

Montoya JG, Liesenfeld O: Toxoplasmosis, *Lancet* 363:1965–1976, 2004.

Ngoungou EB, Bhalla D, Nzoghe A, Darde ML, Preux PM: Toxoplasmosis and epilepsy–systematic review and meta analysis, *PLoS Negl Trop Dis* 9(2), 2015. e0003525.

Petersen E: Toxoplasmosis, *Semin Fetal Neonatal Med* 12:214–223, 2007.

Peyron F, Mc Leod R, Ajzenberg D, et al: Congenital toxoplasmosis in France and the United States: one parasite, two diverging approaches, *PLoS Negl Trop Dis* 11(2), 2017. e0005222.

Remington JS, McLeod R, Thulliez P, et al: Toxoplasmosis. In Remington JS, Klein J, Wilson CB, Baker MD, editors: *Infectious Disease of the Fetus and Newborn Infant*, 6th ed., Philadelphia, 2006, Saunders, pp 946–1091.

Sathekge M, Maes A, Van de Wiele C: FDG-PET imaging in HIV infection and tuberculosis, *Semin Nucl Med* 43(5):349–366, 2013.

Shiadeh MN, Niyyati M, Fallahi S, et al: Human parasitic protozoan infection to infertility: a systematic review, *Parasitol Res* 115:469–477, 2016.

Sullivan Jr WJ, Jeffers V: Mechanisms of Toxoplasma gondii persistence and latency, *FEMS Microbiol Rev* 36:717–733, 2012.

Villard O, Cimon B, L'Ollivier C, et al: Serological diagnosis of Toxoplasma gondii infection, *recommendations from the French National Reference Center for Toxoplasmosis*, *Diagn Microbiol Infect Dis* 84:22–33, 2016.

---

[2]Not commercially available in the United States.

TYPHOID FEVER

Method of
Tamilarasu Kadhiravan, MD

CURRENT DIAGNOSIS

- Typhoid fever typically manifests as an undifferentiated acute febrile illness.
- Soft splenomegaly, normal or low white blood cell count, and elevated liver enzymes are subtle diagnostic pointers.
- Blood culture, drawn before antibiotic administration, is the most useful investigation.
- Consider presumptive treatment in appropriate epidemiologic settings.

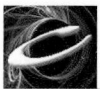

CURRENT THERAPY

- Intermediate susceptibility and resistance to fluoroquinolones are widespread among *Salmonella enterica* Typhi.
- High-dose fluoroquinolones are suboptimal for treating such infections.
- Azithromycin (Zithromax)[1] is the preferred drug for uncomplicated typhoid fever.
- Ceftriaxone (Rocephin)[1] is preferred for treating hospitalized and seriously ill patients.
- Extensively drug-resistant (XDR) typhoid fever, which is resistant to ceftriaxone and fluoroquinolones, is an emerging threat.

---

[1]Not FDA approved for this indication.

Typhoid fever is a bacteremic infection caused by the gram-negative bacillus *Salmonella enterica* serovar Typhi. *S enterica* Paratyphi also causes an illness clinically indistinguishable from typhoid fever. Humans are the only known host of *S enterica* Typhi, and it is transmitted by ingestion of contaminated food or water. Improvement in sanitation and hygiene led to the elimination of typhoid fever from the developed world long before the advent of antibiotics. On the other hand, in parts of the world lacking sanitation, it continues to be an important cause of febrile illness despite the availability of effective antibiotics.

Epidemiology

Typhoid fever is endemic in the developing world, especially the South and South East Asian countries of India, Nepal, Pakistan, Bangladesh, Vietnam, and Indonesia. Annual incidence in endemic settings is typically more than 100 cases per 100,000 population, and it predominantly affects children and young adults. Apart from sick persons with typhoid fever, convalescent carriers and asymptomatically infected food handlers (long-term carriers) are the sources of infection. Potential vehicles of infection include food or water consumed from roadside eateries, ice cubes and ice cream made from contaminated water, and raw vegetables and fruits. In contrast, most cases of typhoid fever in developed countries are imported by travel, especially to the Indian subcontinent.

Pathogenesis and Clinical Features

Following ingestion, the bacilli invade and multiply in the small-intestinal lymphoid tissue before entering the bloodstream. This primary bacteremia leads to widespread seeding of the reticuloendothelial system and intestinal lymphoid tissue, where the infection is amplified and spills over into the circulation. Onset of symptoms usually coincides with this secondary bacteremia. Interestingly, unlike other gram-negative bacteremic infections, septic shock develops relatively late in the course of illness, and the infection can be eminently cured by oral antibiotic therapy.

Abdominal
Paralytic ileus
Intestinal hemorrhage
Intestinal perforation
Secondary peritonitis
Symptomatic liver dysfunction
Acalculous cholecystitis

Extra abdominal
Encephalopathy
Cerebellar dysfunction
Myocarditis
Osteomyelitis and soft tissue abscesses
Multiorgan dysfunction syndrome
Hemophagocytic syndrome
Hemolysis
Glomerulonephritis

Long-term
Gallbladder cancer

Nonetheless, it should be emphasized that any delay in initiating antibiotic therapy increases the risk of complications (Box 1).

During the first week, temperature gradually increases in a stepladder fashion. Localizing symptoms are usually minimal. Anorexia, lassitude, and malaise are often marked. Headache and vomiting are common; however, a supple neck helps rule out meningitis. Abdominal symptoms such as constipation, loose stools, and abdominal pain are not infrequent, but they are nonspecific and often overlooked. Soft, tender enlargement of liver or spleen is seen in about half the patients. Rose spots and relative bradycardia, though classic, are rare. When the infection goes untreated, hypertrophied lymphoid tissue of the Peyer's patches can ulcerate toward the end of the second week, resulting in torrential gastrointestinal bleeding, small intestinal perforation, and secondary bacterial peritonitis. Patients with severe illness can present with a muttering delirium described as *coma vigil*. Untreated typhoid fever often resolves spontaneously in about 4 to 6 weeks. However, the risk of death is high (>10%), and relapses are frequent. Many patients excrete *S enterica* Typhi in feces and urine during convalescence (convalescent carriers), and some of them continue to excrete beyond 1 year (long-term carriers).

Current Pattern of Antimicrobial Susceptibility

Since 1990, a sea change has occurred in the antimicrobial susceptibility of *S enterica* Typhi in endemic countries and elsewhere. Unregulated use of fluoroquinolones initially led to the emergence of *S enterica* Typhi strains with decreased susceptibility. These strains had a subthreshold increase in minimal inhibitory concentration (MIC) that was not detected by conventional disk-diffusion testing. Hence, resistance to nalidixic acid (NegGram)[2] (a quinolone) was often used as a surrogate marker for such strains. Currently, determination of MIC is recommended to identify fluoroquinolone susceptibility. Most infections in endemic countries are now caused by *S. enterica* Typhi with intermediate susceptibility or resistance to fluoroquinolones. Not surprisingly, this change is reflected in far-away geographic locales such as the United States and the United Kingdom. Of late, sporadic instances of resistance to azithromycin and third-generation cephalosporins have been reported. Notably, an ongoing outbreak of extensively drug-resistant (XDR) *S. enterica* Typhi with extended-spectrum β-lactamase–mediated resistance to third-generation cephalosporins has been reported in the Sindh province of Pakistan. In 2019, two-thirds of *S. enterica* typhi isolates from Karachi, Pakistan, were resistant to third-generation cephalosporins. Travel-associated XDR-typhoid cases have been reported from several countries in the Europe and North America.

Diagnosis

Clinical features are nonspecific, and laboratory testing is essential to confirm a diagnosis of typhoid fever. A soft splenomegaly, absence of leukocytosis, mild leukopenia, and modest elevation of transaminases are subtle pointers to a diagnosis of typhoid fever. Blood culture drawn early in the illness before initiation of antibiotics is often fruitful and is the gold standard for the diagnosis of typhoid fever. The time-honored Widal test, which detects agglutinating antibodies to somatic and flagellar antigens of *S enterica* Typhi, adds little to decision making. Initial enthusiasm about rapid serologic tests such as Typhidot and Tubex TF has not been confirmed in community-based studies. None of these tests are sensitive enough to rule out typhoid. In a patient who has nonlocalizing acute febrile illness lasting more than 5 to 7 days in a suggestive epidemiologic setting (residence in or travel to endemic area; outbreaks), it is prudent to treat presumptively for typhoid fever, after reasonably ruling out competing diagnoses such as malaria, dengue, leptospirosis, and rickettsial infection.

Treatment

Fluoroquinolones (ciprofloxacin [Cipro] or ofloxacin [Floxin][1] 7.5 mg/kg twice a day for 5–7 days) were unparalleled in efficacy for treating fully susceptible *S enterica* Typhi strains. However, their use was associated with frequent treatment failures, prolonged defervescence, and higher rates of complications in nalidixic acid-resistant *S. enterica* Typhi (NARST) infections. Given the widespread emergence of reduced susceptibility, fluoroquinolones are no longer considered the drug of choice. Several alternatives have been evaluated in randomized, controlled trials for treating uncomplicated typhoid fever caused by NARST (Table 1). Ease of oral administration, proven efficacy, and safety (under FDA review) make azithromycin (Zithromax)[1] a good first choice for uncomplicated typhoid fever. In hospitalized seriously ill patients and treatment failures, parenteral ceftriaxone (Rocephin)[1] is preferred. Usually, it takes about 4 to 7 days for defervescence after the initiation of antibiotics. Recently, combining oral azithromycin (500 mg qd) with ceftriaxone (2 g qd) for inpatient or cefixime (Suprax)[1] (400 mg qd) for outpatient treatment was found to shorten the fever clearance time by about 7 hours, and fewer patients had persistent bacteremia on Day 3 (17% vs 4%). This clinical trial had certain limitations, and I do not recommend using a combination of antibiotics to treat typhoid fever. Despite in vitro susceptibility, aminoglycosides and first- and second-generation cephalosporins are not effective clinically for treating typhoid fever. Azithromycin (20 mg/kg qd for 7 days)[3] and meropenem (Merrem[1]; 20 mg/kg tid for 14 days) are the only options currently available for the treatment of XDR-typhoid. Antipyretics should be used for symptom relief; ibuprofen (Motrin; 10 mg/kg every 6 hours) is superior to acetaminophen (Tylenol; 12 mg/kg every 6 hours). However, ibuprofen should be avoided when dengue fever is a possibility. A soft, low-residue diet is traditionally advised to prevent intestinal perforation. Such a practice, however, is not founded on scientific evidence. Treatment of *S enterica* Paratyphi infection is identical to that of *S enterica* Typhi infection.

Prevention

Sustained improvement in sanitation and access to safe drinking water are essential to control typhoid fever in endemic areas. Avoiding potentially contaminated food and beverages and being vaccinated before travel decrease the risk of typhoid fever among travelers (see the article on travel medicine). Mass administration of the Vi polysaccharide vaccine (Typhim Vi, Typherix [outside United States]) has been found to confer herd immunity and is a potential tool for the control of typhoid fever in endemic settings.

---

[2]Not available in the United States.

[1]Not FDA approved for this indication.
[3]Exceeds dosage recommended by the manufacturer.

TABLE 1 Outcomes of Alternative Treatments for Nalidixic Acid–Resistant *S enterica* Typhi (NARST) Infection Evaluated in Randomized, Controlled Trials

DRUG	DOSAGE	FEVER CLEARANCE TIME (MEDIAN OR MEAN)	RATE OF TREATMENT FAILURE	RELAPSE RATE	COMMENTS
High-dose ofloxacin (Floxin)[1]	10 mg/kg[3] bid × 7 d	8.2 d	36%	<1%; insufficient data	Not recommended
Gatifloxacin (Tequin)[2]	10 mg/kg qd × 7 d	4.4 d	9%	3%	Serious concerns about dysglycemia; resistance emerging in Nepal
Azithromycin (Zithromax)[1]	10–20[3] mg/kg qd × 7 d	4.4 d	9%	<1%; insufficient data	Effective in XDR-typhoid. Unproven in complicated typhoid fever
Cefixime (Suprax)[1]	10 mg/kg[3] bid × 7 d	5.8 d	27%	9%	High cost; not recommended
Ceftriaxone (Rocephin)[1]	60 mg/kg qd × 7 d	2.8 d	7%	7%	Experts suggest treatment for 10–14 d

Data from Arjyal A, Basnyat B, Nhan HT, et al: Gatifloxacin versus ceftriaxone for uncomplicated enteric fever in Nepal: an open-label, two-centre, randomised controlled trial. Lancet Infect Dis 2016;16:535. Dolecek C, Tran TP, Nguyen NR, et al: A multi-center randomised controlled trial of gatifloxacin versus azithromycin for the treatment of uncomplicated typhoid fever in children and adults in Vietnam. PLoS One 2008;3:e2188; Pandit A, Arjyal A, Day JN, et al: An open randomized comparison of gatifloxacin versus cefixime for the treatment of uncomplicated enteric fever. PLoS One 2007;2:e542; and Parry CM, Ho VA, Phuong le T, et al: Randomized controlled comparison of ofloxacin, azithromycin, and an ofloxacin-azithromycin combination for treatment of multidrug-resistant and nalidixic acid-resistant typhoid fever. Antimicrob Agents Chemother 2007;51:819.
[1]Not FDA approved for this indication.
[2]Not available in the United States.
[3]Exceeds dosage recommended by the manufacturer.

References

Azmatullah A, Qamar FN, Thaver D, et al: Systematic review of the global epidemiology, clinical and laboratory profile of enteric fever, *J Glob Health* 5:020407, 2015.

Basnyat B, Qamar FN, Rupali P, et al: Enteric fever, *BMJ* 372:n437, 2021.

Britto CD, Wong VK, Dougan G, et al: A systematic review of antimicrobial resistance in *Salmonella enterica* serovar typhi, the etiological agent of typhoid, *PLoS Negl Trop Dis* 12:e0006779, 2018.

Chatham-Stephens K, Medalla F, et al: Emergence of extensively drug-resistant *Salmonella* Typhi infections among travelers to or from Pakistan - United States, 2016-2018, *MMWR Morb Mortal Wkly Rep* 68:11, 2019.

Jin C, Gibani MM, Pennington SH, et al: Treatment responses to azithromycin and ciprofloxacin in uncomplicated *Salmonella* typhi infection: a comparison of clinical and microbiological data from a controlled human infection model, *PLoS Negl Trop Dis* 13:e0007955, 2019.

Qamar FN, Yousafzai MT, Dehraj IF, et al: Antimicrobial resistance in typhoidal Salmonella: surveillance for enteric fever in asia project, 2016-2019, *Clin Infect Dis* 71(Supplement_3):S276, 2020.

Qureshi S, Naveed AB, Yousafzai MT, et al: Response of extensively drug resistant *Salmonella* Typhi to treatment with meropenem and azithromycin, in Pakistan, *PLoS Negl Trop Dis* 14:e0008682, 2020.

Vinh H, Parry CM, Hanh VT, et al: Double blind comparison of ibuprofen and paracetamol for adjunctive treatment of uncomplicated typhoid fever, *Pediatr Infect Dis J* 23:226, 2004.

Wijedoru L, Mallett S, Parry CM: Rapid diagnostic tests for typhoid and paratyphoid (enteric) fever, *Cochrane Database Syst Rev*(5), 2017:CD008892.

Zmora N, Shrestha S, Neuberger A, et al: Open label comparative trial of mono versus dual antibiotic therapy for typhoid fever in adults, *PLoS Negl Trop Dis* 12:e0006380, 2018.

VARICELLA (CHICKENPOX)

Method of
Martha Riese, MD

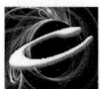

CURRENT DIAGNOSIS

- Historically, varicella has been diagnosed clinically. Symptoms include a pruritic vesicular rash, fever, malaise, abdominal pain, and anorexia.
- Polymerase chain reaction (PCR) testing is available for confirmation of the diagnosis. An open vesicular lesion is swabbed for specimen collection.

CURRENT THERAPY

- For immunocompetent individuals 1 to 12 years of age, treatment is supportive.
- Acyclovir (Zovirax) or valacyclovir (Valtrex) treatment is used to reduce the severity of symptoms and/or risk of complications in those who are younger than 1 year or older than 12 years of age, pregnant women, or for those who are immunocompromised.
- Postexposure prophylaxis with the varicella vaccine (Varivax)[1] is recommended for healthy patients exposed to the virus who do not have evidence of immunity or previous vaccination.
- Varicella zoster immunoglobin (Varizig) administration is recommended for high-risk individuals with exposure history.

[1]Not FDA approved for this indication.

Epidemiology

Varicella infection is caused by the varicella zoster virus (VZV) and is commonly known as chickenpox. This virus is highly contagious and spreads rapidly. Varicella exhibits a seasonality with infections being more common in the winter and spring. Individuals living in tropical climates are typically affected at an older average age than those living in more temperate climates. Historically, prior to the availability of vaccinations, greater than 90% of people were seropositive for varicella by adolescence in temperate areas and less than 5% of adults remained susceptible.

The economic and healthcare burden of varicella is significant. In 1995, the varicella virus vaccine (Varivax) became licensed and available in the United States, beginning an era of reduced morbidity and mortality from the virus. Since the addition of the varicella virus vaccine into the vaccination schedule in the United States in 1996, the overall incidence of the disease has decreased by approximately 92%, and varicella-related deaths have declined by 94%. However, even with the availability of the vaccine and its proven effectiveness at reducing the overall burden of disease, there are still many industrialized countries that have not incorporated it into their national vaccination programs.

Risk Factors
The only risk factor for infection with varicella is exposure to the virus. Adults, immunocompromised patients, infants, and pregnant women are at greatest risk for complications. Specifically, pregnant women, newborns, and the fetus are at high risk for complications.

Following the resolution of the primary infection, the virus remains dormant in the sensory nerve ganglia and can be reactivated at a later time, causing herpes zoster (shingles).

Pathophysiology
The VZV is a double-stranded DNA virus from the Herpesviridae family. The illness is spread by respiratory droplets or direct contact with open vesicular lesions. The virus enters through the respiratory system, mucosa, or conjunctiva. The incubation period is typically 10 to 21 days. The virus replicates in the regional lymph nodes of infected individuals and then is spread throughout the body.

Varicella infection typically confers lifelong immunity, but secondary infections in immunocompetent individuals have been documented on rare occasions. It is thought that subclinical reinfection is common.

Prevention
A live-attenuated varicella virus vaccine, Varivax, has been available since 1995. Currently, in the United States, a two-shot series is recommended for all children and adults who do not have evidence of immunity. The two-shot series of Varivax is more effective than a single dose of the vaccine at preventing infection and complications. A single dose of the vaccine has been shown to prevent infection and reduce the risk of complications, but to a lesser degree than when two shots are administered.

Evidence of immunity is defined as appropriately timed administration of the varicella vaccine, laboratory confirmation of disease, history of diagnosis of varicella or herpes zoster confirmed by a healthcare provider, or birth in the United States before 1980 (although birth prior to 1980 should not be considered sufficient evidence for healthcare workers, pregnant women, or the immunocompromised).

The United States follows the routine childhood vaccination schedule recommended by the Advisory Committee on Immunization Practices (ACIP). In keeping with that schedule, Varivax is recommended for initial administration to healthy children between the ages of 12 and 15 months. The second dose is recommended between ages 4 and 6 years. For children who receive the vaccine series between age 7 and 13 years, the minimum required interval between doses is 3 months. For adolescents over age 13 who have not been previously vaccinated, the first dose should be administered and the second dose should be given 4 to 8 weeks later. The second dose may still be given if more than 8 weeks have lapsed between doses without the need to repeat the series. The varicella vaccine can be safely administered with other vaccines during childhood.

Varicella postexposure prophylaxis with Varivax[1] and/or the varicella zoster immune globulin (Varizig) is recommended to people exposed to active disease who do not have evidence of immunity. The varicella vaccine should optimally be administered to these individuals within 3 to 5 days of exposure to the virus. If the time from exposure exceeds 5 days, the vaccine is still recommended. These individuals should be encouraged to receive the second dose at the appropriate dosing interval.

For individuals without evidence of immunity who are at the highest risk of severe varicella infection and complications, varicella zoster immune globulin may be given following exposure to active disease. The immune globulin should be given within 10

---

[1]Not FDA approved for this indication.

days of exposure for high-risk patients. Patients given the varicella immune globulin should be evaluated for eligibility of future immunization with the varicella vaccine. If they are deemed eligible, an interval of 5 months should lapse prior to the administration of the varicella vaccine.

Varicella immunoglobulin can also be considered for those with contraindications to the varicella vaccine. Contraindications to the varicella vaccine include patients who are pregnant or might be pregnant, malignant neoplasms affecting the bone marrow or lymphatic system, those receiving prolonged immunosuppressive therapy (>2 weeks), moderate or severe concurrent illness, family history of congenital hereditary immunodeficiency, receipt of blood products within the past 3 to 11 months, or history of anaphylactic reaction to gelatin, neomycin, or other components of the vaccine.

Clinical Manifestations
Varicella infection is typically self-limited, with healthy children often having less severe disease than infected adults. Infections often start with a prodrome of fever, chills, malaise, abdominal pain, and pharyngitis that is followed by the appearance of the vesicular pruritic rash on an erythematous base. The lesions have been described as having a "dewdrop on a rose petal" appearance (Figure 1). The rash typically appears on the scalp, face, trunk, and extremities. Lesions may also appear on the mucous membrane of the cornea, conjunctiva, oropharynx, respiratory tract, and vagina. Following the initial prodrome, the first crop of lesions appears as erythematous macular lesions. The lesions commonly transition to papules, then to clear, fluid-filled vesicles, and the vesicles eventually crust over, usually in 1 to 2 days. New crops of lesions continue to appear throughout the course of the illness over approximately 4 to 5 days, ranging between 1 and 7 days. The presence of lesions in different stages is highly characteristic of varicella infection (Figure 2) and helps differentiate the clinical findings of chickenpox from smallpox. Individuals are infectious approximately 1 to 2 days before the onset of the rash until all lesions are crusted over and no new lesions are forming. The stage of the illness when the open vesicles are present is considered to be highly contagious.

Breakthrough infections in previously immunized patients have been documented. These are infections occurring at least 6 weeks following immunization and result from inadequate immunity to the virus. The course of the breakthrough infections in these patients is often shorter and milder with less than 50 lesions. Lesions may not progress to vesicles and or have the typical appearance, potentially making the diagnosis more challenging.

Diagnosis
Historically, the diagnosis of varicella has been based on typical clinical findings. When diagnosing varicella, the history and physical exam are of paramount importance. Noting the characteristics of the rash, including onset and evolution, are helpful in the diagnostic process. The disease is usually self-limiting. An atypical presentation or rash can make the diagnosis based on clinical symptoms difficult. The use of PCR testing is available for confirmation of the diagnosis. An open vesicular lesion is swabbed in order to collect the specimen to be tested. Other sources such as cerebrospinal fluid, blood, saliva, tissue biopsy, and throat swabs may also be used for PCR testing.

Differential Diagnosis
The differential diagnosis of a varicella infection can include hand, foot, and mouth disease; atopic dermatitis; eczema herpeticum; guttate psoriasis; impetigo; viral exanthem; allergic reactions; shingles; and smallpox. Herpes zoster typically presents unilaterally in a dermatomal pattern. Smallpox has been eradicated from natural transmission, but infection via bioterrorism or laboratory exposure must be considered if a suspicious rash is present. The rash seen with smallpox is typically more uniform in appearance and follows a more significant prodrome of symptoms.

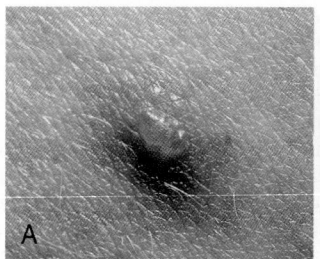 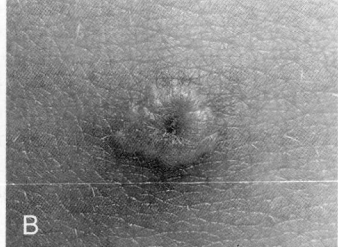 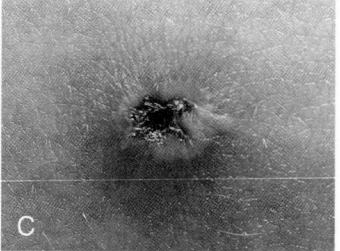

Figure 1 A, "Dewdrop on a rose petal"; a thick-walled vesicle with clear fluid forms on a red base. **B,** The vesicle becomes cloudy and depressed in the center (umbilicated); the border is irregular (scalloped). **C,** A crust forms in the center and eventually replaces the remaining portion of the vesicle at the periphery.

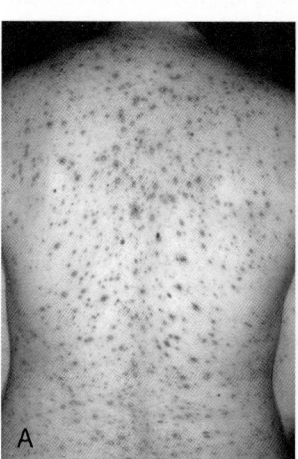 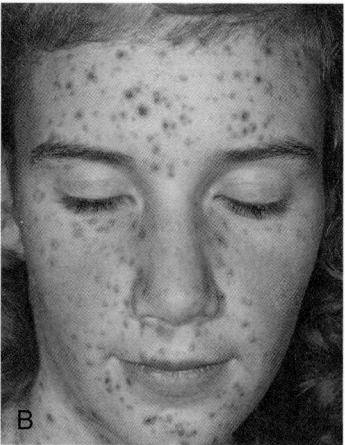

Figure 2 The disease starts with lesions on the trunk (A) and then spreads to the face (B) and extremities.

Treatment

Treatment of varicella infection in healthy children older than 1 year and less than 12 years is symptomatic. Treating fever, malaise, and pharyngitis with ibuprofen or acetaminophen can improve patient comfort. Avoidance of salicylate use is important to reduce the risk of Reye syndrome.

Treatment of adults and children over the age of 12 years involves symptomatic care and antiviral medications such as acyclovir (Zovirax) and valacyclovir (Valtrex). Valacyclovir is more bioavailable and therefore recommended as the first-line treatment. Dosing for valacyclovir is 20 mg/kg up to a maximum of 1000 mg per dose, given three times daily for 5 days. Acyclovir can also be used as treatment, and the recommended dosing for individuals greater than 40 kg is 800 mg five times daily for 5 days. For children over 2 years of age and individuals less than 40 kg, liquid suspension acyclovir (200 mg/5 mL) is dosed 20 mg/kg every 6 hours for 5 days. The maximum dose of acyclovir is 3200 mg daily. If antiviral treatment is deemed necessary it should be started as soon as possible, ideally within 24 hours of rash onset.

For infants less than 12 months of age and immunocompromised individuals, IV antiviral medications are recommended. For adults, dosing of IV acyclovir is 10 to 15 mg/kg every 8 hours for 7 to 10 days. IV acyclovir for infants less than 12 months of age or immunocompromised children is 30 mg/kg/day divided every 8 hours for 7 to 10 days. Ideal body weight should be used to calculate the dosing regimen. With symptomatic improvement, absence of fever for 24 hours, and absence of new lesion development, switching to oral antiviral medication can be considered. For affected individuals with renal impairment, renal dose adjustments are recommended.

Pregnant women with any pulmonary involvement, including upper respiratory symptoms, should be treated with antivirals.

Complications

Approximately 1 in 1000 children with varicella infection will suffer from severe complications. Complications related to varicella infection include pneumonia, secondary bacterial skin or soft tissue infections due to *Staphylococcus aureus* or *Streptococcus pyogenes*, encephalitis, cerebellitis, hepatitis, and even death. Severe complications occur more commonly in immunocompromised individuals, children younger than 1 year, those older than 12 years, adults, and newborns born to mothers that were infected with varicella. Neonates are most susceptible to a severe, even life-threatening disease if the mother develops varicella infection within 5 days prior to delivery or 2 days following birth.

Reye syndrome is another complication that has been associated with varicella infection. This illness presents with symptoms of nausea, vomiting, headaches, excitability, confusion, combativeness, and often progresses to a coma. An association with salicylate administration to febrile children was found to increase the risk of Reye syndrome. Children should not be given salicylates, including aspirin, due to this risk.

Congenital varicella can result in abnormalities of the brain, limbs, and eyes, as well as scarring of the skin and low birth weight. Children with mothers infected during the first and second trimesters have a greater risk of developing congenital varicella syndrome than those infected during the third trimester. Infections during the third trimester increase the risk of disseminated varicella. Infants born to mothers who were infected during pregnancy have an increased risk of developing herpes zoster (shingles) during the first few years of life.

Herpes Zoster
Vaccination

Herpes zoster infections are caused by a reactivation of the latent VZV that has been dormant in the sensory nerve ganglia of individuals who were previously infected with varicella. Patients over the age of 50 or those with a decreased amount of cell-mediated immunity appear to be most susceptible to herpes zoster. Herpes zoster infection typically only affects one side of the body and is distributed within a single dermatome. Disseminated zoster, or disseminated shingles, is characterized by a widespread rash that is not localized to a single dermatome.

There are two vaccines available to help prevent herpes zoster (shingles). Shingrix, a recombinant zoster vaccine, is the currently preferred vaccine and is recommended for individuals over the age of 50 years. Shingrix is given as a two-dose series with doses separated by 2 to 6 months apart. The second vaccine, Zostavax (zoster vaccine live), is a single-dose live-attenuated virus that has been available since 2006 and is approved to prevent shingles in patients ≥50 years of age. Currently, Zostavax has a recommendation from the Centers for Disease Control and Prevention (CDC) for administration to immunocompetent patients who are 60 years of age or older. Zostavax is safe for use in healthy individuals over the age of 60 who are allergic to Shingrix, who prefer Zostavax, or who do not have access to the Shingrix vaccine.

The Shingrix vaccine is preferred over Zostavax as it confers greater efficacy of herpes zoster prevention as well as fewer occurrences of postherpetic neuralgia (PHN)[1]. Shingrix provides

---

[1]Not FDA approved for this indication.

a longer duration of protection. Patients who have had shingles in the past, have had Zostavax previously, or those who are uncertain if they have previously had varicella should still receive the Shingrix vaccine series if they otherwise meet the administration criteria.

Treatment

Treatment of acute herpes zoster with antiviral medication is recommended to aid in diminishing symptoms of the shingles rash, including severity and duration, as well as prevent new lesion formation and decrease viral shedding. Treatment is also thought to potentially decrease the risk of developing PHN.

Dosing regimens for immunocompetent adults include valacyclovir (Valtrex) 1000 mg three times daily for 7 days; famciclovir (Famvir) 500 mg three times daily for 7 days; or acyclovir (Zovirax) 800 mg five times daily for 7 days.

Children who are 11 years of age or younger or those who are immunocompromised with an acute herpes zoster infection should be treated with IV acyclovir 30 mg/kg/day divided every 8 hours for 7 to 10 days. Immunocompromised patients with disseminated herpes zoster should be treated with IV acyclovir therapy. Dosing is 10 mg/kg every 8 hours for 7 days. Ideal body weight should be used to calculate the dose for obese patients.

Treatment has been shown to be most effective if initiated within the first 72 hours of symptom onset. Initiating treatment past 72 hours in immunocompetent adults is recommended if new lesions are still appearing. There is limited evidence available on the efficacy in initiating treatment past 72 hours in immunocompetent patients if new lesions are no longer appearing. Immunocompromised adults should be treated with antiviral medication as soon as possible even if 72 hours have lapsed since the onset of the illness.

Pregnant women should also receive early initiation of treatment regardless of the number of lesions present. Acyclovir is preferred for use in pregnant women; recommended dosing is 800 mg five times daily for 7 days.

Postherpetic Neuralgia

PHN can occur following herpes zoster infection. Symptoms of PHN include severe pain in the area of previous zoster infection even after the rash has resolved. PHN can last for a few days or up to several years. Tricyclic antidepressants, pregabalin (Lyrica), and gabapentin (Neurontin) have the most research to support their use in the reduction of pain from PHN. Some evidence supports the use of topical capsaicin (Zostrix) and lidocaine patches (Lidoderm) in the treatment of herpes zoster. Acetaminophen and nonsteroidal antiinflammatory agents are commonly used, though studies of their effectiveness is limited.

References

Center for Disease Control and Prevention. Shingles Vaccine. Available at https://www.cdc.gov/vaccines/vpd/shingles/hcp/index.html. [Accessed on January 2, 2020].
Center for Disease Control and Prevention. Varicella. Available at https://www.cdc.gov/chickenpox/hcp/index.html. [Accessed on December 27, 2019].
Dooling KL, Guo A, Patel M, et al: Recommendations of the advisory committee on immunization practices for use of herpes zoster vaccines, MMWR Morb Mortal Wkly Rep 67:103–108, 2018.
Leung J, Marin M: Update on trends in varicella mortality during the varicella vaccine era—United States, 1990-2016, Human Vaccines & Immunotherapeutics 14(10):2460–2463, 2018.
Marin M, Guris D, Chaves S, et al: Prevention of varicella: recommendations of the Advisory Committee on Immunization Practices (ACIP), MMWR Recomm Rep 56:1–40, 2007.
Marin M, Leung J, Gershon AA: Transmission of vaccine-strain varicella-zoster virus: a systematic review, Pediatrics 144(3):20191305, 2019.
Marin M, Marti M, Kambhampati A, et al: Global varicella vaccine effectiveness: a meta-analysis, Pediatrics 137(3):e20153741, 2016.
Varicella and herpes zoster vaccines: WHO position paper, June 2014. Recommendations, Vaccine 2016(34):198–199, 2014.
World Health Organization. Immunization, vaccines and biologicals: varicella (2015). Available from http://www.who.int/immunization/diseases/varicella/en/ [Accessed on December 29, 2019].
Wutzler P, Bonanni P, Burgess M, et al: Varicella vaccination- the global experience, Expert Review of Vaccines 16(8):833–843, 2017.

WHOOPING COUGH (PERTUSSIS)

Method of
Raul Davaro, MD

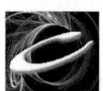

CURRENT DIAGNOSIS

- Pertussis, also known as whooping cough, is an acute respiratory tract infection that has increased in incidence in recent years.
- The diagnosis depends on clinical signs and laboratory testing. Both culture and polymerase chain reaction testing can be used to confirm the diagnosis; serologic testing is not standardized or routinely recommended.

CURRENT THERAPY

- Macrolide antibiotics such as azithromycin are first-line treatments to prevent transmission; trimethoprim/sulfamethoxazole is an alternative in cases of allergy or intolerance to macrolides.
- Current immunization recommendations in the United States consist of administering five doses of the diphtheria and tetanus toxoids and acellular pertussis (DTaP) vaccine to children before 7 years of age and administering a tetanus toxoid, reduced diphtheria toxoid, and acellular pertussis (Tdap) booster between 11 and 18 years of age.

Pertussis is a respiratory infection caused by *Bordetella pertussis*, a gram-negative, pleomorphic aerobic coccobacillus. Infection due to *B. pertussis* affects persons of all ages, with a clinical presentation ranging from a relatively mild-cough illness to a severe illness with pneumonia, seizures, encephalopathy, respiratory failure, and/or death.

Prior to the introduction of whole-cell pertussis vaccines in the United States during the 1940s, the annual number of reported cases often exceeded 200,000. The introduction of childhood pertussis vaccines dramatically altered the epidemiologic landscape of pertussis, with reported cases declining to a nadir of just over 1000 (0.47/100000 population) by the mid-1970s. However, despite substantial declines in disease since the prevaccine era, pertussis remains a significant health problem worldwide, with incidence increasing in several countries in recent years.

Epidemiology

Pertussis is highly contagious and is transmitted via aerosolized droplets through close contact during coughing or sneezing. Studies have identified household members as the source in 75% of cases in infants, mothers being the likely source in almost one-half of these cases. Pertussis shows no seasonality transmission.

During 2000–2016, 339,420 pertussis cases were reported. The majority were in white (88.2%) and non-Hispanic (81.3%) persons, 9.9% were hospitalized, and 0.1% were fatal; however, differences existed by age. Infants had the highest incidence (75.3/100,000 population), accounting for 88.8% of death.

The resurgence of pertussis, probably due to several reasons, including vaccine-driven selection, increased disease awareness and testing, improved diagnostics, and waning immunity.

Transmission

Pertussis is highly contagious and can spread rapidly from person-to-person through contact with airborne droplets. The human nasopharynx can be densely colonized with both commensal bacteria and pathogens, including *B. pertussis*. Infected individuals aerosolize pertussis-containing droplets by coughing or sneezing. Persons with pertussis are most infectious during the mucous producing stage and the first 2 weeks after cough onset.

Pertussis is considered far more contagious than polio, smallpox, rubella, mumps, and diphtheria. Studies showed that one infected person can transmit *B. pertussis* to as many as 12 to 17 other susceptible individuals, while polio and smallpox can be transmitted to 5 to 7, rubella 6 to 7, mumps 4 to 7, and diphtheria 6 to 7 susceptible individuals.

Microbiology and Pathophysiology

Bordetella are small gram-negative, aerobic, nonsporulating coccoid rods. *B. pertussis* infection and disease occur after four important steps: (1) attachment, (2) evasion of host defenses, (3) local damage, and (4) systemic manifestations.

Filamentous hemagglutinin (FHA) and fimbriae (FIM) are two major adhesins and virulence determinants for *B. pertussis*. They are required for tracheal colonization, are highly immunogenic, and are components of certain acellular pertussis vaccines. However, there is likely redundancy in the adhesion role of *B. pertussis* proteins, and it has been suggested that virulence factors such as pertactin (PRN) may mediate attachment in the absence of FHA. Pertussis toxin (PT) also acts as an adhesion and has specific recognition domains for human cilia. Evasion of host defenses occurs primarily through adenylate cyclase toxin (ACT) and PT. PT targets the innate immune system of the lung by inactivating or suppressing G protein–coupled signaling pathways. Through this mechanism of action, PT delays the recruitment of neutrophils to the respiratory tract and targets airway macrophages to promote *B. pertussis* infection.

Immunity

Immunity to pertussis, acquired either from natural infection or through vaccination, is not lifelong. It has been estimated that natural pertussis infection yields 3.5 to 30 years of protection, the estimated protection obtained from the whole-cell pertussis vaccine is 5 to 14 years, and that from the acellular vaccine is 4 to 7 years.

Clinical Symptoms

Pertussis symptoms begin 7 to 10 days after exposure. The disease is characterized by three stages: catarrhal stage, consisting of symptoms indistinguishable from a minor upper respiratory tract infection; paroxysmal stage, named for its characteristic cough consisting of intermittent, sudden bursts of cough, followed by whoop on inspiration and posttussive emesis (the paroxysms of cough are rapid and numerous, occurring up to 15 times in a 24-hour period); and convalescent stage, when paroxysms wane in number and severity. Patients are most contagious during the catarrhal stage. The paroxysmal stage usually lasts 1 to 6 weeks but can be as long as 10 weeks. Almost 80% of adults with confirmed pertussis have an illness involving a cough of at least 3 weeks' duration, and 27% still had a cough after 90 days.

Although symptoms can be prolonged, there is no evidence for chronic infection or long-term carriage of *B. pertussis*. Paroxysms can recur with subsequent respiratory illnesses months after initial illness and are not associated with recurrent isolation of *B. pertussis*. Adolescents and adults frequently have diseases that may not be recognized as pertussis. Whoop is uncommon, but paroxysms of cough and posttussive emesis are common manifestations. A study of adolescents and adults with prolonged cough illness found that 13% to 20% had infections with *B. pertussis*. Pertussis leads to the hospitalization in older children and adolescents in only about 1% to 7% of those affected. Among adults, people older than 65 years are at the highest risk of pertussis hospitalization. Complications also are uncommon in adults,

occurring in about 5%, but can include syncope, rib fractures, pneumonia, and otitis media.

Among immunized patients, especially adolescents and adults, a prolonged cough may be the only manifestation of pertussis. A number of studies have documented that between 13% and 32% of adolescents and adults with an illness involving a cough of 6 days' duration or longer have serologic evidence of infection with *B. pertussis*.

Diagnosis

A positive culture of nasopharyngeal secretions (preferably an aspirate) on selective Regan–Lowe medium is the gold standard for the diagnosis of pertussis. PCR is a rapid test and has excellent sensitivity. However, PCR tests vary in specificity. It is recommended to obtain culture confirmation of pertussis for at least one suspicious case when there is suspicion of a pertussis outbreak. PCR may provide accurate results for up to 4 weeks. After the fourth week of cough, the amount of bacterial DNA in the nasopharynx rapidly diminishes, which increases the risk of obtaining false-negative results. PCR assay protocols that include multiple target sequences allow for speciation among *Bordetella* species.

Treatment

Antimicrobial therapy administered during the catarrhal stage may ameliorate the disease. Antimicrobial therapy is indicated before test confirmation if the clinical presentation is suggestive of pertussis or the patient is at high risk of severe or complicated disease (e.g., is an infant). The duration of treatment for pertussis and postexposure prophylaxis (PEP) is 5 days. After the paroxysmal cough is established, antimicrobial agents have no effect on the course of illness but are recommended to limit the spread of organisms to others. The resistance of *B. pertussis* to macrolide antimicrobial agents has been reported, but rarely. Penicillins and first- and second-generation cephalosporins are not effective against *B. pertussis*.

Trimethoprim-sulfamethoxazole (Bactrim)[1] is an alternative for patients older than 2 months who cannot tolerate macrolides or who are infected with a macrolide-resistant strain, but studies evaluating trimethoprim-sulfamethoxazole as treatment for pertussis are limited (Table 1).

Hospitalized young infants with pertussis should be managed in a setting/facility where these complications can be recognized and managed urgently. Exchange transfusions or leukapheresis have been reported to be life-saving in infants with progressive pulmonary hypertension and markedly elevated lymphocyte counts.

Prevention

In the United States, all vaccines available for preventing pertussis are acellular pertussis formulations combined with tetanus and diphtheria toxoids. Five doses of pertussis-containing vaccine (DTaP [Daptacel, Infanrix]) are recommended prior to entering school: four doses of DTaP before 2 years of age and one dose of DTaP before school entry. Adolescent and adult formulations, known as Tdap vaccines (Adacel, Boostrix), contain reduced quantities of diphtheria toxoid and some pertussis antigens compared with DTaP. A single dose is recommended universally for people 11 years and older, including adults of any age, in place of a decennial tetanus and diphtheria vaccine (Td). Booster doses of Tdap are not recommended for any group of people except pregnant women. The Centers for Disease Control and Prevention (CDC) recommends the use of PEP with antimicrobials in persons at high risk of developing severe pertussis and those who will have close contact with those at high risk of developing severe pertussis.

---

[1]Not FDA approved for this indication.

TABLE 1 Pertussis Treatment

ANTIBIOTIC	DOSING	COMMENTS
Azithromycin (Zithromax)	Children: 10 mg/kg/day for 3 days, or 10 mg/kg on day 1, then 5 mg/kg/day on days 2 through 5 Adults: 500 mg/day for 3 days, or 500 mg on day 1, then 250 mg/day on days 2 through 5	Preferred therapy due to ease of use and tolerability. Preferred agent for infants younger than 1 month Prolongation of the QT interval
Clarithromycin (Biaxin)	Children: 7.5 mg/kg twice daily for 7 days Adults: 500 mg twice daily for 7 days	Fewer adverse effects than erythromycin, but typically more than azithromycin Prolongation of the QT interval CYP3A4 inhibitor; use with caution with other CYP3A4 medications
Erythromycin, delayed release (Ery-Tab)	Children: 40 to 60 mg/kg/day in three or four divided doses for 7 to 14 days Adults: 666 mg three times per day for 7 to 14 days	Gastrointestinal adverse effects limit use Risk of hypertrophic pyloric stenosis in infants CYP3A4 inhibitor; use with caution with other CYP3A4 medications
Trimethoprim/ sulfamethoxazole	Children: 8/40 mg/kg/day divided into two doses for 14 days Adults: one double-strength tablet (160/800 mg) twice daily for 14 days	May be effective for those with intolerance to macrolide antibiotics Caution in pregnancy; contraindicated in infants younger than 2 months, or in mothers breastfeeding infants younger than 2 months

CYP, Cytochrome P450.
From Kline JM, Lewis WD, Smith EA, Tracy LR: Pertussis: A reemerging infection, *Am Fam Physician* 88:507–514, 2013.

References

American Academy of Pediatrics. Pertussis. In: Kimberly DW, Brady MT, Jackson MA, Long SS, eds. *Red Book: 2018 Report of the Committee on Infectious Diseases.* 31st ed. Itasca, IL: AAP.

Ebell MH, Marchello C, Callahan M: Clinical diagnosis of bordetella pertussis infection: A systematic review, *J Am Board Fam Med* 2017; 30:308–319.

Hewlett EL, Edwards KM: Pertussis—not just for kids, *N Engl J Med* 2005; 32:1215–1222.

Kilgore PE, Salim AM, Zervos MJ, Schmitt HJ: Pertussis: microbiology, disease, treatment and prevention, *Clin Microbiol Rev* 2016; 29:449–486.

Kline JM, Lewis WD, Smith EA, Tracy LR: Pertussis: A reemerging infection, *Am Fam Physician* 2013; 88:507–514.

Liang JL, Tiwari T, Moro P, et al: Prevention of pertussis, tetanus, and diphtheria with vaccines in the united states: recommendations of the Advisory Committee on Immunization Practices (ACIP), *MMWR Recomm Rep* 2018; 67(No. RR-2):1–44.

Skoff TH, Hadler S, Hariri S: The epidemiology of nationally reported pertussis in the United States, 2000-2016, *Clin InfecDis* 2019; 68:1634–1640.

YELLOW FEVER

Method of
Lucius M. Lampton, MD

CURRENT DIAGNOSIS

- Yellow fever is a historically important mosquito-borne Flavivirus with high morbidity and mortality.
- Travel to yellow fever–endemic areas in Sub-Saharan Africa and tropical Central and South America is the essential risk factor.
- Symptoms may include abrupt onset of fever, relative bradycardia, headache, and, if severe, jaundice, hemorrhage, and multiorgan failure.
- Diagnosis is with viral culture and serologic tests.
- Although infectious disease experts consider it improbable that yellow fever outbreaks will return to the continental United States, this reemerging disease is threatening to become more prevalent and deadly in tropical South America and Africa. Travel-related cases should be anticipated in the United States and its territories, as well as the possibility of brief episodes of local dissemination in areas bordering the Gulf of Mexico, where the vector, the *Aedes aegypti* mosquito, can be found.

CURRENT THERAPY

- Prevention is key and accomplished by vaccination and mosquito avoidance and control.
- Supportive care is the only treatment.

Epidemiology

Yellow fever is one of the great epidemic diseases of tropical Africa and the Americas. It receives its appellation "yellow" from the symptom of jaundice, which appears in severe disease, and it is caused by an RNA virus, specifically a Flavivirus (a family name derived from yellow fever, with *flavus* Latin for yellow), that is held in natural reservoirs by forest monkeys and spread to people via mosquitoes. The disease, termed an acute hemorrhagic fever, infects humans, all species of monkeys, and certain other small mammals and is transmitted among its hosts by several species of mosquitoes.

There are three types of yellow fever infection: urban, jungle, and intermediate. In urban or classical yellow fever, human-to-human spread occurs by the bite of the *A. aegypti* mosquito, which breeds in urban unpolluted water and bites principally in the daytime. Reinvasion of this mosquito in Central and South America has occurred beginning in the 1970s owing to increases in breeding sites resulting from urbanization and the collapse of vector control efforts. In jungle or sylvatic yellow fever, which was first recognized in 1933, the disease is perpetuated by enzootic infection of mammalians, usually monkeys, disseminated by several different mosquitoes: in South America via the *Haemagogus* and *Sabethes* spp.; in East Africa via *Ae. africanus*; and in West Africa via a variety of species of *Aedes*. Human infection arises by jungle exposure to these mosquitoes. In intermediate or savannah yellow fever, which commonly occurs in Africa, the virus disseminates from mosquitoes to humans residing or working in areas bordering jungles. This cycle also involves spread of the virus from monkey to human or from human to human via the bite of a mosquito.

Yellow fever, also termed Yellow Jack, the Saffron Scourge, fievre jaune, Bronze John, and Black Vomit (the Spanish name is vómito negro), is the deadliest arthropod virus ever to emerge in the Americas. Both the molecular taxonomic research of viral strains and the annals of history reveal an African origin. Most authorities assert it was introduced to the new world by *A. aegypti*–infested slave ships voyaging from West Africa, with its first recognition in the Americas occurring in Yucatan, Mexico, in 1648 (although research suggests the disease was present in the Americas as early as 1498). Over the next two and a half centuries, yellow fever erupted with regularity in American and European port cities, with hundreds of thousands of deaths, earning the virus deserved recognition as one of the worst plagues the world had ever seen. Two of the most significant North American epidemics occurred in Philadelphia in 1793 and in the Mississippi Valley in 1878. American epidemics were the result of the introduction of the mosquito vector and infected humans along routes of trade, especially sea and river ports and rail lines, with particular virulence associated with the Gulf region where *A. aegypti* resided. Early attempts at control focused on quarantine and sanitary measures. The devastation associated with American epidemics was an important impetus in the nation's early public health and sanitation movements for the creation of city, state, and national boards of health.

Although two 19th-century physicians, Josiah Nott and Carlos Juan Finlay, suggested the mosquito was the infectious agent for yellow fever, it was not until 1900 that the work of the US Army Commission in Cuba under Major Walter Reed established that the vector of the urban form of this disease was the *A. aegypti* mosquito, with its viral cause not established until after 1928. Max Theiler developed an attenuated vaccine strain in 1937, which was recognized with a Nobel Prize. In what is acknowledged as one of the most successful campaigns in history against infectious disease, mosquito eradication and control efforts and this vaccine effectively controlled and eliminated urban yellow fever in the Americas and the West Indies, with the last large outbreak occurring in the continental United States in New Orleans in 1905. However, the disease persisted in its jungle form in forest areas in Africa and South America. Vaccine administration remains incomplete in endemic areas, and outbreaks periodically recur. As well, mosquito eradication efforts in both the Americas and Africa have recently slackened, with the resulting resurgence of *A. aegypti* into nearly all of the tropical American countries, placing this region at extraordinary risk for urban outbreaks. While only travel-related cases have been documented in Asia, theoretic anthroponotic dissemination could also take place there in the many areas where the urban vector resides.

Official statistics suggest the incidence of yellow fever fluctuates, with 90% of the 200,000 annual cases reported in Africa. However, authorities warn that these statistics considerably underestimate (owing to underreporting) the true magnitude of epidemics, which field studies estimate as 50 times greater. A frightening prospect associated with failing mosquito control in urban habitats is the potential reemergence of yellow fever similar to the recent rapid resurgence of dengue, which is also transmitted by the vector *A. aegypti*. Experts contend that one of the most profound mysteries of tropical medicine is that this dangerous virus has not emerged more frequently where a susceptible, unimmunized human population and the vector density coexist. However, since the 1980s, a resurgence of yellow fever has been seen across South America and Africa, which augurs potential risk for the United States. While yellow fever outbreaks remain unlikely in the Unites States, travel-related cases should be expected, as well as the possibility of brief urban cycle transmission in the American Southeast.

The 2015–2020 outbreaks in Brazil and Africa portend ominously that yellow fever appears to be moving from its typical rural setting toward urban areas. A large urban outbreak in Angola, which began in December 2015 and subsequently spread to the Democratic Republic of the Congo, resulted in 962 confirmed cases and 393 deaths and included multiple travel-related cases appearing in nonendemic areas internationally such as China. The outbreak in Brazil was first recognized in December 2016, with more than 2251 confirmed cases and 772 deaths noted as of June 1, 2019, including two dozen travel-related

cases. This upsurge of human cases, which is the highest observed in the Americas for decades, reflects the spread into densely populated metropolitan areas, such as Rio de Janeiro and Sao Paulo, which in the past were not considered at risk for transmission. This outbreak has impacted not only Brazil but six other American countries: Bolivia, Colombia, Ecuador, French Guiana, Peru, and Suriname. In the current outbreak, all human cases have been linked only to *Haemagogus* and *Sabethes* mosquitoes.

In response to yellow fever's reemergence in Africa, the World Health Organization (WHO) launched the Yellow Fever Initiative in 2006, vaccinating in mass campaigns more than 105 million people in West Africa and attempting to secure a global vaccine supply. In 2017, the Eliminate Yellow Fever Epidemics (EYE) strategy was initiated with more than 50 partners supporting 40 at-risk countries in the Americas and Africa to prevent, detect, and contain global outbreaks. By 2026, it is projected that 1.38 billion people will be vaccinated against the disease. In March 2018, Brazil's health minister announced that all of the country's 78 million people will be targeted in a large-scale vaccination campaign.

Yellow fever remains the most dangerous arbovirus ever to inhabit the Western Hemisphere. Despite ongoing vaccination and mosquito control efforts in endemic areas, sylvatic and intermediate transmission cycles persist and appear to be expanding toward urban spread. Public health leaders encourage clinicians to utilize heightened suspicion and awareness for the virus, especially among travelers to tropical areas. Recent yellow fever outbreaks underscore boldly the potential threat this disease poses for the international community.

Risk Factors
Travel to yellow fever–endemic areas in Sub-Saharan Africa and tropical Central and South America, between the 15th parallel north and the 15th parallel south, is the essential risk factor.

Pathophysiology
Yellow fever virus has three types or cycles of transmission: urban, jungle (sylvatic), and intermediate (savannah). In urban yellow fever, the virus is spread by the bite of an *A. aegypti* mosquito infected about 2 weeks previously by feeding on a person with viremia. In jungle (sylvatic) yellow fever, the virus is transmitted by various forest canopy mosquitoes that acquire it from wild primates and then disseminate it to humans who are visiting or working in the jungle. Incidence of the disease is highest during months of peak temperature, rainfall, and humidity in South America and during the late rainy and early dry seasons in Africa. In the intermediate (savannah) cycle, which is most common in Africa, transmission of the virus to humans results from humans living or working in jungle border areas, with the virus spread from monkey to human or from human to human by mosquitoes. Humans infected with the virus are infectious to mosquitoes (what is termed being "viremic") shortly before the onset of illness and up to 5 days after onset. Yellow fever is not transmissible by contact, only via a vector's bite.

Prevention
Yellow fever is a mosquito-borne infection that can be prevented by mosquito avoidance and vaccination. Recovery from yellow fever imparts lifelong immunity against the virus.

Mosquito control is an essential component of any strategy to prevent the spread of yellow fever. Before the development of the vaccine and after the mosquito was proven as the vector, eliminating mosquito-breeding sites and decreasing exposure to *A. aegypti* mosquitoes proved successful in ending yellow fever outbreaks in North America and also in the building of the Panama Canal. Today, it remains critical not only to reduce the number of mosquitoes through larvicides and insecticides but also to limit mosquito bites through the use of house screening, mosquito netting, the wearing of protective attire, and the use of insect repellants such as diethyltoluamide (DEET). During jungle outbreaks, mosquito elimination is impractical and evacuation is essential until individuals are immunized and mosquitoes controlled. To prevent further mosquito transmission during outbreaks, infected patients should be isolated in well-screened rooms sprayed with insecticides.

Immunization is the most effective and reliable way to prevent yellow fever in areas in which it is endemic. Live attenuated yellow fever virus vaccine (17D strain) (YF-VAX) should be given (0.5 mL subcutaneously every 10 years) at least 10 days before travel to endemic areas in Africa and Central and South America. A single dose of vaccine gives greater than or equal to 99% protection and confers lifelong immunity. (Although required by some countries, a booster dose of the vaccine is not medically needed.) Although infection is uncommon in most of the endemic areas, vaccination is legally required for entry into many of these countries. The typically well-tolerated vaccine is contraindicated in pregnant women, in individuals with concurrent febrile illness or compromised immunity, and in infants younger than 6 months. If infants aged 6 to 8 months cannot avoid travel to a high-risk location, parents should discuss immunization with their physician, since the vaccine is usually not offered until the age of 9 months. In the United States, the vaccine is given only at US Public Health Service–authorized Yellow Fever Vaccination Centers. The International Certificate of Vaccination is valid for 10 years from 10 days after immunization or immediately after reimmunization.

After the 2016 outbreaks depleted global vaccine supplies, experts suggested as a dose-sparing strategy the utilization of a fractional dose of the vaccine among children 2 years of age or older and among nonpregnant adults.[3] In an observational study, a one-fifth dose of the vaccine induced seroconversion in 98% of recipients. In the 2018 and 2019 outbreaks, mass vaccination campaigns have utilized primarily fractional dosing.

Clinical Manifestations

Yellow fever is characterized by the swift onset of fever, rigors, myalgias, headache, nausea, and vomiting. With an incubation period lasting 3 to 9 days, the illness is typically biphasic, with a two-stage course during which the pulse slows and kidney involvement occurs along with bleeding disorders. Between 5% and 50% of the cases are so mild they are inapparent. In those cases recognized, the pulse is usually rapid initially but by the second day becomes slow for the degree of fever (Faget sign). A tendency to bleed may be seen early in the disease. Often, the face is flushed, with facial edema and conjunctival injection. Restlessness, irritability, and leukopenia are also common. In most cases, this initial period of mild infection resolves after 1 to 3 days, occasionally longer, and the illness concludes with rapid recovery and no sequelae. However, approximately 15% of those infected progress further into the moderate to severe phases. In these cases, the falling fever and remission of symptoms 2 to 5 days after onset are only transitory, and a deadly phase soon begins with renewal of malignant symptoms. This stage of the illness, called intoxication, is marked by the fever returning, and although the pulse remains slow, the blood pressure drops, with resultant renal failure. The flushed face is replaced by a dusky pallor, with swollen, bleeding gums and a pronounced hemorrhagic tendency with telltale black vomit (one of the disease's monikers and classic symptoms) and melena. The skin and eyes may appear yellow (jaundice), the symptom that gave rise to the disease's popular name. (However, this jaundice is generally a symptom of convalescence more than acute disease.) Liver and renal failure (which may progress to acute tubular necrosis) and epigastric tenderness with hematemesis and gastrointestinal hemorrhage often occur. There may be oliguria, albuminuria, disseminated intravascular coagulopathy, backache, dizziness, ecchymoses, myocarditis, agitated delirium, intractable hiccups, seizures, coma, and multiple organ failure. During recovery, bacterial superinfections, particularly pneumonia, may occur.

In terminal cases, death usually transpires within 7 days of onset and is rare beyond 10 days of illness. In patients with intoxication (malignant yellow fever), a 30% to 60% mortality may be seen, with survival depending on the quality of supportive management. At autopsy, the kidneys, liver, heart, and spleen appear to be the organs most impacted by the disease.

Diagnosis

Yellow fever is suspected in patients in endemic areas or returning from them if they develop classic clinical features such as sudden fever with relative bradycardia and jaundice. Mild infection often escapes recognition by the patient or clinician. Complete blood count, urinalysis, liver function tests, coagulation studies, viral blood cultures, and serologic tests should be done. Leukopenia with relative neutropenia is common, as are thrombocytopenia, prolonged clotting, and increased prothrombin time. Bilirubin and aminotransferase levels may be elevated acutely and for several months. Albuminuria, which occurs in 90% of patients, may reach 20 g/L. This finding helps differentiate yellow fever from viral hepatitis. In malignant yellow fever, hypoglycemia and hyperkalemia may occur terminally.

Diagnosis is confirmed by viral culture, serology, the identification of viral antigens and virus-specific immunoglobulin M (IgM) and neutralizing antibodies in serum by several rapid diagnostic methods, or detecting characteristic midzonal hepatocyte necrosis at autopsy. Suspected or confirmed cases must be quarantined and health departments notified. Needle biopsy of the liver during illness is contraindicated because of high risk of hemorrhage.

Differential Diagnosis

Mild yellow fever appears clinically like a broad expanse of other infections presenting with similar symptoms, including dengue, viral hepatitis, malaria, typhus, Q fever, typhoid, Rift Valley fever, leptospirosis, drug-induced syndromes, and toxic causes. Yellow fever may be distinguished from malaria by the findings of conjunctival suffusion or relative bradycardia. The other viral hemorrhagic fevers, which include dengue, Lassa fever, Marburg disease, Ebola, Crimean-Congo hemorrhagic fever, and Bolivian and Argentine hemorrhagic fevers, usually present without jaundice. As well, albuminuria is a reliable hallmark of yellow fever that allows its differentiation from other causes of viral hepatitis.

Treatment

Since no antiviral therapy is currently available, treatment is supportive, focused on aggressive symptom management designed to correct the acid-base imbalance and electrolyte abnormalities caused by emesis, heart failure, and renal derangements. Placement in an intensive care unit is recommended. Transfusions of blood, fresh-frozen plasma, and vitamin K[1] may be utilized with hemorrhagic symptoms. As well, a proton pump inhibitor, H2 blocker, and sucralfate (Carafate)[1] can be helpful as prophylaxis for gastrointestinal bleeding and should be considered in all hospitalized patients. Antipyretics, oxygen, vasopressors, and IV hydration may also be helpful. Avoidance of sedatives and drugs metabolized hepatically is prudent, and medication dosing should be adjusted in the face of declining renal function. Antibiotic therapy for secondary bacterial sepsis is often necessary during the recovery period. Owing to the increased risk of bleeding, avoidance of aspirin and other nonsteroidal antiinflammatory drugs, such as naproxen and ibuprofen, is recommended.

Complications

The majority of those infected with yellow fever will be asymptomatic or experience only mild disease with total recovery. The mortality rates in tropical America range from 45% to 75%, compared with less than 30% in Africa. This difference suggests genetic factors play a role in the course of the illness, as well as the viral strain. The convalescence of a yellow fever patient is usually prolonged and varies from patient to patient. Although uncommon, late death (weeks after the acute illness) can occur

---

[3]Exceeds dosage recommended by the manufacturer.

[1]Not FDA approved for this indication.

as a result of cardiac complications or renal failure. Profound asthenia and fatigue usually last for 1 to 2 weeks, but in some cases can last many months. Jaundice and the elevation of liver enzymes have been known to last an extended period (several months) during convalescence. Survival of an attack imparts life-long immunity against subsequent infection.

References

A Global Strategy to Eliminate Yellow Fever Epidemics 2017–2026, Geneva: World Health Organization; 2018.

Ahuka-Mundeke S, Casey RM, et al: Immunogenicity of fractional-dose vaccine during a yellow fever outbreak—preliminary report, *N Engl J Med* 2018.

Bennett JE, Dolin R, Blaser M: *Mandell, Douglas, and Bennett's Principles and Practice of Infectious Diseases*, 8th ed., Philadelphia, 2015, Elsevier Saunders.

Centers for Disease Control and Prevention. Yellow fever. Available at: https://www.cdc.gov/yellowfever/index.html [accessed July 1, 2021].

Fauci AS, Paules CI: Yellow fever—once again on the radar screen in the Americas, *N Engl J Med* 376:1397–1399, 2017.

Hamer DH, Angelo K, Caumes E, et al: Fatal yellow fever in travelers to Brazil, 2018, *MMWR Morb Mortal Wkly Rep* 67:340–341, 2018.

Kimberlin DW: In *Red Book: 2015 Report of the Committee on Infectious Diseases*, 13th ed., Elk Grove Village, IL, 2015, American Academy of Pediatrics.

Knipe DM, Howley P: *Fields Virology*, 5th ed., Philadelphia, 2007, Lippincott Williams and Wilkins.

Moritz UG Kraemer, et al: Spread of yellow fever virus outbreak in Angola and the Democratic Republic of the Congo 2015–16: a modelling study, *The Lancet Infectious Diseases* 17(3):330–338, 2017.

National Notifiable Diseases Surveillance System (NNDSS): Yellow Fever Case Definition 2019. Available at: https://wwwn.cdc.gov/nndss/conditions/yellow-fever/case-definition/2019/ [accessed July 1, 2021].

Silva NIO, Sacchetto L, de Rezende IM, et al: Recent sylvatic yellow fever virus transmission in Brazil: the news from an old disease, *Virol J* 17(1):9, 2020.

Wilder-Smith A, Monath TP: Responding to the threat of urban yellow fever outbreaks, *The Lancet Infectious Diseases* 17(3):248–250, 2017.

World Health Organization. Yellow fever factsheet. Available at: http://www.who.int/mediacentre/factsheets/fs100/en/ [accessed July 1, 2021].

ZIKA VIRUS DISEASE

Method of
Scott Kellermann, MD, MPH; and Rick D. Kellerman, MD

Zika virus is a mosquito-borne flavivirus. In 1947, researchers at the East African Research Institute in Entebbe, Uganda, were studying yellow fever and placed a caged rhesus macaque in the nearby Zika Forest. The monkey developed a fever and from its serum was isolated a transmissible agent that was first described as Zika virus in 1952. Initially, Zika virus, borne by arboreal mosquitoes such as *Aedes africanus*, infected wild primates and rarely infected humans, even in highly enzootic areas. From its discovery until 2007, there were only 14 confirmed human cases of Zika virus infection, the vertebrate life cycle primarily involving monkey-mosquito-monkey, with rare spillover to humans. Prior to 2007, the virus circulated silently in West Africa. Although endemic in many African and Asian countries, reports of outbreaks on these continents is rare. In 2007, an outbreak was identified in the Yap Islands. In 2013-2014, an outbreak affecting an estimated 30,000 people occurred in French Polynesia. Other isolated outbreaks followed. In 2015-2016, a major outbreak occurred in Brazil and other South American, Central American, and Caribbean countries. The first locally transmitted cases on the United States mainland were reported in 2016. The Zika virus appears to have mutated in character while expanding its geographical range, transforming from a localized endemic, mosquito-borne infection producing only a mild illness to a disease causing explosive outbreaks linked with neurological disorders including Guillain-Barré syndrome and microcephaly. Estimates are that, between October 2015 and January 2016, approximately 1.5 million Brazilians were infected by Zika with 3,500 cases of microcephaly reported within the three poorest states of Paraiba, Pernambuco, and Bahia having the highest incidence. The strain of Zika virus most closely related to the one that emerged in Brazil was originally isolated from patient samples in French Polynesia. In all probability, Zika virus arrived in Brazil in 2014 during the Confederation Cup, when Tahiti's soccer team and its supporters visited a variety of Brazilian venues.

In November 2016, the World Health Organization declared that "The Zika virus and associated consequences remain a significant enduring public health challenge requiring intense action but no longer represent a public health emergency of international concern."

In 2020, 3 US Zika viruses cases were reported, all in travelers. Regarding US territories, 48 cases were reported, all presumed to be through local mosquito-borne transmission.

Epidemiology

Zika virus is transmitted by the daytime-active Aedes mosquitoes, such as *A. aegypti* and *A. albopictus*. With the exception of West Nile virus, which is predominantly spread by culex-species mosquitoes, the arboviruses reaching the Western Hemisphere have all been transmitted by *Aedes* mosquitoes. Millennia ago, North African villagers began storing water in their dwellings, giving arboreal *A. aegypti* a ready medium for depositing their eggs—domestic water-containing vessels. The hatched mosquitoes then fed on humans, evolving into an entirely new maintenance cycle of human–*A. aegypti*–human transmission. Now, thousands of years later, the worst effects of this evolutionary cascade have been seen in the repeated emergence of arboviruses in human ecosystems.

The distribution of *A. aegypti* is more extensive now than ever recorded, extending across all continents including North America.

Another significant Zika virus vector is *Aedes albopictus*, commonly known as the Asian tiger mosquito, named for its white striped legs. *A. albopictus* is of medical importance due to its aggressive daytime human-biting behavior and ability to vector many viruses, including dengue, La Crosse, and West Nile. Figure 1 shows the estimated range of the *Aedes aegypti* and *Aedes albopictus* mosquitoes in the United States.

Most significantly, pregnant mothers may vertically transmit the virus to the developing fetus, potentially resulting in microcephaly. Zika virus has been isolated in semen and vaginal secretions. Male to female as well as female to male sexual transmission of the Zika virus has been reported. Blood transfusions have been a source of transmission outside of the United States. The blood supply in the United States is tested for Zika virus.

Zika has followed a pattern of dispersion analogous to chikungunya, spreading pandemically from west to east. Both viruses now encircle the globe. It appears that both viruses migrated from East Africa to Asia. There is a similar striking movement of Zika and chikungunya from Asia into the Pacific Islands and then to the Americas. Analogous ecological factors might be responsible for their similar spread and may be a key to understanding effective prevention strategies.

Risk Factors

The risk of Zika virus infection for pregnant women is pronounced because of the potential link to microcephaly of the infant. The risk is greatest if the infection is early in pregnancy. There is no evidence that pregnant women are more susceptible to Zika virus infection or that the disease is more severe during pregnancy. Although the transmission of Zika virus is most common due to the bite of an infected mosquito, transmission has also been documented through sexual contact, blood transfusion, laboratory exposure, and both intrauterine and intrapartum transmission. The CDC reports that although Zika virus has been found in breast milk and possible Zika virus infections have been identified in breastfeeding babies, Zika virus transmission through breast milk has not been confirmed. Based on what is known about similar arbovirus infections, once a person has been infected and developed antibodies to Zika virus, they are likely to be protected from a future Zika infection. Based on currently available evidence, once the virus has cleared from the blood of a Zika-infected woman, she is not felt to be at future risk for having a child with a Zika-related birth defect.

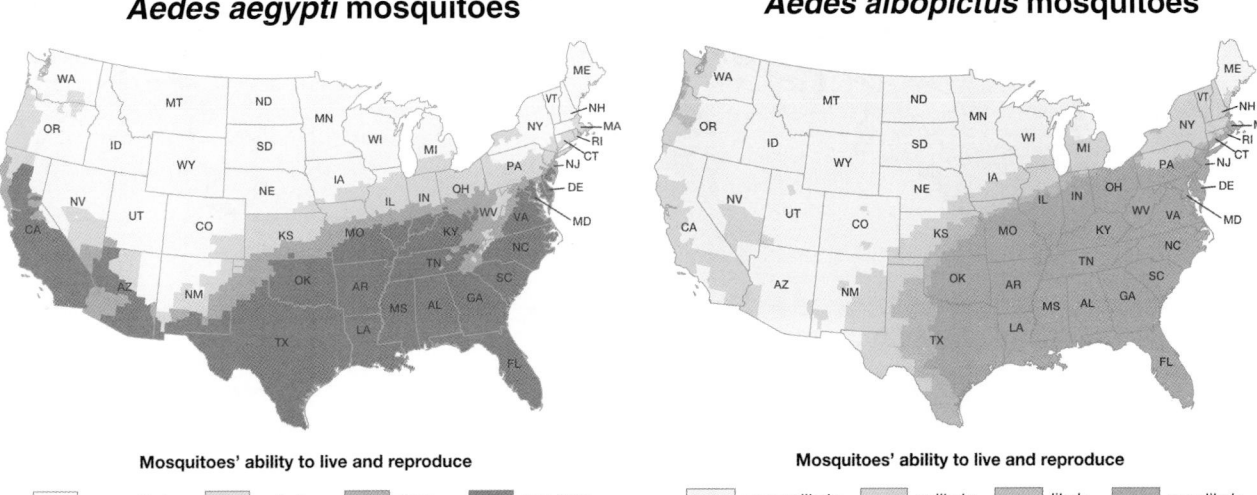

Aedes aegypti mosquitoes

Mosquitoes' ability to live and reproduce

very unlikely   unlikely   likely   very likely

Aedes albopictus mosquitoes

Mosquitoes' ability to live and reproduce

very unlikely   unlikely   likely   very likely

Figure 1 Range of Zika-transmitting mosquitoes in the United States. (Source: https://www.cdc.gov/zika/pdfs/Zika-mosquito-maps.pdf.)

Pathophysiology

The Zika virus is a member of the Flaviviridae virus family, which includes dengue, yellow fever, West Nile, and Japanese encephalitis viruses. Zika is a single-stranded, positive-sense RNA virus that has been fully sequenced. It is one of many arthropod-borne arboviruses. Monkeys are the common vertebrate host of the virus. Arboviruses oftentimes have complex natural transmission cycles involving mammals, birds, and blood-feeding arthropod vectors.

Until recently, only a few arboviruses have caused clinically significant human diseases. These include mosquito-borne alphaviruses such as chikungunya and flaviviruses such as dengue and West Nile. The most historically important of these is the yellow-fever virus, the first recognized viral cause of deadly epidemic hemorrhagic fever.

Prevention

Population-based mosquito control measures are recommended to prevent the spread of Zika virus. Although yellow fever has historically been prevented entirely by aggressive mosquito control, in the modern era vector control has been problematic because of the expense, logistics, public resistance, the development of resistance to the pesticides used and their collateral adverse effects on humans. Although a chemical war against the vector may provide short-term control, programs for improving urban infrastructure and environmental sanitation with a stable supply of potable water would offer more durable results. Among the best preventive measures against Zika virus are house screens, air conditioning, and removal of yard and household debris and containers that provide mosquito-breeding sites, luxuries often unavailable to impoverished residents of crowded urban locales where such epidemics take their greatest toll. Releasing mosquitoes that are sterile or genetically modified to die before they can reproduce is being investigated. Research funded by the Bill and Melinda Gates Foundation has demonstrated the efficacy of Wolbachia in preventing mosquitoes from transmitting viral diseases such at dengue, Zika, chikungunya, and yellow fever.

Because of the association between Zika virus infection and microcephaly in fetuses, the United States Centers for Disease Control and Prevention (CDC) should be consulted for travel guidelines when pregnant women or women considering pregnancy are traveling to affected countries. In some cases, travel may need to be postponed. The CDC website at https://wwwnc.cdc.gov/travel/page/zika-information (Figure 2) contains valuable information regarding areas of the world where risk of exposure to Zika virus is possible. Women who are considering becoming pregnant should consult with their physicians for preconception counseling.

The CDC recommends that women who have had Zika virus exposure through travel or sexual contact and do not have ongoing risks for exposure should wait at least 8 weeks from date of diagnosis, symptom onset (if symptomatic), or last possible exposure before attempting to conceive. During this waiting period, either abstinence should be practiced or barrier contraception with condoms should be used. The 8-week waiting period may decrease the risk of maternal-fetal transmission of the Zika virus.

Zika virus typically remains in the semen for longer periods of time than other body fluids. Accordingly, the CDC recommends waiting at least 3 months from date of diagnosis, symptom onset (if symptomatic), or after the last possible exposure before attempting conception with their partner. During this waiting period, either abstinence should be practiced or barrier contraception with condoms should be used. The recommendation to wait at least 3 months for asymptomatic men is based on the length of time the Zika virus RNA has been detected in semen. The median and 95 percentile for the time until the loss of Zika RNA detection are 42 days and 120 days, respectively, for semen compared to 15 days and 41 days, respectively, for serum and 11 days and 34 days, respectively, for urine. The longest duration of detection of Zika RNA in semen is 370 days, although shedding of infectious Zika virus is believed to be limited to the first few weeks after the onset of illness. There is a lack of evidence that the risk of sexual transmission differs in symptomatic and asymptomatic men.

Between 2015 and July 2018, 52 cases of confirmed sexual transmission of Zika virus infection had been reported in the United States. The longest period from symptom onset in the index case to potential sexual transmission to a partner was between 32-41 days; most reports are of much shorter intervals.

Recommendations for men with possible Zika virus exposure whose partners are pregnant are advised to consistently and correctly use condoms during sex or abstain from sex for the duration of the pregnancy.

Documented reports of sexual transmission have primarily involved transmission from a man to a woman; however, transmission has also been documented from a man to another man and from a woman to a man. If a couple has a female partner and only she travels to an area with risk of Zika, the couple should consider using condoms or not having sex for at least 2 months after the female partner returns, even if she doesn't have symptoms. Pregnant women and men and women who are considering parenthood and who have visited or are considering traveling to areas at risk should consult their physician and reference

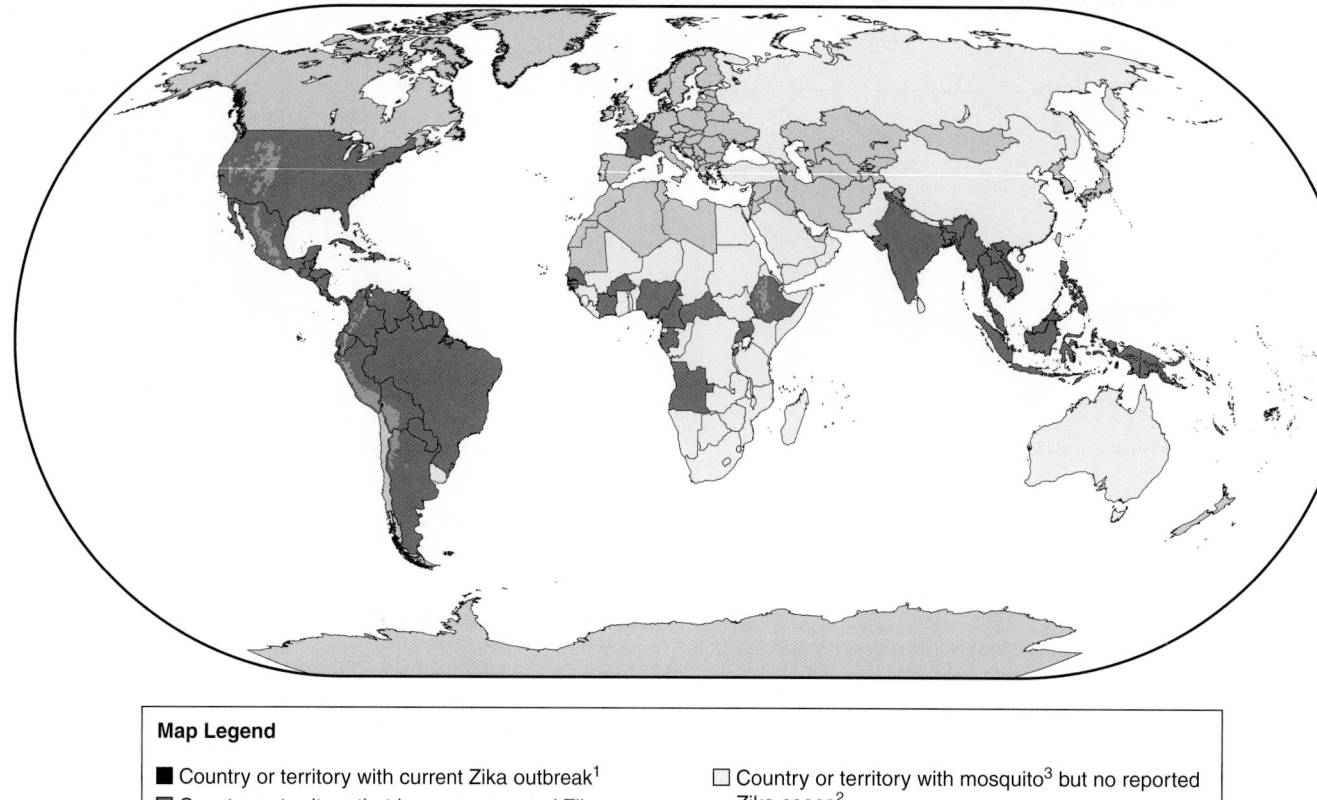

Map Legend

■ Country or territory with current Zika outbreak[1]

■ Country or territory that has ever reported Zika cases[2] (past or current)

■ Areas with low likelihood of Zika infection because of high elevation (above 6,500 feet/2,000 meters)

☐ Country or territory with mosquito[3] but no reported Zika cases[2]

☐ Country or territory with no mosquitoes that spread Zika

[1]No areas are currently reporting Zika outbreaks
[2]Locally acquired, mosquito-borne Zika cases
[3]*Aedes aegypti*

Figure 2 World map of areas with risk of Zika.

the CDC website for travel alerts and pregnancy counseling recommendations.

Avoiding mosquito bites is important for disease control (Table 1). There are hundreds of insect repellants sold in the United States. These insect repellants have different ingredients, different concentrations of ingredients, and different combinations of ingredients. Furthermore, different species of mosquitoes may be differentially repelled by different repellants. Though research is limited, the *Aedes aegypti* and *Aedes albopictus* mosquitoes seem to be most effectively repelled by products that contain at least 25% DEET (N,N-diethyl-m-toluamide), 30% Oil of Lemon Eucalyptus, or 20% picaridin. When applied appropriately, these ingredients may repel mosquitoes for approximately 7 hours and seem to be safe when used during pregnancy. Products with lower concentrations of DEET, Oil of Lemon Eucalyptus, and picaridin are much less effective. Products containing IR3535, 2-undecanone, and products made from natural plant oils such as citronella, lemongrass oil, cedar oil, rosemary oil, cinnamon oil, and geraniol seem to be ineffective against Zika-transmitting mosquitoes. Insect repellents can be used with sunscreen, but the sunscreen should be applied first.

Additional protection from mosquito bites can be achieved by treating outer clothing with permethrin. Permethrin, a derivative of *Chrysanthemum cinerariifolium*, is an insect repellent and insecticide. Though it is poorly absorbed and rapidly inactivated permethrin should not be applied directly to the skin and it should not be used on underclothing. The Environmental Protection

TABLE 1	Prevention of Mosquito Bites

- Remove yard debris (e.g., old tires) and containers that collect water and may provide mosquito breeding sites.
- Wear long-sleeved shirts, long pants, and socks. Tuck pants into socks.
- Apply permethrin to outer clothing.
- Use window screens.
- Use mosquito netting at night if sleeping quarters are not screened.
- Use mosquito netting when children less than 2 months of age—before they can use mosquito repellants—must go outside.
- Apply mosquito repellents directly to exposed skin. When applying mosquito repellents to the face, spray it on the hands, then rub it in. Avoid the eyes and mouth.
- Do not allow young children to apply mosquito repellants themselves. Children who rub mosquito repellant into their own skin are prone to putting their hands into their mouths or touching their eyes.
- Adults should apply mosquito repellant on children by putting the repellant on their own hands and rubbing it into the child's skin.
- To limit the total amount of mosquito repellant that might be absorbed, do not apply to skin under clothing or on skin that is broken (i.e., cuts, rashes).
- Do not use mosquito repellants near food. Wash hands before eating or drinking.
- Wash off mosquito repellant from the skin when it is no longer needed.
- At the end of the day, wash treated skin with soap and water.

Agency (EPA) recommends that clothes treated with permethrin should be washed separately from clothes that are not treated. If washed together, underclothing may absorb permethrin into the fabric which may increase the risk of absorption through the skin. Permethrin-treated clothing will retain repellent activity through multiple washes. The EPA indicates there is no evidence that exposure to permethrin results in adverse effects for pregnant or nursing mothers or adverse developmental effects in their children. Permethrin is listed as pregnancy category B. It can be used on the outer clothing of children older than 2 months of age.

At present no Zika vaccines are available, although Phase 1 and Phase 2 studies are underway, several DNA and mRNA vaccine platforms appear promising.

Clinical Manifestations

The incubation period for Zika virus is estimated to be 3 to 12 days. Serosurvey results from the Yap Islands indicate that only 19% of persons who were infected had symptoms that were attributable to Zika virus. Common symptoms were macular or papular rash (90% of patients), fever (65%), arthritis or arthralgia (65%), nonpurulent conjunctivitis (55%), myalgia (48%), headache (45%), retro-orbital pain (39%), edema (19%), and vomiting (10%). The rash is generally maculopapular and pruritic. Fever, when present, is generally short-term and low-grade. Rarely, immune thrombocytopenia purpura has been linked to Zika. In more than 60 years of observation, severe disease requiring hospitalization is uncommon and case fatality is low.

Diagnosis

In a "pure" Zika epidemic, a diagnosis can be ascertained on clinical grounds. However, dengue and chikungunya have similar clinical presentations and have been epidemic in the Americas, confounding the clinical diagnosis.

The CDC website should be consulted for Zika virus testing recommendations for women who are symptomatic or asymptomatic during pregnancy. Instructions for testing can be found at https://www.cdc.gov/zika/hc-providers/types-of-tests.html.

Cross-reaction with related flaviviruses (e.g., dengue and yellow-fever viruses) is common, complicating the immunologic interpretation of infection. Physicians who deliver an infant suspected of suffering the effects of maternal Zika virus infection should consult the CDC to discuss blood, placental, and umbilical cord sampling. Zika virus infection is a nationally notifiable disease.

Differential Diagnosis

Differential diagnosis encompasses a wide variety of other viral diseases such as dengue, chikungunya, Mayaro virus disease, Ross River fever, Barmah Forest disease, o'nyong-nyong disease, and Sindbis fever. In addition, the CDC lists group A streptococcus, leptospirosis, malaria, rickettsia, rubella, measles, parvovirus, enterovirus, and adenovirus in the differential diagnosis.

Treatment

At present, there is no treatment or vaccine for Zika virus disease. Because symptoms are usually absent or mild, most acutely infected patients do not access the medical system and treat themselves symptomatically. Antiviral medication is ineffective. The mainstays of management are bed rest and supportive care. When multiple arboviruses are co-circulating, testing for a specific viral diagnosis, if available, can be important in anticipating, preventing, and managing complications.

Although the Zika virus has not been associated with hemorrhagic fever, it is probably best to avoid aspirin and nonsteroidal antiinflammatory medications due to their association with hemorrhagic fever syndromes and death when taken for the treatment of similar viruses. The use of aspirin should be avoided in children due to the risk of Reye syndrome. Guidelines for women considering pregnancy and having concerns regarding Zika can be found at the CDC website here: https://www.cdc.gov/pregnancy/zika/women-and-their-partners.html.

Because of the rapidly evolving knowledge about the Zika virus, clinicians are encouraged to freely consult the CDC and WHO websites for clinical guidance.

Monitoring

Pregnant women should be asked about their travel history. Currently the WHO recommends anomaly ultrasound investigations at 18 to 20 weeks' gestation to identify, monitor, or exclude fetal brain abnormalities, particularly microcephaly, for all pregnant women living in areas with ongoing Zika virus transmission. Guidelines for monitoring pregnant females with a potential exposure to Zika virus can be found at https://www.cdc.gov/mmwr/volumes/66/wr/mm6629e1.htm?s_cid=mm6629e1_w.

Complications

The major complication of Zika virus disease is the potential risk of microcephaly as a result of vertical transmission. Amniocentesis has been used to detect the presence of Zika virus in amniotic fluid of women who had ultrasound confirmation of microcephalic fetuses. The virus has been isolated in the brains of newborns and miscarried fetuses. It is unclear whether there may be contributory factors to the development of microcephaly such as nutritional and environmental factors or concomitant infection with other micro-organisms. Other fetal findings have included intracranial calcifications, orbital calcifications, and microphthalmia. It does not appear that the proportion of birth defects differs among mothers who experience symptoms versus those who are asymptomatic.

Microcephaly, other brain abnormalities, and eye anomalies can result from infection during any trimester. A study of pregnancy outcomes in French Territories demonstrated that neurological birth defects occurred in 12.7%, 3.6%, and 5.3% of babies when Zika infection occurred during the first, second, and third trimester, respectively. In a study of pregnancy outcomes in US territories, among pregnancies with confirmed Zika virus infection in the first, second, and third trimesters, the percentages of fetuses or infants with possible Zika-association birth defects was 8%, 5%, and 4%, respectively. According to data in the US Zika Pregnancy and Infant Registry, 5% of pregnancies with suspected Zika virus infection and 10% of pregnancies with laboratory-confirmed Zika infection result in a fetus or newborn with a birth defect, while 15% had a birth defect if the infection occurred in the first trimester. The microcephaly may be subtle. Children may have a craniofacial disproportion and abnormal cranial shape. The fontanelles may be closed or very small and the sutures may be uneven or overlapping. In addition to microcephaly, a phenotypic spectrum has been identified in congenital Zika syndrome. Neurologically, there may be changes in motor activity, severe muscle hypertonia, feeding difficulties, and excessive and inconsolable crying. Musculoskeletal problems include joint immobility, hand and finger contractures, feet contractures and malposition, deep and multiple dimples over joints, abnormal palmar creases and generalized arthrogryposis. Skin on the scalp and other areas of the body may be redundant. Brain imaging may show calcifications, abnormal gyral patterns, enlarged ventricles, and marked decreases in the volume of gray and white matter. The corpus callosum may be thin or absent. The brainstem and cerebellum may be underdeveloped. Seizures, especially in infants between 3 and 6 months of age, may develop and children may exhibit visual problems, hearing loss, and impaired growth. Children exposed to Zika virus in utero who do not have overt signs of Zika virus-associated clinical manifestations or abnormal neuroimaging may have a higher risk of neurodevelopmental delay. The viruses' strong affinity for neural cells may cause neurologic damage that only becomes apparent as children age. Although the full range of birth defects and disabilities associated with Zika virus disease remains to be fully delineated, neural tube defects do not seem to be associated. It is unclear whether infants and children who contract Zika in infancy or early childhood may develop neurologic complications.

Retrospective data from the French Polynesia Zika virus outbreak from October 2013 to April 2014 indicate a close association with Guillain-Barré syndrome. Of the 42 patients diagnosed with Guillain-Barré syndrome, 41 (98%) had anti-Zika virus IgM or IgG, and all (100%) had neutralizing antibodies against Zika virus compared with 54 (56%) of 98 in the control group.

Much still needs to be learned about Zika virus and its geographic spread, transmission, teratogenicity, and long-term complications, including the potential for late onset symptoms in adulthood in previously asymptomatic individuals. A larger issue still to be elucidated in the emergence of Zika and other novel infectious diseases is the role played by urban crowding, ease of international travel, and human encroachments into complex ecosystems.

References

Byrne S: Consumer reports, Mosquito repellents that best protect against Zika. April 16, 2016. http://www.consumerreports.org/insect-repellents/mosquito-repellents-that-best-protect-against-zika/.

Centers for Disease Control and Prevention. Zika virus. Available at https://www.cdc.gov/zika/index.html (accessed June 15, 2019).

del Campo M, Feitosa IM, Ribeiro EM, et al: The phenotypic spectrum of congenital Zika syndrome, *Am J Med Genet* 173:841–857, 2017.

Duffy MR, Chen TH, Hancock WT, et al: Zika virus outbreak on Yap Island, Federated States of Micronesia, *N Engl J Med* 360:2536–2543, 2009.

Environmental Protection Agency: Repellent-treated clothing. https://www.epa.gov/insect-repellents/repellent-treated-clothing#.

Faria NR, Azevedo Rdo S, Kraemer MU: Zika virus in the Americas: Early epidemiological and genetic findings, *Science* 352:345–349, 2016.

Fauci AS, Morens DM: Zika virus in the Americas—yet another arbovirus threat, *N Engl J Med* 374:601–604, 2016.

Honein MA: Recognizing the global impact of Zika virus infection during pregnancy, *N Engl J Med* 378:1055–1056, 2018.

Hoen B, Schaub B, Funk AL, et al: Pregnancy outcomes after ZIKV infection in French territories in the Americas, *N Engl J Med* 378:985–994, 2018.

Kleber de Oliveira W, Cortez-Escalante J, De Oliveira WT, et al: Increase in reported prevalence of microcephaly in infants born to women living in areas with confirmed Zika virus transmission during the first trimester of pregnancy—Brazil, *MMWR Morb Mortal Wkly Rep* 65:242–247, 2016.

Lucey DR, Gostin LO: The emerging Zika pandemic: enhancing preparedness, *JAMA* 315:865–866, 2016.

Lupi E: The efficacy of repellents against Aedes, Anopheles, Culex and Ixodes spp.—a literature review, *Travel Med Infect Dis* 11(6):374–411, 2013.

Musso D: Zika virus transmission from French Polynesia to Brazil (letter to the editor), *Emerg Infect Dis* 21:1887, 2015.

Pattnaik A, Sahoo B, Pattnaik A: Current status of Zika virus vaccines: successes and challenges. https://www.ncbi.nlm.nih.gov/pmc/articles/PMC7349928/.8(2):266, 2020.

Paz-Bailey G, Rosenberg ES, Doyle K: Persistence of Zika Virus in Body Fluids – Final Report, *NEJM* 379:1234–1243, 2018.

Peterson LR, Jamieson DJ, Powers AM, Honein MA: Zika virus, *N Engl J Med* 374:1552–1563, 2016.

Reynolds MR, Jones AM, Petersen EE, et al: Vital signs: update on Zika virus–associated birth defects and evaluation of all U.S. infants with congenital Zika virus exposure – U.S. Zika Pregnancy Registry, 2016, *MMWR* 66:366–373, 2017.

Rodriguez SD, et al: The efficacy of some commercially available insect repellents for Aedes aegypti (Diptera: Culicidae) and Aedes albopictus (Diptera: Culicidae), *J Insect Sci* 15(1):140, 2015.

Shapiro-Mendoza CK, Rice ME, Galang RR, et al: Pregnancy Outcomes After Maternal Zika Virus Infection During Pregnancy – U.S. Territories, January 1, 2016–April 25, 2017, *MMWR* 66:615–621, 2017.

World Health Organization. Zika virus. Available at https://www.who.int/news-room/fact-sheets/detail/zika-virus (accessed June 15, 2019).

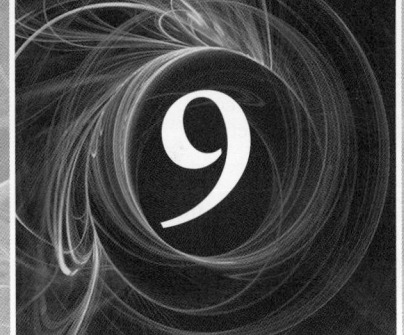

9 Neurological System

ACUTE FACIAL PARALYSIS

Method of
Steven L. Meyers, MD

CURRENT DIAGNOSIS

- Typical cases of acute facial paralysis are diagnosed based on examination and do not require additional evaluation.
- All patients with acute facial paralysis should have a complete neurologic and head and neck examinations.
- The presence of atypical features such as a slowly progressive course, failure to improve, recurrent attacks, or other neurologic findings should prompt additional evaluation with computed tomography (CT) or magnetic resonance imaging (MRI) of the head and a specialist consultation.

CURRENT THERAPY

- Steroid therapy, such as prednisone[1] 60–80 mg daily for 7 days, initiated within 3 days of onset of the facial paralysis, increases the chances of recovery
- The use of antiviral therapy remains controversial without strong evidence of benefit, but valacyclovir (Valtrex)[1] 1000 mg three times daily for 7 days may be beneficial in patients with severe paralysis.
- Eye care with artificial tears, ophthalmic ointments at night, and eye protection should be used in patients with severe facial paralysis.

[1]Not FDA approved for this indication.

Acute facial nerve paralysis, or Bell's palsy, is a common disorder manifesting with the acute to subacute onset of unilateral paralysis of the muscles of facial expression. The Scottish physician Sir Charles Bell described cases of facial paralysis due to trauma in the 1800s, and the idiopathic condition carries his name today. However, there are many possible causes of facial paralysis, and each patient requires a careful history and complete neurologic examination to exclude these possibilities.

Epidemiology and Risk Factors
The annual incidence rate is between 13 and 34 cases per 100,000 population. All age ranges can be affected, but persons between the ages of 15 and 40 years are most commonly affected. Diabetics, pregnant women in the third trimester, and women in the immediate postpartum period are at increased risk. There is no gender, race, or geographic predilection.

Pathophysiology
The seventh cranial, or facial, nerve arises from the pontomedullary junction and runs in close proximity to the eighth cranial nerve to the internal auditory meatus. The nerve then runs through the bony fallopian canal before exiting the skull at the stylomastoid foramen. The labyrinthine portion of the fallopian canal is very narrow, and it is postulated that swelling of the nerve results in compression in this region.

Three branches arise from the facial nerve within the fallopian canal. The greater petrosal nerve arises from the geniculate ganglion, passes to the pterygopalatine ganglion, and eventually supplies innervation to the lacrimal and palatine glands. The second branch is the nerve to the stapedius muscle in the middle ear. The final branch is the chorda tympani, which supplies taste sensation from the anterior two thirds of the tongue.

The pathophysiology of Bell's palsy is uncertain, but a viral cause is the most commonly accepted hypothesis. Many different viruses have been associated with facial paralysis, with herpes simplex virus (HSV) having the strongest evidence. HSV-1 DNA has been detected by polymerase chain reaction assay in endoneural fluid in patients with Bell's palsy undergoing facial nerve decompression.

Herpes zoster is another virus associated with facial nerve paralysis. Herpes zoster oticus (Ramsey Hunt syndrome) is diagnosed when vesicles are seen in the external auditory canal or on the auricle. Other viruses implicated include cytomegalovirus, Epstein–Barr virus, adenovirus, rubella, mumps, influenza B, and coxsackievirus.

The histopathology of the facial nerve supports an inflammatory etiology with findings similar to those seen in herpes zoster infection. The perineurium is edematous, with diffuse infiltration of inflammatory cells between nerve bundles and surrounding the intraneural vessels.

Clinical Manifestations
The clinical presentation of Bell's palsy is typically dramatic and very stereotypical. Pain behind the ear in the region of the mastoid can precede the onset of weakness by hours to days. Weakness of the muscles of facial expression on one side progresses over a period up to 48 hours. Progression over more prolonged periods raises the possibility of a neoplasm affecting the nerve. The degree of weakness can range from quite subtle to complete paralysis of all muscles of facial expression. Typical features include inability to close the eye, sagging of the eyelid, loss of the nasolabial fold, and inability to wrinkle the forehead muscles. Sparing of the forehead muscles suggests a central or upper motor neuron lesion because these muscles receive bilateral innervation. Additional symptoms that may be reported include hyperacusis caused by paralysis of the stapedius muscle, loss of taste in the anterior tongue due to involvement of the chorda tympani, and decreased tearing due to dysfunction of the parasympathetic innervation of the lacrimal gland. However, most patients actually report increased tearing from the affected eye owing to diminished blinking.

Diagnosis and Differential Diagnosis
There is no specific diagnostic test for Bell's palsy. The diagnosis is based on a typical history and examination. Atypical features mandate a search for other causes. A slowly progressive course, parotid gland mass, or involvement in selected branches of the facial nerve can suggest neoplastic compression. Vesicles over the ear or internal auditory canal suggests herpes zoster infection. Patients should be asked about preceding fevers, rashes, and arthralgias, which can prompt evaluation for Lyme disease. However, in the absence of

these features, routine serologic testing is not recommended. Sarcoid is a rare cause of usually bilateral facial paralysis. The onset of facial paralysis in the setting of head injury, particularly in the presence of ipsilateral hearing loss, should prompt imaging of the skull base to rule out a temporal bone fracture (Box 1).

Treatment

Treatment of Bell's palsy can be divided into three categories: general medical therapy, specific medical therapy, and surgical therapy. General medical care includes proper eye care. Reduced blinking and inability to completely close the eye increases the risk of corneal abrasion and ulceration. Artificial tears and ophthalmic ointments can prevent these complications. Patients should be instructed to use proper eye protection to prevent injuries. Facial muscle massage and facial nerve stimulation have no evidence to support their use.

Medical Therapy

Specific medical therapy includes glucocorticoid and antiviral medications. Glucocorticoid therapy has been demonstrated to be effective in both meta-analyses and randomized trials. The two largest trials of glucocorticoid and antiviral therapy demonstrated benefit for steroids but no benefit for antiviral therapy when used either alone or in combination with steroids. Treatment in these trials was begun within 72 hours of onset of paralysis and consisted of relatively high–dose prednisolone (Millipred)[1] 50 to 60 mg daily for 10 days. Antiviral therapy evaluated included acyclovir (Zovirax)[1] 400 mg five times daily for 10 days and valacyclovir (Valtrex)[1] 1000 mg three times daily for 7 days, neither of which showed benefit.

---

[1]Not FDA approved for this indication.

Smaller, lower-quality studies have suggested a benefit of combining antiviral therapy with glucocorticoids, particularly in patients with more severe baseline dysfunction.

Surgical Therapy

Surgical decompression of the facial nerve is not recommended. A 2011 Cochrane review and a 2001 review by the American Academy of Neurology both found no good evidence supporting this treatment modality. Only two small randomized studies showed no differences in outcome between surgical and medical therapy.

Monitoring and Complications

The overall prognosis of Bell's palsy is favorable. In one study of untreated patients, 85% showed signs of recovery within 3 weeks. Ultimately, 71% experienced complete recovery and an additional 13% were felt to have only slight residual weakness. The degree of weakness at onset is an important prognostic indicator: 94% of patients with incomplete paralysis experienced complete recovery. The absence of any improvement, no matter how small, at 3 to 4 months should raise concern regarding the diagnosis and lead to a search for alternative etiologies.

Motor nerve conduction studies, or electroneurography, can be used to help predict prognosis in selected patients. Patients with incomplete lesions that have an excellent prognosis do not require further evaluation. Motor nerve conduction studies involve stimulating the facial nerve electrically and recording muscle responses with surface electrodes over appropriate muscles. The amplitude of the evoked muscle response on the affected side at 10 days can be compared with the unaffected side, giving an estimate of the degree of axonal loss. A 90% drop in amplitude predicts less than complete recovery, and loss greater than 98% predicts significant residual weakness and synkinesis.

In severe cases of facial paralysis, attention to good eye care as previously discussed is important to prevent eye damage and vision loss.

During recovery from severe nerve injury, axonal regrowth may be misdirected, resulting in synkinesis. Voluntary activation of one muscle group can cause activation of other muscles. Attempts at blinking can result in twitching of the mouth, or smiling can cause involuntary blinking. Misdirection of autonomic fibers can result in the syndrome of "crocodile tears," involuntary lacrimation while eating.

Recurrent attacks of facial paralysis on the ipsilateral or contralateral side occur in up to 15% of patients even after many years. Additional recurrences are quite rare, being reported at a rate between 1% and 3%.

References

Engstrom M, Berg T, Stjernquist-Desatnik A, et al: Prednisolone and valaciclovir in Bell's palsy: A randomised, double-blind, placebo-controlled, multicentre trial, *Lancet Neurol* 7:993–1000, 2008.

Gilden DH: Bell's palsy, *N Engl J Med* 351:1323–1331, 2004.

Grogan PM, Gronseth GS: Practice parameter: Steroids, acyclovir, and surgery for Bell's palsy (an evidence based review): Report of the Quality Standards Subcommittee of the American Academy of Neurology, *Neurology* 56:830–836, 2001.

Madhok VB, Gagyor I, Somasundara D, et al. Corticosteroids for Bell's palsy (idiopathic facial paralysis), *Cochrane Database Syst Rev*, 2016, Issue 7, Art. No.: CD001942. https://10.1002/14651858.CD001942.pub5.

Peitersen E: The natural history of Bell's palsy, *Am J Otol* 4:107–111, 1982.

Ronthal M: Bell's palsy: Pathogenesis, clinical features, and diagnosis in adults, *Up to Date*, December 22, 2011. Available at http://www.uptodate.com/contents/bells-palsy-pathogenesis-clinical-features-and-diagnosis-in-adults?source=search_result&search=bell%27s+palsy&selectedTitle=2~26. [accessed 27.08.14].

Ronthal M: Bell's palsy: Prognosis and treatment in adults, *Up to Date*, May 10, 2012. Available at http://www.uptodate.com/contents/bells-palsy-prognosis-and-treatment-in-adults?source=search_result&search=bell%27s+palsy&selectedTitle=1~26. [accessed 27.08.14].

Sullivan FM, Swan IR, Donnan PT, et al: Early treatment with prednisolone or acyclovir in Bell's palsy, *N Engl J Med* 357:1598–1607, 2007.

Yeo SG, Lee YC, Park DC, Cha CI: Acyclovir plus steroid vs steroid alone in the treatment of Bell's palsy, *Am J Otolaryngol* 29:163–166, 2008.

Zandian A, Osiro S, Hudson R, et al: The neurologist's dilemma: A comprehensive clinical review of Bell's palsy, with emphasis on current management trends, *Med Sci Monit* 20:83–90, 2014. https://10.12659/MSM.889876.

ALZHEIMER'S DISEASE

Method of
Katarzyna Wilamowska, MD, PhD; and Janice Knoefel, MD

CURRENT DIAGNOSIS

- There is insufficient evidence on benefits versus harms in screening for cognitive impairment in older adults (Category I).
- Diagnosis of Alzheimer's disease (AD) is clinical, but consider referral to dementia specialist if there are ambiguous findings.

CURRENT THERAPY

- There is no known cure or disease-slowing treatment for AD.
- Acetylcholinesterase inhibitors and NMDA receptor antagonists temporarily improve day-to-day function but do not slow the progression of neuronal cell death.
- Behavioral symptoms of AD are best treated with psychosocial interventions; use pharmacology as a last resort.
- Caregiver training and support is extremely important; it will impact the health of patient and caregiver alike.
- High caregiver burden can result in early institutionalization and poor patient outcomes.

Alzheimer's disease (AD) is considered the most common (60%–80%) individual cause of major neurocognitive disorders (NCDs), previously denominated as dementia. As of 2021, more than 1 in 9 (11.3%) Americans aged 65 or older are living with AD. By 2050, the number of Americans living with AD will double to a projected 12.7 million.

AD is not a result of normal aging (Table 1). There is no cure and, after a prolonged debilitating disease process, AD is fatal. Although we continue to learn more about the pathophysiology of AD, it is known to have indolent asymptomatic deposition of abnormally folded extracellular amyloid-β (Aβ) and clumping tau proteins in the brain that may precede symptoms by more than 20 years. As the disease progresses, amyloid plaques, neurofibrillary tangles, and brain inflammation develop, culminating in neuronal cell death. Research is not yet able to accurately predict the appearance of cognitive symptoms based on these processes.

As with many disorders listed in the DSM-5, dementia carries with it a stigma that may lead patients, family, and friends to avoid or reject the diagnosis. Conversely, a patient with AD, due to the cognitive impact of the disease, may not be aware of their deficits. Diagnosis of AD is often delayed (especially in unbefriended older adults) until the inability for self-care, usually seen as reduction in instrumental activities of daily living (IADLs), brings the patient to the attention of medical professionals.

Screening

Screening for cognitive impairment in older adults continues to be controversial. The US Department of Veterans Affairs, the Canadian Task Force on Preventive Health Care (CTFPHC), the National Institute for Health Care and Excellence (NICE), and the Royal Australian College of General Practitioners (RACGP) recommend against screening for cognitive impairment of asymptomatic older adults. The European Federation of Neurological Societies (EFNS) has no recommendations for asymptomatic individuals, and the US Preventive Services Task Force (USPSTF) states that the current evidence is insufficient to assess the balance of benefits and harms of screening for cognitive impairment in older adults. However, all these organizations encourage screening, work-up, and referrals for cognitive impairment in patients where memory or other cognitive concerns are detected by the patient, knowledgeable informant, or medical practitioner.

On the other hand, the International Association of Gerontology and Geriatrics (IAGG) recommends screening for cognitive impairment of patients with known risk factors for dementia. The Gerontological Society of America (GSA) and the Alzheimer's Association recommend regular screening for cognitive impairment through the Medicare Annual Wellness Visit with coverage for "detection of cognitive impairment" approved by Medicare since 2011.

Risk Factors and Prevention

The strongest risk factors for AD are unmodifiable: age and genetics.

AD is not a normal part of aging, and aging alone does not cause AD. The percentage of Americans with AD increases with age, with the prevalence of AD in those aged 65 to 74 at 5.3%, 75 to 84 at 13.8%, and 85 or older at 34.6%.

TABLE 1	Examples of Changes With Normal Aging vs. Alzheimer's Disease	
COGNITIVE DOMAIN AFFECTED	**NORMAL AGING**	**ALZHEIMER'S DISEASE**
Learning and Memory	Sometimes forgetting names or appointments but remembering them later.	Forgetting important dates or events. Asking for the same information over and over.
Executive Function	Occasional error in balancing a checkbook, omission of a recipe ingredient, taking the wrong turn while driving, making a bad decision once in a while.	Difficulty completing daily tasks, trouble driving to a familiar location, managing a budget, or remembering rules to a favorite game. Poor judgment when dealing with money; victim of financial fraud. Less attention to personal grooming.
Complex Attention	Misplacing things occasionally but able to find them by retracing their steps.	Putting items in unusual places, losing things, unable to retrace steps to find them, may accuse others of stealing.
Language	Sometimes having trouble finding the right word.	Trouble following or joining a conversation. May struggle with vocabulary: word finding, calling things by the wrong name.
Perceptual-motor	Vision changes related to cataracts, glaucoma, age-related macular degeneration.	Difficulty reading, judging distances, determining color/contrast. No longer knows how to use daily household objects (e.g., hairbrush, TV remote, phone)
Social Cognition	Sometimes feeling weary of work, family, and social obligations. Developing very specific ways of doing things and getting upset at change in routine.	Decreased participation in hobbies, social activities, work projects, or sports. Changes in mood and personality; confused, suspicious, depressed, fearful, or anxious. Easily upset.

Several identified genes increase the risk of AD, and people with a first-degree relative (parent or sibling) with AD have a 2.5 lifetime risk of developing AD compared with the general population. AD with mendelian family history is rare and is more likely in early-onset Alzheimer's disease (EOAD, symptom onset before age 65). Of families with EOAD, 86% have a mutation in one of three causative genes: PSEN1 (chromosome 14, most frequent), APP (on chromosome 21, important in trisomy 21 populations), and PSEN2 (chromosome 1, extremely rare).

In late-onset AD, APOE-e4 gene has the strongest impact on risk but by no means is a guarantee of disease development. In fact, recent research suggests lifestyle modifications can decrease the impact of this vulnerability gene marker. Of note, studies of racial or ethnic backgrounds on AD development are inconclusive and, at best, illustrate nonbiologic determinants of health.

Modifiable risk factors include optimizing cardiovascular health, preventing brain cell injuries, decreasing harmful substance exposure, and promoting protective behaviors.

Optimizing cardiovascular health involves controlling hypertension while monitoring for and correcting adverse effects such as cerebral hypoperfusion or falls, controlling hyperlipidemia and diabetes with appropriate treatment, and encouraging smoking cessation.

Preventing brain cell injury starts in early life with consistent helmet use, and with counseling and treatment of substance-use disorders. Treatment of obstructive sleep apnea can prevent injury to brain cells.

The lifetime dose of over-the-counter and prescribed medications with potent anticholinergic action have been shown to increase risk for dementia. Reduction and/or cessation in the use of these medications must be encouraged. Frequently implicated are 1st generation antihistamines, overactive bladder antimuscarinics, muscle relaxants, and tricyclic antidepressants.

Protection includes ameliorating sensory impairment (vision and hearing loss), treating mood disorders, encouraging a healthy diet and exercise, and enhancing brain plasticity in cognitive and social functions. All these behaviors have a transient effect that diminishes once the intervention is abandoned.

Diagnosis
Diagnostic Criteria
Diagnosis of dementia involves meeting the diagnostic criteria for an all-cause major neurocognitive disorder, which necessitates:
- Evidence of cognitive decline from previous functional and performance baseline in a **minimum of two cognitive domains** (complex attention, executive function, learning and memory, language, perceptual-motor, or social cognition)
- Cognitive deficits interfere with patient's ability of independent function
- Deficits cannot be better explained by delirium, affective disturbances, or another disorder

AD diagnosis is clinically classified as **probable** AD or **possible** AD dementia. Core clinical criteria for probable AD dementia are:
- Insidious onset
- Clear-cut history of worsening cognition
- Initial and most prominent cognitive deficits in one of the categories:
  - **Amnestic presentation:** Most common. Presents with impairment in learning and recall of recently learned information. Deficits in other cognitive domains should be present.
  - **Nonamnestic presentation:**
    - **Language presentation:** Deficits in word-finding, but deficits in other cognitive domains should be present.
    - **Visuospatial presentation:** Deficits are in spatial cognition, including object agnosia, impaired face recognition, simultanagnosia, and alexia. Deficits in other cognitive domains should be present.
    - **Executive dysfunction:** The most prominent deficits are impaired reasoning, judgment, and problem solving. Deficits in other cognitive domains should be present.

The diagnosis of probable AD dementia should *not* be applied when there is evidence of other major neurocognitive disorders such as vascular dementia, Lewy body dementia, frontotemporal dementia, primary progressive aphasia, or other active neurologic disease (e.g., Parkinson's disease), nonneurologic comorbidity, or medication use causing substantial cognitive effect (see differential diagnosis section).

Possible AD dementia diagnosis is applied in circumstances of atypical disease course that fulfills the above core diagnostic criteria or in an etiologically mixed presentation.

Differential Diagnoses
The diagnosis of AD must be differentiated from other states of altered cognition (Table 2). Furthermore, in older adults, the presence of delirium, postoperative cognitive dysfunction, post-COVID-19 "brain fog," mild cognitive impairment, or new onset anxiety or mood disorder may be a first sign of future development of major neurocognitive disorder and should trigger closer follow-up.
- Delirium: Develops over a short period of time (hours or days), with change from baseline involving fluctuating levels of attention and awareness throughout the day. Level of activity may range from hyperactive to hypoactive (often underdiagnosed), or mixed. Delirium may be incited by acute infection, change in medical condition, substance intoxication or withdrawal (e.g., drug abuse, over-the-counter or prescribed medications), toxin exposure, or multiple etiologies. Resolution may be acute with correction of underlying cause, but symptoms may persist for weeks or months.
- Postoperative cognitive dysfunction: Develops after receiving anesthesia. Although multifactorial in origin, it is thought to be triggered by the immune/inflammatory response to surgery. Typically affects cognitive domains of learning and memory, and executive function. Resolution typically within 6 months.
- Post–COVID-19 "brain fog": Develops after COVID-19 infection of any severity, including asymptomatic positive tests. Current presumed etiologies include multifactorial delirium, viral-induced immune and inflammatory response, SARS-CoV-2–induced coagulopathy, and direct viral invasion of CNS. Some cases resolve within days or weeks; others have been persistent and may indicate a new cognitive baseline for the patient.
- Mild cognitive impairment (MCI): Insidious onset of symptoms of **minor** neurocognitive disorder where cognitive impairment **does not** interfere with ability to function independently. May affect any cognitive domain and presage development of major neurocognitive disorder. Symptoms may not progress and does not resolve unless substance/medication induced.
- Anxiety or mood disorder: Onset often insidious but may be acute. If new onset of anxiety or depression occurs, it may be the first symptom of a major neurocognitive disorder. Rather than a new onset of mental disorder such as bipolar or attention-deficit/hyperactivity disorder (ADHD), consider chronic undiagnosed disorder with atypical presentation or "new" presentation due to loss of compensatory mechanisms. Resolution depends on appropriate recognition and cognitive/pharmacologic treatment.
- Substance use disorder: Onset may be acute or progressive. Etiology is typically from chronic use but may be brought to medical attention due to discontinuation or overdose. Substances typically indicated are alcohol, stimulants, marijuana, and opioids. Impacts primarily to executive function, memory, and learning domains. Complete resolution of symptoms can occur with prolonged abstinence from substance and correction of nutritional deficiencies, but masked vascular dementia (VaD) may be present as sequelae of chronic substance use. Cannot exclude that presence of neurocognitive changes incited substance use disorder.
- Major neurocognitive disorders that are not Alzheimer's disease: all are progressive and do not resolve. Treatment varies with category and can, in fact, worsen cognitive and behavio-

			CHARACTERISTICS SPECIFIC	
COGNITIVE DISORDER	ONSET	ETIOLOGY	TO DISORDER	TIME TO RESOLUTION

TABLE 2 Differential Diagnosis of Major Neurocognitive Disorder Due to Alzheimer's Disease

COGNITIVE DISORDER	ONSET	ETIOLOGY	CHARACTERISTICS SPECIFIC TO DISORDER	TIME TO RESOLUTION
Delirium	Acute	Multifactorial	Fluctuating levels of attention and awareness	Days, weeks, months
Postoperative cognitive dysfunction	Immediately after anesthesia	Multifactorial Immune/inflammatory response to surgery	Memory and executive function domains most effected	Typically within 6 months
Post–COVID-19 "brain fog"	Positive COVID-19 infection	Multifactorial Viral-induced inflammation Viral-induced coagulopathy Viral invasion of CNS	May affect any cognitive domain	Weeks, months, or persistent
Mild cognitive impairment (MCI)	Insidious	Multifactorial May be reversible if due to substance or medication intoxication Amnestic most common	May affect any cognitive domains; not severe enough to interfere with independent function	Resolves after substance/medication cessation, or persistent
Anxiety or mood disorder	Chronic or new onset	If new onset, consider prodromal neurocognitive disorder or atypical presentation of previously undiagnosed anxiety/mood disorder	Depression: "Pseudodementia" may appear to affect multiple cognitive domains, but upon closer evaluation cognition changes are due to depression Anxiety: suspiciousness, restlessness, insomnia, fearfulness	May improve with combination of cognitive therapy and appropriate medications; recalcitrant disorders may benefit from ECT
Substance use disorder	Progressive due to use, or acute due to overdose or cessation of substance	Alcohol-related brain damage Chronic stimulant use disorder Chronic marijuana use disorder Chronic opioid use disorder	Memory and learning Executive function domains most commonly affected May have VaD component	May improve with cessation of substance and/or repleting nutritional deficiencies, or persistent
Major neurocognitive disorders				
Alzheimer's Disease (AD)	Insidious, most common individual cause of dementia	Misfolded amyloid-β and tau protein deposition leading to neuronal death	Short-term memory loss, language, visuospatial, or executive function most impacted	Progressive
Lewy Body Dementia (LBD): umbrella term for dementia with Lewy bodies and Parkinson's disease dementia	Insidious or pseudoacute in the setting of sleep deprivation	Misfolded α-synuclein (Lewy bodies) deposition in substantia nigra and cortex leading to degradation of dopaminergic neurons	Visual hallucinations, REM sleep disorders; may have bradykinesia, rigidity, or gait changes (see Parkinson's disease chapter) Very sensitive to neuroleptic medications	Progressive
Frontotemporal lobar degeneration (FTLD)	Insidious, symptoms develop earlier in life than AD	Tau and TDP-43 protein inclusions in frontal and temporal lobes Most common cause of dementia in people younger than 60	Behavioral, personality, language changes; memory typically preserved in early disease May have worsening symptoms when treated with cholinesterase inhibitors or NMDA antagonists	Progressive
Vascular dementia (VaD)	Step-wise progression	Cardiovascular risk factors, strokes, infarcts	May affect any cognitive domains; focal findings or gait/balance changes on examination	Progressive
Mixed dementia	Insidious, increases with age	Commonly a combination AD and VaD but can have LBD components	Mixed characteristics of component disorders	Progressive

ral outcomes if misdiagnosed. For brevity, only the most common major neurocognitive disorders are listed in full detail.

- Vascular dementia (VaD): Presentation may affect any cognitive domain, although executive function domain deficits tend to be favored, while memory is initially preserved. Onset of impairment is often abrupt. Patient with cardiovascular risk factors. Physical examination findings are focal in nature (but may be subtle) and often include motor function difficulties, especially slow gait or poor balance. Five percent to 10% of all dementias are of vascular etiology alone.

- Lewy body dementia (LBD): An umbrella term for neurocognitive disorders due to misfolded α-synuclein deposition including Dementia with Lewy Bodies (DLB) and Parkinson's disease dementia (PDD). Presentation characteristic of REM sleep disturbances (acting out dreams), visual hallucinations, and marked visuospatial impairment. Parkinsonian motor symptoms may or may not be present at time of diagnosis (see chapter on Parkinson's disease). Patients in this group are often exquisitely sensitive to neuroleptic medications. Five percent of all patients with dementia are of DLB etiology alone.

- Frontotemporal lobar degeneration (FTLD): Group of disorders that includes behavioral variant FTLD, primary progressive aphasia, Pick's disease, corticobasal degeneration, and progressive supranuclear palsy. Degenerative changes involve tau and TDP-43 protein inclusions preferentially in frontal and temporal lobes leading to marked atrophy. Presentation encompasses marked changes in personality and behavior and/or difficulty producing or comprehending language. Symptoms may worsen when treated with anti-Alzheimer's medications.
- Mixed: Presents as a combination of component neurocognitive disorders with AD, VaD, and, to a lesser degree, LBD. Increases in likelihood with age, with highest likelihood in 85 years and older age group. Over 50% of people with dementia have evidence of more than one type of pathology.
- Other diagnoses to consider: traumatic brain injury, chronic traumatic encephalopathy syndrome, prion disease, Huntington's disease, human immunodeficiency virus (HIV) infection, neurosyphilis, cryptococcosis, brain tumor, subdural hematoma, normal-pressure hydrocephalus, hypoxia secondary to heart failure, hypothyroidism, hypercalcemia, hypoglycemia, temporal arteritis, systemic lupus erythematosus, hepatic or renal failure, metabolic conditions, epilepsy, and multiple sclerosis.

Diagnostic Evaluation
History
Focused history is needed from the patient and at least one knowledgeable informant. Current cognitive and functional difficulties should be discussed, as well as fluctuation of symptoms. Behavior linked to stress, fatigue, or being away from a patient's normal surroundings should also be understood and may clue clinician into treatment needs.

A thorough medication review should be performed with focus on adverse medication effects, goals of care, and deprescribing where possible. Supplements, over-the-counter medications, and herbal remedies need to be evaluated in a nonjudgmental fashion. Reviewing current and past substance use at the same time may reveal more information than if asked separately.

Timeline of the start of functional decline generally precedes presentation to provider by several years. This may be elicited by asking about anecdotes that may have seemed funny or odd at the time (e.g., "Remember when Mom was making her specialty dish and forgot part of the recipe?" or "Remember when Dad took a long time to drive home, even though he was 5 minutes away?"). Any medical illnesses or conditions that may have triggered the decline should be elucidated (e.g., "Mom has never been the same since that infection last year" or "Dad woke up one morning and couldn't see out of his right eye, but he didn't mention it until a few weeks later and it doesn't bother him").

Neurocognitive disorders expose the affected individual to multiple safety concerns, and these must be discussed to detect current problems and to plan for the future. Triggers for further evaluation include "close calls" for motor vehicle accidents, falls, getting lost, or locked out.

Cognitive Status Examination
Although qualitative impressions of cognitive status are helpful in raising suspicions, quantitative evaluation of cognitive status is needed. No single screening tool evaluates all of the cognitive domains: learning and memory, executive function, complex attention, language, perceptual-motor/visuospatial skills, and social cognition. With the limited time of a primary care visit, one is compelled to leverage previsit and office waiting times for questionnaires completed by patient and informant prior to visit, as well as some in-clinic screening tools that may be administered by a medical assistant, nurse, or medical provider (Table 3). These screening tools may aid in the clinical decision making of the provider but need to be interpreted with caution. For example, there may be cases where the patient passes a cognitive screen but fails an entire cognitive domain within the screen, warranting further evaluation.

The Alzheimer's Association "Alzheimer's Disease Pocketcard" mobile app has interactive links to many of the tools listed in this

TABLE 3 Brief List of Self-Administered and Office Screening Tools for Evaluation of Suspected Major Neurocognitive Disorders and Caregiver Burden

TOOL	PREVISIT OR TIME TO ADMINISTER IN OFFICE	PREFERRED PERSON TO ANSWER	COGNITIVE DOMAINS EVALUATED	DESCRIPTION
IADL	Previsit / <5 min	Patient	Executive function, apraxia, agnosia	Independent activities of daily living
ADL	Previsit / <5 min	Patient	Executive function, apraxia, agnosia	Activities of daily living
AD8	Previsit / <5 min	Informant	Memory, executive function, apraxia, agnosia	Good at eliciting early cognitive changes in a variety of dementias; asks informant about judgment, less interest in hobbies, repeats things, trouble using tools, forgets month or year, finances, trouble remembering appointments or daily things
GPCOG	Previsit / <5 min	Patient and Informant	Memory, executive function, aphasia	Recall, orientation, recent news recall; patient questionnaire is paired with an informant questionnaire that asks about memory, finances, wordfinding, ADLs
Short (16 qs) or full (26 qs) IQCODE	Previsit / >10 min	Informant	Memory, executive function, apraxia, agnosia	Asks informant about changes in cognitive function, physical function, patient personality, and behavior
Mini-Cog	<5 min	Patient	Memory, executive function, apraxia	3-item recall plus clock drawing
MIS	<5 min	Patient	Memory	4-item recall

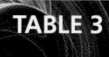

TABLE 3 Brief List of Self-Administered and Office Screening Tools for Evaluation of Suspected Major Neurocognitive Disorders and Caregiver Burden—cont'd

TOOL	PREVISIT OR TIME TO ADMINISTER IN OFFICE	PREFERRED PERSON TO ANSWER	COGNITIVE DOMAINS EVALUATED	DESCRIPTION
SLUMS	6–10 min	Patient	Memory, executive function, aphasia, apraxia, agnosia	Orientation, 5-item recall, math, animals, attention, clock, figures, story
MOCA: may require extra training and licensing	6–10 min	Patient	Memory, executive function, aphasia, apraxia, agnosia	Small trails B, copy figure, clock, naming, verbal fluency, 5-word recall, similarities, orientation, attention
Trail making tests (TMT)	<5 min	Patient	Executive function	Older patients with a TMT-A≥54 seconds or a TMT-B≥150 seconds have a threefold (CI 95% 1.3–7.0) increased risk of performing poorly during driving
Zarit Burden Interview	Previsit /22 questions	Caregiver	Measures perceived social, physical, financial, and emotional burden	Higher scores indicate greater caregiver burden
Revised Memory and Behavior Problems Checklist	Previsit /24 questions	Caregiver	Focused and caregiver reactions to problematic behaviors in patients with dementia	Higher scores indicate greater caregiver burden

chapter and is available for free on iTunes and GooglePlay, or alz.org/hcps where it can be accessed as a web app.

Physical Examination

The neurologic examination should attempt to rule-out Alzheimer's dementia with findings indicative of other major neurocognitive etiologies. Asymmetry in sensation/motor/strength is suggestive of vascular dementia. Tremor and bradykinesia hint at Parkinson's disease syndromes. Abnormalities of eye movement in vertical gaze may signify progressive supranuclear palsy. Peripheral neuropathy, although most likely secondary to diabetes, may indicate B12 deficiency, hypothyroidism, alcoholism, or neurosyphilis.

Laboratory Testing

Reversible or treatable causes of neurocognitive impairment may be revealed by testing complete blood count (CBC), electrolytes including blood glucose, renal function, liver function, thyroid function, syphilis, HIV, and vitamins B12 (cobalamin), B9 (folate), B1 (thiamine), and D (calciferol).

If EOAD is suspected based on family history and early age of presentation, consider genetic counseling prior to testing for PSEN1, PSEN2, or APP. There is currently no clinical benefit to testing for the APOE-e4 gene.

Neuroimaging

Although neuroimaging research continues to move forward on deterministic brain matter changes and correlation to the development of major neurocognitive disorders, these findings do not yet promise diagnosis from neuroimaging alone. At present, there is some controversy as to whether clinical neuroimaging is needed in routine cognitive workups, but we recommend routine brain magnetic resonance imaging (MRI) to rule out stroke, vascular dementia, tumors, or normal pressure hydrocephalus, and perhaps rule in FTLD with focal cortical atrophy.

Of note: There can be significant crossover in presentation between FTLD and AD. As such, Medicare provides conditional reimbursement for a positron emission tomography (PET) for brain amyloid.

When to Refer

Ultimately, the diagnosis of AD in the primary care setting is done clinically after ruling out the above-mentioned differential diagnoses, with more ambiguous cases referred to dementia specialists: geriatricians, geriatric psychiatrists, neurologists, or neuropsychologists. If finding a specialist nearby proves difficult, consider directing your efforts to the closest Alzheimer's Disease Research Center (ADRC).

Treatment

Counseling

Alzheimer's disease is a life-altering diagnosis. Although many patients have heard of AD, they may not know of the progressive debilitation ahead of them. While the patient is decisional, planning and future decisions may be reassuring to both patient and families. It is essential to discuss protection of themselves, their assets, and their wishes pertaining to current and future management of financial, legal, and medical concerns.

Caregiver Support

On average, a person diagnosed with AD survives 4 to 8 years after diagnosis; some may live 20 years. The progressive dependence of patients with AD brings to focus the importance of their caregivers. More than 11 million Americans provide care for people with dementia. They provide emotional support, assist in household tasks and personal care, provide health and medical care at home, navigate healthcare systems, serve as surrogate decision makers, arrange services of community-based organizations, and provide needed information during patient visits.

Eighty-three percent of caregivers are family, friends, and unpaid caregivers, often undertaking this role on the foundation of love or obligation to the care recipient. Most begin this role without adequate training or support. This is not without cost: caregivers report physical, emotional, and financial strain, with 1 in 4 finding it difficult to take care of their own health. Increased caregiver burden correlates with decreases in care recipient quality of life, hastens placement, and increases risk of hospitalization and mortality. (See Table 3 for tools to evaluate caregiver burden.)

Management of Cognitive Symptoms

Until June 2021, Food and Drug Administration (FDA)-approved medications for treatment of AD would only ameliorate symptoms, not alter the progression of the disease. There are two classes of these medications: acetylcholinesterase inhibitors (AChEIs) and NMDA-receptor antagonists (Table 4).

TABLE 4　FDA-Approved Medications for Treating Cognitive Symptoms of Alzheimer's Disease*

	DONEPEZIL (ARICEPT)		RIVASTIGMINE (EXELON)		GALANTAMINE (RAZADYNE)	MEMANTINE (NAMENDA)	COMBINED MEMANTINE-DONEPEZIL (NAMZARIC)
Stage of AD	Mild to moderate	Moderate to severe	Mild to moderate	Mild to moderate	Mild to moderate	Moderate to severe	Moderate to severe
Mechanism	Acetylcholinesterase inhibitor (AChEI)					NMDA receptor antagonist	Shared characteristics of component medications
Route of administration	Tablet; ODT (orally disintegrating tablets)	Tablet	Oral capsules; Oral solution	Patch	Tablet; XR tablet; Oral solution	Tablet; Oral solution	XR tablet
Doses	5 mg, 10 mg; ODT: 5 mg, 10 mg	10 mg, 23 mg	1.5 mg, 3 mg, 4.5 mg, or 6 mg; Oral sol: 2 mg/mL	Patch 4.6 mg/24hr (9 mg rivastigmine); Patch 9.5 mg/24hr (18 mg rivastigmine)	4 mg, 8 mg, 12 mg; Oral sol: 4 mg/mL; XR: 8 mg, 16 mg, 24 mg	5 mg, 10 mg; Oral sol: 2 mg/mL; XR: 7 mg, 14 mg, 21 mg, 28 mg	XR: 7 mg–10mg, 14 mg–10 mg, 21 mg–10 mg, 28 mg–10 mg
Target daily dose	10 mg	23 mg	6 mg BID	9.5 mg/24 hours once daily	Tabs: 12 mg BID; XR: 24 mg QD	10 mg; XR: 28 mg	28 mg–10 mg
Renal impairment	No dose adjustment	No dose adjustment	May be able to tolerate lower doses	No dose adjustment	Do not exceed 16 mg/day; none if CrCl < 9 mL/min	5 mg BID; XR: 14 mg	14 mg–10 mg
Hepatic impairment	Use with caution	Use with caution	May be able to tolerate lower doses	No dose adjustment	Do not exceed 16 mg/day	Use with caution	Use with caution
Frequency	Once daily	Once daily	BID	Daily	Varies	Once daily in evening	Once daily in evening
Minimum interval between dose increases	4–6 weeks between 5 mg and 10 mg	at least 3 months at 10 mg before increasing to 23 mg	2 weeks	4 weeks	4 weeks	1 week	1 week
Administration cautions		23 mg tablet should not be split, crushed, or chewed because this may increase its rate of absorption	Should be taken with meals	The patch should be replaced with a new one every 24 hours. The same site should not be used within 14 days.	Should be taken with meals	XR: do not divide, crush, or chew	Do not divide, crush or chew
Most common adverse effects	Nausea, diarrhea, insomnia, vomiting, muscle cramps, fatigue, and anorexia. May cause bladder outflow obstructions		Nausea, vomiting, anorexia, dyspepsia, and asthenia	Nausea, vomiting and diarrhea	Nausea, vomiting, diarrhea, dizziness, headache, decreased appetite, and weight decreased. May cause bladder outflow obstructions.	Dizziness, headache, confusion, and constipation	Headache, diarrhea, dizziness. May cause bladder outflow obstructions

*See chapter text for aducanumab commentary.

AChEIs increase the available acetylcholine between neuronal synapses, enhancing neurotransmission. These medications are most effective in mild to moderate AD. Donepezil (Aricept), rivastigmine (Exelon), and galantamine (Razadyne) are AChEIs currently approved by the FDA. Historically, the first FDA-approved medication for treating AD was tacrine, but this was withdrawn later due to hepatotoxicity.

NMDA-receptor antagonists function by inhibiting the excitation of NMDA receptors by the neurotransmitter glutamate, preventing influx of Ca^{2+}. This inhibition has the effect of both decreasing excitotoxicity of the neurons involved (reducing symptoms) and restoring the amyloid-β induced Ca^{2+} imbalance (potential neuroprotective role).

On June 7, 2021, aducanumab (Aduhelm) was granted accelerated approval by the FDA for the treatment of any stage of AD. On July 8, 2021, this was narrowed to patients with mild cognitive impairment or mild dementia. This medication is a recombinant human immunoglobulin gamma 1 (IgG1) monoclonal antibody directed against aggregated soluble and insoluble forms of amyloid beta. Because the accumulation of amyloid beta plaques in the brain is part of the AD disease process, there is hope that aducanumab could provide clinical benefit. At this time, aducanumab clinical benefit has not undergone confirmatory testing (efficacy trials were stopped due to futility), and historical drugs that had similar amyloid beta impact have not shown clinical efficacy. This lack of confirmed clinical benefit is a source of controversy as to the appropriateness of the accelerated approval by the FDA. Further data and FDA changes continue to be published while this chapter goes to print.

Treatment with aducanumab involves titrating IV infusions every 4 weeks until the treatment dose of 10mg/kg is achieved at 7th infusion. Treatment monitoring requires a pretreatment MRI (within 1 year), followed by MRI prior to 7th infusion (first full dose) and prior to 12th infusion (6th full dose). The most common adverse effects are Amyloid Related Imaging Abnormalities (ARIA) and hypersensitivity reactions.

Although numerous vitamins and supplements have been studied in prevention and treatment of cognitive behaviors in Alzheimer's disease, the evidence of benefit is inconclusive and not subject to FDA scrutiny.

Multiple studies have shown aerobic exercise has a positive overall effect on cognitive function and may even slow the progression of Alzheimer's disease. Cognitive stimulation (engagement in a range of activities aimed at general enhancement of cognitive and social functioning) has also been shown to have beneficial effects on cognitive function, while music-based therapies and psychological treatment can improve symptoms of anxiety, depression, and quality of life in those suffering from AD. Cognitive training (guided practice of standard tasks designed to engage particular cognitive functions with a range of difficulty levels to suit the individual's level of ability) has been shown to provide a few months of benefit to cognitive function.

Management of Behavioral Symptoms

Behavioral symptoms in AD are the most common reason for acute care appointments, emergency room visits, or psychiatric admissions in persons with major neurocognitive disorders. Although admittedly more difficult to implement, the most effective treatment is nonpharmacologic.

Some behavior disturbances are induced by brain changes due to AD. In early stages of the disease, these are repetition, wandering, and refusing assistance. In moderate AD, pacing, agitation, antisocial or oversexualized behavior, resistance to care, and aggression can be common. Lastly, in late AD, resistance to care and repetitive vocalizations such as moaning or screaming may appear. The disease process notwithstanding, the most common cause of new behavioral symptoms is an environmental trigger, either internal (e.g., infection, pain) or external (e.g., new housing, change in caregivers or daily routine). To manage the behavior, the trigger must be identified.

Patient-centered and adaptive dementia communications skills are key to solving most behavioral symptoms of AD: making eye contact before speaking, using simple language, speaking slowly and clearly, communicating empathy through actions (smiling), asking only one question at a time, and allowing adequate time for the patient to respond (Table 5).

TABLE 5	Initial Treatment of Common Behavioral Symptoms in Alzheimer's Disease			
BEHAVIORAL SYMPTOM	**CONSIDERATIONS**	**TREATMENT**	**FOLLOW-UP**	**CAUTION**
Agitation	Change in patient's environment (most common cause)	If possible, remove the new trigger. If not, caution 3–4 week adjustment period.	1–2 weeks	Reassure caregiver and allow for more frequent contact.
	Lack of caregiver training/knowledge	Provide in office training on redirection, reassurance, de-escalation. Alzheimer's Association offers free online classes on Living with Alzheimer's for Caregivers.	1–2 weeks	Evaluate for caregiver strain as this will have lasting impact on both caregiver and patient health and may lead to early institutionalization of patient.
	Unreported pain	Acetaminophen 500 mg daily. Can slowly scale up to 1000 mg BID. Use the lowest effective dose.	3–4 weeks	Medication review of other APAP containing medications; contraindicated in concurrent hepatic illness
	Infection	Determine source and treat appropriately	After treatment	Many common antibiotics can trigger behavioral issues; review Beers criteria and use with caution
	Drug reaction	Review medications with Beers criteria	1–2 weeks	Due to lower renal and hepatic clearances, drug effect may last longer than expected
Anxiety	Start at half of recommended adult dose, and taper slowly.	Cognitive behavioral therapy, anxiolytics	3–4 weeks	Avoid benzodiazepines or sedative-hypnotics
Depression	Start at half of recommended adult dose, and taper slowly	Cognitive behavioral therapy, antidepressants	3–4 weeks	

Continued

BEHAVIORAL SYMPTOM	CONSIDERATIONS	TREATMENT	FOLLOW-UP	CAUTION
Restlessness/pacing	Ensure proper use of assistive devices or walking buddy	Create an environment that encourages safe walking or other forms of exercise. If patient no longer mobilizes, consider fidget blanket.	At next visit	
Anorexia/cachexia	Due to AD progression: may have lost cognitive domains to prepare food, remember mealtimes, execute coordinated chew/swallow control.	Optimize social supports, deprescribe medications which interfere with eating, provide appealing food and feeding assistance.	At next visit	Avoid appetite stimulants or high-calorie supplements. Do not recommend percutaneous feeding.
Insomnia	Wake-sleep cycle inversions are common in AD; patients have good sleep, just not at hours expected by caregiver	May be corrected with cognitive behavioral therapy, bright light exposure during waking hours, increasing daytime activity, replacing caffeine with decaf, trial of melatonin.[7]	At next visit	Avoid benzodiazepines or sedative-hypnotics
Aggression	See all agitation sections above	Apply all nonpharmacologic interventions possible. As last resort consider AChEI, then antipsychotics/anticonvulsants	1–2 weeks	Avoid benzodiazepines

[7]Available as dietary supplement.

Although it is appropriate to consider anxiolytics and antidepressants in the treatment of anxiety and depression associated with AD, the treatment of agitation and aggression is more nuanced. It is in these cases that we should strive for excellent individualized psychosocial care. Unfortunately, there are times when the patient's agitation and aggression can be extremely distressing to the caregiver and when the medical provider is asked for a prescription. If this is the case for your patient, consider an AChEI as the initial prescription because this medication has been shown to have benefits for apathy, delusions, and purposeless motor behaviors. If a patient has been on a maximal dose of an AChEI for some time and now has new behavioral symptoms, deprescribing should be considered because it may be that the AChEI action has outlived its usefulness.

If AChEI are unsuccessful, antipsychotics (given in order of trial: quetiapine [Seroquel],[1] risperidone [Risperdal],[1] olanzapine [Zyrexa][1]) or anticonvulsants (given in order of trial: carbamazepine [Tegretol],[1] valproate [Depakene][1]) should be carefully considered, starting at half the adult dose and titrating slowly to effect or lack of tolerance to adverse reactions. Thorough documentation of behavioral issues triggering prescription, and deprescription trials should be maintained for these medications. There is a strong national movement to decrease use of antipsychotics in dementia care, especially in nursing homes.

Monitoring

AD is a progressively debilitating neurocognitive disorder with the patient slowly losing the ability to accurately report symptoms or concerns and being increasingly dependent on the care of others. The Reisberg Functional Assessment Staging (FAST) scale was designed to reflect the progressive activity limitations of AD and has been well validated since its initial publication in 1988. Key points of the FAST scale are (1) the scale progresses through all steps in sequence, therefore out of sequence changes should trigger work-up for non-AD causes; and (2) when a patient reaches stage 7, the patient is eligible for hospice benefits.

In addition to monitoring the patient's health and well-being, special attention must be paid to the caregiver's needs, signs of caregiver burn-out, and if, despite all best efforts of the caregiver, the patient requires a higher level of care than can be provided in the current care setting.

References

Alexander GC, Emerson S, Kesselheim AS: Evaluation of aducanumab for Alzheimer disease: scientific evidence and regulatory review involving efficacy, safety, and futility, *J Am Med Assoc* 325(17):1717–1718, 2021. https://doi.org/10.1001/jama.2021.3854.

Alzheimer's Association: Alzheimer's disease facts and figures, *Alzheimers Dement.* 17(3), 2021.

Bruijnen CJWH, Dijkstra BAG, Walvoort SJW, et al: Prevalence of cognitive impairment in patients with substance use disorder, *Drug Alcohol Rev* 38(4):435–442, 2019. https://doi.org/10.1111/dar.12922.

Loy CT, Schofield PR, Turner AM, Kwok JBJ: Genetics of dementia, *Lancet* 383(9919):828–840, 2014. https://doi.org/10.1016/S0140-6736(13)60630-3.

McKhann GM, Knopman DS, Chertkow H, et al: The diagnosis of dementia due to Alzheimer's disease: recommendations from the National Institute on Aging-Alzheimer's Association workgroups on diagnostic guidelines for Alzheimer's disease, *Alzheimers Dement* 7(3):263–269, 2011. https://doi.org/10.1016/j.jalz.2011.03.005.

Milne AC, Potter J, Vivanti A, Avenell A: Choosing wisely: ten things clinicians and patients should question, *Cochrane Database Syst Rev* 2013(2):21–24, 2009.

Nakamura ZM, Nash RP, Laughon SL, Rosenstein DL: Neuropsychiatric complications of COVID-19, *Curr Psychiatry Rep* 23(5), 2021. https://doi.org/10.1007/s11920-021-01237-9.

Patnode CD, Perdue LA, Rossom RC, et al: Screening for cognitive impairment in older adults: an evidence update for the U.S. Preventive Services Task Force, *Agency Healthc Res Qual* 189, 2020. Report No.: 14-05198-EF-1. http://www.ncbi.nlm.nih.gov/pubmed/24354019.

Vaucher P, Herzig D, Cardoso I, Herzog MH, Mangin P, Favrat B: The trail making test as a screening instrument for driving performance in older drivers; a translational research, *BMC Geriatr* 14(1):1–10, 2014. https://doi.org/10.1186/1471-2318-14-123.

[1] Not FDA approved for this indication.

BRAIN TUMORS

Method of
Ryan Merrell, MD

CURRENT DIAGNOSIS

- Subacute to chronic onset of generalized and/or focal neurologic symptoms should alert the physician to order neuroimaging to investigate the possibility of a brain tumor.
- Magnetic resonance imaging (MRI) is preferable to computed tomography (CT) for imaging tumors.
- A biopsy or resection is necessary to diagnose a primary brain tumor or a metastatic tumor of unknown primary origin. The diagnostic yield is increased with a resection.
- Neuroimaging suggestive of meningioma does not require a tissue diagnosis and in many cases can be followed closely with serial neuroimaging.
- If a primary central nervous system (CNS) lymphoma is suspected, corticosteroids should not be given unless absolutely necessary in order not to confound the biopsy diagnosis.

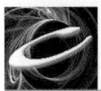

CURRENT THERAPY

- Surgical resection is preferred for patients with most types of brain tumors as long as the resection does not leave the patient with permanent neurologic deficits.
- Whole-brain radiotherapy and stereotactic radiosurgery are the primary treatment modalities for patients with metastatic brain tumors.
- Surgical resection is preferred for patients with large or symptomatic meningiomas that are surgical accessible and in patients who can tolerate surgery.
- Patients with gliomas are treated with fractionated radiotherapy alone or in combination with chemotherapy.
- Patients with primary CNS lymphoma are treated with high-dose methotrexate[1] alone or in combination with other chemotherapy drugs.

[1]Not FDA approved for this indication.

Brain tumors are categorized as metastatic or primary. The incidence and prevalence of metastatic tumors outweigh those of primary tumors up to 10:1. Lung and breast carcinoma make up the majority of metastatic tumors, largely because of their increased prevalence in the population compared with other tumors. Melanoma is a less prevalent malignancy but has a high propensity to metastasize to the brain. Meningioma is usually a benign tumor that is found most often in the fourth through sixth decade, with a female-to-male ratio of 2:1. Gliomas are primary brain tumors that are categorized as high-grade gliomas or low-grade gliomas. High-grade gliomas usually affect patients in the fifth and sixth decades and older, whereas low-grade gliomas usually affect patients in the third and fourth decades. Primary CNS lymphoma is a rare tumor that usually affects patients in the sixth decade and older.

There are very few identifiable risk factors for brain tumors. The histology of the primary neoplasm confers the risk of brain metastases because lung cancer, breast cancer, and melanoma are more likely to metastasize to the brain, whereas colorectal, ovarian, and prostate cancers are less likely to metastasize to the brain. Past exposure to ionizing radiation and a family history of a genetic cancer syndrome are the only known risk factors for primary tumors. Despite much press, cell phone use has not been irrefutably shown to be a risk factor for brain tumors. Immunocompromise such as human immunodeficiency virus (HIV) infection is a well-known risk factor for primary CNS lymphoma.

Brain tumors manifest with the subacute or chronic onset of generalized symptoms such as confusion, headaches, seizures, and nausea or focal symptoms and signs such as visual field deficit, loss of language, unilateral weakness, sensory neglect, or difficulty walking. There are no symptoms or signs specific to any brain tumor because the anatomic location of the tumor in the brain dictates the presentation. These symptoms and signs should prompt neuroimaging with MRI. MRI has largely replaced CT for evaluating brain tumors, although CT serves as a quick screening modality and must be used in patients who have contraindications to MRI. Radiographic features on MRI can predict the type of tumor but cannot accurately confirm the pathology. A tissue diagnosis through a biopsy or surgical resection is necessary to confirm the pathology, except in patients with metastatic tumors with a known primary tumor. The differential diagnosis of mass lesions in the brain includes abscess, demyelinating lesion, inflammatory disease, and other infections such as toxoplasmosis and cysticercosis.

A biopsy or surgical resection provides the definitive diagnosis of the tumor. For most tumors, a resection is preferred when safely possible because the greater amount of tissue obtained avoids the sampling error that can occur with a biopsy. Additionally, maximal surgical debulking can provide significant relief of symptoms. The goal of surgery for all brain tumors is to provide a maximal resection while leaving the patient free of permanent neurologic deficits. Metastatic brain tumors are classified according to the cell of origin. Primary brain tumors are classified according to the World Health Organization (WHO) classification system. Additional molecular classification that can provide prognostic and therapeutic information is often obtained on select primary brain tumors. Oligodendroglioma is a primary brain tumor that has well-characterized chromosomal deletions on the short arm of chromosome 1 and the long arm of chromosome 19 (1p/19q codeletion) that have been shown to predict improved survival and increased sensitivity to treatment. Similarly, O-6-methylguanine-DNA-methyltransferase (MGMT) promoter methylation is a marker that predicts improved survival and may predict improved response to treatment in high-grade glioma.

A major challenge to treating brain tumor is to find drugs that cross the blood-brain barrier. Many chemotherapy drugs used to treat systemic tumors are too large or hydrophilic to cross the blood-brain barrier. Treatments designed to circumvent the blood-brain barrier have only been modestly successful to date.

Metastatic Tumors
Metastatic brain tumors are the most common brain tumors, with as many as 170,000 new cases diagnosed in the United States each year. Metastatic tumors can occur with or without evidence of a primary neoplasm. Findings on brain MRI suspicious for a metastatic tumor should prompt an investigation for a primary malignancy with body imaging (Figure 1). The discovery of a systemic mass that can be biopsied might avoid a brain biopsy or resection in select patients. Occasionally, after an extensive evaluation, no evidence of a primary tumor is found. About 50% of patients have a single metastasis, and the rest have multiple tumors. In general, prognosis is poor, but some patients with less-aggressive primary tumors (melanoma, breast, non–small cell lung carcinoma) can achieve long-term survival. This is particularly true for tumors with targetable mutations such as BRAF in melanoma and epidermal growth factor receptor and anaplastic lymphoma kinase in non-small cell lung cancer. Additionally, immunotherapy has had significant impact in melanoma and other tumors. Clinical trials are evaluating whether treatment with targeted drugs can allow delaying radiotherapy in select patients.

Tumors can metastasize to the nervous system through infiltration of the cerebrospinal fluid (CSF), a process termed *leptomeningeal carcinomatosis* or *carcinomatous meningitis*. Symptoms suggesting leptomeningeal carcinomatosis include altered mental status, headaches, loss of vision, double vision, slurred speech, difficulty swallowing, and lower extremity pain and weakness. Brain MRI can show enhancement of the meninges, and CSF

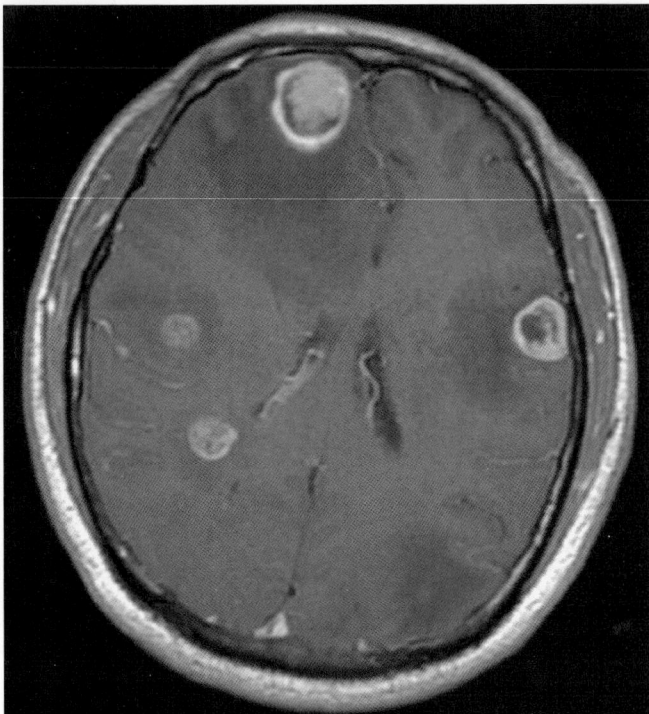

Figure 1 Contrast-enhanced magnetic resonance image shows a multiple enhancing mass with surrounding edema at the gray–white junction, suggesting a metastatic tumor.

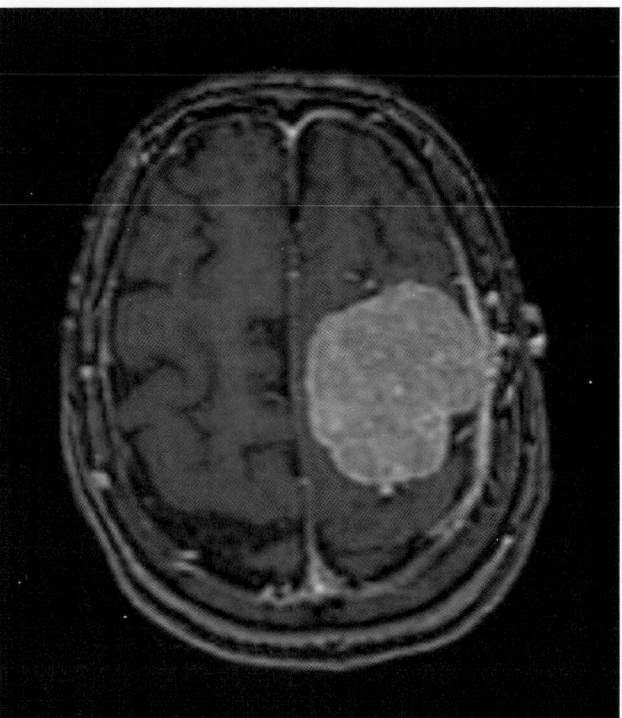

Figure 2 Contrast-enhanced magnetic resonance image shows a homogeneously enhancing mass arising from the dura, with the typical appearance of a meningioma.

from lumbar puncture shows low glucose and elevated protein with malignant cells. A lumbar puncture is not necessary to confirm the diagnosis in a patient with a known primary malignancy and characteristic clinical presentation and MRI findings. The prognosis is poor, on the order of weeks to months. Patients with lymphoma and breast cancer might realize longer survival.

Several factors determine the approach to treatment of metastatic tumors. The age, comorbidities, functional status, degree of neurologic impairment, and extent of the systemic disease determine whether surgery is indicated. Solitary metastases and large symptomatic tumors in patients with multiple tumors are generally resected in patients who are good surgical candidates. Whether a patient undergoes surgical resection or not, radiotherapy is the mainstay of treatment for metastatic tumors.

The two approaches to radiotherapy are whole-brain radiotherapy and stereotactic radiosurgery. In whole-brain radiotherapy, a dose of radiation is fractionated into several treatment sessions and given to the entire brain. In stereotactic radiosurgery, a high dose of radiation is given only to areas of brain involved with tumor and often in one treatment session. The effectiveness of whole-brain radiotherapy versus stereotactic radiosurgery has not been established in large randomized trials. Whole-brain radiotherapy is more suited for patients with multiple metastases or large tumors (more than 3 cm diameter). Stereotactic radiosurgery is indicated for patients with fewer than four metastases, for smaller-volume tumors (less than 3 cm diameter), and for radioresistant tumors such as melanoma. Whole-brain radiotherapy has the advantage of treating the visible and undetectable tumors, but it carries a risk of delayed neurotoxicity that often manifests as cognitive impairment. Recent studies have shown that this cognitive toxicity can be lessened through whole brain radiation with hippocampal sparing and addition of the drug memantine during radiation. Stereotactic radiosurgery has the advantage of local control by treating the visible tumors and carries less risk of delayed neurotoxicity. Stereotactic radiosurgery can be repeated if new tumors develop in areas of brain not previously radiated. The disadvantage of stereotactic radiosurgery is the potential for new tumors to develop in areas of brain not treated.

Treatment of leptomeningeal carcinomatosis involves chemotherapy or radiotherapy. Chemotherapy is often administered directly into the spinal fluid (intrathecal), usually through a ventricular (Ommaya) reservoir. Alternatively, chemotherapy can be given systemically. Common chemotherapeutic agents include methotrexate (Methotrexate PF),[1] cytarabine (Cytarabine PF),[1] and thiotepa.[1] Radiotherapy is usually only used as a salvage treatment after chemotherapy failure or for bulky disease.

Meningiomas

Meningiomas are the most common primary brain tumor, accounting for more than 32% of all tumors. Meningiomas arise from the arachnoid cap cells. They are often discovered incidentally when a patient undergoes neuroimaging for symptoms that are unrelated to the meningioma. The radiographic appearance of meningiomas is one of the most specific of all brain tumors and allows a confident diagnosis without the need for a confirmatory biopsy (Figure 2). The most common radiographic mimicker is a metastatic tumor to the meninges, but usually a patient in this circumstance has a known history of malignancy. Small meningiomas may be followed with serial imaging. Meningiomas that correlate with neurologic deficits or tumors that have grown significantly over time should be treated.

Surgical resection is the preferred treatment if it can be safely accomplished, but it should be avoided in the elderly. Meningiomas are graded WHO I to III; 90% are grade I (benign), and grade III (anaplastic) are the most aggressive and likely to recur. Complete resection is curative in most cases, but some meningiomas recur. If recurrent tumors are large or symptomatic, surgery is the preferred treatment if possible. Radiotherapy, either fractionated or stereotactic radiosurgery, can be used postoperatively to treat residual tumor or to treat tumors that cannot be resected. Meningiomas have an intermediate response to radiotherapy, and grade III tumors often show minimal response.

There is no defined chemotherapy for meningiomas, although several drugs are being actively investigated. Immunotherapy is also being investigated.

---

[1]Not FDA approved for this indication.

TABLE 1	World Health Organization Classification of Common Gliomas in Adults

SUBTYPE	WORLD HEALTH ORGANIZATION GRADE
Low-Grade Gliomas	
Astrocytoma	II
Oligodendroglioma	II
Oligoastrocytoma	II
High-Grade Gliomas	
Anaplastic astrocytoma	III
Anaplastic oligodendroglioma	III
Anaplastic oligoastrocytoma	III
Anaplastic ependymoma	III
Glioblastoma	IV

Gliomas

Gliomas consist of astrocytomas, oligodendrogliomas, and ependymomas, in decreasing order of prevalence. It was once thought that these tumors derived from mutations of normal glial cells, but it is increasingly recognized that gliomas derive from brain tumor progenitor cells. Glioblastoma is the most malignant glioma and accounts for 60% to 70% of all gliomas. Gliomas are classified by the glial cells from which they originate and the histologic features that give them a grade according to the WHO classification (Table 1). Grade III and IV tumors are high-grade gliomas, and grade II tumors are low-grade gliomas. Grade I glioma (pilocytic astrocytoma) is rarely seen in adults. A maximal surgical resection that leaves the patient with minimal neurologic deficits is the preferred initial treatment for all grades of gliomas.

High-Grade Gliomas

Most high-grade gliomas are glioblastoma or anaplastic astrocytoma (WHO grade III); anaplastic oligodendroglioma and anaplastic ependymoma are less common. The brain MRI often shows a ring-enhancing mass centered in the white matter surrounded by edema and causing mass effect (Figure 3). A maximal surgical resection that leaves the patient without permanent neurologic deficits is the goal in high-grade glioma. A maximal resection, younger age, and good performance status are favorable prognostic factors. Methylation of the MGMT promoter correlates with improved survival. High-grade gliomas are aggressive, incurable tumors; the median survival for glioblastoma is 14 to 18 months and for anaplastic astrocytoma is 2 to 2.5 years. The isocitrate dehydrogenase I (IDH 1) mutation is less commonly seen in high grade gliomas and correlates with improved survival.

Treatment of high-grade glioma is based on the histology of the tumor. The standard treatment of glioblastoma consists of fractionated radiotherapy given over 6 weeks with temozolomide (Temodar), an oral chemotherapeutic drug. Temozolomide is given 1 month after the completion of radiotherapy, usually for 6 cycles. Tumor progression occurs on average around 7 months after the original diagnosis for glioblastoma (Table 2). There is no consensus on treatment of anaplastic gliomas, although this is being clarified by two ongoing clinical trials (CATNON and CODEL). Patients with anaplastic astrocytoma are usually treated with 6 weeks of radiotherapy alone followed by adjuvant temozolomide. Patients with glioblastoma and anaplastic astrocytoma are usually treated with 6 months of temozolomide, although some practitioners will treat glioblastoma patients with up to 12 months of temozolomide. Tumor treating fields (TTF) therapy is a cap-like device worn on a shave scalped. TTF delivers radiofrequency pulses to the tumor. Based on the results of a large randomized clinical trial, TTF were approved to add on to the standard therapy of radiation with temozolomide for newly diagnosed glioblastoma.

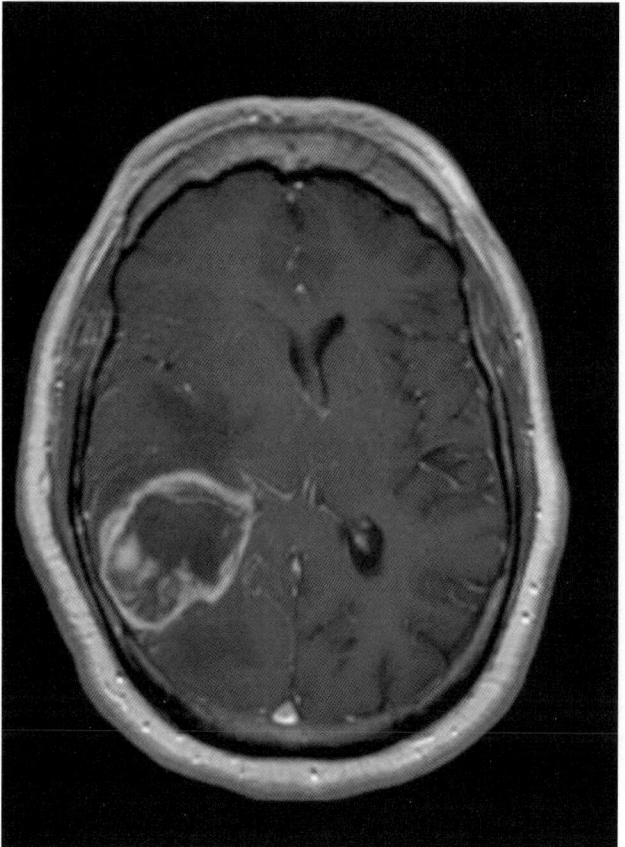

Figure 3 Contrast-enhanced magnetic resonance image shows a ring-enhancing mass with surrounding edema with the typical appearance of glioblastoma.

TABLE 2	Common Chemotherapy for Gliomas

GENERIC NAME	TRADE NAME	DOSE
Temozolomide	Temodar	75 mg/m^2 daily during radiotherapy, $150–200 \text{ mg/m}^2$ after radiotherapy on 5 d per 28 d schedule 50 mg/m^2 daily or 75 mg/m^2 3 wk on, 1 wk off, for recurrent high-grade glioma
Bevacizumab	Avastin	10 mg/kg every 2 wk

Careful consideration should be given to neuroimaging findings suggesting tumor progression within the first 3 to 6 months after radiotherapy because these changes can reflect radiation necrosis (pseudoprogression) rather than true tumor progression.

In the setting of tumor progression, salvage chemotherapy is the mainstay of treatment. Bevacizumab (Avastin), a drug that inhibits blood vessel formation around tumors, is the most common drug that is given at tumor recurrence. Despite showing improvement in progression free survival and symptom control, bevacizumab has never been shown to increase overall survival. Temozolomide given in low dose daily and lomustine (CeeNU) are other approaches for recurrent high-grade glioma. TTF can also be used in the recurrent setting if not used at initial diagnosis. Experimental chemotherapy through a clinical trial is a common option used in recurrent high-grade glioma. Current clinical trials are evaluating targeted therapies and many types of immunotherapy. Occasionally, surgical resection is indicated to improve symptoms, but it has not been shown to improve survival. Surgical resection has been employed more in recent years for clinical trials that require resection of tumor with the local implantation

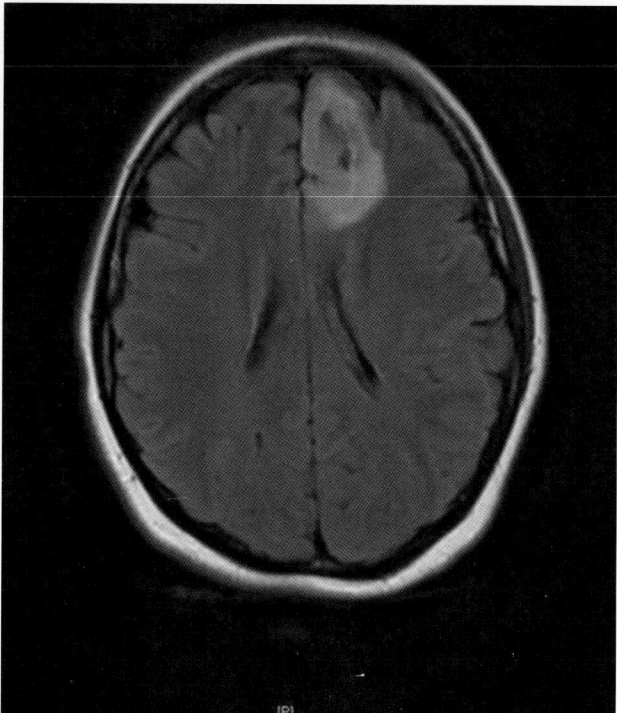

Figure 4 Fluid-attenuated inversion recovery (FLAIR) magnetic resonance image shows a nonenhancing tumor abutting the cerebral cortex with the typical appearance of a low-grade glioma. The tumor proved to be a grade II oligodendroglioma.

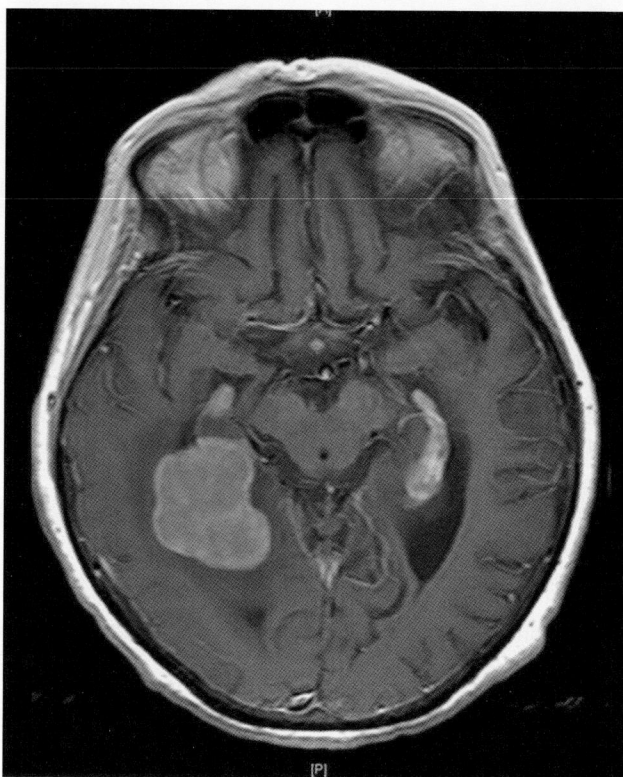

Figure 5 Contrast-enhanced magnetic resonance image shows a homogenously enhancing mass near the surface of the ventricle, suggesting primary central nervous system lymphoma.

722

of a treatment such as immunotherapy. Focused radiation such as stereotactic radiosurgery has not been shown to affect survival.

Anaplastic oligodendroglioma is usually treated with radiation followed by chemotherapy, either PCV (procarbazine [Matulane],[1] CCNU [Lomustine], vincristine[1]) or temozolomide while anaplastic ependymoma is usually treated with radiotherapy alone. Anaplastic oligodendrogliomas with chromosomal 1p/19q codeletions carry better prognosis and response to treatment.

Low-Grade Gliomas

Despite being lower-grade tumors, low-grade gliomas are not benign. The natural history is that patients with low-grade gliomas ultimately progress to high-grade glioma. Low-grade gliomas account for about 15% of all primary brain tumors. Low-grade gliomas are more likely to manifest with seizures than high-grade gliomas. The brain MRI often shows a nonenhancing mass with involvement of white matter and sometimes abutting the cerebral cortex (Figure 4). As in high gliomas, a maximal surgical resection confers a survival advantage in low-grade gliomas. Prognosis varies considerably by tumor histology: Patients with astrocytoma live 5 to 10 years after diagnosis, whereas patients with oligodendroglioma live 10 to 15 years after diagnosis. The isocitrate dehydrogenase I (IDH 1) mutation correlates with improved survival. This mutation is seen in the majority of patients with low-grade glioma.

The results of a randomized clinical trial revealed superior progression free survival and overall survival in patients with low-grade gliomas treated with radiation followed by adjuvant PCV.

In the absence of a head-to-head clinical trial of PCV with temozolomide, many clinicians would use temozolomide in place of PCV because temozolomide is better tolerated. Therefore radiation followed by PCV[1] or temozolomide has become the standard of care for all patients with low-grade gliomas. It still common practice to take a watch and wait approach in select patients with newly diagnosed low-grade glioma who have had

a gross total resection. Clinical trials evaluating IDH inhibitors are ongoing. When patients with low-grade gliomas have findings on neuroimaging that suggest progressive tumor, a surgical resection or biopsy is often conducted to alleviate symptoms and to establish the grade of the tumor. Patients with low-grade gliomas that progress to high-grade glioma are treated similarly to patients with de novo high-grade glioma but with consideration to previous treatments.

Primary Central Nervous System Lymphoma

Primary CNS lymphoma is a rare non-Hodgkin lymphoma that affects the brain, eyes, meninges, and spinal cord and accounts for about 5% of all brain tumors. This tumor is associated with the immunocompromised state, but it has a significant incidence in the immunocompetent. The characteristic radiographic appearance suggests but does not confirm the diagnosis (Figure 5). If primary CNS lymphoma is suspected, corticosteroids should not be given unless they are necessary to reduce increased intracranial pressure. This is because corticosteroids are directly cytotoxic to lymphoma cells, which can confound the tissue diagnosis. Occasionally, the diagnosis can be obtained through CSF testing, but a brain biopsy is often necessary.

Surgical resection has no role in treating this tumor because lymphoma is sensitive to chemotherapy and radiotherapy. The exception is in large tumors causing significant mass effect. Staging tests are necessary to rule out a systemic lymphoma that has metastasized to the CNS. Despite being incurable, primary CNS lymphoma is a more treatable tumor, and many patients live 5 years or longer after diagnosis.

Primary CNS lymphoma is treated with intravenous or intrathecal chemotherapy with or without radiotherapy. Methotrexate[1] is the principal drug used either alone or in combination with other chemotherapy drugs. High doses of methotrexate (3.5–8 g/m²)[3] must be used to overcome the blood-brain barrier. Owing to the

---

[1]Not FDA approved for this indication.

---

[1]Not FDA approved for this indication.
[3]Exceeds dosage recommended by the manufacturer.

potential for renal toxicity, high-dose methotrexate must be given in a setting where kidney function can be carefully monitored (usually the inpatient setting). Some patients with compromised renal function or aversion to hospital stays may not be good candidates for high-dose methotrexate and should be treated with alternative chemotherapy treatments.

Radiotherapy was previously used as an initial treatment, but it is associated with profound cognitive impairment, especially in patients older than 60 years. However, more recent approaches have used lower doses of radiotherapy combined with chemotherapy with less neurotoxicity reported. Opinion is divided about the use of radiotherapy. Chemotherapy can also be used as a salvage treatment. Besides methotrexate, other commonly used chemotherapy drugs include cytarabine,[1] etoposide (Toposar),[1] rituximab (Rituxan),[1] procarbazine (Matulane),[1] and temozolomide (Temodar).[1] In younger patients, an increasingly used treatment at the time of relapse is high-dose chemotherapy with autologous stem cell transplantation. This approach is increasingly being investigated in the newly diagnosed setting. Newer drugs that are being used for salvage therapy include lenalidomide (Revlimid)[1] and ibrutinib (Imbruvica).[1]

---

[1]Not FDA approved for this indication.

References

Ellis TL, Neal MT, Chan MD: The role of surgery, radiosurgery, and whole brain radiation therapy in the management of patients with metastatic brain tumors, *Int J Surg Oncol* 2012:952345, 2012.
Gerstner ER, Batchelor TT: Primary central nervous system lymphoma, *Arch Neurol* 67:291–297, 2010.
Norden AD, Drappatz J, Wen PY: Advances in meningioma therapy, *Curr Neurol Neurosci Rep* 9:231–240, 2009.
Sanai N, Chang S, Berger MS: Low-grade gliomas in adults, *J Neurosurg* 115:948–965, 2011.
Wen PY, Kesari S: Malignant gliomas in adults, *N Engl J Med* 359:492–507, 2008.

GILLES DE LA TOURETTE SYNDROME

Method of
Steve W. Wu, MD; and Donald L. Gilbert, MD, MS

CURRENT DIAGNOSIS

- Multiple motor and one or more vocal tics have been present for some time during the illness, although not necessarily concurrently.
- The tics may wax and wane in frequency but have persisted for more than 1 year since first tic onset.
- Onset occurs before age 18 years.
- The disturbance is not caused by the direct physiologic effects of a substance or a general medical condition.

Gilles de la Tourette syndrome, or Tourette syndrome, was named after French neurologist Georges Gilles de la Tourette, who in 1885 described a series of nine patients with chronic tics. Tourette syndrome is a neuropsychiatric illness that begins in childhood. It is characterized by multiple motor and vocal tics that last for longer than 1 year (see Current Diagnosis box). The prevalence of Tourette syndrome varies greatly among epidemiologic studies, ranging from 0.1% to 3.8%. The prevalence of tic disorders is even higher, especially in children requiring special education.

Simple motor tics are sudden, brief, patterned movements such as eye blinking, facial grimace, head jerk, or shoulder shrug. Complex motor tics can involve a series of simple tics or a seemingly purposeful action, such as jumping, touching, or copropraxia (i.e., performing obscene gestures). Simple vocal tics consist of sounds such as throat clearing, sniffing, and coughing. Patients with complex vocal tics may exhibit echolalia (i.e., repeating others' words), palilalia (i.e., repeating their own words), or coprolalia (i.e., utterance of foul language).

Older children and adolescents often describe a premonitory urge before their tics. Tics can usually be transiently suppressed and are often diminished during focused mental or physical activities. Unlike myoclonus or chorea, tics usually do not affect activities of daily living or occupational or recreational activities. After the brief suppression, the release of the tic often brings relief to the patient. Tic severity commonly worsens during times of emotional stress. Fatigue or illness may also increase tics. Parents often notice more tics when the child is bored or unoccupied with an activity. Tics can occur during light sleep and rapid eye movement (REM) sleep.

Clinical Course

The onset of tics can occur after children are 3 years old, but they usually begin in children 6 to 7 years old. Children often present with motor tics first, followed by the development of vocal tics. Tics often wax and wane in the course of Tourette syndrome. During the early school years, tics often can go unnoticed or be mislabeled as a habit. If tics are noticed by fellow students, bullying is typically not an issue at this age. However, when parents notice the tics, they are often distressed and frequently tell their children to stop the movements.

Tic severity usually increases in the later elementary school years and into adolescence. This is the time when social interference such as bullying begins to occur. By late adolescence and early adulthood, most patients with Tourette syndrome have minimal tics, and some may "outgrow" tics. Because of this pattern, most individuals presenting for medical attention for tics are children.

Patients with Tourette syndrome frequently present with comorbid attention-deficit/hyperactivity disorder (ADHD) and obsessive-compulsive disorder (OCD). They also tend to have more sleep problems, anxiety, and mood disorders.

Diagnosis and Differential Diagnosis

Diagnosis of tic disorders depends on correctly recognizing that the abnormal movements are tics by means of a careful history and thorough physical examination. Laboratory and imaging studies are rarely needed.

Tics may resemble other abnormal movements, such as stereotypy, chorea, ballism, dystonia, and myoclonus. *Stereotypies* are repetitive, simple movements that are suppressible and that usually occur when a child is excited. Stereotypies usually start when the child is younger than 3 years. *Chorea* consists of a sequence of random, continual, involuntary, nonpurposeful, nonrhythmic movements. Choreic movements often flow from one body part to another. *Ballism* is a large-amplitude choreic movement affecting the proximal limb. *Myoclonus* is an involuntary, sudden, shock-like movement. Chorea, ballism, and myoclonus cannot be volitionally suppressed. *Dystonia* is produced by co-contraction of agonist and antagonist muscles, leading to abnormal postures, and its twisting movements typically are slower than tics.

Vocal tics may sometimes lead to the misdiagnosis of asthma, chronic cough, or allergic rhinitis. Other primary tic disorders include Provisional Tic Disorder, Persistent (Chronic) Motor or Vocal Tic Disorder, Other Specified Tic Disorder and Unspecified Tic Disorder (DSM-5).

Tics are nonspecific and may occur in drug-induced movement disorders, after head trauma, and in a variety of neurodevelopmental and neurodegenerative disorders. Complex or atypical cases with multiple comorbidities or multiple abnormalities identified on a general or neurologic examination should be referred for specialist consultation.

A controversial diagnosis in which tics or OCD may occur is called pediatric autoimmune neuropsychiatric disorders associated with streptococcal infections (PANDAS). Criteria for this diagnosis classically include abrupt appearance in prepubertal children of tics or OCD on two or more occasions after documented group A β-hemolytic streptococcal (GABHS) infections. The paradigm for this diagnosis is rheumatic (Sydenham's) chorea; however, PANDAS has no arthritis, carditis, or nephritis and is not thought to be a rheumatic disease. As a result of recent epidemiological studies, the following interventions are not routinely recommended: diagnostic throat cultures and antistreptococcal antibody tests; therapeutic or preventive antibiotics; and immune-modulating therapies such as steroids, intravenous immunoglobulins, or plasmapheresis. Specialty consultation should be considered.

Treatment

There are many factors to consider when treating a patient with Tourette syndrome, including the presence of common symptoms such as inattentiveness, hyperactivity, obsessive or compulsive behaviors, depression, and anxiety (Box 1). When deciding to treat the patient, it is important to prioritize all the neuropsychiatric symptoms and provide accurate educational information. Tics may not always need to be treated medically, and if treatment is needed, tics may not be the first symptom to manage. Daily tic-suppressing medication is considered when there is functional interference, social interference, pain, or classroom or occupational disruption.

The first step in treating Tourette syndrome is educating the patient, parents, and other adult caregivers. Parents, teachers, and other adult caregivers are discouraged from telling the child to stop ticcing because this produces emotional anxiety that may worsen the tics. Educational materials for teachers often promote a conducive environment for the child at school. The patient is encouraged to openly talk about his or her disorder to classmates to promote understanding and minimize bullying. Newer cognitive-behavioral treatments for tic suppression appear to be helpful for children and adolescents, and they should be considered.

Clinical trials enrolling patients with Tourette syndrome are usually small and show small effect sizes. Most commonly used tic-suppressing medications belong to two classes: α_2-adrenergic agonists and dopamine receptor blocking agents (Table 1). Other agents may show modest benefit. Because Tourette syndrome is a chronic, nonfatal disorder, it is prudent to start treatment with medications that carry the least side effects. For this reason, α_2-adrenergic agonists are usually the first-line treatment. Although it is unclear what the second-line agents should be, it is reasonable in many cases to restrict dopamine receptor blocking agents to the most severe cases.

BOX 1 — Therapeutic Approach for Tourette Syndrome

- Educate the patient and family about tics and how tics often diminish spontaneously. Long-term reductions in tics may occur in the late teens, irrespective of pharmacologic therapy.
- Rank the tics, attention-deficit/hyperactivity disorder (ADHD), obsessive-compulsive disorder (OCD), anxiety, mood problems, learning problems, and behavior problems in order of the patient's or the family's perception of severity.
- Consider nonpharmacologic and pharmacologic treatment for each symptom in the order of perceived severity or impairment.
- Provide information to educate teachers and classmates to reduce social impairment.
- If the patient has learning problems, encourage formal assessment through the school or a psychologist. These children may qualify for modified educational methods.
- If ADHD is the most concerning problem, consider treating with clonidine (Kapvay), guanfacine (Intuniv), atomoxetine (Strattera), or methylphenidate (Ritalin). Stimulants are *not* absolutely contraindicated in patients with Tourette syndrome. However, if symptoms of OCD, anxiety, or pervasive developmental disorder are present, ticcing or compulsions may escalate on stimulants. If a patient has done well for months to years on stimulants for ADHD before an exacerbation of tics, it usually is not necessary to discontinue stimulants.
- If behavior problems are the most concerning problem or if a first-degree family member has a bipolar or psychotic disorder, refer the patient to a psychologist or psychiatrist.
- Anxious parents often worsen tic severity. If the family's anxiety is excessive, refer family members to a psychologist.
- If OCD or generalized anxiety disorder is the most severe problem, treatment with a selective serotonin reuptake inhibitor may be considered.
- Do not begin treatment with more than one central nervous system drug simultaneously. Start one, wait 2 to 4 weeks, and then reassess all symptoms before starting the next medication.
- Monitor the benefits and side effects at regular intervals.
- Maintain stable dosing during the school year; consider tapering medications in the summer.
- Consider weaning tic-suppressing medications in the middle to late teen years if tics wane.

TABLE 1 — Therapy for Tics in Tourette Syndrome

MEDICATION	STARTING DOSE	TITRATION	GOAL DOSE
Clonidine (Kapvay)[1]	0.05 mg qhs	0.05 mg every 3–7 d	0.05–0.1 mg tid
Clonidine patch (Catapres-TTS)[1]	Catapres TTS-1 weekly*	Weekly as needed	Catapres TTS-1, TTS-2, or TTS-3 weekly*
Guanfacine (Intuniv)[1]	0.5 mg qhs	0.5 mg every 3–7 d	1–4 mg divided bid
Baclofen (Lioresal)[1]	10 mg qhs	10 mg every 3–7 d	40–90 mg/d divided bid/tid
Clonazepam (Klonopin)[1]	0.5 mg qhs	0.5 mg every wk	1–2 mg bid
Topiramate (Topamax)[1]	25 mg qhs	25–50 mg weekly	50–100 mg bid
Pimozide (Orap)	1 mg qhs	1 mg every 3–5 d	1–4 mg/d divided daily or bid
Haloperidol (Haldol)	0.25–0.5 mg qhs	0.25–0.5 mg every 5–7 d	1–4 mg/d divided daily or bid
Fluphenazine (Prolixin)[1]	0.5 mg qhs	0.5 mg every 3–5 d	1–4 mg/d divided daily or bid
Risperidone (Risperdal)[1]	0.5 mg qhs	0.5 mg every 3–5 d	1–4 mg/d divided daily or bid
Ziprasidone (Geodon)[1]	20 mg qhs	20 mg every wk	20–80 mg/d divided daily or bid
Aripiprazole (Abilify)	1 mg qhs	1 mg every wk	1–20 mg daily or divided bid
Botulinum toxin type A (Botox)[1]	Not applicable	Not applicable	30–300 units in one or more focal sites, injected once every 3 mo

[1]Not FDA approved for this indication.
*The system areas are 3.5 cm² (Catapres TTS-1), 7.0 cm² (Catapres TTS-2), and 10.5 cm² (Catapres TTS-3), and the amount of drug released is directly proportional to the area.

α₂-Adrenergic Agonists

Clonidine (Catapres)[1] and guanfacine (Tenex; Intuniv)[1] are α₂-adrenergic agonists often used to treat tics. Several randomized trials have shown that these agents reduce tic and ADHD symptoms. The main side effects are sedation and lightheadedness due to mild hypotension. Sedation is more common with clonidine. The clonidine patch (Catapres-TTS)[1] may produce less peak sedation, but it commonly produces local skin irritation.

Dopamine Receptor Blocking Agents

Typical and atypical neuroleptics are dopamine receptor blocking agents that can be used to treat tics. Neuroleptics such as pimozide (Orap) and haloperidol (Haldol) can be very effective in tic suppression, but they can cause acute akathisia, dystonic reactions, cognitive blunting, acute anxiety with somatizations and school refusal, sedation, weight gain, metabolic syndrome, and QT prolongation. Monitoring for tardive dyskinesia is also important. Some experts recommend baseline electrocardiograms, particularly for individuals with personal or family history of cardiac arrhythmias. Weight gain and metabolic syndrome should be considered when starting neuroleptics, particularly risperidone (Risperdal)[1] and aripiprazole (Abilify). Some experts recommend obtaining baseline values for weight, blood pressure, fasting glucose, and lipid profile, with follow-up monitoring every 3 months to detect drug-induced metabolic syndrome. Diet modification, routine exercise, or medical therapy may be needed.

Other Tic-Suppressing Medications

Several small, controlled studies show benefit for topiramate (Topamax),[1] baclofen (Lioresal)[1], benzodiazepines,[1] and botulinum toxin type A (Botox)[1] injections for focal, strong tics. Tetrabenazine (Xenazine)[1] has been reported to reduce tics.

Behavioral Therapy

Recent clinical trials show that Comprehensive Behavioral Intervention for Tics, in which the patient learns to increase self-awareness of tics and premonitory urges and to perform antagonistic movements, reduces tics.

Treatment of Comorbid Conditions

ADHD and OCD are common comorbid conditions in Tourette syndrome. These comorbid symptoms are often more debilitating than the tics. Concern about stimulant therapy worsening tics was addressed by the Tourette Syndrome Study Group in the landmark Treatment of ADHD in Children with Tics (TACT) study. In this study, children treated with methylphenidate (Ritalin) had, on average, reduced tic severity, contrary to the widely held belief that stimulants exacerbate tics.

Medical treatment options for ADHD include psychostimulants, α₂=adrenergic agonists guanfacine (Intuniv) and clonidine (Kapvay), and the selective norepinephrine reuptake inhibitor atomoxetine (Strattera). OCD management includes cognitive-behavioral therapy and any of the selective serotonin reuptake inhibitors.

Summary

Tourette syndrome is a complex neuropsychiatric illness with many potential symptoms that may need medical and nonmedical therapies. Cooperation among the primary care physician, neurologist, psychiatrist, and psychologist is imperative for the comprehensive care of severely affected patients. If a patient has mild tics and few or no comorbid symptoms, medical therapy may not be needed. However, if the tics are severe in the presence of many neuropsychiatric symptoms, it is reasonable to refer patients to specialists.

---

[1] Not FDA approved for this indication.

Reference

Martino D, Hedderly T: Tics and stereotypies: a comparative clinical review, *Park Relat Disord* 59:117–124, 2019.

Martino D, Schrag A, Anastasiou Z, et al: Association of group A Streptococcus exposure and exacerbations of chronic tic disorders: a multinational prospective cohort study, *Neurology*, 2021.

Pringsheim T, Okun MS, Muller-Vahl K, et al: Practice guideline recommendations summary: treatment of tics in people with Tourette syndrome and chronic tic disorders, *Neurology* 92(19):896–906, 2019.

Ricketts EJ, Wolicki SB, Danielson ML, et al: Academic, interpersonal, recreational, and family impairment in children with Tourette syndrome and attention-deficit/hyperactivity disorder, *Child Psychiatry and Human Development*, 2021.

Sukhodolsky DG, Woods DW, Piacentini J, et al: Moderators and predictors of response to behavior therapy for tics in Tourette syndrome, *Neurology* 88(11):1029–1036, 2017.

INTRACEREBRAL HEMORRHAGE

Method of
Ronda Lun, MD; and Dar Dowlatshahi, MD, PhD

CURRENT DIAGNOSIS

- Intracerebral hemorrhage is a medical emergency; immediate imaging must be obtained in anyone with acute onset focal neurologic deficits.
- Noncontrast computed tomography (CT) is the gold standard; CT angiography can be helpful for prognostic factors and to rule out underlying vascular malformations.
- Obtain magnetic resonance imaging (MRI) +/– MR venogram (MRV) if etiology of bleed is unclear.

CURRENT THERAPY

- Ensure the airway is protected because level of consciousness could deteriorate rapidly.
- Medical treatment:
  - Hemostasis by correcting coagulopathies
  - Blood pressure (BP) lowering
- Surgical treatment:
  - Posterior fossa decompression for cerebellar hemorrhages
  - Extraventricular drainage for hydrocephalus
  - Evacuation of hematoma may be necessary as a life-saving measure

Introduction

Intracranial hemorrhage (ICH) refers to bleeding within the skull in any intracranial compartment (i.e., subdural, subarachnoid, epidural, or intraparenchymal) (Figure 1). However, the term is commonly used for intraparenchymal hemorrhages specifically, which will be the focus of this chapter. ICH can be further categorized as "spontaneous" or "secondary," with the latter inferring that there is an underlying lesion (i.e., vascular malformation, tumor) or alternative explanation (i.e., trauma) for the bleed (Table 1). Spontaneous ICH is synonymous with hemorrhagic stroke, referring to spontaneous intraparenchymal bleeding in the absence of identifiable secondary causes. It represents 10% to 15% of all strokes and is the second most common subtype after ischemic strokes. Although its incidence has been increasing in recent years, likely as a result of the aging population and increased use of antithrombotic medications, long-term outcomes from ICH have remained largely unchanged, with mortality rates of 50% at 1 year, and loss of functional independence in almost 75% of patients.

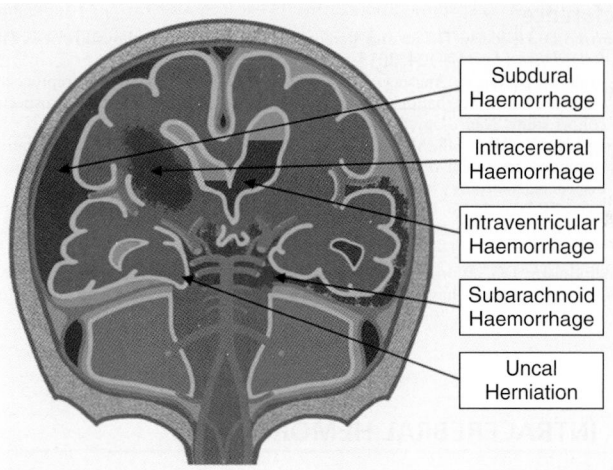

Figure 1 Types of intracranial hemorrhage. From Zebian B, Critchley G: Spontaneous intracranial haemorrhage. Surgery (Oxford) 2015; 33(8):363–368.

Labels:
- Subdural Haemorrhage
- Intracerebral Haemorrhage
- Intraventricular Haemorrhage
- Subarachnoid Haemorrhage
- Uncal Herniation

TABLE 1	Spontaneous vs Secondary Causes of ICH
SPONTANEOUS ICH	**SECONDARY ICH**
Hypertensive vasculopathy	Vascular malformations (dural arteriovenous fistula, arteriovenous malformation, cavernous malformation, capillary telangiectasias)
Cerebral small vessel disease	Cerebral venous thrombosis
Cerebral amyloid angiopathy	Hemorrhagic conversion of ischemic infarct
	Moyamoya disease
	Septic emboli/mycotic aneurysm
	Brain tumors
	Vasculitis (infectious, systemic autoimmune disease, primary CNS)
	Reversible cerebral vasoconstriction syndrome
	Drugs/toxins (cocaine, amphetamines)

Pathophysiology

ICH occurs when an arterial intracranial blood vessel bursts and a hematoma is formed as a result of accumulation of extravasated blood. The hematoma then causes mass effect with compression of adjacent healthy brain tissue, causing neuronal dysfunction and cell death from cytotoxic edema. Hematoma expansion (HE) occurs in up to 1/3 of patients with ICH in the first 6 hours and is a potentially targetable surrogate outcome for improving survival and preventing disability. The risk for hematoma expansion is greatest at within 3 hours after symptom onset, and the predicted probability of HE is inversely associated with time, although delayed expansion after 24 hours can rarely be encountered. Concurrent with the cessation of active bleeding, vasogenic edema will develop and peak over the next 2 to 7 days. Extension of the blood into the ventricular system may cause acute hydrocephalus because of obstruction of venous outflow. Even small volumes of HE are associated with an increased risk for adverse outcomes; the development of a teaspoon of new parenchymal hemorrhage is associated with quadruple the odds of mortality, and the development of even 1 mL of new ventricular hemorrhage has been shown to be associated with increased risk of disability and death. Ultimately, increased intracranial pressure from the mass effect may cause supratentorial herniation, midline shift, and secondary brain injury.

Location of ICH is a helpful predictor in determining the underlying pathogenesis of the ICH. Chronic hypertension is the most common risk factor responsible for subcortical and infratentorial hemorrhages, such as those in the basal ganglia, thalamus, brainstem, and cerebellum. The pathogenesis of hypertensive hemorrhages is attributed to chronic exposure to high pressures in the branching arterioles from major intracranial vessels, resulting in lipohyalinosis of the small arterioles. These relatively fragile vessel walls may then rupture and result in ICH. On the contrary, lobar hemorrhages and convexity subarachnoid hemorrhages in adult patients over the age of 55 are often attributed to cerebral amyloid angiopathy. This disease process is characterized by the deposition of abnormal amyloid beta proteins in the small to medium-sized vessels of the brain, resulting in weakened vascular integrity over time, which increases the risk for arterial rupture. Amyloid-related hemorrhages typically spare the deep gray matter and brainstem, reflecting the distribution of amyloid deposits, most of which are detected only on MRI sequences sensitive for blood byproducts (see Diagnosis section). They are thought to represent clinically silent cerebral microbleeds and are an important risk factor to recognize for increased risk for recurrent ICH.

Although this chapter focuses on arterial ICH, it is important to recognize that bleeding from a ruptured venous blood vessel may occur rarely and that venous hemorrhages are not considered a subtype of ICH. However, it needs to be ruled out as a potential secondary etiology for parenchymal hemorrhage because the treatment and prognosis are drastically different. Counterintuitively, the mechanism by which venous hemorrhages occur is caused by formation of thrombus in the venous drainage of the brain, leading to buildup of intracranial pressure and blockage of cerebral spinal fluid (CSF)/blood outflow from the brain. The backlog of pressure leads to venous infarction, petechial hemorrhage, and ICH. In any patient with a lobar ICH of unknown origin or ICH that crosses typical arterial territories, immediate neuroimaging with CTV or MRV should be pursued to rule out underlying cerebral venous sinus thrombosis as the ultimate culprit.

Clinical Manifestations

Neurologic deficits caused by ICH are sudden in onset, but unlike its ischemic stroke counterpart—where stroke deficits are maximal at onset—neurologic signs and symptoms attributed to ICH tend to worsen with time. As the hematoma expands, patients can rapidly deteriorate, resulting in decreased level of consciousness and requiring intubation. Initial clinical manifestations vary depending on hemorrhage location. The most frequent location for ICH related to chronic hypertension is within the basal ganglia, more specifically the internal capsule/thalamus/putamen/pons. Thus the most common symptomatology includes hemiplegia, hemi-body sensory loss, dysarthria, ataxia, and visual field loss. Cortical bleeds are most frequently associated with cerebral amyloid angiopathy and may clinically manifest with aphasia, apraxia, and hemianopia, in addition to the symptomatology mentioned previously. Epileptic seizures may be seen either at the onset of disease or later, as a manifestation of cortical irritation from blood/scar tissue. Headaches, nausea, vomiting, and decreased level of consciousness are common in the context of increased intracranial pressure (ICP) but may result from other mechanisms such as brainstem compression, development of hydrocephalus, or herniation.

Diagnosis

ICH is a medical emergency. The development of acute neurologic deficits should immediately raise concern for stroke, thus rapid assessment and management are crucial. Initial assessment should prioritize the ABCs of resuscitation—airway, breathing, and circulation—before proceeding with assessment for neurologic deficits. The most commonly used rapid stroke assessment scale is the National Institute of Health Stroke Severity (NIHSS) scale, which can be found in Table 2. However, another frequently used clinical assessment tool is the Glasgow Coma Scale

TABLE 2　NIHSS Stroke Scale

CATEGORY	SCORE/ DESCRIPTION
1a. Level of consciousness (awake, drowsy, comatose, etc.)	0 = alert 1 = drowsy 2 = stuporous 3 = coma
1b. LOC questions (month, age)	0 = answers both correctly 1 = answers one correctly 2 = incorrect
1c. LOC commands (open/close eyes, make fist/let go)	0 = obeys both correctly 1 = obeys one correctly 2 = incorrect
2. Best gaze (eyes open and tracks)	0 = normal 1 = partial hemianopia 2 = complete hemianopia 3 = bilateral hemianopia (blind)
3. Visual fields (introduce visual stimulus to all 4 visual field quadrants)	0 = normal 1 = minor 2 = partial 3 = complete
4. Facial paresis (show teeth, raise eyebrows and squeeze eyes shut)	0 = normal 1 = minor 2 = partial 3 = complete
5a. Motor arm (left) 5b. Motor arm (right) (elevate arm to 90°)	0 = no drift 1 = drift 2 = can't resist gravity 3 = no effort against gravity 4 = no movement X = untestable (joint fusion or limb amputation)
6a. Motor leg (left) 6b. Motor leg (right) (elevate leg 30°)	0 = no drift 1 = drift 2 = Some effort against gravity 3 = no effort against gravity 4 = no movement X = untestable (joint fusion or limb amputation)
7. Limb ataxia (finger-nose, heel-shin)	0 = no ataxia 1 = present in one limb 2 = present in two limbs
8. Sensory (pinprick to face/arm/trunk/leg)	0 = normal 1 = partial loss 2 = severe loss
9. Best language (naming, fluency, reading)	0 = no aphasia 1 = mild to moderate aphasia 2 = severe aphasia 3 = mute
10. Dysarthria (evaluate speech clarity by repeating listed words)	0 = normal articulation 1 = mild or moderate slurring of speech 2 = near unintelligible or worse X = intubated or other physical barrier
11. Extinction and inattention	0 = no neglect 1 = partial neglect (visual, tactile, auditory, spatial, or personal inattention or extinction to bilateral stimulus in one sensory modality) 2 = profound hemi-attention or extinction to more than one modality

(GCS), which is often used to assess indications for intubation in the context of decreased level of consciousness. A threshold of GCS 8 or less is used as an indication for intubation. Immediate neuroimaging should be obtained to confirm the diagnosis and rule out other diseases that may present in a similar manner, including ischemic stroke sand subarachnoid hemorrhage. The

noncontrast CT scan is the gold standard for emergent assessment of ICH. Administration of CT iodinated contrast to facilitate CT angiography may be pursued to look for active contrast extravasation (known as the *spot sign*) and to investigate for underlying lesions such as tumor or vascular malformations. Emergent MRI may be used as the initial imaging modality in select centers, although more commonly MRI is obtained in a delayed fashion to investigate the etiology of the bleed. Useful MRI sequences include T2* susceptibility-weighted images (SWI) or gradient-echo (GRE) sequences, which are sensitive for the detection of deoxyhemoglobin, a byproduct of blood. Additional pursuit of imaging such as CTV or MRV should be considered when there is clinical or radiologic suspicion for CVST. Catheter angiography may be pursued when diagnostic suspicion for underlying vascular malformation is high and no etiology for the ICH can be found.

Therapy

Treatment of ICH is composed of a combination of medical and surgical approaches and generally follows two important principles. During the acute period, stabilizing the hematoma and decreasing the risk for hematoma expansion is crucial and may be achieved through hemostasis and blood pressure (BP) control. Secondly, addressing mass effect and its downstream complications may be done through surgery and osmolar therapies.

Emergency Medical Treatment

The two mainstays of medical treatment in ICH are hemostasis and BP control. Hemostatic abnormalities may not only cause ICH but potentially worsen outcomes if not corrected. Patients with known coagulation factor deficiency or platelet disorders should have replacement of the appropriate factor(s). Patients with significant thrombocytopenia should be considered for platelet transfusion. Those taking vitamin K antagonists (i.e., warfarin) with elevated international normalized ratio (INR) should have their INR corrected rapidly. Either fresh frozen plasma (FFP) or prothrombin complex concentrates (PCC) may be used, although PCC may be superior in achieving a faster INR normalization rate than FFP and is the preferred agent. Vitamin K (phytonadione) needs to be given concurrently because of the short half-life of PCC; the onset of action of vitamin K starts approximately 2 hours after administration and will continue to peak over the next 12 to 14 hours. Other hemostatic factors such as rFVIIa are not currently recommended, although there are ongoing clinical trials evaluating its efficacy in patients presenting in an early time window from symptom onset. Patients taking direct-oral anticoagulants (DOACs) may be eligible for specific reversal agents, such as idarucizumab (Praxbind) for dabigatran (Pradaxa) and andexanet alfa (Andexxa) for factor Xa inhibitors (such as rivaroxaban [Xarelto], edoxaban [Savaysa, Lixiana],[1] or apixaban [Eliquis]). If andexanet alfa is not available, some clinicians may choose to use PCC to reverse factor Xa inhibitors if there is biochemical evidence of activity at time of presentation or confirmed recent ingestion. Patients taking antiplatelet agents prior to development of their ICH should not routinely receive platelet transfusion if their platelet count is normal because it has been found to be harmful rather than beneficial.

Elevated BP is frequently encountered in acute ICH as a result of a variety of physiologic responses. However, high BP is a major risk factor for developing hematoma expansion and thereby worse outcomes after ICH. For patients presenting with systolic blood pressure (SBP) between 150 and 220, lowering the SBP to <140 mm Hg is safe and may be effective for improving functional outcomes at 3 months. However, more aggressive BP lowering may be associated with increased risk for renal insufficiency, and therefore the potential benefit achieved from BP reduction should be balanced with feasibility and maintenance of systemic perfusion pressure to all organs. For those presenting with severely elevated SBP (>220 mm Hg), lowering to 140 mm Hg is practically challenging and may be harmful, thus

---

[1]Not FDA approved for this indication.

many clinicians may choose to target a BP that is 25% lower than the patient's initial SBP instead.

Inpatient Medical Treatment

Medical treatment of ICH should be continued beyond the emergency setting to prevent further complications during hospitalization. Maintenance of normoglycemia and normothermia should be standard of care because hyperglycemia and hypothermia have both been associated with poorer long-term outcomes. Universal dysphagia screening before initiation of an oral diet should be implemented to reduce the risk of aspiration pneumonia, a common complication during the first weeks of hospitalization. To mitigate the risk for urinary tract infections, indwelling foleys should not be inserted without appropriate clinical indication. All patients should have intermittent pneumatic compression devices for prevention of venous thromboembolism (VTE) beginning the day of hospital admission. Once the patient has been deemed clinically and radiologically stable, the patient may be transitioned to a pharmacologic agent for VTE prophylaxis. Osmolar therapies such as hypertonic saline[1] and mannitol (Osmitrol) should be considered in patients with concern for increased intracranial pressure, but these are considered temporizing measures until definitive surgical intervention.

Surgical Management

Although the evidence for indications and timing of surgical treatment of ICH remains somewhat controversial, surgery is often indicated for cerebellar hemorrhages, intraventricular extension, and hydrocephalus. Because of the limitations in room for expansion in the posterior fossa, it is generally accepted that any cerebellar hemorrhage with brainstem compression and/or hydrocephalus and/or neurologic deterioration should have immediate surgical decompression. A threshold of 3 cm in the diameter of the hematoma is commonly used for consideration of surgery. On the contrary, the evidence for supratentorial and deep hemorrhages is much less robust. Hematoma evacuation with decompressive craniotomy/craniectomy may be considered a life-saving measure in deteriorating patients; however, its efficacy for prevention of functional disability has not been well established. In patients with intraventricular hemorrhage causing hydrocephalus and deteriorating level of consciousness, extraventricular drainage (EVD) should be considered. There is limited evidence for irrigation of extraventricular drains with alteplase (Activase)[1] and its use is not routinely recommended based on the current level of evidence. Other surgical interventions such as minimally invasive clot evacuation have demonstrated promising results, and research in this field is active and ongoing. A summary of therapeutic options for ICH are outlined in Table 4.

Monitoring

ICH patients should be cared for in a dedicated stroke or intensive care unit wherever possible, as this has been shown to be associated with better outcomes. Frequent vital sign checks, neurologic assessments with validated scales such as GCS and NIHSS, and continuous cardiopulmonary monitoring should be part of the standard treatment plan. BP monitoring is especially crucial because it is the only therapy that has the potential to improve functional outcomes; thus hypertensive patients should have repeat BP checks every 15 minutes until the desired BP target is achieved and maintained for 24 hours. Electroencephalogram (EEG) monitoring should be considered in any patient who has persistent unexplained decreased loss of consciousness (LOC) caused by frequent subclinical seizures in ICH patients. Continuous monitoring of ICP is not universally indicated but may be considered in patients with evidence of transtentorial herniation, significant intraventricular hemorrhage (IVH), hydrocephalus, or decreased level of consciousness (i.e., Glasgow Coma Scale [GCS] of ≤8).

Complications

Prognostication

ICH patients typically present very severely (i.e., decreased LOC, debilitating deficits), and recovery in ICH tends to be much

[1]Not FDA approved for this indication.

TABLE 3 Glasgow Coma Scale

RESPONSE	SCALE	SCORE
Eye opening response	Eyes open spontaneously	4 points
	Eyes open to verbal command	3 points
	Eyes open to pain	2 points
	No eye opening	1 point
Verbal response	Oriented	5 points
	Confused conversation, but able to answer questions	4 points
	Inappropriate responses, words discernible	3 points
	Incomprehensible sounds or speech	2 points
	No verbal response	1 point
Motor response	Obeys verbal command for movement	6 points
	Purposeful movement to painful stimulus	5 points
	Withdraws from pain	4 points
	Flexion response, decorticate posture	3 points
	Extensor response, decerebrate posture	2 points
	No motor response	1 point
Total possible points		15 points

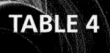

TABLE 4 Components of ICH Score and FUNC Score and Their Associations With Outcomes*

	ICH SCORE	FUNC SCORE
Scoring	Glasgow coma scale: 3–4: 2 points 5–12: 1 point 13–15 0 points	Glasgow coma scale: ≥ 9: 2 points ≤ 8: 0 points
	ICH Volume (cm³): ≥30: 1 point <30: 0 points	ICH Volume (cm³): <30: 4 points 30–60: 2 points >60: 0 points
	Intraventricular hemorrhage: Yes: 1 point No: 0 points	Pre-ICH cognitive Impairment: No: 1 point Yes: 0 points
	ICH location: Infratentorial: 1 point Not infratentorial: 0 points	ICH location: Lobar: 2 points Deep: 1 point Infratentorial: 0 points
	Age (years): ≥80: 1 point <80: 0 points	Age (years): <70: 2 points 70–79: 1 point ≥80: 0 points
	Total: 0–6 (higher score suggests worse prognosis)	Total: 0–11 (lower score suggests worse prognosis)
Association with outcomes in original publication	Association with 30-day mortality: 0: 0% mortality 1: 13% mortality 2: 26% mortality 3: 72% mortality 4: 97% mortality >5: 100% mortality	Association with 90-day functional independence: 0–4: 0% independent 5–7: 13% independent 8: 42% independent 9–10: 66% independent 11: 75% independent

*Prognostication and decisions around withdrawal of care should not be made for at least 48 hours.

TABLE 5	Summary of Therapies in the Treatment of ICH
MEDICAL TREATMENT OPTIONS	
Hemostasis	Known coagulation factor deficiency: replacement of appropriate factors
	Vitamin-K antagonist related ICH: Fresh frozen plasma (FFP) or prothrombin complex concentrates Vitamin K
	DOAC related ICH: Idarucizumab (Praxbind) for dabigatran (Pradaxa) Andexanet alfa (Andexxa) for rivaroxaban (Xarelto), edoxaban (Savaysa, Lixiana),[1] or apixaban (Eliquis) Consider using FFP if andexanet alfa is not available
	Antiplatelet related ICH: Do not give platelet transfusion
	Ongoing trials for rFVIIa: not currently recommended
Blood pressure control	SBP between 150–220 mm Hg: Lowering SBP to 140 mm Hg is safe and may improve functional outcomes Be aware of maintenance of systemic perfusion pressures to other organs (i.e., kidneys) SBP >220 mm Hg: Lowering SBP is still indicated, although practically challenging to 140 mm Hg. Consider lowering SBP by 25% reduction
SURGICAL TREATMENT OPTIONS	
Decompressive surgery	Posterior fossa/cerebellar hemorrhages: Surgery is indicated for any cerebellar hemorrhage with brainstem compression and/ or hydrocephalus and/ or neurologic deterioration Threshold of 3 cm in hematoma diameter for surgical intervention Supratentorial/deep hemorrhages: Surgery may be considered a life-saving measure in deteriorating patients but does not improve functional outcomes
Extraventricular drainage	Indicated for patients with hydrocephalus and decreased level of consciousness Irrigation with alteplase (Activase)[1] is not currently indicated
Minimally invasive surgery	Not currently indicated
PREVENTION OF SECONDARY INJURY AND COMPLICATIONS	
Monitoring	Dedicated stroke unit or intensive care unit with neuroscience expertise Frequent vital sign checks (including blood pressure), neurologic assessments, and continuous cardiopulmonary monitoring if on continuous IV antihypertensives EEG should be considered for decreased level of consciousness Continuous intracranial pressure monitoring may be considered for transtentorial herniation, significant intraventricular hemorrhage (IVH), hydrocephalus, or decreased level of consciousness
Glucose	Maintenance of normoglycemia is recommended
Temperature	Maintenance of euthermia is recommended
Seizure control	Antiepileptics should be considered in those with clinical seizures. It is not routinely recommended as prophylaxis
Dysphagia	Dysphagia assessment needs to be performed before initiation of oral diet to prevent aspiration pneumonia
Urinary tract infection	Foley catheters should not be routinely used
Venous thromboembolism	Intermittent pneumatic compression devices are indicated on first day of hospitalization

[1]Not FDA approved for this indication.

slower than its ischemic stroke counterpart. It is a devastating disease with limited treatment options, and a vital role for the clinician is providing accurate prognostication to family members/patients. The most widely used prognostication tool is the ICH score, which was initially developed to predict 30-day mortality but has since then been validated to predict long-term mortality up to 1 year (Table 3). Other prediction scores include the FUNC score, originally developed to predict the chances of meaningful functional recovery (see Table 3), although its use is less widely implemented. It is generally recommended that prognostication should be deferred to at least 48 to 72 hours after time of presentation to optimally assess the patient's clinical trajectory and to allow time for radiographic stability to ensue.

Acute Neurologic Deterioration
Acute neurologic deterioration is associated with increased risk for long-term disability and mortality and may result from hematoma expansion, seizures, increasing mass effect, development of ventricular hemorrhage, and cerebral herniation. Approximately 1/5 patients will experience early neurologic deterioration. Antiepileptic medications should not be initiated unless a clinical seizure is witnessed or suspected and confirmed with EEG. Important inpatient complications were discussed under "Therapy: Inpatient Medical Treatments."

Long-Term Complications
The long-term sequelae of ICH include physical disability, cognitive impairment, mood disorders, localization-related epilepsy, and increased risk for recurrent ICH. There may be an increased risk for ischemic stroke in patients with a history of ICH caused by avoidance of antithrombotic medications. Important predictors for recurrent ICH include microhemorrhages detected on MRI, uncontrolled hypertension, prior lacunar stroke, older age, and ongoing anticoagulation therapy, although it is still an ongoing, active area

of research. Patients with ICH who require long-term anticoagulation (i.e., atrial fibrillation, mechanical heart valves, hypercoagulable disorders) should be assessed by a neurologist or thrombosis specialist to optimize risk factor control and the risk for future ICH should be weighed against the need for antithrombotic therapy.

Prevention

Primary Prevention

Hypertension is the major modifiable risk factor for hemorrhagic strokes. Uncontrolled hypertension accounts for approximately 74% of ICH worldwide, and treatment of hypertension is effective as both primary and secondary prevention. Use of antithrombotic medication is another modifiable risk factor for ICH. For patients who require long-term anticoagulation for atrial fibrillation or venous thromboembolism, direct oral anticoagulants (DOACs) carry a much lower risk for ICH than warfarin and should be first line therapy unless patients have a specific indication otherwise (i.e., valvular atrial fibrillation, mechanical valve). Patients should not be on antiplatelet agents without appropriate clinical indication because chronic antiplatelet therapy is a known risk factor for ICH.

Secondary Prevention

Hypertension is not only an important risk factor for ICH but is also implicated in other cardiovascular diseases. Treatment of hypertension is effective for attenuating the risk for recurrent hemorrhagic strokes and prevention of ischemic strokes. For patients at a high risk for cardiovascular events who previously experienced an ICH, recent research has shown that antiplatelet therapy may be resumed without an increased risk of recurrent ICH. The decision to start anticoagulants after an ICH, however, is not as clear cut and will depend on the balance of risk for ICH occurrence and clinical indications for requiring anticoagulation. Important factors to consider include the suspected etiology of ICH, control of risk factors prior to the last ICH, age/comorbidities, and patient preference. Lastly, statin therapy is not currently indicated for primary or secondary prevention of intracerebral hemorrhage. Traditionally lower levels of low-density lipoprotein (LDL) have been associated with increased risk for ICH, but research is ongoing to better understand this relationship.

References

Hemphill JC, Bonovich DC, Besmertis L, Manley GT, Johnston SC: The ICH score: a simple, reliable grading scale for intracerebral hemorrhage, *Stroke* 32(4):891–897, 2001, https://doi.org/10.1161/01.str.32.4.891.

Hemphill JC, Greenberg SM, Anderson CS, et al: Guidelines for the management of spontaneous intracerebral hemorrhage: a guideline for healthcare professionals from the American Heart Association/American Stroke Association, *Stroke* 46(7):2032–2060, 2015, https://doi.org/10.1161/STR.0000000000000069.

O'Donnell MJ, Xavier D, Liu L, et al: Risk factors for ischaemic and intracerebral haemorrhagic stroke in 22 countries (the INTERSTROKE study): a case-control study, *Lancet Lond Engl* 376(9735):112–123, 2010, https://doi.org/10.1016/S0140-6736(10)60834-3.

Primary and secondary prevention of ischemic stroke and cerebral hemorrhage: JACC focus seminar, *J Am Coll Cardiol* 75(15):1804–1818, 2020, https://doi.org/10.1016/j.jacc.2019.12.072.

Rordorf G, McDonald C: Spontaneous intracerebral hemorrhage, *Pathogenesis, clinical features, and diagnosis*, 2020. UpToDate. Available at: https://www.uptodate.com/contents/spontaneous-intracerebral-hemorrhage-pathogenesis-clinical-features-and-diagnosis. [Accessed Dec 31, 2020].

Rost NS, Smith EE, Chang Y, et al: Prediction of functional outcome in patients with primary intracerebral hemorrhage: the FUNC score, *Stroke* 39(8):2304–2309, 2008, https://doi.org/10.1161/STROKEAHA.107.512202.

Salman RA-S, Frantzias J, Lee RJ, et al: Absolute risk and predictors of the growth of acute spontaneous intracerebral haemorrhage: a systematic review and meta-analysis of individual patient data, *Lancet Neurol* 17(10):885–894, 2018, https://doi.org/10.1016/S1474-4422(18)30253-9.

Shoamanesh (Co-chair) A, Patrice Lindsay M, Castellucci LA, et al. Canadian stroke best practice recommendations: management of spontaneous intracerebral hemorrhage, 7th Edition Update 2020. *Int J Stroke*. Published online November 11, 2020:1747493020968424, https://doi.org/10.1177/1747493020968424.

Yogendrakumar V, Ramsay T, Fergusson DA, et al: Redefining hematoma expansion with the inclusion of intraventricular hemorrhage growth, *Stroke* 51(4):1120–1127, 2020, https://doi.org/10.1161/STROKEAHA.119.027451.

Ziai WC, Carhuapoma JR: Intracerebral hemorrhage, *Contin Minneap Minn* 24(6):1603–1622, 2018, https://doi.org/10.1212/CON.0000000000000672.

ISCHEMIC CEREBROVASCULAR DISEASE

Method of
Alvaro Cervera, MD, PhD; and Geoffrey A. Donnan, MD

CURRENT DIAGNOSIS

- Early recognition of stroke is crucial to transport patients to hospitals with dedicated stroke units.
- Advanced neuroimaging allows the use of reperfusion therapies with a prolonged time window.

CURRENT THERAPY

- Admission to a stroke unit is the most effective and widely available resource for the majority of patients.
- Thrombolysis and thrombectomy have revolutionized the management of acute stroke, greatly improving the outcome.

Treatment of ischemic stroke has improved significantly in the past few years, and mortality and disability rates owing to this condition have decreased. The management of patients in stroke units and the demonstration of the efficacy of thrombolysis and thrombectomy have been crucial in this achievement. Control of vascular risk factors has decreased the number and severity of events. However, recent studies have found an increased incidence of ischemic stroke in the young. Improved management has included high-quality rehabilitation, which has to start early to improve the recovery (i.e., functional independence) of stroke survivors. The multidisciplinary management of stroke can be improved with specific educational programs aimed at increasing awareness of stroke in the general population and among professionals. The concept of "Time is Brain" has great value in emphasizing that stroke is an emergency. Because the window for the available time-dependent treatments is very narrow, avoiding delay is the major goal in the prehospital phase of acute stroke care. Therefore it is important to transport all stroke patients as soon as possible to the closest hospital with a stroke unit. In rural or remote areas with no stroke unit facilities, telemedicine has proven to be a valid alternative.

Prevention

Lifestyle modification can be a major contributor to reducing the risk of ischemic stroke. Strategies to achieve this protection include avoiding smoking and excessive alcohol consumption, keeping a low/normal body mass index, practicing regular exercise, and having a diet low in salt and saturated fat, high in fruits and vegetables, and rich in fiber. In addition, a Mediterranean diet supplemented with nuts is associated with a decreased risk of vascular events. There is no need to add vitamin supplements to the diet because they have no impact in stroke prevention.

Regular assessment of vascular risk factors (e.g., hypertension, diabetes, and hypercholesterolemia) is important because their control can reduce significantly the incidence of vascular events. In the case of blood pressure, this can be done with diet and pharmacologic therapy, aiming at normal levels of 120/80 mm Hg. After an ischemic stroke, blood pressure should be lowered even in patients with normal blood pressure. Diabetes should be managed with lifestyle modification and pharmacologic therapy as required, and blood pressure needs to be more tightly controlled in these patients (<130/80 mm Hg). The best antihypertensive treatments for diabetics are angiotensin-converting enzyme

TABLE 1	Prevention of Stroke in Patients With Atrial Fibrillation

CHA2DS2-VAS SCALE

RISK FACTOR	SCORE
Congestive heart failure	1
Hypertension	1
Age ≥75	2
Age 65–74	1
Diabetes mellitus	1
Stroke or transient ischemic attack	2
Vascular disease	1
Female sex	1

inhibitors or angiotensin receptor antagonists. Hypercholesterolemia should be managed with lifestyle modification and a statin. After a noncardioembolic ischemic stroke, high-dose statins are beneficial in all patients for secondary prevention.

Postmenopausal hormone replacement therapy should be avoided for the primary or secondary prevention of stroke because it can increase the risk of new vascular events. Other strategies to prevent stroke include the treatment of obstructive sleep apnea with continuous positive airway pressure breathing.

Antithrombotic Therapy

Low-dose aspirin[1] can be used for the primary prevention of stroke in women or of myocardial infarction in men. Nevertheless, its effect is very small, and it cannot be recommended on a population-wide basis. Aspirin is beneficial for the prevention of stroke in patients with asymptomatic carotid stenosis.

In patients with atrial fibrillation, the CHA2DS2-VASc scale (Table 1) is used to decide whether to use anticoagulation. If the score (https://www.mdcalc.com/chads2-score-atrial-fibrillation-stroke-ris) is 2 or more, treatment with oral anticoagulants is indicated. With a score of 1, the decision should be made according to the presence of risk factors, risk of bleeding, and patient choice. If the score is 0, there is no need to start antithrombotic treatment, neither antiplatelets nor anticoagulants. All patients with stroke or transient ischemic attack (TIA) should be anticoagulated, unless strictly contraindicated. Patients with valvular atrial fibrillation require anticoagulation with warfarin, aiming at an international normalized ratio (INR) of 2.0 to 3.0. Patients with prosthetic heart valves should also receive warfarin, and the target INR depends on the prosthesis type. In nonvalvular atrial fibrillation, the treatment options include warfarin (INR 2.0 to 3.0) or a direct oral anticoagulant (dabigatran [Pradaxa], apixaban [Eliquis], rivaroxaban [Xarelto], and edoxaban [Savaysa]). The direct oral anticoagulants are associated with a decreased risk of intracranial hemorrhage when compared with warfarin. Dabigatran (150 mg, twice daily) and apixaban (5 mg, twice daily) have shown to be superior to warfarin in stroke prevention. The dose of the direct oral anticoagulants needs to be adjusted depending on age, renal function, and/or weight.

After an ischemic stroke, all patients should receive antithrombotic therapy. Antiplatelet agents are the first choice unless anticoagulation is required. The most effective regimen is clopidogrel (Plavix) or aspirin plus dipyridamole (Aggrenox). However, low-dose aspirin is a reasonable alternative. During the first 3 weeks after a minor stroke or TIA, the combination

of aspirin plus clopidogrel can be more effective in reducing ischemic events than clopidogrel alone, although the evidence is scarce. However, dual antiplatelet treatment is not recommended in the long term, except if there is an association with unstable angina or non–Q wave myocardial infarction, or if there has been a recent stenting. Anticoagulation is usually indicated for secondary prevention if the stroke cause is cardioembolic and in specific situations, such as aortic arch atheroma or fusiform aneurysms of the basilar artery. However, level 1 evidence is lacking for these approaches.

Management of Carotid Stenosis

In patients with asymptomatic carotid stenosis (≥60%), surgery is indicated only if the risk of stroke is high. Endarterectomy is the treatment of choice if the stenosis is symptomatic (i.e., has been associated with an ipsilateral stroke or TIA), and severe (70% to 99%). Surgery should be performed in centers with a perioperative complication rate of less than 6% and as soon as possible after the last ischemic event.

Endarterectomy may be indicated for certain patients with moderate stenosis (50% to 69%), although it should be performed only in centers with a perioperative complication rate of less than 3% to be effective. In cases of symptomatic carotid lesions, angioplasty plus stenting is a reasonable alternative, mainly in patients younger than 70 years old. If stenting is performed, a combination of clopidogrel and aspirin is required immediately before the procedure and for at least 1 month after to prevent stent thrombosis.

In patients with intracranial atheromatosis and stroke recurrences, intensive medical treatment is the preferred option. Angioplasty and stenting are not recommended.

Management of Patent Foramen Ovale

The presence of a patent foramen ovale (PFO) is associated with cryptogenic stroke in the young. There is evidence that in selected patients with stroke or TIA (<60 years of age, nonlacunar stroke, and exclusion of other causes of stroke) the percutaneous transcatheter closure of the PFO is associated with a significant reduction of new vascular events, although with more frequent atrial fibrillation postprocedure, usually transient. Otherwise, there is no evidence indicating that anticoagulation is more effective than antiplatelets for stroke prevention in patients with PFO.

Management of Acute Ischemic Stroke

All stroke patients should be treated in a stroke unit, because this is associated with a reduction of death, dependency, and the need for institutional care. This effect is present in all stroke patients, irrespective of gender, age, stroke subtype, and stroke severity. Patients with stroke should have a careful clinical assessment, including a neurologic examination. The use of a stroke rating scale, such as the National Institutes of Health Stroke Scale (NIHSS), provides important information about the severity of stroke.

Urgent cranial computed tomography (CT) is mandatory after an ischemic stroke before starting any therapy. Alternatively, magnetic resonance imaging (MRI) or CT perfusion (CTP) can be performed, providing additional information about the selection of patients for mechanical thrombectomy within 6 to 24 hours from symptom onset. However, there is not enough evidence to recommend its routine use in the acute stroke setting.

For the detection and early management of the medical complications of stroke, neurologic status, pulse, blood pressure, temperature, and oxygen saturation should be monitored. Similarly, serum glucose levels need to be monitored and hyperglycemia needs to be treated with insulin accordingly. Normal saline is recommended for fluid replacement during the first 24 hours after stroke. If the patient has a fever, treatment with paracetamol (acetaminophen) may be used while sources of infection are being sought. Reducing blood

---

[1]Not FDA approved for this indication.

pressure is recommended only in patients with extremely high blood pressure or when indicated by other medical conditions. Blood pressure should be lowered gradually, avoiding abrupt changes.

Thrombolysis

All patients suffering an ischemic stroke within 4.5 hours of onset should receive thrombolytic treatment, with intravenous tissue plasminogen activator (tPA [Activase]) unless contraindicated, because it is effective in improving stroke outcome (Box 1). It is very important to start treatment as soon as possible, because pooled analysis has demonstrated that earlier treatment results in a better outcome. Thrombolysis with tPA is effective in all different population subgroups, including the very elderly, even with significant comorbidities. The therapeutic window can be extended up to 9 hours from onset when using advance imaging, such as perfusion-diffusion MRI or CTP. This approach has also been shown to be effective in wake-up strokes. Tenecteplase (TNKase)[1] is an alternative treatment to tPA, with the advantage of being administered in a single bolus (0.25 mg/kg).

Endovascular Thrombectomy

Mechanical thrombectomy using stent retrievers, in addition to thrombolysis, is more effective in improving outcomes than thrombolysis alone in anterior circulation strokes and a large artery occlusion, with a time window of up to 6 hours. This treatment is also effective when there are contraindications for intravenous thrombolysis. In a recent meta-analysis of five major trials (MR CLEAN, ESCAPE, REVASCAT, SWIFT PRIME, and EXTEND IA), endovascular thrombectomy led to significantly reduced disability at 90 days compared with control (odds ratio 2.49), with a number needed to treat of 2.6. All subgroups of patients benefit from this effect. Therefore, health authorities have to implement access to thrombectomy within a reasonable time frame in a network, including stroke centers.

There is recently published evidence indicating that therapeutic window could be extended significantly when using multimodal imaging to select patients who have marked penumbra. Thus, the DAWN trial showed that patients with ischemic penumbra could benefit from thrombectomy up to 24 hours since symptom onset, in comparison with standard care. This result was replicated by the DEFUSE 3 trial, although it included patients up to 16 hours from onset. In Box 2, there is a simplified algorithm for the use of reperfusion therapies in acute ischemic stroke.

Antithrombotic Drugs

All ischemic stroke patients should receive a low dose of aspirin daily. This can be started as soon as possible in patients who have not received reperfusion therapies, but always within 48 hours after onset. However, in patients who received thrombolysis, aspirin should be delayed for 24 hours. The use of other antiplatelet agents during the acute phase of stroke cannot be recommended based on available evidence. Similarly, early administration of unfractionated heparin, low-molecular-weight heparin, or heparinoids is not indicated in patients with acute ischemic stroke.

Treatment of Stroke Complications

Brain edema develops between the second and fifth day after stroke onset and is the cause of early deterioration and death. In

---

[1]Not FDA approved for this indication.

the case of a malignant infarction of the middle cerebral artery, the mortality rate is 80%. In patients younger than 60 years, with this pattern of cerebral infarction, hemicraniectomy has been effective in reducing mortality and severe disability, as shown in the pooled analysis of the DECIMAL, DESTINY, and HAMLET trials. Decompressive hemicraniectomy is also effective in reducing mortality in patients older than 60 years, although the rates of severe disability are very high. Surgery needs to be performed within 48 hours after symptom onset. Surgical decompression is also indicated in the case of large cerebellar infarctions that compress the brainstem.

Stroke-associated infections require appropriate antibiotics, but prophylactic administration is discouraged. Venous thromboembolism is a frequent complication after stroke, but its incidence can be reduced with appropriate hydration and graded compression stockings. If the risk of deep venous thrombosis or pulmonary embolism is high, the use of subcutaneous heparin or low-molecular-weight heparin is beneficial. Early mobilization is an effective way of preventing complications, such as aspiration pneumonia or pressure ulcers. Anticonvulsants are administered only to prevent recurrent seizures but are not used prophylactically.

In the case of urinary incontinence, specialist assessment and management are recommended. Dysphagia is common after stroke and is associated with a higher incidence of medical complications and increased mortality. Malnutrition also predicts a poor functional outcome and increased mortality, and it is important to assess the swallowing capacity and the nutritional status of the patient.

Rehabilitation should be started after admission to the stroke unit. The optimal timing of first mobilization is unclear, but mobilization within the first few days appears to be well tolerated. However, very early mobilization can be associated with a worse outcome, as shown in the AVERT trial. An early, lower-dose, out-of-bed activity regimen is preferable to very early, frequent, higher-dose intervention. It is important to assess cognitive deficits and depression during the patient's hospital stay, because this may require specific intervention, although evidence about the type is lacking.

References

Albers GW, Marks MP, Kemp S, et al: DEFUSE 3 Investigators. Thrombectomy for stroke at 6 to 16 hours with selection by perfusion imaging, *N Engl J Med* 378(8):708–718, 2018.

AVERT Trial Collaboration Group, Bernhardt J, Langhorne P, et al: Efficacy and safety of very early mobilisation within 24h of stroke onset (AVERT): A randomised controlled trial, *Lancet* 386(9988):46–55, 2015.

Campbell BCV, Ma H, Ringleb PA, et al: EXTEND, ECASS-4, and EPITHET Investigators. Extending thrombolysis to 4·5-9 h and wake-up stroke using perfusion imaging: a systematic review and meta-analysis of individual patient data, *Lancet* 394(10193):139–147, 2019.

European Stroke Organisation (ESO): Executive Committee, ESO writing committee: guidelines for management of ischaemic stroke and transient ischaemic attack 2008, *Cerebrovasc Dis* 25:457–507, 2008.

Goyal M, Menon BK, van Zwam WH, et al: Endovascular thrombectomy after large-vessel ischaemic stroke: a meta-analysis of individual patient data from five randomised trials, *Lancet* 387(10029):1723–1731, 2016.

Hacke W, Kaste M, Bluhmki E, et al: Thrombolysis with alteplase 3 to 4.5 hours after acute ischemic stroke, *N Engl J Med* 359:1317–1329, 2008.

Kent DM, Thaler DE: Stroke prevention—Insights from incoherence, *N Engl J Med* 359:1287–1289, 2008.

Nogueira RG, Jadhav AP, Haussen DC, et al: DAWN Trial Investigators. Thrombectomy 6 to 24 hours after stroke with a mismatch between deficit and infarct, *N Engl J Med* 378(1):11–21, 2018.

Powers WJ, Rabinstein AA, Ackerson T, et al: American heart association stroke council. 2018 guidelines for the early management of patients with acute ischemic stroke: a guideline for healthcare professionals from the American heart association/American stroke association, *Stroke* 49(3):e46–e110, 2018.

Vahedi K, Hofmeijer J, Juettler E, et al: Early decompressive surgery in malignant infarction of the middle cerebral artery: a pooled analysis of three randomised controlled trials, *Lancet Neurol* 6:215–222, 2007.

MIGRAINE

Method of
Natalia Murinova, MD

CURRENT DIAGNOSIS

- Migraine is a primary headache disorder with severe one-sided headache associated with nausea, vomiting, and/or light and sound sensitivity.
- Migraine is highly prevalent: it affects more than a billion people worldwide. It is highly disabling and constitutes the second leading cause of years lost to disability.
- The COVID-19 pandemic is a sensitive time for migraineurs, due to an increase in stressors, heightened anxiety, and changes in daily life that often trigger new or worsening migraine.

CURRENT THERAPY

- Acute treatment of migraine
  - Nonspecific
    - Acetaminophen; nonsteroidal antiinflammatory drugs (NSAIDs); antiemetics
  - Specific migraine medication classes
    - FDA approved for acute treatment of migraine with or without aura in adults
    - Triptans, serotonin (5-HT1B, 5-HT1D, 5-HT1F) receptor agonists
    - Ditans, oral serotonin (5-HT1F) receptor agonists
    - Gepants, oral calcitonin gene-related peptide (CGRP) receptor antagonist
- Preventive treatment of migraine
  - Nonspecific therapies
    - Beta-blockers; tricyclics; antiepileptics; *N*-methyl-D-aspartate (NMDA)
  - Specific therapies
    - Anticalcitonin gene-related peptide (CGRP) medications
    - Onabotulinumtoxin A (Botox) injections

Definition

Migraine is a primary headache disorder, not caused by any known structural cause. International Headache Society (IHS) criteria define migraine and explain clinical variability seen in patients.

The headache episode in migraine as defined by IHS has at least two of four defining features (1. one-sided, 2. pulsating, 3. moderate to severe, and 4. aggravated by movement), and at least one of two associated features (1. nausea and/or vomiting, 2. light and sound sensitivity). In its most common form migraine is an episodic recurrent headache lasting 4 hours or longer per episode if left untreated. The frequency varies from rare episodes to everyday headache.

In its more malignant forms, migraine is chronic, daily, non-stop pain with rare or no pain-free time. There is significant clinical variability: unilateral location and pulsating pain is present in around 50% of migraine sufferers. Most patients are disabled from pain; environmental oversensitivity to light, sound, and smell; inability to function; and often transient cognitive dysfunction such as difficulty with concentration. There is a subset of migraine with aura, most commonly the visual symptoms associated with fully reversible visual changes that can mimic transient ischemic attack or stroke.

Many medical providers fail to recognize migraine since they default to the most classic migraine presentation with visual aura with unilateral, pulsating pain with nausea and vomiting. Because migraine can manifest in different ways, this makes diagnosis more challenging. If a patient presents to a medical provider with recurrent moderate-to-severe headaches, migraine diagnosis should be considered. In general, most migraine experts consider a headache migraine unless there is a warning sign or some atypical feature. However, there are a number of neurological disorders that mimic migraine. For example, stroke can present with migraine like headache. The majority of people with "sinus headache" can also suffer from migraine. For patients' safety, other causes of headache and other neurological disorders need to be ruled out. The clinical presentation differs from person to person, and we should consider migraine diagnosis as a possibility in anyone with recurring, disabling headaches and impaired function.

Epidemiology

Migraine affects more than one billion people worldwide. In the United States, migraine affects more than 45 million adults, encompassing 18% to 23% of women and 6% to 9% of men. Onset can occur as early as age 5 years and prevalence peaks in young people, but it can occur at any age. While migraine can be transient, migraine affects people during their most productive years of life. The Global Burden of Disease (GBD) Study 2016 measured how disabling various disorders are across the world, and assessed how disorders affect disability-adjusted life years (DALY). In GBD 2016, migraine was the second-most disabling disorder, after low-back pain. In one study, 88% of patients diagnosed with sinus headache had migraine.

Risk Factors

Migraine is most commonly seen in young white women with family history of migraine. There are many risk factors that can be cumulative for a given individual who presents with migraine. Lifestyle factors that lead to migraine include high-stress work, nutrition (high carbohydrate diet), physical inactivity, and chronic stress. Therefore, a young person with genetic susceptibility to migraine with stress at work, physical inactivity, poor nutrition, and sleep deprivation has increased risk for developing migraine. It is estimated that in 1 year, up to 3% of episodic migraine cases become chronic. Risk factors for migraine chronification are obesity, acute medication overuse, caffeine overuse, stressful life events, depression, and sleep disorders. Comorbid conditions often seen in migraine include anxiety, depression, and insomnia, and these conditions have bidirectional effect.

Pathophysiology

Although migraine was once considered exclusively a disorder of the blood vessels, compelling evidence has led to the realization that a migraine represents a highly choreographed interaction between major inputs from both peripheral and central nervous systems, with the trigeminovascular system and the cerebral cortex among the main players. Migraine was initially thought to be a purely vascular disorder, but it is understood that migraine involves the neurotransmitter calcitonin gene-related peptide (CGRP). The pain of a migraine attack seems to be caused by the release of CGRP in the dura mater, which results in vasodilation and inflammation. Studies have shown that if CGRP is given intravenously to migraine sufferers, most of them have a migraine episode in the next few hours.

Diagnosis and Workup

The main questions are whether the patient presents with headache that meets migraine criteria and whether he or she needs neuroimaging (Table 1). We diagnose migraine using International Headache Society (IHS) criteria (https://ichd-3.org/1-migraine/). Migraine is divided into two major subtypes. Migraine without aura is the most common, characterized by a headache with severe unilateral pain, photophobia, phonophobia and functional impairment. Migraine with aura is most commonly characterized by reversible visual changes that precede and sometimes accompany the migraine pain. The success of migraine treatment depends on making the correct diagnosis. This requires careful headache history, as many patients diagnose themselves with sinus headache or tension-type headache, or other type of headache. Identifying classic symptoms has a high probability

TABLE 1	Precision Questions Helpful in Migraine Diagnosis
1. It this a new kind of headache?	New headache needs further history, make sure this is not a migraine mimic.
2. Use "red flag" questions, such as do you have any other condition such as cancer?	"Red flag" questions are used to exclude secondary headache
3 How many total headache days do you have per month? Lump all headache days.	Total headache days >15 days per month are suggestive of chronic migraine.
4. How long do your headaches last with no treatment?	Duration of headache without therapy should be more than 4 h for migraine diagnosis. With shorter duration, consider other diagnosis, such as trigeminal autonomic cephalgia.
5. What associated symptoms do you have?	For migraine look for associated nausea, light and sound sensitivity.
6. How many days per month do you use an acute therapy for any pain?	Medication overuse headache is commonly seen with chronic migraine, and any medication use for any pain can cause this.

of accurate diagnosis. The headache pattern should distinguish migraine from other primary headaches (tension or cluster headache). The clinical history and neurological examination target need to exclude secondary headache that can present as migraine. In most patients the diagnosis is made using their history and IHS criteria. Diagnostic imaging is not indicated in otherwise healthy migraine patients with normal neurologic examination. Patients with "red flags" such as abnormalities during the neurological examination, fever, unintentional weight loss, history of cancer, transplant or immunodeficiency need further workup with neuroimaging. Which kind of neuroimaging should be performed is a common question: Magnetic resonance imaging (MRI) of the brain with and without contrast is the preferred imaging modality.

Treatment

The pharmacological treatment addresses acute treatment, used for management of acute exacerbations, and preventive treatments that have, shown efficacy in decreasing migraine attacks in the long term. Preventive medications are taken daily for at least several months, sometimes years, to reduce the severity and frequency of migraines before they start.

The treatment strategy for migraines has shifted from using mostly nonspecific pain medications such as aspirin and acetaminophen to migraine-specific therapies such as triptans, ditans, and gepants and other treatments such as neuromodulation (Table 2; Boxes 1–3).

Acute Treatment

Mechanism of Acute Migraine Medications
Migraine pain is considered to be caused by dura mater release of CGRP, with subsequent vasodilation and neurogenic inflammation. Triptans and ergots are agonists of serotonin 5-HT1D receptors, and their activation prevents CGRP release. Agonism at 5-HT1B receptors results in vasoconstriction, which opposes the action of CGRP. Ditans are selective nontriptan oral serotonin (5-HT1F) receptor agonists, which is thought to stop plasma protein release by action of the trigeminal ganglion. 5-HT1F receptors are not present in vessels. Ditans also inhibit trigeminal nucleus caudalis. Ubrogepant (Ubrelvy) and rimegepant (Nurtec ODT) are oral CGRP receptor antagonists.

The American Headache Society (AHS) guideline for acute treatment in 2015 summarized evidence-based assessment of acute treatments for migraine: "The specific medications—triptans and

TABLE 2 Migraine Treatment by Severity and Phenotype

	CLINICAL MIGRAINE PHENOTYPE	STRATEGY	MEDICATION
Increasing migraine severity	Mild to moderate	Acetaminophen	Acetaminophen (Tylenol)[1] 1000 mg
		NSAID	Naproxen sodium (Aleve)[1] 220–660 mg Ibuprofen (Motrin) 800 mg
	Moderate to severe	NSAID+ triptan+ anti-nausea	Naproxen (Aleve) 440 mg+ ondansetron (Zofran)[1] 8 mg ODT+ triptan later for rescue if necessary
		Triptan (5HT1B agonist 5HT1D agonist)	Sumatriptan (Imitrex) (6 mg SQ injection, 20 mg nasal solution, 25 mg, 50 mg and 100 mg oral tablet) Zolmitriptan (Zomig) (2.5 mg, 5 mg nasal solution, oral tablet, oral disintegrating tablet [ODT]) Rizatriptan (Maxalt) (5 mg,10 mg oral tablet, ODT) Naratriptan (Amerge) (1 mg, 2.5 mg PO tablet) Eletriptan (Relpax) (20 mg, 40 mg PO tablet) Almotriptan (Axert) (6.25 mg, 12.5 mg PO tablet) Frovatriptan (Frova) (2.5 mg PO tablet)
		Ditan (5HT1F agonist) Gepant (CGRP antagonist)	Lasmiditan (Reyvow) 50 mg, 100 mg, 200 mg PO tablet Ubrogepant (Ubrelvy) 50 mg, 100 mg PO tablet Rimegepant (Nurtec ODT) 75 mg oral disintegrating tablet
	Severe attack difficult to treat and refractory migraine		Triptan + NSAID+ anti-nausea drug Gepant+ NSAID+ anti-nausea drug Ditan+ NSAID+ anti-nausea drug
			Ketorolac (TORADOL)[1] IM 60 mg Indomethacin[1] oral or rectal Prochlorperazine (COMPAZINE)[1] 5 mg, 10 mg Dexamethasone[1] or prednisone[1]

From Pringsheim T, Davenport W, Mackie G, et al: Canadian Headache Society guideline for migraine prophylaxis, *Can J Neurol Sci* 1;39(2 Suppl 2):S1-59, 2012.
[1]Not FDA approved for this indication.

BOX 1 First-Line Acute Therapy of Migraine

Naproxen (Aleve)[1] 440 mg+ ondansetron (Zofran)[1] 8 mg ODT+ triptan later for rescue if necessary

Triptans:
Sumatriptan (Imitrex) 6 mg SQ injection, 20 mg nasal solution, 25 mg, 50 mg and 100 mg oral tablet
Zolmitriptan (Zomig) 2.5 mg, 5 mg oral tablet; oral disintegrating tablet (ODT); nasal spray
Rizatriptan (Maxalt) 5 mg,10 mg oral tablet, ODT
Naratriptan (Amerge) 1 mg, 2.5 mg oral tablet
Eletriptan (Relpax) 20 mg, 40 mg oral tablet
Almotriptan (Axert) 6.25 mg, 12.5 mg oral tablet
Frovatriptan (Frova) 2.5 mg oral tablet

Ditans:
Lasmiditan (Reyvow) 50 mg, 100 mg, 200 mg oral tablet

Gepants:
Ubrogepant (Ubrelvy) 50 mg, 100 mg oral tablet
Rimegepant (Nurtec ODT) 75 mg oral disintegrating tablet

[1]Not FDA approved for this indication

BOX 2 Steps for Acute Treatment for Migraine Headache

Step 1: Choose options that are not known to lead to medication overuse headache (MOH).
Antiemetics: Ondansetron (Zofran)[1] (tablet, dispersible tablet), prochlorperazine (Compazine)[1] (tablet, suppository), promethazine (Phenergan)[1] (tablet, suppository), metoclopramide (Reglan)[1].
Natural supplements/herbs: Feverfew tea[7], Boswellia[7], magnesium[7].
Anesthetic: Lidocaine nasal spray[1].
Neuromodulation: Cefaly (supraorbital stimulation), Gammacore (vagal nerve stimulation), SpringTMS (transcranial magnetic stimulation).
Nonmedication options: Rest, ice, meditation, biofeedback, distraction, essential oils[7].
Step 2: NSAIDs, longer acting are generally considered less likely to lead to MOH.
Diclofenac (tablet[1], capsule[1], powder), ketorolac[1], naproxen[1], ibuprofen.
Step 3: Limit any acute medications to 1–2 days per week to avoid MOH such as triptans.
Triptans: Sumatriptan (Imitrex) (tablet, nasal spray, injection), rizatriptan (Maxalt) (tablet, dispersible tablet), eletriptan (Relpax), zolmitriptan (Zomig) (tablet, dispersible tablet, nasal spray), almotriptan (Axert), frovatriptan (Frova), naratriptan (Amerge).
Ergotamines: dihydroergotamine DHE 45 injection, Migranal nasal spray

[1]Not FDA approved for this indication.
[7]Available as dietary supplement.

---

dihydroergotamine (nasal spray [Migranal], inhaler[5]) are effective (level A)," whereas "effective nonspecific medications include acetaminophen, NSAIDs, opioids (butorphanol nasal spray)[1] [not recommended], sumatriptan/naproxen (Treximet), and the combination of acetaminophen/aspirin/caffeine (e.g., Excedrin Migraine)" also have level A evidence. "Ergotamine tartrate (Ergomar) and other forms of dihydroergotamine, ketoprofen (Orudis)[1], intravenous and intramuscular ketorolac (Toradol)[1], flurbiprofen (Ansaid)[1], intravenous magnesium (in migraine with aura)[1], and the combination

of isometheptene compounds, codeine/acetaminophen[1], tramadol/acetaminophen (Ultracet)[1], prochlorperazine (Compazine)[1], droperidol (Inapsine)[1], chlorpromazine (Thorazine)[1], and metoclopramide (Reglan)[1] are probably effective (level B)."

[1]Not FDA-approved for this indication.
[5]Investigational drug in the United States.

| BOX 3 | Preventive Medications for Episodic Migraine |

Level A Therapies, Established as Effective and FDA Approved for Episodic Migraine (EM)

Antiepileptic drugs (AEDs): Topiramate (Topamax) (caution if low weight or history of kidney stones), divalproex sodium (Depakote) (caution of weight gain), sodium valproate (Depakene).

Beta-blockers: Propranolol (Inderal), timolol (Blocadren), metoprolol (Lopressor) (the only medication Level A that is not FDA approved).

Specific Preventive Migraine Therapies FDA Approved for EM and CM

Anti CGRP Monoclonal Antibodies: erenumab-aooe (Aimovig), fremanezumab-vfrm (Ajovy), galcanezumab-gnlm (Emgality).

Neuromodulation devices: Cefaly (supraorbital stimulation), Gammacore (vagal nerve stimulation), SpringTMS (transcranial magnetic stimulation)

Level B Therapies, Probably Effective for EM, not FDA Approved for EM

Antidepressants: Amitriptyline, venlafaxine (Effexor XR).

Beta-blockers: Atenolol (Tenormin), nadolol (Corgard).

Level C Therapies, Possibly Effective for EM, not FDA Approved

Calcium Channel Blockers and ACE Inhibitors: Verapamil (Calan), lisinopril (Prinivil).

AEDs: Carbamazepine (Tegretol).

Beta-blockers: Pindolol (Visken).

Antihistamines: Cyproheptadine (Periactin).

Angiotensin-receptor Blockers: candesartan (Atacand), clonidine (Catapres).

It is important to educate patients on appropriate use of acute therapy, since medication overuse headache (MOH) can develop. This is defined as the presence of headache while taking any acute medications for any pain, even if not headache related, more than 15 days per month. MOH is often difficult to treat and is medication- and procedure-refractory. We strongly recommend monitoring days per month of acute medication use and setting a limit on maximum monthly use. An electronic headache diary app, such as https://migrainebuddy.com/, can be helpful in documenting headache days and medication use.

An oral nonopioid analgesic, such as naproxen (Aleve)[1], is often adequate for acute treatment of mild to moderate migraine without nausea or vomiting. Migraine-specific agents should be considered when migraine episodes are moderate to severe. The acute migraine-specific pharmacotherapies include triptans, ergotamines, ditans, and gepants.

Many acute therapies are effective only for some patients and can cause significant side effects. Patients who do not respond to one triptan may respond to another triptan, or a different mode of administration of the same triptan. Note that triptans are contraindicated in patients with vascular risk factors.

- Sumatriptan (Imitrex) (6 mg SQ injections; 20 mg nasal solution; 25 mg, 50 mg, and 100 mg oral tablet)
- Zolmitriptan (Zomig) (2.5 mg, 5 mg nasal solution; oral tablet or oral disintegrating tablet)
- Rizatriptan (Maxalt) (5 mg, 10 mg oral tablet; or oral disintegrating tablet)
- Naratriptan (Amerge) (1 mg, 2.5 mg oral tablet)
- Eletriptan (Relpax) 20 mg, 40 mg oral tablet
- Almotriptan (Axert) (6.25 mg, 12.5 mg oral tablet)
- Frovatriptan (Frova) (2.5 mg oral tablet)

Dihydroergotamine (D.H.E. 45, Migranal) should be considered in patients who are refractory to triptans, although they have the same vascular disease contraindication.

- Dihydroergotamine (D.H.E. 45, 1 mg SQ or IV; Migranal 0.5 mg/nasal spray)

A number of new agents became available in 2020.

- New acute migraine treatment: ditans and gepants

The one approved ditan is lasmiditan (Reyvow), which is an oral serotonin (5hT1F) receptor agonist.

The two approved gepants are ubrogepant (Ubrelvy) and rimegepant (Nurtec ODT), which are oral CGRP receptor agonists. These drugs were approved by the FDA in 2020 for acute migraine treatment with and without aura in adults.

Ditans for Acute Migraine Treatment

Ditans are the only group of medications known to selectively bind serotonin 1F receptor (5-HT1F) on the trigeminal neurons. Ditans do not cause vasoconstriction via the serotonin 1B receptor on blood vessels as triptans do, and therefore are not contraindicated in patients with known vascular risk factors. A majority of patients in clinical studies had at least one cardiovascular risk factor, only a few of the subjects had ischemic heart disease, and none had ischemic events attributed to lasmiditan during the trial within 48 hours. To date, no clinical trials are available that have compared lasmiditan to other acute headache treatments. The most common side effects in clinical trials were dizziness, paraesthesias, and sedation. Cognitive changes and confusion were also reported. Lasmiditan can cause impaired driving ability and there is a drug warning against driving and operating machinery for at least 8 hours after taking this drug. It is important to mention this to the patient. Because of the CNS action, other concomitant CNS depressants should be avoided. Caution is also advised with heart rate-lowering medications. It is not known if ditans can cause serotonin syndrome.

There is no available evidence that supports limiting the use of ditans with SSRIs or SNRIs, due to concerns for serotonin syndrome. However, given the seriousness of serotonin syndrome, caution is warranted, especially in a patient taking other medications, and supplements. No data for pregnancy and breastfeeding are available at this time.

- Lasmiditan (50 mg, 100 mg, or 200 mg PO as a single dose; maximum: 1 dose in 24 hours)

Gepants for Acute Migraine Treatment

Gepants are the only group of oral medications known to selectively bind and antagonize CGRP receptor. Gepants do not cause vasoconstriction, because they do not bind to serotonin 1B receptor on blood vessels as triptans do, and therefore are not contraindicated in patients with known vascular risk factors. CGRP levels tend to increase with migraine, and patients with migraine injected with CGRP develop migraine within 4 hours. No clinical trials are available that have compared gepants to other acute headache treatments. Gepants are well tolerated, and the most commonly reported side effect compared to placebo is nausea in ubrogepant trials. Since gepants are metabolized via CYP3A4 via liver, coadministration with strong inhibitors of CYP3A4 such as ketoconazole and CYP3A4 inducers such as rifampin should be avoided. No data for pregnancy and breastfeeding are available at this time.

- Ubrogepant (50 to 100 mg PO as a single dose; may repeat once based on response and tolerability after ≥2 hours)
- Rimegepant (75 mg PO as a single dose; maximum: 75 mg/24 hours)

Neuromodulation Therapies for Migraine

There are currently several FDA-approved neuromodulation devices for use in migraine, all of which use noninvasive stimulation to modulate brain function. All are considered to have nonsignificant risks and are generally well tolerated by patients. Neuromodulation can be used for acute treatment of migraine. These devices generally require patient payment, although they are generally free of charge for veterans or military active duty.

- Remote electrical neuromodulation (REN) device

- External trigeminal neurostimulation (eTNS) device, Cefaly device
- Single-pulse transcranial magnetic stimulation (sTMS) device
- External vagal nerve stimulation (VNS) device (GammaCore)

Preventive Treatment

There is emphasis on prevention of migraine attacks for many patients, because acute therapy is often less effective in more severe cases. Consider preventive treatments for patients who are disabled by migraine, who are missing work, who are using the emergency room for headache treatment, who have five or more migraine days per month, or who are prone to overusing acute medications. Preventive treatments should also be considered for patients with serious medical problems, such as heart disease or stroke.

Medical providers should consult the American Academy of Neurology (AAN)/AHS guidelines. All guidelines were consistent in their recommendations of treatments for first-line use. All rated topiramate, divalproex/sodium valproate, propranolol, and metoprolol as having the highest level of evidence.

Level A: effective
- Divalproex (Depakote ER)/sodium valproate (Stavzor) 500 to 1000 mg/day
- Metoprolol (Lopressor)[1] 25 to 200 mg/day
- Petasites (butterbur)[7] 50 to 75 mg bid
- Propranolol (Inderal) 40 to 240 mg/day
- Timolol (Blocadren) 10 to 15 mg bid
- Topiramate (Topamax) 25 to 200 mg/day

Level B: probably effective
Should be considered for patients requiring migraine prophylaxis
- Amitriptyline (Elavil)[1] 10 to 150 mg/day
- Fenoprofen (Nalfon)[1] 200 to 600 mg three times per day
- Feverfew[7] 50 to 150 mg bid; 2.08 to 18.75 mg three times per day for MIG-99 preparation
- Ibuprofen (Advil, Motrin)[1] 200 mg twice a day
- Ketoprofen (Orudis)[1] 50 mg three times per day
- Magnesium[1] 600 mg per day
- Naproxen (Naprosyn)[1]/naproxen sodium (Anaprox DS)[1] 500 to 1100 mg/day or naproxen sodium 550 mg twice a day
- Riboflavin (Vitamin B2)[7] 400 mg/day
- Venlafaxine (Effexor ER)[1] 150 mg extended release/day
- Atenolol (Tenormin)[1] 25–100 mg/day

Anti-Calcitonin Gene-Related Peptide Monoclonal Antibodies for Preventive Treatment

Since 2018, CGRP receptor antagonist monoclonal antibodies (mAbs) have been FDA approved for preventive treatment of both episodic and chronic migraine: erenumab-aooe (Aimovig), galcanezumab-gnlm (Emgality), fremanezumab-vfrm (Ajovy), and eptinezumab-jjmr (Vyepti). The first three are intended for self-injection at home. Before covering, most medical insurances require trial of at least three classes of preventive therapies with highest level of evidence including beta-blockers (propranolol or timolol), antiseizure medications (divalproex sodium or topiramate), and tricyclics or SNRIs. They are effective in about one-third of patients with migraine with super-responders, have low side-effect profile, and do not interact with any medications. They are not indicated during pregnancy or breastfeeding due to lack of evidence.
- Erenumab-aooe (Aimovig) 70 mg, 140 mg SQ once a month self-administered by patient
- Fremanezumab-vfrm (Ajovy) 225 mg SQ monthly, or 675 mg every 3 months (quarterly), which is administered as three consecutive subcutaneous injections of 225 mg each

- Galcanezumab-gnlm (Emgality) 240 mg (two consecutive subcutaneous injections of 120 mg each) once as a loading dose, followed by monthly doses of 120 mg injected subcutaneously

Chronic Migraine Treatment

Patients with chronic forms of migraine are especially difficult to treat. They are prone to chronic MOH. Overuse is defined as taking acute medication 15 or more days per month for nonopioid analgesics (including aspirin, NSAIDs, and acetaminophen), and 10 or more days per month for triptans, ergotamines, opioids, and combination analgesics. People can develop MOH at much lower levels of regular medication use. Medical providers should ensure that patients are aware of the risk of MOH and limit medication use well below these levels. We recommend not using acute medication more than 1 to 2 days per week on average, and this includes all acute medications. Neuromodulation is a great option for management of acute exacerbation in patients with chronic migraine because daily use does not lead to rebound and worsening headaches. Always consider preventive medications and lifestyle changes in patients with chronic migraines, because acute medications cause MOH when used 15 or more days per month.

MOH often leads to clinically refractory migraine. Taking acute medications to abort migraine attacks more than 10 days per month can lead to increased neuronal excitability, depletion of central serotonin production and increased release of CGRP. Clinical observation suggests that both preventive and acute treatment for the primary headache usually fail unless the offending medication or medications that caused MOH are stopped.

Treatments for chronic migraine include:
- Topiramate (Topamax)[1] 25 to 200 mg/day
- OnabotulinumtoxinA (Botox)[1] 155 units injections by medical providers every 3 months
- Erenumab-aooe (Aimovig)[1] 70 mg, 140 mg SQ once a month self-administered by patient
- Fremanezumab-vfrm (Ajovy)[1] 225 mg SQ monthly, or 675 mg every 3 months (quarterly), which is administered as three consecutive subcutaneous injections of 225 mg each.
- Galcanezumab-gnlm (Emgality)[1] 240 mg (two consecutive subcutaneous injections of 120 mg each) once as a loading dose, followed by monthly doses of 120 mg injected subcutaneously

Monitoring

Primary care providers should consider regular follow-up of their patients every few months or more frequently until patients are stable and have gained therapeutic success. We recommend adding multimodal therapy at each visit, and this can include exercise, sleep therapy, nutrition therapy, stress reductions, supplements in addition to pharmacotherapy reevaluation. We use the visits to address migraine comorbidities, especially anxiety and sleep. With regular monitoring, medication dose can be optimized for maximum efficacy and the least possible side effects. Acute pharmacotherapy escalation in patients that are not optimally controlled can backfire and lead to development of MOH. When a patient experiences significantly worsening headache on 15 or more days per month and has history of migraine, acute medication frequency of use needs to be assessed. MOH may resolve after the acute medication is stopped; however, in many patients with comorbid anxiety and insomnia, more treatment should be considered. In patients with MOH we should consider preventive therapy and neuromodulation therapy. Compliance with medication therapy can be improved by education offered by caring providers and establishing therapeutic alliance with patients by using motivational interviewing skills.

---

[1]Not FDA approved for this indication.
[7]Available as dietary supplement.

[1]Not FDA approved for this indication.

References

Chou DE, Shnayderman Yugrakh M, Winegarner D: Acute migraine therapy with external trigeminal neurostimulation (ACME): A randomized controlled trial, *Cephalalgia* 39:3–14, 2019.

Dodick DW, Lipton RB, Ailani J, et al: Ubrogepant for the treatment of migraine, *N Engl J Med* 381:2230–2241, 2019.

Goadsby PJ, Wietecha LA, Dennehy EB, et al: Phase 3 randomized, placebo-controlled, double-blind study of lasmiditan for acute treatment of migraine, *Brain* 142:1894–1904, 2019.

Halker Singh RB, Ailani J, Robbins MS: Neuromodulation for the acute and preventive therapy of migraine and cluster headache, *Headache* 59(Suppl 2):33–49, 2019.

Headache Classification Committee of the International Headache S: The International Classification of Headache Disorders, 3rd edition (beta version), *Cephalalgia: Int J Headache* 33(9):629–808, 2013.

Kuca B, Silberstein SD, Wietecha L, Berg PH, Dozier G, Lipton RB: Lasmiditan is an effective acute treatment for migraine: A phase 3 randomized study, *Neurology* 91:e2222–e2232, 2018.

Lipton RB, Croop R, Stock EG, et al: Rimegepant, an oral calcitonin gene-related peptide receptor antagonist, for migraine, *N Engl J Med* 381:142–149, 2019.

Lipton RB, Dodick DW, Silberstein SD, et al: Single pulse transcranial magnetic stimulation for acute treatment of migraine with aura: A randomised, double-blind, parallel-group, sham-controlled trial, *Lancet Neurol* 9:373–380, 2010.

Loder E, Burch R, Rizzoli P: The 2012 AHS/AAN guidelines for prevention of episodic migraine: a summary and comparison with other recent clinical practice guidelines, *Headache: J Head Face Pain* 52:930–945, 2012.

Marmura MJ, Silberstein SD, Schwedt TJ: The acute treatment of migraine in adults: the American headache society evidence assessment of migraine pharmacotherapies, *Headache* 55:3–20, 2015.

Misra UK, Kalita J, Bhoi SK: High-rate repetitive transcranial magnetic stimulation in migraine prophylaxis: a randomized, placebo-controlled study, *J Neurol*1–9, 2013.

Pierelli F, Iacovelli E, Bracaglia M: Abnormal sensorimotor plasticity in migraine without aura patients, *Pain*, 2013.

Pietrobon D, Moskowitz MA: Pathophysiology of migraine, *Ann Rev Physiol* 75:365–391, 2013.

Stovner LJ, Nichols E, Steiner TJ, et al: Global, regional, and national burden of migraine and tension-type headache, 1990–2016: a systematic analysis for the Global Burden of Disease Study 2016, *Lancet Neurol* 17(11):954–976, 2018.

Stovner LJ, Nichols E, Steiner TJ, Vos T. Headache in the Global Burden of Disease (GBD) Studies. In: *Societal Impact of Headache*, 2019, New York, NY: Springer, Cham; 105–125.

Sussman M, Benner J, Neumann P, Menzin J: Cost effectiveness analysis of erenumab for the preventive treatment of episodic and chronic migraine: Results from the US societal and payer perspectives, *Cephalalgia* 38:1644–1657, 2018.

Szperka CL, et al: *Migraine Care in the Era of COVID–19: Clinical Pearls and Plea to Insurers. Headache: J Head Face Pain*, 2020.

Tassorelli C, Grazzi L, de Tommaso M, et al: Noninvasive vagus nerve stimulation as acute therapy for migraine: The randomized PRESTO study, *Neurology* 91:e364–e373, 2018.

Tepper SJ: Debate: Analgesic overuse is a cause, not consequence, of chronic daily headache. Analgesic overuse is a cause of chronic daily headache, *Headache* 42:543–547, 2002.

Vollbracht S, Rapoport AM: The Pipeline in Headache Therapy, *CNS Drugs*1–13, 2013.

Yarnitsky D, Dodick DW, Grosberg BM, et al: Remote electrical neuromodulation (REN) relieves acute migraine: A randomized, double-blind, placebo-controlled, multicenter trial, *Headache* 59:1240–1252, 2019.

MULTIPLE SCLEROSIS

Method of
B. Mark Keegan, MD

CURRENT DIAGNOSIS

- Multiple sclerosis (MS) is an autoimmune demyelinating disease of the central nervous system (CNS).
- Diagnosis is secured from having repeated CNS demyelinating attacks or new CNS demyelinating lesions on magnetic resonance imaging (MRI) or progressive neurologic dysfunction consistent with MS with no better alternative explanation.
- Presence of cerebrospinal fluid (CSF)–specific oligoclonal bands, characteristic of MS, aids diagnosis.

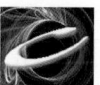

CURRENT THERAPY

- Acute attacks of multiple sclerosis (MS) are treated with high-dose corticosteroids and, in severe cases, plasma exchange.
- Therapy is directed at relapsing-remitting disease with one of the following type 1 interferon β medications: glatiramer acetate (Copaxone), fingolimod (Gilenya), teriflunomide (Aubagio), dimethyl fumarate (Tecfidera), and natalizumab (Tysabri). Therapy for primary progressive MS (progressive disease from onset without prior relapse) is ocrelizumab (Ocrevus).
- Novel MS medications, including further oral medications, and infusion-based monoclonal antibodies are currently under scientific evaluation.

Multiple sclerosis (MS) is an autoimmune inflammatory demyelinating disease of the central nervous system (CNS) that affects approximately 1 million people in the United States alone.

Risk Factors

Women are at least twice as likely as men to develop MS. Other known risk factors for development of MS include ethnicity, genetic background, socioeconomic factors, and environmental exposures. Persons of European ethnicity, particularly those born and reared in extreme northern or southern latitudes, are particularly susceptible to MS although recent data suggest African Americans may have a more severe clinical course. Genetic susceptibility is associated with the major histocompatibility allele, HLA-DRB1, as well as interleukin-2 and interleukin-7 receptors. Low serum vitamin D levels are associated with an increased risk of development of MS and may influence the severity of its clinical course. There are intriguing but as yet unproven associations with infection with Epstein-Barr virus (EBV) (infectious mononucleosis), particularly if EBV is contracted later in adolescence. Exposure to EBV may be necessary but insufficient for developing MS. Comorbid chronic vascular diseases, including hypertension, overweight, and mood disorders complicate and worsen MS disease course. Cigarette smoking is associated with an increased risk for development of MS and is likely associated with an increased severity and clinical course of MS, including that of cognitive impairment.

Pathophysiology

The etiology and pathophysiology of MS as a whole remains uncertain. However, most evidence supports an inflammatory demyelinating disease induced by uncertain environmental factors in a genetically susceptible host. Animal studies, including experimental allergic encephalomyelitis and Theiler murine encephalomyelitis virus, also point to an autoimmune inflammatory demyelinating etiology, possibly associated with viral infection. Studies that suggested chronic cerebrospinal vascular insufficiency having an association with MS have been refuted.

Pathophysiology likely varies among individual patients with MS. Four distinct pathologies in active demyelinating MS lesions have been described. Pattern 1 displays marked macrophage infiltration without humoral abnormalities. Pattern 2 shows distinct humoral abnormalities with complement activation and immunoglobulin (Ig) deposition. Pattern 3 involves primary oligodendrocyte degeneration and early loss of myelin-associated glycoprotein. Pattern 4 reveals oligodendrocyte dystrophy in periplaque white matter. Early studies suggest there could be a therapeutic advantage with different therapies for different types of demyelinating disease.

Prevention

Currently, there is no known way to prevent the development of MS. Patients with a single clinical attack of demyelination and

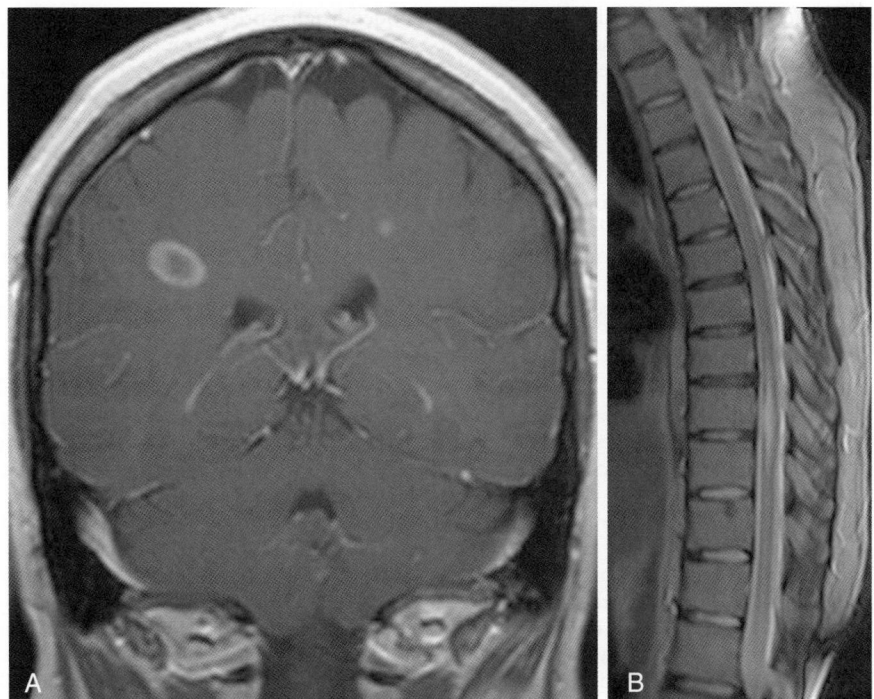

Figure 1 Magnetic resonance image showing brain T_1 gadolinium-enhancing lesions (**A**) and T_2 thoracic spine (**B**) typical of multiple sclerosis.

abnormal magnetic resonance imaging (MRI) ("high-risk" clinically isolated syndrome) have a delayed onset to MS diagnosis with immunomodulatory therapy; however, there is no evidence to support that this prevents the eventual development of MS.

Clinical Manifestations

The clinical course of MS is varied. Approximately 85% of patients present with a relapsing-remitting course. This entails an acute impairment within the CNS, depending on the area of inflammation. A demyelinating cause of a focal neurologic symptom is suggested by an onset over hours to days, with a plateau of impairment over a few weeks. Symptoms then improve either spontaneously or with the use of corticosteroids over a number of days to weeks or longer. Following this, however, symptoms might not completely resolve. Inflammation within the optic nerve (optic neuritis) is heralded by painful, unilateral, central monocular visual deficit (central scotoma). Symptoms of brain stem dysfunction include binocular diplopia, sensory deficits unilaterally on the face and contralaterally on the arm and leg, significant dysarthria, and vertigo. Cerebellar dysfunction is seen with pure ataxia that is typically unilateral. Spinal cord inflammation is indicated by a distinctive, usually gradually rising sensory level of deficit that commonly is accompanied by bowel and bladder impairment and paraparesis or quadriparesis, depending on a thoracic versus cervical level of the lesion.

Progressive forms of MS include secondary progressive MS and primary progressive MS. These are heralded by a slow (months to years) but steady and insidious, progressive neurologic deficit, usually a progressive myelopathy of upper motor neuron gait disorder with spasticity, neurogenic bladder and bowel impairment, and progressive weakness. Occasionally, patients with progressive MS have insidious cerebellar ataxia or dementia in isolation or in association with the myelopathy. Secondary progressive MS is diagnosed when a patient has had a prior history of at least one clinical attack (relapse) with improvement in the past. Primary progressive MS is diagnosed with progressive CNS disease consistent with MS and typical MRI brain scan or spinal lesions from onset without any prior relapse, often with cerebrospinal fluid (CSF) or visual evoked potential abnormalities that support the diagnosis.

Diagnosis

The diagnosis of MS is formalized by the continually revised McDonald criteria. These entail having two or more clinical attacks (relapses) accompanied by two or more objective lesions seen on clinical examination or with evidence for dissemination in space and time diagnosed by further development of new MRI lesions. Additionally, patients with a single clinical attack who have both the presence of MRI gadolinium-enhancing lesions (indicative of acute MS lesions) and nongadolinium-enhancing lesions (indicative of prior MS lesions) are diagnosed with relapsing–remitting MS. Progressive MS is diagnosed when there is progressive CNS disease characteristic of MS for at least 1 year and abnormal brain or spinal cord MRI scan with or without CSF-specific oligoclonal bands (Figure 1). Occasionally, visual-evoked potentials and somatosensory-evoked potentials are used to further document dissemination of MS within the CNS. Serologic investigations are done primarily to rule out MS mimickers depending on and directed by any accompanying systemic symptoms and the clinical setting in individual patients. These may include antinuclear antibodies (ANA for lupus), erythrocyte sedimentation rate, anticardiolipin antibodies, vitamin B12, Lyme serology, and chest imaging for CNS sarcoidosis.

Differential Diagnosis

Other CNS demyelinating diseases can mimic relapsing or progressive MS. Acute disseminated encephalomyelitis (ADEM) is an acute, typically monophasic, and postinfectious CNS inflammatory demyelinating disease. It may be severe; however, if recurrent episodes occur separated by at least 3 months, a diagnosis of relapsing-remitting MS is by far more likely.

Neuromyelitis optica is an autoimmune disease with severe acute attacks but is relatively restricted to the optic nerves and spinal cord. Other brain stem and deep cerebral structures, such as the area postrema, cerebral white matter, and hypothalamus, can also be affected by neuromyelitis optica. Brain MRI scan is usually not consistent with MS, at least early on in the disease, and a specific autoantibody (neuromyelitis optica IgG) directed against the aquaporin 4 water channel is found in most cases.

Clinical syndromes of CNS demyelination with inflammatory myelopathies, inflammatory optic neuritis, and ADEM with serological presence of antibodies to myelin oligodendroglial protein (MOG-Ab) are increasingly recognized.

Optic neuritis may further be mimicked by acute ischemic optic neuropathy. This condition is typically painless, occurs suddenly, and occurs in patients with advanced age and preexisting vascular risk factors.

Progressive myelopathies that mimic primary progressive MS or secondary progressive MS include a compressive myelopathy from cervical spondylosis, disk disease, or neoplastic infiltration; nutritional deficiencies (such as vitamin B12 or copper deficiencies); paraneoplastic disease (e.g., CRMP-5 auto-antibodies); or a vascular progressive cause due to dural arteriovenous fistula.

Treatment

Acute demyelinating MS attacks (relapses) may be treated with high doses of corticosteroids. These may be given orally or intravenously; however, high doses of corticosteroids are necessary and are superior to low doses. For example, a typical regimen is intravenous methylprednisolone (Solu-Medrol) 1000 mg once daily for 3 to 5 days without oral corticosteroid tapering doses. The oral equivalent to this intravenous regimen is prednisone 1000 to 1250 mg orally once daily for 5 days with no oral corticosteroid taper afterward. Gastrointestinal intolerance occurs in some patients, and concomitant use of stomach-protecting agents such as proton pump inhibitors may be recommended. Typical acute corticosteroid side effects include insomnia, irritability, and increased appetite as well as an extremely rare association with avascular hip necrosis. Chronic corticosteroid side effects such as diabetes mellitus, cataracts, weight gain, and cushingoid habitus are more associated with chronic corticosteroid use and not short courses of steroids.

Generally, only MS attacks that are associated with functional impairment (vision loss, diplopia, motor weakness, ataxia) are treated because clinical recovery is hastened, but final clinical recovery is not found to be altered by this therapy. Rarely, patients have very severe acute attacks of MS or other demyelinating disease that does not improve with use of high-dose corticosteroids. In these rare patients, the use of plasma exchange (seven exchanges over approximately 14 days) is recommended. Approximately 45% of patients experience functional recovery within 1 month following plasma exchange. Side effects of plasma exchange therapy include paresthesias related to hypocalcemia, anemia, thrombocytopenia, or complications of central venous access that is required for many patients. Intravenous immunoglobulin (Gammagard)[1] has not yet been shown to improve severe clinical attacks of demyelinating disease.

Chronic parenteral therapy for relapsing–remitting MS includes the use of type 1 β interferons (IFN-β1), glatiramer acetate (Copaxone), natalizumab (Tysabri), alemtuzumab (Lemtrada), or ocrelizumab (Ocrevus) (Table 1). Patients with relapsing-remitting MS may be treated with traditional injectable therapies with preparations of IFN-β1, or glatiramer acetate. Alternatively, oral therapies with fingolimod (Gilenya), siponimod (Mayzent), teriflunomide (Aubagio), and dimethyl fumarate (Tecfidera) are increasingly used as first-line therapies. Cladribine (Mavenclad) is an oral medication for treatment-resistant disease, used as a second-line therapy. Ocrelizumab is approved for treatment of all clinical courses of CNS demyelinating disease, including clinically isolated syndromes, relapsing–remitting MS, and secondary progressive MS. Ocrelizumab also has activity for primary progressive MS, while siponimod is approved for secondary progressive MS with active inflammatory disease. The side-effect profile is well known for traditional injectable agents such as interferons and glatiramer acetate (see Table 1), and they have been safely used for many years. The safety profile for oral therapies seems satisfactory, but their long-term side-effect profile is still being assessed. For fingolimod, first dose monitoring for 6 hours is required to assess heart rate and rhythm and occasional patients have developed progressive multifocal leukoencephalopathy (PML). Teriflunomide may be associated with liver disease and teratogenicity. Dimethyl fumarate is associated with flushing,

gastrointestinal discomfort, and rare patients have developed PML on dimethyl fumarate. Highly active MS therapy may be indicated with natalizumab, alemtuzumab, or ocrelizumab if first-line medications are intolerable, if therapeutic response is suboptimal (continued MS attacks or marked ongoing and new inflammatory disease on MRI despite therapy), or when a concerning clinical onset (severe attack with multiple lesions and incomplete recovery) occurs. The goal of chronic immunomodulatory therapy for MS is a reduction in clinical attacks of MS (between 30% and 60%, depending on the agent) and reduction in new inflammatory MRI lesions (between 40% and 90%, depending on the agent). Patients and health care professionals should realize that the medications are not a cure or for symptomatic benefit (making patients feel better) but specifically for reduction in relapse-related disease.

Natalizumab is clearly associated with the development of PML, a severely impairing, and often fatal, opportunistic brain infection caused by reactivation of dormant John Cunningham virus (JCV). In North America, natalizumab is only available through the TOUCH (Tysabri outreach: unified commitment to health) prescribing program. Risk factors for PML in natalizumab-treated patients include the presence and index value of JCV serum antibody (JCV-AbAB), duration of therapy of at least 2 years, and history of prior immunosuppressive medication therapy (e.g., methotrexate, azathioprine [Imuran]). Seropositivity of MS patients for JCV-AbAB is over 55%. Seroconversion rate from JCV-AbAB negativity to positivity is approximately 2% to 5% per year, and false-negative results are rare (<3%). Currently, no cases of PML have been found in patients persistently seronegative for JCV antibodies. Risk prevalence estimation after 2 years of treatment in JCV Ab-positive patients range from 1:250 for those without history of immunosuppression to 1:90 in those with history of prior immunosuppressive therapy. Mitoxantrone (Novantrone) is a chemotherapy agent that is approved for secondary progressive MS, but given its severe side-effect profile (acute and delayed cardiotoxicity, cases of acute myelogenous leukemia), it is rarely used today. Siponimod (Mayzent) is a selected sphingosine 1 phosphate agonist approved for relapsing forms of MS as well as secondary progressive MS with active disease.

Alemtuzumab (Lemtrada) is a monoclonal antibody (anti-CD52; T and B cells) for relapsing remitting MS with major safety precautions that include development of autoimmune thyroid disease, immune thrombocytopenia, and rarely anti-glomerular basement membrane disease. Daclizumab (Zinbryta) (anti-CD25, IL2 receptor) was withdrawn voluntarily because of case reports of an association with presumably immune-mediated encephalitis. Ocrelizumab ([Ocrevus] anti-CD20 B cells; humanized form) is approved for relapsing-remitting MS and is the only therapy approved for primary progressive MS.

Autologous bone marrow transplantation with stem cell delivery for recovery is under evaluation to determine which cases may respond favorably to it and whether it is equivalent to highly active MS therapies.

Monitoring

Most, if not all, MS patients should be followed by a neurologist at least occasionally. Recommendations for clinical assessment range from 6 to 18 months, depending on clinical activity of relapses and disability. The ideal scheduling of repeat brain MRI scans is controversial and varies depending on MS clinical activity, but general recommendations are every 1 to 2 years.

Complications

MS is one of the main causes for impairment at a young age and trails only acute trauma. Often patients need gait assistance when impairment becomes more severe. This includes the use of a single gait aid, such as a cane or walking stick, or an ankle-foot orthosis for symptomatic foot drop.

Patients often experience symptoms of neurogenic bladder dysfunction, including symptoms of urgency and urge-related incontinence. Bladder stimulants such as caffeine need to be avoided. Patients with this symptom should be investigated for completeness

---

[1]Not FDA approved for this indication.

TABLE 1 Approved Immunomodulatory Therapy for Relapsing-Remitting Multiple Sclerosis

MEDICATION	DOSING	SIDE EFFECTS	MONITORING	ADDITIONAL INFORMATION
Interferon β1a (Avonex)	30 µg IM injection 1 ×/wk	Influenza-like symptoms (fever, chills, arthralgias, myalgias, and headaches), elevated liver function tests, anemia, leukopenia, thrombocytopenia, depression. Localized injection-site rejections	CBC with differential, AST, ALT, ALP, and total bilirubin level every 3 months while on therapy. Thyroid function cascade upon initiation of therapy	Premedication with acetaminophen can ameliorate any postinjection influenza-like symptoms. Ibuprofen and naproxen. Pregnancy category C medication
Interferon β1a (Rebif)	22 µg or 44 µg SC injection 3 ×/wk	Influenza-like symptoms (fever, chills, arthralgias, myalgias, and headaches), elevated liver function tests, anemia, leukopenia, thrombocytopenia, depression. Localized injection-site rejections	CBC with differential, AST, ALT, ALP, and total bilirubin level every 3 months while on therapy. Thyroid function cascade on initiation of therapy	Premedication with acetaminophen can ameliorate any postinjection influenza-like symptoms. Ibuprofen and naproxen. Pregnancy category C medication
Peginterferon β1a (Plegridy)	125 µg SC every 14 days	Influenza-like symptoms (fever, chills, arthralgias, myalgias, and headaches), elevated liver function tests, anemia, leukopenia, thrombocytopenia, and depression. Localized injection-site rejections	CBC with differential, AST, ALT, alkaline phosphatase, and total bilirubin level. Every 3 months while on therapy. Thyroid function cascade on initiation of therapy.	Premedication with acetaminophen may ameliorate any post-injection influenza-like symptoms. Ibuprofen and naproxen. Pregnancy category C medication.
Interferon β1b (Betaseron, Extavia)	250 µg SC injection every other day	Influenza-like symptoms (fever, chills, arthralgias, myalgias, and headaches), elevated liver function tests, anemia, leukopenia, thrombocytopenia, depression. Localized injection-site rejections	CBC with differential, AST, ALT, ALP, and total bilirubin level every 3 months while on therapy. Thyroid function cascade on initiation of therapy.	Premedication with acetaminophen can ameliorate any post-injection flulike symptoms. Ibuprofen and naproxen. Pregnancy category C medication
Glatiramer acetate (Copaxone)	20 mg SC injection daily or 40 mg SC injection 3×/wk	Injection-site reactions (erythema, edema, pruritus, pain), transient chest pain, palpitations, facial flushing, anxiety, shortness of breath	None	Pregnancy category B medication
Fingolimod hydrochloride (Gilenya)	0.5 mg PO once daily	Headache, influenza, diarrhea, back pain, liver enzyme elevations, and cough. New FDA labeling required; investigating unexplained deaths occurring during treatment with fingolimod	Ophthalmologist review before therapy and in 3–4 months for macular edema, repeated annually in those with diabetes mellitus or uveitis. Serology for VZV-IgG to determine immunity CBC with differential, AST, ALT, alkaline phosphatase, and total bilirubin level, ECG ECG before first dose and after 6-h monitoring; first dose must be monitored for 6 h for heart-rate reduction and blood-pressure changes; 6-h monitoring following oral dose must be repeated for patients who discontinue therapy for 14 or more consecutive days. For VZV nonimmune patients, vaccination (2 doses at least 1 month apart) before starting treatment is needed, and treatment may commence 1 month after the second VZV vaccination.	Should not be used in patients with recent MI, unstable angina, stroke, TIA, 2nd- or 3rd-degree AV block, CHF, SSS without cardiac pacing, or QTc >500 ms, or with Class Ia or III antiarrhythmic drugs. Overnight continuous ECG monitoring recommended for those with preexisting cardiac or cerebrovascular disease; recurrent syncope; severe, untreated obstructive sleep apnea; use of β-blockers; or prolonged QTc. Occasional PML Pregnancy category C medication. Caution for redemonstration of severe inflammatory disease on discontinuation.

Continued

Multiple Sclerosis

TABLE 1 Approved Immunomodulatory Therapy for Relapsing-Remitting Multiple Sclerosis—cont'd

MEDICATION	DOSING	SIDE EFFECTS	MONITORING	ADDITIONAL INFORMATION
Siponimod (Mayzent)	The recommended maintenance dosage for most is 2 mg PO once daily • The recommended maintenance dosage in patients with a CYP2C9*1/*3 or *2/*3 genotype is 1 mg PO once daily	Herpes virus infection, upper respiratory infections, fungal skin infections Macular edemaSevere exacerbation of MS rarely reported after discontinuation of a S1P receptor modulator (fingolimod).	CYP2C9 genotype determination. CBC Fundus evaluation (OCT), recent electrocardiogram (within last 6 months), liver transaminase and bilirubin levels. First-dose monitoring is recommended for patients with sinus bradycardia, first- or second-degree (Mobitz type I) atrioventricular (AV) block, or a history of myocardial infarction or heart failure	Concomitant use of siponimod and moderate or strong CYP3A4 inducers (e.g., modafinil, efavirenz [Sustival]) is not recommended for patients with CYP2C9*1/*3 and *2/*3 genotype
Teriflunomide (Aubagio)	7 mg or 14 mg PO once daily	Diarrhea, abnormal liver tests, nausea, influenza, alopecia, potential for hepatotoxicity, may cause significant birth defects if used during pregnancy (pregnancy category X), peripheral neuropathy, transient acute renal failure, and hyperkalemia	CBC monthly for the first 6 months. Liver enzymes Tuberculin skin test Pregnancy test (women of childbearing potential)	Prolonged half-life; recommend removal by activated charcoal or cholestyramine when required. Pregnancy category X medication
Dimethyl fumarate (Tecfidera)	120 mg PO twice daily for 7 days, then 240 mg PO twice daily	Flushing, abdominal pain, nausea, diarrhea	CBC Consider serum. JCV Ab serology	CBC annually PML rarely
Ocrelizumab (Ocrevus)	300 mg³ IV followed by another 300 mg IV in 2 weeks then 600 mg IV q 6 months	Infusion reactions (~34%) Infections respiratory tract, herpes infections Possible increased risk of cancer including breast cancer	CBC Rule out hepatitis B virus before first dose	Approved for CIS, RRMS, SPMS, and PPMS Do not administer if signs of infection delay until infection resolves. Administer vaccines >6 weeks before ocrelizumab infusions Live and live-attenuated vaccines not recommended until B-cell counts recover after discontinuation.
Natalizumab (Tysabri)	300 mg IV once every 28 days	Urticaria and anaphylaxis, headache, arthralgias, nausea, fatigue, depression, infections (urinary tract, pneumonia, herpes simplex or reactivation)	Before treatment: JCV Ab serologic study, head MRI with or without gadolinium, CBC with differential, AST, ALT, alkaline phosphatase, and total bilirubin and pregnancy test if applicable. Every 6 months: JCV Ab serology if seronegative (no need to repeat if JCV Ab is seropositive); head MRI with and without gadolinium every 6 months while on therapy; if PML is suspected, discontinue therapy immediately, PLEX to remove drug, MRI head scan with and without gadolinium with diffusion-weighted imaging; CSF for JCV PCR	Monotherapy approved Risk of PML may be greater in patients with prolonged therapy and those previously treated with immunosuppressive medications. Prescribing professional requires TOUCH enrollment Pregnancy category C medication. Caution for redemonstration of severe inflammatory disease on discontinuation.
Alemtuzumab (Lemtrada)	IV infusion over 4 h × 2 treatment course. First course: 12 mg/day on 5 consecutive days. Second course: 12 mg/day on 3 consecutive days 12 months after the first treatment course	Infusion reactions with anaphylaxis. Autoimmune thyroid disorders, immune thrombocytopenia, antiglomerular basement membrane disease. Malignancies including thyroid cancer, melanoma and lymphoproliferative disorders	CBC with differential, monthly for 48 months after last dose. Creatinine, urinalysis with urine cell counts periodically for 48 months after last dose. Baseline and yearly skin examinations	Premedicate with high-dose corticosteroids, check VZV status and vaccinate those VZV antibody negative

TABLE 1 Approved Immunomodulatory Therapy for Relapsing-Remitting Multiple Sclerosis—cont'd

MEDICATION	DOSING	SIDE EFFECTS	MONITORING	ADDITIONAL INFORMATION
Cladribine (Mavenclad)	2 treatment courses (1.75 mg/kg per treatment course). One treatment course per year for a total of 2 years. Each treatment course is divided into 2 treatment weeks, one at the beginning of the first month and one at the beginning of the second month of the respective treatment year. Each treatment week consists of 4 or 5 days on which a patient receives 10 mg or 20 mg (one or two tablets) as a single daily dose, depending on body weight.	Contraindicated in patients with current malignancy Pregnant women, and women and men of reproductive potential who do not plan to use effective contraception during cladribine dosing and for 6 months after the last dose in each treatment course HIV infection Active chronic infections (e.g., hepatitis or tuberculosis) Women intending to breastfeed on a cladribine treatment day and for 10 days after the last dose	Follow standard cancer screening guidelines CBC 2 and 6 months after the start of each treatment course Monitor CBC annually thereafter If the lymphocyte count at month 2 is below 200 cells per microliter, monitor monthly until month 6 Hold cladribine therapy if the lymphocyte count is below 200 cells per microliter	If VZV-IgG is negative, vaccinate with recombinant zoster vaccine (Shingrix) prior to initiating cladribine Administer live-attenuated or live vaccines at least 4–6 weeks prior to starting cladribine Avoid vaccination with live-attenuated or live vaccines during and after cladribine treatment while the patient's white blood cell counts are not within normal limits.

Ab, Antibody; *ALP*, alkaline phosphatase; *ALT*, alanine aminotransferase; *AST*, aspartate aminotransferase; *AV*, atrioventricular; *BUN*, blood urea nitrogen; *CBC*, complete blood count; *CHF*, congestive heart failure; *CIS*, clinically isolated syndrome; *CSF*, cerebrospinal fluid; *ECG*, electrocardiogram; *FDA*, U.S. Food and Drug Administration; *HIV*, human immunodeficiency virus; *JCV*, John Cunningham virus; *MI*, myocardial infarction; *MRI*, magnetic resonance imaging; *PCR*, polymerase chain reaction; *PLEX*, plasma exchange; *PML*, progressive multifocal leukoencephalopathy; *PO*, by mouth; *PPD*, purified protein derivative; *PPMS*, primary progressive MS; *RRMS*, relapsing-remitting disease; *SPMS*, secondary progressive multiple sclerosis; *SSS*, sick sinus syndrome; *TIA*, transient ischemic attack; *TOUCH*, Tysabri Outreach: Unified Commitment to Health; *VZV-IgG*, varicella zoster virus immunoglobulin G.

of bladder emptying. If there is severe impairment in bladder emptying, urinary catheterization often is recommended. If bladder emptying is complete or only mildly impaired (<100 mL post-void residual), use of medications such as oxybutynin (Ditropan) or tolterodine (Detrol) may be recommended for urge-related symptoms; however, ongoing monitoring of bladder emptying is recommended. Some patients require formal urodynamic evaluation for complex bladder symptoms.

Fatigue is a common MS-related symptom. A complete sleep history to ensure appropriate sleep hygiene is imperative. This includes initiating sleep promptly, maintaining sleep throughout the night, and awakening feeling refreshed. Encouragement of a formal exercise program to facilitate restful sleep and daytime vigor is important. Obstructive sleep apnea, restless legs syndrome, and other parasomnias need to be ruled out as additional contributing factors to fatigue. If sleep hygiene is entirely normal and late afternoon fatigue remains a problem, pharmacologic therapy for MS-related fatigue can proceed. Pharmacologic recommendations are limited but include amantadine hydrochloride (Symmetrel)[1] 100 mg PO twice daily. Modafinil (Provigil)[1] has been shown in some studies to have an effect on MS-related fatigue at a dose of 200 mg PO once daily.

Spasticity associated with upper motor neuron weakness in the lower extremities may be treated with an active daily exercise program directed by physical therapists and physiatrists. Judicious use of baclofen (Lioresal) is helpful (starting at 10 mg once to three times PO daily no more than a maximum of 80 mg/day). Baclofen side effects include drowsiness and liver enzyme elevations. Some patients with significant lower extremity weakness are assisted in their gait by the leg support provided by spasticity, and if spasticity is reduced pharmacologically, this can in fact worsen their gait. Alternatives to baclofen include tizanidine (Zanaflex) and clonidine (Catapres)[1].

MS is a common CNS inflammatory demyelinating disease with heterogenous presentation and prognosis. Relapsing–remitting or attack-related MS is treated with corticosteroids to hasten resolution of acute relapses and chronic immunomodulatory medications such as IFN-β, glatiramer acetate, fingolimod, siponimod, cladribine, teriflunomide, dimethyl fumarate, alemtuzumab, and natalizumab to reduce the number of future clinical attacks and new MRI lesions. Ocrelizumab is the only medication approved for primary progressive MS. Symptomatic care is important in those patients, including the treatment of gait disorder, spasticity, neurogenic bladder dysfunction, and fatigue.

---

[1]Not FDA approved for this indication.

References

Ho PR, Koendgen H, Campbell N, et al: Risk of natalizumab-associated progressive multifocal leukoencephalopathy in patients with multiple sclerosis: a retrospective analysis of data from four clinical studies, *Lancet Neurol* 16:925–933, 2017.

Langer-Gould A, Brara SM, Beaber BE, et al: Incidence of multiple sclerosis in multiple racial and ethnic groups, *Neurology* 80(19):1734–1739, 2013.

Lublin FD, Reingold SC, Cohen JA, et al: Defining the clinical course of multiple sclerosis: the 2013 revisions, *Neurology* 83:278–286, 2014.

Montalban X, Belachew S, Wolinsky JS: Ocrelizumab in primary progressive and relapsing multiple sclerosis, *N Engl J Med* 376:1694, 2017.

Reich DS, Lucchinetti CF, Calabresi PA: Multiple sclerosis, *N Engl J Med* 378:169–180, 2018.

Thompson AJ, Banwell BL, Barkhof F, et al: Diagnosis of multiple sclerosis: 2017 revisions of the McDonald criteria, *Lancet Neurol* 17:162–173, 2018.

Traboulsee AL, Know KB, Machan L, et al: Prevalence of extracranial venous narrowing on catheter venography in people with multiple sclerosis, their siblings, and unrelated healthy controls: a blinded, case-control study, *Lancet* 383:138–145, 2014.

Wallin MT, Culpepper WJ, Campbell JD, et al: The prevalence of MS in the United States, *Neurology* 92(10):e1029–e1040, 2019.

Wingerchuk DM, Banwell B, Bennett JL, et al: International consensus diagnostic criteria for neuromyelitis optica spectrum disorders, *Neurology* 85:177–189, 2015.

MYASTHENIA GRAVIS

Method of
Taylor B. Harrison, MD; and William P. Roche, MD

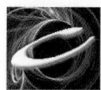

CURRENT DIAGNOSIS

- Myasthenia gravis (MG) is an autoimmune disorder that affects the neuromuscular junction, resulting in fatigable skeletal muscle weakness.
- Diagnosis may be based on clinical history and exam in combination with identification of autoantibodies (Ach-R Abs) or abnormalities on electrodiagnostic testing.
- Myasthenic crisis, defined by respiratory failure, can stem from respiratory or oropharyngeal weakness. It may develop abruptly and typically occurs in the setting of illness, change in medications, or early in the disease course.

CURRENT THERAPY

- Mild symptoms can respond well to anticholinestrase inhibitors such as pyridostigmine (Mestinon).
- A wide range of medications may be used to treat MG, including steroids, nonsteroidal immunosuppressants, as well as intravenous immunoglobulin[1] and plasmapheresis. Thymectomy may be considered in patients with acetylcholine receptor antibodies.
- It is important to recognize that certain medications may worsen MG.
- Myasthenic crisis is a medical emergency, and patients should be treated in the intensive care unit with close respiratory monitoring and possibly intubation. Intravenous immunoglobulin[1] and plasmapheresis are treatment options for myasthenic crisis.

---

[1]Not FDA approved for this indication.

Epidemiology

Myasthenia gravis (MG) is the most common acquired disorder of neuromuscular transmission, with an incidence of 8 to 10 per million annually. The prevalence is 150 to 250 per million, reflecting the disease's low mortality rate. An estimated 700,000 people are living with MG worldwide, with between 36,000 to 60,000 living in the United States.

There exists a bimodal age distribution with two peaks of incidence: the first peak in the second to third decades of life, and a second peak in the seventh to eighth decades. Women predominate in early-onset MG (defined by onset <50 years of age) whereas men predominate with late-onset disease (>50 years of age).

Risk Factors

MG is associated with thymoma: approximately one-third of patients with thymoma will develop myasthenia, and 10% of myasthenic patients have a thymoma. Certain HLA subtypes, which are known to predispose to autoimmune disorders in general, also increase the risk of MG. Other autoimmune disorders are present in about 15% of myasthenic patients, most commonly thyroiditis, followed by systemic lupus erythematosus and rheumatoid arthritis. A small percentage of patients may have a myasthenia-myositis overlap syndrome (Tables 1 and 2).

Pathophysiology

To understand the pathophysiology, a review of normal physiology is needed. In normal muscle contraction, an action potential (AP) travels down a motor nerve to the presynaptic axon

TABLE 1	Medications That May Exacerbate or Precipitate MG

Black box warnings:

Telithromycin (Ketek)[2]

Fluoroquinolones (ciprofloxacin [Cipro], moxifloxacin [Avelox], levofloxacin [Levaquin])

Drugs to avoid:

D-penicillamine (Cuprimine)

Checkpoint inhibitors (ipilimumab [Yervoy], pembrolizumab [Keytruda], nivolumab [Opdivo])

Quinine

IV Magnesium

Use only with caution:

Macrolidess (erythromycin, azithromycin [Zithromax], clarithromycin [Biaxin])

Aminoglycosides (gentamycin [Garamycin], neomycin, tobramycin)

Procainamide (Pronestyl)

Desferrioxamine (Desferal)

Beta blockers (propranolol, metoprolol [Lopressor], carvedilol [Coreg])

Statins (atorvastatin [Lipitor], pravastatin [Pravachol], rosuvastatin [Crestor], simvastatin [Zocor])

[2]Not available in the United States.

TABLE 2	Suggested Medication Monitoring
MEDICATION	**SUGGESTED MONITORING**
Azathioprine (Imuran)	CBC, LFTs weekly for the first month then monthly to every 3 months
Cyclosporine (Sandimmune)	Monthly CBC, LFTs, renal function monthly for 3 months then quarterly Periodic trough level Blood pressure checks
Cyclophosphamide (Cytoxan)	CBC (attention to neutrophil count), electrolytes and renal function, LFTs, UA every 2–4 weeks
Eculizumab (Soliris)	CBC, renal function, LFTs
IVIG (Gammagard)	Renal function monthly, with repeated dosing maybe every 3 months
Methotrexate (Trexall)	CBC, LFTs monthly initially, then at stable dose at least every 3 months
Mycophenolate mofetil	CBC every 2 weeks for first month, then monthly to quarterly
Plasma exchange	Blood pressure and serum calcium
Prednisone	Weight and blood pressure Periodic potassium and HgbA1c Bone density test Periodic eye exam
Rituximab (Rituxan)	CD 20 counts may be considered but varies among providers

CBC, Complete blood count.

terminal. At the axon terminal, the AP triggers voltage-gated calcium channels to open, causing calcium influx. Calcium influx causes synaptic vesicles containing acetylcholine to fuse with the cell membrane, resulting in exocytosis of acetylcholine into the synaptic cleft. Acetylcholine diffuses across the synaptic cleft and binds with nicotinic acetylcholine receptors (AchRs) on the cell membrane of the muscle fiber. The AchRs are ligand-gated ion channels that, once opened, allow cation influx, generating an end plate potential (EPP). When the EPP reaches a threshold value, it triggers voltage-gated sodium channels in the postsynaptic membrane to open, resulting in further cation influx and membrane depolarization, resulting in a muscle fiber AP and muscle fiber contraction. Excess acetylcholine is then broken down by the enzyme acetylcholinesterase (AchE) in the synaptic cleft.

The safety factor is an important concept in understanding the muscle fatigability of MG. The safety factor is the ratio of postsynaptic EPP generated by a quantity of acetylcholine to the threshold required to generate an all-or-none muscle fiber AP and thus muscle fiber contraction. In the healthy state, more acetylcholine is released than is needed to generate a muscle fiber AP. In myasthenia the safety factor is lower, and sufficient acetylcholine may not be released to generate successive APs with repeated contractions. Exercise will result in insufficient neuromuscular transmission over time because of this reduction in safety factor, and as muscle fibers fail to reach threshold to generate an AP, fatigable weakness ensues.

MG is caused by antibodies targeting antigens of the postsynaptic membrane of the neuromuscular junction. In myasthenia gravis, the normal action of acetylcholine at the postsynaptic muscle cell membrane is disrupted by one of several antibody-mediated mechanisms. Most commonly, antibodies are formed against the AchR itself. These AchR antibodies interrupt normal transmission by cross-linking the receptors causing increased turnover or complement-mediated degradation or by inducing conformational changes in the channel, keeping acetylcholine from activating the channel. Other antibodies have been found to cause MG, including antibodies against muscle-specific kinase (MUSK), lipoprotein-related protein 4 (LRP4), or agrin. The postsynaptic cell membrane is folded into secondary synaptic folds, increasing the surface area of the cell membrane, and AchRs are organized in clusters at the peaks of these folds (adjacent to the nerve axon terminal). MUSK, LRP4, and agrin are proteins that participate in AchR clustering on these peaks. Antibody-mediated disruption of the function of these proteins causes reduced AchR concentration on the postsynaptic membrane with reduced safety factor, resulting in a myasthenia phenotype.

Some patients do not have antibodies that are detectable by current serologic testing. These patients are presumed to have antibodies against components of the postsynaptic membrane that have not yet been identified.

Prevention

Although there is no recognized prevention for developing myasthenia, exacerbations (myasthenic crises) are preventable by avoiding certain drugs. In particular, beta blockers, some antibiotics (aminoglycosides, fluoroquinolones, and macrolides), and chelating agents (penicillamine [Cuprimine]) should be avoided in myasthenic patients (see Box 1). Statins should be used cautiously and only at the lowest effective dose.

Clinical Manifestations

Patients with MG will present with weakness of the extraocular, bulbar, axial, or limb muscles. The most characteristic feature of the weakness seen in myasthenia is fatigability; that is, the tendency of a muscle to get weaker with repeated use. Thus, when thinking about weakness from MG, it is important to get a sense of whether the patient's symptoms are exacerbated by exercise, or demonstrate a diurnal fluctuation (with the most typical pattern being weakness that is worse at the end of the day).

Ocular symptoms (ptosis and diplopia) are the first symptoms of myasthenia in approximately 60% of patients, and in 15% to 20% of all myasthenic patients, weakness remains limited to the eye muscles (so-called "ocular myasthenia"). Patients will complain of a drooping eyelid or binocular double vision (that improves with closing one eye) that frequently fluctuates throughout the day or with activity. On physical examination, these patients have ptosis or limitations in extraocular movements that are triggered or exaggerated by sustained upgaze for 60 seconds (so-called "upgaze paresis"). The extraocular manifestations are rarely symmetric, and the ptosis is very often more significant on one side.

Weakness of the limbs tends to be symmetric and usually affects proximal more than distal muscles. Patients will frequently complain of reduced ability to perform repetitive actions of the proximal muscles, such as lifting an arm to comb hair or climbing stairs. On physical examination, fatigability can be demonstrated by having the patient activate the deltoids (arm abduction) or iliopsoas (hip flexion) either against gravity for 2 minutes or against examiner resistance for 5 repetitions of 5 seconds each. Typically, myasthenic patients with weakness of these muscle groups will have a significant decrement in strength between the first repetition and the last. Similar maneuvers can be performed using whichever muscle groups are affected, according to the patient's complaints.

Bulbar weakness manifests as difficulty with speech (dysarthria) or swallowing (dysphagia). These symptoms may also be fatigable; for example, patients may notice more difficulty enunciating toward the end of the day or at the end of a speech, or more trouble swallowing toward the end of a meal or when eating chewy foods such as steak. If shortness of breath is present, it typically improves moving from a supine to sitting position, which helps with diaphragm excursion. Strength of sniff and cough can be easily assessed at the bedside, and weakness of neck flexion may indicate risk for diaphragmatic weakness.

Sensation is not affected in MG. If a patient has sensory loss, static weakness that does not fluctuate with exercise, or other neurologic symptoms aside from weakness, this should prompt the examiner to consider an alternate diagnosis. Deep tendon reflexes are normal in myasthenia gravis.

Diagnosis

It is important to understand the proper diagnostic algorithm for MG, which is based on the combination of clinical history, examination findings, presence of autoantibodies, and results of electrodiagnostic testing. In the setting of a good clinical history and positive examination findings, the presence of pathologic autoantibodies is likely sufficient to confirm the diagnosis. When the clinical history or examination is suggestive but autoantibodies are not present, electrodiagnostic testing is important to confirm a suspected diagnosis, particularly if immunosuppressive or interventional therapies are considered.

Bedside tests to support a diagnosis include the ice pack test and edrophonium. Placement of ice over a ptotic eyelid may lead to clinical improvement, as cool temperature slows down the breakdown of Ach in the synapse due to slowed action of AchE. Edrophonium (Enlon, previously marketed as Tensilon) is a short-acting AchE inhibitor may be used to help confirm a clinical diagnosis. It is best used if the patient has ptosis or extraocular paresis because there is less subjectivity in assessing improvement. Edrophonium is given intravenously (IV) with 0.1 mL of a 10 mg/mL solution administered initially as a test to assess tolerance, and if no unwanted effects are noted, the remainder of the drug is injected and the patient is observed for a clinical response. If a cholinergic reaction occurs, which may include bradycardia or hypotension, then administer 0.5 mg atropine IV.

Laboratory evolution of autoantibodies is standard of care in patients with suspected MG. In generalized MG, Ach-R Abs are generally present in up to 85% of affected individuals with generalized MG. Ach-R Abs may include blocking, binding, as well as modulating antibodies. Of those patients with generalized MG who are seronegative for Ach-R Ab, approximately 30% to 40% are seropositive for MUSK antibodies. In ocular MG, where symptoms are limited to ptosis or binocular diplopia, only about 15% are seropositive for autoantibodies, and if present, those

autoantibodies are Ach-R ab. The vast majority are seronegative and require further evaluation for confirmation of the diagnosis.

Electrodiagnostic testing for a disorder of neuromuscular transmission includes slow repetitive nerve stimulation (RNS). A stimulator is used to depolarize a motor nerve (resulting in an all-or-none nerve AP) and generate a muscle twitch recorded as a compound motor action potential (CMAP). A train of stimuli (between 4 to 6) are performed at a rate of 3 to 5 per second. In MG the dysfunction at the postsynaptic muscle membrane results in some muscle fibers not achieving depolarization sufficient to cause an all-or-none muscle fiber AP, and the size of the overall CMAP (from multiple muscle fibers) is reduced. The threshold for abnormality is a CMAP decrement of >10%, generally between the first and fourth stimuli. If a baseline study at rest is normal, the patient is asked to exercise the muscle for 1 minute, and the study is repeated at 1-minute intervals to assess for the development of decrement. It should be noted that the sensitivity of RNS is increased with the presence of fatigable weakness on examination, because the clinical correlate of a decrement is weakness. Aside from distal hand muscles, trapezius or facial muscles such as nasalis can be studied.

Single fiber electromyography looks for "jitter" or loss of synchronization of individual muscle fibers innervated by a single anterior horn cell in the spinal cord. This is the most sensitive electrodiagnostic test for MG.

Differential Diagnosis

The differential diagnosis for diplopia and ptosis includes cranial nerve palsies: oculomotor (cranial nerve III), trochlear (cranial nerve IV), and abducens (cranial nerve VI). Horner's syndrome may also cause ptosis due to weakness in Mueller's muscle, although other signs such as anisocoria (unequal pupils) that is worsened in the dark is present. Thyroid eye disease may cause any of these symptoms as well. The differential diagnosis for appendicular weakness without sensory loss includes myopathy, pure motor neuropathy, anterior horn cell disease, or a central nervous system pathology involving the motor pathways. These causes of weakness result in static rather than fluctuating weakness.

The main differential diagnosis for fatigable weakness as seen in MG is the Lambert-Eaton myasthenic syndrome (LEMS). LEMS is caused by antibodies against voltage-gated calcium channels on the presynaptic neuromuscular junction and may be paraneoplastic (small cell carcinoma of the lung) or autoimmune. MG and LEMS can be differentiated by the presence of postexercise facilitation of reflexes (after 10 seconds of sustained exercise), as well as antibody and electrodiagnostic testing.

Therapy

Overall, the treatment goal is to achieve freedom from symptoms or functional limitations, recognizing that patients may still have some weakness of some muscles (this is known as minimal manifestation status). Mainstays of treatment include anticholinesterase inhibitors, as well as oral steroids, and a variety of immunosuppressants, as well as intravenous immunoglobulin (IVIG),[1] and plasmapheresis may be used. Broadly, medical therapy can be classified as symptomatic or disease-modifying, the latter with an immunomodulatory effect targeting the underlying disease pathophysiology.

It should be noted that there exists wide variation in therapeutic approaches, and there are limited head-to-head data comparing individual medications. Current treatments, as well as advances in clinical care, have significantly improved the mortality rate of MG and outcomes of myasthenic crisis.

[1]Not FDA approved for this indication.

Symptomatic Therapy

Pyridostigmine (Mestinon) is an AchE inhibitor that increases the amount of acetylcholine in the synaptic cleft by slowing its breakdown by AchE and should be considered as initial therapy. Onset of action is typically within 30 minutes, with benefit generally lasting 3 to 4 hours. As such it is initially dosed 60 mg 3 times daily by mouth and may be increased to 120 mg every 3 to 4 hours while awake, with the total dose typically not exceeding 480 mg/d. It does not penetrate the central nervous system, and most side effects are gastrointestinal. Side effects may include nausea, vomiting, abdominal cramping, diarrhea, sweating, blurred vision, or muscle twitching and cramps. Anticholinergic agents such as glycopyrrolate (Robinul) 1 mg or hyoscyamine sulfate (Levsin)[1] 0.125 mg with each pyridostigmine dose can usually treat these muscarinic side effects effectively. Data suggest that MUSK Ab–positive patients may have a lesser response to acetylcholinersterase therapy when compared with ACH-R–seropositive patients. In the setting of ocular myasthenia, there appears to be more of response in ptosis when compared with diplopia.

Corticosteroids

Corticosteroids, typically prednisone,[1] are a mainstay of immunotherapy and used when pyridostigmine alone does not achieve an adequate treatment response. Two general approaches exist, using either a low-dose or high-dose regimen. Decisions may be dictated by the severity of weakness, presence of significant bulbar dysfunction, or comorbid conditions (such as diabetes). A "low-dose" approach is used with milder disease and includes initiation of 10 to 20 mg daily, and increasing by 5 mg orally weekly to a lower target dose (generally 40–60 mg/d). Oral high-dose (1 mg/kg/d) steroid therapy may be used with moderate-severe weakness and generally has a latency of 2 to 4 weeks before onset of benefit with maximal benefit in 5 to 6 months. It is important to recognize that early clinical deterioration is possible (reported up to 50%) approximately 7 to 10 days after treatment initiation, generally when steroids are dosed at 1 mg/kg/d or higher. In those patients for whom high-dose therapy is introduced, concomitant treatment with either IVIG or plasma exchange (PLEX), discussed herein, may provide protection against early clinical deterioration.

For a patient who has achieved the treatment goal of minimal manifestation on a particular dose of steroids, it is important to consider weaning the dose to reduce side effects. A common approach is a slow taper decreasing 5 mg/d per month on alternate days, with a slower taper once a total dose of 10 mg daily is achieved. Many patients can be maintained on low doses of steroids.

Some patients have an inadequate response to steroids or intolerable side effects or are unable to taper because of recurrence of symptoms. These patients are typically treated with alternative, steroid-sparing, immunomodulatory therapies. Some patients with comorbidities that limit steroid dosing are started on steroids and nonsteroidal immunosuppressant medications concurrently.

Thymectomy

Thymectomy is considered standard of care for those with thymoma, which is present in approximately 15% of patients with generalized MG. A recent study supports thymectomy in Ach-R Ab–positive patients with at least moderately severe disease. Thymectomy patients demonstrated improved outcomes compared with placebo, required less steroids, fewer required steroid-sparing immunosuppressants, and experienced fewer hospitalizations. Thymectomy is controversial for mild symptoms, purely ocular disease, older age (>60 years), and there exist various surgical approaches. It is considered standard of care to pretreat with IVIG or PLEX before surgery if patients are symptomatic.

Other Immunomodulatory Therapies

Azathioprine (Imuran)[1] is a purine analogue that inhibits nucleic acid synthesis, as well as T- and B-cell proliferation. It is a commonly used steroid-sparing immunosuppressant that is considered first-line and has shown efficacy in a randomized clinical trial. Azathioprine allows reduced steroid dose, reduces relapse rate, and prolongs duration of remission. Treatment is generally started at 50 mg daily, increasing by 50 mg every 1 to 2 weeks to approximately 150 to 200 daily (2–3 mg/kg/d), generally in split doses. Onset of action is estimated at 4 to 8 months, and therapy requires regular blood count and liver function monitoring. Side effects include a flulike illness at initiation (reported in up to 10% to 20%, requires cessation), leukopenia, and transaminitis. Thiopurine methyltransferase enzyme testing can be performed, if available, before starting to identify patients at high risk of bone marrow suppression (although monitoring of blood counts is favored by many practitioners).

Intravenous immunoglobulin (IVIG, Gammagard)[1] has been shown to improve weakness in MG. Its mechanism of action is unclear although presumed to stem from neutralizing circulating pathogenic autoantibodies. A dose of 2 g/kg spread over 5 days is a common algorithm for initial treatment, although in patients who previously tolerated it, IVIG could be given as 1 g/kg/d over 2 days. Onset of action is typically within the first week, and benefit may be sustained for 3 to 4 weeks after treatment. Side effects include headache (sometimes severe and related to aseptic meningitis), thrombosis because of increased serum viscosity, and renal failure. Avoidance of sucrose-containing products may decrease risk of renal failure. Slowed infusion rates may help avoid decompensation of heart failure. Patients on maintenance dosing may receive IVIG 1 g/kg every 3 to 4 weeks.

Mycophenolate mofetil (Cellcept)[1] inhibits guanosine nucleotide synthesis that is needed for B and T lymphocytes. Although there have been two negative randomized clinical trials, there are several retrospective reports supporting efficacy and consensus expert opinion is that it remains a treatment option. It is started at 500 mg twice daily and titrated to 1000 to 1500 mg twice daily. Side effects include nausea, vomiting, diarrhea, and leukopenia. It has teratogenic potential and should not be used in pregnancy.

Cyclosporine (Sandimmune)[1] is a calcineurin inhibitor that has suppressed inflammatory cytokines and has multiple effects on T-cell function. It is initiated at approximately 3 mg/kg daily as a twice-daily split dose and may be titrated up to 5 mg/kg/d with a target trough level <300 ng/mL. Onset of action is approximately 2 to 3 months. Side effects include hirsutism, hypertension, clinically significant nephrotoxicity, and increased cancer risk (including dermatologic cancers). Cyclosporine level may be affected by multiple drug interactions, and concomitant medications should be reviewed.

Methotrexate (Trexall)[1] is a folate antimetabolite that may be dosed orally or subcutaneously. A typical oral dose is initiated at 10 mg weekly and titrated to 15 to 25 mg orally once a week. It is recommended that the patient take folate[1] supplementation of approximately at least 1 mg daily. Side effects include stomatitis (folate supplementation may help prevent this), bone marrow suppression, as well as interstitial lung disease (rare). It is important to note that methotrexate is a known teratogen and should be avoided in women of childbearing potential.

Plasmapheresis or PLEX removes plasma from the circulation and replaces it, typically with albumin, with the net effect of removing pathologic autoantibodies and inflammatory

---

[1]Not FDA approved for this indication.

cytokines. Typically five exchanges are performed over a period of 1 to 2 weeks, and benefit is typically observed by the third exchange. PLEX requires placement of a vascath or (if to be used as a maintenance therapy) a permacath. When used as a maintenance therapy, 1 to 2 exchanges are typically performed, at variable intervals, as frequently as weekly. There is a risk of deep venous thrombosis or line infection. Hypotension may occur because of citrate-induced hypovolemia, and it may be associated with hypocalcemia. ACE inhibitors need to be held 24 hours because of bradykinin-related vasodilation.

Rituximab (Rituxan)[1] is a CD20 antibody that has been evaluated in a randomized controlled trial, the results of which are pending. There exists retrospective data to support efficacy, particularly in MUSK Ab patients who have failed initial therapy. It is dosed 325 mg/m^2 weekly for 4 weeks, although it can also be dosed 1 g/m^2 with a second dose 2 weeks later. Dosing may be repeated at 6-month intervals. Side effects include infusion-related symptoms including pruritis, headache, hypotension, nausea, and chills. Rituximab may additionally result in leukopenia, anemia, or thrombocytopenia. Infusion-related symptoms can be pretreated with acetaminophen and diphenhydramine.

Eculizumab (Soliris) is a complement inhibitor that was recently FDA approved for AchR Ab generalized myasthenia gravis. It is dosed at 900 mg weekly for 4 weeks, followed by 1200 mg for the fifth week and thereafter 1200 mg every 2 weeks. Generally only mild infusion reactions are reported, typically managed by pretreatment acetaminophen and diphenhydramine, although there is risk for severe meningococcal infection. Meningococcal immunization is recommended before treatment initiation.

Cyclophosphamide (Cytoxan)[1] is typically reserved for treatment-refractory patients. It may be administered orally with a daily dose ranging from 1.5 to 5 mg daily. Potential side effects of oral cyclophosphamide include cystitis as well as bladder cancer, leading many treating physicians to use IV pulse dosing. A common approach for pulse dosing is 1 gm/m^2 monthly for 6 months (less toxic). Onset of action with pulse dosing is relatively quick, generally about 1 month.

Treatment Considerations in Pregnancy

Pregnancy and postpartum status have been reported to be triggers for worsening of myasthenia. Ideally, prepregnancy planning allows for optimization of clinical status to improve pregnancy outcomes. These patients require expert multidisciplinary care through the postpartum period. In pregnancy the treatment of choice is pyridostigmine, with steroids being the immunosuppressant of choice. Azathioprine[1] and cyclosporine[1] are relatively safe in expectant mothers who are not satisfactorily controlled or cannot tolerate corticosteroids. IVIG[1] and PLEX may also be treatment options.

Transient neonatal myasthenia may affect the newborn infant. This is difficult to predict and requires close attention for signs after delivery. Neonatal critical care support should be readily available for these infants.

Monitoring

After a diagnosis of MG is confirmed, additional testing or monitoring is indicated. The frequency of clinical assessment should be dictated by the severity and nature of the patient's symptoms, as well as the impact of the disease on function.

Patients with MG should be managed in concert with a neurologist. Refractory MG is defined by symptoms that affect function and are unchanged or worse after corticosteroids and at least two other immunosuppressive agents used in adequate doses for adequate duration. Patients meeting criteria for refractory MG should be referred to a physician or medical center with expertise in MG.

Computed tomography of the chest should be performed to screen for thymoma. Assessment of thyroid function is important. If immunomodulatory medications are used for disease control, TB screening should be performed.

Pulmonary and swallowing dysfunction may be encountered. Pulmonary function testing should be performed for patients with symptomatic generalized MG, particularly if there are complaints of dyspnea. Speech therapy referral for a swallow evaluation should be performed if there is concern for dysphagia.

Periodic laboratory monitoring is required with use of immunomodulatory medications, which may vary depending on the specific medication used. Suggested tests and monitoring algorithms are detailed in Box 2.

Complications

The most severe complication of MG is myasthenic crisis, which is defined by worsening of weakness requiring intubation or noninvasive ventilation. Myasthenic crisis may be seen in up to 20% of patients at some point in disease course. Myasthenic crisis is most commonly encountered in the setting of concomitant illness, change in medications, or early in the disease course because maximum weakness occurs in the first year of the disease in 66% of patients. Respiratory failure can result from respiratory muscle weakness, oropharyngeal weakness, or a combination of both. It is important to recognize that new respiratory or swallowing complaints can quickly escalate, and patients with these complaints should be quickly assessed. One can assess diaphragm strength by the force of a strong sniff or cough; patients should be able to count to 20 after a deep breath. Staccato speech or dyspnea that precludes speaking in full sentences is of high concern for myasthenic crisis. Spirometry with forced vital capacity <2 L or negative inspiratory force of <40 cm H$_2$O should be sent to the hospital for further evaluation. Assessment of swallowing function by speech therapy and possible modified barium swallow should be considered in the context of dysphagia for solids and liquids.

IVIG and PLEX have comparable outcomes for the treatment of patients with moderate-to-severe weakness. The response to PLEX may be more predictable than IVIG in severe MG exacerbations, and retrospective data suggests PLEX may be more effective than IVIG in myasthenic crisis. PLEX, however, may be associated with more complications, as well as longer hospital stay and associated hospital costs.

References

Farmakidis C, Pasnoor M, Dimachkie M, Baron R: Treatment of myasthenia gravis, *Neurol Clin* 36:311–337, 2018.

Gilhus NE, Verschuuren JJ: Myasthenia gravis: subgroup classification and therapeutic strategies, *Lancet Neurol* 14:1023–1036, 2015.

Gilhus NE: Myasthenia gravis, *N Engl J Med* 375:2570–2581, 2016.

Myasthenia Gravis Foundation of America. Myasthenia Gravis: A Manual for the Healthcare Provider. Available at http://myasthenia.org/. [accessed April 1, 2018].

Sanders DB, Wilfe GI, Benatar M, et al: International consensus guidance for management of myasthenia gravis, *Neurology* 87:419–425, 2016.

Wilfe GI, Kaminski HJ, Aban IN, et al: Randomized trial of thymectomy in myasthenia gravis, *N Engl J Med* 375:511–522, 2016.

---

[1]Not FDA approved for this indication.

NEUROFIBROMATOSIS (TYPE 1)

Method of
Jason E. Marker, MD, MPA

CURRENT DIAGNOSIS

- Neurofibromatosis type 1 (NF1) can be diagnosed by physicians based on well-defined diagnostic criteria that can be met with a careful history and physical exam.
- Additional testing may be needed in some cases (including genetic testing) to confirm the diagnosis or to provide information that will be important for both short- and long-term management.
- NF1 has important genetic underpinnings, can have extremely variable expression within families, and will evolve in its need for medical intervention throughout the lifetime of the patient.

CURRENT THERAPY

- There is no treatment for NF1. However, there are many therapies for both the common and uncommon manifestations and complications of the condition.
- Many therapies are similar to those used for non-NF1 patients with the same symptoms. However, there are some manifestations where unique therapies are needed, and physicians need to know the difference between these.
- Proper monitoring of the patient aids in the identification of treatable symptoms and allows opportunities for anticipatory guidance and counseling.
- There are several emerging therapies related to the heritability of NF1 that are important for patients of childbearing age to be aware of.

Introduction and Epidemiology

Neurofibromatosis encompasses three distinct genetic entities: NF1, neurofibromatosis type 2 (NF2), and schwannomatosis. Because NF1 is so much more common (incidence of 1:1900 to 1:3000 livebirths) than NF2 (incidence of 1:25,000 to 1:33,000 livebirths) and schwannomatosis (incidence of 1:40,000 to 1:1.7M livebirths), when the word *neurofibromatosis* is used (or the older name, Von Recklinghausen disease), it is generally referring to NF1. NF1 is the primary topic of this chapter.

NF1 is an autosomal dominant genetic disorder and is progressive in that its clinical manifestations evolve over the lifespan. About half of the cases of NF1 are familial and the remainder are the result of new, spontaneous mutations. Life expectancy is reduced by 5 to 15 years and is related to the severity of the clinical manifestations, the emergence of malignant tumors, and excess hypertensive and vascular disease risk. There is no predilection based on race, ethnic origin, or country of birth.

Risk Factors

NF1 is an autosomal dominant condition and affects 50% of the offspring of parents where one parent is affected, making family history the primary predictable risk factor. Advanced paternal age increases the likelihood of a de novo mutation. Eighty percent of newly occurring mutations are believed to come from the paternally derived chromosome.

Pathophysiology

NF1 is the result of mutations in the *NF1* gene (chromosome 17q11.2) that codes for the protein neurofibromin. Neurofibromin is a protein in the GTPase-activating family that stimulates the Ras pathway for tumor suppression. Loss of neurofibromin results in "de-suppression" of tumor growth within susceptible tissues. Although genetic penetrance in NF1 is complete, NF1 is highly variable in its expression (even within families). This is because germline mutations must be coupled with somatic mutations in order for symptoms to manifest clinically.

Several thousand distinct *NF1* mutations have been identified. Many small mutations have demonstrated no genotype-phenotype correlation, while some individuals (1% to 5% of NF1 patients) will have complete loss of the 1.4 to 1.5 Mb of the *NF1* gene and are quite severely affected. Due to the large size of this gene, mutations in the *NF1* gene occur more often than in any other human gene.

Somatic and germline (rare) mosaicism occurs and can result in phenotypically unaffected offspring who could later transmit the mutated gene to their own children.

Prevention

There is no specific prevention for any of the clinical manifestations of NF1. Due to its variable expression, some individuals will simply be more or less affected. To the extent that having a diagnosis of NF1 *could* cause academic challenges, interpersonal hardships, and social isolation, robust anticipatory guidance throughout the lifespan can help these individuals develop proper support systems and personal resilience, preventing some of the morbidity of the disease.

Affected individuals of child-bearing age now have the option of genetic testing of fertilized eggs to select unaffected eggs for implantation. This is an emerging prevention strategy.

Clinical Manifestations

There are a number of clinical manifestations of NF1. Because of the variability of expression of the *NF1* gene, these manifestations may be variably present in any affected individual. The following section on diagnosis will discuss how these clinical manifestations fit into the diagnostic criteria for NF1.

Café-au-lait spots are flat, irregularly shaped, uniformly hyperpigmented macules that appear during the first year of life and then increase in number through childhood. These macules are present in 95% of adults with NF1 but tend to fade and become more indistinct later in life. Among the general population of individuals who do not have NF1, 15% will have one to three café-au-lait macules.

Freckling (primarily in areas of skin apposition like the axillae and inguinal folds) is distinct from café-au-lait macules as the freckles are smaller, more clustered, and generally appear later in childhood than the café-au-lait macules.

Lisch nodules are tan-colored hamartomas of the iris. Lisch nodules do not affect vision and may be seen with simple ophthalmoscopy (although the use of a slit lamp will help identify small nodules and distinguish them from iris nevi). These nodules are seen in up to 90% of adults with NF1, but fewer than 10% of children under 6 years old.

Neurofibromas present as several types of lesions with variable characteristics, risk of pathology, and symptomatology. **Cutaneous peripheral neurofibromas** are benign peripheral nerve sheath tumors that are generally soft, mobile, and fleshy. They may be dermal or epidermal on a broad or pedunculated base. These neurofibromas are nontender, are usually more common on the trunk, and can number from a few to thousands. Cutaneous peripheral neurofibromas do not degenerate into malignant peripheral nerve sheath tumors (MPNSTs). **Plexiform peripheral neurofibromas** can be superficial or deep inside the body. They tend to be more diffuse and involve plaques and tangles of abnormal tissues that can grow into a complex mass. On whole-body scanning, 50% of patients with NF1 will have at least one plexiform neurofibroma. Large plexiform neurofibromas can create symptoms by compressing nearby structures and, unlike cutaneous neurofibromas, they have the capacity to degenerate into MPNSTs. **Nodular neurofibromas** are firm and rubbery. Unlike the cutaneous neurofibromas, they are sometimes tender, often deeper and usually less mobile. They are not as invasive as the plexiform neurofibromas but can undergo degeneration into MPNSTs.

Optic pathway gliomas (OPGs) occur in 15% of children younger than 6 (but rarely in older individuals) and can grow anywhere along the optic tracts. Most individuals are asymptomatic, but advanced tumors can affect vision or even upset the normal function of the hypothalamus with growth rate variations and premature or delayed puberty.

Orthopedic abnormalities are primarily long-bone dysplasias and pseudoarthroses. Anterolateral bowing of the tibia (usually unilateral) in infants and young children can easily go undetected until a pathologic fracture develops at the onset of ambulation. One half of fractures occur during the toddler years. Long-bone pseudoarthrosis has a male predisposition (1.7:1) and NF1 accounts for 50% to 70% of all long-bone pseudoarthroses. Other orthopedic findings in NF1 patients may include short stature (13% have a height less than 2 standard deviations below the mean), scoliosis (10% to 15% of NF1 patients are affected), sphenoid wing dysplasia (leading to facial asymmetry), osteoporosis, and macrocephaly.

Neurologic abnormalities encompass cognitive defects and learning disabilities as well as the risk of seizures. Although profound intellectual disability is rare (the likelihood of having an IQ <70 is similar to the general population), 81% of NF patients will have some impairment in one or more areas of cognitive functioning. While less than half of NF1 patients have a specific learning disability, more than half will have some amount of neuropsychological impairment, including speech articulation problems, AD/HD, or impairment of executive functioning. Seizures occur twice as often in patients with NF1 (prevalence 4% to 6%) as in the general population and can be of any type and occur at any age.

Other manifestations of concern: Rarely, other **central nervous system (CNS) neoplasms** develop. CNS astrocytomas usually arise during childhood and, when not an incidental finding on a scan being done for another purpose, may present with symptoms of increased intracranial pressure. Rare brainstem gliomas are usually symptomatic at presentation. **Malignant peripheral nerve sheath tumors** are highly malignant tumors that can arise from a preexisting plexiform or nodular neurofibromas. The lifetime risk of developing an MPNST in a patient with NF1 is 5% to 13% and most commonly occurs in teenagers and young adults. MPNSTs are usually diagnosed when a plexiform or nodular neurofibroma goes through a period of pain, change in consistency, and rapid growth. **Hypertension**, including hypertension as early as childhood, is common among NF1 patients. Although rare, renal neurovascular lesions can be the cause, and NF1 patients with hypertension should be evaluated for renal artery stenosis.

Diagnosis

The diagnosis of NF1 can be made reliably by a primary care team, but a multidisciplinary team of subspecialists is often involved in the long-term care of these individuals, including during the diagnostic phase. A comprehensive history (including a detailed family history) and examination should be undertaken. Additional testing or referral, as indicated by the initial evaluation, should be pursued to clarify the diagnosis, seek findings amenable to treatment, and facilitate proper anticipatory guidance and patient/family education.

The US National Institutes of Health (NIH) Consensus Conference in 1997 set forth the following diagnostic criteria for NF1:

At least two of the following clinical features must be present to make the diagnosis of NF1:

- Six or more café-au-lait macules greater than 5 mm (prepubertal) or greater than 15 mm (postpubertal) in longest diameter
- Two or more neurofibromas of any type (or a single plexiform neurofibroma)
- Freckling in the axillary or inguinal regions
- Optic glioma
- Two or more Lisch nodules
- A distinctive bony lesion (sphenoid dysplasia or a long-bone dysplasia with or without pseudoarthrosis)
- A first-degree relative with NF1 based on the previous criteria

These NIH criteria are both sensitive and specific, and are met by 97% of NF1 patients by the age of 8 years (100% by the age of 20 years). Nearly half of individuals with a new sporadic mutation fail to meet these criteria by the age of 1 year. Therefore, in an infant with one clinical feature, close observation is needed to determine if other criteria will be met. If, by the age of 4 years, only one criterion is met, referral for a genetic diagnosis may be warranted.

Other specific testing may be needed to make the diagnosis, to determine the extent of involvement of the disorder, or to decide on treatment. These include the following:

- Dermatologic evaluation: If the identification of café-au-lait spots, whether café-au-lait spots meet diagnostic criteria, or the identification of criteria-meeting freckling is in question, referral to Dermatology may be needed. Likewise, the spectrum of neurofibromas is broad and a dermatologist may be needed to properly identify these lesions.
- Lisch nodules: Although occasionally seen with the naked eye or through an office ophthalmoscope, formal ophthalmologic consultation is recommended to look for small Lisch nodules and to assess for optic disk findings suggestive of OPGs or increased intracranial pressure.
- Optic pathway gliomas: Ophthalmologic evaluation is recommended as noted earlier. Brain MRI imaging is not recommended for asymptomatic patients with normal ophthalmologic evaluations.
- Orthopedic abnormalities: Plain radiographs of long bones or CT imaging of craniofacial bones may be needed to identify the diagnostic findings in these areas.
- Neurologic abnormalities: Because new focal seizures could be the result of a new intracranial neoplasm, neuroimaging is warranted with any new seizure activity.
- Other manifestations of concern: MPNSTs are best differentiated from benign plexiform or nodular neurofibromas by positron emission tomography (PET) scan. Evaluating for renal artery stenosis in individuals with new onset hypertension (including children) is indicated.
- Genetic counseling and testing: Genetic testing is usually reserved for cases where the diagnosis remains in question following a thorough history, examination, and nongenetic testing. Additionally, genetic testing may be indicated for family members of the affected individual. Knowing that expression is extremely variable, preconception, embryonic preimplantation, or prenatal (amniocentesis or chorionic villi sampling) testing for individuals in families with NF1 should be considered.

Differential Diagnosis

Because of the well-established diagnostic criteria and availability of genetic testing, the differential diagnosis of NF1 is limited. As noted at the outset, NF2 and schwannomatosis are lumped together with NF1 under the general diagnosis of neurofibromatosis. Schwannomatosis is a complex regional pain syndrome with some common underlying pathophysiology but no overlapping symptoms and unrelated genetics. NF2 will be discussed briefly in the discussion to come.

Legius syndrome includes café-au-lait macules, axillary freckling, and macrocephaly. It does *not* include neurofibromas or CNS tumors, however. Like NF1, Legius syndrome is an autosomal dominant disorder for loss of a tumor suppressor protein, but it affects an entirely different gene.

Constitutional mismatch repair-deficiency syndrome (CMMR-D) is a rare autosomal recessive condition that results in café-au-lait macules (and occasionally axillary freckling and Lisch nodules). Unlike in NF1, individuals with CMMR-D are at risk for hematologic malignancies in infancy and childhood, brain tumors (primarily glioblastomas) in mid-childhood, and colorectal cancer in adolescence and young adulthood. Rhabdomyosarcomas and optic pathway gliomas may occur rarely in CMMR-D.

NF2 is caused by the *NF2* gene on chromosome 22, which encodes for the tumor suppressor protein merlin (or schwannomin), which is a functionally different protein than that produced

by *NF1*. Key differences between NF1 and NF2 include the following points about NF2:
- Few or nonexistent café-au-lait macules
- No Lisch nodules
- No risk of MPNSTs
- Spinal root tumors are schwannomas in NF2 (neurofibromas in NF1)
- No cognitive impairment
- High prevalence of bilateral acoustic schwannomas and resulting hearing loss in 90% to 95% of patients by the age of 30 years
- 60% to 80% have cataracts
- Presence of meningiomas

Noonan syndrome is characterized by short stature and may include café-au-lait macules that may meet the size and number criteria for NF1. Sometimes, the facial features of Noonan syndrome can overlap with the appearance of NF1. However, the webbed neck of Noonan syndrome and the association with pulmonic stenosis are not part of NF1. Although the Ras signaling pathway is involved in Noonan syndrome, the underlying genetics are entirely different.

Surveillance and Therapy

In 2020, the FDA approved oral selumetinib (a kinase inhibitor) for pediatric patients 2 years of age and older with NF1 who have symptomatic, inoperable plexiform neurofibromas. The research that led to this approval showed statistically and clinically significant decreases in the size of these neurofibromas, as well as the pain and disability that often accompanies them. It remains unclear whether selumetinib treatment decreases the likelihood of malignant transformation of plexiform neurofibromas into MPNSTs.

The following areas of surveillance should be undertaken. Where research or expert opinion suggests a proper frequency, it is listed, although shared decision making with the patient/family as well as communication with your medical colleagues will be required to develop appropriate timelines. Therapeutic options are listed here for many of the common issues NF1 patients face, while the management of less common complications is outlined in the next section.

- Yearly examination of the skin for new neurofibromas and any signs of change within an existing neurofibroma should be done. Especially when nodular or plexiform neurofibromas exist (those at risk of malignant transformation), any history of rapid change or new pain should be evaluated thoroughly. A PET scan can distinguish between benign and malignant lesions. Referral to surgical and/or dermatologic colleagues should be made regarding these nodular or plexiform neurofibromas (for biopsy and management decisions) and should be strongly considered for all but the most clear and superficial cutaneous neurofibromas.
- Cutaneous neurofibromas that develop pruritus are often not responsive to antihistamines, although the itching is often improved by the use of gabapentin (Neurontin)[1].
- Yearly blood pressure measurement, even in children and young adults, should be done. Once the diagnosis of essential hypertension is made following testing that excludes the diagnosis of renal artery stenosis, blood pressure should be controlled following standard blood pressure goals and treatment algorithms. Hypertension that becomes hard to control may prompt an evaluation for pheochromocytoma, a rare finding in NF1.
- Growth tracking of weight, height, and head circumference should be done through childhood and adolescence in the usual manner. Additionally, any signs of premature or delayed puberty should be evaluated further. Growth and pubertal abnormalities should prompt an age-appropriate endocrinology referral for additional testing (serum, urine, and/or neuroimaging) and treatments based on these results.

- Neurodevelopmental and academic assessment should be undertaken, involving family members and school personnel when appropriate. Individuals who develop neuropsychiatric and academic problems should undergo formal neurodiagnostic testing, and any identified diagnoses should be treated. These treatments are no different than those used for non-NF1 individuals who carry the same neuropsychiatric diagnosis. Neuroimaging is not indicated in the evaluation of neuropsychiatric conditions unless neurologic deficits exist.
- NF1 patients who develop seizures are treated with the usual seizure management algorithms following neuroimaging to look for new intracranial pathologies. An electroencephalogram (EEG) is not indicated for asymptomatic individuals.
- Evaluation for skeletal changes including scoliosis, facial asymmetry, or long bone abnormalities should be performed yearly during childhood and adolescence, and then at the typical wellness visits into young adulthood (with prompting in these older ages to report any changes that are noticed between visits). Any abnormalities that are encountered should prompt additional imaging and referral to subspecialty care.
- Women with NF1 develop osteoporosis at an earlier age than their non-NF1 peers and should undergo earlier screening in accordance with this fact and with other standard risk factors they may have. When diagnosed, this osteoporosis is treated like it would be for any other patient.
- For unclear reasons, women with NF1 have an increased risk of breast cancer, especially women under the age of 40 (at the age of 70, the risk approximates that of the general population). These are usually invasive ductal carcinomas (the most common type overall) and are managed in the usual way, although these patients need both earlier education about, and screening for, breast cancer.
- Formal ophthalmologic evaluation for visual screening, slit lamp and intraocular examination should take place yearly at least through adolescence, usually in the context of a comprehensive examination. Lisch nodules are nonpathologic and no treatment is needed, but any signs of elevated intracranial pressure or optic disc pathology warrant further testing and management. The optimal frequency of MRI surveillance of an optic pathway glioma is unknown but should be based on symptomatology, size, and rate of progression.
- Brain MRI is not recommended as a routine screening test. It may be a part of the initial diagnostic workup but should not need to be repeated for asymptomatic patients who are otherwise receiving comprehensive surveillance. Of note, "NF-associated bright spots" may be seen on MRI imaging, and the data are inconclusive on the relationship between these spots and any pathologic process. These spots often resolve spontaneously by late childhood.
- Whole body MRI screening or MRI of nonbrain areas of potential concern (such as visible but stable and asymptomatic plexiform or nodular neurofibromas) is not recommended by most authorities. Likewise, screening PET scanning is not recommended.

Management of Complications

The previous section outlines the surveillance of and treatment for most of the common concerns for patients with NF1. Rarely, more significant complications present themselves. These are listed here along with their management plan.

- Symptomatic cutaneous neurofibromas that are cosmetically unacceptable, painful, itchy, or disfiguring will sometimes need to be managed. Once it is clear that the lesions in question are truly simple cutaneous neurofibromas, they may be removed in any manner, including by excision, cryotherapy, laser, or electrodessication.
- Symptomatic plexiform neurofibromas that have not degenerated into MPNSTs that are deemed in need of management or removal should be managed by a multidisciplinary team of surgeons and oncologists who are familiar with this type of tumor. These invasive tumors require nonstandard operative approaches and consideration of emerging chemotherapeutic agents.

---

[1] Not FDA approved for this indication.

- MPNSTs are often due to a co-mutated *SUZ12* gene (which lies contiguous to *NF1*). Individuals with large or complete deletions of the *NF1* gene (those who are generally more severely affected) are at an increased risk of this complication. MPNSTs are usually managed by surgeons and oncologists familiar with NF1 and often involve surgical excision with adjunctive radiation and possibly emerging chemotherapeutic agents.
- Optic pathway gliomas are most commonly found to be low-grade pilocystic astrocytomas. As such, they are often sensitive to the standard oncologic treatments for that type of tumor—but when to observe and when to proceed to treatment is controversial.
- Because the bony architecture of pathologic skeletal lesions is inherently abnormal in these patients, the risk of complications from corrective treatments is higher than in non-NF1 patients. Your local orthopedic colleagues need to be aware of this and obtain tertiary care backup when needed. Amputation is often the best long-term plan for long bone lesions.
- Refractory hypertension in the absence of renal artery stenosis that is ultimately found to be the result of pheochromocytoma should be managed by a multidisciplinary team experienced in the management of this diagnosis. It is managed in the same manner as non-NF1 patients with a pheochromocytoma.
- Short stature is often correctible with growth hormone therapy. However, this treatment is not often used because it compounds the inherent protumorgenic nature of NF1. In extreme cases of short stature when growth hormone is used, clinicians need to be alert to the evolution and potential malignant degeneration of new or existing tumors.
- NF1 patients are at a high risk of psychosocial issues arising from the symptoms they may experience from their NF1, its lack of treatability, and its genetic underpinnings. These symptoms may affect relationship building and reproductive decisions. Extra professional support may be needed, particularly during adolescence.

Although pregnancy is not a "complication" of NF1, its management can certainly be complicated by the diagnosis. Pregnant NF1 patients have increased morbidity (but not mortality) due to hypertensive and vascular complications. These complications should be anticipated and managed by an appropriately trained medical team. Genetic counseling should be recommended, ideally prior to conception, and steps taken to ensure proper evaluation and surveillance for the newborn.

References

Defendi GL: Genetics of neurofibromatosis type 1 and type 2. Available at https://emedicine.medscape.com/article/950151-overview. Accessed 15 November 2018.

Evans DG: Neurofibromatosis type 2. Available at https://www.uptodate.com/contents/neurofibromatosis-type-2. Accessed 15 November 2018.

Food and Drug Administration Package Insert for selumetinib (Koselugo). Available at: https://www.accessdata.fda.gov/drugsatfda-docs/label/2020/213756s000lbl.pdf. Accessed 15 November 2018.

Ferner RE, Huson SM, et al: Guidelines for the diagnosis and management of individuals with neurofibromatosis 1, *J Med Genet* 44:81–88, 2007.

Hart L: Primary care of patients with neurofibromatosis 1, *The Nurse Practitioner* 30(6), 2005.

Hersh JH: Committee on Genetics of the American Academy of Pediatrics: Health Supervision of Children with Neurofibromatosis, *Pediatrics* 121:633–645, 2008.

Human Genetics Society of Australia: *Choosing Wisely Australia: 5 Things Clinicians and Consumers Should Question*, October 2016. Available at http://www.choosingwisely.org.au/getmedia/bbc1ca07-7340-49ca-9e85-ad4c1a7bc197/GESA_Choosing_Wisely_Recommendations.pdf.aspx. Accessed 15 November 2018.

Korf BR: Neurofibromatosis type 1 (NF1): Management and prognosis. Available at https://www.uptodate.com/contents/neurofibromatosis-type-1-nf1-management-and-prognosis. Accessed 15 November 2018.

Korf BR: Neurofibromatosis type 1 (NF1): Pathogenesis, clinical features, and diagnosis. Available at https://www.uptodate.com/contents/neurofibromatosis-type-1-nf1-pathogenesis-clinical-features-and-diagnosis. Accessed 15 November 2018.

Stewart DR, Korf BR, et al: Care of adults with neurofibromatosis type 1: a clinical practice resource of the American College of Medical Genetics and Genomics (ACMG), *Genet Med* 20(7):671–682, 2018 Jul.

Tonsgard JH: Clinical manifestations and management of neurofibromatosis type 1, *Sem Pediatr Neurol, Elsevier* 13:2–7, 2006.

Williams VC, Lucas J, et al: Neurofibromatosis type 1 revisited, *Pediatrics* 123:124–133, 2009.

NONMIGRAINE HEADACHE

Method of
Stephen Ross, MD

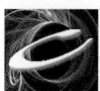

CURRENT DIAGNOSIS

- Evaluation/diagnostic tests should be considered for any patient with headache who also has "red flags" (see Table 2).

CURRENT THERAPY

- Specific therapy for secondary cause of headache should be initiated when identified.
- Symptomatic therapy for nonmigraine headache should be selected based on the headache phenotype.

Evaluation and Diagnosis

Gathering of a thorough history and physical examination (Table 1) facilitates two principal goals of headache management:

1. To determine the need for diagnostic studies to evaluate for potential secondary contributors. The more "red flags" (Table 2) the patient has, the more you must consider this. Depending on the differential diagnosis, evaluation may include brain and/or cervical spine imaging, spinal tap, and blood studies. Specific treatment can be initiated for some identified secondary contributors.
2. To discern dominant headache phenotype (Figure 1) in order to guide symptomatic treatment

The two forms of secondary headache therapy include specific treatment, which addresses underlying etiology, for example, antibiotic for bacterial meningitis, and symptomatic treatment, which is selected based on the dominant headache phenotype. Often headache phenotypes can be segregated into one or more of the following four themes: migrainous (covered in the chapter Migraine Headache), tension-type, cluster-like (trigeminal autonomic cephalalgia [TAC]), and neuralgia. The symptomatic treatment mirrors that used for the parallel primary headache disorders (see the following).

Headache Type and Therapy

For anyone with headache presentation, the first step in evaluation (history and physical) is to discern potential primary versus secondary source of the pain. If there is concern for possible secondary etiology, diagnostic studies should be considered. Symptomatic treatment is similar for primary and secondary etiologies but varies according to the pain phenotype (Table 3). General principles are to start low-dose treatment then titrate up if needed to control pain (understanding that often it can take 3 to 4 weeks before you see benefit of preventive treatments). If the pain is not adequately controlled despite maximum dose or treatment is not tolerated, then consider moving on to a second-line treatment. If there has been some (but not enough) improvement with the first treatment, then a second treatment can be added. If there has been no improvement with the first treatment, taper off the first while adding the second treatment.

Tension-type headache is experienced by almost everyone at some point in their lives. Most do not seek medical evaluation but rather self-manage. Diagnostic criteria are listed in Table 4. The presence or absence of "emotional tension" does not define this condition. Many individuals experience tension-type headache who are not "stressed" and do not have anxiety or depression. If a person is experiencing "stress" or is anxious, this can act as a trigger for tension-type headache, as well as the other primary headache conditions. Tension-type headache has both episodic and chronic forms. Chronic is defined as having symptoms ≥15 days/month for greater than 3 months.

TABLE 1 — Headache Characteristics

Is there more than one type?	Location/radiation	Is there any positional component?	Anything that triggers it?	Any pattern to occurrence? (e.g., always 1 hour after going to bed; or every Spring)
When was the onset?	What does it feel like? (e.g., throbbing, pressure, burning)	Are there any associated features? (e.g., nausea, photophobia, ptosis, lacrimation)	Anything that relieves it?	What treatments have been tried so far? Response to these?
Duration	Frequency	Intensity along with ramp	Any family history of this?	Any change with Valsalva?

TABLE 2 — Headache Red Flags

Onset after age 50 years	"Thunderclap" onset of pain	Positional exacerbation	Onset with recent malignancy, nontrivial head trauma or seizures	Persistent or unexplained vomiting
Worst headache of life	Marked change in pain pattern	Precipitated by Valsalva maneuvers	Unexplained fever	Meningeal signs
First headache of life	Unusual associated features (blindness, diplopia, confusion, weakness)	Lack of response to abortive medications	Blood pressure >180/115 mm Hg	Abnormal neurologic examination

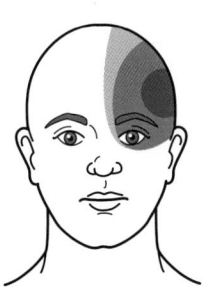

Migraine

Throbbing
Unilateral
Mod-severe
Nausea
Photophobia
Phonophobia
Aura

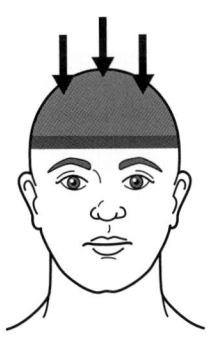

TAC

Unilateral
Orbital/temple
Severe
Ptosis, lacrimation, rhinorrhea, nasal congestion
Restlessness

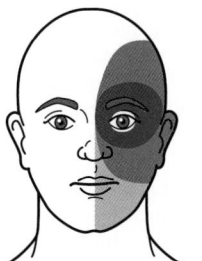

Tension-type

Pressing
Bilateral
Mild-moderate

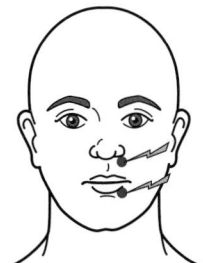

Neuralgiform

Electric/stabbing
Unilateral
Severe
Triggered by innocuous stimuli

Figure 1 Headache phenotypes.

Treatment of Tension Headache

Generally start with physical modalities/relaxation techniques (e.g., local heat, massage, analgesic cream) and/or as needed acetaminophen 325 mg or nonsteroidal antiinflammatory drugs (NSAIDs; e.g., ibuprofen 200 mg, aspirin 325 mg, naproxen 220 mg, diclofenac 50 mg). If this is inadequate, titrate the dose (e.g., acetaminophen 325 mg up to 1000 mg, ibuprofen 200 mg up to 800 mg) and/or referral for additional physical/cognitive modalities (e.g., physical therapy, myofascial release therapy, biofeedback therapy, cognitive behavioral therapy). FDA-approved preventive treatments are lacking. If preventive treatment is needed consider a tricyclic antidepressant (e.g., amitriptyline [Elavil][1] starting with 10 mg or 25 mg at bedtime, titrating up to 150 mg if needed/tolerated). Allow 3 to 4 weeks to assess efficacy before titration to the next dose. Prescreen with electrocardiogram (ECG) and monitor for side effects. Once you reach 100 mg, check amitriptyline blood level and repeat ECG. Alternatives could include venlafaxine [Effexor][1] starting 37.5 mg or 75 mg (two to three times per day or once per day if using the long-acting form) titrating if needed to 225 mg, tizanidine (Zanaflex)[1] starting with 4 mg ½ pill two to three times per day titrating if needed to 2 pills three times per day, baclofen (Lioresal)[1] starting with 5 mg or 10 mg tid titrating if needed up to 20 mg qid, mirtazapine (Remeron)[1] starting with 7.5 mg or 15 mg qhs titrating if needed up to 45 mg.

Cluster-like Headache (Trigeminal Autonomic Cephalalgia)

Cluster-like headaches have three main contrasts to migraine: (1) briefer duration, (2) more likely to have associated ipsilateral autonomic features, and (3) more likely to have agitation/activation during the attack (Box 1). The most common TAC subtype is cluster headache, but even this is 100 times less prevalent than migraine.

A second type of TAC is paroxysmal hemicrania. This has the same diagnostic criteria as cluster headache with one exception, duration. Paroxysmal hemicranias last 2 to 30 minutes.

A third type of TAC is hemicrania continua. This is a unilateral daily constant pain with exacerbations of pain intensity associated with autonomic/activation features similar to cluster headache.

[1]Not FDA approved for this indication.

TABLE 3   Symptomatic Headache Treatment

MIGRAINOUS	TENSION-TYPE	CLUSTER-LIKE	NEURALGIA
See chapter Migraine Headache	Heat, massage, analgesic cream	Sumatriptan (Imitrex SC), zolmitriptan (Zomig)[1], oxygen	Carbamazepine (Tegretol), oxcarbazepine (Trileptal)[1]
	Acetaminophen, NSAID	gammaCore	Topiramate[1], gabapentin (Neurontin), baclofen (Lioresal)[1]
	Physical modalities	Verapamil (Verelan)[1]	Gamma-knife surgery
	Relaxation techniques	Galcanezumab (Emgality)	Microvascular decompression surgery
	Amitriptyline[1]	Topiramate (Topamax)[1], lithium[1]	
	Venlafaxine (Effexor)[1], tizanidine (Zanaflex)[1], baclofen (Lioresal)[1]	For select types—Indomethacin (Indocin)[1]	

[1]Not FDA approved for this indication.

BOX 1   International Headache Society Criteria for Cluster Headache

At least five attacks

Severe unilateral orbital, supraorbital, and/or temporal pain lasting 15–180 min

Either or both of the following:
1. At least one of the following symptoms or signs, ipsilateral to the headache:
   - Conjunctival injection and/or lacrimation
   - Nasal congestion and/or rhinorrhea
   - Eyelid edema
   - Forehead and facial sweating
   - Miosis and/or ptosis
2. A sense of restlessness or agitation

Occurring with a frequency between one every other day and 8 per day

Not better accounted for by another diagnosis

TABLE 4   International Headache Society Criteria for Tension-Type Headache

At least 2 of these 4 characteristics:	Both of the following:
Bilateral location	No nausea or vomiting
Pressing or tightening (non-pulsating) quality	No more than one of photophobia or phonophobia
Mild or moderate intensity	
Not aggravated by routine physical activity such as walking or climbing stairs	

Treatment of Cluster Headache

Triptans or high-flow oxygen are first-line abortive treatments. Preference is given to faster acting agents (e.g., sumatriptan [Imitrex] 6 mg SC injection/20 mg nasal[1] or zolmitriptan [Zomig][1] 5 mg nasal; these may be repeated again in 1 to 2 hours if needed but have a maximum of two doses in a 24-hour period). Oxygen is best administered by nonrebreather face mask at 6 to 12 L/min for 7 to 15 minutes. An alternate abortive treatment is gamma Core, a noninvasive vagus nerve stimulator that may be administered to the anterior neck as a set of three 2-minute stimulations. Other options include IM dihydroergotamine (D.H.E. 45) or 1 mL of 4% intranasal lidocaine[1]. Short-term preventives can include oral steroids or occipital nerve blocks.

First-line preventive treatment is short-acting verapamil[1] starting at 40 to 80 mg oral tid titrating if needed to 480 mg (total daily dose, although there are studies taking the dose up to 720 mg/day[3]). An effective alternative is galcanezumab (Emgality) given as three consecutive 100-mg SC shots each month while cluster headache is active. This is a monthly self-injection that blocks one of the neurotransmitters (calcitonin gene-related peptide [CGRP]) that propagates messages along the pain pathways. Third-line considerations are topiramate (Topamax)[1] or lithium[1]. For refractory cases consider referral to a specialty headache center for sphenopalatine ganglion stimulator.

Paroxysmal hemicranias and hemicrania continua both respond absolutely to indomethacin (Indocin)[1] (25 mg PO tid with meals, if no improvement after 1 week titrate to 50 mg tid, if no improvement after 1 week titrate to 75 mg tid[3], if no improvement after 1 week consider an alternate etiology).

Neuralgia

Neuralgia can be experienced in both primary and secondary headache disorders. An example of this is trigeminal neuralgia that can be primary/idiopathic or secondary (e.g., multiple sclerosis inflammation of the nerve). Neuralgia is often expressed as burning, electric shock, or jolts.

Treatment of Neuralgia

First-line symptomatic treatment for trigeminal neuralgia includes carbamazepine (Tegretol) 100 mg bid titrating up to 1200 mg/day (monitoring level and metabolic panel) or oxcarbazepine (Trileptal)[1] 150 to 300 mg bid titrating up to 2400 mg/day. Second-line agents can include baclofen (Lioresal)[1], pregabalin (Lyrica), gabapentin (Neurontin), topiramate (Topamax)[1], and lamotrigine (Lamictal)[1]. For refractory cases consider referral for Gasserian ganglion percutaneous techniques, which are deep face injections typically performed by pain management. Other treatment options include gamma-knife treatment or microvascular decompression performed by neurosurgeons.

---

[1]Not FDA approved for this indication.
[3]Exceeds dosage recommended by the manufacturer.
*Most of the treatments discussed in this chapter are considered off-label, non-FDA-approved use.

---

[1]Not FDA approved for this indication.

References

Bendtsen L, Evers S, Linde M, et al: EFNS guideline on the treatment of tension-type headache - report of an EFNS task force, *Eur J Neurol* 17:1318–1325, 2010.

Bendtsen L, Zakrzewska JM, Abbott J, et al: European academy of neurology guideline on trigeminal neuralgia, *Eur J Neurol* 26(6):831–849, 2019.

Do TP, et al: Red and orange flags for secondary headaches in clinical practice: SNNOOP10 List, *Neurology* 92(3):134–144, 2019.

Gronseth G, Cruccu G, Alksne J, et al: Practice parameter: the diagnostic evaluation and treatment of trigeminal neuralgia (an evidence-based review): report of the quality standards subcommittee of the American Academy of Neurology and The European Federation of Neurological Societies, *Neurology* 71(15):1183–1190, 2008.

Headache Classification Committee of the International Headache Society (IHS): The international classification of headache disorders, 3rd edition, *Cephalalgia* 38(1):1–211, 2018.

Jensen RH: Tension-type headache - the normal and most prevalent headache, *Headache* 58(2):339–345, 2018.

Kahriman A, Zhu S: Migraine and tension-type headache, *Semin Neurol* 38(6):608–618, 2018.

Robbins MS, Starling AJ, Pringsheim TM: Treatment of cluster headache: the American Headache Society Evidence-Based Guidelines, *Headache* 56(7):1093–1106, 2016.

OPTIC NEURITIS

Method of
Heather E. Moss, MD, PhD; and Tanyatuth Padungkiatsagul, MD

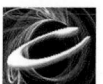

CURRENT DIAGNOSIS

- Vision is impaired, including visual acuity, visual field, and/or color perception.
- Patients typically have eye pain that is worse with eye movement.
- There is a relative afferent papillary defect if only one eye is affected.
- The anterior optic nerve has a normal appearance in two-thirds of affected patients.

CURRENT THERAPY

- Consider IV methylprednisolone (Solu-Medrol, 1 g/day IV for 3 days) followed by oral steroids (1 mg/kg per day for 11 days).
- Avoid low-dose oral steroid monotherapy, as this is associated with a higher relapse rate.
- If brain MRI or blood testing suggest a high-risk, clinically isolated syndrome, consider disease-modifying therapy to delay progression to Multiple Sclerosis (MS) or Neuro-myelitis optica (NMO).
- If the clinical features suggest NMO spectrum optic neuritis, consider IV methylprednisolone and plasma exchange therapy.
- If the patient's history and testing suggest MS-, NMO-, or recurrent MOG-associated disease, consider treatment for these conditions.

Epidemiology

The incidence of optic neuritis is approximately 1 to 5 in 100,000. Though it typically affects women in their fourth decade of life, 1 in 4 patients are male, and patients have been reported ranging from the first to seventh decades of life. Optic neuritis occurs worldwide in persons of various ethnicities.

Optic neuritis can be classified as a clinically isolated syndrome or in association with a disease such as multiple sclerosis (MS) or neuromyelitis optica (NMO). NMO is clinically distinguished by more frequent involvement of the optic nerves and spinal cord and less involvement of the brain than MS and by distinct pathophysiology. A recently identified distinct classification is anti-myelin oligodentrocyte glycoprotein (MOG) associated optic neuritis. Approximately half of patients with optic neuritis as a clinically isolated syndrome develop MS. A small percentage develop NMO.

Risk Factors

A diagnosis of a disease associated with optic neuritis, such as MS or NMO, increases the risk of developing optic neuritis. In one study, more than 70% of patients with MS and 100% of patients with NMO had unilateral optic neuritis at some point. Patients with recurrent MOG-associated flares or persistent elevated serum MOG antibodies may be at risk for recurrent optic neuritis.

Pathophysiology

Most optic neuritis occurs as a result of inflammation causing demyelination of the ganglion cell axons that compose the optic nerve. This is thought to be an immune-mediated process.

Prevention

Disease-modifying therapies have been shown to reduce risk of neurologic relapses in patients with MS or NMO. These therapies presumably also decrease the risk of MS-, NMO-, or recurrent MOG-associated optic neuritis because optic neuritis is a common relapse syndrome in these conditions.

Clinical Manifestations

A typical optic neuritis patient experiences acute or subacute loss of vision characterized by decreased visual acuity, visual field loss, and/or color vision loss, accompanied or preceded by pain in the affected eye that is worse with eye movements. However, 8% of patients do not have pain. Other symptoms include positive visual phenomena in 30% of patients. Other signs include a relative afferent papillary defect in cases where one eye is affected and a mildly swollen optic nerve head in approximately one-third of patients. Optic neuritis in NMO is more likely to have bilateral involvement and severe visual impairment. The spectrum of anti-MOG associated optic neuritis is being defined with initial case series describing a higher prevalence of and more severe optic nerve head swelling than MS or NMO associated optic neuritis.

The natural history of clinically isolated optic neuritis includes resolution of pain 3 to 5 days after onset and nadir of vision 7 to 14 days after onset. Spontaneous improvement in vision is typically evident within 3 weeks, and almost 70% of affected patients recover 20/20 visual acuity even in the absence of treatment. MOG-associated optic neuritis also usually has a favorable final visual outcome. Optic neuritis associated with NMO tends to have less spontaneous recovery of vision and early recognition is important due to benefits of early treatment.

Diagnosis

The diagnosis is based on the clinical presentation. Where there is uncertainty, magnetic resonance imaging (MRI) of the orbits, including fat-saturated sequences (T2 and T1 with and without gadolinium contrast), can help visualize inflammation in the retrobulbar optic nerve. Changes on MRI involving the chiasm or more than 50% of the optic nerve are suggestive of NMO spectrum optic neuritis. Anti-MOG optic neuritis also has distinct imaging features, including perioptic nerve sheath enhancement.

Optic neuritis is often associated with other demyelinating syndromes, most commonly MS. Therefore it is important to screen for historical and current neurologic impairment through history and examination. MRI and/or and cerebrospinal fluid analysis documenting evidence of dissemination in time and space is diagnostic of MS in patients with clinically isolated optic neuritis. In addition, for patients not meeting criteria for MS at time of presentation with clinically isolated optic neuritis, MRI of the brain has been shown to be an important prognostic indicator for development of MS. MRI of the brain showing 0, 1, or more than 3 lesions typical for MS is associated, respectively, with a 25%, 60%, and 78% risk of progression to clinically definite MS.

Less commonly, optic neuritis is associated with other demyelinating syndromes such as NMO. This should be considered in patients with severe vision loss, bilateral involvement, or history of prior optic neuritis or transverse myelitis. A serum antibody (anti-aquaporin 4 or NMO antibody) has been identified as a pathologic agent in this disorder. Testing for this is commercially available with a published sensitivity and specificity of 63% and 99%, respectively. Positive testing for anti-AqP4-IgG in a patient with optic neuritis is diagnostic of NMO per published consensus criteria. A serum antibody (MOG-IgG) is commercially available and aids in the identification of MOG associated optic neuritis.

Differential Diagnosis

Other diagnostic considerations in a patient with unilateral painful vision loss without explanatory pathology evident on ophthalmic examination include other optic neuropathies such as those due to sarcoidosis, lupus, vasculitis, neoplastic, vascular, and infectious causes. Atypical features for optic neuritis such as systemic symptoms, history of cancer, pain that persists beyond 2 weeks, progressive vision loss beyond 14 days, no spontaneous improvement in vision, retinal hemorrhages, cotton-wool spots, or macular exudates should prompt diagnostic evaluation for etiologies other than optic neuritis.

Treatment and Monitoring

The Optic Neuritis Treatment Trial (ONTT) was a randomized trial comparing placebo, oral prednisone, and IV methylprednisolone (1 g/day IV for 3 days) followed by oral prednisone (1 mg/kg per day for 11 days) for acute optic neuritis. IV steroids hastened recovery of vision without affecting final visual outcome compared with placebo treatment. Treatment with low-dose oral prednisone alone (1 mg/kg/day for 14 days) was associated with an increased risk of relapse compared with placebo treatment. The 15-year follow-up results, published in 2008, demonstrated persistence of visual recovery. Studies have demonstrated non-inferiority of high-dose oral steroids (1250 mg prednisone/day for 3 days) to IV methylprednisolone with regards to vision recover following acute optic neuritis.

Many clinicians offer IV or high-dose oral steroid treatment to hasten visual recovery. Monotherapy with low-dose oral prednisone should be avoided. Regardless of the decision to treat or not with steroids, all patients should be monitored closely. Continued progression of vision loss, failure to spontaneously recover vision, or persistent pain should prompt additional diagnostic workup as well as consideration for additional IV steroid therapy for atypical optic neuritis. If this is not effective, plasma exchange has been reported as an effective acute therapy for atypical optic neuritis including NMO-spectrum optic neuritis.

In patients with acute optic neuritis and NMO or acute optic neuritis on the NMO-spectrum, treatment with plasma exchange or rituxamab (Rituxan)[1] should be considered to improve functional visual outcome.

In patients with a clinically isolated syndrome, consideration should be given to institution of disease-modifying therapy for MS based on the type and number of lesions on brain MRI and oligoclonal bands in cerebrospinal fluid. Several clinical trials have shown an association between early treatment with MS therapies and decreased incidence of progression to clinically definite MS in patients with a recent clinically isolated syndrome and clinically silent lesions on brain MRI.

In patients who meet diagnostic criteria for either MS or NMO, consideration should be given to treating the underlying disease. Eculizumab (Soliris) has shown to reduced risk of relapse and increased remission rate in serum anti-aquaporin-4-positive NMO. Decisions regarding chronic therapy following MOG-associated optic neuritis are currently based on recurrence and persistently elevated serum antibody titers.

Complications

Though more than 70% of patients with optic neuritis recover objectively normal visual acuity, many have residual subjective visual disturbances. These often worsen or recur in heat, which is known as Uhtoff's phenomenon.

Complications of steroid therapy include insomnia, agitation, and stomach irritation. Long-term side effects of steroid treatment for this condition are rare owing to the brief period of treatment. Complications of disease-modifying therapies for MS-, NMO-, and MOG-associated disease are reviewed elsewhere.

---

[1] Not FDA approved for this indication.

References

Beck RQ, Cleary PA, Anderson MM, et al: A randomized, controlled trial of corticosteroids in the treatment of acute optic neuritis, The Neuritis Study Group, N Engl J Med 326:581–588, 1992.

Bonnan M, Valentino R, Debeugny S, et al: Short delay to initiate plasma exchange is the strongest predictor of outcome in severe attacks of NMO spectrum disorders, J Neurol Neurosurg Psychiatry. 89:346–351, 2018.

Chen JJ, Flanagan EP, Jitprapaikulsan J, et al: Myelin oligodendrocyte glycoprotein antibody-positive optic neuritis: clinical characteristics, radiologic clues, and outcome, Am J Ophthalmol 195:8–15, 2018.

Cobo-Calvo A, Sepúlveda M, Rollot F, et al: Evaluation of treatment response in adults with relapsing MOG-Ab-associated disease, J Neuroinflammation 16:134, 2019.

Hickman SJ, Ko M, Chaudhry F, et al: Optic neuritis: an update on typical and atypical optic neuritis, Neuro-ophthalmology 32:237–248, 2008.

Merle H, Olindo S, Bonnan M, et al: Natural history of the visual impairment of relapsing neuromyelitis optica, Ophthalmology 114:810–815, 2007.

Morrow SA, Fraser JA, Day C: Effect of treating acute optic neuritis with bioequivalent oral vs intravenous corticosteroids: a randomized clinical trial, JAMA Neurol 75(6):690-6, 2018.

Moss HE: Visual consequence of medications for multiple sclerosis: the good, the bad, the ugly and the unknown, Eye Brain. 29:13–21, 2017.

Optic Neuritis Study Group: The clinical profile of optic neuritis: experience of the optic neuritis treatment trial, Arch Ophthalmol 109:1673–1678, 1991.

Optic Neuritis Study Group: Multiple sclerosis risk after optic neuritis: final optic neuritis treatment trial follow-up, Arch Neurol 65:727–732, 2008.

Optic Neuritis Study Group: Visual function 15 years after optic neuritis, Ophthalmology 115:1079–1082, 2008.

Pittock SJ, Berthele A, Fujihara K, et al: Eculizumab in aquaporin-4-positive neuromyelitis optica spectrum disorder, N Engl J Med 381:614–625, 2019.

Roesner S, Appel R, Gbadamosi J, et al: Treatment of steroid-unresponsive optic neuritis with plasma exchange, Acta Neurol Scand 126(2):103–108, 2012.

Thompson AJ, Banwell BL, Carroll WM, et al: Diagnosis of multiple sclerosis: 2017 revisions of the McDonald criteria, Lancet Neurol. 17:162–173, 2018.

Vodopivec I, Matiello M, Prasad S: Treatment of neuromyelitis optica, Curr Opin Ophthalmol 26(6):476–483, 2015.

Winferchuk DM, Banwell B, Bennett JL, et al: International consensus diagnostic criteria for neuromyelitis optica spectrum disorders, Neurology 85:177–189, 2015.

PARKINSON DISEASE

Method of
Jessica Tate, MD

CURRENT DIAGNOSIS

- Clinical diagnosis based on four cardinal features:
  - Bradykinesia
  - Rigidity
  - Resting tremor
  - Postural instability
- Supportive features: asymmetric onset, response to dopaminergic medication, and presence of nonmotor features such as REM behavior disorder and anosmia.
- Single-photon emission tomography or olfactory testing may aid diagnosis in specific circumstances.

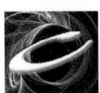

CURRENT THERAPY

- Initial symptomatic treatment with monoamine oxidase-B (MAO-B) inhibitor, dopamine agonist, or carbidopa/levodopa.
  - Carbidopa/levodopa (Sinemet) first line for patients >70; should be initiated in younger patients when severity of motor symptoms warrants it, rather than strict levodopa-sparing approach.
  - Anticholinergic can be used as first-line treatment in younger patients with predominant tremor.
- MAO-B inhibitor, dopamine agonist, or catechol-O-methyltransferase (COMT) inhibitor can be added to levodopa to reduce on-off fluctuations.
- Amantadine (Symmetrel) can reduce levodopa-induced dyskinesias.
- Deep brain stimulation (DBS) is effective for patients with medication-refractory tremor.
- DBS or carbidopa/levodopa enteral suspension (Duopa) is more effective than oral medication alone for patients with severe motor fluctuations.
- Exercise is crucial at all stages and may have neuroprotective benefits.

Epidemiology

Parkinson disease (PD) affects roughly 1% of the population over the age of 60 years and is projected to affect approximately 1.2 million people in the United States by 2030. Updated epidemiologic studies are currently under way. PD is more common in men than women and is suggested to be more common in whites than other racial groups, although this may relate to disparities in healthcare. The average age of onset is in the seventh decade of life, but onset is before age 40 in 3% to 5% of cases. Ninety percent of cases are considered sporadic or idiopathic, whereas approximately 10% are inherited.

Risk Factors

Age is the most significant risk factor. Other proposed risk factors include exposure to pesticides, herbicides, solvents, and well water. Cigarette smoking, coffee consumption, regular exercise, and elevated uric acid levels may be protective. Risk of PD is doubled in first-degree relatives of those affected.

Pathophysiology

The formation of Lewy bodies, intracellular accumulations of the protein α-synuclein, is central to the pathogenesis of PD. This leads to degeneration of dopamine-producing neurons in the substantia nigra pars compacta, setting off a chain of altered signaling in the basal ganglia and ultimately reduced activation of the motor cortex. However, Lewy body deposition and neurodegeneration also occurs in other brain regions, perhaps well before the degeneration of the substantia nigrae. This may explain the myriad nonmotor manifestations of PD, such as early loss of smell and REM behavior disorder, which are under consideration as prodromal symptoms of PD.

Unfortunately, the pathophysiological process that leads to Lewy body formation is not well understood at this time, and several different mechanisms have been proposed. PD is likely caused by a combination of genetic predisposition and environmental factors, which may differ from one individual to another depending on the specific gene or genes responsible. Early disease-modifying interventions, when they become available, are likely to target specific genetic subtypes, and thus genetic testing will likely play a more crucial role in the future diagnosis and treatment of PD.

Clinical Manifestations

The hallmark signs and symptoms of PD are bradykinesia (slow, small-amplitude movement or lack of movement), muscle rigidity (increased resistance to passive movement of the joints that is not velocity-dependent), and resting tremor. Although tremor is a common presenting symptom in PD, some patients with PD *never* develop tremor. The other hallmark symptoms of gait dysfunction and postural instability (loss of postural reflexes crucial to maintaining balance) are uncommon in the early stages of PD but occur later in the disease course.

Loss of dexterity with fine motor tasks, micrographia (small handwriting), hypophonia (soft speech), masked facies (diminished facial expression and reduced blinking), shortened strides, and decreased arm swing while walking are all potential manifestations of bradykinesia.

Rigidity can lead to complaints of stiffness, aching, or cramping. This symptom can lead a patient to explore musculoskeletal causes, such as seeking out a specialist in sports medicine, before realizing it has a neurologic basis. Many physicians believe "cogwheeling" to be specific to a diagnosis of PD. However, cogwheeling typically will not be evident in PD patients without tremor. In addition, patients with essential tremor can exhibit cogwheeling without underlying rigidity.

Parkinsonian tremor most classically starts in one hand, although it can be seen in the jaw and lower extremity as well. It has a slow frequency (4 to 6 Hz) and is visualized with the affected body part at rest. It is often enhanced by distraction (conversation, having the patient perform calculations or name the months backward) and can be temporarily alleviated by concentration or repositioning. When a patient with PD tremor extends an affected upper extremity, the tremor may reappear after a delay. This is referred to as "reemergent rest tremor" and differs from essential tremor, which is typically present immediately on extending the arms.

Early gait changes can include bent posture and shuffling or dragging of the feet, often initially on one side of the body. Later gait changes can include freezing (hesitancy and difficulty initiating a stride with a sensation of feeling stuck to the floor) and festination (a series of small, rapid steps with a sensation of being propelled forward and unable to stop). Postural instability is assessed with the "pull test," in which the examiner stands behind the patient and tugs back firmly on his or her shoulders. An abnormal response is defined by taking two or more steps backward or, in severe cases, by complete lack of response, leading to the examiner catching the patient as he or she falls back.

Diagnosis

The diagnosis of PD is still made clinically in most cases, with a detailed history and neurologic examination. Often, the United Kingdom Parkinson's Disease Society Brain Bank Criteria is used, which requires the presence of bradykinesia along with at least one other cardinal feature as described above. When patients are seen by a movement disorders specialist (a neurologist with additional subspecialty training in PD and related conditions), these clinical features are often objectively scored and tracked over time using a

SYMPTOMS	MANAGEMENT SUGGESTIONS	CONSIDERATIONS
Mood disorders Depression Anxiety disorders	If periodic, optimize PD treatment to minimize on-off fluctuations If more static, typical individualized treatment options including selective serotonin reuptake inhibitors (SSRIs), serotonin and norepinephrine reuptake inhibitors (SNRIs), tricyclic antidepressants (TCAs), counseling, psychotherapy, transcranial magnetic stimulation, etc.	Multiple antidepressants shown to be safe in combination with MAO-B inhibitors, but be aware of rare risk of serotonin syndrome
Sleep disturbances REM sleep behavior disorder (REM-BD) Insomnia Restless leg syndrome (RLS)	For REM-BD, melatonin[7] or clonazepam (Klonopin)[1] at bedtime For insomnia, sleep hygiene counseling, screening for sleep apnea with referral for sleep study if warranted, management of nocturia, treatment of nocturnal stiffness or cramping, etc. For RLS, iron supplementation if ferritin <75, dopamine agonists, gabapentin (Neurontin)[1]	Avoidance of sedative hypnotics due to high risk of adverse effects
Psychosis Illusions Hallucinations Delusions	Lower PD medication dosages *if* possible; discontinuation of other potential offending medications Acetylcholinesterase inhibitors, quetiapine (Seroquel)[1] or clozapine (Clozaril)[1], pimavanserin (Nuplazid)	If acute, requires full medical/neurologic evaluation for infection and other possible causes
Constipation	Hydration, exercise, removal of offending medications if possible PEG 3350 (Miralax)	
Urinary dysfunction	Mirabegron (Myrbetriq) may be helpful for patients without benign prostatic hypertrophy	Urodynamic testing recommended, since multiple factors may be at play (such as BPH) Caution regarding anticholinergics; possible delirium
Orthostatic hypotension	Abdominal binder or compression stockings Midodrine (Proamatine), fludrocortisone (Florinef)[1], or droxidopa (norepinephrine precursor) (Northera)	Extra caution in the hour following levodopa doses Must balance with supine hypertension, which may improve by raising head of bed 30 degrees or a nighttime antihypertensive
Fatigue	Exercise, treatment of depression or sleep disorders if present Avoiding under-medication of PD symptoms Selegiline (Eldepryl), amantadine (Symmetrel) Stimulants such as methylphenidate (Ritalin)[1] (rarely, in extreme cases)	
Drooling	Hard candy or gum RimabotulinumtoxinB (Myobloc) or incobotulinumtoxinA (Xeomin) injections in salivary glands Sublingual atropine[1]	
Weight loss	Monitoring, nutritional supplementation, referral to nutritionist	Associated with negative outcomes in PD including dementia and earlier death; unclear if causal

[1]Not FDA approved for this indication.
[7]Available as a dietary supplement.
MAO-B, Monoamine oxidase type B; *PD,* Parkinson disease.

validated measure such as the Unified Parkinson's Disease Rating Scale. Additional supportive diagnostic criteria are also required, which can include unilateral onset, persistent asymmetry, progression with time, and response to levodopa. Patients also should be questioned about the presence of specific nonmotor symptoms suggestive of PD. These can include loss of smell or presence of REM sleep behavior disorder, which can precede onset of motor symptoms by years or even decades, and autonomic symptoms such as constipation, urinary frequency and urgency, sexual dysfunction, or drooling. These are discussed further in Table 1.

Differential Diagnosis

The differential diagnosis for PD varies somewhat depending on age of onset. In young patients, secondary Parkinsonism should be excluded with testing for Wilson disease. Dopa-responsive dystonia (DRD) can also mimic PD in younger patients. Drug-induced Parkinsonism, usually secondary to dopamine-blocking agents such as atypical antipsychotics or antiemetics, can occur at any age. In older patients, vascular Parkinsonism can resemble idiopathic PD but is secondary to accumulation of significant chronic microvascular ischemic changes, often in the periventricular brain regions, or an accumulation of acute cerebral infarcts over time. These findings can be easily visualized on a noncontrast magnetic resonance imaging (MRI) scan of the brain. An MRI

scan can also reveal disproportionate enlargement of the ventricles that may raise suspicion for normal pressure hydrocephalus, a poorly understood and somewhat controversial condition that can lead to a shuffling gait or freezing of gait resembling PD. Atypical Parkinsonism syndromes include progressive supranuclear palsy (PSP), multiple systems atrophy (cerebellar and Parkinsonian types), corticobasal degeneration, and Lewy body dementia. These conditions can be very difficult to differentiate from idiopathic PD early in their course. Red flags include symmetric onset, lack of response (distinguished from intolerance) to an appropriate dose of levodopa, and early onset of symptoms typically seen in advanced stages of PD such as gait freezing, postural instability, severe autonomic dysfunction such as symptomatic orthostatic hypotension, or hallucinations.

In specific situations, particularly those in which DRD, vascular Parkinsonism, or drug-induced Parkinsonism are suspected, a [123I]FP-CIT single-photon emission tomography scan—known as a DaTscan—can be used to provide supportive information. This scan is designed to detect reduced presynaptic dopamine activity in the caudate and putamen. Uptake is expected to be normal in essential tremor, DRD, drug-induced Parkinsonism, and most cases of vascular Parkinsonism, whereas it is reduced in neurodegenerative Parkinsonism. A major limitation of the DaTscan is its inability to differentiate between PD and atypical Parkinsonism such as PSP.

			SIDE EFFECTS TO	
DRUG CLASS	**MEDICATION NAMES**	**TYPICAL DOSE RANGE**	**CONSIDER**	**COMMENTS**
MAO-B Inhibitors				
	Selegiline (Eldepryl)	5 mg daily to 5 mg BID	Insomnia, confusion, hallucinations	Controversy re: neuroprotective benefits Potential medication interactions (serotonin syndrome)
	Rasagiline (Azilect)	0.5–1 mg daily		
Anticholinergics				
	Benztropine (Cogentin)	0.5 mg daily to 1 mg TID	Dry mouth, cognitive impairment, hallucinations, urinary retention, blurred vision	Useful for tremor, high risk in elderly
	Trihexyphenidyl (Artane)	1 mg daily to 3 mg BID		
Dopamine Agonists				
	Pramipexole (Mirapex)	IR 0.125–1.5 mg TID ER: 0.375–4.5 mg daily	Nausea, leg edema, weight gain, daytime sleepiness, impulse control disorders, hallucinations Patch: skin irritation	Less favorable side effect efficacy profile than levodopa
	Ropinirole (Requip)	IR 0.25–8 mg TID XL: 2–24 mg daily		
	Rotigotine (Neupro)	Transdermal 2–8 mg/24 h		
Oral Levodopa Preparations	Carbidopa/levodopa (Sinemet) C/L controlled release (Sinemet CR)	25/100 mg BID-TID to 50/200 mg BID-TID	Nausea, daytime sleepiness, orthostatic hypotension, hallucinations	Dyskinesias are a long-term complication of therapy

BID, Two times daily; *C/L,* carbidopa/levodopa; *ER,* extended release; *MAO-B,* monoamine oxidase type B; *PD,* Parkinson disease; *TID,* three times daily.

Treatment

Exercise is believed to have neuroprotective benefits and should be strongly encouraged in all stages of PD. Most emphasis has been on cardiovascular forms of exercise, but strength and balance training are likely to be beneficial in this population as well. There are multiple Parkinson's-specific exercise programs appearing nationwide, including stationary cycling, noncombat boxing, and dance.

Symptomatic medication is often initiated either when tremor becomes bothersome, or when motor disability is affecting day-to-day activities. A sizable minority of patients with PD may have medication-refractory tremor, an important point to keep in mind because a patient with isolated tremor and lack of improvement with dopaminergics should not necessarily be considered a nonresponder. Dopaminergics may still be useful to those patients in the future for symptoms such as bradykinesia and rigidity.

For early-stage PD, there are three classes of drugs that are frequently used: monoamine oxidase (MAO)-B inhibitors, dopamine agonists, and levodopa. Levodopa may be chosen as initial therapy in a patient 70 years of age or older because of the lower potential for side effects. In younger patients, it is common to start with an MAO-B inhibitor or dopamine agonist and escalate to levodopa if either of those are poorly tolerated or ineffective. Although a levodopa-sparing strategy has been commonly adopted by clinicians, evidence suggests that earlier initiation of levodopa is associated with better long-term outcomes for patients. Regardless of the patient's age, levodopa should be started when the patient is experiencing disabling symptoms that have not responded to other medication choices. Especially for patients on levodopa, it is best practice to treat with the lowest effective dose to help reduce the risk of dyskinesias. This symptom will be discussed in further detail in the next section. Typical dosages and side effects to consider can be found in Table 2.

Patients with moderate to advanced PD have typically reached a degree of symptom severity that necessitates levodopa. Eventually, they will begin to develop medication fluctuations. These include wearing-off of symptomatic benefits before the next dose, erratic failures of dosages to take effect, and dyskinesias. Dyskinesias are rocking, writhing, or twisting movements that can affect any region of the body. They most commonly occur at the peak of a levodopa dose but, for some patients, can occur at the end of a dose or in a diphasic manner. The pathophysiology behind dyskinesias is not fully understood, but they are believed to be a function of both disease stage and dosage of levodopa. If dyskinesias are not bothersome to the patient, they do not require treatment. If they are bothersome, dosage reduction can be considered but is not always possible due to worsening of motor symptoms. The addition of amantadine (Symmetrel) can be helpful. For early wearing-off, dosing—particularly frequency—of levodopa can be modified, or adjunctive medication can be used such as an MAO-B inhibitor, a dopamine agonist, or a COMT inhibitor. Patients should also be counseled about the potential effect of protein on levodopa absorption and encouraged to space their doses 30 to 60 minutes from meals. For dose failures or abrupt wearing-off, apomorphine can be used to provide rapid onset of symptom relief. Typical dosages and side effects of drugs used for advanced PD are summarized in Table 3. When medication fluctuations are severe, the patient may be considered for an advanced treatment option such as DBS or carbidopa-levodopa enteral suspension (Duopa). The ideal candidate for DBS has idiopathic PD, does not have dementia, and is typically receiving less-than-ideal benefit from medications for one of two reasons. In the first circumstance, levodopa is providing definite symptom reduction, but medication fluctuations have become a significant problem. In the second circumstance, the patient has medication-refractory tremor with or without additional troublesome motor symptoms. The enteral suspension, delivered continuously to the small intestine via a percutaneous endoscopic transgastric jejunostomy (PEG-J) tube and pump, is for patients experiencing significant motor fluctuations with oral medications.

TABLE 3 Medication Choices in Advanced Parkinson Disease.

DRUG CLASS	MEDICATION NAMES	TYPICAL DOSE RANGE	SIDE EFFECTS TO CONSIDER	COMMENTS
MAO-B Inhibitors				
	Selegiline (Eldepryl)	5 mg daily to 5 mg BID	Insomnia, confusion, hallucinations	Adjunct to levodopa
	Rasagiline (Azilect)	0.5–1 mg daily		
	Safinamide (Xadago)	50–100 mg daily		
Dopamine Agonists				
	Pramipexole (Mirapex)	IR 0.125–1.5 mg TID ER: 0.375–4.5 mg daily	Nausea, leg edema, weight gain, daytime sleepiness, impulse control disorders, hallucinations	Adjunct to levodopa
	Ropinirole (Requip)	IR 0.25–8 mg TID XL: 2–24 mg daily		
	Rotigotine (Neupro)	Transdermal 2–8 mg/24 h	Skin irritation	
	Apomorphine (APOKYN)	Subcutaneous 0.2 mL (2 mg) to 0.6 mL (6 mg)	Orthostatic hypotension, nausea	Rapid onset used as rescue medication
	Apomorphine (Kynmobi)	Sublingual 10–30 mg, up to 5 times daily	Orthostatic hypotension, nausea	Rapid onset, used as a rescue medication
COMT Inhibitor	Entacapone (Comtan)	200 mg with each dose of levodopa, up to 8 times daily	Orange urine, diarrhea	Used to prolong levodopa effects Can worsen dyskinesias
	Opicapone (Ongentys)	50 mg at bedtime	Constipation, hypotension, weight loss	Used to prolong levodopa effects Can worsen dyskinesias
Levodopa Preparations				
	C/L (Sinemet) C/L controlled release (Sinemet CR)	Variable—total of 1200–2500 mg levodopa/d	Nausea, daytime sleepiness, orthostatic hypotension, hallucinations	Escalating dosage and frequency in advanced PD to combat wearing-off, must be balanced with side effects
	C/L ER capsules (Rytary)	23.75 mg/95 mg TID—variable		
	C/L/entacapone (Stalevo)	25/100/200 mg TID to 50/200/200 mg 6 times/d	Orange urine, diarrhea	
	Levodopa inhalation powder (Inbrija)	84 mg 1–5 times daily	Cough, upper respiratory infection, nausea, discolored sputum	Used as rescue medication for off periods Contraindicated in patients with lung disease
NMDA Antagonist				
	Amantadine (Symmetrel)	50 mg daily to 100 mg TID	Livedo reticularis, leg edema, insomnia, dry mouth, confusion, hallucinations, myoclonus	Reduces dyskinesias Can also be used for mild, early PD symptoms but now less commonly
	Amantadine ER (Gocovri)	137–274 mg nightly		FDA-approved for PD dyskinesia May reduce off time as well
	Amantadine ER (Osmolex ER)	129–322 mg		

C/L, Carbidopa/levodopa; *COMT,* catechol-O-methyltransferase; *ER,* extended release; *MAO-B,* monoamine oxidase type B; *NMDA,* N-methyl-D-aspartate *PD,* Parkinson disease; *TID,* three times daily.

Monitoring

Swallowing function should be monitored periodically, typically with a modified barium swallow, and modifications in diet and swallowing technique may reduce aspiration risk. A cognitive screening tool such as the Montreal Cognitive Assessment should be administered yearly. Supportive treatment strategies should be used on an ongoing basis, including speech/swallow therapy, physical therapy, and occupational therapy. Therapists with specific training in neurologic disorders should be used when possible. PD-specific programs such as the Lee Silverman Voice Therapy Loud (speech therapy) and Big (physical therapy) programs are particularly helpful.

Complications and Nonmotor Symptoms

Nonmotor symptoms of PD can be more disabling in some cases than the more well-known motor symptoms. These are summarized in Table 1. Depression and anxiety, in particular, affect high numbers of patients with PD. Psychosis is not an inevitable occurrence but affects approximately 50% of patients, usually in more advanced stages of the disease. When PD psychosis is causing fear or agitation, it should be treated with an escalating strategy. Typically, acetylcholinesterase inhibitors will be introduced first, followed by either low-dose quetiapine (Seroquel)[1] or

[1]Not FDA approved for this indication.

pimavanserin (Nuplazid) if symptoms are not stabilized. Pimavanserin is the only drug approved by the Food and Drug Administration for Parkinson's psychosis. Atypical antipsychotics have been associated with an increased risk of death in the elderly, and deaths have also been reported in patients receiving pimavanserin, although causality is not necessarily clear. Risks and benefits must be carefully weighed, but currently these medications may be the only option for a patient experiencing severe psychosis.

The gradual progression of PD is inevitable but highly variable in speed and severity from one individual to another. This is likely dependent on age of onset, other comorbid health conditions, access to expert care, and level of physical activity among other factors. Abrupt worsening of any symptoms of PD should prompt a workup for provoking medical conditions, such as occult urinary tract infection. PD does not directly lead to death, but death can occur in the setting of dysphagia leading to failure to thrive or aspiration pneumonia, or from serious injuries incurred from falls.

References

Bloem BR, de Vries NM, Ebersbach G: Nonpharmacological treatments for patients with Parkinson's disease, *Mov Disord* 30:1504–1520, 2015.

Cumming K, Macleod AD: Early weight loss in parkinsonism predicts poor outcomes: evidence from an incident cohort study, *Neurology* 89:2254–2261, 2017.

de Lau LM, Breteler MM: Epidemiology of Parkinson's disease, *Lancet Neurol* 5:525–535, 2006.

Fahn S, Elton R: Members of the UPDRS Development Committee. In Fahn S, Marsden CD, Calne DB, Goldstein M, editors: *Recent Developments in Parkinson's Disease*, Vol 2. Florham Park, NJ, 1987, Macmillan Health Care Information, pp 15, 3–163. (293–304.

Fox SH, Katzenschlager R, Lim SY, et al: Evidence based medicine publications. International Parkinson and Movement Disorder Society. Available at www.movementdisorders.org/MDS/resources/publications-reviews/EBM-Reviews1.htm. Accessed 15 April 2018.

Gibb WR, Lees AJ: The relevance of the Lewy body to the pathogenesis of idiopathic Parkinson's disease, *J Neurol Neurosurg Psychiatr* 51:745–752, 1988.

Gray R, Ives N, Rick C, et al: Long-term effectiveness of dopamine agonist and monoamine oxidase B inhibitors compared with levodopa as initial treatment for Parkinson's disease (PD MED): a large, open-label, pragmatic randomized trial, *Lancet* 384(9949):1196–1205, 2014.

Jankovic J, Schwartz KS, Ondo W: Re-emergent tremor of Parkinson's disease, *J Neurol Neurosurg Psychiatr* 67:646–650, 1999.

Shrag A, Schott JM: Epidemiological, clinical, and genetic characteristics of early-onset parkinsonism, *Lancet Neurol* 5:355–363, 2006.

REHABILITATION OF THE STROKE PATIENT

Method of
Marlís González-Fernández, MD, PhD; and Dorianne Feldman, MD, MSPT

CURRENT THERAPY

- Stroke rehabilitation improves functional outcomes.
- A comprehensive rehabilitation team composed of physicians, nurses, therapists, and community reintegration professionals can achieve the best outcomes.
- Early evaluation of family support and the home environment is critical to prevent unnecessary institutionalization.
- Evaluation and management of modifiable stroke risk factors, such as smoking, hypertension, and diabetes mellitus, are imperative during stroke rehabilitation to prevent stroke recurrence.
- Rehabilitation of the stroke patient can be hindered by conditions such as pneumonia (usually caused by aspiration), deep venous thrombosis, urinary tract infections, shoulder pain, depression, and spasticity. Early identification and treatment of these conditions are necessary to maximize functional outcomes.

According to the U.S. National Center for Health Statistics, 5.6 million Americans live with disability caused by a previous stroke. Stroke is the leading cause of permanent disability in adults. Conservative estimates suggest that about 45% of stroke patients have moderate to severe disabilities requiring rehabilitation.

The goals of stroke rehabilitation are to maintain and optimize medical management, to maximize functional recovery, to minimize disability, and to improve quality of life and participation in society. The rehabilitative approach endeavors to provide patient-centered care that is organized, comprehensive, and specific to the needs of the stroke patient. The concerted efforts of the patient, family, and rehabilitation team are essential to achieve these goals. Recovery after stroke can be a long and challenging process for the patient and the family. Although functional gains occur most rapidly in the first year after a stroke, additional motor recovery is possible beyond 1 year when patients are involved in targeted rehabilitation programs.

The rehabilitation team is composed of rehabilitation physicians (physiatrists), other physicians such as neurologists and neurosurgeons, rehabilitation nurses, occupational therapists, physical therapists, speech and language pathologists, rehabilitation neuropsychologists, social workers, case managers, nutritionists, vocational counselors, and pharmacists. A goal of the acute inpatient rehabilitation team is to discharge the patient to the least restrictive environment, ideally home. To accomplish this goal, it is critical to evaluate family support and the home environment.

Rehabilitation should start as part of the acute stroke inpatient stay. The decision-making process to determine the appropriate rehabilitation setting after discharge is described in Figure 1. Speech-language pathologists, physical therapists, and occupational therapists evaluate deficits in cognition, communication, deglutition, mobility, and activities of daily living. The severity of deficits in these major areas and the ability of the patient to tolerate therapy determine the appropriate rehabilitation setting.

Stroke patients with mild deficits are able to return home with home or outpatient therapy services. Patients with moderate to severe strokes benefit from more intensive therapy in an institutional setting. Comprehensive inpatient rehabilitation is suitable for patients with moderate to severe deficits who can tolerate intensive rehabilitation (3 hours of therapy per day for 5 days each week or 15 hours of therapy over a 7-day period). If the severity of deficits or medical comorbidities limits the ability of the patient to participate in intensive therapy, alternate settings can be considered.

During the inpatient rehabilitation stage, medical management focuses on secondary stroke prevention in terms of diet; exercise; smoking cessation; and reduction of complications, including optimization of blood pressure control while maintaining cerebral perfusion; prevention and treatment of lipid disorders; and management of poststroke pain, depression, and abnormal muscle tone. During this stage, much of the rehabilitation effort is directed toward educating stroke survivors about complications and the importance of adherence to medical recommendations.

Medical complications, such as deep venous thrombosis and related thromboembolism, pneumonia (usually related to aspiration), skin breakdown, and urinary infections, can hinder a patient's recovery. Early identification of these complications is necessary to maintain progress in the rehabilitation effort. Other complications, such as seizures and cardiac decompensation, are possible and should be monitored.

Stroke often causes significant impairment and activity limitations. Deficits in strength, swallowing, vision, balance, muscle tone, communication, comprehension, cognition, attention, sensory perception, and bladder function are common and can cause difficulty completing activities of daily living, walking, transferring to and from different surfaces, and getting in and out of bed. Post-stroke depression, fatigue, and pain are common and should be addressed to maximize participation in rehabilitative efforts.

Transition to the chronic phase begins after the patient is medically stable and inpatient therapy goals are met. Outpatient therapy services are initiated in conjunction with physiatric, primary care, and neurologic follow-up.

Hemiparesis

Hemiparesis, or one-sided weakness, is one of the most frequent complications after stroke. Recovery of motor function varies. Often, it is limited by muscle atrophy, co-contraction of agonists and antagonists, and abnormal tone. Usually, motor recovery is

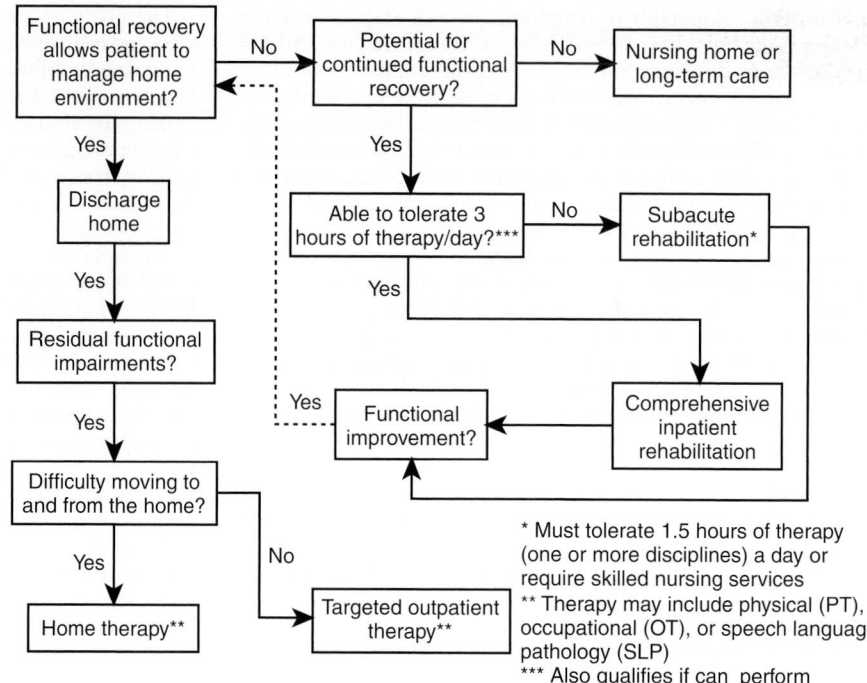

Figure 1 Determination of rehabilitation needs of patients being discharged after an acute stroke.

preceded by the development of patterned muscle movements, or synergies. Synergies occur when select muscles contract in a predictable manner. In the paretic upper extremity, a flexion synergy pattern (i.e., humeral adduction, internal rotation, elbow flexion, forearm pronation, and wrist and finger flexion) is common. In the lower extremity, extension synergies (i.e., hip internal rotation, adduction, extension, knee extension, and ankle extension and inversion) predominate. These patterns can be regarded as functional and nonfunctional. For instance, extension synergy patterns of the lower limb can augment rehabilitation because this position fosters early ambulatory therapy. Conversely, flexion synergy patterns in the upper extremity can significantly impair arm function.

Rehabilitation of the patient with hemiparesis should concentrate on maintaining range of motion and improving strength and posturing. Exercise programs should incorporate functional use of the hemiparetic limb and weight bearing to promote limb recognition, better alignment, muscle elongation, and muscle tone reduction. Bilateral movement in conjunction with sensory training has demonstrated benefit in post-stroke rehabilitation by triggering dual neural networks to be active in both hemispheres to increase motor recovery.

Hemiparesis can lead to contracture, particularly when profound weakness is present, and contracture occurs most commonly in the wrist and ankle. Resting hand splints and solid ankle-foot orthoses can be used to maintain the limb in a neutral position. These devices can be used to prevent loss of motion, control muscle tone, and aid in positioning, particularly when a wheelchair is necessary.

Functional electrical stimulation (FES) has gained increasing interest as a means of enhancing functional movement and strength. Muscle contraction is induced with electrical stimulation. Many products on the market incorporate FES technology for the treatment of footdrop and hand weakness.

Preservation of scapulohumeral positioning is a critical component of rehabilitation. With shoulder weakness, the scapula becomes downwardly rotated, which causes the glenoid fossa to move vertically and result in humeral subluxation. Traditionally, shoulder slings have been prescribed for the hemiplegic shoulder, but their effectiveness in preventing subluxation is questionable.

FES has been used to augment motor return in the hemiplegic shoulder and prevent subluxation. Despite advances in the treatment of the hemiplegic shoulder, it is still unclear which therapeutic interventions should constitute the standard of care.

Constraint-induced therapy (CIT), a therapeutic approach in which the nonparetic limb is restrained, can improve functional movement of the paretic upper extremity in patients with residual hand and wrist movement, even in patients more than 1 year after a stroke. More recently, CIT concepts have been applied to the treatment of aphasia. By limiting the use of nonverbal communication and stimulating verbal output, participants were able to improve language performance and communication.

Weight-supported treadmill training has been proposed to enhance gait training after a stroke. Although a recent clinical trial showed no clear benefit from weight-supported treadmill training on improving gait speed, walking ability, or balance, some advocate for continued research on the effects of this training on overall health, including maintaining bone mass and decreasing insulin resistance.

Dysphagia

Dysphagia after stroke occurs acutely in approximately 50% of stroke patients. Identifying dysphagia in this population is essential for preventing associated morbidity and mortality. Stroke patients with dysphagia are at risk for dehydration, malnutrition, and aspiration pneumonia. As allowed by their overall clinical status and consciousness level, stroke patients should be evaluated as early as possible during their acute hospital stay. Trained clinicians (most commonly speech-language pathologists) should evaluate the patient to make recommendations regarding further dysphagia evaluation or testing and the need for diet modifications or dysphagia rehabilitation.

Hemiplegic Shoulder Pain

Stroke survivors with residual hemiparesis or weakness are at risk for pain syndromes (particularly in the upper extremity), which can significantly limit rehabilitation efforts. These pain syndromes are usually multifactorial. During their rehabilitation, prevention of shoulder pain is key, and interventions should focus on proper positioning, handling, and transfer techniques.

In severe cases, shoulder pain can be accompanied by swollen hands, tenderness, skin changes, erythema, hyperhidrosis, and allodynia. When this occurs, it is referred to as *shoulder-hand syndrome*, a subtype of complex regional pain syndrome (CRPS).

TABLE 1 Neuropharmacologic Agents Commonly Used During Stroke Rehabilitation

DRUG CLASS	DRUG NAME	INDICATION	POTENTIAL PROBLEMS
Benzodiazepines	Diazepam (Valium)	Agitation[1], spasticity	Sedation, confusion, sundowning
	Lorazepam (Ativan)	Agitation[1], seizures	Sedation, paradoxical reactions, confusion, sundowning
Tricyclic antidepressants (TCAs)	Nortriptyline (Pamelor) Amitriptyline (Elavil)	Depression, neuropathic pain[1], central pain[1]	Anticholinergic effects, sedation
Selective serotonin reuptake inhibitors (SSRIs)	Sertraline (Zoloft) Escitalopram (Lexapro) Citalopram (Celexa)	Depression, stimulation[1]	Long titration period, suicidal ideations, serotonin syndrome, syndrome of inappropriate antidiuretic hormone (SIADH), somnolence, seizures
	Fluoxetine (Prozac)	Depression motor recovery[1]	As above for other SSRIs
Stimulants	Modafinil (Provigil) Methylphenidate (Ritalin)	Drowsiness[1], decreased alertness[1], impaired concentration[1], diminished attention[1]	Arrhythmia, seizures, hepatotoxicity, blood pressure changes

[1]Not FDA approved for this indication.

Although the mechanism and cause are unclear, it has been suggested that this process is the result of an overreaction to a neurologic insult and may be inflammatory in nature. In some cases, the pain is severe, resulting in decreased and guarded movements of the limb that limit fuj1nctional use. Shoulder pathology such as rotator cuff strains or tears, bicipital tendonitis, subacromial and subdeltoid bursitis, and glenohumeral subluxation or dislocation contribute to post-stroke shoulder pain and should be treated.

Nonpharmacologic treatment focuses on desensitization techniques, gentle range-of-motion exercises, and physical modalities (e.g., heat, cold, transcutaneous electrical nerve stimulation [TENS], FES). Pharmacologic management includes medications typically used for neuropathic pain syndromes, such as anticonvulsants, tricyclic antidepressants (TCAs), nonsteroidal antiinflammatory drugs, topical agents (e.g., lidocaine [Xylocaine][1], clonidine [Catapres-TTS][1], capsaicin [Zostrix][1]), and injections of steroids or local anesthetics. Antispasmodic medications have been used. When pain relief is not achieved with conservative treatment, sympathetic blocks can be considered. Sympathectomies and spinal cord stimulators can be considered as a last resort.

Spasticity

Spasticity after stroke can significantly impact rehabilitation. The classic upper extremity flexor synergy pattern (i.e., adducted shoulder with flexed elbow, wrist, and fingers) can markedly interfere with the function of the affected arm. Conversely, the classic lower extremity extensor synergy pattern (i.e., extended hip and knee and ankle plantar flexion) can be advantageous for ambulation if plantar flexion can be controlled by physical or pharmacologic agents. If untreated, these patterns can lead to abnormal positioning and contracture.

Treatment of spasticity after stroke should address positioning and exacerbating factors. Splinting or bracing, appropriate wheelchair sitting position, and physical therapy techniques are important to prevent contracture and promote motor recovery. Painful or noxious stimuli can exacerbate spasticity. Shoulder pain, pressure sores, deep venous thrombosis, bladder distention, and constipation are examples of stimuli that can exacerbate spasticity. Pharmacological treatment should take into account the presence of these triggers because spasticity is likely to improve after the stimuli are resolved or relieved.

Pharmacologic treatment of post-stroke spasticity presents some challenges. Effective antispasticity agents such as baclofen (Lioresal) or tizanidine (Zanaflex) can cause somnolence or weaken unaffected muscles, which can significantly affect rehabilitation.

Localized treatments such as botulinum toxins (Botox, Dysport, Myobloc, Xeomin)[1] injections or phenol blocks[1] can be useful, because treatment can be directed toward muscles that are affecting functional use of the limbs. Surgical interventions can be used for patients who have severe spasticity that limits their functional positioning or for patients with the potential for functional grip if tendon lengthening or transfer can be considered.

Cognitive Dysfunction

Stroke patients can experience many cognitive deficits, including visuospatial neglect, cognitive-linguistic deficits, apraxia, memory loss, and attention deficits. Cognitive rehabilitation should concentrate on treatment of the specific deficits of the patient. Visuospatial rehabilitation (including scanning training) is recommended for deficits associated with visual neglect after right stroke. Cognitive-linguistic therapy should be considered for left hemispheric stroke patients with language deficits. Treatment of apraxia should include specific gestural and strategy training.

The use of medications that may impair cognitive function should be limited. Medications that are commonly considered during a stay in a rehabilitative facility that may have a significant impact on cognition and rehabilitation are listed in Table 1.

Depression and Neuropharmacology

Depression is observed in up to one-half of all stroke patients. Depression has been associated with poor functional outcomes and more severe impairments. Vegetative symptoms can have a significant impact on rehabilitative efforts because patient participation in therapy is critical.

Psychoactive drugs can be beneficial and should be considered. Selective serotonin reuptake inhibitors (SSRIs) are recommended in this population because of a better side effect profile and because of the undesirable anticholinergic side effects of TCAs. In patients who are unresponsive to treatment with SSRIs, nortriptyline (Pamelor) may be helpful. In the rehabilitation setting when rapid short-term improvement in symptoms is necessary to increase participation in therapy, the use of psychostimulants (e.g., methylphenidate [Ritalin][1]) may be indicated. Table 1 shows the neuropharmacologic agents commonly used during stoke rehabilitation. Psychotherapy has been associated with modest improvement in post-stroke depression and is considered to be part of a multidisciplinary approach. Research has demonstrated the benefit of the

[1]Not FDA approved for this indication.

[1]Not FDA approved for this indication.

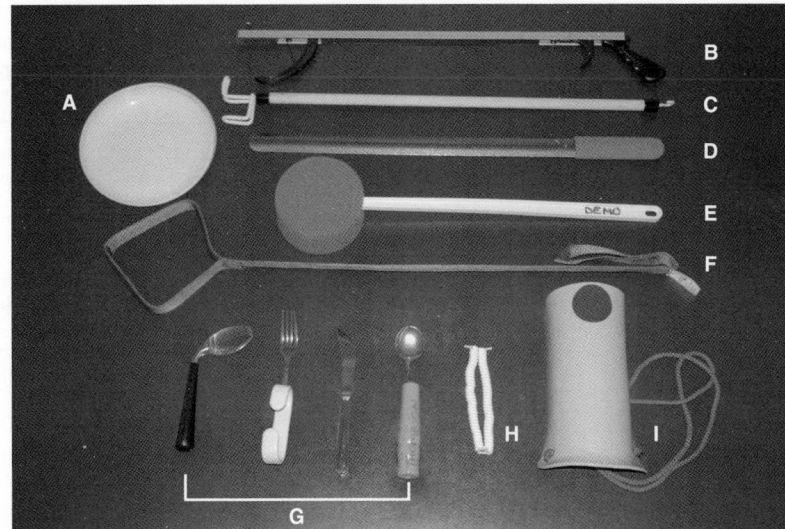

Figure 2 Adaptive equipment commonly used during stroke rehabilitation. The tapered front scoop dish (A) has nonskid feet to keep the plate from sliding. The curved edge simplifies scooping food. The dish is especially suited for patients who have limited flexibility, have decreased motor coordination, or feed using one hand, such as individuals who have had a hemiparetic stroke. The reacher (B) is used to retrieve items from the floor. The long-handled dressing aid (C) is used to reach clothes on the floor or to bring clothes up the paretic side. The long-handled shoehorn (D) facilitates slipping feet into shoes. The long-handle sponge (E) is used to reach the involved side while bathing or when the shoulder range of motion does not allow reaching. The leg lifter (F) and the sound upper limb can be used to assist in moving the paretic lower limb. Adapted feeding utensils (G) are used for patients with grip weakness or difficulties with upper limb range of motion; *left to right*: bent-handle spoon, no-grip fork, rocker bottom knife, and thick-handle spoon. No-tie laces (H) are elastic shoelaces that do not require tying. When using the sock-donning aid (I), the sock slides onto the plastic portion of the device, and the strap is used to pull the sock with the device on the foot.

antidepressant fluoxetine (Prozac)[1] on motor recovery; administration of the drug for 3 months as an adjunct to physical therapy improved motor functioning in post-stroke patients.

Bladder Dysfunction

Bladder dysfunction after stroke depends on the location of the stroke. During the rehabilitation phase, the most common problem is urinary incontinence and urgency associated with uninhibited bladder contraction. Ultrasound bladder scans (usually every 4 hours and after voiding) should be ordered to detect bladder distention and urinary retention. It is standard practice to intervene in cases of bladder volume greater than 500 mL. If volume exceeds this cutoff, intermittent catheterization should be started. Intermittent catheterization is preferable to indwelling catheters because the risk of urinary tract infection is higher with the indwelling catheters. Bladder scans are usually discontinued when postvoiding residual volumes at 3- to 4-hour intervals are low (<150 mL) for a period of 24 to 48 hours.

Mobility and Use of Adaptive Equipment

Activity limitations vary among stroke survivors and can include difficulties with bed mobility, wheelchair propulsion, transfers, gait, stairs, and the basic activities of daily living. The goal of physical therapy and occupational therapy is to maximize functional independence. Addressing mobility limitations is fundamental in stroke rehabilitation because such limitations are related to long-term care needs and independence.

Transfer training comprises learning how to maneuver from one surface or height to another. Ideally, patients should learn to roll and transfer toward their involved and uninvolved sides; however, early mobility efforts are directed to the uninvolved side to minimize the risk of injury.

Gait deviations are common after stroke and interfere with safety and efficiency of locomotion. If an assistive device is needed, the goal of physical therapy is to progress to the least restrictive device possible. Hemiwalkers and wide-based quad canes provide the most stability. An ankle-foot orthosis may be indicated for patients with decreased ankle control and footdrop. Instruction in ascending or descending stairs depends on assistive device requirements. With

weakness, stairs are ascended by initiating movement with the uninvolved or stronger lower extremity. This process is reversed when descending.

For some stroke survivors, functional ambulation is not a realistic goal. In these cases, the wheelchair becomes the primary means of locomotion. Wheelchair prescription requires considerable skill and training and must take into account posturing, body habitus, cognition, physical fitness level, and the home environment. An appropriate wheelchair prescription is required to maximize mobility and prevent complications such as shoulder pain. Physical and occupational therapists should evaluate the patient before providing wheelchair recommendations to vendors. Hemi wheelchairs (i.e., wheelchairs situated closer to the ground) and one-arm drive wheelchairs allow hemiplegic patients to use the uninvolved side for wheelchair propulsion. Lap boards with arm supports can be added to improve hemiparetic arm posturing and sitting symmetry.

For some stroke survivors, the ability to return to driving is considered one of the most important long-term rehabilitation goals. Formal driving rehabilitation programs are available to evaluate and improve driver safety. Driver rehabilitation specialists perform vision, cognitive, and perceptual examinations. Perception tests assess reaction times to visual and auditory stimuli. Values for vision and reaction times are standardized and state-dependent. Specialists should also perform a behind-the-wheel assessment, beginning in a parking lot and progressing to the negotiation of more complex traffic situations. Many modifications can increase independence and assist with a return to driving, including a spinner knob, which can be attached to the steering wheel to allow one-arm control; hand controls for acceleration and braking; left foot pedals to compensate for right foot impairment; and wheelchair lifts.

Adaptive equipment, including bracing, shoe modification, and other tools, increases independence through completion of activities of daily living (e.g., long-handled sponge, reacher, shoe horn, mirror, sock aids) and is extremely beneficial for those with moderate to severe strokes, particularly if hemiparesis is dense (Figure 2). Silverware, pens, and other utensils can be modified for easier maneuverability. Multi Podus boots can be used to prevent plantar flexion contracture development in the hemiparetic limb.

---

[1] Not FDA approved for this indication.

Falls

Falls are common after moderate to severe strokes. In rehabilitation settings, fall prevention usually requires a multimodal approach. Strategies include use of bed-chair alarms, placing those at risk close to the nursing station, wearing skid socks, limiting or refraining from polypharmacy, eliminating slick or irregular floors, and, in some cases, providing a sitter for closer monitoring. Physical and occupational therapists must include general safety and fall recovery as part of the treatment plan.

Visual Impairment

Depending on the location of the stroke, the visual system may be involved. One of the most debilitating visual impairments is visuospatial neglect, a complication of right hemisphere strokes. Left-sided stimuli are not attended to or recognized, and affected individuals must learn to deal with this deficit. Other complications include gaze weakness or paralysis, diplopia, visual field loss, ptosis, tracking disorders, decreased visual acuity, and cortical blindness.

Screening for primary visual skills, including visual acuity, visual fields, and visual tracking, should be done by physiatrists, neurologists, and occupational therapists. If problems are identified, patients should be referred to neuro-ophthalmologists and low-vision rehabilitation programs. Visual acuity problems often can be addressed by incorporating the use of glasses into the therapy session or by changing the prescription. Eye movement disorders and visual field deficits usually lessen as time elapses and may respond to treatment with prisms, head positioning, and unilateral eye occlusion with tape or a patch technique. Prism therapy has also shown promise in treating hemispatial neglect. Patients with continued visual field impairment should be taught eye movement techniques to expand the visual area.

Brain-Based Therapies: Noninvasive Brain Stimulation

Repetitive transcranial magnetic stimulation (rTMS) applies a brief magnetic field to the scalp with enough intensity to penetrate the skull and induce neuronal activation. Some promising results have been seen when rTMS is used after stroke. A second modality, transcranial direct current stimulation (tDCS), applies low-voltage electrical current to stimulate or modify neuronal activity in the brain cortex. The stimulation is applied to discrete areas of the head to target affected areas. Noninvasive brain stimulation has been tested in acute, subacute, and chronic stages of stroke. Studies are evaluating the efficacy of such stimulation therapies on motor recovery, vision impairment, aphasia, and swallowing. Although the side-effect profile of these techniques is positive, more research is necessary to determine the best candidates for treatment and optimal treatment protocols.

Robotics

The aim of robotic technology is to use an adjustable, programmable device to augment mobility in a task-specific manner. Robots can serve in an assistive capacity (perform a desired function) or therapeutic capacity (enhance gait or upper extremity function) and are suitable for this purpose. Robots not only enable more intensive therapy than conventional modes but also incorporate a greater degree of activity repetition. These technologies have shown a small impact on strength gains in the paretic upper extremity. Noninvasive brain stimulation using bilateral tDCS has also been trialed in conjunction with upper extremity robotics in chronic stroke rehabilitation and has demonstrated better results in patients with subcortical strokes as opposed to cortical strokes. The current recommendations are for robotics to be used as an adjunct to traditional rehabilitation interventions.

Virtual Reality

Virtual reality or a computer-devised three-dimensional image has become an increasingly popular rehabilitation therapy for stroke patients. The use of gaming systems that employ this technology are immersive, intensive, and deliver an enjoyable and repetitious means to augment task performance and possibly stimulate upper extremity motor recovery. Additionally, virtual reality gaming can be implemented at home, making it cost effective, available, and adoptable. Current research suggests no superiority when compared to traditional therapies but rather potential efficacy as a supplemental intervention.

Conclusions

Stroke rehabilitation requires the concerted efforts of the patient, family, and medical professionals. A multidisciplinary team with training to address the particular impairments and functional limitations of the stroke patient is critical. The physician's efforts should focus on preventing complications and treating stroke sequelae with the primary goal of improving overall function and participation in society.

References

Bhakta BB: Management of spasticity in stroke, *Br Med Bull* 56:476, 2000.

Chang WH, Kim YH: Robot-assisted therapy in stroke rehabilitation, *J Stroke* 15:174, 2013.

Chollet F, Tardy J, Albucher JF, et al: Fluoxetine for motor recovery after acute ischaemic stroke (FLAME): A randomised placebo-controlled trial, *Lancet Neurol* 10:123, 2011.

Cicerone KD, Dahlberg C, Malec JF, et al: Evidence-based cognitive rehabilitation: Updated review of the literature from 1998 through 2002, *Arch Phys Med Rehabil* 86:1681, 2005.

Feng W, Bowden MG, Kautz S: Review of transcranial direct current stimulation in poststroke recovery, *Topics in Stroke Rehab* 20(1):68–77, 2013.

Hackett ML, Anderson CS, House A, et al: Interventions for treating depression after stroke, *Cochrane Database Syst Rev* CD003437, 2008.

Jones SA, Shinton RA: Improving outcome in stroke patients with visual problems, *Age Ageing* 35:560, 2006.

Kelly-Hayes M, Beiser A, Kase CS, et al: The influence of gender and age on disability following ischemic stroke: The Framingham Study, *J Stroke Cerebrovasc Dis* 12:119, 2003.

Lannin NA, Cusick A, McCluskey A, et al: Effects of splinting on wrist contracture after stroke: A randomized controlled trial, *Stroke* 38:111, 2007.

Laver KE, Lange B, George S: Virtual reality for stroke rehabilitation, *Cochrane Database Sys Rev* (11), 2017.

Legg L, Drummond A, Leonardi-Bee J, et al: Occupational therapy for patients with problems in personal activities of daily living after stroke: Systematic review of randomised trials, *BMJ* 335:922, 2007.

Macko RF, et al: *Stroke Recovery & Rehabilitation*, New York, 2009, Demos Medical Publishing.

Pertoldi S, Di Benedetto P: Shoulder-hand syndrome after stroke. A complex regional pain syndrome, *Eura Medicophys* 41:283, 2005.

Poole D, Chaudry F, Jay WM: Stroke and driving, *Top Stroke Rehabil* 15:37, 2008.

Pruski A, Celnik P: The use of noninvasive brain stimulation, specifically transcranial direct current stimulation after stroke, *Am J Phys Med Rehab* 98(8):735–736, 2019.

Rose T, Nam CS, Chen KB: Immersion of virtual reality for rehabilitation-Review, *Appl Ergonom* 69:153–161, 2018.

Saposnik G, Teasell R, Mamdani M, et al: Effectiveness of virtual reality using Wii gaming technology in stroke rehabilitation: a pilot randomized clinical trial and proof of principle, *Stroke* 41(7):1477–1484, 2010.

Starkstein SE, Mizrahi R, Power BD: Antidepressant therapy in post-stroke depression, *Expert Opin Pharmacother* 9:1291, 2008.

Stein J: Stroke. In Frontera WR, Silver JK, editors: *Essentials of Physical Medicine and Rehabilitation*, Philadelphia, 2002, Saunders, pp 778–783.

Stewart KC, Cauraugh JH, Summers JJ: Bilateral movement training and stroke rehabilitation: A systematic review and meta-analysis, *Journal of the J Neurol Sci* 244(1–2):89–95, 2006.

Straudi S, Fregni F, Martinuzzi C: tDCS and robotics on upper limb stroke rehabilitation: effect modification by stroke duration and type of stroke, *BioMed research international* 2016.

Umphred DA: *Neurological Rehabilitation*, St Louis, 1995, Mosby Elsevier Health Science.

van Wijk I, Algra A, van de Port IG, et al: Change in mobility activity in the second year after stroke in a rehabilitation population: Who is at risk for decline? *Arch Phys Med Rehabil* 87:45, 2006.

Weber LM, Stein J: The use of robots in stroke rehabilitation: A narrative review, *Neuro Rehab* 43(1):99–110, 2018.

Wolf SL, Winstein CJ, Miller JP, et al: Effect of constraint-induced movement therapy on upper extremity function 3 to 9 months after stroke: The EXCITE randomized clinical trial, *JAMA* 296:2095, 2006.

SEIZURES AND EPILEPSY IN ADOLESCENTS AND ADULTS

Method of
José A. Padin-Rosado, MD

CURRENT DIAGNOSIS

- Obtain a thorough clinical history, including a detailed description of the paroxysmal events from the patient and from witness accounts.
- Perform a complete physical and neurologic examination.
- Perform laboratory tests including electrolytes, blood glucose, liver function, and toxicology.
- Obtain a lumbar puncture if signs of infection are present.
- Neuroimaging is strongly recommended. Magnetic resonance imaging (MRI) is the preferred test due to its higher resolution. Head computed tomography (CT) is acceptable in the acute setting to rule out hemorrhage.
- Routine electroencephalography (EEG) with sleep deprivation and activation procedures should be performed as close to the time of occurrence of the paroxysmal event as possible in order to increase the diagnostic yield.

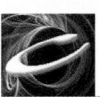

CURRENT THERAPY

- Choose the right medication for the type of epilepsy and epilepsy syndrome.
- Consider the side-effect profile, cost, and drug dosing schedule and adapt to the unique patient characteristics, taking into consideration the patient's comorbidities.
- Aim for monotherapy whenever possible.
- Start low and increase slowly when antiseizure drug (ASD) therapy is being initiated in order to minimize side effects and increase compliance.
- An adequate ASD trial with titration of the medication until clinical effectiveness or side effects occur is recommended.
- When switching from one drug to another, consider overlapping medications to provide protection until the first drug is discontinued.
- If the patient fails two ASD trials either in monotherapy or polytherapy, he or she should be referred to an epilepsy center for evaluation.
- If the patient is seizure free after 2 years of treatment, consider withdrawing ASDs for epilepsies of unknown etiology or epilepsy syndromes known to resolve.

Epilepsy is a disease characterized by an enduring predisposition to generate seizures and by the neurobiologic, cognitive, psychological, and social consequences of this condition. Epilepsy is commonly defined as having two or more unprovoked seizures greater than 24 hours apart. However, as per the classification proposed by the International League Against Epilepsy (ILAE) in 2014, a single seizure can be classified as epilepsy if risk of seizure recurrence is high (see section titled Classification).

A seizure is defined as transient signs or symptoms caused by abnormal excessive synchronous activity of brain neurons. Seizures can be classified as either acute symptomatic (provoked) or unprovoked. Acute symptomatic seizures are associated with a transient systemic or brain insult and will usually not require treatment with antiepileptic drugs because of the transient nature of the precipitant and the associated low risk for development of epilepsy. Unprovoked seizures, on the other hand, may represent the beginning of epilepsy.

Epidemiology

Epilepsy is one of the most common neurologic conditions, affecting more than 50 million people worldwide. The prevalence of epilepsy (number of people with active epilepsy) is approximately 1% in the United States, with 3.4 million people (3 million adults and 470,000 children) suffering from the disease. The incidence of epilepsy (number of new cases of epilepsy) is around 150,000 each year, or 55 per 100,000 population. The incidence is higher in children under the age of 2 and in individuals older than age 65. Men have a slightly higher risk of developing epilepsy than women. African Americans and disadvantaged populations are affected at a higher rate than Caucasians. The lifetime risk of developing a seizure is around 9% to 10%.

Classification
Definition of Epilepsy

In 2014, the ILAE published a practical definition of epilepsy. It classifies epilepsy as a disease of the brain characterized by any of the following criteria: at least two unprovoked or reflex seizures occurring 24 hours apart, one unprovoked or reflex seizure and a probability of recurrent seizures similar to the general recurrence risk (60%) after two unprovoked seizures, occurring over the next 10 years or a diagnosis of an epilepsy syndrome.

In 2017, the ILAE released a major revision of both the classification of the epilepsies and epilepsy syndromes and the classification of seizure types. The classification of the epilepsies and epilepsy syndromes has three levels: (1) classification of the seizure type, (2) classification of the epilepsy type, and (3) diagnosis of an epilepsy syndrome whenever possible. The cause and associated comorbidities are considered at each diagnostic step because these carry treatment implications.

The first step is to classify the type of seizure (Figure 1 and Box 1). It assumes that the patient has been diagnosed with epileptic seizures and then organizes the seizures by where they originate in the brain into either focal onset seizures, formerly known as partial-onset seizure (emanating from networks in one lobe or hemisphere); generalized-onset seizure (seizures engaging bilateral neural networks); and unknown-onset seizures. The term *secondary generalized seizure* is replaced by *focal to bilateral tonic-clonic seizure*, and it is placed in a special category. Then focal-onset seizures can be optionally classified into seizures with preserved awareness as focal aware seizures (formerly known as simple partial seizures) and seizures with impaired awareness as focal impaired awareness seizures (formerly known as complex partial seizures). Focal-onset seizures, generalized-onset seizures, and unknown-onset seizures can be optionally and further subdivided into whether they have associated motor symptoms or other nonmotor symptoms. In some settings, classification into seizure type will be the only attainable level possible for diagnosis because there may be no access to EEG, video, and imaging studies or too little information available to make a higher level of diagnosis.

The second step is to classify the type of epilepsy (Figure 2). This step in the classification assumes that the patient fulfills the diagnosis of epilepsy (ILAE 2014 definition of epilepsy—see earlier) and classifies the epilepsies into focal (focal clinical features and EEG with focal epileptiform abnormalities), generalized (bilateral clinical features and EEG with generalized epileptiform abnormalities), combined generalized and focal (features of both on clinical evaluation and on EEG), and unknown type (either no clinical information available and normal or no EEG available).

The third step is the diagnosis of an epilepsy syndrome whenever possible. A syndrome refers to a cluster of features such as seizure type, EEG findings, and imaging features that tend to occur together and may give information regarding treatment implications and prognosis. Within the generalized epilepsies, a well-known subgroup, known as the idiopathic primary generalized epilepsies, exists and includes four distinct syndromes: childhood absence epilepsy, juvenile absence epilepsy, juvenile myoclonic epilepsy, and generalized tonic-clonic seizures.

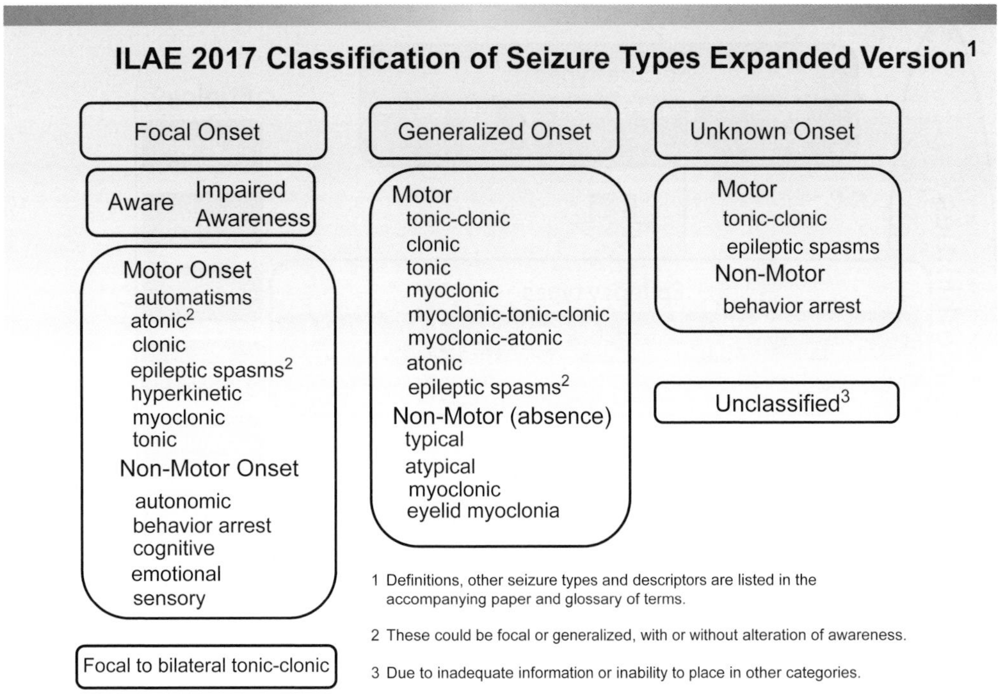

ILAE 2017 Classification of Seizure Types Expanded Version[1]

Focal Onset

Aware | Impaired Awareness

Motor Onset
automatisms
atonic[2]
clonic
epileptic spasms[2]
hyperkinetic
myoclonic
tonic
Non-Motor Onset
autonomic
behavior arrest
cognitive
emotional
sensory

Focal to bilateral tonic-clonic

Generalized Onset

Motor
tonic-clonic
clonic
tonic
myoclonic
myoclonic-tonic-clonic
myoclonic-atonic
atonic
epileptic spasms[2]
Non-Motor (absence)
typical
atypical
myoclonic
eyelid myoclonia

Unknown Onset

Motor
tonic-clonic
epileptic spasms
Non-Motor
behavior arrest

Unclassified[3]

1 Definitions, other seizure types and descriptors are listed in the accompanying paper and glossary of terms.

2 These could be focal or generalized, with or without alteration of awareness.

3 Due to inadequate information or inability to place in other categories.

Figure 1 Classification of seizure types. From Fisher RS, et al: Operational classification of seizure types by the International League Against Epilepsy: Position Paper of the ILAE Commission for Classification and terminology, *Epilepsia* 58:522–530, 2017. *Wylie Journal*: page 525, Figure 2.)

BOX 1	Changes in Seizure Type Classification: 1981–2017

- Change of "partial" to "focal"
- Certain seizures types can be either of focal, generalized, or of unknown onset.
- Seizures of unknown onset may have features that can still be classified.
- Awareness is used as a classifier of focal onset seizures.
- The terms *dyscognitive*, *simple partial*, *complex partial*, *psychic*, and *secondary generalized* were eliminated.
- New focal seizure types include automatisms, autonomic, behavioral arrest, cognitive, emotional, hyperkinetic, sensory, and focal to bilateral-tonic-clonic seizures. Atonic, clonic, epileptic spasms, myoclonic, and tonic seizures can be either focal or generalized.
- New generalized seizure types include absence with eyelid myoclonia, myoclonic absence, myoclonic-tonic-clonic, myoclonic atonic, and epileptic spasms.

From Fisher RS, et al: Operational Classification of seizure types by the International League Against Epilepsy: Position Paper of the ILAE Commision for Classification and Terminology, *Epilepsia* 58:522–530, 2017.

From the moment the patient has been diagnosed with having an epileptic seizure, a cause should be sought. Etiologies include structural etiology (structural abnormality seen on brain MRI that is strongly associated with the development of seizures)—for example, temporal lobe seizures from mesiotemporal sclerosis; genetic etiology (epilepsies with a presumed genetic mutation)—for example, benign familial neonatal epilepsy with mutation in *KNCQ2* or *KNCQ3* (potassium channels); infectious etiology—for example, neurocysticercosis; metabolic etiology—for example, porphyria and pyridoxine-dependent seizures; immune etiology—for example, anti-N-methyl-D-aspartate receptor encephalitis and anti-LGI1 encephalitis; and finally, unknown etiology.

Comorbidities should be considered for every patient with epilepsy at each stage of classification, just as in the case of etiology.

Comorbidities include learning, psychological, and behavioral problems. The term *benign* is replaced by *self-limiting* (likely spontaneous resolution of a syndrome) and *pharmacoresponsive* (the epilepsy syndrome will be controlled with appropriate ASD treatment). This classification is aimed at providing tools for improved diagnosis and understanding of etiology and targeted therapies to the patient's disease.

Diagnosis

The diagnosis of a seizure and epilepsy is largely a clinical one and is highly dependent on the history and physical examination. The clinical history should be obtained from the patient and from a witness. Once the aforementioned information has been obtained, it is analyzed to determine whether indeed the paroxysmal event in question represents a true seizure or a seizure mimicker. If the event of concern represents a seizure, then it is further classified into focal or generalized and into acute symptomatic, a transient phenomenon with lower seizure recurrence, or unprovoked, which confers a higher risk for seizure recurrence and development of epilepsy.

The clinical history is aimed at obtaining a clear description of the prodromal or premonitory state, the preictal state, the ictal state, and the postictal state. The prodromal state occurs hours to days prior to the ictus and is most commonly seen in generalized seizures but may also occur in focal-onset seizures; it consists of behavioral changes, mood swings, fatigue, and changes in sleep patterns. Regarding the preictal period, the patient should be questioned about the presence of warning signs immediately before the seizure onset, also known as auras. An aura is a simple partial seizure or seizure without impaired awareness. An aura points to a focal seizure onset and, according to the description of the aura, we can potentially determine the lobe of onset. For example, a rising gastric sensation and a sensation of déjà vu points to seizure onset in the temporal lobe and visual hallucinations point to onset in the occipital lobe.

At this point the examiner should ask what happened during the event (ictal period). Issues to consider include the level of awareness, the presence of ability to speak, the presence of automatisms (lip smacking, ipsilateral hand automatisms, and contralateral dystonia point to ipsilateral temporal lobe seizures), other behavior, and the duration of the event (true seizures

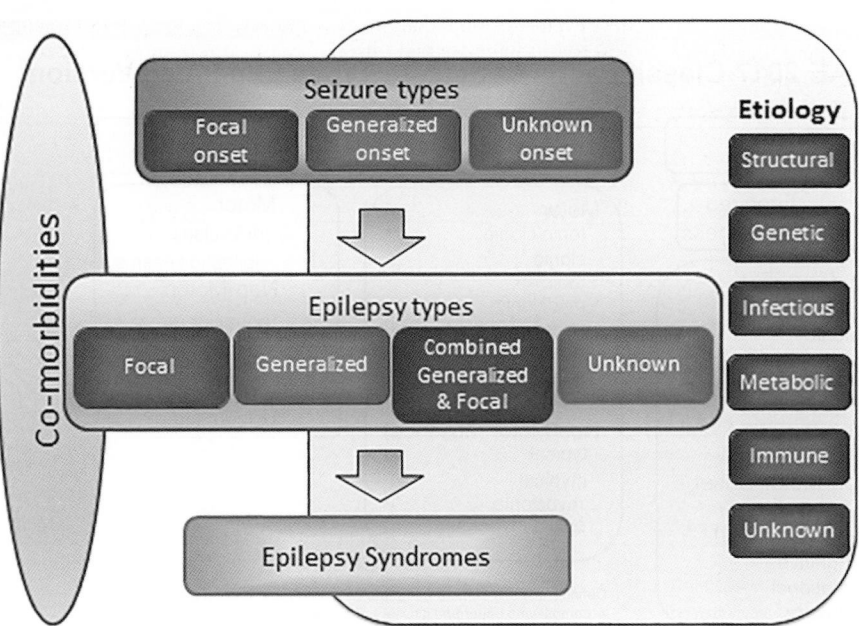

Figure 2 Classification of the epilepsies. From Scheffer IE, et al: ILAE Classification of the Epilepsies: Position paper of the ILAE Commission for Classification and Terminology, *Epilepsia* 58:512–521, 2017. *Wylie Journal*: page 515, Figure 1.

usually last less than 2 minutes, whereas nonepileptic events are usually of longer duration).

The next focus should be on what happened after the event (in the postictal period): whether there was any confusion or fatigue, how long it took the patient to come back to baseline, presence of tongue bites and muscle aches, and urinary incontinence (commonly seen with true seizures). One should also ask about triggers, including sleep deprivation, stress, drug intake, and alcohol withdrawal.

Other information to obtain would include the presence of diurnal variations. For example, frontal lobe seizures usually occur at night, and generalized tonic-clonic and myoclonic seizures most often occur in the morning. If more than one seizure occurs, one should ask about the maximum seizure-free period, seizure frequency (to assess for severity of disease), and response to treatment as well as number of visits to the hospital or the emergency department (ED) and the presence of falls or injuries during seizures to assess for risks and degree of seizure control.

The medical history should include questions regarding the patient's prenatal history and postnatal development to assess for remote symptomatic causes of seizures, history of febrile seizures, history of central nervous system (CNS) lesions (tumors, stroke) and infections, history of brain trauma specifically with associated penetrating injuries with intraparenchymal blood, skull fractures, prolonged loss of consciousness, and family history of epilepsy.

The social history should include questions regarding the patient's level of education and employment. Patients with a higher level of education will usually have a better understanding of their diagnosis and prognosis. Employment is important, because patients at higher risk for the development of subsequent seizures have a higher risk of injury if they work in high-risk jobs (e.g., in construction or other jobs involving the handling of heavy machinery). Patients with altered awareness during a seizure should not be driving. Clinicians should be familiar with the specific state laws regarding driving by patients with seizures and epilepsy. Use of drugs and alcohol is a risk factor for the development of a first provoked seizure, and some illegal drugs may exacerbate or cause seizures. Patients should be discouraged from using illegal drugs and from the excessive intake of alcohol. Review of current medications or newly started medications should be performed to determine whether any can precipitate seizures (e.g., tramadol [Ultram], bupropion [Wellbutrin]).

After the medical history has been obtained, a thorough physical and neurologic examination should be performed. The clinician should look for skin abnormalities such as neurocutaneous manifestations of diseases (e.g., tuberous sclerosis and neurofibromatosis). Test for muscle strength to rule out subtle weakness or postictal Todd paralysis and also lateral tongue/cheek bites, which are commonly seen in true epileptic seizures; also, bruises, scrapes from falls, burns, and muscle and back pain are commonly seen, as are compression fractures caused by convulsive seizures.

Evaluation of a new-onset seizure should be aimed at determining whether the seizure represents an acute symptomatic seizure, usually a transient phenomenon, or an unprovoked seizure.

If the history and examination point to a probable acute symptomatic seizure, life-threatening conditions should be ruled out (hemorrhage, CNS infection, neoplasms) as soon as possible. Basic laboratory tests should be ordered, including a complete blood count, electrolytes (sodium), blood glucose, liver function tests, and toxicology to rule out drug use. If signs of CNS infection are present (fever, nuchal rigidity), a lumbar puncture may be considered. Emergency neuroimaging (usually hydrochlorothiazide [HCT] in the acute setting) should also be performed. If the patient continues to be confused or to have focal deficits not explained by neuroimaging or is not at baseline 30 to 60 minutes after a seizure, emergency EEG or continuous video EEG monitoring should be performed to look for subclinical seizures. If there is evidence of provoking factors (sleep deprivation, alcohol or drug use), neuroimaging is normal, and the patient is back to baseline, the EEG can be delayed and performed in the outpatient setting. The EEG is important, because some patients with symptomatic seizures can also have epileptiform abnormalities perhaps requiring ASD treatment (alcohol withdrawal seizure with focal interictal epileptiform discharges [IEDs] coming from an area of encephalomalacia due to a fall).

Unprovoked seizures are classified into seizures of unknown etiology and seizures with a preexistent brain lesion (remote symptomatic). If the initial workup points to a probable unprovoked seizure, an MRI with epilepsy protocol (3T MRI with 1- to 3-mm slices and coronal fluid–attenuated inversion recovery sequences) interpreted by a neuroradiologist should be performed to rule out subtle lesions such as cortical dysplasias and mesiotemporal sclerosis, which confer higher risk of development of epilepsy. Also, the EEG is of paramount importance to stratify patients at risk for recurrent seizures. The EEG should be performed with sleep deprivation and with activating procedures and as close as possible to the seizure (within 24 hours) to increase the yield of interictal epileptiform abnormalities. There is a 51% chance of recording epileptiform abnormalities if the EEG is performed within 24 hours after a seizure.

Differential Diagnosis

The diagnosis of a seizure or epilepsy can be challenging. There are many paroxysmal conditions, both psychiatric and organic, that may mimic seizures. Of all the seizure mimickers, psychogenic nonepileptic attacks, also known as psychogenic nonepileptic seizures, are most commonly misdiagnosed as epilepsy. The estimated prevalence of psychogenic nonepileptic attacks is 2 to 33 per 100,000, and most patients are younger females. The clinical history and physical examination usually point to the diagnosis of psychogenic nonepileptic attacks. Red flags include poor control on multiple ASDs with a series of normal EEGs, psychiatric history, unusual triggers such as pain and getting upset, diagnosis of chronic pain syndrome and fibromyalgia, seizures in the outpatient clinic or at a physician visit (presence of an audience), and a never-ending list of symptoms on review of systems. Some of these patients also have a history of sexual, emotional, or physical abuse. The physical examination may reveal give-way weakness and histrionic behavior. The gold standard for the diagnosis of psychogenic nonepileptic events is continuous video EEG monitoring. The combination of atypical semiology and the lack of EEG findings during the paroxysmal event enables a definitive diagnosis. Common behaviors seen during a nonepileptic paroxysmal event include position of convenience, ictal eye closure, retained awareness with bilateral motor features resembling a convulsive event, opisthotonic posturing (arched back), pelvic thrusting, crying/weeping, ictal stuttering, baby talk, side-to-side head movements, pseudo-sleep, irregular out-of-phase motor activity ("like a fish out of water"), gradual onset and termination, prolonged attacks, and stop-and-go phenomena.

Syncope is the second most common paroxysmal event misdiagnosed as seizures. Syncope represents a transient lack of blood flow to the brain. Some features are helpful in differentiating syncope from true seizures; these include prodromal symptoms of general malaise, sweating, dizziness, nausea, palpitations and chest pain, and loss of consciousness with rapid recovery after hitting the ground due to rapid brain reperfusion. The challenging part is the fact that many syncopal events show "convulsive-like" behavior, such as clonic phenomena, making the diagnosis more challenging. Syncopal events are usually shorter than typical convulsive seizures and recovery is faster, with no postictal state and usually no tongue bites or urinary incontinence, a feature commonly seen in true convulsive seizures. The most common type of syncope is vasovagal and is precipitated by some situations such as pain or the sight of blood. The other type is reflex syncope due to micturition, cough, Valsalva maneuver, and/or defecation. The EEG shows a typical progression of generalized slowing followed by suppression without any associated ictal features. Cardiac mechanisms should be explored because some could be life-threatening (e.g., Brugada syndrome or other arrhythmias) and would require immediate intervention.

Migraines, especially complicated migraines, and migraine auras cause positive focal symptoms such as visual auras, sensorimotor phenomena, and weakness, which could potentially mimic partial seizures. The course, however, for migraines is in the range of minutes and of seizures in the range of seconds. A complicated migraine may be misdiagnosed as Todd paralysis. Patients with migraines do have history of headaches and retained awareness during the attack; these two features favor the diagnosis of migraines headaches.

Transient ischemic attacks (TIAs) should not be misdiagnosed as seizures because this entity has marked focal negative phenomena (weakness, numbness, aphasia) whereas seizures present mostly positive phenomena (movement, automatisms, jerking). Positive symptoms rarely occur during TIAs (limb-shaking TIA).

Other conditions that may mimic seizures include hypoglycemia, panic attacks, paroxysmal movement disorders, nonepileptic myoclonus, sleep disorders, parasomnias, cataplexia, and hypnic jerks. It important, therefore, to obtain a detailed history, followed by continuous video-EEG monitoring to try to capture these events for final diagnostic purposes, because it is not uncommon to misdiagnose and mislabel these conditions as epilepsy.

Treatment

Treatment should be initiated only if the potential benefit from treatment exceeds the potential for harm. In general, if the patient has an acute symptomatic seizure, treatment with an ASD is usually not necessary because these seizures are caused by a transient and reversible precipitating factor. In these cases it is best to treat the provoking factor (discontinue an offending drug or treating electrolyte abnormality) or allow sufficient time for the acute provoking etiology to resolve.

If an acute symptomatic cause cannot be found, then it is possible that the patient's seizure represents the first unprovoked seizure of an underlying epileptic disorder. About 150,000 adults will have an unprovoked first seizure. Unprovoked seizures are classified into remote symptomatic seizures (preexistent brain lesion) or seizures of unknown etiology. The rate of seizure recurrence after an unprovoked single seizure ranges from 31% to 56% over 2 to 5 years, and most patients will experience a recurrence in the first year. Seizure recurrence rates are significantly higher if there is a prior brain insult (twofold increase), the EEG shows epileptiform abnormalities, there is an abnormality on neuroimaging, and/or if the seizure occurs out of sleep (nocturnal seizure). If any of the aforementioned factors are present, then ASD treatment may be warranted. If ASD treatment is recommended, then patients should be advised that the risk of side effects will range between 7% and 31%, and these are mild and reversible. Patients should be informed that immediate ASD therapy will reduce the risk of seizure recurrence in the first 2 years after the seizure but will not improve the long-term (>3 years) chance of attaining seizure remission. Also, a single seizure can potentially be treated if the consequences of a recurrent seizure will significantly affect quality of life (e.g., driving, work, or general safety). If two or more unprovoked seizures separated by 24 hours occur or if seizure recurrence risk is equal to 60% or more after a single event, then epilepsy is diagnosed and treatment with an antiseizure medication is strongly recommended.

The goal of therapy is complete seizure freedom with no side effects. Around 50% to 60% of patients become seizure free on a single drug. Unfortunately this is not possible in 30% to 40% of patients, necessitating referral to an epilepsy center for evaluation to rule out seizure imitators, evaluate for the presence of possible surgically remediable syndromes, and to try other options including diets and or devices (a vagal nerve stimulator or responsive nerve stimulator).

When a patient is being started on ASD treatment, one should always choose the medication that is effective for the seizure type or epilepsy syndrome. Of all the available ASDs, there are five that have a "broad spectrum" of action (work for both focal and generalized seizures): valproate (Depakote), lamotrigine (Lamictal), levetiracetam (Keppra), topiramate (Topamax), and zonisamide (Zonegran)[1]. A broad-spectrum ASD may be considered if the type of seizure is unknown. All of the available ASDs are effective against focal seizures except ethosuximide (Zarontin); this medication is effective only in the treatment of typical absence epilepsy.

Next, the side-effect profile, cost, and drug dosing schedule must be considered and adapted to the unique patient characteristics, taking into consideration the patient's comorbidities (Tables 1 and 2). For example, drugs with a once-a-day schedule are optimal for patients with a history of prior poor compliance and for the elderly; in patients taking multiple drugs for other comorbidities, the administration of liver enzyme inducers (phenytoin [Dilantin]) should be avoided. If the patient suffers from obesity, topiramate should be considered. In patients with migraine, either valproate or topiramate should be considered, because these drugs are also effective for migraine prophylaxis.

---

[1] Not FDA approved for this indication.

TABLE 1   Dosage and Side-Effect Profile of Commonly Prescribed Antiseizure Drugs

DRUG	HALF-LIFE	INITIAL DOSAGE	MAINTENANCE DOSAGE	INCREMENT	DOSING SCHEDULE	ADVERSE EFFECTS
Carbamazepine (Tegretol)	12–17 h	200 mg bid	600–1800[3] mg	200 mg/week	tid-qid	Hyponatremia, leukopenia, rare aplastic anemia and hepatitis
Gabapentin (Neurontin)	5–7 h	300 mg qd	1200–3600 mg	300 mg q3–7d	tid	60% removed by hemodialysis, prolonged half-life to 51 h with hemodialysis Dosed 300 mg after hemodialysis
Lacosamide (Vimpat)	13 h	50 mg qd	300–600[3] mg	100 mg/week	bid	Extra 50% of dose after each hemodialysis Can prolong PR interval at high doses
Lamotrigine (Lamictal)	25 h alone; 60 h with VPA	6.25–12.5 mg qd–qod	400 mg alone; 100 mg with VPA	12.5–25 mg	bid q2wk	Life-threatening rash, especially with rapid titration and VPA Titration and maintenance doses vary based on other AEDs
Levetiracetam (Keppra)	7 h	500 mg qd	2000–4000[3] mg	500 mg/week	bid	Decrease dose in chronic renal insufficiency, severe hepatic disease
Oxcarbazepine (Trileptal)	9–11 h	300 mg qd	900–2400 mg	300 mg/week	bid	Hyponatremia Fewer side effects than carbamazepine
Phenobarbital	80–100 h	30–60 mg qd	60–120 mg	30 mg q1–2wk	qd–bid	Sedation, Dupuytren contractures, rebound seizures with rapid tapering
Phenytoin (Dilantin)	22 h	200 mg qd	200–300 mg	100 mg/week	qd–bid	Gum hypertrophy, hirsutism, cerebellar ataxia or atrophy, peripheral neuropathy, rare hypersensitivity, hepatitis
Pregabalin (Lyrica)	6 h	50 mg qd	150–600 mg	50 mg q3–7d	bid–tid	Weight gain
Topiramate (Topamax)	21 h	25 mg qd	200–400 mg	25 mg q1–2wk	bid	Cognitive impairment at >400 mg/day, rare kidney stones, glaucoma, oligohidrosis
Valproic acid (Depakene)	9–16 h	250 mg qd	750–3000 mg	250 mg q3–7d	tid–qid	Tremor, weight gain, alopecia, thrombocytopenia Rare hepatitis and pancreatitis Risk of teratogenesis and neural tube defects
Zonisamide (Zonegran)	63 h	100 mg qd	200–400 mg	100 mg q2 wk	bid	Kidney stones, oligohidrosis, rare blood dyscrasias

[3]Exceeds dosage recommended by the manufacturer.

ASD, Antiseizure drug; *bid*, twice a day; *q*, every; *qd*, every day; *qid*, four times a day; *qod*, every other day; *tid*, three times a day; *VPA*, valproic acid

TABLE 2	Choice of Antiseizure Drug in Special Situations	
SPECIAL SITUATION	**DRUG OF CHOICE**	**COMMENTS**
Partial seizures	Carbamazepine, lamotrigine, levetiracetam, oxcarbazepine, topiramate, gabapentin	
Refractory partial seizures	Lacosamide, pregabalin, zonisamide	Second-line treatment
Generalized epilepsies	Lamotrigine, topiramate, valproic acid[1], zonisamide[1]	Avoid valproic acid in women
Absence seizures	Ethosuximide, lamotrigine[1], valproic acid, topiramate[1]	Ethosuximide is the choice only for pure absence seizures and is insufficient in other associated generalized tonic-clonic or myoclonic seizures
Juvenile myoclonic epilepsy	Valproic acid[1], topiramate[1], lamotrigine[1], zonisamide[1], levetiracetam	Avoid valproic acid in women
Myoclonic seizures	Clonazepam, valproic acid[1], levetiracetam	Lamotrigine occasionally exacerbates myoclonic seizures
Women of childbearing potential	Lamotrigine, topiramate, levetiracetam, oxcarbazepine	Avoid enzyme-inducing agents that alter steroid hormones and OCP levels; use OCPs with ≥50 µg of estrogen; OCPs increase the elimination of lamotrigine Significant increased risk of teratogenicity with valproic acid
Elderly patients	Lamotrigine, gabapentin, levetiracetam, topiramate	Avoid polypharmacy and highly protein-bound ASDs and ASDs with high drug–drug interactions
Depression	Lamotrigine[1], topiramate[1]	
Bipolar disorder	Valproic acid[1], carbamazepine, lamotrigine, topiramate[1]	
Migraine	Valproic acid, topiramate	Consider the choice according to sex, side-effect profile, and seizure type
Chronic pain	Pregabalin[1], gabapentin[1]	
Neuropathic pain	Carbamazepine[1], gabapentin[1], pregabalin	

[1]Not FDA approved for this indication.
ASD, Antiseizure drug; *OCP,* oral contraceptive pill.

It is best to aim for monotherapy whenever possible so as to decrease side effects and drug interactions. Titration should begin with a low dose, which is increased slowly to maximize compliance and decrease side effects. If mild side effects occur, reassure the patient, because most are usually transient.

The ASD dosage is increased until freedom from seizure is achieved or side effects occur. In the latter case, the dosage is decreased to the maximal tolerated dose. In switching from one ASD to another, the medications should always overlap. For example, if a new medication is added, one may consider titrating to the effective dosage before decreasing the failed medication. This approach provides some protection against breakthrough seizures during medication transitions.

If polytherapy is needed, consider ASDs with different mechanism of actions ("rational polytherapy")—for example, a sodium channel blocker with a gamma-aminobutyric acid (GABA) enhancer or synergistic mechanisms (e.g., valproate and lamotrigine). Medications with parenteral formulations and a rapid time to therapeutic onset can be considered for rapid control of seizures if the patient is to be discharged from the ED with an adequate therapeutic dose. Drug levels should be obtained when compliance is an issue. Medication levels are a guide and not a goal. The patient's clinical response to an ASD must always be followed.

In general, it is reasonable to consider ASD discontinuation in patients who have been seizure free for 2 years. The reported relapse rate after stopping ASDs is around 41% or less. Factors associated with higher relapse rates include symptomatic epilepsy, age of onset between 10 and 12 years, cognitive delay, abnormal neurologic examination, juvenile myoclonic epilepsy, symptomatic partial epilepsy, abnormal EEG, family history of seizures or epilepsy, poor initial response to drug, and more than one drug before discontinuation. If epileptiform abnormalities are seen and there is worsening of the EEG (increased EEG abnormalities) during discontinuation, relapse rates are higher. Therefore one may consider performing an EEG before and after AED discontinuation.

Characteristics of New Antiseizure Drugs
Felbamate
Felbamate (Felbatol) is effective in the treatment of multiple seizure types, but because of the occurrence of aplastic anemia and hepatic failure, it was briefly withdrawn from the US market in 1994. It is now available only for patients with intractable seizures in whom other medications have failed and when benefits outweigh the risks. Its mechanism of action is blockade of NMDA receptors, modulation of sodium channels, and blockade of calcium channels. The risk for hepatic failure is 14 of 110,000 patients, and it increases with polytherapy.

Gabapentin
Gabapentin (Neurontin) is similar in structure to GABA but it has no effect on the GABA receptor. It enhances glutamic acid decarboxylase (GAD), thereby increasing levels of GABA. This medication has no drug interactions. It is excreted entirely unchanged in kidneys. Gabapentin is used for the treatment of focal seizures with or without secondary generalization. It is ineffective in myoclonus and primary generalized seizures and also at lower dosages. Dosage should be adjusted in patients with renal disease according to creatinine clearance.

Pregabalin

Pregabalin (Lyrica) is an analogue of GABA but, like gabapentin (Neurontin), has no effect on the GABA receptor. It has no drug interactions and is usually well tolerated. The dosage must be adjusted in patients with renal failure, and 50% removed after hemodialysis. It is used as an adjunct in adult patients with focal epilepsies. Common side effects include dizziness, drowsiness, weight gain, dry mouth, and edema.

Lamotrigine

Lamotrigine (Lamictal) works by sodium channel blockade and inhibits release of glutamate. It is a broad-spectrum drug and is used for the adjunctive treatment of focal-onset seizures with or without secondary generalization, crossover to monotherapy, and in LGS. It is also effective in atypical absence[1], tonic/atonic seizures, and in myoclonic seizures, although it may cause exacerbations in some patients with juvenile myoclonic epilepsy. It is one of the preferred drugs to treat elderly patients and pregnant women because of its good safety and pharmacokinetic profile. Lamotrigine levels should be closely watched and will increase significantly with coadministration of valproate; these two medications cause a synergistic therapeutic effect but can also increase adverse reactions (rash). Lamotrigine can cause a rash (5%) if the drug is titrated too quickly; this rash can potentially progress into a life-threatening condition (Stevens-Johnson syndrome [0.1%]), an effect that is more common in children and when valproate is used concomitantly. If rash occurs, the medication should be stopped immediately. Other common side effects include tremor, insomnia, headaches, ataxia, and somnolence. Pregnancy increases lamotrigine clearance by 50%, necessitating dosage adjustments; therefore lamotrigine levels should be monitored before, during, and after pregnancy and dosage should be adjusted accordingly.

Levetiracetam

Levetiracetam (Keppra) is one of the most widely used ASDs because of its good pharmacokinetics, favorable side-effect profile, and multiple formulations, including parenteral and liquid (ease of administration). It is a "broad-spectrum" drug and has a unique mechanism of action (binds to synaptic vesicle protein 2A-SV2A). It does not induce liver enzymes and therefore does not affect the metabolism of other drugs and does not bind to proteins in plasma. This medication must be dosage-adjusted in patients with renal disease and after hemodialysis (add an extra 500 mg). It is one of the few ASDs that decreases the interictal epileptic burden, the other one being Depakote. It is approved as an adjunctive treatment for (1) primary generalized tonic-clonic seizures in adults and children 6 years of age and older with idiopathic generalized epilepsy, (2) focal onset seizures in adults and children 4 years of age and older, and (3) myoclonic seizures in adults and adolescents 12 years of age and older with juvenile myoclonic epilepsy. It is also used off label for prophylaxis in patients after traumatic brain injury and in status epilepticus. Common adverse effects include behavioral changes (avoid in patients with psychiatric conditions), somnolence, asthenia, headache, dizziness, and flulike symptoms. It does not cause any serious idiosyncratic reactions and is safe for the elderly and probably safe to take during pregnancy. Blood levels should be obtained during pregnancy because clearance is then increased, necessitating dosage adjustments.

Brivaracetam

Breviracetam (Briviact) is a chemical analog of levetiracetam, with a similar mechanism of action but a higher affinity (20-fold) for the SV2A receptor. It exhibits linear kinetics with a good side-effect profile, similar to levetiracetam. It is indicated as an adjunctive treatment of focal-onset seizures with or without secondary generalization in adults and children aged 16 years of age and older. It does not have added therapeutic benefit if coadministered with levetiracetam. It may increase serum concentrations of carbamazepine epoxide and phenytoin.

Oxcarbazepine

Oxcarbazepine (Trileptal) is an analogue of carbamazepine but without the toxic epoxide. Thus it is better tolerated than carbamazepine (Tegretol). It is metabolized to a 10-monohydroxy metabolite (MHD), which confers its pharmacologic effect. It is used as monotherapy or adjunctive therapy in focal epilepsies in adults and as monotherapy in the treatment of focal epilepsies in children 4 years of age and older and as adjunctive in children 2 years of age and older. It may exacerbate myoclonic seizures and absence seizures. It interacts with oral contraceptive pills (OCPs), thereby reducing its efficacy. Hyponatremia is rare in children but may be higher in elderly populations. Other side effects include dizziness, fatigue, and headache, which are dose dependent. Patient who develop rash with carbamazepine (Tegretol) may develop rash if treated with oxcarbazepine (Trileptal) because of cross-reactivity.

Tiagabine

Tiagabine (Gabitril) works by reversible inhibition of the GABA-transporter-1, thereby increasing the availability of GABA in the synaptic cleft. It is approved as an add-on medication in the treatment of refractory focal-onset seizures. It can worsen absence seizures and cause status epilepticus in patients with primary generalized epilepsy. Common side effects include tremor, nervousness, dizziness, abdominal pain, diarrhea, and emotional lability.

Topiramate

Topiramate (Topamax) is a broad-spectrum ASD with multiple mechanisms of action. It works by inhibiting sodium conductance and weakly carbonic anhydrase, blocks the alpha-amino-3-hydroxy-5-methyl-4isoxazolepropionic acid (AMPA) glutamate receptor, and enhances GABA. It is approved for the treatment of focal-onset seizures or primary generalized epilepsy as an add-on and in the treatment of LGS. Enzyme inducers (e.g., phenytoin) decrease levels of topiramate by 50%. This medication will need dosage adjustments in patients with renal failure. Topiramate (Topamax) reduces the levels of OCPs, thereby decreasing its effectiveness. Common side effects include word finding difficulties, weight loss (decreased appetite), paresthesias in fingers and mouth, kidney stones, and anhidrosis due to the carbonic-anhydrase effect of this drug, acute myopia in closed-angle glaucoma, ataxia, and tiredness. Usually doses greater than 400 mg are poorly tolerated.

Zonisamide

Zonisamide (Zonegran) is a "broad-spectrum" ASD used in the treatment of focal epilepsy with or without secondary generalization. It is also effective in the treatment of myoclonus in juvenile myoclonic epilepsy (JME)[1] and absence seizures (T-type calcium channel blockade). This ASD has a structure similar to that of the sulfonamides; therefore it is contraindicated in patients with allergies to these antibiotics. It has a long-half life (>60 hours); therefore it can be taken once a day, which increases compliance. The major mechanism of action is by the blockade of sodium channels; it also works on T-type calcium channels and provides weak inhibition of carbonic anhydrase. Enzyme inducers and valproate (Depakote) decrease the half-life. The most common adverse reactions include anorexia with associated weight loss, headache, mental slowing, confusion, ataxia, dizziness, kidney stones (1%) oligohidrosis, and paresthesias (carbonic anhydrase inhibition).

---

[1] Not FDA approved for this indication.

[1] Not FDA approved for this indication.

Vigabatrin

Vigabatrin (Sabril) is a structural analogue of GABA and binds irreversibly to the GABA-T (GABA transaminase), thereby increasing GABA concentrations in the brain. It is indicated for the treatment of epileptic spasms in tuberous sclerosis and in refractory focal-onset epilepsies. It may exacerbate absence seizures and myoclonic seizures and, similarly to tiagabine, may cause generalized spike-and-wave status epilepticus in patients with absence seizures or primary generalized epilepsy. This ASD causes visual field defects (nasal constriction and concentric constriction with preserved central vision), which may be irreversible. Other side effects include fatigue, dizziness, headache, tremor, and double vision.

Rufinamide

Rufinamide's (Banzel's) mechanism of action is probable modulation of sodium channels (prolongation of inactive state of the channel). It is indicated as adjunctive treatment of seizures associated with LGS in both children and adults.

Lacosamide

Lacosamide (Vimpat) has a novel mechanism of action in enhancing the slow inactivation of voltage-gated sodium channels. It is approved for the adjunctive treatment and conversion to monotherapy and monotherapy treatment of focal-onset epilepsies. It is also used off label for the treatment of status epilepticus in the intensive care unit because it is available in an intravenous formulation. This medication does not have significant drug interactions.

Clobazam

Clobazam (Onfi) is a benzodiazepine with a 1,5 substitution instead of the common 1,4 substitution; therefore it has less anxiolytic and sedative effects. It works by binding to the GABA-A receptor. It is approved for the adjunctive treatment of LGS and may also be effective in the treatment of primary or focal seizures with secondary generalized seizures[1] as well as in catamenial epilepsy[1]. It has no significant clinical interactions. Side effects include sedation, dizziness, ataxia, and weakness. No idiosyncratic reactions have been identified.

Perampanel

Perampanel (Fycompa) is a noncompetitive AMPA-receptor antagonist and is indicated in the adjunctive treatment of focal-onset seizures with or without secondary generalization and in primary generalized seizures in adults and adolescents 12 years of age and over. The recommended dose is 8 to 12 mg/day for focal seizures and 8 mg/day for primary generalized seizures. This medication has a black box warning because of potentially severe psychiatric and behavioral reactions (aggressiveness, suicidality, homicidal threats and ideations, and irritability). Common adverse effects include somnolence, headache, dizziness, and fatigue.

Eslicarbazepine

Eslicarbazepine (Aptiom) is a prodrug to s-licarbazepine with a mechanism of action similar to that of oxcarbazepine (Trileptal) sodium channel blockade. It is approved as monotherapy or adjunctive therapy for the treatment of focal-onset seizures. Common adverse effects include dizziness, nausea, diplopia, and headache.

Cenobamate

Cenobamate (Xcopri) reduces repetitive neuronal firing by inhibiting voltage-gated sodium currents. It is also an allosteric modulator of the alpha-aminobutytic acid ion channel. This medication was approved by the FDA as an adjunct or monotherapy for the treatment of focal onset seizures in adults. The recommended initial dosage is 12.5 mg once daily and titrated to the recommended maintenance dose of 200 mg daily. The most common adverse effects seen with this medication are somnolence, dizziness, fatigue, diplopia, and headaches. Avoid administration in patients with familial short QT syndrome and use caution when coadministering with drugs that shorten the QT interval.

Cannabidiol

Cannabidiol (EPIDIOLEX) is the first prescription pharmaceutical formulation of purified CBD oil that was approved for use by the US Food and Drug Administration (FDA) on June 25, 2018, for the treatment of seizures associated with Lennox-Gastaut and Dravet syndromes in patients 2 years of age or older.

The most common side effects of this drug include increase in liver enzymes, especially when used in conjunction with valproate or valpraoate and clobazam; others are decreased appetite, diarrhea, rash, tiredness, rash, sleepiness, and infections.

Special Populations

Women

Epilepsy is one of the most common conditions occurring in women of reproductive age (1.1 million). Women of reproductive age with epilepsy who are taking ASDs should be counseled on the possibility of teratogenicity from ASD therapy and potential interaction with contraception. Some ASDs (enzyme inducers) affect OCPs, leading to decreased effectiveness and unwanted pregnancies. These ASDs are phenobarbital, phenytoin, carbamazepine, oxcarbazepine, eslicarbazepine, felbamate, topiramate (at higher doses >200 mg/day), lamotrigine (doses >300 mg/day), primidone, rufinamide, and clobazam. OCPs can reduce the levels of lamotrigine, leading to breakthrough seizures. In patients taking these ASDs, a second barrier method versus changing to a non–enzyme inducing ASD is recommended. Seizures during pregnancy will remain the same or decrease, but around 15% to 30% of such patients will have an increase in seizure frequency. Most (84% to 92%) women with epilepsy who were seizure free 9 months before pregnancy will remain free of seizures during the pregnancy. Blood levels of lamotrigine, phenytoin, and, to a lesser extent, carbamazepine and possibly levetiracetam and the active oxacarbazepine metabolite, 10-hydroxycarbazepine (MHD), will decrease during pregnancy because of increased clearance; therefore these ASD levels should be monitored and medication dosages adjusted as needed. The risk of seizures to the fetus (especially convulsive seizures) from MHD is higher than the risk to the fetus from ASDs. More than 90% of female patients with epilepsy will deliver a normal baby. The rates of congenital malformations in women with epilepsy taking ASDs is around 4% to 6% (double those of the general population) but remain low. Risk of malformations increases with polytherapy and with higher dosages of ASDs. Valproate/valproic acid is the ASD that carries the highest risk for teratogenicity (6% to 10%), mostly in the form of neural tube defects. It also produces long-term cognitive problems, with a reduction in the child's IQ when the mother has taken valproate (Depakote) during pregnancy. Therefore valproic acid is contraindicated and should not be used as a first-line treatment in women of childbearing potential. Women with epilepsy and of childbearing potential should be supplemented with folic acid at a dose of 0.4 mg/day to decrease the risk of congenital malformations should they become pregnant. Breastfeeding is an important concern in the postpartum period in women taking ASDs. Even though some ASDs (e.g., primidone and levetiracetam) transfer into breast milk, breastfeeding is encouraged. The baby should be monitored for increased sedation if the mother is taking two ASDs.

Elderly Patients

The current world population is aging, and the risk for epilepsy increases dramatically after the age of 65. Recognition of seizures in this group may be more complicated because

---

[1] Not FDA approved for this indication.

the presentation may be atypical. Also, many other conditions may mimic seizures in the elderly, making such a diagnosis a challenging task. The most common seizure type in the elderly is the complex partial seizure, which presents with confusion, staring, change in mental status, and unresponsiveness. The most common cause of epilepsy in this group is cerebrovascular disease. Other conditions that may cause epilepsy include neurodegenerative conditions (Alzheimer disease), head trauma, and brain tumors. When elderly patients are being treated, the pharmacokinetic and pharmacodynamic properties of medications should be considered. Older people have reductions in protein binding, renal elimination, and hepatic metabolism, thereby conferring a higher risk for idiosyncratic reactions and altered kinetics. Gabapentin, lamotrigine, levetiracetam, pregabalin, and oxcarbazepine are usually well tolerated and recommended as first-line treatments in this patient population. AEDs with hepatic enzyme–inducing mechanisms are not recommended in elderly patients because of the potential for interactions with other drugs. Fortunately seizures in this population are easy to control, and monotherapy is usually effective.

Drug-Resistant Epilepsy

Drug-resistant epilepsy (DRE) is defined as the failure of adequate trials of two tolerated, appropriately chosen and used ASDs used in monotherapy or polytherapy to achieve sustained freedom from seizures. DRE affects one-third of patient's living with epilepsy.

These patients should be referred to an epilepsy center for further management, including evaluation by an epileptologist, who will perform a detailed clinical and physical examination and order further diagnostic tests including video EEG monitoring to record the patient's events for final diagnostic purposes and for the evaluation for possible epilepsy surgery. Surgical resection of the epilepsy focus is the only available treatment to cure epilepsy. Seizure freedom rates after temporal lobectomy for mesiotemporal sclerosis is in the range of 70% to 90% and of 40% to 70% in neocortical resections. In patients who are not suitable candidates for epilepsy surgery, dietary treatment or neuromodulation is recommended. Dietary options include the ketogenic diet, the modified Atkins diet, and the low glycemic index diet.

These diets can be used as an add-on therapy in combination with ASDs and devices (vagus nerve stimulator [VNS], responsive neurostimulation system [RNS], and deep brain stimulation [DBS]). The diets have similar seizure-reduction rates (around 50%) in half of these patients. The low glycemic index diet is better tolerated and less restrictive than the modified Atkins diet and the classic ketogenic diet.

Devices approved for the treatment of DRE in the United States include the VNS, RNS, and DBS.

The VNS works by delivering an intermittent mild current to the left vagus nerve. The mechanism of action is unknown but believed to include alterations in the reticular activating system, the central autonomic network, the limbic system, and the diffuse noradrenergic projection system. With long-term use, this device provides greater than 50% seizure reduction in about 50% to 60% of patients, with around 8% becoming seizure free after 2 years. The new SenTiva generator combines traditional VNS therapy with seizure-detection technology via changes in cardiac rhythms.

The responsive neurostimulation system or RNS therapy (Neuropace) was approved by the FDA in 2013 for the treatment of refractory focal-onset seizures. This device continuously monitors and detects abnormal electrical activity that can lead to a seizure and then delivers electrical stimulation to the area of seizure generation to try to abort the seizure. It has two leads, and either subdural or depth electrodes or a combination of both can be used and placed close to or over the epileptogenic zone. These leads are connected to the generator, which is seated on the skull. Treatment with the RNS system is recommended in patients who are not amenable to surgery and have multifocal epilepsy with no more than two discrete seizure onset zones. The median seizure reduction at 5 years was greater than 65%, with 15% of patients achieving seizure freedom.

The DBS was approved by the FDA in 2018 as adjunctive for the treatment of patients with drug-resistant focal onset epilepsy who are 18 years of age or older. This device is particularly useful if the seizure focus is difficult to localize to one or two brain regions. Leads are placed in the anterior nucleus of the thalamus for delivery of electrical stimulation. The Stimulation of the Anterior Nuclei of the Thalamus for Epilepsy (SANTE) trial randomized 110 patients to receive active stimulation vs. sham stimulation; at the end of 5 years, a median reduction in seizures of 69% from baseline was observed and both seizure severity and quality of life improved significantly.

References

Ahmed NS, Spencer SS: An approach to the evaluation of a patient for seizures and epilepsy, *Wisc Med J* 103(1):49–55, 2004.

Benbadis S: The differential diagnosis of epilepsy: a critical review, *Epilepsy Behav* 15:15–21, 2009.

Britton JW: Antiepileptic drug therapy: when to start, when to stop, *Continuum Lifelong Learning Neurol* 16:105–120, 2010.

Fisher RS, Acevedo C, Arzimanaglou, et al: ILAE official report: a practical clinical definition of epilepsy, *Epilepsia* 55:475–482, 2014.

Fisher RS, Cross JH, French JA, et al: Operational classification of seizure types by the international league against epilepsy: position paper of the ILAE commission for classification and terminology, *Epilepsia* 58:522–530, 2017.

Gavvala JR, Schuele SU: New-onset seizure in adults and adolescent: a review, *JAMA* 36:2657–2668, 2016.

Harden CL, Meador KJ, Pennell PB, et al: Management issues for women with epilepsy—focus on pregnancy (an evidence- based review): II. Teratogenesis and perinatal outcomes: Report of the quality standards subcommittee and therapeutics and technology subcommittee of the american academy of neurology and the American epilepsy society, *Epilepsia* 50:1237–1246, 2009.

Harden CL, Pennell PB, Koppel BS, et al: Management issues for women with epilepsy—focus on pregnancy (an evidence- based review): III. Vitamin K, folic acid, blood levels, and breast-feeding: Report of the Quality Standards Subcommittee and therapeutics and technology assessment subcommittee of the American academy of neurology and the american epilepsy society, *Epilepsia* 50:1247–1255, 2009.

Hesdorffer DC, Logroscino G, Benn EKT, et al: Estimating risk for developing epilepsy: a population-based study in Rochester, Minnesota, *Neurology* 76:23–27, 2011.

Krumholz A, Wiebe S, Gronseth G, et al: Practice parameter: evaluating an apparent unprovoked first seizure in adults (an evidence-based review): Report of the quality standards subcommittee of the American Academy of Neurology and the American Epilepsy Society, *Neurology* 69:1996–2007, 2007.

Kwan P, Arzimanoglou A, Berg AT, et al: Definition of drug resistant epilepsy: consensus proposal by the ad hoc Task Force of the ILAE Commission of Therapeutic Strategies, *Epilepsia* 51(6):1069–1077, 2010.

Kwan P, Brodie MJ: Early identification of refractory epilepsy, *N Engla J Med* 342(5):314–319, 2000.

Kwan P, Brodie MJ: Effectiveness of first antiepileptic drug, *Epilepsia* 42(10):1255–1260, 2001.

Ochoa JG: Antiepileptic Drugs. Available at https://emedicine.medscape.com/article/1187334-overview. (Accessed March 22, 2018).

Salanova V, et al: Long-term efficacy and safety of thalamic stimulation for drug resistant partial epilepsy, *Neurology* 84(10):1017–1025, 2015.

Scheffer IE, Berkovic S, Capovilla G, et al: ILAE classification of the epilepsies: Position Paper of the ILAE Commission for Classification and Terminology, *Epilepsia* 58:512–521, 2017.

SLEEP DISORDERS

Method of
Meghna P. Mansukhani, MD; Bhanu Prakash Kolla, MD, MRCPsych; and Erik Kent St. Louis, MD, MS

Sleep is a universal biological imperative for all mammals. Sleep deprivation and sleep disorders are frequent and underappreciated determinants of health status. Sleep is essential for survival, and sleep loss and sleep disorders are associated with major health problems, including cardiovascular, metabolic, neuropsychiatric, and neoplastic disorders, as well as neurobehavioral-associated accidents and risks. Healthy sleep must be regarded along with nutrition and exercise as key pillars for good health.

Recent evidence has suggested that a chief purpose of sleep may be to maintain cerebral metabolic homeostasis, clearing waste products that accumulate during wakefulness such as beta-amyloid, a protein known to abnormally accumulate in Alzheimer's disease. Insufficient sleep quantity appears to be associated with a variety of health problems and may contribute to mortality and dementia risk. Total sleep deprivation, as well as selective deprivation of nonrapid eye movement (NREM) or rapid eye movement (REM) sleep, may be lethal in laboratory animals. Adequate sleep quality is similarly necessary to ensure optimal daytime functioning because basic vigilance, attention and cognitive performance, and overall quality of life are each substantially eroded by disordered sleep, and insufficient sleep and sleep-disordered breathing (SDB) pose significant health hazards. Unfortunately, insufficient sleep quantity and quality is a widespread public health crisis in children and adults worldwide in the developed world, and primary sleep disorders are a highly prevalent cause of morbidity, an important contributor to mortality, and a public health hazard that raises risk for motor vehicle collisions and catastrophic occupational injuries and accidents.

The clinical specialty of sleep medicine initially emerged during the 1970s and 1980s, surrounding growing clinical application of diagnostic polysomnography (PSG). While the main diagnostic use remains evaluation and initial treatment for SDB, PSG and related techniques have tremendous utility for the evaluation of selected patients with nocturnal events, periodic limb movement disorder (PLMD), narcolepsy and related primary central nervous system (CNS) hypersomnias.

In this chapter, we review the classification of common sleep disorders, a practical bedside approach toward interviewing and examining patients with sleep problems, advantages and limitations of diagnostic implements within the sleep laboratory, and summarize diagnostic and therapeutic approaches to common sleep disorders.

The International Classification of Sleep Disorders

The International Classification of Sleep Disorders (ICSD) provides a common nomenclature and taxonomy for disorders of sleep for clinicians and researchers alike. The most current ICSD, ICSD-3, divides sleep disorders into six distinct categories. The ICSD-3 nomenclature is shown in Box 1, and the most common sleep complaints and disorders are presented and discussed in detail throughout this chapter.

Clinical Approach to the Sleep Medicine Patient: The Interview and Examination

The three most common clinical presenting sleep-related complaints are hypersomnia, insomnia, and unusual behaviors or events at night (parasomnias). Hypersomnia, which is excessive sleepiness during waking hours, is often multifactorial and may be related to insufficient sleep quantity, quality, or timing; SDB; sedating medications; or certain medical, psychiatric, or neurologic conditions. Insomnia may be regarded as a problem in initiating or maintaining sleep under conditions that are normally conducive to sleep. Parasomnias are unusual behaviors that are often dangerous to the patient or bed partner during sleep.

Insomnia is a subjective complaint. To some patients it is not at all bothersome to require 20 to 30 minutes to fall asleep, while to others it seems very wrong. While insomnia is fundamentally a subjective symptom, the manifestations follow common patterns. Sleep latency, the time taken to fall asleep, varies significantly, but initial sleep latency longer than 30 minutes may be considered prolonged, once proper sleep-conductive conditions have been established (lights off, dark and quiet sleep environment without distracting stimuli). There is also significant variation in what degree of subjective sleep disruption reflects sleep-maintenance insomnia, as normal individuals may briefly awaken as often as 10 to 15 times each hour, with most such arousals being below the threshold of conscious awareness. Multiple nocturnal awakenings that are disturbing to the patient, especially when there is difficulty reinitiating sleep and prolonged wake after sleep-onset time, may be regarded as sleep-maintenance insomnia. Patients admitting to insomnia should be asked to estimate what amount of their problem is ascribable to an active mind or worries, restless legs, or body pain. Disturbing influences in the sleep environment such as the ambient light, temperature, and noise conditions in the bedroom should be sought. A precise diagnosis is not possible without detailed knowledge of sleep and wake behavior over the entire circadian cycle during a more protracted time, such as 1 to 2 weeks. A sleep diary can be very helpful in gaining needed insights for diagnosis. Increasingly, helpful information about timing and duration of sleep may be logged in applications for personal mobile computing devices.

The patient and physician may at times have difficulty differentiating between hypersomnia and complaints of fatigue (a sense of lacking enough energy to carry out usual daily activities, without the tendency toward dozing or nodding off inadvertently). A quick, incisive bedside test that helps distinguish between hypersomnia and fatigue is the Epworth Sleepiness Scale (ESS), a short questionnaire asking the patient his or her likelihood of dozing inadvertently during usual permissive daytime sedentary settings including reading, watching television, or traveling in a car. An online version is available at http://www.stanford.edu/~dement/epworth.html. Scores over 10 are considered abnormal and indicative of a possible underlying primary sleep disorder and suggest the need for further evaluation. Complaints of hypersomnia must be placed into the context of the sleep history with particular emphasis on the quantity, timing, and quality of sleep.

Patients may also present with complaints of disturbing or unusual activities during sleep (parasomnias). Key diagnostic points in determining the diagnosis for parasomnias include their onset, duration, frequency, time of night, stereotypy, injuries sustained, and whether there is any further behavioral change following the parasomnia episode.

Collateral history obtained from a bed partner may be particularly instructive. Patients should be asked whether they are reported to snore, whether the snoring is intermittent or constant, and if the snoring volume is related to sleeping in a supine position. Disruptive snoring loud enough to be heard outside a closed bedroom door, or witnessed stop-breathing episodes indicating apneas or self-awareness of arousals related to a snort or gasp, are particularly suggestive symptoms of obstructive sleep apnea (OSA). Symptoms such as morning dry mouth and sore throat, frequent morning headaches, or heartburn may indicate a higher likelihood of significant SDB. Patients should be asked about awareness of restless legs symptoms or movements during sleep, and whether they have been told of peculiar sleep-related behaviors or evidence of acting out their dreams, yelling or thrashing in sleep, or exhibiting sleep walking or other amnestic behaviors during sleep.

In addition to a detailed sleep history, taking a thorough general medical history is important because sleep disorders are frequently tightly linked to other diseases. OSA is closely associated with hypertension, coronary artery disease, cerebrovascular disease, atrial fibrillation, obesity, and the metabolic syndrome. Congestive heart failure, even when well compensated, is frequently associated with central sleep apnea syndrome. Restless

BOX 1   The International Classification of Sleep Disorders, 3rd Edition (ICSD-3)

Insomnia
- Chronic insomnia disorder
- Short-term insomnia disorder
- Other insomnia disorder
  Isolated symptoms and normal variants
- Excessive time in bed
- Short sleeper

Sleep-Related Breathing Disorders
The continuum of obstructive sleep-disordered breathing: snoring, Upper-airway resistance syndrome, and obstructive sleep apnea (OSA)

Obstructive sleep apnea (OSA) disorders
- OSA, adult
- OSA, pediatric

Central sleep apnea syndromes
- Central sleep apnea with Cheyne-Stokes breathing
- Central apnea due to medical disorder without Cheyne-Stokes breathing
- Central sleep apnea due to high altitude periodic breathing
- Central sleep apnea due to a medication or substance
- Primary central sleep apnea
- Primary central sleep apnea of infancy
- Primary central sleep apnea of prematurity
- Treatment-emergent central sleep apnea

Sleep-related hypoventilation disorders
- Obesity hypoventilation syndrome
- Congenital central alveolar hypoventilation syndrome
- Late-onset central hypoventilation with hypothalamic dysfunction
- Idiopathic central alveolar hypoventilation
- Sleep-related hypoventilation due to a medication or substance
- Sleep-related hypoventilation due to a medical disorder
- Sleep-related hypoxemia disorder
  Isolated symptoms and normal variants
- Snoring
- Catathrenia

Central Disorders of Hypersomnolence
- Narcolepsy Type I
- Narcolepsy Type II
- Idiopathic hypersomnia
- Kleine-Levin syndrome
- Hypersomnia due to a medical disorder
- Hypersomnia due to a medication or substance
- Hypersomnia associated with a psychiatric disorder
- Insufficient sleep syndrome
  Isolated symptoms and normal variants
- Long sleeper

Circadian Rhythm Sleep-Wake Disorders
- Delayed sleep-wake phase disorder
- Advanced sleep-wake phase disorder
- Irregular sleep-wake rhythm disorder
- Non-24-hour sleep-wake rhythm disorder
- Shift work disorder
- Jet lag disorder
- Circadian rhythm sleep-wake disorder not otherwise specified

Parasomnias
NREM-related parasomnias
- Disorders of arousal (from NREM sleep)
- Confusional arousals
- Sleepwalking
- Sleep terrors
- Sleep-related eating disorder

REM-related parasomnias
- REM sleep behavior disorder
- Recurrent isolated sleep paralysis
- Nightmare disorder

Other parasomnias
- Exploding head syndrome
- Sleep-related hallucinations
- Sleep enuresis
- Parasomnia due to a medical disorder
- Parasomnia due to a medication or substance
- Parasomnia, unspecified
  Isolated symptoms and normal variants
- Sleep talking

Sleep-Related Movement Disorders
- Restless legs syndrome
- Periodic limb movement disorder
- Sleep-related leg cramps
- Sleep-related bruxism
- Sleep-related rhythmic movement disorder
- Benign sleep myoclonus of infancy
- Propriospinal myoclonus at sleep onset
- Sleep-related movement disorder due to a medical disorder
- Sleep-related movement disorder due to a medication or substance
- Sleep-related movement disorder, unspecified

Isolated symptoms and normal variants
- Excessive fragmentary myoclonus
- Hypnagogic foot tremor and alternating leg muscle activation
- Sleep starts (hypnic jerks)

Other Sleep Disorders
- Fatal familial insomnia
- Sleep-related epilepsy
- Sleep-related headaches
- Sleep-related laryngospasm
- Sleep-related gastroesophageal reflux
- Sleep-related myocardial ischemia

Abbreviations: CNS = central nervous system; NREM = non–rapid eye movement [sleep]; REM = rapid eye movement [sleep].

legs syndrome and periodic limb movements in sleep (PLMS) are more common in patients with systemic iron deficiency or renal impairment, or in those with spinal cord or peripheral nerve pathologies. Hypoventilation is more prevalent in patients with neuromuscular disease; advanced obstructive lung disease; kyphosis; and in traumatic, vascular, neoplastic, or degenerative disorders that affect the medullary centers of the brain. Various genetic syndromes such as trisomy-21 produce craniofacial abnormalities predisposing to OSA due to anatomic narrowing of the upper airway.

Physical examination in sleep medicine focuses on signs indicating predisposition or associated sequelae of SDB. Careful inspection of the oropharynx and nares is particularly important because significant oropharyngeal narrowing is the chief anatomic substrate for obstructive SDB, while nasal septal deviation or other nasal obstruction, in addition to a thickened neck and overweight body habitus, may also contribute toward sleep apnea. Careful inspection for signs of neuromuscular disease, such as weakness of cervical flexor or extensor muscles, fasciculations or thoracoabdominal paradox, may help detect the underlying cause for sleep-related hypoventilation. Elevated blood pressure, a cardiac gallop, wet rales, and peripheral edema may be present as signs of systemic hypertension, heart failure, or cor pulmonale associated with untreated SDB.

Diagnostic Tools in the Sleep Laboratory
Polysomnography
Laboratory polysomnography (PSG) is the "gold standard" for formal assessment of suspected SDB, hypersomnia, or parasomnias. PSG is a diagnostic test most often performed in a sleep laboratory; attended by trained technicians; and combining evaluation of sleep, breathing, and movement. During PSG, several polygraphic physiologic variables are analyzed, including electroencephalography (EEG) as well as chin electromyography (EMG) to allow determination of sleep staging, limb EMG leads to analyze periodic leg movements that may disrupt sleep, oronasal airflow measured by a thermistor and nasal pressure sensors, electrocardiography, and respiratory effort measured by inductance plethysmography or piezocrystal monitors. Body position is also analyzed to delineate effects of sleeping position on breathing.

Each 30-second epoch of the PSG is subsequently scored by a sleep technologist as either wake, NREM sleep (N1 or N2 light NREM, or N3 slow wave sleep), or REM sleep according to well-defined guidelines. Sleep architecture, or the composition of sleep by different stages, varies greatly by age, but in middle-aged adults is approximately 60% to 75% N1-N2, 10% to 20% N3, and 15% to 25% REM sleep. Children usually have higher, and elderly individuals have lower, percentages of N3 and REM. Arousals from sleep and their mechanisms, whether due to breathing, movement, or spontaneous causes, are determined. Accordingly, a precise determination of the duration of a patient's total sleep time, sleep efficiency (total time spent asleep divided by time in bed), and disrupting influences on sleep, such as abnormal respiration or movement, may be determined. The effects of confounding medications and medical disorders on sleep architecture, such as selective-serotonin reuptake inhibitors (SSRI) that suppress and delay REM sleep, or benzodiazepines that reduce the N3 and REM amounts and increase sleep stage shifting leading to heightened light NREM N1 and N2, must also be considered.

Attended PSG is advantageous because it allows precise measurement of sleep and relevant cardiorespiratory and neurologic behaviors and allows intervention with therapeutic positive airway pressure (PAP) trials if indicated. Disadvantages of PSG include patient inconvenience, a foreign sleep environment, and expenses due to highly trained personnel and technology. For those patients whose disease severity is difficult to predict, or who may have other complicating medical illnesses that would render interpretation of an out-of-center cardiopulmonary sleep test inaccurate (such as those with significant cardiopulmonary or neurologic diseases), or those who may require noncontinuous PAP modalities, or for those with parasomnia symptoms, attended PSG and treatment design is needed. Split-night PSG remains a cost-effective strategy for many patients.

PSG is currently the only way to actually measure sleep; although the sleep state is currently defined by the variables measured in PSG (EEG, EMG, and EOG), the science of sleep medicine may develop other ways of characterizing the sleep state that are more convenient, precise, and correlate even better with health and disease.

Home Sleep Apnea Testing
PSG is comprehensive, but for patients with characteristic clinical presentations for OSA syndrome, it is often possible to arrive at a diagnosis using a significantly reduced number of recording channels that may be conducted in the home setting. A recent systematic review concluded that many commercially available home monitoring devices do not perform well in sensitivity or specificity. The best out-of-center testing devices use similar measures as PSG but exclude EEG, EMG, or EOG channels needed to score sleep. Thus, these devices typically measure at a minimum airflow using thermistors and nasal pressure transducers, breathing effort using respiratory impedance plethysmography, oxygen saturation using pulse oximetry, and snoring. Using these signals, the frequency of apneas and hypopneas per hour of recording, called the respiratory event index (REI), may be determined.

Some testing devices add markers for sleep, such as actigraphy (see below), position sensors, or pattern recognition of pulse or autonomic variability to estimate sleep time (called peripheral arterial tonometry). Home sleep apnea testing (HSAT) devices are thus far only considered for evaluation of OSA syndrome and are not suitable for diagnostic evaluation of other sleep disorders. Because of limited sensitivity, they are best employed when there is a high pretest probability that the patient has at least moderately severe OSA syndrome. Patients appropriate for HSAT would be those who satisfy three criteria: have a high likelihood of having at least moderately severe OSA, will be good candidates for either autotitrating continuous PAP (CPAP) or an oral appliance, and do not have underlying diseases that either will obscure HSAT or who may have other disorders that require PSG for diagnosis. Because of the poor sensitivity of HSAT, a negative result should be cause for PSG: the patient should have had a high pretest probability for having at least moderately severe OSA.

For medically uncomplicated patients fitting the above criteria, using HSAT followed by APAP most often leads to similar results as attended PSG with CPAP therapy based upon in-lab titration of pressure. This strategy is increasingly being used, largely owing to reduced costs. These good results depend, however, upon expert PAP mask fitting and follow-up. It is best to remember that treatment is chronic and requires ongoing follow-up. More is written about this in the section on OSA below.

Multiple Sleep Latency and Maintenance of Wakefulness Testing
The multiple sleep-latency test (MSLT) provides an objective measure of sleepiness compared with normal individuals lacking primary sleep disorders. The chief clinical indication for MSLT is for evaluation of narcolepsy and related primary CNS hypersomnias such as idiopathic hypersomnia and Kleine-Levin syndrome. A MSLT is carried out during the daytime in a sleep laboratory following nocturnal PSG, with four or five nap opportunities at standard times and intervals, usually at 9:00 and 11:00 AM and 1:00, 3:00, and 5:00 PM. Careful inspection of each nap is subsequently performed to determine the timing of sleep onset relative to commencement of each nap, and whether REM sleep occurs during each nap. A mean sleep latency is then calculated from the average initial sleep latency from each nap. Mean sleep latencies shorter than 8 minutes are considered abnormal and indicative of pathologic excessive daytime sleepiness. Whether or not a sleep-onset REM period (a SOREM, i.e., reaching REM sleep within 15 minutes of sleep onset during a nap) is captured is also considered and tabulated. More than one SOREM is abnormal and is consistent with the diagnosis of narcolepsy.

There are several considerations prior to performing and interpreting a valid MSLT. Patients should be instructed to sleep well for at least 2 weeks preceding the study, to allow at least 6 to 7 hours per night (and when possible, extending time in bed to 8-9 hours), and many sleep specialists document the quantity of sleep before the test with actigraphy monitoring or a sleep diary to ensure adherence to this recommendation and exclude the contaminating influence of insufficient sleep quantity. If it is safe and practically possible to do so, patients should be instructed to taper or discontinue sedative, stimulant, or REM suppressant medications (i.e., opiate analgesics, antidepressants, or other psychotropic or CNS active drugs) with the oversight and permission of other relevant treating primary care, psychiatry, and pain physicians at least 2 weeks prior to MSLT, and certain psychotropic drugs such as fluoxetine (Prozac) with a long elimination half-life should be discontinued for at least a month prior to MSLT to avoid decrease in MSLT sensitivity for delay of REM latency. Patients should undergo a full-night diagnostic PSG the night before a MSLT study to ensure that there is not another primary sleep disorder, such as SDB or PLMD, that could provide an alternative reason for significant sleepiness and to ensure that sufficient sleep quantity of 6 hours or more is obtained.

While the MSLT is designed to assess sleepiness, the maintenance of wakefulness test (MWT) is used to assess the ability to remain awake. The MWT is most useful when an objective measure of the effectiveness of treatment for disorders causing hypersomnolence is needed. The patient is seated in a dim room in a comfortable, semi-reclined position and asked to remain alert but passive for four 40-minute periods that are 2 hours apart. EEG, EOG, and chin EMG are measured, and the signals are analyzed to detect any epochs of unequivocal sleep during each 40-minute period. Normal patients have a mean time to epochs of unequivocal sleep of 30.4 minutes; however, the data is not normally distributed, and 42% of all patients remain awake for the entire 40 minutes on all four opportunities. Since simulated and actual driving performance is compromised with sleep times of 19 minutes or less on MWT, this is a reasonable threshold for the distinction of clinically significant daytime sleepiness, and driving or other safety sensitive tasks should be curtailed when sleep latencies are 19 minutes or shorter.

Actigraphy Monitoring

Wrist actigraphy monitoring is utilized to provide a rigorous estimation of sleep quantity and its circadian pattern. The actigraphy monitor may be worn like a wristwatch and contains an accelerometer that detects movements, which are recorded over time periods lasting up to weeks. The magnitude and pattern of movements may be analyzed and modeled to infer the sleep-wake pattern and provides a graphic representation of the patient's sleep schedule. The test is used in the evaluation of suspected circadian rhythm disorders, to assess response to treatment of insomnia, and for investigating patients with hypersomnia prior to PSG and MSLT to more accurately document the adequacy of sleep prior to the assessment for sleepiness. Recent applications utilizing the accelerometer in smartphones and wrist-worn fitness devices show promise, but most have not been validated as diagnostic tools.

Diagnostic and Therapeutic Approach to Common Sleep Disorders

Insomnia

The insomnia disorders all share three basic components: repeated complaints of insomnia, which may involve difficulties falling asleep, staying asleep, poor sleep quality, or waking undesirably early; an adequate time and opportunity for sleep; and a complaint of resultant daytime impairment. Insomnia is the most common of sleep complaints: nearly 45% of people were affected intermittently within the past year in some large studies, and up to 15% suffer chronic insomnia disorders. Risks for insomnia include female sex, older age, and a psychiatric or medical comorbidity. Chronic insomnia should be distinguished from short-term insomnia, which may occur in anyone occasionally (e.g., the night before an important job interview, or during increased stress). Per the ICSD-3, the sleep disturbance and associated daytime symptoms have to occur at least three times a week for at least three months to meet criteria for chronic insomnia disorder (see Box 1). Insomnia may begin in childhood, continue throughout a patient's lifetime, and appear as a manifestation of neurologic hyperarousal, with demonstrable increases in cerebral metabolism via functional MRI and increases in beta and theta EEG activity as well as generalized increased metabolism and stress hormone production compared with normals in either wake or sleep states. To a lesser extent, these same markers for hyperarousability are seen in other causes of primary insomnia (see Box 1).

In the past, insomnia was classified into primary and secondary, with secondary insomnia being far more common. Secondary insomnia was thought to be a result or accompaniment of an underlying illness. This may be incorrect. For example, it has previously been thought that treatment of secondary insomnia ought to focus on treatment of the underlying disorder. Newer evidence indicates that this approach may be suboptimal for the following reasons: secondary insomnia does not reliably improve when the underlying disorder does; secondary insomnia in general responds to treatment directed at insomnia; and in some cases, the underlying disorder, such as depression, responds better to treatment when the insomnia is addressed directly and concurrently. Furthermore, in several illnesses, such as depression, insomnia may predate the depression by months, and insomnia is a risk factor for future development of many psychiatric illnesses. In addition, primary insomnia was further divided into subtypes of idiopathic insomnia, psychophysiologic (learned) insomnia and paradoxical insomnia (sleep state misperception). Secondary insomnia was also divided into various subtypes such as inadequate sleep hygiene, insomnia due to medical condition, mental disorder, drug or substance. However, it is rare to encounter patients who fit under one of these subtypes exclusively. Most patients with insomnia, primary and secondary, tend to have some diagnostic criteria listed under many of these subtypes. Thus, in the current ICSD-3 insomnia is no longer classified into primary and secondary insomnia and no distinction is made between various etiologic subtypes of primary and secondary insomnia.

Chronic insomnia may be preceded in predisposed individuals by precipitating factors such as illness or stress and may be propagated by behavioral or maladaptive cognitive factors. Some individuals do not appear to require precipitating or propagating factors to develop chronic insomnia and have underlying redisposition toward insomnia. They are prototypic for an underlying predisposition toward insomnia. These individuals manifest insomnia from infancy and persist despite optimization of sleep hygiene and habit. However, in most cases of insomnia, precipitating and/or propagating influences may be found through careful interview and help establish a secure diagnosis.

In these individuals, identifiable precipitating causes that may be traumatic, stressful periods or struggles, medical illness, drugs, or toxins. However, even when the cause is removed, a conditioned response built upon associated and at times maladaptive sleep-related behaviors ensues. Instead of beginning to relax for sleep under permissive circumstances, the affected patient experiences paradoxical arousal as they approach their sleep conditions. The patient under the influence of the precipitating cause may have spent many hours worrying, uncomfortable, clock-watching, or otherwise raising their anxiety levels. Propagating factors include these same behaviors that help maintain sleeplessness once it has begun and may additionally include irregular sleep schedules and the use of drugs. Abuse of alcohol may contribute or be secondary to the sleep disturbance.

Effective treatment strategies for insomnia focus on removing any residual precipitating influences and mitigating or eliminating propagating influences. The main therapies for insomnia are sleep hygiene, behavioral therapies, cognitive therapies, and pharmacologic therapies. Patients often respond best to combined modalities. There is high-level evidence that combined cognitive/behavior therapies (CBT) are at least as effective as pharmacologic therapy for most patients with insomnia. CBT also appears to have enhanced rates of insomnia remission, so these approaches ought generally to be employed first. The addition of hypnotics to CBT has resulted in more rapid remission in some, but not all, studies. Growing recognition of the adverse effect profile of sedative-hypnotic drugs, particularly zolpidem (Ambien), which has been associated with heightened risks of falls and sleep walking, sleep eating, and related amnestic behaviors, has also encouraged a shift toward an earlier application of behavioral approaches to coping with insomnia.

In childhood, the most common causes of insomnia are behavioral. Insomnia may occur when parents fail to establish and enforce an appropriate nightly bedtime, so that their child may subsequently stall and refuse to go to bed in a timely fashion. In other cases, insomnia may occur when a child cannot fall asleep until a usual condition is present, such as being held, rocked, or fed. Appropriate advice and treatments include strict limit-setting for bedtime resistance; maintaining regular sleep schedules with avoidance of napping during the daytimes; and curtailing disrupting influences, such as television watching, gaming, and computer use. Suggesting a nightly cell phone or personal device (i.e., iPod, iPad, or Wii U) check-in procedure is especially helpful in teenage

TABLE 1	Therapeutic Tools for Treating Insomnia	
THERAPY TYPE	**SPECIFIC THERAPIES/COMPONENTS**	**GOALS**
Education/sleep hygiene	Improve knowledge about behaviors that foster or hinder healthy sleep	Improve opportunity and environment for sleep
Behavioral therapies	Stimulus control • Unmodified extinction • Graduated extinction • Positive routines/faded bedtime with response cost • Scheduled awakeningsSleep restriction	Dissociate anxiety or conditioned autonomic response from the process or location of going to sleep
	Relaxation training • Progressive muscle relaxation • Passive relaxation • Autogenic training-biofeedback • Imagery training • Meditation • HypnosisParadoxical intention	Increase pressure for sleep by decreasing the time allotted for sleep, increasing the probability of successful sleep attempts Reduce physiologic and/or cognitive arousal that hinders or disrupts sleep
		Reduce performance anxiety that confounds ability to successfully go to sleep
Cognitive therapies	Cognitive restructuring Decatastrophizing Reappraisal Attention shifting	Decrease unrealistic expectations about sleep, misconceptions, or misattributions regarding causes of insomnia, consequences of insomnia, ability to control sleep; produce a more appropriate and adaptive mind-set
Pharmacologic therapies	Hypnotics Sedating antidepressants Herbal supplements	Enhance sleepiness at appropriate times or to enhance convenience of sleep time and/or duration

children, and caffeinated soda and excessively stimulating activities should be avoided during the evenings. Selected children benefit from incentives such as a patient-parent contract that offers privileges for slightly later bedtimes on weekends after the child adheres regularly to a specified sleep schedule during school nights.

Four considerations for restoring normal sleep hygiene to discuss with all insomnia patients in the office include these three central concepts:

- Maintain a regular sleep schedule. Go to bed and arise at the same time each day. Ideally, the schedule should match the patient's biologic clock, with nocturnal sleep and bedtime/rise time matching their tendency for sleepiness and alertness (sleep education/hygiene).
- Avoid lying sleepless in bed. After 20 to 30 sleepless minutes spent trying to fall asleep, the patient should be instructed to leave the bedroom to pursue a quietly distracting activity, such as reading mundane material or watching a boring television program, and waiting until he or she feels sleepy enough to return to bed. Patients should explicitly avoid reading in bed, listening to the radio in bed, or watching television in bed if they are having difficulty initiating or maintaining sleep. This is a practical form of stimulus control (Table 1).
- Avoidance of clock-watching behavior. Patients should be instructed to remove clocks from their bedrooms or hide the clock face so as to make the insomnia period timeless and of uncertain duration. Falling asleep should not be a race against time, and repetitive checking of the time only serves to reinforce anxiety and further activate the mind (see stimulus control, Table 1). For the same reason, when watching television, discourage patients from watching news shows with scrolling tickertape newsflashes with clock time shown.
- Schedule thinking time earlier in the evening, well in advance of the sleep period. Patients who worry, plan, or think out their problems in bed should be encouraged to schedule a time earlier in the evening, well in advance of their normal bedtime, to attempt to work out these concerns prior to carrying

them into bed. This "constructive worry" or "worry time" represents a practical form of cognitive and stimulus control therapy.

There are numerous other associated issues and behaviors that may be useful for application in selected patients, such as cutting down overall time in bed (sleep restriction), establishing a regular and relaxing bedtime routine (such as by taking a relaxing bath, listening to soothing music, or having a light snack before bed), avoiding daytime naps, avoiding caffeinated beverages after noontime, and establishing a regular morning exercise routine and avoiding evening exercise. It is important for the physician to avoid overloading the patient with too many considerations and tasks at once, however, as the burden of implementing these suggestions then becomes tantamount to too many obtrusive "swing thoughts" during a golf swing. One or two concepts to start with are sufficient, and once mastered and implemented, the patient can gradually phase in other ideas over time. Relaxation training and cognitive behavioral therapy can be very helpful in selected receptive patients who have failed the above typical self-help measures, and as a last resort, periodic or even scheduled chronic pharmacotherapy can also be implemented.

There are now several highly effective and tolerable hypnotic medications available for short-term, intermittent, and chronic use. The class of nonbenzodiazepine receptor agonists (the so-called "Z" drugs, or zolpidem [Ambien], zaleplon [Sonata], and eszopiclone [Lunesta]) are preferred by most sleep specialists but some of them remain costlier than the older generation choices, including the benzodiazepines—which have adverse effects on sleep architecture—as well as diphenhydramine (Benadryl) and trazodone (Desyrel),[1] which each have less specific sleep-promoting effects and more adverse effects and potential for drug-drug interactions, especially in elderly patients. The clinical pharmacology of the most commonly prescribed and most useful hypnotic medications are summarized in Table 2. A concern with each of these may be the potential for habituation of efficacy;

---

[1]Not FDA approved for this indication.

TABLE 2 Clinical Pharmacology of Hypnotic Medications

	MECHANISM OF ACTION	DOSAGE (MG)	DURATION OF ACTION ($T^{1/2}$)	TYPICAL ADVERSE EFFECTS	INTERACTIONS
Diphenhydramine (Benadryl)	H1	25–50	Intermediate (2.4–9.3 h)	Dry mouth, constipation, urinary retention	Nonsignificant
Trazodone (Desyrel)[1]	SRI	50–150	Short (3–6 h)	Dry mouth, dizziness, rash	CYP substrate; several others
Triazolam (Halcion)	BRA	0.125–0.5	Short (1.5–5.5 h)	Tolerance	CYP induction
Temazepam (Restoril)	BRA	7.5–30	Intermediate (8–18 h)	Tolerance	Nonsignificant
Melatonin[2]	MT1–MT2	1–3	Ultra-short (35–50 min)	Hangover type effect	None
Zolpidem (Ambien)	NBRA	5, 10	Short (2–2.6 h)	Amnestic behavior	Numerous
Zaleplon (Sonata)	NBRA	5, 10	Short (1 h)	Headache, amnestic behavior	Several
Eszopiclone (Lunesta)	NBRA	1–3	Intermediate (6 h)	Headache, amnestic behavior, rash possible	Nonsignificant
Ramelteon (Rozerem)	MT1-MT2	8, 16[3]	Short (1–2.6 h)	Hyperprolacti nemia	Ketoconazole (Nizoral), rifampin
Doxepin (Silenor)	H1	3,6	Intermediate (12-15 h)	Dizziness, tachycardia	Nonsignificant
Suvorexant (Belsomra)	Orexin antagonist	10-20	Intermediate (12 h)	Headache, dizziness, abnormal dreams	CYP3A4 inducer
Lemborexant (Dayvigo)	Orexin antagonist	5-10	Intermediate (≤7 h)	Drowsiness, fatigue, headache	CYP3A4 substrate

Abbreviations: $t^{1/2}$=half-life of drug; h=hours; H1=antihistaminergic H1 receptor blocker; SRI=serotonin reuptake inhibitor; BRA=benzodiazepine receptor agonist; CYP substrate=metabolized by cytochrome metabolism, susceptible to enzyme inhibition and elevated serum levels by multiple drugs; CYP induction=cytochrome enzyme inducer, may cause multiple potential drug-drug interactions via this mechanism; NBRA=nonbenzodiazepine benzodiazepine receptor agonist; MT1/MT2=melatonin type 1 and type 2 receptor agonist.
[1]Not FDA approved for this indication.
[2]Available as dietary supplement.
[3]Exceeds dosage recommended by the manufacturer.

fall risk; and the potential to cause sleepwalking, sleep eating, or other amnestic behaviors during sleep. If these adverse effects result, the hypnotic drug should be promptly discontinued with a shift toward the use of cognitive behavioral therapy strategies. In women, zolpidem should be used with particular caution given the slower metabolism of the drug, thereby promoting vulnerabilities to carryover sedation and unpleasant "hangover" type feelings or driving safety risks during the commute the next morning. Pharmacologic therapy of insomnia may be bolstered by the advent of suvorexant (Belsomra), a novel hypocretin antagonist that has a wake-suppressing rather than sleep-promoting mechanism of action. However, it should be noted that the higher doses that were primarily studied were determined as overly sedating and unsafe by the FDA and only the lower doses were approved. Further clinical experience will likely be necessary to establish the role of this medication as a treatment for insomnia.

Sleep-Disordered Breathing

Breathing during sleep is carefully regulated to maintain homeostasis of oxygen, carbon dioxide, and blood pH. The mechanisms and homeostatic set points for ventilation vary systematically between wake, non-REM sleep, and REM sleep. In wake, the resulting ventilatory pattern is governed by careful integration of classic feedback systems designed to keep blood pH at approximately 7.40, arterial $PaCO_2$ at approximately 38 to 45 mm Hg, and PaO_2 greater than approximately 60 mm Hg with cortical influences that govern functions such as speaking, laughing, eating, singing, and other voluntary activities. During non-REM sleep, ventilation is considerably more rhythmic and is governed almost exclusively by the chemoresponsive feedback systems

indicated above; during REM sleep, the chemoresponsive feedback system is further influenced by additional input from REM-influenced neurons, resulting in a less rhythmic and less-carefully regulated metabolic milieu.

Significant deviation from these norms is termed "sleep-disordered breathing" (SDB), and is marked by several distinct event types. Apneas are total or near-total cessations of airflow. Hypopneas are significant declines in tidal volume sufficient to result in significant reduction in oxygenation. Excess effort for breathing may result in arousals from and disturbance of sleep, and are termed respiratory effort-related arousals (RERAs). These types of events are often related as a rate, either as the apnea-hypopnea index (AHI; apneas+hypopneas per hour of sleep), the respiratory disturbance index (apneas+hypopneas+RERAs per hour of sleep), or the REI (apneas+hypopneas per hour of recording when sleep is not measured directly). In addition to these types of SDB, the general baseline minute ventilation may fall to the point where sustained hypoventilation takes place during sleep, termed sleep-related alveolar hypoventilation.

Obstructive SDB: Snoring and OSA

The dynamic upper-airway obstruction, which occurs as a result of sleep in some persons, leads to a continuum of SDB varying from mild snoring to hypopneas to obstructive apneas. The likelihood and extent of upper-airway collapse is determined by the neural input into the dilating upper-airway muscles, influence of sleep state, and upper-airway anatomy. Obstructive events are more likely to occur in REM sleep when muscle tone is lowest, during transitions from lighter non-REM sleep to deep non-REM sleep when sleep is unstable, or when muscle tone is decreased by substances such as alcohol or drugs. The single biggest risk factor for snoring or OSA is obesity, wherein fatty deposition reduces upper-airway dimension, humoral factors reduce net dilating forces of the muscles, and the mechanical effects of obesity reduce lung volumes and the stabilizing effect of tracheal traction on the upper airway. Beyond obesity, many but not all patients have a predisposing anatomy of a narrowed oropharynx, such as a low-lying palate or redundant soft palate tissue, a thickened tongue base, or a narrow hypopharynx, although nasal anatomy with septal deviation or chronic congestion may also aggravate the problem.

Snoring without other symptoms, signs, or polysomnographic evidence of upper-airway obstructions such as hypersomnia, frequent associated arousals, or significant airflow limitation is termed primary snoring. While snoring may be a socially objectionable symptom or disruptive to the patient's sleep partner, snoring in isolation is otherwise not considered to be abnormal and such patients may be reassured if their bed partners are not bothered by their snoring. If treatment is desired, options include relieving nasal obstruction if present, commercially available lubricant throat sprays, mandibular positioning devices, and nasal or upper-airway surgical approaches such as nasal septal repair or uvulopalatopharyngoplasty (UPPP, or UP3 procedure). An otorhinolaryngology consultation may be helpful in determining which surgical approaches may be most beneficial for the individual.

OSA is an extremely common public health problem present in at least 2% to 4% of the general population and has been linked to development of hypertension and is a risk factor for incidental development of stroke, coronary artery disease, congestive heart failure, and atrial fibrillation. OSA has been shown to be associated with a wide variety of endothelial and metabolic abnormalities that favor vascular disease, and when patients with moderate to severe OSA are compared to normals or treated OSA patients, they appear to have a higher mortality and cardiovascular event frequency. Thus, the two main reasons to detect and treat OSA are to improve symptoms and to decrease cardiovascular risks. There are good data to show that treatment of OSA improves symptoms and quality of life. Data regarding the reversal of cardiovascular risk are not as firm, but most experts agree that at least moderate and severe OSA ought to be treated, regardless of symptom severity.

OSA severity is rated by the polysomnographic AHI, the hourly rate of apneas and hypopneas averaged over the total sleep time, or, in the case of HSAT, by the REI. An AHI of 4 per hour or less is considered normal. Mild OSA is diagnosed with an AHI of 5 to 14 per hour, moderate OSA with AHI of 15 to 29 per hour, and severe OSA with AHI being 30 per hour or higher. In most laboratories, correlation of the AHI with specific sleep stages and body positions is usually performed to determine whether positional therapy may be offered, as many patients have OSA only during the supine sleep position (position-dependent OSA), and some manifest OSA only during REM sleep in the supine position.

A form of OSA called the upper-airway resistance syndrome is defined by a clinical complaint of hypersomnia, often accompanied by snoring but without an abnormally high frequency of overt apneas or hypopneas resulting in significant decline in oxygen saturation. PSG confirms repetitive arousals related to the increased respiratory effort (respiratory effort-related arousals, or RERAs, during PSG) required to overcome upper-airway obstruction. Because of the similar pathogenesis and treatment response to relieve upper-airway obstruction, this is considered a variant of OSA.

Therapeutic options for snoring and sleep apnea include reducing nasal congestion or obstruction, positional therapy, nasal continuous positive airway pressure, oral appliances, the nasal expiratory positive airway pressure device, oral pressure therapy (OPT), or surgical management (Table 3). Patients with OSA have higher morbidity from vascular events and higher motor vehicle accident rates. Assessment and appropriate counseling for weight loss, cardiovascular risk factors, and driving while untreated (or extreme caution) should be part of a treatment plan.

Weight loss. Weight loss may reduce soft tissue in the neck, making the oropharynx less compressible. The improvement in lung volumes accompanied by weight loss also favor enhancement of longitudinal traction on the upper airway, the so-called "tracheal tug." About 30% to 40% of patients who are able to achieve substantial weight loss may become cured of their OSA. Careful follow-up is needed because many remissions are not permanent. Alcohol and other substances that reduce upper-airway tone or cause sedation or reduced responsiveness worsen OSA and should be prudently avoided.

Positional therapy. Among the lifestyle or behavioral changes, positional therapy involves employing one or more simple strategies to enforce sleep only in nonsupine body positions, usually on the side. One method is the "tennis ball in T-shirt" approach. The patient wears a snug-fitting T-shirt with a pocket sewn onto the back between the shoulder blades with two or three tennis or wiffle balls inserted into it to discourage the patient from turning onto the back during sleep. Other options include similar commercially marketed shirts or vests (the FDA-approved ZZoma sleep apnea pillow, the "snoring backpack," and similar strategies) and body pillows propped or wedged behind the patient or hugged by the patient. A correctional device for positional sleep apnea is also approved in the European Union. Unfortunately, shoulder or hip pain often limits the application of positional therapy, especially in elderly persons, and long-term adherence or compliance remains poor, with only about one-third of patients able to perpetuate positional therapy strategies in long-term follow-up. Patients with position-dependent OSA should be counseled to be cautious for development of severe OSA problems during any future anticipated prolonged periods of supine sleep, such as postoperative recovery periods following surgery or following a major injury.

Positive airway pressure. The mainstay of treatment for OSA for the majority of patients remains positive airway therapy (PAP). The main components of PAP appliances are the blower unit, which delivers calibrated pressures to hold open the airway; tubing to conduct the pressurized air to the patient; an interface such as a nasal or oronasal mask; and a harness to hold the mask firmly to the patient's face during use. Of the PAP therapies, continuous positive airway pressure (CPAP), which delivers a continuous set pressure between 5 and 20 cm H$_2$O, is usually first tried in the setting of PSG; in many sleep centers, the practice of performing split-night PSG (an initial diagnostic phase followed by a treatment phase of CPAP titration toward an optimal pressure for the individual patient) allows diagnosis and treatment prescription to occur in an efficient manner. If an optimal pressure cannot be determined by laboratory titration or data is not available to guide prescription of a specific pressure for a patient, application of an autotitrating PAP device may be considered, offering flexibility for delivering a relatively wide range of self-adjusting treatment pressures as the patient changes sleep position and enters different sleep stages through the night with accordingly varying apnea severity. Autotitrating PAP has been found to be efficacious in most patients diagnosed with OSA by HSAT. However, close clinical follow-up is needed in all patients who have recently started PAP.

PAP is typically delivered through an interface chosen as most comfortable by the patient, either a nasal mask, nasal pillows, or an oronasal. Nasal pillows, a type of cannula that provides a tight seal within the nares, and a newer tube-like frame that sits in front of and not within the nares are most effective at lower treatment pressures; they may be favored by many patients with claustrophobia but may dislodge at higher pressures or with frequent nocturnal movement. Nasal masks of various types are used in many patients, but if mouth breathing and consequent leak are a problem, a chin strap may be added, or an oronasal face mask may be substituted. Many newer PAP machines offer the feature of pressure relief during exhalation, which may enhance patient tolerability at higher level PAP pressures by "giving way" as the patient expires. Bilevel positive airway pressure (BPAP) may also be employed

TABLE 3	Treatment of Sleep-Related Breathing Disorders		
SLEEP-RELATED BREATHING DISORDER	**TREATMENT MODALITY**		**GOAL**
OSA syndrome	Lifestyle/behavior modification	• Weight loss	Reduced weight may result in improvement airway patency
		• Alcohol avoidance	Alcohol worsens OSA; avoidance of exacerbating factor is encouraged
	Positive airway pressure	• Positional therapy	Enhance airway patency by nonsupine sleeping
		• Continuous positive airway pressure (CPAP)	Counteract collapsing forces in upper airway; "stent" open the upper airway
		• Bilevel positive airway pressure (BPAP)	End expiratory pressure stents open airway; inspiratory pressure enhances minute ventilation or decreases hypopneas
	Upper airway stimulation	Inspire™	Stimulation to upper airway muscles during sleep resulting in increased airway patency
		• Autotitrating positive airway pressure (APAP)	Uses feedback algorithms to adjust pressure in response to airway conditions in order to provide airway patency with minimal mean pressure
	Oral appliances	• Mandibular positioning devices • Tongue retention devices	Enhance airway patency by stabilizing lateral pharyngeal walls and enhancing AP airway dimensions at the velopharyngeal level
	Surgical modification of the upper airway	• Palatal surgeries (uvulopalatopharyngo plasty, others)	Enhance airway patency by reconfiguring soft tissues and/or skeletal structures
		• Maxillo-mandibular advancement	Enhance airway patency by reconfiguring soft tissues and skeletal structures
Central sleep apnea syndromes	Correct underlying disorders (treat heart failure, etc.)	• Various	Reduce stimuli to ventilatory hyperresponsiveness
	Gases	• Oxygen	Reduce responsiveness to variation in CO_2
	Positive airway pressure	• CPAP	Reduce stimulation to ventilate by decreasing lung water, improving V/Q matching, reducing airway resistance
	Transvenous phrenic nerve stimulation (Remede)	• Noninvasive positive pressure ventilation (NIPPV), also referred to as BPAP-ST (Avoid in heart failure patients with ejection fraction<45%)	Provide ventilatory assistance in order to avoid hypercapnia/hypoxemia associated with central apneas or hypopneas, thus reducing hyperventilatory feedback
		• Adaptive servoventilation (Avoid in heart failure patients with ejection fraction<45%)	Provide ventilatory assistance in proportion to needs, reducing or eliminating variability in ventilation and ventilatory drive; avoid hypercapnia/hypoxemia associated with central apneas or hypopneas, thus reducing hyperventilatory feedback.
			Cause diaphragmatic contraction, creating a negative intrathoracic pressure mimicking a normal breathing pattern and augmenting airflow to decrease central apnea.
Hypoventilation syndromes	Positive airway pressure	• Noninvasive positive pressure ventilation (NIPPV), also referred to as BPAP-ST	Provide ventilatory assistance in order to avoid hypercapnia/hypoxemia associated with central apneas or hypopneas
		• Tracheostomy with mechanical ventilation	Provide ventilatory assistance in order to avoid hypercapnia/hypoxemia associated with central apneas or hypopneas, protect or control airway

at higher treatment pressures if CPAP is not well tolerated. Setting a pressure delta ≥4 cm between the inspired and expired pressure may also add a degree of positive pressure ventilation for patients with concurrent sleep-related hypoventilation from an intrinsic pulmonary disease or neuromuscular respiratory muscle weakness.

Oral appliances. Oral appliances may be fitted by a dental sleep specialist. They provide a means of advancing the mandible that pull the tongue base forward slightly, opening the oropharyngeal airway to some degree and obviating some apnea and hypopnea events. The device is most effective for mild to moderate severity and supine position-dependent OSA and generally less predictably effective for most cases of severe OSA. However, the use of oral appliances is increasing due to greater availability of competent dental professionals working with the devices, awareness that for some patients adherence is better with OAs than PAP, and improvements in appliance design that allow enhanced efficacy in some instances. Because oral appliances are less reliably effective in controlling SDB, repeat testing—either with out-of-center sleep testing or PSG after maximal adjustment—is needed to confirm efficacy.

Nasal valve appliances. An expiratory nasal resistance valve appliance (Provent) was approved by the FDA for treatment of OSA. The device may be an alternative for some patients with OSA who fail to tolerate CPAP therapy. The device is a small, disposable oval appliance that is affixed over each of the patient's nares by self-adhesive with an airflow port that offers resistance to expiratory airflow, thereby producing expiratory positive airway pressure and preserving nasal and oropharyngeal airway patency with minimal impedance to inspiratory airflow. The device was proven to significantly reduce polysomnographic AHI and subjective sleepiness on the ESS in a sham-controlled randomized trial. Because they are disposable, a new device must be affixed each night. Appropriate patient characteristics and long-term results are not yet clear, but these may be considered in patients who do not prefer CPAP or oral appliances and are agreeable to follow-up to ensure efficacy.

Oral pressure therapy. A newer option for treatment of mild to moderate OSA is OPT (Winx), which combines an oral appliance with negative intraoral pressure to help keep the tongue and soft palate in a more anterior position, enlarging the retrolingual and retropalatal space. There is as yet limited experience with the device; however, this may be an option for some patients who are averse to or intolerant of other therapies.

Surgery. Surgical modifications of the upper airway are principally of two basic approaches, palatal approaches, tongue-based procedures (genioglossus advancement, hyoid myotomy and suspension, lingualplasty), or maxillomandibular advancement (MMA). Palatal approaches such as UPPP, or "UP3" performed by otorhinolaryngologists are effective for relief of snoring but mostly ineffective for treatment of OSA, especially if severity is moderate or greater in degree. MMA appears to be quite effective in mild to moderate OSA and can even be applied with good effect even in selected severe OSA cases; however, morbidity from perioperative pain is considerable and long-term outcomes remain unclear. A hypoglossal nerve stimulation implant (Inspire) is a novel surgical treatment for PAP-intolerant patients. A recently published randomized controlled trial demonstrated efficacy and reasonable tolerability; however, this device was only recently FDA approved and there is limited clinical experience with it, thus, its future role and scope of use in OSA management remains to be determined.

Central Sleep Apnea Syndrome

Central sleep apnea syndrome results from an unstable ventilatory drive during sleep, resulting in periods of insufficient ventilation and compromise of gas exchange despite a patent oropharyngeal airway. Clinically, patients may share similar symptoms with those with OSA, including snoring, except patients with central sleep apnea more frequently complain of insomnia than hypersomnia. Central sleep apnea has a heterogeneous pathophysiology and may be idiopathic or due to high-altitude-induced periodic breathing, due to Cheyne-Stokes breathing, or narcotic-induced. Neurologic causes—such as brainstem infarction or neurodegenerative disorders, including multiple system atrophy—may also cause central apnea. In heart failure, the presence of central sleep apnea syndrome or Cheyne-Stokes breathing imparts a poor prognosis. A high-quality clinical trial showed that on average, CPAP did not reduce mortality. However, central sleep apnea is often at least partially resistant to treatment with conventional nasal CPAP therapy, and while CPAP may effect improved mean oxygenation, frequent arousals that fragment sleep often continue. However, a recent large multicenter randomized control trial, the SERVE-HF study, showed elevated all-cause and cardiovascular mortality risk in patients with central sleep apnea and symptomatic heart failure with an estimated ejection fraction of ≤45% who were randomized to ASV. Therefore, use of ASV in this patient population is not advised at the current time. Remede, a phrenic nerve stimulator, has recently been approved by the FDA as a treatment option in selected cases with central sleep apnea.

Treatment-Emergent Central Sleep Apnea Syndrome

Treatment-emergent central sleep apnea syndrome is a subtype of central sleep apnea wherein patients have significant obstructive/anatomical problems with ventilation, but also have unstable ventilatory patterns noted in patients with central sleep apnea syndromes. These patients have a clinical and PSG presentation of OSA, but once the upper airway is opened with CPAP, they experience frequent central apneic events that may or may not later resolve with continued exposure to PAP in the home setting. Some patients clearly continue to manifest frequent central sleep apneic events more than five times per hour, leading to the suboptimal outcomes of persisting clinical complaints of hypersomnia and medical risk. Treatment-emergent central sleep apnea syndrome may occur in as many as 4% to 15% of those with OSA. There is emerging evidence that alternative modes of PAP—particularly ASV—may be superior to conventional CPAP for treatment of treatment-emergent central sleep apnea syndrome. A randomized controlled trial recently showed that ASV more reliably relieves SDB, while CPAP fails to control SDB in up to one-third of cases. However, there is also evidence to suggest that treatment-emergent central sleep apnea resolves over time in a substantial number of patients who continue to remain on CPAP therapy.

Sleep-Related Hypoventilation

The causes of hypoventilation during sleep include primary pulmonary parenchymal disorders, neuromuscular conditions affecting bellows musculature, or restrictive physiology of the chest wall accompanying kyphoscoliotic disorders or morbid obesity. While each of these disorders may also ultimately cause daytime hypoventilation, sleep recumbency, especially supine sleep positioning, and REM sleep stage (which leads to relative paralysis of the chest wall and sole dependency on diaphragmatic excursion to drive respiratory effort) often lead to exclusive or initial sleep-related hypoventilation with subsequent medical risk consequent to suboptimal nocturnal oxygenation. Failure to treat significant nocturnal hypoventilation may result in the development of sequelae of hypoxemia such as polycythemia, pulmonary hypertension, and right heart failure, or of hypercapnic respiratory failure. Treatment most often involves use of NIPPV (see Table 4). A newer modality of positive pressure ventilation, volume-assured pressure support ventilation (AVAPS™), consists of a short delivery of a provider-set tidal volume, which, when coupled with a set backup respiratory rate, assures delivery of a minimum minute ventilation, even when changes in the patient's muscular strength or ventilatory load change. These therapies are best titrated in the context of a supervised overnight laboratory polysomnogram under the direction of a sleep or pulmonary medicine specialist. One must be careful not to resort to the potentially dangerous solution of added oxygen therapy alone in severe COPD or neuromuscular etiologies of sleep-related hypoventilation, because as ventilation fails and hypercapnea results, the hypoxic drive to breathe may become the chief factor leading to continued ventilatory effort and oxygen in this context may precipitate acute respiratory failure in some individuals. A morning arterial blood gas on room air following PSG is indicated to assess for potential hypercapnia and assess the impact of ventilatory support. In the context of severe hypercapnia (i.e., Pco_2 of 55 or greater), serial arterial blood gases to monitor the effects of ventilatory support, oxygenation, and accumulating hypercapnia may help determine whether nocturnal mechanical ventilatory support is indicated.

Narcolepsy and Central Disorders of Hypersomnolence

Narcolepsy is the prototypical central disorder of hypersomnolence. Narcolepsy is categorized further as Narcolepsy Type I (previously called narcolepsy with cataplexy) and Narcolepsy Type II (previously called narcolepsy without cataplexy). Cataplexy is a distinctive and highly specific symptom characterized by emotionally provoked muscle atonia intruding into wakefulness that is seen in a minority of patients overall and may

	MECHANISM OF ACTION	DOSAGE (MG)	DURATION OF ACTION ($T\frac{1}{2}$)	TYPICAL ADVERSE EFFECTS	INTERACTIONS
Modafinil (Provigil)	Unknown	100–600[3]	Intermediate (15 h)	Tremor, jitteriness, palpitations, hypertension	Oral contraceptives
Armodafinil (Nuvigil)	Unknown	150–450[3]	Intermediate (15 h)	Tremor, jitteriness, palpitations, hypertension	Oral contraceptives
Pitolisant (Wakix)	Histamine-3 receptor inverse agonist/antagonist	8.9-35.6 mg	Long (8-24 h)	Headache, nausea, insomnia	Antihistamines, oral contraceptives, CYP2D6 inhibitors, CYP3A4 inducers, mirtazapine, TCAs and other QT-prolonging agents
Solriamfetol (Sunosi)	DNRI	75-150 mg	Intermediate (7 h)	Headache, nausea, anxiety, insomnia	Dopamine agonists, CNS stimulants, sympathomimetics, esketamine, MAOIs, SNRIs, bupropion
Methylphenidate (Ritalin)	DNRI	15–100[3]	Short (2–4 h)	Tremor, jitteriness, palpitations, hypertension	Nonsignificant
Methylphenidate SR (Concerta)[1]	DNRI	18–72	Intermediate (3.5 h)	Tremor, jitteriness, palpitations, hypertension	Nonsignificant
Amphetamine/dextroamphetamine (Adderall)	DNRI	15–100[3]	Intermediate (10–13 h)	Tremor, jitteriness, palpitations, hypertension, QTc prolongation	Beware MAOIs, SSRIs, SNRIs, TCAs, bupropion (Wellbutrin)
Dextroamphetamine (Dexedrine)	DNRI	15–100[3]	Long (10–28 h)	Tremor, jitteriness, palpitations, hypertension, QTc prolongation	Beware MAOIs, SSRIs, SNRIs, TCAs, bupropion
Lisdexamfetamine (Vyvanse)[1]	DNRI	20–100[3]	Short (<1 h as prodrug) (10–28 h as dextroamphetamine)	Tremor, jitteriness, palpitations, hypertension, QTc prolongation	Beware MAOIs, SSRIs, SNRIs, TCAs, bupropion
Methamphetamine (Desoxyn)[1]	DNRI	15–100[3]	Intermediate (9–15 h)	Tremor, jitteriness, palpitations, hypertension, QTc prolongation	Beware MAOIs, SSRIs, SNRIs, TCAs, bupropion

[1]Not FDA approved for this indication.
[3]Exceeds dosage recommended by the manufacturer.
Abbreviations: t½=half-life of drug; h=hours; DNRI=dopamine and norepinephrine monoamine reuptake inhibitor; QTc=corrected QT interval; MAOI=monoamine oxidase inhibitor; SSRI=serotonin selective reuptake inhibitor; SNRI=selective norepinephrine reuptake inhibitor; TCA=tricyclic antidepressant (the potential interaction with all these agents is largely theoretical concern for potentiation of serotonin syndrome).

precede but more often follows onset of the main symptom of hypersomnia. In the absence of cataplexy, a diagnosis of Narcolepsy Type I may also be made if cerebrospinal fluid (CSF) hypocretin-1 concentration, measured by immunoreactivity, is <110 pg/mL or <1/3 of mean values obtained in normal subjects with the same standardized assay. In Narcolepsy Type II, there is no cataplexy, and the CSF hypocretin level does not meet the above criteria or has not been measured. In addition to sleepiness and cataplexy, the full clinical pentad of narcolepsy also includes symptoms of sleep paralysis (the inability to move the body upon awakening), hypnogogic hallucinations (the intrusion of dream imagery and mentation into conscious awareness following awakening), and sleep-maintenance insomnia (with frequent nocturnal arousals and difficulty maintaining sleep). However, narcolepsy is most frequently monosymptomatic, with the sole symptom being pervasive, enduring sleepiness and decreased vigilance with a tendency toward dozing off inadvertently in permissive settings and the overwhelming desire to nap during the daytime, especially in the afternoons. Naps are most often highly refreshing; scheduled naps can be utilized to therapeutic advantage or indeed, in rare patients, as the sole treatment for those bent on avoiding stimulant pharmacotherapy. Narcolepsy is relatively uncommon, affecting approximately 1:2000 of the general population. While the etiology of narcolepsy remains unknown, most experts continue to favor a long hypothesized autoimmune cause. Major advances in the understanding of the neurobiology of narcolepsy over the past two decades have included the clear linkage of the HLA DQB1*0602 haplotype in up to 90% patients having narcolepsy with cataplexy, discovery of wake-promoting hypocretin/orexin peptides produced by the perifornical posterolateral hypothalamus, and low to unmeasurable CSF hypocretin in nearly 90% of narcolepsy with cataplexy patients. Within the last few years, epidemic narcolepsy-cataplexy following H1N1 vaccination in Europe and Asia also provided further support for the autoimmune hypothesis of narcolepsy. Unfortunately, these tantalizing discoveries have not yet yielded clear insight into pathogenic mechanisms nor more specific therapies for patients, and the mainstay of treatment for the condition remains the use of older stimulant and wake-promoting medications, or prescribed therapeutic napping, as naps are most often highly refreshing and restorative in narcolepsy patients. Supportive laboratory evidence for narcolepsy includes a relatively normal polysomnogram to exclude other causes of hypersomnia such as OSA or PLMD, followed by a confirmatory MSLT, which demonstrates mean sleep latency shorter than 8 minutes and two or more sleep-onset REM periods during four or five nap opportunities.

Idiopathic hypersomnia is a closely related condition often difficult to distinguish from narcolepsy without cataplexy, although a few nuanced clinical features tend to distinguish it from narcolepsy, chiefly a characteristically reported unrefreshing nocturnal sleep and nap quality. Idiopathic hypersomnia has previously been further subclassified as variants with or without prolonged sleep period, although these phenotypes are overlapping and current diagnostic standards have eliminated this distinction. Other similar enigmatic and poorly understood primary CNS hypersomnias include posttraumatic hypersomnia when there is a history of temporally related antecedent substantial head injury, and recurrent hypersomnia, also known as the Kleine-Levin syndrome, which in addition to hypersomnia includes other neuropsychiatric sequelae such as cognitive and behavioral changes like hypersexuality and hyperphagia. Hypersomnia is also commonly associated with as many as 50% of those with myotonic dystrophy type 1.

The mainstay of treatment for each of these conditions is stimulant and wake-promoting agent therapy, with the goal of improved vigilance and psychomotor functioning. Stimulants and wake-promoting agents range in intensity from lower to higher intensity and efficacy/tolerability options, from modafinil (Provigil) and armodafinil (Nuvigil) on the milder end of the spectrum—although selected narcolepsy patients respond quite well to these drugs—to methylphenidate (Ritalin), and to the amphetamine/dextroamphetamine (Adderall). Relevant clinical pharmacology of the stimulant medications commonly used in clinical practice are summarized in Table 4. Patients with uncontrolled hypersomnias should be cautioned against driving, operating dangerous machinery, or engaging in other similarly dangerous activities or hobbies while they are drowsy, as they may be prone to sudden and unpredictable sleep attacks. Sodium oxybate (gamma hydroxy butyrate) is an FDA approved tightly controlled substance for the treatment of sleepiness and cataplexy in patients with narcolepsy. Sodium oxybate (Xyrem) is usually given in two divided doses, before bedtime and in the middle of the night; it can be dangerous in the setting of uncontrolled OSA or respiratory conditions and central nervous system depressants. Other REM suppressing medications such as tricyclic antidepressants, SSRIs and SNRIs are also used in the treatment of cataplexy.

Circadian Rhythm Sleep Wake Disorders

Circadian rhythm sleep disorders result in misalignment of the timing of the sleep period relative to the desired bed and rise times, resulting in concurrent insomnia and hypersomnia symptoms despite normal total sleep time. The most common circadian rhythm disturbances are actually exogenous influences on the patient and his/her circadian axis, which in these cases is functioning normally but is unable to adjust rapidly enough to the required new temporal milieu. These exogenous disorders include jet lag disorder and shift work disorder, resulting either from imposed transmeridian travel or

alternating work shifts, respectively, that disturb the patient's environmental entraining cues and homeostatic drives for sleep and wakefulness, thereby resulting in misalignment of the patient's endogenous biological sleep drive and typical sleep schedule to the clock time and environment to which they must rapidly adapt.

Jet lag disorder results when an individual crosses across several transmeridian time zones in a single day. Crossing one or two time zones is usually not too difficult for the traveler to accommodate, but crossing three time zones typically causes symptoms of jet lag. Flying eastward is generally much more difficult than flying westward, as patients more easily accommodate phase delay then phase advancing, or "loss" of time. Treatments for jet lag syndrome usually involve efforts to rapidly reentrain the patient to the new environment, and protocols for advance preparation including setting back (for eastward travel) or setting ahead (for planned westward travel) one's daily routine 2 to 3 weeks prior to the trip so that the traveler is already partially reset in his or her circadian routine before departing. Also critical is attempting to rapidly adapt to the new time zone, such as by seeking regular sunlight exposure during the daytime and avoiding light exposure in the evening. Brief use of a hypnotic medication and regular daily doses of melatonin[7] 0.5 to 5.0 mg at bedtime for the first few nights after arrival can help reset the sleep schedule in the new time zone.

Shift-work sleep disorder results from workers who must constantly and regularly alter or rotate their work schedules between different shifts (so-called "swing shifts") or workers who must accommodate a regularly scheduled second or third shift (i.e., shifts other than a day shift). Shift workers often have difficulty adapting and shifting their sleep-wake schedules and develop symptoms of insomnia or hypersomnia. Shift workers must be educated to prioritize regularly obtaining a sufficient quantity of sleep, regardless of their work circumstances. Swing shift workers should also be counseled to avoid working more than five night shifts in a row, as night shift work frequently leads to a greater degree of sleep deprivation over time. Shift workers should also be counseled to avoid rotating swing shifts whenever possible, to strictly avoid scheduling overtime duty, and to avoid long commutes (and to exercise special caution to avoid drowsy driving). Judicious use of caffeinated beverages, or prescribed stimulant therapy with modafinil may be helpful for enhancing vigilance in some patients, but should be used with caution as they might interfere with sleep initiation.

The two most common endogenous circadian disorders are delayed sleep-wake phase disorder (DSWPD) and advanced sleep-wake phase disorder (ASWPD), disorders that are most prevalent in opposite extremes of life. DSWPD is seen most often in adolescents and young adults who are biological night owls in their circadian preference, preferring a delayed bedtime and rise time (i.e., bedtimes well past midnight and subsequent arising times in the late morning or early afternoon). DSWPD patients have an extreme and enduring form of this tendency, however, resulting in persisting misalignment of the patient to societal norms. Adolescent and young adult patients present with profound intractable initial insomnia due to their inability to fall asleep at a conventional bedtime as required for school or most daytime occupations, and profound daytime hypersomnia due to their inability to arise and function in the morning hours. Diagnosis is easily recognized by clinical history and sleep diaries, with or without adjunctive actigraphy to objectively verify the pattern of consistent delayed sleep-phase periods. Contrarily, ASWPD is more common in elderly individuals who are biological larks (i.e., preferring an early bedtime and early rise time by nature). However, the ASWPD elderly are unable to stay awake for desired evening activities (often even unable to go out to dinner with friends), and awaken undesirably early in

---

[7]Available as a dietary supplement.

the morning with a consequent inability to fall back asleep in early morning hours. The presentation can mimic depression, whose hallmark biological sign is often noted to be an early morning awakening; care should be taken to carefully distinguish between these two diagnoses. Treatment of each is difficult; options include specifically timed bright light therapy, with or without light restriction, and timed administration of low dose melatonin. The time of administration differs for the two disorders, and is determined by the patient's own endogenous dim light melatonin onset and arise time, and the phase response curve for light and melatonin administration. Bright light therapy is administered at approximately 2500 lx intensity for at least 30 minutes. The timing of bright light administration is first thing in the morning after arising in DSWPD, where a phase-advancing influence is desired; for ASWPD patients, bright light is prescribed in the late afternoon and early evening hours where it will have a phase-delaying effect. Weeks to a few months of regular therapy are necessary to achieve effect. Adherence is difficult and compliance unable to be verified. Specifically timed melatonin usually given at very low doses for this indication (contrary to its use in higher supraphysiologic doses as a hypnotic agent by many patients in other contexts of insomnia, or its high-dose use in REM sleep behavior disorder [RBD]) may also be administered, but its dose and timing are complicated; it must be given in accordance with the circadian phase response curve to have optimal effects and to avoid complicating the problem. For most patients with DSWPD, immediate release melatonin 0.5 mg should be administered at approximately 1 hour before desired bedtime; in ASWPD, melatonin would instead be given prior to the time point of 8 hours following the patient's usual rise time (so as to have a phase-delaying effect). Adjunctive light restriction is recommended in the late afternoon and evenings for DSWPD to avoid precipitating additional phase delays—such as the avoidance of working with luminescent computer screens or viewing video media from close distance in the late evenings—and some experts advocate the use of commercially available blue light restricting glasses as biologically reasonable, as blue light stimuli in evening hours may exacerbate phase delay and confound other recommended treatment effects. However, the efficacy of blue light restriction currently lacks explicit evidence from large clinical trials. As a last resort, the measure of chronotherapy, a progressive delay of bedtime every few days, is prescribed, with the bed and rise times being progressively and successively delayed until the desired bed and rise times are achieved. Attempts to then entrain the patient on this schedule with the aforementioned measures are again attempted with scheduled bright light and prescribed timed melatonin dosing. This is a lengthier process for DSWPD patients and necessitates work restriction during the approximate 2-week time frame necessary to achieve a turnaround of the desired patient's sleep/wake schedule.

Parasomnias and Other Nocturnal Events

Parasomnias are nocturnal events that disrupt sleep but usually do not appreciably disturb sleep quality. As such, nocturnal events do not typically present with symptoms of insomnia or hypersomnia unless there are other comorbid primary sleep disorders such as OSA, which is a frequent comorbidity presenting along with the parasomnias, especially in adult patients.

Parasomnias may arise from either NREM or REM sleep. The NREM parasomnias are essentially all variations on the theme of disorders of arousal, where the behavioral sleep state lingers into awakening, leaving arousal from sleep incomplete. Consequent clinical manifestations are surprisingly heterogeneous and often age related, with specific syndromes such as sleep terrors (also called night terrors) in children, sleep walking and confusional arousals seen in children and adults, and sleep-related eating behavior seen almost exclusively in adults, especially those receiving zolpidem or other newer prescribed hypnotics.

NREM disorders of arousal are especially common in children in the first decade of life and are regarded as a relatively normal variant (and perhaps in some cases simply representing an exaggerated manifestation of the physiological difficulty in arousing from the characteristically deeper N3 NREM sleep inherent in the developing brain). As such, pediatric parasomnias are frequently outgrown; however, in some patients, they do endure throughout life. In adult patients who present with newly evolved nocturnal events proven to be NREM disorders of arousal, one should be highly suspicious of comorbid primary sleep disorders that provoke arousing events, such as SDB or PLMD.

REM parasomnias include nightmares and RBD. Nightmares are undesirable, disturbing dreams that lead to sudden arousal from sleep with heightened autonomic sequelae of sweating, hypervigilance, tachycardia, and tachypnea. Nightmares and vivid dreaming are present in between 10% and 50% of normal young children and in about 50% of adults, but become abnormally disturbing in content or frequency much less frequently, and the true prevalence of nightmare disorder remains unknown. Patients who present with a chief complaint of frequent nightmares should be reassured as to their biological nature and receive a detailed physical and neurologic history and examination to exclude potential provoking comorbid causes such as a recent medication change in type or dosage, mood or anxiety disorder, or primary sleep disorder such as SDB. If no certain readily reversible triggering cause may be identified, referral for consideration of hypnosis, behavior treatment in the form of imagery rehearsal therapy, or pharmacotherapy with clonazepam (Klonopin)[1] may be helpful in some cases. Nightmares that involve flashbacks of previous traumatic events, most often also with similar daytime flashbacks, suggest the alternative diagnosis of posttraumatic stress disorder (PTSD) and the need for psychiatric evaluation. Recent evidence has suggested that alpha-blocking medications such as prazosin (Minipress)[1] or terazosin (Hytrin)[1] may be helpful in suppressing nightmares associated with PTSD.

RBD is characterized by potentially injurious dream enactment behaviors that mirror frightening dream content (characteristically involving fighting off attackers or defending oneself against assailants). In RBD, bed partners will describe objective witnessed dream enactment manifested by violent limb thrashing movements such as punching or kicking and screaming or shouting vocalization during sleep. While RBD patients rarely leave the bed and sleepwalk, falls or other injurious behavior to self or the bed partner are frequent. Importantly, RBD is strongly associated with future development of neurodegenerative disorders. Elderly patients newly diagnosed with RBD harbor up to an 91.9% risk of developing Parkinsonism within 15–25 years of symptom onset, with a shorter-term risk of 30% to 50%, so that all patients with RBD require serial neurologic examinations and follow-up. RBD in young adults may, however, be caused by antidepressant medications, especially the SSRIs, and removal of the offending drug may lead to resolution of dream enactment in some cases. Diagnosis of RBD is by clinical history as well as confirmatory evidence for increased REM sleep muscle tone evident on polysomnographic electromyogram (EMG) leads in the chin and limbs (known as REM sleep without atonia). Treatment options include melatonin, initially at doses of 3 to 6 mg and gradually titrating toward 12 mg nightly as needed to suppress witnessed injurious behaviors, or clonazepam (Klonopin)[1] 0.5 to 1.0 mg increased to 2 to 3 mg nightly. Great care should be taken to first exclude comorbid OSA prior to use of clonazepam, a potential respiratory and upper-airway suppressant.

Nocturnal epilepsies or psychogenic nonepileptic spells may also arise from sleep or apparent sleep and are additional diagnostic considerations in the differential diagnosis

---

[1]Not FDA approved for this indication.

TABLE 5 | Distinguishing Features of Nocturnal Events

	PREMONITORY SYMPTOMS	BEHAVIORAL CHARACTERISTICS	DURATION	FREQUENCY	EEG/PSG FINDINGS
NREM Parasomnias					
Night terrors	None	Inconsolable screaming	Minutes	1 or less nightly	Arousal from N2-N3
Confusional arousals	None	Confused, amnestic	Seconds to minutes	1 or less nightly	Arousal from N3>N2
Sleepwalking	None	Ambulation, amnesia	Minutes	1 or less nightly	Arousal from N3 » N2
REM Parasomnias					
Nightmares	Dream recall	Arousal, frightened, palpitations	Seconds	Generally 1/nightly	Arousal from REM
RBD	Variable dream recall	Thrashing, complex motor behavior	Seconds to minutes	>1/night, second>first half	REM sleep without atonia
Epilepsies					
BECTS	Facial twitching, hypersalivation	Focal motor or GTC, postictal	Seconds to minutes	>1/night	Arousal from NREM, IEDs EEG pattern
ADNFLE	Bizarre stereotyped motor behavior	Focal motor, bizarre motor	Seconds, < 1 min	1 or multiple attacks/night	Arousal from N2
TLE	Aura variable	CPS, postictal	1–2 min	1 or multiple attacks/night	Arousal from N2
Psychogenic spells	Variable	Variable	often>5 min	1 or multiple attacks/night	Normal awake EEG

Abbreviations: NREM=nonrapid eye movement sleep; N2=stage 2 NREM sleep; N3=stage 3 NREM sleep; REM=rapid eye movement sleep; IEDs=interictal epileptiform discharges; EEG=electroencephalogram; PSG=polysomnogram; BECTs=benign epilepsy of childhood with centro-temporal spikes; ADNFLE=autosomal dominant nocturnal frontal lobe epilepsy; TLE=temporal lobe epilepsy; RBD=REM sleep behavior disorder.

of parasomnias. A high degree of stereotypy (one attack being essentially identical to the next) with multiple attacks within a single night are features suggestive of organic partial extra-temporal (frontal lobe) epilepsy, even in the absence of EEG changes between or during an episode. In children, benign rolandic epilepsy may lead to stereotyped episodes of facial twitching and drooling, with or without secondary generalized tonic clonic seizures. Children or adults with autosomal dominant nocturnal frontal lobe epilepsy (ADNFLE) may present with bizarre brief motor behavior (typically of 10- to 60-second duration) without postictal sleepiness. ADNFLE has recently been mapped in several kindreds as a channelopathy, producing a defect of the neuronal nicotinic acetylcholine receptor. Psychogenic nonepileptic spells are instead characterized by nonstereotypic and often prolonged attacks that arise from a behavior state of apparent sleep that is instead confirmed during video-EEG PSG to represent normal waking EEG background. Distinguishing features for the differential diagnosis of nocturnal events are shown in Table 5.

Sleep-Related Movement Disorders
Sleep-related movement disorders include restless legs syndrome (RLS), periodic limb movement disorder (PLMD), leg cramps, bruxism, rhythmic movement disorder, and others.

RLS and PLMS
Diagnosis of RLS is based completely on a clinical history and typically requires four central elements of the described symptoms: an uncomfortable urge to move the legs, with or without uncomfortable leg sensations; temporary relief by movement; symptoms occurring solely or predominantly at rest; and nocturnal worsening of symptoms. About 50% of patients with RLS will carry a positive family history of the disorder, but positive family history is not necessary for the diagnosis. The nature of the

symptoms as described by the patient may be quite variable with regard to the symptom quality, location or distribution, temporal occurrence, frequency, and severity. RLS symptoms are usually described as uncomfortable, although not really painful, with a sense of a creepy-crawly or prickling discomfort, often below the knees and centered about the shins or calves, but sometimes more proximally in the thighs, or even isolated to the feet and ankles. Symptoms may occur in the arms as well, especially proximally near the shoulders. Augmentation is common, occurring in about 50% of patients treated with dopaminergic drugs and involves a worsening of the symptoms: symptom onset occurs earlier during the day, becomes more intense, and spreads up to the arms. RLS has been linked to deficient iron stores and dopaminergic neurotransmission in the brain and is more common in patients with parkinsonism, multiple sclerosis, epilepsy, and in those with chronic renal insufficiency.

While periodic limb movements of sleep (PLMS) are seen in 80% to 90% of RLS patients, PLMS are not necessary for the diagnosis of RLS. Furthermore, PLMS are also extremely frequent in the general population, seen in 5% to 15% of younger adults and as many as 45% of elderly individuals. PLMD is diagnosed when PLMS is thought to cause daytime hypersomnia in the absence of other sleep disorders.

Nonpharmacologic treatments including warm or cool baths, massage, stretching, or even the application of spontaneous compression devices have been reported to be effective anecdotally and in small case series, but an evidence base for these measures remains poor, and most patients seeking medical care for the symptom have severe enough symptoms to merit pharmacologic treatment.

Iron and pharmacologic treatments for RLS are outlined in Table 6. Iron deficiency, or even low normal body iron stores, may worsen or precipitate symptoms. Measuring a serum ferritin should be considered early in all RLS patients, with iron

TABLE 6 Clinical Pharmacology of Treatments for Restless Leg Syndrome

	MECHANISM OF ACTION	DOSAGE	TYPICAL ADVERSE EFFECTS	INTERACTIONS
Iron Replacement				
Ferrous sulfate[1]	Fe	324 mg, 1 tab every alternate day	Nausea, constipation	None
Ferrous fumarate+vit C[1]	Fe	200/125 mg, 1 tab every alternate day	Nausea, constipation	None
Carbidopa-Levodopa (Sinemet)[1]	DA	25/100 1–2 prn	Nausea, dizziness, ICD	None
Pramipexole (Mirapex)	DA	0.125–1.0 mg[2] qhs	Nausea, dizziness, ICD	None
Ropinirole (Requip)	DA	1–6 mg[2] qhs	Nausea, dizziness, ICD	None
Rotigotine (Neupro Transdermal Patch)	DA	1–3 mg qam	Nausea, dizziness, ICD	None
Gabapentin (Neurontin)[1]	Unknown	300–1200[2] mg qhs	Nausea, dizziness, pedal edema, weight gain	None
Gabapentin Enacarbil (Horizant)	Unknown	600 mg	Nausea, dizziness, pedal edema, weight gain	None
Pregabalin (Lyrica)[1]	Unknown	100–600 mg qhs	Nausea, dizziness, pedal edema, weight gain	None
Tramadol (Ultram)[1] Codeine	MRA MRA[1]	50 mg 400 mg qhs 30–60 mg	Nausea, dizziness Nausea, dizziness	None None
Oxycodone[1]	MRA	5–15 mg	Nausea, dizziness	None

[1]Not FDA approved for this indication.
[2]Exceeds dosage recommended by the manufacturer.
Abbreviations: mg=milligrams; Fe=iron replacement; DA=dopamine agonist; MOR=mu opiate receptor agonist.

replacement therapy begun if serum ferritin values are less than 50 mcg/L. Iron therapy can be constipating or cause GI distress, and the formulation of iron with added vitamin C (Ferrex 150 Plus, Vitelle Irospan) is often better tolerated by those who cannot stomach ferrous sulfate.

Carbidopa-levedopa (Sinemet)[1] may be used for patients with only intermittently disturbing symptoms, but chronic nightly use of carbidopa-levodopa, especially above a dosage of 200 mg daily, may raise the risk of augmentation. For nightly use, the newer dopaminergic agonist medications pramipexole (Mirapex) or ropinirole (Requip) remain a mainstay of treatment. Pramipexole may be initiated at 0.125 to 0.25 mg nightly and titrated every few days to the 0.375 to 0.50 mg range or beyond if needed for symptom control. Doses beyond 1.0 mg[3] are typically not additionally effective and appear to raise augmentation risk. Ropinirole may be initiated at 0.5 to 1.0 mg with gradual upward titration to the 4 to 6 mg[3] range as needed and tolerated. Generally, dosing 1 hour prior to bedtime is sufficient, but if earlier evening or late afternoon symptoms emerge, cautious application of divided doses may be utilized, and some experts advice at least a low morning dosage administered daily to achieve a more chronic steady state of dopamine administration since this may be a sensible strategy to minimize augmentation risk. For either initial first-line therapy, or particularly when patients are beginning to experience earlier symptom onset during the day and may have failed the other short-acting dopaminergic drugs pramipexole and ropinirole, a rotigotine (Neupro) patch has been an advent in RLS management and often may be substituted for those other agents to provide more day-long symptom relief and reduce a growing augmentation tendency. Rotigotine offers several other advantages, as its transdermal delivery system provides continuous day-long release of medication that may minimize peak/trough serum concentration variation and minimize the occurrence of other potential adverse effects. Rotigotine also appears to result in augmentation less frequently than other dopaminergic drugs. All patients receiving dopaminergic agents should be counseled upfront about the approximate 15% idiosyncratic risk of impulse control disorder symptoms (such as pathologic gambling, shopping, or hoarding/punding behaviors), and be forewarned that should such problems result, the medication must be withdrawn and another nondopaminergic drug substituted for symptom control. Typical dose-related adverse effects are also described further in Table 6.

Gabapentin (Neurontin)[1] is increasingly becoming an alternative first-line medication for RLS, dosed 300 to 1200[3] mg every night at bedtime as needed and tolerated. Gabapentin may be the agent of choice in patients with comorbid anxiety, pain and insomnia or in patients who are intolerant, resistant to, or have developed augmentation with dopamine agonist medications. On the other hand a dopamine agonist is still generally the first choice for pharmacologic treatment of RLS in severe cases and may be preferred over gabapentin in patients with comorbid depression, obesity, metabolic syndrome, OSA and history of falls. Gabapentin enacarbil (Horizant) is a prodrug of gabapentin that is better absorbed and carries an indication for RLS, but generic gabapentin is also frequently effective and well tolerated, and there has been no head-to-head trial showing superiority of the more expensive prodrug gabapentin encarbil over that of gabapentin. Other alternatives include clonazepam[1] and tramadol (Ultram).[1] For patients unresponsive to these measures, opiate treatment with oxycodone (Roxicodone)[1] 5 to 15 mg at bedtime, hydromorphone (Dilaudid),[1] or methadone (Dolophine)[1] are often

[1]Not FDA approved for this indication.

[1]Not FDA approved for this indication.
[3]Exceeds dosage recommended by the manufacturer.

effective. A large randomized trial showed that the combination oxycodone-naloxone (Targiniq ER)[1] resulted in substantial improvements in RLS symptoms in patients who had previously shown inadequate response to dopamine agonists. Small case series suggest other alternatives for refractory RLS such as carbamazepine (Tegretol),[1] oxcarbazepine (Trileptal),[1] and lamotrigine (Lamictal).[1] The impact of comorbid OSA should also be considered, as optimization of treatment for SDB may improve both subjective RLS symptoms as well as PLMD frequency in many patients.

Sleep-Related Leg Cramps

Sleep-related leg cramps are a common and enigmatic problem affecting 7% to 10% of children and up to 70% of elderly adults. Unfortunately, despite their extremely common occurrence and impact on the quality of life of cramp sufferers, little is known about the pathophysiology or treatment of this condition. Cramps are painful, involuntary sustained muscle contractions, lasting 2 to 10 minutes and affecting the unilateral or bilateral calves, thighs, or feet, with residual tenderness of the affected muscle lasting up to an hour or longer. The clinical approach to sleep-related leg cramps is to first determine whether they are also present during daytime in addition to sleep. If daytime cramping is prominent, exclusion of a precipitating neuromuscular disorder is paramount, including amyotrophic lateral sclerosis, peripheral neuropathy, myositis, or cramp-fasciculation syndrome. In elderly men, peripheral vascular disease and other systemic medical comorbidities are also common. (The reader is referred to the chapter on neuromuscular disorders for further advice on the diagnosis of these conditions.) A neurologic examination should be conducted on all cramp sufferers, and those having sensorimotor findings, fasciculations, or pathologic reflex findings should be referred for EMG, serum creatinine kinase, or additional blood and urine tests for exclusion of symptomatic causes of neuropathy as appropriate. While additional testing for electrolyte abnormalities such as hypomagnesemia, hypocalcemia, hyponatremia, and hypokalemia can be considered, they are of extremely low yield. When examination findings are normal and cramps are isolated to the sleep state, further diagnostic work-up can usually be avoided. Symptomatic treatment measures for sleep-related leg cramps include tonic water with lemon and advising adequate hydration and nightly stretching of the calves and thighs. Prescription quinine (Qualaquin)[1] carries a FDA black box warning for leg cramp treatment and is essentially no longer used for this indication. For refractory frequent cramp sufferers, a sodium-channel blocking anticonvulsant such as carbamazepine[1], oxcarbazepine[1], or lamotrigine[1] may also be considered.

Sleep-Related Bruxism

Sleep-related bruxism, rhythmic grinding of the teeth during sleep, may lead to significant tooth wear and dental or jaw pain. The condition is usually idiopathic, although it may be associated with psychiatric conditions such as mood or anxiety disorders, especially if it is also present during daytime. Treatment usually involves dental referral for consideration of a fitted mouth guard, although in extreme cases pharmacotherapy with clonazepam[1] or consideration of botulinum toxin (Botox)[1] may be necessary.

Other Sleep-Related Movement Disorders

Sleep-related rhythmic movement disorder usually occurs in patients with psychomotor maldevelopment and involves repetitive head and neck or axial body movements. This behavior is not strictly voluntary and often persists during PSG into deep drowsiness or light NREM sleep, so behavioral treatments alone are often ineffective. Head banging behavior, sometimes into the headboard of the bed, can be injurious at times: a protective helmet or treatment with clonazepam[1] is advisable in some cases. Most other movement disorders, such as organic tremors, myoclonus, or dyskinesias generated by the basal ganglia, are suppressed during sleep but may reemerge during drowsiness or nocturnal awakenings.

Propriospinal myoclonus at sleep onset is characterized by myoclonic jerks having their primary and earliest onset in abdominal and axial muscles prior to spreading to the limbs and may be associated with thoracic spinal cord pathology. Spinal imaging with MRI is advised. Treatment with clonazepam[1] is usual for this uncommon diagnosis, although it is unfortunately often ineffective, and many cases of propriospinal myoclonus are instead found to represent a functional movement disorder.

Isolated Symptoms and Normal Variants

These conditions are felt largely to represent either normal variants or otherwise largely benign disorders. The definition of long and short sleepers are somewhat arbitrary, but may be considered as greater than 10 hours or shorter than 5 hours of habitual sleep. Short or long sleep time are each assumed to be variants of normal behavior in the absence of hypersomnia or nighttime symptoms of insomnia.

Sleep talking, or somniloquy, in isolation is rarely of concern. History is often lifelong in such patients. When sleep talking is newly evolved in an elderly individual or a younger patient receiving antidepressant therapy, RBD should be considered in the differential diagnosis, and the patient should be questioned about other potential evidence for dream enactment behavior. A careful medication history and neurologic examination alone will usually dictate whether further evaluation with PSG may be indicated, but in most cases isolated sleep talking is not a cause for concern.

Sleep starts, hypnic jerks or physiologic myoclonus are near universal in their occurrence and often associated with recent excessive caffeine intake or emotional or physical stress. A history of occurrence of jerks limited to the arms, legs, or axial musculature causing arousal within the first 5 to 10 minutes of sleep, and lacking later recurrence during the night, is typical. Reassurance and avoidance of precipitating factors is advised; however, if hypnic jerks are excessive or recur later in the night, PSG is occasionally necessary to distinguish this benign diagnosis from PLMD or propriospinal myoclonus. Propriospinal myoclonus at sleep onset is characterized by myoclonic jerks having their primary and earliest onset in abdominal and axial muscles prior to spreading to the limbs and may be associated with thoracic spinal cord pathology. Spinal imaging with MRI is advised. Treatment with clonazepam[1] is usual for this uncommon diagnosis.

Other Sleep Disorders

Undesirable influences in the patient's sleep environment can serve to regularly distract or disturb him or her from initiating or maintaining sleep. Typical influences include a bed partner who snores loudly or who causes bed motion due to restless or disturbed sleep; pets who sleep in bed with the patient and cause awakening; environmental noise from neighborhood dogs, car alarms, or neighboring freeway or train way; too much outdoor ambient light; or undesirable household ambient temperature. There is considerable overlap in this category of environmental sleep disturbance with inadequate sleep hygiene, as activating stimuli in the environment may lead the patient toward chronic insomnia and adapting undesirable sleep-related behaviors that serve to further disrupt restful sleep.

Sleep-Related Medical and Neurologic Disorders

Fatal familial insomnia is an exceedingly rare, autosomal dominant variant form of familial Creutzfeldt-Jakob disease, a prion disorder that leads to progressive insomnia and progressive

---

[1]Not FDA approved for this indication.

[1]Not FDA approved for this indication.

cognitive impairment, with death inevitably occurring within 3 years of onset. Aggregate prion protein accumulates in the thalamus and other brain regions, and relentlessly progressive insomnia, panic disorder, hallucinosis, and dementia ensue. Unfortunately, no treatments are currently known for this rare disorder.

Conclusions

Sleep disorders are common and result in significant patient morbidity, daytime dysfunction, and impaired quality of life. Untreated sleep disordered breathing (SDB) may also raise the risk for hypertension, vascular events, and mortality. The most common presenting symptoms of sleep disorders include insomnia, characterized by difficulty initiating and maintaining sleep with poor sleep quality, and hypersomnia, the symptom of excessive daytime sleepiness. Evaluation begins with a detailed history and physical examination, which in select cases may require support and clarification by polysomnography and multiple sleep-latency testing. Fortunately, effective therapies are available for the majority of sleep disorders. Insomnia typically requires behavioral or pharmacologic interventions, while SDB may be effectively treated in most cases with positive airway pressure (PAP) therapy. Primary CNS hypersomnias including narcolepsy require stimulant management in most cases, while most parasomnias benefit from clonazepam.[1] Circadian sleep disorders may require timed light and melatonin therapies. Patients having RLS and PLMD should be evaluated for iron deficiency and may enjoy symptom control through dopaminergic or other alternative symptomatic treatments. The majority of patients with sleep disorders benefit from a careful clinical evaluation and appropriately selected therapies.

---

[1]Not FDA approved for this indication.

References

American Academy of Sleep Medicine: *International Classification of Sleep Disorders: Diagnostic and Coding Manual*, ed 3, Darien, IL, 2014, American Academy of Sleep Medicine. 2014.

Auger RR, Burgess HJ, Emens JS, et al: Clinical practice guideline for the treatment of intrinsic circadian rhythm sleep-wake disorders: Advanced Sleep-Wake Phase Disorder (ASWPD), Delayed Sleep-Wake Phase Disorder (DSWPD), Non-24-Hour Sleep-Wake Rhythm Disorder (N24SWD), and Irregular Sleep-Wake Rhythm Disorder (ISWRD). An update for 2015. An American Academy of Sleep Medicine Clinical Practice Guideline, *J Clin Sleep Med* 11:1119–1236, 2015.

Chesson AL, Anderson WL, Pancer JP, Wise M: Practice parameters for the indications for polysomnography and related procedures: An update for 2005, *Sleep* 28:499–521, 2005.

Collop NA, Tracy SL, Kapur V, et al: Obstructive sleep apnea devices for out-of-center (OOC) testing: Technology evaluation, *J Clin Sleep Med* 7:531–548, 2011.

Costanzo MR, Ponikowski P, Javaheri S, et al: Sustained 12 month benefit of phrenic nerve stimulation for central sleep apnea, *Am J Cardiol* 121(11):1400–1408, 2018.

Johns MW: A new method for measuring daytime sleepiness: The Epworth sleepiness scale, *Sleep* 14:540–545, 1991. Also available online in a patient fillable version at http://www.stanford.edu/~dement/epworth.html.

Kushida CA, Littner MR, Morgenthaler T, et al: Indications for positive airway pressure treatment of adult obstructive sleep apnea patients: A consensus statement, *Chest* 115:863–866, 1999.

Luyster FS, Strollo Jr PJ, Zee PC, et al: Sleep: A health imperative, *Sleep* 35:727–734, 2012.

Morgenthaler TI, Lee-Chiong T, Alessi C, et al: Standards of Practice Committee of the American Academy of Sleep Medicine. Practice parameters for the clinical evaluation and treatment of circadian rhythm sleep disorders, *Sleep* 30:1445–1459, 2007.

Schutte-Rodin S, Broch L, Buysse D, et al: Clinical guideline for the evaluation and management of chronic insomnia in adults, *J Clin Sleep Med* 4:487–504, 2008.

Silber MH, Becker PM, Earley C, et al: Willis-Ekbom Disease Foundation revised consensus statement on the management of restless legs syndrome, *Mayo Clin Proc* 88:977–986, 2013.

St. Louis EK: Key sleep neurologic disorders: Narcolepsy, restless legs syndrome/Willis-Ekbom disease, and REM sleep behavior disorder, *Neurol Clin Pract* 4:16–25, 2014.

Wise MS, Arand DL, Auger RR, et al: American Academy of Sleep Medicine. Treatment of narcolepsy and other hypersomnias of central origin, *Sleep* 30:1712–1727, 2007.

SPORTS-RELATED HEAD INJURIES

Method of
Brandon Hockenberry, MD; Margaret Pusateri, MD; and Christopher McGrew, MD

CURRENT DIAGNOSIS

- Initial evaluation of any sports-related head injury should follow standard emergency medicine procedures.
- Presence of any "red flag" symptoms is concerning for a more serious head injury (skull fracture and intracranial hemorrhage) and requires emergency evaluation.
- If "red flag" symptoms are present and advanced imaging is indicated, a noncontrast computed tomography (CT) scan of the head is the initial study of choice.
- If no "red flag" symptoms are present, one of several validated neuropsychological tests should be administered to evaluate cognitive function (e.g., Sports Concussion Assessment Tool, version 5 [SCAT 5]; https://bjsm.bmj.com/content/bjsports/early/2017/04/26/bjsports-2017-097506SCAT5.full.pdf).
- Ultimately, concussion is still a clinical diagnosis.
- Advanced neuroimaging, fluid biomarkers, genetic testing, helmet sensors, and video surveillance have all been purported as possible prognostic indicators but require further validation.

CURRENT THERAPY

- Blood pressure control is critical for patients with intracranial hemorrhage.
- Small intracranial hemorrhages without midline shift or significant symptoms may be monitored, but surgical decompression is otherwise required.
- For patients requiring sedation, propofol (Diprivan)[1] is often preferred due to its short half-life, which makes it easier to monitor neurologic status.
- Mannitol can also be used to help lower intracranial pressure.
- For posttraumatic seizures, phenytoin (Dilantin)[1] is the preferred medication.
- If there is any concern for concussion, the athlete should immediately be removed from play.
- An athlete should never be allowed to return to play on the same day as the injury.
- After an initial rest period of 24–48 hours, an athlete should begin progressing through return-to-play and return-to-learn protocols (https://www.cdc.gov/headsup/providers/return_to_activities.html).
- In the first 24 hours after injury, acetaminophen is the treatment of choice for associated headaches; nonsteroidal antiinflammatory drugs (NSAIDs) and aspirin can worsen an undiagnosed intracranial hemorrhage.
- If headaches persist longer than 3–5 days, medications that do not pose a risk for rebound headaches (e.g., tricyclic antidepressants) can be used.
- Good sleep hygiene is important for recovery. If insomnia persists for more than 2–3 days after injury, medications can be considered.
- Typical recovery time is up to 2 weeks in adults and 4 weeks in children.
- Access to a multidisciplinary team including physical therapists, neurologists, and psychiatric providers is beneficial for athletes with complicated or prolonged recoveries.
- If an athlete has a history of a learning disability, depression, anxiety, or chronic headaches, recovery can be complicated by an exacerbation of the underlying disease.

---

[1]Not FDA approved for this indication.

Introduction and Epidemiology

Sports-related head injuries include a heterogenous group of insults to the brain caused by either a direct impact to the head or an impact to the body associated with energy transfer into the head.

In the United States, sports are among the leading causes of head injuries. Specifically between the ages of 15 and 24 years, athletic activities are the second leading cause of head injuries; only motor vehicle accidents have a higher incidence. Athletic and recreational activities vary widely in terms of biomechanics and kinetics, resulting in a wide range of associated risks. Many sports are limited by the speed at which an athlete can run (e.g., rugby or soccer), but others allow athletes to compete at much higher speeds, some nearly equivalent to those of motor vehicles (e.g., cycling or skiing). These sports potentially put athletes at a higher risk for more severe head injuries.

Sports- and recreation-related traumatic brain injuries (SRR-TBIs) are monitored by the National Electronic Injury Surveillance System—All Injury Program (NEISS-AIP). According to this program, there were more than 3.4 million visits to emergency departments (EDs) across the United States for SRR-TBIs between 2001 and 2012, or approximately 340,000 per year.

Concussion is by far the most common head injury associated with athletic activity. It is estimated that 1.7 to 3.0 million concussions per year are related to sports and recreational activities. The overall rate is 2.5 concussions per 10,000 athletic events, and concussions make up 5% to 18% of reported injuries in the National Collegiate Athletic Association. It is estimated that 50% of concussions go unreported or undiagnosed. The most common severe head injury is a subdural hematoma, which accounts for greater than 90% of all sport-related catastrophic head injuries. These are most often seen in American football, cheerleading, and skiing/snowboarding and occur in less than 1 per 100,000 athletic events. Fatalities from sports-related head injuries are very rare; however, subdural hematoma is a serious injury. In one study, it was reported that American football players with subdural hematoma had a fatality rate of 8.5% and a 48% rate of suffering permanent neurologic deficits.

Risk Factors

Every athlete is potentially at some risk for a head injury during activity. Many factors contribute to relative risk, with the type of activity being the largest contributing factor. In their younger years, males sustain the most head injuries playing football or wrestling, whereas bicycling and basketball take over top spots after the high school and college years. In females, bicycling and horseback riding contribute the most head injuries. It should be noted that some activities have higher incidence rates of head injuries than the aforementioned activities (e.g., men's/women's ice hockey) but are not as commonly played and therefore do not contribute to the sheer volume of injuries that other activities do. With respect to concussion specifically, men's ice hockey and football have the highest incidence rates (5.5 to 6.5 concussions per 10,000 athletic events) in the high school and college populations. On the women's side, soccer and lacrosse have the highest rates (3 to 3.5 concussions per 10,000 athletic events).

Children and teens are at increased risk for head injuries because they are developmentally immature and more frequently participate in activities that have a higher risk for head trauma. Overall, 70% of all SRR-TBIs are in the age group of 0 to 19 years. In the young athlete, a larger head-to-neck ratio, smaller amount of neck/shoulder musculature, and thinner cranial bones all contribute to an increased chance that a blow to the head will cause a head injury. The active elderly have better balance, fewer falls, and fewer TBIs than their more chronically ill counterparts. Therefore increased age is not an independent risk factor for SRR-TBIs.

At the high school and college levels, males have more concussions than do women in sheer numbers but a lower incidence rate overall. Females may have greater risk because of decreased neck musculature compared with males. Female sex has been associated more commonly with abnormal imaging, surgical

intervention, complication, and death. A history of previous concussion increases risk for future concussions compared with nonconcussed athletes, and the greatest risk for repeat concussion is during the 10-day period after the most recent concussion.

Pathophysiology

The pathophysiology of SRR-TBIs and sports-related concussion (SRC) is multifactorial. Several mechanisms have been identified. Biomechanically, a combination of acceleration, deceleration, and rotational/translational forces directly applied or transmitted to the head affect change at the level of individual cells. Metabolic derangements, neurotransmitter dysfunction, changes in cerebral blood flood, neuroinflammation, microstructural damage, and diffuse axonal injury have all been implicated as potential pathways. Helmet-based measurement studies have attempted to quantify head impacts, providing information on force, frequency, and location. However, results vary widely among athletes diagnosed with concussions. In addition, the accuracy of the data detected by helmet sensors and video surveillance systems has been called into question; it does not necessarily reflect the impact on the brain itself, and there is no evidence to support the use of such systems to attempt to diagnose SRC.

Assessment and Diagnosis of Sports-Related Head Injury

The initial assessment of any sports-related head injury should follow standard emergency medicine procedures. Assessment of the "ABCs" (airway, breathing, and circulation) and evaluation for concomitant cervical spine injury should be the first steps in management. The presence of any red flag symptoms (Box 1) should raise concerns for a serious head injury, such as an intracranial hemorrhage or skull fracture, and requires immediate evaluation in the ED, likely advanced head or neck imaging, and possible specialist consultation. The appropriate emergency action plan should be initiated and the athlete stabilized and transported to the designated medical facility.

Once in the ED, the decision whether to obtain images needs to be made. Some assessment tools have been developed, such as the Pediatric Emergency Care Applied Research Network (PECARN; https://www.mdcalc.com/pecarn-pediatric-head-injury-trauma-algorithm) and Canadian CT Head Injury algorithms. A Glasgow Coma Scale score below 14, palpable skull fracture, or presence of red flag symptoms would all be reasons to image acutely. The initial imaging test of choice after head injury is a noncontrast head CT, which will show fractures, intracranial hemorrhage, midline shifts, and signs of edema. CT with angiography will show decreased blood flow into cerebral vessels because of increased intracranial pressure. However, if increased intracranial pressure due to malignant brain edema or an expanding hematoma is suspected, more invasive intracranial pressure monitoring is a more accurate measure and will be more useful to management (see Box 1).

If no red flag symptoms are present and the athlete does not require emergency medical treatment, he or she should be removed from the field of play if there is any suspicion for

---

BOX 1	Red Flag Symptoms

Persistent vomiting
Seizure
Severe "worst headache of my life"
Focal neurologic deficit
Blurred vision
Slurred speech
Significant drowsiness/poor awakening
Poor orientation to person/place/time
Declining mental status

The presence of any of these symptoms should prompt consideration of emergency department evaluation and head imaging. If no red flags are present, the clinician may be able to send the athlete home safely and follow up in the office the next day.

possible SRC. Several brief neuropsychological tests have been developed to evaluate cognitive function. Examples of practical and validated tests include the SCAT 5 and the Standardized Assessment of Concussion (SAC). The SCAT 5 is broken down into six steps: immediate or on-field assessment, symptom evaluation, cognitive screening, neurologic screening, delayed recall, and decision. In addition to an assessment of the aforementioned red flag symptoms, the immediate or on-field assessment section of the SCAT 5 also includes a review of observable signs (e.g., lying motionless on the playing field, facial injury after head trauma, and blank or vacant look), a memory assessment using the Maddocks Questions (Box 2), a measure of the Glasgow Coma Scale (Table 1), and a cervical spine assessment. It has been found that standard orientation questions (name, location, and year) are not reliable in the immediate assessment of SRC. The Maddocks questions, which focus on sport-specific memory assessment, provide better information to help the examiner determine whether there is a concern for an SRC. Once the initial assessment is complete, if there is any concern for an SRC, the athlete should be removed from the sporting environment and not allowed to return to play on the day of injury.

Diagnosis of SRC remains a clinical diagnosis. Over the past two decades, multiple investigations have focused on the use of advanced neuroimaging (e.g., functional magnetic resonance imaging [f-MRI] and electroencephalogram [EEG]) and body fluid analysis (blood, saliva, and cerebrospinal fluid) as potential tools to aid in the diagnosis of SRCs. (In addition, these modalities have been explored as potential prognostic indicators, attempting to predict clinical recovery or assess the cumulative risk of repetitive trauma.) At this time, advanced neuroimaging, fluid biomarkers, and genetic testing are important research tools but require further validation to determine their ultimate clinical utility in the evaluation and diagnosis of SRC.

Clinical Manifestations

Clinical manifestations after an SRR-TBI and SRC can be varied. The brain itself is a complex organ. Depending on which area is injured, different symptoms may present. With regard to the more serious diseases, such as intracranial hemorrhages or diffuse axonal injury, the athlete is often critically injured, again demonstrating red flag symptoms and signs of increased intracranial pressure. However, SRC is an evolving injury within the acute phase and can often have an initially subtle presentation. Signs and symptoms rapidly change, especially over the first 24 to 48 hours. Classically, symptoms fall into one of four categories: physical (headache, nausea, and dizziness), cognitive (difficulty concentrating and slowed reaction times), emotional (anxiety and irritability), and sleep disturbances (insomnia and hypersomnia). As part of the SCAT 5 and other concussion assessment tools, an in-depth symptom checklist is used to evaluate SRCs both initially and during follow-up. For example, Table 2 outlines the SCAT 5 symptom checklist. It is important to note that there are no specific scoring guidelines that are diagnostic of concussion. The scores are most commonly used to monitor an athlete's recovery, tracking improvement or decline over time. Of note, higher scores at the time of initial injury are associated with longer recoveries.

Treatment

Presence of red flag symptoms listed in Box 1 or a Glasgow Coma Scale score of less than 14 should raise suspicion for a more severe SSR-TBI, such as a skull fracture or intracranial hemorrhage, rather than a typical concussion. If an athlete sustains an SSR-TBI other than concussion, he or she should be evaluated in the ED. In the event of an intracranial hemorrhage of any kind, the largest concern is increasing intracranial pressure. Strict blood pressure control is incredibly important, because an increased blood pressure will increase the pressure in the bleeding vessel and thus the rate and severity of the bleed. Intracranial hemorrhages may be monitored if the bleed is small and not causing a midline shift or significant symptoms. However, definitive treatment with surgical decompression is preferred for subdural and epidural hemorrhages. Most patients will require intubation, sedation, and intracranial pressure monitoring. For sedation, propofol (Diprivan)[1] is the preferred agent at many institutions because it has a short half-life, making it easier to monitor the patient's neurologic status. In the presence of malignant brain edema, mannitol (Osmitrol) can be added to decrease intracranial pressure when strict blood pressure and pain control has failed. For a TBI causing posttraumatic seizure, phenytoin (Dilantin)[1] remains the preferred medication, although many institutions will use older antiepileptic drugs such as valproate (Depakote)[1] or carbamazepine (Tegretol)[1] as treatments of choice.

The current recommendation for the management of SRC is to remove the athlete from play and not allow a return on the same day. The athlete should avoid physical exertion and mental activities that make symptoms worse. After an initial rest period of 24 to 48 hours, the patient should begin progressing

[1] Not FDA approved for this indication.

BOX 2	Memory Assessment: Maddocks Questions

What venue are we at today?
What half is it now?
Who scored last in the game?
What team did you play last week?
Did your team win the last game?

Note: Can be adapted to specific sports as necessary.
These questions help make diagnosis of concussion. No official score cutoff is diagnostic; however, inability to answer them all correctly should raise suspicion for concussion or more severe head injury. Questions can be changed slightly if they are not relevant to a sport, such as swimming.

TABLE 1	Glasgow Coma Scale

BEST EYE RESPONSE (E)	BEST VERBAL RESPONSE (V)	BEST MOTOR RESPONSE (M)
Eye opening spontaneously: 4	Oriented: 5	Obeys commands: 6
Eye opening to voice: 3	Confused: 4	Localizes to pain: 5
Eye opening to pain: 2	Inappropriate words: 3	Flexion/withdrawal from pain: 4
No eye opening: 1	Incomprehensible sounds: 2	Abnormal flexion to pain: 3
	No verbal response: 1	Abnormal extension to pain: 2
		No motor response: 1

Used to rate the severity of head injury. Scores in each category are added for a total of 15 points. Athletes with concussion typically have a Glasgow Coma Scale score of 14 (losing 1 point in the verbal response category) or 15. Scores less than 14 should prompt a visit to the emergency department for head imaging.

to both physical (noncontact) and mental activities. The athlete should return to normal activities of daily living as much as is tolerated without symptom exacerbation. The newest consensus statement on concussion in sport outlines not only a return-to-play protocol but also a return-to-learn protocol. These are outlined in Tables 3 and 4. Children and adolescents should not return to sport until they have fully returned to school. It is important to note that there is no evidence to suggest that any medications or nutritional supplements will improve rate of recovery from concussion. Medications in concussion treatment are primarily used for symptomatic relief.

Monitoring Concussions

After concussion diagnosis, the clinically stable athlete can be sent home if a responsible adult is available to accompany him or her. Sleep is encouraged, and the athlete need not be awakened for evaluation. The athlete should be followed up in a qualified healthcare provider's office within 24 to 48 hours for reevaluation. Follow-up examination should include a symptom severity checklist (see Table 2), history, and neurologic examination at a minimum. Completing a full SCAT 5 evaluation is unnecessary if the athlete had one done at time of injury and still has symptoms. Advanced neuroimaging with MRI is not needed to monitor a concussion and by definition should be normal.

TABLE 2	SCAT 5 Symptoms Checklist
SYMPTOM	**SEVERITY**
Headache	0 1 2 3 4 5 6
"Pressure in head"	0 1 2 3 4 5 6
Neck pain	0 1 2 3 4 5 6
Nausea and/or vomiting	0 1 2 3 4 5 6
Dizziness	0 1 2 3 4 5 6
Blurred vision	0 1 2 3 4 5 6
Balance problems	0 1 2 3 4 5 6
Sensitivity to light	0 1 2 3 4 5 6
Sensitivity to noise	0 1 2 3 4 5 6
Feeling slowed down	0 1 2 3 4 5 6
Feeling like "in a fog"	0 1 2 3 4 5 6
"Don't feel right"	0 1 2 3 4 5 6
Difficulty concentrating	0 1 2 3 4 5 6
Difficulty remembering	0 1 2 3 4 5 6
Fatigue or low energy	0 1 2 3 4 5 6
Confusion	0 1 2 3 4 5 6
Drowsiness	0 1 2 3 4 5 6
More emotional	0 1 2 3 4 5 6
Irritability	0 1 2 3 4 5 6
Sadness	0 1 2 3 4 5 6
Nervous or anxious	0 1 2 3 4 5 6
Trouble falling asleep (if applicable)	0 1 2 3 4 5 6
Total number of symptoms	Of 22
Symptom severity score	Of 132

There is no score cutoff that is diagnostic of concussion; it is simply used to monitor a patient's improvement or decline over time. Higher scores at time of injury are associated with longer recovery times.

SCAT 5, Sports Concussion Assessment Tool version 5.

As the athlete returns to play, close supervision under a qualified healthcare provider such as a certified athletic trainer or physical therapist is ideal but not always possible. When an athlete has progressed through the return-to-play protocol (see Table 3), follow-up with an appropriate qualified healthcare provider should be arranged to obtain full medical clearance to return to full contact activity.

Management of Concussion Complications

Headaches are among the most common symptoms of a concussion and often the symptom that bothers the athlete the most. In the acute period after injury, medications have some potential to mask important symptoms. For the first 1 to 2 hours after the injury, it is important to be able to accurately monitor the patient for a changing clinical picture, which could suggest that the head injury is not a concussion but rather an evolving epidural or subdural hematoma. For the first 24 hours, NSAIDs and aspirin should be avoided because they can thin the blood and potentially make an undiagnosed hematoma become a more significant bleed. Acetaminophen (Tylenol) is the preferred medication for headache in the first 24 hours. After the first day, it is safe to switch to ibuprofen (Motrin), which may have more benefit. If headaches are not improving after 3 to 5 days, it is advisable to switch to another medication that does not pose the risk of creating rebound headaches. Tricyclic antidepressants are a good choice and work very well. Nortriptyline (Pamelor)[1] at a low dose (25 mg/d) is generally well tolerated in children as well as adults and may be stopped abruptly without withdrawal symptoms once the athlete is feeling well and ready to progress back to activities.

Sleep disturbances in athletes with concussion are also very common. Many will not sleep well the first night after injury and want to nap during the day. Other athletes may sleep much more than usual after initial injury. Although there are no clear studies proving the optimal amount of sleep, current trends are to try to return the athlete to normal sleep cycles and daily living as much as possible. An emphasis on sleep hygiene over the first few days is standard. If insomnia persists after 2 to 3 days, medications may be considered. Melatonin[7] is available over the counter, has very few side effects, and is generally well tolerated. The next step would be amitriptyline (Elavil)[1] at a low dose (10– 25 mg/d). This can be especially effective if the athlete has both headaches and poor sleep because it is more sedating than nortriptyline.

A concussion is expected to last no more than 14 days in an adult and less than 4 weeks in the pediatric population. Each individual physician will have a different comfort level treating concussion; however, it is reasonable to consider a referral to a specialty physician once an athlete has passed the normal expected recovery time and is not categorized as a "prolonged concussion." Each city or region will have a different culture about who takes care of the prolonged concussions. Neurologists, sports medicine physicians, and physical medicine and rehabilitation physicians are all well equipped to take care of these athletes. Physical therapists, particularly those who specialize in vestibular rehabilitation, can be very helpful to patients with continued balance problems, concentration difficulties, and other visual symptoms. Last, neuropsychologists can be extremely helpful in difficult cases. Some athletes have complicated clinical histories prior to the injury. Attention-deficit/hyperactivity disorder, depression, anxiety, and chronic headaches can all make the clinical picture very confusing when the athlete is having symptoms such as concentration difficulties, mood swings, insomnia, or headaches that are not

---

[1] Not FDA approved for this indication.
[7] Available as a dietary supplement.

TABLE 3 Graduated Return-to-Play Protocol as Outlined by the Consensus Statement on Concussion in Sport

STAGE	AIM	ACTIVITY	GOAL OF EACH STEP
1	Symptom-limited activity	Daily activities that do not provoke symptoms	Gradual reintroduction of work/school activities
2	Light aerobic exercise	Walking or stationary cycling at slow to medium pace; no resistance training	Increase heart rate
3	Sport-specific exercise	Running or skating drills; no head impact activities	Add movement
4	Noncontact training drills	Harder training drills (e.g., passing drills); may start progressive resistance training	Exercise, coordination, and improved thinking
5	Full-contact practice	After medical clearance, participate in normal training activities	Restore confidence and assess functional skills by coaching staff
6	Return to sport	Normal game play	

Start step 1 after initial 24- to 48-hour period of rest. Each step should take a minimum 24 hours to progress through.

TABLE 4 Example of a Graduated Return-to-Learn Protocol as Outlined by the Consensus Statement on Concussion in Sport

STAGE	AIM	ACTIVITY	GOAL OF EACH STEP
1	Daily activities that do not give the child symptoms	Typical activities of the child during the day as long as he or she does not increase symptoms (e.g., reading, texting, screen time). Start with 5–15 min at a time and build up	Gradual return to typical activities
2	School activities	Homework, reading, or other cognitive activities outside of the classroom	Increase tolerance to cognitive work
3	Return to school part time	Gradual introduction of schoolwork. May need to start with a partial school day or increased breaks during the day	Increase academic activities
4	Return to school full time	Gradually progress school activities until a full day can be tolerated	Return to full academic activities and catch up on missed work

Unlike the return-to-sport protocol, there is no minimum required time for each stage. Some children may be able to tolerate a full school day immediately after injury without difficulty, depending on symptom severity.

improving as expected. It is important to remember that many athletes would not rate their symptom severity score as all zeros at baseline, so expecting them to achieve this goal after injury is impractical. When this scenario is suspected, referral for neuropsychiatric testing can help to divide out which symptoms may be concussion related and which could be more chronic in nature.

Prevention

Helmets have been shown to reduce sports-related skull fractures and intracranial hemorrhages but have not been shown to decrease rates of concussion. Mouth guard use decreases the rate of dental injuries and lip lacerations but has not been definitively proven to decrease the rate of concussion or other brain injuries. Sport-specific rule changes have resulted in reduced rates of head injury. The most prominent and well-studied example is that of youth ice hockey. Introduction of the 2013 Canadian national body checking policy change disallowing body checking in Pee Wee hockey players below the age of 13 years resulted in a 50% relative reduction in injury rate and a 64% reduction in concussion rate in 11-year-old and 12-year-old hockey players in Alberta. Reduction of contact practices in certain team sports such as American football reduces exposure to head injury as well. Finally, epidemiologic evidence has demonstrated that the most likely period for repeat SRC is in the first 10 days after the most recent concussion, so disallowing contact activity during this interval has potential to reduce repeat concussions.

References

Black AM, Hagel BE, Palacios-Derflingher L, et al: The risk of injury associated with body checking among Pee Wee ice hockey players: an evaluation of Hockey Canada's national body checking policy change, *Br J Sports Med* 51:1767–1772, 2017.

Coronado VG, Haileyesus T, Cheng TA, et al: Trends in sports-and recreation-related traumatic brain injuries treated in US emergency departments: The National Electronic Injury Surveillance System—All Injury Program (NEISS-AIP), 2001– 2012, *J Head Trauma Rehabil* 30:185–197, 2015.

Gessel LM, Fields SK, Collins CL, et al: Concussions among United States high school and collegiate athletes, *J Athl Train* 42:495–503, 2007.

Harmon KG, Clugston JR, Dec K, et al: American Medical Society for Sports Medicine position statement on concussion in sport, *Br J Sports Med* 53:213–225, 2019.

Kerr ZY, Roos KG, Djoko A, et al: Epidemiologic measures for quantifying the incidence of concussion in national collegiate athletic association sports, *J Athl Train* 52:167–174, 2017.

McCrory P, Meeuwisse W, Dvorak J, et al: Consensus statement on concussion in sport—the 5th international conference on concussion in sport held in Berlin, October 2016, *Br J Sports Med* 51:838–847, 2017.

Munivenkatappa A, Agrawal A, Shukla DP, et al: Traumatic brain injury: Does gender influence outcomes? *Int J Crit Illn Inj Sci* 6(2):70–73, 2016.

Nagahiro S, Mizobuchi Y: Current topics in sports-related head injuries: a review, *Neurol Med Chir (Tokyo)* 54:878–886, 2014.

Sarmiento K, Thomas K, Daugherty J, et al: Emergency department visits for sports and recreation-related traumatic brain injuries among children—United States, 2010-2016, *MMWR* 68:237–242, 2019; number 10.

Steenerson K, Starling AJ: Pathophysiology of sports-related concussion, *Neurol Clin* 35:403–408, 2017.

TARGETED TEMPERATURE MANAGEMENT (THERAPEUTIC HYPOTHERMIA)

Scott Leikin, DO; Jennifer Wang, DO; and Adel Bassily-Marcus, MD

CURRENT THERAPY

- Targeted temperature management (therapeutic hypothermia) should be considered following resuscitation from cardiac arrest to reduce the risk of anoxic brain injury.
- There does not appear to be a benefit to cooling to a temperature of 33°C when compared to cooling to a temperature of 36°C (97°F).
- There is a paradigm shift of therapeutic hypothermia to preventing fever and instituting a targeted temperature.
- Cooling pads are the most commonly used method to induce hypothermia.

Introduction

Inducing patients to a targeted temperature to reduce anoxic brain injury post cardiac arrest has now become the standard of care at medical institutions around the world. Although the theory has multiple applications for multiple conditions, post cardiac arrest is the most common and studied indication and the focus of this chapter. Although each institution has their own protocol, there are common tenets that are included in each institution's protocols. Current nomenclature is Targeted Temperature Management (TTM) as the theories on ideal temperature for the post cardiac arrest patient have evolved from therapeutic hypothermia. The evolution of TTM is important to understand, as the current theory is fever prevention is where the benefit is and fever is what is associated with poor neurologic outcomes in the post cardiac arrest time period.

The first multicenter, randomized control study on post cardiac arrest care was conducted in Europe and published in the New England Journal of Medicine (NEJM) in 2002. A total of 3551 patients were deemed eligible, but only 275 were included. In the study, 137 were assigned to hypothermia (32 to 34°C as measured by bladder temperature for 24 hours) and 138 to normothermia. To qualify in the study, subjects must have had a witnessed cardiac arrest, with an initial rhythm of ventricular fibrillation (VF) with return of spontaneous circulation (ROSC). The results showed a favorable neurologic outcome in 75/136 patients (55%) in the hypothermia group compared to 54/137 patients (39%) in the normothermia group at 6 months as measured by the Pittsburgh cerebral-performance category. The mortality difference at 6 months was 41% in the hypothermia group and 55% in the normothermia group. This validated the utilization of mild therapeutic hypothermia to improve neurologic outcomes and decrease mortality for witnessed VF cardiac arrest.

In 2002, a NEJM study described survival with good neurologic outcome to hospital discharge in patients who were unconscious after ROSC in out-of-hospital cardiac arrest. In the study, 77 patients were assigned to normothermia or moderate hypothermia (core body temperature of 33°C within 2 hours of ROSC for 12 total hours). Usually, out-of-hospital cardiac arrests have survival rates of only 5% to 35%. The investigators found 21/43 (49%) patients in the hypothermia group survived and had a favorable neurologic outcome compared to 9/34 (26%) in the normothermia group with (P = .046). The authors concluded that moderate hypothermia improved outcomes in patients with coma after ROSC in out-of-hospital cardiac arrest patients.

In 2010, the American Heart Association (AHA) released a class I recommendation for post VF/VT TTM. Pulseless electrical activity/asystole was given a IIb recommendation. TTM is generally defined as a core temperature of 33 to 36°C. Since this recommendation, TTM has been adopted as common practice post cardiac arrest in comatose adult patients.

In May 2011, the Society of Critical Care Medicine published "Targeted temperature management in critical care: A report and recommendations from five professional societies" and determined that TTM with a core body temperature goal of 32 to 34°C be used for post out-of-hospital VF/VT arrest.

In December 2013, the NEJM published a study titled "Targeted Temperature Management at 33°C versus 36°C after Cardiac Arrest." This international multicenter study aimed to determine the optimal temperature associated with improved neurologic outcomes for out-of-hospital cardiac arrest patients. They found no significant 180-day neurologic outcome or mortality difference between the patients in the 33°C arm and the patients in the 36°C arm. There were no adverse effects or benefits to patients cooled to 33°C. The authors concluded that in patients who were unconscious after ROSC was obtained in out-of-hospital cardiac arrest, a temperature of 33°C did not confer a benefit compared to a temperature of 36°C. This shifted the paradigm of therapeutic hypothermia to preventing fever and instituting a targeted temperature.

The International Liaison Committee on Resuscitation and the AHA Emergency Cardiovascular Care Committee and the Council on Cardiopulmonary, Critical Care and Perioperative and Resuscitation reviewed 5045 studies, of which 6 were RCTs and 5 were observational. They recommended: target core temperatures between 32 and 36°C for at least 24 hours and against using pre-hospital cooling with cooled intravenous fluids.

The theoretical benefits of TTM are that it can reduce brain oxygen usage by 6% for every 1°C reduction while also preventing inflammation and cerebral edema. TTM is currently being studied for encephalopathy, bacterial meningitis, cardiogenic shock, traumatic brain injury, and organ donation.

Initiation

With few absolute contraindications, TTM should be considered in all patients who achieved ROSC post cardiac arrest regardless of the underlying rhythm during the cardiac arrest. Many post cardiac arrest patients with ROSC will go to the cardiac catheterization lab for an angiogram and this should not delay the initiation of TTM. Determining the etiology for the cardiac arrest is still extremely important and should not have a bearing on the initiation of TTM. The patient populations in whom TTM is considered a relative contraindication include intracranial hemorrhage, exsanguination, hypotension refractory to multiple vasopressors, severe sepsis, and pregnancy. At our tertiary care academic medical center, the only absolute contraindications are cryoglobulinemia, traumatic injury leading to cardiac arrest, and family refusal or advanced directives that preclude the use of TTM.

Eligibility requires a comatose patient; the patient should not be able to follow commands or respond to noxious stimuli. This is equivalent to a Richmond Agitation Sedation Score of −4 or −5 or Glasgow Coma Scale <8. The patient must have a sustained cardiac rhythm that results in adequate brain perfusion.

The most studied rhythms in cardiac arrest which benefited from TTM were VT or VF. It is uncertain whether pulseless electrical activity and a "nonshockable rhythm" would benefit from TTM but we would advocate that any patient regardless of the underlying rhythm have TTM utilized if ROSC is obtained. This is in line with the 2015 AHA guidelines on post cardiac arrest care and emergency cardiovascular care. The guideline committee came to this conclusion because cohorts who did not receive TTM had such significant neurologic morbidity that the benefits were considered to outweigh the risks. Significant head trauma should be ruled out in patients who present to an emergency department with a noncontrast head computed tomography (CT) scan. Ideally, TTM should be initiated as soon as ROSC is obtained but it is acceptable to initiate it within the first 6 hours, and even up to 12 hours post arrest. We strongly advocate initiating the process as soon as feasible. We would also recommend that pacer pads be applied to the patient's skin and kept in place. The target core temperature should be maintained at the desired temperature for 24 hours. Based on a review of the literature, initiating a core temperature between 32 and 36°C for these patients with external cooling pads is the target.

The most commonly used method to induce hypothermia is with external cooling pads. Once the process is started, the time to target temperature should be within 2 hours. Other less commonly used options include ice bags at the groin, chest, axilla, and neck, and infusing cold saline. Cooled intravenous saline will reduce core temperature by 1°C every 30 minutes. The 2015 AHA guidelines recommend against cooling patients in the prehospital setting with intravenous cooled saline, as survival and neurologic recovery were not shown to be improved in various trials. Urinary catheters with temperature probes are often used to measure core temperature. Other acceptable methods of temperature measurement include esophageal, rectal, central, tympanic, or nasal probes. Axillary and oral temperature measurements are not reliable in measuring core temperature. Potential complications of cooling include electrolyte abnormalities, hyperglycemia, coagulopathy, and arrhythmias.

Maintenance

In TTM, the targeted core temperature should be maintained within 0.5°C for 24 hours. Shivering should be avoided as it creates heat, thereby increasing oxygen demand. Bedside Shivering Assessment Scale (BSAS) should be utilized to help guide therapy for shivering. For sedation purposes, our recommended first-line treatment is propofol (Diprivan) 15 to 20 µg/kg/min. Midazolam (Versed) 1 to 2 mg/h is an alternative. Fentanyl 25 µg/h infusion can be used if adequate sedation is not achieved.

The BSAS treatment algorithm should be utilized to eliminate shivering. In the BSAS, neuromuscular blockade with an agent such as cisatracurium (Nimbex) 0.15 mg/kg IV bolus followed by an infusion of 1 µg/kg/min can be used, although this protocol may mask seizures. The lowest dose that eliminates shivering using agents with a short half life is recommended because hypothermia slows medication metabolism and elimination.

TTM may worsen or cause hemodynamic derangements and arrhythmias, such as hypotension and bradycardia, that are common post cardiac arrest. Maintenance of a mean arterial pressure (MAP) of 80 to 100 mm Hg will help ensure adequate brain perfusion.

TTM patients are mechanically ventilated, and some institutions use esophageal probes to track body temperature, although this is less common, as it is invasive. Oxygen saturation should be maintained at 94% to 96% to avoid hypoxia or hyperoxygenation. Hyperglycemia is common with TTM, so serum glucose should be checked at set intervals, with a goal <180 mg/dL. If serum glucose is persistently >200 mg/dL despite treatment, an insulin drip should be considered. Electrolyte abnormalities, especially hypokalemia, are common during TTM. Therefore, the

serum potassium level should be checked every 4 to 6 hours and replenished if lower than 3.5 meq/L. Rewarming may increase potassium levels.

It has been reported in the literature that up to 66% of TTM patients will develop an infection. Fever and leukocytosis may be present in the absence of infection and are not reliable indicators of infection. A comprehensive plan needs to be developed for every patient when signs of infection are potentially present. Even if a high percentage of patients develop an infection, this has not been shown to affect mortality.

Rewarming

Rewarming should occur 24 hours after achieving the targeted temperature. Rewarming should not occur at a rate that is faster than 0.2°C/h until the patient reaches 37°C; this will likely take between 6 to 12 hours. Once at 37°C, this temperature should be maintained for 48 to 72 hours, as rebound hyperthermia is associated with poor neurologic outcomes. Electrolyte abnormalities such as hyperkalemia, hypoglycemia, and hypotension may occur. Blood pressure should be carefully monitored during the rewarming period.

Post-Therapeutic Hypothermia/Prognosis

The AHA recommends 72 hours before prognosticating neurologic recovery. Presence of at least two of the following: incomplete brain stem reflexes, presence of myoclonus, unreactive electroencephalography (EEG), and absent cortical somatosensory-evoked potentials suggest poor neurologic outcome. A full neurologic examination should be done daily. Involving neurology or neurocritical care is advised to help prognosticate neurologic recovery in post cardiac arrest TTM patients.

References

Badjatia N, Strongilis E, Gordon E: Metabolic impact of shivering during therapeutic temperature modulation the bedside shivering assessment scale, *Stroke* 39(12):3242–3247, 2008, https://doi.org/10.1161/STROKEAHA.108.523654.

Bernard, Gray, Buist: Treatment of comatose survivors of out-of-hospital cardiac arrest with induced hypothermia. *New England Journal of Medicine*, 346:557–563, 2002, https://doi.org/10.1056/NEJMoa003289.

Callaway Clifton W, et al: American heart association guidelines update for cardiopulmonary resuscitation and emergency cardiovascular care, *Circulation* 132(18):S315–S367, 2015, https://doi.org/10.1161/CIR.0000000000000252, 3 Nov. 2015.

Donnino MW, Anderson LW, Berg KM, Reynolds JC: Temperature management after cardiac arrest an advisory statement by the advanced life support task force of the international liaison committee on resuscitation and the american heart association emergency cardiovascular care committee and the council on cardiopulmonary, critical care, perioperative and resuscitation, *Circulation* 132(25):2448–2456, 2015. https://doi.org/10.1161/CIR.0000000000000313.

Friedman OA: *Critical care: targeted temperature management after cardiac arrest*, In JM Orpopello, V Kvetan, SM Pastores. Eds. New York, NY: McGraw Hill, Lange, 2017.

Moler MD, Silverstein FS, Hulubkov R, et al: Therapeutic hypothermia after out-of-hospital cardiac arrest in children, *New Eng Journal of Medicine*, 372:1898–1908, 2015, Available at: https://doi.org/10.1056/NEJMoa1411480.

Nielson MD, PhD, Wetterslev N, MD, PhD, J, & Cronberg, MD, PhD, T: Targeted temperature management at 33°c versus 36°c after cardiac arrest. *New England Journal of Medicine* 369:2197–2206, 2013, Available at: https://doi.org/10.1056/NEJMoa1310519.

Nunnally M, Jaeschke R, Bellingan G: Targeted temperature management in critical care: a report and recommendations from five professional societies, *Critical Care Medicine* 39(5):1113–1125, 2011, https://doi.org/10.1097/CCM.0b013e318206bab2.

T.: Mild therapeutic hypothermia to improve the neurologic outcome after cardiac arrest, *New England Journal of Medicine* 346:549–556, 2002, https://doi.org/10.1056/NEJMoa012689.

Scirica BM: Therapeutic hypothermia after cardiac arrest, *Circulation, Clinician update* 127(2):244–250, 2013, https://doi.org/10.1161/CIRCULATIONAHA.111.076851.

Yunen JR, Tolentino R: *Critical care: chapter: controversies in therapeutic hypothermia*, In JM Oropello, V. Kvetan, SM Pastores. Eds.). New York, NY: McGraw Hill Lange, 2017.

TRIGEMINAL NEURALGIA

Method of
Karlynn Sievers, MD; and Hugh Silk, MD, MPH

CURRENT DIAGNOSIS

The International Headache Society Diagnostic criteria (classic) are as follows:
A. At least three attacks of unilateral facial pain fulfilling criteria B and C
B. Occurring in one or more divisions of the trigeminal nerve, with no radiation beyond the trigeminal distribution
C. Pain having at least three of the following four characteristics:
- Recurring in paroxysmal attacks lasting from a fraction of a second to 2 min
- Severe intensity
- Electric shock-like, shooting, stabbing, or sharp in quality
- Precipitated by innocuous stimuli to the affected side of the face
D. No clinically evident neurologic deficit
E. Not better accounted for by another diagnosis
International Headache Society Diagnostic criteria (secondary)
Same as previous except
F. Secondary trigeminal neuralgia is secondary to another disease process.

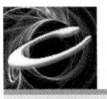

CURRENT THERAPY

- Medications
  - Carbamazepine: start 100 mg twice daily and increase by 200 mg/day to a maximum of 1200 mg/day (number needed to treat = 2)
  - Alternative treatments are available but have not been proven to be as effective (Table 1).
  - For some patients with refractory or severe symptoms, surgical treatment (e.g., microvascular decompression, radiosurgery, alternative invasive procedures) can be helpful.

Epidemiology

The incidence of trigeminal neuralgia is estimated to be 5.9/100,000 women and 3.4/100,000 men. The peak incidence is in patients aged 60 to 70 years. It has also been called "tic douloureux" because of facial spasms that often accompany the disorder.

Risk Factors

Increasing age is a risk factor. Trigeminal neuralgia is rarely diagnosed in patients below 40 years of age. Other risk factors include multiple sclerosis (the incidence of trigeminal neuralgia in this population is 1% to 2%), stroke, and hypertension (especially in women). There is no racial predominance.

Pathophysiology

It is currently hypothesized that trigeminal neuralgia results from demyelination of the fifth cranial nerve, leading to electrical transmission of nerve impulses that are not mediated by neurotransmitters and that generate pain. Demyelination is most commonly caused by aberrant or tortuous blood vessels that cause nerve compression but can also be attributed to sources such as multiple sclerosis or amyloid deposition.

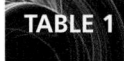
TREATMENT TYPE	EVIDENCE OF EFFECTIVENESS
Medical therapy	
Carbamazepine (Tegretol)	Likely to be beneficial (gold standard)
Oxcarbazepine (Trileptal)[1]	Likely to be beneficial*
Baclofen (Lioresal)[1]	Likely to be beneficial,* particularly in patients with TN caused by MS
Gabapentin (Neurontin)[1]	Unknown effectiveness
Lamotrigine (Lamictal)[1]	Unknown effectiveness
Surgical therapy	
Microvascular decompression	Trade-off between benefits and harms*
Stereotactic radiosurgery	Trade-off between benefits and harms*
Percutaneous destructive radiosurgical techniques	Trade-off between benefits and harms*

*Based on observational studies and/or consensus.
[1]Not FDA approved for this indication.
MS, Multiple sclerosis; *TN,* trigeminal neuralgia.

The most commonly used classification system for trigeminal neuralgia has four categories: classical, symptomatic, secondary, and idiopathic. With classical trigeminal neuralgia, there is no underlying cause for the demyelination other than vascular compression, as described previously. With secondary trigeminal neuralgia, an alternate cause such as multiple sclerosis or tumor is responsible for the demyelination. Symptomatic trigeminal neuralgia is caused by herpes, trauma, or another disorder. A fourth category would include idiopathic trigeminal neuralgia, where there are no radiologic findings that account for the patient's symptoms.

Prevention

There is no known method for the prevention for trigeminal neuralgia.

Clinical Manifestations

Trigeminal neuralgia is a clinical diagnosis made on the basis of recurrent attacks of unilateral facial pain. The pain is intense and is usually described as sharp, shock like, or stabbing. Any of the branches of the trigeminal nerve can be affected, but the maxillary branch is the most common and the ophthalmic branch the least common. The pain lasts for seconds, and most patients are asymptomatic between attacks (though some will have a mild, dull, persistent ache in the area of the affected nerve). Attacks can recur infrequently or hundreds of times per day.

Often, patients have trigger zones that will set off paroxysms of pain with minimal stimulation. Activities such as chewing, teeth brushing, or touching a trigger area can set off attacks; sometimes even minimal stimulation such as a light breeze can trigger an episode. Not all patients have trigger zones; however, the presence of these is nearly pathognomonic for trigeminal neuralgia.

Diagnosis

The diagnosis is clinical, based on the commonly described symptoms listed earlier. Diagnosis of trigeminal neuralgia should be considered in all patients who describe unilateral intense paroxysmal facial pain on three or more occasions. Careful examination of the head and neck and thorough neurologic examination should be performed in all patients. Exam findings are typically normal in patients with trigeminal neuralgia; therefore exam abnormalities should prompt reconsideration of the diagnosis. Sensory abnormalities (including vision or hearing loss), facial muscle weakness, or loss of the corneal reflex are not associated with trigeminal neuralgia and warrant further workup.

Laboratory studies are typically not helpful in making the diagnosis. Temporal mandibular joint or dental radiographs may be helpful to rule out other pathology for those who present with mid or lower face symptoms. Magnetic resonance imaging ([MRI] with and without contrast) of the brain can be helpful in distinguishing between classic and symptomatic trigeminal neuralgia and should be considered in all patients with new onset of symptoms. There is some early evidence that structural MRI techniques can help to identify changes associated with trigeminal neuralgia and to predict those patients who will respond well to surgical intervention, but more research is needed in this area.

Differential Diagnosis

The differential diagnosis includes other types of headaches (migraine, cluster headache, paroxysmal hemicrania), dental sources (cracked teeth, caries, dental abscess), infectious causes (sinusitis, otitis media, postherpetic neuralgia), nervous system pathology (intracranial tumors, multiple sclerosis), temporomandibular joint syndrome, and giant cell arteritis. Many of these other diagnoses will have specific examination findings.

Treatment

Medical treatment should be initiated for all new cases of trigeminal neuralgia. Carbamazepine (Tegretol) has been shown in multiple randomized controlled trials to reduce pain in trigeminal neuralgia and is considered the gold standard for medical treatment. The number needed to treat is 2. Dosing starts at 100 mg twice daily and increases gradually in increments of 200 mg/day to a maximum of 1200 mg/day. Carbamazepine can have side effects such as drowsiness, dizziness, hepatotoxicity, pancreatitis, blood dyscrasias, and ataxia. Consensus opinion is that it has a greater than 50% failure rate for long-term (5 to 10 years) pain control. Oxcarbazepine (Trileptal)[1] can also be used, though the data are not as robust as for carbamazepine (level B for oxcarbazepine vs level A for carbamazepine). Medication should start at 600 mg/day in two divided doses and then be increased to 300 mg every third day to a maximum of 1800 mg. For both medications, testing for the HLA-B*15:02 allele should be considered in at-risk patients (e.g., those of Asian ancestry) to avoid Stevens-Johnson syndrome. Pimozide (Orap)[1] has been promoted as equal to carbamazepine; however, the studies are of low quality with no adverse effect comparison, and pimozide has many potentially serious side effects. Tizanidine (Zanaflex)[1] has been shown to be as effective as carbamazepine but also with low-quality studies. Lamotrigine (Lamictal)[1] can be used in patients who do not tolerate carbamazepine or as an adjunct to those without full benefit from carbamazepine, but the dose must be titrated slowly; therefore it is not as effective for acute pain control. Baclofen (Lioresal)[1] and gabapentin (Neurontin)[1] may be useful in patients with multiple sclerosis who also have trigeminal neuralgia, but evidence is lacking regarding their effectiveness in classical trigeminal neuralgia. Topical lidocaine has been used intraorally for those with significant oral pain from trigeminal neuralgia; however, again, there are

no well-designed studies of its efficacy. A new sodium channel blocker with affinity for the Na$_v$ 1.7 sodium channel is being investigated with some promising evidence of effectiveness, but it is still in clinical trials and not yet available for prescription.

Recent studies have shown some weak data that botulinum toxin A (Botox)[1] can be an effective treatment in reducing both the intensity of pain and frequency of paroxysms in trigeminal neuralgia; adverse events include facial asymmetry and edema or hematoma at the injection site. Alcohol injections[1] and cryotherapy have also been used to treat the pain of trigeminal neuralgia.

For some patients with refractory or severe symptoms, surgical treatment can be helpful. Microvascular decompression and radiosurgery are both common techniques for the treatment of trigeminal neuralgia, with microvascular decompression generally considered to be first-line surgical intervention. Other surgical techniques can include radiofrequency thermocoagulation, glycerol rhizolysis, stereotactic radiosurgery, balloon compression, peripheral nerve section, partial sensory root section, and gamma-knife radiosurgery. Studies have noted sensory side effects, and most evidence for neurosurgical approaches comes from observational studies.

Neuromodulation is an alternative for patients with symptoms refractory to pharmacotherapy who do not want to pursue surgical treatment. Both central and peripheral neuromodulation have been studied, but evidence of effectiveness is very limited.

Treatment for secondary trigeminal neuralgia typically includes treating the underlying cause.

Monitoring

Although there is no standard protocol for monitoring patients with trigeminal neuralgia, the condition is extremely painful, and there have been incidents reported of patients accidentally overdosing on medications or taking their own lives. Therefore it is recommended that patients be monitored at regular intervals to make sure that their pain is controlled and to monitor for side effects from treatment.

Management of Complications

The disease can have relapses and remissions. Medications or alternative treatments should be reinstituted as needed. Tests should be run as needed based on side-effect symptoms, and treatments stopped and others considered based on efficacy and patient tolerance.

---

[1] Not FDA approved for this indication.

References

Gubian A, Rosahl SK: Meta-analysis on safety and efficacy of microsurgical and radiosurgical treatment of trigeminal neuralgia, *World Neurosurg* 103:757–767, 2017.

International Headache Society: International Classification of Headache Disorders (3rd edition – beta version). Available at http://www.ihs-headache.org/ichd-guidelines/ihs-guidelines. (Accessed March 7, 2020).

Khan M, Nishi SE, Hassan SN, et al: Trigeminal neuralgia, glossopharyngeal neuralgia, and mysfascial pain dysfunction syndrome: an update, *Pain Res Manag*7438326, 2017, https://doi.org/10.1155/2017/7438326. Epub 2017 Jul 30. Accessed March 7, 2021.

Krafft R: Trigeminal neuralgia, *Am Fam Physician* 77:1291–1296, 2008.

Obermann, M. Recent advances in understanding/managing trigeminal neuralgia. *F1000Res2019 – Review*. PMID 31069052.

Wiffen PJ, Derry S, Moore RA, et al: Carbamazepine for acute and chronic pain. In *The Cochrane Library*, Issue 8. Chichester, UK, 2013, John Wiley & Sons, Ltd. (Search date 2010).

Zakrzewska JM, Linskey ME: Trigeminal neuralgia, *Am Fam Physician* 94(2):133–135, 2016.

Zakrzewska JM, Linskey ME: Trigeminal neuralgia, *BMJ* 350:h1238, 2015.

Zhang J, Yang M, Zhou M: Non-antiepileptic drugs for trigeminal neuralgia, *Cochrane Database Syst Rev*(12), 2013.

---

[1] Not FDA approved for this indication.

VIRAL MENINGITIS

Method of
Joanna Thomson, MD, MPH; and Samir S. Shah, MD, MSCE

CURRENT DIAGNOSIS

- Typical presentation includes fever, headache, and neck stiffness or pain. Constitutional symptoms include mild lethargy, myalgias, nausea, and vomiting.
- Neonates often present with nonspecific signs and symptoms including lethargy, irritability, and poor feeding.
- Cerebrospinal fluid (CSF) profile should be performed. Results show elevated white blood cell count (often but not always with mononuclear cell predominance), normal to slightly elevated protein, normal glucose, normal to slightly elevated opening pressure, and negative bacterial Gram stain and culture.
- Diagnostic polymerase chain reaction (PCR) and serologic studies can identify the etiologic agent.
- Consider neuroimaging before lumbar puncture if there is concern for increased intracranial pressure or if encephalitis is possible.

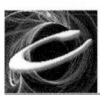

CURRENT THERAPY

- Symptomatic and supportive management includes analgesia, antipyretics, antiemetics, and intravenous fluids.
- Hospitalization is recommended for infants (younger than 1 year), elderly patients (older than 65 years), and immunocompromised patients, as well as for patients presenting with altered mental status, seizures, focal neurologic signs, or the absence of classic viral CSF findings.
- Few medications, with the exception of acyclovir (Zovirax) for HSV, effectively treat viral meningitis.

Epidemiology

The true epidemiology of viral meningitis is unknown because it is not a reportable disease. However, the Centers for Disease Control and Prevention (CDC) estimate 25,000 to 50,000 hospitalizations per year. There is also yearly variation in disease burden. Causes of viral meningitis vary by age group, immune status, season, and geography. There is increased incidence in summer and early fall owing to the high prevalence of enteroviruses and arthropod-borne viruses (arboviruses). Common etiologic agents include enteroviruses, herpes simplex virus (HSV), arboviruses, lymphocytic choriomeningitis virus (LCMV), cytomegalovirus (CMV), varicella zoster virus (VZV), and Epstein–Barr virus (EBV). See Table 1 for features of the common and some less-common viral agents that cause meningitis.

Pathophysiology

Viral infection begins at the mucosal surface of the respiratory tract or gastrointestinal tract, with viral replication occurring in regional lymph nodes. A secondary viremia then occurs that provides access to the central nervous system (CNS). Symptoms of viral meningitis are due to either an immune response to the virus within the CNS (e.g., enterovirus) or direct viral invasion of neural tissue (e.g., HSV1/2).

Prevention

To prevent spread of viral agents responsible for meningitis, hand-washing and other infection-control measures are most important. The infection-control precautions necessary during patient contact depend on mode of transmission of the virus (see Table 1). Vaccines are available for some of the viruses that are known to cause meningitis, including polio (an enterovirus), mumps, measles, and varicella.

Clinical Manifestations

Viral meningitis can be difficult to distinguish from bacterial meningitis. Fever, headache, and neck stiffness and pain are the usual presenting complaints. Headache can be localized to the frontal or retro-orbital areas and may be associated with photophobia. Although neck stiffness and pain are usually present, neck rigidity (positive Kerning's sign or positive Brudzinski's sign) is not always present on examination. Constitutional symptoms can include lethargy, myalgias, and nausea or vomiting. There is often a history of concomitant viral respiratory or gastrointestinal illness at the time of presentation. Seizures can occur with viral causes of meningitis, especially HSV, but should prompt consideration of other diagnostic possibilities.

In contrast to children and adults, neonates often present with nonspecific findings such as lethargy, irritability, and poor feeding. See Table 1 for clinical manifestations associated with specific etiologic agents.

Viral meningitis can also manifest with signs of encephalitis, in which case the encompassing diagnosis is meningoencephalitis. Encephalitis or meningoencephalitis are likely if any of the following are present: altered mental status, seizures, focal neurologic deficits (including aphasia, anosmia, ataxia, cranial nerve deficits, motor weakness, or involuntary movements), or behavioral changes.

Diagnosis

Diagnosis of viral meningitis requires lumbar puncture for CSF studies including cell count, protein, glucose, Gram stain and culture, and specific viral studies. Although a lymphocytic pleocytosis is associated with viral infections, most viral CNS infections initially have a neutrophilic pleocytosis. However, neutrophilic pleocytosis is also associated with bacterial meningitis. In viral meningitis, though CSF protein is normal to slightly elevated, CSF glucose is normal, and no organisms are identified on CSF bacterial Gram stain or culture compared with elevated CSF protein, low CSF glucose, and positive CSF bacterial culture in bacterial meningitis.

Studies to identify a specific virus as the etiologic agent are recommended for patients with severe illness or a complicated course. Viral cultures of CSF are not generally useful given their poor sensitivity, and serologic viral studies require both acute and convalescent titers to demonstrate antibody response to the suspected viral antigen. CSF PCR studies that detect viral DNA or RNA are more sensitive than viral culture and provide more rapid results than serologic viral studies (see Table 1). Multiplex PCR techniques allow for testing of multiple viruses and bacteria with a single CSF sample and a single test. Where available, multiplex PCR may result in considerable savings in time and effort, while improving diagnostic capacity. In some cases, it is useful to perform viral PCR studies on blood (HSV, EBV, CMV, and human herpesvirus [HHV]6), urine (CMV), stool (enterovirus), and skin vesicles (HSV) to further support the diagnosis. However, a positive PCR study from blood, urine, stool, or skin does not provide direct evidence of CNS infection by the same virus. For example, enterovirus isolated from the stool can represent asymptomatic infection or prior infection but may also be isolated from the stool at the same time as concomitant enteroviral meningitis.

Most other testing is not helpful, but further testing (including complete blood count, renal profile, liver function, pancreatic enzymes, and HIV studies) should be guided by the patient's presentation and clinical status.

Neuroimaging (computed tomography [CT] or magnetic resonance imaging [MRI]) should be obtained before lumbar puncture if there is concern for increased intracranial pressure. It is also recommended if symptoms of encephalitis are present (including altered consciousness, seizures, focal neurologic deficits, behavioral changes) to exclude other CNS disease.

TABLE 1	Clinical and Laboratory Characteristics of Viral Meningitis			
VIRUS	**TRANSMISSION**	**KEY CLINICAL FEATURES**	**DIAGNOSIS**	**COMMENTS**
Enterovirus	Fecal-oral	May have rash on exam (e.g., Coxsackie, hand–foot–mouth) Patients with impaired humoral immunity or those <2 wk old can present with a sepsis-like syndrome with multiorgan dysfunction, DIC, cardiovascular collapse	CSF enterovirus PCR	More prevalent in summer and fall
Herpes simplex viruses 1 and 2	Vertical transmission during birth (HSV2), horizontal transmission via contact (HSV1 or HSV2)	10%–30% of adults have symptoms of meningitis with primary HSV2 infection; look for genital vesicular lesions on exam Mollarets meningitis: >3 episodes of fever and meningismus lasting 2–5 d, with spontaneous resolution; episodes may be months to years apart often due to chronic HSV2 CNS infection	CSF HSV1/HSV2 PCR	Meningitis is uncommon with nonprimary HSV2 infection
Arboviruses	Subcutaneous inoculation via mosquito or tick Prevention: Minimize tick and mosquito exposure with personal protection measures including insect repellents and covering exposed skin	Zika virus associated with Guillan-Barré syndrome and in newborn infants microcephaly; sexual transmission is possible	CSF arboviral PCR Zika RT-PCR (performed at CDC Arbovirus laboratory on CSF or serum within first 5–7 days of symptoms); Zika IgM cross reacts with other flaviviruses (e.g., Dengue)	More prevalent in summer and fall Geographic distribution within the United States: Eastern equine encephalitis: Eastern U.S. Western equine encephalitis: Western U.S. St. Louis encephalitis: Across the U.S. (majority of cases in Central and Eastern U.S.) West Nile virus: Across the U.S. California encephalitis (LaCrosse): Midwestern, mid-Atlantic, and Southeastern U.S. Zika virus: Small epidemics have been reported in Southeastern U.S. and Gulf Coast states
Lymphocytic choriomeningitis virus	Virus is present in rodent secretions, feces, and urine Ingestion of contaminated food, exposure of open wounds, or inhalation of aerosolized virus Lab workers, pet owners, and those living in impoverished conditions are highest risk for illness	Accompanied by a flulike illness	Serum LCMV titers (acute and convalescent) CSF findings: May have decreased glucose and WBC count >1000/mL	More prevalent in winter and spring
Cytomegalovirus	Exposure to infected body fluids (e.g., saliva, blood)		CSF CMV PCR	Reactivation of prior infection typically only occurs in the immunosuppressed

VIRUS	TRANSMISSION	KEY CLINICAL FEATURES	DIAGNOSIS	COMMENTS
Epstein–Barr virus	Exposure to infected body fluids (e.g., saliva, blood)	Alice in Wonderland syndrome: altered body image and distortion of visual perception	CSF EBV PCR	Most common neurologic complication with primary infection
HIV	Exposure to contaminated blood or other body fluids (e.g., transfusion, sexual contact, percutaneous blood exposure)	During primary infection, a subset have meningitis or meningoencephalitis May expect thrush and cervical lymphadenopathy	HIV studies	Treatment with HAART
Human herpesvirus 6	Respiratory	Roseola: febrile illness followed by viral exanthem	CSF HHV6 PCR	HHV6 has been demonstrated in the CSF of asymptomatic persons Immunosuppressed persons at risk for symptomatic infection and reactivation
Varicella	Respiratory	Typical vesicular skin lesions of chickenpox on exam CSF pleocytosis has also been demonstrated with reactivation; can also occur in the absence of cutaneous findings of herpes zoster ("zoster sine herpete")	CSF VZV PCR	Rarely diagnosed during acute chickenpox infection; usually a postinfectious complication Other neurologic sequelae of varicella infection are more common than aseptic meningitis; most common is cerebellar ataxia
Mumps	Respiratory	Parotitis on exam is the most prominent sign of infection Aseptic meningitis can precede or follow clinical exam findings CSF profile can demonstrate an unusually high protein with a mild pleocytosis and normal glucose	Serum titers	More common in winter and spring
Measles	Respiratory	CSF pleocytosis in ≤30% of patients with measles; patients are usually without clinical meningitis	Serum titers	In the United States, most cases are imported (e.g., occur in returning travelers)
Influenza	Respiratory	Aseptic meningitis is a less common neurologic complication of influenza infection (encephalopathy is more common)	CSF influenza PCR	More prevalent in winter Increased risk of neurologic complication in young patients and in those with pre-existing medical disease

Abbreviations: CMV = cytomegalovirus; CNS = central nervous system; CSF = cerebrospinal fluid; DIC = disseminated intravascular coagulopathy; HHV = human herpesvirus; HSV = herpes simplex virus; LCMV = lymphocytic choriomeningitis virus; PCR = polymerase chain reaction; VZV = varicella zoster virus; WBC = white blood cell.

Differential Diagnosis

The major item on the differential diagnosis for viral meningitis is bacterial meningitis. The bacterial meningitis score, validated in children 29 days to 19 years, is a clinical prediction rule that identifies patients as at very low risk (0.1%) for bacterial meningitis if they lack all of the following: positive CSF Gram stain, CSF absolute neutrophil count (ANC) of at least 1000 cells/μL, CSF protein of at least 80 mg/dL, peripheral blood ANC of at least 10,000 cells/μL, and a history of seizure before or at the time of presentation. While C-reactive protein (CRP) is not generally useful because it can be high in viral meningitis and low in the initial stages of bacterial disease, elevated serum procalcitonin levels (>0.5 μg/mL in children and >0.2 μg/mL in adults) are more sensitive and specific for distinguishing viral from bacterial meningitis.

Other diagnoses to consider include parameningeal infections (i.e., subdural or epidural empyema, brain abscess), meningitis due to fungi, mycobacteria, rickettsia, mycoplasma, parasites, and other CNS infectious or inflammatory processes including malignancy, drug exposure, rheumatologic disease (e.g., systemic lupus erythematosus), or autoimmune (e.g., anti-NMDA receptor encephalitis).

Treatment

Symptomatic care remains the mainstay of therapy for viral meningitis. Therapy should be directed at pain and fever control (e.g., ibuprofen [Motrin], acetaminophen [Tylenol], ketorolac [Toradol]), management of nausea and vomiting (e.g., ondansetron [Zofran]), and intravenous fluids. Hospitalization is recommended for patients younger than 1 year, the elderly, and the immunocompromised. Patients who present with altered mental status, seizures, focal neurologic signs, or a CSF profile that does not have the classic viral profile should also be hospitalized for clinical management and for antibiotic treatment until bacterial meningitis can be excluded. Advanced care including management of respiratory failure, cardiovascular instability, seizures, disturbed fluid and electrolyte balance, and cerebral edema may be necessary.

Empiric antibiotic coverage may be considered while awaiting CSF culture results in the young, elderly, and immunocompromised, especially if there is suspicion of bacterial meningitis or partially treated bacterial meningitis.

Acyclovir (Zovirax) should be initiated in cases of suspected HSV while waiting PCR confirmation. Dosing of acyclovir is age and weight dependent: 20 mg/kg per dose IV every 8 hours for patients younger than 12 years; 10 mg/kg per dose IV every 8 hours for patients older than 12 years.

In the immunocompromised patient, HHV6 may be treated with foscarnet (Foscavir)[1] or ganciclovir (Cytovene)[1], and CMV may be treated with ganciclovir, valganciclovir (Valcyte), foscarnet, or cidofovir (Vistide). Case reports suggest benefit of such antiviral therapies in the immunocompromised, but no controlled trials have been performed.

Complications

The prognosis of viral meningitis depends on cause and severity of illness as well as age. Non-HSV viral meningitis has low mortality rates in adults and children alike. Mortality and morbidity are associated with other organ system involvement, including meningoencephalitis. Although up to 10% of infants hospitalized with non-HSV viral meningitis experience seizures, altered mental status, or increased intracranial pressure during the acute illness, studies have shown no evidence of long-term neurodevelopmental delay. Most adults recover fully within a week without long-term sequelae. Persistent neurologic sequelae (including headaches, incoordination, concentration difficulties, muscle weakness, and focal neurologic deficits) occur more often in patients with meningoencephalitis.

HSV is associated with high rates of morbidity and mortality. Neonatal isolated CNS HSV has a 4% mortality rate even with acyclovir treatment; mortality is 50% without acyclovir treatment. Unfortunately, acute treatment does not affect morbidity,

as 70% of infants with neonatal CNS HSV infection will suffer from neurodevelopmental impairments. Recent studies have demonstrated improved outcomes in these infants with long-term oral acyclovir suppression therapy. Outside of the neonatal period, CNS HSV infection has a 28% mortality rate with antiviral treatment (70% mortality rate without treatment). Long-term neurologic sequelae occur in two-thirds of survivors who received antiviral therapy, compared with virtually all of those who did not receive treatment.

References

Centers for Disease Control and Prevention. Zika Virus. http://www.cdc.gov/zika/index.html. Accessed February 12, 2016.

Dubos F, Korczowski B, Aygun DA, et al: Serum procalcitonin level and other biological markers to distinguish between bacterial and aseptic meningitis in children: a European multicenter case cohort study, *Arch Pediatr Adolesc Med* 162:1157–1163, 2008.

Hawkes MT, Vaudry W: Nonpolio enterovirus infection in the neonate and young infant, *Paediatr Child Health* 10:383–388, 2005.

James SH, Kimberlin DW, Whitley RJ: Antiviral therapy for herpesvirus central nervous system infections: neonatal herpes simplex virus infection, herpes simplex encephalitis, and congenital cytomegalovirus infection, *Antiviral Res* 83:207–213, 2009.

Khetsuriani N, Quiroz ES, Holman RC, Anderson LJ: Viral meningitis associated hospitalizations in the United States, 1988–1999, *Neuroepidemiology* 22:345–352, 2003.

Kimberlin DW, Lin CY, Jacobs RF, et al: Safety and efficacy of high-dose intravenous acyclovir in the management of neonatal herpes simplex virus infections, *Pediatrics* 108:230–238, 2001.

Kimberlin DW, Whitley RJ, Wan W, et al: Oral acyclovir suppression and neurodevelopment after neonatal herpes, *N Engl J Med* 365:1284–1292, 2011.

Nigrovic LE, Fine AM, Monuteaux MC, et al: Trends in the management of viral meningitis at United States children's hospitals, *Pediatrics* 131:670–676, 2013, [PMID: 23530164].

Nigrovic LE, Kuppermann N, Macias CG, et al: Clinical prediction rule for identifying children with cerebrospinal fluid pleocytosis at very low risk of bacterial meningitis, *JAMA* 297:52–60, 2007.

Rorabaugh ML, Berlin LE, Heldrich F, et al: Aseptic meningitis in infants younger than 2 years of age: acute illness and neurologic complications, *Pediatrics* 92:206–211, 1993.

Rotbart HA: Viral meningitis, *Semin Neurol* 20:277–292, 2000.

Sakushima K, Hayashino Y, Kawaguchi T, et al: Diagnostic accuracy of cerebrospinal fluid lactate for differentiating bacterial meningitis from aseptic meningitis: a meta-analysis, *J Infect* 62:255–262, 2011.

Viallon A, Zeni F, Lambert C, et al: High sensitivity and specificity of serum procalcitonin levels in adults with bacterial meningitis, *Clin Infect Dis* 28:1313–1316, 1999.

Wilson MR, et al: Clinical metagenomic sequencing for diagnosis of meningitis and encephalitis, *N Engl J Med* 380:2327–2340, 2019.

---

[1]Not FDA approved for this indication.

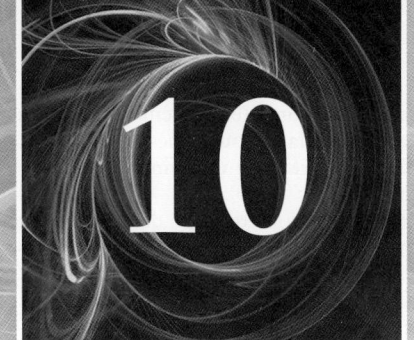

10 Psychiatric Disorders

ALCOHOL USE DISORDER

Method of
David A. Frenz, MD

Unhealthy alcohol use (UAU) is prevalent in the general population and patients seeking healthcare. This chapter will describe its classification, epidemiology, identification, and management in primary care settings.

Classification

UAU represents a continuum of alcohol use associated with negative health consequences, including addiction. This conceptualization has been adopted by the United States Preventive Services Task Force (USPSTF) and is the basis for Screening, Brief Intervention and Referral to Treatment (SBIRT), the contemporary, graded approach to management described in this chapter.

UAU consists of three mutually exclusive categories (Box 1). Hazardous use increases the future risk of negative health consequences; harmful use has already caused adverse health consequences but does not meet criteria for addiction; and alcohol use disorder (AUD), or addiction, is defined by the *Diagnostic and Statistical Manual of Mental Disorders* (DSM-5).

Hazardous use is anchored to binge drinking[a] and weekly consumption limits. A binge is alcohol consumption that results in legal intoxication (blood alcohol concentration [BAC] ≥0.08 gram percent). For healthy adults, this is typically >3 drinks for women and men ≥65 years of age, and >4 drinks for men <65 years of age, where one U.S. standard drink contains 14 grams of ethanol (Table 1). Alcohol intoxication is strongly associated with immediate risks including injuries, suicide, and violence.

Over longer timescales, alcohol is associated with a broad range of conditions including infectious diseases, many cancers, cardiovascular diseases, gastrointestinal diseases, mood disorders and epilepsy. Consuming >7 drinks per week increases all-cause mortality in a linear manner, regardless of gender.

AUD is defined in the DSM-5 as "a problematic pattern of alcohol use leading to clinically significant impairment or distress, as manifested by at least two [criteria], occurring within a 12-month period." DSM-5 outlines 11 criteria such as "alcohol is often taken in larger amounts or over a longer period than was intended" and "recurrent alcohol use resulting in a failure to fulfill major role obligations at work, school, or home." Consumption (frequency and quantity), the defining features of hazardous use, are not part of the construct.

Harmful use exists when alcohol-related harm has occurred but the "problematic pattern" and/or criterion threshold for AUD have not been satisfied.

Epidemiology

Large, population-based surveys have found that 17.1% to 24.4% of Americans binge drink, with considerable regional

---

BOX 1 | The Alcohol-Use Continuum

Low Risk Use, Including No Use
Consumption of alcohol below amounts identified as hazardous; *and* use in circumstances not defined as hazardous (context)
Example: One glass of wine with dinner several days per week

Hazardous Use
Alcohol use that increases the risk for health consequences

Hazardous Consumption
Females; males ≥65 years of age: >3 drinks/day and/or >7 drinks/week
Males <65 years of age: >4 drinks/day and/or >7 drinks/week

Hazardous Context
Example: Alcohol use during pregnancy

Harmful Use
Alcohol use with health consequences in the absence of addiction
Example: College student who sustains a forehead laceration secondary to falling down while intoxicated

Alcohol Use Disorder
Addiction to alcohol per the Diagnostic and Statistical Manual of Mental Disorders
Mild: 2–3 criteria
Moderate: 4–5 criteria
Severe: ≥6 criteria

The shaded portion represents unhealthy alcohol use (UAU).

TABLE 1 | U.S. Standard Drinks: By Definition, One Standard Drink Contains 14 Grams of Ethanol

BEVERAGE	ALCOHOL BY VOLUME	DRINK SIZE
Beer (regular)	5%	12 fl oz
Wine	12%	5 fl oz
Distilled spirits*	40%[†]	1.5 fl oz

Data from U.S. Department of Agriculture and U.S. Department of Health and Human Services. Dietary Guidelines for Americans, 2020–2025 (9th ed). Washington, DC: U.S. Department of Agriculture, 2020, p. 49
*Examples include vodka, gin, whiskey, rum, and tequila
[†]80 proof

variability. This translates into healthcare settings. For example, a cross-sectional study of 2.7 million primary care patients determined that 6.1% exceeded recommended daily consumption limits (male: 8.7%; female: 3.8%).

A similar pattern exists for AUD. The third wave of the National Epidemiologic Survey on Alcohol and Related Conditions (NESARC-III), a cross-sectional survey of American adults, found that 13.9% and 29.1% of the population met criteria for AUD in the preceding year and on a lifetime basis, respectively. Coincidentally, the corresponding prevalence is 13.9% in primary care settings.

| BOX 2 | Two-Step Process for Screening for Unhealthy Alcohol Use (UAU) and Associated Management |

Step 1: Single-Question Screener (SQS)
How many times in the past year have you had X or more drinks in a day?
where X = 4 for females and males ≥65 years of age; and X = 5 for males <65 years of age

Management
0 times: None/done (negative screen)
≥1 times: Proceed to Step 2

Step 2: Alcohol Use Disorders Identification Test (AUDIT)
Administer full-scale AUDIT (10 items)
(https://auditscreen.org/check-your-drinking/)

Management
<8 points: None/done (negative screen)
8–15 points: Brief intervention
16–19 points: Brief intervention and continued monitoring
>19 points: Assess for Alcohol Use Disorder (AUD), initiate treatment if present

Identification

In light of its prevalence and considerable harms, the USPSTF recommends "screening for unhealthy alcohol use in primary care settings in adults 18 years or older, including pregnant women, and providing persons engaged in risky or hazardous drinking with brief behavioral counseling interventions to reduce unhealthy alcohol use."

Various screening instruments exist. The author prefers a two-step process beginning with a single-question screener (SQS)[b] to reduce the testing burden for both patients and clinicians (Box 2). Positive screens are then clarified with the Alcohol Use Disorders Identification Test (AUDIT) (https://auditscreen.org/check-your-drinking/). Both instruments are in the public domain and may be used without formal permission or licensing.

Although patients with UAU can engage in malingering and deception, the SQS's reported sensitivity ranges from 0.73 to 0.88. Its negative predictive value (NPV), which depends on prevalence, is 0.94 to 0.98 when 5% to 15% of those screened have UAU. Said differently, this corresponds to a 2% to 6% false negative classification ("miss rate") at typical base rates in primary care.

Patients with significantly elevated AUDIT scores (>19 points) require careful assessment for AUD. This can be accomplished through structured clinical interviews ("checklists" based on DSM-5 criteria) or referral to a mental health professional for a diagnostic assessment.

Management

Management of UAU depends on patient classification (Box 1). Most patients, including those with AUD, are appropriate for initial treatment in primary care settings.

Brief interventions, motivational enhancement therapy (MET; motivational interviewing) and addiction pharmacotherapy are effective treatments for UAU. The former typically consists of behavioral counseling (focused education and advice) concerning drinking limits and ways to mitigate alcohol-related risks. The National Institute on Alcohol Abuse and Alcoholism (NIAAA) offers a variety of free patient materials to assist with this process.

Motivational interviewing is a person-centered style of counseling for addressing the common problem of ambivalence about changing one's behaviors. A full description of methods and techniques are beyond the scope of this chapter; however, the

literature offers several practical introductions for primary care providers. Systematic reviews have consistently demonstrated its effectiveness for various alcohol-related outcomes, although a recent meta-analysis questioned its efficacy in maintaining abstinence in primary care settings.

Addiction pharmacotherapy, sometimes described as medication-assisted treatment (MAT),[c] is generally reserved for patients with AUD (Box 3). Disulfiram (Antabuse), which was approved by the U.S. Food and Drug Administration in 1951, has generally fallen into disuse secondary to lack of efficacy, medication interactions and potential for various harms.

Naltrexone (ReVia [oral], Vivitrol [IM]) and acamprosate (Campral) both improve drinking outcomes, although with various nuances depending on trial design and type of data analysis. In placebo-controlled trials, acamprosate but not naltrexone increased abstinence, while naltrexone but not acamprosate reduced heavy drinking. Head-to-head trials found differences between the medications; however, they were ultimately equivalent when these data were subject to meta-analysis. Overall, the author selects one medication over the other based on patient preference and factors such as medication compliance and end-organ function.

The literature continues to evolve on the off-label use of medications including baclofen (Lioresal), gabapentin (Neurontin), and topiramate (Topamax). In the author's opinion, these should generally be prescribed in consultation with an addiction medicine specialist after patients have tried and failed adequate therapeutic trials of acamprosate and naltrexone despite robust psychosocial treatments.

Historically, medically managed withdrawal ("detoxication") has occurred in supervised settings. Reliable, carefully selected patients can safely be withdrawn on an ambulatory basis. The author uses the Short Alcohol Withdrawal Scale (SAWS), a patient self-rating scale, to trigger benzodiazepine administration.

Comorbidities

Other mental disorders frequently co-occur[d] with AUD and often precede its onset. In this context, AUA may represent a maladaptive coping mechanism for affective and anxious symptoms, and psychological trauma. Nascent evidence is mixed on treatment priorities and modalities. In the absence of firm guidance, management is empiric and should likely occur in consultation with local mental health experts.

Similarly, medical conditions such as chronic pain syndromes often co-occur with AUD and portend poorer drinking outcomes. Here, too, the literature is incipient, and management should occur in consultation with local experts (e.g., addiction medicine, pain medicine).

Uncertainties and Controversies

Alcoholic Anonymous (AA) formed in the 1930s and continues to play a central role in the recovery community. Its effectiveness has long been debated secondary to defects in trial design such as standardization of interventions, selection bias, blinding and patient attrition. A recent systematic review focused primarily on manualized Twelve-Step Facilitation (TSF), a standardized, professionally delivered treatment that facilitates involvement in AA. It found that TSF improved complete abstinence compared with MET and cognitive behavioral therapy (CBT) and was equivalent for six remaining outcomes such as drinking intensity

---

[b]Also known as the National Institute on Alcohol Abuse and Alcoholism (NIAAA) single-item question or one of the AUDIT-C (consumption) questions.

[c]The author prefers to describe addiction pharmacotherapy as disease-modifying therapy (DMT) because medications are often the primary or sole treatment for addiction, especially for other substance use disorders such as opioid addiction.

[d]There is an old, ungrammatical saw in addiction medicine: "Which came first and which came worse?" Did generalized anxiety disorder (GAD), for example, develop first and then chemical coping and AUD followed? Or, did AUD develop first and anxious symptoms instead represent a substance-induced anxiety disorder? This is often difficult to establish by history and only becomes evident on a post hoc basis.

| BOX 3 | Addiction Pharmacotherapy |

Acamprosate

Brand name: Campral

Usual maintenance dosing: 666 mg by mouth three times per day

Mechanism of action: Postulated to be a gamma-amino butyric acid (GABA) agonist, glutamate antagonist, or both

Elimination: Excreted unchanged in urine

Adverse effects: Principally gastrointestinal, especially diarrhea

Prescribing pearls:

- Obtain baseline renal function test. Moderate impairment does not preclude therapy but requires monitoring. Do not use if eGFR <30 mL/min
- Initiate therapy at usual maintenance dose. Reduce dose to 666 mg two times per day for patients <60 kg. Reduce dose to 333 mg three times per day for eGFR 30–60 mL/min
- Gastrointestinal symptoms, if they develop, generally occur with initiation of treatment and are dose-related and transient. Consider temporary dose reduction (e.g., 333 mg three times per day for 7 days) for severe symptoms that threaten ongoing therapy
- Can be safely used with benzodiazepines and alcohol. May be started during medically managed withdrawal. Patients who resume drinking should be encouraged to continue taking acamprosate

Naltrexone

Brand names: ReVia (oral), Vivitrol (injectable)

Usual maintenance dosing: ReVia 50 mg by mouth daily; Vivitrol 380 mg intramuscularly every 4 weeks

Mechanism of action: Opioid antagonist

Elimination: Extensively metabolized by the liver, primarily excreted in urine

Adverse reactions: Opioid withdrawal syndrome, including precipitated withdrawal if opioid tolerant; hepatotoxicity; injection site reactions

Prescribing pearls:

- Patient must be opioid-free for ≥7 days before initiating therapy. Consider urine toxicology if abstinence cannot be reliably established by history
- Obtain baseline liver function tests. Alcohol-related transaminase elevations are common at baseline and should improve as alcohol consumption decreases. Do not use if transaminases are >5 times normal
- Obtain baseline renal function test. Moderate impairment does not preclude therapy but requires monitoring. Do not use if eGFR <30 mL/min
- Initiate oral therapy at 25 mg per day, titrating to usual maintenance dose over 7–14 days
- Mild opioid withdrawal symptoms, if they develop, generally occur with initiation of treatment, are dose-related and transient (they are likely caused by antagonism of endogenous opioids, e.g., endorphins). Consider temporary oral dose reduction (e.g., 12.5 mg per day for 7 days) for severe symptoms that threaten ongoing therapy
- Repeat liver function tests at 1 month and periodically thereafter
- Can be safely used with benzodiazepines and alcohol. May be started during medically managed withdrawal. Patients who resume drinking should be encouraged to continue taking naltrexone
- Always establish tolerability with the oral formulation before switching to injectable

Data from Center for Substance Abuse Treatment. Incorporating alcohol pharmacotherapies into medical practice. Treatment Improvement Protocol (TIP) Series 49. HHS Publication No. (SMA) 09-4380. Rockville, MD: Substance Abuse and Mental Health Services Administration, 2009.

and alcohol-related consequences. The certainty of evidence was variable and ranged from very low to high, depending on the outcome. None of the studies included a true control condition (e.g., wait list control) or compared TSF to addiction pharmacotherapy. The author takes a "might help, can't hurt" posture but does not consider community-based (peer-led) AA a substitute for treatments for which there is stronger evidence.

The American Society of Addiction Medicine (ASAM) maintains a comprehensive guideline (*The ASAM Criteria*) for assessing patients and matching them to the most appropriate level of care (e.g., outpatient vs. residential treatment) based on their clinical characteristics. It first appeared in 1991 and is widely used by treatment providers and funders (health plans, government agencies). The framework represents expert opinion for which outcome data are sparse. Some have more bluntly noted that matching patients to treatment options based on expert clinician opinion is little better than assigning patients by chance. The author considers *The ASAM Criteria* helpful for risk stratification but gives considerable weight to patient preferences in terms of treatment setting. A carefully supervised trial of office-based addiction treatment (OBAT) is reasonable if a patient is unwilling or unable to pursue a higher level of care, provided imminent danger[e] is absent.

[e]ASAM's doctrine of imminent danger consists of three components: (1) a strong probability that certain behaviors will occur; (2) the likelihood that such behaviors will present a significant risk of serious adverse consequences to the individual and/or others; and (3) the likelihood that such adverse events will occur in the very near future, within hours and days, rather than weeks or months.

References

American Psychiatric Association: *Diagnostic and statistical manual of mental disorders,* ed 5, Arlington, VA, 2013, American Psychiatric Association, p 490ff.

Blondell RD: Ambulatory detoxification of patients with alcohol dependence, *Am Fam Physician* 71(3):495–502, 2005. PMID: 15712624.

Gossip M, Keaney F, Stewart D, et al: A Short Alcohol Withdrawal Scale (SAWS): development and psychometric properties, *Addict Biol* 7(1):37–43, 2002.

Hall K, Gibbie T, Lubman DI: Motivational interviewing techniques—facilitating behaviour change in the general practice setting, *Aust Fam Physician* 41(9):660–667, 2012. PMID: 22962639.

Miller WR, Rollnick S: *Motivational interviewing,* ed 3, New York, 2013, Guilford Press, p 21.

O'Connor EA, Perdue LA, Senger CA, et al: *Screening and behavioral counseling interventions to reduce unhealthy alcohol use in adolescents and adults: an updated systematic review for the U.S. Preventive Services Task Force (Evidence Synthesis, No. 171),* Rockville, MD, 2018, Agency for Healthcare Research and Quality.

O'Connor EA, Perdue LA, Senger CA, et al: Screening and behavioral counseling interventions to reduce unhealthy alcohol use in adolescents and adults: updated evidence report and systematic review for the US Preventive Services Task Force, *J Am Med Assoc* 320(18):1910–1928, 2018. PMID: 30422198.

Saitz R: Unhealthy alcohol use, *N Engl J Med* 352(6):596–607, 2005. PMID: 15703424.

Saitz R, Miller SC, Fiellin DA, Rosenthal RN: Recommended use of terminology in addiction medicine, *J Addict Med* 15(1):3–7, 2021. PMID: 32482955.

Substance Abuse and Mental Health Services Administration: *Systems-level implementation of screening, brief intervention, and referral to treatment. Technical Assistance Publication (TAP) Series 33. HHS Publication No. (SMA) 13-4741,* Rockville, MD, 2013, Substance Abuse and Mental Health Services Administration.

Spithoff S, Kahan M: Primary care management of alcohol use disorder and at-risk drinking. Part 1: screening and assessment, *Can Fam Physician* 61(6):509–514, 2015. PMID: 26071154.

Spithoff S, Kahan M: Primary care management of alcohol use disorder and at-risk drinking. Part 2: counsel, prescribe, connect, *Can Fam Physician* 61(6):515–521, 2015. PMID: 26071155.

Sim MG, Wain T, Khong E: Influencing behaviour change in general practice. Part 1—brief intervention and motivational interviewing, *Aust Fam Physician* 38(11):885–888, 2009. PMID: 19893835.

Sim MG, Wain T, Khong E: Influencing behaviour change in general practice. Part 2—motivational interviewing approaches, *Aust Fam Physician* 38(12):986–989, 2009. PMID: 20369152.

Searight HR: Counseling patients in primary care: evidence-based strategies, *Am Fam Physician* 98(12):719–728, 2018. PMID: 30525356.

The ASAM clinical practice guideline on alcohol withdrawal management, *J Addict Med* 14(3S Suppl 1):1–72, 2020. PMID: 32511109.

US Preventive Services Task Force: Screening and behavioral counseling interventions to reduce unhealthy alcohol use in adolescents and adults: US Preventive Services Task Force recommendation statement, *J Am Med Assoc* 320(18):1899–1909, 2018. PMID: 30422199.

AUTISM

Method of
Rachel Brown, MBBS

CURRENT DIAGNOSIS

- Autism spectrum disorder (ASD) is characterized by the presence of persistent deficits in social communication and social interaction as well as by restricted, repetitive patterns of behavior, interests, or activities
- Symptoms must be present in the early developmental period, cause clinically significant impairment in important areas of functioning, and not be better explained by intellectual disability or global developmental delay.
- ASD may co-occur with intellectual disability, language impairment, with another medical, genetic, environmental, neurodevelopmental, mental or behavioral disorder, or with catatonia.
- Patients with ASD require different levels of support.

CURRENT TREATMENT

- Early identification and intensive intervention is associated with improved outcomes.
- Intervention should start in early childhood and may need to be lifelong. It should focus on improving functional independence through structured education, supported employment and daily living, therapy focused on social skills and communication, and behavioral therapy, especially applied behavioral analysis (ABA).
- Ongoing surveillance and the management of co-occurring medical (sleep, constipation, etc.) and psychiatric (ADHD, anxiety, etc.) conditions is important.
- No biomedical agent reliably improves the core symptoms.
- Stimulants, guanfacine (Intuniv), and atomoxetine (Strattera) have shown benefit for co-occurring ADHD. Treatment of anxiety and depression should follow practice guidelines for those conditions. Antipsychotic agents, such as risperidone (Risperdal) and aripiprazole (Abilify), reduce symptomatic challenging behaviors. However, potential adverse effects include weight gain, sedation, and extrapyramidal symptoms.

Epidemiology

Older epidemiologic studies suggested that autism spectrum disorder (ASD) was a rare disorder, with a prevalence of only 4 in every 10,000 population. With time, estimates of prevalence have steadily increased, and current estimates are 0.6% to 0.7%, with some as high as 1% to 2%. The reasons for the increase are not completely known. Improved awareness of the disorder, especially in those less severely affected, and broader diagnostic criteria have played a significant role. However, a real increase in prevalence remains a possibility. Approximately 45% of individuals with ASD also have intellectual disability.

Studies have consistently shown that males with ASD outnumber females by a factor of at least 2–3 to 1. Older studies placed the male predominance even higher, and there is a suggestion that females have been historically under-recognized. Girls are diagnosed somewhat later in life, and studies suggest that more concurrent behavioral or cognitive problems need to be present in girls for the disorder to be recognized. Around a third of individuals with ASD have a pattern of regression (loss of previously acquired skill) occurring in the second year of life.

Risk Factors, Etiology, and Pathophysiology

The theory that ASD is the consequence of maternal mistreatment has been disproven, and there is no evidence that ASD is caused by vaccination. Both genetic and environmental factors probably play a role. Studies have consistently shown a familial pattern for ASD. Twin studies demonstrate a much higher concordance for monozygotic twins (between 80% and 90%), compared to dizygotic and other siblings, where the risk ranges from around 7% to as high as 20%. The data is somewhat complicated because of the recognition of a so-called "broader autism phenotype" that includes milder but qualitatively similar features to the defining features of autism. Some conditions with known genetic etiology are associated with high rates of ASD. Those include fragile X, Rett, tuberose sclerosis, Down, Angelman, and a variety of others. For the majority of patients with ASD, however, specific syndromes are not present, and the search for a single "autism gene" has been fruitless. Instead, a wide variety of genes are probably associated with ASD susceptibility. Many of the genes are related to transcriptional control, chromatin remodeling, protein synthesis and cellular metabolism, and synapse development and function. Although the estimated heritability of ASD is relatively high, environmental factors also play a part. Recognized risk factors include older maternal and paternal age, gestational hypertension and diabetes, prematurity, and maternal immune activation. Studies of the neurobiology of autism suggest that autism is associated with atypical neural connectivity, and is a problem of neural networks, rather than a structurally discrete abnormality. One commonly reported feature is generalized brain overgrowth in the first 2 years of life, manifested by a larger than average head circumference in a portion of patients with ASD. Studies have also shown some consistent neurologic abnormalities of both white and grey matter in a variety of brain regions, as well as evidence of cortical dysgenesis. Alterations in serotonin and γ-aminobutyric-acid (GABA) systems, as well as oxytocin, vasopressin, and androgens/estrogens are under active investigation. Information about the genetics and neurobiology of this condition are rapidly evolving. It is likely that, in time, ASD may be sub-classified into a number of related conditions, each of which may be diagnosed and treated differently, according to the underlying etiology.

Clinical Manifestations

For the diagnosis of ASD to be made, patients must have both persistent deficits in social communication and interaction as well as repetitive, restrictive behaviors emerging in early childhood (Table 1). Human beings, including children and young babies, are inherently social and interaction seeking. However, in patients with ASD, social approach and interaction is either absent or qualitatively abnormal. In some patients, the onset of abnormality is present from the beginning, while in others there is a period of normal development followed by loss of skills, most commonly in the second year of life. There is a failure of normal back-and-forth conversation and a reduction or absence of normal sharing of interests, affect, and emotion. Normal nonverbal communicative behavior is also abnormal and/or poorly integrated with verbal communication. That means that facial expression may be flat, eye contact disconnected from gestures, such as pointing for

TABLE 1	Examples of Typical Symptoms in Autism Spectrum Disorder
Social impairment	Lack of or abnormalities in eye contact Lack of interest in peers Lack of empathy for others Diminished facial expression Diminished/absent pointing to share enjoyment Abnormal requesting of items, e.g., use of another's hand as a tool Failure to respond to name Poorly developed/absent friendships Difficulties modulating social interactions
Communication	Complete lack of language Absence of babbling Use of stereotyped phrases Idiosyncratic use of language Pronoun reversal Echolalia "Scripting" (e.g. repeating of movie scripts, etc.) Failure to use language for social interaction; unusual prosody Inability to have a back and forth conversation
Repetitive, restricted behaviors	Hand flapping, toe walking, spinning, etc., also known as "stimming" Excessive attachment to inanimate objects Abnormal response to pain, noise, textures, etc. Difficulty with transitions between activities Difficulty with changes in routine

shared enjoyment, and from language, including the requesting of preferred objects. Typical gestures, such as waving bye-bye, playing pat-a-cake, and head shaking may be absent or delayed. Children with ASD have difficulties adjusting to social situations and are either disinterested in peers or experience significant difficulty in making friends and sharing interests, including shared imaginative play. Repetitive, restrictive behaviors typically described include motor abnormalities, sometimes known as "stimming," such as spinning and hand flapping, interests focused on a limited number of play items that are not used for imaginative play, resistance to change and transition, and sensory sensitivity, such as overreaction to loud noises, food textures, and pain. Onset of symptoms must be in "early childhood." Delay in diagnosis may be seen, especially in those with higher intellectual ability, more verbal facility, and in girls. Patients who are not diagnosed in early childhood nonetheless present with deficits in communication and interaction, including social isolation, difficulties in making friends, and focused interests/activities.

Diagnosis
The diagnosis is based on clinical symptoms consistent with the *Diagnostic and Statistical Manual of Mental Disorders,* fifth edition (DSM-5). Symptoms must be present in the early developmental period and cause clinically significant impairment in social, occupational, or other important areas of functioning. ASD may occur with or without accompanying intellectual impairment and language impairment. ASD may be associated with a known genetic or medical condition, with another neurodevelopmental or behavior disorder, and with catatonia. Full evaluation should include a detailed history of presenting symptoms and early development, and observation of the child in a setting where social interaction is required. Although there is no psychological "test" for ASD, validated, structured observation tools may be employed as a component of a detailed diagnostic evaluation. Of these, the most commonly seen is the Autism Development Observation Scale (ADOS), available in multiple versions appropriate for different age groups, and including a version for diagnosis in adults. It is important for practitioners to be aware of local regulations. In some states, access to resources (e.g. early childhood intervention, respite care, applied behavioral analysis, etc.) may only be triggered after specific evaluation requirements are met; those may include assessment by certain kinds of professionals, evaluation in approved settings, or the use of specific tools.

There is a difference between a clinical diagnosis of ASD and a determination that a child is eligible for autism-related educational services. Children with a clinical diagnosis may not necessarily be eligible for special educational services. The latter are determined by assessment for educational need and may be delivered through an Individualized Education Plan (IEP). Families may benefit from advocacy in accessing educational services for social and behavioral difficulties, even when their child is doing well academically. On the other hand, not every child deemed eligible for educational services for autism will have received a formal clinical diagnosis. The latter is important when a child transfers to adult services, when a clinical diagnosis may be necessary to determine eligibility for disability, guardianship, vocational education, or sheltered workshops and group homes.

Differential Diagnosis
DSM-V states that disturbances in development and behavior must not be better explained by intellectual disability or global developmental delay. The latter are the most common differentials. Many individuals with ASD also have intellectual disability. However, to make comorbid diagnoses of ASD and intellectual disability, social communication should be below the general developmental level, and significant repetitive, restrictive activities must be present. Additional differential diagnoses include communication disorders, of which social (pragmatic) communication disorder is the most difficult to distinguish. Language delay is no longer required for the diagnosis of ASD but is very common. Social (pragmatic) language disorder is diagnosed in patients who have deficits in communication but do not have the characteristic repetitive behaviors seen in patients with ASD. Specific sensory deficits in hearing and vision must be excluded. Finally, studies of individuals who have suffered extraordinary and extreme early childhood neglect show that some of these children later demonstrate a pattern of "pseudo-autism."

Screening, Clinical Assessment, Intervention, and Monitoring
Because of the increasing evidence that early intervention for children with ASD may be critical to long term outcomes, routine early screening for ASD is essential. Primary care physicians should follow recommendations for the developmental screening of babies and young children, which include specific screening for ASD at 18 and 24 months. A positive screen should result in a referral for a comprehensive evaluation from a qualified specialist, such as a behavioral pediatrician, child and adolescent psychiatrist, or pediatric neurologist. The comprehensive evaluation will likely be multidisciplinary, and may include evaluations by psychology, speech and language therapy, and occupational therapy. Critical elements include a detailed birth, developmental and medical history, and family medical and psychiatric history, and may include structured interviews of the parent(s). Careful observation of the child is essential and is often supplemented by structured clinical observation. Assessments of adaptive skills should be included, along with intellectual ability and academic and work-related performance where appropriate. Primary care physicians may contribute by completing a full medical examination, including measurement of head circumference, screening for vision and hearing anomalies, careful review for dysmorphology, and assessment for seizure disorder, which is present in 20% of patients with ASD. Children with suspected genetic syndromes should be referred for expert evaluation and follow-up, as should those with suspected specific sensory impairments and seizure disorders. Recommended blood work for children with ASD includes comprehensive blood count, lead level and chromosomal microarray with Fragile X.

There may be a significant delay before the results of a full evaluation become available. However, a child with a significant delay in development should be referred promptly to early intervention, whether or not the diagnosis of ASD has been confirmed.

Every state has an early intervention program for children from birth to 3 years, and older preschool-age school children may be eligible for early childhood special education. Additional referrals for occupational, physical, and speech therapy may also be made, as well as for other enrichment programs, such as Headstart.

As in the management of any other complex medical condition in a child, support for parents and families, and coordination of services is a critical role for primary care. Parent-parent resources may be helpful, both local and internet-based. Although there will be geographic variation in the availability of specific programming, the cornerstone of intervention throughout life should be an individualized program designed to optimize a particular patient's strengths and address deficits, with interventions targeted at maximizing function and quality of life.

Behavioral approaches supplemented by other therapies and interventions supporting social engagement are recommended for children with ASD diagnoses. Programs focus on the development of language and social skills, and reductions in disability and comorbidity, particularly the impairments associated with behavioral disinhibition and aggression. Early intensive behavioral intervention should include applied behavioral analysis, which focuses on the building of discrete skills as well as on diminishing problematic behavioral patterns. Interventions may be delivered through comprehensive programs such as the Early Start Denver Model or TEACCH (Treatment and Education of Autistic and related Communication Handicapped Children), or via a combination of behavioral and educational services and therapy interventions. Programming typically involves parents in the delivery of interventions designed to enhance emotional engagement and communication. Communication is facilitated where necessary through visual scheduling (Picture Enhanced Communication Systems [PECS]), technology enhanced communication, and the use of sign language. Many children with ASD benefit from ongoing special educational interventions, which should target behavioral and social skills training as well as academic interventions. Vocational intervention is recommended for older children, adolescents, and adults. The transition to adult services may be challenging both for patient and family. Planning should start in early adolescence and, besides the transition of medical services if needed, should include careful consideration and planning for appropriate independence and support, including safe driving, options for further education and employment, and the need for possible ongoing guardianship by parents or other relatives. Unemployment is, sadly, very common in adults with ASD, who may become very isolated. Supports should be designed to facilitate their fullest possible engagement with their community, while protecting them, where necessary, from exploitation and abuse.

Patients with ASD may respond in unusual ways to common medical conditions, especially those that are painful and uncomfortable such as dental pain, headache, sinus pain, menstrual cramps, etc. This may be because of unusual response to physical symptoms, because of difficulty in communication, or both. Routine preventive medical and dental visits should be encouraged from early childhood onward. New onset and exacerbations of agitation, irritability, or self-injury in a patient with limited ability to communicate should always prompt a search for a physical cause, including a thorough physical examination.

Certain medical conditions (sleep disturbance; gastrointestinal problems, especially constipation; and seizure disorders) are particularly common in individuals with ASD and are associated with increased likelihood of irritability and behavioral disturbance. Routine surveillance should include attention to these conditions as well as appropriate management and referral. Seizure onset may be in later childhood or adolescence, and poorly controlled seizures are associated with both educational and behavioral deterioration. Some individuals with ASD have very limited dietary intake. Careful enquiry may be followed by blood work if indicated, including blood count, ferritin, vitamin D, and zinc. Referral may be made to a dietician, to behavioral therapy for mealtime related behaviors and/or to occupational therapy if the eating problems are related to problems with texture or swallowing. Many children with ASD have constipation and other gastrointestinal issues such as reflux, diarrhea, and inflammatory bowel disease. These conditions should be monitored and managed aggressively. Finally, sleep difficulties may be prominent, especially in many young children with ASD. Nonpharmacologic approaches (psychoeducation and cognitive-behavioral therapy [CBT]) should be implemented first; these typically include education about the nature and function of sleep and the implementation of good sleep hygiene and bedtime routines. There is some evidence that the use of melatonin as a supplement to sleep-focused CBT may be helpful.

Co-occurring psychiatric disorders are not uncommon in individuals with ASD. Historically, the diagnosis of attention deficit hyperactivity disorder (ADHD) was not possible in patients with ASD, but this changed with the DSM-5. There is suggestive evidence that stimulants, α-2 agonists and atomoxetine (Strattera) are helpful for ADHD, though potentially in a lower percentage of patients and with a higher frequency of side effects compared to the non-ASD population. Anxiety, particularly social anxiety, and generalized anxiety disorders, may present in older children,

TABLE 2	Psychopharmacology in Patients With Autism Spectrum Disorder		
MEDICATION	**TARGET**	**EVIDENCE FOR EFFECTIVENESS**	**RELATED CONSIDERATIONS**
Atypical antipsychotics—risperidone (Risperdal) and aripiprazole (Abilify)	Agitation, aggression, irritability in patients with ASD	Moderate to high, however, side effects may limit utility	Practice guidelines for monitoring; weight gain (for which metformin may be helpful), sedation, extrapyramidal symptoms, and elevated prolactin
SSRI's—citalopram (Celexa)[1], escitalopram (Lexapro), fluoxetine (Prozac)[1], sertraline (Zoloft)[1] and others	Anxiety and mood disorders	Little data for patients with ASD and co-occurring anxiety/depression. Not effective for core ASD symptoms	Common side effects include gastro-intestinal symptoms and increased irritability
Stimulants (methylphenidate [Ritalin], dextroamphetamine [Dexedrine])	ADHD	Well established for ADHD in patients without ASD; moderate evidence for ADHD in patients with ASD	Probably effective in a lower percentage of ASD patients than in uncomplicated ADHD. Side effects include irritability, decreased appetite, insomnia, weight loss, and headache
Melatonin[7]	Sleep disturbance	Some support	Use as an adjunct to CBT for sleep

[1]Not FDA approved for this indication.
[7]Available as dietary supplement.
ADHD, Attention deficit hyperactivity disorder; *ASD*, autism spectrum disorder.

1. Autism Speaks: www.autismspeaks.org
2. The American Academy of Pediatrics official parenting website https://www.healthychildren.org/English/Pages/default.aspx
3. The American Academy of Child and Adolescent Psychiatry: Facts for Families and Medication Guide for Treating Autism Spectrum Disorders: www.aacap.org/AACAP/Families_and_Youth/Home
4. Missouri Family to Family Lifecourse: https://www.lifecoursetools.com/
5. The MIND Institute Autism Distance Education Parent Training: https://health.ucdavis.edu/mindinstitute/centers/cedd/adept.html
6. Centers for Disease Prevention: Learn the Signs. Act Early: https://www.cdc.gov/ncbddd/actearly/milestones/index.html

adolescents, and adults, along with depression and other mood symptoms. CBT is an established treatment in ASD patients without intellectual disability who present with anxiety. There are less data to support the use of CBT in ASD patients who have an intellectual disability and in those who experience mood symptoms rather than anxiety.

Pharmacotherapy

There are currently no pharmacologic interventions available that address the underlying core deficits of autism, though studies targeting the cholinergic, glutaminergic, and oxytocin systems are under way. Psychotropic medication interventions may be used for co-occurring psychiatric conditions, where those are present. Stimulant medications, guanfacine (Intuniv), and atomoxetine may be used for ADHD in patients with ASD. Some supporting data shows efficacy, but in a smaller percentage of ASD than non-ASD patients and with a higher side effect burden. Psychopharmacologic intervention for anxiety and depression should follow clinical guidelines for patients without ASD, including the use of selective serotonin reuptake inhibitors (SSRIs), with awareness that side effects, especially irritability, may be more common (Table 2). Antipsychotic medications have been shown to be effective for symptomatic relief of aggressive, agitated behaviors in adolescents with ASD; however, studies are relatively short term, and the side effects of this group of medications limit their utility. Practice guidelines include specific monitoring for weight gain and associated metabolic abnormalities.

Patients with ASD have been the target of many complementary and alternative interventions (e.g., high dose vitamin regimes, dietary modification such as gluten-casein free diets, omega-3 fatty acids, secretin, chelation, hyperbaric oxygen, antifungal regimes, etc.), none of which have proven efficacy and some of which are frankly dangerous. Patients and their families may need support and guidance in resisting inaccurate, nonscientific claims made by organizations marketing unproven interventions (Table 3).

References

Ameis SH, Kassee C, Corbett-Dick P, et al: Systematic review and guide to management of core and psychiatric symptoms in youth with autism, *Acta Psychiatr Scand* 138(5):379–400, 2018.

American Academy of Child and Adolescent Psychiatry: *Practice Parameter for the Assessment and Treatment of Children and Adolescents with Autism Spectrum Disorder*, Available at: https://www.aacap.org/app_themes/aacap/docs/practice_parameters/autism.pdf 2013

American Academy of Pediatrics Screening Recommendations: Available at: https://www.aap.org/en-us/advocacy-and-policy/aap-health-initiatives/Screening/Pages/Screening-Recommendations.asp

American Psychiatric Association, DSM-5 Task Force: *Diagnostic and Statistical Manual of Mental Disorders: DSM-5*, ed 5, Washington, DC, 2013, American Psychiatric Association.

Lai M-C, Lombardo MV, Baron-Cohen S: Autism, *The Lancet* 383:896–910, 2014.

Sahin M, Sur M: Genes, circuits and precision therapies for autism and related neurodevelopmental disorders, *Science* 350(6263), 2015.

Santosh PJ, Bell L, Fiori F, et al: Pediatric antipsychotic use and outcomes monitoring, *J Child Adolesc Psychopharmacol* 27(6):546–554, 2017.

DELIRIUM

Method of
Tessa E. Rohrberg, MD

CURRENT DIAGNOSIS

- Delirium is a syndrome characterized by the acute onset of cerebral dysfunction with a change or fluctuation in baseline mental status, inattention, and either disorganized thinking or an altered level of consciousness.
- The *Diagnostic and Statistical Manual of Mental Disorders*, Fifth Edition, offers diagnostic criteria for delirium.
- Hyperactive delirium is the most easily recognized subtype and includes symptoms of irritability, restlessness, agitation, or uncooperativeness.
- Hypoactive delirium has been associated with a higher mortality and includes behaviors such as reduced motor activity, apathy, lack of awareness, or lethargy.
- Delirium usually lasts 1–2 weeks, but complications may persist beyond hospitalization.

CURRENT THERAPY

- Prevention is the most effective approach to treatment.
- Antipsychotic medication should not be used prophylactically to prevent delirium.
- Nonpharmacologic therapies are key in management.
- Pharmacologic therapies should be used when nonpharmacologic strategies are not effective or when patients present with a potential for harm to themselves or others.
- Caregivers should be included in a multidisciplinary treatment plan.

Epidemiology

Delirium can be seen in persons of all ages across many clinical settings. Prevalence is affected by patient age, underlying medical diseases, severity of acute insult, and baseline mental status. Although up to 29% of adults may experience delirium during non–intensive care unit (ICU) hospitalization, prevalence is as high as 80% in patients in the ICU with mechanical ventilation and 60% in patients following orthopedic surgery. In addition, up to 80% of patients may experience delirium at the end of life. Delirium may be missed in more than half of the cases. Patients with delirium may have increased length of hospital stay, long-term cognitive impairment, and higher mortality. The costs of delirium and associated complications have been reported up to $150 billion worldwide annually.

Pathophysiology

Although the exact etiology of delirium is unclear, it is often multifactorial and complex. Delirium is a syndrome that results from an acute insult causing cerebral dysfunction. Mechanisms contributing to delirium may include neurotransmitter imbalances and anatomic deficits. Neurotransmitter alterations—including serotonin imbalance, acetylcholine deficiency, dopamine excess, and/or melatonin deficiency—are thought to contribute. These alterations may lead to increased cytokine levels and an inflammatory response that changes the blood-brain barrier and cerebral oxidative metabolism. Higher cortical areas of the brain, such as the prefrontal and nondominant posterior parietal regions, have been implicated by brain imaging in patients with delirium. Other regions thought to be involved include the anterior thalamus, basal ganglia, and temporo-occipital cortex. More research is needed to fully elucidate the stress response and effect of risk factors.

Risk Factors

Many risk factors for developing delirium have been identified; they can be divided into predisposing and precipitating factors. See Table 1 for differentiation of these risk factors. A patient with many predisposing risk factors may experience delirium with only a minor precipitating event, whereas a patient with few predisposing risk factors may require multiple precipitating factors to develop delirium. Medications present a great risk for developing delirium. Those posing a higher risk comprise anticholinergics (including antihistamines, muscle relaxants, and urinary incontinence agents like oxybutynin [Ditropan]), benzodiazepines, dopamine agonists, and meperidine (Demerol); those that pose a moderate-to-low risk include antibiotics, anticonvulsants, antiemetics (metoclopramide [Reglan]), antidizziness agents, antihypertensives, antivirals, corticosteroids, opiates, nonsteroidal antiinflammatory drugs, sedatives, and tricyclic antidepressants.

Clinical Manifestations

The three subtypes of delirium are hyperactive, hypoactive, and mixed. Hyperactive delirium is more commonly recognized in the clinical setting. It typically includes irritability, agitation, restlessness, and uncooperative behaviors. Patients may also have fast or loud speech, combativeness, fast motor responses, nightmares, tangentiality, or persistent thoughts. This subtype is seen in patients experiencing withdrawal from substances of abuse, including drugs or alcohol. Hypoactive delirium may be more difficult to distinguish and thus is associated with more severe complications, including a higher mortality. Hypoactive delirium is frequently found in the elderly and includes sluggishness, apathy, lethargy approaching stupor, lack of awareness, slowed movements, sparse or slow speech, and staring. Metabolic dysfunction—such as hepatic encephalopathy or hypercapnic respiratory failure—may make it more difficult to identify hypoactive symptoms. Delirium may also present with a mixed level of activity and may fluctuate rapidly between hyperactivity and hypoactivity or between normal and disturbed psychomotor activity. Mixed delirium may be misdiagnosed as sundown syndrome.

Diagnosis

The diagnosis of delirium may be missed due to its multifactorial etiology, atypical symptoms of hypoactive delirium, and resemblance to other comorbidities. Diagnosis is dependent on early recognition through routine monitoring. The *Diagnostic and Statistical Manual of Mental Disorders*, Fifth Edition, includes diagnostic criteria for delirium that can be described by the following:

1. A disruption in cognition with inattention, including inability to maintain concentration and awareness of the environment.
2. The disruption from baseline occurs acutely, usually within hours to days, and fluctuates over time.
3. An additional alteration in cognitive processes of memory, orientation, language, or visual perception.
4. The disruption in criteria 1 and 3 cannot be related to another chronic or developing neurocognitive syndrome and cannot happen in a state of unconsciousness or coma.
5. The history, examination, and clinical data indicate that the cognitive disruption results from another medical condition, substance abuse or withdrawal, adverse medication reaction, or exposure to toxins.

The diagnosis of delirium can be further specified as acute (lasting a few hours or days) or persistent (lasting weeks to months), and a hyperactive, hypoactive, or mixed level of activity. Evaluation for the diagnosis of delirium should be done for underlying causes and can be individualized for each patient. Laboratory and radiologic testing usually consists of a complete blood count, comprehensive metabolic panel, urinalysis with microscopy, blood cultures, electrocardiography, and chest radiography. Additional testing might include an arterial blood gas, urine drug screen, serum ammonia, blood alcohol level, computed tomographic (CT) imaging of the head, and cardiac biomarkers. It is important to screen for drug or alcohol withdrawal, as this can present with delirium.

Differential Diagnosis

Many other diseases may closely resemble delirium. Cognitive impairment and mood disorders may be confused with delirium, including dementia or depression. See Table 2 for a comparison of characteristics of these diseases. In the elderly and those with postoperative side effects, it is important to consider urinary and fecal retention. The Critical Illness, Brain Dysfunction and Survivorship (CIBS) Center website (http://www.icudelirium.org) has many mnemonics that can be useful when one is considering other circumstances that mimic delirium. One such mnemonic is "I WATCH DEATH."

Infection	Sepsis, urinary tract infection, pneumonia, HIV
Withdrawal	Alcohol, barbiturates, sedative-hypnotics, opiates
Acute metabolic	Acidosis, alkalosis, electrolyte disturbance, renal or hepatic failure
Trauma	Head injury, heat stroke, postoperative, burns
Central nervous system pathology	Abscess, hemorrhage, subdural hematoma, seizures, encephalitis, meningitis, stroke, tumors, hydrocephalus, syphilis
Hypoxia	Anemia, hypotension, respiratory failure, congestive heart failure, carbon monoxide poisoning
Deficiencies	Vitamin B12, folate, thiamine, niacin
Endocrinopathies	Hypo/hyperthyroid, hypo/hyperglycemia, hyperparathyroidism, adrenal disease
Acute vascular	Hypertensive emergency, pulmonary embolism, arrythmia, myocardial infarction
Toxins/drugs	Anticholinergics, benzodiazepines, alcohol, illicit drugs, pesticides, solvents
Heavy metals	Lead, mercury, manganese

TABLE 1	Risk Factors for Delirium	
PREDISPOSING FACTORS	**PRECIPITATING FACTORS**
Male sex	Dehydration
Age >65 years	Fractures
Previous diagnosis of delirium	Hypoxia
Chronic pain	Infection
Medical comorbidities	Ischemia
Alcohol abuse	Shock
Terminal illness	Recent surgery
Dementia	Urinary or stool retention
Depression	Uncontrolled pain
Elder abuse	ICU environment
Recurrent falls	Sleep deprivation
Malnutrition	Physical restraints or immobility
Polypharmacy	Mechanical ventilation
Sensory impairment	Foley catheter
Pressure ulcers	Coma
Urinary or fecal incontinence	Medications

ICU, Intensive care unit.

TABLE 2 Differential Diagnosis of Delirium

	DELIRIUM	DEMENTIA	DEPRESSION
Features	Confusion and inattention	Memory loss	Sadness, anhedonia
Onset	Acute	Insidious	Slow
Course	Fluctuating, worse at night	Chronic, progressive, stable over course of a day	Single episode or recurrent
Duration	Hours to months	Months to years	—
Consciousness	Altered	Normal	Normal
Attention	Impaired	Normal, except in late stages	May be impaired
Orientation	Fluctuates	Poor	Normal
Speech	Incoherent	Mild errors	Normal or slow
Thought	Disorganized	Impoverished	Normal
Illusions	Common (visual hallucinations)	Rare, except in late stages	Not usually
Psychomotor changes	Yes	No	Yes
Reversible	Usually	Rarely	Possibly

TABLE 3 Prevention and Treatment of Delirium

NONPHARMACOLOGIC	PHARMACOLOGIC
Identify underlying etiology	**Typical Antipsychotics**
Medication review	Haloperidol (Haldol)[1] 0.5–2.0 mg PO q4h or IM q30–60min prn; maximum dose 20 mg q24h
Early mobilization	**Atypical Antipsychotics**
Cognitive reorientation	Risperidone (Risperdal)[1] 0.25–2 mg PO qd–bid
Sensory enhancement	Quetiapine (Seroquel)[1] 25–200 mg PO bid
Pain management	Olanzapine (Zyprexa)[1] 2.5–10 mg PO qd
Cluster activities	Ziprasidone (Geodon)[1] 20–80 mg PO bid
Sleep-wake cycle enhancement	Aripiprazole (Abilify)[1] 10–30 mg PO qd
Family and caregiver support	**Benzodiazepines**
Nutritional and fluid replacement	Lorazepam (Ativan)[1] 0.5–1 mg orally q4h prn
Prevention of constipation	
Restart home psychiatric medications	
Routine use of the Confusion Assessment Method	

[1]Not FDA approved for this indication.

Monitoring

Although many assessment tools exist, the Confusion Assessment Method (CAM) is the most effective screening tool, with a sensitivity of 94% to 100% and a specificity of 90% to 95%. Screening should be performed by a trained health professional and done at least once per shift in patients at moderate to high risk. One should routinely monitor for precipitating factors, including changes in medications, laboratory values, clinical symptoms, and physical examination findings.

Prevention

Prevention is the key to decreasing delirium incidence, hospital costs, and complications. Delirium may be preventable up to 40% of the time. Efforts should involve a multidisciplinary and multicomponent approach. This includes early mobilization, cognitive reorientation activities using calendars and clocks, promotion of normal sleep-wake cycles using protocols that control light and noise stimuli, clustering of patient activities, and improving access to sensory equipment like glasses or hearing aids. Other key interventions include nutrition and fluid replacement, adequate pain management, and the prevention of constipation. Although antipsychotic medications should not be used for the prevention of delirium, home psychiatric medications should be restarted when possible so as to lower the risk for delirium.

Treatment

Treatment of delirium includes the identification and management of the underlying etiologies, assessment of risk factors, and review of the medication list. Delays to initiation of treatment may result in the prolongation of symptoms, the possibility of long-term cognitive impairment, and higher mortality. Treatment is primarily aimed at prevention utilizing the nonpharmacologic measures described earlier. The Hospital Elder Life Program (HELP) is a widely used evidence-based model that uses this approach and involves physicians, nurses, caregivers, family members, and patients. Research has shown that support of family and caregiver involvement can further increase the effectiveness of this model and can contribute to shorter length of hospitalization, reduced healthcare costs, and a decreased incidence of delirium. Pharmacologic therapies are used when nonpharmacologic strategies are not effective. There are currently no antipsychotic medications that are approved by the US Food and Drug Administration for the treatment of delirium. Antipsychotics should be reserved for patients in whom behavioral interventions have failed or are not possible or in those who have a potential for harm to themselves or others. Antipsychotic medications should be used at the lowest effective dose for the shortest possible duration. Haloperidol (Haldol)[1] is the antipsychotic medication used most often for delirium management; however, atypical antipsychotic medications have been shown to be as effective. Haloperidol, risperidone (Risperdal)[1], and quetiapine (Seroquel)[1] are considered the safest when used for delirium. Benzodiazepines

[1]Not FDA approved for this indication.

should not be used for delirium unrelated to alcohol or benzodiazepine withdrawal. Nonopiate medications should be used initially to treat pain in patients diagnosed with delirium. If sedation is required in ICU patients with delirium, studies suggest the use of dexmedetomidine (Precedex) rather than benzodiazepines. See Table 3 for delirium prevention and treatment strategies.

Complications

Delirium is associated with significant long-term complications. Although cognitive impairment following a diagnosis of delirium may improve with time, lasting effects are possible. A longer duration of delirium in critically ill patients has been associated with worse long-term executive function and global cognition. The severity of lasting cognitive impairment has been compared to mild Alzheimer disease or moderate traumatic brain injury. Other complications include the development of mood disorders, loss of function in activities of daily living (ADLs), hospital readmission, longer duration of mechanical ventilation, and increased lengths of stay in the ICU and in hospital. Family members and caregivers may also experience stress in caring for their loved ones with cognitive impairment. Adverse effects of medications used in the treatment of delirium are also impactful and can include extrapyramidal symptoms, QT interval prolongation, insulin resistance, sedation, increased risk of falls, and hypotension. Mortality in patients suffering from delirium is as high as 37% during hospitalization, with a 10% increased risk of death per hospital day. Patients diagnosed with delirium are also up to three times more likely to die at 6 months after discharge. Mortality is greater in those with hypoactive delirium.

References

American Geriatric Society Abstracted Clinical Practice Guideline for Postoperative Delirium in Older Adults. *J Am Geriatr Soc* 63:142-150, 2015.
Critical Illness, Brain Dysfunction, and Survivorship (CIBS) Center. Available at http://www.icudelirium.org. Accessed January 22, 2020.
Delirium. In: American Psychiatric Association: *Diagnostic and Statistical Manual of Mental Disorders*, 5th ed, Arlington, VA, 2013, American Psychiatric Association, pp 596–602.
Downing LJ, Caprio TV, Lyness JM: Geriatric Psychiatry Review: Differential Diagnosis and Treatment of the 3 D's - Delirium, Dementia, and Depression, *Curr Psychiatry Rep* 15:365, 2013, Available at: https://doi.org/10.1007/s11920-013-0365-4, Accessed 27 April 2020.
Hospital Elder Life Program (HELP) for Prevention of Delirium. Available at http://www.hospitalelderlifeprogram.org. Accessed January 29, 2020.
Kalish VB, Gillham JE, Unwin BK: Delirium in older persons: Evaluation and management, *Am Fam Physician* 90(3):150–158, 2014.
Pandharipande PP, Girard TD, Jackson JC, et al: Long-term cognitive impairment after critical illness, *New Engl J Med* 369(14):1306–1316, 2013.
Salluh JIF, Wang H, Schneider EB, et al: Outcome of delirium in critically ill patients: systematic review and meta-analysis, *BMJ* 350:h2538, 2015, Available at: https://doi.org/10.1136/bmj.h2538, Accessed 29 January 2020.
Wang YY, Yu JR, Xie DM, et al: Effect of the tailored, family-involved hospital elder life program on postoperative delirium and function in older adults, *JAMA Internal Medicine* 180(1):17–25, 2019.

DEPRESSIVE, BIPOLAR, AND RELATED MOOD DISORDERS

Method of

Andrei Novac, MD

CURRENT DIAGNOSIS

- Clinical evaluation of mood disorders starts with a thorough psychosocial and medical history.
- Identify symptoms and patterns of the appearance of mood changes.
- Differentiate between unipolar and bipolar symptom patterns.
- Use collateral history, if possible.
- For recent-onset disorder, rule out new medical disorders. Always check thyroid function.

CURRENT THERAPY

- Any underlying medical conditions must be treated simultaneously.
- The mainstay of treatment for all mood disorders remains the combination of pharmacology and psychotherapy.
- Monitor frequently for suicidality.
- Allow at least 2 to 4 weeks for response before a medication switch.
- Switch medication early in cases of intense side effects.
- Monitor for hypomanic switch on medications in undiagnosed bipolarity.

Introduction

Unipolar and bipolar mood disorders are part of a large group of psychiatric conditions referred to as mood or affective disorders. They are among the medical conditions that are most commonly encountered in everyday clinical practice. While current psychiatric texts classify mood disorders in two broad categories (unipolar and bipolar), the clinician has to keep in mind that many mood disorders are mixed and manifest in many co-morbid and atypical forms. Thus, mood disorders and related mood dysregulation encompass a broad range of human experiences: (1) psychiatric disorders, well defined and described in medical texts; (2) a variety of mood syndromes, often comorbid and less well classified and often undiagnosed, which coexist with medical and other psychiatric disorders alike; and (3) mood dysregulation, an aggregate of dispositional traits, at times transient in nature, that are outside clear-cut psychiatric diagnosis but are often related to disturbances of personality. They all deserve particular attention because they can gravely impact the level of functioning, compliance, treatment outcome, and quality of life.

Mood Disorders*

Both the *Diagnostic and Statistical Manual of Mental Disorders*, Fifth Edition (DSM-5), and the ICD-10-CM classify mood disorders into similar types. These include major depressive disorders (unipolar, single episodes, and recurrent), persistent depressive disorder (dysthymia), bipolar I disorder, bipolar II disorder, cyclothymic disorder, and mood disorder due to medical conditions, substance-induced mood disorders, and the "unspecified" unipolar and bipolar disorders. In addition, the DSM-5 has included new clinical entries, such as disruptive mood dysregulation disorder (DMDD), persistent depressive disorder (dysthymia) with intermittent major depressive disorders, and premenstrual dysphoric disorder. The previously entitled "not otherwise specified" syndromes are now called "unspecified mood disorders." New to the DSM-5 are the following *specifiers* that apply to *both* bipolar and unipolar disorders: (1) with anxious distress (a mixture of mood disorder and anxiety disorder), (2) with mixed features, (3) with melancholic features, (4) with atypical features, (5) with psychotic features, (6) with catatonia, (7) with peripartum onset, and (8) with seasonal pattern.

Epidemiology for Unipolar and Bipolar Disorders

Most recent data regarding prevalence comes from the National Comorbidity Survey, which has exposed in detail the rates of subtypes of mood disorders: unipolar, bipolar, and the subthreshold disorders. The lifetime prevalence of any mood disorder was found to be 21.4% (female 24.9%, male 17.5%), with major depression occurring at a lifetime prevalence of 16.9% (female 20.2%, male 13.2%) and 12-month prevalence of 6.8%. Persistent depressive disorder (dysthymia) occurs at a lifetime prevalence of 2.5% (female 3.1%, male 1.8%) and 12-month

---

* In this chapter, no DSM-5 or ICD-10-CM diagnostic codes are included. The clinician is advised to consult the DSM-5 for specific diagnostic codes.

prevalence of 1.5%. The DSM-5 specifies the prevalence for dysthymia as being approximately 0.5% and for the chronic form of major depressive disorder as 1.5%. Bipolar disorders present with a lifetime prevalence of 4.4% (female 4.5%, male 4.3%). If broken down, bipolar I disorder occurs at a lifetime prevalence of 1.0%, and 0.6% of new cases over 12 months. Bipolar II disorder occurs at a prevalence of 1.1% and 0.8%, respectively. Subthreshold bipolar disorder is twice as common at 2.4% lifetime and 1.4% new cases over 12 months.

Risk Factors Common to Unipolar and Bipolar Disorders

For unipolar major depressive disorders, risk factors include gender (women at greater risk), age (18 to 44 years of age at greater risk), marital status (separated and divorced at greater risk), family history (relatives with depression), early parental death, life events (negative stressful events, chronic exposure to stress), low confidence, and urban environments. For bipolar disorder, risk factors are similar. In addition, for bipolar disorder, higher rather than lower socioeconomic status and suburban environments have been cited as risk factors.

Individuals with anxiety disorder, chronic exposure to stress and trauma, substance abuse, psychotic disorders, and chronic medical conditions are all known to be at risk for mood disorders.

Additionally, results from the World Health Organization (WHO) World Mental Health Surveys revealed that 22.9% of adult mood disorders and 31% of anxiety disorders are attributed to childhood adversity. Certain types of adversity, such as frequent childhood bullying, result in a high risk of poor social health and economic outcomes with an increase of suicidality, depression, anxiety disorders, and alcohol dependency, nearly four decades after exposure. In addition, psychiatric symptoms that are present in childhood constitute a risk factor for adult psychopathology, including mood disorders. Anxiety/depression, labile affect, and manic symptoms are all predictors for future onset of bipolar spectrum disorder. Acute and transient psychotic disorder resulted in 28% onset of affective disorder, but only 15% schizophrenia at 1-year follow-up. Finally, a more recently identified risk factor for mood disorders constitutes a gene environment interaction that results in methyltetrahydrofolate reductase (MTHFR) deficiency, and inadequate homocysteine metabolism, a risk factor for depressive disorders. MTHFR activity can be evidenced by readily available genetic testing (i.e., GeneSight). More recently, studies have pointed to the relationship between severity of depression and abnormalities in immune response. Depression has been associated with high levels of C-reactive protein and low levels of fractional exhaled nitric oxide.

Unipolar Depressive Disorder

The DSM-5 reclassifies unipolar depression into: DMDD; Major Depression; Persistent Depressive Disorder (Dysthymia); Pre-Menstrual Dysphoric Disorder; Substance/Medication Induced; Depressive Disorders due to Another Medical Condition; Other Specified Depressive Disorders; and Unspecified Depressive Disorders.

Below, we are first presenting Major Depression as the prototype of most of depression encountered in clinical practice.

Major Depression

The mainstay of major depressive disorder is a major depressive episode. The DSM-5 provides criteria according to a threshold of symptoms, yet all mood disorders have to be understood as lying on a continuum. Therefore, even individuals who do not meet all criteria have to be carefully followed, and in many cases preventive treatment is warranted.

At least five or more of the following symptoms during the same 2-week period are required: (1) depressed mood most of the day, nearly every day (sadness, feelings of emptiness, and tearfulness); (2) marked diminished interest or pleasure in almost all activities; (3) significant weight loss or weight gain or fluctuations in appetite; (4) insomnia or hypersomnia; (5) psychomotor retardation or agitation nearly every day; (6) fatigue or loss of energy; (7) feelings of worthlessness and/or inappropriate guilt; (8) inability to concentrate, think, and make decisions; and (9) recurrent thoughts of death and/or suicidal ideations. These symptoms (1) cause significant distress or impairment in social, occupational, and/or personal functions and (2) are not due to a general medical condition. In the DSM-5, contrary to previous classifications, bereavement and depression are not mutually exclusive. In fact, bereaved individuals can also develop major depression, which would warrant additional medical treatment (see Table 1). The following are some forms of manifestations:

- Major depressive disorder, single episode: Episodes may occur only one time in life or may occur again years later, usually triggered by major stressful events.
- Major depressive disorder, recurrent type: Episodes reoccur at shorter intervals. Often the distance between episodes

TABLE 1	Guidelines to the Differential Diagnoses			
DIAGNOSIS	**SIMILARITIES**	**DIFFERENTIATING DETAILS**	**CLINICAL CLUES**	**TREATMENT RESPONSE**
Major depression (MDD) versus persistent depressive disorder (dysthymia) (PDD)	Depressed mood; depressive cognition (pessimism); and vegetative symptoms (physical)	MDD: Acute or subacute onset; possible recent life stressors; and often more numerous symptoms PDD: May overlap with MDD; chronic, fluctuating course	MDD: Usually a marked drop in functionality PDD: Significant chronic impairment; often symptoms are ego-syntonic; and "personality disorder" flavor	MDD: Antidepressants and/or initial antianxiety medications; consider psychotherapy PDD: Cognitive- behavioral psychotherapy; antidepressants (often long term); sometimes enhancement pharmacology
Mixed mania versus agitated depression	Psychomotor agitation; dysphoria; and mood swings	Mixed mania: Labile affect; often rapid switch with brief euphoric states	Mixed mania: Personal and family history	Mixed mania: Mood stabilizers; caution regarding antidepressants: can cause worsening
		Agitated depression: No euphoric states; severe anxiety, including sympathetic symptoms	Agitated depression: Anxiety symptoms, often subtle, precede depressive symptoms	Agitated depression: Antidepressants and sedating mood stabilizers; avoid long-term tranquilizers
Mania versus cyclothymia	Intermittent states of high energy and euphoria with or without recurrent depression	Mania: Distinct states of high energy; depression is sometimes unnoticed	Mania: More often severe insomnia without fatigue; severity of mania and insomnia directly related	Mania: Mood stabilizers; caution about antidepressants; and atypical antipsychotics if needed

Continued

TABLE 1 Guidelines to the Differential Diagnoses—cont'd

DIAGNOSIS	SIMILARITIES	DIFFERENTIATING DETAILS	CLINICAL CLUES	TREATMENT RESPONSE
		Cyclothymia: Distinct cycling from depression to hypomania	Cyclothymia: May take unpredictable forms; fluctuation of mood and sleep	Cyclothymia: Same as above, according to clinical judgment
Substance abuse disorder versus cyclothymia	Intermittent use of stimulant abuse may mimic cycling mood disorder; may coexist	Substance abuse: Substance abuse tends to escalate	Substance abuse: Look for specific syndromes; drug screen	Substance abuse: Rehabilitation; treat underlying psychiatric symptoms
		Cyclothymia: Cyclothymia may remain constant for years (even lifelong)	Cyclothymia: Negative drug screens; no withdrawals; and no drug culture history	Cyclothymia: Mood stabilizers and/or antidepressants and/or atypical antipsychotics
Personality disorder versus mood disorder	More often overlap; requires concomitant treatment	Personality disorder: Long-term pervasive history since adolescence	Personality disorder: Borderline personality disorder includes mood lability/depressive episodes; often narcissistic personality includes grandiose/hypomanic states	Personality disorder: Acute decompensation; long-term psychotherapy; mood stabilizers; and atypical antipsychotics
		Mood disorder: More often episodic	Mood disorder: More often symptoms are egodystonic	Mood disorder: See treatment of mood disorders
Bereavement versus MDD	May overlap; attention to recent major loss; sometimes similar picture; bereavement and MDD may co-occur	Bereavement: Tends to improve over time	Bereavement: Preoccupation with loss persists	Bereavement: Social support; grief counseling; psychotherapy; and if MDD present, treat as MDD
		MDD: Tends to worsen over time	MDD: Duration of average major depressive episode is 9 months	MDD: See treatment of MDD
Terminal illness–related mood (TIRM) changes versus MDD	May overlap; attention to symptom patterns	MDD has better response to medications	Fear of and preoccupation with death often progress with progression of medical condition	Both warrant trial with antidepressants, recommended prior to any end-of-life decisions
		TIRM dominated by sadness and grief		Experimental only: Treatment with entheogen-enhanced psychotherapy (psilocybin, lysergic acid diethylamide (LSD), methylenedioxymethamphetamine (MDMA))*
Primary mood disorder versus mood disorder arising from medical condition	Clinical picture may be identical	Primary mood disorder: May be triggered by external stressful events	Neurologic, endocrine, infectious, systemic, and blood disorders†	Treat both primary medical condition and mood disorder; treatment same as for primary mood disorder
		Medical condition: Often onset is insidious; sometimes precedes medical condition		

*Not yet approved for use in the United States.
†Medical conditions complicated by mood disorders: Addison disease, AIDS, anemia, brain tumors, chronic pain, complex partial seizures, Cushing disease, cerebrovascular accident, dementia, diabetes mellitus, encephalitis, head trauma, hepatitis, hyperparathyroidism, hyperthyroidism, hypopituitarism, hypothyroidism, infectious mononucleosis, influenza, lupus erythematosus disseminatus, meningitis, multiple sclerosis, pneumonia, porphyria, rheumatoid arthritis, scleroderma, sleep apnea, toxoplasmosis, and others.

shortens with advancement in age. The first few episodes are more likely to be triggered by stressful life events, while in time the condition becomes self-maintained and self-triggered.

- Depressive disorder with catatonic features (motoric immobility, catalepsy, stupor, extreme opposition, posturing, and echolalia).
- Major depression occurring after giving birth may predict further depressive episodes years later. Postpartum depression has also been associated with bipolar disorder.

Depressive disorder can also take a chronic course. Some patients present with *melancholic features* (profound loss of pleasure, depression worse in the morning, early morning awakening, severe psychomotor retardation, severe anorexia, and weight loss). Melancholia may be a predictor of relatively good response to medications. *Atypical depression* features are characterized by inverted functional shift (weight gain and increased appetite, craving for sweets, hypersomnia, leaden paralysis, and long-standing interpersonal rejection sensitivity).

SUBTYPE WITH	PRESENTATION	FEATURES
Anxious distress (with elements of mood disorder and anxiety disorder) 74.6% of MDD	During the majority of days of depressive, manic, or hypomanic episode	Feeling keyed up or tense, feeling restless, unable to concentrate, fear that something awful may happen, etc.
Mixed features 15.5% of MDD	Meets criteria for either mania, hypomania, or depression	With mixed symptoms (if manic, there is associated dysphoria and depression), observable by others
Melancholic features	During the most severe period	Severe anhedonia, worse in the morning, early-morning awakening, psychomotor retardation or agitation, and weight loss or gain
Typical features	During majority of days of a major depressive episode	Inverted functional shift (hypersomnia, hyperphasia, and weight gain), leaden paralysis, and long-standing pattern of interpersonal rejection sensitivity
Psychotic features	The presence of delusions and/or hallucinations	Mood-congruent psychosis (delusions/hallucinations include themes consistent with the type of mood [manic or depressed]) Mood-incongruent psychosis
Catatonia	The presence of catatonia	Catatonic features are present during most of depressive or manic episodes
Peripartum onset	Mania, hypomania, major depression in bipolar I or II disorders	During pregnancy or in the 4 weeks following delivery
Seasonal pattern	At least one type of episode (mania, hypomania, or depression) within a seasonal pattern	Temporal relationship between an episode and a particular time of the year (fall or winter, in bipolar I or II)

Table 2 presents the subtypes (specifiers) of mood disorders according to the DSM-5. These subtypes are encountered both in unipolar and in bipolar mood disorders. Under these new DSM-5 classifications, conditions such as catatonia, seasonal affective disorders (SAD), and atypical depression may occur both in individuals with unipolar disorder and in individuals with bipolar disorders.

Major depression *with psychosis* is more often encountered in inpatient settings. However, early prodromal symptoms, which start with suspicion, paranoid features, or transient perceptive abnormalities, are relatively common. As most of the time, patients with prodromal psychotic features do not volunteer such symptoms, clinicians need to ask, specifically, about the presence of suspicions, "unusual perceptions," which carry a significant, severe prognosis. Such clinical features of psychosis may complicate the treatment regimen. Antidepressive medications alone may sometimes be insufficient or exacerbate some of the psychotic features. In such cases, the addition of antipsychotic medications, frequent monitoring, and psychiatric consultation is necessary. *Seasonal Affective Disorder* is a recurrent type of depression, often combined with bipolar features. Most patients develop major depression of different degrees, between October and February-March, in the northern hemisphere. Clinicians need to specifically inquire about this pattern of occurrence. Curiously, many patients with this subtype of depression have limited awareness of their seasonal pattern. Specific modalities that have emerged in recent years for SAD include light therapy and social rhythm therapy.

Persistent Depressive Disorder (Dysthymia)
Persistent depressive disorder, the new designation for dysthymic disorder, is a chronic form of depression in which the depressed mood has persisted for at least 2 years (in children for at least 1 year), as manifested by at least two of the following symptoms: (1) poor appetite or overeating, (2) insomnia or hypersomnia, (3) low energy or fatigue, (4) low self-esteem, (5) poor concentration or difficulty making decisions, and (6) feelings of hopelessness. These manifestations are distinct from any major depressive episode, there have been no manic symptoms, and there is significant

distress or impairment in social, occupational, or personal functioning. Dysthymia can occur in any age and can co-occur with major depressive disorder.

The following clinical forms have been identified: (1) with pure dysthymic syndrome: no full criteria of major depression have been met in the past 2 years; (2) with persistent major depressive episode: full criteria of a major depressive episode have been present in the past 2 years; (3) with intermittent major depressive episodes, with current episode: full criteria for major depressive episodes are currently met but there have been periods of at least 8 weeks in the last 2 years when major depression criteria have not been met; and (4) with intermittent major depressive episodes, without current episode: no current major depression is identified (only symptoms of dysthymia) but there has been one or more major depressive episode(s) in the past 2 years. Persistent depressive disorder may also qualify for any of the specifiers described in Table 2. (Note: Table 2 specifiers can apply to any of the unipolar and bipolar forms of mood disorders.) The term "minor depression" to distinguish from "major depression" has also been used in earlier contributions. Minor depression refers to two to four symptoms of depression lasting for more than 2 weeks but less than 2 years. This clinical variant falls within the spectrum of persistent depressive disorder (dysthymia). Major depression and persistent depressive disorder (dysthymia) can co-exist. More often, an individual suffering from dysthymia develops major depression as a complication. An earlier literature refers to these complications as "double depression." Such patients necessitate long-term maintenance treatment beyond the acute major depressive episode.

Disruptive Mood Dysregulation Disorder
This condition occurs in childhood or adolescence between the ages of 6 and 18. It is characterized by (1) severe recurrent temper outbursts manifested verbally (verbal rages) and/or behaviorally (physical aggression toward people or property) that are grossly out of proportion in intensity or duration to the situation or provocation; (2) temper outbursts that are inconsistent with developmental level; (3) temper outbursts that occur on average three or more times per week; (4) a mood between temper outbursts that is persistently irritable or angry most of the day, nearly every day,

TABLE 3 Examples of Medications Known to Trigger Depression as a Side-Effect

CLASS	EXAMPLES
Antihypertensives	Clonidine, reserpine, β-blockers
Cardiovascular	Digitalis
Steroids	Prednisone and dexamethasone (Decadron)
Antiarthritic	Indomethacin (Indocin)
Hormonal substitutes	Estrogen, progesterone, testosterone, anabolic steroids, and birth-control pills
Cancer medications	Most chemotherapy combinations, i.e., cycloserine (Seromycin), tamoxifen (Nolvadex), vinblastine (Velban), and vincristine (Vincasar)
Tranquilizers and hypnotics	Diazepam (Valium), triazolam (Halcion), and zolpidem (Ambien)
Analgesics	Codeine, propoxyphene[2], and potentially all opiates
Anti-Parkinson's medication	Levodopa (L-Dopa) and bromocriptine (Parlodel)
Other	Anti-HIV; Medications used in the treatment of hepatitis C

[2]Not available in the United States.

and is observable by others; (5) the previous criteria, which have been present for 12 or more months (with no lapse in symptoms for a duration of 3 or more months); and (6) an age of onset that is before 10 years. Diagnosis should not be made before the age of 6 years or after 18 years.

DMDD was introduced into the DSM-5 for a subgroup of children with mood dysregulation and as an alternative to the diagnosis of childhood bipolar disorder. Some of these patients do move on to develop bipolar disorder. There is a significant overlap between DMDD and the onset of bipolar disorder. In one study of children in psychiatric hospitals, 30.5% met criteria for DMDD by parent report and 15.9% by inpatient unit observation. In clinical practice, young children may present with symptoms of Attention-Deficit Disorder, Hyperactive Type, and comorbid DMDD. Such patients often require careful assessment, complex pharmacologic treatment, and monitoring for possible worsening of bipolar symptoms.

Premenstrual Dysphoric Disorder

• The condition is characterized by the majority of menstrual cycles that include five symptoms. The following symptoms occur in the final week before the onset of menses and begin to improve within a few days after the onset of menses.
• One or more of the following symptoms must be present: (1) marked affective lability (mood swings, feeling suddenly sad or tearful, increased sensitivity to rejection); (2) marked irritability or anger or increased interpersonal conflict; (3) marked depressed mood, feelings of hopelessness, or self-deprecating thoughts; (4) marked anxiety, tension, and/or feelings of being keyed up or on edge.

One or more of the following symptoms must be present to reach a total of five symptoms: decreased interest in usual activities; subjective difficulty in concentration; lethargy; easily fatigued; marked changes in appetite, overeating, or specific food cravings; hypersomnia or insomnia; a sense of being overwhelmed or out of control; physical symptoms such as breast tenderness or swelling, joint or muscle pain, or bloating or weight gain.

Substance/Medication-Induced Depressive Disorder

This diagnosis is used when persistent disturbance in mood predominates the clinical picture and is characterized by depression

and diminished interest or pleasure in activities. These symptoms occur during or soon after substance intoxication or withdrawal or after exposure to a medication. The substance in question has to be known to cause symptoms of depression. Many substances that are abused (illicit and prescription) can cause depression. A 2018 study by Qato, et al., which included 26,000 patients, found that more than one-third of American adults could be experiencing depression due to their prescription medication. Table 1 lists principle groups of medications to be considered when assessing patients with depression.

Depressive Disorder Due to Another Medical Condition

This diagnosis is used when a depressive disorder is triggered by a medical condition (diagnosed by physical examination and laboratory findings) known to cause symptoms of depression. These may include disorders of the central nervous system (CNS), systemic disorders (lupus and cancer), and so forth. Additionally, depression can aggravate many medical conditions, including chronic pain, multiple sclerosis, and cardiovascular disease.

Other Specified Depressive Disorders

These are depressions that do not fully meet the criteria of the previously described conditions. However, they may appear in one of the following forms:

• Recurrent brief depression (symptoms of depression lasting from 2 to 13 days at least once per month) not associated with menstrual cycles
• Short-duration depressive episode (lasting from 4 to 13 days), with at least four symptoms of major depressive episode associated with clinical distress and impaired functioning that persist but never meet criteria of major depression
• Depressive episode with insufficient symptoms (at least one of the symptoms of major depression associated with distress and impairment persisting for at least 2 weeks with no prior history of major depression)

These "other specified depressive disorders" are helpful to clinicians in refining the description of a clinical pattern exhibited by a particular patient.

Unspecified Depressive Disorder

Finally, the previously used designation of "not otherwise specified" now reads "unspecified depressive disorder" (when none of the criteria are fully met, yet the patient is suffering from a mood disorder).

Bipolar Mood Disorders
Manic Episode

A manic episode is characterized by a period of at least 1 week with abnormal and persistently elevated, expansive, or irritable mood. At least three of the following should also be present: (1) inflated self-esteem or grandiosity, (2) decreased need for sleep (yet still feeling rested), (3) more talkative than usual or inability to stop talking, (4) flight of ideas or racing thoughts, (5) distractibility, (6) increase in goal-oriented activities (socially, sexually) or psychomotor agitation, and (7) excessive involvement in pleasurable activities with little regard for consequences (e.g., sexual indiscretions and unwise investments). These symptoms (1) result in marked impairment in most areas of life and (2) are not due to substance abuse or general medical conditions.

Hypomania

A hypomanic episode is similar to, but less intense than, a manic episode. At least three symptoms from the same symptom cluster (inflated self-esteem, decreased need for sleep, excessive talking, racing thoughts, hyperactivity, and increased involvement in pleasurable activities) are required, but the condition is not severe enough to cause marked impairment in social, occupational, and personal functioning, and it does not necessitate hospitalization. However, functional impairment is noticeable over time.

"Bipolar I" disorder requires only one full manic episode for the diagnosis. Usually, individuals with bipolar I disorder also have both manic and depressive episodes, but the depressions

TABLE 4 Other Specified and Unspecified Bipolar Disorders

SUBTYPE	PRESENTATION	FEATURE
Substance/medication-induced bipolar and related disorder	Persistent disturbance of mood characterized by mania, hypomania, with or without depressed mood, which occurs soon after substance intoxication or withdrawal or after administration of a medication	• Substance involved is capable of producing described mood symptoms • Does not occur in the course of delirium • There is significant stress or impairment
Bipolar and related disorder due to another medical condition	• Persistent period of abnormally elevated expansive or irritable mood • Evidence from history, physical examination, and laboratory findings that disturbance is a direct pathophysiologic consequence of another medical condition	• With manic features • With manic or hypomanic-like episode • With mixed features (depression is also present)
Other specified bipolar and related disorder	Symptoms of bipolar disorder, but do not meet full criteria	• Short-duration hypomanic episodes (2–3 days) and major depressive episodes • Hypomanic episodes with insufficient symptoms and major depressive episodes • Hypomanic episode without prior major depressive episode • Short-duration cyclothymia (<24 months)
Unspecified bipolar and related disorders	Patients with bipolar symptoms and clinical distress and impairment; however, the clinician chooses not to specify the reason that the criteria are not met	

can range from severe and disabling to very brief and unnoticed. Therefore, a history of a depressive episode is not required for the diagnosis.

"Bipolar II" disorder is characterized by long periods of hypomania, with occasional major depressive episodes. Such individuals are usually not hospitalized for their hypomania and tend to function relatively well between depressive episodes. Hypomanic states are episodic and exhibit an unequivocal change in functioning that is uncharacteristic for the individual when not symptomatic. These changes are observable by others. Depressions tend to be severe and disabling. Bipolar II disorders do not include full manic episodes.

Mixed States and Rapid Cycling
The particular specifiers for bipolar disorder are mixed states and rapid cycling. *Mixed states* refer to manic or hypomanic episodes with at least three of the following depressive symptoms: prominent dysphoria or depressed mood, diminished interest in activities, psychomotor retardation, fatigue or loss of energy, feelings of worthlessness, and recurrent thoughts of death. Often there is a rapid alternation between mania and depression (rapid cycling). Contingent upon severity, mixed states are usually accompanied by severe impairment. *Rapid cycling* refers to bipolar disorder that includes at least four episodes of illness per year. In addition, bipolar disorders may include any of the specifiers described in Table 2.

Cyclothymic Disorder
Cyclothymic disorder is a cycling mood disorder lasting for 2 years or more and is characterized by numerous periods with hypomanic symptoms and depressive symptoms that do not meet criteria for bipolar disorder or major depression. During a 2-year period (1 year in children and adolescents), hypomanic and depressive periods have been present for at least half the time, and the individual has not been without symptoms for more than 2 months at a time. Criteria for major depression, mania, or hypomanic episodes have never been met. However, in the long run, some patients may develop symptoms of bipolar affective disorder. These symptoms should not be attributable to the effect of a substance (drug abuse and medication) or another medical condition (hyperthyroidism, Cushing disease, etc.). The condition is significantly impairing and includes psychological distress. Cyclothymia has the specifier (subtype) "cyclothymia

with anxious distress." This condition consists of cyclothymia and features of anxious distress as outlined in Table 2. A variety of subclinical forms of *subthreshold cyclothymia* may be encountered in clinical practice. Such patients tend to develop overt symptoms of cyclothymia, or even bipolar disorder, when exposed to a variety of psychosocial stressors, substance abuse, and/or a variety of medications. Finally, Table 4 presents subtypes of bipolar disorder currently listed in the DSM-5 as "other specified bipolar and related disorders" and "unspecified bipolar and related disorder."

Specifiers for Bipolar and Related Disorders
Please refer to Table 2 for specifiers of depressive disorders that apply to bipolar disorders as well.

Diagnosis. When faced with symptoms of mood disorder, a clinician has to decide whether these are transient manifestations related to life circumstances or symptoms of treatable psychopathology. The clinical evaluation of patients with mood disorders starts with a thorough history of the present illness. A thorough medical history is paramount given the numerous medical disorders that present with depression or mania. Mood disorders are, in general, recurrent conditions. Past history will provide not only a suspicion toward a diagnosis but also clues toward clinical manifestations, which, in the cases of depression and mania, are often similar to previous episodes. An early history of childhood behavioral problems can constitute a precursor of mood disorders. The Mental Status Examination provides further clues to the diagnosis. For depressive states, patients often exhibit psychomotor retardation; slow speech; constricted affect; and slow, observable mental activity. For mania and hypomania, the opposite can be observed. Patients show increased psychomotor activity, pressured speech, full or labile affect, and elevated mood. Often, they will appear unrealistically optimistic. In general, the diagnosis of mood disorder is aided significantly by obtaining a collateral history from friends or family members. The value of the Mental Status Examination is enhanced if the clinician knows the patient from before the mood disorder episode. A variety of psychological tests and depression rating scales exist, including the Beck Depression Inventory, the Hamilton Depression Rating Scale, and the Profile of Mood States (POMS) Depression Scale. While extremely useful in quantifying symptoms of depression, psychological testing is time-consuming and not necessary for the initial diagnosis of a mood disorder.

A thorough account of all symptoms present in a patient can point to treatment choice and outcome. Depression symptoms can be classified into at least three major groups:

- Emotional symptoms: sadness, dysphoria, emotional numbness
- Physical symptoms: low energy, sluggishness with difficulties in initiating activities, difficulties concentrating, and sleep and appetite problems
- Cognitive (mental) symptoms: pessimism, loss of enthusiasm, hopelessness, and thoughts of death

Not all three groups of symptoms are present from the beginning. In many individuals, the presence of cognitive symptoms may be a sign of chronicity. At other times, it may have been a premorbid feature or a constant presence between episodes. Cognitive symptoms tend to respond both to medication and to psychotherapy (cognitive-behavioral techniques), and their monitoring is paramount to suicide prevention. If a mood disorder is secondary to a medical condition, the diagnosis will be made both by monitoring for mood symptoms and by pathognomonic medical findings.

Differential Diagnosis

Given the multitude of clinical manifestations, a differential diagnosis both between subtypes of mood disorders and between mood and other psychiatric disorders is necessary. Table 1 presents comparisons and differences between subtypes of mood disorders and guidelines to the differential diagnoses.

Given the frequent overlap of anxiety and mood disorders, it is useful to inquire about the presence of anxiety disorder in a systematic manner. Anxiety disorder symptoms can also be classified into at least three major groups:

- Emotional symptoms: anxiety and/or fear, either fluctuating or in the form of attacks
- Physical symptoms: palpitations, tachycardia, diaphoresis, sweaty palms, sensation of a knot in the throat, muscle tension, shortness of breath, gastrointestinal symptoms, insomnia, and so forth
- Cognitive symptoms: (1) intrusive thoughts (such as "What if…," "I should have…," other specific exaggerated worries), (2) racing thoughts, (3) ruminative thoughts, and so forth

Because of the long-term, chronic, egosyntonic nature of these symptoms, they are often not readily volunteered by the patient unless specifically asked about. Between mood disorders and anxiety disorders, there is a comorbidity of more than 50%, with generalized anxiety, panic disorders, and posttraumatic stress disorders constituting both a risk factor for and a possible complication of mood disorders. Please note that the DSM-5 allows for a specifier "with anxious distress" that can be applied to both unipolar and bipolar mood disorders. Depending on the primary diagnosis, the clinician may choose between adding this specifier or the comorbid separate diagnosis of "anxiety disorder" in addition to mood disorder.

Treatment

Currently, psychopharmacology and psychotherapy are the mainstay of care for mood disorders. As we will see below, a variety of novel treatments (transcranial magnetic stimulation [TMS], ketamine, entheogens) have recently emerged. An accurate initial diagnosis directs the first choice of treatment. Close monitoring of treatment with frequent visits usually predicts better outcome. In general, response is considered to be a 50% reduction of symptoms, while remission refers usually to the absence or only minimal symptoms for 6 months or more. By Tohen and colleagues' opinion, relapse is considered a return of symptoms within 6 months, while recurrence is after 6 months of remission.

Among risk factors for severity, treatment resistance has been a major clinical challenge. Four predictors have been recently identified. They include symptom severity (3.3-fold increase in likelihood for treatment resistance); suicidal risk (a 1.74-fold increase in treatment resistance); comorbid disorder (1.68-fold increase risk); and lifetime number of major depressive episodes (15% increase in treatment resistance per prior episode).

Treatment of Unipolar Depression (Major Depression and Dysthymia)

Given the fact that many depressive disorders occur along a spectrum, the treatment of major depression and dysthymia will be covered together.[†] In addition, a more recent study confirms the fact that comorbidity features, with anxiety, are significant: the anxious/distressed specifier occurs in 74.6% of cases and mixed-features specifier in 15.5% of major depressive disorder patients.

Psychopharmacology

First, a thorough medical workup should be performed in any new case of mood disorder. The National Institutes of Health (NIH)-sponsored STAR*D study (Sequenced Treatment Alternatives to Relieve Depression) recommends the initial choice of a selective serotonin reuptake inhibitor (SSRI) (citalopram [Celexa]). In the study, nonresponders were then switched to sertraline (Zoloft) and/or venlafaxine XR (Effexor XR). In clinical practice, other factors have to be weighed when choosing the first antidepressant. *Prior response history* (italics added) to a specific antidepressant or to an overall treatment modality should take precedence in the first choice of treatment. If such a history is unavailable, any family history of response to a specific treatment should be considered. Response to treatment seems to be similar among blood relatives. Table 5 includes a list of the more common medications used in clinical practice for the treatment of unipolar and bipolar disorder. Given the possibility of manic switch with antidepressants, it is recommended that in bipolar depression, mood stabilizers be started concomitantly with antidepressants.

Although myriad side effects are known to exist for each medication, all SSRIs and serotonin norepinephrine reuptake inhibitors (SNRIs) are generally well tolerated. Any trial of medications should be continued for 4 to 6 weeks before failure is declared. However, clinical judgment in assessing each circumstance, especially regarding suicide risk, is crucial. Often in the initial phase of response, the physical symptom of low energy remits first while cognitive symptoms of depression (persistent thoughts of death) persist. The coexistence of higher energy and thoughts of death may constitute a temporary suicide risk in the initial phase of antidepressant treatment. Currently, biological markers for the prediction of treatment response and side effects are being considered. Psychiatric EEG Evaluation Registry (PEER), by using quantitative EEG technology, compares variations of normal awake EEG readings with a large database of medication responders. Results are available for antidepressants, mood stabilizers, stimulants, second-generation antipsychotics, and so forth. The validity of PEER has been supported by a wealth of published literature; however, more recently the usefulness of PEER has been disputed. The AmpliChip CYP450 Test is a method that predicts side effects by measuring the activity of genes that control the P450 hepatic enzyme system and, implicitly, the ability to metabolize a specific drug. Both methods are promising, but high cost and questions about large individual variability of response, have had so far prevented general use.

Given the risk of suicide, close monitoring during the treatment of major depression is required. The choice of medication and adjustment has to be tailored according to the most dominant initial presentation. For patients with severe insomnia, an SSRI is indicated. If the initial choice (e.g., citalopram

---

[†]The newly introduced DSM-5 diagnosis of disruptive mood dysregulation disorder is a condition of childhood and adolescence. Prior to the publication of the DSM-5, many of these patients were diagnosed as bipolar. Many clinicians prefer to initiate treatment with psychotherapy, which includes addressing a variety of family issues before initiating psychopharmacologic intervention. Premenstrual dysphoric disorder, also newly introduced in the DSM-5, is treated, depending on the intensity of symptoms, by using protocols similar to those utilized in the treatment of dysthymic and/or cyclothymic disorders.

[*]For specifiers and diagnostic codes, please see the DSM-5 and/or ICD-10-CM.

MEDICATION GROUP	MEDICATION	USUAL DAILY DOSE	CAUTIONS
SSRI	Fluoxetine (Prozac) Sertraline (Zoloft) Paroxetine (Paxil) Citalopram (Celexa) Escitalopram (Lexapro) Fluvoxamine (Luvox)*	10–80 mg 25–200 mg 5–60 mg 10–40 mg 5–20 mg 50–300 mg	All can cause sedation, agitation, insomnia, GI side effects, and sexual dysfunction
SSRIs with combined action	Vilazodone (Viibryd) Functions of SSRI and a 5-HT$_{1A}$ receptor agonist Vortioxetine (Brintellix) Functions of SSRI and multiple serotonin receptor agonists and antagonists	10–40 mg 5–20 mg	Same as above
Serotonin-norepinephrine reuptake inhibitor (SNRI)	Venlafaxine XR (Effexor XR) Desvenlafaxine (Pristiq) Levomilnacipran ER (Fetzima)	37.5–225 mg 50–100 mg 40–120 mg	Insomnia, sedation, possible HTN Mydriasis, and urinary hesitation
Dopamine/norepinephrine agonist	Bupropion SR, XL (Wellbutrin SR, XL)	100–450 mg	Agitation, GI side effects, and possible HTN
Stimulants (usually used to enhance effects of other antidepressants)	Methylphenidate (Ritalin)* Dextroamphetamine (Dexedrine)* Amphetamine/dextroamphetamine mixed (Adderall)*	10–60 mg 5–60 mg 5–60 mg	Agitation, insomnia, psychosis, HTN, and seizures
Second-generation neuroleptics	Olanzapine (Zyprexa)* Quetiapine (Seroquel) Aripiprazole (Abilify) Risperidone (Risperdal)* Lurasidone (Latuda) mainly for bipolar disorder Cariprazine (Vraylar)*	2.5–20 mg (in unipolar depression, olanzapine 5 mg, plus fluoxetine 20 mg [Symbyax]) 50–300 mg (up to 800 mg in bipolar disorder) 2–30 mg 0.5–6 mg 20–120 mg/day 1.5–6 mg/day	Metabolic syndrome, sedation Oversedation, metabolic syndrome, and cardiovascular complications in elderly Oversedation, metabolic syndrome, and hyperprolactinemia Somnolence or agitation from akathisia and extrapyramidal symptoms
Tricyclic antidepressants	Amitriptyline (Elavil) Imipramine (Tofranil) Doxepin (Sinequan) Desipramine (Norpramin) Nortriptyline (Pamelor) Maprotiline (Ludiomil) Protriptyline (Vivactil)	50–300 mg 50–300 mg 50–300 mg 50–300 mg 20–200 mg† 100–225 mg 20–60 mg	All can cause anticholinergic effects and sedation; occasional agitation and weight gain
Mixed action (presynaptic and postsynaptic, multiple neurotransmitter action)	Mirtazapine (Remeron) Trazodone (Desyrel) Clomipramine (Anafranil)*	15–30 mg 150–600 mg 50–300 mg†	Sedation, weight gain
MAOI (dietary restrictions are obligatory)	Phenelzine (Nardil) Tranylcypromine (Parnate)	15–90 mg 30–60 mg	Hypertensive crisis, occasional sedation/activation
Mood stabilizers	Lithium carbonate/citrate/ER* Valproate (valproic acid, Depakote ER)* Lamotrigine (Lamictal)/XR* Carbamazepine (Tegretol)*	600–1800 mg (attaining blood level from 0.6 to 1.2 mEq/L) 250–1500 mg (attaining blood level from 50 to 100 mcg/mL) 50–400 mg 200–1000 mg (attaining blood level from 5 to 12 mdg/mL)	Signs of toxicity: tremor, nausea, vomiting, and staggering gait; monitor kidney and thyroid function Oversedation, GI side effects, may affect blood levels of other medications, and weight gain A variety of severe skin rashes, Stevens-Johnson syndrome Monitor blood count for aplastic anemia/agranulocytosis, possible Stevens-Johnson syndrome, and sedation

*Not U.S. Food and Drug Administration approved for this indication.
†Exceeds dosage recommended by the manufacturer.
ER, Extended release; *GI*, gastrointestinal; *HTN*, hypertension; *MAOI*, monoamine oxidase inhibitor; *SSRI*, selective serotonin reuptake inhibitor.

[Celexa], escitalopram [Lexapro], or sertraline [Zoloft]) shows little impact in improving sleep, the temporary addition of a sleep aid is a reasonable choice. Alternatively, some clinicians prefer to avoid hypnotics, which may allow close monitoring of the natural improvement in sleep during the first 2 weeks of SSRI treatment. This in turn may predict a good response. In geriatric patients, long-term SSRI treatment has been found to delay progression from mild cognitive impairment to dementia. For many years, in patients with hypersomnia and hyperphagia—a variant known as "atypical depression"—the first choice was a monoamine oxidase inhibitor (MAOI). Currently, for atypical depression, clinicians prefer as a first choice a norepinephrine/

TABLE 6 Biological Treatments for Medication-Resistant Mood Disorders

TYPE OF INTERVENTION	REPORTED RESPONSE	CURRENT AVAILABILITY
Electroconvulsive therapy (ECT)	50.9%–53.2% remission rate	Common
Transcranial magnetic stimulation (TMS)	41.5%–56.4% response rate, 26.5%–28.7% remission rate	Accepted by several insurance plans
Vagal nerve stimulation (VNS)	53% response rate, 33% remission after 1 year	Rare (neurosurgical)
Deep brain stimulation (DBS)	29% response rate at 1 year	Rare (neurosurgical)
Ketamine (Ketalar) infusion[1]	79% response rate	Very rare (only in selective institutions)
Anterior cingulotomy	33.3% response rate, after 30 months	Very rare (only in selective institutions, neurosurgical)

[1]Not FDA approved for this indication.

TABLE 7 Intervention Options for Phases of Bipolar Disorder

PHASE OF DISORDER	INTERVENTIONS
Acute	Hospitalization if necessary Antipsychotics, tranquilization, and start mood stabilizers
Subacute	Antipsychotics/neuroleptics, mood stabilizers If already medicated, adjust dose
Rapid cycling/mixed	As in acute phase; check thyroid; and medical workup Rule out substance abuse May require treatment indefinitely
Cyclothymia	Mood stabilizers, long term, with or without antidepressants based on history Close initial monitoring May need treatment indefinitely

serotonin reuptake inhibitor (venlafaxine [Effexor], desvenlafaxine [Pristiq]), or a norepinephrine/dopamine active medication (bupropion [Wellbutrin]). Response to medications is often difficult to predict. Again, early in treatment, a thorough medical workup, which should always include a thyroid panel, should be the norm. Sometimes, switches to other classes of antidepressants (dopamine enhancers, tricyclics) are necessary before a result is obtained. Pharmacologic augmentation with mood stabilizers, neuroleptics, and thyroid hormone has been used in cases of treatment-resistant depression. In cases where severe anxiety, insomnia, and poor appetite dominate the picture, the early addition of a second-generation neuroleptic (olanzapine [Zyprexa][1], quetiapine [Seroquel XR], risperidone [Risperdal][1], aripiprazole [Abilify], and, more recently, cariprazine [Vraylar][1]) is recommended (see Table 5). Medication resistance (after several failed trials) dictates the reassessment of diagnosis to further rule out psychiatric and medical comorbidity. For medication-resistant mood disorders, Table 6 presents a list of further biological treatments. Some of these treatments are promising but have yet to be included as routine choices in some of the most difficult-to-treat patients.

Psychotherapy

For mood disorders, cognitive-behavioral, interpersonal and more recently, mindfulness-focused psychotherapy have been considered therapies of choice. Cognitive-behavioral and mindfulness directly address the negative, pessimistic bias

[1]Not FDA approved for this indication.

of the depressive thinking, which is a maintenance factor of depressed mood. The latter addresses social and interpersonal functioning by enhancing coping abilities. Their popularity has been increasing; however, they require special training and supervision. In clinical practice, though, the most readily available therapies remain supportive and insight-oriented psychotherapy. They too complement the effect of pharmacology. Brain imaging studies have revealed that the activity of the subgenual anterior cingulate cortex (Brodmann area 25) predicts the outcome of response to cognitive-behavioral psychotherapy in depression. As a general rule, therapies should have specific goals that need to be discussed with patients at the onset of treatment. This needs to be part of an overall "informed consent" approach to treatment. Given the availability of a variety of clinicians with different levels of expertise that provide psychotherapy, it is important to monitor results and coordinate care. If "split" treatment (pharmacology and psychotherapy provided by different clinicians) is chosen, communication between parties of the treatment team remains a crucial requirement for rapid response and recovery. Other therapeutic measures, such as an increase in physical activity, normalization of sleep, and improvement of social support, are particularly important in promoting recovery.

Neurostimulation

TMS was approved by the FDA in 2008. Over the past 2 years, the majority of insurance plans and Medicare have approved TMS treatment for major depression. It is the treatment modality approved by the FDA that has made the greatest strides in providing neuromodulation treatment for patients with major depressive disorder in over 1000 centers nationwide. Table 6 includes other neuromodulation treatments, which need to be considered when TMS remains ineffective.

Treatment of Bipolar Disorders (Bipolar Type I, Type II, Mixed Type, and Cyclothymia)

The treatment of bipolar disorder has been well refined over the years by a large body of literature. For acute mania, treatment with mood stabilizers and/or antipsychotics has remained the main approach for the past several decades. Severe forms of mania and psychosis usually require hospitalization. Table 7 indicates intervention options for different phases of bipolar disorder.

As indicated in the table, some of the medication choices overlap between different clinical presentations. For chronic forms of bipolarity, such as mixed bipolar and cyclothymic disorder, a variety of new approaches has been developed, including social rhythm therapy. The latter includes monitoring and optimization of social interactions, sleep, and circadian rhythms that seem to benefit bipolar patients. Chronic bipolarity, with its significant impairment and suicide risk, remains a major problem, often requiring multidisciplinary consultations and referral to a tertiary institution. In treatment-resistant cases, employment of electroconvulsive therapy and other novel biological approaches can be

| TABLE 8 | Examples of Mood Syndrome Variants With Different Degrees of Mood Dysregulation as Encountered in the Literature Over the Past Century |

I MSV WITH MANIFESTATIONS OF OTHER PSYCHIATRIC DISORDERS	II MSV WITH UNUSUAL SYMPTOMS (MASKED DEPRESSION)	III MSV AS PART OF OTHER CONDITIONS
Atypical depression	Mood dysregulation and thrill-seeking behavior (gambling, racing, substance abuse, hypersexuality)	Postpartum depression
Subaffective dysthymia		Depression secondary to chronic pain
Hysteroid dysphoria		Substance- and medication-induced mood dysregulation*
Pseudodementia	Reactive overeating	
Pseudoborderline	Isolated sleep disturbance and mood dysregulation	"Organic" mood disorders (due to central nervous system disorders)
Somatic depression		
Underground depression	Atypical facial pain	Vicarious traumatization†
Neurasthenia	Dysphagia	
Mood syndrome as part of personality disorders	Monosymptomatic hypochondriasis	
	Monosymptomatic delusions	
Mood syndromes and depression in schizophrenia		

*Medications more often associated with depression are, among others, reserpine, α-methyldopa (Aldomet), some α- and β-blockers, sedative hypnotics, cimetidine (Tagamet), indomethacin (Indocin), anticancer medications, oral contraceptives, and corticosteroids.
†It has been described as a form of secondary trauma in mental health professionals who treat victims of trauma.
MSV, Mood Syndrome Variant.
Novac and Djenderedjian, unpublished data.

| TABLE 9 | Causes of Mortality in Patients With Bipolar Disease: Index Group Compared to the General Population |

CAUSE OF DEATH	OBSERVED DEATHS (% STUDY GROUP)	EXPECTED DEATHS (% REGISTRAR GENERAL'S* FIGURES)	MORTALITY RATIO (ACTUAL STUDY)
Suicide	15.7	0.67	23.4
Cardiovascular system	42.1	14	3.0
Respiratory system	33.3	1.08	30.8

*Edinburgh Registrar General's Office.
Data from Sharma R, Markar HR. Mortality in affective disorder. *J Affect Disord.* 1994;31:91–96.

lifesaving. Even with partial treatment response, maintenance is paramount. Lifelong maintenance treatment is likely to prevent suicide and further functional deterioration. More recently, suicide prevention both in chronic mood disorders and in personality disorders has been reported with maintenance treatment of lithium carbonate and clozapine (Clozaril)[1]. Among bipolar patients, chronic depression is one of the most treatment-resistant conditions in psychiatry. In any patient with treatment-resistant, undiagnosed bipolar depression, the addition of mood stabilizers may result in the conversion of a treatment nonresponder to a responder. In addition, the value of treatment with lithium carbonate has been recently reiterated in a Finnish study. Lithium carbonate, besides an effective antimanic treatment, can prevent re-hospitalization for bipolar disorder. One 2018 study revealed a significant response when 7000-lux bright white light was administered daily for 4 to 6 weeks, in conjunction with mood stabilizers. The response rate was 68.2% compared to 22.2% in the placebo group. Among the treatment cases, no mood polarity switches occurred. This improvement occurs even in patients who are not diagnosed with SAD. Further replication of these findings may reveal bright light to be a new modality of treatment for bipolar depression, which is readily available and free of significant side effects.

Mood Dysregulation

Mood dysregulation is a broad phenomenon encountered both in clinical and in nonclinical settings. For clinicians, a variety of difficult-to-classify syndromes remain relevant (referred to here as "mood syndrome variants"). These mood syndrome variants present anecdotal but clinically pertinent manifestations collected from the medical literature of the past century. Psychiatric and medical disorders often coexist with different degrees of mood

[5]Investigational drug in the United States.

dysregulation. A more detailed description of each clinical entity in Table 8 is beyond the scope of this chapter. As seen from the table, different forms of mood dysregulation can occur both within and outside DSM diagnoses. For instance, atypical depression has been included in the DSM, whereas other syndromes, such as neurasthenia, remain unclassified. When encountered, any of the listed syndromes should raise suspicion of an underlying mood disorder. A diagnosis of "unspecified depressive disorder" (F32.9) can be made, and the entire mood disorder treatment armamentarium should be considered.

Clinical Course and Prognosis of Mood Disorders

Given the heterogeneity of mood disorders, there is great variation in clinical outcome. Clinical course and outcome depend on whether treatment is available, whether an individual is sensitive or resistant to the treatment, and the degree of compliance. Many individuals with mild and subsyndromal disorders remain undiagnosed, whereas others with severe forms of mood disorders refuse treatment. As a general rule, most untreated mood disorders tend to become chronic. Episodic disorders, such as bipolar I and II and depression, recurrent type, may show more frequent recurrences with advancement in age. Other patients with hyposymptomatic presentations and infrequent episodes may show long-term remissions. Such remissions are favored by stable, low-stress lifestyles. Dyslipidemia, hypertension, type 2 diabetes, coronary vascular disease, and stroke are among the numerous medical complications of chronic mood disorders. Some of these complications are direct side effects of long-term use of psychotropic medications, in particular second-generation antipsychotics. They all contribute to shortened life expectancy of individuals with mood disorders. Table 9 demonstrates the severe impact on life expectancy of bipolar disorder. Mortality comes from suicide, cardiovascular disease, and respiratory disorders. However, treatment can at least partially reverse these trends.

Prevention

Primary prevention of mood disorders requires a concerted effort to educate the public and policymakers for funding of prevention. Depression Awareness Week and other community efforts enhance awareness and decrease stigma. Primary prevention may also include the promotion of general health and healthy work environments and addressing of major social problems, including the avoidance of early trauma and family problems, as well as prevention of excessive stress and trauma in adults. These are all known to be associated with mental illness. Populations at risk need to be identified in primary care settings. Secondary prevention requires the availability of mental health services, including early detection, education about the need for adequate treatment, and continuity of care to prevent impairment. Tertiary prevention would include the continuation of treatment to prevent comorbidity of other psychiatric disorders and catastrophic complications, including suicide. Finally, in the case of mood disorders, quaternary prevention would include long-term follow-up, monitoring of recurrences, and medical comorbidity (accidents, cardiovascular, respiratory, and other medical conditions) to avoid overburdening the health system.

The high medical comorbidity rate recently found among patients with mood disorders varies by medical diagnosis and socioeconomic background. Chronic pain, neurologic conditions, gastrointestinal disorders, cardiovascular disorders, and metabolic syndrome are the most common medical conditions associated with mood disorders. Except for thyroid disorders, the seriousness of the comorbid condition seems to be even higher among patients of lower socioeconomic background. This poses a significant medical and socioeconomic burden of untreated mood disorders.

References

Amare AT, Schubert KO, Klingler-Hoffman M, et al: The genetic overlap between mood disorders and cardiometabolic diseases: A systematic review of genome wide and candidate gene studies, *Transl Psychiatry* 7, 2017. Available at: https://doi.org/10.1038/tp.2016.261.

American Psychiatric Association: *Diagnostic and Statistical Manual of Mental Disorders (DSM-5)*, ed 5, Washington, DC, 2013, American Psychiatric Publishing.

Bartels C, Wagner M, Wolfsgruber S, et al: Impact of SSRI therapy on risk of conversion from mild cognitive impairment to Alzheimer dementia in individuals with previous depression, *Am J Psychiatry* 175:232, 2018.

Binzer S. Multiple Sclerosis. Presented at European Committee for Treatment and Research in Multiple Sclerosis. Abstract 99: 2018; 24(Suppl 2) p. 41.

Cepeda MS, Stang P, Makadia R: Depression is associated with high levels of C-reactive protein and low levels of fractional exhaled nitric oxide: Results from the 2007-2012 National Health and Nutrition Examination Surveys, *J Clin Psychiatry* 77(12), 2016 December.

Connolly KR, Thase ME: If at first you don't succeed: A review of the evidence for antidepressant augmentation, combination and switching strategies, *Drugs* 71:43–64, 2011. Available at: https://doi.org/10.2165/11587620-000000000-00000.

Dobson KS, Dozois DJA, editors: *Risk Factors in Depression*, San Diego, CA, 2008, Academic Press (Elsevier).

Fogel J, Eaton WW, Ford DE: Minor depression as a predictor of the first onset of major depressive disorder over a 15-year follow-up, *Acta Psychiatr Scand* 113(1):36–43, 2006.

Frank E, Kupfer DJ, Thase ME, et al: Two-year outcomes for interpersonal and social rhythm therapy in individuals with bipolar I disorder, *Arch Gen Psychiatry* 62:996, 2005.

Griffiths R, Johnson M, Carducci M, et al: Psilocybin produces substantial and sustained decreases in depression and anxiety in patients with life-threatening cancer: A randomized double-blind trial, *J Psychopharmacol* 30(12):1181–1197, 2016.

Hasin DS, Sarvet AL, Meyers JL, et al: Epidemiology of adult *DSM-5* major depressive disorder and its specifiers in the United States, *JAMA Psychiatry* 75(4):336–346, 2018, https://doi.org/10.1001/jamapsychiatry.2017.4602.

Iosifescu DV, Neborsky RJ, Valuck RJ: The use of the Psychiatric Electroencephalography Evaluation Registry (PEER) to personalize pharmacotherapy, *Neuropsychiatric Dis Treat* 12:2131–2142, 2016. Available at: https://doi.org/10.2147/NDT.S113712.

Janicakk PG. What's new in transcranial magnetic stimulation: Recent developments have enhanced the benefits of this treatment. *Current Psychiatry* 18(3):11-16.

Lahteenvulo M, Tanskanen A, Taipale H, et al: Real-world effectiveness of pharmacologic treatments for the prevention of rehospitalization in a Finnish nationwide cohort of patients with bipolar disorder, *JAMA Psychiatry* 75:347–355, 2018.

Lamers F, van Oppen P, Comijs HC, et al: Comorbidity patterns of anxiety and depressive disorders in a large cohort study: The Netherlands Study of Depression and Anxiety (NESDA), *J Clin Psychiatry* 72:341–348, 2011. Available at: https://doi.org/10.4088/JCP.10m06176blu.

Laursen TM, Musliner KL, Benros ME, et al: Mortality and life expectancy in persons with severe unipolar depression, *J Affect Disord* 193:203–207, 2016.

Merikangas KR, Akiskal HS, Angst J, et al: Lifetime and 12-month prevalence of bipolar spectrum disorder in the national comorbidity survey replication, *Arch Gen Psychiatry* 64:543–552, 2007. Available at: https://doi.org/10.1001/archpsyc.64.5.543.

Metcalf CA, Gold AK, Davis BJ, Sylvia LG, Battle CL: Mindfulness as an intervention for depression, *Psychiatric Annals* 49(1), 2019.

National Comorbidity Survey-Replication: *Appendix Tables: Table 1 and 2.* Available at: http://www.hcp.med.harvard.edu/ncs/publications.php. [Accessed 13 August 2013], 2011.

Qato DM, Ozenberger K, Olfson M: Prevalence of prescription medications with depression as a potential adverse effect among adults in the United States, *JAMA* 319(22):2289–2298, 2018, https://doi.org/10.1001/jama.2018.6741.

Sachs GS, Dupuy JM, Wittmann CW: The pharmacologic treatment of bipolar disorder, *J Clin Psychiatry* 72:704–715, 2011.

Sharma R, Markar HR: Mortality in affective disorder, *J Affect Disord* 31:91–96, 1994.

Siegle GJ, Thompson WK, Collier A, et al: Toward clinically useful neuroimaging in depression treatment: Prognostic utility of subgenual cingulate activity for determining depression outcome in cognitive therapy across studies, scanners, and patient characteristics, *Arch Gen Psychiatry* 69:913–924, 2012. Available at: https://doi.org/10.1001/ archgenpsychiatry.2012.65.

Sit DK, McGowan J, Wiltrout C, et al: Adjunctive bright light therapy for bipolar depression: A randomized double-blind placebo-controlled trial, *Am J Psychiatry* 175:131–139, 2018, https://doi.org/10.1176/appi.ajp.2017.16101200.

Smith D, Court H, McLean G, et al: Depression and multimorbidity in psychiatry and primary care, *J Clin Psychiatry* 75(11):1202–1208, 2014.

Tohen M, Frank E, Bowden CL, et al: The International Society for Bipolar Disorders (ISBD) Task Force report on the nomenclature of course and outcome in bipolar disorders, *Bipolar Disord* 11:453–473, 2009.

Weissman M: The psychological treatment of depression, *Arch Gen Psychiatry* 36:1261–1269, 1979.

DRUG USE DISORDERS

Method of

William M. Greene, MD; and Mark S. Gold, MD

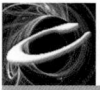

CURRENT DIAGNOSIS

- Screen for substance use in all primary care and emergency settings.
- The clinical interview remains the mainstay of diagnosis.
- Clinicians should have a low threshold for ordering a urine drug test.
- Collateral information should be obtained from family or other sources.
- DSM-5 offers current diagnostic criteria for substance use disorders (Box 1).

CURRENT THERAPY

- Effective pharmacologic and psychosocial treatments exist.
- Formal detoxification is indicated for dangerous withdrawal states or in patients with serious medical comorbidity.
- Pharmacologic relapse prevention options are substance specific, and particularly useful options exist for nicotine and opioids.
- Psychosocial treatments remain the mainstay of substance treatment, and these range along a continuum of intensity from outpatient counseling to long-term residential treatment.
- Patients should be referred to self-help groups (e.g., Narcotics Anonymous) to complement other therapies.
- Indefinite remission is an attainable goal for many—a relapse does not constitute total failure but provides an opportunity to reevaluate the treatment approach.

Epidemiology

Widespread pathologic use of intoxicating substances, both legal and illegal, remains one of the greatest public health concerns facing our nation. According to the 2018 National Survey on Drug Use

BOX 1   DSM-5 Diagnostic Criteria for "Substance Use Disorder"

A problematic pattern of use leading to clinically significant impairment or distress as manifested by two or more of the following in a 12-month period:
- Often taken in larger amounts or longer period than intended
- Persistent desire or unsuccessful efforts to cut down or control use
- Great deal of time spent in activities necessary to obtain, use, or recover from effects
- Craving, or strong desire or urge to use
- Recurrent use resulting in failure to fulfill major role obligations at work, school, or home
- Continued use despite having persistent/recurrent social or interpersonal problems caused or exacerbated by the substance
- Important social, occupational, or recreational activities are given up or reduced because of use
- Recurrent use in situations in which use is physically hazardous
- Continued use despite knowledge of having a persistent/recurrent physical or psychological problem likely to have been caused or exacerbated by the substance
- Tolerance (needing increased amounts for desired effect, or diminished effect with same amount)
- Withdrawal (manifested by characteristic syndrome or taking more to relieve/avoid withdrawal)

Specify current severity:
- Mild: Two to three criteria are met
- Moderate: Four to five criteria are met
- Severe: Six or more criteria are met

and Health, 53.2 million Americans (19.4% of the population) aged 12 years and older used an illicit drug within the preceding year. By order of frequency, these drugs included marijuana, prescription pain relievers, prescription sedatives, hallucinogens, cocaine, prescription stimulants, methamphetamine, and heroin. In addition, 58.8 million Americans (21.5%) aged 12 years and older used tobacco within the previous month, mostly in the form of cigarettes. Each year in the United States, approximately 480,000 people die of an illness attributable to cigarette smoking, making this the foremost cause of preventable death. Overdose deaths have remained a matter of pressing national concern in the United States; opioids were involved in 67.8% of the estimated 70,237 overdose deaths in 2017. Synthetic opioids such as fentanyl accounted for approximately 3000 deaths in 2013; in 2018, they accounted for over 30,000. US life expectancy increases ended in 2010 and started falling in 2014, with fatal overdoses playing a key role in this shift. They rose by almost 387% between 1999 and 2017. Overall, the estimated annual economic cost of tobacco, alcohol, and illicit drugs in the United States is a staggering $740 billion, including costs related to crime, lost work productivity, and health care.

From 1997 to 2019, the rate of past-month cigarette use among 12- to 17-year-olds has steadily dropped from 28.3% to 3.7%. The 2019 Monitoring the Future survey data confirm that cigarette smoking has continued to fall to the lowest rate in the survey's history (i.e., past month use among 12th graders is now at only 5.7%, compared with 36.5% in 1997). Encouraging though these trends may be, they are counterbalanced by the explosive growth of vaping. Among 12- to 17-year-olds, past-month vaping of nicotine has increased from 7.5% in 2017 to 18.1% in 2019. Similarly, past-month vaping of marijuana among 12- to 17-year-olds has increased from 3.6% in 2017 to 10.1% in 2019. Between 2011 and 2019, the number of 12th graders who reported having used any illicit drug at some point in their lives has been holding steady between 47% and 50%. Despite advances in our understanding and treatment of substance use disorders, drug use remains an epidemic, especially in the areas of drugged driving and drug use (including tobacco) in pregnancy.

Diagnosis

The fifth edition of the *Diagnostic and Statistical Manual of Mental Disorders* (DSM-5), published in 2013, eliminated the diagnostic categories of substance abuse and substance dependence. In the interest of consistency and clarity and based on large-population data, they were replaced by a new diagnostic entity: "substance use disorder" (Box 1). It is no longer necessary for the clinician to decide between two different diagnoses. Those familiar with the terminology of DSM-IV will find the new criteria quite familiar, as they essentially represent a combination of the old abuse and dependence criteria with two notable exceptions: one, the legal problem has been eliminated; and two, a craving criterion has been added. When one is diagnosing a substance use disorder, the specific substance for which criteria are met must be listed. In addition, it is also important to document the severity of the disorder based on the number of symptoms present. Examples of specific diagnoses using the new nomenclature would be "alcohol use disorder, moderate" or "alprazolam use disorder, severe." This simpler evidence-based diagnostic schema should eliminate some of the confusion previously surrounding the term "dependence," which was often mistaken to be synonymous with "physiological dependence." It has long been understood, in the context of certain prescribed drugs, that the presence of tolerance and withdrawal is not pathologic in nature; rather, these represent an expected state of neuroadaptation. This fact is reflected in the new criteria for use disorders involving opioids, stimulants, and sedatives. For these three categories, the tolerance and withdrawal criteria are not considered to be met if present when the substance is taken solely under appropriate medical supervision. It should be noted this exception does not apply to cannabis, even if it is "prescribed."

Despite the importance and usefulness of the DSM-5, many patients (and clinicians) may still be left wondering if the problem at hand would appropriately be characterized as "addiction." In a 2011 public policy statement, the American Society of Addiction Medicine offered the following short definition of addiction, which has been well received:

Addiction is a primary, chronic disease of brain reward, motivation, memory and related circuitry. Dysfunction in these circuits leads to characteristic biological, psychological, social and spiritual manifestations. This is reflected in an individual pathologically pursuing reward and/or relief by substance use and other behaviors. Addiction is characterized by inability to consistently abstain, impairment in behavioral control, craving, diminished recognition of significant problems with one's behaviors and interpersonal relationships, and a dysfunctional emotional response. Like other chronic diseases, addiction often involves cycles of relapse and remission. Without treatment or engagement in recovery activities, addiction is progressive and can result in disability or premature death.

Tobacco and Nicotine

Nicotine is the main addictive component in tobacco. It is administered via smoking (e.g., cigarettes, cigars, pipes, bidis, hookah) or in smokeless formulations (e.g., dip, snuff, snus, chew) and now also via vaporization (e.g. electronic cigarettes, vaping devices). Adverse health effects are not equivalent among the different routes of administration; cigarette smoking causes nicotine, affects brain monoamine oxidase (MAO), and other effects in the smoker, some resulting from the smoke and some from the nicotine.

Following administration, nicotine rapidly binds to nicotinic acetylcholine receptors in the central nervous system (CNS), where it acts as a mild psychostimulant and mood modulator in a nonimpairing yet profoundly addictive manner. When the user is tired, smoking has a stimulating effect. When the user is anxious or stressed, smoking exerts a calming effect. Smoking is like an injection without a needle and, given its short half-life, repeated

TABLE 1 Pharmacotherapy for Nicotine Dependence

DRUG	MECHANISM OF ACTION	DOSAGE	INSTRUCTIONS	COMMENTS
Nicotine patch (Nicoderm CQ)	NRT	7 mg, 14 mg, 21 mg	1 patch daily	Tapering of doses recommended to discontinue
Nicotine gum (Nicorette)	NRT	2 mg, 4 mg	Chew slightly then "park" on oral mucosa	Tapering of doses recommended to discontinue
Nicotine lozenge (Commit)	NRT	2 mg, 4 mg	Absorbed through oral mucosa; minimize swallowing	Tapering of doses recommended to discontinue
Nicotine inhaler (Nicotrol Inhaler)	NRT	4 mg/cartridge	6–16 cartridges/day	By prescription only; tedious administration
Nicotine nasal spray (Nicotrol NS)	NRT	0.5-mg/spray	1–2 sprays in each nostril q1h; max 80 sprays/day	By prescription only
Bupropion HCl (Wellbutrin[1], Zyban)	Inhibits reuptake of NE and DA	150-mg SR tab, 300-mg XL tab	300 mg PO (divided qd [XL tab]-bid [SR tab]) daily for 7–12 weeks	Helps with comorbid depression; can help prevent weight gain
Varenicline (Chantix)	Partial agonist at $\alpha_4\beta_2$ nicotinic acetylcholine receptor	0.5 mg, 1 mg	0.5 mg PO qd for 3 days, then 0.5 mg PO bid for 4 days, then 1 mg PO bid for 11 weeks	May smoke during first week; may continue for an additional 12 weeks
Nicotine vaccine (NicVAX)[5]	Antibody sequestration of nicotine	N/A	N/A	In clinical trials

DA, Dopamine; *max,* maximum; *N/A,* not applicable; *NE,* norepinephrine; *NRT,* nicotine replacement therapy; *SR,* sustained release; *XL,* extended release.
[1]Not FDA approved for this indication.
[5]Investigational drug in the United States.

self-administration serves to effectively relieve unpleasant withdrawal symptoms from the nicotine itself. Repeated use quickly leads to both physiologic and psychological dependence.

As with other drugs of abuse, cue-induced cravings play an important role in maintaining the addiction. For example, the smell of the smoke, the sound of a lighter, and the feel of a cigarette on the lips all contribute to an overall process addiction beyond just addiction to the nicotine itself. Tobacco use is also strongly associated with alcohol use, with which it has synergistic toxic effects.

Toxicities from tobacco use are well described and include severe pulmonary disease, cardiovascular disease, and carcinomas of the upper aerodigestive tract and of the bladder. Even secondhand smoke, previously considered harmless, is now correctly regarded as a serious health risk to the nonsmoker and a "drug" itself. Cigarette smoke contains more than nicotine (up to 4700 components, all of which affect the smoker). Additionally, secondhand tobacco exposure in utero can cause serious adverse health effects in the fetus.

Although quitting remains difficult for even the most motivated tobacco users, effective treatments for tobacco use disorder now exist. Clinical trials indicate that a combination of counseling and medications offers the best chance for success and should be offered to patients who are willing to make an attempt to quit. A wide range of nicotine replacement therapies that have been approved by the US Food and Drug Administration (FDA) are readily available and have similar rates of efficacy (Table 1). Patches (Nicoderm CQ), gums (Nicorette), and lozenges (Commit) are available over the counter, but the nasal spray (Nicotrol NS) and inhaler (Nicotrol Inhaler) are available by prescription only. Recently "electronic cigarettes" have gained in popularity, but unlike other nicotine products, they are not yet regulated as drugs by the FDA.

Nonnicotine prescription medications with proven efficacy are available. Bupropion HCl (Wellbutrin) is an antidepressant that was serendipitously noted to dramatically reduce nicotine cravings in some patients; it is now widely used for this purpose (as Zyban). Varenicline (Chantix) was specifically developed to treat tobacco use disorder and represents a considerable advancement, with improved smoking cessation rates. It acts as a partial agonist at the nicotine receptor and effectively serves to satisfy cravings while simultaneously blocking the effects of exogenously administered nicotine. Although probably the most effective agent, varenicline carries a significant risk of psychiatric side effects. The "nicotine vaccine" (NicVAX)[5], a novel approach, failed phase III clinical trials in 2011 and currently does not appear to hold much promise.

Nicotine replacement, bupropion, and varenicline are all considered first-line pharmacotherapy. Bupropion but not varenicline may also be used in combination with nicotine replacement therapies. All pharmacotherapy options are enhanced with the coadministration of counseling or behavioral therapies. Helpful resources for patients interested in quitting include www.smokefree.gov (a government website dedicated to helping people quit smoking), 1-800-QUIT-NOW (a free phone-based services with coaches and educational materials), and a variety of resources available through the American Cancer Society and American Heart Association.

Cannabis

Cannabis (marijuana, pot, weed, grass, ganja, hash) remains the most used illicit drug in the world. As of 2018, 43.5 million Americans aged 12 or older have reported using marijuana during the preceding year (15.9% of the US population). Cannabis is readily harvested from *Cannabis sativa*; typically it is smoked, although it may also be ingested or vaporized. Despite a recent trend whereby states have legalized the use of marijuana for medicinal and recreational purposes, it is still listed as a Schedule I drug by the Drug Enforcement Agency (DEA), which implies a high potential for abuse and no currently accepted medical use. Delta-9-tetrahydrocannabinol (THC) is the active ingredient, which exerts its desired psychoactive effects at CB_1 receptors diffusely throughout the CNS. Marijuana's THC concentration has

---

[5]Investigational drug in the United States.

been steadily increasing as a result of the selective breeding of plants. Annual analysis of the DEA's record of seizures indicates that the average concentration of TCH increased from approximately 1% in 1975 to approximately 10% in 2008. To what extent this makes the drug more dangerous or more addictive remains unclear.

Acute psychoactive effects of cannabis include euphoria, relaxation, heightened sensations, increased appetite, distorted sense of time, slowed reaction time, illusions and hallucinations, paranoia, and anxiety. Acute somatic effects include conjunctival injection, xerostomia, increased heart rate and blood pressure, muscle relaxation, and reduced intraocular pressure. There is no known risk of dangerous overdose, and withdrawal symptoms are generally mild; however, they include irritability, cravings, diminished appetite, and insomnia. Cannabis is now recognized as unequivocally addictive. Users of this drug commonly develop tolerance and demonstrate loss of control and continued use despite negative consequences—the hallmarks of addiction. It is estimated that 1 million Americans sought treatment for cannabis as their primary drug of choice in 2010.

Not surprisingly, with more than 400 chemicals identified in its smoke, cannabis is dangerous with respect to long-term health. Chronic cannabis use is associated with lung cancer, chronic obstructive pulmonary disease, cardiovascular disease, impaired immunity, persistent disruption of memory and attention, and various psychiatric disorders, most commonly anxiety disorders and depressive disorders. There is a growing body of evidence that cannabis abuse can lead to lasting psychosis (i.e., schizophrenia) in predisposed persons.

Currently, treatment of cannabis use disorder remains entirely psychosocial. Various existing drugs (including fluoxetine [Prozac][1], lithium, and buspirone [Buspar][1]) have been investigated. However, well-controlled clinical trials to support their use are lacking. Preliminary data suggest that dronabinol (Marinol)[1] may be of some utility in relieving cravings and withdrawal symptoms without causing intoxication. Rimonabant (Acomplia)[2], a CB$_1$ antagonist previously prescribed for weight loss in Europe, showed promise but has failed to achieve FDA approval because of psychiatric side effects.

Cocaine, Methamphetamine, and Other Stimulants

As a class, cocaine and other stimulants work primarily by enhancing dopamine transmission in a dose-dependent fashion, either directly (amphetamines) or by blocking reuptake (cocaine). Cocaine and a variety of amphetamines (e.g., amphetamine/dextroamphetamine [Adderall], dextroamphetamine [Dexedrine], methamphetamine [Desoxyn], methylphenidate [Methylin, Ritalin]) are available for legitimate medical use as Schedule II drugs. Cocaine (in solution) is still used as a topical anesthetic, and amphetamine derivatives are used to treat attention-deficit/hyperactivity disorder (ADHD), narcolepsy, obesity, and binge-eating disorder[1], Any of these agents may be misused and all carry significant potential for addiction. Even newer "safer" agents such as modafinil (Provigil) and armodafinil (Nuvigil) are associated with use disorders, albeit less commonly than the traditional stimulants.

Prescription stimulant misuse can involve the ingestion of excessive doses to achieve a euphoric high or nonmedical use or diversion of prescriptions (e.g., students sharing medication to facilitate studying). When taken at prescribed doses for an appropriate condition, even methamphetamine is generally safe and effective. In contrast, when it is synthesized in clandestine laboratories and smoked or injected in extremely large quantities, methamphetamine (crystal meth, ice, crank, speed) is alarmingly dangerous. No other commonly abused drug is so strongly associated with permanent brain damage, resembling that seen in victims of traumatic brain injury. As ADHD becomes more recognized and treated, physicians must be aware of the potential for

misuse of their well-intentioned prescriptions. To this end, several recent pharmacologic developments have introduced improved options for treatment. Extended-release formulations of methylphenidate (e.g., Concerta) and amphetamine/dextroamphetamine (Adderall XR) are considered to have less abuse potential than the short-acting formulations. Better still, the formulation of lisdexamfetamine (Vyvanse) includes the amino acid lysine coupled with the amphetamine molecule, consequently acting as a prodrug with the least abuse potential of all ADHD stimulants.

Cocaine and other stimulants induce sympathomimetic effects including tachycardia, hypertension, mydriasis, and diaphoresis. These drugs are commonly associated with seizures, myocardial infarction, hemorrhagic stroke, dyskinesias and dystonias, and psychosis when taken at the doses typically used to achieve euphoria. Withdrawal is generally experienced as a crash and includes fatigue, depressed mood, increased appetite, and cravings. Considered nonaddictive until about 1980, cocaine is now widely recognized as one of the most addictive drugs, particularly in the base form (crack or freebase). MDMA (methylenedioxymethamphetamine), or ecstasy, shares the pharmacodynamic properties of the stimulants combined with serotoninergic effects of the hallucinogens.

Currently no medication has demonstrated efficacy in treating cocaine or stimulant use disorders. Pharmacologic treatment remains symptomatic during the acute withdrawal phase. Stimulant-induced psychosis and mania respond well to traditional psychotropics when warranted; however, to date, no medications have reliably demonstrated efficacy in preventing relapse. A "cocaine vaccine,"[5] which enlists the immune system to develop antibodies rendering cocaine useless, has been studied in humans in a phase III trial that unfortunately has not been successful. In the meantime, traditional psychosocial treatments remain the mainstay of clinical care.

Opioids

Opioids are categorized as endogenous (endorphins, enkephalins, dynorphins), opium alkaloids (morphine, codeine), semisynthetic (heroin, oxycodone [Roxicodone, OxyContin]), or synthetic (methadone [Dolophine], fentanyl [Sublimaze, Duragesic]). The last three categories have a wide range of clinical uses including analgesia, anesthesia, antidiarrhea, cough suppression, detoxification, and maintenance therapy.

Opioids exert their clinical effect at mu, delta, and kappa opioid receptors. The effect on mu receptors is considered the most important, with its activation directly linked to both analgesic and euphoric effects. Most humans subjectively experience opioids with a neutral to aversive response. However, when used in sufficient quantities by genetically vulnerable persons, some users experience energy, relief of emotional pain, and a euphoria many describe as a "total body orgasm." Intoxication manifests with miosis, impaired consciousness, slurred speech, bradycardia, and depressed respiration. Overdose is potentially fatal via respiratory depression, but it is quite amenable to treatment with repeated doses of naloxone (Narcan). The withdrawal syndrome is characterized by a constellation of miserable but not life-threatening symptoms including mydriasis, piloerection, muscle cramps, diaphoresis, vomiting, lacrimation, rhinorrhea, chills, insomnia, cravings, and autonomic hyperactivity.

Since pain was recognized as "the fifth vital sign" in the 1990s, concurrent with heavy marketing campaigns from pharmaceutical companies, the United States experienced a veritable explosion of widespread opioid prescribing for nonmalignant pain. An industry of pain management developed, with the unfortunate side effect of having a sizable proportion of its output being used nonmedically. It is important for prescribers to recognize that the abuse potential of prescription opioids matches—or in some cases even exceeds—that of heroin. Today, oxycodone has a street value of approximately $1.00 per milligram.

Drug Use Disorders

---

[1]Not FDA approved for this indication.
[2]Not available in the United States.

[5]Investigational drug in the United States.

TABLE 2 Useful Medications in Treating Opioid Use Disorders

DRUG	UTILITY	FORMS	ADMINISTRATION	NOTES
Naloxone (Narcan)	Overdose; additive to prevent abuse[1]	SC, IM, IV	0.4–2 mg q2–3 min prn	$T_{1/2}$ = 1 h; wears off quickly
Naltrexone (ReVia, Vivitrol)	Prevention of relapse	PO, IM	ReVia: 50–100 mg PO daily; Vivitrol: 380 mg IM q4wk	Potential for hepatotoxicity; precipitates withdrawal; useful for ETOH as well
Clonidine (Catapres, Catapres-TTS patch)[1]	Withdrawal	PO, transdermal	0.1–0.2 mg PO tid prn; 0.1–0.3 mg q24h transdermal via weekly patch	Monitor for hypotension
Methadone (Dolophine)	Withdrawal; maintenance	PO	Start 20–30 mg PO qd Target 80–120 mg PO qd	Restricted to methadone clinics
Buprenorphine (Subutex, Suboxone [with naloxone], Buprenex injection[1])	Withdrawal; maintenance	SL, IM, IV	Start 2–4 mg SL qd-bid Target 4–32 mg SL daily divided qd-tid	Requires special DEA certification

DEA, Drug Enforcement Administration; *ETOH*, ethanol.
[1]Not FDA approved for this indication.

The most common method of misuse involves simply taking more than prescribed, usually by the appropriate route of administration. Alternatively, individuals with opioid use disorders commonly take their medications via nasal insufflation or inject them intravenously. The extended-release property of certain medications, such as oxycodone (OxyContin), can easily be circumvented by crushing the pills, which greatly enhances the euphoric effect. Even transdermal fentanyl patches (Duragesic) can be misused by any number of methods, such as applying heat to a worn patch, employing complex extraction techniques described online, or simply sucking on the patch itself. If the prescription is used up before its renewal date, the user must either supplement the supply or face the unpleasant effects of withdrawal.

There is no shortage of methods to obtain opioids illicitly. These include seeing multiple prescribers (doctor shopping), purchasing online at foreign "pharmacies," and general trade or purchase on the black market. Also alarming is the growing problem of diversion from hospitals and pharmacies by health care professionals, who are not immune to the disease of addiction. Almost all states have now implemented controlled substance databases (i.e., prescription drug monitoring programs [PDMPs]) aimed at curbing the problem of use disorders involving opioids and other prescription drugs.

Acute detoxification from opioids is achieved by one of two basic strategies: symptomatic treatment with unrelated medications or substitution with a cross-tolerant (opioid) drug with less potential for abuse (Table 2). The first strategy may employ the use of clonidine (Catapres)[1], an α_2-adrenergic agonist, to help with the autonomic component of withdrawal. This is commonly done in combination with other symptomatic treatments on an as-needed basis, using agents such as diazepam (Valium) for anxiety, loperamide (Imodium) for diarrhea, and promethazine (Phenergan)[1] or ondansetron (Zofran)[1] for nausea.

The second strategy typically involves either methadone or buprenorphine (Subutex, with naloxone [Suboxone]). Methadone, a pure mu agonist with a half-life of about 36 hours, is usually started in the 20- to 30-mg range and titrated cautiously by 10 mg every 4 to 7 days. Maintenance therapy with methadone occurs only in the setting of a highly regulated methadone clinic. Buprenorphine, a partial agonist (and kappa antagonist) at the mu receptor, is administered sublingually and has a half-life similar to that of methadone. It was approved in 2002 for office-based treatment of opioid addiction, making pharmacotherapy much more widely available. Caution should be used to avoid administering buprenorphine too soon (before the onset of

[1]Not FDA approved for this indication.

withdrawal syndrome); otherwise acute withdrawal can actually be precipitated. Buprenorphine is available either alone or in combination with naloxone (Suboxone, Zubsolv, Bunavail). Here, the role of naloxone is primarily to deter intravenous use, because naloxone has negligible bioavailability when taken sublingually as prescribed. The FDA has recently approved longer-acting formulations of buprenorphine, including a monthly subcutaneous injection (Sublocade) and a 6-month subdermal implant (Probuphine). These hold promise and give patients more options.

Buprenorphine and methadone are useful in managing acute withdrawal as well as in long-term (months to years) maintenance therapy for preventing relapse to heroin or the opioid of choice. As maintenance therapy, these agents serve to block euphoria, satisfy cravings, and reduce illicit use, with consequent verifiable harm reduction. Buprenorphine, with a built-in ceiling effect because of its unique pharmacology, is much safer than methadone, which is often fatal in overdose. Recent evidence supports the benefit of continuing long-term maintenance therapy indefinitely, as discontinuation is often associated with relapse and other adverse outcomes. Buprenorphine is increasingly being initiated in emergency department settings, and this trend is associated with improved patient outcomes. Increasingly, buprenorphine is being used as an analgesic as well (Butrans Transdermal Patch), and it may be the ideal choice in patients with comorbid pain and addiction who have demonstrated an inability to use other opioids safely.

Also approved for the prevention of opioid relapse is naltrexone, an opioid antagonist, which is available in oral (ReVia) and intramuscular depot formulations (Vivitrol).

Sedative-Hypnotics

This class of drugs includes a wide array of compounds (benzodiazepines, barbiturates, and various related compounds) (Table 3), most of which have at least some potential for abuse. Overall, these medications do much more good than harm and are useful in treating anxiety disorders, insomnia, seizures, and muscle spasms. They are also important in managing withdrawal states and as a component of surgical anesthesia. These drugs act as CNS depressants, and their primary mechanism of action is to enhance inhibitory GABA neurotransmission. The risk of toxicity is by respiratory depression, which is magnified by concomitant use of opioids or other CNS depressants, such as alcohol.

Sedative-hypnotic intoxication and withdrawal states closely resemble those of alcohol except for the more protracted time course of withdrawal. Anxiety, restlessness, insomnia, tremor, nystagmus, tachycardia, and hypertension usually appear 2 to 12 hours after the last dose, and symptoms gradually resolve

TABLE 3	Common Sedative-Hypnotics, Equivalent Dose Conversions	
GENERIC NAME	**TRADE NAME**	**DOSE (mg)**
Benzodiazepines		
Diazepam	Valium	10
Alprazolam	Xanax, Niravam	0.5–1
Lorazepam	Ativan	2
Clonazepam	Klonopin	1–2
Chlordiazepoxide	Librium	25
Clorazepate	Tranxene	7.5
Oxazepam	Serax	10–15
Temazepam	Restoril	15
Triazolam	Halcion	0.25
Flurazepam	Dalmane	15
Barbiturates		
Phenobarbital	N/A	30
Pentobarbital	Nembutal	100
Secobarbital	Seconal	100
Butalbital (with caffeine and aspirin or acetaminophen)	Fiorinal, Fioricet	100
Amobarbital	Amytal	100
Related compounds		
Carisoprodol	Soma	700
Meprobamate	Miltown, Equanil	1200
Chloral hydrate	Noctec	500
Methaqualone[2]	Quaalude	300
Ethchlorvynol[2]	Placidyl	500
Zolpidem	Ambien	20
Zaleplon	Sonata	20
Eszopiclone	Lunesta	3

N/A, Not applicable.
[2]Not available in the United States.

over 1 to 2 weeks. Withdrawal seizures, psychosis, and delirium are fairly common. Detoxification is best accomplished on an inpatient basis and typically involves tapering doses of a long-acting benzodiazepine (e.g., clonazepam [Klonopin], diazepam, clorazepate [Tranxene]) at a rate of about 10% of the initial daily requirement per day. Acute sedative overdose is managed primarily with supportive care and airway management. Flumazenil (Romazicon) 0.2 to 0.5 mg/min IV may be used for acute benzodiazepine overdose, but only with caution because it can precipitate severe acute withdrawal symptoms.

Since their introduction in the 1960s, benzodiazepines, given their enhanced safety profile, have largely replaced barbiturates. However, barbiturates still in common use include phenobarbital and butalbital. Phenobarbital, used mainly for treating seizures, is considered to have a low potential for abuse. Butalbital, compounded with caffeine plus acetaminophen or aspirin (Fioricet, Fiorinal), has moderate abuse potential, typically in combination with other drugs. Carisoprodol (Soma), though not a barbiturate, is metabolized into meprobamate, a barbiturate-like drug. Commonly taken in combination with opioids and other sedatives, carisoprodol is highly abused.

Alprazolam (Xanax) stands out among its peers as the single most abused, most addictive, and yet currently most prescribed sedative-hypnotic. Its rapid onset (T_{max} 1 to 2 hours) and relatively short half-life (6 to 14 hours) contribute to its abuse liability and propensity for withdrawal seizures. Diazepam, historically the most prescribed sedative, also has a relatively rapid onset and significant addictive potential, but its long half-life makes it an ideal agent for use in treating withdrawal from other sedatives. Flunitrazepam (Rohypnol, "roofies") is a benzodiazepine that causes anterograde amnesia. It is now illegal in the United States because of its use in drug-facilitated sexual assaults.

γ-Hydroxybutyric acid (GHB) and baclofen (Lioresal) also act as GABAergic CNS depressants, with intoxication and withdrawal states consistent with the class. Oddly, GHB is considered a Schedule I drug with high abuse potential and no accepted medical use, but when marketed as sodium oxybate (Xyrem), GHB is available as a Schedule III drug (with special restrictions) for use in treating narcolepsy. Baclofen, on the other hand, appears to have rather low addictive potential and may actually play a role in the treatment of alcoholism.[1]

Relatively new drugs—such as zolpidem (Ambien), zaleplon (Sonata), and eszopiclone (Lunesta)—are benzodiazepine-like drugs with CNS depressant activity; they are approved for the short-term treatment of insomnia and have at least some potential for abuse and dependence. Clonazepam (Klonopin) is generally considered to have the lowest potential for euphoria and addiction and is thus the agent of choice if a benzodiazepine must be given to patients with a relative contraindication, such as a history of any drug use disorder.

Conclusion

Despite intensive supply-reduction strategies, improved primary prevention efforts, and the many recent pharmacotherapy advances, drug use disorders remain largely unchanged in their overall scale with the notable exceptions of the increased use of dangerous opioids and increased vaping of nicotine and cannabis. Another notable exception is the significant reduction in tobacco use since the turn of the century. It is estimated that 25% of patients seen in office settings and 50% of those seen in emergency departments have active problems related to substance use. All patients in primary care settings must be screened for tobacco, alcohol, and illicit drug use. Patients should be asked directly about substance use at the initial point of contact (e.g., emergency departments, primary care offices), and clinicians should maintain a healthy degree of skepticism toward patients' responses, remembering that many patients minimize substance use. When any suspicion exists, urine drug screens should be readily utilized without hesitation or fear of communicating mistrust. A variety of affordable quick screen kits are available, which can be sent out for laboratory confirmation of positive results if necessary.

Physicians and other health care professionals are in a unique position to intervene with drug use disorders at the individual level because these disorders are commonly encountered in clinical practice. The problem must first be identified and, depending on the skill set of the primary provider, patients should be treated or referred appropriately. There is an initiative to incorporate formal SBIRT (screening, brief intervention, and referral to treatment) into routine clinical practice. Current procedural terminology (CPT) codes and a reimbursement schedule for screening and brief intervention may be located online at https://www.samhsa.gov/sbirt/coding-reimbursement. Screening may involve the written or verbal assessment of substance use to determine whether the patient exhibits a problematic level of use. The brief intervention aspect of SBIRT targets those with milder substance use disorders and provides effective strategies for intervention before the need for more extensive or specialized treatment arises. Referral to specialized treatment is recommended for patients with

[1]Not FDA approved for this indication.

moderate-to-severe substance use disorders. Data suggest that this approach can be successful in modifying problematic substance use behavior. In addition to formal treatment, physician referral to local 12-step recovery programs (Alcoholics Anonymous, Narcotics Anonymous) has proved beneficial. Ample scientific evidence supports the effectiveness of these programs. Local chapters readily provide physicians with the names and telephone numbers of members willing to welcome newcomers (www.aa.org; na.org).

Physicians are usually well equipped to treat the sequelae of drug use disorders, but they often forget that addiction itself is a treatable disease entity. Treatment ranges in intensity along a continuum that includes medically managed inpatient detoxification, partial hospitalization, intensive outpatient treatment, and outpatient care. The American Society of Addiction Medicine provides patient placement criteria that dictate the appropriate level of treatment based on a multidimensional assessment. Health care professionals should be familiar with the treatment centers in their area; these can place the patient in the appropriate level of care.

It is important to remember that relapse is a characteristic of addiction and does not equate to treatment failure but rather indicates a need for an adjustment in the level of treatment or that of monitoring. Other chronic diseases, such as diabetes and hypertension, necessitate ongoing monitoring and adjustment of treatment interventions as needed, and the same is true of addiction. Recently published data on the treatment and monitoring of recovering physicians (a subgroup of addicts that boasts a 5-year success rate >78%) teach us the lesson that adequate initial treatment coupled with ongoing monitoring is critical. Sustained recovery from a substance use disorder is readily attainable and is characterized by voluntary sobriety, improved personal health, and improved citizenship.

References

American Psychiatric Association: *Diagnostic and Statistical Manual of Mental Disorders*, 5th ed., Washington, DC, 2013, American Psychiatric Publishing.

American Society of Addiction Medicine: Public policy statement: Definition of addiction. August 15, Available at http://www.asam.org/docs/publicy-policy-statements/1definition_of_addiction_long_4-11.pdf, 2011.

Bailey JA, Hurley RW, Gold MS: Crossroads of pain and addiction, *Pain Med* 11:1803–1818, 2010.

DuPont RL, McLellan AT, White WL, et al: Setting the standard for recovery: physicians health programs, *J Subst Abuse Treat* 36:159–171, 2009.

Gold MS, Kobeissy FH, Wang KK, et al: Methamphetamine- and trauma-induced brain injuries: comparative cellular and molecular neurobiological substrates, *Biol Psychiatry* 66:118–127, 2009.

Johnston LD, Miech RA, O'Malley PM, et al: *Monitoring the Future national survey results on drug use 1975-2019: Overview, key findings on adolescent drug use*, Ann Arbor, 2020, Institute for Social Research, University of Michigan.

Kelly JF, Humphreys K, Ferri M: Alcoholics Anonymous and other 12–step programs for alcohol use disorder, *Cochrane Database Syst Rev* (Issue 3):Art. No.: CD012880 2020. https://doi.org/10.1002/14651858.CD012880.pub2.

Office of National Drug Control Policy: *The Economic Costs of Drug Abuse in the United States: 1992–2002*, Washington, DC, 2004, Executive Office of the President, [Publication No. 207303].

Pardo B, Taylor J, Caulkins J P, et al: *The Future of Fentanyl and Other Synthetic Opioids*, Santa Monica, CA, 2019, RAND Corporation, Also available in print form https://www.rand.org/pubs/research_reports/RR3117.html.

Scholl L, Seth P, Kariisa M, et al: Drug and opioid-involved overdose deaths — United States, 2013–2017, *MMWR Morb Mortal Wkly Rep* 67:1419–1427, 2019, https://doi.org/10.15585/mmwr.mm675152e1.

Substance Abuse and Mental Health Services Administration: *Key substance use and mental health indicators in the United States: Results from the 2018 National Survey on Drug Use and Health (HHS Publication No. PEP19-5068, NSDUH Series H-54)*, Rockville, MD, 2019, Center for Behavioral Health Statistics and Quality, Substance Abuse and Mental Health Services Administration. Retrieved from https://www.samhsa.gov/data/.

EATING DISORDERS

Method of

Nandini Datta, PhD; and James Lock, MD, PhD

Bulimia Nervosa

CURRENT DIAGNOSIS

- Binge-eating episodes occur at least once per week for 3 months (eating objectively large quantities of food in a discrete period of time accompanied by a loss of control while eating).
- Compensatory purging episodes occur at least once per week for a period of 3 months (e.g., self-induced vomiting, laxatives, diuretics, excessive and compulsive exercise, enemas) to prevent weight gain.
- Shape and weight are overvalued and impact self-worth and self-esteem.
- Weight is at or above expected range given age, height, and historical growth curves.

CURRENT TREATMENT

- Cognitive behavioral therapy (CBT) is the most evidence-based treatment for bulimia nervosa (BN).
- Interpersonal psychotherapy (IPT) is an appropriate alternative.
- Family-based treatment (FBT) is useful for adolescents with BN.
- Antidepressant treatment (selective serotonin reuptake inhibitors [SSRIs]) may be useful in augmenting psychotherapy or as an alternative in the event that psychotherapy is not effective, refused, or unavailable. It is not as effective as CBT and thus not a front-line approach.

Diagnosis

To diagnose bulimia nervosa (BN), an individual must engage in recurrent binge episodes with compensatory behaviors (e.g., self-induced vomiting, diuretic or laxative use, excessive and compulsive exercise). A binge is a discrete episode of eating a quantity of food that is more than the average person would eat in the same setting, accompanied by a loss of control or feeling as though one cannot stop eating. Nonpurging forms of bulimia occur when an individual uses extreme dietary restriction/fasting and/or exercise as a means of compensating for binge episodes. A disproportionate emphasis on weight and shape in one's self-evaluation is also required in diagnosing BN. DSM-5 criteria require that these episodes occur at a minimum of once weekly for 3 months. Unlike individuals with anorexia nervosa (AN), who may binge and purge, individuals with BN are within range of or above the median body mass index (BMI).

Significant health consequences may accompany BN. Laboratory studies often reveal electrolyte abnormalities, which can lead to cardiac arrhythmias and cardiac arrest in severe cases. Physical examination may detect enamel decay and parotid gland enlargement as a consequence of recurrent vomiting. When ipecac[1] is used to induce vomiting, severe cardiac and skeletal myopathies may develop. Laxative abuse is associated with metabolic acidosis and elevated serum amylase levels. BN has an elevated risk for mortality (crude mortality of 3.9%–6% in an inpatient sample), with many dying by suicide. Most common comorbid psychiatric

---

[1] Not FDA approved for this indication.

diagnoses are mood, anxiety, personality disorders (specifically borderline personality disorder), and substance use disorders.

Epidemiology
BN behaviors typically first occur in middle adolescence (ages 14–16), with onset of full syndrome BN in later adolescence and early adulthood (ages 17–24). The lifetime prevalence estimate of DSM-5 BN ranges from 4% to 6.7%, and while less is known about males, at minimum they are estimated to account for between 10% to 25% of all cases. Symptoms may persist for a number of years, with intermittent periods of remission. A review of existing treatment studies suggests that approximately 45% of patients fully recover, with 27% improving considerably and the remaining 23% exhibiting a chronic course.

Etiology
BN can be explained by a confluence of biologic, sociocultural, psychological, and familial factors. From a biologic standpoint, BN aggregates in families; in twin studies, about half of the variance in heritability can be explained by genetic factors. Serotonin levels may be reduced, and imaging studies show abnormal serotonergic circuitry in the orbital-frontal cortex. Internalization of cultural ideals of beauty may present as a focus on thinness for women, where for males there is often pressure to be muscular with low body fat. Participation in sports where weight and appearance are tied to performance (e.g., gymnastics, wrestling) may increase risk. Early puberty and childhood obesity are common precipitants, as are experiences with peer weight-related teasing. Personality characteristics of individuals with BN may include perfectionism, impulsivity, and instability in interpersonal relationships. Childhood sexual and physical abuse increases the risk for BN.

Treatment
Given the significant physical, social, and emotional consequences associated with BN, effective treatment requires addressing wide-ranging difficulties. Over 70 randomized controlled treatment trials (RCTs) exist for adults with BN, yet only four focus on adolescents. Most studies have examined behavioral therapies, medications, or a combination thereof. CBT is established as the treatment of choice for adults with BN and has been subjected to a large number of RCTs. The underlying assumption of CBT is that bulimic behaviors are maintained by dysfunctional attitudes about shape, weight, and physical appearance, which thereby lead to an overemphasis of these aspects in self-evaluation. Excessive dieting typically ensues, resulting in physiologic and psychological deprivation that increases vulnerability to binge eating. Feelings of guilt and fear about weight gain are mitigated through engaging in purging behaviors. CBT targets this cycle through the use of self-monitoring to increase an awareness of patterns in behaviors, thoughts, and emotions that maintain BN symptoms.

CBT is found to be more effective than no treatment, pill placebo, nondirective supportive psychotherapy, nutritional counseling, stress management, and antidepressant medication therapy. Response to CBT is good, with approximately 50% recovered and 20% with significant reductions in symptoms at the end of treatment. CBT is acceptable and feasible with adolescents; however, a more recent RCT had a 20% rate of abstinence, compared with previous rates of 56% in a case series and 36% in a guided self-help (GSH) version at the end of treatment. Compared with an alternative intervention, interpersonal psychotherapy (IPT), CBT demonstrates a greater probability of remission and reduction in symptoms at the end of treatment. However, these initial differences appear to diminish at a 1-year follow-up, suggesting that, while less efficient, IPT is a viable alternative. IPT was adapted for BN to target interpersonal factors thought to contribute to the development and maintenance of the disorder. IPT has yet to be studied with adolescents.

More recently, CBT has been expanded to address other maintaining features of eating disorders broadly (e.g., interpersonal difficulties, clinical perfectionism, low self-esteem, and mood intolerance). Enhanced CBT (CBT-E) addresses these features and is delivered in a focused or broad (addressing aforementioned maintaining features) format. For individuals with more complex psychopathology, the broad version may be more effective. Further, a novel treatment, integrative cognitive affective therapy for BN (ICAT-BN), may be preferable to CBT-E for individuals with greater affective lability and stimulus seeking behaviors.

Other interventions show promise in the treatment of BN and require further examination. For adolescents, FBT may be helpful, demonstrating higher rates of binge/purge abstinence (40%) than supportive psychotherapy in one study, and higher than CBT (FBT: 39% vs. CBT: 20%) in another. Derived from FBT for AN, parents are supported to directly change dysfunctional eating behaviors. For adults, dialectical behavior therapy (DBT) has been shown to significantly decrease binge/purge episodes when delivered in an individual format. Similar effects were found when an appetite-awareness component was added to standard DBT.

Antidepressants (SSRIs) are the most studied medication treatment for BN. Fluoxetine (Prozac) demonstrates greater reductions in binge eating, purging, and eating-related cognitions than placebo when prescribed at higher doses (60 mg/day). A small pilot study of fluoxetine with adolescents suggests it is acceptable and may decrease BN symptoms. Antidepressants alone are not as effective as when combined with CBT, or as CBT alone.

Binge-Eating Disorder

CURRENT DIAGNOSIS

- Recurrent episodes of binge eating, defined as eating an objectively large amount of food in a discrete period of time with a sense of lack of control during the episode.
- Binge eating is associated with at least three of the following: eating more rapidly than normal; eating until uncomfortably full; eating outside of physical hunger; eating alone because of embarrassment; and subsequent feelings of self-disgust, depression, or guilt.
- There is marked distress associated during a binge eating episode.
- These episodes occur at least once per week over 3 months.
- There is no associated compensatory behavior (e.g., purging), and bingeing does not occur in the context of another eating disorder diagnosis (anorexia or BN).

CURRENT TREATMENT

- CBT and IPT have good evidence of efficacy among adults.
- GSH CBT may be effective for those with less psychopathology.
- DBT requires further study to determine whether good outcomes are sustained over time.
- There is no evidence-based treatment for young patients with binge eating disorder (BED).
- Pharmacologic treatments should be considered as an adjunct to psychotherapy.

Diagnosis
Binge episodes are typically characterized by eating quantities that are larger than others would eat in a similar setting and are accompanied by a feeling of being out of control. Individuals with BED do not engage in compensatory behaviors (e.g., self-induced vomiting, excessive exercise) as in BN. The ICD-11 also recognizes subjective binge episodes, when smaller amounts of food are consumed with loss of control. DSM-5 criteria require that the

episodes occur at a minimum frequency of once per week over a 3-month period. Binge eating (BE) is commonly associated with feelings of guilt and embarrassment and may result in attempts to hide eating. Furthermore, during binge episodes, eating is often rapid and results in feeling uncomfortably full. Most individuals with BED have at least one comorbid psychiatric diagnosis (79% of respondents in one study).

Epidemiology

Lifetime prevalence of BE among adult females was 3% and 3.6% in two separate studies, and 2.1% in males. It occurs at equal rates across ethnic and racial groups. BE most typically onsets in later adolescence or early adulthood, although it does occur in children and is often associated with overweight and obesity, as well as psychological symptoms. Among adolescents with obesity, an estimated 1% meet the criteria for BED, and up to 26% experience BE/loss of control eating. In BED, obesity often predates dieting and subsequent BE, with women having an earlier onset of both dieting and BE. Remission rates in BED are higher than in other eating disorders, although duration and severity is similar to BN.

Etiology

The etiology of BED is unknown. Restrictive dieting, body image dissatisfaction, pressure to be thin, low self-esteem, depressive symptoms, and limited social support increase the risk for the onset of adolescent BE. Increased rates of BE in families suggests there may be a genetic link. Heritability estimates range between .39 and .45. Potential medical causes for BE include CNS tumors, Kleine-Levin syndrome, Kluver-Bucy syndrome, Prader-Willi syndrome, and gastrointestinal pathology, and these causes should be ruled out during assessment. Comorbid psychiatric disorders are common among adults with BED, including mood disorders, anxiety disorders, and, at lesser frequency, substance use disorders and personality disorders. There are high rates of obesity among individuals with BED; however, psychiatric symptoms are linked to the severity of BE rather than obese status.

Treatment

Treatment for adults with BED has received considerable attention in RCTs compared with other eating disorder diagnoses. Most treatments target reduction in BE, psychological symptoms, and weight loss for those who are overweight, as determined by BMI categories. CBT has been applied in multiple formats (group, GSH, CD-ROM delivered, and in combination with medication) and appears to have the highest rates of abstinence. Individual CBT outperformed group CBT in one trial, and a GSH version was more effective in reducing BE than behavioral weight-loss (BWL). CBT targets underlying dysfunctional attitudes and behaviors that maintain BE. An alternative treatment, interpersonal psychotherapy (IPT), is a time-limited psychodynamic therapy targeting interpersonal difficulties that underlie the disorder. IPT is helpful in reducing the frequency of BE. IPT, CBT, and motivational interviewing (MI) all lead to improvements in cognitive restraint, disinhibition, and shape and weight concerns thought to maintain BE.

DBT is another treatment adapted for BED with the aim of targeting affected regulation difficulties formulated to be a maintaining mechanism of BE. Women in a small trial comparing group DBT to a waitlisted group had significantly greater decreases in BE and related eating disorder thoughts and behaviors, with over half abstinent from BE at follow-up. However, compared with supportive psychotherapy, the rate of abstinence, while achieved more quickly in the DBT group, did not differ between the groups at follow-up. Pilot data suggest comprehensive DBT (individual, group, and skills coaching) may be effective.

Pharmacologic treatments targeting BE and weight loss have been tested alone and in combination with psychotherapy. There may be improvement in weight loss with addition of pharmacotherapy. The combination of CBT with topiramate (Topamax)[1]

resulted in greater weight loss and better psychosocial outcomes than CBT with fluoxetine.[1] A high dose of the SSRI escitalopram (Lexapro)[1], anticonvulsants topiramate and zonisamide (Zonegran)[1], lisdexamfetamine (Vyvanse) at a dose of 50 mg or 70 mg, and the selective norepinephrine reuptake inhibitor atomoxetine (Strattera)[1] were each associated with significantly decreased binge eating and weight in separate placebo-controlled trials.

Anorexia Nervosa

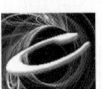

CURRENT DIAGNOSIS

- Persistent restriction of energy (caloric) intake relative to requirements, leading to significantly low weight (e.g., accounting for age, sex, developmental trajectory, and physical health).
- Ongoing behavior interfering with weight gain driven by a fear of becoming fat.
- Disturbance in the perception of shape, weight, overvaluation of weight, and shape in self-evaluation, or lack of acknowledgment of seriousness of low weight.
- Either meets criteria for restricting type, with absence of binge or purge behaviors, or binge eating/purging type.

CURRENT TREATMENT

- FBT for adolescents with AN has the most evidence supporting its efficacy to date.
- AFT may be a helpful alternative.
- There are no first-line treatments for adults with AN.
- CBT may prevent relapse in weight-restored individuals.

Diagnosis

AN is characterized by dietary restriction that is severe enough to lead to seriously low weight, fear of weight gain, and difficulty or inability to accurately perceive shape or weight. Secondary amenorrhea is no longer required for a diagnosis of AN in the DSM-5. Individuals may be classified as AN-restricting subtype or AN-binge/purge subtype. The definition of low weight is less than "minimally normal" among adults or "minimally expected" among children and adolescents. Growth charts normed by age and gender are necessary to calculate expected BMI for individuals under 18 and growth curves may help detect deviations from an individual's growth trajectory. A BMI at or below the 10th percentile is a benchmark reflecting malnourishment associated with AN, and BMI below 18.5 kg/m^2 may be used as guidelines. When an individual meets all criteria for AN, but despite significant weight loss weighs within or above the median BMI range, atypical AN (AAN) may be diagnosed. Otherwise, AAN is associated with the same psychological and physical features of AN.

A wide variety of medical and psychiatric symptoms accompany AN. Potentially life-threatening medical conditions may develop as a result of semistarvation. Vital sign abnormalities (e.g., bradycardia, orthostasis, hypothermia) and amenorrhea are common consequences of malnutrition. Bone loss resulting in osteopenia and, in more severe cases, osteoporosis may occur. Abnormal laboratory findings may occur in some patients with AN who use laxatives, diuretics, and diet pills and who engage in self-induced vomiting.

The lifetime rate of comorbid psychiatric diagnoses among adolescents with AN is approximately 55%. Most commonly, these comorbidities include anxiety disorders (social anxiety, separation anxiety, generalized anxiety and obsessive compulsive disorder [OCD]), depression, and substance abuse. There is significant overlap in OCD symptoms and AN, thus careful consideration

[1]Not FDA approved for this indication.

[1]Not FDA approved for this indication.

must be given to the content of obsessions and compulsions in diagnosis. In AN, obsessional preoccupations are related to eating, food, weight, and shape, and compulsions may appear as calorie counting, excessive exercise routines, and mealtime rituals. Depressive symptoms such as dysphoric thought, low energy, difficulty concentrating, and low self-esteem also manifest in AN and may not indicate a separate depressive disorder.

Epidemiology

Peak age of onset for AN is between 14 and 18 years. Lifetime prevalence of females with a DSM-5 diagnosis of AN in the United States is estimated to be between .8% and 3.6%, based on method of data collection. The incidence of AN among males is less studied, but recent estimates suggest that 1 out of every 4 cases are male. Little is known about the prevalence of AN across racial and ethnic groups. A recent study did not reflect significantly higher rates of AN among non-Hispanic white adolescents compared with Hispanic and non-Hispanic black peers; however, other evidence suggests that it is less common among persons of African origin.

AN has the highest mortality rate of any psychiatric illness, with reports as high as 5% per decade. Rates of chronicity obtained from long-term adult follow-up studies (AN diagnosis persisting greater than 5 years) are estimated between 7% and 15%. Death occurs most commonly secondary to medical complications of starvation or suicide. Prognosis for adolescents with short duration of illness (less than 3 years) is better than adults.

Etiology

The causal mechanisms of AN are multiply determined through the interface of biologic/genetic, psychological, and sociocultural factors. Heritability estimates from twin studies range from 48% to 74%, and family aggregation studies report that AN occurs at about five times the expected rate in affected families. The interactional effect between genes and developmental processes is reflected in studies demonstrating greater heritability among 17-year-old twins compared with 11-year-old twins. Hormonal changes during adolescence could mediate gene expression during puberty, explaining this difference.

Perfectionistic and avoidant personality features are associated with AN and are likely heritable. Neurocognitive features including cognitive rigidity and an overly detailed style of information processing are common and may represent an endophenotype as those who are recovered, as well as unaffected siblings who demonstrate similar cognitive styles. Common developmental challenges associated with adolescence may also precipitate or emerge as a consequence of AN. These include navigating issues of autonomy, self-efficacy, and intimacy. Sociocultural factors including exposure to a Westernized "thin ideal" of beauty for females and an overly muscular ideal for males may be internalized, thereby triggering extreme dieting or exercise. Furthermore, activities where weight or appearance is intertwined with performance may also elevate risk (e.g., gymnastics, ballet, wrestling, figure skating).

Treatment

Given the severity of psychological, social, and health consequences of AN, both close medical monitoring and psychotherapy are the standard of care. In severe cases, inpatient medical monitoring may be required, and standard criteria for hospitalization are available for physicians to treat common consequences of starvation like bradycardia, hypotension, and orthostatic vital sign abnormalities. Findings from RCTs among adults are inconclusive because of dropout rates as high as 50%. Medication trials of antidepressants (serotonin reuptake inhibitors and tricyclics) have high dropout rates and show little to no improvement of weight or eating disorder behaviors. Therefore these should not be used independent of psychotherapy. A recent trial demonstrated an average of 1 lb per month greater weight gain for those taking olanzapine (Zyprexa)[1] than not; however, potential risks, including tardive dyskinesia and metabolic side

effects, need be considered. CBT may help prevent relapse for individuals who are already weight-restored. For underweight individuals, findings are mixed, and nonspecific therapies such as nonspecific supportive clinical management (NSCM) showed better outcomes compared with IPT and CBT at end of treatment. However, improvements in NSCM appear to decline over time, and IPT may catch up to CBT.

Recent treatment studies have focused on improving retention. For example, an enhanced version of outpatient CBT (CBT-E), which employs motivational enhancement strategies, retained 64% of the original sample, improving on previous trends in attrition. Individuals completing treatment had clinically significant improvements in weight and eating disorder psychopathology. When CBT-E was compared with focal psychodynamic therapy and treatment as usual (TAU) in the community, weight gain and improvements in eating disorder symptoms were more rapid. However, focal psychodynamic treatment had the highest rates of recovery at follow-up (35%), though these were only significantly higher than the TAU group.

FBT, otherwise known as *Maudsley family therapy*, has been studied in seven RCTs with superior outcome to other individual therapies. This outpatient treatment empowers parents to disrupt self-starvation and other behaviors that maintain AN. In the initial phase of treatment, parents take full control over managing eating-related behaviors. FBT demonstrates rates of remission ranging from 49% (full remission in weight and eating disorder thoughts and behaviors) to 89% for partial remission. Rates of relapse are about 10% and there is minimal dropout, suggesting it is acceptable to families. FBT delivered in a parent-focused format may be just as effective and preferable to conjoint FBT for families with high levels of expressed criticism.

AFT may be an alternative approach for individuals whose family members are unable to participate. The focus in AFT is on helping an adolescent move toward healthy individuation and increased self-efficacy. AN is conceptualized as an ineffective strategy that the adolescent has adopted in managing common developmental challenges. In AFT, adolescents learn new skills to support eating and weight gain and parents are involved in separated collateral sessions. CBT has also been studied in adolescents; compared with TAU and hospitalization, it appeared to be the most cost-effective approach.

Avoidant-Restrictive Food Intake Disorder

CURRENT DIAGNOSIS

- Disturbance in eating/feeding resulting in persistent failure to meet nutritional and/or energy (caloric) needs.
- The disorder must result in one of the following consequences: significant weight loss or faltering growth; significant nutritional deficiency; dependence on nutritional supplements or enteral feeding; and interference with psychosocial functioning.
- The eating/feeding disturbance is not better explained by another medical or psychiatric condition or by cultural or religious practices.

CURRENT TREATMENT

- There are no established treatments for this new diagnosis, though clinical trials are currently underway.
- CBT or family interventions that employ behavioral strategies are being explored as potential treatment options.

---

[1]Not FDA approved for this indication.

Diagnosis

Avoidant-restrictive food intake disorder (ARFID) is a new diagnosis included in the DSM-5, which reflects the recognition of "food neophobia" or extreme picky eating as challenges. Individuals with ARFID can be of any age and exhibit clinically significant feeding/eating difficulties, which result in failure to meet energy (caloric) or nutritional needs. In response, individuals have low weight or failure to meet expectations for growth, significant nutritional deficiency, a need for enteral feeding or oral nutritional supplementation, and/or impairment in psychosocial functioning. Although there may be failure to thrive or to make expected weight gain/weight loss, ARFID is distinguished from AN by the absence of body image disturbance driving restrictive eating symptoms. Low weight can be determined through clinical judgment and examination of developmental trajectory using growth charts. Nutritional deficiency may be assessed through dietary history, as well as physical examination. Related medical consequences may follow those seen in malnourished individuals with AN (e.g., bradycardia, anemia, hypothermia) and can be life threatening. Individuals with ARFID treated in an inpatient setting are more likely to require nasogastric feeding than those with AN. If limited food intake is better explained by cultural or religious practice, an eating disorder in which there is disturbance in experience of shape/weight, or current physiologic or psychiatric conditions that explain the symptoms, ARFID is not diagnosed. Further, in the event of a coexisting medical diagnosis, food refusal is serious enough to warrant separate clinical attention. Thorough assessment should include examination of feeding, and eating history, psychiatric symptoms, development, and underlying medical causes must be ruled out before making a diagnosis.

Individuals with ARFID often exhibit selective eating, food neophobia, and hypersensitivity to sensory features of food (texture, taste, temperature, appearance). Similar clinical presentations may have varying etiology, requiring individualized treatment plans. In some, development of food avoidance can be traced to a specific aversive event, trauma, or related gastrointestinal problem, or may arise out of a choking, swallowing, or vomiting phobia. Individuals may also have a lack of drive or interest in eating or heightened textural sensitivity, which is also common in autism spectrum disorders.

Epidemiology

No data exist on prevalence, course, and outcome of this disorder. Surveillance studies are underway in the United Kingdom and Canada for related "food avoidance emotional disorder," with overlap in clinical features. In a school-age sample (ages 8–13), prevalence of ARFID was 3.2%. In pediatric inpatient ED programs, rates of ARFID are reported to be between 5% and 14% comprised of a higher proportion of males than other ED diagnoses and tend to be younger. ARFID appears to arise most commonly in infancy and early childhood but can occur at any age and last into adulthood. Preliminary data suggest ARFID occurs at equal rates in males and females. There is no evidence to guide for whom clinical intervention is warranted versus those whose symptoms resolve over time.

In one study, 53% of individuals ages 9 to 22 had at least one co-occurring lifetime psychiatric diagnosis, the most common being an anxiety disorder. Severity of symptoms among those with a sensory sensitivity profile of ARFID was related to increased risk for current and lifetime conduct, neurodevelopmental and disruptive disorders. Increased severity in the fear of aversive consequences profile was associated with increased risk for current and lifetime anxiety, obsessive-compulsive, and trauma-related disorders.

Treatment

There are no systematically studied treatments to date for ARFID; however, behavioral interventions with contingency management have been successfully used among children who have food neophobia in the context of a developmental disability. Given limited data, individualized treatment plans are best derived through assessment of medical history, temperament, psychiatric symptoms, and development. Food avoidance may be treated through use of behavioral strategies (e.g., shaping, chaining, contingency management, extinction) that systematically desensitize individuals to a wider range of foods. Related anxiety management techniques (relaxation training, visualization for mastery) and cognitive strategies derived from CBT may address maintaining psychiatric features. CBT was successfully applied in a case study of young adults with food neophobia, and a transdiagnostic CBT model with family involvement proved useful in a case study of a pediatric patient. Mirtazapine has been used with pediatric patients in two case studies with demonstrated increases in rate of weight gain, improvements in anxiety and eating. In most severe cases of malnutrition, hospitalization for medical stabilization purposes may be needed before outpatient therapy.

References

Bulik CM, Berkman ND, Brownley KA, et al: Anorexia nervosa treatment: a systematic review of randomized controlled trials, *Int J Eat Disord* 40:310–320, 2007.

Call C, Walsh B, Attia E: From DSM-IV to DSM-5: changes to eating disorder diagnoses, *Curr Opin Psychiatry* 26:532–536, 2013.

Couturier J, Isserlin L, Norris M, et al: Canadian practice guidelines for the treatment of children and adolescents with eating disorders, *J Eat Disord* 8(4):1–80, 2020.

Hay P: Current approach to eating disorders: a clinical update: 2020, *Intern Med J* 50:24–29, 2020.

Keery H, et al: Attributes of children and adolescents with avoidant/restrictive food intake disorder, *J Eat Disord* 7:31, 2020.

Kreipe R, Palomski A: Beyond picky eating: avoidant/restrictive food intake disorder, *Curr Psychiatry Rep* 14:421–431, 2012.

Le Grange D, Lock J, editors: *Eating disorders in children and adolescents: a clinical Handbook*, New York, 2011, The Guilford Press.

Peat C, Brownley K, Berkman N, et al: Binge eating disorder: evidence-based treatments, *Curr Psychiatry* 11:32–39, 2013.

Shapiro J, Berkman N, Brownley K, et al: Bulimia nervosa treatment: a systematic review of randomized controlled trials, *Int J Eat Disord* 40:321–336, 2007.

Smink F, van Hoeken D, Hoek H: Epidemiology of eating disorders: incidence, prevalence and mortality rates, *Curr Psychiatry Rep* 14:406–414, 2012.

Steinhausen H, Weber S: The outcome of bulimia nervosa: findings from one-quarter century of research, *Am J Psychiatry* 166:1331–1341, 2009.

Stice E, Marti CN, Rohde P: Prevalence, incidence, impairment and course of the proposed DSM-5 eating disorder diagnoses in an 8-year prospective community study of young women, *J Abnorm Psychol* 122(2):445–457, 2013.

GENERALIZED ANXIETY DISORDER

Method of
Natalie C. Dattilo, PhD; and Andrew W. Goddard, MD

CURRENT DIAGNOSIS

- Generalized anxiety disorder (GAD) is the most common psychiatric disorder seen in the primary care setting.
- GAD is characterized by feelings of dread, negative anticipation, and worry that are difficult to control and may include hypervigilance, excessive reassurance seeking, and behavioral avoidance of anxiety-provoking situations.
- Symptoms of GAD most often include agitation, irritability, restlessness, muscle aches or tension, dizziness, fatigue, racing heart, dry mouth, nausea, decreased sexual desire, sleep or appetite disturbances, and an inability to relax.
- A thorough medical examination and laboratory work may be indicated to rule out underlying physiologic causes, adverse reaction to medication, caffeine or substance use, and drug or alcohol withdrawal.
- Symptoms that are persistent, disruptive, or distressing warrant treatment.
- The Generalized Anxiety Disorder – 7 (GAD-7) is a screening instrument used to assess symptoms of GAD in primary care settings. Scores of 5, 10, and 15 are taken as the cut-off points for mild, moderate, and severe anxiety, respectively. When used as a screening tool, further evaluation is recommended when the score is 10 or greater.

Epidemiology

Anxiety disorders are among the most prevalent psychiatric disorders in the world. In the United States, it is estimated that an anxiety disorder is diagnosed in approximately 16 million adults each year and approximately 30 million meet criteria for an anxiety disorder over the course of their lifetimes. Second to depression, anxiety disorders are the most common mental health problem seen by physicians in the general medical setting. In fact, patients with anxiety are more likely to present initially to a generalist physician office than to a mental health care provider.

Anxiety disorders tend to be chronic and disabling and impose a high individual and societal burden. It has been estimated that the United States spends approximately $40 billion to $60 billion per year for costs associated with anxiety disorders. These include not only direct costs associated with treatment but also indirect costs associated with lost productivity. Thus early detection and treatment is critically important.

Risk Factors

Risk factors associated with anxiety disorders include personal or family history of anxiety; recent increase in stressful life events; lack or perceived lack of social support; ineffective emotional coping strategies; being female; experiencing childhood adversity, including trauma or witnessing a traumatic event; having a chronic health condition or serious illness; having an acute or chronic pain condition; and substance abuse. Having a genetic predisposition to developing an anxiety disorder is likely, although environmental stressors clearly play a role. Research has also shown that patients suffering from anxiety are generally more sensitive to physiologic changes than nonanxious patients. This heightened sensitivity leads to diminished autonomic flexibility, which may be the result of faulty central information processing in anxiety-prone persons.

Pathophysiology

Current evidence suggests that anxiety symptoms are likely caused by dysregulation in the central nervous system fear circuit. Physical and emotional manifestations of this dysregulation can result in a state of hyperarousal. Several neurotransmitter systems have been implicated in the development of this state.

The most commonly considered are the serotoninergic and noradrenergic neurotransmitter systems. Very simply, it is believed that an underactivation of the serotoninergic system and an overactivation of the noradrenergic system are involved, resulting in dysregulation of physiologic arousal and the emotional experience of this arousal. Disruption of the γ-aminobutyric acid (GABA) system has also been implicated because of the response of many of the anxiety-spectrum disorders to treatment with benzodiazepines.

There has also been some interest in the role of corticosteroid regulation and its relation to symptoms of fear and anxiety. Corticosteroids might increase or decrease the activity of certain neural pathways, affecting not only behavior under stress but also the brain's processing of fear-inducing stimuli. The stress response is hardwired into the brain and is most often triggered when survival of the organism is threatened. The stress response, however, can be triggered not only by a physical challenge or threat but also by the mere anticipation (or fear) of threat. As a result, when humans chronically and erroneously believe that a threatening event is about to occur, they begin to experience the physical and psychological symptoms of anxiety and panic.

Finally, a subcortical neural structure, the amygdala, serves an important role in coordinating the cognitive, affective, neuroendocrine, cardiovascular, respiratory, and musculoskeletal components of fear and anxiety responses (fear expression). It is central to registering the emotional significance of stressful stimuli and creating emotional memories. The amygdala receives input from neurons in the sensory cortex. When activated, the amygdala stimulates regions of the midbrain and brainstem, causing autonomic hyperactivity, which can be correlated with the physical symptoms of anxiety.

Prevention

No biological markers are specific enough yet to detect anxiety early, and there is no available evidence to suggest that current medications prove efficacious in preventing these disorders. Therefore, it is important to screen for specific risk factors, such as family history and substance abuse. If a person is anxiety prone, he or she should first be encouraged to adopt healthy lifestyle habits. Exercise has been shown to relieve tension, anxiety, and stress. Patients should avoid stimulants such as caffeine and nicotine, which can exacerbate symptoms. Reducing alcohol intake should be encouraged as well. Educating patients on healthy sleep habits can prevent conditioned (or secondary) insomnia issues. It is also recommended that anxiety-prone persons reduce subjective levels of stress by practicing effective methods of relaxation and other stress management activities, like meditation, yoga, social connection, gratitude journaling, and pleasant event scheduling.

Clinical Manifestations

GAD is characterized by subjective feelings of worry, dread, or anticipation of negative events and can include hypervigilance and avoidance of anxiety-producing situations. Physical symptoms can include jitteriness or shakiness, trembling, muscle aches and tension, sweating, cold or clammy hands, dizziness, or vertigo; fatigue; racing or pounding heart; hyperventilation; sensation of a lump in the throat, choking sensation, or dry mouth; numbness and tingling in the hands, feet, or other body parts; upset stomach, nausea, vomiting, or diarrhea; decreased sexual desire; and sleep and appetite disturbances.

Psychological symptoms include, most predominantly, unrealistic or excessive worry and apprehension, hypervigilance or an inability to relax, distractibility, indecisiveness, and insecurity. Patients often express feelings of impatience, agitation, irritability, and fear. They may ask multiple questions repeatedly in an attempt to quell the anxiety through excessive information or reassurance seeking. In GAD, the worries a patient may express tend to be nonspecific and all-encompassing. They tend to be "worst-case scenario" and "what if?" thinkers. Some patients also exhibit specific phobias such as fear of being far from home or fear of social contact. Patients with GAD may report difficulty falling asleep because they "can't turn their mind off" at night. If a patient reports these symptoms or displays one of several behavioral manifestations of GAD leading to significant distress and/or impairment of function, the condition is unlikely to remit on its own and treatment is warranted.

Diagnosis

A diagnosis of GAD is made when a patient meets the specific diagnostic criteria outlined in the *Diagnostic and Statistical Manual of Mental Disorders, Fifth Edition* (DSM-5). Persons

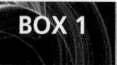

BOX 1	Medical Conditions Often Associated With Anxiety Symptoms

Cardiopulmonary
Angina
Mitral valve prolapse
Pulmonary embolism
Chronic obstructive pulmonary disease (COPD)
Asthma

Endocrine
Hyperthyroidism
Pheochromocytoma
Cushing syndrome
Menopause

Gastrointestinal
Gastroesophageal reflux
Irritable bowel syndrome (IBS)
Gastritis

Neurologic
Dementia
Substance intoxication or withdrawal
Seizure disorder
Migraine

TABLE 1	Pharmacotherapy for the Treatment of Generalized Anxiety Disorder		
DRUG	**STARTING DOSE**	**TARGET DOSE**
Selective Serotonin Reuptake Inhibitors		
Paroxetine (Paxil)*	10 mg qd	10–60 mg qd
Escitalopram (Lexapro)*	5–10 mg qd	10–20 mg qd
Sertraline (Zoloft)	12.5–25 mg qd	50–200 mg qd
Fluoxetine (Prozac)	10 mg qd	20–40 mg qd
Serotonin-Norepinephrine Reuptake Inhibitors		
Venlafaxine (Effexor XR)*	37.5 mg qAM	150–300 mg qAM†
Duloxetine (Cymbalta)*	30 mg qd	60–90 mg qd
Other		
Buspirone (BuSpar)	5 mg bid–tid	10 mg tid

*U.S. Food and Drug Administration indication for generalized anxiety disorder.
†Exceeds dosage recommended by the manufacturer.

with GAD experience uncontrollable, excessive anxiety and worry involving several areas of functioning on most days for at least 6 months. The anxiety must be associated with at least three of the following symptoms: restlessness, fatigue, impaired concentration, irritability, muscle tension, or sleep problems. Patients tend to express chronic excessive nervousness, exaggerated worry, tension, and irritability that appear to have no cause or are more intense than the situation warrants. Physical signs such as headaches, trembling, twitching, or sweating often develop, which lead to further worries. GAD symptoms tend to wax and wane over time, with short-term exacerbations of acute anxiety in response to stress. Symptoms show substantial overlap with those of other medical and psychological disorders, particularly major depressive disorder, substance abuse disorders, and other anxiety disorders, which tends to complicate diagnosis.

Differential Diagnosis

It is important to perform a thorough medical workup when initially assessing the patient with anxiety symptoms. The differential diagnosis can include several organic causes, such as endocrine dysfunction, intoxication or withdrawal, hypoxia, metabolic abnormalities, and neurologic disorders. It is also important to rule out other comorbid psychiatric disorders. Severe depression, bipolar disorder, prodromal schizophrenia, delusional disorder, and adjustment disorder can often be accompanied by severe anxiety. Many organic causes can be ruled out by a thorough history and basic laboratory work, including thyroid-stimulating hormone, urine toxicology, electrocardiogram, complete blood count, and metabolic panel. The most common medical conditions associated with anxiety are presented in Box 1.

The list of drugs suspected of causing anxiety is extensive. Drugs commonly associated with anxiety include stimulants such as amphetamine, cocaine, methamphetamine, and caffeine. Drugs such as lysergic acid diethylamide (LSD) and 3,4-methylenedioxymethamphetamine (MDMA, or "ecstasy") can also cause acute and chronic anxiety. Prescription medications to consider include sympathomimetics, antihypertensives, and nonsteroidal antiinflammatory drugs (NSAIDs).

Treatment and Monitoring

Current practice guidelines indicate that the treatment of an anxiety disorder begins with education. Many people are confused, scared,

or frustrated by the symptoms and behavior and are reassured to know they are not alone and that there are effective interventions. The patient should receive an appropriate medical workup, such as a physical examination, and studies (e.g., electrocardiogram, thyroid-stimulating hormone) when indicated. After ruling out a medical condition, developing a good working alliance with the patient provides a basis for ongoing disease management and prevents unnecessary utilization or overutilization of the medical system, as well as potential exacerbation of symptoms.

A combination of psychotherapy and medication management is recommended as first-line treatment for GAD. CBT has the strongest empirical support to date for the treatment of anxiety. Mindfulness-based stress reduction (MBSR) has an emerging evidence base as an effective alternative or complementary behavioral treatment program for anxiety. Both offer a skills-based approach to treatment. In CBT, the therapist and patient work collaboratively and in an active and problem-solving manner. It is structured and generally short term with an emphasis on reducing symptoms and preventing "flare-ups" by monitoring and changing unhelpful or inaccurate thinking patterns that result in feelings of anxiety and worry. Another critical component of CBT for GAD is learning and applying behavioral relaxation techniques (e.g., diaphragmatic breathing, guided imagery, progressive muscle relaxation) and distress tolerance skills (e.g., mindfulness, acceptance). Volumes of evidence support the efficacy of CBT interventions for GAD, but success requires commitment to treatment on the part of the patient. Its efficacy is also contingent upon the ability of the therapist and the length of time in treatment. Studies show that when compared with patients undergoing monotherapy, patients treated with a combination of CBT and medication experience nearly twice the remission rate.

SSRIs have been shown to be the best-tolerated class of medication, and response rates are significantly higher than placebo for GAD. SSRI medications includes fluoxetine (Prozac),[1] fluvoxamine (Luvox),[1] citalopram (Celexa),[1] escitalopram (Lexapro), paroxetine (Paxil), and sertraline (Zoloft).[1] Some improvement in symptoms should be noted within 3 or 4 weeks, and the dose should be increased if no improvement is seen. In treating any anxiety disorder, SSRIs should be started at low doses and gradually titrated up to therapeutic levels to avoid an initial exacerbation of anxiety. Pharmacotherapy options for the treatment of GAD are presented in Table 1.

---

[1]Not US Food and Drug Administration (FDA) approved for this indication.

Benzodiazepines, which have been commonly used in the past to treat anxiety disorders, are not recommended except in cases of extreme impairment of function and only for very short-term use. The tolerability and lack of addiction potential make the SSRIs more desirable for long-term management, but the delay in response makes short-term symptom relief with a benzodiazepine desirable for those with the greatest impairment. Because of the risk for rebound anxiety when withdrawing from benzodiazepines with short half-lives, such as alprazolam (Xanax), many prefer the longer-acting benzodiazepines, such as clonazepam (Klonopin).[1] However, the addiction potential and the potential for abuse with either drug make this the treatment option of last resort.

If the patient does not respond to the combination of CBT and medication, a reevaluation of symptoms might reveal a comorbid disorder missed on the first examination. Comorbid psychiatric disorders significantly lower the likelihood of recovery from anxiety and increase recurrence rates. Some clinicians try switching to a different SSRI before considering the next step in treatment; however, a referral to a psychiatrist or integrated care consultant for further evaluation and management may be necessary. Treatment-refractory anxiety can be extremely frustrating for the patient, the patient's family, and the treating physician. If benzodiazepine treatment was initiated, this frustration can and does often lead to an increased dependence on the medication and a requirement of increasingly higher doses to achieve the same effect. For long-term gains, therapy in addition to medication treatment should be recommended.

Education is critical to reassure the patient that effective treatment is available, but that patience may be necessary until the right combination of modalities is found. Although all anxiety disorders display a significant amount of chronicity, most patients have an improved outcome with appropriate treatment. Response rates improve when comorbidity is low. Patients with an earlier onset of symptoms (childhood or adolescence) can generally expect a more chronic course and their anxiety symptoms may be more difficult to treat. Patients rarely have a spontaneous remission of symptoms, but most can continue to function despite the symptoms. Nevertheless, time to resolution of symptoms is shortened and overall functioning typically improves with treatment.

Pharmacotherapy often helps to prevent relapse, and rates are improved when effective treatment is continued for 12 months. When considering termination of pharmacologic treatment, the risk for relapse in GAD should be discussed with the patient. When discontinuing the SSRIs, a slow taper is recommended, with close monitoring for withdrawal symptoms (e.g., headache, gastrointestinal upset, restlessness, and other flulike symptoms). Also monitor for rebound anxiety symptoms. If relapse occurs, reinstituting treatment is indicated, and many patients opt for indefinite treatment to maintain remission of symptoms. Lifelong management with pharmacotherapy or psychotherapy, or both, is not unusual for many patients. For many, a maximum reduction of symptoms, rather than a full remission, is an acceptable outcome.

Complications

Untreated anxiety disorders can lead to, or worsen, other mental and physical health conditions, including bruxism (teeth grinding), cognitive impairment, depression, gastrointestinal disorders, headache, insomnia, heart disease, substance abuse, and significantly impaired quality of life.

---

[1]Not FDA approved for this indication.

TABLE 2	Helpful Resources for Family Members and Patients With Anxiety Disorders

ORGANIZATION	WEBSITE
American Family Physician	www.familydoctor.org/condition/generalized-anxiety-disorder
American Psychiatric Association	www.psychiatry.org/patients-families/anxiety-disorders
American Psychological Association	www.apa.org/topics/anxiety
Anxiety Disorders Association of America	www.adaa.org
Association for Behavioral and Cognitive Therapies	www.abct.org
Mental Health America	www.mentalhealthamerica.net/conditions/anxiety-disorders
National Institute of Mental Health	www.nimh.nih.gov/index.shtml

Conclusion

Anxiety disorders are highly prevalent in the United States. GAD is one of the most common psychiatric conditions seen in primary care, second only to major depression. This condition can be disabling and costly to the patient and to the health care system. Despite the prevalence of anxiety disorders, patients often remain undiagnosed and untreated, and patients with unrecognized anxiety disorders tend to be higher utilizers of general medical care. Patients with anxiety disorders can present with multiple somatic complaints and comorbid disorders, causing great effort and expense in identifying the cause of unexplained symptoms. Once an anxiety disorder is identified, patients may be treated using well-tested and efficacious pharmacologic and psychotherapeutic treatments. Helpful resources for patients and families are listed in Table 2.

References

American Psychiatric Association: *Diagnostic and Statistical Manual of Mental Disorders*, ed 5, Washington, DC, 2013, American Psychiatric Association.

American Psychiatric Association: *Practice Guideline for the Treatment of Patients with Panic Disorder*, ed 2, Washington, DC, 2009, American Psychiatric Association.

Campbell-Sills L, Stein MB: *Guideline Watch: Practice Guidelines for the Treatment of Patients With Panic Disorder*, Arlington, VA, 2006, American Psychiatric Association.

Davidson JRT, Feltner DE, Dugar A: Management of generalized anxiety disorder in primary care: Identifying the challenges and unmet needs, *Prim Care Companion J Clin Psychiatry* 12:2010.

Gabbard GO: *Gabbard's Treatment of Psychiatric Disorders*. ed 3, Washington, DC, 2001, American Psychiatric Publishing.

Goddard AW, Coplan JD, Shekhar A, et al: Principles of the pharmacotherapy of anxiety disorders. In Charney DS, Nestler EJ, editors: *The Neurobiology of Mental Illness*, ed 2nd, New York, 2004, Oxford University Press, pp 661–682.

Kessler RC, Berglund P, Demler O, et al: Lifetime prevalence and age-of-onset distributions of DSM-IV disorders in the National Comorbidity Survey Replication, *Arch Gen Psychiatry* 62:593–602, 2005.

Kroenke K, Spitzer RL, Williams JBW, et al: Anxiety disorders in primary care: Prevalence, impairment, comorbidity, and detection, *Ann Intern Med* 146:317–325, 2007.

Lépine JP: The epidemiology of anxiety disorders: Prevalence and societal costs, *J Clin Psychiatry* 63(Suppl. 14):4–8, 2002.

Sadock BJ, Sadock VA: *Kaplan and Sadock's Synopsis of Psychiatry: Behavioral Sciences/Clinical Psychiatry*, ed 10, Philadelphia, 2007, Lippincott Williams & Wilkins.

Spitzer RL, Kroenke K, Williams JBW, Lowe B: A brief measure for assessing generalized anxiety disorder, *Arch Intern Med* 166:1092–1097, 2006.

Stein MB: Attending to anxiety disorders in primary care, *J Clin Psychiatry* 64(Suppl. 15):35–39, 2003.

OBSESSIVE-COMPULSIVE DISORDER

Method of
Rachna Kalia, MD

CURRENT DIAGNOSIS

- Obsessive-compulsive disorder (OCD) is characterized by obsessions (recurrent, persistent, and intrusive unwelcome thoughts, urges, or images) and compulsions (repetitive behaviors or activities that the patient feels forced to perform in response to an obsession).
- Obsessions and compulsions are unwelcome and time-consuming, impair functioning, and usually cause significant anxiety or distress.
- The obsessions or compulsions are not attributable to any toxin, medication, or another medical condition.
- Patients may be unwilling to reveal symptoms of OCD or may lack insight into abnormal thoughts or behaviors.
- Patients with OCD may present with symptoms of depression, another comorbid psychiatric condition, or physical sequelae such as skin damage, fatigue, or insomnia.

CURRENT TREATMENT

- Selective serotonin reuptake inhibitors (SSRIs) and exposure and response prevention (ERP) behavioral therapy are first-line treatments for OCD with good evidence of effectiveness.
- SSRIs, clomipramine (Anafranil), serotonin-norepinephrine reuptake inhibitors (SNRIs), and monoamine oxidase inhibitors (MAOIs) have demonstrated efficacy in the treatment of OCD.
- Effective SSRI therapy often requires high dosages and 8 to 12 weeks of treatment. Long-term adherence is essential. If a patient fails an adequate trial of SSRI monotherapy, a trial of another SSRI is recommended.
- Evidence-based augmentation strategies for treatment-resistant cases include low-dose antipsychotics.
- Comorbid conditions, including depression with suicidal ideation, must be identified and addressed.

Epidemiology

Clinically significant OCD has an estimated lifetime prevalence in US adults of 1.9% to 3.0%. About 2.0% of adults report symptoms that meet criteria for the diagnosis within the prior year. Many more individuals suffer from OCD symptoms that do not reach diagnostic thresholds. Approximately 90% of patients with OCD suffer from at least one additional psychiatric condition, mainly anxiety (75.8%), mood disorders (63.3%), impulse control (55.9%), and substance use disorders (38.6%). Patients report that OCD persists for a mean of 8.9 years. The duration, high morbidity, and significant role impairment place heavy demands on patients and families. The World Health Organization (WHO) ranks OCD as one of the 10 most disabling medical conditions worldwide.

The mean age of onset of OCD is 19.5 years, and new cases are rarely diagnosed after age 35. The majority of childhood and adolescent cases are in males. Nearly a quarter of males report onset before 10 years of age. The onset in females tends to be in adolescence and early adulthood. In adults, the prevalence is approximately equal in men and women. No strong evidence supports racial or ethnic difference in the prevalence of OCD.

Risk Factors, Etiology, and Pathophysiology

Several studies confirm a familial pattern for OCD, especially in childhood-onset forms. Twin studies implicate both genetic and environmental factors. Multiple genes have been implicated, notably areas on chromosomes 9 and 15. Current theory focuses on dysregulation in a network of genes influencing the glutamatergic, serotonergic, and dopaminergic systems, and possibly other parts of the brain, as underlying the development of OCD. The heritability of OCD is estimated to be approximately 40% with the remaining variation attributed to adverse environmental factors. Suggested environmental triggers for OCD include perinatal events, psychosocial stress, trauma, and inflammatory processes, especially streptococcal infection. Neuroimaging and neuropsychiatric studies indicate OCD-related changes in the cortico–striato–thalamo–cortical (CSTC) circuit, known to be critical in evaluating and taking steps to neutralize perceived threats.

Obsessive-compulsive disorder has several subtypes. Some of the childhood-onset forms are comorbid with Tourette's and other chronic tic syndromes. In adults, the common associations with schizophrenia or schizoaffective disorder, bipolar disorder, and eating disorders could indicate that the conditions have overlapping etiologies or that one condition is a risk factor for the other. Clinicians should have an increased awareness of the possibility of OCD in adolescent and young adult patients presenting with a range of psychiatric conditions.

Clinical Manifestations

The core features of OCD are obsessions and compulsions (Table 1). Most patients have both. Obsessions are recurrent, persistent, and intrusive thoughts, urges, or images that are unwelcome and usually cause significant anxiety or distress. Patients attempt to ignore obsessions or to suppress or neutralize them by imposing other thoughts or performing specific activities. Compulsions are repetitive behaviors (e.g., handwashing, organizing, or checking) or activities (e.g., praying, counting, or repeating words silently) that the patient feels forced to perform in response to an obsession. Compulsions are characterized by rigid rules and inflexible behaviors but are not connected in a realistic way with what they are designed to neutralize or prevent and are clearly excessive responses to the intrusive thoughts, urges, or images.

Children may be unable to articulate symptoms and adults may be unwilling to disclose experiences that they recognize as abnormal. Individuals with OCD tend to be secretive about their symptoms, because most of them retain insight into the abnormal nature of their fears or behaviors. The estimated 14% to 30% of patients who have poor insight often have more severe and intractable symptoms. By the time patients present to medical attention, OCD is usually impacting function in society and/or eliciting concern from others about the patient's symptoms. The reported average time from onset of symptoms to diagnosis is 11 years. Other psychiatric conditions are commonly comorbid with OCD, and many patients present or are misdiagnosed as suffering primarily from depression or anxiety. Physical symptoms such as skin damage ("intractable dermatitis") from recurrent handwashing or scratching may be the presenting feature of OCD.

Without intervention, OCD is usually a chronic relapsing condition with adult rates of spontaneous remission estimated at about 20%. Remission in treated patients is associated with shorter duration of symptoms, emphasizing the need for prompt recognition and effective therapy. The risk of suicide is high in patients with OCD, particularly those with depression, posttraumatic stress disorder, or impulse control disorders. One large study reported that 20% made suicidal plans and 11% attempted suicide.

Diagnosis

The diagnosis is based on clinical symptoms consistent with *Diagnostic and Statistical Manual of Mental Disorders*, Fifth Edition (DSM-5) criteria for obsessions and compulsions (see Table 1). The obsessions and compulsions must be time-consuming, often regarded as requiring more than 1 hour per day, or cause clinically significant distress or impairment in social, occupational, or other important areas of functioning. Simple screening questions have been suggested (Table 2). Several more-detailed inventories are available to document symptoms and their impact, but these are of limited use in diagnosis in a primary care setting.

TABLE 1 Examples of Common Obsessions and Compulsions

OBSESSIONS	COMPULSIONS
Contamination or infection ("germophobia")	Avoidance of people or situations perceived as dirty, infectious, or corrupting; excessive cleaning or use of protective materials (surgical gloves, masks, sanitizer)
Control: Fear of losing control of speech or actions in public; making inappropriate comments; doing shameful or hurtful activities in public; inviting ridicule or negative reactions from others	Avoidance of others and public places; guarded behavior and curtailed speech to minimize contact with others
Religious, especially unworthiness, sinfulness, guilt	Praying, ritualizing acts of penance, seeking forgiveness (expression depends on religious belief/tradition of patient)
Sexual: concerns about acting inappropriately or being deviant	Avoidance of sexual situations, materials
Symmetry, correctness, precision	Arranging, ordering, scheduling, checking; "correcting" work of others
Violence; fear of harming others or becoming dangerous	Vigilance, attention to violent incidents, requiring reassurance

TABLE 2 Examples of Screening Questions for Obsessive-Compulsive Disorder

Do you check things repeatedly or wash your hands over and over?
Do you have unpleasant or unusual thoughts that you can't seem to get rid of?
Do you need things symmetrically arranged or always in a certain order?
Do you have trouble discarding things, so that your house is quite cluttered?

TABLE 3 Key Features That Help with Differential Diagnosis

ALTERNATIVE DIAGNOSIS	SYMPTOMS TYPICAL OF OBSESSIVE-COMPULSIVE DISORDER (OCD)	SYMPTOMS TYPICAL OF ALTERNATIVE DIAGNOSIS
Depressive disorders	Focus and content of obsessions is usually broader	Content of depressive ruminations is self-criticism, failures, guilt, regret, or pessimism
Generalized anxiety disorder	Obsessions may not be reality based Rituals may be present	Worries focus on real-life problems, generally more vague Usually no rituals
Posttraumatic stress disorder	Intrusive thoughts are anticipation of future events	Intrusive thoughts are replay of actual events
Schizophrenia, mania	Content is related to OCD Insight usually present	Content is related to persecution, grandiosity, ideas of reference Insight usually absent
Hypochondriasis	Insight usually present Origin is external based	Insight usually absent Origin is misinterpretation of physical signs and symptoms

A diagnosis of OCD also requires eliminating other potential causes of symptoms, as described next.

Differential Diagnosis

Identifying underlying OCD may be challenging in patients presenting with depression, anxiety, or another comorbidity. Some key features help in distinguishing OCD from these conditions (Table 3).

Insight distinguishes OCD from delusions and other features of schizophrenia. An important distinction is between OCD and obsessive-compulsive personality disorder (OCPD). In OCPD, behavior is ego-syntonic, that is, driven by desire or pleasure seeking rather than fear. Clinical OCD also needs to be distinguished from normal individuals who are meticulous and have rigid, inflexible thought processes or from individuals who describe compulsive behaviors such as eating or gambling that are or were pleasurable.

Obsessive-compulsive symptoms can occur in several neurologic conditions such as brain trauma, stroke, encephalitis, temporal lobe epilepsy, Prader-Willi syndrome, Huntington disease, Parkinson disease, carbon monoxide poisoning, or manganese poisoning, but these can usually be identified by the predominant other symptoms.

Treatment and Monitoring

Obsessive-compulsive disorder is a chronic condition with low frequency of spontaneous improvement but high probability of response to therapy if adherence and social support are maintained and comorbidities addressed. Short-term and long-term treatment goals should be established with each patient and those in his or her support system. Goals should focus on management of symptoms to optimize function and quality of life rather than complete resolution of symptoms. Adherence is critical to prognosis. Close follow-up must be secured, especially early in treatment. Given the secretive nature of the illness, the initial presentation may be the only chance to engage these patients in treatment, and must not be missed. Providing patients and families with educational information and access to community resources can help with adherence and social stabilization. Education for patients and others regarding what to expect from pharmacotherapy, including potential adverse effects and the lag period before benefit, can help ease anxiety and improve adherence and prognosis.

Once the diagnosis of OCD has been confirmed, the appropriate setting and strategy for treatment must be decided. The spectrum of treatment settings includes outpatient, adult partial-day programs, residential facilities, and inpatient psychiatric hospitalization. Factors such as suicide assessment, severity of illness, treatment cost, insurance coverage, and social support availability need to be explored to determine the optimal treatment environment.

Both pharmacotherapy and psychotherapy are recommended first-line treatment either alone or in combination (Figure 1). Combined therapy may be more effective than pharmacotherapy alone but has not been shown to be superior to behavioral therapy. Combination therapy may be most useful in patients with a coexisting psychiatric condition for which SSRIs are effective, those with poor response to initial monotherapy, or those who wish to discontinue medication as soon as possible. Practice guidelines recommend use of an approved symptom rating scale to monitor response to therapy, such as the 10-item Yale-Brown Obsessive Compulsive Scale (Y-BOCS).

Pharmacotherapy

SSRIs are first-line treatment agents for OCD (Table 4). Fluoxetine (Prozac), clomipramine (Anafranil), fluvoxamine (Luvox), paroxetine (Paxil), and sertraline (Zoloft) are approved by the U.S. Food

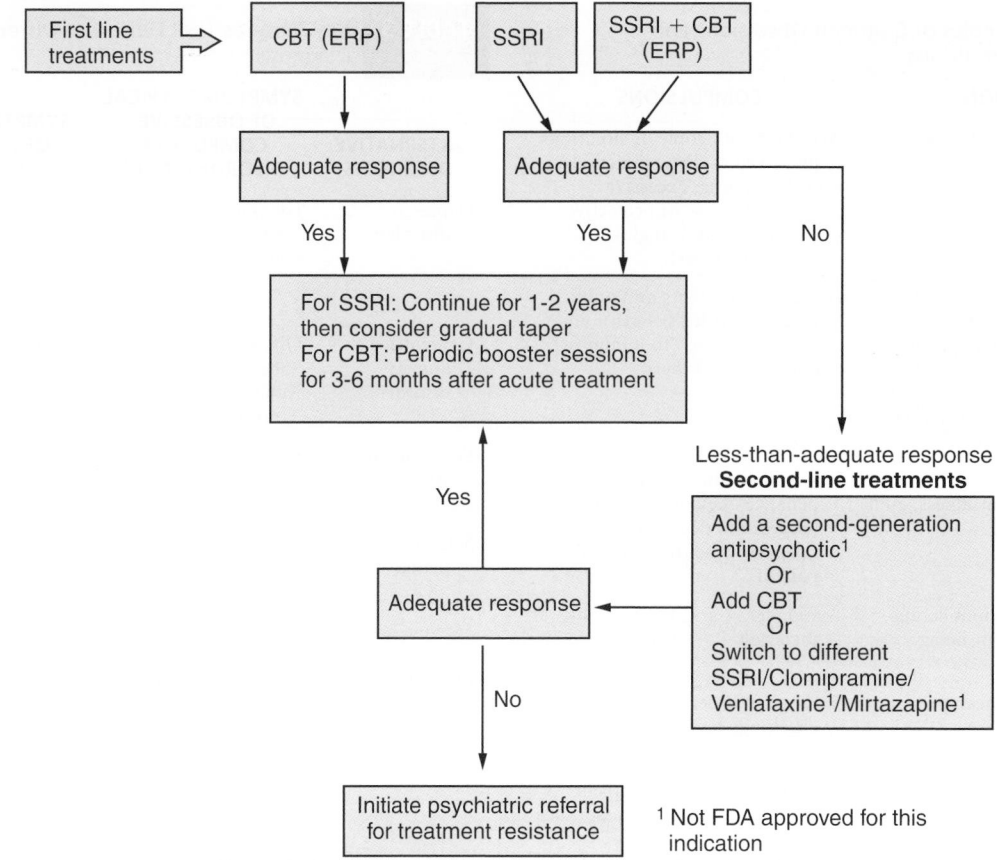

Figure 1 Treatment algorithm for obsessive-compulsive disorder.

TABLE 4 Dosing of Selective Serotonin Reuptake Inhibitors (SSRIs) to Treat Obsessive-Compulsive Disorder

| SSRI | DOSAGE (MG/DAY) | | |
	STARTING	TARGET	USUAL MAXIMAL
Citalopram (Celexa)*	20	40	40
Escitalopram (Lexapro)*	10	20	40†
Fluoxetine (Prozac)	20	40–60	80
Fluvoxamine (Luvox)	50	200	300
Paroxetine (Paxil)	20	40–60	60
Sertraline (Zoloft)	50	200	200

*Not U.S. Food and Drug Administration approved for this indication.
†Exceeds dosage recommended by the manufacturer.

and Drug Administration (FDA) and appear to be equally effective. Medication selection depends on factors including adverse effect profile, cost, concomitant medications, comorbid medical conditions, previous experience with the medication, and patient preference. The selected medication should be initiated at low dose and slowly titrated to effective levels. The optimal response may require a dose exceeding the manufacturer's recommended maximum dose. The "start low, go slow" strategy minimizes adverse effects, especially in older patients, and improves adherence. Common adverse effects include gastrointestinal upset, agitation, insomnia, fatigue, and sexual side effects. Many adverse effects are transitory. Serotonin syndrome is a serious potential risk at high doses. Patients with OCD are at risk of suicide and self-harm, but studies do not indicate increased risk in those treated with SSRIs, including adolescents.

Most patients will not experience substantial improvement for 4 to 6 weeks, and many require 10 to 12 weeks of treatment at optimal dosage. Although full remission of symptoms is reported in only about 10% of patients treated with SSRIs, 40% to 65% improve. The mean improvement in symptoms is 20% to 40%. Effective therapy should be maintained for at least a year and possibly indefinitely. If medication is discontinued, gradual tapering is recommended. Relapse rates in patients who discontinue medication after 2 years of treatment are 25% to 40% and up to 80% after shorter periods of treatment.

If response continues to be inadequate and adherence is confirmed, options include changing the primary agent to clomipramine, venlafaxine (Effexor),[1] or mirtazapine (Remeron),[1] or augmentation with a second-generation antipsychotic agent. Referral to a psychiatric provider with expertise in OCD therapy may be the best option for treatment-resistant cases.

A patient may respond well to a different SSRI, but a full trial of several weeks at adequate dose is necessary before changing medication. Clomipramine is as effective as SSRIs but carries safety concerns. It is strongly serotonergic and anticholinergic and may increase risk of seizure or cardiac arrhythmia. Addition of risperidone (Risperdal)[1] and possibly aripiprazole (Abilify)[1] may benefit some treatment-resistant patients. The efficacy of quetiapine (Seroquel)[1] and olanzapine (Zyprexa)[1] is unclear. All antipsychotic agents require careful monitoring for adverse effects. Medications sometimes used for OCD but with only limited evidence of efficacy include topiramate (Topamax),[1] ondansetron (Zofran),[1] pindolol,[1] buspirone,[1] memantine (Namenda),[1] pregabalin (Lyrica),[1] N-acetylcysteine (Acetadote),[1] naltrexone (Vivitrol),[1] and riluzole (Rilutek).[1]

Psychological Therapy

The strongest evidence for effective behavioral treatment of OCD supports exposure and response prevention (ERP), a form of cognitive-behavioral therapy (CBT) in which patients learn alternative responses to anxiety-provoking stimuli or situations. Weekly or twice-weekly sessions for a total of 20 to 30 hours are recommended followed by monthly "booster" sessions for 3 to 6 months.

[1]Not FDA approved for this indication.

1. Obsessive-Compulsive Foundation: http://www.ocfoundation.org.
2. Obsessive-Compulsive Information Center: http://www.miminc.org/aboutocic.html.
3. Baer L. Getting Control: Overcoming Your Obsessions and Compulsions. New York: Plume Books; 2000.
4. Gravitz HL. Obsessive Compulsive Disorder: New Help for the Family. Santa Barbara, CA: Healing Visions Press; 1998.
5. Steketee GS. Overcoming Obsessive-Compulsive Disorder: Client Manual. Oakland, CA: New Harbinger Publications; 1999.
6. Van Noppen B, Pato M, Rasmussen S. Learning to Live with OCD. New Haven, CT: Obsessive Compulsive Foundation; 2003.

Studies report considerable reduction in symptoms in up to 80% of patients with improvement maintained for up to 5 years. Remote-delivery formats of ERP using the telephone, a computer, or the Internet may provide effective and more accessible alternatives to traditional therapist consultation. ERP therapy not only is first-line treatment for OCD but also has strong evidence of effectiveness as an augmentation strategy to pharmacotherapy.

Cognitive therapy focusing on recognizing and changing interpretation of unrealistic thoughts is also associated with improvement in 60% to 80% of patients with OCD and is a good alternative for those unwilling to undertake ERP.

Other Treatment Options

Deep brain stimulation at the ventral capsule/striatum was approved by the FDA in 2009 for refractory OCD. Good results are reported in about half of patients treated in small trials compared with sham stimulation. Neurosurgical procedures may be recommended for selected patients with intractable OCD. Robust trials of ERP, two or more treatments with different SSRIs, a course of clomipramine, and at least three trials of augmentation therapy are recommended before considering neurosurgical approaches. These include ablative surgeries such as anterior cingulotomy, anterior capsulotomy, subcaudate tractotomy, and limbic leucotomy. These last-resort invasive procedures have had mixed success and carry risk of serious adverse effects. The American Psychiatric Association (APA) warns that they should be performed only at specialist centers.

Table 5 provides a list of educational resources for patients and their families.

References

American Psychiatric Association, DSM-5 Task Force: *Diagnostic and Statistical Manual of Mental Disorders: DSM-5*, ed 5, Washington, DC, 2013, American Psychiatric Association.

Fenske JN, Petersen K: Obsessive-compulsive disorder: Diagnosis and management, *Am Fam Physician* 92:896–903, 2015.

Goodman WK, Alterman RL: Deep brain stimulation for intractable psychiatric disorders, *Ann Rev Med* 63:511–524, 2012.

Goodman WK, Grice DE, Lapidus KAB, Coffey BJ: Obsessive-compulsive disorder, *Psychiatr Clin N Am* 27:257–267, 2014.

Grant JE: Clinical practice: Obsessive–compulsive disorder, *N Engl J Med* 371:646–653, 2014.

Komossa K, Depping AM, Meyer M, et al: Second-generation antipsychotics for obsessive-compulsive disorder, *Cochrane Database Syst Rev*:CD008141, 2010.

Koran LM, Simpson HB. Guideline watch (March 2013): Practice guideline for the treatment of patients with obsessive-compulsive disorder. Available at: http://psychiatryonline.org/pb/assets/raw/sitewide/practice_guidelines/guidelines/ocd-watch.pdf [accessed February 2017].

Pauls DL, Abramovitch A, Rauch SL, Geller DA: Obsessive-compulsive disorder: An integrative genetic and neurobiological perspective, *Nat Rev Neurosci* 15(6):410–424, 2014.

Ponniah K, Magiati I, Hollon SD: An update on the efficacy of psychological therapies in the treatment of obsessive compulsive disorder in adults, *J Obsessive Compuls Relat Disord* 2:207–218, 2013.

Romanelli RJ, Wu FM, Gamba R, et al: Behavioral therapy and serotonin reuptake inhibitor pharmacotherapy in the treatment of obsessive-compulsive disorder: A systematic review and meta-analysis of head-to-head randomized controlled trials, *Depress Anxiety* 31:641–652, 2014.

Ruscio AM, Stein DJ, Chiu WT, Kessler RC: The epidemiology of obsessive-compulsive disorder in the National Comorbidity Survey Replication, *Mol Psychiatry* 15:53–63, 2010.

Veale D, Miles S, Smallcombe N, et al: Atypical antipsychotic augmentation in SSRI treatment refractory obsessive-compulsive disorder: A systematic review and meta-analysis, *BMC Psychiatry* 14:317–330, 2014, https://doi.org/10.1186/s12888-014-0317-5.

PANIC DISORDER

Method of

Cheryl Wehler, MD

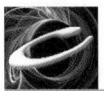

CURRENT DIAGNOSIS

- Panic disorder (PD) is characterized by the presence of multiple untriggered panic attacks.
- These unexpected panic attacks are associated with significant anticipatory anxiety and/or changes in behavior to minimize the consequences or avoid another panic attack.
  - Patients worry about being negatively judged due to visible panic symptoms.
  - Patients worry about dying or "going crazy."
- The panic attacks are not attributable to another medical condition or to the effects of a substance (medication or drug of abuse).
- The panic attacks are not better explained by another mental disorder.
- Patients frequently present with concern about somatic symptoms (e.g., fear of heart attack because of shortness of breath and chest discomfort).
- Assess patients for suicidality, as suicide risk increases with panic attacks or recent diagnosis of panic disorder.

CURRENT THERAPY

- Pharmacology and psychotherapy are effective treatments for PD.
- Selective serotonin reuptake inhibitors (SSRIs), serotonin norepinephrine reuptake inhibitors (SNRIs), tricyclic antidepressants (TCAs), and benzodiazepines have demonstrated efficacy for the treatment of PD.
- The favorable safety profile of SSRIs and SNRIs make them first-line monotherapy agents.
- Although TCAs are effective, their side effects and greater toxicity in overdose limit their clinical utility.
- Monoamine oxidase inhibitors (MAOIs) also appear effective but are reserved for patients who are nonresponders to multiple first-line treatments because of their safety profile limitations.
- Benzodiazepines are not first-line monotherapy but are useful adjuncts to antidepressants if residual anxiety requires additional treatment.
- Although the more rapid response of benzodiazepines (compared with SSRIs/SNRIs) make them attractive, the inevitable physiological dependence make them less so.
- Patients with PD can be sensitive to medication side effects; therefore the adage "start low and go slow" is applicable to dosing.
- Cognitive behavioral therapy (CBT) or CBT with medications are first-line treatments for children and adults with PD.

Epidemiology

The 12-month prevalence estimate for panic disorder (PD) in the general population of the United States and Europe is approximately 2% to 3% in adults and adolescents. Non-Latino Caucasians and Native Americans have significantly higher rates than Latinos, African Americans, and Asian Americans. Adolescent and adult females are approximately twice as likely as males to be affected (although the clinical features of PD do not differ between males and females). The prevalence is highest in adult females. Prevalence rates decline in older individuals. The overall prevalence of PD is low in children (<14 years). PD is associated with the highest number of medical visits among all anxiety disorders.

Risk Factors

Risks factors for PD include a disposition to negativity, experience of childhood physical and sexual abuse, and family history, indicating genetic vulnerability. Respiratory disorders such as asthma are associated with panic disorder. Smoking is a risk factor for panic attacks and PD. PD is associated with social and occupational/physical disability and high economic cost. PD may be comorbid with a variety of other psychiatric diagnoses, such as depression, bipolar affective disorder, and other anxiety disorders.

Diagnosis

PD is defined by the *Diagnostic and Statistical Manual of Mental Disorders,* fifth edition (DSM-V) as recurrent unexpected panic attacks followed by at least 1 month of anticipatory anxiety about having another attack, and a significant change in behavior to avoid another panic attack. A panic attack, the core feature of panic disorder, is an abrupt surge of intense fear/anxiety with concurrent physical and cognitive symptoms (Box 1). To be diagnosed as having PD, a patient must have more than one panic attack that is not the result of an obvious trigger or cue. The best example might be a nocturnal panic attack in which the individual is waking from sleep, with no external cues, in a state of intense fear (panic) and experiencing physical and cognitive symptoms. Expected panic attacks, that is, those for which there is an obvious cue or trigger, also occur in patients with PD. In the United States and Europe, approximately half of individuals with PD experience expected panic attacks as well as unexpected panic attacks. The presence of expected panic attacks does not rule out the diagnosis but is insufficient to make the diagnosis of this disorder.

A thorough diagnostic evaluation, including a complete history and thorough physical examination, is necessary to rule out medical or substance-induced panic attacks and establish the diagnosis of PD. Atypical symptoms or features of a panic attack may be suggestive of a medical illness or pharmacologic substance as the precipitant. A workup that includes laboratory tests such as complete blood cell count, complete chemistry panel (including calcium level), thyroid-stimulating hormone (TSH) level, and urine drug screen may be helpful in determining a medical or substance-related cause. These tests may be followed by a chest radiograph, an electrocardiogram, and cardiac enzymes, as warranted. If the clinical examination or history is suggestive, a Holter monitor, EEG, CT scan, or urine catecholamine assay may be performed.

Clinical Manifestations

In the United States, the median age of onset for PD is 20 to 24 years. PD is rare in childhood but occurs in adolescents; their symptoms are similar to those in adults. Onset after age 45 is unusual. If untreated, the usual course is chronic, and attacks may wax and wane. Some individuals have a chronic course complicated by frequent attacks whereas others have rare episodic symptoms. A minority of individuals have full remission. Caffeine and several other substances can provoke a panic attack.

The severity and frequency of panic attacks vary widely. Individuals who have infrequent panic attacks resemble individuals with more frequent panic attacks with regard to symptoms, demographics, and family history. To be diagnosed with PD, an individual must have more than one full-symptom attack with more than four of the symptoms listed in Box 1. Individuals may, however, have limited-symptom attacks with fewer than four symptoms.

There are three symptomatic facets of PD: acute panic, anticipatory anxiety, and phobic avoidance. Phobic avoidance often includes restricting daily activities to minimize or avoid panic attacks. Panic disorder is associated with other psychopathology, such as other anxiety disorders, particularly agoraphobia.

Although medical illness can precipitate a panic attack, individuals with anxiety, particularly PD, may be hypervigilant and misinterpret mild physical symptoms as harbingers of a catastrophic or fatal illness. Individuals with PD often report feelings of anxiety that are associated with health or mental health concerns.

Panic attacks often contribute to the presentation of other psychiatric illnesses, such as other anxiety disorders and major depression. A thorough history that documents the onset of symptoms, possible triggers, and context of symptoms is critical to establishing the diagnosis of PD. In addition to the history of the present illness and current symptoms, a psychiatric review of symptoms, past psychiatric history, general medical history and current medications, substance use history, family history, and mental status exam are valuable in constructing a psychiatric differential diagnosis and then a final working diagnosis. For instance, an individual with a history of a past trauma presenting with flashbacks, nightmares, and triggered panic attacks may have posttraumatic stress disorder (versus panic disorder).

Suicidal behavior in individuals with anxiety disorders has long been attributed to co-occurring risk factors, such as depression. New research suggests that an anxiety disorder is associated with suicidal ideation and suicide attempts beyond the effects of co-occurring mental disorders. Panic attacks and a recent diagnosis of PD are associated with a higher rate of suicide attempts and suicidal ideation.

BOX 1 DSM-5 Criteria for Panic Disorder

- Recurrent unexpected panic attacks. A panic attack is an abrupt surge of intense fear or intense discomfort that reaches a peak within minutes, and during which time four (or more) of the following symptoms occur:
  Note: The abrupt surge can occur from a calm state or an anxious state.
  - Palpitations, pounding heart, or accelerated heart rate
  - Sweating
  - Trembling or shaking
  - Sensations of shortness of breath or smothering
  - Feelings of choking
  - Chest pain or discomfort
  - Nausea or abdominal distress
  - Feeling dizzy, light-headed, faint, or unsteady
  - Chills or heat sensations
  - Parenthesis (numbness or tingling sensations)
  - Depersonalization (being detached from oneself) or derealization (feelings of unreality)
  - Fear of "going crazy" or losing control
  - Fear of dying
  Note: Culture-specific symptoms (e.g., tinnitus, neck soreness, headache, uncontrollable screaming or crying) may be seen. Such symptoms should not count as one of the four required symptoms [to diagnose PD].
- At least one of the attacks has been followed by 1 month (or more) of one or both of the following:
  - Persistent concern or worry about additional panic attacks or their consequences (e.g., losing control, having a heart attack, "going crazy")
  - A significant maladaptive change in behavior related to the attacks (e.g., behaviors designed to avoid having panic attacks, such as avoidance of exercise or unfamiliar situations)
- The disturbance is not attributable to the physiological effects of a substance (e.g., a drug of abuse, a medication) or another medical condition (e.g., hyperthyroidism, cardiopulmonary disorders)
- The disturbance is not better explained by another mental disorder (e.g., the panic attacks do not occur only in response to feared social situations, as in social anxiety disorder; in response to circumscribed phobic objects or situations, as in specific phobia; in response to obsessions, as in obsessive-compulsive disorder; in response to reminders of traumatic events, as in posttraumatic stress disorder; or in response to separation from attachment figures, as in separation anxiety disorder)

Differential Diagnosis

The differential diagnosis of PD is wide ranging (Table 1). PD is not diagnosed if panic attacks are the direct physiological consequence of another medical condition or substance. Medical conditions that can cause panic attacks include cardiopulmonary conditions such as arrhythmias and asthma or chronic obstructive pulmonary disease (COPD). Endocrine and neurologic disorders such as hyperthyroidism, pheochromocytoma, vestibular dysfunction, and seizures may also cause panic attacks. In addition, central nervous system (CNS) stimulants and withdrawal from CNS depressants may precipitate a panic attack. On the other hand, a panic attack may mimic a wide variety of medical disorders.

Treatment

PD is a common mental disorder. It is associated with social and occupational/physical disability and high economic cost. When symptoms cause significant distress or interfere with functioning, treatment is warranted. Regardless of the modality chosen, the goal of treatment is a reduction in the frequency and severity of panic attacks as well as the resultant anticipatory anxiety and avoidance behaviors.

Research has confirmed the efficacy of multiple psychosocial and pharmacologic interventions in treating PD. Choice of treatment depends on multiple factors, including patient preference; risks and benefits for an individual patient; cost; past treatment history; and co-occurring medical, psychiatric, or substance abuse issues.

Selective serotonin reuptake inhibitors (SSRIs), serotonin norepinephrine reuptake inhibitors (SNRIs), tricyclic antidepressants (TCAs), and benzodiazepines have demonstrated efficacy for the treatment of PD. The favorable safety profile of SSRIs and SNRIs makes them first-line monotherapy agents. Although TCAs are effective, their side effects and toxicity in overdose limit their clinical utility. Monoamine oxidase inhibitors (MAOIs) also appear effective but are reserved for patients who are nonresponders to multiple first-line treatments because of their safety profile. Benzodiazepines are not first-line monotherapy but are useful adjuncts to antidepressants if residual anxiety requires additional treatment (Table 2).

An important consideration when using psychopharmacologic treatments in PD is the side-effect profile of a particular agent. Because patients with PD can be acutely sensitive to medication side effects, it is prudent to start medications at low doses and gradually increase them to therapeutic doses as tolerated. An effective dose is patient dependent—the goal is to prevent (versus respond to) panic attacks. If a decision is made to discontinue a SSRI, SNRI, or TCA, the medication should be gradually tapered when feasible.

TABLE 1 Differential Diagnosis of Panic Attacks

SYSTEM	POSSIBLE DIAGNOSES
Psychiatric	Mood disorder (panic attacks associated with depression or bipolar disorder)
	Anxiety disorders (panic attacks associated with social anxiety, specific phobia, posttraumatic stress disorder, generalized anxiety disorder, obsessive compulsive disorder)
	Agoraphobia
	Psychotic disorder (panic attacks associated with psychosis)
	Somatoform disorder
	Factitious disorder
Cardiac	Myocardial infarction
	Angina
	SVT or other arrhythmia
	Mitral valve prolapse
	Labile hypertension
Respiratory	Asthma
	COPD
	Pulmonary embolus
Neurologic	Seizure disorder
	Vestibular dysfunction
Endocrine	Thyroid disorder
	Hypoglycemia
	Adrenal dysfunction
	Hyperparathyroidism
	Pheochromocytoma
Substance Use	Excess caffeine
	Psychostimulants
Substance Withdrawal	Caffeine
	Nicotine
	Alcohol or sedative
	Opioid

TABLE 2 Pharmacologic Treatments of Panic Disorder

MEDICATION (TRADE NAME)	INITIAL DOSE (MG/DAY)	DOSE RANGE (MG/DAY)
SSRIs		
Citalopram (Celexa)[1]	10–20	20–40
Escitalopram (Lexapro)[1]	5–10	10–20
Fluoxetine (Prozac)	10–20	20–80
Fluvoxamine (Luvox)[1]	50	100–300[†]
Fluvoxamine CR (Luvox CR)[1]	100	100–300
Paroxetine (Paxil)	10–20	20–60
Paroxetine CR (Paxil CR)	12.5–25	25–75
Sertraline (Zoloft)	25	50–200
SNRIs		
Duloxetine (Cymbalta)[1]	30	60–120
Venlafaxine (Effexor)[1]	25–50	150–225
Venlafaxine ER (Effexor ER)	37.5	75–225
TCAs		
Desipramine (Norpramin)	25–50	100–200
Clomipramine (Anafranil)[1]	25	50–150
Imipramine (Tofranil)[1]	25	50–150
Nortriptyline (Pamelor)[1]	10–25	75–150
MAOIs		
Phenelzine* (Nardil)[1]	45[†]	45–75[§]
Benzodiazepines		
Alprazolam (Xanax)	0.25–0.5 tid	5–6
Alprazolam XR (Xanax XR)	0.5–1	3–6
Lorazepam (Ativan)[1]	0.25 tid	2–8[‡]
Clonazepam (Klonopin)	0.25 bid	0.5–2[†]

[1]Not FDA approved for this indication.
*Dietary restrictions required (low-tyramine diet); 2-week washout required before initiation and after termination of monoamine oxidase inhibitor (MAOI) trial.
[†]Divided doses may be given.
[‡]Total daily dosage divided across 2–4 doses/day.
[§]Usually administered tid.

Cognitive behavioral therapy (CBT) and CBT with medications are first-line treatments for children and adults with PD. CBT presents the most evidence of efficacy from random control trials. CBT for panic disorder generally includes psychoeducation, episode monitoring and response, self-awareness of anxious automatic thoughts and beliefs, controlled exposure to fear cues, modification of anxiety-reducing behaviors, and prevention of relapse. Psychosocial interventions, such as CBT, may enhance long-term outcomes by reducing the likelihood of relapse.

References

American Psychiatric Association: *Diagnostic and Statistical Manual of Mental Disorders*, ed 5, Arlington, VA, 2013, American Psychiatric Association.

American Psychiatric Association: *Practice Guideline for the Treatment of Patients with Panic Disorder*, ed 2, Arlington, VA, 2010, American Psychiatric Association.

Craske MG, Kircanski K, Epstein A, et al: Panic disorder: A review of DSM-IV panic disorder and proposals for DSM-V, *Depress Anxiety* 27:93–112, 2010.

Thibodeau MA, Welch PG, Sareen J, Asmundson GJG: Anxiety disorders are independently associated with suicide ideation and attempts: Propensity score matching in two epidemiological samples, *Depress Anxiety* 30:947–954, 2013.

Locke AB, Kirst N, Shultz CG: Diagnosis and management of generalized anxiety disorder and panic disorder in adults, *Am Fam Physician* 91(9):617–624, 2015.

Marchesi C: Pharmacological management of panic disorder, *Neuropsychiatr Dis Treat* 4:93–106, 2008.

Milrod B, Chambless DL, Gallop R, et al: Psychotherapies for panic disorder: a tale of two sites, *J Clin Psychiatry* 9, 2015, Jun (Epub ahead of print).

Stahl SM: *Stahl's Essential Psychopharmacology: The Prescriber's Guide*, ed 5, New York, 2014, Cambridge University Press.

Andrisano C, Chiesa A, Serretti A: Newer antidepressants and panic disorder: A meta-analysis, *Int Clin Psychopharmacol* 28:33–45, 2013.

POSTTRAUMATIC STRESS DISORDER

Method of
Natalie C. Dattilo, PhD

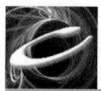

CURRENT DIAGNOSIS

- Posttraumatic stress disorder (PTSD) is quickly becoming one of the most common psychiatric disorders seen in the primary care setting.
- PTSD is diagnosed after a person experiences symptoms for at least 1 month following a traumatic event. However, symptoms may not appear until several months or even years later and can persist as a chronic condition.
- The disorder is characterized by three main types of symptoms: (1) reexperiencing the trauma through distressing recollections, (2) emotional numbness and behavioral avoidance, and (3) increased arousal such as feeling jumpy and easily angered.
- A thorough medical examination and laboratory workup may be indicated to rule out contributing physiologic factors and comorbidities, substance use or misuse, and drug or alcohol withdrawal.
- Symptoms that are persistent, disruptive, or distressing warrant treatment.
- The PTSD Checklist-5 (PCL-5) is a 20-item self-report measure that assesses the 20 *Diagnostic and Statistical Manual of Mental Disorders,* Fifth Edition (DSM-5) symptoms of PTSD. The gold standard for diagnosing PTSD is a structured clinical interview such as the Clinician-Administered PTSD Scale (CAPS-5). When necessary, the PCL-5 can be scored to provide a provisional PTSD diagnosis.

CURRENT THERAPY

- Effective treatments for PTSD include serotonergic antidepressants, certain forms of trauma-based psychotherapy, or a combination of both.
- Educating the patient and family members about treatment options and setting realistic treatment expectations are critical.
- Depending on the patient's preference, treatment may include a selective serotonin reuptake inhibitor (SSRI) starting at low doses with careful titration so as not to exacerbate anxiety or agitation.
- Treatment may also include a trial of cognitive-behavioral therapy, cognitive processing therapy, or prolonged exposure therapy to boost response rates and prevent relapse.
- Refer to or consult with a psychiatrist for patients with severe or particularly complex cases or for patients with a less-than-expected response to treatment.
- Refer to a cognitive-behavioral therapy specialist for patients with a preference for behavioral, skills-based, or nonmedication therapy or for whom pharmacotherapy may be contraindicated.

Epidemiology

In the United States, it is estimated that PTSD is diagnosed in approximately 10.5 million adults (3.5%) each year, and approximately 20.4 million (6.8%) will meet criteria over the course of their lifetimes. The lifetime prevalence of PTSD among men is 3.6% and among women is 9.7%. The 12-month prevalence is 1.8% among men and 5.2% among women. As with depression and anxiety disorders, patients with PTSD are more likely to present initially to a general practitioner's office than to a mental health care provider.

Owing, in part, to increased public awareness, PTSD is quickly becoming one of the most frequently seen clinical problems in primary care. Symptoms frequently overlap with other complaints, such as insomnia, irritability, or pain. Most behavioral symptoms of PTSD are a result of anxiety and hypervigilance, and the clinical presentation shares many phenotypic similarities with other anxiety disorders, such as panic disorder (PD) and generalized anxiety disorder (GAD).

Risk Factors

Risk factors associated with PTSD include exposure to trauma, being female, having lower levels of education and income, being divorced or widowed, having a history of behavioral or psychological problems, family history of behavioral or psychological problems including substance abuse, recent increase in stressful life events, lack or perceived lack of social support, ineffective emotional coping strategies, experiencing childhood adversity or trauma, having a chronic health condition or serious illness, having an acute or chronic pain condition, and substance abuse. Although a genetic predisposition to developing PTSD is likely, environmental stress and early trauma clearly play a role.

Pathophysiology

Our current understanding of PTSD is incomplete; however, several neurobiologic systems have been implicated in the pathophysiology and vulnerability toward developing PTSD after trauma exposure. As in other anxiety disorders, PTSD symptoms are believed to be due to dysregulation of neuronal activity within the central nervous system (CNS), in particular the fear circuit. This dysregulation causes a state of hyperarousal, which gives rise to the physical and emotional manifestations of the condition. Several neurotransmitter systems have been implicated in the genesis of this hyperaroused state. Overstimulation of the CNS and the autonomic sympathetic activity it generates affect the prefrontal cortex and the limbic system (e.g., amygdala, hypothalamus), both of which play an important role in our ability to discern stimuli as aversive or threatening and regulate our stress response.

The two most commonly implicated neurotransmitter systems to date include the serotoninergic and noradrenergic neurotransmitter systems. Very simply, it is believed that an underactivation of the serotoninergic system and an overactivation of the noradrenergic system are involved. These systems interact with other neuronal circuits in various regions of the brain, including the locus ceruleus (LC) and the limbic structures, resulting in a dysregulation of physiologic arousal and the emotional interpretation of this arousal, respectively. Disruption of the γ-aminobutyric acid (GABA) system has also been implicated because of the response of many of the anxiety-spectrum disorders to treatment with benzodiazepines.

There has also been some interest in the role of corticosteroid regulation and its relation to symptoms of fear and anxiety. Corticosteroids might increase or decrease the activity of certain neural pathways, affecting not only an individual's behavior under stress but also how the brain perceives and processes threatening stimuli. The stress response is hardwired into the brain and is most often triggered when survival of the organism is threatened. The stress response, however, can be triggered not only by a physical challenge or threat but also by the mere anticipation (or fear) of threat. As a result, when humans chronically and erroneously believe that a threatening event is about to occur, they begin to experience the physical and psychological symptoms of anxiety and panic.

The hypothalamic–pituitary–adrenal (HPA) axis is another neurocircuit implicated in the initiation of a stress response. The HPA axis assists with the adaptation to stress and the maintenance of homeostasis after challenge. It connects the CNS and the endocrine system, and a dysfunctional HPA axis is associated with numerous psychosomatic and psychiatric disorders. Corticotropin-releasing factor (CRF) is a molecule produced by cells in the hypothalamus in response to physical or psychological stress. Increased levels of CRF in the hypothalamus in response to stress results in the activation of the HPA axis and increased release of cortisol. It is believed that high CRF levels at the time of trauma may facilitate encoding of traumatic memory and enduring anxiety effects. Patients with PTSD exhibit increased cerebrospinal fluid levels of CRF and other abnormalities in the HPA axis system.

Finally, a subcortical neural structure, the amygdala, serves an important role in coordinating the cognitive, affective, neuroendocrine, cardiovascular, respiratory, and musculoskeletal components of fear and anxiety responses. It is central to registering the emotional significance of stressful stimuli and creating emotional memories. The amygdala receives input from neurons in the sensory cortex. When activated, the amygdala stimulates regions of the midbrain and brainstem, causing autonomic hyperactivity, which can be correlated with the physical symptoms of anxiety.

Prevention

No biological markers are specific enough yet to detect which individuals are more likely to develop PTSD after experiencing a trauma, and there is no available evidence to suggest that current medications prove efficacious in preventing this disorder. Therefore it is important to screen for specific risk factors, such as exposure to trauma (either recent or remote), family history of mental health issues, recent increase in stressful life events, or substance abuse. If a person is found to be at risk, but not symptomatic, he or she should first be encouraged to adopt healthy lifestyle habits. Aerobic exercise and other forms of physical activity have been shown to relieve stress and anxiety and improve mood relatively quickly. These patients should also be encouraged to avoid stimulants such as caffeine and nicotine, which can exacerbate symptoms and contribute to insomnia. It is also highly recommended

that anxiety-prone persons manage stress by learning effective methods of behavioral relaxation, applied meditation, and other healthy stress reduction techniques.

Clinical Manifestations

PTSD can manifest in many ways. Behavioral signs may include increased alcohol consumption, change in communication, change in sexual functioning, emotional outbursts, inability to rest or relax, change in appetite, pacing, suspiciousness, self-destructive behavior, or social isolation. Cognitive signs may include changes in alertness, confusion, hypervigilance, memory problems, poor attention and concentration, poor decision making or problem solving, and suicidal ideation. Emotional signs may include agitation, anxiety, apprehension, depression, fear, feeling overwhelmed, grief, guilt, irritability, and loss of emotional control. Sleep is also affected for individuals suffering from PTSD, and they will often report insomnia or nightmares. Other common features include a sense of emotional detachment from others and unwanted or intrusive thoughts; however, these can be difficult for clinicians to identify and patients rarely self-report. Physical symptoms can include chills, difficulty breathing, dizziness, elevated blood pressure, fainting, fatigue, grinding teeth, headaches, muscle tremors, nausea, pain, profuse sweating, rapid heart rate, twitches, and weakness. These symptoms cause significant distress and impairment of function.

Diagnosis

A diagnosis of PTSD is made when the patient meets specific diagnostic criteria as outlined in the DSM-5. In previous versions of the DSM, PTSD was categorized as an anxiety disorder. The diagnosis of PTSD now falls under its own category of mental disorders, called "Trauma and Stressor-Related Disorders," owing to the myriad ways it can present clinically.

PTSD may develop after a person experiences, witnesses, or confronts a physically or psychologically traumatic event. The event may involve actual or threatened death, serious or life-threatening injury or threat of severe injury, or sexual violence or threat of sexual violence. An individual may directly experience the traumatic event; witness, in person, the traumatic event; or learn that the traumatic event occurred to a close family member or close friend. An individual may also develop PTSD after experiencing repeated or extreme exposure to aversive details of the traumatic events. Examples may be first responders collecting human remains or police officers repeatedly exposed to details of child abuse. Note: This does not apply to exposure through electronic media, television, movies, or pictures, unless exposure is work related.

The disorder is characterized by three main types of symptoms: (1) reexperiencing the trauma through distressing recollections, (2) emotional numbness and behavioral avoidance, and (3) increased arousal such as feeling jumpy and easily angered.

A diagnosis of PTSD can be made in adults, adolescents, and children over the age of 6 when one or more of the following reexperiencing symptoms are present:

- Spontaneous or cued recurrent, involuntary, and intrusive distressing memories of the traumatic events (Note: In children repetitive play may occur in which themes or aspects of the traumatic events are expressed.)
- Recurrent distressing dreams in which the content or affect (i.e., feeling) of the dream is related to the events (Note: In children there may be frightening dreams without recognizable content.)
- Flashbacks or other dissociative reactions in which the individual feels or acts as if the traumatic event is recurring (Note: In children trauma-specific reenactment may occur in play.)
- Intense or prolonged psychological distress at exposure to internal or external cues that symbolize or resemble an aspect of the traumatic events
- Physiologic reactions to reminders of the traumatic events

A diagnosis of PTSD can be made in adults, adolescents, and children over the age of 6 when two or more of the following emotional numbness or behavioral avoidance symptoms are also present:

- Inability to remember an important aspect of the traumatic events (not due to head injury, alcohol, or drugs)
- Persistent and exaggerated negative beliefs or expectations about oneself, others, or the world (e.g., "I am bad," "No one can be trusted," "The world is completely dangerous")
- Persistent, distorted blame of self or others about the cause or consequences of the traumatic events
- Persistent fear, horror, anger, guilt, or shame
- Markedly diminished interest or participation in significant activities
- Feelings of detachment or estrangement from others
- Persistent inability to experience positive emotions

In addition to reexperiencing and avoidance, a diagnosis of PTSD can be made in adults, adolescents, and children over the age of 6 when two or more of the following marked changes in arousal and reactivity are also present:

- Irritable or aggressive behavior
- Reckless or self-destructive behavior
- Hypervigilance
- Exaggerated startle response
- Problems with concentration
- Difficulty falling or staying asleep or restless sleep

Finally, the diagnosis is made if the symptoms have been present for at least 1 month and cause clinically significant distress or impairment in functioning.

Differential Diagnosis

It is important to perform a thorough medical workup when initially assessing the patient with PTSD symptoms. Differential diagnoses can include several organic causes, such as endocrine dysfunction, intoxication or withdrawal, hypoxia, metabolic abnormalities, and neurologic disorders. It is also important to consider and rule out any cooccurring psychiatric disorders. Major depression with or without suicidality, bipolar disorder, panic disorder, delusional disorder, polysubstance dependence, and adjustment disorder can often accompany PTSD, in addition to relationship problems and difficulty at work or in social situations.

It is not uncommon for patients with PTSD to report chronic pain or present with "ill defined" or "medically unexplained" somatic symptoms such as headaches, dizziness, tinnitus, and blurry vision or medical issues including diabetes, obesity, and cardiovascular, respiratory, musculoskeletal, neurologic, or gastrointestinal problems. Frequently reported medical comorbidities with PTSD across various studies include cardiovascular disease, especially hypertension, and immune-mediated disorders. Because PTSD is associated with limbic dysfunction and alterations in the HPA axis, neuroendocrine and immune function can be significantly disrupted, and because of its impact on the CNS, pseudo-neurologic symptoms and disorders of sleep–wake regulation are also common.

It is also not uncommon for patients with PTSD to "self-medicate" or cope with their symptoms by drinking alcohol, smoking cigarettes, or using drugs, including cannabis and prescription pain medications or anxiolytics. Studies show that people with PTSD have more issues with drugs and alcohol both before and after being diagnosed with PTSD. In addition, having PTSD increases the risk that one will develop a drinking or drug problem, even in the absence of any prior drug or alcohol use.

Treatment and Monitoring

Current practice guidelines for the treatment of PTSD begin with education. Many people are confused, scared, or frustrated by the symptoms and behavior and are reassured to know they are not alone and that there are effective interventions. The patient should receive an appropriate medical workup, including a physical examination and studies (e.g., electrocardiogram,

thyroid-stimulating hormone) when indicated. In addition to treating any cooccurring or underlying medical conditions, developing a good working alliance with the patient and family provides a basis for ongoing disease management and prevents unnecessary utilization or overutilization of the medical system, as well as potential exacerbation of symptoms.

A combination of psychotherapy and medication management is recommended as first-line treatment for PTSD. Psychological treatments with the most robust empirical support include trauma-focused psychotherapies utilizing exposure techniques, cognitive restructuring, relaxation/stress modulation training, and psychoeducation.

Cognitive-behavioral therapy (CBT) is the most effective non-medication treatment for PTSD. The two types of CBT recommended for PTSD are cognitive processing therapy (CPT) and prolonged exposure (PE). In CPT one examines what he or she is thinking and telling him- or herself about the trauma and decides whether those thoughts are accurate or inaccurate. It can be done individually or in a group. PE works through repeated exposure to thoughts, feelings, and situations the person has been avoiding and helps him or her learn that reminders of the trauma do not have to be avoided. PE is done individually with a therapist. Both CPT and PE offer a skills-based approach to treatment. The therapist and patient work collaboratively and in an active and problem-solving manner. The work structured and generally short term with an emphasis on reducing symptoms. Volumes of evidence support the efficacy of CBT interventions for PTSD, but success requires commitment to treatment on the part of the patient. Its efficacy is also contingent upon the ability of the therapist and the length of time in treatment. Studies show that when compared with patients undergoing monotherapy, patients treated with a combination of CBT and medication experience nearly twice the remission rate.

If combination therapy is initiated owing to symptom severity or patient preference, the SSRIs have been shown to be the best-tolerated class of medications, and response rates are significantly higher than placebo. This class of medication includes fluoxetine (Prozac),[1] fluvoxamine (Luvox), citalopram (Celexa), escitalopram (Lexapro), paroxetine (Paxil), and sertraline (Zoloft). Some improvement should be noted within 3 or 4 weeks, and the dose should be increased if no improvement is seen. In all cases, SSRIs should be started at low doses and gradually titrated up to therapeutic levels to avoid an initial exacerbation of anxiety or agitation. Pharmacotherapy and psychotherapy options for the treatment of PTSD are presented in Tables 1A and 1B.

Benzodiazepines, which have been commonly used in the past to treat anxiety symptoms, are not recommended except in cases of extreme impairment of function, for short-term use only, and only after a thorough substance abuse history has been obtained. The tolerability and lack of addiction potential make the SSRIs more desirable for long-term management, but the delay in response makes short-term symptom relief with a benzodiazepine desirable for those with the greatest impairment. Because of the risk for rebound anxiety when withdrawing from benzodiazepines with short half-lives, such as alprazolam (Xanax), many prefer the longer-acting benzodiazepines, such as clonazepam (Klonopin).[1] However, the addiction potential and the potential for abuse with either drug make this the treatment option of last resort.

If the patient does not respond to the combination of CBT and medication, a reevaluation of symptoms might reveal a comorbid disorder missed on first examination. Comorbid psychiatric disorders significantly lower the likelihood of recovery from PTSD and increase recurrence rates. Many clinicians try switching between SSRIs before considering the next step in treatment, but a referral to a psychiatrist for further evaluation and management may be necessary if this strategy does not work. Treatment-refractory anxiety can be extremely frustrating for both the patient and

---

[1]Not FDA approved for this indication.

TABLE 1A	Pharmacotherapy for the Treatment of Posttraumatic Stress Disorder

DRUG	STARTING DOSE	TARGET DOSE
Selective Serotonin Reuptake Inhibitors		
Paroxetine (Paxil)	10 mg qd	10–60 mg qd
Escitalopram (Lexapro)*	5–10 mg qd	10–20 mg qd
Sertraline (Zoloft)	12.5–25 mg qd	50–200 mg qd
Fluoxetine (Prozac)*	10 mg qd	20–40 mg qd

*Not US Food and Drug Administration approved for this indication.

TABLE 1B	Evidence-Based Psychotherapy for the Treatment of Posttraumatic Stress Disorder

PSYCHOTHERAPY	DESCRIPTION	FORMAT
Trauma-Focused Cognitive-Behavioral Therapy (TF-CBT)		
Cognitive processing therapy (CPT)	Teaches you to reframe negative thoughts about trauma	Weekly individual or group meetings
Prolonged exposure (PE)	Teaches you to gain control by facing your fears	Weekly individual meetings

TABLE 2	Helpful Resources for Patients with Posttraumatic Stress Disorder

ORGANIZATION	WEBSITE
US Department of Veteran Affairs National Center for PTSD	https://www.ptsd.va.gov/index.asp
Anxiety and Depression Association of America (ADAA)	https://www.adaa.org/understanding-anxiety/posttraumatic-stress-disorder-ptsd
National Institute of Mental Health (NIMH)	https://www.nimh.nih.gov/health/topics/post-traumatic-stress-disorder-ptsd/index.shtml
American Academy of Family Physicians (AAFP)	http://www.aafp.org/afp/2000/0901/p1046.html

clinician. This can lead to increased dependence on benzodiazepines and an escalation of doses required for the same effect.

When approaching the start of therapy, the clinician should reassure the patient that effective treatment is available but that patience may be necessary until the right combination of modalities is found. Although PTSD, like all anxiety disorders, displays a significant amount of chronicity, most patients have an improved outcome with appropriate treatment. Response rates improve when comorbidity is low. Patients with an earlier onset of symptoms (childhood or adolescence) can generally expect a more chronic course and may be more difficult to treat. Occasionally, patients can have a spontaneous remission of symptoms and many can continue to function despite their symptoms. However, time to resolution of symptoms is shortened and overall functioning can improve with treatment.

Pharmacotherapy often helps to prevent relapse, and rates are improved when effective treatment is continued for 12 months. When considering termination of pharmacologic treatment, the risk for relapse in all the disorders should be discussed with the patient. When discontinuing the SSRIs, a slow taper is recommended, with close monitoring for withdrawal symptoms (e.g., headache, gastrointestinal upset, restlessness, and other flu-like symptoms). Also monitor for rebound anxiety symptoms. If relapse occurs, reinstituting treatment is indicated, and many patients opt for indefinite treatment to maintain remission of symptoms. Lifelong management with pharmacotherapy or psychotherapy, or both, is not unusual for many patients. For many, a maximum reduction of symptoms, rather than a full remission, is an acceptable outcome.

Complications

Untreated anxiety disorders can lead to, or worsen, other mental and physical health conditions, including bruxism (teeth grinding), cognitive impairment, depression, gastrointestinal disorders, headache, insomnia, heart disease, substance abuse, and significantly impaired quality of life.

Conclusion

PTSD is a highly prevalent psychiatric condition that can be disabling and costly to the patient and to the health care system. Despite the prevalence of PTSD and other mental health disorders, a high percentage of patients often remain undiagnosed and untreated. These untreated patients also tend to be higher utilizers of general medical care. Patients with PTSD often present with multiple somatic complaints and comorbid disorders, causing great effort and expense in identifying the cause of unexplained symptoms. Once PTSD is identified, patients may be treated using well-tested and efficacious pharmacologic and psychotherapeutic treatments. Helpful resources for patients and families are listed in Table 2.

References

American Psychiatric Association: *Diagnostic and Statistical Manual of Mental Disorders*, ed 5, Washington, DC, 2013, American Psychiatric Association.

American Psychological Association: *Clinical Practice Guideline for the Treatment of Posttraumatic Stress Disorder (PTSD) in Adults*, Washington, DC, 2017, American Psychological Association.

Bailey C, Cordell E, Sobin S, Neumeister A: Recent progress in understanding the pathophysiology of posttraumatic stress disorder: Implications for targeted pharmacological treatment, *CNS Drugs* 27:221–232, 2013.

Gabbard GO: Treatment of Psychiatric Disorders, vols. 1–2. 3rd ed, Washington, DC, 2001, American Psychiatric Publishing.

Goddard AW, Coplan JD, Shekhar A, et al: Principles of the pharmacotherapy of anxiety disorders. In Charney DS, Nestler EJ, editors: *The Neurobiology of Mental Illness*, ed 2nd, New York, 2004, Oxford University Press, pp 661–682.

Gupta M: Review of somatic symptoms in post-traumatic stress disorder, *Int Rev Psychiatry* 25:86–99, 2013.

Kessler RC, Berglund P, Demler O, et al: Lifetime prevalence and age-of-onset distributions of DSM-IV disorders in the National Comorbidity Survey Replication, *Arch Gen Psychiatry* 62:593–602, 2005.

Kroenke K, Spitzer RL, Williams JBW, et al: Anxiety disorders in primary care: Prevalence, impairment, comorbidity, and detection, *Ann Intern Med* 146:317–325, 2007.

Lepine JP: The epidemiology of anxiety disorders: Prevalence and societal costs, *J Clin Psychiatry* 63(Suppl. 14):4–8, 2002.

National Comorbidity Survey: NCS-R appendix tables: Table 1. Lifetime prevalence of DSM-IV/WMH-CIDI disorders by sex and cohort. Table 2. Twelve-month prevalence of DSM-IV/WMH-CIDI disorders by sex and cohort. 2005, Available at: http://www.hcp.med.harvard.edu/ncs/publications.php.

Sadock B, Sadock V: *Kaplan and Sadock's Synopsis of Psychiatry: Behavioral Sciences/Clinical Psychiatry*, ed 10, Philadelphia, 2007, Lippincott Williams & Wilkins.

Stein M: Attending to anxiety disorders in primary care, *J Clin Psychiatry* 64:35–39, 2003.

SCHIZOPHRENIA

Method of

Brian J. Miller, MD, PhD, MPH; and Peter F. Buckley, MD

CURRENT DIAGNOSIS

- There are three primary symptom domains in schizophrenia:
  - Positive symptoms (i.e., hallucinations, delusions, disorganized thought, and abnormal psychomotor behavior)
  - Negative symptoms (i.e., restricted affect or avolition/asociality)
  - Cognitive symptoms (i.e., attention, language, memory, and processing speed)
- Symptoms last ≥ 1 month and there are continuous signs of illness for ≥ 6 months.
- There is significant impairment one or more major areas of functioning (work, interpersonal relations, or self-care).
- Rule out that psychosis is not due to a primary mood disorder, schizoaffective disorder, substance intoxication or withdrawal, or a general medical condition.

CURRENT THERAPY

- Antipsychotic medication, with monitoring for medication adherence and side effects.
- Adjunctive medications as needed, including antidepressants, mood stabilizers, benzodiazepines, beta-blockers, and anticholinergics.
- Aggressive monitoring for and management of medical comorbidities, substance use disorders, and suicidality, including collaboration with primary care physician.
- Psychosocial interventions.
- Involvement of family/support system in care.
- Long-term treatment, including outpatient medication management and therapy, with inpatient care for acute crisis intervention/illness exacerbation.

Schizophrenia is a complex, chronic, and often severe psychiatric disorder that is a leading cause of disability worldwide. Although the literal translation of the word schizophrenia is "split mind," patients with this disorder do not have a "split personality" or "multiple personality disorder" (known as dissociative identity disorder). Rather, schizophrenia is a psychotic disorder that interferes with a person's thinking, mood, behavior, and/or interpersonal relations. Schizophrenia often has devastating, lifelong consequences for affected individuals and their families and is associated with an increased risk of premature mortality, including deaths from suicide and cardiovascular disease. In this chapter, the epidemiology and diagnosis of schizophrenia are reviewed. We then discuss pharmacologic and psychosocial treatments for schizophrenia in the context of a chronic disease model. The risks of medical and substance use comorbidity and suicidality are also highlighted.

Epidemiology and Risk Factors

The etiology of schizophrenia is not known, but it is thought to involve interactions between genetic (or epigenetic) and environmental factors, including developmental problems that occur during gestation. The lifetime prevalence of schizophrenia is approximately 1% and is equal in men and women. The usual age of onset is in the late teens or early 20s to late 30s, although schizophrenia can have onset before age 10 (early onset) or after age 45 (late onset). The age of onset is usually younger for men than women.

Several lines of evidence support a genetic contribution to the risk of schizophrenia. There is a 40% lifetime risk of schizophrenia in a child of two parents with schizophrenia. Twin-twin concordance is 50% in monozygotic twins, and 12% in dizygotic twins. A recent genome-wide association study and meta-analysis found that schizophrenia is significantly associated with single nucleotide polymorphisms in the major histocompatibility complex region on chromosome 6p22.1 (which includes several immunity-related genes, particularly complement C4), although numerous other genes have been implicated. There are likely multiple candidate genes that increase the risk of schizophrenia, each with small effect size.

Replicated environmental risk factors for schizophrenia include season of birth (winter), advanced paternal age, prenatal stress throughout gestation (famine and acute maternal stress in the first trimester, prenatal infections with a myriad of different agents, loss of the father in the second or third trimester), obstetric complications (including gestational diabetes, low birth weight, asphyxia), severe childhood abuse, and cannabis use. It remains unclear whether some of these risk factors are causal to schizophrenia or represent early manifestations of disease.

Diagnosis

There are three primary symptom domains in schizophrenia: positive, negative, and cognitive symptoms. Positive symptoms are abnormalities of thought content, including hallucinations (abnormal sensory perceptions in the absence of external stimuli) and delusions (fixed, false beliefs), formal thought disorder (also called disorganized thinking), and abnormal psychomotor behavior (such as catatonia). Hallucinations are most commonly auditory but can occur in any sensory modality. Negative symptoms include impairments in emotional expression (blunted affect), motivation (avolition), social behavior (asociality), speech (alogia), and the ability to experience pleasure (anhedonia). Cognitive symptoms include impairments in attention, language, memory, processing speed, and executive function.

The most commonly used diagnostic criteria for schizophrenia are derived from the *Diagnostic and Statistical Manual of Mental Disorders*, Fifth Edition (DSM-5). These criteria include the presence of two or more characteristic symptoms—delusions, hallucinations, disorganized speech, grossly abnormal psychomotor behavior (such as catatonia), or negative symptoms (i.e., restricted affect or avolition/asociality)—for a significant portion of time during a 1-month period (or less if successfully treated), with continuous signs of the disturbance persisting for at least 6 months. At least one of these two characteristic symptoms should include delusions, hallucinations, or disorganized speech. During this period, there is significant impairment in one or more major areas of functioning, including work, interpersonal relations, or self-care. It must also be established that the disorder is not better accounted for by a primary mood disorder, schizoaffective disorder, substance intoxication or withdrawal, or other general medical condition. From these criteria, it is important to note that delusions and hallucinations, although common, are not required for the diagnosis. Furthermore, although cognitive symptoms are also not required for the diagnosis, they are a tremendous cause of illness-related disability. A diagnosis of schizophrenia is most definitively made by interviewing the patient, obtaining collateral history from family and/or friends, and completing a medical workup (physical examination, routine blood and urine tests). According to DSM-5 (released May 2013), the diagnostic criteria no longer identify subtypes of schizophrenia, primarily because of a lack of utility for clinicians. Also of note, the Psychoses Workgroup for DSM-5 considered the addition of "attenuated psychosis syndrome" (i.e., prodromal or high-risk psychosis) as a diagnostic category. Ultimately, attenuated psychosis syndrome is listed in DSM-5 among conditions that require further research before consideration as a formal disorder. Nevertheless, the early identification of individuals with prodromal or high-risk psychosis, investigation of risk factors and biomarkers that might predict conversion to fulminant psychotic disorder, and early interventions for individuals with prodromal or high-risk psychosis are areas receiving significant attention and effort in the field.

Treatment

At present there is no cure for schizophrenia. Although there is significant clinical heterogeneity within the disorder, schizophrenia is usually a chronic condition that requires long-term treatment. Comprehensive treatment involves outpatient medication management and psychotherapy, psychosocial interventions, involvement of the family/support system, inpatient care for acute crisis intervention/illness exacerbation, and collaboration with primary care physicians. Currently, there is a vigorous research effort for diagnostic, prognostic and theranostic biomarkers in schizophrenia, toward a more "personalized medicine" approach for patients.

Antipsychotic medications play an important role in the pharmacologic management of schizophrenia. So-called first-generation antipsychotics (FGAs) have been in clinical use since the introduction of chlorpromazine (Thorazine) in the 1950s. These agents block the dopamine D2 receptor, and common side effects include extrapyramidal side effects (EPS) (e.g., Parkinsonism, dystonia). The newer or "second-generation antipsychotics" (SGAs), in addition to D2 receptor blockade, are also serotonin 5-HT2 receptor antagonists. While the risk of EPS is lower for SGAs than FGAs, SGAs are associated with a heightened risk of weight gain and the metabolic syndrome. Table 1 provides a more detailed description of antipsychotic medications. The Texas Medication Algorithm Project (TMAP) currently recommends a trial of a single (non-clozapine) SGA for newly diagnosed patients with schizophrenia, or patients never before treated with an SGA. However, neither the TMAP nor the American Psychiatric Association (APA) guidelines for the treatment of schizophrenia preferentially endorse a particular antipsychotic. Clozapine (Clozaril) is primarily used for "treatment-refractory" schizophrenia, usually defined as a lack of/partial response to an adequate trial of monotherapy with two or three different antipsychotics.

Adjunctive medications may also play an important role in the pharmacologic treatment of some patients with schizophrenia. These include antidepressants for depression and anxiety, mood stabilizers for depression or mood elevation, benzodiazepines for anxiety or agitation, beta-blockers for akathisia, and anticholinergics for EPS.

Medication nonadherence is a major treatment issue in patients with schizophrenia at all phases of the illness. Reasons for nonadherence are complex and multifaceted but may include medication side effects, impaired insight into illness, psychopathology in all three symptom domains, lack of efficacy, and comorbid substance use. Over 70% of patients in the Clinical Antipsychotic Trials of Intervention Effectiveness (CATIE) Schizophrenia Trial discontinued medication within the first 18 months of treatment. Medication nonadherence leads to dramatically increased risk of illness relapse, hospitalization, and suicidal behavior and should be routinely assessed in clinical visits. The use of rapid-dissolving oral or long-acting injectable medications may improve adherence in some patients.

Psychosocial interventions are also a cornerstone of the comprehensive treatment of patients with schizophrenia, and when utilized in combination with medication, are more effective than antipsychotics alone. Psychotherapy, including cognitive-behavioral therapy, supportive therapy, and group therapy, promotes improved illness management and medication adherence. Involvement of the patient's family/support system in care, including family-based therapies and psychoeducation, has been shown to increase medication adherence and decrease illness relapse rates. Psychosocial rehabilitation, which may include assertive community treatment, social skills training, vocational rehabilitation, and cognitive remediation, can help maximize patients' psychosocial functioning. There is growing evidence that cognitive remediation therapy in combination with other psychosocial interventions, particularly vocational rehabilitation, can improve real-world functioning for patients with schizophrenia in a relatively short time period.

Although there is no "typical" patient with schizophrenia, the clinical course is often characterized by acute relapses of the illness with the inter-episode absence or attenuation of symptoms. Multiple factors increase a patient's risk of illness relapse, including medication nonadherence, psychosocial stressors, substance use, medical illnesses such as infections, and the natural history of the disorder itself. Hospitalization may be required for acute exacerbations of psychotic symptoms, including hallucinations, delusions, and impaired self-care. Hospitalization may also be required if a patient represents an acute danger to self or others.

The concept of the recovery model and recovery-oriented care is a movement that is currently transforming the delivery of mental health services. Integral to the recovery model are certified peer specialists (CPS). A CPS is a licensed professional who has progressed in their own recovery from mental illness and works to assist patients with schizophrenia and other mental illness in regaining control over their own lives and over their own recovery process. CPSs provide peer support services, serve as consumer advocates, are resources for psychoeducation, and offer the unique perspectives based on their individual experiences.

Comorbidity

Schizophrenia is associated with an increased risk of premature mortality, and cardiovascular disease is a leading cause of death in this patient population. Multiple factors contribute to this risk, including a high prevalence of smoking, poor health habits, poor health care, medication side effects, and (perhaps) the pathophysiology of the disorder itself. SGAs as a class are associated with weight gain and an increased risk of metabolic syndrome. Over 40% of the 1460 patients in the CATIE Schizophrenia Trial met the criteria for metabolic syndrome at baseline. Recommendations for monitoring of patients on SGAs, based on a consensus statement from the American Diabetes Association and the APA, are described in Table 2. Primary care physicians play an important collaborative role with psychiatrists in the detection and management of metabolic disturbances in patients with schizophrenia, in order to minimize the cardiovascular risks associated with these comorbidities.

Patients with schizophrenia are also at an increased risk of suicide, which is also a leading cause of premature mortality. The prevalence of completed suicide in patients with schizophrenia is about 10%, and suicide attempts occur with even greater frequency. Clinicians should routine assess patients for suicidal ideation and, if present, explore risk factors for completed suicide, which include a suicidal plan and intent, previous suicide attempts, a family history of suicide, age, sex, access to lethal means, social isolation, and comorbid substance use. Medications, psychotherapy, and/or hospitalization may be required.

Comorbid substance use disorders predominate in patients with schizophrenia, with an estimated prevalence of 40% to 50%. Common substances of abuse include alcohol, marijuana, and cocaine. Patients with schizophrenia and comorbid substance use are at increased risk of medication nonadherence, illness relapse, hospitalization, suicidal and violent behavior, and an overall poor response to treatment. Furthermore, up to 70% to 90% of patients with schizophrenia are tobacco users, which contribute to the increased risk of medical comorbidity. Clinicians are encouraged to routinely screen for and address substance use in their treatment plans.

Conclusions

Schizophrenia is a complex, heterogeneous, and chronic psychiatric disorder. Comprehensive treatment usually involves long-term medication management and therapy, education for patients and their families, and psychosocial interventions. Primary care physicians play an important collaborative role in the detection and management of medical comorbidities, substance use disorders, and suicidality. Physicians, patients, and families are encouraged to become involved in the National Alliance on Mental Illness (NAMI; www.nami.org), which is a tremendous resource for help, support, education, and advocacy for patients with schizophrenia and other mental illness.

| TABLE 1 | Antipsychotic Medications |

AGENT	MECHANISM OF ACTION*	TYPICAL DOSING	SIDE EFFECTS†	SIDE EFFECTS†	NOTES
First Generation					
Haloperidol (Haldol)	D_2-antagonist	1.5–15 mg/day	EPS/TD Akathisia	NMS Hyperprolactinemia	PO, IM, IV, and long-acting injection formulations
Loxapine (Adasuve)	D_2-antagonist	10 mg/day	Dysgeusia Sedation	Throat irritation	INH formulation; for treatment of acute agitation
Second Generation					
Aripiprazole (Abilify)	Partial D_2-agonist and 5-HT2A antagonist	10–30 mg/day	Weight gain (+) Dyslipidemia (+) Glucose dysregulation (+)	Headache EPS/TD Akathisia	PO, rapid-dissolving PO, IM, transdermal patch, and long-acting injection formulations
Asenapine (Saphris)	D_2-antagonist/5-HT$_2$ antagonist	10–20 mg/day	Weight gain (+) Dyslipidemia (+) Glucose dysregulation (+)	Sedation EPS/TD Akathisia	Rapid-dissolving PO formulation
Clozapine (Clozaril)	D_2-antagonist/5-HT$_2$ antagonist	300–900 mg/day	Weight gain (+++) Dyslipidemia (+++) Glucose dysregulation (++) Agranulocytosis Sedation	Orthostatic hypotension Seizures Myocarditis EPS/TD	PO and rapid-dissolving PO formulations
Iloperidone (Fanapt)	D_2-antagonist/5-HT$_2$ antagonist	12–24 mg/day	Weight gain (++) Dyslipidemia (+) Glucose dysregulation (+)	Dizziness Tachycardia Sedation EPS/TD	PO formulation
Lurasidone (Latuda)	D_2-antagonist/5-HT$_2$ antagonist	40–80 mg/day	Weight gain (+) Dyslipidemia (+) Glucose dysregulation (+)	Sedation Akathisia Nausea EPS/TD	PO formulation
Olanzapine (Zyprexa)	D_2-antagonist/5-HT$_2$ antagonist	5–30 mg/day	Weight gain (+++) Dyslipidemia (+++) Glucose dysregulation (++)	Sedation Dizziness Hyperprolactinemia EPS/TD	PO, rapid-dissolving PO, IM, and long-acting injection formulations
Paliperidone (Invega)	D_2-antagonist/5-HT$_2$ antagonist	6–12 mg/day	Weight gain (+) Dyslipidemia (+) Glucose dysregulation (+)	Tachycardia Headache EPS/TD	PO and long-acting injection formulations Active metabolite of Risperidone (Risperdal)
Quetiapine (Seroquel)	D_2-antagonist/5-HT$_2$ antagonist	200–800 mg/day	Weight gain (++) Dyslipidemia (+) Glucose dysregulation (+)	Sedation Headache Orthostatic hypotension EPS/TD	PO and extended-release PO formulations
Risperidone (Risperdal)	D_2-antagonist/5-HT$_2$ antagonist	2–6 mg/day	Weight gain (++) Dyslipidemia (+) Glucose dysregulation (+)	Sedation Hyperprolactinemia EPS/TD	PO, PO liquid, rapid-dissolving PO, and long-acting injection formulations
Ziprasidone (Geodon)	D_2-antagonist/5-HT$_2$ antagonist	80–160 mg/day	Weight gain (+) Dyslipidemia (+) Glucose dysregulation (+)	Sedation QTc prolongation EPS/TD	PO and IM formulations
Aripiprazole lauroxil (Aristada)	Partial D_2 agonist and 5-HT2A antagonist	441 mg/month or 882 mg/4–6 weeks	Weight gain (+) Dyslipidemia (+) Glucose dysregulation (+)	Headache EPS/TD Akathisia	Long-acting injection formulation
Brexpiprazole (Rexulti)	Partial D2 and 5-HT1A agonist and 5-HT2 antagonist	1–4 mg/day	Weight gain (+) Dyslipidemia (+) Glucose dysregulation (+)	Increased triglycerides EPS/TD Akathisia	PO formulation

Continued

TABLE 1 — Antipsychotic Medications—cont'd

AGENT	MECHANISM OF ACTION*	TYPICAL DOSING	SIDE EFFECTS†	SIDE EFFECTS†	NOTES
Cariprazine (Vraylar)	Partial D2 and D3 agonist	1.5–6 mg/day	Weight gain (+) Dyslipidemia (+) Glucose dysregulation (+)	Headache EPS/TD Akathisia	PO formulation
Lumateperone (Caplyta)	5-HT2A antagonist, partial D2 agonist, D1 receptor–dependent glutamate modulator, serotonin reuptake inhibitor	42 mg/day	Weight gain (+/-) Dyslipidemia (+/-) Glucose dysregulation (+/-)	Headache Somnolence Sedation	PO formulation

Abbreviations: D_2 = dopamine D_2 receptor; +++, severe risk; EPS = extrapyramidal side effects; $5\text{-}HT_2$ = serotonin $5\text{-}HT_2$ receptor; ++ = moderate risk; TD = tardive dyskinesia; + = mild or low risk; NMS = neuroleptic malignant syndrome.

*All first-generation and second-generation antipsychotics have an FDA black box warning for an "association with an increased risk of mortality in elderly patients treated for dementia-related psychosis." All second-generation agents are D_2 and $5\text{-}HT_2$ antagonists; however, many act on multiple receptors, including alpha-adrenergic, beta-adrenergic, histaminergic, muscarinic cholinergic, and D_1, and $5\text{-}HT_1$ receptors.

†EPS and TD are possible side effects with all antipsychotics, but they occur less frequently with second-generation than first-generation drugs.

TABLE 2 — Monitoring Second-Generation Antipsychotic (Excluding Clozapine)

	BASELINE	4 WEEKS	8 WEEKS	12 WEEKS	QUARTERLY	ANNUALLY	IF SYMPTOMS ARISE	EVERY 5 YEARS	OTHER
Personal/family history*	X					X			
Pregnancy test†	X						X		
Weight/BMI	X	X	X	X	X				
Waist circumference	X					X			
Blood pressure	X			X		X			
Fasting glucose/HgbA1C	X			X		X			
Fasting lipid panel	X			X				X	
EKG‡	X						X		
Prolactin	X						X		
CBC with differential§									X

More frequent assessments may be warranted based on clinical status.

*Including obesity, diabetes, hypertension, and dyslipidemia.

†In all women of childbearing age.

‡For patients taking Ziprasidone (Geodon), which may prolong the QTc interval, and Clozapine (Clozaril).

§For patients taking Clozapine (Clozaril). CBC with differential required at baseline, then weekly for 6 months, then every other week for 6 months, then monthly thereafter. Baseline absolute neutrophil count (ANC) must be ≥ 1500/mm³ (or ≥1000/mm³ in patients with benign ethnic neutropenia) due to risk of agranulocytosis.

Schizophrenia

References

American Diabetes Association, American Psychiatric Association, American Association of Clinical Endocrinologists, et al: Consensus development conference on antipsychotic drugs and obesity and diabetes, *J Clin Psychiatry* 65:267, 2020.

American Psychiatric Association: Practice guideline for the treatment of patients with schizophrenia, ed 3, *Am J Psychiatry*, 2020 (in press).

Buchanan RW, Carpenter WT: Schizophrenia and other psychotic disorders. In Sadock BJ, Sadock VA, editors: *Kaplan and Sadock's Comprehensive Textbook of Psychiatry*, ed 8, Philadelphia, 2005, Lippincott Williams and Wilkins, pp 1329–1345.

Buckley PF, Miller BJ, Lehrer DS, et al: Psychiatric comorbidities and schizophrenia, *Schizophr Bull* 35:383, 2009.

Fusar-Poli P, Tantardini M, De Simone S, et al: Deconstructing vulnerability for psychosis: meta-analysis of environmental risk factors for psychosis in subjects at ultra high-risk, *Eur Psychiatry* 40:65–75, 2017.

Laursen TM, Munk-Olsen T, Vestergaard M: Life expectancy and cardiovascular mortality in persons with schizophrenia, *Curr Opin Psychiatry* 25:83, 2012.

Leucht S, Corves C, Arbter D, et al: Second-generation versus first-generation antipsychotic drugs for schizophrenia: a meta-analysis, *Lancet* 373:31, 2009.

Lieberman JA, Stroup TS, McEvoy JP, et al: Effectiveness of antipsychotic drugs in patients with chronic schizophrenia, *N Engl J Med* 353:1209, 2005.

McEvoy JP, Meyer JP, Goff DC, et al: Prevalence of the metabolic syndrome in patients with schizophrenia: baseline results from the Clinical Antipsychotic Trials of Intervention Effectiveness (CATIE), *Schizophr Res* 80:19, 2005.

Messias EL, Chen CY, Eaton WW: Epidemiology of schizophrenia: review of findings and myths, *Psychiatr Clin North Am* 30:323, 2007.

Nelson B, Amminger GP, Yuen HP, et al: Staged treatment in early psychosis: a sequential multiple assignment randomised trial of interventions for ultra high risk of psychosis patients, *Early Interv Psychiatry* 12:292, 2018.

Rodrigues-Amorim D, Rivera-Baltanás T, López M, et al: Schizophrenia: a review of potential biomarkers, *J Psychiatr Res* 93:37–49, 2017.

Shi J, Levinson DF, Duan J, et al: Common variants on chromosome 6p22.1 are associated with schizophrenia, *Nature* 460:753, 2009.

Torrey EF: *Surviving Schizophrenia*, ed 7, New York, 2019, Harper Perennial.

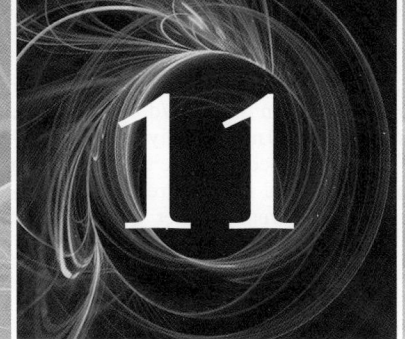

Respiratory System

ACUTE BRONCHITIS AND OTHER VIRAL RESPIRATORY INFECTIONS

Method of
Tomoko Sairenji, MD, MS

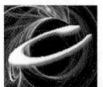

CURRENT DIAGNOSIS

- Most cases of acute bronchitis are caused by viruses and diagnosed clinically.
- Predominant symptom is acute cough, with or without sputum.
- Other diseases such as asthma, pneumonia, chronic obstructive pulmonary disease exacerbation, and heart failure should be ruled out.

CURRENT THERAPY

- Antibiotics are not recommended for most cases of acute bronchitis.
- Dextromethorphan, guaifenesin, and honey may be considered to relieve cough symptoms.
- Patient education: Cough can last 3 weeks or more.

Epidemiology

Acute cough is the most common reason for ambulatory care visits. Acute bronchitis, which is characterized by an acute cough, is most commonly caused by viruses such as rhinovirus, enterovirus, influenza A and B, parainfluenza, coronavirus, coxsackie, and respiratory syncytial virus. Bacterial causes such as *Mycoplasma pneumoniae*, *Chlamydia pneumoniae*, and *Bordetella pertussis* are much less common.

Pathophysiology

Acute bronchitis is caused by an acute inflammatory process in the mucosa of the trachea and bronchi with resultant injury to epithelium of the mucosa.

Clinical Manifestations

Cough is the primary symptom of acute bronchitis, but it can cause other symptoms such as nasal congestion, wheezing, dyspnea, fever, and nonspecific constitutional symptoms.

Diagnosis

Acute bronchitis is diagnosed clinically, characterized by an acute cough with or without sputum production. It is often a diagnosis of exclusion, in which other diseases such as asthma, pneumonia, chronic obstructive pulmonary disease exacerbation, and heart failure are ruled out. Initially, manifestations of acute bronchitis can be identical to the common cold and difficult to distinguish. Patients may have a mildly ill appearance, but fever is less common in bronchitis after the first few days. On auscultation, there may be wheezing or rhonchi that improve with coughing. A patient with a high temperature, otherwise abnormal vital signs, and a more toxic appearance should raise concern for pneumonia or influenza.

Laboratory testing is usually not necessary for the typical patient in the outpatient setting, but it can be done for influenza and pertussis when there is greater suspicion for these diseases.

Imaging such as chest x-rays are not necessary in most cases for patients who have normal vital signs, no bloody sputum, and a normal lung examination. However, it is recommended in those older than 75 years of age, because pneumonia does not always mount a fever or cause tachycardia in the elderly.

Differential Diagnosis
Common Cold/Upper Respiratory Infections (URI)
The common cold can be difficult to differentiate from acute bronchitis. On average, adults have 2 to 4, and young children as many as 6 to 10 episodes annually. It is most commonly caused by rhinoviruses but can also be caused by other respiratory viruses such as coronavirus, influenza, and respiratory syncytial virus and parainfluenza viruses. The symptomatic trajectory of the common cold is sore throat, malaise, and low-grade fever for 1 to 2 days, followed by nasal congestion, rhinorrhea, and cough. Cough can occur in 30% to 40% of cases, and fluid can accumulate in middle ear or sinus cavities. Common cold/URI symptoms are generally the worst on day 3 to 4 and start to improve by day 7. Symptoms that would warrant consideration for more serious disease are respiratory distress, difficulty swallowing, altered mental status, signs suggesting dehydration, stiff neck, rash, or sore throat for more than 5 days. Influenza (high fever with general myalgias), acute bacterial sinusitis (symptoms for more than 10 days without improvement, severe symptoms including fever ≥39°C, and purulent nasal discharge lasting more than 3 consecutive days), streptococcal pharyngitis (absence of cough with tender lymphadenopathy and tonsillar exudates), asthma exacerbations triggered by URI, and infectious mononucleosis (fatigue, fever, sore throat, and adenopathy more severe than typical URI) are other conditions on the differential. Testing is not warranted for the diagnosis of a common cold unless one of these diseases is suspected and needs to be ruled out.

Similar to acute bronchitis, antibiotics are strongly discouraged for the common cold because they provide no benefit in terms of reducing symptom severity or duration. If symptoms are severe, treatment focuses mostly on symptomatic management, of which most can be done using over-the-counter therapies. Rest as well as adequate hydration and nutrition are encouraged but not studied in trials. Acetaminophen and nonsteroidal antiinflammatory drugs can help with fever and discomfort. The combination of antihistamines and decongestants may be more beneficial than either component alone for nasal symptoms. When needed, dextromethorphan may provide symptom relief with cough suppression. Intranasal or inhaled cromolyn sodium[1] may help with rhinorrhea, throat pain, or cough. Various formulations of intranasal cromolyn sodium (NasalCrom) are available over the counter, and oral inhaled cromolyn sodium (Intal) is available by a

---

[1]Not FDA approved for this indication.

prescription. Regular use of vitamin C supplements[1,7] (at least 200 mg/d) may decrease duration of cold symptoms, but they are not effective if started after cold symptoms start. Oral zinc sulfate[1,7] may decrease URI symptom duration and severity, but it is not routinely recommended because of adverse effects (bad taste and nausea).

Croup

Croup affects children with a peak incidence between 6 and 36 months of age, annually affecting 3% of those in this age range. Parainfluenza virus types 1 to 3 constitute 75% of all cases, but infection with many different viruses can produce this illness. Although some cases of croup can be caused by bacteria, it does not change how it is managed.

Croup is diagnosed clinically. Initially, patients experience cold-like symptoms: low-grade fevers and coryza. Inspiratory stridor, hoarseness, and a barking cough are typical findings that follow, peaking between 24 to 48 hours after onset. These symptoms are caused by mucosal inflammatory swelling of the larynx, trachea, and bronchi. Symptoms are often worse at night and can be exacerbated by emotional distress. Most (85%) cases are considered mild, but nasal flaring and retractions, increased respiratory rate, hypoxia, and tachycardia are indicators of more severe croup. Routine radiologic imaging is not encouraged, because the steeple sign that is often associated with croup is actually nonspecific and can be seen in other causes of glottic and subglottic narrowing such as epiglottitis and bacterial tracheitis.

Management of croup is dependent on the severity of the disease. Administration of corticosteroids (single dose of dexamethasone [Decadron][1] 0.6 mg/kg) are recommended for croup of any severity because it reduces return visits and hospitalization rates. Oxygen should be given to children with hypoxia or respiratory distress. Nebulized epinephrine[1] (0.05 mL/kg of racemic epinephrine 2.25% [max dose = 0.5 mL] or 0.5 mL per kg of L-epinephrine 1:1,000 via nebulizer [max dose = 5 mL]) is recommended for moderate or severe croup. It takes effect by vasoconstriction of the upper airway mucosa, leading to decreased edema. It has a quick onset of action, but efficacy wanes after 1 to 2 hours, so monitoring patients beyond 2 hours is recommended.

Humidified air has been commonly used for croup, but it has not been shown to be effective in decreasing croup symptoms or hospital admissions in moderate croup.

Pertussis

Pertussis should be suspected when patients have more than 2 weeks of a characteristic paroxysmal, whooping cough and post-tussive emesis, or recent pertussis exposure. Most pertussis is caused by the bacteria B pertussis. The number of outbreaks and pertussis incidence has increased in recent years. In the early catarrhal stage (1–2 weeks), it is difficult to discern from a common cold. The cough becomes more frequent, and severe bouts characterize the following paroxysmal stage (1–6 weeks, maximum of 10 weeks). Paroxysms of cough can be debilitating and cause post-tussive emesis, weight loss, and other conditions related to severe cough, but there are few symptoms otherwise. After this stage, the cough gradually improves over the course of a few weeks.

Atypical presentations are not uncommon, because those who have acquired immunity can present with a lesser degree of paroxysm. Thus pertussis should be suspected if cough symptoms last more than 3 weeks. Infants may also have atypical presentation of cough without paraoxysmal whooping.

Diagnosis can be confirmed with either culture, polymerase chain reaction (both better for early stages), or serology (accurate in later stage). Efficacy of antibiotics is questionable because treatment does not improve symptoms. However, antibiotics

(Azithromycin [Zithromax][1] is first line—Children: 10 mg/kg/d for 3 days, or 10 mg/kg on day 1, then 5 mg/kg/d on days 2-5; Adults: 500 mg/d for 3 days, or 500 mg on day 1, then 250 mg/d on days 2–5) are still recommended because they eradicate B pertussis from the nasopharynx and may decrease transmission. Immunization is critical to prevent further outbreaks of pertussis.

Bronchiolitis

Bronchiolitis is the most common cause for infant hospitalization of infants. Respiratory syncytial virus is the most common cause of bronchiolitis. Bronchioles become plugged with detached epithelium and inflammatory cells. Onset of upper respiratory symptoms is often soon followed by rapid development of wheezing and labored breathing. Infants with bronchiolitis typically do not have a marked response to asthma treatment with bronchodilators and corticosteroids, despite similar presenting symptoms. Treatment primarily consists of supplemental oxygen and intravenous fluids as needed to prevent dehydration. Palivizumab (Synagis) is used to prevent hospitalization rate for high-risk infants, such as those with premature birth, chronic lung disease, and hemodynamically significant congenital heart disease.

Therapy (or Treatment)
Decreasing Antibiotic Use

Antibiotic use in the treatment of bronchitis is strongly discouraged in all major guidelines, but they are often prescribed regardless of the recommendations. The strongest predictor of whether a patient will receive antibiotics is whether the clinician perceives the patient desires them. Patient education such as setting the expectation that cough from acute bronchitis can last 3 weeks, that antibiotics would not effectively aid in shortening the duration of symptoms, and explaining the undesired consequences of inappropriate antibiotic use such as antibiotic resistance and adverse effects is important. One in five patients treated with antibiotics will experience side effects such as headache, nausea, skin rash, diarrhea, and vaginitis. Patients are more likely to respond to this sort of education if they feel their concerns have been heard and addressed. In some cases, using a delayed prescription strategy wherein patients would need to call for a prescription or agree to pick up antibiotics after a certain number of days may be effective in decreasing antibiotic use. Providing methods for symptomatic management is also important for patients who desire treatment.

Recommended Cough Treatment

Dextromethorphan, guaifenesin, and honey may be considered to relieve cough symptoms. Dextromethorphan (30 mg orally every 6 to 8 hours) is a central-acting antitussive that reduces the cough reflex. In placebo-controlled studies, it was shown to decrease coughs by 19% to 36% (8 to 10 fewer coughs per 30 minutes) compared with placebo. Guaifenesin ([immediate-release] 200 to 400 mg orally every 4 hours) is an expectorant that increases respiratory tract secretions, hence decreasing mucus thickness. Study results vary, but it has been shown to decrease cough frequency and severity compared with placebo. Honey (2.5–10 mL [0.5–2 teaspoons]) has been compared with dextromethorphan, diphenhydramine, and no treatment in children. It was found to be better than no treatment in its effectiveness in decreasing cough severity and frequency and improving sleep quality. Honey would be an option for children older than 1 year, because antitussive use is not recommended in small children.

Cough Treatments that are not Recommended

There is no evidence that centrally acting antitussive codeine[1] has any effect to decrease cough symptoms, and benzonatate (Tessalon Perles), a peripherally acting antitussive has only been shown to be effective in conjunction with guaifenesin. Unfortunately, many over-the-counter therapies do not significantly

---

[1]Not FDA approved for this indication.
[7]Available as a dietary supplement.

impact acute bronchitis symptoms. Clinical trials have shown that ibuprofen (Motrin)[1] and antihistamines are not effective in reducing symptoms of cough. The FDA warns against using cough medications that have antihistamines and antitussives in children younger than 4 years of age because of the high risk for potential harm. Use of beta-agonists is also not recommended, unless the patient presents with wheezing at the time of presentation.

[1]Not FDA approved for this indication.

References

Altunaiji S, Kukuruzovic R, Curtis N, et al: Antibiotics for whooping cough (pertussis), *Cochrane Database Syst Rev* 2007 (3):CD004404.

Barnett ML, Linder JA: Antibiotic prescribing for adults with acute bronchitis in the United States, 1996-2010, *JAMA* 311:2020–2022, 2014.

Ebell MH, Lundgren J, Youngpairoj S: How long does a cough last? Comparing patients' expectations with data from a systematic review of the literature, *Ann Fam Med* 11:5–13, 2013.

Kinkade S, Long N: Acute bronchitis, *Am Fam Physician* 94:560–565, 2016.

Oduwole O, Meremikwu MM, Oyo-Ita A, et al: Honey for acute cough in children, *Cochrane Database Syst Rev*, 2014. Rev (12):CD007094.

Petrocheilou A, Tanou K, Kalampouka E, et al: Viral croup: diagnosis and a treatment algorithm, *Pediatr Pulmonol* 49:421–429, 2014.

Russell KF, Liang Y, O'Gorman K, et al: Glucocorticoids for croup, *Cochrane Database Syst Rev*, 2011. Rev (1):CD001955.

Smith D, McDermott A, Sullivan J: Croup: diagnosis and management, *Am Fam Physician* 97:575–580, 2018.

Smith SM, Fahey T, Smucny J, et al: Antibiotics for acute bronchitis, *Cochrane Database Syst Rev*, 2014. Rev (3):CD000245.

Smith SM, Schroeder K, Fahey T: Over-The-Counter (OTC) medications for acute cough in children and adults in community settings, *Cochrane Database Syst Rev*, 2014. Rev (11):CD001831.

ACUTE RESPIRATORY FAILURE

Method of
Anthony J. Faugno III, MD; and Scott K. Epstein, MD

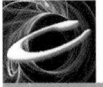

CURRENT DIAGNOSIS

- History and physical examination can give insight into the etiology of hypoxic and hypercapneic respiratory failure but may be insufficient to make a definitive diagnosis and guide therapy.
- An arterial blood gas is mandatory to define severity and whether hypoxic or hypercapneic (or both) respiratory failure is present.
- Additional diagnostic modalities, including chest radiograph, electrocardiogram, cardiac laboratory tests (troponin, brain natriuretic peptide), echocardiography, and selected use of a pulmonary artery catheter, can help identify a specific etiology.

CURRENT THERAPY

- Treatment of acute respiratory failure often begins with nonspecific approaches such as oxygen and mechanical ventilation (noninvasive or invasive).
- The goal of mechanical ventilation is to improve gas exchange and rest the respiratory muscles while waiting for the beneficial effects of specific therapy aimed at the underlying cause (e.g., bronchodilators, antibiotics, and corticosteroids in acute exacerbations of chronic obstructive pulmonary disease [COPD]).
- Noninvasive ventilation avoids many complications associated with invasive ventilation and improves outcomes for patients with acute cardiogenic pulmonary edema and acute exacerbations of COPD.

- High-flow nasal cannula is emerging as the preferred therapy for hypoxic respiratory failure in patients with non-cardiogenic pulmonary edema who do not require urgent intubation.
- Invasive mechanical ventilation can be lifesaving but can cause clinical deterioration if not properly administered.
- Using low tidal volumes (6 mL/kg ideal body weight) can help avoid dangerous dynamic hyperinflation in acute exacerbations of COPD and further lung injury in acute lung injury (e.g., volutrauma, barotrauma).
- Once signs of improvement are evident, focus rapidly shifts to liberating the patient from the ventilator using spontaneous breathing trials to assess the need for ventilatory support followed by airway assessment to determine readiness for extubation.

The respiratory system serves many complex physiologic functions, the most important of which is gas exchange. Using the interface between the alveolar space and capillaries, O_2 is taken up and CO_2 is eliminated. Acute respiratory failure, a life-threatening entity, is present when this system fails, over the course of minutes to hours, resulting in hypoxemia (type I) or hypercapnia (type II), or both. Most patients with acute respiratory failure present with dyspnea, although the correlation with disease severity is poor. Indeed, dyspnea might seem mild in those with baseline chronic respiratory failure, and it might be absent in those with an underlying neurologic process (e.g., drug overdose). Other symptoms and signs such as cough, chest pain, orthopnea, fever, tachypnea, rales, and wheezing are insensitive and nonspecific.

This chapter outlines the general pathophysiology and therapeutic approach to acute respiratory failure by using the examples of three common entities: acute respiratory distress syndrome (ARDS), cardiogenic pulmonary edema (congestive heart failure [CHF]), and acute exacerbation of chronic obstructive pulmonary disease (AECOPD).

Definitions and Pathophysiology
Acute Hypoxic Respiratory Failure
Hypoxic respiratory failure is conventionally defined as an arterial oxygen tension (PaO_2) of less than 60 mm Hg. Because this definition ignores the inspired fraction of oxygen (FiO_2), some favor a PaO_2/FiO_2 ratio of less than 300. To account for the arterial CO_2 tension ($PaCO_2$), others favor an alveolar–arterial (A–a) O_2 gradient greater than 250 mm Hg, using the equation

$$A\text{--}a\ O_2\ gradient = PAO_2 - PaO_2$$
$$= (713 \times FiO_2) - (PaO_2 + PaCO_2/0.8)$$

where 713 is the barometric pressure (760) minus the water vapor pressure. A normal A–a O_2 is less than 10 mm Hg, but this threshold value increases with age. The determination of PaO_2 requires an invasive test, an arterial blood gas. Oxygenation can be continuously monitored noninvasively by pulse oximetry, which provides an estimate of arterial oxygen saturation (SaO_2). In general, an SaO_2 of 0.90 corresponds to a PaO_2 of 60 mm Hg, but the relation depends on temperature, pH, $PaCO_2$, and 2,3-diphosphoglycerate (2,3-DPG). Accuracy is adversely affected by low perfusion states, dark skin pigmentation, nail polish, dyshemoglobins (e.g., carboxyhemoglobin, methemoglobin), intravascular dyes, motion, and ambient light.

Clinicians tend to focus on PaO_2 and SaO_2, but the real parameter of interest is O_2 delivery (DO_2) to organs and tissues. DO_2 depends on cardiac output and O_2 carrying capacity of arterialized blood (CaO_2):

$$DO_2 = CO \times CaO_2$$

where

$$CaO_2 = k\,(Hb \times SaO_2) + 0.003\ PaO_2$$

where k is a constant. DO_2 decreases when cardiac output or hemoglobin is reduced despite a normal PaO_2 and SaO_2. The peripheral response to reduced DO_2 is an increased O_2 extraction ratio (O_2ER), allowing oxygen uptake $\dot{V}CO_2$, an indicator of metabolic demand, to remain constant. Cellular and organ dysfunction occurs when DO_2 and O_2ER are outstripped by metabolic demand. The balance between DO_2 and demand can be estimated by examining the mixed venous O_2 saturation (MvO_2) using the rearranged Fick equation:

$$MvO_2 = SaO_2 - \left(\dot{V}O_2/CO \times Hb \right)$$

When MvO_2 falls below 65% to 75%, imbalance is present. When cellular injury is present, extraction capabilities are limited and cellular hypoxia occurs despite "adequate" DO_2. Under these circumstances, the MvO_2 can be paradoxically normal. These parameters can be determined using a pulmonary artery catheter. The data obtained may be useful in individual patients, but randomized, controlled trials show no benefit when the pulmonary artery catheter is used routinely to guide therapy.

The pathophysiologic mechanisms of type I respiratory failure are listed in Table 1. The most common mechanism is ventilation–perfusion ($\dot{V}/\dot{Q}$) mismatch, characterized by a widened A–a O_2 gradient, a dramatic increase in PaO_2 in response to supplemental O_2, and a variable $PaCO_2$. When areas of low ($\dot{V}/\dot{Q}$) predominate (e.g., reduced ventilation with normal perfusion), the $PaCO_2$ may be low as the patient hyperventilates in an effort (only partially effective) to increase the PaO_2. When areas of high ($\dot{V}/\dot{Q}$) predominate, much ventilation is wasted, and hypercapnia is also present. Areas of lung that are perfused but not ventilated characterize shunt. The resulting fall in PaO_2 depends on the percentage of cardiac output circulating through the shunt and the O_2 content of that blood. Supplemental O_2 has minimal or small effect on PaO_2 because the shunted blood is not exposed to the increased FiO_2. Therefore, treatment is aimed at decreasing shunt by improving ventilation to the affected area or reducing perfusion to that area. When shunt results from a unilateral process (e.g., pneumonia, atelectasis), placing the good lung in the dependent position decreases shunt perfusion, and oxygenation improves.

Acute Hypercapneic Respiratory Failure

Hypercapneic respiratory failure is defined as a $PaCO_2$ greater than 45 mm Hg. The equation used to determine $PaCO_2$ provides insight into the three basic mechanisms underlying hypercapnia:

$$PaCO_2 = k \left(\dot{V}CO_2 \right) / V_E (1 - V_D/V_T)$$

where k is a constant, V_E is total minute ventilation (respiratory rate times tidal volume), and V_D/V_T is the dead space. Therefore, hypercapnia can result from increased CO_2 production $\dot{V}CO_2$,

increased physiologic dead space (V_D/V_T), and decreased minute ventilation (Box 1). Increased $\dot{V}CO_2$ alone is usually insufficient to cause hypercapnia because the respiratory system responds by increasing minute ventilation to keep $PaCO_2$ normal (37 to 43 mm Hg). Conversely, with abnormalities of respiratory muscle function or respiratory drive, or with increased dead space (and diminished reserve), the respiratory response to increased $\dot{V}CO_2$ may be insufficient, and hypercapnia results.

Treatment

Treatment of acute hypoxemic and hypercapneic respiratory failure combines nonspecific (e.g., supplemental O_2, mechanical ventilation) and specific therapy (Boxes 2 and 3).

Oxygen Therapy

In the hospital, 100% O_2 is supplied from a wall source with a regulator determining flow rate in liters per minute. The final delivered oxygen concentration (FiO_2) depends on this flow rate and the amount of room air breathed by the patient. The O_2 flow rate is almost never sufficient to meet all of the patient's ventilatory demands, so varying amounts of room air are entrained to meet these needs. The final inspired oxygen concentration depends on the relative fraction of each gas, total minute ventilation, and the pattern of breathing (including the inspiratory-to-expiratory ratio). O_2 may be administered using nasal prongs, a facial mask, or high-flow devices designed to deliver higher FiO_2 (Table 2). High-flow nasal cannula (HFNC) devices are more capable of meeting the inspiratory flow demands during respiratory distress (in excess of

---

| BOX 1 | Pathophysiologic Mechanisms of Hypercapnia |

Increased Carbon Dioxide Production ($\dot{V}CO_2$)
Fever
Overfeeding
Seizure
Sepsis
Thyrotoxicosis

Decreased Ventilation (V_E)
Depressed respiratory drive
Phrenic nerve injury
Respiratory muscle weakness

Increased Dead Space (V_D/V_T)
Acute exacerbation of chronic obstructive pulmonary disease
Interstitial lung disease (e.g., pneumonia, interstitial fibrosis, etc.)
Pulmonary vascular disease

| TABLE 1 | Pathophysiologic Mechanisms of Acute Hypoxic Respiratory Failure |

MECHANISM	A–A O2 GRADIENT	PACO2	RESPONSE TO 100% O2	CAUSE
Diffusion abnormality	↑	↑ Normal	↑↑	Severe interstitial lung disease ARDS, pneumonia
Hypoventilation	Normal	↑	↑↑↑	Narcotic overdose, obesity hypoventilation syndrome, respiratory muscle weakness
↓ FiO₂	Normal	Usually ↓	↑↑↑	High altitude, smoke inhalation
↓ MvO₂	↑	Usually ↓	↑	ARDS, shock, CHF, PE
Shunt	↑	Usually ↓	None or ↑	ARDS, pneumonia, CHF, atelectasis, PE
$\dot{V}/\dot{Q}$ mismatch	↑	↑, Normal, ↓	↑↑↑	AECOPD, asthma, PE, ARDS, pneumonia

↑, Increased; ↓, decreased; *A–a O2*, alveolar-arterial O_2; *AECOPD*, acute exacerbation of chronic obstructive pulmonary disease; *ARDS*, acute respiratory distress syndrome; *CHF*, cardiogenic pulmonary edema; *FiO2*, fraction of inspired oxygen; *MvO2*, mixed venous oxygen saturation; *PaCO2*, partial pressure of arterial CO_2; *PE*, pulmonary embolism; $\dot{V}/\dot{Q}$, ventilation–perfusion ratio.

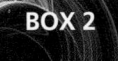 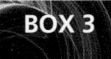

40 L/min) and more reliably deliver the set FiO_2 because they can overcome the entrainment phenomenon. Other reported benefits of HFNC include reduction in respiratory rate and work of breathing and increased end expiratory lung volume. A modest amount of positive end expiratory pressure, approximately 0 to 5 cm H_2O, is supplied by HFNC when breathing with a closed mouth.

Regardless of oxygenation strategy it is important to titrate oxygen support to physiologic endpoints, generally a $SaO_2 > 92\%$. Recent clinical data suggest evidence of potential harm for supraphysiologic blood oxygen tensions, and that an upper limit of supplemental oxygenation should be observed in all patients. The goal here is likely a PaO_2 between 70 and 120 mm Hg with an upper threshold of 98% SaO_2, though this requires further prospective evaluation. In hypercapneic patients (e.g., with AECOPD), high-flow O_2 can lead to worsening hypercapnia and acute respiratory acidosis. The mechanisms are multifactorial: worsening $\dot{V}/\dot{Q}$ matching (increased dead space), decreased intracellular binding of CO_2, and minute ventilation inadequate for the amount of CO_2 produced. Therefore, the goal in these patients is to achieve a PaO_2 of 55 to 60 mm Hg (SaO_2 88% to 90%) with low-flow oxygen (~24% to 28% O_2). If this (often delicate) balance between maintaining tissue oxygenation and avoiding significant respiratory acidosis cannot be achieved, short-term mechanical ventilation may be required.

Mechanical Ventilation

Mechanical ventilation can be delivered noninvasively through a tight-fitting face mask or invasively via an endotracheal tube. The goals of mechanical ventilation are to correct severe arterial blood gas abnormalities, provide respiratory support while specific therapy is used, and unload and rest the respiratory muscles. The ventilator should be set to optimize patient–ventilator interaction and avoid dynamic hyperinflation and intrinsic positive end-expiratory pressure (PEEPi). PEEPi can worsen gas exchange, predispose to barotrauma, and cause hypotension.

Noninvasive Ventilation

Noninvasive ventilation is most commonly applied as continuous positive airway pressure (CPAP), when airway pressure is kept constant throughout the respiratory cycle, or by bilevel positive airway pressure (BiPAP), when inspiratory pressure support actively assists each inspiration. Noninvasive ventilation offers numerous advantages over invasive ventilation, including increased comfort; maintenance of normal swallowing, speech, and cough; less need for sedation; and avoiding the trauma of intubation.

The effective application of noninvasive ventilation starts with carefully explaining the procedure to the patient, followed by selection of a proper-fitting face mask. The mask is placed close to the face to acclimate the patient to high inspiratory flow. The mask is then secured using straps (but not too tightly), and ventilator settings are adjusted to minimize leaks and ensure comfort. The patient is reassessed frequently. Failure to improve within 2 to 4 hours (e.g., reduction in dyspnea, respiratory rate, accessory muscle use, and hypercapnia) signals noninvasive ventilation failure and need for intubation.

Noninvasive ventilation improves outcome (avoids intubation, decreases length of stay, improves survival) in a number of conditions (Table 3). Although randomized, controlled trials show dramatic benefit in AECOPD, other studies show no or uncertain benefit in community-acquired pneumonia, ARDS, pulmonary fibrosis, and routinely after planned extubation. One mechanism for improved outcome is the reduction in infection (pneumonia, sepsis) seen with noninvasive ventilation compared with intubated patients. Noninvasive ventilation should not be used in the presence of respiratory arrest, shock, excessive secretions, inability to protect the airway, an agitated or uncooperative patient, and facial abnormalities that preclude proper application of the mask. Comparison of noninvasive ventilation to high-flow nasal cannula in ARDS suggests evidence of harm in patients with more severe hypoxemia. This phenomenon is hypothesized to be related to ventilator-induced lung injury where tidal volumes are less strictly regulated in noninvasive as compared to invasive ventilation.

TABLE 2 Short-Term Oxygen Delivery Systems

DELIVERY SYSTEM	O2 FLOW RATE (L/MIN)	FIO2 RANGE	COMMENTS
Basic Systems			
Nasal cannula (prongs)	1–6	0.22–0.40	Comfortable
			Facilitates communication and oral intake
			Humidification required at high flow rates
Simple masks	5–6	0.30–0.50	Mask acts as reservoir to increase FiO$_2$
			High flow combats CO$_2$ rebreathing
			Less comfortable
			Must be removed to facilitate communication and oral intake
			Easily displaced with movement
Reservoir Masks			
Nonrebreathing	4–10	0.60–1.00	One-way valve between the mask and the reservoir bag
			Inspired O$_2$ from wall source and reservoir bag
Partial rebreathing	5–10	0.35–0.90	Lacks one-way valve
Venturi masks	4–10	0.24–0.40	Uses Bernoulli principle (fixed amount of entrained room air added to O$_2$)
			Maximum delivered FiO$_2$ can be controlled
			Often used in COPD to avoid excessive FiO$_2$ and risk for hypercapnia
High-flow nasal cannula	10–60	0.21–1	Can overcome room air entrainment, set FiO$_2$ more accurate
			Generates modest amount of positive end expiratory pressure
			Reduces CO$_2$ rebreathing by anatomic dead space washout
			Reduction in work of breathing in select patients

COPD, Chronic obstructive pulmonary disease; *FiO$_2$,* fraction of inspired oxygen.

856

Invasive Ventilation

Invasive mechanical ventilation is delivered via an endotracheal tube. The set parameters include FiO$_2$ and positive end-expiratory pressure (PEEP). For volume-assist control, the clinician chooses respiratory rate and tidal volume. For pressure support, the clinician chooses the inspiratory pressure level above PEEP, and the patient determines respiratory rate. The resulting tidal volume depends on inspiratory pressure level and patient factors including respiratory muscle strength and respiratory system mechanics. Initially the ventilator is set to meet most of the patient's minute ventilation, allowing respiratory muscle rest. Such full support should not be prolonged because diaphragmatic dysfunction can result. Most patients require sedation, but excessive sedation levels are associated with worse outcomes. Therefore, strategies to minimize continuous intravenous sedation using a sedation protocol or once-daily interruption of sedation are recommended.

Invasive mechanical ventilation, especially when prolonged, is associated with numerous complications including ventilator-associated pneumonia, sinusitis, airway injury, thromboembolism, and gastrointestinal bleeding. Therefore, once significant clinical improvement occurs, efforts should focus on rapidly removing the patient from the ventilator. This is achieved by daily screening for readiness (Box 4) followed by a 30- to 120-minute spontaneous breathing trial on minimal or no ventilator support. Patients tolerating the spontaneous breathing trial are extubated if they have a good cough, manageable respiratory secretions, and an adequate mental status to protect the airway. Approximately 25% of patients do not tolerate the spontaneous breathing trial; they should be returned to full ventilator support for 24 hours and undergo careful evaluation for reversible causes. The clinician should consider a more gradual approach to weaning these patients.

Specific Causes of Acute Respiratory Failure
Acute Exacerbation of Chronic Obstructive Pulmonary Disease

Patients with COPD can experience two or three exacerbations per year, especially if they are actively smoking. The best predictor of future exacerbations is a history of previous exacerbations. Other risk factors for exacerbation include serum eosinophilia, pulmonary hypertension and gastric reflux. Hospital mortality ranges from 2% to 11%, rising to 25% for those requiring critical care.

AECOPD is defined by increased sputum volume, purulence, and dyspnea. Physical examination is notable for tachypnea, use of accessory respiratory muscles, diminished breath sounds, prolonged expiratory phase with wheezing, thoraco-abdominal paradox (inward inspiratory abdominal motion), and Hoover sign (inward inspiratory motion of the lower rib cage). The latter two physical signs indicate the presence of dynamic hyperinflation and diaphragmatic dysfunction. AECOPD is further characterized by hypoxemia (resulting from V̇/Q̇ mismatch) and hypercapnia. Patients with more severe underlying disease might demonstrate evidence of acute and chronic respiratory acidosis.

Etiology and Diagnosis

Approximately 50% of AECOPDs result from bacterial infection (e.g., *Pneumococcus* species, *Haemophilus influenzae*, *Moraxella catarrhalis*, and *Pseudomonas* species). The remainder result from viral infection and air pollution. In many cases a cause cannot be identified, although there is increasing appreciation that acute myocardial infarction and pulmonary embolism may be present in up to 25%. Pulmonary embolism may be suggested by a PaCO$_2$ lower than baseline and the need for a higher than expected FiO$_2$ to maintain the SaO$_2$ at greater than 90%. Computed tomographic pulmonary arteriogram is recommended to

TABLE 3 Efficacy of Noninvasive Ventilation in Various Conditions

CONDITION	QUALITY OF EVIDENCE	COMMENT
AECOPD	Strong	↓ Need for intubation
		↓ Nosocomial pneumonia
		↑ Survival
Acute cardiogenic pulmonary edema	Strong	↓ Need for intubation
		↑ Survival
Facilitating weaning in select patients	Strong	↓ Duration of intubation
		Most effective in AECOPD
High risk for extubation failure	Strong	↓ Need for reintubation
Extubation failure in heterogeneous patient population	Moderate	Not effective, two RCTs
Routinely after extubation	Moderate	Not effective, single RCT
Extubation failure in AECOPD	Moderate	Single case-control study
Type I RF, diffuse infiltrates, not ICH	Moderate	↓ Need for intubation
		May ↓ survival, requires close monitoring
Hypoxemic respiratory in ICH with diffuse pulmonary infiltrates	Moderate	↓ Need for intubation
		↑ Survival
Postoperative respiratory failure	Moderate	↓ Need for intubation
		↓ Nosocomial pneumonia
		↑ Survival
Asthma	Weak	Uncertain effect on mortality
		Uncertain effect on intubation
		Benefit may be in ACOS
Obesity hypoventilation	No RCTs	Probably effective in ↓ need for intubation
Do not intubate patients	Observational studies	Most effective with CHF, COPD
Pulmonary fibrosis	Observational studies	Not effective

ACOS, Asthma COPD Overlap Syndrome; *AECOPD,* acute exacerbation of chronic obstructive pulmonary disease; *CHF,* cardiogenic pulmonary edema; *COPD,* chronic obstructive pulmonary disease; *FiO₂,* fraction of inspired oxygen; *ICH,* immunocompromised host; *RCT,* randomized, controlled trial; *RF,* respiratory failure.

BOX 4 Screening Criteria to Assess Readiness to Undergo a Trial of Spontaneous Breathing

Required Criteria
$PaO_2/FiO_2 \geq 150$ *or* $SaO_2 \geq 90\%$ *or* $FiO_2 \leq 40\%$ *and* PEEP ≤5 cm H_2O
Absence of hypotension

Additional Criteria (optional criteria)
Weaning parameters*
- Negative inspiratory force <−20 to −25 cm H_2O
- Respiratory rate (f) ≤35 breaths/min
- Spontaneous tidal volume (V_T) >5 mL/kg
- f/V_T <105 breaths/L per min.

Absence of significant anemia (e.g., Hb ≥8–10 mg/dL)
Absence of fever (e.g., core temperature ≤38.5°C)
Adequate mental status: patient awake and alert or easily aroused.

---
* Recent studies indicate that these parameters are often unnecessary in deciding whether to initiate trials of spontaneous breathing.
Hb, Hemoglobin; *PEEP,* positive end-expiratory pressure.

make the diagnosis, because V̇/Q̇ scanning is nondiagnostic in nearly half of COPD patients, and false-positive high-probability scans occur.

Treatment

Treatment for AECOPD is based on high-quality evidence consisting of numerous randomized, controlled trials and well-performed meta-analyses. Bronchodilator therapy is essential. Nebulized combination therapy (albuterol and ipratropium [DuoNeb]) is effective, but it is not demonstrably superior to single-agent therapy delivered via a metered-dose inhaler. Theophylline should generally be avoided because toxicity outweighs benefits. Antibiotics improve outcome, especially in the presence of fever and increased sputum purulence and volume. Older agents, such as amoxicillin and tetracycline, appear to be less effective than newer macrolides and fluoroquinolones though local resistance patterns should drive antibiotic selection.

Corticosteroids enhance β-agonist activity and counteract the inflammatory state seen in AECOPD. Oral prednisone at a dose of 30 to 40 mg is recommended with a duration of 5 days being noninferior to longer courses. Intravenous therapy (methylprednisolone [Solu-Medrol] 125 mg every 6 hours for 72 hours followed by oral prednisone) should be used in the critically ill patient or when response to oral therapy is suboptimal. There is no role for mucolytic agents or chest physiotherapy during acute exacerbation. Continuation of beta blockers, previously thought to contribute to bronchoconstriction, may in fact be associated with decreased mortality and exacerbations because of impact on COPD comorbidities such as coronary artery disease.

Admission to the intensive care unit (ICU) is indicated for patients with hemodynamic instability, confusion, lethargy and coma, severe dyspnea unresponsive to emergency management, or severely abnormal gas exchange despite initial therapy (PaO_2 <40 mm Hg, $PaCO_2$ >60 mm Hg, pH <7.25). Randomized, controlled trials demonstrate that noninvasive ventilation decreases the risk for intubation and improves survival in AECOPD when there is severe dyspnea, hypoxemia, tachypnea, and significant respiratory acidosis ($PaCO_2$ >45 mm Hg and pH <7.35). Patients who fail noninvasive ventilation or who are not candidates require intubation and mechanical ventilation.

A major risk is the development of dynamic hyperinflation (PEEPi), which occurs when expiratory time is not sufficient to reach functional residual capacity. The resulting air trapping within the thorax can worsen gas exchange, predispose to barotrauma (e.g., pneumothorax), and cause hypotension. PEEPi is minimized by keeping delivered minute ventilation at 5 L/min or less; achieved by lowering tidal volume (e.g., 6 mL/kg ideal body weight) or respiratory rate (8 to 10 breaths/min), or by increasing inspiratory flow rate, allowing more time for expiration. PEEPi is suggested by an elevated plateau pressure or persistent expiratory flow at the time of the next ventilator breath. PEEPi can also increase work of breathing by increasing the patient's inspiratory effort to trigger the ventilator. When extrinsic PEEP is at or just below the PEEPi level, the patient triggers more easily and work of breathing is reduced. The approach to weaning and extubation in AECOPD is similar to that for other conditions, although the risk of failing a spontaneous breathing trial is increased.

Acute Respiratory Distress Syndrome
Etiology and Diagnosis
ARDS is the result of an acute process and is characterized by hypoxemia (PaO_2/FiO_2 <300) with bilateral diffuse alveolar infiltrates, and no evidence of cardiac etiology. Lung injury in this syndrome can result from both pulmonary and extrapulmonary etiologies. Pulmonary causes include pneumonia, gastric aspiration, near drowning, toxic gas inhalation, medication side effects, and lung contusion. Extrapulmonary causes include sepsis, pancreatitis, fat embolism, drug overdose, nonthoracic trauma, and massive transfusion. Conditions that can mimic the clinical findings of ARDS include CHF, diffuse alveolar hemorrhage (DAH), acute cryptogenic organizing pneumonia (COP), and acute eosinophilic pneumonia (AEP). These latter three entities can be diagnosed by bronchoscopy (DAH, AEP) or by open lung biopsy (COP), all of which are treated with high doses of corticosteroids.

Differentiating cardiogenic pulmonary edema from ARDS can be challenging, especially because these conditions can coexist. Physical findings of jugular venous distention and a positive third heart sound, abnormal electrocardiogram (ECG), elevated brain natriuretic peptide (BNP), and positive cardiac enzymes (troponin) point to a cardiac etiology. A chest radiograph showing cardiomegaly, vascular redistribution, widened vascular pedicle, perihilar alveolar infiltrates, and pleural effusions also suggests a cardiac cause. Bedside echocardiography can demonstrate reduced left ventricular function. A pulmonary artery catheter provides definitive evidence of an elevated pulmonary capillary wedge pressure and reduced cardiac output. That said, recent randomized, controlled trials demonstrate no improvement in survival with routine use of the pulmonary artery catheter in ARDS.

Treatment
The first principle of ARDS management is to prevent further lung injury by employing a lung protective ventilation strategy

limiting the transpulmonary pressure, using the plateau pressure as a surrogate. In general this is accomplished by titrating the set tidal volume to 6 to 8 mL/kg of ideal body weight. Once this is achieved the tidal volume is titrated down to achieve a plateau pressure of 30 cm H_2O or less, with lower pressures being more protective. This plateau pressure is measured on the ventilator with an inspiratory hold, and approximates the alveolar pressure. Failing to accomplish this places the lungs at risk for further injury by creating significant shear stress with repeated opening of atelectatic areas (atelectrauma) and overdistending less affected areas (volutrauma, barotrauma). Using small tidal volumes often results in significant hypercapnia, which can have an independent protective effect (permissive hypercapnia). The application of PEEP recruits and opens atelectatic lung, thereby reducing harmful shear forces. The optimal level of PEEP remains uncertain; individual studies have tended to show no mortality benefit of a high PEEP versus a low PEEP ventilatory strategy, however trends in mortality reduction and decreased salvage therapy are seen with a higher PEEP strategy in meta-analysis.

The severity of ARDS is generally subdivided by PaO_2/FiO_2 ratios indicating mild (300 to 200), moderate (200 to 100), and severe (<100) disease; these thresholds correspond to rising risk of mortality. A PaO_2/FiO_2 ratio of less than 150 suggests a higher mortality ARDS phenotype where therapy in addition to lung protective ventilation may provide benefit. Placing the patient in the prone position appears to reduce mortality. The routine use of neuromuscular blockade is controversial with the most recent trial indicating no mortality benefit. Inhaled pulmonary vasodilators, used to optimize V/Q matching, do improve oxygenation but have no impact on mortality. The benefit of extracorporeal membrane oxygenation is yet unclear and is reserved for very severe, high-mortality disease to be used in expert centers. The use of corticosteroids lacked an evidence basis for many years; recent data is suggestive of benefit in a mixed population of ARDS with early use. The clearest benefit of steroids has been seen with treatment of ARDS related to SARs-CoV2 infection, where multiple randomized trials have confirmed a significant mortality benefit.

Cardiogenic Pulmonary Edema
Cardiogenic pulmonary edema occurs in patients with cardiomyopathy or acutely when ischemia is present. Diagnosis is suggested by jugular venous distension, a third heart sound, diffuse rales, abnormal ECG, and a chest radiograph showing cardiomegaly, diffuse alveolar infiltrates, and bilateral pleural effusion. A markedly elevated BNP or pro-BNP further suggests a cardiac etiology.

Therapy consists of oxygen, nitrates, diuretics, afterload reduction, and anti-ischemic therapy if the history or ECG is suggestive. Mechanical ventilation produces positive intrathoracic pressure, which improves cardiac function by decreasing both left ventricular preload and afterload, reversing hypoxemia, and decreasing work of breathing. In hemodynamically stable patients without active ischemia, CPAP at levels of 8 to 12 cm H_2O should be used. A meta-analysis of 15 randomized, controlled trials showed that noninvasive ventilation decreased the need for intubation and improved survival. CPAP and BiPAP appear to be equivalent, although many prefer BiPAP when hypercapnia is present.

Because cardiogenic pulmonary edema is rapidly reversible, intubated patients can often be extubated within 24 hours. That said, the transition from positive pressure ventilation to negative ventilation (e.g., T-piece or extubation) can precipitate pulmonary edema. These patients may benefit from lower periextubation respiratory support to anticipate postextubation pulmonary edema.

References
Acute Respiratory Distress Syndrome: The Berlin Definition, *JAMA* 307(23), 2012.

Acute Respiratory Distress Syndrome Network: Ventilation with lower tidal volumes as compared with traditional tidal volumes for acute lung injury and the acute respiratory distress syndrome, *N Engl J Med* 342:1301–1308, 2000.

Briel M, Meade M, Mercat A, et al: Higher vs lower positive end-expiratory pressure in patients with acute lung injury and acute respiratory distress syndrome: Systematic review and meta-analysis, *JAMA* 303(9):865, 2010.

Ely EW, Baker AM, Dunagan DP, et al: Effect on the duration of mechanical ventilation of identifying patients capable of breathing spontaneously, *N Engl J Med* 335:1864–1869, 1996.

Epstein SK: Complications in ventilator supported patients. In Tobin M, editor: *Principles and Practice of Mechanical Ventilation*, New York, 2006, McGraw Hill, pp 877–902.

Frat J-P, Thille AW, Mercat A, et al: High-flow oxygen through nasal cannula in acute hypoxemic respiratory failure, *N Engl J Med* 372(23):2185–2196, 2015.

Girardis M, Busani S, Damiani E, et al: Effect of conservative vs conventional oxygen therapy on mortality among patients in an intensive care unit: the oxygen-icu randomized clinical trial, *JAMA* 316(15):1583, 2016.

Kress JP, Pohlman AS, O'Connor MF, et al: Daily interruption of sedative infusions in critically ill patients undergoing mechanical ventilation, *N Engl J Med* 342:1471–1477, 2000.

Masip J, Peacock WF, Price S, et al: Indications and practical approach to non-invasive ventilation in acute heart failure, *European Heart Journal* 39(1):17–25, 2018.

Ouellette DR, Patel S, Girard TD, et al: Liberation from mechanical ventilation in critically ill adults: An official American College of Chest Physicians/American Thoracic Society Clinical Practice Guideline, *Chest* 151(1):166–180, 2017.

Rochwerg B, Brochard L, Elliott MW, et al: Official ERS/ATS clinical practice guidelines: noninvasive ventilation for acute respiratory failure, *Eur Respir J* 50(2):1602426, 2017.

Vogelmeier CF, Criner GJ, Martinez FJ, et al: Global strategy for the diagnosis, management, and prevention of chronic obstructive lung disease 2017 report. GOLD Executive Summary, *Am J Respir Crit Care Med* 195(5):557–582, 2017.

ASTHMA IN ADOLESCENTS AND ADULTS

Method of
Matthew A. Rank, MD; and Michael Schatz, MD, MS

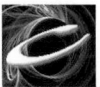

CURRENT DIAGNOSIS

- Confirm the diagnosis by demonstrating an increase in forced expiratory volume in 1 second (FEV₁) by 12% or more after asthma therapy.
- Assess past severity by a history of exacerbations requiring oral corticosteroids, emergency department visits, hospitalization, or intubation.
- Identify environmental exposures, allergic sensitization, and comorbidities that may be aggravating asthma.
- Assess asthma based on symptom frequency, nocturnal awakenings, rescue therapy use, activity limitation, spirometry, and recent exacerbation history.

CURRENT THERAPY

- Nonpharmacologic therapy includes asthma education (especially regarding inhaler technique, self-monitoring, self-management, and importance of adherence to medication), reduction in environmental triggers, addressing any relevant psychosocial issues, and allergen immunotherapy for select patients.
- Preferred step therapy for long-term asthma management is low-dose inhaled corticosteroids, either scheduled or as needed for mild asthma; low- or medium-dose inhaled corticosteroids combined with formoterol¹ scheduled and as needed for moderate asthma; and medium- or high-dose inhaled corticosteroids plus long-acting β-agonists + long-acting muscarinic antagonist for severe asthma, plus additional consideration for other add-on therapies (macrolide antibiotics, biologics, and oral prednisone).
- Asthma exacerbations should be treated with high-dose inhaled β-agonists and early use of systemic corticosteroids.

¹Not FDA approved for this indication.

Asthma is an extremely common chronic medical condition that causes substantial morbidity among its sufferers. In addition to discomfort, asthma can cause sleep disruption, missed school and work, limitations of recreational activities, and acute episodes requiring emergency hospital care. Although the past 40 years have seen the introduction of increasingly effective and convenient medications, recent surveys continue to suggest that asthma remains suboptimally controlled in a substantial proportion of patients. The purpose of this chapter is to describe an approach to assessment and therapy that leads to optimal asthma control. It is based on the Global Strategy for Asthma Management and Prevention (GINA 2021) update and the 2020 Focused Update to Asthma Management from the National Heart Lung Blood Institute but includes recommendations from multiple sources.

Diagnosis

The first step in evaluating a patient with asthma is to confirm the diagnosis. This is particularly important in patients with atypical symptoms or a poor response to asthma therapy. Asthma is confirmed by the demonstration of reversible airways obstruction, which most commonly is an increase in FEV₁ by 12% or more and at least 200 mL after an inhaled bronchodilator for adults, and an increase greater than 12% for adolescents. For some patients, 2 to 4 weeks of chronic inhaled asthma therapy or 2 weeks of oral corticosteroid therapy are necessary to demonstrate reversibility. The latter is particularly important in adults with a history of smoking in whom chronic obstructive pulmonary disease (COPD) is a diagnostic consideration. In patients with normal pulmonary function, asthma can also be confirmed by means of methacholine (Provocholine) or exercise challenge which are two forms of a provocation challenge along with before and after pulmonary function tests. In addition, an elevated fractional exhaled nitric oxide (FENO >50 ppb) can be suggestive of a diagnosis of asthma.

Particularly important masqueraders of asthma include vocal cord dysfunction, panic attacks, hyperventilation, and cough due to postnasal drip, reflux, or angiotensin-converting enzyme (ACE) inhibitor therapy. All of these can also coexist with asthma, so their presence does not exclude asthma. Even when these conditions coexist with asthma, their diagnosis and appropriate therapy usually reduce the patient's respiratory symptoms. Other diagnostic considerations include syndromes of which asthma represents one part: allergic bronchopulmonary aspergillosis, eosinophilic granulomatosis with polyangiitis, and aspirin-exacerbated respiratory disease.

Assessment

Assessment of asthmatic patients involves gathering details of past severity, identifying aggravating factors, and defining current asthma control status.

Current Status

Assessment of the current therapy the patient is actually taking is necessary for understanding the asthma's severity and to appropriately initiate or change therapy. It is particularly important to determine whether the patient is taking long-term control medications, such as inhaled corticosteroids, long-acting β-agonists, leukotriene modifiers, long-acting muscarinic antagonists, oral corticosteroids, or biologics. Both asthma control and risk factors for future exacerbations should be considered. Patients with at least three of the following over the past 4 weeks are defined as uncontrolled in the GINA 2020 guidelines: daytime asthma symptoms more than twice/week, any night waking due to asthma, rescue treatments more than twice/week other than use as pretreatment for exercise, and any activity limitation due to asthma. Other tools to assess asthma control, such as the Asthma Control Test or the Asthma Control Questionnaire, can also be used to determine asthma control (Table 1).

Asthma can be a mild, infrequent illness or a daily severe one. Certain severity markers identify patients who are more likely to experience severe exacerbations or to have symptoms that are more difficult to control and who thus require more careful

TABLE 1	Determining Asthma Control in Patients 12 Years or Older*			
IN THE PAST 4 WEEKS, HAS THE PATIENT HAD:		**WELL CONTROLLED**	**PARTLY CONTROLLED**	**UNCONTROLLED**
Daytime asthma symptoms >2×/week?		None of these	1–2 of these	3–4 of these
Any night waking due to asthma?				
Rescue needed >2×/week other than for pretreatment for exercise?				
Any activity limitation due to asthma?				

*Adapted from GINA 2020 guideline. Can consider using the Asthma Control Test or Asthma Control Questionnaire as other ways to assess asthma symptom control.

TABLE 2	Risk Factors for Future Asthma Exacerbations in Patients 12 Years and Older*
Ever intubated or in intensive care unit for asthma
1 or more severe exacerbations in the past year
Frequent use of rescue inhaler (more than 200 puffs of rescue inhaler per month)
Not adherent to ICS with good technique
Comorbid conditions: obesity, chronic rhinosinusitis, GERD, pregnancy
Psychological or socioeconomic challenges
Low lung function: FEV$_1$ % predicted <60%, high bronchodilator reversibility

FEV1, Forced expiratory volume in 1 second; *GERD,* gastroesophageal reflux disease; *ICS,* inhaled corticosteroid.
*Any of these risk factors increases risk for exacerbations even if an individual has few day-to-day asthma symptoms. The table is adapted from GINA 2019 guidelines.

surveillance. These include histories of asthma hospitalization, especially requiring intensive care or intubation, past requirement for oral corticosteroids, and specific comorbid conditions (Table 2). In patients with prior severe exacerbations, the rapidity of the onset of the exacerbation should be ascertained. Some patients may have minimal day-to-day asthma symptoms but still have a high risk for asthma exacerbations.

Aggravating Factors
Factors that appear to trigger asthma symptoms should be assessed because they may be targets for avoidance therapy. Certain aspects of the patient's environment that can contribute to asthma triggering should be specifically ascertained, including occupational exposures, age of the home, pets, carpeting, visible mold, active or passive smoke, and cockroach exposure. Patients with persistent asthma should have in vitro or skin tests to identify allergic sensitization to pollens, house dust mites, mold spores, animal dander, and cockroaches that can contribute to the maintenance of asthma inflammation or can trigger episodes. The presence of comorbidities that can aggravate asthma, including obesity, rhinitis, sinusitis, gastroesophageal reflux, obstructive sleep apnea, and COPD, should be identified and treated. Finally, psychosocial factors to assess include a history or symptoms of anxiety or depression, attitudes toward asthma and asthma therapy, adherence to therapy, and social support. These may be targets for therapy or may be helpful when creating an effective therapeutic plan and therapeutic alliance.

Long-Term Management
Nonpharmacologic Therapy
The first tenet of nonpharmacologic therapy in the long-term management of asthma is education. Patients need to understand the inflammatory pathophysiology of asthma and the relationships among airway inflammation, bronchospasm, and

symptoms. Patients should be informed that the cause of asthma is unknown and that there is no cure, but triggers can be identified and asthma can be controlled. They should receive education regarding self-assessment, either based on symptoms or peak flow monitoring, and regarding the recognition of early signs of an impending exacerbation.

The next step is to discuss and agree on the goals of therapy. Long-term goals of asthma management include the following:
- Achieve good control of symptoms.
- Maintain optimal pulmonary function.
- Maintain normal activity, including work, school, leisure activity, and exercise.
- Prevent recurrent exacerbations, especially those requiring urgent medical visits.
- Provide pharmacotherapy with minimal or no adverse effects.
- Achieve patient and family satisfaction with asthma care.

The physician should let the patient know that these are the expectations of optimal management and confirm that those are the patient's goals as well.

A very important component of nonpharmacologic therapy is the reduction of relevant environmental triggers. Information should be given regarding environmental control of pollen, mite, mold, animal dander, and cockroach antigens (Box 1) that appear to be relevant based on the history and results of skin or in vitro specific IgE tests. A multifaceted environmental mitigation plan is favored over single interventions. Inhalant allergen immunotherapy should be considered for patients who have persistent asthma when there is clear evidence of a relationship between symptoms and exposure to an allergen to which the patient is sensitive.

Finally, psychosocial issues should be considered and addressed. For many patients, the education and therapeutic alliance described earlier adequately addresses psychosocial concerns. For other patients, poor past adherence requires identifying the barriers to adherence and finding solutions together. Resources for patients with poor social support should be identified. Clinically significant anxiety or depression that can make asthma harder to control should be treated.

Pharmacologic Step Therapy
The main principle of asthma pharmacologic step therapy is to add therapy in steps until control is achieved (step-up) and decrease therapy in reverse steps (step-down) to establish the lowest effective dose necessary to maintain control.

There are two types of asthma medications: quick-relief medications (Table 3) and long-term control medications (Table 4). Systemic corticosteroids can be used either short term to treat an exacerbation (see Table 3) or as long-term maintenance therapy for patients with severe disease (see Table 4). The generally recommended steps of pharmacologic therapy are shown in Table 5. Definitions of low-, medium-, and high-dose inhaled corticosteroids for each of the available preparations are given in Table 6. At each therapeutic step level, the GINA guideline has indicated preferred medications, which generally identify medications with the best balance of efficacy and safety in clinical trials for patients at that level of severity. However, these recommendations are based on population data and must be tailored to individual patient needs, circumstances, and responsiveness to therapy.

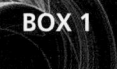

BOX 1   Measures to Control Environmental Factors That Can Make Asthma Worse

Allergens

An approach that considers multiple relevant triggers is most likely to be successful.

Animal Dander

Remove animal from the house or, at a minimum, keep animal out of the patient's bedroom and keep the bedroom door closed.

Dust Mites

Recommended

Encase mattress in a special dust-proof cover.

Encase pillow in a special dust-proof cover or wash it weekly in hot water.

Wash sheets and blankets on the patient's bed in hot water weekly. Water must be hotter than 130°F to kill the mites. Cooler water used with detergent and bleach can also be effective.

Desirable

Reduce indoor humidity to 60% or less.

Remove carpets from the bedroom.

Avoid sleeping or lying on cloth-covered cushions or furniture.

Remove carpets that are laid on concrete.

Cockroaches

Keep all food out of the bedroom.

Keep food and garbage in closed containers.

Use poison baits, powders, gels, or paste (e.g., boric acid). Traps can also be used.

If a spray is used to kill cockroaches, stay out of the room until the odor goes away.

Pollens (from Trees, Grass, or Weeds) and Outdoor Molds

Try to keep windows closed.

If possible, stay indoors, with windows closed, during periods of peak pollen exposure, which are usually during the midday and afternoon.

Indoor Mold

Fix all leaks and eliminate water sources associated with mold growth.

Clean moldy surfaces.

Dehumidify basements if possible.

Tobacco Smoke

Advise patients and others in the home who smoke to stop smoking or to smoke outside the home.

Discuss ways to reduce exposure to other sources of tobacco smoke, such as from daycare providers and the workplace.

Indoor and Outdoor Pollutants and Irritants

If possible, do not use a wood-burning stove, kerosene heater, fireplace, unvented gas stove, or heater.

Try to stay away from strong odors and sprays, such as perfume, talcum powder, hair spray, paints, new carpet, or particle board.

All patients with asthma should have an action plan that describes their pharmacologic self-management. Aspects of pharmacologic self-management include the maintenance medication schedule, rescue therapy doses for increased symptoms, when and how to increase controller medication therapy, when and how to use prednisone, how to recognize a severe exacerbation, and when and how to seek urgent or emergency care. Controller medications may be increased with an upper respiratory infection or with symptoms requiring more than two doses of rescue therapy in 12 hours. Although doubling the dose of inhaled corticosteroids does not appear to generally be sufficient to provide a clinical benefit under these circumstances, quadrupling or quintupling the dose may be helpful. Prednisone is usually needed for patients with incomplete or temporary responses to adequate doses of β-agonists (2–6 puffs with a spacer, waiting at least 1 minute between puffs), substantial interference with sleep every night, requirement for 12 or more puffs of β-agonist in a 24-hour period, or a peak flow less than 60% predicted. Home treatment of exacerbations is further discussed later in this chapter.

Persistent asthma is most effectively controlled with daily long-term control medications, specifically antiinflammatory therapy. For patients receiving long-term control medications, identify their current step of therapy, based on what they are actually taking (see Table 5), and their level of control (see Table 1). Data suggest that the use of antiinflammatory therapy for patients who were previously defined as having mild and intermittent asthma leads to reduced exacerbation risk and can be used as a scheduled or intermittent therapy to reduce exacerbations. In general, step up one step for patients whose asthma is not well controlled. For patients with very poorly controlled asthma, consider increasing by two steps, a course of oral corticosteroids, or both. Before increasing pharmacologic therapy, consider adverse environmental exposures, poor adherence, poor inhaler technique, or comorbidities as targets for intervention. For patients with troublesome or debilitating side effects from asthma therapy, explore a change in therapy.

There are five biologic medications approved for severe asthma not controlled by standard therapy (see Table 4). These biologic medications can be considered for patients with frequent and/or severe asthma exacerbations, poor asthma control, or frequent and/or chronic use of systemic corticosteroids in spite of maximal standard therapy.

Follow-Up

Patients whose asthma is not controlled should be seen every 2 to 6 weeks (depending on their initial level of severity or control) until control is achieved. Once control is achieved, follow-up contact at 1- to 6-month intervals is recommended. These checkups should ensure continued control, identify other changes in the patient's status, and update the patient's action plan.

When well-controlled asthma has been maintained for at least 3 months, a step down in therapy can be considered to determine the minimum amount of medication required to maintain control or reduce the risk for side effects. Reduction in therapy should be gradual because asthma can deteriorate at a highly variable rate and intensity. Doses of inhaled corticosteroids may be reduced by about 25% to 50% every 3 months to the lowest dose possible to maintain control. Many patients with persistent asthma relapse if inhaled corticosteroids are totally discontinued.

Patients should be encouraged to contact their asthma physician for signs of loss of asthma control, such as nocturnal symptoms, increasing β-agonist use, or activity limitation. Consultation with an asthma specialist is recommended if the patient has difficulties achieving or maintaining control of asthma, immunotherapy or an asthma biologic is being considered, the patient requires step 4 care or higher, or the patient has had an exacerbation requiring hospitalization.

Treatment of Exacerbations

Asthma exacerbations are acute or subacute episodes of progressively worsening shortness of breath, cough, wheezing, or chest tightness associated with decreases in expiratory airflow.

Home Management

Patients' action plans should direct their home therapy of asthma exacerbations according to the following recommendations.

Initial therapy should be with inhaled short-acting β-agonists (2–6 puffs by metered-dose inhaler [MDI] or nebulizer). This may be repeated in 20 minutes. With a good response (minimal or no symptoms and peak expiratory flow [PEF] ≥80% predicted or personal best), the patient may continue β-agonists every 3 to 4 hours for 24 to 48 hours. If repeated β-agonists are needed, a short course of oral corticosteroids should be considered.

TABLE 3 Usual Dosages for Quick-Relief Medications for Patients 12 Years and Older

MEDICATION	DOSAGE FORM	ADULT DOSE	COMMENTS
Inhaled Short-Acting β_2-Agonists (SABAs)			
Metered-Dose Inhaler		Applies to All Three SABAs	
Albuterol HFA (Proventil, Ventolin, ProAir)	90 µg/puff, 200 puffs/canister	2 puffs 5 min before exercise	An increasing use or lack of expected effect indicates diminished control of asthma.
Albuterol Breath Activated (ProAir RespiClick, ProAir Digihaler with eModule)	90 µg/puff, 200 puffs/canister	2 puffs q4–6h prn	Not recommended for long-term daily treatment. Regular use exceeding 2 days/week for symptom control (not prevention of EIB) indicates the need for additional long-term control therapy.
Levalbuterol HFA (Xopenex)	45 µg/puff, 200 puffs/canister	2 puffs q4–6h prn	Differences in potencies exist, but all products are essentially comparable on a per-puff basis. May double the usual dose for mild exacerbations. For levalbuterol, should prime the inhaler by releasing 4 actuations prior to use. For HFA, periodically clean HFA activator, as drug may block/plug orifice. Nonselective agents (epinephrine [Primatene Mist], metaproterenol [Alupent]) are not recommended due to their potential for excessive cardiac stimulation, especially in high doses.
Nebulizer Solutions			
Albuterol (AccuNeb, Proventil)	0.63 mg/3 mL 1.25 mg/3 mL 2.5 mg/3 mL 5 mg/mL (0.5%)	1.25–5 mg in 3 mL saline q4–8h prn	May mix with budesonide (Pulmicort) inhalant suspension, cromolyn (Intal) or ipratropium (Atrovent)[1] nebulizer solutions. May double the dose for severe exacerbation.
Levalbuterol (R-albuterol) (Xopenex)	0.31 mg/3 mL 0.63 mg/3 mL 1.25 mg/0.5 mL 1.25 mg/3 mL	0.63 mg–1.25 mg q8h prn	Compatible with budesonide (Pulmicort) inhalant suspension. The product is a sterile-filled, preservative-free, unit-dose vial.
Anticholinergics			
Metered-Dose Inhalers			
Ipratropium HFA (Atrovent)[1]	17 µg/puff, 200 puffs/canister	2–3 puffs q6h	Multiple doses in the emergency department (not hospital) setting provide additive benefits to short-acting β-agonists. Treatment of choice for bronchospasm due to β-blocker. Does not block EIB. Reverses only cholinergically mediated bronchospasm; does not modify reaction to antigen. May be alternative for patients who do not tolerate short-acting β-agonists. Evidence is lacking for ipratropium producing added benefit to β_2-agonists in long-term control asthma therapy.
Ipratropium with albuterol (Combivent Respimat)[1]	20 µg/puff of ipratropium bromide and 100 µg/puff of albuterol, 200 puffs/canister	2–3 puffs q6h	
Nebulizer Solutions			
Ipratropium bromide[1]	0.2 mg/mL (0.02%)	0.5 mg q6h	
Ipratropium bromide with albuterol (DuoNeb)[1]	0.5 mg/3 mL ipratropium bromide and 2.5 mg/3 mL albuterol	3 mL q4–6h	Contains EDTA to prevent discoloration of the solution. This additive does not induce bronchospasm.
Systemic Corticosteroid			
Methylprednisolone (Medrol) Prednisolone (Delta-Cortef, Prelone) Prednisone (Deltasone, Orasone)	2-, 4-, 6-, 8-, 16-, 32-mg tab 5-mg tabs; 5 mg/5 mL, 15 mg/5 mL Prelone 1-, 2.5-, 5-, 10-, 20-, 50-mg tabs; 5 mg/mL, 5 mg/5 mL	Short course (burst): 40–60 mg/day as single or 2 divided doses for 3–10 days	Short courses (bursts) are effective for establishing control when initiating therapy or during a period of gradual deterioration. Action may begin within an hour. The burst should be continued until symptoms resolve. This usually requires 3–10 days but can require longer. There is no evidence that tapering the dose following improvement prevents relapse in asthma exacerbations.
Dexamethasone (Decadron)	0.5-, 0.75-, 1-, 1.5-, 2-, 4-, and 6-mg tablets and 0.5 mg/5 mL and 1 mg/5 mL	0.6 mg/kg as a single dose	Can be considered as an alternative for children presenting to the ED with asthma.

TABLE 3	Usual Dosages for Quick-Relief Medications for Patients 12 Years and Older—cont'd			
MEDICATION	**DOSAGE FORM**	**ADULT DOSE**	**COMMENTS**	
Steroid Injection				
Methylprednisolone acetate (Depo-Medrol)	40 mg/mL 80 mg/mL	240 mg[3],* IM once	May be used in place of a short burst of oral steroids in patients who are vomiting or if adherence is a problem.	

Data modified and updated from the National Asthma Education and Prevention Program (NAEPP) Expert Panel Report 3: Guidelines for the Management of Asthma and 2020: Focused Updates to Asthma Management.
CFC, Chlorofluorocarbon; *EDTA*, edetic acid; *EIB*, exercise-induced bronchospasm; *HFA*, hydrofluoroalkane; *PEF*, peak expiratory flow; *tab*, tablet.
*80 to 120 mg per package insert.
[1]Not FDA approved for this indication.
[3]Exceeds dosage recommended by the manufacturer.

TABLE 4	Usual Dosages for Long-Term Control Medications for Patients 12 Years and Older			
MEDICATION	**DOSAGE FORM***	**ADULT DOSE**	**COMMENTS**	
Systemic Corticosteroids				
Methylprednisolone (Medrol)	2-, 4-, 8-, 16-, 32-mg tab	7.5–60 mg qd in a single dose in a.m. or qod as needed for control	For long-term treatment of severe persistent asthma, administer single dose in a.m. either daily or on alternate days. (Alternate-day therapy may produce less adrenal suppression.)	
Prednisolone (Delta-Cortef, Prelone)	5-mg tab 5 mg/5 mL, 15 mg/5 mL	Short-course (burst) to achieve control, 40–60 mg/day as single or 2 divided doses for 3–10 days	Short courses (bursts) are effective for establishing control when initiating therapy or during a period of gradual deterioration. There is no evidence that tapering the dose following improvement in symptom control and pulmonary function prevents relapse.	
Prednisone (Deltasone, Orasone)	1-, 2.5-, 5-, 10-, 20-, 50-mg tab 5 mg/mL, 5 mg/5 mL			
Inhaled Long-Acting β₂-Agonists			Should not be used for relief of acute symptoms or exacerbations. Use only with ICS.	
Salmeterol (Serevent Diskus)	DPI 50 μg/inhalation	1 inhalation q12h	Decreased duration of protection against EIB may occur with regular use.	
Inhaled Combined Medications*				
Fluticasone and salmeterol (Advair Diskus, Advair HFA and generic)	DPI: 100 μg/50 μg, 250 μg/50 μg, 500 μg/50 μg HFA: 45 μg/21 μg, 115 μg/21 μg, 230 μg/21 μg	1 inhalation bid† 2 puffs bid†	100/50 DPI or 45/21 HFA for patients not controlled on low-to-medium dose ICS. 250/50 DPI or 115/21 HFA for patients not controlled on medium-to-high dose ICS.	
Fluticasone and salmeterol (AirDuo RespiClick, AirDuo Digihaler with eModule)	55 μg/14 μg, 113 μg/14 μg, 232 μg/14 μg	1 inhalation bid		
Budesonide and formoterol (Symbicort and generic)	HFA MDI: 80 μg/4.5 μg, 160 μg/4.5 μg	2 inhalations bid†	80/4.5 for patients not controlled on low-to-medium dose ICS. 160/4.5 for patients not controlled on medium-to-high dose ICS.	
Mometasone and formoterol (Dulera)	50 μg/5 μg, 100 μg/5 μg, 200 μg/5 μg	2 inhalations bid†	100/5 for patients not controlled on low-to-medium dose ICS. 200/5 for patients not controlled on medium-to-high dose ICS.	
Fluticasone furoate/ vilanterol trifenatate (Breo Ellipta)	100 μg/25 μg 200 μg/25 μg	1 inhalation daily	200/25 for patients not controlled on 100/25	
Fluticasone furoate/ umeclidinium/vilanterol (Trelegy Ellipta)	100 μg/62.5 μg/25 μg 200 μg/62.5 μg/25 μg	1 inhalation daily	For patients not controlled on ICS/LABA	
Inhaled Long-Acting Anticholinergic				
Tiotropium (Spiriva Respimat)	1.25 μg or 2.5 μg/actuation	2 puffs daily	Possibly more side effects compared with LABA as add-on therapy to ICS; more effective than placebo when added to ICS; effective when added to ICS/LABA.	
Leukotriene Modifiers				
Leukotriene Receptor Antagonists				
Montelukast (Singulair, generic)	4-mg, or 5-mg chewable tab 10-mg tab	10 mg qhs	Montelukast exhibits a flat dose-response curve. Doses >10 mg do not produce a greater response in adults.	

Continued

MEDICATION	DOSAGE FORM*	ADULT DOSE	COMMENTS
Zafirlukast (Accolate, generic)	10- or 20-mg tab	40 mg/day (20-mg tab bid)	For zafirlukast: Administration with meals decreases bioavailability; take at least 1 h before or 2 h after meals. Zafirlukast is a microsomal p450 enzyme inhibitor that can inhibit the metabolism of warfarin. Doses of this drug should be monitored accordingly. Monitor for signs and symptoms of hepatic dysfunction.
5-Lipoxygenase Inhibitor			
Zileuton (Zyflo)	600-mg tab, immediate-release or extended-release tablets	2400 mg daily (600 mg qid for immediate release or 1200 mg bid for extended release)	Monitor hepatic enzymes (ALT). Zileuton is a microsomal p450 enzyme inhibitor that can inhibit the metabolism of warfarin and theophylline. Doses of these drugs should be monitored accordingly.
Methylxanthines			
Theophylline (Slo-Phyllin, Theobid, Theo-Dur)	Liquids, sustained-release tab, cap	Starting dose 10 mg/kg/day up to 300 mg max Usual max 800 mg/day	Adjust dosage to achieve serum concentration of 5–15 µg/mL at steady-state (≥48 h on same dosage). Due to wide interpatient variability in theophylline metabolic clearance, routine serum theophylline level monitoring is essential. Patient should be told to discontinue if they experience symptoms of toxicity. Various factors (diet, food, febrile illness, age, smoking, and other medications) can affect serum concentration.
Asthma Biologics			
Omalizumab (Xolair)	Subcutaneous (SQ) injection 150 mg/1.2 mL following reconstitution with 1.4 mL sterile water for injection	150–375 mg SQ every 2–4 weeks, depending on body weight and pretreatment serum IgE level	For 6 years and older with moderate to severe allergic asthma not controlled by inhaled corticosteroids. Monitor patient following injections; be prepared and equipped to identify and treat anaphylaxis that may occur. Do not administer more than 150 mg per injection site.
Benralizumab (Fasenra)	30 mg/mL single-dose prefilled syringe, 30 mg/mL autoinjector	30 mg SQ every 4 weeks for first 3 doses, then once every 8 weeks	For 12 years and older with severe eosinophilic asthma.
Mepolizumab (Nucala)	100 mg/mL prefilled syringe, 100 mg/mL autoinjector	100 mg SQ every 4 weeks	For 12 years and older with severe eosinophilic asthma: 100 mg SQ every 4 wks. For 6- to 11-year-olds with severe eosinophilic asthma: 40 mg SQ every 4 wks.
Reslizumab (Cinqair)	Intravenous solution 10 mg/1 mL (10 mL)	3 mg/kg IV over 20–50 min every 4 weeks	For adults with severe eosinophilic asthma.
Dupilumab (Dupixent)	Subcutaneous solution in prefilled syringe: 300 mg/2 mL and 200 mg/1.14 mL; Pen-injector: 300 mg/2 mL	400 mg SQ loading followed by 200 mg every other week OR 600 mg SQ loading followed by 300 mg every other week	For 12 years and older with moderate to severe eosinophilic or corticosteroid-dependent asthma.

ALT, Alanine aminotransferase; *amp,* ampule; *cap,* capsule; *DPI,* dry powder inhaler; *EIB,* exercise-induced bronchospasm; *HFA,* hydrofluoroalkane; *ICS,* inhaled corticosteroid; *LABA,* long-acting β₂-agonist; *max,* maximum; *MDI,* metered-dose inhaler; *SABA,* short-acting β₂-agonist; *tab,* tablet.
*See Table 6 for estimated comparative daily dosages for inhaled corticosteroids.
Data from the National Asthma Education and Prevention Program (NAEPP) Expert Panel Report 3: Guidelines for the Management of Asthma and 2020: Focused Updates to Asthma Management.
†Dose depends on level of severity or control.

With an incomplete response to initial therapy (persistent wheezing and dyspnea and PEF 50%–79% predicted or personal best), oral corticosteroids should be added, β-agonists should be repeated, and the clinician should be contacted that day.

With a poor response (marked wheezing and dyspnea at rest, PEF <50% predicted or personal best), oral corticosteroids should be added, the β-agonist should be repeated immediately, and the patient should call the clinician and usually proceed to the emergency department. For signs of severe distress (e.g., difficulty talking in full sentences, diaphoresis, drowsiness, confusion, or cyanosis), 911 should be called.

Emergency Department and Hospital Management

Assessment should rapidly determine the severity of the exacerbation based on the intensity of symptoms, signs (heart rate, respiratory rate, use of accessory muscles, chest auscultation), peak flow (unless the patient is too dyspneic to perform), and pulse oximetry. Treatment should begin immediately following recognition of an exacerbation severe enough to cause dyspnea at rest, peak flow less than 70% predicted or personal best, or pulse oximetry oxygen saturation less than 95%. While treatment is being given, a brief, focused history, and physical examination pertinent to the exacerbation can be obtained.

In patients with mild to moderate exacerbations (PEF >40% predicted), initial therapy is oxygen to achieve oxygen saturation greater than 93% and inhaled short-acting β-agonists by nebulizer or MDI (4–8 puffs) withholding chamber, which may be repeated up to three times in the first hour. Oral corticosteroids (prednisone 40–80 mg) are recommended if there is no immediate

TABLE 5 Stepwise Approach for Managing Asthma in Patients 12 Years and Older*

STEP	PREFERRED THERAPY	ALTERNATIVE THERAPY
1	As needed short-acting β-agonist (SABA) or as needed low dose ICS-formoterol[1]	
2	Low-dose ICS daily + SABA or Low-dose ICS taken whenever short-acting β-agonist is taken or as needed low-dose ICS-formoterol[1]	
3	Scheduled and as needed low-dose ICS-formoterol[1]	Medium dose ICS + as needed SABA, low dose ICS + (LABA or LTRA or tiotropium) and as needed SABA
4	Scheduled and as needed medium-dose ICS-formoterol[1]	Medium dose ICS + (LABA or LTRA or tiotropium), and as needed SABA
5	Medium to high-dose ICS + LABA+ tiotropium + as needed SABA	Consider add-on therapy with macrolide antibiotics, and/or biologics (anti-IgE, anti-IL5/5R, anti-IL4R). Oral corticosteroids if necessary.

ICS, Inhaled corticosteroid; *LABA*, long-acting β-agonist; *LTRA*, leukotriene receptor antagonist.
*The stepwise approach is meant to assist, not replace, the clinical decision making required to meet individual patient needs. Adapted from GINA 2020 guideline and 2020 NHLBI Focused Update to Asthma Management.
[1]Not FDA approved for this indication.

TABLE 6 Estimated Comparative Daily Dosages for Inhaled Corticosteroids for Patients 12 Years and Older

DRUG	DOSAGE FORM	DAILY DOSE		
		Low (μg)	Medium (μg)	High (μg)
Beclomethasone (QVAR RediHaler)	40 or 80 μg/puff	80–240	>240–480	>480
Budesonide DPI (Pulmicort Flexhaler)	90 or 180 μg/inhalation	180–360	>360–720	>720
Ciclesonide (Alvesco)	80 or 160 μg/actuation	80–160	>160–320	>320
Fluticasone-HFA (Flovent HFA)	MDI: 44, 110, 220 μg/puff	88–264	>264–440	>440
Fluticasone DPI (Flovent Diskus, ArmonAir RespiClick, Arnuity Ellipta)	DPI: 50, 100, and 250 μg/inhalation (Flovent Diskus); 55, 113, and 232 μg/inhalation (ArmonAir RespiClick); 50, 100 and 200 μg/inhalation (Arnuity Ellipta)	100–250	>250–500	>500
Mometasone DPI (Asmanex)	110 or 220 μg/actuation	110–220	>220–440	>440

DPI, Dry powder inhaler; *HFA*, hydrofluoroalkane; *MDI*, metered-dose inhaler.
Data from the National Asthma Education and Prevention Program (NAEPP) Expert Panel Report 3, Guidelines for the Management of Asthma and *Ann Pharm* 43:519, 2009 and GINA 2019.

response to therapy or if the patient had been recently treated with oral corticosteroids.

In patients with severe exacerbations (PEF <40% predicted), initial therapy is oxygen as above, inhaled high-dose short-acting β-agonists (e.g., albuterol 5 mg) and ipratropium (Atrovent 0.5 mg)[1] by nebulizer, and oral or intravenous corticosteroids (prednisone or methylprednisolone [Solu-Medrol] 80 mg). The albuterol may be repeated every 20 minutes or used continuously for 1 hour.

Repeated assessments of symptoms, signs, PEF, and oxygen saturation determine the responsiveness of the exacerbation to therapy. Such assessments should be made in patients presenting with severe exacerbations after the initial bronchodilator treatment and in all patients after three doses of bronchodilator therapy (60–90 minutes after initial treatment). In patients who are improving, short-acting β-agonists may be repeated every hour until a good response is achieved (no distress, PEF >70%). When this response is sustained for at least 60 minutes after the last treatment, the patient may usually be discharged on a course of oral corticosteroids (generally prednisone 40–60 mg for 5–10 days), initiation or continuation of medium-dose inhaled corticosteroids, and arrangement for outpatient follow-up.

In patients who are not improving with the above therapy, adjunctive therapy, such as with intravenous magnesium sulfate[1] (2 g IV over 15–30 minutes) or heliox, may be considered. Noninvasive ventilation or intubation and mechanical ventilation may be required for patients with respiratory failure in spite of treatment.

Summary

Asthma is a very common problem with the potential to cause substantial interference with quality of life. Although there is no cure for asthma, asthma can be well controlled in the majority of patients with proper management and an effective patient-physician relationship. We hope that the method described herein for assessing and managing asthma will assist physicians in helping their patients achieve well-controlled asthma.

---

[1]Not FDA approved for this indication.

References

2020 Focused Update to Asthma Management from the National Heart Lung Blood Institute https://www.nhlbi.nih.gov/health-topics/asthma-management-guidelines-2020-updates.
Global Strategy for Asthma Management and Prevention https://ginasthma.org/gina-reports/.

ATELECTASIS

Method of
Alykhan S. Nagji, MD; Joshua S. Jolissaint, MD; and Christine L. Lau, MD

CURRENT DIAGNOSIS

- Hypoxia
- Tachypnea
- Diminished breath sounds
- Wheezing
- Radiologic signs of atelectasis

CURRENT THERAPY

- Chest percussion or vibration
- Nasotracheal or bronchoscopic suctioning
- Incentive spirometry
- Positive-pressure ventilation
- Ambulation
- Postoperative pain control

Atelectasis refers to the collapse of alveoli that affects segmental or lobar regions of the lung or the entire lung and results in hypoventilation. However, recent studies have suggested that the alveoli are not collapsed but are filled with fluid and foam. These hypotheses are not mutually exclusive; collapsed alveoli and fluid- and foam-filled alveoli may be present concurrently in an atelectatic lung. Although atelectasis is considered a benign condition, early treatment, reversal, and prevention are essential to an overall improved outcome.

Etiology

Compression Atelectasis

Compression atelectasis occurs when the transmural pressure distending the alveolus is reduced to a level that allows the alveolus to collapse. To best illustrate this mechanism, consider the patient who has undergone induction of anesthesia. The diaphragm is relaxed and is displaced cephalad. In the supine position, the pleural pressures increase to the greatest extent in the dependent lung regions and can compress the adjacent lung tissue.

Surfactant Impairment

Surfactant serves to reduce the alveolar surface tension, thereby stabilizing the alveoli and preventing collapse. Reduction in surfactant occurs with certain types of anesthesia. Studies have shown that hyperinflation by means of increased tidal volume, sequential air inflations to the total lung capacity, or even a single cycle of increased tidal volume can increase the release of surfactant, aiding in recruitment and stabilization of alveoli.

Gas Resorption

One mechanism by which gas resorption results in atelectasis involves the patent airway. In regions of the lung with increased ventilation compared to perfusion, which produces a ventilation/perfusion (V/Q) mismatch, there is low alveolar oxygen tension. Increasing the fraction of inspired oxygen (F_{IO_2}) initiates a cascade of events that increases alveolar oxygen tension (P_{AO_2}) and decreases alveolar nitrogen tension (P_{AN_2}), which results in loss of alveolar volume secondary to increased absorption of oxygen.

Another mechanism by which gas resorption leads to atelectasis occurs after complete airway occlusion. In such cases, gas is trapped distal to the obstruction. Gas uptake by the proximal blood flow continues without additional gas inflow. This causes the alveoli to collapse.

Pathophysiology

The trapping of air and hyperinflation of the alveoli are produced from the aforementioned mechanisms. The gases that are trapped are absorbed by the blood perfusing through that region of the lung, which eventually causes collapse of the alveoli. The atelectasis produces alveolar hypoxia and pulmonary vasoconstriction to prevent V/Q mismatching and to minimize arterial hypoxia. This vascular response is effective only if a large part of the lung is not collapsed; otherwise, intrapulmonary shunting occurs.

Clinical Presentation

The signs and symptoms of atelectasis are often nonspecific. The natural course of atelectasis may lead to fever, cough, tachypnea, wheezing, rhonchi, and chest pain. On physical examination, atelectasis may manifest as an area of localized reduced breath sounds with constant wheeze or reduced chest wall expansion or both.

Diagnosis

Chest radiographs aid in the diagnosis of atelectasis. They provide both direct and indirect signs that may indicate an atelectatic etiology for the patient's symptoms.

Direct signs include:
- Displaced pulmonary vessels
- Air bronchograms
- Displacement of intralobar fissures (most reliable sign)

Indirect signs include:
- Pulmonary opacification
- Diaphragmatic elevation
- Hyperexpansion of unaffected lung
- Tracheal, heart, and mediastinal shift toward atelectatic side
- Shift of the hilum toward the collapsed lobe
- Segmental ipsilateral rib approximation

Treatment

Treatment of atelectasis is geared toward the underlying cause. It is important to recognize respiratory distress and to intubate the patient if appropriate.

If the etiology is that of an obstructive atelectasis, chest percussion or vibration and nasotracheal or bronchoscopic suctioning may help in the clearing of secretions. With regard to lung re-expansion, incentive spirometry, continuous or intermittent positive-pressure ventilation, and early ambulation may be used.

Those patients who have a nonobstructive atelectasis caused by a pneumothorax or pleural effusion benefit from tube thoracostomy or thoracentesis. Additionally, appropriate pain management in the postoperative setting allows for proper ventilation.

References

Duggan M, Kavanagh BP: Pulmonary atelectasis: A pathogenic perioperative entity, *Anesthesiology* 102:838–854, 2005.
Duggan M, Kavanagh BP: Atelectasis in the perioperative patient, *Curr Opin Anaesthesiol* 20:37–42, 2007.
Hubmayr RD: Perspective on lung injury and recruitment: A skeptical look at the opening and collapse story, *Am J Respir Crit Care Med* 165:1647–1653, 2002.
Peroni DG, Boner AL: Atelectasis: Mechanisms, diagnosis and management, *Paediatr Respir Rev* 1:274–278, 2000.
Wagner PD, Laravuso RB, Uhl RR, West JB: Continuous distributions of ventilation-perfusion ratios in normal subjects breathing air and 100 per cent O₂, *J Clin Invest* 54:54–68, 1974.

BACTERIAL PNEUMONIA

Method of
Arjun Muthusubramanian, MD, MPH; Alison N. Huffstetler, MD; and Katharine C. DeGeorge, MD, MS

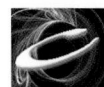

CURRENT DIAGNOSIS

- The clinical diagnosis of pneumonia is aided by patient symptoms of fever, cough, shortness of breath, purulent sputum, or chest pain, and by chest radiography which may demonstrate lobar consolidation, pleural effusion, or cavitary lesions.
- When determining the appropriate treatment setting, use a validated scoring system such as the pneumonia severity index (PSI) or CURB-65 to predict disease severity and risk of death.
- Hospital-acquired pneumonia may be diagnosed in a hospitalized patient who develops a pulmonary infection greater than 48 hours after admission.

CURRENT THERAPY

- Treat outpatients with uncomplicated bacterial pneumonia empirically with high-dose amoxicillin or doxycycline. Only use a macrolide as monotherapy if local pneumococcal resistance is less than 25%.
- Use broad-spectrum antibiotics for empiric treatment of patients with hospital-acquired pneumonia and narrow therapy as soon as possible, based on culture results and sensitivities.
- If a patient has prior respiratory isolation of MRSA or *Pseudomonas aeruginosa*, then presumptive treatment should be initiated and cultures obtained to help guide, and potentially narrow therapy.

Pneumonia (PNA) is a leading cause of death in the United States and accounts for more than 400,000 emergency department (ED) visits annually. PNA often presents with shortness of breath, fever, productive cough, with leukocytosis, and radiographic findings of lobar infiltrate. Diagnosis and treatment should be based on underlying characteristics of the patient and their risk factors. The most common cause of community-acquired pneumonia (CAP) is *Streptococcus pneumoniae*, while hospital-acquired pneumonia (HAP) is more frequently caused by gram-negative bacteria and places patients at a risk for multi-drug resistant (MDR) organisms. Treatment of a non-severe case of PNA in an individual without comorbidities in an outpatient should be empiric and include high-dose amoxicillin or doxycycline; a macrolide should only be used if local pneumococcal resistance is less than 25%. Therapy for inpatients may rely on sputum and blood cultures with targeted antibiotic regimens to reduce cost and complications of therapy. Common treatment regimens for CAP requiring hospitalization include a respiratory fluoroquinolone (such as moxifloxacin [Avelox]) or a beta-lactam (ceftriaxone [Rocephin]) plus a macrolide. Empiric treatment regimens for HAP should be broad and based on local antibiograms, with consideration for coverage for *Pseudomonas aeruginosa* and/or methicillin-resistant *Staphylococcus aureus* (MRSA). Prevention of PNA is essential and pneumococcal vaccines should be routinely provided according to recommended schedules to children and to adults 65 and over.

This chapter discusses diagnosis and treatment of CAP and HAP in adults. While previous guidelines approached healthcare-associated pneumonia (HCAP) and HAP separately, these are now diagnosed and treated as a single disease process (HAP).

Epidemiology

CAP affects approximately 5 to 6 people per 1000 persons per year, with seasonal variance resulting in higher incidence during winter. The associated morbidity and mortality rates are high; in 2015, 16.1 deaths per 100,000 people in the US population were attributed to PNA. Treating these patients comes at a cost of $10.6 to $17 billion in the United States annually. Men are affected more frequently than women, and African Americans more frequently than Caucasians. The very young and elderly (aged ≥65 years) are affected more often than younger adults. Despite our best efforts, advances in medical therapies have not significantly decreased the mortality rate associated with PNA since the advent of penicillin in 1928.

The incidence of HAP is approximately 1.6 to 3.6 cases per 1000 hospital admissions. HAP is a leading cause of hospital-acquired infections (HAIs) and 22% of HAIs are accounted for by HAP. HAP most frequently occurs in patients outside of the intensive care unit (ICU); however, those in the ICU and on mechanical ventilation are at high risk of ventilator-associated pneumonia (VAP). HAP is associated with complications including respiratory compromise, septic shock, acute renal failure, and empyema.

Aspiration PNA is not a separate entity, but rather a subsect that describes the etiology of the particular infection. Microaspiration (aspiration of small amounts of oropharyngeal secretions) is expected in healthy adults during sleep; however, aspiration PNA refers, rather, to large-volume entry of oropharyngeal or upper gastrointestinal contents into the lower respiratory tract (macroaspiration). While 5% to 15% of CAP can be attributed to aspiration PNA, there is no solid data on the contribution of aspiration PNA to HAP.

Etiology
Risk Factors

Predisposing factors for development of PNA include several prescription medications (angiotensin converting enzyme [ACE] inhibitors, antipsychotic medications, glucocorticoids, H-2 blockers, proton pump inhibitors, and sedatives), tobacco use, alcohol use, malnutrition, use of dentures at night, bronchial obstruction due to foreign body, altered mental status due to reversible causes, and pulmonary edema. Nonmodifiable risk factors include immotile cilia, cystic fibrosis, chronic obstructive pulmonary disease (COPD), Kartagener's syndrome, human immunodeficiency virus (HIV), lung cancer, and Young's syndrome.

Community-Acquired Pneumonia Pathogens

Worldwide, *S. pneumoniae* is the leading cause of PNA. In the United States, however, rates of streptococcal PNA have declined following implementation of the pneumococcal vaccine in both adults and children. "Typical" organisms that cause PNA in the United States include *Haemophilus influenza* (although less common following development of the *H. influenza* vaccine in 1987), *S. aureus*, group A streptococcus, *Moraxella catarrhalis*, anaerobes, and aerobic gram-negative bacteria. "Atypical" organisms include *Mycoplasma pneumoniae*, *Legionella* spp., *Chlamydia pneumoniae*, and *Chlamydia psittaci*.

Existing pulmonary infection with influenza, respiratory syncytial virus, human metapneumovirus, adenovirus, and rhinovirus increase the risk of developing a secondary bacterial PNA. Patients admitted to the ICU requiring invasive diagnostic testing frequently become infected with *S. pneumoniae*, but have disproportionate incidence of *Legionella*, *S. aureus*, *H. influenza*, and enteric gram-negative bacilli (*Klebsiella pneumoniae*, *P. aeruginosa*, *Acinetobacter* spp, *M. catarrhalis*). Identification of the organism responsible for CAP is only established in approximately 40% of cases.

Specific patient risk factors, including failure of outpatient therapy, should be considered to identify involved pathogens in CAP. Consider local trends and outbreaks for diagnosis of *Legionella*, *M. pneumoniae*, and *C. pneumoniae*. Alcoholism is frequently linked to anaerobic bacterial PNA, *K. pneumoniae*, *Mycobacterium tuberculosis*, and *S. pneumoniae*. Patients with high risk of aspiration also have higher rates of anaerobic oral flora underlying PNA. Patients with COPD frequently have PNA caused by *C. pneumoniae, H. influenza, Legionella* species, *M. catarrhalis, P. aeruginosa,* and *S. pneumoniae.* Exposure to animals such as bats, birds, or farm animals increases risk of *Histoplasma capsulatum* and *Coxiella burnetii* infections. HIV is a risk factor for *H. influenza, M. tuberculosis,* and *S. pneumoniae* in the early stages and a risk factor for *Pneumocystis jiroveci* in late stages with decreased CD4 count. Travel increases risk for *Blastomyces dermatitidis* and *Coccidioides* species. Severe infections that do not respond to initial therapy should raise concern for possible MRSA infection. When clinical management would be altered by confirmed diagnosis of microbial infection or aforementioned risk factors for particular causative organisms exist, effort should be made for more extensive diagnostic testing.

Hospital-Acquired Pneumonia

Acutely ill, hospitalized patients have a higher risk of aspirating, which accounts for many of the differences in involved pathogens in HAP as compared to CAP. Oropharyngeal colonization with microorganisms that are commonly found in hospitals may occur within 48 hours of admission. Aerobic gram-negative bacilli such as *Escherichia coli, K. pneumoniae, Enterobacter* spp., and *P. aeruginosa* are more commonly identified in patients with HAP, but gram-positive cocci are also identified. HAP, distinct from CAP, places patients at higher risk for MDR pathogens. Prior intravenous (IV) antibiotic use is a strong risk factor for MDR HAP. MRSA is also more common in patients with HAP, primarily due to prior IV antibiotic use as well. MDR *P. aeruginosa* is identified most frequently in patients who have received IV antibiotics, previously on mechanical ventilation, and with a history of COPD, cystic fibrosis, and bronchiectasis.

Diagnosis

Symptoms of PNA most often include fever, cough, shortness of breath, purulent sputum, and chest pain. Physical exam may demonstrate bronchial breath sounds and crackles, although breath sounds may also be entirely normal, especially in the elderly. Oxygen saturation is often reduced, and chest radiography may demonstrate lobar consolidation, pleural effusion, and/or cavitary lesions. Depending on the severity of illness, patients may be treated in the outpatient or inpatient acute care settings, or may require intensive care for ventilatory or vasopressor support.

Community-Acquired Pneumonia

Diagnosis of CAP requires the presence of symptoms (fever, cough, purulent sputum, pleuritis, and/or shortness of breath) plus chest radiographic findings consistent with PNA such as lobar consolidation, pleural effusion, and/or cavitary lesions. Blood oxygen saturation is frequently low and white blood cell counts may be elevated, often with a neutrophilic predominance. Presentation in the elderly may be more subtle, with atypical or absent symptoms, blunted febrile response, and lack of leukocytosis. A patient meets the criteria for severe CAP, as defined by Infectious Diseases Society of America/American Thoracic Society CAP severity criteria, when meeting either one major criterion or three or more minor criteria (Table 1).

Patients diagnosed with bacterial PNA treated in the outpatient setting do not require specific microbial identification; neither noninvasive nor invasive testing is recommended for this population (including blood cultures, endotracheal aspirates, and urine antigen testing).

Expectorated sputum samples for gram stain and culture are not routinely recommended for outpatients. Sputum samples for gram stain and culture should be collected, ideally before initiation of treatment, from those who are hospitalized and who meet one of the following: (1) classified as having severe CAP, (2) being empirically treated for MRSA or *P. aeruginosa,* (3) having prior infection with MRSA or *P. aeruginosa,* or (4) having been hospitalized and have received parenteral antibiotics in the past 90 days. Early gram stain can direct initial empiric therapy, especially with findings of less common pathogens. Sputum samples become lower yield as

TABLE 1	2007 Infectious Diseases Society of America/American Thoracic Society Criteria for Defining Severe Community-Acquired Pneumonia

Minor Criteria

Respiratory rate ≥30 breaths/min

PaO_2/FiO_2 ratio ≤250

Multilobar infiltrates

Confusion/disorientation

Uremia (BUN ≥20 mg/dL)

Leukopenia only due to infection (white blood cell [WBC] count <4000 cells/μL)

Thrombocytopenia (platelet count <100,000/μL)

Hypothermia (core temperature <36°C)

Hypotension requiring aggressive fluid resuscitation

Major Criteria

Septic shock with need for vasopressors

Respiratory failure requiring mechanical ventilation

BUN, Blood urea nitrogen.

the time between treatment initiation and collection of the sample increases. Inadequate samples (<10 inflammatory cells per epithelial cell) should not be sent for gram stain or culture. Nebulized hypertonic saline may be used to induce sputum sample when necessary.

Obtaining blood cultures are recommended for the same population of patients for whom sputum culture collection is indicated. In the general population of patients hospitalized with PNA, false positive blood cultures are common and can increase the duration of hospital stay and potentially misinform treatment decisions. Additionally, false positive blood cultures frequently lead to use of broad-spectrum antibiotics, increasing microbial resistance patterns.

Pneumococcal urinary antigen testing should only be obtained for those with severe CAP. *Legionella* urinary antigen testing routinely should be performed for those with severe CAP or when indicated by epidemiologic factors.

During times of community circulation of influenza, those with CAP should be tested for influenza virus, preferably via nucleic acid amplification. Although biomarkers such as procalcitonin (PCT) can be used to monitor response to therapy, PCT, soluble triggering receptor expressed by myeloid cells 1 (sTREM-1), and C-reactive protein should not be used to guide the diagnosis of bacterial PNA.

Hospital-Acquired Pneumonia

The diagnosis of HAP can be made in hospitalized patients who develop pulmonary infection ≥48 hours after hospital admission. Criteria for HAP require new or progressive findings on chest radiography, fever, leukopenia or leukocytosis, or altered mental status (for patients aged ≥70 years), and new or worsening clinical symptoms or signs consistent with bacterial PNA in the absence of mechanical ventilation.

Similar to the management of CAP, sputum and blood cultures should be obtained only when clinically indicated and biomarkers for diagnostic purposes are not routinely recommended. Low dose computed tomography for diagnosis of HAP may assist in diagnosis.

Treatment Setting

Determination of appropriate treatment setting is important for both patient outcomes and healthcare costs. Inpatient care of PNA can be 25 times as costly as outpatient management and also increases risk of thromboembolic events and superinfection with drug-resistant or virulent organisms. However, inappropriate outpatient management of patients at higher risk of death can lead to potentially avoidable morbidity and mortality.

TABLE 2 — Pneumonia Severity Index

RISK FACTORS	POINTS
Demographics	
Age, men	Age in years
Age, women	Age in years–10
Nursing home resident	+10
Comorbid Conditions	
Active Neoplasm	+30
Liver disease	+20
History of CVA	+10
Chronic heart failure	+10
Chronic renal failure	+10
Physical Exam	
Altered mental status	+20
Respiratory rate elevated >30	+20
Hypotension, SBP <90 mm Hg	+20
Temperature <95°C or >40°C	+15
Tachycardia, pulse >125 bmp	+10
Laboratory and Imaging Findings	
Acidosis, arterial pH <7.35	+30
Hyponatremia, Na <130 mmol/L	+20
BUN ≥30 mg/dL	+20
Glucose ≥250 mg/dL	+10
Hematocrit <30%	+10
PaO_2 <60 mm Hg	+10
Pleural effusion	+10
Total points	

Total points less than 51 indicates low incidence of death from CAP. Patients with increased total points have higher risk of death; the greatest risk for those greater than 130 total points with rate of death for adults diagnosed with CAP of 24.9%.

BUN, Blood urea nitrogen; *CAP,* community-acquired pneumonia; *CVA,* cerebrovascular disease, *SBP,* systolic blood pressure; *Na,* sodium; PaO_2, partial pressure of arterial oxygen.

Several scoring systems have been developed to help predict short-term mortality and need for hospital or ICU admission in patients with bacterial PNA. The following clinical decision aids are the most commonly used:

- *Pneumonia Severity Index (PSI):* Commonly used, well-validated scoring system that evaluates 20 items with emphasis on the age of the patient. Higher PSI scores indicate higher risk of requiring ICU level care or short-term mortality. See Table 2 for details of PSI scoring. Patients classified as risk classes I and II should be managed as outpatients; those with risk class III should be treated in an observation unit or with short-stay hospitalization; risk classes IV and V should be admitted to the hospital.
- *CURB-65:* Severity-of-illness score which incorporates confusion, uremia, respiratory rate, low blood pressure, and age ≥ 65 years into a prognostic model to determine a patient's candidacy for outpatient therapy. A CURB-65 score of ≥2 is indicative of likely need for hospitalization, with consideration for ICU care for those with of scores 3 or greater. This shorter scoring system may be less cumbersome in a busy setting, but the effect on hospital admission rates and patient outcomes have been studied less extensively than the PSI score.
- *SMART-COP:* Assists the physician in determining whether the patient requires ICU level care. The algorithm takes into

TABLE 3 — Risk Factors for Multi-drug Resistant Pathogens in Hospital-Acquired Pneumonia

Risk Factors for MDR Pathogens in Ventilator-Associated Pneumonia (VAP)

Prior intravenous antibiotic use within 90 days

Septic shock at time of VAP
ARDS preceding VAP
Hospitalization greater than or equal to 5 days prior to VAP
Acute renal replacement therapy prior to VAP

Risk Factors for MDR Pathogens in HAP, MRSA in VAP/HAP, and *Pseudomonas* in VAP/HAP

Prior Intravenous antibiotic use within 90 days

ARDS, Acute respiratory distress syndrome; *MDR,* Multi-drug resistant; *MRSA,* methicillin-resistant *Staphylococcus aureus.*

account systolic blood pressure, multilobar chest x-ray findings of infiltrate, albumin, respiratory rate, tachycardia, confusion, oxygenation, and pH and stratifies patients into risk groups that estimate risk of requiring intensive respiratory or vasopressor support.

In addition to clinical judgment, PSI is preferred over CURB-65 in helping guide determination of the need for inpatient management of adults with CAP.

Patients with septic shock requiring vasopressor therapy in the setting of CAP should be admitted to the ICU. If there is clinical concern for impending airway compromise, the patient should be intubated and admitted to the ICU. In several clinical studies, patients who were critically ill and were not initially admitted to the ICU had higher rates of morbidity and mortality.

Treatment

General recommendations for empiric treatment of both CAP and HAP are detailed in Table 4. Antibiotics and supportive care (oxygen, IV fluids, and ventilatory or vasopressor support when necessary) is the mainstay of treatment for both community and hospital-acquired bacterial PNA. Antibiotic selection is guided by several factors:

- Age
- Severity of illness
- Risk of infection by MDR pathogen (Table 3 for risk factors)
- Setting (both timing and location) of PNA onset

Initiation of initial treatment should also be guided by geographic antibiograms, which should be available through local hospitals. The CDC Antibiotic Resistance Patient Safety Atlas provides similar information for the aggregate of hospital-acquired infections. Antibiotic therapy should be narrowed as soon as possible based on culture and subsequent sensitivity results, if culture was obtained.

PCT may be used as an indicator of response to therapy after diagnosis of CAP and HAP based on recent trial data. If PCT measurements decrease to less than 0.1 μg/L, a provider may consider discontinuation of antibiotics.

In addition to antimicrobial therapy for those who require hospitalization, care should be taken to maintain appropriate oral hygiene and to maintain head of bed at 30 to 45 degrees in efforts to minimize risk of aspiration. Serum glucose goal should be less than 180 mg/dL. A few additional considerations exist for patients with severe PNA during hospitalization. These individuals should all receive dual antibiotic therapy, as noted in Table 4. For those who remain hypotensive despite adequate fluid resuscitation, consider screening for occult adrenal insufficiency within 24 hours of admission. Those with hypoxemia or respiratory distress may receive a closely monitored trial of non-invasive ventilation followed by intubation as indicated. Low-tidal volume ventilation (6 mL/kg of ideal body weight) should be utilized.

TABLE 4 Empiric Antibiotic Therapy for Pneumonia for Adults

TYPE OF PNEUMONIA	SETTING	ANTIMICROBIAL THERAPY
Community-Acquired Pneumonia	Outpatient, patient without co-morbidities and without risk-factors for MRSA or *Pseudomonas aeruginosa*[1]	Amoxicillin 1 g 3 times daily OR
		Doxycycline 100 mg 2 times daily OR
		Macrolide (only if local pneumococcal resistance is <25%), such as azithromycin (Zithromax) 500 mg on day 1 followed by 250 mg daily or clarithromycin (Biaxin) 500 mg 2 times daily
	Outpatient, patient with co-morbidities[2]	Respiratory fluoroquinolone[3] OR
		β-lactam[4] PLUS macrolide or doxycycline
	Inpatient, non-severe	Respiratory fluoroquinolone[3] (levofloxacin or moxifloxacin) OR
		Select β-lactam (ampicillin+sulbactam [Unasyn],* cefotaxime [Claforan], ceftriaxone [Rocephin], or ceftaroline [Teflaro]) PLUS macrolide (azithromycin or clarithromycin)
	Inpatient, severe	Select β-lactam (ampicillin+sulbactam,* cefotaxime, ceftriaxone, ceftaroline) PLUS macrolide OR
		Select β-lactam PLUS respiratory fluoroquinolone[3] (levofloxacin or moxifloxacin)
	Prior respiratory isolation of *P. aeruginosa*	ADD piperacillin-tazobactam (Zosyn), cefepime (Maxipime), ceftazidime (Fortaz), imipenem (Primaxin), meropenem (Merrem),* or aztreonam (Azactam) to inpatient regimen
	Prior respiratory isolation of MRSA	ADD vancomycin or linezolid (Zyvox) to inpatient regimen
Aspiration Pneumonia	Outpatient	Amoxicillin/clavulanate (Augmentin) OR clindamycin OR levofloxacin OR moxifloxacin
	Inpatient	β-lactam/β-lactamase inhibitor (ampicillin/sulbactam,* piperacillin/tazobactam) OR carbapenem OR respiratory fluoroquinolone[3] OR 3rd or 4th generation cephalosporin (ceftriaxone, cefepime)
	Inpatient, risk of predominantly anaerobic infection[5]	ADD clindamycin to regimen
	Prior respiratory isolation of MRSA	ADD vancomycin or linezolid to inpatient regimen
Hospital-Acquired Pneumonia	Not at high risk of mortality[6] AND no risk factors for MRSA	Piperacillin/tazobactam OR cefepime OR levofloxacin OR carbapenem (imipenem, meropenem)
	Not at high risk of mortality AND risk factors for MRSA	Select β-lactam (cefepime, ceftazidime, imipenem, meropenem, or piperacillin/tazobactam) OR fluoroquinolone (levofloxacin, ciprofloxacin) OR aztreonam PLUS vancomycin or linezolid
	High risk of mortality, administration of intravenous antibiotics in past 90 days, VAP	Two of select β-lactam (cefepime, ceftazidime, imipenem, meropenem, or piperacillin/tazobactam) OR fluoroquinolone (levofloxacin, ciprofloxacin) OR aminoglycoside (amikacin, gentamicin, tobramycin) OR aztreonam PLUS vancomycin or linezolid

[1]Risk-factors include prior respiratory isolation of MRSA or *P. aeruginosa* OR recent hospitalization and administration of intravenous antibiotics in the last 90 days.

[2]Presence of comorbid conditions (chronic heart, lung, liver, or renal disease; diabetes mellitus; alcoholism; malignancies, asplenia, immunosuppression [iatrogenic or pathologic]), Use of antimicrobials within the past 3 months, High-rate (>25%) of macrolide-resistant *S. pneumonia*.

[3]Respiratory fluoroquinolones include levofloxacin (Levaquin) 750 mg daily, moxifloxacin (Avelox) 400 mg daily, or gemifloxacin (Factive) 320 mg daily.

[4]Amoxicillin/clavulanate (Augmentin) 500 mg/125 mg 3 times daily, amoxicillin/clavulanate 875 mg/125 mg 2 times daily, cefuroxime (Ceftin) 500 mg 2 times daily, cefpodoxime (Vantin) 200 mg 2 times daily.

[5]Risk factors for predominantly anaerobic infection include patients with severe periodontal disease and necrotizing pneumonia or lung abscess.

[6]Risk factors for mortality include need for ventilatory support and septic shock.

*Not FDA approved for this indication.

MRSA, Methicillin-resistant *Staphylococcus aureus*; *VAP*, ventilator associated pneumonia.

Community-Acquired Pneumonia

Patients with suspected CAP should first be risk stratified using one of the PNA severity scoring indices discussed above and in Table 2. If being admitted to the hospital, the first dose of empiric antibiotic (see Table 4) should be administered in the ED as soon as the diagnosis of PNA is made. In addition to the established antibiotics noted in Table 4, the two antibiotics omadacycline (Nuzyra) and lefamulin (Xenleta) were approved in 2018 and 2019, respectively, for the treatment of CAP. Both are available in IV and oral formulations and were shown to be non-inferior to treatment with moxifloxacin (Avelox) in the management of CAP. Patients may be transitioned from IV to oral antibiotics when they are hemodynamically stable, able to tolerate oral medications, and are able to absorb these medications enterally. When possible, an oral antibiotic should be chosen from the same or similar antibiotic class as the IV antibiotic used. Observation of inpatients after transition to oral antibiotics is not necessary as long as the patient is clinically stable and has a safe disposition plan. The recommended duration of antibiotic therapy is at least 5 days, with discontinuation only after the patient has been afebrile for at least 48 to 72 hours and remains clinically stable. Concern for a coexisting extrapulmonary infection may affect antibiotic selection and extend duration of therapy.

If a patient has prior respiratory isolation of MRSA or *P. aeruginosa*, then presumptive treatment should be initiated and cultures obtained to help guide, and potentially narrow therapy. If the patient was recently hospitalized, had IV

TABLE 5	Recommended Vaccinations for the Prevention of Pneumonia	
VACCINE	**POPULATION**	**RECOMMENDATIONS**
Influenza	All persons older than 6 months	Annually If first lifetime dose of influenza vaccine (infants ≥6 months and children≤9 years), 2nd dose should be given 4 weeks after 1st dose
Pneumococcal	All adults	Should receive 1 dose of pneumococcal polysaccharide vaccine (PPSV23 [Pneumovax 23]) at age 65 years or older, at least 5 years after previous dose of PPSV23 (if administered prior to age 65).
	Adults 19–64 years who smoke tobacco or who have chronic heart disease (excluding hypertension), chronic lung disease, chronic liver disease, alcoholism, or diabetes mellitus	1 dose of 23-valent pneumococcal polysaccharide vaccine (PPSV23)
	All immunocompetent adults 65 years and older	Engage in shared clinical decision-making to see if 1 dose of pneumococcal conjugate vaccine (PCV13 [Prevnar 13]) would be appropriate. If both PCV13 and PPSV23 are to be given, PCV13 should be administered first, followed by PPSV23 at least 1 year after PCV13. If they received dose of PPSV23 prior to age 65, dose of PCV13 should be given at least 1 year after 1st dose of PPSV23 and dose of PPSV23 should be given at least 5 years after 1st dose of PPSV23.
	Adults 19 and older with immunocompromising conditions*	Administer 1 dose of PCV13 first and then dose of PPSV23 at least 8 weeks after dose of PCV13 and a second dose of PPSV23 5 years after 1st dose of PPSV23. At age 65 and older, administer one final dose of PPSV23 at least 5 years after previous dose of PPSV23 and at least 8 weeks after dose of PCV13. Only 1 dose of PPSV23 is recommended after age 65 years.
	Adults 19 and older with cerebrospinal fluid leak or cochlear implant	Administer 1 dose of PCV13 first and then dose of PPSV23 at least 8 weeks after the dose of PCV13. At age 65 and older, administer one final dose of PPSV23 at least 5 years after previous dose of PPSV23. Only 1 dose of PPSV23 is recommended after age 65 years.
Haemophilus influenza type B (HiB)	All children younger than 5 years old, unvaccinated older children and adults with certain medical conditions,* people who receive bone marrow transplant	Administer 1 dose of HiB at age 2, 4, 6 (per product) and 12–15 months with minimum of age 6 weeks. Children with one dose at age >15 months need no further doses. For high-risk conditions, children age 12–59 months who previously received 1 or no doses should receive two additional doses of HiB, 8 weeks apart. For children who received two doses before 12 months of age should receive one additional dose. Hib may be given to high-risk adults.

*B- or T- lymphocyte deficiency, complement deficiencies, phagocytic disorders (excluding chronic granulomatous disease), HIV infection, chronic renal failure, nephrotic syndrome, leukemia, lymphoma, Hodgkin disease, generalized malignancy, multiple myeloma, solid organ transplant, iatrogenic immunosuppression, anatomical or functional asplenia.

antibiotics in the past 90 days, and locally validated risk factors for MRSA or *P. aeruginosa*, cultures should be obtained. If managing non-severe PNA, only initiate appropriate coverage if cultures return positive or if rapid nasal polymerase chain reaction is positive for MRSA. If PNA is characterized as severe, then initiate empiric coverage, while awaiting culture results to help guide de-escalation of or continuation of therapy.

Hospital-Acquired Pneumonia
All patients with suspected HAP should be treated with broad spectrum antibiotics (see Table 4). Antibiotic choice should be governed by local antibiograms. The recommendations for further diagnostic testing, including cultures and PCR testing, were described in more detail in the diagnosis section. As described in Table 4, if the patient has risk factors for mortality or for MDR pathogens, then therapy with multiple agents is indicated. However, in selecting antimicrobial coverage, clinicians must weigh the benefit of initiating adequate coverage as soon as possible against the harms of uniform broad-spectrum coverage, such as increased resistance rates, risk of *Clostridium difficile* infection, and adverse drug effects. Whenever MRSA is suspected, treatment with vancomycin or linezolid (Zyvox) should be initiated; daptomycin (Cubicin) should not be used to treat pulmonary MRSA infection.

Prevention
Immunization against influenza, *S. pneumoniae*, and *H. influenza* is the best protection against bacterial PNA in adults and children. Recommended vaccine schedules are described in Table 5. In general, everyone should receive an annual influenza vaccine and individuals should receive *H. influenza* and pneumococcal immunization on a schedule based on age and risk factors. The pneumococcal vaccines have a 44% to 75% efficacy against invasive disease from *S. pneumoniae* for persons 65 and older and have been shown to be cost effective in populations aged 50 years and older. A systematic review demonstrated that the influenza vaccine effectively reduces PNA, hospital admission, and death. Annual influenza immunization is recommended as neuraminidase and hemagglutinin evolve rapidly, and new formulations targeting predicted strains are needed.

References
Centers for Disease Control and Prevention. FastStats - Pneumonia. https://www.cdc.gov/nchs/fastats/pneumonia.htm. Published 2017. Accessed March 10, 2018.

Kalil AC, Metersky ML, Klompas M, et al: Management of adults with hospital-acquired and ventilator-associated pneumonia: 2016 clinical practice guidelines by the infectious disease society of america and the american thoracic society, *Clin Infect Dis* 63(5):61–111, 2016, https://doi.org/10.1093/cid/ciw353.

Kaysin A, Viera AJ: Community- acquired pneumonia in adults: diagnosis and management, *Am Fam Physician* 94(9):698–706, 2016. http://www.aafp.org/afp/2016/1101/p698.html.

Jones RN: Microbial etiologies of hospital–acquired bacterial pneumonia and ventilator–associated bacterial pneumonia, *Clin Infect Dis* 51(S1):S81–S87, 2010, https://doi.org/10.1086/653053.

Mandell LA, Niederman MS: Aspiration pneumonia, *N Engl J Med* 380(7):651–663, 2019, https://doi.org/10.1056/NEJMra1714562.

Mandell LA, Wunderink RG, Anzueto A, et al: Thoracic society consensus guidelines on the management of community-acquired pneumonia in adults, *Clin Infect Dis* 44:S27–S72, 2007, https://doi.org/10.1086/511159.

Metlay JP, Waterer GW, et al: Diagnosis and treatment of adults with community-acquired pneumonia: an officialK clinical practice guideline of the american thoracic society and infectious diseases society of america, *Am J Respir Crit Care Med* 200(7):e45–e67, 2019. https://doi.org/10.1164/rccm.201908-1581ST.

Musher DM, Thorner AR: Community-acquired pneumonia, *N Engl J Med* 371(17):1619–1628, 2014. https://doi.org/10.1056/NEJMra1312885.

Wilson JW, Estes LL: *Mayo Clinic Antimicrobial Therapy: Quick Guide*, 2nd ed., 2012.

Centers for Disease Control and Prevention: *Immunization Schedules*, 2020. https://www.cdc.gov/vaccines/schedules/index.html.

BLASTOMYCOSIS

Method of
John M. Embil, MD; and Donald C. Vinh, MD

CURRENT DIAGNOSIS

- Blastomycosis is most commonly caused by the thermally dimorphic fungi *Blastomyces dermatitidis* and *gilchristii*, which together comprise the *B. dermatitidis* complex.
- *Blastomyces* spp. are endemic to the United States (southeastern and south central states bordering Mississippi and Ohio rivers; upper Midwestern states bordering the Great Lakes) and to Canada (Manitoba and Ontario bordering the Great Lakes; Quebec adjacent to St. Lawrence River).
- Blastomycosis should be suspected in the appropriate clinical context in patients who have resided or traveled to an endemic area.
- Blastomycosis has a broad range of manifestations, mimicking other infectious (e.g., bacteria, mycobacteria) and neoplastic processes.
- Blastomycosis may be asymptomatic, or it can manifest with disease involving the lung, skin, bone and joints, genitourinary system, or central nervous system.
- Diagnosis requires microscopic examination and/or culture of clinical specimens. Blastomyces antigen detection is also useful. Serology has no diagnostic value.

CURRENT THERAPY

- Treatment varies with the severity of disease.
- Long-term suppressive therapy may be required for those who are immunosuppressed.

The *Blastomyces dermatitidis* complex are the thermally dimorphic fungi that most commonly cause blastomycosis. Although novel *Blastomyces* species have been identified, they appear to be much less common than the *B. dermatitidis* complex; these new species have distinct mycological features and may produce atypical presentation of disease. *Blastomyces* spp. exist in mycelial form in the environment but grow as yeast forms at body temperature. Although the *B. dermatitidis* complex is endemic to certain specific regions within North America, numerous cases have been reported from areas where it is not considered endemic. It is presumed that those patients acquired infection in the endemic areas and subsequently presented outside of these geographic locations. However, it is also possible that the natural reservoirs of the fungus are evolving. The clinical manifestations of blastomycosis can be diverse, and therefore this infection should be suspected within the appropriate clinical context in persons with a history of residence or travel to such endemic areas.

Epidemiology

Our knowledge of the exact geographic distribution of *B. dermatitidis* complex is limited by the fact that the fungus cannot be readily recovered from nature; thus, identification of the endemic area has been largely derived from outbreak investigations and small case series. Most epidemiologic studies have depended upon recovery of *B. dermatitidis* in culture from clinical specimens or histologic visualization to establish the diagnosis. In addition, the incidence and prevalence of blastomycosis has been difficult to establish because suitable serologic or skin-prick assays (demonstrating acceptable sensitivity and/or specificity) to confirm infection are lacking. The geographic niche of *Blastomyces* spp. may therefore be greater than is currently believed.

The currently known areas of endemicity for *B. dermatitidis/gilchristii* are the south central and upper midwestern United States, including areas surrounding the Great Lakes. *B. dermatitidis* is also endemic in Wisconsin (1.3 cases per 100,000 population) and Mississippi (1.4 cases per 100,000 population), as well as parts of Missouri, Kentucky, Tennessee, Arkansas, and Alabama. In Canada, the major areas of endemnicity include the province of Manitoba (0.62 cases per 100,000 population), the southern region of Québec (0.46–0.79 cases per 100,000 population), and the Kenora region of the province of Ontario (7.11 cases per 100,000 population). Although most cases of blastomycosis are concentrated in these regions, it should be remembered that persons can acquire infection with *Blastomyces* spp. in these areas but present at a later time to health care providers in locations where blastomycosis is not usually observed. Inquiring about residence or travel to these areas is important to help establish the diagnosis.

Risk factors for acquiring blastomycosis have been defined by case reports, case series, and a small number of case-control studies and have not been conclusively established. Exposure while in endemic regions to soil, decaying wood, or to dust clouds generated by soil disruption is important; however, specific outdoor occupations or activities have not been confirmed. The fungus may also be associated with exposure to river waterways.

Race may be a contributing factor to disease. In one study from Mississippi, African-American race and prior history of pneumonia were independent risk factors for blastomycosis; however, neither environmental nor socioeconomic risk factors were detected. These findings were in contrast to previously noted studies where race and gender were not identified as specific risk factors for acquisition of blastomycosis. One study in Canada noted an increased incidence among the aboriginal population of Manitoba. Thus, it remains unclear if certain ethnic groups are at increased risk for disease or simply reflect differences in exposure.

Immunosuppression may also be an important risk factor, particularly for the tendency to develop severe disease. Blastomycosis has been reported in pregnant women, persons with diabetes mellitus, organ transplant recipients, and persons infected with HIV.

Dogs and humans are the species most commonly affected by *B. dermatitidis* complex. Anecdotally, dogs can serve as a sentinel marker for human disease (i.e., dogs present with systemic infection before their owners), leading to early suspicion of human infections by astute veterinarians. In such cases, it is speculated that humans and their pet dogs have a simultaneous exposure to the same source of fungus and therefore develop synchronous infection. This hypothesis, however, remains to be confirmed, and in a more recent study, canine blastomycosis was not deemed to predict human disease among the human owners. Additional studies are required to establish the relationship between blastomycosis in humans and disease in their pet dogs.

The most common mode of transmission is presumed to be by inhalation of aerosolized conidia from the environment. There are, however, reports of cutaneous blastomycosis occuring after accidental cutaneous inoculation, for example in the laboratory setting during autopsy or after dog bites. The median incubation period, established by reviewing the results of point-source outbreaks, ranges from 30 to 45 days.

Pathophysiology

Following inhalation of conidia into the lungs, the fungus is phagocytosed by alveolar macrophages. The human body temperature allows the fungus to transform to the yeast phase. It is speculated that a process similar to infection with *Mycobacterium tuberculosis* then occurs. The fungus might spread to other organs via the bloodstream and lymphatics. The primary defense against *B. dermatitidis* is through a suppurative response initially with neutrophils, followed by influx of monocytes with establishment of cell mediated immunity, resulting in noncaseating granuloma. The patient with intact immunologic responses can contain the process without progression to clinical disease. Alternatively, the patient can develop a symptomatic pneumonia and then mount a suitable immunologic response and recover. Impaired immunity favors the development of progressive pulmonary disease with or without extrapulmonary manifestations.

It has also been suggested that reactivation of disease can occur at pulmonary or extrapulmonary sites. The pathophysiology of *B. gilchristii* is thought to be similar to that of *B. dermatitidis*. A vaccine that protects humans against infection with *Blastomyces* spp. is unavailable.

Clinical Manifestations

After inhalation of the conidia, an initial infection can occur. Most primary infections (at least 50%) are asymptomatic or mild and usually go unrecognized, resolving spontaneously. In others, a symptomatic pneumonia can develop; recovery can occur either spontaneously or with therapy, without further progression. Some persons develop progressive pneumonia or extrapulmonary manifestations. The type of clinical manifestations (localized, extrapulmonary or disseminated disease) can have a seasonal variation: Persons with manifestations occurring early after exposure (1–6 months) developed localized pneumonia, whereas those who presented later after exposure (4–9 months) tended to have isolated extrapulmonary or disseminated disease. Blastomycosis has been termed "the great mimic," because its clinical manifestations are nonspecific and can be similar to those of many different clinical entities. The most common organ systems involved in blastomycosis, in descending order of frequency, include lung, skin, bone, genitourinary, and central nervous systems (CNS). Box 1 summarizes the key clinical manifestations of blastomycosis.

BOX 1 | Clinical Manifestations of Blastomycosis

Lung

Acute Pneumonia

Acute pneumonia is clinically indistinguishable from bacterial pneumonia.

Patients may present with fevers, chills, dyspnea, and cough, which initially might not be productive but, with time, may be accompanied by sputum production.

Radiographic findings can also be difficult to discern from those due to a bacterial pneumonia.

The radiographic pattern of pulmonary blastomycosis includes the following:

- Lobar infiltrates that mimic bacterial pneumonias
- Cavitary lung lesions and miliary patterns, which can mimic tuberculosis
- Mass lesions that may be mistaken for neoplasms
- Cystic lesions that resemble abscesses

There is no definitive plain radiograph or computed tomographic scan findings characteristic of pulmonary blastomycosis.

The spectrum of clinical pulmonary disease ranges from spontaneous resolution to pneumonia, with or without the acute respiratory distress syndrome; the latter is accompanied by high (50%–89%) mortality rates.

Chronic Pneumonia

A nonresolving pneumonia is one of the hallmarks of pulmonary blastomycosis.

Chronic pneumonia may be associated with fever, chills, weight loss, sputum-producing cough, and hemoptysis.

There is no characteristic radiographic appearance to help establish the diagnosis.

Skin

Cutaneous lesions are the most common extrapulmonary manifestations of blastomycosis. Lesions usually result from dissemination of a primary pulmonary lesion or rarely from direct inoculation.

Lesions can have a number of different appearances, with verrucae (wartlike lesions) and ulcers being the most common

manifestations. The verrucous lesions have a heaped-up appearance with a raw excoriated center. These lesions can mimic squamous cell carcinomas. Cutaneous abscesses may be associated with these lesions.

Ulcerative lesions initially manifest as pustules that eventually erode, producing a bed of granulation tissue that is friable and bleeds when traumatized. Other skin lesions include subcutaneous nodules and isolated abscesses.

Bone and Joint

The most common manifestation of extrapulmonary blastomycosis, after cutaneous disease, is involvement of bones and joints.

Any bone may be involved, although the long bones and axial skeleton are the most commonly affected.

The radiographic findings are indistinguishable from bacterial osteomyelitis and arthritis.

Genitourinary Tract

In the genitourinary tract, the prostate has been reported to be commonly affected by blastomycosis.

Symptoms can mimic prostatitis, and patients can present with obstructive uropathy.

Central Nervous System

The CNS is infrequently affected by *B. dermatitidis*. Infection may occur in isolation or with concomitant non-CNS infection.

CNS blastomycosis can occur in immunocompromised patients (e.g., HIV, solid organ transplant), as well as in patients with little/no risk factors (e.g., diabetes mellitus alone; persons with no underlying co-morbidities).

Clinical manifestations depend on the area of involvement and range from focal neurologic findings (e.g., due to mass lesions in the brain parenchyma) to symptoms of meningitis due to involvement of the meninges.

Radiographically, the findings may be indistinguishable from bacterial processes. Other sites of involvement have been described but are infrequent compared to those summarized above.

Blastomycosis in Special Populations

Children account for a small percentage of the cases of blastomycosis, ranging from 2% to 11%. Children demonstrate a similar spectrum of manifestations as in adults (excluding prostatic disease). The most common symptoms include cough, headache, chest pain, weight loss, fever, abdominal pain, and night sweats. It is postulated that children experience disseminated infection more frequently than do adults.

Although there are few published reports of blastomycosis in pregnancy, disease has been observed in pregnant women, with presumed subsequent intrauterine and perinatal transmission.

Blastomycosis has been reported in persons with advanced HIV and among those who have undergone solid organ transplants. In immunocompromised hosts, it appears that a significant percentage developed rapidly progressive pulmonary disease, leading to respiratory failure and death. For those who are immunocompromised, the reported mortality rate range is 30% to 40%, with death occurring within the first few weeks of disease onset.

Diagnosis

The most reliable technique for confirming the diagnosis of blastomycosis is recovery of the fungus in culture. Alternatively, direct observation of the pathogen by light microscopy or with calcofluor white stain or in histopathologic examination of tissue establishes a presumptive diagnosis. *Blastomyces* spp. are characteristically observed as a thick-walled, broad-based budding yeast. Because colonization does not occur, identification of *B. dermatitidis/gilchristii* should never be considered a contaminant. Serologic assays are extremely variable in their sensitivity and specificity and do not play a role in confirming or excluding the diagnosis, thus limiting their value in therapeutic decision making. A reliable skin test is unavailable, but a urinary antigen detection assay exists that may aid in diagnosis and may be of benefit to follow the efficacy of treatment in established infections. Box 2 summarizes techniques for establishing the diagnosis of blastomycosis.

Treatment

The treatment recommendations for blastomycosis from the Infectious Diseases Society of America (IDSA) are summarized in Table 1. Amphotericin B deoxycholate (Fungizone) is the agent with which there is the greatest experience, particularly for the treatment of patients with severe blastomycosis or for those who have CNS involvement. Lipid preparations of amphotericin B (Abelect, Amphotec, AmBisome)[1] have been shown to be effective in animal models, although clinical trial data are unavailable for these agents in humans. Clinical experience suggests that the lipid formulations are as effective but less toxic than the deoxycholate preparation.

It is generally accepted that in patients with severe disease or CNS involvement, amphotericin B-based products should be used to initiate therapy until the patient is stable, followed by step-down to an azole, specifically itraconazole (Sporanox), to complete the total duration of therapy. Patients on itraconazole should have serum levels of the antifungal drug measured after at least 2 weeks of therapy, targeting a level >1.0mcg/mL and <10.0mcg/mL. Ketoconazole (Nizoral), although once recommended as the agent of choice, is less effective and more toxic than itraconazole. Experience with fluconazole (Diflucan)[1] for the treatment of blastomycosis is limited, although *in vitro* studies have demonstrated that fluconazole is effective against *B. dermatitidis*. Fluconazole does, however, have excellent penetration into the CNS; therefore, fluconazole may be considered as an alternative treatment of CNS blastomycosis. There are also a number of reports of voriconazole (Vfend)[1] being used for the

[1] Not FDA approved for this indication.

successful treatment of CNS blastomycosis, as well as in persons with refractory blastomycosis. A case series of patients with CNS blastomycosis suggested that voriconazole may be the most desirable azole for the management of CNS disease. Similarly, there

| | TREATMENT RECOMMENDATIONS | | |
MANIFESTATION	PRIMARY RECOMMENDATION	ALTERNATIVE RECOMMENDATION	COMMENTS
Pulmonary Infection			
Mild to moderate	Itraconazole (Sporanox) 200mg PO tid × 3 days, then qd or bid × 6–12mo	Fluconazole (Diflucan)[1] 400–800[3] mg/day or ketoconazole (Nizoral) 400–800mg/kg × 6–12mo	For Itraconazole, measure serum levels after at least 2 weeks, to ensure adequate drug exposure. Target level: >1.0mcg/mL and <10.0mcg/mL
Moderate to severe	Lipid formulation of amphotericin B (AmBisome, Abelect, Amphotec)[1] 3–5mg/kg/day OR Amphotericin B deoxycholate (Fungizone) 0.7–1mg/kg/d for 1–2wk or until improvement, followed by itraconazole 200mg PO tid × 3 days then 200mg PO bid × 6–12mo		Amphotericin B toxicity can be attenuated by minimizing the duration of therapy and switching to oral therapy when the patient is stable For Itraconazole, measure serum levels after at least 2 weeks, to ensure adequate drug exposure. Target level: >1.0mcg/mL and <10.0mcg/mL
Disseminated Infection Not Involving the Central Nervous System			
Mild to moderate	Itraconazole 200mg PO tid × 3 days then qd or bid × 6–12mo		
Moderate to severe	Lipid formulation of amphotericin B 3–5mg/kg/d OR Amphotericin B deoxycholate 0.7–1mg/kg/d for 1–2wk or until improvement, followed by Itraconazole 200mg PO tid × 3 days then 200mg PO bid to complete at least 12mo		To minimize toxicity, switching to oral therapy once the patient is stable should be considered Bone and joint infections are usually treated for at least 12mo with itraconazole For Itraconazole, measure serum levels after at least 2 weeks, to ensure adequate drug exposure. Target level: >1.0mcg/mL and <10.0mcg/mL
Central Nervous System Involvement (with or without other manifestations)			
	Lipid preparations of amphotericin B[1] 5mg/kg/d × 4–6wk followed by an oral azole for ≥12mo		It has been suggested that liposomal amphotericin B achieves higher CNS levels than other lipid formulations When switching to oral azole, options include fluconazole[1] 800mg PO qd,[3] itraconazole 200mg PO bid or tid,[3] or voriconazole (Vfend)[1] 200–400[3] mg PO bid Longer durations of therapy may be necessary in the immunocompromised host
Special Populations			
Immunocompromised	Lipid formulation of amphotericin B 3–5mg/kg/d OR Amphotericin B deoxycholate 0.7–1mg/kg/d for 1–2wk or until improvement, followed by Itraconazole 200mg PO tid×3 days then 200mg PO bid to complete at least 12mo		Lifelong suppression with itraconazole 200mg PO qd may be required for those in whom immunosuppression cannot be reversed
Pregnant patients	Lipid formulation of amphotericin B 3–5mg/kg/d		No duration of lipid formulation amphotericin B treatment provided; continue until clinical cure During pregnancy, azoles should be avoided because of potential teratogenicity If the placenta or newborn demonstrates evidence of infection, give amphotericin B deoxycholate 1.0mg/kg/d
Children: mild to moderate	Itraconazole[1] 10mg/kg/d for 6–12mo		Maximum dose of itraconazole should be 400mg/d
Children: moderate to severe	Amphotericin B deoxycholate 0.7–10.0mg/kg/d OR Lipid formulation amphotericin B 3–5mg/kg/d × 1–2wk followed by itraconazole 10mg/kg/d × 12mo		

Modified from Chapman SW, Bradsher RW, Campbell GD, et al: Practice guidelines for the management of patients with blastomycosis. Clin Infect Dis 2000;30:679; and Chapman SW, Dismukes WE, Proia LA, et al: Clinical practice guidelines for the management of blastomycosis: 2008 update by the Infectious Diseases Society of America. Clin Infect Dis 2008;46:1801–12.
[1]Not FDA approved for this indication.
[3]Exceeds dosage recommended by the manufacturer.

are reports on the successful use of posaconazole (Noxafil)[1] and isavuconazole (Cresemba)[1] for blastomycosis. The echinocandins (caspofungin [Cancidas],[1] micafungin [Mycamine],[1] and anidulafungin [Eraxis][1]) have limited activity against *B. dermatitidis* and are not considered appropriate choices.

Table 1 summarizes the therapeutic options for treatment of various types of blastomycosis. Amphotericin B-based therapy is usually the treatment option of choice in persons who have severe disease. Whenever the patient is clinically stable, it is desirable to switch from the potentially toxic amphotericin B to a less-toxic agent (usually an azole). It is important to note that amphotericin B in cumulative doses of 1.5 to 2.5 grams for persons with disseminated blastomycosis, with life-threatening disease, or in those who are immunocompromised or pregnant, can lead to cure without relapses.

In patients with overwhelming pulmonary disease, amphotericin B-based products are the therapeutic agents of choice. Although acute respiratory distress syndrome (ARDS) can complicate the management of these patients, data on the beneficial role of corticosteroids in the management of patients with overwhelming pulmonary disease or ARDS are limited to few case reports. For patients with less-severe pulmonary disease, an alternative to amphotericin B is a 6- to 12-month course of oral itraconazole. A similarly prolonged course of oral itraconazole is also appropriate for persons with bone and joint disease. The precise duration of therapy, however, is unknown and should be individualized. The same is true for cutaneous blastomycosis. For persons with CNS blastomycosis, an initial treatment course of 4 to 6 weeks with intravenous lipid formulation of amphotericin B should be followed with an oral azole to complete at least 12 months of therapy. For those who are immunocompromised, prolonged therapy is also necessary. Patients who are immunosuppressed and in whom the immunosuppression cannot be reversed can require lifelong suppressive itraconazole therapy at 200 mg per day. Additional details for the management of the various stages of blastomycosis should be sought from the most current version of the IDSA guidelines.

References

Bariola JR, Perry P, Pappas PG, et al: Blastomycosis of the central nervous system: a multicenter review of diagnosis and treatment in the modern era, *Clin Infect Dis* 50:797–804, 2010.

Bush JW, Wuerz T, Embil JM, Del Bigio MR, McDonald PJ, Krawitz S: Outcomes of persons with blastomycosis involving the central nervous system, *Diagn Microbiol Infect Dis* 76(2):175–181, 2013.

Chapman SW, Sullivan DC: Blastomyces dermatitidis. In Mandell GL, Bennett JE, Dolin R, editors: *Mandell, Douglas, and Bennett's Principles and Practice of Infectious Diseases*, 7th ed., Philadelphia, 2010, Elsevier, pp 3319–3332.

Chapman SW, Lin AC, Hendricks KA, et al: Endemic blastomycosis in Mississippi: Epidemiological and clinical studies, *Semin Respir Infect* 12:219–228, 1997.

Chapman SW, Dismukes WE, Proia LA, et al: Clinical practice guidelines for the management of blastomycosis: 2008 update by the Infectious Diseases Society of America, *Clin Infect Dis* 46:1801–1812, 2008.

Choptiany M, Wiebe L, Limerick B, et al: Risk factors for acquisition of endemic blastomycosis, *Can J Infect Dis Med Microbiol* 20:117–121, 2009.

Crampton TL, Light RB, Berg GM, et al: Epidemiology and clinical spectrum of blastomycosis diagnosed at Manitoba hospitals, *Clin Infect Dis* 34:1310–1316, 2002.

Litvinov IV, St-Germain G, Pelletier R, Paradis M, Sheppard DC: Endemic human blastomycosis in Quebec, Canada, 1988–2011, *Epidemiol Infect* 141(6):1143–1147, 2013.

Martynowicz MA, Prakash UBS: Pulmonary blastomycosis: An appraisal of diagnostic techniques, *Chest* 121:768–773, 2002.

Meyer KC, McManus EJ, Maki DG: Overwhelming pulmonary blastomycosis associated with the adult respiratory distress syndrome, *N Engl J Med* 329:1231–1236, 1993.

Oppenheimer M, Cheang M, Trepman E, et al: Orthopedic manifestations of blastomycosis, *South Med J* 100:570–578, 2007.

Pappas PG: Blastomycosis in the immunocompromised patient, *Semin Respir Infect* 12:243–251, 1997.

Ward BA, Parent AD, Raila F: Indications for the surgical management of central nervous system blastomycosis, *Surg Neurol* 43:379–388, 1995.

CHRONIC OBSTRUCTIVE PULMONARY DISEASE

Method of
Paresh J. Timbadia, MD; J. Barry Fagan, MD

CURRENT DIAGNOSIS

- Chronic obstructive pulmonary disease (COPD) is a treatable, though not curable, disease.
- Smoking is the most common risk factor for COPD worldwide.
- Sixteen million Americans are diagnosed with COPD. An additional 11 million Americans have COPD but have not been diagnosed.
- Alpha 1 antitrypsin deficiency occurs in 1 in every 1500 to 3000 individuals of European ancestry and is treatable by alpha-1 antitrypsin augmentation.
- Dyspnea, cough, and sputum production are common presenting complaints.
- Examination may reveal use of accessory muscles of ventilation, increased AP diameter, diminished breath sounds, wheezing, rhonchi, or crackles.
- Spirometry is the cornerstone of the diagnosis of COPD. COPD is defined by a reduction in the forced expiratory volume in 1 second/forced vital capacity (FEV_1/FVC).
- The severity of COPD is defined by the FEV_1 percent of predicted; mild (stage 1) FEV_1 >79%; moderate (stage 2) FEV_1 50% to 79%; severe (stage 3) FEV_1 30% to 49%; very severe (stage 4) FEV_1 <30%.

CURRENT THERAPY

- Smoking cessation is the cornerstone of COPD management. Counseling and pharmacotherapy improve quit rates.
- Patients with COPD should receive pneumococcal, influenza, and COVID vaccines.
- Pulmonary rehabilitation improves activity capacity and quality of life and decreases dyspnea and hospitalization.
- Supplemental oxygen is used for resting, nocturnal, or exertional hypoxemia. Supplemental oxygen use prolongs life in those with resting hypoxemia (SpO2 <89%).
- Pharmacotherapy can improve symptoms and decrease exacerbation rate.
- Proper inhaler technique is necessary for maximal benefit from inhaled medications.
- Short-acting beta agonists are appropriate for mild, intermittent symptoms.
- A long-acting beta agonist (LABA), long-acting antimuscarinic (LAMA), or both may be added in patients with more frequent or severe dyspnea.
- Inhaled corticosteroids can decrease exacerbation frequency.
- Attention should be paid to management of retained secretions.
- Noninvasive ventilation can decrease hypercapnia and dyspnea in patients with chronic hypercapnic respiratory failure.
- A selected group of patients with severe disease may benefit from endobronchial valve treatment or surgical interventions, such as lung volume reduction surgery or lung transplantation.
- Exacerbations of COPD in outpatients may be managed with increased frequency of short-acting bronchodilators, systemic corticosteroids, and antibiotics.
- Palliative care is appropriate for patients with severe, refractory symptoms.

Epidemiology

Over 16 million Americans have chronic obstructive pulmonary disease (COPD), but including those undiagnosed, the number may be as high as 24 million. In 2018, overall age-adjusted prevalence of COPD in the United States was 6.6%. The exact prevalence of COPD worldwide is largely unknown, but estimates vary from 7% to 19%. The medical cost of COPD increased to 49 billion in 2020 from 32 billion in 2010. COPD is the fourth leading cause of death in the United States, and third leading cause of death worldwide, causing 3.23 million deaths in 2019. The COPD death rate among men decreased 25% from 57.4 per 100,000 population in 1999 to 42.9 per 100,000 in 2018, while the rate among women has remained relatively stable over this period.

Risk Factors

Smoking is the leading risk factor for COPD in the United States and around the world. In 2018, 13.7% of American adults over age 18 are smokers (15.6% of men and 12% of women), which is approximately 34.2 million people. Globally, some 8 million people use the burning of biomass fuels or coal as their main source of energy for both cooking and heating. This indoor pollution is a significant risk factor for COPD in nonsmoking women and children in the Middle East, Africa, and Asia, and it is estimated to kill 2 million women and children each year. Occupational dusts and chemicals are additional risk factors. Alpha-1 antitrypsin (A1A) deficiency is an important genetic risk factor for COPD. A1A occurs in 1 in every 1500 to 3000 individuals of European ancestry but is less common in Asian and black populations. The metalloproteinase 12 gene is associated with decline in lung function; the relationship between other genes and reduction in lung function is less well understood. It appears that women are more susceptible to the effects of cigarette smoke than men. Other factors possibly playing a role in COPD development include childhood respiratory infections, asthma, and low socioeconomic status.

Pathophysiology

COPD is an inflammatory lung disease caused by an imbalance between proinflammatory cytokines, enzymes, and effector cells, and the pulmonary defense mechanisms. An increase is seen in the number of proinflammatory cells, including circulating neutrophils and CD8 T lymphocytes as well as the number of macrophages in bronchial mucosa. CD8+ cells have the potential to release tumor necrosis factor α, perforins, and granzymes, though the exact role of T lymphocytes in COPD remains unclear. Neutrophils produce proteases, which have the potential to cause alveolar destruction, elastase destruction, and mucus hypersecretion. Macrophages produce proteases and a variety of inflammatory mediators. Cigarette smoke promotes the release of these proinflammatory mediators and also inactivates several antiproteases, causing an inflammation/anti-inflammation imbalance. This imbalance causes a cycle of injury and repair which results in permanent damage to airways, lung parenchyma, and vasculature. The airways become narrowed by increased numbers of goblet cells, increased size of submucosal glands, mucosal thickening, collagen deposition, ciliary dysfunction (promoting retention of secretions within the airway), and destruction of alveolar walls and alveolar support. Loss of pulmonary vascular bed, vascular remodeling, and arterial vasoconstriction lead to hypoxemia from ventilation perfusion mismatch and pulmonary hypertension.

Airway obstruction results in air trapping, hyperinflation, and flattening of the diaphragms. As the diaphragms flatten, the patient requires the use of accessory muscles of ventilation to move air. Airway narrowing or collapse increases the resistance to airflow, increasing the work of breathing and resulting in dyspnea. Lung compliance is decreased at high lung volumes, so breathing at high lung volumes due to hyperinflation also results in dyspnea. Work of breathing is increased at rest in COPD and increases exponentially with activity. Dyspnea often leads to the vicious cycle of decreased activity, deconditioning, and progressive disability.

Diagnosis

Most patients with COPD present to their provider with complaints of dyspnea, cough, and sputum production, or decreased activity capacity. This presentation may be relatively late in the disease course. Many smokers accept their cough as a "smoker's cough." Nonsmokers have a large ventilatory reserve; we breathe about 5 L/min, but our maximum ventilatory volume is approximately 180 L/min. Because of this, especially if the patient is sedentary, they may not notice dyspnea until there has been considerable loss of pulmonary function.

The diagnosis of COPD should be considered in all patients with dyspnea, cough, sputum production, or exposure to risk factors. A careful history should include questions regarding quantity and duration of smoking and exposure to passive smoking or other occupational or environmental exposures. The patient should be asked about activity capacity; activities resulting in dyspnea, cough, and mucus production; and ease or difficulty clearing secretions. The input from a family member or friend is valuable in that the patient may have become desensitized to dyspnea. On observation, the patient may be found in the "tripod" position, resting arms on a surface elevating the clavicles, which places the accessory muscles of ventilation at better mechanical advantage. (This is why patients will often relate that they can walk farther while using a shopping cart, "tripoding" on the cart's handles.) Patients may be observed to be pursed lip breathing, exhaling through pursed lips, elevating the pressure in the airways, stenting them open, and allowing a fuller expiration, decreasing air trapping and hyperinflation. Percussion may reveal evidence of hyperinflation. Auscultation may reveal wheezing or prolonged expiration resulting from airway obstruction, as well as rhonchi from retained secretions in the airways. Normal breath sounds originate in the terminal airways, and emphysematous destruction of these airways results in diminished breath sounds. Emphysema results in increased compliance of the lung, which raises the closing volume (the volume of air within the lung at which airways close). The closing volume may rise above functional residual capacity (the normal end-expiratory volume) causing inspiratory crackles.

Spirometry is the cornerstone of diagnosis of COPD. Airway obstruction is defined by a forced expiratory volume in one second (FEV_1)/forced vital capacity (FVC) of <70%. Patients with airway obstruction may be able to exhale much of their vital capacity (VC), but because of airways narrowing, they cannot do it very quickly, resulting in the low ratio. The degree of obstruction is defined by the FEV_1 percent of predicted value (Table 1). It is recommended that an A1A be obtained in all patients diagnosed with COPD. It is important to note that A1A is an acute-phase reactant and can be elevated during an exacerbation of COPD; it is therefore best to obtain when the patient is clinically stable.

Differential Diagnosis

COPD may be confused with other obstructive airway diseases, most notably asthma. Asthma will most often present at a younger age, though it may be diagnosed during any decade of life. Asthmatics generally have more reversibility and less fixed obstruction, but overlap is seen. Both may have hyperinflation and reduction in forced expiratory flows on pulmonary function

TABLE 1	Chronic Obstructive Pulmonary Disease Staging
SEVERITY	**SPIROMETRY**
Stage I: mild	FEV_1/FVC <70%
	FEV_1 >80%
Stage II: moderate	FEV_1/FVC <70%
	50% ≤FEV_1 <80%
Stage III: severe	FEV_1/FVC <70%
	30% ≤FEV_1 <50%
Stage IV: very severe	FEV_1/FVC <70%
	FEV_1 <30%

FEV_1, forced expiratory volume in 1 second; FVC, forced vital capacity.

TABLE 2 — Smoking Cessation Medications

MEDICATION	DOSAGE AND ADMINISTRATION
Nicotine Transdermal (NicoDerm CQ)	21 mg/24 hours, 14 mg/24 hours, 7 mg/24 hours If >10 cigarettes/D, then use 21 mg/D for 6 weeks, then 14 mg/D for 2 weeks, then 7 mg/D for 2 weeks. If ≤10 cigarettes/D, then use 14 mg/D for 6 weeks, then 7 mg/D for 2 weeks
Nicotine lozenges (Nicorette)	4 mg, 2 mg weeks 1–6, 1 lozenge every 1–2 hours, weeks 7–9 1 lozenge every 2–4 hours, weeks 10–12, 1 lozenge every 4–8 hours
Nicotine gum (Nicorelief, Thrive)	4 mg, 2 mg weeks 1–6, 1 gum every 1–2 hours, weeks 7–9 1 gum every 2–4 hours, weeks 10–12, 1 gum every 4–8 hours
Nicotine inhaler (Nicotrol)	10 mg/cartridge up to 12 weeks, 6–16 cartridges/day up to 12 weeks (if necessary), gradual reduction
Nicotine nasal spray (Nicotrol NS)	0.5 mg/spray each nostril, beginning 1–2/hour, maximum 10/hour, maximum 80 sprays/day up to 8 weeks, then taper up to 6 weeks
Bupropion hydrochloride SR (Zyban)	150 mg per day, first 3 days, then 150 mg bid
Varenicline (Chantix)	Day 1–3, 0.5 mg q day, day 4–7, 0.5 mg bid, day 8–end of treatment, 1 mg bid. Patients who quit at 12 weeks may be treated an additional 12 weeks.

testing, but a reduction in diffusing capacity would be more characteristic of COPD. Exhaled NO will more often be elevated in asthma. Eosinophils are characteristically elevated in the sputum blood and BAL fluid in asthmatics, whereas neutrophils are more commonly elevated in patients with COPD. Considerable overlap occurs in each of these areas. There are a small percentage of patients where COPD and asthma cannot be differentiated; this is called the "overlap syndrome."

Treatment of Stable Chronic Obstructive Pulmonary Disease
The goals of treatment of COPD include improving quality of life, decreasing dyspnea, increasing activity capacity, preventing and treating complications and exacerbations, and prolonging life.

Smoking Cessation
Smoking cessation is the cornerstone of management of COPD. Stopping smoking, along with supplemental oxygen in patients with severe chronic hypoxemia, are the only two interventions that prolong life in patients with COPD. During each clinical interaction with a patient who smokes, it is appropriate to *ask* about their smoking status, *advise* all smokers to quit, *assess* the willingness of the patient to quit, *assist* the patient in quitting, and *arrange* a follow-up visit. Brief counseling alone can improve quit rate. In those patients who express a willingness to attempt to quit, adding pharmacotherapy to counseling is appropriate. Considerations for pharmacotherapy include nicotine replacement therapy, bupropion (Zyban), and varenicline (Chantix) (Table 2). E-cigarettes are not currently recommended to assist with smoking cessation.

Pulmonary Rehabilitation
Pulmonary rehabilitation programs are widely available and can be defined as multidisciplinary programs, which seek to improve the quality of life for patients with COPD or other lung diseases.

Programs vary in content but will always include an exercise and an educational component, supervised by a respiratory therapist. They often meet 2 or 3 times weekly and last about 4 to 12 weeks. The educational component includes information on the disease state, medications used to manage COPD, energy-conserving techniques such as pacing activities, breathing techniques such as pursed-lip breathing, and what steps to take during an exacerbation. Programs may include nutritional advice, smoking cessation education, or psychosocial counseling. The exercise component is tailored to the individual patient and often includes treadmill or stationary bicycle exercise, light weights, arm ergometry, and stretching. Programs stress the importance of maintaining exercise following completion of the program and may offer a phase 3 component for continued exercise. Pulmonary rehabilitation has many proven benefits, including decreased dyspnea, improved quality of life, improved activity capacity, and decreased hospitalization. Pulmonary rehabilitation may be offered to any COPD patient with symptoms of or high risk for exacerbation.

Vaccinations
Annual influenza vaccines are recommended for all patients with COPD. Polysaccharide pneumococcal vaccine (PPSV23 [Pneumovax 23]) are recommended for all patients who smoke and/or have COPD with a repeat dose given 5 years after the first dose. At age 65, pneumococcal conjugate vaccine (PCV13 [Prevnar 13]) is given, since it is more important for those that are immunocompromised, which happens with more advance age. Patients with COPD are at high risk for COVID-19 infection and poor outcomes. COVID-19 vaccination is recommended for all patients with COPD.

Medications
Commonly used medications for the treatment of stable COPD are listed in Table 3. The beta-agonists stimulate beta 2 receptors on airway smooth muscle, causing muscle relaxation and bronchodilation. The short-acting beta-agonists have onset of action in 1 to 3 minutes and duration of action 4 to 6 hours. Because of their quick onset and short duration of action, they are used as "rescue" or prn medications. Some long-acting beta-agonists (e.g., *Formoterol*) also have rapid onset of action, but the duration of action is 12 to 24 hours. Potential side effects of beta-agonists include tremor, tachycardia, and, uncommonly, hypokalemia.

The antimuscarinic bronchodilators bind to muscarinic receptors, which are found on smooth muscle and submucosal glands. Two of these receptors, the M1 and M3 receptors, facilitate acetylcholine transmission which results in bronchoconstriction. Potential side effects of the antimuscarinics include dry mouth and urinary hesitancy. The beta-agonists and antimuscarinics have additive effects on bronchial smooth muscle. Inhaled corticosteroids decrease airway inflammation and have been shown to decrease the frequency of exacerbation of COPD. Unlike asthma, inhaled corticosteroids are not used as sole maintenance therapy in COPD. Potential side effects of the inhaled corticosteroids include a small increase in risk of pneumonia and oral candidiasis. There are now many varieties of inhaler devices. Instruction in the use of the devices and observation of proper technique is necessary to ensure maximal benefit.

In the 2021 Global Initiative for Chronic Obstructive Lung Disease (GOLD) guidelines (Figure 1) (https://www.guidelines.co.uk/respiratory/gold-copd-2021-strategy/45088.article), medication recommendations are dictated by a classification system based on symptom score and exacerbation history. Patients are categorized as having either zero or one exacerbation, not requiring hospitalization, or two or more exacerbations, or at least one exacerbation requiring hospitalization. Symptom severity is based on a symptom scoring scale, such as the Modified British Medical Research Council (mMRC) Dyspnea Scale (Table 4) (https://www.mdcalc.com/mmrc-modified-medical-research-council-dyspnea-scale) and COPD Assessment Test (CAT) (Table 5) (https://www.mdcalc.com/copd-assessment-test-cat). On the CAT, the patient is asked a series of 8 questions,

TABLE 3 Commonly Used Inhaled Medications for Stable COPD

MEDICATION	DOSAGE
Short-acting beta-2 agonist (SABA)	
Albuterol (multiple brands)	2 puffs q 4–6 hours, prn
Levalbuterol (Xopenex)	1–2 puffs q 4–6 hours prn
Ipratropium (Atrovent)	2 inhalations 4 times a day
Albuterol/ipratropium (Combivent Respimat)	1 inhalation 4 times a day
Long-acting beta-2 agonist (LABA):	
Salmeterol (Serevent Diskus)	1 inhalation twice daily
Indacaterol (Arcapta Neohaler)	Inhale contents of one capsule q day
Olodaterol (Striverdi Respimat)	2 puffs once a day, same time of day
Arformoterol (Brovana)	2 mL nebulized twice daily
Formoterol (Perforomist)	2 mL nebulized twice daily
Long-acting antimuscarinic agent (LAMA):	
Tiotropium (Spiriva Handihaler)	2 inhalations of the powder contents of a single Spiriva capsule once daily
Tiotropium (Spiriva Respimat)	2 inhalations once daily
Aclidinium (Tudorza Pressair)	1 inhalation twice daily
Umeclidinium (Incruse Ellipta)	1 inhalation daily
Glycopyrronium Bromide (Seebri Neohaler)	1 capsule inhaled twice daily
Glycopyrrolate (Lonhala Magnair)	1 vial inhaled twice daily
Revefenacin (Yupelri)	1 vial nebulized once daily
Combination medications:	
LABA/LAMA	
Umeclidinium/vilanterol (Anoro Ellipta)	1 inhalation once daily
Olodaterol/tiotropium (Stiolto Respimat)	2 inhalations once daily
Formoterol/glycopyrrolate (Bevespi Aerosphere)	2 inhalations twice daily
Aclidinium/formoterol (Duaklir Pressair)	1 inhalation twice daily
ICS/LABA	
Budesonide/formoterol (Symbicort 160/4.5, 80/4.5)	2 inhalations twice daily
Fluticasone/salmeterol (Advair Diskus 100/50, 250/50, 500/50; Wixela Inhub and AirDuo) (Advair HFA 45/21, 115/21, 230/21)	1 inhalation twice daily 2 inhalations twice daily
Mometasone/formoterol (Dulera 100/5, 200/5)[1]	2 inhalations twice daily
Fluticasone/vilanterol (Breo Ellipta 100/25, 200/25)	1 inhalation once daily
LABA/LAMA/ICS	
Fluticasone/umeclidinium/vilanterol (Trelegy Ellipta 200/62.5,25, 100/62.5/25)	1 inhalation once daily
Budesonide/glycopyrrolate/formoterol (Breztri Aerosphere 160/9/4.8)	2 inhalations twice daily

[1]Not FDA approved for this indication.

grading severity as 0 to 5. The sum of the scores is used to categorize the patient in the GOLD classification grid.

Patients in group A are given a trial of short- or long-acting bronchodilator. The medication is continued if the patient is determined to have benefited from the intervention. Group B patients should be started on a long-acting bronchodilator, either LABA or LAMA. If the patient has continued dyspnea, LAMA and LABA may be used together. For patients with severe dyspnea, treatment may begin with both agents. Initial therapy for group C patients is a LAMA. For patients with persisting exacerbations, adding a LABA is the primary choice. Adding an ICS would be a secondary choice. Recommended initial treatment for group D patients is a LABA/LAMA combination. Consideration could be given to initiating treatment with a LABA/ICS combination, in patients with prominent asthmatic symptoms or an eosinophil count ≥300 cells/microliter. Patients with continuing exacerbations may be switched to a LABA/LAMA/ICS combination. In patients with persisting exacerbations on this treatment, the phosphodiesterase-4 inhibitor roflumilast (Daliresp) 500 mcg/day or prophylactic azithromycin (Zithromax)[1] 250 mg/day or 500 mg on Monday, Wednesday, and Friday have been shown to decrease the frequency of exacerbations.

---

[1]Not FDA approved for this indication.

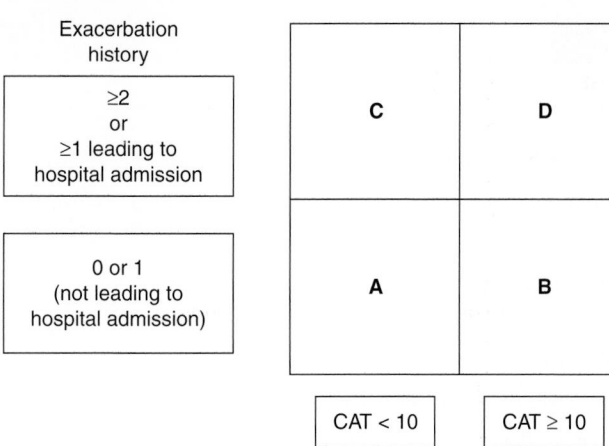

Figure 1 Exacerbation history.

Exacerbation history		
≥2 or ≥1 leading to hospital admission	C	D
0 or 1 (not leading to hospital admission)	A	B
	CAT < 10	CAT ≥ 10
	Symptoms	

TABLE 4	Modified MRC Dyspnea Scale
mMRC Grade 0	I only get breathless with strenuous exercise.
mMRC Grade 1	I get short of breath when hurrying on the level or walking up the hill.
mMRC Grade 2	I walk slower than people of the same age on the level because of breathlessness, or I have to stop for breath when walking on my own pace on the level.
mMRC Grade 3	I stop for breath after walking about 100 meters or after a few minutes on the level.
mMRC Grade 4	I am too breathless to leave the house, or I am breathless when dressing or undressing.

TABLE 5	Chronic Obstructive Pulmonary Disease Assessment Test
I never cough.	0 1 2 3 4 5	I cough all the time.
I have no phlegm (mucus) in my chest at all.	0 1 2 3 4 5	My chest is completely full of phlegm (mucus).
My chest does not feel tight at all.	0 1 2 3 4 5	My chest feels very tight.
When I walk up a hill or one flight of stairs, I am not breathless.	0 1 2 3 4 5	When I walk up a hill or one flight of stairs, I am very breathless.
I am not limited doing any activities at home.	0 1 2 3 4 5	I am very limited doing activities at home.
I am confident leaving my home despite my lung condition.	0 1 2 3 4 5	I am not at all confident leaving my home because of my lung condition.
I sleep soundly.	0 1 2 3 4 5	I don't sleep soundly because of my lung condition.
I have lots of energy.	0 1 2 3 4 5	I have no energy at all.

Sustained release theophylline preparations have a mild bronchodilator effect and may be added to an otherwise maximized regimen, or may be used when cost considerations prohibit the use of long-acting bronchodilators.

Retained secretions may increase dyspnea and hypoxemia. Management may include use of guaifenesin[1] 200 to 400 mg orally every 4 hours as needed, not to exceed 2.4 g/day; potassium iodide (SSKI) 0.3 mL (300 mg) or 0.6 mL (600 mg) diluted in one glassful of water, fruit juice, or milk 3 to 4 times daily, and positive expiratory pressure devices, such as the Acapella.

On follow-up visits, medications may be escalated or de-escalated based on symptoms or exacerbations.

Noninvasive Ventilation

Bilevel ventilation has been used in patients with chronic hypercapnic respiratory failure. Regular use of noninvasive ventilation in this population has shown improvement in walk distance, dyspnea, and hypercapnia by increasing minute ventilation and decreasing work of breathing. Medicare guidelines for prescribing require documented hypercapnia ($PaCO_2$ >51) and a nocturnal oximetry showing desaturation to SaO_2 <89% for at least 5 consecutive minutes during sleep. Initial settings are somewhat empiric, often beginning at IPAP 12 cm H_2O and EPAP 5 cm H_2O. These settings may be adjusted based on comfort and degree of hypercapnia.

Surgical Remedies

Lung volume reduction surgery is a consideration for patients with severe disease meeting certain criteria. The rationale is that removing the most diseased portions of lung in patients with emphysema will decrease hyperinflation, improve ventilation/perfusion matching, and decrease lung compliance. This elevates the diaphragms, placing them at better mechanical advantage, and stents open the airways. Selection criteria come from the National Emphysema Therapy Trial (NETT) and include patients with emphysema who are <75 years old, smoke-free for 6 months, on no more than 20 mg/day of prednisone with functional limitation good compliance, and severe dyspnea despite maximum medical therapy. Laboratory evaluation must demonstrate upper lobe predominant emphysema on chest CT, hyperinflation, low FEV_1 (≤45% predicted; ≥5% predicted if age over 70), and postrehabilitation 6-minute walk >140 m. Exclusionary criteria include morbid obesity, significant comorbidities, previous chest surgery or chest wall deformity that might interfere with the procedure, resting pulmonary hypertension, well-preserved exercise capacity, and significant pleural or interstitial disease.

Lung transplantation may be considered in patients <65 years old (<60 years old for double lung transplant), with FEV_1 <25% predicted and/or $PaCO_2$ >55 mm Hg and/or pulmonary hypertension, especially in patients with progressive disease requiring supplemental oxygen. Exclusionary criteria include other major organ dysfunction, recent malignancy, HIV-positive status, and hepatitis B or C.

An emerging therapy is endobronchial valve therapy in which one-way valves are placed in some airways endoscopically to produce a nonsurgical lung volume reduction. This treatment has been shown to result in improved pulmonary function, exercise capacity, and quality of life in some patients with emphysema.

Supplemental Oxygen

The use of supplemental oxygen in patients with COPD is based on the fact that its use in severely hypoxemic patients helps prevent pulmonary hypertension, cor pulmonale, and premature death. Indications for continuous supplemental oxygen are resting PaO_2 ≤55 mm Hg or PaO_2 56 to 59 mm Hg with evidence of complication, such as pulmonary hypertension or polycythemia. Supplemental oxygen may be prescribed during activity for SaO_2 <89% during activity and may be prescribed during sleep for patients with SaO_2 <89% for at least 5 minutes during sleep.

Treatment of Exacerbations of Chronic Obstructive Pulmonary Disease

COPD exacerbations are defined as an acute increase in symptoms requiring an adjustment in medication. They are defined as mild (requiring only bronchodilator adjustment), moderate (requiring antibiotics and/or oral corticosteroids), or severe (requiring hospitalization or emergency department management). Some factors that help determine the need for hospitalization include severity of symptoms, failure to respond to initial management, increasing hypoxemia or hypercapnia, or mental status changes. Underlying comorbidities or lack of support at home may also contribute to the need for hospitalization. Exacerbations may be triggered by viral or bacterial infections or environmental factors.

An increase in frequency of use of as-needed short-acting beta agonists is initial management for exacerbations. Systemic corticosteroids improve pulmonary function measurement and shorten recovery time. Prednisone 40 mg/day for 5 days is effective and has been shown to have similar effect to intravenous steroid administration. The addition of an antibiotic course, 5 to 7 days, has been shown to improve outcomes in outpatients with either increased dyspnea or increased sputum production plus increased sputum purulence. Antibiotics have been shown to decrease mortality and the incidence of nosocomial infection in patients with exacerbation who require invasive or noninvasive mechanical ventilation.

References

Center for Disease Control and Prevention: Chronic obstructive pulmonary disease. Available at https://www.cdc.gov/copd.

DeCamp M, Lipsom D, Krasna M: The evaluation and preparation of the patient for lung volume reduction surgery, *Proc Am Thorac Soc* 5:427, 2008.

Global Initiative for Chronic Obstructive Pulmonary Disease (GOLD): Global strategy for the diagnosis, management and prevention of COPD 2021. Available at http://www.goldcopd.org.

Hunninghake GM, Cho MH, Tesfaigzi Y, et al: MMP12, lung function and COPD in high risk populations, *N Engl J Med* 361:2599, 2009.

International guidelines for the selection of lung transplant candidates, *Am J Respir Crit Care Med* 158:335, 1998.

Klooster K, Hacken N, Hartman J, et al: Endobronchial valves for emphysema without interlobar collateral ventilation, *N Engl J Med* 373:2325, 2015.

MacNee W: Pathogenesis of chronic obstructive pulmonary disease, *Proc Am Thorac Soc* 2:258, 2005.

Quon BS, Gan WQ, Sin DD: Contemporary management of acute exacerbations of COPD: a systematic review and metaanalysis, *Chest* 133(3), 2008.

Silverman EK, Weiss ST, Drazen EM, et al: Gender-related differences in severe, early onset chronic obstructive pulmonary disease, *Am J Resp Crit Care Med* 162:2152, 2000.

Treating Tobacco Use and Dependence: Available at https://www.ahrq.gov/professionals/clinicians-providers/guidelines-recommendations/tobacco. Accessed February 19, 2017.

Woodhead M, Blasi F, Ewig S, et al: Guidelines for the management of adult lower respiratory tract infections, *Eur Respir J* 133(1), 2008.

World Health Organization: Chronic Respiratory Diseases, Available at: http://www.who.int/respiratory/copd.

COCCIDIOIDOMYCOSIS

Method of
Gregory M. Anstead, MD, PhD

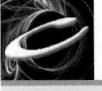

CURRENT DIAGNOSIS

- Maintain a high index of suspicion in patients from endemic areas and travelers
- Diagnostic tests include:
  - Serologic detection of immunoglobulin M and immunoglobulin G antibodies by immunodiffusion, complement fixation, and enzyme immunoassay
  - Culture of sputum, exudates, cerebrospinal fluid, and tissue
  - Direct observation of *Coccidioides* spherules in histopathologic and cytologic specimens
  - Urine antigen enzyme immunoassay

CURRENT THERAPY

Pulmonary Infection

- No risk factors for dissemination; not severe disease—observe
- Risk factors; prolonged symptoms—fluconazole (Diflucan)[1] 400 mg/day or itraconazole (Sporanox)[1] 200 mg twice a day for 3 to 6 months
- Diffuse or severe pneumonia—amphotericin B (Fungizone) 1 mg/kg/day or lipid formulation of amphotericin (Abelcet, AmBisome)[1] 5 mg/kg/day; after improvement, switch to azole; treat for 1 year
- Chronic fibrocavitary disease—azole therapy for at least 1 year; resection in selected cases

Disseminated Disease

- Nonmeningeal, severe disease—amphotericin B 1 mg/kg/day or lipid formulation of amphotericin[1] 5 mg/kg/day; after improvement, switch to azole for 1 to 2 years; consider posaconazole (Noxafil)[1] suspension 200 mg four times daily or tablets 300 mg daily or voriconazole (Vfend)[1] 400 to 600 mg/day daily in refractory cases
- Nonmeningeal, slowly progressive—azole therapy for 1 to 2 years; itraconazole[1] preferred for bony involvement; consider posaconazole[1] or voriconazole[1] (as above) in refractory cases
- Meningeal, central nervous system involvement—fluconazole[1] 800 to 2000 mg/day[3]; intrathecal amphotericin B[1] or voriconazole (Vfend)[1] 200 mg twice daily in refractory cases[1]; shunting for hydrocephalus; consider corticosteroids if vasculitis is present

---

[1]Not FDA approved for this indication.
[3]Exceeds dosage recommended by the manufacturer.

Coccidioidomycosis is caused by soil fungi of the genus *Coccidioides*, divided genetically into *Coccidioides immitis* (California isolates) and *Coccidioides posadasii* (isolates outside California). There are no distinct clinical differences between the two species. *Coccidioides* occurs only in the Western hemisphere, primarily in the southwestern United States (Arizona and parts of California, New Mexico, Utah, Nevada, and Texas) and in northern Mexico, areas characterized by arid to semiarid climates, hot summers, low altitude, alkaline soil, and sparse vegetation. Hyperendemic areas include the San Joaquin Valley of California and Pima, Pinal, and Maricopa Counties in Arizona. *Coccidioides* is also found in parts of Latin America (Guatemala, Honduras, Nicaragua, Argentina, Paraguay, Venezuela, and Colombia). Cases may be observed in nonendemic areas because of travel or reactivation of prior infection. In the United States, an estimated 150,000 cases of coccidioidomycosis occur annually, with the clinical presentation ranging from a self-limited respiratory infection to devastating disseminated disease. The incidence of coccidioidomycosis is increasing in the United States because of rising populations and the resulting construction in the endemic areas. Risk factors for increased severity of coccidioidomycosis include receiving immunosuppressive medications (e.g., corticosteroids, transplant drugs, and tumor necrosis factor–alpha antagonists); pregnancy (esp. the third trimester); genetic factors (i.e., defects in the IL-12/interferon-γ axis and STAT3 pathways, certain ABO blood group and HLA types); and specific races/ethnicities (African Americans, Asian-Pacific Islanders, and Native Americans). Outbreaks may occur after dust storms, earthquakes, droughts, and activities causing soil disruption, such as construction and archeological digs. Persons with occupations involving exposure to soil are also at risk for acquiring coccidioidomycosis.

Coccidioides is dimorphic; in the soil, the organism exists in its mycelial form, which produces barrel-shaped arthroconidia. The usual means of infection is the inhalation of arthroconidia; uncommon routes include direct cutaneous inoculation and organ transplantation. Arthroconidia germinate to produce spherules filled with endospores, the characteristic tissue phase. Spherules rupture to release endospores, which form additional spherules. The spherules become surrounded by neutrophils and macrophages, which leads to granuloma formation. Both B and T lymphocytes are essential for host defense against this pathogen.

Clinical Manifestations

Coccidioidomycosis is asymptomatic in 60% of infected individuals. In the remaining 40%, a self-limited, flu-like illness with dry cough, pleuritic chest pain, myalgias, arthralgia, fever, sweats, anorexia, and weakness develops 1 to 3 weeks after exposure. Primary infection may be accompanied by immune complex–mediated complications, including an erythematous macular rash, erythema multiforme, and erythema nodosum. Acute infection usually resolves without therapy, although symptoms may persist for weeks. In 5% of these patients, asymptomatic pulmonary residua persist, including pulmonary nodules and cavitation. Immunocompromised patients may develop chronic progressive pulmonary infection, with the evolution of thin-walled cavities that may rupture, leading to bronchopleural fistula and empyema formation.

Extrapulmonary disease develops in 1 of every 200 patients and can involve the skin, soft tissues, bones, joints, and meninges. The most common cutaneous lesions are verrucous papules, ulcers, or plaques. The spine is the most frequent site of osseous dissemination, although the typical lytic lesions may also occur in the skull, hands, feet, and tibia. Joint involvement is usually monoarticular and most commonly involves the ankle and knee. Fungemia may occur in immunocompromised patients and carries a poor prognosis.

In coccidioidal meningitis, the basilar meninges are usually affected. Cerebrospinal fluid findings include lymphocytic pleocytosis (often with eosinophilia), hypoglycorrhachia, and elevated protein levels. The mortality rate is greater than 90% at 1 year without therapy, and chronic infection is the rule. Hydrocephalus or hydrocephalus coexisting with brain infarction is associated with a higher mortality rate. Coccidioidomycosis is a great imitator and has many diverse clinical presentations, including immune thrombocytopenia, ocular involvement, massive cervical lymphadenopathy, laryngeal and retropharyngeal abscesses, endocarditis, pericarditis, peritonitis, hepatitis, and lesions of the male and female genitals and urogenital tracts.

Diagnosis

Coccidioidomycosis may be diagnosed by direct observation of spherules in tissues or in wet mounts of sputa or exudates. The growth of Coccidioides in culture usually occurs in 3 to 5 days, with sporulation after 5 to 10 days. Definitive identification is made by DNA probe or exoantigen testing. Laboratory personnel should exercise extreme caution when handling cultures of Coccidioides.

Serologic methods are quite useful in establishing the diagnosis and for monitoring the course of the infection. Immunoglobulin M (IgM) antibodies are present soon after infection or relapse but then wane; quantification does not correlate with disease severity. The IgG antibody appears later and remains positive for months. Rising titers of IgG are associated with progressive disease, and declining titers are associated with resolution. The IgG antibodies can fix complement when combined with coccidioidal antigen and can be detected by immunodiffusion (IDCF); titers of 1:16 or greater suggest disseminated disease. In the cerebrospinal fluid, a positive IDCF of any titer is considered diagnostic of meningitis and is much more sensitive than culture in making the diagnosis. An enzyme immunoassay is also available, but it is less specific. Recently, a specific urinary antigen test became available for the diagnosis of coccidioidomycosis; this assay has a sensitivity of 71% in moderate-to-severe disease, compared with 84% for culture, 29% for histopathologic examination, and 75% for serologic testing.

Treatment

In most patients, primary pulmonary infection resolves spontaneously without treatment. However, all patients require observation for at least 2 years to document resolution of infection and to identify any complications as soon as possible. For patients who have risk factors for disseminated disease (listed earlier), treatment is necessary. Other indications for treatment are severe disease (infiltrates involving both lungs or more than half of one lung; significant hilar or mediastinal lymphadenopathy; complement fixation titers >1:16) and highly symptomatic disease (weight loss >10%; night sweats present for >3 weeks; symptoms present for >2 months).

For diffuse or severe pneumonia, therapy with amphotericin B deoxycholate (Fungizone) 0.5 to 1.5 mg/kg/day, or a lipid formulation of amphotericin B (Abelcet or AmBisome)[1] 2 to 5 mg/kg/day should be given for several weeks, followed by an oral azole, such as itraconazole (Sporanox)[1] 200 mg twice daily or fluconazole (Diflucan)[1] 400 to 800 mg/day. The total duration of therapy should be at least 1 year; for immunosuppressed patients, oral azole therapy should be maintained as secondary prophylaxis. In human immunodeficiency virus (HIV) patients with CD4-positive T-cell counts greater than 250 cells/mm³ who had focal pneumonias that responded to azoles, antifungals may be discontinued. Azole therapy may be used initially for less severe disease. During pregnancy, amphotericin B is the preferred drug, because of the teratogenicity of azoles.

An asymptomatic patient with a solitary nodule or pulmonary cavitation caused by Coccidioides does not require specific antifungal therapy or resection. However, the development of complications from the cavitation, such as hemoptysis or bacterial or fungal superinfection, necessitates initiation of azole therapy. Resection of the cavities is an alternative to antifungal therapy. Rupture of a cavity into the pleural space requires surgical intervention with closure by lobectomy with decortication, in addition to antifungal therapy. For chronic pneumonia, the initial treatment should be an oral azole for at least 1 year. If the disease persists, one may switch to another oral azole, increase the dose if fluconazole was initially selected, or switch to amphotericin B. Resection should be performed for patients with refractory focal lesions or severe hemoptysis.

The treatment of disseminated infection without central nervous system involvement is based on oral azole therapy, such as itraconazole[1] or fluconazole[1] (400 mg/day, or higher in case of fluconazole). If there is little or no improvement or if there is vertebral involvement, treatment with amphotericin B is recommended (dosage as for diffuse pneumonia). Concomitant surgical débridement or stabilization is also recommended. In patients with refractory coccidioidomycosis that has failed to respond to fluconazole, itraconazole, and amphotericin B and its lipid formulations, treatment with posaconazole (Noxafil)[1] suspension 200 mg four times daily with a fatty meal or voriconazole (Vfend),[1] at doses of 400 to 600 mg/day, has been successful. A posaconazole tablet with improved oral bioavailability and an intravenous preparation are now available and likely these new forms of posaconazole are more efficacious. The posaconazole tablet has been dosed at 300 mg/day. Clinical experience with voriconazole is limited.

For coccidioidal meningitis, lifetime treatment with azoles is indicated. Fluconazole,[1] at doses of 800 mg/day or higher,[3] is recommended. There have been a few reports of successful treatment of coccidioidal meningitis with voriconazole (Vfend)[1] 200 mg orally twice daily after a loading dose. Itraconazole is not recommended because of its irregular oral absorption. For patients with increased intracranial pressure at the time of meningitis diagnosis, repeated lumbar punctures are recommended. Obstructive hydrocephalus requires shunting. Intrathecal amphotericin B[1] is now strictly reserved for meningitis

---

[1]Not FDA approved for this indication.

refractory to high-dose azoles or coccidioidal meningitis in the first trimester of pregnancy. In patients with CNS vasculitis with cerebrovascular accident caused by coccidioidomycosis, those that received corticosteroids were less likely to develop additional infarcts compared with those who did not. Reduction of immunosuppression is an important adjunct to antifungal therapy, including the initiation of antiretroviral therapy if the patient has HIV infection. In patients with AIDS and nonmeningeal coccidioidomycosis, antifungal therapy can be discontinued when the CD4 count exceeds 250 cells/mm³.

[1]Not FDA approved for this indication.
[3]Exceeds dosage recommended by the manufacturer.

References

Ampel NM: Coccidioidomycosis: changing concepts and knowledge gaps, *J Fungi (Basel)* 6:354, 2020.

Bays DJ, Thompson GR, Reef S, et al: Natural history of disseminated coccidioidomycosis: examination of the VA-Armed Forces Database, *Clin Infect Dis* ciaa1154, 2020.

Diep AL, Hoyer KK: Host response to *Coccidioides* infection: fungal immunity, *Front Cell Infect Microbiol* 10:581101, 2020.

Donovan FM, Zangeneh TT, Malo J, Galgiani JN: Top questions in the diagnosis and treatment of coccidioidomycosis, *Open Forum Infect Dis* 4:ofx197, 2017.

Gabe LM, Malo J, Knox KS: Diagnosis and management of coccidioidomycosis, *Clin Chest Med* 38:417–433, 2017.

Galgiani JN, Ampel NM, Blair JE, et al: Infectious Diseases Society of America (IDSA) clinical practice guideline for the treatment of coccidioidomycosis, *Clin Infect Dis* 63:e112–e146, 2016.

Hartmann CA, Aye WT, Blair JE: Treatment considerations in pulmonary coccidioidomycosis, *Expert Rev Respir Med* 10:1079–1091, 2016.

Kassis C, Durkin M, Holbrook E, et al: Advances in diagnosis of progressive pulmonary and disseminated coccidioidomycosis, *Clin Infect Dis* 72:968–975, 2021.

Kim MM, Vikram HR, Kusne S, Seville MT, Blair JE: Treatment of refractory coccidioidomycosis with voriconazole or posaconazole, *Clin Infect Dis* 53:1060–1066, 2011.

McCotter OZ, Benedict K, Engelthaler DM, et al: Update on the epidemiology of coccidioidomycosis in the United States, *Med Mycol* 57(Suppl 1):S30–S40, 2019.

Odio CD, Marciano BE, Galgiani JN, Holland SM: Risk factors for disseminated coccidioidomycosis, United States, *Emerg Infect Dis* 23:308–311, 2017.

Stockamp NW, Thompson 3rd GR: Coccidioidomycosis, *Infect Dis Clin North Am* 30:229–246, 2016.

Thompson 3rd GR, Blair JE, Wang S, et al: Adjunctive corticosteroid therapy in the treatment of coccidioidal meningitis, *Clin Infect Dis* 65:338–341, 2017.

Thompson 3rd GR, Lewis 2nd JS, Nix DE, Patterson TF: Current concepts and future directions in the pharmacology and treatment of coccidioidomycosis, *Med Mycol* 157(Suppl 1):S76–S84, 2019.

Van Dyke MCC, Thompson GR, Galgiani JN, Barker BM: The rise of *Coccidioides*: forces against the dust devil unleashed, *Front Immunol* 10:2188, 2019.

CYSTIC FIBROSIS

Method of
Hanna Phan, PharmD; and Cori L. Daines, MD

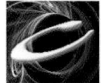

CURRENT DIAGNOSIS

- Cystic fibrosis (CF) is an autosomal recessive genetic disorder that causes dysfunction of the cystic fibrosis transmembrane conductance regulator (CFTR) on the apical surface of epithelial cells leading to inability to move adequate ions, specifically chloride, out of the cell.
- Basic defect leads to thick, dehydrated mucus in the respiratory tract manifesting as chronic cough and recurrent infections.
- Diagnosis is made via a sweat chloride test using quantitative pilocarpine iontophoresis.
- Close to 2000 mutations of CFTR are known, leading to a multitude of clinical phenotypes and severity of disease.

CURRENT THERAPY

- A given patient's overall treatment regimen is often based on various factors, including age, clinical presentation, organ systems involved, disease progression/severity, CFTR genotype, and comorbidities.
- Primary treatment is augmented airway clearance with bronchodilators, mucolytics or mucus hydrators, and mechanical airway vibration.
- For the vast majority of patients, secondary treatment includes use of a CFTR modulator.
- Nutritional therapy consists of enzymes and vitamin replacement for those who are pancreatic insufficient.

Epidemiology

Cystic fibrosis is an autosomal recessive, inherited multisystem disease caused by mutations of the CFTR on chromosome 7. There are currently close to 2000 mutations of CFTR known. Carriage of the gene is highest in individuals of Northern European decent, leading to an incidence of 1 in 3000 non-Hispanic Caucasians in the United States. Incidence is lower in Hispanic Caucasians and those of African descent. There are more than 30,000 individuals with CF in the United States, more than 100,000 individuals worldwide, and approximately 1000 new diagnoses are made each year. Average life expectancy is increasing with new therapies but still varies among countries. In the United States and Canada, life expectancy is well beyond 40 years.

Pathophysiology

Cystic Fibrosis Transmembrane Regulator Genotypes—Genotype/Phenotype

CFTR is a protein in the adenosine triphosphate–binding cassette transporter family that has two transmembrane domains, two nucleotide-binding domains, and a regulatory domain. It shares structural elements with other membrane pumps. Mutations in the gene coding the CFTR fall broadly into six categories. The first category includes premature truncation mutations, leading to no full-length protein. The second category includes the Phe-508del (i.e., F508del) mutation, which is the most common mutation, accounting for 75% of all mutations in the United States. The category II mutations are mutations that result in the cell degrading the CFTR prior to full maturation and function. Class III mutations result in a chloride channel at the cell surface that does not function, or a "gating" mutation. Class IV mutations result in a chloride channel embedded at the cell surface that has decreased and ineffective chloride movement function, and class V mutations are promoter or splicing abnormalities resulting in a reduced number of functional chloride channels at the cell surface. Class VI mutations result in a chloride channel that is not stable on the cell surface and thus, like class V mutations, insufficient quantities of chloride channel at the cell surface.

Understanding the genetics of any given individual with CF is vital in understanding the pathophysiology. Disease manifestation is directly related to the amount of chloride moved at the cell surface. Class I, II, and III mutations result in minimal chloride movement, less than 5% of normal, and "classic" or severe disease phenotype. The presence of one mutation in the class IV, V, or VI category results in greater chloride movement at the surface, typically 10% or more, and a "mild" or "nonclassic" phenotype. Approximately 15% of individuals with CF fall into this latter category and have some preserved chloride channel activity and milder disease phenotype.

Mechanism

CF affects all organs with epithelial cells expressing CFTR, which typically means cells lining a ductal system and the fluid outside that system are affected. In the lungs, the respiratory epithelium is lined with cells that express the CFTR. When the CFTR does not move appropriate amounts of chloride, chloride is trapped inside the cell, which leads to the epithelial sodium channel pumping additional sodium into the cell to balance. The resulting salt inside the cell creates an osmotic gradient across the cell surface and water enters the cell. The water first comes from the periciliary fluid layer, dehydrating the fluid around the cilia, making it difficult for them to beat. Next, water is removed from the outer mucus layer, also dehydrating it, making it thick and viscous. In the sinopulmonary tract, this inspissation of the mucus limits natural mucociliary clearance and leads to inflammation and an advantageous environment for bacterial colonization. Damage to the airways becomes irreversible and leads to a loss of lung function.

A similar issue happens in other organs with any epithelial cell lining a ductal system. In the pancreas, for instance, epithelial cells line the ducts of the exocrine pancreas. The cells pull water from the normal pancreatic excretion, dehydrating it and clogging up the ducts. The enzymes then autodigest the exocrine pancreas, rendering it nonfunctional. The same is true in the biliary ducts of the liver. In the sweat glands, salt and water are trapped in the ducts, making the sweat very salty and leading to the diagnostic test of the sweat chloride test.

Clinical Manifestations
Pulmonary
The tracheobronchial tree in CF has poor mucociliary clearance, as noted previously. People with CF have excessive cough, make mucus, and might wheeze. They have periodic episodes of exacerbation where there is an excessive mucus build-up and bacterial infection. The thick mucus becomes a source of persistent infection with bacteria that are unable to be cleared. Often, the infections are caused by bacteria that are not present in the normal undamaged airway, especially *Staphylococcus aureus* and *Pseudomonas aeruginosa*. When the bacteria become active and the patient experiences an exacerbation, the cough and sputum production will worsen. Exacerbations in children are often triggered by viruses and typical childhood illnesses, and in adults, exacerbations may also be triggered by other environmental factors. With exacerbation, there may be shortness of breath, chest pain, wheezing, dyspnea on exertion or at rest, and fatigue. Other symptoms of a pulmonary exacerbation include weight loss, poor appetite, and fever. Over time, there is progressive loss of lung function owing to infections, mucus, and inflammation. Symptoms become more persistent and bothersome over time, and exacerbations become more common.

Sinuses
The sinuses in CF have the same mucostasis that occurs in the lungs. The mucus impaction leads to chronic sinus congestion and obstruction, persistent infections, and persistent inflammation. Individuals with CF are more likely to develop polyps as well. Symptoms include nasal congestion or drainage, sinus headache, and inability to smell.

Pancreas
Poor growth occurs as a result of insufficient nutrient breakdown and absorption, with malabsorptive, greasy stools occurring owing to this. Owing to malabsorption of fat, fat-soluble vitamins in the diet are also malabsorbed. Individuals with CF can develop significant deficiencies in vitamins A, D, E, and K. In general, the endocrine pancreas that makes insulin is not initially affected in CF. Over time, individuals with CF often develop CF-related diabetes (CFRD) caused by global inflammation of the pancreas. More than 30% to 40% of adults will develop CFRD.

Liver
In the liver, there is inspissation of the bile in the bile duct caused by excessive reabsorption of water from the bile. The resulting blockage of the bile ducts leads to hepatic inflammation. In general, this is asymptomatic for the individual with CF and is found by checking laboratory levels of liver function tests. Occasionally,

this bile blockage is severe and leads to chronic inflammation and biliary cirrhosis of the liver. A small percentage of individuals with CF, typically less than 5%, have fulminant liver failure with portal hypertension, esophageal varices, and splenomegaly, and would need a liver transplant.

Intestines
Excessive reabsorption of fluid in the gut can lead to constipation and even small bowel obstruction. This can also occur when stools are malabsorptive. Some people with CF will have rectal prolapse caused by straining, with either malabsorptive or constipated stools. Other manifestations of CF in the intestines can be a result of medication side effects.

Sweat Gland
Excessive salt is trapped in the sweat, leading to excessive salt loss in the sweat and electrolyte imbalance and dehydration.

Genitourinary
Men with CF generally all have congenital absence of the vas deferens, rendering them naturally infertile. Men still produce sperm but do not have the other structures. Women with CF may have decreased fertility owing to poor nutritional status but, typically, can have children.

Other
CF causes clubbing of the fingers, which is usually more prominent as lung disease progresses. CF-related arthropathies occur in a small percentage of individuals with CF, usually caused by inflammatory markers in circulation that deposit in the joints.

Diagnosis
Because CF is an insidiously progressive disease, it is important to make an early diagnosis and begin therapies as soon as possible. In the United States, the majority of diagnoses are made via newborn screening. Depending on the state, testing involves immunoreactive trypsinogen (IRT) levels with possible genetic panels of mutations. When the state reports a positive newborn screen, the care provider must order/obtain a sweat chloride test on the baby. Diagnoses are then based on the results of the screens. The CF Foundation guidelines state that a positive sweat diagnosis of CF is greater than 30 mmol/L chloride, with 30 to 60 mmol/L chloride being the intermediate zone. Consensus remains that if a child has two mutations, symptoms, and an abnormal sweat chloride (30–60 mmol/L), this is consistent with a diagnosis of CF. Children with symptoms and a sweat chloride greater than 60 mmol/L have CF as well. A secondary diagnosis of CF-related metabolic disorder (CRMS) designates those individuals whose diagnoses are unclear. Those with one mutation and an intermediate sweat (30–60 mmol/L) or those with two mutations and a negative sweat (<30 mmol/L) are followed prospectively for the development of symptoms and should have periodic sweat tests and periodic visits at the CF Center to evaluate for the evolution of symptoms.

As newborn screening has only been widely available for the last 10 to 20 years, children and adults who did not receive newborn screening are still being diagnosed the traditional way, which is the presence of symptoms and a positive sweat test. Here again, a positive sweat means a value of 60 mmol/L, while a value of 30 mmol/L or greater deserves further investigation, such as genetic testing. Sweat tests should be done at certified CF Centers where the testing methodology has been certified by the national Cystic Fibrosis Foundation. Traditional symptomatology per the CF Foundation is represented in the following:
- Very salty-tasting skin
- Persistent coughing, at times with phlegm
- Frequent lung infections, such as pneumonia or bronchitis
- Wheezing or shortness of breath
- Poor growth or poor weight gain in spite of a good appetite
- Frequent greasy, bulky stools or difficulty in bowel movements

- Nasal polyps
- Chronic sinus infections
- Clubbing or enlargement of the fingertips and toes
- Rectal prolapse
- Male infertility

If a diagnosis of CF is suspected owing to symptomatology, no matter what the age or status of newborn screening, a sweat test for definitive diagnosis should be performed.

Treatment
Pulmonary
Nonpharmacologic
Owing to the increased viscosity of the airway secretions and the subsequent obstruction and even mucus plugging in CF, there is a fundamental need for airway clearance or chest physiotherapy as part of chronic care. As a core component of therapy in the pulmonary management of CF, airway clearance or chest physiotherapy helps loosen this mucus, and help with expectoration should be done routinely two to three times per day as part of chronic management in all ages; increased frequency may be necessary during periods of pulmonary exacerbation. Manual physiotherapy or percussion and postural drainage is often the first type introduced into care. Other airway clearance techniques can be used, depending on age, access to devices, and so forth, such as autogenic drainage, active-cycle-of breathing, high-frequency chest compression (e.g., vest) and/or oscillatory positive expiratory pressure (OPEP) devices, and exercise.

Pharmacologic, Chronic Therapy
The selection of chronic medications used in the pulmonary management of CF is currently based on age and clinical need. This is based on current guidelines, US Food and Drug Administration–approved indications for newer agents (e.g., CFTR modulators), and current evidence in cases of off-label medication use. Such pharmacotherapy consists of various medication classes, including bronchodilators, mucolytics, inhaled antibiotics, antiinflammatory agents, and CFTR modulators.

Inhaled medications are used in conjunction with chest physiotherapy to facilitate airway clearance, helping loosen mucus and expectoration, and suppress bacterial growth of pathogens in the airways. The use of a short-acting β-agonist, such as albuterol (Proventil, Ventolin)[1], in either meter dose inhaler or aerosolized or nebulizer form, facilitates mucociliary clearance through bronchodilation and decreases occurrence of bronchospasm from subsequent inhaled therapies such as mucolytics (e.g., hypertonic saline (sodium chloride 7% [HyperSal, PulmoSal]), dornase alfa (Pulmozyme), mannitol inhalation powder (Bronchitol)), and antibiotics. Mucolytics are also fundamental in mucociliary clearance. Nebulized hypertonic saline, most commonly sodium chloride 7% and administered twice a day, increases hydration of sputum through osmotic action, thinning sputum for airway clearance. Dornase alfa breaks down extracellular DNA in sputum, thereby decreasing its viscosity. This nebulized mucolytic is most commonly administered daily, usually following the use of nebulized hypertonic saline in sequence. The use of hypertonic saline and dornase alfa is recommended to help improve lung function and reduce exacerbations. Recently approved as a possible add-on maintenance therapy for persons with CF ages 18 years and older, mannitol inhalation powder (Bronchitol) is a dry powder formulation and thus does not require use of a nebulizer for administration and is dosed twice daily. Because of its acute bronchospasm risk, it should only be used in those who have passed the Bronchitol Tolerance Test, which is administered and performed under supervision. Inhaled corticosteroids with or without a long-acting β agonist are not used to treat CF itself but are appropriate in cases of concurrent asthma.

Some patients with CF may require the use of an inhaled antibiotic to help suppress bacterial burden in the airways and improve patient outcomes such as lung function and exacerbation frequency. Currently, the only FDA-approved inhaled antibiotics are tobramycin inhalation solution (Bethkis, Tobi), tobramycin inhalation powder (Tobi Podhaler), and aztreonam for inhalation solution (Cayston) for patients with CF with *P. aeruginosa*. For those patients who newly acquire *P. aeruginosa*, it is recommended to use an inhaled antibiotic for treatment, with the preferred agent being tobramycin-inhaled solution, for 28 days, in an attempt to eradicate the pathogen. The use of an inhaled antibiotic to prevent the acquisition of *P. aeruginosa* is not recommended. For patients with CF with the persistent presence of *P. aeruginosa* from respiratory cultures, the chronic use of inhaled antibiotics, such as tobramycin or aztreonam, is recommended to improve lung function and reduce exacerbations. For chronic use, the cycling (i.e., on 28 days, off 28 days, etc.) of an inhaled antibiotic is common. The use of continuous inhaled antibiotic therapy, where two different inhaled antibiotics (e.g., tobramycin and aztreonam) are used rotationally, is not routine but has been used by specialists in cases of multidrug-resistant pathogens, advanced or severe lung disease, or patients with frequent acute exacerbations.

Antiinflammatory agents—specifically oral azithromycin and/or high-dose ibuprofen—are also noted in current guidelines. Azithromycin (Zithromax), a macrolide antibiotic, is not used in chronic CF for its antiinfective properties but for its antiinflammatory and immunomodulatory properties. For patients with CF with persistent presence of *P. aeruginosa* from respiratory cultures, the use of chronic azithromycin[1] is recommended to improve lung function and reduce exacerbations. The use in patients with CF who lack the persistent presence of *P. aeruginosa* can be considered to help reduce the frequency of exacerbations. Monitoring for the presence of nontuberculosis mycobacterium (NTM) in respiratory cultures and potential for drug interactions with azithromycin (e.g., medications that may prolong QT interval) is recommended with the use of chronic azithromycin. A less commonly used antiinflammatory agent used among CF centers is high-dose ibuprofen.[1] The therapeutic benefit of slowing the loss of lung function is greatest in children aged 6 to 17 years. This therapy requires therapeutic drug monitoring (i.e., pharmacokinetic assessment of serum ibuprofen levels) and dose adjustment. Subtherapeutic levels can have negative effects on lung function, owing to an increase in inflammatory mediators, and supratherapeutic levels increase the risk for toxicities (e.g., bleeding, nephrotoxicity). This therapy is less common in use, owing to its potential for adverse effects, the need for laboratory monitoring, and the need for pharmacokinetic-based dosing. Routine, chronic use of systemic steroids such as prednisone is not recommended in the chronic management of CF.

CFTR modulators, a newer class of medications, are available for patients with CF with certain CF genotypes. The initial consideration for use and dosing of CFTR modulators is based on age, CF genotype, weight, concurrent therapy, ability to swallow tablets or capsules, and available dosage forms. There are three main types: potentiators, correctors, and amplifiers; however, the latter type is not currently available and is being developed and studied. Ivacaftor (Kalydeco) is a potentiator, increasing chloride movement through the CFTR protein channel. Ivacaftor is intended for patients ≥4 months of age who have the approved genotypes with gating and conducting mutations. Lumacaftor is a corrector, facilitating correct formation and stabilization of CFTR protein. Lumacaftor is combined with ivacaftor as Orkambi for the treatment of CF in patients ≥2 years whose genotype is homozygous Phe508del. Tezacaftor is also a corrector but is longer acting and has some differences compared with lumacaftor with regard to drug interactions and side effects. Like lumacaftor, tezacaftor is combined with ivacaftor as Symdeko for the chronic treatment of CF. Symdeko is approved for patients ≥6 years of age whose genotype is homozygous Phe508del and a number of residual function

Cystic Fibrosis

---

[1]Not FDA approved for this indication.

[1]Not FDA approved for this indication.

mutations. Elexacaftor is also a corrector; however, it binds to a different site on the CFTR protein than tezacaftor. Elexacaftor provides an additive effect in improving cellular processing and trafficking of CFTR, resulting in improved outcomes, including lung function, symptoms (cough, sputum production), exacerbation rate, and nutritional status. Elexacaftor is combined with tezacaftor and ivacaftor as Trikafta and is approved for patients ≥6 years of age who have at least one Phe508del mutation or other approved genotypes. Patients on lumacaftor-ivacaftor (Orkambi) or tezacaftor-lumacaftor (Symdeko) should be considered for transition to elexacaftor-tezacaftor-ivacaftor (Trikafta) when of appropriate age. Currently, tezacaftor-lumacaftor (Symdeko) and elexacaftor-tezacaftor-ivacaftor (Trikafta) are available in tablet blister packs with combination tablets (morning doses) and ivacaftor (evening doses). It is important to make patients/caregivers aware of the different appearing packaging, prescribed dosing, and administration. All of the mentioned CFTR modulators have similar administration and monitoring considerations. Liver function tests aspartate aminotransferase (AST), alanine aminotransferase (ALT), and total bilirubin (T bili) should be done prior to starting therapy, followed by every 3 months for the first year of therapy and annually thereafter. As noncongenital lens opacities or cataracts have been reported in pediatric patients with ivacaftor, a baseline ophthalmologic examination is also recommended in those aged less than 18 years. Follow-up ophthalmologic examinations are recommended, but the frequency is not well defined. Doses should be taken with a fatty meal and with pancreatic enzymes (for those who require the use of pancreatic enzymes as part of CF management). All the listed CFTR modulators are substrates and/or inducers of CYP3A4, and other CYP450 isoenzymes (e.g., CYP2C9), so screening for and managing drug interactions are essential. In addition, dosing modifications or discontinuation may be necessary for moderate or severe hepatic dysfunction.

Pharmacologic, Acute Therapy

Many patients with CF, despite the use of chronic therapies, experience pulmonary exacerbations requiring treatment. In addition to increased frequency of airway clearance or chest physiotherapy, acute pulmonary exacerbations may require the use of systemic antimicrobials. Whenever possible, the selection of systemic antimicrobial agents should be guided by a patient-specific history of respiratory cultures and patient clinical response to past regimens.

When a systemic antimicrobial is required for outpatient management, an oral antibiotic is commonly used, with the duration of most agents being 10 to 14 days. For example, if a given patient has a history of *P. aeruginosa*, use of oral ciprofloxacin (Cipro)[1] or levofloxacin (Levaquin)[1] for 14 to 21 days may be appropriate. Patients who have inhaled antibiotics as part of their chronic regimen may continue treatment cycles during outpatient treatment for acute pulmonary exacerbation. Some CF centers may use home infusion services for intravenous antimicrobials; however, this requires additional logistic considerations, including nursing support, infusion equipment, and laboratory monitoring. In addition, factors related to adherence to airway clearance, social support system at home, and appropriateness of home intravenous access should be considered.

For inpatient management, the use of intravenous antibiotics is more common and the use of oral antibiotic(s) may also be part of the regimen. *P. aeruginosa* is often "double-covered" when possible, specifically when hospitalized and/or requiring intravenous antimicrobials. "Double-coverage" involves the use of two agents active against *P. aeruginosa* from two different antibiotic classes (e.g., beta-lactam and aminoglycoside). The use of both inhaled and systemic (e.g., intravenous) antibiotics of the same class (e.g., aminoglycosides) simultaneously is not common. Another approach is starting intravenous antimicrobials in the inpatient setting, with transition and completion of the therapy course with home infusion services.

There are special instances in which longer courses of medications such as antibiotics or antifungal therapy may be necessary. For example, in the treatment of nontuberculosis mycobacterium (e.g., *Mycobacterium abscessus*), multiple types of antibiotics (e.g., inhaled and oral) may be used for extended durations (e.g., months). In the treatment of allergic bronchopulmonary aspergillosis, antifungal therapy may be used in addition to systemic corticosteroids (e.g., prednisone) for extensive periods of time (e.g., weeks or months). These more complex antimicrobial treatment courses are often managed by specialists (e.g., pulmonary and/or infectious disease specialists).

Nutrition/Gastrointestinal
Nonpharmacologic

Persons with CF often have greater dietary energy intake needs. Consistent, high-calorie dietary intake can be a challenge because of several physiologic factors, including loss of taste or smell caused by chronic sinusitis and chronic gastroesophageal reflux. Behavioral factors may affect nutritional intake, necessitating behavioral intervention by dietitians and/or psychologists. For patients of all ages with continued suboptimal growth, the use of enteral feeding modes may also be necessary. For patients who have chronic constipation or history of distal intestinal obstructive syndrome (DIOS), appropriate hydration and increased fiber content in the diet are recommended.

Infant formulas and breast milk do not provide adequate Na+ for infants with CF. Owing to excessive loss of Na+ through insensible loss, infants are at risk for developing hyponatremic, hypochloremia dehydration. It is recommended that 1/8 teaspoon of table salt be provided from birth and increased with time to ¼ teaspoon by 6 months through 1 year of age, divided throughout the day by feedings. Additional supplementation may be necessary for children and adults living in high-temperature climates and/or involved in considerable physical activities (e.g., sports).

Pharmacologic, Chronic Therapy

For patients who are pancreatic insufficient, the use of pancreatic enzyme replacement therapy (PERT) is needed. There are various brands of PERT that contain various amounts of lipase, protease, and amylase. Pancreatic enzymes should be taken at meal and snack times and in coordination with enteral feeds (when applicable). Dosing of PERT is based on lipase component. Typical pancreatic enzyme initial dosing ranges from 500 to 1500 units of lipase per kilogram body weight per meal, with a maximum of either 10,000 units of lipase per kilogram per day or 2500 units of lipase per kilogram per meal. Enzyme preparations come in a range of concentrations to accommodate all patient needs and minimize the number of capsules required. Given the number of medications a person with CF may require for chronic management, clinicians should be mindful about how many capsules are required per meal or snack when selecting a brand and strength of pancreatic enzyme. When maximal PERT dosing is reached and the individual continues to present with symptoms of malabsorption (e.g., steatorrhea), other etiologies should be investigated. Some clinicians may add an acid suppression agent (e.g., a proton pump inhibitor or H_2 receptor antagonist) to help enhance the activity of pancreatic enzymes through decreasing duodenal acidity; however, the potential risks of long-term acid suppression (e.g., small intestinal bacterial overgrowth [SIBO]) should be considered. A proton pump inhibitor or H_2 receptor antagonist may also be used to treat concurrent gastroesophageal reflux disease.

Supplementation of fat-soluble vitamins (i.e., A, D, E, K) should be provided via specially formulated multivitamins, available in various dosage forms with dosing based on age. Monitoring of vitamin levels is often done at least annually, with adjustments in supplementation of individual vitamins (e.g., vitamin D, cholecalciferol) based on adherence to current treatment, age, and level of deficiency.

For those who have chronic constipation or history of DIOS, chronic use of an osmotic laxative such as over-the-counter

---

[1]Not FDA approved for this indication.

polyethylene glycol 3350 (MiraLAX)[1] may be helpful. Oral *N*-acetylcysteine (Mucomyst)[1] has also been used for the prevention of mucus accumulation in the gastrointestinal (GI) tract of some individuals with DIOS.

Pharmacologic, Acute Therapy

Patients presenting with DIOS often require more aggressive treatment than that of chronic constipation related to CF. Treatment of DIOS may include laxatives at higher doses, use of electrolyte intestinal lavage solution (e.g., GoLYTELY),[1] or hyperosmolar enemas. Oral and/or rectal administration[1] of *N*-acetylcysteine solution has also been used for the treatment of mucus accumulation in the GI tract of some individuals with DIOS.

Monitoring

The monitoring of pulmonary symptoms should be done at each encounter. Spirometry to assess lung function is recommended as part of CF clinic visits to assess changes in forced expiratory volume in one second (FEV_1) relative to baseline. In addition, routine respiratory cultures, including screening for acid-fast bacilli and fungi to monitor for pathogens and susceptibilities are recommended. Nutritional status (e.g., weight, height, weight for length, body mass index) should also be monitored regularly. Annual routine laboratory testing is also done through CF centers and screenings for complications (e.g., CFRD). Recommended monitoring for the various chronic therapies is discussed in the previous section.

Management of Other Complications

In addition to the general manifestation of CF (e.g., pulmonary, growth, and nutrition), complications may appear with age and disease progression. The following are examples and general management approaches. Referral to other specialists, such as endocrinology, gastroenterology, otorhinolaryngology, or transplant (if/when appropriate for advanced disease), may be necessary.

Sinusitis

Treatment of the acute exacerbations of sinusitis can include systemic (e.g., oral) antibiotics, which are also used in pulmonary exacerbations. The use of intranasal irrigations of antimicrobials (e.g., gentamicin)[1] may also be considered, although guidance defining and comparing intranasal irrigation agent selection, formulation, dosing, and monitoring are currently lacking.

Small Intestinal Bacterial Overgrowth

Treatment of SIBO in persons with CF is similar to that of those without CF, including the use of oral antibiotics (e.g., rifaximin [Xifaxan][1]). Nonpharmacologic treatment may include dietary manipulation, such as reducing carbohydrate consumption, resulting in a high-fat, low-carbohydrate diet.

Cystic Fibrosis Related Diabetes

In addition to dietary modifications, when pharmacologic treatment is needed, insulin therapy includes a regimen consisting of long-acting insulin paired with carbohydrate counting and coverage with rapid-acting insulin. Insulin is the most appropriate therapeutic choice because there is a loss of beta-cell function. Acute pulmonary exacerbation or illness may complicate glucose control, especially if systemic corticosteroids are used as part of the management of severe, acute pulmonary exacerbations.

Hepatobiliary Disease

In addition to nutritional support, treatment with oral ursodeoxycholic acid or ursodiol (Actigall)[1] is currently recommended.

---

[1]Not FDA approved for this indication.

References

Borowitz D, Robinson KA, Rosenfeld M, et al: Cystic Fibrosis Foundation evidence-based guidelines for management of infants with cystic fibrosis, *J Pediatr* 155(Suppl 6):S73–S93, 2009.

Farrell PM, White TB, Ren CL, et al: Diagnosis of cystic fibrosis: consensus guidelines from the cystic fibrosis foundation, *J Pediatr* 181S:S4–S15.e1, 2017. https://doi.org/10.1016/j.jpeds.2016.09.064.

Flume PA, Clancy JP, Retsch-Bogart GZ, et al: Continuous alternating inhaled antibiotics for chronic pseudomonal infection in cystic fibrosis, *J Cyst Fibros* 15(6):809–815, 2016.

Flume PA, Mogayzel Jr PJ, Robinson KA, et al: Clinical Practice Guidelines for Pulmonary Therapies Committee. Cystic fibrosis pulmonary guidelines: treatment of pulmonary exacerbations, *Am J Respir Crit Care Med* 180(9):802–808, 2009.

Flume PA, Robinson KA, O'Sullivan BP, et al: Clinical Practice Guidelines for Pulmonary Therapies Committee. Cystic fibrosis pulmonary guidelines: airway clearance therapies, *Respir Care* 54(4):522–537, 2009.

Kapnadak SG, Dimango E, Hadjiliadis D, et al: Cystic Fibrosis Foundation Consensus Guidelines for the care of individuals with advanced cystic fibrosis lung disease, *J Cys Fibr*, 2020. https://doi.org/10.1016/j.jcf.2020.02.015.

Lahiri T, Hempstead SE, Brady C, et al: Clinical practice guidelines from the Cystic Fibrosis Foundation for preschoolers with cystic fibrosis, *Pediatrics* 137(4), 2016.

LeGrys VA, Yankaskas JR, Quittell LM, Marshall BC, Mogayzel PJ: Cystic fibrosis foundation. diagnostic sweat testing: the cystic fibrosis foundation guidelines, *J Pediatr* 151(1):85–89, 2007.

Mogayzel Jr PJ, Naureckas ET, Robinson KA, et al: Cystic fibrosis pulmonary guidelines. Chronic medications for maintenance of lung health, *Am J Respir Crit Care Med* 187(7):680–689, 2013.

Mogayzel Jr PJ, Naureckas ET, Robinson KA, et al: Cystic Fibrosis Foundation pulmonary guideline. pharmacologic approaches to prevention and eradication of initial Pseudomonas aeruginosa infection, *Ann Am Thorac Soc* 11(10):1640–1650, 2014.

Ren CL, Morgan RL, Oermann C, et al: Cystic Fibrosis Foundation Pulmonary Guidelines: use of cystic fibrosis transmembrane conductance regulator modulator therapy in patients with cystic fibrosis, *Ann Am Thorac Soc* 15(3):271–280, 2018.

HISTOPLASMOSIS

Method of
David van Duin, MD, PhD

CURRENT DIAGNOSIS

- The most common symptomatic manifestation of histoplasmosis is acute pulmonary histoplasmosis, which is generally characterized by nonspecific symptoms including fevers, chills, malaise, a nonproductive cough, and chest pain.
- Other presentations of histoplasmosis include chronic pulmonary histoplasmosis, disseminated histoplasmosis in immunocompromised hosts, and extrapulmonary disease such as mediastinal histoplasmosis.
- A multimodality approach to diagnosis, which may include serology, histopathology, antigen testing, and culture, should be considered in the appropriate setting.

CURRENT THERAPY

- Oral itraconazole is the treatment of choice for most forms of histoplasmosis.
- Serum levels of itraconazole are unpredictable and should be monitored during treatment.
- Depending on localization and severity of disease, induction with amphotericin B formulations may be required.
- Careful monitoring of patients during and after treatment is recommended, because relapses are observed in a subset of patients.

Mycology and Pathogenesis

Histoplasma capsulatum var. *capsulatum* and *H. capsulatum* var. *duboisii* are the two varieties of *H. capsulatum* that cause human histoplasmosis. *H. capsulatum* var. *duboisii* is the causative agent of African histoplasmosis, which is characterized by skin, bone, lymph node, and subcutaneous tissue involvement. This chapter focuses solely on the manifestations and treatment of *H. capsulatum* var. *capsulatum,* hereafter referred to as *H. capsulatum.*

H. capsulatum is a thermally dimorphic fungal pathogen, which grows as a mold in the environment, and converts to a yeast at 37°C during infection. During mold growth, *H. capsulatum* forms macroconidia, which are 8 to 15 μm and have thick walls and protuberances, as well as microconidia, which are 2 to 4 μm and have a smooth surface.

Disruption of soil containing *H. capsulatum,* such as during a construction project, results in the aerosolization of microconidia, which are the infectious particles. Inhaled microconidia are phagocytized but are able to survive and convert to yeast phase inside pulmonary macrophages. The resulting dissemination through the reticuloendothelial system is usually quickly contained in immunocompetent hosts, but it can lead to severe disease in the absence of normal immunity. Microconidia can be carried for several miles by air currents. Therefore, persons who are not in the direct vicinity of the disrupted soil are also at risk for developing histoplasmosis.

In tissues, *H. capsulatum* is recognized as 2- to 4-μm oval yeast forms with narrow-based budding. *H. capsulatum* does not have a capsule; the name is derived from the erroneous interpretation by Samuel Darling of an apparent clearing surrounding these yeasts in tissues as a capsule.

Epidemiology

Histoplasmosis is most common in North and Central America, but cases occur worldwide, some in microfoci of infection. Areas of high prevalence include the Mississippi and Ohio River valleys in the United States and Rio de Janeiro State in Brazil. *H. capsulatum* thrives in soil that is enriched with bird or bat guano, and it can be found in high quantities near bird roosts, chicken coops, abandoned old buildings, and bat-infested caves. Because *H. capsulatum* can enter a state of latency and reactivate years later, cases have been described in patients who have a remote history of living in or visiting endemic areas. A complete geographic history and a high index of suspicion are required for the correct diagnosis of such cases in nonendemic areas.

Clinical Manifestations

Most *H. capsulatum* infections are asymptomatic; it is estimated that less than 5% of infections lead to clinical symptoms. The occurrence and severity of a clinical syndrome are thought to be related to the immune status of the host, as well as the size of the infectious inoculum. The most common clinical scenario is acute pulmonary histoplasmosis, but a variety of other symptomatic histoplasmosis syndromes have been described. Also, a substantial number of cases come to clinical attention years after the initial infection during the course of a pulmonary nodule work-up, when malignancy is suspected. Although they are asymptomatic, these cases can lead to anxiety, as well as the morbidity and health care costs associated with radiographic exposures and biopsy procedures.

Acute Pulmonary Histoplasmosis

Most commonly, acute pulmonary histoplasmosis is a self-limited flulike illness. Symptoms are generally nonspecific and include fevers, chills, malaise, a nonproductive cough, and chest pain. Chest radiographs can show diffuse infiltrates in one or more lobes, often with hilar lymphadenopathy. The differential diagnosis includes more common infections such as bacterial and viral pneumonias. Symptoms usually resolve without treatment in 2 to 3 weeks. However, more-severe cases do occur, even in seemingly immunocompetent hosts. In these cases, severe respiratory distress, prolonged symptoms, and even death can occur in the

absence of adequate treatment. This highlights the importance of timely diagnosis and treatment when indicated.

Chronic Pulmonary Histoplasmosis

Some patients with acute pulmonary histoplasmosis fail to clear their infection and go on to develop a chronic pulmonary infection. A subset of these patients has chronic cavitary disease.

Chronic pulmonary histoplasmosis may be arbitrarily defined when the duration of symptoms from pulmonary histoplasmosis exceeds 6 weeks. The classic patient is a white middle-aged to elderly man with chronic obstructive pulmonary disease (COPD). Although these are clearly risk factors for the development of chronic disease, case series have illustrated that even never-smokers without preexisting lung disease are at risk for developing this complication.

A combination of systemic and pulmonary signs and symptoms is usually found in chronic pulmonary histoplasmosis. Fevers, night sweats, weight loss, lack of appetite, subjective loss of energy, and malaise are common systemic symptoms, and pulmonary symptoms include cough, sometimes with minimal hemoptysis, dyspnea, and sputum production. In patients with preexisting lung disease it may be difficult to distinguish these symptoms from baseline symptomatology. Radiology studies classically show cavitary disease without hilar lymphadenopathy. However, nodules, infiltrates, and lymphadenopathy are also seen, especially in nonsmoking women.

Untreated, this form of histoplasmosis can lead to death secondary to respiratory failure. With treatment, prognosis depends on coexisting pulmonary disease, and is generally favorable with regard to microbiological cure. However, relapses occur in up to 20% of cases even after prolonged treatment.

Disseminated Histoplasmosis

Most, if not all, episodes of histoplasmosis have a period of dissemination, during which infected macrophages spread throughout the body via the reticuloendothelial system. In the majority of cases this is a self-limited event, which is quickly contained upon activation of the immune system. However, about 1 in 2000 infections results in progressive disseminated disease. Almost invariably, these cases occur in immunocompromised hosts. Patients at risk for progressive disseminated disease include those with advanced HIV infection, solid organ transplant recipients, patients with hematologic malignancies, and those treated with immunomodulating agents, most notably corticosteroids or tumor necrosis factor α (TNF-α) inhibitors. Infants are also at risk.

Recognition of disseminated histoplasmosis can be challenging. Symptoms include fevers, malaise, anorexia, respiratory symptoms, and weight loss. Laboratory investigations often reveal elevated acute phase reactants, abnormal liver function tests, and pancytopenia. Hepatosplenomegaly and lymphadenopathy occur in about half of cases. Severe cases can be clinically indistinguishable from bacterial sepsis, and patients present with hypotension and multiorgan failure. A potential diagnostic clue to the diagnosis is the presence of mucosal ulcerations, which are generally painful and can occur anywhere in the oral, pharyngeal, or laryngeal mucosa. Various morphologies may be seen, ranging from superficial to verrucous. Adrenal involvement resulting in adrenal insufficiency can occur. These patients present with enlarged adrenals on imaging and clinical symptoms of Addison disease.

Although survival without antifungal therapy has been described, disseminated histoplasmosis is generally fatal if left untreated.

Mediastinal Manifestations of Histoplasmosis

Mediastinal disease can manifest itself as mediastinal fibrosis or granulomatous mediastinitis. Mediastinal fibrosis or fibrosing mediastinitis is an uncommon complication of pulmonary disease, in which extensive fibrotic tissue develops in the mediastinum in response to infection. Men between the ages of 20 and 40 years are at the highest risk for this complication. The fibrosis consists of mature collagen, rather than granulomatous tissue, which encases the structures of the mediastinum and can have a progressive course eventually leading to death. The prognosis depends on the extent of involvement of mediastinal structures. Bilateral disease in which the pulmonary veins are involved is especially associated with poor outcomes. No satisfactory treatment is available.

In contrast, granulomatous mediastinitis, also known as mediastinal granuloma, is characterized by a caseous inflammatory mass of mediastinal lymph nodes. Most patients remain asymptomatic, and cases are often recognized only as an incidental imaging finding. However, a subset of patients develops symptoms related to compromise of mediastinal structures. The prognosis is more benign; usually the process resolves and the involved lymph nodes calcify. The role of treatment in this entity remains unclear.

Central Nervous System Histoplasmosis
Central nervous system (CNS) involvement during *H. capsulatum* infection occurs infrequently. Like other extrapulmonary disease, CNS disease may be seen as a part of progressive disseminated histoplasmosis in about 5% to 10% of disseminated histoplasmosis cases. Additionally, isolated cases in which no other signs of dissemination are found have been reported. CNS histoplasmosis typically results in chronic lymphocytic meningitis, but parenchymal lesions can also be found. Symptoms are similar to those of other chronic infectious meningitides. The typical presentation is a combination of systemic symptoms including fevers, weight loss, and night sweats and localizing symptoms of headache, focal neurologic deficits, or behavioral changes. Treatment failures and relapses are common. Prognosis in the context of adequate treatment is dependent on the degree and the reversibility of immunosuppression.

Other Manifestations of Histoplasmosis
Involvement of all organ systems with *H. capsulatum* has been reported, either in the setting of clinical disseminated histoplasmosis or as an isolated extrapulmonary site of infection.

H. capsulatum as a cause of endovascular and cardiac infections is well established. In endocarditis cases, native and prosthetic valves may be involved. Pericarditis is found in around 5% of patients with pulmonary histoplasmosis, and it appears to represent an immunologic reaction. Consistent with this, symptoms usually resolve with nonsteroidal antiinflammatory drugs (NSAIDs) or corticosteroids. Bone, joint, and skin infections can also occur and can present diagnostic difficulty.

Urogenital involvement is often documented in autopsy series, but it infrequently results in clinical symptoms. Few cases of *H. capsulatum* causing symptomatic prostatitis, nephritis, epididymitis, vaginal and penile ulcers, and ovarian involvement have been reported. Similarly, although autopsy series report gastrointestinal involvement in disseminated histoplasmosis in up to 70% to 90% of cases, specific symptoms attributable to the gastrointestinal tract are much less common. Diarrhea, gastrointestinal bleeding, bowel perforation, or bowel obstruction can result from gastrointestinal histoplasmosis.

Diagnosis
Diagnosing histoplasmosis can be complicated, and the available specific diagnostic tests each have their limitations. If the diagnosis is suspected, using available modalities in combination is generally the right approach. Turn-around time can vary depending on circumstances, and in severe or disseminated cases, empiric therapy may be warranted. Obtaining tissue, when it is feasible to do so, is essential for a pathologic diagnosis.

Histopathology
One of the most useful modalities in reaching a diagnosis is histopathology. Necrotizing or non-necrotizing granulomas are often seen. An experienced pathologist can recognize the specific pattern of yeast forms, mostly inside but also outside of macrophages. The yeast forms are best visualized by a methamine silver stain, such as the Gomori-Grocott methenamine silver stain (GMS). Alternatively, periodic acid–Schiff (PAS) staining may be used. Confusion with other pathogens or, more commonly, staining artifacts can occur, and expert consultation is required in such

cases. Obtaining tissue for histopathology is usually the real challenge, and a careful evaluation of the risk-to-benefit ratio for each individual patient needs to be made.

Cultures
Culture confirmation of histoplasmosis is desirable, but often the yield of cultures is limited. In addition, cultures may be subject to a substantial time delay of several weeks. In disseminated histoplasmosis, cultures are often positive from several sites, including blood and bone marrow. In acute pulmonary histoplasmosis, the yield of respiratory cultures is estimated to be between 9% and 40%, depending on the degree of lung involvement. In mild to moderate cases, cultures are rarely positive. In chronic cavitary lung disease, the yield of culture improves, probably as a reflection of the increased fungal burden in these patients, and cultures can grow *H. capsulatum* in as many as 85% of cases. A positive fungal culture, with microscopic characteristics suggesting *H. capsulatum*, should be confirmed by specific testing. This is usually accomplished by DNA probing.

Serology
Antibody testing can be helpful when used in conjunction with the clinical scenario and other specific testing. The presence of antibodies to *H. capsulatum* may be determined by complement fixation (CF) or immunodiffusion (ID). Immunodiffusion methods evaluate the presence of M and H precipitin bands. Mild acute infections may be characterized by presence of an M band in isolation. Presence of an H band generally indicates more severe or chronic infection and is usually found in combination with an M band. Complement fixation determines the level of antibodies directed against mycelial and yeast antigens separately. For diagnosis, a fourfold rise in either mycelial or yeast CF antibody titer is required.

The incidence of detectable antibodies in persons in endemic areas is much lower than the incidence of positive skin testing, which suggests that detectable antibodies probably wane after exposure to undetectable levels. Therefore, although an isolated antibody titer of 1:32 or greater is not diagnostic, it is very suggestive of histoplasmosis in a patient with a consistent clinical presentation. In addition, any positive titer should lead to additional work-up because a substantial number of patients with confirmed histoplasmosis have antibody titers that are in the low positive range. Antibodies take 2 to 6 weeks to appear, which limits their use in acute cases. Immunosuppressed states clearly diminish the sensitivity of serology, but positive serologies are found in around 50% of disseminated histoplasmosis in immunocompromised patients. Antibody testing may be particularly helpful in CNS histoplasmosis, where cerebrospinal fluid (CSF) cultures are often negative. The finding of detectable anti–*H. capsulatum* antibodies in the CSF is diagnostic in the right clinical setting.

Antigen Detection
A commercial assay is available to determine the presence of polysaccharide antigens shed by *H. capsulatum* in urine or serum. Previously, urine assays appeared to outperform serum assays, but the most recent generation of antigen assays seems to be equivalent in urine and serum. Measuring antigen shedding in bronchoalveolar lavage (BAL) fluid is a new and promising development. Preliminary data indicate that yields from BAL may be increased in pulmonary disease. In general, antigen detection assays are a valuable adjunct to diagnosis and should be obtained in any case in which histoplasmosis is suspected. Because direct shedding is measured, the yield of this test is not diminished in immunocompromised hosts. In limited disease with a minimal fungal burden, antigens are unlikely to be detected.

Treatment
In 2007, the Infectious Diseases Society of America (IDSA) published updated management guidelines for the treatment of histoplasmosis (Table 1). The IDSA emphasizes that all of its guidelines

TABLE 1	2007 IDSA Guidelines for Treating Histoplasmosis				
CLINICAL MANIFESTATION	INDUCTION	DURATION	MAINTENANCE	TOTAL DURATION
Acute Pulmonary				
Mild to moderate <4 weeks	None			
Mild to moderate >4 weeks	None		Itra*	6–12 wk
Moderately severe to severe	AmB†	1–2 wk	Itra*	12 wk
Chronic Pulmonary				
	Itra*	3 day	Itra*	1–2 yr
Disseminated				
Mild to moderate	Itra*	3 day	Itra*	1 yr
Moderately severe to severe	AmB†	1–2 wk	Itra*	1 yr
Granulomatous mediastinitis	Itra*	3 day	Itra*	6–12 wk
CNS	AmB†	4–6 wk	Itra*	1 yr

Abbreviations: AmB = amphotericin B; CNS = central nervous system; ISDA = Infectious Diseases Society of America; Itra = itraconazole.

[1]Not FDA approved for this indication.

*Itraconazole (Sporanox) dosing for mild to moderate disease is 200 mg qd or bid; for all other indications a loading dose of 200 mg tid × 3 d is recommended followed by 200 mg qd or bid, guided by blood levels.

†Amphotericin B, in general liposomal (AmBisome)[1] or lipid formulations (Abelcet)[1] are preferred, but deoxycholate formulation of amphotericin B (Fungizone) may be used as an alternative in the treatment of acute pulmonary histoplasmosis. In CNS histoplasmosis, liposomal amphotericin B[1] is preferred.

"cannot always account for individual variation among patients. They are not intended to supplant physician judgment with respect to particular patients or special clinical situations." Regarding acute pulmonary histoplasmosis, no evidence from clinical trials is available to guide treatment decisions, and the IDSA guidelines are relatively conservative, reserving treatment only for "moderately severe to severe" cases. No explicit definition of severity is provided. Also, when mild to moderate symptoms persist, treatment is not recommended until the patient has been symptomatic for more than 4 weeks. Here, careful clinical judgment is warranted. Although poor long-term outcomes are uncommon in these patients, symptom resolution upon antifungal treatment is the rule. Therefore, some experts treat even mild to moderate acute pulmonary disease with a symptom duration of less than 4 weeks, in contrast to IDSA guideline recommendations.

Recommended induction treatment for the first 1 to 2 weeks in moderately severe to severe acute pulmonary histoplasmosis is a lipid formulation of amphotericin B (AmBisome, Abelcet)[1] 3 to 5 mg/kg IV daily. During induction therapy, methylprednisolone (Solu-Medrol) may be used as needed for respiratory complications. After that, oral itraconazole (Sporanox) can be used (200 mg three times daily for 3 days and then 200 mg twice daily) for a total duration of treatment of 12 weeks. Oral itraconazole for 6 to 12 weeks is the treatment of choice when the decision is made to treat mild to moderate acute pulmonary histoplasmosis.

When itraconazole is used, careful instructions should be given to ensure optimal oral absorption. Using the solution results generally in higher blood levels, but the unpleasant taste can be an issue for patients. To optimize absorption of the capsules, encourage patients to take them with a cola beverage. Because of substantial interpersonal variability in itraconazole metabolism, blood levels remain unpredictable. As a result, levels should be monitored on all patients whose treatment exceeds 2 weeks. In general, blood levels between 1.0 and 10.0 μg/mL are recommended, even though strong evidence for these cutoffs is lacking.

Chronic pulmonary histoplasmosis requires oral itraconazole therapy for 1 to 2 years. As noted earlier, relapses can occur even with prolonged therapy, and some patients require lifelong suppressive therapy. When an asymptomatic pulmonary nodule is found to be a histoplasmoma in the course of a malignancy work-up, no treatment is generally indicated.

In disseminated histoplasmosis with moderately severe to severe symptoms, induction treatment with liposomal amphotericin B[1] (3 mg/kg IV daily) is recommended for the first 1 to 2 weeks. This is followed by oral itraconazole for a total of at least 1 year. When symptoms of disseminated histoplasmosis are mild to moderate, the induction phase can be omitted, and treatment with oral itraconazole for 1 year should suffice. The role of treatment in mediastinal complications of histoplasmosis depends on the etiology. If symptomatic and inflammatory findings predominate, as in granulomatous mediastinitis, treatment with oral itraconazole is warranted. In mediastinal fibrosis, antifungal treatment generally does not improve the prognosis. CNS histoplasmosis should be aggressively treated with liposomal amphotericin B (5 mg/kg daily intravenously) for 4 to 6 weeks, followed by oral itraconazole for at least 1 year.

References

Ashbee HR, Evans EG, Viviani MA, et al: Histoplasmosis in Europe: Report on an epidemiological survey from the European Confederation of Medical Mycology Working Group, *Med Mycol* 46(1):57–65, 2008.

Assi MA, Sandid MS, Baddour LM, et al: Systemic histoplasmosis: A 15-year retrospective institutional review of 111 patients, *Medicine (Baltimore)* 86(3):162–169, 2007.

Cuellar-Rodriguez J, Avery RK, Lard M, et al: Histoplasmosis in solid organ transplant recipients: 10 years of experience at a large transplant center in an endemic area, *Clin Infect Dis* 49(5):710–716, 2009.

Deepe Jr GS: Immune response to early and late *Histoplasma capsulatum* infections, *Curr Opin Microbiol* 3(4):359–362, 2000.

Gugnani HC: Histoplasmosis in Africa: A review, *Indian J Chest Dis Allied Sci* 42(4):271–277, 2000.

Hage CA, Bowyer S, Tarvin SE, et al: Recognition, diagnosis, and treatment of histoplasmosis complicating tumor necrosis factor blocker therapy, *Clin Infect Dis* 50(1):85–92, 2010.

Hage CA, Davis TE, Fuller D, et al: Diagnosis of histoplasmosis by antigen detection in bronchoalveolar fluid, *Chest* 137(3):623–628, 2010.

Hage CA, Wheat LJ, Loyd J, et al: Pulmonary histoplasmosis, *Semin Respir Crit Care Med* 29(2):151–165, 2008.

Kahi CJ, Wheat LJ, Allen SD, Sarosi GA: Gastrointestinal histoplasmosis, *Am J Gastroenterol* 100(1):220–231, 2005.

Kauffman CA: Histoplasmosis: A clinical and laboratory update, *Clin Microbiol Rev* 20(1):115–132, 2007.

Kauffman CA: Diagnosis of histoplasmosis in immunosuppressed patients, *Curr Opin Infect Dis* 21(4):421–425, 2008.

Kauffman CA: Histoplasmosis, *Clin Chest Med* 30(2):217–225, 2009.

Kennedy CC, Limper AH: Redefining the clinical spectrum of chronic pulmonary histoplasmosis: A retrospective case series of 46 patients, *Medicine (Baltimore)* 86(4):252–258, 2007.

Mata-Essayag S, Colella MT, Rosello A, et al: Histoplasmosis: A study of 158 cases in Venezuela, 2000-2005, *Medicine (Baltimore)* 87(4):193–202, 2008.

---

[1]Not FDA approved for this iqudication.

Nosanchuk JD, Gacser A: *Histoplasma capsulatum* at the host–pathogen interface, *Microbes Infect* 10(9):973–977, 2008.

Pasqualotto AC, Oliveira FM, Severo LC: *Histoplasma capsulatum* recovery from the urine and a short review of genitourinary histoplasmosis, *Mycopathologia* 167(6):315–323, 2009.

Thompson 3rd GR, Cadena J, Patterson TF: Overview of antifungal agents, *Clin Chest Med* 30(2):203–215, 2009.

Wheat LJ: Approach to the diagnosis of the endemic mycoses, *Clin Chest Med* 30(2):379–389, 2009.

Wheat LJ, Freifeld AG, Kleiman MB, et al: Clinical practice guidelines for the management of patients with histoplasmosis: 2007 update by the Infectious Diseases Society of America, *Clin Infect Dis* 45(7):807–825, 2007.

Wheat LJ, Kauffman CA: Histoplasmosis, *Infect Dis Clin North Am* 17(1):1–19, 2003. vii.

Wheat LJ, Musial CE, Jenny-Avital E: Diagnosis and management of central nervous system histoplasmosis, *Clin Infect Dis* 40(6):844–852, 2005.

HYPERSENSITIVITY PNEUMONITIS

Method of
David I. Bernstein, MD; and Haejin Kim, MD

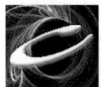

CURRENT DIAGNOSIS

- History of inhalational exposure to an identifiable environmental antigen associated with development of compatible clinical features.
- Objective evidence of acute pneumonitis or chronic pneumonitis with fibrosis based on physical examination, lung function testing, radiographic features, and lung biopsy findings.
- Clinical improvement in symptoms, lung function, and radiographic abnormalities with avoidance of the causative antigen(s).

CURRENT THERAPY

- Avoidance of contact with the offending antigen is essential and is often curative if performed early in the course of the disease.
- Although systemic corticosteroids are often required during the acute phase of hypersensitivity pneumonitis, their impact on disease progression and prognosis has not been determined.

Hypersensitivity pneumonitis (HP), also known as extrinsic allergic alveolitis, is an inflammatory disorder of the lungs mediated by immunologic hypersensitivity to a specific antigen, usually organic in nature. Although more than 200 causative antigens have been implicated, only a small number of individuals develop HP in response to exposure. Table 1 lists common causative agents in HP. Comprehensive lists of causative agents are available.

Pathophysiology

HP is thought to involve primarily delayed type IV (cell-mediated) hypersensitivity and is not mediated by immunoglobulin (Ig)E antibodies. Bronchoalveolar fluid obtained from patients with HP shows a predominant CD8+ lymphocytosis supporting T cell–mediated disease. Viruses are thought to play a role in the development of HP through upregulation of costimulatory molecules on alveolar macrophages and dendritic cells, leading to increased activation of type 1 helper T cells. Adoptive transfer models in animals have shown that CD4+ T cells and cytotoxic T cells are the most important effector cells in experimental HP, rather than cytokines, antibodies, or complement alone.

Clinical Presentation and Diagnosis

The main clinical features for HP are listed in Table 2. HP is diagnosed if the history, physical findings, high-resolution chest CT, and pulmonary function tests indicate infiltrative and restrictive lung disease; exposure is documented to a recognized or new causative agent; and there is significant improvement in symptoms, lung function, and radiographic findings with avoidance of the offending cause. IgG antibody to the offending antigen (serum preciptins) may be demonstrated but is not required for diagnosis. Immediate skin test reactivity is not indicated. These are the most widely accepted criteria, but evidence-based diagnostic guidelines have not been established. The clinician can differentiate acute from chronic HP based on chest CT and lung biopsy findings (see Table 2). A careful home, environmental, and occupational history is essential to identify one or more causative antigens.

Treatment

The primary treatment is cessation of exposure to the sources of offending antigens at home or in the workplace. Effective environmental control measures may include modification of work habits, improvement in ventilation, or change in manufacturing procedures. Systemic corticosteroids are often required and aid in recovery during the acute or subacute phases, but there are no long-term studies of their impact on disease progression or survival rates. Referral to a specialist in hypersensitivity lung diseases is recommended for proper diagnosis and identification of the sources of causative antigens. Individuals with advanced lung

TABLE 1 Hypersensitivity Pneumonitis: Representative Sources and Causative Agents

CONDITION OR PERSONS AT RISK	SOURCE	CAUSATIVE ANTIGENS
Dairy farmers	Hay, grains, silage	Thermophilic actinomycetes
Bird fancier's or pigeon breeder's disease	Avian droppings or feathers	Avian proteins
Humidifier lung	Contaminated water	Thermophilic actinomycetes or other microorganisms
Chemical workers	Polyurethane foam, varnishes, lacquers	Isocyanates
Machine workers	Metalworking fluid	*Pseudomonas fluorescens, Aspergillus niger, Staphylococcus capitis, Rhodococcus* spp., *Bacillus pumilus*
Familial hypersensitivity pneumonitis	Contaminated wood dust in walls	*Bacillus subtilis*
Hot tub lung	Mold on ceiling	*Cladosporium* spp., *Mycobacterium avium*

Modified from Richerson HB, Bernstein IL, Fink JN, et al: Guidelines for the clinical evaluation of hypersensitivity pneumonitis: report of the subcommittee on hypersensitivity pneumonitis, *J Allergy Clin Immunol* 84:839–844, 1989.

TABLE 2	Clinical Features of Hypersensitivity Pneumonitis		
FEATURE	**ACUTE**	**SUBACUTE**	**CHRONIC**
Identification of Source of Exposure to Causative Antigens			
Symptoms	Influenza-like illness ± cough/dyspnea within hours after antigenic exposure	Progressive cough, dyspnea, fatigue, and weight loss	Insidious progression with cough, exertional dyspnea, fatigue, and weight loss
Physical findings	Fever; normal chest examination or bibasilar crackles	Lungs normal or bibasilar crackles	Cyanosis; right-sided heart failure; lungs normal or bibasilar crackles
High-resolution computed tomography	Diffuse ground-glass infiltrates	Reticulation; small centrilobular nodules; air trapping on expiration	Honeycombing, mosaic attenuation, reticular opacities, peribronchiolar interstitial thickening reflecting irreversible pulmonary fibrosis
Pulmonary function testing	↓ FEV$_1$ and FVC (restrictive pattern); ↓ TLC; ↓ PaO$_2$ on exercise challenge; ↓ D$_{LCO}$		
Other findings supportive of a diagnosis of HP	• Improvement with avoidance of environmental exposure to suspect causative antigens • Precipitating antibodies to HP antigens cultured directly from the environment may help identify specific causative microorganisms • BAL lymphocytosis with reduced CD4/CD8 ratio <1 • Surgical lung biopsy: peribronchial interstitial lymphocytic and plasma cell infiltrates and/or noncaseating granulomas; pulmonary fibrosis in advanced cases of chronic HP		

BAL, Bronchoalveolar lavage; *D$_{LCO}$*, carbon monoxide diffusion in the lungs; *FEV$_1$*, forced expiratory volume in 1 second; *FVC*, forced vital capacity; *HP*, hypersensitivity pneumonitis; *PaO$_2$*, arterial partial pressure of oxygen; *TLC*, total lung capacity.
Modified from Richerson HB, Bernstein IL, Fink JN, et al: Guidelines for the clinical evaluation of hypersensitivity pneumonitis: report of the subcommittee on hypersensitivity pneumonitis, *J Allergy Clin Immunol* 84:839–844, 1989.

disease who have undergone lung transplantation for HP have survival rates comparable to individuals with interstitial lung disease.

References

Bernstein D, Lummus Z, Santilli G, et al: Machine operator's lung: A hypersensitivity pneumonitis disorder associated with exposure to metalworking fluid aerosols, *Chest* 108:636–641, 2006.

Girard M, Lacasse Y, Cormier Y: Hypersensitivity pneumonitis, *Allergy* 65:322–334, 2009.

Hanak V, Golbin JM, Hartman TE, et al: High-resolution CT findings of parenchymal fibrosis correlate with prognosis in hypersensitivity pneumonitis, *Chest* 134:133–138, 2008.

Jacobs RL, Andrews CP, Coalson JJ: Hypersensitivity pneumonitis: Beyond classic occupation disease: Changing concepts of diagnosis and management, *Ann Allergy Asthma Immunol* 95:115–128, 2005.

Kern RM, Singer JP, Koth L, Mooney J, et al: Lung transplantation for hypersensitivity pneumonitis, *Chest* 147:1558–1565, 2015.

Lacasse Y, Assayag E, Cormier Y: Myths and controversies in hypersensitivity pneumonitis, *Semin Respir Crit Care Med* 29:631–642, 2008.

Morisset J, Johannson KA, Jones KD: Identification of diagnostic criteria for chronic hypersensitivity pneumonitis: an international modified delphi survey, *Am J Respir Crit Care Med* 197:1036–1044, 2018.

Nogueira R, Melo N, Novais E, et al: Hypersensitivity pneumonitis: Antigen diversity and disease implications, *Pulmonology* 25:97–108, 2019.

Richerson HB, Bernstein IL, Fink JN, et al: Guidelines for the clinical evaluation of hypersensitivity pneumonitis: Report of the subcommittee on hypersensitivity pneumonitis, *J Allergy Clin Immunol* 84:839–844, 1989.

Schuyler M, Gott K, French V: The role of MIP-1alpha in experimental hypersensitivity pneumonitis, *Lung* 182:135–149, 2004.

LEGIONELLOSIS (LEGIONNAIRES' DISEASE AND PONTIAC FEVER)

Method of
Julio A. Ramirez, MD

In the summer of 1976, an outbreak of approximately 182 cases of pneumonia occurred in persons attending the American Legion convention in Philadelphia. One year later, Dr. McDade reported the identification of *Legionella pneumophila*, the bacterium responsible for the infection. Today, the family of Legionellaceae is composed of more than 40 species, with some species having different serogroups. *L pneumophila* causes approximately 85% of all *Legionella* infections. *L pneumophila* serogroup 1 is the single most common member of the family causing clinical infections.

Epidemiology

Legionella is an intracellular organism that lives in natural water. In the aquatic environment, the bacteria live and multiply within freshwater amebae. The number of *Legionella* organisms in the water can increase significantly with appropriate local conditions such as warm temperature, lack of biocides, stagnant water, and presence of amebae and other nutrients. These special conditions can be present in artificial water systems such as cooling towers, whirlpools, decorative fountains, and respiratory therapy devices.

The susceptible host acquires the bacteria from water containing the organism. Infection can be acquired by inhaling aerosols containing *Legionella* organisms or by microaspiration of water contaminated with *Legionella*. The hospitalized patient with *Legionella* pneumonia does not require respiratory isolation because legionellosis is not transmitted from person to person.

Clinical Features

Once *Legionella* organisms reach the respiratory tract, based on the interactions of the organism with the host immune system, the patient can have four possible clinical outcomes: asymptomatic infection, Pontiac fever, Legionnaires' disease, or extrapulmonary disease involving the liver, heart, brain, or other organs. Pontiac fever is a nonpneumonic form of disease characterized by fever, headaches, myalgias, and malaise. The patient has an influenza-like illness, with resolution of disease in a few days without specific antimicrobial therapy. Patients with Legionnaires' disease present with community-acquired pneumonia associated with high fever, gastrointestinal complaints such as diarrhea, and central nervous system complaints such as headaches or mental status changes. Hospital-acquired pneumonia can occur if *Legionella* is present in the hospital water supply.

Diagnosis

The currently available laboratory tests for diagnosis of *Legionella* infections include the direct fluorescent antibody stain (DFA), culture, antigen detection in the urine, antibody detection in serum

TABLE 1 Antibiotic Therapy for Legionella Infections

	ORAL DOSE	IV DOSE
Macrolides		
Azithromycin (Zithromax)	500 mg qd	500 mg qd
Clarithromycin (Biaxin)[1]	500 mg bid	
Erythromycin (Ery-Tab)	500 mg q6h	1 g q6h
Quinolones		
Ciprofloxacin (Cipro)[1]	750 mg bid	400 mg bid
Levofloxacin (Levaquin)	750 mg qd	750 mg qd
Moxifloxacin (Avelox)[1]	400 mg qd	400 mg qd
Rifamycins		
Rifampin (Rifadin)[1]	300 mg bid	300 mg bid
Tetracyclines		
Doxycycline (Vibramycin)[1]	100 mg bid on day 1, then 100 mg qd	100 mg bid on day 1, then 100 mg qd
Omadacycline (Nuzyra)	450 mg qd on day 1 and 2[3], then 300 mg qd	100 mg bid on day 1, then 100 mg qd

[1]Not FDA approved for this indication.
[3]Exceeds dosage recommended by the manufacturer.

by indirect fluorescent antibody testing (IFA), and DNA amplification using the polymerase chain reaction (PCR). The DFA stain can detect all *L pneumophila* serogroups, but a large number of bacteria need to be present in sputum for a positive result. *Legionella* can be cultured from respiratory specimens on selective media composed of buffered charcoal–yeast extract agar. The urinary antigen detection has a specificity greater than 95%; the disadvantage is that the test detects only the antigen of *L pneumophila* serogroup 1. Clinical specimens that have been used to detect *Legionella* by PCR include throat swabs, sputum, tracheal suction, bronchoalveolar lavage fluid, pleural fluid, and lung tissue.

Treatment

In the pulmonary parenchyma, *Legionella* can infect and multiply inside alveolar macrophages, alveolar epithelial cells, and capillary endothelial cells. The poor clinical outcome with β-lactam antibiotics is due to their lack of penetration into cells. Antibiotics with good intracellular penetration that can be used as monotherapy for *Legionella* infections include macrolides, tetracyclines, and quinolones (Table 1). Rifampin (Rifadin)[1] is not used as monotherapy because resistance can rapidly emerge when it is used alone.

Therapy of the patient with severe disease is initiated with intravenous antibiotics. Once the patient reaches clinical stability, the intravenous therapy can be switched to oral therapy. Doses for the most common antibiotics for intravenous and oral therapy are depicted in Table 1. In the nonimmunocompromised patient, the recommended duration of therapy is 7 to 10 days. In immunocompromised patients, because they are at risk for relapsing infection, the recommended duration of therapy is 14 to 21 days.

Several antibiotics have demonstrated clinical efficacy in Legionnaires' disease. Data with several in vitro and animal studies comparing different anti-*Legionella* antibiotics indicate that

[1]Not FDA approved for this indication.

erythromycin (Ery-Tab) is a weak anti-*Legionella* agent. If erythromycin is selected for therapy, it is important to add rifampin to the regimen to increase intracellular killing. From the family of macrolides, azithromycin (Zithromax) is the most active. The best bactericidal activity in the laboratory is achieved with quinolones. Retrospective observational studies indicate that patients treated with levofloxacin (Levaquin) have a shorter time to reach clinical stability and shorter duration of hospital stay. These antibiotics are considered primary anti-*Legionella* agents.

In clinical practice, I treat immunocompromised patients who have severe Legionnaires' disease with a combination of an intravenous quinolone plus an intravenous macrolide (e.g., levofloxacin plus azithromycin). This regimen is based only on the theoretical consideration that synergistic killing may be obtained using a quinolone to alter DNA synthesis and a macrolide to alter protein synthesis.

LUNG ABSCESS

Method of
Dan Schuller, MD

CURRENT DIAGNOSIS

- Lung abscess is usually a complication of aspiration in patients with gingivitis or periodontal disease.
- Mixed aerobic-anaerobic copathogens are common, but sputum cultures are not reliable.
- Lung abscesses are rare in edentulous patients and should prompt evaluation for bronchial obstruction.
- CT scan of the chest is very useful in the diagnostic evaluation.

CURRENT THERAPY

- Prolonged antimicrobial therapy (6–8 weeks) and postural drainage are the cornerstones of therapy.
- Clindamycin (Cleocin) or alternative anaerobic coverage is required even if sputum cultures grow only aerobic bacteria (colonizers or copathogens).
- Percutaneous or bronchoscopic drainage is reserved for selected cases refractory to medical management or at a high risk for complications.
- Surgical resection is seldom needed because of the success of medical therapy.
- Evaluation and management of underlying predisposing conditions should not be neglected.

Definition and Classification

Lung abscess is defined as a focal area of necrosis of the lung parenchyma resulting from microbial infection and usually measuring more than 2 cm in diameter. Smaller or multiple areas of necrosis in contiguous areas are referred to as *necrotizing pneumonia*. Primary lung abscess (80%) is due to direct infection or aspiration. Secondary lung abscess (20%) is secondary to bronchial obstruction, immunodeficiency, pulmonary infarction, trauma, or complications from surgery. Lung abscesses can also be classified according to pathogen (e.g., mixed anaerobic, *Pseudomonas*, mycobacterial, fungal) or duration of symptoms (e.g., chronic with symptoms for more than a month before presentation). If symptoms are present for more than one month, the lung abscess is considered chronic.

Epidemiology and Risk Factors

Most lung abscesses result from aspiration of oral secretions in patients who harbor high bacterial concentrations in the gingival crevices. Periodontal disease, especially gingivitis, is a major predisposing condition, particularly in hosts impaired by altered sensorium due to alcoholism, anesthesia, coma, drug overdose, seizures, or stroke. Because edentulous persons rarely develop lung abscesses, other causes such as malignancy should be carefully sought. Patients with dysphagia, esophageal disease, poor airway protection, or weak cough and respiratory clearance mechanisms are also at risk for developing lung abscess.

Patients whose immune systems are compromised by malignancy, HIV infection, malnutrition, diabetes, chronic use of corticosteroids, or previous organ transplantation are more likely to be infected with aerobic bacteria, mycobacterial or fungal pathogens. These patients are more likely to have multiple abscesses, less response to treatment, and a worse prognosis.

In children, consider secondary causes including foreign body aspiration, congenital cystic adenomatoid malformation, pulmonary sequestration, cystic fibrosis, bronchiectasis, bronchogenic cyst, congenital immunodeficiency, or severe underlying neurologic abnormality.

Lemierre's disease or jugular vein suppurative thrombophlebitis, usually caused by *Fusobacterium necrophorum*, is a rare infection that begins in the pharynx as a tonsillar or peritonsillar abscess and spreads to involve the internal jugular vein, with septic emboli to the lung with secondary cavitations.

Pathophysiology

The understanding of lower airway microbiota in humans as well as the capacity of a microorganism to cause damage in a host has evolved. The development of a lung abscess usually starts when an insult (e.g., inoculum of highly contaminated oral secretions) overcomes the pulmonary mechanisms of defense and begins a process of pneumonitis in the dependent areas affected by aspiration. Depending on the microbiology and the intensity of the inflammatory response, the acute pneumonitis evolves to tissue necrosis after 7 to 14 days and subsequent cavitation. At first, the enclosing wall is poorly defined, but with time and progressive fibrosis it becomes more discrete. When a communication with the airway exists, the suppurative debris from the abscess can partially drain, leaving an air-containing cavity with a radiographic air-fluid level. Occasionally, abscesses rupture into the pleural cavity yielding an empyema or a bronchopleural fistula (Figure 1). Primary abscesses due to aspiration are much more common on the right side than the left and are most often single. The most common locations include the superior segments of the lower lobes and the posterior segment of the right upper lobe.

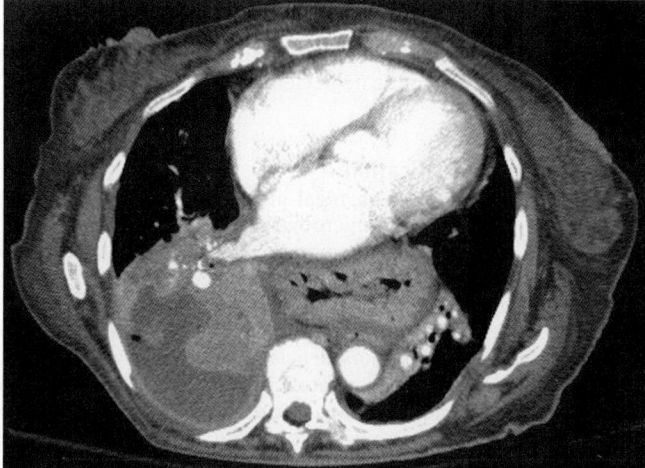

Figure 1 Primary lung abscess in the right lower lobe with rupture into the pleural space causing an empyema.

Clinical Manifestations

Most patients present with insidious symptoms that evolve over a period of weeks to months. Cough productive of copious amounts of putrid, foul-smelling sputum that occurs in paroxysms after changing position are characteristic. Fevers, chills, night sweats, chest pain, dyspnea, general malaise, and fatigue are common. Hemoptysis can vary from blood-streaked sputum to life-threatening hemorrhage. Physical findings can include fever, tachycardia, periodontal disease, halitosis, signs of lung consolidation or pleural effusion, amphoric breath sounds, and occasionally clubbing of the fingers and toes can appear within a few weeks after the onset of an abscess.

Diagnosis

Lung abscess is easily diagnosed when there is a classic clinical presentation with indolent symptoms lasting more than 2 weeks in a host with predisposing risk factors and a chest radiograph revealing a cavitary infiltrate or an air-fluid level. However, numerous pathogens are associated with this syndrome, and attempts to establish microbiological diagnosis and exclude other conditions are warranted.

Computed tomography (CT) scans can be useful for better anatomic definition, to evaluate possible associated conditions such as malignancy, and to rule out pleural involvement. Distinguishing between a lung abscess and an empyema with an associated bronchopleural fistula leading to an air-fluid level can sometimes be challenging, but it is crucial because the management of these conditions is very different. Features that suggest empyema include a lenticular shape or a larger diameter of the air-fluid level on the lateral view of the chest film, an obtuse angle of the cavity with the chest wall, and a split pleural sign with contrast enhancement of the pleura.

Most lung abscesses are caused by anaerobic or mixed aerobic and anaerobic infections. Anaerobic bacteria include *Peptostreptococcus*, *Prevotella*, *Bacteroides* spp., and *Fusobacterium* spp. and are difficult to isolate owing to technical issues and contamination by upper airway flora. Other pathogens, including *Staphylococcus aureus*, *Klebsiella pneumonia*, *Pseudomonas*, *Burkholderia pseudomallei*, *Nocardia*, *Actinomyces*, and mycobacterial or fungal organisms, are more likely to occur in secondary lung abscesses. The bacteriology of lung abscesses may be different in other parts of the world.

Sputum Gram stains and culture should be performed in all patients but interpreted with caution because prior antimicrobial therapy can inhibit growth, and contaminant strains can be misleading. Even when there is abundant growth of a species of aerobic bacteria, treatment should still be directed at covering anaerobes.

In the absence of positive blood or pleural fluid cultures, microbiological confirmation of a lung abscess requires other invasive methods such as a transthoracic needle aspirates (TTNA) or bronchoscopy with bronchoalveolar lavage (BAL) or protected specimen brush (PSB). The best timing for bronchoscopy is controversial because early intervention has the highest diagnostic yield but at the risk of provoking spillage of a relatively contained abscess into additional lobes or the contralateral lung. In patients who are edentulous or in whom there is a high suspicion for malignancy, the indication for bronchoscopic evaluation is almost universal but should be scheduled when the risk for clinical deterioration (e.g., spillage with resultant respiratory failure) has been minimized.

Differential Diagnosis

In addition to the multiple necrotizing infections or an empyema with a bronchopleural fistula (see earlier), there are many noninfectious diseases that can cause cavitary lung lesions and mimic a lung abscess. The differential diagnosis includes neoplasm (primary or metastatic), bullae or cyst with air-fluid level, bronchiectasis, necrotizing vasculitis, or pulmonary infarction. In patients with multiple cavitary lesions, consider septic emboli.

Treatment

Lung abscess is best treated with a prolonged course of adequate antimicrobials and postural drainage. Percutaneous or bronchoscopic drainage and surgery are considered only for selected patients whose disease is refractory to standard care.

Initial empiric antibiotic treatment for a typical community-acquired lung abscess should consist of intravenous clindamycin (Cleocin) 600 to 900 mg every 6 to 8 hours, which has been shown to be superior to penicillin. For patients with a nosocomial or health care–associated lung abscess, additional coverage for enteric gram-negative pathogens including *Pseudomonas aeruginosa* and *Staphylococcus aureus* is appropriate.

Alternative antimicrobial options include ampicillin–sulbactam (Unasyn)[1] 1.5 to 3.0 g IV every 6 hours, piperacillin–tazobactam (Zosyn)[1] 3.35 g IV every 6 hours, cefoxitin (Mefoxin) 2 to 3 g every 6 to 8 hours, or a combination of moxifloxacin (Avelox)[1] 400 mg IV daily and metronidazole (Flagyl) 500 mg IV every 6 to 8 hours. The use of metronidazole as single agent has been associated with a high therapeutic failure rate.

After defervescence and radiographic improvement, parenteral antibiotics can be switched to oral bioequivalent therapy for 6 to 8 weeks or longer depending on the course. Shorter antimicrobial courses are associated with a high rate of relapse. Most experts suggest continuing therapy until there is radiographic resolution or a small stable lesion.

Indications for percutaneous or bronchoscopic drainage include persistent sepsis after 5 to 7 days of antimicrobial therapy, abscesses larger than 4 cm that are under tension or enlarging, and need for mechanical ventilator support. Percutaneous drainage should only be considered when there is a reasonable abscess–pleura symphysis and no associated coagulopathy. Lung resection is rarely needed and is reserved for operable cases refractory to medical treatment.

Postural drainage and chest physiotherapy facilitate removal of pus, relieving symptoms and improving gas exchange. Surgical resection is required in less than 10% of patients whose disease is refractory to medical management.

Finally, evaluation and management of the predisposing conditions leading to aspiration should take place after the patient is stabilized. This can include swallowing assessment, dental work, or oral surgery.

Prognosis

Primary lung abscesses in nonimmunocompromised hosts have cure rates of 90% to 95% with antimicrobial therapy and postural drainage alone. However, in immunocompromised patients and those with bronchial obstruction due to cancer, the mortality has been reported between 20% and 75%.

---

[1]Not FDA approved for this indication.

References

Bartlett JG: Anaerobic bacterial pleuropulmonary infections, *Semin Respir Med* 13:159–164, 1992.

Bartlett JG: The role of anaerobic bacteria in lung abscess, *Clin Infect Dis* 40:923–925, 2005.

Egyud M, Suzuki K: Post-resection complications: abscesses, empyemas, bronchopleural fistulas, *J Thorac Dis* 10:S3408, 2018.

Gudiol F, Manresa F, Pallares R, et al: Clindamycin vs. penicillin for anaerobic lung infections, *Arch Intern Med* 150:2525–2529, 1990.

Hammer DL, Aranda CP, Galati V, Adams FV: Massive intrabronchial aspiration of contents of pulmonary abscess after fiberoptic bronchoscopy, *Chest* 7:306–307, 1978.

Herth F, Ernst A, Becker HD: Endoscopic drainage of lung abscesses. Technique and outcome, *Chest* 127:1378–1381, 2005.

Levinson ME, Mangura CT, Lorber B, et al: Clindamycin compared with penicillin for the treatment of anaerobic lung abscess, *Ann Intern Med* 98:466–471, 1983.

Mandell LA, Niederman MS: Aspiration pneumonia, *N Engl J Med* 380:651–663, 2019.

Mandell LA, Wunderink RG, Anzueto A, et al: Infectious Diseases Society of America/American Thoracic Society consensus guidelines on the management of community-acquired pneumonia in adults, *Clin Infect Dis* 44:S27–S72, 2007.

Mueller PR, Berlin L: Complications of lung abscess aspiration and drainage, *AJR Am J Roentgenol* 178:1083–1086, 2002.

Wang JL, Chen KY, Fang CT, et al: Changing bacteriology of adult community-acquired lung abscess in Taiwan: Klebsiella pneumonia vs anaerobes, *Clin Infec Dis* 40:915, 2015.

LUNG CANCER

Method of
Erin A. Gillaspie, MD, MPH; Amanda S. Cass, PharmD; Jennifer Lewis, MD, MPH; and Leora Horn, MD, MSc

CURRENT DIAGNOSIS

- An improvement in lung cancer outcomes is achievable with use of low-dose computed tomography (CT) for lung cancer screening
- All eligible patients should be screened with an annual low-dose CT scan.
- The accurate staging of lung cancer is crucial in helping to guide treatment recommendations.
- Many patients have no symptoms at the time of diagnosis.
- Tissue diagnosis can be achieved through image-guided endobronchial and surgical biopsies.
- All smokers should be counselled on smoking cessation.

CURRENT THERAPY

- Treatment recommendations are based on stage of cancer and fitness of patient to tolerate surgery.
- Surgically resectable non–small cell lung cancer (NSCLC) is more commonly approached in a minimally invasive fashion.
- Early stage NSCLC is most often treated with definitive surgery with or without chemotherapy.
- Locally advanced NSCLC requires a multimodality treatment regimen often using a combination of radiation, surgery, and systemic therapy.
- Forty percent of patients will have advanced stage of disease at diagnosis, and systemic therapy is the mainstay of treatment.
- All patients with Stage IV disease should have molecular and PD-L1 testing to help guide therapy.
- Routine disease monitoring is important both after curative-intent treatment and during treatment for incurable disease.
- Small cell lung cancer (SCLC) is aggressive and the mainstay of treatment is systemic therapy combined with radiation in early stage disease or immunotherapy in advanced disease.

Epidemiology

Lung cancer is the leading cause of cancer-related mortality in the United States among both men and women. The overall incidence rate is decreasing, more rapidly among men, largely due to the declining use of tobacco. Lung cancer is predominantly a disease of older individuals, aged 65 to 84 with average age at diagnosis of 70. There is an equal distribution in lung cancer incidence among African Americans and Caucasians as a whole. However, the highest incidence is among African American males and Caucasian females. Incidence and mortality rates among Hispanics and Native and Asian Americans are approximately 40% to 50% of that of Caucasians. The majority (79%) of cases are diagnosed at locally advanced or advanced stages of disease, which accounts for the relatively poor overall survival (OS). The 5-year OS is 18.6%; local, 30% regional, and 5% distant.

Epithelial lung cancers are divided into four major cell types: small cell lung cancer (SCLC), adenocarcinoma, squamous cell carcinoma, and large cell carcinoma; the latter three types are collectively known as non–small cell lung cancers (NSCLCs). All histologic types of lung cancer can develop in current and former smokers, although squamous and small cell carcinomas are most commonly associated with heavy tobacco use. It is essential to distinguish histologically between SCLC and NSCLC because these subtypes have different natural histories and therapeutic approaches. In addition, the molecular subtype of NSCLC has become an important part of treatment planning because some chemotherapeutic agents perform quite differently in squamous cell cancers versus adenocarcinoma. Further, patients with adenocarcinoma are more likely to harbor tumor mutations making them candidates for targeted therapy.

Risk Factors

Tobacco use (cigarettes, cigars, and pipes) is by far the greatest risk factor for lung cancer, accounting for approximately 80% to 90% of lung cancer deaths. Risk increases as a function of both quality and duration of tobacco exposure. Environmental tobacco smoke (ETS) or second-hand smoke is also an established cause of lung cancer.

Radon gas is the second most common risk factor. Prolonged exposure to low-level radon in homes might impart a risk of lung cancer equal or greater than that of ETS.

Additional risk factors include asbestos, radiation, agent orange, chromium, cadmium, and arsenic. Individuals with occupations in rubber manufacturing, roofing, paving, and chimney sweeping are also felt to be at an increased risk for developing lung cancer. Finally, family history of lung cancer is a risk factor, but the exact genetic driver remains unclear. Notably, the incidence of lung cancer in never smokers is increasing for reasons that are also unclear.

Prevention

Smoking cessation is the cornerstone of lung cancer prevention. Stopping tobacco use before middle age avoids more than 90% of the lung cancer risk attributable to tobacco. Moreover, smoking cessation in individuals with an established diagnosis of lung cancer is associated with improved survival and decreased toxicities from therapy.

The combination of smoking cessation counseling with medications leads to a higher likelihood of successful quit attempts. US Food and Drug Administration (FDA) approved medications include nicotine replacement therapy (nicotine patches [NicoDerm CQ], lozenges [Nicorette], gum [Nicorelief, Nicorette], spray [Nicotrol NS]), varenicline (Chantix), and bupropion (Zyban). Nicotine patches, which provide longer periods of nicotine replacement, should be used in combination with gum or lozenges to treat short-term cravings. The results of a multicenter, double-blinded, randomized controlled trial, the Evaluating Adverse Events in Global Smoking Cessation Study (EAGLES trial), compared varenicline, bupropion, nicotine patch, and placebo in more than 8000 smokers and found that the efficacy of each medication was higher than placebo. The results of this trial also demonstrated that there was no increase in neuropsychiatric symptoms in smokers exposed to varenicline, leading the FDA to remove the black box warning.

Patients must want to stop smoking and must be willing to work hard to achieve the goal of smoking abstinence to achieve success. Counseling using the 5 As remains the recommended five major steps in intervention (Table 1). A shortened version, the 3 As, is an alternative for busy clinicians and involves **asking** and recording smoking status, **advising** patient of health benefits, and **acting** on patient's response.

TABLE 1	The 5As of Smoking Cessation Counseling
Ask	Ask and record smoking status
Advise	Advise smokers on benefit of stopping in a personalized, appropriate manner
Assess	Assess motivation to quit
Assist	Assist in smokers' quit attempt
Arrange	Arrange follow up with cessation services

Early Detection

Clinicians have an important opportunity to improve lung cancer outcomes through early detection. Increasing evidence demonstrates a mortality benefit when screening high-risk individuals with low-dose computed tomography (LDCT). Lung cancer screening with LDCT is recommended by the US Preventive Services Task Force (USPSTF) for individuals aged 55 to 80, current or former smokers who have quit within the past 15 years, and smokers who have at least a 30 pack-year history of smoking. Medicare covers LDCT screening for a similar group of high-risk individuals, differing only in the upper age limit (ages 55 to 77). These policy decisions were made following the results of the National Lung Screening Trial (NLST).

The NLST was a large, multicenter, randomized controlled trial performed in the United States that compared annual chest x-ray (CXR) to LDCT in 53,454 patients who were considered high-risk for the development of lung cancer. This trial was terminated early when it met its primary endpoint of achieving a 20% relative reduction in lung cancer mortality favoring the LDCT arm. Nearly twice as many early stage 1A cancers were detected in the LDCT group compared with the CXR group (40% vs. 21%). The overall rates of lung cancer death were 247 and 309 deaths per 100,000 person-years in the LDCT and CXR groups, respectively. Compared with the CXR group, the rate of death in the LDCT group from *any* cause was reduced by 6.7% (95% CI, 1.2 to 13.6; $P = .02$). A common critique of the NLST is the high false positive rate. However, across 3 rounds of screening in the LDCT arm, only 24.2% of screening exams were positive and went on to require additional imaging or biopsy. The interpretation of screening LDCT continues to improve through the use of the American College of Radiology's structured reporting system, Lung-RADs, which has further decreased the false positive rate.

More recently, the Danish-Belgium Lung Cancer Screening Trial (NELSON) found a 26% relative reduction in lung cancer mortality when screening high-risk individuals with LDCT compared with no screening, further supporting the role for annual LDCT scans in high-risk individuals as part of health maintenance.

Clinical Manifestations

The size, location, and the manifestation of paraneoplastic syndromes determine the clinical presentation of most patients with lung cancer. Most patients with early stage disease are asymptomatic and their cancer is discovered incidentally on CXR or CT scans (Table 2).

TABLE 2	Clinical Signs and Symptoms of Lung Cancer

TUMOR LOCAL EFFECTS	DISTANT METASTASIS EFFECTS	PARANEOPLASTIC SYNDROME
Cough	Bone pain	Hypercalcemia
Dyspnea	Headache	SIADH
Hemoptysis	Nausea and vomiting	Lambert-Eaton syndrome
Chest pain	Seizure	Cerebellar ataxia
Hoarseness	Weight loss	Encephalitis
SVC syndrome	Fatigue	Cachexia/anorexia
Postobstructive pneumonia	Abdominal pain	Cushing syndrome
Pleural effusion	Spinal cord compression	
Pericardial effusion	Pathologic fracture	

SIADH, Syndrome of inappropriate antidiuretic hormone secretion; *SVC,* superior vena cava.

Peripheral tumors may invade the chest wall and can present with pain. Centrally located tumors may cause symptoms from direct invasion or compression of mediastinal structures. Symptoms may include cough, hemoptysis, wheezing, stridor, or even postobstructive pneumonia. Patients may present with diaphragmatic paralysis due to phrenic nerve invasion, superior vena cava (SVC) syndrome with facial edema, bluish discoloration of the upper chest, and shortness of breath. They may even have dysphagia from esophageal compression. Mediastinal lymph node involvement can cause disruption of the recurrent laryngeal nerve, leading to hoarseness. Tumors arising in the superior sulcus, so-called Pancoast tumors, can result in a lower brachial plexopathy and Horner syndrome. Pleural effusion may also be the presenting sign for lung cancer and can cause pain, dyspnea, or cough (see Table 2).

Symptoms from metastatic disease may be the first sign of malignancy. Frequent sites of metastasis include supraclavicular and cervical lymph nodes, bone, brain, liver, and adrenal glands. Brain metastases occur in 10% to 30% of patients. Symptoms include seizures, nausea and vomiting, headache, or focal neurologic dysfunction. Bony metastases present with pain, pathologic fracture, or spinal cord compression. Liver metastases can cause biliary obstruction and jaundice; however, this is not particularly common. Constitutional symptoms may include anorexia, weight loss, weakness, fever, and night sweats.

Lung cancers are notable for ectopic production of hormones leading to several paraneoplastic syndromes. These are most commonly described in SCLC; however, it can occur in rare cases of NSCLC as well. The most common paraneoplastic syndromes in NSCLC are tumor cachexia and hypercalcemia. The causes of tumor cachexia are not well characterized. Hypercalcemia is mediated by the production of parathyroid hormone–related peptide (PTHrP). The peptide stimulates release of calcium from bones, resulting in an elevation in calcium in the blood and osteopenia. This syndrome is treated effectively with bisphosphonate therapy. Hypertrophic pulmonary arthropathy can occur with NSCLC or SCLC and is characterized by digital clubbing and periostitis of the long bones that are demonstrable on plain x-rays.

Paraneoplastic syndromes unique to SCLC include Lambert-Eaton myasthenic syndrome (LEMS), syndrome of inappropriate antidiuretic hormone (SIADH), and Cushing syndrome. A patient presenting with LEMS should always be ruled out for malignancy; 50% of patients who present with this syndrome have cancer, and in 95% of those cases, it is SCLC. Another paraneoplastic syndrome related to SCLC is SIADH. SIADH generally resolves within 1 to 4 weeks of initiating chemotherapy. During this period, serum sodium can usually be managed and maintained above 128 mEq/L via fluid restriction. Demeclocycline (Declomycin)[1] can be a useful adjunctive measure when fluid restriction alone is insufficient. Vasopressin receptor antagonists also have been used in the management of SIADH but are costly and have increased unique toxicities such as liver injury.

Cushing syndrome due to ectopic production of adrenocorticotropic hormone (ACTH) by SCLC and pulmonary carcinoids results in electrolyte disturbances rather than classic changes in body habitus. Treatment with standard medications such as metyrapone[1] and ketoconazole (Nizoral)[1] is largely ineffective.

Cerebellar degeneration may be associated with anti-Hu, anti-Yo, or P/Q channel autoantibodies. Cutaneous manifestations such as dermatomyositis are rare. Thrombosis including Trousseaus syndrome, marantic endocarditis, and coagulopathies are also uncommon and are usually associated with a worse prognosis.

Diagnostic Techniques

Once lung cancer is suspected, tissue biopsy is required to make a definitive diagnosis. In patients with suspected metastatic disease, a biopsy of a distant site of disease is preferred for tissue confirmation because it provides additional staging information.

Several methods can be considered depending on the location of the tumor, and the technique should be tailored to the location of the primary tumor and the presence of mediastinal nodal involvement or metastatic disease. Transbronchial biopsy can be performed for centrally located tumors, and the yield may be increased by using endobronchial ultrasound (EBUS) techniques. Mediastinal nodal involvement or direct extension into the mediastinum may be evaluated by bronchoscopy paired with endoscopic ultrasound (EUS) or surgically by mediastinoscopy.

For peripheral lesions, a CT-guided needle biopsy may be considered. This route of biopsy is associated with a risk of pneumothorax that requires intervention in approximately 5.6% of cases.

The advent of navigational bronchoscopy has allowed interventional pulmonologists to sample nodules in the periphery of the lungs with very high yield. If equivocal results are obtained, transthoracic biopsies using a minimally invasive approach (video-assisted thoracoscopic surgery [VATS] or robotic-assisted thoracoscopic surgery [RATS]) may be used as both diagnostic and therapeutic options. For patients presenting with a pleural or pericardial effusion, cytologic examination of the fluid can establish the diagnosis.

The tenets of biopsy are the same no matter the method chosen: there should be adequate tissue for diagnosis, histologic subtyping, and molecular testing. If sufficient tissue is not obtained to further classify the subtype of lung cancer, additional procedures to obtain sufficient tissue are often warranted, particularly in patients with advanced stage disease.

Staging

The accurate staging of lung cancer is crucial in guiding treatment recommendations (Tables 3 and 4). Staging makes use of imaging modalities combined with biopsy to help determine size, location, and histology of a lesion. A complete history and physical examination along with assessment of performance status is important in evaluating a patient's ability to tolerate therapy (Figure 1).

Imaging

Computed tomography (CT) scanning is a standard part of the workup for lung cancer and determining the candidacy for resection. Although excellent in delineating the extent of the primary lesion disease and some sites of metastatic disease, it is the least sensitive and specific modality for the identification of lymph node involvement or distant metastatic disease. CT scan of the chest should always be obtained with extension through the adrenal glands, a common site of metastatic disease.

Positron emission tomography (PET) scans play an important role in both nodal and extrathoracic staging. PET scans attempt to identify sites of malignancy based on glucose metabolism by measuring the uptake of ^{18}F-fluorodeoxyglucose (FDG). Rapidly dividing cells will preferentially take up ^{18}F-FDG and appear as a "hot spot." Combined ^{18}F-FDG PET-CT imaging has been shown to improve the accuracy of staging in NSCLC compared with visual correlation of PET and CT on either study alone. A standardized uptake value (SUV) of greater than 2.5 on PET is considered highly suspicious for malignancy. False negatives can be seen in diabetes, in lesions less than 8 mm, and in slow-growing tumors (e.g., carcinoid tumors or well-differentiated adenocarcinoma). Confirmation of PET scan abnormalities with tissue diagnosis remains important because this modality of imaging also carries the risk of false-positive upstaging; particularly in regions where histoplasmosis is prevalent.

Mediastinoscopy was once considered the gold standard diagnostic technique for the assessment of mediastinal lymph nodes. Mediastinoscopy can evaluate level lymph node stations 2R, 4R, 2L, 4L, and 7, and can send whole lymph nodes for analysis. This has been replaced in many centers by EBUS, which is less invasive and offers the ability to sample both N1 and N2 nodes. Review of available publications reveals a median sensitivity of 89% for EBUS and a very low risk of complications. In addition, rapid onsite evaluation (ROSE) of cytological samples confirms adequacy at the time of procedure to enhance overall yield.

[1]Not FDA approved for this indication.

TABLE 3 TNM Staging

PRIMARY TUMOR (T)		LYMPH NODES (N)		DISTANT METASTASIS (M)	
T0	No evidence of primary tumor	N0	No regional lymph nodes involved	M0	No distant metastases
Tis	Carcinoma in situ	N1	Ipsilateral lymph node peribronchial and/or ipsilateral hilar or intrapulmonary lymph nodes involved	M1	Distant metastases present
T1	Tumor ≤3 cm, surrounded by lung or visceral pleura without bronchoscopic evidence of invasion more proximal than lobar bronchus	N2	Ipsilateral mediastinal or subcarinal lymph nodes involved	M1a	Separate tumor nodule(s) in contralateral lobe; pleural or pericardial nodule(s) or malignant pleural or pericardial effusion
T1a	Tumor ≤1 cm	N3	Contralateral mediastinal or hilar lymph nodes or ipsilateral or contralateral scalene or supraclavicular lymph nodes involved	M1b	Single extrathoracic metastasis
T1b	Tumor >1 cm but ≤2 cm			M1c	Multiple extrathoracic metastases in one or more organs
T1c	Tumor >2 cm but ≤3 cm				
T2	Tumor >3 cm but ≤5 cm or with any of the following: involves main bronchus but does not involve carina, invades visceral pleura, associated with atelectasis or obstructive pneumonitis				
T2a	Tumor >3 cm but ≤4 cm				
T2b	Tumor >4 cm but ≤5 cm				
T3	Tumor >5 cm but ≤7 cm or with any of the following: separate tumor nodule(s) in same lobe as primary or directly invades				
T4	Tumors >7 cm in greatest dimension or any tumor that invades the mediastinum, diaphragm, heart, great vessels, recurrent laryngeal nerve, carina, trachea, esophagus, spine or separate tumor in a different lobe of the ipsilateral lung				

A magnetic resonance imaging (MRI) with contrast of the brain is mandatory in all patients with SCLC. In patients with NSCLC, an MRI of the brain should also be performed in patients with nodal involvement, stage IV disease, or any neurologic symptoms.

Assessing Treatment Candidacy

After establishing the stage of cancer, a meticulous evaluation should be performed prior to recommending therapy (see Figure 1). Workup should include history and physical examination, blood work including a complete blood count, renal function and liver function tests, pulmonary function tests, nutritional assessments, and cardiac clearance in patients being selected for surgery. Assessment of a patient's performance status has important prognostic and therapeutic implications and should be noted in all patients.

In patients who are being considered for surgery, smokers should be counseled to stop immediately. In addition to helping to reduce the risk of perioperative pulmonary complications and death, it will also help to reduce the long-term consequences related to tobacco abuse.

Assessment of Cardiovascular Risk

Major cardiac-related adverse events occur in approximately 2% to 3% of patients after pulmonary resection. The thoracic revised cardiac risk index is a validated tool that can be used to help guide which patients should be sent for additional preoperative consultation. Patients who score more than 1.5 on the cardiac index, or those describing limited exercise capacity or recent diagnosis of active heart disease all warrant evaluation by a cardiologist.

Assessment of Pulmonary Function

Patients undergoing pulmonary resection commonly have several coexisting conditions and exposures that can affect pulmonary function. It is therefore essential to ensure adequate pulmonary reserve prior to proceeding with resection. Most surgeons will request a spirometry and measurement of diffusion capacity for carbon monoxide (DLCO) for all patients undergoing pulmonary resection. These are calculated as a percentage of the predicted value. The forced expiratory volume in 1 second (FEV_1), measured during spirometry, determines the mechanical function of the lung, that is, the airflow limitations of medium to large airways. The DLCO value provides a gross estimate of the function at the alveolar-capillary membrane. The DLCO (the actual and predicted postoperative percentage) has been shown in various studies to be the most important predictors of perioperative complications and mortality.

A postoperative predicted FEV_1 or DLCO of less than 60% should prompt additional testing such as a shuttle walk test or stair-climbing exercise. If the postoperative predicted DLCO is less than 30% to 40%, this denotes an increased risk and warrants a formal cardiopulmonary exercise test with measurement of maximal oxygen consumption. This quantitative assessment has established thresholds associated with surgical risk. A ventilation-perfusion scan may also be helpful in patients with heterogeneous, underlying lung disease.

Surgical Approach to Lung Cancer

The approach to surgery and extent of pulmonary resection is determined by the size and location of the tumor and experience of the surgeon.

TABLE 4	Staging Groups		
STAGE	**T**	**N**	**M**
Stage 0	Tis	N0	M0
Stage IA1	T1a	N0	M0
Stage IA2	T1b	N0	M0
Stage IA3	T1c	N0	M0
Stage IB	T2a	N0	M0
Stage IIA	T2b	N0	M0
Stage IIB	T1a to c	N1	M0
	T2a	N1	M0
	T2b	N1	M0
	T3	N0	M0
Stage IIIA	T1a to c	N2	M0
	T2a to b	N2	M0
	T3	N1	M0
	T4	N0	M0
	T4	N1	M0
Stage IIIB	T1a-c	N3	M0
	T2a to b	N3	M0
	T3	N2	M0
	T4	N2	M0
Stage IVA	Any	Any	M1a
	Any	Any	M1b
Stage IVB	Any	Any	M1c

Open Lobectomy

The majority of pulmonary resections continue to be performed in open fashion via thoracotomy and often involve dividing muscle and taking out a portion of a rib.

Surgery is performed with a special endotracheal tube (a double-lumen tube) that allows the operative lung to be collapsed while maintaining ventilation to the contralateral lung. After thoracotomy, the chest is inspected to rule out metastatic disease and confirm that the tumor is resectable.

Surgery begins with the removal of N1 and N2 lymph nodes, which are sent to pathology. A lobectomy is performed by isolating the arteries, vein, and bronchus associated with the lobe and dividing each along with the fissure that connects the upper, middle (right), and lower lobes. Once the lobectomy is completed, the remaining lung is reinflated to fill the pleural space, and chest tubes are positioned to help drain fluid and air while the patient recovers.

Lung resections carry a significant risk of perioperative morbidity, with 37% of patients experiencing some form of postoperative complication—atrial arrhythmia and prolonged air leak being the most common. Other complications can include infection, bleeding, hypoxia, and death.

Video-Assisted Thoracoscopic Surgery Lobectomy

Most academic medical centers have transitioned to a minimally invasive approach for the majority of pulmonary resections—VATS or robotic resections as described later.

A VATS lobectomy is conducted in similar fashion to an open lobectomy but utilizes two to three small ports in the chest, each measuring approximately 1 cm, and a slightly larger utility incision measuring 3 cm through which the specimen is removed. VATS differs from open surgery in both the length of incisions as well as minimal disruption or division of muscle fibers and there is no rib spreading. A camera and special instruments have been designed to make the surgery possible.

Comparison of outcomes shows that both open surgery and VATS provide equal cancer-specific outcomes. Both VATS and open surgery have similar patterns of postoperative complications, although VATS occurs at a lesser rate. Additional benefits of VATS include earlier recovery, earlier discharge, less pain, less impact on pulmonary function, better quality of life, and increased delivery of adjuvant therapy.

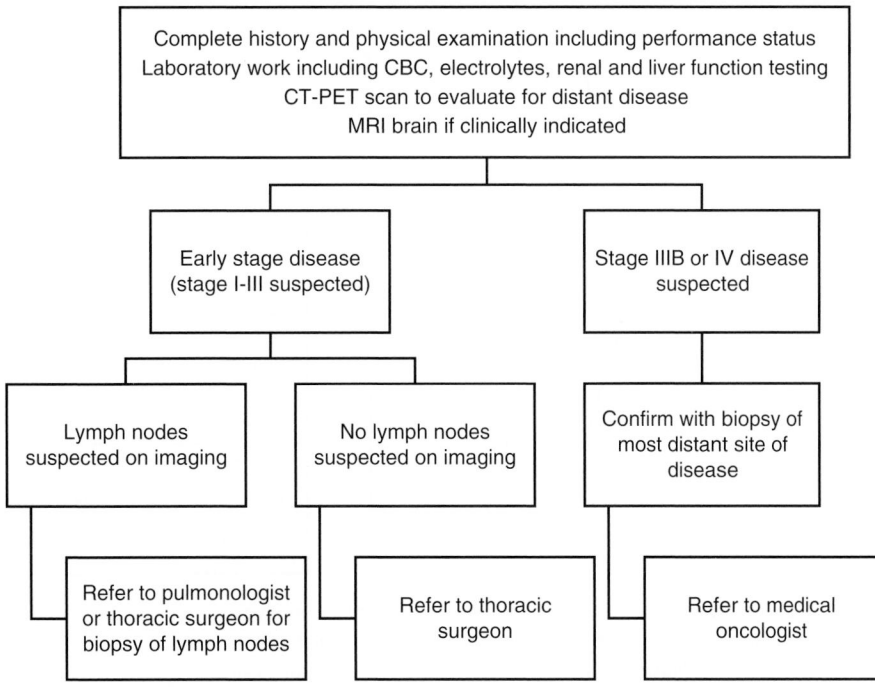

Figure 1 Approach to diagnosis. *CBC*, Complete blood count; *PS*, performance status.

Robotic Lobectomy

Robotic lobectomies were first performed in 2003, and the use of this technology has continued to increase with time. Much like VATS, robotic lobectomy is performed through small (8 mm) incisions.

This newer technology has several advantages over traditional thoracoscopic surgery in that it provides a three-dimensional, high definition visualization compared with only a two-dimensional view in thoracoscopic surgery. In addition, the instruments have 9 degrees of freedom and include the ability to staple and seal vessels.

Robotic surgery also boasts the same patient benefits as VATS.

Extent of Resection: Lobar Versus Sublobar Resection

Lobectomy has long been considered the standard of care and the optimal oncologic procedure for the management of resectable lung cancer. More limited resections (including segmentectomy or wedge resection) were thought to be associated with higher risk of recurrence and historically were reserved for patients with limited cardiopulmonary reserve.

The advent of CT screening for lung cancer and improvements in imaging technology have led to the identification of earlier stage cancers (<2 cm), and partially solid lesions or completely ground glass lesions. This has prompted a renewed interest in the possibility of more limited resection that preserves more pulmonary function and thereby a patient's ability to undergo subsequent resections if required.

The recommended extent of resection remains highly controversial. Investigators have not been able to definitively define the ideal tumor size or histology for a sublobar resection. Detractors argue that most evidence supporting sublobar resections comes from single-institution, retrospective analysis with pooled histology and surgical technique (wedge or segmentectomy), resulting in confounded results that may not be broadly disseminated.

Treatment: Non–Small Cell Lung Cancer

Stage I and II Lung Cancer

Surgery is considered the treatment of choice for stage I and II NSCLC (Figure 2; see Table 3). Based on the eighth edition staging system, this includes tumors that are node negative and up to 7 cm in size, tumors that involve the chest wall, and pericardium or satellite nodules in the same lobe. Surgery is also performed for patients who have smaller tumors up to 5 cm or tumors involving the main bronchus and ipsilateral, hilar nodes.

Operative mortality rates for patients undergoing pulmonary resection are lower if the resection is performed by a high-volume surgeon (>70 procedures per year), and surgeons who have had dedicated thoracic surgical training.

Comprehensive pathologic staging is just as important at the time of surgery as it is in the workup of a patient. Lymph nodes should be sampled from N2 stations (on the right side, stations 4R, 7, and 9R; on the left side, stations 5, 6, 7, and 9L) and N1 stations (stations 10 through 14) at the time of surgery. There is notably a 6% to 8% rate of occult N2 disease discovered at the time of final pathology for patients with T1 tumors and negative preoperative assessments.

There is currently no clear role for neoadjuvant chemotherapy in these patients; however, adjuvant chemotherapy is recommended for tumors that are determined on final pathology to be greater than 4 cm or in patients with lymph node involvement. The benefit of adjuvant chemotherapy was firmly established in 2008 by a landmark meta-analysis (the Lung Adjuvant Cisplatin Evaluation Study [LACE]) that demonstrated a 5.4% improvement in 5-year survival for patients treated with surgery followed by adjuvant chemotherapy compared to surgery alone.

The benefit was primarily confined to patients with stage II or IIIA disease, with only a modest benefit in patients with tumors less than 4 cm. Additionally, adjuvant chemotherapy showed no benefit in patients with an Eastern Cooperative Oncology Group (ECOG) score of 2. In 2011, the NSCLC Collaborative Group

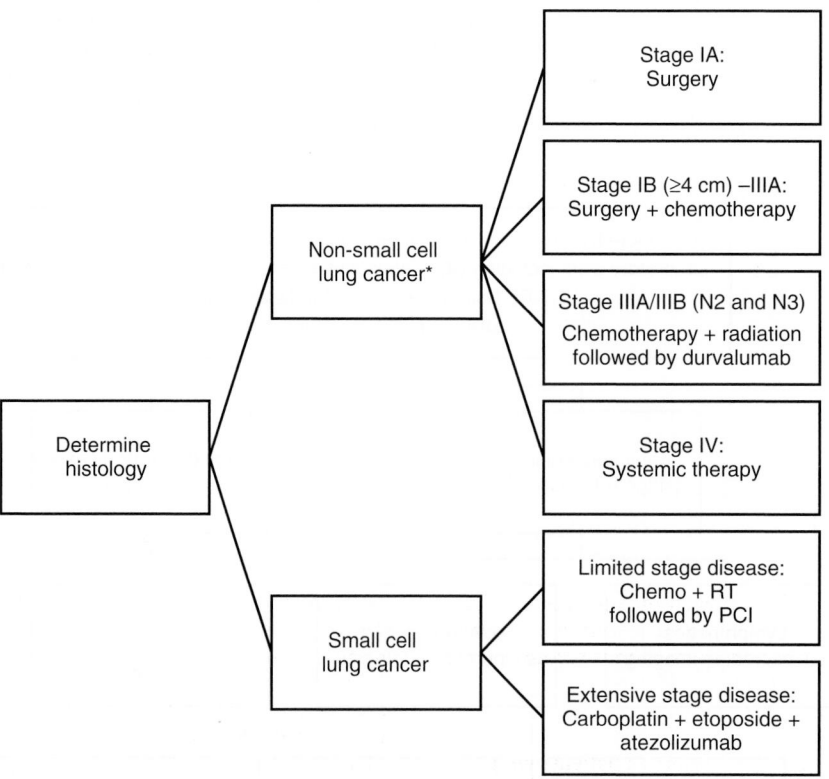

* For patients with stage IV NSCLC knowledge of histologic subtype,
PD-L1 and molecular testing are essential for selecting systemic therapy

Figure 2 General treatment algorithm for lung cancer.

compiled a postoperative chemotherapy meta-analysis and reported a similar survival benefit in patients with stage II disease. There is no role for adjuvant chemotherapy in patients with stage IA NSCLC. In patients with stage IB NSCLC and high-risk features, adjuvant chemotherapy may be considered, although this concept remains controversial.

The optimal platinum-based chemotherapy regimen remains unclear. Positive trials used platinum doublets, with debatably the best trial data coming from cisplatin (Platinol)[1] and vinorelbine (Navelbine). However, a 2015 meta-analysis from the Cochrane Database showed clear benefit from adjuvant chemotherapy irrespective of the regimen used. The E1505 trial assessed the addition of bevacizumab (Avastin) to cisplatin-based chemotherapy. While this trial demonstrated no benefit in OS, a post hoc analysis compared the different platinum doublet regimens (pemetrexed [Alimta], gemcitabine [Gemzar], docetaxel [Taxotere], and vinorelbine) and found no difference in either overall or disease-free survival but noted cisplatin and pemetrexed were associated with improved tolerance and were preferred among physicians for patients with non-squamous NSCLC.

If a decision is made to proceed with adjuvant chemotherapy, treatment should be started within 6 to 12 weeks after surgery, assuming the patient has fully recovered, and should be administered for no more than four cycles. Although a cisplatin-based chemotherapy is the preferred treatment regimen, carboplatin (Paraplatin)[1] can be substituted for cisplatin in patients who are unlikely to tolerate cisplatin for reasons such as reduced renal function, presence of neuropathy, or hearing impairment.

Postoperative radiation is usually reserved for patients in whom there is a concern for residual disease (i.e., patients with positive margins on final pathology) or in patients with N2 disease. In patients where both chemoradiotherapy is indicated postoperatively, concurrent rather than sequential treatment with chemotherapy and radiation is preferred.

In patients with stage I and II disease who either refuse or are not suitable candidates for surgery, stereotactic body radiation therapy (SBRT) is a treatment option for patients with tumors that are ≤5 cm. Treatment is typically administered in three to five fractions delivered over 1 to 2 weeks and is associated with a disease control rate of approximately 90% and 5-year survival rates of up to 60%. Cryoablation is another technique occasionally used to treat small, isolated tumors (i.e., ≤3 cm). However, very little data exist on long-term outcomes with this technique.

Locally Advanced Lung Cancer

The treatment of locally advanced lung cancer is complex and requires a multidisciplinary approach.

T3N1 Tumors

T3N1 is a relatively infrequent stage of lung cancer but surgery has a well-defined role as the primary treatment for these tumors. T3 lung cancers range in size from 5 to 7 cm or invade structures that can be routinely taken en bloc with the lung: the chest wall, pericardium, or a single phrenic nerve. Often, hilar nodal involvement is discovered at the time of resection. The surgical goal is an en bloc resection with microscopically negative margins.

Surgical resection should be followed by adjuvant chemotherapy as described previously. If a complete resection is not technically feasible then concurrent chemoradiation is recommended as described in the following section.

Stage IIIA Tumors

This is a heterogenous group that comprises patients with:
(1) small tumors (T1–T2) with ipsilateral mediastinal lymph node involvement (N2)

(2) large tumors (T3–T4) with ipsilateral lymph node involvement (N1)

(3) large tumors (T4) without any lymph node involvement (N0).

We will discuss some of the nuances of this complex group in the following subcategories: N2 disease, T4 tumors, and superior sulcus tumors.

N2 Disease

The optimal management of N2 disease is perhaps the most challenging and controversial area in thoracic oncology. Tumor characteristics and nodal burden of disease as well as performance status play an important role in determining who should be considered for surgery. Patients with clinical stage I or II disease who are discovered to have N2 positive nodes at the time of resection should undergo lobectomy with mediastinal lymphadenectomy and then be referred for adjuvant chemotherapy as described previously. In most cases, pathologic involvement of mediastinal lymph nodes is documented preoperatively, and a multimodality approach is recommended because these patients are at high risk for local and distance recurrence.

Patients who are deemed surgically resectable, the optimal combination and order of treatments remain debated. Some centers favor neoadjuvant chemotherapy and others a neoadjuvant chemoradiotherapy (6000 cGY).

The Intergroup 0139 study sought to help define the roles of therapy for N2 disease. The trial found no definitive survival benefit with surgery after neoadjuvant chemoradiation compared to definitive chemoradiation therapy alone. The study outcomes were confounded by a very high mortality rate in patients undergoing pneumonectomy that likely impacted this outcome. Subgroup analysis did show a trend toward survival benefit in patients undergoing lobectomy as a part of trimodality treatment.

More contemporary studies (mostly single institution) have demonstrated significantly higher median survival and freedom from recurrence compared with the INT0139 trial for trimodality therapy. Vyfhuis et al. achieved a median survival of 60 months with trimodality therapy compared with 20-month survival for bimodality (chemotherapy and radiation) in surgically resectable patients.

Patients with stage IIIA disease that are not surgical candidates or patients with stage IIIB disease are treated with concurrent chemoradiation therapy. In patients with a good ECOG performance status, the preferred regimen is with cisplatin[1] and etoposide (Toposar)[1] is the preferred therapeutic combination. However, carboplatin (Paraplatin)[1] and paclitaxel (Taxol) are often substituted for patients who cannot tolerate cisplatin-based chemotherapy for reasons stated previously.

The randomized, placebo-controlled, phase III trial, PACIFIC, demonstrated a significant improvement in progression-free survival (PFS) and OS in patients treated with concurrent chemoradiation followed by 1 year of therapy with the immune checkpoint inhibitor durvalumab (Imfinzi) compared to placebo. Benefit was seen across all tumor histologies and irrespective of PD-L1 status. This trial has established this as a new standard of care for patients with locally advanced, unresectable disease. There is no role for durvalumab in patients treated with trimodality therapy.

Esophagitis and pneumonitis are the two most common toxicities associated with concurrent chemoradiation.

T4 Tumors

T4 tumors are locally aggressive with invasion of critical mediastinal structures such as the pulmonary artery, heart, aorta, SVC, trachea, esophagus, spine, or diaphragm. Surgery can be considered as part of a multimodal therapy plan in high-volume centers with dedicated thoracic surgeons. Meticulous preoperative planning and in some cases multidisciplinary surgical approach is necessary to ensure complete resection.

---

[1]Not FDA approved for this indication.

[1]Not FDA approved for this indication.

Superior Sulcus Tumors

Superior sulcus tumors, also known as Pancoast tumors, arise from the apical segment of the right upper or left upper lobe. These tumors may invade any of the structures in the apex of the chest: brachial plexus, subclavian artery, subclavian vein, musculature, ribs, paravertebral sympathetic chain, or spinal nerve roots. Patients may present with shoulder pain, Horner syndrome, or neurologic complications of the upper extremity.

As with other locally advanced tumors, multidisciplinary approach is the mainstay of management of superior sulcus tumors. Complete staging is important to help determine resectability. MRI is often used in conjunction with other imaging modalities to better assess chest wall invasion and neurologic involvement.

Treatment with neoadjuvant chemoradiotherapy followed by surgery results in superior survival for patients with N0 or N1 disease. Surgery is generally completed 3 to 5 weeks after completion of chemoradiotherapy and involves an en bloc resection of the tumor, chest wall, and any other involved structures with subsequent reconstruction.

Patients with unresectable disease (medical inoperability, positive mediastinal nodes) should be offered concurrent chemoradiation followed by durvalumab consolidation as described previously.

Stage IIIB

Stage IIIB includes any tumors with contralateral mediastinal nodal involvement or large tumors (>5 cm) with ipsilateral mediastinal nodal involvement. These tumors are considered inoperable because surgery has not been shown to confer any survival benefit. These patients should be treated with concurrent chemoradiation therapy followed by durvalumab.

Stage IV

Approximately 57% of patients present with stage IV disease at the time of diagnosis and have an overall 5-year relative survival of around 5.8%. Moreover, a significant proportion of patients who present with early stage NSCLC will relapse despite initial curative-intent therapy. For patients who have relapsed, the treatment approach is similar to that used for patients with stage IV disease. Systemic therapy depends on a patient's performance status, histology, and PD-L1 and molecular status. ECOG performance status is also an important factor to help determine the treatment approach for a patient, as patients with an ECOG performance status of 3 or 4 have been shown to not respond well to chemotherapy and have a high likelihood of toxicity. These patients should receive best supportive care and palliative radiation if indicated. Of note, in patients receiving systemic therapy, the early application of palliative care in conjunction with chemotherapy is associated with improved survival and a better quality of life. Treatment of stage IV NSCLC can be divided into three pathways: (1) immune sensitive (PD-L1 status), (2) oncogenic driver directed, and (3) nonbiomarker-driven, histology-based treatment.

Chemotherapy

Chemotherapy has been an important therapeutic option for decades in the treatment of patients with stage IV NSCLC. Historically, platinum-based regimens with cisplatin[1] or carboplatin[1] in combination with another agent have been considered the standard of care and confer a survival benefit in patients with stage IV disease.

Treatment recommendations have continued to evolve over the years. Histology of the NSCLC has come to be very important in treatment consideration; phase III trials have demonstrated cisplatin[1] and pemetrexed to be superior to cisplatin[1] and gemcitabine (Gemzar) in patients with nonsquamous NSCLC, while cisplatin and pemetrexed had a lower PFS and similar OS

when compared to cisplatin and gemcitabine in patients with squamous cell histology. Other studies have confirmed the benefit of pemetrexed in nonsquamous NSCLC and have shown its limited activity in squamous cell NSCLC. This survival difference is thought to be related to the differential expression of thymidylate synthase (TS), one of the targets of pemetrexed, with higher expression of TS being reported with squamous cancers. Importantly, bevacizumab (Avastin), a monoclonal antibody that targets vascular endothelial growth factor (VEGF), was also established as unsafe to administer in patients with squamous NSCLC and is FDA approved in combination with carboplatin and paclitaxel as a first-line option only in non-squamous NSCLC patients.

Immunotherapy

Immune checkpoint inhibitors have increasingly become part of the first-line treatment paradigm in patients with metastatic NSCLC without a driver mutation. These agents appear to have less efficacy in patients with driver mutations such as EGFR and ALK, reinforcing the importance of molecular testing prior to treatment initiation. Checkpoint inhibitors exert antitumor effects by inhibiting negative T-cell regulators. Regardless of histology, all patients with advanced stage lung cancer should have PD-L1 testing prior to embarking on therapy.

A randomized phase III trial demonstrated a superior response rate and PFS and OS when pembrolizumab (Keytruda) was compared to platinum-based chemotherapy in patients with tumors that were PD-L1 ≥50%, which led to its FDA approval in this setting. This result was seen irrespective of tumor histology. Based on the Keynote 042, this indication was expanded to include patients with PD-L1 of ≥1%. Its use in patients with PD-L1 of 1% to 49% is controversial due to a subgroup analysis showing no benefit of pembrolizumab compared to chemotherapy, while positive results were seen in trials with combination chemotherapy and immunotherapy.

In the phase III trials Keynote 189 and Keynote 407, combination therapy with platinum (cisplatin or carboplatin)-pemetrexed and pembrolizumab in non-squamous NSCLC and carboplatin-taxane (paclitaxel or nab-paclitaxel) and pembrolizumab in squamous cell NSCLC was superior to chemotherapy alone in patients regardless of PD-L1 status. Patients in both trials who were treated with a regimen containing pembrolizumab have improved PFS and OS. However, the additive benefit of chemotherapy to patients with tumors that are PD-L1 ≥50% to pembrolizumab alone remains unclear beyond small subset analyses from the aforementioned trials. Combination chemotherapy with carboplatin, paclitaxel, bevacizumab, and atezolizumab (Tecentriq) has also been shown to be superior to carboplatin, paclitaxel, and bevacizumab in patients regardless of PD-L1 status and is also FDA approved as a first-line treatment option for non-squamous NSCLC based on the IMpower 150 trial. Although this regimen is not preferred, it is important to note that this trial included patients with EGFR and ALK mutations. Numerous other trials are currently ongoing evaluating the use of immunotherapy in NSCLC, both alone and in combination with other immunological agents, chemotherapy, targeted therapy, and radiotherapy.

Targeted Therapy

Molecular testing for driver mutations has become increasingly important for the treatment of patients with NSCLC. Driver mutations are most commonly seen in patients who are young, never smokers with non-squamous NSCLC. Multiple driver mutations have been detected in more than 50% of patients with non-squamous NSCLC (Figure 3), with targeted therapy available for patients with EGFR, ALK, ROS-1, NTRK, and BRAF mutations. Although not FDA-approved, there are commercially available agents that can be used in patients with MET and RET mutations, with new agents currently being evaluated in clinical trials. In addition, promising agents are in clinical trials for patients with KRAS mutations. In patients who harbor a mutation and are

---

[1]Not FDA approved for this indication.

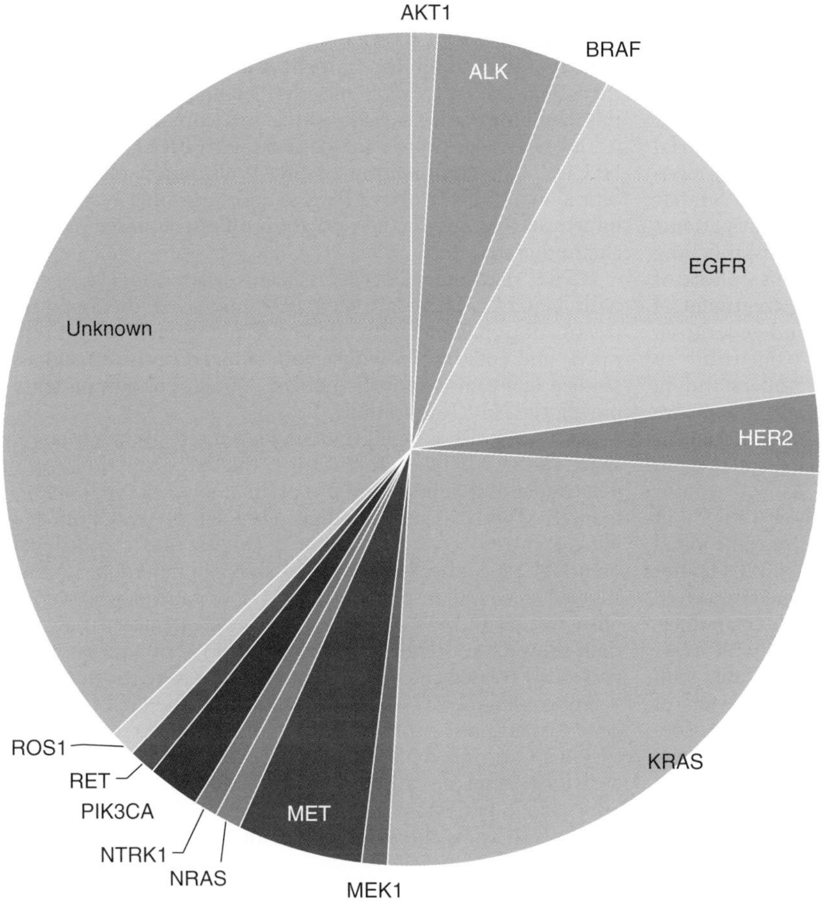

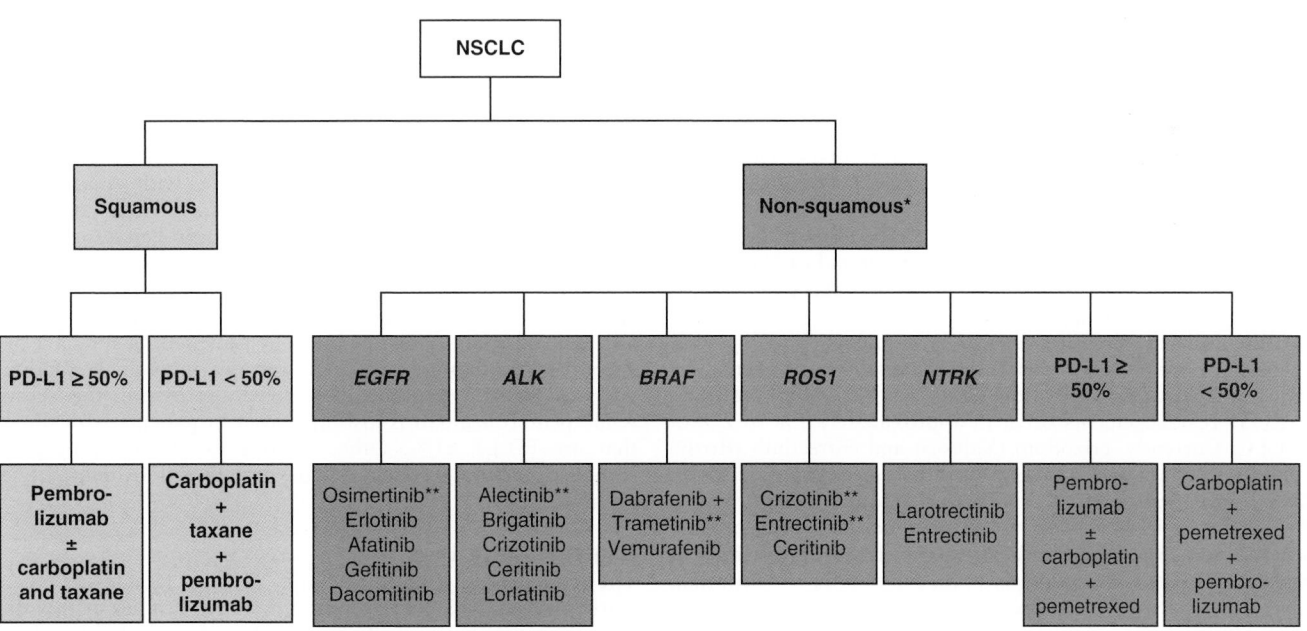

Figure 3 Molecular mutations in non-squamous, non–small cell lung cancer.

Frequency of Driver Mutations	
AKT1	1%
ALK	3-8%
BRAF	3-4%
EGFR	10-35%
HER2	2-4%
KRAS	15-25%
MEK1	1%
MET	4%
NRAS	1%
NTRK1	2-3%
PIK3CA	1-3%
RET	1-2%
ROS1	1%
Unknown	20-40%

Figure 4 Treatment algorithm for metastatic non–small cell lung cancer.

also strongly PD-L1 positive, the presence of the mutation should drive selection of therapy (Figure 4).

EGFR mutations have been reported in approximately 15% of North American patients with metastatic nonsquamous NSCLC, of which 90% are exon 19 deletions or exon 21 L858R point mutations. First- and second-generation *EGFR* tyrosine kinase inhibitors (TKIs) erlotinib (Tarceva), gefitinib (Iressa), and afatinib (Gilotrif) are approved as first-line therapy based

on clinical trials demonstrating have all shown increased PFS in patients with *EGFR* mutated NSCLC when compared to chemotherapy in treatment-naïve patients with *EGFR* mutation-positive NSCLC. Despite the observed PFS benefits, a majority of patients eventually develop therapeutic resistance. Furthermore, approximately 50% of patients who develop acquired resistance to *EGFR* TKI therapy acquire a second site mutation occurring within exon 20 (i.e., T790M). Consequently, osimertinib

(Tagrisso), a third-generation mutant-specific *EGFR* inhibitor that irreversibly binds to the kinase domain of *EGFR*, was initially approved for use only in patients who develop an *EGFR T790M* mutation during a treatment with a first- or second-generation *EGFR* TKI. Osimertinib has now been approved for first-line use based on results from FLAURA, a phase III, trial that compared osimertinib to erlotinib or gefitinib in the first-line setting for patients with *EGFR*-positive NSCLC. Similar response rates were seen between treatment groups, but patients treated with osimertinib had improved PFS and OS, establishing osimertinib as the preferred first-line option for this cohort of patients. Osimertinib also demonstrated improved treatment of brain metastasis, an Achilles heel of first- and second-generation TKI agents. Unavoidably, patients treated with osimertinib in the first-line setting will develop resistance, and understanding of these resistance mechanisms remains important. There are several ongoing trials that are examining these resistance mechanisms and looking at the most effective treatment strategies in patients at the time of progression.

ALK-positive NSCLC accounts for approximately 3% to 7% of patients diagnosed with NSCLC. Crizotinib (Xalkori) was the initial *ALK* TKI to gain accelerated approval by the FDA in 2011 after two open-label, randomized phase III trials demonstrated improved response rates and PFS with crizotinib compared with chemotherapy in both the first- and second-line setting for patients with *ALK*-positive disease. Similar to *EGFR* TKI therapy, patients treated with crizotinib will predictably develop resistance, with almost 50% of patients developing brain metastases at the time of progression. Later generation *ALK* TKIs have been developed to overcome these resistance mechanisms, better penetrate the CNS penetration, and improve side-effect profiles. Ceritinib (Zykadia), a second-generation *ALK* TKI, was initially approved for patients who had progressed on or had proved intolerant to crizotinib. Subsequently, it was approved as a front-line therapy option, demonstrating superior PFS compared to chemotherapy in patients with *ALK*-positive NSCLC. More recently, alectinib (Alecensa) and brigatinib (Alunbrig) demonstrated superior PFS and central nervous system (CNS) control compared to crizotinib in patients with *ALK*-positive NSCLC, with alectinib receiving FDA approval and considered the preferred option as front-line therapy for *ALK*-positive NSCLC. Lorlatinib (Lorbrena), a third-generation *ALK* TKI, is also approved in patients who have progressed on a prior ALK inhibitor. Its unique structure maintains activity against the most common resistance mechanism that develops in patients treated with a first- or second-generation *ALK* TKI, G1202R. The optimal sequencing of *ALK* TKIs has yet to be determined, but testing for resistance mechanisms at the time of progression is becoming increasingly important and can help guide therapy for second-line treatment with an oral agent rather than switching to chemotherapy.

Structurally the ROS-1 oncogene is homologous to the ALK oncogene, which has been helpful in the discovery of agents targeting ROS-1, with many of the *ALK* TKIs also inhibiting ROS-1. ROS1 rearrangements occur in approximately 1% to 2% of NSCLC. Currently, crizotinib (Xalkori) and entrectinib (Rozlytrek) are the only two FDA-approved therapies for patients with ROS-1 mutations and are the preferred options for first-line therapy for patients with ROS-1 positive NSCLC. Lack of CNS penetration is a known barrier of treatment with crizotinib but newer ROS-1 TKIs including ceritinib, entrectinib, and lorlatinib have shown activity in the CNS.

BRAF mutations occur in approximately 2% to 3% of NSCLC patients, and more than 50% of these are V600E. Due to prior success in *BRAF*-mutated melanoma, three *BRAF*-target regimens have been studied in NSCLC, vemurafenib (Zelboraf)[1], dabrafenib (Tafinlar), and dabrafenib plus the MEK-inhibitor trametinib (Mekinist). Dabrafenib and vemurafenib have demonstrated promising results in phase II trials. As seen in the melanoma literature, concurrent downstream inhibition of MAPK/

extracellular signal-related kinase (MEK) was proposed to delay tumor resistance to *BRAF* inhibition. Dabrafenib in combination with the MEK inhibitor trametinib had response rates of more than 60% and PFS of 9 months, leading to FDA approval of this combination and establishing this combination as the preferred treatment option for patients with BRAF V600E positive NSCLC. The combination of BRAF inhibition plus MEK inhibition maintains longer PFS and more durable responses with improved tolerability and toxicity profiles compared to cytotoxic chemotherapy.

NTRK rearrangements have been reported in 1% of patients with NSCLC. There are two FDA-approved therapies for the treatment of patients with an *NTRK* mutation, larotrectinib (Vitrakvi) and entrectinib, which both showed positive results when studied in a tumor agnostic patient population with patients harboring the *NTRK* mutation.

MET exon 14 skipping mutations, caused by mutations in the splice site of MET, are found to be the oncogenic driver in up to 4% of adenocarcinomas and 2% of squamous cell carcinomas. Capmatinib (Tabrecta) and tepotinib (Tepmetko) were both recently FDA approved based on phase II studies that enrolled patients with NSCLC and a MET exon 14 skipping mutation. Capmatinib showed an overall response rate in 41% of patients who were previously treated and 68% of patients who were treatment naive. Tepotinib showed an overall response rate in 43% of patients who were previously treated and 43% of patients who were treatment naïve.

Approximately 1%–2% of patients with NSCLC have RET gene fusions, and patients are younger and have no smoking history with advanced disease and adenocarcinoma histology. Selpercatinib (Retevmo) and pralsetinib (Gavreto) were recently FDA approved in patients with NSCLC with a RET gene fusions based on phase II trials showing an overall response rate of 64% and 57%, respectively.

Second-Line Therapy and Beyond

Second-line therapy for advanced NSCLC was almost never recommended until a seminal study in 2000 showed that docetaxel (Taxotere) improved survival compared to supportive care alone. Over a decade later, docetaxel and ramucirumab (Cyramza) received FDA approval after a phase III trial found the combination to impart a modest improvement in response rate, OS, and PFS compared with docetaxel alone. Ramucirumab binds to the VEGF receptor but it is important to note that safety concerns seen with bevacizumab (Avastin) in patients with squamous histology were not reported. In patients who have not received a platinum agent for advanced disease who progresses on a first-line TKI or pembrolizumab (Keytruda) should be considered for a platinum-based doublet as their second-line therapy, not single agent docetaxel or docetaxel and ramucirumab. If a patient has not received immunotherapy in the first-line setting and have progressed on platinum-based chemotherapy, nivolumab (Opdivo), and atezolizumab (Tecentriq) received approval in this setting, while pembrolizumab is also approved in patients with tumors that are PD-L1 ≥1%. Other options for disease progression include gemcitabine (Gemzar) or pemetrexed (Alimta), if not given previously.

Oligometastatic Disease

The concept of oligometastatic disease (single-site metastatic disease) was first proposed in 1995. Studies at this time described patients with disease in the adrenal gland or brain as actually having a relatively favorable prognosis. For these lesions, the standard of care includes surgical resection of both the primary and metastasis if they present synchronously or resection of the recurrence (metachronous disease). Generally, for synchronous disease (primary tumor and metastatic disease identified at the same time), the metastatic site is treated first. If this is not able to be successfully addressed, there is no benefit to resecting the primary. Third-line therapy and beyond is reasonable for patients with a good performance status and can tolerate another agent.

---

[1]Not FDA approved for this indication.

Treatment Small Cell Lung Cancer

SCLC, which accounts for 15% to 20% of new lung cancer cases, is an aggressive disease characterized by rapid growth and early widespread metastasis. The primary etiologic agent responsible for SCLC is tobacco smoke. The aggressive nature of SCLC is underscored by its high mutational burden, including loss of expression of the tumor suppressor genes *p53* in 70% to 80% and retinoblastoma in almost 100% of tumors. Although there is a shift in recommendations for the staging of SCLC, most patients are still diagnosed using the traditional staging system of limited stage disease (LS) and extensive stage disease (ES). At the time of diagnosis, approximately 30% of patients have limited-stage disease (LS-SCLC), defined as tumors confined to the hemithorax that can be encompassed in a tolerable radiation port, while about 70% of patients have extensive-stage disease (ES-SCLC), defined as the presence of overt metastatic disease by imaging or physical examination. Chemotherapy with or without radiotherapy is the treatment of choice for most patients. While initially extremely responsive to treatment, the majority of patients relapse and develop chemotherapy-resistant disease, with a median survival of 12 to 20 months for patients with LS disease and 7 to 11 months for patients with ES disease.

For decades, first-line therapy consisted of four to six cycles of platinum-based chemotherapy with either cisplatin[1] or carboplatin (Paraplatin)[1] plus either etoposide (Toposar) or irinotecan (Camptosar)[1] followed by observation. In LS-SCLC, cisplatin is preferred to carboplatin in combination with etoposide and chemotherapy is generally combined with radiation as described later. However, carboplatin can be substituted for cisplatin to decrease incidence of nephrotoxicity and nausea and vomiting.

Recently, IMpower 133, a phase III trial in patients with ES-SCLC demonstrated superior OS when atezolizumab (Tecentriq) was combined with carboplatin and etoposide for four cycles followed by maintenance atezolizumab compared to carboplatin and etoposide alone, making combination chemotherapy with a checkpoint inhibitor a new treatment option for patients with this disease. Additionally, an interim analysis of the phase III trial CASPIAN trial also showed improved OS with the addition of durvalumab (Imfinzi) to a platinum-etoposide regimen plus durvalumab maintenance when compared to a platinum-etoposide regimen alone.

Although up to 80% of patients will respond to first-line chemotherapy, the majority will eventually relapse, and topotecan (Hycamtin) is the only approved agent in the second line. Nivolumab (Opdivo) has also received FDA approval in the third-line setting, but this was in patients who had not received a checkpoint inhibitor in the first-line setting.

Radiation therapy is also an important component in the therapeutic armamentarium for patients with SCLC. Patients with LS-SCLC are generally treated with concurrent chemoradiation therapy with four cycles of chemotherapy and radiation added with either cycle one or two of therapy. For patients who are not candidates for concurrent chemoradiation therapy, sequential therapy can also be considered with radiation after chemotherapy. Prophylactic cranial irradiation (PCI) has been shown to decrease brain metastases and improve OS in patients with LS-SCLC and should be considered in patients who have responded well to initial therapy. Long-term toxicities, including deficits in cognition, have been reported after PCI, and for many patients observation with an MRI every 3 months has been adopted as standard of care. In patients with ES-SCLC, thoracic radiation can be considered although has not been shown to improve OS. Similarly, a large phase III trial in patients with ES-SCLC without brain metastases following chemotherapy demonstrated no improvement in OS for patients treated with PCI compared to observation. The role of radiotherapy in ES-SCLS is generally confined to palliation of symptoms such as pain from bone metastases.

Surgery has for many decades played a very limited role in the treatment of SCLC due to its propensity to metastasize. The pendulum is beginning to shift for early-stage, node-negative SCLC. More contemporary studies have demonstrated that surgery may play a beneficial role in a select group of patients.

Invasive mediastinal staging should be performed for patients without evidence of metastatic disease. In node-negative patients with T1 and T2 tumors, a lobectomy followed by adjuvant chemotherapy should be offered to medically fit patients. The 5-year survival in this group of patients is 40% to 50%.

Monitoring

Routine disease monitoring is important both after curative treatment and during treatment for incurable disease.

Non–Small Cell Lung Cancer

The National Comprehensive Cancer Network (NCCN) guidelines have clear recommendations for the follow up of NSCLC and SCLC divided by stage, and these are summarized in the following.

After completion of curative therapy for stages I and II, a history and physical examination along with a chest CT (+/–) contrast every 6 months for the first 2 to 3 years should be performed. If after 2 to 3 years there are no findings that would require alternative monitoring, the patient can be transitioned to annual history, physical examination, and a low-dose, noncontrast CT scan of the chest.

Patients with Stages I and II who were treated with radiation rather than surgery should be followed by a slightly more aggressive regimen. Patients should have a history and physical examination along with a chest CT (+/–) contrast every 3 to 6 months for the first 3 years, then every 6 months for the next 2 years. At that time, if there are no findings that would require alternative monitoring, the patient can be transitioned to annual history, physical examination, and a low-dose, noncontrast CT scan of the chest.

Patients with stages III and IV oligometastatic disease should likewise be followed with history and physical examination along with a chest CT (+/–) contrast every 3 to 6 months for the first 3 years, then every 6 months for the next 2 years. If there are no findings that would require alternative monitoring, the patient can be transitioned to annual history, physical examination, and a low-dose, noncontrast CT scan of the chest.

Any residual or new radiographic abnormalities will require consideration of more frequent imaging. Please note that a PET, CT, and brain MRI are not routinely indicated as part of surveillance; however, they should be tailored to each patient and their primary sites of disease.

Symptoms of shortness of breath, cough, wheezing, new bone pain, headache, or constitutional symptoms should prompt immediate evaluation with imaging to rule out disease recurrence, and the patient's primary oncologist should be contacted.

While patients are being treated with palliative system therapy, scans are routinely obtained every 6 to 8 weeks while on chemotherapy or every 8 to 9 weeks while on immunotherapy.

Small Cell Lung Cancer

SCLC has a distinct follow-up recommendation. Patients who were diagnosed and treated for LS disease should have follow-up with history and physical, CT scan of the chest/abdomen every 3 months for the first year and every 6 months for the subsequent 2 years. At that time, the patients may transition to annual examinations and imaging. MRI scans of the brain are essential as well and are recommended every 3 to 4 months for year 1 and every 6 months for year 2.

Patients with ES will have more frequent follow- ups. A history and physical with CT scans of the chest/abdomen should occur every 2 months for the first year, every 3 to 4 months for years 2 and 3, every 6 months in years 4 and 5, and then annually. Monitoring of the brain is the same as for LS, with an MRI scan of the

---

[1]Not FDA approved for this indication.

brain recommended every 3 to 4 months for year 1 and every 6 months for year 2.

Any patient, regardless of type of cancer, should have a survivorship plan created as part of follow-up. These plans apply to survivors across the continuum of care. This comprehensive, individualized plan includes the aforementioned cancer-specific follow-up but also highlights important nutritional considerations, physical activity, and immunizations. Patients should be encouraged to continue routine screening for other malignancies and routine health maintenance. Ongoing smoking cessation should be encouraged.

Summary

The treatment of cancers is rapidly changing with the advent of immunotherapy, targeted therapy, localized radiation treatments, and minimally invasive surgical approaches. The intricacies of treatment, now more than ever before, demand a multidisciplinary approach to ensure that patients are provided with the best possible care to optimize both their quantity and quality of life.

References

Antonia SJ, Villegas A, Daniel D, et al: Durvalumab after chemoradiotherapy in stage iii non-small-cell lung cancer, *N Engl J Med* 377(20):1919–1929, 2017.

Gaissert HA, Ferenandez FG, Crabtree T, et al: The Society of thoracic surgeons general thoracic surgery database: 2017 update on research, *Annals Thor Surg* 104(5):1450–1455, 2017.

Gandhi L, Rodrigues Abreu D, Gadgeel S, et al: (Keynote-189). Pembrolizumban plus chemotherapy in metastatic non-small cell lung cancer, *NEJM* 327:2078–2092, 2018.

Horn L, Mansfield AS, Szczęsna A, et al: IMpower133 Study Group: First-line atezolizumab plus chemotherapy in extensive-stage small-cell lung cancer, *N Engl J Med* 379(23):2220–2229, 2018.

Paz-Ares L, Luft A, Vincente D, et al: (Keynote-407). Pembrolizumab plus chemotherapy for squamous non-small cell lung cancer, *NEJM* 379:2040–2051, 2018.

Peters S, Camidge RC, Shaw AT, et al: Alectinib versus crizotinib in untreated alk-positive non–small-cell lung cancer, *N Engl J Med* 377:829–838, 2017.

Reck M, Rodriguez-Abreu D, Robinson AG, et al: Pembrolizumab versus chemotherapy for PD-L1-positive non-small-cell lung cancer, *N Engl J Med* 375(19):1823–1833, 2016.

Soria JC, Ohe Y, Vansteenkiste J, et al: Osimertinib in untreated egfr-mutated advanced non-small-cell lung cancer, *N Engl J Med* 378:113–125, 2018.

Spyratos D, Zarogoulidis P, Ket al. Porpodis, et al: Preoperative evaluation for lung cancer resection, *J Thorac Dis* 6(Suppl)1:S162–166, 2014.

The National Lung Screening Trial Research Team: Reduced lung-cancer mortality with low-dose computed tomographic screening, *NEJM* 365:395–409, 2011.

OBSTRUCTIVE SLEEP APNEA

Method of
Omar G. Ahmed, MD; and Masayoshi Takashima, MD

CURRENT DIAGNOSIS

Symptoms
- Excessive daytime fatigue and somnolence
- Morning headaches
- Loud snoring and gasping for air
- Witnessed apneic episodes following loud snoring
- Frequent nocturia with no other underlying etiology
- Hypertension

Clinical Signs and Risk Factors
- Central obesity with body mass index (BMI) >30 kg/m²
- Large neck circumference (>17 inches in men; >16 inches in women)
- Being male or a postmenopausal female
- Use of sedatives or alcohol before going to bed
- Family history of sleep apnea
- Craniofacial abnormalities: retrognathia, micrognathia, congenital malformations

CURRENT THERAPY

- Gold standard for treatment is positive airway pressure
- Weight loss, smoking cessation, avoidance of sedatives
- Improvement of sleep hygiene and sleep schedule
- Minimally invasive procedures (i.e., oral appliances, palatal stents, radiofrequency turbinate reductions) may be beneficial for a select patient population
- Surgical therapy is usually reserved for patients not tolerating or unable to use CPAP or BiPAP
- Implants for muscle stimulation
- Initial procedures are focused on decreasing upper airway resistance to improve compliance with CPAP or BiPAP
- Identification of anatomic sites of obstruction is critical to successful surgical outcomes

BiPAP, Bilevel positive airway pressure; *CPAP,* continuous positive airway pressure.

Sleep-disordered breathing encompasses the spectrum from upper airway resistance syndrome to obstructive sleep apnea (OSA). OSA is characterized by episodes of partial or complete upper airway collapse leading to cessation or reduction of airflow. Such events lead to oxygen desaturation and sleep fragmentation, causing excessive daytime sleepiness, morning headaches, depression, memory loss, impaired alertness, decreased libido, and reduced cognitive function. Nighttime symptoms are often more telling, and obtaining a sleep history from a bed partner is exceptionally helpful. The most common symptoms include loud snoring, restless sleep, choking or gasping episodes, and frequent awakening from sleep. Nocturnal perspiration, nocturia, and symptoms of nocturnal gastroesophageal reflux are also commonly associated with severe OSA.

As the severity of OSA typically increases with age, nightly hypoventilation and activation of the sympathetic nervous system lead to pathophysiologic derangements, such as hypertension, ischemic heart disease, myocardial infarction, stroke, arrhythmia, and premature death. An apnea-hypopnea index (AHI) of greater than 5 has been shown to be associated with increased risk of cerebrovascular accident. An AHI greater than 20 is associated with increased mortality. Patients with oxygen desaturation below 90% have an elevated incidence of cardiac arrhythmia. These potentially severe consequences, along with a patient's decreased quality of life, substantiate the need for early recognition and treatment.

Definitions of terms related to sleep apnea are listed in Box 1.

Epidemiology

On the basis of available population-based studies, the prevalence of OSA among adults between 30 and 60 years of age is estimated to be 6% for women and 13% for men. This represents relative increases over the last two decades of 14% to 55% among subgroups divided by age, gender, and body mass index (BMI). OSA remains undiagnosed in 70% to 80% of patients because their symptoms are often vague, and OSA must be diagnosed with polysomnography.

Risk Factors

When controlling for gender and BMI, patients over age 50 have an increased prevalence of OSA secondary to decreased muscle tone.

Obesity (BMI >30 kg/m²) is a risk factor for OSA. A 10% increase in weight is associated with a sixfold increase in risk for development of OSA, and a 10% weight loss is associated with a 26% decrease in AHI. Patients undergoing bariatric surgery on average have postsurgical reductions in AHI of 29 events per hour. There is evidence of a potential link between OSA and insulin resistance.

Approximately 30% of hypertensive persons have OSA and up to 50% of OSA patients have hypertension. Resistant hypertension, which is defined as blood pressure greater than 140/90 mmHg despite therapy with at least three different antihypertensive classes, is especially prevalent in the OSA population. It is estimated that 90% of male patients and 77% of female patients with resistant hypertension have OSA. A dose-effect relationship between OSA severity and severity of hypertension has been established. Mechanisms for hypertension center around hypoxemia and hypercapnia leading to increased oxidative stress, decreased nitric oxide secretion, and increased catecholamine, angiotensin II, aldosterone, renin, and endothelin-1 secretion.

Male patients are nearly twice as likely to have OSA as female patients. Estrogen and progesterone might play a protective role because population-based studies have demonstrated that postmenopausal women have a two- to threefold increased risk of OSA compared to premenopausal women.

African Americans and Asians are at greater risk for OSA than Caucasians. Being African American is an independent risk factor for severe sleep-disordered breathing, with an odds ratio of 2.55 compared with Caucasians. Asians have a narrower cranial base, a higher Mallampati score, smaller thyromental distance, and steeper thyromental plane than Caucasians, which might account for their increased risk.

Pathophysiology

Airway obstruction leading to OSA can occur anywhere along the pathway from the nostrils, soft palate, base of tongue, hypopharynx, and the epiglottis. The airway lacks skeletal structure and is vulnerable to influences, such as muscle tone, fat deposition, and tissue redundancy.

Prevention

Lifestyle modification can prevent OSA. Patients should adopt a healthy and athletic lifestyle to develop good muscle tone and weight loss, avoid sedatives and alcohol at bedtime, establish regular sleeping patterns, avoid the supine sleeping position, and elevate the head when sleeping.

Diagnosis

Definitive diagnosis of OSA is made by polysomnography. Mild OSA is defined as an AHI of 5 to 15 per hour; moderate OSA is an AHI of 15 to 30 per hour; and severe OSA is an AHI greater than 30 per hour. There are several types of polysomnograms patients can obtain, ranging from Level 1 to 3. Level 1 sleep studies are performed in a sleep laboratory with a technician in attendance. It assesses at least seven channels of data (but usually 16+), including respiratory, cardiovascular, and neurological parameters. Level 1 sleep studies have long been the gold standard of diagnoses of sleep-disordered breathing and other sleep disorders. Patients spend the night in a sleep laboratory during which multiple physiologic variables are continuously monitored. These include electroencephalogram (EEG), electrooculogram (EOG), electromyogram (EMG), oronasal airflow, chest wall effort, body position, snore volume, electrocardiogram (ECG), and oxyhemoglobin saturation. Laboratory testing also includes a complete accounting of sleep variables, monitoring of cardiac rhythm, and assessment of possible restless legs syndrome (RLS) or periodic limb movements (PLMs) during sleep. This information enables the clinician to determine the severity of the condition and identifies potentially relevant comorbidities.

Level 2 sleep studies use the same equipment as Level 1 but do not have a technician in attendance. These are rarely offered or ordered. In recent years, Level 3 sleep studies have grown in popularity. These tests use portable monitors that allow sleep studies to be performed in a patient's home. Level 3 studies only measure three channels of data: oximetry, airflow, and respiratory effort. A thorough diagnostic study requires at least 6 hours of sleep, allowing assessment of variability related to sleep stages.

If there are sufficient apneas or hypopneas during the first half of the study (ideally 4 hours of diagnostic testing, with a minimum of 2 hours if an AHI >40 is confirmed), a split-night study may be performed, in which the second half of the night (minimum of 3 hours of sleep) is devoted to titration of continuous positive airway pressure (CPAP) therapy. If the criteria for a split-night sleep study are not achieved during the night, a second night for titration study is ordered. The split-night protocol is a cost-effective use of laboratory resources that is particularly well suited for patients with severe OSA.

A meta-analysis comparing Level 1 and 3 studies showed that Level 3 portable sleep studies displayed good diagnostic performance compared to Level 1 in-lab sleep studies in adult patients with high pre-test probability of moderate or severe OSA, and no unstable comorbidities. For patients suspected to have other types of sleep disorders, a Level 1 sleep study remains the gold standard.

According to the Institute for Clinical Systems Improvement (ICSI), polysomnography should be performed in patients with symptoms of OSA and one or more of the following: cardiovascular disease, hypertension, coronary artery disease, obesity, sleep complaints, type 2 diabetes mellitus, recurrent atrial fibrillation, and large neck circumference.

Treatment

Initially, patients should be counseled to avoid practices that can potentially worsen the severity of OSA. CNS depressants taken before sleep (alcohol, sleep medications, pain medications) can worsen upper airway collapse during sleep and should be discouraged. Weight loss and maintenance should always play a role in the treatment of these patients. Myofunctional therapy, which is a series of isometric and isotonic exercises of the oral cavity and pharyngeal muscles, is designed to increase upper airway tone. Oral pressure therapy uses a mouthpiece to generate negative pressure to gently pull the palate forward, opening the retropalatal airway. End positive airway pressure (EPAP) therapy uses nasal appliances to increase expiratory resistance and prevent pharyngeal collapse.

In patients with positional OSA, defined as greater than a two-fold difference in AHI between supine and nonsupine positions, avoiding the supine position during sleep may suffice to normalize ventilation during sleep. There are several commercial devices worn around the neck or back that gently vibrate when a patient is supine. Nightly compliance rates are 75% to 96%.

Continuous Positive Airway Pressure Therapy
CPAP remains the therapeutic mainstay for primary treatment of OSA. It serves as a pneumatic stent for the upper airway and is effective in reducing the physiologic abnormalities measured on polysomnography. Additionally, CPAP is thought to augment lung volumes and elicit a reflex that increases tone in the upper airway musculature. Overall, it has been shown to reduce AHI, improve quality of life, and reduce cardiovascular risk.

There are many manufacturers of CPAP devices and many interfaces that help maximize comfort with treatment. Expiratory pressure release (EPR) is available through several CPAP manufacturers. EPR does not seem to compromise the effectiveness of CPAP therapy and improves the patient's sense of comfort with therapy, but it does not seem to systematically improve the level of adherence. Automatically adjusting positive airway pressure (APAP) is similar to CPAP, but instead of delivering a constant pressure, APAP adjusts delivered pressure breath to breath.

Bilevel respiratory-assist devices deliver alternating levels of positive airway pressure and may be considered an alternative therapeutic option when standard CPAP is not tolerated or when oxygen saturation is not raised sufficiently with standard CPAP. In some cases of severe OSA (in particular among patients with underlying pulmonary conditions), supplemental oxygen can be used in conjunction with CPAP therapy.

The main disadvantage with positive airway pressure treatment is poor compliance. CPAP adherence rates—defined as at least 4 hours per night—70% of nights are between only 39% and 50% overall CPAP compliance. Treatment is effective as long as the patient uses the device for the entire night, every night. APAP, CPAP desensitization, and the use of integrated heated humidifiers helped improve adherence to therapy.

Oral Appliances
Oral appliances worn in the mouth during sleep can help maintain a patent airway, especially in patients with significant positional sleep apnea who sleep supine and experience airway collapse secondary to the tongue falling posteriorly. In general, there are two types of appliances, mandibular-advancement appliances and tongue-retaining devices. The mandibular-advancement appliances are currently used more often and have been more widely studied. They require viable dentition for retention and they are fitted to the maxillary and mandibular dentition to enable the protrusion of the mandible, therefore increasing oropharyngeal patency. The most common side effect is drooling. Temporomandibular joint pain might limit the viability of this therapy, and chronic use of the appliance can result in a change of the dental occlusion. A dentist with expertise in sleep medicine should ideally implement and monitor this type of treatment.

Surgical Procedures
If patients are not tolerating CPAP and a significant upper airway anatomic obstruction is identified, surgery should be considered. A variety of procedures help stabilize the retropalatal region, and others are intended to stabilize the retrolingual airway (Box 2). Sleep surgery has been shown to be most effective when addressing multiple levels of obstruction. Procedures are often combined for maximum effectiveness, such as septoplasty, turbinate reduction, tonsillectomy,

---

| BOX 2 | Treatments for Obstructive Sleep Apnea |

Nasal Obstruction
Septoplasty
Rhinoplasty or nasal valve surgery
Turbinate reduction
Adenoidectomy

Retropalatal Obstruction
Tonsillectomy
Uvulopalatopharyngoplasty
Z-palatoplasty
Lateral pharyngoplasty
Palatal stents
Radiofrequency soft palate surgery

Retrolingual Obstruction
Transoral robotic-assisted base of tongue reduction
Lingual tonsillectomy
Genioglossus advancement
Hyoid suspension
Tongue base suspension
Upper airway stimulation device (hypoglossal nerve stimulator)
Maxillomandibular advancement

---

uvulopalatopharyngoplasty, and genial tubercle advancement. With the advent of transoral robotic surgery (TORS), surgeons are now able to access the posterior oropharynx, base of tongue, and hypopharynx more easily, and procedures to address these areas are more common.

It is challenging to predict which patients are likely to have a successful surgical outcome. Much of this difficulty is associated with accurately identifying the site(s) of obstruction. The current gold standard is drug-induced sleep endoscopy (DISE), a procedure that examines the upper airway while the patient is in a drug-induced (propofol [Diprivan][1] or dexmedetomidine [Precedex]), sleep-resembling state. As the patient snores and obstructs, a flexible fiberoptic scope is passed through the nose to evaluate the upper airway for the site of obstruction. The advantage of a DISE in comparison to assessing the airway while awake is it can more naturally evaluate sites of obstruction during sleep. DISE has shown to alter surgical treatment plans in 50% of OSA patients. The VOTE system is the most commonly used scoring system that evaluates the four major anatomical areas for potential obstruction, including the velum (palate), oropharyngeal walls (lateral), tongue, and epiglottis. Both the extent and configuration of collapse are noted. Although there is no clear consensus that DISE improves surgical outcomes for sleep surgery, there are retrospective studies that have shown benefit. Patients with anterior-posterior palatal collapse on DISE compared to concentric collapse had better outcomes following UPPP. Another study found DISE helped identify patients with significant oropharyngeal lateral wall collapse and complete base of tongue obstruction. These features were inversely correlated with surgical success.

In recent years, the development of new implantable devices that allow for upper airway stimulation has offered a new solution for patients with specific anterior-posterior collapse of the upper airway. The upper airway stimulation device monitors respiratory patterns and stimulates primarily tongue muscles to protrude during inspiration, relieving OSA.

A substantially more invasive procedure, the maxillomandibular advancement, has been shown to be very effective in a number of case series. However, the only definitive surgical cure is tracheostomy, which completely bypasses the upper airway but is not without its comorbidities.

Monitoring

The patient's response to therapy needs to be monitored. In the case of CPAP therapy, monitoring of CPAP adherence is critical, because subjective reports are inaccurate. Resolution of excessive sleepiness is the desired outcome for patients who are symptomatic at baseline. If excessive sleepiness remains problematic despite documentation of desirable CPAP adherence, treatment with modafinil (Provigil) 100 to 400 mg in the morning might be considered. Other potential conditions affecting sleep need to be monitored and, if necessary, treated. Often, other conditions, such as poor sleep hygiene, RLS, PLMs, or psychophysiologic insomnia, interfere with adequate response to therapy.

For patients who undergo surgery, retesting is indicated. The interval at which retesting should be done depends on the type of surgery that was performed. Retesting 3 months following the surgical intervention is adequate in most cases.

References

Al Lawati NM, Patel SR, Ayas NT: Epidemiology, risk factors, and consequences of obstructive sleep apnea and short sleep duration, *Prog Cardiovasc Dis* 51:285–293, 2009.

Ancoli-Israel S, Klauber MR, Stepnowsky C, et al: Sleep-disordered breathing in African-American elderly, *Am J Respir Crit Care Med* 52:1946–1949, 1995.

Ashrafian H, Toma T, Rowland SP, et al: Bariatric surgery or non-surgical weight loss for obstructive sleep apnoea? A systematic review and comparison of meta-analysis, *Obes Surg* 25(7):1239–1250, 2015.

Cai A, Wang L, Zhou Y: Hypertension and obstructive sleep apnea, *Hypertens Res* 39:391–395, 2016.

Caples SM, Rowley JA, Prinsell JR, et al: Surgical modifications of the upper airway for obstructive sleep apnea in adults: a systematic review and meta-analysis, *Sleep* 33(10):1396–1407, 2010.

Dedhia RC, Strollo PJ, Soose RJ: Upper airway stimulation for obstructive sleep apnea: Past, present, and future, *Sleep* 38:899–906, 2015.

El Shayeb M, Topfer LA, Stafinski T: Diagnostic accuracy of level 3 portable sleep tests versus level 1 polysomnography for sleep-disordered breathing: a systematic review and meta-analysis, *CMAJ* 186(1):E25–E51, 2014. https://doi.org/10.1503/cmaj.130952.

Fujita S, Conway W, Zorick F, Roth T: Surgical correction of anatomic abnormalities in obstructive sleep apnea syndrome; Uvulopalatopharyngoplasty, *Otolaryngol Head Neck Surg* 89(6):923–934, 1981.

Heiser C, Steffen A, Boon M, et al: Post-approval upper airway stimulation predictors of treatment effectiveness in the ADHERE registry, *Eur Respir J* 53, 2019.

Hsin-Ching L, Friedman M, Hsueh-Wen C, et al: The efficacy of multilevel surgery of the upper airway in adults with obstructive sleep apnea/hypopnea syndrome, *The Laryngoscope* 118:902–908, 2008.

Institute for Clinical Systems Improvement (ICSI): *Diagnosis and Treatment of Obstructive Sleep Apnea in Adults*, Bloomington, MN, 2008, Institute for Clinical Systems Improvement.

Levendowski DJ, Seagraves S, Popovic D, Westbrook PR: Assessment of a neck-based treatment and monitoring device for positional obstructive sleep apnea, *J Clin Sleep Med* 10:863–871, 2014.

Li KK, Powell NB, Kushida C, et al: A comparison of Asian and white patients with obstructive sleep apnea syndrome, *Laryngoscope* 109:1937–1940, 1999.

Peppard PE, Young T, Palta M, et al: Longitudinal study of moderate weight change and sleep-disordered breathing, *JAMA* 284:3015–3021, 2000.

Peppard PE, Young T, Palta M, et al: Prospective study of the association between sleep-disordered breathing and hypertension, *N Engl J Med* 342:1378–1384, 2000.

Punjabi NM: The epidemiology of adult obstructive sleep apnea, *Proc Am Thorac Soc* 5:136–143, 2008.

Quan SF, Howard BV, Iber C, et al: The Sleep Heart Health Study: Design, rationale, and methods, *Sleep* 20:1077–1085, 1997.

Sher AE, Schechtman KB, Piccirillo JF: The efficacy of surgical modifications of the upper airway in adults with obstructive sleep apnea syndrome, *Sleep* 19(2):156–177, 1996.

Soares D, Sinawe H, Folbe AJ, et al: Lateral oropharyngeal wall and supraglottic airway collapse associated with failure in sleep apnea surgery, *Laryngoscope* 122:473–479, 2012.

Strollo PJ, Soose RJ, Maurer JT, et al: Upper-airway stimulation for obstructive sleep apnea., *N Engl J Med* 370:139–149, 2014.

Vilaseca I, Morello A, Montserrat JM, et al: Usefulness of uvulopalatopharyngoplasty with genioglossus and hyoid advancement in the treatment of obstructive sleep apnea, *Arch Otolaryngol Head Neck Surg* 128:435–440, 2002.

Wang Y, Sun C, Cui X, et al: The role of drug-induced sleep endoscopy: predicting and guiding upper airway surgery for adult OSA patients, *Sleep Breath* 22:478–482, 2018.

PLEURAL EFFUSION AND EMPYEMA

Method of
Timothy M. Millington, MD; and David J. Finley, MD

CURRENT DIAGNOSIS

- At least 200 mL of pleural fluid must be present to be seen on chest x-ray.
- Decubitus x-ray or CT may be needed to assess for loculations or atelectatic lung.
- Pleural fluid evaluation by laboratory studies (pH, glucose, LDH, protein), cytology, and microbiology can usually determine the etiology of an effusion.
- Repeat chest CT after drainage or directed inspection of the pleural space may be needed in cases where malignancy is suspected.

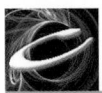

CURRENT THERAPY

- Most transudative effusions will resolve with treatment of the underlying medical process.
- Exudative effusions may be managed by serial thoracentesis, per-cutaneous drainage, or pleurodesis, depending on the etiology
- Pleural space infection is treated with a combination of instilled fibrinolytics and surgical drainage.
- Malignant pleural effusions frequently recur after drainage, and the most durable treatment strategy is surgically-directed talc pleurodesis or indwelling pleural catheter.

Pleural effusions have multiple etiologies, which makes diagnosis and management a common clinical issue. Although the amount of fluid produced varies significantly, an average 0.1 to 0.2 mL/kg is maintained within the pleural space. Production of fluid is matched with removal during normal physiologic states, but aberrations of this homeostasis with local or systemic diseases lead to the formation of an effusion. Symptoms are related to the volume of fluid and the etiology of the fluid accumulation, including both benign and malignant processes. Secondary infection of a pleural effusion, known as an empyema, is a significant complication that necessitates aggressive treatment of both the underlying cause and the empyema itself.

Symptoms are variable and include dyspnea, orthopnea, cough, and chest discomfort, although patients can be asymptomatic, even with very large effusions. Dullness to percussion and decreased breath sounds are often hallmarks of effusions, but these signs are also seen with lung masses and consolidative pneumonias. A clinical history, physical examination, and imaging studies are often needed in combination to diagnose an effusion.

Etiology

Many local and systemic illnesses are associated with the formation of a pleural effusion. Clinical history can indicate the most common cause of the effusion, but diagnostic procedures are often necessary to delineate the etiology. Determination of an exudative or transudative effusion can point out possible disease that may be the cause (Box 1).

Fluid that is low in total protein is a transudative effusion, which is most commonly caused by decreased oncotic pressure or increased capillary hydrostatic pressure. Transudative effusions can also be caused by fluid traversing the diaphragm, as seen in patients with ascites.

Exudative effusions are high in total protein (pleural fluid-to-serum ratio >0.5) and often have an elevated cell count. Increased capillary permeability and decreased lymphatic clearance, usually due to a local or systemic inflammatory illness, produce exudative

BOX 1 Etiologies of Transudative and Exudative Effusions

Transudative
Congestive heart failure
Cirrhosis
Pulmonary emboli
Peritoneal dialysis
Renal disorders
Myxedema
Sarcoidosis

Exudative
Malignancy
Infection
Drugs (e.g., nitrofurantoin [Marcodantin, Macrobid],
    methotrexate [Trexall])
Chylothorax
Pulmonary emboli
Gastrointestinal diseases (e.g., pancreatitis)
Collagen vascular disease (e.g., rheumatoid arthritis)
Asbestos exposure
Trauma (e.g., hemothorax, chest surgery)
Postpericardiectomy or postmyocardial infarction syndrome
Pleuropericarditis

effusions. The causes are varied, but the most common causes are malignancy, infection, and pulmonary emboli.

Diagnosis

Imaging

Approximately 200 to 500 mL of pleural fluid is necessary before it can be visualized on a posteroanterior upright chest x-ray, usually as blunting of the costophrenic angle. A lateral decubitus chest x-ray is more sensitive, often discerning fluid with as little as 100 mL present; layering of the fluid confirms that it is free flowing. Loculations can be seen on x-ray but may be mistaken for lung or pleural masses. Large effusion can completely opacify the hemithorax where the effusion is located. Distinguishing pleural fluid from atelectatic lung due to airway occlusion can be challenging and, in such cases, drainage should not be attempted until ambiguity is resolved by additional imaging studies.

Ultrasound is useful in defining the location and extent of an effusion and can also identify loculated effusions, pleural thickening, and masses. When used to help guide thoracentesis, it can increase diagnostic accuracy and yield and decrease complications.

Chest computed tomography (CT) has distinct advantages over x-ray and ultrasound, although without intravenous contrast it may still be difficult to differentiate pleural fluid from consolidated lung. The utility of chest CT to detect masses is significantly decreased when there is a large effusion associated with compressive atelectasis. Imaging with CT after initial drainage of a large effusion is recommended to obtain the most information regarding the possible etiologies of the effusion and aid in operative planning for treatment of an empyema. It also delineates pleural masses and helps differentiate pleural disease from lung pathology (e.g., loculated effusion vs. lung abscess).

Thoracentesis

It is often difficult to discern the cause of an effusion solely based on the patient's clinical presentation and image studies. Also, when concerned about a malignant process or an infected effusion, these studies do not give enough information to make a definitive diagnosis. Thoracentesis is the diagnostic procedure of choice, allowing drainage of the fluid to relieve symptoms for the patient and provide a specimen for evaluation. Ultrasound should be employed to help guide thoracentesis, especially if the effusion is small or loculated. Care must be taken when draining

a large amount of fluid in one setting due to the risk of reexpansion pulmonary edema. If a patient becomes symptomatic during the procedure (persistent cough, significant pleuritic pain, or shortness of breath), no more fluid should be removed at that time. Coagulopathy is a contraindication to thoracentesis due to the risk of intrathoracic bleeding. If the fluid appears cloudy, bloody, or milky then leaving a drainage catheter in place following thoracentesis should be strongly considered. Imaging should be obtained after all drainage procedures to document resolution and ensure that no pneumothorax is present. Pneumothorax after thoracentesis may be iatrogenic but may also reflect inability of a trapped lung to fully expand (ex vacuo pneumothorax) and warrants additional work-up.

Pleural Fluid

The initial evaluation of pleural fluid is done at the bedside by inspecting the fluid for color, viscosity, and odor. These simple steps can point the clinician toward the correct diagnosis. In addition to bedside evaluation, the fluid should be sent for the following laboratory studies: pH, glucose, lactate dehydrogenase (LDH), protein, cytology, Gram stain, and culture (including fungal and viral). Serum pH, protein, LDH and glucose should be sent at the same time.

Light's criteria are helpful in differentiating between an exudative and transudative effusion (Box 2). The sensitivity and specificity of Light's criteria is 82% to 90%.

Transudative effusions rarely need any further intervention, and the goal of treatment is directed at the underlying condition (see Box 1). For exudative effusions, the cause of the effusion dictates the treatment. Incorporating the clinical picture and radiographs with the pleural fluid chemistry studies, cytology, and cultures, the diagnosis is often obtained. Malignant effusions can have positive cytology, but they are more likely to have a pleural fluid glucose level less than 60 mg/dL and to be bloody. An elevated amylase level is seen in esophageal perforation, pancreatitis, and malignant effusions. Chylothorax can be definitively diagnosed if the triglyceride level is more than 110 mg/dL within the pleural fluid. Finally, pH, glucose, and cultures are useful in the treatment of patients with a presumed infected pleural effusion (empyema).

Up to 25% of patients will not have a definitive diagnosis based on the clinical scenario and pleural fluid evaluation. These patients can require further diagnostic testing, including repeat thoracentesis or evaluation of the chest cavity via video-assisted thoracoscopic surgery (VATS) with pleural biopsies.

Treatment

After initial evacuation of pleural fluid effusion, treatment is directed at preventing reaccumulation. In the case of hepatic hydrothorax, cardiogenic effusion or effusion related to renal insufficiency, the effusion should resolve with appropriate medical treatment of the underlying disease. Esophageal perforation and chylothorax generally require addressing the primary process with endoscopic, interventional, or surgical approaches. Special cases in which surgical management may be indicated include malignant and infectious effusions.

Malignant Pleural Effusion

Palliation of malignant pleural effusions is accomplished either by pleurodesis or palliative indwelling catheter. Both strategies are more likely to be successful in patients being treated with appropriate chemotherapy.

The most effective strategy for chemical pleurodesis is thoracoscopically directed spray talc pleurodesis, which will achieve resolution in about 85% of cases. A VATS approach has the added advantage that directed pleural biopsies may be obtained, with a significantly higher sensitivity for diagnosing pleural metastatic disease than fluid cytology alone. Bedside pleurodesis via tube thoracostomy can be attempted but is less likely to be successful.

For very high output malignant effusions or if incompletely lung expansion occurs, a tunneled indwelling long-term silicone-elastic catheter (PleurX) may be placed either operatively or percutaneously. This tube may be drained with a closed suction canister either on a regular schedule or as needed for symptoms. Regular drainage of malignant effusion achieves spontaneous pleurodesis in the majority of cases in about 6 weeks.

Infected Pleural Space and Empyema

A parapneumonic effusion (exudative effusion in the setting of pulmonary infection) is seen in 20% to 40% of patients admitted for pneumonia, of whom 10% to 20% will develop a complicated parapneumonic effusion or empyema (pus in the pleural space). Progression to empyema is most often due to delay in treatment and leads to longer hospital stays and increased morbidity and mortality. Other causes of infected effusions are trauma, thoracic surgical procedures, perforated esophagus, systemic infection, and transdiaphragmatic spread.

Parapneumonic effusions can be separated into three stages: exudative (stage I), fibropurulent (stage II), and organizational (stage III). Stage I effusions are free flowing, sterile reactive exudates and often do not reaccumulate after initial drainage. Although small, minimally symptomatic stage I effusions may resolve with appropriate antibiotics, it is difficult to determine the stage of an effusion clinically and at a minimum thoracentesis is indicated in most cases. Careful consideration should always be given to leaving a drainage tube in case a more advanced parapneumonic effusion is diagnosed.

Stage II effusions, or complicated parapneumonic effusions, are more viscous with lower glucose level and pH. Multiple pockets of loculated fluid with proteinaceous septations may be present. Complete drainage of all loculations is required to prevent progression to empyema or organized effusion and a chest drain (image-guided percutaneous catheter or thoracostomy tube) should be left behind in all cases. Early surgical intervention with thoracoscopic adhesiolysis may be considered if loculations are present. Alternatively, combination therapy with intrapleural tissue plasminogen activator (t-PA) and deoxyribonuclease (DNase) improves fluid drainage and reduces the need for surgical intervention. Complete drainage of all loculated pockets is of paramount importance and surgery may still be necessary after treatment with fibrinolytics.

Complicated parapneumonic effusions may go unrecognized and be treated late, particularly in patients with other medical or social comorbidities such as diabetes mellitus, dementia, developmental delay, and intravenous drug use. The result is progression to frank intrapleural pus, or empyema. Complete evacuation of the effusion is now required, and initial tube thoracostomy is indicated although often insufficient. If the patient does not improve promptly or the space is not completely drained, then surgery is recommended. The initial attempt at drainage should be thoracoscopic although conversion to thoracotomy may be required. Multiple large-bore chest tubes should be left in place until drainage has resolved. In the presence of frank pus, fibrinolytic therapy is less likely to be of benefit, although it may be considered in patients who are medically unable to tolerate surgery.

If infected fluid is evacuated but a residual cavity remains, then chronic infection is likely. This risk is greatly increased by the presence of a bronchopleural fistula, either arising from a lung abscess or due to surgical complication. In these situations, long-term drainage with an open thoracostomy or Eloesser flap, may be required to eradicate the infection. Ultimate obliteration of the space may require a rotational muscle flap.

If the pleural space is incompletely drained but adequately sterilized with antibiotics, the effusion may progress to the organizational stage. This is characterized by heavy fibrin deposit with the formation of a thick peel throughout the pleura with loculations and trapping of the lung, preventing re-expansion. Patients may report significant dyspnea and pulmonary function tests will show a restrictive pattern. Classic CT findings include thickened pleura with multiple loculations. Decortication, either via VATS or thoracotomy, is required to completely remove the peel off the parietal and visceral pleura. A robotic-assisted approach increases the likelihood of successful minimally invasive decortication.

References

Davies Helen E, et al: Effect of an indwelling pleural catheter vs chest tube and talc pleurodesis for relieving dyspnea in patients with malignant pleural effusion: the TIME2 randomized controlled trial, *JAMA* 307(22):2383–2389, 2012.

de Campos JR, Vargas FS, de Campos Werebe E, et al: Thoracoscopy talc poudrage: A 15- year experience, *Chest* 119:801–806, 2001.

Feller-Kopman David, Light Richard: Pleural disease, *N Engl J Med* 378(8):740–751, 2018.

Luh SP, Chen CY, Tzao CY: Malignant pleural effusion treatment outcomes: Pleurodesis via Video- Assisted Thoracic Surgery (VATS) versus tube thoracostomy, *Thorac Cardiovasc Surg* 54:332–336, 2006.

Luh SP, Hsu GJ, Cheng- Ren C: Complicated parapneumonic effusion and empyema: Pleural decortication and video- assisted thoracic surgery, *Curr Infect Dis Rep* 10:236–240, 2008.

Rahman NM, Chapman SJ, Davies RJ: Diagnosis and management of infectious pleural infection, *Treat Respir Med* 5:295–304, 2006.

Rahman Najib M, et al: Intrapleural use of tissue plasminogen activator and DNase in pleural infection, *N Engl J Med* 365(6):518–526, 2011.

PNEUMOCONIOSIS: ASBESTOSIS AND SILICOSIS

Method of
David N. Weissman, MD

CURRENT DIAGNOSIS

- History of inhalation of mineral or metal dust
- Respiratory symptoms such as cough and dyspnea
- Spirometry and lung volumes show restriction or mixed obstruction/restriction in advanced disease
- Interstitial lung disease can usually be demonstrated by chest imaging. Biopsy is usually unnecessary in the setting of good exposure history and typical findings on chest imaging.
- No other likely cause of interstitial lung disease is present

CURRENT THERAPY

- Treatment is symptomatic and similar to that for other patients with chronic lung disease
- Give pneumococcal and influenza vaccinations.
- Provide empiric treatment with short- and long-acting inhaled bronchodilators and inhaled corticosteroids when they are found to provide symptomatic relief.
- Give supplemental oxygen therapy if pulmonary hypertension is present or to prevent pulmonary hypertension if O_2 saturation is less than 88% at rest, with exercise, or with sleep.
- Consider lung transplantation in the setting of end-stage lung disease.

TABLE 1   Representative Pneumoconioses

SOURCE	MAIN CLINICAL FEATURES	OCCUPATION	DUST
Crystalline silica	Silicosis, COPD, increased susceptibility to TB, lung cancer, autoimmune diseases	Mining, stone cutting, pottery, foundry work, artificial stone countertop work	Free crystalline silica (SiO_2)
Asbestiform fibers	Asbestosis, bronchogenic carcinoma, mesothelioma, various forms of benign pleural disease	Insulation, shipbuilding, construction, some mining (e.g., vermiculite mining in Libby, MT)	Various asbestiform fibers
Coal	Coal workers' pneumoconiosis, COPD	Coal mining	Coal mine dust
Hard metal	Hard metal lung disease (cobalt lung), asthma	Machinists, metal workers	Hard metal, composed primarily of tungsten carbide and cobalt

COPD, chronic obstructive pulmonary disease; TB, tuberculosis.

The pneumoconioses are a group of interstitial fibrotic lung diseases predominantly associated with occupational exposures. They are caused by inhalation of mineral or metallic dust particles small enough to penetrate into the deep lung (respirable size range) (Table 1). These agents interact with pulmonary target cells, including alveolar macrophages and alveolar epithelial cells, to activate a cascade of inflammatory mediators including growth factors. Although exposure to these dusts can induce other types of respiratory disease as well, the final common pathway leading to pneumoconiosis is alveolar epithelial cell damage and interstitial fibrosis. This chapter focuses on silicosis and asbestosis, two common forms of pneumoconiosis.

Asbestosis

Asbestos is composed of strong, heat-resistant fibers of hydrated magnesium silicate classified morphologically as serpentine (chrysotile) or amphibole (crocidolite [riebeckite asbestos], amosite [cummingtonite-grunerite asbestos], anthophyllite asbestos, actinolite asbestos, and tremolite asbestos). In addition, certain asbestiform fibers (winchite, richterite, erionite) can cause adverse health effects identical to those of asbestos. Fiber dimensions and persistence in tissues are key determinants of toxicity. There is a dose–response effect between the quantity of asbestos inhaled and the severity of fibrotic lung disease. Asbestos is also a carcinogen, and increasing exposure is associated with increased risk for lung cancer, mesothelioma, ovarian cancer, and laryngeal cancer.

Although asbestos is no longer mined in the United States, importation of asbestos-containing products continues. Exposures also continue to occur, especially in construction and renovation (due to reservoirs of asbestos that are still present in many older buildings), the heating trades (where asbestos is often encountered), and with exposure to older or imported asbestos-containing automotive friction products such as brake linings and clutch facings. Workers exposed to asbestos can carry it home on their clothing, resulting in exposure of family members. Living near geological formations prone to asbestos formation in California has been implicated as a risk factor for mesothelioma.

The Occupational Safety and Health Administration (OSHA) permissible exposure limit (PEL) for asbestos is 0.1 fiber per cc air. This limit was based in part on the limits of the analytical methodology used in exposure assessment. Exposure to the PEL every day over a 45-year working lifetime has been estimated to be associated with an increased risk of cancer (lung, mesothelioma, and gastrointestinal) of 336 cases per 100,000 exposed persons and an increased risk of asbestosis of 250 cases per 100,000 exposed persons.

Asbestosis causes symptoms of dyspnea and cough. Latency between initial exposure and disease onset is related to exposure intensity. In the United States, this period is generally about two or more decades. The disease can lead to chronic respiratory failure. Effects of smoking add to the severity of the disease and can cause obstructive findings in addition to the expected decreased lung volume and diffusion capacity associated with fibrotic lung diseases. Bibasilar inspiratory crackles on auscultation, finger clubbing, and bibasilar small, irregular parenchymal opacities on chest x-ray with extension to mid- and upper-zones with advancing disease are characteristic.

The International Labour Organization (ILO) has established a system for classification (grading) of radiographs for the presence of radiographic abnormalities in lung parenchyma and pleura that are associated with pneumoconiosis, as well as their severity. The ILO classification system is widely used in epidemiology, surveillance, administrative, and legal settings. The small opacity profusion grades of 0/1 and 1/0 are often considered as defining the boundary between normal and abnormal lung parenchyma.

High-resolution computed tomography (CT) is the most sensitive imaging method for suspected asbestosis. Findings associated with asbestos exposure include lower lobe or diffuse irregular opacities, bronchial wall thickening, rounded atelectasis, and pleural abnormalities such as pleural plaques and diffuse pleural thickening. The presence of pleural plaques on radiography (particularly bilateral calcified pleural plaques); or uncoated asbestos fibers or fibers coated with an iron-rich proteinaceous material (asbestos bodies) in sputum, bronchoalveolar lavage, or lung biopsy help differentiate asbestosis from idiopathic pulmonary fibrosis.

Criteria for Diagnosis

Diagnosis is supported by radiographic chest imaging or lung biopsy findings of interstitial lung disease compatible with asbestosis; documentation of exposure to asbestos by history, the presence of pleural plaques (bilateral pleural plaques are essentially pathognomonic for asbestos exposure), or the presence of asbestos bodies or an excessive burden of uncoated asbestos fibers in lung biopsy tissue or possibly via bronchoalveolar lavage or sputum; and no other likely explanation for the diffuse fibrotic lung disease.

Asbestos-Related Benign Pleural Disease

Pleural plaques are characteristic forms of localized parietal pleural thickening that are usually bilateral and asymmetrical, involve the lower lung fields or the diaphragm, and spare the costophrenic angles and apices. Pleural plaques are a marker for exposure to asbestos and are often associated with other asbestos-related conditions. Pleural plaques generally result in minimal reductions in forced vital capacity and do not degenerate into malignant lesions.

In contrast, diffuse visceral pleural thickening can result in adhesions between the visceral and parietal pleura with major decreases in forced vital capacity and respiratory insufficiency sufficient for consideration of decortication.

Benign pleural effusions can occur in the first decade after asbestos exposure and contain erythrocytes and a mixed inflammatory cell infiltrate of lymphocytes, neutrophils, and eosinophils. The thickened visceral pleura and adjacent atelectatic lung tissue can result in a pleural-based area of rounded atelectasis, simulating a lung mass on chest radiography. CT can reveal the comet sign, a pleural band connecting the apparent mass to an area of thickened pleura.

Lung Cancer and Malignant Mesothelioma

Exposure to all forms of asbestos increases the risk of lung cancer. The peak risk occurs at about 30 to 35 years after the onset of exposure. Tobacco smoking increases this risk in a supra-additive fashion, increasing risk to a level greater than for asbestos or smoking alone. In contrast, smoking does not further increase the asbestos-associated risk for malignant mesothelioma. Asbestos-associated malignant mesothelioma can also affect the peritoneum (and sometimes the pericardium), but when it affects the pleura, this disease manifests with dyspnea, chest pain, and bloody pleural effusion (most often unilateral). A latency period of 30 years or longer after initial exposure is common. Biopsy and specialized immunohistochemical stains are typically required to distinguish malignant mesothelioma from benign mesothelial proliferations and various carcinomas such as adenocarcinomas. It is currently unclear when to screen asbestos-exposed individuals at increased risk for lung cancer with low-dose chest computed tomography.

Treatment

Treatment of asbestosis is symptomatic and similar to that for other patients with chronic lung disease (Box 1). Lung transplantation should be considered in the setting of end-stage lung disease. Treatment of benign pleural disease is also symptomatic; as already noted, decortication is an option for managing severe cases of diffuse visceral pleural thickening. Depending on extent of disease, mesothelioma may be treated with surgery, radiation, chemotherapy, or some combination of these. In general, prognosis is poor. Mesothelioma-associated malignant pleural effusion can require palliation through procedures such as pleurodesis, pleurectomy, and decortication. Asbestos-associated lung cancer is managed in the same fashion as lung cancer occurring without a history of exposure to asbestos.

Silicosis

Silicosis is a fibrosing interstitial lung disease resulting from the inhalation of crystalline silicon dioxide (silica) in dust of respirable size. The commonest form of crystalline silica is quartz, which is the main component of sand and is present in most rocks. Noncrystalline (amorphous) silica, like that in diatomaceous earth or glass, does not cause silicosis. However, heating amorphous silica, as occurs in foundries when molten metal is poured into clay castings, can convert amorphous silica into cristobalite, a hazardous form of crystalline silica. Mining, stone cutting, sandblasting, and foundry work are all examples of trades associated with exposure to respirable dust containing crystalline silica. The International Agency for Research on Cancer (IARC) has designated crystalline silica as a Group 1 human lung carcinogen.

In 2016, OSHA established a new PEL for respirable crystalline silica of 0.05 mg/m^3. It also established requirements for engineering and administrative controls, personal protective equipment, and medical surveillance including periodic chest radiography and spirometry obtained at least every 3 years. Reporting of silicosis cases to public health authorities is required in some states.

Radiographic Patterns of Silicosis

Three main radiographic patterns of silicosis have been described. Two are nodular interstitial patterns and one is an alveolar-filling pattern. The *simple* pattern is associated with nodules that are smaller than 10 mm and that are predominantly rounded and in the upper lung zones. *Progressive massive fibrosis* (PMF) is found in more advanced interstitial disease. It is associated with multiple coalescent larger nodules, upper lobe fibrosis, upward retraction of the hila, and compensatory hyperinflation of the lower lobes. The large upper-zone opacities can cavitate, sometimes in the setting of superimposed mycobacterial infection. Hilar adenopathy can occur in association with either pattern, sometimes with an egg-shell pattern of hilar node calcification. A third radiographic pattern is an alveolar-filling process. Overwhelming silica exposure over a short period can cause a pathologic response called *silicoproteinosis*, in which alveoli become flooded with proteinaceous fluid. The condition resembles idiopathic pulmonary alveolar proteinosis. The radiographic alveolar filling pattern favors the lower lung zones and is not necessarily associated with the changes of simple silicosis or PMF.

Silicosis Syndromes

Three syndromes of silicosis can be defined based on clinical course and radiographic pattern. Chronic silicosis develops slowly, usually 10 to 30 years after first exposure. It most often has the simple radiographic pattern, but it can be associated with PMF.

Accelerated silicosis develops more rapidly, within 10 years after first exposure. It is associated with higher intensity exposures and can be associated with either the simple or PMF radiographic patterns. Accelerated silicosis is differentiated from chronic silicosis by its more rapid course. Patients with accelerated courses are at greater risk for developing PMF. The clinical presentations of chronic and accelerated silicosis are variable but include cough, dyspnea, and a variety of chest findings ranging from a normal chest examination to crackles, rhonchi, or wheezing. PMF is associated with more severe symptoms and respiratory impairment. Findings compatible with both restrictive and obstructive lung disease (decreased forced vital capacity [FVC], forced expiratory volume at 1 sec [FEV$_1$], FEV$_1$/FVC,

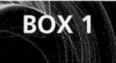
Patients

Stop further exposure to silica or asbestos.
  Stop smoking, avoid exposure to tobacco products.

Physicians

Provide early treatment of respiratory infections with antibiotics.

Give pneumococcal and influenza vaccinations.

Maintain a high index of suspicion and provide early evaluation of symptoms for lung, laryngeal, and ovarian cancers and mesothelioma in asbestos-exposed patients.

Maintain a high index of suspicion for pulmonary infection with *Mycobacterium tuberculosis,* nontuberculous mycobacteria, and fungi in silica-exposed patients.

Screen silica-exposed patients for latent tuberculosis infection. Treat latent infections with one of the currently-approved drug protocols.

Provide empiric treatment with short- and long-acting inhaled bronchodilators and inhaled corticosteroids when they are found to provide symptomatic relief.

Give supplemental oxygen therapy if pulmonary hypertension is present or to prevent pulmonary hypertension if O$_2$ saturation is less than 88% at rest, with exercise, or with sleep.

Consider lung transplantation in the setting of end-stage lung disease.

diffusion capacity) can occur, potentially leading to cor pulmonale and respiratory failure.

Acute silicosis is associated with very intense exposures to silica, leading to symptoms within a few weeks to a few years after exposure. Intense exposure results in lung injury caused by flooding of alveoli with proteinaceous material, or silicoproteinosis. As already noted, the radiographic appearance is that of an alveolar-filling pattern favoring the lower lung zones. Patients present weeks to a few years after exposure with cough, weight loss, fatigue, and occasional pleuritic chest pain, crackles on auscultation, and progression to respiratory failure often complicated by mycobacterial infection.

Criteria for Diagnosis

The diagnosis of silicosis is predicated on a history of exposure to respirable crystalline silica, typical chest x-ray findings, and the lack of a more likely diagnosis. High-resolution CT detects changes of silicosis with greater sensitivity than chest radiography. Lung biopsy is seldom required for diagnosis in the setting of a good exposure history and typical findings on chest imaging.

Treatment

Treatment is symptomatic and similar to that for other patients with chronic lung disease (see Box 1). Experimental therapies such as oral corticosteroid therapy and whole-lung lavage have been reported, but clinical benefit is unclear. Lung transplantation should be considered for patients with end-stage lung disease.

All forms of silicosis, as well as substantial exposure to crystalline silica in the absence of silicosis, are associated with an increased risk of pulmonary tuberculosis and fungal infections. Patients should be evaluated for latent tuberculosis infection by tuberculin skin testing or with an interferon gamma release assay. A positive tuberculin skin test in a patient with a history of substantial silica exposure of at least 10 mm of induration should be considered evidence of tuberculosis infection, regardless of previous immunization with bacille Calmette-Guérin. If testing for latent tuberculosis infection is positive, an evaluation for active tuberculosis should be performed and active disease treated. If active tuberculosis is not present, treat for latent infection. As in other settings, treatment for active or latent infection should be provided using one of the drug treatment protocols recommended by the Centers for Disease Control and Prevention. Vaccination for influenza should be provided annually. In addition, adults with silicosis should be vaccinated with 13-valent pneumococcal conjugate vaccine (PCV13, Prevnar 13) and 23-valent pneumococcal polysaccharide vaccine (PPSV23, Pneumovax 23) according to current Centers for Disease Control and Prevention recommendations.

Disclaimer

The findings and conclusions in this report are those of the authors and do not necessarily represent the views of the National Institute for Occupational Safety and Health or the Centers for Disease Control and Prevention.

References

American Thoracic Society: Diagnosis and initial management of nonmalignant diseases related to asbestos, *Am J Respir Crit Care Med* 170(6):691–715, 2004.
CDC (Centers for Disease Control and Prevention). 2016. Recommended vaccines by age. Available at: https://www.cdc.gov/vaccines/vpd/vaccines-age.html, accessed 3/14/2017.
Department of Labor: Mine Safety and Health Administration: 30 CFR Parts 56, 57, and 71. Asbestos exposure limit; proposed rule, *Fed Reg* 70:43950–43989, 2005.
Leung CC, Yu IT, Chen W: Silicosis, *Lancet* 379(9830):2008–2018, 2012.
Miller A: Radiographic readings for asbestosis: misuse of science—validation of the ILO classification, *Am J Ind Med* 50:63–67, 2007.
Oksa P, Wolff H, Vehmas T, Pallasaho P, Frilander H, editors: *Asbestos, Asbestosis, and Cancer—Helsinki Criteria for Diagnosis and Attribution 2014*, Tampere, 2014. (Juvenes Print.
Petsonk EL, Rose C, Cohen R: Coal mine dust lung disease. New lessons from old exposure, *Am J Respir Crit Care Med* 187(11):1178–1185, 2013.

PULMONARY HYPERTENSION

Method of
Dan Schuller, MD; and Anthony Peter Catinella, MD, MPH

CURRENT DIAGNOSIS

- Pulmonary arterial hypertension (PAH) is a type of pulmonary hypertension (PH) based on restricted flow because of vascular wall remodeling and increased pulmonary vascular resistance. PH does not equal PAH.
- The clinical presentation of PH is subtle and nonspecific with dyspnea, fatigue, and exercise limitation. A high index of suspicion is required.
- Echocardiography is the recommended initial screening test.
- Right heart catheterization, preferably at an expert center, should be obtained before initiation of specific PAH treatments.
- PAH is a diagnosis of exclusion.
- Multimodality risk stratification with combination of functional class assessment, echocardiography, exercise testing (6-minute walk test), B-type natriuretic peptide, and hemodynamic parameters are required at the time of initial diagnosis and for longitudinal monitoring.

CURRENT THERAPY

- Early referral to a PH expert center is recommended
- General measures and supportive care include avoiding pregnancy and high altitude travel, influenza, COVID-19, and pneumococcal immunizations, supplemental oxygen for hypoxemia, diuretics and electrolyte replacement when needed, correction of anemia and optimal evaluation, and management of associated comorbidities.
- There are now 12 Food and Drug Administration (FDA)–approved drugs for the treatment of PAH.
- With a few exceptions, PAH patients at low or intermediate risk should be treated with upfront combination therapy with endothelin receptor antagonists (ERAs) and phosphodiesterase-5 inhibitors (PDE5i).
- In high-risk PAH patients, combination therapy including intravenous prostanoid and referral for lung transplantation is recommended.
- PAH requires a multidimensional approach to care that includes rehabilitation, psychosocial, spiritual support, and palliative care.

Definition and Classification

In 2018, a revised hemodynamic definition of pulmonary hypertension (PH) became a mean pulmonary arterial pressure (mPAP) greater than 20 mm Hg rather than the prior level of 25 mm Hg. This is a hemodynamic definition based on measurements taken during right heart catheterization at rest, as the criterion standard. Based on Ohm's law, resistance is directly proportional to a pressure gradient and inversely proportional to flow. Thus the pulmonary vascular resistance (PVR) is calculated by dividing the pressure gradient (mPAP minus venous pressure as measured by the pulmonary capillary wedge pressure or PCWP) by the cardiac flow rate using the cardiac output or CO:

$$PVR = (mPAP - PCWP)/cardiac\ output\ (CO)$$

Rearranging the equation to calculate the mPAP yields MPAP = (PVR × CO) + PCWP. From this simple equation, different hemodynamic profiles leading to PH can be distinguished (Figure 1). PH can occur because there is an increase in PVR (or precapillary PH), an increase in PCWP (or postcapillary PH), an increase in

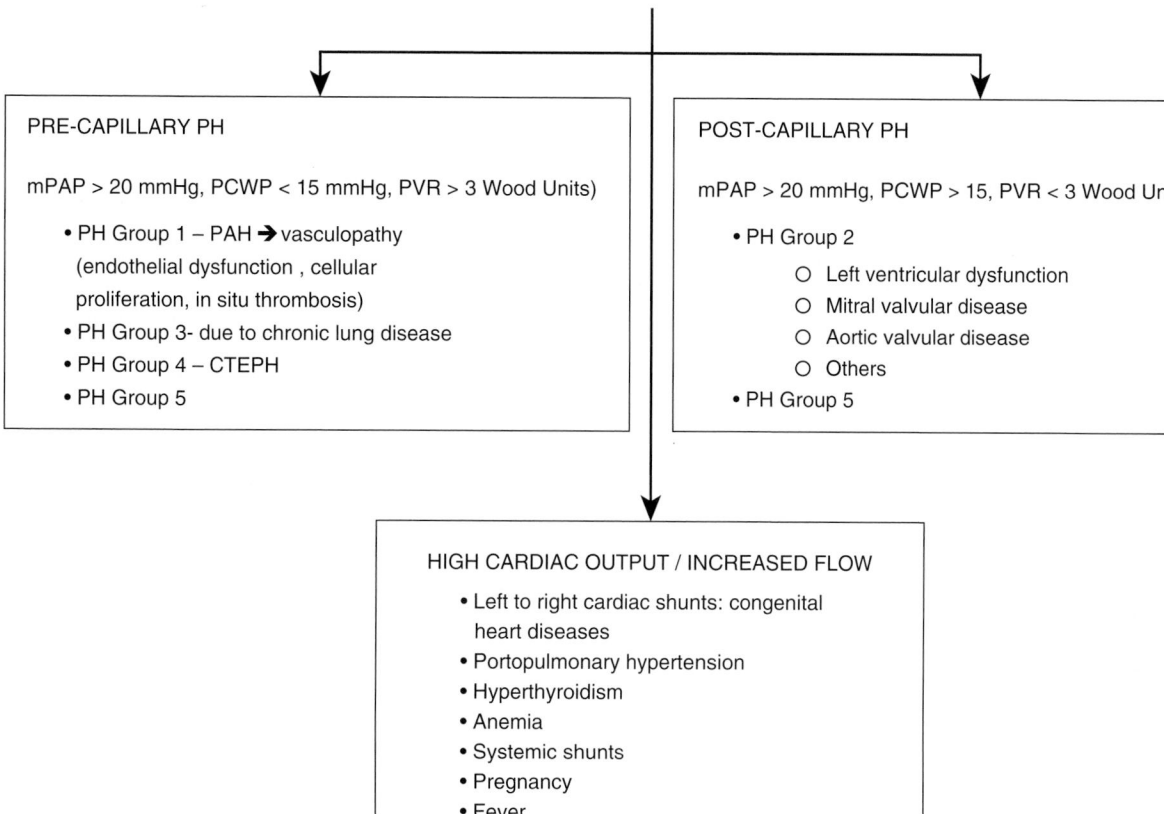

HEMODYNAMIC PROFILES IN PULMONARY HYPERTENSION

Pulmonary Arterial Pressure = (Pulmonary Vascular Resistance) (Cardiac Output) + Wedge Pressure

PRE-CAPILLARY PH

mPAP > 20 mmHg, PCWP < 15 mmHg, PVR > 3 Wood Units)

- PH Group 1 – PAH ➔ vasculopathy (endothelial dysfunction , cellular proliferation, in situ thrombosis)
- PH Group 3- due to chronic lung disease
- PH Group 4 – CTEPH
- PH Group 5

POST-CAPILLARY PH

mPAP > 20 mmHg, PCWP > 15, PVR < 3 Wood Units

- PH Group 2
  - ○ Left ventricular dysfunction
  - ○ Mitral valvular disease
  - ○ Aortic valvular disease
  - ○ Others
- PH Group 5

HIGH CARDIAC OUTPUT / INCREASED FLOW

- Left to right cardiac shunts: congenital heart diseases
- Portopulmonary hypertension
- Hyperthyroidism
- Anemia
- Systemic shunts
- Pregnancy
- Fever

Figure 1 Hemodynamic profiles in pulmonary hypertension.

flow (high cardiac output state), or any combination of these. Isolated precapillary PH occurs when the mPAP is greater than 20 mm Hg to define the PH state, and the PVR is elevated (≥3 Woods unit) while the PCWP is normal (≤15 mm Hg). Likewise, isolated postcapillary PH occurs when the mPAP is greater than 20 mm Hg and the PCWP is greater than 15 mm Hg while the PVR is normal at less than 3 Woods unit. Commonly, one finds combined pre- and postcapillary PH with all values abnormally elevated.

Understanding these equations permits appropriate classification, which has therapeutic implications, and for insight into sudden clinical worsening with progression of the natural history of the underlying conditions. For instance, a patient with idiopathic PH can have an increase in pulmonary pressures caused by progression of the disease (precapillary) or from interval development of a high output state such as fever, anemia or pregnancy, or from interval development of fluid overload or left ventricular dysfunction (postcapillary).

PH is classified into five groups (Box 1) based on common underlying mechanisms or pathophysiology. Only PH Group 1 is designated as pulmonary arterial hypertension (PAH) with restricted flow caused by vascular wall remodeling and increased PVR. PH Group 2 is caused by left heart disease, a common condition that elevates pulmonary venous pressures; this group represents the highest proportion of PH patients in the United States. PH Group 3 is caused by chronic intrinsic lung diseases with chronic hypoxia and/or hypercapnia as a common mechanism; in patients with mild to moderate chronic obstructive pulmonary disease (COPD), the prevalence of PH is about 20% and increases to 50% in more advanced cases of the disease. PH Group 4 is predominantly caused by chronic thromboembolic disease, which

causes obliteration of the pulmonary vascular bed by chronic organized thrombus leading to increased PVR. PH Group 5 consists of heterogeneous conditions with multifactorial mechanisms that affect PH.

PAH is a rare, progressive, incurable disease of the small pulmonary arteries characterized by precapillary PH, vascular cell proliferation, aberrant remodeling, and thrombosis in situ (Figure 2). This group is amenable to specific PAH therapies. PAH is further subdivided into categories because of various etiologies and risk factors linked to a common pathogenesis but with significant variability in presentation, natural history, and response to treatment.

In the United States, almost half of the cases of PAH are idiopathic, whereas approximately 25% are associated with connective tissue disease (predominantly scleroderma), nearly 10% with congenital heart disease, 5% with liver disease (porto-pulmonary hypertension), and 5% with drugs or toxins (e.g., methamphetamine [Desoxyn], dasatinib [Sprycel], or appetite suppressants). Schistosomiasis is a rare parasitic infection in the United States, but it is endemic in 74 countries. Worldwide, 85% of persons infected with schistosomiasis are in sub-Saharan Africa and the disease represents the most common cause of PAH worldwide.

Heritable PAH has been associated with a number of genetic mutations (predominantly the bone morphogenetic protein receptor type 2 [*BMPR2*] gene, activin receptor-like kinase type 1 [*ALK1*], and endoglin) and accounts for almost 3% of cases in the United States. It is transmitted as an autosomal-dominant trait, with incomplete penetrance estimated to be approximately 10% to 20%. Genetic anticipation, distinguished by decreasing age of disease onset, has been reported in families affected with heritable PAH.

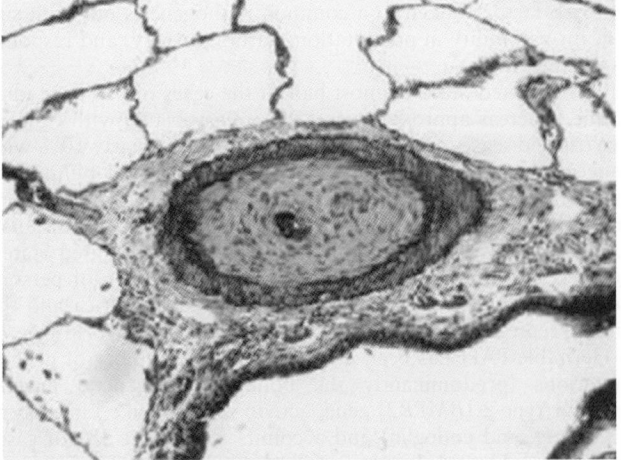

BOX 1 · Clinical Classification of Pulmonary Hypertension

Group 1: Pulmonary arterial hypertension (PAH)
Idiopathic PAH (IPAH)
Heritable PAH
Drug- and toxin-induced PAH
PAH associated with:
 Connective tissue disease
 HIV infection
 Portal hypertension
 Congenital heart disease
 Schistosomiasis
PAH long-term responders to calcium channel blockers
PAH with overt features of venous/capillaries pulmonary
 veno-occlusive disease (PVOD)/ pulmonary capillary
 hemangiomatosis (PCH) involvement
Persistent pulmonary hypertension (PH) of the newborn
 syndrome

Group 2: Pulmonary hypertension caused by left heart disease
PH caused by heart failure with preserved left ventricular
 ejection fraction (LVEF)
Valvular heart disease
Congenital/acquired cardiovascular conditions leading to
 postcapillary PH

Group 3: Pulmonary hypertension caused by lung diseases and /or hypoxia
Obstructive lung disease
Restrictive lung disease
Other lung disease with mixed restrictive/obstructive pattern
Hypoxia without lung disease
Development lung disorders

Group 4: Pulmonary hypertension caused by pulmonary artery obstructions
Chronic thromboembolic PH
Other pulmonary artery obstruction

Group 5: Pulmonary hypertension with unclear and/or multifactorial mechanism
Hematologic disorders
Systemic and metabolic disorders
Other

Figure 2 Typical advanced pulmonary arteriopathy in idiopathic pulmonary arterial hypertension. Note the proliferative changes in all three vessel layers, including intimal hyperplasia, medial hypertrophy, and adventitial fibrosis. From Broaddus VC, Mason RJ, Ernst JD, et al: *Murray & Nadel's Textbook of Respiratory Medicine,* 6 ed, Elsevier, 2016.

Clinical Manifestations

The initial symptoms of PAH are often subtle and nonspecific; mean time between symptom onset and PAH diagnosis is approximately 2 years. Patients often report progressive or exertional breathlessness, fatigue, and exercise limitation. With progression, patients may present with near syncope or syncope, palpitations, or anginal chest pain. Early detection requires a high index of suspicion because attribution to conditions such as asthma or "being out of shape" is a common error that can contribute to delay in diagnosis. Failure to respond to typical treatments for heart failure or asthma may be an important clue. Dysphonia or hoarseness caused by compression of the recurrent laryngeal nerve (Ortner's syndrome), which is caused by an enlarged pulmonary artery, occurs in less than 1% of patients. Early physical findings of PH may be nonspecific and include an accentuated pulmonary component of the second heart sound (P2) and a midsystolic ejection murmur. Physical findings in more advanced cases that involve right ventricular failure include a right parasternal lift, right ventricular gallop, diastolic murmur of pulmonary regurgitation, jugular venous distention, lower extremity edema, ascites, and signs of low cardiac output, including cool extremities. A murmur of tricuspid regurgitation may be audible, and this murmur intensifies with inspiration, unlike that of mitral regurgitation. Patients with suspected PH may also exhibit signs of associated conditions, such as telangiectasias, Raynaud's phenomenon, sclerodactyly, calcinosis, or malar erythema in connective tissue diseases; evidence of liver cirrhosis or portal hypertension; venous insufficiency or varicosities suggestive of possible thromboembolic disease; and obvious signs of underlying cardiac or respiratory diseases, including obstructive sleep apnea. Suggestive electrocardiographic findings include right axis deviation greater than 110°, which has a positive predictive value between 72% and 93% and a negative predictive value between 26% and 65%. Other associated findings include right atrial enlargement and right ventricular hypertrophy.

Diagnosis

The diagnostic evaluation is aimed at screening high-risk individuals, excluding secondary causes of PH, and evaluating possible associated conditions. In addition, various elements of the comprehensive examination are useful for subsequent risk stratification, which is required to select the best therapeutic option and assess prognosis. PAH is always a diagnosis of exclusion.

After reviewing pertinent previous medical records and performing a complete history and physical examination, the pivotal test in the diagnostic algorithm by the primary care provider or non-PH expert center is a transthoracic echocardiogram (TTE) to assess the probability of PH. An echocardiogram has an intermediate or high risk for PH based on a peak tricuspid regurgitation velocity 2.9 m/s or greater or right ventricular systolic pressure ≥35 mm Hg. In one series, TTE had a sensitivity of 87% (95% confidence interval [CI] 84.8%, 90.0%) and specificity of 66% (95% CI 60.7%, 71.6%). After a positive screen, a decision has to be made as to whether to fast track the referral of the patient to a PH expert center or to advance locally the diagnostic evaluation with additional testing aimed at diagnosing common causes of PH and ruling out chronic thromboembolic pulmonary hypertension (CTEPH). A comprehensive evaluation may include chest film, electrocardiogram, TTE, ventilation-perfusion lung scan, pulmonary function testing, 6-minute walk test, serologic evaluation (HIV, antinuclear antibodies [ANA], BNP, and others), and right-side cardiac catheterization for hemodynamic assessment and vasoreactivity testing. Depending on the results, additional, contingent tests may include a transesophageal echocardiogram, stress echocardiogram, "bubble" echocardiogram, computed tomography (CT) scan of the chest with or without pulmonary angiogram, coagulopathy profile, blood gases, overnight oximetry, polysomnography, or a cardiac magnetic resonance imaging (MRI). During cardiac catheterization, additional interventions, such as exercise or fluid challenges, pharmacologic interventions with vasoactive agents, and/or a left-side cardiac catheterization, may be useful to secure a definitive diagnosis, assess potential mixed etiologies, and determine the hemodynamic profile for risk stratification.

Vasoreactivity testing in patients with PAH can be accomplished with the use of inhaled nitric oxide,[1] intravenous epoprostenol sodium (Flolan),[1] or intravenous adenosine (Adenocard).[1] A positive vasodilator response is defined as greater than 10% decrease in mPAP to an absolute value of less than 40 mm Hg with no decrease in cardiac output. Patients who show acute vasoreactivity should be considered for a high-dose calcium channel blocker titration challenge under hemodynamic monitoring in an intensive care setting. For the minority of patients that demonstrate a favorable response to either oral diltiazem (Cardizem)[1] or nifedipine (Procardia),[1] the selection of drug and dosing will depend on the cumulative dose of the acute challenge, their heart rate, and hemodynamic tolerance.

Novel diagnostic tools that are being investigated for PAH but are not universally available yet include V/Q single photon emission CT (SPECT) and dual-energy CT (DECT), three-dimensional dynamic contrast enhanced MRI, parametric MRI mapping, intravascular ultrasound, and optical coherence tomography.

Risk Stratification

In addition to the etiologic classification of PAH, the World Health Organization (WHO) also uses a functional classification for patients with PH, modeled after the New York Heart Association classification for heart failure. PAH patients are classified by severity of dyspnea and limitation of physical activity:

Class I includes patients with no limitation on physical activity. Routine physical activities do not cause increased dyspnea, chest pain, fatigue, or presyncope.

Class II includes patients with mild limitation of physical activities. These patients are comfortable at rest, but routine physical activities result in increased dyspnea, chest pain, fatigue, or syncope.

Class III includes patients with marked limitation of physical activities. They are comfortable at rest, but activities that are less than ordinary result in dyspnea, chest pain, fatigue, or palpitations.

Class IV includes patients unable to perform any physical activity without symptoms. Dyspnea or fatigue may be present at rest, and discomfort increases with any activity.

Low-risk criteria associated with a good prognosis include WHO functional class I–II, 6 MWT distance greater than 440 m, right atrial pressure (RAP) less than 8 mm Hg, Cardiac Index ≥2.5 L/min/m².

Adverse PAH prognostic factors include PAH associated with connective tissue disease, human immunodeficiency virus (HIV), heritable or porto-pulmonary hypertension; men greater than 60 years; renal insufficiency with eGFR less than 60 mL/min/1.73 m²; WHO functional class III or IV; systolic blood pressure less than 110 mm Hg; heart rate greater than 96 BPM; all-cause hospitalization within 6 months; 6 MWT distance less than 165 m; brain natriuretic peptide (BNP) test greater than 800 pg/mL or NT pro BNP ≥1100 pg/mL; pericardial effusion; diffusion capacity (DLCO) less than 40% of predicted; and RAP >20 mm Hg.

Treatment

General supportive measures for patients with PH are listed in Box 2. The overall goals of therapy are to prevent clinical worsening, decrease hospital admissions, improve quality of life (decreased symptoms), WHO functional class (increased activity level), improve hemodynamics, 6-minute walk results, and optimize survival. For PH diagnostic groups 2 to 3, early and correct identification of the underlying conditions is paramount to prevent misclassification and provide optimal treatment, such as effective diuresis of heart failure, correction of hypoxemia for

---

[1]Not FDA approved for this indication.

COPD, use of CPAP for OSA, and so forth. Cases consistent with mixed PH where the PVR is increased and believed to be out of proportion for the underlying PH Group 2 or 3 disorder usually require referral to a PH expert center. PAH specific therapies are not FDA approved for these patients and may lead to the development of pulmonary edema in PH Group 2 or worsening gas exchange in PH Group 3 patients.

Patients with CTEPH–PH Group 4 require therapeutic anticoagulation and consideration for pulmonary thromboendarterectomy at a center of expertise. Riociguat (Adempas), an activator of nitric oxide causing vasodilation is indicated and FDA approved for patients with inoperable or persistent/recurrent CTEPH.

Specific PAH therapy is usually started for symptomatic patients in WHO functional class II, III, or IV if they showed no acute vasoreactivity or if they did not maintain an acceptable sustained response to calcium channel blockers. Nonresponders to acute vasoreactivity testing who are at low or intermediate risk should be treated with initial oral combination therapy with an endothelin receptor antagonist (ERA) and a phosphodiesterase-5 inhibitor (PDE5i).

Currently available therapeutic choices include ERAs such as ambrisentan (Letairis), bosentan (Tracleer), or macitentan (Opsumit); PDE-5i's such as sildenafil (Revatio) or tadalafil (Adcirca); soluble guanylate cyclase stimulator, riociguat (Adempas); prostacycline analog agents (PCAs) such as intravenous epoprostenol (Flolan, Veletri), intravenous or subcutaneous treprostinil (Remodulin), inhaled treprostinil (Tyvaso), oral treprostinil (Orenitram); oral selective prostacycline receptor agonist, selexipag (Uptravi), or inhaled iloprost (Ventavis). Use of these medications should be done under the auspices of or at an expert referral center.

Based on the global experience over the last three decades and more than 40 randomized controlled trials preformed on nearly 10,000 patients we have learned the following: (a) In treatment-naïve PAH patients, any monotherapy is better than placebo and associated with an improvement in exercise capacity and outcome; (b) in treatment-naïve and newly diagnosed (incident) PAH patients, initial combination therapy improves symptoms, exercise capacity, and outcomes compared with monotherapy; and (c) in already treated (prevalent) PAH patients, sequential combination therapy improves exercise capacity, hemodynamics and outcomes compared with patients who continue on background therapy.

In therapy-naïve (incident) PAH patients, initial combination therapy with ambrisentan and tadalafil was associated with a significant lower risk of clinical-failure events that was defined as the first occurrence of a composite of death, hospitalization for worsening PAH, disease progression, or unsatisfactory long-term clinical response. On the other hand, bosentan added to sildenafil therapy in patients with PAH was not superior to sildenafil monotherapy in delaying the time to the first morbidity/mortality event. This discrepancy observed between two different drug combinations within the same categories of drugs may be explained by the known drug-drug interaction where bosentan significantly decreases the plasma concentration of sildenafil, but sildenafil increases the plasma concentrations of bosentan.

In a long-term event-driven trial of predominantly prevalent patients with symptomatic PAH, macitentan monotherapy or added to background therapy significantly reduced morbidity and mortality.

In a randomized, double-blind trial, riociguat significantly improved exercise capacity and secondary efficacy endpoints including PVR, NT-pro BNP, WHO functional class, time to clinical worsening, and dyspnea scores.

Among PAH patients who remained symptomatic on monotherapy with bosentan or sildenafil, inhaled treprostinil improved exercise capacity and quality of life and was usually well tolerated.

In a large, event-driven trial of predominantly prevalent patients with PAH on background therapy, the oral selective prostacyclin receptor (IP) agonist selexipag reduced the risk of death or complications from PAH. In nonvasoactive and treatment-naïve patients at high risk, initial combination therapy including IV PCA is recommended. Intravenous epoprostenol receives the strongest recommendation for high-risk patients because it has reduced the 3-month rate of mortality, even as monotherapy. Referral for lung transplantation should also be considered.

The decision regarding initial therapy must be individualized and incorporates many factors and determinants of risk, including WHO functional class, progression of symptoms, hemodynamic assessment, 6-minute walk test, biomarkers of severity, comorbidities, access to emergent care, and psychosocial support.

Surgical options for advanced cases of PAH including balloon graded atrial septostomy and lung transplantation are beyond the scope of this chapter but remain important treatment options for patients with refractory disease.

Monitoring

Goal-directed therapy has been described, calling for periodic assessment every 3 to 6 months and possible escalation of therapy. This approach has been associated with improved survival, with specific goals that include clinical stability, WHO functional class II, a 6-minute walk distance of greater than 400 m, and near-normal RAP and cardiac output.

Health coaching, goal setting, and periodic evaluation of advanced directives should always be incorporated in the longitudinal monitoring of PAH patients.

The optimal management of the PH patients requires a holistic, multidimensional approach that incorporates shared decision making integrating medical care, rehabilitation, psychosocial support, spiritual support, palliative care, education, and participation in support groups.

Special Situations
Pregnancy

The effect of pulmonary hypertension on pregnancy, although substantial, has been altered by recent treatments. Current guidelines recommend counseling of pregnant women and their partners on the outcomes associated with pulmonary hypertension with discussion of possible termination of the pregnancy, and the need for vigilant avoidance of pregnancy using contractive practices. However, some recent studies suggest current treatment modalities are having some impact on better outcomes. The ROPAC study by Silwa et al. demonstrated maternal and neonatal mortality was substantially lower than previously reported (4.6% and 2.7%, respectively). No maternal deaths occurred during gestation and most occurred at least 1 week after delivery. Most of the maternal deaths occurred in those with more severe pulmonary arterial hypertension. In a more recent meta-analysis of 19 studies, Jha et al. published in 2020 a maternal mortality rate of 11.5 per 100 pregnancies, with 81.6% occurring in the early postpartum period.

Physicians caring for pregnant patients with pulmonary hypertension should consult an obstetrician, maternal fetal medicine specialist, pulmonologist, and geneticist if first-trimester termination is not an option.

COVID-19

The COVID-19 pandemic has altered the standard of care for patients with PAH with most healthcare systems adapting to new recommendations from healthcare agencies to minimize exposure risks to patients and healthcare providers. The evaluation and initiation of treatments for new PAH patients has been more challenging as a result of difficulties accessing some testing such as pulmonary function, nuclear medicine ventilation scans or elective invasive hemodynamic evaluations.

The initiation of specific PAH therapies and the up-titration of riociguat (Adempas), selexipag (Uptravi), and prostacyclines that traditionally relied on specialized nurse educator visits were less available because of travel and socially distancing restrictions and have adapted to increasingly use telehealth platforms.

COVID-19 vaccination is strongly recommended for patients with pulmonary hypertension because they represent a high-risk population group.

References

Al-Naamani K, Hijal T, Nguyen V, Andrew S, Nguyen T, Huynh T: Predictive values of the electrocardiogram in diagnosing pulmonary hypertension, *Int J Cardiol* 127(2):214–218, 2008.

Arunachalam A, Chaisson NF, Tonelli AR: Methods to improve the yield of right heart catheterization in pulmonary hypertension, *Respir Med*, 2020. Available at. https://doi.org/10.1016/j.yrmex.2020.100015.

Aryal SR, Moussa H, Sinkey R, et al: Management of reproductive health in patients with pulmonary hypertension, *Am J Obstet Gynecol MFM* 2:100087, 2020.

Barnes H, Yeoh HL, Fothergill T, et al: Prostacyclin for pulmonary arterial hypertension, *Cochrane Database Syst Rev* 5(5):CD012785, 2019.

Benza RL, Gomberg-MaitandM, Elliot G, et al: Predicting survival in patients with pulmonary arterial hypertension. the reveal risk score calculator 2.0 and comparison with ESC/ERS- based risk assessment strategies, *Chest* 156(2):323–333, 2019.

Boucly A, Weatherald J, Savale L, et al: Risk assessment, prognosis and guideline implementation in pulmonary arterial hypertension, *Eur Respir J* 50(2):1700889, 2017.

Broderick-Forsgren K, et al: Improving on the diagnostic characteristics of echocardiography for pulmonary hypertension, *Int J Cardiovasc Imaging* 33(9):1341–1349, 2017.

Farha S: COVID-19 and pulmonary hypertension, *Cleve Clin J Med*, 2020.

Frost A, Badesch D, Gibbs JSR, et al: Diagnosis of pulmonary hypertension, *Eur Respir J* 53(1):1801904, 2019.

Galiè N, Barberà JA, Frost AE, et al: Initial use of ambrisentan plus tadalafil in pulmonary arterial hypertension, *N Engl J Med* 373(9):834–844, 2015.

Galie N, Humbert M, Vachiery JL, et al: 2015 ESC/ERS guidelines for the diagnosis and treatment of pulmonary hypertension, *Eur Heart J* 37(1):67–119, 2016.

Ghofrani HA, Galiè N, Grimminger F, et al: Riociguat for the treatment of pulmonary arterial hypertension, *N Engl J Med* 369(4):330–340, 2013.

Jha N, Jha AK, Mishra SK, Sagili H: Pulmonary hypertension and pregnancy outcomes: systemic review and meta-analysis, *Eur J Obstet Gynecol Reprod Biol* 253:108–116, 2020.

HoeperMM, Bogaard HJ, Condliffe R, et al: Definitions and diagnosis of pulmonary hypertension, *J Am Coll Cardiol* 62(25 Suppl), 2013 Dec 24. D42–50.

Klinger JR, Elliot CG, Levine DJ, et al: Therapy of pulmonary arterial hypertension in adults: update of the chest guidelines and expert panel report, *Chest* 155(3):565–586, 2019.

Konstantinides SV: Trends in pregnancy outcomes in patients with pulmonary hypertension: still a long way to go, *Eur J Heart Fail* 18:1129–1131, 2016.

Kovacs G, Avian A, Foris V, et al: Use of ECG and other simple non-invasive tools to assess pulmonary hypertension, *PloS One* 11(12):e0168706, 2016.

McLaughlin V, Channick RN, Ghofrani HA, et al: Bosentan added to sildenafil in patients with pulmonary arterial hypertension, *Eur Respir J* 46(2):405–413, 2015 Aug.

McGoon MD, Ferrari P, Armstrong I, et al: The importance of patient perspectives in pulmonary hypertension, *Eur Respir J* 53(1):1801919, 2019.

McLaughlin VV, Benza RL, Rubin LJ, et al: Addition of inhaled treprostinil to oral therapy for pulmonary arterial hypertension: a randomized controlled clinical trial, *J Am Coll Cardiol* 55(18):1915–1922, 2010.

McLaughlin VV, Channick RN, Ghofrani HA, et al: Bosentan added to sildenafil therapy in patients with pulmonary arterial hypertension, *Eur Respir J* 46(2):405–413, 2015.

Pulido T, Adzerikho I, Channick RN, et al: Macitentan and morbidity and mortality in pulmonary arterial hypertension, *N Engl J Med* 369(9):809–818, 2013.

Raina A, Humbert M: Risk assessment in pulmonary arterial hypertension, *Eur Respir Rev* 25(142):390–398, 2016.

Rich S, Kaufmann E: High dose titration of calcium channel blocking agents for primary pulmonary hypertension: guidelines for short-term drug testing, *J Am Coll Cardiol* 18:1323–1327, 1991.

Ryan JJ, Melendres-Groves L, Zamanian RT, et al: Care of patients with pulmonary arterial hypertension during the coronavirus (COVID19) pandemic, *Pulm Circ* 10(2):1–7, 2020.

Sahay S, Farber HW: Management of hospitalized patients with pulmonary arterial hypertension and COVID-19 infection, *Pulm Circ* 10(3):1–5, 2020.

Simonneau G, Montani D, Clermajer DS, et al: Haemodynamic definitions and updated clinical classification of pulmonary hypertension, *Eur Respir J* 53(1):1801913, 2019.

Sitbon O, Channick R, Chin KM, et al: Selexipag for the treatment of pulmonary arterial hypertension, *N Engl J Med* 373(26):2522–2533, 2015.

Sliwa K, van Hagen IM, Budts W, et al: Pulmonary hypertension and pregnancy outcomes: data from the Registry of Pregnancy and Cardiac Disease (ROPAC) of the European Society of Cardiology, *Eur J Heart Fail* 18:1119–1128, 2016.

Tapson VF, Jing ZC, Xu KF, et al: Oral treprostinil for the treatment of pulmonary arterial hypertension in patients receiving background endothelin receptor antagonist and phosphodiesterase type 5 inhibitor therapy (the FREEDOM-C2 study): a randomized controlled trial, *Chest* 144(3):952–958, 2013.

SARCOIDOSIS

Method of
W. Ennis James, MD; and Marc A. Judson, MD

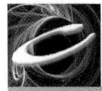

CURRENT DIAGNOSIS

- The diagnosis of sarcoidosis is one of exclusion.
- Tissue biopsy, confirming noncaseating granulomatous inflammation, is required in most cases.
- Initial evaluation should include screening for dangerous organ involvement.

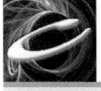

CURRENT THERAPY

- Many cases of sarcoidosis do not require treatment.
- Treatment is typically indicated when sarcoidosis results in impaired quality of life or involves potentially dangerous organs.
- Corticosteroids are the most commonly used initial therapy but are associated with significant side effects.

Sarcoidosis is a multisystem granulomatous disease of unknown cause. The lung is most commonly affected, but any organ may be involved. The natural course of sarcoidosis is variable, ranging from an asymptomatic state to a progressive disease causing significant organ dysfunction that may be life threatening. This variability in organ involvement and disease presentation often makes the diagnosis of sarcoidosis problematic.

Epidemiology

Sarcoidosis occurs worldwide and affects all races and ages. Although the disease has been thought to be most common between ages 20 and 40, analyses from large databases have revealed that the incidence and prevalence of the disease are greatest between ages 45 and 65. There is an earlier onset of disease in African Americans and males. A large analysis from an American national healthcare database found an incidence of 17.8 per 100,000 in African Americans and 8.1 per 100,000 in Caucasians, and a prevalence of 141 per 100,000 in African Americans and 50 per 100,000 in Caucasians. Incidence and prevalence rates were lower in Hispanic Americans than Caucasians and lower still in Asian Americans. The highest prevalence of sarcoidosis is found in whites in Scandinavia and in persons of African descent in the United States. The relative risk for having sarcoidosis increases significantly if a family member has it as well. In the United States, nearly 20% of African Americans with sarcoidosis have an affected first-degree relative, compared with 5% in whites.

The clinical presentation and severity of sarcoidosis vary among racial and ethnic groups. The disease tends to be more severe in African Americans, whereas Caucasians are more likely to be asymptomatic at presentation. Extrathoracic manifestations are more common in certain populations, such as ocular and cardiac sarcoidosis in Japanese populations, chronic uveitis and lupus pernio in African Americans, and erythema nodosum in Europeans. There is increasing evidence that genetic polymorphisms affect the risks and manifestations of the disease. This is consistent with the current theory that sarcoidosis does not have a single cause but is the result of an abnormal host (granulomatous) response to one of many potential antigens in a genetically susceptible person.

Immunopathogenesis

The exact immunopathogenesis of sarcoidosis is unknown, but it is thought to be similar to that of other granulomatous diseases. That is, antigen-presenting cells (APCs), usually either macrophages or dendritic cells, process and present an antigen via a human leukocyte antigen (HLA) class II molecule to T lymphocytes and their receptors. These T lymphocytes are usually of the CD4 T-helper 1 (T_H1) class. The antigen involved in this reaction is unknown, and there may be many antigens that are each associated with a specific HLA class II molecule and T-cell receptor. This could explain the inability to determine one specific cause of sarcoidosis and the varied phenotypic expressions of the disease.

The interaction of APCs and T lymphocytes activates the APCs to produce tumor necrosis factor α (TNF-α) and other cytokines. A proliferation of CD4 T_H1 lymphocytes also ensues, which results in the secretion of interferon-γ (IFN-γ), interleukin (IL)-2, IL-12, and other cytokines. These cytokines activate and recruit monocytes and macrophages and transform them into giant cells, which are important building blocks of the granuloma. Recent evidence suggests that an additional factor leading to this series of immunologic events is the persistence of antigen, possibly related to the production of soluble AA amyloid fibrils, that prevents antigen degradation.

The typical sarcoidosis lesion is a noncaseating (nonnecrotic) granuloma. The sarcoid granuloma consists of a compact core of macrophage-derived epithelioid and multinucleated giant cells surrounded by a perimeter of monocytes, lymphocytes, and fibroblasts. Granulomas can resolve spontaneously or with therapy; however, they can also persist and lead to persistent hyalinization and fibrosis. The development of such fibrosis can cause permanent organ damage and in large part determines the prognosis.

Clinical Features and Clinical Course
Pulmonary Sarcoidosis
Between 30% and 60% of patients with pulmonary sarcoidosis are asymptomatic, and the disease is detected incidentally on chest x-ray. Some patients present with nonspecific pulmonary symptoms, such as dyspnea, cough, wheezing, and chest pain. Respiratory failure from sarcoidosis is extremely rare at presentation. Unlike many other interstitial lung diseases, crackles are rarely heard on chest auscultation. Abnormalities on the chest radiograph occur in more than 90% of patients with pulmonary sarcoidosis. Bilateral hilar adenopathy occurs in 50% to 85% at disease presentation, and 25% to 50% have parenchymal infiltrates. Sarcoid granulomas have a predilection for

TABLE 1 Chest Radiograph Stages of Sarcoidosis

RADIOGRAPHIC STAGE	BILATERAL HILAR LYMPH NODE ENLARGEMENT	PARENCHYMAL DISEASE
I	Yes	No
II	Yes	Nonfibrotic
III	No	Nonfibrotic
IV	No or yes	Fibrotic

Adapted from Judson MA, Baughman RP: Sarcoidosis. In Baughman RP, du Bois RM, Lynch JP, Wells AU, (eds): *Diffuse Lung Disease: A Practical Approach*. London, Arnold, 2004, p 10929.

BOX 1 Factors Associated with a Poor Prognosis in Sarcoidosis

Symptomatic at presentation
African American race
Extrathoracic disease
Stage II to III versus stage I on chest x-ray
Age >40 years
Splenic involvement
Lupus pernio
Disease duration >2 years
Forced vital capacity <1.5 L
Stage IV chest x-ray or aspergilloma
Pulmonary hypertension

Data from Judson MA, Baughman RP: Sarcoidosis. In Baughman RP, du Bois RM, Lynch JP, Wells AU, (eds): *Diffuse Lung Disease: A Practical Approach*. London, Arnold, 2004, p 109–29.

the bronchovascular bundles, subpleural locations, intralobular septa, and the airways.

A radiographic staging system was developed several decades ago (Table 1). Groups of patients with higher radiographic stages have more-severe pulmonary dysfunction, lower remission rates, and greater mortality. However, there is significant overlap among these groups, and stages are highly inaccurate predictors of outcomes for individual patients.

Advanced pulmonary stage IV (fibrocystic) sarcoidosis displays destruction of the lung architecture, with upward traction of the hila, lung distortion, upper-lobe volume loss, fibrocystic disease, honeycombed cysts, and decreased lung volumes. Aspergillomas can develop in these large cystic lesions and may be associated with life-threatening hemoptysis. Bronchiectasis from airway distortion also can occur and is an additional potential cause of hemoptysis.

The majority of patients with pulmonary sarcoidosis have a vital capacity of greater than 70% of predicted at diagnosis. Pulmonary function and the chest radiographic findings are often discordant and often do not correlate with symptom severity. In pulmonary sarcoidosis patients with a normal lung parenchyma (stage I), the vital capacity, diffusing capacity, partial pressure of arterial oxygen (PaO_2) at rest, PaO_2 with exercise, and lung compliance are abnormal in 20% to 40% of cases. Patients with abnormal lung parenchyma have abnormal pulmonary function tests 50% to 70% of the time. Patients with stage IV fibrocystic sarcoidosis tend to have the most severe pulmonary dysfunction.

Sarcoidosis is an interstitial lung disease with a restrictive ventilatory defect often found on spirometry. It is underappreciated, however, that endobronchial involvement is common in sarcoidosis, and therefore airflow obstruction may be the major abnormality found on pulmonary function testing. Wheezing may be the prominent presenting symptom of sarcoidosis, and many cases of sarcoidosis are misdiagnosed as asthma. Airflow obstruction is also common in chronic pulmonary sarcoidosis, where it is caused by airway distortion from fibrosis. The cause of dyspnea in pulmonary sarcoidosis is multifactorial. It may be the result of abnormalities of gas exchange or lung mechanics, weakness of the respiratory muscles, obesity from corticosteroid therapy, pulmonary hypertension, or sarcoidosis involvement of the heart.

Only 3% to 5% of patients die of sarcoidosis. In the United States, 75% of these deaths are the result of complications of advanced pulmonary fibrosis including pulmonary hypertension, infection, and life-threatening hemoptysis, which may result from the development of aspergillomas. Despite these potential complications, the overall prognosis is favorable in patients stage IV sarcoidosis with a 10-year survival of over 80% . Staging systems, including one that incorporates the lung function, pulmonary artery to ascending aorta diameter ratio greater than 1, and the presence of greater than 20% fibrosis on imaging, can be useful predictive of mortality. Other organs that result in fatalities from sarcoidosis are the heart and the central nervous system (CNS). In Japan, death from sarcoidosis is more commonly caused by cardiac than pulmonary involvement.

Patients who present with Löfgren syndrome or with asymptomatic bilateral hilar adenopathy on chest radiograph have a good prognosis. African Americans tend to have a worse prognosis than Caucasians, with lower forced vital capacity and are more likely to develop new organ involvement within 2 years of diagnosis. Box 1 lists risk factors associated with a poor prognosis.

Extrapulmonary Sarcoidosis

The extrapulmonary manifestations of sarcoidosis can predominate in many patients. Extrapulmonary disease can affect the prognosis and treatment options for sarcoidosis.

The eyes and skin are the most common extrapulmonary organs involved with sarcoidosis. Ocular manifestations occur in 25% to 50% of patients; anterior uveitis is the most common manifestation. Symptoms of anterior uveitis include red eyes, painful eyes, and photophobia. However, one-third of patients with anterior uveitis from sarcoidosis have no ocular symptoms. In addition, an intermediate or posterior uveitis can cause vision problems or can be asymptomatic. For these reasons, all patients with sarcoidosis should undergo an eye examination by an ophthalmologist. Other ocular manifestations of sarcoidosis include conjunctivitis, keratoconjunctivitis sicca (dry eyes), scleritis, and optic neuritis.

Skin lesions in sarcoidosis can be classified into two categories: specific lesions that demonstrate noncaseating granulomas on biopsy and nonspecific lesions that do not (Figure 1). The specific skin lesions are often papular and have a predilection for areas of previous scars and tattoos. Lupus pernio is a type of specific skin lesion causing disfiguring lesions on the face, often with erythema and significant induration. These lesions have a predilection for the nose, cheeks, medial and lateral sides of the eyes, and lateral sides of the mouth. Lupus pernio lesions are relatively recalcitrant to therapy and often respond only partially to corticosteroids. The most common nonspecific skin lesion is erythema nodosum, which is often seen with an acute sarcoidosis presentation of fever, arthritis (especially in the ankles), pulmonary symptoms, and bilateral hilar adenopathy on chest radiograph. This syndrome is known as *Löfgren syndrome* and tends to have a good long-term prognosis.

Cardiac and neurologic sarcoidosis can be life threatening and are therefore important to recognize. Cardiac involvement is detected clinically in 5% of sarcoidosis patients during life but in 25% at autopsy. Cardiac sarcoidosis can cause left ventricular dysfunction, cardiac arrhythmias, and sudden cardiac death. All patients with sarcoidosis should be screened for cardiac sarcoidosis. Such screenings should include an electrocardiogram (ECG), as well as eliciting symptoms of left ventricular dysfunction (e.g., orthopnea, peripheral edema) and cardiac arrhythmia (e.g., palpitations, sensation of skipped heartbeats, syncope). Transthoracic echocardiography (TTE) and Holter monitoring have been recommended by some as appropriate additional screening tests. Patients with significant symptoms, abnormal ECG, or TTE should undergo more definitive testing for the diagnosis

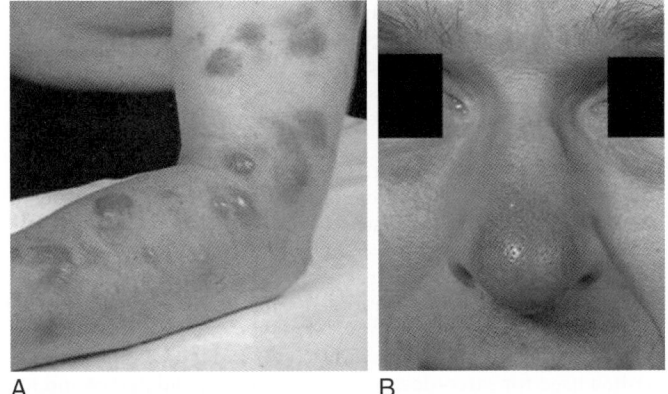

Figure 1 Skin lesions of sarcoidosis. (A) Sarcoid lesions may occur at any site, and they may take nodular, papular, or plaque forms. Biopsy is often necessary for diagnosis. (B) *Lupus pernio* is the term used to describe a dusky-purple infiltration of the skin of the nose, cheeks, or ears in chronic sarcoidosis. (From Forbes CD, Jackson WF: *Color Atlas and Text of Clinical Medicine*, 3rd ed. London, Mosby, 2003, with permission).

of cardiac sarcoidosis. Such testing includes advanced imaging, such as cardiac positron emission tomography (PET) or magnetic resonance imaging (MRI) with and without contrast to identify features. The diagnosis of cardiac sarcoidosis is typically made noninvasively, based on a combination of a typical clinical presentation coupled with the detection of characteristic findings on advanced imaging after other possible etiologies have been excluded. Because myocardial involvement is patchy, endomyocardial biopsy is diagnostic in less than 25% and is not commonly performed to make the diagnosis of cardiac sarcoidosis.

Clinically apparent neurosarcoidosis occurs in less than 10% of sarcoidosis patients. Palsy of the seventh cranial nerve is the most common manifestation of neurosarcoidosis, and it often predates the diagnosis of the disease. Sarcoidosis can affect any part of the peripheral nervous system and CNS and can cause a cranial nerve palsy, mononeuropathy or polyneuropathy, aseptic meningitis, seizures, mass lesions in the brain and spinal cord, hydrocephalus, and encephalopathy. Brain and spinal cord MRI with contrast is the imaging test of choice to evaluate potential CNS sarcoidosis in patients with a compatible clinical presentation.

Sarcoidosis causes clinically apparent peripheral lymphadenopathy in more than 10% of patients. The spleen may be involved in up to 50% of patients, but it is usually asymptomatic and rarely causes hypersplenism.

Bone involvement is occasional, usually occurring as small cysts or cortical defects found in the small bones of the hands and feet. An acute sarcoid arthritis often is present at disease onset and has a good prognosis. This is commonly found in the ankles of patients who present with Löfgren syndrome. Chronic sarcoid arthritis is rare. It is usually a nondestructive arthropathy of the shoulders, wrists, knees, ankles, and small joints of the hands and feet.

Sarcoidosis of the sinuses is underappreciated. It can occur in the nasopharynx, hypopharynx, larynx, or any of the sinuses and is known as *sarcoidosis of the upper respiratory tract*. Sarcoidosis of the upper respiratory tract is often relatively recalcitrant to therapy.

Histologic evidence of hepatic sarcoidosis is present in 50% to 80% of sarcoidosis patients, although most of these patients are asymptomatic and have normal liver function tests. Hepatomegaly, abdominal pain, and pruritus are the most common symptoms associated with hepatic sarcoidosis but are present only in 15% to 25% of patients with hepatic involvement. Elevation of the serum alkaline phosphatase is the most common liver function test abnormality.

Hypercalcemia or hypercalciuria leading to nephrolithiasis, resulting in renal dysfunction, can occur with sarcoidosis. These phenomena are the result of the enzyme 1α-hydroxylase in activated macrophages that convert 25-hydroxyvitamin D to 1,25-dihydroxyvitamin D, the active form of the vitamin. This results in increased gut absorption and increased renal excretion of calcium that can cause nephrolithiasis. Patients with sarcoidosis-associated hypercalcemia typically have low 25-hydroxyvitamin D levels with 1,25-dihydroxyvitamin D levels that are elevated or at the upper limits of normal in combination with a low or low-normal parathyroid hormone.

Sarcoidosis rarely involves the thyroid, kidney, breast, genitourinary (GU) tract, and gastrointestinal (GI) tract.

Patients can have constitutional symptoms such as fever, night sweats, weight loss, malaise, and fatigue at presentation. These symptoms occasionally are associated with hepatic sarcoid involvement but may be a sign of the systemic nature of the disease, presumably from cytokine release, rather than specific organ involvement. A small fiber neuropathy may occur with sarcoidosis and cause pain or autonomic dysfunction.

Diagnosis and Initial Workup

The diagnosis of sarcoidosis requires a compatible clinical picture, histologic demonstration of noncaseating granulomas, and exclusion of other diseases capable of producing a similar histologic and clinical picture. It is prudent to bear a healthy degree of skepticism in the diagnosis and evaluate the patient closely for additional clues supporting an alternative diagnosis. Mycobacterial and fungal diseases must always be considered as alternative causes of granulomatous inflammation. Therefore stains and cultures of tissue specimens for mycobacteria and fungi always should be obtained when the diagnosis of sarcoidosis is considered. Hypersensitivity pneumonitis, a granulomatous lung disease from inhalation of bioaerosols, is another disease that may mimic sarcoidosis. Bioaerosols from hot tubs and birds are the most common causes of hypersensitivity pneumonitis, and clinicians should specifically inquire about these two exposures in individuals who are being evaluated for sarcoidosis. Sarcoidosis is a systemic disease, so signs or symptoms of extrathoracic disease such as uveitis, skin lesions, or an elevated serum alkaline phosphatase concentration should be sought. Because of the varied clinical presentation of sarcoidosis, there is no single diagnostic algorithm.

It is prudent to select a biopsy site associated with less morbidity, such as the skin if a lesion is present. Transthoracic needle aspiration under ultrasound guidance (EBUS-TBNA) of mediastinal lymph nodes via bronchoscopy has a high yield for the diagnosis of pulmonary sarcoidosis and has supplanted mediastinoscopy at many centers. Transbronchial lung biopsy has a diagnostic yield of 40% to more than 90% in pulmonary sarcoidosis. Endobronchial biopsy has a 40% to 60% sensitivity and adds to the yield of transbronchial biopsy.

Bronchoalveolar lavage (BAL) with examination of lymphocyte populations has been used in the evaluation of possible pulmonary sarcoidosis. In sarcoidosis, there is an increased number of BAL lymphocytes, and these are predominantly CD4+. It has been proposed that an increase in BAL lymphocytes and a BAL CD4/CD8 ratio greater than 3.5 makes the diagnosis of sarcoidosis highly likely.

Although serum angiotensin-converting enzyme (ACE) often is elevated in active sarcoidosis, the specificity and sensitivity of this test are inadequate for it to be used diagnostically. Serum ACE may be used as supportive evidence for the diagnosis, and it also may be used in some instances to follow disease activity.

Gallium-67 (^{67}Ga) scanning is cumbersome because it takes several days to complete and is infrequently used as a diagnostic test. However, bilateral hilar uptake and right paratracheal uptake (lambda sign) coupled with lacrimal and parotid uptake (panda sign) with ^{67}Ga strongly suggest a diagnosis of sarcoidosis. Fluorodeoxyglucose PET scanning (outside the CNS) and MRI studies using contrast (CNS and cardiac) have essentially replaced 67Ga scanning for detecting sarcoidosis activity.

Ideally, the diagnosis of sarcoidosis requires a demonstration of noncaseating granulomas in at least one organ. However, certain clinical presentations are so specific for the diagnosis of sarcoidosis that the diagnosis may be accepted without tissue biopsy. Extreme caution must be used in these situations to ensure that there is no clinical information that would suggest an alternative

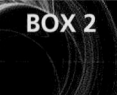

BOX 2 Clinical or Laboratory Findings That Strongly Support a Diagnosis of Sarcoidosis Without a Tissue Biopsy

- Löfgren syndrome
- Heerfordt syndrome (uveoparotid fever)
- Asymptomatic bilateral hilar adenopathy on chest x-ray
- ^{67}Ga scan showing a lambda sign and a panda sign

diagnosis that should prompt a tissue biopsy. Clinical or laboratory findings that strongly support the diagnosis of sarcoidosis without a tissue biopsy are listed in Box 2.

Treatment

Therapy is often not mandatory for sarcoidosis because the disease can remit spontaneously. Systemic antisarcoidosis therapy is indicated for potentially dangerous disease and for disease causing significant quality-of-life impairment. Potentially dangerous organ involvement includes neurosarcoidosis, cardiac sarcoidosis, renal sarcoidosis, hypercalcemia that does not respond to dietary measures, and ocular sarcoidosis that does not respond to topical (eyedrop) therapy. Therapy should also be considered when the disease is progressive and at risk of resulting in long-term morbidity. In general, treatment is discouraged for asymptomatic stage I pulmonary sarcoidosis, elevations of serum liver function tests, or specific levels of ACE.

The decision to treat sarcoidosis can be problematic, because the disease has a variable prognosis that must be weighed against the potential side effects of therapy. It is often most prudent to monitor patients without therapy if they are asymptomatic or have only mild organ dysfunction. For pulmonary sarcoidosis, asymptomatic patients and those with mild disease that might spontaneously remit usually are not treated. For patients with clinical findings that predict spontaneous remission (e.g., erythema nodosum), the benefits of treatment often are offset by the toxicity of therapy. Often these patients can be managed with supportive therapy such as nonsteroidal antiinflammatory drugs (NSAIDs) for arthralgias and fever and bronchodilators and inhaled corticosteroids for wheezing and cough.

It is recommended that patients with mild to moderate pulmonary sarcoidosis be observed for 2 to 6 months, if possible. Patients who improve will have avoided the toxicity of corticosteroids, and patients who deteriorate over this period should be considered for treatment. Patients with pulmonary dysfunction who neither improve nor deteriorate during the observation period may be given a corticosteroid trial, or they may be observed further. Patients with severe pulmonary dysfunction or pulmonary symptoms causing significant impairment should be treated.

Corticosteroids often are used to treat sarcoidosis, but the dose, duration of therapy, and methods by which one can assess effectiveness have not been standardized. Topical corticosteroid therapy should be used whenever possible in an attempt to minimize systemic complications. This includes corticosteroid eye drops for anterior sarcoid uveitis and corticosteroid creams and injections for localized skin lesions. Pulmonary sarcoidosis usually is treated initially with 20 mg/day of prednisone or its equivalent. Higher doses may be required for neurosarcoidosis and cardiac sarcoidosis. The patient usually is evaluated within 2 to 12 weeks for a response with the goal of tapering corticosteroids down to the lowest effective dose (ideally <10 mg/day) as quickly as possible. This dose is usually continued for at least 6 months. Patients failing to respond to therapy within 3 months are unlikely to respond to a more protracted course of therapy or a higher dose.

The relapse rate after corticosteroid therapy is withdrawn may be as high as 70%, and therefore patients need to be followed closely as the corticosteroid dose is tapered and discontinued. In some patients, there may be recurrent relapses requiring long-term low-dose therapy. On occasion, the chronic prednisone dose needed to prevent relapse is less than 5 mg/day. Patients who relapse after corticosteroids have been withdrawn should be retreated with corticosteroids. Alternative agents, such as corticosteroid-sparing agents, to control the disease in a patient on a chronic low dose of prednisone should be considered. On occasion, alternative agents may completely replace corticosteroid therapy. In general, corticosteroid-sparing agents should not be considered unless the patient requires more than 7.5 mg/day of prednisone to control the disease.

Methotrexate (Rheumatrex)[1] and hydroxychloroquine (Plaquenil)[1] are the most-studied alternative sarcoidosis medications. They are usually used as corticosteroid-sparing agents but at times can be used as replacement therapy. Methotrexate is most useful for pulmonary, skin, joint, and eye sarcoidosis. Hydroxychloroquine is often used for sarcoidosis of the skin, joints, and nerves and for hypercalcemia from sarcoidosis. Azathioprine (Imuran)[1] may be useful for sarcoid uveitis, but usually it is added to corticosteroid plus methotrexate in this instance. Leflunomide (Arava)[1] has also been shown to be useful in the treatment of pulmonary and extrapulmonary sarcoidosis. Monoclonal antibodies against TNF-α, such as infliximab (Remicade)[1] and adalimumab (Humira)[1], are useful agents in sarcoidosis patients with severe disease and/or who fail to respond to the aforementioned treatments. Minocycline (Minocin)[1] and doxycycline (Vibramycin)[1] may be useful for skin sarcoidosis. Cyclosporine (Sandimmune)[1] is ineffective for pulmonary sarcoidosis; cyclophosphamide (Cytoxan)[1] may have a potential role in refractory neurosarcoidosis.

Therapy should also be considered for the nongranulomatous aspects of the disease. Sarcoidosis-associated small fiber neuropathy may respond to medications for neuropathic pain, monoclonal antibodies against TNF-α, or intravenous immunoglobulin[1]. Sarcoidosis-associated fatigue may benefit from a physical training program, neurostimulants, or monoclonal antibodies against TNF-α.

---

[1]Not FDA approved for this indication.

References

Baughman RP, Culver DA, Judson MA: A concise review of pulmonary sarcoidosis, *Am J Respir Crit Care Med* 183:573–589, 2011.

Baughman RP, Field S, Costabel U: Sarcoidosis in America: analysis based on health care use, *Ann Am Thorac Soc* 13:244–252, 2016.

Baughman RP, Nunes H, Sweiss NJ, et al: Established and experimental medical therapy of pulmonary sarcoidosis, *Eur Respir J* 41(6):1424–1438, 2013.

Baughman RP, Teirstein AS, Judson MA, et al: Clinical characteristics of patients in a case control study of sarcoidosis, *Am J Respir Crit Care Med* 164:1885–1889, 2001.

Birnie DH, Sauer WH, Bogun F, et al: HRS Expert Consensus Statement on the Diagnosis and Management of Arrythmias Associated with Cardiac Sarcoidosis, *Heart Rhythm* 11:1304–1323, 2014.

Chen ES, Song Z, Willett MH, et al: Serum amyloid A regulates granulomatous inflammation in sarcoidosis through Toll- like receptor-2, *Am J Respir Crit Care Med* 181:360–373, 2010.

Hamzeh N, Steckman D, Sauer W, Judson MA: Pathophysiology and clinical management of cardiac sarcoidosis, *Nature Rev Cardiol* 12:278–288, 2015.

Hunninghake GW, Costabel U, Ando M, et al: ATS/ERS/WASOG statement on sarcoidosis, *Am J Respir Crit Care Med* 160:736–755, 1999.

Judson MA: The clinical features of sarcoidosis: a comprehensive review, *Clinic Rev Allerg Immunol* 49:63–78, 2015.

Judson MA: The diagnosis of sarcoidosis, *Clinics Chest Med* 29:415–427, 2008.

Judson MA, Costabel U, Drent M, et al: The WASOG Sarcoidosis Organ Assessment Investigators. The WASOG Sarcoidosis Organ Assessment Instrument: an update of a previous clinical tool, *Sarcoidosis Vasc Diff Lung Dis* 31:19–27, 2014.

Lower EE, Baughman RP: Prolonged use of methotrexate in refractory sarcoidosis, *Arch Intern Med* 155:846–851, 1995.

Nardi A, Brillet P, Letoumelin P, et al: Stage IV sarcoidosis: comparison of survival with the general population and cause of death, *Eur Respir J* 38:1368–1373, 2011.

Tavee JO, Karwa K, Ahmed Z, et al: Sarcoidosis-associated small fiber neuropathy in a large cohort: Clinical aspects and response to IVIG and anti-TNF alpha treatment, *Respir Med* 126:135–138, 2017.

Tremblay A, Stather DR, MacEachern P, et al: A randomized controlled trial of standard vs endobronchial ultrasonography-guided transbronchial needle aspiration in patients with suspected sarcoidosis, *Chest* 136:340–346, 2009.

TUBERCULOSIS AND OTHER MYCOBACTERIAL DISEASES

Method of
Laura Elyse Shevy, MD; and Parisa Mortaji, MD

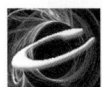

CURRENT DIAGNOSIS

- Latent tuberculosis (TB) infection is diagnosed in an asymptomatic person previously exposed to TB who has a positive tuberculin skin test or interferon-γ release assay.
- A positive tuberculin skin test (TST) or interferon-γ release assay (IGRA) does not distinguish latent tuberculosis infection (LTBI) from TB disease.
- The gold standard for diagnosing active pulmonary TB disease is acid fast bacilli (AFB) culture on respiratory specimens; AFB smear and nucleic acid amplification testing are also useful in diagnosis.
- All patients with LTBI or TB disease should undergo HIV testing.

CURRENT THERAPY

- LTBI: rifamycin-based regimen for 3 to 4 months.
- Treatment of TB disease should be done in conjunction with the local public health department.
- Drug-susceptible pulmonary TB disease: isoniazid (INH) + rifampin (RIF) + pyrazinamide (PZA) + ethambutol (EMB) for 2 months, followed by 4 months of INH + RIF.
- Drug-susceptible extrapulmonary TB disease is typically treated as per pulmonary TB disease but treatment and duration vary based on anatomic site(s) involved.
- Treatment of drug-resistant TB disease should be done in consultation with a TB expert.

Overview

Mycobacterial diseases occur worldwide and cause significant morbidity and mortality. These organisms comprise *Mycobacterium tuberculosis* complex, the causative pathogen in tuberculosis disease and latent tuberculosis infection; *Mycobacterium leprae* complex, the etiologic agent of Hansen's disease (leprosy); and around 80 pathogenic species of nontuberculous mycobacteria. This chapter mainly focuses on the diagnosis and management of tuberculosis, with a brief overview of Hansen's disease, and some infections caused by nontuberculous mycobacteria.

Tuberculosis

Mycobacterium tuberculosis, the bacteria responsible for tuberculosis (TB) disease and latent tuberculosis infection (LTBI), affects people in every country. It is the leading cause of infectious diseases mortality by a single pathogen worldwide, and it is the ninth leading cause of death overall. An estimated 2 billion people, or 25% of the global population, are thought to be infected with *M. tuberculosis*. The majority of individuals who become infected remain asymptomatic and develop LTBI. Risk factors for TB infection include overcrowding, congregate healthcare and incarceration facilities, poverty, human immunodeficiency virus (HIV) and AIDS, malnutrition, excessive alcohol use, tobacco use, drug use, silicosis, end-stage renal disease, diabetes mellitus, malignancy, and other immunosuppressive disorders and medications. TB disproportionately affects racial and ethnic minorities and people experiencing homelessness.

Pathophysiology

M. tuberculosis is an aerobic, non–spore forming, acid-fast staining, slow-growing bacillus. There are at least nine species in the genus *Mycobacterium* that comprise *M. tuberculosis* complex, although not all are pathogenic to humans. The majority of TB infections worldwide are caused by *M. tuberculosis* sensu stricto; in West Africa, up to 50% of cases are caused by *M. africanum*. Humans are the only known reservoir of *M. tuberculosis*. Transmission occurs from person to person via aerosolized droplets, which can remain suspended in the air for several hours. For this reason, the proximity, frequency, and duration of exposure are some of the most important factors in infection transmission. Other general factors include immune status of the exposed individual, infectiousness of the person with TB disease, and environmental factors.

Primary infection occurs after inhalation of the tubercle bacilli, which establish in the midlung zone terminal air spaces and are engulfed by alveolar macrophages. When the tubercle bacilli destroy the macrophages, pneumonitis develops. The bacilli are released and travel via lymphatics to regional lymph nodes and can then spread hematogenously throughout the body. The most commonly affected sites that uptake infected cells and allow for bacilli multiplication include the apical posterior lung, lymph nodes, kidneys, long bones, vertebrae, and brain/eyes/meninges. These sites may become nidi of infection either during the acute infection or after a latent period.

The majority of infections are contained through the host's cell-mediated immune response 3 to 9 weeks after transmission. The initial immunologic cascade encapsulates the bacilli and creates granulomas—protective shells that keep the tubercle bacilli in check. This leads to infection latency. Such people with latent TB infection are not symptomatic of TB disease and are not contagious to others.

A minority of people may develop significant infection in the area of initial pulmonary transmission (the Ghon complex) and necrosis and radiographically visible calcification of draining regional lymph nodes (the Ranke complex). This may progress to pneumonia, also known as "progressive primary disease," and occurs most often in children, older adults, and patients living with HIV.

Progression from LTBI to TB disease occurs in about 5% to 10% of immune competent patients, usually within the first 2 years after infection or under certain medical conditions. Tubercle bacilli multiply rapidly and when no longer contained by the immune response cause TB disease. Pulmonary TB disease is most commonly seen in the lung apices (Figure 1). Reactivation of infection can occur throughout the body, with common extrapulmonary infections including pleural empyema, lymphadenitis, genitourinary infection, vertebral osteomyelitis, meningitis, uveitis, and pericarditis.

Prevention

Prevention of TB disease transmission is mainly through rapid identification and airborne isolation of patients with suspected or confirmed disease and prompt initiation of treatment. In countries with a high prevalence of TB, the bacille Calmette-Guerin (BCG) vaccine is often administered. This live, attenuated vaccine is derived from *Mycobacterium bovis* and has shown to be effective at preventing severe infection, mainly in children.

Clinical Manifestations

TB can cause two conditions: latent TB infection and active TB disease. By definition, a person with LTBI has no symptoms of TB disease. TB disease may be pulmonary or extrapulmonary. Clinical features of pulmonary TB disease may include fever, drenching night sweats, weight loss, anorexia, malaise, pleuritic chest pain, productive cough, and hemoptysis, typically with several weeks of symptoms. Clinical manifestations of extrapulmonary TB disease are myriad and are manifestations of the involved organ systems as outlined above.

Principles of Diagnosis

Of utmost importance, latent TB must be distinguished from active TB disease. Treatment for latent TB infection and TB

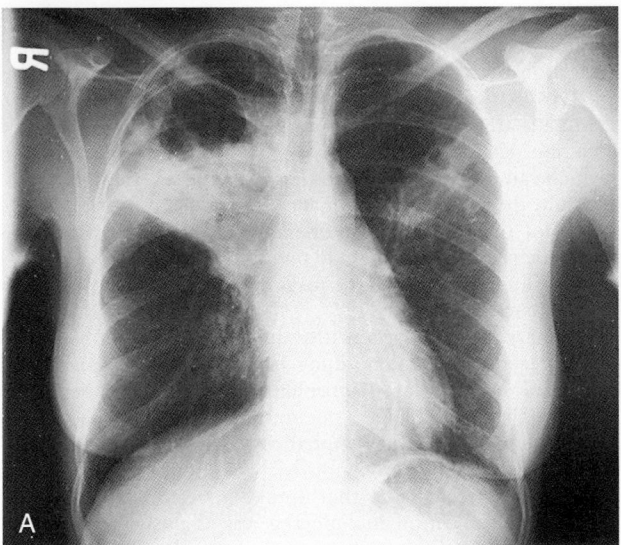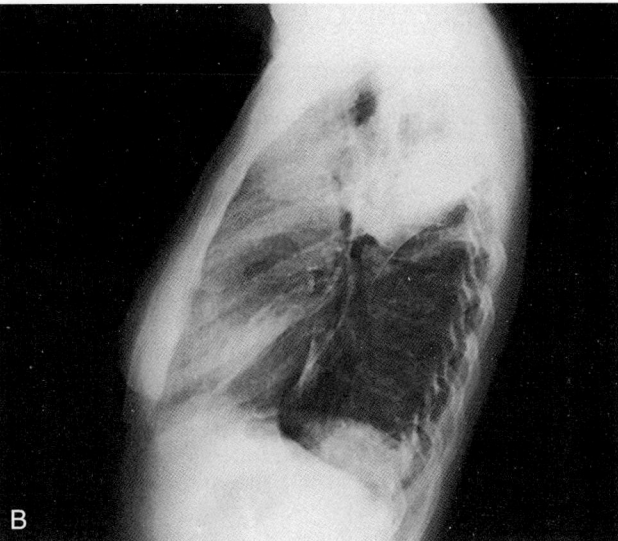

Figure 1 Posteroanterior (A) and left lateral (B) chest x-rays showing typical reactivation (postprimary) tuberculosis in the adult. Bilateral upper lobe fibrocavitary disease affects predominantly the apical and posterior segments of the right upper lobe. From Weller PF, Guerrant RL, Walker DH: *Tropical Infectious Diseases: Principles, Pathogens and Practice*, 3rd ed., Elsevier; 2011.

disease differ greatly. Treating for LTBI when active TB disease is present can induce drug resistance, lead to increased morbidity and mortality, and potentially increase risk of transmission. Typically a test for previous TB exposure is performed—the tuberculin skin test (TST) and/or an interferon-γ-release assay (IGRAs). The following must be performed: a full history and physical to evaluate current symptoms and signs of disease; past medical and social history to evaluate for risk factors for infection and progression from infection to TB disease if infection is present; medications for possible drug–drug interactions if treatment is warranted; and so on. A chest radiograph should be performed to evaluate for active pulmonary involvement (i.e., airspace opacities, pleural effusions, parenchymal cavitary lesions). Sputum for other respiratory specimens, and/or sampling of other infected sites, is performed for diagnostic testing as outlined in the following.

Diagnosis
Latent Tuberculosis Infection
There are two methods to diagnose LTBI: the TST (Tubersol) and IGRAs. TST is an intradermally injected protein precipitate of heat-inactivated tubercle bacilli—purified protein derivative (PPD)—or tuberculin. In people with previous TB infection and cell-mediated immunity, intradermal PPD induces a delayed-type hypersensitivity reaction characterized by induration. The test is interpreted via transverse diameter measurement of the induration (not erythema) after 48 to 72 hours. The TST therefore requires two clinical visits for TST placement and subsequent interpretation. Table 1 outlines interpretation of the TST based on risk group. False positive results can occur in people who have received BCG vaccination or who have infections with nontuberculous mycobacteria (NTM).

IGRAs are blood tests and measure T-cell release of interferon-γ in response to stimulation with highly TB-specific antigens. False positive results do not occur from previous BCG vaccination and are much less likely to occur in setting of NTM infections, which make them more specific than TST. Two commercially available IGRAs include the QuantiFERON-TB Gold Plus (QFT-Plus) and the T-SPOT®TB test (T-Spot). If available and feasible, the IGRA should be used over TST, especially if the patient has a history of receiving the BCG vaccine, is unlikely to return to have the TST interpreted, or has a high likelihood of TB infection.

Due to limited data on IGRA testing reliability in children, TST is the recommended method of testing for children under 5 years old. The American Academy of Pediatrics (AAP) recommends that either a TST or an IGRA be used in children 2 years of age and older. For children previously vaccinated with BCG—regardless

of age—IGRA is preferred to avoid a false-positive TST result caused by the previous BCG vaccination.

Of extreme importance to recognize is that neither TST nor IGRA can distinguish TB disease from LTBI. A true positive TST or IGRA only indicates the person has, at some point, been exposed to and developed some cell-mediated immunity against *M. tuberculosis*. TST and IGRAs cannot be used alone to diagnose active TB disease.

Active Tuberculosis Disease
Active pulmonary TB disease is diagnosed in the presence of symptoms and/or signs of TB disease and by obtaining three sputum specimens 8 to 24 hours apart for acid-fast bacilli (AFB) smears, cultures, and nucleic acid amplification testing when available. Rapid molecular rifampin (Rifadin, Rimactane)/INH susceptibility testing should be performed, when available, for specific patient populations. *M. tuberculosis* typically takes about 3 to 8 weeks for visible growth on solid media and 10 to 20 days for liquid broth culture growth. Nucleic acid amplification testing (NAAT) uses real-time polymerase chain reaction (PCR) amplification to aid in detection of *M. tuberculosis* genetic material. However, culture remains the gold standard for diagnosis, and susceptibility testing should be performed on the initial positive culture. If a person cannot produce sputum, hypertonic saline can be used to induce sputum production. As a last resort, flexible bronchoscopy can be pursued to obtain respiratory specimens. If a respiratory specimen is positive by AFB smear but negative by NAAT, it is unlikely that the positive smear result represents active TB disease. In a patient in whom suspicion for TB disease is intermediate-high, if a respiratory specimen AFB smear is negative but NAAT is positive, a presumptive diagnosis of TB disease can be given. However, a negative NAAT is not sufficient to exclude pulmonary TB disease.

Active extrapulmonary disease requires sampling of potentially affected fluid or tissues. Cell counts and chemistries should be measured on amenable fluid specimens including pleural, cerebrospinal (CSF), ascitic, and synovial fluids. Adenosine deaminase can be measured on pleural, CSF, ascitic, and pericardial fluids. AFB smear microscopy, culture, NAAT, and histopathology should be performed on available specimens. False negative AFB smears and NAAT are not uncommon and should not be used to exclude diagnosis of active TB disease.

Principles of Treatment
Treatment of both LTBI and TB disease should be patient-centered, with care tailored to the patient's social situation,

TABLE 1	Interpreting Tuberculin Skin Testing (TST) Results	
RISK OF INFECTION **DEGREE OF INDURATION**		**POSITIVITY BY RISK GROUP**
≥5 mm		• People living with HIV • Recent contacts of people with infectious TB disease • People who have fibrotic changes on chest radiograph • Recipients of solid organ transplants • Other immunosuppressed patients (e.g., patients on prolonged therapy with corticosteroids >15 mg per day of prednisone, patients on TNF-α antagonists)
≥10 mm		• People born in countries where TB disease is common, including Mexico, the Philippines, Vietnam, India, China, Haiti, Guatemala, and other countries with high rates of TB • People who inject or use drugs • Mycobacteriology laboratory workers • People who live or work in high-risk congregate settings (e.g., nursing homes, homeless shelters, or correctional facilities) • People with certain medical conditions that place them at high risk for TB (e.g., silicosis, diabetes mellitus, severe kidney disease, certain types of cancer, and certain intestinal conditions) • People who are <90% of ideal body weight • Children <5 years of age • Infants, children, and adolescents exposed to adults in high-risk categories
≥15 mm		• Individuals without known TB risk factors

Adapted from American Thoracic Society: Targeted tuberculin testing and treatment of latent tuberculosis infection. *MMWR Recomm Rep* 49:1–51, 2000.

medical comorbidities, and clinical condition. Directly observed therapy (DOT), the practice of observing the patient physically ingest antituberculous medications, is a widely implemented standard of practice in TB programs in the United States and has been shown to significantly improve treatment success compared with self-administered therapy. Thus DOT is recommended for routine treatment of patients with all forms of TB as feasible.

The purpose of treating LTBI is to prevent progression to TB disease in those individuals at high risk for infection and progression to disease.

The objectives of treating TB disease are to cure the individual patient, decrease risk of morbidity and mortality from disease, reduce transmission of *M. tuberculosis* to other people, and prevent development of drug resistance during antituberculous therapy.

The treatment of multidrug resistant (MDR) TB disease (defined as resistance to INH and rifampin [Rifadin, Rimactane]) and extensively drug resistant (XDR) TB disease (resistance to INH, rifampin [Rifadin, Rimactane], levofloxacin [Levaquin[1]], and at least one second-line injectable agent) is complicated, and therapy should be pursued in consultation with a TB expert.

Treatment
Latent Tuberculosis Infection
The decision to initiate prophylactic therapy for latent TB infection is a risk-benefit decision based on the patient's likelihood of infection and likelihood of progression from LTBI to TB disease. The risk of progression from LTBI to TB disease in an immunocompetent host is 5% to 10% over a lifetime. People with diabetes have a 30% lifetime risk. People living with HIV have a 7% to 10% risk per year of progressing from LTBI to TB disease. Studies have demonstrated benefit in decreasing incidence of TB disease by treating LTBI in people who are under 5 years old, living with HIV, otherwise immunosuppressed (e.g., corticosteroid use >15 mg/prednisone or equivalent/day, use of immunosuppressive drugs such as tumor necrosis factor (TNF)-α inhibitors), household contacts of or have had recent exposure to a person with active TB disease, residents of high-risk congregate health facilities, persons with abnormal chest radiographs consistent with previous TB, and people with silicosis, among other conditions. Treatment regimens are outlined below. It is advisable to consult

a TB expert if the patient is a contact of an individual with known drug-resistant TB disease.

In 2020, the National Tuberculosis Controllers Association (NTCA) and Centers for Disease Control and Prevention (CDC) updated guidelines for treatment of LTBI for persons living in the United States. There are now three preferred regimens, all rifamycin-based, of 3 to 4 months' duration. These regimens are preferred due to their effectiveness, safety profile, and high treatment success rate. Some potential downsides of these regimens include increased cost over alternatives, adverse drug effects and potential for significant drug-drug interactions (including warfarin, oral contraceptives, antifungals, HIV antiretroviral therapy, among others). If drug–drug interactions preclude use of a preferred regimen, alternative regimens of daily isoniazid (Nydrazid) (INH) monotherapy for 6 or 9 months' duration can be used. Daily INH regimens are effective, but caution should be used due to the increased risk of hepatotoxicity, and the potential to induce drug resistance from the longer treatment duration. From 25 to 50 mg of pyridoxine (vitamin B6)[1] should be added for those people at risk of developing peripheral neuropathy such as pregnant women or people with diabetes mellitus, chronic kidney disease, malnutrition, HIV, alcohol use disorder, or other conditions; 100 mg dose is recommended for people who already have peripheral neuropathy. If daily INH cannot be used, rifabutin (Mycobutin)[1] may substitute for rifampin (Rifadin, Rimactane) in one of the three preferred regimens, as the former has fewer drug interactions (Table 2).

Drug-Susceptible Pulmonary Tuberculosis Disease
The preferred treatment regimen for drug-susceptible pulmonary TB disease includes an intensive treatment phase with 2 months of isoniazid (Nydrazid) (INH), rifampin (Rifadin, Rimactane) (RIF), pyrazinamide (Zinamide) (PZA), and ethambutol (Myambutol) (EMB), followed by a continuation phase of 4 months of INH and RIF. If drug susceptibilities are available prior to starting treatment, EMB can be omitted; as soon as susceptibility to INH and RIF are confirmed, ethambutol (Myambutol) can be discontinued. The CDC recommends continuous daily dosing of the above agents rather than intermittent dosing for both the intensive and continuation phase of treatment. Pyridoxine,[1] or

---

[1]Not FDA approved for this indication.

[1]Not FDA approved for this indication.

TABLE 2   Preferred Treatment Regimens for Latent Tuberculosis Infection

PREFERRED REGIMENS	DURATION OF THERAPY	DOSAGES	FREQUENCY OF ADMINISTRATION
INH* + RPT	3 months	Adults and children aged >12 years: INH: 15 mg/kg; 900 mg maximum dose RPT: 10–14 kg: 300 mg 14–25 kg: 450 mg 25–32 kg: 600 mg 32–49.9 kg: 750 mg ≥50 kg: 900 mg maximum dose Children ages 2–11 years: INH: 25 mg/kg; maximum dose 900 mg RPT: as above	Once weekly
RIF	4 months	Adults: 10 mg/kg, maximum dose 600 mg Children: 15–20 mg/kg, maximum dose 600 mg	Daily
INH + RIF	3 months	Adults: INH: 5 mg/kg, maximum dose 300 mg RIF: 10 mg/kg, maximum dose 600 mg Children: INH: 10–20 mg/kg, maximum dose 300 mg RIF: 15–20 mg/kg, maximum dose 600 mg	Daily

INH, Isoniazid (Nydrazid); *RIF*, rifampin (Rifadin, Rimactane); *RPT*, rifapentine (Priftin).

*Vitamin B6 (pyridoxine)[1] is given in conjunction with INH for those at risk for developing—or already suffering from—peripheral neuropathy per text above.

[1]Not FDA approved for this indication.

Adapted from Sterling TR, Njie G, Zenner D, et al: Guidelines for the treatment of latent tuberculosis infection: Recommendations from the National Tuberculosis Controllers Association and CDC, 2020. *MMWR Recomm Rep* 69(No. RR-1):1–11, 2020.

vitamin B6, should be given throughout the duration of INH administration as discussed above. It is highly advised these regimens are given by DOT. If this frequency of DOT is difficult to achieve, alternative regimens can be used as outlined in the Official American Thoracic Society/Centers for Disease Control and Prevention/Infectious Diseases Society of America Clinical Practice Guidelines: Treatment of Drug-Susceptible Tuberculosis.

Drug-Susceptible Extrapulmonary Tuberculosis Disease

The treatment regimens for drug-susceptible extrapulmonary TB disease largely follow that of pulmonary TB disease with 2 months of intensive phase INH, RIF, PZA, EMB, followed by a continuation phase with INH and RIF. The duration of the continuation phase, however, depends on anatomic site involved. Disease that is treated with a standard 6-month regimen, as for pulmonary TB disease above, include tuberculous pericarditis, lymphadenitis, pleural, genitourinary, peritoneal, military, and other disseminated disease.

There has been some controversy in the literature about adjunctive corticosteroid use for TB pericarditis to prevent development of constrictive pericarditis: current ATS/CDC/IDSA guidelines do not recommend routine use of steroids in TB pericarditis, but consideration to steroid use can be given to patients with large pericardial effusion, high levels of inflammatory cells/markers in the pericardial fluid, or those with early signs of constriction.

TB meningitis is treated for 2 months with the standard four-drug regimen (INH, RIF, PZA, EMB) in adults, followed by 7 to 10 months of INH and RIF for drug-susceptible disease. In pediatric patients, the American Academy of Pediatrics recommends initial 2 months of treatment with INH, RIF, PZA, and either ethionamide (Trecator), if possible, or an aminoglycoside, followed by INH and RIF for the 7 to 10 month consolidation phase. Optimal treatment duration of TB meningitis is not well known. Serial lumbar punctures may be of utility to help define total duration. Adjunctive steroids are recommended in the acute illness as they have been demonstrated to provide mortality benefit in clinical trials; steroids should be tapered over 6 to 8 weeks.

Bone and joint infection is typically treated with 9 months total duration, up to 12 months in setting of extensive hardware. Spinal TB disease with TB meningitis is treated as for meningitis above.

Multidrug-Resistant TB

Resistance in *M. tuberculosis* develops through spontaneous point mutations. MDR TB is defined as that which is resistant to both INH and RIF. XDR TB is a subset of MDR TB with additional resistance to a fluoroquinolone and a second-line injectable agent. MDR and XDR TB can be acquired as the primary infection, or resistance can develop while on therapy for a previously susceptible TB isolate. Acquisition of primary drug-resistant TB is influenced by geographic area where infection was acquired. Risk factors for development drug resistance while on therapy include incomplete medication adherence, inadequate drug absorption or dosing, and single-drug treatment. Consultation with a TB expert is advised if MDR or XDR TB is suspected or confirmed.

Tuberculosis Disease in Special Circumstances
Sputum/Culture-Negative Tuberculosis

Sputum/culture-negative pulmonary TB is defined as failure to isolate organisms in the setting of high clinical suspicion of disease. Potential etiologies for negative cultures include low bacillary populations, inadequate sputum specimens, or overgrowth of cultures with other microorganisms. If clinical suspicion is high, treatment should be initiated with reevaluation every 2 to 3 months.

Tumor Necrosis Factor-α Inhibitors

Patients being treated with TNF-α inhibitors are at increased risk for reactivation of latent TB and death from disseminated TB disease. Patients who are being considered for initiation of these drugs should have clinical evaluation for TB exposure/disease, IGRA testing (or TST if IGRA is not available), and radiographic chest imaging prior to initiation of anti-TNF-α therapy. All patients should receive treatment for LTBI if identified, and if no absolute contraindications exist, TNF-α inhibitor initiation delayed at least a month into the start of LTBI treatment if feasible.

Patients Living With HIV

Patients living with HIV are at high risk for developing TB infection; with a 20- to 40-fold increased risk compared with the general population. TB infection can occur at any CD4 T lymphocyte cell count, and a direct correlation between degree of immunodeficiency and TB infection risk exists. There are many potential complications of treating TB in patients living with HIV, and it is highly advised that treatment be done in conjunction with a specialist in treating HIV and TB. There are numerous drug–drug interactions between rifamycins and many classes of HIV antiretroviral therapy (ART). Patients with HIV-related TB disease are at risk for immune reconstitution inflammatory syndrome (IRIS), a paradoxical worsening of signs and symptoms of infection after initiation of ART. Finally, even with treatment, these patients are at increased risk for reinfection with TB compared with the general population.

The timing of ART initiation for HIV in setting of TB infection is complicated and beyond the scope of this text, and management by an HIV/TB treatment expert is highly advised. At all CD4 counts, people with HIV without active TB disease have significantly improved outcomes with early initiation of ART. However, there are some opportunistic infections for which early initiation of ART is potentially injurious, including patients with both HIV and TB meningitis.

When TB occurs in patients already on ART, treatment for TB should be started immediately and ART modified to prevent any drug interactions while still working toward virologic suppression.

In patients who have already been on ART, the standard 6-month TB treatment regimen should be used for drug-susceptible TB (Table 3). If ART has not yet been initiated, the continuation phase of TB therapy should be extended by 3 months, for a total of 7 months. ART should be initiated in the first 2 weeks if the CD4 count is <50 cells/uL and by 8 to 12 weeks if the CD4 count is 50 or greater, the exception being in the setting of TB meningitis as above, in which case ART should be held until 8 weeks of TB treatment have been completed.

The most up-to-date TB treatment recommendations for persons living with HIV infection can be found in the AIDSinfo guidelines "Guidelines for the Prevention and Treatment of Opportunistic Infections in Adults and Adolescents with HIV." Consultation with, and evaluation and management by, an expert in HIV and TB treatment is highly advised for patients with these complicated clinical presentations.

Monitoring and Complications

All patients diagnosed with LTBI or TB disease should have baseline HIV testing. If the patient has risk factors for hepatitis B and/or C, baseline serologies should be checked as well.

All patients should be advised of the potential minor and serious adverse effects of their medication regimens (Table 4). Patients taking rifampin (Rifadin, Rimactane) should be warned about the innocuous orange/rust-colored staining of body fluids (urine, sweat, tears). The most common adverse effects of the first-line agents are outlined below.

Rash is a major adverse effect of all four of the first-line agents and can be due to various mechanisms and of various severities. A pruritic rash without associated symptoms can be managed symptomatically with antihistamines. A petechial rash may indicate thrombocytopenia from rifamycin hypersensitivity and warrants permanent discontinuation of the rifamycin. Rash associated with fever, mucus membrane involvement, or generalized erythema is more likely to suggest Steven-Johnson syndrome or toxic epidermal necrolysis and warrants prompt discontinuation of all medications and consultation with a dermatologist.

The most serious adverse drug event associated with isoniazid (Nydrazid), pyrazinamide (Zinamide), and rifampin (Rifadin, Rimactane) is drug-induced liver injury (DILI). DILI should be suspected if the ALT level is at least three times the upper limit of normal in the presence of hepatitis symptoms or at least five times the upper limit of normal in the absence of symptoms. An asymptomatic increase in ALT concentration occurs in nearly 20% of patients, and in this case therapy should be continued.

TABLE 3 Preferred Regimens for Drug-Susceptible Pulmonary TB Disease

INTENSIVE PHASE	DURATION	ADULT DOSAGE FOR DAILY ADMINISTRATION
INH* RIF PZA EMB	7 days per week for 8 weeks OR 5 days per week for 8 weeks	INH: 5 mg/kg (typically 300 mg) RIF: 10 mg/kg (typically 600 mg) PZA: 30–40 mg/kg EMB: 15–25 mg/kg

CONTINUATION PHASE	DURATION	ADULT DOSAGE FOR DAILY ADMINISTRATION
INH RIF	7 days per week for 18 weeks OR 5 days a week for 18 weeks	INH: 5 mg/kg (typically 300 mg) RIF: 10 mg/kg (typically 600 mg)

DOT, Directly observed therapy; *EMB*, ethambutol (Myambutol); *HIV*, human immunodeficiency virus; *INH*, isoniazid (Nydrazid); *PZA*, pyrazinamide (Zinamide); *RIF*, rifampin (Rifadin, Rimactane).
*Vitamin B6 (pyridoxine)[1] is given in conjunction with INH for those at risk for developing—or already suffering from—peripheral neuropathy per text above.
[1]Not FDA approved for this indication.

TABLE 4 Major Adverse Effects of First-Line Medications for the Treatment of Tuberculosis Disease

FIRST-LINE MEDICATIONS	MOST COMMON ADVERSE SIDE EFFECTS
INH	Hepatotoxicity Rash Drug-induced lupus Peripheral neuropathy
Rifamycins (RIF, RPT, RFB)	Hepatotoxicity Rash GI upset Thrombocytopenia Hypersensitivity reactions
PZA	Hepatotoxicity Rash GI upset Gout
EMB	Optic neuritis Rash

EMB, Ethambutol (Myambutol); *INH*, isoniazid (Nydrazid); *PZA*, pyrazinamide (Zinamide); *RFB*, rifabutin (Mycobutin); *RIF*, rifampin (Rifadin, Rimactane); *RPT*, rifapentine (Priftin).

Latent Tuberculosis Infection

For routine LTBI treatment in an otherwise healthy patient, apart from HIV and viral hepatitis serologies as above, no other baseline or serial laboratory monitoring is necessary. Patients who have/are at risk to have chronic liver disease, use alcohol regularly, are pregnant, are within 3 months postpartum, or have HIV should have baseline alanine aminotransferase (ALT), aspartate aminotransferase (AST), bilirubin, and alkaline phosphatase checked. Liver tests as above should be considered for patients of advanced age, those with chronic medical conditions, and those taking multiple chronic medications. Active viral hepatitis and end-stage liver disease are relative contraindications to the use of INH, RIF, or RPT in LTBI treatment.

While on LTBI treatment, the patient should have a minimum of once monthly medical assessments. During visits, the patient should be evaluated for development of symptoms/signs of TB disease, adherence to LTBI treatment regimen, and symptoms/signs of adverse effects. Serial liver tests, as above, should be monitored in those who have baseline abnormal LFTs, are at risk for hepatitis, or who develop symptoms/signs of hepatitis while on therapy. Treatment should be discontinued if any of the liver enzymes are greater than three times the upper limit of normal in presence of hepatitis symptoms or five times the upper limit of normal in an asymptomatic individual. For liver enzyme elevations less than three times the upper limit of normal in a symptomatic patient, treatment continuation can be considered provided there is close clinical and laboratory monitoring.

At completion of therapy, patients should be provided documentation of their initial TST or IGRA, treatment regimen and duration, and date of treatment completion. They should be advised to present such documentation if TB testing is required in the future, as IGRAs and TSTs are likely to remain positive despite successful LTBI treatment. Patients should be reminded that treatment for LTBI greatly decreases the risk of progression to TB disease but does not eliminate it 100%, and counseling on the symptoms/signs of TB disease and when/how to seek further care should be provided.

Active Tuberculosis Disease

Within a week of diagnosis, a treatment and monitoring plan specific to the patient should be developed in collaboration with the local department of health. As previously mentioned, all patients should have baseline HIV testing and viral hepatitis testing as indicated. All patients should have a baseline assessment of platelets, creatinine, ALT, AST, bilirubin, alkaline phosphatase, and a diabetes screen as recommended by the American Diabetes Association. Those patients for whom ethambutol (Myambutol) is included in treatment regimen should have a baseline Snellen test for visual acuity as well as color discrimination tests.

While on therapy, patients should be seen monthly and evaluated for treatment response and any adverse medication effects. Repeat laboratory testing should be done periodically if laboratory abnormalities were present at baseline, or if the patient develops symptoms/signs of adverse drug effects. Patients taking ethambutol (Myambutol) should be asked at each visit about vision changes and undergo monthly color discrimination tests.

During treatment of pulmonary TB disease, sputum, or other specimens for AFB/culture should be obtained at least monthly until cultures convert from positive to negative. If treatment has been continued for at least 2 months and the patient remains culture-positive, repeat drug susceptibility testing should be performed. Repeat chest radiographs can be pursued if there is clinical worsening or failure of symptoms to improve.

Treatment failure can occur for a number of reasons including medication nonadherence, unrecognized drug resistance, malabsorption, drug–drug interactions, or laboratory error (erroneously positive culture in a patient who is otherwise clinically well). The standard of care should be to add two to three new drugs. A single new agent should never be added to a failing regimen as it can lead to amplification of drug resistance as well as acquired resistance to the newly added drug.

The treatment of TB disease can be complicated, especially in patients who have HIV, are pregnant, have chronic liver disease and other comorbid conditions, have or develop drug-resistant TB, or develop serious adverse reactions to therapy. Clinicians who do not have experience with such complicated circumstances should consult a TB expert.

Nontuberculous Mycobacteria

NTM are a diverse group of environmental bacteria found worldwide. NTM are species other than *M. tuberculosis* and *M. leprae* complex. Not all NTM species are pathogenic to humans. *Mycobacterium avium* complex (MAC) is the most prevalent NTM causing human infection, and pulmonary disease is its most common presentation. NTM infections most often present as pulmonary infections in hosts with altered local or systemic immune function. Extrapulmonary infections can occur in both immune competent and immune suppressed hosts and include infections of lymph nodes, skin/soft tissue, bone, and prosthetic devices and catheters; disseminated infections occur almost exclusively

in patients with advanced immunosuppression (e.g., patients with stage III HIV). Diagnosis of NTM infections requires a clinical syndrome supported by imaging and microbiologic data. Treatment varies by species and susceptibility patterns and typically requires a multidrug regimen to prevent development of drug resistance. Management of these complicated infections should be undertaken in conjunction with an expert in nontuberculous infection diagnosis and treatment.

Pathophysiology

As above, nontuberculous mycobacterial infections are typically acquired through contact with contaminated soil, water, dust, vegetable matter, or less commonly through zoonotic spread. NTM are not part of normal human flora. Pulmonary infections have been associated with inhalation or microaspiration from contaminated recirculating water systems, as have some skin and soft tissue infections been directly correlated to such aqueous sources. However, the ubiquitous presence of these organisms in nature makes it difficult to determine where a specific person's infection was acquired. Human-to-human transmission does not occur with the rare exception of pulmonary infections transmitted between persons with cystic fibrosis.

Host risk factors for infections include immunosuppression, especially corticosteroid use, uncontrolled HIV, TNF-α antagonist use, certain inherited disorders of immune suppression, and other systemic immunosuppressive states and medications; gastroesophageal reflux disease (GERD); and chronic pulmonary disease such as cystic fibrosis, bronchiectasis, and chronic obstructive pulmonary disease. Some activities that have been associated with NTM infections include use of hot tubs, saunas, steam rooms, and prolonged showers; cleaning swimming pools and fish tanks; waxing hair removal and pedicures at nail salons; and tattooing and other cosmetic procedures.

Prevention

When possible, reversing/treating causes of immunosuppression can help prevent nontuberculous mycobacterial infections. Prompt initiation of effective ART for patients with HIV and CD4 T lymphocytes <50/mm^3, for example, can help prevent MAC and other NTM infections, without need for prophylaxis with macrolides. Previous practice guidelines for people with HIV and CD4 T lymphocytes <50/mm^3 included initiation of azithromycin (Zithromax) for MAC prophylaxis. Due to the rapid viral suppression observed with current HIV ART, such patients who are starting effective ART no longer require MAC prophylaxis. For patients with chronic lung disease, it is reasonable to avoid exposure to potentially aerosolized NTM such as with recirculating water systems (hot tubs, steam rooms, prolonged showers, swimming pools) and aerosolized soil exposure. For patients with chronic lung disease and known NTM pulmonary colonization or disease, it is advisable to limit systemic and inhaled steroids as much as feasible. Like with *M. tuberculosis*, TNF-α inhibitors increase risk for NTM infection, and more aggressive disease progression and should be avoided when possible for susceptible patients. Avoiding nonsterile and nonregulated tattooing, cosmetic procedures, etc., can also help prevent some NTM infections.

Clinical Manifestations

Infections have a wide variety of presentations and largely depend on anatomic site of infection, host immune response, and infecting NTM species. Pulmonary infections comprise 80% of NTM infections. Pulmonary infections typically occur in people with underlying lung disease or immunosuppression and in some with chest wall deformities. Presentation is usually subacute or chronic and includes cough; other symptoms may include cough, shortness of breath, low-grade fevers, night sweats, weight loss, anorexia, and fatigue.

Cervicofacial lymphadenitis ("scrofula") is the most common extrapulmonary manifestation of MAC and is typically seen in children. This presents with typically painless, unilateral, firm lymph node swelling in the mandibular or jugular regions. Systemic symptoms are uncommon in the immune-competent host. Notably when seen in adults, cervicofacial lymphadenitis is more likely to be due to *M. tuberculosis* than NTM.

Various NTM different species cause skin and soft tissue infections, usually due to direct inoculation after traumatic wound, injections, and cosmetic procedures; rarely cutaneous manifestations of systemic disease can be seen. Lesions can appear as ulcers, papules, nodules, eschars, sporotrichoid lesions, or plaques with local swelling. Tenderness, erythema, swelling may be present and systemic symptoms are often absent.

Multiple species of NTM have been found to cause bone and joint infection. Injuries and implanted prosthetic devices (e.g., prosthetic joints) are risk factors for such infections. Patients may present with pain, swelling, erythema, purulent drainage, and pathologic fractures, with or without systemic symptoms.

Disseminated NTM infections occur in immunocompromised hosts and may present with fevers, chills, sweats, weight loss, and fatigue. Pancytopenia due to bone marrow and splenic involvement can lead to shortness of breath and pallor, easy bleeding/bruising, and superimposed infections due to neutropenia. Gastrointestinal involvement may cause diarrhea, abdominal pain, and hepatosplenomegaly.

Healthcare-associated infections also occur, especially in the setting of implanted prosthetic devices/material and intravascular catheters and after cosmetic procedures including mammoplasty and tattooing.

Diagnosis

The diagnosis of pulmonary NTM disease requires pulmonary symptoms, radiographic evidence of disease, exclusion of other diagnoses, and microbiologic criteria: Positive culture results from at least two sputum specimens or positive culture from at least one bronchial wash or lavage or lung tissue with granulomatous inflammation and >1 positive sputum or bronchial wash culture. AFB smears are notoriously insensitive. Colonization of the airways can occur with NTM, so a single positive sputum culture is not diagnostic of disease. Patients who don't meet all of the criteria should be followed closely over time, as NTM pulmonary disease may still develop.

Diagnosis of extrapulmonary NTM infections is typically through AFB culture(s) performed on the involved tissue or body fluid in the setting of a compatible clinical syndrome. NTM can colonize nonsterile areas in the body, so the presence of a positive AFB culture without an associated clinical syndrome must be interpreted cautiously. NTM lymphadenitis is best diagnosed by excisional lymph node biopsy for AFB culture and histopathology, as aspiration of NTM infected lymph nodes can lead to fistula formation. Explanted prosthetic devices can be sonicated and AFB culture performed on fluid. Tissue biopsies of affected areas may demonstrate noncaseating granulomatous changes on histopathology, with or without AFB seen on smear, and AFB culture is still necessary for diagnosis and treatment.

Disseminated MAC is diagnosed by isolation of the organism in AFB blood culture or other sterile site such as bone marrow, liver, or spleen. When available, direct detection of MAC in blood by PCR may be as sensitive and specific as culture, with results available in hours as opposed to weeks.

Drug susceptibility testing done on the mycobacterial species isolated is necessary to help guide treatment decisions.

Treatment

Treatment of NTM infections is, with few exceptions, complicated and requires input or management by specialists in NTM infections. NTM have intrinsic resistance to many antibiotics and can develop resistance on therapy. Treatment therefore typically requires two or three antimicrobial agents for a prolonged period of time, often 6 months to a year. If underlying immune suppression can be mitigated (e.g., holding or decreasing doses of immunosuppressive agents), such modifications should be made. Specific treatments vary for the different anatomic sites affected,

species of NTM involved, antibiotic susceptibility patterns, host immune status, and the patient's tolerance for specific antimicrobials, prolonged duration, and the potential adverse effects. For pulmonary NTM disease, not all patients who meet diagnostic criteria need to be treated: Some people will have spontaneous resolution without antimicrobial therapy; when treated, duration is quite prolonged; treatment requires multiple drugs with various side effect profiles; treatment may require months of intravenous antibiotics; and pulmonary infection has a significant rate of relapse/recurrence.

Mycobacterium leprae *Complex*

Hansen's disease, also known as leprosy, is an indolent mycobacterial infection largely affecting skin and nerves caused by *Mycobacterium leprae* complex (*Mycobacterium leprae* and lepromatosis). It is an underdiagnosed disease due to its insidious onset of symptoms, the stigma associated with diagnosis and the healthcare system, and misrecognition of symptoms especially in areas of low prevalence. According to the World Health Organization (WHO), in 2019 there were 202,256 new cases diagnosed globally, with prevalence of 22.9 per million people. The majority of cases are reported from India, Brazil, and Indonesia. Untreated, Hansen's disease leads to significant morbidity and very impaired quality of life. The psychosocial stigma associated with the disease, however, is often felt by patients to be worse than the physical symptoms and must be addressed from time of initial evaluation through and beyond treatment.

Pathophysiology

Hansen's disease is a granulomatous infection caused by *Mycobacterium leprae* and *lepromatosis*, which comprise *M. leprae* complex. These organisms are gram-positive AFB that cannot be grown in culture. They replicate slowly, and average disease incubation period is 5 years. Though incompletely understood, transmission is felt to be person-to-person through nasal and respiratory secretions. Nine-banded armadillos in the southeastern United States, red squirrels in Scotland and England, chimpanzees, and macaques have all been found to carry *M. leprae* or *M. lepromatosis*, so zoonotic transmission is also implicated, though less frequently.

More than 95% of people worldwide are felt to have immunity to *M. leprae* complex, so in actuality, Hansen's disease is not very transmissible. Clinical and histopathologic disease occurs on a continuum, classified into five types by the Ridley-Jopling schema, depending on degree of host cell-mediated immune response to *M. leprae* complex. Disease types range from polar tuberculoid form (TT) with a strong immune response including well-formed granulomas, few bacilli, and more classic clinical manifestations, to the polar lepromatous type (LL) with minimal cell-mediated immune response, foamy macrophages without granulomas, and many bacilli seen on histopathology. LL clinical manifestations are less commonly recognized and are described below. Borderline tuberculoid (BT), midborderline (BB), and borderline lepromatous (BL) types have various degrees of both cell-mediated and humoral response.

Prevention

As with TB, the mainstay of prevention of Hansen's disease is early diagnosis and treatment of infected patients. There is currently no FDA approved vaccine to prevent infection with *M. leprae* complex. BCG vaccine[1]—that given in endemic regions to prevent severe TB disease in children—when given to household contacts of people with Hansen's disease may decrease risk of transmission of *M. leprae* complex. Additionally, in household contacts of infected patients, BCG vaccination decreases likelihood of developing multibacillary disease.

Patients with Hansen's disease who have hypoesthetic lesions are at risk to develop injuries, such as burns and ulcers, in the

---

[1]Not FDA approved for this indication.

insensate areas. Daily checks for foot wounds, avoiding walking barefoot, use of protective silicone gloves when cooking, and so on are important in the prevention and early detection and management of injury.

Clinical Manifestations

As *M. leprae* complex cannot be grown in culture, a high degree of clinical suspicion is necessary to pursue diagnosis. *M. leprae* complex requires cooler temperatures for growth and therefore has a predilection for cooler areas of the body including skin, cutaneous nerves, ears, and nose, including septum, eyes, larynx, and testes. Presentations vary according to degree of immune response to the bacilli. Cutaneous manifestations can include macules, patches, papules, or nodules. Lesions can be hypopigmented or reddish. The skin may be thick, scaly, or dry appearing. The hypopigmented areas are often hypoesthetic. Injuries to hypoesthetic areas are common and cause painless ulcers, burn wounds, lacerations, etc. Wounds may become infected. There may be madarosis: loss of the eyebrows and/or eyelashes. Thickening and nodularity of skin on the face can lead to a "leonine facies" appearance. Involvement of the nasal bridge can cause a "saddle nose" deformity. Perforation of the nasal septum can occur. Laryngeal involvement can lead to hoarseness. Eye involvement can include episcleritis and iridocyclitis. Lagophthalmos can occur leading to keratitis, corneal opacities, ectropion, entropion, and trichiasis. Neural involvement can lead to not only anesthetic areas but also thickened peripheral nerves, peripheral neuropathy, claw hand, foot drop, or paralysis of an extremity.

A particular area of concern that significantly affects patients living with Hansen's disease is the associated stigma and negative beliefs surrounding Hansen's disease, due to historic, religious, and social implications. Thus one must consider psychological burden associated with this infection when relaying diagnosis and throughout the patient's care.

Diagnosis

There are two main schema used for diagnosis: a binary clinical classification schema devised by the WHO for use where histopathology is not readily available and the histopathologic and clinical spectrum of the Ridley-Jopling classification. The WHO schema divides disease into multibacillary and paucibacillary, depending on number of skin lesions visible. The Ridley-Jopling schema classifies disease on a spectrum as outlined above and is based on skin biopsy for histopathology and Fite stain. Additional methods of identification of *M. leprae* complex include identification of the bacilli DNA in tissue biopsies by nucleic acid amplification techniques such as PCR.

Treatment

Using multidrug regimens, Hansen's disease is curable. Early recognition and treatment are key to preventing disability. The most active antimicrobial agents used to treat Hansen's disease include dapsone, rifampin (Rifadin, Rimactane),[1] and clofazimine (Lamprene). Other agents with efficacy include some fluoroquinolones, minocycline (Cleeravue-M, Dynacin, Minocin, Myrac, Solodyn, Ximino),[1] and clarithromycin (Biaxin).[1] As in other mycobacterial infections, multidrug regimens are imperative to prevent emergence of drug resistance and increase cure rates. Glucose-6-phosphate dehydrogenase (G6PD) deficiency testing should be performed prior to starting dapsone and the drug avoided if deficiency is present. Clofazimine (Lamprene) can only be obtained in the United States through the National Hansen's Disease Program (NHDP) in Louisiana. The NHPD is the sole facility in the United States dedicated to Hansen's disease diagnosis, treatment, and research. Consultation with their expert physicians and pharmacists is highly recommended. There are many resources available to patients and healthcare providers alike through the NHDP, including review of histopathology specimens, consultation regarding molecular diagnosis

of *M. leprae* complex, antimicrobial therapy free of costs for patients, and educational materials for physicians and patients to improve understanding of the disease and help prevent injury and disability. Finally, resources are available through NHDP for surgical care and rehabilitation of patients referred for digit or limb threatening wounds. Contact information can be found at https://www.hrsa.gov/hansens-disease/index.html.

Monitoring

G6PD deficiency testing should be performed prior to starting dapsone, and the drug avoided if deficiency is present. Patients should be monitored frequently while on therapy for potential adverse effects of various medications including anemia, QTc prolongation (clofazimine [Lamprene] and clarithromycin [Biaxin]), and skin discoloration (minocycline). Treatment efficacy is indicated by resolution of skin lesions and lack of new skin or nerve lesions. Patients should be monitored closely and educated about the signs and symptoms of reversal reactions, which can occur before, during, and even after therapy. At every visit, examination of all extremities should be performed to evaluate new and existing wounds.

Complications

Complications of Hansen's disease itself stem from injuries to hypoesthetic areas as above (largely hands and feet) and complications of peripheral neuropathy such as claw hand and foot drop. Evaluation and management by occupational and physical therapists and appropriate surgical referrals are often indicated.

As mentioned above, G6PD levels should be checked prior to initiation of dapsone and the drug avoided if patient is deficient in the enzyme, otherwise hemolytic anemia may develop. CBC with differential and ECG for QTc should be evaluated at baseline and periodically while on clofazimine (Lamprene) therapy.

Before, during, or even after therapy, pathologic immune reactions including reversal reactions and erythema nodosum leprosum can occur. Rarely, specific reversal reactions can be life threatening. Reversal reactions are inflammatory states, and measurement of biomarkers of inflammation can be helpful for evaluation and monitoring. Reversal reactions are treated with various immunosuppressing agents and consultation with the experts at NHDP is recommended.

References

American Thoracic Society: Targeted tuberculin testing and treatment of latent tuberculosis infection, *MMWR Recomm Rep (Morb Mortal Wkly Rep)* 49:1–51, 2000.

Bennett J, Dolin R, Blaser M: Infections cause by nontuberculous mycobacteria other than Mycobacterium avium complex. In Bennett J, Dolin R, Blaser M, editors: *Mandell, Douglas, and Bennett's Principles and practice of infectious diseases*, 9 ed, Elsevier, pp 3049–3058, 2020.

Bennett J, Dolin R, Blaser M: *Mycobacterium avium* complex. In Bennett J, Dolin R, Blaser M, editors: *Mandell, Douglas, and Bennett's Principles and practice of infectious diseases*, 9 ed, Elsevier, pp 3035–3048, 2020.

Bennett J, Dolin R, Blaser M. *Mycobacterium leprae* (leprosy). In Bennett J, Dolin R, and Blaser M, editors: Mandell, *Douglas, and Bennett's Principles and practice of infectious diseases*, 9 ed, Elsevier, pp. 3022-3034, 2020.

Bennett J, Dolin R, Blaser M: Mycobacterium tuberculosis. In Bennett J, Dolin R, Blaser M, editors: *Mandell, Douglas, and Bennett's Principles and practice of infectious diseases*, 9 ed, Elsevier, pp 2985–3021, 2020.

Daley CL, Iaccarino JM, Lange C, et al: Treatment of nontuberculous mycobacterial pulmonary disease: an Official ATS/ERS/ESCMID/IDSA clinical practice guideline, *Clin Infect Dis* 71(4):e1–e36, 2020.

Daley CL, Winthrop KL: *Mycobacterium avium* complex: Addressing Gaps in diagnosis and management, *J Infect Dis* 222(S4):S199–S211, 2020.

Dheda K, Barry 3rd CE, Maartens G: Tuberculosis, *Lancet* 387(10024):1211–1226, 2016 (Erratum in: Lancet 2016; 387(10024):1162).

Lewinsohn DM, Leonard MK, LoBue PA, et al: Official American Thoracic Society/Infectious Diseases Society of America/Centers for Disease Control and Prevention clinical practice guidelines: diagnosis of tuberculosis in adults and children, *Clin Infect Dis* 64(2):e1–e33, 2017.

Leon KE, Jacob JT, Franco-Paredes C, et al: Delayed diagnosis, leprosy reactions, and nerve injury among individuals with Hansen's disease seen at a United States clinic, *Open Forum Infect Dis* 3(2):ofw063, 2016. Available at: https://academic.oup.com/ofid/article/3/2/ofw063/2399323. [Accessed 17 May 2021].

Nahid P, Dorman SE, Alipanah N, et al: Official American Thoracic Society/Centers for Disease Control and Prevention/Infectious Diseases Society of America clinical practice guidelines: treatment of drug-susceptible tuberculosis, *Clin Infect Dis* 63(7):e147–e195, 2016.

---

[1]Not FDA approved for this indication.

Nahid P, Mase SR, Migliori GB, et al: Treatment of drug-resistant tuberculosis. An Official ATS/CDC/ERS/IDSA clinical practice guideline [published correction appears in Am J Respir Crit care med. 2020 Feb 15;201(4):500-501], *Am J Respir Crit Care Med* 200(10):e93–e142, 2019.

National Hansen's Disease (Leprosy) Program Caring and Curing Since 1894. Available at: https://www.hrsa.gov/hansens-disease/index.html. [Accessed 06/17/2021].

Office of AIDS Research Advisory Council, Centers for Disease Control and Prevention, National Institute of Health, HIV Medicine Association (HIV-MA) of the Infectious Diseases Society of America (IDSA). Guidelines for the Prevention and Treatment of Opportunistic Infections in Adults and Adolescents with HIV. Available at: https://clinicalinfo.hiv.gov/en/guidelines/adult-and-adolescent-opportunistic-infection/whats-new-guidelines [accessed 06/18/2021].

Sterling TR, Njie G, Zenner D, et al: Guidelines for the treatment of latent tuberculosis infection: recommendations from the National Tuberculosis Controllers Association and CDC, 2020, *MMWR Recomm Rep (Morb Mortal Wkly Rep)* 69(No. RR-1):1–11, 2020.

World Health Organization. Leprosy (Hansen's Disease). Available at: https://www.who.int/news-room/fact-sheets/detail/leprosy [accessed 06/19/2021].

VENOUS THROMBOEMBOLISM

Method of
Moniba Nazeef, MD; and John P. Sheehan, MD

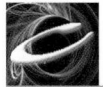

CURRENT DIAGNOSIS

- A comprehensive history is the most important diagnostic tool to assess risk factors including recent surgery, bedridden state, trauma, orthopedic procedure, or active cancer.
- Moderately high–sensitivity D-Dimer assays (>85% sensitivity) can be used to exclude venous thromboembolism (VTE) if there is low clinical probability but should be combined with imaging in all other cases.
- Venous compression ultrasonography (CUS) is a noninvasive, affordable, and widely available test for the diagnosis of deep vein thrombosis (DVT). Computed tomography pulmonary angiography (CTPA) is the current gold standard for the diagnosis of pulmonary embolism (PE).

CURRENT THERAPY

- The choice of initial therapy is frequently guided by the clinical scenario. Initial therapy includes unfractionated heparin (UFH), low-molecular-weight heparin (LWMH), fondaparinux (Arixtra), or the direct oral anticoagulants (DOACs) rivaroxaban (Xarelto) or apixaban (Eliquis)
- The traditional heparin-warfarin regimen has been increasingly supplanted by the use of direct oral anticoagulants (DOAC).
- Standard treatment for a new episode of DVT or pulmonary embolism (PE) is 3 to 6 months of therapeutic anticoagulation. The recommended duration of anticoagulation for VTE requires individualized analysis of the clinical presentation and patient specific factors that weigh both recurrence and bleeding risk.

Venous thromboembolism (VTE) is a significant health problem, with surveillance data suggesting that 60,000 to 100,000 people die of VTE each year in the United States. Approximately 50% to 60% of this disease burden is associated with a recent hospitalization, underscoring the importance of VTE prophylaxis. VTE is comprised of superficial vein thrombosis (SVT), deep venous thrombosis (DVT), and pulmonary embolism (PE). DVT typically starts in the deep veins of the lower extremities and progresses proximally. If untreated, a clot can break off and travel to the lungs where it is trapped in the pulmonary circulation, resulting in PE. DVT confined to the deep veins of the calf is termed *isolated distal DVT*, whereas involvement of the popliteal or more proximal veins is termed *proximal DVT*. SVT represents thrombosis in the superficial veins of the legs or arms and rarely progresses to DVT. The focus of this chapter is to understand the risk factors, diagnosis, treatment, and prevention of DVT and PE.

Pathophysiology/Risk Factors

Venous blood flow is maintained by a delicate homeostatic balance of prothrombotic and antithrombotic factors. Virchow's triad describes the major factors leading to VTE from a pathophysiologic standpoint: (1) intrinsic hypercoagulability, (2) endothelial damage, and (3) venous stasis. Most often, a combination of these factors leads to the development of VTE. Based on the presence or absence of typical clinical risk factors, VTE occurrences can be considered either provoked (e.g., post-surgical) or unprovoked (spontaneous). Furthermore, provoking risk factors may be transient/reversible (e.g., estrogen use) versus nontransient/irreversible (e.g., lower extremity paresis), which has implications for decisions regarding duration of anticoagulant therapy Table 1.

Acquired Risk Factors

Certain clinical conditions shift the balance between procoagulant and anticoagulant factors to promote thrombosis. These conditions include surgery, pregnancy and puerperium, inflammation, active cancer, major trauma, specific medications, and a variety of conditions that lead to immobility. A more comprehensive list is provided in Table 1. Many of these clinical conditions cause multiple changes relevant to VTE risk. For example, surgical interventions may induce endothelial damage, immobilization leading to venous stasis, platelet activation, and trigger inflammatory responses that increase fibrinogen, factor VIII, and von Willebrand factor levels. Orthopedic procedures involving the lower limbs and abdominopelvic surgeries in cancer patients are especially high risk from a VTE standpoint. Active cancer is associated with 20% of all VTE and involves a variety of mechanisms leading to hypercoagulability, including increased tissue factor

TABLE 1	Risk Factors for Venous Thromboembolism

Transient/Reversible

Surgery (esp. lower limb orthopedic surgery)
General anesthesia >30 min
Immobility due to surgical or medical condition
Oral contraceptives/hormone replacement therapy
Pregnancy, puerperium
Major trauma
Acute inflammation
Indwelling venous catheters
Heparin induced thrombocytopenia
May-Thurner sydrome
Travel-associated thrombosis
Medications including tamoxifen, L-asparaginase, immunomodulatory agents (lenalidomide), EPO

Permanent/Non-Reversible

Active cancer
Antiphospholipid syndrome
Myeloproliferative neoplasms
Paroxysmal nocturnal hemoglobinura (PNH)
Lower extremity paresis from neurologic disease
Sickle cell disease
Nephrotic syndrome
Active autoimmune conditions (SLE, IBD, ITP,TTP)
Chronic infection/inflammation
Morbid obesity (BMI > 40)

EPO, Erythropoietin; SLE, systemic lupus erythematosus; IBD, inflammatory bowel disease; ITP, immune thrombocytopenic purpura; TTP, thrombotic thrombocytopenic purpura.

expression, venous obstruction, indwelling catheters, reduced mobility, and chemotherapy.

Pregnancy and the puerperium, oral contraceptives (OC), and hormone replacement therapy (HRT) are important VTE risk factors in women. OC and HRT are associated with a number of changes in hemostatic protein levels and platelet function that appear globally prothrombotic. Higher estrogen content is associated with increased thrombotic risk and is modulated by a combination with specific progestins. Additionally, there is a higher risk of VTE in OCP users with a positive family history, suggesting an underlying genetic predisposition.

A variety of conditions that involve prolonged immobilization enhance VTE risk. Cast immobilization of the lower extremity, paresis after neurologic events, multiple trauma, orthopedic surgeries, travel-associated immobility (>4–6 hours) or a bedridden state due to a variety of medical or surgical conditions result in stasis that promotes venous thrombosis. Many of these clinical situations are also associated with an inflammatory state that concomitantly increases intrinsic hypercoagulability of the blood. Venous wall injury may occur via a variety of mechanisms, including surgical interventions, indwelling intravenous catheters, trauma, and vasculitis.

Genetics of Venous Thromboembolism

Although acquired clinical risk factors are critical to assessing risk, the genetic contribution to VTE is also substantial, with heritability of VTE estimated at 40% to 47%. Like many complex phenotypes, VTE has a multigenic basis in which most individual alleles make relatively small contributions to overall risk. Factor V Leiden and the prothrombin G20210A polymorphism are examples of such alleles (2- to 4-fold relative risk). At least 17 genes have been identified that harbor VTE-associated variants. Importantly, family history remains an independent risk factor even after excluding known gene variants associated with thrombophilia, suggesting that unidentified genes also contribute to VTE risk. Deficiencies of the coagulation inhibitors antithrombin, protein C, and protein S are rare conditions with a more substantial effect on the relative risk of VTE (10- to 20-fold increase) but tend to be diagnosed erroneously in the setting of acute thrombosis. The multigenic basis of VTE has implications for thrombophilia testing that include: (1) identification of minor alleles (e.g., FV Leiden) is not helpful for prediction of VTE recurrence risk; (2) a careful family history is generally more valuable than a thrombophilia evaluation; and (3) the *absolute* risk for carriers of thrombophilic alleles is generally quite small and does not justify indefinite anticoagulation. A robust estimate of individual genetic risk requires systematic screening of all known VTE risk genes or whole genome/exome sequencing approaches that are not routinely available. Thus current thrombophilia testing rarely contributes to clinical decision making in patients with VTE. Testing should never be pursued for provoked events and is best limited to selected situations such as presentations at a young age (<30 years) or known thrombophilic traits occurring in the context of a family history of VTE. A thorough personal and family history is generally sufficient to determine the likelihood of an underlying inherited hypercoagulable state.

Epidemiology and Natural History

The exact incidence of VTE is unknown, but it is estimated that about 300,000 to 600,000 Americans are affected by VTE each year. VTE incidence appears ~30% higher in African Americans and ~70% lower in Asian and Native American populations relative to Caucasians. Importantly, the incidence of VTE increases with age, particularly after age 50. Whereas overall VTE is slightly more common in men, women have an increased incidence before age 40 based on the impact of pregnancy and contraceptives. In older age groups, the frequency of PE is increased relative to DVT. Finally, the incidence of VTE has been increasing steadily since the mid-1980s, which may, in large part, represent the increased use and enhanced sensitivity of computed tomography (CT) scans and magnetic resonance imaging (MRI).

The natural history of VTE is impacted by the underlying clinical risk factors, provoked versus unprovoked nature of the event, reversibility of risk factors, and location/nature of the thrombotic event. In general, untreated thrombi tend to extend proximally, break off, and embolize to the pulmonary circulation, where they may result in infarction and pulmonary hypertension. The risk of PE is increased for proximal versus distal involvement with DVT. More than 75% of VTE starts in the calf veins, and 20% to 30% of these cases progress to involve proximal veins in the leg or pelvis. Approximately 50% of patients with untreated symptomatic proximal DVT develop symptomatic PE, whereas the incidence of asymptomatic PE is even higher. Importantly, 10% of symptomatic PE is rapidly fatal, and 30% of patients with untreated symptomatic nonfatal PE will have a fatal recurrence. Thus recognition of PE is of the utmost clinical importance. Anticoagulant therapy inhibits thrombus growth and largely prevents interval recurrence, whereas endogenous thrombolysis may result in partial or complete resolution of the thrombus. Uncommonly, progressive thrombosis in the presence of anticoagulation may occur in high-risk situations such as metastatic malignancy or the antiphospholipid syndrome.

The risk of VTE recurrence after stopping anticoagulation varies significantly based on clinical presentation. About 20% to 40% of VTE episodes are unprovoked in nature, which is associated with a substantially higher recurrence rate. For unprovoked clots, recurrence rate is estimated to be ~10% in one year, ~30% in 5 years, and approaches ~40% in 10 years. In contrast, the recurrence risk of VTE associated with surgery (a transient risk factor) is less than 3% per year. Recurrences tend to occur in a similar site to the initial event, which is particularly important in the case of PE, as 25% of pulmonary embolism presents as sudden death. In contrast, the risk of recurrent VTE is much smaller in isolated distal (calf) DVT compared with proximal DVT and PE.

Long-Term Complications of VTE
Postthrombotic Syndrome (PTS)
About 20% to 50% patients with DVT develop some degree of PTS within the subsequent 1–2 years. Chronic venous obstruction, inflammation, endofibrosis, and valvular dysfunction contribute to the chronic venous insufficiency of PTS. Risk factors for PTS include persistent DVT symptoms after one month, extensive or recurrent DVT, inadequate anticoagulation, and advanced age. Manifestations include chronic leg edema, pain, heaviness, erythema, and venous ulcers that may result in significant disability. PTS is largely non-reversible, emphasizing the importance of DVT prevention. Graduated compression stockings provide symptomatic relief by preventing pooling of blood in the lower extremities, but do not prevent PTS. In the 5% to 10% of patients with severe PTS, active supportive care and consultation with vascular surgery, dermatology, or vein specialists should be sought early to avoid development of debilitating venous ulcers.

Chronic Thromboembolic Pulmonary Hypertension (CTEPH)
CTEPH is a long-term complication of PE affecting 3% to 4% patients despite adequate anticoagulation. CTEPH is characterized by progressive pulmonary hypertension and right-side heart failure due to remodeling of pulmonary vasculature by thrombotic material. Patients with large central or extensive pulmonary emboli, hemodynamic compromise, and right heart dysfunction at diagnosis are at highest risk. Chronic progressive dyspnea with exertion is the most common symptom, and the clinician must have a high clinical suspicion based on patient's history of PE. An echocardiogram revealing elevated pulmonary arterial hypertension should trigger evaluation with a VQ scan. The presence of chronic mismatched segmental perfusion defects on the VQ scan is diagnostic of CTEPH. If anatomically feasible, treatment of choice is pulmonary endarterectomy, which can reverse the hemodynamic and functional abnormalities. Early recognition and referral to a specialized surgical treatment center are critical to patient outcomes. Lifelong anticoagulation is recommended for all patients with CTEPH.

Diagnosis of Deep Venous Thrombosis

The diagnosis of DVT proceeds via determination of clinical probability, D-dimer screening, and confirmatory imaging.

Clinical Features

Diagnosis begins with evaluation of the clinical scenario for VTE risk factors and suspicious physical exam findings. Suggestive features in the patient's recent history include recent surgery or bedridden state, trauma or orthopedic procedure, active cancer, and other typical risk factors (**Table 1**). Classic symptoms of DVT include limb swelling, pain, and erythema. On exam, unilateral calf swelling, pitting edema, dilated veins, and tenderness on palpation can be seen. The clinical probability becomes stronger when more of these findings are present. Risk stratification systems such as the Wells model (Table 2) use these clinical features to rapidly classify patients as high (~60% thrombosis), moderate (~25%), or low (~5%) risk for DVT. Differential diagnosis of DVT includes trauma, cellulitis, osteomyelitis, chronic venous insufficiency, arterial ischemia, ruptured Baker's cyst, hematoma, and superficial thrombophlebitis. Because neither history nor physical examination findings are specific for DVT, D-dimer screening and objective imaging must be pursued if sufficient clinical suspicion exists. A simplified algorithm for diagnosis of DVT is provided (Figure 1).

D-Dimer Screening

D-dimer is a specific fibrin degradation product generated by plasmin cleavage of cross-linked fibrin clot, formed by thrombin and Factor XIII activity. D-dimer represents a useful screening tool based on excellent sensitivity and a high negative predictive value for VTE. However, D-dimer lacks specificity, as it is increased in a variety of conditions, including acute inflammation, recent surgery or trauma, pregnancy, DIC, advanced age, or cancer. The level of clinical suspicion also impacts interpretation of D-dimer results. Specific D-dimer assays vary in sensitivity and specificity, although qualitative testing has largely been replaced by enzyme-linked immunosorbent assay–based quantitative assays. More recently, highly sensitive assays (>95% sensitivity) using latex-enhanced immunoturbidimetric immunoassays provide rapid quantitation for use in the diagnosis of VTE. Point-of-care (POC) testing with specified cutoff values are also available. Thus the clinician should be familiar with the type of D-dimer testing available locally. Highly sensitive assays have a good negative predictive value to rule out VTE without further testing. Moderately high–sensitivity assays (>85% sensitivity) can be used to exclude VTE if there is low clinical probability but should be combined with imaging in all other cases. Qualitative or semiquantitative assays are generally not reliable for excluding thrombosis. Finally, if clinical suspicion for DVT or PE is high, a negative D-dimer should not be used to rule out VTE, and appropriate imaging should be pursued to confirm the diagnosis.

Imaging

Ultrasonography

Venous compression ultrasonography (CUS) is a noninvasive, affordable, and widely available test for the diagnosis of DVT. The deep veins are assessed by use of a compression probe with lack of compressibility in a venous segment indicative of thrombus. Duplex technology or color-coded Doppler scanning visualizes blood flow to allow accurate identification of deep veins. Lack of flow plus non-compressibility increases diagnostic accuracy and also facilitates diagnosis in veins that cannot be compressed (e.g., pelvic and subclavian veins). Venous ultrasonography has an excellent sensitivity and specificity (~94%) for diagnosis of proximal limb DVT. The common femoral, femoral, and trifurcation

TABLE 2	Wells Model for Predicting Pretest Probability of Deep Vein Thrombosis	
CLINICAL VARIABLE		**POINTS**
Active cancer (treatment ongoing or within previous 6 months or palliative)		1
Recently bedridden >3 days or major surgery within 4 weeks		1
Pitting edema confined to the symptomatic leg		1
Dilated superficial veins (non-varicose)		1
Previous documented DVT		1
Paralysis, paresis, or recent plaster immobilization of the 1 lower extremities		1
Localized tenderness along the distribution of the deep 1 venous system		1
Calf swelling 3 cm greater than asymptomatic side measured 10 cm below tibial tuberosity		1
Alternative diagnosis at least as likely as DVT		-2

Clinical probability by interpretation of total score: >2 points, high; 1 or 2, moderate; <1, low.

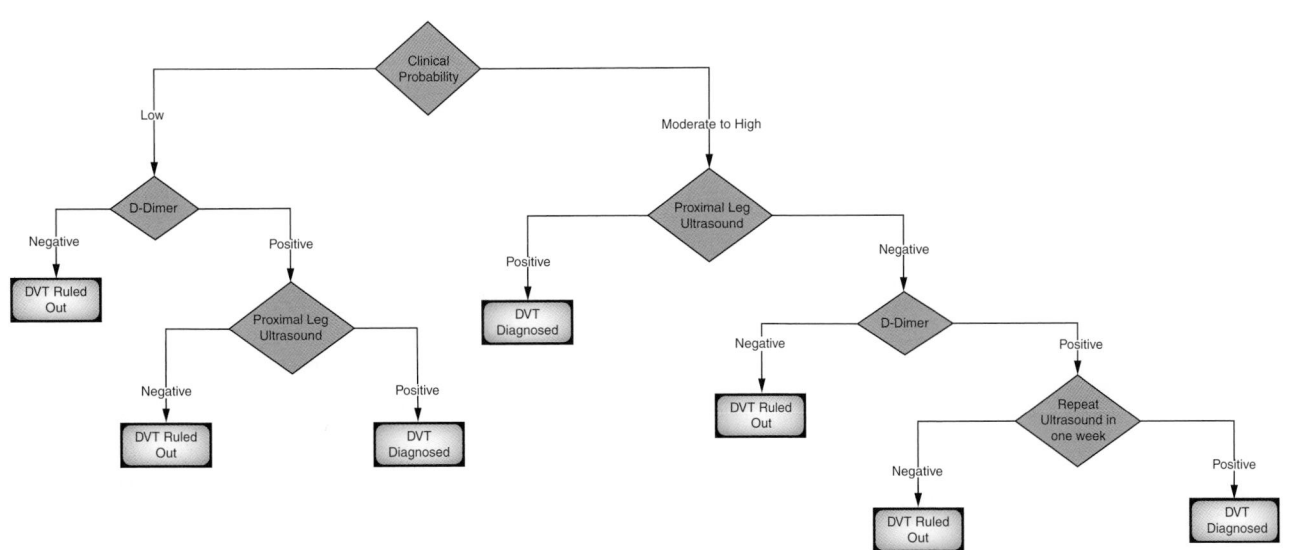

Figure 1 Suggested diagnostic algorithm for diagnosis of deep venous thrombosis (DVT).

of calf veins are readily visualized. In most cases, a negative test is sufficient to rule out proximal VTE. Currently two methods for CUS are used: (1) the two point compression technique, which only evaluates the proximal veins in the groin and popliteal fossa; and (2) whole-leg ultrasound scanning evaluating both proximal and distal veins. The sensitivity and specificity of CUS for calf vein DVT is significantly lower and highly operator dependent. Therefore many centers only perform the proximal vein assessment, which is reliable, reproducible, and efficient. If clinical suspicion remains high after a negative proximal vein ultrasound scan, repeat ultrasound scanning should be performed in about a week to assess for proximal extension in the deep venous system. If negative, no further testing is needed. A negative whole-leg CUS test result essentially rules out DVT and does not need follow-up testing. However, this approach is time consuming, may lead to increased diagnosis of calf vein thromboses, and potential overtreatment. The 3-month incidence of symptomatic proximal venous thrombosis in patients with a normal initial test are comparable at ~1% for both approaches. For upper extremities, compression ultrasonography is about 86% sensitive and specific.

Contrast Venography
Previously the gold standard for diagnosis of DVT, contrast venography is rarely used because it is invasive and requires contrast exposure. CT and MR venography have a sensitivity and specificity of >90% for DVT in lower extremities. However, these studies are also not widely used for diagnosis because of increased cost, radiation, and contrast exposure. CT and MR venography are useful to define anatomy in patients with multiple recurrent DVT (evaluation by CUS is problematic), an indeterminate abnormality on ultrasound scanning, or a thrombus diagnosed in the setting of very low clinical suspicion.

Diagnosis of PE
Similar to DVT, the diagnosis of PE requires determination of clinical probability, consideration of D-dimer testing, and confirmatory imaging.

Clinical Features
A patient presenting with risk factors for VTE and antecedent history of DVT should raise the suspicion for pulmonary embolism. The most common symptoms of PE are shortness of breath and chest pain. Pleuritic chest pain is typical, but PE may also present with substernal pressure or be confused with musculoskeletal pain. Other symptoms may include cough and hemoptysis. Clinical signs include tachypnea, tachycardia, and hypoxia. The findings of DVT in the lower extremities increase the probability of PE. The Well's model for PE provides a useful framework to estimate the pretest probability using these variables (Table 3).

Chest X-Ray, Electrocardiography, and Troponin
Chest x-ray should be performed in all suspected cases. The classical "Hampton's hump" or peripheral wedge-shaped opacity corresponding to a large pulmonary infarct is seldom appreciated and not very sensitive or specific. However, a chest x-ray is useful in assessing for other conditions such as pneumonia, pneumothorax, and pulmonary edema that can present in similar fashion. Electrocardiography (EKG) should be performed in anyone presenting with chest pain to rule out myocardial infarction. Evidence of right heart strain on EKG has predictive and prognostic value in assessment of pulmonary embolism. Similarly, a troponin level is usually obtained in evaluation for myocardial ischemia. An elevated troponin level in the absence of EKG evidence of ischemia can be suggestive of myocardial injury in the setting of massive or submassive PE.

Ventilation/Perfusion (V/Q) Scanning
V/Q scans have largely been replaced by computed tomography pulmonary angiography (CTPA). However, V/Q scans remain

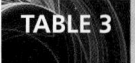

TABLE 3	Wells Model for Predicting Pretest Probability of Pulmonary Embolism	
CLINICAL VARIABLE		**POINTS**
Clinical signs and symptoms of DVT (minimum leg swelling and pain with palpation of the deep veins		3
An alternative diagnosis is less likely than PE		3
Heart rate >100 beats/min		1.5
Immobilization or surgery in the previous 4 weeks		1.5
Previous DVT/PE		1.5
Hemoptysis		1
Active Cancer (treatment ongoing or within previous 6 months or palliative)		1

Clinical probability by interpretation of total score: >6 points, high; 4 to 6, moderate; <4, low.

useful in selected patients with significant renal insufficiency (to avoid contrast dye) and young or pregnant females (to avoid radiation exposure). This technique uses inhaled and intravenous radioisotopes to evaluate ventilation and circulation in the pulmonary parenchyma and vasculature, respectively. A normal perfusion scan in the setting of a normal chest x-ray excludes PE. The addition of a ventilation scan increases specificity by accounting for other pulmonary disorders. A normal chest x-ray and ventilation scan in areas with multiple large perfusion defects that involve >75% of a segment (V/Q mismatch) is associated with >80% probability of PE and considered a high-probability V/Q scan. An intermediate-probability scan usually requires further diagnostic evaluation because it is considered nondiagnostic in most situations. Three-dimensional single-photon emission CT (SPECT) is now used by many centers in place of planar VQ scans. SPECT may be more accurate than planar VQ scanning, resulting in fewer nondiagnostic studies.

Computed Tomography Pulmonary Angiography
Computed tomography pulmonary angiography (CTPA) is the modality of choice for diagnosis of PE. It is a relatively noninvasive procedure that can provide prompt diagnosis of PE. With recent advancements, the availability of thin-slice scans provides a detailed analysis of pulmonary vasculature that increases the sensitivity for detecting thrombi at the subsegmental and peripheral arterial level. In contrast to V/Q scanning, CTPA provides detailed visualization of the lung parenchyma, which can detect peripheral pulmonary infarctions and alternative diagnoses. When required, the CTPA examination can be extended to include the iliac veins, providing a detailed view with a single contrast exposure. CTPA has excellent sensitivity and specificity for diagnosis of lobar and segmental PE. Diagnostic accuracy is lower at the subsegmental level, and results should be interpreted in the context of clinical probability, proximal lower extremity ultrasound results, and D-dimer level. A simplified algorithmic approach to diagnosis of PE is provided (Figure 2). CTPA use is limited by costs, exposure to potentially nephrotoxic contrast dye, and chest radiation. It should be avoided in younger women because of the associated increased risk of breast cancer.

Pulmonary Angiography
Formerly the gold standard for the diagnosis of PE, pulmonary angiography is an invasive procedure that has been replaced by CTPA and is now very rarely performed.

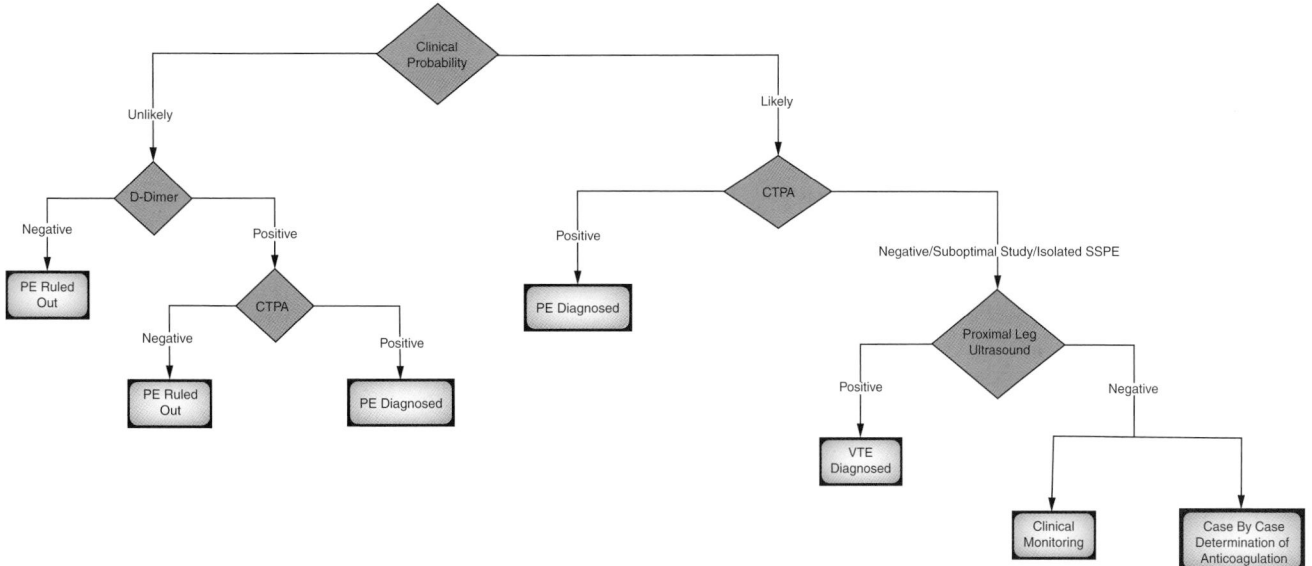

Figure 2 Suggested diagnostic algorithm for diagnosis of pulmonary embolism (PE). *CTPA*, computed tomography pulmonary angiography; *SSPE*, subsegmental pulmonary embolism.

Magnetic Resonance Angiography

Pulmonary contrast-enhanced magnetic resonance angiography (CE-MRA) is emerging as a useful alternative to CTPA in select patients such as younger females and those with severe iodinated contrast allergy. Currently, CE-MRA has limited availability and usefulness that is dependent on the expertise and experience of the available radiologists.

Diagnosis of Recurrent DVT

The diagnosis of recurrent DVT can be challenging, because signs and symptoms of PTS in the affected extremity can obscure the diagnosis. Clinical assessment of the probability for recurrent DVT is less well standardized than initial episodes; however, many predictive factors are expected to be shared. The clinician should assess for the presence of ongoing clinical risk factors, attempt to discern between chronic and acute signs and symptoms, and consider D-dimer testing. A negative D-dimer test can be used to exclude recurrent DVT, although the accuracy of this approach has not been well studied. If D-dimer testing is positive or has not been done, CUS is performed. The finding of non-compressibility of an ipsilateral femoral or popliteal vein segment, which was previously unaffected, can be considered diagnostic. For diagnosing recurrent DVT in a previously affected vein segment, an increase in thrombus diameter of at least 4 mm on serial CUS in combination with a D-dimer measurement can serve as helpful criteria. This diagnosis requires the expertise of an experienced radiologist with the previous ultrasound available for comparison. In practice, comparison with previous CUS is difficult, given the operator-dependent characteristics of the test. If comparison with the previous examination is equivocal or unavailable, CT or MR venography may be considered. An intraluminal filling defect suggests acute rather than remote thrombosis. Alternatively, a patient with initially equivocal CUS findings can undergo serial repeat examinations to detect DVT extension.

Treatment of Venous Thromboembolism
Anticoagulation Therapy for VTE

Patients with newly diagnosed VTE should be promptly initiated on therapeutic anticoagulation. In the absence of a severely symptomatic lower extremity, high thrombus burden pulmonary embolism with right ventricular dysfunction or significant cardiovascular comorbidity, management is predominantly outpatient. In the presence of PE, a simplified pulmonary embolism severity index (sPESI) is often used to assess appropriateness for outpatient therapy. The sPESI score includes the following factors (1 point each): age >80, history of cancer, chronic cardiopulmonary disease, pulse >110 beats/min, systolic blood pressure <100 mm Hg, arterial oxygen saturation <90%. Patients with a sPESI score ≥1 are considered "high risk" and should be considered for initial inpatient management.

Choice of Initial Anticoagulant Therapy

The choice of initial therapy is frequently guided by the clinical scenario. Initial therapy includes unfractionated heparin (UFH), low-molecular-weight heparin (LWMH), fondaparinux (Arixtra), or the direct oral anticoagulants rivaroxaban (Xarelto) or apixaban (Eliquis) (Table 4). Therapeutic UFH is administered intravenously (IV) and demonstrates complex pharmacokinetics (both hepatic and renal clearance) that requires laboratory monitoring of drug effect (aPTT or anti–factor Xa activity). Thus UFH therapy requires hospital admission and has largely been replaced by other options. UFH may still be appropriate for patients experiencing inpatient VTE events, especially if a need for invasive procedures is anticipated (half-life, 1–2 hours). The therapeutic target range for UFH is a 1.5- to 2.5-fold increase over the baseline aPTT or 0.3–0.7 U/mL anti–factor Xa activity. In contrast, LMWH is administered subcutaneously and primarily cleared by the kidneys, resulting in predictable pharmacokinetics. Subcutaneous administration facilitates outpatient treatment and predictable pharmacokinetics allow weight-based dosing without laboratory monitoring. Fondaparinux (synthetic pentasaccharide) is exclusively cleared by the kidneys with a long half-life (17–21 hours) that allows for once-daily, weight-adjusted subcutaneous dosing. Fondaparinux similarly does not require routine laboratory monitoring, but caution is warranted in patients with mild renal insufficiency where drug accumulation may increase bleeding risk. Heparin therapy (UFH, LWMH, or fondaparinux) for VTE is administered for a *minimum* of 5 days followed by transition to longer-term oral anticoagulation with an oral vitamin K antagonist (VKA) or a direct oral anticoagulant (DOAC). Alternatively, rivaroxaban or apixaban can be initiated immediately after VTE diagnosis and bypass the need for heparin therapy (see below).

Historically, vitamin K antagonists (VKA) are the primary oral anticoagulants for the long-term treatment of VTE. Warfarin (Coumadin) is the VKA used almost exclusively in the United States. Warfarin and other VKA inhibit vitamin K-dependent γ-carboxylation of the coagulation zymogens (proenzymes). This post-translational modification is required for both efficient protein secretion and function (membrane binding) of

	TABLE 4	Drugs for the Treatment of VTE		
DRUG	**DOSING**	**ELIMINATION**	**HALF-LIFE**	**MONITORING**
UFH	80 units/kg IV bolus, then 18 units/kg/hour initial infusion rate	Complex, hepatic/renal metabolism	1–2 hours	APTT Anti-FXa activity
LMWH	Dalteparin (Fragmin): 200 U/kg SQ QD Enoxaparin (Lovenox): 1 mg/kg SQ BID	Predominantly renal	3–5 hours	None required*
Fondaparinux (Arixtra)	5.0 mg SQ QD (<50 kg) 7.5 mg SQ QD (50–100 kg) 10 mg SQ QD (>100 kg)	Renal	17–21 hours	None required*
Warfarin (VKA) (Coumadin)	Initially 5 mg po QD, broad range (2.5–10 mg)	Extensive hepatic metabolism, Renal excretion for metabolites	Pharmacokinetics: 20–60 hrs, variable †Pharmacodynamics: 42–72 hours	PT/INR (2.0–3.0)
Dabigatran (Pradaxa)	Parenteral anticoagulant × 5-10 days, then dabigatran 150 mg po BID	>80% renal, 20% biliary Pro-drug	12–17 hours 14–17 hours (elderly)	None required
Rivaroxaban (Xarelto)	15 mg po BID × 21 days; then 20 mg po QD	66% renal, 33% biliary CYP450 substrate	5–9 hours 9–12 hours (elderly)	None required
Apixaban (Eliquis)	10 mg po BID × 7days, then 5 mg po BID	25% renal, 75% biliary CYP450 substrate	8–15 hours	None required
Edoxaban (Savaysa)	Parenteral anticoagulant × 5–10 days, then edoxaban 60 mg po QD (30 mg < 60 kg)	35% renal, 60% biliary	10–14 hours	None required
Betrixaban (Bevyxxa)‡	160 mg first dose, then 80 mg po QD for 35–42 days‡	11% renal 85% biliary	19–27 hours	None required

UFH, Unfractionated heparin; LMWH, low-molecular-weight heparin.
*Anti-FXa activity can be used in selected circumstances such as pregnancy and extremes of body weight (BW) (BW <45 kg or >100 kg).
†Pharmacodynamics of coagulation protein recovery most relevant to in vivo effect of VKA.
‡Betrixaban FDA approved for VTE prophylaxis only.

coagulation factors VII, IX, X, and II. Vitamin K is oxidized during γ-carboxylation of these coagulation factors, and warfarin inhibits enzymatic regeneration of the reduced form of vitamin K, creating a functional deficiency. This mechanism of action is the basis for (1) the reversibility of the warfarin by administration of the reduced form of vitamin K, (2) the reduction in warfarin effect by dietary vitamin K, and (3) the enhancement of the warfarin effect by many antibiotics, as bacterial flora are a major source of vitamin K. Warfarin also undergoes extensive metabolism by the liver, which provides multiple opportunities for drug interactions. Thus genetic variation in liver metabolism, variable dietary vitamin K intake, and numerous potential drug interactions generate substantial individual variation in warfarin dose requirements.

Warfarin (2.5- to 10-mg initial dose) is usually started the same day as heparin, overlapped with parenteral heparin therapy for a *minimum* of 5 days and discontinued once a therapeutic warfarin level is obtained on two consecutive days. The warfarin effect is monitored by the international normalized ratio (INR), which represents a prothrombin time (PT) that has been corrected for specific reagent sensitivity. The target INR for VTE treatment is 2.0 to 3.0. The pharmacodynamic effects of warfarin on the INR are primarily determined by the in vivo half-lives of the relevant coagulation factors. Thus the full effect of a warfarin dose change on the INR is usually not seen for 48 to 72 hours, correlating with the half-life of factors IX, X, and prothrombin (factor II). This delayed effect necessitates overlap with heparin therapy for at least 5 days, or longer if further warfarin dose titration is required to reach a therapeutic INR. Initial warfarin dosing should be conservative (2.5 mg daily) if enhanced sensitivity is expected, including patients that are elderly (>65 years old), low

body weight (<45 kg), hypoalbuminemic (<2 g/dL), on antibiotic therapy or have poor oral intake.

The traditional heparin-warfarin regimen has been increasingly supplanted by the use of direct oral anticoagulants (DOAC). DOACs are orally available, low-molecular-weight compounds that directly inhibit the active site of either factor Xa (rivaroxaban [Xarelto], apixaban [Eliquis], edoxaban [Savaysa]), or thrombin (dabigatran [Pradaxa]). In general, these drugs possess predictable pharmacokinetics and relatively short half-lives, allowing fixed once- or twice-daily oral dosing without routine monitoring. Both rivaroxaban and apixaban are approved for initial use after the VTE diagnosis with a more intensive dose regimen that tapers to the standard maintenance dose after 21 days for rivaroxaban or 7 days for apixaban (Table 4). Edoxaban and dabigatran are approved for continued treatment of VTE at their standard maintenance dose after 5 to 10 days of a parenteral anticoagulant (usually LWMH). Differences in clearance mechanisms have implications for clinical usage. For instance, dabigatran is heavily dependent on renal clearance and can accumulate with increased bleeding risk in patients with significant renal insufficiency (CrCl <30 mL/min). In contrast, apixaban dosing is less affected by renal insufficiency but should not be used in patients with significant liver dysfunction or biliary stasis.

Comparison of Warfarin Versus DOACs
DOACs demonstrate equivalent efficacy to the traditional combination of LMWH and warfarin in the treatment of VTE. Advantages of the DOACs include rapid onset of action, predictable dose response, no monitoring requirement, elimination of parenteral

TABLE 5	Reversal Agents		
DRUG	**REVERSAL AGENT**	**DOSING**	**COMMENTS**
Heparin	Protamine*	1–1.5 mg/100 U UFH IV	Hypersensitivity reactions, less effective vs. LMWH
Warfarin	4 factor PCC (Kcentra) FFP Vitamin K	25–50 U/kg IV 2–4 liters 1–10 mg oral or IV	Dose depends on INR, PCC favored over FFP Volume overload, Transf rxn Reversal takes 6–24 hours
Dabigatran	Idarucizumab (Praxbind)	2.5 g IV for 2 doses (within 15 min)	Drug specific monoclonal Fab fragment
Rivaroxaban Apixaban Edoxaban[1] Betrixaban[1]	Andexanet alfa (Andexxa)[1] 4 factor PCC[†]	800 mg IV bolus @ 30 mg/min, then 960 mg infusion @ 8 mg/min 50 U/kg IV	Reverses factor Xa active site inhibitors

*FDA approved for treatment of heparin overdose. Off-label uses: heparin neutralization (adults); intracranial hemorrhage associated with heparin or LMWH; LMWH overdose (adults).
[†]Evidence for reversal of factor Xa inhibitors by PCC is low quality.
[1]Not FDA approved for this indication.

therapy (rivaroxaban and apixaban), no significant diet interactions, limited drug interactions, and an overall safety signal equivalent to or better than warfarin. Meta-analysis of DOAC trials demonstrate that fatal bleeding, intracranial hemorrhage (ICH), and clinically relevant, non-major bleeding are reduced with DOACs compared to warfarin. The rate of GI bleeding was similar. Given the potentially life-changing nature of ICH, the lower rate with DOACs is particularly significant. Disadvantages of DOACs include cost, inability to monitor compliance with routine coagulation testing, the impact of renal function on drug clearance, and lack of widely available reversal agents. The relatively short half-lives of DOACs and recent development of reversal agents (Table 5) partially overcomes the reversibility advantage for warfarin. Largely based on safety profile and ease of use, recent guidelines provide a weak recommendation for DOACs over warfarin in patients without cancer.

Cancer-Associated Thrombosis

VTE associated with cancer accounts for ~20% of all cases and clearly is a heterogeneous patient population. Treatment of cancer-associated thrombosis is problematic in that patients are at increased risk for both VTE recurrence and bleeding complications. In addition to the multiple drug interactions that complicate VKA use in cancer patients, LMWH demonstrates significantly lower rates of recurrent VTE relative to VKA therapy. Thus LMWH for the first 6 months after the event has been the standard recommendation. The role of DOACs in cancer-associated thrombosis continues to evolve. Meta-analysis of subgroups from the large DOAC VTE trials demonstrates no difference in VTE recurrence or major bleeding compared with LMWH for primarily low-risk cancer patients. Subsequent comparison of edoxaban and dalteparin (Hokusai Trial) in a broader population of active cancer patients demonstrated a lower rate of VTE recurrence but higher rate of major bleeding. A randomized study comparing rivaroxaban to dalteparin (SELECT-D) demonstrated similar findings with reduced VTE rate and increased non-major bleeding in the DOAC arm. The increased bleeding was primarily observed in patients with upper GI or urothelial cancers in both studies. Ongoing studies will further address the role of DOACs in this setting. Duration of therapy is generally at least 6 months, but may be modified based on disease response, bleeding risk, and prognosis.

Special Considerations in the Acute Management of Venous Thromboembolism (VTE)

Although the vast majority of patients diagnosed with venous thromboembolism (VTE) should be promptly initiated on therapeutic anticoagulation, a limited number of acute presentations may require a modified approach. These presentations include the following:

Massive Pulmonary Embolism (PE) With Hemodynamic Instability

Patients presenting with hemodynamically unstable PE (SBP < 90 mmHg for 15 minutes, requiring vasopressors or overt shock) are at high risk for right heart failure and death. The focus for these patients should be resuscitation (IV fluids, pressors, oxygenation, and airway control) and rapid confirmation of diagnosis (perfusion scan or CT pulmonary angiography). If highly unstable, then bedside ECHO may be used for a presumptive diagnosis based on right ventricular findings. Prompt thrombolytic therapy (tPA [Activase] 100 mg IV) or consideration of emergency endovascular therapy should be pursued, with the former being more readily available.

Patients who present with worsening right heart failure, pre-resuscitation cardiopulmonary arrest, free-floating thrombus, or high thrombus burden in the absence of systemic hypotension may also be considered for thrombolytic therapy. Many institutions have a pulmonary embolism response team (PERT) to facilitate decision making and institution of therapy. However, for the majority of patients presenting with evidence of right ventricular dysfunction (by ECHO or CT) without systemic hypotension (i.e., "sub-massive" or intermediate risk PE), the use of thrombolytic therapy remains controversial. This controversy stems from both heterogeneity in patient selection for these trials and the inability to demonstrate long-term benefits over anticoagulation alone.

Broader use of thrombolytic therapy is primarily limited by the increased risk of major bleeding (9.2%) versus anticoagulation (3.4%), which includes a 1.5% incidence of intracranial bleeding. Contraindications include previous intracranial hemorrhage, known intracranial vascular lesion or malignancy, ischemic stroke within 3 months, suspected aortic dissection, active bleeding or bleeding diathesis, and closed head/facial trauma within 3 months. Relative contraindications include poorly controlled hypertension, recent surgery (14 days), and pregnancy. The use of combined modalities (catheter-based fibrinolysis, pharmacomechanical clot dissolution) and lower doses of tissue plasminogen activator (tPA 50 mg IV) may modulate the bleeding risk, but currently broader application of thrombolytic therapy remain controversial.

Extensive Proximal Vein Lower Extremity Thrombosis

Proximal iliac vein thrombosis is often highly symptomatic and may result in severe postthrombotic syndrome (PTS). Rarely, compromise of the arterial supply may occur, as described for phlegmasia alba dolens ("milk leg") and phlegmasia cerulea dolens. The former describes a swollen, white extremity with early compromise of arterial flow secondary to extensive DVT. The latter is an advanced stage characterized by severe swelling, cyanosis, and blue discoloration of the extremity—a precursor of venous gangrene. These entities are emergencies that require prompt anticoagulation, elevation, and consideration of endovascular intervention. The presence of bilateral proximal iliac vein thrombosis should prompt evaluation for IVC thrombus or agenesis, particularly in younger patients. Catheter-directed thrombolysis and endovascular approaches have been pursued in proximal iliofemoral venous thrombosis in an attempt to reduce the risk of severe PTS. Recent studies have been unable to demonstrate that the desired benefit in PTS reduction outweighs the increased risk of bleeding. Thus the routine use of thrombolytic therapy for proximal iliofemoral venous thrombosis cannot be recommended, and patient selection for this approach remains controversial.

Spontaneous Proximal Upper Extremity Thrombosis

The majority of upper extremity DVT is related to intravenous catheters, malignancy, or thrombophilia. Spontaneous upper extremity DVT in the absence of provocation is rare. This entity (Paget-Schroetter syndrome) tends to occur in a younger, often adolescent population with a recent history of exercise or strenuous activity usually involving the dominant upper extremity. This presentation in the absence of usual VTE risk factors should prompt an evaluation for venous thoracic outlet syndrome (TOS). Because of the younger age of these patients and significant disability associated with PTS in the upper extremity (particularly the dominant hand), the initial approach has included thrombolysis (within 14 days), anticoagulation, and evaluation for venous TOS. However, no rigorous comparison of these approaches or combinations of approaches has been undertaken. If evidence for venous TOS is demonstrated, first rib resection on the affected side is often recommended. In the absence of a predisposing anatomical abnormality, an underlying thrombophilic state or occult malignancy should be considered.

VTE Presenting With Paradoxical Embolism

The occurrence of arterial embolism, most commonly cryptogenic stroke, in the presence of DVT and a right-to-left shunt (i.e., patent foramen ovale or PFO) suggests the diagnosis of paradoxical embolus. Standard anticoagulation for VTE is recommended, followed by PFO closure when complete. If indefinite anticoagulation is planned, the additional benefit of PFO closure is unclear.

Acute Venous Thromboembolism With Contraindication to Anticoagulation

Occasional patients diagnosed with acute VTE will have an absolute contraindication to anticoagulation. Placement of a temporary IVC filter may be considered in these patients to provide short-term protection from PE. However, the vast majority of contraindications to anticoagulation are temporary and definitive anticoagulation therapy should be instituted as soon as feasible. IVC filter use is associated with increased risk of lower extremity DVT. Evaluation for IVC filter removal should be planned within 3 to 6 months, depending on the clinical scenario.

Isolated Subsegmental Pulmonary Embolism and Incidental VTE

The enhanced sensitivity of current CT scanners and extensive use of CT angiography has led to an increased diagnosis of isolated subsegmental PE. Treatment of isolated subsegmental PE (where proximal DVT has been excluded) is controversial as the natural history and benefit of anticoagulation is unclear. If an isolated subsegmental defect occurs in a clinical context that is high risk for recurrent VTE (e.g., malignancy), therapeutic anticoagulation is preferred. Alternatively, for an isolated subsegmental PE occurring in a patient that is otherwise low risk for VTE recurrence, clinical surveillance is preferred. Based on the frequency of diagnostic and staging CT scans in cancer patients, an incidental diagnosis of VTE is not an uncommon finding. Although outcome data are limited in this setting, incidental VTE appears to have similar effects on mortality and risk of VTE recurrence. Because the outcomes for incidental and symptomatic VTE in cancer patients appear similar, most cases of incidental VTE should be treated similar to symptomatic VTE.

Special Circumstances for Anticoagulant Monitoring

The predictable dose responses for LMWH, fondaparinux and the DOACs allow use without monitoring. However, select circumstances exist where monitoring may be desirable. LMWH is the preferred anticoagulant in pregnancy, but weight-based dosing may not be as accurate during pregnancy. Periodic confirmation of therapeutic target levels (0.5–1.2 U/mL anti–factor Xa activity) 4 hours after subcutaneous injection is often recommended. Likewise, the accuracy of weight-based LMWH dosing with a body weight <45 kg or >100 kg is not extensively validated. Confirmation of therapeutic peak levels in these individuals is recommended. Similarly, a need for DOAC drug levels may arise when assessing compliance, bleeding with potential drug overdose, or for an emergent procedure. DOACs directed against factor Xa (rivaroxaban, apixaban, and edoxaban) are monitored with an anti–factor Xa activity assay using a drug-specific standard curve. Significant dabigatran drug effect is excluded with a normal thrombin time. Alternatively, dabigatran drug effect can be detected by prolongation of the APTT or more specialized coagulation tests. The INR is not sensitive to dabigatran.

Reversal Agents

Acute reversal of anticoagulation may be required for drug overdose with clinically significant bleeding or emergent procedures. If the situation is non-emergent, holding warfarin (4–5 days depending on INR) or DOACs (2–3 days depending on renal function) is preferable. If urgent reversal is required, specific agents exist for UFH, warfarin, and, more recently, DOACs (Table 5). Although UFH overdose may be reversed with dose-adjusted protamine, the short half-life of UFH and potential toxicity of protamine often mitigate against use. Protamine[1] is most commonly used to reverse high-dose UFH after cardiopulmonary bypass. LMWH overdose may also be treated with protamine, but significantly less effectively. Warfarin is fully reversed by administration of 4 factor prothrombin complex concentrate (PCC) or fresh frozen plasma (FFP). The 4-factor PCC dose is modified based on the INR and favored over FFP, which may be complicated by volume overload and transfusion reactions. Immediate reversal with PCC or FFP should be followed with 5 to 10 vitamin K by the oral or IV route. Vitamin K takes 6 to 24 hours to act but is critical to maintaining anticoagulant reversal because the PCC or FFP effect will wane based on plasma half-life of the coagulation factors. Notably, high doses of vitamin K can result in relative warfarin resistance for the ensuing 1 to 2 weeks. Lower doses of vitamin K (1–2 mg) may be appropriate for less serious bleeding where early reinitiation of warfarin is anticipated. Highly specific agents for the reversal of DOACs are now available. Dabigatran is rapidly reversed by administration of idarucizumab (Praxbind), a humanized monoclonal Fab fragment that neutralizes the parent drug and major metabolites. DOACs targeting factor Xa (rivaroxaban, apixaban, edoxaban, betrixaban [Bevyxxa]) may be rapidly reversed with andexanet alfa (Andexxa), a truncated, inactive form of recombinant factor Xa that acts as a decoy for small molecules targeting the factor Xa active site. Andexanet alfa was approved for life-threatening bleeding in patients treated with rivaroxaban and apixaban based on an open label, single group study (ANNEXA-4). Given the relatively short half- lives of the DOACs, the high cost, and association with increased risk of thromboembolic events for andexanet alfa, it should be reserved for truly emergent procedures or life-threatening anticoagulant-related bleeding.

---

[1] Not FDA approved for this indication.

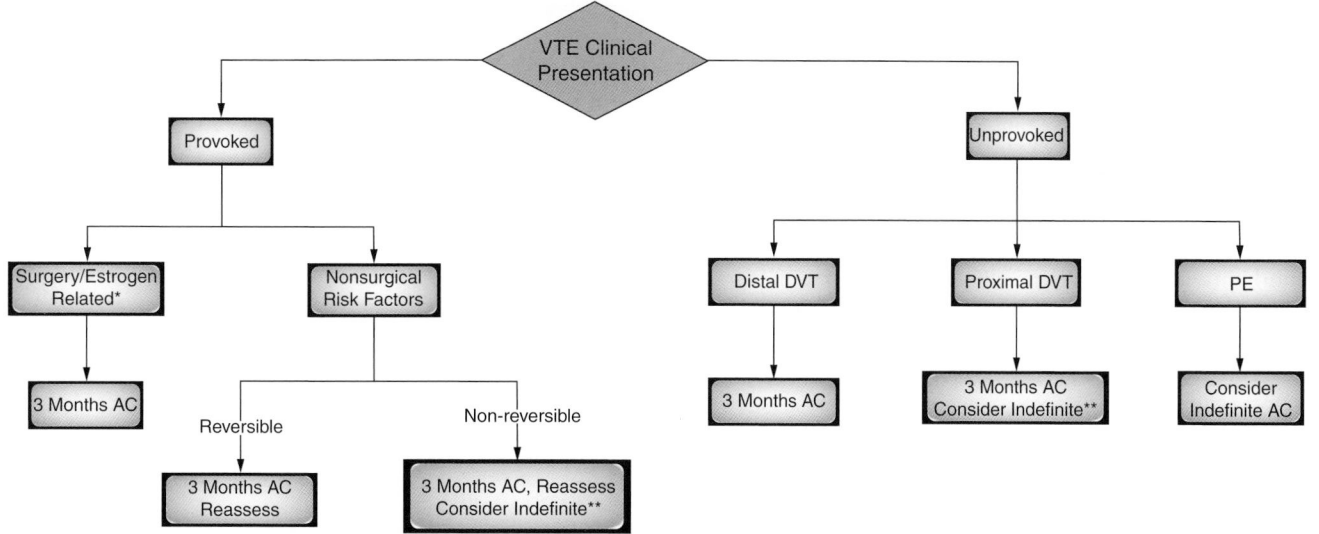

Figure 3 Suggested algorithm for treatment of VTE. AC = anticoagulation. *Estrogen- related includes oral contraceptives, hormone replacement therapy, pregnancy and puerperium. **Indefinite anticoagulation includes reduced dose DOAC options after initial 3 months therapeutic AC.

Duration of Anticoagulation

Standard treatment for a new episode of DVT or PE has traditionally been 3 to 6 months of therapeutic anticoagulation. The recommended duration of anticoagulation for VTE requires individualized analysis of the clinical presentation and patient specific factors that weigh both recurrence and bleeding risk (Figure 3).

Clinical Presentation

Recurrence risk varies widely based on clinical presentation (see Natural History). The key distinction is between events that occur in the absence (unprovoked) versus the presence (provoked) of established VTE risk factors (Table 1). The majority of cases with clinical risk factors present may be categorized as transient/reversible (e.g., surgery, estrogen) or permanent/nonreversible (e.g., dense hemiplegia secondary to stroke). Surgery is a major transient risk factor for VTE with a low recurrence risk (3% at 5 years). Three months of anticoagulation is sufficient for this population, while shorter durations are associated with increased risk of recurrence. Estrogen-related events have a similarly low risk of recurrence if re-exposure is avoided. A second category of VTE events occurs in association with a nonsurgical transient risk factor (leg injury, significant medical illness, travel-associated) and demonstrates an intermediate recurrence risk (15% at 5 years). This subgroup is substantially more heterogeneous than the surgical group, with a variety of triggering factors and broader recurrence risk estimates. VTE events associated with nonreversible clinical risk factors may require extended anticoagulation with periodic reassessment of risks and benefits. Unprovoked VTE demonstrates a high risk of recurrence (30% at 5 years) and, in many respects, behaves as a chronic disease. Finally, patients with an underlying malignancy represent ~20% of VTE cases but are usually excluded from natural history studies. Cancer-associated thrombosis demonstrates a 15% annualized recurrence risk with longer-term risk more difficult to estimate based on competing mortality from the underlying cancer. These patients have concomitant increased bleeding risk, complicating the risk–benefit analysis for anticoagulation.

Thrombus Site

Thrombus location significantly influences recurrence risk, with more proximal events demonstrating higher rates of recurrence. Patients with isolated distal or calf vein DVT are half as likely to have recurrent events compared to proximal DVT or PE. Patients presenting with proximal DVT have similar recurrence risk to patients with PE. However, patients initially presenting with PE are substantially more likely to have a PE recurrence relative to patients presenting with DVT only. This finding takes on particular importance when one considers the cause specific mortality rate associated with PE is greater than 10%. Thus patients presenting with unprovoked PE deserve particular attention with regard to consideration of indefinite anticoagulation.

Standard Versus Indefinite Anticoagulation

Clinical presentation categorizes patients with regard to recurrence risk, which is critical to the decision between standard (3 months) and indefinite anticoagulation (Figure 3). This decision is also influenced by bleeding risk and requires clinical judgment. As above, VTE associated with surgical or estrogen-related provoking factors and distal DVT (provoked or unprovoked) should be treated with therapeutic anticoagulation for 3 months. Conversely, most patients with unprovoked proximal DVT or PE should be considered for indefinite therapy based on their substantial recurrence risk, unless they also have high bleeding risk. There is little rationale for arbitrary extended periods of anticoagulation beyond the standard 3 to 6 months, unless awaiting resolution of a risk factor (e.g., extended immobilization). Prolongation of anticoagulation beyond 6 months in patients with unprovoked VTE delays but clearly does not prevent recurrence. A number of strategies, including postanticoagulation D-dimer testing (3–5 weeks) and risk stratification models, have attempted to identify patients with unprovoked VTE for which anticoagulation may be safely stopped. Post-anticoagulation D-dimer testing is the most established strategy, further stratifying these patients into high (8.8%) and low (3.0%) first-year recurrence rates. Conversely, the presence of persistent or multiple antiphospholipid antibodies increases recurrence risk (1.8- to 4.5-fold) for patients presenting with unprovoked VTE. Alternative approaches to risk reduction in unprovoked VTE include indefinite anticoagulation with reduced intensity DOACs or daily ASA. ASA reduces recurrence risk by ~1/3 in unprovoked VTE but is inferior to reduced dose rivaroxaban and apixaban (EINSTEIN CHOICE, AMPLIFY-EXT).

VTE associated with nonsurgical risk factors is more problematic with regard to definitive assessment of recurrence risk. Patients who suffer VTE with minor provocations may have a recurrence rate that approaches unprovoked VTE. These patients should be treated for at least 3 months and reassessed. Clinical factors that may impact a decision for indefinite anticoagulation include underlying cardiopulmonary disease (decreased ability to tolerate recurrence), ongoing inflammation (inflammatory bowel disease, autoimmune disease, chronic infections), prolonged immobilization (stroke), and male sex. For patients with a prolonged but ultimately reversible risk factor (i.e., stroke immobility improving with physical therapy), prolongation of anticoagulation until resolution of the underlying risk factor is reasonable. Similarly, travel-associated thrombosis may be a recurring risk that requires an intermittent prophylaxis plan. Bleeding risk assessment is important to decisions regarding recommended duration of therapy. Major risk factors for bleeding on anticoagulation include: advanced age, previous bleeding history, cancer, renal or liver failure, previous stroke, diabetes mellitus, nonsteroidal inflammatory drugs or antiplatelet therapy, comorbidity and reduced functional capacity, recent surgery, frequent falls, and alcohol (Table 6). Additional risk assessment tools (e.g., HAS-BLED score) exist, primarily validated for warfarin therapy.

Clinical Decision Making

Particularly for clinical situations with modest evidence, shared decision making between physician and patient is desirable in determining the duration of anticoagulant therapy. Medical comorbidities affecting bleeding or fall risk in the elderly, patient anxiety about recurrent VTE events, and occupational/lifestyle risks for trauma may substantially impact anticoagulation decisions. Family history should be obtained with particular attention to first-degree relatives affected by VTE, including unprovoked events and age of presentation. Questions regarding the underlying cause for a VTE event often drive requests for thrombophilia evaluations. These requests generally fail to acknowledge the complex, multigenic basis for VTE and rarely contribute to clinical decision making (see "Genetics of Venous Thromboembolism"). The clinical presentation and family history are substantially more useful than identification of minor thrombophilia traits, which are poor predictors of VTE recurrence. Finally, when a decision is made to pursue indefinite anticoagulation, periodic reassessment of this decision is important. The risk-to-benefit ratio of anticoagulation may change as the patient's medical history evolves. The hematology consultant serves an important role in facilitating difficult anticoagulation decisions.

Prevention of Venous Thromboembolism

About 60% of VTE events are associated with recent hospitalization or surgery, and up to 70% of these cases are preventable. However, less than half of hospitalized patients receive appropriate prophylactic measures. Given the significant morbidity and mortality associated with VTE, primary prophylaxis strategies in high-risk situations are of great medical importance and may provide a cost savings. Risk stratification of patients based on surgery or medical illness, patient characteristics (previous VTE, active cancer, duration of immobility, etc.), and bleeding risk impact recommendations for pharmacologic and mechanical prophylaxis. Pharmacologic agents include LMWH, fondaparinux, low-dose UFH, VKA, and DOACs. The focus in this section is primarily on heparin and DOACs given the available evidence. Mechanical prophylaxis includes graduated compression stockings (GCS) that are >15mm Hg at the ankle or intermittent pneumatic compression devices (IPCs). IPCs enhance lower extremity deep vein blood flow and may increase fibrinolytic activity. These modalities can be used alone or in combination for patients with high bleeding risk who cannot use pharmacologic prophylaxis. IPCs are considered more effective than GCS alone, particularly after orthopedic surgery.

General Surgery

For general surgery patients, well-established risk assessment tools such as the Caprini or Rogers scores stratify patients by VTE risk to identify those who would benefit from pharmacologic prophylaxis. In general, if the risk of VTE is moderate to high and bleeding risk is low, pharmacologic prophylaxis with

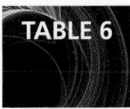

TABLE 6 Risk Factors for Bleeding With Anticoagulant Therapy and Estimated Risk of Major Bleeding in Low-, Moderate-, and High-Risk Categories

Risk Factors

Age >65 y

Previous bleeding

Cancer

Metastatic cancer

Renal failure

Liver failure

Thrombocytopenia

Previous stroke

Diabetes

Anaemia

Antiplatelet therapy

Poor anticoagulant control

Comorbidity and reduced functional capacity

Recent surgery

Frequent falls

Alcohol abuse

Nonsteroidal antiinflammatory drug

Categorization of Risk of Bleeding

	ESTIMATED ABSOLUTE RISK OF MAJOR BLEEDING		
	LOW RISK (0 RISK FACTORS)	MODERATE RISK (1 RISK FACTOR)	HIGH RISK (≥2 RISK FACTORS)
Anticoagulation 0–3 mo			
Baseline risk (%)	0.6	1.2	4.8
Increased risk (%)	1.0	2.0	8.0
Total risk (%)	1.6	3.2	12.8
Anticoagulation after first 3 mo			
Baseline risk (%/y)	0.3	0.6	≥2.5
Increased risk (%/y)	0.5	1.0	≥4.0
Total risk (%/y)	0.8	1.6	≥6.5

Data from the 9th Edition of the Antithrombotic Guideline (AT9).

LMWH or low-dose UFH should be given. If the bleeding risk is high, intermittent pneumatic compression with or without GCS should be used. Ideally, the minimal duration of prophylaxis is 5 to 10 days but varies widely based on duration of bed rest, inpatient stay, and comorbid conditions. In patients with active cancer undergoing abdominopelvic surgery, prophylaxis should be extended to 4 weeks after surgery.

Orthopedic Surgery

Orthopedic procedures are associated with high risk of VTE, especially those involving the lower extremities and pelvic region. For patients undergoing total hip or total knee arthroplasty, pharmacologic prophylaxis using LMWH, UFH, DOACs, or adjusted-dose warfarin should be used if no

TABLE 7	Risk Factor Stratification and Prophylaxis Options	
RISK STRATIFICATION	**RECOMMENDED PROPHYLAXIS**	**DURATION**
Low Risk		
Same-day surgery Medical illness in a fully mobile patient	Early mobilization	-
Moderate Risk		
Most general surgery procedures	LMWH UFH IPC/GCS with or without pharmacologic prophylaxis as appropriate	5–14 days
Most acute medical illnesses	LMWH UFH Betrixaban^	Duration of inpatient stay Extended duration beyond hospitalization may be appropriate for very-high-risk patients in whom bleeding risk is low
High Risk		
Hip or knee replacement surgery	LMWH UFH Fondaparinux Rivaroxaban Apixaban Dabigatran* Adjusted dose Warfarin	At least 10–14 days Extended duration up to 4 weeks preferred ASA may be used subsequently for extended duration of therapy
General surgery with active cancer, previous VTE	LMWH** UFH Adjusted dose Warfarin	Extended duration (4 weeks) for abdominopelvic surgeries in cancer patients
Major Trauma, Spinal cord injury	IPC with or without GCS, use pharmacologic prophylaxis when appropriate	

Abbreviations: DVT: deep venous thrombosis; GC: graduated compression; IPC: intermittent pneumatic compression; LMWH: low-molecular-weight heparin; UFH: unfractionated heparin; VTE: venous thromboembolism.
^^Usually started postoperatively and adjusted to achieve an international normalized ratio of 2.0–3.0
^FDA approved for patients hospitalized for acute medical illness at high risk of VTE
*FDA approved for VTE prevention after hip replacement surgery
**Off-label use in cancer patients

contraindication exists. LMWH is quite effective and safe with the benefit of long-term experience with these agents. Low-dose DOACs have shown comparable efficacy to enoxaparin in this population with a similar low absolute risk of bleeding. Low-dose apixaban (2.5 mg twice daily), rivaroxaban (10 mg daily), and dabigatran (150 mg daily) appear safer than higher doses. Prophylaxis should continue at least 10 to 14 days, and prolongation up to a month should be considered for major orthopedic surgery. Low-dose aspirin has been shown to be effective for extended prophylaxis after initial acute phase of therapy (~5 days) with standard anticoagulant in patients undergoing total hip or knee arthroplasty; however, anticoagulants are generally favored for high-risk patients. IPCs should be used during the inpatient stay in addition to pharmacologic prophylaxis. If bleeding risk is high, IPCs should be used until pharmacologic agents can be safely administered. For arthroscopic procedures of the knee and other low-risk procedures, prophylaxis is generally not indicated unless other risk factors exist. A summary of available agents and recommendations for prophylaxis is provided (Table 7).

Acute Medical Illness

For hospitalized patients with medical illnesses, the risk of VTE is ~8 fold higher than the general population. Patients expected to be hospitalized with reduced mobility >3 days, a previous history of VTE, active infection or malignancy, recent surgery or trauma, heart failure or respiratory failure should be considered for prophylaxis. The Padua score is a prospectively validated risk assessment model that stratifies patients into groups with high (~11%) or low (0.3%) incidence of VTE. Current prophylaxis options for medical patients include LMWH, low-dose UFH, and fondaparinux. When bleeding risk is considered moderate to high, mechanical prophylaxis using IPCs or GCS should be used until it is safe to add anticoagulants. For low-risk patients admitted for short duration or remaining ambulatory, withholding prophylaxis may be appropriate. Clinical context and bleeding risk assessment should also impact these decisions.

Although pharmacologic prophylaxis is typically limited to the acute illness during the inpatient stay, analysis of population-based data suggests that ~75% of VTE events occur well after discharge, at a median of almost 3 weeks. Furthermore, increased compliance with inpatient prophylaxis over time has not resulted in the expected decrease in the rate of VTE. The effect of extended DOAC prophylaxis (35–42 days) has been examined in medical patients for apixaban, rivaroxaban, and betrixaban. Reduced-dose apixaban and rivaroxaban demonstrated similar VTE prevention to standard enoxaparin prophylaxis but increased bleeding events. Evaluation of betrixaban in a select patient group (elevated D-dimer and elderly) demonstrated modestly better VTE prevention relative to enoxaparin, with an increase in nonmajor but not major bleeding. Extended prophylaxis is an area of ongoing investigation with unresolved issues that include appropriate patient selection and discerning the impact of specific anticoagulants versus prophylaxis duration on outcomes.

References

Chatterjee S, Chakraborty A, Weinberg I, Kadakia M, Wilensky RL, Sardar P, et al: Thrombolysis for pulmonary embolism and risk of all-cause mortality, major bleeding, and intracranial hemorrhage: a meta-analysis, *JAMA* 311(23):2414–2421, 2014.

Connors JM: Thrombophilia testing and venous thrombosis, *N Engl J Med* 377:1177–1187, 2017.

Heit JA, Crusan DJ, Ashrani AA, Petterson TM, Bailey KR: Effect of a near-universal hospitalization-based prophylaxis regimen on annual number of venous thromboembolism events in the US, *Blood* 130:109–114, 2017.

Kearon C, Akl EA, Ornelas J, Blaivas A, Jimenez D, Bounameaux H, et al: Antithrombotic therapy for VTE disease: CHEST Guideline and Expert Panel Report, *Chest* 149:315–352, 2016.

Kearon C, Parpia S, Spencer FA, Baglin T, Stevens SM, Bauer KA, et al: Antiphospholipid antibodies and recurrent thrombosis after a first unprovoked venous thromboembolism, *Blood* 131:2151–2160, 2018.

Konstantinides SV, Vicaut E, Danays T, Becattini C, Bertoletti L, Beyer-Westendorf J, et al: Impact of thrombolytic therapy on the long-term outcome of intermediate-risk pulmonary embolism, *J Am Coll Cardiol* 69:1536–1544, 2017.

Raskob GE, van Es N, Verhamme P, Carrier M, Di Nisio M, Garcia D, et al: Edoxaban for the treatment of cancer-associated venous thromboembolism, *N Engl J Med* 378:615–624, 2018.

Vedantham S, Goldhaber SZ, Julian JA, Kahn SR, Jaff MR, Cohen DJ, et al: Pharmacomechanical catheter-directed thrombolysis for deep-vein thrombosis, *N Engl J Med* 377:2240–2252, 2017.

Weitz JI, Lensing AWA, Prins MH, Bauersachs R, Beyer-Westendorf J, Bounameaux H, et al: Rivaroxaban or aspirin for extended treatment of venous thromboembolism, *N Engl J Med* 376:1211–1222, 2017.

Zoller B, Ohlsson H, Sundquist J, Sundquist K: A sibling based design to quantify genetic and shared environmental effects of venous thromboembolism in Sweden, *Thromb Res* 149:82–87, 2017.

VIRAL AND MYCOPLASMAL PNEUMONIAS

Method of
Cheston B. Cunha, MD; and Burke A. Cunha, MD

 CURRENT DIAGNOSIS

Influenza (human, avian, swine)
- Mild influenza A or B presents acutely with headache, fever, sore throat, plus/minus rhinorrhea.
- Severe influenza A presents with an acute onset (patients often able to name the hour the influenza began) and rapidly become bed bound.
- Headache, myalgias, and prostration may be severe.
- With swine influenza, gastrointestinal symptoms (e.g., nausea/vomiting or diarrhea) may be prominent.
- Auscultation of the lungs is quiet, disproportionate to the degree of respiratory distress. Influenza is an interstitial process and not alveolar, which explains the absence of rales.
- With severe influenza, patients rapidly become hypoxemic. Hypoxemia is accompanied by an A-a gradient >35, which indicates a interstitial oxygen diffusing defect.
- Severe tracheobronchitis is common and manifested by hemoptysis.
- Relative lymphopenia with monocytosis occurs early followed by thrombocytopenia and later leukopenia. Low titer elevations of cold agglutinins are not infrequent (≥1:18).
- Patients may have chest pain exacerbated by breathing mimicking pleuritic chest pain. This is the result of direct intracostal muscle involvement with the influenza virus, which results in myositis and pain on inspiration.
- The chest radiograph in early influenza in mild to moderate cases is normal or near normal, with minimal, if any, increase in interstitial markings. The chest radiograph in fulminant cases shows symmetrical bilateral patchy infiltrates without pleural effusion in 48 hours.
- Severe influenza A is accompanied by severe hypoxemia cyanosis, and may be followed by an early fatal outcome.
- Influenza pneumonia most often presents alone without bacterial superinfection, but bacterial infection may accompany (e.g., MSSA/CA-MRSA) or follow influenza (e.g., *S. pneumoniae* or *H. influenzae*).
- Purulent sputum with influenza indicates concurrent bacterial pneumonia usually caused by *S. aureus* (methicillin-susceptible *Staphylococcus aureus* [MSSA]/methicillin-resistant *Staphylococcus aureus* [MRSA]). Bacterial pneumonia following influenza (after 1–2 weeks), is suggested by leukocytosis, focal or segmental pulmonary infiltrates, and purulent sputum; the pathogens are not *S. aureus,* but most commonly are *S. pneumoniae* or *H. influenzae.*
- A laboratory diagnosis may be made by multiplex polymerase chain reaction (PCR) of respiratory secretions.

COVID-19
- COVID-19 is caused by a novel β-coronavirus (different than the novel β-coronaviruses causing severe acute respiratory syndrome [SARS] and Middle East respiratory syndrome [MERS]) identified as SARS-CoV-2.
- Common nonspecific laboratory abnormalities include leukopenia, relative lymphopenia, thrombocytopenia, and mildly elevated serum transaminases.
- Chest x-ray (CXR) early resembles that of influenza pneumonia (i.e., essentially unremarkable, without definite/discreet infiltrates).
- As COVID-19 pneumonia progresses, the CXR shows bilateral interstitial fuzzy/fluffy peripheral infiltrates.

- Chest computed tomography (CT) scans may show bilateral peripheral infiltrates with or without consolidation.
- Diagnosis of COVID-19 is by reverse transcription PCR (RT-PCR) of respiratory tract specimens or antigen testing. RT-PCR usually becomes positive early in the disease course (days).
- COVID-19 seems to preferentially affect adults, with relative sparing of young children. Elderly patients with advanced lung/cardiac disease are particularly predisposed to severe disease/complications.

Mycoplasma pneumoniae
- In a patient with community-acquired pneumonia (CAP) who has a dry, nonproductive cough without severe headache or myalgias, the most likely diagnosis is *M. pneumoniae. M. pneumoniae* CAP is commonly accompanied by nonexudative pharyngitis and/or loose stools or watery diarrhea.
- The temperature is usually less than 102°F (38.9°C) and is not accompanied by frank rigors or pleuritic chest pain.
- Relative bradycardia and elevations in the serum transaminases are not features of *M. pneumoniae* CAP.
- Respiratory viruses are often associated with mild elevations of cold agglutinins (≤1:16) but *M. pneumoniae* is the only pathogen causing CAP associated with highly elevated cold agglutinin titers (≥1:64). Elevated cold agglutinin titers occur in up to 75% of patients with *M. pneumoniae*, and occur early and transiently.
- In a patient with CAP, elevated cold agglutinin titers (>1:8) effectively rule out the typical pathogens, as well as *Legionella* species and *C. pneumoniae.*
- Elevated *M. pneumoniae* ELISA IgG titers indicate past exposure/infection and not current infection or co-infection with another pathogen.
- In the absence of an antecedent respiratory tract infection (e.g., nonexudative pharyngitis, otitis, etc., in the preceding 3 months), the presence of an increased *M. pneumoniae* ELISA IgM titer is diagnostic of acute infection.

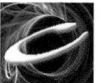 **CURRENT THERAPY**

Viral Influenza
- The aim of therapy is to inhibit the influenza virus and prevent its attachment/spread to uninfected respiratory epithelial cells.
- The neuramidase inhibitors shorten the course of influenza by 1 to 2 days and have antiviral activity. These agents are active against both influenza A and B.
- Most strains of human and avian flu, but not swine flu, are resistant to amantadine (Symmetrel) or rimantadine (Flumadine).
- Amantadine and rimantadine may have an important therapeutic effect in severe influenza A by increasing distal airway dilation and increasing oxygen action.
- Peramivir (Rapivab) may be useful in those unable to take oral neuraminase inhibitors.

COVID-19
- Effective therapy for hospitalized patients with COVID-19 pneumonia is with remdesivir (Veklury) 200 mg (IV) for the first dose, then 100 mg (IV) q24h for 5 to 10 days.
- Dexamethasone[1] 6 mg IV/ PO daily for 10 days should be considered in patients who are hospitalized and require supplemental oxygen.

Mycoplasma pneumoniae
- The agents active against *M. pneumoniae* are macrolides, tetracyclines, quinolones, and ketolides. β-Lactam antibiotics are not active against *M. pneumoniae* because it does not contain a bacterial cell wall.

- Goals of therapy of *M. pneumoniae* CAP are to eradicate the infection, decrease the shedding of *M. pneumoniae* in respiratory secretions posttherapy, and to prevent post-treatment asthma.
- Therapy is equally efficacious with macrolides, doxycycline (Vibramycin), or a respiratory quinolone intravenously, orally, or in combination for 1 to 2 weeks.
- The mode of administration is determined by the severity of the CAP and the setting. Outpatients are usually treated orally. Patients hospitalized with severe CAP are initially treated intravenously and then changed to an oral agent.
- Macrolide resistance to *M. pneumoniae* has been described in children and reported in adults.

---

[1]Not FDA approved for this indication.

Influenza pneumonia is the most important cause of viral pneumonia in adults. Influenza A is the predominant type of influenza found in adults, and influenza B is more common in children. Influenza A has the potential for severe disease, occurs seasonally, and is the predominant type involved in influenza pandemics. *M. pneumoniae* CAP was first recognized decades ago as distinctive from bacterial and viral pneumonias. It was originally described by Eaton as "Eaton agent" pneumonia caused by a pleuropneumonia-like organism (PPLO), later shown to be caused by *M. pneumoniae*. *M. pneumoniae* is a common cause of pneumonia in all age groups, but the peak incidence of *M. pneumoniae* CAP is in young adults. *M. pneumoniae* CAP is a common cause of ambulatory CAP.

The term *atypical pneumonia* was first applied to viral pneumonias because the clinical laboratory and radiologic findings were different from those caused by typical bacterial pulmonary pathogens. In influenza pneumonia, the clinical findings are confined to the trachea, bronchi, lung parenchyma, and central nervous system. *M. pneumoniae* CAP is a systemic infection with a pulmonary component. Over the years, atypical pneumonia has come to refer to pneumonia caused by systemic nonviral/nonbacterial pathogen agents that have a pulmonary component. Viral pneumonias are no longer considered atypical pneumonias. Atypical pneumonias may be divided into nonzoonotic and zoonotic atypical CAPs. Nonzoonotic CAPs are most commonly caused by *M. pneumoniae*, *Chlamydia pneumoniae*, or *Legionella* species, whereas the three most common zoonotic atypical pneumonias are caused by *Chlamydia psittaci* (psittacosis), *Francisella tularensis* (tularemia), or *Coxiella burnetii* (Q fever). All of the atypical pneumonias are distinct clinical entities that may be differentiated on the basis of their characteristic pattern of extrapulmonary organ involvement. Although some viruses may occasionally have extrapulmonary manifestations (i.e., influenza, adenovirus with viral pneumonias), the primary clinical features are confined to the lungs. *M. pneumoniae* is a critical cause of nonzoonotic atypical CAP, particularly in the ambulatory setting. *M. pneumoniae* CAP may be severe in patients with impaired host defenses or those with severe, preexisting cardiopulmonary disease.

Influenza (Human, Avian, and Swine)
Viral influenza pneumonia affects children and adults. Influenza B is the primary cause of mild influenza in children and adults. Influenza A is primarily an infection of adults that may be mild to severe. Influenza A has the potential for pandemic spread (e.g., swine influenza [H_1N_1]).

Influenza occurs during the winter months, usually peaking in February. Influenza is spread by aerosolized droplet infection from person to person and via fomites. Influenza A is classified into subtypes based on hemagglutinin (H) and neuramidase (N) surface proteins. An important characteristic of the influenza A virus is antigenic drift, which refers to minor changes in surface protein shift in the neuramidase or hemagglutinin receptors. With influenza A, these surface receptor proteins are important in cellular adherence of the influenza virus and spread of influenza

from respiratory epithelial cells. The vaccine for the flu season most often includes the influenza hemagglutinin and neuramidase types seen at the end of the preceding year's season. Prevention of attachment and spread of the virus is helpful in controlling the spread of influenza; vaccine protection conferred by specific antibody response to influenza A is highly protective (approximately 80% in noncompromised hosts).

During the years when influenza B has been prevalent, vaccines for the subsequent year contain an influenza B component.

Clinical manifestations of influenza A in adults varies considerably from mild to fatal infection. Mild infection is usually manifested as an acute febrile illness characterized by headache and myalgias with dry, unproductive cough and rhinorrhea. Mild influenza may be caused by influenza A or B and usually resolves in a few days without complications in normal hosts who have good cardiopulmonary function.

Severe influenza A (human, avian, swine) occurs in normal healthy adults and may be fatal. The onset of severe influenza A (human, avian, swine) is sudden, and the patient often recalls the exact hour of onset. The patient is febrile, with early/extreme prostration rendering the patient bedridden. Fever rapidly rises and may be accompanied by chills. Neck soreness, severe headache, and myalgias are typical. Sore throat, eye pain, conjunctival injection, and hemoptysis are frequently present. Chest pain worsened by deep inspiration is not truly pleuritic but rather reflects influenza A myositis of the intracostal muscles. Shortness of breath is related to the degree of hypoxemia. Severe influenza A causes an oxygen diffusion defect as manifested by an increased A-a gradient (>35). Profound hypoxemia may be accompanied by cyanosis. Hypotension caused by hypoxemia and vascular collapse may follow. The course of fulminant viral influenza A is of short duration.

Physical findings are few in viral influenza (i.e., conjunctival suffusion). Auscultation reveals absolutely quiet lungs because the infectious process is interstitial and not alveolar. Routine blood tests are usually unremarkable except for leukopenia, relative lymphopenia, and thrombocytopenia. Atypical lymphocytes are not present, but low titers of cold agglutinins may be present. Cold agglutinins (if present) have titers less than or equal to 1:18. In fatal cases, a pale blue hue of the skin may be noted, and there may be bleeding from multiple orifices before death. The chest radiograph in uncomplicated influenza A is unremarkable, with minimal perihilar bilateral increased prominence of interstitial markings possible. In severe influenza A pneumonia, the chest radiograph shows bilateral symmetrical perihilar infiltrates without pleural effusions in <48 hours.

Patients may die from severe influenza A without superimposed bacterial pneumonia. Most deaths during the 1918–1919 pandemic were young military recruits who died of influenza A pneumonia without bacterial pneumonia. Influenza may be complicated by bacterial pneumonia. Bacterial pneumonias complicating influenza may occur concurrently at presentation or may occur after an interval of improvement 1 to 2 weeks after the presentation of influenza. Influenza A presenting concurrently with bacterial pneumonia is caused by *Staphylococcus aureus*. In contrast to influenza alone, MSSA/CA-MRSA is manifested by an increase in fever, shaking chills, leukocytosis, purulent sputum, localized rales on auscultation, bacteremia, and focal/segmental infiltrates on chest radiograph that rapidly cavitate in less than 72 hours. Alternatively, patients with influenza A may develop a secondary bacterial infection 1 to 2 weeks later. Secondary bacterial pneumonia is less severe and is usually caused by *Streptococcus pneumoniae* or *Haemophilus influenzae*.

Viral influenza-like illnesses (ILIs) most often present during the winter months or influenza season. For clinical and therapeutic purposes, it is important to differentiate influenza A from viral ILIs in hospitalized adults. Some clinical features may point to a specific ILI viral etiology, but a specific viral diagnosis can be made by viral respiratory PCR of nasopharyngeal swab specimens. The only viral ILI likely to mimic influenza A presenting with a fulminant severe viral CAP is MERS. The mimics of ILIs are presented (Table 1). The main nonviral mimic of influenza A in hospitalized adults is Legionnaire's disease (LD). LD may be differentiated from influenza A and other viral ILIs by CXR findings and characteristic nonspecific laboratory tests. With LD CAP, the CXR shows one or more nonfocal infiltrates. Fever, usually greater than 102° F, is accompanied by relative bradycardia. With LD, the ESR is highly elevated (>90 mm/h), the ferritin is highly elevated (>2 times normal), and the serum phosphorus is decreased early, as is serum sodium. Although an elevated CPK and mild transaminitis often accompany LD, these findings are not uncommon in influenza A and some viral ILIs. There are few infections that may mimic the dry, productive cough of *M. pneumoniae* CAP. Pertussis is most likely to mimic mycoplasma. Pertussis, unlike mycoplasma, is not accompanied by watery diarrhea. The distinguishing laboratory feature of *M. pneumoniae* CAP is elevated cold agglutinins not found with pertussis. The key non-specific laboratory finding in pertussis is marked lymphocytosis (Table 2).

COVID-19 emerged from Wuhan, China in 2019 and spread worldwide early in 2020, resulting in a pandemic.

TABLE 1	Mimics of Influenza A in Hospitalized Adults Presenting with Influenza-like Illnesses (ILIs)		
INFLUENZA-LIKE ILLNESSES (ILIS)	**CHEST FILM FEATURES**		**CLINICAL CLUES**
MERS	Ill-defined infiltrates (early) Bilateral dense interstitial nodular infiltrates (late) Severe cases often develop ARDS		Recent travel to Middle East or contact with MERS case Dry cough and sore throat Hemoptysis (in some) Diarrhea (common) WBC count normal, thrombocytopenia Elevated LDH
COVID-19	CXR: Ill-defined infiltrates (early) Bilateral, peripheral dense interstitial infiltrates. Severe cases often develop ARDS		Fever and dry cough Diarrhea (common) Myocarditis (late, in some) ARDS (in some) Leukopenia Relative lymphopenia Thrombocytopenia Mildly elevated serum Transaminases (early) Elevated CPK (in some) Elevated D-dimer may herald coagulopathy
RSV	Clear CXR (early) Bilateral ill-defined infiltrates on CXR (late) Chest CT: GGO (non-specific)		Antecedent/concurrent rhinorrhea Hoarseness Lymphocyte/monocyte ratio >2
HPIV-3	Clear CXR (early) Bilateral ill-defined infiltrates on CXR (late)		Hoarseness Prolonged lymphocyte/monocyte ratio <2 Monocytosis
EV-D86	Clear CXR (early) Bilateral ill-defined infiltrates on CXR (late)		Diarrhea (common) Flaccid paralysis
Legionnaire's disease	Rapidly progressive, asymmetric, ill-defined infiltrates on CXR Consolidation and small pleural effusions (common) Cavitation (rare)		High fevers (>102 °F) Highly elevated ESR (>90 mm/h) Ferritin (>2 xn) Leukocytosis with relative lymphopenia Elevated CPK (in some) Mild transient elevated transaminases common (early) Microscopic hematuria (early)

Abbreviations: MERS = Middle East respiratory syndrome; COVID-19: Coronavirus disease; RSV = respiratory syncytial virus; HPIV = human parainfluenza virus; EV = enterovirus; GGO = ground gloss opacity; CXR = chest x-ray; ARDS = acute respiratory distress syndrome.

TABLE 2	Mimics of Mycoplasma pneumoniae in Community Acquired Pneumonia (CAP) Hospitalized Adults		
MYCOPLASMA CAP MIMICS	**CHEST FILM FEATURES**		**CLINICAL CLUES**
C. pneumoniae	Ill-defined lower lobe infiltrates (often ovoid) No consolidation, cavitation or effusion		No seasonal predisposition Hoarseness Protracted dry cough Mycoplasma-like illness that doesn't respond to erythromycin Wheezing (in some) No diarrhea No cold agglutinins Rhinorrhea proceeds dry cough (1–2 weeks)
Pertussis	Perihilar illdefined infiltrates ("shaggy heart" sign) No consolidation, cavitation or effusions		Protracted dry cough Persistent cough (without typical "whoop" of children) Afebrile or minimal fevers Marked lymphocytes (> 60%) No cold agglutinins

COVID-19 is caused by a novel β-coronavirus (different than the novel β-coronaviruses causing SARS and MERS) identified as SARS-CoV-2. SARS-CoV-2 is thought to have been contracted from wild animals in food markets. COVID-19 spreads rapidly via airborne transmission, and may be spread from asymptomatic individuals.

Patients most commonly present with fever, headache, sore throat, dry cough, shortness of breath, and diarrhea (in some).

Clinically, the spectrum of COVID-19 ranges from asymptomatic cases to symptomatic cases. Symptomatic COVID-19 most often presents as a mild ILI; in more severe cases, it presents as a viral pneumonia (not unlike influenza pneumonia). Severe COVID-19 pneumonias have severe hypoxemia caused by an oxygen diffusion defect (high A-a gradient). Fatal cases are due to ARDS and/or myocarditis. Common nonspecific laboratory abnormalities include leukopenia, relative lymphopenia, thrombocytopenia, and mildly elevated serum transaminases. Serum LDH or CPK are often elevated. Elevated D-dimers also present frequently and may herald a subsequent coagulopathy.

Early CXR resembles that of influenza pneumonia (i.e., essentially unremarkable without definite/discrete infiltrates). As COVID-19 pneumonia progresses, the CXR shows bilateral Interstitial peripheral infiltrates. CXR demonstrates no/small bibasilar effusions. Chest CT scans may show bilateral nodular infiltrates with or without consolidation. Cavitation is not a feature of COVID-19 pneumonia. Co-infection or superinfection is a rare occurrence in COVID-19.

Diagnosis of COVID-19 is by RT-PCR of respiratory tract specimens. A positive RT-PCR result may be present early in the disease course, although it may not become positive for a few days. If clinical suspicion is high, serial testing may reveal RT-PCR + after 2 to 3 repeat tests. The RT-PCR should not be used as a test of cure. RT-PCR + may persist for 1 to 2 weeks after clinical recovery, although transmission should not occur during this time period. Antibody testing may become positive after several weeks.

COVID-19 seems to preferentially affect adults, with relative sparing of young children. Elderly patients with advanced lung/cardiac disease are particularly predisposed to severe disease/complications.

Anti-Influenza Therapy

Therapy of viral influenza is directed at inhibiting viral replication and preventing further infection of respiratory epithelial cells. The neuramidase inhibitors zanamivir (Relenza), oseltamivir (Tamiflu), and peramivir (Rapivab) have anti-influenza A and B activity. Neuramidase inhibitors decrease the severity and duration of influenza symptoms by 1 to 2 days. Current flu strains are resistant to amantadine and rimantadine, but these drugs may still be useful to increase peripheral airway dilation and oxygenation, which may be of critical importance in severe influenza A with severe hypoxemia. Mild influenza A/B may be treated with neuramidase inhibitors. Mild cases of influenza A should be treated at the onset of the illness. For severe influenza A, neuramidase inhibitors provide optimal anti-influenza therapy (Table 3). For human and avian influenza (H_5N_1), these antiviral drugs may be ineffective, but are effective against swine influenza.

COVID-19 Therapy

At the time of writing, optimal therapy of COVID-19 continues to evolve. Effective therapy for hospitalized patients with COVID-19 pneumonia who require oxygen is remdesivir (Veklury) 200 mg (IV) for the first does, then 100 mg (IV) q24h for 5 to 10 days. Monoclonal antibodies continue to be studied, but seem to reduce rate of hospitalization, particularly in high risk patients. Dexamethasone has a role in limiting mortality in patients admitted with COVID-19 who require supplemental oxygen. Interlukin inhibitors (IL-6 in particular) may have a role in select patients with COVID-19. Vaccines have begun to play a critical role in prevention of COVID-19, although the increasing number of genetic variants may blunt the effectiveness of existing vaccines.

Mycoplasma Pneumoniae

M. pneumoniae is a common cause of ambulatory CAP. It affects all age groups, and in normal hosts with intact cardiopulmonary function, *M. pneumoniae* CAP is usually a mild, self-limiting infection. However, *M. pneumoniae* derives its importance from difficulty in diagnosis, the necessity for non–β-lactam therapy, and because of its effect on peripheral airways.

M. pneumoniae CAP is one of the nonzoonotic causes of CAP (the others being *Legionella* and *Chlamydia pneumoniae*). *M. pneumoniae* is an atypical pneumonia that is a systemic infectious disease with a pulmonary component. It may be distinguished from other atypical pneumonias by its characteristic pattern of extrapulmonary organ involvement. *M. pneumoniae* CAP most closely resembles *C. pneumoniae* CAP clinically, but is very different from LD in terms of its epidemiology, age distribution, pattern of extrapulmonary organ involvement, and severity.

Clinically, *M. pneumoniae* presents as a subacute febrile illness. Temperatures rarely exceed 102°F (38.9°C). Rigors are not a feature of *M. pneumoniae* CAP, but patients may complain of chilly sensations. Mild headache and/or myalgias are not uncommon. The most common presenting symptom in *M. pneumoniae* CAP is the prolonged, nonproductive, dry cough. Patients with *M. pneumoniae* CAP often complain of or have mild nonexudative pharyngitis. Rhinorrhea and conjunctivitis are not features of *M. pneumoniae* CAP. Watery diarrhea is commonly present in *M. pneumoniae* CAP, but abdominal pain is not a clinical finding. Other extrapulmonary manifestations are uncommon or rare (e.g., meningoencephalitis, pericarditis, hemolytic anemia, glomerular nephritis, Guillain-Barré syndrome, erythema multiforme). *M. pneumoniae* has a distinctive pattern of extrapulmonary organ involvement that does not include cardiac involvement (relative bradycardia) or hepatic involvement, including normal serum glutamate-oxaloacetate transaminase (SGOT) or serum glutamate-pyruvate transaminase (SGPT). The distinguishing laboratory feature of *M. pneumoniae* CAP is elevated cold agglutinin titers. Although a variety of infectious and noninfectious diseases are associated with cold agglutinin elevations, they are usually of low titer (i.e., <1:16). There are no pulmonary infections presenting as CAP that are associated with high elevations of cold agglutinin titers (i.e., ≥1:64). Although elevated cold agglutinins occur early in up to 75% of patients with *M. pneumoniae* CAP, they are still diagnostically important when present. In a patient with CAP and a cold agglutinin titer greater than or equal to 1:64, the diagnosis of *M. pneumoniae* CAP is very likely.

M. pneumoniae may be differentiated from the typical bacterial pneumonias because of the presence of extrapulmonary findings, including nonexudative pharyngitis, loose stools or watery diarrhea, erythema multiforme, and high cold agglutinin. Patients with typical bacterial CAP usually have a more acute onset of presentation, a productive cough, and temperatures that may exceed 102°F (38.9°C), often accompanied by chills. Patients with typical pneumonia often have pleuritic chest pain, which is not a feature of *M. pneumoniae* CAP. Among the atypical pneumonias, the zoonotic pneumonias (i.e., tularemia, psittacosis, Q fever) may be eliminated from consideration if there is a recent zoonotic contact history with the appropriate vector.

C. pneumoniae CAP resembles closely *M. pneumoniae* CAP. *C. pneumoniae* may be distinguished by the absence of cold agglutinins and the presence of hoarseness, which is a feature of *C. pneumoniae* CAP but not *M. pneumoniae* CAP. Loose stools or watery diarrhea are not usual features of *C. pneumoniae* CAP. The most common clinical problem is differentiating *Legionella* from *Mycoplasma* CAP; this may be done by appreciating the differences in the pattern of extrapulmonary organ involvement with each of these pathogens. *Legionella* may be clinically differentiated from *Mycoplasma* by acuteness of onset or severity, the presence of relative bradycardia, temperatures greater than 102°F (38.9°C), and the presence of abdominal pain. From a laboratory standpoint, highly elevated cold agglutinin titers argue strongly against the diagnosis of *Legionella* and point to *M. pneumoniae*. Nonspecific laboratory tests in a patient with CAP that suggest *Legionella* and argue against *M. pneumoniae* include otherwise unexplained hypophosphatemia, hyponatremia, microscopic hematuria, and increased creatinine. *Legionella* does not affect the upper respiratory tract as does *Mycoplasma* (e.g., nonexudative pharyngitis). Ear findings are not a feature of Legionnaires' disease but are common in *M. pneumoniae* CAP. The finding most likely to cause confusion between *M. pneumoniae* and *Legionella pneumophila* is the presence of loose stools or watery diarrhea, which is found in both.

M. pneumoniae may be cultured from the throat in viral culture media, but the diagnosis is usually made serologically. An elevated enzyme-linked immunosorbent assay (ELISA) or enzyme immunoassay (EIA) IgM titer suggests acute or recent infection, but an elevated IgG titer indicates past exposure but not acute infection. Elevated IgG titers regardless of degree of elevation are not diagnostic of current infection with *M. pneumoniae* and only indicate previous antigenic exposure. *M. pneumoniae* ELISA IgM levels may take up to 3 months to decrease. Therefore, clinicians should take into account recent antecedent respiratory illness to properly interpret elevated IgM titers, including patients with nonexudative pharyngitis within 3 months prior to the presentation of CAP. The combination of an increased *M. pneumoniae* IgM titer and highly elevated cold agglutinin titers is virtually diagnostic of acute infection. Cold agglutinin titers are elevated transiently early and rapidly fall; the simultaneously elevated cold agglutinins and IgM titers of *M. pneumoniae* indicate active or current infection. In patients with CAP caused by another organism (e.g., *S. pneumoniae*), the presence of elevated *Mycoplasma* IgG titers does not indicate co-infection but only preexisting serologic exposure to *M. pneumoniae*.

M. pneumoniae Therapy

M. pneumoniae has a predilection for the respiratory epithelial cells and resides on their surface. Mycoplasmas have no definite cell wall like the typical pathogens causing CAP. Their position on the surface of the respiratory epithelium and their absence of a cell wall necessitates the therapeutic approach, which includes non–β-lactam antibiotics with the capacity to penetrate into the *Mycoplasma* organisms. Traditionally, macrolides and tetracyclines have been used successfully to treat *M. pneumoniae*. Both tetracyclines and macrolides are effective against *Mycoplasma* because they interfere with intracellular protein synthesis at the ribosomal level. Tetracyclines penetrate intracellularly better than macrolides, with the exception of penetration into the alveolar macrophage, which is relevant in *Legionella* but not *M. pneumoniae* infections. Macrolides and tetracyclines are both active against *Mycoplasma*. Patients treated with macrolides or tetracyclines defervesce rapidly over 24 to 48 hours. Clinical defervescence manifests by an increased feeling of well-being and a decrease in fever. The dry cough persists during and after therapy regardless of the anti-*Mycoplasma* antimicrobial used.

There are important differences in the shedding rates of *Mycoplasma* from respiratory epithelial cells posttherapy when using tetracyclines instead of macrolides. Tetracycline therapy is associated with a more rapid decrease in shedding. Tetracyclines with better ability to penetrate intracellularly, such as doxycycline (Vibramycin), are the most rapid at decreasing *Mycoplasma* shedding, which is an important public health consideration. Mycoplasmas are transmitted by aerosolized droplet infection. Because patients with *Mycoplasma* have a prolonged cough, organisms not eliminated from respiratory epithelial cells may be aerosolized during coughing for weeks following the acute infection, spreading the infection to susceptible individuals via aerosolized droplets. The aim of therapy is to rapidly treat the patient's pneumonia and extrapulmonary sites of involvement. The secondary goal is to rapidly decrease shedding and aerosolization to prevent the spread of *Mycoplasma* to other individuals. An additional therapeutic goal is to decrease the incidence of post-*Mycoplasma* asthma seen in some patients. *M. pneumoniae* CAP may exacerbate preexisting asthma, but may also cause permanent post-CAP asthma in some individuals.

Until recently, doxycycline was the most active antimicrobial to use against *M. pneumoniae*. Currently, the "respiratory quinolones," levofloxacin (Levaquin) and moxifloxacin (Avelox), are highly active anti–*M. pneumoniae* antimicrobials. The respiratory quinolones and doxycycline penetrate cells efficiently and interfere with intracellular enzymes or protein synthesis of intracellular organisms. Respiratory quinolones and doxycycline are highly effective anti-*Mycoplasma* agents and rapidly decrease shedding of *M. pneumoniae* in respiratory secretions.

Therapy for *M. pneumoniae* is ordinarily 1 to 2 weeks. Patients who have impaired cardiopulmonary disease or are immunocompromised may require 2 full weeks of therapy. In patients with borderline cardiopulmonary function, *M. pneumoniae* as with other relatively low virulence pathogens may present as severe CAP. Antimicrobial therapy for typical or atypical CAP should be directed against the presumed pathogen and not based on co-morbidities. Normal healthy hosts are treated with the same antimicrobial as patients hospitalized with severe CAP. Patients hospitalized with compromised cardiopulmonary function caused by severe *M. pneumoniae* CAP are most often initially treated intravenously with doxycycline (Vibramycin), a macrolide, or a respiratory quinolone. Most patients with *M. pneumoniae* CAP present in the ambulatory setting, which permits therapy with oral doxycycline, a macrolide, or a respiratory quinolone (Table 4).

References

Ali NJ, Sillis M, Andrews BE, et al: The clinical spectrum and diagnosis of *Mycoplasma pneumoniae* infection, *Q J Med* 58:241–251, 1986.

Cunha BA: Hepatic involvement in *Mycoplasma pneumoniae* community-acquired pneumonia, *J Clin Microbiol* 3:385–386, 2003.

Cunha BA: Influenza: Historical aspects of epidemics and pandemics, *Infect Dis Clin North Am* 18:141–155, 2004.

Cunha BA: The atypical pneumonia: Clinical diagnosis and importance, *Clin Microbiol Infect* 12(12–24), 2006.

Cunha BA: *Pneumonia essentials*, ed 3, Sudbury, MA, 2010, Jones & Bartlett.

Cunha BA: *Antibiotic essentials*, ed 14, New Delhi, 2015, Jaypee Medical Publishers.

Cunha BA, Corbett M, Mickail N: Human parainfluenza virus type 3 (HPIV-3) viral community-acquired pneumonia (CAP) mimicking swine influenza (H1N1) during the swine flu pandemic, *Heart Lung* 40:76–80, 2011.

Cunha BA, Pherez FM, Strollo S, Syed U, Laguerre M: Severe swine influenza A (H1N1) versus severe human seasonal influenza A (H3N2): clinical comparisons, *Heart Lung* 40:257–261, 2011.

Cunha BA, Raza M: During influenza season: all influenza-like illnesses are not due to influenza: dengue mimicking influenza. *J Emerg Med* 2015;48:e117–20.

Cunha CB, Opal SM: Middle East respiratory syndrome (MERS): a new zoonotic viral pneumonia. , *Virulence* 5:650–654, 2014.

Cunha CB: The first atypical pneumonia: the history of the discovery of Mycoplasma pneumoniae, *Infect Dis Clin North Am* 24:1–5, 2010.

Debré R, Couvreur J: Influenza: Clinical features. In Debré R, Celers J, editors: *Clinical Virology: the evaluation and management of human viral infections*, Philadelphia, 1970, WB Saunders, pp 507–515.

File TM, Tan JS: *Mycoplasma pneumoniae* pneumonia. In Marrié TJ, editor: *Community-acquired pneumonia*, New York, 2001, Kluwer Academic/Plenum Publishers, pp 487–500.

Foster CB, Friedman N, Carl J, Piedimonte G: Enterovirus D68: a clinically important respiratory enterovirus, *Cleve Clin J Med* 82:26–31, 2015.

Hammerschlag MR: *Mycoplasma pneumoniae* infections, *Curr Opin Infect Dis* 14:181–186, 2001.

Hurt AC, Selleck P, Komadina N, et al: Susceptibility of highly pathogenic A(H5N1) avian influenza viruses to the neuraminidase inhibitors and adamantanes, *Antiviral Res* 73:228–231, 2007.

Louria DB, Blumenfeld HL, Ellis JT: Studies on influenza in the pandemic of 1957–1958. II. Pulmonary complications of influenza, *J Clin Invest* 38:213–265, 1959.

Lu QB, Wo Y, Wang HY, Wei MT, Zhang L, Yang H, et al: Detection of enterovirus 68 as one of the commonest types of enterovirus found in patients with acute respiratory tract infection in China, *J Med Microbiol* 63:408–414, 2014.

Marrie TJ: Empiric treatment of ambulatory community-acquired pneumonia: always include treatment for atypical agents, *Infect Dis Clin North Am* 18:829–841, 2004.

Murray HW, Masur H, Senterfit LS, Roberts RB: The protean manifestations of *Mycoplasma pneumoniae* infection in adults, *Am J Med* 58:229–242, 1975.

Nisar N, Guleria R, Kumar S, et al: Mycoplasma pneumoniae and its role in asthma, *Postgrad Med J* 83:100–104, 2007.

Recovery Collaborative Group, Horby P, Lim WS, et al: Dexamethasone in hospitalized patients with COVID-19 - preliminary report, *N Engl J Med*, 2020.

Yang Y, Guo F, Zhao W, Gu Q, Huang M, Cao Q, et al: Novel avian-origin influenza A (H7N9) in critically ill patients in China, *Crit Care Med* 43:339–345, 2015.

VIRAL RESPIRATORY INFECTIONS

Method of
Robert C. Welliver Sr., MD

CURRENT DIAGNOSIS

- Rapid diagnostic kits are available for many common respiratory viruses. These tests are used increasingly to establish that antibiotic therapy is not necessary in many patients with febrile respiratory illnesses or with lower respiratory tract infections.
- The presence of wheezing on physical examination virtually excludes bacterial infection from consideration in subjects with lower respiratory disease.

CURRENT THERAPY

- The management of most viral respiratory infections consists of rest, adequate caloric and fluid intake, and management of fever and malaise.
- Corticosteroids are essential in the management of croup.
- Specific antiviral therapy is available only for influenza virus infection, and beneficial effects have been more readily achieved in prevention rather than treatment.

Viral infections of the respiratory tract are among the most common infections in humans, and they account for significant morbidity at all ages. Infants and young children can sustain six to eight such infections annually, and adults have an average of nearly two such infections per year.

Rhinoviruses are the most commonly identified etiologic agents and cause illness year-round. Other common causative agents during winter months include influenza viruses and respiratory syncytial virus, and enteroviruses predominate in summer months. The parainfluenza viruses also commonly cause respiratory infection, particularly in autumn (type 1) and late spring or summer (type 3). Coronaviruses, metapneumoviruses, adenoviruses, and other agents are identified less often.

Although each of these agents can cause a common cold, some viral infections are associated with characteristic patterns of respiratory disease. Most of these viruses can also exacerbate asthma, cystic fibrosis, and chronic obstructive pulmonary disease (COPD).

Common Colds

Colds are the most common of the viral respiratory illnesses. Pharyngitis is usually the earliest sign of a cold, beginning a few days after infection has taken place. Nasal congestion and clear or slightly cloudy rhinorrhea usually follow within 24 to 48 hours. Cough occurs in approximately 30% to 40% of those infected, and fluid can accumulate in middle ear or sinus cavities that have become blocked as a result of mucosal swelling. Ear and sinus cavity infections occur when this fluid is trapped for a week or more. Treatment with antibiotics is ineffective before this time, and they are ineffective especially in the absence of other clinical signs of ear and sinus infections.

Colds are a frequent cause of missed school and work, and even of mild morbidity, but they are rarely serious in otherwise healthy persons. The most appropriate approach to treatment therefore entails rest, with adequate nutrition and hydration. Agents that inhibit the activity of cyclooxygenase probably represent the most effective form of pharmacologic intervention. These compounds include acetaminophen (Tylenol) and the nonsteroidal anti-inflammatory agents (NSAIDs) such as ibuprofen (Motrin). They are effective in reducing fever and, perhaps more importantly in most colds, reducing malaise, headache, and pharyngitis.

Nasal congestion and some rhinorrhea during colds are related to dilation of blood vessels in the nose and sinuses. Vasoconstrictors have therefore been used extensively to attempt to reverse these symptoms. Oral decongestants such as pseudoephedrine (Sudafed) have minimal effect on nasal congestion, and can result in systemic hypertension, anxiety, and difficulty sleeping. The propensity for these compounds to cause cardiac arrhythmias in the very young child has led to recommendations against their use in the first year or two of life. Nasal sprays containing vasoconstricting agents such as oxymetazoline (Afrin) can result in mild temporary relief of nasal obstruction. However, the use of these compounds for more than 3 or 4 days can result in rebound vasodilation and paradoxically increased rhinorrhea.

Numerous investigations have evaluated the role of antihistamines in colds. The release of histamine itself is not associated with fever, cough, or malaise, so effects on these symptoms would not be expected. Furthermore, nasal congestion and discharge may be more related to the release of kinins, and not histamine. Indeed, the administration of antihistamines in adults and, particularly, in children has not demonstrated strikingly positive results. As many as 40% of subjects treated with placebo report beneficial effects. Side effects of histamine use, primarily sedation and dry mouth, are commonly encountered.

Cough can be one of the most irritating symptoms during colds. Cough during colds is principally caused by secretions entering the airway (postnasal drip) and not by inflammation of the airway itself. Therefore, it is not surprising that cough suppressants, especially codeine, have little effect on cough induced by colds. Antihistamines have also been found to be ineffective in relief of cough during colds.

Influenza-Like Illness

The influenza syndrome is defined as the abrupt onset of fever, headache, and striking degrees of malaise and prostration, often with intense myalgia. Respiratory symptoms can occur concurrently, but they might not be prominent features. The principal cause is, of course, influenza virus, although infection with many other viruses can cause similar (although not as intense) symptoms. The illness is generally self-limited, and most symptoms resolve over 4 or 5 days. Lassitude can persist for up to 2 weeks.

Influenza virus infection and influenza-like illness are best treated symptomatically, relying on rest, adequate intake of fluids and calories, and appropriate analgesic therapy. Compounds referred to as *M2 inhibitors* such as amantadine (Symmetrel) and rimantadine (Flumadine) have been approved for therapy. Positive outcomes from therapy with these agents are observed only when therapy is instituted within 48 hours after the onset of symptoms, and benefits are not striking. In recent years, resistance to M2 inhibitors has been commonly observed among circulating epidemic strains of influenza virus.

More recently, inhibitors of the activity of influenza viral neuraminidase have been used in treatment and prevention of influenza virus infection in adults and children. The first such compound released, zanamivir (Relenza), was administered by inhalation but was unpopular because of its irritating effects on the airway. An oral compound, oseltamivir (TamiFlu), has been used to prevent and to treat influenza virus infection. As with M2 inhibitors, it is believed that treatment should be started within the first 48 hours of symptoms and that prophylaxis should be instituted within 48 hours of exposure. Treatment with oseltamivir shortens the duration of subsequent illness by only about 24 hours. Treatment can prevent some of the complications of influenza infection, including pneumonia. The drug may be more effective as a therapeutic agent, because it may be up to 90% effective in preventing culture-positive symptomatic influenza illness. The recommended dose for adults is 75 mg orally every 12 hours for 5 days. In children, the appropriate dose based on body weight is 30 mg twice daily for children weighing less than 15 kg, 45 mg twice daily for children weighing 15 to 23 kg, 60 mg twice daily for children weighing 23 to 40 kg, and 75 mg twice daily for children weighing more than 40 kg. The principal side effect is nausea, which can be reduced by taking the drug with food.

A new type of antiviral (baloxavir marboxil [Xofluza]) was released for treatment of influenza infections in 2018. This drug acts by a different mechanism than previous antivirals used to treat influenza infections. The advantages are that it is given as a single dose for the entire course of treatment, and reduces the duration of influenza illness by approximately 24 hours. It does not seem more effective than oseltamivir in reducing influenza-related symptoms. The appropriate doses are 40 mg for individuals age 12 years or greater and weighing less than 40 kg (88 lbs.) to less than 80 kg (176 lbs), and 80 mg for individuals weighing greater than or equal to 80 kg (176 lbs.).

In 2009, a novel H1N1 strain of influenza caused a worldwide pandemic. At the time of this writing, both this epidemic H1N1 strain as well as the seasonal influenza A/H3N2 and type B strains continue to circulate in the world. The considerable majority of these epidemic and seasonal strains continue to show sensitivity to oseltamivir, while most are resistant to M2 inhibitors. All strains continue to show sensitvity to zanamivir.

Croup

Croup is defined by the occurrence of hoarseness or laryngitis, a deep, brassy or barking cough, and inspiratory stridor. Airway obstruction in croup is caused by constriction in the subglottic area, often noted on radiographs by a steeple-shaped narrowing of the air column in this region. Affected children are usually afebrile and nontoxic in appearance.

Parainfluenza virus type 1 is the primary cause of croup, although infection with many different viruses can produce this illness, and influenza virus can cause a particularly severe form of croup. Bacterial secondary infection occurs uncommonly, but it can result in fever and severe obstruction of the airway. Administration of dexamethasone (Decadron)[1] at 0.6 mg/kg either orally or intramuscularly markedly reduces the rate of hospitalization, admission to the intensive care unit, and intubation for croup.

Bronchiolitis

Bronchiolitis represents the most common cause for hospitalization of infants in developed countries. Infants present with a history of several days of upper respiratory symptoms, followed by the rapid onset of wheezing and labored breathing. Respiratory syncytial virus (RSV) is the most common cause and is the agent found in the most severe cases that result in respiratory failure. Contrasting with asthma, obstruction of the airway in bronchiolitis is a result of plugging of bronchioles with detached epithelium and inflammatory cells. Mucus plugging and constriction of smooth muscle are not prominent. Also in contrast with asthma is the absence of a sustained response to bronchodilators and corticosteroids among infants with bronchiolitis.

Therapy of bronchiolitis primarily consists of administration of supplemental oxygen and replacement of fluid deficits as needed. Ribavirin (Virazole)[1] is a compound with antiviral activity against RSV, but controlled studies have not demonstrated meaningful differences in outcomes between treated and untreated subjects. The compound is quite expensive and must be delivered via a special aerosol generator.

Palivizumab (Synagis), a preparation consisting of a monoclonal antibody against the fusion protein of RSV, has proved to be effective in reducing the rate of hospitalization for RSV infection by approximately 50% when given to high-risk infants. Infants who may be considered candidates for therapy include those with chronic lung disease, those born prematurely, and those with hemodynamically significant congenital heart disease. Doses of palivizumab (15 mg/kg) are given on a monthly basis throughout the local RSV season, usually November through March.

References

Akerlund A, Klint T, Olen L, Runderantz H: Nasal decongestant effect of oxymetazoline in the common cold: An objective dose-response study in 106 patients, J Laryngol Otol 103:743–746, 1989.

Buckingham SC, Jafri HS, Bush AN, et al: A randomized, double-blind, placebo-controlled trial of dexamethasone in severe respiratory syncytial virus (RSV) infection: Effects on RSV quantity and clinical outcome, J Infect Dis 185:1222–1228, 2002.

Curley FJ, Irwin RS, Pratter MR, et al: Cough and the common cold, Am J Respir Crit Care Med 138:305–311, 1988.

Flores G, Horwitz RI: Efficacy of β₂-agonists in bronchiolitis: A reappraisal and meta-analysis, Pediatrics 100:233–239, 1997.

Johnson DW, Jacobson S, Edney PC, et al: A comparison of nebulized budesonide, intramuscular dexamethasone, and placebo for moderately severe croup, N Engl J Med 339:498–503, 1998.

Muether PS, Gwaltney Jr JM: Variant effect of first- and second-generation antihistamines as clues to their mechanism of action on the sneeze reflex in the common cold, Clin Infect Dis 33:1483–1488, 2001.

Randolph AG, Wang EL: Ribavirin for respiratory syncytial virus lower respiratory tract infection, Arch Pediatr Adolesc Med 150:942–947, 1996.

Tavorner D, Danz C, Economos D: The effects of oral pseudoephedrine on nasal patency in the common cold: A double-blind single-dose placebo-controlled trial, Clin Otolaryngol 24:47–51, 1999.

Treanor JJ, Hayden FG, Vrooman PS, et al: Efficacy and safety of the oral neuraminidase inhibitor oseltamivir in treating acute influenza: A randomized controlled trial. US Oral Neuraminnidase Study Group, JAMA 283:1016–1024, 2000.

Van Voris LP, Betts RF, Hayden FG, et al: Successful treatment of naturally occurring influenza A/USSR/77 H1N1, JAMA 245:1128–1131, 1981.

[1]Not FDA approved for this indication.

[1]Not FDA approved for this indication.

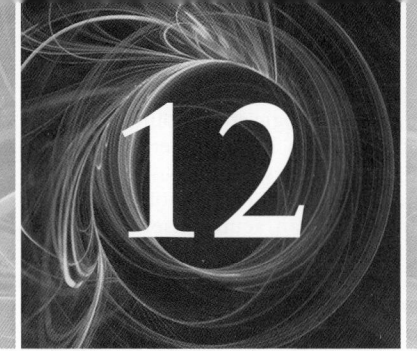

12 Rheumatology and the Musculoskeletal System

AXIAL SPONDYLOARTHRITIS

Method of
Atul Deodhar, MD, MRCP; and Sonam Kiwalkar, MD

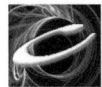

CURRENT DIAGNOSIS

- Axial spondyloarthritis (axSpA) is an umbrella term that includes ankylosing spondylitis (AS) and nonradiographic axial spondyloarthritis (nr-axSpA). The presence or absence of definitive sacroiliitis on radiographs differentiates AS (also called radiographic axSpA) from nr-axSpA. The latter is a condition with the same clinical features and similar disease burden as AS except that definitive radiographic features of sacroiliitis are lacking.
- In the absence of diagnostic criteria, the diagnosis of AS is made by the presence of definitive sacroiliitis on sacroiliac (SI) joint x-ray plus either chronic (>3 months) inflammatory back pain or restriction in spinal movements or chest expansion (Modified New York Criteria for Classification of AS).
- Because definitive sacroiliitis may take up to 10 years to appear on a radiograph from the start of chronic inflammatory back pain (the most common first symptom), early or mild disease can be missed.
- When AS is suspected with features of inflammatory back pain, usually starting before age 45, along with other clinical features of spondyloarthritis—such as uveitis, psoriasis, enthesitis, asymmetric peripheral inflammatory arthritis, family history of spondyloarthritis, high C-reactive protein (CRP), inflammatory bowel disease, a good response to nonsteroidal antiinflammatory drugs (NSAIDs)—but an x-ray of the SI joints is negative or uncertain for definitive sacroiliitis, magnetic resonance imaging (MRI) of the SI joints and/or human leukocyte antigen (HLA)-B27 typing may help in making the diagnosis of axSpA.

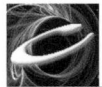

CURRENT THERAPY

- Nonpharmacologic interventions include active physical therapy, self-directed physical exercise, patient education, and smoking cessation.
- NSAIDs are the first line of pharmacologic treatment.
- In those who are not responding adequately to NSAIDs, treatment with tumor necrosis factor-α inhibitors (TNFi) or interleukin-17 inhibitors (IL-17i) is recommended.
- Retrospective analysis in cohorts of patients with AS using long-term TNFi has shown a reduced rate of new bone formation in the spine, although no pharmaceutical agents have shown "disease modifying" ability in prospective studies to date.
- Conventional synthetic antirheumatic drugs such as sulfasalazine (Azulfidine)[1] or methotrexate[1] can be used to treat peripheral arthritis in axSpA patients, but they do not have efficacy in axial disease.

[1]Not FDA approved for this indication.

Definition and Spectrum of the Disease

Axial spondyloarthritis (axSpA) is an umbrella term that includes ankylosing spondylitis (AS) and nonradiographic axial spondyloarthritis (nr-axSpA). The presence or absence of definitive sacroiliitis on radiographs differentiates AS (also called radiographic axSpA) from nr-axSpA.

AxSpA is a chronic, immune-mediated inflammatory disorder involving the sacroiliac (SI) joints, the spine, and often the hips. In some, spinal bony fusion develops gradually over several years and may lead to reduced spine and neck flexibility. The axial skeleton is always involved, and involvement of the peripheral joints occurs in approximately 30% of patients. Enthesitis is a common occurrence. Extraarticular manifestations (EAMs) include osteoporosis, psoriasis, acute anterior uveitis, and inflammatory bowel disease (IBD) (i.e., Crohn disease or ulcerative colitis).

Epidemiology

Based on the 2009 to 2010 National Health and Nutritional Examination Survey (NHANES), the estimated prevalence of axSpA in the US population is about 1.0%, of which 0.5% of patients are reported to have AS. The prevalence of nr-axSpA is thus assumed to be the other 0.5%, as pelvic radiographs and SI magnetic resonance imaging (MRI) examinations were not carried out in this population-based study.

The prevalence of axSpA varies with the geographic region and, in general, depends on the prevalence of human leukocyte antigen (HLA)-B27. Prevalence of HLA-B27 is less than 1% in Japan, 3% in African Americans, and more than 20% in some native populations of eastern Siberia and Alaska; it is 8% in western Europe and 10% to 16% in Scandinavian countries. AxSpA is thus rare in the Japanese and African American populations. The prevalence of axSpA is about 0.5% in persons of European descent and 1.4% in those of Scandinavian ancestry, whereas it rises to 2% to 3% in natives of eastern Siberia and Alaska. The risk of axSpA is increased among those with an affected first-degree relative. The male-to-female ratio is 2:1 for the diagnosis of AS. In contrast, there is hardly any difference in the prevalence of nr-axSpA among males and females.

Pathogenesis

Genetics plays a major role in the pathogenesis of spondyloarthritis, and the *HLA-B27* gene has a major association with AS. *HLA-B27* is present in about 70% to 90% of patients with AS in most ethnic groups. The risk of disease in family members of patients with AS is 63% in monozygotic twins, 20% in dizygotic twins, 8.2% in first-degree relatives, 1% in second-degree relatives, and 0.7% in third-degree relatives. The overall contribution to AS heritability by *HLA-B27* is estimated to be approximately 20%. Some other genes associated with AS—such as endoplasmic reticulum aminopeptidases (*ERAP-1* and *ERAP-2*) and interleukin-23 receptor (*IL-23R*)—have been implicated to play a role in the pathogenesis.

The following hypotheses have been put forth to explain the role of *HLA-B27* in the pathogenesis of AS:
1. Arthritogenic peptide presentation. Certain antimicrobial peptides have molecular mimicry to self-peptides found in the joints, and it is hypothesized that *HLA-B27* presents these to cytotoxic T cells. The activated T-cell lymphocytes then lead to autoreactivity, arthritis, and spondylitis.

2. HLA-B27 heavy chain homodimer. The heavy chains of the HLA-B27 molecule can form homodimers when they are expressed on the cell surface, resulting in their recognition by natural killer cell receptors. This can enhance the survival and proliferation of CD-4 T cells and increase the production of IL-17 in vivo.

3. HLA-B27 misfolding and unfolded protein response. HLA-B27 assembly takes place in the endoplasmic reticulum (ER) before it is expressed on the cell surface. The misfolded HLA-B27 molecules accumulate in the ER, leading to cellular stress secondary to the unfolded protein response. This then activates the IL-23/IL-17 pathway of inflammation.

4. HLA-B27 shaping of the human gut microbiome. The human body contains a large community of commensals and symbiotic bacteria, fungi, and viruses called microbiota. The term *microbiome* refers to the genomes of these microorganisms. The composition of the gut microbiome is influenced by genes and other environmental factors. It is postulated that HLA-B27 predisposes to AS by influencing gut microbiome. Studies have shown that the microbiota composition of patients with AS differs from that of rheumatoid arthritis patients as well as healthy controls. Further, *HLA-B27*–positive healthy individuals have a microbiome that differs from that of *HLA-B27*–negative subjects.

In animal models of spondyloarthritis, *HLA-B27* transgenic rats and mice, when raised in a germ-free environment, did not develop spondyloarthritis but rather a spondyloarthritis-like disease when they were housed in a typical laboratory environment, suggesting a role for microbes in the pathogenesis of spondyloarthritis. More than 60% of patients with AS have subclinical acute or chronic intestinal inflammation. This loss of architectural and functional integrity in the intestinal epithelium enables the passage of microbial products into the submucosa and then into systemic circulation. Innate and adaptive immune cells recognize these microbial products and produce proinflammatory cytokines. These microbial products and the immune cells travel from the gut to distant sites, such as peripheral joints and entheses, causing inflammation.

Clinical Manifestations

The most common manifestations of axSpA include chronic inflammatory low back, hip, and/or buttock pain. The typical characteristics of inflammatory back pain include age of onset less than 40 years, insidious onset without any identifiable cause, improvement with exercise or activity and no improvement with rest, and pain in the second half of the night. Neck pain is rarely the presenting feature due to involvement of the cervical spine; when this is present, it is more commonly seen in women.

The limitation of spinal motion is initially the result of axial inflammation and later is secondary to the ossification of ligamentous structures, bony fusion of apophyseal joints, and outer fibers of the annulus fibrosus of the intervertebral disks, leading to the development of syndesmophytes.

Hip involvement is seen in up to 40% of patients. The typical symptoms are pain in the groin or radiation of pain to the medial thigh or the knee. Hip involvement is associated with significant functional impairment. Other peripheral joints—such as the ankles, knees, shoulders, and, to a lesser extent, the sternoclavicular joint, the temporomandibular joint, and small joints of the hands and feet—may also be involved.

Enthesitis is a classic feature of axSpA. Enthesitis presents as pain, stiffness, and tenderness at the sites of insertions of ligaments, muscles, or tendons to a bone. Typical areas of enthesitis include the Achilles tendon, plantar fascia attachment to the calcaneum, costochondral junctions, and the paraspinal muscle attachment to the pelvic rim. Diffuse swelling of toes or fingers, called dactylitis ("sausage digits"), is occasionally seen in axSpA.

EAMs associated with axSpA include psoriasis, IBD, uveitis, and osteoporosis. A large epidemiologic study found that 42% of axSpA patients had one or more EAMs; uveitis was present in 27%, IBD in 10%, and psoriasis in 11%. Uveitis seen in association with axSpA presents as eye discomfort during the prodromal phase followed by an acute onset of eye redness, pain, photophobia, and miosis. The usual characteristics of uveitis associated with axSpA are acute in onset, unilateral, and involving the anterior part of the uvea. Even though overt IBD is seen in only 10% of axSpA patients, more than 60% have subclinical mucosal inflammation in the gut.

Diagnosis

Within the United States, there is a significant delay of 10 to 14 years in the diagnosis of axSpA from symptom onset. There are many reasons for this, including the commonality of back pain in the general population and the rarity of axSpA as a cause of back pain. There are no specific physical findings or laboratory tests to diagnose axSpA; the diagnosis is based on pattern recognition and clinical reasoning. Patients with back pain are generally seen by nonrheumatologists who may not be familiar with features of inflammatory back pain and may not suspect axSpA. In the optimal clinical setting with a patient complaining of onset of chronic (>3 months) inflammatory back pain starting before age 45 years, the presence of other features of spondyloarthritis (as described earlier), a positive HLA B-27 test, and a plain x-ray of the SI joint showing sacroiliitis, the diagnosis of AS would be straightforward. Radiographic findings such as sclerosis; joint erosions; or widening, narrowing, or ankylosis of the SI joint suggest sacroiliitis.

During this early stage of disease (also known as nr-axSpA), MRI scan (without contrast) of the SI joints may show evidence of active inflammation and may also show structural changes such as sclerosis, fatty metaplasia, or erosions that aid in making the diagnosis. The required sequence of MRI imaging and the features that suggest a diagnosis of nr-axSpA include the following:

1. T1-weighted sequence. Structural changes such as erosions and ankylosis can be seen. Fat metaplasia appears hyperintense.

2. Fat-suppressed T2-weighted (short-TI inversion recovery [STIR]) sequence, osteitis, representing active inflammation and reported as bone marrow edema, appears hyperintense.

When the clinical suspicion of axSpA is high but an x-ray of the SI joints is negative or inconclusive for sacroiliitis, the presence of the features previously noted on MRI of the SI joints may help in confirming a diagnosis of nr-axSpA.

The changes of inflammation on STIR imaging (i.e., "osteitis") can be seen in professional athletes, military recruits, and even in normal individuals because of mechanical stress ("false-positive MRI"). It is therefore important to emphasize that ruling out common causes of back pain, pattern recognition, and clinical reasoning is the key to a diagnosis of axSpA.

Plain radiographs of the spine may show characteristic changes in AS. Romanus lesions or the "shiny corner sign" and squaring of the vertebral body are seen due to erosions at the attachments of the spinal ligaments at the vertebral corners in early disease. This is followed by ossification of the outer layer of annulus fibrosus, leading to syndesmophyte formation on plain x-ray. In the late stages, ankylosis of the spine, also known as bamboo spine, may be seen in a small percentage of AS patients. The role of low-dose computed tomography (CT) in the diagnosis of axSpA is currently being researched.

An elevated erythrocyte sedimentation rate (ESR) or C-reactive protein (CRP) is seen in only 30% to 40% of patients with active AS.

Differential Diagnosis

Chronic nonspecific back pain is common in the general population (19% according to the NHANES study); hence mechanical causes of back pain should be considered first.

Diffuse idiopathic skeletal hyperostosis (DISH) is sometimes mistaken for "bamboo spine of AS." DISH is a noninflammatory condition affecting the spine. It is more commonly seen in obese, diabetic males, often greater than 50 years of age. Radiographically, DISH is characterized by calcification of the anterior longitudinal ligament involving at least four contiguous vertebral bodies, sometimes referred to as "flowing osteophytes." The flowing osteophytes are bulky and typically appear on the right side of the spine. SI joints are not involved in patients with DISH.

Osteitis condensans ilii (OCI) can be mistaken for sacroiliitis but is usually an asymptomatic benign disorder of multiparous women. OCI is characterized by radiographic findings of a triangular area of dense sclerosis on the lower and inferior part of iliac side of the SI joint. OCI is not associated with erosions or ankylosis of the SI joints.

Inflammatory back pain with sclerotic changes on SI joint x-ray can also be seen in conditions such as (1) postpartum insufficiency fracture of the sacrum; (2) septic sacroiliitis from tuberculosis, brucellosis, fungi, and other infectious agents; and (3) rarely malignancies such as acute lymphoblastic leukemia.

Treatment

The goals of treatment of axSpA are to reduce symptoms, improve and maintain spinal flexibility and normal posture, reduce functional limitations, and decrease complications of the disease. The mainstay of treatment has been NSAIDs, exercise and physical therapy, biologics such as tumor necrosis factor-α inhibitors (TNFi) and interleukin-17 inhibitors (IL-17i), and small molecules such as Janus kinase inhibitors (JAKi).

Treatment of axSpA can be divided into nonpharmacologic, pharmacologic, and surgical interventions.

Nonpharmacologic interventions: These include active physical therapy (on land or aquatic), self-directed physical exercise, patient education, and smoking cessation. These are recommended at all stages of the disease.

Pharmacologic interventions: Box 1 outlines pharmacologic interventions for the treatment of axSpA.

In clinical practice, most of the treatment recommendations for nr-axSpA are extrapolated from studies based on AS. Based on a 52-week placebo-controlled trial, certolizumab pegol (Cimzia) was approved by the FDA for the treatment of nr-axSpA in the United States.

The use of biologics and small molecules has been associated with an increased risk of serious infections. While bacterial infections are seen in both classes of drugs, herpes zoster is seen mostly with JAKi while reactivation of latent tuberculosis is mostly seen with TNFi. Therefore, screening for latent tuberculosis should be performed before these therapies are initiated.

Some of the side effects of TNFs and IL-17s include injection-site reactions with subcutaneous preparations or infusion reactions with infliximab (Remicade) or golimumab (Simponi). Some of the other adverse effects of TNFi are the development of demyelinating disease, worsening of heart failure, recurrence of lymphoma or malignant melanoma, and paradoxical development of psoriasis-like skin lesions. Some of the adverse events of IL-17is include leukopenia, candidiasis, and the development or worsening of IBD. Adverse effects of JAKi include nasopharyngeal infections and increased risk of blood clots.

Surgical interventions: Total hip arthroplasty should be considered in patients with refractory hip pain or functional decline in the presence of radiographic evidence of structural damage. Spinal corrective osteotomies are occasionally necessary for fixed kyphotic deformities seen in advanced AS but should be undertaken only in centers of expertise.

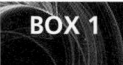

BOX 1 Pharmacologic Interventions for the Treatment of Ankylosing Spondylitis

1. NSAIDs are used in full doses either continuously or on an "as required" basis depending on the severity of symptoms, comorbidities, and patient preferences. No particular NSAID is preferred over any other.
2. If patients continue to have symptoms despite a 4-week trial of full-dose NSAIDs, therapy is escalated to TNFi. Currently five TNFi agents are approved for the treatment of AS (and for nr-axSpA in certain countries):
   a. Soluble receptor of TNF—Etanercept (Enbrel) 50 mg, SC injection once weekly
   b. TNFi monoclonal antibodies
      i. Adalimumab (Humira) 40 mg SC every 2 weeks
      ii. Golimumab (Simponi) 50 mg SC once a month or (Simponi Aria) 2 mg/kg intravenous (IV) at weeks 0, 4, and then every 8 weeks thereafter
      iii. Certolizumab pegol (Cimzia) 200 mg SC twice a month or 400 mg SC once a month
      iv. Infliximab (Remicade) 5 mg/kg IV infusion every 6 weeks
   c. No TNFi is preferred over any other except in patients with concomitant uveitis or IBD, where monoclonal antibodies are preferred over soluble receptor TNFi.
3. In case of secondary failure of TNFi (failing after initial benefit), an alternative TNFi can be used. In case of primary failure of TNFi (no response), an IL-17i, secukinumab (Cosentyx) can be used. Secukinumab is given SC as 150 mg at weeks 0, 1, 2, 3, and 4, followed by 150 mg or 300 mg every 4 weeks. Ixekizumab (Taltz), another IL-17i, can also be used. It is given subcutaneously as 160 mg once, followed by 80 mg every 4 weeks.
4. JAKi such as tofacitinib (Xeljanz)[1] 5 mg two times a day or upadacitinib (Rinvoq)[1] 15 mg once a day can be used in case of secondary failure of TNFi. These agents have shown promising results in phase II and phase III trials.
5. Conventional synthetic DMARDs like sulfasalazine (Azulfidine),[1] up to 3 g/day, and methotrexate,[1] up to 25 mg/week, are effective in the treatment of peripheral joint involvement but not of axial disease in AS.
6. Local glucocorticoid injections for enthesitis or intraarticular injections for active peripheral arthritis can provide relief for flareups. However, injection of inflamed weight-bearing tendons such as the Achilles tendon is not recommended due to the risk of rupture. Systemic glucocorticoids do not have any benefit in AS and should be avoided.

[1]Not FDA approved for this indication.
AS, Ankylosing spondylitis; *DMARDs,* disease-modifying antirheumatic drugs; *IBD,* inflammatory bowel disease; *IL-17i,* interleukin-17 inhibitors; *NSAIDs,* nonsteroidal antiinflammatory drugs; *SC,* subcutaneous; *TNFi,* tumor necrosis factor-α inhibitors.

Monitoring

Patients should be monitored regularly for disease activity, functional impairment, and medication safety. The frequency of monitoring is individualized. Assessment of disease activity can be done by the following methods:

1. Use of the Bath Ankylosing Spondylitis Disease Activity Index (BASDAI): This is a patient-administered questionnaire with six questions answered on a visual analog scale of 0 to 10. A BASDAI score of equal to or greater than 4 is indicative of active disease. Clinically significant improvement is defined as an absolute change of equal to or greater than 2.
2. Use of the Ankylosing Spondylitis Disease Activity Score (AS-DAS): It incorporates three questions used in the BASDAI, a patient global assessment of disease activity, and CRP. An AS-DAS score of below 1.3 is defined as inactive disease, 1.3 to

2.1 is low disease activity, 2.1 to 3.5 is high disease activity, and greater than 3.5 is very high disease activity. A reduction of equal to or greater than 1.1 in ASDAS is considered a significant improvement.

Structural damage due to axSpA can be measured by the modified Stoke Ankylosing Spondylitis Spine Score. This score correlates with disease activity as measured with ASDAS.

Functional impairment can be measured by the Bath Ankylosing Spondylitis Functional Index. This is a patient-administered questionnaire that includes 10 activities of daily living. The Bath Ankylosing Spondylitis Metrology Index is an index of spinal and hip mobility in patients with AS. It includes lateral lumbar flexion, tragus-to-wall distance, modified Schober test, maximal intermalleolar distance, and cervical rotation.

The ESR and CRP may be useful in monitoring disease activity. MRI of the SI joints or spine is expensive and is not indicated to monitor disease activity of AS. Spine x-rays are not used for monitoring purposes in daily practice, although they may be used to counsel patients about lifestyle changes (such as stopping smoking) or to start biologic therapy.

Complications

The prevalence of osteoporosis is approximately 25% after 10 years of axSpA. Vertebral fractures are seen in about 10% of patients with AS. The lower cervical spine is the most commonly involved area, where there is often also neurologic compromise. One should consider vertebral fractures in patients with neck and back pain that has changed in intensity or character from baseline. Another rare complication is the cauda equine syndrome from long-standing AS owing to the inflammation of the lumbosacral nerve roots caused by arachnoiditis. Cardiac manifestations include aortic valve insufficiency and conduction abnormalities. Pulmonary manifestations are rare and include chest expansion restriction from ossification of costovertebral joints and upper lobe–predominant interstitial lung disease. Patients with AS can have IgA nephropathy or, in late stages, renal amyloidosis if the disease is left untreated. Cardiovascular disease is being recognized as a common comorbidity in patients with AS and is linked to chronic inflammation. All patients with AS should be counseled about the traditional risk factors for cardiovascular disease, and appropriate treatment should be instituted if necessary.

References

Bennett AN, McGonagle D, O'Connor P, et al: Severity of baseline magnetic resonance imaging-evident sacroiliitis and HLA-B27 status in early inflammatory back pain predict radiographically evident ankylosing spondylitis at eight years, *Arthritis Rheum* 58(11):3413–3418, 2008. https://doi.org/10.1002/art.24024.

Braun J, Sieper J: Ankylosing spondylitis, *Lancet (London, England)* 369(9570):1379–1390, 2007. https://doi.org/10.1016/S0140-6736(07)60635-7.

Brophy S, MacKay K, Al-Saidi A: The natural history of ankylosing spondylitis as defined by radiological progression, *J Rheumatol* 29(6):1236–1243, 2002.

de Winter JJ, van Mens LJ, van der Heijde D: Prevalence of peripheral and extra-articular disease in ankylosing spondylitis versus non-radiographic axial spondyloarthritis: a meta-analysis, *Arthritis Res Ther* 18(1), 2016 https://doi.org/10.1186/s13075-016-1093-z.

Deodhar A, Mease PJ, Reveille JD, et al: Frequency of axial spondyloarthritis diagnosis among patients seen by us rheumatologists for evaluation of chronic back pain, *Arthritis Rheum* 68(7):1669–1676, 2016, https://doi.org/10.1002/art.39612.

Reveille JD: Genetics of spondyloarthritis - beyond the MHC, *Nat Rev Rheumatol* 8(5):296–304, 2012. https://doi.org/10.1038/nrrheum.2012.41.

Reveille JD, Witter JP, Weisman MH: Prevalence of axial spondylarthritis in the United States: estimates from a cross-sectional Survey, *Arthritis Care Res* 64(6):905–910, 2012. https://doi.org/10.1002/acr.21621.

Rudwaleit M, Khan MA, Sieper J, et al: Commentary: the challenge of diagnosis and classification in early ankylosing spondylitis: do we need new criteria? *Arthritis Rheum* 52(4):1000–1008, 2005. https://doi.org/10.1002/art.20990.

Van Der Heijde D, Ramiro S, Landewé R, et al: 2016 update of the ASAS-EULAR management recommendations for axial spondyloarthritis, *Ann Rheum Dis*, 2017. https://doi.org/10.1136/annrheumdis-2016-210770.

Ward MM, Deodhar A, Gensler LS, et al: 2019 Update of the American College of Rheumatology/Spondylitis Association of America/Spondyloarthritis Research and Treatment Network recommendations for the treatment of ankylosing spondylitis and nonradiographic axial spondyloarthritis, *Arthritis Care Res*, 2019. https://doi.org/10.1002/acr.24025.

BURSITIS AND TENDINOPATHY

Method of
Kyle Goerl, MD

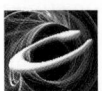

CURRENT DIAGNOSIS

Tendinopathy
- Tendinitis is an inflammatory condition only present within the first weeks of a tendon injury.
- Tendinosis is a degenerative condition usually developing weeks after the initial injury.
- The diagnosis is typically made clinically with a thorough history and physical examination.
- Most tendinopathies occur secondary to overuse, and can be acute, chronic, or recurrent.
- Tendinopathies are usually characterized by pain, possible swelling, and dysfunction of the affected tendon.
- If the diagnosis is in question, magnetic resonance imaging and ultrasound are helpful diagnostic aides.

Bursitis
- Bursitis is an inflammatory reaction of a bursa.
- Bursitis is typically the result of overuse or trauma, but systemic illnesses can also cause bursitis.
- The olecranon, prepatellar, and trochanteric bursa are particularly susceptible to traumatic bursitis because of their location immediately under the skin with minimal subcutaneous fat for protection.
- Bursitis rarely occurs alone, so a search should be conducted for an associated condition such as tendinopathy or a tendon tear.
- Imaging studies demonstrate that lateral hip pain is usually tendinopathy, not "trochanteric bursitis," a term that should be reserved for image-proven bursitis.
- Septic bursitis usually only affects the olecranon and prepatellar bursa, and care must be taken to distinguish it from aseptic bursitis.
- Common pathogens in septic arthritis include *Staphylococcus aureus* and β-hemolytic *Streptococcus*.
- If the diagnosis of septic bursitis is in question, aspiration should be performed, and the aspirate sent for Gram stain, cell count and differential, culture and crystal analysis, and blood should be sent for culture, complete blood count, C-reactive protein, and erythrocyte sedimentation rate.

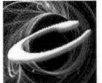

CURRENT THERAPY

Tendinopathy
- Given that tendonitis is an inflammatory condition, NSAIDs should be considered. Ice, activity modification, and rest are also effective.
- Tendinosis is not an inflammatory condition, so NSAIDs are not usually a part of the treatment regimen.
- Tendinosis responds well to physical therapy and, in particular, eccentric exercises. Deep tissue massage with tools is also an effective treatment modality.
- Steroid injections can be effective for short term pain relief, but not for long-term healing, and should not be a routine part of the treatment plan. Steroid injections can be considered if the patient is in too much pain to perform physical therapy.
- Injections of blood products such as whole blood and platelet-rich-plasma, prolotherapy and sclerotherapy have

varying levels of evidence supporting their effectiveness, but are reasonable alternatives to surgery.
- When conservative measures fail, more invasive procedures such as tenotomy, tendon scraping, and open débridement should be considered, but are rarely needed.

Bursitis
- Early treatment should include NSAIDs, ice, activity modification, and rest.
- If an associated condition like tendinopathy is discovered, appropriate treatment should target that condition as well, and typically involves physical therapy.
- In the event of septic bursitis, antibiotic treatment should be initiated. Parenteral medication should be heavily considered, given the high failure rate of oral antibiotics.
- Surgery is rarely needed for bursitis.

Tendinopathy

Background
Tendon is a connective tissue used to attach muscle to bone. Normal tendon tissue is dense and has a highly regular and fibrillar pattern. Tendinopathy is the term used to describe a clinical syndrome typically resulting from overuse of a tendon. Traditionally the term tendonitis has been used to describe all tendon injuries, but the suffix "–itis" indicates the presence of inflammation, and inflammation is only present early on in the tendinopathy disease process. Inflammation may have resolved and inflammatory cells may no longer be present, but the patient may still have pain. At that point the disease process has changed from one of inflammation to a degenerative problem more appropriately termed tendinosis (Table 1).

Tendinopathies are characterized by pain, swelling, and impairment of functional activities of the affected region. They can be acute, chronic, or recurrent. The diagnosis is usually clinical based on history and physical examination. Typically, there is a history of repetitive motion, which can be anything from painting a wall to playing a sport like tennis. If this historical information is lacking, then a systemic medical condition should be considered.

With repetitive activities and inadequate recovery time tenocytes will begin producing inflammatory substances, and the load-bearing matrix of the tendon will begin to breakdown and become fibrotic. The collagen matrix becomes disorganized with fibers separating and healing in an erratic, disorganized manner. There is an increase in mucoid ground substance, hypercellularity, and pathologic vessel and sensory afferent nerve formation. The abnormal nerve formation likely contributes to the sensation of pain. This histopathological degenerative process is more appropriately called tendinosis. The degenerative mechanism appears to be multifactorial, with contributions from:
1. Classic inflammatory mediators like interleukins, prostaglandins, and substance P.
2. Altered load bearing on a tendon as in shoulder impingement.
3. Systemic influences such as aging.

Tendinopathy is occurring at higher rates in the developed world secondary to an increase in recreational sport participation. Lower extremity tendons, like the Achilles and patellar tendons, bear a large amount of tensile force (Table 2). Thirty percent of runners will suffer Achilles tendinopathy in their lifetime, with an odds ratio of 31:2 when compared with age matched controls, and repetitive exposure is a risk factor. One in 3 patients with Achilles tendinopathy do not participate in sports. With respect to patellar tendinopathy, jumping sports like volleyball and basketball are risk factors. Historically, most lateral hip pain was labeled "trochanteric bursitis." Research using imaging techniques, including magnetic resonance imaging (MRI) and ultrasound (), has concluded that lateral hip pain around the greater trochanter is more likely caused by tendon tears or tendinopathy of the gluteus medius and gluteus minimus muscle-tendon complex than inflammation of the trochanteric bursa. Rarely is there an actual bursitis present, so the diagnosis "trochanteric bursitis" should no longer be used regularly unless there is documented bursitis on an imaging study. This is important because the patient is more likely to benefit long-term from physical therapy (PT) as opposed to nonsteroidal antiinflammatory drugs (NSAIDs), or steroid injections, attributable to the underlying pathology being more likely tendon related than bursa related. Without an imaging study, the better term for lateral hip pain at this time is greater trochanteric pain syndrome (GTPS).

Many upper extremity tendons, such as those of the wrist, are adapted to gliding through synovial sheaths. The most commonly affected tendons in the upper extremity are the rotator cuff, specifically the supraspinatus tendon, and the common extensor tendon (more precisely the extensor carpi radialis brevis) involved in lateral epicondylopathy, commonly known as *tennis elbow*. Despite names like tennis elbow and golfer's elbow, upper extremity tendinopathies (see Table 2) are more likely the result of repetitive motion from work or hobby related activities. When sports are a cause of upper extremity tendinopathy, they are typically sports requiring overhead motion like baseball, volleyball, and tennis. Up to 35% to 50% of adult tennis players will develop an elbow tendinopathy during their lifetime. A common cause of tendinopathy in the wrist is De Quervain tenosynovitis. De Quervain tenosynovitis affects the first dorsal compartment of the wrist containing the abductor pollicis longus and extensor pollicis brevis tendons. As the term "tenosynovitis" suggests, this condition results in irritation and swelling of not only the tendons themselves, but also of the synovial sheath encapsulating those tendons.

Some patients will develop tendinopathies without repetitive activity. Diseases of glucose metabolism and atherosclerosis are associated with a higher incidence of tendinopathy. Some common medications are also associated with tendinopathy including statins, fluoroquinolone antibiotics, and steroids, especially when steroids are injected intratendinously, which should be avoided.

Evaluation
On physical examination the affected tendon will sometimes appear swollen, and it is typically tender to palpation. The affected tendon-muscle complex may exhibit restricted flexibility, and stretching it or activating it against resistance may reproduce the patient's pain.

TABLE 1	Tendinopathy Progression	
	TENDONITIS	**TENDINOSIS**
Pathology	Inflammatory	Degenerative
Timing	Days to weeks	Weeks to years
Imaging	Typically unnecessary	Radiographs initially Ultrasound or magnetic resonance imaging for persistent symptoms

TABLE 2	Common Tendinopathy Sites

Upper Extremity
- Rotator cuff (especially supraspinatus)
- Medial epicondyle
- Lateral epicondyle (especially extensor carpi radialis brevis)
- First dorsal compartment of the wrist (De Quervain)

Lower Extremity
- Gluteus medius and gluteus minimus
- Iliopsoas
- Patellar
- Achilles

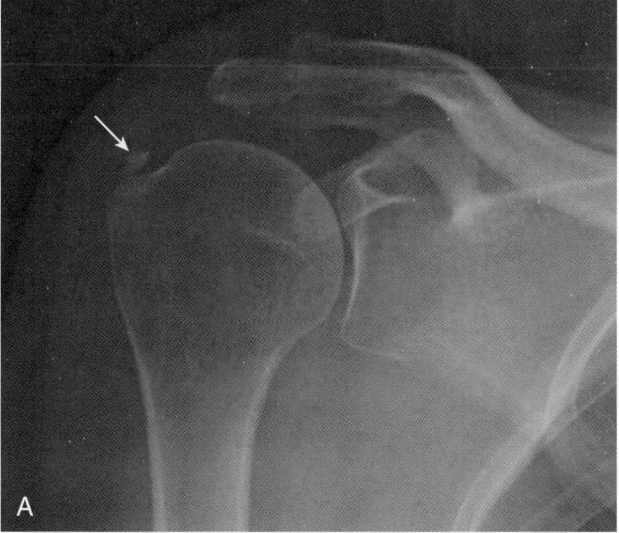

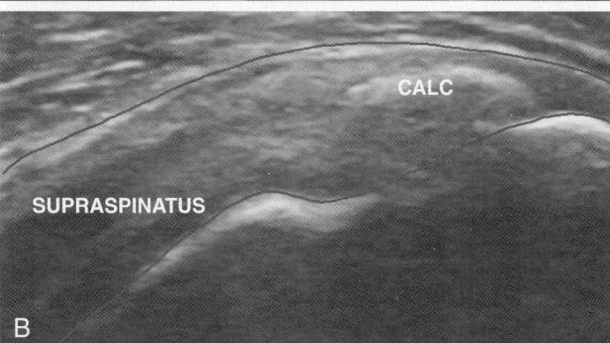

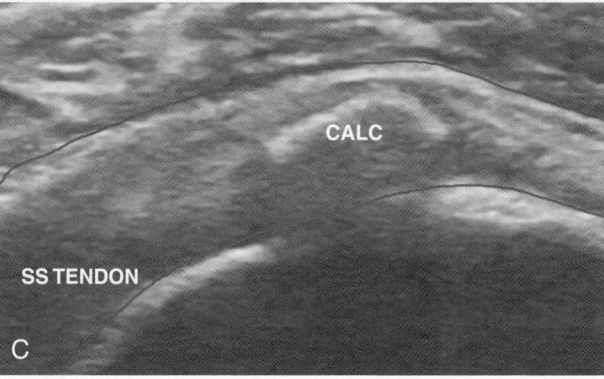

Figure 1 **A,** AP of the patients shoulder demonstrating a calcific lesion near the humeral head. **B,** Long axis view; **C,** short axis view both by ultrasound of the same patient's supraspinatus tendon *(outline)* near its attachment at the humeral head. The humeral cortex shows as hyperechoic on the bottom of the tendon. The calcification is noted to be within the tendon near the attachment. Acoustic shadowing is noted underneath the calcification, which prevents viewing the entire calcific structure and the underlying humeral cortex. *Abbreviations:* CALC=calcification, SS=supraspinatus.

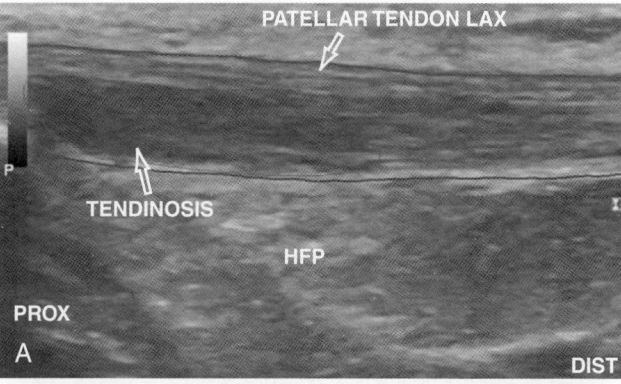

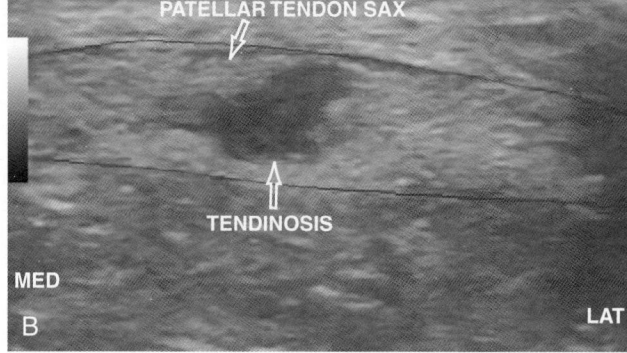

Figure 2 **A,** Long axis view; **B,** short axis view both by ultrasound of a patellar tendon *(outline)* demonstrating tendinosis as evidence by the hypoechoic heterogeneous region outline, which represents the degeneration and irregularity of tendinosis. *Abbreviations:* DIST=distal, HFP=Hoffa's fat pad, MED=medial, LAT=lateral, LAX=long axis, P=patella, PROX=proximal, SAX=short axis.

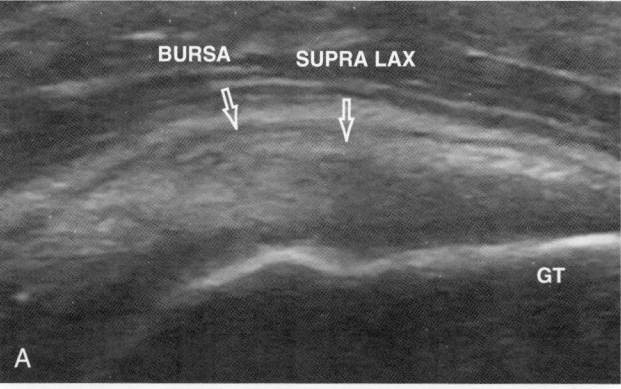

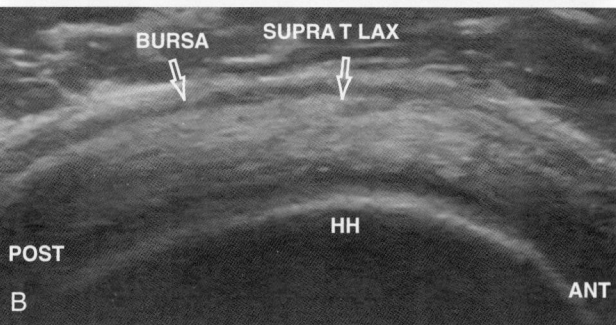

Figure 3 **A,** long axis view; **B,** short axis view both by ultrasound of a supraspinatus tendon with a subacromial-subdeltoid bursitis. The tendon is hyperechoic and fibrillar, which is in contrast to the overlying hypoechoic bursa. *Abbreviations:* ANT=anterior, GT=greater tuberosity, HH=humeral head, LAX=long axis, POST=posterior, SAX=short axis, SUPRA T=supraspinatus tendon.

When the diagnosis of a tendinopathy is in question, imaging can be helpful. Radiographs of the affected area should be considered, to look for abnormalities such as large calcifications within tendons (Figure 1, *A*). When the diagnosis is in question or the patient has failed a course of physical therapy, advanced imaging should be considered. This is usually accomplished by either ultrasound or MRI. Ultrasound can reveal thickening or structural changes within the tendon consistent with degeneration and other abnormalities such as calcification. As tendinopathies are commonly associated with bursitis, bursal thickening consistent with bursitis may also be seen (Figures 1, *B-C,*2, and 3). Similar findings may be demonstrated on MRI (Figure 4).

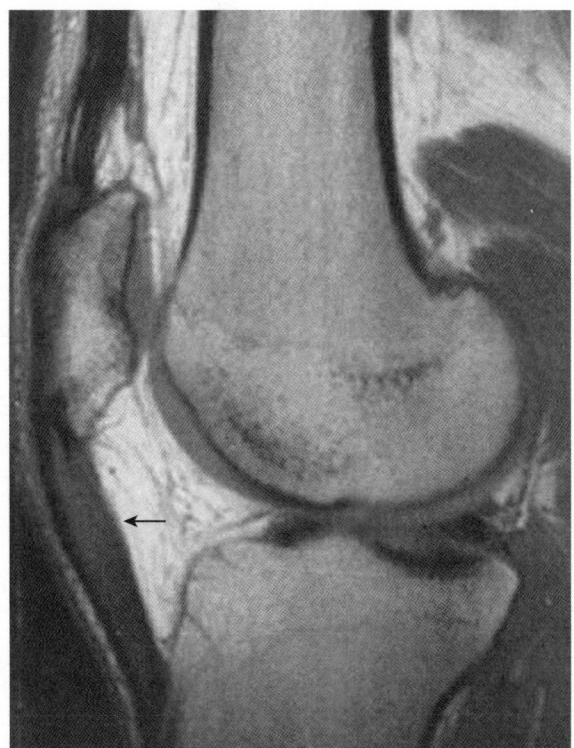

Figure 4 MRI appearance of tendinopathy. Sagittal T1-weighted image of the knee in a professional basketball player demonstrates abnormal signal and increased size in the patellar tendon, consistent with severe tendinopathy *(arrow)*. The tendon is normally devoid of signal. (From Grainger RG, Allison DJ, Adam A, Dixon AK. Grainger and Allison's Diagnostic Radiology, 4th ed. Philadelphia: Churchill Livingstone; 2001.)

Determining which imaging modality to use can be challenging. MRI is considered the gold-standard for diagnosing tendinopathies and has the advantage of demonstrating an anatomic overview of the affected area, in addition to providing soft tissue contrast. However, in trained hands, the advantages of ultrasound include ease of use, point-of-care examination, dynamic evaluation of the tendon and muscles, better resolution than MRI, and guidance for injections and procedures.

Prevention

Prevention is always the best option. Tendons do not respond well to acute changes in routine or long periods of rest. This should be kept in mind by athletes during the off-season, someone taking on a new labor job on an assembly line, or a secretary with a new work space. These "potential patients" should be eased into their new routines, because all of these scenarios are classic setups for the development of a tendinopathy. Maintaining activity during the offseason and preparing one's self for changes in the workplace will help to mitigate the risk of tendinopathy development.

Treatment

Medications are rarely employed in the treatment of tendinosis because the patient usually does not present to the clinician's office until long after the disease process has begun. If the patient is caught early enough, for example within a week or two of the offending event (eg, lateral epicondylitis a week after painting a house), then the disease process is still likely an inflammatory one, and appropriately termed a tendonitis. In this case, NSAIDs are appropriate to try to stop the inflammatory process and ultimately try to prevent it from progressing to a degenerative process. Other effective treatments for tendonitis include activity modification, rest, and ice. However, if the patient has had pain for months, the process has likely progressed to tendinosis. The use of NSAIDs has been shown to negatively affect the repair mechanism involved in tendinosis, thus they should be used cautiously in this situation.

Expectations about healing tendinosis should be addressed early. To begin with, tendon healing takes significant time and effort on the part of the patient. Additionally, many of the treatment modalities used to heal tendons will produce a reasonable amount of pain in and of themselves. This is actually a good thing as it indicates the patient is working hard enough to heal and that the healing process is occurring. It is not uncommon to have minor setbacks during the rehabilitation process. There should be an overall trend from a state of disease to health, but the path to recovery is not typically linear. The initial management of tendinopathy should be rehabilitation through PT. The patient should be informed that the "work" of PT is not done at the therapist's office, but it is done at home on their own. Failing to adhere to the treatment program will almost ensure a lack of recovery.

The exercises performed in PT aim to reorganize the degenerative matrix, reduce tenocyte activity, improve tendon compliance, and provide analgesia. Specifically, eccentric exercises have proven to be an effective treatment. An eccentric exercise is one that strengthens the muscle-tendon complex while lengthening the complex. For example, if a patient is being treated for lateral epicondylosis, the eccentric exercise would be to move the wrist from extension to flexion against resistance, lengthening the common extensor tendon. Strengthening exercises also work to hypertrophy the muscle, which is commonly atrophied after long periods of abnormal use from compensatory movement by the patient to try to reduce pain. The time needed for the exercises to work well is 3 months, which correlates with the time needed to form new fibroblasts, the presumed mechanism by which eccentric exercises work.

PT exercises should be done bilaterally as there is a proven crossover effect for tendinopathies, whereby exercising the non-affected side actually improves the affected side. Adding static stretching to eccentric exercises has been shown to improve outcomes over eccentric exercises alone in patellar tendinopathy, and should be included in an effective rehabilitation program. Before releasing an athlete back to sports activity, the final components of an optimal rehabilitation program includes explosive concentric movements (e.g., weightlifting or box jumps), higher eccentric loading exercises (e.g., jumping from an elevated surface like a box and landing on the ground), and sports-specific movements like sprinting and cutting.

The other treatment modality commonly employed by a physical therapist in tendinosis is deep soft tissue massage with tools. These tools are used to scrape along the pathologic tendon, which promotes blood flow and inflammation leading to the breakdown of the degenerative tissue and ultimately healing of that tissue.

When these conservative measures fail, more aggressive treatment methods should be considered. It is important to point out that the following treatment options are supported by limited high quality evidence, but are nonetheless reasonable alternatives to a surgical procedure. Less invasive methods include extracorporeal shockwave therapy and low-intensity pulsed ultrasound. Glyceryl trinitrate patches are sometimes used to promote blood flow, and have been shown to provide some pain relief. Injections are common treatment modalities in tendinopathies. Steroid injections are commonly used, but usually provide short-term pain relief at best. There is evidence for long-term negative effects of steroids, so they should be used judiciously. A reasonable time to try a steroid injection is when the patient is experiencing so much pain that they are unable to perform therapy. Ultrasound guidance in the hands of a trained physician can help ensure that the injection is placed properly, and specifically not intratendinously. Other treatment options requiring a more trained physician, such as a sports medicine specialist, include prolotherapy, sclerotherapy, and biological blood product injections. Prolotherapy, the injection of hypertonic glucose, is thought to work by inducing a local inflammation-repair mechanism. In sclerotherapy, a sclerotic agent, typically polidocanol, is injected to degrade the tendinopathy pain generators, namely the abnormal vessels and sensory nerves within the tendinopathic tissue. Blood products, including whole blood and platelet-rich-plasma, are used with the intent to deliver a high concentration of growth factors to the tendinopathic tissue, where blood flow is typically low.

If the tendinopathy does not respond to these treatment options, then more invasive measures are typically considered. A tenotomy procedure uses a sharp object, typically a large bore needle, to repetitively fenestrate the degenerated portion of tendon tissue, as noted on ultrasound guidance, to cause bleeding, and stimulate tissue healing. There is a newer technique, whereby the outside of tendon is scraped with a needle or scalpel. The procedure is guided by increased color Doppler signal on ultrasound indicating high vascularity and presumed nerve formation. The recovery from these techniques is usually a minimum of 6 weeks, so they should be reserved for recalcitrant cases. Finally, an open procedure can be performed to remove macroscopically abnormal tissue through an incision in the tendon; unfortunately the recovery for this sort of a procedure is in the time frame of 4 to 12 months.

Bursitis
Background
Bursas are fluid filled sacs designed to reduce friction between various tissues including bones, skin, tendons, and muscles. Typically, there is little fluid within a bursa, but with irritation from overuse or trauma, the bursa may swell with fluid leading to pain and dysfunction. This is referred to as bursitis because of the inflammatory nature of the condition.

There are multiple locations in the body where bursitis more commonly occurs, including the shoulder, elbow, hip, and knee. Bursitis usually develops from either trauma or overuse, but systemic illnesses like rheumatoid arthritis, diabetes mellitus, gout or pseudogout, and immunosuppression may also lead to bursitis. Bursas that are more susceptible to traumatic bursitis include the prepatellar, olecranon, and trochanteric bursas; they are closer to the skin and have little subcutaneous fat over them, thus they are more likely to sustain a direct impact. Both the olecranon and prepatellar bursa are also at risk for chronic irritation and trauma. Olecranon bursitis is seen in patients who frequently rest on their elbows, as in desk workers and truck drivers. Prepatellar bursitis is seen in patients who kneel for work like carpet layers and house cleaners.

Septic bursitis is rare, and it most commonly affects the olecranon and prepatellar bursa. This occurs via direct inoculation from the traumatic event. The most common organisms isolated are *Staphylococcus aureus* followed by β-hemolytic *Streptococcus*, with about 10% being polymicrobial infections.

The other bursas in the body are more susceptible to overuse injuries. The bursas around the shoulder most commonly affected include the subacromial-subdeltoid bursa, and the scapulothoracic bursa. Athletes who perform overhead movements in sports like baseball, softball, tennis, volleyball, and swimming are at greater risk for irritating these bursas. Of course, athletes are not the only people at risk for bursitis. Manual laborers working with their arms, especially when flexed or abducted regularly can also develop bursitis around the shoulder.

The hip and pelvis have multiple bursas, but the more commonly affected include the bursas around the greater trochanter and iliopsoas. As stated in the tendinopathy section, lateral hip pain is rarely caused by "trochanteric bursitis," but there are bursa present under the gluteus maximus, gluteus medius, and gluteus minimus muscle-tendon complexes. Bursitis in this region is rarely found without an associated problem like gluteal tendinopathy, or iliotibial (IT) band syndrome. In fact, it is likely that one of these underlying problems led to the bursitis. There is also a bursa under the iliopsoas muscle as it crosses the iliopectineal eminence and anterior hip joint.

Rare causes of knee bursitis include irritation of the suprapatellar bursa, deep infrapatellar bursa, pes anserine bursa, semimembranosus bursa, and medial collateral ligament bursa (Voshell bursa). Bursitis at these locations is almost always from chronic overuse. In the ankle, the retrocalcaneal bursa may also be irritated from overuse.

Evaluation
Evaluation of a patient with suspected bursitis should always begin with a thorough history. Usually the clinician will discover a history of either trauma or overuse, but the patient should also be questioned about the presence of systemic illness. Physical exam of the affected region should include inspection for erythema and swelling. Warmth may be noted on palpation. Range of motion may be limited, but is not a consistent finding. Strength is rarely affected. The appearance of decreased strength may only reflect pain, not true weakness. True weakness would suggest an associated concern like tendinopathy or a tendon tear.

Patients with the presenting symptom of shoulder pain should be evaluated for rotator cuff tendinopathy and scapulothoracic dysfunction and winging, which predispose the athlete to impingement and bursitis. For patients complaining of hip pain, another symptom they may complain of is snapping. The patient should be questioned if the snap is reliably reproducible. If so, then have the patient demonstrate the snap. Snapping laterally is typically the gluteus maximus muscle or the iliotibial band snapping over the greater trochanter, and this is a risk factor for bursitis. If the snapping is anterior in the hip, it is likely the iliopsoas tendon snapping over the iliopectineal eminence or anterior femoral head, which can lead to iliopsoas bursitis.

For the olecranon and prepatellar bursas, special attention must be given to the fact that they are more likely to develop into a septic bursitis from a bacterial infection. If there is evidence of an abrasion over these particular areas, the physician needs to ensure there is not an associated infection. Erythema, progressive swelling, and painful range of motion may point towards the presence of an infection, but these symptoms are often present in aseptic bursitis as well, making the diagnosis difficult. Fever may be present, but its absence does not rule out infection. If there is any concern for infection, the bursa needs to be aspirated and fluid sent for cell count and differential, crystal analysis, gram stain, and culture before starting antibiotics. Blood should also be sent for a complete blood count, C-reactive protein, erythrocyte sedimentation rate, and cultures.

Imaging is not always necessary to diagnose bursitis. Swelling and erythema over a known bursa may be enough to make a diagnosis, but if the diagnosis is in question, then imaging typically begins with radiographs. Radiographs can evaluate for bony abnormalities that may suggest an underlying reason for bursitis. For example, spurring on the undersurface of the acromion can be a risk factor for subacromial-subdeltoid bursitis. Radiographs can also be used to rule out fracture or to evaluate for a foreign body, especially in the setting of olecranon or prepatellar bursitis.

Further evaluation is typically done with either MRI or ultrasound. MRI offers the advantage of global assessment of the affected region, in addition to allowing enhancement of soft tissues. In skilled hands, ultrasound is an effective tool to demonstrate bursitis throughout the body (see Figure 3). Ultrasound also has the distinct advantage of real-time imaging during a dynamic examination of the affected tissue. If aspiration or injection is needed, ultrasound can help guide the procedure. Both MRI and ultrasound modalities are useful in assessing for associated diagnoses like tendinopathy.

Treatment

Bursitis treatment usually begins with conservative measures like rest or activity modification, NSAIDs, compression, padded splinting, and ice. If the bursitis is acute, it is typically responsive to these basic treatments. As stated previously in this chapter, it is common to find associated problems with the bursitis. These include rotator cuff tendinopathy, gluteal tendinopathy, and iliotibial band syndrome. It is imperative that these issues be treated as well or the bursitis will likely reoccur. This typically requires a home exercise plan usually best directed by a physical therapist.

If these problems fail to respond to this conservative approach, including rehabilitation, then a steroid injection can be considered. There is reasonable evidence that doing the injection under ultrasound guidance will lead to better outcomes, especially for the subacromial-subdeltoid bursa, but blind injections are certainly reasonable if ultrasound is not available. Research reveals that steroid injections for greater trochanteric pain syndrome demonstrate clinically relevant relief at 3 months postinjection when compared with usual care, but that difference disappears by 12 months. This is a common finding with steroid injections. Thus, it is reasonable to consider a steroid injection for pain relief, especially if the patient is unable to participate in PT, but it is unlikely to "fix" the patient's problem long-term.

For olecranon and prepatellar bursitis, the clinician must first differentiate between septic and aseptic bursitis. If the bursa is infected, following aspiration and lab collection, antibiotics must be initiated. The decision about whether to use oral versus parenteral antibiotics and whether admission is warranted depends upon the severity of the infection and the reliability of the patient. Oral therapy should be used cautiously, as treatment failure has been seen in up to 39% to 50% of patients. The duration of antibiotic treatment is usually 10 to 14 days. Surgical intervention is rarely necessary, but should be considered in patients who fail to respond to incision and drainage and appropriate antibiotics, if there is suspicion of a foreign body, or there is an inability to adequately drain the bursa.

With aseptic bursitis of the prepatellar and olecranon bursas, the clinician should resist the urge to aspirate and inject with steroids. Aspiration and injection is a possible treatment option, but should only follow a failed conservative approach. The reason for this is that once drained, the bursa is likely to fill with fluid again quickly, and there is a risk for an iatrogenic infection. Steroids are also known to cause skin atrophy. A 6- to 8-week trial of the conservative approach is reasonable.

References

Ackermann PW, Renstrom P: Tendinopathy in sport, *Sports Health* 4:193–201, 2012.

Chang A, Miller TT: Imaging of tendons, *Sports Health* 1:293–300, 2009.

Long SS, Surrey DE, Nazarian LN: Sonography of greater trochanteric pain syndrome and the rarity of primary bursitis, *Am J Roentgenol* 201:1083–1086, 2013.

Reilly D, Kamineni S: Olecranon bursitis, *J Shoulder Elbow Surg* 25:158–167, 2016.

Scott A, Docking S, Vicenzino B, et al: Sports and exercise-related tendinopathies: a review of selected topical issues by participants of the second International Scientific Tendinopathy Symposium (ISTS) Vancouver 2012, *Br J Sports Med* 47:536–544, 2013.

Seroyer ST, Nho SJ, Bach BR, et al: Shoulder pain in the overhead throwing athlete, *Sports Health* 1:108–120, 2009.

Williams BS, Cohen SP: Greater trochanteric pain syndrome: a review of anatomy, diagnosis and treatment, *Anesth Analg* 108:1662–1670, 2009.

Wu T, Song HX, Dong Y, Li JH: Ultrasound-guided versus blind subacromial-subdeltoid bursa injection in adults with shoulder pain: A systematic review and meta-analysis, *Semin Arthritis Rheum* 45:374–378, 2015.

COMMON SPORTS INJURIES

Method of
Andrew S.T. Porter, DO

CURRENT DIAGNOSIS

- Lateral Ankle Sprain—Pain over lateral ankle ligament(s) with localized swelling. Often associated with laxity and pain with anterior drawer and/or talar tilt test. Obtain x-rays based on the Ottawa ankle and foot rules.
- Medial Ankle Sprain—Less common than lateral ankle sprain. Pain in the deltoid ligament with localized swelling. Obtain x-rays based on Ottawa ankle and foot rules.
- High Ankle Sprain—Syndesmotic injury. Pain with squeeze test and/or dorsiflexion with external rotation.
- Osteochondral Ankle Injuries—Most commonly seen in the talar dome. Associated with an ankle inversion injury and ankle pain. Often have a joint effusion and soft tissue swelling and can have mechanical symptoms (catching, locking, crepitus, and a feeling of giving way). Obtain x-rays initially and then magnetic resonance imaging (MRI) to grade degree of injury.
- Anterior Cruciate Ligament (ACL) Injuries—Most common after noncontact injuries. Physical examination reveals a diffuse knee effusion, positive Lachman, and/or anterior drawer test. Obtain x-rays then MRI for further evaluation.
- Posterior Cruciate Ligament (PCL) Injuries—Occur with varus/valgus stress with the knee in full extension. Physical examination reveals a positive posterior drawer and sag sign. Obtain x-rays then MRI for further evaluation.
- Medial Collateral Ligament (MCL) Injuries—Occur with valgus stress or twisting with or without contact. Physical examination reveals localized effusion and a positive valgus stress testing and tenderness to palpation along the MCL. Graded 1 to 3.
- Osteochondral Knee Injuries—Most commonly seen in the femoral condyle. Associated with a knee injury. Knee pain and, often, mechanical symptoms of the knee. Palpation of the femoral condyles with the knee in flexion reproduces pain. Obtain x-rays initially and then MRI to grade degree of injury.
- Mallet Finger—Disruption of the extensor mechanism insertion into the distal phalanx.
- Jersey Finger—Occurs after avulsion of the flexor digitorum profundus tendon from its insertion on the distal phalanx.
- Proximal Interphalangeal (PIP) Joint Dorsal Dislocation—Injury to the volar plate with or without an avulsion fracture.
- Scaphoid Fracture—Pain over the scaphoid with or without a fall on an outstretched hand injury is a scaphoid fracture until proven otherwise. Obtain wrist x-rays with a scaphoid view.
- Tendinosis—Repetitive chronic tendon injuries result in scarring, disorganization of fibers, degeneration, and are without an inflammatory component.
- Stress Fractures—Most often seen in active patients as a result of excessive stress on normal bone from overactivity or normal stress on a bone that is deficient (osteoporotic, poor nutrition, or in female athlete triad). History is positive for bone pain, and physical examination reveals tenderness to palpation in the affected bone and often a positive tuning fork test, hop test, and fulcrum test. Obtain x-rays first, then MRI or bone scan if needed.
- Spondylolysis/Spondylolisthesis—Most often seen in young athletes with insidious onset low back pain and history of repetitive extension. Positive stork test. X-rays initially, and if negative, may proceed with limited CT and SPECT scan or MRI.

CURRENT THERAPY

- Lateral Ankle Sprain—Treat with RICE (rest, ice, compression, elevation) and early rehab. Return to play (RTP) is generally 1 to 4 weeks and is based on functional progression. RTP with ankle brace.
- Medial Ankle Sprain—Treat with RICE and early rehab. RTP with ankle brace.
- High Ankle Sprain—Treat with RICE and boot for 1 to 3 weeks and then rehab. RTP takes a longer time compared with lateral ankle sprain.
- Osteochondral Ankle Injuries—Degree of injury is graded via MRI, and this guides treatment and RTP.
- ACL Injuries—ACL tears often need reconstruction that is individualized in active patients who require knee stability.
- PCL Injuries—Isolated PCL injuries often heal conservatively with protected weight bearing in an extension brace and knee rehab.
- MCL Injuries—Often heal conservatively with bilateral hinged knee brace and knee rehab. Generally, RTP in 2 to 6 weeks.
- Osteochondral Knee Injuries—Degree of injury is graded via MRI, and this guides treatment and RTP.
- Mallet Finger—Treat with continuous full-extension stack splinting of the distal interphalangeal joint for 6 weeks and then nighttime splinting and activity splinting for 6 weeks.
- Jersey Finger—Treatment is referral to orthopedic surgeon for surgical intervention.
- PIP joint dorsal dislocation—Reduce dislocation and obtain x-rays. Treat with progressive extension blocking splint with 30° to 40° of flexion and decrease by 10° per week.
- Scaphoid Fracture—If x-rays with scaphoid view are negative, place in a short-arm thumb spica cast and follow up in 2 weeks. If x-rays remain negative but pain persists, obtain a CT or MRI. Treat nondisplaced scaphoid fractures with short-arm thumb spica cast: proximal-third fractures 12 to 20 weeks, middle-third fractures 10 to 12 weeks, and distal-third fractures 4 to 6 weeks.
- Tendinosis—Treat by creating inflammation to facilitate healing.
- Stress Fractures—Treat with general treatment for stress fractures plus specific treatment based on stress fracture site.
- Spondylolysis/Spondylolisthesis—Treat with extension blocking brace, rest, rehabilitation with core strengthening and lower extremity flexibility, and gradual RTP.

Ankle Injuries

The ankle is the most common joint injured in athletes. Ankle sprains are common, as they represent 25% of all sports-related injuries. The Ottawa ankle and foot rules help in the decision to obtain x-rays (Box 1). In general, treatment will consist of RICE (rest, ice, compression, elevation), early mobilization, and rehab. Prevention of ankle injuries is important and consists of ankle braces, ankle taping, neuromuscular training program, and regular sport-specific warm-up exercises.

Lateral Ankle Sprain

The most common ankle sprain is a lateral inversion sprain that results from landing on an inverted foot with or without plantarflexion. The lateral ankle ligaments are the anterior talofibular ligament (ATFL), calcaneofibular ligament, and the posterior talofibular ligament. The ATFL is the most commonly sprained ligament. Lateral ankle sprains are most commonly treated with RICE initially, then early ambulation, range of motion, progression into strengthening, and then proprioception rehabilitation. Proprioception rehabilitation includes balancing on one leg and performing balancing exercises on a wobble board. For example, patients can balance on one leg when brushing their teeth.

BOX 1 Ottawa Ankle and Foot Rules

- An ankle x-ray series is indicated if there is pain in the malleolar zone and any of these findings are made:
  - Tenderness over the lateral malleolus
  - Tenderness over the medial malleolus
  - Inability to bear weight four steps immediately after the injury or in the emergency department or physician's office
- A foot x-ray series is indicated if there is pain in the midfoot zone and any of these findings are made:
  - Tenderness over the base of fifth metatarsal
  - Tenderness over the navicular bone
  - Inability to bear weight four steps immediately after the injury and in the emergency department or physician's office

---

*X-rays are indicated if any of these criteria are met.
Data from Bachmann and colleagues (2003) and Tiemstra (2012).

Athletes should return to play (RTP) with a lace-up/velcro ankle brace after injury with or without taping. This added stability will help prevent future ankle injuries and also decrease the severity of ankle injuries. Most athletes will RTP in a few days to 4 weeks; this return is based on pain, obtaining full active range of motion and full strength, and functional stability.

Medial Ankle Sprain

Medial ankle ligament sprains are rare, account for < 10% of ankle injuries, and are often accompanied with a lateral malleolar fracture or syndesmotic injury. The medial ankle ligament is the deltoid ligament and is injured via external rotation or eversion. These ankle sprains are treated similarly to lateral ankle sprains.

High Ankle Sprain

High ankle sprains, also known as syndesmotic ankle sprains, occur through forced external rotation of a dorsiflexed foot most commonly but also occur by forced internal rotation of a fixed plantar flexed foot. The syndesmotic ligaments connect and stabilize the distal tibia to the distal fibula. The syndesmotic ligaments are the anterior tibiofibular ligament, posterior tibiofibular ligament, transverse tibiofibular ligament, interosseous ligament, and the interosseous membrane. Palpate the fibular head for pain. Pain on palpation of the fibular head might indicate a maisonneuve fracture, a fracture of the proximal third of the fibula associated with syndesmotic disruption. A high ankle sprain has a longer healing time compared to a lateral ankle sprain. Often these need immobilization with a boot or cast for 1 to 4 weeks to help with healing before beginning rehab. RTP after a high ankle sprain depends on pain, achieving a full active range of motion, full strength, and functional stability. Incomplete healing of a high ankle sprain can result in distal tibia and fibula instability.

Osteochondral Ankle Injuries

Osteochondral injuries are injuries to the articular surface of a joint. These injuries range from small undisplaced depressions and cracks in the osteochondral surface to small pieces of articular cartilage and bone that break off of the articular surface and float within the joint. Osteochondral injuries occur most commonly on weight-bearing articular surfaces. In osteochondral injuries, osteonecrosis of subchondral bone occurs, resulting in separation of cartilage and subchondral bone from underlying, well-vascularized bone. The term *osteochondral lesion* (OCL) is favored over the previously used term *osteochondritis dessicans* because there might not be an inflammatory component of the injury. OCLs are often associated with repeated trauma or overuse in athletes. OCLs typically present with pain in the affected joint and can develop with a specific injury or over several months in highly active athletes. OCLs are more

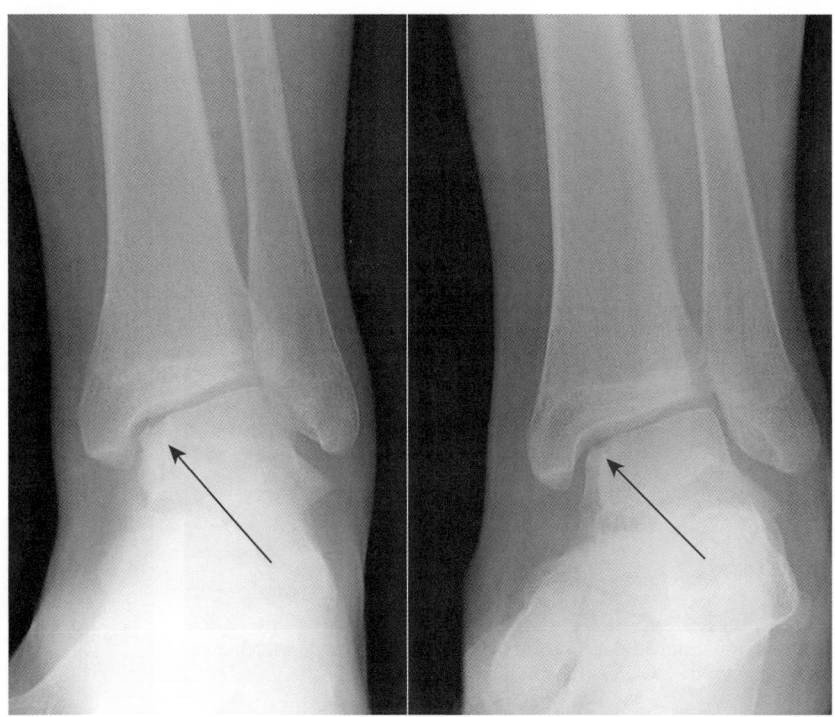

Figure 1 X-rays of the left ankle, AP and mortise views, which demonstrate a grade 2 osteochondral lesion (OCL) along the medial talar dome.

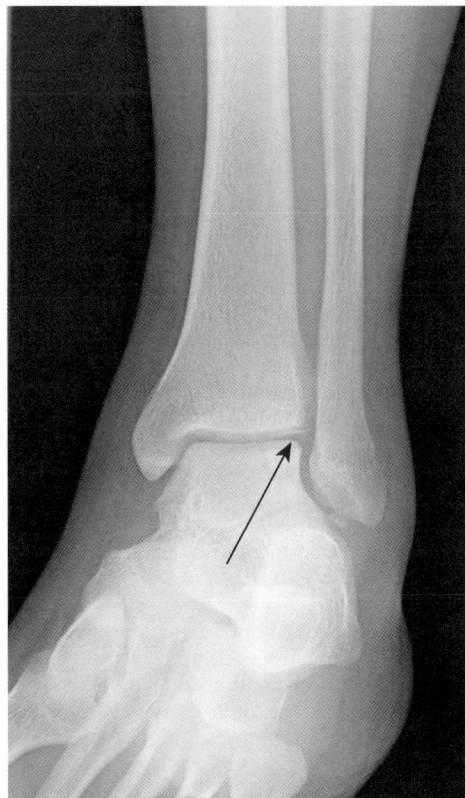

Figure 2 X-ray of the left ankle, mortise view, which demonstrates a grade 4 OCL along the lateral talar dome.

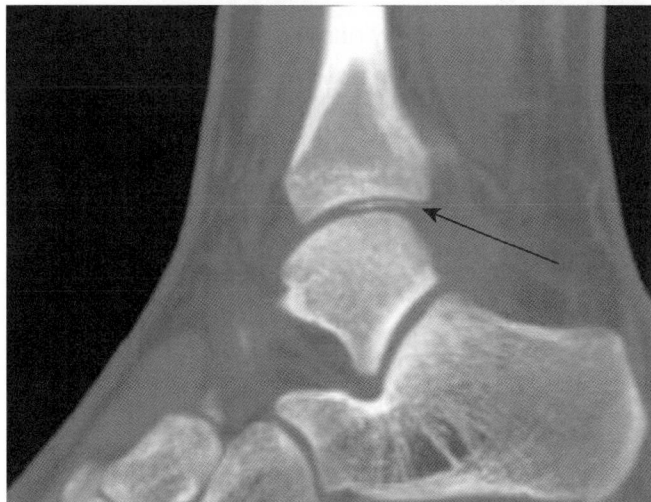

Figure 3 CT scan without contrast. Sagittal image of ankle, which demonstrates a grade 4 OCL of the talar dome.

common in younger patients with open physes (growth plates) and are referred to as juvenile OCLs. Adult OCLs describe this condition in skeletally mature patients.

Osteochondral injuries are a cause for pain in up to 25% of ankle injuries and need to be considered when a patient presents with ankle pain. Acute osteochondral injuries in the ankle most commonly affect the talar dome (Figures 1–3) but can also be found in the distal tibia (Figure 4). OCLs are first evaluated by x-rays (see Figures 1 and 2) and then graded by magnetic resonance imaging (MRI) (Table 1). CT scan (see Figure 3) is sometimes utilized as well. Grade 1 to 3 juvenile OCLs and grade 1 to 2 adult OCLs are treated conservatively. Conservative treatment consists of no weight bearing (NWB) in a cast or boot for 6 to 10 weeks followed by partial weight bearing (PWB) to full weight bearing (FWB) over 2 to 6 weeks, followed with an ankle brace for 3 months, and ensuring adequate calcium and vitamin D intake to facilitate healing. Nonsteroidal antiinflammatory drugs (NSAIDs) should be avoided because they can slow bone healing, and OCLs are probably not an inflammatory process. For grade 4 juvenile OCLs, grade 3 and 4 adult OCLs, and those that have not clinically healed with conservative care operative treatment is required. Operative treatment options depend on OCL size and type and include removal of the OCL followed by transchondral drilling and microfracture to stimulate fibrocartilage

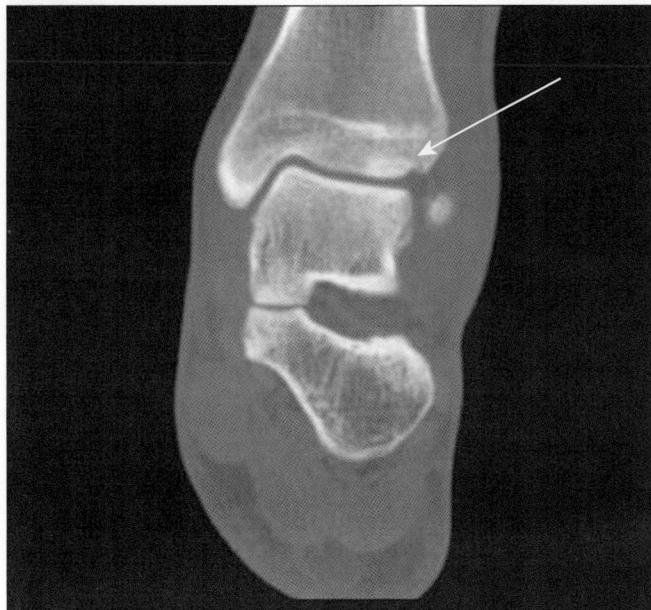

Figure 4 CT scan without contrast. Coronal image of ankle, which demonstrates a grade 1 OCL of the distal lateral tibia.

TABLE 1	Classification of Osteochondral Lesions	
STAGE	**PLAIN X-RAY FINDINGS**	**MRI FINDINGS**
1	Depressed osteochondral fragment	Articular cartilage thickening and low signal changes in subchondral bone
2	Osteochondral fragment attached by bone	Articular cartilage breached, no synovial fluid around fragment
3	Detached nondisplaced fragment	Articular cartilage breached, synovial fluid around fragment
4	Displaced fragment	Loose foreign body

formation, fixation of the OCL with an osteochondral allograft, osteochondral autograft transfer, and autologous chondrocyte implantation.

Knee injuries—The knee joint lacks intrinsic bone stability, so most stability is from the major knee ligaments.

Anterior Cruciate Ligament Injuries

The anterior cruciate ligament (ACL) is the key stabilizer of the knee and is one of two major intraarticular knee ligaments, the other being the posterior cruciate ligament (PCL). Most ACL tears occur from noncontact injuries. Women experience ACL tears up to nine times more often than men do. The main function of the ACL is to prevent excessive anterior tibial translation relative to the femur. Patients who sustain an injury to their ACL often describe hearing a pop, feeling instability in their knee, experiencing pain immediately after the injury, and develop an associated knee effusion. On-the-field evaluation is ideal in an ACL injury, as the hamstrings will often start to tighten up shortly after the injury, preventing anterior tibial translation. This will prevent an isolated test of the ACL and give the false impression that an ACL endpoint is present when in fact the ACL is completely torn. The anterior drawer (Figure 5) and Lachman test (Figure 6) are the main physical examination tests to evaluate the ACL. Obtain x-rays and then MRI if an ACL tear is suspected. The blood supply to the ACL is poor and is provided by the middle geniculate artery off of the popliteal artery. Because of the poor blood supply, ACL tears often need reconstruction if

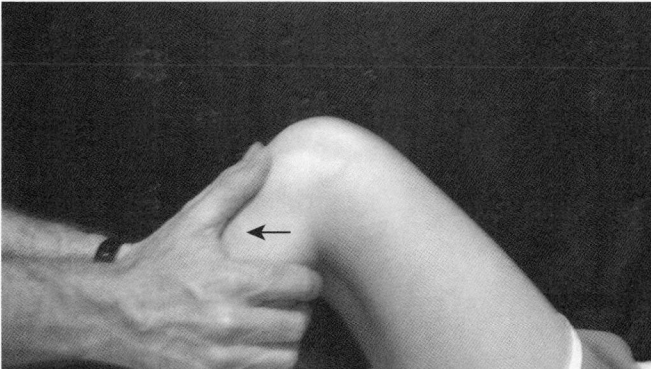

Figure 5 Anterior drawer test for ACL laxity. Patient's knee is flexed 90°. Examiner applies anterior force to the tibia in relation to the patient's femur to evaluate for laxity.

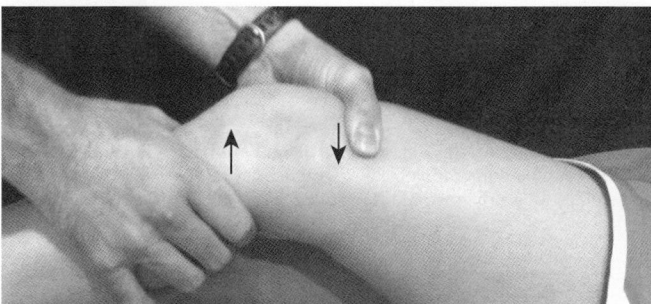

Figure 6 Lachman test for ACL laxity. Patient's knee is flexed 20°–30°. Examiner grasps the distal femur and proximal tibia and applies anterior force to the tibia and posterior force to the femur to evaluate for ACL laxity.

athletes want to return to a high level of activity and knee stability is needed. ACL reconstruction timing is important and often will occur 3 to 4 weeks after injury to allow for swelling to decrease, ROM and strength to improve, and inflammation to decrease. Also during this presurgical time, it is important to have patients perform pre-hab (presurgical rehabilitation), focusing on AROM and knee strengthening. A knee effusion will cause the quadriceps muscles to weaken and atrophy. Hamstring tendon autograft, patella tendon autograft, quadriceps tendon autograft, and allograft are all used for ACL reconstruction. Each graft has advantages and disadvantages and should be discussed with the orthopaedic surgeon before reconstruction and individualized for each patient. Continuing to participate in high-level activity after an ACL tear if undiagnosed can lead to a knee dislocation and further intraarticular knee injury.

PCL Injuries

The PCL is the other major intraarticular knee ligament. Isolated PCL injuries are much less common than ACL injuries and make up only 3.5% of ligamentous knee injuries in sports, with the remaining 96.5% of PCL injuries associated with multiligamentous knee injuries. PCL injuries, unlike ACL injuries, are the result of external forces (e.g., a soccer player sliding into the goal post and tearing his or her PCL). The main function of the PCL is to resist posterior tibial translation. Posterior drawer testing (Figure 7) and a sag sign test (Figure 8) are the physical examination tests used to evaluate the PCL. Obtain x-rays then MRI if a PCL tear is suspected. The blood supply to the PCL is better than the blood supply to the ACL. Isolated PCL injuries (grades 1 and 2) are treated conservatively because surgical reconstruction has not been shown to be helpful. Conservative treatment consists of protected weight bearing in an extension brace followed by quadriceps rehabilitation and ROM exercises. RTP is generally 4 to 6 weeks after a PCL injury. Surgical intervention is recommended for associated injuries to the ACL, medial collateral ligament (MCL), and posterior lateral corner (grade 3 PCL injury).

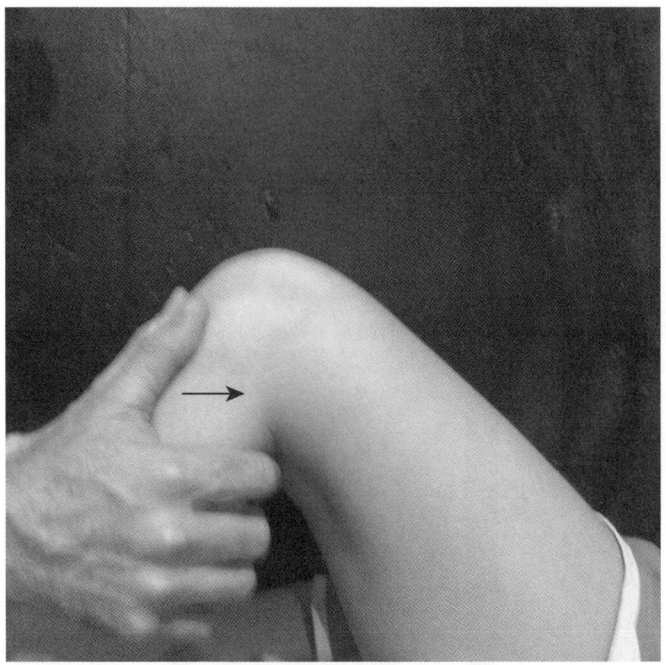

Figure 7 Posterior drawer test for PCL laxity. Patient's knee is flexed 90°. Examiner applies posterior force to the tibia in relation to the patient's femur to evaluate for laxity.

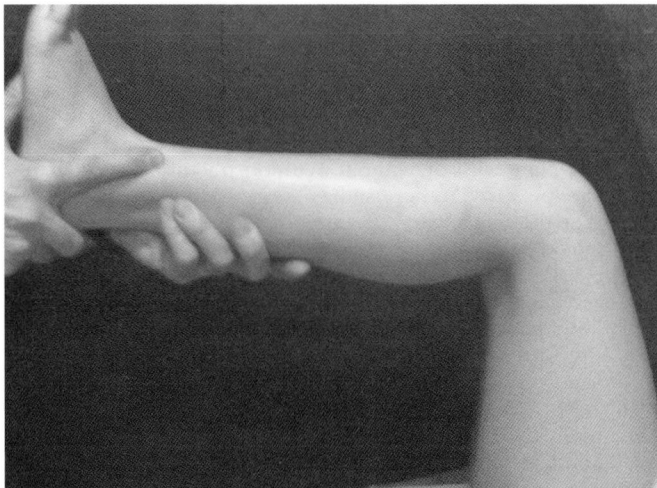

Figure 8 Sag sign test for PCL laxity. Examiner views the tibia condyles from the lateral side to evaluate for a posterior sag (displacement) in the appearance that would indicate a PCL injury.

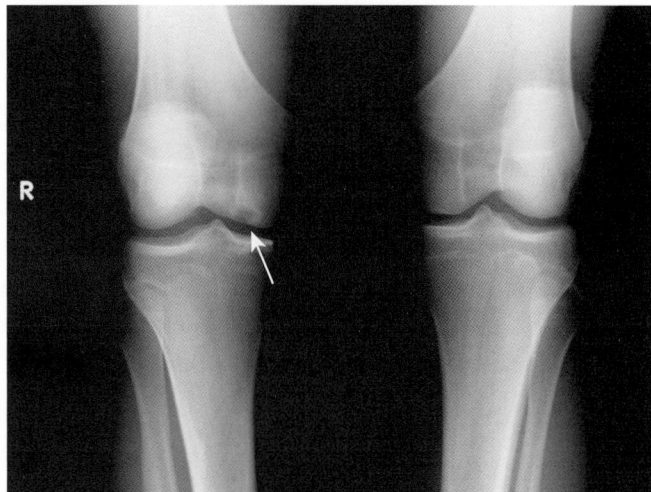

Figure 9 X-ray of the bilateral knees, AP view, which demonstrates a grade 1 OCL along the right knee medial femoral condyle.

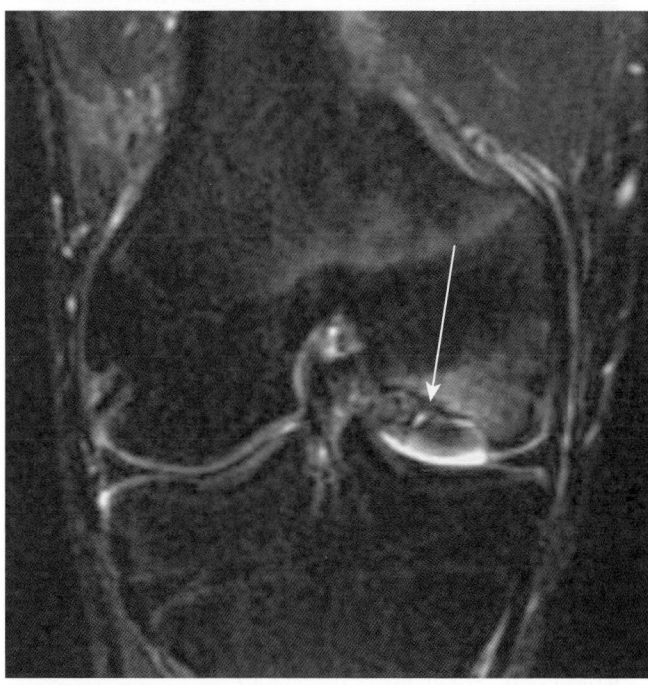

Figure 10 Magnetic resonance imaging (MRI) of the right knee, without contrast. Coronal T2 fat saturation image, which demonstrates a grade 4 OCL of the medial femoral condyle.

MCL Injuries

The MCL is an extraarticular ligament that resists knee valgus forces. An MCL sprain results from a valgus stress to a partially flexed knee. Athletes will present with localized pain and swelling along the medial aspect of the knee. Most MCL injuries are isolated ligament injuries, but more severe MCL injuries can involve tears of the medial meniscus and ACL, commonly referred to as the "terrible triad." The MCL is examined by palpation and valgus stress testing at 0° and 30° of knee flexion. MCL injuries are graded 1, 2, or 3 depending on severity of injury. A patient with a grade 1 MCL sprain has pain in the MCL but no valgus stress testing laxity. A grade 2 MCL sprain has valgus stress testing laxity but a solid endpoint. A grade 3 MCL sprain has no endpoint with valgus stress testing. Thankfully, the MCL has a rich vascular supply and can often heal conservatively. Treatment consists of RICE for the first 1 to 2 weeks and a bilateral hinged knee brace to facilitate healing. Weight bearing and ROM and strengthening exercises are started when they are tolerable. RTP after an MCL injury depends on the grade and generally takes 2 to 6 weeks.

Osteochondral Knee Injuries

Osteochondral injuries occur in the knee as well as in the ankle. Osteochondral injuries of the knee most commonly affect the lateral aspect of the medial femoral condyle but can be found anywhere along the medial or lateral femoral condyle, patella, or trochlea. History is significant for knee pain, with or without swelling and mechanical symptoms (catching, locking, crepitus, and feeling of giving way). On palpation, patients can have pain in the affected area with knee flexion with or without crepitus. Obtain x-rays initially (Figure 9) and then grade the OCL severity by MRI (Figure 10). CT scans are also utilized sometimes. Grade 1 to 3 juvenile knee OCLs and grade 1 to 2 adult knee OCLs are

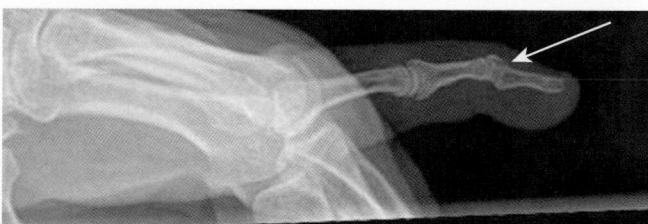

Figure 11 X-ray of the left hand, lateral view, which demonstrates a mallet finger of the fifth finger. Note the flexion of the DIP joint and avulsion fracture of the distal phalanx that involves about 30% of the joint space.

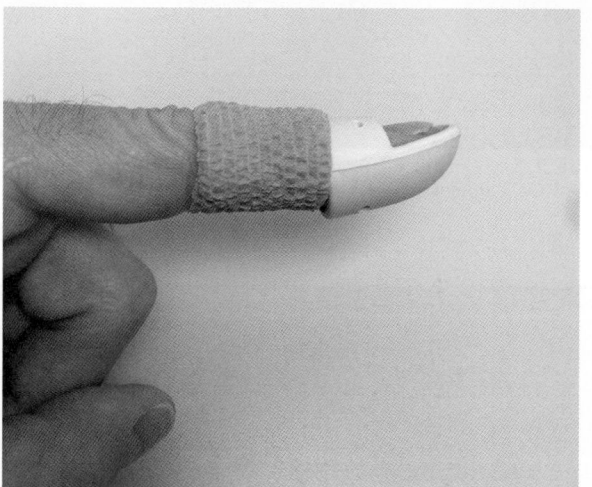

Figure 12 Stack splint with Coban wrap added for stability that immobilizes the DIP joint at neutral to 5° of hyperextension.

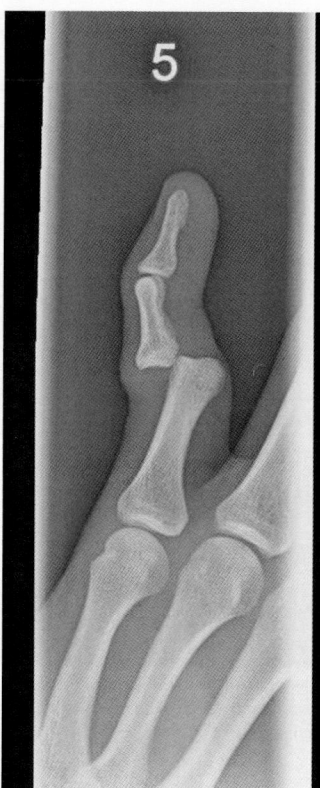

Figure 13 X-ray of the left hand, oblique view, which demonstrates a proximal interphalangeal (PIP) joint dorsal and lateral dislocation.

treated conservatively. Grade 4 juvenile OCLs, grade 3 to 4 adult OCLs and all OCLs that have failed conservative care are treated operatively.

Hand Injuries
Mallet Finger
A mallet finger occurs after forced flexion of an actively extended distal interphalangeal (DIP) joint, resulting in disruption of the extensor mechanism insertion into the distal phalanx. Patients with a mallet finger are unable to actively extend the DIP joint. This injury can be associated with an avulsion fracture (Figure 11). For acute injuries, general treatment consists of continuous extension splinting of the DIP joint (0° to 10° of hyperextension) for at least 6 weeks. The 6-week clock starts over if the DIP joint is allowed to flex at all during the initial 6 weeks of treatment or if, at the end of the 6 weeks, the mallet finger is not completely healed. After the initial 6 weeks, it is recommended to continue with nighttime splinting and activity splinting for another 6 weeks to ensure adequate healing and avoidance of surgery. To perform this splinting, a stack splint is well tolerated and is protective (Figure 12). Orthopaedic referral is indicated if the patient is unable to obtain full passive extension of the DIP joint or if the avulsion fracture involves over 30% of the joint space.

Jersey Finger
A jersey finger results from the avulsion of the flexor digitorum profundus tendon from its insertion on the distal phalanx. This commonly occurs in football and rugby players when the tip of their flexed finger is caught in a jersey and the DIP joint of the finger is then forcefully extended. After this injury occurs, the patient is unable to actively flex the DIP joint. Treatment is urgent referral to an orthopaedic surgeon for surgical intervention.

Proximal Interphalangeal Joint Dorsal Dislocation
Proximal interphalangeal (PIP) joint injuries are the most common joint injuries in sports. Most PIP dislocations are dorsal and result from hyperextension with an axial load. Dislocations are described by the position of the distal fragment in relation to the proximal fragment. PIP dorsal dislocations cause injury to the volar plate with or without avulsion fracture. Pre-reduction x-rays are preferred if they can be obtained promptly (Figure 13). X-rays of the finger with at least one view being a true lateral view should be obtained to rule out fracture. However, many PIP dorsal dislocations occur on the playing field and it is reasonable to reduce these dislocations, buddy tape the affected finger, and allow the patient to RTP with x-rays obtained after the athletic competition. Reduction is usually uncomplicated and is performed urgently via hyperextending the joint, applying traction in plane with the finger, then flexing the joint. Post reduction films are a necessity (Figure 14). Stability testing of the collateral ligaments should be performed after the reduction. Full flexion and extension of the PIP joint will be possible if the joint is stable. A stable joint without a large avulsion fragment should be treated with a progressive extension blocking splint (Figures 15 and 16). Start with 30° to 40° of flexion and decrease by 10° per week over 3 to 4 weeks, then buddy tape the injured finger with activity PRN (8). Some PIP dorsal dislocations have a lateral component to them and these are treated similar to pure dorsal dislocations (see Figure 13). Orthopaedic surgeon referral is indicated if there is a large avulsion fracture or the joint is unstable.

Scaphoid Fracture
The scaphoid bone is the most common carpal bone that is fractured and is a common injury that is encountered in primary care. Interestingly, scaphoid fractures occur most commonly in young men. Scaphoid fractures occur less commonly in young children and the elderly because of the relative weakness of the distal radius compared with the scaphoid in these age groups. Often a scaphoid fracture is caused by a FOOSH (fall on an outstretched hand) injury. On physical examination, if the patient has pain over the scaphoid tubercle or in the anatomical snuffbox with or without a history of a FOOSH injury, the clinician needs to have a high index of suspicion for a scaphoid fracture when evaluating the wrist

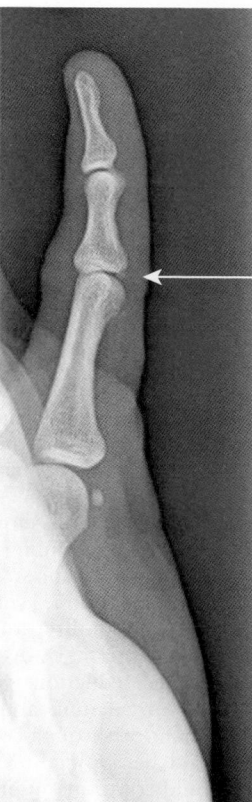

Figure 14 X-ray of the left hand, lateral status postreduction view, which demonstrates a relocated proximal interphalangeal (PIP) joint. Note the avulsion fracture of the middle phalanx.

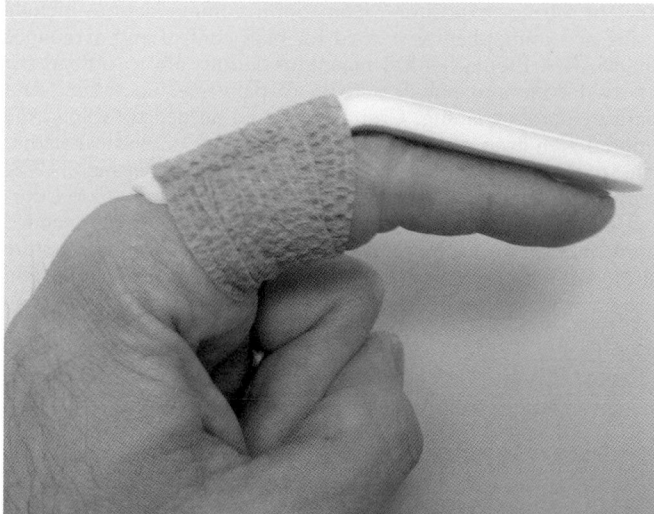

Figure 15 Dorsal extension blocking splint at 30°–40° of flexion at the PIP joint. Note that there is no pressure over the PIP joint volar plate and that flexion and extension at the DIP joint is possible.

x-rays. Obtain the standard wrist x-rays (AP, lateral, and oblique views) plus a dedicated scaphoid view (AP with ulnar deviation) and be aware that early imaging with x-rays is often unrevealing for a scaphoid fracture (Figure 17). If a fracture is not seen on x-rays, the clinician needs to have a high index of suspicion for a scaphoid fracture, place the patient in a short-arm thumb spica cast, and have the patient follow up in 2 weeks. If repeat x-rays remain negative and the patient continues to have scaphoid pain, proceed with an MRI of the wrist with T2 fat saturation views or a CT scan. If a scaphoid fracture is noted on imaging, the location

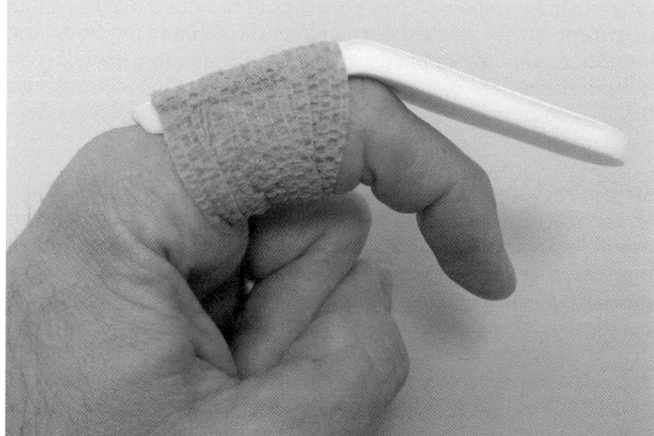

Figure 16 Dorsal extension blocking splint at 30°–40° of flexion at the PIP joint. This figure illustrates the freedom of motion that is possible at the PIP joint (full flexion and limited extension) and the DIP joint (full flexion and extension).

of the scaphoid fracture will guide treatment. Because the blood supply to the scaphoid is distal to proximal, scaphoid fractures are harder to heal than other carpal fractures. Nondisplaced middle-third or proximal-third scaphoid fractures are treated with a long- or short-arm thumb spica cast with the wrist at 20° to 30° of extension and the thumb in slight extension and abduction for 10 to 20 weeks. Middle-third fractures should be immobilized for 10 to 12 weeks. Proximal-third fractures should be immobilized from 12 to 20 weeks. It is much easier to regain flexion in the wrist after casting than it is to regain extension. If the elbow is incorporated in the cast, it should be casted at 90° of flexion. A long-arm cast may decrease healing time, but it does not improve nonunion rates. A nondisplaced distal-third fracture should be treated in a short-arm thumb spica cast for 4 to 6 weeks. For displaced fractures or non-healing fractures, a referral to an orthopedic surgeon is recommended. Use acetaminophen for pain control and avoid nonsteroidal antiinflammatory drugs (NSAIDs) because NSAIDs can impair bone healing. Ensure adequate energy availability via diet and adequate calcium and vitamin D intake, and avoid tobacco exposure to help heal the fracture. Bone health and bone nutrition are a part of the big picture in fracture healing.

Overuse Injuries
Tendinosis
The paradigm and management of tendon overuse injuries is changing. The term *tendinitis* is generally used to refer to painful overuse tendon conditions and implies that inflammation is present. However, the most common pathology in chronic painful tendons is tendinosis. Tendinosis occurs after repetitive injuries to a tendon results in intertendinous scarring, disorganization of tendon fibers, and degeneration. Tendinosis does not have an inflammatory component. Early on in a tendon injury, there is inflammation resulting in tendinitis, but after about 6 weeks this generally evolves into tendinosis. Early activity modification and treatment of tendinitis with NSAIDs and rehabilitation may prevent the development of tendinosis. Tendinosis is a problematic condition that affects many active people, young and old. To address these more chronic tendon injuries, healing is facilitated by creating an inflammatory response. To create inflammation, treatments such as eccentric strengthening (Figure 18), deep soft tissue massage with tools (e.g., gua sha or Graston, or ASTYM) (Figure 19), nitroglycerin patches (Nitro-Dur),[1] and musculoskeletal ultrasound-guided percutaneous needle tenotomy (with or without injection of autologous blood, prolotherapy, or platelet-rich plasma) have all been utilized and have been shown to be effective (Table 2). It is important to avoid NSAIDs when trying to create inflammation because NSAIDs will prevent the

Not FDA approved for this indication.

inflammatory response. This concept of tendinosis diagnosis and treatment can be utilized for tendons throughout the body and is most commonly applied to the Achilles tendon, patella tendon, iliotibial (IT) band, piriformis, gluteus medius, hamstrings, biceps, common elbow flexor tendon, and common elbow extensor tendon.

Stress Fractures

Stress fractures occur when osteoclastic activity overwhelms osteoblastic activity. Bone injury unfolds over a continuum of time, starting with normal bone that progresses to stress reaction, then stress fracture, and finally fracture if the bone continues to be injured. This can occur as a result of excessive stress on normal bone from overactivity or normal stress on a bone that is deficient (osteoporotic, poor nutrition, or in female athlete triad).

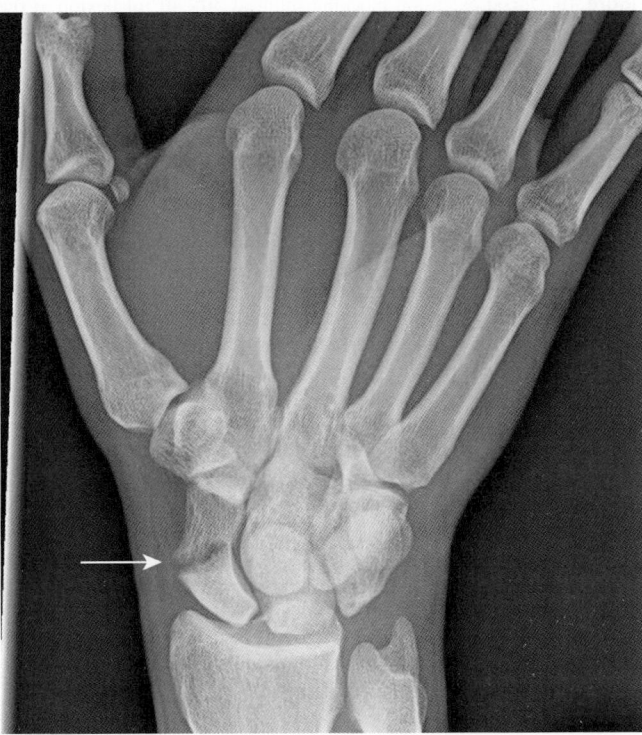

Figure 17 Scaphoid view x-ray (AP view with ulnar deviation) is important to obtain in addition to your standard wrist views (AP, lateral, and oblique) when scaphoid fracture is suspected. This scaphoid fracture was not seen on the x-rays on the day of the injury. Patient continued to have wrist pain and then presented 10 weeks later, and x-rays were obtained demonstrating the scaphoid fracture.

Stress fractures are common injuries in athletes and occur most often in the lower extremities. Running sports account for 69% of stress fractures. Stress fractures should be considered in someone who is active, presents with bone pain, and who performs repetitive activities with limited rest or with a recent increase in activity. Physical examination tests to perform in the area of interest are palpation, the tuning fork test, the fulcrum test, and the hop test (Table 3). If a stress fracture is suspected, x-rays should be obtained, keeping in mind that it takes 2 to 3 weeks for signs of stress fracture (i.e., periosteal reaction, callus formation, fracture line) to show up on an x-ray, and often stress fractures do not show up on x-rays. If x-rays are negative and a diagnosis is needed to help guide care and RTP, a bone scan or MRI with T2 fat saturation views (Figures 20 and 21) should be obtained. The bone scan and MRI are equally sensitive, but an MRI is more specific and avoids patient radiation exposure. An MRI is more expensive. Because a bone scan can stay positive for up to 18 months, clinical progress should not be monitored with a bone scan.

To prevent stress fractures, athletes should distribute loading forces on the bone with cross training and biomechanical adjustments (i.e., orthotics, proper shoes, stretches, strengthening, running mechanics), consume sufficient calories to maintain adequate energy availability, and ensure appropriate intake of calcium and vitamin D. A study by Lappe of female Navy recruits showed reductions in stress fractures in those consuming 2000 mg of calcium[1] and 800 IU vitamin D[1] daily, either as a supplement or through consumption of dairy products. Tobacco should be avoided. Additionally, women of child bearing age should try to maintain regular menses by consuming adequate calories and avoiding a negative energy balance.

General treatment for stress fractures can be grouped into nutrition, medication, and biomechanical recommendations. Nutrition recommendations include optimizing energy availability in the diet, ensuring adequate calcium and vitamin D intake, and avoidance of tobacco exposure. Medication recommendations include using acetaminophen as needed for pain control and avoidance of NSAIDs. Biomechanical recommendations are to offload the affected bone and reduce activity to pain-free functioning and pain-free cross-training. Crutches may be needed to offload the injured area even more than a walking boot/cast or steal shank. The patient may require complete non-weight bearing (NWB) with the overall goal being to obtain pain-free ambulation during the initial treatment. Tables 4 and 5 outline recommended guidelines for protected weight bearing for specific stress fracture sites. Additional recommendations are to begin a rehabilitation program when tolerated and to stretch and strengthen supporting

Not FDA approved for this indication.

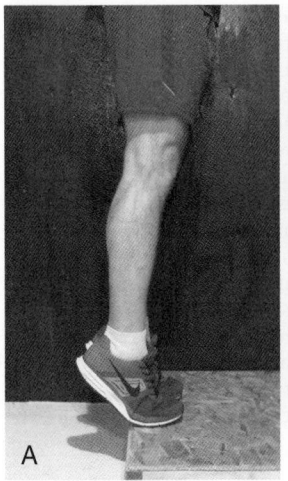
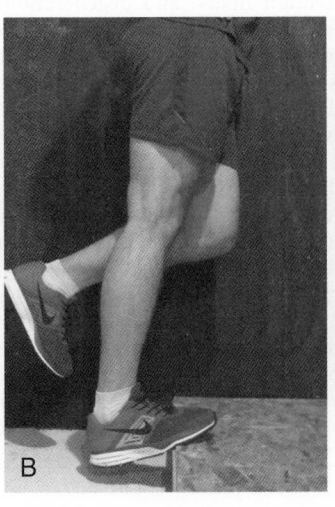
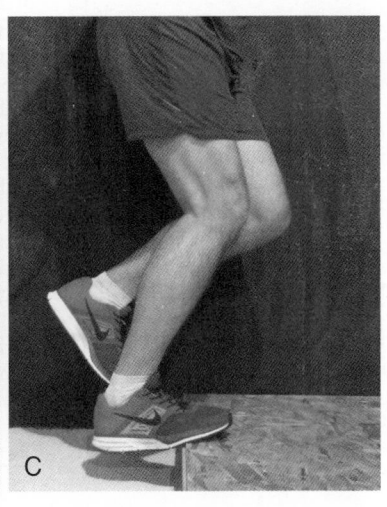

Figure 18 Eccentric exercises for Achilles tendinosis. (**A**) Patient begins with the injured leg straight and the ankle in flexion. The assistance of the uninjured leg was utilized to get in this starting position. (**B**) The ankle of the injured leg (right leg, in this case) is slowly lowered in a controlled fashion to full dorsiflexion to eccentrically strengthen (while lengthening the calf muscles) the right Achilles tendon. The left leg is then brought back down, and full plantarflexion in both ankles is performed, recruiting the uninjured leg to assist with getting back to position (**A**). (**C**) The eccentric exercise from (**B**) is repeated with the knee bent at 45°.

structures. Start a gradual increase in activity when the patient is pain-free.

Because of their propensity for delayed healing and nonunion, certain stress fractures are considered high risk, necessitate prompt treatment, and may ultimately require surgical fixation.

Low-risk stress fractures have a lower incidence of delayed healing and nonunion. High-risk stress fractures that appear stable and nondisplaced can be treated nonoperatively with close follow-up. Consider referral to an orthopaedic surgeon for failed

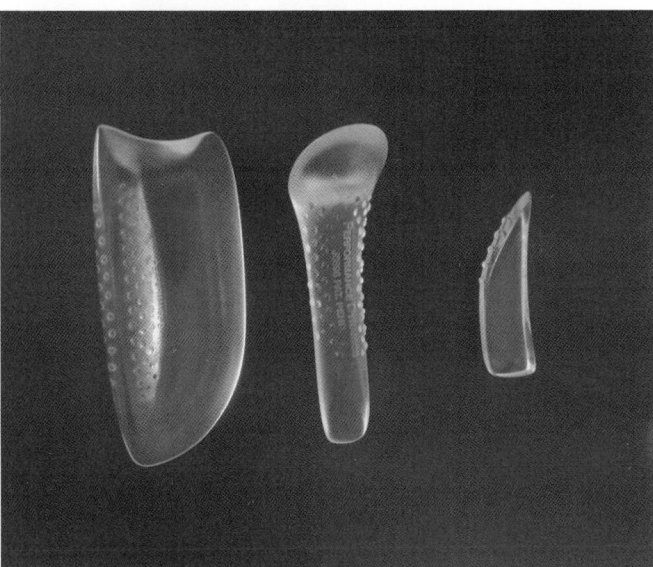

Figure 19 ASTYM® tools.

TABLE 2	Treatment of Tendinosis
TREATMENT MODALITY	**DESCRIPTION**
Deep soft tissue massage with tools (gua sha, Graston, ASTYM) (Figure 19)	One to three times per week for 4–6 wk; most common with athletic trainer certified or physical therapist
Nitroglycerin patches (Nitro-Dur)[1]	0.1 mg/h patch, apply Q24 h to a different location on tendon for at least 6 wk
Eccentric strengthening (Figure 18)	3 sets of 15 exercises, twice daily, for 12 wk
Musculoskeletal ultrasound-guided percutaneous needle tenotomy with or without autologous blood injection, prolotherapy, or platelet-rich plasma	Referral to primary care sports medicine physician

[1]Not FDA approved for this indication.

TABLE 3	Stress Fracture Physical Exam Tests
PHYSICAL EXAM TEST	**POSITIVE TEST**
Palpation	Pain over affected bone with palpation
Stork test (Figure 22)	Back extension with rotation while standing on one leg increases pain in the pars interarticularis region
Fulcrum test	Pain in fracture site while applying a bending force (e.g., over the exam table) to distal extremity while proximal extremity is kept relatively immobilized
Hop test	Hopping 10 times on affected leg reproduces pain at fracture site
Tuning fork test	Vibrating tuning fork over fracture site results in pain at site

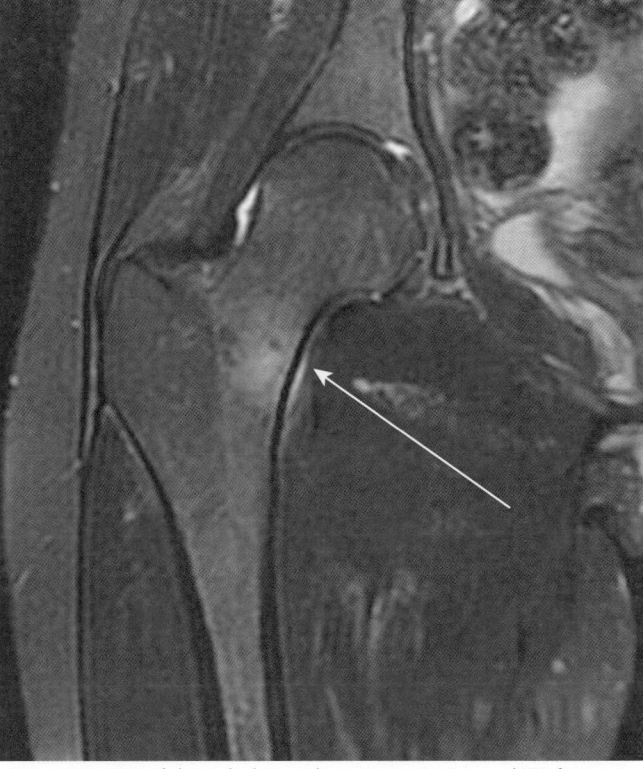

Figure 20 MRI of the right hip without contrast. Coronal T2 fat saturation image demonstrates a compression-sided femoral neck stress fracture (note surrounding bone edema in white).

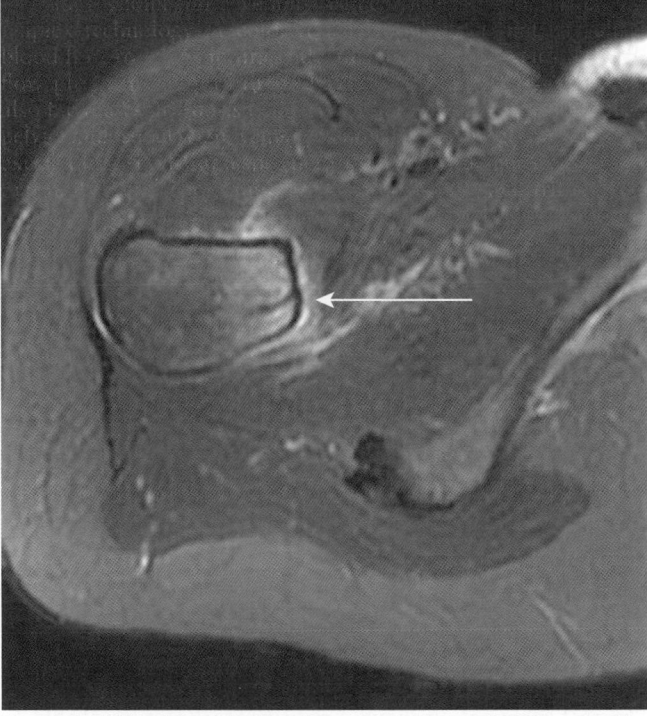

Figure 21 MRI of the right hip without contrast. Axial T2 fat saturation image that demonstrates a compression sided femoral neck stress fracture (note edema in white and probable fracture line in black that measures up to 11 mm).

TABLE 4	High-Risk Stress Fracture Initial Treatment
HIGH-RISK STRESS FRACTURE	**INITIAL TREATMENT (IF STABLE AND NONDISPLACED)**
Femoral neck (compression side) (Figures 20 and 21)	NWB for 6–8 wk then PWB to FWB over next 6–8 wk
Anterior tibia (tension side)	NWB for 6–8 wk then PWB to FWB over next 6–12 wk
Medial malleolus	Pneumatic lower leg boot for 6–8 wk
Navicular	NWB cast/boot for 6 wk then 6-wk RTP progression
Base of fifth metatarsal (Jones)	NWB cast/boot 6–8 wk
May consider surgery for quicker RTP	
Sesamoids	NWB cast/boot 6 wk

Abbreviations: NWB = non-weight bearing; PWB = partial weight bearing; FWB = full weight bearing.

TABLE 5	Low-Risk Stress Fracture Initial Treatment
LOW-RISK STRESS FRACTURE	**INITIAL TREATMENT**
Sacrum/pelvis	WBAT 7–12 wk
Femoral shaft	WBAT 6–8 wk
Posterior medial tibia (compression side)	WBAT boot 2–12 wk (longer time with cortical break) then transition to pneumatic tibial brace
Fibula	WBAT 1–4 wk
Metatarsal (2nd–5th)	Steel shank/walking boot 3–6 wk

Abbreviations: WBAT = weight bearing as tolerated.

conservative treatment. Biomechanical forces along the bone with activity are used to classify tibia and femur stress fractures. For example, during running, the tibia and femur have different forces exerted on different parts of the bone. The tibia compresses posteriorly, so there is more compression along the posterior tibia and more tension along the anterior aspect of the tibia. The femoral neck compresses inferiorly and medially with running, so there is more compression along the inferior medial aspect of the femoral neck and more tension along the superior lateral aspect of the femoral neck. These variable forces on different parts of the bone affect the potential for delayed healing and nonunion.

Spondylolysis and Spondylolisthesis

Spondylolysis is a nondisplaced stress fracture of the pars interarticularis. Spondylolisthesis occurs when there is bilateral spondylolysis with listhesis (slippage) of the vertebral body. Spondylolisthesis is graded 1 to 4 depending on how much slippage is present with each grade, accounting for 25% (i.e., grade 1 = 0–25%).

When a young athlete presents with low back pain, spondylolysis needs to be considered: this can be the cause of their pain up to 47% of the time. Spondylolysis is an overuse injury caused by repetitive hyperextension and/or rotation and has increased incidence in ballet dancers, gymnasts, divers, soccer players, and football linemen. L5 is the most common level for a spondylolysis. The history is significant for insidious onset of deep pain in the low back exacerbated by extension. Physical examination shows a positive Stork test (see Table 3), often with reproduction of pain on the side of weight bearing (Figure 22). If history and physical exam are suggestive of a pars interarticularis injury, x-rays of the lumbar spine, including

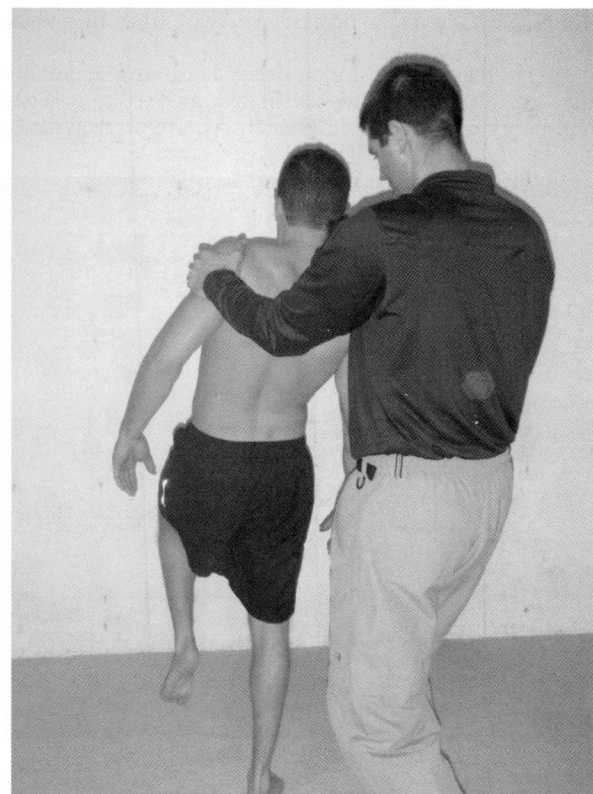

Figure 22 Stork test: To assess localized spondylolysis pain, a single leg hyperextension rotation test (stork test) is performed. The patient stands on one leg and hyperextends and rotates the spine. Reproduction of the patient's pain is suggestive of a spondylolysis.

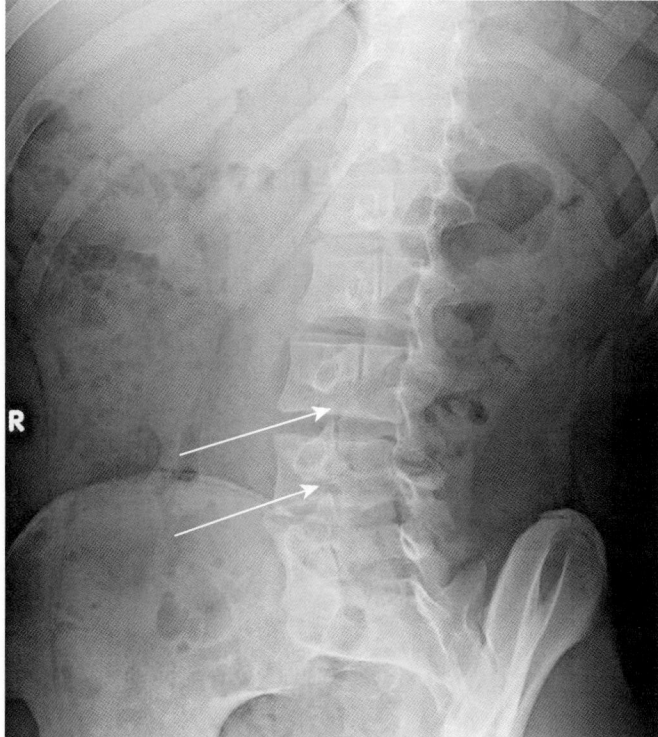

Figure 23 Oblique view x-ray of the lumbar spine, which demonstrates a L3 and L4 spondylolysis.

oblique views, should be obtained. Oblique view x-rays provide the best view to identify a spondylolysis even though they only demonstrate spondylolysis about 30% of the time when it is present (Figure 23). If x-rays are negative, proceed with

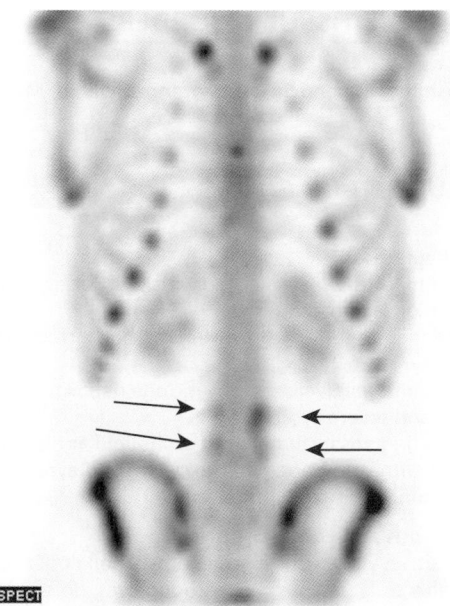

Figure 24 SPECT scan lumbar spine, PA view, which demonstrates an acute bilateral L3 and L4 spondylolysis.

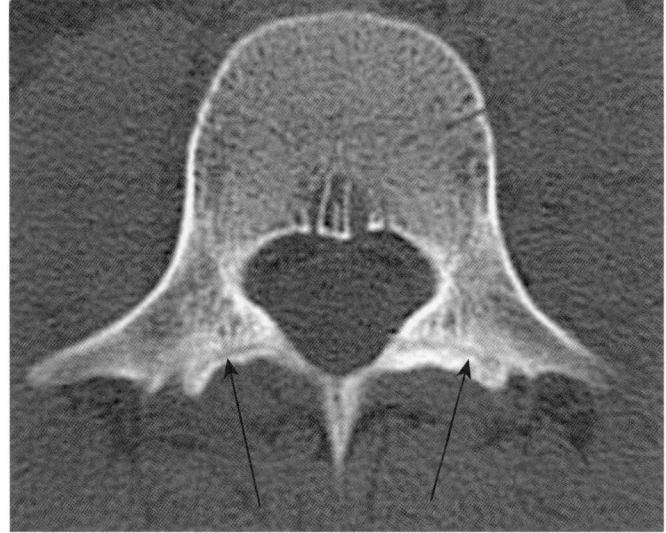

Figure 25 CT scan without contrast. Axial image at L3 shows bilateral pars interarticularis fractures that appear acute with jagged and nonsclerotic fracture edges.

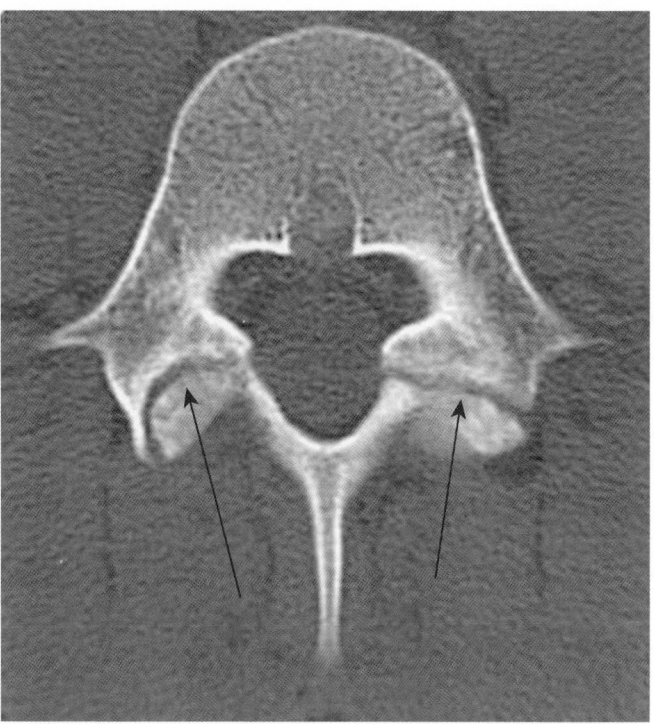

Figure 26 CT scan without contrast. Axial image at L4 shows bilateral pars interarticularis fractures. Right L4 pars fracture appears more chronic in appearance, with sclerotic fracture edges on the lateral aspect. Left L4 pars fracture appears more acute, with more jagged-appearing edges.

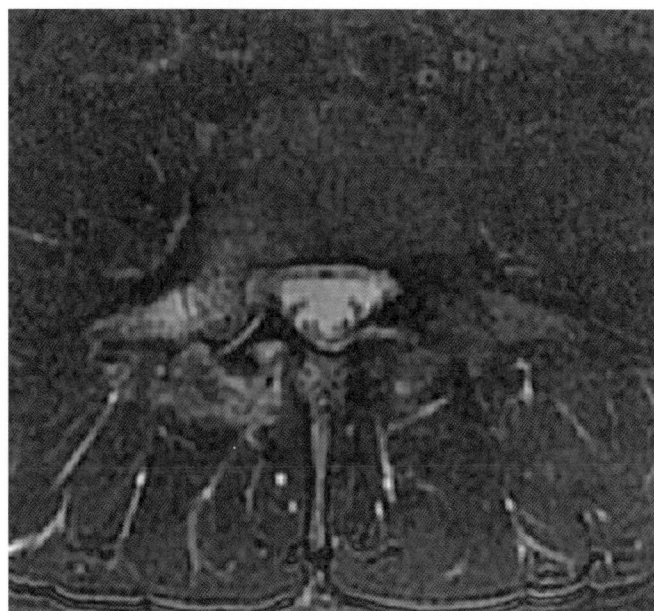

Figure 27 MRI lumbar spine without contrast. Axial T2 fat saturation image at L5 that demonstrates a right L5 spondylolysis signified by right pars interarticularis bone edema in white at L5.

MRI or with SPECT scan. If the SPECT scan is positive (Figure 24), then proceed with limited CT scan (Figures 25 and 26). If radiation exposure is a concern, or if high-definition MRI is readily accessible, thinly sliced stacked axial cuts with T2 fat saturation views in all planes using a high-definition MRI is the test of choice (Figure 27). A spectrum of recommended treatments and conservative approaches that allow for a prompt and safe RTP are reasonable. For acute spondylolysis, the recommended treatment consists of a warm and form-extension-blocking back brace worn all day except for showering and bathing (23–24 hours per day) for the first month of treatment in conjunction with rest from activity. During the second month, use of the brace during the day with rehabilitation is suggested. Rehabilitation consists of core strengthening and lower extremity flexibility. The third month consists of a gradual return to activity, continuing core strengthening and flexibility, and wearing the brace with activity. When treating spondylolysis, a healed pars interarticularis injury is defined as pain-free activity that may include bony union of the pars interarticularis stress fracture or fibrous nonbony union. Generally, the patient should wear the brace for at least 1 year with activity and sometimes longer depending on the severity of

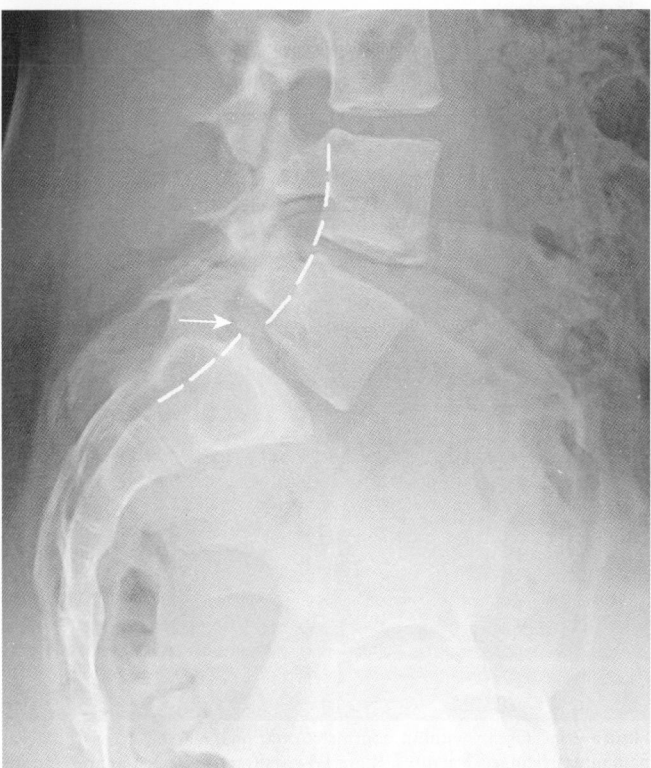

Figure 28 Lateral view x-ray of the lumbar spine, which demonstrates a grade 1 L5 spondylolisthesis.

injury. Utilize acetaminophen for pain, avoid NSAIDs, ensure adequate energy availability, maximize calcium and vitamin D intake, and avoid tobacco exposure to facilitate bone healing.

The general goal for spondylolisthesis treatment is to prevent further slippage; treatment is similar to that for spondylolysis. Surgical referral is indicated for grade 2, 3, or 4 spondylolisthesis (Figure 28).

References

Almekinders LC: Anti-inflammatory treatment of muscular injuries in sports, *Sports Med* 15:139–145, 1993.

Bachmann LM, Kolb E, Koller M, et al: Accuracy of Ottawa ankle rules to exclude fractures of the ankle and mid-foot: systematic review, *Br Med J* 326:417–424, 2003.

Beynnon BD, Johnson RJ, Brown L: Knee. In DeLee JC, Drez D, Miller MD, editors: *DeLee & Drez's Orthopaedic Sports Medicine Principles & Practice*, 3rd ed., Philadelphia, 2009, Elsevier, pp 1579–1847.

Gellman H, Caputo RJ, Carter V, et al: Comparison of short and long thumb-spica casts for non-displaced fractures of the carpal scaphoid, *J Bone Joint Surg Am* 71:354–357, 1989.

Haskell A, Mann RA: Foot and ankle. In DeLee JC, Drez D, Miller MD, editors: *DeLee & Drez's Orthopaedic Sports Medicine Principles & Practice*, 3rd ed., Philadelphia, 2009, Elsevier, pp 1865–2205.

Kaeding C, Best TM: Tendinosis: Pathophysiology and nonoperative treatment, *Sports Health* 1:284–292, 2009.

Lappe J, Cullen D, Haynatzki G, et al: Calcium and vitamin D supplementation decreases incidence of stress fractures in female navy recruits, *J Bone Miner Res* 23:741–749, 2008.

Leggit JG, Meko CJ: Acute finger injuries: part I. Tendons and ligaments, *Am Fam Physician* 73:810–816, 2006.

Liem BC, Truswell HJ, Harrast MA: Rehabilitation and return to running after lower limb stress fractures, *Curr Sports Med Rep* 12:200–207, 2013.

Purcell L, Micheli L: Low back pain in young athletes, *Sports Health* 1:212–222, 2009.

Simon AM, Manigrasso MB, O'Connor JP: Cyclo-oxygenase 2 function is essential for bone fracture healing, *J Bone Miner Res* 17:963, 2002.

Tiemstra JD: Update on acute ankle sprains, *Am Fam Physician* 85:1170–1176, 2012.

CONNECTIVE TISSUE DISORDERS

Method of
Molly A. Hinshaw, MD; and Susan Lawrence-Hylland, MD

CURRENT DIAGNOSIS

Lupus Erythematosus

- The erythematous-violaceous and variably pruritic, tender, or scaly eruption is photosensitive.
- Mild to moderate systemic involvement may include arthritis and pleurisy.
- Severe systemic involvement may include nephritis, cerebritis, vasculitis, and severe cytopenias.
- Associated findings include antiphospholipid antibodies associated with thromboembolism or stroke, Raynaud's phenomenon, and sicca symptoms.

Dermatomyositis and Polymyositis

- Photosensitive, violaceous-erythematous, poikilodermatous, and variably scaly patches occur around eyes, on extensor extremities (especially over joints), upper back, scalp, and dystrophic nail folds with prominent telangiectasias.
- Patients may have or develop myositis or pulmonary involvement.
- Age-appropriate cancer screening is required for adults.

Scleroderma

- Patients have firm, variably pruritic, and indurated plaques.
- Localized scleroderma (i.e., morphea or asymmetric sclerotic plaques) may be seen.
- Limited systemic sclerosis is characterized by symmetric sclerosis of distal extremities, and patients may have systemic disease.
- Diffuse systemic sclerosis is characterized by symmetric sclerosis of the trunk and proximal extremities, and patients may have systemic disease.
- Sclerodactyly (i.e., thickening of skin of digits) may occur in patients with systemic sclerosis.
- Pulmonary, cardiac, and gastrointestinal screening should be done for patients with systemic sclerosis.
- Patients with systemic sclerosis should be evaluated and monitored for renal crisis.
- Raynaud's phenomenon may develop in patients with systemic sclerosis.

CURRENT THERAPY

Lupus Erythematosus

- Patients should be counseled on photoprotection measures.
- Localized cutaneous disease is treated with medium- to high-potency topical corticosteroids, and intralesional triamcinolone acetonide 10 mg/mL (Kenalog-10) is added if needed.
- Mild to moderate systemic involvement is treated with low- to medium-potency prednisone 5 to 20 mg/day and with antimalarials.
- Severe disease is treated with prednisone 1 mg/kg/day with a taper based on clinical response. Steroid-sparing agents include azathioprine (Imuran),[1] mycophenolate mofetil (CellCept),[1] methotrexate (Rheumatrex),[1] and cyclophosphamide (Cytoxan).[1]
- Thromboembolism or stroke is treated by anticoagulation with warfarin (Coumadin), aspirin, or heparin.
- Sicca syndrome is treated with frequent water intake, saliva replacement, artificial tears, routine dental care, and pilocarpine (Salagen).

Dermatomyositis and Polymyositis

- Patients should be counseled on photoprotection measures.
- Medium-potency topical corticosteroids and calcineurin inhibitors are used for cutaneous disease.
- Prednisone 1 mg/kg/day is first-line therapy for muscle or pulmonary disease.
- Methotrexate[1] 10 to 25 mg/week is a steroid-sparing agent used for muscle involvement.
- Hydroxychloroquine (Plaquenil)[1] 200 mg/day is used for persistent skin involvement.

Scleroderma

- For localized scleroderma, UVA[1] 20 to 60 J/cm^2 or psoralen plus UVA (PUVA) is used to resolve established lesions; high-potency corticosteroids and calcipotriene (Dovonex)[1] may help to reduce pruritus and inflammation in new lesions; and systemic prednisone[1] or methotrexate[1] may be used for rapidly progressive new lesions.
- Treatment of systemic sclerosis is primarily aimed at limiting complications.
- Physical therapy is used for contractures.
- Systemic sclerosis is treated with cyclophosphamide (Cytoxan),[1] mycophenolate mofetil (CellCept),[1] methotrexate[1] 10 to 25 mg/week, and photopheresis.
- Renal crisis is treated with captopril (Capoten)[1] 6.25 mg three to six times/day and titrated to effect.
- Raynaud's is treated with warming techniques, calcium channel blockers, antiadrenergic agents, antiplatelet drugs, and topical vasodilators.

---

[1]Not FDA approved for this indication.

Lupus Erythematosus

Lupus erythematosus is an autoimmune connective tissue disease that may localize to the skin or involve several organ systems. A complete review of systems with evaluation of positive findings is necessary to thoroughly assess patients for signs of systemic lupus as defined by the American Rheumatism Association. Cutaneous lupus erythematosus manifests in chronic, subacute, and acute forms. A punch biopsy from within an erythematous lupus lesion is useful for confirming the diagnosis.

Clinical Features

Discoid lupus and tumid lupus are the two forms of chronic cutaneous lupus erythematosus. Discoid lupus lesions are tender or pruritic, erythematous to violaceous, scaly plaques that typically occur on sun-exposed skin. The lesions resolve with scarring, and when the lesions affect the scalp, they cause scarring alopecia. Tumid lupus manifests as pruritic, erythematous to violaceous, nonscaly plaques that typically preferentially affect the face and trunk.

The lesions of subacute cutaneous lupus erythematosus occur as erythematous to violaceous, scaly macules and as annular or polycyclic patches. These lesions are commonly located on sun-exposed skin and heal without scarring.

Acute cutaneous lupus erythematosus is exemplified by malar erythema (i.e., butterfly rash) and by poikiloderma (i.e., hyperpigmentation, telangiectasias, and epidermal atrophy). It is a manifestation of systemic lupus erythematosus (SLE). Cutaneous lesions may be widespread. In addition to the American Rheumatism Association criteria, patients with SLE may also develop Raynaud's phenomenon, hypercoagulability, and overlap syndromes with Sjögren's disease, dermatomyositis, and other conditions.

Hydrochlorothiazide (HydroDIURIL), terbinafine (Lamisil), minocycline (Minocin), procainamide (Pronestyl), hydralazine (Apresoline), and isoniazid (Nydrazid) are a few of the pharmaceutical agents that cause drug-induced lupus. This disease manifests with synovitis, photosensitivity, and positive serology results, and it may have cutaneous lesions that do not necessarily abate with cessation of the medication.

Management

Prevention

All patients with lupus erythematosus should be counseled on photoprotection, including protecting skin from sunlight and avoiding sun exposure during peak hours (i.e., between 10 AM and 2 PM). Ultraviolet A and B wavelengths may cause lupus to flare. Broad-spectrum sunscreen with an SPF of 30 or higher and that contains titanium, zinc, Mexoryl (L'Oreal), or Helioplex (Neutrogena) should be used whenever patients are outdoors. Photoprotective clothing, available from multiple vendors, is useful for limiting sun exposure.

Patients with lupus are relatively immunosuppressed by their disease. Vaccinations should be kept up to date, although there is a debate about the necessity and safety of vaccination against meningococcal disease (Neisseria meningitidis) (Menactra, Menomune), varicella-zoster virus (Zostavax), and Streptococcus (Pneumovax).

Treatment of Cutaneous Lupus Erythematosus

Medium-potency topical corticosteroids should be used for lupus localized to the skin, and they are used as adjunct treatment for patients with systemic lupus. Use of triamcinolone 0.1% cream (Flutex) for lesions on the head and neck until symptoms subside or up to 2 weeks continuously is an appropriate starting strength. Ointment-based vehicles are useful for lesions on the trunk and extremities. They are also the vehicles of choice on the scalp of patients of African American descent. Foam or liquid- or lotion-based corticosteroids work well in the scalp of other ethnic groups and can be used on the trunk and extremities. If lesions persist, the corticosteroid can be occluded, or intralesional injections with triamcinolone can be repeated monthly as needed. Intralesional triamcinolone acetonide at concentrations of 5 mg/mL (Kenalog) can be injected into lesions on the face or neck and doses of 10 to 20 mg/mL (Kenalog-10, Kenalog) into lesions on the trunk or extremities. Intralesional corticosteroids may cause mild discomfort, atrophy of the skin or subcutis, or stretch marks. Topical calcineurin inhibitors such as pimecrolimus (Elidel)[1] or tacrolimus (Protopic)[1] may be used for maintenance treatment but are not recommended for new or active lesions because they do not work quickly. Recurrent or refractory cutaneous lesions require systemic treatment.

Treatment of Systemic Lupus Erythematosus

Antimalarials, including hydroxychloroquine (Plaquenil),[1] are disease-modifying agents that limit the progression of lupus. Hydroxychloroquine, chloroquine (Aralen),[1] and quinacrine[2] (at compounding pharmacies) raise the pH of inflammatory cells, inhibiting inflammatory pathways that cause end-organ damage in patients with SLE.

Hydroxychloroquine is typically used first at 200 mg daily for 2 weeks and then increased to 400 mg daily. Patients need laboratory monitoring and a baseline and then yearly eye examination because the medication may be deposited in the retina over time. Hydroxychloroquine exerts its effects within 2 to 3 months of beginning treatment. Its effects are diminished in smokers.

Depending on end-organ involvement in SLE, immunosuppression with systemic corticosteroids such as prednisone at doses of 1 mg/kg/day is appropriate. Steroid-sparing drugs such as methotrexate (Rheumatrex),[1] acitretin (Soriatane),[1] or mycophenolate mofetil (CellCept)[1] are added. After signs of inflammation subside, prednisone is tapered.

Treatment of Musculoskeletal Manifestations

Arthralgia is a common complaint that can usually be managed with acetaminophen or nonsteroidal antiinflammatory drugs (NSAIDs). For true arthritis unresponsive to the previously described measures, hydroxychloroquine[1] 200 mg twice daily can be added. After that, treatments similar to those used for rheumatoid arthritis can be added, although the antitumor necrosis factor agents usually are

---

Not FDA approved for this indication.
Not available in the United States.

avoided in lupus. Methotrexate[1] 7.5 to 25 mg PO once weekly may be used along with folic acid[1] 1 mg daily to help limit side effects. Routine toxicity monitoring includes frequent complete blood cell counts and liver tests. Azathioprine (Imuran)[1] 0.5 to 2 mg/kg can be used with frequent monitoring of complete blood cell counts and liver tests. A sample for testing the thiopurine methyltransferase activity level should be drawn before initiating therapy because a genetic deficiency can lead to severe pancytopenia. Leflunomide (Arava)[1] 10 to 20 mg PO once daily can be used with frequent blood cell counts and liver tests. Low-dose glucocorticoids (prednisone 5–10 mg/day) may be used as a bridge to steroid-sparing therapy and to treat intermittent flares.

Treatment of Hematologic Manifestations

Autoimmune cytopenias are common and are often a defining feature of SLE. Lymphopenia (absolute lymphocyte count <1500 cells/microliter) does not require therapy. Hemolytic anemia in SLE is the result of antierythrocyte antibodies that activate complement, and it is treated with prednisone at a dose based on clinical severity. Typically, 1 mg/kg/day, or approximately 60 mg, is used for 4 to 6 weeks, with gradual tapering as long as the response is maintained. For severe hemolytic anemia, pulse methylprednisolone (Solu-Medrol) 1 g IV for 3 consecutive days can be tried, followed by the previously described standard dosing. For patients who do not respond to glucocorticoids or are unable to taper prednisone to low doses, other treatments can be used. They may include azathioprine[1] 1.5 to 2.5 mg/kg/day, mycophenolate mofetil[1] 1000 to 2000 mg/day in divided doses, danazol (Danocrine)[1] 300 to 600 mg/day in divided doses, intravenous immunoglobulin,[1] or rituximab (Rituxan)[1] 375 mg/m[2] weekly for four doses.

Immune thrombocytopenia results from antiplatelet antibodies that identify platelets for early destruction. Treatment is indicated when patients have signs or symptoms of spontaneous bleeding or when the platelet count drops below 50,000/mL. The initial treatment approach with glucocorticoids is similar to that used for hemolytic anemia. For patients with chronic thrombocytopenia or for those who cannot achieve an acceptable long-term dose of prednisone, steroid-sparing agents, including azathioprine,[1] mycophenolate mofetil,[1] danazol,[1] rituximab,[1] and intravenous immunoglobulin[1] can be used in doses similar to those used for hemolytic anemia. Dapsone,[1] cyclosporine (Sandimmune, Neoral),[1] and cyclophosphamide (Cytoxan)[1] have also been used.

Thrombotic thrombocytopenia purpura may occur in SLE, and it must be differentiated from immune thrombocytopenia because treatment requires emergent plasmapheresis. Manifestations of thrombotic thrombocytopenia purpura include fever, microangiopathic hemolysis, and central nervous system and renal abnormalities.

Antiphospholipid antibodies include the lupus anticoagulant, anticardiolipin antibodies, and β2-glycoprotein. They are associated with coagulopathy, thrombocytopenia, late-trimester miscarriage, and heart valve abnormalities. Antiphospholipid antibodies that can be determined with blood testing but are not associated with thromboembolism do not require treatment. Low-dose aspirin[1] may be considered but has not been shown to prevent future thrombosis. Hydroxychloroquine[1] 200 mg twice daily has been shown to reduce the risk. Patients with antiphospholipid antibodies who develop thromboembolism need lifelong treatment with warfarin (Coumadin). A goal international normalized ratio (INR) remains controversial because different studies advocate for high-intensity warfarin (INR >3) or low-intensity therapy (INR >2). For women who have suffered a miscarriage determined to be related to antiphospholipid antibodies, low-dose aspirin and heparin 5000 units SQ twice daily may increase the likelihood of a successful pregnancy.

Treatment of Renal Manifestations

Many patients with SLE have mild to severe renal involvement. Diagnosis by renal biopsy is important to establish the type of kidney involvement. Lupus nephritis is considered one of the more severe manifestations of the disease, and treatment is aimed

at preventing renal failure. Treatment should be coordinated with a rheumatologist or nephrologist.

Class I disease requires no specific therapy. The class IIb pattern with more than 1 g of proteinuria can be treated with moderate-dose prednisone (20 mg/day for 6 weeks to 3 months), followed by tapering. Class III and IV patterns of disease have the same prognosis and are treated similarly with high-dose prednisone (1 mg/kg/day) for at least 6 weeks before tapering, based on clinical response, by 10 mg a week to a maintenance of 10 to 15 mg/day. In addition to prednisone, cytotoxic therapy is initiated with cyclophosphamide[1] 0.5 to 1 g/m[2] of body surface area monthly for 6 months and tapered to every 3 months, based on clinical response, for a total of 2 to 3 years. Cyclophosphamide has serious toxicities, including hemorrhagic cystitis, bone marrow suppression, infertility, teratogenicity, and increased risk of malignancy. 2-Mercaptoethane sulfonate sodium (Mesna)[1] can be given with each infusion to minimize bladder toxicity. Class V disease can be treated with prednisone alone, similar to class IIb disease, unless there are coexisting features of class III or IV disease, for which treatments outlined previously should be implemented.

An acceptable alternative to cyclophosphamide for class III and IV disease is mycophenolate mofetil[1] 2 to 3 g/day in divided doses combined with corticosteroids (dosing outlined earlier). This appears to be an effective therapy with fewer side effects than traditional therapy.

Treatment of Nervous System Manifestations

Neuropsychiatric involvement is common in patients with lupus. Symptoms can range from mild to severe and include headache, aseptic meningitis, neuropathy, myelopathy, cognitive dysfunction, seizures, cerebritis, and stroke. A thorough evaluation is necessary to define the cause of nervous system dysfunction and differentiate it from a medication side effect. For seizures, antiepileptic therapy is used, preferably in coordination with a neurologist. Lupus cerebritis and transverse myelitis are two of the more serious manifestations that need to be treated emergently with aggressive immunosuppression in coordination with a rheumatologist or neurologist. Treatment includes high-dose corticosteroids and cyclophosphamide,[1] similar to treatment for lupus nephritis.

Dermatomyositis and Polymyositis
Clinical Features

Dermatomyositis may affect skin and muscle. Cutaneous dermatomyositis manifests with violaceous erythema of characteristic areas, including the periorbital skin (i.e., heliotrope rash), upper back (i.e., shawl sign), dorsal hands (i.e., Gottron's papules), scalp, lateral thighs (i.e., Holster sign), and periungual skin, where dilated capillary loops and erythema are observed. Patients may report muscle weakness. As in lupus, a punch biopsy of an actively inflamed cutaneous lesion shows characteristic features.

Evaluation of patients with cutaneous dermatomyositis is not complete without assessment for systemic involvement. Serum aldolase is the most specific marker for myositis, and it can be used as a measure of response to treatment. Creatinine kinase and alanine aminotransferase levels may be elevated but are not specific indicators. An electromyogram shows dampening of signals, and a muscle biopsy shows a characteristic pattern of myositis. Inflammatory lung disease, diagnosed by the characteristic pattern on chest computed tomography, bronchoalveolar lavage, or biopsy, may be life limiting and therefore should be treated aggressively, similar to lung disease in scleroderma. Adult patients should have age-appropriate cancer screening because dermatomyositis is a paraneoplastic phenomenon in 10% to 50% of patients.

Some patients present with characteristic cutaneous dermatomyositis but no systemic involvement (i.e., dermatomyositis sine myositis). The risk of concurrent or subsequent cancer development is thought to be increased. These patients require monitoring for systemic involvement that may develop over time.

Not FDA approved for this indication.

Not FDA approved for this indication.

Treatment

Patients with dermatomyositis need photoprotection similar to patients with lupus. Periodic evaluation by clinical examination and review of systems allows for early intervention for developing visceral or muscle involvement.

Cutaneous dermatomyositis is treated the same as lupus (see earlier). Dermatomyositis with systemic involvement is initially treated with immunosuppression using prednisone at doses of 1 mg/kg/day. Steroid-sparing agents are incorporated early in the disease and include antimalarials (methotrexate,[1] azathioprine,[1] and mycophenolate mofetil[1]) at doses that are used in treating lupus.

Scleroderma
Clinical Features

Scleroderma is a sclerosing condition of skin or viscera, or both. The cause is unknown, but transforming growth factor-β plays a role. Type I and III collagens are excessively produced, as are other substances, including glycosaminoglycans, tenascin, and fibronectin.

Cutaneous scleroderma without Raynaud's phenomenon or clinically relevant systemic involvement is also known as *morphea*. Morphea has different distribution patterns, including guttate, linear, segmental, or diffuse distribution, but it is always characterized by indurated plaques that are inflammatory initially, have an advancing inflammatory ("lilac") border as they progress, and then become hyperpigmented. The cutaneous lesions may restrict movement of joints and can cause restricted growth of underlying structures, particularly when they develop in childhood.

Systemic sclerosis may affect the respiratory, renal, cardiovascular, genitourinary, and gastrointestinal systems and vascular structures. Raynaud's phenomenon may be the first presenting symptom of systemic sclerosis, and it can be severe, leading to digital ulcerations and autoamputation. The American College of Rheumatology has defined criteria for the diagnosis.

Tests for antinuclear antibodies are positive in approximately 95% of patients, who typically present with a homogeneous or speckled pattern. A nucleolar pattern is more specific for systemic sclerosis. Anticentromere antibodies are present in 60% to 90% of patients with limited disease but are rare in diffuse disease. Topoisomerase I (Scl-70) antibodies are positive in 30% of patients with diffuse disease and are associated with pulmonary fibrosis. Anti-PM-Scl antibodies are present in overlap syndromes and are associated with myositis and renal involvement.

Treatment
Treatment of Limited Scleroderma

For limited scleroderma, treatment with topical medium-potency corticosteroids such as triamcinolone 0.1% ointment (Kenalog) plus calcipotriene (Dovonex)[1] 0.005% cream or intralesional triamcinalone[1] 20 mg/mL may slow progression of active lesions or improve the pruritus and cutaneous stiffness that typify cutaneous scleroderma. For rapidly evolving disease, prednisone[1] 1 mg/kg/day and methotrexate[1] 15 to 20 mg/week may help slow progression of disease. UVA[1] given over 36 treatments at doses of 30 to 60 mJ/cm² or PUVA (oral methoxsalen [8-MOP] 10 mg taken 2 hours before treatment with UVA light) can soften the existing plaques of morphea.

Treatment of Systemic Sclerosis: Raynaud's Phenomenon

First-line treatment for Raynaud's phenomenon is preventive, with cold avoidance and the use of warming techniques. If pharmacotherapy is required, extended-release calcium channel blockers such as nifedipine (Procardia XL)[1] starting at 30 mg/day or amlodipine (Norvasc)[1] starting at 5 mg/day may be useful. If this is not helpful, the α-blocker prazosin (Minipress)[1] 1 mg three times daily or the angiotensin receptor blocker losartan (Cozaar)[1]

50 mg daily may be helpful. Antiplatelet therapy with low-dose aspirin[1] (81 mg/day) or dipyridamole (Persantine)[1] 50 to 100 mg three or four times daily may be useful. Topical vasodilators such as nitroglycerin ointment (Nitro-Bid)[1] applied to the base of the affected finger three times daily can be helpful in refractory disease. Digit-threatening ischemia may be treated with an intravenous prostaglandin such as alprostadil (Prostin VR)[1] or iloprost (Ilomedine),[5] which require peripheral or central access. Patients with severe recurrent digital ischemia may ultimately benefit from surgical sympathectomy.

Treatment of Gastrointestinal Manifestations

The most common gastrointestinal manifestation is esophageal reflux caused by esophageal dysmotility. Proton pump inhibitors such as omeprazole (Prilosec)[1] 20 mg twice daily should be used and may prevent the development of esophageal strictures. Prokinetic drugs such as metoclopramide (Reglan)[1] 10 mg four times daily can be helpful. Erythromycin[1] 500 mg three or four times daily can help esophageal and gastric hypomotility. Small bowel hypomotility can lead to bacterial overgrowth, resulting in malabsorption and diarrhea. Rotating antibiotics that include metronidazole (Flagyl),[1] ciprofloxacin (Cipro),[1] and amoxicillin/clavulanate (Augmentin)[1] can be used.

Treatment of Pulmonary Manifestations

Inflammatory lung disease occurs commonly in patients with scleroderma and can be life limiting. Cyclophosphamide[1] at doses of up to 2 mg/kg/day for up to 2 years may slow progression of pulmonary disease. Pulmonary hypertension occurs more commonly in limited systemic sclerosis than in diffuse disease. Symptomatic patients may receive treatment with prostacyclin analogues, which require continuous infusions. The endothelin receptor antagonist bosentan (Tracleer)[1] can be given orally starting at 62.5 mg twice daily. Liver tests should be monitored frequently. At this point, care is typically coordinated with a cardiologist to monitor disease progression and treatment response. Anticoagulation for pulmonary hypertension may improve survival because of the frequent occurrence of pulmonary arterial thrombosis.

Treatment of Renal Manifestations

Angiotensin-converting enzyme (ACE) inhibitors (e.g., captopril [Capoten[1]] beginning at 6.25 mg three to six times daily and titrated for blood pressure control) have dramatically reduced the incidence of renal failure and death due to renal crisis. Avoidance of prednisone at doses greater than 15 mg/day is also important in reducing the risk of renal crisis.

Investigational drug in the United States.

Not FDA approved for this indication.

References

Atzeni F, Bendtzen K, Bobbio-Pallavicini F, et al: Infections and treatment of patients with rheumatic diseases, *Clin Exp Rheumatol* 26(Suppl. 48):S67–73, 2008.

Dziadzio M, Denton CP, Smith R: Losartan therapy for Raynaud's phenomenon and scleroderma, *Arthritis Rheum* 42(12):2646–2655, 1999.

Ginzler EM, Dooley MA, Aranow C, et al: Mycophenolate mofetil or intravenous cyclophosphamide for lupus nephritis, *N Engl J Med* 353(21):2219–2228, 2005.

Iorizzo LJ, Jorizzo JL: The treatment and prognosis of dermatomyositis: An updated review, *J Am Acad Dermatol* 59:99–112, 2008.

Matucci-Cerinic M, Steen VD, Furst DE, et al: Clinical trials in systemic sclerosis: Lessons learned and outcomes, *Arthritis Res Ther* 9(Suppl. 2):S7, 2007.

Nihtyanova SI, Denton CP: Current approaches to the management of early active diffuse scleroderma skin disease, *Rheum Dis Clin North Am* 34:161–179, 2008.

Pisoni CN, Sanchez FJ, Karim Y, et al: Mycophenolate mofetil in systemic lupus erythematosus: Efficacy and tolerability in 86 patients, *J Rheumatol* 32:1047–1052, 2005.

Steen VD: The many faces of scleroderma, *Rheum Dis Clin North Am* 34:1–15, 2008.

Subcommittee for Scleroderma Criteria of the American Rheumatism Association Diagnostic and Therapeutic Criteria Committee: Preliminary criteria for the classification of systemic sclerosis (scleroderma), *Arthritis Rheum* 23:581–590, 1980.

Tan EM, Cohen AS, Fries JF, et al: The 1982 revised criteria for the classification of lupus erythematosus, *Arthritis Rheum* 25:1271–1272, 1982.

Wallace DD: *Lupus Erythematosus*, ed 7, Philadelphia, 2006, Lippincott Williams & Wilkins2006.

FIBROMYALGIA

Method of
Timothy Sowder, MD; Jeffrey Michael Foster, DO; and Andrea L. Nicol, MD, MSc

CURRENT DIAGNOSIS

- Fibromyalgia (FM) is a common condition, seen in 2% to 8% of the population, depending on the diagnostic criteria used.
- Hallmark symptoms of FM typically include widespread body pain, cognitive difficulties ("fibro fog"), poor sleep, and fatigue. Other associated symptoms may also include headaches, abdominal or pelvic pain, and symptoms of depression or anxiety.
- FM may occur independently of any other medical conditions, but is also known to associate with other painful conditions such as osteoarthritis and autoimmune disorders such as lupus and rheumatoid arthritis.
- No blood tests or imaging modalities are useful for diagnosing FM; however, tender point examination and questionnaires are available for aiding in diagnosis.

CURRENT THERAPY

- Treatment should be multidisciplinary and focus on symptom management, lifestyle modifications, and psychological interventions.
- A variety of on-label and off-label medications are available to mechanistically address the altered pain processing underlying FM.
- Physical therapy, exercise, and psychological treatments such as cognitive behavioral therapy are of the utmost importance in adequate management of FM symptoms.
- Seeing patients frequently to monitor medications, address side effects, and provide motivational interviewing and care is important to providing optimal patient pain relief and minimizing poor outcomes.

Epidemiology

The global prevalence of fibromyalgia (FM) has been estimated to be 2.7% (4.2% female, 1.4% male), but studies have produced varying results. Historically, studies have been conducted using the 1990 American College of Rheumatology (ACR) diagnostic criteria, which required pain to be present on palpation of at least 11/18 tender points to confirm a diagnosis of FM. Using these criteria, prevalence estimates range from 0.4% to 8.8% with 2.0% in the USA (3.4% of females and 0.5% of males, ratio ~7:1). The problems with these criteria include difficulty reproducing tender points, significantly higher rates in women (possibly due to increased number of tender points in women or a higher pressure pain threshold in males), and a strong correlation with various measures of distress and negative affect. In 2010 the ACR released updated criteria that do not require a tender point assessment. These new criteria have yielded prevalence estimates of 7.7% in women and 4.9% in men for a ratio of 1.6:1, which is similar to that seen in other chronic pain conditions. The prevalence is similar in different countries, cultures, and ethnic groups; there is no evidence that FM has a higher prevalence in industrialized countries and cultures. There are also concerns about underdiagnosis of FM with only 12% to 28% of subjects identified during population-based surveys as fulfilling the ACR 1990 criteria having ever been diagnosed with FM.

Risk Factors

There are both genetic and environmental risk factors associated with the development of FM. FM has been thought to affect mostly women with initial studies predicting that women were up to seven times more likely to develop FM. More recent studies using updated criteria have found less of a discrepancy but still indicate an increased risk with women being 1.5 to 2 times more likely to be affected than men. FM can affect people of all ages, including children. Many patients are diagnosed when they are young or middle aged, but studies show that prevalence rises with age, peaking in people greater than 60 years old. It is postulated that perhaps widespread chronic pain in older patients is more likely to be attributed to osteoarthritis or other degenerative conditions instead of FM, however, the two conditions are known to coexist. Patients diagnosed with certain conditions like rheumatoid arthritis and lupus have been noted to be more likely to develop FM than others. Obesity, poor sleep, low physical activity levels, and decreased job or life satisfaction are potentially modifiable risk factors. There are many other conditions associated with FM, though the degree of contribution to actual disease development has yet to be determined. Individuals with FM are more likely to have psychiatric disorders, including depression, anxiety, obsessive-compulsive disorder, and posttraumatic stress disorder. A history of childhood, adolescent, or adulthood abuse or traumatic events have also been linked with the development of FM and other centralized pain syndromes. Maladaptive cognitive features are poor prognostic factors for FM and can include catastrophizing and fear-avoidance of movement and activity. Lower education and other indicators of lower social status have been thought to place patients at an increased risk for FM, though other studies did not find a significant difference in developed and wealthy areas versus rural and poor areas.

Pathophysiology

FM can be thought of as a centralized pain state, where "centralized" refers to amplification of pain emanating from the central nervous system. Evidence suggests that dysfunction in central nervous system pain processing mechanisms underlie this condition and include central amplification of pain and nonpainful stimuli (including auditory, visual, and olfactory). Typical manifestations of central amplification include allodynia (pain resulting from a non-noxious stimulus) and hyperalgesia (increased sensitivity to a painful stimulus), and temporal summation (progressive increase in the pain response to repetitive painful stimulus). This term "centralized pain" does not exclude that an individual's peripheral nervous system and its nociceptive input may be contributing to the patient's overall pain symptoms, but rather that they feel greater levels of pain than would be normally expected based on the degree of peripheral nociceptive input. However, it must be noted that many patients with FM do not have any identifiable structural or functional abnormalities in the periphery that would explain their widespread pain and associated symptoms. The concept of central amplification helps describe the heterogenous clinical features of FM as many of the same neurotransmitters that control sensory sensitivity and pain also control mood, memory, fatigue, and sleep. A variety of quantitative research methods have been employed to establish that central amplification is involved in the pathophysiology of FM, including quantitative sensory testing and functional, chemical, and structural brain neuroimaging. Functional magnetic resonance imaging (MRI) has corroborated that nonnoxious stimuli such as mild pressure activates brain regions involved in pain processing compared with healthy controls. It has also been found that endogenous pain inhibitory pathways do not effectively operate in patients with FM. This defective inhibition is postulated to exist due to altered homeostasis of inhibitory and excitatory neurotransmitters.

Clinical Manifestations

The patient with FM can experience a wide variety of symptoms, including pain, fatigue, sleep disturbance, cognitive dysfunction, and mood alterations. These patients typically present with chronic widespread pain for at least 3 months that is not fully explained by injury or inflammation. This pain is typically identified as being "all over," but drawings by patients show various localized areas of pain, which may migrate in intensity from time to time. Somatic pain is typically the dominant feature; however, visceral pain (including abdominal and pelvic pain) and headaches are also commonly seen. Most frequently, the affected areas include the shoulders, arms, lower back, buttocks, and thighs. Widespread pain in the joints is also common. The patients most generally experience pain that is throbbing, achy, and tender. This pain is often accompanied by generalized hypersensitivity, allodynia, and hyperalgesia, which is indicative of the underlying central amplification. Other symptoms can include numbness, tingling, burning, cramps, and sensitivity to light and sound. Exacerbating factors for these patients' pain include emotional distress, weather changes, sleeping problems, and strenuous activity. A total of 70% to 90% of patients with FM sleep fewer hours, have more frequent waking, and report nonrestorative sleep. They also suffer from significant fatigue, weakness, and stiffness that are worse in the morning and improve as the day progresses. A total of 76% of patients report mental confusion, forgetfulness, and concentration difficulties. This cognitive dysfunction is frequently described as being more bothersome than their widespread pain. These symptoms are so pervasive and disruptive that they are commonly referred to as "fibro fog." In addition, there is an affective component to the cognitive dysfunction that is usually described by patients as feeling fatigued and exhausted all the time, irrespective of how much sleep they get. Depression, anxiety, and posttraumatic stress disorder are comorbidities with high prevalence in this patient population, and their various symptoms can also be present in the patient with FM.

Diagnosis

FM is a condition with distinctive clinical characteristics that allow for it to be diagnosed in the primary care setting. Although many practitioners may have concern that the diagnosis of FM is controversial or that it may label patients in a negative manner, studies suggest that the opposite is true. Establishing the diagnosis of FM can actually provide substantial validity and relief for patients for their previously unexplained symptoms. Prompt diagnosis is a vital component of effective FM management and is linked with patients having greater satisfaction in health, which in turn leads to decreased health care utilization and its associated costs.

In the clinical setting, FM should be considered as a diagnosis in any patient presenting with chronic widespread or multifocal pain. It is commonly comorbid in patients with other chronic pain syndromes, those with thyroid dysfunction, and patients with rheumatic diseases. There exists other co-occurring pain syndromes that have been linked to the same pathophysiology as FM that may also spark a clinicians' suspicion for FM such as irritable bowel syndrome, interstitial cystitis, migraine headache, temporomandibular disorder, and chronic pelvic or genitourinary pain (e.g., interstitial cystitis, vulvodynia). It is very important to note that FM should *not* be considered a diagnosis of exclusion.

A thorough history including asking about pain during childhood and adolescence, other comorbid pain symptoms, a history of childhood or adulthood abuse, or other traumatic events will help elucidate whether FM should be considered in the differential diagnosis. An excellent physical exam including musculoskeletal, neurologic, assessment of tenderness or significant pain to palpation, and allodynia should always be performed. Laboratory tests are not necessary or useful to establish the diagnosis of FM, besides possibly helping sort through the differential diagnoses. Basic laboratory evaluation may include vitamin D levels, thyroid panels, erythrocyte sedimentation rate, C-reactive protein, and blood count or blood chemistries to guide an assessment of potentially treatable causes of diffuse musculoskeletal pain. Detailed serologic studies are not necessary unless the patient has other signs and symptoms of other potential comorbid diseases. No imaging studies are specific in diagnosing FM, and one must be careful in performing radiographs or other imaging studies, as these can have findings that are associated with the degenerative aging process, but may not be the actual cause of the patient's ongoing pain symptoms.

The 1990 ACR tender point exam has been historically used to "diagnose" FM; however, it was originally developed to be used for research and was never intended to be used in clinical practice. Revised versions of diagnostic criteria were published in 2010 and again in 2016. These revised criteria do not require a tender point exam to elucidate a diagnosis and may be ascertained with a self-report questionnaire (Table 1). These criteria rapidly assess widespread pain symptoms and associated symptoms of poor sleep, cognitive difficulties, fatigue, and mood problems. Once diagnosed, treatment for FM can be initiated immediately, even if further tests or referrals to specialists are pending.

Differential Diagnosis

While the diagnosis of FM can be difficult and time-consuming, providing the patient with an answer to their issues can decrease healthcare costs by decreasing biological testing and imaging, decreasing the number of visits, and decreasing the number and dosage of drugs prescribed. With such a wide variety of possible symptomatic expressions of FM, it is important to address the differential diagnoses in a systematic way. Arthralgias are commonly seen in osteoarthritis and spondyloarthritis, but are also seen in rheumatic diseases like rheumatoid arthritis, Sjögren syndrome, systemic lupus erythematous, and polymyalgia rheumatica. Inflammatory, metabolic, and drug-induced myopathies and myalgias should also be ruled out. Myofascial pain syndrome, tendonitis, and bursitis are common pathologies that cause pain in localized areas. Neurologic disorders such as multiple sclerosis and myasthenia gravis should be considered in addition to radiculopathies, and both peripheral and compressive neuropathies that could complicate the picture. Viral infections and Lyme disease should be considered as potential infectious causes. Endocrinopathies like hypothyroidism, Cushing syndrome, and hyperparathyroidism can cause weakness, but are unlikely to cause the significant widespread pain seen in FM. There are other disorders that frequently overlap or co-occur with FM that should be optimally treated in conjunction. These include depression, anxiety, obsessive-compulsive disorder, posttraumatic stress disorder, tension headaches, migraines, temporomandibular disorder, chronic fatigue syndrome, irritable bowel syndrome, interstitial cystitis (painful bladder syndrome), chronic prostatitis, and vulvodynia. It is important for any clinician to distinguish that the patient's symptoms are not explained by another pathology or systemic disorder because treatment of these entities can vary greatly. However, the 2016 Revised Fibromyalgia Criteria does not exclude the diagnosis of FM if other conditions are present. Each of these problems should be considered as variables and optimally treated when attempting to diagnose this complex syndrome.

Treatment

FM is best approached by using an integrated, multidisciplinary approach where pharmacologic and nonpharmacologic treatments are provided in parallel. Engaging and motivating the patient toward their treatment goals as an active participant

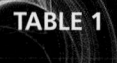
TABLE 1 — American College of Rheumatology 2016 Revised Fibromyalgia

Criteria

A patient satisfies modified 2016 fibromyalgia criteria if the following three conditions are met:

(1) Widespread pain index (WPI) ≥ 7 and symptom severity scale (SSS) score ≥ 5 OR WPI of 4–6 and SSS score ≥ 9.
(2) Generalized pain, defined as pain in at least 4 of 5 regions, must be present. Jaw, chest, and abdominal pain are not included in generalized pain definition.
(3) Symptoms have been generally present for at least 3 months.

Ascertainment

(1) WPI: note the number of areas in which the patient has had pain over the last week. In how many areas has the patient had pain? Score will be between 0 and 19.
Left upper region (Region 1)
  Jaw, left
  Shoulder girdle, left
  Upper arm, left
  Lower arm, left
Right upper region (Region 2)
  Jaw, right
  Shoulder girdle, right
  Upper arm, right
  Lower arm, right
Left lower region (Region 3)
  Hip (buttock, trochanter), left
  Upper leg, left
  Lower leg, left
Right lower region (Region 4)
  Hip (buttock, trochanter), right
  Upper leg, right
  Lower leg, right
Axial region (Region 5)
  Neck
  Upper back
  Lower back
  Chest
  Abdomen
(2) SSS score
  Fatigue
  Waking unrefreshed
  Cognitive symptoms
For the each of the 3 symptoms above, indicate the level of severity over the past week using the following scale:
  0 = No problem
  1 = Slight or mild problems, generally mild or intermittent
  2 = Moderate, considerable problems, often present and/or at a moderate level
  3 = Severe: pervasive, continuous, life-disturbing problems
  The SSS score: is the sum of the severity scores of the 3 symptoms (fatigue, waking unrefreshed, and cognitive symptoms) (0–9) plus the sum (0–3) of the number of the following symptoms the patient has been bothered by that occurred during the previous 6 months:
(1) Headaches (0–1)
(2) Pain or cramps in lower abdomen (0–1)
(3) And depression (0–1)

The final symptom severity score is between 0 and 12

The fibromyalgia severity (FS) scale is the sum of the WPI and SSS

A diagnosis of fibromyalgia is valid irrespective of other diagnoses. A diagnosis of fibromyalgia does not exclude the presence of other clinically important illnesses.

---

comorbid mood or psychiatric disturbances. Forming treatment teams can be very useful and should include clinicians with expertise in exercise/physical activity (e.g., physical therapists), patient education, and pain psychology.

Most comprehensive guidelines on treatment of FM generally recommend that all patients should receive education on their condition, the importance of being an active participant in their care, and that setting reasonable and attainable goals and expectations for treatment. Patients need to be informed that instead of searching for treatments to cure the condition, that management of the condition should focus on pain reduction (not complete pain relief), increased physical functioning, and improved quality of life. This management should rely heavily on stress reduction, exercise and physical activity, adequate sleep, and improving function through cognitive restructuring (e.g., reducing catastrophizing, increasing self-efficacy). Pharmacologic treatments can be effective in alleviating some of the symptoms of FM, but rarely will patients achieve significant improvements without embracing these essential self-management strategies.

In the United States, there are three drugs currently approved by the US Food and Drug Association (FDA) for the treatment of FM: (1) pregabalin (Lyrica), (2) milnacipran (Savella), and (3) duloxetine (Cymbalta). These drugs mechanistically treat FM through either increasing the activity of inhibitory neurotransmitters (milnacipran and duloxetine) or to decrease the activity of excitatory neurotransmitters (pregabalin). Table 2 highlights the FDA-approved medications in the pharmacologic treatment of FM. Careful initiation and titration are recommended to improve patient compliance and response, given the incidence of side effects or drug-drug interactions. There are a variety of commonly utilized drugs other than those listed previously, although none of them have an FDA approval for the FM indication. These other medications have been shown in a variety of research studies to provide pain and symptom relief in FM and include gabapentin (Neurontin)[1], tricyclic antidepressants (e.g., nortriptyline [Pamelor][1], amitriptyline [Elavil][1]), cyclobenzaprine (Flexeril)[1], and venlafaxine (Effexor)[1]. Basic analgesics such as acetaminophen and nonsteroidal antiinflammatories (NSAIDs) have little evidence supporting effectiveness for FM. Other emerging therapies such as low-dose naltrexone (ReVia, Vivitrol)[1] warrant further investigation and should only be used in refractory cases by those who are familiar with its use. There exists no evidence that mu-opioid agonists are helpful in the long-term treatment of FM and ultimately increase central amplification overtime, thereby increasing the potential for worsening pain and functioning whilst placing the patient at risk for dependence and addiction. Clinicians and patients should recognize that in many cases, treatment with pharmacologic agents may be ineffective. The choice of drug should always be discussed with the patient and should focus on targeting the most bothersome symptoms. Oftentimes multiple types of drugs/drug combinations are needed. If a drug is trialed and does not lead to clinically meaningful relief after four weeks at the full recommended dose, it should be tapered or stopped, and an alternative drug trialed.

Nonpharmacologic treatment for FM consists of psychological and educational interventions, in addition to physical modalities and should be an integral part of a comprehensive FM treatment plan. Education should be a foundational intervention applied immediately with diagnosis or early in the patient's treatment plan, and should consist of information on the underlying pain mechanisms causing clinical pain and associated symptoms (e.g., central nervous system pain and sensory amplification) and information on the nature of the condition (e.g., nonprogressive, chronic, and lifelong with episodic flares, risk of other comorbid conditions). This will provide a strong foundation to then add psychological therapies, which are typically behavioral based and focused on acceptance theories. Cognitive behavioral therapy has been shown

in their care is vital for success. As stated before, FM can be diagnosed and treated in the primary care setting. Referral to specialists should only be necessary when pain is refractory to therapy (e.g., comprehensive pain management clinic), those in whom the diagnosis is uncertain (e.g., to a rheumatologist or neurologist depending on symptoms), or those with significant

TABLE 2	Comparison of FDA-approved Pharmacologic Therapies for Fibromyalgia				
DRUG	**DATE OF FDA APPROVAL**	**MECHANISM OF ACTION**	**AVAILABLE STRENGTHS**	**DOSING**	**COMMON SIDE EFFECTS**
Duloxetine (Cymbalta)	June 16, 2008	Serotonin norepinephrine reuptake inhibition	20 mg; 30 mg; 60 mg	• 60 mg/day recommended total dose (doses higher than 60 mg rarely helpful for pain) • Start 30 mg/day for 1 week or longer and then may increase to 60 mg/day	Dry mouth, somnolence, nausea, constipation, decreased appetite, hyperhidrosis
Milnacipran (Savella)	January 14, 2009	Serotonin norepinephrine reuptake inhibition	12.5 mg; 25 mg; 50 mg; 100 mg; convenience starter pack	• Convenience starter pack dosing: Start 12.5 mg daily × 1 day, then 12.5 mg bid × 2 days, then 25 mg bid × 4 days, then 50 mg bid • Max dose 100 mg bid (200 mg/day)	Nausea, constipation, hot flush, hyperhidrosis, vomiting, palpitations, increased heart rate, dry mouth, hypertension
Pregabalin (Lyrica)	June 21, 2007	Non-selective alpha-2-delta calcium channel blocker	25 mg; 50 mg; 75 mg; 100 mg; 150 mg; 200 mg; 225 mg; 300 mg	• Start at 75 mg bid (can start much lower in sensitive or older patient population) • May increase to 150 mg bid within 1 week • Max dose 225 mg bid (450 mg/day)	Dizziness, somnolence, dry mouth, peripheral edema, blurred vision, weight gain, abnormal thinking/cognitive difficulties

to be effective for the treatment of FM and focuses on the link between pain, mood, thoughts, and behavior, and trying to unravel negative coping mechanisms such as catastrophizing and poor self-efficacy. Mind-body therapies, including stress reduction, biofeedback, and mindfulness, have also shown good benefit for FM.

Physical activity, including active and passive modalities, is perhaps the most important nonpharmacologic treatment for FM. Physical therapy, including warm-water aquatherapy, can be utilized initially to help patients improve their conditioning and obtain education on how to incorporate movement and activity into their daily lives. Among different exercise interventions, aerobic exercise has been shown to be the most beneficial. Patients should start with low-to-moderate intensity activities (such as walking, stationary cycling, or swimming). Over time, patients can increase their intensity and duration over time to a goal of at least 20 min/day at least two to three times weekly. It is important to counsel patients on pacing themselves and that initially they may have more soreness or pain as they gradually build their physical conditioning and strength. Continuation of the exercise regimen is of paramount value as ongoing exercise has been associated with maintenance of improvements in FM. Passive forms of physical activity such as balneotherapy (heated spa treatments), manipulation, massage, transcutaneous electrical stimulation,

and ultrasound have only weak evidence to support their use. Complementary and alternative medicine options that may be considered include acupuncture, yoga, tai chi, and qi gong meditation, but there are few high-quality evidence studies to support their use as first-line therapy.

Monitoring

No laboratory or imaging monitoring is required in the treatment of FM. Regular/frequent outpatient engagement with patients is recommended—to discuss the comprehensive care plan and focus on patient goals for treatment, as increased outpatient engagement has been shown to reduce morbidity and mortality (including risk of suicide) in patients with FM.

References

Arnold LM, Gebke KB, Choi EHS: Fibromyalgia: management strategies for primary care providers, *Int J Clin Pract* 70(2):99–112, 2016.
Borchers AT, Gershwin ME: Fibromyalgia: A critical and comprehensive review, *Clinic Rev Allerg Immunol* 49:100–151, 2015.
Clauw DJ: Fibromyalgia: A clinical review, *JAMA* 311(15):1547–1555, 2014.
Perrot S: Fibromyalgia: A misconnection in a multi-connected world?, *Eur J Pain*, 2019. https://doi.org/10.1002/ejp.1367. Available at: [Epub ahead of print].
Rahman A, Underwood M, Carnes D: *Fibromyalgia*. BMJ 348:g1224, 2014.
Talotta R, Bazzichi L, Di Franco M, et al: One year in review 2017: fibromyalgia, *Clin Exp Rheumatol* 35(Suppl. 105):S6–S12, 2017.
Wolfe F, Clauw DJ, Fitzcharles M, et al: 2016 Revisions to the 2010/2011 fibromyalgia diagnostic criteria, *Semin Arthritis Rheum* 46(3):319–329, 2016.

JUVENILE IDIOPATHIC ARTHRITIS

Method of
Ashley Cooper, MD

CURRENT DIAGNOSIS

- Juvenile idiopathic arthritis (JIA) is a clinical diagnosis. JIA is diagnosed when objective signs of arthritis persist in a child for at least 6 weeks in the absence of another identifiable cause.
- Children who present with musculoskeletal pain without accompanying objective signs of joint inflammation (swelling or painful, limited range of motion) are unlikely to have arthritis. In many children with JIA, swelling and joint limitation are more prominent than pain.
- Laboratory testing has limited value in diagnosing JIA. In some cases, no laboratory tests are needed to make the diagnosis. When clinically indicated, laboratory tests are used to exclude other causes of arthritis such as infection (including Lyme disease in endemic areas), malignancy, or underlying systemic autoimmune disease.
- The antinuclear antibody (ANA), rheumatoid factor (RF), and anticitric citrullinated peptide (anti-CCP) have prognostic but *not* diagnostic value in JIA. These tests should not be drawn to evaluate musculoskeletal pain in children in the absence of objective signs of arthritis.

CURRENT THERAPY

- Medical therapy is individualized for each child based on severity and number of affected joints and comorbidities. The goal of treatment is to completely control joint inflammation to minimize symptoms and prevent damage.
- Many rheumatologists use a step-up treatment approach, titrating medication until inactive disease is achieved. In children with severe arthritis, early combination therapy is sometimes used. With appropriate use of currently available medications, most children with JIA can achieve clinically inactive disease.
- Current treatment options include scheduled nonsteroidal antiinflammatory drugs (NSAIDs), intraarticular corticosteroid injections, disease-modifying antirheumatic drugs (DMARDs, most commonly methotrexate), and biologic response modifiers (such as antitumor necrosis factor alpha, anti-interleukin-1, or anti-interleukin-6 therapy).
- With the currently available medications, many children with JIA do not require systemic corticosteroids. Steroids should not be prescribed to a child presenting with joint pain or swelling of unclear etiology.
- Optimal timing and approach to medication discontinuation in patients who have achieved inactive disease are unclear. Relapse rates are high after medication discontinuation in most JIA subtypes.
- A partnership between the child's rheumatologist and primary care provider is key to safe use of immune-modulating medications. Optimal management includes:
  - Medication toxicity monitoring with periodic laboratory studies;
  - Prompt evaluation of infectious symptoms in immunosuppressed patients;
  - Administration of age-appropriate vaccines (with avoidance of live virus vaccines in patients on immunosuppression);
  - Counseling of adolescents to avoid alcohol while on methotrexate and pregnancy while on teratogenic medications.

- Children with JIA should remain physically active and be allowed to continue participating in sports and leisure activities as tolerated. Physical and/or occupational therapy is indicated for patients with limited mobility, deconditioning, or compromised activities of daily living.
- Regular screening for uveitis is an essential part of JIA management to allow prompt treatment of this sight-threatening complication.

Juvenile idiopathic arthritis (JIA) is an umbrella term that encompasses multiple forms of chronic, immune-mediated arthritis that begin in childhood. The classification system currently used for JIA was established in 1995 by the International League of Associations for Rheumatology (ILAR). By replacing the term *juvenile rheumatoid arthritis* with *juvenile idiopathic arthritis* and defining additional subtypes, the ILAR criteria better reflect the clinical heterogeneity among children with arthritis. Absence of the term "rheumatoid" from the current nomenclature appropriately highlights that most cases of juvenile arthritis are not simply early onset rheumatoid arthritis (RA), as only 5% of all children with JIA have rheumatoid factor (RF) positive polyarticular disease.

The subtypes of JIA are summarized in Table 1 and include oligoarticular, polyarticular (RF negative and RF positive), enthesitis-related (a childhood-onset spondyloarthropathy closely related to ankylosing spondylitis), psoriatic, and systemic arthritis.

Although each of these conditions has a distinct phenotype, the presence of chronic inflammatory arthritis is the unifying feature and sine qua non of JIA. A careful history and physical exam are the most important tools in diagnosis. A complete exam of all joints should be performed in children with possible JIA as the pattern of affected joints impacts disease classification. Additional affected joints are often identified on exam that have not been apparent to patients and parents. Common pitfalls in diagnosis of arthritis in children include the following:

- *Diagnosing JIA in the absence of objective clinical signs of arthritis (joint inflammation).* Most children who present to the primary care office with joint pain (even chronic pain) do not have JIA. Isolated pain in the absence of objective findings of arthritis such as swelling predicts against JIA or other chronic rheumatic disease.
- *Attempting to rule in JIA with laboratory studies.* ANA tests can be positive in up to 30% of healthy children, and the most common cause of a positive RF in children is recent viral infection. Due to the high frequency of positive results in children without rheumatic disease, these tests should not be drawn to evaluate for arthritis in the setting of normal exam findings.
- *Attempting to rule out JIA with laboratory studies.* Arthritis is a clinical diagnosis. If a child presents with chronic joint swelling, limited range of motion or contractures, one should not be falsely reassured by normal labs. Many children with arthritis have completely normal inflammatory markers and a negative ANA, and 95% of children with JIA are RF negative.

Risk Factors/Prevention

All JIA subtypes are generally thought to result from an aberrant immune response to an environmental trigger in a genetically predisposed person. A monozygotic twin concordance of 25% to 40% and increased autoimmunity in family members of children with JIA suggest a significant genetic contribution to disease development. Recent genome-wide association studies have revealed susceptibility loci for JIA, though differences in genetic factors exist between clinical JIA subtypes. Strong genetic associations are rare for most JIA subtypes and many identified risk loci are associated with multiple autoimmune diseases. The exception is that 80% to 90% of children with enthesitis-related arthritis (ERA) are human leukocyte antigen (HLA) B27 positive. Testing for specific HLA alleles currently has no diagnostic utility in JIA. For the interested reader, Hersh and Prahalad recently

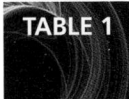

TABLE 1	International League of Associations for Rheumatology Classification Criteria for Juvenile Idiopathic Arthritis

JIA CLASSIFICATION CRITERIA

JIA Definition:
Inflammatory arthritis in at least one joint that begins before age 16, persists at least 6 weeks, and has no other identifiable cause.

JIA SUBTYPE	DESCRIPTION
Oligoarthritis	Arthritis affects 1–4 joints in the first 6 months
• Persistent	Never extends beyond 4 joints
• Extended	Extends to affect 5 or more joints after first 6 months
Polyarthritis	Arthritis affects 5 or more joints in the first 6 months
• RF negative	
• RF positive	
Enthesitis-Related Arthritis	Arthritis and enthesitis, OR Arthritis or enthesitis with at least 2 of the following: • Signs of sacroiliitis, • Positive HLA-B27, • Onset in a boy age 6 or older, • Acute anterior uveitis, • HLA-B27-related disease in a first-degree relative.
Psoriatic Arthritis	Arthritis and psoriasis, OR Arthritis and at least 2 of the following: • Dactylitis, • Nail pitting or onycholysis, • Psoriasis in a first-degree relative.
Systemic JIA	Arthritis in at least 1 joint with at least 2 weeks of fever that is daily for at least 3 days, with at least one of the following: • Evanescent erythematous rash, • Generalized lymphadenopathy, • Hepatomegaly and/or splenomegaly, • Serositis.
Undifferentiated	Fulfills criteria for no category or 2 or more categories

JIA, Juvenile idiopathic arthritis.
Data from Petty RE, Southwood TR, Manners P, et al. International League of Associations for Rheumatology classification of juvenile idiopathic arthritis: second revision, Edmonton, 2001. *J Rheumatol*. 2004;31(2):390–392.

reviewed the genetics of JIA, and Yasin and Schulert published a detailed review of the genetics and pathophysiology of systemic JIA (SJIA).

There is no known prevention for JIA.

Pathophysiology

Synovitis in JIA is characterized by synovial hypertrophy, edema, and hypervascularity. A mixed inflammatory infiltrate of T and B lymphocytes, plasma cells, macrophages, and dendritic cells is found in the synovial lining of affected joints. Infiltrating mononuclear cells produce proinflammatory cytokines and chemokines that contribute to bone and cartilage erosion and perpetuate recruitment of inflammatory cells.

SJIA is uniquely characterized by significant innate immune activation, including increased production of the proinflammatory cytokines interleukin-1 (IL-1) and 6 (IL-6). Some experts suggest that SJIA may be better classified as an autoinflammatory disease.

Given their unique clinical phenotypes, the epidemiology, clinical manifestations, diagnosis, and management of the JIA subtypes will each be discussed separately. Some general principles of diagnosis and management reviewed in "Current Diagnosis and Therapy", previously discussed, and introduced in the oligoarticular JIA section are applicable to all JIA subtypes.

Oligoarticular Juvenile Idiopathic Arthritis
Epidemiology

Oligoarticular JIA is the most common JIA subtype, comprising 40% to 50% of all cases, with an incidence of approximately 1 in 10,000 children per year. Peak age of onset is 1 to 4 years, with a female predominance. It is most commonly seen in children of Northern European descent.

Clinical Manifestations

Children with oligoarticular JIA present with arthritis in one to four joints, without spread to more than four joints in the first 6 months of disease. Oligoarthritis typically affects large joints in an asymmetrical pattern. The most common presentation is arthritis of a single knee. Swelling is the predominant symptom, often with little or no apparent pain early in the disease course. Affected joints may have a limited range of motion or contractures. A relatively painless limp is common, and is sometimes the first symptom apparent to parents. Stiffness is worse in the morning or after inactivity, though may be difficult for children to describe. Children with oligoarthritis may experience a persistent oligoarticular course (limited to four or fewer affected joints throughout the child's life) or an extended articular course (spread to five or more joints after the first 6 months of disease).

Diagnosis

A careful history and exam are key to diagnosis. Persistent joint swelling for more than 6 weeks, joint contracture, and/or gait disturbance are the most common presenting symptoms of oligoarticular JIA. Physical exam reveals joint effusion or thickened synovium indicating joint inflammation. Some children may also have warmth, decreased range of motion, contracture, or pain with range of motion on exam. Atrophy of adjacent muscles can be seen in chronic arthritis. Children with oligoarticular JIA are otherwise well-appearing. Severe pain (especially with nighttime waking), extremely red or hot joints, *migratory* swelling, fevers, rash, pallor, or a generally ill-appearing child suggest an alternative diagnosis.

All forms of JIA are diagnosed on the basis of objective signs of arthritis, a history of at least 6 weeks of persistent symptoms, and exclusion of alternative diagnoses *as appropriate based on the patient's clinical picture*. As there is no single test that can confirm the diagnosis of JIA, the value of lab testing is limited to excluding other diagnoses and for prognostic purposes in confirmed cases of JIA (see "Complications"). Radiographs have limited diagnostic value with the exception of detecting other conditions such as malignancy. MRI or musculoskeletal ultrasound can be useful in cases of equivocal or challenging physical exam (such as in obese patients).

Differential Diagnosis

In some patients with a classic clinical picture, no specific workup for other diagnoses is needed. Prompt evaluation by a pediatric rheumatologist is key to confirming the presence of arthritis, determining an appropriate individualized workup, and rapidly initiating treatment if a diagnosis of JIA is established.

Features that suggest the need to evaluate for alternative diagnoses include the following:

- Atypical demographics (age, ethnicity)—may suggest a different JIA subtype such as ERA in older children (see "Enthesitis-Related Arthritis").
- Travel history—may suggest the need to evaluate for Lyme arthritis or tuberculosis in patients residing in or traveling to endemic areas.
- Atypical clinical features—severe pain, constitutional symptoms such as weight loss, fevers, fatigue, or an ill appearance should prompt consideration of infection, malignancy, inflammatory bowel disease, or systemic collagen vascular disease such as lupus in a child with arthritis. Acute, subacute, or migratory arthritis suggests an infectious or postinfectious cause (including rheumatic fever). Episodic joint swelling, especially after trauma, may suggest a bleeding disorder or intra-articular vascular malformation.

Treatment

Treatment of JIA aims to completely control joint inflammation to control symptoms and mitigate the risk of joint damage. In oligoarticular JIA, either scheduled nonsteroidal antiinflammatory drugs (NSAIDs) or intraarticular corticosteroid injections are used as first line therapy. NSAIDs must be administered at anti-inflammatory doses on a scheduled basis to control inflammation, and may take 6 to 8 weeks to be effective. Naproxen (Naprosyn) is often preferred due to twice daily dosing and available liquid formulation. Steroid joint injections can control inflammation rapidly and are often used for patients with contractures or severe arthritis to more rapidly restore physical function. Intraarticular steroid injections should not be repeated more frequently than every 3 months. In patients with arthritis refractory to NSAIDs or steroid injections, traditional or biologic disease modifying antirheumatic drugs (DMARDs), such as methotrexate (Trexall) and tumor necrosis factor (TNF) inhibitors, can be used (some are off-label) in a stepwise fashion until disease control is achieved. DMARDs should be prescribed and monitored by a rheumatologist.

Monitoring

JIA disease control is monitored by a rheumatologist on the basis of history and physical exam. The frequency of follow-up visits varies depending on the patient's disease course and medications. Assessments of functional status should be performed to identify patients who would benefit from physical and occupational therapy service or school accommodations. Eye screening for uveitis is a critical part of JIA monitoring (see "Complications"). Medication toxicity monitoring depends on the medication used:

- Daily NSAIDs: complete blood count (CBC), comprehensive metabolic panel (CMP), and urinalysis every 6 to 12 months.
- Methotrexate: CBC and CMP at baseline, 1 month after starting or dose escalation, and then every 3 months on stable doses. Urine pregnancy screening should be considered in girls of reproductive age.
- Biologic DMARDS: Similar lab screening to methotrexate, with some variation depending on medication. Testing for tuberculosis should be performed prior to starting biologic medications.

Patients on immunosuppressive medications should be evaluated promptly for symptoms of infection. They should avoid live virus vaccines, but receive all other age-appropriate vaccinations including an annual flu vaccine.

Complications

Articular complications include joint limitation, contractures, and muscle atrophy, leading to chronic disability and pain, though these complications are less common with currently available treatments. A complication of arthritis unique to the growing child is local growth disturbance, most commonly seen as leg length discrepancy as a result of knee arthritis. Inflammation near the open growth plate can cause overgrowth of the affected limb in young children or premature growth plate closure leading to a shorter limb in adolescents.

Chronic anterior uveitis is a common complication of JIA, particularly oligoarticular and RF negative polyarticular JIA. Chronic uveitis is treatable but carries a high risk of morbidity including cataract, glaucoma, synechiae (adhesions leading to an irregular pupil), band keratopathy (corneal calcium deposits), and blindness. Chronic uveitis is often completely asymptomatic until damage has occurred. Because it can only be detected by slit lamp exam performed by an eye doctor, regular screening is critical to early detection, treatment, and prevention of permanent damage. Uveitis is more likely to occur early in the course of disease, in patients who are ANA positive, and who have an early age of arthritis onset. Well-established screening recommendations guide the frequency of eye exams, ranging from every 3 to 12 months, depending on risk factors. Risk stratification for uveitis is the only use of ANA testing in patients with JIA. Uveitis may occur independent of active arthritis, so eye screening is a critical

part of health maintenance for people with JIA throughout their lives. All children diagnosed with uveitis should see an ophthalmologist with experience treating uveitis. Topical corticosteroids are first-line therapy for anterior uveitis, though long-term use is not advisable given the risk of cataracts and glaucoma. Methotrexate[1] and the TNF inhibitors adalimumab (Humira) and infliximab (Remicade)[1] are used widely in children with refractory uveitis. Some patients require more aggressive treatment for uveitis than for arthritis.

Polyarticular Juvenile Idiopathic Arthritis
Epidemiology

Polyarticular arthritis has two subtypes. RF negative polyarthritis has two peaks of onset (at 1 to 4 years and in adolescence) and comprises 20% of all JIA. It is more common in girls and occurs in all ethnicities. RF positive polyarthritis makes up only 5% of JIA, has a peak onset of 9 to 11 years, and is more common in girls and in nonwhites.

Clinical Manifestations

Children with polyarthritis present with evidence of arthritis (swelling, morning stiffness, pain, limited range of motion) in five or more joints. Young children may present with gait disturbance or loss of milestones, while older children may present with prolonged morning stiffness or difficulty with activities of daily living and fine motor tasks. Large and small joints in the extremities are affected (often symmetrically). Long-standing disease can produce bony overgrowth of the small joints in the hands or joint deformities including wrist subluxation and boutonniere deformities of the fingers. Arthritis of the cervical spine (presenting with limited extension) and temporomandibular joint (TMJ; presenting with decreased mouth opening, jaw deviation, or micrognathia) are common and cause significant morbidity. Mild to moderate systemic symptoms, including fatigue and weight loss, may be present; however, high grade fevers should not occur.

Diagnosis

Diagnosis hinges on the presence of arthritis in five or more joints on physical exam (typically with some degree of wrist and hand involvement), at least 6 weeks of symptoms, and exclusion of other causes. There are no confirmatory tests; however, in patients with polyarticular JIA diagnosed clinically, the RF and anticitric citrullinated peptide (anti-CCP) have prognostic value. RF and anti-CCP positivity are associated with a more severe, erosive course. Some children with polyarticular JIA have normal inflammatory markers, while others have a moderately elevated erythrocyte sedimentation rate (ESR) and anemia of chronic disease. These findings are more useful for assessing overall health and monitoring response to therapy than in establishing an initial diagnosis, as they are nonspecific.

Differential Diagnosis

Reactive arthritis may present with polyarticular joint swelling, but is typically acute in onset and characterized by more pain than is seen in JIA. The arthritis of acute rheumatic fever is typically exquisitely painful and has a unique migratory pattern. While patients with polyarticular JIA may experience an *additive* arthritis pattern early in the disease course, *migratory* arthritis (i.e., swelling resolving completely in one joint and moving to another) is not seen in JIA. In patients with extreme pain, bone pain, pallor, or severe fatigue, malignancy such as leukemia or neuroblastoma should be considered.

Polyarthritis can occur as a manifestation of other underlying autoimmune diseases, including systemic lupus erythematosus, mixed connective tissue disease, or inflammatory bowel disease. The best approach to evaluating for these conditions is a thorough history and physical exam. Oral ulcers, Raynaud phenomenon, or malar or discoid rashes raise concern for lupus. Because ANA tests are nonspecific and have a high positive rate in both the healthy and JIA populations, an ANA test in isolation is not helpful in evaluating for lupus unless it is negative (which essentially excludes lupus). In cases in which the history or physical raises concern for lupus, using a combination of several laboratory studies is more helpful. A reasonable initial workup for lupus when clinical suspicion is high includes an ANA, specific lupus antibodies (Smith, double-stranded DNA), ESR, C3 and C4 levels, CBC to evaluate for cytopenias, a urinalysis, creatinine, and blood pressure measurement.

Inflammatory bowel disease can present with inflammatory arthritis. Inflammatory bowel disease (IBD) should be considered in patients with significant oral ulcers, chronic abdominal pain and/or diarrhea, weight loss, significantly elevated ESR, or anemia.

Treatment
The goals of treatment are the same as for oligoarticular disease, although children with polyarticular JIA often require more aggressive medical therapy to attain inactive disease. Scheduled NSAIDs are often started first line or in conjunction with other medications for pain relief, but rarely are effective as monotherapy. Intraarticular steroid injections may be used in combination with systemic therapy for severely affected or critical joints, but monotherapy with steroid injections is not a viable approach to treating this disease.

Most children with polyarticular JIA require treatment with DMARDs for disease control. There are two general approaches to initiation of medications: step-up therapy and early aggressive (combination) therapy. The choice of approach may be driven by provider and/or patient preference or severity of disease. In a step-up approach, methotrexate is most commonly used as the first DMARD. Methotrexate (10 to 15 mg/m^2 or 0.4 to 1 mg/kg) once weekly is administered orally or subcutaneously, with subcutaneous dosing preferred by many pediatric rheumatologists on the basis of possible improved absorption and mitigation of side effects.

Biologic medications shown to be effective in JIA refractory to methotrexate include TNF inhibitors (etanercept [Enbrel], adalimumab [Humira], golimumab [Symponi], and infliximab [Remicade][1]), the IL-6 inhibitor tocilizumab (Actemra), the T cell costimulation inhibitor abatacept (Orencia) and the Janus kinase inhibitor tofacitinib [Xeljanz]. Selection of an initial biologic medication can be driven by a variety of factors including patient/parent preference, logistics of administration, side effects, comorbid medical conditions, and (in our current health system) insurance restrictions. The anti-CD20 medication rituximab (Rituxan)[1] is sometimes used in patients with RF positive disease, usually after failure of other medications.

Early aggressive approach, such as first-line combination therapy with methotrexate and a TNF inhibitor with or without adjunctive NSAIDs, intraarticular steroid injections, or a short oral steroid bridge, is sometimes used. With earlier aggressive use of DMARDs, treatment with systemic corticosteroids can now be limited to short courses or avoided altogether in most children. While systemic steroids can produce rapid improvements in pain, symptoms return quickly after discontinuation and their side effect profile makes long-term use unacceptable. Systemic steroids should *never* be initiated in a child presenting with musculoskeletal pain of unknown etiology, given the danger of corticosteroids in undiagnosed infection or malignancy.

Monitoring
Monitoring of clinical disease and medications (NSAIDs, methotrexate, TNF inhibitors) is the same as described for oligoarthritis. Other biologic medications have similar monitoring requirements, including testing for latent tuberculosis (TB) prior to initiation. Some biologics have additional recommended laboratory monitoring parameters. Given the expertise needed to safely prescribe and monitor DMARDs, these medications should only be prescribed to children with JIA by a rheumatologist. In patients with systemic inflammation or anemia at presentation, these labs should be followed as adjunctive markers of disease activity, but normalization should not falsely reassure that arthritis is well

controlled if the joint exam indicates otherwise. Children with polyarticular JIA who develop fever while on immunosuppression should be assessed promptly for infection.

Complications
Articular complications in polyarticular JIA include joint contractures, deformities, growth disturbances, and progressive, erosive disease. Cervical spine, TMJ, hip, and wrist involvement are associated with higher morbidity. Fortunately, with earlier aggressive treatment, severe joint destruction and severe physical disability are now less common. Surgical interventions are sometimes required for patients with severe micrognathia (mandibular distraction or reconstruction techniques), joint destruction (joint replacements), or severe growth disturbances (limb inequality procedures).

Children with polyarticular JIA can also develop chronic uveitis. Similar to oligoarticular JIA, age of onset, duration of disease, and ANA status are risk factors for development of uveitis and direct frequency of eye screening. The exception is that uveitis is rare in RF positive polyarticular JIA; thus eye screening is needed only once yearly in this subtype.

Enthesitis-Related Arthritis
Epidemiology
ERA is the only JIA subtype more common in boys, makes up 9% to 19% of all JIA, and has a peak age of onset of 10 to 13 years.

Clinical Manifestations
ERA is a childhood form of spondyloarthropathy and closely related to ankylosing spondylitis. Spondyloarthropathies are characterized by axial arthritis, although in children peripheral arthritis precedes axial disease, sometimes by years. Peripheral arthritis in ERA preferentially affects the lower extremities, often asymmetrically. Arthritis of the hips and sacroiliac joints, tenosynovitis (inflammation of tendon sheaths), and *enthesitis* (inflammation at the bony insertions of tendons, ligaments, or fascia) are common findings. *Tarsitis,* diffuse swelling of the dorsum of the foot, is relatively unique to ERA. Pain is more prominent in ERA than other JIA subtypes. Axial arthritis develops in some patients in late adolescence or adulthood. Uveitis in ERA is acute and symptomatic (with a red, photophobic eye), distinct from uveitis in other forms of JIA.

Diagnosis
ERA usually presents as monoarthritis or oligoarthritis in the lower extremities (hips, knees, ankles). Diagnosis is made on the basis of arthritis on exam with a history supporting a chronic course. HLA-B27 positivity can support the diagnosis, though the HLA-B27 is not a diagnostic test (as some ERA patients are B27 negative and many B27 positive individuals are healthy). Though most children do not have sacroiliitis or spinal arthritis at presentation, findings of inflammatory spinal arthritis on radiographs or magnetic resonance imaging strongly suggest this diagnosis.

Differential Diagnosis
School-aged children with ERA often present with arthritis of a single knee or ankle. In addition to the diagnostic considerations outlined above for oligoarthritis, ERA must be distinguished from oligoarticular JIA itself. Clues to diagnosis in this clinical scenario are older age (recall that the peak age of onset of oligoarticular JIA is age 1 to 4), male gender, and supporting clinical features if present (tenosynovitis, enthesitis, acute uveitis).

In children presenting with hip symptoms, infectious and orthopedic conditions (including slipped capital femoral epiphysis or Perthes) should be considered. Rarely, older adolescents present with sacroiliitis. Low back stiffness, worse in the morning, helps distinguish from infectious and orthopedic conditions, though imaging is usually required to make this distinction with confidence. The vast majority of children with chronic low back pain have mechanical rather than inflammatory pain.

Treatment

The general approach to treatment of ERA is similar to polyarticular JIA, though for patients with sacroiliitis or spinal arthritis, TNF inhibition should be considered early in the disease course.

Monitoring

Monitoring is very similar to polyarticular JIA with a few exceptions:

1. Children with ERA should be monitored closely for development of axial arthritis. This may include a combination of the following approaches: querying symptoms of inflammatory back pain, eliciting sacroiliac pain on exam, measuring spine mobility (with a modified Schober test), and/or imaging sacroiliac joints with x-ray or magnetic resonance imaging (MRI).
2. Eye exams are only required once yearly and as indicated based on symptoms as uveitis in ERA is usually symptomatic.

Complications

Acute uveitis occurs in some patients with ERA, and often responds to topical corticosteroids. Patients who develop a red or photophobic eye should be evaluated promptly by an eye doctor. Arthritis of the spine, sacroiliac joints, and hips can be difficult to control, sometimes leading to joint destruction, even in the setting of prompt and aggressive therapy. In adulthood, these patients are at risk for progressive, ascending ankylosis of the spine.

Juvenile Psoriatic Arthritis

Epidemiology

Juvenile psoriatic arthritis comprises approximately 10% of JIA, is more common in girls, and has two peaks of onset: preschool and late childhood.

Clinical Manifestations

Psoriatic arthritis usually presents with peripheral joint involvement and can occur in a monoarticular, oligoarticular, or polyarticular pattern. Both small and large joints can be affected, often in an asymmetrical pattern. *Dactylitis,* or a sausage digit, is a unique feature of psoriatic arthritis not seen in other forms of JIA. Dactylitic fingers and toes exhibit diffuse swelling that extends beyond individual joints. Arthritis of the distal interphalangeal (DIP) joints is also unique to psoriatic arthritis among children with JIA. There is some clinical overlap between psoriatic arthritis and ERA. Enthesitis and tenosynovitis are prevalent features and sacroiliitis can occur in up to 30% of adolescents. Nail changes, including pitting, horizontal ridges, and onycholysis, are common, and overt psoriasis occurs in about half of children. Both chronic uveitis (with risk factors similar to patients with oligo- and polyarticular JIA) and acute uveitis (in HLA-B27 positive patients) can occur.

Diagnosis

Unlike adults, children with psoriatic arthritis often present with arthritis prior to skin disease. In patients with chronic arthritis and psoriasis, the diagnosis is relatively straightforward. In those with chronic arthritis without psoriasis, clinical clues to diagnosis include dactylitis, psoriatic nail changes (pitting or onycholysis), or a first-degree relative with psoriasis.

Differential Diagnosis

Depending on the pattern of joint involvement, differential diagnosis includes other forms of JIA (oligoarticular, polyarticular, ERA) and other conditions listed previously in the differential of these JIA subtypes. Small joint involvement or dactylitis help distinguish psoriatic from oligoarticular JIA in young children with less than five affected joints.

Treatment

The treatment approach is similar to polyarticular JIA, though for patients with sacroiliitis, enthesitis, or dactylitis, TNF inhibition has the most well-established efficacy.

Monitoring

Monitoring is similar to other forms of JIA including eye screening for chronic uveitis described for oligo- and polyarthritis and monitoring for axial arthritis described for ERA. In addition, patients who have not developed skin manifestations should be monitored for development of psoriasis.

Complications

Articular and ocular complications are similar to other JIA subtypes, though children with psoriatic arthritis often have poorer functional outcomes and lower rates of remission off medication than those with oligo- or polyarticular JIA.

Systemic Juvenile Idiopathic Arthritis

Epidemiology

SJIA occurs in children of all ages and into adulthood (Still disease in adults). It is the only form of JIA that affects boys and girls equally. SJIA makes up 10% to 20% of JIA. It occurs in all ethnicities, with increased prevalence in some Asian countries including Japan.

Clinical Manifestations

SJIA is characterized by fever, rash, and arthritis. Fevers in SJIA are high grade, typically spiking once (quotidian) or twice (double quotidian) daily with return to normal temperature between fevers. The rash seen in SJIA is salmon-colored or erythematous, macular or urticarial, sometimes with associated Koebner phenomenon. A unique feature of the SJIA rash is its *evanescent* nature: it appears with fever and resolves or fades during afebrile periods. The arthritis in SJIA can affect any number of joints, in any pattern, and is not always present at disease onset. In some patients, the latent period between onset of systemic features and arthritis is weeks or months. Many patients exhibit nonspecific symptoms, including fatigue, irritability, and myalgia during fevers.

Children with SJIA have significant systemic inflammation during periods of disease activity. Profoundly elevated white blood count, platelet count, ESR, CRP, and anemia are common.

SJIA is truly a systemic disease, with some patients exhibiting lymphadenopathy, hepatosplenomegaly, and serositis (pleural or pericardial effusions). The most feared complication of SJIA is macrophage activation syndrome (MAS; see "Complications").

Diagnosis

SJIA is diagnosed based on the presence of quotidian fevers, evanescent Stills rash, arthritis, and systemic inflammation, with exclusion of similar conditions. SJIA often leads to inpatient evaluation, given patients' high grade fevers and ill appearance. Children who lack arthritis at the time of presentation are challenging to diagnose. In practice, SJIA is often presumptively diagnosed before arthritis has been present for 6 weeks (and sometimes in the absence of arthritis), as the severity of this disease can necessitate urgent treatment.

Differential Diagnosis

SJIA has a broad differential diagnosis that includes infectious (viral, bacterial), oncologic (leukemia, neuroblastoma), and inflammatory conditions (Kawasaki, polyarteritis nodosa, inflammatory bowel disease, among others). Involvement of infectious disease and oncology consultants can help exclude these mimics, particularly if treatment with corticosteroids is being considered. Additional workup, including infectious studies and bone marrow biopsy, is appropriate in cases of diagnostic uncertainty.

Treatment

The treatment paradigms have evolved more for SJIA than any other JIA subtype over the last decade. Traditionally, children with SJIA were treated with systemic corticosteroids, resulting in the full spectrum of anticipated morbidities (growth delay, infections, osteoporosis, etc.). Traditional DMARDs and TNF inhibitors are significantly less effective than for other JIA subtypes.

Targeted therapy with inhibition of IL-1 (with anakinra [Kineret][1] or canakinumab [Ilaris]) or IL-6 (with tocilizumab [Actemra]) is the emerging standard of care, though optimal timing of these medications is unclear. Many pediatric rheumatologists are now using IL-1 or IL-6 blockade first line or after a failed NSAID trial to avoid or minimize corticosteroids. Systemic corticosteroids continue to have a role in severe disease or MAS. Other treatments for MAS include cyclosporine (Neoral)[1] and etoposide (Toposar)[1].

Monitoring

Monitoring is similar to polyarticular JIA, with a few exceptions. As uveitis is rare in SJIA, eye exams are needed only annually. Laboratory markers of systemic inflammation are useful in monitoring disease activity and evaluating for impending MAS, which can develop even when disease otherwise appears well controlled. Given the serious and life-threatening nature of this disease, all children with SJIA should be followed closely by a pediatric rheumatologist or an adult rheumatologist with experience managing SJIA.

Complications

Articular complications of SJIA are similar to polyarticular JIA, though the arthritis of SJIA is often aggressive and destructive. There is emerging evidence that earlier treatment with targeted biologics may prevent progression to chronic polyarthritis.

MAS is a serious complication of SJIA, characterized by unregulated production of proinflammatory cytokines, macrophage proliferation, and hemophagocytic activity in the bone marrow and other organs. MAS is a potentially fatal rheumatologic emergency. It is often suspected on the basis of rapidly worsening clinical status and the development of continuous fever. Laboratory findings include a profoundly elevated ferritin, elevated lactate dehydrogenase and transaminases, falling blood cell counts, and paradoxically low or falling ESR and fibrinogen in the setting of other signs of systemic inflammation. MAS is currently considered a secondary form of hemophagocytic lymphohistiocytosis (HLH).

Not FDA approved for this indication.

References

Aeschlimann FA, Chong S, Lyons TW, et al: Risk of serious infections associated with biologic agents in juvenile idiopathic arthritis: a systematic review and meta-analyses, *J Pediatr* 204:162–171, 2019.

Clarke SLN, Sen ES, Ramanan AV: Juvenile Idiopathic arthritis-associated uveitis, *Pediatric Rheumatol Online J* 14:27, 2016.

Crayne CB, Beukelman T: Juvenile idiopathic arthritis: oligoarthritis and polyarthritis, *Pediatr Clin N Am* 65:657–674, 2018.

Hersh AO, Prahalad S: Genetics of juvenile idiopathic arthritis, *Rheum Dis Clin N Am* 43:435–448, 2017.

Lee JJL, Schneider R: Systemic juvenile idiopathic arthritis, *Pediatr Clin N Am* 65:691–709, 2018.

Petty RE, Southwood TR, Manners P, et al: International League of Associations for Rheumatology classification of juvenile idiopathic arthritis: second revision, Edmonton, 2001, *J Rheumatol* 31(2):390–392, 2004.

Shoop-Worrall SJW, Kearlsey-Fleet L, Thomson W, Verstappen SMM, Hyrich KL: How common is remission in juvenile idiopathic arthritis: a systematic review, *Semin Arthritis Rheum* 47:331–337, 2017.

Wong KO, Bond K, Homik J, Ellsworth JE, Karkhaneh M, Ha C, Dryden DM: Antinuclear antibody, rheumatoid factor, and cyclic-citrullinated peptide tests for evaluating musculoskeletal complaints in children: Comparative Effectiveness Review No. 50, *Agency for Healthcare Research and Quality*, 2012. Available at https://effectivehealthcare.ahrq.gov/sites/default/files/pdf/musculoskeletal-complaints-tests-children_research.pdf. Accessed 1 January 2019.

Yasin S, Schulert GS: Systemic juvenile idiopathic arthritis and macrophage activation syndrome: update on pathogenesis and treatment, *Curr Opin Rheumatol* 30:514–520, 2018.

OSTEOARTHRITIS

Method of
Rachel Chamberlain, MD; Jacob Christensen, DO; and Christopher Bossart, MD

CURRENT DIAGNOSIS

- Risk factors for osteoarthritis (OA) include age, gender, genetics, and anatomic factors, which are nonmodifiable; modifiable risk factors include body mass index (BMI), tobacco use, trauma, physical activity, and muscle strength.
- OA is diagnosed using both clinical and radiologic information.
- Clinical signs and symptoms include joint pain, crepitus, mild swelling, and joint line tenderness to palpation. Symptoms wax and wane and may be related to activity but can be present at varying times of day.
- The Kellgren-Lawrence Classification system can help determine the grade of OA, but the ultimate determination of the severity is based on clinical factors.

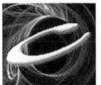

CURRENT THERAPY

- First-line therapy for OA includes exercise, physical therapy, and weight loss (if the patient is overweight or obese).
- Nonsteroidal antiinflammatory drugs (NSAIDs) are the best studied pharmacologic treatment for OA pain. Their use must be balanced by their side effects and the patient's comorbid conditions.
- Injections of corticosteroids may be used for OA pain management, but their pain relief effects are not long term.
- Hyaluronic acid injections can be considered in patients with mild to moderate OA of the knee, but this is an expensive therapy and evidence of effectiveness is mixed.
- No current treatment either in systemic medications or injections alters the course of OA. Research in the long-term benefits of biologic agents is ongoing.
- Total joint replacement is an expensive but definitive treatment for many patients with OA. The referring clinician should consider the patient's overall health and help optimize the patient's health for a successful outcome when referring for a total joint replacement.

Osteoarthritis (OA), also known as degenerative joint disease, is the most common form of arthritis worldwide. OA is a significant cause of morbidity, disability, and decreased quality of life. It is one of the leading contributors to global years lived with disability (YLDs) by Global Disease Burden studies. It is the leading cause of lower extremity disability. OA affects about one in eight people in the United States, or 27 to 31 million, and about 250 million people worldwide, with the most commonly affected joints being the knees, hips, hands, feet, and spine. As the age of the population and the rates of obesity increase, the economic impact of OA also increases. It is estimated that OA costs 1% to 2.5% of GDP in developed countries, with the majority of cost for treatment (85%) coming from joint replacement surgeries.

OA has been previously characterized pathologically by varying levels of cartilage involvement. One may find fissures and microfibrillations in mild or early disease, and erosive destruction of the joint surfaces may be seen in more advanced disease. However, it is recognized that the effects of OA can be seen throughout the entire joint including the bone, synovium, menisci, and ligaments.

Pathogenesis

The pathogenesis of OA remains unclear. For decades, the traditional belief was that OA was a "wear and tear" condition associated with the cumulative stress of aging. This theory has not been shown to be true, or at least it is not an accurate depiction of "the whole story." Research investigating other possible mechanisms is gaining traction. More recent research areas of focus include what role inflammatory mediators, genetics, metabolic factors, proteases, and biomarkers may play in the development of OA.

Risk Factors

Despite the pathogenesis of OA being unclear, a number of factors have been identified to be associated with increased risk. These risk factors include age, gender, body mass index (BMI), genetics, tobacco smoking, trauma, chronic overuse, anatomic factors, and muscle strength.

Age—There is a clear correlation between aging and development of OA. It is also clear that the aging of joint tissues and the development of OA are separate and distinct processes. There are a number of aging changes within the joint that may contribute to development of OA including: thinning of articular cartilage, reduced hydration, accumulation of advanced glycation end-products (AGEs), and abnormal calcification ("chondrocalcinosis"). Based on population based radiographic surveys from the Framingham study, the prevalence of knee OA in patients aged 63 to 94 was 33%, and symptomatic knee OA was 9.5%.

Gender—OA is more common in women than men. Some have postulated that the correlation between age and OA explains the why OA is more common in the postmenopausal years; however, there is some evidence to suggest decreased estrogen exposure in women could also be a contributing factor.

BMI—Being overweight or obese has been well documented as a strong risk factor for development of OA. This is likely both related to increased mechanical forces and metabolic changes associated with obesity. Weight loss has also been shown to reduce the risk of developing knee OA.

Genetics—Twin studies have shown a genetic contribution of about 40% to 70% depending on the site of OA. There exists substantial heterogeneity depending on the site of involvement, and there is also racial variation, which makes studying this genetic component more difficult.

Trauma and chronic overuse—Trauma, which includes both major injuries and surgery, increases the risk of OA. For example, history of anterior cruciate ligament (ACL) tear in the knee is associated with increased risk of OA development regardless of whether surgical reconstruction is done. The mechanism for this is not completely understood. Chronic overuse as is seen in some occupations carries an increased risk of development of OA. For example, professional soccer players have an increased risk of developing knee OA, and professional baseball pitchers have a higher risk of developing elbow OA.

Biomechanical factors—Joint structural abnormalities may increase the risk of developing OA. The understanding of the role of muscle strength in OA is expanding. It is known that patients with knee and hip OA have reduced muscle strength in the surrounding muscles. However, it has been thought previously that this was a consequence of the symptoms of OA causing decreased activity, muscle atrophy, and subsequent weakness. There is more recent evidence to suggest that muscle weakness may actually predate the onset of knee OA.

Clinical Features

OA is characterized clinically by insidious onset, usage-related joint pain, which can be accompanied by mild stiffness. Pain can be present at varying times of day. Mild swelling may be present in OA; however, large effusion and history of trauma or injury should prompt further workup. Patients may complain of limitation in range of motion, as well as a sensation of giving way or buckling (particularly in knee OA). Tenderness to palpation along the joint lines is a common physical exam finding. Joint deformity is a sign of advanced disease. Symptoms are typically slowly progressive as is the disease course.

OA severity can be graded based on radiographic criteria or a combination of radiographic criteria and symptom severity. Perhaps the most commonly used radiographic criteria is the Kellgren-Lawrence method, classifying OA severity into grades 0 to 4 based on presence of joint space narrowing, osteophyte formation, and sclerosis of subchondral bone (Table 1). This method is certainly useful, though it should be mentioned that there are limitations to this method—namely, that there is somewhat poor correlation between radiographic findings and symptoms. It is estimated that up to 50% of people with radiographic findings of OA do not have any symptoms.

Current Therapy

Treatment for OA is individualized based on patient symptoms, values, needs, goals, and response to therapies. There is no single treatment for OA, which reliably and consistently manages symptoms on its own. Therefore, a combination of therapeutic approaches is used in order to optimize function, minimize pain, and in some cases modify the process of damage to the joint. In general, safer treatments should be considered first before trying other treatments with higher risk profiles. Treatments can be placed into four categories: nonpharmacologic, pharmacologic, nonsurgical, and surgical interventions.

Nonpharmacologic Therapies

Nonpharmacologic therapies represent the mainstay of treatment for OA initially. These therapies include education, exercise, weight management, braces, assistive devices, psychologic therapies, manual medicine, and alternative therapies.

Education—It is important to inform patients about their diagnosis, the modifiable risk factors for their specific case, and their expected prognosis. Information should be provided regarding the various treatment options including their risks, benefits, costs, and alternatives. Doing this helps encourage active shared decision making and combat some of the common misconceptions about OA management. Patient involvement in setting goals and self-managing their condition improves adherence and can make a significant difference in patients' view of their disease.

Exercise—The goal of exercise therapy is reduction in pain and improvement in joint function. Various forms of exercise exist, and physical activity in general should be encouraged, providing it is done with patient symptoms as a guide. The forms of exercise with the best evidence for improvement, particularly in knee OA, are aerobic exercise and resistance strength training. Perhaps the most readily available form of aerobic exercise is walking, and formal walking programs have been shown to significantly improve OA symptoms, as well as quadriceps strength. Aquatic exercise has also been shown to be beneficial, and has the added benefit of decreased weight-bearing stress on joints.

Weight loss—In overweight and obese patients (BMI > 25), a reduction of 10% of baseline body weight has been shown to

TABLE 1	Kellgren Lawrence Radiographic Classification of Osteoarthritis of the Knee
Grade 1	Doubtful joint space narrowing, possible osteophytic lipping
Grade 2	Definite osteophytes, possible joint space narrowing
Grade 3	Moderate osteophytes, definite joint space narrowing, some sclerosis, possible bone-end deformity
Grade 4	Large osteophytes, marked joint space narrowing, severe sclerosis, definite bone ends deformity

Data from Kellgren JH, Lawrence JS. Radiological assessment of osteo-arthrosis. *Ann Rheum Dis.* 1957;16:494–502.

decrease OA-related joint pain. This is true of patients with knee and hip OA, but may also be beneficial in patients with OA of the hands in light of evidence that increased BMI is a risk factor for development of hand OA. Again, this may be partially related to metabolic changes.

Braces and assistive devices—Walking aids, such as a walking stick or cane, as well as knee braces for patients with joint malalignment, may be helpful, and should be considered as an adjunct treatment in appropriate patients. OA of the thumb is particularly amenable to splinting to improve pain.

Psychologic therapies—Chronic pain from OA can have significant effects on a patient's ability to function. Often as patients feel less able to perform the activities they enjoy, their mood is adversely affected, which in turn negatively affects their pain symptoms. There is some evidence that psychological interventions, such as cognitive behavioral therapy, are helpful in this regard.

Manual medicine—Manual techniques, whether performed by a physical therapist, doctor of osteopathic medicine (DO), massage therapist, or chiropractor, typically focus on improvement/maintenance of range of motion as well as joint mobility. There is some limited evidence to suggest manual manipulation may improve pain scores, particularly when combined with exercise therapy. However, more research in this area is needed.

Alternative therapies—There is currently insufficient evidence to recommend the use of acupuncture, therapeutic ultrasound, and neuromuscular electrical stimulation for treatment of OA.

Pharmacotherapy

Despite the fact that nonpharmacologic agents are first line, many patients with OA require drug therapy. Although no available medications predictably reverse or halt the inexorable progression of the disease, some medications do reduce pain and inflammation, enhancing the patient's quality of life.

Analgesics—The most common nonnarcotic analgesic agent currently used for OA is acetaminophen (Tylenol). The recommended dose for OA is 1 g administered every 8 hours or three to four times daily (not to exceed 4 g/day). However, even at a high dose, studies are mixed if acetaminophen is effective for OA pain. Adverse effects are rare, but caution must be exercised in patients who have preexisting renal or liver conditions. Duloxetine (Cymbalta) 60 mg daily is approved by the US Food and Drug Administration (FDA) for mild to moderate pain resulting from OA. In a double-blind, randomized, placebo-controlled study of patients with chronic pain due to OA of the knees, there was significant improvement with duloxetine versus the placebo. In treating OA, the regular use of opioids is not recommended or supported. Tramadol (Ultram) is commonly used, particularly in patients who have contraindications to nonsteroidal antiinflammatory drugs (NSAIDs), but we suggest caution in prescribing even this medication given potential for tolerance. While for years it has been suggested that opioids improve quality of life and function in patients with chronic pain from OA, there is no evidence to support this in OA. Opioids may be needed occasionally for intense pain, but the benefits are limited compared to the risks of tolerance, opioid misuse, addiction, overdose, and death.

Nonsteroidal antiinflammatory drugs—Pain in OA patients is often not adequately controlled with pure analgesics, whereas NSAIDs in adequate dosage can provide significant clinical improvement. The 2013 AAOS Guidelines on nonsurgical management of knee OA recommend NSAIDs with a strong strength of recommendation. If simple analgesics fail to provide adequate relief, one of the many currently available NSAIDs may be tried. Clinical trials with naproxen (Anaprox), diclofenac (Voltaren), and sulindac (Clinoril) showed significantly greater improvement when compared with high-dose acetaminophen. The chief limiting factor in the use of NSAIDs is the possible induced gastric pathologic changes, disturbed renal function, and potential increased cardiac events. In addition, many patients with OA may be on other platelet inhibiting medications and interactions should be taken into consideration. For patients ages 75 and above, topical NSAIDs are advised over oral given less toxicity and adverse effects. Cost and compliance also must be given consideration. Many of the NSAIDs are now available in dosage forms that can be given once or twice daily, which helps overcome the issue of noncompliance.

Cyclooxygenase 2 inhibitors—COX-2 inhibitors block prostaglandin synthesis and inflammatory mediators without the COX-1 effect of inhibiting gastric mucosal protection. In the United States, the COX-2–specific inhibiting NSAID that is FDA approved is celecoxib (Celebrex). It is equivalent to the older nonselective NSAIDs with regard to therapeutic effectiveness, but the risk of gastrointestinal injury and adverse effects on platelet aggregation is lessened. The risk of renal side effects is probably comparable with that of the conventional NSAIDs. A trial assessing the effect of celecoxib on cardiovascular events found a slightly higher risk of cardiovascular events, but primarily only at higher doses (400 mg/day or greater). In addition, celecoxib can be used with low-dose aspirin (81 mg) daily and anticoagulants, including warfarin. It is important to take into consideration that the cost of Celebrex is several times that of traditional NSAIDs.

Glucosamine and chondroitin sulfate—Glucosamine and chondroitin sulfate are over-the-counter dietary supplements that have gained moderate press touting their possible symptom-modifying effects. However, there is no significant evidence demonstrating that either of these used alone or in combination prevents or reduces arthritis in the knee. A Cochrane review shows mild improvement in pain scores at short-term follow-up with glucosamine compared with placebo, however only with certain preparations of the product. At this point, multiple organizations including the American College of Rheumatology and American Academy of Orthopedic Surgeons cannot recommend their use in treating OA.

Turmeric—Turmeric[7] has been used for treatment of many inflammatory disease processes, including OA, with modest improvement in pain. Curcumin[7] is the primary constituent within turmeric, and there is thought that regular intake can protect joints in individuals with OA. The studies to date are small and limited in number, but they do show modest reduction in pain among those with OA. Larger studies would be needed in order for a definitive recommendation to be made but given its low side effect profile and risk of adverse effects it seems to be a reasonable addition to treatment. However, turmeric may interact with other antiplatelet therapies, and this should be considered individually for each patient.

Disease-modifying drugs—To date, there are no known medications that reliably slow or stop the disease process of OA, and disease modifying antirheumatic drugs (DMARDs) are not recommended in the treatment of OA.

Intra-articular Injections

Corticosteroid injections (CSI)—Early in symptomatic OA it is preferable to attempt to control symptoms by nonpharmacologic therapy and with oral therapy, rather than by local injection. CSI are commonly used for OA. Steroids are strong antiinflammatory medications, and there is reasonable evidence that CSI decreases pain in the short term. There remain concerns that CSI may damage cartilage and therefore hasten the advancement of OA. Clinical trials remain mixed. However, when noninvasive therapies are not controlling OA pain or a patient has an OA flare, CSI can provide relief. CSI is thought to be relatively safe to be given three to four times per year, although this is an expert opinion and not based in sound evidence. The remote risk of introducing infection from the procedure is minimized by adhering to a meticulous aseptic technique. CSI is thought to be less problematic than systemic steroids when it comes to side effects such as raising blood sugar, but caution should be used in patients with diabetes, particularly uncontrolled DM. While arthrocentesis of

---

Available as dietary supplement.

a painful arthritic joint is commonly done, there is little evidence that this is an effective therapy, particularly after the short term.

Hyaluronic acid—Intra-articular hyaluronic acid (HA) injections have been approved by the FDA since 1997 as a medical device for OA of the knee. The clinical use of intra-articular HA in painful OA of the knee was introduced in Europe in the 1990s. The mechanism of action of HA is not completely understood, but it is thought to restore normal viscoelastic properties to the pathologically altered synovial fluid. Other possible beneficial effects include protection of the chondrocytes, antiinflammatory effects, and possible improvement of the mechanics of joint motion. Unfortunately, in non-industry-funded studies, head-to-head comparisons often fail to show superiority over cortisone and placebo injections. In addition, HA does not change the course of OA. Numerous preparations of FDA-approved HA products are in wide use in the United States. Initially, all HA products were extracted from rooster combs; however, that is no longer the case. In approximately 2% to 8% of patients injected with avian derived product, a subsequent pseudoseptic reaction can occur, mimicking an infected joint. Newer HA products are not animal-derived preparations but rather are developed from biological fermentation of streptococcal bacteria. In the United States, these products are only approved for knee OA. Drawbacks of intra-articular HA products include mixed evidence, cost, and less efficacy in patients with morbid obesity or severe (Kellrgan Lawrence Grade 4) OA.

Platelet rich plasma (PRP)—PRP injections have become popular in recent years. However, as many of these procedures are not covered by insurance, their use has been limited secondary to the expense of these treatments. There are some studies suggesting increased efficacy in functional improvement when compared to HA products. However, the data are still lacking, and it is hard to make clear conclusions at this point.

Stem cells—Stem cell injections have become an intriguing area of research. The thought that intra-articular injections of stem cells can help improve/restart chondrogenesis, and regeneration of damaged cartilage is actively being researched. However, a recent systematic review of the literature shows only a low level of evidence for its use, all of which were studies deemed to be at high risk for bias. At this time, it is not considered a mainstay treatment for OA in the United States.

Surgical Management of Osteoarthritis

Surgical management of arthritis varies by which joint is affected, with knee arthritis being most common, followed by hip. Knee arthroscopy should not be used to manage knee OA and/or degenerative meniscus tears in the setting of OA, as there is little to no improvement compared with exercise. Additionally, arthroscopic partial meniscectomy for degenerative meniscus tears may increase risk of developing OA. Hemiarthroplasty can be considered in patients with unicompartmental knee arthritis, and may carry less risks than total knee arthroplasty (TKA). In addition, a valgus-producing proximal tibial osteotomy may be beneficial in patients with symptomatic medial compartment knee OA. Total joint arthroplasty is an expensive surgery, though often well covered by insurance companies. The surgeries carry significant risks, including cardiovascular events, deep vein thrombosis, and prosthesis infection, which can lead to long hospitalizations for intravenous antibiotics and repeat surgeries. Not all patients have the pain relief and function improvement expected from total joint arthroplasty (TJA).

When referring a patient to orthopedic surgery for consideration of a total hip or knee arthroplasty, the clinician may be able to help prepare the patient to optimize their surgical outcome. This includes, but is not limited to, helping a patient with smoking cessation, weight loss, and diabetes control. Ideally, a patient would be tobacco/nicotine free for at least 8 weeks prior to surgery, would have a BMI less than 40, and would have a hemoglobin A1C ≤7.0. In addition, the referring clinician should take into consideration that patients with chronic pain and/or opioid use, depression and anxiety, liver cirrhosis/hepatitis C, and other chronic conditions may not have optimal outcomes from total joint replacement. It is acceptable to delay total knee arthroplasty up to 8 months to improve these modifiable risk factors without decreasing the patient's benefit from total joint arthroplasty. Arthroplasty procedures are also performed for arthritis of the shoulder, elbow, wrist, thumb, and ankle with varying degrees of evidence for pain and quality of life improvement. Surgical techniques and prostheses are undergoing advancements and improving patient outcomes for the less commonly done arthroplasty surgeries, and clinicians can expect this technology to continue to advance in the future.

Conclusions

OA remains a very common source of pain and disability throughout the world and also carries a significant financial burden. The pathophysiology of OA is more complex than previously believed, and is not fully understood. OA has both modifiable and nonmodifiable risk factors. Nonmodifiable risk factors include age, gender, and genetic risk/family history. Modifiable risk factors include weight loss in patients who are overweight or obese, eliminating tobacco exposure, trauma and overuse, and control of metabolic syndrome.

Nonpharmacologic therapy for OA is first-line treatment and includes education and management of patient expectations, weight loss, exercise, and physical therapy. Braces and assistive devices, cognitive behavioral therapy, manual therapy, and alternative therapy may also be considered but have less definitive evidence.

Pharmacologic therapy is usually required for OA, with acetaminophen being first line. Clinicians should educate patients on high dose acetaminophen and safe amounts to take to achieve therapeutic effect without danger to liver. NSAIDs are often more effective at controlling pain from OA, but do carry a higher risk profile for gastrointestinal bleeding, renal dysfunction, and cardiovascular events. Herbal medications such as glucosamine chondroitin and turmeric may also be beneficial but studies are mixed. Opioids should be avoided in management of OA pain, as there is no evidence that they improve function and quality of life (as previously proposed) but do carry very serious side effects.

Nonsurgical interventions such as intra-articular injections can be beneficial in managing pain from OA. It is important to counsel patients that none of the current injection therapies have data that they change the course of the disease process; they only help control pain and improve function. Corticosteroid injections often give the patient good pain relief but are often not long lasting. HA injections may also be beneficial, but many studies show equivocal pain improvement compared with cortisone and the cost is much greater. Studies are still ongoing at biologic agent injections such as PRP and stem cell therapies, and data is mixed. It is unclear if these expensive, non-FDA-approved therapies are beneficial at this time.

Total joint arthroplasty is the definitive treatment for OA, with the best data in hip followed by knee arthroplasty. These surgeries carry significant risks, especially in the older population that OA most commonly affects. In addition, surgery is very expensive and associated with significant time loss from work. Patients' chronic medical conditions should be well controlled prior to a total joint arthroplasty, to minimize risks of poor outcomes or adverse effects.

References

American Academy of Orthopedic Surgeons: Management of Osteoarthritis of the Hip Evidence-Based Clinical Practice Guideline, Available at: https://www.aaos.org/uploadedFiles/PreProduction/Quality/Guidelines_and_Reviews/OA%20Hip%20CPG_3.13.17.pdf. Accessed 15 March 2019.

Bartels EM, Juhl CB, Christensen R, et al: Aquatic exercise for the treatment of knee and hip osteoarthritis, *Cochrane Database of Systematic Reviews*, 2016. Available at: https://doi.org/10.1002/cca.1312.

Brown GA: AAOS Clinical Practice Guideline: Treatment of osteoarthritis of the knee: evidence-based guideline, *Journal of the American Academy of Orthopaedic Surgeons* 21(9):577–579, 2013, Available at: https://doi.org/10.5435/jaaos-21-09-577.

Conaghan, P. I56. DMARDs in Osteoarthritis: What is the evidence? *Rheumatology*, 53(suppl_1):i12–i13, 2014, Available at: https://doi.org/10.1093/rheumatology/keu061.003

Dadabo J, Fram J, Jayabalan P: Noninterventional therapies for the management of knee osteoarthritis, *The Journal of Knee Surgery* 32(01):046–054, 2018, Available at: https://doi.org/10.1055/s-0038-1676107.

Dai WL, et al: Efficacy of platelet-rich plasma in the treatment of knee osteoarthritis: a meta-analysis of randomized controlled trials, *Arthroscopy* 33(3):659–670.e1, 2017 Mar, Available at: https://doi.org/10.1016/j.arthro.2016.09.024. Epub 2016 Dec 22. Review PubMed PMID: 28012636.

Fransen M, Mcconnell S, Harmer AR, Esch MV, Simic M, Bennell KL: Exercise for osteoarthritis of the knee, *Cochrane Database of Systematic Reviews*, 2015, Available at: https://doi.org/10.1002/14651858.cd004376.pub3.

Henrotin Yves, et al: Curcumin: a new paradigm and therapeutic opportunity for the treatment of osteoarthritis: curcumin for osteoarthritis management, *SpringerPlus* 2(1), 2013, Available at: https://doi.org/10.1186/2193-1801-2-56.

Hochberg MC, Altman RD, April KT, et al: American College of Rheumatology 2012 recommendations for the use of nonpharmacologic and pharmacologic therapies in osteoarthritis of the hand, hip, and knee, *Arthritis Care & Research* 64(4):465–474, 2012, Available at: https://doi.org/10.1002/acr.21596.

Kohn MD, Sassoon AA, Fernando ND: Classifications in Brief: Kellgren-Lawrence Classification of Osteoarthritis, *Clin Orthop Relat Res* 474(8):1886–1893, 2016, Available at: https://doi.org/10.1007/s11999-016-4732-4.

Lin KY, et al: Intra-articular injection of platelet-rich plasma is superior to hyaluronic acid or saline solution in the treatment of mild to moderate knee osteoarthritis: a randomized, double-blind, triple-parallel, placebo-controlled clinical trial, *Arthroscopy* 35(1):106–117, 2019 Jan, Available at: https://doi.org/10.1016/j.arthro.2018.06.035. PubMed PMID: 30611335.

McGrory B, Weber K, Jevsevar D, Sevarino K: Surgical management of osteoarthritis of the knee, *Journal of the American Academy of Orthopaedic Surgeons* 24(8), 2016, Available at: https://doi.org/10.5435/JAAOS-D-16-00159.

Moyer RF, Birmingham TB, Bryant DM, et al: Valgus bracing for knee osteoarthritis: a meta-analysis of randomized trials, *Arthritis Care & Research* 67(4):493–501, 2015, Available at: https://doi.org/10.1002/acr.22472.

Nakagawa Yasuaki, et al: Short-term effects of highly-bioavailable curcumin for treating knee osteoarthritis: a randomized, double-blind, placebo-controlled prospective study, *Journal of Orthopaedic Science* 19(6):933–939, 2014, Available at: https://doi.org/10.1007/s00776-014-0633-0.

Oneill TW, Mccabe PS, Mcbeth J: Update on the epidemiology, risk factors and disease outcomes of osteoarthritis, *Best Practice & Research Clinical Rheumatology* 32(2):312–326, 2018, Available at: https://doi.org/10.1016/j.berh.2018.10.007.

Pas HI, Winters M, Haisma HJ, et al: Stem cell injections in knee osteoarthritis: a systematic review of the literature, *Br J Sports Med* 51(15):1125–1133, 2017 Aug, Available at: https://doi.org/10.1136/bjsports-2016-096793. Epub 2017 Mar 3. Review PubMed PMID: 28258177.

Sanders TL, Pareek A, Kremers HM: Long-term follow-up of isolated ACL tears treated without ligament reconstruction, *Knee Surgery, Sports Traumatology, Arthroscopy* 25(2):493–500, 2016, Available at: https://doi.org/10.1007/s00167-016-4172-4.

Siemieniuk RAC, Harris IA, Agoritsas T, et al: Arthroscopic surgery for degenerative knee arthritis and meniscal tears: a clinical practice guideline, *BMJ* 357, 2017https://doi.org/10.1136/bmj.j1982.

Sihvonen R, Paavola M, Malmivaara A, et al: *Br J Sports Med* 54:1332–1339, 2020.

Smithers CJ, Young AA, Walch G: Reverse shoulder arthroplasty, *Curr Rev Musculoskelet Med* 4(4):183–190, 2011, Available at: https://doi.org/10.1007/s12178-011-9097-4.

Towheed TE, Maxwell L, Anastassiades TP, et al: Glucosamine therapy for treating osteoarthritis, *Cochrane Database Syst Rev* (2)CD002946, 2005 Apr 18. Review PubMed PMID: 15846645.

Tsoukas D, Fotopoulos V, Basdekis G, Makridis KG: No difference in osteoarthritis after surgical and non-surgical treatment of ACL-injured knees after 10 years, *Knee Surgery, Sports Traumatology, Arthroscopy* 24(9):2953–2959, 2015, Available at: https://doi.org/10.1007/s00167-015-3593-9.

OSTEOPOROSIS

Method of

Alexei O. DeCastro, MD; Scott Bragg, PharmD; and Peter J. Carek, MD, MS

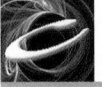

CURRENT DIAGNOSIS

- Recommend evaluation of risk factors for falls and osteoporotic fractures.
- Recommend screening for osteoporosis with bone mineral density (BMD) testing in women age 65 years and older.
- Recommend screening for osteoporosis in postmenopausal women younger than 65 years at increased risk of osteoporosis.
- Current evidence is insufficient to recommend screening for osteoporosis in men.
- Determination of BMD is helpful for those with clinical osteoporotic fractures to determine the severity of the disorder and to help guide future treatment decisions.
- Consider clinical and laboratory workup of secondary causes of osteoporosis in patients with osteoporosis.
- Current evidence is insufficient to recommend routine vertebral fracture assessment and trabecular bone scores, although they may improve fracture risk assessment.

CURRENT THERAPY

- Recommend a comprehensive nutritional assessment targeting normal body weight and adequate ingestion of calcium and vitamin D.
- Evidence does not support taking calcium and vitamin D for primary prevention of osteoporotic fracture in adults over age 50. For secondary prevention, recommend at least 1200 mg/day of calcium and 800 to 1000 IU/day of vitamin D. Dietary sources are preferred, but supplements may be necessary to meet goals.
- Weight-bearing and muscle-strengthening exercises are important tools to reduce the risk of falls and fracture.
- Pharmacologic osteoporosis treatment may reduce fracture risk in patients with a clinical diagnosis of osteoporosis (i.e., hip or vertebral fractures without major trauma) or radiographic evidence of osteoporosis (i.e., BMD T-scores ≤–2.5 at the lumbar spine, femoral neck, or total hip).
- Pharmacologic treatment may also reduce fracture risk in patients with low bone mass and high 10-year fracture risk. The 10-year fracture risk is high if the 10-year hip fracture probability is ≥3% or if the 10-year probability of a major osteoporosis-related fracture is ≥20%. To access fracture risk, use the fracture risk assessment tool (FRAX) from the US-adapted algorithm from the World Health Organization.
- Treatment of premenopausal women and men younger than 50 years old with osteoporosis therapy is controversial. Z-scores ≤–2.0 indicate osteoporosis. However, osteoporosis treatment is often reserved for glucocorticoid-induced osteoporosis in patients at high fracture risk or patients with multiple fragility fractures.
- The drugs currently approved by the US Food and Drug Administration (FDA) for treating osteoporosis include alendronate (Fosamax), ibandronate (Boniva), risedronate (Actonel), zoledronic acid (Reclast), calcitonin (Miacalcin), raloxifene (Evista), denosumab (Prolia), teriparatide (Forteo), abaloparatide (Tymlos), and romosozumab (Evenity).

Osteoporosis is a skeletal disease characterized by low bone mass and structural deterioration of bone tissue, which is associated with decreased bone strength and increased susceptibility to fractures. Its clinical relevance is increasing because healthcare professionals are caring for more older adults and because of the high morbidity and mortality associated with the disease. Osteoporosis is asymptomatic until the patient has a fracture, so identifying patients at high fracture risk and prevention is important. Once a vertebral fracture is present, patients may develop back pain, height loss, and/or thoracic kyphosis. Hip fractures are associated with thigh or groin pain and typically limit a patient's mobility. Primary or secondary prevention of fracture in patients with osteoporosis is a challenge because screening can be difficult and treating osteoporosis has many risks and benefits.

The World Health Organization (WHO) has defined osteoporosis as a condition in which bone mineral density (BMD) assessed by dual-energy x-ray absorptiometry (DEXA) at the lumbar spine or hip is decreased. Osteoporosis is seen in postmenopausal women or men over age 50 with a BMD of 2.5 standard deviations (SDs) below normal (T-score $\leq$−2.5) compared with young-adult reference population. Low bone mass, previously known as osteopenia, is a milder degree of bone loss seen in the same populations (T-score of −1.0 to −2.4). Although the risk of fracture increases significantly with decreasing BMD, large observational studies have demonstrated that osteoporotic fractures can occur across a wide spectrum of BMDs. Thus osteoporotic fractures may be caused by low bone quantity and poor bone quality, a component not measured by DEXA scans. Qualitative determinants of bone strength include trabecular bone scores, microcracks, mineralization defects, bone geometry, cell death, changes in bone size, and changes in bone turnover. Even though a low BMD defines osteoporosis, a fragility fracture (i.e., fracture without trauma or a low-trauma fall) may clinically diagnose osteoporosis.

The U.S. Preventive Services Task Force (USPSTF) recommends screening for osteoporosis in women greater than 65 years old and in women younger than 65 who are at equal or increased risk of osteoporosis compared with an average 65-year-old woman (Grade B recommendation). To identify patients at increased risk, multiple decision support tools exist, but the most widely used tool is the fracture risk assessment tool (FRAX), which helps calculate the 10-year risk of a hip fracture and a major osteoporotic fracture. The FRAX considers several major independent risk factors including BMD of the femoral neck, previous fracture history, family history of fracture, age, sex, ethnicity, glucocorticoid use, alcohol abuse, current smoking status, and possible secondary osteoporosis causes. Despite these recommendations, many women with osteoporosis go unrecognized and untreated. In one study from an insurance claims database, less than 50% of women with a fragility fracture had an osteoporosis diagnosis within 1 year of the fracture and less than 30% were treated with pharmacologic therapy.

Epidemiology

Osteoporosis is the most common metabolic disorder of the skeleton. Based on 2010 data in the United States, approximately 8 million women and 2 million men had osteoporosis, and another 43 million people had low bone mass. The estimated prevalence of osteoporosis is highest in Mexican Americans, followed by non-Hispanic Whites, and lowest in non-Hispanic Blacks. Worldwide, 200 million women suffer from osteoporosis, and those women have an estimated 65% lifetime risk of a fragility fracture. In men with osteoporosis, the estimated lifetime risk of a fragility fracture is 42%. Hip fractures are the most feared fragility fracture because they cause a mortality rate of 10% to 20% at 12 months, and up to 25% of those with hip fractures require long-term nursing care.

Screening

Considering risk factors for osteoporosis is important at annual well visits or during all visits in high-risk individuals. Nonmodifiable risk factors are genetic background, advancing age, female sex, low socioeconomic status, being Hispanic American or non-Hispanic White, personal history of fracture, and family history of fracture in a first-degree relative. Modifiable risk factors consist of low body weight, hormonal deficiencies, smoking, alcohol abuse, inactive lifestyle, and a diet low in calcium and vitamin D.

In addition, certain medications affect skeletal homeostasis and increase fracture risk. Routine assessment and minimizing high-risk medications (e.g., glucocorticoids, immunosuppressive medications, anticonvulsants, sex hormone deprivation therapy, proton pump inhibitors), when possible, can lower fracture risk. Other comorbid illnesses (e.g., chronic kidney disease, hyperthyroidism, rheumatoid arthritis) increase the risk of secondary osteoporosis, so better control of the underlying condition and frequent screening may be necessary.

Several decision support tools are available to help identify patients who are at high risk for osteoporosis and fracture. The most common risk assessments include FRAX, the simple calculated osteoporosis risk estimation, the osteoporosis self-assessment tool, and the osteoporosis risk assessment instrument. However, many clinicians prefer using FRAX because it incorporates easy-to-identify risk factors, helps determine the appropriateness of a DEXA, and provides a 10-year absolute fracture risk. FRAX uses readily available information such as age, body mass index, parental fracture history, comorbid conditions that cause secondary osteoporosis, and tobacco and alcohol use. The FRAX tool also incorporates DEXA results but does not require this information to estimate fracture risk. The USPSTF recommends screening with a DEXA scan in all women 65 years and older and postmenopausal women less than 65 years old if their 10-year fracture risk with FRAX is 9.3% or higher. The other decision support tools to assess the need for a DEXA scan may be reasonable as well because they rely on fewer factors and have comparable sensitivity.

The National Osteoporosis Foundation (NOF) and the International Society for Clinical Densitometry recommend screening all men 70 years and older and men 50 to 69 years of age based on risk factors. However, the USPSTF guidelines state that insufficient evidence is available to support screening for osteoporosis in men. Other screening risk assessments, such as vertebral imaging and trabecular bone scores, may be considered in addition to DEXA scans to help identify asymptomatic vertebral fractures or to quantify bone microarchitecture. These techniques may help better characterize 10-year fracture risk or guide pharmacologic treatment decisions, although neither vertebral imaging nor trabecular bone scores are discussed in the USPSTF guidelines because of limited data with these screening modalities.

The optimal rescreening interval remains unclear after an initial DEXA scan. Most guidelines recommend rescreening after 2 to 3 years of antiresorptive therapy or in high-risk individuals not taking therapy. In patients receiving antiresorptive therapy, a baseline DEXA and a repeat at 3 years may be a cost-effective strategy to minimize the number of DEXA scans if a patient improves as expected and is then able to start a drug holiday. There is some evidence that waiting for 15 years to rescreen is a reasonable strategy in low-risk individuals with an initial normal T-score. Shared decision making should be used to determine when to stop screening because evidence has not identified a clear time to stop, and patient risk factors vary significantly.

Pathophysiology

Although osteoporosis is often thought of as synonymous with decreased BMD, this association is not always present. Several factors can lead to decreased bone strength, including small bone size, increased length of the femoral neck, cortical porosity, decreased viability of osteocytes, and others.

Peak bone mass typically occurs in an individual's third decade of life. Differences in the peak bone mass may be secondary to genetic, hormonal, and environmental variables. Increases in body size and skeletal load also play a role in determining peak bone mass. Physical activity during childhood also enhances bone mass, whereas chronic diseases during childhood may decrease BMD. The contribution of genetic variants is unclear because osteoporosis is a polygenic disease and the individual genetic variants seem to have small effect on BMD and fracture risk. BMD correlates strongly with fracture risk, but other factors also influence fracture risk. As an example, Mexican Americans and Asian

Americans have lower BMDs than non-Hispanic Whites or non-Hispanic Blacks; however, Asian Americans and non-Hispanic Blacks have lower hip fracture rates compared with Mexican Americans and non-Hispanic Whites.

Age-related bone loss is a significant factor in the development of osteoporosis. Bone resorption begins to overtake bone formation with advancing age. Hormonal deficiency causes bone loss because testosterone and estrogen help determine bone homeostasis (i.e., osteoclast-induced bone resorption vs. osteoblast-supported bone formation). In women, rapid estrogen loss after menopause initially affects trabecular bone density. After a few years, bone loss continues to occur more slowly and primarily affects cortical sites. This slower phase is associated with a decreased number of osteoblasts and a slower bone formation rate. Men, however, are less likely to develop bone loss because of greater bone gain during puberty and no sudden loss of sex hormones. In addition, there is evidence that aging itself is an independent risk factor for bone loss. Other contributing factors include loss of muscle strength and coordination, which increase the risk for falls and fragility fractures.

Clinical Manifestations

There are typically no clinical manifestations of osteoporosis until a patient actually has a fracture. The signs and symptoms associated with osteoporosis correspond to direct or indirect manifestations of these fractures. Patients may have height loss, back pain, and thoracic kyphosis after experiencing a vertebral fracture. Moreover, manifestations from thoracic kyphosis could include dyspnea, from pulmonary restrictive lung disease, or constipation. Significant pain is often seen with both vertebral fractures and hip fractures although some patients may present with asymptomatic vertebral fractures that can be clinically inconspicuous. Functional disability is common after a fracture and many times requires rehabilitation to improve long-term functional status.

Diagnosis

Osteoporosis can be diagnosed after a fragility fracture (i.e., low-trauma fracture of appendicular or axial bones, excluding the skull) or radiographically. The initial evaluation includes a history to assess for clinical risk factors for fracture, evaluation for secondary conditions that contribute to bone loss, a physical examination, basic laboratory tests, and assessment of medications that increase fracture risk. Most cases of osteoporosis are diagnosed by a DEXA scan of the total hip, femoral neck, or lumbar spine, with a T-score of −2.5 or below. Bone mass measurements by DEXA must be interpreted in relation to the patient's age, ethnicity, fracture history, family background, previous medication use, timing of menopause, and other concomitant disorders.

Other techniques for measuring bone mass include ultrasound of the calcaneus, wrist, and finger; computed tomography of the spine; or peripheral quantitative computed tomography of the wrist and tibia. However, these tests have limited availability, increase radiation exposure, and are expensive so they are rarely used. Alternatively, DEXA scans give a precise estimate of BMD, are widely available, and are cost-effective tools.

DEXA results are expressed as a T-score and a Z-score. The WHO established the T-score as an SD difference between an individual's BMD and a sex- and ethnicity-matched young-adult reference population. The T-score should be used in the evaluation of men age 50 and older and postmenopausal women. The T-score provides an indication of the risk for developing fractures because of the association of fractures with decreasing BMD. A T-score that is −2.5 SD or more is diagnostic of osteoporosis; a T-score that is between −1.0 and −2.4 SD below the mean is defined as low bone mass, also known as *osteopenia*. A T-score of −2.5 SD or below plus a fragility fracture is termed *severe osteoporosis*. BMD measurements may be different across various bone sites in the same patient. These discrepancies may likely be related to differences in skeletal compartments (trabecular vs. cortical) at distinct sites. To classify the degree of osteoporosis use the lowest T-score from the lumbar spine, femoral neck, or total hip.

The Z-score is the SD difference between the patient's BMD and a reference population matched for age, sex, and ethnicity. A low Z-score of −2.0 SD or below indicates osteoporosis and can identify patients in need of further workup or even osteoporosis treatment. Z-scores should be used in the evaluation of adult men younger than age 50, premenopausal women, and children. Less evidence exists for characterizing the severity of disease or need for osteoporosis treatment in these populations, making patient care decisions difficult. For example, there is no great way to compare the BMD of a child to an adult who has achieved peak bone mass or to determine at what Z-score treatment is warranted. Further research is needed to identify appropriate groups to screen with Z-scores and whether osteoporosis treatment changes patient-oriented outcomes.

Biochemical markers reflect the activity of the bone-remodeling unit. Urinary pyridinoline and deoxypyridinoline are two common bone turnover markers. However, their roles in the management of osteoporosis are not clear. Future use of these biochemical markers may be helpful in determining risk and for monitoring patients treated with medications for osteoporosis.

Differential Diagnosis

Because an osteoporosis diagnosis is relatively straightforward, the differential focuses on a comprehensive workup of potential secondary causes of osteoporosis. If evaluation does not support a clear secondary cause, there is currently little evidence for additional testing in postmenopausal women. However, in premenopausal and perimenopausal women, additional testing may help identify important risk factors not easily assessed by a history and physical examination. More than 50% of men with vertebral fractures have secondary causes of osteoporosis. Common causes of osteoporosis in men are long-term use of glucocorticoids, hypogonadism, alcohol abuse, myeloma, and comorbid causes (e.g., celiac disease, hyperthyroidism, hyperparathyroidism). When screening for secondary causes of osteoporosis, note these recommendations are expert opinion suggestions.

Prevention

Prevention of osteoporosis is important because bone loss with aging is difficult to correct. Lower peak bone mass established in early adulthood may determine bone strength and fracture risk decades later. Therefore prevention starts with good nutrition, maintenance of a healthy body weight, and weight-bearing exercise to optimize bone mass during bone-forming years. Quitting smoking and avoiding excessive alcohol intake are other important lifestyle factors to emphasize with patients. Medications that may be harmful to bone health should be monitored and stopped when possible. Prevention with antiresorptive treatment in patients with low bone mass may increase BMD, restore bone strength, and reduce fracture risk in high-risk patients.

Calcium and vitamin D are both physiologically vital in bone formation. However, studies are conflicting on the benefits of calcium and vitamin D[1] for primary prevention of fracture in older adults. Several studies with high potential for bias have shown increases in BMD and reduction of fracture risk in high-risk adult patients given both calcium and vitamin D. As a result, the NOF recommends 1200 mg of elemental calcium and 800 to 1000 IU of vitamin D daily for postmenopausal women. However, recent studies with low potential for bias do not support calcium or vitamin D to reduce the risk of fractures or to increase BMD in older adults when used in primary prevention. Concerns about renal adverse events, particularly nephrolithiasis, exist with excessive dietary and/or supplemental calcium. There is also theoretical concern that excessive calcium administration could increase the risk of myocardial infarction via coronary calcification, although there are no strong data supporting this concern.

Not FDA approved for this indication.

Treatment

Nonpharmacologic Therapy

Nondrug therapy includes addressing risk of falls, diet, exercise, and smoking. Vision deficits, gait abnormalities, cognitive impairment, dizziness, and balance problems are common but preventable causes of falls. Performing a formal home safety evaluation and modifying the patient's living environment by improving lighting and removing loose rugs can enhance safety. Physical therapy evaluation and treatment can address both balance and gait issues. Regular physical activity with aerobic, weight-bearing, and resistance exercises are effective in increasing spine BMD. Patients should exercise at least 30 minutes three times per week. However, there is no evidence that high-intensity exercise provides greater benefit. Frequent medication assessment is also important and may reduce the risk of falls if stopping unnecessary or potentially inappropriate medications like those outlined by the Beers Criteria.

Ensuring adequate nutrition is an initial approach in treating osteoporosis, especially calcium and vitamin D. Studies showing the efficacy of calcium on fracture primary prevention are mixed, with some meta-analyses showing benefit and others showing no effect. Although primary prevention benefit is unclear, adequate calcium and vitamin D consumption should be encouraged when used with bisphosphonates and denosumab (Prolia) to reduce the risk of hypocalcemia and to ensure optimal effectiveness. Because optimal doses are not established, a daily intake of at least 1200 mg of calcium and 800 to 1000 IU of vitamin D[1] is recommended for all women with osteoporosis by the NOF based on historic recommended dietary amounts. Calcium and vitamin D supplements are often used because of low dietary consumption and reduced vitamin D creation with decreased sun exposure with aging. Both calcium carbonate and calcium citrate can be used, but caution should be used because of constipation and gastrointestinal upset.

The appropriate vitamin D level remains unclear, with mixed evidence and different experts advocating for different goal values. Some studies suggest that a serum 25-hydroxyvitamin D level of at least 30 ng/mL is needed to reduce falls and to improve physical function in the elderly. However, many experts advocate for treating only severely low 25-hydroxyvitamin D values <20 ng/mL because of mixed evidence with slightly low vitamin D values. In patients with confirmed vitamin D insufficiency, administration of 50,000 IU of oral ergocalciferol (vitamin D_2 [Drisdol])[1] once-weekly for 8 to 12 weeks was thought to be safe and effective. However, a more recent study has shown that high-dose vitamin D may increase the risk of falls, so these high intermittent doses should be reevaluated. A repeat serum 25-hydroxyvitamin D value is controversial considering no clear ideal value is known.

Pharmacologic Treatment

All drugs approved by the FDA for osteoporosis reduce vertebral fracture risk. The antifracture effects of these medications are due to an increase in BMD and an improvement in qualitative measures of bone strength. The drugs approved by the FDA to treat or prevent osteoporosis are noted in Table 1.

The mechanisms of each class of osteoporosis agent are slightly different and primarily work through decreasing bone resorption by inhibiting osteoclasts or increasing bone formation by stimulating osteoblasts. The bisphosphonates (e.g., alendronate [Fosamax], risedronate [Actonel], ibandronate [Boniva], zoledronic acid [Reclast]) impair osteoclastic resorption through the inhibition of farnesyl diphosphate synthase, a key enzyme that supports osteoclast activity. Raloxifene (Evista), conjugated equine estrogen (Premarin), and bazedoxifene/conjugated equine estrogen (Duavee) inhibit osteoclastogenesis through blocking the receptor activator of nuclear factor κB ligand/osteoprotegerin (OPG) system expressed on osteoblasts that signal the production of osteoclasts. Denosumab (Prolia), a monoclonal antibody, works similarly to estrogen by inhibiting the receptor activator of nuclear factor κB ligand system for osteoclast formation. Calcitonin (Miacalcin) works through a different mechanism by inhibiting osteoclast activity through the calcitonin receptor. Parathyroid hormones (i.e., teriparatide [Forteo], abaloparatide [Tymlos]) stimulate osteoblast bone formation, increasing calcium absorption in the gastrointestinal tract and promoting renal tubular calcium reabsorption. Lastly, romosozumab (Evenity), a new class of monoclonal antibody, inhibits sclerostin, which is a protein that regulates bone metabolism. By inhibiting sclerostin, romosozumab will increase osteoblast activity and reduce osteoclast activity.

TABLE 1 Osteoporosis Treatment Dosing and Effectiveness on Fracture Risk Reduction

MEDICATION	ROUTE	DOSE	CLINICAL EVIDENCE OF EFFICACY		
			VERTEBRAL	HIP	NONVERTEBRAL
Alendronate (Fosamax)	Oral	Oral 10 mg daily or 70 mg weekly	+	+	+
Risedronate (Actonel)	Oral	5 mg daily or 35 mg weekly	+	+	+
Zoledronic acid (Reclast)	IV	5 mg yearly	+	+	+
Ibandronate (Boniva)	Oral	150 mg monthly	+	–	–
	IV	3 mg every 3 months	+	–	–
Denosumab (Prolia)	SubQ	60 mg every 6 months	+	+	+
Abaloparatide (Tymlos)	SubQ	80 mcg daily	+	–	+
Teriparatide (Forteo)	SubQ	20 mcg daily	+	–	+
Romosozumab (Evenity)	SubQ	210 mg monthly	+	+	+
Raloxifene (Evista)	Oral	60 mg daily	+	–	–
Bazedoxifene/ conjugated equine estrogen (Duavee)[1]	Oral	20/0.45 mg daily	+	–	–
Conjugated equine estrogen (Premarin)[1]	Oral	0.3–1.25 mg daily	+	+	+
Calcitonin (Miacalcin)	Nasal	200 IU daily	+	–	–
	IM or SubQ	100 IU daily	+	–	–

IM, Intramuscular; *IU*, international units; *IV*, intravenous; *SubQ*, subcutaneous.
[1]Not FDA approved for this indication.

There are different approved indications for bisphosphonates in patients with osteoporosis. Alendronate (Fosamax) and risedronate (Actonel) are approved for the prevention and treatment of postmenopausal osteoporosis, treatment of osteoporosis in men, and treatment of glucocorticoid-induced osteoporosis. Ibandronate (Boniva) is approved only for prevention and treatment of postmenopausal females with osteoporosis. Daily and intermittent doses of ibandronate have demonstrated benefit on reducing only vertebral fractures, which limits its use because other bisphosphonates have better evidence at reducing vertebral, nonvertebral, and hip fractures. Zoledronic acid (Reclast), an intravenous (IV) bisphosphonate, is approved for once-yearly treatment of postmenopausal osteoporosis or alternatively can be administered once every other year if used to prevent osteoporosis. Zoledronic acid is the only osteoporosis therapy shown to reduce all-cause mortality and may be a preferred option in those who cannot tolerate or are nonadherent with oral therapy. In patients with an osteoporotic hip fracture, it is essential that they receive treatment with a bisphosphonate after surgery to modify the subsequent risk of fracture at any site. There have been concerns that bisphosphonates started soon after surgery could disrupt bone remodeling and fracture healing, but current evidence shows that early administration of bisphosphonates does not delay fracture healing. Therefore they should be given soon after surgery to reduce subsequent fractures.

The ideal duration of bisphosphonate therapy is unknown. Low-risk patients may consider discontinuing therapy after 3 to 5 years once the risks and benefits are weighed. Low-risk patients are typically defined as those that have a T-score that improves into an osteopenia or normal range and have not had recent fragility fractures. In low-risk individuals, benefits from the initial bisphosphonate course may last for another 5 years or longer. High-risk patients (e.g., patients with a T-score still below −2.5, having recent fragility fractures) could have the continued benefit of reducing vertebral fractures with bisphosphonates up to 10 years, but other types of fractures do not seem to be reduced and the risk of long-term complications (e.g., atypical fractures, osteonecrosis of the jaw, atrial fibrillation, myocardial infarction, esophageal cancer) may increase.

Side effects of oral bisphosphonates include esophageal and gastric irritation, musculoskeletal pain, and hypocalcemia. They must be taken with a full glass of water, and a 30- to 60-minute wait is required before eating or reclining to lower the risk of gastrointestinal adverse effects. Intravenous bisphosphonates are associated with hyperthermia, episcleritis, uveitis, and hypocalcemia. Atypical femur fractures with bisphosphonates, particularly alendronate, appear rare but are seen more frequently when used longer than 5 years. Young women are particularly prone to these fractures, which often require surgical intervention. Prodromal symptoms that have been linked to this syndrome include proximal femur pain and evidence of previous stress fracture or cortical thickness on x-ray. Osteonecrosis of the jaw is the other most feared complication with long-term bisphosphonate use, but again it is very rare. The actual incidence of both atypical fractures and osteonecrosis of the jaw are difficult to predict because these are largely point estimates from cohort studies with so few events seen in randomized trials.

Denosumab (Prolia) is a monoclonal antibody approved for treatment of men and postmenopausal women with osteoporosis who are at high risk for fracture. It is given as a subcutaneous injection every 6 months. Similar to alendronate, risedronate, and zoledronic acid, denosumab may significantly reduce the risk of vertebral, nonvertebral, and hip fractures compared with placebo. The safety profile of denosumab has been demonstrated in long-term trials, although there was a reported modest increase in skin infections with continued use. Long-term risks of atypical fractures and osteonecrosis of the jaw have been reported with denosumab similar to bisphosphonates, so it is recommended to reevaluate the need for continued treatment after 3 to 5 years.

Conjugated equine estrogen (Premarin) is an effective therapy at reducing all types of fractures, but is often reserved for women unable to use other options because of potential serious consequences. These complications include thromboembolism, stroke, myocardial infarction, and some types of cancer. Raloxifene (Evista), on the other hand, improves BMD and reduces the risk of vertebral fractures but not nonvertebral or hip fractures. Unfortunately, raloxifene can exacerbate the vasomotor symptoms of menopause and increase the risk of thromboembolic events. Raloxifene may be considered in postmenopausal women with osteoporosis who cannot tolerate bisphosphonates, have no vasomotor symptoms, have a low risk of venous thromboembolism, and have a high breast cancer risk. A combination of bazedoxifene (a new selective estrogen receptor modulator) with conjugated equine estrogens (Duavee) has been approved for prevention of postmenopausal osteoporosis and treatment of vasomotor symptoms associated with menopause. It might prove to be an alternative to raloxifene, but it is still associated with many of the serious precautions seen with estrogen therapy.

Parathyroid hormones (i.e., teriparatide [Forteo], abaloparatide [Tymlos]) have recognized antifracture effects on both vertebral and nonvertebral sites. Currently, therapy with either treatment should be limited to 2 years and reserved for patients at the highest fracture risk or refractory to other antiresorptives. There are slight differences in FDA indications with teriparatide being approved for postmenopausal women, men, or in patients with glucocorticoid-induced osteoporosis, whereas abaloparatide has only been approved for postmenopausal women. Parathyroid hormone analog therapy can only be used for 2 years based on concerns for osteosarcoma, which has only been seen in laboratory animals exposed to high doses. Consequently, parathyroid hormones are contraindicated in patients with risk of osteosarcoma, such as those with Paget's disease of the bone, previous skeletal radiation, or unexplained elevations of alkaline phosphatase. Adverse effects may include orthostatic hypotension, hypercalcemia, nausea, arthralgia, risk of renal stones, and leg cramps. In addition to its approved indications, some experts recommend using one of the anabolic options in patients who experience an atypical fracture or patients who have not improved on bisphosphonates. No evidence exists for combining anticatabolic and anabolic classes of drugs at the same time. However, it is recommended that after a period of 2 years of using parathyroid hormones, sequential therapy with an antiresorptive should be started to avoid posttreatment bone loss.

Romosozumab (Evenity) is a monoclonal antibody that works by binding and inhibiting sclerostin. Sclerostin is a glycoprotein that inhibits osteoblast bone formation and, to a lesser degree, increases osteoclast bone resorption. There is robust evidence showing better effectiveness at reducing hip, vertebral, and nonvertebral fractures when compared head-to-head with alendronate over 24 months. The FDA rejected romosozumab at first because of concern for increasing the risk of myocardial infarction and stroke, but it was approved in April 2019 for postmenopausal women at high fracture risk. The increased risk of cardiovascular events is still a concern, but long-term safety studies are ongoing. Romosozumab should be reserved for patients at high fracture risk because of safety concerns and high costs. When romosozumab is used, it is given as two consecutive subcutaneous injections (total dose of 210 mg) once every month for up to 1 year. If osteoporosis therapy remains warranted after 12 monthly doses, consider sequential therapy with another antiresorptive medication.

References

Barrionuevo P, Kapoor E, Noor A, et al: Efficacy of pharmacological therapies for the prevention of fractures in postmenopausal women: a network meta-analysis, *J Clin Endocrinol Metab* 104(5):1623–1630, 2019.

Bilezikian JP: Efficacy of bisphosphonates in reducing fracture risk in postmenopausal osteoporosis, *Am J Med* 122(2 Suppl):S14–S21, 2009.

Bischoff-Ferrari HA, Dawson-Hughes B, Orav EJ, et al: Monthly high-dose vitamin D treatment for the prevention of functional decline: a randomized clinical trial, *JAMA Intern Med* 176(2):175–183, 2016.

Bischoff-Ferrari HA, Dawson-Hughes B, Staehelin HB, et al: Fall prevention with supplemental and active forms of vitamin D: a meta-analysis of randomised controlled trials, *BMJ* 339:b3692, 2009.

Bolland MJ, Leung W, Tai V, et al: Calcium intake and risk of fracture: systematic review, *BMJ* 351:h4580, 2015.

By the 2019 American Geriatrics Society Beers Criteria® Update Expert Panel: American geriatrics society 2019 updated AGS Beers Criteria® for potentially inappropriate medication use in older adults, *J Am Geriatr Soc* 67(4):674–694, 2019.

Chen SJ, Chen YJ, Cheng CH, et al: Comparisons of different screening tools for identifying fracture/osteoporosis risk among community-dwelling older people, *Medicine (Baltim)* 95(20), 2016:e3415.

Eastell R, Rosen CJ, Black DM, et al: Pharmacological management of osteoporosis in postmenopausal women: an endocrine society clinical practice guideline, *J Clin Endocrinol Metab* 104(5):1595–1622, 2019.

Final Recommendation Statement: *Osteoporosis to prevent fractures: screening*, U.S. Preventive Services Task Force, 2019. https://www.uspreventiveservice staskforce.org/Page/Document/RecommendationStatementFinal/osteoporos is-screening1.

Fink HA, MacDonald R, Forte ML, et al: Long-term drug therapy and drug holidays for osteoporosis fracture prevention: a systematic review. In *Comparative effectiveness review No. 218. (Prepared by the Minnesota evidence-based practice center under contract No. 290-2015-00008-I) AHRQ publication No. 19-EHC016-EF*, Rockville, MD, 2019, Agency for Healthcare Research and Quality.

Gourlay ML, Fine JP, Preisser JS, et al: Bone-density testing interval and transition to osteoporosis in older women, *N Engl J Med* 366(3):225–233, 2012.

Hippisley-Cox J, Coupland C: Predicting risk of osteoporotic fracture in men and women in England and Wales: prospective derivation and validation of QFracture scores, *BMJ* 339:b4229, 2009.

Jeremiah MP, Unwin BK, Greenawald MH, Casiano VE: Diagnosis and management of osteoporosis, *Am Fam Physician* 92(4):261–268, 2015.

Karinkanta S, Piirtola M, Sievanen H, et al: Physical therapy approaches to reduce fall and fracture risk among older adults, *Nat Rev Endocrinol* 6(7):396–407, 2010.

Ketteler M, Block GA, Evenepoel P, et al: Diagnosis, evaluation, prevention, and treatment of chronic kidney disease–mineral and bone disorder: synopsis of the kidney disease: improving global outcomes 2017 clinical practice guideline update, *Ann Intern Med* 168(6):422–430, 2018.

Khosla S, Melton LJ: Clinical practice: osteopenia, *N Engl J Med* 356(22):2293–2300, 2007.

Lyles KW, Colon-Emeric CS, Magaziner JS, et al: Zoledronic acid and clinical fractures and mortality after hip fracture, *N Engl J Med* 357(18):1799–1809, 2007.

Moyer V: To supplement or not to supplement: the U.S. Preventive Services Task Force recommendations on calcium and vitamin D, *Ann Intern Med* 158(9):691–696, 2013.

Nguyen ND, Ahlborg HG, Center JR, et al: Residual lifetime risk of fractures in women and men, *J Bone Miner Res* 22(6):781–788, 2007.

Ralston SH, Uitterlinden AG: Genetics of osteoporosis, *Endocr Rev* 31(5):629–662, 2010.

Rosen CJ: Clinical practice. Postmenopausal osteoporosis, *N Engl J Med* 353(6):595–603, 2005.

Rosen CJ: Bone remodeling, energy metabolism, and the molecular clock, *Cell Metab* 7(1):7–10, 2008.

Saag K, Petersen J, Brandi ML, et al: Romosozumab or alendronate for fracture prevention in women with osteoporosis, *N Engl J Med* 377(15):1417–1427, 2017.

Schousboe JT, Taylor BC, Fink HA, et al: Cost-effectiveness of bone densitometry followed by treatment of osteoporosis in older men, *J Am Med Assoc* 298(6):629–637, 2007.

Uitterlinden AG, Ralston SH, Brandi ML, et al: The association between common vitamin D receptor gene variations and osteoporosis: a participant-level meta-analysis, *Ann Intern Med* 145(4):255–264, 2006.

Weaver J, Sajjan S, Lewiecki EM, Harris ST: Diagnosis and treatment of osteoporosis before and after fracture: a side-by-side analysis of commercially insured and Medicare Advantage osteoporosis patients, *J Manag Care Spec Pharm* 23(7):735–744, 2017.

Wells GA, Cranney A, Peterson J, et al: Alendronate for the primary and secondary prevention of osteoporotic fractures in postmenopausal women, *Cochrane Database Syst Rev* 1:CD001155, 2008.

Wright NC, Looker AC, Saag KG, et al: The recent prevalence of osteoporosis and low bone mass in the United States based on bone mineral density at the femoral neck or lumbar spine, *J Bone Miner Res* 29(11):2520–2526, 2014.

Zhao J, Zeng X, Wang J, Liu L: Association between calcium or vitamin D supplementation and fracture incidence in community-dwelling older adults, *J Am Med Assoc* 318(24):2466–2482, 2017.

PAGET'S DISEASE OF BONE

Method of
Ian R. Reid, MD

CURRENT DIAGNOSIS

- Suspect the presence of Paget's disease in those patients with bone pain, bone deformity, isolated elevation of alkaline phosphatase, or lytic/sclerotic lesions on radiographs.
- Paget's disease is diagnosed from plain radiographs.
- Bone scintigraphy identifies the affected bones and allows some assessment of disease activity.
- Biochemical markers of bone turnover allow more precise assessment of turnover and response to therapy.
- Serum total alkaline phosphatase activity is the most cost-effective marker, although bone-specific alkaline phosphatase and procollagen type I N-terminal propeptide (PINP) are marginally more sensitive.

CURRENT THERAPY

- Zoledronate (zoledronic acid, Reclast) 5 mg given as a single infusion over 15 minutes; retreatment is seldom required within 5 years.
- Alendronate (Fosamax) 40 mg/day for 6 months; retreatment may be required between 2 and 6 years.
- Risedronate (Actonel) 30 mg/day for 2 months; retreatment may be required between 1 and 5 years.

Paget's disease is a focal skeletal condition in which one or more bones has a clearly circumscribed area of increased turnover (Figure 1A). Either osteoblasts or osteoclasts may predominate at a given time, resulting in sclerosis or lysis, respectively. Areas that are initially lytic often become sclerotic later, and it is common to see both changes within the same bone (see Figure 1B). Unaffected areas of the skeleton are completely normal, in marked contrast to some rare congenital conditions which are sometimes (inappropriately) referred to as early-onset or juvenile Paget's disease. Such conditions (e.g., familial expansile osteolysis, idiopathic hyperphosphatasia) have different etiologies, clinical presentations, and responses to treatment when compared to Paget's disease.

Etiology

Within pagetic bone, there is a loss of the usual tight control of bone cell function, and the bone-resorbing cells (osteoclasts) and bone-forming cells (osteoblasts) both exhibit overactivity. In the case of osteoclasts, this leads to local areas of bone loss, which can result in deformity or fracture. Osteoblast overactivity leads to the random laying down of new bone, which is disorganized in its structure, mechanically inadequate, and prone to deformity. Osteoblast overactivity can also lead to bone expansion, resulting in bone pain, premature arthritis (if it affects articular surfaces), and nerve compression (e.g., in the spine or skull). Figure 1B shows the effects of osteoblast and osteoclast overactivity on the structure of an affected tibia. The disease progresses along a long bone at a rate of about 1 cm per year, so most patients have had active disease for 1 or more decades before presentation. Typically, the disease progresses until the entire bone is involved. However, Paget's disease does not spread from one bone to another, so the number of affected bones remains constant throughout the disease course.

Paget's disease sometimes runs in families, and about 10% of patients are reported to have an affected relative. This observation has led to much work seeking genetic associations of the

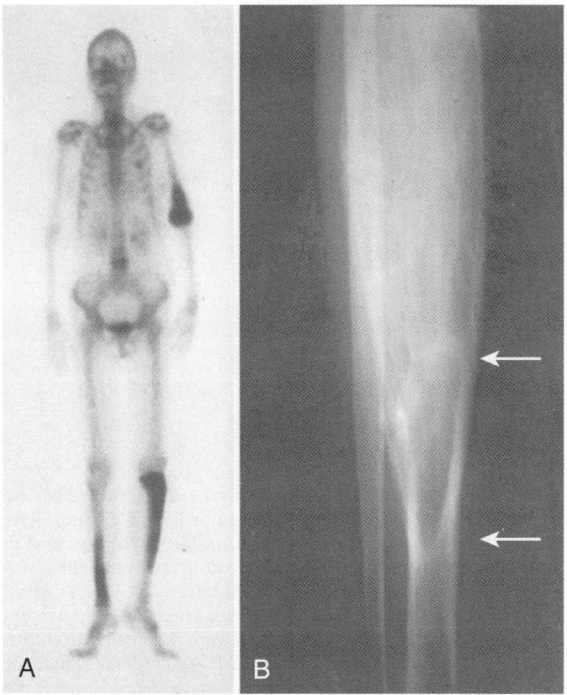

Figure 1 **A,** Bone scintigram in a patient with Paget's disease, demonstrating the multifocal nature of the condition and the presence of normal bone at other sites. **B,** Tibia affected by Paget's disease. The upper tibia is of increased density and width as a result of osteoblast overactivity, whereas the lower part of the affected bone shows a lytic region *(between arrows)* resulting from osteoclastic bone resorption. Below this, the bone is normal. Copyright I. R. Reid, used with permission.

condition. It is now apparent that mutations of the gene for sequestosome 1 are associated with Paget's disease in some families. Other research has focused on possible environmental causes, and a slow viral infection has been suggested. Evidence that the prevalence of Paget's disease has decreased in recent decades would be consistent with altered exposure to an environmental agent. However, both the genetic and environmental hypotheses fail to account for the focal nature of the condition, which in some ways resembles a benign neoplasm.

Altered gene expression in osteoblasts and bone marrow stromal cells from pagetic bone has been demonstrated recently, including increased levels of dickkopf-1, interleukin-1, and interleukin-6. These changes are likely to result in stimulation of osteoclast proliferation and inhibition of osteoblast growth, leading to development of the characteristic lytic bone lesions. This work suggests that the key abnormality may reside in the osteoblast, rather than the osteoclast, as was assumed in the past. Uncertainties remain regarding the primary abnormality giving rise to this condition.

Epidemiology

Paget's disease is classically a condition of older adults, most patients being older than 60 years of age at diagnosis. There is a male preponderance in some studies. It is overwhelmingly a condition of individuals with European forebears, particularly from the United Kingdom and Western Europe (excluding Scandinavia), where about 6% to 7% of the older population is affected. Among older white Americans, the prevalence is about 2%. There is evidence that prevalence and disease severity are both declining, possibly reflecting change in an environmental etiologic factor. It is extremely uncommon in individuals with predominantly Asian or Polynesian ancestry, although it is observed in some black populations.

Clinical Presentation

The most common symptoms attributable to Paget's disease are bone and joint pain. The bone pain is typically worse at rest and may trouble patients particularly at night. With skull involvement, pounding headaches can result. If Paget's disease leads to deformity of joint surfaces, premature arthritis occurs. This is particularly common at the hips. Deformity in long bones can occur, and involvement of the

radius or weight-bearing bones of the lower limb often manifests in this way. Microfractures, which can be very painful, sometimes occur over the convexity of a deformed, weight-bearing bone. These can progress to complete fractures. Fractures can also occur through an area of active lytic disease in a weight-bearing bone.

Deafness is a common manifestation of Paget's disease and is caused by involvement of the bones of the middle ear or compromise of the eighth cranial nerve. More rarely, other neurologic syndromes can arise from nerve entrapment, including paraplegia as a result of spinal cord involvement.

Some pagetic patients are asymptomatic and are diagnosed because of an incidental finding of elevated circulating levels of alkaline phosphatase. The diagnosis may also result from an incidental radiographic finding, such as in studies of the urinary tract. Commonly, only one or two bones are involved, although disease may be more widespread. The pelvis, vertebral bodies, long bones, and skull are the most common sites, but almost any bone can be involved.

Diagnosis

Serum alkaline phosphatase, the most widely available marker of osteoblast activity, is usually elevated; however, if only one bone is involved, this test can be normal. In any patient with an elevation of alkaline phosphatase, it is important to determine whether this is coming from liver or bone. This question is usually addressed by other liver function tests, although assays of bone-specific alkaline phosphatase and of other osteoblast-specific markers (e.g., procollagen type I N-terminal propeptide [PINP]) are available. If the elevation of alkaline phosphatase is bony in origin, it is important to rule out other bone conditions such as metastatic cancers (e.g., breast, prostate). This is usually done by identifying the sites of skeletal abnormality on a bone scintigram and then obtaining plain radiographs of the abnormal areas.

Paget's disease has a characteristic appearance on plain radiographs, showing either bony rarefaction or sclerosis (depending on whether the osteoclastic or osteoblastic phase is predominating), disorganization of trabecular architecture, and the other abnormalities already discussed (e.g., deformity). Bone biopsy is not usually necessary to confirm the diagnosis.

Other biochemical markers of osteoblast or osteoclast activity, such as breakdown products of bone collagen, have been used in Paget's disease. Total alkaline phosphatase, bone alkaline phosphatase, PINP or N-terminal telopeptide of type I collagen (NTX) identified more than 95% of pagetic subjects in one cohort of pagetic subjects, although the poorer precision of NTX reduced its utility in monitoring the effects of treatment. Osteocalcin, C-telopeptide of type I collagen, and urinary free deoxypyridinoline are less useful for assessment of baseline activity and monitoring response to therapy. Total alkaline phosphatase remains the most widely used test because of its low cost and wide availability.

Treatment

Treatment of Paget's disease almost always relies on the potent bisphosphonates, primarily zoledronate (Reclast). These compounds have a very high affinity for the bone surface, where they remain for years. They are ingested by osteoclasts when bone is resorbed and inhibit a key enzyme in the mevalonate pathway, farnesyl pyrophosphate synthase. This results in disruption of the osteoclast cytoskeleton and cell death. Bisphosphonates are preferentially taken up at sites of high bone turnover, which accounts for their utility as bone scintigraphy agents, and therefore target active pagetic bone.

The preferred treatment at present is the potent intravenous bisphosphonate zoledronate (Reclast, generic), which is administered in a single dose of 5 mg over 15 minutes. It has been compared with the standard 2-month course of risedronate (Actonel) in two randomized, controlled trials. At 6 months, 96% of patients receiving zoledronate had a therapeutic response, compared with 74% of those randomized to risedronate ($P < 0.001$). Alkaline phosphatase levels normalized in 89% of patients in the zoledronate group and in 58% of those in the risedronate group ($P < 0.001$). Zoledronate showed a more rapid onset of action and superior effects on quality-of-life measures. Perhaps the most impressive data with zoledronate have been those from the open follow-up of responders in these studies. Six years after drug administration, relapse had occurred in 0.7% of those receiving zoledronate but in 20% of risedronate-treated patients. Therefore, zoledronate produces much more sustained responses to therapy than have hitherto been possible.

Potent oral bisphosphonates such as alendronate (Fosamax, generic) and risedronate (Actonel, generic) have been widely used, but are usually less effective than zoledronate. These are administered daily over periods of 2 to 6 months and produce good disease control. The duration of treatment chosen in the pivotal clinical trials was arbitrary to some extent, and individual patients may require longer or shorter initial courses to achieve remission. Oral bisphosphonates have a very low bioavailability. Therefore, they must be taken in a fasting state, with a glass of water, and at least 30 minutes before consumption of food or other fluids. Positively charged ions (including calcium supplements, antacids, and mineral supplements) bind avidly to bisphosphonates and impair their absorption, so they must be taken at a different time of day. Potent bisphosphonates can cause irritation to the upper gastrointestinal tract and should not be prescribed to patients with inflammation or ulceration in that region. Patients should remain upright for 30 minutes after taking oral bisphosphonates to minimize the risk of reflux and associated esophagitis or ulceration.

The injectable bisphosphonate pamidronate (Aredia, generic) has been used in the past for treatment of Paget's disease. It is typically given as a series of infusions of 60 to 90 mg, each administered over a period of 1 to 2 hours. Pamidronate produces partial or complete remissions of disease activity that last for up to several years. The first administration of the drug may be accompanied by mild flu-like symptoms, which settle over 24 to 48 hours and usually do not recur. Their resolution can be hastened by the use of paracetamol (acetaminophen, Tylenol) or similar agents.

Potent bisphosphonates can cause mild hypocalcemia, which is usually asymptomatic and not a cause for concern. However, in patients with marked vitamin D deficiency, hypocalcemia can be more severe and sustained. Therefore, it is important to ensure that patients are vitamin D sufficient before receiving these drugs—a serum 25-hydroxyvitamin-D level greater than 40 nmol/L is more than adequate. Many physicians prescribe calcium to patients receiving bisphosphonate therapy (given in the evening if the oral bisphosphonate is given in the morning) as a further protection against hypocalcemia.

In the past, the weak bisphosphonate etidronate (Didronel) was used to treat Paget's disease. This is much less effective than the agents discussed previously. If used in high doses or for more than a few months, it carries the risk of producing osteomalacia, which can lead to bone pain and fractures. Therefore, it no longer has a place in the treatment of Paget's disease. Calcitonin (Miacalcin Injection) has also been relegated to an historical role only, because its efficacy is much less than that of the potent bisphosphonates and its effects are rapidly reversed after cessation of therapy. Denosumab (Prolia)[1] has some efficacy, but also appears to be inferior to zoledronate.

There are several philosophical approaches to Paget's disease management, none of which is strictly evidence based. There is general agreement that patients with symptoms attributable to Paget's disease should receive treatment. This is clear-cut in patients who have bone pain at the site of a pagetic lesion, but it is a common observation that antipagetic drugs can produce variable degrees of improvement in pain from joints adjacent to pagetic bone. Patients with neurologic complications from spinal cord or other nerve entrapments also improve with antipagetic therapy.

Treatment aimed at preventing complications of Paget's disease is variably endorsed, because there is no clinical trial evidence that treatment prevents the progression of deformity, the development of pagetic symptoms, or fracture. However, it is clear that treatment leads to a restoration of normal bone histology (Figure 2) and radiographic healing of lytic lesions and that, in the absence of such intervention, both bone lysis and deformity progress. It seems unreasonable to withhold safe therapies that are able to halt histologic and radiologic disease progression. Therefore, many experienced physicians endorse the provision of antipagetic therapy for individuals with lytic lesions in long bones; lesions at sites that are likely to lead

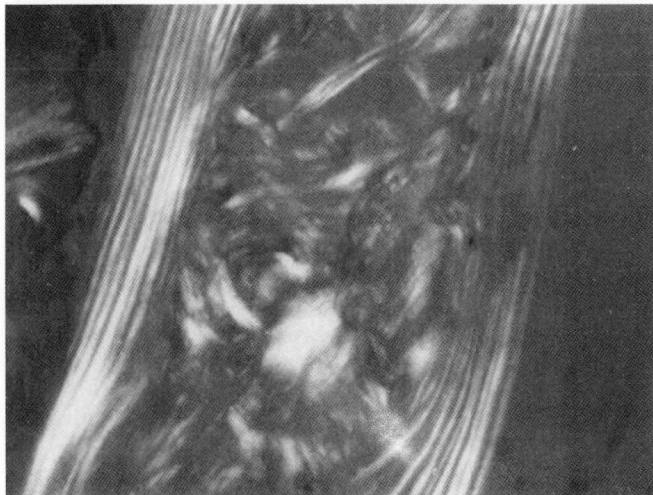

Figure 2 Section of a bone trabecula affected by Paget's disease, viewed under polarized light to show orientation of lamellae. In the center of the trabecula, the collagen fibers are chaotically laid down (woven bone), consistent with active Paget's disease. Over the outer surfaces, collagen is organized in parallel lamellae, indicating the restoration of normal bone microarchitecture after treatment with alendronate. Reprinted with permission from: Reid IR, Nicholson GC, Weinstein RS, et al: Biochemical and radiologic improvement in Paget's disease of bone treated with alendronate: A randomized, placebo-controlled trial. Am J Med 1996;101:341–48.

to neurologic complications, arthritis, or deformity; or involvement of the skull that could compromise hearing. Expert opinion also supports the use of antipagetic therapy before elective surgery on pagetic bone, because this approach reduces the vascularity of pagetic bone and results in less perioperative blood loss. On the other hand, Paget's disease in asymptomatic patients whose future risk of complications is thought to be low (e.g., with involvement of the ilium) is commonly managed without specific pharmaceutical intervention, although the availability of a safe, single-dose treatment with zoledronate is increasing the inclination to treat.

When providing treatment targeted at these goals, it is important to consider how adequacy of therapy can be judged. In the case of patients with pain, maximal relief of pain is an important endpoint. Lytic lesions should be treated and monitored with sequential radiographs until healing is apparent. Activity at other sites can be assessed indirectly with biochemical markers of bone turnover, although these are much less sensitive in patients with monostotic disease. In this context, there can be considerable residual activity at a single affected site without the markers being abnormal. Bone scintigrams provide the most sensitive method of assessing local disease activity.

In the past, Paget's disease caused substantial morbidity in the elderly population. However, it is now possible to achieve adequate and sustained disease control with use of intravenous zoledronate. Prompt use of these agents, when indicated, can be expected to halt disease progression and to effectively prevent the development of significant complications from this condition.

References

Kanis JA: *Pathophysiology and Treatment of Paget's Disease of Bone*, London, 1991, Martin Dunitz.

Miller PD, Brown JP, Siris ES, et al: A randomized, double-blind comparison of risedronate and etidronate in the treatment of Paget's disease of bone, *Am J Med* 106:513–520, 1999.

Ralston SH, Langston AL, Reid IR: Pathogenesis and management of Paget's disease of bone, *Lancet* 372:155–163, 2008.

Reid IR, Davidson JS, Wattie D, et al: Comparative responses of bone turnover markers to bisphosphonate therapy in Paget's disease of bone, *Bone* 35:224–230, 2004.

Reid IR, Lyles K, Su GQ, et al: A single infusion of zoledronic acid produces sustained remissions in Paget disease: data to 6.5 years, *J Bone Miner Res* 26(9), 2011. 2261–70.

Reid IR, Miller P, Lyles K, et al: Comparison of a single infusion of zoledronic acid with risedronate for Paget's disease, *N Engl J Med* 353:898–908, 2005.

Reid IR, Nicholson GC, Weinstein RS, et al: Biochemical and radiologic improvement in Paget's disease of bone treated with alendronate: A randomized, placebo-controlled trial, *Am J Med* 101:341–348, 1996.

Singer FR, Bone III HG, Hosking DJ, et al: Paget's disease of bone: an Endocrine Society Clinical Practice Guideline, *J Clin Endocrinol Metab* 99(12):4408–22, 2014.

¹Not FDA approved for this indication.

POLYMYALGIA RHEUMATICA AND GIANT CELL ARTERITIS

Method of
Mark A. Matza, MD, MBA; and Sebastian H. Unizony, MD

CURRENT DIAGNOSIS

Primary Polymyalgia Rheumatica
- Age is greater than 50 years.
- Symptoms include pain and stiffness involving the shoulder and hip girdles, and sometimes the neck and lower back. Symptoms are worse after immobilization (e.g., morning) and improve with activities.
- Constitutional symptoms such as fever, fatigue, and weight loss can be present. Peripheral arthralgias or arthritis (e.g., wrists) occasionally occur.
- Only 15%–20% of patients with primary or isolated polymyalgia rheumatica (PMR) develop giant cell arteritis (GCA).
- Upon disease onset, acute-phase reactants (erythrocyte sedimentation rate and C-reactive protein concentration) are typically elevated but can rarely be normal.
- Ultrasound can be used to assess for synovitis, tenosynovitis, or bursitis in the shoulders and hips.

Giant Cell Arteritis
- Age is greater than 50 years.
- Acute-phase reactants (erythrocyte sedimentation rate and C-reactive protein concentration) are elevated in approximately 95% of the cases before treatment with glucocorticoids is initiated.
- Symptoms include new-onset headaches (often temporal), scalp tenderness, jaw or tongue claudication, and vision impairment such as diplopia, amaurosis fugax, episodic blurry vision, and/or blindness.
- Approximately 50% of patients with GCA also have PMR symptoms.
- Constitutional symptoms such as fever, fatigue, and weight loss are often present. In addition, about 10% of GCA cases present only with fever and without other cranial or PMR manifestations.
- Temporal arteries may be prominent, beaded, or tender on examination, but they may also be normal. Vascular bruits and decreased pulses can be auscultated in the presence of large-vessel disease.
- Temporal artery biopsy is the diagnostic test of choice for patients presenting with cranial symptoms, but false-negative results may occur.
- Ultrasound can also be diagnostic in the appropriate clinical scenario when hypoechoic circumferential mural thickening (i.e., halo sign) is identified in the temporal arteries.
- Noninvasive cross-sectional imaging, including computed tomography angiography, magnetic resonance angiography, or positron emission tomography, can be used to evaluate for large-vessel involvement (e.g., aorta, subclavian arteries, axillary arteries).

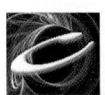

CURRENT THERAPY

Primary Polymyalgia Rheumatica
- Prednisone at a dose of 15–20 mg/day (or equivalent glucocorticoid) is used initially. The starting dose should be continued for 1 full month to suppress the disease effectively and then tapered to 10 mg by the end of month 2 of treatment. Prednisone can then be tapered off at the rate of 1 mg/month for a total prednisone duration of approximately 1 year.
- Should symptoms recur with tapering, the glucocorticoid dose should be increased temporarily, followed by a new tapering attempt.
- Methotrexate[1] and tocilizumab (Actemra)[1] can be considered for relapsing patients or patients at high risk for glucocorticoid toxicity (e.g., poorly controlled diabetes mellitus).

Giant Cell Arteritis
- Treatment should not be delayed while awaiting confirmatory testing (e.g., temporal artery biopsy), given the risk of blindness (15%–20%) in untreated patients.
- Prednisone[1] at a dose of 1 mg/kg or approximately 60 mg (or equivalent glucocorticoid) should be started immediately if the diagnosis is suspected.
- Pulse dose methylprednisolone[1] (1 g daily for 3 days) should be considered if vision changes occur (e.g., amaurosis fugax, monocular permanent vision loss).
- Tocilizumab (Actemra) is an effective drug for remission maintenance and glucocorticoid-sparing in GCA patients both with new-onset and relapsing disease.
- Once the disease activity is controlled, glucocorticoids are tapered off gradually.
- In patients receiving only glucocorticoids, tapers usually last 12 to 24 months, but relapses are common (up to 70% of cases), requiring dose adjustments and prolongation of glucocorticoid therapy.
- In patients receiving tocilizumab, glucocorticoid tapers are typically shorter (e.g., 6 months), and disease relapses are seen in only approximately 30% of the patients within 1 year.
- Approximately 40% of GCA patients in remission after treatment with tocilizumab (162 mg weekly) for 1 year may be able to discontinue tocilizumab and remain in remission for at least 2 more years.
- The use of low doses of aspirin[1] to prevent ischemic complications of GCA is controversial.
- Prophylaxis for glucocorticoid-induced osteoporosis with bisphosphonates, calcium, and vitamin D should be considered in all patients receiving glucocorticoids.
- Immunizations according to the national guidelines (influenza and pneumococcus) should be administered to all GCA patients, especially when they receive glucocorticoids and tocilizumab.

[1]Not FDA approved for this indication.

Primary polymyalgia rheumatica (PMR) and giant cell arteritis (GCA) are related and often overlapping systemic inflammatory disorders that typically affect patients older than 50 years of age. Women are more commonly affected than men, and Caucasians more so than African Americans, Asians, and Hispanics. Symptoms range from proximal muscle aching in primary PMR to blindness in GCA. Both conditions are characterized by elevated serum inflammatory markers (erythrocyte sedimentation rate [ESR] and C-reactive protein [CRP]). Most patients quickly respond to glucocorticoids (e.g., prednisone), but many of them fail to maintain long-term disease control during or after glucocorticoid tapers. Interleukin (IL)-6 receptor blockade with tocilizumab (Actemra) in combination with up to 6 months of prednisone has demonstrated efficacy for remission maintenance, glucocorticoid sparing, and quality-of-life improvement in GCA randomized clinical trials. Preliminary evidence suggests that tocilizumab[1] might also be beneficial in some patients with primary PMR.

Primary Polymyalgia Rheumatica
Clinical Presentation
Primary or isolated PMR is characterized by symmetric proximal joint pain and stiffness (i.e., shoulders and hips). The lifetime

Not FDA approved for this indication.

risks for primary PMR in women and men older than 50 years of age are 2.4% and 1%, respectively. Disease onset can be acute or subacute, but patients sometimes delay seeking medical attention for days to weeks. Symptoms are classically worse early in the morning and after periods of immobilization (e.g., a "long commute"). Morning stiffness is generally prolonged greater than 45 minutes. Involvement of the peripheral joints (e.g., wrists, knees, and ankles) is rare. Weight loss, fatigue, anorexia, and low-grade fever can be seen. Physical examination is usually unrevealing. However, some patients may demonstrate tenderness and limited active range of motion of the shoulder and hip girdles, but synovitis (e.g., joint swelling, effusion, or erythema) is absent. Range of motion with passive limb movements is typically better.

Apart from occurring in isolation (i.e., primary PMR), PMR symptoms can be seen in nearly 50% of patients with GCA (as discussed later).

Diagnosis

Diagnosis is made based on the clinical presentation and the exclusion of other conditions (e.g., rheumatoid arthritis, GCA, and regional noninflammatory rheumatisms [such as rotator cuff tendinopathy]). Almost all patients demonstrate increased serum ESR and/or CPR at disease onset before treatment is started. Patients have negative rheumatoid factor and anti-CCP antibodies. The response to glucocorticoids (e.g., prednisone) is also often a telling indication of PMR: most patients experience dramatic clinical improvements within 24 to 48 hours. Ultrasound can be used to detect synovitis, tenosynovitis, or bursitis in the shoulders and hips. GCA occurs in approximately 15% to 20% of patients with primary PMR. Therefore, these patients should be queried closely to detect any symptoms that suggest GCA—namely headaches, scalp tenderness, jaw claudication, and visual disturbances.

A minority of patients with presentations of PMR eventually declare their true underlying disorder to be rheumatoid arthritis. Such patients can convert from seronegative to seropositive (i.e., positive rheumatoid factor or anti-CCP antibodies) at some point during follow-up. The presence of distal joint symptoms (e.g., small joints of the hands) might help predict the evolution to rheumatoid arthritis (RA), but the development of RA cannot be predicted if seronegative at baseline. Rarely, late-onset spondyloarthritis initially can be confused with PMR.

Treatment

Patients with primary PMR are treated with glucocorticoids. Prednisone at a dose of 15 to 20 mg is often used to induce disease remission. Symptoms should dramatically improve within 1 to 2 days. Infrequently, patients require higher doses (e.g., 25 to 30 mg) over a longer period (e.g., 5 to 7 days) to achieve clear responses. However, in cases that do not demonstrate classic responses to glucocorticoids, ruling out other conditions (e.g., GCA) is mandatory. The initial glucocorticoid dose is maintained for about 4 weeks to ensure clear sustained resolution of the clinical manifestations and normalization of the inflammatory marker values. A gradual glucocorticoid taper is then begun to maintain the disease in remission. Patients usually taper the daily prednisone dose by 2.5 to 5 mg every 2 to 4 weeks until the dose of 10 mg is achieved. Subsequently, the taper progresses at a rate of 1 to 2.5 mg every 2 to 4 weeks until glucocorticoid discontinuation. The total duration of the treatment in the absence of a disease flare is about 12 to 18 months. Unfortunately, many patients relapse and require an increased prednisone dose and renewed tapering attempt once the disease is again controlled.

Most patients can eventually taper off prednisone completely; however, in some, a low dose of prednisone may be required to prevent the recurrence of symptoms. For patients with primary PMR who require excessive prednisone exposure to maintain disease control, methotrexate[1] or IL-6 blockade therapy with tocilizumab (Actemra)[1] should be considered.

Not FDA approved for this indication.

Giant Cell Arteritis
Clinical Presentation

GCA is the most frequent form of primary vasculitis in adults. The disease causes granulomatous inflammation in the large arteries, including the aorta and its primary branches—particularly the vessels of the head and neck. The epidemiology of GCA is identical to the one of primary PMR, with the exception that GCA is three times less frequent. The lifetime risks for GCA in women and men older than 50 years are 1% and 0.5%, respectively. The incidence of GCA increases with each decade and peaks around 73 years of age.

The onset of GCA is often subacute or acute. The most frequent clinical manifestations of this condition can be divided into four not mutually exclusive categories: cranial manifestations, PMR symptoms, constitutional symptoms, and signs and symptoms of large artery involvement.

The cranial manifestations of GCA include headache, jaw claudication, scalp tenderness, temporal artery abnormalities (e.g., prominent arteries, palpable beading, decreased pulsation, or tenderness), and visual symptoms (e.g., diplopia, amaurosis fugax, transient blurred vision, and blindness). The most frequent cranial manifestation is headache (60% to 70% of cases), which may involve not only the temporal region but also other cranial locations. The only unique feature of the GCA-related headache is that it is new for the patient. Jaw claudication, which is reported by 30% to 50% of patients, is very specific of GCA. Typically, patients with jaw claudication notice pain when eating foods that require vigorous chewing, such as meats. Jaw pain is exertional and resolves with mandibular rest. Less frequently, patients may report tongue or pharyngeal pain during mastication and swallowing.

About one-third of patients with GCA have visual manifestations, including diplopia, blurred vision, amaurosis fugax, and the most serious GCA complication—permanent vision loss or blindness. Unlike the slowly progressive blurred vision seen in elderly patients with cataracts, the blurred vision reported by GCA patients is usually monocular (although it can be bilateral), acute, and short lived (e.g., minutes to hours). Blindness, which develops in 8% to 20% of patients, occurs in greater than 90% of the cases before GCA is suspected and treatment with glucocorticoids is initiated. This complication can develop abruptly but, more often, is preceded by episodes of blurred vision or amaurosis fugax. By the time blindness occurs, most patients have increased inflammatory markers in serum and also report other clinical manifestations (headaches, jaw claudication, PMR symptoms, etc.). The mechanism of vision loss in GCA is in the great majority of the cases ischemia of the head of the optic nerve (so-called anterior ischemic optic neuropathy). Unfortunately, blindness is generally irreversible.

Approximately 50% of patients with GCA also have PMR symptoms. In addition, most patients with GCA and primary PMR report nonspecific manifestations such as fever, malaise, fatigue, anorexia, or weight loss. At times, fever is the only presenting symptom of GCA, and high clinical suspicion is required to order confirmatory tests to make the diagnosis (e.g., temporal artery biopsy). Finally, despite the fact that nearly all patients have some degree of large-vessel involvement at least histologically, only about 30% of patients develop clinical manifestations related to it. Vascular inflammation can cause structural damage of the walls of elastic arteries, leading to dilation and dissection, as well as narrowing of the lumens of muscular arteries resulting in stenosis, occlusion, and distal ischemia. The most frequently affected vessels include the thoracic and abdominal aorta, and the vertebral, carotid, subclavian, axillary, and brachial arteries. Signs and symptoms related to the involvement of limb arteries may include extremity claudication, decreased peripheral pulses, blood pressure asymmetries, and vascular bruits. Involvement of the vertebral and, less often, the carotid circulation may cause transient ischemic attack and stroke. Aortic disease may lead to aortic aneurysm (mainly in the thoracic aorta) and less frequently aortic dissection. In most patients, however, large artery inflammation and subsequent arterial damage are clinically silent and only detected by vascular imaging.

Diagnosis

GCA is diagnosed based on a combination of clinical presentation, laboratories, imaging, and biopsy. The temporal arteries may be bulging, irregular, or tender on examination; however, they may also be normal, even if temporal artery biopsy subsequently confirms the presence of GCA. The laboratory hallmark of GCA is the elevation of the inflammatory markers ESR and CRP, which is seen in ~95% of untreated patients with new-onset disease. Although elevation of the inflammatory markers is highly sensitive for the diagnosis of GCA, the specificity of these tests is low (~30%).

A characteristic pattern of inflammation in a temporal artery, with granulomatous infiltrates composed of lymphocytes, macrophages, and giant cells, is the most specific test for the diagnosis of GCA. Because skipped lesions (i.e., diseased segments alternating with normal-appearing tissue) are common, multiple sections of biopsies of at least 1 to 2 cm should be examined to increase the diagnostic yield. In addition, simultaneous or sequential bilateral temporal artery biopsies may decrease the false-negative biopsy rate in up to 13% of cases.

Vascular imaging (i.e., ultrasound, MRA, CTA, and PET) has been increasingly incorporated into the care of patients with GCA. Changes suggestive of vasculitis can be found in the arterial walls and/or lumens. Characteristic mural lesions may include circumferential wall thickening or edema, contrast enhancement, and ^{18}fluorine-2-deoxy-D-glucose (FDG) uptake. Luminal lesions may include stenosis, occlusion, and aneurysmal dilatation. Temporal artery ultrasound scanning may reveal a characteristic "halo sign," caused by edema within and around the blood vessel wall. Several studies and meta-analyses have estimated the sensitivity (55% to 100%) and specificity (75% to 100%) of the halo sign for the diagnosis of GCA compared with clinical diagnosis as the gold standard.

Treatment

Treatment with high-dose glucocorticoids should not be delayed to obtain a temporal artery biopsy or ultrasound. A dose of prednisone[1] 1 mg/kg or approximately 60 mg (or prednisone equivalent) should be initiated promptly when a diagnosis of GCA is considered. Lower doses (e.g., 40 mg/day) can be used for individuals who are frail and elderly. If visual involvement has occurred, pulse dose methylprednisolone[1] 1000 mg daily for 3 days can be initiated, followed by high-dose oral glucocorticoids. The optimal duration of a prednisone taper in GCA is not certain. In one randomized clinical trial, the percentage of patients achieving sustained disease remission at 1 year was essentially the same regardless of whether patients received a 6-month or 12-month prednisone taper. Sustained remissions were achieved in only 14% and 18% of patients, respectively. Thus, although high-dose glucocorticoids are effective at controlling GCA and inducing remission in most patients, the great majority of patients experience disease flares whenever prednisone is tapered to a lower dose (e.g., <15 mg/day) or discontinued.

The interleukin-6 receptor blocker tocilizumab (Actemra) is now approved worldwide for the treatment of GCA in combination with glucocorticoids. The addition of tocilizumab leads to substantial improvement in the rate of glucocorticoid-free remissions at 1 year and a reduction in the cumulative prednisone dose by approximately 50%. Tocilizumab can be administered either intravenously (8 mg/kg each month)[1] or subcutaneously (165 mg each week). The high rate of treatment failure with regimens involving prednisone alone suggests that all patients without contraindications to tocilizumab (e.g., history of diverticulitis) should be treated with the combination

---

Not FDA approved for this indication.

of tocilizumab and prednisone initially, followed by an aggressive prednisone taper designed to discontinue prednisone within 4 to 6 months. In a trial of the interleukin-6 receptor blocker tocilizumab, 42% of patients who completed 1 year of weekly tocilizumab in disease remission were able to discontinue treatment and maintain treatment-free remissions for at least 2 more years. Some patients, on the other hand, may require ongoing tocilizumab or even tocilizumab plus prednisone to maintain disease control. Patients who are not able to discontinue prednisone entirely can usually be controlled well with the combination of tocilizumab and low-dose prednisone.

Aspirin[1] (81 mg/day), which has been shown in some retrospective studies and a meta-analysis to reduce the incidence of vision loss, should be considered in all patients without contraindications. Prophylaxis for glucocorticoid-induced osteoporosis with bisphosphonates, calcium, and vitamin D should be implemented, particularly since GCA tends to afflict elderly individuals, many of whom have significant comorbidities at baseline, including osteoporosis. Prophylaxis for *Pneumocystis jiroveci* pneumonia may also be considered in appropriate clinical circumstances, particularly when prolonged or recurrent courses of high-dose glucocorticoids are required in patients with underlying chronic pulmonary conditions (e.g., emphysema).

References

Akiyama M, Kaneko Y, Takeuchi T: Tocilizumab in isolated polymyalgia rheumatica: A systematic literature review, *Semin Arthritis Rheum*, 2020.

Buttgereit F, Dejaco C, Matteson EL, Dasgupta B: Polymyalgia rheumatica and giant cell arteritis: a systematic review, *JAMA* 315(22):2442–2458, 2016.

Dasgupta B, Cimmino MA, Maradit-Kremers H, et al: 2012 provisional classification criteria for polymyalgia rheumatica: a European league against rheumatism/American College of Rheumatology collaborative initiative, *Ann Rheum Dis* 71(4):484–492, 2012.

Hoffman GS: Giant cell arteritis, *Ann Intern Med* 165(9):ITC65–ITC80, 2016.

Kermani TA, Schmidt J, Crowson CS, et al: Utility of erythrocyte sedimentation rate and C-reactive protein for the diagnosis of giant cell arteritis, *Semin Arthritis Rheum* 41(6):866–871, 2012.

Koster MJ, Matteson EL, Warrington KJ: Large-vessel giant cell arteritis: diagnosis, monitoring and management, *Rheumatology (Oxford)* 57(suppl 2):ii32–ii42, 2018.

Lally L, Forbess L, Hatzis C, Spiera R: Brief report: a prospective open-label phase IIa trial of tocilizumab in the treatment of polymyalgia rheumatica, *Arthritis Rheumatol* 68(10):2550–2554, 2016.

Ruediger C, Nguyen L, Black R, et al: Efficacy of methotrexate in polymyalgia rheumatica in routine rheumatology clinical care, *Intern Med J*, 2020.

Soriano A, Muratore F, Pipitone N, et al: Visual loss and other cranial ischaemic complications in giant cell arteritis, *Nat Rev Rheumatol* 13(8):476–484, 2017.

Stone JH, Tuckwell K, Dimonaco S, et al: Trial of tocilizumab in giant-cell arteritis, *N Engl J Med* 377(4):317–328, 2017.

PSORIATIC ARTHRITIS

William Tillett, MBChB, PhD; and Laura C. Coates, MBChB, PhD

CURRENT DIAGNOSIS

- Psoriatic arthritis (PsA) is a form of inflammatory arthritis genetically associated with the spondylarthritides (SpA) (e.g., ankylosing spondylitis, reactive arthritis [ReA], inflammatory bowel disease [IBD], arthritis).
- It is usually diagnosed in the presence of psoriasis (personal or family history), negative rheumatoid factor, and other typical features such as dactylitis and nail involvement.
- Presentation is highly heterogeneous with potential involvement in multiple domains (arthritis, enthesitis, dactylitis and axial disease, skin plaques, and nail dystrophy), as well as SpA-related extraarticular manifestations (IBD and uveitis).

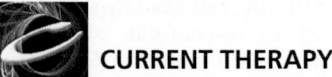

CURRENT THERAPY

- Therapy of PsA aims to control musculoskeletal inflammation (arthritis, enthesitis, dactylitis, and axial disease) and cutaneous manifestations (skin plaques and nail dystrophy).
- Treatment usually follows a step-up approach with non-steroidal antiinflammatory drugs (NSAIDs), topical therapies (for skin plaques), conventional synthetic disease-modifying antirheumatic drugs (DMARDs; e.g., methotrexate [Trexall], leflunomide [Arava][1]) and biologics (inhibitors of tumor necrosis factor [TNF], interleukin [IL]-12/23, IL-17, IL-23) and targeted synthetic DMARDs (apremilast [Otezla] and Janus kinase [JAK] inhibitors).
- PsA is commonly associated with comorbidities such as depression and increased cardiovascular risk with elements of the metabolic syndrome, which may have an impact on therapeutic choice.

[1]Not FDA approved for this indication.

Epidemiology

Psoriatic arthritis (PsA) is a destructive inflammatory arthritis occurring in up to 20% people with psoriasis. Psoriasis affects approximately 2% to 3% of the US population. The exact prevalence of PsA among the general population has been difficult to estimate due to the heterogeneous nature of the disease and variety of different classification criteria. The lowest prevalence estimates come from Japan (0.001%) and highest from Italy (0.42%). Data from recent studies have been more consistent with prevalence estimates of 0.16% in North America and 0.19% in the United Kingdom. PsA affects men and women equally and can develop at any age but typically occurs in the 10 to 15 years after the diagnosis of psoriasis, usually between the ages of 30 and 50 years. The incidence of developing PsA among people with psoriasis is approximately 2% per year. In a recent prospective study of patients with psoriasis, 51 of 464 patients developed PsA over an 8-year follow-up period.

Risk Factors

A number of risk factors have been identified that appear to increase the risk of developing PsA. The presence of human leukocyte antigen (HLA)-B27 is an established genetic risk factor. Increased rates of PsA are seen among those with more severe psoriasis (relative risk [RR] 5.4 $P = 0.006$). The site of psoriasis may also be important, and some reports suggest that intergluteal and scalp psoriasis confer an increased risk of developing PsA. Nail psoriasis (pitting, onycholysis, subungual hyperkeratosis, and oil drop discoloration) is also associated with an increased likelihood of developing PsA. Nail dystrophy occurs in 80% of patients with PsA but only 20% patients with psoriasis alone. Obesity is a well-documented risk factor for developing both psoriasis and PsA. The higher the body mass index (BMI), the higher the risk of developing arthritis. Alcohol is a potentially modifiable risk factor with associated increased rates of both psoriasis and arthritis. Data relating to smoking as a risk factor are mixed, with reports suggesting both increased risk and a potentially protective effect.

Pathophysiology

Genetics

The exact etiology of PsA remains uncertain. Genetics are known to play a central role. However, the number of genes identified do not account for the strong heritability seen clinically. Approximately 40% of people with PsA will have a first-degree relative with the condition. PsA appears to have a stronger association with HLA-B and HLA-C alleles, whereas psoriasis is associated with HLA-C. HLA-Cw6, B57, DR7, and B17 are all associated with early-onset psoriasis. HLA-B7, HLA-B27, DR4, 38, and DR7 are associated with PsA. HLA-B39, B27, and DR7 are

associated with more progressive/destructive disease, whereas HLA-B22 appears to be protective.

Immunopathology

Tissue-specific autoantibodies have not yet been identified. The inflammatory arthritis is characterized by hypervascularity, hypertrophy/tissue proliferation, and inflammatory cell infiltrate. Lymphocytes (particularly Th17 cells) and dendritic cells are known to play an important role. The cytokine profile for PsA shows a predominance of tumor necrosis factor (TNF)-α, interleukin (IL)-1, and IL-10.

Infection and Trauma

The temporal link between infections and the development of PsA raises the possibility of a pathologic role of bacteria or viruses. There are higher rates of both psoriasis and PsA in human immunodeficiency virus (HIV) endemic areas, and psoriasis is often more extensive among patients with HIV. The gut microbiome is an area of current interest where disturbance of the normal microbiota is being investigated as a possible immunologic trigger. Finally, a small number of epidemiologic studies have made the association with trauma and the subsequent development of PsA, but reports are inconclusive.

Prevention

There are no known strategies to prevent the development of PsA. Preventive strategies focus on early diagnosis and prevention of damage accumulation, loss of function, and disability. The treatment of comorbid conditions, predrug-treatment screening, and drug dose optimization to minimize drug exposure are important prevention strategies.

Early diagnosis and treatment strategies focus on the prevention of damage and subsequent disability. Untreated inflammation results in damage to the articular surface and surrounding tissues with subsequent loss of movement, pain, limitation of function, and reduced quality of life. Erosion of the surface of the bone, narrowing of the joint space, and new bone formation (osteoproliferation) cause pain, reduced movement, and physical dysfunction. Observational studies have suggested that delay of diagnosis by as little as 6 months results in more damage and worse physical function.

In the United Kingdom, annual screening of patients with psoriasis for arthritis is recommended using the Psoriasis Epidemiology Screening Tool (PEST) questionnaire. The questionnaire asks patients with psoriasis if they have ever had pain in their joints, if a doctor has ever told them they have arthritis, if they have had nail pitting, if they have had pain in their heel, and if they have ever had a completely sausage-like swelling of a finger or toe without reason. A score of 3 or more is positive.

Clinical Manifestations

PsA is classified with the seronegative spondyloarthropathies that include axial spondyloarthritis (axSpA), reactive arthritis (ReA), and inflammatory bowel disease (IBD) arthritis. The seronegative spondyloarthropathies share many of the clinical and genetic features, such as HLA-B27 association, enthesopathy (inflammation at the tendon and ligament insertion to the bone), association with uveitis, spondyloarthritis, and asymmetric peripheral arthritis.

The classical patterns of PsA are listed in the following points, although there is often overlap between these groups:
- Polyarthritis (five or more joints)
- Oligoarthritis (four or fewer joints)
- Monoarthritis (one joint)
- Spondyloarthritis (axial disease)
- PsA mutilans (digital shortening/telescoping due to onycholysis)

Polyarthritis is the most common form occurring in approximately 60% cases, whereas mutilans only occurs in 5% of cases.

The signs of PsA are heterogeneous and include the following:

Psoriasis—In its most common plaque form, the skin lesions of psoriasis are characterized by scaly plaques on the extensor surfaces. Psoriasis can be hidden in the scalp, ear, natal cleft, and umbilicus. Most patients develop their psoriasis before developing arthritis, but a small proportion, approximately 10%, will develop psoriasis after their arthritis. A proportion of patients present with musculoskeletal symptoms but are unaware they have skin psoriasis, which can be subtle in sites such as the hairline, intergluteal region, behind the ear, or umbilicus. Other patterns of psoriasis include guttate (small spots that can be widespread), palmar-plantar (palms and soles), and inverse (affecting the flexural creases).

Nail dystrophy—Pitting (fine pits), onycholysis (lifting of the distal nail plate), hyperkeratosis (thickening of the nail plate), and oil drop discoloration (salmon-colored spots) are the most common nail manifestations of psoriasis. Other features include leukonychia, Beau lines, and longitudinal ridging. Nail pitting can be clinically subtle but a helpful sign to distinguish PsA from other types of arthritis. Nail dystrophy itself is associated with an increased risk of developing arthritis and can be the only manifestation of psoriasis.

Joint disease—Inflammatory arthritis is the hallmark of PsA. The joints appear swollen and hot and are stiff and painful. The recognized patterns of joint involvement are inflammatory polyarthritis (five or more joints involved, which may be symmetric or asymmetric in distribution), oligoarticular (fewer than 5 joints), monoarticular (one joint), axial (spondyloarthritis), and mutilans (digital shortening due to onycholysis).

Enthesitis—Inflammation at the insertion of the tendon or ligament to the bone (rather than the mid-portion of the tendon, which is more likely to be an overuse tendinopathy) may be a sign. Many sites can be affected by enthesitis. However, the most readily assessable are the Achilles insertion to the calcaneus, the lateral epicondyle of the elbow, and the medical condyle of the femur. Enthesitis is not commonly seen in rheumatoid arthritis and can be a useful distinguishing sign. The assessment of enthesitis can be challenging, as many entheseal insertions correlate anatomically with myofascial tender points seen in fibromyalgia. Ultrasound can be helpful to examine for sonographic features of enthesitis, such as insertional hypervascularity, osteoproliferation, and erosion.

Dactylitis—Also known as "sausage finger," dactylitis is the swelling of an entire digit. Dactylitis occurs on 50% of patients with PsA at some point in their disease. The inflammation is at the joint, tendon, and extracapsular tissues.

Spondyloarthritis—Spondyloarthritis affects up to 50% of patients with PsA, but cohort studies have suggested only half of these patients have symptoms of inflammatory back pain. Inflammatory back pain typically occurs before the age of 40 years, will wake people in the second half of the night, are characteristically stiff in the morning, and feel better with exercise and nonsteroidal antiinflammatory drugs. The radiographic features are of sacroiliitis (sclerosis, erosions, and fusion), which can be asymmetrical, and syndesmophytes (bone formation, which can be fine or chunky), which can flow between vertebrae, causing fusion.

Other manifestations include uveitis (approximately 30% patients, RR 3.5 compared with the general population), metabolic syndrome (elevated BMI, hypertension, and dyslipidemia), IBD (Crohn disease, RR 2.9 compared with the general population), and depression.

Diagnosis

In the absence of specific antibodies, the diagnosis of PsA remains clinical. The Classification Criteria for Psoriatic Arthritis (CASPAR) criteria were developed for use in clinical trials to ensure a consistent trial population and have also been shown to apply in the clinical setting as diagnostic criteria (Box 1).

Differential Diagnosis

The other seronegative spondyloarthropathies are in the primary differential diagnosis.

The absence of an infectious trigger or concurrent IBD discount ReA and IBD arthritis. The presence or history of psoriasis (or a first-degree relative with psoriasis) is the most useful distinguishing feature in differentiating from axSpA.

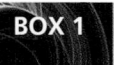

BOX 1 The Classification Criteria for Psoriatic Arthritis Criteria

Confirmed inflammatory articular disease (joint, spine, or entheseal) with at least three points from the following features:
1. Current psoriasis (two points)
2. A past personal history or family history of a first-or second-degree relative with psoriasis (one point each)
3. Dactylitis (one point)
4. Juxtaarticular new bone formation (ill-defined ossification near joint margins—excluding osteophyte formation—on plain hand and feet radiographs; one point)
5. Rheumatoid factor negativity (one point)
6. Psoriatic nail dystrophy (onycholysis, pitting, and hyperkeratosis observed on current physical examination; one point)

Osteoarthritis is a common and clinically challenging differential, particularly in the hands. Young age of onset, the presence of nail psoriasis at the affected ray, and radiographic features of PsA are the most useful distinguishing features.

Gout is an important differential for two reasons. First, a history of a swollen toe is often mistaken as gout (or podagra). Second, uric acid is commonly mildly elevated in patients with PsA. A careful history and examination for other clinical features of PsA can be helpful, such as history of psoriasis, nail dystrophy at the affected toe, enthesitis, or axial symptoms. Ultrasound to examine for sonographic features of crystal deposition or aspiration to examine for crystals may be required. Concurrent gout and PsA are rare but recognized.

Investigations to support the diagnosis include:
- Rheumatoid factor (RhF) and anticyclic citrullinated peptide (ACPA or anti-CCP) are usually negative.
- Inflammatory markers such as C-reactive protein (CRP), plasma viscosity (PV), and erythrocyte sedimentation rate (ESR) can often be normal and do not exclude inflammatory joint disease.
- Plain radiographs can be helpful to distinguish PsA from rheumatoid arthritis (RA) or osteoarthritis (OA). The plain radiographic features of PsA are erosions, joint space narrowing, osteoproliferation (bone formation), ankyloses (fusion), and, in the mutilans form of the disease, osteolysis (bone resorption).
- Magnetic resonance imaging (MRI) and ultrasound are both frequently used to assess for spondyloarthritis and articular and entheseal inflammation, respectively.

Therapy (or Treatment)

The treatment of PsA aims to control inflammation related to the disease to improve symptoms, maximize function, and prevent long-term complications. Different therapies may be chosen dependent on the domains of disease (arthritis, skin, nails, enthesitis, dactylitis, axial disease) that are active in any one individual patient. In general, treatment of PsA follows a step-up approach with treatment escalated in case of nonresponse to the previous therapy. Ideally treatment should follow a treat-to-target approach where a treatment target, such as minimal disease activity (MDA), is reassessed at each visit, and therapy is assessed if the target is not met. This approach has been shown to improve disease control in the tight control of PsA (TICOPA) trial.

Nonsteroidal antiinflammatory drugs are used frequently to help manage pain and stiffness but do not seem to have a significant effect on the disease course. Particularly in the early stages of disease or in the case of disease flares, parenteral steroids (intraarticular or intramuscular) are used to control inflammation quickly, although there can be a risk of psoriasis flare on withdrawal of systemic steroids. The mainstay of therapy in PsA are disease-modifying antirheumatic drugs (DMARDs), which are grouped into three categories:

1. Conventional synthetic DMARDs (methotrexate, sulfasalazine [Azulfidine],[1] leflunomide [Arava][1])
2. Biologic DMARDs (TNF inhibitors, IL-12/23, -17, or -23 inhibitors)
3. Targeted synthetic DMARDs (phosphodiesterase 4 [PDE-4] and Janus kinase [JAK] inhibitors)

Conventional synthetic DMARDs (csDMARDs) are commonly used to treat skin psoriasis and peripheral arthritis. The use of these drugs is based on their efficacy in psoriasis and in rheumatoid arthritis, although the data supporting their efficacy in PsA are relatively lacking. The most commonly used csDMARD is methotrexate, although the placebo-controlled MIPA (Methotrexate In PsA) trial did not show a significant effect of methotrexate over placebo. Many rheumatologists discounted these data due to flaws in the study design (low target dose used, poor completion rate). Interestingly in the supplementary data from the study, it seemed that patients with polyarticular disease responded much better to methotrexate than those with oligoarthritis. This may be due to a differential response in different forms of arthritis, but it most likely relates to the sensitivity of the outcome measures used. There is, however, proven efficacy for the use of methotrexate in psoriasis, so this drug is useful to manage patients with both peripheral arthritis and active psoriasis. Sulfasalazine (Azulfidine)[1] is also commonly used and does have a number of studies supporting its efficacy. However, a Cochrane review in 2000 summarized the results of these studies and concluded that while it was effective, the effect size was relatively small. Leflunomide (Arava)[1] is the conventional DMARD with the strongest trial data. The TOPAS study in 2004 confirmed efficacy of leflunomide versus placebo but came shortly before breakthrough trials with biologic therapies with superior results.

Despite the mixed data on the csDMARDs and their effect on clinical measures of disease activity, none of them have any proven effect on disease progression in the form of radiographic damage. Observational studies have suggested that early use of therapies and higher dosages used in more recent years may be associated with less radiographic damage, but this has not been formally tested. There is very limited data in treating other domains of PsA, such as enthesitis and dactylitis, where only small open label studies are available. In axial PsA, as in other axial spondylarthritides, there is no evidence of efficacy of conventional drugs, and treatment algorithms rely on biologic therapies.

A number of biologic DMARDs (bDMARDS) have proven efficacy in PsA and have been licensed for use in this condition. There are five different TNF inhibitors (adalimumab [Humira], certolizumab [Cimzia], etanercept [Enbrel], infliximab [Remicade], and golimumab [Simponi]), which have all shown efficacy across the key domains of PsA, including arthritis, enthesitis, dactylitis, skin, and nails. They have all shown long-term efficacy and retardation of radiographic damage, confirming their effect on structural progression. In most of the studies, around 50% of the patients were also receiving a concomitant csDMARD (usually methotrexate). However, in PsA, in contrast to rheumatoid arthritis, there has not been a significant difference in efficacy seen with combination treatment over monotherapy biologics. Recently a randomized trial addressed this point, comparing methotrexate monotherapy, etanercept monotherapy, and the combination in a placebo-controlled trial. This study confirmed superiority of both etanercept arms over methotrexate monotherapy but did not find a difference in effect with concomitant use of csDMARDs.

As a secondary outcome in the PsA studies, there has been a significant difference seen in enthesitis and dactylitis using clinical measures. In the PsA studies and in specific psoriasis studies, the efficacy of TNF inhibitors has been proven for both skin and nail disease. As yet, there are no specific studies in axial PsA, but data in axSpA and/or ankylosing spondylitis has confirmed the efficacy of TNF inhibitors for spinal symptoms.

A number of IL inhibitors have been licensed for the treatment of PsA. Ustekinumab (Stelara; a p40 antibody that blocks the action of IL-12 and IL-23) is particularly effective for psoriasis, with proven superiority over TNF inhibitors. It also has evidence of efficacy for peripheral arthritis, enthesitis, and dactylitis. Surprisingly, however, despite a small positive open label study, a randomized trial in axSpA was halted early, with no evidence of efficacy over placebo. Thus the phenotype of disease must be considered when choosing a therapy.

IL-17A inhibitors (secukinumab [Cosentyx] and ixekizumab [Taltz]) are now licensed for PsA and ankylosing spondylitis, providing an alternative biologic option for those with PsA. These drugs showed even higher responses in skin psoriasis, with head-to-head studies confirming superiority over ustekinumab and TNF inhibitors. Additional drugs targeting the Th17 pathway are in development. Bimekizumab[5] blocks both IL-17A and IL-17F and has positive phase II trial results. Further studies will show if dual blockade is superior to blocking IL-17A alone. Brodalumab (Siliq),[1] a human antibody against the IL-17 receptor, would also block different forms of IL-17 and has positive phase II data in PsA.

A number of specific IL-23 inhibitors are also in development, with guselkumab (Tremfya) licensed for use in PsA. These bind to the p19 subunit, providing specific blockade of IL-23 only, and have been shown to have impressive efficacy in skin psoriasis. Phase II and phase III trial data are available in PsA, with evidence of efficacy in peripheral arthritis, but again studies in ankylosing spondylitis and axSpA have been halted due to lack of efficacy in the spinal domain.

In recent years, a third class of drugs, the targeted synthetic DMARDs (tsDMARDs), have also become available for the treatment of PsA. Apremilast (Otezla) is a PDE-4 inhibitor with proven modest efficacy in the treatment of peripheral arthritis, psoriasis, enthesitis, and dactylitis, but not in axial SpA. Although responses seem lower than the biologic drugs, apremilast has a very reassuring safety profile with no requirement for regular blood monitoring. The other group of tsDMARDs in development focus on targeting the JAK pathway. Tofacitinib (Xeljanz) and upadacitinib (Rinvoq) are licensed for treatment of peripheral arthritis, with comparable improvements in arthritis, enthesitis, and dactylitis outcomes to adalimumab, which was included in both studies as either an internal control or head-to-head comparison. Tofacitinib shows modest efficacy on skin psoriasis with seemingly higher responses seen in the upadacitinib[1] PsA trial, although they are not specifically licensed for psoriasis. Studies in ankylosing spondylitis suggest that JAK inhibitors are also efficacious for axial disease. Other JAK inhibitors, with different selectivity for JAK pathways, are in phase II and phase III studies.

In all cases, the aim of treatment should be to minimize disease activity. The choice of therapy can be difficult, as there are few head-to-head comparison studies and many of the newer biologic or tsDMARDs appear to have similar efficacy in arthritis. In cases with significant psoriasis, an argument could be made for IL-12/23, IL-17, or IL-23 inhibitors, where superior efficacy has been shown in psoriasis and PsA trials. For those with axial disease, proven efficacy is limited to TNF, IL-17 inhibitors, and JAK inhibitors. In other cases, the choice of medication often depends on comorbidities, where therapies may be contraindicated (IL-17 inhibitors worsening active IBD) or helpful (TNF inhibitors).

Monitoring

Monitoring of PsA may include assessment of clinical disease activity measures, patient-reported outcomes, laboratory tests, and imaging. The majority of day-to-day disease monitoring consists of clinical outcome measures, often combined with patient-reported outcomes.

Not FDA approved for this indication.

Not FDA approved for this indication.
Investigational drug in the United States.

Ideally all domains of disease should be assessed to allow optimal choice of therapy. To assess arthritis, a full 68/66 joint count is required, rather than reduced joint counts used in rheumatoid arthritis. Dactylitis is usually evident when joints are examined. Enthesitis can be assessed clinically looking for tenderness and swelling at the site of key tendon attachments. In cases of doubt, ultrasound imaging can be helpful to look for inflammation and increased blood flow. Although rheumatologists are focused on musculoskeletal signs, when treating patients with PsA, they should also assess skin and nail manifestations. This can be a relatively brief assessment, such as a body surface area of skin psoriasis affected; it is important not to underestimate the impact of skin involvement on patient's quality of life.

Multiple patient-reported outcomes are available to measure the patient perspective in PsA, including questionnaires assessing pain, function, work disability, and other impacts. The majority of these are research tools, and they are often combined with physician-assessed clinical measures to form composite scores. In clinical practice, some questionnaire may be used to assess the patient perspective and encourage dialogue with patients.

As mentioned previously, treatment recommendations now state that a treat-to-target approach should be implemented in routine care of PsA. Recommendations state that the treatment target should ideally be remission with the alternative target of low disease activity if remission is not feasible. Additional recommendations on treat-to-target have highlighted that the target of therapy should include both musculoskeletal and skin manifestations of disease. Thus the MDA criteria have been recommended for the target of treatment, as these include measures of arthritis, psoriasis, enthesitis and patient-reported pain, global activity, and functional ability.

Management of Complications

PsA is associated with a number of comorbidities. It is part of the spectrum of spondyloarthritis and has associated extraarticular manifestations (EAMs), including potential overlap with IBD and uveitis. The involvement of these other systems is important to recognize to aid diagnosis and then comanage patients to optimize outcome. Often therapies for PsA are also licensed for treatment of EAMs, allowing treatment of the disease as a whole.

Other comorbidities, not directly related to the disease complex, are also prominent in patients with psoriasis and PsA. Depression and anxiety are prevalent in up to half of the population and are important to address to maximize quality of life and also to aid adherence to therapy. Patients with psoriasis and PsA also have a much higher risk of metabolic syndrome and associated cardiovascular comorbidity. There are higher rates of obesity, diabetes, hypertension, hyperlipidemia, and associated complications such as nonalcoholic fatty liver disease and cardiovascular events. The cardiovascular risk seems to be higher in those with severe active disease and provides another argument for effective control of inflammation. Beyond controlling disease, patients need support and interventions to manage their other risk factors such as weight, smoking, blood pressure, and lipid control.

References

Charlton R, Green A, Shaddick G: On behalf of the PROMPT study group. Risk of uveitis and inflammatory bowel disease in people with psoriatic arthritis: a population-based cohort study, *Ann Rheum Dis* 77:277–280, 2018.

Coates LC, Kavanaugh A, Mease PJ, et al: Group for research and assessment of psoriasis and psoriatic arthritis: treatment recommendations for psoriatic arthritis 2015, et al. *Arthritis Rheum* 68(5):1060–1071, 2016.

Coates LC, Moverley AR, Let al. MP, et al: Effect of tight control of inflammation in early psoriatic arthritis (TICOPA): a UK multicentre, open-label, randomised controlled trial, *Lancet* 386(10012):2489–2498, 2015.

Ogdie A, Weiss P: The epidemiology of psoriatic arthritis, *Rheum Dis Clin North Am* 41(4):545–568, 2015.

Taylor W, Gladman D, Helliwell P: Classification criteria for psoriatic arthritis: development of new criteria from a large international study, *Arthritis Rheum* 54:2665–2673, 2006.

Tillett W, Charlton R, Nightingale Aal, et al: Interval between onset of psoriasis and psoriatic arthritis comparing the UK Clinical Practice Research Datalink with a hospital-based cohort, *Rheumatology* 56(12):2109–2113, 2017.

Van den Bosch F, Coates L: Clinical management of psoriatic arthritis, *Lancet* 391(10136):2285–2294, 2018.

Veale DJ, Fearon U: The pathogenesis of psoriatic arthritis, *Lancet* 391:2273–2284, 2018.

RHEUMATOID ARTHRITIS

Method of
Megan Krause, MD

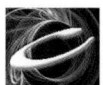

CURRENT DIAGNOSIS

- Clinical diagnosis based on combination of history, examination, and supporting laboratory studies.
- Presentation is typically chronic symmetric polyarticular inflammatory arthritis.
- While not required for diagnosis, supporting laboratory studies include positive rheumatoid factor (RF), positive anticitrullinated protein antibodies (ACPA), elevated C-reactive protein (CRP), and elevated sedimentation rate (ESR).
- Radiographs can be normal at diagnosis. Findings of periarticular osteopenia and erosions are supportive of diagnosis of rheumatoid arthritis (RA).

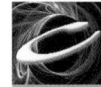

CURRENT THERAPY

- Methotrexate (Otrexup, Rasuvo, Rheumatrex) initial dose typically 10 to 15 mg weekly with an increase based on disease activity up to 25 mg weekly orally or subcutaneously in conjunction with daily folic acid[1] 1 mg orally daily.
- Hydroxychloroquine (Plaquenil) 5 mg/kg orally per day with maximum of 400 mg daily.
- Sulfasalazine (Azulfidine-EN) initially dose typically 500 mg orally once daily or 500 mg twice daily, increasing up to goal dose of 1000 to 1500 mg twice daily.
- Leflunomide (Arava) 10 to 20 mg orally once daily.
- Azathioprine (Imuran) initial 1 mg/kg/day orally with increasing dose based on response to maximum of 2.5 mg/kg/day.
- Janus kinase inhibitors
  - Tofacitinib (Xeljanz) immediate release 5 mg orally twice daily or extended release 11 mg orally once daily.
  - Baricitinib (Olumiant) 2 mg orally once daily.
  - Upadacitinib (Rinvoq) 15 mg orally once daily.
- Tumor necrosis factor (TNF) inhibitors
  - Adalimumab (Humira) 40 mg subcutaneous every other week.
  - Certolizumab (Cimzia) 400 mg subcutaneous at week 0, 2, and 4, then 200 mg every other week or 400 mg every 4 weeks.
  - Etanercept (Enbrel) 50 mg subcutaneous every week.
  - Golimumab (Simponi, Simponi Aria)
    - Simponi: 50 mg subcutaneous every 4 weeks
    - Simponi Aria: 2 mg/kg intravenous at week 0, 4, and then every 8 weeks
  - Infliximab (Remicade) 3 mg/kg intravenous at week 0, 2, and 6 and then every 8 weeks but, if persistent disease activity, dose can be adjusted between 3 and 10 mg/kg every 4 to 8 weeks.
- Interleukin 6 (IL6) receptor inhibitors
  - Tocilizumab (Actemra)
    - Subcutaneous: if less than 100 kg: 162 mg every other week, increase to weekly if persistent disease activity; if more than 100 kg: 162 mg every week.
    - Intravenous: 4 mg/kg every 4 weeks, can be increased to 8 mg/kg every 4 weeks if persistent disease activity.
  - Sarilumab (Kevzara) 200 mg subcutaneous every 2 weeks.
- T cell co-stimulation inhibitors
  - Abatacept (Orencia)
    - Subcutaneous: 125 mg once weekly (with or without IV loading dose).
    - Intravenous: if less than 60 kg: 500 mg; if 60 to 100 kg: 750 mg; if more than 100 kg: 1000 mg with initial dosing at week 0, 2, and 4, and then every 4 weeks.

- B cell inhibitor
  - Rituximab (Rituxan) 1000 mg IV day 1 and 15, subsequent doses can be repeated at 24 weeks.
- Interleukin 1 receptor inhibitor
  - Anakinra (Kineret) 100 mg subcutaneous every day.

[1]Not FDA approved for this indication.

Epidemiology

Individuals can develop rheumatoid arthritis (RA) at any age, but a peak incidence is between 50 and 75 years. Women are affected at a frequency of two to three times greater than men. It is estimated that the prevalence is approximately 1% in the United States.

Risk Factors

The exact pathogenesis of RA is not completely understood. It is likely the consequence of the interplay of multiple factors, including genetic predisposition and epigenetic factors, along with environmental exposures that result in the systemic inflammatory process. The environmental factors are diverse and are likely not the same in all individuals. Cigarette smoking has been identified as a significant risk factor. Periodontal disease also is associated with development of RA. Silica is an example of an associated occupational exposure.

Multiple genetic risk factors have been identified. The shared epitope, referring to a specific sequence at the HLA-DRB1 locus, which is involved with antigen presentation, has been one of the most studied. Other genetic factors have been identified but individually contribute a small increase in risk.

Pathophysiology

The combination of genetics, epigenetic factors, and environmental exposures lead to downstream consequences of loss of tolerance to self. Both the innate and adaptive immune systems are activated in this process. Diverse immune cells including T cells, B cells, macrophages, and dendritic cells are involved in the pathogenesis. The production of cytokines contributes to the wide variety of downstream tissue targets that lead to the diverse clinical manifestations of RA. While RA frequently is diagnosed based on presentation of inflammatory arthritis, the production of cytokines and interplay of multiple cell types leads to the multiorgan dysfunction.

Prevention

It is not understood how to prevent the development of RA. Limiting known risk factors such as smoking and maintaining periodontal health would be reasonable recommendations.

Clinical Manifestations

Articular Manifestations

Classically, individuals will present with symmetric inflammatory polyarthritis (affecting five or more joints) frequently affecting the wrists, metacarpophalangeal joints (MCPs), proximal interphalangeal joints (PIPs), and metatarsophalangeal joints (MTPs). Both small and large joints can be affected. The distal interphalangeal joints (DIPs) and lumbar spine are spared.

On examination, the joints can be warm, erythematous, swollen, and tender. Range of motion of joints is frequently limited. The synovitis on exam can be described as boggy in contrast to bony hypertrophic changes of osteoarthritis.

Extraarticular Manifestations

One of the consequences of the systemic nature of RA is that the symptoms are not limited to the joints. The extraarticular manifestations can have significant impact both in terms of morbidity and mortality. High clinical suspicion is required, and evaluation is necessary to differentiate toxicity of medications versus a manifestation of RA. More data are required to understand how the advances in therapy will impact extraarticular manifestations.

Individuals with RA can develop subcutaneous nodules, which sometimes can be independent of disease activity. Rarely, individuals can develop a paradoxical increase in rheumatoid nodules with methotrexate.

Individuals can present with significant dryness of the mouth consistent with secondary Sjögren syndrome. Some of these individuals will have positive autoantibodies, such as SSA/Ro and SSB/La.

Pulmonary manifestations can be quite varied and have important implications for treatment. Pleural disease can be seen and can include pleural effusions and pleurisy. Pulmonary nodules can also be present. Interstitial lung disease can present in wide ranging patterns, including usual interstitial pneumonia (UIP), nonspecific interstitial pneumonia (NSIP), organizing pneumonia, and constrictive bronchiolitis.

Cardiac manifestations can include accelerated coronary artery disease. If the joint symptoms preclude significant exertion, patients may not present with classic angina. Pericardial disease can range from pericarditis, pericardial effusion, and constrictive pericarditis. Depending on the location, rheumatoid nodules affecting the heart can be associated with valve dysfunction and conduction abnormalities.

Episcleritis and scleritis can be associated with RA. A dreaded ocular complication of RA is peripheral ulcerative keratitis and corneal melt; this requires emergent ophthalmologic evaluation.

Frequently hematologic abnormalities can be associated with RA. Anemia of chronic disease, leukocytosis, and thrombocytosis can be frequently seen. A minority of individuals will develop Felty syndrome, which includes clinical manifestations of splenomegaly, leukopenia (frequently neutropenia), and frequent infections.

Entrapment syndromes such as carpal tunnel syndrome can be a presenting symptom of RA or develop over the course of the disease. In the case of carpal tunnel syndrome, it is the result of compression of the median nerve due to swelling of the flexor tendons.

RA can affect the cervical spine. The atlantoaxial joint can be prone to subluxation, which can result in myelopathy. A high clinical suspicion is required, as individuals may not present with neck pain and joint damage can obscure examination findings such as reflexes.

An increasingly rare manifestation is vasculitis secondary to RA. This can have multiple manifestations but can include cutaneous ulcers and mononeuritis multiplex.

Diagnosis

Rheumatoid arthritis is a clinical diagnosis based on the pattern of clinical and laboratory findings. Rarely at presentation, individuals can present with monoarticular (one joint) or oligoarticular (two to four joints), but typically when observed over time, individuals will have polyarticular involvement.

Tests to aid diagnosis include the RF, which refers to an immunoglobuin M (IgM) directed against immunoglobulin G (IgG). It is a nonspecific test and can be elevated related to age, as well other diseases that can mimic RA, such as hepatitis C. ACPA have the advantage of being more specific than RF with specificity as high as 95%. Individuals are considered to have seropositive RA when either RF or ACPA is positive; this occurs in approximately 70% to 80% of individuals. Acute phase reactants including CRP and ESR, when elevated, are supportive of the diagnosis but not required for the diagnosis. Anemia of chronic disease, thrombocytosis, and leukocytosis can also be supportive of the diagnosis but are nonspecific.

The American College of Rheumatology (ACR) and European League Against Rheumatism (EULAR) have developed classification criteria. Domains included the pattern of joint involvement, serology status (RF and ACPA), acute phase reactants (CRP and ESR), and duration of symptoms (cutoff of 6 weeks).

At presentation, x-rays can be normal. The earliest abnormality in RA on x-ray evaluation of the joints includes soft tissue swelling and periarticular osteopenia. Additional changes on x-rays include symmetric joint space narrowing and marginal erosions. If erosions are present at diagnosis, this is associated with a worse prognosis.

Differential Diagnosis
The differential diagnosis is broad for RA. Multiple infections can cause polyarticular joint pain. Viral etiologies can include hepatitis B, hepatitis C, and HIV. Parvovirus B19 can also be a mimic of RA; joint pain can be a prominent feature in adults in contrast to children who rarely have joint involvement. Typically the arthritis of parvovirus B19 will resolve spontaneously over a few weeks. Travel history is also an important element of the history; for example, Chikungunya and Dengue can present with arthritis symptoms. Rubella, both the illness and vaccine, can be associated. Bacterial infection such as endocarditis and Lyme disease can present with oligoarticular/polyarticular joint pain. Rheumatic fever is also in the differential and can present with migratory joint pain.

Inflammatory arthritis can be a manifestation of other systemic rheumatologic conditions including seronegative spondyloarthritis (psoriatic arthritis, arthritis secondary to inflammatory bowel disease, reactive arthritis, and ankylosing spondylitis/axial spondyloarthritis). The pattern of involvement can be helpful, as seronegative spondyloarthritis frequently presents in an asymmetric, large joint predominant, and lower extremity predominant fashion. Inflammatory arthritis can develop secondary to connective tissue disease such as systemic lupus erythematosus and systemic sclerosis. ANCA-associated vasculitis can also present with arthritis. Paraneoplastic syndromes can present with joint pain including hypertrophic osteoarthropathy.

Treatment
The goals of treatment of RA are to address both the short term and long term complications of RA. The overarching principle is "treat to target." The goal of therapy should be to achieve clinical remission or low disease activity. The treatment approach must be individualized and consider the comorbidities of the patient. The significant cost of the medications must also be considered in therapy decisions.

Analgesics and Nonsteroidal Antiinflammatory Drugs
Analgesics and nonsteroidal antiinflammatory agents can be utilized to help address breakthrough pain. However, these agents should not be the foundation of treatment. Their role can be used to help control symptoms while a maintenance strategy with conventional disease-modifying antirheumatic drugs (DMARDs) and/or biologics is being established, as there is delay to the full clinical benefit of these medications. Since these medications do not alter the natural history of the disease, they should not be used in isolation.

In patients with extensive damage related to RA, these medications can have a role in helping address pain. DMARDs and biologics are unable to address pain related to damage.

Glucocorticoids
Glucocorticoids are frequently used due to their rapid onset of action, which distinguishes them from DMARDs and biologics. These are frequently utilized at initial diagnosis or with flares of established disease. However, the side effects of corticosteroids limit their use. Corticosteroids should not be utilized in isolation to treat RA. Corticosteroids can be given in multiple administration forms, including oral, intramuscular, and intraarticular. The choice of which to use is dependent on the individual patient's scenario.

Conventional Disease Modifying Antirheumatic Drugs
Conventional DMARDs are immunosuppressants with the goal of inducing and maintaining remission of patients with RA.

Methotrexate
Methotrexate (Otrexup, Rasuvo, Rheumatrex), in the absence of contraindications, is typically the first-line medication utilized

for RA. The exact mechanism specifically for RA is incompletely understood. Methotrexate inhibits dihydrofolate reductase which results in reduction of DNA synthesis and, as a result, cell replication. However, this is not the role in isolation as daily folic acid[1] is prescribed to help counter the side effects and does not reverse the therapeutic benefit. Methotrexate also increases the release of adenosine which leads to reduction of inflammation.

Methotrexate can be given in both oral and subcutaneous administration forms. Typically, the starting dose is 10 to 15 mg weekly with titration depending on clinical response, up to 25 mg weekly. At higher doses, gastrointestinal absorption can be limited, and this can be a situation to prefer the subcutaneous form.

Common side effects can include oral ulcers, nausea, fatigue, increased infection risk, cytopenias, and hepatotoxicity. Methotrexate requires routine blood monitoring specifically for cytopenia and hepatotoxicity. The toxicity of methotrexate is increased in the setting of renal dysfunction, and in this setting there should be consideration of dose reduction versus choosing an alternative agent.

Methotrexate is a teratogen. The recommendation is to wait 3 months from stopping methotrexate before trying to conceive.

Hydroxychloroquine
Hydroxychloroquine (Plaquenil) has multiple mechanisms of action including inhibition of antigen presentation via interference of toll-like receptors and acidification of lysosomes.

It is an oral medication with the dose range of 200 to 400 mg daily. It is a weight-based regimen, and when using real body weight, the dose is 5 mg/kg with the maximum of 400 mg daily.

Side effects can include photosensitive rash, hypoglycemia, hearing loss, and retinal toxicity. Hydroxychloroquine can deposit in the retina which can ultimately lead to vision loss if not identified. Individuals are recommended to have routine eye examinations so changes related to hydroxychloroquine, including bull's eye maculopathy, can be identified and hydroxychloroquine can then be discontinued if necessary. Eye comorbidities, such as macular degeneration, may complicate the ability to monitor for hydroxychloroquine toxicity and would need to be discussed with patient's eye provider.

Sulfasalazine
The exact mechanism of action of sulfasalazine (Azulfidine-EN) in RA is not currently well understood.

It is an oral medication that is utilized twice daily. The dose is typically started at 500 mg once or twice daily with titration of dose to 1000 to 1500 mg twice daily.

Side effects include rash, gastrointestinal side effects, cytopenias, and hepatoxicity. Laboratory monitoring is required to monitor for cytopenia and hepatotoxicity.

Leflunomide
Leflunomide (Arava) inhibits dihydroorotate dehydrogenase, which results in the reduction of pyrimidine synthesis and ultimately reduction of cellular replication.

It comes in an oral form. A loading dose is not required and frequently not used, as it can result in a side effect of diarrhea. Leflunomide has a very long half-life due to its entrance in the enterohepatocyte circulation.

Side effects include diarrhea, cytopenias, hepatoxicity, and increased infection risk. It requires routine laboratory monitoring for cytopenia and hepatoxicity. It is contraindicated in pregnancy.

A cholestyramine (Questran)[1] washout procedure can be utilized to eliminate leflunomide when needed for a time sensitive scenario, such as a woman wanting to pursue pregnancy.

Azathioprine
Azathioprine (Imuran) is an inhibitor of purine synthesis and as a result of cellular replication.

Not FDA approved for this indication.

It is an oral medication and the dosing is weight based. Azathioprine is typically started at 1 mg/kg/day and can be escalated up to a maximum of 2.5 mg/kg/day.

Side effects can include cytopenias, rash, nausea, diarrhea, and pancreatitis. Azathioprine requires routine monitoring for cytopenias and hepatotoxicity. A thiopurine methyltransferase (TPMT) level can be checked prior to initiation for assessment of the metabolism of azathioprine. If there are reduced levels of TPMT activity, then one would need to consider using a reduced dose or an alternative agent.

Azathioprine has been less commonly used as other agents have become available. Interstitial lung disease secondary to RA is one scenario in which it is still utilized.

Synthetic Disease Modifying Antirheumatic Drugs
Janus kinase (JAK) Inhibitors
Tofacitinib (Xeljanz), baricitinib (Olumiant), and upadacitinib (Rinvoq) are targeted small molecules that inhibit Janus kinases (JAKs). Inhibition blocks intracellular signaling of cytokine receptors and results in decreased gene activation.

Both are oral medications. Side effects can include cytopenia, hepatotoxicity, cardiovascular risk, and cholesterol elevation. Routine lab monitoring is required to monitor for these complications. There are rare reports of bowel perforation, and currently there is a recommendation to avoid in the setting of diverticulitis.

Biologics
Biologics refer to the complex chemical structure of these medications. Biologics can be used in combination with conventional DMARDs.

TNF Inhibitors
TNF inhibitors inhibit the effect of TNF alpha, a proinflammatory cytokine. There are five different TNF inhibitors: etanercept (Enbrel), adalimumab (Humira), certolizumab (Cimzia), golimumab (Simponi), and infliximab (Remicade). Etanercept has a component of the TNF receptor, allowing it to bind TNF alpha, and prevents it from binding to TNF receptors. The remaining are monoclonal antibodies targeting TNF alpha. Etanercept, adalimumab, certolizumab, and golimumab come in a subcutaneous form. Golimumab and infliximab are available as an infusion. Biosimilars, referencing their similar structure and as a result function but not identical to their corresponding biologic, are now available for some of the TNF inhibitors (e.g., Avsola [infliximab-axxq], Inflectra [infliximab-dyyb], and Renflexis [infliximab-abda] are biosimilars to infliximab).

Side effects include injection site/infusion reactions. Patients must be counseled on infection risk to wide-ranging organisms, ranging from bacterial, viral, fungal, and mycobacterial. Individuals must undergo tuberculosis testing prior to initiation of therapies. There were initial concerns regarding lymphoma in the setting of TNF inhibitor use, but it is likely that the underlying RA drives the risk primarily. TNF inhibitors can be associated with exacerbations of congestive heart failure. Multiple sclerosis would be a contraindication to TNF inhibitors.

Interleukin 6 Receptor Inhibitor (Tocilizumab and Sarilumab)
Tocilizumab (Actemra) and sarilumab (Kevzara) are both interleukin 6 (IL6) receptor inhibitors, which prevents activation of the receptors of IL6. This prevents the downstream activation of targets of IL6, a proinflammatory cytokine.

Tocilizumab comes as both infusion and subcutaneous versions. Sarilumab comes as a subcutaneous version.

Side effects include cytopenia, particularly neutropenia and thrombocytopenia, hepatotoxicity, and elevated cholesterol. Routine monitoring is necessary. Injection site/infusion reactions are also a risk. The infection concerns are similar to TNF inhibitors, with the risk pertaining to diverse organisms. Due to rare reports of bowel perforations, it is recommended to be avoided in the setting of diverticulitis.

T Cell Coactivation Inhibition
Abatacept (Orencia) prevents T cell coactivation by binding the costimulating signal (CD80/86) on antigen presenting cells and preventing it from binding T cells. Administration forms include subcutaneous injection and intravenous infusions. Side effects include injection/infusion site reactions. Infection risk is also a concern with abatacept. Higher rates of chronic obstructive pulmonary disease (COPD) exacerbations have been described with patients on abatacept.

B Cell Inhibition
Rituximab (Rituxan) depletes B cells by targeting CD20, which is present on B cells.

It is an intravenous medication. The timing of subsequent doses is typically every 6 months.

The risks of rituximab include infusion reactions. Infection risk is a concern with rituximab, particularly considering the long timeframe of effect. Careful attention must be given to prevent hepatitis B reactivation. Even in patients with evidence of natural immunity via cleared infection, they would be a candidate for hepatitis B reactivation prophylaxis. Progressive multifocal leukoencephalopathy (PML) related to JC virus has been reported in patients receiving rituximab for the indication of RA. The risk is very low, and in multiple reports, patients were also on additional immunosuppressants such as chemotherapy.

Interleukin 1 Inhibition
Anakinra (Kineret) is an inhibitor of the IL1 receptor preventing the downstream activation of IL1, a proinflammatory cytokine. Risks are similar to other biologics in terms of infection, injection site reaction, cytopenia, and nausea. It is a daily subcutaneous injection.

Combination Therapy
Combination therapy is frequently utilized for treatment of RA. An indication to proceed with combination therapy is when disease activity is persistent despite therapeutic dosing with a single agent. A frequently used combination therapy is termed "triple therapy." This refers to the combination of methotrexate, sulfasalazine, and hydroxychloroquine. A single biologic can be utilized in combination with conventional DMARDs, most frequently methotrexate. Two biologics are not recommended to be utilized together, due to concern with increased infection risk.

Choice of Therapy
Multiple factors must be weighed in terms of the choice of therapy for RA. If there are no contraindications, methotrexate is typically used as the first choice. If there is an insufficient response to a maximized dose of methotrexate, including use of subcutaneous methotrexate, then combination therapy is frequently utilized. If methotrexate is unable to be tolerated, then leflunomide could be considered in its place. The combination therapy to be utilized with methotrexate could include triple therapy versus methotrexate in combination with a biologic or synthetic DMARD (JAK inhibitors). Triple therapy has been compared with methotrexate plus biologic therapy in multiple studies and overall thought to be equivalent in terms of achieving clinical response. The choice between the two is dependent on discussion with the patient. Consideration for the forms of administration would need to be taken into account. Comorbidities of the patient can restrict choices. Another consideration is cost and insurance coverage for different medications. Currently, there is not available testing to inform choice of therapy in a personalized manner beyond consideration of comorbidities.

When patients have consistently achieved clinical remission, there can be consideration for reduction in treatment. There is increased risk of flare of disease when reducing medications. Patients would need to be counseled regarding this risk and monitored closely.

Special Scenarios
Pregnancy
As RA can affect women of childbearing age, understanding the goals in terms of pregnancy must be understood for patients with

RA. Methotrexate and leflunomide would be contraindicated in the setting of pregnancy. Methotrexate is associated with known congenital abnormalities. The recommendation would be to stop methotrexate 3 months prior to contraception. Leflunomide has a much longer half-life and the level could be checked and, if elevated, then could use cholestyramine washout. If there is a possibility of pregnancy, then hydroxychloroquine or sulfasalazine are frequently used options in this setting. TNF inhibitors have been utilized in pregnancy. The recommendations would be to stop TNF inhibitors over the course of pregnancy with the specific TNF inhibitors having different recommendations; certolizumab is not thought to cross the placenta due to its chemical structure, and in some individuals, this is continued throughout the pregnancy. Less information is available about the safety of other biologics in pregnancy and, if possible, would be avoided until further information is known.

Patients frequently have improvement in their clinical symptoms during pregnancy, which emphasizes the importance of an individualized approach during pregnancy. Patients should be counseled on the risk for flare in the postpartum setting.

Breastfeeding
Data is limited regarding the effects of medications for RA and breastfeeding. The potential benefits of breastfeeding would need to be weighed with potential risk. Methotrexate and leflunomide are avoided during breastfeeding. An individualized approach is necessary in conjunction with the patient and obstetrician.

Malignancy
Data is limited regarding the ideal choice of therapy in the setting of a history of malignancy. DMARDs are frequently preferred over biologics in the setting of prior malignancy. Specifically in the setting of lymphoproliferative disorders, if a biologic is indicated due to disease activity, rituximab is preferred over other biologic choices. Individualized decisions must be made in conjunction with the patient and their hematologist/oncologist.

Preoperative Management
Due to the risk of atlantoaxial instability in RA, particularly in long-standing disease, patients prior to surgery should be screened for this complication. Cervical spine x-rays with flexion and extension views would be recommended. The results should be reviewed with an anesthesiologist to assist with planning for positioning during surgery.

Management of immunosuppressant medications must be reviewed with the surgeon and take into account the nature of surgery as well as the pharmacokinetics of the immunosuppressants. Data are limited on the ideal management of immunosuppressants in this setting. Guidelines have been published in the setting of total hip and knee arthroplasty.

Monitoring
There are two components of monitoring for patients with RA. The first is to assess for disease activity both from the standpoint of the joints as well as extraarticular manifestations. From the joint perspective, there are multiple disease activity scores that can be utilized. Some rely solely on patient reported outcomes. Others are a combination of patient reported outcomes, exam findings, and provider global assessment. Swollen joint counts and tender joint counts are frequently utilized. Specifically for laboratory monitoring of disease activity, ESR and CRP can be utilized but do not trend with disease activity in all patients. ACPA and RF do not trend with disease activity and thus the values do not need to be repeated if positive.

Separately, drug toxicity must be assessed including clinical symptoms and laboratory monitoring. In addition, monitoring for development of infection is also necessary.

Management of Complications
If drug toxicity develops, depending on the nature of toxicity, the medication dose should either be reduced or discontinued. If the side effect likely reflects a class effect, consider an agent in a different drug class. If infection occurs while on immunosuppressant therapy, these medications should be held at least until the infection has resolved. Restarting would be dependent on the clinical scenario, including the nature of the infection and the specific treatment for RA.

References

Aletaha D, Neogi T, Silman AJ, et al: 2010 Rheumatoid Arthritis Classification Criteria: an American College of Rheumatology/European League Against Rheumatism Collaborative Initiative, *Arthritis Rheum* 62:2569–2581, 2010.

Aletaha D, Smolen JS: Diagnosis and management of rheumatoid arthritis: a review, *JAMA* 320:1360–1372, 2018.

Anderson J, Caplan L, Yazdany J, et al: Rheumatoid arthritis disease activity measures: American College of Rheumatology recommendations for use in clinical practice, *Arthritis Care Res (Hoboken)* 64:640–647, 2012.

Goodman SM, Springer B, Guyatt G, et al: 2017 American College of Rheumatology/American Association of Hip and Knee Surgeons guideline for the perioperative management of antirheumatic medication in patients with rheumatic diseases undergoing elective total hip or total knee arthroplasty, *Arthritis Care Res* 69:1111–1124, 2017.

Hochberg M: *Rheumatology*, Seventh edition, Philadelphia, PA, 2019, Elsevier. 2019.

Singh JA, Saag KG, Bridges Jr SL, et al: 2015 American College of Rheumatology guidelines for the treatment of rheumatoid arthritis, *Arthritis Care Res (Hoboken)* 68:1–25, 2016.

Smolen JS, Landewe R, Bijlsma JS, et al: EULAR recommendations for the management of rheumatoid arthritis with synthetic and biologic disease-modifying antirheumatic drugs: 2016 update, *Ann Rheum Dis* 76:960–977, 2017.

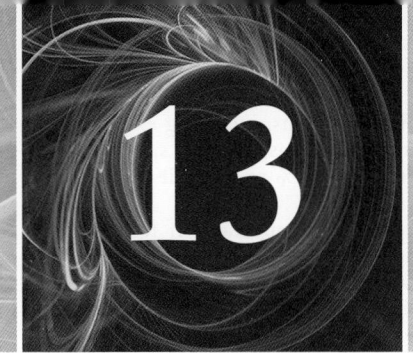

13 Sexually Transmitted Diseases

CHLAMYDIA TRACHOMATIS

Method of
Tracy L. Williams, MD

CURRENT DIAGNOSIS

- Screen all sexually active woman 25 years of age or younger for *C. trachomatis* annually regardless of symptoms per the CDC recommendations.
- Symptomatic patients should be tested regardless of gender.
- Reinfection with *C. trachomatis* is common.
  - Retest all patients who have a history of *C. trachomatis* or *N. gonorrhea* at 3 to 6 months following treatment, regardless of whether their partner(s) were treated.
  - If the patient does not follow up at 3 to 6 months, then retest upon presentation for medical care within the first 12 months posttreatment.
- Patients who screen positive for *C. trachomatis* need to be screened for gonorrhea, syphilis, and HIV.
- Perform test of cure on pregnant patients at 3 to 4 weeks posttreatment and repeat in 3 to 6 months, preferably in the third trimester if the pregnant woman was diagnosed during the first trimester.
- Rescreen pregnant patients for other sexually transmitted infections (STIs) 3 months posttreatment including gonorrhea, syphilis, and HIV.

CURRENT THERAPY

- Azithromycin (Zithromycin) 1 g orally in a single dose or doxycycline (Vibramycin) 100 mg orally twice a day for 7 days are the recommended regimens for nonpregnant patients and for presumptive treatment for *C. trachomatis*.
- All of the patient's recent sexual partners need referral and treatment.
  - The patient's last sexual contact should be referred and treated if it has been more than 60 days since the patient had a sexual partner.
  - The partner needs to be treated for *C. trachomatis* even if his or her personal STI results are negative.
- Counsel patients and their partners to abstain from sexual contact until 7 days after one-dose therapy or after the final dose of the 7-day regimen.
- The CDC recommends patients who test positive for *N. gonorrhea* only be treated for *C. trachomatis* when coinfection is not excluded.

Epidemiology

Chlamydia trachomatis is the most common notifiable sexually transmitted infection (STI) in the United States, with an incidence of over 1.8 million cases per year according to the Centers for Disease Control and Prevention (CDC) in 2018. Women age 15 to 19 years are the most commonly affected, followed by women age 20 to 24. The incidence of *C. trachomatis* has steadily climbed yearly since it became a federally mandated notifiable disease; part of this is an artifact of improved screening practices that are discovering disease in asymptomatic patients.

C. trachomatis costs an estimated $2.4 billon annually. Cost-benefit analyses have consistently shown prioritizing screening efforts in asymptomatic women to be cost-effective.

Risk Factors

The risk of contracting *C. trachomatis* increases with: multiple sexual partners; unprotected sex including vaginal, oral, and anal intercourse; anal-receptive intercourse; and men having sex with men. The risk increases in the presence of other coinfections including human immunodeficiency virus (HIV) or herpes simplex virus (HSV). African Americans have a fourfold higher incidence compared to their white counterparts (13% versus 2.4%, respectively).

Pathophysiology

Chlamydia trachomatis is an obligate intracellular parasite. It is found only in human cells, but can live on fomites for up to 30 hours. Previous infections do not yield protection against future infections with *C. trachomatis*. *C. trachomatis* does not infect the squamous epithelium of the vaginal vault, but can infect the urethra, the squamocolumnar junction of the cervix, the rectal mucosa, and the oropharynx.

Prevention

Prevention depends on screening of asymptomatic patients, who make up a large portion of the infected population. The United States Preventive Task Force (USPSTF) recommends annual screening of all sexually active women younger than 25 years of age and for older women at increased risk.

The CDC and the USPSTF found insufficient evidence to recommend routine screening of men based on cost-effectiveness, efficacy, and practicality, but screening of symptomatic men or men in areas with high prevalence of *Chlamydia*, including men having sex with men, men in correctional facilities, and men visiting STI clinics, is recommended. Overall, screening of men is recommended so long as it does not detract resources from the screening of women. Symptomatic patients should be tested regardless of gender.

Men who have sex with other men are at high risk for bacterial and viral STI. The CDC STI screening recommendation in this group is an annual test for urethral infection with *C. trachomatis* and *N. gonorrhea*. The preferred methodology is testing the urine using nucleic acid amplification technique (NAAT). Men who have receptive anal intercourse are recommended to have annual anal screening for both *C. trachomatis* and *N. gonorrhea*. Men who have oral receptive sex are also advised to have pharyngeal screening for *N. gonorrhea* but not *C. trachomatis*. The NAAT is only Food and Drug Administration (FDA)–approved on urine in the above scenarios but is used off-label in laboratories that have met all regulatory requirements.

Patients who screen positive for *Chlamydia* need to be screened for other STIs, including gonorrhea, syphilis, and HIV.

Abstinence and monogamous relationships are ideal to help prevent the transmission of *C. trachomatis*. Safer sex practices to limit the spread of *C. trachomatis* include the consistent use of condoms. Epidemiologic studies show that people often base their decision to use condoms on their perception of their partner's risk. Given the high prevalence of asymptomatic *C. trachomatis* infections in certain American populations, selective condom use is not an effective strategy.

Clinical Manifestations

Most infections are asymptomatic. However, some women will report vaginal discharge, postcoital or intermenstrual bleeding, or lower abdominal pain. Men are more commonly symptomatic than women and may report dysuria or urethral discharge.

Untreated *C. trachomatis* in women has significant health sequelae. Approximately 40% of women with untreated *Chlamydia* go on to develop pelvic inflammatory disease (PID). Women with PID may become infertile (20%), develop debilitating chronic pelvic pain (18%), or suffer ectopic pregnancy (9%).

Men do not tend to suffer as severe sequelae from *C. trachomatis*. The most common illness is urethritis, but men may also suffer epididymitis, proctitis, and conjunctivitis. Reactive arthritis is also more common in men.

Diagnosis

Tests used for detection of *C. trachomatis* can be divided into molecular (NAAT, DNA probing, and hybrid capture), antigen detection (direct immunofluorescence and enzyme immunoassay), and cell culture.

The most reliable method of testing for *C. trachomatis* is NAAT. It is FDA-approved for use on vaginal/endocervical secretions, male intraurethral swabs, and first-catch urine. It is not FDA-approved for rectal or orophyngeal use but is used off label in laboratories as described above. The primary benefit of NAAT is the lack of a need for viable organisms to induce a positive test result; this increases its sensitivity to more than 95% because of the ability to detect *C. trachomatis* even if only one copy of the targeted RNA or DNA is present. Its specificity is also desirable at 99%.

C. trachomatis cell culture is used as the reference standard for all testing but has many limitations, including expense, long turnaround time (72 hours), and transport and specimen storage requirements. Its sensitivity is 80% to 85%. It is not readily available.

Limiting barriers to screening is important. If testing in the clinic is difficult to arrange, self-collected vaginal swab specimens perform at least as well as other approved specimens using NAAT. First-catch urine NAAT testing is also more acceptable to many patients, particularly asymptomatic men and women who do not otherwise need a pelvic examination.

Differential Diagnosis

Infection with *Chlamydia* is often asymptomatic but is included in the differential diagnosis of various organ system complaints. It should be ruled out in any sexually active patient presenting with urethritis, mucopurulent cervicitis, epididymitis, and proctitis. There is significant overlap in the symptoms caused by *C. trachomatis* with *N. gonorrhea*, so testing for both bacteria with NAAT is preferred. Other agents that are included in the differential diagnosis after *C. trachomatis* and *N. gonorrhea* have been ruled out include: *Trichomonas vaginalis*, HSV, adenovirus, *Mycoplasma* species, and *Ureaplasma*. More specifically, persistent urethritis after treatment with doxycycline (Vibramycin) can be caused by infection with *T. vaginalis* or doxycycline-resistant *Urea urealyticum* or *Mycoplasma genitalium*.

C. trachomatis should be ruled out in newborn infants with conjunctivitis in the first 30 days of life or pneumonia at 1 to 3 months of life, especially if they were born to mothers with untreated chlamydial infections.

Treatment

Recommendations for treatment regimens are summarized in Box 1. The benefit of using single-dose azithromycin (Zithromycin) is the ability to directly observe the patient taking the therapy.

BOX 1 | *Chlamydia trachomatis:* Recommended Treatment Regimens by Clinical Syndrome

Cervicitis or urethritis or for presumptive treatment in nonpregnant patient*
- Azithromycin (Zithromycin) 1 g orally in a single dose
or
- Doxycycline (Vibramycin) 100 mg orally twice a day for 7 days

Alternative regimens (one of the following)
- Erythromycin base (E-Mycin) 500 mg orally four times a day for 7 days
or
- Erythromycin ethylsuccinate (EES) 800 mg orally four times a day for 7 days
or
- Levofloxacin (Levaquin)[1] 500 mg orally once daily for 7 days
or
- Ofloxacin (Floxin) 300 mg orally twice a day for 7 days

Pregnant patient with cervicitis or urethritis*
- Azithromycin 1 g orally in a single dose
or
- Amoxicillin 500 mg orally three times a day for 7 days

Alternative regimens
- Erythromycin base 500 mg orally four times a day for 7 days
or
- Erythromycin base[†] 250 mg orally four times a day for 14 days
or

- Erythromycin ethylsuccinate 800 mg orally four times a day for 7 days
or
- Erythromycin ethylsuccinate[†] 400 mg orally four times a day for 14 days

Epididymitis
- Ceftriaxone (Rocephin) 250 mg IM in a single dose
  plus
- Doxycycline 100 mg orally twice a day for 10 days

Ophthalmia neonatorum or C. trachomatis pneumonia
- Erythromycin base or ethylsuccinate 50 mg/kg/day orally divided into 4 doses daily for 14 days[‡]

Recommended regimen for children who weigh <45 kg
- Erythromycin base or ethylsuccinate 50 mg/kg/day orally divided into 4 doses daily for 14 days

Recommended regimen for children who weigh ≥45 kg but who are <8 years old
- Azithromycin 1 g orally in a single dose

Recommended regimens for children aged ≥8 years
- Azithromycin 1 gram orally in a single dose
or
- Doxycycline 100 mg orally twice a day for 7 days

Inpatient and outpatient PID
- Please refer to PID chapter for treatment regimens

Providers should consult the Centers for Disease Control and Prevention's website at http://cdc.gov/std/treatment for up-to-date treatment recommendations.
*Consider concurrent treatment for gonococcal infection if prevalence of gonorrhea is high in the patient population under assessment.
[1]Not FDA approved for this indication
[†]The lower-dose and longer-treatment option with erythromycin can be considered if gastrointestinal tolerance is an issue.
[‡]Infants <6 weeks of age who are treated with erythromycin should be followed for signs and symptoms of infantile hypertrophic pyloric stenosis.

The 7-day course of doxycycline (Vibramycin) has comparable cure rates to azithromycin, but decreased compliance.

Presumptive treatment for *C. trachomatis* should be considered for high-risk patients with cervicitis. High-risk patients include women up to 25 years old, those with new or multiple sexual partners, those who engage in unprotected sex, especially if follow-up cannot be ensured, and those for whom a relatively insensitive diagnostic test is used in place of NAAT.

The CDC only recommends presumptive treatment for *C. trachomatis* for patients being treated for *N. gonorrhea* when coinfection is not excluded. Coinfection is common, as illustrated in a study that found 20% of men with *N. gonorrhea* and 42% of women with *N. gonorrhea* were also infected with *C. trachomatis*. Cotreatment is also recommended in the hope that it will impede the development of antimicrobial-resistant *N. gonorrhea*.

Chlamydia trachomatis is a reportable infectious disease. The patient is instructed to refer all of his or her sexual partners for testing and treatment if they have had sexual contact during the previous 60 days. If the patient has not been sexually active for the last 60 days, then the patient is to refer his or her most recent sexual contact. The patient's recent sexual partners should be treated empirically even if their personal STI evaluation returns negative results. The patient and his or her sexual partners should be counseled to abstain from sexual activity for 7 days post treatment. Reinfection, rather than recurrence, is the more common etiology of repeat *C. trachomatis* infection.

Expedited partner therapy is an option in certain cases. This entails the patient delivering the antibiotic to his or her partner(s) without a physician first seeing the patient. Patients are to give their partners written materials on the importance of following up with a physician if any signs of complications occur (e.g., pelvic pain in women or testicular pain in men). It can be used effectively in certain situations but is not routinely recommended in men who have sex with men because of the high risk for coexisting infections, especially undiagnosed HIV infection, in their partners. Please refer to the CDC website (www.cdc.gov/std/ept) to check on legality in individual states. In general, utilizing the traditional patient-physician model is preferred.

Infants born to women with untreated *C. trachomatis* infection are at increased risk for vertical transmission. Prophylactic treatment with oral erythromycin (E-Mycin) for *C. trachomatis* is not recommended. The state-mandated standard erythromycin eye ointment (Ilotycin) that all newborns receive is still indicated. Overall, infants born to infected mothers need to be closely monitored for any signs and symptoms of infection and treated appropriately.

Intrauterine devices (IUDs) have regained popularity in the United States after they were implicated in causing PID in the 1970s. The IUD has evolved and now the risk of PID appears increased only in the first three weeks postinsertion. If *C. trachomatis* or PID is contracted with an IUD in place, practitioners must decide if the IUD should be removed. Research has found insufficient evidence to mandate removal, but close follow-up is mandatory.

Monitoring

Repeat testing is recommended for all patients, including pregnant women, treated for *C. trachomatis* at 3 months regardless of the treatment status of the patient's partner(s) because reinfection is so common. If the patient does not follow up at 3 months, he or she should be retested upon presentation for medical care within the first 12 months posttreatment.

Test of cure, which is testing at 3 to 4 weeks posttreatment, is recommended only for pregnant patients. Testing for cure earlier than 3 to 4 weeks increases the rate of false positive results. The pregnant woman who is treated for *C. trachomatis* during the pregnancy also qualifies to be rescreened in the third trimester for *N. gonorrhea*, HIV, and syphilis in addition to *C. trachomatis*.

Complications

C. trachomatis is a major public health concern because it results in serious health complications and sequelae. In women it can cause PID, endometritis, ectopic pregnancy, infertility, salpingitis, and perihepatitis (Fitz-Hugh-Curtis syndrome). In men it is associated with postgonococcal or nongonococcal urethritis and epididymitis. Reactive arthritis can occur in both men and women.

C. trachomatis is especially problematic in pregnancy because it is associated with an increased risk of preterm labor and preterm premature rupture of membranes. Infants born to women infected with *Chlamydia* risk suffering pneumonia and conjunctivitis.

C. trachomatis pneumonia can present as an afebrile pneumonia often with a staccato cough without wheezing between 1 and 3 months of life. *C. trachomatis* conjunctivitis, also known as ophthalmia neonatorum, is uncommon in the United States, but worldwide it is the number one cause of blindness. It usually presents within the 5th and 12th day of life but can present at up to 1 month of age. State-mandated prophylactic eye ointment given to babies at birth mainly helps prevent gonococcal ophthalmia; it does not prevent perinatal transmission of *Chlamydia* from mother to infant. Therefore the screening of pregnant women and ultimate treatment of their *Chlamydia* during pregnancy is the best method of preventing complications in newborn infants.

References

Bebear C, de Barbeyrac B: Genital *Chlamydia trachomatis* infections, *Clin Microbiol Infect* 15:4–10, 2009.

Blas MM, Canchihuaman FA, Alva IE, et al: Pregnancy outcomes in women infected with *Chlamydia trachomatis*: a population-based cohort study in Washington State, *Sex Transm Infect* 83:314–318, 2007.

Centers for Disease Control and Prevention (CDC). Sexually Transmitted Disease Surveillance 2018. Available at: https://www.cdc.gov/std/stats18/ [accessed March 7, 2021].

Centers for Disease Control and Prevention (CDC). Sexually transmitted diseases treatment guidelines 2015. MMWR Recomm Rep 2015;64(No. 3):[55–60].

Honey E, Augood C, Templeton A, et al: Cost effectiveness of screening for *Chlamydia trachomatis*: a review of published studies, *Sex Transm Infect* 78:406–412, 2002.

Johnson RE, Newhall WJ, Papp JR, et al: Screening tests to detect *Chlamydia trachomatis* and *Neisseria gonorrhoeae* infections—2002, *MMWR Recomm Rep* 51(RR-15):1–38, 2002.

Kramer A, Schewebke I, Kampf G: How long do nosocomial pathogens persist on inanimate surfaces? A systematic review, *BMC Infect Dis* 6:130, 2006.

LeFevre ML: U.S. Preventive Services Task Force. Screening for chlamydia and gonorrhea: U.S. Preventive Services Task Force recommendation statement, *Ann Intern Med.* 161(12):902–910, 2014.

Lyss SB, Kamb ML, Peterman TA, et al: *Chlamydia trachomatis* among patients infected with and treated for *Neisseria gonorrhoeae* in sexually transmitted clinics in the United States, *Ann Intern Med* 139:178–185, 2003.

St. Cyr S, Barbee L, Workowski KA, et al: Update to CDC's Treatment Guidelines for Gonococcal Infection, 2020. MMWR Morb Mortal Wkly Rep, 69:1911–1916, 2020.

CONDYLOMATA ACUMINATA

Method of
M. Chantel Long, MD

CURRENT DIAGNOSIS

- Condylomata acuminata are usually flesh-colored, brown, or gray and can be flat, plaquelike, or exophytic papules, giving them the classic "cauliflower" appearance.
- The lesions may be single or multiple and can range in size from minute to several centimeters in diameter.
- When the appearance of the lesion is typical, confirmatory tests are usually unnecessary.
- Suspicious lesions or uncertain diagnoses warrant biopsy to rule out malignancy.

CURRENT THERAPY

- In the absence of dysplasia, treatment of subclinical human papilloma virus infection is not recommended.
- The goal of therapy is to eliminate symptoms, namely clinically apparent warts, rather than address the underlying HPV infection.
- Common treatment options include podofilox (Condylox), imiquimod (Aldara, Zyclara), sinecatechins (Veregen), podophyllin resin (Podocon-25), trichloroacetic acid (Tri-Chlor), cryotherapy, and surgery.

Epidemiology

Condylomata acuminata, commonly known as genital warts, is a sexually transmitted disease caused by the human papilloma virus (HPV). It is estimated that 20 million people are infected with HPV in the United States, with the highest prevalence in adolescents and young adults. Lifetime incidence of HPV infection is greater than 50% and appears to be increasing, making it the most common sexually transmitted disease.

Risk Factors

Risk factors associated with HPV infection include sex with an infected partner, early age at first sexual intercourse, multiple sexual partners, history of sexually transmitted infections, cigarette smoking, and lack of condom use. The majority of patients whose sexual partner has condyloma will themselves develop condyloma within 3 months. An even larger percentage of people are believed to develop subclinical infection.

Pathophysiology

About 90% of warts are caused by HPV types 6 and 11; condyloma can be coinfected with types 16, 18, 31, 33, 35, and 45, which have oncogenic potential. Genital skin appears to be less susceptible to the oncogenic potential of HPV compared to the transformation zones of the cervix and anal canal.

The virus is easily transmitted via sexual contact. Vertical transmission and autoinoculation are possible. The average incubation period between infection and appearance of condyloma ranges from 3 months to several years. Condyloma can persist or recur after therapy, undergo malignant transformation, or spontaneously regress.

Prevention

Prevention options include HPV vaccination, abstinence, routine condom use, and limiting sexual partners. Once patients have condyloma, they should be encouraged to use condoms consistently. Educate patients that condoms can decrease transmission but might not completely prevent infection.

Two HPV vaccine series are currently available in the United States. Gardasil is a quadrivalent HPV vaccine indicated for male and female patients aged 9 to 25 years for prevention of cervical cancer and genital warts. Cervarix is the bivalent vaccine indicated for female patients aged 9 to 25 years for prevention of cervical cancer.

Clinical Manifestations

Most genital warts are asymptomatic on presentation, although patients can present with complaints of a "bump." Localized irritation, pruritus, pain, or bleeding can occur, and symptoms may vary based on the location and size of the lesions. Usually, the warts appear flesh-colored, brown, or gray and can be flat, plaquelike, or exophytic papules, giving them the classic "cauliflower" appearance. The lesions may be single or multiple and range in size from minute to several centimeters in diameter. Flat HPV lesions might not be grossly visible.

The majority of HPV infections are either subclinical or unrecognized. Clinically apparent disease might represent only a small portion of the actual infected area.

Diagnosis

When the clinical appearance of the lesion is typical, confirmatory tests are usually unnecessary. The entire anogenital tract should be examined because of the widespread nature of HPV. A magnifying glass and anoscopy may be helpful for thorough detection and examination. Application of dilute 3% to 5% acetic acid solution to the skin surface can help detect subtle HPV lesions by producing an acetowhitening of the condyloma; however, this is not a specific test and is not routinely recommended. Pap smears or tissue biopsy can provide histopathologic confirmation of the diagnosis. Biopsy is recommended to rule out malignancy in any suspicious lesions, such as large or rapidly growing condyloma; pigmented, atypical, friable, bleeding, or ulcerated lesions; sites of previous treatment failure; areas of recurrence; acetowhite lesions; or lesions in immunocompromised patients. Although costly and not recommended, HPV identification via DNA testing can be performed.

Differential Diagnosis

Table 1 outlines the differential diagnosis for condylomata acuminata.

TABLE 1	Differential Diagnosis
LESION	**APPEARANCE**
Verruca vulgaris	Occurs anywhere Tends to be thicker, drier, and hyperkeratotic
Molluscum contagiosum	Occurs anywhere Smooth, round papules with central umbilication
Seborrheic keratoses	Occurs anywhere Multiple waxy, rough, hyperpigmented papules
Condyloma latum	Moist, rounded, white papules of syphilis
Pearly penile papules	Smooth, uniform, small, 1–2mm at corona, benign
Vestibular papillae	Both sides of vulva, female equivalent of pearly penile papules
Lichen planus	Purplish, pruritic rash or flat-topped polygonal papules
Nonpigmented nevi	Occurs anywhere Flat or raised, reddish or flesh colored

	DRUG	USE ON	ADVANTAGES	DISADVANTAGES	INSTRUCTIONS

TABLE 2 Treatment Regimens

DRUG	USE ON	ADVANTAGES	DISADVANTAGES	INSTRUCTIONS
Patient Applied				
Podofilox 0.5% gel or solution (Condylox)	Moist warts	Relatively inexpensive	Avoid in pregnancy Avoid on mucous membranes Do not exceed 10cm^2 area Do not exceed 0.5mL daily; can have systemic side effects	Apply bid × 3d, then 4d off Repeat weekly May use for 4–6 cycles
Imiquimod 5% cream (Aldara)	Dry or moist warts		Avoid with large warts >10cm^2 Requires compliance Hypo- or hyperpigmentation of treated skin can occur	Apply nightly on dry warts Apply every other night on moist warts Use up to 16wk Wash off after 6–10h
Sinecatechins 15% ointment (Veregen)	Dry warts		Avoid in pregnancy Avoid in immunocompromised patients	Apply tid Use up to 16wk Do not wash off
Provider Applied				
Podophyllin resin (Podocon-25, Podofilm)	Moist warts	Use on large warts May use on urethral meatus	Avoid in pregnancy Do not exceed 10cm^2 area Do not exceed 0.5mL daily; can have systemic side effects	Apply thin layer with cotton tip Allow to air dry Repeat weekly Leave on for 4h Do not cover May leave on overnight if tolerated
Trichloroacetic acid (TCA) (Tri-Chlor 80%)	Small, few Moist warts	May use on vagina, cervix May use on anal warts May use in pregnancy	Avoid with dry and large warts	Apply sparingly with cotton tip Air dry Repeat weekly to every other week Do not allow to "run" on normal skin Neutralize with soap or sodium bicarbonate
Cryotherapy	Small, few, flat Dry or moist	May use in pregnancy May use liquid nitrogen in vagina, meatus, anus	Avoid with large warts Avoid cryoprobe use in vagina or anus	Freeze q1–2wk Freeze 1–2mm border May offer/need local anesthesia
Surgery	Small or large Dry or moist	May use on anal warts Use on large warts and large treatment areas	Avoid in patients with bleeding disorder	Scissors, shave biopsy, punch excision, curettage, cautery, laser
Interferon-α-2b injections (Intron A)	Refractory warts		Expensive Flulike side effects	Multiple intralesional injections Several times a week Often requires specialty referral
Laser vaporization	Refractory warts	May use on intraurethral and large warts as well as large treatment areas	Expensive	Requires specialty referral

Condylomata Acuminata

1009

Treatment

In the absence of dysplasia, the Centers for Disease Control and Prevention recommends no treatment of subclinical HPV infection. The goal of treatment is to eliminate symptoms, namely clinically apparent warts, rather than address the underlying HPV infection. Current treatments do not eradicate the virus.

Ideally, treatment of condyloma should continue until all warts are gone. A repeated course of therapy is often required to achieve a wart-free state. Recurrence may be due to latent HPV in the surrounding normal tissue, HPV reinfection, or improper selection or use of a therapy modality. Nearly all treatment regimens have similar efficacy and rates of intolerance and toxicity. All are known to cause local pain and irritation. Any given treatment has a 40% to 80% rate of wart clearance and up to a 50% recurrence rate. It is unknown whether eliminating warts will decrease infectivity of current or future sexual partners.

The factors to consider when deciding on treatment include location and size of the warts, the patient's tolerance and preference, cost, convenience, and the clinician's preference. Patient-applied options allow the patient greater control; however, this requires good compliance, and the warts must be accessible by the patient or caregiver. Provider-applied treatments are good choices for large treatment areas. Data regarding the efficacy of using more than one modality at a time are lacking. It is common practice for health care providers to combine treatment modalities. Table 2 outlines current therapy regimens. Topical fluorouracil (Efudex)[1] is no longer recommended. Failure to respond after four treatments or failure to clear within 3 months warrants a change in therapy modality and possible reevaluation of the diagnosis.

Advise patients to abstain from sexual activity while undergoing treatment for genital warts.

Monitoring

Counseling of patients regarding prevention and recognition of condyloma as well as screening and treatment of sexual partners should be part of the comprehensive management plan. One

---

[1]Not FDA approved for this indication.

should consider testing for other sexually transmitted diseases because they often coexist with HPV. Encourage patients to discuss their HPV diagnosis with sexual partners. Asymptomatic partners likely harbor a subclinical infection, and examination for genital warts is appropriate if lesions are suspected. Discuss the need for smoking cessation and regular physician examinations, including Pap smears, as ways to prevent early HPV-related neoplasm.

Complications

Anogenital HPV infection with high-risk genotypes is associated with squamous cell carcinoma of the cervix, vagina, vulva, penis, and anus. Persistent HPV infection is the most important risk factor for development of cervical intraepithelial neoplasia and cancer.

References

American Academy of Pediatrics. Human papillomavirus. In: Pickering LK, Baker CJ, Kimberlin DW, Long SS, editors. Red Book: 2009 Report of the Committee on Infectious Diseases. 28th ed. Elk Grove Village, IL: American Academy of Pediatrics; 2009. p. 477–483.

Centers for Disease Control and Prevention: *Epidemiology and Prevention of Vaccine-Preventable Diseases. The Pink Book*, ed 12, Washington, DC, 2011, Public Health Foundation.

Centers for Disease Control and Prevention: 2010 Sexually transmitted diseases treatment guidelines, *MMWR* 59:1–5, 2010. 69–78.

Centers for Disease Control and Prevention. Human papillomavirus: HPV information for clinicians. Available at www.cdc.gov/std/hpv/Provider6-2005/ApF1-DesignA.pdf [accessed August 6, 2015].

Gilbert SM, Lambert SM, Weiner D: Extensive condylomata acuminata of the penis: Medical and surgical management, *Infect Urol* 16:65–76, 2003.

Kodner CM, Nasrat S: Management of genital warts, *Am Fam Physician* 70:2335–2342, 2004.

GENITAL ULCER DISEASE: CHANCROID, GRANULOMA INGUINALE, AND LYMPHOGRANULOMA

Method of
Todd Stephens, MD

Chancroid, granuloma inguinale, and lymphogranuloma venereum (LGV) are important genital ulcer diseases that should be included in the differential diagnosis of patients presenting with anal or genital ulcers with or without inguinal adenopathy. Syphilis and herpes simplex virus testing should be considered on all such patients because of similarities in clinical presentation. Testing or treatment for other potential sexually transmitted infections (STIs), including HIV, should be considered given the high risk for concomitant infection.

Chancroid

History

Chancroid, also called soft sore, was first distinguished from the hard chancre of syphilis by Ricord in 1838. Ducrey, in Naples, demonstrated that inoculation of material from the chancroid ulcer into the skin of the forearm could reproduce the ulcer, and he went on to identify the causative organism, which bears his name.

Epidemiology

Chancroid is an important cause of genital ulceration in most countries of the developing world, accounting for about 10 million cases annually. Chancroid was diagnosed in 60% of patients who had genital ulcers and who presented to STI clinics in Africa before the HIV epidemic. Now, herpes simplex lesions represent a higher percentage. The prevalence of this disease is highest among commercial sex workers, and the presence of chancroid lesions significantly increases the risk of transmission of HIV. Although generally rare in industrialized countries, there have been several well-documented outbreaks in urban centers of North America, particularly among men who have sex with men.

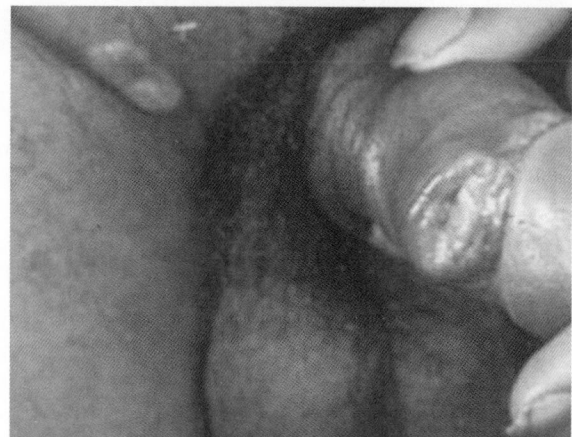

Figure 1 Chancroid. This photo shows an early chancroid ulcer on the penis along with accompanying regional inguinal adenopathy. (Courtesy of Dr. Pirozzi, Centers for Disease Control and Prevention.)

Etiology

Chancroid is caused by *Haemophilus ducreyi*, a small anaerobic Gram-negative bacillus that forms streptobacillary chains on Gram stain and grows only on enriched media.

Clinical Features

After an incubation of 3 to 7 days, a papule appears that soon ulcerates, leaving a soft ulcer with an undermined edge and a purulent base. Vesicles are not seen. About half of patients develop unilateral inguinal adenopathy (Figure 1). Both the adenopathy and the lesions are very painful. Lesions can be single or multiple, and atypical presentations occur. Kissing lesions often occur on adjacent cutaneous surfaces. Not infrequently, a giant ulcer develops with several smaller satellite ulcers around the periphery, which can mimic the ulcerative phase of herpes simplex. More than half of the lesions occur on the prepuce, particularly in uncircumcised men. In women, the majority of lesions are on the fourchette, labia, and perianal area. Adenopathy can progress to bubo formation with tender, overlying erythema. These buboes can rupture and produce inguinal abscesses.

Diagnosis

Gram stain of smears obtained from the ulcer base has been advocated in the past for diagnosis, but this lacks both sensitivity and specificity. The preferred diagnostic modality is swabs for culture from the ulcer base or undermined edge. These are plated directly on enriched media (GC agar and Mueller-Hinton agar base) and incubated for 72 hours in an atmosphere of 5% carbon dioxide at 33°C. Polymerase chain reaction (PCR) and immunochromatography tests are also available.

Treatment

The Centers for Disease Control and Prevention (CDC) recommend a syndromal management approach in which a positive diagnosis is suggested if the patient has one or more painful ulcers and no evidence of syphilis or herpes simplex virus. Ulcers with painful adenopathy are pathognomonic (Table 1 lists antimicrobial treatment). The safety and efficacy of azithromycin (Zithromax) for pregnant and lactating women have not been established. Ciprofloxacin (Cipro)[1] is contraindicated during pregnancy and lactation. No adverse effects of chancroid on pregnancy outcome have been reported. Serologic testing for syphilis, HIV, and other appropriate STIs should be performed. Chancroidal ulcers should be kept clean with regular washing in soapy water and kept dry. Fluctuant buboes might require incision and drainage, which is preferable over needle aspiration. Treatment of all sexual partners within 60 days should be

[1]Not FDA approved for this indication.

TABLE 1 Clinical Features and Treatment Summary of Chancroid, Granuloma Inguinale, and Lymphogranuloma Venereum

FEATURES AND TREATMENT	CHANCROID	GRANULOMA INGUINALE	LYMPHOGRANULOMA VENEREUM
Clinical Features			
Incubation period	3–7 days	3–40 days	1–28 days
Primary lesion	Papule	Papule	Papule or vesicle
Ulcerative lesion painful	Yes	No	No
Lymphadenopathy	Yes (unilateral)	No	Yes (unilateral or bilateral)
Base	Purulent	Raised, easily bleeds	Nonvascular
Border	Round, raised, undermined edges	Irregular, expansion along skin folds	Irregular, ragged
Treatment			
Treatment of choice (any of the options listed)	Azithromycin (Zithromycin) 1g Ciprofloxacin (Cipro)[1] 500mg bid × 3d Ceftriaxone (Rocephin)[1] 250mg IM once	Azithromycin[1] 1g PO once a week or 500 mg qd for >3 weeks until all lesions have completely healed Doxycycline (Vibramycin) 100mg bid × 3 wks	Azithromycin[1] 1g weekly × 3wk Doxycycline 100mg bid × 3wk
Alternative treatment (any of the options listed)	Erythromycin (Ery-Tab)[1] 500mg qid × 7d	Azithromycin[1] 1g PO qwk × 3 wk Erythromycin[1] 500mg qid × 3 wk Ciprofloxacin[1] 750mg bid × 3 wk Ceftriaxone[1] 1 gm IM daily for at least 3 weeks and until all lesions have completely healed.	Erythromycin[1] 500mg qid × 3wk

[1]Not FDA approved for this indication.

pursued, and treatment is similar to that for the source patient. Patients should not engage in sexual activity until the ulcers are healed.

Granuloma Inguinale (Donovanosis)

History
Granuloma inguinale was first recognized in India, where Donovan observed, in an oral lesion of the disease, the bodies that bear his name. There is considerable confusion about terminology between this disease and LGV, because various similar synonyms have been used inconsistently. Adding to the confusion, Donovan's name is associated with two tropical diseases that he discovered: leishmaniasis, with the discovery of intracellular protozoan inclusions that bear his name (Leishman-Donovan bodies), and granuloma inguinale (whose intracellular inclusions were believed to be caused by protozoa but are now known to be caused by bacteria).

Epidemiology
Endemic areas are localized to a few specific areas of the tropics, particularly India, Papua New Guinea, Brazil, and the eastern part of South Africa, particularly Durban. Commercial sex workers and men are primarily involved.

Etiology
The disease is caused by an encapsulated Gram-negative coccobacillus *Klebsiella granulomatis* (previously known as *Calymmatobacterium* or *Donovania granulomatis*).

Clinical Features
A firm, painless papule or nodule is the presenting sign of granuloma inguinale. The incubation period is variable from 3 to 40 days from inoculation. This nodule quickly ulcerates, and the base is highly vascular, is beefy red, and bleeds easily. Lymphadenopathy is not part of the clinical presentation of this disease, distinguishing granuloma inguinale from chancroid and LGV. However, the ulcer can be easily confused with chancroid, condyloma lata, ulcerated verrucous warts, and squamous carcinoma. Untreated, the ulcers slowly expand, particularly along skin folds

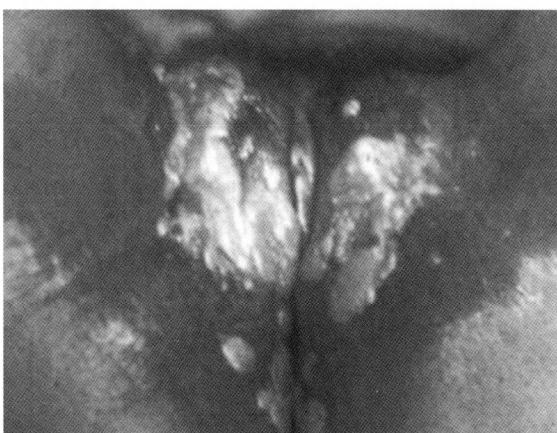

Figure 2 Granuloma inguinale. (Source: NEHC http://www.nhec.med.navy.mil/hp/sharp/std_pictures.htm)

toward the inguinal region or anus (Figure 2). The ulcers are flat and raised and have slightly hypertrophic margins, but the bases are typically free of pus and necrotic debris. Less-common presentations include extragenital lesions involving the neck and mouth; cervical lesions that resemble carcinoma; and involvement of the uterus, tubes, and ovaries, producing hard masses, abscesses, or frozen pelvis.

Diagnosis
Diagnosis requires the demonstration of intracellular Donovan bodies from Giemsa or Wright staining of smears taken from a swab of the ulcer base or from biopsy material.

Treatment
See Table 1 for antimicrobial treatment. Treatment should be continued until lesions are resolved and, if possible, a little longer to reduce the risk of relapse.

Lymphogranuloma Venereum

History
LGV was first differentiated from syphilis in 1906 by Wasserman, though the first full description of the disease was given by Durand, Nicolas, and Favre in 1913. In 1925, Frei developed an intradermal skin test that gave positive responses in most LGV patients. The term "tropical bubo" was associated with the disease later.

Epidemiology
LGV is largely confined to the tropics and is not a common STI. The global overall incidence is in a decline. It is seen more commonly in men, but since 2004, there has been a resurgence manifesting as proctitis in North America and Europe among HIV-positive men who have sex with men.

Etiology
LGV is a chlamydial infection caused by the invasive L1, L2, and L3 serovars of *Chlamydia trachomatis*, an intracellular gramnegative bacterium.

Clinical Features
LGV is essentially a systemic disease whose natural course is divided into three distinct phases. The initial phase of LGV is normally an inconspicuous genital lesion beginning as a typically small, painless papule or vesicle occurring 1 to 28 days after inoculation. This papule or vesicle quickly ulcerates and heals without a scar, and it often goes unrecognized by the patient (Figure 3). However, the second phase of LGV is the development of increasingly painful lymphadenopathy, often with fever and malaise. The lymphadenopathy progresses to bubo formation over 1 to 2 weeks. When a sexually active adult patient presents with an inguinal bubo not associated with genital ulcers, LGV is an important diagnosis to consider. The infected nodes are usually unilateral (bilateral in a third of cases) and often coalesce into a matted mass that can project outwards above or below the inguinal ligament, producing the pathognomonic groove sign present in 20% of patients with LGV. The buboes are likely to rupture, forming multiple sinuses. Untreated, LGV can cause extensive lymphatic damage, resulting in elephantiasis of the genitalia. Anal involvement, likewise, can lead to perirectal abscesses, fistulas, and rectal strictures. These complications represent the late phase of LGV.

Diagnosis
The diagnosis of LGV can only be confirmed using PCR methods of smears, scrapings, or aspirated material. Alternatively, the ability to perform micro-immunofluorescence serology testing using a fluorescein-conjugated monoclonal antibody and viewing the slide with a fluorescence microscope can demonstrate the inclusion bodies within the cytoplasm of macrophages. Gram staining by itself lacks appropriate sensitivity or specificity. Additional laboratory findings include leukocytosis, elevated erythrocyte sedimentation rate, and increases in immunoglobulin G and cryoglobulins.

Treatment
Antimicrobial treatment is summarized in Table 1. Needle aspiration or incision and drainage of fluctuant buboes may be required for symptomatic relief but are not routinely recommended for treatment because drainage can delay healing. Fistula openings should receive sterile dressings. One of the primary goals of treatment of LGV is to prevent long-term complications such as anogenital strictures or fistulas. Plastic surgical operations may be of benefit in cases with extensive rectal strictures or elephantiasis of the genitalia. However, these surgical interventions should only

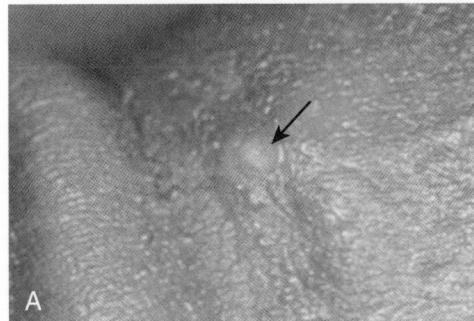
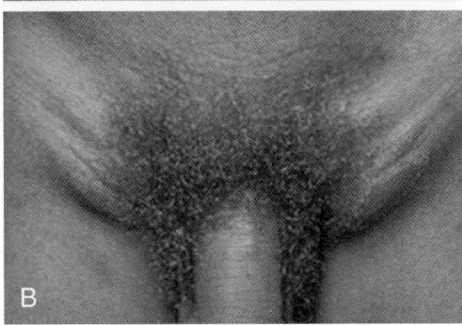

Figure 3 Lymphogranuloma venereum. **A,** Small ulcerative lesion near corona of penis *(arrow)*. **B,** Bilateral inguinal adenopathy, with developing groove sign as adenopathy expands above and below the inguinal ligament. (A courtesy Ronald Ballard, Reproduced with permission from The Diagnosis and Management of Sexually Transmitted Infections in South Africa, 3rd ed., Johannesburg, South African Institute for Medical Research, 2000. **B** courtesy Connexions (http://cnx.org/content/m14883/latest/Case_10-pres1-1.jpg).)

be performed after a prolonged course of antibiotics. Scars should be monitored to detect malignant change.

Management of Sex Partners
Any person having had sexual contact with a patient with LGV within 60 days before the onset of the patient's symptoms should be examined and presumptively treated with azithromycin[1] 1gram orally as a single dose or doxycycline 100mg orally twice a day for seven days. Symptomatic patients should be treated with longer treatment regimens.

---

[1]Not FDA approved for this indication.

References
Centers for Disease Control and Prevention: Sexually Transmitted Diseases Treatment Guidelines, 2021, Granuloma Inguinale (Donovanosis). Available at https://www.cdc.gov/std/treatment-guidelines/donovanosis.htm.

Centers for Disease Control and Prevention: Sexually Transmitted Diseases Treatment Guidelines, 2015, *MMWR Recomm Rep* 64(No. RR-3):1–137, 2015. Available at http://www.cdc.gov/std/tg2015/toc.htm.

Habif T: In *Clinical Dermatology*, Philadelphia, 2004, Mosby, pp 325–329.

Leppard B: In *An Atlas of African Dermatology*, Oxon, UK, 2002, Radcliffe Medical Press, p 69, 151, 237.

Ndinya-Achola JO, Kihara AN, Fisher LD, et al: Presumptive specific clinical diagnosis of genital ulcer disease (GUD) in a primary health care setting in Nairobi, *Int J STD AIDS* 7(3):201–205, 1996.

O'Farrell N: Granuloma Inguinale. In Ryan E, Hill D, Solomon T, editors: *Hunter's Tropical Medicine and Emerging Infectious Diseases*, ed 10, Canada, 2020, Elsevier, pp 531–533.

Richens J, Mabey DC: Sexually transmitted infections (excluding HIV). In Cook GC, Zumla AI, editors: *Manson's Tropical Diseases*, ed 22, London, 2009, Saunders, pp 403–434.

Ronald A: Chancroid. In Hunter GW, Strickland GT, Magill AJ, editors: *Hunter's Tropical Medicine and Emerging Infectious Diseases*, ed 8, Philadelphia, 2000, WB Saunders, pp 367–369.

GONORRHEA

Method of
John Brill, MD, MPH

CURRENT DIAGNOSIS

- Gonorrhea is caused by the gram-negative diplococcus *Neisseria gonorrhoeae*.
- Asymptomatic gonococcal infections are common in men and women, particularly in extragenital locations.
- Molecular tests are more sensitive than culture for diagnosis, particularly in extragenital locations.
- All patients diagnosed with gonorrhea should be tested for other sexually transmitted infections, including human immunodeficiency virus (HIV).
- Annual screening for *N. gonorrhoeae* infection is recommended for all sexually active women aged less than 25 years and for older women at increased risk for infection.

CURRENT THERAPY

- Ceftriaxone (Rocephin) 500 mg IM is the first-line treatment for gonorrhea, with the addition of Doxycycline (100 mg PO BID × 7 days) if concomitant chlamydia has not been ruled out. Persons weighing over 150 kg should be given a dose of ceftriaxone 1.0 g IM.
- The higher dosing of ceftriaxone compared with prior recommendations reflects a small increase in resistance. Doxycycline is now preferred over azithromycin due to a sevenfold increase in azithromycin resistance from 2014 to 2018.
- Only immunoglobulin E–mediated allergic reaction to penicillin (PCN) or cephalosporins (anaphylaxis, Stevens-Johnson syndrome, or toxic epidermal necrolysis) should contraindicate the use of ceftriaxone. Due to limited options, infectious disease consultation is recommended in this situation.

Epidemiology

Gonorrhea (GC) is the second most common reportable human infection in the United States, with 583,405 cases reported in 2018, a 63% increase since 2014. After a historic low in 2009, rates have progressively increased in all US regions, with western US states showing the greatest increase over the last 5 years (79.9%) (Figure 1). Cases in men who have sex with men (MSM) drive most of this escalation (Figure 2). The actual number of cases is estimated to be at least double that reported because of asymptomatic cases and underreporting. Regional rates vary widely from 43 (Vermont) to 611 (District of Columbia) per 100,000 population (Figure 3). The estimated annual US healthcare cost related to GC infections is $162 million.

Risk Factors

Risk factors for infection include unprotected intercourse, adolescent and young adult age, new/multiple sexual partners, and exchanging sex for money or drugs (Figure 4). Gonococcal infection is strongly associated with other STIs. In fact, at a county population level, the human immunodeficiency virus (HIV) infection rate carries the highest association with GC rates, superseding all other socioeconomic and demographic risk factors. Additional risk factors for gonorrhea include inconsistent condom use among persons who are not in mutually monogamous relationships, previous or coexisting STIs, and exchanging sex for money or drugs. Military recruits, incarcerated persons, and persons receiving care at public STI clinics are also at high risk. A significant ethnic disparity in GC rates is seen, with rates in Black men 8.9 times higher than those in White men and Black women

and 8.4 times higher than in White women in 2016; however, these proportions have been decreasing since 2011.

Pathophysiology

N. gonorrhoeae infects noncornified epithelial cells such as the urethra, endocervix, rectum, oropharynx, and conjunctiva. The bacteria divide by binary fission every 20 to 30 minutes, thus the rapid emergence of symptoms. *N. gonorrhoeae* attaches to different types of mucus-secreting epithelial cells via a number of alterable structures located on the surface of gonococci and additionally uses several mechanisms to counter the immune system. *N. gonorrhoeae* is primarily spread by infected secretions (oral, urethral) coming into contact with mucosal surfaces. Mother-to-child transmission is well established, hence, the recommendation to treat all newborns prophylactically with erythromycin (Ilotycin) 0.5% ophthalmic ointment.

Screening and Prevention

The US Preventive Service Task Force recommends annual screening for *N. gonorrhoeae* infection in all sexually active women aged less than 25 years and in older women at increased risk for infection (e.g., those who have a new sex partner, more than one sex partner, a sex partner with concurrent partners, or a sex partner who has an STI)—a "B" recommendation. The US Preventive Service Task Force concludes that the current evidence is insufficient to assess the balance of benefits and harms of screening for gonorrhea in men—an "I" recommendation. A 2021 draft update maintains the same recommendations.

MSM without consistent condom use are at high risk for gonorrhea infection; the Centers for Disease Control and Prevention (CDC) recommends that sexually active MSM be screened at least annually at anatomic sites of exposure. Mucosa that is infected by GC is more susceptible to HIV, even in asymptomatic states, raising the impetus for screening and treatment. Because the bacterium is an obligate human pathogen with adult transmission only via sexual contact, avoidance of intimate contact with an infected person is the optimal mode of prevention. Male latex condoms, used correctly and consistently, are highly effective at preventing GC transmission; polyurethane male and female condoms are effective when intact but have higher breakage rates.

Clinical Manifestations

The most common symptom of genital GC infection is a mucopurulent urethritis or cervicitis. In men, genital GC typically manifests with urethral discharge and dysuria 2 to 5 days after exposure; however, approximately 30% of urethral infections are asymptomatic. About half of genitally infected women will show symptoms, most commonly vaginal discharge, dysuria, and itching, generally 5 to 10 days after exposure. The great majority of rectal and pharyngeal infections are asymptomatic. GC can also present as ocular and disseminated infection. Except for neonatal infections, believed to arise from perinatal transmission, diagnosis of gonococcal infection in infants and children should trigger a sexual abuse investigation, including multisite testing.

Diagnosis

Laboratory diagnosis of GC can be made by gram staining of urethral secretions in symptomatic men, by culture of endocervical or urethral specimens, or by nucleic acid amplification testing (NAAT) of urine or the target location. Gram staining of urethral discharge showing leukocytes with intracellular gram-negative diplococci is extremely specific and sensitive. Gram staining is not sensitive enough to rule out infection in symptom-free men or in extraurethral locations. NAAT has largely replaced culture and appears to be more than twice as sensitive as culture in extragenital locations. The increased sensitivity of NAATs is due to their ability to produce a positive test result from as little as a single copy of the target DNA. False-positive test results can occur with NAAT, especially if NAAT has not been cleared by the US Food and Drug Administration (FDA) for use with these specimens or if it is ordered too soon after treatment because NAATs do not

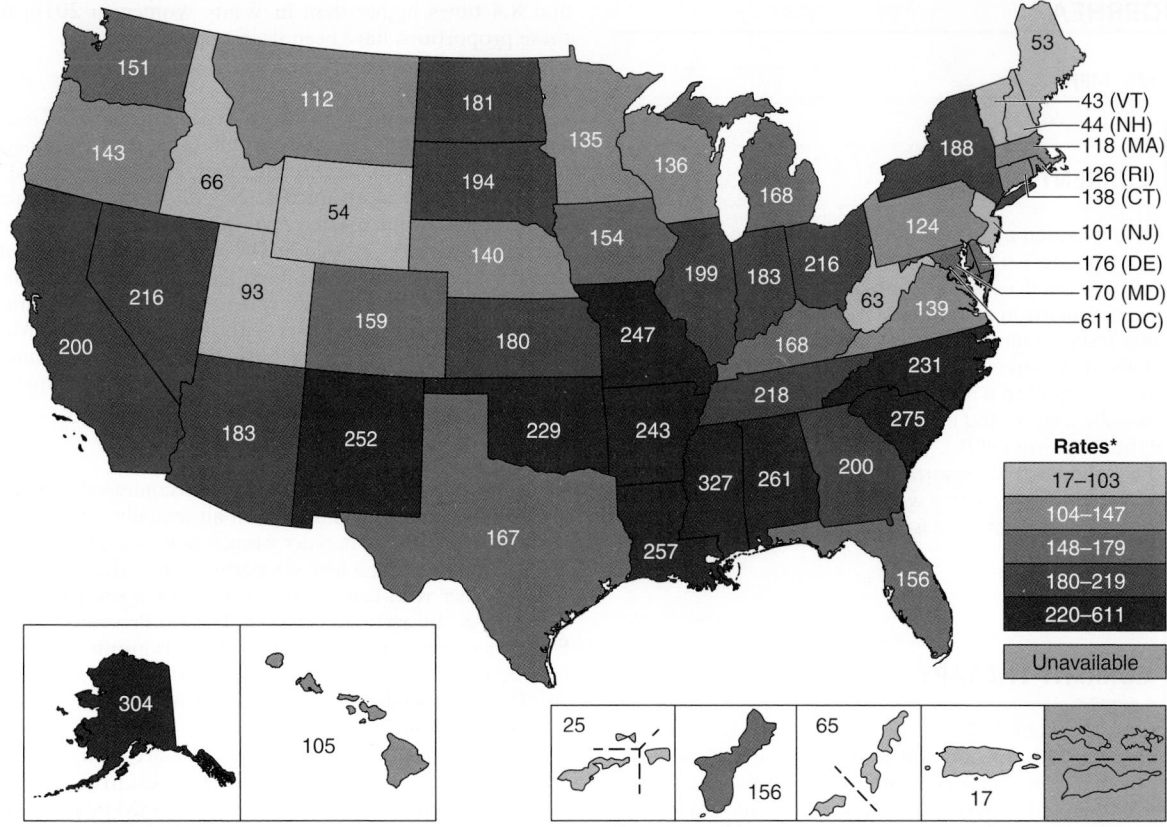

Figure 1 Gonorrhea—Rates of reported cases by state and territory, United States, 2018. From CDC: Sexually Transmitted Disease Surveillance 2018. https://www.cdc.gov/std/stats18/gonorrhea.htm. Accessed March 21, 2021.

require viable organisms. Although this higher sensitivity has allowed the use of less invasively collected specimens, such as first-catch urine, specific site testing (pharyngeal or rectal specimens) will detect up to 80% more infections than urine screening alone, highlighting the importance of a careful exposure history and consideration of multiple-site screening in high-risk populations. Recent literature has also demonstrated that approved self-collection vaginal swabs are accurate and highly acceptable to patients.

Differential Diagnosis

Differential diagnosis of gonorrheal genital infections includes *Chlamydia trachomatis* (CT), *Mycoplasma genitalium*, *Trichomonas vaginalis*, and herpes simplex infection. In women, yeast vaginitis and bacterial vaginosis should be considered. Coinfection is common and cannot be ruled out on clinical grounds; therefore cotesting for CT and *Trichomonas* should be done in all patients, and all patients should be offered testing for HIV, syphilis, and hepatitis.

Gonococcal conjunctivitis is typically purulent and unilateral but again cannot be distinguished clinically from other bacterial infections. Because gonococcal eye infections in adults generally result from autoinoculation, this diagnosis should prompt testing at other exposure sites.

Therapy

The 2020 CDC guidelines recommend a single intramuscular dose of ceftriaxone (Rocephin) 500 mg for the treatment of uncomplicated gonorrhea in persons weighing less than 150 kg, with the addition of oral doxycycline (100 mg BID for 7 days) if concomitant

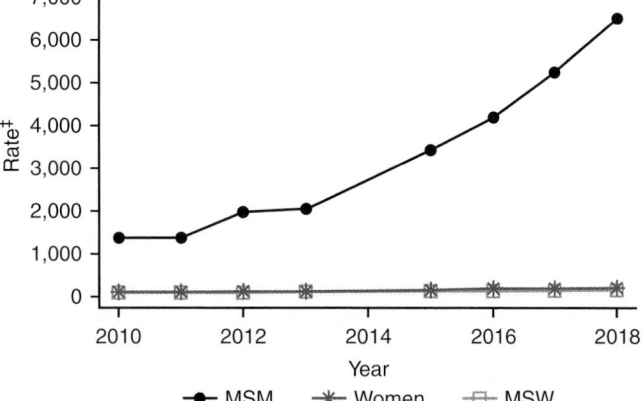

Figure 2 Gonorrhea—Estimated rates of reported gonorrhea cases by MSM, MSW, and women. STD Surveillance Network (SSuN), 2010 to 2018. From CDC: Sexually Transmitted Disease Surveillance 2018. https://www.cdc.gov/std/stats18/gonorrhea.htm. Accessed March 21, 2021.

chlamydial infection has not been excluded. For persons weighing over 150 kg, a single 1 g IM dose of ceftriaxone should be used. During pregnancy, azithromycin (Zithromax) 1 g as a single dose is recommended to treat chlamydia or as concomitant therapy to ceftriaxone if chlamydial infection has not been excluded. If administration of IM ceftriaxone is not available, a single 800 mg oral dose of cefixime (Suprax) is an alternative regimen.

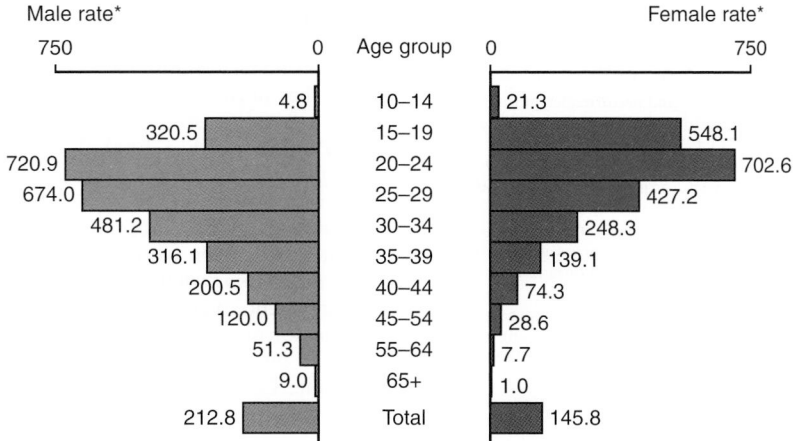

Male rate*

	Age group	
4.8	10–14	21.3
320.5	15–19	548.1
720.9	20–24	702.6
674.0	25–29	427.2
481.2	30–34	248.3
316.1	35–39	139.1
200.5	40–44	74.3
120.0	45–54	28.6
51.3	55–64	7.7
9.0	65+	1.0
212.8	Total	145.8

Female rate*

* Per 100,000.

Figure 3 Rates of reported gonorrhea cases by age group and sex, United States, 2018. From CDC: Sexually Transmitted Disease Surveillance 2018. https://www.cdc.gov/std/stats18/gonorrhea.htm. Accessed March 21, 2021.

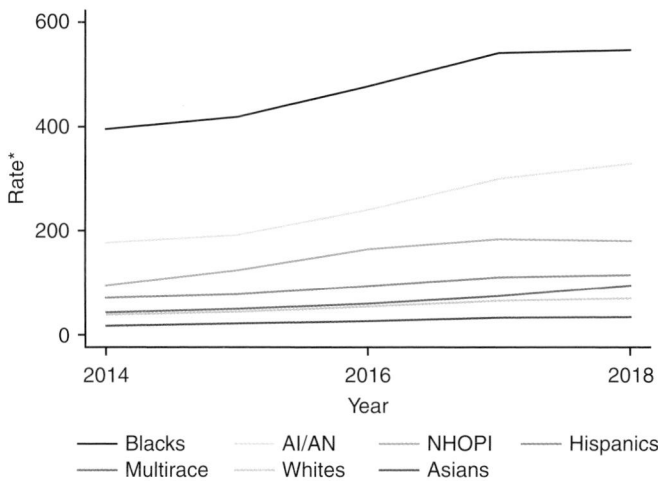

* Per 100,000.

Figure 4 Gonorrhea—Rates of reported cases by race/ethnicity, United States, 2014 to 2018. From CDC: Sexually Transmitted Disease Surveillance 2018. https://www.cdc.gov/std/stats18/gonorrhea.htm. Accessed March 21, 2021.

The higher dosing in ceftriaxone in the 2020 CDC guidelines reflects a small increase of Minimum Inhibitory Concentration (MIC) of isolates versus the 250 mg dose suggested previously, while azithromycin resistance increased over sevenfold between 2014 and 2018, leading to the recommended switch to doxycycline.

Data are limited regarding alternative regimens for treating gonorrhea among persons who have either a cephalosporin- or immunoglobulin E–mediated penicillin allergy (e.g., Stevens-Johnson syndrome, anaphylaxis). Infectious disease consultation is recommended.

Expedited partner therapy (EPT) is a strategy of treating sex partners of patients with GC or chlamydia without examining the partner. EPT is advocated by the CDC to decrease reinfection rates, particularly where the likely alternative is no care. In 2019 all US states and territories except South Carolina allowed EPT as an exception to scope-of-practice legislation requiring an established clinician-patient relationship. A challenge for EPT with gonorrhea is the need for parental administration of the preferred therapy, ceftriaxone. If oral therapy seems to be the only option for a partner to be treated, cefixime[1] 800 mg (Suprax, two 400-mg single-dose tablets) should be used, again in conjunction with

doxycycline 100 mg BID × 7 days if chlamydial infection has not been excluded.

Monitoring

The 2020 CDC monitoring guidelines contained several changes from prior recommendations:

- Because reinfection is common, occurring in 7% to 12% of patients, men and women with gonorrhea should be retested 3 months after treatment of the initial infection, regardless of whether they believe that their sex partners were successfully treated.
- If the 3-month retesting does not occur, clinicians should retest whenever the individual next presents for care within 1 year of initial treatment.
- A test-of-cure is needed 7 to 14 days after treatment for people who are treated for a throat infection, as ceftriaxone levels are more variable in the pharynx.
- Pregnant women treated early in pregnancy should have a test of cure as well as retest in third trimester.
- Those with persistent symptoms 3 weeks or more after treatment should have a test of cure.

Testing with NAAT in a shorter interval after treatment may result in false-positive test results because of the presence of DNA fragments. In this situation, testing should be repeated for CT and *Trichomonas* to reduce the potential for false-negative initial test results. For continued symptomatic genital infections despite appropriate therapy, culture with sensitivity testing is recommended.

Management of Complications

In men younger than 40, GC causes about 30% of cases of epididymitis, marked by unilateral testicular pain and swelling. Uncommon male complications of *N. gonorrhoeae* include inguinal lymphadenitis, penile edema, periurethral abscess or fistula, accessory gland infection (Tyson glands), balanitis, urethral stricture, and perhaps prostatitis. Female complications of gonorrhea are more frequent and burdensome; they include pelvic inflammatory disease, potentially leading to infertility or ectopic pregnancy. Disseminated gonococcal infections may occur in up to 2% of untreated patients. Certain gonococcal strains are more likely to cause disseminated gonococcal infections. Although patients are bacteremic, many appear nontoxic. Symptoms and signs may include fevers, myalgias, arthralgias, asymmetric polyarthritis, and a characteristic dermatitis consisting of a small number (<30) of skin lesions on the distal extremities that begin as papules and progress to pustules and ulcerations. Rarely, meningitis and endocarditis may occur. Hospitalization and consultation with an infectious disease specialist are recommended.

---

[1]Not FDA approved for this indication.

References

Andreatos N, Grigoras C, Shehadeh F, et al: The impact of HIV infection and socioeconomic factors on the incidence of gonorrhea: a county-level, US-wide analysis, *PLoS ONE [Electronic Resource]* 12(9):e0183938, 2017.

Arias M, Jang D, Gilchrist J, et al: Ease, comfort, and performance of the HerSwab vaginal self-Sampling device for the detection of *Chlamydia trachomatis* and *Neisseria gonorrhoeae, Sex Transm Dis* 43:125–129, 2016.

CDC: *Sexually transmitted disease surveillance 2018,* Atlanta, GA, 2019, US Department of Health and Human Services, CDC. https://www.cdc.gov/std/stats18/STDSurveillance2018-full-report.pdf.

Grov C, Cain D, Rendina HJ, Ventuneac A, Parsons JT: Characteristics associated with urethral and rectal gonorrhea and chlamydia diagnoses in a US national sample of gay and bisexual men: results from the One Thousand Strong Panel, *Sex Transm Dis* 43:165–171, 2016.

St Cyr S, Barbee L, Workowski KA, Bachmann IH, Pham C, Schlanger K, Torrone E, Weinstock H, Kersh EN, Thorpe P: Update to CDC's treatment guidelines for gonococcal infection, *MMWR (Morb Mortal Wkly Rep)* 69(50):1911–1916, 2020, https://doi.org/10.15585/mmwr.mm6950a6.

United States Preventive Services Task Force: Final Recommendation Statement: *Chlamydia and Gonorrhea Screenings.* Available at www.uspreventiveservice rvice-staskforce.org/Page/Document/RecommendationStatementFinal/chlamydia- and-gonorrhea-screening. Accessed Mar 21, 2021

NONGONOCOCCAL URETHRITIS

Method of
Shannon Dowler, MD

CURRENT DIAGNOSIS

- The gold standard for rapid diagnosis of nongonococcal urethritis (NGU) in a clinic setting is a Gram stain of urethral discharge positive for greater than 2 WBC/hpf and negative for gram-negative diplococci (diagnostic for *Neisseria gonorrhea*). Microscopic diagnosis of this nature is often immediately available only in dedicated sexual health clinics.
- The majority of patients with NGU present to primary or urgent care, so clinical presentation in a male with symptoms of penile discharge and/or dysuria, with a positive sexual history, is adequate for presumptive diagnosis while awaiting confirmatory testing.
- A urine sample (the first portion of urine stream results in the highest yield) should be sent for nucleic-acid amplification testing (NAAT).
- It is important to take a thorough sexual history and test exposed extragenital sites of infection (such as the throat and anus).
- In adolescents and young adults, a test of reinfection is recommended 12 weeks after treatment. In select patients where there is concern for nonadherence, or in pregnant patients with positive NAAT, test of reinfection/cure (TOR/C) is recommended in 4 weeks. All patients with a positive NAAT should have TOR/C in 3 to 4 months.
- Patients with recurrent infection or persistent symptoms should be evaluated for reinfection, drug resistance, or causes of NGU other than *Chlamydia*, such as *Trichomonas vaginalis* or *Mycoplasma genitalium*.

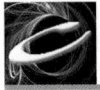

CURRENT THERAPY

- If immediate test results are not available, empiric treatment to cover both *Chlamydia trachomatis* and *Neisseria gonorrhea* is recommended with ceftriaxone (Rocephin) 500 mg IM × 1 (1 g for patients ≥150 kg) and doxycycline 100 mg BID × 7 days. An alternate regime in place of doxycycline is azithromycin (Zithromax) 1 g PO × 1.
- Stocking medications for the immediate treatment of *C. trachomatis* and *N. gonorrhea* in the clinic is best practice and strongly recommended.
- Expedited partner therapy (EPT) is recommended, though local state law should dictate this practice. Guttmacher Institute maintains an active database of EPT rules by state.

Epidemiology

There are several etiologies of NGU in the United States, the most common being *Chlamydia trachomatis*. In 2019, the CDC estimates that in the United States there were 1.8 million *C. trachomatis* infections reported—up 19% from 2015. This represents yearly increases since 2000. The second most common cause is *Mycoplasma genitalium*, an infection that is increasingly recognized as a contributor to NGU. Only in 2019 was the first FDA-approved diagnostic laboratory test for *M. genitalium* available commercially. Men who have sex with women are at higher risk for *Trichomonas vaginalis* than men who have sex with men, and the prevalence varies geographically. Historically poor testing options for men have made it difficult to quantify the prevalence of NGU due to *T. vaginalis*, though new tests are now readily available. Other less common causes include *Ureaplasma urealyticum*, herpes simplex virus (HSV), and adenovirus.

Risk Factors

The risk factors for NGU include sexual activity without using barrier method protection, younger age (<25 years), high-risk sexual partners, multiple sex partners, and a history of sexually transmitted disease (STD). Other contributing factors include low socioeconomic status and racial and ethnic minority status.

Pathophysiology

NGU as a broad term describes the inflammation of the male urethra usually caused by infection other than *Neisseria gonorrhea*. Inflammation as a result of the infection causes a penile discharge that ranges in consistency from mucoid to mucopurulent and a range of dysuric symptoms from none to marked burning. While the cause of NGU is most often bacterial (e.g., *C. trachomatis* and *M. genitalium*), it can also be caused by protozoa, *T. vaginalis*, viral etiologies (HSV), and other etiologies.

Prevention

The mainstay of public health primary prevention efforts includes the education of adolescents and young adults about the inherent risks of unprotected sex, multiple partners, and high-risk sexual partners. Efforts at "abstinence-only" education have resulted in poor outcomes. Encouraging the use of barrier methods, limiting the number of sexual partners, and avoiding high-risk partners are primary prevention strategies. Secondary prevention is geared toward making sexual health clinics widely available and affordable for all people, regardless of insurance status, and ensuring primary care practices are equipped for screening for, treatment of, and education on signs and symptoms of infection.

Clinical Manifestations

Most men with NGU present with symptoms of dysuria and urethral discharge. Dysuria can range from intermittent and episodic discomfort to persistent pain. Discharge ranges from clear to mucoid to mucopurulent. Frankly purulent and abundant discharge should alert the clinician to strongly consider *N. gonorrhea*. Many men may not be aware of discharge, so asking questions about "crusting" on the penis or underwear can be helpful. The clinical examination is critical. "Milking" the penis can allow for urethral discharge to manifest at the tip of the penis. At times, the urethral meatus can be inflamed and red. In men with *T. vaginalis*, the symptoms are often more mild and vague, such as "a tingling feeling" or "itching inside the penis" with urination; discharge is less common. Clinicians should pay attention to the presence of significant findings such as enlarged lymph nodes, ulcers, warts, rashes, and scrotal/testicular pain, as patients may present with more than one infection.

Diagnosis

While Gram stain of the urethral discharge is the gold standard for immediate diagnosis, this modality is rarely available in standard clinical practice. If Gram stain is available, the absence of gram-negative diplococci and the presence of greater than 2 WBC/hpf suggest a diagnosis of NGU. For all patients, further testing by nucleic-acid amplification testing (NAAT) should be undertaken.

A urine sample should be collected after physical examination (ideally limited to the "first" portion of the stream). The NAAT test has high specificity and sensitivity, and results are often available in hours or within a day for many labs. There is not an indication for culture of any causes of NGU. In men who have sex with women, *T. vaginalis* should be strongly considered as an etiology, and testing for *T. vaginalis* is now available to add to *N. gonorrhea* and *C. trachomatis* NAAT tests. Alternatively, a urine sample can be spun for microscopy, and in experienced labs, *T. vaginalis* can be diagnosed with microscopy. Wet prep testing is not a reliable test for *T. vaginalis* in men. In January 2019, the first FDA-approved NAAT for *M. genitalium* was introduced to the US market. Current CDC guidelines do not routinely recommend screening for *M. genitalium* at this time, though with the availability of new, rapid testing guidelines, it should be monitored. For patients who have refractory or recurrent symptoms, the diagnosis of *M. genitalium* should be considered, but testing is indicated for patients with persistent or recurrent symptoms when NAAT testing is negative for other etiology.

Increasingly, nongenital sites of asymptomatic infection are being identified, particularly in the throat and anus. A thorough sexual history should include sites of sexual contact, and screening should be performed at those sites when a patient presents with symptoms or risk for sexually transmitted infections. Routine screening should also include sampling from extragenital sites. Numerous studies have confirmed that many patients with negative urine NAATs will have asymptomatic *C. trachomatis* or *N. gonorrhea* infections in other sites of sexual contact.

Therapy/Treatment

Patients with characteristic symptoms who have a Gram stain performed that rules out *N. gonorrhea* should be treated for NGU empirically with doxycycline 100 mg BID × 7 days. This guidance in the 2021 CDC STI guidelines reflects a significant change. Alternatively, azithromycin (Zithromax) 1 g by mouth in one dose can be given; unfortunately, due to emerging drug resistance, this should be reserved for patients where the likelihood of treatment non-adherence is very high. In the absence of Gram stain testing availability, empiric treatment coverage with both azithromycin and ceftriaxone (Rocephin) should be considered in patients with a history of recent infection, high-risk contacts, or symptoms of urethritis. All clinical locations that test and treat for sexually transmitted infections should maintain a supply of oral azithromycin and metronidazole (Flagyl), as well as intramuscular ceftriaxone to provide immediate treatment and reduce barriers to care such as transportation to a pharmacy, pharmaceutical insurance coverage, cost, and concerns about confidentiality, particularly in younger patients.

If trichomonas is suspected, new guidelines recommend men receive a one time 2 g dose of metronidazole but women receive 500 mg BID × 7 days, a marked change from prior guidelines. Of note, the new guidelines also disabuse the historical potential for the interaction between alcohol and metronidazole and no longer list this as a contraindication. Additional regimens are available at the free-of-charge STD treatment guidelines page on the CDC website (cdc.gov). The STD treatment guideline app is an excellent public source tool for treatment guidelines.

If a patient presents with persistent symptoms despite appropriate treatment, the clinician must consider reinfection or drug resistance. If the patient had negative tests for *N. gonorrhea* and *C. trachomatis*, the clinician should consider empiric treatment for *T. vaginalis* with metronidazole 2 g PO ×1 or tinidazole (Tindamax) 2 g PO ×1 if the patient is a male who has sex with females. The possibility of *M. genitalium* should be considered in patients with NGU, particularly those with recurrent or persistent symptoms. *M. genitalium* has developed rapid drug resistance, with more than a third of infections now resistant to azithromycin. Performing NAAT testing for recurrent or persistent symptoms in the absence of a confirmatory *C. trachomatis* or *N. gonorrhea* result should be undertaken. The guidelines for treatment are different based on whether resistance testing is available from your lab. If it is not available, the recommended treatment is doxycycline 100 mg BID × 7 days followed by moxifloxacin (Avelox)[1] 400 mg daily for 7 days. CDC recommends testing partners for *M. genitalium* and treating if positive; alternatively, if testing not an option for partners of positive cases, then the same drug regimen can be used.

All patients treated for NGU should be advised to abstain from sex for 1 week to allow for clearance of infection. Known sexual partners should be treated with expedited partner therapy when allowed by state law. The patient should not resume sexual activity until the partner is adequately treated. Positive tests should be reported to the health authority as indicated by state law.

Monitoring

Partner treatment is recommended for all confirmed causes of NGU. Test of reinfection closely after treatment (4 weeks) is recommended in high-risk patients and test of cure after treatment (3 months) for all patients with a positive NAAT for *C. trachomatis* or *N. gonorrhea*. TOR/C is not routinely recommended for *T. vaginalis*.

Complications

Untreated *C. trachomatis* infection in men can cause epididymitis, prostatitis, and reactive arthritis. Autoinoculation to the eyes is a potential complication in untreated urethral infections and requires immediate treatment.

---

[1]Not FDA approved for this indication.

References

BASHH Guidelines. https://www.bashhguidelines.org/current-guidelines/urethritis-and-cervicitis/mycoplasma-genitalium-2018/ (Accessed April 18, 2020)

Centers for Disease Control and Infection. Emerging Infectious Diseases: Increasing Macrolide and Fluoroquinolone Resistance in *Mycoplasma genitalium*. May 2017. wwwnc.cdc.gov/eid/article/23/5/16-1745_article (Accessed April 28. 2020).

Centers for Disease Control and Prevention. Chlamydia. July 30, 2019. gov/std/stats18/chlamydia.htm (accessed April 18, 2020).

Guttmacher Institute. Partner Treatment of STIs. Guttmacher.org/state-policy/explore/partner-treatment-stis (accessed April 18, 2020)

US Food and Drug Administration: FDA permits marketing of first test to aid in the diagnosis of a sexually-transmitted infection known as *Mycoplasma genitalium*, January 23, 2019. https://www.fda.gov/news-events/press-announcements/fda-permits-marketing-first-test-aid-diagnosis-sexually-transmitted-infection-known-mycoplasma. (accessed 28 April 2020).

SYPHILIS

Method of
Jennifer Frank, MD

CURRENT DIAGNOSIS

- Serologic testing includes both nontreponemal-specific testing (VDRL and RPR) and treponemal-specific testing (FTA-Abs [fluorescent treponemal antibody absorption] and TP-PA [*Treponema pallidum* particle agglutination]).
- Cerebrospinal fluid testing (VDRL [Venereal Disease Research Laboratory], protein, cell count) is performed to diagnose neurosyphilis.

CURRENT THERAPY

- Penicillin is first-line therapy for all types and stages of syphilis.
- Penicillin is the only recommended treatment for pregnant women and for congenital syphilis. Penicillin-allergic patients should undergo desensitization.

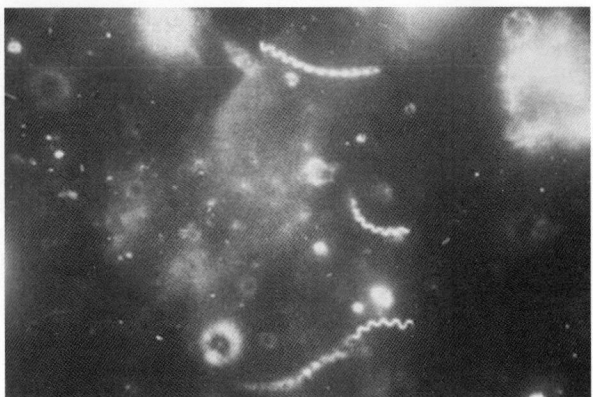

Figure 1 *Treponema pallidum* on darkfield microscopy.

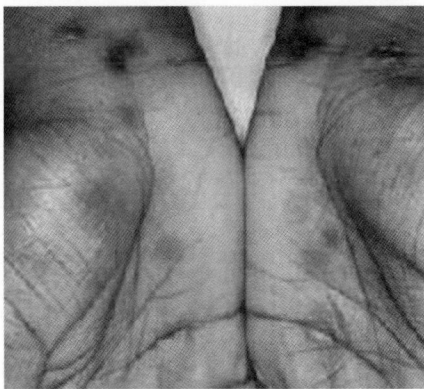

Figure 2 Syphilis skin lesion.

Epidemiology

The rate of primary and secondary syphilis reached a low point (2.1 per 100,000) in 2000 and has increased since that time, reaching a rate of 10.8 per 100,000 in 2018; this represented a 14.9% increase from 2017 and is the highest rate since 1993. The recent increase in rates has occurred in both men and women, in all regions, in all age groups between 15 years and older, and in all ethnicities. Men who have sex with men (MSM) have the highest rates of primary and secondary syphilis. Seventy-two percent of states saw an increased rate from 2016 to 2017; the West continues to have the overall highest rate. Congenital syphilis is also increasing with a rate of 33.1 cases per 100,000 live births in 2018, a 39.7% increase from 2017; this represents a steady increase since 2012 and mirrors the increased rates among women.

Risk Factors

MSM and HIV-positive persons are at highest risk for primary and secondary syphilis. Other risk factors include living in the certain geographic areas in the United States or an urban area, and being born to a mother infected with syphilis.

Pathophysiology

Syphilis is caused by infection with the spirochete *Treponema pallidum* subspecies *pallidum* (Figure 1). The average incubation period is 21 days (range 3-90 days). Primary infection manifests with signs and symptoms at the site of infection; secondary and tertiary syphilis manifest with systemic signs and symptoms. Syphilis is primarily sexually transmitted but may be transmitted perinatally or through nonsexual cutaneous transmission Previous infection does not confer long-term immunity.

Prevention

Prevention includes both avoiding initial infection and preventing disease progression through early detection and treatment. Transmission of syphilis can be reduced (although not eliminated) by using condoms. Screening for syphilis in pregnancy combined with treatment of infected women reduces perinatal transmission. Screening high-risk populations may prevent spread of infection.

Screening

The US Preventive Services Task Force recommends screening people at increased risk for syphilis. Screening HIV-infected men or MSM every 3 months increases rates of detection. All pregnant women should be screened for syphilis at the first prenatal visit. Women at increased risk should be rescreened in the third trimester, at delivery, and after any potential exposure to an infected partner.

Clinical Manifestations

Primary syphilis manifests as a chancre at the site of inoculation. The chancre, a painless ulcer with sharp borders, is usually solitary and associated with regional lymphadenopathy. Atypical presentations include extragenital location (most commonly oral or anal) and the presence of pain or multiple lesions.

Secondary syphilis characteristically manifests with a generalized rash with variable features four to eight weeks after onset of primary syphilis (Figure 2). The palms and soles are affected in the majority of patients. Typically, the rash is maculopapular or papulosquamous and nonpruritic. Other clinical manifestations include highly infectious flat lesions (condyloma lata), fever, malaise, sore throat, headache, myalgias, alopecia, and, rarely, renal, bone, eye, or liver involvement. Latent syphilis, by definition, has no clinical manifestations. Ocular syphilis can occur during any stage of syphilis and has been reported in 20 states in the last few years. Patients with syphilis should be screened for any visual symptoms or eye complaints.

Tertiary syphilis, which is rare, is a late manifestation in untreated people and includes neurosyphilis, cardiovascular, and gummatous disease. Gummas are nodular lesions that vary in size and location. They can ulcerate and cause local tissue destruction. Cardiovascular syphilis most commonly manifests as aortitis of the ascending aorta. The clinical manifestations of neurosyphilis are numerous and include meningitis with or without vascular involvement, dementia, tabes dorsalis (posterior column involvement with ataxia and bowel and bladder dysfunction), and ocular or otologic involvement.

Congenital syphilis has early (birth to 2 years) and late (2 to 20 years) clinical manifestations. Early signs include hepatosplenomegaly, rash, fever, neurosyphilis, pneumonitis, rhinitis, generalized lymphadenopathy, hepatitis, ascites, hematologic disease, renal disease, periostitis, and osteochondritis. Late manifestations (present in 40% of untreated patients) include skeletal deformities, neurologic disease (deafness), dental abnormalities, and ocular abnormalities.

Diagnosis

Diagnosis of primary syphilis may be optimally diagnosed by specific testing of the skin lesion or exudate as it can take several weeks for treponemal antibodies to develop. There are three methods for testing of exudate: direct fluorescent antibody testing, PCR testing, and darkfield microscopy; all have limited availability. Serologic testing is done using nontreponemal (VDRL or RPR) and treponemal testing (multiple types, including FTA-ABS and TPPA) because both tests have limitations; it may take several weeks for antibodies to develop. Nontreponemal testing may be falsely positive with other medical conditions, but antibody titers correlate with disease activity and therefore can indicate response to treatment. Nontreponemal tests usually become nonreactive after successful treatment. A serofast reaction can occur in which the nontreponemal test stays reactive. Treponemal tests are specific for syphilitic infection but usually stay reactive regardless of treatment or disease status. Treponemal test antibody titers do not match the level of disease activity and therefore cannot be used to monitor treatment response. Reverse sequence testing has been used in which a treponemal specific test is the initial screening test, followed by a non-treponemal test. Reverse sequence testing has a higher

TABLE 1 CDC Recommendations for Treatment of Syphilis

	RECOMMENDED PENICILLIN TREATMENT	
STAGE	PENICILLIN	DOSAGE
Primary and secondary syphilis	Benzathine penicillin G (Bicillin LA)	2.4 million U IM once
Early latent syphilis (acquired within previous 12 mo)	Benzathine penicillin G	2.4 million U IM once
Late latent syphilis	Benzathine penicillin G	2.4 million U IM weekly × 3 doses
Tertiary syphilis	Benzathine penicillin G	2.4 million units IM weekly × 3 doses
Neurosyphilis	Aqueous crystalline penicillin G *or* Continuous infusion *or* Procaine penicillin (Wycillin) *plus* Probenecid	3–4 million U q4h 18–24 U daily IV × 10–14 d (preferred) 2.4 million U IM 500 mg PO qid
Congenital Syphilis		
Proven or highly probable disease	Aqueous crystalline penicillin G *or* Procaine penicillin G	100,000–150,000 U/kg/d (divided 50,000 U/kg/dose) IV q12h × first 7 d of life, then q8h for total of 10 d of treatment 50,000 U/kg/dose IM daily × 10 d
Normal examination but mother inadequately treated	Aqueous crystalline penicillin G *or* Procaine penicillin G *or* Benzathine penicillin G	100,000–150,000 U/kg/d (divided 50,000 U/kg/dose) IV q12h × first 7 d of life, then q8h for total of 10 days of treatment 50,000 U/kg/dose IM daily × 10 d 50,000 U/kg/dose IM once
Normal examination, serologic titers ≤4× the maternal titer, and mother adequately treated during pregnancy	Benzathine penicillin G	50,000 U/kg/dose IM once

Abbreviation: CDC = Centers for Disease Control and Prevention.

false-positive rate with the initial screening step of testing but identifies more cases of syphilis, particularly early infection, previously treated infection, or long-standing infection. If reverse sequence screening is used, a third treponemal specific test using different antigens should be used to confirm the results.

Neurosyphilis is diagnosed based on clinical signs and symptoms using laboratory testing to support a clinical diagnosis. No single test can be used to diagnose all patients with neurosyphilis, which means that neurosyphilis is usually diagnosed by a combination of serologic testing, testing of cerebrospinal fluid (CSF), and clinical evaluation. Laboratory testing includes reactive serologic testing; cerebrospinal fluid (CSF) VDRL (Venereal Disease Research Laboratory) testing, which is specific but not sensitive; and CSF positive for white blood cells or protein, or both. The CSF FTA-ABS (fluorescent treponemal antibody absorption) test is sensitive but less specific than CSF VDRL testing. Patients with latent, tertiary, or neurosyphilis should be tested for HIV infection.

Differential Diagnosis

Syphilis, which can affect every organ system, has historically been called the great mimicker. Syphilis is on the differential diagnosis of, most commonly, conditions causing genital ulcers or lesions, conditions causing systemic rashes affecting the palms and soles, conditions causing ocular and otologic manifestations (uveitis, sudden visual changes, hearing loss), and conditions causing dementia, meningitis, or ataxia.

Treatment

Penicillin G is the preferred treatment for all stages of syphilis; other forms of penicillin (oral penicillin, combinations of benzathine and procaine [Bicillin CR]) are not effective. The stage and extent of clinical disease determine which preparation is used, the dosage, and the length of treatment (Table 1). In penicillin-allergic

patients, antibiotic alternatives exist for all types and stages of syphilis except for syphilis in pregnancy and congenital syphilis.

Neurosyphilis is ideally treated with penicillin. Alternative treatment of primary and secondary syphilis and early latent syphilis includes doxycycline (Vibramycin) 100 mg orally twice a day or tetracycline 500 mg orally four times daily for 14 days. Ceftriaxone (Rocephin)[1] 1 g daily IM or IV for 10 to 14 days is also used, although data is limited regarding optimal dose and treatment duration. Azithromycin (Zithromax)[1] 2 g orally as a single dose may be used when treatment with both penicillin and doxycycline is contraindicated, although treatment failures have been reported and azithromycin is not appropriate treatment for MSM, HIV-infected patients, or in pregnancy. Penicillin-allergic patients with late latent syphilis can be treated with doxycycline 100 mg orally twice daily or tetracycline 500 mg orally four times daily for 28 days, recognizing that there is limited data to support this treatment. Treatment of pencillin-allergic patients with tertiary syphilis should be done is consultation with a specialist. Ceftriaxone[1] 2 g given IV or IM daily for 10 to 14 days has been described for the treatment of neurosyphilis in penicillin-allergic patients.

The Jarisch-Herxheimer reaction is an acute febrile reaction (with accompanying headache, myalgias, and other symptoms) occurring within 24 hours of treatment of syphilis. It is more common in early stages of syphilis and rare in newborns.

Monitoring

No definite criteria exist for either cure of syphilis or treatment failure. It is recommended that nontreponemal antibody titers be followed every 6 months, and patients should be periodically reexamined for clinical signs or symptoms of syphilitic

---

[1]Not FDA approved for this indication.

infection. Treatment failure is probable in patients with either persistent or recurrent clinical signs or symptoms or a sustained fourfold increase in nontreponemal antibody titer (compared to maximum titer at time of treatment). Treatment failure is possible if nontreponemal antibody titers fail to decline fourfold within 6 months after treatment. Suspected treatment failure warrants retesting for neurosyphilis and HIV infection. Patients with HIV infection, with congenital syphilis, who are pregnant, or who have neurosyphilis warrant closer and more-specific laboratory and clinical follow-up. Full recommendations can be found in the Centers for Disease Control and Prevention (CDC) treatment guidelines (http://www.cdc.gov/std/tg2015/syphilis.htm).

Complications

Complications of syphilis are primarily related to neurologic involvement, tertiary syphilis, or late manifestations of congenital syphilis.

References

ACOG. Clinical Practice: Syphilis Resurgence Reminds Us of the Importance of STD Screening and Treatment during Prenatal Care. Available at https://www.acog.org/About-ACOG/ACOG-Departments/ACOG-Rounds/May-2017/Syphilis-Resurgence.

Cantor AG, Pappas M, Daeges M, Nelson HD: Screening for syphilis: updated evidence report and systematic review for the US Preventive Services Task Force, *JAMA* 315:2328–2337, 2016.

Centers for Disease Control and Prevention. 2015 Sexually Transmitted Diseases Treatment Guidelines. Available at: http://www.cdc.gov/std/tg2015/syphilis.htm.

Centers for Disease Control and Prevention: Discordant results from reverse sequence syphilis screening, United States, 2006–2010, *MMWR Morbid Mortal Wkly Rep* 60:133–137, 2011.

Centers for Disease Control and Prevention, Association of Public Health Laboratories: Laboratory diagnostic testing for *Treponema pallidum*, Expert Consultation Meeting Summary Report, January 13–15, 2009, Atlanta, GA. Available at: http://www.aphl.org/aphlprograms/infectious/std/Documents/ID_2009Jan_Laboratory-Guidelines-Treponema-pallidum-Meeting-Report.pdf. 2009.

Centers for Disease Control and Prevention: Clinical Advisory: Ocular Syphilis in the United States. Available at, https://www.cdc.gov/std/syphilis/clinicaladvisoryos2015.htm, 2015.

Centers for Disease Control and Prevention. 2018 Sexually Transmitted Disease Surveillance. Available at https://www.cdc.gov/std/stats18/syphilis.htm.

Centers for Disease Control and Prevention: Discordant results from reverse sequence syphilis screening: five laboratories, United States, 2006–2010, *MMWR Morb Mortal Wkly Rep*. 60(5):133–137, 2011.

Kent ME, Romanelli F: Reexamining syphilis: an update on epidemiology, clinical manifestations, and management, *Ann Pharmacother* 42:226–236, 2008.

Koss CA, Dunne EF, Warner L: A systematic review of epidemiologic studies assessing condom use and risk of syphilis, *Sex Trans Dis* 36:401–405, 2009.

Lautenschlager S: Cutaneous manifestations of syphilis, *Am J Clin Dermatol* 7:291–304, 2006.

Marra CM: Update on neurosyphilis, *Curr Infect Dis Rep* 11:127–134, 2009.

New York City Department of Health and Mental Hygiene, and the New York City STD PreventionTraining Center: The diagnosis and management of syphilis: an update and review. March 2019. www.nycptc.org.

Woods CR: Congenital syphilis—persisting pestilence, *Pediatr Infect Dis* 28:536–537, 2009.

USPSTF: Syphilis Infection in Nonpregnant Adults and Adolescents: Screening; June 2016.

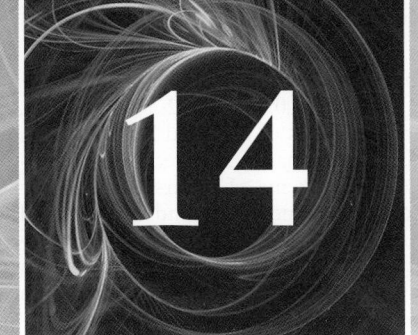

14 Skin Disease

ACNE VULGARIS

Method of
Lisa M. Johnson, MD; and Daniel J. Van Durme, MD, MPH

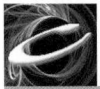

CURRENT DIAGNOSIS

- Acne vulgaris (AV) is primarily found in teenagers and young adults and is characterized by microcomedones that develop into open and closed comedones (blackheads and whiteheads), inflammatory papules and pustules, or nodules and cysts.
- AV lesions are primarily on the face, neck, upper arms, back, and chest.
- Acneiform lesions are typically found in various stages, with many patients having a predominant type.

CURRENT THERAPY

- Acne therapy targets abnormal hyperkeratinization, excess sebum production, colonization by *Propionibacterium acnes*, and inflammation. Therapy involves prevention of new lesions and control over a long period of time with response generally seen in 6 to 8 weeks.
- Numerous topical and oral medications have demonstrated efficacy for patients with acne; there is little evidence for which is best.
- Benzoyl peroxide is an excellent starting agent because of extensive safety and efficacy studies, its demonstrated benefit in controlling *P. acnes*, and some benefits in controlling abnormal keratinization and inflammation.
- Topical retinoids should also be considered starting agents because of their demonstrated benefits in controlling abnormal keratinization leading to microcomedones, a primary lesion in acne.
- Topical antibiotics such as clindamycin (Cleocin-T) and erythromycin (Akne-Mycin) should be used in combination with topical retinoids for more efficacy or with benzoyl peroxide to decrease the likelihood of bacterial resistance.
- Oral antibiotics such as the class of tetracycline should be used if acne is widespread or unresponsive to topical agents.
- Oral contraceptives have proven benefits for most types of acne.
- Oral isotretinoin (Accutane, Claravis) can be very effective and even cures many patients, but the teratogenic and other side effects are profound and mandate use with extreme caution.

Acne (or acne vulgaris [AV]) and rosacea (previously called *acne rosacea* and sometimes *adult acne*) are often thought of together. However, they actually represent different pathophysiologic processes and require different therapeutic approaches.

Epidemiology
Acne is a chronic inflammatory dermatosis that is most common in adolescents, affecting approximately 85% of teenagers with the average age of onset being 11 to 12 years of age, peaking at ages 15 to 17. It can occur, however, in most age groups and can persist into adulthood. It is typically worse in male patients. The severity varies widely. There is no mortality associated with acne, but there is often significant physical and psychological morbidity, such as permanent scarring, poor self-image, depression, and anxiety. More severe forms of acne are found in those with a genetic predisposition and those with earlier onset.

Prevention
There is some evidence to suggest that high glycemic index diets may be associated with acne. In 2007, a randomized controlled trial with 23 Australian males, aged 15 to 25 years, examined the impact of a low glycemic diet on acne. Those randomized to follow the low glycemic load (LGL) diet had significant improvement in acne severity, a significant reduction in weight and body mass index (BMI), a significant decrease in free androgen index, and improved insulin sensitivity at the end of 12 weeks. The study was limited by its small sample size and the fact that both the intervention and control groups lost weight.

There is some evidence that dairy products (particularly skim milk) might contribute to acne, but others have questioned the strength of these studies. Although some small preliminary studies have examined the role of antioxidants (including oral zinc), probiotics, and fish oil on acne, the existing evidence is not strong enough, at this time, to support any recommendations regarding these dietary factors.

Pathophysiology
The pathophysiology of acne involves androgens as a major contributing factor, and thus acne starts with puberty. Four intersecting pathophysiologic processes are involved in acne, and the sequence and degree of contribution of each factor is still under study. The lesions begin with abnormal keratinization of the pilosebaceous glands that are more concentrated on the face, neck, and trunk. The keratin that lines the opening of the glands becomes more cohesive; this blocks the gland from being able to adequately excrete the sebum, and the plugged opening dilates. This leads to a closed comedone (whitehead) or open comedone (blackhead). Additional factors include the proliferation of the gram-positive *Propionibacterium acnes* (*P. acnes*) and an increase in inflammatory mediators, such as cytokines, leukotrienes, lymphocytes, and macrophages, which lead to the papules and pustules of inflammatory acne. Finally, the abnormal and excess production of sebum, particularly triggered by androgens, can play a key role as well, notably in nodulocystic acne.

Diagnosis
Diagnosis is generally straightforward, especially in teenagers. Dermatologic lesions include open and closed comedones, pustules, inflammatory papules, nodules, and cysts. Lesions are primarily found on the face, neck, upper arms, back, and chest. They are typically found in various stages, and many patients have a predominant type.

Clinical Manifestations
Clinical manifestations include open and closed comedones (blackheads and whiteheads), inflammatory papules and pustules, and, in severe cases, nodules and cysts. There are several proposed classification schemes to help identify the numbers and

types of lesions. Perhaps the most useful combines an estimate of the numbers of lesions with a descriptor of the lesions and location. Thus a patient can have mild (few lesions) papulopustular acne of the face and severe (many lesions) comedonal acne on the back and shoulders. This classification helps identify optimal treatment and provides a better description to assess response to therapy.

Differential Diagnosis

Differential diagnosis should include drug-induced acne (especially from steroids), which can be identified by seeing all lesions at nearly the same stage of development. Rosacea should also be considered in the differential diagnosis of AV, though the age of onset and symptomatology are usually distinguishing.

Treatment

The topical therapy of AV includes the use of agents that are available over the counter or via prescription. Therapy choice may be influenced by age of the patient, site of involvement, extent and severity of disease, cost, and patient preference. Topical therapies may be used as monotherapy in combination with other topical agents or in combination with oral agents in both initial control and maintenance.

Additionally, it is key to set realistic expectations about how acne can be controlled with the regular use of a variety of agents and how it can take 6 to 8 weeks to see improvement. If these issues are not addressed, the likelihood of adherence and long-term improvement are low.

Commonly used topical acne therapies include benzoyl peroxide, salicylic acid, antibiotics, combination antibiotics with benzoyl peroxide, retinoids, retinoid with benzoyl peroxide (BP), retinoid with antibiotic, azelaic acid, and sulfone agents.

BP is an antibacterial agent that kills *P. acne* through the release of free oxygen radicals and is also mildly comedolytic. No resistance to this agent has been reported, and the addition of BP to regimens of antibiotic therapy enhances results and may reduce development of drug resistance. BP is available as topical washes, foams, creams, or gels and can be used as leave-on or wash-off agents. Strengths available for acne therapy range from 2.5% to 10%. Benzoyl peroxide therapy is limited by skin irritation, staining and bleaching of fabric, and uncommon contact allergy. Total skin contact time and formulation can also affect efficacy. Lower concentrations (e.g., 2.5–5%), water-based, and wash-off agents may be better tolerated in patients with more sensitive skin. Results may be noted in as soon as 5 days.

Topical antibiotics for acne accumulate in the follicle and have been postulated to work through antiinflammatory mechanisms and via antibacterial effects. These agents are best used in combination with BP, which increases efficacy and decreases the development of resistant bacterial strains. Monotherapy with topical antibiotics in the management of acne is not recommended because of the development of antibiotic resistance.

Clindamycin 1% solution or gel is currently the preferred topical antibiotic for acne therapy. Topical erythromycin in 2% concentration is available as a cream, gel, lotion, or pledget but has reduced efficacy in comparison with clindamycin because of resistance of cutaneous *Staphylococci* and *P. acnes*.

Topical retinoids (tretinoin [Retin-A, Renova, Avita], adapalene [Differin], or tazarotene [Tazorac]) are all extremely effective for abnormal keratinization and comedone development and thus treat existing lesions and prevent the development of new lesions. These can be irritating and come in a variety of strengths. Patients might need to start at the lowest strength with every-other-day dosing and work up to the highest strength needed and tolerated. Some formulations of tretinoin (primarily generic products) are not photo stable and should be applied in the evening. All are contraindicated in pregnancy.

Topical retinoids enhance other topical acne regimens and allow for maintenance of clearance after discontinuation of oral therapy. Retinoids are ideal for comedonal acne and, when used in combination with other agents, for all acne variants. Three

topical agents are available that contain retinoids in combination with other products: adapalene 0.1%/ BP 2.5% (Epiduo), approved for use in patients ≥9 years of age, and 2 agents with fixed combination clindamycin phosphate 1.2%/tretinoin 0.025% gel (Veltin, Ziana), approved for patients ≥12 years of age.

Salicylic acid preparations are comedolytic and can be used for patients who cannot tolerate either benzoyl peroxide or topical retinoids, although salicylic acid preparations have not been shown to be as effective. Azelaic acid 20% cream (Azelex) is mildly effective as a comedolytic, antibacterial, and antiinflammatory agent; it is also a category B in pregnancy.

The sulfone agent, dapsone 5% gel (Aczone), is available as a twice-daily agent for the therapy of AV. In clinical trials, topical dapsone showed modest to moderate efficacy, primarily in the reduction of inflammatory lesions. Combination with topical retinoids may be indicated if comedonal components are present. Topical dapsone may be oxidized by the coapplication of BP, causing orange-brown coloration of the skin, which can be brushed or washed off.

Topical dapsone 5% gel is pregnancy category C and has efficacy and safety data down to patients 12 years of age. Aluminum chloride[1] possesses antibacterial activity and therefore has been investigated in the treatment of acne. There is some evidence to suggest the efficacy of sodium sulfacetamide (Klaron, Ovace Plus). Topical niacinamide (nicotinamide)[7] 2% to 4% gel is available over the counter.

For patients with moderate inflammatory and comedonal lesions, it can be appropriate to start both BP and topical retinoids at the initial visit; however, the applications should be separated in time because the BP will inactivate the retinoid. An effective regimen (if tolerated) is a BP wash in the morning and topical retinoid at bedtime.

Antibiotics should be added if response to topical BP and retinoids is inadequate at the 6- to 8-week follow-up visit. Topical clindamycin (Cleocin-T) and erythromycin (Akne-Mycin) have demonstrated efficacy and be used twice a day at the same time as the BP. There are also combination agents that conveniently add the two agents into a single preparation: clindamycin 1% plus BP 5% gel (BenzaClin, Duac) and erythromycin 3% plus BP 5% gel (Benzamycin). They are more expensive, however.

Oral antibiotics should be started if the acne is moderate to severe, if it is too widespread to reasonably cover with topical antibiotics, or if there is an inadequate response after 6 to 8 weeks of topical antibiotics. The tetracycline class of antibiotics should be considered first-line therapy in moderate to severe acne, except when contraindicated because of other circumstances (i.e., pregnancy, <8 years of age, or allergy).

Minocycline in an extended-release form (Ximino) appears safest (at 1 mg/kg once daily), but no dose response was found for efficacy. Doxycycline appears effective in the 1.7 to 2.4 mg/kg dose range. Subantimicrobial dosing of doxycycline (i.e., 20 mg twice daily [immediate release] to 40 mg daily [delayed release]) has also shown efficacy in patients with moderate inflammatory acne. Adverse events with the tetracycline class vary with each medication. Photosensitivity can be seen with the tetracycline class, doxycycline being more photosensitizing than minocycline. Doxycycline is more frequently associated with gastrointestinal disturbances. Doxycycline is primarily metabolized by the liver and can be used safely in most patients with renal impairment. Minocycline has been associated with tinnitus, dizziness, and pigment deposition of the skin, mucous membranes, and teeth. Minocycline-induced skin pigmentation is more common in patients taking higher doses for longer periods of time. The rare serious events associated with minocycline include autoimmune disorders, such as drug reaction with eosinophilia and systemic symptoms (DRESS), drug-induced lupus, and other hypersensitivity reactions. Finally, pseudo tumor cerebri is a rare phenomenon associated with the tetracycline class of antibiotics.

---

[1] Not FDA approved for this indication.
[7] Available as dietary supplement

Erythromycin[1] and azithromycin[1] have also been used in the treatment of acne. Azithromycin has been primarily studied in the treatment of acne with different pulse dosing regimens ranging from 3 times a week to 4 days a month, with azithromycin being an effective treatment in the time span of usually 2 to 3 months. However, a recent study compared using azithromycin 3 times per month to daily doxycycline use and showed that doxycycline had superior results. The macrolide class of antibiotics is most commonly associated with gastrointestinal disturbances. Erythromycin is associated with a higher incidence of diarrhea, nausea, and abdominal discomfort than azithromycin.

TMP-SMX (trimethoprim-sulfamethoxazole [Bactrim, Septra DS])[1] taken twice daily also has side effects to consider but can be useful when other agents are not tolerated. The adverse events of TMP/SMX include gastrointestinal upset, photosensitivity, and drug eruptions. Multiple skin reactions have been observed with patients on this medication, the most severe eruptions being Stevens-Johnson syndrome and toxic epidermal necrolysis. Other adverse effects can include blood dyscrasias, such as neutropenia, agranulocytosis, aplastic anemia, and thrombocytopenia. Although these are rare adverse events, patients on long-term therapy with this medication should be periodically monitored with a complete blood cell count.

Penicillins and cephalosporins are sometimes used in the treatment of acne and can be used as an alternative treatment when circumstances dictate. In particular, these medications represent a useful option in patients who may be pregnant or who have allergies to the other classes of antibiotics.

All oral agents should be used in combination with BP and/or a topical retinoid but not in combination with topical antibiotics. If significant improvement is noted, oral agents should be decreased after 3 to 4 months or stopped in order to attempt maintenance control with topical agents. Limiting systemic antibiotic use is urged because of the reported associations of inflammatory bowel disease, pharyngitis, *C. difficile* infection, and the induction of *Candida vulvovaginitis*.

Combined oral contraceptives can be very helpful in female patients with moderate acne because of their antiandrogenic effects, which decrease sebum production. There are currently four combined oral contraceptives (COCs) approved by the FDA for the treatment of acne. They are ethinyl estradiol/norgestimate (Ortho Tricyclen), ethinyl estradiol/norethindrone acetate/ferrous fumarate (Estrostep Fe, Tilia Fe, Tri-Legest Fe), ethinyl estradiol/drospirenone (Yasmin, Yaz), and ethinyl estradiol/drospirenone/levomefolate (Beyaz, Rajani).

COC use is associated with cardiovascular risks. Venous thromboembolic events (VTEs) have been the center of an ongoing debate regarding COCs. Traditionally, higher doses of ethinyl estradiol have been linked to increased risks of VTE. However, in recent years, some progestins have been implicated as risk factors for VTE. A recent Cochrane meta-analysis evaluated 25 publications reporting on 26 studies focused on oral contraceptives and venous thrombosis. The analysis concluded that all COC use increases the risk of VTE compared with nonusers. The relative risk of venous thrombosis for COCs with 30 to 35 micrograms of ethinyl estradiol and gestodene desogestrel, cyproterone acetate, or drospirenone was similar and about 50% to 80% higher than for COCs with levonorgestrel. To put this increased risk into perspective, it is important to note that the baseline risk of VTE in nonpregnant, nonusers of COCs is 1 to 5 per 10,000 woman-years. Users of COCs have a VTE risk of 3 to 9 per 10,000 woman-years. Users of drospirenone containing COCs have a VTE risk of about 10 per 10,000 woman-years. Pregnant women have a VTE risk between 5 and 20 per 10,000 woman-years, and women within 12 weeks postpartum have a VTE risk of between 40 and 65 per 10,000 woman-years.

Oral isotretinoin (Accutane, Claravis) has demonstrated marked benefit for patients with severe recalcitrant acne, even inducing a full remission. It is a potent teratogen; therefore every woman of child-bearing potential taking isotretinoin should be carefully counseled regarding various contraceptive methods (including long-acting reversible contraception) that are available. Isotretinoin has a host of other significant side effects, including cheilitis, epistaxis, photosensitivity, and many others. Prescribed at 0.5 to 2 mg/kg per day over 20 weeks, it is like chemotherapy for acne. It is extremely tightly regulated, and both prescribers and patients must register with the iPledge program to write for the medicine and to receive the prescriptions. See www.ipledgeprogram.com. When all the precautions are managed, it can be an extremely effective option for the patients with the worst cases of acne.

References
Gannon M, Underhill M, Wellik KE: Which oral antibiotics are best for acne? *J Fam Pract* 60:290–292, 2011.
Knutsen-Larson S, Dawson AL, Dunnick CA, et al: Acne vulgaris: pathogenesis, treatment, and needs assessment, *Dermatol Clin* 30:99–106, 2012.
Strauss JS, Krowchuk DP, Leyden JJ, et al: Guidelines of care for acne vulgaris management, *J Am Acad Dermatol* 56:651–663, 2007.
Titus S, Hodge J: Diagnosis and treatment of acne, *Am Fam Physician* 86:734–740, 2012.
Zaenglein AL, Pathy AL, Schlosser BJ, et al: Guidelines of care for the management of acne vulgaris, *J Am Acad Dermatol* 74(Issue 5):945–973, 2016. e33.

ATOPIC DERMATITIS

Method of
Peck Y. Ong, MD

CURRENT DIAGNOSIS

- Itch must be present for the diagnosis of atopic dermatitis. In addition, the diagnosis must include three or more of the following criteria (U.K. Working Party's Diagnostic Criteria for Atopic Dermatitis):
  - History of generalized dry skin
  - Visible flexural dermatitis
  - Onset of the skin condition before 2 years (not used for patients younger than 4 years)
  - History of itchy skin involving the following areas: elbows, behind knees, front of ankles, or around the neck
  - History of asthma or allergic rhinitis (or for children younger than 4 years, history of atopic disease in a first-degree relative)

CURRENT THERAPY

- Bathe or shower for 10 to 20 minutes daily and pat dry gently.
- Follow immediately by applying an emollient on unaffected areas and an antiinflammatory medication on affected areas.
- Use topical corticosteroids as a first-line antiinflammatory medication; alternative medications are topical calcineurin inhibitors, topical phosphodiesterase 4 inhibitor or dupilumab (Dupixent).
- Avoid environmental triggers such as extreme heat, humidity, or dryness.
- Avoid food allergens that may cause anaphylaxis. Consult an allergist regarding the interpretation of serum-specific IgE tests or food challenge.
- Treat skin infection only when clinical signs are present (e.g., oozing, impetigo).
- Severe, generalized infection or vesicular lesions may indicate herpes simplex virus infection; persistent fever may indicate invasive *S. aureus* infection.

---

[1] Not FDA approved for this indication.

Atopic dermatitis (AD) is a chronic inflammatory skin disease that is characterized by itch and a predilection of eczema on extensor areas in young infants or flexural areas in older children and adults. In the United States, AD affects about 15% of children and 2% of adults. For more than 85% of patients, AD begins during the first 5 years, but 50% of the children with AD improve significantly or outgrow the disease by age 7. The persistence of AD depends on various factors: early onset, severity, family history of AD, personal history of asthma, and food or inhalant allergies.

The itch associated with AD causes significant discomfort in these patients and often leads to sleep loss and to poor school or work performance. The quality of life of children with generalized AD is worse than that for children with diabetes, epilepsy, asthma, cystic fibrosis, or renal disease. The maternal stress in taking care of children with moderate to severe AD is equivalent to that associated with care of children with diabetes, Rett syndrome, profound deafness, or the need for enteral feeding.

Pathophysiology

AD is caused by a combination of genetic and environmental factors. Patients with AD have a defective skin barrier. This leads to a loss of skin hydration and susceptibility to environmental triggers. There is evidence that the skin barrier defects of AD are caused by genetic mutations. Studies have shown that many AD patients carry a genetic mutation in filaggrin, a protein with important barrier function.

Potential external triggers of AD include microbial pathogens and environmental allergens. Almost 100% of AD skin lesions are colonized by *Staphylococcus aureus*, which may produce toxins that trigger immune response in the skin. As a result, AD patients produce an increased amount of pro-allergic cytokines, such as interleukin-4 (IL-4), IL-5, and IL-13, in their skin. These cytokines lead to an increased infiltration of inflammatory T cells and eosinophils. IL-4 and IL-13 also are important for the production of serum IgE, the level of which is elevated in AD patients.

Diagnosis and Clinical Assessment

Most AD patients can be diagnosed by clinical history and physical examination. Typical presentation includes itch, dryness, flexural dermatitis, early age of onset, and atopy such as multiple food allergies. Patients with generalized eczema or adult-onset eczema can present as a diagnostic challenge. The differential diagnosis includes immunodeficiency (e.g., hyper-IgE syndrome, Omenn syndrome), malignancy (e.g., cutaneous T-cell lymphoma), zinc deficiency (i.e., acrodermatitis enteropathica), and celiac-associated dermatitis (i.e., dermatitis herpetiformis) (Table 1). AD children seldom present with failure to thrive, unless they are under severe dietaryrestriction. Failure to thrive should therefore prompt further investigation. Punch skin biopsies may be needed when the diagnosis is still unclear.

The prevalence of mild, moderate, and severe AD is 80%, 18%, and 2%, respectively. Most patients with mild to moderate disease have flexural, extensor, or facial involvement, whereas patients with severe disease often present with total-body involvement with or without erythroderma (Figure 1). Validated scales for assessing the severity of AD include Scoring of Atopic Dermatitis (SCORAD) and Eczema Area and Severity Index (EASI). These scoring systems or a simplified diagram documenting the extent of dermatitis are useful for more objective follow-up of the patient's progress.

Management of Atopic Dermatitis and Associated Conditions

Daily Maintenance Care

Changes in humidity can adversely affect AD symptoms. Dry conditions lead to increased transepidermal water loss and dry AD skin. Extreme heat, humidity, and sweating may lead to

TABLE 1	Differential Diagnoses of Atopic Dermatitis
DISEASE CATEGORY	**DIFFERENTIAL DIAGNOSES**
Dermatologic diseases	Contact dermatitis, seborrheic dermatitis, psoriasis, dyshidrotic eczema, eosinophilic pustular folliculitis, ichthyosis vulgaris
Neoplastic diseases	Cutaneous T-cell lymphoma, Langerhans cell histiocytosis
Immunodeficiencies	Hyper-IgE syndrome, severe combined immunodeficiency, Omenn syndrome, IPEX (immune dysregulation, polyendocrinopathy, enteropathy X-linked) syndrome
Infectious diseases	Scabies, cutaneous candidiasis, tinea versicolor
Nutritional deficiencies	Acrodermatitis enteropathica (zinc deficiency), essential fatty acid deficiency, biotin deficiency
Multisystemic disorders	Netherton syndrome, dermatitis herpetiformis

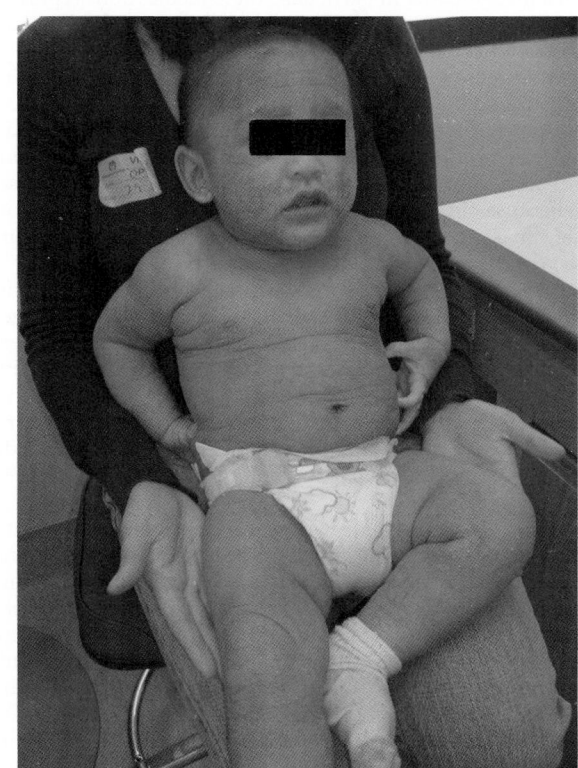

Figure 1 Generalized atopic dermatitis.

irritation of AD skin. AD patients are at increased risk for contact or irritant dermatitis, which may occur with over-the-counter topical skin medications that contain multiple ingredients. Wool or synthetic acrylic fabrics may also be irritating to AD skin.

To improve barrier function, AD patients should bathe or shower for 10 to 20 minutes once or twice daily, followed immediately by gently drying the skin and applying an emollient on the unaffected areas and a topical antiinflammatory medication on the affected areas. A petrolatum-based emollient is recommended in infants and young children because of its occlusive property. In older children and adults, the ointment may not be tolerated well because of its greasy feel, and another emollient or moisturizer may be chosen based on the patient's preference or experience.

Itch may continue to be a problem even if the rash has improved. The mechanisms of itch in AD are not fully understood but do not appear to be mediated solely by histamine. The use of first-generation antihistamines (diphenhydramine [Benadryl][1] and hydroxyzine [Vistaril]) in AD largely depend on their sedative effects and are best used at bedtime. The second-generation, nonsedating antihistamines such as loratadine (Claritin)[1] and cetirizine (Zyrtec)[1] have not proved helpful in treating AD. Low-dose doxepin has been used anecdotally to treat itching in AD.

Topical and Systemic Medications

The first-line medication for AD is a topical corticosteroid (TCS). For mild AD, a TCS with group VI and VII potency (Table 2) may suffice. However, for moderate to severe AD, a TCS with at least group III to V potency is chosen to increase efficacy and to shorten the duration of need for these medications.

The use of TCS is confronted with various obstacles, including rare side effects such as skin atrophy, but mostly patients' or parents' misunderstanding of TCS. Studies have shown that twice-daily use of fluticasone propionate (Cutivate) 0.05% cream (group V) and desonide (DesOwen, Tridesilon) 0.05% ointment or aqueous gel (group V and VI, respectively) continuously up to 1 month in young children with AD results in no significant adverse effect. It is therefore important to clarify for patients or parents the safety and side effects based on the potency of the TCS.

Topical calcineurin inhibitors (TCI) (pimecrolimus [Elidel] 1% cream and Protopic/tacrolimus ointment) are alternative nonsteroidal antiinflammatory medications for AD. Elidel is indicated for mild to moderate AD in patients older than 2 years, whereas 0.03% and 0.1% Protopic are indicated for moderate to severe AD in patients 2 to 15 years old and in patients 16 years old or older, respectively. Both Elidel and Protopic have an FDA black box warning saying that their long-term use may be associated with cancer risk. However, a recent large longitudinal study has failed to confirm this risk. These medications continue to be useful alternatives for skin areas that are prone to atrophy, including the face, axillae, and groins.

A third class of topical medication, phosphodiesterase 4 inhibitor (crisaborole [Eucrisa] 2% ointment), has been approved by the FDA for patients 2 years and older with mild to moderate AD. A biologic dupilumab (Dupixent), which targets IL-4 and IL-13, has also been approved by the FDA for patients 6 years and older with moderate to severe AD.

Wet-wrap treatment, phototherapy, and systemic immunosuppressive therapies (e.g., cyclosporine [Sandimmune, Neoral],[1] azathioprine [Imuran],[1] methotrexate [Trexall],[1] and mycophenolate mofetil [CellCept])[1] are alternatives, but not approved by FDA, for severe AD patients. Because of the potential serious adverseeffects associated with these treatments, referral to an allergist or dermatologist is recommended before their initiation.

Systemic corticosteroids usually are not recommended for AD because of their known adverse effects, including stunted growth in children, adrenal suppression, osteoporosis, and cataracts. A rebound of AD symptoms is common after the medication is stopped. If a systemic corticosteroid is used, it should be tapered over a short period (e.g., a week) while topical antiinflammatory treatment is intensified.

The efficacy and side effects of the following medications have not been established in AD: intravenous immunoglobulin (IVIG),[1] anti-IgE (omalizumab [Xolair]),[1] probiotics,[7] montelukast (Singulair),[1] Chinese medicinal herbs,[7] and fish oils.[1]

---

[1]Not FDA approved for this indication.
[7]Available as a dietary supplement.

TABLE 2 Classification of Topical Corticosteroids Based on Potency

GROUP	TOPICAL CORTICOSTEROIDS
I (most potent)	Clobetasol propionate 0.05% (Temovate) (cream, ointment, gel), betamethasone dipropionate, augmented 0.05% (Diprolene) (cream, ointment), diflorasone diacetate 0.05% (Psorcon) (ointment)
II	Amcinonide 0.1% (Cyclocort) (ointment), betamethasone dipropionate 0.05% (Diprosone) (ointment), mometasone furoate 0.1% (Elocon) (ointment), halcinonide 0.1% (Halog) (cream), fluocinonide 0.05% (Lidex) (gel, cream, ointment), desoximetasone (Topicort) (0.05% gel, 0.25% cream, 0.25% ointment)
III	Fluticasone propionate 0.005% (Cutivate) (ointment), amcinonide 0.1% (Cyclocort) (lotion, cream), diflorasone diacetate 0.05% (Florone) (cream), betamethasone valerate 0.1% (Valisone) (ointment)
IV	Flurandrenolide 0.05% (Cordran) (ointment), mometasone furoate 0.1% (Elocon) (cream), triamcinolone acetonide 0.1% (Kenalog) (cream), fluocinolone acetonide 0.025% (Synalar) (ointment), hydrocortisone valerate 0.2% (Westcort) (ointment)
V	Flurandrenolide 0.05% (Cordran) (cream), fluticasone propionate 0.05% (Cutivate) (cream), hydrocortisone butyrate 0.1% (Locoid) (cream), fluocinolone acetonide 0.025% (Synalar) (cream), desonide 0.05% (Tridesilon) (ointment), betamethasone valerate 0.1% (Valisone) (cream), hydrocortisone valerate 0.2% (Westcort) (cream), prednicarbate 0.1% (Dermatop) (cream)
VI	Alclometasone dipropionate 0.05% (Aclovate) (cream, ointment), fluocinolone acetonide 0.01% (Synalar) (solution, cream) (Derma-Smoothe/FS Oil), Desonide 0.05% (Tridesilon) (cream and aqueous gel)
VII (least potent)	Hydrocortisone 1%/2.5% (lotion, cream, ointment).

Data from Stoughton RB. Vasoconstrictor assay—specific applications. In Maibach HI, Surber C, editors. *Topical Corticosteroids*. Basel, Switzerland: Karger, 1992, pp 42–53.

Food Allergies

At least 30% of children with moderate to severe AD have one or more food allergies, compared with 4% to 6% of the general population. Accurate diagnosis of food allergies in AD patients is crucial because it can prevent life-threatening anaphylaxis or unnecessary food restriction.

The diagnosis of food allergy involves history taking and food challenge. History taking is helpful in the diagnosis of food allergy in most patients. It is often useful to begin by asking the patients whether they have any problems or reactions with any of the seven food allergens: milk, egg, peanut, wheat, soybean, seafood, and tree nuts. These foods account for more than 90% of food allergies. Almost all food allergic reactions occur in the first hour. AD patients may complain of immediate worsening of itching after ingestion. Symptoms of anaphylactic reactions include throat-clearing, cough, shortness of breath, vomiting, dizziness, fainting, and headache, which may be attributed to hypotension. Most food allergic reactions also manifest with skin symptoms, including hives, swelling, or generalized itching.

Skin tests and serum specific IgE are useful in the context of negative or undetectable test results because they have a negative predictive value of more than 95%. The level of a positive test result (i.e., skin test wheal size or serum-specific IgE level), which correlates with the chance of a reaction, should be interpreted in the context of a clinical reaction. Consider consultation with an allergist regarding food challenge if there are still concerns regarding positive serum-specific IgE. More accurate epitope-specific IgE assays may be available to clinicians in the near future.

Patients with confirmed food allergy should avoid any amount of the food allergen. Parents or patients should be instructed to read food allergen labels carefully. All packaged foods in the United States are required to label the contents of milk, eggs, peanuts, wheat, soybeans, fish, shellfish, or tree nuts. Organizations, such as the Food Allergy Research & Education, can provide patients and parents with useful information on potential hidden food allergens and alternative food sources.

AD children often have multiple food allergies, including cow's milk and soy, and the use of a hydrolyzed or amino acid–based formula can provide an alternative source of nutrition. For these patients, consultation with a dietitian can be helpful in managing food avoidance and nutrition needs.

Patients or parents of children with anaphylactic reactions should be prescribed and instructed on the use of an epinephrine autoinjector (EpiPen or Auvi-Q 0.15 mg for patients who weigh more than 15 kg but less than 30 kg; 0.3 mg for patients who weigh 30 kg or more, while Auvi-Q 0.1 mg for patients who weigh 7.5–15 kg).

Infants with severe AD who consume peanut products early have a 86% relative risk reduction in the development of peanut allergy. For any infants with AD under a year, clinicians should consider introducing peanut products early in their diet according to the guidelines of National Institute of Allergy and Infectious Disease, or consult an allergist.

Infections
Most AD patients are colonized by *S. aureus* on their skin lesions or in their nostrils. The frequency of colonization increases with AD severity. Exacerbation of AD is frequently associated with secondary *S. aureus* skin infections. Other common skin pathogens in AD include group A β-hemolytic *Streptococcus* and herpes simplex virus (HSV), which causes eczema herpeticum (Figure 2). Many reports have documented invasive *S. aureus* infections such as bacteremia, septic arthritis, osteomyelitis, and endocarditis in AD patients. Persistent fever or focal limb pain should alert the physician to the possibility of these infections.

The reasons for the high rate of bacterial colonization and skin infections in AD are not completely understood. A defective skin barrier and decreased cutaneous innate immunity (i.e., deficiency in natural skin antibiotics) likely contribute to the frequency of skin infections in patients with AD.

Because of the concern about increasing bacterial resistance, antibiotics are not recommended unless clinical infection is confirmed. The use of dilute bleach in treating AD remains controversial.

Inhalant Allergies and Asthma
Eighty-five percent of AD infants have concurrent respiratory allergies or are at risk for allergic rhinitis or asthma. However, whether inhalant allergens lead to a worsening of AD remains controversial. Randomized, double-blind, placebo-controlled studies have shown positive and negative effects of house dust mites (HDM) as a trigger for AD symptoms. Because there is no serious side effect associated with the use of HDM-proof bed and pillow encasings, unless cost is an issue, these encasings are recommended for AD patients with HDM sensitization. Further research is needed to confirm the role of inhalant allergens, including furry pets and pollens, as triggers for AD.

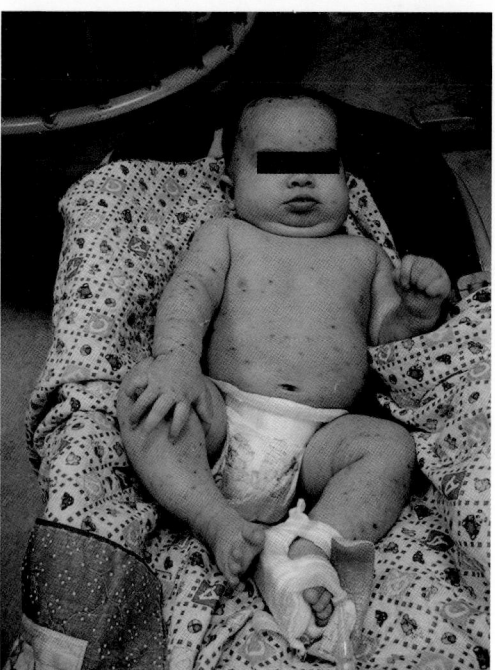

Figure 2 Eczema herpeticum.

Investigational Treatments for Atopic Dermatitis
Because of the concern about potential side effects associated with existing therapies of AD, several agents are being investigated for the treatment of AD. They include anti-IL-13, anti-IL-31 receptor, and Janus kinase (JAK) inhibitors. Anti-IL-31 receptor is a potential anti-itch medication for AD, whereas topical or oral JAK inhibitors are potential nonsteroidal alternatives. With improved understanding of the pathophysiology of AD, treatments for AD are likely going to be more target-specific in the future.

References
Beattie PE, Lewis-Jones MS: A comparative study of impairment of quality of life in children with skin disease and children with other chronic childhood diseases, *Br J Dermatol* 155:145–151, 2006.

Beck LA, Thaçi D, Hamilton JD, et al: Dupilumab treatment in adults with moderate-to-severe atopic dermatitis, *N Engl J Med* 371:130–139, 2014.

Chopra R, Vakharia PP, Sacotte R, Silverberg JI: Efficacy of bleach baths in reducing severity of atopic dermatitis: a systematic review and meta-analysis, *Ann Allergy Asthma Immunol* 119(5):435–440, 2017.

Du Toit G, Roberts G, Sayre PH, et al: Randomized trial of peanut consumption in infants at risk for peanut allergy, *N Engl J Med* 372:803–813, 2015.

Eichenfield LF, Basu S, Calvarese B, et al: Effect of desonide hydrogel 0.05% on the hypothalamic-pituitary-adrenal axis in pediatric subjects with moderate to severe atopic dermatitis, *Pediatr Dermatol* 24:289–295, 2007.

Elias PM: Barrier-repair therapy for atopic dermatitis: corrective lipid biochemical therapy, *Expert Rev Dermatol* 3:441–452, 2008.

Faught J, Bierl C, Barton B, Kemp A: Stress in mothers of young children with eczema, *Arch Dis Child* 92:683–686, 2007.

Friedlander SF, Hebert AA, Allen DB: for the Fluticasone Pediatrics Safety Study Group: Safety of fluticasone propionate cream 0.05% for the treatment of severe and extensive atopic dermatitis in children as young as 3 months, *J Am Acad Dermatol* 46:387–393, 2002.

Paller AS, Fölster-Holst R, Chen SC, et al: No evidence of increased cancer incidence in children using topical tacrolimus for atopic dermatitis, *J Am Acad Dermatol* 83(2):375–381, 2020. Aug.

Suprun M, Sicherer SH, Wood RA, et al: Early epitope-specific IgE antibodies are predictive of childhood peanut allergy, *J Allergy Clin Immunol* 146(5):1080–1088, 2020.

Togias A, Cooper SF, Acebal ML, et al: Addendum guidelines for the prevention of peanut allergy in the United States: report of the National Institute of Allergy and Infectious Diseases-sponsored expert panel, *J Allergy Clin Immunol* 139:29–44, 2017.

Wang V, Boguniewicz J, Boguniewicz M, Ong PY: The infectious complications of atopic dermatitis, *Ann Allergy Asthma Immunol* 126(1):3–12, 2021.

BACTERIAL DISEASES OF THE SKIN

Method of
Karissa Gilchrist, MD

CURRENT DIAGNOSIS

- The large variety of bacterial skin infections can usually be distinguished by history, physical exam, and clinical presentation.
- Bacterial infections can range from those affecting the superficial layers of skin to the deep layers and soft tissue.
- Many infections are precipitated by a breach in the normal skin barrier.
- Infection can vary in severity depending on how extensive and invasive it is.
- Deep infection can lead to systemic toxicity.
- Necrotizing infection can rapidly progress and cause extensive tissue damage and even death.

CURRENT THERAPY

- Antibiotic therapy is selected based on knowledge of the most likely causative pathogen or based on culture results.
- When a loculated abscess is identified, procedural incision and drainage should be performed.
- Broad-spectrum empiric antibiotic coverage should be initiated when a rapidly progressing necrotizing infection is suspected.
- Delay in surgical consultation and debridement of necrotizing infection may result in tissue damage, limb loss, and/or death.
- Tissue culture of necrotizing infection can guide antibiotic choice.

Bacterial infections of the skin can manifest in a broad range of clinical presentations. Bacterial skin diseases can occur both superficially and in the deep layers. They can also range from mild to aggressive and life-threatening infection. Skin infections have increased in prevalence and severity in part due to the development of resistant bacterial organisms. For this reason, it is critical for clinicians to be able to promptly recognize and manage bacterial infections of the skin.

Common Infections

Cellulitis

Cellulitis is an acute bacterial skin infection that causes poorly demarcated areas of erythema, warmth, tenderness, and edema of the skin involving the deep dermal and subcutaneous layers. Depending on the extent of edema and inflammation, the affected skin may develop bullae, ecchymosis, or maceration. Cellulitis may occur on any area of the skin but is typically found on the lower extremities and is almost always unilateral. Cellulitis develops when there is a break in the skin and pathogens are able to breach the surface. It most commonly arises from infection with streptococci. *Staphylococcus aureus* is a less common cause of cellulitis but should be considered in special circumstances such as bite wounds, penetrating trauma, intravenous drug use, or in immunocompromised patients (Table 1).

Culture or biopsy of the affected skin is not routinely recommended for the diagnosis of cellulitis. Cultures often yield negative or unhelpful results as the rapidly spreading skin manifestations may be more likely related to a strong inflammatory response to the inciting pathogen and may not be representative of the bacterial load. Blood cultures may be considered if there are systemic signs of infection. Diagnosis of cellulitis should be made clinically. Labs and imaging may be obtained to help distinguish

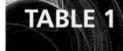

TABLE 1	Primary Pathogen for Common Bacterial Skin Infections
DIAGNOSIS	**ORGANISM**
Cellulitis	Streptococci (*Staphylococcus aureus* less common)
Impetigo	*S. aureus* Group A beta-hemolytic streptococci
Folliculitis	*S. aureus* Gram-negative bacteria
Abscess	*S. aureus*, predominantly MRSA

MRSA, Methicillin-resistant *S. aureus*.

cellulitis from other diagnoses and rule out complications such as underlying abscess, deep venous thrombosis, osteomyelitis, or necrotizing fasciitis. Stasis dermatitis is commonly mistaken for cellulitis and can be differentiated by its bilateral appearance and lack of skin trauma.

In the treatment of mild cases of uncomplicated nonpurulent cellulitis without systemic signs of infection, an oral antibiotic agent that is active against streptococci—such as cephalexin (Keflex), dicloxacillin[1], or amoxicillin/clavulanate (Augmentin)—should be used. If the patient has a penicillin allergy, clindamycin can be used as an alternative. The typical treatment duration is 5 days, but this may be extended in the case of residual symptoms. In patients who fail oral antimicrobial treatment or in those with systemic signs of infection, an intravenous regimen with an agent such as cefazolin (Ancef), ceftriaxone (Rocephin), or clindamycin should be considered. In cases where there is increased risk of methicillin-resistant *S. aureus* (MRSA) infection, such as penetrating trauma or intravenous drug use, intravenous vancomycin should be added (Table 2).

Erysipelas

For some, the term *erysipelas* is synonymous with cellulitis. However, erysipelas refers to infection that is limited to the upper dermis; cellulitis extends into the deeper dermis. The borders of the erysipelas rash are more clearly demarcated than those of cellulitis. Erysipelas is always nonpurulent. The treatment outlined earlier for cellulitis can be applied to erysipelas with antibiotics targeted against streptococci and, if systemic signs or symptoms are present, parental agents can be used.

Impetigo

Impetigo is a common bacterial skin infection that can occur at any age but is most commonly seen in children. It is most prevalent in hot, humid conditions and is highly contagious. It is transmitted by direct contact and may develop secondarily after a disruption of the skin occurs from an insect bite or other underlying disease such as eczema or psoriasis.

Impetigo can be classified into two major categories: bullous and nonbullous. Bullous impetigo is a result of *S. aureus* infection. Strains of this organism produce a factor that cleaves the junction between the epidermal and dermal skin layers. This causes a delicate vesicle to form, which may break open, leaving behind a crusted erosion. Nonbullous impetigo is most commonly caused by *S. aureus*, group A beta-hemolytic streptococci, or a combination of both (see Table 1). This form of impetigo typically begins as erythematous papules or pustules. These lesions develop a discharge that dries and forms a classic honey-colored crust.

Treatment for both bullous and nonbullous impetigo consists of antibiotic therapy aimed at both staphylococcal and streptococcal organisms (see Table 2). Either topical or oral antibiotics can be used for treatment of impetigo depending on the severity and extent of infection. Topical treatment with mupirocin

---

[1]Not FDA approved for this indication.
[2]Not available in the United States.

TABLE 2 Suggested Antibiotic Agents for Common Bacterial Skin Infections

DIAGNOSIS	ANTIBIOTIC
Cellulitis	• Cephalexin (Keflex) • Dicloxacillin[1] • Amoxicillin/clavulanate (Augmentin) Alternative: • Clindamycin Severe infection: • Cefazolin (Ancef) • Ceftriaxone (Rocephin) MRSA risk factors: • Vancomycin
Impetigo	Mild cases: • Topical mupirocin (Bactroban) Severe or extensive cases: • Cephalexin (Keflex) • Dicloxacillin[1] MRSA risk factors: • Doxycycline • Clindamycin • Trimethoprim/sulfamethoxazole (Bactrim DS)[1]
Folliculitis	Suspected *S. aureus*: • Topical mupirocin (Bactroban)[1] or clindamycin[1] • Cephalexin (Keflex) • Dicloxacillin Suspected *Pseudomonas*: • No treatment • Ciprofloxacin (Cipro)[1]
Abscess	• Trimethoprim/sulfamethoxazole (Bactrim DS)[1] • Clindamycin

MRSA, Methicillin-resistant *S. aureus*.
[1]Not FDA approved for this indication.

(Bactroban) ointment 2% three times daily for 5 days can be effective for mild cases of impetigo. Over-the-counter topical bacitracin[1] or triple antibiotic ointments are not as effective as mupirocin in the treatment of impetigo. If an oral agent is desired for more severe or extensive cases, therapy should consist of an antibiotic medication that is active against *S. aureus*, such as cephalexin (Keflex) or dicloxacillin[1] for 7 days. *S. aureus* isolates from impetigo are typically methicillin-susceptible *S. aureus* (MSSA); however, if MRSA is suspected or confirmed with direct culture of an impetiginous lesion or its drainage, treatment with doxycycline, clindamycin, or sulfamethoxazole-trimethoprim (Bactrim DS)[1] for 7 days is recommended.

Ecthyma

Ecthyma is a form of impetigo that infects deeper layers of the skin into the dermis. Lesions appear as "punched out" ulcerations with an overlying crust and surrounding erythematous edema. Ecthyma differs from impetigo in that it heals with scarring due to the deep skin involvement. The principal pathogen causing ecthyma is group A streptococcus (GAS). Treatment of ecthyma differs from that of impetigo and always requires oral antibiotic therapy. Penicillin is the first-line choice of antibiotic agent. With both impetigo and ecthyma, care should be taken to use contact precautions and frequent handwashing to prevent spread.

Ecthyma Gangrenosum

Ecthyma gangrenosum is a skin eruption that classically arises in immunocompromised patients with *Pseudomonas aeruginosa* bacteremia. An ecthyma gangrenosum lesion typically begins as an erythematous macule or pustule and quickly develops into a gangrenous ulcer. This lesion results from bacterial invasion of the vascular wall and subsequent tissue ischemia and necrosis.

There may be one single eruption or several. Lesions can occur in any location, with the axilla and genital regions most commonly affected. Although it is possible for lesions to occur in an immunocompetent patient without any signs of systemic illness, the presence of ecthyma gangrenosum should definitely raise the clinician's suspicion for bacteremia, especially with *P. aeruginosa*. Treatment involves empiric antibiotic therapy with an antipseudomonal agent. Blood cultures should be obtained, and lesions can be swabbed for culture to help guide antibiotic narrowing.

Folliculitis

Folliculitis is the infection and inflammation of hair follicles. It typically presents as erythematous papules or pustules in hair follicles. As with most inflammatory skin diseases, pruritus is the most frequent symptom. Lesions may be painful. Folliculitis is typically infectious, with the most common etiology being bacterial. It can also be caused by viral, fungal, or parasitic infection. Bacterial folliculitis is most frequently caused by *S. aureus* but may also result from infection with gram-negative bacteria (see Table 1). Multiple factors may predispose a patient to develop folliculitis; these include underlying immunodeficiency, frequent scratching (from underlying eczema or other pruritic skin disease), nasal colonization with *S. aureus*, shaving in the opposite direction of hair growth, hyperhidrosis, or prolonged use of topical corticosteroids. Exposure to underchlorinated heated water is the classic risk factor for developing "hot tub folliculitis," which is caused by *P. aeruginosa* infection. In this example of gram-negative folliculitis, pustules appear on the areas of hair-bearing skin that were exposed to the contaminated water. Onset may occur up to 48 hours after exposure.

Diagnosis is typically made clinically, and the distribution of lesions may be suggestive of a pathogenic etiology. Folliculitis occurring primarily on the face or scalp is most likely due to *S. aureus*. Culture of pustule contents may be considered if the diagnosis is unclear. Pseudomonal folliculitis is often self-limiting but may necessitate treatment with oral ciprofloxacin (Cipro)[1] in the setting of immunodeficiency or in severe cases. Topical mupirocin (Bactroban)[1] or topical clindamycin[1] is an effective treatment for cases of superficial folliculitis thought to be caused by *S. aureus*. In very mild and localized cases of *S. aureus*, lesions may even resolve spontaneously. If the disease is extensive, refractory to topical treatment, or appears to involve the deep areas of the follicles, an oral antibiotic should be used for treatment. First-line agents include cephalexin (Keflex) or dicloxacillin treatment for 7 to 10 days. If MRSA is suspected or confirmed on culture, oral trimethoprim/sulfamethoxazole (Bactrim DS)[1], clindamycin, or doxycycline should be used for treatment (see Table 2). It is important to try to minimize or eliminate any predisposing factors identified in order to prevent recurrence.

Abscess

An abscess is a collection of pus within the skin or soft tissue. It presents as an erythematous, painful nodule that is fluctuant, sometimes with an overlying pustule. *S. aureus* is responsible for the majority of abscesses (see Table 1), with a large portion being due to methicillin-resistant strains (MRSA). Immunosuppression or any disruption of the normal skin barrier may predispose a patient to develop one or multiple abscesses. Procedural incision and evacuation of the abscess debris should be performed for treatment. Care should be taken to probe the cavity and release loculated areas within the abscess. Proper wound care should follow with application of a dry gauze dressing with or without packing of the wound space. Systemic antibiotics should be used in addition to incision and drainage in cases of multiple lesions, abscesses larger than 2 cm, immunosuppression, signs of systemic toxicity, refractory lesions, extensive surrounding cellulitis, or presence of implanted medical devices. It is reasonable to forgo antibiotic therapy in an otherwise healthy patient with a single small abscess, especially in the setting of numerous antibiotic

[1]Not FDA approved for this indication.

allergies. However, there is now evidence to suggest that treatment with trimethoprim/sulfamethoxazole (Bactrim DS)[1] or clindamycin for any patient who has undergone incision and drainage may improve cure rates and decrease the risk of recurrence (see Table 2).

Furuncle and Carbuncle

When an abscess forms at the base of a hair follicle, it is referred to as a furuncle. This is different from folliculitis, where infection does not extend deeper than the epidermis. A carbuncle develops when several furuncles occur in multiple adjacent follicles and the infection coalesces into a larger mass of pus. Carbuncles commonly occur on the back of the neck and in the axilla. As in the case of cutaneous abscesses, the principal pathogen for furuncles and carbuncles is *S. aureus*. Many furuncles will rupture spontaneously, allowing the pus to drain. The application of moist heat may also help to encourage spontaneous drainage. Carbuncles and larger furuncles should be treated with incision and drainage.

Invasive Infections

Necrotizing Soft Tissue Infection

Necrotizing cellulitis is an aggressive, rapidly spreading life-threatening bacterial infection of the skin. When there is involvement of the fascia or muscle, the descriptive term becomes *necrotizing fasciitis* or *necrotizing myositis*, accordingly. These infections result in significant tissue destruction and have a high mortality rate. Necrotizing infections may be precipitated by varying degrees of disruption of the skin barrier due to anything from insect bites to intravenous drug use or major penetrating trauma. Diabetes increases the risk of developing a necrotizing soft tissue infection.

Necrotizing infection presents as skin erythema, edema, and warmth with underlying crepitus that develops quickly over the course of hours and progresses rapidly. Skin findings are usually associated with severe pain, which may be out of proportion to findings on examination. Signs of systemic toxicity, such as fever or hemodynamic instability, may also appear. Delayed clinical recognition can result in extensive tissue damage, limb loss, or death. Prompt surgical consultation should be made if a necrotizing soft tissue infection is suspected. If the diagnosis is unclear, a computed tomography scan may be helpful in revealing the presence of gas in the soft tissues, but it should not delay surgical intervention. Treatment should include emergent surgical debridement as well as empiric antibiotic administration. Care should be taken to provide hemodynamic support as needed. Blood cultures would ideally be obtained prior to the administration of antibiotics. Empiric therapy should consist of a polymicrobial approach with a combination of agents aimed at treating MRSA, aerobes, and anaerobes (Table 3). Antibiotic therapy can be tailored according to culture results from tissue obtained during surgical debridement.

Fournier Gangrene

Fournier gangrene is a form of necrotizing soft tissue infection involving the perineal region. It is typically seen in middle-aged adults, particularly those who have diabetes mellitus. Potential predisposing factors may include recent urologic procedures, chronic use of an indwelling urinary catheter, or urethral trauma. However, this condition can develop without these risk factors. Cutaneous and systemic findings are similar to those of other necrotizing soft tissue infections, and prompt surgical debridement with broad-spectrum empiric antibiotic coverage is critical.

Invasive Group A Streptococcal Infection with Toxic Shock Syndrome

GAS is a common cause of superficial skin infections, as outlined earlier in this chapter. However, this pathogen can sometimes lead to invasive disease and result in necrotizing infection. Toxic shock syndrome is a complication that may arise when invasive

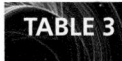

TABLE 3 Suggested Antibiotic Agents for Invasive Bacterial Skin Infections

DIAGNOSIS	ANTIBIOTIC
Necrotizing soft tissue infection Group A streptococcal infection with toxic shock syndrome	1. Vancomycin, linezolid (Zyvox), or daptomycin (Cubicin) plus 2. Piperacillin-tazobactam (Zosyn) or a carbapenem or Ceftriaxone (Rocephin) plus metronidazole(Flagyl) or Fluoroquinolone plus metronidazole (Flagyl)
Invasive	1. Clindamycin plus 2. Penicillin
Staphylococcal scalded skin syndrome	Intravenous oxacillin, nafcillin, cefazolin (Ancef), or vancomycin
Tularemia	Mild or moderate disease: • Oral fluoroquinolone or doxycycline Severe disease: • IV/IM gentamicin[1] or IM streptomycin

[1]Not FDA approved for this indication.

GAS produces a toxin that induces the subsequent release of inflammatory cytokines. Skin manifestations include induration and erythema of the affected areas, eventually giving rise to hemorrhagic skin sloughing. It is often associated with signs of systemic toxicity and multiorgan failure. Toxic shock syndrome may also develop as a result of invasive postpartum endometritis. It is a rapidly progressive disease and prompt treatment should be provided along with hemodynamic support. Antibiotic treatment includes coverage with both clindamycin and penicillin (see Table 3). Clindamycin has the additional benefit of helping to suppress the toxin-mediated inflammatory response. Dual coverage with penicillin is important due to potential clindamycin resistance.

Staphylococcal Scalded Skin Syndrome

Staphylococcal scalded skin syndrome is a complication that can arise from any infection caused by *S. aureus*, such as impetigo, for example. It typically occurs in children and develops as a result of exotoxins produced by the bacteria. Skin findings include painful erythema and desquamation; the mucous membranes are spared. Fever and generalized malaise usually accompany the cutaneous findings. Diagnosis can usually be made clinically; however, culture of the suspected primary infection can be collected for confirmation. One should keep in mind that areas of desquamation or bullae in scalded skin syndrome will be sterile, as these lesions are a result of the exotoxins and not direct bacterial infection. Therefore culture of these areas is unlikely to be helpful.

Patients with staphylococcal scalded skin syndrome are typically treated in an inpatient setting with intravenous antibiotics and supportive care. First-line antibiotic agents include oxacillin, nafcillin, cefazolin (Ancef), and vancomycin (see Table 3). Clindamycin is not a recommended first-choice agent due to high rates of resistance.

Tularemia

Tularemia is an uncommon infection caused by *Francisella tularensis*; it occurs after exposure to an infected insect or animal, most commonly a tick or rabbit. Clinical manifestations vary in severity. The most common form of tularemia is ulceroglandular disease. Symptom onset typically occurs within 3 to 5 days following exposure and begins with nonspecific constitutional symptoms such as fever, headache, myalgias, and generalized malaise. Cutaneous manifestations commonly begin with a single erythematous ulceration with or without a central eschar. Location of the skin lesion is based on the site of inoculation, and the anatomic distribution of findings is regional. Rarely, there may be multiple skin lesions. Ulceroglandular tularemia is associated with localized tender lymphadenopathy. Glandular tularemia has the same characteristics as ulceroglandular tularemia without the ulcerations.

When tularemia is suspected clinically, serology should be sent for diagnosis. It generally takes 2 weeks for antibodies to *Francisella* to reach diagnostic levels, and serology may need to be repeated if clinical suspicion is high. Polymerase chain reaction (PCR) testing can be completed more rapidly depending on lab availability of the test. Blood or tissue cultures are rarely positive; if such specimens are collected, laboratory staff should be notified in advance of tularemia suspicion in order to optimize conditions for culture growth as well as for infection control precautions. Treatment consists of selecting an effective antibiotic regimen. In general, an oral fluoroquinolone or doxycycline would be a reasonable initial treatment for patients with mild or moderate disease. If the infection is severe, intravenous or intramuscular gentamicin[1] or intramuscular streptomycin is recommended (see Table 3). Of note, *F. tularensis* has the potential to be used as a bioterrorism agent, as it is easily disseminated and infection can occur at low exposure. In such a case, recognition and reporting are critical.

---

[1]Not FDA approved for this indication.

References

Daum RS, Miller LG, Immergluck L, et al: A placebo-controlled trial of antibiotics for smaller skin abscesses, *N Engl J Med* 376:2545–2555, 2017.

Handler MZ, Schwartz RA: Staphylococcal scalded skin syndrome: diagnosis and management in children and adults, *J Eur Acad Dermatol Venereol* 28:1418–1423, 2014.

Jeng A, Beheshti M, Li J, Nathan R: The role of beta-hemolytic streptococci in causing diffuse, nonculturable cellulitis: a prospective investigation, *Medicine (Baltimore)* 89:217–226, 2010.

Luelmo-Aguilar J, Santandreu MS: Folliculitis: recognition and management, *Am J Clin Dermatol* 5:301–310, 2004.

Pereira LB: Impetigo – review, *An Bras Dermatol* 89:293–299, 2014.

Raff AB, Kroshinsky D: Cellulitis: a review, *JAMA* 316:325–337, 2016.

Snowden J, Simonsen KA: Tularemia. In *StatPearls*. Treasure Island (FL), StatPearls Publishing, 2020.

Stevens DL, Bisno AL, Chambers HF, et al: Practice guidelines for the diagnosis and management of skin and soft tissue infections: 2014 update by the Infectious Diseases Society of America, *Clin Infect Dis* 59:e10–52, 2014.

AUTOIMMUNE BULLOUS DISEASES

Method of
Dominic J. Wu, MD; and Anand Rajpara, MD

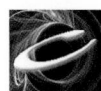

CURRENT DIAGNOSIS

- There is a significant overlap between the major autoimmune bullous diseases, which include pemphigus vulgaris, bullous pemphigoid, dermatitis herpetiformis, linear IgA bullous disease, and more.
- Biopsy is usually required for diagnosis, including routine hematoxylin and eosin stain (H&E) histology and other special tests including direct immunofluorescence (DIF), indirect immunofluorescence (IIF), and ELISA.
- Preferred biopsy sites include edge or entire intact blister/bulla (H&E), perilesional "normal" appearing skin (DIF).
- Different staining patterns on DIF, salt-split skin, and IIF can help differentiate between diseases that appear similar on routine histology.
- It is important to evaluate for other causes of blistering disease, including infectious causes such as bullous impetigo, herpes simplex virus, varicella zoster virus, and noninfectious causes such as severe contact allergic dermatitis, poison ivy dermatitis, and others.

CURRENT THERAPY

- Immunosuppressive medications are the mainstay treatment for autoimmune bullous diseases.
- Specific treatments for each diagnosis are listed under each section. Many of the treatment regimens are not Food and Drug Administration (FDA)–approved treatments and should only be attempted by experienced clinicians familiar with each medication and their side effect profiles and monitoring parameters.
- Traditional first-line therapy is with oral corticosteroids to induce remission, with or without adjunctive steroid-sparing therapy.
- Topical corticosteroids should be attempted for milder cases of bullous pemphigoid prior to initiation of systemic corticosteroids because of side effects and risks for systemic steroids and efficacy of topicals.
- Adjunctive steroid-sparing therapy may help clinicians lower and eventually taper the doses of corticosteroids.
- Patients on higher doses of corticosteroids and/or longer courses of treatment with corticosteroids may require prophylaxis or treatment of osteoporosis and peptic ulcer disease.
- Early involvement of relevant specialties is critical given the complex nature of the disease and treatment options.

Epidemiology

The autoimmune bullous diseases are a heterogenous group of diseases, mostly occurring in the elderly. Please see each section for specific epidemiologic comments.

Pathophysiology

Specific antibodies and pathophysiology will be discussed under specific diseases discussed in this chapter.

Diagnosis

There is significant clinical overlap between the major autoimmune bullous diseases. In addition to obtaining a detailed clinical history, biopsies are usually required for diagnosis. Ideal sample sites for routine histology (H&E) are of the blister/bullae (intact if possible, or the edge of the bulla), and normal-appearing perilesional skin for direct immunofluorescence (DIF). Punch biopsies (usually 4 mm punch tool) or deeper shave biopsies are common biopsy methods. Specific staining patterns are noted under each individual disease entity below. Indirect immunofluorescence (IIF) may also be helpful, although it is beyond the scope of this chapter and will not be discussed in detail.

Pemphigus

Pathophysiology

In normal skin tissue, epithelial cells are held together by adherens and desmosome protein junctions. In pemphigus diseases, different desmosomal proteins are targeted by autoantibodies, causing a loss of connection between adjacent cells, resulting in splitting of skin layers. The causes of pemphigus diseases vary, including idiopathic, drug-induced cases (traditionally penicillamine and ACE inhibitors such as captopril), underlying conditions such as thymoma, myasthenia gravis, autoimmune thyroiditis, and more. Epidemiologic studies have shown higher incidence in people of Jewish ancestry. Certain genetic predispositions have also been identified, including HLA-DRB1, HLA-DR4, and HLA-DR6.

The pemphigus group of bullous diseases includes (1) pemphigus vulgaris and pemphigus vegetans, (2) pemphigus foliaceus and pemphigus erythematosus, and (3) paraneoplastic pemphigus. Pemphigus vulgaris and pemphigus vegetans are caused by circulating IgG autoantibodies, primarily against desmoglein 3 (Dsg3), which is mostly found on the lower portion of the epidermis. Desmogleins are desmosomal cadherin proteins that form desmosomes, which join cells together. Patients with pemphigus foliaceus have autoantibodies directed against desmoglein 1 (Dsg1). As its name denotes, paraneoplastic pemphigus is a paraneoplastic syndrome associated with an underlying neoplastic disorder (most frequently non-Hodgkin's lymphoma, CLL, Castleman's disease, thymoma, sarcoma, and Waldenström's macroglobulinemia). In paraneoplastic pemphigus, patients may have circulating autoantibodies against nearly all the different components of the desmosome junction including plakin family proteins and both Dsg1 and Dsg3.

Clinical Manifestations

Pemphigus vulgaris presents with painful flaccid skin blisters/bullae and erosions in the oral cavity. Oral involvement is typically seen in cases of pemphigus vulgaris, which can be quite helpful in distinguishing between pemphigus foliaceus (typically no oral involvement) and other autoimmune bullous diseases such as bullous pemphigoid, in which a smaller subset of patients have oral mucosal involvement. Nikolsky sign (shearing of skin with slight pressure or rubbing of perilesional skin) and Asboe-Hansen (pressure placed on intact bulla results in spreading of bulla to surrounding skin) are both found in cases of pemphigus vulgaris.

Pemphigus foliaceus (including the Brazilian endemic variant Fogo Selvagem and pemphigus erythematosus) typically present with impetigo-like crusted erosions involving the face, scalp, and upper trunk. Blisters tend to be more superficial and fragile, creating what is frequently described as a cornflake-like scale and crust. Nikolsky sign also is typically positive. Pemphigus foliaceus typically spares mucosal surfaces, differentiating it from pemphigus vulgaris.

Paraneoplastic pemphigus presents as a more severe-appearing form of pemphigus. In addition to pemphigus vulgaris-like skin findings, paraneoplastic pemphigus typically presents with severe mucosal involvement with extensive crusted stomatitis extending onto the vermillion lip and scarring conjunctivitis. There may also be erosions in the esophagus, genitalia, and nasopharynx. Palms and soles may also be affected, distinguishing this entity from pemphigus vulgaris.

Diagnosis

In addition to classic clinical findings, biopsy is usually required to confirm diagnosis with routine H&E histology, DIF, and other workup as indicated (including IIF, ELISA, and immunoprecipitation/immunoblotting).

Pemphigus vulgaris biopsies initially show eosinophilic spongiosis, followed by suprabasilar acantholysis without keratinocyte necrosis. Classically, one would also expect to find a tombstoning pattern of vertically oriented keratinocytes of the basal layer attached to the basement membrane zone (BMZ). DIF shows intercellular IgG deposition (with or without C3) in a chicken-wire appearance, with greater concentration in the lower epidermis.

Pemphigus foliaceus and its variants appear similarly to pemphigus vulgaris on histology, but on DIF one would expect to find higher concentration of IgG +/- C3 deposition in the upper epidermis. Pemphigus erythematosus may also have granular to linear IgG and C3 deposition along the BMZ.

Paraneoplastic pemphigus histology demonstrates intercellular IgG and C3 deposition, in addition to linear IgG and C3 deposition along the BMZ. Gold standard of diagnosis of paraneoplastic pemphigus is immunoprecipitation or immunoblotting for antibodies against plakin proteins, and ELISA detection of anti-DsG antibodies.

Treatment and Monitoring

Pemphigus can be a severe and deadly disease requiring immunosuppressive treatment. Because of the complex nature of the disease and treatment, early involvement of relevant specialists including but not limited to dermatology, rheumatology, gastroenterology, otolaryngology, oral medicine, and ophthalmology is critical. Clinicians prescribing immunosuppressive medications must be comfortable and familiar with the medications, including their side effect profile and monitoring parameters.

First-line treatment of pemphigus diseases is systemic corticosteroids for rapid disease control in conjunction with steroid-sparing immunosuppressive medications such as azathioprine (Imuran),[1] mycophenolate mofetil (CellCept),[1] or rituximab (Rituxan only for pemphigus vulgaris). Although numerous systemic steroids may be used, most frequently clinicians use prednisone 1 mg/kg/day. Higher doses of prednisone (100–150 mg daily) may sometimes be needed for more severe diseases, but prolonged use of higher doses may result in greater morbidity and mortality. In our practice, we aim to taper patients completely off of corticosteroids within 3 to 6 months. However, low-dose regimens such as prednisone 5 mg daily may be required for several years. For patients on long-term corticosteroid therapy vitamin D, calcium supplementation, and especially bisphosphonate therapy can help prevent or treat osteoporosis, while H_2 blockers (e.g., famotidine [Pepcid][1], ranitidine [Zactac][2]) or PPIs (e.g., omeprazole [Prilosec][1]) are recommended to prevent or treat peptic ulcer disease in patients taking concomitant nonsteroidal antiinflammatory drugs (NSAIDs).

Corticosteroid therapy should be initiated in combination with a steroid sparing agent because these agents typically take 3 to 6 months to take full effect. First-line steroid sparing agents include azathioprine[1] (2–3 mg/kg/day based on the patient's thiopurine methyltransferase [TPMT] levels), mycophenolate mofetil[1] (1–1.5 g twice daily), and rituximab (Rituxan only for pemphigus vulgaris). In our practice we dose rituximab IV 1000 mg once every 2 weeks for 2 doses, followed by maintenance dose of 500 mg at months 12 and 18, and every 6 months thereafter based on clinical response. Milder cases may be treated with dapsone[1] (25 mg daily for 1 week, then increase dose in 25 mg increments weekly based on clinical response up to maximum 100 mg daily), niacinamide[1] (nicotinamide), and tetracycline.[1] Topical corticosteroids such as triamcinolone 0.1% ointment or clobetasol. 0.05% ointment twice daily may be helpful in milder cases for pruritic or painful skin lesions. Second-line steroid-sparing agents with varying levels of efficacy described include methotrexate[1] (10–25 mg once weekly with folic acid supplementation[1] on days not taking methotrexate), cyclophosphamide,[1] and TNF-a inhibitors.[1] Severe refractory cases may be treated with IV immunoglobulin (IVIG)[1] therapy, or with rituximab or cyclophosphamide,[1] with or without plasmapheresis.

Treatment response should be monitored with IIF or ELISA levels, which can help detect quantitative levels of circulating antibodies.

Patients with paraneoplastic pemphigus may also have improvement in cutaneous lesions with systemic steroids, with or without adjunctive steroid-sparing agents. Excision of benign neoplasms such as thymomas and localized Castleman's disease may lead to resolution within months. Cases of paraneoplastic pemphigus from underlying malignancies are highly recalcitrant to treatment and carry a poor prognosis of up to a 90% mortality rate.

Bullous Pemphigoid
Pathophysiology

Bullous pemphigoid (BP) is the most common autoimmune blistering disorder and typically affects elderly patients. Patients with BP have circulating autoantibodies against different proteins, along the BMZ. The most common and important antigenic targets in BP include IgG autoantibodies targeted against the hemidesmosomal proteins BP180 (also referred to as BPAG2 and type XVII collagen) and BP230 (also referred to as BPAG1). BP180 is the primary mediator of BP. Complement activation causes eosinophilic and neutrophilic infiltration to the tissues, release of mediators and degradatory enzymes resulting in subepidermal blisters. Drug-induced cases of BP are most frequently

---

[1] Not FDA approved for this indication.
[2] Not available in the United States.

because of furosemide, ACE inhibitors, NSAIDs, and antibiotics including cephalosporins, beta-lactams, and D-penicillamine.

Clinical Manifestations

BP initially presents as pruritic urticarial papules and plaques on the trunk, abdomen, and flexures of extremities. This progresses to tense fluid-filled blisters and bullae on a urticarial base. Patients often complain of intense pruritus. After the bullae and blisters rupture, denuded areas of erosions and crusted areas remain.

Diagnosis

In addition to clinical findings and history, biopsy is required for diagnosis. On histology, lesions of the urticarial phase demonstrate eosinophilic spongiosis with eosinophils lining up at the dermoepidermal junction (DEJ). During the bullous phase, lesions demonstrate subepidermal split with numerous eosinophils in the blister cavity and dense inflammation in the dermis. DIF is the most sensitive test for BP and shows linear IgG and C3 deposition along the DEJ. Salt-split skin DIF is a special type of modified DIF study that uses NaCl solution to split the biopsy specimen at the lamina lucida, allowing for localization of the bound antibodies. BP antibodies classically show staining on the top of the blister cavity. Unlike in pemphigus vulgaris, IIF levels do not correlate well with BP disease activity and are not useful for determining treatment response.

Treatment

Although BP carries lower mortality risk compared with pemphigus vulgaris, treatment is indicated for its significant morbidity.

There have not been many controlled trials performed for BP therapies, and recommendations tend to be based on consensus opinion and clinician experience. Most frequently used first-line therapy includes high-potency topical corticosteroids or systemic corticosteroids and steroid-sparing immunosuppressive medications. Some studies have shown that topical clobetasol propionate (Temovate, Clobex) 0.05% may have better response than oral prednisone 0.5–1 mg/kg/day, with fewer side effects. Although prednisone has traditionally been the standard approach to oral therapy, side effects should be weighed highly, and topical steroids should be attempted first in mild to moderate cases. Dapsone[1] (see pemphigus vulgaris section on treatment) or tetracycline[1] (500 mg four times daily) given with niacinamide[1] (500 mg three times daily) may also be efficacious as first-line treatment. There have been increasing reports of successful treatment with dupilumab (Dupixent)[1] (600 mg subcutaneous injection loading dose, followed by 300 mg every other week) and prednisone. We have implemented this successfully in patients with BP in our institution.

Immunosuppressive medications may be necessary in severe or recalcitrant cases. Azathioprine[1] and mycophenolate mofetil[1] have shown similar efficacy. Rituximab,[1] methotrexate,[1] cyclophosphamide,[1] IVIG,[1] and cyclosporine[1] (4–5 mg/kg/day) are potentially effective second-line options. IVIG may be especially helpful in steroid-resistant cases. Dosing regimens for these medications are similar to those of pemphigus. There have been several case reports of omalizumab (Xolair)[1] (monoclonal anti-IgE antibody) showing good response in some patients.

In our practice, for patients with severe bullous pemphigoid and no contraindications, we start prednisone at 0.5 mg/kg/day along with mycophenolate mofetil. We aim to taper the patient off of steroids in 3 to 6 months while increasing mycophenolate mofetil to a max dose of 1.5 gm twice daily if needed. For patients with mild to moderate disease, or in patients with severe disease but contraindications to corticosteroids and/or immunosuppressants, we treat with topical steroids in conjunction with doxycycline/nicotinamide, IVIG, and/or dapsone.

Denuded, eroded areas tend to heal spontaneously and may not require further treatment other than appropriate wound care. BP is considered a chronic condition, although some cases may be self-limited over a period of about 5 years. High levels of BP180 at the time of discontinuing therapy are associated with a higher risk of relapse.

Mucous Membrane Pemphigoid

Pathophysiology

Mucous membrane pemphigoid (MMP), also referred to as *cicatricial pemphigoid*, is a rare autoimmune bullous disease with numerous targets in the anchoring filament zone including epiligrin (also referred to as laminin 332), $\alpha_6\beta_4$ integrin (specifically the β_4 subunit), and c-terminus of BP180. Antiepiligrin MMP has a strong association with underlying malignancy, most frequently adenocarcinoma. Patients with antibodies against the $\alpha_6\beta_4$ integrin may have exclusive ocular involvement. MMP most frequently affects the elderly, with a female predominance.

Clinical Manifestations

As its name denotes, MMP mostly involves the mucosa, most commonly the oral and conjunctival mucosa. Patients with oral involvement present with numerous painful chronic erosions of the oral mucosa including the gingiva, buccal mucosa, palate, and lips. Eye involvement is typically bilateral, initially presenting as a relatively nonspecific conjunctivitis, which progresses to fibrosis and eventual formation of adhesions of the bulbar and palpebral conjunctiva (symblepharon), ectropion, dry eyes, and inward facing eyelashes (trichiasis). Skin involvement is less common and tends to be more limited. The most common extramucosal sites include the scalp, face, neck, and upper trunk. Skin lesions may heal with atrophic scars, which may help distinguish this entity from BP.

Diagnosis

In addition to clinical history[1] and examination findings, biopsy is required for diagnosis including routine histology, DIF, and salt-split skin. IIF may also be helpful. Routine histology findings are similar to BP with fewer eosinophils. DIF staining shows linear IgG, IgA, +/- C3 deposition along the BMZ. Salt-split skin testing shows an epidermal staining pattern, except for antiepiligrin, which shows dermal staining pattern.

Treatment

For patients with mild, limited oral disease, treatment with topical triamcinolone acetonide (Oralone) 0.1% dental paste twice daily to oral lesions can be quite effective. Dapsone[1] (start 25 mg daily and titrate slowly based on response after 1 week) is our first-line systemic treatment for mild-moderate oral mucosal disease. Limited cutaneous disease can be treated with topical corticosteroids such as triamcinolone 0.1% ointment or clobetasol 0.05% ointment twice daily to affected areas on the body. Tetracycline[1] (500 mg four times daily) with niacinamide[1] (500 mg three times daily) may also be effective.

In patients with more severe oral disease and/or ocular disease, treatment with systemic steroids and cyclophosphamide is often needed. Most frequently oral prednisone 1 mg/kg/day is started with cyclophosphamide[1] (1–2 mg/kg/day), and therapy may continue after clinical remission for maintenance. Clinicians should attempt to taper prednisone after remission is achieved if possible, although some patients may continue to require low doses of prednisone to prevent recurrence. Ocular disease may result in scarring, and early involvement of an experienced ophthalmologist is essential.

MMP is a chronic condition which may result in scarring, disfigurement, and even blindness.

---

[1] Not FDA approved for this indication.

Linear IgA Bullous Dermatosis/Chronic Bullous Disease of Childhood
Pathophysiology
Adult-onset linear IgA bullous dermatosis (LABD) is a rare autoimmune subepidermal bullous disease affecting elderly patients greater than 60 years old. Chronic bullous disease of childhood (CBDC) is typically a self-limited bullous disease affecting young children beginning around 2 or 3 years old and may remit by teenage years. Patients with LABD/CBDC have circulating IgA autoantibodies targeting antigens derived from BPAG2, and some patients may have both IgA and IgG autoantibodies. Medication-induced LABD/CBDC is most frequently caused by vancomycin, followed by penicillin and cephalosporin antibiotics, captopril, NSAIDs, phenytoin, and many more offending medications.

Clinical Manifestations
Both adult-onset LABD and CBDC present with tense blisters/bullae and urticarial plaques that may be arranged in an annular or polycyclic formation, often described as *crown of jewels arrangement*. Individual lesions may appear quite similar to that of bullous pemphigoid and dermatitis herpetiformis. The most frequently affected sites include the trunk, flexures of extremities, groin, buttocks, and the face (in children). Patients may or may not have mucosal involvement.

Diagnosis
Biopsies of early urticarial lesions may show diffuse neutrophilic infiltrate along the BMZ. Biopsies of bullous lesions show subepidermal blisters/bullae filled with neutrophils and a neutrophil-predominant infiltrate in the papillary dermis. DIF of perilesional skin is the gold standard for diagnosis and shows linear IgA deposition along the BMZ. Salt-split skin testing may show epidermal staining.

Treatment
Dapsone[1] is considered first-line therapy for cases of LABD and CBDC. We recommend starting at 25 mg daily, which may be increased weekly by increments of 25 mg based on clinical response (maximum dose varies by age). Second-line agents for those who cannot tolerate dapsone include colchicine[1] (up to 0.6 mg two times daily in pediatric patients and up to three times daily in adult patients) and sulfapyridine[2] (500 mg twice daily starting dose, titrated appropriately based on clinical response).

In cases of drug-induced LABD/CBDC, the offending medication should be discontinued. Lesions are expected to resolve within a few weeks of stopping the medication.

Epidermolysis Bullosa Acquisita
Pathophysiology
Epidermolysis bullosa acquisita (EBA) is a very rare acquired bullous disease, most commonly found in adults of East Asian and African American descent. It is frequently associated with inflammatory bowel disease (especially Crohn's disease), multiple myeloma, systemic lupus erythematosus, diabetes mellitus, hepatitis C infection, and other underlying diseases.

Patients may have IgG autoantibodies targeting type VII collagen, which is a major component of anchoring fibrils in the basement membrane zone.

Clinical Manifestations
The noninflammatory, or mechanobullous, variant of EBA is the most commonly recognized subtype. Patients present with hemorrhagic bullae and erosions on trauma-prone sites including the dorsal hands and feet, elbows, and knees. Lesions may heal with scarring, milia, and nail dystrophy. Inflammatory EBA clinically is indistinguishable to BP. Lesions of inflammatory EBA may also heal with scarring and milia. Patients may also have oral and ocular erosions which may appear similarly to MMP.

Diagnosis
In addition to clinical findings, biopsy is required for diagnosis of EBA to distinguish it from other subepidermal bullous diseases. Routine histology shows subepidermal blisters with varying degrees of neutrophilic and eosinophilic infiltrates. DIF of perilesional skin shows linear IgG and C3 deposition along the BMZ. Unlike BP, DIF of EBA lesions tend to show more linear IgG deposition rather than C3. Salt-split skin technique shows dermal staining.

Treatment Options
Some patients may have good response to prednisone (0.5–1 mg/kg/day), with or without dapsone. Dapsone[1] monotherapy may also be effective for patients (initiated at 25 mg daily and increased appropriately based on clinical response). This dose should be maintained for several months prior to tapering attempts. Colchicine[1] (0.6 mg twice to thrice daily) may be effective. Patients with resistant or severe disease may have more rapid relief with cyclosporine[1] (4–5 mg/kg/day). Other agents with reported success include rituximab,[1] IVIG,[1] infliximab (Remicade),[1] minocycline,[1] plasmapheresis, and PDE-4 inhibitors.[1]

Unfortunately, cases of EBA tend to be quite resistant to treatment relative to BP and other subepidermal bullous diseases. The disease is usually chronic and waxes and wanes. Patients should avoid trauma as much as possible because it may contribute to further blister formation. The inflammatory subtype of EBA may have better response to therapy compared with the mechanobullous noninflammatory subtype.

Dermatitis Herpetiformis
Pathophysiology
Dermatitis herpetiformis (DH) is a chronic and relapsing bullous disease which is strongly associated with celiac disease. People of Northern European descent are most commonly affected, and it is quite rare in patients of Asian and African American descent. More than 97% of patients with DH and celiac disease have one or both HLA-DQ2 and HLA-DQ8 alleles. In addition to celiac disease, DH is also associated with other autoimmune conditions including Hashimoto's thyroiditis, type 1 diabetes mellitus, and pernicious anemia.

Gluten is a grain protein found in many foods containing wheat, rye, and barley. Gluten is broken down into gliadin during digestion, which is then transported across the gastrointestinal (GI) mucosa to the lamina propria, where it binds with tissue transglutaminase 2 (TTG2). This complex is recognized by HLA-DQ2 or HLA-DQ8 on antigen presenting cells (APCs) and activating the T-cell and B-cell activated autoinflammatory cascade to form IgA autoantibodies against TTG2 or the TTG2-gliadin complex. These bound IgA antibodies lead to neutrophil recruitment, resulting in damage to intestinal villi. Epitope spreading (diversification of epitope specificity) results in production of IgA autoantibodies against epidermal transglutaminase (TTG3), which then binds to TTG3 within dermal papillae. Neutrophils recruited by this process release elastase and other proteolytic enzymes, resulting in the formation of subepidermal blisters seen in DH.

Clinical Manifestations
Patients with DH classically present with extremely pruritic herpetiform vesicles on an urticarial base. The vesicles can be ruptured very easily, so excoriations, rather than intact vesicles, are more frequently seen on examination. Lesions are typically

[1] Not FDA approved for this indication.
[2] Not available in the United States.

distributed on the symmetric extensor extremities (elbows and knees), buttocks, back, neck, face, and scalp. A minority of approximately 20% of patients with DH have symptomatic gastrointestinal disease; however, the majority of patients have evidence of gluten-sensitive enteropathy on gastrointestinal biopsy samples.

Diagnosis

Clinical history can be particularly helpful in cases of DH. A history of worsening of disease with gluten-containing diets is a useful clue, although patients are not always aware of their specific dietary habits unless they keep a careful food diary.

Biopsy samples should be obtained on early blisters if possible. Routine histology shows subepidermal bullae most pronounced above the dermal papillae, and neutrophilic infiltrates in the dermal papillae. These findings can be quite similar to LABD, so DIF testing and serologic testing can be helpful. DIF of perilesional skin shows granular IgA deposits with or without C3 deposition in the dermal papillae. Serologic testing for DH and celiac disease can be helpful, including serum antitissue transglutaminase or antiendomysial antibodies (present in approximately 80% of patients with DH and greater than 95% of patients with celiac disease); however, it is important to keep in mind that tests can also be falsely negative if the patient has been keeping a gluten-free diet. Patients with IgA deficiency may also have falsely negative testing for anti-TTG antibodies, so IgA levels should be assessed concurrently.

Treatment Options

Dapsone is the treatment of choice in patients with DH. Patients tend to have a rapid response to dapsone (within 2–3 days) with improvement in cutaneous disease. The usual dose of dapsone in DH is to start at 50 mg daily and increase in increments of 25 mg based on clinical response to a maximum of to a maximum of 100–200 mg daily. Typically, patients are well controlled on 50–100 mg daily. Patients do not typically see an effect on their GI disease, if present. Prior to initiating dapsone, it is important to evaluate for G6PD deficiency. Sulfapyridine[2] is an effective second-line therapy with less risk of hemolysis.

Gluten-free diets (avoiding wheat, rye, and barley) can be effective to control both cutaneous and gastrointestinal disease. It may also reduce the risk of development of GI lymphomas associated with celiac disease. DH is typically a lifelong, chronic, relapsing disease. It is important to involve relevant specialties including dermatology, nutrition, and gastroenterology to help manage patients with DH.

---

[2] Not available in the United States.

References

Abdat R, Waldman RA, et al: Dupilumab as a novel therapy for bullous pemphigoid: a multicenter case series, *J Am Acad Dermatol* 83(1):46–52, 2020.

Bolotin D, Petronic-Rosic V: Dermatitis herpetiformis, *J Am Acad Dermatol* 64(6):1017–1033, 2011.

Cizenski JD, Michel P, et al: Spectrum of orocutaneous disease associations: immune-mediated conditions, *J Am Acad Dermatol* 77(5):795–806, 2017.

Feliciani C, Joly P, et al: Management of bullous pemphigoid: the European Dermatology Forum consensus in collaboration with the European Academy of Dermatology and Venereology, *Br J Dermatol* 172(4):867–877, 2015.

Gouveia R, Teixeira A, et al: Linear immunoglobulin A bullous dermatosis, *J Pediatr* 170:338, 2016. e1.

Kirtschig G, Murrell D, et al: Interventions for mucous membrane pemphigoid/cicatricial pemphigoid and epidermolysis bullosa acquisita: a systematic literature review, *Arch Dermatol* 138(3):380–384, 2002.

Murrell DF, Peña S, et al: Diagnosis and management of pemphigus: recommendations of an international panel of experts, *J Am Acad Dermatol* 82(3):575–585, 2020.

Mutasim DF: Management of autoimmune bullous diseases: pharmacology and therapeutics, *J Am Acad Dermatol* 51:859–877, 2004.

Wojnarowska F, Kirtschig G, et al: Guidelines for the management of bullous pemphigoid, *Br J Dermatol* 147:214–221, 2002.

CONTACT DERMATITIS

Method of

James A. Yiannias, MD; Genevieve L. Egnatios, MD; and Heidi E.K. Mullen, DO

CURRENT DIAGNOSIS

- Gather a detailed history on skin exposures, including the use of these items:
  - Irritants
  - Alkalis: soaps, detergents, cleansers
  - Acids
  - Hydrocarbons: petroleum, oils
  - Solvents
  - Potential allergens including
    - Metals: nickel sulfate; cobalt chloride (e.g., jewelry, makeup, personal products)
    - Fragrances: balsam of Peru (Myroxylon pereirae; fragrance); fragrance mix
    - Methylisothiazolinone, methylchloroisothiazolinone (preservatives)
    - Benzalkonium chloride (preservative)
    - Formaldehyde and formaldehyde-releasing preservatives such as quaternium-15
    - Topical antibiotics such as neomycin, bacitracin
- Examine the skin for the location and pattern of eruption:
  - Eyelid: nail polish
  - Postauricular scalp: perfume
  - Perioral area: chewing gum, toothpaste
  - Trunk: dyes, clothing finish
  - Wrist: nickel, chrome
  - Waistline: rubber
  - Feet: shoes
  - Wounds: topical antibiotic ointment
- Perform patch testing:
  - T.R.U.E. TEST with 35 allergens (note: two common allergens, benzalkonium chloride and propolis, are not included in this panel)
  - Customized series with 70 or more allergens

CURRENT THERAPY

- Avoid irritants and allergens, using the prepared patient handout.
- Consult the SkinSAFE shopping list of skin care products free of the top 10 most common allergens (if patch testing is not performed).
- Consult a customized SkinSAFE shopping list of skin care products free of the patient's contact allergens, based on patch test results.
- Topical corticosteroids can be applied.
- Hydrocortisone 2.5% (Hytone) can be applied twice daily on the face, neck, axillae, groin, and intertriginous areas.
- Triamcinolone 0.1% (Kenalog) can be applied twice daily on the body.
- For severe reactions, short-term, higher-potency steroids can be applied (e.g., clobetasol [Clobex] 0.05% twice daily).
- Sedating antihistamines can be taken: doxepin (Sinequan)[1] 10 to 20 mg qhs.
- Steroid-sparing topical agents can be applied: tacrolimus 0.1% (Protopic),[1] pimecrolimus 1% (Elidel),[1] crisaborole 2% (Eucrisa).[1]
- For severe, acute episodes, systemic corticosteroids can be taken in a several-week tapering course (e.g., prednisone 60 mg for 5 days, 40 mg for 5 days, and 20 mg for 5 days).

- Longer-term systemic therapy is possible for severe or recalcitrant disease.
- Phototherapy is suggested, with narrowband ultraviolet B.
- Azathioprine (Imuran)[1] can be taken 1 to 3 mg/kg qd.
- Mycophenolate mofetil (CellCept)[1] can be taken 2 to 3 g qd.
- Methotrexate[1] can be taken 10 to 25 mg per week.
- Cyclosporine (Neoral)[1] can be taken 2.5–5 mg/kg qd short term.
- Dupilumab (Dupixent)[1] can be taken by injection at 600 mg initially and then 300 mg every other week.

[1]Not FDA approved for this indication.

Dermatitis typically manifests as papules and vesicles with weeping and oozing that can become lichenified and scaly when chronic. When this clinical picture is secondary to an exogenous substance coming into contact with the skin, it is termed *contact dermatitis*. Further delineation leads to irritant versus allergic contact dermatitis, although in practice these often overlap.

Irritant contact dermatitis is not an allergic process. It represents damage to the skin from repeated and cumulative exposure to an agent. Irritants do not require prior sensitization. A decreased barrier function of the skin—for example, with frequent handwashing—can predispose to the condition or exacerbate it. Examples include alkalis (in soaps, detergents, and cleansers), acids (in germicides, dyes, and pigments), hydrocarbons (in petroleum and oils), and solvents.

Allergic contact dermatitis is an immunologic process classified as a type IV cell-mediated delayed hypersensitivity reaction. Poison ivy is a classic example. It requires an initial exposure to the contactant in which sensitization occurs but without outward physical effect. Subsequent exposure can elicit a striking response that is independent of the amount of the contactant.

From 1994 to 2016 the most common contact allergens have changed little. Based on studies performed by the North American Contact Dermatitis Group (NACDG) and the Mayo Clinic Contact Dermatitis Group (MCCDG), the allergens most consistently in the top 10 were nickel sulfate, balsam of Peru, fragrance mix, quaternium-15, neomycin, bacitracin, formaldehyde, and cobalt chloride (Box 1). However, in the past few years, two additional preservatives have gained prominence: methylisothiazolinone (MI) and benzalkonium chloride. Common sources of exposure to nickel include costume jewelry, snaps, zippers, and other metal objects. Balsam of Peru and fragrance mix are markers for fragrance sensitivity. Sources of exposure to formaldehyde include skin care products, household products, and the resins in plastics and clothing. Quaternium-15 is a formaldehyde-releasing preservative and may be found in items such as skin care products, paper, inks, and photocopier toner. Neomycin and bacitracin are topical antibiotics available alone and in combination with polymyxin (Neosporin), antifungals, and corticosteroids. Cobalt is found with other metals, including zinc, and in items such as jewelry, crayons, hair dye, and antiperspirants. MI is a common preservative found in personal care products and may be used in combination with another preservative, methylchloroisothiazolinone (MCI/MI). Benzalkonium chloride is commonly used in the healthcare field as a cleanser, an antiseptic, and a preservative but is also found in personal care products such as wipes and an increasing number of skin care products.

Others less consistently in the top 10 during that period were methyldibromo glutaronitrile, gold sodium thiosulfate, potassium dichromate, *p*-phenylenediamine, thiuram mix, methylisothiazolinone/methylchloroisothiazolinone (MCI/MI), and propolis. Methyldibromo glutaronitrile is a preservative and can be found in healthcare and personal products. Clinically relevant sources of gold may be found in jewelry and dental appliances. Potassium dichromate is used in cement, leather, and steel surfaces. Permanent hair dyes are the usual source of *p*-phenylenediamine. Thiuram mix is in rubber and some personal products. Propolis is another marker of fragrance sensitivity.

BOX 1   Top 10 Most Common Allergens

North American Contact Dermatitis Group
- Nickel sulfate
- Methylisothiazolinone (MI)
- Fragrance mix
- Formaldehyde 2%
- Methylchloroisothiazolinone/methylisothiazolinone (MCI/MI)
- Balsam of Peru
- Neomycin
- Bacitracin
- Formaldehyde 1%
- *p*-Phenylenediamine

Mayo Clinic Contact Dermatitis Group
- Nickel sulfate
- MI
- Balsam of Peru
- Neomycin
- Cobalt chloride
- Benzalkonium chloride
- Fragrance mix I
- Potassium dichromate
- Bacitracin
- MCI/MI

Data from DeKoven JG, Warshaw EM, Zug KA, et al: North American Contact Dermatitis Group patch test results: 2015-2016. *Dermatitis* 29:297–309, 2018; Veverka KK, Hall MR, Yiannias JA, et al: Trends in patch testing with the Mayo Clinic standard series, 2011-2015. *Dermatitis* 29(6):310–315, 2018.

Each year since 2000, the American Contact Dermatitis Society has designated an allergen of the year, designed to spotlight allergens, common or not, that are rising in significance. For 2021, acetophenone azine was chosen. Acetophenone azine is found in shin pads and footwear that contain cushioning foam made of ethyl vinyl acetate. Other designated allergens of the year have been alkyl glucosides, cobalt chloride, benzophenones, MI, acrylates, dimethyl fumarate, neomycin, mixed dialkyl thioureas, nickel, fragrance, *p*-phenylenediamine, corticosteroids, cocamidopropyl betaine, bacitracin, thimerosal, gold, disperse blue, propylene glycol, nonallergen parabens, and isobornyl acrylate. Alkyl glucosides are surfactants that are pervasive in consumer products, including cosmetics. Benzophenones, such as oxybenzone, are chemical ultraviolet light filters that are found in sunscreens and personal care products. Artificial nails, dentures, and bone cement contain acrylates, but these substances are only allergenic when in the liquid, powder, or paste forms. Dimethyl fumarate is a biocide in furniture, shoes, and textiles. It is often placed in little paper packets with these items. Rubber products and shoe glue are common sources of mixed dialkyl thioureas. Shampoos often contain cocamidopropyl betaine as a lathering agent. Thimerosal is a preservative for medications and personal care products, including contact lens solution. Disperse blue is a fabric dye. Patients with an allergy to disperse dyes may also react to *p*-phenylenediamine. Propylene glycol is a common ingredient in personal care products, topical corticosteroids and other medications, and foods. Parabens are preservatives commonly found in cosmetics, foods, pharmaceuticals, dentifrices, and suppositories. Isobornyl acrylate, an adhesive, is often used in medical devices, such as insulin pumps, and can also be found in acrylic nails.

Diagnosis

The evaluation of a patient with suspected contact dermatitis begins with the history. Specific questions directed at the patient's occupation, hobbies, and home routine will be helpful. Examination should note the location and pattern of the eruption. Although eyelid dermatitis may be seen in the atopic patient, nail polish may be the source of the offending allergen. Dyshidrotic

Introduction

Eczema, also known as dermatitis, is an inflammation of the skin due to dryness, irritation, or possible external allergy. Eczema/dermatitis is not contagious.

Some skin care products contain fragrance even though the package says "fragrance free" or "unscented." Therefore, please choose the skin care products as listed below by their *exact brand name*.

Suggestions

Soaps/Cleansing
- Vanicream cleansing bar
- Free and Clear liquid cleanser
- Aveeno moisturizing bar for dry skin fragrance Free or Aveeno advanced care body wash
- Oilatum unscented soap
- Neutrogena original formula fragrance-free (bar or liquid)

  Any of the shampoos listed in this brochure may be used as your hand or body soap.
- Vanicream shave cream for sensitive skin

Moisturizers
- Vanicream, Vanicream Lite
- Aveeno daily moisturizing lotion fragrance Free
- Plain Vaseline, Vaniply
- DML unscented
- Use moisturizers twice daily.
- All of the above are OK to use on the face.
- After showering, blot excess water with hands and apply cream. Do not use a towel to dry.
- Robathol bath oil

Deodorants
- Almay unscented antiperspirants
- Plain cornstarch from the grocer can be used.

Shampoo
- Free and Clear shampoo and conditioner
- DHS clear shampoo and DHS conditioner
- If you have dandruff, use DHS sal shampoo or Neutrogena T-SAL shampoo (not T-Gel).
- Conditioners can be used as "leave on" hair gel.

Hairspray
- Fragrance-free hairspray such as Free and Clear hairspray
- Caution: Hairsprays labeled as "unscented" may not be fragrance free.

Laundry and Home Care
- Unscented laundry detergents (Tide free, Cheer free and gentle, All free clear, Arm & Hammer unscented, Wisk free, Purex unscented)
- Wash all new clothes and linens five times before using.
- Old clothes and fabrics are preferred.
- Use white vinegar in rinse cycle to help remove soap.

Hand, Nail, and General Skin Care Tips
- Wear cotton gloves under rubber/vinyl gloves for any activities where hand-wetting is expected.
- Trim nails short. Long nails are dangerous to skin, especially when sleeping.

Sunscreens
- Vanicream sunscreen #30 or #60

Make-ups/cosmetics
- If you would like a list of make-ups and cosmetics that are free of the most common allergy-causing ingredients, ask your provider about a "virtual patch testing" printout from our Mayo CARD program.

Avoid

Soaps/Cleansing
- No hot water (use lukewarm).
- Avoid hot tubs.
- No rubbing alcohol.

Moisturizers
- No creams, lotions, oils or powders other than those recommended in this brochure.
- No Neosporin, triple antibiotic, or bacitracin antibiotic ointments.

Fragrances
- No perfumes, colognes, after shave, or pre-shave on any part of body/clothing.

Laundry and Home Care
- No fabric softener in washer.
- Bounce unscented fabric softener sheets in dryer if desired.
- No washing machine water softener such as Calgon (in-house water softeners are acceptable).
- White vinegar may be used as a general household cleaner.

Hand, Nail, and General Skin Care Tips
- No wetting of hands more than five times a day.
- Avoid tight-fitting clothes unless your doctor has advised you to wear a pressure garment such as support hose.
- No scrubbing! No loofah! No pumice stone!
- Do not pull off dead skin. Snip with scissors instead.

Figure 1 Sample of prepared handout (used at Mayo Clinic Arizona) with recommendations for the patient on hypoallergenic skin care products.

eczema occurs as vesicles along the lateral aspects of the fingers, whereas eczematous changes along the dorsal hands are more commonly due to an allergen. Other distributions as clues include postauricular scalp (perfume), perioral area (chewing gum, toothpaste), trunk (dyes or clothing finish), wrist (nickel or chrome), waistline (rubber), feet (shoes), and history or presence of wounds (topical antibiotic ointment).

Patch testing can confirm or reveal a contact allergy. It involves placement of allergens against the skin of the patient's back for 48 hours. An initial reading is then done, with follow-up readings typically at 96 hours. Prepared series include the thin-layer, rapid-use epicutaneous test (T.R.U.E. TEST), which consists of 35 allergens and 1 negative control (https://www.truetest.com); customized series, such as the NACDG Standard Series with 70 allergens and the Mayo Clinic's Standard Series with 73 allergens, must be manually assembled. The majority of dermatologists performing patch testing use T.R.U.E. TEST. Note that benzalkonium chloride, MI, and propolis are not included in that panel. Overall, the NACDG estimates that 25% to approximately 40% of allergic reactions would have been missed by the T.R.U.E. TEST based on their data for 2015 to 2016.

In addition to ascertaining degree of positivity, relevance must be determined. This involves collaborating with patients to assess the likelihood that they are currently exposed to the positive antigen.

Treatment

Ideally, the allergen or allergens will be identified and avoided. Realistically, compliance is a challenge. To assist patients in avoiding antigens in skin care products, SkinSAFE was created in 1999. It includes approximately 14,392 ingredients and 55,891 individual over-the-counter and prescription skin care products. Once the patient's allergens have been identified with patch testing, they can be entered into the database, and a list of products free of those substances is generated. The patient should be reminded that even small and infrequent exposures can perpetuate the eczema.

Topical corticosteroids applied twice daily are helpful in hastening resolution and may also be used for disease control when the allergen is unknown. Low-potency corticosteroids such as 2.5% hydrocortisone (Hytone) are recommended for the thinner skin of the face, neck, axillae, groin, and intertriginous areas. Midpotency steroids such as triamcinolone 0.1% (Kenalog, Kenonel) are appropriate for the thicker skin of the body. Short-term use of higher-potency steroids may be necessary if the reaction is severe. If there is significant pruritus, sedating antihistamines such as doxepin (Sinequan)[1] 10 to 20 mg taken nightly 2 hours before bedtime can provide relief. Steroid-sparing topical immunomodulators such as tacrolimus (Protopic),[1] pimecrolimus (Elidel),[1] and crisaborole (Eucrisa)[1] may be helpful adjuncts. Treatment for severe acute episodes can entail a several-week tapering course of systemic corticosteroids, especially if the eruption is widespread. Other longer-term systemic therapies for severe or resistant disease include phototherapy or systemic immunosuppressants such as azathioprine (Imuran),[1] mycophenolate mofetil (CellCept),[1] methotrexate,[1] cyclosporine (Neoral),[1] or dupilumab (Dupixent).[1]

It may take many weeks before the skin reverts to a normal appearance despite successful avoidance of antigens. A prepared handout with concrete recommendations for the patient on truly hypoallergenic skin care is beneficial. A sample of that used at Mayo Clinic Arizona is shown in Figure 1.

If patch testing is not performed, an initial approach may be to instruct the patient on avoiding the most common contact allergens via a handout and prescribing symptomatic treatment including topical and oral therapies. SkinSAFE can generate a shopping list of products free of the top 10 allergens as identified by the NACDG and the MCCDG. Patients may access SkinSAFE independently (at https://www.skinsafeproducts.com, Apple App Store, or Google Play Store under "SkinSAFE") to generate this list or build customized lists free of fragrances, common preservatives, parabens, nickel, lanolin, coconut, and topical antibiotics.

---

[1]Not FDA approved for this indication.

In 35% of patients, simply using products free of the top 10 allergens can prompt clearance. Some physicians follow these measures for several months, especially if the eruption is mild, before pursuing formal patch testing.

An excellent primer for the physician interested in learning more about contact allergy diagnosis and management is *Contact and Occupational Dermatology*.

References

Aerts O, Herman A, Mowitz M, et al: *Isobornyl acrylate*, Dermatitis, 2020. https://doi.org/10.1097/DER.0000000000000549. [Epub ahead of print].

Bruze M, Zimerson E: Dimethyl fumarate, *Dermatitis* 22:3–7, 2011.

Castanedo-Tardana MP, Zug KA: Methylisothiazolinone, *Dermatitis* 24:2–6, 2013. https://doi.org/10.1097/DER.0b013e31827edc73.

DeKoven JG, Warshaw EM, Belsito, et al: North American contact dermatitis group patch test results 2013-2014, *Dermatitis* 28:33–46, 2017. https://doi.org/10.1097/DER.0000000000000225.

DeKoven JG, Warshaw EM, Zug KA, et al: North American contact dermatitis group patch test results: 2015-2016, *Dermatitis* 29:297–309, 2018. https://doi.org/10.1097/DER.0000000000000417.

Heurung AR, Raju SI, Warshaw EM: Benzophenones, *Dermatitis* 25:3–10, 2014. https://doi.org/10.1097/DER.0000000000000025.

Jacob SE, Scheman A, McGowan MA: Allergen of the year: propylene glycol, *Dermatitis*, 2017. https://doi.org/10.1097/DER.0000000000000315.

Macneil JS: *Henna tattoo ingredient is allergen of the year*, Skin & Allergy News, 2006. Available at: http://www.skinandallergynews.com/index.php?id=372&cHash=071010&tx_ttnews%5Btt_news%5D=559.

Marks JG, Elsner P, DeLeo VA: In *Contact and occupational dermatology*, 3 ed, Mosby, 2002.

Nelson SA, Yiannias JA: Relevance and avoidance of skin care product allergens: pearls and pitfalls, *Dermatol Clin* 27:329–336, 2009.

Raison-Peyron N, Sasseville D: Acetophenone azine, *Dermatitis* 32:5–9, 2021.

Sasseville D: Acrylates, *Dermatitis* 23(3–5), 2012. https://doi.org/10.1097/DER.0b013e31823d5cd8.

Splete H: *Dermatologists name isobornyl acrylate contact allergen of the year*, Dermatology News, 2019. Available at: https://www.mdedge.com/dermatology/article/195656/contact-dermatitis/dermatologists-name-isobornyl-acrylate-contact.

Thin-layer rapid-use epicutaneous test (T.R.U.E. TEST). https://www.smartpractice.com/shop/wa/category?cn=Products-T.R.U.E.-TEST&id=508222&m=SPA. Accessed March 20, 2021.

Veverka KK, Hall MR, Yiannias JA, et al: Trends in patch testing with the Mayo Clinic standard series, 2011-2015, *Dermatitis* 29(6):310–315, 2018. https://doi.org/10.1097/DER.0000000000000411.

Warshaw EM, Belsito DV, Taylor JS, et al: North American contact dermatitis group patch test results: 2009 to 2010, *Dermatitis* 24:50–59, 2013.

Warshaw EM, Maibach HI, Taylor JS, et al: North American contact dermatitis group patch test results: 2011-2012, *Dermatitis* 26(1):49–59, 2015. https://doi.org/10.1097/DER.0000000000000097.

Wentworth AB, Yiannias JA, Keeling JH, et al: Trends in patch test results and allergen changes in the standard series: a Mayo Clinic 5-year retrospective review. January 1, 2006, through December 31, 2010, *J Am Acad Dermatol* 70:269–275, 2014. e4. https://doi.org/10.1016/j.jaad.2013.09.047.

Yiannias J: *Virtual patch testing: data driven empiric contact allergen avoidance*, Baltimore, MD, 2013, American College of Allergy, Asthma and Immunology Annual Scientific Meeting. November 11, 2013.

CUTANEOUS T-CELL LYMPHOMAS, INCLUDING MYCOSIS FUNGOIDES AND SÉZARY SYNDROME

Method of
Gary S. Wood, MD

CURRENT DIAGNOSIS

For Cutaneous T-cell Lymphomas, obtain the following:
- History: duration and pace of lesion development
- Skin examination: extent of patches, plaques, tumors, and ulcers
- Extracutaneous examination: status of lymph nodes, liver, and spleen
- Laboratory: complete blood cell count, differential, and lesional biopsy results
- Imaging: CT or fused PET/CT scans of the chest, abdomen, and pelvis (not needed for early stage mycosis fungoides)

CURRENT THERAPY

Guidelines Are Primarily for Mycosis Fungoides and Sézary Syndrome:
- Stages IA–IIA: skin-directed therapy with potent topical corticosteroids, topical mechlorethamine (Valchlor), or phototherapy; radiation therapy or topical bexarotene (Targretin) in selected cases
- Stages IIB–IVB: skin-directed therapy plus one or more systemic therapies, such as interferon alfa-2b (Intron A),[1] bexarotene (Targretin), romidepsin (Istodax), or methotrexate; photopheresis for erythrodermic cases
- Combination therapies are often used in intermediate- and advanced-stage disease.
- Multiagent chemotherapy is usually not an effective long-term treatment strategy.

[1]Not FDA approved for this indication.

Cutaneous T-Cell Lymphomas
Classification
Virtually every subtype of T-cell lymphoma involves the skin primarily or secondarily. The principal types of primary cutaneous T-cell lymphomas (CTCLs) recognized in the World Health Organization and European Organization for Research and Treatment of Cancer classification include mycosis fungoides (MF) and its leukemic variant, the Sézary syndrome (SS); CD30+ large cell lymphoma and lymphomatoid papulosis (LyP); CD30- large cell lymphoma; and pleomorphic CD4+ small or medium cell variants (Table 1). All other primary CTCLs comprise only a few percent of the total. This discussion focuses on MF and SS because they account for up to 75% of primary cutaneous cases.

Standard Diagnosis and Staging Methods
The evaluation of CTCL patients begins with a thorough clinical history and physical examination. Key elements of the history include the pace and nature of disease development, the presence or absence of spontaneous regression of lesions, prior therapy, and ingestion of drugs (e.g., anticonvulsants, antihistamines, other agents with antihistaminic properties) that have been associated with pseudolymphomatous skin eruptions that can mimic CTCLs. The review of systems should establish the presence of

TABLE 1	Simplified Classification of Primary Cutaneous T-Cell Lymphoma	
CTCL TYPE	**PROPORTION OF PRIMARY CTCL (%)**	**5-YEAR SURVIVAL RATE (%)**
MF and variants	60	85
SS	3	35*
CD30+ large cell/LyP	25	<95
Pleomorphic small/medium cell**	8	99
Miscellaneous	<1	Variable

Abbreviations: CTCL = cutaneous T-cell lymphoma; MF = mycosis fungoides; SS = Sézary syndrome.
Complete classification in Willemze R, Cerroni L, Kempf W, et al. The 2018 update of the WHO-EORTC classification for primary cutaneous lymphomas. *Blood* 133(16):1703–1714, 2019.
*The 5-year survival rate depends on the criteria used to define SS, and it may be as low as 10%.
**Now regarded as a lymphoproliferative disorder, not lymphoma.

lymphoma-associated constitutional symptoms (e.g., fever of unknown origin, night sweats, weight loss, fatigue). In addition to general aspects, the physical examination should document the type and distribution of skin lesions and whether there is lymphadenopathy, hepatosplenomegaly, or edema of extremities (i.e., potential sign of lymphatic obstruction).

Histopathologic analysis of representative lesional skin biopsy specimens is the primary means of confirming the clinical diagnosis. Biopsy specimens should be deep enough to include the deepest portions of the cutaneous lymphoid infiltrates because these areas often exhibit the most diagnostic features. Putative extracutaneous involvement should be confirmed by biopsy if it is relevant to clinical management.

Routine blood tests include a complete blood cell count, differential review, and general chemistry panel. A "Sézary prep" is used to assess peripheral blood involvement.

Internal nodal and visceral involvement by lymphoma usually is assessed with chest radiography, computed tomography (CT), or combined positron emission tomography and CT (PET/CT) scans of the chest, abdomen, and pelvis. These radiologic studies usually are not needed for patients with early forms of MF (i.e., nontumorous skin lesions without evidence of extracutaneous involvement assessed by physical examination); however, they are usually obtained during the work-up of other types of CTCLs. The role of immunopathologic and molecular biologic assays in the diagnosis and staging of CTCLs is discussed later.

An algorithm for the diagnosis of early MF has been proposed by the International Society for Cutaneous Lymphomas (ISCL) (see Pimpinelli et al. in References). It relies on a combination of clinical, histopathologic, immunopathologic, and clonality criteria. This differs from former approaches that have been based primarily on histopathologic criteria.

Mycosis Fungoides, Sézary Syndrome, and Variants
Clinical Features

MF classically manifests as erythematous, scaly, variably pruritic, flat patches or indurated plaques, often favoring the most sun-protected areas. The patches or plaques may progress to cutaneous tumors and involvement of lymph nodes or viscera, although this usually does not occur as long as the skin lesions are reasonably well controlled by therapy. SS manifests as total-body erythema and scaling (i.e., erythroderma), generalized lymphadenopathy, hepatosplenomegaly, and leukemia. Large-plaque parapsoriasis is essentially the prediagnostic patch phase of MF. Lesions may exhibit poikiloderma (i.e., atrophy, telangiectasia, and mottled hyperpigmentation and hypopigmentation) and have then been referred to as *poikiloderma atrophicans vasculare*.

Follicular mucinosis refers to a papulonodular eruption in which hair follicles are infiltrated by T cells and contain pools of mucin. In hairy areas, this may result in alopecia. Follicular mucinosis may exist as a lesional variant of MF (i.e., follicular MF) or as a clinically benign entity (i.e., alone or associated with other lymphomas).

Granulomatous slack skin is a variant of MF that manifests with pendulous skin folds in intertriginous areas. Lesional skin biopsy specimens contain atypical T cells in a granulomatous background.

Pagetoid reticulosis manifests as a solitary or localized, often hyperkeratotic plaque containing atypical T cells that are frequently confined to a hyperplastic epidermis. Some authorities regard it as a variant of unilesional MF, whereas others think it is a distinct entity.

Other variants of MF include hypopigmented, palmoplantar, bullous, and pigmented purpuric forms. The latter form shows clinicopathologic overlap with the pigmented purpuric dermatoses. *Tumor d'emblée* MF is an outmoded concept used in the past to refer to supposed cases of MF that manifested as cutaneous tumors in the absence of patches or plaques. Most experts now prefer to classify such cases as other forms of CTCL, depending on their histopathologic features.

Histopathologic and Cytologic Features

A well-developed plaque of MF contains a bandlike, cytologically atypical lymphoid infiltrate in the upper dermis that infiltrates the epidermis as single cells and cell clusters known as Pautrier's microabscesses. The atypical lymphoid cells exhibit dense, hyperchromatic nuclei with convoluted, cerebriform nuclear contours and scant cytoplasm. The term *cerebriform* comes from the brain-like ultrastructural appearance of these nuclei. In more advanced cutaneous tumors, the infiltrate extends diffusely throughout the upper and lower dermis and may lose its epidermotropism. In the earlier patch phase of the disease, the infiltrate is sparser, and lymphoid atypia may be less pronounced. In some cases, it may be difficult to distinguish early patch-type MF from various types of chronic dermatitis. The presence of lymphoid atypia and absence of significant epidermal intercellular edema (i.e., spongiosis) help to establish the diagnosis of early MF.

Involvement of lymph nodes by MF begins in the paracortical T-cell domain and may progress to complete effacement of nodal architecture by the same types of atypical lymphoid cells that infiltrate the skin. These cells can be seen in low numbers in the peripheral blood of many MF patients; however, those with SS develop gross leukemic involvement, usually defined as at least 1000 tumor cells/mm^3. These cells are known as Sézary cells, and they are traditionally detected by manual review of the peripheral blood smear (the so-called Sézary prep). They may also be defined by various immunophenotypic criteria.

Immunophenotyping

Cellular antigen expression is usually assessed by immunoperoxidase methods for tissue biopsy specimens and by flow cytometry for blood specimens. Almost all cases of MF or SS begin as phenotypically and functionally mature CD4$^+$ T-cell neoplasms of skin-associated lymphoid tissue (SALT). MF and SS express homing markers consistent with "effector memory" and "central memory" T cells, respectively. They express the SALT-associated homing molecule cutaneous lymphocyte antigen (CLA) and most mature T-cell surface antigens, with the exceptions of CD7 and CD26, which are often absent. As disease progresses, the tumor cells often dedifferentiate and lose one or more mature T-cell markers, such as CD2, CD3, or CD5.

Cases typically express the α/β form of the T-cell receptor. At least in advanced cases, the cytokine profile is consistent with the T_H2 subset of CD4$^+$ T cells (i.e., production of interleukin [IL]-4, IL-5, and IL-10 rather than T_H1 cytokines such as IL-2 and interferon-γ). Expression of the high-affinity IL-2 receptor (CD25, TAC) ranges widely, with most cases showing a variable minority of lesional CD25$^+$ cells. Tumor cells can be induced to express a regulatory T-cell phenotype (Treg) in vitro. MF cases that express CD8$^+$ or other aberrant phenotypes occur occasionally but behave like conventional cases. They should not be confused with rare aggressive CTCLs exhibiting cytotoxic T-cell differentiation.

In addition to tumor cells, MF and SS lesions contain a minor component of immune accessory cells (i.e., Langerhans cells and macrophages) and CD8$^+$ T cells with a cytolytic phenotype. This presumed host response correlates positively with survival and tends to decrease as lesions progress. A favorable response to therapy such as photopheresis appears to correlate with normal levels of circulating CD8$^+$ cells.

Molecular Biology

Well-developed MF or SS is a monoclonal T-cell lymphoproliferative disorder. Southern blotting or polymerase chain reaction (PCR) assays demonstrate monoclonal T-cell receptor gene rearrangements. The greater sensitivity of PCR assays allows the demonstration of dominant clonality in many patch-type lesions of MF. These assays sometimes detect dominant clonality in lesional skin showing only chronic dermatitis histopathologically. These cases are called *clonal dermatitis* and may represent the earliest manifestation of MF because several have progressed to histologically recognizable MF within a few years. However, some cases of clinicopathologically defined early-phase MF lack a detectable monoclonal T-cell population until later in their clinical course. Next generation high throughput T-cell receptor sequencing is emerging as a more sensitive and quantitative alternative to other molecular assays of T-cell clonality.

In addition to aiding initial diagnosis, gene rearrangement analysis has facilitated staging and prognosis. Because some patients without MF or SS can have low levels of circulating Sézary-like cells and because not all cases of peripheral blood involvement in MF or SS exhibit morphologically recognizable tumor cells, the demonstration of dominant clonality that matches the clone in lesional skin has proved to be a useful diagnostic adjunct. The same holds true for assessing lymph node involvement. T-cell receptor gene rearrangement analysis of MF and SS lymph nodes is more sensitive than histopathology and possesses at least some prognostic relevance.

TNMB Staging

Although several proposed methods have used a weighted extent approach to more accurately determine the MF or SS tumor burden, the preferred approach is the tumor–node–metastasis–blood (TNMB) system, which is detailed in Tables 2 and 3. The original tumor (skin), lymph nodes, and metastasis (visceral organs) version of this system has been modified by the ISCL to incorporate the extent of blood involvement (B classification) into the staging process. Table 2 shows the TNMB classification relevant to MF and SS, and Table 3 shows how this information is used to determine the stage of disease. The prognostic relevance of this staging system has been supported by numerous studies, and use of the TNMB helps to guide the selection of therapies. For example, early-stage MF is the most amenable to control with topically directed treatments, whereas advanced MF or SS with extracutaneous involvement usually requires systemic therapies or topical plus systemic combinations.

Treatment

Treatment guidelines for CTCL published by the National Comprehensive Cancer Network can be found at www.nccn.org. Rather than cure, which is attained in less than 10% of cases, the goal of MF and SS therapy is to reduce the impact of the skin disease on quality of life. For most patients, this is achieved by reducing pain, itch, and infection and improving clinical appearance. Appearance is affected by the disfigurement of the eruption and by the profound degree of scale shedding in some patients. Because the natural history of early-stage MF predicts a virtually normal life span, the goal of treatment must be directed at quality of life. For more advanced stages, prolongation of life expectancy may be a reasonable treatment goal.

Regardless of presentation, relief of symptoms should be addressed early. For dryness and scaling, the use of emollient ointments is indicated. These include petrolatum, Aquaphor, and commercially available shortening such as Crisco (an inexpensive alternative).[1] For modest dryness, creams (e.g., Nivea, Cetaphil, Eucerin) can be adequate and more acceptable to patients. Mild superfatted soaps such as Dove and Oil of Olay are recommended. Soap substitutes such as Cetaphil are also acceptable. Pruritus can be addressed with oral agents such as hydroxyzine (Atarax) or diphenhydramine (Benadryl)[1] 2 to 5 mg/kg/day and divided into four daily doses. Antipruritics work better when used on a regular basis rather than on an as-needed basis. Nonsedating antihistamines tend to be less effective. Measures to reduce dryness also help to reduce pruritus. Secondary infection needs to be treated with appropriate antibiotics. Their selection is guided by results of skin cultures but usually involves coverage of gram-positive organisms.

Phototherapy

Two main phototherapeutic regimens are used to treat CTCLs. Ultraviolet B radiation (290–320-nm broad band or 311-nm

---

[1]Not FDA approved for this indication.

TABLE 2	TNMB Classification of Mycosis Fungoides and Sézary Syndrome

Skin (T)

T1	Patches and/or plaques; <10% body surface area
T2	Patches and/or plaques; ≥10% body surface area
T3	Tumors with/without other skin lesions
T4	Generalized erythroderma

Lymph Nodes (N)

N0	Not clinically enlarged; histopathology not required
N1	Clinically enlarged; histopathologically negative
N2	Clinically enlarged; histopathologically equivocal
N3	Clinically enlarged; histopathologically positive

Visceral Organs (M)

M0	No involvement
M1	Involvement

Peripheral Blood (B)

B0	Atypical cells ≤5% of lymphocytes
B1	Atypical cells >5% of lymphocytes
B2	Atypical cells ≥1000/mm^3

T1 and T2 can be subclassified as patch only vs. plaque +/– patch. N and B categories can be subclassified as clone positive or negative. For updates, see www.nccn.org.

TABLE 3	TNMB Staging System for Mycosis Fungoides and Sézary Syndrome

STAGE	SKIN	LYMPH NODES	VISCERA	BLOOD
IA	T1	N0	M0	B0–1
IB	T2	N0	M0	B0–1
IIA	T1–2	N1–2	M0	B0–1
IIB	T3	N0–2	M0	B0–1
IIIA	T4	N0–2	M0	B0
IIIB	T4	N0–2	M0	B1
IVA-1	T1–4	N0–2	M0	B2
IVA-2	T1–4	N3	M0	B0–2
IVB	T1–4	N0–3	M1	B0–2

Modified from Olsen E, Vonderheid E, et al: Revisions to the staging and classification of mycosis fungoides and Sézary syndrome: A proposal of the International Society for Cutaneous Lymphomas (ISCL) and the cutaneous lymphoma task force of the European Organization of Research and Treatment of Cancer (EORTC). Blood 2007;110(6):1713–1722. For updates, see www.nccn.org.

narrow band) can be used for patients with patches but not those with well-developed plaques or tumors. Seventy percent of patients achieve total clinical remission, usually within about 3 to 5 months. Another 15% achieve partial remission. Narrow-band UVB usually is more effective than broadband UVB and achieves maximal responses more rapidly. A synthetic form of hypericin

(SGX301)[5] applied topically and activated by visible fluorescent light has undergone clinical trials and is currently being evaluated by the FDA.

Psoralen–ultraviolet A (PUVA) photochemotherapy uses oral 8-methoxypsoralen (8-MOP)[1] 0.6 mg/kg as a photosensitizer before UVA (320–400 nm) exposure. Sixty-five percent of patients with patch or plaque disease achieve complete remissions, and 30% have partial responses to this modality. For most patients, maximal responses are achieved within 3 months, and after 5 months, it is unlikely that further improvement will be gained. Limitations of these modalities include actinic damage, photocarcinogenesis, retinal damage (if eyes are not protected), and the inconvenience of getting to phototherapy centers. PUVA also has the risk of nausea and a theoretical risk of cataract induction without proper eye protection.

During the clearing phase of treatment, phototherapy treatments usually are administered three times per week. After resolution of skin lesions, treatment frequency is usually tapered gradually to once weekly for UVB and once every 4 to 6 weeks for PUVA. These maintenance regimens are often continued for months to years because abrupt cessation of phototherapy is commonly associated with rapid relapse, which is probably related to the persistence of microscopic disease after clinical clearing.

Topical Therapy

Like phototherapeutic regimens, topical therapies are appropriate for disease confined to the skin (stage I). Topical corticosteroids are frequently used for CTCLs, often before diagnosis. Low-potency formulations are useful on the face and skin folds. Medium-potency preparations are appropriate for the trunk and extremities. High-potency formulations are useful for recalcitrant lesions; however, prolonged use of such potent agents can cause local atrophy and adrenal suppression. Roughly half of patients achieve complete remissions, and most others have partial remissions. Response duration varies widely with the individual pace of disease and patient compliance. Topical corticosteroids are particularly useful as a means to relatively quickly ameliorate severe signs and symptoms and as an adjuvant therapy in combination with other primary treatments.

Mechlorethamine (nitrogen mustard, HN$_2$, Mustargen) is applied topically in an aqueous solution or in an ointment, such as Aquaphor. Although these forms are not FDA approved for this indication, a 0.016% gel formulation (Valchlor) is now commercially available and FDA approved. The aqueous form is prepared at home and involves a daily dose totaling 10 mg in 60 mL water. The ointment form is prepared by a pharmacist in 1-pound lots at a concentration of 10 mg mechlorethamine per 100 g ointment. Only the amount of ointment needed to apply a thin layer is used. Either formulation is usually applied at bedtime to lesional skin for limited disease or to the entire skin surface (excluding the head unless it is also involved) for more extensive disease. It is then showered off every morning using soap and water. Results are similar to those from PUVA. Advantages include therapy at home and availability in all regions of the country. Disadvantages are daily preparation (aqueous form only), daily application, and possible allergic contact dermatitis (more common with the aqueous preparation). Maximal efficacy is expected within 6 months. Mild flare-ups of disease may occur during the first few months of treatment and probably represent inflammation of subclinical skin lesions, analogous to the clinical accentuation of actinic damage during topical therapy with 5-fluorouracil (Efudex). As with phototherapy, topical mechlorethamine is tapered gradually after remission is achieved in an effort to delay clinical relapse.

Carmustine (BCNU, BiCNU)[1] is applied to the total skin surface as an alcohol/aqueous solution (10–20 mg in 60 mL).[6] Complete responses are seen in 85% of patients with stage IA disease (<10% involvement) and 50% of patients with stage IB disease

(>10% involvement). Another 10% of patients obtain partial responses. Advantages include those described for nitrogen mustard and reports of success with application only to lesional skin. Disadvantages include skin irritation followed by telangiectasia formation and possible bone marrow suppression necessitating blood monitoring.

A topical gel formulation of the retinoid X receptor (RXR)–specific retinoid, bexarotene (Targretin), is useful for localized or limited skin lesions. The principal side effect is local irritation.

Radiotherapy

Conventional radiotherapy for mycosis fungoides therapy has been used for approximately 100 years. It is useful in the treatment of isolated, particularly problematic lesions such as recalcitrant tumors or ulcerated plaques. In addition to benefit from the photons delivered by radiotherapy, electron beam therapy (0.4 Gy per week for 8–9 weeks) is also useful for CTCL therapy. An approximately 85% complete response rate of skin disease with a median duration of 16 months is expected with electron beam therapy. An advantage is an excellent rate of complete response. Disadvantages include limited access to required equipment and expertise and cutaneous toxic effects, such as alopecia, sweat gland loss, radiation dermatitis, and skin cancers. As with other skin-directed therapy, the benefit for internal disease is limited. Cumulative toxicity also limits the number of courses a patient may receive. Localized electron beam therapy is also useful for treating cases of limited-extent MF and in treating selected problematic MF lesions in patients who are otherwise responding to therapy. After completion of total-skin electron beam therapy, patients require maintenance therapy such as topical mechlorethamine[6] or phototherapy to prolong remission. Low dose radiotherapy is emerging as an effective alternative to conventional regimens.

Apheresis-Based Therapy

Leukapheresis and particularly lymphocytapheresis (6000–7000 mL of blood treated three times per week initially, then according to response) have been used in the treatment of SS patients. Benefit has been reported in several case reports and small case series; however, response rates are not possible to determine. Photopheresis (i.e., extracorporeal photochemotherapy) describes an apheresis-based therapy in which circulating lymphocytes are first exposed to a psoralen (orally or extracorporeally) and then exposed to UVA extracorporeally. In contrast to leukapheresis, in which leukocytes are discarded, all cells are returned to the patient's circulation during photopheresis. Response rates in erythrodermic patients are 33% to 50%, and median survival for SS patients is prolonged from 30 months to more than 60 months. In recent years, extracorporeal photochemotherapy has been used increasingly in conjunction with one or more systemic therapies to enhance efficacy. The toxicity of the systemic agents is diminished because they are often used in combination at reduced doses.

Cytokine Therapy

Interferon alfa-2a (Roferon-A)[2] or alfa-2b (Intron-A)[1] (1 to 100 × 10^6 units) is given subcutaneously or intralesionally every other day to once weekly. A standard starting dose is 3 × 10^6 units three times per week. Response rates are approximately 55%, with complete responses occurring in 17% of patients. Advantages include the relative ease of delivery. Disadvantages include anorexia, fever, malaise, leukopenia, and risk of cardiac dysrhythmia. Interferon alfa-2a or alfa-2b combined with narrow-band UVB or PUVA is effective for many patients with generalized skin lesions unresponsive to phototherapy alone.

Tumor-Associated Antigen-Directed Therapies

Various specific tumor-associated antigens have been targeted with antibody-based therapy. The response rate typically is low, and response durations are short. Less specific targets are CD4, CD5, and IL-2 receptors. Of this class of agent, the most promising is denileukin diftitox (Ontak, DAB389 IL-2) (9–18 μg per/kg/day IV on 5 consecutive days, every 3 weeks). This agent is a fusion protein combining IL-2 and diphtheria toxin. Cells bearing the IL-2 receptor (in the lesions of at least one half of MF patients) bind and internalize the drug. The drug also may destroy Treg cells that are CD25[+] and suppress immune responses. Inside the cell, the toxin portion of the molecule disrupts protein synthesis, leading to cell death. Approximately 10% of patients achieve complete responses, and total response rates of near 40% have been reported. Half of responders and 20% of nonresponders experienced decreased pruritus. Adverse events include capillary leak syndrome, flulike symptoms, and allergic reactions. Combination therapy with denileukin diftitox and multiagent chemotherapy is being explored for advanced disease. Alemtuzumab (Campath)[1] is an antibody directed against CD52. It has shown benefit in advanced-stage disease. This agent can be used alone or in conjunction with multiagent chemotherapy. Brentuximab vedotin (Adcetris)[1] is an anti-CD30 antibody linked to the microtubule toxin monomethyl auristatin E. It can be effective in those cases of MF that express sufficient CD30. Mogamulizumab (Poteligeo) is an antibody directed against CCR4. It is approved for relapsed or refractory MF or SS after at least one other systemic therapy. Pembrolizumab (Keytruda)[1] is an antibody directed against PD1. It can be of benefit for relapsed or refractory MF or SS.

Systemic Chemotherapy

Various regimens of single-agent and multiagent chemotherapy have been used in the treatment of MF and SS. Oral methotrexate, chlorambucil (Leukeran)[1] with or without prednisone,[1] and etoposide (VePesid)[1] have shown therapeutic activity. The best response has been in erythrodermic patients treated with methotrexate (5 to 125 mg weekly),[3] who have shown a 58% response rate. The combination of low-dose methotrexate and interferon alfa has been reported to yield a high response rate in advanced-stage MF and SS.

The use of multiagent regimens is controversial because of the small number of patients treated with any given regimen. There is even some evidence that for some populations of CTCL patients, survival may be reduced. For individual patients with advanced disease, however, cyclophosphamide (Cytoxan),[1] doxorubicin (Adriamycin),[1] vincristine (Oncovin),[1] and prednisone[1] (CHOP regimen) can provide some short-term palliation. In some cases, CHOP has successfully eradicated large cell transformation of MF and returned patients to their more clinically indolent patch or plaque baseline disease. Idarubicin (Idamycin)[1] in association with etoposide, cyclophosphamide, vincristine, prednisone, and bleomycin (Blenoxane)[1] (VICOP-B regimen) has demonstrated response rates of 80% (36% complete response rate) for patients with stage II through IV disease and 84% for MF patients, with a median duration of response longer than 8 months. Other regimens have been used with more modest success.

Several purine nucleoside analogues have been used for CTCL treatment, including erythrodermic variants. These include 2-chlorodeoxyadenosine (cladribine [Leustatin],[1] with a response rate of 28%), 2-deoxycoformycin (pentostatin [Nipent],[1] with a response rate of 39%), and fludarabine (Fludara).[1] Toxicities include pulmonary edema, bone marrow and immune suppression, and neurotoxicity.

Retinoids

Retinoids have therapeutic activity against MF and SS alone and in combination with other therapies, such as interferon alfa or PUVA (the latter combination is called Re-PUVA). Arotinoid,[5] acitretin (Soriatane),[1] and 13-cis-retinoic acid (isotretinoin [Accutane])[1] have various degrees of efficacy, and they typically are used in conjunction with other modalities. A newer RXR-specific retinoid, bexarotene, has an overall response rate of about 40% and can be used alone or in combination with phototherapy and other systemic agents such as interferon alfa-2. Disadvantages of bexarotene therapy include signs of hypothyroidism and vitamin A toxicity, particularly hyperlipidemia.

Enzyme Inhibitors

Vorinostat (Zolinza) is the first histone deacetylase inhibitor to be FDA approved for MF and SS. The overall response rate approaches 40% using a standard oral dose of 400 mg/day. Side effects include gastrointestinal symptoms, thrombocytopenia, and cardiac conduction abnormalities. Rhomidepsin (Isotodax) is an intravenously administered histone deacetylase inhibitor recently approved by the FDA for MF and SS. Forodesine[5] is a purine nucleoside phosphorylase inhibitor that preferentially affects T cells because they contain relatively high concentrations of this enzyme. Forodesine has undergone clinical trials for MF and SS in the United States and appears to have a response rate of about 40%.

Miscellaneous Therapies

Various other therapies have been tried for MF and SS with modest success. Nonmyeloablative allogeneic stem cell transplantation has led to favorable responses in some patients; however, the total number treated is small. Cyclosporine (Sandimmune)[1] has been used for MF and SS. Transient improvement is followed by worsened survival due to immunosuppression, and it is not a recommended therapy. Thymopentin[5] has given excellent results in SS patients (i.e., 40% complete response rate and 35% partial response rate, with a median duration of response of 22 months). The lack of follow-up reports in recent decades leaves the status of this therapy in question.

Selection of Therapy

Initial choices among conventional treatments for MF and SS depend on the types of lesions and the stage of disease. Disease subsets are followed by recommended initial treatments in parentheses: unilesional or localized MF (local radiation therapy), patch MF (broad- and narrow-band UVB, PUVA, mechlorethamine), patch/plaque MF (PUVA, mechlorethamine), thick plaque/tumor MF (electron beam radiation therapy, interferon alfa-2, bexarotene, histone deacetylase inhibitors), erythrodermic MF/SS (photopheresis), and nodal or visceral MF or SS (interferon alfa-2, bexarotene, histone deacetylase inhibitors, experimental systemic therapies, systemic chemotherapy).

Second-line therapeutic choices often involve interferons, retinoids, or histone deacetylase inhibitors, usually in combination with primary modalities. Multimodality combinations, often at reduced doses, are used commonly to treat patients with stage IIB or more advanced disease. Medium-potency topical corticosteroids, such as 0.1% triamcinolone cream or ointment (Kenalog),[1] are useful adjuncts to many different therapies. The optimal use of newer therapeutic agents in various subtypes and stages of MF and SS is still being established. Evidence-based guidelines for MF and SS therapy have been developed by the National Comprehensive Cancer Network (NCCN) (www.nccn.org).

Lymphoproliferative Disorders Associated with Mycosis Fungoides and Sézary Syndrome
Types and Clinical Features

Patients with MF or SS are at increased risk for large T-cell lymphomas, lymphomatoid papulosis, and Hodgkin's disease. Molecular biologic analysis has shown that these disorders and MF often share the same clonal T-cell receptor gene rearrangement

---

[1]Not FDA approved for this indication.
[2]Not available in the United States.
[3]Exceeds dosage recommended by the manufacturer.

[5]Investigational drug in the United States.

when they arise in the same individual. As a consequence, they are considered to be subclones of the original MF tumor clone. The development of large T-cell lymphoma in a patient with MF or SS is referred to as *large cell transformation of MF*. This occurs in up to 20% of cases in some series and is associated with a median survival of only 1 to 2 years. One half of these large T-cell lymphomas are CD30[+]; however, the generally favorable prognosis of primary cutaneous CD30[+] anaplastic large cell lymphoma may not extend to these secondary forms of CD30[+] lymphoma. These patients may need to be treated with systemic chemotherapy such as CHOP or with experimental systemic therapies appropriate for advanced-stage CTCL.

Lymphomatoid papulosis manifests as recurrent, usually generalized crops of spontaneously regressing, erythematous papules that can exhibit crusting or vesiculation before resolution. It is the clinically benign end of a disease continuum that has primary cutaneous CD30[+] anaplastic large cell lymphoma at its other extreme. Intermediate forms of disease can occur. Histopathologically, lesions contain a mixed-cell infiltrate, including large, atypical T cells that resemble Reed-Sternberg cells and their mononuclear variants (so-called type A) or large MF-type cells (so-called type B). Type A cells are CD30[+]. A type C form is also recognized. It has sheets of type A cells histologically mimicking CD30[+] large T-cell lymphoma but is different from it clinically. A type D variant containing CD8[+] CD30[+] large atypical cells has also been described recently, as well as a few other rare subtypes. All types of lymphomatoid papulosis behave similarly. Patients with lymphomatoid papulosis sometimes respond to tetracycline[1] or erythromycin[1] (500 mg PO bid), presumably on the basis of antiinflammatory activity. Most cases improve within 1 month with low-dose methotrexate (10–20 mg PO every week). PUVA and narrow-band UVB given three times per week are other therapeutic options.

Treatment

In most cases, non-MF/SS CTCLs are treated with radiation therapy (with or without complete surgical excision) if they are localized or with various multiagent systemic chemotherapy regimens if they are generalized. The roles of other agents remain to be defined, except that studies have proved that methotrexate (10–40 mg PO every week) is effective therapy for most cases of primary cutaneous CD30[+] anaplastic large cell lymphoma. Therapies being investigated for this lymphoma include anti-CD30 antibodies, alone or conjugated to toxins. One of these antibody conjugates (brentuximab vedotin [Adcetris]) is FDA approved for primary cutaneous anaplastic large cell lymphomas and CD30+ MF. Denileukin diftitox[2] has been reported to be effective against some subcutaneous panniculitic T-cell lymphomas.

[1]Not FDA approved for this indication.
[2]Not available in the United States.

References

Olsen E, Vonderheid E, et al: Revisions to the staging and classification of mycosis fungoides and Sézary syndrome: A proposal of the International Society for Cutaneous Lymphomas (ISCL) and the cutaneous lymphoma task force of the European Organization of Research and Treatment of Cancer (EORTC), *Blood* 110(6):1713–1722, 2007.

Pimpinelli N, Olsen EA, Santucci M, et al: Defining early mycosis fungoides, *J Am Acad Dermatol* 53(6):1053–1063, 2005.

Richardson SK, Lin JH, Vittorio CC, et al: High clinical response rate with multimodality immunomodulatory therapy for Sézary syndrome, *Clin Lymphoma Myeloma* 7(3):226–232, 2006.

Vonderheid EC, Bernengo MG, Burg G, et al: Update on erythrodermic cutaneous T-cell lymphoma: Report of the International Society for Cutaneous Lymphomas, *J Am Acad Dermatol* 46(1):95–106, 2002.

Willemze R, Jaffe ES, Burg G, et al: WHO-EORTC classification for cutaneous lymphomas, *Blood* 105(10):3768–3785, 2005.

Wood GS, Greenberg HL: Diagnosis, staging, and monitoring of cutaneous T-cell lymphoma, *Dermatol Ther* 16(4):269–275, 2003.

CUTANEOUS VASCULITIS

Method of
Molly A. Hinshaw, MD; and Susan Lawrence-Hylland, MD

CURRENT DIAGNOSIS

- Cutaneous vasculitis can be limited to skin (leukocytoclastic vasculitis) or associated with systemic disease.
- Perform punch biopsy of intact, nonulcerated skin lesion.
- "Vasculitis" on skin biopsy describes vessel appearance and is not a clinical diagnosis.
- Thorough review of systems and physical examination are necessary to evaluate for systemic vasculitis.

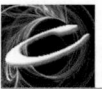

CURRENT THERAPY

Leukocytoclastic Vasculitis
- First identify instigating factors: infection, medications.
- Care is symptomatic. Lesions typically remit without treatment.
- If needed, short course of prednisone may be given and tapered over 3 to 6 weeks.

All Forms of Vasculitis
- Treat underlying systemic vasculitis.

Vasculitis is an inflammatory-mediated destruction of blood vessels. The systemic vasculitides have historically been differentiated by their involvement of small, medium, or large blood vessels. Names used to describe isolated cutaneous vasculitis have included hypersensitivity vasculitis and leukocytoclastic vasculitis (LCV). In 1990, the American College of Rheumatology proposed five criteria for the classification of hypersensitivity vasculitis: age older than 16 years, possible drug trigger, palpable purpura, maculopapular rash, and skin biopsy showing neutrophils around vessel. At least three out of five criteria yield a sensitivity of 71% and specificity of 84%. In 1994, a new nomenclature proposed at the Chapel Hill International Consensus Conference in North Carolina further classified vasculitis (Box 1). The term "hypersensitivity vasculitis" was not used, because most vasculitides that would have previously been in this category fall into either microscopic polyangiitis or cutaneous LCV. LCV is vasculitis restricted to the skin without involvement of vessels in other organs. Cutaneous vasculitis may be a clue to systemic vasculitis and guides the clinician to a comprehensive evaluation (Table 1).

Vasculitis can affect almost any organ, and once affected, end organs can become dysfunctional. Such dysfunction may be as innocuous as cutaneous, tender, transient papules or as devastating as a stroke. A thorough evaluation of the patient with a complete review of systems, physical examination, laboratory evaluation, and clinical follow-up allows a distinction to be made between the different forms of vasculitis.

Leukocytoclastic Vasculitis

Epidemiology

LCV is common. The incidence and prevalence are unknown. Mean age of onset ranges from 34 to 49 years of age. The female-to-male ratio ranges from approximately 2:1 to 3:1.

Risk Factors

LCV is often secondary to a known trigger including infection, drug ingestion, or malignancy. LCV can also be a presenting feature of autoimmune disease.

<table>
<tr><td>**BOX 1**</td><td colspan="2">Chapel Hill Consensus 1994 Classification of Vasculitis</td></tr>
</table>

Large-Vessel Vasculitis
Giant cell arteritis
  Takayasu's arteritis

Medium-Vessel Vasculitis
Classic polyarteritis nodosa
  Kawasaki's disease

Small-Vessel Vasculitis
Churg-Strauss syndrome
  Cutaneous leukocytoclastic vasculitis
  Essential cryoglobulinemia
  Henoch-Schönlein purpura
  Microscopic polyangiitis (polyarteritis)
  Wegener's granulomatosis

Pathophysiology

LCV is best characterized as immune complex–mediated inflammatory destruction of the postcapillary venules of any organ. The exact mechanisms of vascular destruction is unknown.

Clinical Manifestations

LCV typically manifests as nonblanchable macules that evolve to papules or, less commonly, pustules and ulcers (Figure 1). Clues to the diagnosis include a monomorphous, ruddy-brown appearance owing to leakage of hemosiderin pigment from vessels. Lesions measure a few millimeters to a few centimeters in diameter. LCV is often localized to the lower extremities but may be diffuse. Pruritus, pain, or burning of the skin lesions are indicators that the patient might have a vasculitis extending beyond LCV.

Diagnosis

To confirm a clinical impression of LCV, perform a punch biopsy in the center of a nonulcerated cutaneous lesion that is less than 24 to 48 hours old and submit the sample in 10% formalin (standard medium). It is important to biopsy an intact, nonulcerated active lesion (Figure 2) because ulcers can show histologic features simulating vasculitis regardless of whether the patient has true vasculitis or not.

Pathology reveals a mononuclear or polymorphonuclear inflammation of the small blood vessels (called LCV), most prominent in the postcapillary venules. The appearance may be necrotizing or non-necrotizing.

Differential Diagnosis

LCV manifests as erythematous papules or occasionally as papulopustules that can simulate a variety of entities (see Table 1). The review of systems and physical examination should be directed to evaluate for diseases that have cutaneous vasculitis as a component of their presentation (see Table 1). All patients with LCV should have a urinalysis to evaluate for hematuria as a sign of kidney involvement, with subsequent evaluation and management if identified.

Treatment

The primary goal in the management of LCV is to identify and treat instigating factors, including infection and medications. Supportive treatment includes resting, elevating legs, and wearing support hose. When review of systems, physical examination, and urinalysis do not reveal associated systemic diseases, treatment of LCV is generally not necessary. Lesions typically remit without treatment. In rare patients with symptomatic, extensively pustular, or progressive lesions, a short course of prednisone[1] dosed at 1 mg/kg/day initially and tapered over 3 to 6 weeks may be used,

---

[1]Not FDA approved for this indication.

TABLE 1	Diseases with Cutaneous Vasculitis as a Component of Their Presentation	
DISEASE	**SKIN LESIONS**	**CLUES AND CONFIRMATION**
Urticarial vasculitis	Individual lesions look like urticaria but last >24 h; typical urticaria last a few hours, always <24 h Pruritus, burning of skin lesions	May be associated with connective tissue disease, medications, low complement, viral infections (e.g., hep B, hep C, EBV) Skin biopsy
Henoch-Schönlein purpura	Wheals progress to petechia, ecchymoses and palpable purpura Lesions are in gravity-dependent or pressure-dependent areas such as legs or the buttocks in toddlers	Arthralgia or arthritis, hematuria, abdominal pain, melena Skin biopsy and DIF for IgA
Essential mixed cryoglobulinemia	Palpable purpura	Peripheral neuropathy, GN Hep C positive Serum cryoglobulins
Wegener's granulomatosis	Palpable purpura, hemorrhagic lesions, petechiae, skin ulcers	c-ANCA >80% Pulmonary hemorrhage, GN Biopsy affected organ
Churg-Strauss syndrome	Maculopapular rash, palpable purpura, hemorrhagic lesions, subcutaneous nodules, livedo reticularis or Raynaud's disease	ANCA (50%) Asthma, allergic rhinitis Eosinophilia >1.5 × 10⁹/L Pulmonary infiltrates, pulmonary neuropathy Biopsy affected organ
Microscopic polyangiitis	Palpable purpura, hemorrhagic lesions, petechiae, skin ulcers, splinter hemorrhages	p-ANCA >60% Pulmonary hemorrhage, GN Biopsy affected organ
Polyarteritis nodosa	Livedo reticularis, tender nodules, skin ulcers, bullae or vesicles	Hypertension, elevated creatinine, abdominal pain, constitutional symptoms (fever) Abnormal angiogram Biopsy affected organ

Abbreviations: c-ANCA = classic antineutrophil cytoplasmic antibody; DIF = direct immunofluorescence; EBV = Epstein-Barr virus; GN = glomerulonephritis; hep = hepatitis; Ig = immunoglobulin; p-ANCA = protoplasmic-staining antineutrophil cytoplasmic antibody.

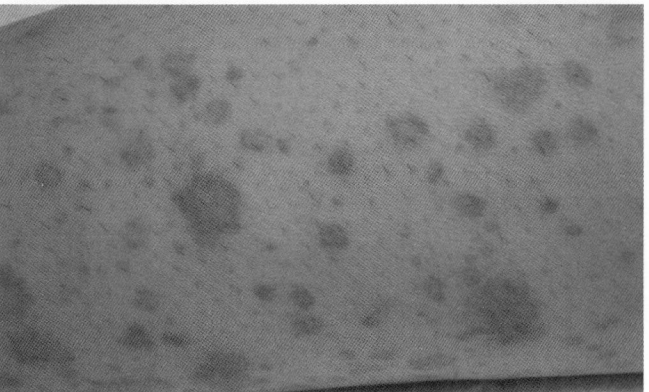

Figure 1 Leukocytoclastic vasculitis: palpable, purpuric, nonblanching, erythematous to ruddy-brown thin papules. Additional secondary changes include small pustules (pustular vasculitis) or shallow, small ulcerations.

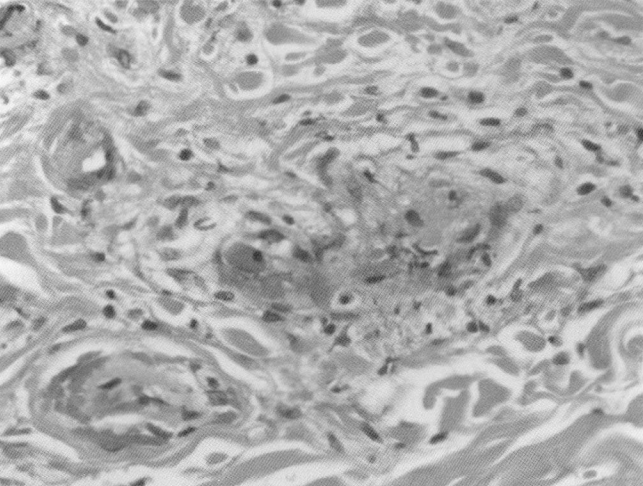

Figure 2 Biopsy of intact clinical lesion of leukocytoclastic vasculitis. Histology shows destruction of postcapillary venules with fibrin deposition, degenerate inflammatory cells, and extravasated erythrocytes.

to a systemic process can include fever, arthralgias, myalgias, anorexia, abdominal pain, pulmonary abnormalities, or neurologic symptoms.

Skin biopsy may aid in the diagnosis of a systemic vasculitis (Henoch-Schönlein purpura), but biopsy of an affected end organ may be necessary to confirm a diagnosis. Pathology focuses on the confirmation of vasculitis in a small, medium, or large vessel.

Aside from Henoch-Schönlein purpura, treatment of systemic vasculitis is typically much more aggressive than treatment of LCV and should be pursued in conjunction with involvement of a rheumatologist, nephrologist, or pulmonologist. Systemic disease leads to severe complications including renal failure, pulmonary damage, permanent vascular disease, or neurologic insult depending on the viscera affected.

References

Gayraud M, Guillevin L, le Toumelin P, et al: Long-term followup of polyarteritis nodosa, microscopic polyangiitis, and Churg-Strauss syndrome: Analysis of four prospective trials including 278 patients, *Arthritis Rheum* 44:666–675, 2001.

Hannon CW, Swerlick RA: Vasculitis. In Bolognia J, Jorizzo J, Rapini R, editors: Dermatology, vol 1. St Louis, 2003, Mosby, pp 381–402.

Hoffman GS, Kerr GS, Leavitt RY, et al: Wegener granulomatosis: An analysis of 158 patients, *Ann Intern Med* 116:488–498, 1992.

Jennette JC, Thomas DB, Falk RJ: Microscopic polyangiitis (microscopic polyarteritis), *Semin Diagn Pathol* 18:3–13, 2001.

Jenette JC, Falk RF, Andrassy K, et al: Nomenclature of systemic vasculitides. Proposal of an international consensus conference, *Arthritis Rheum* 37(2):187–192, 1994.

DISEASES OF THE HAIR

Method of
Dirk M. Elston, MD

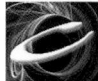

CURRENT DIAGNOSIS

- A sudden increase in shedding most commonly represents telogen effluvium.
- Hair thinning is more likely to represent pattern alopecia.
- Scarring alopecia generally requires a biopsy for diagnosis.
- Most medically significant hirsutism results from polycystic ovarian syndrome.
- New-onset virilization suggests the possibility of a tumor.

CURRENT THERAPY

- Pattern alopecia in men is treated with oral finasteride (Propecia), topical minoxidil (Rogaine), or both.
- Pattern alopecia in women is treated with antiandrogens (such as spironolactone [Aldactone][1]) and oral[1] or topical minoxidil. Platelet-rich plasma injections may be of benefit in both men and women.
- Alopecia areata can require intralesional corticosteroid injections, topical immunotherapy, or therapy with agents such as methotrexate (Trexall)[1] or Janus kinase (JAK) inhibitors.
- A scalp biopsy is critical to guide therapy in scarring alopecia.
- Hirsutism may be treated with laser epilation or systemic antiandrogens. Topical eflornithine (Vaniqa) can slow regrowth of hair.

[1]Not FDA approved for this indication.

although no controlled trials have been performed using oral corticosteroids for isolated LCV. Rapid steroid taper can lead to rebound. Systematic evaluation of the use of other medications, such as colchicine[1] or dapsone,[1] to treat isolated LCV has not been performed.

Monitoring
Patients with LCV are at risk for recurrent or chronic vasculitis. In addition, apparent LCV can occur as a systemic disease that is not recognizable at the first episode. Patients with persistent or recurrent LCV require follow-up to ensure disease clearance, to monitor for medication side effects, and to evaluate for evolving disorders known to be associated with cutaneous vasculitis (see Table 1).

Complications
Isolated LCV generally resolves without sequelae. However, pustular or ulcerative LCV may be complicated by local sequelae such as cutaneous ulcerations and scars.

Cutaneous Vasculitis Associated with Systemic Vasculitis
Cutaneous vasculitis may be a component of the presentation of multiple diseases (see Table 1). When a clinician reads a pathology report from a biopsy of a skin lesion that states "vasculitis," it is important to realize that this term is a descriptor of the histopathology. It is the clinician's challenge to determine whether "vasculitis" is as potentially innocuous as LCV or part of a more severe systemic disease. Symptoms that are clues

Epidemiology
Hair disorders are common, with more than half of the population affected by pattern alopecia and the prevalence of hirsutism varying significantly by ethnicity.

Risk Factors
Most causes of alopecia and hirsutism are genetically determined.

Pathophysiology

Pattern alopecia relates to increased sensitivity to dihydrotestosterone. Telogen effluvium relates to an alteration in the normal hair cycle, with many hairs shedding synchronously. Alopecia areata represents an inflammatory insult directed against melanocytes in the hair bulb. There is strong evidence that the disease is mediated by Th1 lymphocytes. Polycystic ovarian syndrome is an insulin-resistance syndrome resulting in excess production of androgens.

Prevention

Little can be done to prevent hair disorders, so the focus is generally on diagnosis and treatment.

Clinical Manifestations

Pattern alopecia manifests with apical scalp thinning. In men, receding of the hairline at the temples is typical, whereas women demonstrate widening of the part but retain the anterior hairline. Telogen effluvium manifests with diffuse shedding of telogen hairs (hairs with a nonpigmented bulb). Alopecia areata typically occurs with patchy hair loss. Shed hairs demonstrate tapered fracture at the base. Syphilitic alopecia resembles alopecia areata but often affects smaller areas, with only partial hair loss, resulting in a moth-eaten appearance. Scarring alopecia shows permanent areas of smooth alopecia lacking follicular openings.

Polycystic ovarian syndrome manifests with evidence of anovulation and excess androgen production. Signs of virilization suggesting a possible tumor include new onset of hirsutism, deepening of the voice, change in body habitus, and clitoromegaly.

Diagnosis

Alopecia

The first step is to determine whether a hair shaft abnormality exists (Box 1). This is particularly important in Black patients, in whom trichorrhexis nodosa is a common cause of hair loss. Trichorrhexis nodosa results from overprocessing of the hair. Hair density is normal at the level of the scalp, but hairs break off, leaving patches of short hair.

The next step is to determine whether telogen effluvium exists. Telogen effluvium manifests with increased shedding of hairs with a blunt nonpigmented bulb (Figure 1), and it commonly follows an illness, surgery, delivery, or crash diet by 3 to 5 months. Hairs can often be easily extracted with a gentle hair pull or 1 minute of combing. The presence of tapered fracture suggests alopecia areata, syphilis, or heavy metal poisoning. Alopecia areata can result in diffuse hair loss, but it more commonly manifests with well-defined round patches of hair loss. The skin is either normal or salmon pink. Syphilis more often shows a moth-eaten pattern of alopecia (Figure 2).

Most patients with hair loss need only limited laboratory testing or none at all. Thyroid disorders and iron deficiency are common, and testing for them is relatively inexpensive. I recommend them when telogen effluvium is present. Their presence can also accelerate the course of pattern alopecia, and it is reasonable to test for them in women with this disorder. Thyroid-stimulating hormone is the best screen for thyroid disorders. The role of iron deficiency in telogen hair loss is controversial, but iron deficiency is common, easily established, and inexpensive to correct. Iron status also serves as an indicator of overall nutritional status. Although a low ferritin level proves iron deficiency, ferritin behaves as an acute phase reactant and a normal level does not rule out iron deficiency. Therefore, I recommend measurement of ferritin, serum iron, iron binding capacity, and saturation.

A scalp biopsy is required in any patient with scarring alopecia. It may also be necessary in other patients if history and physical examination do not establish a diagnosis and the alopecia is progressive. The scalp biopsy should be performed with a 4-mm biopsy punch oriented parallel to the direction

---

BOX 1 Diagnosis of Alopecia

Trichodystrophy
Types
- Trichorrhexis nodosa
- Inherited trichodystrophies
- Fractures

Causes
- Alopecia areata
- Chemotherapy
- Heavy metal

Determine Type
Anagen Effluvium
Tapered fractures can be caused by
- Alopecia areata
- Chemotherapy
- Heavy metal
Loose anagen can be caused by
- Loose anagen syndrome
- Easily extractable anagen in scarring alopecia

Telogen Effluvium
Increased shedding of club hairs can be caused by
- Diet, illness
- Pregnancy
- Medication
- Papulosquamous disorders
- Pattern alopecia

Diagnosis
Laboratory Studies
- Iron
- Thyroid-stimulating hormone
- Endocrine studies in virilized women

Biopsy
Nonscarring types
- Telogen effluvium
- Pattern alopecia
- Alopecia areata
Scarring types
- Lupus erythematosus
- Lichen planopilaris
- Folliculitis decalvans

Other Permanent Alopecia
- Idiopathic pseudopelade
- Morphea

---

of hair growth. Collagen hemostatic sponge (Gelfoam and others) can be placed into the resulting hole to stop bleeding and eliminate the need for sutures. The biopsy should be done in a well-established but still active area of inflammation if one can be identified. A combination of vertical and transverse sections increases the diagnostic yield and is usually recommended. In patients with scarring alopecia, half of the vertically bisected specimen should be sent for direct immunofluorescence. An additional biopsy of an end-stage scarred area can demonstrate characteristic patterns of scarring with an elastic tissue stain. This can help distinguish among causes of scarring alopecia such as lupus erythematosus (Figure 3), lichen planopilaris, pseudopelade, and folliculitis decalvans.

Hirsutism

Patients with *new-onset* virilization should be evaluated to rule out an ovarian or adrenal tumor. Ovarian and adrenal imaging

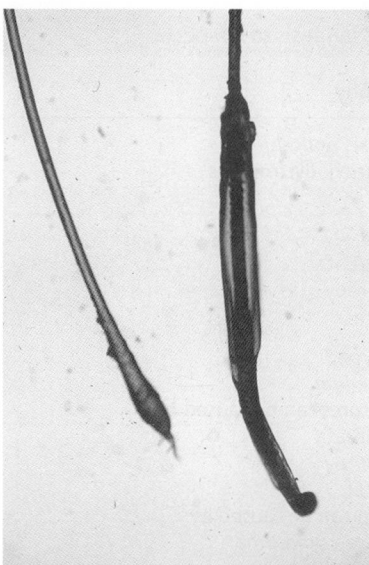

Figure 1 Telogen hair on *left*, anagen hair on *right* for comparison.

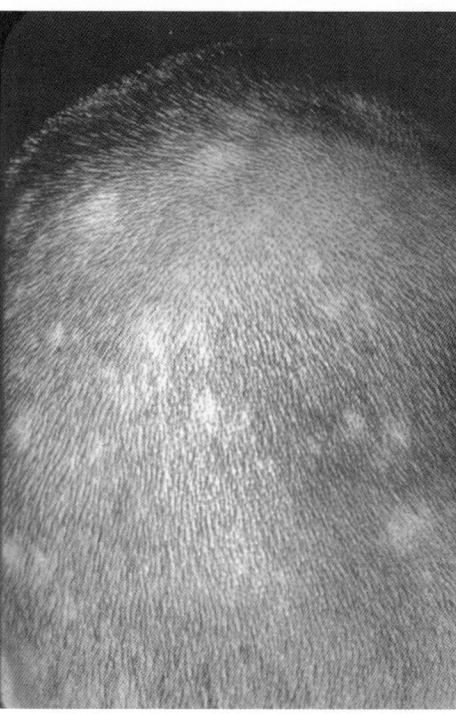

Figure 2 Moth-eaten syphilitic alopecia.

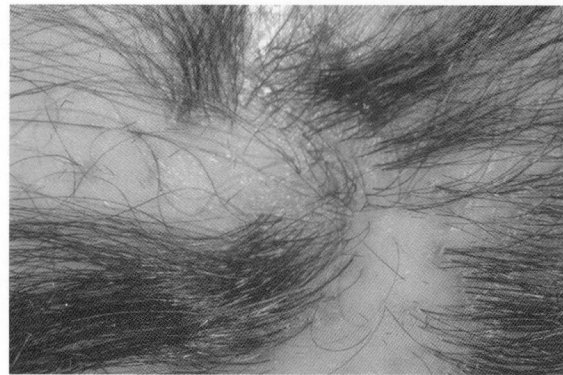

Figure 3 Scarring alopecia secondary to chronic cutaneous lupus erythematosus.

Differential Diagnosis

Syphilis can mimic alopecia areata, and serologic testing should be performed in any sexually active patient with a new diagnosis of alopecia areata. Correct diagnosis of scarring alopecia depends of a thorough examination for other cutaneous signs of lupus erythematosus or lichen planus as well as the results of a skin biopsy.

Tinea capitis can occur as inflammatory boggy areas with hair loss (kerion) or with subtle seborrheic-type scale and black-dot areas of hair loss. A potassium hydroxide (KOH) examination can be performed by rubbing the affected area with moist gauze and examining broken hairs that cling to the gauze.

Hirsutism should be distinguished from hypertrichosis. Hirsutism is a male pattern of hair growth occurring in a woman and is hormonal in nature. Hypertrichosis is excess hair growth that occurs outside of an androgen-dependent distribution. It can be found in metabolic disorders such as porphyria or may be a sign of internal malignancy (Figure 4).

Nonclassic 21-hydroxylase deficiency accounts for up to 10% of patients with medically significant hirsutism. Screening with a baseline morning 17-OH-progesterone is associated with many false positive results. A stimulated 17-OH-progesterone is more specific, but the results of testing seldom affect management because outcomes with dexamethasone (Decadron)[1] are no better than with spironolactone (Aldactone).[1]

Treatment
Alopecia

Telogen effluvium commonly resolves spontaneously once the cause has been eliminated. Poor diet and papulosquamous diseases of the scalp such as seborrheic dermatitis and psoriasis can perpetuate a telogen effluvium and should be treated. The importance of a diet containing adequate protein and trace minerals should be emphasized. Deficiencies and thyroid abnormalities should be addressed. Seborrheic dermatitis responds to topical corticosteroids. Medicated shampoos containing selenium sulfide (Selsun Blue) or zinc pyrithione (T-gel Daily Control) can be helpful. Scalp psoriasis can require more potent topical steroids such as fluocinonide solution (Lidex) and calcipotriene (Dovonex) applied on weekends or daily. Systemic agents such as methotrexate (Trexall)[1] at doses of 7.5 to 20 mg once weekly may be required to control severe scalp psoriasis.

Pattern alopecia in men is mediated by dihydrotestosterone (DHT). Men with pattern alopecia may be treated with daily topical minoxidil 2% to 5% (Rogaine), oral minoxidil (Loniten)[1] in doses from 0.5 to 5 mg daily, and oral finasteride (Propecia) at a dose of 1 mg daily. In women, the pathogenesis

studies and a total testosterone level are the best screens. A total testosterone more than 200 ng/dL or dehydroepiandrostenedione sulfate (DHEAS) more than 8000 ng/dL suggests tumor. In patients with physical signs of Cushing disease, a 24-hour urine cortisol should be obtained. Most patients with *chronic* medically significant hirsutism have polycystic ovarian syndrome (PCOS). The diagnosis is established by means of history and physical examination, and the most important laboratory tests are serum lipids and fasting glucose to establish associated cardiac risk factors. A clinical diagnosis of PCOS requires the presence of hirsutism, acne or pattern alopecia, and evidence of anovulation (fewer than nine periods per year or cycles longer than 40 days). Ratios of luteinizing hormone (LH) to follicle-stimulating hormone (FSH) have poor sensitivity and specificity for diagnosing PCOS. Imaging for ovarian cysts seldom affects management.

---

[1]Not FDA approved for this indication.

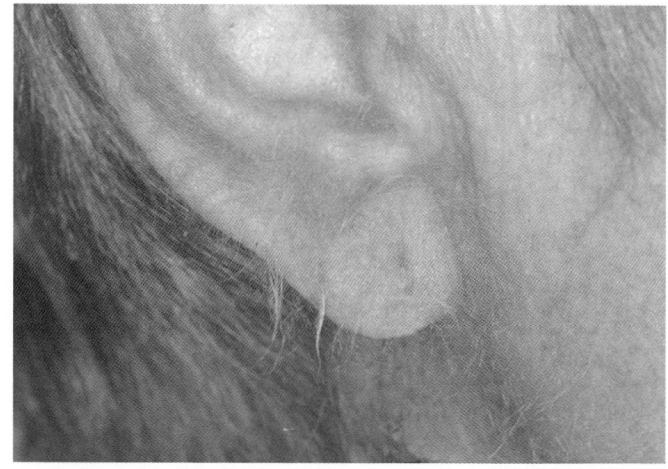

Figure 4 Malignant hypertrichosis secondary to ovarian cancer.

is complex, and adrenal androgens may play a larger role. Finasteride[1] is of less benefit in the majority of women with pattern alopecia. Spironolactone[1] 100 mg twice daily can be helpful and may be combined with oral minoxidil.[1] In women of childbearing potential, spironolactone should always be used in conjunction with an oral contraceptive. Side effects are uncommon but can include urinary frequency, irregular periods, dyspareunia, and nausea. Most patients demonstrate a minor increase in serum potassium. Those with kidney failure are at risk for life-threatening potassium retention. Topical 2% minoxidil can also be of benefit, and some women derive added benefit from the 5% formulation. All patients with pattern alopecia should be evaluated for superimposed causes of telogen effluvium such as inadequate diet and seborrheic dermatitis.

Tinea capitis is often overlooked in adults and Black children, in whom the manifestations of inflammation can be subtle. Black dot and seborrheic tinea are common in Black children. Patchy hair loss is an important clue to the diagnosis. Treatment is summarized in Table 1.

Localized patches of alopecia areata respond to intralesional injections of triamcinolone hexacetonide (Aristospan) (2.5–5 mg/mL) given once per month. Approximately 0.1 mL/cm^2 is injected to a maximum of 3 mL during any one session. Minoxidil solution produces slow regrowth in some patients who cannot tolerate other treatments. Anthralin (Dritho-Scalp 0.5%)[1] is sometimes used in children. It is applied 30 minutes before showering. It can stain skin and anything else it touches.

Topical immunotherapy with dinitrochlorobenzene (DNCB)[1], squaric acid dibutylester (SADBE),[1] or diphenylcyclopropenone (DPCP)[1] is more effective than either minoxidil or anthralin. DNCB is mutagenic in the Ames assay and none of the topical immunotherapies are currently approved for human use. A 2% solution of the sensitizer is applied to the arm in acetone to induce initial sensitization. Subsequently, diluted solutions, starting at about 0.001%, are applied weekly to the scalp with a cotton-tipped applicator. Roughly 20% to 60% of patients have responded to this regimen in various studies.

Tofacitinib (Xeljanz)[1] and other JAK inhibitors are often effective in patients with refractory alopecia areata. Biologic agents have shown mixed results. Methotrexate[1] in psoriatic doses (7.5–20 mg weekly for an adult) can be effective. Sulfasalazine (Azulfidine)[1] is sometimes effective in doses ranging from 500 to 1500 mg three times a day.[3] Patients should be encouraged to read about new therapies on the National Alopecia Areata Foundation website (https://www.naaf.org).

Early, aggressive therapy for discoid lupus erythematosus is recommended to prevent permanent scarring. Topical corticosteroids are rarely sufficient. Intralesional injections are performed in a manner similar to that described above. Initial control of severe disease can be achieved with a single 3-week tapered course of oral prednisone at a dose of 60 mg daily for the first week, 40 mg daily for the second week, and 20 mg daily for the third week. Intralesional steroid injections or a systemic steroid-sparing agent are required for maintenance therapy. Systemic agents that can be effective include antimalarials, dapsone,[1] methotrexate,[1] mycophenolate mofetil (CellCept),[1] and thalidomide (Thalomid).[1] I generally begin treatment with hydroxychloroquine (Plaquenil)[1] at a dose of 400 mg daily for an adult. Dapsone is used at a dose of 100 mg daily for an adult. Thalidomide has been used effectively at doses of 50 to 100 mg daily, but peripheral neuropathy and teratogenicity limit its use. Mycophenolate mofetil is used at a dose of 1 g twice daily, and methotrexate is used at doses of 7.5 to 20 mg weekly. Background pattern (androgenetic) alopecia should be treated as well.

End-stage cicatricial alopecia is best treated by scalp reduction and hair transplantation. The disease can flare up in response to surgery, and it is best to plan a 3-week tapered course of prednisone[1] or a month of cyclosporine (Neoral)[1] to help prevent the flare.

Lichen planopilaris is treated in a manner similar to lupus, except that hydroxychloroquine[1] is of less benefit and oral retinoids (acitretin [Soriatane][1] at doses of 25 to 50 mg daily) are more likely to be successful. Topical calcineurin inhibitors can be effective in achieving and maintaining remission. A few months of pioglitazone (Actos)[1] can induce remission in a subset of patients and the frontal fibrosing alopecia variant can respond to dutasteride (Avodart).[1] Patients should be aware of the risks associated with each of these treatments, including bladder cancer and hypospadias in a male fetus. Mycophenolate mofetil (CellCept)[1] 1 g twice daily or a JAK inhibitor may be effective when other treatments fail, and excimer laser can also be effective for lichen planopilaris. It is contraindicated in lupus erythematosus.

Folliculitis decalvans manifests with crops of pustules that result in permanent scarring. Patients respond to weekend applications of clobetasol (Clobex, Olux) together with prolonged use of antistaphylococcal antibiotics such as doxycycline (Doryx)[1] 100 mg twice daily.

---

[1]Not FDA approved for this indication.
[3]Exceeds dosage recommended by the manufacturer.

---

[1]Not FDA approved for this indication.

Hirsutism

Treatment options include laser epilation, eflornithine (Vaniqa) cream to reduce the rate of hair growth, or spironolactone[1] at a starting dose of 100 mg twice daily as described for pattern alopecia. Cyproterone acetate is used in some countries but is not available in the United States. Other options that are less commonly used include insulin sensitizers, flutamide (Eulexin),[1] metformin (Glucophage),[1] and leuprolide (Lupron)[1] plus estrogen.[1]

Monitoring

Patients treated with topical or intralesional corticosteroids should be monitored for cutaneous atrophy. Patients on JAK inhibitors should have quarterly evaluations of blood count, chemistries, and lipids. Those on hydroxychloroquine should be monitored for ocular toxicity, including corneal deposits and retinal damage, although these are very rare at usual doses. They should also be monitored periodically for thrombocytopenia, agranulocytosis, and hepatitis. Patients beginning dapsone therapy should be screened for G6PD deficiency. Potential side effects include hemolysis, methemoglobinemia, and neuropathy. Monitoring includes periodic blood count assessment and measurement of strength and sensation. Mycophenolate mofetil can produce pancytopenia, and blood counts should be monitored. Methotrexate is cleared by the kidneys, and kidney function should be assessed at baseline. Periodic assessment of liver-function tests and blood count is warranted, as is a yearly chest radiograph. I also monitor procollagen 3 terminal peptide levels quarterly to assess the risk of hepatic fibrosis. Patients on antiandrogen therapy should be monitored for dyspareunia resulting from vulvar atrophy.

Complications

Patients with pattern alopecia and PCOS have a greater risk of metabolic syndrome with cardiac complications. They should be evaluated for lipid abnormalities and glucose intolerance and treated appropriately.

[1]Not FDA approved for this indication.

References

Brown J, Farquhar C, Lee O, et al: Spironolactone versus placebo or in combination with steroids for hirsutism and/or acne, *Cochrane Database Syst Rev* (2)CD000194, 2009.

Buzney E, Sheu J, Buzney C, Reynolds RV: Polycystic ovary syndrome: a review for dermatologists: Part II. Treatment, *J Am Acad Dermatol* 71(5):859.e1–859.e15, 2014.

Durdu M, Ozcan D, Baba M, Sec͵kin D: Efficacy and safety of diphenylcyclopropenone alone or in combination with anthralin in the treatment of chronic extensive alopecia areata: a retrospective case series, *J Am Acad Dermatol* 72:640–650, 2015.

Elston DM, Ferringer T, Dalton S, et al: A comparison of vertical versus transverse sections in the evaluation of alopecia biopsy specimens, *J Am Acad Dermatol* 53(2):267–272, 2005.

Fukumoto T, Fukumoto R, Magno E, Oka M, Nishigori C, Horita N: Treatments for alopecia areata: a systematic review and network meta-analysis, *Dermatol Ther* 25:e14916, 2021, https://doi.org/10.1111/dth.14916. Epub ahead of print 33631058.

Gentile P, Garcovich S, Scioli MG, et al: Mechanical and controlled prp injections in patients affected by androgenetic alopecia, *J Vis Exp* 27(131), 2018.

Giordano S, Romeo M, di Summa P, et al: A meta-analysis on evidence of platelet-rich plasma for androgenetic alopecia, *Int J Trichology* 10(1):1–10, 2018.

Ramadan WM, Hassan AM, Ismail MA, El Attar YA: Evaluation of adding platelet-rich plasma to combined medical therapy in androgenetic alopecia, *J Cosmet Dermatol* 12, 2021, https://doi.org/10.1111/jocd.13935. Epub ahead of print 33438346.

Somani N, Turvy D: Hirsutism: an evidence-based treatment update, *Am J Clin Dermatol* 15(3):247–266, 2014.

Vano-Galvan S, Pirmez R, Hermosa-Gelbard A, et al: Safety of low-dose oral minoxidil for hair loss: a multicenter study of 1404 patients, 00418-7 *J Am Acad Dermatol* S0190-9622(21)00418-7, 2021, https://doi.org/10.1016/j.jaad.2021.02.054. Epub ahead of print 33639244.

Waśkiel-Burnat A, Kołodziejak M, Sikora M, et al: Therapeutic management in pediatric alopecia areata: a systematic review, *J Eur Acad Dermatol Venereol* 25, 2021, https://doi.org/10.1111/jdv.17187. Epub ahead of print 33630354.

DISEASES OF THE MOUTH

Method of
Lisa Simon, MD, DMD; and Hugh Silk, MD, MPH

CURRENT DIAGNOSIS

High-risk conditions
- Ludwig angina: Spread of infection most commonly from a mandibular molar into the sublingual and submaxillary spaces that surround the airway, causing urgent respiratory compromise.
- Cavernous sinus thrombosis: Ascending infection and thrombosis of intracranial vessels that can be caused by a maxillary dental infection. Requires urgent neurologic and neurosurgical evaluation.
- Lesions concerning for oral cancer: Most commonly squamous cell carcinoma (SCC), may present as sessile or fungating, with red or white shading. Usually asymptomatic, may feature fixed, painless lymph nodes. Associated with alcohol and tobacco use.

Common conditions
- Dental caries: Most common infectious disease globally, near 100% prevalence. Dental pain indicates that the tooth will require root canal therapy or extraction to resolve the infection.
- Periodontal disease: Inflammatory loss of the tooth's attachment structure, which can cause pain, tooth mobility, and eventual tooth loss.

Oral ulcers
- Acute ulcers most likely infectious (herpes simplex virus [HSV], Coxsackie) or aphthous ulcers, tend to resolve within 7 to 10 days.
- Chronic ulcers will appear more desquamative and widespread within the oral cavity. They are more likely to be due to a dermatologic condition (pemphigus vulgaris, mucous membrane pemphigoid, lichen planus) and should prompt investigation of other dermatologic findings.

Oral lesions and masses
- Cessation of triggering activity (e.g., use of chewing tobacco) and evaluate for resolution.
- Refer for biopsy if lesions persist for more than 14 days.

Xerostomia
- Perception of dry mouth, which can make speaking and swallowing more difficult and predisposes patients to rampant dental decay.
- Associated with polypharmacy, especially drugs with known anticholinergic properties.
- Can also be due to autoimmune destruction of salivary glands from Sjögren disease or SICCA syndrome.

Osteonecrosis of the jaw
- Antibiotics for purulent exudate.
- Refer to oral surgeon or oral medicine specialist for monitoring and possible resection of necrotic bone.

Antibiotic prophylaxis for dental procedures
- For infective endocarditis prevention, this is necessary only in individuals with prosthetic valves or implants, unrepaired cyanotic congenital heart disease or repair with residual defect, history of cardiac transplant with valvular regurgitation, or history of infective endocarditis.
- No prophylaxis necessary for individuals with prosthetic joints.
- Prophylaxis necessary only for procedures that involve manipulating the gingiva.
- Prophylaxis can be taken up to 2 h after a procedure with equivalent efficacy.

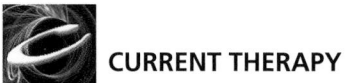
Management of painful odontogenic or periodontal infections
- Definitive resolution requires dental treatment.
- Penicillin VK 500 mg qid or amoxicillin[1] 500 mg tid for 7 days
- If penicillin allergic: clindamycin[1] 300 mg qid for 7 days

Management of oral ulcers
- For herpetic ulcers: Treat as early as possible with acyclovir (Zovirax) 400 mg tid for 5 to 10 days
- For aphthous ulcers or other autoimmune etiologies: If focal, triamcinolone 0.1% in orabase (Kenalog Orabase), apply topically after each meal and at bedtime; if extensive, dexamethasone (Decadron)[1] 0.5 mg/5 mL elixir, rinse for 2 min after each meal and at bedtime, then expectorate.
- Pain relief can be achieved with diphenhydramine (Benadryl)[1] liquid 12.5 mg/5 mL blended 1:1 with a coating agent such as Kaopectate[1] or Maalox[1]; can be used to rinse every 2 h.

Management of oral candidiasis
- Clotrimazole (Mycelex) troches five times a day for 14 days
- Nystatin (Mycostatin 100,000 U/mL), 400,000 to 600,000 U, rinse daily for 14 days; may soak denture overnight if applicable
- For angular cheilitis or focal infection: Nystatin/triamcinolone 1% (Mycolog) cream daily for 14 days

Management of xerostomia
- Reduce or stop medications that cause xerostomia
- Ensure access to water or ice chips throughout the day
- Sialologues such as Biotène rinse or gel
- Cholinergic agonist such as pilocarpine (Salagen) 5 to 10 mg tid before meals

Management of osteonecrosis
- Antibiotics for purulence (see infections, earlier).
- Chlorhexidine gluconate (Peridex) rinse to reduce bacterial burden (*off-label use*): Rinse with 15 mL bid and expectorate.
- Pain medication if needed; avoid opioids when possible.
- Refer to oral surgeon or oral medicine provider for extensive necrosis and possible resection.

Antibiotic prophylaxis for dental procedures
- Amoxicillin[1] 2 g 30 to 60 min before procedure
- If penicillin allergic: Clindamycin[1] 600 mg, cephalexin (Keflex)[1] 2 g, azithromycin (Zithromax)[1], or clarithromycin (Biaxin)[1] 500 mg

[1]Not FDA approved for this indication.

Caries

Dental caries are the most prevalent infectious disease in the world, affecting more than 90% of the population. Caused primarily by the acidogenic species *Streptococcus mutans* and lactobacilli, fermentation of dietary sugars produces acids that create holes in the teeth. Diets high in sugar—including both fermentable carbohydrates, sugary foods, and sugar-sweetened beverages—increase caries risk.

The prevalence and severity of caries has decreased substantially in the United States since the introduction of fluoride into community water sources. For pediatric patients ages 6 months to 16 years who primarily drink well water or reside in communities without water fluoridation, fluoride supplementation should be offered according to the guidelines set by the American Academy of Pediatrics.

Saliva is basic in nature and can reduce acid in the mouth and remineralize teeth to counteract the caries process. Consequently individuals with xerostomia, a common side effect of many medications, are at higher risk of caries, which are more likely to develop at the base of the tooth (the cervical aspect) in xerostomic mouths (see xerostomia, further on) (Figure 1).

Caries initially appear as chalky white spots on the tooth enamel. Eventually, decay will expand into a visible lesion, which may appear dark yellow, brown, or black. Interproximal decay (caries between the teeth) may be visible only radiologically until quite advanced. Patients may report sensitivity to sweet foods, progressing to sensitivity to hot and cold. Spontaneous pain caused by tooth decay indicates that the bacterial infection has spread to the neurovascular supply within the tooth (the pulp) and should be managed as a dental abscess (see later).

Patients with visibly carious dentition should be urged to visit a dentist as promptly as possible. If available, topical 5% sodium fluoride varnish can be applied off label by a provider to slow the progression of caries. Patients should also be counseled to reduce the quantity and frequency of dietary sugar intake.

Prevention includes twice daily brushing of teeth with proper technique and fluoridated toothpaste, daily flossing, and limiting sugary drinks and snacks. Children should be assisted with brushing until approximately age 8 and should use only a smear of fluoride-containing toothpaste until age 3. Fluoride should be offered (as noted previously) in communities with nonfluoridated water, and fluoride varnish should be offered at medical visits until age 6. Everyone with teeth should visit a dental provider regularly for cleanings, radiographs, and advice, usually twice annually, more or less based on risk. Individuals without teeth should still have regular dental visits to evaluate denture fit.

Periodontitis

Periodontal disease is a polymicrobial infection of primarily anaerobic, gram-negative pathogens within the *periodontium*, the attachment apparatus between the tooth and the alveolar bone. Proliferation of bacteria in the periodontal space causes local inflammation, which leads to sensitive and friable gingival tissue and eventual tooth mobility from inflammatory damage to the periodontal ligament and bone. Periodontal disease is extremely common, present in approximately 40% of all adults worldwide and in 20% of middle-aged US adults, and prevalence increases with age. Patients with diabetes are at especially high risk of periodontal disease. Severe congenital forms of periodontal disease are known to be caused by disorders of neutrophil adhesion.

Accumulation of bacteria near or within the periodontal space may initially present with gingivitis, or inflammation of the gingiva without bone or attachment loss. Patients may report friable gingiva (bleeding when eating, brushing, or flossing the teeth) and sensitivity. As the disease progresses, the loss of bone will cause the teeth to appear to lengthen. Teeth with reduced attachment may become spaced apart or splayed due to the impact of repeated occlusal forces on unstable teeth. In advanced stages, teeth may be freely mobile on examination. The gingiva will appear boggy and friable, and bleeding or suppuration may be noticed when the teeth or gingiva are manipulated. Patients presenting with an acute onset of new bleeding and expansile gingiva should be evaluated for a hematologic abnormality suggestive of malignancy prior to referral for dental treatment.

Definitive diagnosis, including the severity of the periodontal disease and whether individual teeth can be maintained or must be extracted, must be made by a dentist using clinical exam and radiographic findings. Dental professionals will perform probing to evaluate loss of attachment between bone and tooth. The primary treatment to prevent further attachment loss is *scaling and root planing* to remove the bacterial concretions below the gingiva that are causing the inflammatory response.

Topical and occasionally systemic antibiotic therapy may be prescribed by a dental professional as part of surgical treatment for periodontitis. Patients presenting with an acute abscess (e.g., fluctuant swelling, pain, constitutional symptoms) should be managed in the same manner whether the abscess is periodontal or dental in origin, as noted in the section titled "Odontogenic Infections," later.

Prevention of periodontitis is similar to caries prevention in terms of dental hygiene, diet, and professional dental care. For adults, electric toothbrushes may reduce plaque and gingivitis compared

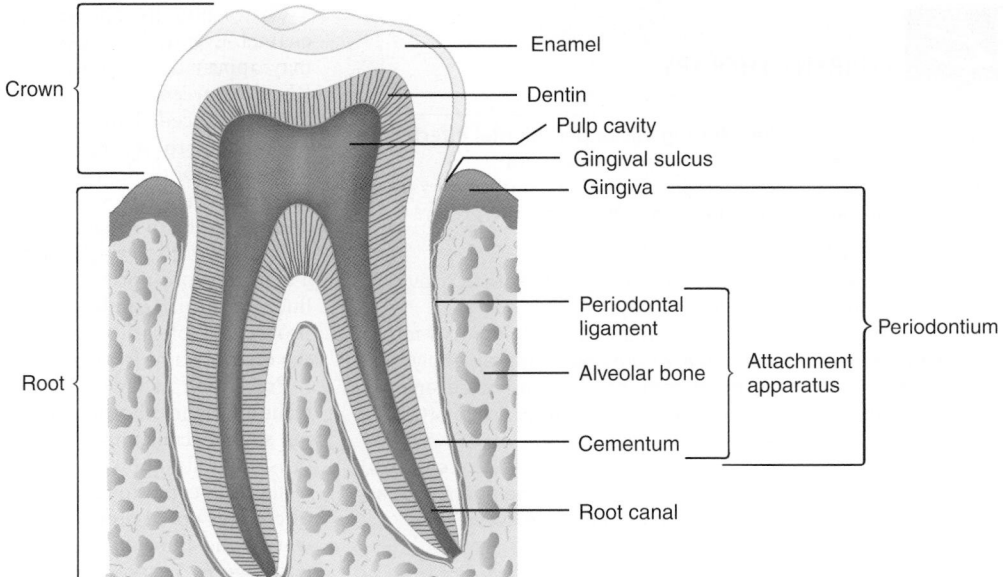

Figure 1 Basic anatomy of the tooth and periodontium. (From Walls R, et al: *Rosen's Emergency Medicine: Concepts and Clinical Practice*, ed 9. Philadelphia, 2018, Elsevier.)

Labels in figure: Crown, Root, Enamel, Dentin, Pulp cavity, Gingival sulcus, Gingiva, Periodontal ligament, Alveolar bone, Cementum, Attachment apparatus, Periodontium, Root canal

with manual toothbrushing, especially for patients with manual dexterity limitations. Tobacco use also contributes to periodontal disease; thus avoidance or cessation should be encouraged.

Necrotizing Ulcerative Gingivitis

An uncommon presentation of gingival disease is necrotizing ulcerative gingivitis (NUG), also referred to as Vincent angina or "trench mouth" for its prevalence among young soldiers during World War I. More common in young people, NUG presents with fever, malaise, and severe gingival pain without loss of bone or attachment. It is caused by mixed bacterial infection that includes anaerobes. Clinical exam will reveal exquisitely tender gingiva throughout the mouth, possibly more severe in the anterior teeth, with inflammation and the appearance of "punched out" gingival papillae between the teeth, with a fetid odor.

Patients require source control in the form of dental scaling, but topical antibiotic treatment with chlorhexidine gluconate (Peridex) as well as empiric treatment with penicillin or metronidazole (Flagyl)[1] can dramatically improve symptoms. Individuals presenting with NUG should be evaluated for a potential underlying source of immunocompromise, such as human immunodeficiency virus (HIV) infection. Other risk factors include nutritional deficiencies and stress.

Odontogenic Infections

Progression of untreated dental disease, both periodontitis and dental caries, can result in focal infection. Infection may be due to a periodontal abscess or spread of infection from a necrotic tooth into the supporting bone. Patients will often have globally poor dentition on exam and report a history of prior dental pain that may have resolved spontaneously.

Patients most often present with severe localized pain that may be worse at night. Involved teeth may be localized by evaluating for focal fluctuance, tooth mobility, or pain produced by percussion of the tooth with a tongue depressor. Visible drainage of exudate through a fistula or the gingival cuff of a tooth may be associated with relief of pain due to reduced buildup of pressure.

Most dental infections do not result in systemic compromise; however, providers should be proactive in ruling out more serious complications. Ludwig angina is a form of airway compromise resulting from spread of infection, most commonly from the mandibular molars, into the submandibular and submaxillary fascial spaces that ring the trachea, causing urgent airway compromise. Patients will appear acutely ill with trismus, submandibular swelling, and difficulty managing secretions. Patients require imminent transfer to a tertiary care facility for airway management and surgical source control. Cavernous sinus thrombosis, most commonly resulting from the ascending infection from maxillary anterior teeth, initially manifests with loss of the nasolabial fold, periorbital swelling, and ophthalmoplegia; it can lead to vision loss, elevated intracranial pressure, and stroke and requires urgent transfer. Descriptions of these two conditions are given in Table 1.

For stable patients, evidence of systemic spread such as fever, tachycardia, or descending lymphadenopathy are indications for antibiotic treatment. Although not medically indicated, patients who do not have timely access to a dentist may benefit from antibiotic prescription as a palliative measure to reduce infection burden and pain until they can receive treatment. Most infections are polymicrobial, with a predominance of aerobic, gram-positive organisms and a low prevalence of antibiotic resistance. A 1-week course of penicillin VK, amoxicillin, or clindamycin[1] for patients with penicillin allergy should be enough to provide several weeks of pain relief.

For acute pain relief, patients should be offered a local anesthetic injection if possible. Bupivacaine (Marcaine, Sensorcaine, generic) provides the longest-lasting relief, but lidocaine with 1:100,000 epinephrine can also be effective. Combined analgesia with a nonsteroidal antiinflammatory drug (NSAID) and a non-NSAID is effective in reducing dental pain, and adult patients without contraindications may take up to 800 mg tid of ibuprofen and 1000 mg tid of acetaminophen concurrently for relief. Providers may consider short courses (3 days) of opioid analgesia for unremitting pain.

Definitive treatment of all oral infections requires source control, whether from extraction of the involved tooth, root canal treatment, or periodontal therapy. Referral to a dentist as soon as feasible should be a primary goal, and it should be emphasized to patients that infection will recur even if their symptoms resolve transiently.

Oral Ulcers

Ulcerated lesions within the oral cavity may be due to multiple possible etiologies, including infectious or autoimmune causes. The likely etiology can often be determined by a careful history and physical exam.

About 90% of the population is ultimately infected with oral herpes simplex virus (HSV), most commonly HSV-1, with rarer infection by HSV-2. Initial presentation of HSV infection (primary herpetic gingivostomatitis) is more likely involve severe

---

[1]Not FDA-approved for this indication.

TABLE 1	Complications of Dental Infection Requiring Emergent Transfer and Their Clinical Presentation
Ludwig angina	• History of toothache in a mandibular molar • Fever and malaise, submandibular swelling, trismus, drooling, muffled voice, elevated floor of mouth, stridor
Cavernous sinus thrombosis	• History of toothache in a maxillary tooth • Fever and malaise, loss of nasolabial fold, periorbital swelling, confusion, obtundation

ulceration of the oral mucosa as well as constitutional symptoms such as fever. Adults are more likely to present with nonspecific symptoms such as pharyngitis, whereas children are more likely to have the classic presentation. If ulceration is severe enough to prevent adequate fluid intake, those presenting with more severe symptoms should be evaluated for risk of dehydration. Symptoms generally resolve within 1 to 2 weeks without severe complications such as encephalitis.

Following initial infection, HSV remains dormant in the sensory nerve ganglia, with rate and severity of recurrence varying considerably among individuals. Recurrence may be activated by periods of stress, including local trauma or systemic illness. Recurrent HSV-related ulcerations favor fixed keratinized tissue such as the gingiva or lips (herpes labialis). Symptoms typically present with a prodromal burning or tingling sensation followed by the appearance of painful small vesicles that rupture. The ulcer may appear purple or gray on the periphery, and a yellow layer of keratin overlying the ulcer may be present. Patients who present with prodromal symptoms may have a shortened course if they are prescribed acyclovir (Zovirax), either as a capsule or a topical cream, very early in the presentation of symptoms. Patients with repeat recurrence may benefit from a "pill in pocket" approach to treatment. Recurrence is usually seen one to six times a year and generally becomes less severe and frequent with time. If recurrences are frequent, antivirals can be given orally for suppression with the patient reevaluated annually. Treatment of first episodes requires a longer duration of treatment with oral antivirals.

Aphthous stomatitis is an immune complex–mediated condition that can also result in recurrent oral ulceration. Patients may similarly report that ulcers are induced by stress or local trauma and share a similar prodrome of pain or pruritus at the site of ulcer formation. Ulcers are most commonly less than 10 mm in size, though they can be larger. Aphthous ulcers may be distinguished from HSV-related ulcers due to their predilection for less keratinized oral surfaces such as the buccal, sublingual, and palatal mucosa and for presenting with multifocal lesions. Ulcers resolve within 7 to 10 days without treatment. Aphthous ulcers can be quite painful, and patients may find relief from topical benzocaine 20% (Orabase or Orajel), although patients should be cautioned to forego excessive use in order to avoid the risk of methemoglobinemia. Exceedingly painful ulcers may resolve more quickly with topical corticosteroids. Triamcinolone 0.1% in orabase (Kenalog Orabase) can be applied topically after each meal and at bedtime; if ulcers are extensive, dexamethasone (Decadron)[1] 0.5 mg/5 mL elixir can be prescribed as a rinse for 2 minutes (and then expectorated) after each meal and at bedtime.

Symptomatic relief of oral ulcers from any cause may be obtained from a mouth rinse with a combination of diphenhydramine (Benadryl)[1] and a coating agent such as bismuth subsalicylate (Kaopectate)[1] or aluminum/magnesium antacid (Maalox)[1]. This formulation is sometimes colloquially referred to as "magic mouthwash."[6]

Several other conditions may initially present with oral ulceration. Simple trauma such as biting the buccal mucosa can lead to a local ulceration. Oral lichen planus may present with oral

ulcerations or peeling of keratinized gingiva around the teeth as well as reticulated white "Whickham striae" on the mucosa. Generalized sloughing of the mucous membranes should prompt high concern for a systemic source and demands a more complete dermatologic exam. Onset within weeks of beginning a new medication could indicate the onset of Stevens-Johnson syndrome or toxic epidermal necrolysis, which may present first with mucosal involvement. Mucous membrane pemphigoid or pemphigus vulgaris may also present with mucosal sloughing. Such presentations should be referred for biopsy and further workup. Behçet disease also presents with genital and oral ulcerations; there are usually multiple ulcers and systemic symptoms, including eye inflammation, skin ulcers, and arthralgias. Coxsackie virus presenting as "hand, foot, and mouth disease" is usually more obvious, as many of the lesions are outside of the mouth on and around the lips and the classic round lesions on the hands, feet, and occasionally the buttocks. Coxsackie is also much more common in children and rare in adults.

Last, mucositis may be induced by chemotherapy or head and neck radiation. Such ulcerations are often widespread and exquisitely painful and may impair patients' ability to take in adequate fluids and nutrition. These symptoms should be managed jointly with a patient's oncology team, including prevention, which can involve the following treatments: aloe vera, amifostine (Ethyol), granulocyte colony stimulating factor (G-CSF), honey, keratinocyte growth factor, polymyxin/tobramycin/amphotericin (PTA)[1], antibiotic pastille/paste[6], and sucralfate (Carafate)[1].

Oral Soft Tissue Lesions

Lesions within the oral cavity can be extremely heterogenous in appearance, ranging from fungating to sessile, white to red and even pigmented, and ulcerated or smooth. White coloration often indicates increased keratinization, whereas increased red shading indicates increased vascularity. Oral SCC is the most common malignancy of the oral cavity, representing 90% of all intraoral cancers. Malignant lesions are more likely to manifest with raised/irregular borders, be fixed or indurated, be painless, and feature painless lymphadenopathy. The highest-risk sites for malignant transformation are the lateral aspect of the tongue, the floor of the mouth, and the junction of the hard and soft palate. Both alcohol and tobacco use are risk factors, and both behaviors together increase the risk of SCC up to 300-fold. Rising rates of HPV infection have increased the prevalence of HPV-associated SCC of the throat (including tonsils and base of tongue); however, there has not been a similar rise in rates of oral SCC. The HPV vaccine may help to reduce oropharyngeal cancer rates.

Detection of an intraoral lesion should prompt examination for possible traumatic causes (e.g., a recent burn or tongue bite) and removal of potential causative factors (e.g., smoking cessation). Bilateral lesions are more likely to be benign and this can be a reassuring finding. Any lesion that fails to resolve after 2 weeks of observation should be biopsied and/or referred for definitive diagnosis. The differential diagnosis for common oral soft tissue lesions is listed in Table 2.

Treatment of oral squamous cell carcinoma (SCC) is multidisciplinary and often requires both surgical resection/excision as well as chemotherapy and radiation. Five-year survival rates remain around 60%. Unfortunately, no preventive measures have been widely successful, with even routine oral examination being given a designation of insufficient evidence to support implementation ("I") and not recommended by the US Preventive Services Task Force.

Lesions that may appear benign, such as leukoplakia or erythroplakia, should be monitored closely and biopsied if not resolving. Mild forms of these lesions will resolve on their own, whereas persisting lesions can be precancerous. They are often thickened, painless, on the buccal mucosa (inside cheek), on the tongue or

---

[1]Not FDA approved for this indication.
[6]May be compounded by pharmacists.

---

[1]Not FDA-approved for this indication.
[6]May be compounded by pharmacists.

TABLE 2 Differential Diagnosis of Common Oral Soft Tissue Lesions

Red or White Lesions

Traumatic/frictional keratosis	Benign thickening of keratin layer due to repeated trauma
Leukoedema	Variant of normal; bilateral whitening of the buccal mucosa, which disappears when the mucosa is stretched
Oral candidiasis	Fluffy white patches that will reveal an erythematous base when scraped
Oral papilloma	Related to infection with low-risk HPV strain; may be fungating or pedunculated, most commonly on tongue
Oral lichen planus	Reticulations, Wickham striae, and desquamation of buccal mucosa and gingiva
Leukoplakia/ erythroplakia/ erythroleukoplakia	Irregular, usually unilateral change in coloration, risk of malignant transformation, biopsy needed
Squamous cell carcinoma	May appear as white, red, or ulcerative lesion; biopsy any lesion that persists after 2 weeks

Ulcerations

Aphthous ulcers	Immune-mediated ulcers on nonkeratinized oral mucosa
Herpetic ulcers	Ulcers most prominent on gingiva and lips
Angular cheilitis	Ulcerations at corners of the lips; may be associated with nutrient deficiency or with ill-fitting dentures; treat with antifungal cream in addition to managing underlying cause
Mucous membrane pemphigoid	Desquamation of gingiva; associated with desquamation of other body mucosal surfaces
Pemphigus vulgaris	Desquamation of mucosa to vermillion border; may present months or years before presentation on the skin

HPV, Human papillomavirus.

floor of mouth, and either white or red in color. The smoking of tobacco is a risk factor for these lesions.

Oral Candidiasis

Oral candida infections are heterogenous in presentation. Other than in extremely rare cases, all are caused by *Candida albicans*, which is also a common colonizer of asymptomatic individuals. Recent antibiotic use is a risk factor, as is uncontrolled diabetes and the use of inhaled corticosteroids. Of note, although immunocompromised patients are at higher risk, oral candidiasis is *not* considered indicative of immunocompromise.

Most commonly, patients will report the presence of white patches that may appear on the buccal mucosa and palate. Such patches can be scraped away with a tongue depressor or gauze, and irritated, bleeding tissue will be present beneath. Patients may report some mouth dryness, irritation, or discomfort when swallowing, but they will not be constitutionally ill.

In addition to the more classic presentation of oral thrush, candida may colonize macerated tissue in contact with dentures (atrophic candidiasis), or in the moist regions at the labial corners (angular cheilitis). Atrophic candidiasis may be asymptomatic, or patients may report worsening discomfort with denture use. The candida infection will be evident as a bright red outline in the shape of the patient's dental prosthesis. White patches are usually not present.

Angular cheilitis may cause pain with wide mouth opening and will reveal erythematous, sometimes weeping tissue at the corners of the mouth. Although angular cheilitis is associated with some B vitamin deficiencies, it can also be caused by ill-fitting dentures, causing the collapse of the facial tissues and producing a moist environment suitable for fungal superinfection. A nutritional history and evaluation for other signs or symptoms of nutrient deficiency can rule out the need for further evaluation; regardless, a topical antifungal treatment should be prescribed. New properly fitting dentures and vitamin supplementation are the other necessary treatments.

The choice of anticandidal treatment should be based on the extent of infection. More widespread infection such as thrush or atrophic candidiasis should be treated with clotrimazole (Mycelex) troches or nystatin (Mycostatin) pastilles or rinse. Nystatin rinse is more suitable for patients with xerostomia, who may find the troches difficult to dissolve, and for patients who wear dentures, who should be instructed to soak their dentures overnight in the nystatin solution in addition to receiving intraoral treatment. For patients with angular cheilitis, a nystatin ointment or clotrimazole cream applied to the affected area may be more comfortable. Systemic antifungals such ketoconazole (Nizoral) or fluconazole (Diflucan) should be considered only for immunocompromised patients or those who cannot tolerate topical treatment.

To prevent the development of candidiasis, patients with partial or complete dentures should be advised to brush their dentures twice daily and to remove them during sleep, when they can be soaked in an over-the-counter denture cleansing solution or a mouthwash such as Listerine. Dentures should not be brushed or cleaned with toothpaste, which can scratch the surface. Management of xerostomia can prevent the development of candidiasis in these patients (see later). Individuals using corticosteroid inhalers should be advised to rinse their mouths with water after use and expectorate. There is some evidence that probiotic prescription concurrently with oral antibiotics may reduce risk of candidiasis development, especially for denture wearers.

Xerostomia

Xerostomia refers to the subjective feeling of a dry mouth due to reduced salivary flow. This may be due to autoimmune conditions such as SICCA or Sjögren syndrome or a history of head and neck radiation but is more commonly due to the anticholinergic effects of numerous medications, with polypharmacy putting individuals at particularly high risk. Behavioral factors such as tobacco, marijuana, and methamphetamine (Desoxyn) use can also increase risk.

As saliva plays a critical role in remineralizing the dentition after acidic insults from dietary sugar intake, xerostomia is associated with higher caries risk; widespread caries at the base of the tooth nearest the gingiva is a common finding. Saliva also has antibacterial and antifungal properties, thus xerostomia places patients at higher risk for oral infections.

Patients may report a feeling of "cotton mouth," which makes it difficult or even painful to eat, swallow, or talk. Physical exam will reveal dry, shiny oral tissues with thickened, ropy white saliva that may aggregate at the corners of the lips. Severity of reported symptoms may not correlate fully with physical findings.

Patients for whom the xerostomia is possibly a pharmacologic adverse reaction should undergo a thorough medication review, with reduction in dose or elimination of any unnecessary medications, especially those with known anticholinergic side effects. Following this and for individuals with a known cause of xerostomia (e.g., head and neck radiation), treatment is symptomatic. Many patients report improvement with frequent small sips of water throughout the day. Symptoms should first be managed with over-the-counter salivary replacement rinses or gels (such as Biotène). Sucking candy can increase salivary flow, although it is essential to select sugar-free candies. Patients should be advised to avoid sugar-rich foods, including sugar-sweetened beverages, if at all possible, given their heightened caries risk.

If this fails to cause improvement, off-label prescription of a cholinergic agonist such as cevimeline (Evoxac), pilocarpine (Salagen), or bethanechol (Urecholine) can be considered. Although these medications successfully increase salivary output, the inevitability of undesired cholinergic agonism causing excessive sweating, gastritis, and other symptoms often results in discontinuation of the medications. Patients considering systemic treatment with a cholinergic agonist should be warned of these adverse effects as well as the increased risk of acute angle-closure glaucoma.

Osteonecrosis of the Jaw

Osteonecrosis of the jaw (ONJ) most commonly occurs in individuals with a history of head and neck radiation or with bisphosphonate exposure. Intravenous bisphosphonates put patients at much higher risk of ONJ (95% of cases) compared with those on an oral bisphosphonate regimen. Because it has a relatively lower vascular supply, the mandible is more prone to osteonecrosis.

Individuals should be warned of the risk of ONJ and advised to complete necessary dental work, especially dental extractions, prior to beginning radiation or bisphosphonate therapy when appropriate. Due to the prolonged half-life of bisphosphonates, drug holidays prior to dental treatment for patients already taking them are not recommended. Patients with a history of head and neck radiation in need of oral surgery, especially in the mandible, may benefit from adjunctive hyperbaric oxygen therapy, which may require close collaboration with the treating dentist or oral surgeon.

Lesions may appear spontaneously due to occlusal forces. Patients may report an area of roughness or mild discomfort, most commonly on the medial aspect of the mandible, near the tongue. Alternately, patients may present with nonhealing sockets after a tooth extraction or other dental procedure. Such areas of necrosis may expand over time. Diagnosis is empiric but may benefit from confirmation by an oral medicine practitioner or oral surgeon.

Management is largely symptomatic. Patients should be prescribed antibiotics if the area is purulent (see the earlier section titled "Odontogenic Infections"), and extensive areas of necrosis may need to be resected. Chlorhexidine gluconate (Peridex) rinses may assist with reducing the bacterial burden within the areas of necrosis, thus reducing rates of superinfection.

Antibiotic Prophylaxis Before Dental Procedures

Changes to guidelines by the American Dental Association and the American Heart Association within the last 5 years have greatly restricted recommendations for the use of antibiotic prophylaxis prior to dental procedures. Currently, the only patients who require antibiotic prophylaxis for the prevention of infectious endocarditis are those with prosthetic valves or prosthetic materials used for valve repair, a history of cardiac transplant with ongoing valvular regurgitation, unrepaired cyanotic congenital heart disease or repaired heart disease with a residual defect or regurgitation adjacent to a prosthetic patch or device, and individuals with a prior history of infective endocarditis. Children within 6 months of repair of a congenital cardiac condition or with a residual defect should also be prescribed prophylactic antibiotics. Patients without these conditions who may have received antibiotic prophylaxis in the past should be reassured that the potential risks of antibiotic prescription (including *Clostridium difficile* infections) outweigh the extremely low risk of infective endocarditis caused by dental procedures.

It is currently not recommended that patients with a history of prosthetic joint replacement receive prophylactic antibiotics.

Only those dental procedures that involve manipulation of the gingiva (e.g., a dental cleaning or dental extraction) require antibiotic prophylaxis. Patients should be advised to discuss the necessity of prophylaxis with their dentist, who may also be the prescriber of any necessary antibiotics. One dose of antibiotic should be taken 30 to 60 minutes before the procedure. In the event they forget to take a dose before a dental appointment, patients should also be informed that the prophylactic efficacy of antibiotics is equivalent up to 2 hours after a dental procedure.

Amoxicillin[1] is the antibiotic of choice for most patients. For those with an allergy to penicillins, cephalexin (Keflex)[1], clindamycin[1], azithromycin (Zithromax)[1], or clarithromycin (Biaxin)[1] can be used, though care should be taken for potential cross-reactivity of cephalosporins in penicillin-allergic patients. Generally doses are as follows: amoxicillin 2 g; if penicillin allergic, clindamycin 600 mg, cephalexin 2 g, azithromycin or clarithromycin 500 mg.

---

[1]Not FDA approved for this indication.

References

Cochrane Oral Health. Available at: https://oralhealth.cochrane.org/ Accessed January 20, 2020.

Lockhart PB, Tampi MP, Abt E, et al: Evidence-based clinical practice guideline on antibiotic use for the urgent management of pulpal- and periapical-related dental pain and intraoral swelling: A report from the American Dental Association, *J Am Den Assoc* 150(11):906–921, 2019.

Neville BW, Damm DD, Allen CM, Chi AC: *Oral & Maxillofacial Pathology*, ed 4, Missouri, 2015, WB Saunders, Elsevier.

Nishimura RA, Otto CM, Bonow RO, et al: 2017 AHA/ACC focused update of the 2014 AHA/ACC guideline for the management of patients with valvular heart disease: A report of the American College of Cardiology/American Heart Association Task Force on clinical practice guidelines, *Circulation* 135:e1159–e1195, 2017.

Plemons JM, Al-Hashimi I, Marek CL: American Dental Association Council on Scientific Affairs managing xerostomia and salivary gland hypofunction: executive summary of a report from the American Dental Association Council on Scientific Affairs, *J Am Den Assoc* 145(8):867–873, 2014.

Reamy BV, Derby R, Bunt CW: Common tongue conditions in primary care, *Am Fam Physic* 81(5):627–634, 2010.

Sollecito TP, Abt E, Lockhart PB, et al: The use of prophylactic antibiotics prior to dental procedures in patients with prosthetic joints: Evidence-based clinical practice guideline for dental practitioners--a report of the American Dental Association Council on Scientific Affairs, *J Am Den Assoc* 146(1):11–16 e8, 2015.

Stephens MB, Wiedemer JP, Kushner GM: Dental problems in primary care, *Am Fam Physic* 98(11):654–660, 2018.

DISEASES OF THE NAIL

Method of
Jonathon Firnhaber, MD, MAEd, MBA

CURRENT THERAPY

Ingrown nail
- Ingrown nails with mild acute inflammation may be treated with antiseptic soaks and a moderate-potency topical steroid. The distal anterior tip and lateral edges of the ingrown toenail can be elevated with cotton or wool to allow the nail to advance without further penetrating the nail fold.
- Ingrown nails with moderate or greater inflammation generally require surgical intervention. Partial nail plate removal is performed under local anesthesia.
- If the ingrown nail is recurrent, liquid phenol or a radiofrequency surgical electrode can be used to permanently ablate the lateral portions of the nail matrix and germinal tissue.

Onychomycosis
- Physicians should not prescribe oral antifungal therapy for suspected onychomycosis without confirmation of infection.
- Terbinafine (Lamisil) is the preferred agent for onychomycosis. It offers a higher cure rate and fewer drug interactions than alternative antifungal agents.
- Topical agents for onychomycosis offer limited efficacy as primary treatments. Efficacy may be improved by thorough debridement of the affected nail or nails prior to treatment and at multiple points during treatment.
- The risk of recurrent onychomycosis may be reduced by preventing and treating tinea pedis.

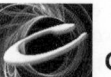

CURRENT DIAGNOSIS

Onychomycosis
- The vast majority of onychomycosis is caused by dermatophytes, typically *Trichophyton rubrum* and *Trichophyton mentagrophytes*.
- Dermatophyte onychomycosis typically presents with invasion of the hyponychium or lateral nail folds, causing onycolysis, nail plate thickening, and subungual debris.
- Superficial white onychomycosis is also caused by dermatophytes and presents as a powdery white discoloration of the nail surface.
- Nondermatophyte organisms are responsible for 10% to 20% of cases of onychomycosis but may be clinically indistinguishable from disease caused by common dermatophytes.
- *Candidal* onychomycosis is uncommon and may present as proximal nail changes in association with paronychia.
- Accurate diagnosis of onychomycosis depends on the collection of an adequate sample for evaluation. The affected nail plate and subungual debris should be sent for fungal culture.

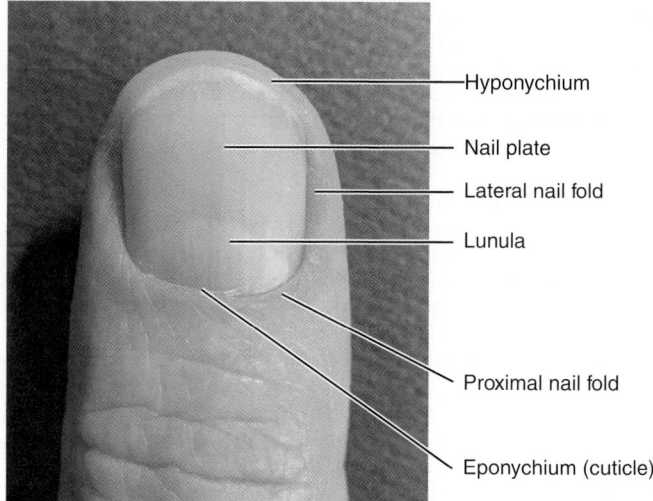

Figure 1 Surface anatomy of the nail unit.

Nail Anatomy

The nail unit includes several clinically important components (Figure 1). The nail plate is made of keratin, which is hard and translucent. The skin of the lateral and proximal nail folds surrounds the nail plate, and the proximal nail fold overlies the matrix. The keratin layer of the proximal nail fold extends over the nail plate to form the cuticle. The tip of the proximal nail fold has capillary loops, which are typically inapparent but may become visible in connective tissue diseases such as systemic lupus erythematosus (SLE) and scleroderma.

The nail plate is primarily synthesized by the matrix epithelium. The distal aspect of the nail matrix is visible as the lunula and is continuous with the nail bed. The nail bed extends from the distal nail matrix to the hyponychium and consists of parallel longitudinal ridges. Splinter hemorrhages, which are visible through the nail plate, represent bleeding at the base of these ridges. The hyponychium begins at the distal edge of the nail bed and is a short segment of keratinized skin that is not covered by the nail plate.

Fingernails grow 0.5 to 2 mm per week and thus take approximately 6 months to grow from the proximal matrix to the distal free edge. Toenails grow much more slowly, taking 12 to 18 months for complete replacement of the nail. Although nails grow continuously, their growth rate slows with age and with decreased capillary perfusion.

Noninfectious Nail Disorders

Psoriasis

Clinical Features and Diagnosis

Although multiple inflammatory skin diseases may affect the nail unit, nail changes are seen in up to 90% of patients with psoriasis over the course of their disease. Nail involvement typically occurs in conjunction with skin disease and is particularly common in patients with psoriatic arthritis involving the distal digits. Nail changes may, however, occur as an isolated finding and support a diagnosis of psoriasis when skin changes are equivocal or absent.

Nail psoriasis has multiple presentations, depending on the portion of the nail unit that is affected. Most commonly, nail matrix psoriasis presents as nail plate pitting. More extensive nail matrix involvement leads to leukonychia (white discoloration of the nail) and loss of integrity of the nail plate, with crumbling and fragmentation. Psoriasis of the hyponychium leads to an accumulation of scaly yellow debris that may elevate the nail plate. Psoriasis of the nail bed may trigger irregular separation of the nail plate and nail thickening, resulting in yellow discoloration of the nail plate. Both

of these changes may be mistaken for onychomycosis, and onychomycosis may occur in psoriatic nails, emphasizing the importance of verifying the presence of a fungal infection prior to treatment.

Treatment

Topical treatments for psoriatic nail disease include high-potency topical steroids, vitamin D analogues, and topical retinoids; however, relatively poor penetration of the nail plate by these agents limits their potential benefit. Systemic therapy is rarely indicated for nail disease without skin or joint involvement.

Onychogryphosis

Onychogryphosis, or "ram's horn nail," affects the great toes and causes marked thickening, discoloration, and curvature of the nail plate. The condition may be triggered by repeated minor trauma from poorly fitting shoes and can eventually make it impossible for the patient to wear shoes. This deformity may be complicated by pain, distal onycholysis, subungual hemorrhage, or onychomycosis. Treatment primarily involves mechanical debridement of the thickened nail plate with a high-speed rotary burr. Surgical removal of the entire nail is associated with prolonged healing of the nail bed, which is generally not well tolerated. Onychogryphosis is more commonly seen in older patients and is also associated with self-neglect, homelessness, dementia, and peripheral vascular disease.

Pincer Nails

Inward deformation of the lateral edges of the nail plate results in a tube- or pincer-shaped nail. The nail bed is drawn into and pinched by the nail, often causing significant pain. Triggers for pincer nails include onychomycosis, psoriasis, and local tumors. Most commonly, however, biomechanical or arthritic changes cause the nail matrix to widen, and the nail ultimately becomes too wide for the nail bed. In extreme cases, removal of the medial, lateral, or both nail margins with ablation of the associated nail matrix, in a manner similar to treatment of an ingrown nail, is indicated to relieve the compression of the nail bed.

Spoon Nails

Spoon-shaped nails, with lateral elevation and a central depression of the nail plate, is termed koilonychia. Although spoon nails may be seen in healthy children and adults, the spontaneous onset of spoon nails is associated with iron deficiency anemia and may be seen in 50% of patients with idiopathic hemochromatosis. The spoon deformity resolves once the anemia has been corrected.

Beau Lines

Beau lines are transverse depressions in the nail plate that arise from the temporary interruption of nail growth within the nail matrix. Acute systemic events may trigger Beau lines in all nails, whereas localized trauma or paronychia will limit the finding to the traumatized nail or nails. The grooves have been associated with multiple systemic conditions including zinc deficiency, pemphigus, Raynaud disease, and myocarditis as well as with illnesses accompanied by high fever, such as rheumatic fever, measles, mumps, hand-foot-and-mouth disease, and malaria. They may also be triggered by chemotherapeutic agents cytotoxic to the nail matrix.

The distance of a Beau line from the proximal nail fold can allow the clinician to estimate the time of the triggering event based on an average growth rate of 3 mm per month for fingernails and 1 mm per month for toenails.

Habit-Tic Deformity
Habit-tic deformity is triggered by chronic biting or picking at a section of the proximal nail fold, usually of the thumb. The resulting nail plate deformity consists of a longitudinal band of horizontal grooves that often extend from the proximal nail fold to the tip of the nail. Habit-tic deformity may be confused with Beau lines associated with chronic paronychia or chronic eczema of the proximal nail fold. Habit-tic deformity produces closely spaced sharp grooves, whereas Beau lines tend to be more smooth and undulating. Formal treatment is not necessary, and the deformity resolves once the chronic irritation ceases and the nail grows out.

Ingrown Nail
Clinical Features and Diagnosis
Ingrown nails (onychocryptosis) are common, painful conditions, most often affecting the great toe. The nail plate of the great toe extends several millimeters beyond the medial and lateral nail folds. In properly trimmed nails, its margin should be apparent at the distal portion of the nail. Excessive or improper trimming of the lateral nail plate will often leave behind a sharp spike of nail that is covered by the lateral nail fold. Lateral pressure from poorly fitted shoes or trauma may exacerbate the problem. The nail pierces the lateral or medial nail fold and enters the dermis, acting as a foreign body. Initial pain and swelling give way to a robust inflammatory response with edema, purulent drainage, and granulation tissue surrounding the penetrating nail.

Treatment
Ingrown nails with mild acute inflammation may be treated conservatively with antiseptic soaks and a moderate-potency topical steroid. If visible, the distal anterior tip and lateral edges of the ingrown toenail can be elevated from the adjacent soft tissue with cotton or wool, which both withdraws the foreign body and allows the nail to advance without further penetrating the nail fold. If collodion is available, it can help fix the cotton or wool in place, so that it will require less frequent replacement. Antibiotics are of limited value, as purulent drainage is associated with the foreign body reaction and is less indicative of an acute bacterial infection.

Ingrown nails with greater-than-mild inflammation generally require surgical intervention. The toe is anesthetized with 1% or 2% lidocaine without epinephrine, either with a digital block or local infiltration of the proximal and lateral nail fold. A narrow periosteal elevator is inserted under the ingrown nail parallel to the lateral nail fold and advanced with upward pressure against the nail plate to minimize risk of damage to the underlying nail bed. The surgeon must ensure that the periosteal elevator is fully advanced to the base of the nail plate, which is 3 to 5 mm proximal to the proximal nail fold. Once the elevator reaches the base of the nail, a sudden decrease in resistance will be noted and care should be taken to not advance it further into the toe. The elevated nail is clipped longitudinally, again taking care to include the most proximal portion of nail, and removed. Residual granulation tissue can be removed with iris scissors or a curette.

If the ingrown nail is recurrent, liquid phenol can be used to permanently ablate the lateral portions of the nail matrix and germinal tissue. Once the nail bed has dried, a phenol-soaked cotton swab is applied for 3 minutes, followed by a thorough wash with 70% isopropyl alcohol, which neutralizes the phenol. Alternatively, a radiofrequency surgical electrode can be used to cauterize the nail matrix and germinal tissue. A flattened tip coated with Teflon on one side is used to protect the proximal nail fold. Regrowth of the nail occurs in up to 25% of patients following phenol cauterization, but the rate of regrowth is less than 5% with radiofrequency cauterization.

Subungual Hematoma
Subungual hematoma is most often caused by direct trauma to the nail plate, which causes bleeding and separation of the nail plate from the nail bed. Hematomas that are fully contained under the nail plate can be exquisitely painful. Drainage, whether spontaneous or by clinician intervention, relieves the pain immediately. The quickest and most effective method of draining the hematoma is by puncturing the nail plate with a hot-tip electrocautery or with a red-hot paperclip tip, taking care not to advance the instrument into the nail bed. Anesthesia is not required for this procedure. Trephination of the nail with a fine-point scalpel blade or large-bore needle tip can be painful, as pressure is required to puncture the nail. Trauma to the proximal nail fold or underlying nail matrix can cause bleeding that is not apparent until the nail plate emerges from the nail fold with blood stains. Staining will be present until the nail fully grows out.

Acute Paronychia
Trauma or manipulation of the proximal and lateral nail fold may trigger acute, painful swelling and erythema of the proximal and/or lateral nail folds, which is termed acute paronychia. Most superficial infections will present with a collection of purulent material about the cuticle or lateral nail fold. These superficial abscesses can quickly be drained with a 1- to 2-mm nick from the tip of an 18- or 21-gauge needle or #11 scalpel blade. Alternatively, the instrument may be inserted between the proximal nail fold and the nail plate, lifting the nail fold to achieve drainage. Neither anesthesia nor oral antibiotics are required. More diffuse erythema and swelling without any superficial abscess suggest a deeper infection. Antibiotics active against *Staphylococcus* and a deeper incision may be required. Acute and chronic paronychias are distinctly different processes.

Chronic Paronychia
Chronic paronychia is triggered by chronic exposure to contact irritants and moisture. Clinically, it presents with tenderness, mild erythema, and mild swelling about the proximal and lateral nail folds of most or all fingers. Typically, many or all fingers are involved simultaneously. The primary pathophysiologic change is separation of the cuticle from the nail plate, which allows bacteria and fungal organisms to colonize the space between the nail plate and proximal nail fold. Manipulation of the cuticle further disrupts the barrier and accelerates the process. Culture of purulent material expressed from the proximal nail fold may show polymicrobial growth and will often include *Candida*. In this case, *Candida* is a colonizer rather than a true pathogenic cause of chronic paronychia, and it disappears once the integrity of the cuticle barrier has been restored. If the colonizing organisms include *Pseudomonas aeruginosa*, the nail plate may develop a green discoloration. The nail plate itself is not infected but may develop Beau lines as a result of the chronic inflammation.

Chronic paronychia is slow to resolve; its treatment hinges on eliminating exposure to contact irritants, limiting exposure to moisture, and treatment of the associated inflammation and infection. Low- to midpotency topical steroid creams may be used for 2 to 4 weeks. Because of the broad polymicrobial colonization typical of chronic paronychia, oral or topical antibiotics are unlikely to affect the time to resolution. Topical antifungal agents, such as ciclopirox (Loprox)[1] applied to the

---

[1]Not FDA approved for this indication.

proximal nailfold two or three times per day, or oral fluconazole (Diflucan)[1] 200 mg daily for 1 to 4 weeks, may help to mitigate the chronic inflammation.

Myxoid Cysts

Digital mucous, or myxoid, cysts present as solitary dome-shaped nodules 2 to 6 mm in diameter located at the distal interphalangeal joint (DIP) or proximal nail fold. They are contiguous with the DIP joint capsule and contain synovial fluid, which is viscous, gelatinous, and clear to light yellow in color. Myxoid cysts most commonly occur in the 40- to 70-year age group and are twice as common in women as in men. When the lesion extends to the proximal nail fold, it can compress the matrix, causing a longitudinal groove on the nail plate. Myxoid cysts may be triggered by a reactive process or by herniation of the synovium; they are typically associated with a joint affected by osteoarthritis. Although most lesions are asymptomatic and do not require intervention, they may cause pain or decreased range of motion. In those cases, simple incision and drainage with the tip of a large-bore needle often provides relief. Recurrent lesions may require excision by a hand surgeon.

Nail Infections

Fungal Nail Infections

Clinical Features and Diagnosis

Tinea of the nails, or tinea unguium, affects 2% to 14% of the general population; prevalence increases with age.

About 90% of toenail and virtually all fingernail onychomycosis is caused by dermatophytes, typically *Trichophyton rubrum* and *Trichophyton mentagrophytes*. *Epidermophyton* and *Microsporum* species are less frequent causes. The most common clinical presentation of dermatophyte onychomycosis is fungal invasion of the hyponychium or lateral nail folds, which causes onycholysis, nail plate thickening, and subungual debris. Fungus may also invade the nail plate from above; superficial white onychomycosis causes a powdery white patchy discoloration of the nail surface. Least commonly, fungus will invade through the proximal margin, giving the appearance of infection emerging from beneath the nail as it grows. This presentation—proximal subungual onychomycosis—is a marker for lack of resistance to dermatophyte infection and is more prevalent in individuals with immunodeficiency.

Dermatophytes invade normal keratin, whereas molds invade altered keratin. Onychomycosis, therefore, can be caused by other fungal species, including *Candida* and nondermatophyte molds such as *Acremonium*, *Alternaria*, *Aspergillus*, *Fusarium*, *Onycholiza*, *Scopulariopsis*, and *Scytalidium* species. Nondermatophyte organisms are responsible for 10% to 20% of cases of onychomycosis. The distinction is important because treatment may differ from that for dermatophyte infection. Candidal onychomycosis is uncommon and may present as proximal nail changes in association with paronychia or as onycholysis with typical nail plate thickening and subungual debris. Nondermatophyte infection most commonly presents with distal-lateral subungual onychomycosis and may be difficult to distinguish from typical dermatophyte onychomycosis.

At least half of patients with onychomycosis will experience some degree of pain or discomfort. As a result, patients may choose less than ideal footwear or have difficulty with ambulation, increasing the risk of falls, particularly among the elderly. Additionally, dystrophic nails may disrupt the surrounding cutaneous barrier, creating a point of entry for skin bacteria or leading to toe or foot ulceration.

Accurate diagnosis of onychomycosis depends on the collection of an adequate sample for evaluation. The onycholytic portion of the affected nail plate should be trimmed as far proximally as possible. Subungual debris is then collected from the nail bed using a curette, taking care to sample from different parts (proximal and distal) of the infected nail. Fungi collect in the nail plate and in the cornified cells of the nail bed. Superficial nail samples are unlikely to produce a high fungal yield.

All national guidelines recommend that physicians not prescribe oral antifungal therapy for suspected onychomycosis without confirmation of infection. Direct microscopy of nail scrapings using potassium hydroxide (KOH) can quickly confirm the presence of fungal hyphae, but the procedure does not identify the exact infectious organism. Formal culture may take 4 weeks or longer to produce a result and offers a sensitivity of only about 50%.

Treatment

Oral antifungal agents—including terbinafine (Lamisil), itraconazole (Sporanox), and fluconazole (Diflucan)[1]—penetrate keratinizing tissue and produce higher drug levels in the nail plate than in plasma. Therapeutic levels may remain in the nails for at least a month after the discontinuation of therapy. Periodic debridement of the infected nail during the course of treatment may increase the cure rate. Treatment with systemic antifungals must be weighed against the risk of hepatic toxicity and the potential for interactions with multiple other medications.

Despite adequate treatment, recurrence of onychomycosis is seen in 40% to 70% of patients and is more likely in patients with extensive involvement of the proximal nail, immunosuppression, or peripheral vascular disease. Oral antifungal agents for onychomycosis are outlined in Table 1.

Three topical drugs for onychomycosis are available in the United States: ciclopirox (Penlac), efinaconazole (Jublia), and tavaborole (Kerydin). Fingernails are treated daily for 24 weeks; toenails are treated daily for 48 weeks. Once weekly, the lacquer should be removed with acetone and any residual diseased nail material filed or clipped away. Complete cure rates typically do not exceed 15% but may be enhanced by thorough debridement of a thickened, lytic nail prior to treatment.

Toenails take 12 to 18 months to be replaced; fingernails take 4 to 6 months for the same process. Therefore, immediately after completion of therapy, the nail will not appear to be completely

---

[1]Not FDA approved for this indication.

TABLE 1	Oral Antifungal Agents for Onychomycosis		
DRUG	**DOSING**	**INDICATIONS**	**POTENTIAL COMPLICATIONS**
Terbinafine (Lamisil)	250 mg daily for 12 weeks (toenails); 6 weeks (fingernails)	First-line treatment for typical dermatophytes	Hepatic toxicity
Itraconazole (Sporanox)	200 mg bid for 7 days, then 21 days off for two courses (8 weeks total) (fingernails); 200 mg daily for 12 weeks (toenails)	Preferred for nondermatophyte molds Treatment option for *Candida*	Hepatic toxicity Multiple drug interactions Lower cure rate than terbinafine
Fluconazole (Diflucan)[1]	150–300 mg weekly for 6 months	Treatment of choice for *Candida*	Hepatic toxicity Multiple drug interactions Lower cure rate than terbinafine

[1]Not FDA approved for this indication.

normal. Rather, a proximal segment of newly formed, fungus-free, and normal-appearing nail will be present and will gradually extend distally as a new nail is produced.

The risk of recurrent onychomycosis may be reduced by preventing and treating tinea pedis. Prolonged use of a topical antifungal agent, such as terbinafine (Lamisil), may prevent nail reinfection after successful treatment with oral medication. Avoidance of trauma to the tips of the nails from tight-fitting shoes may also decrease the risk of recurrence. Foot powder and the use of moisture-wicking socks can limit the moisture surrounding the foot, preventing the warm, dark, moist environment that is conducive to fungal growth.

Pseudomonas Nail Infection

Pseudomonas is the bacterium that is most likely to infect the nail unit, and such infections are characterized by blue-green discoloration beneath the nail and onycholysis. Typically, only one nail is involved. Risk factors include chronic nail trauma, nail disease such as psoriasis, and chronic paronychia. Topical treatment, such as fluoroquinolone or aminoglycoside solutions, or antiseptic soaks with dilute bleach or chlorhexidine (Hibiclens), are often curative. Response rates are enhanced by trimming away any diseased or lytic nail prior to treatment.

Periungual Verrucae

Verruca vulgaris—common warts—are caused by human papillomavirus infection and can involve the periungual and subungual skin of the nail unit. Fingers are more commonly affected than toes. Periungual verrucae present the same as warts at other cutaneous sites, with a hyperkeratotic papule, associated thrombosed capillaries, and disruption of epidermal architecture. Verrucae do not typically involve the nail matrix, but lesions of the proximal nail fold can compress the matrix and lead to nail plate dystrophy.

Periungual verrucae are notoriously difficult to treat. Topical agents are appropriate initial therapeutic options for periungual verrucae, typically including the use of a keratolytic such as salicylic acid. Success rates with topical agents are enhanced with occlusion of the lesion, but several months of daily treatment may be required. Cryotherapy is an additional first-line option and is more efficacious if the lesion is debulked with scissors or scalpel prior to treatment. Longer freeze times may also improve efficacy. Aggressive cryotherapy at the proximal nail fold may damage the underlying nail matrix and lead to permanent nail dystrophy. Intralesional treatment with candida antigen[1], mumps antigen[1], or bleomycin[1] has demonstrated success in the treatment of refractory periungual verrucae. Surgical approaches such as excision and electrosurgery have a moderate potential for scarring and are associated with higher recurrence rates. Squamous cell carcinoma of the nail unit presents as a hyperkeratotic lesion that may be indistinguishable from a wart. Therefore lesions that are recalcitrant to conventional therapy warrant biopsy.

[1]Not FDA approved for this indication.

References

de Berker D: Clinical practice. Fungal nail disease, *New Engl J Medicine* 360(20):2108–2116, 2009.

de Berker D: Nail anatomy, *Clin Dermatol* 31(5):509–515, 2013.

Biesbroeck LK, Fleckman P: Nail disease for the primary care provider, *Med Clin N Am* 99(6):1213–1226, 2015.

Gupta AK, Versteeg SG, Shear NH: Onychomycosis in the 21st century: an update on diagnosis, epidemiology, and treatment, *J Cutan Med Surg* 21(6):525–539, 2017.

Lipner S, Scher R: Evaluation of nail lines: Color and shape hold clues, *Cleve Clin J Med* 83(5):385–391, 2016.

Maddy AJ, Tosti A: Hair and nail diseases in the mature patient, *Clin Dermatol* 36(2):159–166, 2018.

Westerberg DP, Voyack MJ: Onychomycosis: Current trends in diagnosis and treatment, *Am Fam Physician* 88(11):762–770, 2013.

ERYTHEMA MULTIFORME

Method of
Chad Douglas, MD, PharmD

CURRENT DIAGNOSIS

- Acute cutaneous target-like papules, plaques, and bullae
- Oral mucosal lesions can be present
- Predominance in young adults
- Most often associated with acute or chronic herpes simplex virus (HSV-1) infection
- Less commonly associated with medications such as sulfonamide and penicillin antibiotics

CURRENT THERAPY

- Treat any underlying infection and discontinue any potential offending medications
- Mild disease: symptomatic care with oral antihistamines, topical corticosteroids
- Severe and persistent disease: prednisone, cyclosporine (Neoral and Sandimmune)[1] azathioprine (Imuran)[1]
- Recurrent episodes: prophylaxis with HSV antiviral agents

[1]Not FDA approved for this indication.

Epidemiology

Erythema multiforme (EM) is an acute, mucocutaneous, immune-mediated hypersensitivity disorder. This rare self-limiting disorder has an estimated incidence of 0.01% to 1% and predominately occurs in young adults between the ages of 20 and 40. Up to 20% of cases occur in children and adolescents.

Risk Factors

Erythema multiforme is most commonly associated with viral, fungal, and atypical bacterial infections. More than 60% of infection-associated cases of erythema multiforme occur with herpes simplex virus (HSV), most commonly HSV-1. Mycoplasma pneumonia is the second most common infectious organism associated with erythema multiforme and up to 5% of patients with this atypical pneumonia develop EM. Most cases of recurrent erythema multiforme are associated with acute HSV infections or reactivation of chronic HSV infections. The second most common cause of erythema multiforme are medications. Medication accounts for 10% to 20% of erythema multiforme cases and is referred to as drug-induced EM (DIEM). The most common medication classes in DIEM are sulfonamides, penicillins, nonsteroidal antiinflammatory agents, and aromatic amine anticonvulsants such as carbamazepine (Tegretol), phenytoin (Dilantin), and phenobarbital. Drug-induced erythema multiforme is considered a separate and distinct entity from hypersensitivity and cutaneous adverse drug reactions such as maculopapular erythema, Stevens-Johnson syndrome (SJS), and toxic epidermal necrolysis (TEN).

Pathophysiology

The pathophysiology of erythema multiforme has been extensively delineated in herpes-associated EM (HAEM). HSV DNA fragments are transported to distant skin sites by peripheral blood mononuclear cells. HSV genes within these fragments express various enzymes including DNA polymerase that leads to recruitment of CD4+ TH1 cells. These CD4+ TH1 cells release interferon-gamma (INF-gamma) that initiates an inflammatory cascade with the sequestration of circulating monocytes, natural killer (NK) cells, and lymphocytes as well as recruitment of autoreactive T-cells. This extensive immune response leads to keratinocyte destruction. In contrast, the pathophysiology of drug-induced erythema multiforme involves tumor necrosis factor α (TNF-α) production that leads to epidermal destruction. Human leukocyte antigen polymorphisms have not been extensively characterized in DIEM, as they have been in more classic immune-mediated cutaneous drug hypersensitivity reactions such as SJS and TEN.

Prevention

There is no current prevention for erythema multiforme; however, the knowledge of infectious agents and medications that can cause EM can help one identify patients who could be at risk for development of this condition. Future studies in the advancement of pharmacogenetics may potentially identify human leukocyte antigen polymorphisms that could predispose patients to HAEM or DIEM.

Clinical Manifestations and Diagnosis

Erythema multiforme is a self-limited eruption that most often appears in a symmetric distribution on distal extremities with frequent involvement of dorsal surfaces of the hands and extensor surfaces of extremities. Prodromal syndrome such as fever, chills, malaise, and arthralgia can occur but are rare. Lesions often burn or itch and progress from distal areas of the body toward proximal regions. Initial lesions are usually sharply demarcated red or pink macules that can resemble hives or early stages of SJS. Unlike hives, these lesions become fixed and do not migrate. Mucosal involvement and skin sloughing is less common than with SJS. The macules become popular and may gradually enlarge into plaques that are several centimeters in diameter. Lesions often contain three concentric zones including a central darker red region, a pale pink edematous zone, and a peripheral red ring. These characteristic "target" or "iris" lesions may only contain a central dark red region with a lighter peripheral ring and may not appear until several days after onset of the eruptions. Lesions of multiple morphology are usually present, thus the name "multiforme." Mucosal lesions, when present, are red and edematous and often involve blister formation. These lesions are usually limited to the oral cavity and affect the lips, inside of cheeks, and the tongue. Typically, lips are swollen with hemorrhagic crusting. Erythema multiforme associated with mycoplasma pneumonia may present with mucosal lesions alone without cutaneous manifestations. Diagnosis is most often made clinically in patients with characteristic lesions and a preceding or concurrent infection that is known to be commonly associated with EM. A clinical diagnosis can also be made in patients with characteristic lesions who are taking a commonly associated medication. Rarely, a skin biopsy is needed to rule out other conditions, although there is no single diagnostic histologic feature specific to erythema multiforme. Erythema multiforme usually resolves spontaneously within 3 to 5 weeks.

Differential Diagnosis

Early erythema multiforme lesions can resemble urticaria, drug eruptions, viral exanthem, maculopapular erythema as well as early stages of Stevens-Johnson syndrome and toxic epidermal necrosis. Bullous lesions may resemble bullous pemphigoid and target lesions may resemble pityriasis rosea or vasculitis.

Treatment

Although erythema multiforme is self-limiting, early identification and treatment of the causative infectious agent or immediate discontinuation of an offending medication can reduce the severity and duration of the condition. Symptomatic treatment with oral first-generation antihistamines (diphenhydramine [Benadryl] 25 to 50 mg po q 6 hours prn or hydroxyzine [Atarax] 25 to 100 mg po q 6 hours prn) and mid-potency topical corticosteroids (triamcinolone [Kenalog] 0.1% cream) will usually suffice for mild disease. More severe disease including cases with mucosal involvement as well as recurrent EM can be treated with prednisone, cyclosporine (Neoral, Sandimmune),[1] or azathioprine (Imuran)[1]. The use of dapsone[1] and antimalarial agents in severe disease has demonstrated varying success. Recurrent erythema multiforme is most often associated with HSV-1, and herpes viral suppressive therapy with acyclovir (Zovirax)[1] or valacyclovir (Valtrex)[1] has been shown to be effective. Valacyclovir (Valtrex) is given once daily until the patient is recurrence free for 4 months. The valacyclovir (Valtrex) dose is then reduced with eventual discontinuation. Although reintroduction of an offending medication does not frequently cause recurrence of erythema multiforme, caution should still be advised when considering the future use of such medication or other medications within the same drug class.

Monitoring and Complications

Mucosal involvement may limit a patient's ability to eat or drink and close monitoring is advised in such cases. This can be of particular concern in pediatric patients. Skin lesions are usually not associated with scarring but postinflammatory hyperpigmentation can occur and often take several months to resolve.

[1] Not FDA approved for this indication.

References

Anquier-Durant A, Mockenhaupt M, et al: Correlations between clinical patterns and causes of erythema multiforme majus, Stevens-Johnson syndrome, and toxic epidermal necrolysis: results of an international prospective study, *Arch Dermatol* 138(8):1019–1024, 2002 Aug.

Aurelian L, Ono F, Burnett J: Herpes simplex virus (HSV)-associated erythema multiforme (HAEM): a viral disease with an autoimmune component, *Dermatol Online J* 9(I), 2003.

Kokuba H, Aurelian L, Burnett J: Herpes simplex virus associated erythema multiforme (HAEM) is mechanistically distinct from drug-induced erythema multiforme: interferon-gamma is expressed in HAEM lesions and tumor necrosis factor-alpha in drug-induced erythema multiforme lesions, *J Invest Dermatol* 113:808–815, 1999.

Lamoreux MR, Sternbach MR, Hsu WT: Erythema Multiforme, *Am Fam Physician* 74(11):1883–1888, 2006 Dec 1.

Ono F, Sharma BK, Smith CC, et al: CD34+ Cells in the peripheral blood transport herpes simplex virus DNA fragments to the skin of patients with erythema multiforme (HAEM), *J Invest Dermatol* 124:1215–1224, 2005.

Sokumbi O, Wetter DA: Clinical features, diagnosis, and treatment of erythema multiforme: a review for the practicing dermatologist, *Int J Dermatol* 51:889–902, 2012.

Svensson CK, Cowen EW, Gaspari AA: Cutaneous drug reactions, *Pharmacol Rev* 53(3):357–379, 2001 Sep.

FUNGAL INFECTIONS OF THE SKIN

Method of
Therese Holguin, MD; Sabah Osmani, MD; and Kriti Mishra, MD

CURRENT DIAGNOSIS

- Dermatophyte infections
  - Nonhair-bearing (glabrous) skin diagnostic techniques include scraping of the leading edge of scale with glass slide onto glass slide, cover slip, and applying 10% potassium hydroxide (KOH) to edge of coverslip. Heat the bottom of the slide slightly, clean off with tissue, and view under microscope without condenser. Counterstaining with chlorazol black E or Parker blue-black ink may help visualize hyphae.
  - Hair-bearing skin may require a tissue biopsy with special fungal stains to confirm diagnosis.
  - Culture of scale, hair, and nail fragments sent to the laboratory in a sterile urine cup and clearly marked "for dermatophyte culture" is an additional testing method. Nail fragments can be sent in formalin for periodic acid-Schiff (PAS) staining (a quick-turnaround test).
- Tinea versicolor
  - Stratum corneum removal with a glass slide against a glass slide and KOH examination as above is done for diagnosis. Cultures require a special media, and the laboratory needs notification that this is the organism suspected.
- Candida cutaneous infections
  - Unroofing a pustule by scraping gently with a 15 blade and spreading contents onto a glass slide for KOH evaluation will review the characteristic yeast and pseudohyphae. Culture is usually not necessary.

- Dermatophyte infections
  - Nonhair-bearing skin mild infections are treated with topical agents if severe and widespread; systemic and topical agents together will provide higher cure rate. Prevent reinfection of feet by wearing sandals when possible, especially in public places, alternating shoes, and keeping feet dry. For groin infections, dry well after showering and put socks on before underwear.
  - Hair-bearing skin and hair infections require systemic therapy for cure. Nail infections may be cured with newer topical agents.
- Tinea versicolor
  - Topical treatment with topical agents such as selenium sulfide lotion applied for 10 minutes for 2 weeks, neck to knees, is a cheap and effective treatment. Systemic agents may be needed for resistant cases. Prevention may require maintenance therapy with topical agents during warm and humid months.
- Candida cutaneous infections
  - Topical agents such as nystatin or ketoconazole cream are an effective choice. Prevention of intertrigo is somewhat successful if care to dry thoroughly after showering in body fold areas is done routinely. Zinc-talc shake lotion may be used once or twice daily.

Dermatophyte (tinea) infections are a group of filamentous fungal infections of the skin, hair, and nails and can be noninflammatory or inflammatory. The route of acquisition for dermatophytes is either person-to-person (anthropophilic) or from animals (zoophilic). Geophilic dermatophytes grow in soil and are a rare source of infection in humans. The causative organisms are of three genera: *Microsporum*, *Trichophyton*, and *Epidermophyton*.

Dermatophytoses are the most common fungal infections worldwide, affecting 20% to 25% of the world population. The predominant agents have changed over time by geography and population based on migration of populations, hygiene practices, and therapeutic breakthroughs (griseofulvin [Gris-PEG]). Clinical classification is based on site of infection. Tinea pedis refers to infection of the feet, tinea manuum the hands, tinea cruris the groin, and tinea corporis the skin excluding already mentioned sites plus scalp and nails. Tinea unguium (onychomycosis) refers to nail infection, tinea barbae to beard area, tinea faciei the face, and tinea capitis the scalp and hair. Virulence of the infection is dependent on underlying factors suppressing immunity (diabetes, cancer, HIV infection). Dissemination can be seen in the immunosuppressed.

Superficial infections of the skin and mucous membranes caused by yeasts are caused by *Candida* species. Also common are infections due to lipophilic yeast fungus *Malassezia*.

Superficial Mycoses Dermatophytes

Tinea Capitis

The populations most at risk are children, with boys more commonly than girls. The onset of puberty and change in the relative composition of unsaturated fatty acids in sebum is protective. African Americans and Hispanics have an increased incidence of *Trichophyton tonsurans*. Pet exposure is associated with infections of *Microsporum canis*. Infection with *Trichophyton schoenleinii (favus)*, still seen in less-developed countries, is of characteristic cup-shaped crusts, or scutula. Inflammatory presentations are most often seen in zoophilic infections. Patches of alopecia are common.

Tools for diagnosis include potassium hydroxide (KOH) preparation of scale or hair tweezed from affected patch to be

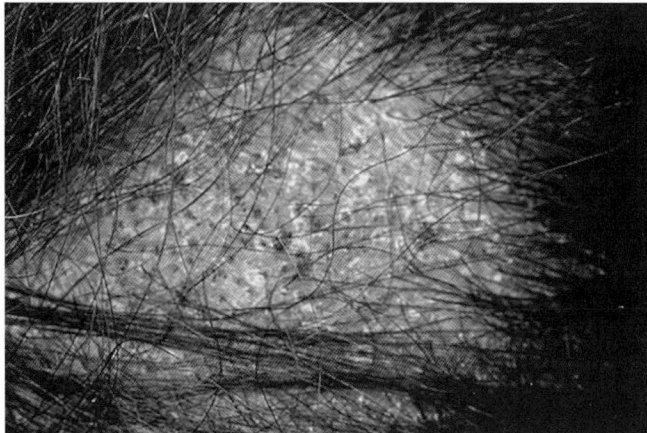

Figure 1 Black dot tinea.

examined microscopically. The Wood's light will show fluorescence with ectothrix infections (organism on outside of shaft) but not endothrix infections (spores on inside of shaft). Samples for culture are obtained by rubbing a wet cotton-tipped applicator over the affected area and applying this or pulled hairs onto the dermatophyte test medium or other medium if species identification is required in resistant cases. The differential diagnosis includes seborrheic dermatitis, psoriasis, folliculitis, pediculosis, secondary syphilis, discoid lupus erythematosus, lichen planus, lichen simplex chronicus, trichotillomania, alopecia areata, and other inflammatory follicular conditions.

Tinea Faciei and Barbae

Frequently misdiagnosed, infection of the face or beard is rare. Beard infections (tinea sycosis or barber's itch) can be deep and inflammatory and are seen in agricultural workers, especially those working with farm animals. Discoid lupus is a commonly mistaken diagnosis, and biopsies are sometimes required to differentiate.

Tinea Corporis

"Ringworm" is a layperson's descriptive term of the characteristic clinical findings of dermatophyte infections. The term accurately portrays the appearance of an erythematous annular plaque with a scaly, raised, leading edge (Figure 2). Severe infections may herald new HIV infection or be secondary to topical immunosuppressant such as calcineurin inhibitors or, more commonly, steroids. KOH examination sampling should be taken from the leading edge. The differential diagnosis includes pityriasis rosea, impetigo, inflammatory dermatoses such as psoriasis and seborrheic dermatitis, and syphilis.

Tinea Cruris

More common in men and when humidity is high, "jock itch" or "crotch itch" involves the upper thigh, intertriginous area, and peripheral spread into the perineum and perianal areas. The scrotum is rarely involved. The usually well-defined border may display scale, papules, or pustules.

The differential diagnosis includes a bacterial infection, erythrasma, candidiasis, intertrigo, psoriasis, and dermatitis. Morphology of the rash and expected involvement of other cutaneous sites is useful to eliminate these possible diagnoses. The origin of the infection is believed to be autoinoculation from tinea pedis or onychomycosis.

Tinea Manuum and Pedis

A classic finding of "one hand and two feet" involvement is useful to lead one to consider tinea manuum (Figure 3). The organism involved in the infection determines the amount of inflammation resultant. Whereas *Trichophyton rubrum* produces a dry scale with erythema of hands and feet (moccasin-type), *Trichophyton interdigitale* (previously known as *Trichophyton mentagrophytes*) often leads to a painful, itchy, blistering eruption of the feet. Other signs of *T interdigitale* include interdigital maceration and superficial infection of the toenails with a distinct white

Fungal Infections of the Skin

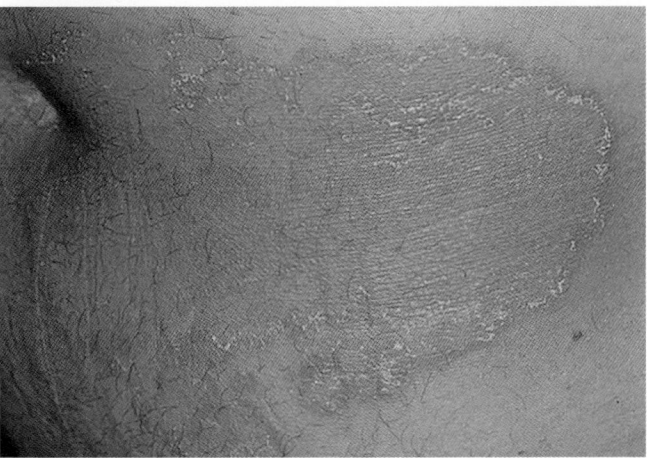

Figure 2 Tinea corporis.

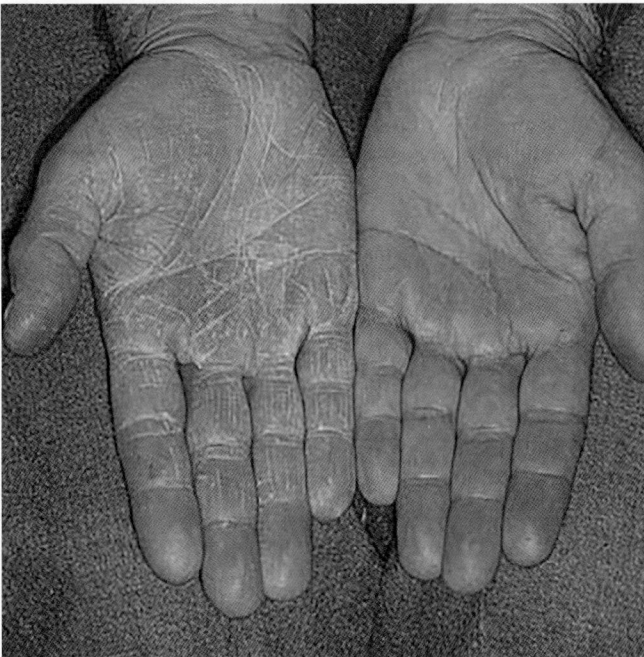

Figure 3 Tinea manuum.

appearance (white superficial onychomycosis). Toe-web infection with gram-negative bacteria may be consequential. Hyperhidrosis is often a precursor to this type of infection. An idiopathic reaction "dermatophytid" is a fairly common pruritic rash of small blisters involving the palms and sometimes the sides of the feet.

Onychomycosis

Fungal infections of the nail are caused by dermatophytes (tinea unguium), yeasts, and nondermaphytic molds. It is common in the general population, accounting for 50% of skin fungal infections. Risk factors include advanced age, diabetes, circulatory disorders, and family history. There are three major subtypes of onychomycosis: distal lateral subungual onychomycosis, white superficial onychomycosis, and proximal subungual onychomycosis. Distal lateral subungual onychomycosis is the most common subtype and is caused by the anthropophilic dermatophytic fungus, *T. rubrum*. Symptoms include an initial discoloration of the distal corner of the nail that may be white, gray, or brown caused by accumulation of keratinous debris under the nail that eventually spreads to involve the entire nail. Other common features are onycholysis, or splitting of the nail from the bed, nail thickening, and impaired nail growth. The diagnosis typically involves KOH, mycologic laboratory confirmation (culture), and biopsy. Yeast onychomycosis is most commonly caused by

Candida albicans and typically involves fingernails of hands frequently exposed to moisture. Nondermaphytic molds primarily involve toenails. Though not life threatening, onychomycosis can significantly impair an individual's quality of life with concerns such as issues cutting the nails and cosmetic disfigurement.

Pityriasis Versicolor

This superficial fungal infection of the skin is caused by a dimorphic lipophilic fungus, *Malassezia* species, which is part of the physiologic skin flora. Certain environmental, genetic, and immunologic factors can predispose the fungus to convert to its pathogenic hyphal form and development of disease. It grows best in warm, humid climates; thus there has been a higher prevalence reported in tropical climates. Furthermore, potential hormonal changes during adolescence can increase sebum production and allow for *Malassezia* to thrive, and the prevalence is even further increased in active adolescents. The pathophysiology may also be related to an impaired immune system.

The diagnosis is usually made clinically, but the presentation may vary; it classically consists of a well-demarcated rash with fine scale and thin plaques. The rash may be hyperpigmented, hypopigmented, or erythematous. Typically, the rash appears on the torso but may become widespread. The lesions may be mildly pruritic or asymptomatic. If KOH is performed on skin scrapings, numerous spores and hyphae can be visualized ("spaghetti and meatball" appearance). Treatment options include topical antifungals, including azoles and terbinafine, selenium sulfide (antidandruff), and zinc pyrithione (Head & Shoulders). Oral azole antifungals can be used; systemic treatment is not first-line therapy because of side effects.

Candidiasis

A dimorphic commensal fungus inhabiting the skin, mouth, and reproductive tract, candidiasis, is found in up to 70% of healthy individuals. *Candida* infection of the skin usually involves moist or occluded areas such as the groin, axillae, and diaper area in the young. Candidal intertrigo classically presents as erythematous and macerated plaques with peripheral scaling. Satellite lesions help differentiate candidal lesions from other conditions. Skin lesions are typically nontender but may develop central pallor or become hemorrhagic in patients with thrombocytopenia. Primary treatment is topical azole and polyene (nystatin) antifungals that are well tolerated. Adjunct therapy with low-dose topical corticosteroids may be used for associated pruritus and pain. Systemic antifungal therapy is rarely used but may be used for refractory disease.

Treatment
Tinea Capitis
First-line treatment for tinea capitis is systemic griseofulvin, but terbinafine may also be considered. Terbinafine may be more effective than griseofulvin in treating *T. tonsurans*, whereas griseofulvin may be more effective against *Microsporum*. Fluconazole and itraconazole are additional options that have demonstrated less evidence-based efficacy.

Pediatric Dosages (>2 years)

Griseofulvin

- Microsize ([Grifulvin V, generic] 500 mg tablets): 20 to 25 mg/kg/day × 6 to 12 weeks (daily max 1000 mg/day)
- Ultramicrosize ([Gris-PEG, generic] 125 mg, 250 mg tablets): 10 to 15 mg/kg/day × 6 to 12 weeks (daily max 750 mg/day)
- Griseofulvin microsize suspension ([Grifulvin V, generic] 125 mg/5 mL): 15 to 25 mg/kg/day × 2 to 12 weeks

Terbinafine ([Lamisil, generic] 250 mg tablets)[1]

- 10–20 kg: 62.5 mg/day × 4 to 6 weeks
- 20–40 kg: 125 mg/day × 4 to 6 weeks
- >40 kg: 250 mg/day × 4 to 6 weeks

---

[1] Not FDA approved for this indication.

Terbinafine (Lamisil granules) (not available in the United States)

- <25 kg: 125 mg/day × 4 to 6 weeks
- 25–35 kg: 165.5 mg/day × 4 to 6 weeks
- >35 kg: 250 mg/day × 4 to 6 weeks

Fluconazole oral suspension ([Diflucan, generic][1] 10 mg/mL, 40 mg/mL)

- Continuous: 6 mg/kg/day × 20 days (daily max 400 mg)
- Pulse: 6 mg/kg/day, once per week × 8 to 12 weeks

Itraconazole (Sporanox)[1]

- Continuous:
- Oral suspension (10 mg/mL): 5 mg/kg/day × 4 weeks
- Pulses (3 pulses)
- Oral suspension: 3 mg/kg/day, 1 week/month × 2 to 3 months
- Capsules (100 mg): 5 mg/kg/day, 1 week/month × 2 to 3 months

Adult Dosages

Terbinafine (Lamisil)[1]

- 250 mg/day × 4 to 6 weeks

Fluconazole (Diflucan)[1]

- 50 mg/day × 4 to 7 weeks, or
- 150 mg/week × 4 weeks

Itraconazole (Sporanox)[1]

- 100–200 mg/day × 4 weeks

Topical therapies can also be helpful used twice-weekly in conjunction with systemic treatment. These include antifungal shampoos like selenium sulfide (antidandruff), ciclopirox (Loprox), and zinc pyrithione (Head & Shoulders).

Tinea Corporis, Tinea Cruris, Tinea Pedis, Tinea Mannum, Tinea Faciei, Tinea Barbae

Topical treatments should be used for 2 to 6 weeks once or twice daily. Options include terbinafine (Lamisil), butenafine (Lotrimin-Ultra), naftifine (Naftin), clotrimazole (Lotrimin), econazole (Spectazole), ketoconazole (Nizoral), sertaconazole (Ertaczo), luliconazole (Luzu), eberconazole (Ebernet).[2] Begin therapy with topical treatment and reserve systemic treatment for widespread, resistant, or severe disease. If necessary:

Pediatric Dosages (all are off-label and not FDA approved)

Terbinafine (tablets)[1]

- <20 kg: 62.5 mg/day × 2 weeks
- 20–40 kg: 125 mg/day × 2 weeks
- >40 kg: 250 mg/day × 2 weeks

Itraconazole[1]

- 5 mg/kg/day divided qd-BID × 2 weeks (max 200 mg/day)

Griseofulvin (dosages listed are for age >2 to adolescent)

- Microsize: 10 to 20 mg/kg/day × 2 to 8 weeks
- Ultramicrosize: 5 to 15 mg/kg/day divided qd-BID
- (Max: 750 mg/day)

Adult Dosages (all are off-label and not FDA approved)

- Terbinafine[1]
- 250 mg/day × 2 to 4 weeks

Itraconazole[1]

- 200 mg/day × 1 week

Fluconazole[1]

- 150–300 mg/week × 2 to 4 weeks (pulse dosing)

Griseofulvin

- Microsize: 500 to 1000 mg/day × 2 to 4 weeks
- Ultramicrosize: 375 to 500 mg/day × 2 to 4 weeks

Terbinafine 250 mg + itraconazole 200 mg × 3 weeks[1] (resistant cases)

Tinea Unguium

Children may respond completely to antifungal topical lacquer or solutions without systemic therapy. Lacquers, such as Amorolfine (Curanail, Loceryl, Locetar, Odenil) (not available in the United States), are debrided and reapplied daily. Hydrolacquers, such as ciclopirox (Penlac) may also be used and are removable with washing and reapplied daily. Topical solutions, like efinaconazole (Jublia) and tavaborole (Kerydin), are used for 48 to 60 weeks.

If systemic therapy is required—and in all adult cases—first-line treatment is terbinafine. Systemic treatment in conjunction with lacquers has been associated with higher cure rates. Additionally, conventional oral therapy followed by topical for maintenance may help prevent recurrence.

If there is no response to treatment or the patient cannot tolerate the medication, itraconazole may be used. Fluconazole[1] has not been shown to be as effective and requires long duration of treatment (up to 6 months) and is therefore not a preferred treatment. Griseofulvin is not recommended. Lasers and photodynamic therapy if available are considered third-line options. Surgical options include chemical (40%–50% urea compound) or surgical nail avulsion.

Pediatric Dosages

Terbinafine (Ages 2+)

- <20 kg: 62.5 mg/day
- 20–40 kg: 125 mg/day
- >40 kg: 250 mg/day × 6 weeks for fingernails, × 12 weeks for toenails

Itraconazole

- Continuous: 200 mg/day × 6 weeks for fingernails, × 12 weeks for toenails
- Pulse: 200 mg BID, 1 week/month × 2 months for fingernails, × 3 months for toenails

Adult Dosages

Terbinafine

- Continuous: 250 mg/day × 6 weeks for fingernails, × 12 weeks for toenails
- Pulse (for toenails): 250 mg BID × 4 weeks, no treatment × 4 weeks, 250 mg BID × 4 weeks (12 weeks total)

Itraconazole

- Continuous: 200 mg/day × 6 weeks for fingernails, × 12 weeks for toenails
- Pulse: 200 mg BID 1 week/month × 2 months for fingernails, × 3 months for toenails

Additional Comments

Before beginning systemic antifungal therapy, obtain a baseline CBC and liver function tests. Repeat laboratories if therapy lasts >6 weeks.

Griseofulvin is contraindicated in pregnancy and there are restrictions for becoming pregnant or fathering after medication course is complete. Patients should avoid alcohol during treatment. Griseofulvin is more effectively absorbed with fatty foods like peanut butter, yogurt, ice cream, and so on. (Therapeutic failures have been noted due to lack of absorption.)

Itraconazole has negative inotropic effects and can lead to QT prolongation.

[1]Not FDA approved for this indication.

[2]Not available in the United States.

Ketoconazole[1] has risks of fatal liver damage and adrenal insufficiency and is generally not recommended.

[1]Not FDA approved for this indication.

References

Asz-Sigall D, Tosti A, Arenas R: Tinea unguium: diagnosis and treatment in practice, *Mycopathologia* 182:95–100, 2017.

Chen X, Jiang X, Yang M, et al: Systemic antifungal therapy for tinea capitis in children: an abridged cochrane review, *J Am Acad Dermatol* 76:368–374, 2017.

Gupta A, Foley K, Versteeg S: New antifungal agents and new formulations against dermatophytes, *Mycopathologia* 182:127–141, 2017.

Gupta AK, Kogan N, Batra R: Pityriasis versicolor: a review of pharmacological treatment options: expert opinion on pharmacotherapy, *Expert Opin Pharmacother* 6:165–178, 2005.

Hay R: Tinea capitis: current status, *Mycopathologia* 182:87–93, 2017.

Kyriakis KP, Terzoudi S, Palamaras I, et al: Pityriasis versicolor prevalence by age and gender, *Mycoses* 49:517–518, 2006.

Nenoff P, Krüger C, Ginter-Hanselmayer, et al: Mycology—an update. Part 1: Dermatomycoses: Causative agents, epidemiology and pathogenesis, *J Dtsch Dermatol Ges* 12:188–209, 2014.

Perlroth J, Choi B, Spellberg B: Nosocomial fungal infections: epidemiology, diagnosis, and treatment, *Med Mycol* 45:321–346, 2007.

Priyanka S, Mala B, Gurvinder P, et al: Evaluation of efficacy and safety of oral terbinafine and itraconazole combination therapy in the management of dermatophytosis, *J Dermatol Treat*, 2019, https://doi.org/10.1080/09546634.2019.16
12835.

Solís-Arias MP, García-Romero MT: Onychomycosis in children: a review, *Int J Dermatol* 56:123–130, 2017.

KELOIDS

Method of
Leslie A. Greenberg, MD

CURRENT DIAGNOSIS

- Clinical characteristics: firm, raised, papular, plaque-like, nodular, and tumorous scar tissue that extends beyond the initial wound borders. May be painful or pruritic and disfiguring.
- Location: more commonly found on ears, upper back and chest, and upper arms.
- Cause: results from an abnormal healing process after skin trauma or inflammation.
- Histologic characteristics: abnormally functioning dermal fibroblasts and overproduction of extracellular matrix result in markedly thickened bundles of hyalinized collagen arranged in a haphazard fashion.

CURRENT THERAPY

Medical Therapies
- Intralesional corticosteroids (triamcinolone acetonide [Kenalog])
- Interferon alfa (IFN-alfa2b [Intron A])[1]
- Intralesional fluorouracil (5-FU, Adrucil)[1]

Surgical Therapies
- Cryotherapy
- Primary excision

Physical Modalities
- Pressure therapy
- Radiation therapy
- Laser therapy

Miscellaneous Therapies
- Silicone gel sheeting or gel

[1]Not FDA approved for this indication.

Keloids are common, benign fibroproliferative lesions resulting from altered wound healing caused by abnormalities of fibroblast function and extracellular matrix overproduction. Lesions may be painful and severely disfiguring—at times, limiting range of motion. Histologically, keloids are foci of brightly eosinophilic-staining collagen bundles laid haphazardly.

Keloids may be papular, plaque-like, nodular, or tumorous. The term *keloid* is derived from the Greek word meaning "tumor-like." A keloid extends beyond the site of injury. Keloids tend to shrink over time but rarely resolve.

Epidemiology

Keloids occur more commonly in people of African and Asian descent. There may be a familial or genetic contribution to keloid development as an autosomal dominant inheritance with incomplete penetrance. Keloids may be intentionally induced for cosmetic purposes. For example, the ancient Olmec of Mexico in pre-Columbian times are one ethnic group that has used keloid scarification as an intentional means of decoration.

Pathophysiology

Unlike scars, keloids are made up of markedly thickened bundles of collagen that are arranged in a haphazard fashion. Normal scar tissue formation, in contrast, consists of fibrillary bundles of collagen that are aligned parallel to the skin surface.

The pathogenesis of keloid formation is unknown. Fibroblast proliferation and increased collagen synthesis are due to the overexpression of growth factors. Growth factor production fails to self-regulate and does not turn off once the wound is well healed. Alteration of programmed fibroblast apoptosis has been implicated. It has been suggested that keloid fibroblasts fail to undergo physiologically programmed cell death and thereby produce extra connective tissue. Genetic factors are likely involved, and studies have identified four susceptibility loci.

Keloids represent the end stage of an inflammatory process that starts after a traumatic disruption of skin integrity. Over a period of weeks, abnormally functioning fibroblasts replace the granulation tissue associated with the early stages of healing. At that point, a distinctive morphologic scar or keloid may be noticeable. After a keloid is fully formed, it may look the same for years or it may enlarge over time.

Risk Factors

Certain populations are at higher risk to develop keloids. Dark-skinned individuals, such as those of Asian, African, and Hispanic descent, have a 15-fold increased risk to develop keloids compared with light-skinned individuals. Skin insults such as lacerations, secondarily infected skin lesions, surgery, or ear piercings challenge the body's healing processes and may result in keloids, although keloids may also form without an inciting trauma. Keloids are more commonly found on the ears, upper back and chest, and upper arms. Ongoing tension or movement across the wound healing site may predispose to keloid formation. Genetics is a factor, as there are reports of familial cases with varied modes of inheritance, indicating multiple genetic disorders that may influence keloid formation. Patients with specific rare inherited conditions like Goeminne syndrome and Rubinstein-Taybi syndrome are at increased risk of keloid formation. Age affects the propensity to make a keloid with the highest incidence in individuals aged 10 to 20 years. Keloids are rarely found in newborns or older adults.

Prevention

The best treatment is prevention of unnecessary trauma or surgery, including ear piercing and elective cosmetic surgery. Early treatment of acne helps decrease inflamed pustules and papule formation, which, when located at the posterior neck, may become acne keloidalis nuchae. Patients with acne keloidalis nuchae should avoid shaving the neck region and instead should use scissors to trim hair no shorter than one-eighth of an inch. Consider varicella vaccination (Varivax)[1] to decrease keloid risk of chickenpox

[1]Not FDA approved for this indication.

lesions. Lack of ultraviolet (UV) B light may increase the risk of keloid formation. In fact, using UV A1 phototherapy may be a promising treatment of keloids. Other environmental preventive measures are to keep the wound moist, as well as avoid sun exposure and tension on the wound.

Clinical Manifestations

Keloids are firm, rubbery, raised, papular, plaque-like, nodular, and tumorous scar tissue that extends beyond the initial wound borders. Lesions may develop as early as 1 month after injury, or may begin to form 1 year after an inflammatory incident. Frequently, lesions are pruritic, are tender to palpation, and may be the source of sharp, shooting pains. Location is more often on the ears, jaw, neck, shoulders, upper back, and presternal chest. Keloids may be disfiguring and, in rare instances (e.g., location over a joint), may impair function. Keloids do not spontaneously regress.

Diagnosis

The clinical diagnosis of a keloid is usually apparent. Rarely is histologic confirmation necessary. Lesions may continue to grow for weeks to months. Keloids on the ears, neck, and abdomen tend to be pedunculated, whereas those on the central chest and extremities are usually raised with a flat surface. Most keloids are round, oval, or oblong, with regular margins; however, some have a claw-like configuration with irregular borders.

Differential Diagnosis

Hypertrophic scars appear different than keloids because the wound healing is linear, stays within the boundaries of the original wound site, and may be transiently indurated or tender to palpation. Hypertrophic scars are as prevalent in light- or dark-skinned individuals and as a rule tend to flatten significantly over time without treatment.

Giant cell fibroblastoma is a low-grade sarcoma considered a juvenile form of dermatofibrosarcoma protuberans. It is uncommon and locally aggressive. Histology shows multinucleated cells with hyperchromatic nuclei and infiltrating sheets of spindle-shaped fibroblasts.

Lobomycosis is a chronic fungal infection occurring in tropical areas of Latin America. It appears as localized slow-growing nodules in exposed skin.

Dermatofibrosarcoma protuberans is an uncommon, locally aggressive cutaneous soft tissue sarcoma that may present as a plaque-like area of cutaneous thickening that can be violet–red or blue at the margins. Rarely, this may arise within a preexisting scar or tattoo. Definitive diagnosis usually requires a core needle or incisional biopsy.

Treatment

Goals of therapy should be discussed with the patient. Often goals are cosmetic and functional improvement, reduction of scar volume, and relief of pain and itching at the site. Consider taking pretreatment photographs for comparison purposes.

Intralesional Corticosteroid

Injections of intralesional corticosteroids are considered first-line therapy for keloids. A systematic review showed that up to 70% of cases respond with flattening of lesions, though the recurrence rate is up to 50% at 5 years. For local anesthesia, apply liquid nitrogen for 10 to 15 seconds or lidocaine-prilocaine cream (EMLA) under occlusion for 1.5 hours before injection. Do not use liquid nitrogen for more than 30 seconds or permanent hypopigmentation may result. Use triamcinolone acetonide (Kenalog) 10 mg/mL. Space injections approximately 0.5 to 1.0 cm apart. Use a ½-inch, 30-gauge Luer-Lok (twist-on) needle with bevel directed up toward the skin and a tuberculin syringe to allow injection under pressure. Wear a face shield to avoid contact with back-pressure spray. Inject within the bulk of the lesion with enough triamcinolone to make the keloid blanch, usually 0.1 to 0.5 mL. Multiple injections may be needed. Injections may be given monthly until the desired degree of involution and/or symptomatic relief is achieved. If no change

occurs after one injection with triamcinolone acetonide 10 mg/mL, increase the strength to 40 mg/mL (Figure 1). If no change occurs after three or four injections, consider referral to a plastic surgeon or dermatologist for surgical excision.

Surgical Excision

Surgical excision of a keloid may help aesthetically and symptomatically, though lesions tend to recur and may result in more extensive scarring. After excision, immediately inject the base of the surgical site in multiple sites with triamcinolone acetonide 20 mg/mL. Use a 30-gauge needle and then occlude the excision site with a pressure dressing such as Elastoplast. Corticosteroid injections should then be repeated at 2-week intervals over a course of 3 to 4 months.

Silicone Gel Sheeting

The use of silicone sheeting may be effective for the treatment of symptoms such as pain and itching for established keloids. It may also be used early in wound healing to prevent keloids at the site of new injuries. In some trials, silicone sheeting was effective in 70% to 80% of cases to avoid keloid formation. Sheeting is placed on top of the keloid, taped into place, and left on for 12 to 24 hours per day. The sheet is washed daily and replaced every 10 to 14 days. Consider effectiveness after 2 to 6 months of therapy. Over-the-counter and prescription self-drying silicone gel formulations are an alternative for exposed or larger areas.

Cryosurgery

Cryotherapy can be used in conjunction with intralesional corticosteroids. This is widely available, is effective, and has an excellent safety profile. A 10- to 30-second freeze-thaw cycle can be repeated up to three times per treatment session and repeated every 4 to 6 weeks until a response occurs. One major permanent side effect is hypopigmentation, which may be most apparent in darker-skinned patients.

Pressure Therapy

When pressure (to an area of possible keloid formation) is applied early in the healing process, it may decrease keloid formation. This is thought to occur due to decreases in oxygen

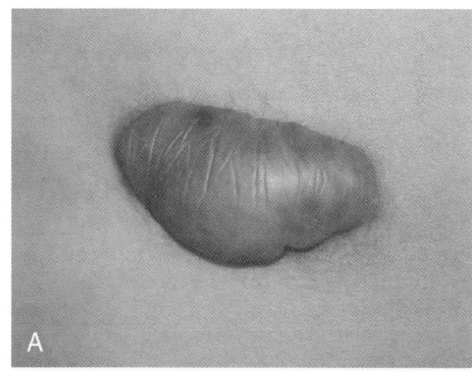
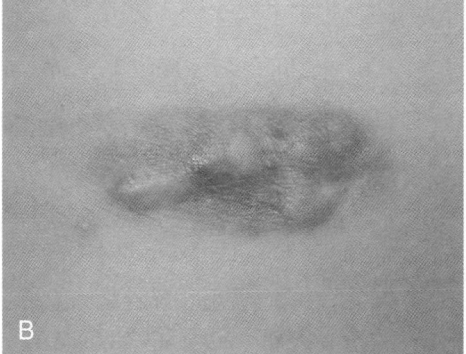

Figure 1 (A) A keloid on the back. (B) The scar after four intralesional injections of corticosteroid 10 mg/mL at 4 weeks apart. Note side effects of skin atrophy and hypopigmentation. Reprinted with permission from Manuskiatti W: Current management of hypertrophic scars and keloids. *Siriraj Hosp Gaz* 55:249–258, 2003.

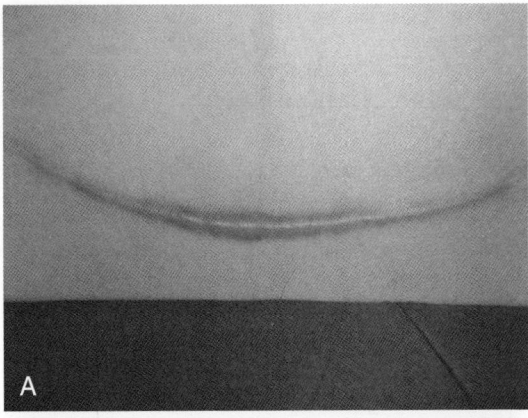

Figure 2 (A) A scar developing after cesarean section. (B) The scar after two pulsed dye laser treatments 8 weeks apart.

tension of the wound by occluding small blood vessels and decreasing fibroblast proliferation. The optimal pressure should be 20 to 30 mm Hg for 12 to 24 hours per day for 6 to 12 months. Zimmer splints are inexpensive, molded earring-like pressure therapy that may be an effective treatment for keloids following ear piercing.

Intralesional 5-Fluorouracil

Intralesional 5-fluorouracil (FU) has been used for scars that do not respond to intralesional corticosteroids. Schedule intralesional injections of 5-FU (Adrucil)[1] 50 mg/mL with a volume of 0.5 to 2.0 mL per session for every 4 weeks up to 12 weeks. Intralesional 5-FU has been shown to improve keloids by 50% and is considered to work best on small keloids. Injections may be painful and may cause hyperpigmentation. 5-FU can be mixed with triamcinolone acetonide for keloids resistant to triamcinolone alone: 0.1 mL of triamcinolone acetonide 40 mg/mL can be mixed with 0.9 mL of 5-FU 50 mg/mL and injected weekly for 8 weeks. A pulsed dye laser has been used in combination with intralesional injection of a mixture of 5-FU and steroid with cumulative beneficial effect (Figure 2).

Surgical Excision

Surgical excision of keloids may be indicated if conservative therapies alone are unsuccessful. Excision is associated with keloid recurrence of up to 100%.

Postoperative Radiation Therapy

Low-dose radiation therapy may be highly effective in reducing keloid recurrence if done immediately after surgical excision. However, there is no universally accepted radiation dose or modality for the postoperative treatment of keloids.

Monitoring

Surveillance of scars during wound healing is important to alert the provider that keloids may be forming. Appropriate, focused, and timed treatment can then be performed. In a patient with keloid history, using prophylactic therapy may be instituted when a new wound is incurred. Close follow-up monitoring is vital during immediate and aggressive treatment.

Complications

Patients should be advised that keloids can be recalcitrant to all types of therapy. If a keloid recurs (especially if ablative methods such as electrosurgery are used), it may be more disfiguring than the original lesion. Trauma to the keloid may predispose the lesion to erosion and localized bacterial infection.

References

Asilian A, Darougheh A, Shariati F: New combination of triamcinolone, 5-fluorouracil, and pulsed-dye laser for treatment of keloids and hypertrophic scars, *Dermatol Surg* 32:907, 2006.

Derm101.com. Scars, keloids, and anetodermas. Available at www.derm101.com/clinical-atlas/scars-keloids-and-anetodermas (accessed August 2, 2016).

Kelly AP: Update on the management of keloids, *Semin Cutan Med Surg* 28:71–76, 2009.

Kontochristopoulos G, Stefanaki C, Panagiotopoulos A, et al: Intralesional 5-fluorouracil in the treatment of keloids: an open clinical and histopathologic study, *J Am Acad Dermatol* 52(3 Pt 1):474, 2005.

Medscape.com. Keloid and hypertrophic scar differential diagnosis. Available at http://emedicine.medscape.com/article/1057599-differential; [accessed 06.10.17].

Nakashima M, Chung S, Takahashi A, et al: A genome-wide association study identifies four susceptibility loci for keloid in the Japanese population, *Nat Genet* 42:768, 2010.

Shaffer JJ, Taylor SC, Cook-Bolden F: Keloidal scars: a review with a critical look at therapeutic options, *J Am Acad Dermatol* 46:63, 2002.

Van Leeuwen MC, van der Wal MB, Bulstra AE, et al: Intralesional cryotherapy for treatment of keloid scars: a prospective study, *Plast Reconst Surg Glop Open* 3:e437, 2015.

MELANOMA

Method of
Geoffrey Gibney, MD; and Vesna M. Petronic-Rosic, MD, MSc, MBA

CURRENT DIAGNOSIS

- ABCDEs:
  - **A**symmetry of lesion.
  - **B**order irregularity, bleeding, or crusting.
  - **C**olor change or variegation.
  - **D**iameter larger than 6mm or growing lesion.
  - **E**volving: Surface changes or symptomatic.
- The "ugly duckling" sign: A mole that looks or feels different compared to surrounding moles.
- Total-body photography and dermoscopy.
- Excisional biopsy with narrow margins.
- Interpretation by physician experienced in the microscopic diagnosis of pigmented lesions.
- Molecular analyses (rarely).
- Appropriate staging workup.
- Genetic testing when appropriate (rarely).

CURRENT THERAPY

- Early diagnosis and appropriate surgical therapy is the gold standard.
- Complete excision must be achieved with appropriate margins based on tumor thickness.
- Sentinel lymph node biopsy may be offered to patients with melanoma 0.8 to 4 mm thick, or any melanoma thickness if ulceration is present, with clinically unaffected regional nodes and without distant metastases.
- Dissection of the lymph node basin is not routinely offered to patients with micronodal metastases, although it can be offered in select patients.
- Dissection of the lymph node basin is offered to patients with macronodal metastases.
- Adjuvant therapy is offered for resected stage III and IV disease.
- Stage IV treatment depends on location and extent of metastatic disease and may include surgical resection, radiation therapy, and/or systemic therapy.

Melanoma is a malignancy of pigment-producing cells (melanocytes). Melanocytes are located predominantly in the skin but are also found in the eyes, ears, gastrointestinal tract, leptomeninges, and oral and genital mucous membranes.

Epidemiology

Even though melanoma accounts for less than 5% of skin cancer cases, it causes the most skin cancer deaths. The American Cancer Society's most recent estimates for melanoma in the United States for 2020 are 100,350 new cases, with 6,850 deaths. The prevalence of melanoma in the United States doubled over three decades from 1982 to 2011, from 11.2 per 100,000 population to 22.7 per 100,000. The overall melanoma incidence rate has continued to increase, but may be starting to decrease in recent birth cohorts. The lifetime risk for developing melanoma is about 1 in 28 for males and 1 in 41 for females. More notable, the melanoma mortality rates dropped by 7% and 5% to 6%, respectively, annually in men and women aged 20 to 64 years and aged 65 years and older from 2013 to 2017. Mortality rates remain higher in blacks compared to all races combined.

Risk Factors

A large number of nevi is the strongest risk factor for melanoma in persons of European ancestry. Atypical mole syndrome is another risk factor. Exposure to ultraviolet light is a major risk factor, especially in persons who have fair hair and skin, who have solar damage, who had sunburns and short, sharp bursts of sun exposure in childhood, and who used tanning beds. Tanning beds appear more detrimental when used before the age of 20 years. The International Agency for Research on Cancer has classified indoor tanning devices as "carcinogenic to humans" based on extensive review of scientific evidence. Familial risk factors include mutations in *CDKN2A(p16INK4a)*, which are associated with increased risks for both melanoma and pancreatic cancer; they are transmitted in an autosomal dominant fashion and account for approximately 20% to 50% of familial melanoma cases. In recent years, mutations in *BRCA1*-associated protein 1 (BAP1), shelterin complex, microphthalmia-associated transcription factor (MITF), and phosphatase and tensin homolog (PTEN) have also been associated with melanoma and internal organ cancers. Organ transplant recipients have an increased risk for melanoma. Genodermatoses with a defect in DNA repair (such as xeroderma pigmentosum) increase risk for melanoma.

Pathophysiology

Transformation of normal melanocytes into melanoma cells likely involves a multistep process of progressive genetic mutations that alter cell proliferation, differentiation, and death and affect susceptibility to the carcinogenic effects of ultraviolet radiation. Primary cutaneous melanoma can develop in preexisting melanocytic nevi, but more than 60% of cases likely appear de novo.

Melanomas arising in skin that is chronically sun damaged show molecular features that distinguish them from melanomas arising in skin that is not sun damaged. In particular, the tumor mutational burden is highest in melanoma arising from sun exposed areas, which is associated with response to immunotherapies. In addition, activating somatic mutations in the *BRAF* gene are seen in 40% to 60% of cutaneous melanoma, leading to constitutive activation of the MAPK pathway. Additional common mutations include *NRAS* (28%), *P53* (15%), *NF1* (14%), *CDKN2A* (13%), and *PTEN* (9%). The genetic makeup of non–sun exposed acral melanoma differs from cutaneous melanoma, with a lower frequency of *BRAF* mutations and the presence of *KIT* mutations in up to 12% of patients. Genetic studies have shown that 50% of familial melanomas and 25% of sporadic melanomas may be associated with mutations in the tumor suppressor gene p16. Linkage studies have identified chromosome 9p21 as the site of the familial melanoma gene.

Prevention

Early detection of thin cutaneous melanoma is the best means of reducing mortality. Patients with a history of melanoma should be educated regarding sun-protective clothing and sunscreens, skin self-examinations for new primary melanoma, possible recurrence within the surgical scar, and screening of first-degree relatives, particularly if they have a history of atypical moles.

Clinical Manifestations

Early signs of melanoma include the ABCDEs:
- Asymmetry of lesion
- Border irregularity, bleeding, or crusting
- Color change or variegation
- Diameter larger than 6 mm or growing lesion
- Evolving: Surface changes or symptomatic

The "ugly duckling" sign is also useful to recognize lesions that look or feel different compared to surrounding moles.

Lentigo maligna (melanoma in situ) begins as an irregular tan brown macule that slowly expands on sun-damaged skin of elderly persons. Long-term cumulative sun exposure confers the greatest risk. Progression to invasive lentigo maligna melanoma is estimated to be 30% to 50%.

Superficial spreading melanoma, the most common type in light skin, represents approximately 70% of all melanomas. Peak incidence is in the fourth and fifth decade. Superficial spreading melanoma can arise in a preexisting melanocytic nevus that slowly changes over several years; it most commonly affects intermittently sun-exposed areas with the greatest nevus density (upper backs of men and women and lower legs of women). Pigment varies from black and blue-gray to pink or gray-white, and the borders are irregular. Absence of pigmentation often represents regression.

Nodular melanoma represents 15% of all melanomas. The median age at onset is 53 years. Clinically, a uniform blue-black, blue-red, or red nodule usually begins de novo and grows rapidly. About 5% are amelanotic. The most common sites are the trunk, head, and neck.

Acral lentiginous melanoma accounts for 10% of melanomas overall but is the most common type among Japanese, African Americans, Latin Americans, and Native Americans. The median age is 65 years, with equal gender distribution. It occurs on the palms or soles or under the nails and is on average 3 cm in diameter at diagnosis. Clinically, the lesion is a tan, brown-to-black, flat macule with color variegation and irregular borders. It does not appear to be linked to sun exposure.

Diagnosis

Excisional biopsy with narrow margins is recommended for diagnosis. Incisional biopsy is acceptable when suspicion for melanoma is low, the lesion is large, or it is impractical to perform a complete excision. It is believed not to be detrimental if subsequent therapeutic surgery is performed within 4 to 6 weeks. Dermoscopy and total body photography are adjunctive noninvasive diagnostic techniques. Routine laboratory tests and imaging studies are not required for asymptomatic patients with primary cutaneous melanoma 4 mm or less in thickness for initial staging or routine follow-up. Indications for such studies are directed by a thorough medical history and complete physical examination.

Histologic interpretation should be performed by a physician experienced in the microscopic diagnosis of pigmented lesions. Molecular analyses for evidence of gene mutations, DNA copy-number abnormalities, or changed protein expression are useful adjunctive tools in the assessment of histologically ambiguous primary melanocytic tumors. It is now known that melanomas from sun-damaged skin, non-sun-damaged skin, or mucosal or acral surfaces harbor distinct molecular phenotypes.

The new revised American Joint Committee on Cancer (AJCC) staging system was published in 2017. Key changes in the eighth edition of the AJCC Cancer Staging Manual include:

1. tumor thickness measurements to be recorded to the nearest 0.1 mm, not 0.01 mm;

2. definitions of T1a and T1b are revised (T1a, <0.8 mm without ulceration; T1b, 0.8-1.0 mm with or without ulceration or <0.8 mm with ulceration), with mitotic rate no longer a T category criterion;

3. pathological (but not clinical) stage IA is revised to include T1bN0M0 (formerly pathologic stage IB);

4. the N category descriptors "microscopic" and "macroscopic" for regional node metastasis are redefined as "clinically occult" and "clinically apparent";

5. prognostic stage III groupings are based on N category criteria and T category criteria (i.e., primary tumor thickness and ulceration) and increased from three to four subgroups (stages IIIA-IIID);

6. definitions of N subcategories are revised, with the presence of microsatellites, satellites, or in-transit metastases now categorized as N1c, N2c, or N3c based on the number of tumor-involved regional lymph nodes, if any;

7. descriptors are added to each M1 subcategory designation for lactate dehydrogenase (LDH) level (LDH elevation no longer upstages to M1c);

8. a new M1d designation is added for central nervous system metastases.

This evidence-based revision of the AJCC melanoma staging system will guide patient treatment, provide better prognostic estimates, and refine stratification of patients entering clinical trials.

Five-year and ten-year survival rates based on the TNM classification range from 99% and 98% for patients with stage IA melanomas to 82% and 75%, respectively, for patients with stage IIC melanomas based on the AJCC 8th edition (Table 1). This dataset included patients dating as far back as 1998, which likely underrepresents the current melanoma-specific survival given the development of highly effective targeted and immune checkpoint therapies in the past decade.

Differential Diagnosis

The differential diagnosis includes melanocytic nevus, angioma, pigmented basal cell carcinoma, pyogenic granuloma, seborrheic keratosis, Kaposi's sarcoma, and hematoma (especially for acral lentiginous melanoma).

Treatment

Early diagnosis combined with appropriate surgical therapy is curative in most patients. For melanoma in situ, wide excision with 0.5 to 1.0 cm margins is recommended; lentigo maligna histologic subtype may require >0.5 cm margins to achieve histologically negative margins because of characteristically broad subclinical extension. Surgical margins for invasive melanoma should be at least 1 cm and up to 2 cm clinically measured around the primary tumor; clinically measured surgical margins do not need to correlate with histologically negative margins. Margins may be modified to accommodate individual anatomic or functional considerations. The recommended margins are:

Tumor Thickness	Clinically Measured Surgical Margin	Strength of Recommendation	Level of Evidence
In situ	0.5–1.0 cm	C	III
≤1.0mm	1 cm	A	I
1.01–2.0mm	1–2 cm	A	I
≥2.0mm	2 cm	B	I, II, III

Strength of Recommendations: A, B, C Level of Evidence: I, II, III (https://www.aad.org/practicecenter/quality/clinical-guidelines/melanoma/surgical-management, accessed 07.01.2019)

The recommended deep margin is muscle fascia. Wider margins and Mohs' micrographic surgery can reduce the risk of contiguous subclinical spread for the desmoplastic variant of melanoma.

Sentinel lymph node biopsy (SLNB) provides accurate staging information for patients with clinically unaffected regional nodes and without distant metastases. The status of SLN is the most important prognostic indicator for disease-specific survival in patients with primary cutaneous melanoma; however, the SLNB has not demonstrated an improvement in overall survival (MSLT1 study). Candidates for SLNB include patients with newly diagnosed primary cutaneous melanoma with a depth of at least 0.8 mm or presence of ulceration and who are clinically node-negative and have no clinical evidence of metastatic disease. In cases of positive SLNB, completion lymph node dissection has not demonstrated a survival advantage over observation and nodal surveillance in two large randomized prospective studies (DeCOG-SLT and MLST2 studies). This has been practice-changing in that most melanoma patients with positive SLNB are now managed by observation/nodal surveillance, although completion lymph node dissection may be offered to select patients and remains an option within the NCCN guidelines. In patients with clinically detected regional nodal metastases (palpable and positive cytology or histopathology), therapeutic lymph node dissection of the involved basin is indicated in the absence of distant metastases.

For resectable local or in-transit recurrences, excision with a clear margin is recommended. For numerous or unresectable in transit metastases, isolated limb perfusion or infusion with melphalan, intralesional injection with the oncolytic viral therapy talimogene laherparepvec (TVEC), or systemic targeted or immune checkpoint therapy are generally considered.

Radiotherapy is indicated in select patients with lentigo maligna melanoma, as an adjuvant in patients where re-resection of positive margins/recurrence is not feasible, for management of solitary/oligometastatic metastases (especially for brain metastases), and for palliation of symptomatic tumor sites.

Numerous adjuvant therapies have been investigated for the treatment of locoregional cutaneous melanoma following complete surgical removal. The current US Food and Drug Administration (FDA) approved agents include interferon alfa-2b (Intron A high dose and pegylated formulations [Peg-Intron]), anti-cytotoxic T-lymphocyte antigen-4 (CTLA-4) therapy (ipilimumab [Yervoy]), anti-programmed cell death 1 (PD-1) therapy (nivolumab [Opdivo] and pembrolizumab [Keytruda]), and BRAF targeted therapy (dabrafenib [Tafinlar] plus trametinib [Mekinist] in BRAF V600 mutant melanoma only). Interferon and ipilimumab are now seldom used since the more recent approval of the anti-PD-1 and BRAF targeted therapies, which are generally well tolerated and reduce relapse rates by 43% to 53% in patients with resected stage III melanoma. Of note, nivolumab is also approved as adjuvant therapy for resected stage IV melanoma.

Metastatic melanoma is an aggressive, immunogenic, and molecularly heterogeneous disease. In the last decade, treatment of melanoma took a dramatic turn with the discovery of targeted therapy aimed at the BRAF mutations in the mitogen-activated protein kinase (MAPK) pathway and immune checkpoint inhibitors. In 2011, the FDA approved ipilimumab, an anti-CTLA-4 antibody for metastatic melanoma therapy. Since then, novel monoclonal antibody agents that inhibit PD-1—pembrolizumab and nivolumab—were approved in 2014, followed by the nivolumab plus ipilimumab combination therapy in 2015. An additional class

TABLE 1	Melanoma Specific Survival by AJCC 8th Edition.	
STAGE	**5 YEAR SURVIVAL**	**10 YEAR SURVIVAL**
Stage I		
IA	99%	98%
IB	97%	94%
Stage II		
IIA	94%	88%
IIB	87%	82%
IIC	82%	75%
Stage III		
IIIA	93%	88%
IIIB	83%	77%
IIIC	69%	60%
IIID	32%	24%

of immunotherapy, the intralesional oncolytic viral therapy T-VEC (talimogene laherparepvec, Imlygic), received approval in 2015. Its use is limited to patients with palpable unresectable metastatic melanoma. The selective *BRAF* inhibitor vemurafenib (Zelboraf) was also approved in 2011 for the treatment of patients with advanced *BRAF* V600 mutant melanoma. Additional *BRAF* targeted regimens were subsequently approved, with the combination *BRAF* plus MEK inhibitors now the standard approach based on improvement in survival over monotherapy. The three approved *BRAF* plus MEK inhibitor regimens include dabrafenib [Tafinlar] plus trametinib [Mekinist], vemurafenib [Zelboraf] plus cobimetinib [Cotellic], and encorafenib [Braftovi] plus binimetinib [Mektovi]. Long-term survival of patients has dramatically improved with the new classes of *BRAF* targeted and anti-PD-1 therapies. Historically, approximately 10% of patients with advanced unresectable melanoma were alive at 5 years. The most recent prospective studies with dabrafenib plus trametinib, pembrolizumab, nivolumab, and nivolumab plus ipilimumab have shown 5-year survival rates of 34%, 43%, 44%, and 52%, respectively.

Although melanoma has traditionally been regarded as a near uniformly fatal malignancy, personalized treatment of this cancer relies on the recognition of its genetic heterogeneity and our ability to pharmacologically target these specific and recurrent changes. Recent advances in the treatment of melanoma have come from the understanding that melanoma is a large family of molecularly distinct diseases. Emerging evidence suggests that different melanoma subtypes may each be driven by diverse mechanisms of progression, associated with differing mechanisms of tumor escape and specific immunosuppression, innate immune cell activation, and altered T-cell trafficking into tumor sites that in turn modulate response to immunotherapies.

Monitoring

Most metastases occur in the first 1 to 3 years after treatment of the primary tumor, and an estimated 4% to 8% of patients with a history of melanoma develop another primary melanoma, usually within the first 3 to 5 years following diagnosis. The risk of new primary melanoma increases in the presence of multiple dysplastic nevi and family history of melanoma. Consider cancer genetics consultation in patients with three or more melanomas in aggregate in first-degree or second-degree relatives on the same side of the family, families with three or more cases of melanoma or pancreatic cancer on the same side of the family, and (in low-incidence countries) patients with three or more primary melanomas.

The frequency of dermatologic monitoring is as follows:
- For patients with stage IA to IIA: every 6 to 12 months for 5 years, then every year as needed.
- For patients with stage IIB to IIC: every 3 to 6 months for 2 years, then every 3 to 12 months for 3 years, then every year as needed.

Follow-up visits for all patients should include a thorough medical history, review of systems, complete skin examination, and examination of lymph nodes. In patients at high risk for metastatic disease or with an abnormal examination, appropriate imaging studies, laboratory studies, or biopsies may be indicated. Evidence to support the use of routine imaging and laboratory studies in asymptomatic resected stage I to II melanoma patients with a normal physical examination remains controversial and is left to the discretion of the physician.

Complications

Metastasis may occur locally in the regional lymph node basins, or it can occur distally in the skin (away from the melanoma scar), the remote lymph node(s), the viscera, and skeletal and central nervous system sites.

References

Abbasi NR, Shaw HM, Rigel DS, et al: Early diagnosis of cutaneous melanoma: revisiting the ABCD criteria, *JAMA: The Journal of the American Medical Association* 292:2771–2776, 2004.
Cancer Genome Atlas N: Genomic classification of cutaneous melanoma, *Cell* 161:1681–1696, 2015.

Gershenwald JE, Scolyer RA, Hess KR, et al: Melanoma staging: evidence-based changes in the American joint committee on cancer eighth edition cancer staging manual, *CA: A Cancer Journal for clinicians* 67:472–492, 2017.
Guy Jr GP, Thomas CC, Thompson T, et al: Vital signs: melanoma incidence and mortality trends and projections - United States, 1982-2030, *MMWR Morb Mortal Wkly Rep* 64:591–596, 2015.
Kwak M, Farrow NE, Salama AKS, et al: Updates in adjuvant systemic therapy for melanoma, *Journal of Surgical Oncology* 119:222–231, 2019.
Larkin J, Chiarion-Sileni V, Gonzalez R, et al: Five-Year Survival with Combined Nivolumab and Ipilimumab in Advanced Melanoma, *The New England Journal of Medicine* 381:1535–1546, 2019.
National Comprehensive Cancer Network (NCCN) Clinical Practice Guidelines in Oncology. Cutaneous Melanoma. Version 2.2020. nccn.org.
Robert C, Grob JJ, Stroyakovskiy D, et al: Five-Year Outcomes with Dabrafenib plus Trametinib in Metastatic Melanoma, *The New England Journal of Medicine* 381:626–636, 2019.
Sladden MJ, Balch C, Barzilai DA, et al: Surgical excision margins for primary cutaneous melanoma, *The Cochrane Database of Systematic Reviews* CD004835, 2009.
Soura E, Eliades PJ, Shannon K, Stratigos AJ, Tsao H: Hereditary melanoma: Update on syndromes and management: Genetics of familial atypical multiple mole melanoma syndrome, *Journal of the American Academy of Dermatology* 74:395–407, 2016; quiz 408-310.
Wong SL, Faries MB, Kennedy EB, et al: Sentinel Lymph Node Biopsy and Management of Regional Lymph Nodes in Melanoma: American Society of Clinical Oncology and Society of Surgical Oncology Clinical Practice Guideline Update, *Journal of Clinical Oncology: Official Journal of the American Society of Clinical Oncology* 36:399–413, 2018.
Yeh I, Jorgenson E, Shen L, et al: Targeted Genomic Profiling of Acral Melanoma, *Journal of the National Cancer Institute* 111:1068–1077, 2019.

NEVI

Method of
Jane M. Grant-Kels, MD; and Michael Murphy, MD

CURRENT DIAGNOSIS

Benign Melanocytic Lesions
- Symmetrical
- Sharply demarcated border
- Uniform color
- Diameter usually 6 mm or less and stable

Malignant Melanocytic Lesions
- Asymmetrical
- Poorly circumscribed border
- Variegated in color
- Diameter often >6 mm and increasing (changing or evolving)

CURRENT THERAPY

- Acquired melanocytic nevus: No treatment is required unless the lesion is asymmetrical or has an irregular border, change or variegation in color, or change in diameter. Symptomatic lesions should be biopsied.
- Recurrent melanocytic nevus: No treatment required if the original biopsy was benign.
- Halo melanocytic nevus: No treatment, but excision is recommended if atypical clinical features are identified.
- Congenital melanocytic nevus: Removal based on melanoma risk, cosmetics, and functional outcome. If not excised, routine follow-up with the use of photography, dermoscopy, and computer assistance is recommended.
- Blue nevus: No treatment, but excision is recommended if atypical clinical features are identified.
- Spitz nevus: If clinically unusual, a complete excisional biopsy is recommended.
- Dysplastic nevus: If only one lesion is present, excision may be considered. Patients with many dysplastic nevi require close surveillance, with removal of any lesion suspicious for melanoma.

Melanocytic nevi, or moles, are benign neoplasms composed of melanocytes. Melanocytic nevus cells are derived from melanocytes. Compared with melanocytes, nevus cells are not dendritic, are larger, and contain more abundant cytoplasm, often with coarse melanin granules. Nevus cells tend to aggregate into groups or nests. Melanocytic nevi are extremely common and can be found on almost everyone, anywhere on the cutaneous surface. This article discusses the most common types of melanocytic nevi: acquired melanocytic nevi, recurrent melanocytic nevi, halo melanocytic nevi, congenital melanocytic nevi (CMN), blue nevi, Spitz nevi, and dysplastic melanocytic nevi.

Melanocytic nevi demonstrate both heterogeneous clinical and molecular characteristics, but share common "driver" mutations with melanoma. Acquired melanocytic nevi and dysplastic nevi commonly harbor oncogenic mutations in BRAF, which is the predominant oncogene in melanoma. CMN and blue nevi frequently exhibit NRAS mutations and GNAQ/GNA11 mutations, respectively. Spitz nevi and atypical Spitz tumors often show HRAS and BAP1 alterations, in addition to rearrangements in other kinase genes. These early "driver" mutations are believed to initiate the development of benign melanocytic nevi.

Acquired Melanocytic Nevi

Acquired melanocytic nevi are subdivided into junctional, compound, and intradermal types based on the location of the nevus cells. By definition, these lesions are not present at birth but can begin to appear in early childhood, usually after 6 to 12 months of age. Peak ages of appearance of melanocytic nevi are 2 to 3 years of age in children and 11 to 18 years in adolescents. Although nevi can appear at any age, it is relatively unusual for new melanocytic nevi to develop in middle-aged or older adults. With time, nevi can spontaneously regress. Consequently, patients in their ninth decade of life usually demonstrate few melanocytic nevi. An average white adult has 10 to 40 melanocytic nevi, but African Americans have far fewer, averaging only 2 to 8.

The number and location of melanocytic nevi have been shown to be associated with sun exposure, immunologic factors, and genetics. Consequently, melanocytic nevi are most numerous on the sun-exposed skin of the head, neck, trunk, and extremities, but they are only rarely found on covered areas such as the buttocks, female breasts, and scalp. Evidence suggests that patients with an increased number of melanocytic nevi (>50) might have an increased risk of melanoma.

Melanocytic nevi appear in a sequential fashion. Junctional melanocytic nevi arise during childhood as flat, dark macules. Histologically, an increase in single or nested melanocytes is located at the dermoepidermal junction. With time, some of the junctional nests of melanocytes migrate into the dermis (compound melanocytic nevi). Clinically, compound melanocytic nevi are elevated and less heavily pigmented than junctional melanocytic nevi. Ultimately, all of the nevus cells migrate into the dermis (intradermal melanocytic nevi), resulting in the development of a tan or skin-colored dome-shaped papule. Melanocytic nevi can be flat or elevated and even polypoid, papillomatous, or verrucous, and can demonstrate a range of color from skin-tone to black, but they are characteristically uniform in color, symmetrical, well margined, and usually smaller than 6 mm in diameter.

All melanocytic lesions of clinical concern should be examined with a dermatoscope—a handheld instrument with a magnified lens and a light source similar to an ophthalmoscope. This instrument allows evaluation of colors and microstructures not visible to the naked eye, helps determine whether pigmented lesions are melanocytic or nonmelanocytic, and aids in distinguishing whether melanocytic pigmented lesions are likely to be malignant. Used by an experienced physician with proper training, the dermatoscope improves diagnostic accuracy by 20% to 30%. Another useful technology is reflectance confocal microscopy (RCM), as it safely offers noninvasive imaging of skin lesions at cellular-level magnification and is reported to reduce unnecessary biopsies by 50% to 60%. RCM utilizes a low-energy laser light that focuses on a specific area of tissue; the magnitude of back-scattering of light depends on the differences in refractive indices of various structures in the skin. The horizontal images of the skin afford review of a lesion up to 8 mm × 8 mm in diameter and extend 200 to 300 µm into the skin.

It is unnecessary to surgically remove all melanocytic nevi because they are benign neoplasms of melanocytes. However, indications for removal include ABCDE (asymmetry, irregular border, variegation or change in color, change in diameter, or evolving), symptoms (e.g., pruritus), evidence of inflammation or irritation, cosmetic issues, and patient anxiety. Melanocytic nevi on acral, genital, or scalp skin that appear benign do not require surgical removal. Shave biopsies are appropriate therapy for lesions considered clinically benign. However, if a lesion is being removed because of concern regarding the possibility of malignancy, an excisional biopsy (biopsy of choice) or incisional biopsy (including a deep scoop) that extends to the subcutaneous tissue is indicated. All melanocytic lesions should be submitted to a dermatopathologist for histologic review. A history of recent sun exposure or trauma should be conveyed to the dermatopathologist because such external trauma can induce reactive atypical histologic findings.

Recurrent Melanocytic Nevi

Recurrent melanocytic nevi are melanocytic nevi that have previously been incompletely removed (either iatrogenically or traumatically) and have recurred weeks to months later. Irregular brown pigmentation is clinically noted within the scar site. If the original biopsy demonstrated a benign melanocytic nevus, re-treatment is unnecessary unless the aforementioned indications are present. However, these nevi can demonstrate pseudomelanomatous histologic features. Therefore if the repigmented area is excised, the dermatopathologist should be notified of the clinical history and, if possible, the slides from the original biopsy should be obtained and reviewed to ensure that the lesion is not histologically misdiagnosed.

Halo (Melanocytic) Nevi

Halo (melanocytic) nevi are melanocytic nevi in which a white rim or halo has developed. This phenomenon most commonly occurs around compound or intradermal nevi and is histologically associated with a dense, bandlike inflammatory infiltrate. The white halo area is histologically characterized by diminished or absent melanocytes and melanin. Approximately 20% of patients with halo nevi also exhibit vitiligo.

Although a halo can develop around many lesions in the skin, the most important differential diagnosis is between a halo nevus and melanoma with a halo. The halo and the central melanocytic proliferation of halo nevi are symmetrical, round or oval, and sharply demarcated. Halo nevi most commonly occur in adolescence as an isolated event, but approximately 25% to 50% of affected persons have two or more.

The clinical course of halo nevi is variable. With time, the halo can repigment while the central nevus persists. Alternatively, the melanocytic nevus can regress completely and leave a depigmented macule that can persist or repigment over months or years.

Halo nevi do not require surgical excision unless atypical clinical features suggest the possibility of an atypical melanocytic lesion. It is advisable (particularly in adults, in whom halo nevi are less common) to perform a complete cutaneous examination with and without the aid of a Wood's lamp to rule out any associated atypical pigmented or regressed lesions. All patients should be advised to use sunscreens or protective clothing because of the increased risk of sunburn in the depigmented halo region.

Congenital Melanocytic Nevi

By definition, CMN are present at birth. Arbitrarily, they have been classified into small (<1.5 cm), medium (1.5 to 20 cm), and large (>20 cm) lesions. Terms such as *bathing trunk* or *garment-type* nevi refer to CMN that cover a significant portion of the cutaneous surface.

The approximate incidence of small congenital nevi is 1% of all live births. Large congenital nevi are rare and reported in only 1 in 20,000 births. Histologically, some congenital nevi have distinguishing histologic features (melanocytic nevus cells that extend into the deeper dermis as well as the subcutis and melanocytic nevus cells arranged periadnexally, angiocentrically, within nerves, and interposed between collagen bundles). However, these features have been identified in some acquired melanocytic nevi and are absent in some congenital nevi (especially small ones). In addition, the history obtained from the patient or their parents is often inaccurate. Consequently, it can be very difficult in some cases to distinguish a small congenital nevus from an acquired nevus.

Congenital nevi can give rise to dermal or subcutaneous nodular melanocytic proliferations. The vast majority of these lesions, particularly in the neonatal period, are biologically benign, despite a worrisome clinical presentation and atypical histologic features. Genetic analysis has shown that benign melanocytic proliferations within congenital nevi harbor aberrations qualitatively and quantitatively different from those seen in melanoma.

Patients with multiple CMN (two or more, of any site or size) are at risk for extracutaneous (i.e., endocrine, metabolic, neurological) manifestations, termed *CMN syndrome*. The primary significance of congenital nevi is related to the potential risk for progression to melanoma. Essentially, the larger the nevus, particularly if accompanied by multiple small CMN, the greater the risk of progression to melanoma. Historically, even small nevi were estimated to exhibit a lifetime melanoma risk of 5%. However, recent prospective studies suggest that small and medium congenital nevi are associated with a low risk that may approximate the risk of acquired nevi. Conversely, large congenital nevi have a lifetime risk of melanomatous progression of approximately 6.3%. Up to two-thirds of melanomas that arise within these giant congenital nevi have a nonepidermal origin (arising mainly in the deep dermis and subcutis with high Breslow thickness on presentation), thus making clinical observation for malignant change difficult. Approximately 50% of these melanomas occur in the first 5 years of life, 60% in the first decade, and 70% before 20 years of age. Patients with large congenital nevi, especially those that involve posterior axial locations (head, neck, back, or buttocks) and are associated with satellite congenital nevi, are at increased risk for neurocutaneous melanosis (melanosis of the leptomeninges) and primary central nervous system (CNS) melanoma. Recent data suggest that in up to one-third of these patients, the primary melanoma develops within the CNS rather than the skin. The risk of melanoma appears to be higher in those with congenital abnormalities of the CNS (12% vs. 1% to 2% without CNS changes).

For large congenital nevi that involve a posterior axial location, screening magnetic resonance imaging (MRI) is indicated to characterize congenital disease, if any, and act as a baseline should the child present with new neurological symptoms at a later stage. If clinical symptoms or MRI indicate neurocutaneous melanosis, excision of the large nevus should be postponed until 2 years of age (the median age of neurologic symptoms). Patients with neurocutaneous melanosis have a greater than 50% mortality rate within 3 years. The risk and morbidity of multiple, staged excisions of a large CMN is not appropriate in patients with symptomatic neurocutaneous melanosis. All other large CMN are candidates for excision as soon as general anesthesia is considered a relatively safe risk. Other issues that need to be considered before undertaking staged excisions include cosmetic issues, functional outcome, and psychosocial issues. The staged excisions are usually started after 6 months of age for nevi on the trunk and extremities and later for those on the scalp to allow closure of the fontanelle. If removal is not undertaken, follow-up with monthly self-examination, photography, dermoscopy, confocal laser microscopy, and computer assistance are recommended.

For small congenital nevi, routine excision is not always recommended because the risk of melanoma is lower, and if it occurs, it usually arises within the epidermis after puberty. If the lesions are not excised, follow-up by alternating visits to a dermatologist and primary care physician along with serial photography are indicated. Inasmuch as small congenital nevi typically enlarge with the growth of the child and can change in appearance with time, educating families on benign, predictable changes in contradistinction to potentially alarming changes is extremely important. If a lesion enlarges or changes suddenly or if parental anxiety or cosmetic issues arise, excision should then be contemplated for even small congenital nevi. Elective excision is best done when the patient is approximately 8 years old. With the use of topical anesthetic cream EMLA (eutectic mixture of local anesthetics: 2.5% lidocaine plus 2.5% prilocaine) or topical 4% lidocaine (ELA-Max), children of this age are usually cooperative and unscathed by the procedure.

Blue Nevi

Blue nevi occur primarily on the face and scalp, in addition to the dorsal surfaces of the hands and feet, as well-circumscribed, slightly raised or dome-shaped bluish papules that are usually less than 1 cm in diameter. Although these lesions are usually acquired in childhood and adolescence, rare congenital lesions have been reported. Histologically, blue nevi demonstrate a combination of intradermal spindle or dendritic melanin-pigmented melanocytes and melanophages with dermal fibrosis. The blue appearance of these lesions is a function of both the depth of the melanin in the dermis and the Tyndall phenomenon: longer wavelengths of light penetrate the deep dermis and are absorbed by the lesional melanin, and shorter wavelengths (e.g., blue) are reflected back. Blue nevi that are clinically stable and that do not demonstrate atypical features do not require removal.

Spitz Nevi

Nevi of large spindle and epithelioid cells (Spitz nevi) are relatively uncommon. In Australia, an annual incidence of 1.4 per 100,000 people has been recorded. Most Spitz nevi are noted in children and adolescents: One-third occur before the age of 10 years, one-third between the ages 10 to 20 years, and one-third past the age of 20 years. Rarely, lesions can occur in patients older than 40 years. Seven percent of Spitz nevi have been reported as congenital.

Four clinical types of Spitz nevi are recognized: light-colored soft Spitz nevi that can resemble a pyogenic granuloma; light-colored hard Spitz nevi that can resemble a dermatofibroma; dark Spitz nevi that must be distinguished from other melanocytic lesions, including melanoma; and disseminated or agminated Spitz nevi. Spitz nevi are typically smaller than 6 mm in diameter and dome shaped, with a smooth pink or tan surface and sharp borders. Although they can occur anywhere on the cutaneous surface except mucosal or palmoplantar areas, they are most commonly seen on the face (especially in children) and legs (especially in women). Spitz nevi in adults are usually more heavily melanized than those in children.

Dermatoscopy or epiluminescent microscopy (examination of lesions with enhanced light and a dermatoscope) helps magnify the images in vivo and can assist in establishing the clinical diagnosis of some Spitz nevi. Histologically, the lesion can demonstrate features similar to those of melanoma, which earned the lesion its original designation by Sophie Spitz as a melanoma of childhood. Because Spitz nevi can be histologically difficult to distinguish from melanoma, if a biopsy is performed on a lesion because of parental, cosmetic, or transitional concern, complete excision with clear margins is recommended. Spitz nevi show fundamental genomic differences compared with melanoma, consistent with the generally benign behavior of these lesions. Spitz nevi typically demonstrate no or only a very restricted set of chromosomal aberrations (i.e., 11p gain in a subset of Spitz nevi). A distinct subset of atypical Spitz tumors is characterized by BRAF mutation and loss of BAP1 expression.

Dysplastic Melanocytic Nevi

Dysplastic melanocytic nevi, or Clark's nevi, or nevi with architectural disorder and cytologic atypia, can occur sporadically as an isolated lesion or lesions or as part of a familial autosomal dominant syndrome. When such lesions occur sporadically, they are considered a marker for a patient who is at increased risk of melanoma (6% risk vs. an approximate 0.6% risk in the normal white population in the United States). In association with a family history or personal past medical history of melanoma, patients with dysplastic melanocytic nevi should be considered to have a significant risk of melanoma. One first-degree family member with melanoma is associated with a lifetime risk of melanoma of 15% for the patient with dysplastic melanocytic nevi. Two or more first-degree family members with melanoma place a patient with dysplastic melanocytic nevi at a lifetime risk of developing melanoma that approaches 100%. Less commonly, dysplastic melanocytic nevi can progress to melanoma. Such progression has been documented by serial photography. However, these data are confounded by the fact that clinically and histologically dysplastic melanocytic nevi may be difficult to distinguish from an early melanoma.

Dysplastic melanocytic nevi are clinically distinguished from common acquired melanocytic nevi by a diameter usually larger than 6 mm, an irregular border, asymmetry, and variable color with possible shades of brown, red, pink, and black; dysplastic melanocytic nevi can be flat, with or without a raised center (fried egg appearance). The lesions begin to appear in mid-childhood and early adolescence. New lesions can appear throughout the patient's life. In addition to the back and extremities, these lesions can occur on sun-protected areas, including the scalp, buttocks, and female breasts. Dysplastic melanocytic nevi can be few or numerous, with hundreds of lesions.

Histologically, dysplastic melanocytic nevi show both architectural disorder: extension of the junctional component beyond the dermal component (shouldering); bridging of nests between adjacent rete ridges; papillary dermal concentric and lamellar fibroplasia; and a variable lymphocytic infiltrate with vascular ectasias. They also show cytologic atypia of melanocytes: increased nuclear size, hyperchromasia, dispersion, or variation of nuclear chromatin patterns, and the presence of nucleoli. Although there is some discordance in the histologic grading of dysplastic melanocytic nevi among expert dermatopathologists, there is some evidence to support the use in clinical practice of a two-tier grading system: Grade A are dysplastic melanocytic nevi with mild or moderate cytologic atypia, and grade B are dysplastic melanocytic nevi with severe cytologic atypia. The probability of having a personal history of melanoma in any given patient with dysplastic melanocytic nevi correlates with the grade of cytologic atypia in melanocytic nevi cells. In addition, the presence of severe cytologic atypia in dysplastic melanocytic nevi correlates with a significantly greater risk of melanoma development (19.7%) compared with moderate (8.1%) or mild (5.7%) cytologic atypia.

Management of these patients is difficult. Dysplastic melanocytic nevi are not uncommon. Reportedly, as many as 4.6 million people in the United States have one or more sporadic dysplastic melanocytic nevi. Familial dysplastic melanocytic nevi are estimated to involve 50,000 patients in the United States. The risk of melanoma for these patients is probably on a continuum and correlated with their family history of melanoma or dysplastic melanocytic nevi, personal history of melanoma, number of acquired and dysplastic melanocytic lesions, and history of sun exposure. Removal of all dysplastic melanocytic nevi is inappropriate inasmuch as the chance of any single lesion becoming malignant is small and, in addition, the melanoma can arise de novo.

In cases of mild and moderate dysplastic nevi with microscopically positive margins and no concerning residual clinical lesion, observation, rather than reexcision, is a reasonable management option. All severely dysplastic nevi should be reexcised. Partial biopsy of any pigmented lesion that is suspicious for melanoma can lead to delayed melanoma diagnosis and is discouraged.

Management includes patient education and total body photography for comparison at future skin examinations. Patients should avoid the sun and use sunscreens and protective clothing. These patients should have regular biannual or quarterly examinations of the entire integument, including the oral, genital, and perianal mucosa, the scalp, and an ophthalmologic examination. Comparison with the previous total body photographs and use of the dermatoscope can be helpful. Any lesions that are suspicious

for melanoma should be excised. Examination of first-degree family members (parents, siblings, and children) of patients with melanoma or dysplastic melanocytic nevi is recommended to identify other persons at high risk.

References

Argenziano G, Catricala C, Ardigo M, et al: Dermoscopy of patients with multiple nevi, *Arch Dermatol* 147:46–49, 2011.
Arumi-Uria M, McNutt NS, Finnerty B: Grading of atypia in nevi: correlation with melanoma risk, *Mod Pathol* 16:764–771, 2003.
Bauer J, Bastian BC: Distinguishing melanocytic nevi from melanomas by DNA copy number changes: comparative genomic hybridization as a research and diagnostic tool, *Dermatol Ther* 19:40–49, 2006.
de Snoo FA, Kroon MW, Bergman W, et al: From sporadic atypical nevi to familial melanoma: risk analysis for melanoma in sporadic atypical nevus patients, *J Am Acad Dermatol* 56:748–752, 2007.
Ferrara G, Soyer HP, Malvehy J, et al: The many faces of blue nevus: a clinicopathologic study, *J Cutan Pathol* 34:543–551, 2007.
Gelbard AN, Tripp JM, Marghoob AA, et al: Management of Spitz nevi: a survey of dermatologists in the United States, *J Am Acad Dermatol* 47:224–330, 2002.
Goodson AG, Florell SR, Boucher KM, et al: Low rates of clinical recurrence after biopsy of benign to moderately dysplastic melanocytic nevi, *J Am Acad Dermatol* 62:591–596, 2010.
King R, Hayzen BA, Page RN, et al: Recurrent nevus phenomenon: a clinicopathologic study of 357 cases and histologic comparison with melanoma with regression, *Mod Pathol* 22:611–619, 2009.
Kinsler VA, O'Hare P, Bulstrode N, et al: Melanoma in congenital melanocytic naevi, *Br J Dermatol* 176:1131–1143, 2017.
Naeyaert JM, Brochez L: Dysplastic nevi, *N Engl J Med* 349:2233–2240, 2003.
Price HN, Schaffer JV: Congenital melanocytic nevi: when to worry and how to treat: facts and controversies, *Clin Dermatol* 28:283–302, 2010.
Que K, Grant-Kels JM, Longo C, Pellacani G: Basics of confocal microscopy and the complexity of diagnosing skin tumors: new imaging tools in clinical practice, diagnostic workflows, cost-estimate and new trends, *Dermatol Clinics* 34:367–375, 2016.
Roh MR, Eliades P, Gupta S, Tsao H: Genetics of melanocytic nevi, *Pigment Cell Melanoma Res* 28:661–672, 2015.
Sommer LL, Barcia SM, Clarke LE, Helm KF: Persistent melanocytic nevi: a review and analysis of 205 cases, *J Cutan Pathol* 38:503–507, 2011.
Tetzlaff MT, Reuben A, Billings SD, et al: Toward a molecular-genetic classification of spitzoid neoplasms, *Clin Lab Med* 37:431–448, 2017.

NONMELANOMA CANCER OF THE SKIN

Method of
Julia Dai, MD; and Diana Bolotin, MD, PhD

CURRENT DIAGNOSIS

- Skin cancers are polymorphous in appearance, ranging from small papules and plaques to nodules and tumors of different colors, sizes, and consistencies.
- The surface may be smooth, scaly, ulcerated, or crusted.
- A common feature is that all of these skin neoplasms grow continuously and relapse when superficially treated.
- The distinction between skin cancers and benign neoplasms or inflammatory dermatoses may be difficult for the nondermatologist to make.

CURRENT THERAPY

- For the majority of nonmelanoma skin cancers, localized treatments are sufficient and include cryotherapy, immunotherapy, topical chemotherapy, and photodynamic therapy.
- Surgical techniques include electrodesiccation and curettage, simple excision, and Mohs micrographic surgery, which offers intraoperative confirmation of complete tumor removal and maximal cure rates.
- The Mohs procedure is indicated for more-aggressive tumors, for tumors in certain anatomic locations, and in immunosuppressed patients.
- Rarely, sentinel lymph node dissection and adjuvant therapies, such as radiation and chemotherapy, are warranted.

Nonmelanoma skin cancer (NMSC) is a heterogeneous group of skin malignancies that includes basal cell cancer (BCC) and squamous cell cancer (SCC). These are the most common skin cancers and NMSC in the stricter sense of the definition (Figure 1). The more-inclusive use of the term NMSC also includes malignant neoplasms of adnexal, fibrohistiocytic, and vascular origin, as well as Merkel cell carcinoma and metastatic tumors. The vast majority of NMSCs are slowly growing and locally invasive neoplasms that are often diagnosed and treated by dermatologists. Management of the more aggressive tumors often requires a team approach to diagnosis, treatment, and clinical follow-up (Table 1).

Basal Cell Carcinoma

BCC accounts for the majority of NMSC seen in the United States and is increasingly diagnosed in younger patients. Light skin complexion and history of ultraviolet (UV) light exposure are the predominant risk factors for BCC in the majority of the population. Intermittent intense UV light exposures early in life, but not cumulative UV light exposure, pose the highest risk factor for developing BCC later in life. Other risk factors for BCC include exposure to ionizing radiation, psoralen photochemotherapy, arsenic, and smoking. A history of BCC also increases one's risk for developing a subsequent BCC. Immunosuppression, especially in recipients of solid-organ transplants, presents a significant risk factor for BCC. Inherited genodermatoses such as Gorlin, Bazex, and Rombo syndromes, xeroderma pigmentosum, and some forms of albinism are predisposing factors for BCC as well. Mutations in *PTCH1* that are found in Gorlin syndrome have been shown to be an early event underlying BCC pathogenesis.

Clinically, BCC is most commonly found on the head and neck region, though any part of the body can develop this tumor. The presentation varies depending on the histologic subtype of the tumor. Although many histologic variants of BCC exist, the most common subtypes are superficial, nodular and micronodular, morpheaform, and metatypic. The histologic heterogeneity results in variable clinical findings. Superficial BCC typically forms an erythematous scaly patch or plaque. Nodular BCC is the more classic-appearing lesion, a pink pearly nodule with or without central crust or ulcer. Unlike these subtypes, morpheaform BCC clinically resembles an ill-defined scar; it is the most histologically aggressive variant with a tendency for deep local invasion. Metatypic BCC is also known as basosquamous carcinoma, because it has histologic features of both BCC and SCC, though it is distinguished from the latter by molecular markers. This subtype also has a tendency for more-aggressive growth.

Although it is potentially locally destructive, BCC rarely metastasizes. Successful treatment of this tumor involves its local eradication. A number of treatment options exist and depend on the histologic subtype of the tumor. For small, superficial tumors, a nonsurgical approach can suffice, though nonsurgical treatment often carries a higher risk of recurrence than surgical treatment. Nonsurgical options include topical 5-fluorouracil (Efudex 5%), topical imiquimod (Aldara), liquid nitrogen cryotherapy, photodynamic therapy, and local radiation therapy.

Electrodesiccation and curettage (ED&C) is an option that has a high cure rate for small and superficial tumors (95% to 98%). Standard excision with adequate margins is an appropriate surgical treatment providing good cure rates, especially for tumors with nonaggressive histologic pattern. Mohs micrographic surgery (MMS) offers the advantage of precise margin examination during excision and therefore carries the lowest overall rate of recurrence. This tissue-sparing procedure is also advantageous in terms of reconstruction on cosmetically sensitive regions. MMS is indicated to treat recurrent tumors, those in immunosuppressed patients, aggressive histologic variants, and BCCs located on certain areas of the face known to carry a higher risk of recurrence.

Although locally advanced and metastatic BCCs are uncommon, treatment with targeted molecules such as vismodegib (Erivedge) have demonstrated clinical efficacy.

Squamous Cell Carcinoma

Cutaneous SCC is the second most common skin malignancy. Its incidence is rising among both men and women in the United States. Development of SCC is intimately linked to the cumulative ultraviolet radiation exposure of the patient via a mechanism that combines DNA damage with immunosuppression. History of ionizing radiation exposure is a risk factor as well. Similar to BCC, occupational exposures such as arsenic can also predispose one to SCC. Patients with xeroderma pigmentosum or oculocutaneous albinism also are at higher risk for SCC.

Chronic inflammation or injury can predispose to epidermal malignant transformation. Examples of this phenomenon are SCC developing within scars from burns, in chronic ulcers and skin overlying osteomyelitis, and in persistent lichen sclerosus or lichen planus. These tumors have a more-aggressive behavior and higher rates of metastasis.

Human papilloma virus (HPV) predisposes to SCC. Verrucous carcinoma, a well-differentiated subtype of SCC, has a well-documented association with HPV types 6 and 11.

Transplant patients are at high risk for SCC that correlates with the degree of immunosuppression. In fact, SCC development is up to 250 times greater in the immunosuppressed compared to the general population, whereas BCC increases to a lesser extent with immunocompromise. A more common association between HPV and SCC has been noted in the immunocompromised population and might account for the disproportional increase of SCC over BCC in this population.

As with BCC, history of previous SCC has been found to be a risk factor for developing a subsequent SCC. This risk appears especially pronounced in smokers.

Unlike BCC, SCC often has a precursor lesion: actinic keratosis. Histologically, actinic keratosis demonstrates partial thickness atypia of the epidermis, and patients often describe it as waxing and waning. Full-thickness histologic atypia is seen in SCC in situ (Bowen disease), whereas invasive SCC penetrates the basement membrane to invade underlying dermis. Histologically, the degree of differentiation of SCC tends to correlate with its clinical behavior. Well-differentiated lesions tend toward local invasion, as opposed to poorly differentiated SCC, which more commonly is infiltrative.

The typical clinical presentation of SCC is that of a hyperkeratotic pink plaque. More-advanced lesions may be nodular and can ulcerate. In most cases, SCC shows only local invasion; however, perineural invasion and rarely metastasis are more likely with SCC than BCC. The central face, temples, and scalp present high-risk zones for recurrence and metastasis.

Treatment of SCC involves modalities similar to those used for BCC. Cryotherapy is the mainstay of treatment for actinic keratosis. Topical treatment with 5-fluorouracil (Carac 0.5%, Fluoroplex 1%, Fluorouracil 2 or 5%, Efudex 5%) alone or in combination with calcipotriol (Dovonex)[1]; imiquimod (Aldara or Zyclara); ingenol mebutate (Picato); or photodynamic therapy is often used as field therapy to depopulate large regions of the skin of actinic keratosis lesions. Continued sun protection has been shown to be of benefit to prevent progression from actinic keratosis to SCC, especially in the immunocompromised population. Systemic retinoids, such as acitretin (Soriatane)[1] and nicotinamide[7] have also been used for the prevention and reduction of NMSC, particularly in high-risk populations. SCC in situ may be treated with ED&C. Excision with a clear surgical margin is often used in treatment of SCC on the trunk or extremities, but MMS yields the highest cure rates, especially in high-risk areas such as the face and scalp. Adjuvant radiotherapy, surgical excision, and targeted approaches with anti-PD-1 monoclonal antibodies may be used alone or combination for more-aggressive tumors. Overall, the prognosis for a patient

---

[1]Not FDA approved for this indication.
[7]Available as dietary supplement

with cutaneous SCC depends heavily on location, degree of histologic differentiation, invasion, and metastasis.

Neoplasms of Adnexal Origin

The adnexal structures of the skin include the pilosebaceous unit as well as apocrine and eccrine glands and ducts. A great number of benign and malignant tumors of adnexal origin occur in the skin. Most of the adnexal malignancies are rare. Sebaceous carcinoma and microcystic adnexal carcinoma (MAC) are two of the more common adnexal carcinomas that have an aggressive nature and may be subtle at presentation.

Sebaceous Carcinoma

Sebaceous carcinoma is an aggressive malignancy that is most commonly found on the head and neck region. More specifically, it is one of the more common tumors of the eyelid and periocular

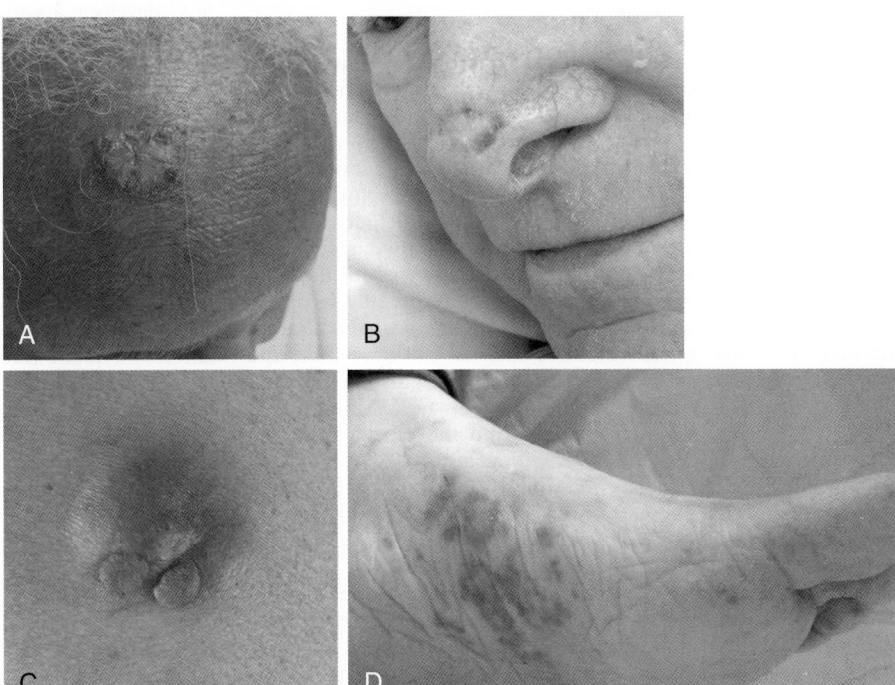

Figure 1 Clinical images of skin cancers. (A) Squamous cell carcinoma in sun-exposed skin of a 102-year-old African American woman. (B) Depressed scarlike appearance of a morpheaform basal cell carcinoma on the nose. (C) This firm tumor on the abdomen is a dermatofibrosarcoma protuberans. (D) Violaceous plaques on the instep in an elderly Greek man typical for endemic Kaposi sarcoma.

TABLE 1	Overview of Therapeutic Modalities for the Management of Skin Cancers	
THERAPEUTIC MODALITY	**NEOPLASM**	**COMMENT**
Cryotherapy	AK, SCC in situ Superficial BCC Kaposi sarcoma	Versatile, but operator dependent
Topical 5-fluorouracil (Efudex)	AK, SCC in situ Superficial BCC	Will treat preclinical AK
Topical imiquimod (Aldara)	AK Superficial BCC	Flulike adverse effects can occur
Photodynamic therapy	AK, SCC in situ Superficial BCC	SCC and BCC are off-label uses
Electrodesiccation and curettage	AK, SCC BCC	
Excision	All	
Mohs micrographic surgery	BCC, SCC MAC, sebaceous carcinoma DFSP, AFX Angiosarcoma EMPD, MCC	Preferred for certain types of invasive tumors (e.g., morpheaform BCC), on high-risk regions (e.g., nose, lip), and settings (e.g., recurrence, immunosuppressed patient)
Radiation therapy	BCC, SCC Kaposi sarcoma, angiosarcoma MCC Inoperable tumors	Careful risk-to-benefit evaluation

AFX, Atypical fibroxanthoma; *AK,* actinic keratosis; *BCC,* basal cell carcinoma; *DFSP,* dermatofibrosarcoma protuberans; *EMPD,* extramammary Paget disease; *MAC,* microcystic adnexal carcinoma; *MCC,* Merkel cell carcinoma; *SCC,* squamous cell carcinoma.

area. Due to its nonspecific clinical presentation it is often treated as chalazion before biopsy and diagnosis. Population-based risk factors associated with development of sebaceous carcinoma include older age and European ethnicity. History of irradiation- and immunosuppression predisposes to sebaceous carcinoma development, similar to BCC and SCC. Sebaceous carcinoma is one of the cutaneous neoplasms characteristic of Muir-Torre syndrome, which results from mutations in DNA mismatch repair genes and is associated with multiple sebaceous neoplasms and internal malignancy.

Clinical diagnosis of sebaceous carcinoma is difficult, and therefore progressive or nonresolving eyelid lesions require biopsy. Treatment of sebaceous carcinoma is primarily surgical. Wide local excision with 5- to 6-mm margins or MMS is indicated. A lower rate of recurrence with MMS (11.1%) has been shown as compared to local excision (32%). Close follow-up is indicated to monitor for recurrence and metastasis.

Microcystic Adnexal Carcinoma
MAC is another adnexal malignancy with predilection for the head and neck. In the United States it is most prevalent in the white population and on the left side of the body, suggesting UV irradiation as a risk factor. Although it can be seen in a wide age range of patients, older patients have a higher risk of developing MAC. The low incidence of this tumor makes it difficult to evaluate other risk factors, though cases have been reported in immunosuppressed patients and those with a history of radiation therapy.

Clinically, MAC occurs as a slowly growing, pink- to flesh-colored ill-defined plaque. Paresthesia and/or numbness are common complaints and have been attributed to the high degree of perineural invasion by this tumor. MAC is a locally aggressive tumor with an unpredictable pattern of infiltrative growth. Histologically, MAC exhibits both pilar and sweat duct differentiation, deep invasion with a desmoplastic stromal response, and perineural invasion.

Surgical excision is the standard of care treatment for MAC, and radiation as an adjunct therapy is reported in a few cases. Because this tumor can extend for centimeters subclinically, MMS is favored as the first-line surgical treatment because it allows complete examination of the surgical margins intraoperatively and has been reported to have a lower recurrence rate than standard excision.

Fibrohistiocytic Malignancies
Fibrohistiocytic tumors of the skin are derived from the mesenchymal tissue and range from those of intermediate malignant potential to aggressive pleomorphic sarcomas. Of these overall rare malignancies, dermatofibrosarcoma protuberans (DFSP) and atypical fibroxanthoma are more frequently encountered.

Dermatofibrosarcoma Protuberans
DFSP is the most common fibrohistiocytic malignancy of the skin. It occurs at various ages ranging from infancy to older adulthood. The pathogenesis of DFSP involves a translocation between chromosomes 17 and 22 that fuses the collagen type 1 α1 gene (COL1A1) with the platelet-derived growth factor B-chain gene (PDGFB). This fusion gene results in overexpression of PDGFB, which acts as a potent growth stimulant for mesenchymal cells. In general slowly growing, DFSPs are locally invasive and infiltrative rather than metastatic. Therefore, treatment of this tumor is primarily surgical.

A high recurrence rate has been noted in a number of studies and is attributed to the infiltrative growth of the tumor. MMS reduces recurrence rates, and is often recommended. DFSP is thought to be a radiosensitive tumor, and adjunctive radiation therapy has been successful used both pre- and postoperatively. The discovery of COL1A1-PDGFB fusion has led to trials of imatinib (Gleevec) therapy as an adjunct to surgery for

DFSP. So far, a limited number of clinical reports have demonstrated regression of DFSPs during treatment with imatinib. Larger studies and long-term follow-up are needed to determine whether this warrants a change to the current treatment recommendations.

Atypical Fibroxanthoma
Atypical fibroxanthoma is a low-grade sarcoma of the skin. This locally invasive tumor favors sun-damaged skin of the head and neck region in older adults. Patients with xeroderma pigmentosum have a higher risk for developing atypical fibroxanthoma. It has a nonspecific clinical presentation, and a biopsy with histopathology is needed for diagnosis. Histologically, this tumor often exhibits marked pleomorphism and frequent mitoses. Often immunohistochemical staining is necessary for definitive diagnosis. Surgery is the treatment of choice for atypical fibroxanthoma. Either wide local excision or MMS may be used, though lower recurrence rates have been reported with MMS. Despite the pleomorphic microscopic appearance, this tumor rarely metastasizes, and the prognosis with appropriate treatment is favorable.

Vascular Malignancies
Vascular neoplasms of the skin are rare. Kaposi sarcoma (KS) and angiosarcoma, both increasingly encountered in healthy older adults as well as immunosuppressed patients, are discussed here.

Kaposi Sarcoma
Controversy exists regarding the nature of cell proliferation seen in KS. Some regard it as a true malignancy, and others view it as a reactive proliferation. Four types of KS exist: KS of elderly men of Jewish and Mediterranean origin, African endemic KS, immunosuppression-associated KS, and AIDS-associated KS. Infection with human herpesvirus 8 (HHV 8) is involved in the pathogenesis of all types of KS. Clinical findings include non-blanching purpuric patches and plaques that can progress to nodules with ulceration. KS can be isolated to the skin or can become disseminated to the lymph nodes and viscera. Diagnosis is established with histopathology and immunostaining. Management of KS is complex owing to the varied clinical course of the four subtypes. In cases of localized lesions, surgery, cryotherapy, or laser treatment may be useful. Radiotherapy can also be used for localized disease. Patients with disseminated KS are generally treated with chemotherapy. In AIDS-associated KS, institution of HIV medications has been shown to effect resolution of KS.

Angiosarcoma
Angiosarcoma is a more rare but aggressive vascular cutaneous malignancy that tends to metastasize and carries a poor prognosis. Clinically, angiosarcoma favors the head and neck area of elderly men; it can also arise within sites of previous radiation therapy or chronic lymphedema. No association between angiosarcoma and HHV8 has been found. Patients present with an asymptomatic enlarging purpuric plaque that can eventually develop a nodular component. Angiosarcoma may have multifocal involvement that is often not appreciated clinically. The treatment for angiosarcoma involves wide local excision and postoperative radiation. The overall prognosis is poor, and distant metastasis-free 5-year survival rates range between 20% and 37%.

Other Nonmelanoma Skin Cancers
Merkel Cell Carcinoma
Merkel cell carcinoma (MCC) is a rare but often fatal NMSC that derives from cutaneous neuroendocrine cells. Fair skin and a history of exposure to UV light are risk factors for developing MCC. Like many other NMSCs, MCC favors the head and neck and is much more common in the elderly. Immunosuppression appears to be a risk factor for MCC development because its incidence is significantly increased in patients with AIDS and recipients of organ transplants. Polyomavirus has been implicated in the pathogenesis of MCC.

This malignancy is often metastatic upon presentation. Clinically, it occurs as a nonspecific, red asymptomatic papule or nodule. A biopsy with immunohistochemical analysis is diagnostic. The therapy for MCC involves surgery with wide local excision or MMS. Sentinel lymph node biopsy can be performed for staging purposes but should be considered on a case-by-case basis. MCC is sensitive to radiation therapy, which is a recommended adjuvant treatment for patients with lymph node involvement. Palliative chemotherapy often produces a response; however, recurrence is common. Preliminary data indicates a promising signal with checkpoint immunotherapy in patients with advanced disease, though prognosis remains poor for metastatic disease or lymph node involvement.

Paget Disease

Paget disease refers to intraepidermal spread of adenocarcinoma. Two types are seen in the skin: mammary Paget disease and extramammary Paget disease (EMPD). Mammary Paget disease is most commonly seen in women and has a strict association with adenocarcinoma of the breast. The lesions are usually unilateral scaly red plaques that favor the nipple. Often the underlying tumor is not clinically present but is detected through imaging. Other dermatoses of the nipple can resemble mammary Paget disease, and therefore definitive diagnosis requires biopsy and immunohistochemistry. Surgical excision along with appropriate treatment of the breast cancer is the recommended treatment. Prognosis depends on the extent of breast cancer at diagnosis, though it appears to be worse for breast cancer patients with mammary Paget disease than those without.

EMPD consists of two types of disease: type I disease, which is associated with distant adenocarcinoma, and type II, primary cutaneous EMPD. Both are very rare but, like mammary Paget disease, have a female predominance. Most commonly EMPD is found in the genital or perianal region; however, other areas of the skin can be affected less frequently. Clinically, EMPD manifests as a well-demarcated red plaque that can become erosive. Long-standing disease can spread from the groin to the trunk, mimicking an inflammatory dermatosis. Definitive diagnosis is based on biopsy findings, and further work-up includes extensive screening for associated internal malignancy. Treatment relies on surgical excision with wide margins. MMS can be used to examine margins intraoperatively. Prognosis for type I EMPD depends on the extent of underlying tumor, but that for type II is favorable.

Cutaneous Metastases

Metastasis to the skin often heralds the systemic spread of an internal malignancy. Primary malignancy underlying the skin metastasis tends to differ by sex and age. In men, lung cancer is the most common source of skin metastasis, whereas breast cancer is the more common primary tumor in women. The head and neck are favored as sites of skin metastasis in men but the trunk is favored in women.

The clinical presentation of skin metastasis is varied and often nonspecific. A new, asymptomatic cutaneous or subcutaneous nodule may be the reason for a biopsy that reveals metastasis of an unknown primary tumor. Diagnosis is made by histopathology and appropriate molecular staining. Specific clinical patterns of metastasis may be encountered. Inflammatory carcinoma can be seen with cutaneous breast cancer metastases. Occasionally, neoplastic infiltration leads to localized areas of alopecia. Zosteriform distribution of skin metastasis has been reported with breast, colon, or SCC.

Leukemia cutis refers to skin involvement with acute myelogenous leukemia, chronic myelogenous leukemia, myelodysplastic syndromes, chronic lymphocytic leukemia, or adult T-cell lymphoproliferative diseases. In rare cases, skin involvement precedes bone marrow disease and is termed *aleukemic leukemia cutis*. In chronic leukemias, skin involvement tends to predict disease progression into the acute phase. Children appear to have a higher incidence of leukemia cutis as compared to adults but have a better overall prognosis.

Metastatic skin tumors are distinguished from primary cutaneous malignancies histologically. Treatment is always geared toward the primary malignancy. Regardless of type of neoplasm or site of metastasis, spread of an internal malignancy to the skin carries a poor prognosis.

References

Alam M, Ratner D: Cutaneous squamous-cell carcinoma, *N Engl J Med* 344(13):975–983, 2001.

Billings SD, Folpe AL: Cutaneous and subcutaneous fibrohistiocytic tumors of intermediate malignancy: An update, *Am J Dermatopathol* 26(2):141–155, 2004.

Buitrago W, Joseph AK: Sebaceous carcinoma: The great masquerader: Emerging concepts in diagnosis and treatment, *Dermatol Ther* 21(6):459–466, 2008.

Chen L, Aria AB, Silapunt S, Migden MR: Emerging nonsurgical therapies for locally advanced and metastatic nonmelanoma skin cancer, *Dermatol Surg* 45(1):1–16, 2019.

Cho-Vega JH, Medeiros LJ, Prieto VG, Vega F: Leukemia cutis, *Am J Clin Pathol* 129(1):130–142, 2008.

Christenson LJ, Borrowman TA, Vachon CM, et al: Incidence of basal cell and squamous cell carcinomas in a population younger than 40 years, *JAMA* 294(6):681–690, 2005.

Cumberland L, Dana A, Liegeois N: Mohs micrographic surgery for the management of nonmelanoma skin cancers, *Facial Plast Surg Clin North Am* 17(3):325–335, 2009.

Dasgupta T, Wilson LD, Yu JB: A retrospective review of 1349 cases of sebaceous carcinoma, *Cancer* 115(1):158–165, 2009.

Dubina M, Goldenberg G: Viral-associated nonmelanoma skin cancers: A review, *Am J Dermatopathol* 31(6):561–573, 2009.

Eisen DB, Michael DJ: Sebaceous lesions and their associated syndromes: Part I, *J Am Acad Dermatol* 61(4):549–560, 2009.

Fan H, Oro AE, Scott MP, Khavari PA: Induction of basal cell carcinoma features in transgenic human skin expressing Sonic Hedgehog, *Nat Med* 3(7):788–792, 1997.

Feng H, Shuda M, Chang Y, Moore PS: Clonal integration of a polyomavirus in human Merkel cell carcinoma, *Science* 319(5866):1096–1100, 2008.

Hussein MR: Skin metastasis: A pathologist's perspective, *J Cutan Pathol* 37(9):e1–320, 2010.

Kamino H, Jacobson M: Dermatofibroma extending into the subcutaneous tissue. Differential diagnosis from dermatofibrosarcoma protuberans, *Am J Surg Pathol* 14(12):1156–1164, 1990.

Kanitakis J: Mammary and extramammary Paget's disease, *J Eur Acad Dermatol Venereol* 21(5):581–590, 2007.

Karagas MR, Stukel TA, Greenberg ER, et al: Risk of subsequent basal cell carcinoma and squamous cell carcinoma of the skin among patients with prior skin cancer. Skin Cancer Prevention Study Group, *JAMA* 267(24):3305–3310, 1992.

Lee DA, Miller SJ: Nonmelanoma skin cancer, *Facial Plast Surg Clin North Am* 17(3):309–324, 2009.

Lehmann P: Methyl aminolaevulinate-photodynamic therapy: a review of clinical trials in the treatment of actinic keratoses and nonmelanoma skin cancer, *Br J Dermatol* 156(5):793–801, 2007.

Lemm D, Mugge LO, Mentzel T, Hoffken K: Current treatment options in dermatofibrosarcoma protuberans, *J Cancer Res Clin Oncol* 135(5):653–665, 2009.

Maddox JS, Soltani K: Risk of nonmelanoma skin cancer with azathioprine use, *Inflamm Bowel Dis* 14(10):1425–1431, 2008.

Marcet S: Atypical fibroxanthoma/malignant fibrous histiocytoma, *Dermatol Ther* 21(6):424–427, 2008.

McGuire JF, Ge NN, Dyson S: Nonmelanoma skin cancer of the head and neck. I: Histopathology and clinical behavior, *Am J Otolaryngol* 30(2):121–133, 2009.

Mendenhall WM, Mendenhall CM, Werning JW, et al: Cutaneous angiosarcoma, *Am J Clin Oncol* 29(5):524–528, 2006.

Prieto VG, Shea CR: Selected cutaneous vascular neoplasms, A review, *Dermatol Clin* 17(3):507–520, 1999, viii.

Rockville Merkel Cell Carcinoma Group: Merkel cell carcinoma: Recent progress and current priorities on etiology, pathogenesis, and clinical management, *J Clin Oncol* 27(24):4021–4026, 2009.

Rubin AI, Chen EH, Ratner D: Basal-cell carcinoma, *N Engl J Med* 353(21):2262–2269, 2005.

Schwartz RA, Micali G, Nasca MR, Scuderi L: Kaposi sarcoma: a continuing conundrum, *J Am Acad Dermatol* 59(2):179–206, 2008.

Smeets NW, Krekels GA, Ostertag JU, et al: Surgical excision vs Mohs' micrographic surgery for basal-cell carcinoma of the face: Randomised controlled trial, *Lancet* 364(9447):1766–1772, 2004.

Spencer JM, Nossa R, Tse DT, Sequeira M: Sebaceous carcinoma of the eyelid treated with Mohs micrographic surgery, *J Am Acad Dermatol* 44(6):1004–1009, 2001.

Ulrich C, Jurgensen JS, Degen A, et al: Prevention of non-melanoma skin cancer in organ transplant patients by regular use of a sunscreen: A 24 months, prospective, case-control study, *Br J Dermatol* 161(Suppl. 3):78–84, 2009.

Wetter R, Goldstein GD: Microcystic adnexal carcinoma: a diagnostic and therapeutic challenge, *Dermatol Ther* 21(6):452–458, 2008.

Yu JB, Blitzblau RC, Patel SC, et al: Surveillance, Epidemiology, and End Results (SEER) database analysis of microcystic adnexal carcinoma (sclerosing sweat duct carcinoma) of the skin, *Am J Clin Oncol* 33(2):125–127, 2010.

PAPULOSQUAMOUS ERUPTIONS

Method of
Tam T. Nguyen, MD

CURRENT DIAGNOSIS

- Psoriasis can be clinically described as erythematous plaques with silvery white scales.
- Severity is rated as mild (< 5% body surface area [BSA]), moderate (5%–10% BSA), or severe (>10% BSA).
- Most cases are mild chronic plaques involving the extensor surfaces.
- Involvement of scalp and palmar and plantar surfaces is classified as severe.
- Psoriasis is commonly comorbid with several conditions, including cardiovascular disease, depression, and metabolic disorders.

CURRENT THERAPY

- Class I/II (super-potent) topical steroid is the mainstream treatment of mild to moderate psoriasis.
- For moderate to severe cases, systemic treatment with methotrexate is the gold standard.
- Narrowband ultraviolet B (UVB) remains a safe treatment option for all patients including children and pregnant women.
- Several immunomodulators or biologicals including etanercept (Enbrel) have been proved very effective therapy. Biologicals can be given as monotherapy or in combination with other modalities for very recalcitrant cases.
- Treatment of comorbid conditions is paramount.

Epidemiology

Psoriasis, a common chronic idiopathic inflammatory disorder, affects 2% to 3% of Americans. The number of persons affected by this condition has more than doubled from 1970 to 2000. It is a chronic disorder that can involve many organ systems including skin, mucosa, the gastrointestinal tract, and joints. Although the onset of psoriasis can occur at any age, there is a bimodal distribution peaking in young adults in their early 20s and again in persons in their 50s. There is an equal prevalence among male and female patients, but the incidence is higher in men among younger adult populations.

Risk Factors

There is a strong family history and association with HLA-Cw6, HLA-B13, and HLA-B27. Psoriatic genes appear to be located on four key genes called pSOR1-4, which show an autosomal dominant pattern. There are about 36 gene loci associated with psoriasis. The genome-wide association study (GWAS) showed that the genes STAT3 and STAT5 regulate the cytokines associated with psoriasis. In addition to the genetic etiology, environmental triggers, such as drugs, infection, and stress, also have a role in the pathogenesis of the psoriasis. Psychogenic stress from home and school is especially common in pediatric cases. Lithium and β-blockers are two well-known triggers of psoriasis. Certain conditions, such as Crohn's disease and multiple sclerosis, predispose patients to developing psoriasis.

Pathophysiology

Even though the exact mechanism is unknown, psoriasis is a disease of T cells that leads to abnormal epidermal differentiation and hyperproliferation. Normal skin has epidermal turnover of about 21 to 28 days, but psoriatic skin turns over every 3 to 4 days. Several cytokines, including IL-12 and IL-23, are part of the immune-mediated disease.

Diagnosis

Although most psoriatic lesions have characteristic scaly and silvery plaques, the lesions can be misleading. Refer to Box 1 for the differential diagnosis. Psoriasis has several subtypes including erythrodermic, pustular, and vulgaris. Psoriasis vulgaris has several subtypes including chronic plaque, guttate (Figure 1), and inverse psoriasis. More than 80% to 90% of psoriasis cases are the chronic plaque psoriasis. Therefore this chapter focuses on this subtype.

Severity of psoriasis is classified based on the body surface area (BSA) involved. There are several severity instruments, such as Koo-Menter Psoriasis, for assessing the severity. One of the best validated tools is the Psoriasis Area Severity Index (PASI). These instruments are used to classify the condition according to coverage of body surface area (BSA) as either mild (< 5% of BSA), moderate (5%–10% of BSA), or severe (>10% of BSA). BSA can be estimated using the rule of 9s. Each upper extremity and the head is 9%, and the chest, back, and each lower extremity are 18%. For children, similar rules apply, except that each lower extremity is 13.5%. When the lesions involve difficult regions such as hands, feet, face, scalp, and genitalia, they are treated as severe regardless of the amount of BSA they cover.

Fortunately, more than 70% to 75% of cases are classified as mild to moderate, and there is no need for blood work. However, when psoriasis is associated with comorbidities, such as depression and heart disease, or when systemic medications cause serious side effects, it may be reasonable to get basic laboratory tests such as a complete blood count with platelet (CBC), chemistry, liver function tests (LFTs), cholesterol panel, hepatitis B and C, uric acid, and erythrocyte sedimentation rate (ESR). For patients at high risk, consider HIV testing. Also, consider evaluating for tuberculosis with a PPD test. These laboratory tests are even more crucial when considering treating with immunosuppressants like methotrexate (Trexall) and biological agents. Liver biopsy should be done if methotrexate is used at a cumulative dose of 3.5 to 4g. Equally important, patients' quality of life needs to be assessed, which can be done with an instrument called the Dermatology Life Quality Index (DLQI).

Differential Diagnosis

The differential diagnosis of psoriasis is lengthy and can be tricky. Box 1 lists the differential diagnosis of psoriasis.

Clinical Manifestations

Most presentations of psoriasis are asymptomatic. When symptomatic, the most common clinical manifestation is pruritus. Other possible symptoms include fever and malaise, especially for more extensive disease. When psoriasis involves the joints, patients can have pain and stiffness in the involved joints; many of these cases involve the distal interphalangeal joints. On physical examination, the lesions are well-circumscribed dark pink to red plaques with silvery to white scales (Figures 2 and 3). Scales can be absent in certain locations, such as the intertriginous area (gluteal folds) (Figures 4 and 5). The margins are sharp and distinct, especially over extensor surfaces such as the elbows and knees (see Figure 2). Lesions also can involve the sacral area, nails, scalp, and the genitalia. If psoriasis forms under a nail, onycholysis (lifting of the nail plate) can occur with pitting and subungual keratosis.

When the scales are removed, several distinctive minute blood droplets appear, called the Auspitz sign. Use caution when removing the scales because it can be painful. When new lesions form at a site of trauma, it is called the Koebner phenomenon. Diagnosis can be made clinically. However, when in doubt, biopsy the lesion, which will show a thickened epidermis with an absent granular cell layer. The stratum corneum is hyperkeratotic, with classic infiltration of neutrophils.

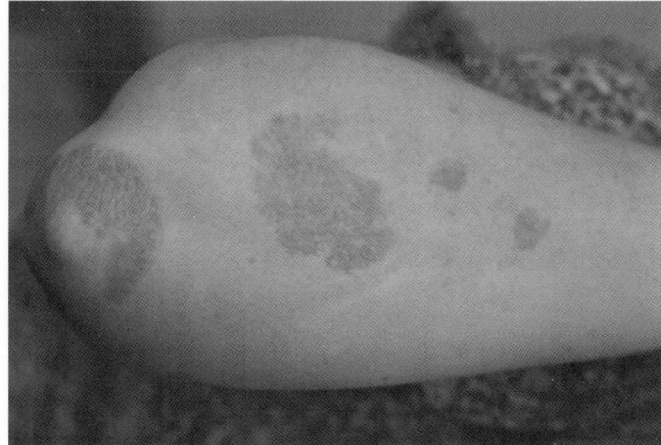

Figure 2 Chronic plaque psoriasis on the extensor surfaces.

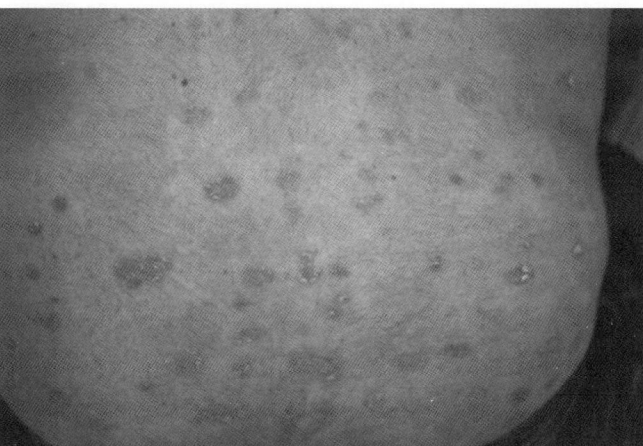

Figure 1 Guttate psoriasis with droplike, discrete papules and small plaques with scales.

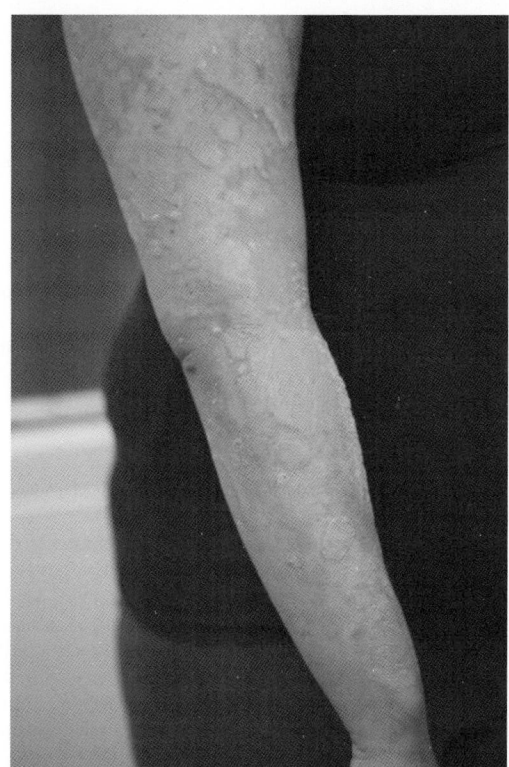

Figure 3 Chronic plaque psoriasis with classic silvery scales.

If this inflammatory process affects the joints, psoriatic arthritis ensues. Although this article does not discuss psoriatric arthritis, it is important to recognize when it occurs. Unlike rheumatoid arthritis, the distal interphalangeal (DIP) joints are regularly involved, but it can affect any joints. Psoriatric arthritis only occurs in 4% to 42% of patients with psoriasis. Diagnosis can be made with the CASPAR criteria, which evaluates five possible presentations, including having psoriasis, nail dystrophy, negative rheumatoid factor, dactylitis, and radiographic evidence.

Treatment

Corticosteroids remain the mainstay for psoriasis therapy; they reduce inflammation, decrease mitosis, and reduce erythema. Because most cases are mild to moderate, the first-line therapy to consider is topical corticosteroids. Even for severe cases that require systemic treatment, topical steroids should still be considered as a first-line adjuvant therapy. Because psoriatic lesions are thickened, it is critical to go directly to super-potent steroids (class I), such as clobetasol (Clobex) (refer to Box 2 for steroid potency). When the localized lesions are lichenified and do not respond to potent topical corticosteroids, using steroid-impregnated tapes (flurandrenolide tape [Cordran]), which function as an occlusive wrap, can help. However, for areas of thinner skin, such as mucosa and lesions on the face, use less-potent topical steroids. Use caution when using class 1 steroids owing to all the potential side effects, including skin atrophy, hypopigmenta

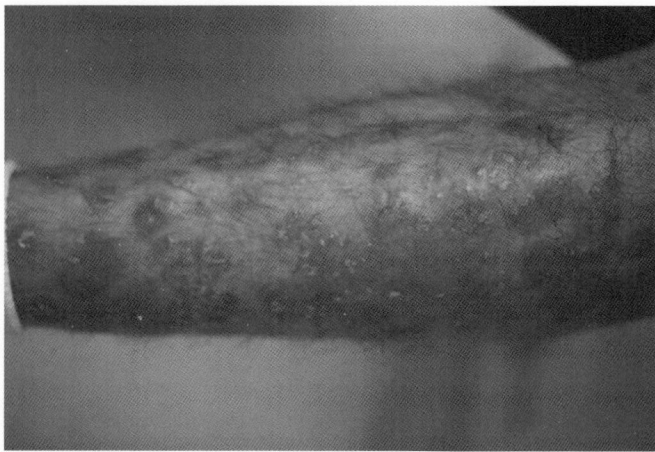

Figure 4 Chronic plaque psoriasis with limited scales.

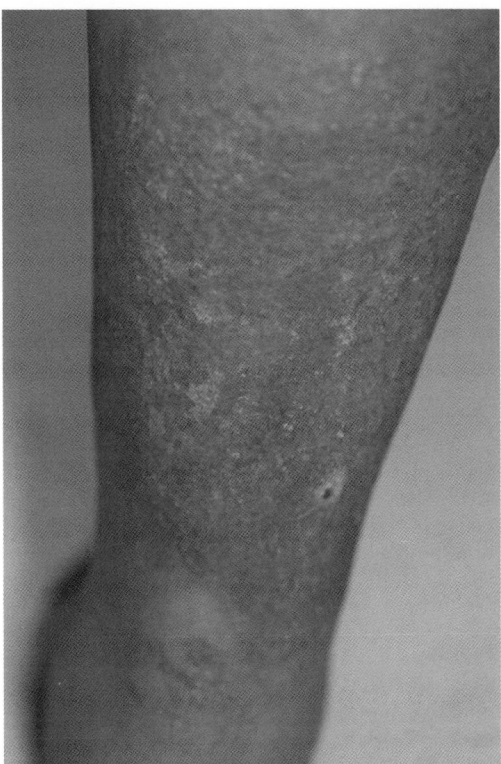

Figure 5 Chronic plaque psoriasis without scales.

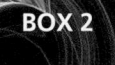
Class 1: Super Potent
Clobex lotion 0.05%, clobetasol propionate
Cormax cream or solution, 0.05%, clobetasol propionate
Diprolene gel or ointment, 0.05%, bethamethasone dipropionate
Olux foam, 0.05%, clobetasol propionate

Class 2: Potent
Elocon ointment, 0.1%, mometasone furoate
Florone ointment, 0.05%, diflorasone diacetate
Halog ointment/cream, 0.1%, halcinonide
Lidex cream, gel, ointment, 0.05%, fluocinonide

Class 3: Upper Mid-Strength
Cutivate ointment, 0.005%, fluticasone propionate
Cyclocort cream/lotion, 0.1%, amcinonide
Lidex-E cream, 0.05%, fluocinonide
Maxivate cream/lotion, 0.05%, betamethasone dipropionate
Valisone ointment, 0.1%, betamethasone valerate

Class 4: Mid-Strength
Aristocort cream, 0.1%, triamcinolone acetonide
Cordran ointment, 0.05%, flurandrenolide
Elocon cream, 0.1%, mometasone furoate
Kenalog cream, ointment, spray, 0.1%, triamcinolone acetonide

Class 5: Lower Mid-Strength
DesOwen ointment, 0.05%, desonide
Diprosone lotion, 0.1%, betamethasone dipropionate
Kenalog lotion, 0.1%, triamcinolone acetonide
Synalar cream, 0.025%, fluocinolone acetonide

Class 6: Mild
Derma-Smoothe/FS Oil, 0.01%, fluocinolone acetonide
DesOwen cream, 0.05%, desonide
Synalar cream/solution, 0.01%, fluocinolone acetonide
Tridesilon cream, 0.05%, desonide

Class 7: Least Potent
Topicals with hydrocortisone, dexamethasone[6], methylprednisolone[6], and prednisolone[6]

[6]May be compounded by pharmacists.

tion, telangiectasis, striae, and potential systemic absorption. In addition to the possible side effects, tachyphylaxis (reduced efficacy with prolonged use) can occur. Therefore it is crucial to limit the use of potent topical steroids to less than 12 weeks.

One way to reduce the use of topical steroids is by using the vitamin D_3 analogue class, such as calcipotriene (Dovonex). This class of drugs inhibits epidermal proliferation and stimulates cellular differentiation. It is considered as effective as medium-potency corticosteroids, without the side effects. However, one drawback is that it takes about 8 weeks to be effective. Therefore it should not be used for acute psoriatic eruptions. More often it is used in combination with topical steroids, since topical calcipotriene in combination with high dose topical steroids like betamethasone (Enstilar) works better than either alone. It is generally well tolerated topically, but about 10% of patients experience burning and itching or hypercalcemia.

Other topical applications include tazarotene (Tazorac) and anthralin (Dritho-Crème HP 1%, Dritho-Scalp 0.5%). Tazarotene is an acetylenic retinoid and can be as effective as high-potency topical corticosteroids. However, its use is limited owing to the side effects of erythema, burning, pruritus, and peeling. Therefore it is best to combine it with corticosteroids to reduce the irritation. In addition, tazarotene can stain clothing, and it is less popular owing to the side effects (redness and irritation on skin as well as staining) and the feel and smell of the solutions. However, it is a good alternative to topical corticosteroids.

For a limited number of thickened lesions, consider intralesional steroid injections, such as a single intralesional injection of a mid-potency steroid (e.g., triamcinolone acetonide or Kenalog-10, 5–10 mg/mL). Most injected plaques clear completely and remain in remission for months. However, as with other steroid injections, side effects of skin atrophy and telangiectasis can occur. Therefore the face and intertriginous areas should not be injected because of the increased risk of side effects.

For severe and recalcitrant cases, systematic medications are needed. One of the gold standards in the United States and many other countries is methotrexate (Trexall) because it is available as a generic. Its exact mechanism is unknown; initially it was believed to inhibit proliferation, but more-recent studies describe an antiinflammatory property. The most common serious side effect of this drug is hepatotoxicity (as many as 33% of patients show some liver disease). Therefore it is crucial to screen for alcohol dependency, liver disease, and obesity. Standard practice is to check baseline CBC and liver function enzymes, and then repeat these laboratory tests after 1 month of therapy. Methotrexate is highly teratogenic; hence it is absolutely contraindicated in pregnancy. After stopping the medication, men should wait at least 3 months and women should wait one ovulatory cycle before attempting to conceive.

There are two methods for initiating methotrexate. Most patients start at an initial dose of 7.5mg (3 tabs of 2.5mg) weekly; in pediatric cases dosage[1] is 0.2 to 0.7 mg/kg weekly. Others start at a higher dosage of 0.4 to 0.5 mg/kg weekly. Unfortunately, there is no current study to compare the two methods. With either dosing regimen, do not exceed 30 mg per week. Methotrexate depletes the body's storage of folic acid, so it is important to supplement folic acid 1mg daily except the day when methotrexate is taken. The methotrexate can be titrated upward every 2 to 4 weeks.

Unlike methotrexate, which can take several weeks before it becomes effective, cyclosporine (Neoral), a calcineurin inhibitor, is rapidly effective for severe cases. It is dosed at a low dose of 2 to 5 mg/kg/day divided into two doses and increased slowly every

[1]Not FDA approved for this indication.

2 to 4 weeks. Maintenance dosage is about 3 to 5 mg/kg/day. A main concern for this drug is nephrotoxicity. As long as the use of cyclosporine is limited to 1 year, it is generally safe. However, kidney function still needs to be monitored regularly. Cyclosporine has been associated with an increased risk of squamous cell carcinoma, especially when the patient has a history of psoralen plus ultraviolet A (PUVA) therapy.

Although not FDA-approved, azathioprine (Imuran) has been a successful systemic medication for psoriasis. Generally, it is initially dosed at 0.5 mg/kg. If there is cytopenia, then the dosage can be increased by 0.5 mg/kg/day every 4 to 6 weeks as needed. Another dosing method is based on thiopurine methyltransferase (TPMT) levels. If the TPMT is less than 5.0 U, do not use azathioprine. If the level is between 5 and 13.7 U, the maximum daily dose should be 0.5 mg/kg/daily. If the TMPT level is between 13.7 and 19.0 U, then the maximum daily dose may be increased to 1.5 mg/kg. There is only one FDA-approved phosphodiesterase type-4 inhibitor (PDE4), apremilast (Otezla). Taken orally twice a day, this drug inhibits PDE4 leading to increased intracellular cAMP levels.

Acitretin (Soriatane) and isotretinoin (Claravis)[1] are retinoids, which are vitamin A derivatives. Although acitretin is more commonly used, either may be used and requires a period of 3 to 6 months to achieve results. However, these retinoids are generally less effective than methotrexate and cyclosporine. Though they are less effective and a longer time is required for this class of agents to work, their main benefits include no malignancy potential and no immunosuppression. Therefore these drugs are safe in patients with HIV and other immunosuppressive conditions. Unfortunately, acitretin and isotretinoin are highly teratogenic. Both male and female patients need to be drug free for 1 year for isotretinoin and 3 years for acitretin before they conceive. For other possible treatment agents, refer to Box 3.

In recent years, immunomodulators or biologicals have revolutionized the treatment course of psoriasis. Generally, criteria for this class of therapy are PASI greater than 10 and failure of other therapies or a contraindication to other therapies such as methotrexate. Most agents are limited to 1 to 2 years of use because most studies have not been evaluated beyond 2 years. Tuberculosis should be evaluated (PPD and possibly chest x-ray) before starting these biologics. All the medications in this class should be avoided in pregnancy. Alefacept (Amevive)[2] and efalizumab (Raptiva) are T-cell inhibitors. Efalizumab (Raptiva) was withdrawn from the market in 2009 owing to reported cases of progressive multifocal leukoencephalopathy. Another class is tumor necrosis factor (TNF).

Etanercept (Enbrel), one of the first TNF inhibitors, should not be used in patients with multiple sclerosis. Four monoclonal antibodies include infliximab (Remicade), adalimumab (Humira), certolizumab (Cimzia), and golimumab (Simponi)[1], and all are TNF inhibitors. In recent years, a new class of biologics that inhibit interleukin (IL)-12 and IL-23 has shown promising results. Ustekinumab (Stelara) was first approved within this class, followed by guselkumab (Tremfya), tildrakizumab (Ilumya), and risankizumab (Skyrizi) in 2019 and mirikizumab in 2020. Secukinumab (Cosentyx), a new biological for plaque psoriasis is a recombinant, high-affinity, fully humanized IgG monoclonal antibody that selectively binds and neutralizes interleukin-17A (IL-17A). Additional three IL-17A inhibitors, ixekizumab bimekizumab, (Taltz) bimekizumab, and brodalumab (Siliq), have been approved for use. Currently, bimekizumab and mirikizumab are investigational drugs in the US.

Etanercept (Enbrel) blocks TNF-α. It is generally dosed at 50mg SC twice weekly for 12 weeks and then 50mg weekly. Patients can self-administer the drug; laboratory monitoring is not required. There are limited data beyond 2 years. Etanercept is the preferred drug for children. Infliximab (Remicade) blocks both soluble and bound TNF-α. Its dosage is 3 to 5 mg/kg IV on weeks 0, 2, and 6, and then every 6 to 8 weeks. Medication generally is infused over 2 hours. It is approved for 1 year. In a comparative study, infliximab was found to be superior to methotrexate. TNF does not appear to increase the risk of herpes zoster but could be associated with an increase in melanoma.

Adalimumab (Humira) blocks both soluble and bound TNF-α. Initiate the dose at 40mg SC every 2 weeks, although some patients require dosing every 7 to 10 days. Alternatively, the initial dose may be 80mg followed by 40mg. Patients may self-administer the injections. As with infliximab, before initiating treatment, obtain a PPD (and consider chest x-ray as well). Antibodies can develop within the first 28 weeks, which will decrease the efficacy of the drug. Both infliximab, which has been in use for many years, and adalimumab have limited long-term safety data beyond 1 year. Some data suggest an increase in cancer risk beyond 1 year. Adalimumab is FDA approved for psoriatic arthritis.

Alefacept (Amevive)[2], a T-cell inhibitor, is dosed at 15mg IM or IV once a week for 12 weeks. Its efficacy follows the rule of thirds: It works well in about one-third of cases, does not work at all in one-third of cases, and the rest fall in between. After a cycle of 12 weeks, the courses may be repeated as needed. However, it is crucial initially to monitor T-cell counts biweekly. A newer agent, ustekinumab (Stelara), has been shown to improve lesions in 66% to 76% of cases. It is initially dosed at 45 to 90mg SC at weeks 0 and 4, depending on body weight. Maintenance is every 12 weeks. Besides ustekinumab, another Il-12/IL-23 inhibitor, guselkumab (Tremfya), was approved in 2017 and is dosed at 100 mg/mL SC in weeks 0 and 4, then every 8 weeks.

When these therapies are contraindicated, one alternative is phototherapy. This is the reason many patients report decreased symptom severity during the summer months due to the natural UV light. Phototherapy started with photochemotherapy with oral or topical psoralens combined with UVA light (PUVA). Although phototherapy is very effective for psoriasis, even in very thick lesions, recent studies have shown an increased risk of skin cancer. Therefore PUVA has become less popular since the advent of UVB radiation treatment, especially with narrow-band UVB (NB-UVB). NB-UVB is equally effective as PUVA and does not have the risk of skin cancer. The exact mechanism is unknown, but it is believed to affect DNA and to suppress IL-17 and IL-23, creating photoproducts that interfere with cell cycle progression. NB-UVB is first-line course of therapy for pregnant and pediatric patients. There are two methods for initiating NB-UVB phototherapy: the skin type protocol, which is easier to execute; and the minimum erythema dose (MED), which is more detailed but more accurate. Refer to Table 1 for treatment protocols. Both protocols generally require 30 to 35 treatments with the optimal frequency of three times a week.

[1]Not FDA approved for this indication.
[2]Not available in the United States.

[1]Not FDA approved for this indication.
[2]Not available in the United States.

TABLE 1 Methods for Initiating Narrow-Band Ultraviolet B (NB-UVB) Therapy and Subsequent Dosing of Phototherapy

THERAPY	MED NB-UVB PROTOCOL						MED NB-UVB PROTOCOL
	TYPE 1	TYPE 2	TYPE 3	TYPE 4	TYPE 5	TYPE 6	
Initial dose	130 mJ/cm^2	220 mJ/cm^2	260 mJ/cm^2	330 mJ/cm^2	350 mJ/cm^2	400 mJ/cm^2	Start with 50%–70% MED The starting dose should be based on the provider's comfort and the patient's history of response to light; e.g., start closer to 70% if the patient has a history of tanning and start closer to 50% if the patient has a history of burning; most centers start at 70%

SUBSEQUENT DOSES

Severe erythema	No treatment. When burn resolves, decrease by 50% of last dose and then increase dose by 10%						
Mild erythema	Same dose	Same dose	Same dose	Same dose	Same dose	Same dose	Decrease dose by 20%
Barely perceptible erythema	—	—	—	—	—	—	Same (erythmogenic) or slight decrease (suberythmogenic)
No erythema: increase dose by	15 mJ/cm^2	25 mJ/cm^2	40 mJ/cm^2	45 mJ/cm^2	60 mJ/cm^2	65 mJ/cm^2	20%

DOSING SCHEDULE

Optimal schedule	3 ×/wk (M, W, F) is the optimal schedule because less is not as effective and more does not improve the resolution. Subsequent treatments should not be less than 24 hours from the last treatment. For the treatment of eczema, no clear guideline to the frequency. Some use 5 ×/wk.

DOSE ADJUSTMENTS FOR MISSED DAYS

MISSED DAYS	DOSE ADJUSTMENT
1–7	Increase doses per skin type
8–11	Same dose
12–14	Decrease by 2 treatments' worth
15–20	Decrease by 25%
21–27	Decrease by 50%
28 +	Start over

Given all the treatment options (refer to Box 4), the choice of the treatment regimen depends on several factors. First, the severity of the psoriasis must be determined as well as the social and emotional impact of the condition. Another consideration is financial, including the insurance coverage, copayment, and deductibles. The lowest-cost treatment is methotrexate, and alefacept is the highest. The patient's conveniences and preferences should be discussed. If the severity is only mild to moderate without much emotional impact, topical steroid and vitamin D analogue should be considered the first options. Other topicals include tar (Balnetar, Psoriasin, Scytera), anthralin (Dritho-Crème HP, Dritho-Scalp), and tretinoin (Retin-A)[1]. If the degree is severe and/or the patient has emotional impact, systemic medications should be used. Most insurance plans will probably require that the patient try at least one oral medication before employing the biologicals. If systemic therapy is used, consider combining it with phototherapy (if possible). If there is no improvement within 2 to 4 months, the regimen should be changed to biologicals. Other combinations may be employed for better resolution.

For healthy patients, any of these therapies may be tried. Unfortunately, there are limitations with children, pregnant women, and patients trying to conceive. For pediatric patients, topical agents should be tried first, followed by UVB monotherapy. If the plaques are still recalcitrant, add either methotrexate (Trexall) or phototherapy. If phototherapy is not available and topical agents have failed, consider using methotrexate or cyclosporine (Neoral). Other options for pediatric patients include adalimumab (Humira) and etanercept (Enbrel). For pregnant women and patients trying to conceive, first try topical agents followed by UVB (ideally narrowband). This combination remains the safest option. If stronger options are needed, the only class B drugs are systemic steroids, adalimumab (Humira), alefacept (Amevive)[2], infliximab (Remicade), and ustekinumab (Stelara). An absolute contraindication in this population is the retinoid class, such as isotretinoin (Claravis)[1] and acitretin (Soriatane).

[1]Not FDA approved for this indication.

[1]Not FDA approved for this indication.
[2]Not available in the United States.

BOX 4 Treatment Options for Psoriasis

Topical
Steroid
Tar (e.g., Balnetar, Psoriasin, Scytera)
Anthralin (Dritho-Crème HP, Dritho-Scalp)
Calcipotriene (Dovonex)
Calcitriol (Vectical)
Adapalene (Differin)[1]
Tazarotene (Tazorac)
Tretinoin (Retin-A)[1]
Calcineurin inhibitors (pimecrolimus [Elidel][1], tacrolimus [Protopic][1])

Oral or Systemic
Methotrexate (Trexall)
Acitretin (Soriatane)/Isotretinoin (Claravis)[1]
Cyclosporine (Neoral)
Mycophenolate mofetil (Cellcept)[1]

Immunomodulators
Alefacept (Amevive)[2]
Etanercept (Enbrel)
Infliximab (Remicade)
Adalimumab (Humira)
Ustekinumab (Stelara)
Secukinumab (Cosentyx)
Ixekizumab (Taltz)
Brodalumab (Siliq)

Phototherapy
UVA
UVB

[1]Not FDA approved for this indication.
[2]Not available in the United States.

Complications

Patients suffering from psoriasis cope with the physical appearance of their lesions as well as the associated mental anguish associated with many other chronic ailments. Furthermore, psoriasis is associated with other chronic diseases, such as abdominal obesity, metabolic syndrome, and atherogenic dyslipidemia. Weight loss can improve the appearance of psoriatic plaques. Patients with psoriasis are more likely to have coronary artery disease, elevated blood pressure, obesity, and insulin resistance. Treating psoriasis decreases the cardiovascular risks. There is an increased risk of malignancy, such as lymphoma. Substance abuse and smoking are common among these patients as well.

References

Ahlehoff O, et al: Cardiovascular disease event rates in patients with severe psoriasis treated with systemic anti-inflammatory drugs: a Danish real-world cohort study, *J Intern Med* 273:197–204, 2012.

American Academy of Dermatology Work Group, Menter A, Korman NJ, Elmets CA, et al: Guidelines of care for the management of psoriasis and psoriatic arthritis: section 6. Guidelines of care for the treatment of psoriasis and psoriatic arthritis: case-based presentations and evidence-based conclusions, *J Am Acad Dermatol* 65(1):137–174, 2011.

Callen JP, Krueger GG, Lebwohl M, et al: AAD: AAD consensus statement on psoriasis therapies, *J Am Acad Dermatol* 49(5):897–899, 2003.

Dubertret L: Retinoids, methotrexate and cyclosporine, *Curr Probl Dermatol* 38:79–94, 2009.

Foulkes AC, Grindlay DJ, Griffiths CE, Warren RB: What's new in psoriasis? An analysis of guidelines and systematic reviews published in 2009–2010, *Clin Exp Dermatol* 36(6):585–589, 2011 Aug quiz 588–9.

Gottlieb A, Korman NJ, Gordon KB, et al: Guidelines of care for the management of psoriasis and psoriatic arthritis: section 2, *Psoriatic arthritis: overview and guidelines of care for treatment with an emphasis on the biologics, J Am Acad Dermatol* 58(5):851–864, 2008.

Herrier RN: Advances in the treatment of moderate-to-severe plaque psoriasis, *Am J Health Syst Pharm* 68(9):795–806, 2011.

Jensen P, Zachariae C, Christensen R, et al: Effect of weight loss on the severity of psoriasis: a randomized clinical study, *JAMA Dermatol* 149:795–801, 2013.

Johnson-Huang LM, Suárez-Fariñas M, Sullivan-Whalen M, et al: Effective narrow-band UVB radiation therapy suppresses the IL-23/IL-17 axis in normalized psoriasis plaques, *J Invest Dermatol* 130(11):2654–2663, 2010.

Kalb RE, Strober B, Weinstein G, Lebwohl M: Methotrexate and psoriasis: 2009 National Psoriasis Foundation Consensus Conference, *J Am Acad Dermatol* 60:824–837, 2009.

Kimball AB, Gladman D, Gelfand JM, et al: National Psoriasis Foundation: National Psoriasis Foundation clinical consensus on psoriasis comorbidities and recommendations for screening, *J Am Acad Dermatol* 58:1031–1142, 2008.

Kuhn A, Patsinakidis N, Luger T: Alitretinoin for cutaneous lupus erythematosus, *J Am Acad Dermatol* 67(3):e123–6, 2012.

Menter A, Gottlieb A, Feldman SR, et al: Guidelines of care for the management of psoriasis and psoriatic arthritis: section 1. Overview of psoriasis and guidelines of care for the treatment of psoriasis with biologics, *J Am Acad Dermatol* 58:826–850, 2008.

Ormerod AD, Campalani E, Goodfield MJ: BAD Clinical Standards Unit: British Association of Dermatologists guidelines on the efficacy and use of acitretin in dermatology, *Br J Dermatol* 162:952–963, 2010.

Trueb RM: Therapies for childhood psoriasis, *Curr Probl Dermatol* 38:137–159, 2009.

Tsoi LC, et al: Identification of 15 new psoriasis susceptibility loci highlights the role of innate immunity, *Nat Genet* 44:1341–1348, 2012.

PARASITIC DISEASES OF THE SKIN

Method of
Andreas Katsambas, MD, PhD; and Clio Dessinioti, MD, MSc, PhD

 CURRENT DIAGNOSIS

Cutaneous Amebiasis
- Purulent, foul-smelling nodules, ulcers, cysts, sinuses
- Microscopic identification of *Entamoeba histolytica* in stool or biopsy samples
- Molecular methods

Cutaneous Leishmaniasis
- Ulcerated nodule (i.e., volcano sign)
- Identification of *Leishmania* parasites by direct examination or culture from the lesion aspirate or biopsy
- Montenegro skin test
- In vitro lymphocyte proliferation assay
- Polymerase chain reaction

Trypanosomiasis
Chagas' Disease
- Chagoma: painful erythematous nodule
- Regional adenopathy
- Cardiomyopathy, megaesophagus, megacolon
- Microscopic examination of *Trypanosoma cruzi* in blood, lymph node biopsy, or skin biopsy or culture

African Sleeping Sickness
- Trypanosome chancre: painful, inflammatory nodule
- Regional adenopathy
- Fever, generalized pruritic eruption with erythematous annular plaques
- Central nervous system involvement
- Microscopic identification of *Trypanosoma brucei* in chancre fluid, lymph node aspirates, blood, bone marrow, cerebrospinal fluid

Cutaneous Toxoplasmosis
- Roseola, urticaria, prurigo-like nodules
- Isolation of *Toxoplasma gondii* in the skin

Ascariasis
- Urticaria
- Identification of adult worm or eggs in stool

Cutaneous Larva Migrans
- Creeping eruption
- Intense pruritus

Cysticercosis
- Subcutaneous nodules
- Isolation of *Taenia solium* in skin lesion
- Serologic tests

Dracunculiasis
- Ruptured blister with prolapsing worm

Filariasis
Lymphatic Filariasis
- Fever with lymphangitis and lymphadenitis
- Chronic pulmonary infection
- Progressive lymphedema leading to massive tissue thickening, especially of the legs and scrotum (i.e., elephantiasis)
- Microscopic identification of microfilariae in blood

Onchocerciasis (River Blindness)
- Subcutaneous nodules, dermatitis, "leopard skin," "lizard skin," lymphedema
- Identification of microfilariae in skin snips
- Blindness

Loiasis (Calabar Swellings)
- Pruritus, localized subcutaneous swellings
- Serpiginous lesion on the conjunctivae
- Microscopic identification of microfilariae in blood

Schistosomiasis (Snail Fever)
- Pruritic papules, edema
- Fever, lymphadenopathy, diarrhea
- Bilharziasis cutanea tarda: pruritic, grouped papules
- Identification of the eggs in stool, urine, biopsy of affected tissues
- Enzyme-linked immunosorbent assay (ELISA) tests

Cercarial Dermatitis (Swimmer's Itch)
- Extremely pruritic erythematous macules, papules, vesicles on body areas exposed to infested water

Human Scabies
- Pruritus worsening at night
- Papules, excoriations, nodules, burrows on genitals, interdigital spaces, axillae, wrists
- Microscopic identification of mites or eggs or feces from burrows or papules

Pediculosis
Pediculosis Capitis
- Intense pruritus of the scalp
- Nape dermatitis
- Identification of lice and nits on the hair

Pediculosis Corporis (Vagabond's Itch)
- Intense pruritus, erythema, urticarial lesions, papules, nodules, and excoriations
- Identification of lice and nits on clothing

Pediculosis Pubis
- Pruritus
- Blue macules
- Identification of lice and nits on pubic hair

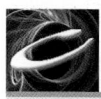

CURRENT THERAPY

Cutaneous Amebiasis
- Metronidazole (Flagyl) 750 mg PO three times daily for 7 to 10 days, or
- Tinidazole (Tindamax) 2 g once PO daily for 5 days, followed by iodoquinol (Aloquin) 650 mg PO three times daily for 20 days or paromomycin (Humatin) 25 to 35 mg/kg/day PO in three doses for 7 days

Cutaneous Leishmaniasis
- Sodium stibogluconate (Pentostam)[10] 20 mg/kg/day IV or IM for 20 days, or
- Meglumine antimoniate (Glucantime)[1] 20 mg/kg/day IV or IM for 20 days, or

- Miltefosine (Impavido) 2.5 mg/kg/day PO (up to 150 mg/day) for 28 days, or
- Topical paromomycin, a formulation of 15% paromomycin and 12% methylbenzethonium chloride in soft white paraffin (Lesheutan)[1,6] applied twice daily for 10 days or
- Pentamidine (Pentam 300)[1] 2 to 3 mg/kg IV or IM daily or every second day for four to seven doses

Trypanosomiasis
Chagas' Disease (American Trypanosomiasis)
- Nifurtimox (Lampit)[10] 8 to 10 mg/kg/day PO in three or four doses for 90 to 120 days, or
- Benznidazole (Radanil, Rochagan)[10] 5 to 7 mg/kg/day PO in two doses for 60 to 120 days

East African Sleeping Sickness
- Suramin (Germanin)[10] 100 to 200 mg (test dose) IV, then 1 g IV on days 1, 3, 7, 14, 21
- For late disease with involvement of the central nervous system, melarsoprol (Mel-B)[10] 2 to 3.6 mg/kg/day IV for 3 days; after 7 days, 3.6 mg/kg/day for 3 days; repeat after 7 days

West African Sleeping Sickness
- Pentamidine (Pentam 300)[1] 4 mg/kg/day IM for 10 days, or
- Suramin (Germanin)[10] 100 to 200 mg (test dose) IV, then 1 g IV on days 1, 3, 7, 14, 21
- For late disease with involvement of the central nervous system, melarsoprol (Mel-B)[10] 2.2 mg/kg/day IV for 10 days, or
- For late disease with involvement of the central nervous system, eflornithine (Ornidyl)[10] 400 mg/kg/day IV in four doses for 14 days

Cutaneous Toxoplasmosis
- Self-limited disease; treatment not needed in healthy, nonpregnant persons
- For pregnant women or immunocompromised patients: pyrimethamine (Daraprim) 25 to 100 mg/day PO for 3 to 4 weeks (plus leucovorin 10–25 mg with each dose of pyrimethamine) and sulfadiazine[1] 1 to 1.5 g PO four times daily for 3 to 4 weeks

Ascariasis
- Albendazole (Albenza)[1] 400 mg PO once, or
- Mebendazole (Vermox) 100 mg PO twice daily for 3 days or 500 mg once, or
- Ivermectin (Stromectol)[1] 150 to 200 µg/kg PO once

Cutaneous Larva Migrans
- Ivermectin (Stromectol)[1] 200 µg/kg PO once; a second dose may be needed, or
- Albendazole (Albenza)[1] 400 mg daily PO for 3 days
- Topical thiabendazole[2] 10% to 15% applied three times daily for 5 to 7 days for a limited number of lesions

Dracunculiasis
- Slow extraction of the worm, which is facilitated by metronidazole (Flagyl)[1] 250 mg PO three times daily for 10 days

Filariasis
Lymphatic Filariasis
- Diethylcarbamazine (DEC, Hetrazan)[10] 6 mg/kg/day PO in three doses for 12 days, or
- Ivermectin (Stromectol)[1] 200 µg/kg PO once together with albendazole (Albenza)[1] 400 mg PO once; kills only the microfilaria, not the adult worms
- For patients with microfilaria in the blood, DEC as follows: day 1: 50 mg; day 2: 50 mg three times daily; day 3: 100 mg three times daily; days 4 through 14: 6 mg/kg in three doses

Onchocerciasis
- Ivermectin (Stromectol) 150 µg/kg PO once for 6 to 12 months, until asymptomatic
- DEC: contraindicated because it may lead to blindness

Loiasis
- DEC[10] 6 mg/kg/day PO in three doses for 12 days
- For patients with microfilaria in the blood, DEC as follows: day 1: 50 mg; day 2: 50 mg three times daily; day 3: 100 mg three times daily; days 4 through 14: 9 mg/kg in three doses

Schistosomiasis
- Praziquantel (Biltricide) 40 mg/kg/day[3] in two doses for 1 day (*S. haematobium* and *S. mansoni*) and 60 mg/kg/day[3] in three doses for 1 day (*S. japonicum, S. mekongi*)

Human Scabies
- Permethrin (Acticin, Elimite) 5% cream rinse, applied for 10 hours; a second application 7 to 10 days later, or
- Benzyl benzoate 25% solution[6] applied topically; second application 7 to 10 days later, or
- Crotamiton 10% (Eurax) applied twice daily for 2 days; second application 7 to 10 days later
- Sulfur 6% to 10% ointment in petrolatum[6]
- Ivermectin (Stromectol)[1] 200 µg/kg PO once: treatment of choice for crusted scabies

Pediculosis
Pediculosis Capitis
- Malathion (Ovide) 0.5% lotion, applied for 8 to 12 hours before being washed off; approved for children older than 6 years, or
- Permethrin (Nix) 1% lotion, applied to shampooed hair and washed off after 10 minutes; second application 7 to 10 days later; approved for children older than 2 years
- Pyrethrins with piperidyl butoxide (RID) applied for 10 minutes
- Benzyl benzoate 25% solution[6]
- Lindane shampoo: for recalcitrant disease, associated with serious reactions not to be used in children
- Ivermectin 0.5% lotion (Sklice), apply to dry hair and scalp then rinse off after 10 minutes

Pediculosis Corporis
- Disinfection of clothes

Pediculosis Pubis
- Same treatment as pediculosis capitis: three times daily

---

[1]Not available in the United States.
[2]Not available in the United States.
[3]Exceeds dosage recommended by the manufacturer.
[6]May be compounded by pharmacists
[10]Available in the United States from the Centers for Disease Control and Prevention.

Parasitic diseases are a common cause of morbidity and mortality, particularly in tropical and developing countries. They may be caused by protozoa, helminths, or arthropods. Because of the immigration of persons from tropical and subtropical countries worldwide and the travel of people from industrialized to tropical regions, parasitic diseases may be found in temperate climates. Skin lesions may provide important diagnostic clues for parasitic infections, and they are reviewed in the following sections, along with updated treatment guidelines.

Diseases Caused by Protozoa
Cutaneous Amebiasis
Intestinal amebiasis is caused by *Entamoeba histolytica*, which may rarely invade the skin and cause cutaneous amebiasis. The disease is transmitted by ingestion of food or water contaminated with cyst forms of the parasite and through fecal exposure during sexual contact.

Cutaneous amebiasis develops at the site of the invasion of the parasites into the skin from an underlying amebic abscess, usually at the perianal area or the abdominal wall. Cutaneous findings include purulent, foul-smelling nodules, cysts, and sinuses, which are associated with regional adenopathy and dysentery. Skin lesions grow rapidly and may lead to death if left untreated.

Diagnosis of cutaneous amebiasis is confirmed by microscopic identification of *E. histolytica* in the stool and in aspirates or biopsy samples obtained during colonoscopy, during surgery, or from the border of an ulcer. Treatment of choice for extraintestinal amebiasis is oral metronidazole (Flagyl) 750 mg PO three times daily for 7 to 10 days or tinidazole (Tindamax). Tinidazole was FDA approved in 2004 for the treatment of intestinal amebiasis in adults (2 g/day for 3 days) and children older than 3 years, and it appears to be as effective as, and better tolerated than, metronidazole. Either treatment should be followed by iodoquinol (Aloquin) 650 mg PO three times daily for 20 days or paromomycin 25 to 35 mg/kg/day PO divided in three doses for 7 days.

Leishmaniasis
Leishmaniasis results from the infection with intracellular protozoan parasites belonging to the genus *Leishmania*. Leishmania parasites are transmitted to humans and other mammalian hosts (e.g., dogs, rodents) during feeding by infected female phlebotomine sandflies that serve as vectors. The parasites exist as promastigotes in the midgut of sandflies and as amastigotes (i.e., Leishman-Donovan bodies) within macrophages of humans and other mammals. Based on the extent and the severity of involvement in the human host, leishmaniasis may be clinically classified as cutaneous leishmaniasis, diffuse cutaneous leishmaniasis, mucocutaneous leishmaniasis, and visceral leishmaniasis.

Cutaneous leishmaniasis (New World or Old World form) begins as a small erythematous papule at the site of the bite of the sandfly, which evolves into an ulcerated nodule with a raised and indurated border (i.e., volcano sign) (Figure 1). The lesions gradually heal with a depressed scar. Diffuse cutaneous leishmaniasis is characterized by widespread cutaneous involvement without visceralization. Mucocutaneous leishmaniasis (known as espundia in South America) affects the skin, the mucosa, and the cartilages of the upper respiratory tract (especially the nose and the larynx) and may result in severe disfigurement. Visceral leishmaniasis results from the involvement of the bone marrow, spleen, and the liver, and it may lead to death if left untreated. It manifests with fever, splenomegaly, pancytopenia, and wasting. Post–kala azar dermal leishmaniasis may appear within a year after visceral disease independent of treatment, and it is characterized by macules, papules, and nodules, which are usually hypopigmented.

Diagnosis of leishmaniasis is based on finding the parasites in the skin from the lesion aspirate or biopsy by direct examination or culture. The leishmanin (Montenegro) skin test shows past and current infections, and it detects the inflammatory response in the skin after injection of phenol-killed parasites into the dermis. A past or current infection is also documented by an in vitro lymphocyte proliferation assay that requires a drop of blood from a finger prick. Polymerase chain reaction (PCR) techniques maybe used to identify different *Leishmania* species. Circulating antibody levels are not considered a useful diagnostic sign.

Cutaneous leishmaniasis is usually self-limited and may not require treatment. Treatment of cutaneous leishmaniasis is indicated in case of numerous lesions or when lesions affect the face to avoid scarring. Therapies include sodium stibogluconate (Pentostam)[10] 20 mg/kg/day IV or IM for 20 days. Meglumine antimoniate (Glucantime)[2] 20 mg/kg/day IV or IM for 20 days or miltefosine (Impavido) for 28 days may be used. In 2014, FDA approved oral miltefosine for the treatment of cutaneous leishmaniasis caused by *L. braziliensis, L. paramensis,* and *L. guyanensis* in adults and adolescents who are not pregnant or breastfeeding. The FDA-approved treatment regimen for persons who weigh from 30 to 44 kg is one 50-mg oral capsule of miltefosine twice a day (total of 100 mg per day) for 28 consecutive days. The approved regimen for persons who weigh at least 45 kg (99 pounds) is one 50-mg capsule three times a day (total of 150 mg per day) for 28 consecutive days. Miltefosine is contraindicated

---

[2]Not available in the United States.
[10]Available in the United States from the Centers for Disease Control and Prevention.

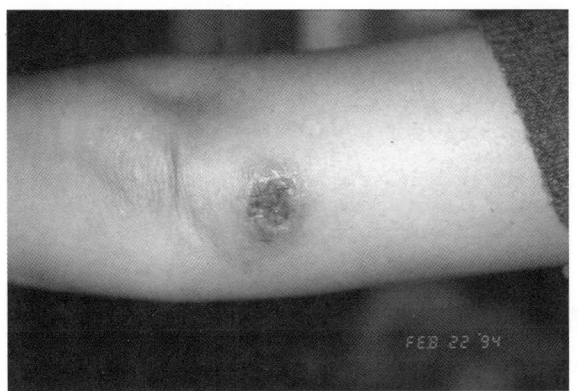

Figure 1 Cutaneous leishmaniasis is characterized by an ulcerated nodule with a raised and indurated border (i.e., volcano sign).

in pregnant women during treatment and for 5 months thereafter. Alternatively, intralesional injections of antimonials 1 mg/kg once weekly, cryotherapy, local heat, oral ketoconazole (Nizoral)[1], topical amphotericin B[2], pentamidine (Pentam)[1] 2 to 3 mg/kg IV or IM daily or every second day for four to seven doses, or topical paromomycin[1,6] (applied twice daily for 10–20 days) may be used.

The production of antileishmanial antibodies does not correlate with resolution of the disease. Infection and recovery are associated with lifelong immunity to reinfection by the same species of *Leishmania*, although interspecies immunity may also exist.

Trypanosomiasis

There are three types of trypanosomiasis:

- American trypanosomiasis or Chagas' diseases, caused by *Trypanosoma cruzi*
- East African sleeping sickness, caused by *Trypanosoma brucei rhodesiense*
- West African sleeping sickness, caused by *Trypanosoma brucei gambiense*

American trypanosomiasis (i.e., Chagas' disease) is caused by the parasite *T. cruzi*, and it is endemic in Central and South America. The disease is transmitted by the bite of infected "cone-nosed" insects, by transfusion of infected blood, by organ transplantation, and across the placenta. During the acute stage, Chagas' disease manifests with a painful erythematous nodule, known as chagoma, which is associated with regional adenopathy. The chronic stage manifests with cardiomyopathy, megaesophagus, and megacolon. Diagnosis is confirmed by microscopic identification of the parasite in fresh anticoagulated blood, in blood smears, by lymph node biopsy or skin biopsy, or by culture. Treatment includes benznidazole (Radanil, Rochagan)[10] 5 to 7 mg/kg/day PO in two doses for 60 to 90 days or nifurtimox (Lampit)[10] 8 to 10 mg/kg/day PO in three or four doses for 90 to 120 days.

African trypanosomiasis (i.e., East and West African sleeping sickness) occurs in Africa and is transmitted by the bite of infected male and female tsetse flies. It manifests with a highly inflammatory, painful, red or violaceous, indurated nodule surrounded by an erythematous halo, called trypanosome chancre, at the site of the inoculation of the parasites. There is regional adenopathy. Later, the chancre resolves spontaneously, and the patient has fever, malaise, a generalized pruritic eruption with erythematous annular plaques or urticarial lesions, and central nervous system (CNS) involvement with personality changes, apathy, somnolence, coma, and death. Diagnosis is based on the identification of trypanosomes by microscopic examination in chancre fluid, affected lymph node aspirates, blood, bone marrow, or in the late stages of infection, cerebrospinal fluid.

Treatment of East African sleeping sickness consists of suramin (naphthylamine sulfonic acid, Germanin)[10] 100 to 200 mg (test dose) IV and then 1 g IV on days 1, 3, 7, 14, and 21. For late disease with CNS involvement, melarsoprol B (a trivalent organic arsenical, Mel-B)[10] is used in the following dosage regimen: 2 to 3.6 mg/kg/day IV for 3 days; after 7 days, 3.6 mg/kg/day for 3 days; and the latter repeated after 7 days. For West African sleeping sickness, treatment of choice is pentamidine isethionate (Pentam 300)[1] 4 mg/kg/day IM for 10 days or suramin (Germanin)[10] as used for East African sleeping sickness. For late disease with involvement of the CNS, eflornithine (Ornidyl)[10] 400 mg/kg/day IV in four doses for 14 days is used.

Cutaneous Toxoplasmosis

Systemic toxoplasmosis (congenital or acquired) is caused by the parasite *Toxoplasma gondii*, and it usually is transmitted from contact with infected cats. The disease may also be acquired by eating raw or undercooked meats from infected animals. Cutaneous involvement is rare. It manifests with punctate macules or ecchymoses in the congenital form, and the acquired form manifests with roseola and erythema multiforme lesions, urticaria, prurigo-like nodules, and maculopapular lesions. Diagnosis of cutaneous toxoplasmosis is confirmed by isolation of the parasite in the skin. Treatment is not needed for healthy nonpregnant patients because symptoms resolve in a few weeks. Treatment for pregnant women or immunocompromised patients includes pyrimethamine (Daraprim) 25–100 mg/d PO for 3–6 wks together with sulfadiazine[1] 1–15 g PO qid for 3–6 wks. Leucovorin[1] should be taken with each dose of pyrimethamine.

Diseases Caused by Helminths

Ascariasis

Ascariasis is caused by *Ascaris* species, mainly *Ascaris lumbricoides*. It is transmitted by the ingestion of eggs in soil contaminated with human feces. Skin involvement of ascariasis manifests with urticaria. Diagnosis is based on finding the adult worm or eggs in the feces. Treatment includes albendazole (Albenza)[1] 400 mg PO once or mebendazole (Vermox) 100 mg PO twice daily for 3 days (or 500 mg once) or ivermectin (Stromectol)[1] 150 to 200 μg/kg PO once.

Cutaneous Larva Migrans

Cutaneous larva migrans is also known as creeping eruption, with the first term describing a syndrome and the second a clinical sign found in various conditions. The syndrome cutaneous larva migrans is caused when various nematode larvae (i.e., hookworms, such as *Ancylostoma braziliense*, *Ancylostoma caninum*, *Bunostomum phlebotomum*) of dogs, cats, and other mammals penetrate and migrate through the skin. Cutaneous larva migrans is transmitted by skin contact to soil contaminated with animal feces. In humans, larvae are unable to reach internal organs and eventually die. Cutaneous larva migrans manifests with intensely pruritic, papular lesions, which evolve as the larvae migrate to a characteristic linear, minimally elevated, serpiginous tract that moves forward in an irregular pattern. Diagnosis is easily made clinically and is supported by a travel history or by possible exposure in an endemic area.

Treatment of choice consists of ivermectin (Stromectol)[1] at a single dose of 200 μg/kg. In case of treatment failure, a second dose usually suffices. Ivermectin has an excellent safety profile, without any notable adverse events, and it has been used in millions of individuals in developing countries during onchocerciasis and filariasis control operations. It is contraindicated in children who weigh less than 15 kg (or are younger than 5 years) and in pregnant or breast-feeding women. Alternatively, repeated courses of oral albendazole (Albenza)[1] 400 mg daily for 3 days

---

[1]Not FDA approved for this indication.
[2]Not FDA approved for this indication.

---

[1]Not FDA approved for this indication.
[6]May be compounded by pharmacists.
[10]Available in the United States from the Centers for Disease Control and Prevention.

may be used. Treatment with oral thiabendazole (Mintezol)[2] 50 mg/kg daily for 2 to 4 days has been associated with adverse events such as dizziness, nausea, vomiting, and intestinal cramps, and it is therefore not recommended. In the absence of multiple or widespread lesions, topical treatments may be considered, such as topical thiabendazole[2] 10% to 15%, applied three times daily for 5 to 7 days, which has similar efficacy with oral ivermectin and no adverse events.

Cysticercosis

Cysticercosis is caused by the larval stage (i.e., cysticerci) of the pork tapeworm *Taenia solium*, and it is the most common helminthic infection of the CNS. It is transmitted by ingesting eggs in food, in water, or on hands contaminated with human feces. Cutaneous manifestations are subcutaneous nodules that occur mainly on the extremities and trunk. There may be involvement of the CNS (i.e., seizures), eye, intestines, skeletal muscle, heart, kidneys, lung, and liver. Diagnosis is confirmed by isolation of the parasite in a nodule and by serologic tests.

Treatment options include surgery, albendazole (Albenza) 400 mg PO twice daily for 8 to 30 days, or praziquantel (Biltricide)[1] 100 mg/kg/day PO in three doses for 1 day and then 50 mg/kg/day in three doses for 29 days. Any cysticercocidal drug may cause irreparable damage when used in the presence of ocular or spinal cysts.

Dracunculiasis

Dracunculiasis is caused by the nematode *Dracunculus medinensis*. It is transmitted by drinking water with copepods (i.e., tiny aquatic arthropods) infected with the larvae of *D. medinensis*. In the human stomach, copepods release the larvae that mature and migrate to the skin, causing an erythematous papule or blister. The blister ruptures, and the female worm can often be seen prolapsing through the skin. Treatment includes extraction of the worm combined with wound care. Metronidazole (Flagyl)[1] 250 mg PO three times daily for 10 days may be efficacious and facilitates removal of the worm.

Filariasis

Filariasis is caused by nematodes (i.e., roundworms) that inhabit the lymphatics and subcutaneous tissues. The most common filarial infections include lymphatic filariasis, onchocerciasis, and loiasis.

Lymphatic Filariasis

Lymphatic filariasis is caused by *Wuchereria bancrofti, Brugia malayi,* and *Brugia timori,* and it is transmitted by mosquitoes. Adult worms result in a chronic inflammatory cell infiltrate around lymphatic vessels, causing their dilatation, hypertrophy, and obstruction. Many patients are asymptomatic, but some may develop fever with lymphangitis and lymphadenitis, chronic pulmonary infection, and progressive lymphedema leading to massive tissue thickening, especially of the legs and scrotum (i.e., elephantiasis). The overlying skin is thickened. Diagnosis is based on microscopic identification of the microfilariae in the blood and affected tissues.

Treatment consists of diethylcarbamazine (DEC, Hetrazan)[10] in the following regimen: 50 mg on day 1, 50 mg three times daily on day 2, 100 mg three times daily on day 3, and 6 mg/kg in three doses on days 4 through 14. Prophylaxis with DEC 500 mg/day for 2 days each month is effective against *W. bancrofti* infection for travelers in endemic areas.

Onchocerciasis

Onchocerciasis (i.e., blinding filariasis) is caused by the filarial nematode *Onchocerca volvulus,* which is transmitted by the blackflies *Simulium.* It may manifest with subcutaneous onchocercid nodules, acute or chronic dermatitis, depigmentation (i.e., leopard skin), and skin atrophy (i.e., lizard skin), and in later stages, it may manifest with lymphadenopathy and lymphedema. The microfilariae have a predilection for the eyes, and the infection can lead to blindness (i.e., river blindness). Diagnosis is based on identification of microfilariae in skin snips.

Treatment consists of ivermectin (Stromectol) 150 µg/kg PO every 6 to 12 months until asymptomatic. DEC is contraindicated as it may lead to blindness.

Loiasis

Loiasis (i.e., Calabar swellings) is caused by the parasite *Loa loa,* which is transmitted by deerflies (*Chrysops*). Cutaneous manifestations include pruritus, urticaria, and Calabar swellings, which are erythematous, warm, subcutaneous swellings associated with the migration of the worm through the subcutaneous tissues. Occasionally, there is subconjunctival migration of the adult worm, producing a migrating serpiginous lesion on the conjunctivae. Diagnosis is confirmed by identification of microfilariae in the blood by microscopic examination.

DEC[10] is the treatment of choice in the following regimen: 50 mg on day 1, 50 mg three times daily on day 2, 100 mg three times daily on day 3, and 9 mg/kg/day in three doses on days 4 through 14. Ivermectin (Stromectol)[1] may cause encephalopathy in patients with a heavy *L. loa* infection. Prophylaxis with DEC is effective for *L. loa* in adults who travel in endemic areas.

Schistosomiasis

Schistosomiasis (i.e., snail fever) in humans is caused mainly by the trematodes *Schistosoma haematobium, Schistosoma japonicum,* and *Schistosoma mansoni.* All trematodes have a life cycle that involves the snail as an intermediate host. The infective cercariae leave the snail, swim, and penetrate the human skin, causing a pruritic papular dermatosis. The disease is transmitted by exposure to contaminated water with live cercariae or by drinking infested water. Skin findings of acute schistosomiasis include pruritic schistosomal dermatitis due to a hypersensitivity response to the cercariae and edema of the face, extremities, genitals, and trunk. Schistosomal fever (i.e., Katayama fever), lymphadenopathy, and diarrhea may also develop. Late skin findings (i.e., bilharziasis cutanea tarda) appear in patients with visceral disease and include firm, pruritic, grouped papules. Secondary infection, ulceration, and development of squamous cell carcinoma may follow. Diagnosis is confirmed by identification of the eggs in the urine or stool, by biopsy of affected tissues, or by enzyme-linked immunosorbent assay (ELISA).

Treatment includes praziquantel (Biltricide) 40 mg/kg/day[3] in two doses for 1 day (for *S. haematobium* and *S. mansoni*) or 60 mg/kg/day[3] in three doses for 1 day (for *S. japonicum*).

Cercarial Dermatitis

Cercarial dermatitis (i.e., swimmer's itch) is caused by cercariae (i.e., larvae) of nonhuman schistosomes that penetrate the skin and die without invading other tissues. It is transmitted by contact with fresh or salt water contaminated with cercariae. It manifests with extremely pruritic, erythematous macules of sudden onset, which evolve into papules, vesicles, and urticarial lesions located on parts of the body directly exposed to the water, while sparing clothed areas. Cercarial dermatitis is a self-limited disease, and treatment is symptomatic with topical steroids and oral antihistamines.

Diseases Caused by Arthropoda
Human Scabies

Scabies is a common skin infestation caused by the mite *Sarcoptes scabiei,* which is an obligate human parasite. Scabies is transmitted by direct contact with an infested individual or by

[1]Not FDA approved for this indication.
[2]Not available in the United States.
[10]Available in the United States from the Centers for Disease Control and Prevention.

[1]Not FDA approved for this indication.
[3]Exceeds dosage recommended by the manufacturer.

contact with bedding and clothing. The incubation period for scabies is about 3 weeks, and reinfestation results in symptoms within 1 to 3 days. Scabies is characterized by pruritus that usually worsens at night. Papules, nodules, excoriations, and burrows may be found. Lesions are usually located on interdigital spaces, wrists, ankles, axillae, waist, and genitals. Scabies manifests as red-brown nodules that represent a hypersensitivity response. In adults, the head is usually spared, whereas the involvement of the scalp, palms, and soles is common in infants.

Crusted or Norwegian scabies manifests with hyperkeratotic papules or plaques of the hands and feet (often with nail involvement) and an erythematous scaly eruption on the face, neck, scalp, and trunk. Because pruritus is often absent, this disease can be misdiagnosed as psoriasis, eczema, or an adverse drug reaction. Lesions contain thousands of mites and are highly contagious. Crusted scabies mainly affects immunocompromised patients (e.g., patients with human immunodeficiency virus infection), mentally retarded persons, or debilitated patients.

Diagnosis is based on the microscopic identification of mites or their eggs or feces from burrows or papules. Treatment should be applied from the neck down in adults, and in infants, application should include the scalp and face (avoiding the eyes and mouth).

Treatment includes 5% permethrin (Elimite) applied for 10 hours and repeated after 1 week. A 25% benzyl benzoate solution[6] is also efficacious in adults, and because of low toxicity, it is recommended in a lower concentration (10%) for children older than 4 months and for women during pregnancy. Sulfur ointments in petrolatum[6] at concentrations of 6% to 10% may be used for scabies in children and pregnant women. Alternative treatments for scabies include crotamiton 10% (Eurax) applied once daily for 2 days, or ivermectin (Stromectol)[1] as a single- or two-dose regimen of 200 µg/kg/dose can be used. Aggressive treatment with ivermectin at a single dose of 200 µg/kg, repeated after 2 weeks with or without topical 5% permethrin cream (two applications, 1 week apart) and keratolytics (5% salicylic acid ointment[1] applied twice daily) is the treatment of choice for crusted scabies. All sexual and close personal and household contacts within the preceding 6 weeks should be treated simultaneously. Bedding and clothing should be decontaminated (i.e., machine washed and dried using the hot cycle or dry cleaned) or removed from body contact for at least 3 days, because the mite dies when separated from the human host.

Pediculosis

Pediculosis (i.e., lice) is a contagious dermatosis, caused by lice, which are blood-sucking, wingless insects and are obligate human parasites. Two species of lice infest humans causing three clinical forms of infestation: *Pediculus humanus capitis* (i.e., head louse), *Pediculus humanus corporis* (i.e., body louse), and *Phthirus pubis* (i.e., pubic louse). The body louse is the only louse that can carry human disease, including rickettsioses and epidemic typhus.

Pediculosis Capitis

Pediculosis capitis is caused by *P. humanus capitis*, and it is transmitted by close contact or by fomites with combs, brushes, towels, and hats. It manifests with pruritus (due to the saliva of the louse), excoriations, nape dermatitis, secondary bacterial infection, and cervical and suboccipital lymphadenopathy. Diagnosis is based on identification of lice and eggs or nits on the hair and on fluorescence of nits with Wood's light. Visible nits are deposited on the hair shaft, close to the scalp. After adequate treatment, nits found at 1.0 to 1.5 cm from the scalp are not alive.

Topical pediculicides should be applied according to the package instructions. Treatment includes malathion (Ovide) 0.5% lotion applied for 8 to 12 hours or permethrin (Nix) 1% cream rinse applied to shampooed hair for 10 minutes. A second application with permethrin is recommended 1 week later to kill hatching progeny. Alternatively, pyrethrins with piperidyl butoxide (RID) can be applied and washed off after 10 minutes. Benzyl benzoate 25% solution[6] is mainly a scabicide, but it may also be used as a pediculicide. Ivermectin lotion 0.5% (Sklice) was approved by the FDA in 2012 for treatment of head lice in persons 6 months of age and older, using a fine-toothed comb. Bedding, clothing, and headgear should be decontaminated (as for scabies) or removed from body contact for 2 weeks. Information for managing head lice can be found at the National Pediculosis Association web site (http://www.headlice.org).

Pediculosis Corporis

Pediculosis corporis (i.e., vagabond's itch) is caused by *P. humanus corporis*, which lives and reproduces in the lining of clothes and leaves the clothing only for feeding from the skin. This disease is usually found among vagabonds. Transmission occurs mainly through contact with contaminated clothing or bedding. Clinical manifestations include pruritus, excoriations, and small, red macules that usually occur on the back. Clothes should be examined carefully for lice.

Treatment is the same as for pediculosis capitis. Dry heat or washing in hot water followed by ironing is effective in killing the lice and their ova in clothing. Items that cannot be washed should be removed from body contact for 2 weeks.

Pediculosis Pubis

Pediculosis pubis is caused by *P. pubis* and affects the pubic hair. However, if left untreated, it may also affect very hairy regions of the chest, abdomen, axillary region, and especially in children, the eyelashes, edge of the scalp, and eyebrows. Patients present with pruritus. Useful diagnostic signs include small, blue-gray macules on the trunk, thighs, and axillae (i.e., taches bleuâtres or maculae ceruleae) due to conversion of bilirubin to biliverdin by the saliva of the louse and a brown "dust" found on underclothing due to the excreta of the insects. *P. pubis* is transmitted mainly by sexual contact, but it also may be transmitted by clothing or from parents to children.

Patients with pubic lice should be evaluated for other sexually transmitted diseases. Treatment of pediculosis pubis is the same as for pediculosis capitis. Bedding and clothing should be decontaminated (as for scabies) or removed from body contact for 2 weeks. Attention should be paid to treating sexual partners within the previous month because they are a common cause of reinfestation. For infested eyelashes and eyebrows, ophthalmic-grade petrolatum ointment may be used two to four times daily for 10 days, and lice and nits should be carefully removed from the eyelashes with forceps.

References

Centers for Disease Control (CDC): Disease exposure while traveling, Available at: http://www.cdc.gov/travel/ (accessed August 15, 2014).

Centers for Disease Control (CDC): Leishmaniasis, Available at: http://www.cdc.gov/parasites/leishmaniasis/health_professionals/index.html#tx (accessed March 1, 2015).

Centers for Disease Control: Malathion, Available at: http://www.cdc.gov/parasites/lice/head/gen_info/faqs_malathion.html (accessed March 1, 2015).

Gorkiewicz-Petkow A: Scabicides and pediculicides. In Katsambas AD, Lotti TM, editors: *European Handbook of Dermatological Treatments*, 2nd ed., Berlin, 2003, Springer, pp 775–779.

Goyal NN, Wong GA: Psoriasis or crusted scabies, *Clin Exp Dermatol* 33:211–212, 2008.

Heukelbach J, Feldmeier H: Epidemiological and clinical characteristics of hookworm-related cutaneous larva migrans, *Lancet Infect Dis* 8:302–309, 2008.

Klaus SN, Frankenburg S, Dhar AD: Leishmaniasis and other protozoan infections. In Freedeberg IM, Eisen AZ, Wolff K, et al: , editors: *Fitzpatrick's Dermatology in General Medicine*, 6th ed., New York, 2003, McGraw-Hill, pp 2215–2224.

Lucchina LC, Wilson ME: Cysticercosis and other helminthic infections. In Freedeberg IM, Eisen AZ, Wolff K, et al: editors: *Fitzpatrick's Dermatology in General Medicine, 6th ed.*, New York, 2003, McGraw-Hill, pp 2225–2259.

Paller AS, Mancini AJ: Bites and infestations. In *Hurwitz Clinical Pediatric Dermatology*, Philadelphia, 2006, Saunders, pp 479–501.

Stone SP: Scabies and pediculosis. In Freedeberg IM, Eisen AZ, Wolff K, et al: , editors: *Fitzpatrick's Dermatology in General Medicine*, 6th ed., New York, 2003, McGraw-Hill, pp 2283–2289.

Tsoureli-Nikita E, Campanile G, Hautmann G, et al: Pediculosis. In Katsambas AD, Lotti TM, editors: *European Handbook of Dermatological Treatments*, 2nd ed., Berlin, 2003, Springer, pp 775–779.

Wadowski L, Balasuriya L, Harper HN, et al: Lice update: new solutions to an old problem, *Clin Dermatol* 33:347–354, 2015.

---

[1]Not FDA approved for this indication.
[6]May be compounded by pharmacists.

PIGMENTARY DISORDERS

Method of

Rebat M. Halder, MD; and Ahmad Reza Hossani-Madani, MD, MS

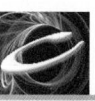

CURRENT DIAGNOSIS

Hyperpigmentation

- Ephelides: Multiple, small (1–4 mm), light- to dark-brown macules with poorly defined margins that occur on sun-exposed areas of the body.
- Solar lentigines: Light-brown to dark-brown macular hyperpigmented lesions that are induced by natural or artificial sources of radiation and that can coalesce; they are located on face, neck, forearms, and hands.
- Melasma: Arcuate or polycyclic light- to dark-brown macules that coalesce into patches on face, neck, or forearms.
- Postinflammatory hyperpigmentation: Dark patches or macules with indistinct margins at the location of an inciting inflammatory event.

Hypopigmentation

- Pityriasis alba: Round, well-defined, pale macules with fine overlying powdery white scales, ranging in size from 0.5 to 5 cm in diameter, that transition to smooth, hypopigmented macules.
- Vitiligo: Sharply demarcated, depigmented, milky-white macules in a localized or generalized distribution.
- Idiopathic guttate hypomelanosis: Multiple circular, smooth, small macules that are porcelain white, with occasional black dots, found on sun-exposed areas of upper and lower extremities.
- Postinflammatory hypopigmentation: Off-white or tan macules with ill-defined borders at the site of an inciting inflammatory event.

CURRENT THERAPY

Hyperpigmentation

- Ephelides: Hydroquinone 4% (Blanche, Melpaque HP, Skin Bleaching-Sunscreen) plus maximum UVA-blocking sunscreen in the morning and tretinoin 0.025% cream (Retin-A)[1] in the evening
- Solar lentigines: Hydroquinone 4% plus tretinoin 0.025% cream (Retin-A)[1] in the evening; cryotherapy; laser therapy.
- Melasma: Monotherapy with hydroquinone 4% twice daily or tretinoin 0.025%[1] in the evening; double therapy with hydroquinone 4% twice daily plus tretinoin 0.025%[1] in the evening; triple therapy with fluocinolone acetonide 0.01% plus hydroquinone 4% plus tretinoin 0.05% (Tri-Luma Cream) in the evening; cysteamine cream (Cyspera)[2] once daily.
- Postinflammatory hyperpigmentation: Treat inciting event; hydroquinone 4% alone or in combination with low-potency topical steroid; cysteamine cream (Cyspera)[2] once daily.

Hypopigmentation

- Pityriasis alba: Emollients, lubricants, sunscreen; tacrolimus 0.1% ointment (Protopic)[1] twice daily or low-potency non-halogenated steroid for face and medium-potency steroid for body; phototherapy (UVB) for extensive disease.
- Vitiligo: In patients with less than 20% body surface area (BSA) involvement, treat with cover-up cosmetics, topical (potent or very potent steroid or calcineurin inhibitor trial for less than 2 months), phototherapy (UVB), or excimer laser. If local treatment fails, a surgical grafting approach may be used if the patient has less than 20% BSA involvement. For patients with more than 20% BSA involvement, phototherapy (UVB) is preferred. For patients with more than 50% BSA or disfiguring facial involvement, depigment with monobenzyl ether of hydroquinone (monobenzone 20% [Benoquin]), 4-methoxyphenol, or Q-switched ruby laser (694 nm).
- Idiopathic guttate hypomelanosis: Cryotherapy; dermabrasion; surgical minigrafting; intralesional steroids.
- Postinflammatory hypopigmentation: Cosmetics; topical corticosteroids; topical PUVA.

---

[1]Not FDA approved for this indication.
[2]Available through dispensing clinics or online.

Definition

The word *chromophore* is defined as elements that impart color to the skin. Hyperchromias describe abnormally darker skin, and hypochromias describe abnormally lighter skin. Pigmentation refers to melanotic causes of skin color change, differentiating it from skin color changes as a result of blood, carotene, bilirubin, or other causes. Hyperpigmentation refers to an increase in melanin production, melanocyte number, or both in the skin. Hypopigmentation refers to decrease of melanin, melanocytes, or both in the skin. Depigmentation refers to the absence of both melanin and melanocytes. Deposition of melanin in the epidermal layers visibly appears as a yellow to brownish hue. Dermal deposition appears as blue or blue-gray, with mixed epidermal and dermal melanin deposition appearing gray or blue-brown.

Evaluation

A thorough history and visual inspection of the pigmentary disorder can provide useful clues to the diagnosis, particularly recognition of pigmentary patterns (diffuse, circumscribed, linear, or reticulated). Further examination may be achieved by using the Wood's lamp to differentiate epidermal from dermal melanin.

General Recommendations for All Pigmentary Disorders

Broad-spectrum sunscreen with an SPF of 30 is recommended, in addition to wearing protective clothing. Avoiding prolonged sun exposure is also desired.

Hyperpigmentation

Ephelides

Description

Ephelides (freckles) are multiple, small (1–4 mm), light- to dark-brown macules with poorly defined margins that occur on sun-exposed areas of the body (face, upper back, arms). They are more commonly found in children (fading with age), fair-skinned persons, and those with red or blonde hair (especially those of Celtic ancestry). A relationship has been shown between painful sunburns in youth and development of ephelides, and the macules become darker with greater UV exposure. They are thought to be genetic in origin, following an autosomal dominant pattern, and are strongly associated with variants in the melanocortin-1-receptor (MC1R). Ephelides are significant because they are associated with an increased risk of melanoma and nonmelanoma skin cancer, perhaps serving as a marker for sun susceptibility.

Treatment

Although treatment is not necessary, modalities include either hydroquinone 4% (Blanche, Melpaque HP, Skin Bleaching-Sunscreen) plus maximum ultraviolet A (UVA)-blocking sunscreen in the morning and tretinoin 0.1% cream (Retin-A)[1] in the evening. Other therapies have included cryotherapy, lasers, and chemical peels.

Solar Lentigo (Lentigo Senilis Et Actinicus)

Description

Solar lentigines are pigmented spots that share morphologic similarities with ephelides, making differentiation difficult. They are

---

[1]Not FDA approved for this indication.

defined as light-brown to dark-brown macular hyperpigmented lesions induced by natural or artificial sources of radiation, which can coalesce. The incidence increases with age, and more than 90% of white persons older than 50 years demonstrate lesions. They appear most often on the face, neck, forearms, and hands. They can occur in nonclassic locations in those receiving phototherapy (such as the penis). Histologically, they differ from ephelides by the presence of epidermal hyperplasia, increased melanocyte number, and elongation of the rete ridges.

Treatment
Although treatment is not necessary, two different modalities have been used: physical therapies and topical therapies. Physical therapies include cryotherapy and lasers, and topical treatments include retinoids or combinations of agents. Liquid nitrogen may be used with a cotton swab for 5 to 10 seconds to induce lightening. Recurrence rates may be as high as 55% at 6 months. Side effects include atrophy with longer cryoprobe application, postinflammatory hyper- or hypopigmentation, and pain. The Q-switched Nd:YAG (1064 nm) laser, among others, has been used with success.

Melasma
Description
Melasma is a hypermelanosis of the face, neck, and forearms that occurs with a higher incidence in women of African American, Latin American, and Asian descent. It appears on sun-exposed areas as arcuate or polycyclic macules that coalesce into patches. Epidermal melanin deposition causes a brownish appearance, and dermal melanin appears bluish. Combined epidermal and dermal melanin deposition appears gray. It is distributed in a central facial (65%), malar (20%), or mandibular (15%) pattern. More commonly seen in women and those with darker skin, it can also be found in men. Contributing factors include a genetic predisposition, pregnancy, oral contraceptive use, endocrine dysfunction, hormonal treatment, UV light exposure, cosmetics, and phototoxic drugs.

Treatment
First-line treatment for melasma consists of broad-spectrum sunscreen with greater than SPF 30 coverage in addition to monotherapy with hydroquinone 4% twice daily or tretinoin 0.025% (Retin A)[1] nightly. Double therapy with hydroquinone 4% twice daily plus tretinoin 0.025%[1] nightly may prove efficacious after an unsuccessful trial of monotherapy. If that fails, triple therapy may be attempted, with fluocinolone acetonide 0.01%, hydroquinone 4%, and tretinoin 0.05% (Tri-Luma) once daily being effective. Side effects of triple therapy include erythema, desquamation, burning, dryness, and pruritus at the site of application; telangiectasia; perioral dermatitis; acne breakouts; and hyperpigmentation. Cysteamine cream (Cyspera)[2] once a day can be used as an alternative to hydroquinone. Chemical peels, superficial and medium depth, and Q-switched 1064 nm Nd:YAG laser or intense pulsed light (IPL) may also be used for patients whose topical treatments have failed.

Postinflammatory Hyperpigmentation
Description
Postinflammatory hyperpigmentation is a very common condition that occurs as a result of a previous or ongoing inflammatory process, most commonly acne vulgaris, atopic dermatitis, infections, and phototoxic reactions, and as a result of treatment with topical medications, chemical peels, and lasers. Postinflammatory hyperpigmentation occurs more commonly in persons with darker skin pigmentation and appears as dark patches or macules with indistinct margins at the location of the inciting inflammatory event.

Treatment
Primary treatment is aimed at treating the inciting cause of the hyperpigmentation. Additional effective therapies include 4% hydroquinone alone or in combination with a topical steroid.

Broad-spectrum sunscreen should also be employed. Cysteamine cream (Cyspera)[2] can be used as an alternative to hydroquinone.

Hypopigmentation or Depigmentation
Pityriasis Alba
Description
Pityriasis alba is a childhood or adolescent condition that affects all races. It begins as an erythematous macule with ill-defined borders. The erythema fades after a few weeks, leaving two or three round, well-defined, paler macules with overlying fine powdery white scale, ranging in size from 0.5 cm to 5 cm in diameter. These eventually transition to smooth, hypopigmented lesions, which are generally located on the face. The pathogenesis of this disorder is unknown.

Treatment
Pityriasis alba is thought to be a self-limited skin disease. However, general treatment guidelines include use of emollients and lubricant, use of sunscreen, and decreasing sun exposure. Lesions limited to the face may be treated with hydrocortisone 1%[1] or other mild, nonfluorinated steroid. More potent steroids may be used for lesions on the body, including hydrocortisone valerate 0.2% (Westcort)[1] or alclometasone dipropionate 0.05% (Aclovate).[1] However, these can lead to atrophy if used over an extended period. Newer, nonsteroidal, effective alternatives include tacrolimus 0.1% ointment (Protopic)[1] twice daily. Side effects include a burning sensation that fades over time. Extensive disease that is not amenable to topical therapy might benefit from phototherapy (UVB).

Vitiligo
Description
Persons with vitiligo acquire sharply demarcated, depigmented macules in a localized or generalized distribution. These macules appear milky white compared with the surrounding normally pigmented skin. Lesions can increase in size. There is no predilection for race or sex, and three-quarters of patients generally present before the age of 30 years.

Treatment
General recommendations include the use of sunscreen, avoidance of the sun, and use of protective clothing. Treatments for localized vitiligo (<20% of body surface area) include cover-up cosmetics, a 2-month trial of topical treatment (potent or very potent corticosteroid or calcineurin inhibitor), excimer laser, or topical PUVA. Adults who have failed treatments for localized vitiligo may be considered for narrow-band UVB or surgical treatment, which includes split-skin grafting, transfer of suction blisters, or autologous epidermal suspensions added to dermabraded skin. Surgical candidates should have localized, limited involvement and should not demonstrate lesion enlargement or Koebner phenomenon for 12 months prior to treatment. Patients with more than 20% body involvement may be considered for narrow-band UVB (311 nm). Those with greater than 50% body involvement or disfiguring facial involvement may be considered for complete depigmentation with monobenzyl ether of hydroquinone 20% (monobenzone 20% [Benoquin]). Children are generally not offered surgical treatment.

Idiopathic Guttate Hypomelanosis
Description
This is an acquired, asymptomatic leukoderma with multiple, circular, smooth, small macules that have a porcelain-white color. Brown dots are occasionally observed within the macules. The macules increase in number with age, but they generally do not increase in size. They are most commonly located on sun-exposed areas of the upper and lower extremities.

Treatment
Treatments have included cryotherapy, dermabrasion, surgical minigrafting, and intralesional steroids; however, none of these have shown consistent acceptable results. Phototherapy has not been shown to be effective.

---

[1] Not FDA approved for this indication.
[2] Available through dispensing clinics or online.

[1] Not FDA approved for this indication.
[2] Available through dispensing clinics or online.

Postinflammatory Hypopigmentation

Description

Postinflammatory hypopigmentation is the result of an inciting inflammatory event leading to lesions that are off-white or tan, with ill-defined borders. This entity is noticed more commonly in those with darker skin.

Treatment

Hypopigmentation resolves with treatment of the underlying condition. Cosmetic cover-ups may be useful. Topical corticosteroids, tacrolimus 0.1% ointment (Protopic),[1] and phototherapy may also be used in patients who have lesions in cosmetically distressing areas.

---

[1] Not FDA approved for this indication.

References

Cestari T, Arellano I, Hexsel D, Ortonne JP: Melasma in Latin America: option for therapy and treatment algorithm, *J Eur Acad Dermatol Venereol* 23:760–772, 2009.

Gupta AK, Gover MD, Nouri K, Taylor S: The treatment of melasma: a review of clinical trials, *J Am Acad Dermatol* 55:1048–1065, 2006.

Halder RM, Richards GM: Management of dyschromias in ethnic skin, *Dermatol Ther* 17:151–157, 2004.

Halder RM, Richards GM: Topical agents used in the management of hyperpigmentation, *Skin Therapy Lett* 9:1–3, 2004.

Hexsel DM: Treatment of idiopathic guttate hypomelanosis by localized superficial dermabrasion, *Dermatol Surg* 25:917–918, 1999.

Lin RL, Janniger CK: Pityriasis alba, *Cutis* 76:21–24, 2005.

Nordlund JJ, Boissy RE, Hearing VJ, et al: In *The pigmentary system: physiology and pathophysiology*, 2 ed, Blackwell Publishing, 2007.

Nordlund JJ, Cestari TF, Chan F, Westerhof W: Confusions about color: a classification of discolorations of the skin, *Br J Dermatol* 156(Suppl 1):S3–S6, 2007.

Ortonne JP, Pandya AG, Lui H, Hexsel D: Treatment of solar lentigines, *J Am Acad Dermatol* 54:S262–S271, 2006.

Ploysangam T, Dee-Ananlap S, Suvanprakorn P: Treatment of idiopathic guttate hypomelanosis with iquid nitrogen: light and electron microscopic studies, *J Am Acad Dermatol* 23:681–684, 1990.

Rigopoulos D, Gregoriou S, Charissi C, et al: Tacrolimus ointment 0.1% in pityriasis alba: an open-label randomized, placebo-controlled study, *Br J Dermatol* 155:152–155, 2006.

Taylor SC, Burgess CM, Callender VD, et al: Postinflammatory hyperpigmentation: evolving combination treatment strategies, *Cutis* 78:S6–S19, 2006.

PREMALIGNANT SKIN LESIONS

Method of
Daniel Stulberg, MD; and Katarzyna Wilamowska, MD, PhD

CURRENT DIAGNOSIS

Actinic Keratoses
- Scaly white or flesh-colored lesions often with palpably rough surface
- Individuals with light skin and hair color are at high risk
- Most common on face, hands, and sun-exposed skin

Actinic Cheilitis
- Scale, thickening or fissures on the lips
- Lower lip more commonly involved than upper lip

Porokeratoses
- Macular lesions with slight scale or rice-paper appearance and hyperkeratotic border
- Disseminated superficial actinic porokeratoses (DSAP) predominant type–autosomal dominant transmission

Human Papillomavirus Disease
- Verrucous or papular flesh-colored lesions
- Genital, perineal, perirectal, or oral locations are at risk of malignancy

Atypical Nevi
- Multiple irregularly pigmented nevi in the familial atypical mole and melanoma syndrome
- Numerous, often raised nevi, especially with shades of red, brown, and black

CURRENT THERAPY

Actinic Keratoses or Cheilitis
- Cryosurgery first line if limited number of lesions
- Topical medications for extensive actinic change with multiple lesions
- 5-fluorouracil (Carac, Efudex) typically 2–3 weeks, although multiple protocols/variations
- Diclofenac sodium (Solaraze) longer protocol, less effective
- Imiquimod (Aldara, Zyclara) longer protocol, less effective
- Ingenol mebutate (Picato) 3-day course limited by maximum of 25-cm² treatment area and expense of medication
- Less commonly, laser, curettage, retinoids, photosensitizing medications followed by light therapy

Porokeratoses
- See treatment options for actinic keratoses

Actinic keratoses are the most common precancerous skin lesions seen in usual practice. If untreated, it is estimated that from 0.1% to 10% of these lesions will progress to squamous cell carcinoma that requires significantly more aggressive treatment. Fortunately, effective treatment is available, although it can cause significant discomfort. Risk factors for developing actinic keratoses are similar to those of developing basal cell carcinoma (BCC), squamous cell carcinoma (SCC), and, to a certain extent, melanoma skin cancer. These risk factors include lighter skin colors, family history of actinic keratoses or nonmelanoma skin cancer, exposure to sunlight, ultraviolet radiation, use of tanning beds, and immunosuppression from disease, or immunosuppressant medications to prevent organ transplant rejection.

There are several other conditions or situations that can increase risk of precancerous and cancerous skin lesions. The first is arsenic. This is rare in developed countries and, other than avoiding arsenic exposures, is treated as outlined below for actinic keratoses. The human papilloma virus (HPV) can lead to papillomatous lesions and genital and oropharyngeal. Individuals with the familial atypical mole and melanoma syndrome (FAMMS), previously called atypical nevus syndrome, have multiple abnormal-appearing nevi and a family history of melanoma. Patients with atypical nevi and more than one first-degree relative with melanoma have a risk of melanoma approaching 100%.

Actinic keratoses should be treated to reduce the risk of progression to squamous cell carcinoma unless the patient has a limited life expectancy and the clinician determines that, based on the condition of the patient and their comorbidities, the discomfort of treatment would outweigh the benefits for the patient. Avoiding sun exposure and using broad-brimmed hats, sunscreen, and protective clothing while outdoors can reduce the risk of additional lesions. Unfortunately, because of the long lead time between sun exposure and onset of disease, most patients will continue to develop more actinic keratoses due to the underlying skin damage. Patients should be counseled regarding the occurrence of additional precancerous and cancerous skin lesions and should be examined every 6 to 12 months, or even more frequently depending on the amount of disease burden, their individual risk factors, and clinical judgment.

There are several rare inherited genetic disorders that predispose patients to precancerous and cancerous cutaneous lesions, grouped under genodermatoses. Xeroderma pigmentosum (XP) is an autosomal recessive disorder where homozygotes have severe sun sensitivity due to inability to repair sun-damaged DNA, leading to development of BCCs, SCCs, and melanomas in early childhood. Basal cell nevus syndrome, another autosomal dominant disorder, is characterized by developmental anomalies and tumors, especially BCCs, starting in the fourth decade of life. Oculocutaneous albinism results from a group of autosomal recessive disorders of melanin biosynthesis. This deficiency leads to reduced or absent pigmentation of skin, hair, and eyes, leading to early photodamage.

Nevus sebaceous presents as a waxy yellow or brown congenital plaque or plaques. Around the time of puberty the plaque can thicken and develop into benign or, less commonly, malignant tumors. In addition to these specific disorders, patients with chronic ulceration, burn scars, radiation therapy fields, and inflammatory conditions including discoid lupus, lichen planus, lichen sclerosis, and lymphedema are at risk of developing skin cancers in affected areas.

Actinic Keratoses and Actinic Cheilitis
Clinical Manifestations
Actinic keratoses (AKs) are an abnormal proliferation of keratinocytes and a precursor of squamous cell carcinoma. Over time, 0.1% to 10% of the lesions will progress to squamous cell carcinoma. AKs present as rough or scaly white or flesh-colored lesions, often with a slightly erythematous base (Figure 1). A combination of visual inspection of the skin and tactile examination is useful to diagnose these lesions. Often they are easier to identify by gently palpating the patient's skin for their characteristic rough surface on sun-exposed areas. If there is significant underlying erythematous thickened tissue, the clinician should consider whether the lesion has already progressed to squamous cell carcinoma, and potentially proceed with biopsy (Figure 2). Patients frequently note that they have scratched off a lesion but it returns over time, and many patients who have had multiple AKs become very adept at pointing them out to their clinician.

Actinic cheilitis is the same precancerous process when it occurs on the lips. It is more common on the lower lip, which catches the sun's rays more directly. The lip becomes rough, or the patient notes that it is always chapped. Dyshidrotic chapped lips can be in the differential diagnosis. A trial of topical lip balm may be initiated, and if the rough surface does not resolve, actinic cheilitis is the likely diagnosis. If there is ulceration or significant thickening of the lip, biopsy should be performed because of the possibility of squamous cell carcinoma of the lip.

Treatment
For patients with a limited number of lesions, destruction with cryosurgery is a quick and effective treatment with success rates generally above 95%. Cryosurgery can be performed using a

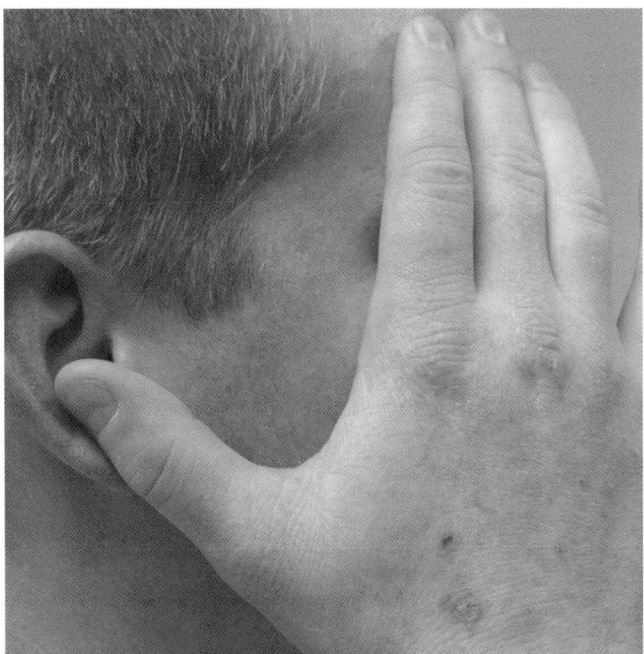

Figure 1 Early onset of actinic keratoses in young man with high-risk skin type.

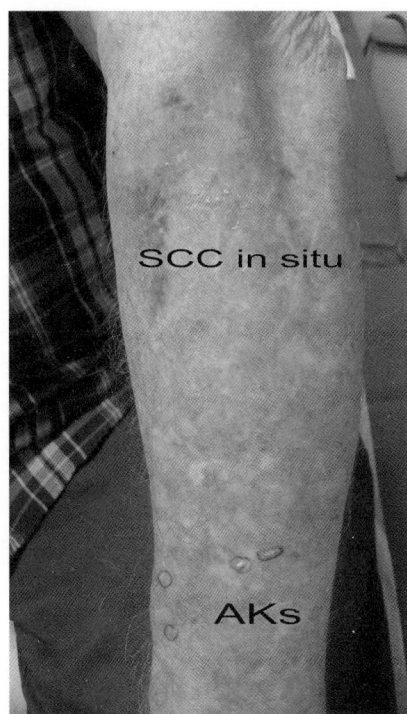

Figure 2 Sun-damaged skin with multiple actinic keratoses and squamous cell carcinoma in situ, a.k.a. Bowens disease.

variety of tools. Liquid nitrogen spray devices provide the coldest temperatures and fastest treatment in clinical practice. Other useful options include nitrous oxide spray devices, evaporative refrigerant liquids, mechanically cooled metal probes via refrigerant technology or compressed nitrous oxide or carbon dioxide devices or using a swab dipped in liquid nitrogen. Treatment protocols vary based on the instrument. For liquid nitrogen spray, there are multiple sized apertures available and freezing protocols based on clinician preference and lesion size. One protocol is to hold the spray tip 1 to 2 cm from the AK, spray until the lesion is frozen and keep frozen for 6 seconds, allow the lesion to thaw, and repeat the cycle. For clinical efficiency it is useful to treat several lesions in succession to allow the earlier lesions to thaw before repeating the freeze (Figure 3). Counsel the patient that the cold spray does cause discomfort and even feels like a burning or stinging sensation. After treatment, the lesions typically become erythematous, have slight swelling, and sometimes will blister. If they blister, topical petrolatum and an adhesive bandage may be used to protect the healing wound. If lesions do not resolve after adequate cryosurgery, consider biopsy for possible squamous cell carcinoma, which will require more aggressive treatment. Patient discomfort of cryosurgery varies. Most individuals will tolerate up to 15 lesions, although some patients will only tolerate cryosurgery of a few lesions, and some will tolerate treatment of dozens of lesions. Patients can return for additional cryosurgery on subsequent visits, or, if they have a very high density of lesions, topical agents may be more efficient to treat large areas with multiple lesions. The lips can be treated with cryosurgery or topical agents for actinic cheilitis. Because of the risk of swelling and discomfort, a lighter freeze protocol may be useful for the lips.

Topical chemotherapy with 5-fluorouracil (Carac, Efudex) has been used to treat AKs successfully for decades. It is particularly useful for field or blanket therapy in patients with multiple lesions and is very effective in clearing more than 90% of the lesions in treated areas. There are multiple variations in treatment protocols, and it is manufactured in 0.5% and 5% topical creams and 2% and 5% topical solutions. One option is to apply 5% 5-fluorouracil to the affected areas twice daily for 2 weeks until there is significant inflammation, often erosions and exudate (Figures 4 and 5). If there has been no reaction, the treatment can

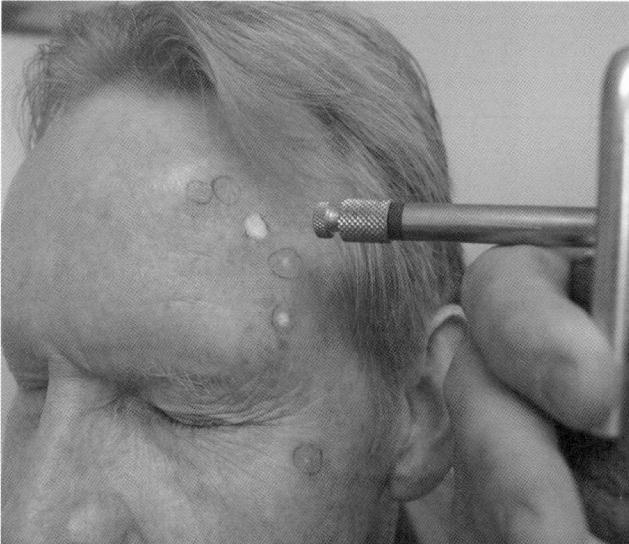

Figure 3 Treating multiple actinic keratoses with cryosurgery.

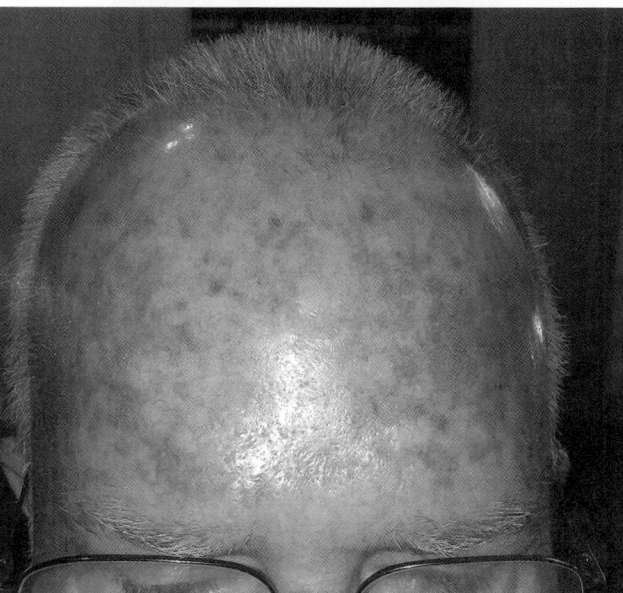

Figure 4 BID 5-fluorouracil at 3 weeks.

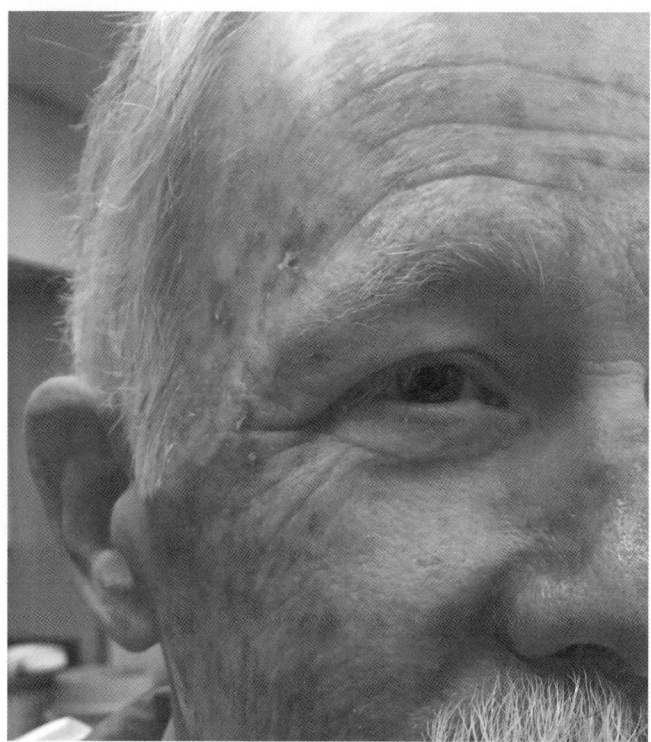

Figure 5 Daily 5-fluorouracil at 5 weeks.

be extended out to 3 weeks. There is significant discomfort with this treatment protocol, which can be lessened by not treating the patient's entire affected areas all at once. Starting with treatment of one forearm and allowing that to heal before proceeding to the next forearm can be a useful way of starting and allowing the patient to get some familiarity with its use before starting it on a portion of their face or scalp. Treating the entire face or scalp can be very uncomfortable, so treating only one portion at a time and waiting until that heals before treating another area may be helpful. Because of photo sensitivity and increased risk of sunburn, it is preferable to perform treatment during the winter months or use strict sun avoidance. The 0.5% 5-fluorouracil formulation may be better tolerated on the lips for actinic cheilitis. Patients should be counseled to expect significant inflammation. It may also be useful to advise them that as a topical chemotherapy, this medication targets the lesions and typically does not cause inflammation of unaffected skin.

Because of the amount of inflammation with 5-fluorouracil, other topical treatments have been developed. They cause less inflammation but unfortunately also have lower efficacy rates. These other treatments include topical imiquimod (Aldara,

Zylara), diclofenac (Solaraze), and ingenol mebutate (Picato). Imiquimod is used at bedtime twice a week for 16 weeks. Diclofenac is used twice daily for 8 to 12 weeks and is typically better tolerated. Both of these are less effective than topical 5-fluorouracil. Ingenol mebutate is used once daily for only 3 days. Its use is limited currently by its high cost and only being approved to use for 25cm^2, approximately a 2″ × 2″ area, which is extremely small compared with the large amount of skin usually affected by AKs and an efficacy of less than 50%.

Outside of typical primary care practices, several other options exist. Photodynamic therapy can be used after a sensitizing application of aminolevulinic acid (Levulan) or methyl aminolevulinate (Metvixia). Nonselective chemical peels, dermabrasion, and ablative lasers can be used for field therapy to an entire area, treating both lesions and unaffected skin in the treatment field. Individual lesions may be treated with laser, trichloroacetic acid (Tri-Chlor),[1] or curettage.

Nicotinamide[1,7] 500mg orally BID has been shown to reduce the rate of developing additional lesions in patients already affected by actinic keratoses. The medication needs to be continued to maintain its effect.

Porokeratoses
Clinical Manifestations

Although much less common than actinic keratoses, porokeratoses also have malignant potential. Disseminated superficial actinic porokeratoses, like AKs, present on sun-exposed areas. They usually present as atrophic or rice-paper–appearing lesions surrounded by a slightly raised border (Figure 6). The plaque form (i.e., Mibelli's porokeratosis) is large and progressive, and the linear type may be generalized or segmental. Both of these types often manifest very early in life. Malignant transformation occurs mostly commonly in the linear type, followed by the Mibelli type. It is rare in the disseminated type and has not been reported in the punctate type.

---

[1]Not FDA approved for this indication.
[7]Available as a dietary supplement.

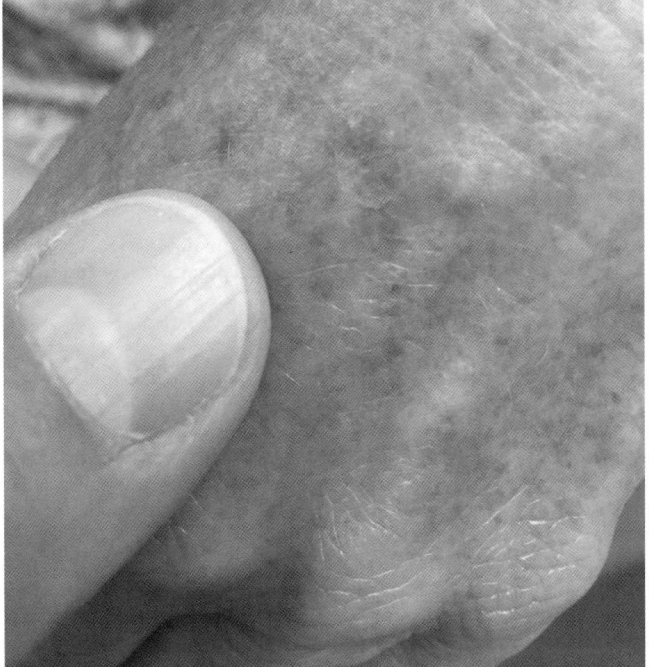

Figure 6 Porokeratosis with rice-paper appearance and peripheral ridge a.k.a. cornoid lamella.

Treatment

Disseminated superficial porokeratosis can be treated with locally destructive methods as outlined above for actinic keratoses and surgical excision.

Management of Complications

Treatment with cryosurgery is expected to cause local inflammation including possible vesicles and erosions. Topical petrolatum under an adhesive dressing or applied multiple times per day if used without a dressing can facilitate moist wound healing. Cryosurgery can cause hypopigmentation, which can be cosmetically distressing for patients with darker skin types and can predispose to sunburn in any skin type. Inflammation from topical medications for actinic keratoses can be soothed by application of petrolatum. Secondary infections, impetigo, and cellulitis are uncommon but possible after cryosurgery or inflammation associated with topical products. Antibiotics to cover methicillin-resistant *Staphylococcus aureus* and *Streptococcus spp.*, should be prescribed if needed. Reactivation of herpes labialis can occur when treating the lips. Prophylactic antiviral therapy may reduce the risk of an outbreak in patients with history of herpes labialis.

References

Ameluz for actinic keratoses: *Med Lett Drugs Ther* 58(1509):155–156, 2016.
Bolognia JL, Jorizzo J, Schaffer JV, editors: *Dermatology*, New York, 2012, Elsevier.
Damian DL: Nicotinamide for skin cancer chemoprevention, *Australas J Dermatol* 58:174–180, 2017.
de Berker D, McGregor JM, Hughes BR: British Association of Dermatologists Therapy Guidelines and Audit Subcommittee. guidelines for the management of actinic keratoses, *Br J Dermatol* 156:222–230, 2007.
James WD, Berger TG, Elston DM, editors: *Andrews' Diseases of the Skin—Clinical Dermatology, 11th ed*, Philadelphia, 2011, Saunders.
Martin G: The impact of the current United States guidelines on the management of actinic keratosis: is it time for an update? *J Clin Aesthet Dermatol* 3(11):20–25, 2010.
Philipp-Dormston WG, Müller K, Novak B, NMSC-QoL Study Group, et al: Patient-reported health outcomes in patients with non-melanoma skin cancer and actinic keratosis: results from a large-scale observational study analyzing effects of diagnoses and disease progression, *J Eur Acad Dermatol Venereol.*, 2017 Nov 17.
Poulin Y, Lynde CW, Barber K, et al: Canadian non-Melanoma Skin Cancer Guidelines Committee. Non-melanoma skin cancer in Canada Chapter 3: Management of Actinic Keratoses, *J Cutan Med Surg* 19:227–238, 2015.
Wood GS, Gunkel J, Stewart D, et al: Nonmelanoma skin cancers. In Abeloff MD, Armitage JO, Niederhuber JE, Kastan MB, editors: *Abeloff's Clinical Oncology*, 4th ed, Philadelphia, 2008, Churchill Livingstone.

PRESSURE INJURY

Method of
Rebecca M. Wester, MD

CURRENT DIAGNOSIS

- In April 2016, the National Pressure Ulcer Advisory Panel redefined the definition: pressure injury replaces the terms "pressure ulcer," "decubitus ulcer," and "bed sores."
- Pressure injury develops from pathologic changes in combination with localized skin and underlying soft tissue damage, typically over a bony prominence or associated with a medical device. Skin can be intact or have an open ulcer.

CURRENT THERAPY

- Treatment is based on the stage and characteristics of the pressure injury.
- Nutrition and pressure relief are important interventions.
- Host-specific factors have profound effects on the healing process and have a greater influence than what is put on the wound.

Epidemiology

Most pressure injuries develop during acute hospitalizations, in spite of the adoption of national pressure ulcer prevention guidelines. Prevalence rates for pressure injuries have changed little over the past two decades. Hospitalized patients in intensive care or undergoing cardiovascular or hip surgery have higher rates.

End-stage skin failure occurs when hypoperfusion occurs at the end of life. The prevalence of pressure injuries is 11% to 18% for palliative care patients, nearly double in comparison with hospital rates. Pressure injuries impose a significant burden, not only on the patient but also on the entire health care system. To put it into perspective, the cost of treating 10 pressure injuries is equivalent to 5 knee replacements, 6 hip replacements, 9 pacemakers, or 5 bypass operations.

Risk Factors

External factors that lead to the development of pressure injuries include pressure, shearing forces, friction, and moisture. Interaction of these external factors with host-specific factors such as immobility, sensory loss, incontinence, reduced perfusion, and compromised nutritional status culminates in tissue damage. Decreased skin perfusion resulting from hypotension, anemia, shock, or peripheral artery disease is increasingly recognized as an important cause of pressure ulcers. Other risk factors are cerebrovascular disease, cardiovascular disease, recent lower extremity fractures, medications, and diabetes.

Pressure ulcer risk assessment. The Braden and Norton scales are commonly used for pressure risk assessment. These scales assess risk factors such as physical and mental condition, mobility, moisture, continence, and nutrition. However, they are weak predictors of risk of ulcers and may be no better at reducing risk than clinical judgment.

Pathophysiology

Pressure alone is not sufficient to cause an ulcer; it's the addition of the confounding host-specific factors that ultimately leads to tissue damage. Superficial lesions are primarily the result of moisture and friction. Exposure to moisture in the form of perspiration, urine, or feces can lead to skin maceration. Friction occurs when patients are dragged across an external surface. This results in an abrasion with damage to the most superficial layer of skin. Friction contributesmostly to stage 2 pressure injuries, with limited contributions to stage 3 to 4 pressure injuries because it does not cause the necrotic changes associated with deep tissue injury. Pressure injuries are greatest over bony prominences where weight-bearing points come in contact with external surfaces and immobilization devices. Pressure over a bony prominence tends to result in a cone-shaped distribution, with the most affected tissues located deep, adjacent to the bone–muscle interface. Thus the extent of injury to deep tissues is often much greater than perceived from the visible ulcer on the skin surface. Typically, stage 3 to 4 pressure injuries start as a deep tissue injury that may then progress to the surface. There is little evidence to suggest that a stage 4 pressure injury develops as a gradual progression from stage 1 to stage 4.

Differential Diagnosis

Besides pressure injuries, other chronic skin ulcers are arterial ulcers, venous stasis ulcers, and diabetic ulcers: arterial ulcers occur in distal digits or over bony prominences, venous stasis ulcers occur on the lateral aspect of the lower leg in the setting of chronic edema, and diabetic ulcers occur in regions of callous formations. Traumatic injuries such as abrasions, skin tears, or burns are not pressure injuries; nor are surgical incision sites. Only pressure injuries are staged; never stage a wound that arises from a different etiology.

Diagnosis

Staging is done according to the National Pressure Ulcer Advisory Panel Pressure Injury Staging System:

Stage 1: Nonblanchable erythema of intact skin. May appear differently in darkly pigmented skin. Color changes do not include purple or maroon discoloration; this indicates deep tissue injury.

Stage 2: Partial-thickness skin loss with exposed dermis. The wound bed is viable, pink or red, and moist, and may also present as an intact or ruptured serum-filled blister. Adipose (fat) is not visible and deeper tissues are not visible. Granulation tissue, slough, and eschar are not present. This stage should not be used to describe moisture-associated skin damage (MASD) including incontinence-associated dermatitis (IAD), intertriginous dermatitis (ITD), medical adhesive–related skin injury (MARSI), or traumatic wounds (skin tears, burns, abrasions).

Stage 3: Full-thickness skin loss. Adipose (fat) is visible in the ulcer and granulation tissue and rolled skin edges are often present. Slough or eschar may be visible. The depth of tissue damage varies by anatomic location; areas of significant adiposity can develop deep wounds. Undermining and tunneling may occur. Fascia, muscle, tendon, ligament, cartilage, and bone are not exposed. If slough or eschar obscures the extent of tissue loss, then it is an unstageable pressure injury.

Stage 4: Full-thickness skin and tissue loss. Exposed or directly palpable fascia, muscle, tendon, ligament, cartilage, or bone is in the ulcer. Slough or eschar may be visible. Rolled edges, undermining, and tunneling often occur. Depth varies by anatomic location. If slough or eschar obscures the extent of tissue loss, then it is an unstageable pressure injury.

Unstageable: Obscured full-thickness skin and tissue loss. The extent of tissue damage within the ulcer cannot be determined because it is obscured by slough or eschar. If slough or eschar is removed, a stage 3 or 4 pressure injury will be revealed. Stable eschar (dry, adherent, intact, without erythema or fluctuance) on the heel or ischemic limb should not be softened or removed.

Deep tissue injury: Persistent, nonblanchable, deep red, maroon, or purple discoloration. May appear as a dark wound bed or blood-filled blister. Pain and temperature skin changes often precede skin color changes. Discoloration may appear differently in darkly pigmented skin. The wound may evolve rapidly from intense or prolonged pressure and shear forces at the bone–muscle interface. The wound may evolve rapidly to reveal the actual extent of injury or may resolve without tissue loss. If necrotic tissue, subcutaneous tissue, granulation tissue, fascia, muscle, or other underlying structure is visible, then it

is a full-thickness pressure injury (unstageable or stage 3 or 4). Do not use deep tissue injury to describe vascular, traumatic, neuropathic, diabetic, or dermatologic conditions.

Medical device–related pressure injury: Results from the use of devices designed and applied for diagnostic or therapeutic purposes. The resultant pressure injury generally conforms to the pattern or shape of the device. The injury should be staged using the staging system.

Mucosal membrane pressure injury: Found on mucous membranes in patients with a history of a medical device in use at the location of the injury. Owing to the anatomy of the tissue, these ulcers cannot be staged.

Therapy

Pressure relief. Position the patient frequently at fixed intervals to relieve pressure over compromised areas. There is no evidence to suggest an optimal interval at which to reposition patients, although every 2 hours is recommended based on expert opinion. Advanced static support surfaces (mattress overlays and foam, gel, or air mattresses) rather than standardized hospital mattresses should be used to prevent pressure injuries in high-risk patients. Check the pressure-relieving devices for "bottoming out" by inserting your hand (palm up) between the device and the bed under the patient's sacral area. The device is considered ineffective if you are unable to slide your hand freely. For immobile individuals, offload the heels by "floating the heels" with pillows under the patient's legs.

Pain. Dressing changes hurt. Use individualized pain management.

Assessment of nutrition/hydration. Pressure injuries occur in sicker individuals in whom overall intake may be reduced by coexisting illness. If adequate dietary intake is compromised, supplemental vitamins/minerals at the recommended daily allowance (RDA) should be considered. Protein supplementation may improve outcomes in the treatment of pressure ulcers, as per current guidelines. However, a 2014 Cochrane review concluded that there is no clear evidence that nutritional interventions (i.e., dietary supplementation) reduce the number of people who develop pressure injuries or help the healing of existing pressure injuries. There is no evidence to support the use of vitamin C or zinc to treat pressure injuries in patients who are not deficient in these nutrients. There is no difference in healing rates associated with supratherapeutic doses of vitamin C or zinc. The decision to use tube feeding must consider the patient's wishes, overall goal of care, and complications of tube feeding. Recent studies surprisingly observed that the use of tube feedings increased the incidence of pressure injuries and was associated with poorer healing. Tube feeding is associated with agitation, increased use of physical and chemical restraints and worsening of ulcers in individuals with severe dementia.

Removal (débridement) of necrotic tissue. Débridement by any of several methods (Table 1) may improve the time to a clean wound bed, but the effect of débridement on the time to healing remains to be determined.

Promotion of healing (reepithelialization). Pressure injuries should be cleansed with saline or tap water, and slough and necrotic tissue débrided (see Table 1). The choice of a particular

---

TABLE 1   Débridement Methods

Mechanical: Wet-to-dry dressings; removes both devitalized and viable tissues; causes pain

Surgical (sharp): Scalpel, scissors, or forceps to remove devitalized tissue; quick and effective by skilled clinician; should be used when infection is suspected; causes pain

Enzymatic: Topical débriding agent to dissolve the necrotic tissue; appropriate when there are no signs or symptoms of local infection

Autolytic: Synthetic dressing to allow the devitalized tissue to self-digest from the enzymes found in the ulcer fluids; recommended for those who cannot tolerate débridement; may take a long time to be effective; commonly used with palliative wounds

Biosurgery: Larvae to digest devitalized tissue; quick and effective; good option for those who cannot tolerate surgical débridement; limited by access to larvae

TABLE 2	Pressure Injury Dressing Types	
DRESSING	**RECOMMENDATIONS**
Hydrocolloid	Light to moderate exudate ulcers
	Clean stage 2 or shallow (noninfected) stage 3 ulcers
	Consider using filler dressing beneath in deep ulcers to fill dead space
Transparent film	Partial thickness with minimal exudate ulcers or closed wounds
	Consider for autolytic débridement
	Consider as secondary dressing with alginate or other wound filler that will likely remain in the ulcer for an extended time (3–5 days)
	Do not use on moderately to heavily exudative ulcers
	Do not use as cover dressing over enzymatic débriding agents
Hydrogel	Full thickness with minimal or no exudate (stage 3 or 4) ulcers
	Consider use on shallow, minimally exudate ulcer
	Consider amorphous hydrogel for granulating noninfected ulcers
	Consider for dry ulcer beds
Alginate	Full thickness with moderate to heavy exudate ulcers with cavities (stage 3 or 4)
	Consider in clinically infected ulcer with concurrent treatment for the infection
Foams	Exudate stage 2 and shallow stage 3 ulcers
	Avoid using single small piece pf foam in exudate ulcer with cavities
	Consider gelling foam in heavily exuding ulcers
Silver impregnated	Clinically infected or heavily colonized. Avoid prolonged use; discontinue when wound infection is controlled

dressing depends on the wound characteristics, such as amount of exudate, dead space, or wound infection. A hydrocolloid, foam, or other nonadherent dressing that promotes a moist wound environment should be used (Table 2). Follow manufacturer recommendations regarding frequency of dressing changes.

Monitoring

Measurement. After staging the pressure injury, measure the length, width, and depth of ulcers. Document the presence of exudate, necrotic tissue, eschar, slough, undermining, and tunneling. Presence of healing tissue (pink granulation or epithelialization) should be recorded as well. Measurement frequency depends onthe patient's care location, whether it's the hospital, a long-term care facility, or home care.

Infection. All pressure ulcers are colonized with bacteria. Never swab a chronic ulcer. The presence of bacteria alone does not indicate active infection, only colonization. Edema, odor, and purulent discharge are nonspecific. Worsening pain, erythema at wound edges, and warmth are signs of advancing cellulitis. Fever or delirium may be the only signs of infection. Systemic rather than topical antibiotics should be used to treat an infected pressure ulcer. Consider osteomyelitis when bone is exposed.

References

The cost of pressure injuries. Available at http://www.cobro.co.nz/cms/the cost of pressure injuries [accessed February 14, 2017].

Don't recommend percutaneous feeding tubes in patients with advanced dementia; instead offer oral assisted feeding. Available at http://www.choosingwisely.org [accessed February 14, 2017].
Langer G, Fink A: Nutritional interventions for preventing and treating pressure ulcers, *Cochrane Database Syst Rev* 6:CD003216, 2014.
Lyder CH: *Pressure ulcers and wound care. Geriatric Review Syllabus: A Core Curriculum in Geriatrics Medicine*, ed 8th, New York, 2013, American Geriatrics Society.
National Pressure Ulcer Advisory Panel. Available at http://www.npuap.org [accessed January 3, 2017].
Raetz JG, Wick KH: Common questions about pressure ulcers, *Am Fam Physician* 92(10):888–894, 2015.
Thomas DR: Clinical management of pressure ulcers, *Clin Geriatr Med* 29:397–413, 2013.
Thomas DR: Does pressure cause pressure ulcers? An inquiry into etiology of pressure ulcers, *J Am Med Dir Assoc* 11:397–405, 2010.

PRURITUS ANI AND VULVAE

Method of
Muhammad Ahmad Ghazi, MD

CURRENT DIAGNOSIS

- Anogenital pruritis is primarily idiopathic; most secondary etiologies can be divided into dermatologic, anogenital conditions, and systemic causes.
- Good history and physical examination are important for accurate diagnosis.
- Laboratory tests and procedures to diagnose the cause of pruritis ani and vulvae should be tailored to individual patients based on their presentation.

CURRENT THERAPY

- Initial treatment is usually conservative, and clinicians should focus on reassurance, education about hygienic practices, regular bowel movements, avoidance of moisture and irritants, and a trial of topical corticosteroids.
- Anogenital conditions such as hemorrhoids, fissures, skin tags, and fistulas—if present—must be treated first.
- Pruritus vulvae secondary to lichen planus, lichen sclerosus, and lichen simplex chronicus usually require superpotent topical steroid treatment.
- Refractory cases of pruritus ani may benefit from injectable treatments of methylene blue.[1]
- Suspicious lesions of vulva and perineum that are resistant to initial treatment must be biopsied to rule out malignancy.

[1]Not FDA approved for this indication.

Pruritus ani and vulvae is not a disease per se; rather, it is a symptom or manifestation of an underlying disease or the result of poor personal hygienic practices. Pruritus is derived from the Latin *prurire*, which means "to itch." Pruritis ani is literally an unpleasant sensation leading to scratching the skin around the anal opening. Anogenital pruritus is a commonly ignored skin condition. Symptoms range from mild to severe and can be complicated by sleep disturbances, anxiety, depression, and social embarrassment. Pruritus ani and vulvae can be primary, in which case there is no identifiable cause, or be secondary to an underlying condition. Most of the secondary causes are anorectal, including hemorrhoids, fistulas, and fissures. Psoriasis, lichen sclerosus, and lichen simplex chronicus are common secondary dermatological causes of pruritus in the vulvar region.

Epidemiology

Pruritus ani is a common condition with an estimated prevalence of 1% to 5% of the population. It affects all ages and both genders. Male to female prevalence of pruritus ani is about 4:1. Symptoms are worse at night and in warm, moist climates. Pruritus vulvae is seen in women of all ages. Young females usually present with an infectious etiology while the primary disease is more common in postmenopausal women. Genital pruritus in men is rare and usually presents with balanitis.

Risk Factors

Poor personal hygiene, chronic diarrhea, obesity, high-risk sexual behaviors, and immunodeficiency states predispose a person to pruritus in the anogenital area. Heat, sweating, and tight undergarments may exacerbate the condition. A proposed list of causative factors is included in Boxes 1 and 2.

Pathophysiology

The itching sensations of pruritus ani and vulvae are mediated by unmyelinated C fibers, which are distributed densely in the perineal region at the dermal-epidermical junction of the skin. Irritants in stool (exotoxins, intestinal lysosymes, endopeptidase, trypsins) and increased alkalinity of certain foods such as tomatoes, chocolate, and caffeine contribute to the perianal itching that precedes scratching. The itch-scratch cycle is mediated by several mechanical and inflammatory mediators, including histamine, kallikrein, bradykinin, trypsin, serotonin, and neuropeptides. The resulting nerve impulse is carried via spinothalamic tract to the thalamus, where the itching sensation is perceived. Intestinal transit time and altered anal sphincter pressure are influenced by certain foods that predispose people to perianal seepage and pruritus.

Pruritus vulvae is the result of increased permeability of the dermis resulting from a structurally thin strateum corneum as compared to the rest of the vulvar skin. Factors aggravating the pruritus include constant friction, rubbing, anatomic location, occlusion, moistness, fear of uncleanliness in women, and excessive washing. The most common cause of pruritus vulvae is

---

BOX 1 Common Causes of Pruritus Ani

Acute
Idiopathic up to 25% of cases
Fecal contamination:
Poor hygiene
Fecal incontinence
Anal sphincter dysfunction
Anorectal pathology: 10% to 50% of cases
Hemorrhoids, perianal fissures, pilonidal sinus, perianal abscess, rectal prolapse, polyps, and papilloma
Mechanical factors:
Excessive washing, rubbing, synthetic undergarments
Infectious:
Erythrasma (corynebacterium infection), Candida, dermatophytosis, herpes simplex, human papilloma virus, HIV, syphilis
Parasitic:
Scabies, pinworm
Dermatoses:
Allergic or contact dermatitis, psoriasis, drug eruptions
Dietary factors:
Tomatoes, chilis, coffee, beer, soda, dairy, chocolate, tea, citrus fruits

Chronic
Dermatoses:
Allergic or contact dermatitis, psoriasis, lichen planus, lichen simplex chronicus, lichen sclerosis, Hailey-Hailey disease
Inflammatory:
Inflammatory bowel disease (ulcerative colitis and Crohn's disease)
Malignant:
Anal squamous cell cancer
Extramammary Paget's disease
Lymphoma/leukemia
Metabolic:
Diabetes mellitus, chronic liver disease and chronic kidney disease, celiac disease, iron deficiency anemia, hypovitaminosis A, B, D, E
Miscellaneous:
Hyperhidrosis
Neuropathic pruritus
Psychogenic (anxiety related)

BOX 2 Common Causes of Pruritus Vulvae in Women

PREPUBERTAL AGE
Poor hygiene
Sensitization of vulvar skin: soaps, deodorants
Contact dermatitis
Parasitic infestations: Pinworms (Enterobius vermicularis), pediculosis, scabies
Bacterial infections (Group A beta hemolytic infections and Escherichia coli)
Vaginal candidiasis (rare in this age group)
Lichen sclerosis
Suspected child sexual abuse (based on evidence of genital trauma)

REPRODUCTIVE AGE
Vaginitis
Trichomonas
Bacterial vaginosis
Candidiasis
Rarely tinea cruris
Herpes simplex type II
HIV, syphilis
Dermatitis
Atopic dermatitis
Contact dermatitis
Psoriasis
Lichen planus
Lichen simplex chronicus
Lichen sclerosis
Seborrheic dermatitis
Pregnancy
Vulvar itching is worsened because of vulvar engorgement; pregnancy also predisposes women to vaginal discharge and candidiasis
Systemic diseases: Diabetes, renal and liver diseases
Miscellaneous
Vulvar intraepithelial neoplasia (HPV)
Mechanical trauma
Idiopathic

POSTMENOPAUSAL AGE
Urinary or fecal incontinence
Menopause: Lack of estrogen leads to loss of skin elasticity and makes it prone to itching
Atrophic vaginitis
Lichen sclerosis
Paget's disease of vulvae
Vaginal malignancy (squamous cell cancer)

---

vulvar dermatitis or eczema, which affects one-third to half of all women presenting with this complaint. Dermatitis or eczema can be endogenous and the result of familial disposition, and it manifests as atopic dermatitis. Exogenous dermatitis such as contact dermatitis can be allergic, given that a trigger (allergen) might induce an immune response or contact irritant dermatitis. Common irritants include soaps, shampoos, vaginal creams, alcohol, tea tree oil,[7] douches, vaginal hygiene products, vaginal contraceptives, sanitary pads, nylon underwear, and toilet paper. Chemical allergens contributing to contact dermatitis in the genital area include benzocaine, neomycin, ethylenediamide, propylene glycol, latex dyes, nickels, semen, lanolin, perfumes, and tampons.

Clinical Manifestations

Perianal and vulvar itching, erythema, excoriations, fissures, hemorrhoids, pinworms, and fecal incontinence may be noticed on inspection of the perineal area. In the acute phase, skin redness of varying degrees is visible. Excoriations from the skin from itching may be present. Fissures in the labial folds may be present. Superinfection with yeast or bacteria may complicate the presentation.

Chronic anogenital dermatitis usually presents as erythema of varying degrees, and papillae appear in the labial folds. Hypo- or hyperpigmentation of the skin or thickening of the labial skin

---

[7]Available as dietary supplement.

might develop over time, causing "lichenification," which leads to lichen simplex chronicus.

Diagnosis of Pruritus Ani and Vulvae

A detailed history of bowel habits and personal hygiene (including products used, such as perfumes); dietary habits (e.g., caffeine consumption); and previous medical, psychiatric, and surgical history help elucidate the cause of pruritus ani. The patient should be asked about personal or family history of hives, asthma, conjunctivitis, or atopy when allergic dermatitis is suspected. Other relevant questions of history include recent use of antibiotics, clothing preferences, family history of cancers, other family members with similar symptoms (pinworms and scabies), rectal bleeding, change in bowel habits, or sexual preference (anal receptive intercourse). For pruritus vulvae, the patient should be asked about any history of itching, burning sensation, vaginal discharge, postcoital bleeding, or dysperunia. Rarely, elderly patients with lumbosacral radiculopathy may experience perianal itching as a result of neurological deficits.

Physical Examination

Inspection with a bright light and a chaperone is recommended. Palpation includes a digital rectal exam and a female pelvic examination in case of pruritus vulvae. Wet preparation of vaginal secretions for Candida, bacterial vaginosis, potassium hydroxide testing, and cultures for *Neisseria gonorrhoeae* and chlamydia are recommended. Microscopic examination of scrapings will help to differentiate the parasitic and fungal infections.

Laboratory Tests

Laboratory tests should not be done routinely in all cases and should be tailored to the patient's history and physical examination. Below is a list of laboratory tests that should be considered when diagnosing possible causes of anogenital pruritus:
1. CBC (complete blood count) helps to differentiate between parasitic and infectious cases and diagnoses anemia (a possible cause of chronic pruritus ani)
2. Chemistry profile (to identify systemic causes such as hepatic and kidney diseases)
3. Urinalysis to screen for infection and systemic diseases such as diabetes
4. DNA polymerase chain reaction probe for gonorrhea and chlamydia
5. Cellophane tape test to look for pinworms
6. Stool for ova and parasites
7. Test for diabetes mellitus and HIV if suspected
8. Anal Pap smear for HPV is indicated if there is a history of anal receptive intercourse

Procedures

Anoscopy and proctoscopy are indicated to diagnose hemorrhoids and perianal fistulae. Colposcopic examination of the perineum may provide a detailed view of local pathology.

Colonoscopy is indicated for patients over 40 with a family history of colon cancers. Patch testing should be performed to diagnose allergic contact dermatitis. A skin biopsy is indicated in case of ulcerated skin lesions, refractory cases, and suspicious lesions to rule out malignancy. A 3 to 6 mm punch biopsy is recommended.

Differential Diagnosis

A broad range of clinical problems can be enumerated in the differential diagnosis, including (but not limited to) allergic skin reactions, infections, parasitic infestations, chronic liver disease, diabetes, and neoplasms; chronic conditions such as psoriasis or dermatitis; infections such as condylomata accuminata; and skin cancers such as Bowen's disease, squamous cell cancer, Paget's disease, or melanoma.

Prevention and Treatment

General Principles of Treatment

The goal of treatment should be the resolution of symptoms, restoration of skin anatomy, and prevention of recurrence. The most important step in the management of pruritus ani and vulvae is reassurance and patient education (Figure 1). An informed and educated patient tends to deal with symptom-related anxiety better. To identify and treat the cause, it should be understood that pruritus ani and vulvae are commonly idiopathic, and conservative measures are usually sufficient to treat the condition. However, secondary causes need to be identified and treated.

Anorectal conditions such as hemorrhoids, fistulas, and fissures may require surgical treatment and consultation. Antidiarrheals should be used in cases of loose stool. A high-fiber diet should be started.

Women presenting with vulvar pruritus should be screened and treated for vaginal infection (e.g., one dose of oral fluconazole [Diflucan] 150 mg for vulvovaginal candidiasis; metronidazole [Flagyl] 500 mg oral twice daily for 7 days for bacterial vaginosis). Dermatological conditions such as psoriasis and dermatitis are treated with topical steroids. Hormone replacement therapy can be used in cases of menopause. Topical estrogen creams are better alternatives for symptomatic relief.

Patients should be instructed to gently cleanse the perianal area twice daily and after each bowel movement. Sitz baths with plain warm water are recommended for perianal pruritus. The perianal area should be patted dry after washing. Patients with vulvar pruritus should avoid tight undergarments, jeans, and panty hose. The use of laundry detergents, bubble baths, feminine douches, or sprays containing protease should be discouraged. Women with a predisposition to vulvar dermatitis should wear loose pants. Panty liners should be avoided and replaced with tampons or cotton cloth. Vulvae should be washed gently; women should avoid vigorous rubbing or cleaning. Patients with vulvar pruritus should use a bland moisturizer as a soap substitute to avoid irritation resulting from chemicals. The vulva should be dried before wearing underwear, and excessive perspiration should be controlled with talcum powder. Patients should be encouraged to manage incontinence and maintain an ideal body weight. Cornstarch should be avoided, as it can lead to bacterial colonization and exacerbation of symptoms.

Dietary modifications (for anal pruritus) are imperative, including limitations on the consumption of chocolate, tea, coffee, citrus fruits, and alcoholic beverages. Eating yogurt is recommended, especially while on antibiotics, to prevent diarrhea and worsening of perianal seepage.

Emollients such as aqueous creams or petrolatum or emulsifying ointments treat itching and dry skin, which can prevent erosion and ulcer formation. These agents can be used irrespective of the etiology of pruritus. Zinc oxide (Desitin) cream is used topically to prevent excoriations in cases of perianal and vulvar pruritus. Combination products such as zinc oxide/bacitracin (rash relief antibacterial), zinc oxide/menthol (Calmoseptine), and zinc oxide/miconazole (Vusion) are available and can be used for symptomatic relief. Topical anesthetics (lidocaine 5% [L-M-X5 Anorectal, Topicaine 5]) may be used twice a day to help with acute symptoms. Topical benzocaine (Vagisil Anti-Itch Creme) should be avoided, as it is a strong irritant and allergen. Cool compresses and gel packs can help. Ice should not be used, as it can cause frostbite.

Antihistamines should be used to improve sleep, and patients should wear cotton gloves at night to prevent itching while asleep. Nails should be cut short, and nail varnish should be avoided. Sedating antihistamines might help (e.g., hydroxyzine [Vistaril] 50 mg PO at bedtime; doxepin [Sinequan][1] 10 to 100 mg at bedtime; citalopram [Celexa][1] 20 to 40 mg during the daytime). Citalopram can also help with underlying anxiety symptoms, but caution is advised in the elderly and patients at risk of arrhythmias, because citalopram can cause QT interval prolongation. Any suspicious lesions of the vulvae and perineum should be biopsied to rule out underlying malignancy.

Pharmacologic Treatments

For mild pruritus ani, 1% to 2.5% hydrocortisone (Hydrocort) topical ointment is effective. Pramoxine (Prax, Senna Sensitive)

---

[1]Not FDA approved for this indication.

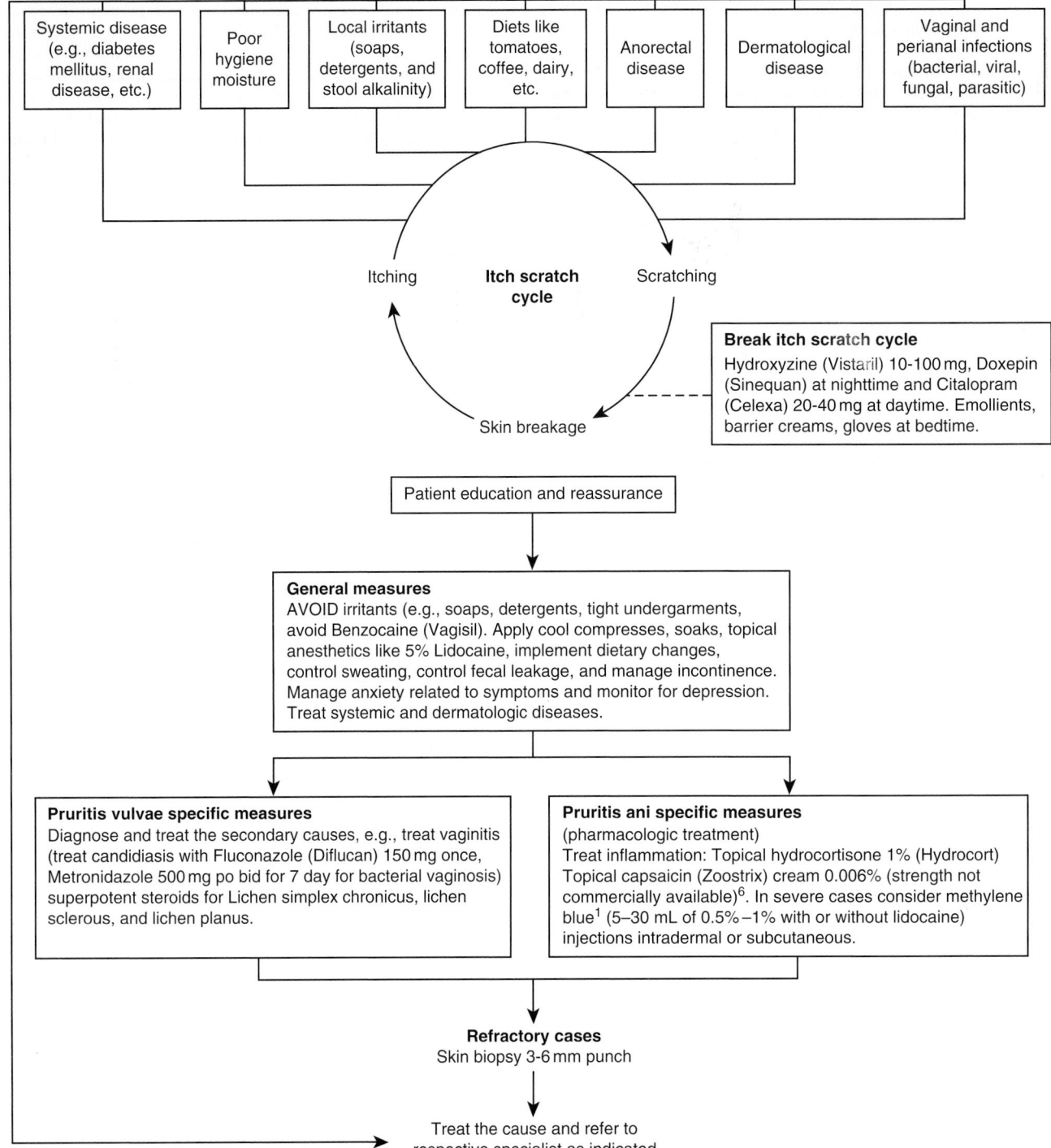

Figure 1 Pathogenesis and management of pruritus ani and vulvae. [1]Not FDA approved for this indication. [6]May be compounded by pharmacists.

can also be used alone or in combination with topical hydrocortisone cream (Analpram-HC, Pramosone). 1% Hydrocortisone/1% iodoquinol (Vytone) can be used as an antiinflammatory treatment for external use in the anal and vulvar area. Topical capsaicin cream 0.006%[6] has been used in cases of refractory itching and can be combined with topical hydrocortisone cream to avoid hypersensitivity. This strength of capsaicin cream is not commercially available.[6] Mild topical corticosteroid ointments are sufficient to treat the perianal pruritus, and superpotent steroids should be avoided, as the skin is thin and there is a risk of ulcer formation. Methylene blue[1] injections are reserved for long-standing, intractable pruritus ani. Methylene blue 0.5% to

1% 5 to 30 mL mixed with normal saline and local anesthetics is injected intradermally, subcutaneously, and intracutaneously in the perianal skin to produce hypoesthesia. This treatment may be repeated, and studies report a success rate of 80% to 90%. Possible complications associated with methylene blue injections include cellulitis, transient urinary incontinence, urinary retention, skin abscess and skin necrosis. Long term effectiveness of these injections need further prospective studies.

For moderate vulvar disease, 0.1% triamcinolone (Kenalog) ointment is recommended. For severe cases and thickened skin, the superpotent steroid topical clobetasol (Temovate) or halobetasol (Ultravate) 0.05% ointments can be used. The use of these superpotent steroid creams should be limited and reserved for the resistant cases of pruritus vulvae, lichens

---

[6]May be compounded by pharmacists.

simplex chronicus, lichen sclerosus, or resistant lichen planus. Vulvar lichen and lichen planus should be treated over the long term with superpotent steroids for adequate response and treatment. A very thin layer of steroid cream should be used, and patients should be educated about the side effects of the medication before starting the treatment. For vulvar lichen planus and lichen sclerosus, superpotent steroids are used topically once or twice daily for 2 to 3 months; three times a week for 1 month; then once or twice per week for the long term. For lichen simplex chronicus, treatment is twice daily for 2 weeks and then once daily for 2 weeks. It then moves to three times per week.

Topical calcineurin inhibitors 1% pimecrolimus cream (Elidel)[1] or 0.03% to 1% tacrolimus ointment (Protopic)[1] may be used for refractory cases as steroid-sparing agents. A common side effect of these agents is a burning sensation, so their use is controversial in cases of lichen sclerosis and lichen planus. Lichen sclerosis has 2-5% increased risk of developing squamous cell cancer, therefore clinical monitoring is recommended every 6–12 months and suspicious lesions must be biopsied.

In cases of neuropathic pruritus ani and vulvae, amitriptyline (Elavil)[1] 10 to 150 mg at bedtime is suggested. Other options are gabapentin (Neurontin)[1] 300 to 3600 mg up to three times a day (maximum daily dose is 3600 mg); pregabalin (Lyrica)[1] 75 to 400 mg/day; and mirtazapine (Remeron)[1] 7.5 to 15 mg at bedtime. In resistant and rare cases in which none of the above mentioned treatments is effective, radiation treatment may be indicated to destroy nerve endings. Naltrexone[1], an opioid antagonist has shown effectiveness in reducing itching episodes after one week of treatment in a case study. Case reports suggest treatment of perianal atopic dermatitis resistant to other treatments may respond to dupilumab (Dupixent)[1], which is a monoclonal antibody. Treatment should be reserved for biopsy confirmed cases of atopic dermatitis in consultation with dermatologist. Several experimental treatments, such as laser phototherapy, alcohol injection therapy, radiation, and surgery, have not been studied and are not recommended routinely.

Complications

Pruritus ani and vulvae can lead to myriad complications, including lichenification, skin excoriations, ulcers, secondary bacterial infections, and abscess formation.

Referral

For undiagnosed and resistant skin conditions, patients should be referred to a dermatologist. Persistent anal itching, a change in bowel habits, and rectal bleeding should prompt a referral to a gastroenterologist and colorectal specialist. Pruritus vulvae with vaginal bleeding and weight loss are indications for referral to a gynecologist.

Monitoring and Prognosis

Most cases of pruritus ani and vulvae are treated with general measures that lead to a full recovery. Long-term use of corticosteroids should be discouraged, and periodic monitoring for side effects, including skin erosions and bleeding, is advisable based on reported symptoms. The idiopathic disease usually persists and depicts a relapsing remitting course.

---

[1]Not FDA approved for this indication.

References

Al-Ghnaniem R, Short A, Pullen A: 1% Hydrocortisone ointment is an effective treatment of pruritus ani: A pilot randomized controlled crossover trial, *Int J Colorectal Dis* 22:1463–1467, 2007.
Family Practice Notebook: Pruritus vulvae. Available at http://www.fpnotebook.com/gyn/vulva/vlvrprts.htm, 2013 (accessed December 14, 2013).
Jones DJ: ABC of colorectal disease. Pruritus ani, *BMJ* 1305:575–577, 1992.
Margesson LJ: Overview of treatment of vulvovaginal disease, *Skin Therapy Lett* 16:5–7, 2011.
Margesson L, Danby WF: Pruritus ani and vulvae. In *Conn's Current Therapy 2013*: Philadelphia, 2012, Elsevier, pp 276–278.
Markell KW, Billingham RP: Pruritus ani: Etiology and management, *Surg Clin North Am* 90:125–135, 2010.
Mentes BB: Intradermal methylene blue injection for the treatment of intractable idiopathic pruritus ani: Results of 30 cases, *Tech Coloproctol* 8:11–14, 2004.
Reidy T, Rafferty JF: Management of pruritus ani. In *Current Surgical Therapy*, Philadelphia, 2011, Elsevier Mosby, pp 243–246.
Siddiqi S, Vijay V, Ward M, et al: Pruritus ani, *Ann R Coll Surg Engl* 90:457–463, 2008.
Stermer E, Sukhotnic I, Shoul R: Pruritus ani: An approach to an itching condition, *J Pediatr Gastroenterol Nutr* 48:513–516, 2009.
Weichert GE: An approach to the treatment of anogenital pruritus, *Dermatol Ther* 17:129–133, 2004.
Yang EJ, Murase JE: Recalcitrant anal and genital pruritis treated with dupilumab, *Int J Womens Dermatol* 4:223–226, 2018.

PYODERMA GANGRENOSUM

Method of
Dominic J. Wu, MD; and Anand N. Rajpara, MD

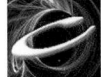

CURRENT DIAGNOSIS

- Pyoderma gangrenosum (PG) is a chronic inflammatory and ulcerative skin disease of uncertain etiology that is commonly mistaken for skin infection.
- Diagnosis of PG is typically a diagnosis of exclusion. Thorough workup to exclude other causes of ulcerative diseases (e.g., infection, malignancy, vascular) is paramount.
- There is no uniformly accepted diagnostic algorithm, and many have been proposed. A recent Delphi consensus set of diagnostic criteria is becoming more widely adopted.
- Recent diagnostic criteria require biopsy of the ulcer edge demonstrating neutrophilic infiltrate as the major criterion, while ruling out infection is no longer an absolute requirement.

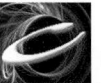

CURRENT THERAPY

- There is no established gold standard treatment regimen.
- Goals of therapy should include reducing inflammation, reducing pain, and controlling any contributing underlying diseases.
- Due to the nature of the disease and complex medical treatments, it is important to involve relevant consultants early on, such as dermatology, rheumatology, gastroenterology, rheumatology, ophthalmology, etc.
- For mild, localized disease, consider topical and/or intralesional corticosteroids.
- For moderate to severe cases, the first-line systemic agents are historically systemic corticosteroids and cyclosporine (Neoral, Sandimmune).[1]
- Alternative treatment options that have shown success include tumor necrosis factor-α (TNF-α) inhibitors such as infliximab (Remicade)[1] and adalimumab (Humira),[1] mycophenolate mofetil (CellCept),[1] IVIG,[1] tetracyclines,[1] and more.
- Avoid debridement and surgical procedures due to risk of pathergy.
- Appropriate wound care is essential, including selection of appropriate dressings. Less exudative wounds can be treated with hydrogels and films. More exudative lesions should be managed with more absorptive dressings such as hydrocolloids and alginates. Consider involvement of wound care specialists.

[1]Not FDA approved for this indication.

Pathophysiology and Epidemiology

Pyoderma gangrenosum (PG) is a chronic ulcerative inflammatory neutrophilic dermatosis of uncertain etiology that is often misdiagnosed as severe skin infection. It is a relatively rare condition with incidence estimated at approximately 3 to 10 cases per million people per year, but it is not uncommonly encountered in dermatology clinic. It most frequently presents in young to middle-aged female adults between 20 to 50 years of age. Although its exact etiology is unknown and 25% to 50% of patients have idiopathic disease, it is frequently associated with numerous systemic diseases including inflammatory bowel disease (ulcerative colitis, Crohn disease), malignancy, granulomatosis with polyangiitis, Behçet disease, and more. This association suggests a possible underlying immunologic abnormality. PG is also a component of multiple genetic conditions including PAPA (pyogenic arthritis, PG, acne), PASH (PG, acne, hidradenitis suppurativa), and PAPASH (pyogenic arthritis, PG, acne, hidradenitis suppurativa) syndromes. Pathergy, even from minor trauma, may result in initiation and aggravation of PG lesions.

Clinical Manifestations

The clinical appearance of PG can often mimic other skin diseases, especially ulcerative infectious skin diseases, vascular diseases, and malignancies. The classic most characteristic clinical subtype is ulcerative PG. In addition, there are three other main clinical subtypes including pustular, bullous, and vegetative. The initial lesion of classic PG (ulcerative) typically begins as a painful solitary nodule or pustule that ruptures and undergoes necrosis, resulting in the formation of an ulcer. The most frequent location of PG is on the lower extremities (especially the pretibial region); however, it can appear anywhere including mucous membranes. The center of the classic PG ulcer is frequently coated with purulent material and granulation tissue. The edge of the ulcer is characteristically dusky to violaceous, irregular, undermined, and overhanging (Figure 1). Pustular PG is more commonly seen in patients with underlying inflammatory bowel disease and presents with multiple pustules with surrounding erythema to violaceous rim. These pustules may or may not rupture to form a more classic-appearing PG ulcer. Bullous, or atypical PG, is most commonly seen in patients with underlying lymphoproliferative disorders such as leukemia or multiple myeloma. Lastly, vegetative PG presents with more superficial ulcerations without significant central purulence and undermined borders.

Although the ulcer of PG is not infectious in itself, it may become secondarily infected, resulting in increased purulence and malodor.

Diagnosis

The clinical, laboratory, and histologic findings in PG are rather nonspecific; thus a diagnosis of PG is typically a diagnosis of exclusion. A detailed history of the lesion including evolution, pain, pathergy, and any associated underlying conditions are critical. General approach to workup includes biopsy of ulcer edge demonstrating neutrophilic infiltrate, and broad workup should be considered to exclude other causes including complete blood count (CBC; underlying hematologic disorder), bacterial and fungal cultures, herpes simplex virus (HSV)/varicella zoster virus (VZV) PCR, antinuclear antibody (ANA) (underlying autoimmune conditions—systemic lupus erythematosus, collagen vascular disorders), antineutrophil cytoplastic antibodies (ANCA; granulomatous vasculitis), hypercoagulability studies (vascular etiology), rheumatoid factor, urinalysis, serum and/or urine protein electrophoresis, chest imaging, and colonoscopy (evaluate for inflammatory bowel disease [IBD]). Other laboratories including comprehensive metabolic profile, hepatitis panel (which can also be helpful in evaluating for cryoglobulinemia), and tuberculosis screening are also helpful in preparation of potential treatment with immunosuppressive agents. Individual clinicians may choose varying levels of workup, depending on clinical suspicion and patient history.

Numerous diagnostic criteria and algorithms have been proposed, although they have not been uniformly accepted. Previously, diagnostic criteria required excluding all other diagnoses including infection, which is challenging and often results in delayed treatment. A recent Delphi consensus of international experts proposed and validated a set of diagnostic criteria as below:

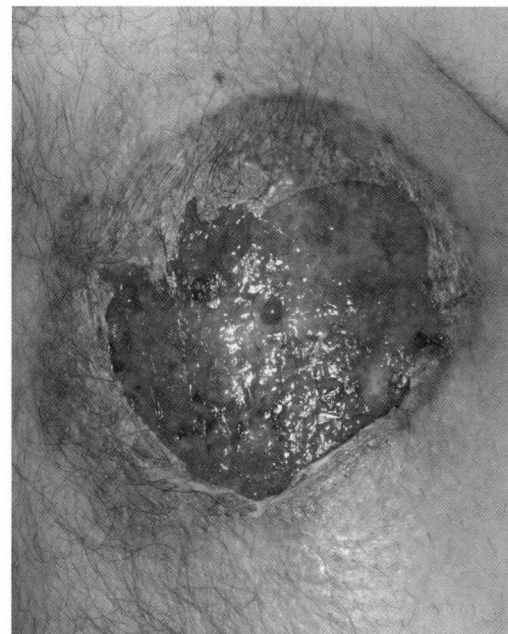

Figure 1 Classic ulcer of pyoderma gangrenosum with dusky to violaceous, irregular, undermined border. From James WD, et al: *Andrews' Diseases of the Skin*. Philadelphia: Elsevier; 2019.

Major criterion:

- Biopsy of ulcer edge demonstrating a neutrophilic infiltrate

Minor criteria:

- Exclusion of infection
- History of pathergy
- Personal history of IBD or inflammatory arthritis
- History of papule, pustule, or vesicle that rapidly ulcerated
- Peripheral erythema, undermining border, and tenderness at site of ulceration
- Multiple ulcerations (at least one occurring on an anterior lower leg)
- Cribriform or "wrinkled paper" scar(s) at sites of healed ulcers
- Decrease in ulcer size within 1 month of initiating immunosuppressive medication(s)

Diagnosis of PG requires the major criterion and four or more minor criteria. These criteria are becoming more widely adopted in academic institutions.

Differential Diagnosis

It is important to consider and exclude alternative diagnoses when evaluating a patient with possible PG. PG can mimic ulcerative infections such as herpes simplex virus, ecthyma gangrenosum, chancroid, deep fungal infections, sporotrichosis, atypical mycobacterial infection, necrotizing fasciitis, syphilis, and Buruli ulcer. Vascular disorders to consider include venous or arterial ulcerations, vasculitides including granulomatosis with polyangiitis, polyarteritis nodosa, cryoglobulinemia, and so on.

Therapy

There is no one-size-fits-all treatment for PG, and the goal of therapy is primarily to reduce the inflammatory process, promote healing, reduce pain, and treat any contributing underlying medical conditions. Debridement and surgical therapy should be avoided if possible due to pathergy and potential for worsening disease. Surgical therapy in other areas of the body should also be avoided if possible due to risk of developing similar lesions at other sites. It is important to involve relevant consultants as soon as possible based on the patient's case, including dermatology, ophthalmology, rheumatology, oncology, gastroenterology, and so on.

First-line therapy includes local high-potency topical corticosteroids such as clobetasol propionate 0.05% (Clobex, Temovate) twice a day and/or systemic corticosteroids such as prednisone 0.5 to 1 mg/kg/day divided in two to three doses, with slow taper over weeks to months. Colchicine[1] 0.6 mg PO three times a day has shown success as monotherapy or used in conjunction with corticosteroids. Cyclosporine (Neoral, Sandimmune)[1] 2.5 to 5 mg/kg/day divided twice a day has been demonstrated to lead to rapid improvement in pain and improvement in ulceration. Combination therapy with systemic corticosteroids and cyclosporine has also demonstrated success. Milder localized disease can be treated with intralesional corticosteroid injections such as with triamcinolone acetonide (Kenalog) 10 mg/mL into the ulcer edge or high-potency topical corticosteroids.

Alternative therapies utilized with success for moderate to severe disease include infliximab (Remicade)[1] 5 mg/kg IV at weeks 0, 2, and 6; adalimumab (Humira)[1] 80 mg SC loading dose, followed by 40 mg SC weekly or every other week; mycophenolate mofetil (Cellcept)[1] 750 mg to 1.5 g PO twice a day; dapsone[1] 50 to 150 mg daily; sulfasalazine (Azulfidine) 0.5 to 6 g PO daily divided in 3 to 4 doses, methotrexate[1] 2.5 to 25 mg PO, SC, or IM weekly, and more. The authors have also seen success with intravenous immunoglobulin (IVIG)[1] 1.5 to 3 g/kg IV monthly given over 2 to 5 days, although this can be incredibly expensive and is generally used as adjuvant therapy. IVIG is also an option for treatment if there is secondary infection and immunosuppressive therapies with TNF-α inhibitors are contraindicated.

Tetracycline antibiotics such as minocycline (Minocin)[1] 200 to 300 mg/day divided in 2 doses have also been reported to show success in treatment of PG, thought to be related to their anti-inflammatory properties by reducing chemotaxis of neutrophils.

Appropriate wound care for PG ulcers is essential, depending on the clinical appearance of the lesion. Wound care specialists should be utilized if possible. Occlusive dressings are often utilized to increase the rate of healing by promoting angiogenesis, promoting collagen synthesis, and acting as a barrier against secondary infection. Hydrogels and films such as Tegaderm may be used in lesions with minimal exudate. In more exudative lesions, more absorptive dressings such as hydrocolloids, foams, and alginates would be more appropriate. Examples of these dressings that are frequently utilized for ulcer management include DuoDERM and SeaSorb. It is important to note that these dressings, especially alginates, may be associated with foul odor due to their reaction with healing tissue and may not actually be an indicator of secondary infection. Avoid wet-to-dry dressings, as this debridement may incite pathergy and cause aggravation of the wound.

Monitoring

PG tends to be a chronic and recurrent disease. Ulcers may take many months to heal, and it is essential to monitor for any signs of developing infection. Patients and clinicians should monitor for increased pain, increased purulence, fevers, increased erythema and/or streaking—all of which can be indicators for secondary infection. Topical and oral antimicrobials may be helpful; however, this may lead to antibiotic resistance and should be utilized only if secondary infection is confirmed.

Adequate control of any contributing underlying conditions is essential, and patients should be advised that trauma and elective surgical procedures may trigger the development of future PG lesions.

Many of the treatments utilized in the management of PG also have their large range of adverse side effects, and it is important to monitor patients closely when they are taking these medications. For example, systemic corticosteroids are the most commonly employed agents in PG. More severe or resistant lesions may require prolonged therapy and at higher doses, which can lead to increased adverse side effects. These patients should be closely monitored, and consider recommending supplemental calcium, vitamin D, proton pump inhibitors if indicated, and even bisphosphonates. The duration of

treatment is case-dependent and should be determined based on clinical response and any concerning side effects.

[1]Not FDA approved for this indication.

References

Ahronowitz I, Harp J, Shinkai K: Etiology and management of pyoderma gangrenosum: a comprehensive review, *Am J Clin Dermatol* 13(3):191–211, 2012.

Braswell SF, Kostopoulos TC, Ortega-Loayza AG: Pathophysiology of pyoderma gangrenosum (PG): an updated review, *J Am Acad Dermatol* 73(4):691–698, 2015.

Brooklyn T, Dunnill G, Probert C: Diagnosis and treatment of pyoderma gangrenosum, *BMJ* 333(7560):181–184, 2006.

Cummins DL, Anhalt GJ, et al: Treatment of pyoderma gangrenosum with intravenous immunoglobulin, *Br J Dermatol* 157(6):1235–1239, 2007.

Davis MDP, Moschella SL: Neutrophilic Dermatoses: pyoderma gangrenosum. In Bolognia JL, et al: *Dermatology 2018*, ed 4, Philadelphia, 2018, Elsevier, pp 459–463.

Maverakis E, Ma C, et al: Diagnostic criteria of ulcerative pyoderma gangrenosum: a Delphi consensus of international experts, *JAMA Dermatol* 154(4):461–466, 2018.

Neill BC, Seger EW, et al: The 5 P's of pyoderma gangrenosum, *J of Drugs in Dermatol* 18(12):1283, 2019.

Patel F, Fitzmaurice S, et al: Effective strategies for the management of pyoderma gangrenosum: a comprehensive review, *Acta Derm Venereol* 95(5):525–531, 2015.

ROSACEA

Method of
Lisa M. Johnson, MD; and Daniel J. Van Durme, MD, MPH

CURRENT DIAGNOSIS

- Rosacea is a chronic inflammatory disease of the skin that predominantly affects the convexities of the central face (cheeks, chin, nose, and central part of forehead). It most commonly occurs in adults aged 30 to 50 years.
- Rosacea is a clinical diagnosis.
- Transition to a phenotype-based approach to the diagnosis, classification, and management of rosacea from the traditional subtype-based approach is occurring, allowing more individualized management of symptoms that most concern a patient.
- Two cutaneous phenotypes may be considered independently diagnostic of rosacea: (1) fixed centrofacial erythema in a characteristic pattern that may periodically intensify, or (2) phymatous changes.
- The presence of two or more major phenotypes (flushing, telangiectasia, inflammatory lesions, and ocular manifestations) may be considered diagnostic of rosacea.
- Common exacerbating factors that intensify signs and symptoms include alcohol, heat, spicy foods, and sunlight.

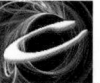

CURRENT THERAPY

- Therapy is best chosen based on severity and predominant manifestation(s).
- Avoidance of known triggers is key for all types,
- Brimonidine tartrate 0.33% gel (Mirvaso, Onreltea) and oxymetazoline hydrochloride 1% cream (Rhofade) are useful for facial flushing. Ivermectin cream (Soolantra) and metronidazole gel (Metrogel, Rosadan) can be effective for papules and pustules. Isotretinoin (Accutane, Claravis)[1] can be effective in treating very severe and refractory rosacea.
- Ocular rosacea can be treated with increased eyelid hygiene, adding topical or oral antibiotics if needed.
- Rhinophyma (sebaceous gland hypertrophy and fibrosis) needs surgical management.

[1]Not FDA approved for this indication.

Rosacea is well established as a chronic cutaneous syndrome, encompassing various combinations of potential signs and symptoms that

[1]Not FDA approved for this indication.

manifest primarily on the convexities of the central face (cheeks, chin, nose, and central part of forehead). Signs and symptoms are often characterized by repeated remissions and exacerbations. Rosacea is commonly diagnosed in certain demographic groups, and in epidemiologic studies of Whites, its prevalence has been 10% or higher. Although it has been most frequently observed in patients with fair skin, rosacea has also been diagnosed in Asians, Latin Americans, African Americans, and Africans. The disorder is identified more often in women than in men, and although it may occur at any age, the onset typically occurs at any time after age 30.

Diagnosis

The classification of rosacea was updated in 2016 and modified in 2019 by the global ROSacea COnsensus panel (ROSCO). This panel recommended transitioning to an individualized phenotype-based approach to the diagnosis, classification and management of rosacea rather than the traditional subtype-based approach. By focusing on individual lesions rather than a group of dermatologic characteristics constituting a subtype, treatment can be tailored to the signs and symptoms that most concern an individual patient.

Diagnostic Phenotypes

The panel identified two phenotypes as independently diagnostic of rosacea: (1) centrofacial erythema associated with periodic intensification, and (2) phymatous changes. Phymatous changes include patulous follicles, skin thickening or fibrosis, glandular hyperplasia, and a bulbous appearance of the nose. Rhinophyma is the most common form, but other phymas may occur.

Major Phenotypes

Flushing transient erythema, telangiectasia, inflammatory lesions, and ocular manifestations were major phenotypes commonly identified in patients with rosacea but were not considered individually diagnostic. In the absence of one of the two diagnostic phenotypes, the presence of two or more of these major phenotypes may be considered diagnostic.

Secondary Phenotypes

Secondary signs and symptoms of rosacea may appear with one or more diagnostic or major phenotypes and include burning or stinging, edema, and a dry appearance.

Ocular Rosacea

Ocular rosacea can occur in the context of mild, moderate, or severe dermatologic disease and may also appear in the absence of diagnostic skin manifestations. Ocular signs strongly suggestive of ocular rosacea include lid margin telangiectases, interpalpebral conjunctival injection, spade-shaped infiltrates in the cornea, and scleritis and sclerokeratitis.

Treatment

One key aspect of management is to have the patient maintain a careful diary for the purpose of determining and then avoiding his or her own triggers. Common triggers include alcohol, heat, certain foods, sunlight, stress, and menstruation, among others. Broad-spectrum sunblock (UVA and UVB) should be used daily, along with application of moisturizers for dry skin and drying applications for oily skin, and gentle cleansing of the whole face. Cosmetics with a red-neutralizing green pigment can help appearance.

Brimonidine tartrate 0.33% gel (Mirvaso, Onreltea) is a selective alpha2-adrenergic receptor agonist with vasoconstrictive activity and has been approved for the treatment of persistent (nontransient) facial erythema in adults 18 years and older with rosacea, along with oxymetazoline hydrochloride 1% cream ([Rhofade] an alpha1A-adrenoreceptor agonist that also activates alpha2-receptors at higher concentration).

Patients with mild to moderate papules and pustules benefit from topical 1% ivermectin cream (Soolantra), which is applied to the face once daily, and topical antibiotics such as metronidazole 0.75% to 1% cream, lotion, or gel (MetroCream 0.75%, Noritate 1% cream, MetroLotion 0.75%, Rosadan 0.75% gel,

Metrogel 1% or azelaic acid 20% cream [Azelex][1] or 15% gel [Finacea]) applied once or twice daily. Persistent telangiectasias can be effectively treated with laser therapy and intravascular aethoxysklerol ([Asclera] 0.5%–1%)[1] injections.

Patients affected by mild phymata benefit from tetracycline[1] therapy. Standard therapies for advanced phymata are ablative (destructive) laser and dermato-surgery. Low-dose isotretinoin (Accutane, Claravis)[1] appears to reduce phymata by its antiinflammatory capacity and by lessening the number of sebaceous glands and inhibiting their proliferation.

There is no US Food and Drug Administration (FDA)–approved therapy for facial edema. Immunomodulators such as isotretinoin[1] and dapsone (oral or topical [Aczone gel])[1] or combination therapies with doxycycline (Oracea)/prednisolone have been tried, but the therapeutic value is unclear.

Both prescribers and patients must register with the iPledge program to prescribe and to receive the prescriptions for isotretinoin. See www.ipledgeprogram.com.

Ocular rosacea can often be controlled with increased eyelid hygiene, washing with warm water and baby (no-tears) shampoo twice a day along with artificial tears. Long-term consumption of omega-3 fatty acids[7] may improve meibomian-gland dysfunction. Topical ophthalmic cyclosporine drops (Restasis)[1] applied as one drop to the eye twice daily (12 hours apart) demonstrate statistically significant improvement in common signs and symptoms compared with artificial tears. If severe, it can be treated with systemic tetracycline.[1] If it persists, ophthalmology referral is necessary.

---

[1]Not FDA approved for this indication.
[7]Available as a dietary supplement.

References

Buddenkotte J, Steinhoff M: Recent advances in understanding and managing rosacea, *F1000Res* 7:F1000 Faculty Rev-1885, 2018, https://doi.org/10.12688/f1000research.16537.1. Published 2018 Dec 3.
Gallo RL, Granstein RD, Kang S, Mannis M, Martin S, Tan J, Thiboutot D: Standard classification and pathophysiology of rosacea: the 2017 update by the National Rosacea Society Expert Committee, *J Am Acad Dermatol* 78(1):148–155, 2018.
Goldgar C, Keahey DJ, Houchins J: Treatment options for acne rosacea, *Am Fam Physician* 80:461–468, 2009.
Powell FC: Clinical practice: rosacea, *N Engl J Med* 352:793–803, 2005.
Schaller M, Almeida LMC, Bewley A, et al: Recommendations for rosacea diagnosis, classification and management: update from the global ROSacea COnsensus 2019 panel, 182(5):1269–1276, 2020.
Tan J, Almeida LMC, Bewley A, et al: Updating the diagnosis, classification and assessment of rosacea: recommendations from the global ROSacea COnsensus (ROSCO) panel, *Br J Dermatol* 176:431–438, 2017.
Wollina U: Rosacea and rhinophyma in the elderly, *Clin Dermatol* 29:61–68, 2011.

STEVENS-JOHNSON SYNDROME AND TOXIC EPIDERMAL NECROLYSIS

Method of
Scott Worswick, MD

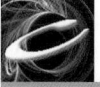

CURRENT DIAGNOSIS

- A diagnosis of toxic epidermal necrolysis (TEN) can be rendered when the body surface area (BSA) involved contains more than 30% denuded skin.
- A diagnosis of Stevens-Johnson Syndrome (SJS) can be rendered when less than 10% of the BSA involves denuded skin.
- SJS-TEN overlap is diagnosed when the involved BSA is between 10% and 30% BSA.
- Patients with SJS, SJS-TEN overlap, and TEN should have involvement of not only the cutaneous surface but also at least one mucosal region (most commonly the oral mucosa). Cases do exist with no mucosal involvement but this is rare and should prompt consideration of an alternate diagnosis.
- A thorough drug history and skin biopsy (ideally using the fresh-frozen technique) are essential when considering a diagnosis of SJS or TEN.

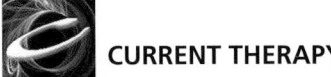

CURRENT THERAPY

Epidemiology

Toxic epidermal necrolysis (TEN) is a rare diagnosis, only afflicting approximately one patient per million per year (most studies cite this incidence rate, though one study from the United States did cite an incidence rate as high as 12.7 per year). Stevens-Johnson Syndrome (SJS) and SJS-TEN overlap affect approximately five per million patients per year. The overall mortality varies greatly among different studies but is currently estimated to be ~25% for TEN. It can affect patients of any age, and most data regarding therapy are stratified by age into pediatric and adult cohorts. There are some experts who feel there may be a viral trigger or co-factor for the disease because prevalence increases in the spring.

Risk Factors

Common implicated agents include sulfonamide antibiotics as well as more recently described penicillin and cephalosporin antibiotics, aromatic anticonvulsants, allopurinol (Zyloprim), and nonsteroidal antiinflammatory drugs (NSAIDs). Numerous other medications have been reported to trigger the disease and some other common offending agents include the anti-programmed death-1 and anti-cytotoxic T-lymphocyte-associated protein 4 chemotherapeutic agents, dapsone and nevirapine (Viramune). The most important intervention is to determine and remove the offending agent as some studies cite an increase in mortality of 34% per day if the offending agent is not removed from the patient's regimen.

Certain tests can be performed after hospitalization in selected cases to determine the most likely offending agent if unknown. For example, patch testing can be done, and in the case of carbamazepine-induced SJS-TEN, has a sensitivity greater than 70%. Likewise, if multiple drugs are suspected as potential inciting agents, it may be worth checking the patient's human leukocyte antigen (HLA) types and correlating this with his/her ethnicity to make an educated guess about likely agent (if a patient has three potential inciting agents including allopurinol, the patient is of Asian descent, and HLA-typing reveals positive HLA-B5801, it could be concluded with a higher level of certainty that allopurinol is the most likely agent).

Less common triggers include vaccines such as MMR and less commonly the meningococcal, varicella and influenza vaccines, herpes, and ultraviolet light. These are more likely to be implicated in patients with target lesions or low body surface area (BSA) involvement and are exceedingly rare in patients diagnosed with full-blown TEN. An important trigger to consider in the work-up is mycoplasma, which can be responsible for causing mycoplasma-induced rash and mucositis (MIRM). MIRM is a clinical mimicker common in pediatric patients, which is characterized by lower BSA but worse mucosal involvement (typically involving two sites and usually including the ocular mucosa in dramatic fashion).

In addition to the causes of SJS and TEN described previously, there are risk factors that seem to predispose patients to the disease. These include: HIV (some studies cite a thousand-times increased chance of developing TEN among HIV-positive patients, even when controlled for the number and type of medications these patients were exposed to), lupus, female gender, Asian or African ethnicity, patients undergoing brain cancer treatment with corticosteroids and radiation, and certain HLA types. For example, one recent meta-analysis found that certain HLA-B subtypes predispose Asian patients to the development of carbamazepine-induced TEN, including HLA-B1502, HLA-B4001, HLA-B4601, and HLA-B5801. Other studies have identified HLA-B1502 as a risk factor for aromatic anticonvulsant-induced TEN among various Asian populations, HLA-B5801 as a risk factor for allopurinol-induced TEN among Asians, HLA-C0401 for nevirapine-induced TEN among patients in Malawi, and HLA type B3802, A29, B12, and DR7 as a risk factor among Europeans for sulfonamide-induced TEN.

Pathophysiology

As described previously, an immunologic basis for the development SJS and TEN is hypothesized given the fact that certain HLA types among certain groups predispose them to development of the disease. There currently exist four theories to explain how small drugs might interact with HLA and T-cell receptors (TCRs) to initiate a chain of events leading to SJS/TEN.

In the hapten theory (which has been validated in the case of penicillin-induced drug reactions), it is presumed that the drug molecule combines with an endogenous peptide and this is presented to the HLA molecule and recognized by the TCR. In the p-i model (pharmacologic interaction with the immune receptors), which has been validated in carbamazepine-HLA-B1502 interactions, the drug itself binds directly, reversibly, and noncovalently to HLA and/or TCR. In the altered peptide repertoire model, it is proposed that the drug binds to the peptide-binding groove of the HLA molecule thereby altering the overall binding ability of the HLA molecule. Lastly, in the altered TCR repertoire model, it is suggested that some drugs (such as sulfamethoxazole) can bind directly to the TCR (but not with the HLA molecule) and thereby alter the conformation of the TCR giving them the ability to bind to self-HLA.

Regardless of the type of interaction that allows a drug to alter the way HLA and TCR react to self, patients with TEN exhibit increased activity of natural killer (NK) cells and specific T lymphocytes (NK T-cells and CD* + cytotoxic T-cells). These cells mediate keratinocyte cell death via a cascade of events including Fas–FasL binding and procaspase-8 activation, increased tumor necrosis factor-α and interferon-γ levels, and activation of the perforin-granzyme-granulysin apoptosis pathway.

Differential Diagnosis

Patients with SJS and TEN typically complain of skin pain before the eruption begins. A prodrome consisting of low-grade fever, malaise, and/or flu-like symptoms is not uncommon. Within days some degree of mucosal involvement (which can take the form of dusky erythema, bullae/vesicles, denuded mucosal surface(s), dysuria, ocular erythema, pain with defecation, or pain with swallowing) is almost universal, while the extent of cutaneous involvement can vary dramatically but should include either a dusky erythema with eventual vesicles, bullae, or denuded skin, or less commonly targetoid lesions. The majority of patients with SJS and TEN present with painful red-purple (dusky) patches or macules that progress over the span of a few days. Areas that began with dusky erythema develop superimposed bullae, vesicles, or denuded skin.

Most patients with SJS and TEN do not present with typical targets on cutaneous exam. Such lesions are characterized by a small red central papule surrounded by a white ring and finally most peripherally by another ring of erythema. These lesions characterize erythema multiforme, which is much more commonly the result of herpes rather than drug allergy. However, there are rare reported cases of SJS and TEN that do include or are even dominated by cutaneous typical or atypical targets.

The main differential diagnosis for patients with classic dusky erythema, mucosal involvement, and skin pain includes acute graft-versus-host disease (GVHD), bullous lupus, generalized fixed drug eruption (FDE), cutaneous burns, paraneoplastic pemphigus (PNP), in pediatric patients MIRM, and in infants infection with the Chikungunya virus. The majority of these entities can be ruled out by clinical history alone, as patients with acute GVHD should have had a recent transplant and patients with PNP a concurrent malignancy. Dramatic mucosal involvement, in any age group, should prompt work-up for mycoplasma; when MIRM is suspected it should be treated with empiric antibiotics and in severe cases IVIG[1]. Patients with a known malignancy (particularly chronic lymphocytic leukemia [CLL], lymphoma, Castleman disease, sarcoma, or thymoma) and/or of older age and with significant mucosal disease should have, in addition to a biopsy, a direct immunofluorescence (DIF) performed and serum drawn for indirect immunofluorescence and ELISA performed to rule out PNP. It is important to check a DIF as well in any patients with joint pain or other symptoms suggestive of systemic lupus erythematosus (SLE), as well as antinuclear antibody (ANA), anti-Sjogren's syndrome–related antigen (SSA), and anti-Sjogren's Syndrome Type B (SSB), anti-dsDNA and anti-Smith. Likewise, if you are evaluating an infant who has no medication exposure and is from an endemic area, it is important to check serum titers for the Chikungunya virus.

Diagnosis

Determining the inciting agent is as important as making a quick diagnosis of TEN. A thorough drug history is essential including prn medication usage (frequently patients do not report their NSAID use or a recent antibiotic exposure). If SJS or TEN is suspected and the inciting agent is known, it is important to immediately inform the patient and his/her family of the suspected allergy and add it to the patient's medication allergy list. Dermatology should be consulted and when possible/necessary will ideally perform a skin biopsy to be processed emergently using the fresh-frozen technique (results can be ready within 30 minutes). Hematoxylin and eosin staining will also be done on permanent sections (and these results are available 1 to 3 days later depending on the site/lab).

After making a diagnosis of SJS or TEN, a practitioner can employ a scoring system called SCORTEN to estimate the patient's mortality. In this system a patient receives one point if he/she is aged above 40 years, BSA greater than 10%, history of concurrent malignancy within 2 years, serum blood urea nitrogen greater than 28 mg/dL, glucose greater than 252 mg/dL, bicarbonate level less than 20 mEq/L, and heart rate more than 120 beats per minute during the first 24 hours. With each increasing point, mortality increases such that a score of 2 confers an expected mortality of 12%; a score of 3 equates to a 35% mortality; a score of 4 with a 58% mortality; and a score of 5 or higher with an expected 90% chance of mortality.

Therapy
Medical Therapy

Classic therapy for SJS and TEN was with systemic corticosteroids but this has fallen out of favor in the United States due to recent meta-analyses suggesting no improvement in outcomes. Likewise, IVIG[1] was a mainstay of therapy in the early 21st century, but a large review from Europe found a worsened mortality in patients given IVIG compared with those given steroids or supportive care alone. Other data are conflicting with some studies suggesting that a 4-day dose of daily 1 g/kg IV[1] provides a mortality benefit, with other studies finding no improvement.

More recent success seems to have come from the utilization of etanercept (Enbrel)[1] or cyclosporine (Neoral, Sandimmune)[1] in the treatment of this disease. In 2014 a group from Italy treated 10 patients with one 50 mg subcutaneous dose and found not only a 0% mortality despite an expected mortality of 47%, but also decreased time to re-epithelialization. Likewise, in 2018 a

Taiwanese group found an improved mortality benefit of etanercept over corticosteroids among 96 patients.

Similarly, data emerging in the last decade have suggested that cyclosporine also confers a mortality benefit. In 2010 a British case series found a 0% mortality in patients receiving 3 mg/kg per day orally despite a predicated ~30% mortality based on SCORTEN. Another study cites a significantly decreased time to re-epithelialization (3.67 days) among patients who survived after receiving cyclosporine at a dose of 3 to 4 mg/kg per day.

Adjuvant Mucosal Therapies

Patients with SJS/TEN can suffer from long-term skin/hair/nail complications including post-inflammatory hyperpigmentation, photosensitivity (70% of patients according to one study), chronic pruritus, eruptive nevi, nail changes, hypertrophic scars, and telogen effluvium. They also have a significant morbidity when their mucosal surfaces are severely involved with disease. Ocular complications can include ectropion, trichiasis, ankyloblepharon, corneal scarring, and even blindness. To some extent these complications are minimized by a choice of systemic therapy to mediate disease (i.e., either etanercept or cyclosporine). However, other measures can also be employed including amniotic membrane grafting by ophthalmology (which has been shown in a randomized controlled trial to improve multiple ocular outcome measures), topical steroid application, oxygen therapy, and bronchodilators. Likewise, urogenital sequelae occur in about one in four patients and can include adhesions leading to dyspareunia or even total vaginal fusion. Therefore involvement of gynecology or urology in the care of any patient with genital SJS/TEN is essential.

Monitoring

It is important to remember that the cutaneous examination of a patient with TEN differs greatly depending on the time of exam relative to the onset of eruption. With onset it is possible the patient will only complain of pain and have no skin lesions whatsoever. Within days a typical exam would include florid oral mucosal involvement with areas of skin showing dusky erythematous macules or patches. Over the next few days, most of the cutaneous lesions will evolve and become vesicles, bullae, or entire surfaces will denude. Monitoring for efficacy of chosen therapy means being aware of what is expected in terms of progression (that some or all areas that were dusky will denude), and ensuring that no new dusky areas develop.

The most common cause of death in patients with TEN is infection, so checking daily white blood cell counts and following vitals every 2 to 4 hours if not more frequently is essential. Fevers can occur simply as the result of the disease process itself, but any fever should prompt blood, urine, and sputum cultures. Prophylactic antibiotics have not been shown to improve outcomes but when an infection is suspected it must be treated immediately.

References

Canavan TN, Mathes EF, Friedan I, et al: Mycoplasma pneumonia-induced rash and mucositis as a syndrome distinct from Stevens-Johnson syndrome and erythema multiforme: A systematic review, *JAAD* 72(2):239–245, 2015.

Chahal D, Aleshin M, Turegano M, et al: Vaccine-induced TEN: A case and systematic review, *Dermatology, Online Journal* 24(1), 2018.

Chen CB, Abe R, Pan RY, et al: An updated review of the molecular mechanisms in drug hypersensitivity, *Journal of Immunology Research*, 2018.

Conner C, McKenzie E, Owen C: The use of cyclosporine for SJS-TEN spectrum at the University of Louisville: A case series and literature review, *Dermatology Online Journal* 24(1), 2018.

Lee HY, Walsh SA, Creamer D: Long-term complications of SJS/TEN: The spectrum of chronic problems in patients who survive an episode of SJS/TEN necessitates multidisciplinary follow-up, *British Journal of Dermatology* 177:924–935, 2017.

Paradisi A, et al: Etanercept therapy for TEN, *JAAD* 71(2):278–283, 2014.

Schneck J, et al: Effects of treatment on the mortality of SJS and TEN: A retrospective study on patients included in the prospective EuroSCAR Study, *JAAD* 58(1):33–40, 2008.

Valeyrie-Allanore L, Wolkenstein P, Brochard L, et al: Open trial of ciclosporin treatment for SJS and TEN, *British Journal of Dermatology* 163(4):847–853, 2010.

Wang CW, Yang LY, Chen CB, et al: Randomized, controlled trial of TNF-alpha antagonist in CTL-mediated severe cutaneous adverse reactions, *J Clin Invest* 128(3):985–996, 2018.

Wang Q, Sun S, Xie M, et al: Association between the HLA-B alleles and carbamazepine-induced SJS/TEN: A meta-analysis, *Epilepsy Research* 135:19–28, 2017.

---

[1]Not FDA approved for this indication.

SUNBURN

Method of
Kamille S. Sherman, MD

CURRENT DIAGNOSIS

- Typically a first-degree or second-degree burn occurring on sun-exposed or ultraviolet (UV)-exposed (e.g., tanning bed) skin within 4 hours to 2 days of exposure
- May be demarcated from unaffected skin by an obvious boundary where protective clothing prevented the sun or UV exposure, with the burned area having a consistent, continuous appearance

CURRENT THERAPY

- Over the counter nonsteroidal antiinflammatory drugs (NSAIDs) or acetaminophen at doses as directed by the manufacturer on the packaging can relieve pain and decrease inflammation but will not change long-term damage to the skin. Some experts recommend a short-term course of oral steroids if a large area of skin is sunburned.
- Cool the skin, either with a cool bath/shower or apply a cool, damp towel or wear cool, damp flannel clothing over the affected area.
- Drink plenty of water to prevent dehydration or rehydrate if mildly dehydrated.
- Do not break any blisters on the skin.
- Do not apply benzocaine or other "-caine" types of products, as they can irritate the skin, cause allergic reactions, or precipitate methemoglobinemia.
- Apply a soothing moisturizer, such as aloe vera[7] or calamine, PRN. This may be in lotion or gel form.
- As skin heals, apply hydrating moisturizers.
- As healing occurs, avoid reinjury/reexposure of affected skin to sun or UV light.
- Assess for secondary infection and treat if necessary.
- Review patient medication list, as some over-the-counter and prescription drugs and herbal remedies increase sensitivity to UV light.

[7]Available as dietary supplement.

Epidemiology

In a study of 31,162 US adults, using the 2015 National Health Interview Survey (NHIS) Cancer Control Supplement, a total of 34.2% of adults experienced sunburn in 2015. Of those experiencing sunburn, 16.3% experienced one sunburn, 9.9% experienced two sunburns, 3.4% experienced three sunburns, and 4.6% experienced four or more sunburns. There is epidemiologic evidence suggesting that the harmful effects of UV radiation exposure from typical doses of sunlight vary over the course of the life span, with some evidence of a window of biologic vulnerability in childhood that translates into increased skin cancer risk later in life.

Risk Factors

"Sun sensitivity" was assessed using two questions in the 2015 NHIS Cancer Control study. One question asked what would happen to the respondent's skin if, after several months of not being in the sun, the individual went out in the sun for an hour without sunscreen, a hat, or protective clothing (short exposure). The second question asked the individual what would happen if he or she were out in the sun repeatedly, such as every day for 2 weeks, without sunscreen, a hat, or protective clothing (i.e.,

repeated exposure). About half of individuals who described themselves as "sun sensitive" indicated they would experience sunburn (50.2%).

Non-Hispanic white individuals are more likely to experience sunburn than other racial/ethnic groups. Adults who self-reported skin that tended to burn after repeated sun exposure were more likely to become sunburned as compared with individuals who easily develop tans. Behaviors associated with sunburn include use of self-applied tanning products, aerobic activity, binge drinking in the past 30 days, and overweight or obesity. An increase in the number of sunburns an individual experiences is directly related to an increase in the risk of skin cancer.

Approximately 50.2% of adults aged 18 to 29 years reported having experienced sunburn, as did 14.8% of adults aged 66 years or older.

The level of UV protection afforded by clothing can vary widely based on color, material, and weave of the fabric. The US Preventive Services Task Force (USPSTF) reports that indoor tanning before age 35 years, or more than 10 tanning sessions over a lifetime and for longer than 1 year, have been linked to increased skin cancer risk.

Pathophysiology

UV radiation (both A and B) from both solar and artificial sources has been classified as a human carcinogen by national and international organizations. UVA damage is associated with "aging," whereas UVB is associated with "burning." UVB rays are responsible for directly damaging skin cell DNA by inducing the formation of thymine-thymine cyclobutane dimers. As the body generates a DNA repair response to these dimers, inflammatory markers lead to vasodilation, edema, and pain, which manifest as classic-appearing sunburn. UVB light also activates peripheral nociceptors by causing an increase in chemokines.

Prevention

The most frequently used sun protection behaviors among US adults include staying in the shade (37.1%) and using sunscreen (31.5%). About one-fourth of those engaging in sun-protective behaviors wear long clothing to the ankles (28.4%). Less frequent behaviors include regular use of long-sleeved shirts (12.3%) and wide-brimmed hats (14.2%). Women are more likely to use shade (41.3%) and sunscreen (40.2%) as protective behaviors, whereas men are more likely to wear long clothing to the ankles (34.3%) and to use shade (30.7%).

The sun protection factor (SPF) is a relative measure of the fraction of sunburn-producing UV rays that reach the skin. Assuming correct application, "SPF 20" means that one-twentieth of the burning radiation will reach the skin. The effectiveness of a sunscreen can be calculated by multiplying the SPF by the length of time it takes a user to suffer a burn without sunscreen. For example, if a person develops a sunburn in 20 minutes when not wearing a sunscreen, using an SPF 30 sunscreen would protect the individual for about 10 hours. Because the intensity and wavelength distribution of UVB rays varies throughout the day and by latitude, the effectiveness of sunscreen also varies. Direct exposure to the sun should be avoided between the hours of 10 A.M. and 4 P.M. A broad-spectrum sunscreen with SPF of at least 30 should be applied 30 minutes before sun exposure and every 90 minutes thereafter, even if the product is labeled "water resistant."

There are many suggestions regarding the appropriate use of sunscreen, although the NHIS found that sunscreen users were actually more likely to experience sunburn. This probably happens because sunscreen users are out in the sun more frequently than those who do not use sunscreen regularly.

Along with recommending staying in the shade, the American Cancer Society uses a slogan popularized in Australia as one of that country's skin cancer prevention strategies: "Slip! Slop! Slap! ... and Wrap!" The phrase is a way to remind individuals to slip on a shirt, slop on sunscreen, slap on a hat, and wrap on sunglasses to protect eyes and sensitive skin from the sun's harmful rays.

Clinical Manifestations

Sunburn appears most often as a first-degree burn—an injury affecting the epidermis and associated with erythema, pain, and mild swelling followed by skin peeling. More severe sunburn may lead to second-degree burns, in which blisters accompany the erythema and swelling. Second-degree sunburns hurt more significantly and affect both the epidermis and dermis. These burns can take several weeks to heal.

Diagnosis

The diagnosis is based largely on the history of sun exposure coupled with the classic appearance and distribution of sunburn.

Differential Diagnosis

The differential diagnosis of sunburn includes autoimmune diseases such as systemic lupus erythematosus and dermatomyositis; bacterial infections such as staphylococcal scalded skin syndrome, cellulitis, and erysipelas; and dermatologic diseases such as rosacea, acne, stasis dermatitis, and seborrheic dermatitis. There are also congenital ichthyotic conditions. Other solar reactions caused by the sun's rays include solar urticaria, photoallergic type IV sensitivity reactions, and phototoxic reactions.

Treatment

Treatment for sunburn is largely supportive. Oral analgesics, such as nonsteroidal antiinflammatory drugs and/or acetaminophen, provide some relief. Cool bathing, cool towels, and flannel clothing moistened with cool water can provide some comfort. Moisturizing topical products such as aloe vera or calamine may provide comfort. Some experts recommend steroid usage, either topical or orally, although consensus on their use is mixed and steroids are usually reserved for patients with extensive areas of sunburn. Treatment of secondary skin infections, especially if broken blisters are infected, includes antibiotic usage for common skin pathogens. The avoidance of local anesthetic creams and sprays containing "-caine" derivatives is standard advice. "Caines" can irritate the skin, cause allergic reactions, and precipitate methemoglobinemia. Opioids for pain associated with sunburn should be avoided except in the most unusual circumstances. Adequate water intake to prevent or reverse dehydration is encouraged. In the rare case of extensive sunburn with large areas of blistering accompanied by massive fluid loss and electrolyte imbalances, intravenous rehydration may be considered as well as transfer to a burn unit. Avoiding another sunburn, especially before the first one appears "healed," is important. The DNA damage caused by sunburn is not reversible. There are no topical or systemic agents that are FDA approved to reverse UV damage to the skin.

Monitoring and Complications

Most sunburns are self-limited and will heal over a number of days to weeks, at least appearing "healed" to casual inspection. Patients who suffer severe sunburn should be warned to watch for the development of secondary infections. The underlying DNA changes in the skin are linked to the development of skin cancers, including melanoma. The USPSTF recommends "counseling young adults, adolescents, children, and parents of young children about minimizing exposure to UV radiation for persons aged 6 months to 24 years with fair skin types to reduce their risk of skin cancer."

The USPSTF concludes that current evidence is insufficient to assess the balance of benefits and harms of counseling adults about skin self-examination. Evaluation of suspicious skin lesions should be undertaken by physicians, with monitoring and/or removal of suspicious lesions.

Skin cancer is the most common type of cancer in the United States. Although invasive melanoma accounts for 2% of skin cancer types, it is responsible for 80% of skin cancer deaths. Basal and squamous cell carcinoma, the two predominant types of nonmelanoma skin cancer, represent the vast majority of skin cancers. About 5.4 million basal and squamous cell skin cancers are diagnosed in the United States each year; they occur in an estimated 3.3 million Americans, as some people have more than one. About 8 out of 10 of these are basal cell cancers. About 2000 people die from basal or squamous cell skin cancers in the United States annually. There will be an estimated 100,350 new cases of melanoma skin cancer in 2020. The 5-year survival rate for melanoma, according to the American Cancer Society, is 92%. Treatment for skin cancer can include surgery and radiation therapy, as well as some newer forms of nonsurgical treatment such as novel topical drugs, photodynamic therapy, and laser surgery.

References

Guerra KC, Crane JS: Sunburn. [Updated 2019 Nov 25]. In: StatPearls [Internet]. Treasure Island.

Holman DM, Ding H, Guy GP, et al: Prevalence of sun protection use and sunburn and association of demographic and behavioral characteristics with sunburn among us adults, *JAMA Dermatol* 154(5):561–568, 2018 May, Published online 2018 Mar 14.

US Environmental Protection Agency: Sun safety. Available at https://www.epa.gov/sunsafety. [Accessed 13 January 2020].

US Food and Drug Administration: Sunscreen: how to help protect your skin from the sun. Available at https://www.fda.gov/Drugs/ResourcesForYou/Consumers/BuyingUsingMedicineSafely/UnderstandingOver-the-CounterMedicines/ucm239463. [Accessed 2 December 2019].

U.S. Preventive Services Task Force: Final recommendation statement: skin cancer prevention: behavioral counseling. Available at https://www.uspreventiveservicestaskforce.org/Page/Document/RecommendationStatementFinal/skin-cancer-counseling2. [Accessed 2 December 2019].

URTICARIA AND ANGIOEDEMA

Method of
Joyce M.C. Teng, MD, PhD

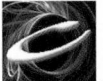

CURRENT DIAGNOSIS

- Acute and chronic urticaria have the same features, including erythematous, edematous papules or wheals with central pallor that last less than 24 to 48 hours.
- Laboratory assessments are not recommended for acute urticaria in the absence of evidence suggesting underlying systemic illness.
- Limited laboratory studies are indicated for chronic urticaria only if there are signs of systemic disease.
- Serum measurements of C4 and C1-esterase inhibitor are the recommended initial tests if hereditary or acquired angioedema are suspected.
- Skin biopsy should be considered to rule out urticarial vasculitis if an individual lesion is painful and persists for more than 2 to 3 days with accompanying ecchymosis or petechiae.

CURRENT THERAPY

- Primary treatment of urticaria and angioedema is removal of triggering factors and initiation of therapy for symptomatic relief.
- Oral antihistamines are the cornerstones of therapy. The application of first-generation H_1-antihistamines may be limited by central nervous system and anticholinergic side effects.
- Nonsedating second generation antihistamine are often used as first line therapy. Higher dose can be used when symptoms are not controlled.
- Anti-IgE therapy, omalizumab (Xolair), has been approved for patients over 12 years of age with chronic idiopathic urticaria. Systemic corticosteroids and immunosuppressive therapy, especially cyclosporine (Neoral),[1] have been used successfully in cases that are refractory to the maximum dose of antihistamines.
- Fresh-frozen plasma infusions along with standard airway precautions have been recommended for angioedema patients with laryngeal edema.
- A subcutaneous C1 esterase inhibitor injection (Haegarda) has been used successfully to prevent attack in hereditary angioedema.

[1]Not FDA approved for this indication.

Urticaria, or hives, is a common cutaneous eruption that occurs in up to 25% of the general population sometime during their lives (Bailey, 2008). It is characterized by transient, circumscribed, pruritic, erythematous papules or plaques, often with central pallor. Individual lesions often coalesce into large wheals on the trunk and extremities that may resolve over a few hours without leaving any residual skin changes. The process is mediated by mast cells in the superficial dermis, and skin changes often resolve within 30 min to 24 hr.

Angioedema is a similar process occurring in deep dermis or subcutaneous tissue. Angioedema may occur independently, accompanied by urticaria, or as a component of anaphylaxis. It is characterized by localized swelling that develops over minutes to hours and resolution may take up to 72 hours. Common locations of angioedema include the mucosa and areas with loose connective tissue, such as the face, eyes, lips, tongue, and genitalia. Patients usually do not have pruritus, but they may have pain and a sensation of warmth. Angioedema is usually a benign process that resolves without sequelae unless it involves the larynx. African Americans are disproportionately affected, representing up to 40% of the hospital admissions for angioedema.

Classification

Urticaria can be classified as acute or chronic, depending on the duration. Acute urticaria usually lasts for less than 6 weeks and can be spontaneous or triggered by infection, medication, insect bite, and food (Table 1). The chronic form, lasting more than 6 weeks, accounts for approximately 30% of cases of urticaria, and no clear causes can be identified in more than 80% of these cases. Stress however has been identified as a trigger in some of the cases. Depending on the triggers, chronic urticaria can be classified as cold, heat, solar, delayed pressure, vibratory, cholinergic, contact, or aquagenic urticaria. A significant number of patients with chronic urticaria may have persistent symptoms for more than 10 years. Approximately 40% of patients with chronic urticaria have associated angioedema, although the incidence of laryngeal edema is low.

Diagnosis

Urticaria is diagnosed clinically in most cases. A detailed history, physical examination, and complete review of systems are essential for diagnosing patients with urticaria and angioedema. The history should include the distribution and characteristics of lesions (e.g., pain, pruritus), duration of skin eruption, accompanying angioedema, airway involvement and other associated systemic symptoms (e.g., fever, arthralgia, swelling joints, refusal to walk by children). Patients should also be questioned about changes in dietary habits, stress, recent exposures, infection, and newly administered medications, including antibiotics, over-the-counter analgesia, and hormones. Patients who suffer from recurrent angioedema should be asked about their use of angiotensin-converting enzyme (ACE) inhibitor medications.

Laboratory assessment is usually not helpful in diagnosing patients with acute urticaria who lack any history or clinical findings to suggest an underlying disease process. A limited number of diagnostic tests are indicated in the evaluation of patients with chronic urticaria when there is sign of systemic disease associated, such as a complete blood cell count with differential white blood cell count, an erythrocyte sedimentation rate (ESR) or C-reactive protein (CRP) determination, a thyroid-stimulating hormone (TSH) level, antithyroglobulin and antimicrosomal antibodies, antinuclear antibodies (ANA), folate, B12, ferritin, liver function test, and hepatitis B and C serologies. A detailed review of systems may help to narrow the focus of the screening test.

A skin biopsy of an early lesion should be performed to rule out urticarial vasculitis if the affected individual has skin lesions that are painful and last for more than 2 to 3 days with residual ecchymosis or petechiae. In patients with angioedema, prominent edema of the interstitial tissue may be demonstrated by biopsy. It is associated with antibodies against C1q, which leads to persistent complement activation and low serum C3, C4. Serum measurements of C4 and C1-esterase inhibitor are recommended initial tests if hereditary or acquired angioedema is suspected. Hereditary angioedema is caused by deficiency (type I) or dysfunction (type II) of C1-esterase inhibitor protein. A C1q level should be obtained to screen for the acquired form of angioedema if the affected individual is middle-aged. Additional constitutional symptoms and extracutaneous manifestations are often present in patients with autoinflammatory syndromes such as Schnitzler's syndrome, cryopyrin-associated periodic syndrome (CAPS), Muckle-Wells syndrome (MWS), neonatal-onset multisystem inflammatory disease (NOMID) and, rarely, hyper-IgD syndrome (HIDS) and tumor necrosis factor receptor alpha-associated periodic syndrome (TRAPS).

Treatment

More than two thirds of cases of urticaria are self-limited. Spontaneous remission of chronic urticaria and angioedema is also common. The primary objective of management is to identify and discontinue the offending trigger. A patient presenting with angioedema must first be assessed for signs of airway compromise. Medical therapy is indicated for those who are symptomatic.

Antihistamines remain the first-line therapy for most patients with urticaria, because the primary complaint of pruritus is predominantly mediated by histamine released from mast cells. First-generation antihistamines such as hydroxyzine (Atarax or Vistaril 1 mg/kg (max 25 mg/dose) for children and 25–50 mg every 6 hours in adults), diphenhydramine (Benadryl 25–50 mg every 6 hours), cyproheptadine (Periactin 4 mg three times daily), and chlorpheniramine[1] (Chlor-Trimeton 4 mg every 6 hours) are potent and have the quickest onset of action. However, the treatments are often limited by their sedating and anticholinergic side effects. Many first-generation antihistamines are available over the counter, providing accessible first-line therapy for patients. Patients with urticaria that lasts for several days should be considered for treatment using second-generation antihistamines such as loratadine (Claritin[1] 10 mg twice daily[3]), desloratadine[1] (Clarinex 5 mg twice daily[3]), cetirizine[1] (Zyrtec 10 mg twice daily[3]), levocetirizine[1] (Xyzal 5 mg daily), and fexofenadine[1] (Allegra 180 mg twice daily[3]). If urticaria is not adequately controlled, the second generation antihistamine dosage can be at least doubled. Doxepin (Sinequan),[1] an H_1- and H_2-receptor antagonist, is seven times more potent than hydroxyzine in suppression of wheal and flare responses. Because of its central nervous system side effects, combined use of doxepin with a first-generation antihistamine should be restricted. Topical 5% doxepin cream (Zonalon)[1] may help to suppress pruritus in patients with localized urticaria. Anti-IgE

TABLE 1 Mechanisms in Urticaria and Angioedema

DISORDER	CAUSES
Immunoglobulin-mediated urticaria	Ig-E mediated: food, medication, insect bites, contact allergen, aeroallergens, other causes Urticaria associated with autoimmunity: antinuclear antibodies (ANAs), thyroid autoantibodies, other causes
Direct activation of mast cell degranulation	Physical stimuli: exercise, heat, cold, pressure, aquagenic, solar radiation, etc. Other agents: opiates, antibiotics (e.g., vancomycin [Vancocin]), radiocontrast, ACTH (Cortrosyn), muscle relaxants
Complement-mediated	Viral infections, parasites, blood transfusion
C1-esterase inhibitor deficiency	Genetic and acquired angioedema, paraproteinemia
Reduced kinin metabolism	Angiotensin-converting enzyme (ACE) inhibitors
Reduced arachidonic acid metabolism	Aspirin

[1]Not FDA approved for this indication.
[3]Exceeds dosage recommended by the manufacturer.

treatment using omalizumab (150–300 mg per month) for chronic urticaria refractory to high-dose antihistamine therapy has been approved by the FDA for patients over 12 years of age in US. While the treatment is highly effective, safe, and suitable for long-term use, it has a high cost.

Systemic prednisone at 30 to 40 mg in a single morning dose is sufficient to suppress acute urticaria in adults. Tapering should be gradual over a 3- to 4-week period by decreasing the dosage 5 mg every 3 to 5 days to minimize rebound. Alternate-morning dosing when reaching 20 mg daily may help to minimize the steroid side effects. Methylprednisolone (Solu-Medrol 40 mg) should be given intravenously as initial therapy to patients with angioedema. This may be followed by a tapering oral course. Chronic therapy with systemic steroids is to be avoided. Three months of off-label treatment with cyclosporine (Neoral)[1] at 3 to 5 mg/kg can be given safely to patients who are refractory to corticosteroid or omalizumab therapy. Close monitoring for hypertension and renal insufficiency is necessary during the treatment.

Leukotriene inhibitors such as zileuton (Zyflo[1] 600 mg four times daily), zafirlukast (Accolate[1] 20 mg twice daily), and montelukast (Singulair[1] 10 mg once daily) may be effective for patients with autoimmune urticaria.

Proper management of underlying autoimmune thyroid disease or autoimmune collagen vascular diseases has been beneficial for patients with associated urticaria. Life-threatening angioedema triggered by angiotensin-converting enzyme (ACE) inhibitors has been successfully treated with infusion of fresh-frozen plasma. Hereditary angioedema can be prevented with tranexamic acid[1] or modified androgens. Intravenous C1-esterase inhibitor (Cinryze) or icatibant (Firazyr), a bradykinin B2 antagonist, can be administered to prevent acute attacks. Subcutaneous injection of C1-esterase inhibitor (Haegarda) has been approved by FDA in 2017 to prevent hereditary angioedema attacks. Treatments with methotrexate[1], warfarin (Coumadin),[1] plasmapheresis, colchicine,[1] hydroxychloroquine (Plaquenil),[1] anti-TNF-alpha,[1] interferon,[1] and intravenous immunoglobulin (Baygam)[1] have been reported for severe, refractory[1] urticaria. Vitamin D[1] supplementation can also be beneficial in reducing symptoms in patients with a deficiency. These treatments are administered only by specialists on an individual basis. Non-pharmacotherapeutic means such as frequent use of skin emollients, avoidance of hot shower, scrubbing, and excessive sun exposure should also be recommended as part of management plans.

[1]Not FDA approved for this indication.

References

American Academy of Allergy, Asthma and Immunology response to the EAACI/GA 2 LEN/EDF/WAO guideline for the definition, classification, diagnosis, and management of Urticaria 2017 revision, 74(2):411–413, 2019.

Bailey E, Shaker M: An update on childhood urticaria and angioedema, *Curr Opin Pediatr* 20(4):425–430, 2008.

Champion RH, Roberts SO, Carpenter RG, Roger JH: Urticaria and angio-oedema. A review of 554 patients, *Br J Dermatol* 81(8):588–597, 1969.

Joint Task Force on Practice Parameters: The diagnosis and management of urticaria: A practice parameter. Part II. Chronic urticaria/angioedema, *Ann Allergy Asthma Immunol* 85(2):521–544, 2000.

Kaplan AP, Joseph K, Maykut RJ, et al: Treatment of chronic autoimmune urticaria with omalizumab, *J Allergy Clin Immunol* 122(3):569–573, 2008.

Lin RY, Cannon AG, Teitel AD: Pattern of hospitalizations for angioedema in New York between 1990 and 2003, *Ann Allergy Asthma Immunol* 95(2):159–166, 2005.

Longhurst H, Cicardi M, Craig T, et al: Prevention of hereditary angioedema attacks with a subcutaneous C1 inhibitor, *N Engl J Med* 376(12):1131–1140, 2017 Mar 23.

Maurer M, Rosen K, Shieh HJ: Omalizumab for chronic urticaria, *N Engl J Med* 386:2530, 2013, https://doi.org/10.1056/JEJMc1305687.

Maurer M, Rosen K, Hsieh HJ, et al: Omalizumab for the treatment of chronic idiopathic or spontaneous urticaria, *N Engl J Med* 368:924–935, 2013.

Nizami RM, Baboo MT: Office management of patients with urticaria: An analysis of 215 patients, *Ann Allergy* 33(2):78–85, 1974.

Powell RJ, Du Toit GL, Siddique N, et al: BSACI guidelines for the management of chronic urticaria and angio-oedema, *Clin Exp Allergy* 37(5):631–650, 2007.

Saini SS, Bindslev-Jensen C, Maurer M, et al: Efficacy and safety ofomalizumab in patients with chronic idiopathic/spontaneous urticaria who remain symptomatic on H1 antihistamines: a randomized, placebo-controlled study, *J Invest Dermatol* 135:67–75, 115, 2015.

VENOUS ULCERS

Method of
Jose A. Jaller, MD; and Robert S. Kirsner, MD, PhD

CURRENT DIAGNOSIS

- Venous ulcers are the most common cause of lower-extremity ulceration.
- Valvular incompetence, vein distention, muscular weakness, and/or a decrease in the range of motion of the ankle may lead to venous insufficiency.
- The mechanism of cutaneous ulceration resulting from venous insufficiency remains unclear.
- The typical location for a venous ulcer is on the medial malleolus.
- Complications of chronic venous ulcers are cellulitis and less often squamous cell carcinoma.
- Compression is the gold standard of treatment of venous disease.

CURRENT THERAPY

- Compression therapy is used to deliver a graded compression of 30–40 mm Hg at the ankle. Arterial disease should be excluded prior to full compression.
- Systemic medications as adjuvant therapy to compression bandages include aspirin[1], pentoxifylline (Trental), or micronized purified flavonoid fraction (Daflon 500 mg)[2].
- Other treatments, along with compression, include engineered skin, placental and skin grafts, electrical stimulation, locally derived growth factors, and venous surgery.
- The lifelong use of elastic compression stockings (30–40 mm Hg) is the mainstay of prevention.

[1]Not FDA approved for this indication.
[2]Not available in the United States.

Ulcers resulting from venous insufficiency are the most common cause of leg ulceration. The Wound Healing Society classifies wounds as *acute* if they sustain restoration of anatomic and functional integrity in an orderly and timely process and *chronic* if they do not. Venous leg ulcers (VLUs) are more frequently seen in the elderly population; however, about 1 in 5 primary VLUs occur in patients under 40 years of age. Personal or family history of venous disease, obesity, smoking, advanced age, female sex, hypertension, and leg injuries are strong risk factors to the development of VLUs.

Epidemiology

Venous insufficiency affects approximately 5% of the world's population and about 2% of the American population. VLUs affect 1% to 2% of adults in the United States, accounting for over 2 million lost workdays annually. The associated pain, inability to perform daily activities, and social stigma due to the appearance and odor of the wounds drastically diminish patients' quality of life. Moreover, the high cost of treatment, time off work, and hospital admissions forge a massive economic burden in the healthcare system. Seventy percent of all leg ulcers result solely from venous disease, and an additional 20% of patients have mixed arterial and venous disease. A recent report that used claims data from 2013 private and governmental insurance companies revealed that wounds and ulcers had the highest direct US healthcare cost of all skin diseases ($12 billion) and caused approximately 21% of all deaths related to skin condition, second only to cutaneous cancers.

Pathophysiology

In the lower extremities, the venous system comprises the deep and superficial veins. Blood flows from the superficial to the deep veins through the communicating or perforating veins to ultimately reach the heart. Veins contain unidirectional valves that prevent blood return or reflux. During calf muscle relaxation, the pressure difference (high pressure in the superficial veins) allows blood flow from the superficial to deep veins. When a healthy individual contracts the calf muscles, a high pressure develops in the deep vein system, allowing blood to flow from the deep veins to the heart. If the calf muscle contraction is restricted or the one-way valves are deficient, the system fails to adequately return venous blood to the heart, leading to venous hypertension (also known as sustained ambulatory high pressure).

The pathway to developing an ulcer due to venous insufficiency is unclear, albeit several hypotheses have been considered since the beginning of the 20th century. Patients with chronic venous disease can develop ulcers in their lower extremities for a different reason (e.g., trauma), but given their venous disease and suboptimal wound healing capacity, these lesions can develop into VLUs. In the early 1980s, Browse and Burnard suggested that venous hypertension could lead to endothelial distention, causing extravasation of fibrinogen into the interstitial fluid, which results in "pericapillary fibrin cuff" formation around the capillary vessels. Fibrin cuffs act as a barrier to diffusion of oxygen and nutrients, causing ischemia and ulcer formation. A few years later, Coleridge-Smith and colleagues suggested that venous hypertension could lead to decreased capillary perfusion, resulting in leukocyte trapping. The trapped leukocytes release proteolytic enzymes, which result in free radical formation and capillary damage. The increased capillary permeability causes extravasation of fibrinogen and other metabolites, which leads to the formation of a fibrin cuff around the capillaries and ultimately ischemia.

Further studies supported the presence of increased levels of monocyte aggregation. Claudy and colleagues showed that leukocyte activation caused release of tumor necrosis factor alpha (TNF-α), ultimately leading to pericapillary fibrin cuff formation. In 1993, Falanga and Eaglstein observed that fibrin cuffs were discontinuous around capillaries and therefore did not form a barrier to oxygen and nutrients causing ischemia. They also postulated the "trap" hypothesis, which suggests that venous hypertension causes endothelial cell distention leading to extravasation of macromolecules (i.e., α_2-macroglobulin and fibrinogen) into the dermis. Moreover, α_2-macroglobulin can bind to growth factors, such as TNF-α and transforming growth factor beta (TGF-β), making them unavailable for wound repair. Patients with venous disease may have other factors that contribute to venous ulcer formation, such as systemic alteration in fibrinolysis and arteriovenous shunting. Despite all previously conducted studies and hypotheses, further research is needed to explain the mechanism of cutaneous ulceration resulting from venous insufficiency.

Evaluation and Diagnosis

VLUs are diagnosed clinically; however, blood flow imaging, pathology, and microbiologic cultures can aid to rule out other conditions. Clinical signs, such as wound location, associated venous disease, and past personal history of venous ulcers, are paramount for the diagnosis. VLUs are typically located on the lower leg, particularly in the medial lower leg or medial malleolus. The ulcer usually begins as a blister or erosion on the skin that hinders healing and develops into a full-thickness lesion, or ulcer. Ulcer borders are irregular and usually smooth. The base of the ulcer may be covered with granulation tissue, yellow slough, or both. Venous ulcers are associated with the presence of pigmentation, erythema, dermatitis, edema, and induration (i.e., lipodermatosclerosis) of the surrounding skin and with varicose veins in the lower leg. Hemosiderin deposition resulting from red blood cell extravasation and iron-related stimulation of melanocytes cause the surrounding hyperpigmentation.

Lipodermatosclerosis is caused by sclerosis of the dermis and subcutaneous tissue. The presence of lipodermatosclerosis has been associated with a greater impairment of fibrinolysis in patients with venous ulcers and may be a poor prognostic factor for restriction of leg movement. Other known prognostic factors are duration and size of the ulcer and history of venous surgery. Ulcers present for longer than 6 months and larger than 5 cm in diameter tend to be more refractory to therapy.

A diagnosis of venous ulcers may be based on clinical presentation. The findings of a lower leg ulcer associated with lipodermatosclerosis or varicose veins, or both, suggest a venous ulcer. Other common findings include atrophie blanche (i.e., porcelain white scars with telangiectasia and dyspigmentation) and dermatitis. Venous dermatitis is associated with erythema, eczema, pruritus, and scaling of the skin. Contact dermatitis surrounding the ulcer may result from the use of topical agents.

Even though venous insufficiency can be confirmed with a variety of techniques, including duplex ultrasound or plethysmography, the presence or absence of arterial disease is a more important factor dictating treatment and prognosis. Compression should be used with caution in patients with peripheral arterial disease (PAD). Also, sharp debridements should be avoided as much as possible in patients with PAD. These patients might need evaluation by a vascular surgeon for possible revascularization of the affected vessel.

A simple, noninvasive measurement to assess peripheral arterial disease is the ankle brachial index (ABI). This value is calculated by dividing the systolic pressure in the ankle by the systolic pressure in the arm. An ABI of less than 0.9 indicates peripheral vascular disease and represents an independent risk factor for vascular disease in other vascular beds, such as the coronary arteries. Care must be taken with diabetic or elderly patients who may have a falsely negative ABI value. All patients with an abnormal ABI value should be further evaluated. Consider a vascular consultation, magnetic resonance angiography (MRA), angioplasty, and stent bypass.

To aid in the exclusion of any underlying disease (e.g., hematologic disease, diabetes), initial laboratory tests should include complete blood cell (CBC) count with a differential count, chemistry panel, hemoglobin A1C, prealbumin and albumin determinations, liver function tests, and levels of homocysteine, proteins C and S, antithrombin III, and factor V Leiden.

Several vascular studies help in the diagnosis and severity of venous disease. Color duplex ultrasound is usually the initial study done to assess venous reflux in the lower extremities. Continuous-wave Doppler studies may yield false-negative results because it may be difficult to differentiate between the superficial and deep venous system. Air plethysmography and photoplethysmography are helpful in evaluating venous reflux and calf muscle dysfunction. Invasive venography is the gold standard to assess venous reflux, but it is used only as a last resort because of its invasive properties.

The CEAP classification was developed in 1994 by the American Venous Forum (AVF) to standardize the diagnosis and treatment of venous disease. It was based on clinical manifestations (C), etiologic factors (E), anatomic distribution of disease (A), and underlying pathophysiologic findings (P).

Complications

Main complications of long-term or chronic venous ulcers are cellulitis, osteomyelitis, and squamous cell carcinoma. A finding of exposed tendon or bone, in addition to suggesting an underlying osteomyelitis, suggests an ulcer with a nonvenous cause.

Radiographs and biopsy for histology and culture are appropriate first steps in evaluation. Consult an orthopedic surgeon for further analysis and treatment, which may include a bone biopsy and bone débridement.

Treatment

Compression is the gold standard of treatment of venous disease. After arterial disease has been excluded, reversal of the effects of venous hypertension through compression bandages and leg elevation is the cornerstone of therapy.

The goal of compression therapy is to deliver sustained graded compression with 30 to 40 mm Hg at the ankle. These bandages are applied circumferentially from the toes to the knees (involving the heel) with the foot dorsiflexed. The optimal method to deliver this pressure is through multilayered elastic compression dressings. Elastic compression dressings deliver compression during ambulation (i.e., walking) and at rest, accommodate to reduction in edema, and are superior to single-layered dressings. Inelastic compression (short-stretch compression) may deliver similar results but appear to require greater sophistication by those applying them to accomplish this. Inelastic bandages, which do not deliver compression at rest, may be advantageous[1] in patients with arterial disease or patients who do not tolerate full compression (e.g., elderly). Highly pressured compression stockings are as effective as compression wrappings; however, patients' compliance is a significant limitation. Additionally, studies have reported that any leg exercise or physical activity, in addition to compression therapy, may lead to increased VLU healing outcomes.

Systemic medication as adjuvant therapy to compression bandages, such as pentoxifylline[1] (Trental 400 to 800 mg three times daily[3]), aspirin[1], or micronized purified flavonoid fraction (MPFF, Daflon 500 mg[2] [diosmin[7] 90% and hesperidin[7] 10%]) have shown to be superior to compression bandages alone with regard to the rate of healing. The use of pentoxifylline as adjuvant therapy to compression in venous ulcers has been shown to be very beneficial.

Wound bed preparation was proposed as a way to help the healing process. It is a multistep process that improves the wound bed by removing necrotic and fibrinous wound tissue, increasing the amount of granulation tissue, and decreasing edema, chronic wound fluid (i.e., exudate), and bacterial burden.

The decision of which wound dressing to use will depend on the amount of wound drainage. Occlusive dressings should be used for dry to mildly exudative wounds, providing a moist environment for healing. A variety of types of occlusions may be used, and the choice depends on several factors, including the location of the wound and the amount of fibrinous slough and exudate present. Foam, gel, and calcium alginate dressings are highly absorbent dressings and should be used for moderate-to-severe exudating wounds. Sharp wound debridement should be performed to remove any devitalized tissue. Fear of excessive infection with the use of occlusive dressings is unfounded. Topical antiseptics and cleansing agents should be used with caution because they may increase the time required for healing. Topical agents such as cadexomer iodine (Iodosorb), silver-impregnated dressings, and topical anesthetics are alternatives that do not prolong healing. These topical agents should be considered when the wound appears contaminated, but not infected. Wound infections should be treated like cellulitis, with systemic antibiotics.

Up to 50% of venous ulcers may be refractory to compression therapy alone. This refractory subset may be predicted by baseline characteristics (size and duration) and by a decrease in size with 2 to 4 weeks of treatment (Figure 1). Other available treatments include tissue-engineered skin, autologous skin, electrical stimulation, treatment with locally delivered growth factors, and venous surgery. Three categories exist for skin grafts: autologous, allogeneic (cultured), and artificial (tissue-engineered skin). Three different techniques have been used for autologous skin grafts: epidermal skin graft (only epidermis and no dermis), split-thickness skin graft (all the epidermis and a portion of the dermis), and full-thickness skin graft (complete dermis and epidermis). The use of artificial, or bioengineered grafts, has risen in the past decades.

Apligraf is a bilayered engineered living skin composed of keratinocytes and fibroblasts from neonatal foreskin that is approved by the US Food and Drug Administration for treatment of venous leg and diabetic neuropathic foot ulcers. Likewise, other synthetic skin grafts have used animal tissue to generate this sophisticated dressing. Surgical treatment of incompetent superficial and perforator veins along with standard of care (i.e., compression) reduce the risk of recurrence.

After healing occurs, patients with venous insufficiency are at risk for recurrence. The lifelong use of elastic compression stockings (30 to 40 mm Hg) is the mainstay of therapy, but early intervention after recurrence is critical. Health professionals need to understand the importance of further research to ultimately minimize the psychological, physical, and socioeconomic impact that ulcers caused by venous insufficiency have on patients and society.

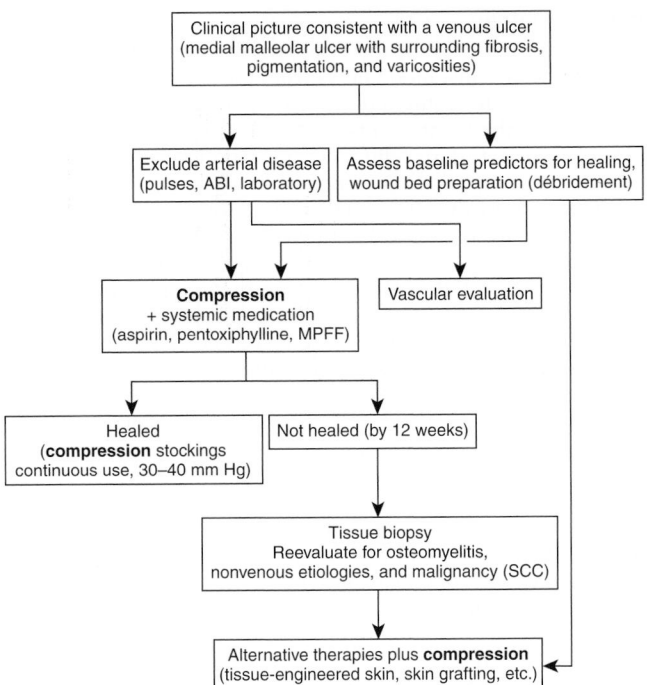

Figure 1 Simplified algorithm for the diagnosis and treatment of patients with venous ulcers. *ABI*, Ankle-brachial index; *MPFF*, micronized purified flavonoid fraction; *SCC*, squamous cell carcinoma.

---

[1]Not FDA approved for this indication.
[2]Not available in the United States.
[3]Exceeds dosage recommended by the manufacturer.
[7]Available as dietary supplement.

References

Abbade LP, Lastória S: Venous ulcer: Epidemiology, physiopathology, diagnosis and treatment, *Int J Dermatol* 44:449–456, 2005.

Browse NL, Burnand KG: The cause of venous ulceration, *Lancet* 2:243–245, 1982.

Claudy AL, Mirshahi M, Soria C, et al: Detection of undegraded fibrin and tumor necrosis factor alpha in venous leg ulcers, *J Am Acad Dermatol* 25:623–627, 1991.

Coleridge-Smith PD, Thomas P, Scurr JH, et al: Causes of venous ulceration: A new hypothesis? *Br Med J* 296:1726–1727, 1988.

Falanga V, Eaglstein WH: The trap hypothesis of venous ulceration, *Lancet* 341:1006–1008, 1993.

Jull A, Arroll B, Parag V, Waters J: Pentoxyphilline for treating venous leg ulcers, *Cochrane Database Syst Rev* (3:CD001733, 2007.

Jull A, Slark J, Parsons J: Prescribed exercise with compression vs compression alone in treating patients with venous leg ulcers: a systematic review and meta-analysis, *JAMA Dermatol* 154(11)1304–11, 2018.

Kirsner R: Wound bed preparation, *Ostomy Wound Manage* (Feb. Suppl.):2–3, 2003.

Kirsner RS: Exercise for leg ulcers: "working out" the nature of venous ulcers, *JAMA Dermatol* 154(11):1257–9, 2018.

Kirsner RS, Falanga V: Techniques of split-thickness skin grafting for lower extremity ulcerations, *J Dermatol Surg Oncol* 19:779–783, 1993.

Kirsner RS, Pardes JB, Eaglstein WH, Falanga V: The clinical spectrum of lipodermatosclerosis, *J Am Acad Dermatol* 28:623–627, 1993.

Lazarus GS, Cooper DM, Knighton DR, et al: Definitions and guidelines for assessment of wounds and evaluation of healing, *Arch Dermatol* 130:489–493, 1994.

Lim HW, Collins SAB, Resneck JS Jr., et al: The burden of skin disease in the United States, *J Am Acad Dermatol* 76 (5):958–972.e952, 2017.

Olin JW, Beusterien KM, Childs MB, et al: Medical costs of treating venous stasis ulcers: Evidence from a retrospective cohort study, *Vasc Med* 4:1–7, 1999.

Phillips TJ, Machado F, Trout R, et al: Prognostic indicators in venous ulcers, *J Am Acad Dermatol* 43:627–630, 2000.

Singer AJ, Tassiopoulos A, Kirsner RS: Evaluation and management of lower-extremity ulcers, *N Engl J Med* 377(16):1559–1567, 2017.

Trent JT, Falabella A, Eaglstein WH, Kirsner RS: Venous ulcers: Pathophysiology and treatment options, *Ostomy Wound Manage* 51:38–54, 2005.

VIRAL DISEASES OF THE SKIN

Method of
Sylvia L. Brice, MD

CURRENT DIAGNOSIS

Herpes Simplex Viruses 1 and 2
- Clinical: Grouped vesicles or erosions, especially in perioral or anogenital location
- Laboratory: Tzanck smear, viral culture, antigen detection, PCR, gG-based type-specific serology

Varicella-Zoster Virus
- Clinical: Papules, pustules, vesicles in diffuse (varicella) or dermatomal (herpes zoster) distribution
- Laboratory: Tzanck smear, antigen detection, viral culture, PCR

Hand-Foot-and-Mouth Disease
- Clinical: Papulovesicles on oral mucosa, hands, feet following fever, constitutional symptoms
- Laboratory: PCR

Parvovirus B19
- Clinical: "Slapped cheeks" reticular erythema on trunk or extremities following fever, constitutional symptoms; arthralgias, arthritis, purpuric eruptions; transient aplastic crisis, fetal hydrops
- Laboratory: B19 specific IgM serology, PCR

Molluscum Contagiosum
- Clinical: Few to multiple 1- to 4-mm umbilicated flesh-colored papules
- Laboratory: Histopathology if clinical appearance atypical

Orf
- Clinical: One to several solid to vesicular nodules on hands, forearms; history of exposure to sheep, goats, cattle
- Laboratory: Histopathology if clinical appearance atypical; PCR

Abbreviation: NSAID = nonsteroidal antiinflammatory drug.

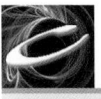

CURRENT THERAPY

Herpes Simplex Viruses 1 and 2
- Acyclovir (Zovirax), valacyclovir (Valtrex), famciclovir (Famvir)
- For acyclovir resistance: foscarnet (Foscavir),[1] cidofovir (Vistide)[1]

Varicella-Zoster Virus
- Acyclovir, valacyclovir, famciclovir
- For acyclovir resistance: foscarnet,[1] cidofovir[1]

Hand-Foot-and-Mouth Disease
- Supportive care

Parvovirus B19
- Supportive care, IVIg (Gammagard)[1]

Molluscum Contagiosum
- Surgical or chemical methods of destruction
- Immunomodulators (imiquimod [Aldara],[1] cimetidine [Tagamet][1])

Orf
- Self-limited

[1]Not FDA approved for this indication.
Abbreviation: HSV = herpes simplex virus; IVIg = intravenous immunoglobulin.

Herpes Simplex Viruses 1 and 2

Herpes simplex virus types 1 and 2 (HSV-1 and HSV-2) are the most closely related members of the human herpesvirus family, and the skin lesions they produce are clinically indistinguishable. Clusters of tense blisters on an erythematous base often quickly evolve into erosions or ulcerations with associated crusting. Lesions can develop at any mucocutaneous site but are typically found in the perioral or anogenital regions. Both HSV-1 and HSV-2 are transmitted by direct mucocutaneous contact with an infected host. Following viral replication in the skin or mucosa, intact viral nucleocapsids travel via sensory neurons to the corresponding dorsal root ganglia to establish latency. Later, a variety of stimuli can trigger reactivation. The virus travels back along the sensory neurons to the mucocutaneous surface to replicate and induce active or subclinical infection. In the case of subclinical infection, no active skin lesions are evident, but infectious particles are present, a state known as asymptomatic shedding. Although the viral titer is much lower than during clinically active disease, asymptomatic shedding of the virus in oral and genital secretions is thought to be responsible for the majority of cases of HSV transmission.

Primary, initial nonprimary (also known as first episode), and recurrent are terms used to further define the nature of the HSV infection. A *primary* infection refers to a patient's first infection with either type of HSV at any site. These patients are seronegative initially but subsequently develop HSV type-specific antibodies. A patient who is already infected with one HSV type and then develops an infection with the alternate type experiences an *initial nonprimary* or first-episode infection (e.g., the first episode of genital herpes in a patient with a prior history of orofacial herpes). These patients are seropositive for one type-specific HSV antibody (e.g., HSV-1) and later develop antibodies specific for the alternate HSV type (e.g., HSV-2). A *recurrent* infection is one that occurs at a site of prior infection. These patients are seropositive for HSV-1 or HSV-2, or both. Because most primary infections, whether oral or genital, are asymptomatic, the first evidence of disease often represents a recurrent or initial nonprimary infection.

Orofacial Herpes Simplex Virus Infection

Orofacial HSV, also known as herpes labialis, fever blisters, or cold sores, is commonly acquired during childhood or adolescence. Symptomatic primary disease usually takes the form of gingivostomatitis with or without additional lesions on the cutaneous perioral surfaces. Fever, malaise, and tender lymphadenopathy may also be present. In recurrent episodes, clusters of blisters erupt along the vermillion border of the lips, and subsequent erosions and crusting persist for several days up to 2 weeks. Lesions can develop anywhere in the perioral area, especially on the cheeks. In men, a viral folliculitis of the beard area (herpetic sycosis) may be mistaken for a bacterial process because it is often pustular. The presence of a prodrome and recurrence in the same site are clues to the correct diagnosis. Although recurrent intraoral lesions of HSV can occur, they are uncommon in immunocompetent persons. Exposure to ultraviolet light is a common trigger factor for herpes labialis, as is fever or intercurrent infection.

Genital Herpes Simplex Virus Infection

When symptomatic, primary genital herpes often involves bilaterally distributed lesions in the anogenital area with associated fever, inguinal adenopathy, and dysuria or urinary retention. Aseptic meningitis can also occur. The lesions often persist for 2 to 3 weeks or longer. Nonprimary infections are usually less severe and have fewer constitutional symptoms. Recurrent episodes tend to be milder and shorter in duration. Often, there is a prodrome of tingling or burning followed by the development of localized vesicles that can quickly rupture, leaving nonspecific erosions or ulcerations. The lesions may be anywhere within the anogenital region but tend to recur close to the same area in subsequent episodes. The time between exposure and development of primary disease is estimated to be from 3 to 14 days. However, more often the first clinical indication of disease is a recurrence, which can occur weeks to years after the initial infection. Prior infection with HSV-1 provides some protection against acquisition of HSV-2.

Based on seroepidemiologic evidence, it is estimated that approximately 17% of the United States population aged 14 to 49 years are infected with HSV-2. In most of these persons, this disease has not been officially diagnosed and they are unaware that they are infected. Nevertheless, they experience asymptomatic shedding and unknowingly transmit the disease to sexual partners. Interrupting this cycle of transmission has become a major focus among health care providers who work with these patients. A combination of patient education and appropriate use of systemic antiviral agents may be gradually having some impact on this epidemic. Recommendations for patients with genital herpes include avoiding sex with uninfected partners when active lesions or prodromal symptoms are present and routinely using latex condoms to minimize transmission during periods of asymptomatic shedding. Chronic suppressive doses of oral antiviral agents (Table 1), including acyclovir (Zovirax), valacyclovir (Valtrex), and famciclovir (Famvir), significantly reduce the frequency of clinical recurrences as well as the rate of asymptomatic shedding and may be recommended together with these other practices to reduce the risk of transmission.

Although HSV-2 is the etiologic agent in a majority of cases of genital herpes infections, an increasing number of genital herpes infections are caused by HSV-1. Symptomatic recurrences and asymptomatic shedding are less frequent with genital HSV-1 infection than with genital HSV-2 infection, and this distinction becomes important for patient counseling and prognosis.

Other Mucocutaneous Herpes Simplex Virus Infections

Eczema herpeticum, also known as Kaposi's varicelliform eruption, represents a cutaneous dissemination of HSV usually seen in patients with atopic dermatitis or other underlying skin disease. Herpetic vesicles develop over an extensive mucocutaneous surface, most often the face, neck, and upper trunk, presumably spreading from a recurrent oral HSV infection or asymptomatic shedding from the oral mucosa. Eczema herpeticum can also develop in the presence of genital HSV. As with other HSV infections, eczema herpeticum may be recurrent. In addition, patients can develop localized, recurrent HSV in previously involved areas. Because of the extensive and inflammatory nature of the process and the possible secondary bacterial infection, the underlying viral etiology may be obscured. A history of eczema and recurrent HSV in the patient and careful observation for the grouped vesicles or erosions can be key to the correct diagnosis.

Herpetic whitlow refers to HSV infection of the hand, usually one or more distal digits. Previously thought to be limited to health care professionals with exposure to oral secretions of their patients, it is now recognized that autoinoculation from orolabial or genital HSV contributes to a significant number of cases.

Herpes gladiatorum is a problem seen most commonly in athletes who participate in close contact sports such as wrestling. Typically transmitted from active herpes labialis or asymptomatic shedding in oral secretions of an infected opponent, herpes gladiatorum often affects the head, neck, or shoulders and may be recurrent. In the wrestler with frequent outbreaks, chronic suppressive therapy may be recommended.

Diagnosis

Viral culture remains a common and acceptable method for diagnosing HSV infection. This method is sensitive when specimens are obtained from lesions that have not yet become too dry or crusted, usually during the first 2 to 3 days after onset. An adequate sample, obtained by unroofing the blister and swabbing the base, increases the likelihood of an accurate result. Antigen detection tests can remain positive even after lesions have dried, as long as the specimen includes epithelial cells and not just debris. For this method, a scraping from the lesion is usually smeared on

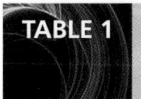

TABLE 1 Recommendations for Systemic Antiviral Treatment of Mucocutaneous Herpes Simplex Virus Infection

EPISODE	DRUG	DOSAGE
Genital Herpes Simplex Virus		
Primary or first episode	Acyclovir	Mild to moderate: 400 mg PO tid[3] or 200 mg PO 5 ×/d × 7–10 d Severe: 5 mg/kg IV q8h × 5 d
	Valacyclovir	1 g PO bid × 7–10 d
	Famciclovir[1]	250 mg PO tid × 10 d
Recurrent episode (start at prodrome)	Acyclovir	400 mg PO tid × 5 d[3] or 800 mg PO bid × 5 d[3] or 800 mg PO tid × 2 d[3]
	Valacyclovir	500 mg PO bid × 3 d *or* 1 g daily × 5 d
	Famciclovir	1 g PO bid × 1 d *or* 125 mg PO bid × 5 d
Chronic suppression	Acyclovir	>6 outbreaks per year: 400 mg PO bid *or* 200 mg PO tid Adjust up or down according to response
	Valacyclovir	6–10 outbreaks per year: 500 mg PO qd ≥10 outbreaks/year: 1 g PO qd
	Famciclovir	≥6 outbreaks/year: 250 mg PO bid
Orofacial Herpes Simplex Virus		
Primary or first episode	Acyclovir[1]	15 mg/kg 5 ×/d × 7 d
	Valacyclovir[1]	1 g bid × 7 d
	Famciclovir[1]	500 mg bid × 7 d
Recurrent episode (start at prodrome)	Acyclovir[1]	400 mg PO 5 ×/d × 5 d
	Valacyclovir	2 g PO bid × 1 d
	Famciclovir	1500 mg in 1 dose
Chronic suppression	Acyclovir[1]	400 mg PO bid-tid
	Valacyclovir[1]	500 mg–1 g PO qd
Orolabial or Genital Herpes Simplex Virus in Immunosuppressed Patients		
Recurrent or suppressive	Acyclovir[1]	400 mg PO tid *or* 5–10 mg/kg IV q8h
	Valacyclovir	500 mg–1 g PO bid
	Famciclovir	500 mg PO bid

[1]Not FDA approved for this indication.
[3]Exceeds dosage recommended by the manufacturer.

a glass slide to be sent to the laboratory. Not all antigen detection methods are designed to distinguish HSV-1 from HSV-2.

Polymerase chain reaction (PCR) is highly sensitive and has become routinely available for diagnosis of mucocutaneous HSV infections. PCR may also be useful for detection of asymptomatic shedding.

The Tzanck smear (cytologic detection) is both insensitive and nonspecific but may be of use in some clinical settings. It does not differentiate HSV types or HSV from varicella-zoster virus (VZV).

Serologic testing for HSV was previously of limited use because it could not reliably differentiate HSV-1 from HSV-2. Because they share significant genetic homology, HSV-1 and HSV-2 code for a number of common proteins that are not antigenically distinct. However, they also code for type-specific proteins that can be used to differentiate them. Current tests based on detecting type-specific viral glycoprotein G (gG-based, type-specific assays) are accurate and should be requested for this purpose. A positive HSV-2 serology may be useful in confirming the diagnosis of genital herpes in a patient with a negative viral culture or with unrecognized or asymptomatic disease. Alternatively, a negative serology can help exclude the diagnosis of HSV in a patient with chronic, nonspecific oral or genital symptoms.

Varicella Zoster Virus

VZV, another member of the human herpesvirus family, produces two specific patterns of disease in the skin. The primary infection results in varicella, also known as chickenpox, a widespread vesicular eruption usually seen in the pediatric population. Following the primary infection, VZV establishes latency in the dorsal root ganglia until some later point, when reactivation can occur. The ensuing unilateral dermatomal distribution of blisters, often preceded by neuralgic pain, is known as herpes zoster or shingles. Herpes zoster is especially common in patients older than 50 years, but it may be seen at any age. It is also seen more commonly in immunocompromised patients, such as organ transplant recipients or patients infected with HIV. Herpes zoster is no longer considered a marker for underlying cancer, and evaluation for occult malignancy in an otherwise asymptomatic patient is not indicated. A single recurrence of herpes zoster, usually in the same dermatome, may occur, but this is uncommon in immunocompetent individuals. Additional recurrences, however, suggest a dermatomal form of HSV, and laboratory assessment for this possibility may be indicated.

The most common dermatomes involved with herpes zoster are in the thoracolumbar (T3-L2) and trigeminal (V1) regions. Skin lesions typically evolve from papules to vesicles and pustules, and then to crusted erosions, before healing approximately 2 to 4 weeks after onset. The associated neuropathic pain commonly persists after the lesions have healed. Pain that continues for more than 3 months after the skin lesions resolve is referred to as postherpetic neuralgia, one of the most common and debilitating complications of this infection.

Several clinical presentations of herpes zoster deserve additional attention. Ophthalmic zoster, with lesions along the tip, side, or base of the nose indicating involvement of the nasociliary branch of the trigeminal nerve (Hutchinson's sign), may be associated with increased risk for ocular complications. Prompt initiation of a systemic antiviral agent (Table 2) and evaluation by an ophthalmologist are recommended. Disseminated zoster, with more than a few lesions outside the primary and immediately adjacent dermatomes, can indicate visceral involvement and its associated complications. The term *zoster sine herpete* describes patients with neuropathic pain resembling zoster but without any skin lesions. The diagnosis can be supported by demonstration of increased IgG antibody titers between the acute and convalescent phases. Chronic zoster is seen predominantly in HIV-infected persons. Single or multiple warty growths can persist for weeks or months in areas of skin previously involved by typical lesions of varicella or herpes zoster. Chronic zoster is often resistant to acyclovir. Tissue biopsy and viral cultures, with further testing for antiviral resistance, may aid in assessment.

Herpes Zoster

Diagnosis

Diagnosis of herpes zoster is often made on clinical grounds alone. A Tzanck smear can provide additional support of the viral etiology. With atypical presentations, however, the diagnosis is best confirmed by real time PCR. An antigen detection method can be used if active blisters are present. Both are rapid and differentiate VZV from HSV. Viral cultures is insensitive but may be required if there is a need to assess possible antiviral resistance. Basic VZV serology is rarely useful for diagnosis.

Treatment

There are three systemic antiviral agents routinely used for the treatment of HSV and VZV infections: acyclovir, valacyclovir, and famciclovir. All three are highly effective and generally well tolerated. Because they inhibit only actively replicating viral DNA, they have no impact on latent infection. Recommendations for antiviral treatment of mucocutaneous HSV infections and herpes zoster, localized topical measures, and available formulations are outlined in Tables 1 to 5. Optimal antiviral dosage schedules for less-common HSV infections, such as herpetic whitlow, have not been determined. The doses outlined in Table 1 for either episodic or chronic suppressive therapy can be used as a guideline in these cases.

Acyclovir became available more than 25 years ago and continues to be widely used. Inside an infected host cell, acyclovir must be phosphorylated—first by a virally encoded enzyme (thymidine kinase) and then by host-cell enzymes—to the active form of the drug, acyclovir triphosphate. As a nucleotide analogue, acyclovir triphosphate is incorporated into replicating viral DNA, abruptly terminating further synthesis of that viral DNA chain. Acyclovir triphosphate also interferes with viral DNA replication by directly inhibiting viral DNA polymerase. Valacyclovir is an oral prodrug of acyclovir and has a much higher bioavailability. After ingestion, valacyclovir is rapidly metabolized to acyclovir, and the subsequent mechanism of action is as just described. Famciclovir is an oral prodrug of penciclovir (Denavir), designed for greater bioavailability. Similar to acyclovir, penciclovir must first be phosphorylated by viral thymidine kinase and then by cellular enzymes to penciclovir triphosphate. In this active form, penciclovir triphosphate interferes with viral DNA synthesis and replication by inhibiting viral DNA polymerase. Famciclovir has greater bioavailability and a longer intracellular half-life than acyclovir. For all three agents, the required activation by viral thymidine kinase and the preferential inhibition of viral DNA synthesis contribute to the highly specific antiviral activity.

If taken as recommended, acyclovir, valacyclovir, and famciclovir are generally comparable in their safety and effectiveness. Valacyclovir and famciclovir offer the convenience of less-frequent dosing. Dosing for all three should be adjusted in the presence of renal insufficiency (see Table 5).

TABLE 2	Recommendations for Systemic Antiviral Treatment of Herpes Zoster	
	DOSAGE	
DRUG	**IMMUNO-COMPETENT PATIENTS**	**IMMUNO-SUPPRESSED PATIENTS**
Acyclovir	800 mg PO 5 × per d × 7–10 d	800 mg PO 5 × per d × 10 d* 10 mg/kg/dose IV q8h × 7–10 d*
Valacyclovir	1 g PO tid × 7 d	1 g PO tid × 10 d*
Famciclovir	500 mg PO tid × 7 d	500 mg PO tid × 10 d*

*Continue until there are no new lesions for 48 h.

TABLE 3	Topical Treatment Options for Mucocutaneous Herpes Simplex Virus and Varicella Zoster Virus Infections
TREATMENT	**COMMENT**
Cool, moist compresses using tap water or aluminum acetate 1:20 to 1:40 (Burow's solution, Domeboro, Bluboro)	Good for moist, oozing lesions to accelerate drying. Apply wet dressing to involved skin and cover with a dry cloth to allow evaporation
Calamine lotion or similar shake lotion containing alcohol, menthol, and/or phenol; Aveeno colloidal oatmeal	Useful as drying and antipruritic agent. May be applied after wet dressing
Bacitracin,[1] Polysporin, mupirocin[1] (Bactroban)	Use if there is concern for localized secondary bacterial infection
2% Viscous lidocaine, compounded suspensions[1,6] (e.g., Kaopectate[1] or Maalox,[1] diphenhydramine,[1] lidocaine)	Useful for temporary pain relief of oral or genital mucosal involvement
Acyclovir ointment	Used together with systemic antiviral agents, may be of benefit to immunocompromised individuals for localized HSV
Penciclovir (Denavir) cream	Can decrease the duration of lesions in herpes labialis by half a day if applied every 2h while awake for 4 days beginning at the first sign of disease
Acyclovir buccal tablet (Sitavig) 50 mg	Can decrease the duration of herpes labialis by 0.8 days if single tablet is applied within 1 hour of prodromal symptom

[1]Not FDA approved for this indication.
[6]May be compounded by pharmacists.
Abbreviation: HSV = herpes simplex virus.

TABLE 4	Formulations of Acyclovir, Valacyclovir, and Famciclovir			
DRUG	**ORAL**	**TOPICAL**	**INTRAVENOUS**
Acyclovir	200, 400, 800 mg; 50 mg buccal tablet	5% Ointment (5g, 15g, 30g); 5% cream (5g)	Yes
Valacyclovir	500 mg, 1 g	No	No
Famciclovir	125, 250, 500 mg	No	No
Penciclovir (Denavir)	No	1% cream (1.5g, 5g)	No

TABLE 5	Recommended Antiviral Dose Modification in Patients with Impaired Renal Function				
CREATININE CLEARANCE (ML/MIN)	**GENITAL HERPES SIMPLEX VIRUS**			**HERPES ZOSTER**	**HERPES LABIALIS**
	INITIAL	**RECURRENT**	**SUPPRESSION**		
Acyclovir (Zovirax)					
>25	200 mg 5 ×/d	200 mg 5 ×/d	400 mg q12h	800 mg 5×/d	
10–24	200 mg 5 ×/d	200 mg 5 ×/d	400 mg q12h	800 mg q8h	
<10	200 mg q12h	200 mg q12h	200 mg q12h	800 mg q12h	
Valacyclovir (Valtrex)					
>50	1g q12h	500 mg q12h	500 mg-1 g q24h	1g q8h	2g PO bid for 1 d
30–49	1g q12h	500 mg q12h	500 mg-1 g q24h	1g q12h	1g PO bid for 1 d
10–29	1g q24h	500 mg q24h	500 mg q24-48h	1g q24h	500 mg bid for 1 d
<10	500 mg q24h	500 mg q24h	500 mg q24-48h	500 mg q24h	500 mg single dose
Famciclovir (Famvir)					
>60		125 mg q12h	250 mg q12h	500 mg q8h	
40–59		125 mg q12h	250 mg q12h	500 mg q12h	
20–39		125 mg q24h	125 mg q12h	500 mg q24h	
<20		125 mg q24h	125 mg q24h	250 mg q24h	
>60		1g bid × 1d			1500 mg single dose
40–59		500 mg bid × 1 d			750 mg single dose
20–39		500 mg single dose			500 mg single dose
<20		250 mg single dose			250 mg single dose

Although antiviral therapy does not decrease the incidence of postherpetic neuralgia, all three agents decrease the time for lesion healing and shorten the overall duration of pain if initiated within 48 to 72 hours after the onset of herpes zoster. Valacyclovir and famciclovir appear to be more effective than acyclovir for this purpose, presumably because of easier dosing. An otherwise healthy person younger than 50 years who has discrete involvement on the trunk and mild to moderate pain might benefit minimally or not at all from this intervention, especially if it is initiated after 72 hours of lesion onset. However, patients who are older than 50 years, are immunosuppressed, have involvement in the ophthalmic distribution, or have more-extensive lesions or severe pain should receive systemic antiviral therapy, even if the 72-hour deadline has expired. Adequate pain control, often requiring opiates, is also important.

The addition of systemic corticosteroids to the antiviral regimen is not recommended for uncomplicated herpes zoster. Corticosteroids may be of benefit in herpes zoster complicated by facial paralysis, cranial polyneuropathy, or acute retinal necrosis. Corticosteroids should not be used without concomitant systemic antiviral therapy.

Vaccination with a herpes zoster vaccine substantially reduces the incidence of both herpes zoster and postherpetic neuralgia. There are two herpes zoster vaccines available. The live attenuated vaccine (ZVL/Zostavax) has been in use since 2006 and is given as a single intramuscular injection. The Zoster Vaccine Recombinant, Adjuvanted (RZV/Shingrix) received FDA approval in October 2017, for immunocompetent adults 50 years and older. RZV is a non-live recombinant glycoprotein E vaccine and requires 2 doses given intramuscularly 2–6 months apart. The U.S. Advisory Committee on Immunization Practices (ACIP) currently recommends the use of RZV for immunocompetent adults aged 50 years or older for the prevention of herpes zoster and related complications. The ACIP also recommends RZV for adults aged 50 years or older who previously received the live-attenuated herpes zoster vaccine (ZVL/Zostavax) and either RZV or ZVL for adults aged 60 years or older (RZV is preferred).

Despite widespread use of these antiviral agents, antiviral resistance is rarely a problem in the immunocompetent population. However, it does arise in the setting of immunosuppression. The basis for the resistance is most commonly a mutation in the gene coding for thymidine kinase. Less often there is a mutation in the viral DNA polymerase. In either case, all three standard drugs become ineffective. Alternative antiviral agents available for treatment of acyclovir-resistant HSV and VZV infections include foscarnet (Foscavir)[1] and cidofovir (Vistide).[1]

Hand-Foot-and-Mouth Disease

Hand-foot-and-mouth disease is typically a disease of childhood. The most common etiologic agent is a nonpolio enterovirus, Coxsackie A16, and transmission is via the oral–oral or fecal–oral route. It is highly contagious. Several days after exposure, a prodrome of low-grade fever, malaise, abdominal pain, or respiratory symptoms can develop, followed by the appearance of papulovesicles on the palate, tongue, or buccal mucosa. Similar lesions can subsequently develop on the feet and hands. The eruption persists for 7 to 10 days and then resolves. Treatment is symptomatic. Nail dystrophies including onychomadesis (separation of the proximal portion of the nail plate from the nail bed) and Beau's lines (horizontal grooves in the nail plate) may be seen 2–4 weeks later.

Since 1997, outbreaks of hand-foot-and-mouth disease caused by enterovirus 71 have been reported in Asia and Australia. Although hand-foot-and-mouth disease associated with Coxsackie A16 infection is typically a mild illness, hand-foot-and-mouth disease caused by enterovirus 71 has shown a higher incidence of neurologic involvement, including fatal cases of encephalitis.

An atypical hand-foot-and-mouth disease with more widespread cutaneous involvement has been reported as associated with Coxsackievirus A6. There is a predilection for areas commonly involved in atopic dermatitis, such as the antecubital and popliteal fossae and this presentation may be confused with eczema herpeticum or VZV infection. Diagnosis of these more atypical cases may require laboratory assessment. This could include antigen detection or PCR to exclude HSV and VZV. Reverse Transcription PCR (RT-PCR) of vesicle fluid, oropharyngeal swab or stool specimen may be used to confirm the enterovirus infection.

Parvovirus B19

Cutaneous manifestations of parvovirus B19 infection include the childhood exanthem known as erythema infectiosum (fifth disease) and, less commonly, petechial or purpuric eruptions. The virus is transmitted primarily via respiratory secretions and, to a much lesser extent, through blood or blood products. The host cells for viral replication are erythroid progenitor cells, which subsequently undergo cell lysis.

A child with erythema infectiosum typically develops a low-grade fever and nonspecific upper respiratory symptoms approximately 2 days before the onset of rash. The rash has been described as having a slapped-cheeks appearance, with prominent redness over the malar eminences. This is followed by a pink-to-red lacy or reticular eruption over the trunk and extensor surfaces of the arms and legs. The rash usually lasts a week to 10 days but can transiently recur over months in response to precipitating factors such as sunlight, exercise, and bathing. Diagnosis of erythema infectiosum is usually made on clinical grounds, and treatment is symptomatic. By the time the rash appears and the diagnosis has been made, the child is no longer infectious. Much less commonly parvovirus B19 infection may manifest as a papular-purpuric eruption with edema, erythema, and patecchiae in a "gloves and socks" distribution on the hands and feet.

Infection with parvovirus B19 in older adolescents and adults often manifests with arthralgias or arthritis rather than a rash. In certain patient populations, parvovirus B19 infections may be associated with complications including transient aplastic crisis, chronic anemia, and hydrops fetalis. In these less-typical presentations, serology (anti-B19 IgM or documented seroconversion) may be needed for diagnosis. Intravenous immunoglobulin (IVIg [Gamimune N])[1] is used successfully for treatment of chronic or persistent infection in immunosuppressed patients.

Molluscum Contagiosum

Molluscum contagiosum are benign umbilicated papules caused by infection with the *Molluscipoxvirus*, a member of the poxvirus family. Lesions are limited to the mucocutaneous surface and typically appear in clusters on the face, trunk, and skin fold areas in children and on thighs, lower abdomen, and suprapubic areas in sexually active adults. Large numbers of lesions in an extensive distribution may be seen in the immunosuppressed population.

Transmission routinely occurs by skin-to-skin contact with an infected host, but transmission from contaminated fomites has been reported. Autoinoculation commonly occurs. Diagnosis is usually based on clinical examination, but histopathology of atypical lesions may be used for confirmation.

Because molluscum contagiosum tends to be self-limited, treatment is not always recommended, but it can reduce the risk of autoinoculation and transmission to others. Treatment modalities are primarily aimed at destroying the lesions, similar to those used for verruca vulgaris (Table 6). In the case of sexual transmission, evaluation for other sexually transmitted diseases may be indicated.

Orf and Milker's Nodules

Orf (also known as ecthyma contagiosum) and milker's nodules are caused by the closely related *Parapoxvirus*, a member of the poxvirus family. The virus responsible for orf is widespread in

Viral Diseases of the Skin

1113

---

[1] Not FDA approved for this indication.

[1] Not FDA approved for this indication.

TABLE 6	Treatment Options for Molluscum Contagiosum
TREATMENT	**COMMENT**
Cryotherapy (liquid nitrogen)	Freeze individual lesions for 5–10 sec Repeat PRN in 2–3 wk
Curettage	Entire lesion may be removed using a curette; this results in bleeding Removal of central core with toothpick or other pointed instrument is also effective
Cantharidin (Cantharone)[1]	Blister-inducing agent: Apply to lesion with toothpick, air dry Cover with tape or adhesive bandage Patient to wash area after 24 h (or sooner if significant pain)
Podophyllin (25% in tincture of benzoin)[1]	Cytotoxic agent: Apply to lesion with toothpick Patient to wash off after 4–6 h Contraindicated in pregnancy
Podofilox (Condylox 0.5% gel or solution)[1]	Done by patient: Apply bid for 3 consecutive d/wk × 2–4 wk Contraindicated in pregnancy
Salicylic acid/lactic acid (Occlusal, Duofilm)[1]	Done by patient: Apply daily
Imiquimod (Aldara) 5% cream[1,2]	Done by patient: Apply daily 5 consecutive d/wk Leave on overnight Continue for 8–12 wk
Cimetidine (Tagamet)[1]	30 mg/kg/d PO × 6–12 wk Can boost cell-mediated immunity
Candida antigen (Candin)[1]	Intralesional injection 0.3 mL[3]

[1]Not FDA approved for this indication.
[2]Not available in the United States.
[3]Exceeds dosage recommended by the manufacturer.

sheep and goats, whereas the virus causing milker's nodules is found in cattle. Transmission to humans is by direct contact with infected animals or recently vaccinated animals and is usually seen several days and up to 2 weeks after exposure. Preexisting skin trauma or other disruption of the normal cutaneous barrier enhances the risk of transmission. Barrier precautions and proper hand hygiene are important preventive measures.

Orf and milker's nodules most commonly appear as one to several nodules on the dorsal aspect of the hands or forearms. Lesions evolve through several clinical stages over a period of 3 to 5 weeks, ranging from solid red nodules to vesicular, exudative, or wartlike tumors. As with other poxvirus infections, lesions of orf often demonstrate central umbilication. Regional lymphadenopathy and lymphangitis are commonly seen.

Diagnosis is based on a history of exposure and clinical examination. Tissue biopsy for histopathology or electron microscopy may also be used. Orf virus infection can resemble skin lesions associated with potentially life-threatening zoonotic infections such as tularemia, cutaneous anthrax, and erysipeloid. Should this be a concern, definitive diagnostic testing using PCR is available through the Centers for Disease Control and Prevention (CDC).

In general, the lesions of orf are self-limited, resolving within 4 to 6 weeks, and treatment is not routinely required. However, immunocompromised persons can develop more progressive and destructive lesions requiring therapeutic intervention such as topical cidofovir[1,6] or imiquimod (Aldara).[1]

[1] Not FDA approved for this indication.
[6] May be compounded by pharmacists.

Reference

Advisory Committee on Immunization Practices Recommended Immunization Schedule for Adults Aged 19 Years or Older—United States, 2018, *MMWR* 67(5):158–160, 2018.

Bergqvist C, Kurban M, Abbas O: Orf virus infection, *Rev Med Virol* 27(4), 2017.

Centers for Disease Control and Prevention: Sexually Transmitted Diseases Treatment Guidelines, 2010. MMWR 59(RR-12), 2010. , http://www.cdc.gov/STD/treatment/2010.

Cernik C, Gallina K, Brodell RT: The treatment of herpes simplex infections: an evidence-based review, *Arch Intern Med* 168(11):1137–1144, 2008.

Dayan RR, Peleg R: Herpes zoster - typical and atypical presentations, *Postgrad Med* 129(6):567–571, 2017.

Gnann JW, Whitley RJ: Genital herpes, *N Engl J Med* 375:666–674, 2016.

Nassef C, Ziemer C, Morrell DS: Hand-foot-and-mouth disease: a new look at a classic viral rash, *Curr Opin Pediatr* 27(4):486–491, 2015.

Qiu J, Soderlund-Venermo M, Young NS: Human parvoviruses, *Clin Microbiol Rev* 30(1):43–113, 2017.

Sacks HS: Review: Adjuvant recombinant subunit vaccine prevents herpes zoster more than live attenuated vaccine in adults ≥ 50 years, *Ann Intern Med* 170(4), 2019.

van der Wouden JC, van der Sande R, Kruithof EJ, et al: Interventions for cutaneous molluscum contagiosum, *Cochrane Database Syst Rev* 17(5):CD004767, 2017.

WARTS (VERRUCAE)

Method of
M. Chantel Long, MD

CURRENT DIAGNOSIS

- Common warts: rough, hyperkeratotic, firm papules usually found on the extremities.
- Flat warts: small, flat, pink or flesh-colored papules on the face, arms, or legs.
- Plantar and palmar warts: callus-like lesions that disrupt skin lines on the soles or palms.
- Mosaic warts: large clusters of warts.
- Filiform warts: small, finger-like lesions on the face.
- Genital warts: flesh to brown colored, flat or exophytic, found in the anogenital region.
- Differential diagnoses: seborrheic keratoses, molluscum contagiosum, keratoacanthoma, squamous cell carcinoma, acrochordon, amelanocytic melanoma, calluses, and corns.

CURRENT THERAPY

- Approximately 20% of warts spontaneously resolve within 3 months and 60% within 2 years in a healthy person.
- Salicylic acid and dimethyl ether.
- Cryotherapy.
- Cantharidin (Cantharone).[1,6]
- Surgical removal.
- Pulsed-dye laser.
- Immunotherapy: topical imiquimod (Aldara),[1] intralesional *Candida* antigen (Candin).[1]
- Photodynamic therapy.

[1]Not FDA approved for this indication.
[6]May be compounded by pharmacists.
Note: Cantharidin and Candin are not FDA approved. Aldara is approved for genital and perianal warts only.

Verrucae, commonly known as cutaneous warts, are benign skin growths caused by the human papillomavirus (HPV). Cutaneous warts are divided into common warts, plantar warts, flat warts, and genital warts. Common warts account for 70% of all cutaneous warts. Two-thirds of untreated common warts spontaneously regress within 2 years, but previously infected individuals have a higher rate of developing new warts than those who were never infected.

Epidemiology

It is estimated that 10% of the general population has cutaneous warts, and warts are one of the most common reasons for dermatologic visits. Transmission occurs through direct contact with an infected person or indirectly through fomites. As a result, warts are seen with greater frequency among groups of people in close contact, such as schoolchildren. Thus, warts are more common in adolescents with a frequency estimated as high as 20%. Since the extent of infection is determined by the immune response, warts are also more common in immunocompromised patients. Auto-inoculation is possible by scratching the lesions, often leading to a linear pattern.

Pathophysiology

Warts are caused by HPV. More than 100 genotypes of HPV have been identified, and the virus is prevalent. HPV causes both clinical and subclinical infections and plays a role in certain cutaneous malignancies, including squamous cell carcinoma. It is found in the basal layer of the epidermis but replicates in the superficial, well-differentiated layer of the skin. The cellular proliferation gives rise to thick, hyperkeratotic lesions generally known as warts. The warts can occur anywhere on the skin or mucous membranes.

Clinical Manifestations

Most warts are asymptomatic, though patients often present with complaints of a "bump." Usually, the warts appear flesh-colored, brown, or gray and can be flat to exophytic, giving them the classic "cauliflower" appearance. The lesions may be single or multiple and may range in size from miniscule to several centimeters in diameter. Localized irritation, pruritus, pain, or bleeding may occur. Symptoms vary based on the location and size of the lesions.

Several types of warts occur with variations in appearance, site of infection, and the specific type of HPV involved. Common warts (verrucae vulgaris) are white to flesh-colored, rough, hyperkeratotic, raised, and firm, usually found on the extremities. They disrupt normal skin lines on the fingers and toes and are most associated with HPV types 1, 2, and 4. Flat warts (verrucae plana) are caused by HPV types 3, 10, or 28 and are tan to flesh colored. They are small, 1 to 3 mm in diameter, flat, sharply demarcated growths that appear in large numbers on the face, arms, or legs. They usually occur in a linear arrangement related to local trauma, such as shaving. Butcher warts are associated with HPV type 7 and have a thick, raised, exophytic appearance. They are most common in workers who regularly handle raw meat or fish. Plantar and palmar warts (verrucae plantaris and verrucae palmaris) are hard, thickened, callus-like lesions that disrupt skin lines on the soles or palms. They are associated with HPV types 1, 2, 4, 27, and 57. They are usually flesh colored, covered with callus, and can be painful, especially when located on pressure points. If warts coalesce into a plaque, this is termed a *mosaic* wart. Filiform warts are slender, finger-like growths most commonly seen on the face, especially around the eyelids, nose, and mouth. Periungual warts are common warts impinging on and growing under toenails or fingernails. Genital warts (condyloma acuminatum) are flesh colored to brown, flat or exophytic lesions, occurring in anogenital regions. Mucosal papillomas are warts that occur on mucous membranes, usually in the mouth or vagina, and tend to be white in color.

Epidermodysplasia verruciformis is a rare, autosomal recessive disorder that leads to widespread reddish brown, flat papules on the trunk, hands, face, and extremities. These warts have malignant potential, especially on sun-exposed areas. It is estimated that one-third may become malignant. These patients present in childhood. Chronically infected with multiple types of HPV, including types 3, 5, 8, 9, 12, 14, 15, 17, 19 to 25, 36 to 38, 47, 49, and 50, the warts have lifelong persistence. Another related disease is verrucous carcinoma. This is a slow-growing variant of squamous cell carcinoma that occurs in the oral mucosa, anogenital region, or plantar surface. These warts are associated with HPV types 6 and 11.

Risk Factors

Risk factors most associated with verrucae include immunosuppression and close contact. Due to their decreased immune response, immunocompromised hosts are at increased risk not only for infection, but also for malignant transformation of the warts. Pregnancy, previous wart infection, and handling raw meat or fish are also known risk factors.

Differential Diagnosis

The differential diagnosis of warts includes seborrheic keratoses, molluscum contagiosum, keratoacanthoma, squamous cell carcinoma, acrochordon, amelanocytic melanoma, porokeratosis, calluses, and corns.

Diagnosis is based on clinical findings. When the clinical appearance of the lesion is typical, no other confirmatory tests are usually necessary. Paring down the stratum corneum, or outer layer of skin, may reveal black dots, which are thrombosed or bleeding capillaries, and helps confirm the diagnosis. If needed, tissue biopsy can provide histopathologic confirmation. In immunocompromised patients, biopsy is recommended to rule out squamous cell carcinoma in any suspicious lesions, which includes large or rapidly growing, pigmented, atypical, friable, bleeding, or ulcerated lesions.

Treatment

Approximately 20% of warts spontaneously resolve within 3 months and 60% within 2 years in a healthy person. Therefore, treatment is not always necessary. Current treatments do not eradicate the virus and do not guarantee resolution. Most patients seek treatment because of the physical appearance, discomfort, or interference with daily and social functioning, especially if located on the palms, digits, or soles. The American Academy of Dermatology established reasoning for wart treatment, including the desire of the patient; for symptoms of pain, bleeding, itching, or burning; for disabling or disfiguring lesions; for large numbers or large size of lesions; for a desire to prevent spread to unblemished skin; and because of a concomitant immunocompromised condition. Immunosuppressed patients are at higher risk for developing numerous warts and require treatment to prevent progression to squamous cell carcinoma. It is often more difficult to eradicate warts in an immunosuppressed host.

Many therapeutic modalities are available for the treatment of warts. No single therapy is universally effective. Warts can resolve, recur, shrink, or grow despite therapy. It is likely that all wart therapies work by triggering an immune response to the presence of papillomavirus in the skin. Treatment of warts must be individualized and often more than one modality is needed to achieve resolution. Conservative, less painful, and less expensive treatments are preferred.

Treatment methods are divided into the categories of home remedies, over-the-counter treatments, and office-based therapies. Office-based treatments include destructive methods, surgical or laser procedures, immunologic intervention, and combination therapy.

Home Remedies

Home remedies include applications of tea tree oil,[7] garlic extract,[7] duct tape,[1] and hyperthermic therapy. One study comparing cryotherapy with duct tape occlusion of common warts showed resolution in 85% of the children treated by occlusion, compared with 60% in the liquid nitrogen group. Proper protocol involves covering the wart with duct tape, which is left in place for 6 days. Then the site should be soaked, pared down with an emery board, and left uncovered overnight. This is repeated for a total of eight cycles. Another common home remedy is hyperthermic therapy. This involves immersing the affected area in a 45°C water bath for 30 minutes three times per week. It is a safe and inexpensive option.

---

[1]Not FDA approved for this indication.
[7]Available as dietary supplement.

Over-the-Counter Treatment

The most common over-the-counter option used by patients is one of the salicylic acid products, such as Compound W, Duofilm, Occlusal-HP, and Mediplast. These keratolytic products are offered as a solution, gel, cream, or pad in concentrations from 10% to 60%. They can be quite successful when used consistently and as directed in motivated patients. Repeated application, with pumice stone or callus file use, results in cure rates of 60% to 80%, but takes several weeks to work.

More recently, several over-the-counter wart-freezing therapies have become available. One such option is dimethyl ether, marketed as Compound W Freeze Off or Dr. Scholl's Freeze Away. These are available in aerosol form for wart treatment, which can be repeated every 2 weeks. Dimethyl ether achieves a temperature of –57°C, which is markedly higher than the –196°C temperature obtained with liquid nitrogen. This results in a more shallow depth of destruction. Because salicylic acid and dimethyl ether treatments destroy the infected epidermis and cause an immune reaction, they can be irritating and tedious, prompting many patients to seek medical care.

Office-based Treatment

Office-based treatments are largely destructive, immunomodulating, or both. Destructive treatments include cryosurgery, surgical excision, laser therapy, or repeated application of topical chemotherapy agents, such as salicylic acid, cantharidin (Cantharone),[1,6] podophyllin (Podocon),[1] or 5-fluorouracil (Efudex).[1] The most commonly used physician office-based treatment is cryotherapy with liquid nitrogen. It can be applied by a cotton-tipped applicator or cryogun. The wart and a 1 to 2 mm margin are frozen for 10 to 30 seconds. The freeze should be repeated once after a thaw of 20 seconds. If the warts are thick, they can initially be pared down. The patient is told that a blister will result and should be left intact if possible. Treatment should be repeated every 3 to 4 weeks until normal skin markings return. Cryotherapy has demonstrated a 60% to 80% cure rate. If warts persist beyond 3 months of therapy, another method of treatment should be selected.

Another option is cantharidin (Cantharone) in a 0.7% colloidal solution. It is a chemical derived from blister beetles that is painless on application and well tolerated by children. It causes epidermal necrosis with blistering after application and occlusion for 8 hours. It is applied in the office and repeated every 4 weeks. Although not Food and Drug Administration (FDA) approved, it is a commonly used technique and can be compounded by a pharmacist. It is useful for treatment of common, periungual, and plantar warts in children, and the cure rate approaches 80%. Unfortunately, an occasional "donut wart," a ring of new warts surrounding the cleared original site, occurs.

Surgery is used for large, solitary warts, and is more direct. Large common warts of the hands or extremities are more easily treated if they are debulked surgically. This method is not recommended for plantar warts because of scarring. Surgical removal followed by electrodesiccation and curettage is effective but requires local anesthesia and can result in scarring.

Other destructive methods of wart removal usually are reserved for resistant, multiple lesions, or recalcitrant warts in immunosuppressed patients. This often requires specialty referral. Acids, including bichloroacetic and trichloroacetic acid (Tri-Chlor),[1] should be applied by a skilled practitioner because they are known to cause pain on application, ulceration, and even scarring. Laser therapy, most often with a pulsed-dye laser (PDL) or carbon dioxide (CO_2) laser, provides selective photothermolysis of blood vessels within the wart, which compromises blood supply and results in necrosis. The PDL method is less aggressive and less painful than CO_2 vaporization. These treatments cause minimal damage to normal skin. Overall, both therapies are generally well tolerated, but local anesthesia may be necessary. Although more expensive, these methods have cure rates ranging from 45% to 90%. Photodynamic therapy (PDT) is useful for patients with multiple recalcitrant warts, especially patients who are immunosuppressed. PDT involves a topical photosensitizer applied by a trained provider. It is activated by visible light, resulting in tissue destruction. Studies of this method have been promising.

Immune modulation alone or in combination with destructive methods is helpful in treating resistant warts. The self-applied immunomodulator imiquimod (Aldara) was initially approved for treatment of genital warts. It is also used anecdotally to treat flat and common warts by inducing cytokines, including interferon production, at the site of application. A thin coat is applied at bedtime and then washed off after 6 to 10 hours. It is usually applied three times weekly and combined with cryotherapy or salicylic acid.

Intralesional immunotherapy, which includes *Candida* antigen (Candin),[1] interferon alfa-2b (Intron A),[1] bleomycin,[1] and MMR vaccine,[1] is an effective option for treatment in some patients. *Candida* antigen injection (Candin) is considered a first-line therapy in children with large or multiple warts and a second-line therapy for patients with resistant warts. It is well tolerated. *Candida* antigen is commercially available as a 1:1000 dilution. Using a 30-gauge needle and tuberculin syringe, one can inject 0.2 to 0.3 mL directly into the wart. Pretesting is unnecessary, side effects are minimal, and more than 75% of patients treated with a series of three injections have clearing of the injected and distant warts. Intralesional interferon alfa-2b (Intron A) has been used successfully to treat genital warts and warts that have not responded to conventional therapies. The clearance rate varies from 36% to 62%, but it requires multiple injections in a physician's office, is expensive, and can cause systemic adverse effects such as flu-like symptoms. Intralesional bleomycin is effective but expensive and causes severe pain. The MMR vaccine is used off-label for intralesional injection and often combined with lidocaine for comfort.

Other topical immunomodulators, such as squaric acid dibutylester (SADBE)[1,6] or diphencyprone,[1,7] are contact sensitizers that induce an allergic dermatitis through type IV hypersensitivity reactions. Although time consuming, treatment with SADBE is well tolerated and a good choice for recalcitrant warts in children. Other topical products available for off-label treatment include retinoids, formaldehyde compounds, and 5-fluorouracil (Efudex).[1] These agents interfere with epidermal proliferation, effect a nonspecific antiviral action, or inhibit mitosis, leading to keratinocyte and viral death. All of these choices usually require specialty referral.

Oral immunomodulation with high-dose cimetidine (Tagamet)[1] has been proposed. It is postulated to enhance cell-mediated immune response. Evidence has been anecdotal. Daily doses of 30 to 40 mg/kg have been used divided twice a day to four times a day for 8 to 12 weeks.

To ensure resolution and no recurrence of warts, the patient and practitioner must often make compromises in regard to convenience, discomfort, and scarring. The factors to consider when deciding on treatment include wart location and size, patient tolerance and preference, cost, convenience, and clinician preference. Patient-applied options allow the patient greater control; however, this requires good compliance and the warts must be accessible by the patient or caregiver. Provider-applied treatments are good choices for large treatment areas. Data regarding the efficacy of using more than one modality at a time are lacking. It is common practice for health care providers to combine treatment modalities. Table 1 outlines current therapy regimens.

Patient Education

Counseling of patients regarding the goal and length of treatment is necessary. Patients should be educated that current treatments do not eradicate HPV, and therefore the objective of therapy is elimination of symptoms. They also need to understand that a repeated course of therapy is often required and it may take weeks to months to achieve desired results. Each treatment should be reviewed in detail, including risks and benefits. Subsequently, the management should be tailored depending on the wart, patient, and practitioner.

---

[1]Not FDA approved for this indication.
[6]May be compounded by pharmacists.

[1]Not FDA approved for this indication.
[6]May be compounded by pharmacists.

TABLE 1 Treatment Regimens

DRUG	AVAILABLE AS	MECHANISM OF ACTION	DISADVANTAGES	INSTRUCTIONS
Patient Applied				
Salicylic acid (Compound W, Duofilm, Occlusol-HP, or Mediplast)	Solution, gel, lotion, cream, plaster, pad 10%–60% concentration	Keratolytic that destroys the infected epidermis while irritation stimulates an immune response	Local irritation Requires multiple applications Requires compliance Wart may need to be pared down to increase penetration	Apply nightly until clear, usually for weeks to months
Dimethyl ether (Compound W, Freeze Off, Dr. Scholl's Freeze Away)	OTC in spray canister	As above	Local irritation Requires compliance Blistering may occur	May treat every 2 weeks Total of four treatments per wart advised
Retinoids (Accutane, Retin-A, Soriatane)[1]	Soriatane (10 and 25 mg tabs), Accutane (10, 20, and 40 mg tabs), Retin-A cream/gel	Antimitotic that interferes with epidermal proliferation	Systemic with mucocutaneous dryness, elevated triglycerides, abnormal liver enzymes Avoid use in pregnancy Local irritation and dryness	Take PO daily If topical form, apply nightly
Imiquimod (Aldara)[1]	Cream 5%	Immunomodulator that mediates cytokines	Irritation, erythema, pruritus, scarring, hyperpigmentation	Apply 3 times/wk on mucosal skin Apply daily on keratinized skin
Cimetidine (Tagamet)[1]	Tablets (200, 300, 400 mg) Liquid (300 mg/5 mL)	Immunomodulator that may enhance immune response	Unclear efficacy Diarrhea Many drug-drug interactions	30–40 mg/kg daily, divided bid–qid for 8–12 weeks
Provider Applied				
Cryotherapy	Cryogun or cotton-tip application	Destroys infected dermis, induces inflammation, and leads to stimulated immune response	Pain, erythema, blistering, hypopigmentation, scarring Onychodystrophy if not careful with periungual warts	Freeze for 10–30 seconds with a 1–2 mm border, allow to thaw, then repeat May offer/need local anesthesia May repeat every 3–4 weeks
Candida antigen injections (Candin)[1]	1:1000 dilution	Immunomodulator	Discomfort	Intralesional injection of 0.2–0.3 mL
Trichloroacetic acid (TCA)[1]	Solution, up to 50%	Destroys infected epidermis; best for mucosal surfaces	Pain	Apply sparingly with cotton tip, air dry Repeat weekly to every other week Do not allow to "run" on normal skin Neutralize with soap or sodium bicarbonate
Cantharidin (Cantharone)[1]	Colloidal solution 0.7%, compounded	Destroys epidermis, leads to blister formation Is painless, good for kids	Avoid on face Blistering will occur	Apply with fine applicator to wart only and have patient wash off after 6–8 hr
Surgery		Surgical removal	Avoid if bleeding disorder Often requires anesthesia Scarring	Surgical excision followed by curettage and cauterization
Interferon alpha-2b (Intron A)[1] injections		Immunomodulator	Expensive Flu-like side effects	Multiple intralesional injections several times a week Often requires specialty referral
Laser vaporization		Destroys epidermis	Expensive Requires local anesthesia	Requires specialty referral

[1]Not FDA approved for this indication.
Abbreviations: bid=twice a day; OTC=over-the-counter; PO=orally; qid=four times a day.

References

Cockayne S, Hewitt C, Hicks K, et al: Cryotherapy versus salicylic acid for the treatment of plantar warts: a randomized controlled trial, *BMJ* 342:d3271, 2011.

Kwok CS, Holland R, Gibbs S: Efficacy of topical treatments for cutaneous warts: a meta-analysis and pooled analysis of randomized controlled trials, *Br J Dermatol* 65:233–246, 2011.

Leung L: Recalcitrant nongenital warts, *Aust Fam Physician* 40–42, 2011.

Simonart T, De Maertelaer V: Systemic treatments for cutaneous warts: a systematic review, *J Dermatolog Treat* 23:72–77, 2012.

Yelverton CB: Warts. In *Manual of dermatologic therapeutics*, Philadelphia, 2007, Lippincott Williams & Wilkins, pp 233–240.

15

Urogenital Tract

ACUTE KIDNEY INJURY

Method of
Sarah Burns, DO, MS

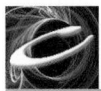

CURRENT DIAGNOSIS

- Acute kidney injury (AKI) is a common diagnosis seen in the outpatient setting, in the emergency department, and in hospitalized patients.
- AKI is defined by increase in serum creatinine by ≥0.3 mg/dL within 48 hours, increase ≥1.5 times the baseline creatinine within 7 days, or oliguria.
- Identify the underlying cause of AKI, denoted by pathophysiologic etiology (prerenal, intrinsic, and postrenal) to determine therapy.

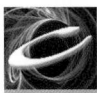

CURRENT THERAPY

- Treat any reversible causes identified.
- Ensure hemodynamic stability.
- Correct any imbalances in electrolytes or in acid-base standing.
- Avoid nephrotoxins and renally dose all medications if glomerular filtration rate (GFR) is decreased.
- Prompt consultation to specialists to determine whether renal replacement treatment is appropriate.

Background/Definitions

Acute kidney injury (AKI) is a diverse syndrome defined by a sudden decrease in kidney function shown by a rise in serum creatinine and/or decrease in urine output. This sudden decrease in renal function affects fluid balance, electrolyte balance, acid-base balance, and waste elimination. The older term *acute renal failure* has been supplanted by AKI. The term *AKI* reflects a lack of strict separation between normal renal function and complete failure of the kidneys.

Previously there was no standard definition for diagnosing AKI, and there were more than 30 different definitions in the literature. In 2004 Risk, Injury, Failure, Loss, and End Stage Kidney Disease (RIFLE) criteria were proposed, evolving into the AKI Network (AKIN) criteria in 2007. In 2012 these validated criteria were adapted into international clinical practice guidelines released by Kidney Disease: Improving Global Outcomes (KDIGO). Although KDIGO criteria are widely used in research, there are parts of the definition that have not been validated. However, most experts endorse the use of KDIGO criteria for the diagnosis and management of AKI.

KDIGO criteria denote AKI when there is an increase in serum creatinine greater than or equal to 0.3 mg/dL within 48 hours, or an increase greater than or equal to 1.5 times the baseline creatinine within 7 days, or a decrease in urine volume to less than 0.5 mL/kg/h over 6 hours. To further describe the severity of AKI, there are stages (Table 1) describing the amount of change in serum creatinine from baseline. Multiple studies have demonstrated that increasing severity of AKI is associated with increased mortality and worse kidney function in the future.

Epidemiology

AKI is commonly found in hospitalized patients, and the incidence appears to be increasing over time in the United States. A 2013 meta-analysis for all hospitalized patients worldwide showed an overall incidence of AKI in 21.6% of patients. With the KDIGO definition, this study showed that 1 in 5 adults and 1 in 3 children worldwide experience AKI during a hospital stay. A 2015 multinational cross-sectional study of AKI in intensive care unit (ICU) patients showed AKI occurred in 57.3% of ICU patients. Additionally, it has been observed that rises in serum creatinine are associated with adverse patient outcomes, increased mortality, longer length of hospital stay, and higher healthcare costs. AKI also has been shown to be an independent risk factor for mortality.

There are multiple factors, based on several observational studies, that may affect the chance of developing AKI. These factors vary between individuals, and it is not clear why one factor would cause an individual to develop an AKI and another not to. As delineated by KDIGO clinical practice guidelines, the following increase the risk of AKI: critical illness, sepsis, shock, burns, trauma, major surgery including cardiac surgery, nephrotoxic drugs, iodinated radiocontrast agents, and poisonous animals and plants. KDIGO clinical practice guidelines indicate that certain patient populations are susceptible to AKI, and they include the following: volume depletion, older age, female sex, black race, chronic kidney disease (CKD), other chronic diseases (including heart, lung, and liver), diabetes mellitus, cancer, and anemia.

Etiology

The causes of AKI can be broadly divided by the pathophysiologic etiology, specifically prerenal, intrinsic, and postrenal causes (Box 1). Prerenal AKI from renal hypoperfusion is the most common cause of AKI in the community setting. Acute tubular necrosis (ATN; an intrinsic etiology) is the most common cause of hospital-acquired AKI. Although the cause of AKI is traditionally classified by the portion of the kidney affected, it should be noted that diseases may cross these pathophysiologic boundaries. Therefore AKI may be multifactorial.

Prerenal

Prerenal AKI is caused by renal hypoperfusion caused by a decrease in the arterial volume. Recall that autoregulation will help maintain the kidney's glomerular filtration rate (GFR) by blunting changes in blood flow by various mechanisms. Ultimately, autoregulation can only compensate for a degree in decreased renal perfusion. For example, in those with CKD, these autoregulatory mechanisms are diminished which increases the susceptibility of developing an AKI on CKD. Decreased arterial volume occurs in renal vasoconstriction, which is caused by sepsis (early in course), hepatorenal syndrome, iodinated contrast, medications such as norepinephrine or vasopressin, nonsteroidal antiinflammatory drugs, and angiotensin-converting enzyme inhibitors. Intravascular

TABLE 1 Staging of Acute Kidney Injury (Based on Kidney Disease: Improving Global Outcomes).

STAGE	SERUM CREATININE	URINE OUTPUT
1	≥0.3 mg/dL increase OR 1.5–1.9 times baseline	<0.5 mL/kg/h for 6–12 h
2	2–2.9 times baseline	<0.5 mL/kg/h for ≥12 h
3	3 times baseline OR Increase in creatinine to ≥4 mg/dL OR Starting renal replacement therapy	<0.3 mL/kg/h for ≥24 h OR Anuria for ≥12 h

volume depletion reduces the arterial volume to the kidneys and is caused by gastrointestinal losses, hemorrhage, diuretic use, cirrhosis, nephrotic syndrome, and burns. Renal hypoperfusion is also caused by reduction in cardiac output, which is seen in shock, pericardial disease, heart failure, pulmonary embolism, pulmonary hypertension, and sepsis. Systemic vasodilation is another cause of renal hypoperfusion and is caused by sepsis, cirrhosis, anaphylaxis, and drugs. Increased abdominal pressure as seen in abdominal compartment syndrome can be another cause of prerenal AKI.

The clinical presentation of prerenal AKI is variable and dependent on the cause. The cause should be investigated first with an excellent history and physical examination. Prerenal causes may be suspected in patients with dehydration, gastrointestinal losses such as vomiting or diarrhea, sweating, other insensible losses, increased ostomy output, bleeding, dizziness, or syncope. Prerenal causes should be suspected in patients with chronic medical conditions, such as heart failure or cirrhosis. All medications (current, recently used, prescribed, over the counter) should be investigated in every patient suspected to have an AKI from any cause. Further work-up is discussed below. Prerenal AKI may improve rapidly if the underlying cause is treated, if the volume status is improved, and/or if the offending medication is removed.

Intrinsic

Intrinsic AKI can be divided into the component of the kidney that is affected, which includes diseases of the vasculature, the glomeruli, the tubules, and the interstitium. Vascular causes are uncommon and include those that affect the small vessels and those that affect the large vessels. Small vessels are affected by vasculitides, scleroderma, and malignant hypertension. Large vessels are affected by aneurysms, infarct from aortic dissection, venothrombosis, and atheroembolism especially in the setting of recent vascular surgery or arterial catheterization.

Glomerular diseases originate from inflammation of the vessels and the glomeruli and may be a manifestation of an infection, of a vasculitis, or of a rheumatologic disorder. Glomerular diseases are divided into nephritic and nephrotic diseases, determined by less than 3 g of proteinuria per day or more than 3 g of proteinuria per day, respectively. Rapid progressive glomerulonephritis (RPGN) is an acute cause of AKI that may be seen in the hospital and always presents with a nephritic pattern. Nephrotic patterns of AKI are rarely encountered in hospitalized patients.

Tubular and interstitial diseases commonly cause AKI specifically from damage caused by ischemia, endogenous or exogenous nephrotoxins, medications, or infections. Tubulointerstitial diseases include ATN, acute interstitial necrosis, cast nephropathy, acute urate nephropathy, crystalline nephropathy, and acute phosphate nephropathy. The most common AKI in hospitalized patients is caused by ATN. ATN occurs from prolonged renal hypoperfusion and tissue ischemia or from endogenous or exogenous nephrotoxic exposure. Common endogenous nephrotoxins include hemolysis, rhabdomyolysis,

tumor lysis syndrome, and multiple myeloma. Common exogenous nephrotoxins include radiocontrast, aminoglycosides, ethylene glycol, cisplatin, and methotrexate. Common nephrotoxins associated with AKI are listed in Box 2. Cast nephropathy is attributable to excess immunoglobulin light chains in multiple myeloma. Excess cellular contents released into circulation after chemotherapy can cause acute urate nephropathy in tumor lysis syndrome, less common nowadays with the prophylactic use of allopurinol (Zyloprim) or rasburicase (Elitek) prior to chemotherapy administration. Intravenous acyclovir (Zovirax) causes crystalline nephropathy. Oral sodium phosphate solution (Fleet) given for a bowel preparation for colonoscopy can cause acute phosphate nephropathy through an unclear mechanism.

The clinical presentation of intrinsic AKI is variable and dependent on the cause. The cause should be investigated first with an excellent history and physical examination. Vascular causes of intrinsic AKI should be suspected in recent vascular surgery, recent arterial catheterization, anticoagulation, atheroembolic disease, flank pain, or trauma. Glomerular causes of intrinsic AKI should be suspected in patients with systemic lupus erythematosus, systemic sclerosis, rash, arthritis, HIV infection, hepatitis C viral infection, cough, sinusitis, hematuria, hemoptysis, or weight loss. ATN should be suspected in patients with exposure to nephrotoxins, hypotension, trauma, or exposure to radiocontrast agents. AIN should be suspected in medication use or if there is a rash, fever, infection, or arthralgias. Further work-up is described in the following. Management and prognosis are variable and depend on the underlying cause.

Postrenal

Postrenal AKI is caused by obstruction of any cause in the urinary tract, within the kidney itself or from the ureter, bladder, bladder neck, or urethra. The most common cause is caused by obstruction of the bladder neck, either structural or functional, such as seen in benign prostatic hyperplasia. Other causes include extrinsic compression from metastatic cancer, neurogenic bladder, or retroperitoneal fibrosis, or intrinsic obstruction from calculi, crystals, or blood clots.

The clinical presentation of postrenal causes of AKI with variable urine output from anuria to polyuria, hematuria (if clots are present or malignancy is suspected), dysuria, urgency, increased frequency, weak stream, nocturia, spinal cord injuries, or longstanding poorly controlled diabetes. An excellent history and physical examination will start the investigation of the cause. It is important to diagnosis and treat postrenal causes promptly to avoid long-term damage and improve the chance for recovery.

Approach to Diagnosis

The cause of AKI should always be approached in a patient-centered manner. The diagnostic work-up will depend on clinical context, severity, and duration of AKI in addition to comorbid conditions. For patients in the outpatient setting with new onset or rapidly worsening GFR, close follow-up is warranted, and these patients should likely be hospitalized for daily monitoring

BOX 1 Etiology of Acute Kidney Injury by Pathophysiology

Prerenal Causes
- Hypovolemia caused by true or effective intravascular volume depletion
  Hemorrhage of any cause, gastrointestinal (GI) losses (diarrhea, vomiting), diuretics, burns, cirrhosis, nephrotic syndrome
- Diminished cardiac output or pump failure
  Shock, pericardial disease, heart failure, pulmonary embolism, pulmonary hypertension, and sepsis
- Systemic vasodilation
  Sepsis, cirrhosis, anaphylaxis, and drugs
- Vasoconstriction of renal vessels
  Sepsis (initially), hepatorenal syndrome, iodinated contrast, medications such as norepinephrine (Levophed) and vasopressin, nonsteroidal antiinflammatory drugs, and angiotensin-converting enzyme inhibitors
- Increased abdominal pressure
  Abdominal compartment syndrome

Intrinsic Causes
- Intrinsic renal vascular disease
  Small: vasculitides, thrombotic thrombocytopenic purpura, scleroderma, atheroembolic disease, and malignant hypertension
  Large: infarct from aortic dissection, systemic thromboembolism, renal artery aneurysm, and renal vein thrombosis
- Intrinsic renal glomerular disease
  Nephritic: proliferative glomerulonephritis (e.g., rapidly progressive glomerulonephritis)

Nephrotic: nonproliferative glomerulonephritis
- Intrinsic tubular and interstitial disease
  Acute tubular necrosis
  Angiotensin-converting enzyme inhibitors/angiotensin II receptor blockers plus nonsteroidal antiinflammatory drugs, radiocontrast or other nephrotoxins, after cardiac surgery, sepsis/shock or prerenal state, and rhabdomyolysis
- Acute interstitial nephritis
  Nonsteroidal antiinflammatory drugs, aspirin, omeprazole (Prilosec), thiazide diuretics, furosemide, allopurinol (Zyloprim), penicillin, vancomycin, and cephalosporins
- Cast nephropathy
  Multiple myeloma
- Acute urate nephropathy
  Tumor lysis syndrome
- Crystalline nephropathy
- IV acyclovir (Zovirax)
- Acute phosphate nephropathy after phosphate bowel prep

Postrenal Causes
- Extrinsic
  Benign prostatic hyperplasia
  Metastatic cancer
  Retroperitoneal fibrosis
  Neurogenic bladder
- Intrinsic
  Calculi
  Crystals
  Blood clots

BOX 2 Common Nephrotoxic Medications Associated With Acute Kidney Injury

- Vancomycin
- Aminoglycosides
- Penicillin
- Piperacillin and tazobactam (Zosyn)
- Cephalosporins
- Heme pigments
- Cisplatin
- Radiocontrast
- Pentamidine (Pentam)
- Foscarnet (Foscavir)
- Cidofovir (Vistide)
- Tenofovir (Viread)
- IV immunoglobulin
- Mannitol
- Synthetic cannabinoids
- Nonsteroidal antiinflammatory drugs
- Angiotensin-converting enzyme inhibitors
- Aspirin
- Omeprazole (Prilosec)
- Thiazide diuretics
- Furosemide (Lasix)
- Allopurinol (Zyloprim)

acute, acute on chronic, or chronic process. Once an acute process is identified, the evaluation of AKI should be categorized into prerenal, intrinsic, or postrenal cause to determine further work-up and ultimately treatment. At minimum, the clinician should obtain urinalysis, urine microscopy, laboratory studies including complete blood count, and metabolic panel with creatinine and electrolytes. Prerenal causes are more suggestive when blood urea nitrogen (BUN):creatinine ratio is greater than 20, when urine specific gravity is elevated, or when urine sodium is low. A renal ultrasound may be useful to obtain to assess for postrenal causes including obstruction, and can specifically give information on cortical thickness, differences in densities in cortex and medulla, integrity of the collecting system, and kidney size. Postvoid residual may be considered and placement of urinary catheter if obstruction is suspected. Although a patient's urine output is an important clinical indicator, it is not necessarily kidney specific. Urine output may increase, decrease, or maintain irrespective of the insult affecting the kidneys. Trends in urine output can be useful when determining possible causes of AKI.

Measurements of fractional excretion of sodium (FeNa) or urea (FeUr) have not consistently been shown to have clear clinical correlations. FeNa is defined by the following formula:

$$FeNa = \frac{100 \times (\text{urinary sodium} \times \text{serum creatinine})}{(\text{serum sodium} \times \text{urinary creatinine})}$$

FeNa less than 1% suggests prerenal and FeNa greater than 2% suggests ATN. Despite the claims that a FeNa calculation can determine prerenal AKI versus ATN, there is no absolute FeNa value that is always diagnostic of prerenal disease. There are many limitations in using FeNa, including that there are other causes of AKI that have a calculated FeNa of less than 1% (including some occasions of ATN). Additionally, single measurements of creatinine may be

of laboratory studies and clinical status, especially if urgent or emergent treatment is warranted.

Careful review of the medical record can aid in determining trends in serum creatinine, assisting in the determination of an

misleading, given that serum creatinine can vary even in a given day. Patients with CKD have impaired sodium handling and in the setting of prerenal disease, will have a FeNa that is greater than 1%. However, this FeNa value should not preclude the clinician from addressing the underlying issue (for example, hypovolemia causing prerenal AKI in a patient with known CKD) solely based on a FeNa percentage. FeNa is not sensitive or specific enough in the inpatient population and therefore is not generalizable to the average hospitalized patient. The entirety of a patient's presentation should allow the clinician to determine the cause of AKI.

Approach to Treatment

The cause of AKI will determine the treatment. If history and examination are pointing toward prerenal volume depletion as the mechanism of AKI, then intravenous fluids should be administered. This does not apply to prerenal AKI from heart failure or cirrhosis. Hypovolemia and hypotension should be addressed with balanced crystalloid solutions (for example, lactated Ringer's), which will reduce the risk of severe hyperchloremic metabolic acidosis that can occur with saline solutions. The optimal rate of infusion of fluids depends on the clinical status of the patient and comorbidities with expert recommendation to consider 1 to 3 L of fluid to start and to avoid volume overload. Concern for sepsis or infection should be treated appropriately including cultures as indicated, intravenous fluid resuscitation, and antibiotics. Urinary obstruction should be treated and depending on the site of obstruction, a patient may need placement of a urinary catheter or percutaneous nephrostomy tube. Depending on the patient's GFR, any medication given should be renally dosed. All nephrotoxic insults should be avoided. Diuretics should be used in the setting of volume overload, such as in acute decompensated heart failure causing AKI, and it should be noted that diuretics do not specifically affect AKI recovery or have a survival benefit. If there are life-threatening abnormalities or imbalances caused by AKI including volume overload, hyperkalemia, acidemia, or uremia, then prompt consultation is warranted to a nephrologist and likely to a critical care specialist. In these cases, renal replacement therapy or another hemodialysis modality will likely be considered. The ideal timing to starting dialysis in patients with AKI is unknown, and the mortality benefit to early initiation of dialysis also is unclear. As already mentioned, in patients with acute decompensated heart failure, diuretics are used and inotropes may also be necessary to achieve improvement in renal perfusion in the setting of decreased cardiac output. In patients with liver disease and concomitant AKI, hepatorenal syndrome may be considered as the underlying cause of AKI; however, it is a diagnosis of exclusion and is treated in the ICU with norepinephrine (Levophed)[1] or on the general medical floor with midodrine (Proamatine)[1], octreotide (Sandostatin)[1], and albumin[1]. Acute interstitial nephritis should be treated with the withdrawal of the inciting medication or agent, and if there is no improvement in some days, patients may benefit from glucocorticoids. ATN has no one specific treatment, as it is dependent on the underlying cause (ischemia or nephrotoxins).

Prognosis and Outcomes

AKI is associated with adverse patient outcomes, increased mortality, longer length of hospital stay, and higher healthcare costs. The duration of AKI tends to vary between 7 and 21 days. Some patients with AKI recover kidney function within days and some require dialysis for months. After an episode of AKI, patients are at increased risk for CKD and end-stage renal disease (ESRD). Patients with CKD who experience AKI are more likely to advance to ESRD. Some patients may never return to their baseline kidney function. Irreparable decline in kidney function is more likely in patients of advanced age, those with CKD, and those with heart failure. Mortality rates range from 16% to 50% according to stage of AKI and also depend on cause of

AKI, concurrent comorbid conditions such as sepsis, lung or liver failure, and cerebrovascular events. Patients who are discharged after a hospitalization during which AKI occurred warrant close follow-up. The KDIGO clinical practice guideline, in their expert opinion, recommended that clinicians evaluate patients 3 months after AKI for resolution of AKI or new onset CKD or worsening of preexisting CKD.

Developing Issues—Biomarkers

The aim of AKI biomarkers is to excel in early diagnosis, to assess risk accurately, to assess treatment response, and to evaluate prognosis. There are over 20 biomarkers available to date that can be divided into functional biomarkers, tubular enzymes, damage biomarkers, and preinjury phase biomarkers in the evaluation of AKI. Nearly all biomarkers can be affected by at least one factor. The urine biomarker NephroCheck (insulin-like growth factor-binding protein [IGFBP7] and tissue-inhibitor of metalloproteinases 2 [TIMP2]) is FDA approved and commercially available. Despite validation in the prediction of onset of severe AKI in the critical care setting, this test has limitations including that it can commonly lead to false positive results (especially if used in patients that are low risk for AKI) and cannot be used in the outpatient setting. Given the heterogeneity of AKI, it is evident that no one biomarker is entirely specific for AKI. Biomarkers are but one factor in risk assessment in AKI, and there are newer developments related to monitoring and evaluating AKI risk progression. These include electronic alert systems, machine learning algorithms and artificial intelligence, in addition to models based on renal angina index, furosemide stress test, or biomarkers. Additional study is needed to validate and to standardize risk models to better intervene upon AKI to improve outcomes.

References

Alge JL, Arthur JM: Biomarkers of AKI: a review of mechanistic relevance and potential therapeutic implications, *Clin J Am Soc Nephrol* 10(1):147–155, 2015. https://doi.org/10.2215/CJN.12191213.

Balogun R: Fractional excretion of sodium, urea, and other molecules in acute kidney injury - UpToDate. https://www-uptodate-com.libproxy.unm.edu/contents/fractional-excretion-of-sodium-urea-and-other-molecules-in-acute-kidney-injury?search=fena&source=search_result&selectedTitle=1~40&usage_type=default&display_rank=1#H791015361.

Cooper CM, Fenves AZ, Cooper CM: Before you call renal: acute kidney injury for hospitalists, *J Hosp Med* 10(6), 2015. Available at: 10.1002/jhm.2325.

Hoste EAJ, Bagshaw SM, Bellomo R, et al: Epidemiology of acute kidney injury in critically ill patients: the multinational AKI-EPI study, *Intensive Care Med* 41(8):1411–1423, 2015. Available at: 10.1007/s00134-015-3934-7.

Levey AS, James MT: Acute kidney injury, *Ann Intern Med* 167(9):ITC66, 2017. https://doi.org/10.7326/AITC201711070.

Oh DJ: A long journey for acute kidney injury biomarkers, *Ren Fail* 42(1):154–165, 2020. https://doi.org/10.1080/0886022X.2020.1721300. PMID: 32050834; PMCID: PMC7034110.

Ostermann M, Joannidis M: Acute kidney injury 2016: diagnosis and diagnostic workup, *Crit Care* 20(1):299, 2016. https://doi.org/10.1186/s13054-016-1478-z.

Ostermann M, Bellomo R, Burdmann EA, et al: Conference participants. Controversies in acute kidney injury: conclusions from a kidney disease: improving global outcomes (KDIGO) conference, *Kidney Int* 98(2):294–309, 2020. https://doi.org/10.1016/j.kint.2020.04.020. Epub 2020 Apr 26. PMID: 32709292.

Pahwa AK, Sperati CJ: Urinary fractional excretion indices in the evaluation of acute kidney injury: urinary excretion indices in AKI, *J Hosp Med* 11(1):77–80, 2016, https://doi.org/10.1002/jhm.2501.

Rahman M, Shad F, Smith MC: Acute kidney injury: a guide to diagnosis and management, *Acute Kidney Injury* 86(7):9, 2012.

Sharfuddin AA, Weisbord SD, Palevsky PM, Molitoris BA: *Acute kidney injury. Brenner and Rector's the Kidney*, Philadelphia, PA, 2016, Elsevier, pp 958–1011. e19. http://www.clinicalkey.com/#!/content/book/3-s2.0-B978145574836500031X.

Susantitaphong P, Cruz DN, Cerda J, et al: World incidence of AKI: a meta-analysis, *CJASN* 8(9):1482–1493, 2013. https://doi.org/10.2215/CJN.00710113.

Wald R: Changing incidence and outcomes following dialysis-requiring acute kidney injury among critically ill adults: a population-based cohort study-clinical key, *Am J Kidney Dis* 65(6):870–877, 2015.

Wasung ME, Chawla LS, Madero M: Biomarkers of renal function, which and when? *Clin Chim Acta* 438:350–357, 2015. https://doi.org/10.1016/j.cca.2014.08.039.

Yu MK, Kamal F, Chertow GM: Updates in management and timing of dialysis in acute kidney injury, *J Hosp Med* 7, 2019. Available at: 10.12788/jhm.3105.

Section 2: AKI definition, *Kidney Int Suppl* 2(1):19–36, 2012, https://doi.org/10.1038/kisup.2011.32.

---

[1] Not FDA approved for this indication.

CHRONIC KIDNEY DISEASE

Method of
Catharine Do, MD; and Mark Unruh, MD, MS

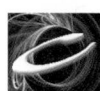

CURRENT DIAGNOSIS

- The estimated glomerular filtration rate (eGFR) is the generally accepted, best index of kidney function. Normal eGFR varies according to age, sex, and body size; in young adults, it is approximately 125 mL/min per 1.73 m² and declines with age.
- Chronic kidney disease (CKD) is defined as GFR < 60 mL/min/1.73 m² as well as elevated markers of kidney damage. The most common marker of kidney damage is urine albumin.
- The most common method to access GFR is serum creatinine combined with CKD-EPI equation. If possible, determine the underlying cause of CKD and consider referral to a nephrologist for management if GFR < 30 mL/min/1.73 m²

CURRENT THERAPY

- Initiate treatment to delay or prevent disease progression, including an angiotensin-converting enzyme inhibitor (ACEI) or an angiotensin receptor blocker (ARB) to reduce blood pressure to < 130/80 mm Hg and urine total protein excretion to as low as possible but at least < 1 g/day.
- Prevent or treat biochemical or clinical abnormalities including serum potassium, calcium, bicarbonate, calcium, phosphorous, parathyroid hormone, and hemoglobin.
- Evaluate for presence of comorbid conditions such as hypertension, diabetes, and cardiovascular disease.

Chronic kidney disease is the term used to describe patients with decrease in glomerular filtration rate (GFR) or kidney damage such as albuminuria; there are different levels of CKD. CKD has been classified by cause, kidney function, and severity of albuminuria. *Kidney damage* is defined as structural or functional abnormalities of the kidney, initially without decreased GFR, which over time can lead to decreased kidney function. Markers of kidney damage include abnormalities in the composition of the blood or urine or structural abnormalities in imaging tests. *End-stage renal disease (ESRD)* or *kidney failure* is the term used to describe patients who have advanced renal failure requiring renal replacement therapy (i.e., either hemodialysis/peritoneal dialysis or transplantation). CKD has been associated with higher costs of care and risk of death.

Most chronic kidney disease demonstrates an inexorable progression. The rate of decline could be estimated as much as 7-10 mL/min/year in those with an untreated diabetic nephropathy. Electrolyte homeostasis, causes of progressive decline in function, and manifestations of kidney failure are similar enough across the different pathologies that we can think of common underlying routes to progression, symptoms, and hopefully amelioration of CKD. These interventions often do not reverse kidney disease; rather, they slow the progression of kidney disease. Therefore earlier diagnosis and treatment may delay kidney death so that a patient can avoid undergoing dialysis, transplantation, and the complication of kidney failure.

Prevalence of Chronic Kidney Disease
Estimates are that there are 30 times as many subjects with chronic kidney disease as compared to ESRD. Approximately 14.7% of the US adult population is thought to have some form of chronic kidney disease. Of note, the majority of those with

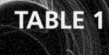

TABLE 1	Risk Factors for the Development or Progression of Kidney Disease

Albuminuria
Hypertension
Episodes of acute kidney injury
Underlying cause of kidney disease (e.g., diabetic nephropathy)
Obesity
Hyperlipidemia
Smoking
High-protein diet
Metabolic acidosis
Hyperphosphatemia
Hyperuricemia
Hyperglycemia

stage 1 and 2 kidney disease may not even be aware of their kidney disease. Furthermore, more than 75 million are thought to have an increased risk of developing CKD. Only a fraction of patients understand that they have CKD, so it is crucial that to convey this to them so that they can take steps to slow the progression of CKD.

Risk Factors for CKD
The non-modifiable risk factors are important for risk stratification by screening and for understanding the pathophysiology of CKD progression (Table 1). These risk factors include age and ethnicity, which are risk factors for many kidney diseases. For example, African-American patients with diabetes have a two-to-three-fold higher risk of developing kidney failure compared to white patients. Modifiable risk factors are important for both understanding disease progression and as a possible option for prevention or therapy. For example, the heavy consumption of analgesics has been associated with the development of kidney failure. The number of patients that develop kidney disease and at risk for developing kidney disease will increase with the increasing prevalence of diabetes and aging of the population.

Approach to the Diagnosis of Chronic Kidney Disease
In clinical practice, the serum creatinine and blood urea nitrogen (BUN) concentrations are commonly used as indicators of GFR. The laboratory measurement of creatinine and urea is accurate and reliable, although normal values may vary slightly from lab to lab. Creatinine production varies with muscle mass, and therefore changes in lean body weight influence the serum creatinine level. For example, a body builder may have an elevated Cr but normal renal function and vice versa for a cachectic elderly woman with muscle atrophy. When using the plasma creatinine to assess GFR, it is also important to keep in mind the semi-logarithmic relationship between the serum creatinine concentration and GFR. Kidney Disease International Global Outcomes (KDIGO) Guideline on Chronic Kidney Disease currently recommends using the Chronic Kidney Disease Epidemiology (CKD-EPI) 2009 creatinine equation: The CKD-EPI equation is currently the most accurate way to estimate GFR from serum creatinine.

CKD-EPI CREATININE EQUATION:

$$\text{GFR} = 141 \times \min(S_{cr}/\kappa, 1)^\alpha \times \max(S_{cr}/\kappa, 1)^{-1.209} \times 0.993^{\text{Age}} \times 1.018 \text{ [if female]} \times 1.159 \text{ [if black]}$$

where: S_{cr} is serum creatinine in mg/dL,
κ is 0.7 for females and 0.9 for males,
α is −0.329 for females and −0.411 for males,
min indicates the minimum of S_{cr}/κ or 1, and
max indicates the maximum of S_{cr}/κ or 1.

Formulas derived from studies of large groups of patients—such as those by Cockroft and Gault and the Modification of Diet in Renal Disease (MDRD) in which GFR was correlated with other factors (e.g., body weight, age, and serum albumin)—are sufficiently accurate to use for clinical purposes.

The recent classification of CKD includes a measure of albuminuria. A spot albumin/creatinine ratio serves as a very important biomarker. Higher levels of albuminuria are linked to progression of CKD, higher frequency of acute kidney injury, higher rates of dialysis, and higher risk of death.

There are novel estimating equations that use a range of new biomarkers to estimate kidney function. The most widely used is Cystatin C, which can be used to estimate GFR in patients with extremes of age or body habitus. Cystain C is a low-molecular-weight cysteine protease inhibitor produced in all nucleated cells and has a constant level of production but rises with poor renal function. Hence, Cystatin C may serve to improve the estimates of GFR in a number of settings. However, Cystatic C levels are affected by thyroid disease and inflammation. so providers should interpret this biomarker with caution in these settings.

Management of Chronic Kidney Disease
Staging of CKD

The purpose of CKD staging is to guide management, including stratification of risk for progression and complications of CKD. Staging of CKD should be done according to Figure 1 and Table 2 and based on:

- Cause of disease
- Six categories of eGFR (G stages)
- Three levels of albuminuria (A stages)

The GFR is the generally accepted best index of kidney function. Chronic kidney disease (CKD) is defined as GFR less than 60 mL/min per 1.73 m² as well as markers of kidney damage. In the United States the most common marker of kidney damage is urine albumin. Other markers are kidney cysts or pathologic changes in the kidney, for example. The severity of CKD is also determined by the level of GFR.

CKD Stage 3 (moderately decreased GFR)

Stage 3 CKD (a GFR of 30 to 59 mL/min per 1.73 m²) has been subdivided into GFR stages 3a (G3a – GFR 45 to 59 mL/min per 1.73 m²) and 3b (G3b – GFR 30 to 44 mL/min per 1.73 m²) to more accurately reflect the continuous association between lower GFR and risk for mortality and adverse kidney outcomes.

CKD Stage 4 (Severely decreased GFR)

GFR 15–29 mL/min per 1.73 m²

CKD Stage 5 (Kidney failure)

G5 – GFR < 15 mL/min per 1.73 m² or treatment by dialysis

Referral to a nephrologist is recommended when eGFR < 30 mL/min per 1.73m² and/or urine albumin creatinine ratio is > 300 mg/g, with earlier referral recommended in specific cases. Early referral to a nephrologist is associated with improved outcomes once patients initiate dialysis.

General Approach to Treatment of Chronic Kidney Disease

Treatment of CKD is divided according to modalities that are specific to the underlying disorder and those that are used to treat all patients with CKD.

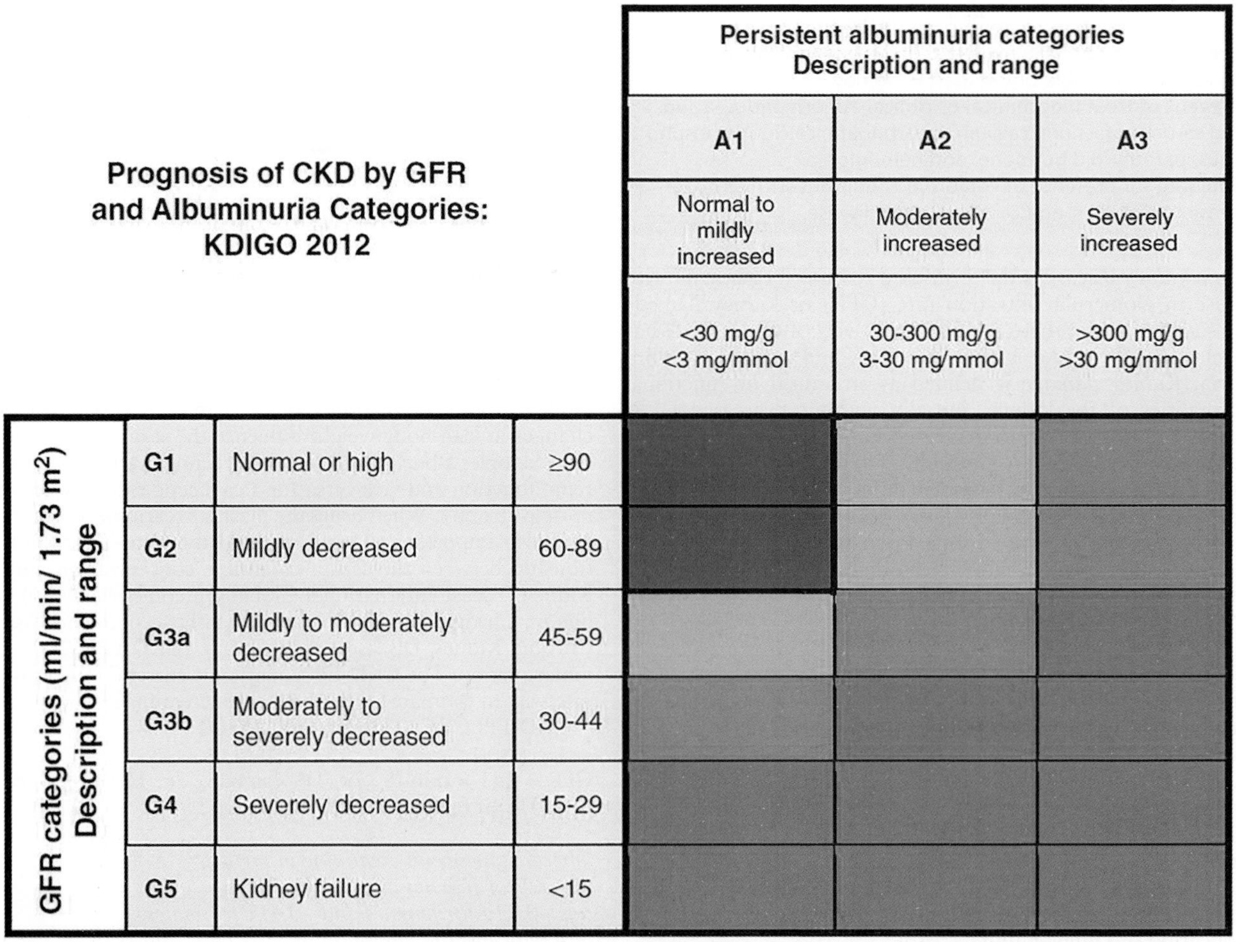

Prognosis of CKD by GFR and Albuminuria Categories: KDIGO 2012

			Persistent albuminuria categories Description and range		
			A1	A2	A3
			Normal to mildly increased	Moderately increased	Severely increased
			<30 mg/g <3 mg/mmol	30-300 mg/g 3-30 mg/mmol	>300 mg/g >30 mg/mmol
GFR categories (ml/min/ 1.73 m²) Description and range	G1	Normal or high	≥90			
	G2	Mildly decreased	60-89			
	G3a	Mildly to moderately decreased	45-59			
	G3b	Moderately to severely decreased	30-44			
	G4	Severely decreased	15-29			
	G5	Kidney failure	<15			

Very dark gray (G1/G2 and A1): low risk (if no other markers of kidney disease, no CKD); Light gray (G3a and A1; G1/G2 and A2): moderately increased risk; Medium gray (G3b and A1; G3a and A2; G1/G2 and A3): high risk; Medium dark gray (G4/G5 and A1; G3b/G4/G5 and A2; G3a/G3b/G4/G5 and A3): very high risk.

Figure 1 Prognosis of CKD by GFR and albuminuria.

The physician treating the patient with CKD has two goals: preventing or delaying progression of CKD and alleviating the electrolyte and hormonal abnormalities that can lead to symptoms or complications. The provider can use the CKD classification system shown in Figure 1 to educate patients and highlight the need for adhering to strategies to slow the rate of CKD progression.

Strategies to Slow Progression of CKD

Since we have a better understanding of the progression of kidney disease, we can effectively slow progression. Rather than losing 10ml/min/year of kidney function as an untreated Type 1 diabetic, those with adequate disease control can forestall the need for dialysis by slowing the rate of progression anywhere from 2 to 6 mL/min/year. This makes a dramatic difference to the individual and to society in terms of quality of life and costs to the health care system. Treat the underlying cause by identifying reversible factors such as volume depletion, uncontrolled hypertension, obstructive uropathy and nephrotoxins.

Blood Pressure Management

In addition to the use of an ACE-I or ARB, management of hypertension in CKD first entails salt-depleting therapy with a salt-restricted diet and diuretic therapy (Table 3). Patients frequently require additional therapy to combat the enhanced vasoconstriction and to attempt to slow the rate of CKD progression. The KDIGO Blood Pressure guidelines have recommended a target blood pressure of < 130/80 for those with advance kidney disease. Among patients with diabetes and CKD, these guidelines recommended a blood pressure target < 140/90 based largely on results from the ACCORD study. Lastly, there is a real opportunity to improve care due to gaps in awareness, treatment, and control of BP among patients with CKD. Although BP treatment has been shown to slow progression of CKD, there is a substantial number of CKD patients with poor BP control. Around 30% of CKD patients are not aware of their BP. Of those that are aware, substantial portions are untreated. Few of those that are treated, are controlled. Only one-fifth of the patients with CKD stages 3–4 have awareness, treatment, and control of BP.

Angiotensin- Converting Enzyme Inhibitors and Angiotensin Receptor Blockers

Angiotensin- converting enzyme inhibitors (ACE-Is) and angiotensin receptor blockers (ARBs) are preferred anti-hypertensive agents for the treatment of blood pressure among patients with CKD, particularly patients with albuminuria. Ang II plays a key role in the progression of glomerulosclerosis, and there is a large amount of experimental data in both animals and people that blocking AngII mitigates progressions. This is thought to be due to a reduction in the glomerular capillary hypertension, reduction in proteinuria, and a diminution of the Ang II fibrosing effects. ACE-I and ARB both are likely to delay progression of kidney disease and have cardiovascular benefits. Some

TABLE 2	Chronic Kidney Disease Classification Based on Glomerular Filtration Rate and Albuminuria

GFR STAGES	EGFR (ML/MIN/1.73M2)	TERMS
G1	>90	Normal or high
G2	60–89	Mildly decreased
G3a	45–59	Mildly to moderately decreased
G3b	30–44	Moderately to severely decreased
G4	15–29	Severely decreased
G5	<15	Kidney failure (add D if treated by dialysis)

ALBUMINURIA STAGES	ALBUMIN/CREATININE RATIO (MG/G)	TERMS
A1	<30	Normal to mildly increased
A2	30–300	Moderately increased
A3	>300	Severely increased

*Chronic kidney disease is defined as either GFR ≤60 mL/min/1.73 m^2 for ≥ 3 months or structural or functional abnormalities manifested by presence of markers of kidney damage in blood, urine, or imaging studies.†Uremic symptoms include nausea, vomiting, anorexia, metallic taste, pericarditis, peripheral neuropathy, central nervous system changes including difficulty with concentration, and seizures.

TABLE 3	Recommendations for the Treatment of Patients With CKD

BLOOD PRESSURE CONTROL IN CKD	MAINTAIN BLOOD PRESSURE < 130/80 MM HG < 140/90 FOR DIABETIC CKD
Reduce proteinuria by administering angiotensin-converting enzyme inhibitors (ACEIs) or angiotensin receptor blockers (ARBs)	Decrease urine protein excretion as low as possible, at least < 1 g/day
Control phosphate concentration with phosphate binders, using non–calcium-containing binders when possible	Maintain serum phosphate toward the normal range in CKD
Maintain vitamin D level by administration of vitamin D analogs	Maintain 25-OH vitamin D levels at 30 ng/mL by administration of cholecalciferol (D$_3$) or ergocalciferol (D$_2$)
Prevent hyperparathyroidism with vitamin D analogs or calcimimetics	Maintain parathyroid levels between 150–600 (2–9 × normal)
Correct anemia with erythropoiesis-stimulating agents and iron replacement as needed	Maintain hemoglobin between 10 and 11 mg/dL. Keep iron saturation (iron/TIBC) > 20%
Administer diuretics to control hypertension and volume overload	Maintain euvolemia when possible
Control serum potassium with dietary restriction, diuretics, and/or potassium exchange resin as necessary	Maintain serum potassium < 5.0 mEq/L
Prevent malnutrition with adequate calories and protein intake	Maintain protein intake between 0.6 and 1 g/kg in CKD and between 1 and 1.3 g/kg on dialysis
Control metabolic acidosis with administration of sodium bicarbonate or sodium citrate	Maintain serum bicarbonate > 22 mEq/L but < 26 mEq/L

studies have examined the possibility of using both together in treatment of chronic kidney disease, with results suggesting more harm than benefit owing to higher rates of hyperkalemia and acute kidney injury among patients receiving dual therapy. The ACE/ARBs substantially delay progression of kidney failure. There does not appear to be a point where you should discontinue ACE/ARB medications unless after starting these medicines there is a significant rise in creatinine. When an ACE-I or ARB causes a rise in creatinine > 30%, the agent should be held to investigate potential renal artery stenosis or volume depletion.

Dietary Protein Restriction

The role of dietary protein restriction in renoprotective strategies for CKD patients remains controversial. Kidney Disease Improving Global Outcomes (KDIGO) suggests daily restriction in protein intake to 0.8 g/kg for CKD patients, although a very-low-protein diet has been associated with increased mortality over the long term. One study had shown a benefit with nuts and other healthy protein foods in reducing the progression and mortality from CKD.

In spite of the fact that inconclusive results of the largest controlled clinical trial done to investigate protein restriction in CKD, the Modified Diet in Renal Disease (MDRD) study, a benefit of moderate protein restriction was suggested by a long-term follow-up analysis. Several prior and subsequent studies and meta-analyses appear to support the role of low protein in retarding progression of CKD and delaying initiation of maintenance dialysis therapy.

Overall, most experts believe that, despite the absence of observed benefit in the MDRD trial, systematic reviews suggest that protein restriction may be beneficial, and the balance of evidence suggests a benefit of moderate dietary protein restriction. Limiting protein intake is also associated with favorable laboratory and metabolic effects, including reduction of blood urea nitrogen levels, uremic toxins, and acid load, in addition to reduced phosphorus load with better control of metabolic bone disorders. Protein restriction may be particularly effective in diseases characterized by hyperfiltration, such as diabetes and certain glomerulopathies.

In patients with CKD, a balanced and individualized dietary approach based on low-protein diet should be carefully monitored, with periodic follow-up for adequate caloric intake and surveillance to optimize protein malnutrition with body weight as well as serum albumin.

Avoid Nephrotoxic Medications

Avoid nephrotoxins and note that both prescription and over-the-counter medications can have delterious kidney effects. The most concerning nephrotoxins over the counter are NSAIDS, antacids, proton pump inhibitors, and a number of herbal medications (licorice, Cat's Claw). Several prescription medications can be deleterious to the kidney. Noteworthy are the calcineurin inhibitors such as cyclosporine (Sandimmune) and tacrolimus (Prograf), which cause progressive renal insufficiency. We know this because solid-organ transplants have a high rate of kidney failure. Other medications such as aminoglycosides and amphotericin (Fungizone) or the use of IV contrast have detrimental effects on the hospitalized patient.

Clinical Manifestations of Kidney Failure

P. A. Piorry coined the word *urémie* in 1847 to indicate problems caused by "contaminating the blood with urine." The basic abnormality is the presence of waste products that are not being eliminated by the kidney. In current use, the term *uremia* reflects a clinical syndrome associated with loss of kidney function. Uremic symptoms in advanced CKD result both from kidney excretory failure (retention of urea, certain hormones, polyamines, trace elements, serum proteases, so-called "middle molecules," pyridine derivatives, B_2-microglobulin, etc.) and from the loss of metabolic and endocrine functions

TABLE 4	Signs and Symptoms of Kidney Failure

CARDIOVASCULAR COMPLICATIONS	ENDOCRINE DISORDERS
Hypertension	Secondary hyperparathyroidism
Ischemic cardiac disease	Glucose intolerance (uremic diabetes)
Pericardial disease	Hyperlipidemia
Congestive heart failure	Sexual dysfunction/infertility

Hematologic Abnormalities	Immunologic Defects
Anemia	Lymphocytopenia, leukopenia
Bleeding tendency	Decreased antibody responses
	Decreased cell-mediated response
	Increased susceptibility to infection

Neuropsychiatric Abnormalities	Dermatologic Abnormalities
Peripheral neuropathy	Pruritus, uremic pigmentation,
CNS disturbances	uremic frost, calciphylaxis, nail changes
Seizures	
Sleep disorders	
Musculoskeletal Abnormalities	Gastrointestinal Abnormalities
Bone disease	Anorexia, nausea, vomiting
Myopathies	Upper tract disease: gastritis, duodenitis,
Carpal Tunnel Syndrome	

normally performed by the kidney. Uremia is thought to be in part due to protein intake, since a low-protein diet mitigates some of the symptoms. While we know that some of the uremic toxins are partially dialyzable, the exact etiology of uremia remains unknown.

Uremia also relates a loss of metabolic and endocrine functions normally performed by the intact kidney. Hence, kidney failure is a multisystem disorder (see Table 4). The measurement of kidney function can be variable, and that degree of variability makes it difficult to use as the only factor in clinical decision making. Therefore, as CKD progresses, clinicians tend to regularly assess the subjective symptoms associated with uremia. In particular, uremia has been described in the following systems: neurologic (sleep, memory), GI (appetite, nausea, dysguesia), and dermatologic (itching). If the severity of these symptoms cannot be managed by symptomatic therapy, then that would be an indication for starting dialysis. Furthermore, if a dialysis patient has these symptoms, it may reflect an inadequate treatment, and the dialysis dose will have to be increased. Of note, the usual physical signs of kidney failure can be rapidly assessed during an exam: blood pressure, pericardial rub, edema, and crackles on lung exam.

Measures Designed to Treat Comorbidity in Kidney Disease
Anemia (Table 5)
Anemia may be managed in patients with CKD by first ruling out other causes of anemia such as GI bleeding and iron deficiencies. Iron deficiency is common in patients with CKD and may be evaluated with a total iron saturation (TSAT) and ferritin. Low ferritin (<100ng/mL) and TSAT (<20) in patients with moderate to advanced CKD indicate an absolute iron deficiency. Iron

TABLE 5	Factors to Consider in the Management of Patients With CKD

Contributors to the loss of kidney function
Hypertension
Diabetes mellitus
Dietary salt intake
Proteinuria
Metabolic acidosis
Complications of chronic kidney disease
Anemia
Platelet dysfunction
Abnormal bone and mineral metabolism (e.g., secondary
   hyperparathyroidism)
Lipid abnormalities (elevated cholesterol and triglycerides)
Metabolic acidosis
Volume overload
Electrolyte disturbances (e.g., hyperkalemia)
Cardiovascular disease

deficiency may be treated using the oral or intravenous route. After iron stores are restored, if the anemia persists and other causes are ruled out, then a erythropoiesis-stimulating agent (ESA) such as erythropoietin (Procrit, Epogen) may be used. For CKD patients, the uses of ESAs are shown to reduce the need for blood transfusions and modestly improve quality of life. The risks of ESA use include an increase in cardiovascular events, hypertension, and cancer progression. For CKD patients the recommendations are to initiate therapy if the Hgb are below 10g/dL with an individualized decision for a target based on risks and benefits. In many cases, providers target a hemoglobin between 10 mg/dL and 11 mg/dL and avoid exceeding levels > 12 mg/dL.

Metabolic Acidosis

Metabolic acidosis develops in CKD when the eGFR drops below 30 mL/min. Recent studies have linked metabolic acidosis in CKD to protein wasting, loss of bone, and sympathetic activation. Observational studies have also linked metabolic acidosis to a higher rate of CKD progression and increased risk of death. There are a large number of ongoing studies testing whether oral sodium bicarbonate supplementation in CKD preserves renal function, and bicarbonate supplementation has been widely adopted for metabolic acidosis in CKD. A standard dose used in clinical trials for CKD patients has been sodium bicarbonate 1 mEq/kg/day. The supplemental bicarbonate may be titrated up or down depending on serum bicarbonate and symptoms. If bicarbonate is not tolerated by patients, then clinicians could try Shohl's solution (citric acid/sodium citrate), as citrate is converted to bicarbonate by the liver. Currently, a reasonable target serum bicarbonate for patients with moderate to advanced CKD would be > 22mEq/L and < 26mEq/L.

Divalent Ion Metabolism

CKD is associated with abnormalities of divalent ions (Ca^{++}, P) and of the hormones that regulate the concentration of these minerals in body fluids. It is of note that the dysregulation of these divalent ions has also attracted attention as a possible source of cardiovascular disease, since those with CKD are found to have calcium deposition and a calcification of heart valves. Lastly, failed management of divalent ions may lead to calcific uremic arteriolopathy, or calciphylaxis. Calciphylaxis is a rare syndrome characterized by the development of painful nodules in the soft tissue that indurate and ulcerate. This disorder has no uniformly effective treatment and has a high mortality rate. Serum phosphorus is controlled by administration of phosphate binders usually starting with calcium citrate (Citracal) or acetate (PhosLo). If these are not successful or if patients have elevated serum calcium levels, then sevelamer (Renagel) or lanthanum (Fosrenol) can be used alone or in combination with calcium binders. Physicians should aim to maintain serum phosphorus levels between 2.7 and 4.6 mg/dL in CKD stage 3 and 4 and between 3.5 and 5.5 mg/

dL in CKD stage 5. Defining the target PTH level in the setting of CKD remains a challenge because of end-organ resistance to PTH. Parathyroid hormone levels should be maintained between 150 and 600 pg/mL (2–9 × normal) in end-stage renal disease and patients on dialysis. Suppression of parathyroid hormone secretion can be achieved by administration of various vitamin D analogs in combination with calcimimetic agents such as cinacalcet (Sensipar). Serum calcium levels should be monitored closely. Low 25-OH vitamin D levels have been documented in a large number of individuals both with and without renal failure. In patients with renal impairment this can contribute to the abnormal 1,25-OH vitamin D levels. Measurement of 25-OH vitamin D levels should be obtained in all patients with CKD and estimated GFR less than 60 mL/min/1.73 m^2. If levels are below 30 ng/mL, ergocalciferol (D_2) or cholecalciferol (D_3) should be given at sufficient doses to maintain it above this level.

Hyperkalemia

The clinical consequence of hyperkalemia includes cardiac toxicity, muscle weakness, and death. The target potassium concentration for patients with CKD should remain in the normal range, and patients should be monitored during treatment with ACEIs or ARBs. Management of a high serum potassium in patients with CKD should include a low-potassium diet. If there is a sudden increase, it may be due to use of salt substitutes, large amounts of juice, or eating high-potassium foods. It may be helpful to get a nutrition consult to help the patient maintain a low-potassium diet and have a nutritionist be aware of differences in diverse foods, since both noni and coconut juice are high in potassium. In addition, review medications for those associated with hyperkalemia and consider decreasing the dose of ACEI or ARB. Diuretics also may be used to decrease serum potassium levels in CKD, with loop diuretics the most widely used for patients with an eGFR <30 mL/min. Lastly, potassium binding agents may be used to control serum potassium levels in patients with advanced CKD. The potassium exchange resin, sodium polystyrene sulfonate (Kayexalate), or one of the newer exchange resins patiromer (Veltassa) decreases serum potassium levels.

Volume Overload

Sodium retention contributes to hypertension and edema among patients with CKD. In order to adequately address volume overload, both the intake and sodium excretion may need to be addressed in patients with CKD. Patients should adhere to a low-sodium diet, which is often complicated by other dietary restrictions (low-potassium, low-phosphate, ADA diet). Given the complexity of diet in CKD, use of a nutritionist with expertise in kidney-related diets can help both volume overload and the other complications of CKD. In addition to sodium restriction, patients may need to use a diuretic for blood pressure and volume management. In the setting of an eGFR <30 mL/min, loop diuretics are often used to address volume overload. The loop diuretics such as furosemide (Lasix) should be dosed frequently enough to maintain a negative sodium balance. If the loop diuretic at higher doses is not adequately addressing volume overload, then an additional distal tubule diuretic such as metolazone (Zaroxolyn) may be used to increase urinary sodium excretion. It should be noted that increasing sodium excretion may cause acute kidney injury of CKD patients, particularly in the setting of ACEI/ARB and other diuretics. In this case, the patients will often respond to reducing the diuretic dose with close monitoring.

Chronic Kidney Disease–Mineral Bone Disorder (CKD-MBD)

Chronic kidney disease–mineral bone disorder (CKD-MBD) is a systemic disorder of mineral and bone metabolism associated with CKD due to hyperphosphatemia from diminished kidney phosphorus excretion and hypocalcemia due to impaired kidney production of active 1, 25-(OH)2 D leading to secondary hyperparathyroidism. Elevations in serum fibroblast growth factor 23 (FGF23), metabolic bone disease, soft tissue calcifications, and other metabolic derangements are associated with morbidity and mortality in CKD. The management of CKD-MBD is complex due to homeostatic system and multiple treatment options without definitive randomized trials. The ideal strategy should be normalizing serum calcium, phosphate, PTH, and metabolic acidosis while minimizing the risks associated with the therapies. The various treatment options for hyperphosphatemia and secondary hyperparathyroidism include dietary phosphorus restriction, phosphate binders, calcitriol (Rocaltrol) or other active vitamin D analogues, calcimimetics, adequate hemodialysis, and parathyroidectomy. The optimal PTH level in the setting of CKD remains a challenge and has not been prospectively determined. KDIGO guidelines recommend that PTH be kept between two to nine times the upper limit of normal for the assay.

Cardiovascular Disease

While >10 million American adults are estimated to have a GFR <60 mL/min (i.e., CKD 3 or worse), far fewer are on dialysis or have received a transplant. Why is there a disparity between the number receiving renal replacement therapies and the number with CKD? Most patients with CKD die from cardiovascular disease (CVD) prior to requiring dialysis or transplantation. On dialysis, the risk of death from CVD remains 10–100 times higher than the general population. A 25-year-old man on hemodialysis has approximately the same risk of dying from heart disease as an 80-year-old without CKD. Traditional risk factors account for only a portion of the CVD risk associated with CKD. Traditional risk factors include age, diabetes, lipids, hypertension, and smoking, among others. Many nontraditional risk factors are believed to play a role in increasing CVD risk in CKD. Some of these risk factors are anemia, volume overload, hyperparathyroidism, calcium/phosphate disturbances, uremia, and malnutrition/inflammation often associated with CKD. The exact role these nontraditional risk factors play is an actively researched area. In general, consider patients with CKD high-risk patients for CVD, and CKD is considered by some to be a coronary equivalent. Data indicate that patients with lower GFRs (<45 mL/min) and microalbuminuria/proteinuria carry a very high CVD risk (~ equivalent to a prior history of coronary disease). This is important when seeing a patient in the emergency room for chest pain or when evaluating a patient pre-operatively for surgery, etc. Treatment focuses on optimizing management of known CVD risk factors and being alert for harbingers of active CVD. Those caring for CKD patients must address CVD risk management. Primary prevention focuses on blood pressure, exercise, +/- aspirin, +/- statins. The data available for cardiovascular risk management is limited in part owing to the exclusion of patients with significant CKD in many large studies. Hence, the utility of ASA and statins (if any) in this setting is not well established. CKD patient's often present with atypical symptoms of CVD, a high index of suspicion is important.

The Effect of Sodium Glucose Co-Transporter 2 Inhibitors on Chronic Kidney Disease

Novel oral hypoglycemic agents sodium glucose co-transporter 2 (SGLT2) inhibitors have expanded pharmacotherapeutic options for the treatment of type 2 diabetes mellitus (DM). SGLT2 receptor expression is limited to the renal proximal tubule. These receptors reabsorb filtered urinary glucose, contributing to hyperglycemia. SGLT2 inhibitors lower serum glucose by preventing renal reuptake of glucose, producing an osmotic diuresis, thus lowering blood glucose. The hypoglycemic effects of urinary glucose enrichment depends on renal function, and thus are limited in those with advanced chronic kidney disease below eGFR of 30 mL/min/m². SGLT2 inhibitors include canagliflozin (Invokana), empagliflozin (Jardiance), and dapagliflozin (Farxiga), among many. These agents have pleotropic effects such as protective cardiovascular and renal benefits in addition to their hypoglycemic effects. Studies of SGLT2 inhibitors including CREDENCE, EMPA-REG, and CANVAS have shown cardiovascular benefits of these agents, leading to their preference as second-line medications for the treatment of type 2 DM in those with established cardiovascular disease. The renal protective benefits as seen with canagliflozin include reduction in loss of renal function as well as reduction in albuminuria, both important in the treatment of diabetic nephropathy. These agents are thought to prevent hyperfiltration observed in diabetic nephropathy. In addition, blood pressure lowering was also observed with SGLT2 inhibitor treatment with the mechanism ascribed to osmotic diuresis. Whether all SGLT2 inhibitors confer renal protective effects remains to be seen. A small reduction in GFR can occur after starting an SGLT2 inhibitor. This is common and should be followed. It is not a reason to stop the drug. For now, these novel medications are welcome additions to classic renin-angiotensin-aldosterone blockade agents commonly used to treat and slow the progression of diabetic nephropathy.

References

Fox CS, Matsushita K, Woodward M, Bilo HJ, et al: Associations of kidney disease measures with mortality and end-stage renal disease in individuals with and without diabetes: a meta-analysis, Chronic Kidney Disease Prognosis Consortium, *Lancet* 380(9854):1662–1673, 2012.

Furuki T, Kobayashi K, Toyoda M, et al: The influence of long-term administration of SGLT2 inhibitors on blood pressure at the office and at home in patients with type 2 diabetes mellitus and chronic kidney disease, *J Clin Hypertens* 22(12):2306–2314, 2020.

Ingelfinger JR, Rosen CJ: Clinical credence - SGLT2 inhibitors, diabetes, and chronic kidney disease, *N Engl J Med* 380(24):2371–2372, 2019.

Kalantar-Zadeh K, Fouque D: Nutritional management of chronic kidney disease, *N Engl J Med* 377(18):1765–1776, 2017.

KDIGO: 2017: clinical practice guideline update for the diagnosis, evaluation, prevention, and treatment of chronic kidney disease–mineral and bone disorder (CKD-MBD), *Kidney Int Suppl (2011)* 7(1):1–59, 2017.

KDOQI: Clinical practice guidelines and clinical practice recommendations for diabetes and chronic kidney disease, *Am J Kidney Dis* 49:S12–S54, 2007.

Klahr S, Levey AS, Beck GJ, et al: The effects of dietary protein restriction and blood-pressure control on the progression of chronic renal disease. Modification of Diet in Renal Disease Study Group, *N Engl J Med* 330:877–884, 1994.

Kovesdy CP, Appel LJ, Grams ME, et al: Potassium homeostasis in health and disease: a scientific workshop cosponsored by the National Kidney Foundation and the American Society of Hypertension, *Am J Kidney Dis* 70(6):844–858, 2017.

Kraut JA, Madias NE: Metabolic acidosis of CKD: an update, *Am J Kidney Dis* 67(2):307–317, 2016.

Levey AS, Stevens LA, Schmid CH, et al: A new equation to estimate glomerular filtration rate, *Ann Intern Med* 150:604–612, 2009.

Loniewski I, Wesson D: Bicarbonate therapy for prevention of chronic kidney disease progression, *Kidney Int* 85(3):529–535, 2014.

Milder YM, Stocker SL, Samocha-Bonet D, Day RO, Greenfield JR: Sodium-glucose cotransporter 2 inhibitors for type 2 diabetes-cardiovascular and renal benefits in patients with chronic kidney disease, *Eur J Clin Pharmacol* 75(11):1481–1490, 2019.

Navaneethan SD, Schold JD, Arrigain S, et al: Serum bicarbonate and mortality in stage 3 and stage 4 chronic kidney disease, *Clin J Am Soc Nephrol* 6(10):2395–2402, 2011.

Neal B, Perkovic V, Matthews DR: Canagliflozin and cardiovascular and renal events in type 2 diabetes, *N Engl J Med* 377(21):2097–2099, 2017.

Perkovic V, Jardine MJ, Neal B, et al: Canagliflozin and renal outcomes in type 2 diabetes and nephropathy, *N Engl J Med* 380(24):2295–2306, 2019.

Pfeffer MA, Burdmann EA, Chen CY, et al: A trial of darbepoetin alfa in type 2 diabetes and chronic kidney disease, *N Engl J Med* 361(21):2019–2032, 2009.

Raphael K: Metabolic acidosis in CKD: core curriculum 2019, *Am J Kidney Dis* 74(2):263–275, 2019.

Toyama T, Neuen BL, Jun M, et al: Effect of SGLT2 inhibitors on cardiovascular, renal and safety outcomes in patients with type 2 diabetes mellitus and chronic kidney disease: a systematic review and meta-analysis, *Diabetes Obes Metab* 21(5):1237–1250, 2019.

Webster AC, Nagler EV, Morton RL, Masson P: Chronic kidney disease, *Lancet* 389(10075):1238–1252, 2017.

Wright Jr JT, Williamson JD, Whelton PK, et al: A randomized trial of intensive versus standard blood pressure control, *N Engl J Med* 374(23):2284, 2016.

MALIGNANT TUMORS OF THE UROGENITAL TRACT

Method of
Danica May, MD; and Moben Mirza, MD

 CURRENT DIAGNOSIS

Prostate cancer

- Prostate cancer is the most common cancer diagnosis for men in the United States.
- Screening with prostate-specific antigen (PSA) and digital rectal exam (DRE) should be offered starting at age 55 and ending at age 70 for the average risk patient. For higher risk patients (African American patients or strong family history of prostate cancer), screening should be discussed starting at age 40.
- Prostate cancer risk factors include African ancestry, family history, as well as Lynch syndrome and other genetic mutations.
- Transrectal ultrasound (TRUS)-guided biopsy is the diagnostic test for prostate cancer and may be indicated for patients with elevated PSA or abnormal DRE.
- Staging involves cross-sectional abdominal and pelvic imaging as well as bone scan for patients with high risk cancer.

Benign and malignant renal rumors

- Most patients with renal cell carcinoma (RCC) are diagnosed incidentally on imaging work-up for other symptoms or complaints. The classic triad of a palpable mass, hematuria, and flank pain is a relatively rare presentation.
- Risk factors for RCC are smoking, obesity, hypertension, and genetic syndromes such as von Hippel-Lindau disease, Birt-Hogg-Dube syndrome, and tuberous sclerosis complex.
- Most malignant renal masses are renal cell carcinoma, but lymphoma, metastases from other malignancies, and other renal malignancies should be considered in the differential as treatment options will vary.
- Benign masses include oncocytoma, angiomyolipoma (AML), renal cysts, and adenomas among others.
- Staging of renal masses involves abdominal imaging with CT scan or MRI. Chest imaging should be obtained. Laboratory analysis should include a CBC, CMP, and urinalysis. CT-guided core renal mass biopsy may be obtained after urologic consultation.

Urothelial cell carcinoma

- Urothelial cell carcinoma can affect the renal pelvis, ureter, bladder, or urethra, though most cases occur in the bladder.
- The average patient is older than age 60 and may have significant medical comorbidities.
- Risk factors include smoking, radiation, certain chemical exposures, and Lynch syndrome.
- Microscopic or gross hematuria is the most common presentation. Patients may also present with urgency, frequency, dysuria, flank pain, or have hydronephrosis discovered on imaging.
- Work-up involves a CT urogram for patients with adequate renal function and cystoscopy.
- Tumors discovered in the bladder should be resected endoscopically for diagnosis and staging. Tumors in the renal pelvis or ureters can be biopsied ureteroscopically.

Primary carcinoma of the prostate and urethra

- Primary urethral malignancies typically consist of urethral or squamous cell carcinoma.
- Patients often present with hematuria, and overall survival remains poor.
- Studies are lacking on this rare disease state, but treatment depends on stage, disease location, and histology.

Penile cancer

- Penile cancer is a rare malignancy with poor prognosis for men with advanced stage disease.
- Presentation often involves an ulceration or palpable mass, and biopsy is the key to diagnosis.
- The vast majority of penile lesions are squamous cell carcinomas.
- Risk factors for penile cancer involve chronic inflammation, tobacco use, lack of neonatal circumcision, STDs, HPV infection specifically with subtypes 6, 16, and 18, and phimosis.
- Staging scans involve chest, abdomen, and pelvis imaging with attention paid to the inguinal lymph nodes.

Testicular cancer

- Testicular cancer is diagnosed in men with a median age of 33 years and has excellent outcomes at 5 years.
- Risk factors for testicular cancer include undescended testis and a personal or family history of testicular cancer.
- The majority of testicular cancers are germ cell tumors, which include seminoma and non-seminoma.
- Germ cell tumors can also present in extra-testicular locations such as the retroperitoneum or mediastinum.
- Men with a testicular mass should undergo an ultrasound and intratesticular masses that are concerning for malignancy should be removed via radical orchiectomy. Sperm banking should be offered.
- Serum tumor markers include beta-hCG, AFP, and LDH. Staging, pathology, and tumor markers dictate next management steps.

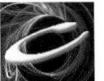 **CURRENT THERAPY**

Prostate cancer

- Treatment options depend on PSA, Gleason grade, clinical stage, and the patient's overall health and life expectancy. Men with limited life expectancy may be good candidates for watchful waiting. Active surveillance is an option for men with low-risk and some men with favorable intermediate risk prostate cancer.
- Treatment options for clinically localized prostate cancer include radical (typically robotic) prostatectomy and radiation therapy in the form of external beam or brachytherapy with or without androgen deprivation therapy.
- The cornerstone of treatment for men with nodal or metastatic disease involves androgen deprivation therapy.
- Other treatment options include chemotherapy, immunotherapy, or newer secondary hormone therapies.
- Following definitive therapy, follow up for men treated for prostate cancer involves regular PSA monitoring every few months for 5 years and then yearly after that.

Benign and malignant renal tumors

- Surgery remains a mainstay of treatment for localized renal cell carcinoma. Partial or radical nephrectomy can be performed taking into consideration the clinical stage, tumor location, patient's overall health, renal function, presence or absence or a contralateral kidney, and genetic syndromes predisposing the patient to future malignancies.
- Ablative therapy and active surveillance are options for small renal masses.
- Simple renal cysts do not require treatment. Complex or enhancing cysts should be treated based on their risk of malignancy.
- Follow up for patients treated for renal cell carcinoma involves periodic laboratory analysis as well as cross-sectional abdominal and chest imaging.

- Systemic therapy options for patients with metastatic renal cell carcinoma have increased drastically with the newest treatments including immune checkpoint inhibitors.
- The treatment of angiomyolipomas (AMLs) is often based on size and is directed toward prevention of the complication of retroperitoneal hemorrhage. Embolization or surgical removal has traditionally been proposed at a 4-cm size, although larger AMLs can be safely observed.

Urothelial cell carcinoma

- Treatment options depend on stage, grade, and tumor location.
- Superficial low-grade bladder tumors can be managed with resection and periodic surveillance cystoscopy.
- Patients with superficial high-grade cancer or cancers invasive into the lamina propria (T1) diagnosed on initial resection may be offered a repeat resection. Treatment following this often involves induction and maintenance intravesical Bacillus Calmette-Guérin (BCG) therapy. Patients with high-grade T1 bladder cancer should be counseled and offered radical cystectomy. These patients should have periodic cystoscopy and upper tract imaging as indicated.
- The standard of care for patients with muscle invasive (T2) bladder cancer is cisplatin-based neoadjuvant chemotherapy followed by radical cystectomy. Patients ineligible for cisplatin-based chemotherapy should undergo immediate radical cystectomy.
- For patients who are unwilling or unfit for radical cystectomy, chemoradiation therapy can be offered.
- Upper tract tumors of the renal pelvis or ureter are managed by grade as well as clinical stage. The pathologic stage may not be accurately established prior to definitive treatment.
- Nephroureterectomy should be offered for patients with upper tract urothelial cell carcinoma. Other options can include endoscopic management with tumor ablation or partial resection of the ureter if tumor location is amenable. Cisplatin-based neoadjuvant or adjuvant chemotherapy should be considered.

Primary urothelial carcinoma of the prostate and urethra

- Superficial urothelial tumors (Tis, Ta, T1) of the urethra can be resected or biopsied followed by intravesical BCG therapy.
- The surgical treatment for men with T2 proximal urethral cancer involves removal of the bladder and prostate with urethrectomy. More distal disease involving the pendulous urethra can be managed with a distal urethrectomy or partial penectomy.
- Women are often treated with cystectomy and urethrectomy.
- Patients with higher stage urethral cancer may be offered neoadjuvant or adjuvant chemotherapy or radiation therapy.

Penile cancer

- Organ sparing approaches include topical therapy, laser therapy, Mohs surgery, glansectomy, radiation therapy, or wide local excision and are most utilized in patients with superficial or properly selected penile cancer patient with T1 disease.
- More aggressive tumors should be treated with partial or total penectomy.
- Higher risk patients need to undergo inguinal node dissection and pelvic node dissection should be considered for highly selected patients.
- Neoadjuvant chemotherapy should be considered for bulky, bilateral, or fixed inguinal lymphadenopathy.

Testicular cancer

- Following radical orchiectomy, imaging of the chest, abdomen, and pelvis is key for staging. Repeat tumor markers should also be collected as persistent tumor marker elevation after orchiectomy changes treatment.
- Patients with localized seminoma with normal tumor markers can undergo surveillance, chemotherapy, or radiation therapy.

- For patients with more advanced disease, treatment options should include chemotherapy or radiation therapy.
- In patients with pure seminoma and a residual retroperitoneal mass, further work-up with a PET/CT scan can aid in characterization of residual disease.
- Radiation therapy is not a standard treatment for men with non-seminoma testicular cancer.
- Patients with localized non-seminoma with normal tumor markers can undergo observation, chemotherapy, or retroperitoneal lymph node dissection (RPLND).
- For patients with more advanced disease, treatment options should include chemotherapy and/or surgical resection.
- Residual retroperitoneal masses in the patient treated for non-seminoma testicular cancer should be removed via RPLND.
- Follow up for all patients with testicular cancer includes surveillance with chest, abdominal, and pelvic imaging as well as periodic tumor markers.

Prostate Cancer

Background

Prostate cancer is the most common cancer diagnosis among men in the United States. It accounts for over 191,000 new cases in 2020 and is the third most common overall malignancy after breast and lung/bronchus cancers. It is a relatively indolent cancer with 97.8% 5-year relative survival. Family history of prostate cancer, particularly among first-degree relatives, is a well-known risk factor for developing prostate cancer. Known genetic alterations include both germline as well as somatic mutations. Common mutations include BRCA1/2, ATM, MLH1, MSH2, MSH6, and PMS2, among many others. Syndromes linked to prostate cancer include Lynch syndrome and hereditary breast and ovarian cancer (HBOC) syndrome. Other risk factors for development of prostate cancer include increasing age, African American ancestry, smoking, and Ashkenazi Jewish heritage.

Diagnosis

Prostate cancer is most often diagnosed in a localized and asymptomatic state via screening. Rarely, prostate cancer is detected at a locally advanced state with symptoms of pelvic pain, urinary retention, or ureteral obstruction with hydronephrosis. The minority of men are diagnosed in the metastatic state, with the most frequent complaint being bone pain from metastases. The utilization of prostate-specific antigen (PSA) blood testing has drastically changed the diagnosis of prostate cancer from a historically predominantly metastatic state to a localized and potentially curable state in the current era. In 2012, the US Preventive Services Task Force released a grade D recommendation against the use of PSA-based screening for any man. This recommendation was modified in 2018 to allow for informed decision making for prostate cancer screening in men aged 55 to 69. The American Urological Association recommends individualized prostate cancer screening for men aged 40 to 54 who are at higher risk, shared decision-making for men aged 55 to 69, and cessation of screening for men aged 70 or older or those men with life expectancy less than 10 to 15 years. Screening of prostate cancer with PSA should not be dismissed with the assumption that prostate cancer is an indolent cancer. Screening can lead to diagnosis and appropriate risk stratification.

The basis of prostate cancer screening is serum PSA as well as digital rectal exam (DRE). While PSA is only produced by the prostate, it is not specific to malignant versus benign cells, and there are a variety of causes of elevated PSA. Benign causes of elevated PSA include benign prostate hypertrophy, prostatitis, instrumentation of the urethra such as catheterization or utilization of cystoscopy, and urinary tract infections. One of the

TABLE 1 Risk Stratification and Staging Workup

NCCN RISK GROUP	CLINICAL/PATHOLOGIC FEATURES	IMAGING
Very low	T1c AND Gleason score ≤6/grade group 1 AND PSA <10 ng/mL AND Fewer than 3 prostate biopsy fragments/cores positive, ≤50% cancer in each fragment/core AND PSA density <0.15 ng/mL/g	Not indicated
Low	T1–T2a AND Gleason score ≤6/grade group 1 AND PSA <10 ng/mL	Not indicated

Favorable intermediate	T2b–T2c OR
	Gleason score 3 + 4 = 7/grade group 2 OR PSA 10–20
	  ng/mL AND
	Percentage of positive biopsy cores <50%
		Bone imaging: not recommended for staging
		Pelvic ± abdominal imaging: recommended if nomogram
		  predicts >10% probability of pelvic lymph node
		  involvement

Unfavorable intermediate	T2b–T2c OR
	Gleason score 3 + 4 = 7/grade group 2 or Gleason score
	  4 + 3 = 7/grade group 3 OR
	PSA 10–20 ng/mL
		Bone imaging: recommended if T2 and PSA >10 ng/mL
		Pelvic ± abdominal imaging: recommended if nomogram
		  predicts >10% probability of pelvic lymph node
		  involvement

High	T3a OR
	Gleason score 8/grade group 4 or Gleason score 4 + 5 =
	  9/grade group 5 OR
	PSA >20 ng/mL
		Bone imaging: recommended
		Pelvic ± abdominal imaging: recommended if nomogram
		  predicts >10% probability of pelvic lymph node
		  involvement

Very high	T3b–T4 OR
	Primary Gleason pattern 5 OR
	>4 cores with Gleason score 8–10/grade group 4 or 5
		Bone imaging: recommended
		Pelvic ± abdominal imaging: recommended if nomogram
		  predicts >10% probability of pelvic lymph node
		  involvement

NCCN, National Comprehensive Cancer Network; *PSA,* prostate-specific antigen.
From Partin AW: *Campbell-Walsh-Wein Urology,* ed 12, Elsevier, 2021.

difficulties of PSA utilization is that there is no cutoff normal level. In fact, 6.6% of men with a PSA of 0.5 ng/mL or less were found to have prostate cancer with rates increasing to 26.9% in men with PSA of 3.1 to 4.0 ng/mL. In general, PSA increases with age. Some men may have an abnormal DRE, which can prompt further work-up. Worrisome findings including induration or nodules palpable within the prostate.

Following screening with PSA and DRE, further work-up includes a prostate biopsy. The vast majority of prostate biopsies are performed with transrectal ultrasound (TRUS) to help with volumetric and anatomical surveys. The majority of prostate cancer is detected in the peripheral zone, so the standard 12-core biopsy template targets this area in a systematic fashion. Prostatic volume as well as anatomy such as large intravesical lobes should be noted as this information can be helpful in surgical planning.

Prostate MRI is an increasingly utilized tool in men with various clinical situations including elevated PSA with a prior negative biopsy, performance of active surveillance (AS; further discussed below), staging, and surgical planning, as well as in men whose pathology appears discordant with their rectal examination or PSA level. Multiparametric MRI gives not only detailed anatomic information, but also functional assessment of various tumor regions. This information can then be used for an MRI-guided biopsy or more commonly fusion biopsy via platforms that fuse concerning MRI findings with real-time TRUS biopsy for improved lesion targeting.

The vast majority of prostate cancers are adenocarcinomas. Prostate biopsy pathology is based on Gleason grading system 1 to 5, with 5 reflecting poorly differentiated and most aggressive cells. The grading system is translated into a score that adds the most common and second most common grading pattern to yield a score between 2 and 10. Further classification into a Gleason group between 1 and 5 informs appropriate risk classification. In general, low-risk prostate cancer consists of Gleason 6 prostate cancer (Gleason group 1), while intermediate risk prostate cancer consists of Gleason 7 prostate cancer (Gleason group 2 and 3). High-risk prostate cancer includes Gleason sums 8, 9, and 10 prostate cancer (Gleason groups 4 and 5). Risk groups also take into account clinical stage, PSA levels, and biopsy core

positivity. TNM staging is used for prostate cancer. Prostate cancer diagnosed either surgically via a transurethral resection of the prostate or via TRUS biopsy is stage T1. T2 is organ-confined prostate cancer, while T3 is defined as extra-prostatic extension. Finally, T4 involves invasion of surrounding structures including the bladder, pelvic floor or sidewall, or rectum (Table 1). Grade, stage, and risk group are instrumental in treatment decisions.

Current recommendations include germline testing for patients with positive family history of prostate cancer; high-risk, regional, or metastatic prostate cancer; Ashkenazi Jewish ancestry; or intraductal histology. Various genetic alterations necessitate genetic counseling as well as change some treatment options. Staging imaging should be carried out for certain men diagnosed with prostate cancer. Current recommendations include pelvic imaging with or without abdominal imaging via CT or MRI as well as a radionuclide bone scan in men with unfavorable intermediate, high risk, and very high-risk disease.

Treatment

Treatment decisions for men diagnosed with prostate cancer depend on a series of factors including risk group, staging, and clinical node status on imaging, as well as the patient's overall health and life expectancy. In patients with limited life expectancy, observation may be utilized. Observation of known prostate cancer involves monitoring the patient with eventual initiation of palliative androgen deprivation therapy (ADT) for symptomatic or imminently symptomatic disease. On the other hand, AS may be utilized for patients with very low risk or low risk disease, and the properly selected favorable intermediate risk disease patient with adequate life expectancy. AS involves periodic assessment of PSA, DRE, and surveillance biopsies. Prostate MRI may also be utilized in an AS algorithm. AS aims to allow for early disease reclassification with ability to perform definitive treatment at that point. Approximately two-thirds of men on AS will be able to avoid treatment and the associated side effects. Another effect of AS is less overtreatment of small, indolent prostate cancers.

The preferred treatment for very low risk and low risk prostate cancer patients with adequate life expectancy is AS. Other options in the properly selected patient population include external beam radiation therapy (EBRT) or brachytherapy, radical prostatectomy (RP), or observation. As previously mentioned, AS remains an option for patients diagnosed with favorable intermediate risk prostate cancer. This cohort of men may also be treated with EBRT or brachytherapy as well as RP. Treatment recommendations for men with unfavorable intermediate risk prostate cancer include RP, EBRT combined with ADT, or EBRT and brachytherapy boost with ADT. For men with high risk or very high risk prostate cancer, treatment recommendations include EBRT and ADT with or without docetaxel (Taxotere) chemotherapy, EBRT with brachytherapy and ADT, or RP. In men with regional lymphadenopathy, the cornerstone of treatment is ADT. This may be combined with EBRT or abiraterone (Zytiga).

Following definitive treatment, patients should be monitored with PSA and DRE every 3 to 6 months. Following RP, PSA should be undetectable as all prostate and prostate cancer tissue has theoretically been surgically removed. Men treated with EBRT or brachytherapy should have a decline in PSA to a low, steady level. In men with detectable or rising PSA after RP, repeat imaging including bone imaging, CT, MRI, C-11 choline, F-18 fluciclovine PET/CT, or PET/MRI may be utilized to assess for sites of disease recurrence. If no metastases are detected, observation or EBRT with or without ADT are treatment options. When metastases are detected, ADT combined with apalutamide (Erleada), docetaxel (Taxotere), abiraterone (Zytiga), enzalutamide (Xtandi), or EBRT to the primary tumor in the setting of low volume metastases are treatment options. Most men with metastatic prostate cancer initially have castration-naïve prostate cancer and respond to medical or surgical (orchiectomy) castration. A rising PSA in the setting of castrate level testosterone indicates the advent of castration-resistant prostate cancer (CRPC), and ADT should be continued indefinitely. Once castration resistance has been identified, bone health should be prioritized with utilization of denosumab (Xgeva) or zoledronic acid (Zometa) in the setting of bone metastases. Therapy options include abiraterone (Zytiga), docetaxel (Taxotere), enzalutamide (Xtandi), sipuleucel-T (Provenge), radium Ra 223 dichloride (Xofigo) for symptomatic bone metastases, or mitoxantrone (Novantrone) for palliation in men who cannot tolerate other therapies. Painful bony metastases can be palliated with EBRT.

Benign and Malignant Renal Tumors
Background
Kidney and renal pelvis cancers account for 4.1% of all new cancer cases at more than 73,000 cases in the United States in 2020 leading to 14,830 deaths. The 5-year relative survival from 2010 to 2016 is approximately 75%. The majority of kidney masses are detected incidentally on cross-sectional imaging for other chief complaints, and the median age at diagnosis is 64 years. These tumors can be primary renal cell carcinoma (RCC), metastases from second primaries such as breast, lung, ovarian, or melanoma as well as lymphoma deposits, or benign renal tumors such as oncocytoma, angiomyolipoma (AML), renal cysts, leiomyoma, and adenomas. RCC subtypes include clear cell, chromophobe, papillary, collecting duct, translocation, and medullary carcinoma. The majority of tumors are clear cell RCC, which comprise 70% of RCC subtypes.

Hereditary syndromes predisposing patients to RCC include von Hippel-Lindau (VHL) disease, hereditary papillary renal carcinoma (HPRC), hereditary leiomyomatosis and renal cell carcinoma (HLRCC), tuberous sclerosis complex (TSC), and Birt-Hogg-Dube (BHD) syndrome, among others. Other risk factors include smoking, obesity, and hypertension.

Diagnosis
Rarely patients with RCC present with a triad of symptoms including hematuria, a flank mass, and flank pain. More commonly, patients are found to have a renal mass on imaging performed for other indications and the frequency of incidental detection has increased with widespread abdominal imaging. In

the patient with a renal mass, laboratory analysis should include a CBC, CMP, and urinalysis. Cross-sectional abdominal imaging with CT or MRI with contrast should be obtained if not already performed. A chest x-ray is required to complete staging but chest CT, bone scan, brain MRI, and core-needle biopsy may also be obtained. Patients who present with multiple renal masses or young age (<46 years old) may be referred for genetic evaluation. Core-needle biopsy of renal masses may be indicated in patients with unclear etiology of their renal mass such as concern for an infiltrating mass like lymphoma, AS guidance, or in combination with ablation strategies.

TNM stage and histologic grade are important for prognosis and treatment guidance in the patient with RCC. Stage T1 tumors are tumors ≤7 cm in greatest dimension and are limited to the kidney. T2 tumors are greater than 7 cm but ≤10 cm and are limited to the kidney. T3 disease involves invasion into major veins including the renal vein or vena cava or invasion into perinephric tissue, while T4 disease is invasion beyond Gerota's fascia. Histologic grade is graded as G1 through G4 with increasing dedifferentiation.

Renal cysts are a very common benign finding and are graded via Bosniak classification with scores ranging from I to IV. Simple cysts are defined as thin-walled cysts without septa, calcifications, or solid component and lack enhancement. As the Bosniak score increases, so does the complexity and malignancy risk of the cyst with Bosniak IV cysts defined as cysts with enhancing soft tissue components and thick or irregular walls or septa. Oncocytomas are the most common benign, enhancing mass and are associated with BHD syndrome. They are often diagnosed on pathology as diagnosis via imaging characteristics can include hypervascularity with a central scar but are not definitive findings. AMLs are common manifestations in patients with TSC but are often easily diagnosed on CT or MRI due to the presence of macroscopic fat, which has negative Hounsfield units. While benign, AMLs are the leading cause of spontaneous retroperitoneal hemorrhage and intervention is targeted toward prevention of this outcome. A cutoff size of 4 cm has been suggested, at which point treatment via surgery or embolization may be offered and discussed. Treatment should be tailored to patient circumstances. Patients with TSC and multiple or enlarging AMLs may be offered everolimus (Afinitor), an mTOR inhibitor for size reduction. While other benign renal lesions do occur, they are relatively rare and beyond the scope of this chapter.

Treatment
Surgery remains a mainstay of treatment for localized RCC. Surgical options include removal of the whole kidney via radical nephrectomy or removal of the mass with preservation of the remaining healthy parenchyma via partial nephrectomy. In general, partial nephrectomy is the approach of choice for stage T1 tumors, especially if tumors are less than 4 cm with a favorable location within the kidney. Radical nephrectomy may be indicated based on tumor size, clinical stage, and anatomy but can be associated with decreased renal function. Concomitant lymph node dissection has not been shown to improve oncologic outcomes. The adrenal gland should be removed for large upper pole tumors or abnormal appearance on staging imaging. Other treatment options include AS or ablative techniques. AS is preferable for elderly patients with comorbidities and small renal masses or in patients who prefer to avoid intervention. Periodic imaging is performed with intervention for enlarging masses. Ablative techniques involve microwave, cryoablation, or thermal ablation and are again most utilized in small renal masses less than 3 cm. Advanced RCC can extend into the renal vein, vena cava, or even the right atrium. Depending on the level of tumor thrombus, cardiothoracic surgery may need to be involved with resection to allow for utilization of vascular bypass. Follow up for patients is dependent on stage but involves periodic laboratory analyses as well as chest and abdominal imaging.

Some patients who present with metastatic disease may ultimately undergo a cytoreductive nephrectomy with resection of the primary tumor followed by systemic therapy. In general, this is offered to patients with lung-only metastases, good performance status, and good prognostic features. Patients who do not fit these criteria should undergo a biopsy and be evaluated for systemic therapy. In addition, some patients with localized disease treated with a partial or radical nephrectomy will develop systemic disease and should also consider systemic therapy. Tumor histology determines treatment options with clear cell being the most common histology. Systemic therapy for RCC is rapidly evolving with a shift from the cytokine era to targeted therapies consisting of tyrosine kinase inhibitors (TKIs), mammalian target of rapamycin inhibitors (mTORs), and immune checkpoint inhibitors. Systemic therapy for favorable risk patients with clear cell histology includes axitinib (Inlyta) with pembrolizumab (Keytruda), pazopanib (Votrient), or sunitinib (Sutent), while poor or intermediate risk patients with clear cell histology should be offered ipilimumab (Yervoy) with nivolumab (Opdivo), axitinib (Inlyta) with pembrolizumab (Keytruda), or cabozantinib (Cabometyx). Patients with non-clear cell histology should be offered enrollment into a clinical trial or sunitinib (Sutent).

Urothelial Cell Carcinoma
Background
Urothelial cell carcinoma is a malignancy that can affect the renal pelvis, ureter, bladder, and urethra, although the majority of cases are bladder cancer. In 2020, in the United States an estimated 81,400 new cases of bladder cancer will be diagnosed with nearly 18,000 deaths. Urothelial cell cancer is a male predominant disease and affects the elderly with a median age of diagnosis of 73 with many patients having significant medical comorbidities. Modifiable risk factors include smoking, pelvic radiation, chemical exposure, obesity, and diabetes mellitus. Lynch syndrome is associated with upper tract urothelial cell carcinomas.

Diagnosis
The most common presenting sign of urothelial cell carcinoma is microscopic or gross hematuria but can also include lower urinary tract complaints, hydronephrosis on imaging, or flank pain. Work-up for hematuria involves upper tract imaging frequently with a CT urogram, a CT of the abdomen and pelvis with pre-contrast, post-contrast, and delayed images, as well as cystoscopy. If tumors are found in the bladder and cross-sectional imaging has not been performed, a CT or MRI of the abdomen and pelvis should be obtained. Next steps involve endoscopic resection of the tumors for pathological analysis and staging. Upper tract, which includes renal pelvis or ureteral tumors, may be visualized during ureteroscopy with biopsy allowing for differentiation of low versus high grade tumor cells as well as identification of location and volume of tumor for future treatment guidance. Chest imaging as well as laboratory tests complete staging.

Stage and grade are key to guide treatment decisions for patients with urothelial cell carcinoma with grade designated as low or high. TNM staging of bladder cancer is broken up into Ta, Tis, T1, T2, T3, and T4. Ta is noninvasive while Tis is urothelial carcinoma in situ. T1 involves invasion into lamina propria, T2 invades muscularis propria, T3 invades perivesical tissue, and T4 invades prostatic stroma, uterus, vagina, pelvic wall, abdominal wall, or seminal vesicles. TNM staging is similar for the renal pelvis and ureter with T3 defined as invasion into peripelvic fat, renal parenchyma, or periureteral fat and T4 defined as invasion into adjacent organs or through the kidney into perinephric fat.

Most bladder, ureter, and renal pelvis tumors are urothelial cell carcinomas. Subtypes also known as variant histology include nested, microcystic, micropapillary, plasmacytoid, clear cell, sarcomatoid, squamous, and lymphoepithelioma-like. Distinct and more rare types of genitourinary tract malignancies of the urothelium include squamous cell, adenocarcinoma, and small cell carcinoma.

Treatment
Bladder
Once bladder cancer has been diagnosed, appropriate pathologic and radiologic staging should be completed. Pathology determines need for repeat transurethral resection of bladder tumor

(TURBT) with recommendations for second resection for Ta high-grade tumors and any T1 tumors. Patients with Ta low-grade tumors may be observed. For patients with high-grade T1 disease, a radical cystectomy should be offered. Patients with Tis, Ta high-grade, and T1 disease should be offered intravesical therapy usually with Bacillus Calmette-Guérin (TICE BCG) or BCG therapy (Figure 1). Treatment options for muscle invasive or T2 disease are quite different and the gold standard is platinum-based neoadjuvant chemotherapy followed by radical cystectomy (Figure 2). Prior to treatment for muscle invasive bladder cancer (MIBC), a CBC, CMP, and chest imaging should be obtained. A bone scan is indicated if concern for bony metastases exists. A radical cystectomy involves removal of the bladder, prostate, and seminal vesicles for men. A radical cystectomy in females involves removal of the bladder often with concomitant removal of the uterus, ovaries, anterior vagina, and urethra. A urinary diversion is then formed with the majority of patients receiving an ileal conduit with abdominal stoma. Continent diversions are also options. Cisplatin-based neoadjuvant chemotherapy with dose dense methotrexate[1], vinblastine[1], doxorubicin (Adriamycin), and cisplatin (ddMVAC) or gemcitabine (Gemzar)[1] with cisplatin (GC) are the current recommendations. If patients are unable to tolerate chemotherapy, immediate radical cystectomy should be performed. Adjuvant chemotherapy is recommended for adverse pathologic features including stage T3-T4 or node positive disease if not given in a neoadjuvant fashion. Finally, chemoradiotherapy with bladder preservation may be selected by some patients. Ideal candidates should not have hydronephrosis or extensive carcinoma in situ. Concurrent radiation therapy with radio sensitizing chemotherapy such as cisplatin and 5-FU (fluorouracil)[1] are administered. The patient's bladder should be reassessed after 2 to 3 months with surgical consolidation as a consideration for residual muscle invasive disease. In patients who present with concern for nodal involvement or metastases, options include neoadjuvant therapy followed by consolidative cystectomy or systemic therapy alone. In the locally advanced or metastatic patient population who are cisplatin ineligible, gemcitabine (Gemzar)[1] with carboplatin (Paraplatin)[1], atezolizumab (Tecentriq)[1], or pembrolizumab (Keytruda)[1] are the preferred regiments.

Upper Tract Urothelial Cell Carcinoma
The treatment of upper tract urothelial cell carcinoma follows the same basic principles as treatment of bladder cancer. As previously mentioned, ureteroscopy with biopsy of tumor allows for grade determination though is much less likely to accurately diagnose stage due to the limited ability to obtain specimens via a ureteroscope. The gold standard for nonmetastatic upper tract disease involves a radical nephroureterectomy with bladder cuff removal. Platinum-based neoadjuvant chemotherapy should be considered for patients with lymphadenopathy, large high-grade tumors, sessile tumors, or concern for parenchymal invasion. For some small, papillary, unifocal, low-grade tumors, management may involve endoscopic management with laser ablation of tumor and periodic surveillance ureteroscopy or cross-sectional imaging. Distal ureteral tumors can at times be managed with a distal ureterectomy with ureteral reimplant.

Primary Carcinoma of the Prostate and Urethra
Background
Primary carcinoma of the prostate or urethra is quite rare. Prostatic urethral histology is most often urothelial in origin while the remaining urethral primary malignancies are predominantly squamous cell carcinoma. Overall survival is relatively poor at 42% at 5 years. Due to the low incidence, a lack of data and studies of ideal management for these patients are lacking. Stage, disease location, histology, and tumor size remain important prognostic factors.

---

[1]Not FDA approved for this indication.

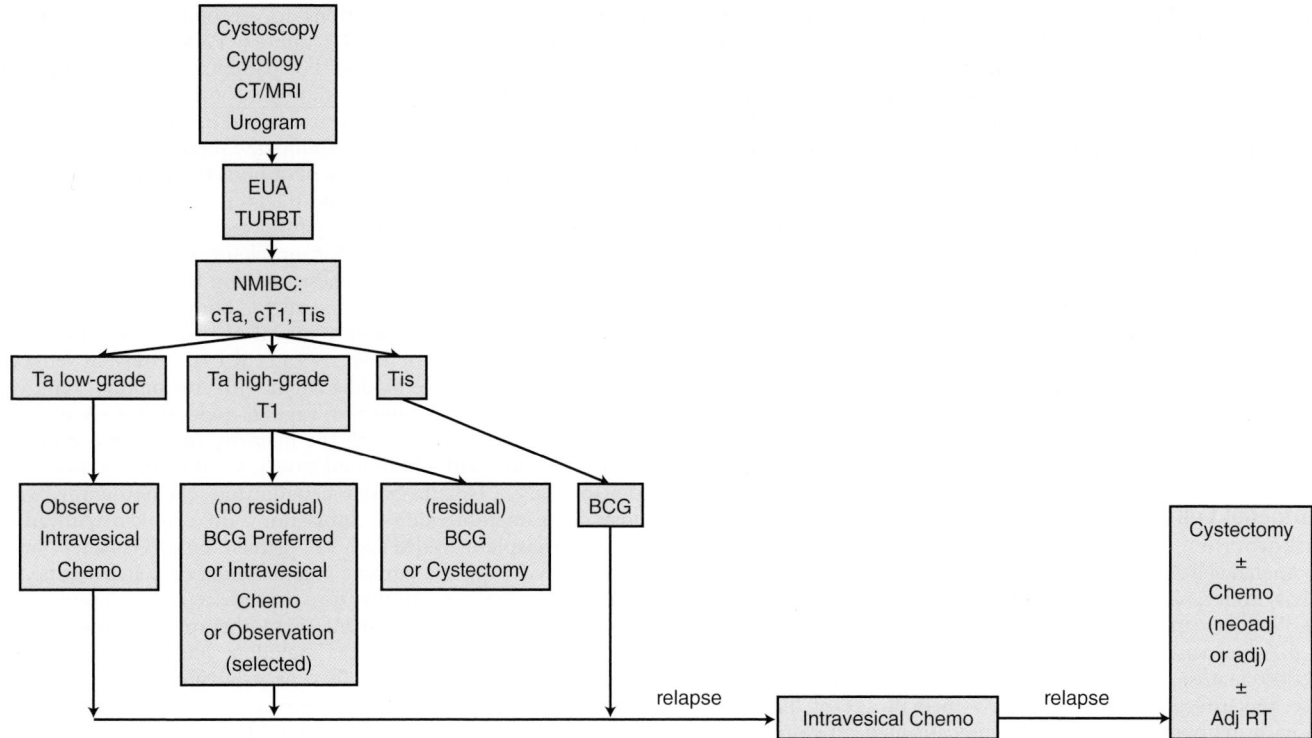

Figure 1 Management algorithm for non-muscle-invasive bladder cancer. *BCG*, Bacillus Calmette-Guerin; *Chemo*, chemotherapy; *CT*, computed tomography; *EUA*, examination under anesthesia; *NMIBC*, non-muscle-invasive bladder cancer; *MRI*, magnetic resonance imaging; *RT*, radiotherapy; *TURBT*, transurethral resection of bladder tumor. From LaRiviere MJB, Brian C, Christodouleas JP: Bladder cancer. In *Gunderson & Tepper's Clinical Radiation Oncology*, 2020, Elsevier.

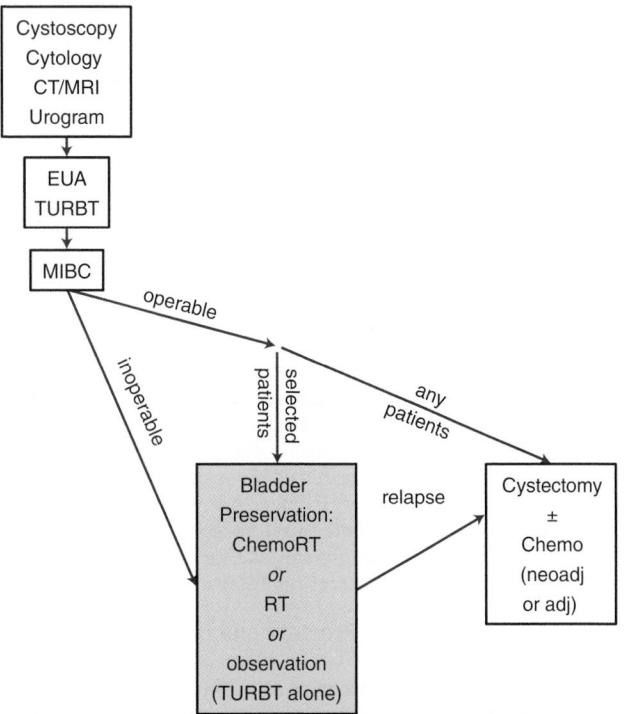

Figure 2 Management algorithm for muscle-invasive bladder cancer. *adj*, Adjuvant; *Chemo*, chemotherapy; *ChemoRT*, chemoradiotherapy; *CT*, computed tomography; *EUA*, examination under anesthesia; *MIBC*, muscle-invasive bladder cancer; *MRI*, magnetic resonance imaging; *neo-adj*, neoadjuvant; *RT*, radiotherapy; *TURBT*, transurethral resection of bladder tumor. From LaRiviere MJB, Brian C, Christodouleas JP: Bladder cancer. In *Gunderson & Tepper's Clinical Radiation Oncology*, 2020, Elsevier.

Diagnosis

Initial work-up involves DRE in men with cystoscopy and transurethral or transvaginal resection or biopsy of the tumor. Cross-sectional imaging with MRI or CT of the pelvis assists with tumor staging as well as assesses for concomitant lymphadenopathy, while chest imaging assesses for metastases.

Treatment

As with urothelial malignancies of the bladder, Tis, Ta, or T1 urothelial cell carcinoma of the male prostate or urethra and female urethra should be followed by a repeat resection and subsequent BCG treatment[1]. In men, proximal urethral disease (prostatic or bulbar urethra) stage T2 or higher is ideally managed with a urethrectomy with cystoprostatectomy. T2 urothelial disease of the pendulous urethra can be managed with a distal urethrectomy or partial penectomy. Adverse pathology or positive margins may be further managed with chemotherapy or chemoradiotherapy. In women, T2 urethral urothelial malignancies should be managed with chemoradiotherapy, urethrectomy with cystectomy, or distal urethrectomy if tumor location is amenable. In more advanced disease stages including T3–T4 or palpable inguinal lymphadenopathy, systemic therapy with or without concomitant radiation followed by consolidative surgery are guideline recommendations.

Penile Cancer

Background

Penile cancer remains a rare disease in North America and Europe, with approximately 2200 cases diagnosed and 440 deaths in 2020 in the United States. It remains a highly lethal disease if not caught at a very early stage. Once disease has spread to pelvic lymph nodes, 5-year survival rates are 0%. As with prostate and bladder malignancies, increasing age is a risk factor for penile cancer with

---

[1]Not FDA approved for this indication.

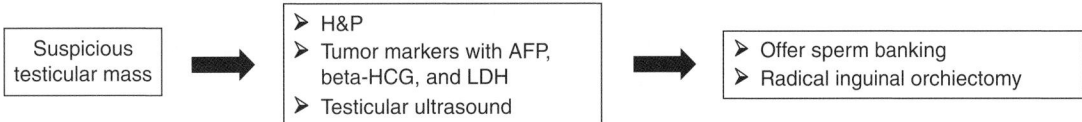

Figure 3 Management algorithm for suspicious testicular mass.

a median age of diagnosis of 68 years in the United States. Other risk factors include phimosis, which also limits examination and early detection as well as tobacco use, chronic inflammation, balanitis, lichen sclerosis, poor hygiene, STDs (specifically HIV and HPV), and lack of neonatal circumcision. Key HPV types include 6, 16, and 18. Histology of penile cancer is overwhelmingly squamous cell carcinoma with subtypes including verrucous, papillary squamous, warty, and basaloid. Verrucous histology carries the most favorable prognosis with more aggressive variants including sarcomatoid and adenosquamous. Tumor grade is designated as grade 1 to 4 with 1 being well differentiated and grade 4 being poorly or undifferentiated.

Diagnosis

A careful physical examination is key for men who present with penile lesions, while care should be taken to observe lesion characteristics including location, size, and consistency, as well as perform an inguinal lymph node examination to assess for lymphadenopathy. Staging utilizes the TNM staging system with Tis defined as carcinoma in situ, Ta as non-invasive squamous cell carcinoma, T1 as superficial invasion substratified based on lymphovascular/perineural invasion and high versus low grade, T2 with corpus spongiosum or urethral invasion, T3 with corpora cavernosal invasion, and T4 as invasion into surrounding structures such as the bony pelvis, prostate, or scrotum. Tissue should be obtained for pathologic analysis. MRI or ultrasound can assess with anatomic characterization of the tumor.

Treatment

Organ sparing approaches for management of penile cancer include topical therapy, laser therapy, Mohs surgery, glansectomy, and wide local excision. Topical therapies include imiquimod (Aldara)[1] and 5-FU (Efudex)[1]. Organ sparing approaches can be primary treatment options for patients with Tis, Ta or the properly selected patient with T1 penile cancer. Low-grade T1 tumors can also be treated with radiation therapy. If location or size preclude less aggressive therapies, partial penectomy may be necessary. Higher-grade T1 tumors often necessitate partial or total penectomy with intraoperative frozen sections to ensure negative margins. T2 tumors or greater should be treated aggressively with partial or total penectomy, although radiotherapy or chemoradiotherapy are also options. Patients with low risk pathology, Tis-T1a penile cancer, should undergo inguinal lymph node surveillance while higher risk pathology, T1b or greater penile cancer, necessitates cross-sectional imaging of the chest, abdomen, and pelvis with inguinal lymph node dissection or dynamic sentinel node biopsy. In low risk patients with palpable lymphadenopathy, biopsy should be performed with node dissection performed for positive nodes with or without neoadjuvant chemotherapy. For palpable inguinal lymphadenopathy larger than 4 cm, fixed lymph nodes smaller than 4 cm, or bilateral lymphadenopathy, patients should receive neoadjuvant chemotherapy if medically suitable followed by inguinal lymphadenectomy with or without pelvic lymphadenectomy. Other treatment options include radiation therapy or chemoradiotherapy. Adjuvant chemotherapy should be offered for patients with multiple positive nodes or extranodal extension. Finally, adjuvant radiation therapy should be offered to the patient with positive pelvic nodes. For patients who present with metastases, systemic chemotherapy, radiation therapy, or chemoradiotherapy are options. The preferred chemotherapy regimen is TIP with

paclitaxel (Taxol)[1], ifosfamide (Ifex)[1], and cisplatin (Platinol)[1]. Patients with recurrence should be referred for a clinical trial or treatment with pembrolizumab (Keytruda)[1].

Testicular Cancer
Background

Testicular cancer is predominantly a disease of younger men with median age at diagnosis of 33 years of age. An estimated 9,610 new cases will be detected in 2020 with 440 deaths. Testicular cancer has a high 5-year survival rate of 95%. Risk factors include a family history of testicular cancer, personal history of testicular cancer, or undescended testicle. The majority of testicular tumors are germ cell tumors consisting of seminoma and nonseminoma. Seminomas are the more common subtype and carry a more favorable prognosis. Nonseminomas can be comprised of choriocarcinoma, embryonal carcinoma, yolk sac tumors, and teratoma. Germ cell tumors that originate outside the testicle may be located in the retroperitoneum or mediastinum and follow similar treatment recommendations.

Diagnosis

Men with testicular cancer often present with painless testicular enlargement or a mass. They may at times experience pain, which can be confused with epididymitis or orchitis. Ultrasound examination is the next step with findings of an intratesticular mass necessitating collection of serum tumor markers including AFP, beta-hCG, and LDH.

Staging follows the TNM classification. Tis tumors are germ cell neoplasia in situ, T1 tumors are limited to the testis without lymphovascular invasion (LVI), T2 tumors are limited to the testis with LVI or invade hilar soft tissues or epididymis, T4 tumors invade the spermatic cord, and T4 tumors involve scrotal invasion. Nodal metastases are classified based on size, and metastases are divided into non-retroperitoneal nodal disease/pulmonary metastases or non-pulmonary metastases. Finally, the S stage is based on post-orchiectomy tumor markers.

Treatment

Once an intratesticular mass is identified on physical exam or trans-scrotal ultrasound, radical inguinal orchiectomy is the next step (Figure 3). Sperm banking should be offered to any patient who wishes to preserve future fertility before radical orchiectomy and certainly prior to any systemic therapy or retroperitoneal lymph node dissection. Following orchiectomy, chest imaging and a CT scan of the abdomen and pelvis should be obtained with repeat post-operative tumor markers. For patients with T1 to T4 localized pure seminoma with normal tumor markers, treatment following orchiectomy can include surveillance (which is preferred), carboplatin (Paraplatin)[1], or radiation therapy. For patients with pure seminoma and retroperitoneal lymphadenopathy less than 5 cm in maximum dimension, options include chemotherapy with a regimen of bleomycin, etoposide (Toposar), and cisplatin (Platinol) or etoposide (Toposar) with cisplatin, as well as radiation therapy to the retroperitoneum. For patients with bulkier retroperitoneal lymphadenopathy, non-regional lymphadenopathy, or metastases, chemotherapy is recommended. PET/CT scans may be obtained in the patient with residual post-chemotherapy masses with resection if PET positive.

Non-seminomatous testicular cancer is managed differently than seminoma, and radiation therapy is not indicated. For patients without lymphadenopathy and normal tumor markers, options include surveillance, chemotherapy regimens as previously described for pure seminoma, and RPLND. For patients with enlarged lymph nodes in the retroperitoneum, treatment options include chemotherapy or RPLND. Treatment should be focused on chemotherapy for patients with bulky retroperitoneal lymphadenopathy, non-retroperitoneal lymphadenopathy, or metastases. Patients who undergo chemotherapy with residual masses larger than one centimeter on follow up CT scans should undergo surgical resection. Follow up for patients treated for testicular cancer can include periodic tumor markers, CT scan of the abdomen and pelvis, and chest x-ray.

Early urologic consultation should be considered for several common clinical conditions to prevent delayed diagnosis. Patients with elevated PSA or hematuria may frequently be treated with antibiotics for presumptive prostatitis or urinary tract infections. These patients should instead be promptly referred to a urologist to prevent delayed diagnosis of prostate cancer or urologic malignancy. In addition, patients with testicular masses may not seek work-up and treatment in a timely fashion. Upon presentation, a prompt ultrasound should be obtained. Initial empiric treatment with antibiotics for presumed orchitis or epididymitis can be avoided for intratesticular masses seen on ultrasound to allow for expedient orchiectomy.

References

"Cancer Stat Facts." Retrieved 6/12/2020, 2020, from https://seer.cancer.gov/stat facts/.

LaRiviere MJB, Brian C, Christodouleas John P: Bladder Cancer. *Gunderson & Tepper's Clinical Radiation Oncology. ClinicalKey*, Elsevier, 2020.

"NCCN Guidelines." NCCN Guidelines for Treatment of Cancer by Site. Retrieved 6/25/20202, 2020.

Thompson IM, et al: "Prevalence of prostate cancer among men with a prostate-specific antigen level < or =4.0 ng per milliliter, *N Engl J Med* 350(22):2239–2246, 2004.

Taneja SSB, Marc A: In *Active Management Strategies for Localized Prostate Cancer. Campbell-Walsh-Wein Urology. A. W. Partin. ClinicalKey*, Elsevier, 2020.

NEPHROLITHIASIS

Method of
William J. Somers, MD

CURRENT DIAGNOSIS

- Renal calculi can present acutely or more often are discovered as an incidental finding on an unrelated radiologic study.
- Ureteral calculi present with either acute onset of excruciating flank pain or a gradual onset preceded by generalized abdominal discomfort.
- Renal colic pain can radiate from ipsilateral flank to lower abdomen, often mimicking pain from cholecystitis, appendicitis, or ovarian conditions such as torsion or ruptured ovarian cysts.
- Physical exam will reveal an anxious patient experiencing sharp, excruciating costovertebral pain. Pain commonly occurs in waves. Percussion of the flank reveals exquisite tenderness. The patient cannot find a comfortable resting position.
- Computed tomography (CT) scan without intravenous contrast (CT stone protocol) is the definitive diagnostic study. Abdominal plain film and renal ultrasonography are not as accurate as CT.
- Urinalysis may demonstrate either microscopic or gross hematuria. Pyuria in the absence of bacteriuria is common and does not always indicate infection.
- Nausea, vomiting, and low-grade fever are common. Temperature over 101°F suggests infection and is an acute urologic emergency.

CURRENT THERAPY

- Low calcium diets may contribute to the development of kidney stones.
- Asymptomatic renal stones can be managed electively with observation or surgical intervention.
- Once the acute episode is controlled with intravenous analgesics, and the patient is discharged from the emergency room, ureteral obstruction can be managed with oral analgesics, liberal oral fluid intake, and expectant observation if the patient is afebrile and the stone is 5 mm or less in size.
- A follow-up renal ultrasound should be obtained 2 weeks after the first presentation of symptoms. If hydronephrosis persists or if the stone has not passed, refer the patient to a urologist.
- Fever and/or leukocytosis, regardless of a clean urine, indicates possible pyonephrosis, a surgical emergency, and the patient should be hospitalized for definitive treatment.
- Patients who are calcium stone formers should be encouraged to maintain a low sodium, low protein, normal calcium diet, and increase oral intake of fluids to 2 L daily.
- Patients who are recurrent calcium stone formers should be offered thiazide diuretics in addition to maintaining the dietary measures to limit stone formation.
- Patients who form uric acid stones should be encouraged to maintain a liberal oral intake of fluids and try to maintain an alkaline urine with potassium citrate (Urocit-K).

Pathophysiology

Urine exists in four states: **undersaturated**, in which no crystals will form; **metastable**, a state where concentration of salts is high but urine inhibitors prevent supersaturation; **saturated**, where addition of salts will not dissolve; and **supersaturated**, which is an unstable solution and crystals can form spontaneously. Urine is generally in a supersaturated state.

The generally accepted theory describing stone formation begins with spontaneous crystallization in a supersaturated urine. This tiny crystal nucleus then attaches to a cell membrane in the collecting tubule. This nidus then attracts other crystals and cell debris forming a tiny calcification, which gradually grows larger as these particles continue to adhere to the mass. Some of these calcifications break off and proceed to the collecting system or remain in the renal tubules indefinitely.

Another theory suggests that spontaneous crystallization occurs at damaged sites along the nephron. Crystals attach to the damaged cell wall, remain fixed in place, and attract further crystal accumulation. Initial cell damage is believed to occur from high calcium oxalate levels based on studies that implicate oxalate as the sole cause for renal tubule cell damage. Pak 1976 showed that the calcium oxalate concentration is four times higher in urine than its solubility in water. This higher concentration may have an adverse effect on the cells, an interesting but as yet unproved theory.

Historically Randall plaques were believed to provide a base for crystal nucleation in the collecting system. These plaques are located in the loop of Henle just below the urothelium in the renal papillae. As they grow, they erode through the urothelium forming a nidus for crystal attachment and growth.

Since a supersaturated salt solution will spontaneously generate crystal formation, there must be some inherent factors that inhibit crystal formation. Citrate, magnesium, and pyrophosphates are the major stone inhibitors naturally found in urine. Citrate is the major inhibitor. Citrate complexes with calcium, reducing its availability and thus preventing spontaneous precipitation of calcium oxalate as well as inhibiting the calcium crystal nucleation. Magnesium binds to oxalate, also reducing its availability to bind with calcium.

Other inhibitors such as Tamm-Horsfall proteins have been identified, but their role is not fully understood.

Calcium Stones

Calcium stones are the most common type of stone in the United States. Hypercalciuria is the first step in stone formation. Thirty percent to 40% of calcium is absorbed in the small intestine, and about 10% from the colon. The kidney filters 270 mmol of calcium daily and absorbs all except for approximately 4 mmol. The active form of vitamin D is the most potent stimulator of intestinal calcium absorption. Calcium transport is regulated at three sites: intestine, bone, and kidney. Low calcium intake stimulates increased calcium absorption, which stimulates parathyroid hormone (PTH). PTH regulates the conversion of 25-hydroxyvitamin D to 1,25-dihydroxyvitamin D or calcitriol. PTH also stimulates the mobilization of calcium from bone through the action of osteoclasts and increases the absorption of calcium from renal tubules.

The classic model for hypercalciuria describes three types:
1. Absorptive hypercalciuria, the most common form, occurs in 55% of stone formers and is caused by increase in intestinal absorption of calcium. Absorptive hypercalciuria can be categorized as Type 1, in which urinary calcium remains high despite a low calcium diet, and Type 2, in which urinary calcium is normalized on a low calcium diet.
2. Resorptive hypercalciuria, identified in approximately 5% of stone formers, is usually seen in patients with hyperparathyroidism. Excessive PTH secretion causes increased production of calcitriol (1,25-dihydroxyvitamin D) which causes increased intestinal absorption of calcium. These patients present with hypercalciuria, hypercalcemia, and reduced phosphatemia. Patients with serum calcium levels above 10 should be evaluated for hyperparathyroidism.
3. Renal hypercalciuria, commonly referred to as renal leak hypercalciuria, is caused by a defect in calcium reabsorption in the proximal tubule. It is characterized by high fasting urine calcium levels, normal serum calcium levels, and elevated PTH.

Other causes for hypercalcemia include sarcoidosis, granulomatous diseases, malignancy, and glucocorticoid use. Malignancy is the most common cause for hypercalcemia in hospitalized patients. Of the malignancies, lung and breast are most common. It is believed the tumors produce cytokines and other factors which cause bone destruction through the action of osteoclasts, resulting in bone destruction and subsequent hypercalcemia. Glucocorticoids stimulate the release of PTH. Nephrolithiasis is common in patients with Cushing syndrome.

Calcium Stones and Calcium and Vitamin D Supplementation

If a patient develops de novo kidney stones while taking calcium and vitamin D supplements, order a 24-hour urine collection for calcium, phosphorus, uric acid, and citrate. If this demonstrates hypercalciuria, refer to a nutritionist for dietary guidance. Suggest that dietary calcium is a more natural way of increasing calcium levels, whereas calcium supplements could increase the risk. I would also question the need for taking both supplements.

Oxalate

Oxalates cause increased urinary saturation of calcium oxalate, which in turn can cause calcium oxalate stone formation. Primary hyperoxaluria is an autosomal recessive disorder responsible for end-stage renal failure before the age of 15 in 50% of young patients.

Enteric hyperoxaluria is the most common cause of acquired hyperoxaluria. It is associated with chronic diarrheal conditions, loss of large segments of small bowel, and intrinsic bowel disease. Loss of fat absorption in these patients results in increased oxalate absorption. Oxalate readily binds to calcium, which can ultimately initiate stone formation.

Renal Tubular Acidosis

Renal tubular acidosis (RTA) describes a defect in urinary acidification resulting in a metabolic acidosis. Hypokalemia, elevated urine pH, hypocitraturia, and hypercalciuria can lead to stone formation. There are three common types of RTA. Type 1, or distal, RTA patients are at high risk for stone formation. Calcium phosphate stones are associated with Type 1 patients which should prompt the physician to further diagnostic testing. Treatment can decrease the rate of stone formation. Type 2, or proximal, RTA is not associated with nephrolithiasis. Type 4 RTA is not commonly associated with stones, but they can occur.

Uric Acid Stones

Uric acid stones are unique in that they can be dissolved medically. Uric acid is the end product of purine metabolism. Humans lack the enzyme uricase which is the final step in the metabolism of uric acid to allantoin. Uric acid is not readily soluble in normally acidic urine. Hyperuricosuria is found in patients with gout, type 2 diabetes, and Lesch-Nyan syndrome. Alkalinizing urine is the primary treatment for asymptomatic uric acid renal stones.

Prevention

The time-honored key to prevention for all stones is increased water intake. Multiple studies have shown increasing oral intake of fluids to produce a 2 to 2.5 L daily urine output is the most efficient and least expensive way to prevent most stones. Additional measures include a low salt diet, limiting protein, and avoiding foods with high oxalate content.

When available, the stone should be analyzed to provide a diagnosis and a specific plan tailored to the type of stone and underlying pathologic cause if present. A complete medical history should be obtained which can identify an underlying cause such as hyperparathyroidism, Cushing syndrome, type 2 diabetes, antiviral medication, and so on. The American Urological Association has published guidelines for prevention and management of nephrolithiasis, which are summarized in the following.

Common misconceptions about the type of fluid patients should be drinking include avoiding alcohol, coffee, colas, wine, and beer. Only one study reported a decrease in the recurrence rate when patients avoided colas but the rate was so low it was not clinically significant. In general, there is no definite consensus on avoidance of certain fluids or the selection of certain fluids to help prevent recurrent calcium oxalate stones. Neither water hardness nor grapefruit juice are associated with stone formation. Carbonated water beverages may have a slight benefit against stone formation. Vitamin D replacement does not appear to be a risk factor for stone formation.

Contrary to popular belief, a low-calcium diet is associated with an increase in calcium oxalate stones. It is believed that low calcium intake results in increased oxalate absorption from the gut and higher levels of urinary oxalate. Recommendations suggest daily calcium intake of 1 to 2 g. A low-sodium diet has been shown to decrease urinary calcium excretion but in general, compliance with a low-sodium diet is difficult. A high-oxalate diet has been shown to increase stone recurrence. Patients should be counseled to limit foods high in oxalate. Oxalate content of various foods is readily available through online searches. Here again, a 1- to 2-g daily intake of calcium seems to offset the risk of stone recurrence in these patients with high urinary oxalate levels. Calcium supplements in older women may lead to a higher risk of stone disease, but there are conflicting reports. If a patient is taking supplements, baseline 24-hour urine collections should be obtained to monitor urinary calcium levels and make dietary adjustments as needed. Since urinary citrate is a stone inhibitor, patients should be encouraged to add fruits and vegetables to their diet. There is no hard evidence that drinking lemonade or adding lemon to tap water prevents recurrent stone formation. Animal protein intake contributes to an acidic urine, which promotes stone formation. Patients should limit their weekly intake of meats, cheese, eggs, and fish.

There are no definitive studies demonstrating a beneficial effect of reducing a high purine diet with lower uric acid stones formation. But in general, patients with recurrent calcium or uric acid stones and a diet high in purines may benefit from reducing their intake of high purine foods. These include various seafoods, shellfish, water fowl, organ meats, game meats, pork, and poultry. Simply restricting red meats without limiting other high purine foods is not beneficial.

For those patients who have failed dietary measures or those that continue to form stones after altering their diets, medical therapy is indicated.

Thiazide diuretics are the gold standard for treatment of recurrent calcium oxalate stones. Chlorthalidone[1] 25 mg daily, hydrochlorothiazide[1] 50 mg daily, and indapamide[1] 2.5 mg daily are all well tolerated. (Patients should be monitored for hypokalemia.) Potassium citrate (Urocit-K) 10 to 20 mEq daily can be prescribed for patients with recurrent calcium oxalate stones, uric acid stones, and cystine stones. Sodium citrate is an alternate choice but risks creating a higher urinary calcium load. A baseline 24-hour urinary citrate level and follow-up study 6 months later will determine if therapy is effectively raising urinary citrate levels. Uric acid stones can be dissolved with aggressive urinary alkalinization using potassium citrate. Patients with hyperuricosuria and recurrent calcium oxalate or uric acid stones should be offered allopurinol (Zyloprim) 300 mg daily. Patients with cystine stones should be managed with high fluid intake, urinary alkalinization with potassium citrate, and reduction in sodium and protein intake. Thiol drugs should be prescribed if dietary measures fail. Alpha-mercaptopropionyl glycine (tiopronin, Thiola) 800 mg daily in 3 divided doses is the standard treatment. An alternative preparation D-penicillamine (Cuprimine) is associated with more severe side effects and should be a second-line choice.

Struvite stones occur in the presence of chronic urinary infection. Treatment of the stone with sterilization of the urinary tract is the best option. If surgery is not an option, suppressive antibiotic therapy may help.

According to one recent study only one in three patients will follow recommendations to prevent recurrent stones.

Diagnosis

A CT scan without intravenous contrast is the most accurate way of diagnosing renal and ureteral stones. It is the first choice for suspected renal or ureteral stones. An abdominal plain film is an unreliable and inaccurate diagnostic tool. It should never be ordered in an acute situation. Small 1- to 2-mm stones are difficult to see on plain films. Uric acid stones, cystine stones, and triamterene stones are radiolucent and seldom visible on plain films. Renal ultrasound is a good tool to identify and follow hydronephrosis but it does not accurately identify renal stones and cannot be used to follow ureteral stones. It too does not play a role in the acute situation. A CT stone protocol is readily available in medical centers and outpatient facilities. It can be performed in less than 15 minutes and no preparation is required. Diagnosis is instantaneous and accurate. MRI has been used to diagnose ureteral stones in pregnant females but interpretation is dependent on the experience of the radiologist and his or her familiarity with the technique. It is not frequently used for this purpose.

Differential Diagnosis

Asymptomatic nephrolithiasis is usually discovered as an incidental finding on an unrelated radiological study. Intense renal

shadowing on abdominal ultrasound is suggestive for renal stone. A calcification overlying the renal shadow on an abdominal plain film can suggest renal stone, but the differential includes arterial calcifications, stomach or intestinal contents, calcified lymph nodes, renal cell tumors, cholelithiasis, etc. Pelvic calcifications seen on plain films can be ascribed to phleboliths, ovarian calcifications, prostate calcifications, appendoliths, vascular calcifications, bladder stones, and so on. Needless to say, plain films should not be expected to provide an accurate diagnosis. Unless the renal stone is obstructing the renal pelvis, it does not cause pain. Patients who present with back pain and nonobstructing renal stones should not be treated for renal colic. Further diagnostic evaluation is indicated.

In contrast to asymptomatic renal stones, ureteral stones almost always present with dramatic onset of excruciating pain. The diagnosis is almost instantaneous. Renal colic is localized to either costovertebral area. Nausea and vomiting are common. Pain is not relieved by changing position. As the stone progresses distally the pain can mimic multiple acute abdominal conditions. The differential diagnosis of right lower quadrant abdominal pain includes:
- Acute appendicitis
- Ovarian conditions (e.g., rupture, ectopic pregnancy)
- Incarcerated inguinal hernia
- Cholecystitis
- Testicular torsion
- Diverticulitis, but very rarely

The differential for left lower quadrant pain is the same as for right lower quadrant pain, with the exception of appendicitis and cholecystitis, for obvious reasons. Diverticulitis is more commonly seen in the descending colon than in the ascending colon.

Treatment
Renal Stones
Asymptomatic renal stones pose a dilemma whether to treat or not. One of the largest retrospective studies evaluated the natural history of these stones based on location, and size of the stone. In more than 3 years of active observation, they found 60% of stones remained asymptomatic, 7% passed spontaneously, and 20% were operated on for pain. Less than 30% of the stones caused renal colic. Most studies determined lower pole stones did not pass spontaneously but grew faster in size than stones in the upper collecting system. These upper pole stones also passed more spontaneously. Patients should be offered treatment of renal stones if larger than 5 mm and in the upper pole of the kidney. Lower pole stones can be followed if the patient is not anxious to have treatment or if the stone has been present for years without change in size or location. Stones 10 mm or larger should be treated regardless of position. These stones could pass spontaneously and will require emergency surgery. All staghorn calculi should be treated unless comorbidities prevent surgical intervention. Autonephrectomy is the ultimate outcome for untreated staghorn calculi.

Once a decision is made to treat a renal stone, the next step is to decide which method is best for the patient. Factors to consider are size of the stone, stone composition, location, number of stones, and body habitus.

Rigid and flexible ureteroscopy with holmium laser disintegration of stones is rapidly replacing electrocorporeal shockwave lithotripsy (ESWL) for both ureteral and renal calculi. The success rate for stone destruction and removal is higher than ESWL. ESWL is indicated for renal and ureteral stones less than 20 mm. However the clearance rate after ESWL is only 60%.

Percutaneous nephrostolithotomy (PNL) is the best choice for these larger stones. All staghorn and partial staghorn calculi should be treated by PNL.

Medical dissolution treatment should be offered to patients with uric acid or cystine stones. Unfortunately, compliance to a medical and dietary regimen is dismal and most will need surgical intervention.

[1]Not FDA approved for this indication.

Ureteral Stones

It is generally accepted that stones less than 5 mm will pass spontaneously over 3 months. Most stones pass sooner than that.

The following is a general guide for treatment of the acute episode:

- CT stone protocol to identify the number, size, and location of the stone(s)
- Intravenous narcotic and antiemetic if necessary
- Urinalysis to evaluate for bacteria. Pyuria and hematuria are common and not signs of infection. If bacteria are present obtain culture and begin empiric antibiotics.
- Abdominal plain film. If the stone is visible this will provide a way to follow the stone.
- CBC, electrolytes
- Hydronephrosis will be present but does not dictate treatment.

Once pain is controlled, the patient is able to tolerate fluids by mouth, laboratory tests are acceptable, and the patient can be discharged with oral narcotics and possibly an alpha blocker. Oxycodone 5 mg PO q4-6 hours is a good choice for pain control. Tamsulosin (Flomax)[1] 0.4 mg PO daily has been shown in many studies to assist in spontaneous stone passage, but recent research has called this into question.

A randomized double-blind, placebo-controlled clinical trial study published in 2018 found no benefit for prescribing tamsulosin for stones less than 9 mm.

A Cochrane review meta-analysis published just before the previously mentioned study came to the conclusion that alpha blockers likely increase stone clearance rates but also slightly increase the risk of major adverse advents—retrograde ejaculation, lightheadedness, and hypotension. They also found alpha-blockers to be less effective in stones less than 5 mm.

Urologic dogma holds that stones less than 5 mm have spontaneous passage rates of higher than 90%. Stones in the distal ureter have a 98% passage rates. I believe most urologists doubt 9-mm stones will pass with or without the concomitant use of tamsulosin unless the patient has passed these large stones previously. Surgical intervention, either ureteroscopy or ESWL, is usually the preferred treatment option.

Since there is no clear choice, I believe a 6-week course of tamsulosin is reasonable. The patient should be followed every 2 weeks. If the stone has not passed by then, surgical intervention should be discussed with the patient.

Patients with any of the following signs and/or symptoms should be admitted and urologic consultation obtained as soon as possible:

- Fever and leukocytosis, or signs of sepsis
- Solitary kidney
- Uncontrolled pain or vomiting
- Bilateral ureteral stones
- Stones larger than 5 to 7 mm
- Uretero-pelvic junction stones larger than 5 mm

The choice to insert a ureteral stent depends on the urologist and his or her assessment of the situation. There are no strict rules, but insertion of stent is left to the discretion of the urologist.

Once the patient is discharged, he/she should be encouraged to drink as much fluids as possible and strain the urine for the stone. If the stone is visible on plain film, the patient should return to the office in 2 weeks for a renal ultrasound and abdominal plain film. If the stone is progressing and the patient is not experiencing significant pain, observation can continue. If the renal sonogram demonstrates increasing hydronephrosis, urologic consultation is indicated.

If the stone has not passed within 30 days, urologic consultation should be obtained. It is not uncommon for a patient to pass the stone and not see it in the urinary stream. Renal sonogram is very useful to identify resolution of the hydro nephrosis in these cases.

Once the patient collects the stone, it should be sent for analysis. A follow-up renal sonogram should be obtained 6 to 8 weeks after passage to identify any residual silent hydronephrosis. If hydronephrosis is present, urologic consultation should be obtained.

Complications

The most serious complication of nephrolithiasis is pyonephrosis, infected urine behind an obstructing stone. This is a urologic emergency requiring immediate drainage of the obstructed kidney. A percutaneous nephrostomy is the quickest way to achieve drainage.

Stones can become lodged in the ureter and remain asymptomatic. They eventually become impacted. The urothelium surrounds and covers the stone, trapping it in place over time. Silent hydronephrosis continues until the kidney eventually becomes atrophic and nonfunctioning. This is the reason why either a CT or renal sonogram must be obtained 6 to 8 weeks after patient passes a stone or is no longer symptomatic.

Failure to identify treatable conditions such as hyperparathyroidism, hyperuricemia, and cystinuria contribute to recurrent stone formation and morbidity associated with stone passage.

Surgical complications from ureteroscopy include pain, hemorrhage, infection, ureteral perforation, and ureteral avulsion. Ureteral avulsion should never occur and is the most feared complication by every urologist. Ureteral stents can usually manage any other ureteral complication.

Complications from ESWL include hemorrhage, perirenal hemorrhage, failure to disintegrate the stone, and retained stone fragments. Some studies have shown an association between uncomplicated ESWL and delayed onset of diabetes and hypertension.

Monitoring

Stone patients should have yearly radiologic studies for at least the first 5 years after they present with a stone. There is a 50% chance they will develop another stone during that time. CT is the most accurate but abdominal plain films are useful if the stone(s) are visible. There is no place for renal sonogram for monitoring patients. If the stone burden increases over time urologic consultation should be obtained.

If a 24-hour urine collection is obtained and dietary or medical treatment is recommended the metabolic evaluation should be repeated 6 months later to determine if the plan is effective. Not surprisingly, most patients will not comply with the recommendations. Periodic 24-hour metabolic evaluations every few years is a good way to remind patients to self-monitor their fluid intake and modify their diets if necessary. Symptomatic pregnant women should be managed conservatively unless they develop urinary tract infection or a nonprogressive stone.

References

Assimos D, et al: Surgical management of Stones. American Urological Association/Endourological Society Guideline, Part 1, *J Urol* 196:1153–1160, 2016.

Campschroer T, et al: Alpha-blockers as medical expulsive therapy for ureteric stones: a Cochrane systematic review, *BJU Int* 122(6):932–945, 2018.

Kidney Stones, American Urological Association July 2016.

Meltzer AC, Burrows PK, Wolfson AB, et al: Effect of tamsulosin on passage of symptomatic ureteral stones: a randomized clinical trial, *JAMA Intern Med* 178(8):1051–1057, 2018, https://doi.org/10.1001/jamainternmed.2018.2259.

Medical Management of Kidney Stones: AUA Guideline March 2014, Pearle, M et. al.

---

[1]Not FDA approved for this indication.

PRIMARY GLOMERULAR DISEASE

Method of
Saeed Kamran Shaffi, MD, MS

CURRENT DIAGNOSIS

- Hematuria, proteinuria, hypoalbuminemia, hyperlipidemia, and elevated blood urea nitrogen and creatinine levels are the main laboratory abnormalities seen in patients with primary glomerular diseases.
- Our ability to diagnose some of the glomerular diseases and to monitor their disease-activity has improved with the recent discovery of disease-specific serum and kidney biopsy markers.

CURRENT THERAPY

- The goals of management of a primary glomerular disease patient are:
  - To diagnose the glomerular abnormality
  - To slow the progression of chronic kidney disease and subsequent development of end-stage kidney disease
  - To manage and ameliorate the glomerular disease symptoms
  - To prevent complications of primary glomerular diseases and the therapies used for their management, such as infection, thrombosis, coronary vascular disease, osteoporosis, and trace metal deficiencies

Clinical Presentation

The clinical presentation of the primary glomerular diseases can be grouped into syndromes, which are listed in Box 1.

Nephrotic syndrome: The disease-defining symptoms of the nephrotic syndrome are >3.5 g/day of proteinuria in adults, serum albumin of <3 g/L, and edema. Hyperlipidemia and thrombophilia are often present.

Sub-nephrotic proteinuria: These patients have proteinuria of <3.5 g/day without hypoalbuminemia, edema, and hyperlipidemia.

Acute nephritic syndrome: Nephritic syndrome presents as microscopic hematuria, which is defined as >3 red blood cells (RBC) per high-power field (HPF). Patients with the nephritic syndrome also have a varying amount of proteinuria and may have an elevated creatinine level indicating a decline in the glomerular filtration rate (GFR).

Asymptomatic microhematuria: Hematuria is seen on urine analyses; however, these patients do not develop progressive kidney dysfunction.

Rapidly progressive glomerulonephritis (RPGN): Rapidly progressive glomerulonephritis is a syndrome associated with a rapid decline in renal function over the course of a few days, weeks, or months. On the kidney biopsy, RPGN presents as glomerular crescents which form due to the disruption of the glomerular basement membrane with fluid spillage in the Bowmans space resulting in extracapillary cellular proliferation and crescent formation.

Slowly progressive nephritic syndrome: Some of the glomerular diseases have a smoldering course with persistent hematuria and proteinuria that may eventually lead to CKD and end-stage kidney disease.

Causes of primary glomerular diseases: Table 1 lists the causes of primary glomerular diseases.

Diagnosis of the Primary Glomerular Diseases

Glomerular disease is suspected when a clinician notices hematuria, proteinuria, or an abnormal blood urea nitrogen or creatinine level. It is paramount to rule out other conditions which can present with similar abnormalities.

Hematuria: It is imperative to differentiate between the glomerular and nonglomerular hematuria (Box 2 and Figure 1).

Proteinuria: Proteinuria is often seen in primary glomerular diseases. Urinary protein and albumin excretion in an adult should not exceed 150 mg/day, and 30 mg/g, respectively. Reduction in proteinuria—especially when sustained longitudinally—is associated with better clinical outcomes. In clinical practice, a spot urine protein to creatinine (P/C) ratio or albumin to creatinine ratio is often used for the assessment of the proteinuria; however, the concordance between the spot and the 24-hour urine collection is poor. On the other hand, 24-hour urine collection is cumbersome, is not feasible in children, and is associated with significant under- and overcollection even in highly motivated patients. Therefore, a morning first void spot urine (P/C) ratio is adequate for proteinuria surveillance; however, a 24-hour urine collection for proteinuria assessment should be considered when the use of therapeutic agents that can cause significant morbidity is being contemplated for proteinuria reduction.

GFR assessment: The best method to estimate GFR in patients with glomerular diseases is not known. Assessment of the longitudinal trends in the estimated GFR (eGFR) in this population may provide the clinicians with a better guide of renal status than a single value in isolation.

Kidney biopsy: Apart from a few situations such as serum anti-phospholipase A 2 receptor positivity in a high biopsy risk patient and steroid responsive nephrotic syndrome in children, which is almost always due to minimal change nephropathy, a kidney biopsy is essential for the diagnosis of primary glomerular diseases. Kidney biopsy not only provides a definitive diagnosis of the primary glomerular abnormality in most of the patients but also informs the clinician of the prognosis by quantifying the degree of the irreversible changes such as glomerulosclerosis, interstitial fibrosis, and tubular atrophy.

General Management of Primary Glomerular Diseases

Primary glomerular diseases may manifest as signs and symptoms (Box 3) which can be debilitating.

Treatment of Primary Glomerulonephritis

Edema: Dietary sodium restriction (1.5 to 2 g or 60 to 80 mmol/day) is the first step for edema management due to nephrotic syndromes. Oral loop diuretics (Table 2) should be used if the sodium restriction does not ameliorate the symptoms. Use of diuretics with better oral bioavailability and longer half-life may be more effective in edema management (see Table 2). Gut wall edema in patients with severe nephrotic syndrome may preclude effective diuresis with orally administered diuretics in which case intravenous loop diuretics alone or combined with a thiazide diuretic (e.g., metolazone [Zaroxolyn]) may be tried. Use of loop diuretics with intravenous albumin (Albuminar)[1] to maximize diuresis is controversial with some reports showing beneficial while others showing equivocal results; this strategy can be considered in patients with severe diuretic resistance.

Hypertension: Optimal control of hypertension in patients with a glomerular disease may decrease cardiovascular morbidity and mortality, and slow CKD progression. There is limited evidence for sodium restriction and angiotensin-converting enzyme inhibitors (ACEi) or angiotensin receptor blockers (ARBs) use to achieve a goal BP target of <125/75 mm Hg in patients with >1g/day of proteinuria.

Hyperlipidemia: Patients with primary glomerular diseases are at a higher risk of developing hyperlipidemia and cardiovascular

---

[1] Not FDA approved for this indication.

| BOX 2 | Signs of Glomerular Hematuria. |

>22% dysmorphic* RBCs on optical and >40% on phase contrast microscopy

In the setting of hematuria and dysmorphic RBCs, an immunoreactive albumin excretion of >0.59 mg/mg total protein excretion is strongly suggestive of glomerular hematuria

The newer generation of the urine analysis machines (sediMAX) automate the phase-contrast microscopy detection of dysmorphic RBCs without loss of precision

*Red blood cells in the glomerular hematuria develop membrane abnormalities when they pass through the inflamed glomerular membranes and are called dysmorphic. A certain type of dysmorphic RBC, with characteristic membrane blebs called acanthocytes, are strongly correlated with glomerular hematuria.

| TABLE 1 | Causes and Clinical Presentation of the Primary Glomerular Diseases |

CAUSES OF PRIMARY GLOMERULAR DISEASE	PRESENTATION
Minimal change disease	Nephrotic syndrome
Primary focal segmental glomerulosclerosis	Usually nephrotic syndrome, rarely nephritic syndrome
Primary membranous glomerulonephritis	Nephrotic syndrome
IgA nephropathy	Usually nephritic syndrome, sometimes microscopic hematuria or gross hematuria
Postinfectious glomerulonephritis	Nephritic syndrome
Membranoproliferative glomerulonephritis due to alternate complement pathway abnormalities (dense deposit disease and C3 glomerulonephritis)	Nephritic syndrome
Fibrillary glomerulonephritis	Nephritic or nephrotic syndrome
Thin basement membrane disease	Asymptomatic microscopic hematuria

events. Hyperlipidemia should be treated aggressively to the same targets as the general population.

Hypercoagulable states: Patients with glomerular diseases are at significant risk of thromboembolism due to the alterations in the pro-coagulant and anticoagulant factors. The incidence of thromboembolism has been reported as high as 8% to 44%, and 5% to 62% in nephrotic syndrome and membranous glomerulonephritis, respectively. Anticoagulation should be considered in patients with a low serum albumin (below 2 to 2.5 g/dL) along with one of the following: >10 g/d of proteinuria; BMI of >35 kg/m^2; family history and genetic disposition of thromboembolism; New York Heart Association Class III or IV congestive heart failure; recent abdominal or orthopedic surgery; prolonged immobilization. The Chapel Hill group has devised an online calculator (https://www.med.unc.edu/gntools/) to aid the clinicians in deciding about the use of anticoagulation in patients with membranous glomerulonephritis.

Case-reports have described aspirin[1], warfarin (Coumadin)[1], low-molecular–weight heparin,[1] or direct-acting oral anticoagulant (DOAC) use for thromboembolism prevention in patients with nephrotic syndrome. Expert opinion suggests starting anticoagulation with low-dose, low-molecular–weight heparin, followed by introduction of warfarin. When therapeutic INR is achieved, stop heparin. Alternatively, low-molecular–weight heparin with aspirin has been suggested for a period of 3 months before introducing warfarin if proteinuria does not resolve.

Chronic kidney disease: Studies have shown that complete remission of proteinuria is associated with preservation of renal function and end-stage kidney disease. Disease-modifying therapies, which will be described later, should be used to prevent the development of renal fibrosis which is irreversible.

Trace metal deficiency: Patients with primary glomerular diseases who have nephrotic syndrome may have deficiencies of iron, copper, zinc, and selenium. Twenty-five hydroxyvitamin D [25-(OH)D] deficiency, which is extremely common in patients with nephrotic syndrome, is due to urinary loss of 25(OH)D, and is often difficult to treat unless the patient achieves complete remission. Treatment of 25(OH)D deficiency is outlined in Box 4 and is similar to that in the general population.

Endocrine abnormalities: Loss of hormone-binding proteins and albumin in patients with proteinuric glomerular diseases leads to various endocrine abnormalities. Low T4 levels are seen in approximately 50% of nephrotic syndrome patients with preserved renal function due to urinary loss of thyroid-binding globulin; however, these patients are usually euthyroid due to their preserved ability to convert T4 to T3. On the other hand, glomerular disease patients with low GFRs have a diminished T3 level due to diminished conversion of T4 to T3; however, unlike other chronic illnesses, the conversion of T4 to metabolically inactive reverse T3 (rT3) is not enhanced.

Risk of infections: Chronic kidney disease, nephrotic syndrome, and use of the immunosuppressive medications are some of the risk factors that increase the propensity to develop infections in patients with primary glomerular diseases. Patients should be up to date on their vaccinations to mitigate infection risk (Box 5).

Pneumocystis jirovecii prophylaxis should be administered to patients who are on >20 mg of prednisone and/or on immunosuppressive medications that affect the T cells such as corticosteroids and cyclophosphamide (Cytoxan).

Therapy of Specific Glomerular Diseases
Minimal-Change Disease

Minimal-change disease is the most common cause of nephrotic syndrome in children (90%) and is rare adults (10%). No abnormality is detected on light microscopic evaluation of the kidney; however, the electron microscopy shows diffuse foot process effacement. A child presenting with nephrotic syndrome is assumed to have a minimal-change disease and does not require a kidney biopsy. In adults, minimal-change disease is a rare occurrence and is usually diagnosed with a kidney biopsy. Most cases of minimal-change disease are idiopathic, although secondary causes such as drugs (nonsteroidal antiinflammatory drugs [NSAIDs]), hematological malignancies, and thymoma are associated with this condition. Therapy of minimal-change disease is shown in Box 6.

Primary Focal Segmental Glomerulosclerosis

Primary focal segmental glomerulosclerosis is a pathological term denoting patchy glomerulosclerosis and is thought to be due to an unknown permeability factor which causes proteinuria, hypertension, and kidney dysfunction. This condition should be

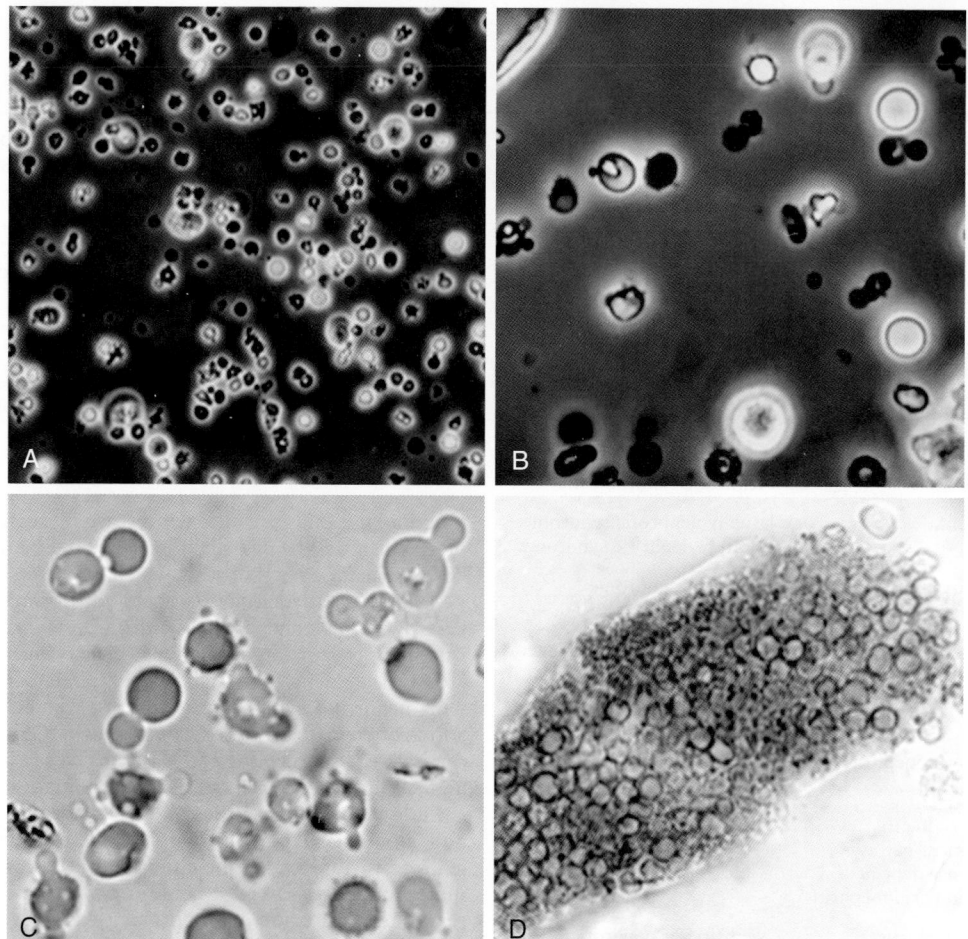

Figure 1 A and B. Acanthocytes: phase contrast microscopy, unstained; C. Acanthocytes: brightfield microscopy, unstained; D. RBC cast: brightfield microscopy, unstained. (Courtesy of Jay R. Seltzer, M.D. Chief of Nephrology - Missouri Baptist Medical Center - St. Louis Missouri.)

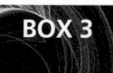

BOX 3	Abnormalities Seen in the Primary Glomerular Diseases

Edema
Hypertension
Hyperlipidemia
Hypercoagulable state
Chronic kidney disease
Trace metal and vitamin deficiencies
Endocrine hormonal abnormalities
Infection risk

differentiated from the secondary glomerulosclerosis (focal or global) which is a sequela of kidney injury. Reduction in proteinuria is associated with better renal survival and is the goal of therapy. Box 7 shows the therapies used for the management of primary focal segmental glomerulosclerosis.

Primary Membranous Glomerulonephritis

Idiopathic membranous glomerulonephritis is the second most common cause of nephrotic syndrome in the US adults. This condition is characterized by diffuse subepithelial deposits seen on kidney biopsy. Our understanding of the pathophysiology of the idiopathic membranous glomerulonephritis was revolutionized in 2009 with the discovery of elevated M-type phospholipase-A(2) receptor [PLA2R], an antigen expressed in the human podocytes, antibody in the serum and the immune deposits in the glomeruli of the vast majority of patients. Antibodies against thrombospondin type 1 domain-containing 7A (THSD7A) have been found in PLA2R negative idiopathic membranous patients (2% to 4%).

Serum anti-PLA2R and THSD7A antibody levels are measured by commercial laboratories and are used to monitor idiopathic membranous glomerulonephritis disease activity—a rise in titer is associated with relapse while a fall is associated with remission. Box 8 details the treatment strategies used for the management of primary membranous glomerulonephritis.

IgA Nephropathy

IgA nephropathy is the leading cause of glomerulonephritis worldwide. A multi-hit hypothesis has been proposed in the pathogenesis of IgA nephropathy, with mistracking of the poorly O-glycosylated galactose deficient IgA1 (Gd-IgA1) into the circulation, thought to be derived from the mucosal B-cells, production of IgG and IgA antibodies against Gd-IgA1, formation and deposition of mesangial immune complexes, and activation of the complement system resulting in immune-mediated injury leads to kidney damage. The antigen-antibody complexes deposit in the kidneys and cause a mesangial (M) and endocapillary (E) proliferative glomerulonephritis which can lead to glomerulosclerosis (S) and tubular atrophy (T). At times, IgA nephropathy can also present as crescentic glomerulonephritis (C). The MEST-C classification of the kidney biopsy provides useful information regarding disease prognostication. The secondary cause of IgA nephropathy such as HIV and cirrhosis should be ruled out. IgA nephropathy often has a smoldering course presenting as a nephritic syndrome with progressive loss of kidney function that may lead to end-stage kidney disease. Recently, it has been shown that decreasing proteinuria to <1 g/day results in better renal survival and has become one of the goals of therapy. Box 9 shows the therapeutic options for IgA nephropathy.

Many new therapeutic options are being developed for the management of IgA nephropathy. A phase 3 clinical trial to

NAME	RELATIVE POTENCY	ORAL BIOAVAILABILITY	HALF-LIFE (HOURS)	ELIMINATION ROUTE	COMMENTS
Furosemide (Lasix)	1	~60%	~1.5	~65% renal, 25% metabolism	Renal disease prolongs half-life
Bumetanide (Bumex)	40	~80	~0.8	~62% renal, 38% metabolism	Liver disease prolongs half-life
Torsemide (Demadex)	20	~80%	~3.5	~20% renal, 80% metabolism	Liver disease prolongs half-life

TABLE 2 Pharmacokinetics of Loop Diuretics

BOX 4 Treatment of Vitamin D Deficiency in Primary Glomerular Diseases

25(OH)D level less than 12 ng/mL: treat with 50,000 international units (IU) of vitamin D2 (ergocalciferol)[1] or vitamin D3 (cholecalciferol)[1] orally once a week for 6 to 8 weeks followed by 800–1000 IU/day of vitamin D3 for maintenance therapy. Higher doses of daily vitamin D3 may be necessary if the levels remain low (<30 ng/mL) 3 months after therapy initiation.

25(OH)D levels between 12 and 20 ng/mL: treat with 800–1000 IU/day of vitamin D3. Repeat levels in 3 months. Higher vitamin D3 doses may be necessary if the levels are below the normal range (30–50 ng/mL).

25(OH)D level between 20 and 30 ng/mL: treat with 600–800 IU of vitamin D3 daily.

[1]Not FDA approved for this indication.

BOX 5 Recommended Immunization in Patients With Glomerular Diseases

Hepatitis A vaccine (Havrix, VAQTA)
Hepatitis B vaccine (Engerix-B, Recombivax HB)
Haemophilus influenzae type B conjugate vaccine (Hib [ActHIB, Hiberix])
Annual trivalent inactivated influenza vaccine
1 dose thirteen-valent pneumococcal conjugate vaccine (PCV13 [Prevnar 13]) followed in 8 weeks by a 23-valent pneumococcal polysaccharide vaccine (PPSV23 [Pneumovax 23]), then repeat PPSV23 in 5 years since the last dose; at age 65 years or older, administer 1 dose PPSV23 at least 5 years after the most recent PPSV23
Meningococcal Vaccine against sero-group (A, C, W and Y; Menactra, Menveo)[1]

[1]Not FDA approved for this indication.

BOX 6 Minimal-Change Disease Therapy

Prednisone 1 mg/kg (maximum 80 mg) or alternate-day single dose of 2 mg/kg (maximum 120 mg) for 4–16 weeks. Taper slowly in 6 months if complete remission (proteinuria <300 mg/g) is achieved in 4 weeks.

Most patients respond to corticosteroids but 25% of treated patients have frequent relapses and 30% become steroid dependent (two relapses during or within 2 weeks of completing steroid therapy). No response to steroids in 8–16 weeks should be considered steroid resistance.

Second-line agents are calcineurin inhibitors, oral cyclophosphamide (Cytoxan), or rituximab (Rituxan)[1]

[1]Not FDA approved for this indication.

BOX 7 Primary Focal Segmental Glomerulosclerosis Therapy

First line: Prednisone 1 mg/kg q day or 2 mg/kg every alternate day. Continue high-dose steroids for 4–16 weeks until complete remission is achieved, followed by a taper in 6 months.

Second line: Calcineurin inhibitors for patients who cannot tolerate prednisone.

Third line: Patients with frequently relapsing primary FSGS may respond to rituximab (Rituxan)[1]

Fourth line: Mycophenolate mofetil (MMF [CellCept]).[1]

Adrenocorticotropic hormone (ACTH) gel (Corticotropin [HP Acthar]).[1]

[1]Not FDA approved for this indication.

BOX 8 Primary Membranous Glomerulonephritis Therapy

Watchful waiting for 6 months with maximization of ACEi or ARB. Factors associated with low likelihood of achieving spontaneous remission are persistence of >4 g/day of proteinuria with no response to antihypertensive/antiproteinuric therapy in 6 month; presence of life threatening nephrotic syndrome; greater than 30% increase in serum creatinine; and a high anti-PLA2R antibody titer.

Oral cyclophosphamide[1] and prednisone with or without intravenous methylprednisolone (Solumedrol) pulses in alternate months for 6 months. Some centers use cyclophosphamide and prednisone together for 3 months, while others eliminate prednisone altogether.

Calcineurin inhibitors are as effective as cyclophosphamide in inducing remission; however, the risk of relapse after medication discontinuation is high.

Rituximab[1] has similar rates of complete remission as cyclophosphamide, however, the complete remission rate is lower. Furthermore, rituximab-treated patients are less likely to develop adverse events than cyclophosphamide-treated groups.

[1]Not FDA approved for this indication.
ACEi, Angiotensin-converting enzyme inhibitors; *ARB,* angiotensin receptor blockers.

---

study the effects of a molecule that inhibits the lectin-binding pathway of the complement system is currently being conducted. Another trial studied the effects of oral budesonide (Entocort EC)[1] in patients with IgA nephropathy and showed that this agent reduced proteinuria significantly compared to placebo and a phase 3 study is currently being planned.

Postinfectious Glomerulonephritis

Acute postinfectious glomerulonephritis presents as nephritic syndrome, acute kidney injury, and low serum complement levels

[1]Not FDA approved for this indication.

BOX 9 — IgA Nephropathy Therapy

Maximum ACEi/ARB therapy to bring the proteinuria to <1 g/day. If eligible, patients should be provided information about the currently ongoing clinical trials for IgA nephropathy.

Patients who continue to have >1 g/day of proteinuria, despite maximum ACEi/ARB inhibition for >6 months with a BP of <125/75 mm Hg, should receive a 6-month course of corticosteroids if their eGFR is >50 mL/min/1.73 m². Recent data show that patients with eGFR <50 mL/min/1.73 m² may benefit from corticosteroid therapy; however, they may experience higher serious adverse events.

Patients with IgA nephropathy in whom >50% glomeruli show crescents should be treated with corticosteroids and cyclophosphamide.[1]

[1]Not FDA approved for this indication.
ACEi, Angiotensin-converting enzyme inhibitors; *ARB*, angiotensin receptor blockers; *eGFR*, estimated GFR.

BOX 10 — Dense Deposit Disease (DDD) and C3 Glomerulonephritis (C3GN) Therapy

Patients with >500–1000 mg/g of proteinuria should receive ACEi/ARB therapy.

Patients with severe disease and a known autoantibody have been treated with plasma exchange, rituximab[1], and eculizumab (Soliris)[1].

Patients with a genetic defect have been treated with plasma exchange with fresh frozen plasma.

Patients with rapidly progressive glomerulonephritis should be treated with plasma exchange, corticosteroids, and cyclophosphamide[1] or mycophenolate mofetil[1].

[1]Not FDA approved for this indication.
ACEi, Angiotensin-converting enzyme inhibitors; *ARB*, angiotensin receptor blockers.

and is more common in children and young adults. This condition was classically described in the convalescence of scarlet fever, but other bacteria, viruses, and protozoa can also cause this condition. Kidney biopsy shows diffuse proliferative glomerulonephritis with prominent mesangial and subepithelial deposits that on immunofluorescence microscopy show positivity for C3 and IgG. It can also present as crescentic glomerulonephritis which portends a poor prognosis. The treatment of renal failure due to postinfectious glomerulonephritis is symptomatic. The primary infection that caused postinfectious glomerulonephritis should be treated appropriately if present at the time of diagnosis. Children have an excellent prognosis with the recovery of kidney function in the vast majority of the patients. However, adults with this condition have a poor renal prognosis with 30% of the patients developing CKD. The outcomes are particularly worse for patients with severe proteinuria with two out of three patients developing progressive kidney dysfunction.

Membranoproliferative Glomerulonephritis due to Alternate Complement Pathway Abnormalities

Membranoproliferative glomerulonephritis (MPGN) is a pathological phenotype seen on kidney biopsy characterized by endocapillary proliferative glomerulonephritis, increased mesangial matrix, and thickening of the glomerular basement membranes. Various infectious, autoimmune, vascular, and neoplastic processes can lead to this type of glomerular injury. MPGN is now classified on the basis of disease mechanism rather than the histological findings with an emphasis of staining intensity of C3 and IgG on immunofluorescence microscopy. Presence of both C3 and IgG point toward an immune-complex-mediated process. Predominant C3 staining on immunofluorescence with minimal IgG staining indicates abnormalities in the alternate complement pathway that cause dense deposit disease (DDD) and C3 glomerulonephritis (C3GN). These are rare conditions affecting children and young adults and present as nephritic syndrome, renal function abnormalities, and hypertension. Laboratory data abnormalities include low C3 levels with normal C4 levels (alternate complement pathway abnormality), presence of antibodies (C3 nephritic factor, anti-factors H, B, or I), gene mutations of the alternate complement pathway proteins (complement factor H and I-related protein gene mutations), diminished serum factors that regulate the alternate complement pathway (serum factor H, B, I, and serum membrane cofactor protein [MCP]), and elevated terminal complement pathway constituents (C5b-9). Treatment options for DDD and C3GN are listed in Box 10.

Fibrillary Glomerulonephritis

Fibrillary glomerulonephritis is an uncommon condition primarily affecting adults. Kidney biopsy shows amyloid-like deposits; however, they are Congo-Red negative and thus are not truly amyloid. Electron-microscopy shows characteristic findings of randomly organized fibrils sized 10 to 30 nm. One-third of the patients with fibrillary glomerulonephritis have another disorder such as autoimmune disease, malignancy, and monoclonal gammopathy. Recently, our understanding of the pathophysiology of idiopathic fibrillary glomerulonephritis improved significantly with the identification of DnaJ homolog subfamily B member 9 (DNAJB9)—a member of the molecular chaperone gene family—in fibrillary deposits. Almost all the patients with fibrillary glomerulonephritis showed positive immunohistochemistry to DNAJB9 while all the patients with amyloidosis were negative. The disease usually presents as nephritic syndrome. The prognosis is generally poor with most of the patients developing end-stage kidney disease. Antiproteinuric therapy with ACEi/ARB and immunosuppression have been tried with variable results with the patients with milder disease (non-nephrotic range proteinuria and preserved eGFR) more likely to achieve complete remission.

References

Agrawal S, Zaritsky JJ, Fornoni A, Smoyer WE: Dyslipidaemia in nephrotic syndrome: mechanisms and treatment, *Nat Rev Nephrol* 14(1):57–70, 2018 Jan.

Cattran DC, Kim ED, Reich H, et al: Membranous nephropathy: quantifying remission duration on outcome, *J Am Soc Nephrol JASN* 28(3):995–1003, 2017 Mar.

Floege J, Barbour SJ, Cattran DC, et al: Management and treatment of glomerular diseases (part 1): conclusions from a Kidney Disease: Improving Global Outcomes (KDIGO) Controversies Conference, *Kidney Int* 95(2):268–280, 2019 Feb.

Harris RC, Ismail N: Extrarenal complications of the nephrotic syndrome, *Am J Kidney Dis Off J Natl Kidney Found* 23(4):477–497, 1994 Apr.

Improving Global Outcomes (KDIGO) Glomerulonephritis Work Group: Kidney Disease: KDIGO Clinical Practice Guideline for Glomerulonephritis, *Kidney Inter Suppl* 2:139–274, 2012.

Lee T, Biddle AK, Lionaki S, et al: Personalized prophylactic anticoagulation decision analysis in patients with membranous nephropathy, *Kidney Int* 85(6):1412–1420, 2014 Jun.

Nasr SH, Vrana JA, Dasari S, et al: DNAJB9 is a specific immunohistochemical marker for fibrillary glomerulonephritis, *Kidney Int Rep* 3(1):56–64, 2017 Aug 8.

Ponticelli C, Glassock R: *Treatment of primary glomerulonephritis*, North America, 2009, ESCCO eBook Subscription Academic Collection.

Radice A, Trezzi B, Maggiore U, et al: Clinical usefulness of autoantibodies to M-type phospholipase A2 receptor (PLA2R) for monitoring disease activity in idiopathic membranous nephropathy (IMN), *Autoimmun Rev* 15(2):146–154, 2016 Feb.

Reich HN, Troyanov S, Scholey JW, Cattran DC: Remission of proteinuria improves prognosis in IgA nephropathy, *J Am Soc Nephrol* 18(12):3177–3183, 2007 Dec 1.

Rovin BH, Caster DJ, Cattran DC, et al: Management and treatment of glomerular diseases (part 2): conclusions from a Kidney Disease: Improving Global Outcomes (KDIGO) Controversies Conference, *Kidney Int* 95(2):281–295, 2019 Feb.

PYELONEPHRITIS

Method of
Patricia D. Brown, MD

CURRENT DIAGNOSIS

- Abrupt onset of fever, flank pain, and costovertebral angle tenderness with or without symptoms of cystitis are classic presenting features.
- Patients with lower UTI symptoms or laboratory evidence of UTI accompanied by flank pain, fever, or signs of systemic toxicity such as GI complaints should be managed as having APN.
- Urinalysis with microscopic examination should be performed in all patients with suspected APN. Absence of pyuria is strong evidence against the diagnosis.
- A urine culture should be obtained in all patients with APN. Blood cultures should be obtained in those who are hospitalized.
- Patients should be categorized into those with uncomplicated and those with complicated infections.

Abbreviation: APN = acute pyelonephritis; GI = gastrointestinal; UTI = urinary tract infection.

CURRENT THERAPY

- Hospitalization is recommended for patients unable to tolerate oral intake, those with severe pain, and those with signs of severe sepsis. Hospitalization is generally recommended for patients with complicated infections and for all pregnant women.
- Parenteral regimens for hospitalized patients include an aminoglycoside, third-generation cephalosporin, or fluoroquinolone, with oral switch therapy selected on the basis of culture and susceptibility data.
- Initial empiric therapy for outpatients is a fluoroquinolone.
- Imaging is not recommended for patients with uncomplicated infections. Pre- and postcontrast computed tomographic scans should be obtained in those who fail to respond within 72 hours to appropriate antibiotic therapy.

Acute pyelonephritis (APN) is a urinary tract infection (UTI) that involves the renal parenchyma, also referred to as *upper tract UTI*. Most episodes of APN occur as a result of ascending infection from the bladder; patients with APN might or might not have symptoms of concomitant cystitis. Rarely, pyelonephritis occurs secondary to hematogenous seeding of the kidney as a result of infection elsewhere, most commonly endocarditis due to *Staphylococcus aureus* or disseminated fungal infection.

Epidemiology
Surprisingly little is known about the epidemiology of APN. Similar to cystitis, APN (and hospitalization for APN) is more common in women than men; men have been reported to have higher in-hospital mortality. In contrast to cystitis, risk factors for pyelonephritis are not well defined. A study of nonpregnant women 18 to 49 years of age found risk factors for APN included factors known to be risk factors for acute cystitis, including frequency of sexual intercourse, recent UTI, diabetes, and maternal UTI history. The incidence of bacteremia in patients with APN is reported to be 11% to 53% in various studies; risk factors for bacteremia are not well established. In one study, age greater than 65 years, vomiting, pulse greater than 110 beats per minute, segmented neutrophils greater than 90%, and pyuria with greater than 50 leukocytes per high-powered field were independent risk factors for bacteremia in women with uncomplicated APN.

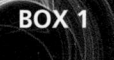

Similar to lower UTI, APN can be further classified into complicated or uncomplicated infection. The factors that make an episode of APN a complicated UTI are outlined in Box 1.

Clinical Presentation
The classic presenting features of APN include abrupt onset of fever, flank pain, and costovertebral angle tenderness with or without symptoms of lower UTI including dysuria, urgency, and frequency. Unfortunately, there is no single constellation of signs or symptoms that is pathognomonic for APN. When localization studies have been performed on patients with symptoms of acute cystitis, 30% to 50% have been shown to have APN. Women who present with symptoms that have been present more than 7 days and those with a recent history of UTI are more likely to have APN. Flank pain is reported in approximately one-half of patients with APN but also occurs in almost 20% of patients with cystitis. Fever is present in one half of patients with APN, but less than 5% of patients with cystitis. Nausea, vomiting, and diarrhea occur commonly in patients with APN, and gastrointestinal (GI) symptoms can dominate the presenting complaints.

In general, patients who present with lower urinary tract symptoms or laboratory evidence of urinary tract infection accompanied by fever, flank pain or tenderness, or signs of systemic toxicity, such as GI symptoms, should be treated for APN.

The diagnosis can be particularly challenging in the frail elderly patient, because symptoms such as frequency, urgency, and incontinence are often chronic in this patient population and unrelated to active UTI. Change in mental status may be the only presenting complaint. Because the prevalence of bacteriuria in this patient population is high, particularly among those with chronic indwelling catheters, UTI must be a diagnosis of exclusion.

Acute pelvic inflammatory disease can have a presentation similar to APN. Pelvic examination should be performed on all sexually active women to exclude this diagnosis.

The differential diagnosis of APN is outlined in Box 2.

Diagnosis
Urinalysis, ideally with microscopic examination, using a clean-catch, midstream specimen, should be performed in all patients with suspected APN. Pyuria is a key finding in the diagnosis of UTI, and the absence of pyuria is strong evidence against a diagnosis of APN. Direct microscopic examination under high power of the urinary sediment from a centrifuged specimen should reveal more than 10 leukocytes per high-powered field. The presence of white blood cell (WBC) casts is highly specific for localization of the infection to the kidney, but it is inadequately sensitive to exclude the diagnosis of APN. The dipstick test for leukocyte esterase is used as a rapid screening test to detect significant pyuria; the sensitivity is reported to be 75% to 96%, with

BOX 2 Differential Diagnosis of Acute Pyelonephritis

- Appendicitis
- Cholecystitis
- Diverticulitis
- Gastroenteritis
- Herpes zoster
- Musculoskeletal pain, including vertebral disorders
- Ovarian cysts, tumors
- Pancreatitis
- Perforated viscus
- Pelvic inflammatory disease
- Pneumonia
- Renal stones, renal vein thrombosis, renal infarction

a specificity of 94% to 98%. Because of the lower range of the reported sensitivity of the dipstick test, microscopic examination to exclude significant pyuria should be obtained in patients with suspected APN.

The presence of nitrite in the urine, detected by a dipstick test, has a reported sensitivity of 35% to 85% and a specificity of 92% to 100% for UTI. Microscopic examination of a gram-stained, centrifuged urine specimen revealing at least one bacterium per oil-immersion field correlates with more than 10^5 colony-forming units (cfu)/mL of bacteria, with a sensitivity of 95%. Although this is the standard definition of significant bacteriuria, it has been shown that women with UTI can have levels of bacteriuria as low as 10^2 cfu/mL.

Although the microbiology of APN has remained predictable, significant changes in antimicrobial susceptibility patterns have occurred. Therefore, in contrast to recommendations for acute uncomplicated cystitis, a urine culture should be obtained in all patients with suspected APN. The need to obtain blood cultures has been debated, because blood cultures rarely yield a pathogen different from what was isolated from the urine. Bacteremia has been reported in 11% to 53% of patients hospitalized with APN. Bacteremic patients have a longer length of stay, and one report suggests that this is due to a longer time to resolution of fever. Many experts continue to recommend that blood cultures be obtained as part of the diagnostic evaluation of patients who are ill enough to require hospitalization; blood cultures are not necessary for those who will be managed as outpatients.

The role of diagnostic imaging in the management of APN is discussed later. In some cases with an atypical presentation, imaging may be helpful to confirm the diagnosis of APN. In this setting, pre- and postcontrast computed tomography (CT) is the imaging procedure of choice in adults.

Microbial Etiology

Most cases of APN are caused by *Escherichia coli*. Other enterobacteriaceae, including *Klebsiella* species and *Proteus* species, are also occasionally implicated. Other gram-negative pathogens such as *Pseudomonas*, *Serratia*, *Enterobacter*, and *Acinetobacter* should be considered in health care–associated infections. *Enterococcus* is an uncommon pathogen in community-acquired infections, but it must be considered in health care–associated infections, including vancomycin-resistant enterococci. Other gram-positive pathogens include *Streptoccocus agalactiae* and *Staphylococcus* species. Although a common cause of acute cystitis in young women, *Staphylococcus saprophyticus* is a rare cause of pyelonephritis; the finding of *Staphylococcus aureus* in a urine culture should always prompt a search for an extrarenal source of infection that might have served as a source of hematogenous seeding. A Gram stain of the urine is a simple and rapid test to exclude a gram-positive pathogen as the etiology of APN and guide the initial selection of empiric therapy.

The emergence of resistance to trimethoprim-sulfamethoxazole (TMP-SMX [Bactrim]) among *E. coli* has had a major impact on the approach to initial empiric antimicrobial therapy for APN.

It is clear that the prevalence of resistance varies depending on geographic region, and clinicians often do not have access to meaningful local resistance data. Recent reports of increasing fluoroquinolone resistance among uropathogens are of great concern, although overall resistance rates in North America remain low. Also concerning is the increasing prevalence of extended-spectrum β-lactamase (ESBL) *E.coli* and *Klebsiella* species, although these are mainly a concern in health care-associated infections in the U.S. Risk factors for infection with ESBL producing organisms are poorly defined however recent infection or colonization with an ESBL producing organism should be considered a risk factor for this pathogen. Other potential risk factors include older age, frequent antibiotic use in the preceding year and recent APN in patients with underlying diabetes. Carbapenemase-producing Enterbacteriaceae are also now reported in health care-associated complicated infections.

Treatment

The first decision in the management of patients with APN is whether or not the patient requires hospitalization. Although prospective randomized trials are lacking, several retrospective studies as well as several prospective nonrandomized trials suggest that outpatient management is safe for many patients. Hospitalization should be considered for patients who cannot tolerate oral intake or who have severe pain or signs of severe sepsis. A strategy of initial management in the emergency department or an observation unit with an initial dose of parenteral antibiotic therapy, intravenous fluids, and symptomatic treatment of nausea and pain may be used in select patients to avoid hospital admission. Patients who will be treated as outpatients should have a stable social situation and the ability to contact the physician and return promptly if their symptoms worsen. Hospitalization is generally recommended for patients with complicated infections. Most experts believe that pregnant women with APN should always be hospitalized.

There are surprisingly few prospective randomized trials of the treatment of pyelonephritis. For patients who require hospitalization, parenteral therapy with an aminoglycoside, a third-generation cephalosporin, or a fluoroquinolone is recommended. At my institution we discourage fluoroquinolones for this indication because there are other effective alternatives and we wish to minimize the use of these very broad-spectrum agents in the hospital setting. Although resistance to TMP-SMX among uropathogenic *E. coli* appears to have leveled off and might actually be decreasing, this agent should not be used for empiric therapy of APN. If a ESBL-producing organism is suspected, empiric therapy should include a carbapenem. Because risk factors for ESBL-producing organisms are not well defined, consideration for coverage of these pathogens should be given in all patients with APN who have severe sepsis or septic shock. Multi-drug resistant pathogens may require treatment with newer B-lactam/B-lactamase inhibitor drugs such as ceftazidime-avibactam (Avycaz), ceftolozane-tazobactam (Zerbaxa), or meropenem-vaborbactam (Vabomere).

If a gram-positive pathogen is suspected or suggested by the results of urine Gram stain, ampicillin or ampicillin-sulbactam (Unasyn) with or without an aminoglycoside can be used. Patients should receive intravenous therapy until they are clinically improving and able to reliably tolerate oral intake; oral therapy can be chosen based on the results of urine culture and susceptibility data. TMP-SMX, a fluoroquinolone, and ampicillin are all potential candidates for oral switch therapy. The narrowest spectrum, least expensive agent to which the isolated pathogen is susceptible should be chosen. Despite in vitro susceptibility data, first- and second-generation cephalosporins have a poor track record in the treatment of APN and are generally not recommended, with the exception of pyelonephritis in pregnancy.

Bacteremic patients might take longer to respond but do not require more prolonged parenteral therapy. The total duration of therapy for pyelonephritis is generally 14 days. Seven days of therapy with ciprofloxacin for uncomplicated APN has been shown to be effective as has 5 days of therapy with high-dose (750 mg daily) levofloxacin, and these regimens are endorsed by the current guidelines. Longer courses of therapy may be required for select patients with complicated pyelonephritis. For outpatients, initial empiric therapy with a fluoroquinolone is recommended, with adjustment of therapy, if needed, based on the results of urine culture. All of the currently available fluoroquinolones can be used, with the exception of moxifloxacin (Avelox), which does not achieve adequate levels in the urine. Although it is useful in the treatment of cystitis, norfloxacin (Noroxin) is not recommended for the treatment of APN because it does not achieve sustained tissue or serum levels. Suggested antimicrobial dosing regimens for APN are outlined in Box 3.

Imaging

Imaging is generally not needed in patients with uncomplicated APN. For patients with complicated infections (e.g., history of stones, prior renal surgery), renal ultrasound with abdominal plain films is considered an acceptable alternative to excretory urography. For patients with diabetes or other immunocompromise and for patients who fail to respond after 72 hours of appropriate antibiotic therapy, pre- and postcontrast CT is the imaging procedure of choice.

Follow-up

Most patients will respond to appropriate antibiotic therapy. Follow-up urine cultures to document microbiological response are not recommended in patients who have responded clinically.

References

Foxman B, Klemstine KL, Brown PD: Acute pyelonephritis in US hospitals in 1997: hospitalization and in-hospital mortality, *Ann Epidemiol* 13:144–150, 2003.

Gupta K, Hooton TN, Naber K, et al: International clinical practice guidelines for the treatment of acute uncomplicated cystitis and pyelonephritis in women: a 2010 update by The Infectious Diseases Society of America and the European Society for Microbiology and Infectious Diseases, *Clin Infect Dis* 52:e103–e120, 2010.

Kim KS, Kim K, Jo YH, et al: A simple model to predict bacteremia in women with acute pyelonephritis, *J Infect* 63:124–130, 2011.

Nikolaidis P, Dogra VS, Goldfarb S, et al: ACR appropriateness criteria–acute pyelonephritis, *J Am Coll Radiol* 15(11S):S232–S239, 2018.

Pappas PG: Laboratory in the diagnosis and management of urinary tract infections, *Med Clin North Am* 75:313–325, 1991.

Sandberg T, Skoog G, Hermansson AB, et al: Ciprofloxacin for 7 days versus 14 days in women with acute pyelonephritis: a randomised, open-label and double-blind, placebo-controlled, non-inferiority trial, *Lancet* 380:484–490, 2012.

Scholes D, Hooton TM, Roberts PL, et al: Risk factors associated with acute pyelonephritis in healthy women, *Ann Intern Med* 142:20–27, 2005.

TRAUMA TO THE GENITOURINARY TRACT

Method of
Anna Faris, MD; and Yooni Yi, MD

The genitourinary tract is involved in about 10% of trauma cases. The kidney, followed by the bladder and urethra, are the most commonly involved genitourinary organs. In most cases, injury to the genitourinary tract is not isolated, and the initial evaluation of urologic injuries should consider the context of the patient's associated injuries and triage more pressing or life-threatening issues. Still, early involvement of the urologist is prudent to help plan further interventions. The spectrum of genitourinary injuries is widespread, and management can range from immediate repair to temporization with delayed reconstruction. The goal of a urologist in the trauma setting is to establish urinary drainage in order to optimize kidney function, minimize hemorrhage, and control urinary extravasation to reduce associated complications such as infection or ileus.

Renal Trauma

Renal injury occurs in 1% to 5% of all trauma cases. Blunt impact accounts for the majority of renal injuries (82% to 95%) and causes damage secondary to direct organ injury or disruption of the kidney from its attachments (e.g., renal hilum and ureteropelvic junction). Penetrating trauma most commonly is caused by stabbing or gunshot wounds. The damage from penetrating injury can be limited to the tract of the stab wound, or it can be more extensive secondary to necrosis from energy transfer and the blast effect of high-velocity bullets. The history is crucial in the diagnosis of renal injury and should include the mechanism of trauma as well as any preexisting kidney disease or condition that might contribute to worsening renal function. Hematuria has a very poor correlation with degree of injury because disruption of the ureteropelvic junction, arterial disruption or thrombosis, and other severe injuries can exist in a setting with no hematuria.

The American Association for the Surgery of Trauma (AAST) classifies renal injuries into five grades (Figs. 1 and 2):
- Grade 1: Nonexpanding subcapsular hematoma/contusion with absence of parenchymal injury
- Grade 2: Less than 1 cm laceration into the renal cortex, not extending into the collecting system, with a nonexpanding hematoma confined to the perirenal fascia
- Grade 3: Greater than 1 cm laceration, extending through the renal cortex and medulla but not the collecting system
- Grade 4: Laceration extending to the collecting system with urinary extravasation or a segmental vascular injury with contained hematoma; renal artery thrombosis
- Grade 5: Shattered kidney or renal pedicle avulsion

With evolving imaging technology and endovascular management techniques, one group attempted to simplify injury severity grades 4 and 5 as follows:
- Grade 4: Parenchymal laceration involving the collecting system, lacerations of the collecting system with urinary extravasation, renal pelvis laceration and/or complete ureteral pelvic disruption; vascular segmental injuries
- Grade 5: Vascular compromise of the main renal arteries or veins such as laceration, avulsion, or thrombosis

Renal injury should be suspected in any trauma patient who has a penetrating injury with flank ecchymosis, broken ribs, gross or microscopic hematuria (≥3 red blood cells per high-power field), a blunt injury with gross hematuria, or a blunt injury with microscopic hematuria and shock (systolic blood pressure <90 mm Hg). In addition, imaging of the urinary tract should be obtained in children who have more than 50 red blood cells per high-power field even in the absence of hypotension.

In a stable patient, radiographic evaluation should consist of computed tomographic (CT) scanning with intravenous contrast and delayed images showing opacification of the collecting

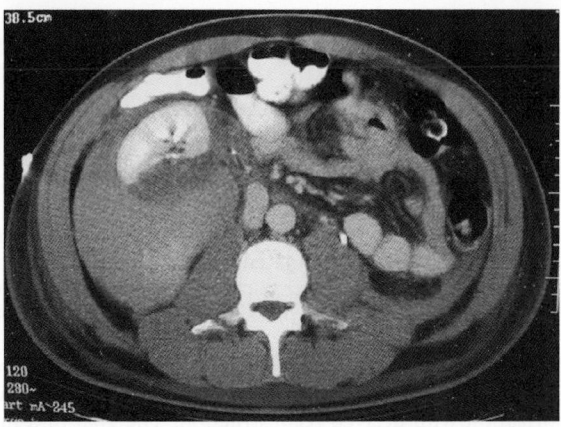

Figure 1 Computed tomography scan demonstrating large right perirenal hematoma and thrombosed posterior segmental artery. This was classified as a grade IV renal injury.

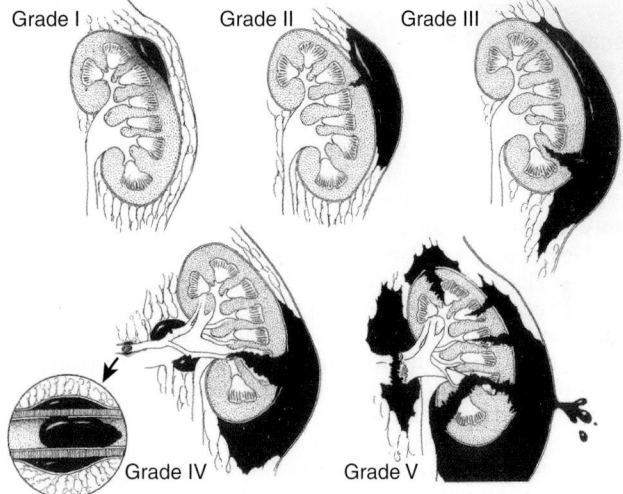

Figure 2 American Association for the Surgery of Trauma grading system for traumatic renal injuries: grade I, renal contusion and subcapsular hematoma; grade II, cortical laceration and perirenal hematoma; grade III, laceration into medulla or segmental renal artery thrombosis without a parenchymal injury; grade IV, laceration involving the collecting system, with or without a devascularized segment and contained vascular injury; grade V, renal artery thrombosis, avulsion of the renal pedicle, and shattered kidney. (From McAninch JW [ed]: Traumatic and Reconstructive Urology. Philadelphia, WB Saunders, 1996.)

system and ureters (CT urogram). In the absence of a CT scan in a patient who is transported directly to the operating room for exploration, an intraoperative single-film intravenous pyelogram can be performed to confirm that two functioning kidneys are present; however, the poor quality of the images makes them unreliable for staging purposes.

Kidney exploration is indicated for the patient who is hemodynamically unstable despite resuscitation in whom renal injury is thought to be the reason for a life-threatening and persistent hemorrhage. If there are findings of a large perirenal hematoma (>4 cm) and/or notable vascular contrast extravasation in the setting of a Grade 3–5 injury and hemodynamic instability, intervention should be performed. Another absolute indication for renal exploration and revascularization is renal artery hilar avulsion or renal artery thrombosis when bilateral or in a solitary kidney. In patients undergoing exploratory laparotomy for associated injuries, renal exploration should be performed only in the presence of an expanding or pulsatile hematoma. Exploration of a nonexpanding, nonpulsatile hematoma is associated with a higher rate of nephrectomy and should be avoided. Almost all other injuries can be managed conservatively or with minimally invasive methods. Patients with bleeding specifically limited to segmental renal vessels and who are stable can be taken for angioembolization. This minimally invasive procedure is only appropriate at institutions with skilled and available interventional radiologists.

Increasing rates of conservative management have greatly decreased rates of nephrectomy, with current practice revealing 80% of high-grade injuries managed conservatively. The factors most predictive of nephrectomy are grade of injury and penetrating injury.

Nonoperative management consists of supportive care with intravenous hydration, antibiotics, bedrest, and serial measurements of hemoglobin and hematocrit. Patients can ambulate after they are clinically stable, gross hematuria has resolved, and the hemoglobin and hematocrit have been relatively constant over 24 hours.

Routine early follow-up imaging for grades 1 to 3 blunt renal injury is unnecessary. Any imaging should be motivated by a change in the patient's clinical situation or laboratory values. Follow-up imaging is indicated within 48 hours of initial injury for patients with grade 4 or 5 injuries. Imaging is also prudent in cases with concern for worsening urinoma or hematoma that might require further intervention. Clinical signs such as worsening flank or abdominal pain, abdominal distension, fevers, and/or continued drop in blood counts can alert clinicians to such complications. Additionally, there should be periodic monitoring of blood pressure following renal trauma.

Ureteral Trauma

Trauma to the ureter is rare (1% of all genitourinary trauma). This is most likely because of its position in the retroperitoneum and bony pelvis protection, its relatively small caliber, and its mobility. The etiology of ureteric trauma is mostly iatrogenic occurring secondary to gynecologic, general surgery, and urologic procedures. Ureteral injury should be suspected in all cases of penetrating trauma to the abdomen, especially with high-velocity projectiles, because of the blast effect.

The AAST has classified ureteric injuries into five grades of severity:
- Grade 1: Hematoma only
- Grade 2: Injury involving less than 50% of the circumference of the ureter
- Grade 3: Injury involving greater than or equal to 50% of the circumference of the ureter
- Grade 4: Complete transection with less than 2 cm of devascularization
- Grade 5: Complete transection with more than 2 cm of devascularization

The diagnosis usually is made intraoperatively if a high suspicion of ureteric injury is present or postoperatively by imaging obtained for investigation of fistula formation or clinical signs of upper tract obstruction. Hematuria is not a sensitive marker for ureteral injury; therefore, lack of hematuria does not portend a lack of ureteral injury. For non-iatrogenic injuries, imaging should be obtained in patients who had rapid deceleration or penetrating injuries to the flank. Imaging modalities used are usually intravenous pyelography, CT scanning with intravenous contrast and delayed images (CT Urogram), and retrograde pyelography. Findings indicative of ureteral injury include contrast extravasation, ureteral narrowing, and delayed peristalsis (Fig. 3). Alternatively, the ureters may be interrogated intraoperatively by using direct inspection, injection of intravenous methylene blue[1], or by passing a ureteral catheter (if it passes easily, an injury is unlikely).

Grade 1 and 2 injuries can be managed initially by placement of a ureteral stent. If grade 2 or 3 injuries are identified immediately during exploration for a suspected ureteric injury, they can be managed by primary closure of the ureteric injury over an internal stent and placement of an abdominal drain as long as there is no associated thermal injury or necrosis. Grade

---

[1] Not FDA-approved for this indication.

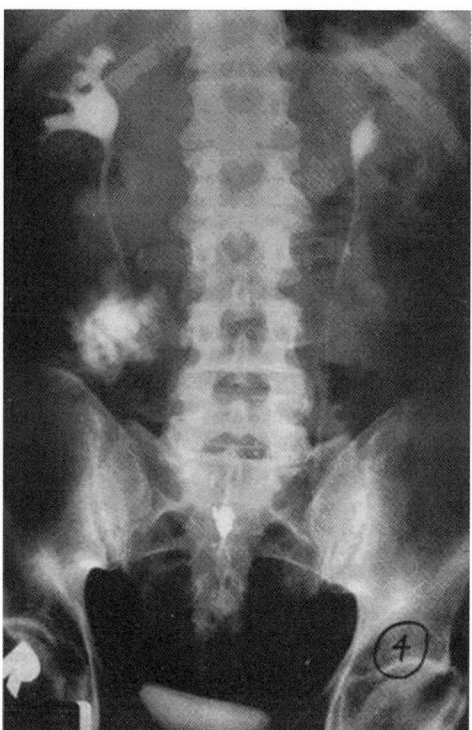

Figure 3 Intravenous pyelogram demonstrating extravasation of urine from right mid-ureter.

3 through 5 injuries usually require debridement of nonviable ends with re-anastomosis over an internal ureteral stent or more complicated surgical procedures involving mobilization of the bladder and reimplantation of the ureter into the bladder. In an unstable patient, ureteral repair may be managed with temporary urinary drainage and a definitive repair in a delayed fashion. If internal ureteral stent placement is not possible, percutaneous nephrostomy tubes can be placed. An additional drain may be required if the urine leak is not contained by nephrostomy tubes alone. The type of ureteral repair depends on the amount of devitalized tissue and the location of the injury (proximal, mid, or distal ureter). Ureteroureterostomy, transureteroureterostomy, ureterocalicostomy, renal autotransplantation, ureteroneocystostomy with or without Boari flap or psoas hitch, and bowel interposition are all treatment options for various degrees of ureteral injuries.

Bladder Trauma

Blunt trauma accounts for 51% to 86% of bladder injuries resulting from external trauma, and approximately 70% (35% to 90%) of those patients have associated pelvic fractures. The most common cause of blunt trauma is motor vehicle crashes. Penetrating trauma accounts for 14% to 49% of traumatic bladder injuries. The incidence of iatrogenic injury varies by procedure but is highest for hysterectomy and other obstetric and gynecologic procedures. In cases of blunt trauma, injury should be suspected in patients who have pelvic fractures, suprapubic pain, inability to void, ileus or abdominal distention. For iatrogenic injuries, urine in the field, visible laceration of the bladder, or gas distention of the urinary drainage bag in laparoscopic surgery warrants further investigation. It is important to delineate whether a bladder injury involves intraperitoneal or extraperitoneal rupture. Intraperitoneal rupture occurs at the level of the bladder dome, where the muscular support is weakest (Figs. 4 and 5).

The diagnostic test of choice is a CT cystogram, in which the bladder is filled with contrast to capacity (350 to 400 mL instilled by gravity). Passive filling of the bladder by clamping of the catheter is associated with unacceptably high rates of false-negative tests. Plain film cystography is an alternative, but a single anteroposterior film is insufficient; post-drainage films and, preferably,

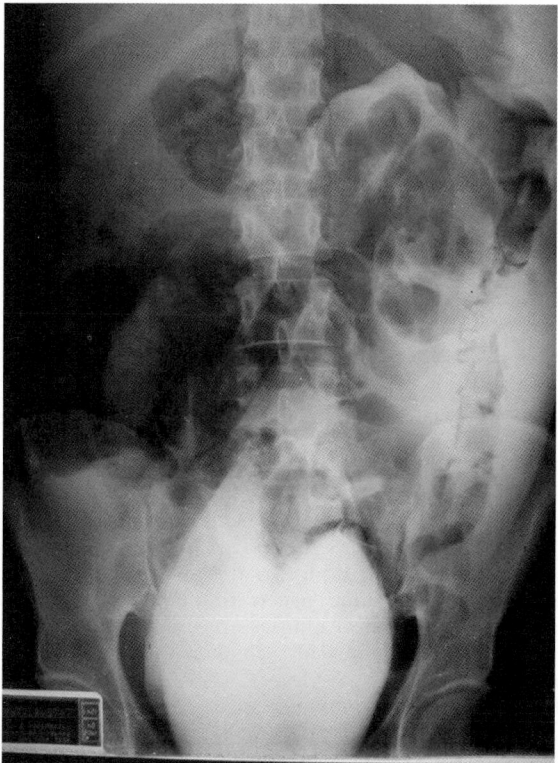

Figure 4 Intraperitoneal bladder rupture. Note contrast extravasating from the dome of the bladder and outlining the small intestine as well as the left colon.

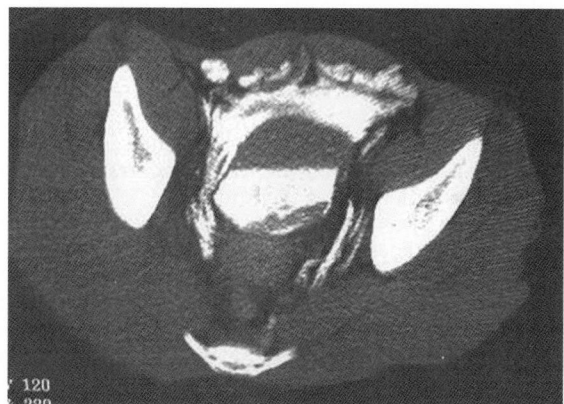

Figure 5 Extraperitoneal bladder rupture seen on computed tomographic cystogram.

oblique views should be obtained as well. In both settings, retrograde urethrography should be performed, if there is a suspicion of urethral injury, before placement of a Foley catheter.

Most extraperitoneal bladder ruptures can be managed with Foley catheter drainage for 7 to 10 days. Bladder neck involvement, concomitant vaginal or rectal injuries, presence of bone fragments in the bladder, or bladder wall entrapment necessitate surgical intervention. Intraperitoneal ruptures should be managed with surgical exploration because of the associated ileus and peritonitis caused by urine leak. It is recommended that penetrating bladder injuries are explored and repaired because of the risk of necrosis. Bladder repair is performed with a multiple-layer closure and catheter drainage for 7 to 10 days.

Urethral Trauma

Traumatic injury to the urethra occurs in 1.5% to 10% of patients who sustain a pelvic fracture. Female urethral injuries are very rare. The male urethra is anatomically divided into a

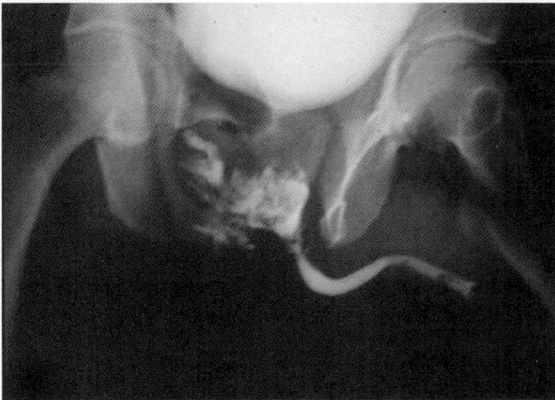

Figure 6 Retrograde urethrogram diagnostic of partial bulbar urethral transaction resulting from straddle injury.

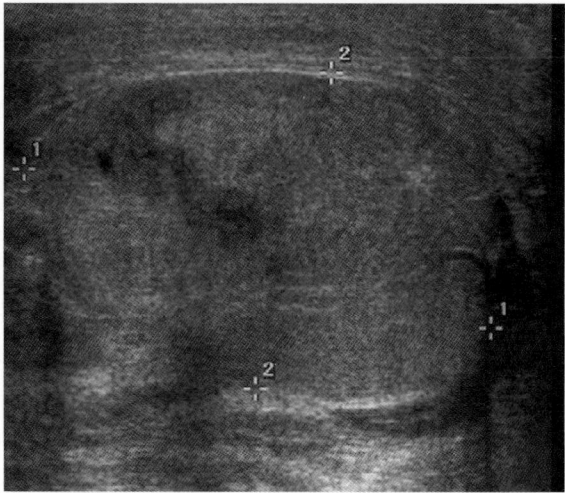

Figure 7 Testis ultrasound image demonstrating heterogeneous architecture characteristic of testicular rupture.

posterior portion (prostatic and membranous urethra) and an anterior portion (bulbous urethra, penile/pendulous urethra, and fossa navicularis). Injury to the anterior urethra occurs mostly from blunt trauma, penetrating injuries, or instrumentation. Posterior urethral injuries are usually associated with pelvic fractures but can occur secondary to blunt, penetrating, or iatrogenic injury.

Classic signs of urethral injury include blood at the meatus, a high-riding prostate on rectal examination, inability to void, or perineal or scrotal ecchymosis. Imaging is indicated with any of these signs. The imaging study of choice is a retrograde urethrogram, and it should be performed before placement of a urethral catheter is attempted. In the absence of any signs, the diagnosis is most frequently made when retrograde urethrography is performed to investigate difficulty with urethral catheter placement (Fig. 6).

The AAST grading system does not distinguish between anterior or posterior injury but classifies urethral injuries as follows:

- Grade 1: Contusion and blood at the meatus with normal urethrogram
- Grade 2: Stretch injury with no extravasation of contrast
- Grade 3: Partial disruption with contrast extravasating at the injury site but still reaching the bladder
- Grade 4: Complete disruption with contrast not reaching the bladder; urethral defect of less than 2 cm
- Grade 5: Complete disruption with urethral defect greater than 2 cm or complex injury involving the bladder neck, prostate, rectum, or vagina

Grade 1 and 2 injuries can be managed conservatively by the placement of a urethral catheter. Management of grade 3 urethral injury should initially emphasize stabilization of the patient because extensive bleeding could be present in cases of severe injury to the pelvis. Placement of a catheter may be attempted even if there is a suspicion of partial urethral injury. If this is met with difficulty, a suprapubic tube may be placed.

In cases of complete disruption, prompt urinary drainage should be established by placement of a suprapubic tube catheter. This can help facilitate a primary realignment or repair with delayed urethroplasty. Primary realignment involves endoscopic passage of a guidewire across the defect and placement of a catheter over the guidewire. Immediate open repair is rarely indicated unless complex injury extends into the bladder neck, rectum, or vagina. Immediate exploration is recommended for anterior urethral injuries associated with penetrating trauma or penile fractures. Female urethral injuries are optimally treated at initial presentation to decrease the risk of incontinence. Physicians should continue to follow patients for at least 1 year, monitoring for complications such as incontinence, erectile dysfunction, and stricture formation.

Trauma to the External Genitalia

Injury to the scrotum is most frequently secondary to blunt trauma and can cause a hematoma, ecchymosis, or testicular injury. Scrotal swelling and patient discomfort can make separation of testicular injury from extratesticular scrotal trauma difficult on physical examination. In the case of blunt scrotal injuries, a scrotal ultrasound should be performed in most patients with suspicion of testicular rupture. A heterogeneous echo pattern in the testicular parenchyma on ultrasonography suggests testicular injury (Fig. 7). Visualization of a tear in the tunica albuginea is less accurate. Ultrasound studies with Doppler additionally provide information about any compromise in testicular blood flow. In the setting of penetrating scrotal injury, surgical exploration is recommended.

Scrotal exploration should be performed whenever testicular injury is suspected. If the tunica is ruptured and there is extrusion of seminiferous tubules, the extruded tubules should be debrided, hemorrhage controlled, and the tunica closed. Testicular salvage rates are highest when the scrotum is explored acutely compared to delayed exploration. Another indication for scrotal exploration is a large hematocele; evacuation of the hematoma can decrease the morbidity associated with protracted recovery and resolution of the hematoma and can occasionally identify a manageable source of bleeding. Scrotal exploration should also be performed in cases of inconclusive ultrasound findings or whenever the clinical suspicion for testicular injury is high.

Trauma to the penis can range in severity from a contusion to complete amputation. In cases of penile amputation, stabilization of the patient is important, and the need for transfusion should be addressed. Immediate microreimplantation is the management technique of choice if available. The severed penile segment should be immediately placed in a normal saline bag over ice to help preserve the fragment for reimplantation.

A penile fracture occurs after blunt injury to the erect penis rupturing the tunica albuginea. Such injuries are usually incurred during sexual intercourse and patients often report a "crack" or a "pop" followed by pain and detumescence. The hematoma is usually limited to the penis, unless the injury also involves Buck fascia, causing ecchymosis and bruising that involves the scrotum as well. Surgical exploration, closure of the fascial defect, and repair of any associated urethral injury should be done acutely. In cases of unclear history or physical examination, the provider may consider penile ultrasound or penile MRI for more conclusive evidence of a penile fracture. It is also important to rule out associated urethral injury, which occurs in 10% to 22% of the cases.

In females, blunt trauma to the vulva is rare. Injuries to genitalia can be associated with sexual assault and must be evaluated in that context. Consequently, vaginal smears should be taken, and the vagina should be thoroughly inspected under anesthesia with a speculum.

Trauma resulting in skin loss, such as burns, large abrasions, and avulsions, should be explored and debrided in an effort to stage the injury and decrease the risk of complications such as Fournier gangrene and urinoma. Delayed reconstruction can be performed after stabilization and proper delineation of viable versus nonviable tissues. The reconstructive options include mobilization of local flaps or skin grafts.

Conclusion

Critical considerations when treating urogenital trauma include patient stability, mechanism of injury, and maintaining broad differentials for organ involvement. Appropriate imaging in the hemodynamically stable patient is crucial to avoid missing injuries that can risk severe complications such as uncontrolled bleeding, urine leaks, and infections. Guidelines have migrated towards more conservative treatments demonstrating success in select cases such as decreased nephrectomy rates and improved urethral healing without strictures. Early involvement of a urologist to guide proper workup and management can help optimize recovery outcomes.

References

Buckley JC, McAninch JW: Revision of current American Association for the Surgery of Trauma renal injury grading system, *J Trauma* 70(1):35–37, 2011.

Coccolini F, Moore EE, Kluger Y, et al: Kidney and uro-trauma: WSES-AAST guidelines, *World J Emerg Surg* 14:54, 2019.

Keihani S, Yizhe MS, Presson AP, et al: Contemporary management of high-grade renal trauma, *J Trauma Acute Care Surg* 84(3):418–425, 2018.

Lumen N, Kuehhas FE, Djakovic N, et al: Review of the current management of lower urinary tract injuries by the, *EAU Trauma Guidelines Panel* 67(5):925–929, 2015.

McGeady JB, Breyer BN: Current epidemiology of genitourinary trauma, *Urol Clin North Am* 40(3):323–334, 2013.

Morey AF, Brandes S, Dugi DD, et al: Urotrauma: AUA guideline, *J Urol* 192(2):327–335, 2014.

Phonsombat S, Master VA, McAninch JW: Penetrating external genital trauma: A 30-year single institution experience, *J Urol* 180(1):192–195, 2008, discussion 195–196.

Serafetinides E, Kitrey ND, Djakovic N, et al: Review of the current management of upper urinary tract injuries by the EAU Trauma Guidelines Panel, *Eur Urol* 67(5):930–936, 2015.

URETHRAL STRICTURE DISEASE

Method of
Hadley Wyre, MD; and Sable Shew, MD

CURRENT DIAGNOSIS

- Perform a thorough history and physical examination, delineating past trauma, instrumentation, and sexual history, as well as a complete genitourinary examination.
- Patients with urethral stricture will commonly present with obstructive symptoms of weak urinary stream, straining to urinate, and even frank urinary retention.
- In-office testing consists of urinalysis and urine culture for evaluation of infection, as well as uroflowmetry and postvoid residual bladder ultrasound to evaluate urine flow rate and emptying ability.
- Retrograde urethrogram remains the gold standard for diagnosis of urethral stricture disease.

CURRENT THERAPY

- In the acute setting of urinary retention, the ideal management would be placement of a suprapubic tube to avoid manipulation of the stricture; however, dilation and catheter placement may be appropriate or necessary in some patients.
- Depending on the patient, goals of care should be delineated regarding treatment of stricture disease; that is, definitive therapy versus chronic management of stricture symptoms.
- Endoscopic treatments are available and include urethral dilation and direct visualization internal urethrotomy; however, repeat attempts at these approaches have a low long-term success rate.
- Surgical management includes both anastomotic and augmentation urethroplasty—both of which are more invasive than endoscopic approaches but are known to have improved long-term patency rates.

Urethral stricture disease affects 0.6% of the male population and can be classified in multiple ways: anterior versus posterior, benign versus malignant, extrinsic versus intrinsic, and congenital versus acquired. The urethra is a conduit for urine from the bladder to outside of the body. In males, the anterior urethra (region encircled by corpus spongiosum) begins at the meatus and includes the fossa navicularis, penile urethra, and bulbar urethra—strictures here are the result of scarring of the urethral epithelium and surrounding spongy tissue, termed spongiofibrosis. As this scarring narrows the urethral lumen, symptoms become noticeable. Typically, the urethral lumen must narrow to less than 14 French for this scarring to be the cause of any voiding symptoms. Anterior urethral stricture can be secondary to iatrogenic injury, infections, penile/perineal trauma, pelvic fractures, and self-instrumentation. In the posterior urethra, including the membranous urethra, prostatic urethra, and bladder neck, narrowing is termed contracture or stenosis and is the result of a distraction injury sustained during pelvic trauma or prior surgical procedures of the prostate (Figure 1).

Diagnosis

Often patients with strictures will present with obstructive voiding symptoms including weak or intermittent stream, postvoid dribbling, straining to urinate, or overt urinary retention. Nonobstructive symptoms include postvoid fullness, urinary tract infections, and pelvic pain. A thorough history, including a detailed social/sexual history, and physical examination should be done, and any prior trauma to or instrumentation of the genitourinary tract noted. The physical examination should be comprehensive, with the genital examination examining for palpable strictures in the anterior urethra.

Laboratory workup should include urinalysis and urine culture for evaluation of infection, as well as a basic metabolic panel to evaluate for any renal function compromise. It is possible to perform an assessment of voiding symptoms in a clinic setting with the use of postvoid ultrasound and uroflowmetry. Once the patient has voided to completion, an ultrasound measurement of postvoid residual urine volume can objectively estimate the patient's ability to evacuate and alert the provider to overt retention. Uroflowmetry is the measurement of flow rate of urine—findings that suggest significant stricture include an elongated voiding time and a low maximal flow rate, essentially flattening the flow curve to a plateau appearance.

The gold standard in urethral stricture diagnosis remains the retrograde urethrogram. Radiocontrast is administered via catheter in a retrograde fashion, filling the urethra and opacifying it—this study is especially helpful for evaluating the length, location,

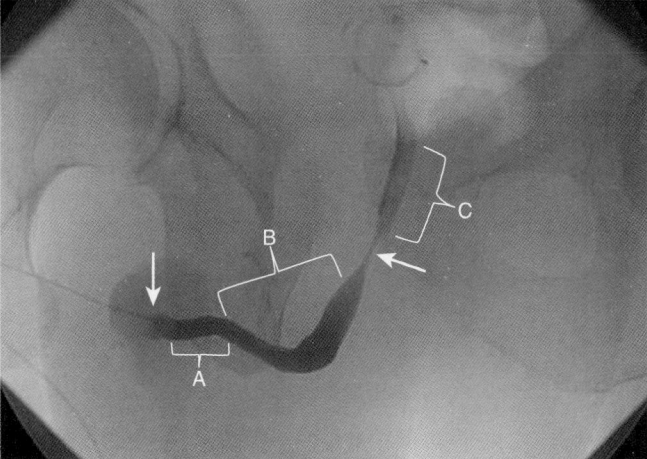

Figure 1 Anatomy of male urethra. (A) Penile urethra. (B) Bulbar urethra. (C) Prostatic urethra. White arrow by A=fossa navicularis; white arrow between B and C=membranous urethra.

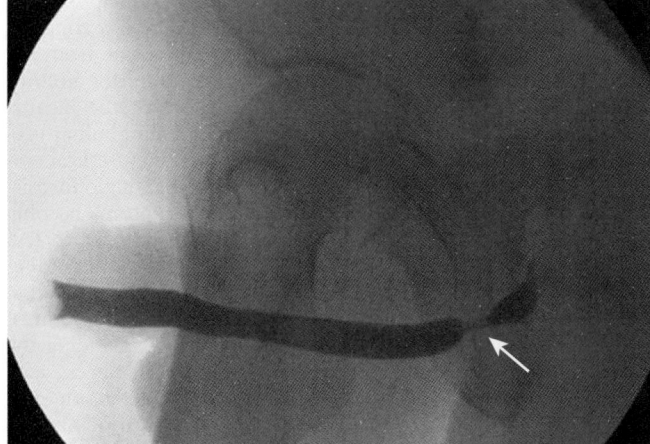

Figure 2 Bulbar urethral stricture visualized on retrograde urethrogram.

and severity of strictures in the anterior urethra. Additionally, an antegrade study, or voiding cystourethrogram, can be performed to allow for visualization of the bladder neck, prostatic urethra, and membranous urethra. In addition to cystoscopic evaluation for direct visualization of the stricture, ultrasound of the penis/perineum can be used to further delineate characteristics of the stricture. Biopsy is occasionally performed to rule out malignancy as a cause of the stricture (Figure 2).

Acute Treatment

Acutely, the main complication from a urethral stricture is frank urinary retention, which may be associated with a decline in renal function. Typically a urethral catheter cannot be placed because of obstruction from the stricture. In the setting of overt urinary retention, a suprapubic tube is often placed at the bedside or in the operating room to allow for rapid decompression of the urinary system without manipulating the stricture. There are times where suprapubic tube placement may not be possible, and it is therefore reasonable to dilate the stricture and place a urethral catheter to drain the urine. However, manipulation of the stricture can lead to an increase in the length of the stricture and complexity of the eventual repair.

Long-Term Treatment

Multiple modalities exist for the treatment of urethral stricture disease, with varying success rates and complication rates. A thorough discussion between the patient and provider, considering the patient's goals for either cure or symptom management,

life expectancy, and stricture qualities, is vital to ensuring that an appropriate care plan is developed. Prior to proceeding with any treatment, it is essential to evaluate the urethra proximal to and distal to the stricture with the modalities mentioned earlier; this is to ensure removal of all affected tissue and prevent recurrence.

Conservative management with urethral dilation is appropriate as a first attempt at treatment of a short stricture with minimal spongiofibrosis, with the ultimate goal of stretching rather than tearing tissue to open the lumen without increasing the scarring present. Direct visualization internal urethrotomy (DVIU) is opening of a stricture—by laser, cold knife, or hot knife—to release the scar and allow the urethra to heal at a larger diameter over a catheter. Long-term success rates for DVIU have been reported at 20% to 30% for short strictures with minimal spongiofibrosis. It is important to note that the success rate of repeat DVIU is close to 0%, and after failure, the patient should be referred for definitive surgical repair.

Surgical management includes operations to excise the scar and perform urethral anastomosis, and tissue transfer reconstruction with harvesting of distant tissue—typically oral mucosa—for urethral augmentation. Anastomotic urethroplasty is best for short strictures, 1 to 2 cm in length, while augmentation urethroplasty can be utilized for much longer defects. For any type of urethral reconstruction, restricture is the most common complication, as well as sexual dysfunction and ejaculatory dysfunction. Other treatment options include long-term suprapubic tube drainage, perineal urethrostomy, and urinary diversion, depending on each patient's individual case and discussion with the patient's surgeon. Regardless of modality, clinicians should monitor patients for symptomatic recurrence of strictures.

References

Albers P, Fichtner J, Bruhl P, et al: Long-term results of internal urethrotomy, *J Urol* 156:1611–1614, 1996.

Andrich DE, Mundy AR: The nature of urethral injury in cases of pelvic fracture urethral trauma, *J Urol* 165:1492–1495, 2001.

Bhargava S, Chapple CR, Bullock AJ, et al: Tissue-engineered buccal mucosa for substitution urethroplasty, *BJU Int* 93:807–811, 2004.

Fichtner J, Filipas D, Fisch M, et al: Long-term outcome of ventral buccal mucosa onlay graft urethroplasty for urethral stricture repair, *Urology* 64:648–650, 2004.

Hudak SJ, Atkinson TH, Morey AF: Repeat transurethral manipulation of bulbar urethral strictures is associated with increased stricture complexity and prolonged disease duration, *J Urol* 187(5):1691–1695, 2012.

Kellner DS, Fracchia JA, Armenakas NA: Ventral onlay buccal mucosal grafts for anterior urethral stricture: Long-term followup, *J Urol* 171:726–729, 2004.

McCallum RW, Colapinto V: The role of urethrography in urethral disease. Part I. Accurate radiological localization of the membranous urethra and distal sphincters in normal male subjects, *J Urol* 122:607–611, 1979.

McCammon KA, Zuckerman JM, Gerald HJ: Surgery of the penis and urethra. In Wein A, et al: 11th edition,, Campbell-Walsh UrologyPhiladelphia, 2016, Elsevier, pp 907–945.

Rosen MA, Nash PA, Bruce JE, et al: The actuarial success rate of surgical treatment of urethral strictures, *J Urol* 151:370, 1994.

URINARY INCONTINENCE

Method of
Simon Patton, MD; and Renee M. Bassaly, DO

CURRENT DIAGNOSIS

- Urinary incontinence is broadly categorized as stress urinary incontinence or urgency urinary incontinence.
- The diagnosis can often be determined by a careful history and physical examination but can be aided with noninvasive methods such as a bladder diary.
- It is important to rule out any other potential causes of incontinence including urinary tract infection, urinary retention, or medication side effect.

- Modest weight loss has been shown to help both forms of incontinence and is an important first-line therapy.
- Urgency urinary incontinence can initially be managed with lifestyle modifications including timed voiding and avoidance of bladder irritants, as well as physical therapy. Further options include medications (anticholinergics or B$_3$ agonists).
- Third-line therapy for urgency urinary incontinence includes sacral neuromodulation, botulinum toxin injections, and tibial nerve stimulation.
- Stress urinary incontinence can be managed conservatively with home Kegel exercises or formal pelvic floor training with physical therapy. Mechanical urethral support using a disposable tampon-like device or incontinence pessary is another non-invasive option.
- Surgical management of stress urinary incontinence is midurethral slings, principally using synthetic mesh. I would include Burch and autologous sling.

Epidemiology

Urinary incontinence is a very common problem particularly in the female population, with incidence roughly twice that of male patients (30% vs. 17%). The exact incidence may be difficult to know, however, because this is a sensitive subject that patients may not volunteer unless solicited. The annual cost of treating incontinence is estimated to be $24 billion, and annually 260,000 women undergo surgery for stress incontinence.

Risk Factors

Risk factors vary between genders. Women are at greater risk due to anatomic differences, principally a shorter urethral length. Other risk factors include increased age, parity, obesity, diabetes, smoking, and pelvic radiation. In male patients a history of prostate surgery or an enlarged prostate are potential risk factors. Urinary tract symptoms including incontinence may represent manifestations of neurologic disorders including history of stroke, multiple sclerosis, or spinal cord injury.

Pathophysiology

The bladder consists of a smooth muscular reservoir (the detrusor muscle), two inlets (the ureters), and an outlet (the urethra). Urine from the kidneys enters the bladder via the ureters and exits via the urethra, which is itself a muscular tube consisting of smooth and striated muscle. Bladder function has two phases: storage and emptying. During the storage phase, the bladder collects urine; this phase involves relaxation of the detrusor muscle and contraction of the urethral muscle, all of which is under sympathetic and voluntary control. The emptying phase involves relaxation of the urethral muscles and contraction of the detrusor, which is mediated by the parasympathetic system. Under normal circumstances, emptying is voluntarily initiated in the adult.

In women, the bladder and urethra are supported by the anterior vaginal wall, which, in turn, is suspended by connective tissue attachments from the pelvic floor muscles. Continence is maintained when the urethral closure pressure exceeds the detrusor pressure. Adequate support from the anterior vaginal wall is required to maintain this relationship during periods of increased intraabdominal pressure. Consequently, urinary continence depends on the relative relaxation of the detrusor, the contraction of urethral muscles, and the support of the anterior vaginal wall. Incontinence can ensue when these relationships are disrupted.

Prevention

The pelvic floor musculature plays an important role in the maintenance of continence, and as such, pelvic floor physical therapy directed at these muscles has been shown to improve continence in both postmenopausal women and younger postpartum women, at least in the short term. Physical therapy in the male population has not been studied as a prevention strategy. One modifiable risk factor for incontinence is obesity, and even a modest weight loss of 10% has been shown to help improve continence status.

Clinical Manifestation

Urinary incontinence can be a sign, symptom, as well as a diagnosis. Urinary incontinence falls into two broad categories: stress incontinence and urge incontinence. Stress urinary incontinence occurs when urethral closure pressure cannot increase sufficiently to compensate for a sudden increase in intraabdominal pressure, as from laugh, cough, or Valsalva maneuver. Urgency urinary incontinence occurs when an unintended bladder contraction creates an insuppressible urge to void, leading to urinary leakage. When patients have signs or symptoms of both stress and urge incontinence, it is referred to as *mixed urinary incontinence*.

Diagnosis

Diagnosis rests principally on a careful history and physical examination. A thorough history is important to solicit what causes a patient to leak. Leakage with laughing, coughing, sneezing, exercise, or similar exertion would most likely be stress urinary incontinence. Leakage associated with an urge that is difficult to defer is likely urgency urinary incontinence. If patients have both symptoms, then they likely have mixed urinary incontinence. If a patient complains of symptoms of mixed incontinence, a careful history to determine which is most bothersome is important. If the patient has difficulty knowing what has caused their leakage, a 3-day bladder diary recording liquid consumed, times and amounts voided, and leakage events with associated symptoms can help with diagnosis and treatment.

Other pertinent components to a thorough history include surgery to the spinal cord, bladder neck, or pelvic floor, which may lead to obstruction; neurologic disease (e.g., multiple sclerosis or a spinal cord lesion); or psychiatric disease (e.g., dementia, which may limit the ability to recognize a need to void). Musculoskeletal function, with emphasis on mobility, should be reviewed. A detailed medication history will identify any medications that may affect urine output or bladder function. It is important to also elicit any other symptoms that may coexist with incontinence and signal pelvic floor dysfunction, including nocturia, fecal incontinence, or constipation.

After a thorough history, a detailed physical examination is necessary. A focused genitourinary examination includes inspection of the external genitalia. Eliciting reflexes from the S2-S4 nerve roots will help determine whether there is any neurologic component. In female patients, perform a pelvic examination and look for any prolapse or pelvic masses and note whether any atrophy is present. Palpation of the urethra allows for evaluation of any urethral masses or possible diverticula. Lastly, assessment of pelvic floor musculature is important, evaluating for any pain or discomfort in the levator ani muscles and assessing the patient's ability to perform a proper Kegel exercise. In males, performance of a digital rectal examination is recommended to evaluate for any prostatic masses or hypertrophy.

The physical examination provides an opportunity for diagnosis as well; asking the patient to cough or perform a Valsalva maneuver allows for the direct visualization of stress incontinence if present. Additionally, this provides an opportunity in female patients to evaluate for prolapse and assess urethral mobility. Historically, this was done by placing a cotton swab in the urethra to observe for hypermobility seen with >30 degrees of mobility on strain from baseline. However, because of patient discomfort, this test is not routinely performed. After completing the physical examination, one must perform a urinalysis to rule out any infectious etiology and at times perform a post-void residual (either with a bladder scan or with catheterization) to evaluate for any possible voiding dysfunction. If the patient has a more complex history because of prior urologic surgery, neurologic disease, or is difficult to diagnose on history and physical alone, then complex urodynamic testing may be indicated.

Differential Diagnosis

The differential diagnosis for urinary incontinence includes stress urinary incontinence, urgency urinary incontinence, and a mixture of the two as mentioned above. Other causes of undesired leakage of urine include overflow (due to urinary retention), functional (due to impaired mobility or mental capacity), as well as a fistula or diverticulum. A patient with a fistula most commonly presents with the complaint of constant persistent urinary leakage. In the industrialized world these generally form after genitourinary surgery, whereas in developing countries trauma from childbirth is the primary cause. A diverticulum may present with a painful anterior vaginal wall mass as well as irritative voiding symptoms such as urinary frequency, urgency, dysuria, and postvoid dribbling. Other causes of lower urinary tract symptoms such as urgency, frequency, and dysuria include urinary tract infection, uncontrolled diabetes, or urinary tract malignancy.

Therapy

Stress Urinary Incontinence

Nonsurgical options for treatment of stress urinary incontinence include strengthening of the pelvic musculature through Kegel exercises and mechanical support of the urethra. Kegel exercises may be performed by the patient at home, although some patients may have difficulty identifying the muscles to perform them properly. Formal training with a pelvic floor physical therapist can help the patients learn to identify the muscles (sometimes using biofeedback devices) and contract them appropriately. Proper contraction of the levator ani muscles provides improved support for the bladder and urethra and helps decrease leakage.

Mechanical support of the urethra and bladder neck can be accomplished using an incontinence pessary or a disposable incontinence tampon. Pessaries are ring-shaped silicone devices with a knob that is meant to sit under the urethra. Patients are fitted for the correct size in the office. Patients must be followed up for at 3 to 6 month intervals to ensure the pessary has not caused any erosions or excoriations. This can be avoided by teaching patients how to insert and remove the pessary themselves or prescribing a vaginal estrogen cream in postmenopausal patients. A disposable option is available over the counter as well. It comes in three sizes, and the patients can fit themselves at home with the starter pack. Once they find the correct size, it can be placed when the patient desires and may be kept in place for up to 8 hours. Some patients choose this option if they only have stress incontinence during certain times (i.e., exercise).

If conservative therapies do not adequately address their complaints, surgical options are available. The general principle of restoring support to the urethra is the same as in conservative therapies. This can be accomplished by placing a sling under the urethra. The sling material can be lightweight polypropylene mesh or fascia (either autologous or cadaveric). The most commonly used type is the synthetic mesh and it is placed either retropubically or through the obturator membrane. Both methods have been shown to have a high rate of satisfaction with a low complication rate.

Stress incontinence in men is much less common but can also be treated with slings placed at the bulbar urethra. Artificial urinary sphincters can also be implanted that compress the urethra and can be controlled by the patient.

Urgency Urinary Incontinence

Lifestyle modifications are a good first-line therapy for patients with urgency urinary incontinence. Drinking an appropriate amount of fluids and avoiding foods and beverages that are known to irritate the bladder can provide significant relief. Additionally, performing timed voiding can help retrain the bladder. Formal training with a pelvic floor physical therapist has also been shown to significantly decrease incontinence episodes. It is important to note, however, that just performing Kegel exercises is often not adequate in these patients and can in fact worsen their symptoms if they already have tightly held, nonrelaxing pelvic floor musculature.

Pharmacologic therapy consists of anticholinergic medications or beta 3 agonists. Anticholinergic medications target the muscarinic receptors on the bladder; however, they are not specific and can cause significant dry mouth, dry eyes, and constipation, side effects that lead to a high discontinuation rate. Patients are unable to take this class of medication if they have closed-angle glaucoma. Additionally, there have recently been some concerns raised about long-term use leading to cognitive decline. The beta 3 agonists also work to slow down detrusor contractions but do so by targeting a different receptor. They have been shown to raise blood pressure and so are precluded in patients with uncontrolled severe hypertension; all patients should routinely check their blood pressure after starting one of these medications.

Third-line therapies for urgency urinary incontinence include sacral neuromodulation, tibial nerve stimulation, and intradetrusor injection of botulinum toxin A. Sacral neuromodulation has been approved by the Food and Drug Administration for this indication, as well as fecal incontinence and voiding dysfunction. It consists of a lead placed in the S3 foramen and connected to a pacemaker-like device that is implanted in the adipose of the buttocks. Patients are then able to control some of the settings (including program and amplitude) from an external device. The sacral nerve roots can also be stimulated via the tibial nerve. Treatments involve a small, acupuncture-sized needle placed in the tibial nerve followed by 30 minutes of stimulation. These are carried out at weekly treatments for 12 weeks followed by monthly maintenance therapy. Botulinum toxin A, a neurotoxin that works by decreasing the presynaptic release of acetylcholine, can be injected directly into the detrusor muscle. A risk of this treatment is urinary retention, which requires that patients be able to perform self-catheterization.

Mixed Urinary Incontinence

If a patient presents with components of both stress and urgency, eliciting first which symptom is the most bothersome allows for appropriate tailoring of treatment. It is important to remind patients that even a modest weight loss of 10% can help reduce bothersome urinary symptoms by up to 60%. As noted above, physical therapy can help address both type of incontinence as a valuable first-line therapy.

Overflow Incontinence

If a patient is diagnosed with overflow incontinence, then management is directed at maintaining an empty bladder through self-catheterization. In male patients, if the retention is due to prostatic hypertrophy, then pharmacologic therapy with α-agonists or 5α reductase inhibitors may be warranted. If medication fails to improve their symptoms, then surgical treatment with ablation (microwave or radiofrequency) or resection is indicated.

Complications

Urinary incontinence can cause significant morbidity in terms of financial as well as psychological burdens on patients. In addition to causing rashes and skin breakdown, incontinence also leads to depression, isolation, anxiety, depression, and increased risk of falls. Incontinence is one of the leading causes of institutionalization in the elderly. As the population ages, the incidence of incontinence will continue to increase, making its diagnosis and treatment increasingly important.

References

Abrams P, Cardozo L, Fall M, et al: The standardisation of terminology of lower urinary tract function: report from the Standardisation Sub-committee of the International Continence Society, *Neurourol Urodyn* 21:167–178, 2002.

AUGS: Consensus Statement: Association of Anticholinergic Medication Use and Cognition in Women With Overactive Bladder, *Female Pelvic Med Reconstr Surg* 23:177–178, 2017.

Hay-Smith EJ, Herderschee R, Dumoulin C, Herbison GP: Comparisons of approaches to pelvic floor muscle training for urinary incontinence in women, *Cochrane Database Syst Rev*, 2011;12: CD009508.

Hersh L, Salzman B: Clinical management of urinary incontinence in women, *Am Fam Physician* 87:634–640, 2013, Review. Erratum in: Am Fam Physician 2013;88:427.

Hu TW, Wagner TH, Bentkover JD, et al: Costs of urinary incontinence and overactive bladder in the United States: a comparative study, *Urology* 63:461–465, 2004.

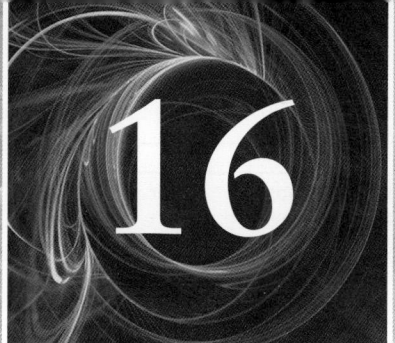

16 Men's Health

BENIGN PROSTATIC HYPERPLASIA

Method of
Judd W. Moul, MD

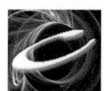

CURRENT DIAGNOSIS

- Benign prostatic hyperplasia (BPH) is an extremely common condition in aging men, characterized by prostate gland growth that can obstruct the flow of urine and cause urinary symptoms.
- Diagnosis of BPH is usually based on symptoms of weak urine stream, hesitancy, intermittent stream, nocturia, and dribbling. These symptoms are generally called *lower urinary tract symptoms* (LUTS).
- Additional diagnostic aids include digital rectal examination (DRE), urinary flow rates and post void residual (PVR) measurements, PSA blood test, cystoscopy, and sometimes urodynamic testing.

CURRENT THERAPY

- Medical therapies include alpha blocker agents (most commonly tamsulosin) and five-alpha reductase inhibitors (finasteride or dutasteride), sometimes used individually or together.
- Surgical therapy includes transurethral resection of the prostate (TURP) using electrocautery or laser devices, and open or robotic simple prostatectomy for men with very large gland size.
- More recent minimally-invasive surgical approaches include Uro-Lift, REZUM, prostate artery embolization (PAE), and various laser techniques such as laser enucleation procedures (such as HOLEP).
- Therapy is individualized based on degree of urinary symptoms, patient bother, and the size of the prostate.

Benign prostatic hyperplasia (BPH) is a disease process characterized by the increased growth of prostatic cells within the prostate gland, which sits at the base of the bladder and surrounds and fuses with the urethra. These glandular changes may result in changes in urinary flow, collectively known as lower urinary tract symptoms (LUTS). The presence of LUTS such as weak stream, increased frequency and urgency of urination, nocturia, and the feeling of incomplete bladder emptying occurring secondary to prostate enlargement are more accurately characterized as benign prostatic obstruction (BPO); however, most clinicians routinely and acceptably apply the BPH diagnosis. Although many other disease processes (i.e., congestive heart failure, poorly controlled diabetes, renal failure, and many others) can contribute to LUTS in males, BPH is a leading contributor to urinary dysfunction in older males and is known to significantly affect quality of life.

Epidemiology

BPH is generally considered a disease of the aging male, with associated symptoms uncommon before the age of 40 years. By ages 60 years and 85 years, the histologic prevalence of BPH at autopsy is 50% and 90%, respectively. Likewise, the associated LUTS increase with age. At age 70 years, about 40% of men report LUTS; by age 75 years, the incidence of LUTS increases to 50%.

Pathophysiology

Although BPH is common, we know very little about its true pathophysiology. Current thought attributes BPH to an "awakening" of senescent epithelial and smooth muscle cells of the prostatic transition zone. Before the 1980s, BPH was generally thought of as a static condition of a gradually growing prostate gland causing progressive bladder outlet obstruction, following the "donut hole" analogy that the prostate is like a donut surrounding the bladder neck and outlet. With aging and prostate growth, the donut hole gets smaller, causing progressive obstruction. In the era when surgical treatment via transurethral resection of the prostate (TURP) was the only effective treatment, this simple static explanation was sufficient. We now know that BPH has both a static obstructive and a dynamic component under neural control. In addition, the contribution of the bladder to LUTS has been well recognized as a key contributor to the dynamic component of BPH and LUTS.

Specifically, the static growth and proliferation of the periurethral tissue in BPH is thought to be driven by androgens, as men castrated before puberty do not develop BPH. Testosterone, the main male hormone, is converted to the more active metabolite dihydrotestosterone (DHT) by the enzyme 5α-reductase in the prostatic stromal and epithelial cells. 5α-Reductase occurs in two forms, types 1 and 2. However, only type 2 is present in the prostate and genitalia. This is critical for understanding one of the two main classes of medical therapy for BPH—the 5α-reductase inhibitors (5-ARIs), medications that block the conversion of testosterone to DHT.

The dynamic component of BPH and LUTS is attributed to autonomic input to the smooth muscles in the lower urinary tract, including the bladder, prostate, and urethra. These areas have a large concentration of α_1-adrenergic receptors that, when stimulated, cause increased smooth muscle tone. This physiology then leads to increased urethral resistance and contributes to the obstructive symptoms of BPH, leading to the basis for the other main class of drugs to treat BPH—the α_1-adrenergic blockers.

Symptoms

LUTS include urinary frequency, decreased force and caliber of the urinary stream, hesitancy, straining to void, urgency, and nocturia. The degree of impact may range from minimal "bother" to frank urinary retention with renal failure. Most urologists now use a standardized self-administered questionnaire, such as the International Prostate Symptom Score (IPSS) (Figure 1), designed to elicit symptoms and bother in a typical male population with suboptimal health-seeking behavior.

It is now very common for men to be referred to urology for a collection of age-related issues including elevated prostate-specific antigen (PSA), LUTS, BPH, and erectile dysfunction (ED). Commonly, the PSA or ED brings the patient to the attention of the healthcare system for the first time in years and may be the first opportunity to influence men on healthy living and health

International Prostate Symptom Score (I-PSS)

Patient Name: _____ Date of birth: _____ Date completed _____

In the past month:	Not at all	Less than 1 in 5 times	Less than half the time	About half the time	More than half the time	Almost always	Your score
1. Incomplete emptying How often have you had the sensation of not emptying your bladder?	0	1	2	3	4	5	
2. Frequency How often have you had to urinate less than every two hours?	0	1	2	3	4	5	
3. Intermittency How often have you found you stopped and started again several times when you urinated?	0	1	2	3	4	5	
4. Urgency How often have you found it difficult to postpone urination?	0	1	2	3	4	5	
5. Weak stream How often have you had a weak urinary stream?	0	1	2	3	4	5	
6. Straining How often have you had to strain to start urination?	0	1	2	3	4	5	
	None	1 Time	2 Times	3 Times	4 Times	5 Times	
7. Nocturia How many times did you typically get up at night to urinate?	0	1	2	3	4	5	
Total I-PSS score							

Score   1–7: *Mild*   8–19: *Moderate*   20–35: *Severe*

Quality of life due to urinary symptoms	Delighted	Pleased	Mostly satisfied	Mixed	Mostly dissatisfied	Unhappy	Terrible
If you were to spend the rest of your life with your urinary condition just the way it is now, how would you feel about that?	0	1	2	3	4	5	6

Figure 1 The International Prostate Symptom Score (IPSS) questionnaire. Available from the Urological Sciences Research Foundation at: http://www.usrf.org/questionnaires/AUA_SymptomScore.html. Accessed April 18, 2020.

maintenance as they enter their middle or older age. Recognizing this, all healthcare providers should keep this in mind and try to perform a broader men's health assessment while the patient is available.

Diagnosis

The diagnosis of BPH is generally made based on symptoms or the IPSS standardized questionnaire, self-administered by the patient, combined with a digital rectal examination, PSA blood test, urinalysis, and, in some cases, a transrectal ultrasound or cystoscopy. The differential diagnosis can include urinary tract infection (UTI), prostatitis, urinary stones in the lower urinary tract, urethral stricture disease, neurogenic or overactive bladder, prostate or bladder cancer, and even congestive heart failure. Some common medications, such as over-the-counter cold medicines containing α-adrenergic agents, can exacerbate LUTS and can even put a man into acute urinary retention if he has underlying BPH.

A properly performed digital rectal examination is critical to master in the diagnosis of BPH. Because the posterior prostate gland is located adjacent to the rectum and about 3 to 5 cm internal to the anus, the experienced clinician can gain valuable information from this examination. We prefer the patient to bend over the examining table with toes pointed slightly inward, the knees bent slightly forward and the forehead and arms/elbows resting on the table. The examiner uses a liberally lubricated gloved index finger to palpate the posterior side of the prostate for size estimate and for any induration or nodularity that might indicate the presence of prostate cancer. In such a case, referral to a urologist would be mandatory.

The size of the prostate is measured either by estimating the weight in grams or the volume in cubic centimeters. Models have been developed to teach clinicians how to gauge size and consistency. In general, a normal-size prostate is 20 to 25 g (or cm^3) in middle-aged men. A size of 25 to 30, 30 to 50, and greater than 50 g (or cm^3) is a general guide to mild, moderate, and severe BPH. However, size does not necessarily correlate with symptoms, and both symptom score and size estimate should be reported. The size gauges the histologic condition and the symptoms indicate the LUTS and the bother index, which are both important for individualized treatment.

The laboratory assessment should include a urinalysis to rule out hematuria. Like an abnormal digital rectal examination, a urinalysis that shows persistent red blood cells should prompt referral to a urologist for cystoscopic and upper urinary tract assessment. A urinalysis suggesting UTI should be followed up with a urine culture. If the patient presents in acute or chronic urinary retention and especially if there is a high postvoid or post-catheter residual bladder volume, a serum creatinine and blood urea nitrogen should be obtained. Severe BPH sometimes causes hydronephrosis and renal insufficiency; rarely, it causes renal failure. In-office bladder ultrasound scanners are very useful to quickly assess residual urine.

Contemporary diagnosis of BPH involves obtaining a PSA result. The latest guidelines from the American Urological Association (https://www.auanet.org) regarding the use of PSA testing are very helpful. Although the traditional upper limit of normal for PSA testing has been 4.0 ng/mL, recent guidelines are based more on changes in PSA levels over time, considering that most men with BPH will have prior PSA results. In the specific setting of using PSA to help manage BPH, the best data come from the Proscar Long-Term Efficacy and Safety Study (PLESS), where a PSA of 0 to 1.3 ng/mL, 1.4 to 3.2 ng/mL, and greater than 3.2 ng/mL was associated with small, medium, and large prostate glands (assuming that prostate cancer has been ruled out) and predicted therapeutic response to finasteride (Proscar) (see later).

Treatment

Treatment of BPH is always individualized to the patient and involves evaluation of symptoms and bother along with objective findings from examination and laboratory results. Current treatments range from periodic monitoring with a surveillance-only approach to the treatment of extreme cases with open or robotic enucleation surgery.

Active Surveillance and Watchful Waiting

For many men, especially those with lower symptom scores and little bother, annual monitoring with digital rectal examination, PSA, urinalysis, and symptom assessment are all that is required. Many men are happy to be reassured that they do not have clinically significant prostate cancer and are glad to hear that no immediate treatment is necessary.

Complementary and Alternative Medicine

The use of complementary and alternative medicine supplements is very common and physicians should ask patients about their use, just as they ask about prescription medications. There are now many "prostate" and "men's health" supplements containing a variety of chemicals, including zinc, saw palmetto,[7] vitamin E,[1] vitamin D[1], and selenium,[7] among others. Aside from a few European clinical trials of saw palmetto, the use of supplements to help BPH is speculative. One challenge is quality assurance of dose and ingredients of these agents, which are not regulated by the US Food and Drug Administration (FDA). Although it was not done to investigate BPH, the NIH-funded Selenium and Vitamin E Cancer Prevention Trial (SELECT) to determine whether vitamin E or selenium, or both, would prevent prostate cancer is illustrative. Neither supplement had any effect on prostate cancer (or BPH to our knowledge). With the lack of robust trial data for the plethora of supplements, the answer from evidence-based medicine is clear.

Medical Therapy
α-Blocker Medications

The use of oral α-adrenergic blocking agents to treat BPH has been commonplace since the 1980s. These agents are directed at the dynamic component of BPH and LUTS by relaxing the smooth muscle tissue in the bladder neck and prostate. In simple terms, they relax the bladder outlet, resulting in better urinary flow.

Initial agents, such as prazosin (Minipress),[1] were not selective blockers and were also used to treat hypertension. Furthermore, these early agents were not long acting and had to be taken multiple times per day, which severely limited their practical clinical utility. The next generation in the class were doxazosin (Cardura) and terazosin (Hytrin), which were longer-acting agents dosed only once a day. However, they were not selective and also lowered blood pressure, so titration was necessary. The third- and current-generation agents are selective blockers that treat BPH but do not lower blood pressure when used at recommended doses. The three in this class are tamsulosin (Flomax), alfuzosin (Uroxatral), and silodosin (Rapaflo).

In general, clinicians use α-blockers in men with smaller prostate glands (≤30–35 g or cm3), in younger men, and in patients where rapid effect is needed. Side effects of this class can include headache, dizziness, asthenia, drowsiness, and retrograde ejaculation, with alfuzosin reported to have the lowest rate of retrograde ejaculation among these drugs. The α-blockers are also now frequently used to relieve the dysfunctional voiding, which is believed to contribute significantly to some cases of prostatitis.

5α-Reductase Inhibitors

The 5α-reductase inhibitors have been available since the early 1990s. Finasteride (Proscar) was the first agent in this class (5 mg/day) and is a type 2 inhibitor. Dutasteride (Avodart; 0.5 mg/day) is a type 1 and type 2 inhibitor that was approved in 2002. Both drugs prevent the conversion of testosterone to the more active metabolite DHT in the prostate. This inhibition results in involution of BPH tissue and prostatic shrinkage. On average, most men achieve a reduction of 20% to 40% in prostate size after at least 6 months of use. In general these agents are most effective in men with prostate glands more than 30 g (or cm3) in size. Both drugs are expected to result in lower PSA levels by about 50% after 6 months of use. It is critical to take this into account when a patient is being screened for prostate cancer. If the PSA level does not fall by about half and the patient has been compliant with medication, he should be referred for urologic evaluation. In following up on men taking finasteride or dutasteride, PSA is generally doubled in assessing risk for prostate cancer. However, the PSA velocity or doubling time and other prostate cancer screening tools are still valid as long as the effect on PSA is appreciated.

Two key clinical trials are important. The Medical Therapy of Prostate Symptoms (MTOPS) trial showed that the combination of an α-blocker (doxazosin) and a 5α-reductase inhibitor (finasteride) was more effective than either alone or than placebo in treating BPH and LUTS. The Prostate Cancer Prevention Trial (PCPT), in a large 7-year study, showed that finasteride lowered the rate of prostate cancer by 25% over placebo. The Reduction by Dutasteride of Prostate Cancer Events (REDUCE) trial confirmed the prostate chemoprevention benefit of this class of drugs, showing that dutasteride also lowered the rate of prostate cancer by 23% over placebo. In 2010, the FDA ruled that dutasteride would not be approved for prostate cancer prevention, citing safety concerns in this prevention setting. In 2013, the long-term follow-up of the PCPT showed that there was no excess mortality associated with long-term finasteride use compared with placebo, proving the long-term safety of this therapy.

Urologists frequently use 5α-reductase inhibitors to treat chronic hematuria due to an enlarged prostate after exclusion of more worrisome etiologies such as renal or bladder cancer; they may also prescribe these agents before prostate surgeries or procedures for BPH to lessen surgical bleeding.

Minimally Invasive Procedures

In the past 35 years, a series of minimally invasive procedures have appeared in practice with the goals of reducing prostatic obstruction while preserving sexual function with normal

---

[1]Not FDA approved for this indication.
[7]Available as dietary supplement.

erections and ejaculation. Balloon dilation, transurethral microwave therapy (TUMT), and transurethral needle ablation (TUNA) have all fallen from favor due to lack of durable effect in improving LUTS. Two newer minimally invasive procedures have, however, shown durability in multiyear randomized clinical trials. The prostatic urethral lift procedure (UroLift) utilizes small, permanently implanted anchors placed cystoscopically that physically retract and compress the obstructing lobes of the prostate and can provide almost immediate improvement in flow rates and symptom scores. Alternatively, water vapor thermal therapy (Rezum) utilizes radiofrequency-generated water vapor (103°C) injected cystoscopically into the prostate tissue, resulting in gradual resorption of the treated tissue and significant improvements in flow rates and symptom scores over the course of weeks following the procedure. Both procedures carry the benefits of very low rates of ED and retrograde ejaculation; however, whether either procedure will provide long-lasting relief of LUTS similar to more invasive surgical procedures remains unknown. Prostatic artery embolization (PAE) has shown promise in several studies as a minimally invasive therapy for BPH; however, the 2018 American Urologic Association guidelines have recommended against PAE as therapy for bothersome LUTS outside of a clinical trial setting. High-intensity focused ultrasound was granted FDA approval in 2015 for ablation of prostate tissue but has not gained wide use for BPH management and is more frequently utilized in the treatment of prostate cancer.

Surgical Therapy

TURP remains the gold standard treatment for men who have failed to improve on medical therapy, who dislike or are intolerant of medication side effects, or who have developed urinary retention, renal failure secondary to BPH, or large bladder calculi. TURP is associated with relatively low rates of incontinence and ED; however, retrograde ejaculation is an expected and permanent outcome for most men undergoing this surgery. Evolutions of the traditional TURP procedure now utilize saline irrigation, thereby reducing the risk of hyponatremia during the procedure. Several laser technologies (Greenlight, Holmium, or Thulium) utilized for the enucleation or vaporization of prostate tissue have resulted in reduced hospital stays, transfusion rates, and duration of catheterization compared with TURP and are recommended treatment options for medically complex cases calling for anticoagulant therapy. Aquablation utilizes a transurethral water jet to ablate prostate tissue under ultrasound guidance. Finally, for men with severe BPH and very large glands (>150 g), simple prostatectomy performed robotically or via a small suprapubic incision remains a valuable and highly effective surgical treatment. As with radical prostatectomy used for the treatment of prostate cancer, open or robotic prostatectomy for BPH should be performed by urologic surgeons who are highly experienced in this area.

Summary

With the widespread acceptance of medical therapies for BPH in the 1980s and 1990s, treatment paradigms rapidly shifted away from surgical treatment for bothersome voiding symptoms. A growing number of studies have suggested an association between medical therapies for LUTS and the development of dementia. These studies are controversial and preliminary; however, it is common in our practice to encounter elderly men who are using two or three medications for the management of symptoms. With increasing awareness of the risks of polypharmacy and with the advent of new minimally based procedures for BPH, many of which can be performed in office, the pendulum seems to be swinging back toward the earlier consideration of surgical treatment for BPH.

References

Barkin J: Benign prostatic hyperplasia and lower urinary tract symptoms: evidence and approaches for best case management, *Can J Urol*(Suppl 18)14–19, 2011.

Biester K, Skipka G, Jahn R, et al: Systematic review of surgical treatments for benign prostatic hyperplasia and presentation of an approach to investigate therapeutic equivalence (non-inferiority), *BJU Int* 109:722–730, 2012.

Dahm P, Brasure M, MacDonald R, et al: Comparative effectiveness of newer medications for lower urinary tract symptoms attributed to benign prostatic hyperplasia: a systemic review and meta-analysis, *Eur Urol* 71:570–581, 2017.

Djavan B, Kazzazi A, Bostanci Y: Revival of thermotherapy for benign prostatic hyperplasia, *Curr Opin Urol* 22:16–21, 2012.

Gravas S, Bachmann A, Reich O, et al: Critical review of lasers in benign prostatic hyperplasia (BPH), *BJU Int* 107:1030–1043, 2011.

Lepor H, Kazzazi A, Djavan B: α-Blockers for benign prostatic hyperplasia: the new era, *Curr Opin Urol* 22:7–15, 2012.

Nicholson TM, Ricke WA: Androgens and estrogens in benign prostatic hyperplasia: past, present and future, *Differentiation* 82:184–199, 2011.

Roehrborn C, Barkin J, Gange S, et al: Five year results of the prospective randomized controlled prostatic urethral L.I.F.T. study, *Can J Urol* 24(3):8802–8813, 2017.

Roehrborn C, Gange S, Gittelman M, et al: Convective thermal therapy: durable 2-year results of randomized controlled and prospective crossover studies for treatment of lower urinary tract symptoms due to benign prostatic hyperplasia, *J Urol* 197(6):1507–1516, 2017.

Slater S, Dumas C, Bubley G: Dutasteride for the treatment of prostate-related conditions, *Expert Opin Drug Saf* 11:325–330, 2012.

EPIDIDYMITIS AND ORCHITIS

Method of
Robin A. Walker, MD

CURRENT DIAGNOSIS

- Subacute or gradual onset of scrotal pain and swelling that occasionally radiates to the lower abdomen. It is typically unilateral; however, inflammation can spread to the opposite testicle.
- Fever and urinary tract symptoms (e.g., dysuria, frequency, urgency, hematuria) may be present.
- The testicle should be in normal position with the cremasteric reflex intact (rule out torsion).
- Pain is relieved by elevation of testicle (Prehn sign).
- Ultrasound with Doppler is readily available and has high sensitivity and specificity for ruling out testicular torsion; however, referral to urology should not be delayed if torsion is suspected.
- Urinalysis should be obtained, preferably on first-void urine.
- Urine should be sent for culture, especially when a sexually transmitted disease (STD) is not suspected.
- Nucleic acid amplification assays for gonorrhea and chlamydia can be run on urine or urethral specimens.

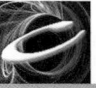

CURRENT THERAPY

- Sexually active men 14 to 35 years old: ceftriaxone(Rocephin)[1] 250 mg IM once and doxycycline (Vibramycin)[1] 100 mg BID for 10 days. Azithromycin (Zithromax)[1] 1 g PO for one dose may be substituted for doxycycline if compliance is questionable.
- Oral cephalosporins and fluoroquinolones are no longer recommended for gonococcal infections.
- For older men or when enteric organisms are thought to be the most likely cause: ceftriaxone 250 mg IM once plus either levofloxacin (Levaquin)[1] 500 mg PO bid for 10 days or ofloxacin (Floxin)[1] 300 mg PO bid for 10 days.
- Cultures, if obtained, should be followed and treatment adjusted accordingly.
- Patients should follow up in 2 to 3 days. Pain should improve in 1 to 3 days with treatment. Failure to improve should elicit reevaluation of the diagnosis and therapy, and consideration should be given to other causes, such as a testicular tumor/cancer, abscess, infarction, tuberculosis (TB), or fungal pathogens.
- Sexual partners should be referred for evaluation and treatment if there was intercourse in the preceding 60 days from onset of symptoms.
- Education should occur regarding prevention of STDs.

[1]Not FDA approved for this indication.

Epidemiology

Epididymitis is most common in males 18 to 35 years of age but can occur in all ages. There are approximately 600,000 cases per year in the United States, which accounted for 1 in 144 outpatient visits by men (2002 data).

In men 35 years of age or younger who are sexually active, the most common pathogens are *Chlamydia trachomatis* and *Neisseria gonorrhoeae*. In those older than 35 years, the cause is most likely a urinary tract pathogen, such as *Escherichia coli*. In men who perform insertive anal intercourse, coliform bacteria are common causative agents. Other less common pathogens include TB, fungal infections, and viruses. Cytomegalovirus has been identified as a cause in HIV patients.

In boys ages 2 to 13, the incidence is approximately 1.2 per 1000 and is most commonly a postinfectious inflammatory reaction to pathogens such as enteroviruses, adenoviruses, and mycoplasmal pneumonia. If a bacterial pathogen is isolated, a urologic workup for any anatomic abnormalities is warranted.

Other uncommon noninfectious causes of epididymitis include vasculitides and medications such as amiodarone (Pacerone).

Orchitis is less common than epididymitis and is most often associated with concurrent epididymitis, occurring in approximately 60% of men with epididymitis. In prepubertal boys, orchitis is usually a sequala of mumps infection. Between 20% and 30% of men with mumps develop orchitis.

Risk Factors

The predominant risk factor for epididymitis is unprotected sexual intercourse. Additionally, trauma from strenuous physical activity, bicycle or motorcycle riding, and prolonged sitting can predispose to epididymitis. Risk factors in prepubertal boys and men over age 35 are related to anatomic abnormalities (e.g., prostatic obstruction, posterior urethral valves, meatal stenosis), recent instrumentation, or urogenital tract surgery (e.g., vasectomy). In prepubertal boys, recent infections can predispose to a postinfectious inflammatory reaction in the epididymis.

Pathophysiology

Infective epididymitis is usually caused by the retrograde ascent of pathogens, most commonly bacterial. Noninfectious epididymitis can be autoimmune or can be associated with known syndromes (e.g., Behçet disease) or a side effect of medications, most notably amiodarone (Pacerone). If symptoms last longer than 3 months, the patient meets the diagnostic criteria for chronic epididymitis.

Clinical Manifestations

The typical presentation is a subacute onset of unilateral scrotal pain. Any acute onset of pain requires careful consideration of possible testicular torsion. The pain in epididymitis can radiate to the lower abdomen. Fever and urinary tract symptoms such as increased frequency, dysuria, and hematuria are frequently present. The cremasteric reflex is preserved and the testicle should be in its normal anatomic position. The epididymis is tender, swollen, and often indurated. Pain is relieved on testicular elevation (Prehn sign). Over time, scrotal wall erythema and a reactive hydrocele may appear and infection can spread from the epididymis to the testicle (orchitis) as well as to the opposite testicle.

Epididymitis secondary to noninfectious causes tends to have a more gradual onset of symptoms.

Viral orchitis from mumps is characterized by an abrupt onset of unilateral testicular pain with swelling that typically occurs between 4 and 7 days after the development of parotitis. About 75% of patients with orchitis will also have fever and one-third will complain of dysuria.

Diagnosis

Diagnosis can be made by a careful history and physical examination; however, laboratory testing can help to confirm epididymitis. Urine should be obtained for analysis and culture, preferably from a first-void sample. The presence of leukocyte esterase and 10 or more white blood cells (WBCs) per high-power field is suggestive of urethritis, helping to differentiate it from testicular torsion.

Nucleic acid amplification tests for *N. gonorrhoeae* and *C. trachomatis* should be run on all sexually active men 35 years of age or younger and those over age 35 who are at increased risk. These can be run on urine or urethral samples. A Gram stain of urethral discharge should demonstrate five or more WBCs per high-power field. Gonococcal infection is established by the presence of WBCs containing intracellular gram-negative diplococci. Depending on risks, consideration should be given to testing for the presence of other STDs.

Color Doppler ultrasound is a readily availability study with a sensitivity and specificity for testicular torsion ranging between 89% and 100%. However, imaging should not delay immediate referral to a specialist if torsion is clinically suspected.

Differential Diagnosis

- Testicular torsion: duration less than 6 hours, absence of cremasteric reflex, diffuse testicular tenderness. Elevation of the testis usually exacerbates discomfort.
- Orchitis: testicular tenderness and swelling, normal cremasteric reflex.

Therapy/Treatment

In sexually active men between the ages of 14 and 35, empiric treatment should be started for suspected epididymitis before laboratory results are available. The current recommended regimen is ceftriaxone (Rocephin)[1] 250 mg IM once plus doxycycline (Vibramycin)[1] 100 mg PO bid for 10 days. If compliance is questionable or the patient is allergic to doxycycline, azithromycin (Zithromax)[1] 1 g PO once can be substituted. The Centers for Disease Control and Prevention no longer recommends fluoroquinolones or oral cephalosporins for the treatment of gonococcal infections.

For men 35 year of age or older when a coliform pathogen is suspected, treatment consists of ceftiraxone (Rocephin) 250 mg once plus either levofloxacin (Levaquin)[1] 500 mg PO for 10 days or ofloxacin (Floxin)[1] 300 mg PO bid for 10 days.

Most patients can be treated in the outpatient setting. Inpatient treatment is recommended for suspicion of abscess, intractable pain, signs of sepsis, or failure of outpatient care. Symptomatic care consists of pain control with supportive garments, analgesics, rest, and cold packs.

Orchitis, when not associated with epididymitis infection, is typically treated in a supportive manner with hot or cold packs, rest, nonsteroidal antiinflammatory drugs (NSAIDs), and scrotal elevation. Symptoms from virus-associated orchitis typically resolve in 3 to 10 days.

Complications

Complications include sepsis, abscess, formation, extension of infection, and infertility.

---

[1]Not FDA approved for this indication.

References

Centers for Disease Control and Prevention. Sexually transmitted diseases treatment guidelines; 2015. Available at https://www.cdc.gov/std/tg2015/epididymitis.htm [accessed 09.28.20].

Centers for Disease Control and Prevention: Update to CDC's sexually transmitted diseases treatment guidelines, 2010; oral cephalosporins no longer recommended treatment for gonococcal infections, *MMWR Morb Mortal Wkly Rep*, 61:590–594, 2012.

Centers for Disease Control and Prevention: Update to CDC's sexually transmitted diseases treatment guidelines, 2006; fluoroquinolones no longer recommended for treatment of gonococcal infections, *MMWR Morb Mortal Wkly Rep*, 56:332–336, 2007.

Kaver I, Matzkin H, Braf ZF: Epididymo-orchitis: a retrospective study of 121 patients, *J Fam Pract* 30:548–552, 1990.

Remer EM, Casalino DD, Arellano RS, et al: ACR appropriateness criteria; acute onset of scrotal pain—without trauma, without antecedent mass, *Ultrasound Q* 28:47–51, 2012.

Trojian TH, Lishnak TS, Meiman D: Epididymitis and orchitis: an overview, *Am Fam Physician* 79:583–587, 2009.

ERECTILE DYSFUNCTION

Method of
Aleksandr Belakovskiy, MD; Joel J. Heidelbaugh, MD; and Karl T. Rew, MD

CURRENT DIAGNOSIS

- Questionnaire
- Sexual Health Inventory for Men (SHIM) [also called International Index of Erectile Function (IIEF-5)] https://www.baus.org.uk/_userfiles/pages/files/Patients/Leaflets/SHIM.pdf
- Assessment of risk factors
- Tobacco use
- Diabetes
- Hypertension
- Hyperlipidemia
- Obesity
- Iatrogenic causes
- Psychogenic causes
- Physical exam including vitals, body mass index (BMI), genital exam, and assessment for secondary sex characteristics
- Relationship between erectile dysfunction, endothelial dysfunction, and coronary heart disease

CURRENT THERAPY

- Lifestyle modifications including tobacco cessation, weight-loss, increased exercise
- Sexual health counseling
- Medication modification if taking medications knownto contribute to erectile dysfunction
- Pharmacotherapy (Table 1)
- Oral phosphodiesterase type 5 (PDE-5) inhibitors:avanafil (Stendra), sildenafil (Viagra), tadalafil (Cialis), and vardenafil (Levitra, Staxyn)
- Prostaglandin: alprostadil; either by intracavernosal injection(Caverject, Edex) or as an intraurethral suppository (Muse)
- Requires a test dose in the office and instruction ontechnique for proper administration
- Vacuum erectile devices
- Penile implants

Erectile dysfunction is the inability to attain or maintain a penile erection sufficient for sexual satisfaction.

Epidemiology
Numerous studies have investigated the prevalence of erectile dysfunction in men of various ages. Based on the most recent studies, worldwide prevalence increases with age. For men under age 40 the prevalence is 1% to 10%; for ages 40 to 49 it is 2% to 15%; for men ages 50 to 59 it is mixed, ranging from 15% to 40%; for ages 60 to 69 it is 20% to 40%; and for men 70 and older it is 50% to 100%. Among men in the United States the prevalence is 22% overall. This is higher than the 16% prevalence for seven other countries found in a study comparing the United States to Brazil, Mexico, United Kingdom, Germany, France, Italy, and Spain. Accurate diagnosis of erectile dysfunction has varied over time, with current literature favoring the use of validated questionnaires such as the Sexual Health Inventory for Men (SHIM; https://www.baus.org.uk/_userfiles/pages/files/Patients/Leaflets/SHIM.pdf).

Risk Factors
A number of medical conditions can predispose to erectile dysfunction. Numerous studies have demonstrated the correlation between cardiovascular disease and the incidence of erectile dysfunction. Risk factors that predispose to cardiovascular disease also play similar roles in erectile dysfunction, including increasing age, diabetes, hypertension, hyperlipidemia, tobacco use, and obesity.

Certain classes of medications can contribute to the development of erectile dysfunction. One of the most common is the antidepressants, specifically selective serotonin reuptake inhibitors (SSRIs) and serotonin norepinephrine reuptake inhibitors (SNRIs). Common antihypertensive medications can also contribute to or exacerbate erectile dysfunction, including beta blockers, alpha blockers, calcium channel blockers, and thiazides. Other medication classes that should be considered in patients with erectile dysfunction include opiates, first-generation antihistamines, and benzodiazepines.

Risk factors for psychogenic erectile dysfunction should also be evaluated. Psychogenic erectile dysfunction can occur at any age, but it is frequently seen in men under age 40, and it often occurs in men with anxiety, stress, depression, or a history of sexual abuse. Assess for healthy sexual partnerships by asking about performance anxiety and sexual desire discrepancy, both of which are common contributors to erectile dysfunction. Clues that erectile dysfunction may have a psychogenic component include the ability to have normal erections with masturbation, and the continued presence of nocturnal erections. If needed for evaluation, nocturnal tumescence testing can be performed.

Tobacco, alcohol, opioids, and substances such as marijuana and cocaine can cause erectile dysfunction. All substance use should be assessed. Many other health issues can contribute to erectile dysfunction, including a history of prostate or pelvic surgery, radiation therapy, or trauma; gonadal, thyroid, or other diseases that affect hormone levels; testicular pain; and chronic diseases that affect general health and well-being.

Pathophysiology
The pathophysiology of erectile dysfunction depends on the etiology of the condition. Many men have multiple potential causes. Psychogenic erectile dysfunction is due to nonorganic causes, while individuals with risk factors for cardiovascular disease primarily have etiologies stemming from vascular disease. Iatrogenic erectile dysfunction due to medication use or prior surgery may be caused by inhibition of the parasympathetic nervous system or other mechanisms of action.

Erectile dysfunction can be a warning sign of silent cardiovascular disease. The relationship between erectile dysfunction and the risk factors for coronary heart disease was noted in the Massachusetts Male Aging Study. The endothelial dysfunction that can precede the clinical stage of atherosclerotic disease is recognized as an additional risk factor for erectile dysfunction in men without symptoms of cardiovascular disease. Endothelial function is mediated by nitric oxide, which is also the mechanism responsible for the vascular dilatation required to obtain and maintain an erection. A man with erectile dysfunction should be considered at risk for cardiovascular disease until proven otherwise.

Prevention
Erectile dysfunction prevention is centered around treating modifiable risk factors. Treatment of overweight and obesity with dietary changes and increased aerobic exercise can aid in the prevention of erectile dysfunction. For tobacco users, cessation should be strongly encouraged. Bupropion (Zyban) and varenicline (Chantix) can be used for smoking cessation with limited risk of exacerbating erectile dysfunction. Nicotine replacement therapy can be used as a bridge to help with tobacco cessation. Appropriate treatment of comorbid diseases, including diabetes, hypertension, and hyperlipidemia can also aid in prevention. Sexual health counseling that focuses on good partner communication and healthy relationship dynamics can help prevent psychogenic erectile dysfunction.

Clinical Manifestations

Many men are uncomfortable mentioning problems of sexual function. Some men will report erectile dysfunction without providing information on the specifics of their concern. It is important for physicians to proactively ask about sexual function, and to clarify if a patient's concern is with achieving or maintaining an erection, or if it may be related to ejaculation or low libido. Low libido can be secondary to stress, mood disorders, hypogonadism, or other causes. The evaluation and potential treatments will differ based on the specific concern. Questionnaires such as the SHIM (https://www.baus.org.uk/_userfiles/pages/files/Patients/Leaflets/SHIM.pdf) can provide additional information to help distinguish the specific clinical manifestation.

Diagnosis

The history provides the majority of information needed for the diagnostic evaluation, including a review of known medical and surgical history, use of medications and substances, an assessment of current relationship satisfaction, and a questionnaire such as the SHIM. The history should include risk factor evaluation, assessment for any history of cardiovascular disease, diabetes, hypertension, hyperlipidemia, or mood disorders, as well as a review of medications that might contribute to erectile dysfunction. A physical exam should also be performed, including evaluation of blood pressure, body mass index, secondary sex characteristics, and a genital exam.

The role of laboratory studies is limited. In individuals who lack secondary sex characteristics, as well as those with refractory symptoms despite PDE-5 inhibitor use, check a morning total testosterone to assess for hypogonadism. Limited evidence supports obtaining a morning total testosterone in all men with erectile dysfunction. If the initial morning total testosterone is low, it should be repeated at least once in several months to confirm the diagnosis. If morning testosterone levels are normal in a patient with high likelihood of hypogonadism, a free testosterone or bioavailable testosterone can be checked to help account for the effects of sex hormone–binding globulin. If evidence of hypogonadism is found, additional testing to distinguish primary versus secondary hypogonadism should be done. Hemoglobin A1c and a lipid panel may be helpful if there is a suspicion for underlying diabetes, hyperlipidemia, or cardiovascular disease contributing to erectile dysfunction. If a review of symptoms elicits a suspicion for hypothyroidism, checking a thyroid stimulating hormone level may be indicated. Consultation with a urologist, endocrinologist, or men's health specialist may be helpful when the etiology is unclear.

Differential Diagnosis

In men presenting with concern for erectile dysfunction, the differential diagnosis is geared toward deciphering the underlying cause. As previously mentioned, there are numerous potential contributing factors to erectile dysfunction. It is important to assess for both organic and psychogenic causes. The history should include asking about nocturnal tumescence, as well as the ability to achieve and maintain an erection with and without a partner. If erectile dysfunction occurs regardless of situation, this is more likely to indicate an organic etiology. If it occurs primarily with a partner, further evaluation of the relationship is indicated. As mentioned above, numerous factors can predispose to erectile dysfunction, and related diagnoses may include cardiovascular disease, tobacco use, diabetes, hypertension, hyperlipidemia, obesity, and metabolic syndrome. Medications should also be reviewed, because they can cause iatrogenic erectile dysfunction in some patients.

Therapy (or Treatment)

Lifestyle modifications play an important role in both the prevention and treatment of erectile dysfunction. Weight reduction for overweight or obese men (BMI >25 kg/m²) and increased exercise for all men can improve SHIM scores. Underlying illnesses such as hyperlipidemia, hypertension, and diabetes should be adequately controlled in order to decrease their potential impact on erectile dysfunction. Another important consideration is tobacco cessation; current or former smoking increases the risk of erectile dysfunction. Sexual health counseling is often helpful for individuals and couples dealing with erectile dysfunction, no matter what the etiology is. Referral to a mental health professional or sexuality expert may be beneficial.

Pharmacologic treatment begins with oral PDE-5 inhibitors. They prevent the breakdown of cyclic guanosine monophosphate (cGMP) and allow increased nitric oxide levels, causing smooth muscle relaxation of the corpora cavernosa, and helping to sustain an erection. This requires a functional libido as well as intact vasculature in order to achieve an erection. There are four PDE-5 inhibitors currently approved in the United States for treatment of erectile dysfunction: avanafil (Stendra), sildenafil (Viagra), tadalafil (Cialis), and vardenafil (Levitra, Staxyn) (see Table 1). There are no significant differences in safety or benefit among these medications. Tadalafil has a longer duration of action than the others.

PDE-5 inhibitors are usually taken on an as-needed basis, with onset of effects typically within about 1 hour of ingestion. The lowest effective dose should be used to reduce the risk of adverse reactions. Higher doses do not lead to a linear increase in beneficial effect, but can increase the risk of adverse reactions. Tadalafil, because of its longer duration of action, can be taken daily at a lower dose with similar efficacy to as-needed dosing. The duration of adverse effects may be longer with daily use.

The most common adverse reactions to PDE-5 inhibitors include headache, flushing, dyspepsia, dizziness, nasal congestion, visual disturbance, and myalgias. Overall, these adverse reactions tend to be mild to moderate in nature and are similar across all four medications. Special consideration should be given to individuals who take nitrate-containing medications; the combination of a PDE-5 inhibitor with nitrates can cause severe hypotension that may be life threatening.

Testosterone is not an effective monotherapy for erectile dysfunction. However, for men with confirmed hypogonadism, the combination of a PDE-5 inhibitor with testosterone replacement may be effective.

If patients do not have adequate symptom relief with lifestyle modification, sexual health counseling, and oral PDE-5 inhibitor use, the prostaglandin alprostadil (Caverject, Edex, Muse) can be considered. Alprostadil works by relaxing arterial smooth muscle and is available in intraurethral and injectable preparations (see Table 1). The intraurethral formulation (Muse) is a dissolvable suppository placed in the urethra with an applicator. The injectable form (Caverject, Edex) is injected directly into one side of the corpora cavernosa. Alprostadil can be used as a single agent or in combination with a PDE-5 inhibitor. If the patient is amenable to a trial of alprostadil, an in-office test dose should be administered to find the lowest effective dose and to teach proper administration technique. Some patients may not be suitable candidates if they are not comfortable with injections or intraurethral insertion. Alprostadil should be avoided in patients who have sickle cell anemia or other risk factors for priapism.

If pharmacological therapies are ineffective or contraindicated, patients may elect to use a vacuum erectile device. These prescription devices are placed over the penis and a vacuum pump removes air from inside the device, creating an influx of blood into the penis and leading to an erection. A ring is then slid from the base of the vacuum tube onto the penis to constrict the outflow of blood and maintain the erection. To avoid ischemic injury, the ring should only be used for up to 30 minutes. Adverse effects of vacuum erectile devices may include the erect penis feeling cool or cold to the touch due to the restricted blood flow, and bending at the base of the penis due to the application of the constricting ring. Overall, these devices have a fairly high satisfaction rate. Caution should be used when considering a vacuum erectile device for patients who are taking anticoagulants or have bleeding disorders.

For patients with erectile dysfunction refractory to the above treatments, surgical implantation of a penile prosthesis can be offered. Penile prostheses come in several forms, including inflatable devices and persistently semirigid implants. Patients and

TABLE 1 Pharmacotherapy for Erectile Dysfunction

GENERIC NAMES	BRAND NAMES	SIZES	TYPICAL DOSING	COMMENTS
Oral Phosphodiesterase Type 5 (PDE-5) Inhibitors				
avanafil	Stendra	50-, 100-, 200-mg tablet	50–200 mg by mouth once daily as needed, 1 h before sexual activity	Use lowest effective dose. Contraindicated with nitrates.
sildenafil	Viagra	25-, 50-, 100-mg tablet	25–100 mg by mouth once daily as needed, 1 h before sexual activity	Use lowest effective dose. Contraindicated with nitrates.
tadalafil	Cialis	2.5-, 5-, 10-, 20-mg tablet	5–20 mg by mouth once daily as needed, 1 h before sexual activity OR 2.5–5 mg by mouth once daily without regard to sexual activity	Use lowest effective dose. Contraindicated with nitrates. Has a longer duration of action than other PDE-5 inhibitors.
vardenafil	Levitra Staxyn	5-, 10-, 20-mg tablet 10-mg oral dissolving tablet	5–20 mg by mouth once daily as needed, 1 h before sexual activity	Use lowest effective dose. Contraindicated with nitrates. Available as a 10 mg oral dissolving tablet (Staxyn)
Prostaglandin				
alprostadil injectable	Caverject20 mcg/mL, 40 mcg/mL vials	Caverject Impulse10 mcg/0.5 mL, 20 mcg/0.5 mL prefilled syringesEdex 10 mcg/mL, 20 mcg/mL, 40 mcg/mL cartridges	Initiate dose at 1.25 or 2.5 mcg intracavernosally and titrate does with no more than 2 doses per 24 hours (maximum dose: 40 mcg [Edex], 60 mcg [Caverject]). Self administration: maximum 3 times/week with 24 hours between doses	Provide an in-office test dose and instruction in proper technique for administration. Use lowest effective dose.
alprostadil intraurethral	Muse	125-, 250-, 500-, 1000-mcg urethral suppositories	Initiate dose at 125 or 250 mcg intraurethrally and titrate dose on separate occasions in physician's office. Maximum 2 suppositories per 24 hours for self-administration	Provide an in-office test dose and instruction in proper technique for administration. Use lowest effective dose.

their partners should be counseled regarding risks and benefits to ensure realistic postsurgical expectations. Risks include scarring, penile shortening, recurrent infections, and mechanical failure requiring removal.

Monitoring
A validated questionnaire such as the SHIM (https://www.baus.org.uk/_userfiles/pages/files/Patients/Leaflets/SHIM.pdf) is a simple and reliable tool for monitoring ongoing symptoms. A periodic clinical evaluation, including a review of all supplements and medications, can be helpful to identify potential causes of symptoms and any adverse reactions.

Management of Complications
The majority of adverse reactions with PDE-5 inhibitors are mild to moderate in nature and can be limited by using the lowest effective dose. PDE-5 inhibitors are contraindicated in patients taking nitrates because of the significant risk of life-threatening hypotension. If accidentally ingested, the patient should be monitored by healthcare professionals. The risk also depends on which specific agent was ingested, as the duration of action differs between medications. While the risk of prolonged erection (priapism) is low with PDE-5 inhibitors, men with erections lasting greater than 4 hours should seek emergency attention.

The major potential complication of alprostadil is a prolonged erection lasting greater than 4 hours, which will require emergent urological treatment. Penile fibrosis is also a risk that has been reported in 4.9% of patients using alprostadil at 4 years.

Treatment with exogenous testosterone impairs spermatogenesis and should be avoided in men who are trying to conceive or are interested in future fertility.

The major complication of vacuum erectile devices is ischemic injury, generally when the constricting ring is left in place for greater than 30 minutes at a time. Any suspicion for ischemic injury should also prompt emergent urologic intervention.

Patients with penile implants are prone to recurrent infections or mechanical failure, potentially requiring removal of the device.

References
Burnett AL, Nehra A, Breau RH, et al: Erectile dysfunction: AUA Guideline, *J Urol* 200(3):633–641, 2018 Sep, https://doi.org/10.1016/j.juro.2018.05.004. Epub 2018 May 7.

Buvat J, Büttner H, Hatzimouratidis K, et al: Adherence to initial PDE-5 inhibitor treatment: randomized open-label study comparing tadalafil once a day, tadalafil on demand, and sildenafil on demand in patients with erectile dysfunction, *J Sex Med* 10(6):1592–1602, 2013.

Costa P, Grandmottet G, Mai HD, Droupy S: Impact of a first treatment with phosphodiesterase inhibitors on men and partners' quality of sexual life: results of a prospective study in primary care, *J Sex Med* 10(7):1850–1860, 2013.

Ghanem HM, Salonia A, Martin-Morales A: SOP: physical examination and laboratory testing for men with erectile dysfunction, *J Sex Med* 10(1):108–110, 2013.

Khayyamfar F, Forootan SK, Ghasemi H, Miri SR, Farhadi E: Evaluating the efficacy of vacuum constrictive device and causes of its failure in impotent patients, *Urol J* 10(4):1072–1078, 2014.

Martin-Morales A, Haro JM, Beardsworth A, Bertsch J, Kontodimas S: Therapeutic effectiveness and patient satisfaction after 6 months of treatment with tadalafil, sildenafil, and vardenafil: results from the erectile dysfunction observational study (EDOS), *Eur Urol* 51(3):541–550, 2007.

Mccabe MP, Sharlip ID, Lewis R, et al: Incidence and prevalence of sexual dysfunction in women and men: a consensus statement from the Fourth International Consultation on Sexual Medicine 2015, *J Sex Med* 13(2):144–152, 2016.

Mulhall JP, Trost LW, Brannigan RE, et al: Evaluation and management of testosterone deficiency: AUA Guideline, *J Urol* 200(2):423–432, 2018 Aug, https://doi.org/10.1016/j.juro.2018.03.115. Epub 2018 Mar 28.

Rosen RC, Fisher WA, Eardley I, et al: The multinational Men's Attitudes to Life Events and Sexuality (MALES) study: I. Prevalence of erectile dysfunction and related health concerns in the general population, *Curr Med Res Opin* 20(5):607–617, 2004.

Selvin E, Burnett AL, Platz EA: Prevalence and risk factors for erectile dysfunction in the US, *Am J Med* 120(2):151–157, 2007.

PROSTATE CANCER

Method of
William G. Nelson, MD, PhD

CURRENT DIAGNOSIS

- Serum prostate-specific antigen (PSA) testing, with or without digital rectal examination (DRE), can be used for prostate cancer screening for men beginning at age 50 years until age 70 years.
- Prostate cancer screening carries significant risks of overdiagnosis and overtreatment of clinically insignificant prostate cancers.
- The diagnosis of prostate cancer is usually made via ultrasound-guided transrectal core needle biopsies that sample the prostate; magnetic resonance imaging (MRI) is increasingly used to direct core biopsies to regions of the prostate suspicious for harboring aggressive prostate cancers.
- Histologic grade (Gleason score) and anatomic stage provide prognosis needed for treatment decision making. Several different tumor-based molecular biomarker tests can add further prognostic information.
- Metastatic prostate cancer can be evaluated using ^{99m}Tc-methylene diphosphonate (MDP) of ^{18}F-sodium fluoride (NaF) bone scans, abdominopelvic computed tomography (CT) scan or MRI, and ^{11}C-choline, ^{18}F-fluciclovine, or ^{68}Ga-PSMA positron emission tomography (PET) studies.
- Germline genetic testing for DNA repair gene variants, along with tumor testing for DNA repair gene defects, tends to accompany diagnosis of high-risk localized, loco-regionally advanced, and metastatic prostate cancer.

CURRENT THERAPY

- Options for management of localized prostate cancer include active surveillance, radical prostatectomy, external beam radiation therapy, brachytherapy, and proton radiotherapy.
- Androgen deprivation therapy (ADT) using gonadotrophic hormone-releasing hormone analogs is a mainstay of systemic prostate cancer treatment.
- CYP17 inhibitors and androgen receptor antagonists can be used to further ablate androgen signaling.
- Taxane chemotherapy, given along with ADT for hormone-sensitive metastatic prostate cancer or at the time of progression to castration-resistant prostate cancer (CRPC), improves survival.
- The α–particle-emitting calcium mimetic ^{223}Ra can palliate painful, bony metastases.
- Poly(ADP-ribose) polymerase (PARP) inhibitors may be effective in up to 20% of men with CRPC who carry germline and/or somatic mutations in homologous recombination repair genes (*BRCA1, BRCA2, ATM,* and others).
- Immune checkpoint blockade may be of benefit for men with mismatch repair-deficient prostate cancer.

Prostate cancer comprises the most commonly diagnosed cancer among men in the United States, with an estimated 248,530 new cases and 34,130 deaths expected for 2021. Some 1 in 8 men can expect to be diagnosed with prostate cancer at some point during life, though the risk of dying from the disease is only about 1 in 41. African American men suffer disproportionately with the disease, exhibiting more than twice the age-adjusted mortality as Caucasians.

The prostate itself is a male sex accessory gland located adjacent to the rectum in the pelvis and surrounding the urethra to supply secretions to the ejaculate. Why it should spawn so many cancers has proven enigmatic. The prostate can be divided into three zones, a *peripheral zone* where most prostate cancers arise, a *transition zone* near the urethra prone to benign enlargement (benign prostatic hyperplasia/hypertrophy [BPH]), and a *central zone*. Under the influence of the male androgenic hormones testosterone (T) and dihydrotestosterone (DHT), normal epithelial cells produce the serine protease prostate-specific antigen (PSA; encoded by the gene *KLK3*). The appearance of PSA in the bloodstream tends to indicate epithelial barrier dysfunction within the prostate, attributable to three highly prevalent conditions in aging men in the United States: inflammation (prostatitis), BPH, or prostate cancer. Blood testing for PSA has emerged as a common screening tactic for prostate cancer, necessarily confounded by the near ubiquitous coexistence of prostatitis and BPH.

Most men present with prostate cancer apparently confined to the prostate gland, often detected by PSA screening. Though usually indolent, when aggressive, prostate cancer tends to spread to bony sites, causing pain by undermining bone architecture through stimulating osteoblastic activity, a phenomenon readily evident via ^{99m}Tc-methylene diphosphonate (MDP) of ^{18}F-sodium fluoride (NaF) bone scanning. Men dying of prostate cancer also manifest metastasis to lymph nodes, liver, the dura, and elsewhere.

Men diagnosed with prostate cancer today confront a large and often confusing array of treatment options. The typical man diagnosed with the disease is at least 65 years of age or older; the risks and benefits associated with different treatment choices in this age range are relevant not only for prostate cancer specialty care but for general medical care as well. The 5-year survival for a man with localized prostate cancer is >95%, underscoring the need for balancing prostate cancer treatment selection with other health priorities.

Epidemiology

Heredity plays as significant a role in prostate cancer development as for any other common cancer. Analyses of concordance for prostate cancer between monozygotic (identical) versus dizygotic (fraternal) twins have consistently found excess prostate cancers among the identical twins despite similar environmental exposures, leading to the estimate that as many as 42% of prostate cancer cases may be attributable to inheritance. Two sets of inherited susceptibility genes merit special attention for prostate cancer treatment. Germline defects in DNA double-strand break repair genes, such as *BRCA1, BRCA2, ATM, PALB2, FANCA, RAD51D,* and *CHEK2,* or in DNA mismatch repair genes, such as *MSH2, MLH1,* MSH6, and *PMS2,* may increase the risk of developing prostate cancer or of exhibiting metastatic prostate cancer progression. Defective DNA repair in prostate cells has important treatment implications. When germline DNA repair gene defects are accompanied by somatic alterations at the remaining allele, crippling of DNA double-strand break repair can serve as an indication for treatment with poly(ADP-ribose) polymerase (PARP) inhibitors, while loss of DNA mismatch repair constitutes an indication for treatment with immune checkpoint inhibitors. With a growing role in prostate cancer treatment decision making, both germline testing and tumor tissue testing for DNA repair gene defects have become increasingly common for men with the disease. Of course, the detection of defective DNA repair genes in the germline of a man with prostate cancer should also alert his physician to consider cascade genetic testing of relatives, as abnormal repair gene carriers could be at risk for breast, ovarian, colorectal, or other cancers.

Evidence for a critical contribution of the environment to prostate cancer is as strong as is the case for an impact of heredity. Prostate cancer incidence and mortality vary widely throughout the world, and migrants from low-risk regions to high-risk regions tend to adopt higher prostate cancer predilection within a single generation. Whether the high rates of prostate cancer in the United States reflect ingestion of food carcinogens, such as the heterocyclic amines and polycyclic aromatic hydrocarbons in overcooked meats (known to cause prostate cancer in rodents), or reflect inadequate intake of tomatoes and cruciferous vegetables, replete with antioxidant micronutrients (known to protect against prostate cancer in model studies), has not been established. Whatever the etiology of the disease, prostates removed at autopsy from high-risk parts of the world display an astonishing abundance both of chronic inflammation and of undiagnosed prostate cancers. And, in rodent models, exposures that cause prostate cancer also trigger chronic prostatic inflammation, connecting the two disease processes. In the United States, asymptomatic prostatitis arises in nearly all men as they age, leading to the appearance of proliferative inflammatory atrophy (PIA) lesions, the earliest histologic precursors to prostate cancer. In turn, small prostate cancers ultimately appear in as many as 64% of men age 60 to 70 years. Fortunately, the majority of these cancers pose little threat to health or to life. Nonetheless, this reservoir of indolent asymptomatic disease in the midst of chronically inflamed prostates complicates prostate cancer screening, early detection, and treatment, leading to significant overdiagnosis and overtreatment of the disease.

Risk Factors

Key risk factors for prostate cancer include age, family history, African ancestry, a diet rich in saturated fats and red meats, and a sedentary lifestyle—all features that may motivate the use of prostate cancer screening as a part of routine primary care. The most widely used screening strategies feature blood testing for PSA with or without digital rectal examination (DRE), usually beginning at age 50 to 55 years or earlier for African American men, for men with a strong family history, or for men known to be carriers of prostate cancer risk genes. Unfortunately, even though the benefits of screening for reducing prostate cancer progression to metastasis and prostate cancer mortality have been demonstrated in a large randomized trial, prostate cancer screening remains highly controversial. The United States Preventive Services Task Force (USPSTF) formally recommends that men aged 55 to 69 years discuss the potential benefits and harms of prostate cancer screening with their physician before pursuing PSA testing and rectal examination (assigning a grade C). For men aged 70 years and older, the USPSTF recommends against prostate cancer screening (grade D).

Pathophysiology

Nearly all of the exposures that can cause prostate cancers in laboratory mice and rats, ranging from charred meat carcinogens to estrogens to various "hit-and-run" infectious agents, trigger chronic inflammatory changes in prostate tissues that lead to PIA. Some fraction of PIA lesions, likely those exhibiting morphologic atypia and containing somatic genome alterations, in turn progress to prostatic intraepithelial neoplasia (PIN) and to prostate cancer.

The normal prostate contains an epithelium able to contribute secretions to the ejaculate. The epithelium features (1) basally located cells, expressing cytokeratins K5 and K14, and p63; (2) columnar secretory cells, expressing the androgen receptor (AR), PSA, cytokeratins K8 and K18, and prostate-specific membrane antigen (PSMA); and (3) neuroendocrine cells, producing chromogranin A, neuron-specific enolase, and synaptophysin. PIA lesions arising in response to epithelial damage give rise to "intermediate cells" that express markers characteristic of both basal and luminal cells. The cellular target of transformation is likely such an "intermediate cell"; the resultant PIN or prostate cancer cells exhibit many of the phenotypic characteristics of columnar secretory cells, including the expression of AR, PSA, and PSMA, and acquire expression of new gene products, such as α-methylacyl-CoA racemase (AMACR). For this reason, many prostate pathologists use immunohistochemical staining for basal cells (antibodies against cytokeratins K5/K14 and p63) and for neoplastic prostate cells (antibodies against AMACR) to aid in prostate cancer diagnosis; prostate cancer cells tend to be cytokeratin K5/K14-negative, p63-negative, and AMACR-positive.

Prostate cancer cells acquire a number of somatic genome and epigenome alterations. Fusion translocations of an androgen-regulated gene, *TMPRSS2*, to genes encoding various members of the E26 transformation-specific (ETS) family of transcription factors are the most common somatic genetic changes in prostate cancers. Somehow, these gene fusions allow prostate cancer cells to coopt androgen signaling to drive neoplastic transformation and malignant progression. As a result, interference with androgen signaling forms the foundation for most advanced prostate cancer treatments. When such translocations are not present, other somatic alterations, such as mutations in *SPOP*, are more frequent. Hypermethylation of *GSTP1*, encoding detoxification enzyme for carcinogens and oxidants, can be detected in >90% of cases. DNA methylation changes at other loci are also very common. The somatic defects in genes and gene function somehow allow prostate cancer cells to proliferate, escape terminal differentiation, and survive to grow in ectopic sites, such as in bones, lymph nodes, and other organs. Two notable somatic gene defects, mutations or deletions in *TP53* and in *PTEN*, have been consistently associated with malignant prostate cancer progression.

Prevention

There are no established drugs that prevent prostate cancer, although there have been three very large randomized clinical trials of agents for prostate cancer prevention. One such trial aimed to test predictions from epidemiologic studies and earlier small clinical trials that inadequate intake of the micronutrients selenium and vitamin E might lead to increased prostate cancer risk. The trial, called Selenium and Vitamin E Cancer Prevention Trial (SELECT), enrolled men 55 years or older (50 years or older for African Americans) with an unremarkable DRE and a serum PSA of 4.0 ng/mL or less to treatment with the micronutrients for 7 to 12 years (randomized to 200 μg selenomethionine[7] daily, 400 IU α-tocopherol[7] daily, the combination, or neither). Unfortunately, the study failed to show any reduction in prostate cancer, instead revealing a slight increase in prostate cancer incidence among men taking vitamin E. As a result, high-level intake of selenium, vitamin E, and other nutritional supplements for the purpose of prostate cancer prevention should be discouraged.

The two other large randomized trials tested the propensity for the 5α-reductase inhibitors finasteride (Proscar)[1] and dutasteride (Avodart)[1] to prevent prostate cancer development. In one of the studies, called the Prostate Cancer Prevention Trial (PCPT), finasteride (5 mg daily or a placebo) was given to healthy men age 55 years and older, with a normal DRE and a serum PSA of 3.0 ng/mL or less, for 7 years. During the trial, men with increasing PSA values or an abnormal DRE were subjected to prostate biopsy. At the end of the trial, biopsies were planned for all of the men. The results were a decrease in prostate cancer detection from 24.4% of men receiving a placebo to only 18.4% of men treated with finasteride, but an increase in more aggressive high-grade prostate cancers in men receiving finasteride versus placebo from 6.4% to 5.1%.

Similar results were encountered with dutasteride in the other trial, called Reduction by Dutasteride of Prostate Cancer Events (REDUCE), where men with an elevated serum PSA between 2.5 to 10.0 ng/mL and a recent negative prostate biopsy were given dutasteride (0.5 mg daily) or a placebo for 4 years, with prostate biopsies obtained after 2 and 4 years on study. Overall, prostate cancer was reduced from 25.1% to 19.9% for men taking dutasteride, but high-grade prostate cancer was increased in these men from <0.1% to 0.5%. Data from PCPT and REDUCE clearly indicated that 5α-reductase inhibitors are better at preventing low-grade cancers than high-grade cancers. Whether the development of high-grade cancers was actually increased in either trial, or whether these cancers were just more easily detected, has been controversial, and the US Food and Drug Administration (FDA)

---

[1]Not FDA approved for this indication.
[7]Available as dietary supplement.

has not approved either finasteride or dutasteride for prostate cancer prevention. In 2019, long-term follow-up of participants in the PCPT revealed no increases in prostate cancer mortality accompanying finasteride treatment, likely affirming the general safety of 5α-reductase inhibitor treatment for BPH and male pattern baldness and reanimating discussions about how 5α-reductase inhibitors might be used to lower the overall burden of prostate cancer in some way.

Clinical Manifestations

Most men present for prostate cancer care after a diagnosis triggered by prostate cancer screening and are thus initially asymptomatic. Local progression of the disease can result in lower urinary tract symptoms of voiding obstruction or irritation, in urinary tract infections and urosepsis, in erectile dysfunction, in hematospermia, and in diminished ejaculate volume. Metastatic prostate cancer dissemination most often involves the skeleton, resulting in bone pain and low blood counts, and involves pelvic lymph nodes and nearby lymphatics, resulting in lower extremity edema or retroperitoneal fibrosis, respectively.

Diagnosis

Prostate cancer diagnosis is typically made using transrectal ultrasound (TRUS)-guided prostate biopsy. The technique involves the repeated firing of an 18-gauge needle from a spring-loaded gun through a port on the TRUS probe. To sample prostate tissue, the biopsy needle passes through the rectum into the prostate, and fluoroquinolone antibiotics are typically administered before the biopsy procedure. Hematuria and/or hematospermia occur commonly after prostate biopsy. Hospital admissions, usually the result of an infection, are rare but can be needed in up to 7% of men with significant comorbidities. Importantly, TRUS does not delineate the locations of prostate cancers within the prostate. For this reason, the numbers and sites of biopsies placed during a prostate biopsy procedure, typically 10 to 12 directed laterally into the peripheral zone of the gland, are designed to minimize the chance of missing life-threatening high-grade cancers.

Increasingly, magnetic resonance imaging (MRI) has been employed to better direct prostate biopsies, hoping to reduce detection of low-grade cancers that pose little threat to life and to more accurately sample high-grade disease. Multiparametric MRI (mpMRI) incorporates T2-weighted anatomic imaging, diffusion-weighted imaging, and contrast enhancement to highlight suspicious areas in the prostate for biopsy. The technique generates a standardized "suspicion" score for individual lesions, using the Prostate Imaging–Reporting and Data System (PI-RADS). The magnetic resonance (MR) image itself can then be used to direct TRUS biopsies via coregistration (or "fusion") of the acquired mpMRI data with real-time TRUS. Biopsies obtained by MRI/TRUS fusion are becoming more widespread, especially for men who need a repeat biopsy because of a persistently elevated or rising serum PSA.

The histologic grade and anatomic stage of newly diagnosed prostate cancer carry important prognostic information useful for treatment planning. Recently, prostate cancer grade "groups" (1, best prognosis and 5, worst prognosis) have been introduced into clinical practice as risk tools for localized prostate cancer. These "groups" are derived from Gleason scoring as conducted by an expert genitourinary pathologist. The Gleason score represents the sum of the two most common histologic patterns of growth exhibited by the cancer within the prostate; the pattern designations range from pattern 3 to pattern 5 (there are no patterns 1 or 2), providing Gleason scores from 6 to 10. The disease stage focuses on the extent of tumor in the prostate itself (T1, not palpable by DRE; T2, palpable by DRE; T3, extending outside the prostate itself; and T4, invading adjacent pelvic structures), in regional lymph nodes (N0, no lymph node metastases; N1, lymph node metastases), and in distant sites (M0, no distant metastases; M1, metastases). Staging tools include a number of imaging modalities, including abdominopelvic computed tomography (CT) or MR images and nuclear medicine scans for soft tissue and for bone, using ^{11}C-choline, ^{18}F-fluciclovine, or ^{18}F-sodium fluoride. New nuclear medicine scans targeting PSMA, expressed by normal and neoplastic prostate cells, are under development. FDA approval has been granted for ^{68}Ga-PSMA positron emission tomography (PET)-CT (or PET-MRI) scanning for prostate cancer detection in lymph nodes or for identifying site of recurrence in the setting of a rising serum PSA after local treatment.

Differential Diagnosis

The critical issue surrounding the diagnosis and staging of many men with prostate cancer is whether the disease is at risk to progress to threaten life or whether it is so indolent as to not need treatment. Most men with indolent disease indicated by a Gleason score of 6 (grade group 1) do not need immediate treatment, and many may never need treatment. Instead, these men can be monitored using *active surveillance*, with serum PSA tests twice yearly, DREs each year, and MR images and/or prostate biopsies as necessary or after 2 to 4 years. This surveillance strategy aims to detect higher Gleason score prostate cancer if it appears. Gleason score greater than 7 (grade groups 2–5) tends to be an indication for curative local disease treatment with surgery or radiation therapy. Deferring aggressive local therapy as part of active surveillance appears safe, and as a result, active surveillance has become a common approach to prostate cancer care. By avoiding aggressive intervention until and unless necessary, active surveillance is distinct from observation or watchful waiting approaches, which are typically reserved for men with significant comorbidities and limited life expectancy.

Therapy

For localized prostate cancer with Gleason score greater than 7 (grade groups 2–5), curative treatments include radical prostatectomy, interstitial brachytherapy, and external beam radiation therapy. Most radical prostatectomies these days are performed using a robot-assisted laparoscopic approach. Urinary incontinence and erectile function after the procedure vary greatly between surgeons, with as many as 20% of men describing some level of urine leakage 2 years after radical prostatectomy, and at least 26% of men reporting significant sexual dysfunction a year after surgery. Ideally, following surgery, the serum PSA should fall to an undetectable level and remain so in perpetuity if the procedure resulted in prostate cancer cure. Two-thirds of men subjected to radical prostatectomy remain free of PSA recurrence 15 years after surgery. A rising serum PSA after surgery is a sign that prostate cancer has recurred or persisted somewhere. Nonetheless, such a PSA rise may not herald imminent overt metastasis or death. In one analysis, only 30% of men with a rising serum PSA postsurgery had suffered with metastatic prostate cancer by 8 years after the initial PSA increase. The rate of serum PSA rise can be informative; a rapid doubling of serum PSA values is usually associated with a greater threat of symptomatic disease progression.

Prostate brachytherapy provides for direct irradiation of localized prostate cancer, via implantation of radioactive sources into the prostate using image guidance. The procedure itself is fairly convenient, able to be completed as an outpatient within a couple of hours using spinal anesthesia. The most common radioactive sources used are ^{125}I (iodine) and ^{103}Pd (palladium) and as many as a hundred seeds might be implanted. In general, though the ^{125}I seeds decay more slowly than the ^{103}Pd seeds, prostate brachytherapy implants are essentially inert by 10 months after insertion into the prostate. Complications of brachytherapy for prostate cancer differ from those of radical prostatectomy and of external beam radiotherapy, with irritative voiding symptoms reported by at least half of men in the first few months after implant placement. These symptoms tend to abate after a year or so, persisting in some 15% to 20% of men. Long-term side effects can include urethral stricture, incontinence, erectile dysfunction, and rectal irritation. Relative contraindications to prostate brachytherapy include large prostate size (requires a lot of seeds or use of androgen deprivation to shrink the prostate), preimplant obstructive urinary symptoms (greatly worsen after implantation), and history of transurethral surgery for symptomatic BPH (tends to lead to incontinence).

A series of technical innovations have improved both the efficacy and safety of external beam radiation therapy, including CT-based treatment planning, the use of multileaf collimators in modern linear accelerators, and improvements in treatment planning software. Three-dimensional conformal radiation therapy (3D-CRT) allows creation of more accurate target volumes using reconstructions of pelvic CT images, better sparing vulnerable structures such as the bladder and the rectum. Intensity-modulated radiation therapy (IMRT) even further optimizes dose distribution for prostate cancer treatment, by controlling the intensity of radiation dose, in addition to the shape of the volume designated for treatment. Despite more accurate deposition of radiation doses to the prostate, side effects of external beam radiation therapy remain mostly rectal toxicity (early irritation and late rectal bleeding), late urethral strictures, and erectile dysfunction. External beam radiation can also be used as adjuvant therapy for prostate cancer with positive surgical margins after radical prostatectomy or as salvage therapy for local prostate cancer recurrence after surgery.

Proton beam radiotherapy has become available at a limited number of treatment centers. The physical properties of protons allow them to deposit energy very precisely, with little radiation dose to skin and little radiation scatter to nearby tissues. This behavior is ideal for cancers located in close proximity to sensitive structures in the body, such as at the base of the skull, near the eye, and elsewhere. For prostate cancer, proton radiotherapy has emerged as an effective treatment for localized disease, but whether this approach offers an improvement over conventional external beam radiation using 3D-CRT with IMRT awaits the results of an ongoing randomized clinical trial.

Systemic approaches to prostate cancer include agents targeted at androgen signaling, taxane chemotherapy, radiopharmaceuticals, PARP inhibitors, and immune checkpoint inhibitors. Disruption of androgen signaling has been a mainstay of advanced prostate cancer care for seven decades. Originally accomplished by surgical removal of the testes, and later by the administration of estrogens, androgen deprivation therapy (ADT), involving a reduction in circulating testosterone levels to <50 ng/mL, is now more commonly achieved by inhibition of pituitary gonadotropin production, using luteinizing hormone–releasing hormone (LHRH) analogs that cause suppression of testosterone production. Injectable LHRH analogs are all available in long-acting depot formulations (goserelin [Zoladex] 10.8 mg depot every 3 months, leuprolide [Lupron Depot] 22.5 mg depot every 3 months, and triptorelin [Trelstar] 3.75 mg depot monthly) and antagonists (degarelix [Firmagon] 240 mg depot initially followed by 80 mg depot monthly). An oral LHRH antagonist, relugolix [Orgovyx or Relumina] 360 mg initially followed by 120 mg daily, has also become available. The benefits of ADT are evident in most men by a decline in the serum PSA, a shrinkage of metastatic cancer deposits, and improvements in symptoms, such as bone pain, that accompany metastatic prostate cancer progression. Side effects often include hot flashes, bone loss, reduced libido, decreased muscle mass, increased fat, and fatigue. An increased risk for cardiovascular disease is also suspected, and ADT may prolong the QT/QT$_c$ interval by electrocardiography.

Ultimately, most men on ADT for advanced prostate cancer progress to castration-resistant prostate cancer (CRPC). Nonetheless, the prostate cancers in many men with CRPC remain addicted to androgen signaling and continue to produce PSA, which requires an activated AR. In this setting, two strategies have emerged to ablate androgen signaling more completely. One involves the use of the AR antagonists enzalutamide ([Xtandi] 160 mg daily), apalutamide ([Erleada] 240 mg daily), and darolutamide ([Nubeqa] 600 mg twice daily). Each is approved by the FDA for CRPC; enzalutamide is approved for CRPC with or without overt metastases, whereas apalutamide and darolutamide are approved for CRPC without overt metastases (enzalutamide and apalutamide are also approved to give along with ADT for castration-sensitive

metastatic prostate cancer). A second approach involves inhibition of adrenal steroid biogenesis to further reduce circulating levels of androgenic hormones. Abiraterone ([Zytiga] 1000 mg daily with 5 mg prednisone twice daily), a CYP17 inhibitor, suppresses extragonadal androgen production and provides an effective treatment for CRPC. Abiraterone must be administered along with replacement corticosteroids (5 mg prednisone twice daily). Blood testing for circulating prostate cancer cells expressing the AR mRNA splice variant V7 (AR-V7) for men with CPRC can predict resistance to AR antagonists and abiraterone, steering men instead toward taxane chemotherapy. Also, both AR antagonists and abiraterone are being explored in combination with LHRH analogs in clinical trials as initial systemic hormone treatment for high-risk localized prostate cancer.

ADT can be used as adjuvant therapy along with prostate radiotherapy, as initial treatment for prostate cancer recurrence manifest as a rapidly rising serum PSA in the absence of overt metastases following surgery or radiotherapy, and as treatment for established metastatic prostate cancer, with or without taxane chemotherapy. Of these three indications, the use of ADT for men with disease recurrence after primary therapy remains somewhat controversial. The concern is that the benefits may not be much better than waiting to initiate ADT until overt metastases can be detected, while the hazards, including bone loss, possible risk for cardiovascular complications, and poor quality-of-life are significant. Careful monitoring of PSA rises and periodic use of imaging studies may allow for introduction of ADT before symptoms of metastatic prostate cancer appear. ^{68}Ga-PSMA PET-CT or PET-MRI scanning for prostate recurrence in the setting of a rising serum PSA can aid in treatment planning and timing. Another tactic for ADT I this setting has been intermittent administration. Intermittent ADT appears to control prostate cancer progression as well as continuous ADT and to provide some minor improvement in quality-of-life. Finally, a novel strategy now in clinical trials for men with advanced prostate cancer exposed to ADT for at least 6 months is the administration of androgenic hormones. This approach can lower serum PSA levels in more than half of men treated and improve quality-of-life.

Of all of the cytotoxic chemotherapy drugs used for advanced prostate cancer, agents targeting intracellular microtubules have exhibited disproportionate activity. Prostate cancer cells tend to have low growth rates, rendering most antineoplastic drugs that interfere with cell replication less effective than for other cancers. Taxane drugs, including docetaxel (Taxotere) and cabazitaxel (Jevtana), disrupt microtubule function in both replicating and nonreplicating cells. In nonreplicating prostate cancer cells, the taxane drugs may hinder the trafficking of AR and other critical gene regulatory proteins into the cell nucleus, triggering apoptosis. Both docetaxel (75 mg/m^2 every 3 weeks given along with prednisone 10 mg daily) and cabazitaxel (25 mg/m^2 every 3 weeks given along with prednisone 10 mg daily) are effective treatments for CRPC, able to lower serum PSA, reduce measurable volumes of cancer seen on imaging studies, and prolong disease survival. Docetaxel toxicity includes significant neutropenia, ankle edema, peripheral neuropathy, hair loss, and nail changes. Cabazitaxel, which was more effective than docetaxel for multidrug-resistant tumor cells in preclinical studies and better able to penetrate the blood–brain barrier, was initially used to treat docetaxel-resistant CRPC. In that setting, cabazitaxel caused more substantial neutropenia than docetaxel and was associated with more diarrhea and asthenia. A randomized trial comparing docetaxel to cabazitaxel as first-line treatment for metastatic CRPC revealed similar overall survival for either treatment, and docetaxel remains the preferred first-line chemotherapy option. Six doses of docetaxel given every 3 weeks is now frequently used along with ADT for men with metastatic hormone-sensitive prostate cancer, significantly prolonging overall survival compared with ADT alone in two large randomized clinical trials. In addition to the taxanes docetaxel and cabazitaxel, the topoisomerase poison mitoxantrone (Novantrone) is approved by the FDA as an agent capable of improving quality-of-life for men with CRPC.

Palliation of symptomatic bone metastases in men with CRPC can be achieved using the α–particle-emitting calcium mimetic ^{223}Ra. The agent has a brief half-life ($t_{1/2}$ = 11.4 days) and a marked proclivity for skeletal uptake; an estimated 40% to 60% of administered ^{223}Ra ends up in bones. ^{223}Ra (50 kBq/kg) is typically given in six injections at 4-week intervals. Side effects include nausea, vomiting, diarrhea, leg swelling, and low blood counts. More recently, ^{177}Lu- and ^{225}Ac-labeled PSMA ligands have been introduced into the care of men with CRPC. Early trials hint at marked beneficial treatment responses. Nonetheless, significant xerostomia resulting from salivary gland toxicity (a site of PSMA expression) bedevils the use of these agents so far. Attempting to optimize radiolabeled PSMA ligand dosing to limit salivary gland damage, to prevent radioisotope uptake by the salivary gland, and to improve treatment for salivary gland dysfunction, postradioactive PSMA ligand administrations are ongoing.

The up to 20% of men with CRPC who carry germline and/ or somatic mutations in homologous recombination repair genes (*BRCA1*, *BRCA2*, *ATM*, *PALB2*, *FANCA*, *RAD51D*, and *CHEK2*) may derive significant benefit from treatment with PARP inhibitors. PARPs are enzymes that contribute to several steps in DNA repair. Inhibition of PARP in cells with homologous recombination deficiency results in "synthetic lethality" and apoptosis. This phenomenon has been exploited successfully for the treatment of ovarian and breast cancers carrying defective homologous recombination repair genes. The PARP inhibitors olaparib ([Lynparza] 300 mg twice daily), rucaparib ([Rubraca] 600 mg twice daily), and niraparib ([Zejula][1] 300 mg daily) have all shown early evidence of activity in the treatment of CRPC with deficient homologous recombination repair; olaparib and rucaparib are FDA approved for CRPC in the setting of homologous recombination repair gene defects. Common side effects of PARP inhibitors include gastrointestinal symptoms and fatigue.

Two additional systemic treatment approaches merit attention. First, for CRPC arising in the setting of DNA mismatch repair deficiency, like other cancers with DNA mismatch repair defects, the immune checkpoint inhibitor pembrolizumab ([Keytruda][1] 200 mg every 3 weeks) can be effective at achieving significant and durable treatment responses. Major side effects include "autoimmune breakthrough events" such as colitis, pneumonitis, and hypophysitis. Immune checkpoint inhibitor therapy otherwise shows very little activity against prostate cancers. Second, for men with CRPC manifest as small cell neuroendocrine cancer, treatment with chemotherapy doublet regimens like cisplatin or carboplatin and etoposide may be helpful.

Monitoring

Men treated for clinically localized prostate cancer by surgery or radiation therapy are monitored for cancer recurrence principally by serum PSA testing every 6 to 12 months and by DRE yearly. A newly detectable or rising serum PSA can trigger a more complete evaluation using bone scans, abdominopelvic CT or MRI, and ^{11}C-choline, ^{18}F-fluciclovine, or ^{68}Ga-PSMA PET. ^{18}F-deoxyglucose PET imaging is not helpful. If necessary, a prostate biopsy may be undertaken in the setting of disease recurrence after radiation therapy.

Metastatic prostate cancer treatment can be monitored using serial serum PSA determinations and repeated imaging at known and/or symptomatic sites of disease. In addition, whether used for nonmetastatic or metastatic prostate cancer, ADT carries a substantial risk of osteoporosis. As such, men should be subjected to dual energy x-ray absorptiometry (DEXA) scanning. For men with a low fracture risk, calcium (1000 mg) and vitamin D (400 IU) supplements may suffice, but for men facing a higher probability of bone fracture, treatment with agents such as denosumab ([Prolia] 60 mg every 6 months), zoledronic acid ([Reclast][1] 4 mg no more often than monthly), or alendronate ([Fosamax][1] 70 mg once weekly) should be considered along with calcium and

vitamin D. Men receiving ADT should also be screened for diabetes and for cardiovascular disease, conditions that are common among men in the age range for prostate cancer.

Management of Complications

Men who are survivors of prostate cancer face a number of health challenges that comprise long-term side effects of the treatment(s) they received. Surgery tends to disrupt urinary and sexual functions. Stress incontinence may be the most common urinary problem, though more severe incontinence can occur. Urinary symptoms, such as urgency, frequency, and nocturia can arise; sometimes these symptoms herald the appearance of a urethral stricture at the site of the anastomosis of the bladder neck to the urethra during surgery. Urethral strictures related to scarring can be distinguished from cancer recurrence and treated via dilation by a urologist. Sexual problems include difficulties achieving erections sufficient for intercourse and a change in sexual experience attributable to lack of ejaculation and to differences in orgasms. Frank discussions about sexual function after primary prostate cancer treatment can aid in sexual recovery. Some urologists have attempted to use phosphodiesterase type 5 inhibitors (sildenafil [Viagra][1] 50 mg, vardenafil [Levitra][1] 10 mg, and tadalafil [Cialis][1] 5 mg) early after surgery to augment restoration of erectile function. These drugs have also been used successfully by some men to improve erections months and years after surgery. Radiation therapy late effects can also include urinary and sexual difficulties, and can involve the rectum in inflammation, pain, bleeding, and incontinence. Minor rectal symptoms can be alleviated using stool softeners, but more severe complications require the attention of a gastroenterologist or colorectal surgeon. Hyperbaric oxygen may help some men with radiation proctitis as a late effect of prostate cancer treatment.

ADT causes a diverse collection of long-term side effects, including loss of libido, erection problems, hot flashes, weight gain and obesity, mood changes/depression, anxiety/distress, gynecomastia, anemia, osteoporosis, diabetes/metabolic syndrome, and decreased lean muscle mass. Increased physical activity and dietary changes appropriate for obesity can be helpful. Careful attention and screening for psychological stress and depression should be a routine aspect of prostate cancer survivorship care. Even men likely cured of prostate cancer by surgery or radiation therapy frequently suffer with significant "PSA anxiety" around the time of follow-up vigilance to detect disease recurrence. Hot flashes, which occur in as many as 40% of men on ADT, can be treated using selective serotonin reuptake inhibitors such as paroxetine ([Paxil][1] 10 to 20 mg daily), serotonin and norepinephrine uptake inhibitors such as venlafaxine ([Effexor XR][1] 75 mg daily), or the anticonvulsant gabapentin ([Neurontin][1] 600 mg or more daily).

---

[1]Not FDA approved for this indication.

References

Antonarakis ES, Feng Z, BJet al. T, et al: The natural history of metastatic progression in men with prostate-specific antigen recurrence after radical prostatectomy: long-term follow-up, *BJU Int* 109:32–39, 2012.

De Marzo AM, Platz EA, Sutcliffe S, et al: Inflammation in prostate carcinogenesis. *Nat Rev Cancer* 7:256–269, 2007.

Mateo J, Carreira S, Sandhu S, et al: DNA repair defects and olaparib in metastatic prostate cancer, al. *N Engl J Med* 373:1697–1708, 2015.

Nelson WG, Antonarakis ES, Carter HB, De Marzo AM, DeWeese TL: Prostate cancer. In Niederhuber JE, Armitage JO, Doroshow JH, Kastan MB, Tepper JE, editors: *Abeloff's clinical oncology*, 6 ed, Churchill Livingstone, 2018.

Nelson WG, De Marzo AM, Isaacs WB: Prostate cancer, *N Engl J Med* 349:366–381, 2003.

Nuhn P, De Bono JS, Fizazi K, et al: Update on systemic prostate cancer therapies: management of castration-resistant prostate cancer in the era of precision oncology, *Eur Urol* 75:88–99, 2019.

Sanda MG, Dunn RL, Michalski J, et al: Quality of life and satisfaction with outcome among prostate-cancer survivors, *N Engl J Med* 358:1250–1261, 2008.

Siegel RL, Miller KD, Fuchs HE, et al: Cancer statistics, 2021, *CA Cancer J Clin* 71:7–33, 2021.

Viswanathan SR, Ha G, Hoff AM, et al: Structural alterations driving castration-resistant prostate cancer revealed by linked read genome sequencing, *Cell* 174:433–447, 2018.

---

[1]Not FDA approved for this indication.

PROSTATITIS

Method of
Charles R. Powell, MD

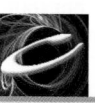

CURRENT DIAGNOSIS

- The workup for prostatitis begins with a thorough history and physical as well as a urinalysis and urine culture. Diagnosis is based on symptoms (Figure 1) and tenderness on digital rectal examination. There is a controversial role for prostate massage and culture of expressed prostatic secretions.
- Urinalysis and midstream urine culture are important to distinguish bacterial from nonbacterial causes but is not necessary for the diagnosis of prostatitis.
- Prostatitis is categorized as acute or chronic. It has been further characterized by the United States National Institutes of Health (NIH) National Institute of Diabetes, Digestive, and Kidney disorders (NIDDK) into four categories: acute bacterial, chronic bacterial, chronic pelvic pain syndrome (also called chronic nonbacterial prostatitis), and asymptomatic (Table 1).
- Chronic prostatitis is defined as duration longer than 3 months and typically manifests with pelvic pain and lower urinary tract symptoms.

CURRENT THERAPY

- The majority of prostatitis falls under the category of chronic prostatitis/chronic pelvic pain syndrome, and monotherapy has not proven effective.
- Fluoroquinolone antibiotics are first-line therapy for acute and chronic *bacterial* prostatitis, which are thought to comprise <10% of all cases. Ciprofloxacin (Cipro) and levofloxacin (Levaquin) have demonstrated cure rates of 73% to 75% in one randomized controlled trial (RCT) with culture-proven prostatitis.
- Trimethoprim/sulfamethoxazole (Bactrim)[1] can be considered first-line therapy, but local antibiotic resistance patterns should be considered prior to empiric treatment.
- First-generation cephalosporins, doxycycline (Vibramycin),[1] tetracycline,[1] azithromycin (Zithromax),[1] and clarithromycin (Biaxin)[1] are all second-line agents.
- Acute prostatitis may require inpatient admission and intravenous (IV) antibiotics depending on the severity and presence of sepsis. Urinary retention may require suprapubic tube urinary drainage as a foley catheter may worsen prostate inflammation.
- The role of antibiotics in the treatment of *chronic pelvic pain syndrome* is less clear. Treatment directed at *specific phenotypes* has improved outcomes. The UPOINT treatment philosophy has garnered much interest in the urologic community and is used to phenotype subjects and to direct multimodal therapy.

[1]Not FDA approved for this indication.

Epidemiology

The prevalence of prostatitis is approximately 8.2% (range, 2.2%–9.7%). It accounts for 8% of visits to urologists and up to 1% of visits to primary care physicians. In 2000, the estimated cost to diagnose and treat prostatitis was $84 million, not including pharmaceutical spending.

Risk Factors

The risk factors for prostatitis include urinary tract infection, elevated post-void residual (urinary retention), recent history of prostate biopsy, urinary catheterization, unprotected anal intercourse, recent urethral instrumentation such as cystoscopy, and condom catheter use.

Pathophysiology

Prostatitis is commonly associated with infection, but can also describe noninfectious chronic pelvic pain as well as asymptomatic histologic evidence of sterile inflammation. The causes for acute and chronic *bacterial* prostatitis include prior genitourinary infections such as epididymitis/orchitis, infection resulting from prostate needle biopsy, and recent urinary tract infection. Other predisposing factors include obstruction of urine from urethral stricture, benign prostatic hyperplasia (BPH), or neurogenic causes. A causative organism can be found in <10% of prostatitis cases. The causative organisms include *Escherichia coli* (most common at 65%–80% of infections), *Pseudomonas aeruginosa*, *Serratia* species, *Klebsiella* species, and *Enterobacter aerogenes*. Gram-positive organisms include enterococci. Organisms isolated from patients with recent history of lower urinary tract instrumentation or manipulation exhibit more resistance to ciprofloxacin (Cipro) and cephalosporins. For these patients, ciprofloxacin is often inadequate. A combination of cephalosporins and aminoglycosides is appropriate. Patients with a history of human immunodeficiency virus (HIV) infection should prompt investigation for atypical pathogens. The cause of chronic pelvic pain syndrome/chronic nonbacterial prostatitis (National Institutes of Health [NIH] category 3) is less well understood, as is asymptomatic prostatitis (NIH category 4).

Prevention

Prophylactic antibiotic dose is appropriate prior to urologic procedures, particularly prostate needle biopsy according to the American Urological Association Best Practice Statement for Urologic Surgery (https://www.auanet.org). Preprocedure rectal swabs to assess resistance patterns are now considered in select cases where resistance is more likely.

Clinical Manifestations

Figure 1 details some symptoms of prostatitis, separated by domain.

Diagnosis

Diagnosis of acute and chronic bacterial prostatitis is primarily based on history, physical examination, urine culture, and urine specimen testing pre- and postprostatic massage. If acute bacterial prostatitis is suspected, prostatic massage should not be performed as this might be harmful. Sexually active men younger than 35 years and older men who engage in high-risk sexual behaviors should be tested for *Neisseria gonococcus* and *Chlamydia trachomatis* as well. The presence of leukocytes in the semen, first voided urine, midstream urine, expressed prostatic secretions, or postprostatic massage urine did not correlate with symptoms when studied in a prospective manner. Bacterial localization studies, such as the Meares-Stamey 4-glass test, are useful in subcategorizing type 3 chronic pelvic pain syndrome but have unclear significance in the acute clinical setting.

Differential Diagnosis

The differential diagnosis of prostatitis includes acute cystitis, BPH, prostate cancer, urinary tract stones, bladder cancer, prostatic abscess, enterovesical fistula, foreign body within the urinary tract, voiding dysfunction, and inflammatory conditions of the bladder such as interstitial cystitis/painful bladder syndrome.

Therapy (or Treatment)

Treatment depends on the NIH National Institute of Diabetes, Digestive, and Kidney disorders (NIDDK) prostatitis classification category. For those with acute prostatitis, oral ciprofloxacin

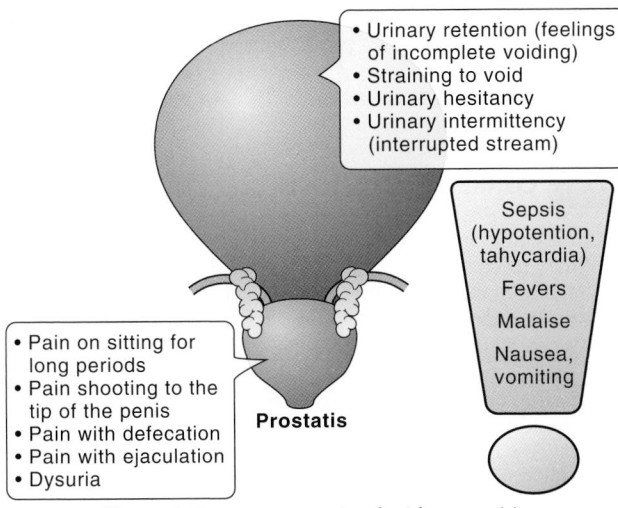

- Urinary retention (feelings of incomplete voiding)
- Straining to void
- Urinary hesitancy
- Urinary intermittency (interrupted stream)

Sepsis (hypotention, tahycardia)

Fevers

Malaise

Nausea, vomiting

Prostatis

- Pain on sitting for long periods
- Pain shooting to the tip of the penis
- Pain with defecation
- Pain with ejaculation
- Dysuria

Figure 1 Symptoms associated with prostatitis.

TABLE 1	National Institutes of Health Consensus Classification of Prostatitis
CATEGORY	**DESCRIPTION**
I. Acute bacterial prostatitis	Acute infection of the prostate gland with positive urine or semen cultures. Symptoms present for less than 3 months
II. Chronic bacterial prostatitis	Chronic infection of the prostate gland with positive urine or semen cultures. Symptoms present for greater than 3 months
III. Chronic pelvic pain syndrome	Chronic pelvic pain in the absence of bacterial infection localized to the prostate. Symptoms present for greater than 3 months
A. Inflammatory	Significant WBC count in the prostatic secretions, urine, or semen
B. Noninflammatory	Insignificant WBC count in the prostatic secretions, urine, or semen
IV. Asymptomatic prostatitis	WBC count elevated and/or bacteria in the prostatic secretions, urine, semen, or histologic specimens of prostate tissue

WBC, White blood cell.

(Cipro)[1] 500 mg orally, twice daily for 4 to 6 weeks or levofloxacin (Levaquin)[1] 500 mg orally, once daily for 4 to 6 weeks is appropriate for nonseptic appearing patients. Trimethoprim/sulfamethoxazole (Bactrim, Septra),[1] 160 mg/800 mg orally twice daily for 4 to 6 weeks is also appropriate, depending on local antibiotic resistance patterns. Patients appearing septic (hypotension, tachycardia, high fevers) should be admitted to the hospital and started on broad-spectrum antibiotics such as ampicillin 2 g intravenous every 6 hours and an aminoglycoside such as gentamicin 1 mg/kg intravenous every 8 hours. Aminoglycosides should be monitored and adjusted based on serum peak and trough levels. Aminoglycosides should be used cautiously in patients with azotemia. Prostatic abscess should be considered if patients do not improve within 24 to 48 hours. Prostatic abscesses are urologic emergencies and can be drained with transurethral resection of the prostate, ultrasound-guided transrectal needle drainage, or computed tomography (CT)-guided needle drainage. Urinary retention should be treated with suprapubic catheter drainage in cases of acute prostatitis. Chronic bacterial prostatitis (CBP) is treated with the same oral agents as acute bacterial prostatitis. For the treatment of chronic pelvic pain syndrome (CPPS), antibiotics play a less clear role, but fluroquinolone antibiotics used empirically for 4 to 6 weeks have been effective in previously untreated patients. There is little value to repeated courses of antibiotics if the first course is not effective. There is conflicting evidence for alpha blockers such as tamsulosin (Flomax 0.4 mg orally once per night).[1] The interested reader is referred to a review article by Nickel and Shokes 2010, wherein a multidisciplinary approach is advocated taking into account a more detailed six-domain phenotype with therapy directed at the relevant phenotype(s). This is known as UPOINT. These phenotype domains include urinary (broken down into voiding and storage symptoms), psychosocial (subdivided into depression and catastrophizing), organ specific (divided into bladder and prostate), infection (noted in the urine or expressed prostatic secretions), neurologic (divided into focal and systemic), and tenderness (muscle). Categorizing patients according to these domains may allow clinicians to personalize treatment using a multimodal approach involving physical therapy, psychiatry, and medication.

Other therapies have been described with low-quality evidence for efficacy. These are included below as an alternative treatment option for patients who do not respond to the interventions and strategies outlined above. The 5-alpha reductase inhibitors (finasteride [Proscar®][1]) have demonstrated slight improvement over placebo in two underpowered randomized controlled trials (RCTs), but carry a 10% to 15% risk of adverse events including "partial impotence." Chronic opioid therapy (COT) is appealing to some, but as the United States Centers for Disease Control (CDC) has noted, the harms outweigh the benefits for most causes of chronic pain. Its use should be discouraged. Celecoxib (Celebrex®)[1] has demonstrated no benefit over placebo in one RCT utilizing the NIH-Chronic Prostatitis Symptom Index (CPSI) instrument as the validated endpoint. Allopurinol (Zyloprim)[1] has demonstrated a slight benefit versus placebo in an underpowered RCT that utilized a nonvalidated questionnaire as the clinical endpoint. Pentosan Polysulfate (Elmiron®)[1] has demonstrated a slight benefit in the NIH-CPSI quality-of-life domain compared with placebo, but not in other endpoints. Twenty-two of 100 men (22%) withdrew from the study due to adverse events such as diarrhea, headache, and nausea. Transurethral microwave therapy (TUMT) of the prostate, a treatment for BPH, has been noted in one very small RCT (n = 20) comparing sham treatment versus TUMT reported 7/10 patients having at least 50% improvement, measured by nonvalidated "global assessment" endpoint. Transurethral resection of the prostate (TURP) has also been discussed but no RCT exists having the intent to treat men with chronic prostatitis. It is an untested option for men in whom all other treatment modalities have failed, but it has a long history of ameliorating obstructive and irritative lower urinary tract symptoms (LUTS), which often accompany CPPS. Investigators have noted some nonrandomized benefit to administration of 200 units onabotulinumtoxin A (Botox) directly into the prostate. They report that 72% of 42 nonrandomized men responded at 3 months, compared with 0% who underwent cystoscopy alone. The improvement fell to 37% at 12 months, not surprising since the medication loses efficacy 6 to 12 months after administration.

[1]Not FDA approved for this indication.

[1]Not FDA approved for this indication.

Monitoring

Monitoring is based on symptoms. In cases of acute prostatitis treated with appropriate antibiotics, persistent fevers should prompt a workup for prostatic abscess. The NIH-CPSI patient-reported questionnaire can be used to quantify symptoms over time. It is available online at http://eprovide.mapi-trust.org/instruments/national-institute-of-health-chronic-prostatitis-symptom-index. PSA testing plays no role in the treatment or monitoring of prostatitis but should be considered if risk factors for prostate cancer are present such as a prostate nodule or family history. PSA testing is affected by acute inflammation and should be postponed until a few months after the symptoms of prostatitis have resolved.

Complications

Acute prostatitis can progress to urosepsis and hypotension. CBP might have the ability to progress to chronic pelvic pain syndrome and become a source of pain for years.

References

Abdel-Meguid TA, Mosli HA, Farsi H, et al: Treatment of refractory category III nonbacterial chronic prostatitis/chronic pelvic pain syndrome with intraprostatic injection of onabotulinumtoxinA: a prospective controlled study, *Can J Urol* 25(2):9273–9280, 2018.

Bowen DK, Dilubanza E, Schaefer A: Chronic bacterial prostatitis and chronic pelvic pain syndrome, *BMJ Clin Evid* 8:1802, 2015.

Bundrick W, Heron SP, Ray P, et al: Levofloxacin versus ciprofloxacin in the treatment of chronic bacterial prostatitis: a randomized double-blind multicenter study, *Urology* 62:537–541, 2003.

Collins M, Stafford RS, O'Leary MP, et al: How common is prostatitis? A national survey of physician visits, *J Urol* 159(4):1224–1228, 1998.

Ha US, Kim ME, Kim CS, et al: Acute bacterial prostatitis in Korea: clinical outcome, including symptoms, management, microbiology and course of disease, *Int J Antimicrob Agents* 31(Suppl 1):S96–S101, 2008.

Krieger JN, Lee SW, Jeon J, et al: Epidemiology of prostatitis, *Int J Antimicrob Agents* 31(Suppl 1):S85–S90, 2008.

Leskinen M, Lukkarinen O, Marttila T: Effects of finasteride in patients with inflammatory chronic pelvic pain syndrome: a double-blind, placebo-controlled, pilot study, *Urology* 53:502–505, 1999.

Litwin MM, Fowler FJ, Nickel JC, et al: *Prostatatitis: the National Institutes of Health chronic prostatitis symptoms Index (NIH-CPSI)*. Retrieved 12/26/2012, 2012, from http://www.prostatitis.org/nih-cpsi.html.

Litwin M, McNaughton-Collins M, Fowler FJ, et al: The National Institutes of Health chronic prostatitis symptom index: development and validation of a new outcome measure. Chronic Prostatitis Collaborative Research Network, *J Urol* 162(2):369–375, 1999.

Nickel JC, Downey J, Pontari MA, et al: A randomized placebo-controlled multicentre study to evaluate the safety and efficacy of finasteride for male chronic pelvic pain syndrome (category IIIA chronic nonbacterial prostatitis), *BJU Int* 93:991–995, 2004.

Nickel JC, Forrest JB, Tomera K, et al: Pentosan polysulfate sodium therapy for men with chronic pelvic pain syndrome: a multicenter, randomized, placebo controlled study, *J Urol* 173:1252–1255, 2005.

Nickel JC, Shoskes DA: Phenotypic approach to the management of the chronic prostatitis/chronic pelvic pain syndrome, *BJU Int* 106(9):1252–1263, 2010.

Nickel J, Sorensen R: Transurethral microwave thermotherapy for nonbacterial prostatitis: a randomized double-blind sham controlled study using new prostatitis specific assessment questionnaires, *J Urol* 155:1950–1955, 1996.

Persson B, Ronquist G, Ekblom M: Ameliorative effect of allopurinol on nonbacterial prostatitis: a parallel double-blind controlled study, *J Urol* 155:961–964, 1996.

Pontari MA, Joyce GF, Wise M, et al: Prostatitis, *J Urol* 177(6):2050–2057, 2007.

Roberts RO, Lieber MM, Rhodes T, et al: Prevalence of a physician-assigned diagnosis of prostatitis: the Olmsted County study of urinary symptoms and health status among men, *Urology* 51:578–584, 1998.

Schaeffer AJ, Knauss JS, Landis JR, et al: Leukocyte and bacterial counts do not correlate with severity of symptoms in men with chronic prostatitis: the National Institutes of Health Chronic Prostatitis Cohort Study, *J Urol* 168(3):1048–1053, 2002.

Sharp VJ, Takacs EB, Powell CR: Prostatitis: diagnosis and treatment, *Am Fam Physician* 82(4):397–406, 2010.

Wolf JS, Carol J, Dmochowski RR, et al: "*Urologic Surgery Antimicrobial Prophylaxis.*" Transrectal prostate biopsy, 2008. Retrieved 12/26/2012, 2012, from http://www.auanet.org/content/media/antimicroprop08.pdf.

Zhao WP, Zhang ZG, Li XD, et al: Celecoxib reduces symptoms in men with difficult chronic pelvic pain syndrome (Category IIIA), *Braz J Med Biol Res* 42:963–967, 2009.

URINARY TRACT INFECTIONS IN THE MALE

Method of
Donald A. Neff, MD

CURRENT DIAGNOSIS

- Urinary tract infection (UTI) can involve any portion of the urinary tract.
- Infection at any site in the urinary tract places the entire system at risk.
- UTIs can be broadly categorized as uncomplicated or complicated.
- Although uncommon, men can have uncomplicated UTI.
- Urologic evaluation is recommended for UTI in young boys.
- Detailed workup of uncomplicated UTI in the adult male is usually not needed.
- Urinalysis is useful to establish presumptive diagnosis.
- Urine culture with sensitivities is helpful to document infection and guide therapy.
- Repeat urine culture after treatment is unnecessary in uncomplicated infections.
- Screening urine cultures in asymptomatic individuals should be avoided.

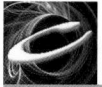

CURRENT THERAPY

- The goal of treatment is elimination of infection from the urinary tract.
- Prompt initiation of treatment can prevent the spread of infection to other portions of the urinary tract.
- Management of complicated UTI should include imaging of the upper urinary tract.
- Efforts should be made to control underlying risk factors in patients with complicated UTI.
- For complicated UTI, repeat culture after treatment may be helpful to document clearance of infection.

Definitions

Standardized terminology is helpful for communications between providers.

Bacteriuria: Presence of bacteria in the urine. This may be symptomatic or asymptomatic. Asymptomatic bacteriuria may not require treatment.

Pyuria: Presence of white blood cells (WBCs) in the urine. Suggests infection or inflammatory response of the urothelium. Sterile pyuria is lack of bacterial growth in presence of WBCs in the urine and should warrant further investigation to determine the underlying cause.

Urinary tract infection (UTI): Inflammatory response of urothelium to bacterial invasion

Uncomplicated UTI: Infection in a healthy patient with anatomically and functionally normal urinary tract. These infections respond promptly to appropriate treatment.

Complicated UTI: Infection associated with an anatomically or functionally abnormal urinary tract. The host may be immunocompromised. Risk factors for complicated UTI include male gender, advanced age, diabetes, immunosuppression, recent antibiotic use, the presence of an indwelling urinary catheter, recent instrumentation, and recent hospitalization.

Colonization: Presence of bacteriuria in the urine and absence of inflammatory response. Often seen in patients with indwelling urinary catheters. Generally, colonization does not require treatment. Overtreatment of the colonized urinary tract will select for bacterial resistance.
Isolated UTI: Infection in patient with no or remote prior history
Recurrent UTI: Infection that occurs after successful treatment of a prior infection. May be bacterial persistence or reinfection. Persistence is suggested by growth of the same organism. Reinfection usually shows growth of different types of organisms.
Unresolved UTI: Generally due to bacterial persistence. Repeated infection with same organism with similar resistance profile.

Introduction

Urinary tract infections (UTIs) are one of the most common bacterial infections in humans. UTI is defined as an inflammatory response of the urothelium to bacterial invasion. Infections of the urinary tract encompass a wide variety of diagnoses depending on the specific anatomic site of infection, the common denominator being bacterial invasion of genitourinary organs and tissues. Any site within the urinary tract may be involved including the kidney (pyelonephritis), ureters (ureteritis), bladder (cystitis), prostate (prostatitis), epididymis (epididymitis), and urethra (urethritis). Once any part of the urinary tract is infected, the remaining portions of the system are placed at risk for further bacterial invasion. Due in part to the relative rarity of UTI in adult males, evaluation and management of UTI in this population is hampered by lack of high-quality empirical data with which to guide treatment decisions.

Incidence and Epidemiology

UTI in males is not a reportable disease. Therefore, true incidence is difficult to assess in the United States. For both sexes, UTI accounts for 7 million office visits and 400,000 hospitalizations annually. In men, UTI accounts for 0.6% of all office visits. During infancy, the incidence of symptomatic UTIs is higher in boys than in girls, primarily related to circumcision status. Bacteria adhere to the inner prepuce, allowing easier access to the meatus followed by ascending infection. Neonatal circumcision reduces the rate of UTI in boys by over 90%. After the neonatal period, symptomatic UTI is uncommon until middle age. The incidence then increases to approach 10% by age 61, 14% in ages 61 to 70, 26% in ages 71 to 80, and 42% over age 81.

Pathophysiology

In the modern era most infections of the urinary tract occur via the ascending route. This begins with colonization of the perineum, most commonly with fecal bacteria. These bacteria then move from the perineal area to the urethra and to the bladder, ureter, and eventually the kidney. Fecal flora is a common source with *Escherichia coli* being the most common cause of UTIs. *E. coli* accounts for 85% of community acquired and 50% of hospital acquired infections. Hematogenous seeding does occur; however, this is much less likely in anatomically and physiologically normal individuals. The kidney may be secondarily infected by *Staphylococcus aureus* or *Candida fungemia* in this manner. In certain geographic areas, tuberculosis of the urinary tract is still seen and reaches these organs hematogenously. These types of infection are facilitated by prior renal damage or obstruction of the urinary tract.

Adherence of bacteria to the uroepithelium is an essential step in the pathogenesis of UTI. Bacterial virulence factors such as adhesins, type-1 pili, and P pili facilitate adherence to receptors on uroepithelial cells. Some individuals are genetically predisposed to infection, with increased uroepithelial receptivity to adherence of bacteria resulting in increased susceptibility to infection. Once within the bladder, uropathogenic bacteria are internalized into the intracellular space of superficial urothelial cells. In this space, the bacteria are more protected from the immune response and form intracellular bacterial communities, eventually forming protective biofilms. Bacteria then escape from the intracellular space into the urinary lumen, where they readhere and reinvade the uroepithelium. Once the inoculum is sufficient, a host immune response occurs. This response involves multiple cell types including neutrophils, macrophages, and other immunocytes along with associated cytokines. This inflammatory response results in the symptoms of UTI. Indeed, the levels of certain inflammatory factors have been correlated with the severity of symptoms.

The urinary tract has natural defenses in place to resist adherence and ascension of bacteria. Normal urogenital flora form a barrier to colonization by uropathogenic bacteria. Inhibitory urinary factors include osmolality, urea, organic acid concentration, and pH. Uromodulin is a protein present in the urine that binds to type-1 pili, preventing binding of bacteria to the urothelium. Regular and complete emptying of the bladder helps to expel bacteria and keep bacterial inoculum low.

Clinical Manifestations

The specific clinical symptoms of UTI depend on the anatomic site of infection. Urethritis presents with dysuria, urinary urgency and frequency, and penile discharge. The penis may be tender or swollen. Associated inguinal lymphadenopathy may be present. Epididymitis usually presents as unilateral testicular pain that is gradual in onset. The scrotum is swollen, warm, and erythematous. Scrotal cellulitis may be present. Acute prostatitis includes fevers, chills, dysuria, and pelvic pain. Urinary hesitancy and weak stream are often seen due to swelling of the prostate gland and increased resistance of flow through the prostatic urethra. Cystitis is associated with dysuria, urinary urgency, and urinary frequency. There may be associated suprapubic pain or gross hematuria. Pyelonephritis is associated with the classical triad of fevers, chills, and flank pain. In older adults, symptoms may not be as clear. Generalized abdominal pain, increased confusion, and altered mental status may be the presenting signs of UTI in these individuals.

An important consideration is the entity of asymptomatic bacteriuria. In this instance bacteria are able to be identified in a noncontaminated urine culture. However, there is no associated immune response, or the clinical symptoms mentioned above. Indeed, urine is not sterile as has been previously thought, with a normal urinary microbiome present that is difficulty to detect on routine culture media.

Prevalence of asymptomatic bacteriuria increases with age and can be seen in up to 15% of men over age 75. In general, asymptomatic bacteriuria should not be treated. The 2019 guidelines of the Infectious Diseases Society of America (IDSA) recommend screening and treatment of men for asymptomatic bacteria only in patients undergoing invasive urologic procedures. Inappropriate treatment of asymptomatic bacteria contributes to antimicrobial resistance.

Differential Diagnosis

The differential diagnosis of UTI should be focused on the anatomic location of symptoms. Urethritis can be caused by multiple organisms, and sexually transmitted diseases should be considered. Lower urinary tract symptoms (urgency, frequency) associated with cystitis can also be seen with bladder stones or bladder tumors. Flank pain may result from urinary tract obstruction due to stone, trauma, or musculoskeletal sources. Sterile pyuria should prompt investigation for stone, tuberculosis, and malignancy. Sterile pyuria may also be associated with nonurologic diagnosis such as appendicitis, diverticulitis, or autoimmune diseases.

Clinical Evaluation

The foundation for evaluation of a patient with UTI remains a thorough history and physical examination. A detailed surgical history is helpful to determine risk factors for complicated UTI. A urinalysis is essential in the evaluation of urinary symptoms and can provide information for a preliminary diagnosis.

Normal urine should be free of bacteria and inflammation. False negatives can occur early in the clinical course or when a patient has taken antimicrobial therapy prior to obtaining the urine specimen. False positives may be caused by contamination or over-the-counter remedies such as phenazopyridine (positive nitrites). The decision to send a urine culture should be based on the overall clinical picture. For an uncomplicated UTI, a urine culture is helpful but not required unless the patient fails to improve with treatment. If symptoms fail to improve, or if the patient has risk factors for complicated UTI, a culture is strongly recommended to determine the underlying organism and antimicrobial sensitivities. Proper collection and storage of the urine specimen can minimize the potential for false results.

Localization of bacteria to differentiate the source of an infection within the lower urinary tract of males can be challenging. The Meares-Stamey four-glass urinary tract localization test has been well described. First, the patient is asked to void 5 to 10 cc into a sterile container (VB1). A second, midstream specimen is then obtained (VB2). A prostatic massage is then performed by digital rectal examination (DRE), and the expressed fluids are collected (EPS). Finally, the postprostate massage urine is collected. The four specimens are then sent separately for culture and sensitivity. VB1 represents urethral flora, VB2 represents bladder urine flora, EPS and VB3 represent prostatic flora. The four-glass test can be expensive, cumbersome, and is often of low diagnostic yield. An alternate approach is a modified Meares-Stamey two-glass test, which is easier and less costly to perform. This is performed by collecting a urine specimen premassage and then a second specimen post-massage. The premassage specimen represents bladder flora, and the post-massage specimen represents the prostatic flora.

Due to the rarity of urinary infection in boys outside of the neonatal period, urologic investigation is essential for the evaluation of UTI in the pediatric population to rule out structural abnormalities. These include vesicoureteral reflux, posterior urethral valves, congenital ureteropelvic junction obstruction, ureterocele, and megaureter. Referral to a pediatric urologist should be considered. Early diagnosis and therapy will help prevent scarring and preserve renal function. A history of constipation should be elucidated, as bowel-bladder dysfunction places boys at risk of UTI. The optimal imaging approach to the pediatric patient is controversial. The combination of renal-bladder ultrasound and voiding cystourethrogram (VCUG) has traditionally been used to assess both the upper and lower urinary tracts. In the modern era, provided the renal bladder ultrasound is normal, VCUG may be safely deferred. A nuclear medicine scan can be useful to determine differential renal function and identify the presence of obstruction of the upper urinary tract.

For adults, the use of radiographic investigations is again based on the unique clinical picture of a given patient. For uncomplicated UTI, particularly in otherwise healthy men whose infections resolve easily, detailed investigations, including imaging, are often not necessary. Complicated infections require further investigation to search for a nidus or anatomic abnormality. These include patients with a recurrent or unresolved infection or patients with aforementioned risk factors. Computed tomography (CT) urography is a complete study of the upper urinary tract and includes a noncontrast phase, a nephrographic phase, and delayed images to evaluate the upper urinary drainage system. This study allows for assessment of renal stones, masses, impaired or altered drainage, and is the imaging study of choice in patients with normal renal function. For patients with poor renal function, renal-bladder ultrasound is a reasonable alternative. Measurement of post-void residual is helpful to determine whether retention of urine is causing urinary stasis.

Treatment

Elimination of the infecting organism from the urinary tract is the goal of therapy for UTI. There is limited data to guide duration of treatment of UTI in males, with many treatment strategies extrapolated from studies done in females. Although traditionally men have been considered to always have complicated UTIs, an afebrile man with a first UTI and no complicating factors can be considered to have an uncomplicated UTI.

In general, empirical selection of antimicrobial therapy should be selected to target the pathogen being treated, with local resistance patterns taken into consideration. Uncomplicated infections should be anticipated to resolve promptly with appropriate therapy. Duration of therapy for these types of infections in men is not well established, but 5 to 7 days of treatment is reasonable depending on the agent chosen. Prompt initiation of broad spectrum therapy in complicated UTIs will help prevent further dissemination of the infection and the development of sepsis. Treatment can later be tailored to the results of culture and sensitivities. These infections require longer duration of therapy, 10 to 14 days. In the setting of multidrug-resistant isolates, parenteral therapy may be required for the duration of treatment. For patients with bacterial persistence after treatment, a thorough urologic evaluation should be made, followed by an attempt to eliminate the source of bacteria if possible.

Monitoring and Prevention

In most patients with UTI, routine repeat culture of urine after therapy is not indicated. However, if patients thought to have uncomplicated UTI do not improve as expected, a urine culture should be obtained to guide therapy. Similarly, rapid recurrence of symptoms after initial improvement should prompt repeat urine culture. Antibiotic prophylaxis in males is generally not warranted, and prevention should be directed at elimination or treatment of the underlying cause if possible. For example, initiation of medications in patients with incomplete bladder emptying due to BPH, or treatment of an infected urinary stone would be of higher yield than suppressive antibiotics.

Management of Complications

Complications in patients with UTI should be managed according to the clinical setting. The decision to admit a patient to the hospital is dictated by multiple factors. Nontoxic patients who can take PO medications may be safely managed as outpatients. Immunosuppressed or diabetic patients may warrant admission for observation. These patients and those with other risk factors for complicated UTI may progress rapidly to sepsis, and admission to the intensive care unit (ICU) may be necessary. Patients who develop perinephric or prostatic abscess will require either percutaneous or surgical drainage.

Special Considerations

Patients with chronic indwelling catheters will nearly always be colonized. Screening cultures are not indicated and should be avoided. In general, bacterial colonization of the urinary tract should not be treated unless symptoms develop. It is often counterproductive to attempt clearance of bacteria in this population as overtreatment will select for bacterial resistance. Further, elimination of benign colonizing bacteria from the urinary tract in these individuals often allows more virulent bacteria to establish residence. Antimicrobial prophylaxis is not indicated. Treatment strategies in these individuals should be focused on the underlying factors leading to the need for catheter drainage. These include institution of clean intermittent catheterization when possible, or more frequent changing of the catheter if necessary.

Another special consideration is the presence of a bacterial UTI in an obstructed urinary system. This most commonly occurs when a kidney stone causes ureteral obstruction in the setting of pyelonephritis. These patients can rapidly progress to sepsis.

Prompt drainage of the affected renal unit either by ureteral stent or by percutaneous nephrostomy tube, along with institution of appropriate antimicrobial therapy, is essential in the management of these patients.

References

Detweiler K, et al: Bacteria and urinary infections in the elderly, *Urol Clin North Am* 42(4):561–568, 2015.

Foxman B: Epidemiology of urinary tract infections: incidence, morbidity, and economic costs, *Am J Med* 113(Suppl 1A):5S–13S, 2002.

Nicolle L: Asymptomatic bacteriuria: when to screen and when to treat, *Infect Dis Clin North Am* 17(2):367–394, 2003.

Nicolle L: Uncomplicated urinary tract infection in adults including uncomplicated pyelonephritis, *Urol Clin North Am* 35:1–12, 2008.

Nicolle L, et al: *Clinical Practice Guideline for the Management of Asymptomatic Bacteriuria: 2019 update by the Infectious Diseases Society of America*, Available at: https:// https://www.idsociety.org/practice-guideline/asymptomatic-bacteriuria/. Accessed February 28, 2021.

Schappert SM: Ambulatory care visits of physician offices, hospital outpatient departments, and emergency departments: United States, 1995, *Vital Health Stat* 13:1–38, 1997.

Simmering JE, et al: *The increase in hospitalizations for urinary tract infections and the associated costs in the United States, 1998–2011 open forum infectious diseases. 2017 winter*, 4(1). Available at: https://www.ncbi.nlm.nih.gov/pmc/articles/PMC5414046/. Accessed February 28, 2021.

Subcommittee on Urinary Tract Infection: Reaffirmation of AAP Clinical Practice Guideline: the diagnosis and management of the initial urinary tract infection in febrile infants and young children 2–24 months of age, *Pediatrics* 138(6), 2016.

Schaeffer MD Anthony J, et al: Infections of the urinary tract. In Wein AJ, editor: *Campbell-Walsh Urology* Elsevier, pp 237–303, 2015.

17 Women's Health

ABNORMAL UTERINE BLEEDING

Method of
Sarina Schrager, MD, MS

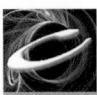

CURRENT DIAGNOSIS

- Anovulation and pelvic structural abnormalities are the most common causes of abnormal vaginal bleeding in reproductive-age women.
- All women with abnormal bleeding should have a pregnancy test.
- A pelvic ultrasound will detect many structural causes of abnormal bleeding.
- Either a pelvic ultrasound or endometrial biopsy is appropriate for evaluation of postmenopausal bleeding.

CURRENT THERAPY

- Unstable women with acute heavy vaginal bleeding should be admitted to hospital for intravenous (IV) estrogen therapy (Premarin) or surgical intervention.
- Treatment of anovulatory bleeding includes ovulation induction if a woman desires pregnancy and hormonal cycle control if she does not.
- Anovulatory women are at risk for endometrial hyperplasia or carcinoma due to unopposed estrogen and should have regular progesterone-induced withdrawal bleeds.
- Treatment of menorrhagia can include nonsteroidal antiinflammatory drugs (NSAIDs), tranexamic acid (Lysteda), or insertion of a levonorgestrel intrauterine device (IUD) (Mirena).

Epidemiology

Abnormal vaginal bleeding is a common complaint in primary care. The prevalence of some type of abnormal bleeding is between 10% and 30% among women of reproductive age. Anovulatory bleeding is more common in women who are perimenopausal and who are overweight. The estimated direct and indirect costs of abnormal bleeding are $1 billion and $12 billion annually, respectively. Abnormal bleeding is also a common reason for women to be referred to gynecologists and is an indication for up to 25% of all gynecologic surgery.

Pathophysiology

Normal menstrual bleeding is defined as regular vaginal bleeding that occurs at intervals from every 21 to 35 days. A normal menstrual cycle is ovulatory, with two distinct phases: the follicular phase and the luteal phase. The follicular phase is the first half of the cycle. The luteal phase occurs after ovulation, when the corpus luteum develops in anticipation of a possible pregnancy. Table 1 defines vocabulary to describe different patterns of abnormal bleeding.

TABLE 1	Causes of Abnormal Uterine Bleeding (ACOG)
PALM (structural causes)	**COEIN (non-structural causes)**
Polyp	Coagulopathy
Adenomyosis	Ovulatory dysfunction
Leiomyoma	Endometrial
Malignancy and hyperplasia	Iatrogenic
	Not yet classified

TABLE 2	Signs and Symptoms of Ovulatory Cycles	
Regular cycle length		Presence of premenstrual stress (PMS) symptoms
Dysmenorrhea		Mittelschmerz (pain at ovulation)
Changes in cervical mucus		Biphasic temperature curve
Premenstrual breast tenderness		Positive test result from luteinizing hormone (LH) predictor kit

The pathologic abnormality in anovulatory cycles is a lack of ovulation, which produces an unopposed estrogen state. The luteal phase of the menstrual cycle is dominated by progesterone, which is only produced after ovulation. This lack of progesterone contributes to irregular endometrial growth and nonuniform bleeding. In a normal cycle, the entire endometrium sloughs off during menstruation. In an anovulatory cycle, different sections of endometrium outgrow their blood supply at different times and bleed erratically. Anovulatory bleeding (also referred to as dysfunctional uterine bleeding) is unpredictable in timing and amount of bleeding.

The most common structural abnormalities that cause abnormal bleeding are endometrial polyps, leiomyomas, adenomyosis, and hyperplasia or malignancy.

Abnormal bleeding is also common in women who use hormonal contraception, usually due to endometrial abnormalities from exogenous hormones. Women who take combination estrogen/progestin contraception often have intermenstrual bleeding for the first 3 months of treatment. Missed pills are a very frequent cause of abnormal bleeding. In women using progestin-only methods, the abnormal bleeding usually is caused by progestin-induced endometrial atrophy.

Diagnosis

All women with abnormal bleeding should have a thorough history and physical examination and a pregnancy test. If the pregnancy test is negative, the next step is to determine whether her cycles are ovulatory or anovulatory. Table 2 describes characteristics of ovulatory cycles. Laboratory evaluation includes looking for causes of anovulation (Table 3), assessing for anemia with a hemoglobin and hematocrit level, and consideration of getting a pelvic ultrasound to look for structural abnormalities.

In menorrhagia, evaluation for a coagulation disorder (most commonly von Willebrand disease), liver failure, or chronic renal

TABLE 3	Causes of Anovulatory Cycles

Hypothalamic
- Weight loss
- Eating disorders
- Female athlete triad
- Chronic illness
- Stress
- Excessive exercise

Polycystic ovary syndrome

Thyroid disorders

Hyperprolactinemia

Idiopathic chronic anovulation

Medication-induced (i.e., after discontinuation of hormonal contraceptives)

TABLE 4	Clinical Evaluation of a Woman With Abnormal Bleeding

OVULATORY BLEEDING	ANOVULATORY BLEEDING
History, physical examination, pregnancy test	History, physical examination, pregnancy test

In menorrhagia:
• Consideration of liver function tests, BUN/Cr, CBC, coagulation profile
  • Pelvic ultrasound to exclude uterine fibroids
  • Sonohysterogram to exclude polyps or adenomyosis
  • Endometrial biopsy (especially if age >45) to exclude endometrial hyperplasia
	Laboratory studies:
	• TSH
	• Prolactin
	• CBC (if acute bleeding episode or frequent heavy bleeding)
	• Consideration of endometrial biopsy (especially if age >45) to exclude hyperplasia or malignancy
	• Evaluation for other symptoms of PCOS

In intermenstrual bleeding: • Pap smear, cervical cultures	Screen for eating disorder, stress, female athlete triad

Abbreviations: BUN/Cr=blood urea nitrogen/creatinine; CBC=complete blood count; Pap=Papanicolaou smear; PCOS=polycystic ovary syndrome; TSH=thyroid-stimulating hormone.

TABLE 5	Treatment Options for Abnormal Vaginal Bleeding

Anovulation: cycle control with estrogen/progestin contraception, DMPA, levonorgestrel IUD (Mirena), or scheduled progestin-induced withdrawal bleeds, ovulation induction with clomiphene citrate (Clomid), and referral to gynecologist if pregnancy desired

Acute bleeding episode—outpatient: administration of high-dose OCPs (up to 4 per day) for 5–7 days with subsequent continuous cycling with OCPs for at least 1 month, administration of oral estrogen to acutely stop bleeding, or administration of oral progesterone to acutely stop bleeding

Acute bleeding episode—inpatient: IVF, supportive care, IV estrogen therapy, consultation for surgical intervention

Menorrhagia—treatment with NSAIDs, tranexamic acid (Lysteda), insertion of levonorgestrel IUD, referral for endometrial ablation or surgical treatment of structural abnormality

On combination estrogen/progestin contraception: supportive care for first 3 months, assessment of adherence to pill regimen, add supplemental estrogen, change to a method with a higher dose of estrogen or a different class of progestin

On progestin-only contraception: add supplemental estrogen or combination oral contraceptive pill and NSAID to decrease bleeding

Abbreviations: DMPA=depot medroxyprogesterone acetate (Depo-Provera); IUD=intrauterine device; IV=intravenous; IVF=in vitro fertilization; NSAID=nonsteroidal antiinflammatory drug; OCP=oral contraceptive pill.

(OCPs), estrogen, cyclic progesterone, NSAIDs, or tranexamic acid (Lysteda) is indicated. Women with structural abnormalities causing menorrhagia should be referred for possible surgical treatment.

Treatment of women with ovulatory bleeding is indicated if the woman is anemic or is bothered by her bleeding pattern. However, treatment of anovulation with some type of progesterone is necessary to reduce the risk of endometrial hyperplasia or carcinoma. All women with chronic anovulation should have regular progesterone-induced withdrawal bleed. OCPs, monthly cycling of progesterone, and continuous administration of progestin contraception (e.g., depot medroxyprogesterone acetate [Depo-Provera] or levonorgestrel IUD [Mirena]) are all effective treatments (Table 5).

Treatment of women with abnormal bleeding on OCPs involves education and support to try to get them through the first 3 months on the pills. After that, consideration of supplemental estrogen, changing to a higher dose of an estrogen pill, changing to a pill with a different class of progestin, use of a supplemental NSAID to decrease the amount of bleeding, decreasing the hormone free interval, or changing to a nonhormonal type of contraception are all potential treatments.

References

Abdel-Aleem H, d'Arcangues C, Vogelsong KM, et al: Treatment of vaginal bleeding irregularities induced by progestin only contraceptives, *Cochrane Database Syst Rev*(4), 2007. CD003449.

ACOG: Practice bulletin no 128: Diagnosis of abnormal uterine bleeding in reproductive-aged women, *Obstet Gynecol* 120:197–206, 2012.

ACOG: Practice bulletin no. 136. Management of abnormal uterine bleeding associated with ovulatory dysfunction. *Obstet Gynecol* 122(1):176–185, 2013.

Ely JW, Kennedy CM, Clark EC, et al: Abnormal uterine bleeding: a management algorithm, *J Am Board Fam Med* 19:590–602, 2006.

Liu Z, Doan QV, Blumenthal P, et al: A systematic review evaluating health-related quality of life, work impairment, and health-care costs and utilization in abnormal uterine bleeding, *Value Health* 10:183–194, 2007.

Naoulou B, Tsai MC: Efficacy of tranexamic acid in the treatment of idiopathic and non-functional heavy menstrual bleeding: a systematic review, *Acta Obstet Gynecol* 91:529–537, 2012.

Schrager S: Abnormal bleeding associated with hormonal contraception, *Am Fam Physician* 65:2073–2080, 2002. 2083.

Sweet MG, Schmidt-Dalton TA, Weiss PM, et al: Evaluation and management of abnormal uterine bleeding in premenopausal women, *Am Fam Physician* 85:35–43, 2012.

failure is also indicated. Evaluation in an acute bleeding episode (usually due to anovulatory bleeding) should include a hemoglobin and hematocrit if the bleeding is heavy assessment of volume status, and an endometrial biopsy. Postmenopausal bleeding is related to an increased risk of endometrial hyperplasia and cancer and should be evaluated with a transvaginal ultrasound to look at the endometrial thickness (under 4 mm is reassuring) or an office endometrial biopsy. Table 4 describes the steps in evaluation of a woman with abnormal bleeding.

Treatment

If a woman presents with heavy bleeding and exhibits any signs or symptoms of hypovolemia, she should be admitted to the hospital and either treated with IV conjugated estrogen (Premarin) to stop the bleeding or have a surgical procedure (such as dilation and curettage). If the bleeding is heavy but the woman is stable and her hemoglobin and hematocrit are close to normal, outpatient treatment with high-dose oral contraceptive pills

AMENORRHEA

Method of
Colleen Loo-Gross, MD, MPH

CURRENT DIAGNOSIS

- In the absence of physiologic causes (e.g., pregnancy, lactation, and menopause), four conditions account for the majority of amenorrhea cases: polycystic ovary syndrome, hypothalamic amenorrhea, hyperprolactinemia, and primary ovarian insufficiency.
- Most causes of amenorrhea can be identified through a detailed history, physical examination, and laboratory evaluation.
- Müllerian agenesis is the most common cause of anatomic malformations associated with amenorrhea.
- In the evaluation of amenorrhea, it is important to exclude physiologic causes such as pregnancy and lactation, as well as potential iatrogenic causes (e.g., hormonal contraception, chemotherapy and radiation therapy, and medications that may cause hyperprolactinemia).
- Initial laboratory evaluation should include follicle-stimulating hormone (FSH), thyroid-stimulating hormone (TSH), and prolactin levels.
- In amenorrheic women less than 40 years of age, an elevated FSH level in the menopausal range indicates primary ovarian insufficiency.
- A low or normal FSH value in amenorrhea without evidence of anatomic cause suggests chronic anovulation, most commonly attributed to hypothalamic amenorrhea or polycystic ovary syndrome.
- In cases of elevated prolactin level (with no evidence of thyroid disease), MRI is warranted to assess for a possible pituitary tumor.

CURRENT THERAPY

- The underlying cause of amenorrhea should be treated accordingly.
- For those with an estrogen deficient state, cyclic hormone therapy may be indicated, and adequate calcium and vitamin D intake are essential to reduce the risk of osteoporosis.
- Fertility considerations should be addressed in all causes of amenorrhea.
- Psychosocial support, such as counseling services and peer support groups, is an important aspect of management.

Amenorrhea is defined as the absence of menses. Its prevalence, when not related to pregnancy or lactation, is approximately 3% to 4% among premenopausal women. Amenorrhea is further categorized into primary amenorrhea (prior to menarche) and secondary amenorrhea (following menarche). Evaluation for primary amenorrhea should be initiated when menarche has not occurred by 15 years of age, or sooner for females without onset of menses within 5 years of thelarche. Evaluation should also be considered when thelarche has not occurred by 13 years of age. Secondary amenorrhea is the lack of menses for 3 months in females with preceding regular cycles or 6 months in those with irregular menstrual cycles.

Etiology

There are a number of potential etiologies of amenorrhea. In the absence of physiologic causes (e.g., pregnancy, lactation, and menopause), four conditions account for the majority of amenorrhea cases: polycystic ovary syndrome (PCOS), hypothalamic amenorrhea, hyperprolactinemia, and primary ovarian insufficiency. The approximate frequency of common causes of primary and secondary amenorrhea are shown in Tables 1 and 2. Other considerations may also include adrenal disease, adrenal hyperplasia, chronic disease, Cushing syndrome, androgen-secreting tumors, central nervous system infections, and a history of trauma (such as traumatic brain injury).

With primary amenorrhea, anatomic defects and chromosomal abnormalities (with associated primary ovarian insufficiency) are often causative factors. Anatomic abnormalities may cause amenorrhea due to obstruction along the genital outflow tract. With Müllerian agenesis, incomplete development of the Müllerian duct embryologically results in a range of defects due to agenesis or atresia of the uterus and/or vagina, though ovarian function is usually unaffected. Müllerian agenesis is a common cause of primary amenorrhea among females who present with normal signs of adrenarche and breast development. In primary ovarian insufficiency, amenorrhea occurs as the result of ovarian follicle depletion or dysfunction. It comprises 2% to 10% of cases of amenorrhea.

Excluding pregnancy, the most common causes of secondary amenorrhea are hypothalamic amenorrhea and PCOS. Functional hypothalamic amenorrhea occurs in the presence of hypothalamic-pituitary-ovarian axis suppression, without evidence of organic cause. In these cases, the regulatory pulsatile secretion of gonadotropin-releasing hormone (GnRH) is affected, leading to abnormally low levels of estrogen.

Evaluation

Most causes of amenorrhea can be identified through a detailed history, physical examination, and laboratory evaluation. It is important to exclude physiologic causes of amenorrhea such as pregnancy and lactation, as well as potential iatrogenic causes (for example, hormonal contraception, chemotherapy and radiation therapy, and medications that may cause hyperprolactinemia such as antipsychotics, antidepressants, opiates, and metoclopramide [Reglan]). The incidence of amenorrhea is approximately 12% in women taking antipsychotic medications, due to the resultant increase in prolactin levels.

History

Obtaining a detailed history is an important component in the evaluation of amenorrhea. The presence of vasomotor symptoms, such as hot flashes, may be indicators of primary ovarian insufficiency, whereas reports of headache or vision changes may prompt further evaluation for possible central nervous system tumor or empty sella syndrome. Women with anatomic causes of amenorrhea, such as transverse vaginal septum, imperforate hymen, and isolated absence of the vagina or cervix, may report cyclic pelvic pain, which occurs due to blood accumulation behind the outflow tract obstruction and in some cases, associated endometriosis. Anosmia may be an indication of the rare Kallmann syndrome, which presents with amenorrhea due to GnRH deficiency and is associated with abnormal development of the olfactory bulb.

Additional history details should include assessment of mood and stress, weight changes, nutrition and eating patterns, and exercise routines, with evaluation for a possible eating disorder or other cause of an overall energy deficit. Abnormal historical findings such as these may be suggestive of functional hypothalamic amenorrhea. It is also important to assess for signs or symptoms of thyroid disease and of other potential chronic medical conditions.

Family history may also provide useful information. A positive family history for delayed menarche may suggest constitutional delay of puberty as the cause of amenorrhea, though this is considered a diagnosis of exclusion. A family history of primary ovarian insufficiency is also worth noting, given the related genetic predisposition. Moreover, early menopause in family members is a risk factor associated with primary ovarian insufficiency.

TABLE 1	Common Causes of Primary Amenorrhea	
CATEGORY		**APPROXIMATE FREQUENCY (%)**
Breast development present		30
Müllerian agenesis		10
Androgen insensitivity		9
Transverse vaginal septum		2
Imperforate hymen		1
Constitutional delay of puberty		8
No breast development: high FSH		40
46,XX		15
46,XY		5
Abnormal karyotype		20
No breast development: low FSH		30
Constitutional delay of puberty		10
Prolactinoma		5
Kallmann syndrome		2
Other CNS etiology		3
Stress, weight loss, eating disorders		3
Polycystic ovary syndrome		3
Congenital adrenal hyperplasia		3
Other		1

CNS, Central nervous system; FSH, follicle-stimulating hormone.
Adapted from Practice Committee of American Society for Reproductive Medicine. Current evaluation of amenorrhea. *Fertil Steril.* 2008;90:S219–S225.

TABLE 2	Common Causes of Secondary Amenorrhea	
CATEGORY		**APPROXIMATE FREQUENCY (%)**
Low or normal FSH		66
Stress, weight loss, eating disorders		
Non-specific hypothalamic causes		
Chronic anovulation, including PCOS		
Hypothyroidism		
Cushing syndrome		
Pituitary tumor, empty sella, Sheehan syndrome		
Gonadal failure: high FSH		12
46,XX		
Abnormal karyotype		
Hyperprolactinemia		13
Anatomic		7
Asherman syndrome (intrauterine synechiae)		
Other hyperandrogenic states		2
Ovarian tumor		
Non-classic congenital adrenal hyperplasia		
Undiagnosed		

FSH, Follicle-stimulating hormone; PCOS, polycystic ovary syndrome.
Adapted from Practice Committee of American Society for Reproductive Medicine. Current evaluation of amenorrhea. *Fertil Steril.* 2008;90:S219–S225.

Physical Examination

About 15% of those with primary amenorrhea have an abnormality noted on genital examination. Both internal and external genitalia should be examined. A shortened vagina is associated with conditions such as Müllerian agenesis (which may present with a range of defects resulting from incomplete embryologic development of the Müllerian duct), imperforate hymen, transverse vaginal septum, cervical atresia, or other uterine anomalies. In some cases, the vagina may appear as no more than a small dimple.

Additional physical findings may also help guide the evaluation of amenorrhea. Dysmorphic features should be noted, such as a webbed neck or short stature, which may be suggestive of Turner syndrome. Galactorrhea may warrant evaluation for a pituitary tumor. Clinical evidence of self-induced vomiting may be suggestive of a hypothalamic etiology of amenorrhea.

The physical examination should further assess for secondary sexual characteristics, such as the presence of pubic hair and also breast development, which is an indicator of endogenous estrogen effect. Conversely, the presence of thin vaginal mucosa is a sign of low endogenous estrogen level. Signs of hirsutism, acne, and male pattern alopecia are indicators of androgen excess, which may suggest hyperandrogenic etiologies of amenorrhea such as PCOS. Body mass index (BMI) also helps to differentiate PCOS from other causes of amenorrhea (such as functional disorders of the hypothalamus) given its typical presentation with obesity.

Laboratory Studies

When the etiology of amenorrhea is not evident after completing a thorough history and physical examination, additional assessment is warranted. Initial laboratory evaluation should include levels of follicle-stimulating hormone (FSH), thyroid-stimulating hormone (TSH), and prolactin. Abnormal thyroid levels should be managed accordingly. An elevated prolactin level without apparent cause necessitates further investigation with diagnostic imaging of the pituitary gland.

In amenorrheic women less than 40 years of age, an elevated FSH level in the menopausal range indicates primary ovarian insufficiency. The FSH level should be repeated at least 1 month following the initial result for confirmation. For women less than 30 years of age with identified primary ovarian insufficiency, a karyotype should be obtained to assess for possible chromosomal abnormality. Karyotype analysis may be considered for those over 30 years of age as well. In cases when the cause is not identified, particularly in women who also have a family history of primary ovarian insufficiency, premutation carrier testing for the fragile X gene (*FMR1*) should be considered.

A low or normal FSH value in amenorrheic women without evidence of anatomic cause suggests chronic anovulation, most commonly attributed to hypothalamic amenorrhea or PCOS. In principle, hypothalamic amenorrhea would be associated with low estradiol levels, and PCOS would more often be associated with normal estradiol levels. However, estradiol levels fluctuate and testing is not recommended to help distinguish between these diagnoses. Similarly, the progesterone challenge test for withdrawal bleeding is not considered a reliable indicator of estrogen levels, given both high false positive and false negative rates.

Imaging Studies
In certain situations, further evaluation with imaging may be indicated, such as the use of ultrasound, magnetic resonance imaging (MRI), or hysteroscopy to assess for a potential anatomic abnormality. Examples include the absence of the uterus in primary amenorrhea, as may be seen with Müllerian agenesis and 46,XY conditions like androgen insensitivity syndrome, or the presence of intrauterine synechiae (Asherman syndrome) in those with prior procedural instrumentation of the uterus. In cases of an elevated prolactin level (with no evidence of thyroid disease), MRI is warranted to assess for a possible pituitary tumor, which is present in 50% to 60% of women with hyperprolactinemia.

Diagnoses and Management
Anatomic Causes
Müllerian agenesis is the most common cause of anatomic malformations associated with amenorrhea, comprising approximately 10% of primary amenorrhea cases. In addition to malformations along the genital tract, over half of Müllerian agenesis cases may also present with other congenital abnormalities, such as urinary tract or skeletal defects (e.g., scoliosis, vertebral arch anomalies, and wrist hypoplasia). Thus, it is important to assess for the presence of coexisting congenital anomalies in those with Müllerian agenesis. Renal ultrasound and spinal X-ray imaging should be considered in these women.

A less common cause of anatomical defects in the uterus or vagina is complete androgen insensitivity, which accounts for 5% of primary amenorrhea. Other anatomic defects leading to primary amenorrhea include transverse vaginal septum (2% of cases), imperforate hymen (1% of cases), and isolated absence of the vagina or cervix. In women with prior history of procedural interventions involving the uterus or cervix, intrauterine synechiae (Asherman syndrome) and cervical stenosis should also be considered as potential etiologies of amenorrhea. In cases of Asherman syndrome, treatment often involves hysteroscopy for lysis of the intrauterine adhesions.

Women with Müllerian agenesis typically present with normal secondary female sexual characteristics, in the setting of anatomic defects in all or some aspects of the uterus and vagina. Women with complete androgen insensitivity may also present with vaginal defects, though in addition they have a family history suggestive of androgen insensitivity, lack of pubarche, and may present with inguinal hernias or masses containing testes. Complete androgen insensitivity is an X-linked recessive condition and is confirmed by an elevated serum testosterone level in the male range and karyotype analysis (46,XY). Of note, complete androgen insensitivity confers an increased risk of gonadal malignancy, and treatment includes gonadal removal, typically after completion of growth and breast development. Hormonal replacement therapy is indicated following prophylactic gonadal removal for the maintenance of bone health.

The first-line treatment for Müllerian agenesis includes vaginal dilation to achieve elongation, a nonsurgical, patient-controlled therapy that has a success rate above 90%. Surgery to create a vagina is much less commonly required and reserved for rare cases. Psychosocial support is another important aspect of treatment for these individuals. Fertility considerations should also be addressed. In those with Müllerian agenesis who desire children, options may include assisted reproductive technology with gestational surrogacy or adoption. With regard to ongoing care, routine cervical cancer screening is not typically indicated given the absence of a cervix in these women.

Primary Ovarian Insufficiency
Persistently elevated FSH levels in the menopausal range indicate impaired ovarian function, consistent with primary ovarian insufficiency. Other terms to describe this condition have been previously used, including premature ovarian failure, premature menopause, and primary ovarian failure. This condition may affect 1% to 5% of women, though the etiology is not always known.

Congenital causes are a factor in some cases of primary ovarian insufficiency, with certain chromosomal abnormalities leading to gonadal dysgenesis, an example being Turner syndrome (45,X). Chromosomal abnormalities are identified in 50% of adolescents without comorbidities who present with primary amenorrhea and in 13% of women 30 years of age or younger who present with secondary amenorrhea. With regard to management, it is important to remember that the incidence of gonadal malignancy is up to 25% for women with a Y chromosome. Accordingly, in 46,XY women with lack of gonadal function as evidenced by elevated FSH levels and absence of hormone secretion, gonadal removal is indicated at the time of diagnosis.

Primary ovarian insufficiency has shown associated genetic predisposition, and premutation carrier testing for fragile X syndrome should be considered in these women when another cause has not been identified. Among those with a normal karyotype, 6% of women with primary ovarian insufficiency are found to have premutation of the *FMR1* (fragile X) gene. Additionally, primary ovarian insufficiency may also be seen with various endocrinopathies, such as hypoparathyroidism and hypoadrenalism, or autoimmune disease. Specifically, approximately 4% of cases have adrenal or ovarian antibodies, and autoimmune disorders may be found in up to 40% of women with primary ovarian insufficiency, most commonly thyroid disease.

For women with primary ovarian insufficiency, infertility should be addressed, though up to 10% may have temporary remission with spontaneous conception. It is unclear whether oral contraceptives are as effective in this population, so alternative methods such as barrier contraception or intrauterine device options are more appropriate for pregnancy prevention. Genetic predisposition for this condition should also be addressed. Consultations with reproductive endocrinology and fertility specialists are indicated when pregnancy is desired, as options are limited beyond donor *in vitro* fertilization. Psychosocial counseling and support should be offered as well.

Annual visits are recommended in those with primary ovarian insufficiency. Given the increased cardiovascular risk associated with the early estrogen deficient state, steps should be taken to ensure optimized cardiovascular health, including routine screening for hypertension and a lipid panel at least every 5 years. Furthermore, hormonal treatment until the typical age of menopause is appropriate both to support bone health as well as to develop and maintain secondary sexual characteristics. The estrogen deficient state in this condition poses risk to the attainment of peak bone mass. Thus, weight-bearing exercise as well as adequate calcium (1300 mg per day) and vitamin D (400 to 1000 IU per day) intake are also important aspects of management to reduce the risk of osteoporosis. With regard to hormone therapy in these cases, additional potential benefits include decreased risk of ischemic heart disease, less cardiovascular mortality, and vasomotor symptom control. Of note, combined oral contraceptives provide higher levels of hormones than are necessary for this purpose and are not recommended in this setting. A more appropriate regimen would include daily estradiol (e.g., 100 μg dose in transdermal [Alora, Dotti, Minivelle, Vivelle] or oral form [Estrace], though the latter confers a relatively higher thromboembolism risk), with 12 days of cyclic progesterone monthly (e.g., medroxyprogesterone acetate [Provera] 10 mg). For those still undergoing pubertal growth and maturity, specialized care is recommended, as hormone therapy should begin with estrogen before the introduction of progesterone, with the purpose of mimicking hormonal levels associated with development.

Hyperprolactinemia and Pituitary Causes
Another potential etiology of amenorrhea or oligomenorrhea is an elevated prolactin level, which inhibits the release and thus the effect of gonadotropins. Specifically, the presence of hyperprolactinemia suppresses GnRH secretion. When hyperprolactinemia is identified, in the absence of other potential causes such as medications or thyroid disease, an MRI of the head is warranted for further evaluation. Among women who present with amenorrhea and elevated prolactin, 50% to 60% are associated with a pituitary tumor. Additionally, pituitary disorders including Sheehan

syndrome, pituitary gland necrosis, and empty sella syndrome may also be causes of anovulation and amenorrhea, as well as other pituitary or central nervous system tumors and organic diseases.

Regarding treatment for hyperprolactinemia, dopamine agonists may be used to aid in decreasing prolactin levels, regardless of the presence of pituitary tumor. This has an effect on the subsequent restoration of menses. In cases of pituitary adenoma, surgical resection may be warranted.

Hypothalamic Amenorrhea

The most common cause of chronic anovulation is functional hypothalamic amenorrhea, often associated with stress, weight loss, poor nutrition, and strenuous exercise. In these cases, suppression of the normal hypothalamic-pituitary-ovarian axis occurs as a result of an overall energy deficit, though the exact pathophysiology remains unclear. A much less common cause of hypothalamic amenorrhea is isolated gonadotropin deficiency, such as that seen in Kallmann syndrome (primary GnRH deficiency).

Multidisciplinary care should be considered in the approach to treatment of functional hypothalamic amenorrhea. Appropriate nutrition rehabilitation and reduction of strenuous exercise are important aspects of management for these women, and restoration of menses usually occurs following correction of the energy deficit. Furthermore, treatment should address stress reduction and psychosocial health, which may also play a role in the resumption of menses. As for pharmacologic management, evidence suggests that the use of leptin may help restore GnRH pulsatility and thus ovulation and menses, given its regulatory role in hypothalamic dysfunction. For those with hypothalamic amenorrhea desiring pregnancy, treatment options for ovulation induction may be pursued, typically with GnRH or gonadotropin therapy.

Similar to primary ovarian insufficiency, hypothalamic amenorrhea is associated with an estrogen deficient state, so affected women are at increased risk for osteoporosis. Bone density screening may be considered. In addition to nutrition rehabilitation and a decrease of strenuous activity, it is important to ensure adequate calcium and vitamin D intake with supplementation. Cyclic hormone therapy at physiologic doses may be considered for optimizing bone health, such as in cases where correction of the underlying cause of hypothalamic amenorrhea is not easily achieved. However, the potential beneficial effects on bone density in these cases are limited in the absence of appropriate nutrition rehabilitation. Furthermore, the use of bisphosphonates in the premenopausal population is not recommended given the limited data available and concern for potential teratogenic risks. Thus, treatment should primarily focus on addressing the underlying cause of hypothalamic amenorrhea.

Polycystic Ovary Syndrome

Chronic anovulation and amenorrhea may also occur with PCOS, though these women are more likely to present with oligomenorrhea. The presence of obesity and concomitant signs of androgen excess help distinguish PCOS from hypothalamic amenorrhea. Typically, a higher BMI is associated with PCOS, while normal or low BMI is more often associated with functional hypothalamic amenorrhea. According to the Rotterdam Consensus Criteria from 2003, the diagnosis of PCOS requires at least two of the following: (1) signs of androgen excess, (2) the presence of polycystic ovaries, and (3) ovulatory dysfunction. However, the 2006 Androgen Excess Society criteria for PCOS differ slightly from these guidelines, specifically requiring hyperandrogenism as one of the diagnostic conditions, along with ovarian dysfunction (oligo-anovulation and/or polycystic ovaries) and exclusion of other androgen excess or related disorders. The evidence of hyperandrogenism may be established by clinical findings (e.g., hirsutism, acne, male pattern alopecia) or laboratory measurement. Generally, serum androgen levels in those with PCOS do not exceed twice the upper limit of normal range, so further investigation for other etiologies of hyperandrogenism would be warranted in these cases.

The management of women with PCOS includes monitoring for insulin resistance and glucose intolerance, dyslipidemia, and cardiovascular risk, with subsequent interventions as indicated for any identified comorbidities. Treatment also involves healthy lifestyle modifications directed at dietary changes, exercise, and weight loss, given the association of PCOS with obesity. Furthermore, low-dose combined oral contraceptives are recommended to reduce the risk for endometrial cancer in the setting of chronic anovulation. Pharmacotherapy with metformin (Glucophage)[1] is another important treatment consideration, which may provide beneficial effects on ovulation, menstrual abnormalities, and androgen levels, in addition to its known effects on improving glucose tolerance.

---

[1]Not FDA approved for this indication.

References

American College of Obstetricians and Gynecologists: Committee Opinion No. 728. Müllerian agenesis: diagnosis, management, and treatment, *Obstet Gynecol* 131:e35–42, 2018.

American College of Obstetricians and Gynecologists: Committee Opinion No. 605. Primary ovarian insufficiency in adolescents and young women, *Obstet Gynecol* 123:193–197, 2014.

Gordon CM: Clinical practice: Functional hypothalamic amenorrhea, *N Engl J Med* 363(4):365–371, 2010.

Klein DA, Poth MA: Amenorrhea: An approach to diagnosis and management, *Am Fam Physician* 87(11):781–788, 2013.

Practice Committee of American Society for Reproductive Medicine: Current evaluation of amenorrhea, *Fertil Steril* 90:S219–S225, 2008.

BACTERIAL INFECTIONS OF THE URINARY TRACT IN WOMEN

Method of
Kinder Fayssoux, MD

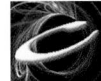

CURRENT DIAGNOSIS

- Acute cystitis is the most common urologic disorder in women.
- *Escherichia coli* and *Staphylococcus saprophyticus* are the causative agents for 80% of community acquired urinary tract infections (UTIs).
- *E. coli* is also the most common uropathogen in the nosocomial setting.
- Anatomic risk factors include short urethra, the proximity of the urethra to the anus, and the colonization of the periurethral mucosa with bowel flora.
- Other risk factors include previous UTI, sexual intercourse, and, separately, the use of spermicide, pregnancy, diabetes, incontinence, cystocoele, and incomplete emptying of the bladder and dysfunctional voiding (defined as abnormal bladder emptying in the absence of neurologic disease).
- Postmenopausal women are also at increased risk if they are estrogen deficient.
- Acute cystitis typically presents with abrupt onset of dysuria, increased frequency, and/or urgency. Less frequently a patient will present with hematuria, suprapubic discomfort, or back/costovertebral angle pain. If a fever is present, it is usually less than 38.9°C (102°F).
- Acute pyelonephritis can evolve from either asymptomatic bacteriuria or from an ascending bladder infection.
- Symptoms usually include fever usually greater than 38.9°C (102°F) with chills, nausea/vomiting, dysuria, increased frequency, urgency, and costovertebral angle (CVA) tenderness (usually unilateral).
- *E. coli* is the major pathogen in acute pyelonephritis and treatment depends on severity and pregnancy status.

- Empiric therapy for uncomplicated UTIs should be dependent on the most recent antibiotic guidelines and the uropathogen resistance patterns in a community.
- In a community with >20% incidence of resistant *E. coli*, nitrofurantoin (Macrobid) 100 mg bid for 7 days is the treatment of choice with quinolones as second-line therapy.
- In a community with <20% *E. coli* resistance, trimethoprim/sulfamethoxazole 160/800 (Bactrim DS) PO twice daily for 3 days is also acceptable as first-line therapy with quinolones still considered as second-line therapy.
- Phenazopyridine (Pyridium), a smooth muscle relaxant, can be prescribed for spasm relief.
- Fungal UTIs or candiduria should be treated with fluconazole (Diflucan) 200 mg daily for 2 weeks.
- Outpatient treatment guidelines for acute pyelonephritis are the same as for uncomplicated UTI except the duration of antimicrobial therapy is longer (10–14 days).
- Inpatient treatment for acute pyelonephritis is typically IV levofloxacin (Levaquin) (750 mg daily) or ampicillin (1 g every 6 h).
- Acute pyelonephritis should resolve in 48 to 72 hours, if patients are not getting better, imaging should be undertaken with ultrasound or CT scan to assess for renal abscess or urethral obstruction.

Acute Cystitis (Urinary Tract Infection)

Acute cystitis is the most common urologic disorder among women. It represents 4% of all outpatient visits. Of these visits, 52% present to a primary care clinic and 23% to the emergency department. The annual health care costs associated with urinary tract infections (UTIs) are roughly 1.6 billion and climbing. Antimicrobial prescriptions for UTIs account for 15% of all outpatient prescriptions. One-third of all women will have at least one symptomatic UTI by age 24, with more than half of all women having at least one during their lifetime.

Acute cystitis can be defined as uncomplicated or complicated. Uncomplicated cystitis is defined as a UTI in patients with normal urinary tract anatomy without a contributing medical condition such as diabetes mellitus, neurogenic bladder, pregnancy, renal insufficiency, immune deficiency, recent antibiotic use, recent genitourinary instrumentation, spinal cord injury, ureteral obstruction, or nephrolithiasis. Complicated cystitis is defined as a UTI in patients with abnormal urinary tract anatomy or with one of the aforementioned medical conditions. These patients generally require urine culture as part of the initial work-up to guide antimicrobial therapy and often additional condition specific evaluation and treatment.

Acute cystitis is caused by ascending bacteria of perineal/urethral/fecal origin through the urethra into the bladder and renal systems. *Escherichia coli* and *Staphylococcus saprophyticus* are the causative agents for 80% of community acquired UTIs (complicated and uncomplicated). *E. coli* is also the most common uropathogen in the nosocomial setting. Other known uropathogens include *Pseudomonas spp*, *Klebsiella spp*, *Proteus*, *Corynebacterium urealyticum*, and *Providencia*. Fungal UTIs caused by *Candida spp*, *Aspergillus spp*, and *Cryptococcus neoformans* are also increasingly encountered. These are usually caused by indwelling urinary devices and seen more frequently in diabetics. Other populations prone to fungal UTIs include patients who are immunocompromised, hospitalized, or elderly.

There are numerous risk factors for acute cystitis, several specific to women. Risk factors unique to women include several related to their anatomy. These anatomic differences are the primary reason for the increased incidence of UTI in women when compared to men and include the female's relatively short urethra (when compared to the male counterpart), the proximity of the urethra to the anus, and the colonization of the periurethral mucosa with bowel flora.

Other risk factors include previous UTI, sexual intercourse, and, separately, the use of spermicide, pregnancy, diabetes, incontinence, cystocoele, and incomplete emptying of the bladder and dysfunctional voiding (defined as abnormal bladder emptying in the absence of neurologic disease). Postmenopausal women are also at increased risk if they are estrogen deficient.

Dysfunctional voiding has an unknown etiology and results in increased external sphincter activity during voluntary voiding which results in reflux, increasing chances of UTI.

Commonly advised behavioral modifications thought to decrease the risk of UTI (e.g., postcoital voiding, increased fluid intake, avoidance of urinary holding, douching, front-to-back wiping, proper tampon/sanitary napkin use, and loose/cotton underwear) have been supported by the literature.

Acute cystitis typically appears as an abrupt onset of dysuria, increased frequency, and/or urgency. Less frequently a patient will present with hematuria, suprapubic discomfort, or back/costovertebral angle pain. If a fever is present, it is usually less than 38.9°C (102°F).

Obtaining a good history that assesses for risk factors and symptoms is important in diagnosing acute cystitis. In a woman who presents with one or more symptoms of UTI (dysuria, frequency, urgency, hematuria), the probability of infection is already 50%. A urine dipstick is a useful diagnostic test, with a positive (+) nitrite or leukocyte esterase result increasing the chances of infection. The combination of positive nitrite *and* leukocyte esterase results has the highest diagnostic correlation with UTI. Physical examination findings may include suprapubic tenderness or costovertebral angle tenderness, although these are unlikely in an uncomplicated UTI scenario.

The gold standard for diagnosis of acute cystitis is a culture that has 10^2 to 10^3 colony-forming units of a single uropathogen from a clean catch or catheterized urine specimen. However, research has shown that, for uncomplicated cystitis, ordering cultures and sensitivities makes little difference in treatment while increasing cost of care. Thus, it is reasonable to start empiric treatment without a culture and sensitivities in a patient presenting with uncomplicated UTI.

The differential diagnosis for an uncomplicated UTI includes:
- Vaginitis/vaginal infections: can cause dysuria
  - *Gardnerella*, *Candida albicans*, and *Trichomonas*
- Urethritis: can cause dysuria/frequency
  - STDs (*Chlamydia trachomatis*, gonorrhea, herpes simplex)
  - Pelvic floor spasm (leads to urethral spasm/irritability)
- Interstitial cystitis
- Malignancy
- Renal tuberculosis

Differentiating between sexually transmitted infections (STI), vaginal infections, and UTIs can be difficult because symptoms and signs commonly overlap. History elements that should prompt a pelvic examination and laboratory evaluation for pathogens are complaints of a vaginal discharge or vaginal irritation/pruritus. Persistent hematuria should raise the concern for underlying malignancy or renal tuberculosis, and further evaluation should be done.

Empiric therapy for uncomplicated UTIs should be dependent on the most recent antibiotic guidelines and the uropathogen resistance patterns in a community. In a community with >20% incidence of resistant *E. coli*, nitrofurantoin (Macrobid) 100 mg bid for 7 days is the treatment of choice with quinolones as second-line therapy. In a community with <20% *E. coli* resistance, trimethoprim/sulfamethoxazole 160/800 (Bactrim DS) PO twice daily for 3 days is also acceptable as first-line therapy with quinolones still considered as second-line therapy. Phenazopyridine (Pyridium), a smooth muscle relaxant, can be prescribed for spasm relief and is usually only necessary for the first 24 hours after treatment is initiated. Fungal UTIs or *candiduria* should be treated with fluconazole (Diflucan) 200 mg daily for 2 weeks.

For a complicated UTI, a culture must always be obtained and the patient should be evaluated in the context of his or her specific comorbid condition before treatment.

Acute Pyelonephritis

Acute pyelonephritis can evolve from either asymptomatic bacteriuria or from an ascending bladder infection. Although it can progress from an uncomplicated cystitis, it more commonly presents from a complicated cystitis in the setting of other medical conditions such cholelithiasis, urinary obstruction, malformations, or pregnancy.

Symptoms usually include fever usually greater than 38.9°C (102°F) with chills, nausea/vomiting, dysuria, increased frequency, urgency, and CVA tenderness (usually unilateral). These symptoms can present on a spectrum from mild to severe. *E. coli* is the major pathogen, and treatment depends on severity and pregnancy status. Pregnant patients or patients with moderate to severe nausea/vomiting that would interfere with oral antibiotic treatment should be hospitalized and have blood cultures done in addition to urine culture. Patients with mild symptoms and the ability to tolerate oral antibiotics can be treated as on an outpatient basis with a urine culture obtained before initializing treatment. Outpatient treatment guidelines are the same as for uncomplicated UTI, except the duration of antimicrobial therapy is longer (10–14 days). Inpatient treatment is typically IV levofloxacin (Levaquin 750 mg daily) or ampicillin (1 g every 6 h). Once the inpatient is able to tolerate oral antibiotics and the infection is felt to be controlled, he or she can be switched to oral antibiotics and discharged to complete a 14-day course of treatment as an outpatient.

Symptoms should resolve in 48 to 72 hours; if patients are not getting better, imaging should be undertaken with ultrasound or CT scan to assess for renal abscess or urethral obstruction.

Urethritis

Urethritis usually has a gradual onset and is accompanied with milder symptoms of dysuria, frequency, urgency, or hematuria. It can also occur with a vaginal discharge and complaints of dyspareunia and vaginal pruritus depending on cause. Chalmydial, gonorrheal, candidal and trichomonal urethritis is usually accompanied by a vaginal discharge. Candidal urethritis can also be associated with pruritus and dyspareunia. If urethritis is suspected, a pelvic examination and further laboratory work-up is necessary.

Asymptomatic Bacteriuria

Asymptomatic bacteriuria is defined as the presence of 100,000 microorganisms/milliliter of urine without any symptoms of cystitis.

No screening should be performed in healthy nonpregnant women, elderly living in the community, diabetic women, institutionalized elderly, or persons with spinal cord injury. Pregnant women are the exception. They should be screened; positive cultures need to be treated, as there is an increased likelihood of asymptomatic bacteriuria turning into UTI or pyelonephritis because of vesicoureteral reflux and urinary stasis resulting from increased progesterone levels.

Recurrent Cystitis

Recurrent cystitis is defined as at least three episodes of uncomplicated UTI with one or more documented positive (+) cultures in 12 months. It can be due to relapse or reinfection. Relapse is defined as infection occurring with the same organism as a previous UTI. Reinfection is when symptoms return after treatment and a completely symptom-free interval along with a negative urine culture or when the second infection is caused by a different organism. Most recurrent cystitis tends to be caused by reinfection.

In patients presenting with recurrent cystitis, an age-based evaluation is a good place to start. Adolescents who are not sexually active should be evaluated for congenital abnormalities. Premenopausal females should be questioned about the temporal relationship of the onset of UTI to increased frequency/recent sexual intercourse, spermicide use (with or without condom or diaphragm), or renal stones. Postmenopausal females should be evaluated for decreased estrogen/vaginal atrophy, incontinence, incomplete bladder emptying, cystocoeles, and prolapse.

If a complete and thorough evaluation is done, complicating factors are ruled out, modifiable factors are treated, and recurrent cystitis still remains a problem, then treatment should be considered. Treatment options include continuous antibiotics, postcoital therapy, or self- initiated treatment at the first sign or symptom of an infection.

Gross hematuria or persistent microscopic hematuria should increase suspicion for an underlying malignancy. Also, recurrent cystitis symptoms in a setting of negative cultures may suggest mycobacterial infection or interstitial cystitis.

Catheter Associated Urinary Tract Infection

Catheter-associated UTI is defined as a UTI in a patient who had an indwelling urethral catheter within 48 hours of onset of infection. Indwelling urinary catheters and clean intermittent catheterization are associated with the highest rates of bacteriuria; after 1 month of either there is almost 100% risk of bacteriuria. Formation of a bacterial biofilm on the catheter is thought to be the mechanism of infection in this setting.

No treatment is recommended for asymptomatic patients, and neither prophylactic antibiotics nor routine UA and culture are recommended for this population. For symptomatic patients, the first step is to determine whether the catheter can be removed. If it cannot, then it should be replaced. In addition, a blood and urine culture (taken from a new catheter) should be obtained. Initial treatment is the same as for an uncomplicated UTI as discussed earlier. Confirmation of susceptibility should be confirmed with culture results.

References

Litza JA, Brill JR: Urinary tract infection, *Primary Care Clinical Office Practice* 37:491–507, 2010.

Minardi D, d'Anzeo G, Cantoro D, et al: Urinary tract infections in women: Etiology and treatment options, *Int J Gen Med* 4:333–343, 2011.

Finer G, Landau D: Pathogenesis of urinary tract infections with normal female anatomy, *Lancet* 4:631–634, 2004.

Foster RT: Office gynecology uncomplicated urinary tract infections in women. Obstet Gynecol Clin 35:235–48.

Berek JS: *Berek and Novak's Gynecology*, Philadelphia, 2012, Lippincott. p. 570–71.

Essentials evidence plus: Urinary tract infection (adults), Available at http://essentialevidenceplus.com, accessed August 16, 2016.

Essentials evidence plus: Urethritis (female), http://essentialevidenceplus.com, Accessed August 16, 2016.

Bent SN, Nallamothu BK, Simel DL, et al: Does this woman have an acute uncomplicated urinary tract infection? *JAMA* 287:2701–2710, 2002.

Wagenlehner F, Weidner W, Naber K: An updated on uncomplicated urinary tract infections in women, *Curr Opin Urol* 19:368–374, 2009.

Dielubaza EJ, Schaeffer AJ: Urologic issues for the internist- urinary tract infections in women. Med Clin North Am 95:27–41.

Giesen LG, Cousins G, Dimitrov BD, et al: Predicting acute uncomplicated urinary tract infections in women: A systematic review of the diagnostic accuracy of symptoms and signs, *BMC Fam Pract* 11:78, 2010. Available at http://www.biomedcentral.com/1471-2296/11/78, accessed August 16, 2016.

BENIGN BREAST DISEASE

Method of
Lauren Nye, MD

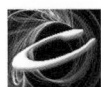

CURRENT DIAGNOSIS

- Mammography is used for breast cancer screening, and it is recommended to begin screening in women at average risk for breast cancer between ages 40 and 50.
- Benign breast disease may present with an abnormality on screening breast imaging or with a breast symptom such as a breast mass or nipple discharge.
- Nonproliferative breast lesions are not associated with an increased risk of breast cancer.
- Proliferative breast lesions without atypia are associated with a slightly increased risk for breast cancer, whereas proliferative lesions with atypia are associated with a significantly increased risk for breast cancer.
- Factors contributing to a woman's breast cancer risk include family history, personal health history, and modifiable lifestyle factors.

CURRENT THERAPY

- Some benign breast lesions do not need any further intervention after diagnosis; others may require surgical excision to rule out malignancy.
- Women at high risk for breast cancer may warrant additional breast screening or begin screening at an earlier age.
- Women at high risk for breast cancer should be counseled on risk reduction strategies, including lifestyle modification.
- Chemoprevention agents include tamoxifen, raloxifene (Evista), and aromatase inhibitors.

Breast health is an important aspect of women's health care; it includes breast cancer screening and evaluation of breast concerns. Benign breast disease can be identified on a biopsy done for an abnormal screening test, a palpable breast mass, nipple discharge, or other breast concerns. Benign breast disease may be associated with an increased risk for breast cancer. Women at high risk for breast cancer should be considered for additional breast cancer screening recommendations and risk reduction strategies.

Presentation and Workup

Patients can present with benign breast disease after an abnormality detected on screening imaging or after workup for breast symptoms such as a palpable mass, breast pain, or spontaneous nipple discharge. In women who are considered at average risk for breast cancer based on medical and family history, screening includes history and physical examination by their health care provider, clinical breast examination, and breast imaging. Breast awareness should be encouraged, but formal breast self-examinations in average-risk women have not been shown to have a breast cancer mortality benefit, although in women who performed self-breast examinations, a greater number of benign breast lesions were detected.

Breast Cancer Screening

Women at average risk for breast cancer should begin screening mammography between age 40 and 50. The 2016 updated recommendations of the US Preventive Services Task Force (USPSTF) recommend biennial screening mammography for women ages 50 to 74; the decision to start screening mammography prior to age 50 should be individualized. The 2015 American Cancer Society (ACS) breast cancer screening guidelines for women at average risk include a strong recommendation to begin screening mammography at age 45 and a qualified recommendation to begin at age 40, continuing as long as the woman is in good overall health and life expectancy is 10 years or greater. The most updated recommendation from the National Comprehensive Cancer Network (NCCN) and the American College of Radiology (ACR) is for annual screening mammography beginning at age 40. The standard for breast cancer screening is the digital mammogram; however, in recent years digital breast tomosynthesis has become more prevalent and available to women at breast imaging centers. Digital breast tomosynthesis has both a higher breast cancer detection rate and a lower recall rate compared with the digital mammogram for breast cancer screening. In women with heterogeneously dense breast or dense breast tissue on screening mammogram, the risks and benefits of supplemental screening with bilateral breast screening ultrasound or breast MRI should be discussed as high breast density limits mammogram sensitivity.

Normal and abnormal findings on breast imaging are reported using the universal classification system by the ACR's classification: the Breast Imaging Reporting and Data System (BI-RADS). Table 1 includes the BI-RADS categories, the risk of malignancy, and the recommended follow-up. BI-RADS 0 indicates an incomplete assessment and that further workup is needed, typically with additional imaging recommendations. BI-RADS 3 lesions are considered probably benign based on appearance; a mammogram and/or ultrasound in 6 months is recommended for follow-up. BI-RADS 4 and BI-RADS 5 lesions are suspicious or highly suggestive of malignancy, respectively, and a biopsy of the lesion is recommended.

Palpable Breast Mass

In patients who present with a palpable breast mass, workup is determined by patient age, menopausal status, and degree of suspicion of breast mass. Fig. 1 outlines the algorithm for evaluation of a woman with a breast mass. In women younger than age 30 with a mass of low clinical suspicion, it would be appropriate to consider observation over one to two menstrual cycles prior to moving on to ultrasound imaging if the mass persists. If no mass is detected on ultrasound, short-term clinical follow-up is recommended. Diagnostic mammography with ultrasound may be considered in women younger than age 30 who have a mass of high clinical suspicion or increased breast cancer risk. In postmenopausal women and women 30 years of age and older, a clinically palpable breast mass should be evaluated with a diagnostic mammogram and ultrasound. A clinically suspicious mass without a radiographic correlate on imaging should be evaluated for palpation-guided biopsy of the mass. A patient identified to have a simple cyst on imaging can return to age-appropriate breast screening. A solitary complicated cyst should be aspirated or be followed in short-term follow-up for stability. Multiple complicated cysts are considered a benign finding and do not require aspiration or short-term follow-up. Routine cytology of aspirated fluid is not recommended. If the mass persists after aspiration of a complicated cyst or if initial imaging shows a mass of high clinical suspicion or a complex cystic and solid mass, ultrasound-guided biopsy of the mass is recommended.

The sonographic description of a simple cyst is a round or oval circumscribed mass with acoustic enhancement and lacking any solid components or Doppler signals. A nonsimple cyst may be complicated or a complex cystic and solid mass. A complicated cyst is round or oval and circumscribed but may show low-level internal echoes without demonstrating vascular flow, whereas a complex cystic and solid mass may have thick septations, thick and irregular walls, and an internal solid component; it may display internal echoes, internal blood flow, and lack of posterior wall enhancement.

Nipple Discharge

Some women may present with nipple discharge without a palpable mass. Concerning features for pathologic nipple discharge

TABLE 1	Breast Imaging Reporting and Data System Mammography Classification		
BI-RADS CATEGORY	**DEFINITION**	**RISK FOR MALIGNANCY**	**RECOMMENDED FOLLOW-UP**
0	Incomplete assessment	N/A	Further imaging
1	Negative study	N/A	Routine mammogram screening
2	Benign	N/A	Routine mammogram screening
3	Probably benign	≤ 2%	Repeat imaging in 6 months
4	Suspicious	>2%–95% depending on degree of suspicion	Biopsy recommended
5	Highly suggestive of malignancy	≥ 95%	Biopsy recommended
6	Known biopsy-proven malignancy	N/A	Appropriate action should be taken

BI-RADS, Breast Imaging Reporting and Data System.

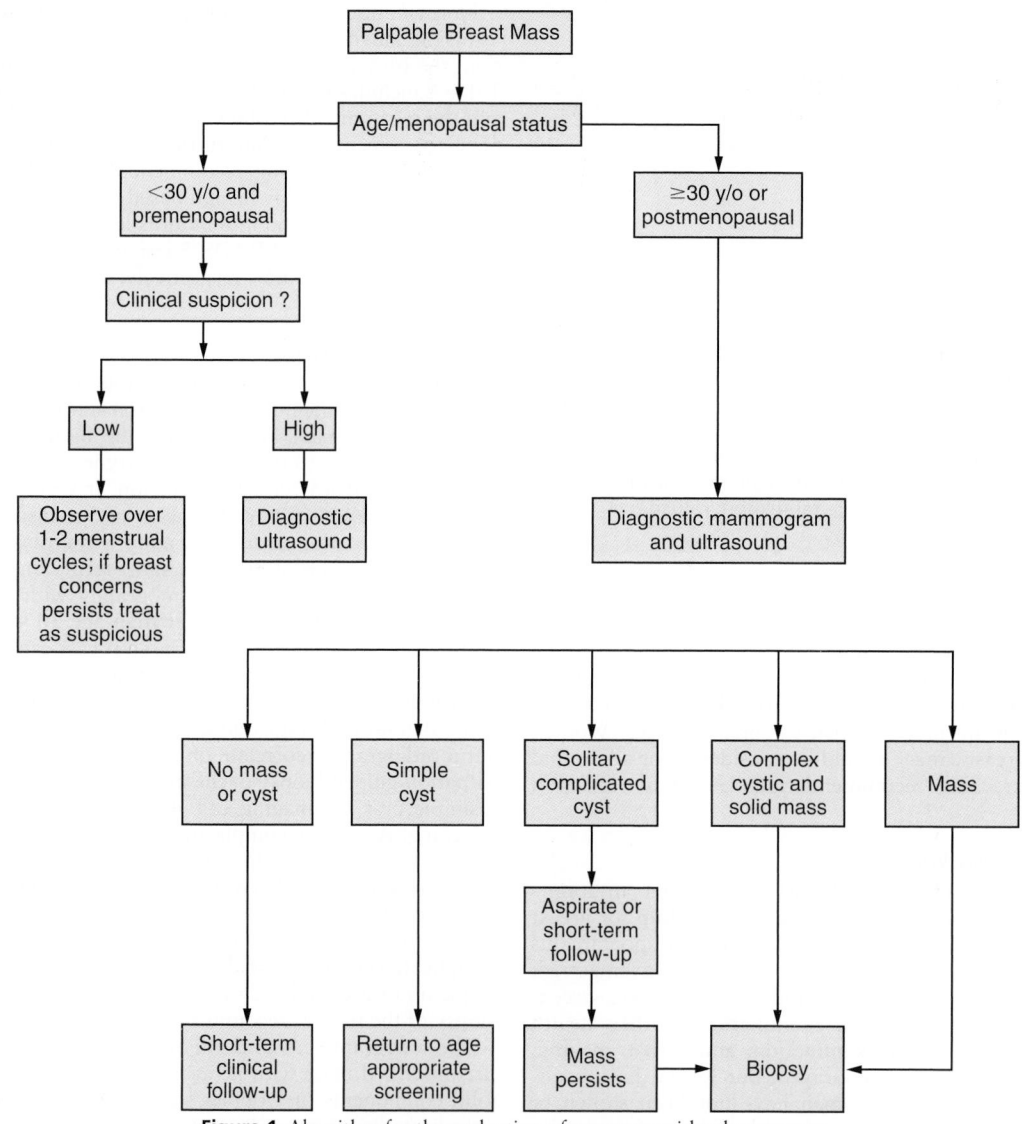

Figure 1 Algorithm for the evaluation of a woman with a breast mass.

include a spontaneous unilateral single-duct discharge that is reproducible on examination and discharge that is clear, serous, sanguineous, or serosanguinous. Nonspontaneous nipple discharge or multiduct discharge is likely physiologic and the most common cause is duct ectasia. Women should be educated on avoiding further breast compression to elicit the discharge, ensure that they are up to date on age-appropriate breast cancer screening, and review potential medications that could cause nipple discharge. In women with spontaneous pathologic single-duct nipple discharge, the most common etiology is an intraductal papilloma. The most common malignant explanation would be ductal carcinoma in situ (DCIS). The workup should include diagnostic mammography and ultrasound for women 30 years of age or older and at least a diagnostic ultrasound in women younger than age 30. Suspicious or highly suspicious imaging findings warrant biopsy. If initial imaging does not explain the

TABLE 2	Benign Breast Lesions	
NONPROLIFERATIVE LESIONS	PROLIFERATIVE LESIONS WITHOUT ATYPIA	PROLIFERATIVE LESIONS WITH ATYPIA
Apocrine metaplasia	Fibroadenomas	Atypical ductal hyperplasia
Breast cysts	Microglandular adenosis	Atypical lobular hyperplasia
Columnar cell change	Moderate or florid usual ductal hyperplasia	
Duct ectasia	Papilloma	
Fibrosis	Radial scar	
	Sclerosing adenosis	

nipple discharge, a ductogram or magnetic resonance imaging (MRI) may be considered for further evaluation. In some cases duct excision may be recommended; otherwise the patient should have short-term follow-up with clinical breast examination and imaging.

Benign Lesions

Benign breast diseases can be categorized as nonproliferative, proliferative without atypia, proliferative with atypia, and miscellaneous other conditions such as fat necrosis, various types of mastitis, pseudoangiomatous stromal hyperplasia, fibrous mastopathy, amyloid deposits, and dermatologic conditions. Table 2 outlines the benign breast lesions. A study by Dupont and Page in the 1980s and a review by Hartmann et al. in 2005 found that nonproliferative breast disease was not associated with an increased risk for breast cancer. Proliferative breast disease without atypia is associated with a slightly increased risk for breast cancer but less than two times the average population risk. Proliferative breast disease with atypia is associated with a significantly increased breast cancer risk that can be four to five times higher than the average population risk.

Nonproliferative Lesions

Nonproliferative breast lesions are also known as fibrocystic disease or change and include duct ectasia, fibrosis, and apocrine metaplasia. In women without a significant family history of breast cancer, nonproliferative breast lesions are not associated with an increased breast cancer risk. In the study by Dupont and Page including 3303 patients with benign breast disease, only 2.2% of the patients with nonproliferative lesions had breast cancer at a mean follow-up of 17 years. The Hartmann study of 9087 women followed for a median of 15 years found that the strength of family history was an independent risk factor; in women with nonproliferative lesions, the relative risk of breast cancer was 1.27. No increased risk was found in women with no family history.

Ductal ectasia and breast cysts are common findings. Occasionally the ectatic ducts are surrounded with periductal inflammation, which can occur in nonlactating women when the duct becomes congested with debris. This can lead to periductal mastitis that requires treatment with antibiotics. Breast cysts are most common in perimenopausal women but can occur in premenopausal women and postmenopausal women on hormone replacement therapy. Breast cysts may present in women with fibrocystic breast disease, which women may report as nodular breast tissue and is caused by microcystic formation and stromal proliferation of the breast. Apocrine metaplasia, in which acini and cysts are lined with large columnar cells that resemble the apocrine sweat glands, is not an uncommon finding. The individual cells are large, with abundant granular eosinophilic cytoplasm. The apical aspects of these cells have a rounded protrusion into the cyst

spaces. Columnar cell change is characterized by enlargement of the terminal duct lobular units and dilated acini without atypia.

Proliferative Lesions Without Atypia

Proliferative breast lesions without atypia include fibroepithelial lesions such as fibroadenomas, moderate or florid usual ductal hyperplasia, microglandular and sclerosing adenosis, papillomas, and radial scars. Proliferative breast lesions without atypia are associated with a slightly increased risk of breast cancer compared with the average risk of the population, with the relative risk estimated between 1.8 and 1.9. These lesions are not currently considered to put a woman at high risk for breast cancer unless other risk factors are present, such as family history.

Fibroadenomas are benign processes containing glandular and fibrous tissue. Fibroadenomas were originally classified as nonproliferative lesions (including in the Hartmann study) but are now typically considered proliferative breast lesions. Simple fibroadenomas without associated proliferative disease are not associated with an increased risk for breast cancer, while complex fibroadenomas and those with coinciding proliferative disease are associated with a slight increase in breast cancer risk. Fibroadenomas are most common in young premenopausal women and can fluctuate in size with changes in hormones. They do not routinely need to be excised unless they are enlarging or have associated symptoms, such as tenderness.

The normal number of epithelial linings within the breast is two. Epithelial hyperplasia has a spectrum of changes from mild to severe, presenting with an escalating scale of complexity. Usual ductal hyperplasia (UDH) is an increased number of cells within the duct that will vary in size and shape but will appear benign and without atypia. Microglandular adenosis and sclerosing adenosis are lesions with an increased number of glandular elements within fibrous stroma. Microglandular and sclerosing adenosis may be associated with microcalcifications and/or a mass on mammography.

Classic papillomas are masslike lesions that occur within large ducts close to the subareolar area. Histologically, they are composed of arborizing fronds of fibrovascular stroma lined by epithelial cells with a stalk attaching the mass to the wall of the cyst within which they arise. They can appear as a mass on mammography or present with unilateral nipple discharge. Papillomas can be associated with hyperplasia with and without atypia or DCIS; in those cases, surgical excision is recommended to rule out malignancy.

Radial scars or complex sclerosing lesions are a pathologic diagnosis but can cause abnormalities on breast imaging including mass, nonmass enhancement, or architectural distortion. Histologically, they have a central fibroelastic core with radiating and branching ducts and lobules at the periphery. The etiology of these lesions is unknown. Depending on the size and presentation, surgical excision may be recommended to rule out underlying malignancy.

Proliferative Lesions with Atypia

Proliferative lesions with atypia include atypical ductal hyperplasia (ADH) and atypical lobular hyperplasia (ALH). These atypical hyperplasia lesions are characterized by an abundance of monotonous-appearing epithelial cells partially filling a duct and/or lobule. The presence of atypical hyperplasia is a risk factor for future breast cancer and is associated with a relative risk of breast cancer between four and five times the general population risk. The risk of breast cancer over the 25 years following a biopsy demonstrating atypical hyperplasia is estimated at 30%. The number of foci of atypia present in the specimen can stratify the risk, with one focus being a lower risk compared to three or more foci of atypia. These patients should be managed in a multidisciplinary fashion to include assessment of concordance between radiology and pathology. The standard management for atypical hyperplasia including ADH and ALH is surgical excision to rule out underlying malignancy; however, select patients who have concordance with imaging may be appropriate for screening in lieu of surgical excision.

Miscellaneous Benign Breast Conditions

Pseudoangiomatous stromal hyperplasia (PASH) is a lesion of a stromal proliferation with anastomosing spaces, with the dense hyalinized stroma intermixed with glandular components. These spaces could appear as vascular structures to the untrained pathologist. PASH may appear similar to an angiosarcoma but can be differentiated by the lack of atypia and mitosis. PASH can present with a palpable mass, with a mammogram abnormality, or as an incidental finding. Historically this lesion commonly underwent excision; however, depending on the size of the lesion, concordance with imaging, and other risk factors, PASH may be appropriately monitored with follow-up imaging.

Fat necrosis is secondary to trauma or injury to the breast. Fat necrosis typically presents with a painless breast mass and appears as an ill-defined dense mass on breast imaging. A biopsy is recommended to rule out malignancy; however, no further treatment is necessary.

High-Risk Evaluation and Management

The lifetime risk of breast cancer for women in the United States is approximately one in eight. There are elements of a woman's personal or family history that may increase her risk for breast cancer and potentially warrant additional screening and management. Risk factors that contribute to a women's lifetime risk of breast cancer include family history of breast and/or ovarian cancer, genetic mutations associated with hereditary breast cancer, reproductive history, personal history of multiple breast biopsies or a breast biopsy showing atypical hyperplasia or lobular carcinoma in situ (LCIS), and dense breast tissue on mammography. Women who received thoracic radiation prior to age 30 are also at an increased risk for breast cancer. Modifiable risk factors for breast cancer include increased body mass index, sedentary lifestyle, alcohol intake, and hormone replacement therapy with estrogen and progesterone. Breast cancer risk assessment tools are available to estimate a woman's risk and include the Breast Cancer Risk Assessment Tool (previously referred to as the Gail model) and family history–based models such as, BRCAPRO, and Tyrer-Cuzick. In 2019, the USPSTF updated recommendations for BRCA-related cancer risk and recommended women with a family history of breast, ovarian, tubal, or peritoneal cancer and previously treated survivors of any of those cancers should be assessed for genetic risk.

Women considered at high risk for breast cancer include those with a Gail Model 5-year breast cancer risk of greater than or equal to 1.7%, a lifetime risk of breast cancer of greater than 20% based on a family history–based model, or a history of thoracic radiation prior to age 30, as well as women harboring a deleterious genetic mutation associated with breast cancer or a personal history of atypical hyperplasia or lobular carcinoma in situ. Women at high risk for breast cancer may be eligible for additional screening including earlier age at initiation of screening/imaging and consideration of an annual breast MRI.

Women at high risk for breast cancer should be counseled on screening recommendations and risk reduction strategies. Lifestyle modifications associated with decreased breast cancer risk include breastfeeding, achieving a healthy body mass index, limiting alcohol consumption, and exercising regularly. Some women may be considered for risk-reducing surgery. Chemoprevention may also be an option for women at high risk for breast cancer.

Chemoprevention

Risk-reducing agents, also known as chemoprevention, are appropriate to consider in women with atypical hyperplasia, LCIS, or a 5-year breast cancer risk of greater than or equal to 1.7%. Risk-reducing agents include tamoxifen, raloxifene (Evista), and the aromatase inhibitors (exemestane [Aromasin][1] and anastrozole [Arimidex][1]). Chemoprevention is taken daily for 5 years and associated with a potential risk reduction of 40% to 65%. No survival benefit has been demonstrated in women who take chemoprevention, and the risks and benefits of each therapy should be discussed. Tamoxifen is a selective estrogen receptor modulator (SERM) and is the only agent available for premenopausal women. Tamoxifen should not be recommended to women who are currently pregnant or considering future pregnancy owing to potential teratogenic effects. The National Surgical Adjuvant Breast and Bowel Project (NSABP) Breast Cancer Prevention Trial (NSABP P-1) of tamoxifen 20 mg daily for 5 years verses placebo included both pre- and postmenopausal women at high risk for breast cancer and demonstrated a reduced risk of invasive breast cancer of 49%. In this study tamoxifen was associated with an increased rate of endometrial cancer, deep vein thrombosis, pulmonary embolism, and stroke, and these events were more frequent in women over the age of 50. Raloxifene is a second-generation SERM. The STAR trial (NSABP P-2) randomized postmenopausal women at high risk for breast cancer to 5 years of tamoxifen 20 mg daily versus raloxifene 60 mg daily. Raloxifene was demonstrated to be as effective as tamoxifen at reducing the risk of invasive breast cancer but not noninvasive breast cancer. Raloxifene was associated with a lower rate of venous thromboembolic events and endometrial cancer. Aromatase inhibitors were studied in postmenopausal women for breast cancer prevention in the MAP.3 (exemestane) and IBIS-II (anastrozole) trials. Exemestane 25 mg daily for 5 years was associated with a 65% relative reduction in annual incidence of breast cancer compared with placebo. Anastrozole 1 mg daily for 5 years reduced the incidence of estrogen receptor–positive breast cancers by over 50% compared with placebo with a hazard ratio (HR) of 0.47. In both trials, musculoskeletal complaints and vasomotor symptoms were more common in the aromatase inhibitor groups. Vaginal dryness and decreased libido are also common side effects of aromatase inhibitors. There is potential for a decrease in bone mineral density while taking an aromatase inhibitor; however, no increased fracture rate was seen in either trial. In postmenopausal women, age and comorbidities along with bone health should be considered when a risk-reducing agent is being selected.

References

Ciatto S, Houssami N, Bernardi D, et al: Integration of 3D digital mammography with tomosynthesis for population breast-cancer screening (STORM): a prospective comparison study, *Lancet Oncol* 14(7):583–589, 2013, https://doi.org/10.1016/S1470-2045(13)70134-7. 23623721.

Cuzick J, Sestak I, Forbes JF, et al: Investigators I-I. Anastrozole for prevention of breast cancer in high-risk postmenopausal women (IBIS-II): an international, double-blind, randomised placebo-controlled trial, *Lancet* 383(9922):1041–1048, 2014, https://doi.org/10.1016/S0140-6736(13)62292-8. 24333009.

Dupont WD, Page DL: Risk factors for breast cancer in women with proliferative breast disease, *N Engl J Med* 312(3):146–151, 1985, https://doi.org/10.1056/NEJM198501173120303, PubMed PMID: 3965932.

Fisher B, Costantino JP, Wickerham DL, et al: Tamoxifen for prevention of breast cancer: Report of the National Surgical Adjuvant Breast and Bowel Project P-1 Study, *J Natl Cancer Inst* 90(18):1371–1388, 1998, PubMed PMID: 9747868.

Goss PE, Ingle JN, Ales-Martinez JE, et al: Investigators NCMS. Exemestane for breast-cancer prevention in postmenopausal women, *N Engl J Med* 364(25):2381–2391, 2011, https://doi.org/10.1056/NEJMoa1103507. 21639806.

Hartmann LC, Sellers TA, Frost MH, et al: Benign breast disease and the risk of breast cancer, *N Engl J Med* 353(3):229–237, 2005, https://doi.org/10.1056/NEJMoa044383. 16034008.

Oeffinger KC, Fontham ET, Etzioni R, et al: American Cancer Society. Breast cancer screening for women at average risk: 2015 guideline update from the American Cancer Society, *JAMA* 314(15):1599–1614, 2015, https://doi.org/10.1001/jama.2015.12783, PMCID: PMC4831582. PubMed PMID: 26501536.

Siu AL, USPST Force: Screening for breast cancer: US Preventive Services Task Force Recommendation Statement, *Ann Intern Med* 164(4):279–296, 2016, https://doi.org/10.7326/M15-2886. PubMed PMID: 26757170.

Thomas DB, Gao DL, Ray RM, et al: Randomized trial of breast self-examination in Shanghai: final results, *J Natl Cancer Inst* 94(19):1445–1457, 2002. PubMed PMID: 12359854.

Vogel VG, Costantino JP, Wickerham DL, et al: National Surgical Adjuvant Breast and Bowel Project. Effects of tamoxifen vs raloxifene on the risk of developing invasive breast cancer and other disease outcomes: the NSABP Study of Tamoxifen and Raloxifene (STAR) P-2 trial, *JAMA* 295(23):2727–2741, 2006, https://doi.org/10.1001/jama.295.23.joc60074. 16754727.

---

[1]Not FDA approved for this indication.

BREAST CANCER

Method of
Lauren Nye, MD

CURRENT DIAGNOSIS

- Mammography is used for breast cancer screening, and it is recommended to begin screening in women at average risk for breast cancer between ages 40 and 50.
- Women with an elevated risk for breast cancer may be considered for additional high-risk screening that can include breast magnetic resonance imaging (MRI) or other supplemental screening in addition to annual mammography.
- Individuals with a palpable breast mass or breast symptom concerning for malignancy and those with an abnormal screening mammogram need diagnostic breast imaging.
- Women with diagnostic breast imaging that is suspicious or highly suggestive of malignancy should undergo core needle biopsy.

CURRENT THERAPY

- Breast cancer is a heterogeneous disease and requires a multidisciplinary approach and multimodality therapy.
- The treatment of early-stage breast cancer may include local therapy such as surgery and radiation as well as systemic therapy including chemotherapy, endocrine therapy, and biologic therapy.
- Metastatic breast cancer is treated with systemic therapy; the goal of treatment is disease control and preserving quality of life.
- Breast cancer survivors may have multiple long-term complications of therapy that need to be addressed, including vasomotor symptoms, osteoporosis, lymphedema, and increased cardiac risk factors as well as psychosocial distress and financial toxicity.

Overview

Breast cancer is the most common cancer and the third leading cause of death among women in the United States. It is a heterogeneous disease for which a personalized approach is important in the evaluation and treatment of each individual. Furthermore, the multidisciplinary team is vital in the management of breast cancer and can include a medical oncologist, surgical oncologist, plastic surgeon, radiation oncologist, pathologist, supportive services, and the patient's personal physician. At the conclusion of treatment and active surveillance, the patient typically returns to his or her primary care physician for continued survivorship care.

Epidemiology

It is estimated that there were 281,550 new cases of breast cancer in 2021. The estimated deaths from breast cancer in the same year were 43,600, accounting for 6.8% of all cancer deaths. Female breast cancer is most commonly diagnosed among women from 55 to 64 years of age, with the median age at diagnosis of 62. Although rare, male breast cancer comprises 1% of all breast cancer cases in the United States. The incidence of breast cancer has risen slowly by 0.3% annually, whereas the mortality rate has been falling by 1.8% each year. The 5-year relative survival rate improved by 16% over 30 years, from 74% in 1980 to 90.9% in 2010. Despite the improvement in mortality for most individuals, there remains a breast cancer mortality disparity for African American women diagnosed with breast cancer.

Risk Factors

Well-recognized risk factors for breast cancer include older age, female sex, white race, obesity, high exposure to hormones (either exogenous or endogenous), personal and family history of breast cancer, inherited genetic mutations, benign breast disease (e.g., atypical hyperplasia and LCIS), previous history of radiation therapy to the chest, as well as lifestyle factors such as alcohol consumption and obesity.

Individuals who carry a *BRCA1* or *BRCA2* mutation are at a significantly higher risk for developing breast cancer. In a 2017 case-control study by Couch et al. of more than 65,000 women with breast cancer, genetic mutations associated with an increased risk of breast cancer were identified in 10.2% of cases. The most common gene mutations identified included *BRCA1*, *BRCA2*, *ATM*, *CHEK2*, *PALB2*, *BARD1*, and *RAD51D*. Individuals with a strong family history of cancer should be considered for genetic counseling and testing for appropriate risk stratification.

Risk Reduction

For women at an average risk for breast cancer, lifestyle modifications including regular aerobic exercise, maintaining a healthy weight, and limiting alcohol are most important for breast cancer risk reduction. In addition, complying with breast cancer screening recommendations provides an opportunity for early detection and decreased mortality. Women at average risk for breast cancer should begin screening mammography between age 40 and 50. The US Preventive Task Force (USPSTF) updated recommendations in 2016 recommend biennial screening mammography for women aged 50 to 74 years. The decision to start screening mammography prior to age 50 should be individualized. The 2015 American Cancer Society (ACS) breast cancer screening guidelines for women at average risk include a strong recommendation to begin screening mammography at age 45 and a qualified recommendation to begin at age 40 and continue as long as the patient remains in good overall health and has a life expectancy of 10 years or greater. The most updated recommendations from the National Comprehensive Cancer Network (NCCN) and the American College of Radiology (ACR) are for annual screening mammography beginning at age 40. The standard for screening breast imaging is the digital mammogram; however, in recent years digital breast tomosynthesis has become more prevalent and available to women at breast imaging centers. Digital breast tomosynthesis has both a higher breast cancer detection rate and lower recall rate compared with the digital mammography for breast cancer screening.

Women who are at an increased risk for breast cancer may be considered for additional screening and risk reduction measures. Factors that increase a women's risk include having a known genetic mutation associated with hereditary breast cancer, having a family history of breast cancer in a first- or second-degree relative, especially premenopausal breast cancer or male breast cancer, having a personal history of a breast biopsy with atypical hyperplasia or lobular carcinoma in situ, having a personal history of chest radiation before age 30, or having a high breast density. Several breast cancer assessment tools are available for the evaluation of personalized breast cancer risk (e.g., Breast Cancer Risk Assessment Tool, Tyrer-Cuzick, BRCAPRO models). Women with a lifetime risk of breast cancer greater than 20% on a family history–based model or women with a genetic mutation or prior chest radiation may be eligible for additional annual screening with breast MRI. Certain high-risk populations may benefit from risk-reducing therapies such as chemoprevention and risk-reducing mastectomy, especially for carriers of high-penetrance mutations.

Clinical Manifestations

Women with ductal carcinoma in situ (DCIS) and early-stage breast cancer may be asymptomatic. The most common symptoms of breast cancer include the following:
- New palpable mass in the breast or axilla
- Skin changes such as dimpling, erythema, irritation, edema, thickening, peau d'orange (Fig. 1)
- Nipple retraction

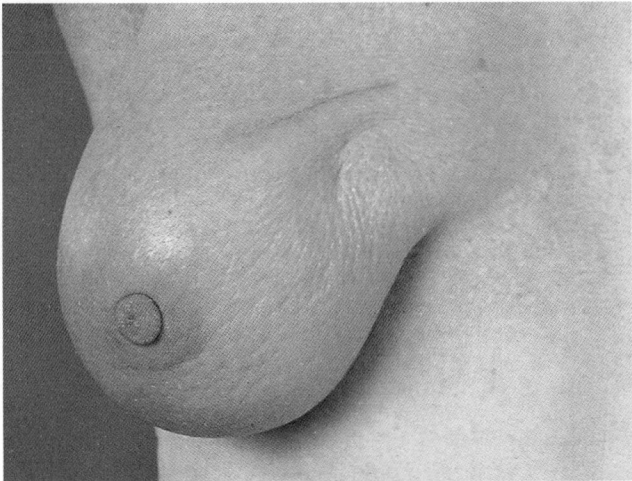

Figure 1 Peau d'orange of the breast.

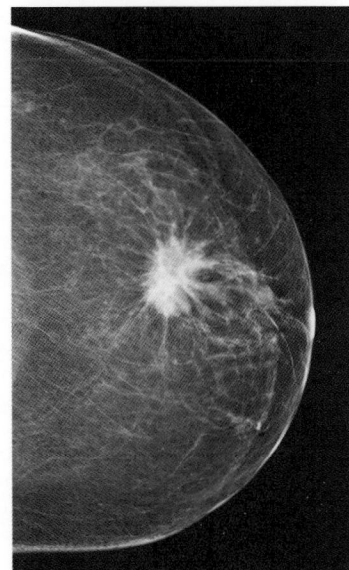

Figure 2 Breast cancer on mammogram.

- Abnormal nipple discharge
- New asymmetric appearance of breast

Differential Diagnosis

Differential diagnoses include benign conditions such as fibroadenoma, papilloma, breast cyst, and mastitis as well as malignant conditions such as breast lymphoma, sarcoma, neuroendocrine tumors, leukemia, and skin metastasis from breast or other primary tumors.

Diagnosis

Once breast malignancy is suspected clinically, either by palpation or breast imaging (Fig. 2), further evaluation is warranted. Women with an abnormal mammogram should undergo further diagnostic imaging, which may include diagnostic mammography, ultrasonography, or breast MRI. Normal and abnormal findings on breast imaging are reported using the universal classification system of the American College of Radiology (Breast Imaging Reporting and Data System [BI-RADS]). BI-RADS 0 indicates an incomplete assessment and that further workup is needed, typically with additional imaging. BI-RADS 1 and BI-RADS 2 lesions are negative or benign, respectively. BI-RADS 3 lesions are considered probably benign based on appearance; a mammogram or ultrasound scan in 6 months is recommended for follow-up. BI-RADS 4 and BI-RADS 5 lesions are suspicious or highly suggestive of malignancy, respectively, and a biopsy of the lesion is recommended. Core needle biopsy is the recommended approach for tissue sampling. The pathology report from a biopsy of a primary breast cancer will typically include the histology and tumor prognostic markers. These histologic subtypes of breast cancer include ductal, lobular, mixed, metaplastic, as well as the more favorable histologic subtypes of tubular, mucinous, and papillary.

Once breast cancer has been diagnosed, appropriate clinical staging is done, directed by a medical oncologist or surgical oncologist. This may include further breast imaging to characterize the extent of the tumor, axillary staging with ultrasound to assess for abnormal-appearing lymph nodes, and clinical examination with consideration of whole-body staging with computed tomography (CT) scan of the chest, abdomen, and pelvis depending on the size and lymph node involvement of the primary lesion. Bone scanning or positron emission tomography (PET/CT) may also be considered in some circumstances. Staging of the breast cancer is done in accordance with the American Joint Committee on Cancer (AJCC) staging system. The most updated version, the *AJCC Cancer Staging Manual*, Eighth Edition, was published in December 2017 and includes anatomic stage groups, clinical prognostic stage groups, and pathologic prognostic stage groups. All patients should have a clinical prognostic stage documented as part of their treatment plan, and those with surgery as initial treatment may also have a pathologic prognostic stage. The updated staging guidelines also include biomarker testing results within the staging system.

Pathophysiology

Breast cancer is a heterogeneous disease. Malignant cells arise from neoplastic proliferation of epithelial cells in the ducts or lobules of the breast. If neoplastic cells are confined within the duct or lobule, the lesion is termed *ductal* or *lobular in situ*, respectively. DCIS is a precursor lesion that can potentially develop into invasive carcinoma. Invasive carcinoma is classified into four distinct molecular subtypes: luminal A, luminal B, basal-like, and HER2 enriched. More frequently we use the tumor receptor markers of the breast cancer to guide therapy, namely estrogen receptor (ER), progesterone receptor (PR), and HER2 overexpression. Hormone receptor–positive breast cancer (meaning progesterone- or estrogen receptor–positive) is the most common type of breast cancer, comprising more than 65% of all breast cancers. In general it has a less aggressive course with a long survival, even in the metastatic setting. In contrast, hormone receptor–negative and HER2-negative breast cancer—also known as triple negative breast cancer (TNBC)—tends to be more aggressive and has a much poorer outcome, especially in the advanced setting. Although the natural course of HER2-overexpressed disease tends to be aggressive, HER2-positive breast cancer now has a longer survival time since the advent of effective HER2-directed therapies.

Treatment

Breast cancer is a complex disease that requires multidisciplinary management as well as a tailored therapy plan depending on the stage, histologic subtype, and prognostic tumor marker status. Current modalities for treating breast cancer include local therapy such as surgery and radiation therapy as well as systemic therapy including chemotherapy, endocrine, and biologic therapy.

Early-stage breast cancer is treated with surgery (lumpectomy or mastectomy) with or without radiation therapy. Women who undergo lumpectomy and radiotherapy have equivalent survival outcomes to those receiving mastectomy. Axillary lymph nodes are typically evaluated by sentinel lymph node biopsy and/or axillary lymph node dissection depending on initial clinical findings and lymph node involvement with metastases on pathologic review. For selected cases, preoperative (neoadjuvant) treatment with chemotherapy or endocrine therapy are used. Neoadjuvant chemotherapy is indicated for inoperable or locally advanced breast cancer such as inflammatory breast cancer, extensive primary tumor extending to the chest wall or skin, bulky or matted axillary lymph nodes, and extra-axillary lymph node involvement. In the setting of operable breast cancer, neoadjuvant systemic treatment may be recommended to optimize surgical outcomes or to allow for assessment of tumor response on surgical pathology to guide adjuvant systemic therapy.

After definitive surgical management, adjuvant systemic therapy may be offered to reduce the risk of local and distant recurrence. Chemotherapy is considered for those at high risk for recurrence, characterized by large tumor size, positive lymph nodes, high-grade histology, or a triple negative (hormone receptor–negative, HER2-negative) breast cancer. For hormone receptor–positive, HER2-negative, axillary node–negative breast cancer, the 21-gene recurrence score is widely used to evaluate for the potential benefit of adjuvant chemotherapy. HER2-positive breast cancer is treated with HER2-directed biologic agents along with chemotherapy followed by maintenance therapy with anti-HER2 agents such as trastuzumab (Herceptin), pertuzumab (Perjeta), and ado-trastuzumab emtansine (Kadcyla). When an anthracycline chemotherapy or HER2 antibody therapy is indicated, baseline cardiac function evaluation by either echocardiogram or multigated acquisition scan must be obtained before treatment and will be regularly monitored during the treatment with HER2-directed therapies. Radiation therapy, if indicated, is typically offered after chemotherapy.

After local treatment of hormone receptor–positive breast cancer with or without chemotherapy, adjuvant endocrine therapy is recommended for a minimum of 5 years with either a selective estrogen-receptor modulator (SERM) such as tamoxifen (Nolvadex), an aromatase inhibitor such as anastrozole (Arimidex), letrozole (Femara), or exemestane (Aromasin). In general, the choice of endocrine therapy agents is based on the menopausal state and side-effect profiles. Aromatase inhibitors need to be combined with ovarian suppression in premenopausal women. Adjuvant endocrine therapy is associated with an approximate 50% reduction in breast cancer recurrence.

Locally recurrent disease without distant metastasis can be managed with a curative intent. Combination of local therapies and systemic treatment may be used depending on the clinical scenario. Metastatic (stage IV) breast cancer with distant metastasis is not curable and is managed with the intent of disease control while maintaining quality of life and requires systemic therapy. Local therapies such as surgery and radiation therapy are indicated for palliative purposes when appropriate. Hormone-positive metastatic breast cancer can be treated with endocrine therapy as first-line treatment if there is no evidence of visceral crisis. Cyclin-dependent kinase (CDK4/6) inhibitors have emerged as promising agents for hormone receptor–positive, metastatic disease. In combination with endocrine therapy, CDK inhibitors demonstrated longer progression-free survival, and in some cohorts an overall survival benefit. In patients with a somatic (tumor) PIK3CA mutation, the PI3Kα inhibitor, alpelisib (PIQRAY), is approved in combination with fulvestrant (Faslodex) for individuals after an endocrine-based regimen. An mTOR inhibitor can be also used in this setting in combination with endocrine therapy. The mTOR inhibitor is known to overcome endocrine resistance, although toxicity (e.g., mucositis and gastrointestinal side effects) may limit its use.

Metastatic HER2-positive breast cancer is treated with HER2-directed agents and chemotherapy. Additional strategies include drug antibody conjugates (ado-trastuzumab emtansine [Kadcyla], fam-trastuzumab deruxtecan-nxki [Enhertu]) or dual HER2 blockade such as trastuzumab (Herceptin) and pertuzumab (Perjeta) or lapatinib (Tykerb) or neratinib (Nerlynx) with chemotherapy, which demonstrate superior progression-free survival compared with a single HER2 agent added to chemotherapy. Biosimilars for trastuzumab are now available. For HER2-positive and hormone receptor–positive disease, dual HER2-targeted therapy combined with an aromatase inhibitor may be beneficial.

The first immunotherapy approved for the treatment of breast cancer is atezolizumab (Tecentriq) in combination with nab-paclitaxel (nanoparticle albumin-bound paclitaxel [Abraxane]) for metastatic triple negative breast cancer with PDL-1 tumor expression. Immunotherapy overall is better tolerated than chemotherapy but has a unique profile of potential toxicities including colitis, pneumonitis, dermatologic reactions, and endocrinopathies along with less common immune mediated adverse events.

Although single chemotherapy is preferred for metastatic disease, combined chemotherapy may be indicated for diseases with high tumor burden or in visceral crisis. Management of metastatic breast cancer may also include germline genetic testing for a *BRCA1* or *BRCA2* mutation and/or genomic testing of the tumor to identify potential molecular targets unique to the individual or tumor. In 2018, the US Food and Drug Administration (FDA) approved olaparib (Lynparza) and talazoparib (Talzenna), which are a poly-ADH ribose polymerase inhibitors, for the treatment of metastatic HER2-negative, *BRCA*-associated breast cancer. Further targeted therapies may be explored in the setting of a clinical trial.

For patients with bone metastasis, bone-targeted therapies such as denosumab (Xgeva) and intravenous bisphosphonates are given to reduce skeletal-related events, such as pathologic fractures. Patients with poor dentition or oral hygiene who need future dental procedures during treatment are at increased risk for osteonecrosis of the jaw; thus dental evaluation is important before bone-directed therapy is initiated.

Monitoring and Survivorship

The majority of breast cancer patients are treated with curative intent and gain long-term survival. The risk of recurrence, however, is a realistic concern for many years after definitive therapy, especially for women with locally advanced or node-positive disease. Once the patient has completed definitive treatment, careful history taking and physical examination become the most important aspects of surveillance. Patients are advised to schedule an office visit up to four times yearly for the first 5 years and then annually. Monitoring for recurrence by laboratory and radiologic tests should be kept minimal in the nonmetastatic setting unless clinically indicated otherwise.

Women should continue to undergo annual screening mammography for their remaining breast tissue. If they were receiving high-risk screening with a breast MRI based on a genetic mutation, this may also be continued after breast cancer treatment. Annual gynecologic assessment is recommended for women on tamoxifen because of the associated increased risk of uterine cancer, which typically presents with abnormal bleeding in postmenopausal women. Patients on an aromatase inhibitor should have a bone mineral density completed at baseline and then annually while receiving treatment. Bone-modifying agents such as intravenous bisphosphonates or RANK ligand inhibitors may be used for management or prevention of osteoporosis while on aromatase inhibitor therapy.

In addition, women receiving adjuvant endocrine therapy may experience menopause-related symptoms such as vasomotor symptoms, vaginal dryness, and sexual dysfunction. Patients are encouraged to discuss these symptoms with their physicians because they can frequently be managed with nonhormone-based approaches. Venlafaxine (Effexor)[1], oxybutynin (Ditropan)[1], and gabapentin (Neurontin)[1] have demonstrated efficacy in management of hot flashes, as well as cognitive behavioral therapy acupuncture and avoiding triggers. Vaginal moisturizers and lubricants can be applied to help alleviate symptoms of vaginal dryness. Laser therapy may also be considered in some circumstances.

Long-term complications after definitive treatment may include lymphedema and self-image issues after surgery, skin changes after radiation therapy and persistent neuropathy, prolonged hair loss, fatigue, cognitive impairment, and a small risk of developing leukemia and myelodysplastic syndrome after chemotherapy.

Heart disease remains the leading cause of death among US women. Those who have undergone treatment for breast cancer may be at a higher risk for myocardial events depending on their baseline risk factors and the treatment they received. Accumulating evidence suggests that lifestyle modifications including regular exercise, achieving a healthy body mass index, limiting alcohol intake, and abstaining from tobacco products lead to optimal outcomes for breast cancer survivors.

---

[1] Not FDA approved for this indication.

References

American Cancer Society: *Cancer Facts & Figures*, 2021.

Baselga J, Cortes J, Kim SB, et al: Pertuzumab plus trastuzumab plus docetaxel for metastatic breast cancer, *N Engl J Med* 366:109–119, 2012.

Couch FJ, Shimelis H, Hu C: Associations between cancer predisposition testing panel genes and breast cancer, *JAMA Oncol* 3(9):1190–1196, 2017.

Davies C, Pan H, Godwin J, et al: Long-term effects of continuing adjuvant tamoxifen to 10 years versus stopping at 5 years after diagnosis of oestrogen receptor-positive breast cancer: ATLAS, a randomized trial, *Lancet* 381(9869):805–816, 2013.

Finn RS, Crown JP, Lang I, et al: The cyclin-dependent kinase 4/6 inhibitor palbociclib in combination with letrozole versus letrozole alone as first-line treatment of oestrogen receptor-positive, HER2-negative, advanced breast cancer (PALOMA-1/TRIO-18): a randomized phase II study, *Lancet Oncol* 16(1):25–35, 2015.

Fisher B, Anderson S, Bryant J, et al: Twenty-year follow-up of a randomized trial comparing total mastectomy, lumpectomy, and lumpectomy plus irradiation for the treatment of invasive breast cancer, *N Engl J Med* 347:1233–1241, 2002.

Noone AM, Howlander N, Krapcho M, et al: SEER Cancer Statistics Review, 1975-2015, National Cancer Institute. Bethesda, MD, https://seer.cancer.gov/csr/1975_2015/, based on November 2017 SEER data submission, posted to SEER website, April 2018.

Slamon DJ, Leyland-Jones B, Shak S, et al: Use of chemotherapy plus a monoclonal antibody against HER2 for metastatic breast cancer that overexpresses HER2, *N Engl J Med* 344:783–792, 2001.

Sparano JA, Gray RJ, Makower DF, et al: Prospective validation of a 21-gene expression assay in breast cancer, *N Engl J Med* 373:2005–2015, 2015.

Verma S, Miles D, Gianni L, et al: Trastuzumab emtansine for HER2-positive advanced breast cancer, *N Engl J Med* 367:1783–1791, 2012.

CANCER OF THE ENDOMETRIUM

Method of
Locke Uppendahl, MD; and Boris Winterhoff, MD

CURRENT DIAGNOSIS

- The high incidence of uterine cancer in developed countries reflects increased obesity rates.
- The progression from atypical hyperplasia to adenocarcinoma is a consequence of prolonged, unopposed estrogen exposure.
- Approximately 90% of women with uterine cancer report abnormal uterine bleeding, with postmenopausal bleeding the most common.
- Over 95% of uterine cancers are diagnosed in women 40 years or older.
- In most uterine cancer cases, the tumor is confined to the uterine corpus at the time of diagnosis and portend a good prognosis.
- Uterine carcinomas are classified into two broad histologic categories: the estrogen related endometrioid (Type I) and nonestrogen related (Type II) tumors.

CURRENT THERAPY

- Comprehensive surgical staging with total hysterectomy, bilateral salpingo-oophorectomy, and bilateral pelvic and para-aortic lymphadenectomy is a critical component for the diagnosis and management of all endometrial cancers.
- The utility and extent of lymph node dissection in endometrial cancer is controversial.
- The decision for adjuvant therapy is based on the risk of relapse and persistent disease.
- Surgery alone is usually curative for women with early-stage, low-risk disease.
- Adjuvant vaginal brachytherapy is recommended for early-stage endometrial cancers that demonstrate pathologic features known to increase risk of vaginal cuff recurrence, such as high-grade, deep myometrial invasion, cervical involvement, or presence of lymphovascular space invasion.
- Women with advanced-stage (stage III or IV) or recurrent endometrial cancer are frequently treated with systemic, platinum-based chemotherapy

Epidemiology

In the United States, uterine cancer is the most common gynecologic malignancy of the female genital tract, with an estimated 65,620 new cases and 12,590 deaths expected for 2020. Approximately 1 in 35 women will develop invasive cancer over their lifetime, with an average age of diagnosis of 62 years. The high incidence observed in developed countries is attributable to increased obesity rates and other risk factors.

Uterine cancer is one of the few malignancies where survival has not improved since the mid-1970s. In fact, death rates for uterine cancer rose in 2011 through 2015 by 2% per year. The 5-year survival rate for all stages is 22% lower for black women compared to white women. This large disparity likely reflects a delay in diagnosis in this population.

Classification

Uterine cancers arising from the lining of the uterus are called endometrial carcinoma and are classified into two broad histologic categories: the estrogen related endometrioid (Type I) and nonestrogen related (Type II) tumors.

Type I tumors

Type I tumors are the predominant form of endometrial cancer, comprising approximately 80% of new diagnoses. They include tumors of endometrioid histology and often arise in the background of atypical endometrial hyperplasia. Type I tumors are more indolent, diagnosed at earlier stages, occur in younger women, and overall portend a favorable prognosis. Patients with high-grade (grade 3) endometrioid adenocarcinoma have a less favorable prognosis. The average age at diagnosis is approximately 62 years old, with nearly 70% of the tumors confined to the uterus at time of diagnosis.

Recent, comprehensive genomic characterization has identified a number of genetic alterations associated with type I tumors. The loss of function in the DNA mismatch repair (MMR) enzymes MLH1, MSH2, MSH6, and PMS2 results in the inability to properly detect and repair abnormal DNA sequences. This leads to mutations in genes that have microsatellite repeats. Microsatellite instability (MSI) is found in approximately one-third of type I tumors and can be as a result of germline or sporadic mutations. Other commonly mutated genes include *PTEN*, *CTNNB1*, *PIK3CA*, *ARID1A*, and *KRAS*.

Type II tumors

In contrast to type I tumors, other endometrial cancers are unrelated to unopposed estrogen exposure. Type II cancers include clear cell and serous histology tumors. They are diagnosed more frequently among older, non-obese, non-white women and portend an unfavorable prognosis due to the later stage in diagnosis and the aggressive nature of the tumor.

Serous carcinoma of the endometrium represents ~10% of endometrial carcinomas but accounts for 40% of all endometrial cancer-related deaths. They often invade deep into the myometrium and demonstrate the ability for early peritoneal spread. Uterine serous carcinomas are molecularly distinct and are characterized by high genomic instability (high copy number alterations), low mutational burden, and *TP53* mutations. Newer evidence demonstrates dysregulation of the *Her2/neu* oncogene in 27% of cases. Clear cell carcinomas, another rare but aggressive subtype, represent ~5% of endometrial carcinomas. The 5-year overall survival rates for serous and clear cell carcinomas are 41% and 65%, respectively. Recently, genomic characterization identified approximately 25% of grade 3 endometrioid tumors cluster with serous carcinomas, with very high somatic copy-number alterations. Nearly 90% of these tumors have *TP53* mutations. Novel mutations in *TAF1* have been implicated in a subset of clear cell carcinomas.

Risk Factors

Type I tumors are strongly linked to long-term, unopposed exposure to estrogen. Therefore risk factors include any excessive exogenous (hormonal therapy, tamoxifen [Nolvadex]) or endogenous (obesity, chronic anovulation, estrogen-secreting tumors) estrogen exposure to the uterine lining. In the United States, the high prevalence of obesity has increased the incidence of uterine cancer over the past two decades. A BMI 25 to < 30 kg/m² confers a relative risk of 1.5 to develop endometrial cancer, compared to 7.1 for BMI > 40 kg/m². Other risk factors for type I tumors include nulliparity, diabetes mellitus, and hypertension.

Tamoxifen (Nolvadex) is a selective-estrogen receptor modulator (SERM) used in the treatment and prevention of breast cancer. The drug functions as an antagonist in the breast but has agonist effects on the endometrium. The risks of endometrial cancer associated with tamoxifen, although very low, are well documented in the literature.

Lynch / Hereditary Non-Polyposis Colorectal Cancer (HNPCC) syndrome is caused by mutations in DNA mismatch-repair genes *MLH1, MSH2, MSH6,* and *PMS2.* The lifetime risk of developing colorectal and endometrial cancer is 25–50% and 15–71% (depends on mutated gene), respectively.

Pathophysiology

The World Health Organization (WHO) has recently clarified the classification of endometrial hyperplasia, differentiating between only two categories: (1) hyperplasia without atypia and (2) atypical hyperplasia / endometrioid intraepithelial neoplasia. Multiple studies have demonstrated the progression of atypical hyperplasia to adenocarcinoma is a consequence of prolonged, unopposed estrogen exposure.

Prevention

Over 95% of uterine cancers are diagnosed in women 40 years or older. Therefore abnormal uterine bleeding in these women should prompt evaluation with endometrial biopsy or dilatation and curettage (D&C). Depending on age and reproductive desire, women with endometrial hyperplasia may be treated with removal of estrogen stimulus, the periodic use of progestins, or by hysterectomy to prevent the onset of uterine cancer. For women with atypical hyperplasia, hysterectomy is the treatment of choice, because coexistent adenocarcinoma may be present in 40% of cases. In addition, this group of women carries a 30% risk of developing invasive carcinoma later in life. Finally, women with a uterus should never receive estrogen-only hormone replacement therapy (HRT). The addition of a progestin to HRT can prevent endometrial hyperplasia and subsequent endometrial cancer.

Despite no current scientific evidence, women diagnosed with Lynch syndrome should consider annual screening with endometrial sampling and transvaginal ultrasound, beginning between ages of 30 and 35 years. Hysterectomy with or without oophorectomy is an option after childbearing to deter the risk of endometrial cancer.

Clinical Manifestations

Abnormal uterine bleeding is often the only presenting symptom in women diagnosed with endometrial cancer. Upwards of 90% of women diagnosed with endometrial cancer report abnormal uterine bleeding, with postmenopausal bleeding the most common. However, postmenopausal bleeding has many etiologies, and only ~15% of these women will have endometrial cancer.

For pre- and perimenopausal women, the diagnosis is more challenging and often delayed. For this group of women, intermenstrual bleeding, prolonged, heavy bleeding, or the absence of menses for several months interrupted with episodes of bleeding warrants investigation.

Finally, Papanicolaou smears demonstrate malignant cells in only ~50% of women with underlying endometrial cancer. This highlights the ineffectual screening method of indirectly sampling the endometrium. To date, no screening method for the general population is recommended.

Diagnosis

Diagnosis of endometrial cancer is confirmed with a histological specimen. All women suspected of having uterine cancer due to abnormal uterine bleeding should have their endometrium sampled via biopsy. Most often, this can be done in the clinic with a rigid or flexible catheter. With this technique, reported detection rates for postmenopausal and premenopausal are 99.6% and 91%, respectively. However, there is approximately a 10% false-negative rate with endometrial biopsy. Therefore a negative biopsy result in women highly suspicious for endometrial cancer should undergo exam under anesthesia and curettage. Finally, transvaginal ultrasound demonstrating an endometrial thickness of 5 mm or more in a postmenopausal woman requires endometrial sampling.

Women taking tamoxifen should be counseled about the increased risk of endometrial cancer and to report any abnormal vaginal bleeding so they can be thoroughly evaluated. However, no evidence supports the screening of asymptomatic women with ultrasound or serial endometrial sampling.

Staging

Due to the high incidence of lymph node metastases, the Cancer Committee of the International Federation of Gynecology and Obstetrics (FIGO) replaced a clinical staging system with a surgical staging system in 1988. The current, updated in 2009 FIGO staging system is detailed in Table 1.

Treatment

Comprehensive surgical staging with exploration of the abdominal cavity, total hysterectomy with bilateral salpingo-oophorectomy, and bilateral pelvic and para-aortic lymphadenectomy are critical components for the diagnosis and management of all endometrial cancers. For type II tumors, meticulous surgical staging with the addition of collection of peritoneal washings for cytology, omentectomy ± peritoneal biopsies is required, since metastatic disease is often only identified microscopically. In cases with gross metastatic disease, cytoreductive surgery may be required. Surgical staging can be performed by laparotomy, laparoscopy, or robotically assisted procedure.

TABLE 1	Carcinoma of the Endometrium
Stage I: Tumor confined to uterine corpus	
IA	Tumor limited to endometrium or < 50% myometrial invasion
IB	≥50% myometrial invasion
Stage II: Extension to cervical stroma	
II	Cervical stromal invasion
Stage III: Local and/or regional spread	
IIIA	Tumor invades serosa and/or adnexa
IIIB	Vaginal and/or parametrial extension
IIIC1	Pelvic lymph node involvement
IIIC2	Para-aortic lymph node involvement
Stage IV: Distant spread	
IVA	Tumor invades bladder and/or rectal mucosa
IVB	Distant metastases, including abdominal spread and/or inguinal lymph nodes

Tumor grade, cell type, and presence/absence of malignant cytology in pelvic washings should be reported along with stage.

The utility and extent of lymph node dissection in endometrial cancer is controversial. Different strategies, including universal, selective, and sentinel lymph node mapping, are currently used. The universal method performs uniform comprehensive surgical staging for nearly all patients with endometrial cancer. This method allows for the most complete information postoperatively to make adjuvant decisions, but a significant percentage of women will develop lymphedema secondary to the nodal dissection. A common selective approach involves avoiding lymph node dissection in patients who have grade 1 or 2 endometrioid histology with < 50% myometrial invasion and tumor size < 2 cm, since these patients have < 1% risk of nodal metastases. Finally, an alternative approach utilizing sentinel lymph node mapping with indocyanine green dye is becoming more popular. Early studies have demonstrated promising results in decreasing morbidity while optimizing the pathological assessment of nodes in these women. Regardless the strategy, the presence of pelvic or para-aortic lymph node metastases remains one of the most important prognostic factors for endometrial cancer.

Following surgery, women are stratified by age and pathologic features to determine their risk for recurrence and the need for adjuvant therapy.

Adjuvant Therapy

The decision for adjuvant therapy is difficult and is based on the risk of relapse and persistent disease. In general, women with stage IA, grade 1 or 2 endometrioid adenocarcinoma have a favorable prognosis, and no adjuvant radiation is necessary following surgery. Early-stage endometrial carcinomas with risk factors for recurrence, stage II-IV cancers, and all serous and clear cell carcinomas often require adjuvant therapy in the form of radiation, chemotherapy, or a combination of both.

Early-Stage Disease

Surgery alone is usually curative for women with early-stage, low-risk disease. Women with early-stage, high-risk or high-intermediate risk factors are often recommended adjuvant radiation. The treatment can be in the form of external beam radiation therapy or vaginal brachytherapy. All serous and clear cell carcinomas of the uterus are recommended to receive adjuvant platinum-based combination chemotherapy regardless of stage. Adjuvant systemic therapy in patients with high-risk, early-stage endometrioid carcinoma remains controversial.

Metastatic Disease

Approximately 10–15% of patients will present with metastatic disease at presentation. Surgical cytoreduction is the preferred treatment approach if complete resection is achievable because it is associated with improved progression-free and overall survival. This would be followed by adjuvant platinum-based combination chemotherapy. The most common regimens are carboplatin (Paraplatin)[1] plus paclitaxel (Taxol)[1] or the triple drug combination of cisplatin (Platinol)[1], doxorubicin (Adriamycin)[1], and paclitaxel.

Patients who are not candidates for surgical cytoreduction either due to grossly metastatic disease or too poor a surgical candidate have a poor prognosis, with 5-year relative survival of < 20%. These patients should be offered systemic chemotherapy generally with palliative intent. Radiation therapy to achieve local control in the pelvis to palliate bleeding, discharge, and pain is often performed.

Recurrent Disease

Local recurrences, distance metastases, and simultaneous local and distant metastases are found in 50%, 29%, and 21%, respectively. Isolated vaginal recurrences are often salvaged with either surgery or radiation.

Distant recurrent endometrial cancer portends a poor prognosis. Systemic chemotherapy is given with a palliative intent,

with the most active agents including platinums, taxanes, and anthracyclines.

Combination Chemotherapy and Radiation Therapy. Several studies have evaluated combining chemotherapy and radiation therapy in advanced-stage endometrial cancer. Most recently, a randomized phase III trial compared cisplatin and tumor volume directed irradiation followed by four cycles of chemotherapy (experimental arm) against six cycles of chemotherapy (control arm). While the overall survival is immature, the study reported no increase in recurrence-free survival in optimally debulked, stage III or IV endometrial cancer.

Our experience involves using a "sandwich" method of irradiation between rounds of chemotherapy for advanced or recurrent endometrial cancer. The phase II trial demonstrated an overall 5-year survival of 79% with acceptable toxicity. The optimal sequencing of chemotherapy and radiation warrants further development.

Hormone Therapy

Prior to endometrial cancer, the risk of endometrial hyperplasia and the development into carcinoma can be significantly reduced with administration of a progestin. After the development of carcinoma, patients whose tumors test positive for estrogen receptor (ER) and progesterone receptor (PR) are associated with longer survival, with PR being a stronger predictor than ER. However, the role of adjuvant progestins in stage I or II endometrial cancer has not been demonstrated to be of value and may worsen cardiovascular disease. Progestins are commonly used in advanced or recurrent well-differentiated endometrial cancers. Oral megestrol acetate (Megace) and medroxyprogesterone acetate (Provera)[1] are two of the most commonly used progestins.

The SERM tamoxifen[1] has been used to treat patients with recurrent endometrial cancer, with response rates seen in ~22% of patients. The aromatase inhibitors anastrozole (Arimidex)[1] and letrozole (Femara)[1] were investigated in recurrent and metastatic endometrial cancer and demonstrated minimal activity.

Targeted Therapy

Multiple novel agents are being evaluated in clinical trials for use in treatment against endometrial cancer. Bevacizumab (Avastin)[1] is a monoclonal antibody directed against vascular endothelial growth factor (VEFG) that is active in endometrial cancer. Recent randomized trials demonstrated a benefit with the addition of bevacizumab to carboplatin and paclitaxel in first-line and second-line treatment of advanced, metastatic, and recurrent endometrial cancer. Results from phase 3 trials are needed prior to adopting as standard of care.

Pembrolizumab (Keytruda) is an immune checkpoint inhibitor that has FDA approval for the use in advanced solid tumors demonstrating MMR deficiency or MSI. In patients with endometrial cancer, it is often used following progression on platinum-based chemotherapy in women with MMR or MSI tumors. In the fall of 2019, the FDA approved two new therapeutic agents, lenvatinib (Lenvima), a combination of the inhibitors of VEGFR1, VEGFR2, and VEGFR3 kinases, and a humanized monoclonal antibody, pembrolizumab (Keytruda), for microsatellite-stable (MSS) tumors.

Trastuzumab (Herceptin)[1] and lapatinib (Tykerb)[1] are anti–human epidermal growth factor 2 (HER2) are investigational agents being tested as single agents and in combination with chemotherapy in some endometrial cancers, although the results thus far are not encouraging. The mechanistic Target of Ramamycin (mTOR) inhibitors everolimus (Zortress)[1] and ridaforolimus (MK-8669)[5] have been used to treat advanced-stage and recurrent endometrial cancers, with mixed response.

Monitoring

Surveillance recommendations for endometrial cancer are stratified by risk of recurrence, and most women diagnosed and treated

---

[1]Not FDA approved for this indication.

[1]Not FDA approved for this indication.
[5]Not available in the United States.

for endometrial cancer will fall into the low-risk category. High risk for recurrence is defined as advanced stage or grade 3 endometrioid, serous, or clear cell histology. Follow-up recommendations for low-risk women involve a history and physical examination, including a speculum and pelvic examination, scheduled every 6 months for the first 2 years, then yearly. Women with high risk of recurrence should have the same follow-up recommendations at intervals of 3 months for the first 2 years, every 6 months in years 2–5, then yearly. Pap test/cytology, CA 125, and routine radiographic imaging are not recommended. Women suspected of recurrence should have imaging performed.

References

The American College of Obstetricians and Gynecologists Committee Opinion no. 631: Endometrial intraepithelial neoplasia, *Obstet Gynecol* 125(5):1272–1278, 2015.

de Boer SM, et al: Adjuvant chemoradiotherapy versus radiotherapy alone for women with high-risk endometrial cancer (PORTEC-3): final results of an international, open-label, multicentre, randomised, phase 3 trial, *Lancet Oncol* 19(3):295–309, 2018.

Geller MA, et al: A phase II trial of carboplatin and docetaxel followed by radiotherapy given in a "Sandwich" method for stage III, IV, and recurrent endometrial cancer, *Gynecol Oncol* 121(1):112–117, 2011.

Kandoth C, et al: Integrated genomic characterization of endometrial carcinoma, *Nature* 497(7447):67–73, 2013.

Pecorelli S: Revised FIGO staging for carcinoma of the vulva, cervix, and endometrium, *Int J Gynaecol Obstet* 105(2):103–104, 2009.

Salani R, et al: An update on post-treatment surveillance and diagnosis of recurrence in women with gynecologic malignancies: Society of Gynecologic Oncology (SGO) recommendations, *Gynecol Oncol* 146(1):3–10, 2017.

CANCER OF THE UTERINE CERVIX

Method of
Lucybeth Nieves-Arriba, MD; and Peter G. Rose, MD

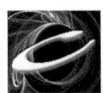

CURRENT DIAGNOSIS

- New recommendations for cytology screening recommend starting screening at 21 years of age.
- Initial workup must include a biopsy.
- Imaging techniques including magnetic resonance imaging and positron emission tomography–computed tomography can assist in treatment planning.

CURRENT THERAPY

- Despite recent availability of human papillomavirus (HPV) vaccination (Gardasil[2], Gardasil 9, Cervarix[2]) and advances in screening, cervical cancer remains a significant global health problem, especially in underserved populations.
- Improved understanding of the disease has allowed more conservative treatment of selected patients with early-stage disease.
- For advanced and high-risk cervical cancer, chemoradiation has had a significant impact on survival.

[2]Not available in the United States.

Epidemiology

Worldwide, cervical cancer is the fourth most common cancer in women. It is the greatest cancer killer of young women and the most common cause of death from cancer in women in the developing world. Worldwide in 2018, among the 570,000 new cases of cervical cancer, the highest incidence rates were in Africa, Central and South America, and Asia. In the United States, it is estimated that approximately 13,240 new cases were diagnosed and 4170 patients died from cervical cancer in 2018. Significant disparities in incidence and stage at time of diagnosis have been identified among different ethnic groups—African Americans, Asian Americans, European Americans, and Latin Americans—in the United States. Factors that increase the risk of cervical cancer include early age at first coitus, multiple sexual partners, history of sexually transmitted diseases, low socioeconomic status, cigarette smoking, immunosuppression, and Fanconi syndrome.

Pathophysiology

Cervical cancer occurs secondary to viral transformation of the surface (epithelial) cells by high-risk types of the human papillomavirus (HPV), and it is the only gynecologic cancer that can be prevented by regular screening. Persistent infection with high-risk HPV has been identified as the essential factor in the pathogenesis of the majority of cervical cancers. The virus's ability to transform human epithelium has been associated with the expression of two viral gene products, E6 and E7, which interact with p53 (a tumor-suppressor protein) and retinoblastoma protein (pRB), respectively, and affect control mechanisms of the cell cycle.

The prevalence of genital HPV infection in the world is estimated to be 400 million. Data from the National Health and Nutrition Examination Survey (NHANES) estimate the prevalence of HPV infection among girls and women in the United States aged 14 to 59 years is 26.8%. In about 90% of cases, the high-risk HPV infection is cleared by the immune system within 16 months. HPV infections in girls and younger women are more likely transient and therefore less likely to be associated with significant cervical lesions.

Prevention and Screening

Advances in molecular biology have allowed the development of viral-like particles using the L1 protein (major immunogenic capsid protein) of the HPV virus. Currently approved HPV vaccines include: Gardasil (2006)[2], Cervarix (2009)[2], and Gardasil 9 (2014). These vaccines are approved to use in girls/boys and women/men between the ages of 9 and 26 years. The FDA expanded its approval in 2018 to include men and women between 27 and 45 years old. Awareness of the importance of HPV vaccination has increased but vaccination rates for US adolescents are still not at goal with only 48.6% vaccinated as of 2017.

The current standard screening algorithm in the United States for preventing cervical cancer is presented in Table 1. Women with abnormal cytology are referred for a colposcopic examination. The colposcopic examination is used to guide biopsies of the exocervix, and in most cases an endocervical biopsy is also performed. The biopsy results then determine the type of follow-up and or therapy required.

Staging

The International Federation of Gynecology and Obstetrics (FIGO) defined the most commonly accepted staging of cervical cancer. This staging is based on a careful clinical examination and the results of specific radiologic studies and procedures. FIGO's latest update (2009) is summarized in Table 2.

In cervical cancer, primary lesions initially progress to lymphatics in the parametrium and pelvic nodes and then extend laterally to the pelvic side wall, bladder, and rectum. The two major spread patterns identified in cervical cancer include direct extension and lymphatic spread.

[1]Not available in the United States.

| TABLE 1 | Cervical Cytologic Screening Guidelines from the American College of Obstetricians and Gynecologists |

AGE (YEAR)	RECOMMENDATION FOR CYTOLOGIC SCREENING	COMMENTS
Younger than 21	Avoid screening	
21 to 29	Screen every 3 years	
30 to 65 or 70	May screen every 3 years	This recommendation applies only to women with 3 consecutive cytologic tests; exceptions include women with HIV infection, compromised immunity, a history of cervical intraepithelial neoplasia grade 2 or 3, or exposure to DES in utero.
	Screen every 5 years	Pap + HPV co-testing use
Between 65 and 70	May discontinue screening	This recommendation applies only to women with ≥3 consecutive negative cytologic tests and no abnormal tests in the preceding 10 years; exceptions include women with multiple sexual partners.

DES, Diethylstilbestrol.
Adapted from American College of Obstetricians and Gynecologists (ACOG). Cervical cancer screening and prevention. American College of Obstetricians and Gynecologists (ACOG); (ACOG practice bulletin; no. 168); 2016.

Diagnosis

The initial workup for cervical cancer depends on whether a cervical lesion is visible. Patients without a visible cervical lesion require a cone biopsy to diagnose stage IA1 or IA2 tumor. Patients with a cervical lesion are assessed by history and physical examination and possibly by examination under anesthesia for biopsy, cystoscopy, sigmoidoscopy, and conventional imaging (chest x-ray, intravenous pyelogram). Other imaging modalities including computed tomography (CT), magnetic resonance imaging (MRI), and fluorodeoxyglucose positron emission tomography (FDG-PET) are useful in evaluating nodal or other metastatic sites but are not incorporated in the FIGO staging system owing to their limited availability worldwide. MRI performed significantly better than CT in detecting parametrial invasion, presence of bladder or rectal invasion, and identification of women suitable for fertility-preserving surgery. PET-CT is the most sensitive modality in identifying nodal metastasis or metastatic disease assisting with radiotherapy planning and evaluation of metabolic response to therapy. A 3-month post-therapy PET scan is highly predictive of long-term survival outcome.

Treatment

Multiple factors including tumor stage, size, histologic features (lymphovascular space invasion [LVSI], nonsquamous components, and depth of cervical stromal invasion), and evidence of lymph node metastasis influence the choice of treatment for cervical cancer. Patients with stage IA1 cervical cancer have undergone a cone biopsy and pathology demonstrates 3 mm of invasion or less, less than 7 mm width, no LVSI,

| TABLE 2 | Revised FIGO Staging for Carcinoma of the Cervix |

STAGE	CRITERIA
Stage I	
I	The carcinoma is strictly confined to the cervix
IA	Invasive carcinoma, which can be diagnosed only by microscopy, with deepest invasion ≤5 mm and largest extension ≥7 mm
IA1	Measured stromal invasion of ≤3 mm in depth and extension of ≤7 mm
IA2	Measured stromal invasion of >3 mm in depth and extension of >7 mm
IB	Clinically visible lesions limited to the cervix or preclinical cancers greater than stage IA
IB1	Lesion >5 mm depth of stromal invasion and <2 cm greatest dimension
IB2	Lesion 2 cm to <4 cm in greatest dimension
1B3	Lesion >4 cm in dimension
Stage II	
II	Cervical carcinoma invades beyond the uterus, but not to the pelvic wall or to the lower third of the vagina
IIA	Without parametrial invasion
IIA1	Clinically visible lesion ≤4 cm in greatest dimension
IIA2	Clinically visible lesion >4 cm in greatest dimension
IIB	With obvious parametrial invasion
Stage III	
III	The tumor extends to the pelvic wall and/or involves lower third of the vagina and/or causes hydronephrosis or nonfunctioning kidney
IIIA	Tumor involves lower third of the vagina, with no extension to the pelvic wall
IIIB	Extension to the pelvic wall and/or hydronephrosis or nonfunctioning kidney
IIIC1	Pelvic lymph node metastasis only
IIIC2	Para-aortic lymph node metastasis
Stage IV	
IV	The carcinoma has extended beyond the true pelvis or has involved (biopsy proven) the mucosa of the bladder or rectum; a bullous edema, as such, does not permit a case to be allotted as stage IV
IVA	Spread of the growth to adjacent organs
IVB	Spread to distant organs

Adapted from Bhatla N, Berek JS, Cuello Fredes M, et al. Revised FIGO Staging for carcinoma of cervix uteri. Int J Gynaecol Obstet. 2019;145:129–135.

and negative margins. Patients with this extent of disease can safely be treated with a less-radical hysterectomy, an extrafascial hysterectomy. Pelvic lymphadenectomy is not recommended owing to the low risk of pelvic node metastasis (<1%). In patients who desire to retain fertility, a cone biopsy may be considered. Wright and colleagues reported on 1409 women from the SEER database who were younger than 40 years and had stage IA1 cancer. The 5-year survival was 98% among 568 who underwent cone biopsy alone versus 99% among 841 who underwent hysterectomy.

TABLE 3   Randomized Trials of Cisplatin-Based Chemoradiation

TREATMENT	STAGE	SURVIVAL			SIGNIFICANCE
		TYPE	PERCENTAGE (%)		
Gynecology Oncology Group 85					
RT/5-FU* infusion/bolus cisplatin*	IIB-IVA	3 y PFS	67		P = .033
RT/oral HU*			57		
Gynecology Oncology Group 109					
Rad hyst/RT	IA2-IIA	Est. 4-y	63		P = .003
Rad hyst/RT/cisplatin*/5-FU*			80		
Radiation Therapy Oncology Group 9001					
RT	IIB-IVA	DFS	40		P < .001
RT/5-FU*/cisplatin*			67		
Gynecology Oncology Group 120					
RT + cisplatin*	IIB-IVA	3-y PFS	67		P < .001
RT + cisplatin*/5-FU*/HU*			64		
RT + HU*			47		
Gynecology Oncology Group 123					
RT + TAH	IB2	3 y PFS	74		P < .001
RT + cisplatin* + TAH			83		
Di Silvestro et al.					
RT + cisplatin	IB2-IVA	3 y PFS	64		P = .7869
RT + cisplatin + TPZ			63		
Pearcey et al.					
RT + cisplatin*	IB-IVA >5 cm	5-y DFS	62		P = .42
RT			58		

DFS, Disease-free survival; *5-FU*, fluorouracil (Adrucil); *HU*, hydroxyurea; *PFS*, progression free survival; *rad hyst*, radical hysterectomy; *RT*, radiotherapy; *TAH*, total abdominal hysterectomy.
*Not FDA approved for this indication.

Patients with stage IA2 to IB1 are generally treated with radical hysterectomy; in patients who are not candidates for surgery owing to comorbidities, radiation therapy is used. In patients with high-risk criteria after surgery—positive surgical margin, parametrial involvement, and positive pelvic nodes—cisplatin-based[1] chemoradiation, based on a positive randomized trial, is recommended. Those with intermediate risk factors including tumor size, cervical stromal invasion, and lymphovascular invasion had an improved progression-free survival with adjuvant radiation.

Radical trachelectomy—laparoscopic, vaginal, or open—in conjunction with lymphadenectomy is a reasonable alternative treatment for select young patients with stage IA2 and IB1 who desire to maintain their childbearing capacity. The criteria used for patient selection include early-stage cervical cancer with a lesion less than 2 cm, no lymphovascular invasion, and no lymph node metastasis. Reports comparing radical trachelectomies with matched controls identified increased complications (25% vs. 3%) and overall less-radical dissection.

Treatment of stage IB2 cancer of the cervix varies depending on the bulkiness and shape of the lesion. Surgery and chemoradiation therapy have advantages and disadvantages. Finan and colleagues reported that up to 72% of patients with stage IB2 disease who were treated with surgery received adjuvant radiation owing to high-risk factors identified in pathologic evaluation of specimens. In a randomized Gynecologic Oncology Group trial, 94% of patients with IB2 cervical cancer who underwent radical hysterectomy had high or intermediate risk factors warranting adjuvant radiation.

In 1999 the National Cancer Institute (NCI) initiated a clinical alert recommending that concurrent cisplatin-based chemotherapy be given with radiotherapy to women with cervical cancer based on five randomized studies, and this established a new standard of care (Table 3).

It is estimated that approximately 35% of patients with invasive cervical cancer will have recurrent or persistent disease, with most recurrences occurring in the first 2 years following primary therapy. Recurrence can be expected in 10% to 20% of patients treated with radical hysterectomy in contrast to 30% to 50% treated for more-advanced disease primarily with radiation plus concurrent chemotherapy. The site

[1] Not FDA approved for this indication.

TABLE 4 Phase III Trials Comparing Cisplatin Doublets and Cisplatin Alone to Treat Metastatic or Recurrent Cervical Carcinoma

STUDY	STAGE	RESPONSE RATE (%)	PROGRESSION-FREE SURVIVAL (MO)	OVERALL SURVIVAL (MO)
Gynecology Oncology Group 110				
Cisplatin[1]	IVB or recurrent	18	3.2	8
Cisplatin/mitolactol[8]		21	3.3	7.3
Cisplatin/ifosfamide (Ifex)[1]		31	8.3	4.6
Significance		$P = .004$	$P = .003$	$P = .835$
Gynecology Oncology Group 149				
Cisplatin/bleomycin[1]/ ifosfamide	IVB or recurrent	31	5.1	8.4
Cisplatin/ifosfamide		32	4.6	8.5
Significance		$P = .42$	$P = .495$	$P = .79$
Gynecology Oncology Group 169				
Cisplatin	IVB or recurrent	19	2.8	8.8
Cisplatin/paclitaxel (Taxol)[1]		36	4.8	9.7
Significance		$P = NS$	$P = NS$	$P = NS$
Gynecology Oncology Group 179				
Cisplatin	IVB or recurrent	13	2.9	6.5
Cisplatin/topotecan (Hycamtin)[1]		27	4.6	9.4
Cisplatin/methotrexate[1]/ vinblastine (Velban)[1]/ doxorubicin (Adriamycin)[1]				
Significance		$P = .004$	$P = .014$	$P = .017$
Gynecology Oncology Group 204				
Cisplatin/paclitaxel versus cisplatin/vinorelbine (Navelbine)[1]			HR[†] = 1.35	NR
Cisplatin/gemcitabine (Gemzar)[1]			HR[†] = 1.43	NR
Cisplatin/topotecan	IVB or recurrent		HR[†] = 1.28	NR
Gynecology Oncology Group 240				
Cisplatin/paclitaxel	IVB or recurrent	45%	5.9	13.3
Paclitaxel/topotecan		27%		
Cisplatin/paclitaxel/ Bevacizumab		50%	8.2	17.0
Paclitaxel/topotecan/ Bevacizumab		47%	HR = 0.67	HR = 0.71

NR, Not reported; *NS*, not significant.
[1]Not FDA approved for this indication.
[8]Orphan drug in the United States.
[†]Hazard ratio for PFS for experimental arms to cisplatin/paclitaxel.

of the recurrence can direct further treatment. Patients with central pelvic recurrences after surgery are candidates for curative radiation; after primary treatment with radiation therapy patients may be candidates for curative radical surgery (exenteration). Prognosis is more favorable for patients undergoing exenteration when there is a small (<3 cm) central recurrence, no sidewall involvement, and longer than 2 years of disease-free interval. Those with small recurrences limited to the cervix or upper vagina can occasionally be treated with radical hysterectomy and upper vaginectomy.

However, most recurrences are distant, involving the lung, bone, abdominal cavity, and supraclavicular lymph nodes. Recurrences within irradiated areas have a poor response to therapy (0% to 5%). Recurrences in the nonirradiated areas respond better to chemotherapy, with response rates of 25% to 70%. The use of chemotherapy in the treatment of recurrent cervical cancer is challenging because agents are only moderately active and patients can present with renal impairment secondary to obstructive uropathy, resulting in altered excretion with increased toxicity from chemotherapeutic agents. Table 4 compares results of randomized chemotherapy trials for the treatment of recurrent cervical cancer.

New treatment strategies for recurrent disease include immunotherapy with multiple ongoing trials at this time.

Conclusion

Adherence to current screening guidelines should allow early cervical cancer or precancerous detection. However, most patients with cervical cancer have not participated in regular screening and present with a variety of disease extents.

References

American Cancer Society: Cancer facts and figures. Available at http://www.cancer.org/Research/CancerFactsFigures/CancerFactsFigures/index. [Accessed 28 May 2019].

American College of Obstetricians and Gynecologists (ACOG): Cervical Cancer Screening and Prevention. Practice Bulletin #168. ACOG, *Obstet Gynecol* 128, 2016. e111-30.

Bhatla N, et al: Revised FIGO staging for carcinoma of the cervix uteri, *Int J Gynaecol Obstet* 145:129–135, 2019.

Bloss JD, Blessing JA, Behrens BC, et al: Randomized trial of cisplatin and ifosfamide with or without bleomycin in squamous carcinoma of the cervix: A Gynecologic Oncology Group study, *J Clin Oncol* 20:1832–1837, 2002.

Covens A, Shaw P, Murphy J, et al: Is radical trachelectomy a safe alternative to radical hysterectomy for patients with stage IA-B carcinoma of the cervix? *Cancer* 86:2273–2279, 1999.

DiSilvestro PA, Ali S, Craighed PS, et al: Phase III randomized trial of weekly cisplatin and irradiation versus cisplatin and tirapazamine and irradiation in stages IB2, IIA, IIB, IIIB and IVA cervical carcinoma limited to the pelvis: a Gynecologic Oncology Group study, *J Clin Oncol* 32(5):458–464, 2014.

Dunne EF, Unger ER, Sternberg M, et al: Prevalence of HPV infection among females in the United States, *JAMA* 297(8):813–819, 2007.

Finan MA, Decesare S, Fiorica JV, et al: Radical hysterectomy for stage IB1 vs IB2 carcinoma of the cervix: does the new staging system predict morbidity and survival? *Gynecol Oncol* 62(2):139–147, 1996.

Keys HM, Bundy BN, Stehman FB, et al: Cisplatin, radiation, and adjuvant hysterectomy compared with radiation and adjuvant hysterectomy for bulky stage IB cervical carcinoma, *N Engl J Med* 340(15):1154–1161, 1999. Erratum in N Engl J Med 1999;341(9):708.

Long 3rd HJ, Bundy BN, Grendys EC, et al: Randomized phase III trial of cisplatin with or without topotecan in carcinoma of the uterine cervix: A Gynecologic Oncology Group study, *J Clin Oncol* 23(21):4626–4633, 2005.

Monk BJ, Sill MW, McMeekin DS, et al: Phase III trial of four cisplatin-containing doublet combinations in stage IVB, recurrent, or persistent cervical carcinoma: A Gynecologic Oncology Group study, *J Clin Oncol* 27(28):4649–4655, 2009.

Moore DH, Blessing JA, McQuellon RP, et al: Phase III study of cisplatin with or without paclitaxel in stage IVB, recurrent, or persistent squamous cell carcinoma of the cervix: A Gynecologic Oncology Group study, *J Clin Oncol* 22(15):3113–3119, 2004.

Morris M, Eifel PJ, Lu J, et al: Pelvic radiation with concurrent chemotherapy compared with pelvic and para-aortic radiation for high-risk cervical cancer, *N Engl J Med* 340(15):1137–1143, 1999.

National Cancer Institute: Cervical cancer. Available at: http://www.cancer.gov/cancertopics/types/cervical. [Accessed 27 May 2019].

Omura GA, Blessing JA, Vaccarello L, et al: Randomized trial of cisplatin versus cisplatin plus mitolactol versus cisplatin plus ifosfamide in advanced squamous carcinoma of the cervix: A Gynecologic Oncology Group study, *J Clin Oncol* 15(1):165–171, 1997.

Pearcey R, Brundage M, Drouin P, et al: Phase III trial comparing radical radiotherapy with and without cisplatin chemotherapy in patients with advanced squamous cell cancer of the cervix, *J Clin Oncol* 20(4):966–972, 2002.

Peters 3rd WA, Liu PY, Barrett 3rd RJ, et al: Concurrent chemotherapy and pelvic radiation therapy compared with pelvic radiation therapy alone as adjuvant therapy after radical surgery in high-risk early-stage cancer of the cervix, *J Clin Oncol* 18(8):1606–1613, 2000.

Rose PG, Bundy BN, Watkins EB, et al: Concurrent cisplatin-based radiotherapy and chemotherapy for locally advanced cervical cancer, *N Engl J Med* 340(15):1144–1153, 1999.

Tewari KS, Sill MW, Long HR, et al: Improved survival with bevacizumab in advance cervical cancer, *N Engl J Med* 370(8):734–743, 2014.

Whitney CW, Sause W, Bundy BN, et al: Randomized comparison of fluorouracil plus cisplatin versus hydroxyurea as an adjunct to radiation therapy in stage IIB-IVA carcinoma of the cervix with negative para-aortic lymph nodes: A Gynecologic Oncology Group and Southwest Oncology Group study, *J Clin Oncol* 17(5):1339–1348, 1999.

Wright JD, Nathavithrana R, Lewin SN, et al: Fertility-conserving surgery for young women with stage IA1 cervical cancer: Safety and access, *Obstet Gynecol* 115(3):585–590, 2010.

CONTRACEPTION

Method of
Rachel A. Bonnema, MD, MS

CURRENT THERAPY

- Combined estrogen and progesterone methods (e.g., pills, patch, ring) are effective and commonly used. They provide excellent cycle control and decreased rates of ectopic pregnancy, pelvic inflammatory disease, and endometrial and ovarian cancer, and they can be used in extended-cycle methods for patients who desire fewer than 12 periods per year.
- The use of estrogen has been associated, albeit rarely, with the development of deep vein thrombosis, myocardial infarction, and stroke; estrogen should not be used in smokers older than 35 years and in patients with diabetes with end organ damage, coronary artery disease, migraines with aura, or a known hypercoagulable condition.
- For women with a contraindication to estrogen, progestin-only methods are safe to use.
- Long-acting reversible contraception (LARC) such as an implant or intrauterine device (IUD) is safe and extremely effective and should be considered in all women, including nulliparous women.

Nearly half of all pregnancies in the United States are unplanned, a rate higher than the rate in other developed countries. Primary care physicians need up-to-date knowledge on contraceptive counseling for women to provide the best match between patient and contraceptive method, in part because providers frequently need to supply contraceptives to women who have particular medical comorbidities. Newer contraceptive preparations are now available, including a vaginal ring that can be reused for up to 1 year, a progestin-only pill with a wider window for missed pill.

Nonhormonal Methods

Nonhormonal methods of contraception include barrier methods and the copper intrauterine device (IUD). These methods are safe, easily available, inexpensive, and reversible. Common barrier methods include male and female condoms, spermicides, vaginal sponges, diaphragms, and cervical caps (Table 1). Only condom use has been consistently found to protect against sexually transmitted diseases including HIV, and condom use may reduce risks of cervical cancer as well. Barrier methods have the lowest efficacy rates of all contraceptive methods, and users should also be counseled about emergency contraception (EC). The copper IUD is an extremely effective form of long-acting reversible contraception (LARC) and is a particularly attractive option for a woman with contraindications to hormone use desiring effective contraception.

Combined Hormonal Contraception

Combined hormonal contraception (CHC) contains estrogen (ethinyl estradiol) and a progestin and works primarily by preventing the surge of luteinizing hormone and thereby preventing ovulation. CHC can be delivered as an oral contraceptive pill (OCP), as a vaginal ring (NuvaRing, Annovera), or as a transdermal patch (Xulane). Risks, benefits, side effects, and contraindications of CHC are thought to be largely similar across delivery methods.

There are many noncontraceptive benefits to CHC, including first-line treatment for dysfunctional uterine bleeding, dysmenorrhea, and menorrhagia. Benefits in addition to menstrual control include reduction in the risks for, and symptoms of, endometriosis, ovulatory pain, ovarian cysts, benign breast disease, premenstrual syndrome, and premenstrual dysphoric disorder. CHC also reduces risk of ovarian and endometrial cancers; these risk reductions extend for years after stopping CHC. The most common side effects of CHC are outlined in Table 2. The risk of venous thromboembolism (VTE) may be higher in obese patients, smokers, and those who use certain

TABLE 1 Nonhormonal Contraception

| | BARRIER METHODS | | | INTRAUTERINE DEVICE |
	CONDOM (MALE/FEMALE)	DIAPHRAGM OR CERVICAL CAP	SPONGE	COPPER IUD
Duration	Female condom can be inserted up to 8 h before intercourse; male condoms must be changed with each act of intercourse	Can be placed up to 6 h before intercourse and should be removed within 6 h after	Can be left in for 30 h and through multiple acts of intercourse	Approved for up to 10 years
Typical-use failure rate*	15%	15%	15%	Less than 0.1%
Side effects and considerations	High failure rates: condom can break or slip Acceptability by partner may be limited	Requires expert fitting Needs to be refitted after childbirth Requires dexterity and self-placement by patient Use with spermicide increases efficacy but can lead to risk of UTIs, increased risk of toxic shock syndrome, and potential increased risk of HIV transmission	May increase risk of UTIs Use with spermicide increases efficacy but can lead to risk of UTIs, increased risk of toxic shock syndrome, and potential increased risk of HIV transmission	Bleeding and cramping with menses initially Low risk of ectopic pregnancy, premature delivery, perforation, or expulsion Avoid with active infection, undiagnosed genital bleeding, cervical cancer, or Wilson disease
Consider in:	Patients at risk for STIs Patients without access to medical care and who are looking for nonhormonal, reversible, and convenient methods of contraception	Women who are looking for nonhormonal, reversible, and convenient methods of contraception	Women who are looking for nonhormonal, reversible, and convenient methods of contraception Patients without access to medical care	Women with contraindication to hormones or who desire hormone-free, long-acting, reversible contraception Women in need of EC followed by long-term effective contraception

EC, Emergency contraception; *HIV*, human immunodeficiency virus; *IUD*, intrauterine device; *UTI*, urinary tract infection.
*Trussel J. Contraceptive failure in the United States. *Conception* 83:397–404, 2011.

progestins such as desogestrel or drospirenone. This risk is lower, however, than the risk of VTE associated with pregnancy, and the absolute risk of VTE among CHC users remains small.

CHCs can be used safely by those with a range of medical conditions, including well-controlled hypertension, uncomplicated diabetes, migraines *without* aura when less than age 35, and a family history of breast cancer, to name a few. CHC use is contraindicated in patients who have a history of migraine headache with aura at any age, or in those over age 35 with any migraine, owing to elevated risk for stroke. Owing to the increased risk of a cardiovascular event, CHC is also contraindicated in patients with moderate hypertension, diabetes with end organ damage, or known cardiovascular disease and in those who smoke after age 35 years. Other contraindications include a personal history of breast cancer, an estrogen-dependent tumor, unexplained vaginal bleeding, stroke, known thromboembolic disorder, or known VTE. Elevated risk of VTE and negative effect on lactation restrict the use of CHC in the first 6 weeks after delivery.

Combined Oral Contraceptive Pills

There are dozens of formulations of OCPs, which differ by their estrogen dosage, progestin type and dosage, and hormone delivery schedule. OCPs can be monophasic, where each pill contains the same amount of hormones, or multiphasic, where pills contain different amounts of hormones throughout the monthly cycle. The different formulations offer patients options in cycle length, hormone levels, duration of withdrawal bleeding, and side effect profile. Education should include taking their pill at the same time each day; this becomes even more critical in OCPs containing lower dosages of estrogen (20 µg). If a pill is missed, it should be taken as soon as remembered. If 2 days of pills are missed, the regimen includes two pills daily for 2 days in a row with a backup method utilized. If 3 days of pills are missed, the pill pack should be discarded and a backup method utilized. At that point, it should be discussed whether to start a new pack or to change contraceptive methods.

Traditional OCP regimens include 21 days of hormones, followed by 7 days of placebo pills during which menses occur. For those who desire fewer days of menses or fewer than 12 menses per year, extended-cycle OCP regimens can be offered that shorten the placebo period to 4 days, offer a placebo week every 4 months, or eliminate the placebo week altogether. Extended-cycle regimens have other benefits, including decreased hormone withdrawal symptoms such as headaches, tiredness, bloating, excessive bleeding, or menstrual pain.

In addition to estrogen dose and scheduling, it is also important to consider the progestin component, which theoretically may affect libido, weight gain, acne, and hirsutism. These choices, however, must be balanced with the potential increased risk for VTE; levonorgestrel-containing OCPs have a long track record and are associated with a lower risk of VTE than other progestins such as desogestrel, gestodene, and drospirenone.

Contraceptive Patch

Norelgestromin/ethinyl estradiol (Xulane) is a thin transdermal patch delivering a daily dose of 35 µg/d ethinyl estradiol and 150 µg/d norelgestromin. Patches should be changed weekly for 3 weeks on "patch change day" followed by a patch-free week during which menses occur. Only one patch should be worn at a time, and no more than 7 days should pass during the patch-free week. The patch has decreased efficacy in women who weigh more than 90 kg. Most of the noncontraceptive benefits, side effects, cardiovascular risks, and contraindications are similar to those of other forms of CHC, but there may be an increased risk of VTE in patch users compared with users of OCPs. Studies are controversial as to the actual increase in risk associated with

TABLE 2 Hormonal Contraception

	COMBINATION ESTROGEN-PROGESTIN		PROGESTIN-ONLY			
	TRADITIONAL (OCPS, PATCH, SA/EE RING)	**EXTENDED CYCLE (OCPS, ENG/EE RING)**	**PILL**		**INJECTION**	**IMPLANT/IUD**
			NORETHINDRONE	**DROSPIRENONE (SLYND)**		
Duration Reversibility	Daily pill Immediate	Daily pill or monthly ring Immediate	Daily pill with no hormone-free interval Immediate	Daily with 4 day hormone-free interval Immediate	3 months Variable	3–6 years Immediate
Typical-use failure rate*	9%	9%	9%		6%	0.05%–0.8%
Side effects†	Spotting, nausea, headache, breast tenderness, VTE, stroke, MI	Similar to traditional with increased risk for unpatterned bleeding	Unpatterned bleeding, or absence of bleeding; headaches, nausea, mood changes, breast tenderness		Unpatterned bleeding, or absence of bleeding; weight gain, depression, reversible decrease in BMD	Unpatterned bleeding, or absence of bleeding
Consider in:	Women with dysmenorrhea, menorrhagia, irregular menstrual periods, acne, hirsutism, or polycystic ovary syndrome	Women who do not desire monthly periods. Offers particular benefit for women with estrogen withdrawal symptoms, dysmenorrhea, or endometriosis	Women with contraindication to estrogen, hypercoagulable states, dysmenorrhea, migraine with aura, or breast-feeding		Women with contraindication to estrogen, seizure disorder, hypercoagulable states, dysmenorrhea, migraine with aura, or breast-feeding	Women with contraindication to estrogen, seizure disorder, hypercoagulable states, dysmenorrhea, migraine with aura, or breast-feeding

BMD, Bone mineral density; *IUD*, intrauterine device; *MI*, myocardial infarction; *OCP*, oral contraceptive pill; *VTE*, venous thromboembolism.
*Trussell J. Contraceptive failure in the United States. *Contraception* 83:397–404, 2011.
†Note: For all combination methods, must have no contraindication to estrogen.

patch use but did prompt the updating of the drug label to indicate a higher risk of VTE. Of note, the VTE risk associated with patch use is lower than that associated with pregnancy.

Vaginal Ring

Contraceptive vaginal rings (CVR) deliver hormones directly through the vaginal epithelium for highly effective contraception without the need for daily dosing. There are currently two CVRs that are US Food and Drug Administration (FDA)-approved for use in the United States. Etonogestrel/ethinyl estradiol (NuvaRing) is a soft plastic ring that is inserted vaginally by the patient, usually for 3 weeks and then removed for 1 week at which time menses occur. A new ring is inserted 7 days after the last was removed even if bleeding is not complete. The ring releases 15 µg of ethinyl estradiol and 0.12 mg of etonogestrel daily for 3 to 5 weeks, so it can be kept in longer than 3 weeks for those desiring the benefits of extended-cycling use discussed previously. Each ring releases approximately half the level of hormones as the average OCP without affecting efficacy. If the ring falls out (as occurs rarely), it can be rinsed and reinserted without a change in efficacy. Most find the ring easy to insert and remove and comfortable to retain during intercourse.

A newer ring containing a year's contraception with segesterone acetate (SA) and ethinyl estradiol (EE) is now available. The SA/EE ring (Annovera) is used for 21 days followed by a 7-day use-free interval for up to 13 consecutive cycles. Unlike the NuvaRing, no data are available on extended periods of continuous use with the same SA/EE ring; during counseling, special emphasis should be placed on the increased pregnancy risk for patients who remove the ring for more than 2 hours. Both rings available are highly effective, similar to other combined hormonal methods, and have excellent cycle control. The vaginal ring has been associated with an increase in leukorrhea. Otherwise, its noncontraceptive benefits, side effects, cardiovascular risks, and contraindications are similar to those of other forms of CHC.

Progestin-Only Contraceptives

Progestin-only contraceptives are particularly beneficial for those with a contraindication to estrogen because progestin-only methods have decreased medical risks associated including no increased risk of stroke, myocardial infarction, or VTE. All progestin-only methods have a similar method of action: Ovulation is variably inhibited, cervical mucus is thickened, and the endometrial lining undergoes histologic alterations making implantation less likely. Owing to the fact that many of the progestin-only methods are long acting, they tend to have lower failure rates as opposed to CHCs (see Table 2). All progestin-only methods are appropriate for breast-feeding.

Pill

There are now two progestin-only pills (POPs) available in the United States. Norethindrone pills are taken without a hormone-free interval and fertility returns immediately on discontinuation. In fact, most experts believe fertility can return in as little as 3 hours after a missed dose; thus patients should be counseled to use a backup method if 3 or more hours late in taking her dose. Given this small window for error, this method should be prescribed only to patients who can adhere closely to a daily pill schedule. Additionally, counseling should include that while taking norethindrone pills normal menstrual patterns may include anything from amenorrhea to menometrorrhagia. This unpatterned bleeding is likely one of the greatest obstacles to wider use of progestin-only oral contraception.

A new POP contraceptive contains drospirenone 4 mg (Slynd) and is available in a 24-day supply of hormone and a 4-day supply of placebo, allowing for a timed withdrawal bleed. The drospirenone-only pill maintains contraceptive efficacy even with 24-hour delayed or missed-pill errors; patients can be counseled to take a missed tablet as soon as remembered if within 24 hours or with the next scheduled dose if more than 24 hours late. Although intermenstrual bleeding rates are still high, the menstrual profile may be more tolerable compared with other POPs.

Owing to the fact that POPs have demonstrated no significant negative effects on breastfeeding, POPs can be prescribed immediately postpartum. POPs may have similar effects as other progestin-only methods in decreasing the frequency of sickle cell crises; however, unlike depot medroxyprogesterone acetate (DMPA, Depo-Provera) injections, certain anticonvulsants may lower effectiveness of the POP, so other methods may be more beneficial in patients with seizure disorders.

Injectable

The intramuscular DMPA injection (Depo-Provera 150 mg) is given every 12 weeks and has a typical-use failure rate of 6%. A lower dose of DMPA (104 mg in Depo-SubQ Provera) has been approved for subcutaneous injection. Patients with seizure disorders are particularly good candidates for DMPA injections because, unlike other forms of contraception, the efficacy of DMPA is not affected by enzyme-inducing antiepileptic drugs. Depo-Provera may also decrease seizure frequency, providing additional benefit. DMPA reduces serum estradiol levels, which can adversely affect bone health. There is a clear association between DMPA use and decreased BMD; however data has shown the BMD loss to be reversible with discontinuation of use and there is no increased risk of fracture with use of DMPA. The World Health Organization has recommended that there be no restriction on the use of Depo-Provera in ages 18 to 45. According to recent consensus guidelines, clinicians should advise patients about the risk for BMD loss but can reassure them about reversibility with discontinuation.

Intrauterine System

The levonorgestrel intrauterine system (LNG-IUS) is a highly effective contraceptive method long considered to be reversible sterilization owing to its excellent efficacy in preventing pregnancy and quick return to fertility after its removal. There are now multiple formulations of LNG IUS that prevent pregnancy for 3 to 6 years (Skyla, Kyleena, Mirena, Liletta), categorized by the amount of levonorgestrel that they contain: 52 mg in Mirena and Liletta, 19.5 mg in Kyleena, or 13.5 mg in Skyla. The LNG-IUS is ideal for those who require highly effective contraception and is particularly beneficial for patients requiring a progestin-only contraception. Its relatively low cost over time is another factor for patients to consider. Numerous studies have confirmed the effectiveness of the LNG-IUS for reduction of menstrual blood loss in menorrhagia, leiomyomas, and pain caused by endometriosis; Mirena received FDA approval for the indication of menorrhagia and has been shown to decrease menorrhagia for those on anticoagulation. Insertion of the LNG-IUS requires a trained provider. At the time of placement, cramping and pain may occur; a rare complication of placement is uterine wall rupture. Many will likely develop amenorrhea, though may experience initial irregular bleeding and spotting.

Implant

There is one single-rod subdermal implant available in the United States called Nexplanon that is a highly effective long-term contraceptive containing the progestin etonogestrel (ENG). The rod is implanted in the upper arm and remains active for 3 years. ENG does not cause a hypoestrogenic state and thus is not considered to have any significant effect on BMD. ENG implantation can be done as a simple procedure by a trained provider under local anesthetic with a preloaded, disposable applicator. Patients experience a quick return to normal cycles after implant removal, and there have been no reports of infertility after removal. Similar to other progestin-only forms of contraception, irregular bleeding is the major side effect of the ENG implant. The most common bleeding pattern associated with the implant is infrequent, irregular bleeding. This remains an important counseling point since the highest rate of discontinuation is during the first 8 to 9 months of use, primarily owing to frequent bleeding.

Permanent

Permanent birth control methods include vasectomy and female sterilization by various procedures. These methods are highly effective (typical failure rate 0.15%–0.5%); however, they are permanent and can be associated with regret. Each sterilization procedure has advantages and disadvantages that should be considered by the patient before choosing which one to use.

Emergency Contraception

Familiarity with EC is critical both for those having unprotected sex and for those who are using methods with higher failure rates. EC use has not been shown to reduce compliance with other first-line methods. EC primarily acts by inhibiting or delaying ovulation and works before implantation; if a fertilized egg has already implanted, EC will not work. EC includes pills (composed of estrogen + progestin, progestin only, and antiprogestins) and copper IUD placement (inserted up to 5 days after unprotected intercourse)[1]; EC pills are most effective when taken in the first 12 hours but have gradually decreasing effectiveness for up to 120 hours after intercourse. The most accessible form of EC in the United States contains levonorgestrel only (Plan B One Step) and is over the counter without age restrictions.

Counseling

When counseling patients about their contraceptive choices, it is important that providers are aware of their role in giving information and allowing patients to make informed decisions. The only effective contraceptive is one that a patient is willing to use consistently and correctly, and the choice of contraception is ultimately the patient's decision. Providers must educate patients regarding the advantages and disadvantages of each method that is medically appropriate for them. Discussing a patient's preferences for menstrual frequency and tolerance for scheduled and unscheduled bleeding is important in deciding which contraceptive will best fits a patient's needs. Providers should counsel patients on expected side effects as well as expectant management strategies. Every effort should be made to remove barriers to initiation, including having no requirement for a pelvic examination or Pap smear before initiation. Using the conversation about contraceptives to also discuss safe sex is ideal.

---

[1]Not FDA approved for this indication.

References

ACOG Committee on Practice Bulletins—Gynecology: ACOG practice bulletin. No. 73: use of hormonal contraception in women with coexisting medical conditions, *Obstet Gynecol* 107:1453–1472, 2006.

Baker C, Creinin MD: Contraception update, *OBG Manage* 32(10):10–18, 2020.

Curtis KM, Tepper NK, Jatlaoui TC, et al: U.S. Medical eligibility criteria for contraceptive use, 2016, *MMWR Recomm Rep* 65(No. RR-3):1–104, 2016. https://doi.org/10.15585/mmwr.rr6503a1.

Finer LB, Zolna MR: Unintended pregnancy in the United States: incidence and disparities, 2006, *Contraception* 84:478–485, 2011.

Lanza LL, McQuay LJ, Rothman KJ, et al: Use of depot medroxyprogesterone acetate contraception and incidence of bone fracture, *Obstet Gynecol* 121:593–600, 2013.

Parkin L, Sharples K, Hernandez RK, et al: Risk of venous thromboembolism in users of oral contraceptives containing drospirenone or levonorgestrel: nested case control study based on UK General Practice Research Database, *BMJ* 340:d2139, 2011.

Petitti DB: Combination estrogen-progestin oral contraceptives, *N Engl J Med* 349:1443–1450, 2003.

Spencer AL, Bonnema RA, McNamara MC: Helping women choose appropriate hormonal contraception: update on risks, benefits, and indications, *Am J Med* 122:497–506, 2009.

Trussel J: Contraceptive failure in the United States, *Contraception* 83:397–404, 2011.

World Health Organization: Cardiovascular disease and use of oral and injectable progestogen-only contraceptives and combined injectable contraceptives. Results of an international, multicenter, case-control study. World Health Organization Collaborative Study of Cardiovascular Disease and Steroid Hormone Contraception, *Contraception* 57:315–324, 1998.

DYSMENORRHEA

Method of
Linda Speer, MD

CURRENT DIAGNOSIS

- Primary dysmenorrhea (painful menses without underlying pathology) is common among adolescents and young women. It usually begins shortly after menarche.
- Diagnosis of primary dysmenorrhea can be made based on typical history of crampy pelvic pain during the first 1 to 3 days of the menstrual cycle. Pelvic examination is not required.
- Secondary dysmenorrhea (with underlying pathology) should be considered in cases that do not match the typical history, begin later in life, and/or are refractory to treatment.
- The most common cause of secondary dysmenorrhea is endometriosis. The clinical standard for diagnosis of endometriosis is laparoscopic confirmation. Ultrasound imaging is useful in some cases.

CURRENT THERAPY

- Nonsteroidal antiinflammatory drugs (NSAIDs) are well-established first-line therapy for treatment of primary dysmenorrhea. None has been confirmed as superior to others.
- Cyclooxygenase-2 (COX-2) inhibitors are effective and have fewer gastrointestinal side effects but may be less effective than NSAIDs.
- Oral contraceptives and the levonorgestrel intrauterine system (Mirena)[1] reduce dysmenorrhea.
- Other effective therapies include topical heat, high-frequency transcutaneous electrical nerve stimulation (TENS), and several herbal preparations.
- Treatments for endometriosis as a secondary cause of pelvic pain and dysmenorrhea include hormonal suppression of the endometrial tissue, conservative laparoscopic surgical debulking, and hysterectomy in selected cases.

[1]Not FDA approved for this indication.

Dysmenorrhea is defined as painful menses. Primary dysmenorrhea occurs without underlying pathology, typically beginning soon after menarche. It is common in adolescent girls, with prevalence ranging from 20% to 90% depending on measurement methods; about 15% of adolescents describe their dysmenorrhea as severe. The median duration of each episode is 2 days beginning with the onset of menses. During adolescence, dysmenorrhea leads to high rates of school absence and activity nonparticipation. According to representative national survey data in the United States, 14% of adolescent girls aged 12 to 17 years frequently miss school because of menstrual cramps.

A prospective cohort study showed that the prevalence and severity of dysmenorrhea was lower at 24 years of age than at 19 years of age. At 24 years of age, 67% of the women still experienced dysmenorrhea, and 10% reported pain severity that limited daily activity. The prevalence and severity of dysmenorrhea were reduced in women who were parous at 24 years and nulliparous at 19 years, but they were unchanged in women who were still nulliparous or women who had had a miscarriage or abortion.

There is a significant correlation between the severity of dysmenorrhea and the amount of menstrual flow. Survey data demonstrate that depression and anxiety are associated with menstrual pain and suggest that loss of social support is a significant contributor to menstrual symptoms. The severity of dysmenorrhea is not associated with height, weight, or regularity of the menstrual cycle. A relationship to smoking has been found inconsistently.

Secondary dysmenorrhea typically starts later in life after the onset of an underlying causative condition, most often endometriosis. The association between dysmenorrhea and endometriosis is uncertain for women with minimal disease. However, based on a study of more than 1000 women with laparoscopically confirmed endometriosis, chronic pelvic pain, dyspareunia, and dysmenorrhea are in fact related to the extent of endometriosis.

Diagnosis

For adolescents who present with complaints typical for primary dysmenorrhea, treatment may be started empirically without a pelvic examination or diagnostic studies. Sexually active adolescents and young women should be screened for chlamydia and gonorrhea, which can be done with either urine or a genital sampling.

For adolescents and women who do not have a history consistent with primary dysmenorrhea or who are refractory to treatment, endometriosis may be suspected. The gold standard for diagnosis is laparoscopy and biopsy. Ultrasound may also be useful, especially to identify endometriomas.

Treatment

Nonsteroidal Antiinflammatory Drugs

A Cochrane review of randomized, controlled trials (RCTs) concluded that among women with primary dysmenorrhea, NSAIDs were significantly more effective for pain relief than placebo or acetaminophen (Tylenol). No specific NSAID was shown to be superior to others for either pain relief or safety. However, the available evidence had little power to detect such differences, because most individual comparisons were based on few small trials. In one study in which diclofenac (Voltaren) 100 mg was compared with placebo for treatment of primary dysmenorrhea, the authors found that leg strength and aerobic capacity were maintained at the level found during luteal phase when women took diclofenac for dysmenorrhea, but they were reduced during menses in the placebo group.

COX-2 Inhibitors

Several COX-2 inhibitors have been evaluated for treatment of dysmenorrhea in RCTs. Celecoxib (Celebrex) 200 mg was compared with naproxen sodium (Naprosyn) 550 mg and placebo for treatment of dysmenorrhea and found to be superior to placebo but not as effective as naproxen. Etoricoxib (Arcoxia)[5] 120 mg daily was found to be better than placebo and equivalent to mefenamic acid (Ponstel) for treatment of primary dysmenorrhea with less nausea and epigastric pain than mefenamic acid.

Oral Contraceptives

In a systematic review of NSAIDs and oral contraceptives (OCs) for treatment of dysmenorrhea that included 10 placebo-controlled RCTs of NSAIDs, two RCTs of OCs and six prospective observational studies of OCs, the authors concluded that both are effective. In a study of women with laparoscopically proven endometriosis, low-dose ethinyl estradiol and norethisterone (norethindrone) decreased dysmenorrhea associated with endometriosis as compared with placebo (with pain assessment on a verbal rating scale from 0 to 3). There was also a significant reduction in volume of endometriomas with OCs but not placebo.

Levonorgestrel Intrauterine System

The levonorgestrel intrauterine system (LNG-IUS), Mirena, reduces menstrual bleeding and dysmenorrhea, which can be a desirable side effect for women desiring long-term contraception. In an uncontrolled case series of women treated with LNG-IUS for adenomyosis, dysmenorrhea diminished continuously during the 3-year study from a mean 78 mm to a mean 12 mm on a

[5]Investigational drug in the United States.

100-mm visual analog scale. Overall satisfaction with treatment was 73%. Depot medroxyprogesterone acetate[1] (Depo-Provera) is similarly effective, but it is less likely to be well tolerated owing to unpredictable bleeding, weight gain, and mood changes.

Transcutaneous Electrical Nerve Stimulation
In a study comparing transcutaneous electrical nerve stimulation (TENS) with interferential current for treatment of dysmenorrhea, each group received application of the modality for 20 minutes while experiencing dysmenorrhea. Both groups improved significantly from baseline without significant difference between them. High-frequency TENS has been found to be effective for the treatment of dysmenorrhea in a number of small trials. Low-frequency TENS does not appear to be effective.

Topical Heat and Infrared Light
Two meta-analyses have concluded that topical heat is likely an effective therapy based on several small low-to-moderate-quality studies. In a trial comparing far-infrared emitting belt versus placebo belt for treatment of primary dysmenorrhea, both with concurrent application of topical heat, both groups improved, and the duration of the analgesic effect was significantly longer in the group treated with the infrared belt.

Complementary and Alternative Medicine Approaches
Herbal
Several herbal remedies have been studied in RCTs for treatment of dysmenorrhea and found to be effective as compared with placebo or NSAIDs. They include *Psidii guajava* extract[7] 6 mg/day, French maritime pine bark extract (pycnogenol),[7] ginger root powder[7] 250 mg 4 times daily, salix extract (willow bark) 400 mg daily, and cinnamon one 1000 mg capsule daily. A pilot study of oral lactobacillus capsules (probiotic)[7] suggests that it may also be helpful.

Acupressure and Acupuncture
The evidence for the effectiveness of acupuncture is not conclusive. In unblinded studies women experience clinically relevant reduction in pain scores, a mean of more than 10 points on a 100-point scale, which could be due to placebo effect. In fact, in a well-designed RCT of electro-acupuncture at the Sanyinjiao point (the point expected to be related to uterine pain) compared to an unrelated nonacupoint or no acupuncture, the only significant differences were with the no-acupuncture group as measured with a visual analogue rating scale.

Adequate blinding is also an issue among studies of acupressure. For example, in an RCT comparing auricular seed acupressure versus adhesive tape only for treatment of primary dysmenorrhea the acupressure group (but not the tape only group) had instructions to massage the seed 15 times, three times daily for 20 days. Menstrual pain decreased significantly in the acupressure group. Several other studies suggest that acupressure at the Sanyinjiao point or Taichong point is more effective than no intervention or inadequately blinded control groups. Because acupressure is a low-cost and harmless intervention, it may be worth considering even if the pain reduction is a placebo response. It appears to be less effective than analgesics.

Yoga and Other Physical Activity
Yoga is another alternative approach with low cost and little risk that may be worth considering despite weak evidence for effectiveness. In one unblinded RCT, three yoga poses (cat, cobra, and fish) were studied for treatment of primary dysmenorrhea. Participants randomized to the intervention group were told to do the yoga poses during luteal phase and complete a questionnaire regarding menstrual characteristics. The control group was asked to complete the questionnaire only. There was significant reduction in intensity and duration of pain in the yoga group compared with baseline and with the control group.

Two meta-analyses have concluded limited quality evidence suggests that physical activity interventions reduce the duration and intensity of primary dysmenorrhea, perhaps more than oral analgesics. Further study is needed to determine what physical activity regimens are most beneficial.

Spinal Manipulation
Overall there is no evidence to suggest that spinal manipulation is effective in the treatment of primary and secondary dysmenorrhea.

Surgical Treatment
Surgical treatment may be considered in severe and refractory cases of pelvic pain including dysmenorrhea. Laparoscopic uterosacral nerve ablation (LUNA, n=35) alone has been compared with LUNA plus presacral neurectomy (n=32). There were no differences between groups for relief of dysmenorrhea at 3-, 6-, and 12-month follow-up, but more surgical complications were experienced with neurectomy.

Treatment of Endometriosis
Treatment of endometriosis may start with use of NSAIDs, hormonal contraceptives, and/or LNG-IUS.[1] However, often endometriosis is diagnosed after those first-line therapies have failed. Debulking of the ectopic endometrial tissue during laparoscopy can relieve pain.

Other treatments involve hormonal suppression of endometrial tissue. Danazol is a 19-nortestosterone derivative with a long history of use for treatment of endometriosis pain at a dosage of 400 to 800 mg daily for 6 months, but it is often poorly tolerated owing to androgenic side effects. Oral progestin regimens (medroxyprogesterone acetate[1] [DepoProvera] up to 100 mg daily[3] or norethindrone [Aygestin] up to 15 mg daily) may be used to suppress menses for a 6-month course. Other accepted therapies include gonadotropin-releasing hormone (GnRH) agonist analogues such as leuprolide (Lupron). Aromatase inhibitors have been shown to be effective in a systematic review of several small RCTs. Etonogestrel subdermal implant[1] (Nexplanon) has been evaluated in an uncontrolled case series and found to be associated with pain relief.

In severe refractory cases, hysterectomy may be considered.

---

[1]Not FDA approved for this indication.
[3]Exceeds dosage recommended by the manufacturer.

References

Alonso C, Coe CL: Disruptions of social relationships accentuate the association between emotional distress and menstrual pain in young women, *Health Psychol* 20:411–416, 2001.

Andersch B, Milsom I: An epidemiologic study of young women with dysmenorrhea, *Am J Obstet Gynecol* 144:655–660, 1982.

Armour M, Smith CA, Steel KA, Macmillan F: The effectiveness of self-care and lifestyle interventions in primary dysmenorrhea: a systematic review and meta-analysis, *BMC Complement Altern Med* 19:22, 2019.

Bazarganipour F, Lamyian M, Heshmat R, et al: A randomized clinical trial of the efficacy of applying a simple acupressure protocol to the Taichong point in relieving dysmenorrhea, *Int J Gynaecol Obstet* 111:105–109, 2010.

Brown J, Crawfort TJ, Datta S, Prentice A: Oral contraceptives for pain associated with endometriosis, *Cochrane Database Syst Rev* CD001019, 2018.

Brown J, Pan A, Hart RJ: Gonadotrophin-releasing hormone analogues for pain associated with endometriosis, *Cochrane Database Syst Rev* (12):CD008475, 2010.

Carroquino–Garcia P, Jimenez–Rejano JJ, Medrano–Sanchez E, et al: Therapeutic exercise in the treatment of primary dysmenorrhea: A systematic review and meta-analysis, *Phys Ther* 99:1371-80, 2019.

Chantler I, Mitchell D, Fuller A: Diclofenac potassium attenuates dysmenorrhea and restores exercise performance in women with primary dysmenorrhea, *J Pain* 10:191–200, 2009.

Daniels S, Robbins J, West CR, Nemeth MA: Celecoxib in the treatment of primary dysmenorrhea: Results from two randomized, double-blind, active- and placebo-controlled, crossover studies, *Clin Ther* 31:1192–1208, 2009.

Doubova SV, Morales HR, Hernández SF, et al: Effect of a *Psidii guajavae folium* extract in the treatment of primary dysmenorrhea: A randomized clinical trial, *J Ethnopharmacol* 110:305–310, 2007.

Harlow SD, Park M: A longitudinal study of risk factors for the occurrence, duration and severity of menstrual cramps in a cohort of college women, *Br J Obstet Gynaecol* 103:1134–1142, 1996.

Jahangirifar M, Taebi M, Dolatian M: The effect of cinnamon on primary dysmenorrhea: A randomized, double-blind clinical trial, *Complement Ther Clin Pract* 33:56–60, 2018.

Jensen JT: Noncontraceptive applications of the levonorgestrel intrauterine system, *Curr Womens Health Rep* 2:417–422, 2002.

---

[1]Not FDA approved for this indication.
[7]Available as dietary supplement.

Juang CM, Chou P, Yen MS, et al: Laparoscopic uterosacral nerve ablation with and without presacral neurectomy in the treatment of primary dysmenorrhea: A prospective efficacy analysis, *J Reprod Med* 52:591–596, 2007.

Jo J, Lee SH: Heat therapy for primary dysmenorrhea: A systematic review and meta-analysis of its effects on pain relief and quality of life, *Sci Rep* 8:16252, 2018.

Kashefi F, Ziyadlou S, Khajehei M, et al: Effect of acupressure at the Sanyinjiao point on primary dysmenorrhea: A randomized controlled trial, *Complement Ther Clin Pract* 16:198–202, 2010.

Khodaverdi S, Mohammedbeigi R, Khaled M, et al: Beneficial effects of oral lactobacillus on pain severity in women suffering from endometriosis: A pilot placebo-controlled randomized clinical trial, *Int J Fertil Steril* 13:178–183, 2019.

Klein JR, Litt IF: Epidemiology of adolescent dysmenorrhea, *Pediatrics* 68:661–664, 1981.

Lee CH, Roh JW, Lim CY, et al: A multicenter, randomized, double-blind, placebo-controlled trial evaluating the efficacy and safety of a far infrared-emitting sericite belt in patients with primary dysmenorrhea, *Complement Ther Med* 19:187–193, 2011.

Liu CZ, Xie JP, Wang LP, et al: Immediate analgesia effect of single point acupuncture in primary dysmenorrhea: A randomized controlled trial, *Pain Med* 12:300–307, 2011.

Matthewman G, Lee A, Kaur JG, Daley AJ: Physical activity for dysmenorrhea: a systematic review and meta-analysis of randomized controlled trials, *Am J Obstet Gynecol* 219, 2018. 255e.1–e.20.

Marjoribanks J, Ayeleke RO, Farquhar C, Proctor M: Nonsteroidal anti-inflammatory drugs for dysmenorrhoea, *Cochrane Database Syst Rev* (7): CD001751, 2015.

Mirbagher-Ajorpaz N, Adib-Hajbaghery M, Mosaebi F. The effects of acupressure on primary dysmenorrhea: A randomized controlled trial. Complement Ther Clin Pract 2011;17:33–26.

Moen MH, Stokstad T: A long-term follow-up study of women with asymptomatic endometriosis diagnosed incidentally at sterilization, *Fertil Steril* 78:773–776, 2002.

Momoeda M, Taketani Y, Terakawa N, et al: Is endometriosis really associated with pain? *Gynecol Obstet Invest* 54(Suppl. 1):18–21, 2002.

Nawathe A, Patwardhan S, Yates D, et al: Systematic review of the effects of aromatase inhibitors on pain associated with endometriosis, *BJOG* 115:818–822, 2008.

Ozgoli G, Goli M, Moattar F: Comparison of effects of ginger, mefenamic acid, and ibuprofen on pain in women with primary dysmenorrhea, *J Altern Complement Med* 15:129–132, 2009.

Proctor ML, Smith CA, Farquhar CM, Stones RW: Transcutaneous electrical nerve stimulation and acupuncture for primary dysmenorrhoea, *Cochrane Database Syst Rev* 2(1):CD002123, 2002.

Proctor ML, Hing W, Johnson TC, Murphy PA: Spinal manipulation for primary and secondary dysmenorrhoea, *Cochrane Database Syst Rev* (3):CD002119, 2006.

Raisi Dehkordi Z, Rafaieian-Kopaei M, Hosseina-Baharanchi FS: A double-blind controlled crossover study to investigate the efficacy of salix extract on primary dysmenorrhea, *Complement Ther Med* 44:102–109, 2019.

Rakhshaee Z. Effect of three yoga poses (cobra, cat and fish poses) in women with primary dysmenorrhea: A randomized clinical trial. *J Pediatr Adolesc Gynecol* 2011;24:192–6.

Ranong CN, Sukcharoen N: Analgesic effect of etoricoxib in secondary dysmenorrhea: A randomized, double-blind, crossover, controlled trial, *J Reprod Med* 52:1023–1029, 2007.

Selak V, Farquhar C, Prentice A, Singla A: Danazol for pelvic pain associated with endometriosis, *Cochrane Database Syst Rev* (4):CD000068, 2007.

Sheng J, Zhang WY, Zhang JP, Lu D: The LNG-IUS study on adenomyosis: A 3-year follow-up study on the efficacy and side effects of the use of levonorgestrel intrauterine system for the treatment of dysmenorrhea associated with adenomyosis, *Contraception* 79:189–193, 2009.

Strinić T, Buković D, Pavelić L, et al: Anthropological and clinical characteristics in adolescent women with dysmenorrhea, *Coll Antropol* 27:707–711, 2003.

Sundell G, Milsom I, Andersch B: Factors influencing the prevalence and severity of dysmenorrhoea in young women, *Br J Obstet Gynaecol* 97:588–594, 1990 .

Suzuki N, Uebaba K, Kohama T, et al: French maritime pine bark extract significantly lowers the requirement for analgesic medication in dysmenorrhea: A multicenter, randomized, double-blind, placebo-controlled study, *J Reprod Med* 53:338–346, 2008.

Telimaa S, Puolakka J, Rönnberg L, Kauppila A: Placebo-controlled comparison of danazol and high-dose medroxyprogesterone acetate in the treatment of endometriosis, *Gynecol Endocrinol* 1:13–23, 1987.

Tugay N, Akbayrak T, Demirtürk F, et al: Effectiveness of transcutaneous electrical nerve stimulation and interferential current in primary dysmenorrhea, *Pain Med* 8:295–300, 2007.

Wang MC, Hsu MC, Chien LW: Effects of auricular acupressure on menstrual symptoms and nitric oxide for women with primary dysmenorrhea, *J Altern Complement Med* 15:235–242, 2009.

Witt CM, Reinhold T, Brinkhaus B, et al: Acupuncture in patients with dysmenorrhea: A randomized study on clinical effectiveness and cost-effectiveness in usual care, *Am J Obstet Gynecol* 198:166, 2008. e1–8.

Wong CL, Lai KY, Tse HM. Effects of SP6 acupressure on pain and menstrual distress in young women with dysmenorrhea. *Complement Ther Clin Pract* 2009;16:64–9.

Yisa SB, Okenwa AA, Husemeyer RP: Treatment of pelvic endometriosis with etonogestrel subdermal implant (Implanon), *J Fam Plann Reprod Health Care* 31:67–70, 2005.

ENDOMETRIOSIS

Method of
Zachary Kuhlmann, DO

CURRENT DIAGNOSIS

- Clinical symptoms associated with endometriosis include chronic pelvic pain, dysmenorrhea, dyspareunia, and infertility.
- A pelvic sonogram may be helpful to aid in diagnosis of endometriosis. Care should be taken to exclude other gynecologic and non-gynecologic etiologies of pain.
- Diagnostic laparoscopy may reveal powder burn–like lesions, adhesions, endometriomas, or other signs of endometriosis on inspection.
- The gold standard to make a pathologic diagnosis of endometriosis requires a tissue biopsy of a suspected lesion.

CURRENT MANAGEMENT

- Initial therapy for endometriosis includes NSAIDs, progesterones, combined OCPs, danazol (Danocrine), GnRH agonists, and GnRH antagonists.
- Diagnostic laparoscopy with excision or ablative techniques are often used to treat endometriosis.
- It is reasonable to consider empiric medical therapy with a GnRH agonist before surgery in some situations.
- Hysterectomy with bilateral salpingo-oophorectomy is definitive surgical treatment for endometriosis.

Endometriosis is a common and benign gynecologic condition diagnosed when endometrial tissue is found outside the uterus. Common places for endometrial tissue to implant include the peritoneum and ovaries, although endometriosis can occur outside the pelvis as well. Other locations for endometriosis to be found include the rectovaginal septum, bowel, bladder, pleura, abdominal wall, and even the brain in rare cases. Endometriosis is an estrogen-dependent, inflammatory disorder.

Epidemiology

Endometriosis affects between 5% to 10% of women of reproductive age. Women who experience infertility may have a prevalence of endometriosis of up to 50%, and women with chronic pelvic pain may experience a prevalence of endometriosis well over 80%.

Risk Factors

There appears to be an inheritable component for endometriosis. Women who have a first-degree relative affected by endometriosis may have a 6 to 7 times higher incidence than women without an affected relative. Other risk factors for endometriosis include menarche before age 11 and extremes of cycle length (either short or long cycles). Women who breastfeed for long durations, women who have more children, and women who exercise regularly may see a reduction in their risk of endometriosis.

Pathophysiology

There are many theories regarding the origin of endometriosis. Perhaps the most popular hypothesis proposes that retrograde menstruation allows for endometrial tissue to be passed back through the fallopian tubes and implant into the pelvis. Another theory suggests that coelemic metaplasia occurs. In this theory, it is thought that the differentiation of mesothelial

TABLE 1 Differential Diagnosis for Chronic Pelvic Pain Based on Organ Systems

GYNECOLOGIC	GASTROINTESTINAL	URINARY	MUSCULOSKELETAL
Endometriosis	Irritable bowel syndrome	Urinary tract infection	Fibromyalgia
Adenomyosis	Diverticuli	Interstitial Cystitis	Ankylosing spondylitis
Cervicitis	Crohn's	Malignancy	Arthritis
Leiomyoma	Ulcerative Colitis	Renal lithiasis	Muscle strains
Ovarian cysts	Gastroenteritis		
Pelvic adhesive disease	Hemorrhoids		
Hydrosalpinx/tubal disease			
Pelvic congestion syndrome			

cells into endometrial cells results in endometriosis lesions. It is also thought that hematogenous or lymphatic spread is a plausible explaination forendometriosis. Endometrial cells may be deposited from the vascular or lymphatic vessels onto tissues outside the uterus. One final theory for the etiology of endometriosis involves bone marrow. Cells originating from the bone marrow may differentiate into endometrial tissue outside the uterus.

No matter how endometriosis originates, the immune system plays a pivotal role in the disease process. Endometriosis is associated with an overproduction of estrogen, prostaglandins, and cytokines. Estrogen is overproduced by an increase in aromatase activity. Cyclooxygenase-2 (COX-2) activity is also increased, which stimulates prostaglandin production. Endometriosis is also associated with progesterone resistance, and that magnifies the effect of estrogen in an already estrogen-rich environment. This inflammatory cascade leads to an increase in cytokines and macrophages. The cytokines increase the presence of macrophages and lymphocytes in the peritoneum.

The chronic inflammation identified in endometriosis may cause pain by stimulating the nerve endings or affect the neural innervations of the uterus. Fallopian tube function and sperm function may be adversely affected by the inflammatory cytokines. Also, the fallopian tubes may be completely blocked in some cases of endometriosis.

Clinical Manifestations

Many clinical symptoms have been associated with endometriosis. Cyclical pain is often described with endometriosis. Some of the more commonly recognized symptoms include dysmenorrhea, chronic pelvic pain, dyspareunia, and infertility. Dysmenorrhea can be described as primary or secondary. The dysmenorrhea with endometriosis is classically described as secondary dysmenorrhea because it is associated with a pathologic diagnosis. Primary dysmenorrhea is when there is painful menstruation in the absence of pelvic pathology. Examples of chronic pelvic pain with endometriosis may include other visceral symptoms such as dyschezia or dysuria. Hematuria, diarrhea, constipation, and chronic back pain may all be symptoms associated with endometriosis.

Interestingly, the extent of disease may not necessarily correlate with the severity of symptoms. Some women with a small foci of endometriosis may have excruciating symptoms, whereas others with extensive endometriosis may only experience mild symptoms.

Exam findings consistent with a diagnosis of endometriosis may include uterosacral ligament nodulartiy/tenderness and presence of an adnexal mass. Tenderness in the cul-de-sac with a fixed and immobile uterus may also indicate presence of endometriosis. Cyclical hemoptysis has been reported with endometriosis. Endometriotic implants have also been located in scars, so the presence of cyclical pain in an abdominal incision may lead to suspicion of endometriosis.

Diagnosis/Differential Diagnosis

The diagnosis of endometriosis is made surgically. The gold standard to make a diagnosis of endometriosis is to have a pathologic specimen from a tissue biopsy of a suspected lesion. Histology will reveal endometrial glands and stroma and inflammation. If a biopsy is not performed, surgical findings consistent with an endometriosis diagnosis include lesions that look like black powder burns and nonclassical red or white lesions. Endometriomas have also been described as a classic surgical finding of endometriosis. Endometriomas are an ovarian structure filled with endometriosis and are colloquially described as chocolate cysts because when they rupture, it appears as though chocolate syrup flows out of the cyst. Endometriomas appear on sonographic imaging as cysts with homogenous internal echoes. Although rare, endometriosis can sometimes be found in the bladder. If bladder involvement is suspected, such as the case of cyclical hematuria, a cystoscopy may be of benefit for diagnosis. Although surgery remains the mainstay of diagnosis for endometriosis, some studies suggest there is a low correlation between the severity of symptoms, the amount of endometriosis visualized on surgical inspection, and diagnostic histologic findings.

Pelvic imaging may be helpful in the evaluation of endometriosis, especially in the presence of an adenxal mass. In patients with pelvic pain or disorders of menstruation, a sonogram is usually the preferred imaging modality for the pelvis. Computed tomography (CT) may help delineate the size and characteristic of an adnexal mass and is likely most useful to rule out other pathology or surrounding organ involvement. The usefulness of magnetic resonance imaging (MRI) is limited in the evaluation of endometriosis and should be reserved for extreme cases where specific organ involvement such as the bladder or bowel is suspected. MRI may also be useful in evaluating specific musculoskeletal conditions.

There is no good serum marker to make the diagnosis of endometriosis. CA-125 levels may be elevated in endometriosis, but there are many other inflammatory conditions that cause an elevation in CA-125 levels.

When initially evaluating for endometriosis, one should consider a thorough differential diagnosis for causes of chronic pelvic pain. Table 1 lists the differential diagnosis for chronic pelvic pain. A basic approach to the patient with chronic pelvic pain should include a detailed history and physical, urinalysis, gonorrhea/chlamydia cultures, consideration of pelvic sonogram, and serum or urine beta human chorionic gonadotropin (Bhcg). If after careful evaluation, endometriosis is at the top of the differential diagnosis for the patient's pelvic pain, then discussion with the patient regarding empiric treatment or diagnostic workup should occur.

Medical Therapy

The goal of medical intervention for endometriosis is the treatment of pain. A reasonable approach to treating the patient with suspected endometriosis is to give a trial of empiric medical therapy. Although endometriosis is a surgical diagnosis, some patients with suspected endometriosis may wish to avoid surgery. Medical therapy is usually preferred for those patients who would like to preserve fertility and who are interested in delaying childbearing while managing their symptoms.

The combined oral contraceptive pill (OCP) is a usual first-line therapy for the treatment of suspected or diagnosed endometriosis. A 3- to 6-month trial with empiric treatment with OCPs is a reasonable time frame to assess effectiveness of medical treatment. OCPs should be avoided in patients that have contraindications to OCPs including pregnancy, history of thrombosis, liver disease, migraine with aura, uncontrolled hypertension, and those patients that smoke and are over the age of 35 years.

Other medications used to treat endometriosis include danazol (Danocrine), nonsteroidal anti-inflammatory drugs (NSAIDs), progestins, and gonadotropin releasing hormone (GnRH) agonists and antagonists. NSAIDs may improve the pain and dysmenorrhea associated with endometriosis. Danazol is an effective treatment for endometriosis. The side effect profile for danazol limits its use. Danazol has been associated with masculinizing symptoms, which can include acne and hair growth. Danazol should be avoided in pregnancy because the masculinizing effects could be detrimental to a female infant.

Physicians commonly prescribe progestins in three different ways to treat endometriosis: injectable, oral, or intrauterine. Injectable medroxyprogesterone (Depo-SubQ Provera 104) is approved by the Food and Drug Administration (FDA) for the treatment of endometriosis. Depo-Provera's side effects may include weight gain, bleeding, amenorrhea, and slow return to fertility. Patients using Depo-Provera may initially experience irregular bleeding but often develop amenorrhea after the second dose is administered. Return to fertility after Depo-Provera is discontinued can also pose a problem. Oral agents such as norethindrone acetate (Aygestin) have also been approved by the FDA for the treatment of endometriosis. The levonorgestrel-containing intrauterine device (IUD) (Mirena)[1] is approved only for contraception and the treatment of menorrhagia, but it may still be an effective treatment for endometriosis.

The GnRH agonists are among the most effective medications available to treat endometriosis. The side effects of GnRH agonists include menopausal-like symptoms such as vaginal dryness, hot flashes, and osteopenia. The addition of add-back therapy may help ameliorate some of the GnRH agonist symptoms. Typically, add-back therapy involves the use of progestins concurrently with a GnRH agonist. Practice patterns vary; some providers may start add-back therapy immediately when a patient is started on a GnRH agonist. It is recommended that add-back therapy be initiated after 6 months of GnRH agonist use if it was not started previously. In addition to progestins, the combination of progestins and estrogen have been used for add-back therapy. The maximum duration of GnRH agonist treatment is typically 12 months. Another class of medication to treat endometriosis is the GnRH antagonist, currently available as elagolix (Orilissa). Advantages to this medication are that it is in an oral form and available in multiple doses. Studies showed estradiol suppression in a dose dependent manner. Common side effects include hot flashes, headaches, and nausea. Although add-back therapy is widely used in GnRH agonists, it has not been studied with the GnRH antagonists. When using this medication, consideration of a nonhormonal contraception would be recommended.

Surgical Therapy

The goal of surgery for endometriosis is to relieve pain and/or infertility. One of the first questions the provider must answer is when to perform surgery. Surgery may be indicated if medical treatment has failed. Other times, the severity of symptoms or presence of large endometriomas may direct a provider to consider surgery sooner.

Laparoscopy is a common surgical approach for patients with confirmed or suspected endometriosis. At the time of laparoscopy, the surgeon can assess the uterus, ovaries, and surrounding viscera for pathology. When endometriosis is encountered on laparoscopy, common approaches are to excise or ablate the lesions. Excision of endometriosis allows for a pathologic diagnosis. If the provider elects to ablate the lesions, this can be performed through electrocautery or laser. In addition to diagnosing and treating endometriosis, further evaluation of patients with infertility can be done at the time of laparoscopy. Tubal function can be assessed through a chromotubation where dye is passed through the fallopian tubes to prove the tubes are patent. Although laparotomy allows for thorough evaluation of the pelvis, it is usually reserved for cases of confirmed endometriosis where the extent of adhesions and distorted anatomy makes laparoscopy unsafe.

Endometriomas present an array of challenges when noted at the time of surgery. The decision to drain the cyst versus perform a cystectomy during surgery must be made by the surgeon. A general approach is to use a "3-centimeters (cm) rule" to help guide management decisions. Patients with an endometrioma greater than 3 cm may benefit from cystectomy, whereas endometriomas less than 3 cm may be managed by drainage and ablation. Although removing the endometrioma through cystectomy may confer a decreased risk or recurrence, the risk of damaging healthy ovarian tissue is ever present. Other confounders to consider are future fertility plans of the patient, severity of symptoms, and previous treatments for endometriosis.

In a patient who has completed childbearing or has no desire for future fertility, hysterectomy with a bilateral salpingo-oophorectomy (BSO) may be considered for treatment of endometriosis. Studies suggest that hysterectomy alone is less effective at curing pain than hysterectomy with a BSO. Although hysterectomy with BSO offers definitive treatment for endometriosis, surgery does not guarantee resolution of pain. Many routes may be considered for surgery, including laparoscopic, robotic-assisted laparoscopic, or laparotomy with a total abdominal hysterectomy/BSO. Although vaginal hysterectomy is a common and preferred route of surgery, the distorted anatomy and presence of adhesions often associated with endometriosis tends to discourage many surgeons from performing vaginal hysterectomies for endometriosis.

Monitoring

Patients diagnosed with endometriosis may require frequent monitoring of symptoms. Routine visits with a physician may help determine the effectiveness of current treatment regimens. Physicians should consider what the patient's goals of treatment are: Does the patient want resolution of pain or infertility or both? Individualized plans may help each patient achieve their goals of treatment. As with any diseases involving chronic pain, care should be taken to regularly assess patients with endometriosis for depression.

References

ACOG Practice Bulletin Number 114. Management of Endometriosis. 2010.

Bulun SE: Endometriosis, *N Engl J Med* 360:268–279, 2009.

Cramer DW, Missmer SA: The epidemiology of endometriosis, *Ann N Y Acad Sci* 955:11–22, 2002.

Davis L, Kennedy SS, Moore J, Prentice A: Oral contraceptives for pain associated with endometriosis, *Cochrane Database Syst Rev* 2007;(3):Cd001019.

Dlugi AM, Miller JD, Knittle J: Lupron depot (leuprolide acetate for depot suspension) in the treatmemnt of endometriosis: a randomized, placebo-controlled, double-blind study, *Fert Steril* 54:419–427, 1990.

Guidance LC, Kao LC: Endometriosis, *Lancet* 364:1789–1799, 2004.

Olive DL, Pritts EA: The treatment of endometriosis: a review of the evidence, *Ann N Y Acad Sci* 955:360–372, 2002.

Pittaway DE, Fayez JA: The use of CA-125 in the diagnosis and management of endometriosis, *Fertil Steril* 46:790–795, 1986.

Rawson JM: Prevalence of endometriosis in asymptomatic women, *J Reprod Med* 36:513–515, 1991.

Ripps BA, Martin DC: Endometriosis and chronic pelvic pain, *Gynecol Clin North Am* 20:709–717, 1993.

Surrey E, Taylor HS: Long-term outcomes of elagolix in women with endometriosis, *Obstetrics and Gynecology* 132:147–160, 2018.

Sutton CJ, Ewen SP, Whitelaw N, Haines P: Prospective, randomized, double blind, controlled trial of laser laparoscopy in the treatment of pelvic pain associated with minimal, mild, and moderate endometriosis, 62:696–700, 1994.

Walter AJ, Hentz JG, Magtibay PM, Cornella JL, Magrina JF: Endometriosis: correlation between histologic and visual findings at laparoscopy, *Am J Obstet Gynecol* 184:1407–1411, 2001.

[1]Not FDA approved for this indication.

FEMALE SEXUAL DYSFUNCTION

Method of
Melissa Hague, MD

CURRENT DIAGNOSIS

- Sexual pain is a common cause of distress for women and their partners, with up to 50% of women experiencing distress at some point in their lifetime.
- Women may present with a complaint of decreased libido, but on further questioning may have significant pain with sex that is causing or contributing to decreased desire.
- Always ask about relationship stress, pain, and ability to achieve climax when discussing sexual distress with female patients.
- Many medications interfere with libido, as does a patient's lifestyle and overall health status.
- Like many medical concerns, female sexual dysfunction is a complex, multifactorial problem that should be addressed with a holistic multidisciplinary approach.

CURRENT THERAPY

- You cannot treat decreased libido in a patient who is having sexual pain without addressing the source of the pain.
- Determine the cause of sexual pain; once this has been adequately addressed, you may consider a treatment plan for decreased libido.
- Consider the approach to sexual pain from the outside working in. Start with skin or vulvar causes, such as lichen sclerosis, atrophy, or herpes. Work in toward the pelvic floor and consider muscle or nerve pain as a cause. Once you have considered these as a source of pain and not found a problem, you can consider a bimanual exam and see if pain occurs with cervical or uterine motion, or if there is evidence of pelvic mass.
- Realize that patients who have suffered sexual trauma, such as abuse or rape, will need a multidisciplinary approach that may include a physician, physical therapist, and counselor or sex therapist to help them with pain and libido concerns.
- Physical therapists trained in the treatment of pelvic floor dysfunction are an essential part of the team approach to treatment of patients with neuromuscular pelvic floor pain or dyspareunia.
- Mindfulness is a tool used by therapists to help patients struggling with anorgasmia to improve the sexual experience.
- Engaging the partner in developing a treatment plan for sexual pain or decreased libido is important to obtain endorsement from the patient. This is especially the case if you are recommending abstaining from sex for a period of time to allow for healing.

Epidemiology

The prevalence of female sexual function concerns in the primary care clinic is difficult to quantify. Depending on which article you read, the prevalence is between 30% and 100% throughout the lifespan of a woman. The emotional toll that low libido, sexual pain, and anorgasmia take on women and their partners is significant. Patients experiencing sexual pain may be hesitant to discuss their concerns, or may have had a negative experience with a health care provider in the past when they tried to discuss concerns. On average, patients see more than six health care providers before the source of their sexual pain or libido concerns are adequately addressed. The occurrence of sexual concerns is higher in patients with depression, chronic pain, cancer diagnosis, bowel or bladder problems, and arthritis, as well as in the postmenopausal years.

The general topic of female sexual function can be difficult to address in the primary care setting. When a patient presents for an annual exam, for example, and she says she is having pain with intercourse, it can cause anxiety on the part of the practitioner. This is often not a visit that can be accomplished in a 10-minute slot, so do not hesitate to tell the patient that you want to make sure you have adequate time to address her concerns. If this was not the reason for her visit, consider asking her to schedule a visit when you have more time available so that you can best help her. Having a basic knowledge about a systematic approach to female sexual pain can help the practitioner have confidence in discussing this area of distress with women and their partners. We will approach this from two different areas of concern: decreased libido and sexual pain.

Pathophysiology, Diagnosis, Treatment: Decreased Libido

If a patient comes in complaining of decreased sex drive, you must consider many issues and life concerns that can impact intimacy. At the heart of hypoactive sexual desire disorder (HSDD) is an imbalance between excitatory (dopamine and norepinephrine) and inhibitory (serotonin) neurotransmitters in key regions of the brain. The difficulty in women is that libido is impacted by psychosocial factors, such as relationship concerns; physical concerns, such as obesity or arthritis; medical conditions; and medications. In research that includes women complaining of decreased libido, 30% may improve with placebo alone. This tells us how important addressing the psychosocial problems can be. The first question to consider is very simple and very powerful, "Do you like your partner?" This sole question can open up lines of communication and help sort out the cause of decreased desire (Box 1). If the patient indicates that her relationship is not currently rewarding or that she does not get along well with her partner, there is no pill that will solve desire concerns. Help the patient see that intervention in the form of counseling from a qualified provider may provide the best treatment for sexual concerns, or at least offer a good starting point. Make sure to follow your first question with the next question, "Does sex hurt?" If a woman has sexual pain, she may avoid sexual encounters. Helping the patient understand that sexual pain is not normal and is treatable may help her open up to you about the other important considerations for diagnosis, including onset, duration, circumstances in which the pain occurs, and associated factors. You may also need to assess her willingness and desire to address the problem of pain. Some women are resistant to discussing their pain due to a history of poor medical encounters

---

BOX 1   Decreased Libido Diagnosis

Psychological: Do you like your partner?

If they do not have a good relationship, you have an opportunity to point them to resources in your community to help them. Consider referral to a local marriage and family therapist or sex therapist to intervene.

Physical: Does sex hurt?

If a woman is experiencing sexual pain she will also suffer from low libido, as her brain is trying to protect her body from further trauma. Once you discover there is pain, work toward diagnosis or referral to a specialist. Set the expectation that until her pain has been addressed you do not expect her to have an improvement in libido.

Neurologic: Are you able to achieve climax?

If a woman is unable to orgasm, she may have lower desire. Acknowledging her lack of climax and the distress it is causing is the first step in helping her decide if she wishes to explore this area further with a specialist.

with physicians, previous trauma, or a foundational religious and/or cultural belief system surrounding sex. As stated previously, treatment for this condition is best guided by a careful history and discussion with the patient. If libido has been a concern for a significant period of time, encourage the patient to see a qualified counselor. Creating a list of resources available in your area is helpful to have on hand. If the patient previously had what she considers a good sex drive and this is a new problem, consider new medications, trauma, or recent events that may have triggered the onset of pain. See the list of medications impacting libido (Box 2). Although this is not exhaustive, if the patient is on more than one medication that affects sex drive, you may need to work with her to adjust medications. If she is premenopausal and not on any medications, treatment for HSDD includes psychosocial intervention, lifestyle adjustment, and medications. Lifestyle adjustments may include changing her schedule so there is time for intimacy, as many patients are too busy to allow for adequate time for arousal and a positive sexual experience. Also keep in mind the positive effect exercise has on sex drive—both directly, by increasing norepinephrine; and indirectly, by improving stamina and self-image. Dietary considerations are also important, as women who are overweight or obese may suffer from low libido due to self-image, fatigue from hyperinsulinemia or diabetes, and gastrointestinal or other issues. Currently, there are two FDA-approved treatments for HSDD: flibanserin (Addyi), which is a daily medication, and bremelanotide (Vyleesi), which is an episodic injectable medication. Both need to be prescribed by physicians experienced with the medication, indications, and potential side effects. Many other medications have been used to improve libido (see Box 2). Another consideration in women being treated for depression is to switch them from an inhibitory medication to one that may have a positive effect on libido. Encouraging patients to have open communication with their partners about what leads to pleasure and what does not is essential when addressing desire and arousal.

BOX 2   Treatment of Decreased Libido

May inhibit desire or arousal
- SSRIs
- Antipsychotics
- Benzodiazepines
- TCAs
- Lithium
- Phenytoin (Dilantin)
- Trazodone (Desyrel)
- OCP
- Narcotics
- Beta blockers
- Digoxin
- Spironolactone (Aldactone)
- Antihistamines
- Anticholinergics

May improve desire or arousal
- Flibanserin (Addyi)
- Bremelanotide (Vyleesi)
- Buspirone (BuSpar)
- Bupropion (Wellbutrin)
- Naltrexone/bupropion (Contrave)
- SNRIs
- Transdermal testosterone
- Topical (vulvar/vaginal) estrogen
- Topical (vulvar) testosterone
- Hormonal therapy in postmenopausal women

OCP, Oral contraceptive pill; *SNRIs,* serotonin–norepinephrine reuptake inhibitors; *SSRIs,* selective serotonin reuptake inhibitors; *TCAs,* tricyclic antidepressants.

Pathophysiology, Diagnosis, Treatment: Sexual Pain

Dyspareunia can have many origins. The layered approach described by Dr. Coady is a systematic way to consider evaluation and also helps us understand the pathophysiology of this often complex problem (Box 3). Consider that the pain can be due to skin concerns or changes, neurologic problems, muscle pain, bowel conditions, bladder pain, medications (such as chemotherapy), and medical problems, such as endometriosis or enlarged uterus. A careful history and exam are the most important diagnostic tools when helping discern the cause for sexual pain.

There are many different ways to evaluate a patient for pain with sex, and specifically, pain with intercourse. When you take a history in a patient complaining of sexual pain it is important to glean from her the duration, inciting factors, alleviating factors, previous treatment, and what she thinks is causing the pain. Understanding if she has primary (never had a sexual encounter without pain) or secondary (new onset, previous pain-free encounters) dyspareunia is also important. Primary sexual pain can be caused by a history of sexual trauma, tight hymenal ring, skin-level concerns such as atrophy, herpes, or lichen sclerosis, pelvic floor muscle pain, or internal pain such as endometriosis, ovarian cysts, or other pelvic organ pathology. Secondary sexual pain can include the same causes but may be easier to treat depending on the sequence of events that led to the patient's onset of pain. When taking a history of the patient's pain, it is important to ask her if the pain is only on penetration or if it occurs through the entire encounter. Pain that only occurs with deeper penetration may more likely be pelvic floor muscle pain or endometriosis, whereas pain that occurs with any touch points you toward vulvar causes such as lichen sclerosis or atrophic changes.

Once you have gathered a careful history, it is important to perform a careful exam. Start with a very careful inspection of the vulva. Note the presence of labia minora—if absent or blunted, this may be consistent with atrophy. Note the clitoral hood—if it is retracted or adhesions are noted, the patient may have lichenification. A bright light and magnification (such as a colposcope) are often helpful in careful visualization. If no abnormalities are noted on careful inspection, look at the introitus. Patients with localized provoked vestibulodynia (LPV) may have an area of erythema at the 6 o'clock position of the introitus, just external to the hymenal ring. Show the patient a cotton swab and tell her you are going to touch areas on the vulva and you want her to tell you if anything hurts. With light pressure (depressing about 1 mm), touch the patient's thigh, slowly working inward to the labia. Touch the clitoris, the area around the urethra, and the area just external to the hymenal ring. Lastly, touch the area around the anus, as the rectal branch of the pudendal nerve could be the cause of the pain. If she has significant pain on palpation with the swab along Hart line, note the location of the pain and consider referral to a specialist who can address LPV. If the exam is normal and her pain does not appear to be external, do a careful exam of the pelvic floor. One way to do this is to insert one finger and gently palpate the muscles of the pelvic floor one at a time. A careful review of the anatomy of this area is helpful. If you are not comfortable evaluating for pelvic floor pain, referral to a sexual pain specialist or pelvic floor physical therapist is appropriate. If the patient does not seem to have pain on palpation of the pelvic floor muscles, performing a

---

BOX 3   Sexual Pain Pathophysiology

Causes of Sexual Pain: The Layered Approach
Surface layer: lichen sclerosis, herpes, atrophy
Nerve layer: localized provoked vestibulodynia, pudendal neuralgia
Myofascial layer: chronic pain or acute, secondary to injury
Organ layer: ovarian cyst, endometriosis
Body-wide systems: gastrointestinal, psychological (history of trauma or abuse)

bimanual exam can be helpful; however, great care must be taken to avoid further trauma. I do not often do a bimanual exam on patients with a complaint of sexual pain as their pain is often elicited by the previously described exam. A speculum is rarely useful for these patients and should be avoided if they are complaining of pain with intercourse, as you may cause her more pain and further discourage the patient from seeking medical help.

Your treatment plan for sexual pain must be guided by the differential diagnosis you develop following a careful history and exam. For skin concerns, clobetasol topical is the treatment for lichenification that includes lichen sclerosis and lichen simplex chronicus. If nerve or pelvic floor muscle pain is noted, sending the patient to a qualified physical therapist is a good first step. If this fails, or if the patient desires medication to help with the discomfort while working with a therapist, vaginal diazepam (Valium) can be utilized. The patient uses 10 mg at HS and is encouraged to use this as needed to help with more severe discomfort, as many of the patients who have dyspareunia also have generalized pelvic floor pain that may interfere with sleep or daily living activities. If physical therapy does not provide relief, a sexual medicine specialist may perform dry needling or trigger point injections to help with the pain. If the cause does not seem to be related to either skin or pelvic floor pain, an ultrasound may help to identify ovarian masses or uterine enlargement and the patient may need referral to a gynecologist for surgical intervention. In cases of gastrointestinal dysfunction, such as constipation or diarrhea, consider treatment of this dysfunction as it could lead to improvement in dyspareunia.

A Note About Atrophy

When considering atrophic or hypoestrogenic changes many clinicians think of a postmenopausal woman. When it comes to sexual pain, however, do not forget that atrophy can be seen in premenopausal women in the setting of cancer treatment, postoophorectomy patients, and patients who have been on combined oral contraceptive pills for a period of time. Each of these patients may require a unique approach to treatment. For instance, if a woman is experiencing atrophy due to treatment of a nonhormonal cancer, such as leukemia, treating her with systemic or local hormonal therapy is likely the most appropriate approach. If she is currently being treated for breast cancer, discussing a treatment plan with her oncologist is important. Keep in mind that vaginal estrogen has a long-established safety record in breast cancer patients due to the low absorption. If you do not have experience in this area, helping your patient connect with a gynecologist or sexual medicine physician who *does* treat cancer survivors is essential. In the meantime, encourage her to use adequate vaginal lubrication and moisturizers. Lubrication that is water based is not often sufficient for a severely atrophic patient and oil-based lubrication, such as coconut oil, olive oil, or a commercially available product meant for sensitive tissues, is much superior. Encourage women to use moisturizers not just for intercourse, but also post-bathing, swimming, or exercising. Be aware that many patients who are breastfeeding or are taking combination oral contraceptives may also experience atrophic changes that cause pain during sexual encounters. For these patients, a small amount of topical vulvar hormones applied to the introitus is often quite effective in relieving symptoms.

References

American College of Obstetricians and Gynecologists Committee on Gynecologic Practice Committee Opinion 659, *The use of vaginal estrogen in women with a history of estrogen-dependent breast cancer*, March, 2016, reaffirmed 2018.
Coady D: Chronic sexual pain: a layered guide to evaluation, *Contemporary OB/GYN* 60:18–28, 2015.
Goldstein A, editor: *Female sexual pain disorders evaluation and management*, Hoboken, 2009, Wiley-Blackwell.
Goldstein AT, Belkin ZR, Krapf JM, et al: Polymorphisms of the androgen receptor gene and hormonal contraceptive induced provoked vestibulodynia, *J Sex Med* 11:2764–2771, 2014.
Shifren JL, Monz BU, Russo PA, et al: Sexual problems and distress in United States women: Prevalence and correlates, *Obstet Gynecol* 112:970–978, 2008.
Stein A: *Heal pelvic pain: a proven stretching, strengthening, and nutrition program for relieving pain, incontinence, ibs, and other symptoms without surgery*, New York, 2009, McGraw Hill, pp 785–802.

INFERTILITY

Method of
Michael P. Diamond, MD; and Jessica Rachel Kanter, MD

CURRENT DIAGNOSIS

- Infertility is defined as the inability to conceive with regular intercourse after 12 months in couples in which the female partner is younger than 35 or after 6 months in couples in which the female partner is over 35.
- The incidence of infertility is increasing.

CURRENT THERAPY

- Assisted reproductive technologies are being used with increasing frequency and with increasing success rates.

Epidemiology

Infertility is defined as the failure to conceive after 12 months of regular, unprotected intercourse. In couples where the female partner's age exceeds 35 years, evaluation may begin after just 6 months of infertility, and in those over 40 years, more immediate evaluation may ensue, owing to the time-sensitive nature of the problem. In some circumstances, diagnostic evaluation and therapeutic intervention are warranted at an earlier time. Infertility affects approximately 15% of couples. Many of these patients present to their primary care physician. Timely evaluation and potential referral to an infertility subspecialist are prudent.

Risk Factors

There are numerous risk factors that contribute to infertility. The most common is age. However, it is necessary to evaluate other potential contributing factors to infertility, as these may help to narrow the differential diagnosis and achieve a more targeted subsequent treatment plan. For example, a history of sexually transmitted infections (STIs), especially chlamydia, and episodes of pelvic inflammatory disease have been associated with tubal factor infertility in women. Metabolic disorders such as obesity and polycystic ovarian syndrome, which may lead to anovulation, are an increasingly more prevalent concern and a major risk factor for infertility. Finally, certain genetic diseases such as fragile X, Turner syndrome, cystic fibrosis, and Klinefelter disease may also lead to inability to conceive or difficulty in conceiving.

Pathophysiology

The pathophysiology of infertility should be grouped first by male and female factors and then by the component of their respective reproductive tracts. One must not discount the fact that multiple factors may coexist, including etiologies of infertility in both partners of a heterosexual couple. Unexplained infertility has been reported to be accountable for 8% to 28% of infertility in couples; however, in intensively evaluated couples, the rate is likely to be 25%.

Prevention

Some etiologies of infertility may be preventable. Many cases of tubal factor infertility may be prevented by protecting against the transmission of STIs. Barrier contraception is essential to prevent STIs, particularly in high-risk individuals with an early age of coitarche and/or those with multiple sexual partners. Even with highly efficacious forms of contraception such as intrauterine devices, long-acting injectable progestins, and progestin-containing subdermal implants, providers must counsel their patients that barrier contraception is still of the utmost importance in preventing STI transmission.

There are also various medical therapies, particularly those related to cancer treatment, that may be detrimental to fertility. In these cases, oncofertility consultation prior to treatment will optimize fertility preservation. For men, sperm cryopreservation is a relatively easy, noninvasive method. For women, oocyte or embryo preservation, experimental approaches to medically induce ovarian suppression, ovarian transposition, and experimental ovarian tissue cryopreservation are all helpful tools for women undergoing gonadotoxic chemotherapy or radiation therapy.

Finally, fertility should also be considered when managing tubal ectopic pregnancy in women. Medical therapy, when not contraindicated, is an excellent option in the compliant patient with an ectopic pregnancy. When surgery is necessary, salpingostomy may be considered, when possible, in lieu of salpingectomy, in an attempt to preserve tubal function—particularly in the setting of a damaged or absent contralateral fallopian tube.

Clinical Manifestations
Infertile patients generally present with failure to conceive after a variable time of home intercourse. The definition of infertility is subdivided into primary and secondary infertility. Primary infertility means the patient has not borne children in the past. Secondary infertility means the patient has successfully procreated in the past.

Diagnosis
The diagnosis of infertility begins with a thorough history and physical examination. It is important to remember that a history must be obtained from both partners during this evaluation. The male partner assessment begins with a semen analysis. Semen analysis should be performed after 2 to 5 days of abstinence for optimal results. Textbooks often suggest two semen analyses, preferably separated in time by at least 1 month.

Female partner assessment should focus on ovulatory function, ovarian reserve, and structural abnormalities. Initial evaluation should include determination of ovarian reserve by hormonal evaluation of antimüllerian hormone (AMH) or cycle day 2 to 5 follicle-stimulating hormone (FSH). A thyroid-stimulating hormone (TSH) may also be considered, especially if ovulatory dysfunction is suspected, as thyroid dysfunction is common in women. Ovulation may be confirmed with a midluteal progesterone level. Other labs may be ordered if clinically indicated, such as androgens in women with hirsutism. Tubal patency is assessed by sono-hysterosalpingogram or hysterosalpingogram. These imaging tests also allow assessment of the uterine cavity for uterine contour and any abnormalities, including fibroids or polyps. Sonography may also be useful in identifying müllerian anomalies or anomalies of the basic structure of the uterus. Magnetic resonance imaging remains the gold standard for identifying müllerian anomalies; however, 3D ultrasonography has demonstrated promising and more cost-effective results in recent literature. In cases where other pelvic pathologies such as endometriosis and adhesions are suspected, diagnostic laparoscopy may be considered. Chromotubation during laparoscopy may be performed to assess fallopian tube patency. Finally, for both partners, karyotype analysis may be considered.

Differential Diagnosis
When determining a differential diagnosis, both male and female factors must be considered.

Male Factors
Male factor infertility is a component of infertility in approximately 40% to 50% of couples. The most common etiologies of male factor infertility are oligospermia and azoospermia. The etiologies leading to these diagnoses are broad and varied, and include genetic conditions such as cystic fibrosis (leading to congenital absence of the vas deferens).

Female Factors
Female factors for infertility are numerous and most easily subdivided by system.

Ovulatory Dysfunction
Inability to produce a viable oocyte each month can be related to several factors. First, anovulation may occur, meaning oocytes are present in the ovaries but none are released on a regular basis. This can be related to hormonal ovarian suppression or metabolic disturbances. Alternatively, an oocyte may not be produced secondary to a paucity of oocytes owing to age, genetic factors, or prior insults to the ovaries, such as radiation therapy. In addition to the aforementioned AMH and day 3 FSH and serum estradiol to assess ovarian function, ultrasound may be employed to evaluate antral follicle count—another marker of ovarian reserve.

Tubal Factor
The fallopian tubes are responsible for transporting the oocyte from the ovaries to the uterine cavity. For this to occur, at least one fallopian tube must be patent. Perhaps the most common etiology of tubal factor infertility is a history of pelvic inflammatory disease, with one of the most common inciting agents being *Chlamydia trachomatis*. *C. trachomatis* is particularly problematic in women, as the initial infection may be asymptomatic. Other tubal infertility may arise from prior tubal ligation, other tubal surgery, history of ectopic pregnancy, or scarring of the tubal lumen.

Uterine Factor
Irregularities within the uterine cavity may also lead to infertility, generally secondary to poor implantation of the fertilized embryo. Some such etiologies may be present from birth—namely müllerian anomalies. The abnormally shaped uterine cavity in these anomalies reduces the opportunity for normal implantation and embryo growth.

During the course of a woman's life, she may develop benign intrauterine growths, including polyps and leiomyomas that can reduce the opportunity for normal embryo implantation. Finally, prior uterine surgery may damage the endometrium and myometrium, as in Asherman syndrome, or cause uterine cavity scarring, known as *synechiae*.

Combined
One must not forget that multiple etiologies in a wide variety of combinations may be at play in female factor infertility.

Unexplained
Perhaps the most frustrating of all diagnoses is unexplained infertility. In couples who have had a negative fertility workup, a specific etiology of infertility is never revealed. There is new, burgeoning research in the area of sperm microRNA that may identify male factor infertility in men with otherwise normal semen analyses. Although not currently in wide use, such studies may be of great utility in the future.

Prior Diagnosis
As the field of infertility is becoming understood to an increasingly greater degree, there are prior diagnoses that have fallen out of favor. One such diagnosis is cervical factor insufficiency. It was previously evaluated by the postcoital test, in which a sample of cervical mucus would be taken after intercourse and was evaluated for the presence of motile sperm. This test has fallen out of favor owing to subjectivity, lack of reproducibility, and poor correlation with future fertility.

Also out of favor is the prior diagnosis of luteal phase deficiency (LPD), previously defined as inadequate endogenous progesterone production during the luteal phase of the menstrual cycle. No clinical tests have proven reliable for LPD; nor have any treatments demonstrated any significant improvement in treating infertility.

Treatment

The mainstay of therapy is first treating underlying disorders such as obesity, thyroid disease, and so forth. Other known causes of infertility that require surgical management may include intrauterine pathology (e.g., polyps, fibroid tumors) or removal of a hydrosalpinx—a distally blocked fallopian tube filled with serous fluid.

With a normal male partner semen analysis, the first step in intervention is generally an oral agent to induce ovulation combined with intrauterine insemination. Options for induction include clomiphene citrate (Clomid) and off-label use of letrozole, an aromatase inhibitor. If this fails, therapy can proceed to treatment with injectable gonadotropins (i.e., FSH and luteinizing hormone) to stimulate the development of ovarian follicles and ovulation with intrauterine insemination or in vitro fertilization. Various additional procedures may be considered if in vitro fertilization is pursued, including assisted hatching of the embryo with the hope to increase implantation rates; intracytoplasmic sperm injection to increase fertilization rates of the oocytes, particularly in the setting of male factor infertility; and preimplantation genetic screening to evaluate for embryonic genetic anomalies, particularly in women of advanced maternal age.

Monitoring

To reduce the risks associated with ovulation induction and ovarian stimulation, monitoring of serum estradiol and follicular development is performed. Monitoring provides the ability to minimize the occurrence of multiple gestation and complications associated with ovarian hyperstimulation syndrome.

---

[1]Not FDA approved for this indication.

References

Gelbaya TA, Potdar N, Jeve YB, Nardo LG: Definition and epidemiology of unexplained infertility, *Obstet Gynecol Surv* 69(2):109–115, 2014.

Infertility Workup for the Women's Health Specialist: ACOG committee opinion summary, number 781, *Obstetrics & Gynecology* 133(6):e377–e384, 2019.

Jodar M, Sendler E, Moskovtsev SI, et al: Absence of sperm RNA elements correlates with idiopathic male infertility, *Sci Transl Med* 7(295):295–296, 2015, https://doi.org/10.1126/scitranslmed.aab1287.

Practice Committee of American Society for Reproductive Medicine: Diagnostic evaluation of the infertile female: A committee opinion, *Fertil Steril* 98(2):302–307, 2012.

Practice Committee of American Society for Reproductive Medicine: Current clinical irrelevance of luteal phase deficiency: A committee opinion, *Fertil Steril* 103(4):e27–e32, 2015.

Sharlip ID, Jarow JP, Belker AM, et al: Best practice policies for male infertility, *Fertil Steril* 77(5):873–882, 2002.

MENOPAUSE

Method of
Andrew M. Kaunitz, MD; and JoAnn E. Manson, MD, DrPH

CURRENT DIAGNOSIS

- In women who meet clinical criteria for menopause who present for management of vasomotor symptoms (VMS), checking follicle-stimulating hormone (FSH) and estradiol levels is not necessary. However, if no recent level is available, checking a thyroid-stimulating hormone (TSH) level to rule out thyroid disease is appropriate.
- Occasionally, nonmenopausal conditions can masquerade as menopausal VMS.
- Although genitourinary syndrome of menopause (GSM) can be presumptively diagnosed based on a characteristic history, a pelvic examination can help exclude other vulvovaginal conditions that can present with similar symptoms.
- Although laboratory assessment is not necessary to establish that GSM is present, vaginal pH is typically higher than 5.0.

CURRENT THERAPY

- Estrogen represents the most effective therapy for VMS and related symptoms.
- Oral and transdermal estrogen have similar efficacy in treating menopausal VMS.
- Estrogen plus progestin therapy (EPT) is appropriate when treating menopausal symptoms in women with an intact uterus.
- For healthy women younger than age 60 or within 10 years of menopause onset with bothersome symptoms, the benefits of systemic hormone therapy (HT) are likely to outweigh risks.
- Conjugated estrogen (CE) 0.45 mg combined with the selective estrogen receptor modulator bazedoxifene 20 mg (Duavee) (without concomitant use of a progestational agent) is approved to treat VMS and prevent osteoporosis in women with an intact uterus.
- Low-dose paroxetine mesylate (Brisdelle) 7.5 mg is the only nonhormonal formulation approved to treat VMS. Off-label use of venlafaxine (Effexor) is also effective in treating VMS. However, these agents are less effective than standard-dose HT.
- Arbitrary discontinuation of systemic HT when women turn 65 is not evidence based. Although controversial, extended use of systemic HT may be appropriate in well-counseled women for treatment of persistent VMS, prevention of bone loss, and prevention/treatment of atrophic genital changes. Women considering extended use of systemic HT should be aware that with a longer duration of EPT, the risk of breast cancer increases. If GSM/atrophic changes represent the only indication for HT, local low-dose vaginal estrogen is appropriate and highly effective.

Epidemiology

Menopause, the permanent cessation of menstruation caused by loss of ovarian function, occurs at a mean age of 51 to 52 years. With increases in life expectancy, currently more than 50 million US women are 50 years of age or older.

Risk Factors

Spontaneous menopause represents a natural event. Spontaneous menopause occurs at a younger age in women who smoke or undergo hysterectomy with ovarian conservation. Chemotherapy, radiation therapy, or bilateral oophorectomy can induce menopause.

Clinical Manifestations and Pathophysiology

Often described by women as hot flashes or night sweats, VMS represent the most bothersome symptoms of menopause and the most common reason women present for care at the time of the menopausal transition. VMS often include a sudden sensation of heat in the face, neck, and chest and persist for several minutes or less. VMS may cause flushing, chills, anxiety, and sleep disruption. VMS are caused by estrogen withdrawal and are associated with pulsatile luteinizing hormone secretion and decreased endorphin concentration in the hypothalamus, as well as increased release of norepinephrine and serotonin. VMS occur in almost three-quarters of women during the late perimenopausal transition and are more prevalent among the groups listed in Box 1. The median duration of moderate to severe VMS is approximately 10 years.

GSM, also known as vulvovaginal or genital atrophy, signifies the progressive changes in the vulva, vagina, and urethra resulting from estrogen deficiency. GSM, which characteristically causes vaginal dryness and pain with sex, represents a common condition that adversely impacts health, sexuality, and quality of life in menopausal women.

Diagnosis

Although FSH levels increase and estradiol levels decline in menopausal women, such testing is not necessary when late perimenopausal or postmenopausal women report characteristic VMS as described previously. Because thyroid disease is common in women and can cause symptoms that mimic VMS, checking a TSH level is appropriate in women seeking treatment for VMS.

Although GSM can be presumptively diagnosed based on a characteristic history, a pelvic examination can help exclude other vulvovaginal conditions that can present with similar symptoms (see the next section). Physical examination findings characteristic of GSM are listed in Box 2. Although laboratory assessment is not necessary to establish that GSM is present, vaginal pH is typically higher than 5.0.

Differential Diagnosis

Nonmenopausal conditions that can masquerade as menopausal VMS include anxiety disorders, thyroid disease, autoimmune conditions, carcinoid syndromes, diabetic autonomic dysfunction/hypoglycemia, insulinoma/pancreatic tumors, epilepsy, infections, tuberculosis, mast cell disorders, and new-onset hypertension, as well as the use of certain selective serotonergic reuptake inhibitors or serotonin-norepinephrine reuptake inhibitors.

Lichen sclerosus, chronic candidiasis, contact dermatitis, and lichen planus represent vulvar conditions that might be confused with GSM.

Therapy

Estrogen represents the most effective therapy for VMS and related symptoms. Higher doses are more effective; oral and transdermal formulations have comparable efficacy. Many estrogen formulations/doses are also approved for the prevention of osteoporosis. Because estrogen-only therapy (ET) in women with an intact uterus increases the risk of endometrial neoplasia, estrogen-progestin therapy (EPT) is appropriate when treating VMS in women with a uterus. In the United States the most commonly used oral estrogens for systemic treatment of VMS are estradiol (E2, Estrace) and conjugated equine estrogens (CEE, Premarin). Standard doses of these estrogens are 1.0 mg and 0.625 mg, respectively; lower and higher doses are available. Weekly and twice-weekly skin patches and other transdermal E2 formulations are available; estradiol patches releasing 0.05 mg and 0.0375 mg daily are considered standard dose; and lower- and higher-dose patches are available. A 3-month vaginal systemic E2 ring (Femring) for treatment of VMS is also available; the ring releasing 0.05 mg E2 daily is considered the standard dose.

In the United States the progestational agents most commonly prescribed to accompany systemic ET in women with an intact uterus are medroxyprogesterone acetate (MPA [Provera], available in 2.5-mg, 5-mg, and 10-mg doses) and micronized progesterone (Prometrium) in 100-mg and 200-mg capsules. Micronized progesterone is formulated with peanut oil. With standard-dose estrogen, an appropriate daily dose of MPA or micronized progesterone used continuously is 2.5 mg and 100 mg, respectively. Because micronized progesterone has a hypnotic effect, it should be taken at night. A variety of oral estrogen–progestin formulations, all of which have demonstrated endometrial safety, are available in different doses and combine CEE with MPA (Prempro); E2 or ethinyl E2 with norethindrone acetate (Activella, Femhrt); or E2 with drospirenone (Angeliq), norgestimate (Prefast), or progesterone (Bijuva). Transdermal estrogen–progestin combination formulations combine E2 with norethindrone acetate (CombiPatch) or levonorgestrel (Climara Pro). The North American Menopause Society has posted tables listing all formulations approved in the United States or Canada for treating menopausal symptoms (http://www.menopause.org/docs/default-source/professional/nams-ht-tables.pdf?sfvrsn=18.pdf). Although off-label use of testosterone can increase sexual desire in menopausal women, efficacy is achieved only with supraphysiologic doses, which may cause hyperandrogenic adverse effects.

CE 0.45 mg combined with the selective estrogen receptor modulator bazedoxifene 20 mg (Duavee; without the concomitant use of a progestational agent) is approved to treat VMS and prevent osteoporosis in women with an intact uterus and does not increase the incidence of uterine bleeding or endometrial hyperplasia. This novel combination formulation may be useful for women with an intact uterus who choose not to use progestin, including those intolerant of progestin side effects.

Among US women using HT, approximately one-third are using compounded HT; most users are not aware these formulations are not evaluated or approved by the US Food and Drug Administration (FDA). FDA-approved HT is preferable to compounded HT, unless a specific FDA-approved formulation is not available.

Nonhormonal therapy with paroxetine (Paxil),[1] escitalopram (Lexapro),[1] citalopram (Celexa),[1] venlafaxine (Effexor),[1] desvenlafaxine (Pristiq),[1] gabapentin (Neurontin),[1] and pregabalin (Lyrica)[1] are more effective than placebo but less effective than HT in treating VMS. Low-dose paroxetine mesylate (Brisdelle) 7.5 mg is the only nonhormonal formulation approved to treat VMS. Lowering the ambient temperature, use of fans, wearing layered clothing, and avoiding tobacco, alcohol, and caffeine represent commonsense measures for women bothered by VMS. In a clinical trial, clinical hypnosis was found more effective than placebo in addressing VMS. Although over-the-counter herbal formulations, including soy and black cohosh, have been widely used to treat VMS, these have not been found to be more effective than placebo.

When clinicians identify GSM, they should advise women that (unlike VMS) without proactive management, GSM progresses. If severe symptoms are not present, recommending use of over-the-counter lubricants (or substances such as coconut or olive oil) for sexual activity, as well as regular use of vaginal moisturizers, is helpful. Such women should also be advised that regular sexual activity may help improve symptoms and prevent progression. If other indications for systemic HT such as treatment of VMS or prevention of osteoporosis are present, systemic HT is effective in treating GSM. However, if GSM represents the only indication for HT, local low-dose vaginal estrogen is appropriate and highly effective. Vaginal estrogen also reduces the risk of recurrent urinary tract infections and overactive bladder symptoms in menopausal women. In the United States, two low-dose creams, estradiol (Estrace and generics) and CEE (Premarin), are available. Although package labeling provides instructions for

---

[1]Not FDA approved for this indication.

patients regarding dose and schedule, in practice, most women use a fraction of an applicator vaginally (and often also benefit from digital application to vestibular tissues) one to three times weekly. Some women find the use of vaginal estrogen creams to be messy. Vaginal tablets (Vagifem and generics) equivalent to 10 mcg E2 are inserted vaginally with an applicator nightly for 2 weeks, then twice weekly for maintenance. Vaginal 4 mcg or 10 mcg E2 inserts (Imvexxy) are placed digitally nightly for 2 weeks, then twice weekly for maintenance. The 3-month low-dose E2 vaginal ring (Estring) releases 7.5 mcg E2 daily. An oral systemic selective estrogen receptor modulator, ospemifene (Osphena), improves symptoms of GSM; some users report VMS. In late 2016, the FDA approved vaginal dehydroepiandrosterone (DHEA, prasterone; Intrarosa) for the treatment of GSM.

Monitoring

For most women using systemic HT, the monitoring of serum estrogen levels is not indicated. However, when women continue to report bothersome symptoms despite escalating HT doses, monitoring can be useful. In contrast to fluctuating serum estrogen levels in women using oral estrogen, transdermal ET results in relatively steady-state levels; serum E2 levels of 40 to 100 pg/mL represent a reasonable target range for menopausal women age 50 or older. Serum E2 levels as high as 120 pg/mL may be appropriate for younger menopausal women.

Side Effects of Systemic Hormone Therapy

Breast tenderness, bloating, and uterine bleeding represent common side effects of ET. Although lowering the ET dose may reduce side effects, this may cause VMS to increase. Progestins cause dysphoria in some women. Prescribing a different progestin, prescribing progestins sequentially, off-label use of a progestin intrauterine device (Skyla, Kyleena, Mirena, Liletta), or use of the CEE/bazedoxifene combination formulation (Duavee) or antidepressant therapy may be helpful in this setting.

Safety of Hormone Therapy

Findings from the Women's Health Initiative (WHI) study of oral CEE and MPA, CEE alone, and other recent randomized clinical trials have helped clarify the benefits and risks of combination estrogen–progestin and estrogen-alone therapy. A 2013 WHI report detailed findings from the two HT trials with a median 13 years of cumulative follow-up. Since initial findings of the WHI were first published in 2002, use of systemic HT has dramatically decreased, owing to misinterpretation of WHI findings, which has generated anxiety and confusion among clinicians and women. Importantly, absolute risks of adverse events related to hormone therapy were much lower for younger women (ages 50–59) than for older women (Figure 1). Overall, for healthy women with bothersome VMS younger than age 60 and/or within 10 years of menopause onset, the benefits of HT for women outweigh risks.

With respect to coronary heart disease (CHD), HTs impact varies by age of users. Among women who initiate HT before age 60 and/or within 10 years of menopause, HT does not increase (and may reduce) risk. In contrast, among women older than age 60 and/or more than 10 years following menopause onset, initiating HT appears to increase CHD risk.

With respect to stroke, the WHI found that CEE alone or with MPA increased risk; however, for women younger than age 60, the absolute increase in risk was small (see Figure 1).

With respect to venous thromboembolism (VTE), including pulmonary embolism, oral estrogen with or without progestin increases risk, particularly within 2 years of HT initiation.

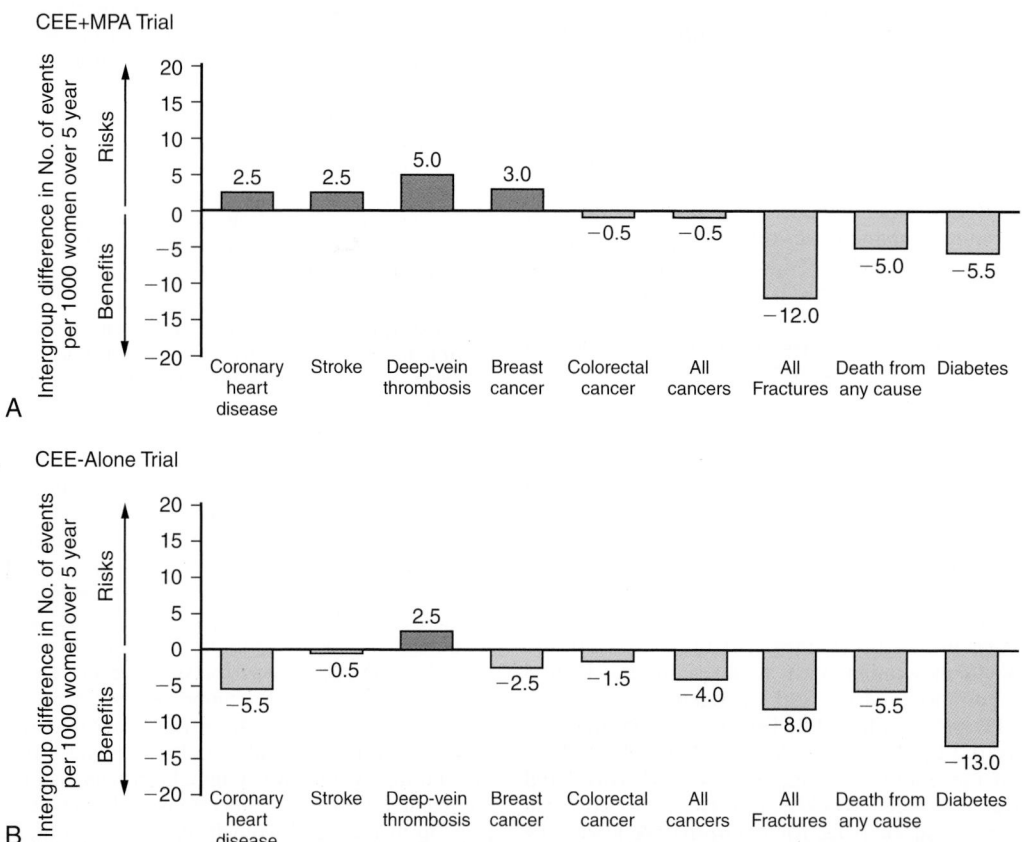

Figure 1 Benefits and risks of the two hormone therapy formulations evaluated in the Women's Health Initiative. Results are shown for the two formulations, conjugated equine estrogens (CEEs) alone (B) or in combination with medroxyprogesterone acetate (A; MPA), for women 50 to 59 years of age. Risks and benefits are expressed as the difference in the number of events (number in the hormone therapy group minus the number in the placebo group) per 1000 women over 5 years. Data from Manson JE, Chlebowski RT, Stefanick ML, et al. Menopausal hormone therapy and health outcomes during the intervention and extended poststopping phases of the Women's Health Initiative randomized trials. *JAMA* 310:1353, 2013.

Absolute risks of VTE are higher for women initiating HT more than 10 years following menopause onset. Observational studies have consistently found that in contrast to oral HT, HT with transdermal (e.g., skin patch) estrogen elevates VTE risk less (if at all) compared with oral HT. Because oral estrogen and body mass index represent independent risk factors for VTE, transdermal estrogen is preferable for most women at elevated baseline VTE risk, including obese women. Personal and familial risk of cardiovascular disease, stroke, and VTE should be considered when initiating HT. Low-dose vaginal estrogen has not been found to elevate the risk of CHD, stroke, VTE, breast or endometrial cancer. With respect to breast cancer risk, WHI results diverged, with increased risk in the CEE-plus-MPA group and borderline reduced risk in the CEE-alone group. With 13 years of follow-up, a modest elevation of risk (hazard ratio [HR] 1.28) persisted in the CEE-plus-MPA group in all participant age strata. To put the elevated risk of breast cancer observed among women randomized to CEE plus MPA into perspective, the attributable risk with combination hormone therapy is less than one additional case of breast cancer diagnosed per 1000 users of combination hormone therapy annually. Another way to put this elevated HR into perspective is to recognize that the HR of 1.28 is slightly higher than that seen with one daily glass of wine, and less than that noted with two daily glasses. With long-term follow-up of WHI participants randomized to CEE alone, a significantly reduced risk of breast cancer (HR = 0.79) emerged over this time period. During cumulative 18-year follow-up of participants in the WHI hormone therapy trials, all-cause mortality rates did not differ appreciably between the intervention and control groups in the overall cohort. The HR for all-cause mortality among women assigned hormone therapy compared with those assigned placebo was 0.99 (95% confidence interval [CI], 0.94–1.03) in the overall pooled cohort; HRs were 1.02 (95% CI, 0.96–1.08) with CEE + MPA and 0.94 (95% CI, 0.88–1.01) with CEE alone. In a 2019 report, women with prior bilateral oophorectomy and randomized to estrogen-alone in their 50s, compared with those randomized to placebo, were found to have a statistically significant 32% reduction in all-cause mortality during long-term follow up. With more than 20 years of follow-up of WHI participants in the two randomized trials, prior randomized use of CEE alone, compared with placebo, among women who had a previous hysterectomy, was associated with a significantly lower breast cancer incidence and lower breast cancer mortality. In contrast, prior randomized use of CEE plus MPA, compared with placebo, among women who had an intact uterus, was associated with a significantly higher breast cancer incidence but no significant difference in breast cancer mortality.

Although trials up to 2 years in duration found that CEE plus bazedoxifene did not increase risk of breast cancer, long-term trials are needed. In women with *BRCA1* or 2 mutations, limited observational data suggest that use of HT does not increase breast cancer risk, suggesting that mutation carriers should not defer risk-reducing salpingo-oophorectomy, owing to concerns that HT to treat VMS would be unsafe.

Low-dose vaginal ET may be used as long as needed, including indefinitely; routine use of concomitant progestin therapy for endometrial protection is not recommended. In the absence of reported spotting or bleeding, routine endometrial surveillance during the use of vaginal ET is not recommended. However, clinicians should recognize that endometrial safety data for currently marketed formulations are based on 1-year trials, with no trials assessing the safety of longer-term administration available.

Current package labeling for low-dose vaginal estrogen, as for all systemic HT formulations, includes a boxed warning that refers to endometrial cancer, myocardial infarction, stroke, invasive breast cancer, pulmonary emboli, and dementia. This warning reflects safety concerns associated with findings from clinical trials of systemic HT, and does not reflect current evidence regarding local low-dose vaginal estrogen.

A personal history of breast cancer is listed as a contraindication to use of all systemic and local low-dose vaginal HT (other contraindications to the use of HT are listed on package labeling). However, one study found that use of the low-dose estrogen vaginal ring does not cause persistently elevated serum estradiol levels in breast cancer survivors using aromatase inhibitors; some oncologists prescribe this ring off-label to treat symptomatic atrophy in breast cancer survivors (including those using aromatase inhibitors), periodically checking serum estradiol levels. Nonetheless, many oncologists caution against the use of vaginal HT in breast cancer survivors. In package labeling for vaginal DHEA (Intrarosa), a personal history of breast cancer is not listed as a contraindication, although current or past history of breast cancer is listed in the Warning and Precautions section.

Extended Use/Discontinuation of Systemic Hormone Therapy

Although controversial, extended use of systemic HT may be appropriate for the treatment of persistent VMS, prevention of bone loss, and prevention/treatment of GSM in selected, well-counseled women. Extended use of systemic HT should not be confused with the initiation of systemic HT by women older than age 60 or more than 10 years following menopause onset—a practice that is known to be associated with an elevated risk of CHD (see the previous section on safety). Women considering extended use of systemic HT should be aware that with longer duration of EPT, the risk of breast cancer increases. Since older age is an independent risk factor for VTE, the use of transdermal estrogen formulations should be considered in this setting. Arbitrary discontinuation of systemic HT when women turn 65 is not evidence based.

When women discontinue systemic HT, a loss of bone mass and progression of GSM/atrophic genital changes occur. The likelihood of recurrent VMS in this setting appears similar with abrupt and gradual (dose-tapering) discontinuation of HT.

Financial Disclosure

Dr. Kaunitz has served on advisory boards for Mithra and Pfizer. His department receives research funding from Mithra. Dr. Manson does not report any potential conflicts of interest.

References

Bhupathiraju SN, Grodstein F, Stampfer MJ: Vaginal estrogen and chronic disease in the nurses' health study, *Menopause* 26, 2019.

Chlebowski RT, Anderson GL, Aragaki AK, et al: Association of menopausal hormone therapy with breast cancer incidence and mortality during long-term follow-up of the Women's Health Initiative randomized clinical trials, *J Am Med Assoc* 324:369, 2019.

Kaunitz AM, Manson JE: Clinical expert series: management of menopausal symptoms, *Obstet Gynecol* 126:859, 2015.

Manson JE, Aragaki AK, Bassuk SS, et al: For the WHI Investigators. Menopausal estrogen-alone therapy and health outcomes in women with and without bilateral oophorectomy: a randomized trial, *Ann Intern Med* 171:406, 2019.

Manson JE, Aragaki AK, Rossouw JE, et al: Menopausal hormone therapy and long-term all-cause and cause-specific mortality: the Women's Health Initiative randomized trials, *J Am Med Assoc* 310:927, 2017.

Manson JE, Chlebowski RT, Stefanick ML, et al: Menopausal hormone therapy and health outcomes during the intervention and extended poststopping phases of the Women's Health Initiative randomized trials, *J Am Med Assoc* 310:1353, 2013.

Manson JE, Kaunitz AM: Menopause management: getting clinical care back on track, *N Engl J Med* 374:803, 2016.

Melisko ME, Goldman ME, Hwang J, et al: Vaginal testosterone cream vs estradiol vaginal ring for vaginal dryness or decreased libido in women receiving aromatase inhibitors for early-stage breast cancer: a randomized clinical trial, *JAMA Oncol* 3:313–319, 2017.

North American Menopause Society: Approved prescription products for menopausal symptoms in the United States and Canada. Available at: http://www.menopause.org/docs/default-source/professional/nams-ht-tables.pdf?sfvrsn=18.pdf.

North American Menopause Society: The 2017 hormone therapy position statement of the North American Menopause Society, *Menopause* 24:728–753, 2017.

Trabuco EC, Moorman PG, Algeciras-Schimnich A, et al: Association of ovary-sparing hysterectomy with ovarian reserve, *Obstet Gynecol* 127:819, 2016.

Vinogradova Y, Coupland C, Hippisley-Cox J: Use of hormone replacement therapy and risk of venous thromboembolism: nested case-control studies using the QResearch and CPRD databases, *BMJ* 364, 2019.

OVARIAN CANCER

Method of
Mihae Song, MD; and Zenas Chang, MD, MS

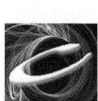

CURRENT DIAGNOSIS

- The US Preventive Services Task Force (USPSTF), the American College of Obstetricians and Gynecologists (ACOG), and the Society of Gynecologic Oncologists (SGO) recommend against the routine screening of low-risk asymptomatic women with transvaginal ultrasonography or serum tumor marker testing.
- Women at high risk (presenting with an identified *BRCA* gene mutation or a family history of cancer suggestive of a hereditary cancer syndrome) should be referred for formal genetic counseling and testing. Current National Comprehensive Cancer Network guidelines recommend screening this population with transvaginal ultrasonography every 6 months with serum CA 125 levels.
- Patients with persistent and progressive abdominal symptoms should be evaluated for ovarian cancer. A pelvic exam and imaging studies (transvaginal ultrasonography) may be helpful in identifying a pelvic mass. Findings such as an elevated CA 125 (in a postmenopausal woman), a nodular or fixed pelvic mass, ascites, or evidence of abdominal or distant metastasis warrant referral or consultation with a gynecologic oncologist.

CURRENT THERAPY

- Asymptomatic women at high risk for ovarian cancer due to a hereditary cancer syndrome should be referred for consideration of a prophylactic bilateral salpingo-oophorectomy (BSO). The timing of this procedure may depend on the cancer syndrome and the patient's reproductive wishes. Referral to a gynecologic oncologist for this discussion may be appropriate.
- Ovarian cancer is treated with a combination of surgical debulking and chemotherapy. The sequence of treatment depends on the clinical status of the patient and whether or not the disease can be resected. Conventional chemotherapy remains the backbone of adjuvant treatment; myelosuppression, fatigue, and neuropathy are some of the most common side effects during treatment.

Epidemiology

Ovarian cancer is the second most common type of female reproductive cancer, but the leading cause of death from gynecologic cancer. There are approximately 22,000 new cases of ovarian cancer per year in the United States, with almost 14,000 deaths yearly. There are several histologic subtypes of ovarian cancer, including epithelial (arising from the surface epithelium of the ovary), sex cord-stromal (arising from the cells that support and surround the oocytes), and germ cell tumors (derived from primordial oocytes). In women under 20 years of age, germ cell tumors are the most common, while epithelial ovarian cancer occurs most commonly in women over 50 years of age. The stage at diagnosis and prognosis vary significantly based on histology. Epithelial tumors account for the vast majority of cases and deaths from ovarian cancer.

Epithelial ovarian cancer has a low prevalence of approximately 1 case per 2500 women per year, with an approximate 1.3% lifetime risk for developing ovarian cancer. Average age at the time of diagnosis is approximately 63 years. Because of a lack of accurate screening tests and vague presenting symptoms, approximately 75% of patients are diagnosed with advanced-stage disease, with an average 5-year survival of 20% to 30%. Caucasian women have the highest incidence rate of ovarian cancer.

The remaining subtypes of ovarian cancer are rare but more likely to be benign. In contrast to epithelial ovarian cancer, most patients with malignant sex cord-stromal neoplasms are diagnosed at an earlier stage and age. Incidence is as low as 0.2 per 100,000 women. Germ cell tumors occur predominantly in young women between 10 and 30 years of age. These neoplasms are primarily limited to one ovary but tend to grow rapidly compared to epithelial or sex cord-stromal tumors. Young women of Asian/Pacific Islander and Hispanic descent are more likely to develop germ cell tumors than Caucasians.

Risk Factors

Significant risk factors for epithelial ovarian cancer are age, early menarche, late menopause, hereditary cancer syndromes, nulliparity, endometriosis, and asbestos. Age and each additional year of ovulation (early menarche/late menopause, nulliparity) are hypothesized to increase risk due to trauma to the ovarian epithelium, which can lead to malignant transformation. Other factors are controversial and include menopausal hormone therapy, obesity, polycystic ovary syndrome, intrauterine devices, talc, cigarette smoking, diet, or infertility and infertility treatments. Systemic reviews of these factors do not currently show clear associations with an increased risk of ovarian cancer.

Approximately 15% to 20% of ovarian cancer cases may be due to hereditary cancer syndromes. More than half of women with an inherited ovarian cancer will have a deleterious mutation in *BRCA1/2* or have Lynch syndrome (mutations in *MLH1, MSH2, MSH6, PMS2*). Other rare hereditary syndromes such as Li-Fraumeni *(TP53)*, Cowden *(PTEN)*, or Peutz-Jeghers *(STK11)* syndromes can also increase the risk for ovarian cancer. The lifetime risk of ovarian cancer can vary significantly by mutation, with an estimated 40% risk for *BRCA1*, 15% risk with *BRCA2*, and 11% to 24% risk with Lynch syndrome (depending on genotype). As medical genetic counseling and testing rates increase, additional genes *(BRIP1, RAD51C, RAD51D, PALPB2)* continue to be identified that may increase the risk for ovarian cancer.

BRCA1/2 mutations are inherited in an autosomal dominant pattern and markedly increase susceptibility to breast and ovarian cancer, with some increased risk for tumors in prostate, male breast, and pancreas. Certain ethnic groups such as Ashkenazi Jewish (2.5%), Icelandic (0.6%), and French Canadian have increased rates of *BRCA* mutations, although *BRCA* mutations have also been identified in Hispanic and African American populations as well. The risk for ovarian cancer under 40 years is low; however, women with *BRCA* mutations tend to have a younger average age at the time of diagnosis (age 50 for *BRCA1*; age 60 for *BRCA2*). Therefore, discussion of risk-reducing BSO in these women is recommended (see Prevention, later) to reduce ovarian as well as breast cancer risk.

Lynch syndrome is also inherited in an autosomal dominant fashion and is similarly associated with the development of multiple cancer types—primarily colon and endometrial cancer. Ovarian cancer is less common than endometrial cancer in these women, but surveillance for gynecologic malignancies is recommended, with risk-reducing surgery indicated at the completion of childbearing and/or by a certain age (see Prevention, later).

Pathophysiology

Approximately 95% of malignant ovarian cancers are epithelial ovarian cancers. The most common subtype of epithelial ovarian cancers is high-grade serous carcinoma, which comprises approximately 70% of cases. The remaining 30% are considered rare and include histologies, including low-grade carcinoma, mucinous carcinoma, clear cell carcinoma, and endometrioid carcinoma. High-grade serous carcinomas are more likely to present at an advanced stage (III or IV, with intraabdominal spread), whereas the rare subtypes are more likely to present in early stages (stage I or II, limited to the pelvis).

High-grade serous ovarian cancer, fallopian tubal carcinoma, and primary peritoneal carcinoma are considered a single clinicalentity due to shared clinical behavior and treatment. Embryologically, the coelomic epithelium differentiates into a variety of cell types, including those found in the fallopian tube, uterus, cervix, and ovarian stroma. Historically, the ovary was the presumed source, as most patients would present with large ovarian masses at the time of diagnosis. Current evidence suggests that there may be more than one mechanism for carcinogenesis, including malignant transformation of the ovarian surface epithelium, tubal neoplasia that leads to metastasis to the ovary, or malignant transformation from endometriosis or endosalpingiosis. These carcinomas generally demonstrate genetic instability, grow and metastasize rapidly, but are more chemosensitive. Even though most high-grade serous ovarian cancer patients are diagnosed at an advanced stage, the majority will respond to chemotherapy and enter remission. Unfortunately, many of these patients will then recur and eventually succumb to their disease.

Low-grade serous tumors account for less than 5% of all cases of ovarian carcinoma and are typically diagnosed at advanced stages as well. However, they share characteristics with borderline ovarian neoplasms (tumors of low malignant potential). Borderline tumors are intermediate lesions between benign cysts and malignant tumors, with characteristics of atypical proliferation and can recur, but are noninvasive. Low-grade tumors may arise from a prior borderline tumor, are invasive, but are relatively indolent. Once diagnosed, primary surgery is the recommended approach, as low-grade serous ovarian cancers are rather chemoresistant.

Clear cell and endometrioid carcinoma differ from serous tumors in that they may arise from foci of preexisting endometriosis. Mucinous carcinomas of the ovary may arise from a mucinous borderline tumor. These subtypes are generally diagnosed at earlier stages but generally behave more aggressively if metastatic. At advanced stages, there is worse overall survival when compared with high-grade serous carcinoma; this is generally thought to be due to resistance to chemotherapy.

Sex cord-stromal neoplasms include granulosa cell and Sertoli-Leydig cell neoplasms. Compared to epithelial neoplasms, they are more likely to produce sex steroid hormones, present with early-stage disease, and rarely metastasize to the lymph nodes. Prognosis due to early-stage disease is generally favorable.

Germ cell tumors include a variety of benign and malignant neoplasms. The most common germ cell tumor is a mature cystic teratoma (dermoid), which is benign. Dysgerminomas are the most common malignant ovarian germ cell tumor, but other malignant subtypes include yolk sac tumors, immature teratomas, and embryonal carcinomas. These subtypes are often chemosensitive, with an excellent prognosis if diagnosed early.

Prevention

No routine screening for ovarian cancer in the general population is recommended. Due to the low prevalence of ovarian cancer, the sensitivity, specificity, positive predictive value, and negative predictive value of transvaginal ultrasonography and serum tumor markers (CA125) have been unreliable and does not reduce ovarian cancer mortality. Due to the high false-positive rate, this can lead to moderate to substantial harm from unnecessary surgical interventions in women who do not have cancer (US Preventive Services Task Force [USPSTF] recommendations). This was recently evaluated by the large, randomized Prostate, Lung, Colorectal, and Ovarian (PLCO) Cancer Screening Trial, which found that annual screening of postmenopausal women with both CA 125 and TVUS compared with usual care did not reduce mortality in the general population. The

incidence of ovarian cancer was not different for women who were screened, and the majority of women were still diagnosed with advanced-stage disease.

Factors that may decrease the risk of epithelial ovarian cancer include BSO, tubal ligation/salpingectomy, hysterectomy, oral contraceptive use, breastfeeding, and parity. BSO is the most effective risk-reducing strategy; however, women may still develop peritoneal carcinoma at a rate of approximately 1%. Due to the role of tubal neoplasia in epithelial ovarian cancer, tubal ligation (regardless of the technique used) has been associated in large epidemiologic studies with an approximate 20% decrease in risk of ovarian cancer. Studies on the effect of opportunistic salpingectomy (removal of fallopian tubes in average-risk women undergoing pelvic surgery for another indication) without oophorectomy are currently ongoing. A meta-analysis of hysterectomy without BSO similarly showed a 20% reduction in the risk of ovarian cancer. Prolonged oral contraceptive use has also been shown to reduce the risk of ovarian cancer, with a meta-analysis showing more than 50% reduction in risk among average-risk women with greater than 10 years of use. Due to the rarity of sex cord-stromal and germ cell tumors, protective factors are less clear.

Women with a significant family history for breast (notably male breast cancer), uterine, ovarian, or colon cancer should be referred for genetic counseling and possible genetic testing. Expert opinion suggests screening for women at high risk for a hereditary ovarian cancer with transvaginal ultrasound and CA125 every 6 months—starting at age 30 for BRCA patients, or 5 to 10 years before the earliest age of first diagnosis of ovarian cancer in the family. Screening for Lynch patients may begin at age 30 to 35 or 5 to 10 years before the earliest age of first diagnosis of any Lynch-related cancer in the family.

In women with a known BRCA mutation, risk-reducing BSO is recommended at completion of childbearing, between 35 and 40 years in women with BRCA1, or 40 to 45 years in women with BRCA2. BSO has been shown to decrease ovarian cancer risk as well as mortality in these patients; however, there remains a baseline 1% risk for developing primary peritoneal cancer. Hysterectomy is not routinely recommended as part of the risk-reducing procedure. While general gynecologists may be able to perform this procedure, referral to a gynecologic oncologist, if available, is recommended, as there are specific protocols for pathologic review, as well as for the management of abnormal findings. In women who have not completed childbearing, oral contraceptive use has been shown to have potentially up to a 5% decrease in ovarian cancer risk per year of use. There is some theoretical concern that hormonal contraception may increase the risk of breast cancer in these patients; however, in the large meta-analysis available, there is no evidence supporting increased risk in current users or in the first 10 years after cessation of use. Use of other contraceptives, such as the patch or vaginal ring, have not yet been studied in this context.

ACOG, SGO, and the American College of Gastroenterology recommend risk-reducing total hysterectomy with BSO for women with Lynch syndrome after completion of childbearing or by age 40 to 45. The remaining risk for peritoneal cancer of 1% following BSO is extrapolated from studies in women with BRCA mutations.

Clinical Manifestations

Patients with ovarian cancer may present with a wide variety of symptoms (Box 1). Most commonly, women will present in the outpatient setting with vague symptoms such as pelvic or abdominal pain, or gastrointestinal symptoms such as abdominal enlargement (from ascites or from mass effect), bloating, early satiety, or changes in bowel habits. Occasionally, incidental findings of a pelvic mass or signs of more advanced disease (peritoneal spread, lymphadenopathy) may be identified at the time of imaging performed for other indications. Acute presentations are typically due to widely metastatic disease, causing conditions such as bowel obstruction or pleural effusions that may require prompt intervention. Postmenopausal bleeding may be a presenting symptom but is more likely to be associated with uterine pathology. Of note, young patients with signs of precocious puberty, abnormal vaginal bleeding, or hirsutism (likely due to abnormal hormone production) should be evaluated for possible sex cord-stromal neoplasms. Rarely, patients may present with paraneoplastic syndromes with neurologic findings, hemolytic anemia, or nephrotic syndromes.

Diagnosis

Patients with persistent and progressive abdominal symptoms should be evaluated for ovarian cancer. A pelvic exam and imaging studies (transvaginal ultrasonography) may be helpful in identifying a pelvic mass. Composition of the mass (mixed cystic and solid), as well as the presence of thick septations, mural nodules, or papillary excrescences on imaging, would increase suspicion for malignancy. Other diagnostic findings (Box 2), such as an elevated CA125 (in a postmenopausal woman), a nodular or fixed pelvic mass on exam, or evidence of ascites, abdominal, or distant metastasis on imaging warrants referral or consultation with a physician trained to stage and debulk ovarian cancer, such as a gynecologic oncologist. Aspiration or biopsy of a cystic pelvic mass is not generally recommended. Needle biopsy of a solid metastatic lesion or paracentesis for cytology may be considered for diagnosis.

Differential Diagnosis

Due to the varied and nonspecific symptoms on presentation, the differential diagnosis is broad. If an adnexal mass is identified, different gynecologic as well as gastrointestinal or urologic causes should be considered. These may include benign or malignant conditions (Box 3).

Therapy

Historically, ovarian cancers have been treated, regardless of histology, with a combination of chemotherapy and surgery. Referral to a gynecologic oncologist for management is recommended. The backbone of chemotherapy is a platinum agent in combination with a taxane. Newer data suggest benefit for potential combinations with other agents, such as the antiangiogenic agent bevacizumab or poly(ADP-ribose) polymerase

(PARP) inhibitors. Immunotherapy has had limited efficacy in ovarian cancer at this time. All patients with a diagnosed ovarian cancer should also be referred for genetic counseling and for genetic testing.

Monitoring

During chemotherapy, myelosuppression, fatigue, and neuropathy (from a combination of a taxane and platinum agent) are some of the most common side effects. Management of these symptoms will be in coordination with the treating oncologist or potentially with palliative care. Neuropathy, difficulties with memory and concentration ("chemo brain"), and fatigue may improve in the first year after completion of therapy, but some symptoms may persist long term, with effects on quality of life. The etiology of cognitive dysfunction and fatigue is not well understood, but these patients may respond to cognitive behavioral therapy and exercise.

Current SGO recommendations for post-treatment surveillance include a thorough evaluation of symptoms and physical examination. For years 0 to 2 after completion of treatment, surveillance visits are scheduled every 3 to 4 months. For years 2 to 3, visits are every 4 to 6 months; and for years 3 to 5, they are every 6 months. After 5 years, yearly visits with a gynecologic oncologist or general gynecologist are appropriate. No Pap tests or cytology studies are indicated during this time, and routine CA125 levels upon each visit are optional. No routine radiographic imaging (chest XR, PET or CT scans, MRI, or ultrasounds) is recommended during surveillance, due to insufficient data to support this use. If recurrence is suspected due to symptoms, CT scans or CA125 may be useful prior to repeat consultation with a gynecologic oncologist.

References

Buys SS, Partridge E, Black A, et al: Effect of screening on ovarian cancer mortality: the Prostate, Lung, Colorectal and Ovarian (PLCO) Cancer Screening Randomized Controlled Trial, *JAMA* 305(22):2295, 2011.

Eskander R, Berman M, Keder L: Practice Bulletin No 174: Evaluation and Management of Adnexal Masses, *Obstet Gynecol* 128(5):e210–e226, 2016.

Matteson KA, Gunderson C, Richardson DL: Committee Opinion No. 716: The Role of the Obstetrician-Gynecologist in the Early Detection of Epithelial Ovarian Cancer in Women at Average Risk, *Obstet Gynecol* 130(3):e146–e149, 2017.

Salani R, Khanna N, Frimer M, et al: An update on post-treatment surveillance and diagnosis of recurrence in women with gynecologic malignancies: Society of Gynecologic Oncology (SGO) recommendations, *Gynecol Oncol* 146(1):3–10, 2017.

Schorge JO, Modesitt SC, Coleman RL: SGO white paper on ovarian cancer: etiology screening and surveillance, *Gynecol Oncol* 119(1):7–17, 2010.

Yoon SH, Kim SN, Shim SH, et al: Bilateral salpingectomy can reduce the risk of ovarian cancer in the general population: a meta-analysis, *Eur J Cancer* 55:38–46, 2016.

PELVIC INFLAMMATORY DISEASE

Method of
Amy E. Curry, MD

CURRENT DIAGNOSIS

- Pelvic inflammatory disease is a clinical diagnosis based on suspicious clinical findings in a woman who is at risk.
- Patients may be asymptomatic. Symptoms may range from nonspecific complaints including lower abdominal pain, vaginal discharge, dyspareunia, and irregular uterine bleeding to high fever, vomiting, and lower abdominal tenderness with rebound.
- Physical examination findings may include vaginal and endocervical discharge, as well as cervical motion, uterine and adnexal tenderness, and adnexal fullness.
- Cultures should be performed for *Chlamydia trachomatis* and *Neisseria gonorrhoeae*, the two most commonly implicated organisms, though a variety of infectious agents may be causative.

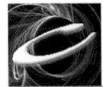

CURRENT THERAPY

Empiric treatment for pelvic inflammatory disease (PID) should be initiated in any woman at risk for sexually transmitted infections if:
- Pelvic or lower abdominal pain is present;
- Cervical motion tenderness OR uterine tenderness OR adnexal tenderness is found on pelvic examination;
- No other cause for the pain can be identified.

Inpatient therapy for PID:
- There is no designation of Regimen A or B. Cefotetan (Cefotan) 2 g IV every 12 hours OR cefoxitin (Mefoxin) 2 g IV every 6 hours PLUS doxycycline (Vibramycin) 100 mg PO/IV every 12 hours.

  OR
- Clindamycin (Cleocin) 900 mg IV every 8 hours PLUS gentamicin (Garamycin) 2 mg/kg of body weight loading dose followed by 1.5 mg/kg of body weight IV/IM every 8 hours. A single daily dose of 3 to 5 mg/kg of body weight IV/IM can also be used.
- Alternate regimen: ampicillin/sulbactam (Unasyn) 3 g IV every 6 hours PLUS doxycycline (Vibramycin) 100 mg PO/IV every 12 hours.

Outpatient therapy for PID:
- Ceftriaxone (Rocephin) 250 mg IM single dose PLUS doxycycline (Vibramycin) 100 mg PO every 12 hours for 14 days WITH/WITHOUT metronidazole (Flagyl) 500 mg PO every 12 hours for 14 days.

  OR
- Cefoxitin (Mefoxin) 2 g IM and probenecid (Benemid) 1 g PO both given concurrently as a single dose PLUS doxycycline (Vibramycin) 100 mg PO every 12 hours for 14 days WITH/WITHOUT metronidazole (Flagyl) 500 mg PO every 12 hours for 14 days.

  OR
- Other parenteral third-generation cephalosporins: either ceftizoxime (Cefizox) 1 g IM single dose OR cefotaxime (Claforan) 1 g IM single dose PLUS doxycycline (Vibramycin) 100 mg PO every 12 hours for 14 days WITH/WITHOUT metronidazole (Flagyl) 500 mg PO every 12 hours for 14 days.
- Alternative treatment options are available for those who have penicillin or cephalosporin allergy.

Pelvic inflammatory disease (PID) is a polymicrobial infection of any or all of the upper genital tract organs in women. It is initiated by a community-acquired sexually transmitted agent and can involve the uterus, fallopian tubes, and ovaries, as well as adjacent pelvic structures.

Epidemiology
In the United States, the diagnosis of PID accounted for 90,000 initial visits to physician offices between 2007–2016 and 4.4% of women (2.5 million) 18 to 44 years of age reported a history of PID based on 2013-2014 survey data.

Risk Factors
The single greatest risk factor for PID is a history of multiple sex partners. Other risk factors include 15 to 25 years of age, a male partner with symptoms of a sexually transmitted infection (STI) such as dysuria or urethral discharge, history of previous STI or PID, inconsistent use of condoms, African American ethnicity, and use of vaginal douching. Any phenomenon that disrupts the mucus barrier of the endocervical canal can also potentially facilitate PID, such as menses, bacterial vaginosis, or intrauterine instrumentation. Accordingly, the risk of an intrauterine device causing PID usually occurs during the first 3 weeks following insertion and rarely thereafter.

Pathophysiology
PID occurs when bacteria from the vagina ascend into the normally sterile environment of the upper genital tract. This typically occurs in the setting of a *Neisseria gonorrhoeae* or *Chlamydia trachomatis* infection. Ascending bacteria can include anaerobes, especially those implicated in bacterial vaginosis, group A and B *Streptococcus*, *Escherichia coli*, *Klebsiella*, *Proteus mirabilis*, *Haemophilus influenzae*, *Peptococcus*, genital *Mycoplasma*, *Actinomycosis*, and cytomegalovirus. Methicillin-resistant *Staphylococcus aureus* has been reported to cause PID, but rarely. Once present, this polymicrobial infection can remain asymptomatic or cause endometritis, salpingitis, oophoritis, peritonitis, perihepatitis, or tubo-ovarian abscesses.

Clinical Presentation
PID may be asymptomatic. It may have an indolent presentation of low-grade fever, weight loss, and nonspecific abdominal pain. A more symptomatic presentation of PID includes bilateral lower quadrant abdominal pain, recent onset of dyspareunia, abnormal vaginal bleeding, and vaginal discharge. On physical examination, the patient may have fever, decreased bowel sounds, diffuse lower abdominal tenderness with rebound tenderness, and/or right upper quadrant tenderness. During the pelvic examination, purulent vaginal or endocervical discharge, vaginal mucosa redness, and cervical irritation or friability may be noted. Cervical motion pain or tenderness of the adnexa or uterus during the bimanual examination is strongly suggestive of PID.

There are several diagnostic findings that support the diagnosis of PID: the presence of abundant white blood cells or clue cells in vaginal or cervical mucus; the presence of an STI, especially gonorrhea or chlamydia; an elevated erythrocyte sedimentation rate or C-reactive protein; an elevated serum white blood cell count; evidence of endometritis on endometrial biopsy; findings of thickened, fluid-filled fallopian tubes, free fluid in the pelvis, or a tubo-ovarian abscess on transvaginal sonography or magnetic resonance imaging; or evidence of pelvic organ inflammation on laparoscopic exploration.

Diagnosis
Unfortunately, no single element of the history, finding on physical examination, laboratory test result, or diagnostic procedure has both the sensitivity and the specificity to help the clinician accurately diagnose PID. Consequently, PID remains a diagnosis based primarily on clinical suspicion in at-risk women.

Differential Diagnosis

The differential diagnosis of PID includes ectopic pregnancy, inflammatory bowel disorders, ovarian cysts and cyst rupture, ovarian torsion, appendicitis, endometriosis, proctitis, urinary tract infections, diverticulitis, constipation, or functional pain related to current or past abuse.

Treatment

The 2015 Centers for Disease Control and Prevention (CDC) treatment guidelines for PID are outlined in the Current Diagnosis and Current Therapy boxes. These guidelines recommend empiric treatment for PID in all at-risk women who meet the criteria listed and encourage health care providers to "maintain a low threshold for the diagnosis" and treatment of PID due to "the potential for significant damage to the reproductive health of women."

Treatment guidelines are based on the patient's need for inpatient versus outpatient care. The Pelvic Inflammatory Disease Evaluation and Clinical Health (PEACH) trial demonstrated no difference in the reproductive outcomes of women with mild-to-moderate PID who were randomized to inpatient treatment versus those randomized to outpatient treatment.

Indications for inpatient treatment of PID include the following: pregnancy; failed trial or intolerance to oral medications; signs of severe PID such as high fever, nausea, vomiting, or intractable abdominal pain; complicated PID (e.g., peritonitis, perihepatitis); and pelvic abscesses. The need for surgical intervention or diagnostic exploration to rule out other abdominal pathology would alsomandate inpatient treatment. In those patients requiring inpatient treatment, any one of the parenteral antibiotic regimens as outlined above may be administered, depending on the patient's history of allergies and the cost and availability of treatment options. When possible, the use of oral doxycycline (Vibramycin) is preferred over intravenous (IV) infusion due to the pain of IV infusion and the similar bioavailability of the oral form as compared to IV administration. Treatment should also include appropriate analgesia, antiemetics, antipyretics, IV fluids, and rest. Patients may be transitioned from parenteral to oral therapy after 24 hours of sustained clinical improvement including lack of fever. Further completion of a total of 14 days of treatment with oral medications is recommended. Those patients treated with any of the inpatient regimens or the alternative regimen should be transitioned to oral doxycycline (Vibramycin) 100 mg every 12 hours. Those treated with clindamycin (Cleocin) and gentamicin (Garamycin) should be transitioned to oral doxycycline (Vibramycin) 100 mg every 12 hours or oral clindamycin (Cleocin) 450 mg every 6 hours. If a tubo-ovarian abscess is present, in addition to surgical consultation, the patient should be transitioned preferably to oral clindamycin (Cleocin) 450 mg every 6 hours for a total of 14 days of treatment. Alternatively, oral doxycycline (Vibramycin) 100 mg every 12 hours with oral metronidazole (Flagyl) 500 mg every 8 hours for a total of 14 days of treatment may also be used.

In patients not meeting criteria for inpatient treatment, any of the outpatient treatment regimens as outlined above may be used, the choice being again dependent on the cost and availability of treatment options. The addition of metronidazole (Flagyl) is recommended due to cephalosporin limitations in anaerobic coverage and in the case of *Trichomonas* or bacterial vaginosis infections. The addition of metronidazole (Flagyl) is also recommended if there is a history of recent uterine instrumentation.

Of note, the CDC recently updated their guideline for treatment of uncomplicated urogenital gonorrhea infections to ceftriaxone 500 mg IM dose × 1 for patients <150 kg and 1 gm IM × 1 for patients ≥150 kg. The PID treatment guidelines have not been updated, however. Routine use of quinolones is no longer recommended in empiric treatment of PID due to increasing resistant *N. gonorrhoeae*. If a cephalosporin allergy exists and inpatient treatment with clindamycin (Cleocin) and gentamicin (Garamycin) is not available, risk for gonorrhea is low, cultures are obtained and follow-up is available, levofloxacin (Levaquin) 500 mg PO every 24 hours or ofloxacin (Floxin) 400 mg PO every 12 hours or moxifloxacin (Avelox) 400 mg PO every 24 hours with metronidazole (Flagyl) 500 mg PO every 12 hours for 14 days may be used.

In patients with a history of penicillin allergy, a careful reaction history should be taken to assess the risk of using a cephalosporin in the empiric treatment of PID. There is negligible cross-reactivity between penicillins and third-generation cephalosporins. If a cephalosporin cannot be safely used, the patient can be admitted for treatment with parenteral clindamycin (Cleocin) and gentamicin (Garamycin).

Regardless of the treatment regimen used, patients should be advised to abstain from intercourse until treatment is completed and they are free of symptoms. In patients with an intrauterine device (IUD), there are inconclusive data to recommend its removal, unless clinical improvement does not occur, but close clinical follow-up is warranted. There is no difference in the treatment regimens for PID in women with a history of HIV.

Patient Monitoring and Counseling

Patients treated with an outpatient regimen should be evaluated for clinical improvement within 48 to 72 hours. If no improvement is noted, the patient should be hospitalized for parenteral antibiotics and further diagnostic evaluation. All patients should be counseled on the need to complete the full course of antibiotic treatment to decrease the potential complications of PID. Patients should be informed of the cause of their infection, if known, and the need for any sexual partners to be tested and treated. Testing for HIV, syphilis, and hepatitis B and C should also be offered. If the patient is an appropriate candidate, immunization against hepatitis B (Engerix-B, Recombivax HB) and human papillomavirus (Gardasil 9) should also be offered. In order to decrease future PID episodes, patients should be advised on the need for safe sex practices and the recommendation for future routine screening for chlamydia and gonorrhea.

Complications

Complications of PID include recurrence of the infection, infertility secondary to fallopian tube scarring, chronic pelvic pain, and ectopic pregnancy. Extension of the infection can also occur, potentially causing pelvic abscesses, peritonitis, and perihepatitis (Fitz-Hugh-Curtis syndrome).

References

Campagna JD, Bond MC, Schabelman E, Hayes BD: The use of cephalosporins in penicillin-allergic patients: a literature review, *J Emerg Med* 42(5):612–620, 2012.
Curry A, Williams T, Penny M: Pelvic inflammatory disease: diagnosis, management, and prevention, *Am Fam Physician* 100(6):357–364, 2019.
Kreisel K, Torrone E, Bernstein K, Hong J, Gorwitz R: Prevalence of pelvic inflammatory disease in sexually experienced women of reproductive age United States, 2013–2014, *MMWR Morb Mortal Wkly Rep* 66(3):80–83, 2017.
Ness RB, Soper DE, Holley RL, et al: Effectiveness of inpatient and outpatient treatment strategies for women with pelvic inflammatory disease: results from the pelvic inflammatory disease evaluation and clinical health (PEACH) randomized trial, *Am J Obstet Gynecol* 186:929–937, 2002.
St. Cyr S, Barbee L, Workowski KA, et al: Update to CDC's treatment guidelines for gonococcal infection, 2020, *MMWR Morb Mortal Wkly Rep* 69:1911–1916, 2020.
Tepper NK, Steenland MW, Gaffield ME, Marchbanks PA, Curtis KM: Retention of intrauterine devices in women who acquire pelvic inflammatory disease: a systematic review, *Contraception* 87(5):655–660, 2013.
Workowski KA, Bolan GA: Centers for Disease Control and Prevention. Sexually transmitted diseases treatment guidelines, 2015. {published correction appears in *MMWR Recomm Rep* 64(33):924, 2015} *MMWR Recomm Rep* 64(RR-03), 1–137, 2015.

PREMENSTRUAL SYNDROME

Method of
Ellen W. Freeman, PhD

CURRENT DIAGNOSIS

- Confirm that symptoms occur premenstrually and abate following menses.
- Confirm that symptoms are clinically significant and impair daily activities and/or cause problems for the woman.
- Obtain a medical history and conduct a physical examination to determine that other disorders are not causing the symptoms.
- Assess depression, stress, substance abuse, and other diagnoses that could cause the symptoms.
- Ask the woman to maintain a daily symptom report for two or more menstrual cycles to confirm the reported symptoms and their relation to the menstrual cycle.
- Perform laboratory tests only as needed to confirm general good health or rule out other suspected conditions.

CURRENT THERAPY

SSRI	Range Studied (mg)	Mean Dose (mg/d)
Citalopram (Celexa[1])	10–30	20
Escitalopram (Lexapro[1])	10–20	15
Fluoxetine (Prozac,[1] Sarafem*)	10–60	20
Paroxetine (Paxil[1])	10–30	20
Paroxetine-CR* (Paxil-CR)	12.5, 25	NA[†]
Sertraline (Zoloft*)	50–150	75
SNRI		
Venlafaxine (Effexor[1])	37.5–200	112.5

[1]Not FDA approved for this indication.
*FDA approved for the indication of premenstrual dysphoric disorder (PMDD).
[†]Not applicable because of fixed-dose study.

The premenstrual syndromes (PMS) are characterized by mood, behavioral, and physical symptoms that occur from several days to 2 weeks before menses and remit with the menstrual flow. The term *PMS* as used by clinicians and the general public is generic, imprecise, and commonly applied to numerous symptoms. Included symptoms range from the mild and normal physiologic changes of the menstrual cycle to clinically significant symptoms that limit or impair normal functioning. In recent years, randomized controlled trials and other well-designed studies have defined diagnostic criteria for PMS and identified effective treatments for this disorder.

Based on scientific evidence at this time, serotonergic antidepressants are considered the primary treatment for clinically significant PMS, and particularly its severe form termed *premenstrual dysphoric disorder* (PMDD). This review focuses on PMS and its treatment with serotonergic antidepressants. It is not a comprehensive review of all treatments or associated literature. Other recent reviews may guide the reader to further information and other treatments for PMS and PMDD.

Symptoms

Numerous symptoms were traditionally attributed to PMS. This plethora is related in part to the absence of a clear diagnosis that distinguishes PMS from other comorbid conditions. Many

disorders, both physical and psychiatric, are exacerbated premenstrually or occur as a comorbid disorder with PMS. When a careful diagnosis is made to distinguish PMS from other conditions, a much smaller group of symptoms appear to be typical of the disorder (Box 1).

Mood symptoms are usually the main complaint (irritability, anxiety, tension, mood swings, feeling out of control, depression), but behavioral symptoms (e.g., decreased interest, fatigue, poor concentration, poor sleep) and physical symptoms, most commonly breast tenderness and abdominal swelling, are also present. Multiple studies suggest that irritability is the cardinal symptom of PMS. Although depressive symptoms such as low mood, fatigue, sleep difficulties, and poor concentration are frequent complaints of women with PMS, the growing evidence indicates that PMS is not a simple variant of depression but has distinct mechanisms that differ from those of depressive disorders.

Prevalence

Surveys indicate that PMS is among the most common health problems reported by reproductive-age women. Current estimates from epidemiologic data indicate that up to 30% of women experience severe and clinically significant premenstrual symptoms, although only 6% to 8% of menstruating women meet the stringent and predominantly dysphoric criteria for PMDD.

Morbidity

The morbidity of PMS is related to its severity, chronicity, and resulting distress that affect work, personal relationships, or daily activities. The level of impairment is significantly above community norms and similar to that of other health problems such as major depressive disorder. Studies consistently demonstrate that the greatest impairment or distress resulting from PMS is in relationships with the partner or children and in the effectiveness of work.

Etiology

The etiology of PMS remains undefined, although the monthly cycling of the reproductive hormones appears to have an essential role in the disorder. While circulating levels of the hormones are in normal range, the dominant theory is that some women have an underlying vulnerability to the normal fluctuations of one or more of these hormones. It is further believed that PMS involves central nervous system–mediated interactions of the reproductive steroids with neurotransmitters. A current review of the genetic etiology found only limited evidence for the genetic basis of PMDD, with both familial and candidate gene studies having negative or conflicting results. The principal research evidence at this time supports the involvement of reproductive hormones, serotonergic dysregulation, and possibly dysregulation of GABAergic receptor functioning. Recent evidence suggested a pathophysiological role of beta-adrenergic mechanisms in the clinical pain of PMS.

Diagnosis

A diagnosis of PMS is determined primarily by the *timing* and the *severity* of the symptoms. These factors, together with an assessment of whether other physical or psychiatric disorders may account for the symptoms, are more important for the diagnosis than the particular symptoms, which are typically nonspecific and must be assessed for their relationship to the menstrual cycle.

Box 2 lists the diagnostic criteria for PMS presented by the American College of Obstetricians and Gynecologists. These criteria indicate that PMS symptoms must be experienced during the 5 days before menses and abate during the menstrual flow. The symptoms should cause identifiable impairment or distress, be confirmed by prospective reports recorded daily by the woman for at least two to three consecutive menstrual cycles, and not be accounted for by other disorders.

To diagnose PMS, a medical history should be obtained and a complete physical with gynecologic examination performed. PMS is understood to occur in ovulatory menstrual cycles; cycles that are irregular or outside the normal range are an indication for further gynecologic investigation. Comorbid conditions such as dysmenorrhea, endometriosis, uterine fibroids, pelvic inflammatory disease, thyroid disorders, migraine, diabetes, mood disorders, substance abuse, and numerous other possibilities should be identified. It may be difficult to determine whether the symptoms under investigation are an exacerbation of a comorbid condition or superimposed on another condition. In either case, the usual recommendation is to treat the ongoing condition first, then reassess and possibly add treatment for the symptoms that arise premenstrually.

The diagnostic criteria for PMDD are listed in the *Diagnostic and Statistical Manual of Mental Disorders, Fifth Edition (DSM-V)* and are intended to diagnose a severe, dysphoric form of PMS. Importantly, the Food and Drug Administration (FDA) has approved medications only for the indication of PMDD and not for the indication of PMS at the present time. Briefly, the PMDD criteria require 5 of 11 *listed* symptoms including at least one mood symptom. Physical symptoms, regardless of the number, are considered a single symptom in meeting the diagnostic criteria. The 11 PMDD symptoms are depressed mood, anxiety or tension, mood swings, anger or irritability, decreased interest, concentration difficulties, fatigue, appetite change or food cravings, sleep disturbance, feeling overwhelmed, and physical symptoms. At least five of these symptoms must *each* be severe premenstrually and abate with the menstrual flow. The symptoms must markedly interfere with functioning, be confirmed by daily symptom reports for at least two menstrual cycles, and not be an exacerbation of another physical or mental disorder.

No laboratory test identifies PMS or PMDD and none should be routinely performed for diagnosis. Laboratory tests that indicate or confirm other possible disorders are useful if suggested by the individual woman's symptom presentation or medical findings.

The key diagnostic tool for evaluating premenstrual symptoms is the daily symptom report. The diagnostic criteria for both PMS and PMDD include a daily symptom report that is maintained by the woman for at least two menstrual cycles to confirm that the woman's reported symptoms are linked to the menstrual cycle in the requisite pattern. Numerous symptom reports appropriate for this diagnosis are identified in the medical literature. It is important that the ratings indicate the severity of each symptom (and not simply check the presence or absence of symptoms).

It is informative to use two visits for the diagnostic evaluation. Although counterintuitive, seeing the patient following menses when PMS symptoms have abated is instructive. If symptoms are absent, it provides strong evidence for the diagnosis. If symptoms are present in the follicular phase, the type and severity of the symptoms are important diagnostic information for identifying other physical or mental disorders that may be the primary focus of treatment.

Treatment

Selective Serotonin Reuptake Inhibitors

Serotonergic antidepressants are the primary treatment for severe PMS and PMDD at this time. Modulating serotonergic function is consistent with a leading theoretical view that the normal gonadal steroid fluctuations of the menstrual cycle are associated with an abnormal serotonergic response in vulnerable women. A meta-analysis of randomized controlled trials of selective serotonin reuptake inhibitors (SSRIs) in treatment of PMS and PMDD determined that these drugs were an effective first-line therapy, with both a statistically significant and clinically meaningful difference from placebo. The FDA has approved fluoxetine (Sarafem), sertraline (Zoloft), and controlled-release paroxetine (Paxil CR) for the indication of PMDD. Other randomized, placebo-controlled, double-blind trials show efficacy of citalopram (Celexa[1]), escitalopram (Lexapro[1]), venlafaxine (Effexor[1]) (a selective serotonin-norepinephrine reuptake inhibitor [SNRI]), and clomipramine (Anafranil[1]) (a tricyclic antidepressant) for treatment of PMS and PMDD, but they are not FDA approved for this indication.

Effective doses of SSRIs are consistently at the low end of the dose range for depressive disorders in all reports of PMS and PMDD treatments. Significant response is often seen in the first menstrual cycle of treatment, with smaller increments with or without dose adjustments in the second and third treatment cycles. If there is not sufficient response in the first treated menstrual cycle, the dose should be increased in the next cycle unless precluded by side effects.

Side effects are common with the initiation of an SSRI but are usually transient and abate within 1 to 2 weeks of continued treatment. The most common side effects include headache, nausea, insomnia, fatigue or lethargy, diarrhea, decreased concentration, dizziness, and decreased libido or delayed orgasm. The sexual side effects of SSRIs have received considerable attention, although it is often difficult to determine the extent to which sexual effects are related to the medication or to preexisting conditions. The incidence of decreased sexual interest or delayed orgasm in the few published reports of PMS patients is approximately 9% to 16%, which is notably lower than the rates reported with the use of SSRIs by depressed patients. Another important issue is the lack of any well-controlled clinical trials of SSRI treatment for PMS and PMDD in adolescents. Whether SSRIs are safe and effective for this indication in women younger than 18 years is not demonstrated.

Luteal Phase Dosing

The use of medication only in the symptomatic luteal phase of the menstrual cycle is particularly important in PMS because of the cyclic pattern of the symptoms, which occur only in the premenstrual phase and abate following menses. Efficacy of luteal phase administration of the SSRIs is demonstrated in multiple trials: three large multicenter, randomized, placebo-controlled

---

[1]Not FDA approved for this indication.

trials that examined fluoxetine (Sarafem), paroxetine (Paxil), and sertraline (Zoloft); a trial that directly compared continuous and luteal phase administration of sertraline; and multiple preliminary studies.

Luteal phase administration of an SSRI is typically initiated 14 days prior to the expected onset of menstrual bleeding and concluded within several days of bleeding, using a taper for increased doses. As with continuous dosing, the SSRI doses are usually at the low end of the dose range.

A preliminary study compared symptom-onset dosing (mean of 6 days before menses) to luteal-phase dosing and found no difference between the two dosing regimens in improvement overall, although there was suggestion that women with more severe symptoms may respond better to full luteal-phase dosing. A recent RCT of sertraline in symptom-onset dosing suggested greater improvement with sertraline compared to placebo, but results were inconsistent and varied with the symptom scale. Importantly, however, this study showed that cessation of symptom-onset treatment was not associated with discontinuation symptoms.

Side effects may be less frequent with an intermittent dosing regimen because they may not occur when not taking the medication. However, some women experience recurring side effects when dosing is resumed.

Insufficient Response to Selective Serotonin Reuptake Inhibitors

Approximately 60% of PMS and PMDD patients in controlled studies respond well to an SSRI. There are no clear predictors of response. An adequate trial of an SSRI for PMS and PMDD is at least two menstrual cycles at a dose level of demonstrated efficacy, with a third cycle when there is partial response. If a woman has an insufficient response or unacceptable side effects, it is reasonable to try another SSRI. Although the SSRIs are similar in their structure and have similar response rates and side-effect profiles, an individual patient may respond better to one SSRI versus another.

Other approaches to a poor treatment response include augmenting the SSRI with another medication to address the non-responding symptoms, but there is no systematic information on this in PMS or PMDD treatment. Switching to another class of medication, such as anxiolytics, is suggested, but no data indicate whether nonresponders to SSRIs will respond to another class of medication. Nonresponse may also be related to other comorbid disorders. A thorough review of the diagnosis and adjustments of the premenstrual doses of medication for both the primary disorder and PMS should be considered before pursuing other treatments.

Other Treatments
Hormonal

In spite of the evidence for hormonal involvement in PMS and PMDD, traditional oral contraceptives (OCs) do not show efficacy for the disorder. However, some data indicate that shortening or omitting the placebo week in the traditional OC pill pack may effectively treat PMS and PMDD. The FDA has approved the oral contraceptive YAZ (ethinyl estradiol 20 mcg/drospirenone 3 mg), a 24/4-day combination pill, to treat PMDD. The continuous daily use of an OC (without a hormone-free interval) suppresses ovulation-related hormone cyclicity. Continuous daily levonorgestrel 90 mcg/ethinyl estradiol 20 mcg (Amethyst[1]) has been evaluated for continuous use up to one year and may be useful for managing the symptoms of PMDD. A Cochrane review of estrogen preparations for management of PMS found only five randomized controlled trials out of more than 500 reports. The evidence was considered low-quality, inconclusive with regard to effectiveness, and too limited to provide answers regarding the safety of these preparations for the indication of PMS.

Gonadotropin-releasing hormone (GnRH) agonists such as depot leuprolide (Lupron)[1] and buserelin[2] (Suprefact) are effective for PMS and PMDD but are of limited usefulness because of the risks associated with low estrogen levels that result from these treatments. Although add-back therapy using low-lose estrogen and progesterone together with the GnRH agonist did not appear to reduce efficacy in a meta-analysis, there are no definitive data on the safety and efficacy of this approach in long-term treatment. The historic use of progesterone has failed to show efficacy for the mood and behavioral symptoms of PMS in numerous controlled trials.

Anxiolytics

Alprazolam (Xanax)[1] and buspirone (Buspar)[1] showed modest efficacy for PMS in some studies but not others. Although these medications offer an alternative to antidepressants, the response rates appear much lower, and it is not known whether a PMS patient who does not respond to antidepressants will respond to an anxiolytic. The risk of dependency with alprazolam should be considered. Dosing should be strictly limited to the luteal phase, and the patient should have no history of substance abuse.

Nonpharmacologic

Calcium supplementation[1] (500 mg daily; 600 mg twice daily) reduced PMS symptoms significantly more than placebo in several clinical trials. Improved symptoms included anxiety, depression, water retention, and somatic changes. Calcium offers a dietary supplement approach that may be beneficial for some women with PMS, although there are no predictors of which women will respond well to this therapy. Vitex agnus castus (chasteberry[7]) appears to be a safe and effective treatment for PMS or PMDD in randomized controlled trials. Other complementary and alternative therapies may be helpful for some women, but there is no consistent evidence of their efficacy for PMS.

Behavioral treatments that facilitate coping or reduce stress may reduce PMS symptoms. Cognitive-behavioral therapy is effective for PMS, and in one study it was as effective as the SSRI fluoxetine after 6 months of treatment.

Treatment Duration

The published studies of treatment efficacy for PMS and PMDD are based on acute treatment of 2 to 3 months' duration. Several investigations suggest that PMS symptoms are likely to return within several months after medication is stopped. It also appears that PMS symptoms do not resolve spontaneously but continue for many years. These observations of PMS as a chronic condition and the swift return of symptoms following the cessation of medication suggest that treatment can be expected to be long term. In a controlled study that compared 4 months to 1 year of SSRI treatment, approximately half of the patients who improved with SSRI treatment relapsed within 6 to 8 months after discontinuing medication. Longer treatment was marginally better at preventing relapse. Patients with more severe symptoms before treatment were the most likely to relapse, while patients who experienced symptom remission with treatment were least likely to relapse.

Conclusions

The SSRIs are currently the first-line treatment for severe PMS and PMDD. Continuous dosing and luteal phase dosing regimens are similarly effective for these disorders when the symptoms are clearly limited to the luteal phase of the menstrual cycle. Hormonal treatments have lacked consistent scientific evidence of their efficacy or safety or both for PMS treatment. Several new oral contraceptives that decrease or omit the placebo interval, calcium supplementation, and cognitive behavioral therapy may provide an effective alternative to antidepressant medications. Evidence indicates that long-term maintenance of the medication may be required for PMS and PMDD.

---

[1]Not FDA approved for this indication.

[2]Not available in the United States.
[7]Available as dietary supplement

References

American College of Obstetricians and Gynecologists: *Guidelines for women's health care: a resource manual*, 4th ed., Washington, DC, 2014, American College of Obstetricians and Gynecologists,. 2014.

American College of Obstetricians and Gynecologists: *Patient Education FAQ057*, Washington, DC, 2015, American College of Obstetricians and Gynecologists,. 2015.

American Psychiatric Association: *Diagnostic and statistical manual of mental disorders*, 5th ed, Arlington, VA, 2013, American Psychiatric Association.

Armour M, Ee CC, Hao J, et al: Acupuncture and acupressure for premenstrual syndrome, CD005290 *Cochrane Database Syst Rev* (8), 2018. Aug.

Freeman EW: Luteal phase administration of agents for the treatment of premenstrual dysphoric disorder, *CNS Drugs* 18(7):453–468, 2004.

Freeman EW, Rickels K, Sammel MD, et al: Time to relapse after short-term or long-term treatment of severe premenstrual syndrome with sertraline, *Arch Gen Psychiatry* 66(5):537–544, 2009.

Ismaili E, Walsh S, O'Brien PMS, et al: Fourth consensus of the International Society for Premenstrual Disorders (ISPMD): auditable standards for diagnosis and management of premenstrual disorder, *Arch Womens Ment Health*, 19(6):953–958, 2016.

Marjoribanks J, Brown J, O'Brien PMS, et al: Selective serotonin reuptake inhibitors for premenstrual syndrome (Review), *Cochrane Libr* 6:21–32, 2013.

McEvoy K, Osborne LM, Nanavati J, et al: Reproductive affective disorders: a review of the genetic evidence for premenstrual dysphoric disorder and postpartum depression, *Curr Psychiatry Rep* 94(19):94–106, 2017.

Naheed B, Kuiper JH, Uthman OA, et al: Non-contraceptive oestrogen-containing preparations for controlling symptoms of premenstrual syndrome, CD010503 *Cochrane Database of Syst Rev* (3), 2017. Mar.

Pearce E, Jolly K, Jones LL, et al: Exercise for premenstrual syndrome: a systematic review and meta-analysis of randomized controlled trials, 20X10132 *BJGP open* (3), 2020. Aug 4.

Whelan AM, Jurgens TM, Naylor H: Herbs, vitamins and minerals in the treatment of premenstrual syndrome: a systematic review, *Can J Clin Pharmacol* 16:c407–c429, 2009.

UTERINE LEIOMYOMA

Method of
James W. Haynes, MD; and Theodore T. Tsaltas, MD

CURRENT DIAGNOSIS

- Uterine leiomyomas are the most common pelvic tumors in women.
- Risk factors include African American ethnicity, family history, obesity, decreased physical activity, nulliparity, and early menarche.
- Exact pathophysiologic mechanism is unknown but tumors consist of swirls of smooth muscle cells and fibroblasts.
- The primary clinical manifestations of uterine fibroids include heavy menstrual bleeding and pelvic pain.
- Ultrasonography is the primary diagnostic test of choice when fibroids are suspected.
- Differential diagnoses includes adenomyosis, ectopic pregnancy, endometrial polyp, endometriosis, pregnancy, endometrial carcinoma, uterine sarcoma, and metastatic disease.

CURRENT THERAPY

- Therapy for uterine leiomyomas is based on symptoms, uterine size, and future fertility desires.
- Nonsurgical treatment options include nonsteroidal antiinflammatory drugs, oral contraceptives, progestational, and gonadotropin-releasing hormonal pharmaceutical agents.
- Indications for surgical treatment include uterine size >12 weeks, anemia from menometrorrhagia, soiling of clothing or bedding from menometrorrhagia, intractable dysmenorrhea or dyspareunia, and urinary or bowel obstruction.
- The definitive treatment option is hysterectomy with laparoscopic/robotic vaginal route being preferred.
- Other viable surgical interventions include myomectomy, uterine artery embolization, radio frequency focused ablation, and endometrial ablation.

Epidemiology

Uterine leiomyomas (fibroids) are the most common pelvic tumors in women. Approximately 30% to 50% of premenopausal women have ultrasound evidence of fibroids without symptoms. Leiomyomas rarely occur prior to puberty and incidence increases with age, peaks at age 50, and decreases after menopause. African American women have a two- to threefold incidence compared with Caucasian, Asian, and Hispanic women who have similar frequencies of fibroids. African American women have an earlier onset of disease with an average age of onset 5 years earlier compared with Caucasian women. Additionally, African American women have larger and more numerous fibroids compared with Caucasian women.

Risk Factors

Box 1 includes risk factors for uterine fibroid development. Consumption of vegetables and fruits, dark-meat fish, vitamin D, and vitamin A, as well as physical activity, are associated with a decreased risk of fibroids. Data is conflicting with respect to oral contraceptives and smoking, while breastfeeding, vitamin C, vitamin E, and folates have no association with the development of fibroids.

Pathophysiology

Uterine leiomyomas consist histologically of smooth muscle cells and fibroblasts that ultimately form round, hard tumors. The exact pathologic mechanism of disease is unknown but a smooth muscle cell mutation has been hypothesized.

Prevention

There are currently no proven therapies that prevent uterine fibroid formation. Identification of the genes responsible for fibroid growth in patients genetically predisposed to fibroids could possibly lead to genomic-mediated prevention of fibroids.

Clinical Manifestations

About 50% to 80% of uterine fibroids are asymptomatic. Heavy menstrual bleeding and pelvic pain are the most common symptoms associated with uterine fibroids. Additional symptoms include secondary dysmenorrhea, abdominal distention, pelvic pressure, urinary symptoms (urgency, frequency, incontinence, hydronephrosis), bowel dysfunction including constipation, back pain, dyspareunia, and infertility.

Diagnosis

Physical examination of the abdomen and pelvis may elucidate an enlarged uterus secondary to uterine fibroids. Transvaginal ultrasonography is 90% to 99% sensitive in the detection of uterine fibroids but may miss small or subserosal fibroids. Hysteroscopy or sonohysterography increase diagnostic sensitivity for subserosal myomas.

BOX 1	Uterine Fibroid Risk Factors

African American descent
First-degree relative with uterine fibroid
Early menarche
Less than three obstetric deliveries
Five years since last birth
Obesity
Metabolic syndrome
Decreased physical activity
Childhood trauma
Beef, red meat, ham
Vitamin D deficiency
Alcoholic beverages (especially beer)
Caffeine intake (younger women)
Hormone replacement therapy

Differential Diagnosis

Diagnostic possibilities in patients presenting with symptoms of uterine fibroids include adenomyosis, ectopic pregnancy, endometrial polyp, endometriosis, pregnancy, endometrial carcinoma, uterine carcinosarcoma, uterine sarcoma, and metastatic disease.

Treatment of Myomas

Myomas are benign lesions, hence, there is no a priori requirement for treatment. Management is based on symptoms and patient's wishes. Three parameters control recommendations: uterine size, severity of symptoms, and the patient's interest in childbearing.

There are a limited number of options for management:
- Definitive surgery
  - Hysterectomy (various methods)
- Palliative/uterine conserving surgery
  - Myomectomy (open or laparoscopic)
  - Hysteroscopic myomectomy
  - Uterine artery embolization
  - Radiofrequency focused ablation
- Symptomatic treatment
  - Nonsteroidal antiinflammatory drugs (NSAIDs)
  - Oral contraceptives
  - Progestational agents
  - Gonadotropin-releasing hormone (GnRH) agonists
  - Endometrial ablation

The indicators for surgical intervention include the following:
- Uterine size >12 weeks (>14 weeks for some insurers to cover)
- Anemia from menometrorrhagia
- Soiling of clothing or bedding from menometrorrhagia
- Intractable dysmenorrhea or dyspareunia
- Urinary or bowel obstruction

The choice of procedure is strongly constrained by a patient's desire for future childbearing. This precludes hysterectomy and procedures that destroy the endometrial cavity to stop bleeding, such as endometrial ablations. Uterine conservation may prove impossible or have marked complications if the number of myomas is large. Of note, surgical intervention for subfertility is indicated in selected cases but the data related to optimal methods of management is limited and inconclusive.

Hysterectomy

While multiple newer treatments have been introduced, hysterectomy remains the single most common management. It is definitive, ending mass impingement symptoms, bleeding, pain, urinary frequency, and constipation with a single intervention. Recurrence of myomas is extremely rare after hysterectomy.

The route of hysterectomy remains under debate. When possible, a vaginal hysterectomy is the preferred route, as it has the lowest morbidity of all types. More than two-thirds of hysterectomies for myomas are still done by open abdominal route, despite laparoscopy and robotic surgery having been repeatedly demonstrated as equivalent or superior for blood loss and complications.

Surgical complications of hysterectomy are common, but significant complications are rare. The most common problems are urinary tract infection (~25%) and superficial wound disruptions. More serious complications include deep venous thrombosis and pulmonary embolism, anaerobic pelvic cellulitis, and pneumonia. Organ injury to bowel, bladder, blood vessel, or ureter occurs in approximately 1/500 cases, 1/1000 for vaginal procedures. Bleeding sufficient to require transfusion occurs in about 1% of hysterectomies.

Myomectomy

Myomectomy is the procedure of choice for symptomatic myomas in women desiring fertility preservation. Myomas may be removed abdominally, vaginally, laparoscopically, or via hysteroscopy, depending on their size and location. Myomectomy does not necessarily lead to future cesarean delivery, but if cavity integrity is violated or there is an extensive dissection it then becomes mandatory.

Laparoscopic procedures are much less invasive but require significant skill. Closure of myomectomy defects is also difficult and time consuming. Hystereoscopic resection is an elegant technique applicable only to intracavitary myomas.

Between 40% and 75% of patients undergoing myomectomy will have a future hysterectomy. Complication rates from open myomectomy are significantly higher than for hysterectomy, accounted for by fever and blood loss.

Uterine Artery Embolization

Uterine artery embolization (UAE) now accounts for approximately 3% of myomectomies. The method uses injectable microspheres placed under fluoroscopic guidance. It is effective for isolated myomas of moderate size (up to 5 cm), although lesions up to 9 cm have been treated by UAE. It is an outpatient procedure done in interventional radiology suites without entering the abdominal cavity.

There are several significant problems with UAE that have limited its broad application. Inflammatory mediators released by myoma necrosis can cause substantial cramping and bowel symptoms. Lesion defects cannot be closed, leading to uterine wall defects with secondary placental implantation abnormalities and uterine rupture in pregnancy. Vascular anatomy is quite variable, and microspheres can be injected into any of the branches of the internal iliac. This can lead to necrosis of bladder, buttock, or vulva. Limitations in available facilities as well as trained and experienced operators, combined with the significant complications, has limited usage of UAE.

Radiofrequency Ablation

This technique uses focused, high frequency radio wave or ultrasound to cause mechanical destruction of myomas. It is an uncommon technique because of limited facilities and experienced practitioners. It does not have the potentially disfiguring complications of UAE but does have all its other problems, as well as risk of destruction of normal uterine tissue.

Observation

Since myomas are benign, they may be observed if indications for hysterectomy noted above are not met. In this setting the goal is symptom control. Cramping can be managed with NSAIDs. Acetaminophen (Tylenol) has less than 30% of the peripheral antiinflammatory activity of ibuprofen (Advil, Motrin) so that ibuprofen, aspirin, and other NSAIDs are much preferred. The individual drug choice relies with the patient and practitioner.

Bleeding can be improved with oral contraceptives, progestational agents, or tranexamic acid (Lysteda). In pooled results, tranexamic acid was more effective than medroxyprogesterone injection (Depo-Provera)[1] used over an equivalent time, reducing menstrual blood loss by 30%. Depo-Provera also provides contraception and uterine mass shrinkage at the expense of breakthrough bleeding. Progestational intrauterine devices are a possible option for bleeding control without causing systemic side effects. While appealing, like other medical management options, these devices do not alter the course of the myoma.

GnRH agonists are extremely effective in effecting uterine mass shrinkage. Volume reduction up to 70% is possible with a 3-month course. Myoma reexpansion is, however, prompt and returns to original size. GnRH agonists are thus not suitable for treatment of myomas. Rather, they are best used to shrink myomas prior to surgery, making their removal easier and faster. Since Depo-Provera achieves almost as much shrinkage, few insurers cover GnRH agonists for this purpose.

---

[1]Not FDA approved for this indication.

Managing Complications

Complications other than pain and bleeding are uncommon. Uterine mass and distortion can become so great as to obstruct venous return from the legs and pelvis, leading to deep venous thrombosis. Obstipation can occur, requiring manual disimpaction. More frequently, but still uncommon, urinary obstruction with retention or inability to void is possible.

The most frequent problem during observation of myomas is degeneration. Myomas are monoclonal tumors and thus have only a single, primary blood supply. If their growth outstrips available perfusion, the myocytes undergo necrosis. This can be quite painful. Management consists of NSAIDs, heavy hydration, rest, and occasional use of opioids. If initial interventions fail, inpatient management may be necessary for pain control. Intramuscular ketorolac (Toradol) materially reduces pain and can be used in an outpatient setting.

Leiomyomatosis peritonealis disseminata is a very rare condition where myomatous change occurs along the smooth muscle of the internal iliac arterioles. It can produce pelvic congestion, altered perfusion, and deep venous thrombosis. Management is by hysterectomy followed by GnRH agonists for 3 to 6 months. Complete resolution is the norm.

Myomas do not undergo malignant degeneration, but the frequency of uterine sarcoma is generally expressed as a proportion of all myoma cases. Uterine sarcomas are rare, with incidental discovery in a myomatous uterus in about 1/1000 myomatous uteri. Early epidemiologic studies on power morcellators indicated a rate of sarcoma in myomatous uteri of up to 1%. Larger studies have clearly shown this is a massive overstatement. Many hospitals are accordingly again allowing use of power morcellation for myomectomy and laparoscopic removal of large hysterectomy specimens.

Some situations with myomas require prompt attention. Sudden, rapid uterine growth in a woman over 40 years of age should prompt consideration for sarcoma. Similarly, such tumors should not be morcellated but removed intact, either by open surgery or a laparoscopy with minilap.

Myomas can be confused with thecoma-fibromas, a benign ovarian tumor. The thecoma-fibroma is usually stone hard and heavily calcified on ultrasound but can be so large and firm that it cannot be distinguished from a myoma. Laparoscopy can distinguish the lesions.

References

Al-Hendy A, Myers ER, Stewart E: Uterine Fibroids: burden and unmet medical need, *Semin Reprod Med* 35:473–480, 2017.

Alternatives to hysterectomy in the management of leiomyomas, *Obstet Gynecol* 96, 2008.

De La Cruz MD, Buchanan EM: Uterine fibroids: diagnosis and treatment, *Am Fam Physician* 95(2):100–107, 2017.

Emanuel MH, Wamsteker K, Hart AA, Metz G, et al: Long-term results of hysteroscopic myomectomy for abnormal uterine bleeding, *Obstet Gynecol* 93(5):743–748, 1999.

Keder L, Olsen M, editors: *Gynecologic Care*, Cambridge University Press, 2018.

Keller JM, Gaba ND: Vaginal hysterectomy, chapter 10.

Keder L, Olsen M, editors: *Gynecologic Care*, Cambridge University Press, 2018. Cronin B: Abdominal hysterectomy, Chapter 11.

Keder L, Olsen M, editors: *Gynecologic Care*, Cambridge University Press, 2018. Tsaltas, T: Laparoscopic hysterectomy, Chapter 12.

Lumsden MA, Hamoodi I, Gupta J, Hickey M: Fibroids: diagnosis and management, *BMJ* 35:h4887, 2015.

Metwally M, Raybould G, Cheong YC, et al: Surgical treatment of fibroids for subfertility, *Cochrane Database Syst Rev* (1)CD003857, 2020.

Palomba S, Zupi E, Falbo A, Russo T, et al: A multicenter randomized, controlled study comparing laparoscopic versus minilaparotomic myomectomy: reproductive outcomes, *Fertil Steril* 88(4):933–941, 2007.

Pavone D, Clemenza S, Sorbi F, Fambrini M, Petraglia F: Epidemiology and risk factors of uterine fibroids, *Best Pract Res Clin Obstet Gynaecol* 46:3–11, 2018.

Spies JB, Bruno J, Czeyda-Pommersheim F, Magee ST, et al: Long-term outcome of uterine artery embolization of leiomyomata, *Obstet Gynecol* 106(5):933–939, 2005.

Tanos V, Berry KE: Benign and malignant pathology of the uterus, *Best Pract Res Clin Obstet Gynaecol* 46:12–30, 2018.

Wallach EE, Vlahos NF: Uterine myomas: an overview of development, clinical features, and management, *Obstet Gynecol* 104(2):393–406, 2004.

VULVAR NEOPLASIA

Method of
Christine Conageski, MD

CURRENT DIAGNOSIS

- Most cystic lesions are benign. Excision is reserved for symptomatic cysts and suspicious Bartholin's gland cysts, especially in women older than 40 years of age.
- All solid lesions should be biopsied for diagnostic purposes.
- Multifocal disease requires multiple biopsies to rule out invasive disease.
- Most premalignant and malignant lesions cause pruritus, discomfort, or a noticeable lesion.
- The vagina and cervix in women with dysplastic or malignant vulvar lesions should be evaluated.

CURRENT THERAPY

- Benign solid lesions should be excised.
- After ablative treatment of vulvar intraepithelial neoplasia (VIN), excise any residual lesions to rule out occult invasive disease.
- Avoid podophyllin and 5-fluorouracil in women of reproductive potential.
- Rule out synchronous neoplasms in women with Paget's disease.
- Invasion more than 1 mm requires radical excision and lymph node evaluation.

The female external genitalia includes the mons pubis, labia majora, labia minora, clitoris, perineal body, and the structures of the vaginal introitus or vestibule. Whether benign or malignant, vulvar neoplasms are uncommon, occur at all ages, and have varying characteristics. Therefore liberal use of biopsies is usually required for diagnosis and treatment decisions.

Benign Cystic Neoplasms

Benign cystic lesions of the vulva include Bartholin's duct cyst, sebaceous and epidermal inclusion cysts, mucinous cysts, Skene duct cysts, and cysts of the canal of Nuck. Bartholin's duct cyst, located in the posterior labia near the vaginal introitus, is most common. Treatment is usually not required in asymptomatic young women (<40 years). If the cyst is symptomatic or infected, however, drainage, marsupialization or use of a Word catheter, is indicated. Bartholin's gland carcinomas are rare, especially in women younger than 40 years of age. But if the mass feels firm or nodular, it should be biopsied.

Sebaceous and epidermal inclusion cysts are also common. They are prone to infection but rarely malignant. If an infection develops, they should be incised and drained. Mucinous cysts are rare and possibly arise from the minor vestibular glands. They are located anteriorly on the vulva, typically on the inner labia minora. Skene duct cysts are located next to the urethra. Excision of these cysts is necessary only if symptomatic.

Cysts of the canal of Nuck are located in the anterior portion of the labia majora at the termination of the insertion of the round ligament. These cysts represent herniation of the peritoneum through the inguinal canal and contain peritoneal fluid. If symptomatic, excision must be accompanied by closure of the fascial defect to prevent recurrence.

Benign Solid Neoplasms

The benign solid tumors of the vulva include fibromas, myomas, lipomas, hidradenomas, syringomas, myoblastomas, vestibular adenomas, and angiomas, among others. Benign pigmented lesions, such as nevi and seborrheic keratoses, may occasionally be found. Malignancy is rare, but most should be excised for diagnostic and therapeutic purposes.

Condyloma Acuminatum

Vulvar condyloma acuminatum is a sexually transmitted verrucous lesion of the vulva caused by human papilloma virus (HPV), most frequently types 6 and 11. These lesions are warty growths that frequently cover large areas of the vulva. Smoking and immunosuppression are risk factors. Representative biopsies should be obtained to document disease and rule out malignancy. Wide local excision can be used for small lesions, although these growths are usually best treated by ablation to avoid morbdity associated with excision.

Chemical ablative techniques include self or provider-administered medications. Self-administered medications include topical podofilox (0.5%, Condylox) or imiquimod (5%, Aldara). Podofilox is applied twice daily for 3 days, repeated weekly for 4 weeks and imiquimod is applied three times per week for up to 16 weeks. It is primarily an immune modulator. Providers may instead choose in-office application of trichloroacetic acid (Tri-Chlor), 5-fluorouracil[1] (1%, Fluoroplex or 5%, Efudex),[1] or podophyllin. Podophyllin and 5-fluorouracil should not be used in women who could become pregnant. Surgical ablative therapies include CO_2 laser vaporization and use of the Cavitron ultrasonic aspirator (CUSA), especially for extensive disease.

Intraepithelial Neoplasms of the Vulva

Vulvar Intraepithelial Neoplasia

Vulvar intraepithelial neoplasia (VIN) is a dysplastic condition of the squamous epithelium whose incidence is increasing, especially in younger women. There are two pathologically distinct types of VIN, usual and differentiated types.

The usual type has a strong association with HPV infections and thus shares similar risk factors with cervical intraepithelial neoplasias (CIN). These risk factors include early first intercourse, multiple sexual partners, smoking, and immunosuppression. Up to 22% of women have concurrent CIN lesions and up to 71% have had a previous, concominant or subsequent history of vaginal intraepithelial neoplasia. Differentiated VIN is not associated with HPV and is found in relation to vulvar dermatoses such as lichen sclerosus. Differentiated VIN typically occurs in older women with a mean age of 67 years compared to 47.8 years in usual type VIN. Symptoms of both types include pruritus (most common), pain, a noticeable lesion, and discoloration. Most patients with HPV-related disease have multifocal lesions. Typical findings are raised white, gray, red, or mottled lesions; application of 4% acetic acid for several minutes can help identify faint lesions and outline abnormal vascular patterns. Diagnosis of VIN is made by punch biopsies through full thickness of the epithelium to rule out invasion. Usual and differentiated VIN have very different cancer progression risks, 5.7% for HPV-mediated VIN and 32.8% for differentiated VIN. Differentiated VIN, also, has a shorter time to progression, 22.8 months compared to 41.4 months.

Treatment of VIN can be categorized into excisional and ablative therapies. Management should be individualized to each patient taking into account risk of progression, distribution of disease and histologic features on biopsy. Often a combination of medical and surgical management is appropriate. Patients at risk for microinvasion (unifocal disease, raised lesions, older age, and prior radiation) should have the lesion excised completely if possible. Skinning vulvectomy is rarely used because of psychological and sexual consequences related to scarring and disfigurement.

The ablative therapies can be divided into mechanical and chemical. The mechanical method most commonly used is the CO_2 laser, although use of the CUSA is also described. Both can ablate large or multifocal lesions successfully with an excellent cosmetic and functional outcome. The chemical method most commonly used is topical 5-fluorouracil (5%, Efudex).[1] Because of its teratogenic potential, it should not be used in women who could become pregnant. It canbe applied on two consecutive nights weekly for

TABLE 1	Recurrence of Vulvar Intraepithelial Neoplasia III
TREATMENT METHOD	**% RECURRENCE**
Chemical ablation	20–40
Mechanical ablation	20–40
Wide local excision	
Negative margin	15–25
Positive margin	30–45

10 weeks. An alternative ablative therapy is use of imiquimod[1] (Aldara), as described earlier. Because of the irritation caused by these topical therapies, many patients have problems with treatment compliance. Residual disease should be excised to rule out invasion.

Patients with VIN frequently have recurrent disease, regardless of the treatment method used (Table 1). Continued smoking increases this risk, so patients should be counseled in smoking cessation. In those patients whose cancers recur and are retreated, subsequent 5-fluorouracil prophylaxis, with a single application biweekly, is used successfully to minimize further recurrences.

Paget's Disease

Paget's disease of the vulva is an uncommon condition characterized by a patchy, eczematoid lesion that frequently covers much of the vulva. Most patients are postmenopausal and present with complaints of pruritus. Although Paget's disease is an in situ disease process, 15% to 25% of patients have an underlying malignancy, usually an adenocarcinoma of the apocrine glands but occasionally an invasive Paget's. In addition, up to 30% of patients have a synchronous adenocarcinoma of the breast, colon, rectum, or upper genital tract. Screening for these cancers is therefore recommended. To assess for invasion, the lesion should be excised via wide local excision or simple vulvectomy with at least 5 mm of the adjacent subcutaneous tissue. Achieving negative margin status is frequently difficult. However, the risk of recurrence is approximately 30% whether margins are negative or positive. Thus expectant management, reserving treatment for symptomatic recurrences, is usually recommended.

Invasive Vulvar Lesions

Less than 5% of gynecologic cancers arise on the vulva. Over 90% are squamous cell carcinomas. The etiology of this type appears mixed. The differentiated type is more common, occurs in older women (age 60–69, mean age 65) and is associated with vulvar dystrophies. The classic or usual type is predominantly associated with HPV-16. These women are slightly younger (age 45–52 years) and present with earlier stage disease. Other histologic types are melanomas (5%–10%), basal cell carcinomas (2%–3%), adenocarcinomas (1%), and sarcomas (1%–2%). Most patients present with a combination of symptoms, including pruritus, discomfort, and complaints of a mass. Examination frequently reveals a suspicious lesion, which should be biopsied for diagnosis. Vulvar cancers typically spread by local extension and lymphatic dissemination. Factors that influence dissemination include tumor size (Table 2), depth of invasion (Table 3), lymphovascular space invasion, and tumor grade. Staging is surgical and classified using the tumor, nodes, and metastasis (TNM) system as well as the International Federation of Gynecology and Obstetrics (FIGO) system (Table 4).

Squamous Cell Carcinomas and Adenocarcinomas

Surgical management of squamous cell carcinomas and adenocarcinomas depends on the size, depth of invasion, and location of the lesion. The vulvar lesion is managed with a radical excision. Management of the groins is based on depth of invasion. Lesions with invasion of less than 1 mm (Stage IA) have minimal risk of lymphatic spread (<1%) and do not require lymphadenectomy. All others require surgical assessment of the lymph nodes. Lesions

---

[1]Not FDA approved for this indication.

[1]Not FDA approved for this indication.

TABLE 2	Incidence of Regional Node Metastases by Tumor Diameter
TUMOR DIAMETER (CM)	**% POSITIVE INGUINAL NODES**
<1	1–15
5–20	
25–35	
35–50	
≥50	≥50

TABLE 3	Incidence of Regional Node Metastases by Depth of Tumor Invasion
DEPTH OF INVASION (MM)	**% POSITIVE INGUINAL NODES**
<1	1–5
1–3	10–15
3–5	15–30
5–10	30–45

less than 2 cm in size of the primary tumor, greater than 2 cm from the vulvar midline and are of squamous histology require only unilateral lymphadenectomy. Those without these characteristics or have palpable lymph nodes of the contralateral side require bilateral assessment. This surgical approach is associated with significant morbidity including disfigurement, wound breakdown, and problems with lymphocysts and chronic lymphedema. For patients with very large lesions or lesions in sensitive areas such as the clitoris, preoperative radiation, followed by less radical excision of residual disease, may minimize problems with the vulvar wound. Current investigations are ongoing in the use of sentinel lymph node dissections as a method of minimizing the groin morbidity without sacrificing survival. Positive vulvar margins or metastases to lymph nodes are managed with postoperative radiation. Survival depends on stage at diagnosis (Table 5).

Verrucous Carcinoma

Verrucous carcinoma is a large exophytic tumor that resembles giant condyloma acuminatum. It is a variant of squamous carcinomas but has an excellent prognosis because of the lack of metastases. Verrucous carcinomas have a high tendency to recur and should be managed with radical local excision.

Malignant Melanoma

Malignant melanoma is the second most common vulvar malignancy. Most patients have disease on the mucosal surfaces of the vulvar introitus, clitoris, and labia minora. The vulvar lesion is treated by radical excision, but management of the groins is controversial. The risk of spread is significant with a tumor thickness greater than 0.75 mm, but survival at 5 years is only approximately 10% with groin node metastases. Some argue against node dissection for this reason. However, given some long-term survivors with modern melanoma therapy, either lymphadenectomy or sentinel lymph node dissection, as is done for other cutaneous melanomas, appears indicated.

Basal Cell Carcinoma

Basal cell carcinomas typically occur in elderly white women, are commonly located on the labia majora, and have characteristics similar to basal cell carcinomas at other sites. Treatment is wide local excision only because metastases are rare. Basal cell carcinomas are prone to local recurrence, however. A malignant squamous component must be ruled out because it should be managed as a squamous cell carcinoma.

TABLE 4	Staging Vulvar Carcinoma	
TNM CATEGORIES	**FIGO STAGES**	
T Primary tumor		
T0		No evidence of primary tumor
Tis		Carcinoma in situ
T1	I	Confined to vulva
T1a	IA	Lesions ≤2 cm in size, confined to the vulva or perineum and with stromal invasion ≤1 mm
T1b	IB	Lesions >2 cm in size OR any size with stromal invasion >1.0 mm, confined to the vulva or perineum
T2	II	Tumor of any size with extension to adjacent perineal structures (lower/distal 1/3 urethra, lower/distal 1/3 vagina, anal involvement)
T2	III	Tumor of any size with or without extension to adjacent perineal structures (lower/distal 1/3 urethra, lower/distal 1/3 vagina, anal involvement) with positive inguino-femoral lymph nodes
T3	IVA	Tumor of any size with extension to any of the following: upper/proximal 2/3 of urethra, upper/proximal 2/3 vagina, bladder mucosa, rectal mucosa, or fixed to pelvic bone
T3	IVB	Any distant metases including pelvic lymph nodes
TNM CATEGORIES	**FIGO STAGES**	
N Regional lymph nodes		
N0		No lymph node metastases
N1		One or two regional lymph nodes with the following features:
N1b	IIIAi	One lymph node metastasis, ≥ 5 mm
N1a	IIIAii	One to two lymph node metastases, < 5 mm
N2	IIIB	Regional lymph node metastasis with the following features:
N2b	IIIBi	Two or more lymph node metastases, ≥ 5 mm
N2a	IIIBii	Three or more lymph node metastases, <5 mm
N2c	IIIC	Lymph node metastasis with extracapsular spread
N3	IVA	Fixed or ulcerated regional lymph node metastasis
TNM CATEGORIES	**FIGO STAGES**	
M Distant metastases		
M0		No distant metastases
M1	IVB	Distant metastasis (including pelvic lymph node metastasis)

Abbreviations: TNM = tumor, node, metastasis; FIGO = International Federation of Gynecology and Obstetrics.

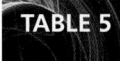

TABLE 5 Survival Rate by FIGO Stage for Patients With Invasive Squamous Cell Vulvar Cancer

FIGO STAGE	OVERALL SURVIVAL (PERCENT)		
	One year	Two years	Five years
I	96.4	90.4	78.5
II	87.6	73.2	58.8
III	74.7	53.8	43.2
IV	35.3	16.9	13.0

Abbreviation: FIGO = International Federation of Gynecology and Obstetrics.

Sarcomas

Leiomyosarcoma is the most common vulvar sarcoma and usually arises in the labia majora. Malignant fibrous histiocytoma is the second most common. Management of these lesions is radical vulvar excision.

References

Beller U, Quinn MA, Benedet JL, et al: Carcinoma of the vulva, *Int J Gynaecol Obstet* 95:S7, 2006.

Garland SM: Imiquimod, *Curr Opin Infect Dis* 16:85–89, 2003.

Homesley HD, Bundy BN, Sedlis A, et al: Prognostic factors for groin node metastasis in squamous cell carcinoma of the vulva (a Gynecologic Oncology Group study), *Gynecol Oncol* 49:279–283, 1993.

Hording U, Junge J, Lundvall F: Vulvar intraepithelial neoplasia III: a viral disease of undetermined progressive potential, *Gynecol Oncol* 56(2):276, 1995.

Krebs HB: The use of topical 5-fluorouracil in the treatment of genital condylomas, *Obstet Gynecol Clin North Am* 14(2):559–568, 1987.

Modesitt SC, Waters AB, Walton L, et al: Vulvar intraepithelial neoplasia III: Occult cancer and the impact of margin status on recurrence, *Obstet Gynecol* 92(6):962–966, 1998.

Phillips GL, Bundy BN, Okagaki T, et al: Malignant melanoma of the vulva treated by radical hemivulvectomy, a prospective study of the Gynecologic Oncology Group, *Cancer* 73:2626–2632, 1994.

Tebes S, Cardosi R, Hoffman M: Paget's disease of the vulva, *Am J Obstet Gynecol* 187:281–284, 2002.

Trimble CL, Trimble EL, Woodruff JD: Diseases of the vulva. In Hernandez E, Atkinson BE, editors: *Clinical Gynecologic Pathology*, Philadelphia, 1995, WB Saunders, pp 1–90.

Van de Nieuwehnof, et al. Vulvar squamous cell carcinoma development after diagnosis of VIN increases with age. *Eur J Canc* 45:851, 2009.

Wright VC, Chapman WB: Colposcopy of intraepithelial neoplasia of the vulva and adjacent sites, *Obstet Gynecol Clin North Am* 20(1):231–255, 1993.

VULVOVAGINITIS

Method of
Heather L. Paladine, MD, MEd; and Urmi Desai, MD, MS

CURRENT DIAGNOSIS

- The most common causes of vulvovaginitis are bacterial vaginosis, candidal vulvovaginitis, and *Trichomonas* infection.
- Vulvovaginitis should be diagnosed by a combination of patient history, physical exam findings, and office-based or laboratory testing. Patients should not be treated presumptively based on history and examination.
- Bacterial vaginosis is diagnosed based on at least three of four of the Amsel criteria: fishy vaginal odor spontaneously or with KOH testing; vaginal pH above 4.5; thin, homogeneous vaginal discharge; and clue cells on saline microscopy.
- Vulvovaginal candidiasis is diagnosed based on symptoms of a thick whitish discharge, itching, and/or discomfort together with budding or pseudohyphae on KOH microscopy or positive fungal culture.
- The gold standard for *Trichomonas* diagnosis is nucleic acid amplification testing.

CURRENT TREATMENT

- Treatment of bacterial vaginosis is recommended for symptomatic women, and both oral and topical metronidazole (Flagyl tablet[1], MetroGel (75%) or topical clindamycin (Cleocin 2%) are first-line treatments for both pregnant and nonpregnant women.
- First-line treatment for symptomatic women with vulvovaginal candidiasis includes either oral fluconazole (Diflucan) or topical azole therapy for nonpregnant women; for pregnant women, topical therapy is preferred.
- First-line therapy for *Trichomonas* infection includes a one-time dose of metronidazole for both pregnant and nonpregnant patients.
- Patients should be adequately counseled about treatment regimens for vaginitis, including discussion of disulfiram-like reactions with alcohol consumption when taking metronidazole and tinidazole (Tindamax), potential weakening of condoms by oil-based topical therapies, and the importance of avoidance of sexual intercourse until treatment of bacterial vaginosis or *Trichomonas* is complete.

[1]Not FDA approved for this indication.

Epidemiology

The term *vulvovaginitis* includes conditions that result in irritation of the vagina or vulva, causing symptoms of itching, burning, pain, odor, or discharge. Vulvovaginitis is a common condition in women's health, accounting for about 10% of office visits each year and affecting almost every woman at some point in her life. The three most common causes of vulvovaginitis are bacterial vaginosis (BV, accounting for up to 50% of cases in which a diagnosis is made), vulvovaginal candidiasis (VVC, accounting for 30% of cases), and *Trichomonas* (accounting for 15% to 20% of cases). The remaining diagnoses include genitourinary syndrome of menopause (GSM, formerly called atrophic vaginitis), inflammatory vaginitis, and allergic/irritant vaginitis. A specific cause is not found in up to 30% of patients.

Risk Factors

Risk factors for vulvovaginitis vary by condition. Although BV is not a sexually transmitted infection, it occurs almost exclusively in women of reproductive age who are sexually active and more commonly in women with new or multiple sexual partners. BV is found more often in women who smoke cigarettes or douche.

VVC is more common in women who are immunosuppressed, such as those who have HIV or diabetes, or are pregnant. Recent antibiotic use is also a risk factor.

Trichomonas is a sexually transmitted infection and is more likely to occur in women who have other sexually transmitted infections, who have multiple sexual partners, or who have had unprotected intercourse. As with many sexually transmitted infections, disparities exist in the prevalence of *Trichomonas*, with infections more commonly occurring in nonwhite, low-income, and formerly incarcerated people.

Pathophysiology

In women of reproductive age, the normal vaginal environment is acidic, with a pH of less than 4.6. This is thought to be due to the prevalence of lactobacilli, which produce lactic acid, as part of the normal vaginal flora; however, the exact mechanism is unclear. BV represents a shift in the normal vaginal flora to anaerobic bacteria. The mechanism of this shift is also not entirely clear but is associated with risk factors such as douching and intercourse, which may change the vaginal pH.

VVC is caused by infection with species of candidal fungi, most commonly *Candida albicans*. Some 10% to 30% of women may have candida organisms among their normal vaginal flora.

TABLE 1	Diagnosis of Vulvovaginitis			
CONDITION	**SYMPTOMS**	**EXAM FINDINGS**	**PH**	**MICROSCOPY FINDINGS**
Normal	Discharge changes with menstrual cycle	Thin clear or whitish discharge	Normal (4–4.5)	Epithelial cells, lactobacilli
Bacterial vaginosis	Fishy odor, vaginal discharge, vaginal discomfort/dyspareunia	Homogenous gray/white discharge	Elevated (≥4.6)	Clue cells on wet mount
Vulvovaginal candidiasis	Vulvar irritation or itching, vaginal discharge	Vulvar excoriations or erythema Thick, clumpy white discharge	Normal (4–4.5)	Pseudohyphae or budding yeast on KOH exam
Trichomonas	Foul-smelling discharge, vaginal pain or discomfort	Cervical inflammation with "strawberry cervix," yellow-green frothy vaginal discharge	Elevated (≥4.6)	Mobile trichomonads on wet mount, white blood cells
Genitourinary syndrome of menopause (formerly atrophic vaginitis)	Vulvar itching, vaginal pain or discomfort, dyspareunia, vaginal dryness	Vulvar excoriations, clear vaginal discharge, thin friable mucosa with loss of vaginal rugae	Elevated (≥4.6)	May have white blood cells, parabasal cells, decreased lactobacilli
Irritant/allergic vaginitis	Vulvar or vaginal discomfort or pain	Vulvar or vaginal erythema, fissures, lichenification	Elevated (≥4.6)	May have white blood cells, parabasal cells, decreased lactobacilli
Inflammatory vaginitis	Vulvar or vaginal discomfort, pain or burning; Vaginal discharge	Purulent vaginal discharge Vaginal erythema or rash	Elevated (≥4.6)	Many white blood cells, parabasal cells, decreased lactobacilli

Candidal infections result from an interaction between biologic, genetic, and environmental factors leading to differences in the host immune response, host susceptibility, and the virulence of different strains of *Candida*.

Trichomonas is a protozoan infection. The risk factors as already described are similar to those for other sexually transmitted infections.

Prevention

Although previous studies have defined risk factors for BV, it is not known whether avoiding these risk factors (such as douching or unprotected intercourse) will reduce the risk. Studies that have looked at the prevention of recurrent BV through treatment with probiotics such as lactobacilli or other methods to maintain an acidic vaginal pH have not been conclusive.

Routine testing for conditions such as HIV or diabetes is not recommended in women with VVC unless she has other risk factors. Women who are prone to develop VVC after taking antibiotics can use topical or oral antifungal medications during their treatment with antibiotics. Although probiotics are commonly used for the prevention and treatment of VVC, they have not been well studied.

Trichomonas is a sexually transmitted infection; therefore prevention includes condom use or being in a monogamous relationship.

Clinical Manifestations

Table 1 includes symptoms and physical examination findings for the common causes of vulvovaginitis. These symptoms can cause significant feelings of shame, distress, and decreased quality of life, especially in women with recurrent infections.

Diagnosis

The diagnosis of vulvovaginitis is unreliable based on history and physical examination findings alone and should include office-based or laboratory testing to confirm. There is a risk of misdiagnosis or delay in diagnosis with presumptive treatment, as patients may get temporary relief of vulvovaginal symptoms with topical antifungals even if they do not have a fungal infection. Although newer laboratory tests have become available for the

TABLE 2	Amsel Criteria
CRITERION	**POSITIVE RESULT**
Vaginal discharge	Thin homogeneous discharge
Odor of discharge	Fishy odor on testing with KOH
Vaginal pH	pH ≥4.6
Microscopy	Clue cells on saline microscopy

Three positive criteria are needed for a diagnosis of bacterial vaginosis.

diagnosis of BV and VVC, the American College of Obstetricians and Gynecologists continues to recommend testing with history, examination, microscopy, and pH testing unless microscopy is not available. The newer tests include DNA testing for *Gardnerella vaginalis* or the presence of vaginal sialidase activity for the diagnosis of BV and DNA testing for *Candida* species. The newer tests are also less cost effective. Table 1 also includes pH and microscopy findings for causes of vulvovaginitis.

BV is traditionally diagnosed via the Amsel criteria (Table 2), although Gram stain is considered the gold standard. A positive diagnosis requires three out of four criteria: fishy vaginal odor or positive odor on testing of vaginal discharge with 10% potassium hydroxide (KOH); vaginal pH above 4.5; a thin, homogeneous vaginal discharge; and clue cells (epithelial cells with adherent bacteria (Fig. 1) on microscopic examination of vaginal discharge with normal saline (wet mount).

VVC is diagnosed based on the combination of clinical signs and symptoms and either microscopy or fungal culture of vaginal discharge. Microscopy has a sensitivity of 50% to 70% for candidal vulvovaginitis; therefore fungal culture is recommended when microscopy is negative in a patient with typical symptoms. Fig. 2 demonstrates microscopy results with KOH that are positive for yeast. Fungal culture can also identify non-*albicans* species of *Candida*, which may be more difficult to treat.

Nucleic acid amplification testing is recommended for the diagnosis of *Trichomonas*, as microscopy is only 50% to 60%

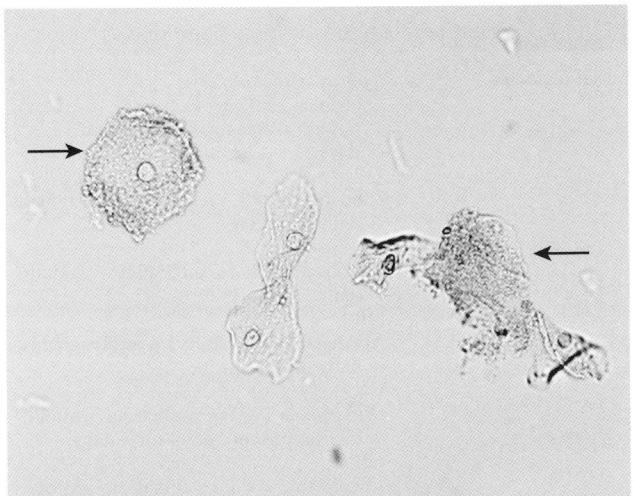

Figure 1 Clue cells on saline microscopy. (From Brunzel: *Fundamentals of Urine & Body Fluid Analysis*, Fourth Edition. Elsevier, 2018.)

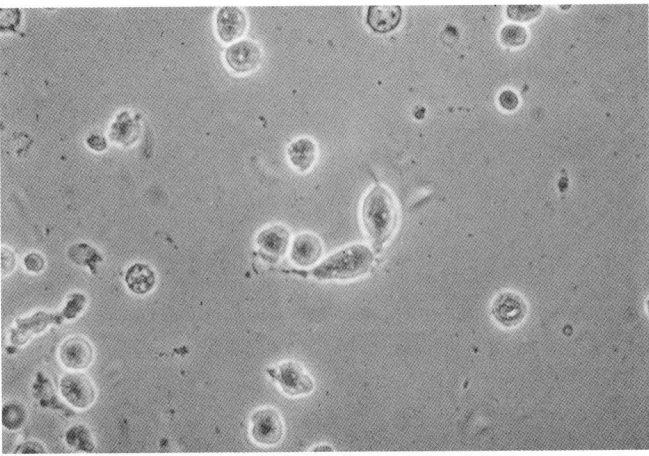

Figure 3 *Trichomonas* on saline microscopy. (From Mandell GL, Bennett JE, Dolin R: *Principles and Practice of Infectious Diseases*, Seventh Edition, Churchill Livingstone Elsevier, 2010.)

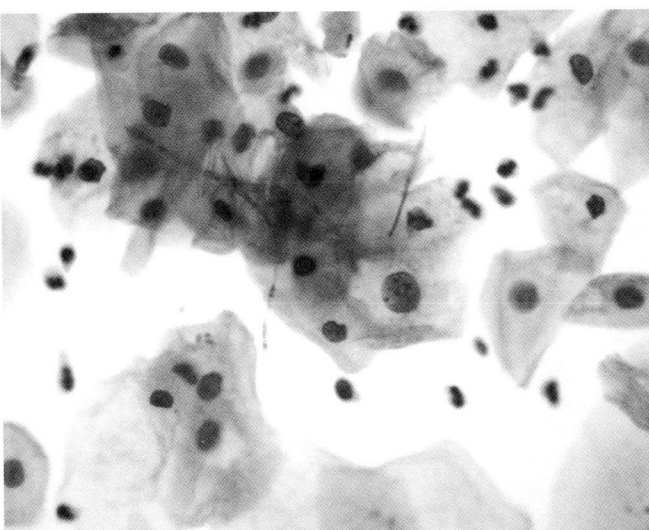

Figure 2 Candidal pseudohyphae on KOH microscopy. (From Herran CP, Nucci MR: *Gynecologic Pathology: A Volume in the Series Foundations in Diagnostic Pathology*, Second Edition. Elsevier, 2021.)

sensitive. Commercial DNA probe tests are also available, as well as a point-of-care antigen detection test. Sensitivities may be lower with the newer tests, although this varies by test. Fig. 3 shows positive saline microscopy for *Trichomonas*.

Differential Diagnosis

In addition to BV, VVC, and *Trichomonas*, other less common conditions can result in vulvovaginal symptoms. GSM was formerly known as atrophic vaginitis and results from a decrease in estrogen levels following menopause. Women who are breast-feeding or using progestin-only contraception also have a relative estrogen deficiency and may experience similar symptoms. GSM is characterized by vaginal dryness and discomfort and may also include urinary tract symptoms and clear vaginal discharge. GSM is a presumptive diagnosis made on characteristic examination findings in a postmenopausal woman once other causes of vaginitis have been excluded.

Vulvovaginitis may be caused by a reaction to irritant or allergen exposure. Triggers can include latex (used in condoms), spermicides, and chemicals in sanitary pads or toilet paper. This is also a diagnosis of exclusion. In unclear cases, referral to an allergist for patch testing may be helpful.

Inflammatory conditions are thought to be underdiagnosed and may be responsible for many of the cases of vulvovaginitis that were not previously given a diagnosis. They occur more commonly in women who are perimenopausal. The patient has a purulent vaginal discharge with vulvovaginal erythema or rash, and microscopy characteristically demonstrates many white blood cells. The etiology is thought to be autoimmune.

Treatment

Bacterial Vaginosis

Treatment of bacterial vaginosis is recommended to alleviate symptoms but may also be helpful in reducing susceptibility to other sexually transmitted diseases including HIV and those caused by *Chlamydia trachomatis, Neisseria gonorrhoeae,* and *Trichomonas vaginalis.* Treatment also reduces the risk of recurrence. Additionally, in pregnant women, treatment has been associated with potential decreases in adverse outcomes including late miscarriages and poor neonatal outcomes, although it may not have a significant impact on the prevention of preterm labor, as may have been thought in the past. Treatment is recommended for all symptomatic women. Both initial oral and topical therapies are acceptable treatments in pregnancy.

Initial and alternative treatment regimens are presented in Table 3; considerations in choosing regimens include patient preference and cost. Of note, secnidazole (Solosec) is a newer oral agent that provides for one-time dosing; however, it may be cost-prohibitive for patients. If the metronidazole (Flagyl)[1] oral regimen is prescribed, patients should be counseled on potential disulfiram-like reaction with alcohol consumption for 24 hours following completion of medication, and similarly for 72 hours following completion of tinidazole (Tindamax). Patients should also be counseled that oil-based topical therapies including clindamycin may weaken latex condoms or diaphragms. Additionally, to prevent recurrent infection, patients should be counseled to avoid sexual intercourse until after completion of therapy and to avoid douching.

Vulvovaginal Candidiasis

The rationale for the treatment of vulvovaginal candidiasis is relief of symptoms. Treatment regimens for VVC are listed in Table 4 for initial treatment and treatment of recurrence. In non-pregnant patients, the choice between oral and topical azoles can be based on patient preference. Those patients who are prescribed topical therapies should be counseled that topical azole preparations may be oil based and can weaken latex condoms. Topical

---

[1]Not FDA approved for this indication.

TABLE 3	Treatment of Bacterial Vaginosis
Initial regimens	Metronidazole (Flagyl)[1] 500 mg PO bid for 7 days or metronidazole 0.75% gel (MetroGel), one full applicator (5g) intravaginally daily for 5 days Or clindamycin 2% cream (Cleocin), one full applicator (5 g) intravaginally hs for 7 days
Alternative regimens	Secnidazole (Solosec) 2 g PO once Tinidazole (Tindamax) 2g PO daily for 2 days Or tinidazole 1g PO once daily for 5 days Or clindamycin[1] 300 mg PO bid for 7 days Or clindamycin ovules 100 mg intravaginally hs for 3 days
Pregnancy	Either oral or vaginal regimens suggested in initial treatment section
Treatment of recurrence	First recurrence: retrial of same regimen or trial of alternative initial regimen Multiple recurrences: Metronidazole 0.75% gel, intravaginally twice weekly for 4 to 6 months[3]

[1]Not FDA approved for this indication.
[3]Exceeds dosage recommended by the manufacturer.

therapies may cause local irritation or hypersensitivity reactions, although systemic effects are not of concern. Oral azoles can cause nausea, abdominal pain, headache, and rarely elevations in liver function tests. For pregnant patients, only topical therapies should be prescribed.

For those with severe VVC or with immunocompromise, longer treatment may be necessary, such as a 7- to 14-day course.

For recurrent VVC (four or more episodes within a year), longer duration of initial therapy followed by maintenance therapy is recommended. Non-*albicans* VVC should also be considered and appropriate diagnostic testing performed to guide treatment, which may include a 7- to 14-day course of an azole topical or oral regimen (other than fluconazole [Diflucan]), and potentially a 2-week course of treatment with boric acid[6] if recurrent.

Trichomonas

The rationale for the treatment of *Trichomonas* infection includes a decrease of symptoms and reduced transmission to sexual partners. *Trichomonas* infection in pregnant women is associated with adverse outcomes including preterm birth and low–birth weight infants; however, treatment has not shown a definite reduction in these outcomes. For patients with HIV, *Trichomonas* infection is associated with pelvic inflammatory disease; thus screening and treatment can help to prevent this complication. Regimens for initial therapy and treatment of recurrence are listed in Table 5. Patients should be counseled regarding a potential disulfiram-like reaction with alcohol consumption for 24 hours following the completion of oral metronidazole and similarly for 72 hours following tinidazole. A 7-day course as opposed to a single-dose regimen is preferred for patients with HIV infection, as the single-dose regimen has been shown to be less effective.

Persistent or recurrent *Trichomonas* infection is often due to reinfection. When patients are being counseled about treatment, they should be advised to avoid intercourse until treatment is completed, symptoms have resolved, and partners have been treated. All patients diagnosed with *Trichomonas* should be asked to inform partners of the need for presumptive treatment. Additionally, patients should be retested within 3 months of diagnosis to ensure adequate treatment and address potential reinfection. In cases where treatment-resistant infection is suspected, a 1-week

[6]May be compounded by pharmacists.

TABLE 4	Treatment of Vulvovaginal Candidiasis
Initial regimens	*Topical azole therapy:* Clotrimazole (Gyne-Lotrimin) 1% cream 5 g intravaginally daily for 7 to 14 days OR Clotrimazole 2% cream 5 g intravaginally daily for 3 days OR Miconazole 2% cream 5 g intravaginally daily for 7 days OR Miconazole 4% cream 5 g intravaginally daily for 3 days OR Miconazole 100 mg vaginal suppository, one suppository daily for 7 days OR Miconazole 200 mg vaginal suppository, one suppository for 3 days OR Miconazole 1200 mg vaginal suppository, one suppository for 1 day OR Tioconazole (Vagistat) 6.5% ointment 5 g intravaginally in a single application *Prescription intravaginal agents:* Butoconazole (Gynazole) 2% cream (single-dose bioadhesive product), 5 g intravaginally in a single application OR Terconazole (Terazol) 0.4% cream 5 g intravaginally daily for 7 days OR Terconazole 0.8% cream 5 g intravaginally daily for 3 days OR Terconazole 80 mg vaginal suppository, one suppository daily for 3 days OR fluconazole (Diflucan) 150 mg PO once
Alternative regimens	N/A
Pregnancy	Topical azole therapy applied intravaginally for 7 days
Treatment of recurrence	Topical azole therapy for 7 to 14 days OR fluconazole 150 mg every third day for three doses[3] For maintenance: Oral fluconazole (100, 150, or 200 mg) weekly for 6 months[3]; consider topical treatment if oral is not feasible

[3]Exceeds dosage recommended by the manufacturer.

TABLE 5	Treatment of *Trichomonas* Infection
Initial regimens	Metronidazole (Flagyl) 2 g PO, single or divided dose on same day OR tinidazole (Tindamax) 2 g PO once
Alternative regimens	Metronidazole 500 mg PO bid for 7 days[3]
Pregnancy	Metronidazole 2 g PO once
Treatment of recurrence	Trial of metronidazole, 500 mg bid for 7 days[3] If metronidazole 500 mg bid for 7 days fails: Trial of metronidazole, 2 g daily for 7 days[3] If above regimens fail: Consider susceptibility testing (contact Centers for Disease Control and Prevention)

[3]Exceeds dosage recommended by the manufacturer.

regimen should be attempted. If the infection still persists, further testing should be implemented according to guidance from the Centers for Disease Control and Prevention.

Noninfectious Vaginitis

Treatment of genitourinary syndrome of menopause includes low-dose vaginal estrogen therapy or topical lubricant therapy for less severe symptoms. Inflammatory vaginitis is still not well understood, although long-term maintenance therapy with topical clindamycin[1] or steroids may be helpful.

---

[1]Not FDA approved for this indication.

References

American College of Obstetricians and Gynecologists: Vaginitis in nonpregnant patients. ACOG Practice Bulletin No. 215, *Obstet Gynecol* 135:e1–e17, 2020.

Anderson MR, Klink K, Cohrssen A: Evaluation of vaginal complaints, *JAMA* 291(11):1368–1379, 2004.

Centers for Disease Control and Prevention: Sexually Transmitted Diseases Treatment Guidelines, *MMWR Recomm Rep* 64(No. RR-3):1–137, 2015, 2015.

Rahn DD, Carberry C, Sanses TV, et al: Vaginal estrogen for genitourinary syndrome of menopause: a systematic review, *Obstetr Gynecol* 124(6):1147, 2014.

Reichman O, Sobel J: Desquamative inflammatory vaginitis, *Best Prac Res Clin Obstetr Gynaecol* 28(7):1042–1050, 2014.

Sobel JD: Recurrent vulvovaginal candidiasis, *AJOG* 214(1):15–21, 2016.

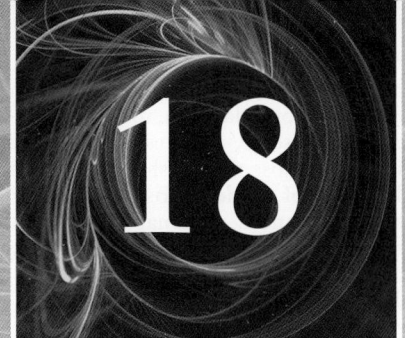

18 Pregnancy and Antepartum Care

ANTEPARTUM CARE

Method of
Matthew K. Cline, MD; and Natawadee Young, MD

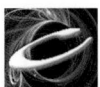

CURRENT DIAGNOSIS

- Pregnancy evaluation should begin 3 to 6 months before conception with optimization of underlying medical conditions, update of immunizations, and commencement of prenatal vitamins with 400 μg of folic acid.[1]
- Preconception counseling with a specialist in high-risk pregnancies should be considered in all patients with underlying medical conditions, such as diabetes and hypertension.
- Early ultrasound (< 13 weeks) assists with establishment of accurate estimated date of confinement and is an essential task in the first prenatal visit.
- The first prenatal visit should include a review of the medical and obstetric histories, current medications, allergies, herbal remedies, supplements, and tobacco, alcohol, and drug use.
- Prenatal laboratory studies should be done at the first visit after a pregnancy is confirmed with a urine pregnancy test. These studies include hemoglobin, platelet count, type and screen, rubella status, hepatitis B screening, syphilis screen, and a urine culture. All women should be screened for HIV. High-risk patients should be screened for hepatitis C, gonorrhea, and chlamydia.
- Genetic screening should be offered based on ethnic history.
- Offer aneuploidy screening to all women in the first trimester along with counseling about risks and benefits. These tests aid in diagnosis of chromosome abnormalities. If a patient opts for a first-trimester screen, it is important to perform an alpha-fetoprotein (AFP) screen in the second trimester to screen for neural tube defects. All women should be offered amniocentesis or chorionic villous sampling for genetic testing with appropriate counseling.
- Appropriate weight gain in pregnancy depends on maternal body mass index (BMI) before pregnancy. In patients with a normal BMI, a 25- to 30-pound weight gain is recommended. Underweight patients are encouraged to gain 30 to 35 pounds, and overweight patients are encouraged to gain no more than 20 pounds.
- Prenatal visits should begin at 8 to 12 weeks' gestation and continue monthly until 28 weeks. Visits should then be every 2 weeks until 36 weeks and then weekly. Each visit should include assessment of maternal weight, blood pressure (BP), fundal height measurement, documentation of fetal heart tones, and review of symptoms of preterm labor and preeclampsia.
- All patients should undergo a glucose challenge test at 24 to 28 weeks. This is done nonfasting by administering a 50-g load of glucose and obtaining a serum sample 1 hour after administration. A level greater than 140 mg/dL is considered abnormal, and a 3-hour glucose tolerance test is indicated (which is done after a 12-hour fast with a 100-g oral glucose load). If a woman demonstrates abnormalities in two of the four values, gestational diabetes is diagnosed.

[1]Not FDA approved for this indication.

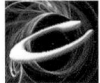

CURRENT THERAPY

- Administration of the inactivated influenza vaccine (Fluzone, Fluvirin, Fluarix) is recommended in all pregnant patients, regardless of trimester, who will be pregnant (or up to 3 months postpartum) during the flu season.
- Additionally, administer Tdap vaccine (Adacel, Boostrix) in each pregnancy given between 27 and 36 weeks or immediately postpartum in order to decrease rates of pertussis in this age group.
- An updated listing of vaccination recommendations throughout pregnancy (including international travel) can be found at www.cdc.gov/vaccines/pregnancy/hcp/guidelines.html
- Folic acid supplementation[1] should begin before conception. The recommended dose is 400 μg daily and is usually given as a prenatal vitamin. In patients with a previous pregnancy complicated by a neural tube defect, 4 mg daily[3] is recommended to decrease the chance of recurrence of a neural tube defect.
- All patients with HIV should be treated with appropriate HAART (highly active anti-retroviral therapy) for the patient and her HIV viral type throughout the pregnancy.
- Intrapartum zidovudine (Retrovir) is recommended for all patients with HIV whose HIV RNA load is ≥ 50 copies/ml or who have concerns with adherence to HAART therapy. Consideration of cesarean delivery is appropriate based on viral load evaluation.

[1]Not FDA approved for this indication.
[3]Exceeds dosage recommended by the manufacturer.

Antepartum Care

Ideally, antepartum care commences 3 to 6 months before conception with the recommendation that women who are sexually active and not using contraception should begin taking daily multivitamin or folic acid supplements. The most convincing trials of this were performed in Europe and China when it was concluded that women of reproductive age should take multivitamin supplements containing 0.4 mg of folate daily to reduce the incidence of neural tube defects. Women with histories of children with neural tube defects or other anomalies should increase this dose to 4 mg[3] of folate in the periconceptional period to reduce risks of recurrence.

Preconception counseling should also include an accurate assessment of preexisting maternal medical conditions. This is the ideal time to stress changes in factors that respond to early intervention: quitting smoking, refraining from alcohol or drug abuse, treating gum disease, and avoiding teratogens. Alcohol is a known teratogen. Immunization status should be reviewed and vaccines should be administered as appropriate. Special consideration is given to patients with thyroid disease. Concern focuses on associations with low intelligence quotients (IQs) in children conceived by hypothyroid mothers. Patients with diabetes should be counseled that the increased risk of birth defects is directly related to the level of glucose control at conception.

[3]Exceeds dosage recommended by the manufacturer.

- Current disease involving renal, cardiac, or endocrine systems
- Fetal anomalies (in previous pregnancies or first-degree family relatives)
- History of preterm delivery
- Incompetent cervix or recurrent miscarriages
- Isoimmunization
- Known carrier of genetic disorder
- Multiple gestation
- Placenta previa after 28 weeks
- Prior intrauterine fetal demise or stillbirth
- Systemic diseases such as hypertension, diabetes, or asthma
- Third-trimester bleeding

High-risk obstetric referrals may be offered to women with potential for obstetric complications suggested by conditions listed in Box 1. Identification of the high-risk patient is critical to minimizing adverse outcomes.

In most cases, a woman's pregnancy is a normal event that is complicated by potentially dangerous disease in a minority of cases. The physician who manages pregnant patients must follow the normal changes that occur during antepartum care, so that abnormalities can be recognized and treated appropriately. Additionally, routine prenatal care offers multiple opportunities for patient education, primary intervention, and appropriate monitoring of the low-risk pregnancy in the setting of the family and community. For some women, antepartum care is part of their own continuum in a long-term primary care relationship with caregivers.

Timeline of Routine Antepartum Care
First Visit and Early Care
History
After pregnancy is confirmed, it is extraordinarily important to determine the duration of pregnancy and the estimated date of confinement (EDC). Further care is heavily predicated on this estimate. The history begins with ascertaining the first day of the last normal menstrual period and calculating the EDC by assuming duration of pregnancy averages 280 days (40 weeks). Because a first-trimester dating ultrasound (US) is accurate to within 5 days at confirmation or determination of an accurate EDC, its value cannot be overestimated.

The documentation of prior obstetric history includes prior complications, route of delivery, and estimated birth weights. Maternal medical disorders are often exacerbated by pregnancy; cardiovascular, renal, and endocrine disorders require evaluation and counseling concerning possible treatments required. A history of previous gynecologic surgery, including cesarean delivery, is important to consider. A family history of twinning, diabetes mellitus, familial disorders, or hereditary disease is relevant.

Current medications (prescription and nonprescription) are reviewed, along with any herbals or supplements. Certain prescription medications are known teratogens and should be discontinued. Examples include isotretinoin (Accutane), tetracycline (Sumycin), quinolone antibiotics (ciprofloxacin [Cipro], levofloxacin [Levaquin]), "statin" cholesterol-lowering medications such as atorvastatin (Lipitor) and rosuvastatin (Crestor) and warfarin (Coumadin). Angiotensin-converting enzyme (ACE) inhibitors and angiotensin receptor blockers (ARBs) should not be used in pregnancy because they can be associated with fetal renal agenesis.

It is important to determine the pregnant patient's risks for developing preeclampsia during the first trimester prenatal visit because starting low dose aspirin (81 mg) between 12 to 28 weeks (ideally before 16 weeks' gestation) can prevent morbidity and mortality from preeclampsia. One or more of the following high-risk factors is an indication for beginning low dose aspirin after 12 weeks: a history of previous preeclampsia, multifetal gestation, renal disease, autoimmune disease, diabetes, and chronic hypertension. Consideration of low dose aspirin should be given for patients with more than one of moderate-risk factors for preeclampsia including obesity, advanced maternal age, history of low birth weight infants or adverse birth outcomes, and low socioeconomic status or African American race.

Open discussion of substance abuse (alcohol, tobacco, and illicit drugs) is an integral part of the patient interview. Counseling patients about smoking cessation is vital in early pregnancy. Smoking increases the risk of fetal death or damage in utero. It is also associated with increased risk of placental abruption and placenta previa, each of which put both mother and child at risk, along with premature birth. The interest that pregnant women have in delivering a healthy infant can be a potent motivator for change at this point.

Opioid use in pregnancy has escalated in the last decade. Early screening for opioid use, misuse, and for opioid use disorder along with brief intervention and referral is recommended for all pregnant women. Pregnant women with opioid use disorder should be referred to psychosocial resources and to a qualified clinic or treatment center that is able to assist in managing the patient with methadone or buprenorphine throughout the pregnancy and postpartum period. Medically assisted withdrawal is currently not recommended in pregnancy due to the high risk for relapse and the associated harms that occur with addiction. Patients and care teams should be prepared for the risk of neonatal abstinence syndrome if there is continued opioid or other illicit drug use during pregnancy.

Domestic Violence Screening and Counseling
Pregnancy is also a time of increased incidence of domestic or intimate partner violence, and because of this, it is appropriate to screen patients about the safety of their homes and relationships starting at the first prenatal visit. The United States Preventive Services Task Force (USPSTF) gives screening for domestic or intimate partner violence a "B" rating, supporting its use in routine prenatal care. A large evidence review supports benefit to patients being screened with one of many possible screening tools. The Personal Violence Screen consists of three "Yes" or "No" questions that can be quickly administered to a patient in private, and a positive result is one or more "Yes" responses:
1. Have you been hit, kicked, punched, or otherwise hurt by someone in the past year?
2. Do you feel unsafe in your current relationship?
3. Is there a partner from a previous relationship who is making you feel unsafe now?

A positive screen should be followed by specific referral to local resources for the patient to reach a safe environment and continued support. Each office should evaluate local resources and have a prepared contact list for these patients to use as their next step to safety.

Examination
Physical examination begins with a thorough general examination to assess maternal well-being, including BMI and BP. The BMI is calculated by dividing weight in kilograms by height in meters squared. The BMI of a patient is categorized as underweight (under 19.8), normal weight (19.8 to 25), overweight (25 to 30), or obese (over 30).

Breast examination may be significant for changes in pregnancy that result from hormonal responses by the mammary ducts. These changes include engorgement and vascular prominence, occasionally resulting in mastodynia. Enlargement of areolar sebaceous glands occurs between 6 and 8 weeks' gestation.

A pelvic examination is performed with attention to the adequacy of pelvis and evaluation for adnexal masses. Numerous changes in the pelvic organs occur in pregnancy. For example, congestion of the pelvic vasculature (Chadwick's sign) causes

TABLE 1	U.S. Preventive Services Task Force Recommendations for Pregnancy

Grade A = The USPSTF recommends the service. There is high certainty that the net benefit is substantial. Screening/actions in pregnancy in this category include the following:
- Screen for hepatitis B infection in all pregnant women.
- Screen for HIV infection in all pregnant women.
- Screen for syphilis in all pregnant women.
- Screen for cervical cancer in all women between 21 and 65 who have a uterus.
- Ask about smoking and provide augmented, pregnancy-tailored counseling for those who smoke and are pregnant.
- All women planning or capable of pregnancy should take 400–800 µg of folic acid daily.
- Screen all women at the first visit by Rh(D) typing and antibody screen.

Grade B = The USPSTF recommends the service. There is high certainty that the net benefit is moderate or there is moderate certainty that the net benefit is moderate to substantial. Screening/actions in pregnancy in this category include the following:
- Screen for asymptomatic bacteriuria at 12 to 16 weeks or at first prenatal visit.
- Screen for chlamydia in pregnant women 24 and younger or at high risk.
- Screen for gonorrhea if at high risk of infection.
- Provide intervention during pregnancy and after birth to support breast-feeding.
- Screen for alcohol misuse and provide behavioral counseling interventions to reduce its misuse.
- For women at high risk of preeclampsia, start low-dose aspirin[1] at 81 mg/day after 12 weeks of gestation.
- Screen for gestational diabetes mellitus (GDM) in asymptomatic pregnant women after 24 weeks of gestation.
- Screen for depression in pregnant and postpartum women.
- Screen women of childbearing age for intimate partner violence (IPV), such as domestic violence, and provide or refer women who screen positive to intervention services.
- Screen throughout pregnancy for preeclampsia by blood pressure measurement.
- Repeat Rh(D) antibody testing for all unsensitized women at 24-28 weeks.

Grade C = Clinicians may provide this service to selected patients depending on individual circumstances. However, for most individuals without signs or symptoms there is likely to be only a small benefit from this service.

Grade D = The USPSTF recommends against the service. There is moderate or high certainty that the service has no net benefit or that the harms outweigh the benefits.
- Screen for bacterial vaginosis in asymptomatic pregnant women at low risk for preterm birth.
- Screen for herpes simplex with serology in asymptomatic pregnant women.

Grade I = The USPSTF concludes that the current evidence is insufficient to assess the balance of benefits and harms of the service.
- Screen for iron deficiency anemia in asymptomatic pregnant women.
- Screen for illicit drug use in pregnancy.
- Screen for elevated blood lead levels in asymptomatic pregnancy women.

Listing of all topics is available at https://www.uspreventiveservicestaskforce.org/BrowseRec/Index/browse-recommendations.
Abbreviation: USPSTF = U.S. Preventive Services Task Force.
[1]Not FDA approved for this indication.

bluish discoloration of the vagina and cervix. Softening of the cervix due to increased vascularity of the cervical tissue (Goodell's sign) can occur as early as 4 weeks.

Portable devices using Doppler will reliably detect fetal heart tones at a normal rate of 120 to 160 beats per minute as early as 11 weeks.

Laboratory Studies

Routine laboratory studies and screenings in pregnancy are listed in Table 1, along with their USPSTF level of recommendation.

Other Studies

Aneuploidy screening for common chromosomal abnormalities should be offered to all women, with counseling about risks and benefits. Current strategies include either cell free DNA aneuploidy screening or the more traditional maternal serum biomarker tests (PAPP-A/b-HCG) with or without nuchal translucency measurement. Invasive diagnostic testing for fetal chromosomal disorders through either chorionic villus sampling or amniocentesis is offered to all women, but especially if patients have increased risk or if the screening tests are abnormal. Second trimester screening for neural tube defects with maternal serum alpha fetoprotein is offered to all women. Second trimester fetal anatomy ultrasound evaluation is also offered around 20 weeks of gestation. Women may decline all screening and testing options after informed counseling.

Cell-free DNA screening was utilized primarily after 10 weeks in high-risk women such as those with prior aneuploidy, or older than age 35. However, there is now evidence using cell-free DNA screening in the general population, and results appear to be comparable. It has the highest detection rate (DR) for Down syndrome in high-risk women (98% DR with positive screening rates of less than 0.5%, positive predictive value of 93%). Positive predictive values are lower for trisomy 18 (64%), trisomy 13(44%), and sex chromosome aneuploidies (39%). However, it must be emphasized that for younger or low-risk women, false positive rates will be higher because of a lower pretest probability in these populations. In addition, the test cannot distinguish between fetal and maternal DNA, and causes of false positive screening tests can include placental mosaicism, a resorbing twin, or even maternal malignancy or aneuploidy. For this reason, ACOG recommends diagnostic testing with CVS or amniocentesis after a positive cell-free DNA screen prior to decisions about termination of the pregnancy. Cell-free DNA screening testing after a positive first trimester screen can also add additional information prior to diagnostic invasive tests. Appropriate pre and posttest counseling is important due to these evolving issues.

Chorionic villus sampling (CVS) (done at 10–12 weeks' gestation) or amniocentesis (performed at 14–16 weeks' gestation) should be offered to women older than 35 years, to those with abnormal first-trimester screens or second trimester "quad" screens, and to those with significant family history of genetic disease. From either test, fetal cells grown in culture may be subjected to chromosomal, metabolic, or DNA study for trisomy 13, 18, or 21 or abnormal numbers of sex chromosomes. CVS cannot be used for diagnosis of neural tube defects, but amniocentesis can accurately diagnose open neural tube defects or open abdominal defects by measuring amniotic fluid AFP.

Patients with tuberculosis exposure may be assessed for active tuberculosis with skin testing (if not vaccinated with Bacillus Calmette-Guérin [BCG]) and chest x-ray with abdominal shielding. Serologic assessment for toxoplasmosis, cytomegalovirus, and varicella immunity are not routinely indicated.

Currently it is recommended that all pregnant couples of Caucasian background be screened for being carriers of cystic fibrosis genes. Additionally, screening for genetic disorders should be undertaken if concern exists based on racial or ethnic background (hemoglobinopathies, β-thalassemia, α-thalassemia, Tay-Sachs disease) or familial background (cystic fibrosis, fragile X, Duchenne's muscular dystrophy).

Education

Several areas are appropriate for routine education during the first prenatal visit, and may be provided by handouts, nursing instruction, or directly by the physician. These will vary based on the patient's individual knowledge and prior experience, but at a minimum should include discussions of the following:
- Common discomforts of pregnancy and safe methods to relieve them
- Foods to avoid during pregnancy and safe food preparation
- Avoidance of tobacco, ethanol, and nonprescribed drugs throughout pregnancy

- Limitations on travel and importance of proper seatbelt use
- Danger signs of pregnancy and reasons to call or be seen after hours
- Availability of birth education classes, tours, and other educational resources

Follow-up

Follow-up visits are scheduled once monthly until 28 weeks' gestation, and then patients are followed twice monthly until 36 weeks. Visits are then scheduled at weekly intervals until delivery. At each visit, weight, BP, fetal heart tones, and fundal height are noted. In the last 6 weeks of pregnancy, assessing fetal position is also appropriate.

Interval history includes questions about diet, sleeping patterns, and fetal movement. Warning signs such as bleeding, contractions, leaking of fluid, headache, or visual disturbances are reviewed.

15 to 20 Weeks' Gestation

Interval History

At each visit, it is appropriate to ask about specific symptoms: headache, dysuria, swelling, vaginal discharge, any bleeding, pelvic pain, and nausea or vomiting. The nausea and vomiting of the first trimester usually begins to decrease after 12 to 14 weeks. By this point in the pregnancy, the patient is usually feeling well. The other items above, if present, may indicate reasons for a targeted examination to evaluate for the cause, such as a speculum examination with wet prep for an increased symptomatic discharge (though the physiologic discharge of pregnancy has often become evident by this point, it should be asymptomatic).

Alpha-Fetoprotein and Aneuploidy Testing

For patients who received first-trimester aneuploidy screening, maternal serum AFP testing should be offered for all pregnancies at 16 to 20 weeks as a means of screening for open neural tube defects. High levels of AFP are associated with various fetal anomalies, including neural tube defects, multiple gestations, and ventral wall defects. Unexplained elevation of AFP has been associated with poor fetal growth, fetal loss, and preeclampsia. In cases with unexplained elevation of AFP, maternal and fetal surveillance should be increased. Low levels of AFP are associated with increased risk of Down syndrome.

For those who did not have the first trimester screen, a "quad screen" with multiple analytes can be done at this time to screen for aneuploidy such as trisomy 21, 18, and 13 as well. The interpretation of this test depends on the gestational age; even if timed correctly, it is known to have a moderate level of false-positive results. Therefore the first step after an abnormal AFP or quad screen is to refer for a detailed ultrasound to confirm gestational age and assess fetal anatomy. If the results of the screening remain abnormal, definitive testing via amniocentesis is recommended.

Physical Findings

Interval changes in the physical examination now include the start of colostrum secretion, which can begin as early as 16 weeks' gestation. The mother might detect fetal movements (quickening) at around 18 to 20 weeks. The uterus is palpable at 20 weeks at the umbilicus.

Chloasma is darkening of the skin over the forehead, bridge of the nose, or cheekbones and is more obvious in those with dark complexions. It can begin to manifest at this time, and is intensified by exposure to sunlight. Darkening of the skin in the areolae and nipples becomes more accentuated. A darkened line appears in the lower midline of the abdomen from the umbilicus to the pubis (linea nigra). The basis of these changes is stimulation of melanophores by increased melanocyte-stimulating hormone.

At 15 to 20 weeks, abdominal enlargement can appear more rapid as the uterus rises out of the pelvis and into the abdomen.

Ultrasonography

Sonography has long established itself as the single most useful technology in monitoring pregnancy and diagnosing complications. It is for this reason that an anatomic US is offered at 18 to 20 weeks to evaluate growth, placentation, amniotic fluid volume, and fetal anatomy. If earlier dating of the pregnancy is uncertain, this is an opportunity to confirm or refute prior estimates. If anomalous conditions are discovered or the patient has a history of diabetes, advanced maternal age, or has prior children with anomalies, more comprehensive US becomes necessary.

20 to 35 Weeks' Gestation

Interval History

This period in the middle trimester of the pregnancy is often the time when patients feel their best: the challenges of nausea and vomiting from the first trimester are usually past. Patients should be asked about diet and activity, fetal activity (which should continue to increase throughout this period), and any symptoms that might suggest preeclampsia, such as hand or face swelling, visual changes, or severe headaches. Vaginal secretions do increase during this period but any bleeding or leakage of a large amount of fluid, along with any uterine rhythmic contractions, should also prompt a call or evaluation of the patient.

Physical Findings

The uterus should be palpable at the umbilicus at 20 weeks, and from this period until 34 weeks the measurement in centimeters from the fundus to the symphysis pubis should correspond to the gestational age in weeks. Measurements that are more than 2 cm below the expected size should raise suspicion for oligohydramnios, intrauterine growth restriction, fetal anomalies, or an abnormal fetal position. Conversely, measurements more than 2 cm larger than expected may indicate multiple gestation, polyhydramnios, or fetal macrosomia. These rules apply for the gestational ages of 20 to 34 weeks. Either situation can be evaluated with maternal US examination and consultation with a maternal-fetal-medicine specialist.

New physical examination findings at this time include the onset of stretch marks (striae) of the breasts and abdomen. These are caused by separation of underlying collagen tissue, a response to increased adrenocorticosteroid. The ligamentous structures of the pelvis also undergo slight but definite relaxation of the joints, a progesterone effect. As the uterus enlarges, it often rotates to the right. Braxton-Hicks contractions, characterized as painless uterine tightening, increase in regularity. The fetal outline can be easily palpated through the maternal abdominal wall.

Laboratory Studies

Increased surveillance for preeclampsia should occur in any patient with a previous history of preeclampsia or chronic hypertension predating the pregnancy. Newer guidelines require only two blood pressures 4+ hours apart that are 140/90 or greater for the diagnosis of preeclampsia along with 1+ urinary protein, a urinary protein to creatinine ratio of 0.3 or greater, or >300 mg of protein in a 24-hour urine collection. Further evaluation for patients with elevated BP (>140/90) should include evaluation for symptoms or findings that are consistent with severe features: headaches, visual changes, pulmonary edema, RUQ pain or epigastric pain, BP of 160 or higher systolic or 110 or higher diastolic on two occasions 4 hours apart, or laboratory evidence of thrombocytopenia (platelets below 100,000), liver transaminases elevated to at least twice the normal level, a serum creatinine that has doubled or is greater than 1.1. If any severe feature is present, the diagnosis of preeclampsia does not require proteinuria. Once the diagnosis of preeclampsia is made, management will be based on gestational age as well as presence of severe features. For additional details, please see chapter "Hypertension in Pregnancy."

A complete blood count (to screen for anemia) and a nonfasting 1-hour glucose tolerance test (after ingestion of 50 g of glucose) are scheduled to detect patients at risk for developing gestational diabetes at 24 to 28 weeks. If the screening test is abnormal, a

3-hour test is performed with 100 g of glucose to confirm the diagnosis. Two or more abnormal values on this test are considered diagnostic of gestational diabetes mellitus.

A repeat Rh antibody is checked at 28 weeks' gestation in Rh-negative mothers. Those who remain unsensitized at 28 weeks' gestation receive a first dose of Rho(D) immune globulin (RhoGAM) of 300 µg to prevent maternal isoimmunization to fetal red blood cells. (This should also be given at any point after the first 12 weeks of pregnancy in the setting of significant maternal trauma in an Rh-negative mother. If there is suspicion of a significant fetal-maternal hemorrhage, a Kleihauer-Betke test can be used to quantitate the amount of fetal blood in the maternal circulation in order to increase the dose of RhoGAM appropriately.)

Follow-up

Return visits at 2-week intervals are initiated beginning at 28 weeks, and the patient is oriented to the labor and delivery ward. Precautions are given regarding the onset of conditions listed in Box 2. The onset of any of these should prompt immediate medical attention.

36 to 41 Weeks' Gestation

Physical Findings

Patients often note increased vaginal discharge at this time in their pregnancy, a physiologic consequence of hormone stimulation. The discharge consists mainly of epithelial cells and cervical mucus and is treated with reassurance. Discharge accompanied by itching, burning, or malodor should be evaluated with a wet prep and any abnormalities treated.

Laboratory Studies

Vaginal and rectal rapid molecular tests are collected to evaluate for the presence of group B streptococci (GBS) at 36 0/7 to 37 6/7 weeks. GBS organisms are implicated in preterm labor, amnionitis, endometritis, and wound infection. If tests are positive, the patient will be given antibiotic prophylaxis during active labor to protect the newborn against vertical transmission and the resulting infection that could occur. If a patient has a positive urine testing during the pregnancy of over 100,000 colony-forming units of GBS, she is treated at the time of that culture but also assumed to be heavily colonized and given intrapartum antibiotics without performing the vaginal/rectal cultures at 36 0/7 to 37 6/7 weeks.

Follow-up

Follow-up visits are planned on a weekly basis with emphasis on weight gain, BP, and signs of preeclampsia. Review of precautions regarding infection, pregnancy loss, and symptoms of preeclampsia completes the visit.

Late Term and Postterm Gestation

About 6% of pregnancies continue beyond 42 weeks and are considered postterm. The period between 41 0/7 and 41 6/7 weeks is named late term pregnancy. Due to increased perinatal morbidity and mortality beginning at 41 0/7 weeks, guidelines recommend elective induction of labor at 41 weeks after shared decision-making with patients. Should the patient decline induction, then experts recommend fetal surveillance twice weekly between 41 and 42 weeks gestation with nonstress testing, amniotic fluid measurement, or the biophysical profile, followed by induction of labor at 42 weeks gestation.

Common Concerns of the Antenatal Period

Bleeding

About one-half of pregnant women experience some form of bleeding during the pregnancy; often this is benign. Patients also have a heightened awareness of symptoms that previously may have gone unnoticed in the nonpregnant state. Efficient and competent evaluation, followed by compassion and reassurance when prudent, allays many fears and provides clear direction. Spotting due to bleeding at the implantation site occurs from the time of implantation (about 6 days after fertilization) until 29 to 35 days after the last menstrual period in many women. Usually, cardiac activity on US and appropriate β-hCG levels confirm a viable early pregnancy. First-trimester bleeding may be a sign of spontaneous miscarriage or ectopic pregnancy and deserves further evaluation, often with a pelvic examination and US. Vaginal bleeding in late pregnancy is covered in other chapters.

Nausea

Nausea is a common symptom that occurs in most pregnancies. It is heightened before 14 weeks' gestation and is largely benign. The etiology is not well understood but likely is related to elevating levels of β-hCG. Nausea of pregnancy can occur at any time during the day. Aggravating factors vary with the individual patient; success varies with interventions designed to reduce symptoms.

Uncomplicated nausea may be responsive to small nonfatty portions at mealtime. Pyridoxine (vitamin B_6)[1] tablets 12.5 mg three times daily with 12.5 mg of doxylamine (Unisom)[1] twice a day are safe in pregnancy and may be helpful. A combination product of doxylamine 10 mg and pyridoxine 10 mg (Diclegis) is approved by the FDA for the treatment of nausea and vomiting of pregnancy in women who do not respond to conservative management. Antiemetic drugs in the outpatient setting are the next step; ondansetron (Zofran, FDA category B)[1] 4 to 8 mg up to three times a day and meclizine (Antivert, FDA category B)[1] 12.5 to 25 mg three times a day are agents with the best safety profile.

Inability to control protracted vomiting in conjunction with clinical dehydration can require hospitalization for IV fluids and treatment of hyperemesis gravidarium. Extreme nausea and vomiting that persists beyond 18 to 20 weeks' gestation may be a sign of multiple gestation, thyroid disease, molar pregnancy, or liver or pancreatic disease.

Nutrition and Weight Gain

The mother's nutrition is a vital factor in the development of the fetus from preconception through the postpartum period. Therefore, the pregnant woman should be advised to eat a balanced diet and should be informed of the additional 300 kcal/day needed during pregnancy. The American College of Obstetricians and Gynecologists (ACOG) recommends a target weight gain of 22 to 27 pounds (10–12 kg) during pregnancy. It also advises that underweight women might need to gain more and obese women should gain less. Nutritional requirements for protein are 80 g/day, for calcium are 1500 mg/day, for iron are 30 mg/day, and for folate are 0.4 mg/day (4 mg/day in some cases, such as those patients with previous baby with neural tube defects). Patients with seizure disorders managed with valproic acid (Depakene) or carbamazepine (Tegretol) are also at risk for birth defects and might benefit from the higher dose of folate.

---

[1]Not FDA approved for this indication.

Heartburn

Heartburn in the form of reflux esophagitis is caused by the enlarging uterus displacing the stomach and by progesterone's relaxation of the lower esophageal sphincter. Treatment consists of taking antacids, decreasing exacerbating factors such as spicy foods, eating more frequently but in smaller quantities, limiting eating before bedtime, and taking H_2-blockers.

Urinary Symptoms

Urinary frequency, nocturia, and bladder irritability are common complaints due to progesterone-mediated relaxation of smooth muscle and subsequent altered bladder function. Later in pregnancy, urinary frequency becomes even more prominent from pressure on the bladder by the enlarging uterus and the fetal presenting parts, such as when the fetal head descends into the pelvis.

Dysuria, however, is often a sign of infection that requires antibiotic treatment. Bacteriuria combined with urinary stasis from altered bladder function predisposes the patient to pyelonephritis. Although simple urinary tract infections are treated on an outpatient basis, pyelonephritis remains the most common nonobstetric cause for hospitalization during antenatal care.

Patients with a diagnosis of pyelonephritis require hospitalization, aggressive fluid replacement, and IV antibiotics until they remain afebrile for longer than 24 hours. Close monitoring of maternal respiratory status is important because these women are at risk for acute respiratory distress syndrome (ARDS) and renal failure as well as a significant increase in preterm labor and delivery. All patients should complete a 14-day course of antibiotic treatment. After treatment has been completed, suppressive therapy should be continued until delivery.

Infection

Two infections of special note are HIV and bacterial vaginosis (BV). HIV transmission to the newborn can be reduced significantly with appropriate infectious disease and maternal-fetal medicine specialty management. Although all symptomatic pregnant women with BV should be treated, evidence is inconclusive for screening and treating asymptomatic women, even those with a high risk history of prior preterm delivery or PPROM. Because of well-documented safety and efficacy of oral[1] and vaginal metronidazole, and vaginal clindamycin cream, any of these three are considered first-line for treatment in pregnancy.

Chlamydia trachomatis is an obligate intracellular bacterium and is the most common sexually transmitted bacterial infection in women of reproductive age. It may be associated with urethritis, mucopurulent cervicitis, and acute salpingitis, or it may be clinically silent. Perinatal transmission is clearly associated with neonatal conjunctivitis (leading to blindness) and pneumonia and is likely associated with preterm delivery, premature rupture of membranes, and perinatal mortality. Diagnosis is confirmed by nucleic acid amplification testing (NAAT) during routine screening. Doxycycline should be avoided in pregnancy, and erythromycin is associated with gastrointestinal upset, so treatment with azithromycin (Zithromax 1000 mg as single dose) is often the best choice in pregnancy.

Gonococcal infection is associated with concomitant chlamydia infection in about 40% of infected pregnant women. It is usually limited to the lower genital tract, including the cervix, urethra, and periurethral or vestibular glands. Because of an association between gonococcal cervicitis and septic spontaneous abortion, and because preterm delivery, premature rupture of membranes, and postpartum infection are more common with gonococcal infection, routine cultures are appropriate at the first antenatal visit. Because some strains have rendered some β-lactam drugs ineffective for therapy, the recommendation for uncomplicated gonococcal infection is intramuscular ceftriaxone (Rocephin) 250 mg plus azithromycin (Zithromax) 1 g orally as a single dose.

Vaginosis due to *Candida albicans* can become symptomatic with caseous white discharge and vaginal itching or burning, and it may be associated with red satellite lesions on the vulva. Marked inflammation of the vagina and introitus may be noted. Topical application of over-the-counter antifungal creams such as miconazole nitrate (Monistat) or nystatin (Mycostatin) is generally helpful in controlling the imbalance of vaginal flora, but this requires a 7-day regimen to achieve adequate cure rates. A single dose of fluconazole (Diflucan), 150 mg by mouth, is another appropriate choice, but only after the first trimester.

Trichomonas vaginalis can be found in 20% to 30% of pregnant patients, but only a small number complain of discharge or irritation. This flagellated, oval, motile organism can be seen on normal saline wet prep and is evident clinically by presence of a foamy or greenish discharge accompanied by multiple cervical petechiae. The CDC now recommends highly sensitive and specific nucleic acid amplification test (NAAT) in testing for trichomonads (95.3–100% sensitive, 93.2–100% specific for the APTIMA T. vaginalis test), as wet prep microscopy is rather insensitive (51–65%). There are also several new point-of-care tests that are now FDA-approved using antigen detection or DNA hybridization probe technology that have results available in as little as 10 minutes (OSOM Trichomonas rapid test) to 45 minutes (Affirm VP III). Treatment is oral metronidazole (Flagyl) as a single 2-g dose for the patient and her partner (though most states support expedited partner treatment, each practitioner will need to individualize this approach).

Rubella, also known as German measles, is directly responsible for spontaneous miscarriage and severe congenital malformations. Although large epidemics of rubella are nonexistent in the United States because of immunization, the disease can still affect up to 25% of susceptible women. Absence of rubella antibody indicates susceptibility. Vaccination involves an attenuated live virus (MMR) and therefore is avoided in pregnancy. Vaccination of nonpregnant susceptible women (including those during the postpartum period) and hospital personnel continues to be the mainstay of therapy. Detection by immunoglobulin M (IgM)–specific antibody confirms recent infection.

Varicella-zoster virus, the etiologic agent of childhood chickenpox, is a DNA herpes virus that remains latent in the dorsal root ganglia and may be reactivated years later to cause herpes zoster or shingles. Infection early in pregnancy can lead to severe congenital malformations, including chorioretinitis, cerebral cortical atrophy, hydronephrosis, and cutaneous and bony leg defects. Varicella-zoster immunoglobulin (VariZIG) (30–40 kg: 500 U; ≥40.1 kg: 625 U) can attenuate varicella infection if given to an exposed, nonimmune pregnant woman within 96 hours of her exposure to a patient with active varicella.

Genital herpes simplex virus (HSV) can present at any gestational age and is characterized by multiple, painful genital ulcers or vesicles; the diagnosis can be confirmed (if not in labor) through use of PCR laboratory testing. If active genital lesions are noted in labor, cesarean delivery is indicated because the fetus is at risk for acquiring the virus during passage through the birth canal. For HSV outbreaks remote from term, acyclovir (Zovirax) and its derivatives can shorten the course of an outbreak. For those with a history of active herpes during or preceding pregnancy, prophylaxis with acyclovir or similar approved antiviral medications from 36 weeks onward can decrease the chance of an outbreak at term and the need for a cesarean delivery.

Influenza can occur during pregnancy, and because the risk of secondary complication such as pneumonia is increased during the antepartum period, influenza vaccination is recommended for all patients in any trimester who are pregnant or up to 3 months postpartum during the local influenza season. Rapid testing of nasal or throat swabs can ascertain the diagnosis of influenza. Though oseltamivir (Tamiflu) and zanamivir (Relenza) are both FDA category C in pregnancy, no toxic effects have been observed in animal trials, so these are the preferred agents. These agents need to be started as soon as possible to provide the most benefit in symptom duration and severity.

---

[1]Not FDA approved for this indication.

Varicose Veins

Pressure by the enlarged uterus on venous return from the legs and progesterone-mediated vasodilation can lead to prominent varicosities and edema of the legs or vulva. Any concern for deep vein thrombosis should be ruled out with duplex ultrasound imaging. Benign varicosities almost invariably return to normal after delivery, thus limiting the need for intervention in the antepartum period, though their symptoms may be decreased through the wearing of support hose. Edema of the lower extremities is common, responds to elevation, and must be differentiated from facial or hand edema accompanying preeclampsia. Hemorrhoids are manifestations of the varicosities of the rectal veins. Treatment focuses on stool softeners, sitz baths, and over-the-counter topical preparations. If a hemorrhoid becomes firm and tender, evaluation for possible treatment by opening and removing the thrombus can provide immediate relief.

Constipation

Bowel transit time and relaxation of intestinal smooth muscle are both increased due to progesterone effects, resulting in overall slowing of bowel function. If pronounced, this can lead to constipation. Dietary management of this condition is centered on recommendations for increased fluids and high-fiber foods; stool softeners, such as docusate (Colace), can also be used in pregnancy. Enemas and laxatives are not recommended.

Upper Extremity Discomfort

Periodic numbness and tingling of the fingers is due to exacerbations of carpal tunnel compression exacerbated by tissue edema. Splinting of the affected hand at night may help, along with stretching exercises of the wrist and neck that can be done throughout the day. Most of these symptoms resolve after delivery.

Backache and Pelvic Discomfort

Endocrine relaxation of ligamentous structures coupled with an offset center of gravity create exaggerated lordotic spinal curve, joint instability, and back pain. Most women experience some form of this discomfort as pregnancy progresses. Advice given for improvements in posture, local heat, acetaminophen (Tylenol), and massage may be helpful. Minimizing the time spent standing can have a positive effect. Round ligament pain usually occurs during the second trimester and is described as sharp bilateral or unilateral groin pain. It may be exacerbated by change in position or rapid movement and might respond to similar measures. These routine aches and pains of pregnancy must be differentiated from rhythmic cramping pains originating in the back or uterus. The latter may be a sign of preterm labor requiring appropriate evaluation.

Leg Cramps

Leg cramps in the form of recurrent muscle spasms in pregnancy are believed to be due to lower levels of serum calcium or higher levels of serum phosphorus. The calves are most commonly involved and attacks are more frequent at night and in the third trimester. There are no data from controlled trials to show benefit over placebo for treatment targeted toward reduced phosphate and increased calcium or magnesium intake. Local heat, putting the affected muscle on stretch, acetaminophen, and massage can be helpful in acute events.

Intercourse

In general, intercourse is considered safe in pregnancy. The exception to this rule is found in patients who have a known placenta previa, are experiencing uterine bleeding, or have postcoital cramps and spotting. It may be wise to avoid intercourse in couples who are at risk for special circumstances. Firmer recommendations can be made in instances of placenta previa or known rupture of membranes; in these instances intercourse should not occur.

Dental Care

Ideally, women should have dental care completed before conception. However, dental procedures under local anesthesia may be carried out at any time during the pregnancy. Use of nitrous oxide inhalants is to be avoided, however. Long procedures should be postponed until the second trimester. Antibiotics are appropriate as needed for dental infections and in cases of rheumatic heart disease or mitral valve prolapse with regurgitation.

X-rays, Ionizing Radiation, and Imaging

The adverse effects of ionizing radiation are dose dependent, but there is no single diagnostic procedure that results in a dose of radiation high enough to threaten the fetus or embryo. Diagnostic radiation of less than 5000 mrad is considered by ACOG to have minimal teratogenic risk, and if medically indicated, x-ray imaging may be performed safely (with appropriate abdominal shielding). Patients receiving dental x-rays are additionally protected by a lead apron. Still, the need for x-ray films should be evaluated for risks and potential benefits in the individual pregnant patient to conservatively protect the mother and fetus from theoretical genetic or oncogenic risk. Magnetic resonance imaging (MRI) is considered safe due to its mechanism of action, which is a nonionizing form of radiation. Radioactive iodine (^{131}I) is contraindicated in pregnancy.

Immunization

Live virus vaccines must be avoided during pregnancy because of possible effects on the fetus. These include measles, mumps, rubella (MMR), yellow fever (YF-Vax), and varicella (Varivax) vaccinations. The risks to the fetus from the administration of rabies vaccine (RabAvert, IMOVAX) are unknown.

Diphtheria and tetanus toxoid with pertussis (Tdap) is recommended between 27 and 36 weeks by the CDC and ACIP to decrease the risk of whooping cough in the newborn infant. The hepatitis B vaccine (Engerix B, Recombivax HB) series is safe and may be given in pregnancy to women at risk. The inactivated influenza vaccine (Fluzone, Fluvirin, Fluarix) is also recommended in all women during any trimester they will be pregnant during the flu season (or up to 3 months postpartum during flu season).

Tests of Fetal Well-Being

A primary goal in antepartum care is the competent management of patient care extended to both mother and baby in order to reduce the risk of fetal demise after 24 weeks, ensure optimal conditions for term delivery after 37 weeks, and intervene for evolving conditions threatening the well-being of either patient. Any pregnancy that may be at increased risk for antepartum fetal compromise is a candidate for tests of fetal well-being performed weekly, beginning at 28 to 32 weeks. Some conditions requiring antepartum testing are listed in Box 3.

Nonstress Test

The nonstress test (NST) consists of fetal heart rate monitoring in the absence of uterine contractions. A reactive tracing is one in which heart rate accelerations of 15 beats/min above the baseline of 120 to 160 beats/min are of at least 15 seconds' duration. Two of these accelerations must be observed in a 20-minute period.

BOX 3 Conditions That Prompt Enhanced Fetal Surveillance

- Decreased fetal movements
- Fetal growth restriction
- Hypertensive disorders
- Insulin-dependent diabetes mellitus
- Multiple gestation with discordant fetal growth
- Oligohydramnios or polyhydramnios
- Postterm pregnancy
- Prior loss or stillbirth

False-positive nonreactive tracings are more common before 28 weeks' gestation.

Biophysical Profile

The biophysical profile (BPP) consists of an NST with ultrasound observations. A total of 10 points is given for the following elements (2 points each):

- Reactive NST
- Presence of fetal breathing movements of 30 seconds or more in 30 minutes
- Fetal movement defined as three or more discrete body or limb movements within 30 minutes
- Fetal tone defined as one or more episodes of fetal extremity extension and return to flexion
- Quantification of amniotic fluid volume, defined as a pocket of fluid that measures at least 2 cm by 2 cm

The results of a BPP are usually reported out of 8 points if done without the NST, and out of 10 points if done with an NST. Scores of 8 or 10 points (out of 10) are considered reassuring, with retesting indicated in 4 to 7 days depending on the original indication for the testing. A score of 6 points is borderline; testing should be repeated in 24 hours. Scores of 4 or 2 points are nonreassuring and should prompt additional testing, treatment, or planning for delivery depending on the setting.

References

ACOG Committee Opinion No: 743. Low-dose aspirin use during pregnancy, *Obstet Gynecol* 132(1):44–52, 2018.

ACOG Committee Opinion No: 797. Prevention of group B streptococcal early-onset disease in newborns, *Obstet Gynecol* 35(2):51–72, 2020.

American College of Obstetricians and Gynecologists: *Compendium of selected publications*, Atlanta, 2012, American College of Obstetricians and Gynecologists.

American College of Obstetricians and Gynecologists: Screening for fetal aneuploidy. Practice Bulletin 163, *Obstet Gynecol* 127(5):e123–e137, 2016.

Centers for Disease Control and Prevention: Guidelines for Vaccinating Pregnant Women. Available at www.cdc.gov/vaccines/pregnancy/hcp/guidelines.html. [Accessed 2 May 2020].

Centers for Disease Control and Prevention: Sexually transmitted diseases treatment guidelines. Available at https://www.cdc.gov/std/tg2015/toc.htm, 2015. [Accessed 2 May 2020].

Committee Opinion No: 711. Opioid use and opioid use disorder in pregnancy, *Obstet Gynecol* 130(2):81–94, 2017.

McParlin C, O'Donnell A, Robson SC, et al: Treatments for hyperemesis gravidarum and nausea and vomiting in pregnancy: a systematic review, *JAMA* 316(13):1392–1401, 2016.

Middleton P, Shepherd E, Crowther CA: Induction of labour for improving birth outcomes for women at or beyond term, *Cochrane Database of Systematic Reviews* 5:CD004945, 2017, https://doi.org/10.1002/14651858, CD004945.pub4.

Nelson HD, Bougatsos C, Blazina I: Screening women for intimate partner violence: a systematic review to update the U.S. Preventive Services Task Force Recommendation, *Ann Intern Med* 156:796–808, 2012, W279–82.

Zolotor A, Carlough M: Update on prenatal care, *Am Fam Physician* 89(3):199–208, 2014.

ECTOPIC PREGNANCY

Method of
Christina M. Kelly, MD

CURRENT DIAGNOSIS

- Vaginal bleeding and abdominal pain in the first trimester of pregnancy raise concern for ectopic pregnancy, but a normal intrauterine pregnancy (IUP) or early pregnancy loss could exist.
- High-resolution transvaginal ultrasound (TVUS) and measurement of serum β–human chorionic gonadotropin (hCG) are the best initial steps in determining whether a pregnancy is ectopic.
- A single hCG value is not diagnostic of pregnancy location, viability, or gestational age. It can determine whether the level is in the discriminatory zone.

- If the hCG is above the discriminatory zone (3000–3500 mIU/mL), absence of a gestational sac with a yolk sac or embryo visualized in the uterus is highly suggestive of a nonviable gestation, either an early pregnancy loss or an ectopic pregnancy.
- If the initial hCG is below the discriminatory zone and there is no ultrasound evidence of ectopic pregnancy, patients should be followed up with repeat hCG levels every 48 hours. There is not a universal method to predict an expected minimal rise for serial hCG levels for a viable IUP. Rather, it is dependent on the initial hCG level. Updated guidelines about the appropriate hCG patterns help guide decision making and determine whether additional diagnostic interventions are needed.
- If definitive findings of an intrauterine or ectopic pregnancy are not present on TVUS in a pregnant patient with a positive hCG level, a pregnancy of unknown location exists. Serial monitoring is needed to either establish a definitive diagnosis or reasonably exclude an IUP before an ectopic pregnancy is diagnosed and treated. Uterine aspiration can be considered to confirm the diagnosis of early pregnancy loss or ectopic pregnancy based on the presence or absence of chorionic villi.

CURRENT THERAPY

- Surgical management of ectopic pregnancy is indicated when a patient is hemodynamically unstable, exhibits signs of intraperitoneal bleeding, reports symptoms concerning for a ruptured ectopic mass, or has a contraindication to methotrexate.
- For a patient who is clinically stable and has a nonruptured ectopic pregnancy, either surgical or medical management of ectopic pregnancy are safe and effective options. For the patient to make an informed choice, a shared decision-making model can be used that reviews the risks for and benefits of both approaches and considers the clinical features of the ectopic pregnancy, stability of the patient, future fertility plans, and additional patient characteristics that would preclude one approach or the other.
- Medical management with systemic methotrexate (not approved by the Food and Drug Administration) requires regular patient follow-up for laboratory and office visits until hCG levels are undetectable.
- Medical management with methotrexate is most effective when ectopic pregnancies are less than 4 cm on TVUS,
- Pretreatment hCG levels are less than 5000 mIU/mL, and fetal cardiac activity is not detected on TVUS.
- Expectant management of ectopic pregnancy may be considered in special circumstances, such as an asymptomatic and informed patient with reliable social resources in the setting of decreasing hCG levels that indicate pregnancy resolution.

An ectopic pregnancy is a potentially serious threat to the general and reproductive health of a pregnant person. Despite vast improvements in the clinical care of patients with ectopic pregnancy over recent years, diagnostic challenges and therapeutic controversies regarding this condition still exist. The objective of this chapter is to provide an overview of the epidemiology, diagnosis, and contemporary management of ectopic pregnancy. The chapter focuses on ectopic pregnancies that implant in the fallopian tube, which represent greater than 95% of all ectopic pregnancies.

Epidemiology

Of all pregnancies in the United States, approximately 1% to 2% are diagnosed as ectopic. The current incidence of ectopic pregnancy is difficult to calculate accurately because of the lack of tracking in both the hospital and outpatient settings, but recent studies estimate that over the last 25 years, it has increased six-fold. This rise may be the result of enhanced diagnostic capabilities, increased incidence of sexually transmitted infections and other risk factors, expanded use of infertility treatments, and heightened awareness of health professionals.

Ectopic pregnancy is the leading cause of maternal mortality in the first trimester of pregnancy in the United States, accounting for 2.7% of pregnancy-related deaths, and there should be continued high suspicion for at risk patients. However, the ectopic-related mortality rate is declining despite the increase in incidence. Between 1980 and 2007, 876 deaths were attributed to ectopic pregnancy, which represented a 56.6% decline in mortality rate between 1980 to 1984 and 2003 to 2007. However, age and racial disparities still persist. The ectopic pregnancy mortality ratio was 6.8 times higher for Black people compared with whites and 3.5 times higher for patients over 35 years old compared with those younger than 25 years old.

Pathophysiology

Damage to the fallopian tube and fallopian tube dysfunction are the primary factors associated with development of ectopic pregnancy. Normal embryo transport can be disrupted by damage to the structural integrity of the mucosal portion of the fallopian tube. Intratubal scarring secondary to infection or trauma could lead to trapping of a conceptus within intratubal adhesions or diverticula. Alteration of the hormonally mediated events leading to implantation, as sometimes occurs in treatments for infertility, offers another mechanism for consideration. A change in the estrogen-to-progesterone ratio could theoretically affect smooth muscle activity in the fallopian tube, immobilizing ciliary activity.

Risk Factors

Half of all patients with ectopic pregnancy will not report any known risk factors; therefore the absence of risk factors should not decrease clinical suspicion. However, identification of clinical and historical risk factors for ectopic pregnancy could aid in early diagnosis. The most significant historical risk factors include prior ectopic pregnancy, prior fallopian tube surgery, infertility treatment, and hospitalization for pelvic inflammatory disease (PID). History of prior ectopic pregnancy is the strongest of these. Major clinical risk factors include pain or moderate-to-severe vaginal bleeding at presentation. Less significant risk factors are tobacco use and age >35 years old. Up to 53% of pregnancies that occur with a copper or progestin-releasing intrauterine device (IUD) in place are ectopic; however, the overall failure rate IUDs is less than 1%.

Diagnosis and Clinical Manifestations

Although some patients present acutely with a ruptured ectopic pregnancy and hemoperitoneum, the vast majority (up to 80%) of ectopic pregnancies are diagnosed in stable patients who can be managed in the outpatient setting. Therefore reproductive-age people who present with symptoms of vaginal bleeding or abdominal discomfort need to be tested for pregnancy. If a patient is found to be pregnant, then their pregnancy needs to be differentiated as an ectopic pregnancy, a nonectopic gestation at risk for early pregnancy loss (EPL), or a normally developing IUP. The use of TVUS and hCG assays represent the current standard for this differentiation and for accurate and timely diagnosis of ectopic pregnancy.

Transvaginal Ultrasonography

Evaluating a patient with suspected ectopic pregnancy properly with TVUS requires an understanding of the findings typical of normal and abnormal pregnancies. The earliest ultrasonographic finding of a normal IUP is the gestational sac surrounded by a thick echogenic ring, located eccentrically within the endometrial cavity. On average, the gestational sac is seen on TVUS 5 weeks after the first day of the last menstrual period. The gestational sac grows and follows an approximate developmental timeline, which is represented by the following findings on TVUS: a yolk sac seen within the gestational sac at 5.5 weeks of gestation, an embryonic (fetal) pole at 6 weeks gestation, and cardiac activity at 6.5 weeks gestation.

A definitive IUP can be diagnosed by TVUS when a gestational sac with a yolk sac or embryo with or without cardiac activity is seen. A normal-appearing gestational sac should not solely be used to diagnose an IUP because it can be simulated by a pseudo- gestational sac and intrauterine fluid collection, which occurs in 8% to 29% of patients with ectopic pregnancy. The pseudogestational sac likely represents bleeding into the endometrial cavity by the decidual cast. The presence of an adnexal gestational sac with a fetal pole and cardiac activity is the most specific but least sensitive sign of ectopic pregnancy, occurring in only 10% to 17% of cases. Adnexal rings (fluid sacs with thick echogenic rings) that have a yolk sac or nonliving embryo are accepted as specific signs of ectopic pregnancy and are visualized in ectopic pregnancies 33% to 50% of the time.

A critical concept in the evaluation of early pregnancy by TVUS is that of the hCG discriminatory zone, or the level at or above which an examiner should see a normal intrauterine gestation, if present. In the setting of an hCG level above the discriminatory zone and no intrauterine pregnancy on ultrasound, an ectopic pregnancy or an abnormal intrauterine pregnancy is highly likely. The exact hCG discriminatory value varies somewhat based on the institution, ultrasound machine, ultrasonographer's experience, and hCG assay used. The value used should be conservatively high—at least 3000 mIU/mL and up to 3500 mIU/ mL—to minimize the risk of misdiagnosing a desired IUP as an ectopic pregnancy and treating it as such.

Hormonal Assays

Many patients with suspected ectopic pregnancy will present with a hCG below the discriminatory zone and have an ultrasound that does not provide a definitive diagnosis of an intrauterine or extra-uterine gestation (7%–20%). This is a pregnancy of unknown location (PUL), and serial monitoring is needed to establish a definitive diagnosis. Repeat hCG measurements are indicated at least every 48 hours to evaluate the appropriateness of hormonal trends along with serial TVUS studies. Comparing serial measurements of hCG from an individual patient to accepted patterns of hCG trends in early pregnancy helps distinguish an ectopic pregnancy from a viable IUP or a spontaneous EPL.

When evaluating serial hCG levels and predicting an expected minimal rise between values for a viable IUP, current evidence demonstrates there is not a universal trend that applies to all pregnancies at all gestations. Rather, it depends on the initial hCG level. Previous data showed that approximately 99% of viable intrauterine pregnancies are associated with a ≥53% increase in β-hCG values every 2 days. For pregnancies with an initial hCG value below 1500 mIU/mL, this calculation could apply. However, for pregnancies with higher initial hCG values, a laxer calculation should be used. One study suggests the following for an expected minimal rise for different initial hCG levels: 49% for levels <1500 mIU/mL, 40% for levels 1500 to 3000 mIU/mL, and 33% for levels >3000 mIU/mL. This represents a more conservative approach to incorporating invasive diagnostic procedures when following hCG values to prevent the interruption of normal pregnancies.

Patients with symptomatic first-trimester pregnancies, nondiagnostic ultrasound, and a hCG level that is declining (when the initial value is below the discriminatory zone) should also be followed with serial hCG levels until resolution to distinguish a resolving EPL from an ectopic pregnancy. Fifty percent of patients with ectopic pregnancies will present with declining hCG levels. Research describing the expected elimination of hCG in spontaneous EPL indicate that the minimum rate of decline ranges from 12% to 35% at 2 days to 34% to 84% at 7 days. Faster rates of decline occur with higher initial hCG levels. When the serial decline in hCG is in the range associated with spontaneous EPL, continued follow-up surveillance is indicated. If the hCG decline is slower than expected for an EPL, an ectopic pregnancy must be highly suspected.

Uterine Aspiration

The patient presenting with either (1) initial hCG below the discriminatory zone followed by an abnormal rise or decline or (2) initial hCG value at or above the discriminatory zone with no detectable intrauterine pregnancy has an abnormal pregnancy. The only exception to the rule for the second scenario would be if a multiple gestation had been conceived. The challenge for the clinician is then to determine whether the pregnancy is an abnormal IUP or an ectopic pregnancy. Office uterine vacuum aspiration or dilation and curettage in the operating room can help confirm the diagnosis of early pregnancy loss or ectopic pregnancy based on the presence or absence of chorionic villi. However, before this is considered, a progressing IUP must be reasonably excluded through serial monitoring with TVUS and hCG levels.

Uterine aspiration may spare some patients from receiving methotrexate[1]. If chorionic villi are present in the uterine aspiration specimen, then a failed IUP is confirmed. No further treatment is indicated. If chorionic villi are absent, hCG levels need to be monitored starting at 12 to 24 hours after the procedure to determine whether they increase, plateau, or decrease appropriately. The hCG trend after uterine aspiration determines whether medical management of ectopic pregnancy with methotrexate should be implemented. The patient's preference, development of symptoms, and level of clinical suspicion for ectopic pregnancy also play an important role in whether methotrexate is given.

There is debate in the literature on whether uterine aspiration is needed before methotrexate is given to treat ectopic pregnancy. Empiric treatment of suspected ectopic pregnancy without the performance of uterine vacuum aspiration or dilation and curettage could result in inappropriate treatment of up to 40% of patients. Performing uterine aspiration could delay treatment of an ectopic pregnancy; however, the risk of tubal rupture for these patients is low (1.7%).

Treatment and Therapeutic Monitoring

Surgery has long been the mainstay of treatment for ectopic pregnancy, but medical management is a widely used alternative. Both are safe and effective treatment options for patients who are clinically stable. The choice of any treatment depends on factors such as clinical presentation, the risks of either surgery or medical management to the patient, and future fertility plans.

Surgical Management

Patients with hemodynamic instability caused by a ruptured ectopic pregnancy require laparotomy and salpingectomy of the involved fallopian tube owing to extensive tubal damage. Most patients with ectopic pregnancy who are stable can be safely treated with laparoscopy. For patients with an unruptured ectopic pregnancy, surgical options include tube-sparing salpingostomy or removal of the fallopian tube (salpingectomy).

The decision between salpingostomy and salpingectomy depends on the location of the ectopic pregnancy within the fallopian tube, the extent of the damage to the fallopian tube, and the patient's desire for future fertility. Ideal candidates for salpingostomy include patients who have an ectopic pregnancy in the ampulla or infundibulum of the fallopian tube. Salpingectomy is reserved for patients with isthmic ectopic pregnancies, tubal rupture, or an ipsilateral recurrent ectopic pregnancy. Patients who have completed childbearing might be better candidates for salpingectomy than salpingostomy.

With respect to future fertility, subsequent IUP, and repeat ectopic pregnancy, a systematic review and meta-analysis of two randomized controlled trials (RCT) and 16 cohort studies showed that for the RCTs, there was not a difference between salpingectomy and salpingostomy for the likelihood of a subsequent IUP and repeat ectopic pregnancy. For the cohort studies, salpingectomy was associated with a lower likelihood of subsequent IUP. The cohort studies also found a higher risk for repeat ectopic pregnancy among pregnant people treated by salpingectomy with risk factors for future infertility (previous ectopic pregnancy, endometriosis,

history of infertility, history of tubal surgery, pregnancy conceived with in-vitro fertilization, known hydrosalpinx or tubal occlusion, or intraoperative identification of contralateral tubal pathology).

Medical Management

Methotrexate (MTX) is a folic acid antagonist that impairs DNA synthesis and cellular replication targeting rapidly proliferating cells such as trophoblasts. It can be used for medical management of ectopic pregnancy in patients who have a confirmed or high clinical suspicion of ectopic pregnancy, an unruptured mass, and no contraindication to the medication.[1]

Absolute contraindications to medical management of ectopic pregnancy are listed in Table 1. Among the most important of these is the inability of the patient to comply with follow-up after initiation of therapy. Without the ability to monitor the response to MTX and provide additional doses if deemed appropriate, opportunities to prevent ectopic rupture could be missed. To ascertain whether a patient is eligible for MTX therapy, a comprehensive laboratory and medical evaluation should first be performed, including a complete blood count and renal and liver function tests Treatment failure occurs when the hCG level decline is deemed inadequate and surgery is required. In some cases, medication failure presents as tubal rupture requiring emergent surgery.

Relative contraindications in Table 1 pertain to patient characteristics that reduce the odds of successful treatment. The strongest predictor for the efficacy of MTX treatment is an initial hCG concentration >5000 mIU/mL, and it is associated with a failure rate of 14.3% or higher.

Three methotrexate treatment regimens exist: single-dose, two-dose, and multidose regimens (Table 2). These designations refer more to the number of intended doses in the protocol rather than the actual number or doses received by all patients. For any of the protocols, once hCG levels have declined by at least 15% between interval assessments, no additional doses of medication are required, but hCG must still be followed until complete resolution to ensure treatment efficacy. A systematic review and meta-analysis of six RCTs demonstrated that the single-dose and multiple-dose regimens have similar success rates, and the difference between the single-dose and double-dose regimens was not statistically significant. More side effects occurred with the multiple-dose regimen compared with single-dose and double-dose. The definition of successful treatment with MTX is resolution of the ectopic pregnancy without surgery, and the success rate ranges from 70% to 95% depending on the initial hCG level and treatment protocol.

The biggest risk of medical management with MTX is ectopic pregnancy rupture. There is also the risk of fetal death or teratogenic effects if an IUP occurs shortly after treatment, and patients should be counseled to wait one ovulatory cycle after hCG levels are undetectable before attempting pregnancy again.

Side effects of MTX therapy occur in up to 30% of patients; however, most of these resolve rapidly and are generally of minor consequence. Abdominal pain is common early in treatment and is of concern as a possible indicator of tubal rupture. A potential cause of this pain in nonacute patients can be tubal miscarriage. Additional potential side effects include nausea, vomiting, diarrhea, gastritis, stomatitis, and liver transaminitis. Serious side effects such as alopecia and neutropenia can occur but are extremely rare.

Reproductive success after successful MTX therapy appears similar to that after salpingostomy. The most critical predictors of fertility after ectopic pregnancy treated by any conservative means are the condition of the contralateral fallopian tube and the presence of additional ectopic risk factors.

Expectant Management

Because numerous ectopic pregnancies resolve spontaneously, there has been great interest in considering expectant management

---

[1]Not FDA approved for this indication.

[1]Not FDA approved for this indication.

TABLE 1 Contraindications to Medical Management of Ectopic Pregnancy With Methotrexate

	ACOG*	ASRM†
Absolute contraindications	Intrauterine pregnancy; breastfeeding; laboratory evidence of immunodeficiency; preexisting blood dyscrasias (bone marrow hypoplasia, leukopenia, thrombocytopenia, or clinically significant anemia); known sensitivity to methotrexate; active pulmonary disease; peptic ulcer disease; clinically significant hepatic, renal, or hematologic dysfunction; hemodynamically unstable patient; inability to participate in follow-up	Breast-feeding; evidence of immunodeficiency; moderate-to-severe anemia, leukopenia, or thrombocytopenia; sensitivity to methotrexate; active pulmonary or peptic ulcer disease; clinically important hepatic or renal dysfunction; intrauterine pregnancy
Relative contraindications	Ectopic mass >4 cm by TVUS; embryonic cardiac activity by TVUS; high initial hCG concentration (>5,000 mIU/mL)	Ectopic mass >4 cm detected by TVUS; embryonic cardiac activity detected by TVUS; patient declines blood transfusion; patient is not able to participate in follow-up; high initial hCG level (>5000 mIU/mL)

TVUS, transvaginal ultrasound; hCG, β–human chorionic gonadotropin.
*Data are from the American College of Obstetricians and Gynecologists (ACOG).
†Data are from the American Society for Reproductive Medicine (ASRM).

TABLE 2 Methotrexate[1] Protocols for Treatment of Ectopic Pregnancy

	SINGLE DOSE	TWO DOSE	MULTIDOSE
Day 1	Check hCG value. Administer first dose of MTX 50 mg/m^2 IM.	Check hCG value. Administer first dose of MTX 50 mg/m^2 IM.	Check hCG value. Administer first dose of MTX 1 mg/kg IM followed by leucovorin[1] 0.1 mg/kg IM on day 2. Check hCG on day 2.
Day 4	Check hCG value.	Check hCG value. Administer second dose of MTX 50 mg/m^2 IM.	Administer second dose of MTX (day 3) and leucovorin (day 4). Check hCG on day 4.
Day 7	Check hCG value looking for 15% decrease between days 4 and 7. If >15% fall, check hCG weekly until not detectable in serum. If <15% fall, administer second dose of MTX 50 mg/m^2 IM.	Check hCG value for 15% decrease between days 4 and 7. If >15% fall, check β-hCG weekly until not detectable in serum. If <15% fall, administer third dose of MTX 50 mg/m^2 IM.	Continue administering doses of MTX and leucovorin (i.e., course 3 days 5 and 6 and course 4 days 7 and 8) until hCG values have declined by 15%. Do not exceed 4 courses. If >15% decline, check hCG weekly until not detectable in serum.
Day 11		Check hCG value for 15% decrease between days 7 and 11. If >15% decline, check hCG weekly until not detectable in serum. If <15%, administer fourth dose of MTX 50 mg/m^2 IM.	
Weekly surveillance	If follow-up hCG value plateau or rise, consider surgical intervention or repeat dose of MTX as additional therapy.	If follow-up hCG value plateau or rise, consider surgical intervention or repeat dose of MTX as additional therapy.	If follow-up hCG value plateau or rise, consider surgical intervention or repeat dose of MTX as additional therapy.

hCG, β–human chorionic gonadotropin; IM, intramuscular; MTX, methotrexate.
[1]Not FDA approved for this indication.

in selected patients. Expectant management includes close monitoring of symptoms, determination of hCG levels every 48 hours, and serial TVUS. The likelihood of successful ectopic resolution is highest in the presence of a nondiagnostic ultrasound and hCG values below the discriminatory zone.

References

ACOG: Practice bulletin No. 193 interim update: tubal ectopic pregnancy, *Obstet Gynecol* 131:e91–e103, 2018.

Barnhart KT, Guo W, Cary MS, et al: Differences in serum human chorionic gonadotropin rise in early pregnancy by race and value at presentation, *Obstet Gynecol* 128:504–511, 2016.

Barnhart K, van Mello NM, Bourne T, et al: Pregnancy of unknown location: a consensus statement of nomenclature, definitions, and outcome, *Fertil Steril* 95:857–866, 2011.

Barnhart KT, Sammel MD, Gracia CR, Chittams J, Hummel AC, Shaunik A: Risk factors for ectopic pregnancy in women with symptomatic first-trimester pregnancies, *Fertil Steril* 86:36–43, 2006.

Connolly A, Ryan DH, Stuebe AM, Wolfe HM: Reevaluation of discriminatory and threshold levels for serum beta-hCG in early pregnancy, *Obstet Gynecol* 121:65–70, 2013.

Hendriks E, Rosenberg R, Prine L: Ectopic pregnancy: diagnosis and management, *Am Fam Physician* 101(10):599–606, 2020. PMID: 32412215.

Insogna IG, Farland LV, Missmer SA, Ginsburg ES, Brady PC: Outpatient endometrial aspiration: an alternative to methotrexate for pregnancy of unknown location, *Am J Obstet Gynecol* 217:185.e1–185.e9, 2017.

Menon S, Colins J, Barnhart KT: Establishing a human chorionic gonadotropin cutoff to guide methotrexate treatment of ectopic pregnancy: a systematic review, *Fertil Steril* 87:481–484, 2007.

Ozcan MCH, Wilson JR, Frishman GN: A systematic review and meta-analysis of surgical treatment of ectopic pregnancy with salpingectomy versus salpingostomy, *J Minim Invasive Gynecol* 28(3):656–667, 2021. https://doi.org/10.1016/j.jmig.2020.10.014. Epub 2020 Oct 24. PMID: 33198948.

Yang C, Cai J, Geng Y, Gao Y: Multiple-dose and double-dose versus single-dose administration of methotrexate for the treatment of ectopic pregnancy: a systematic review and meta-analysis, *Reprod Biomed Online* 34(4):383–391, 2017. https://doi.org/10.1016/j.rbmo.2017.01.004.

HYPERTENSION IN PREGNANCY

Method of
Leah Peterson, MD

CURRENT DIAGNOSIS

- Hypertensive disorders of pregnancy are a major cause of morbidity and mortality for women and infants
- Hypertensive disorders of pregnancy are divided into four categories:
  ○ Gestational hypertension
  ○ Chronic hypertension
  ○ Chronic hypertension with superimposed preeclampsia
  ○ Preeclampsia–eclampsia
- Preeclampsia can be diagnosed by the presence of hypertension and end-organ damage, even in the absence of proteinuria.

CURRENT THERAPY

- Blood pressure readings ≥160/105 require pharmacologic treatment.
- Nifedipine (Procardia), labetalol (Trandate), and methyldopa are approved for treatment of hypertensive disorders in pregnancy.
- Patients with gestational hypertension and preeclampsia should be monitored with regular labs, sonograms, and antenatal testing.
- Delivery is the definitive treatment for preeclampsia.
- Hypertensive disorders in pregnancy are an indication for early delivery. Delivery time is based on severity of maternal symptoms and estimated gestational age of the fetus.
- Magnesium sulfate injection is indicated in severe preeclampsia, for the prevention of eclampsia. It is also the preferred agent for treatment of eclampsia.
- Hypertensive disorders of pregnancy can present in the postpartum period.
- Preeclampsia is associated with increased risk for cardiovascular disease later in life.
- Initiation of daily low-dose aspirin[1] late in the first trimester is indicated for prevention of preeclampsia in certain high-risk women.

[1]Not FDA approved for this indication.

Epidemiology

Hypertensive disorders complicate nearly 10% of pregnancies (Box 1) and their incidence is increasing. Preeclampsia causes 50,000–60,000 deaths per year worldwide, in addition to causing significant maternal and fetal morbidity in hundreds of thousands of others. Some of these outcomes can be prevented or improved on through implementation of the updated recommendations in clinical practice.

Pathophysiology

The precise mechanism for the development of preeclampsia is unknown. A major component in the development of preeclampsia is the excessive placental production of antagonists to both vascular epithelial growth factor (VEGF) and transforming growth factor β (TGF-β). These antagonists to VEGF and TGF-β disrupt endothelial and renal glomerular function resulting in edema, hypertension, and proteinuria. In addition, there appears to be a heritable component, and oxidative stress and abnormal

placental implantation can further increase the risk of developing the disease.

Prevention

In women with history of a delivery at less than 34 0/7 weeks' gestation, or with history of preeclampsia in multiple pregnancies, daily low-dose aspirin therapy is suggested. Low-dose aspirin is not associated with increased bleeding or placental abruption. Supplementation with vitamin C[1] or E[1] is not recommended in the prevention of preeclampsia. Supplementation of calcium[1] in women with preeclampsia is only indicated in those who are calcium-deficient. Bed rest and salt restriction are not recommended for prevention of preeclampsia.

Diagnosis

Isolated hypertensive disease diagnosed prior to 20 weeks of gestation is classified as chronic hypertension. Gestational hypertension is defined as the onset of hypertension (≥140/90 on two occasions at least 4 h apart), after 20 weeks' gestation, in the absence of proteinuria or other criteria for preeclampsia.

Preeclampsia is a hypertensive disorder that is multisystemic in nature and is specific to pregnancy. It presents after the 20th week of gestation, and typically near term. Traditionally, diagnosis of preeclampsia has been based on new onset hypertension and the presence of proteinuria. Clinically significant proteinuria is defined as ≥300 mg on a 24-h urine, or a spot microalbumin/creatinine ratio ≥0.3. The use of dipstick quantification of proteinuria is discouraged unless no other method is available. Urinary protein levels are not correlated with outcome severity and are not themselves considered a severe feature.

There are some women who present with hypertension and signs of systemic disease in the absence of proteinuria. The presence of end-organ damage, as noted in Table 1, combined with onset of hypertension after 20 weeks' gestation is sufficient for a diagnosis of severe preeclampsia, even in the absence of proteinuria. The presence of any one of these features may signal impending eclamptic seizure. In addition to seizure and maternal end-organ damage, complications from preeclampsia include intrauterine growth restriction, placental abruption, and fetal demise.

Management

Chronic hypertension is associated with intrauterine growth restriction, placental abruption, and progression to preeclampsia. Treatment of chronic hypertension is indicated if blood pressure (BP) is consistently greater than 160/105, and approved treatment agents include methyldopa, nifedipine (Procardia), and labetalol (Trandate). It is essential to avoid overtreatment,

[1]Not FDA approved for this indication.

TABLE 1	Diagnostic Criteria for Preeclampsia
Blood pressure	• Greater than or equal to 140 mm Hg systolic or greater than or equal to 90 mm Hg diastolic on two occasions at least 4 h apart after 20 weeks of gestation in a woman with a previously normal blood pressure
	• Greater than or equal to 160 mm Hg systolic or greater than or equal to 110 mm Hg diastolic, hypertension can be confirmed within a short interval (minutes) to facilitate timely antihypertensive therapy
and	
Proteinuria	• Greater than or equal to 300 mg per 24-h urine collection (for this amount extrapolated from a timed collection) or • Protein/creatinine ratio greater than or equal to 0.3[a] • Dipstick readying of 1+ (used only if other quantitative methods not available)

Or in the absence of proteinuria, new-onset hypertension with the new onset of any of the following:

Thrombocytopenia	• Platelet count less than 100,000/mL
Renal insufficiency	• Serum creatinine concentrations greater than 1.1 mg/dL or a doubling of the serum creatinine concentration in the absence of other renal disease
Impaired liver function	• Elevated blood concentrations of liver transaminases to twice normal concentration
Pulmonary edema	
Cerebral or visual symptoms	

[a]Each measured as mg/dL
American College of Obstetricians and Gynecologists. Hypertension in pregnancy. 2013. Available at http://www.Acog.org/Resources-And-Publications/Task-Force-and-Work-Group-Reports/Hypertension-in-Pregnancy.

TABLE 2	Contraindications to Expectant Management
Deliver immediately if:
Uncontrollable severe hypertension
Eclampsia
Pulmonary edema
Disseminated intravascular coagulation (DIC)
Abruption
Non-reassuring fetal heart tones
Intrapartum fetal demise

TABLE 3	Signs and Symptoms of Magnesium Toxicity	
	MANIFESTATIONS	LEVEL (MG/DL)
Loss of patellar reflex		8–12
Double vision		8–12
Feeling of warmth, flushing		9–12
Somnolence		10–12
Slurred speech		10–12
Muscular paralysis		15–17
Respiratory arrest		15–17
Cardiac arrest		30–36

to prevent adverse fetal outcomes from decreased perfusion. Therefore the goal is to keep BP below 120/80 with treatment. Angiotensin-converting enzyme (ACE) inhibitors, angiotensin receptor blockers (ARBs), and atenolol (Tenormin) should not be used in pregnancy due to fetal risk. Women with chronic hypertension should also be monitored with serial ultrasound after fetal viability.

Gestational hypertension is managed with expectant monitoring and delivery at 37 weeks. BP should be measured twice weekly, and patient should have weekly assessment of LFTs and platelet count to assess for development of preeclampsia. Antihypertensive therapy should be initiated for BP ≥160/105. Additionally, the patient should have once-weekly nonstress testing.

Preeclampsia should be managed similarly to gestational hypertension, with the addition of regular sonograms for fetal growth, and twice-weekly fetal nonstress testing. Delivery should occur at 37 weeks, and should occur at 34 weeks if patient develops severe features.

In the event that the patient develops preeclampsia with severe features prior to 34 weeks, steroids (12 mg betamethasone [Celestone][1] IM q12h×2 doses, or 6 mg dexamethasone [Decadron][1] q12h×4 doses) can be given and delivery can be postponed for 48 h, unless maternal or fetal instability develops. Contraindications to expectant management in this scenario are noted

[1]Not FDA approved for this indication.

in Table 2. If severe features are noted prior to fetal viability, delivery should occur immediately. Expectant management is not recommended due to maternal risk.

In addition, magnesium sulfate ($MgSO_4$) is indicated in preeclampsia with severe features. Administration of $MgSO_4$ has been shown to prevent eclamptic seizures and placental abruption in these patients. Patients with preeclampsia without severe features should be monitored closely, and $MgSO_4$ should be started if severe features develop. $MgSO_4$ is given as a 4–6-g intravenous loading dose, followed by a maintenance infusion of 1–2 g/h. Women with normal renal function do not require serum magnesium testing, but all women receiving $MgSO_4$ should be monitored closely for signs of magnesium toxicity by serial evaluations of reflexes, respiratory rate, and urinary output. Signs and symptoms of magnesium toxicity are noted in Table 3.

Inpatient management for 72 h postpartum is recommended for women with gestational hypertension or preeclampsia. Blood pressure levels decrease in most women, but if blood pressure remains >150/100 on two occasions 4 h apart, an antihypertensive regimen should be started. If level is <160/100, BP should be rechecked 15 min later, and antihypertensive treatment should be started within 60 min. Oral nifedipine or labetalol, and intravenous labetalol or hydralazine (Apresoline) are commonly used agents. Nonsteroidal antiinflammatory drugs (NSAIDs) should be avoided in the patient with hypertension that persists past 24 h postpartum, as they may worsen BP.

Preeclampsia may begin in the postpartum period, so all patients should be counseled about signs and symptoms prior to discharge. In addition, preeclampsia is a risk factor for future cardiovascular disease. In women who delivered prior to 37 weeks or have history of recurrent preeclampsia, yearly assessment of BP, lipids, fasting glucose, and body mass index (BMI) is suggested.

Complications

HELLP syndrome (hemolysis, elevated liver enzymes, and low platelet count occurring in association with preeclampsia) occurs in 20% of pregnancies complicated by preeclampsia with severe features. HELLP syndrome is diagnosed by the presence of LFTs >2× normal, hemolysis (lactate dehydrogenase >600U/L, damaged erythrocytes noted on peripheral smear, or bilirubin >1.2 mg/dL, and platelets <100,000). Diagnosis of HELLP can be difficult, as 12–18% of patients with the disorder are normotensive, and 13% do not have proteinuria. Evaluation for HELLP syndrome includes a complete blood count and LFT testing. A DIC panel should also be considered if platelet count is <50,000.

Patients with HELLP should receive MgSO$_4$ from admission until 24–48h postpartum. Platelet transfusion is indicated if counts are <20,000 prior to vaginal delivery or <50,000 prior to cesarean delivery, or in women with abnormal bleeding. Corticosteroids have been shown to increase platelet counts in women with HELLP syndrome but have not been shown to improve maternal or fetal outcomes, except for the benefit of improving fetal lung function prior to 34 weeks' gestational age. Because the condition is often progressive and associated with sudden deterioration of both maternal and fetal condition, prompt delivery is indicated if the HELLP presents later than 34 weeks.

Eclampsia is a life-threatening complication of preeclampsia, defined as new-onset grand mal seizures in a woman with preeclampsia. Seizures typically last 60–90 seconds, and may be followed by a postictal state. During an eclamptic seizure, the fetus often becomes hypoxic and bradycardic. Eclampsia can occur antepartum, intrapartum, or postpartum. It can be preceded by a wide range of symptoms, and can occur even in the absence of proteinuria or hypertension. Eclampsia is often preceded by persistent headache, visual changes, altered mental status, and upper abdominal pain.

MgSO$_4$ is the drug of choice in treating eclampsia, both for the initial convulsion and for prevention of subsequent ones. The dosing regimen is a 6-g loading dose given over 15–20min, followed by a maintenance infusion of 2g/h for at least 24h after the convulsion. No other anticonvulsants should be given in attempt to shorten or abolish the initial convulsion. Care should be taken to protect the airway, reduce risk of aspiration, and prevent maternal injury. Ten percent of eclamptic women will have a second convulsion after receiving magnesium. If this occurs, an additional 2-g dose should be given intravenously over 3–5 min.

References

American College of Obstetricians and Gynecologists: *Hypertension in pregnancy*. 2013, Available at http://www.Acog.org/Resources-And-Publications/Task-Force-and-Work-Group-Reports/Hypertension-in-Pregnancy.

Duley L, Gülmezoglu AM, Henderson-Smart DJ, Chou D: Magnesium sulphate and other anticonvulsants for women with pre-eclampsia, *Cochrane Database Syst Rev*(11)CD000025, 2010.

Hart L, Sibai BM: Seizures in pregnancy: epilepsy, eclampsia, and stroke, *Semin Perinatol* 23:207–224, 2013.

Leeman L, Dresand LT, Fontaine P: Hypertensive disorders of pregnancy, *Am Fam Physician* 93(2):121–127, 2016.

Sibai BM: Diagnosis, controversies, and management of the syndrome of hemolysis, elevated liver enzymes, and low platelet count, *Obstet Gynecol* 103:981–991, 2004.

POSTPARTUM CARE

Tara J. Neil, MD

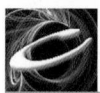

CURRENT DIAGNOSIS

- The postpartum period consists of the period from delivery of the infant until 6 to 8 weeks postpartum.
- Postpartum hemorrhage is a medical emergency and is usually caused by uterine atony.
- Fever during the postpartum period is typically caused by endometritis or mastitis.

CURRENT THERAPY

- Continue to monitor and check for resolution of any complications or medical conditions that arise during pregnancy.
- Uterine atony responds to massage and medications. Providers should be familiar with the medications and their dosages.
- Postpartum contraception counseling should be started immediately and all forms can be used by 6 weeks postpartum.
- Breastfeeding is the preferred nutrition for newborns and success is dependent on provider counseling and encouragement.

BOX 1 Causes of Postpartum Hemorrhage

- Uterine atony
- Vaginal or cervical laceration
- Coagulation disorder
- Uterine inversion
- Retained placenta/products

Postpartum care encompasses the period after delivery of infant and placenta until 6 to 8 weeks after delivery. The hormonal and physiologic systems that underwent changes during pregnancy return to normal during this time. During the initial 24 to 48 hours, most patients are monitored in the hospital for possible complications after delivery.

Postpartum Hemorrhage

Postpartum hemorrhage is defined as blood loss greater than 500 mL after vaginal delivery or greater than 1000 mL after cesarean section. It is the major cause of maternal morbidity and mortality worldwide. Practitioners should be prepared to diagnose and treat the cause.

Some common causes of hemorrhage are identified in Box 1, including the most common cause: uterine atony. Once abnormal bleeding is identified, resuscitation measures should be started, including intravenous (IV) access, nursing assistance, starting fluid resuscitation with crystalloids or blood products, and anesthesia if needed. In addition, administration of tranexamic acid (Cyklokapron)[1] 1000 mg IV has been shown to decrease mortality regardless of the cause of bleeding. The uterus should be examined using a bimanual examination and vigorous massage. If the uterus is boggy, the medications listed in Table 1 can be used to improve uterine tone and decrease bleeding. If the bladder is full, a catheter should be placed. Careful inspection of the cervix, vaginal walls, and perineum should be performed to identify other sources of hemorrhage. If bleeding is not slowed or the cause of hemorrhage not identified, manual exploration of the uterus can be performed with proper anesthesia to check for retained products. Surgical treatment with dilation and curettage and hysterectomy can also be used if manual exploration and medical management do not control bleeding. If the patient is hemodynamically stable and the resources are available, embolization of the uterine arteries can also control bleeding.

---

[1]Available as dietary supplement.

TABLE 1	Medications Used to Treat Uterine Atony		
MEDICATION	**ADMINISTRATION**	**FREQUENCY**	**SPECIAL CONSIDERATIONS**
Oxytocin (Pitocin)	10 units IM 10–40 units in 1000 mL of IV solution	Once Continuous to maintain uterine tone	Should not be given directly in IV
Methylergonovine maleate (Methergine)	0.2 mg IM/IV 0.2 mg PO	Repeat every 2–4 h as needed 3–4 times daily for maximum of 7 days	Contraindicated in hypertension
Carboprost tromethamine (Hemabate)	0.25 mg IM	Repeat every 15–90 min. Maximum dose 2 mg	Contraindicated in active cardiac, renal, pulmonary, and liver disease. Use cautiously in asthmatics.
Misoprostol (Cytotec)[1]	800–1000 µg rectally[3]	One-time dose	

[1]Not FDA approved for this indication.
[3]Exceeds dosage recommended by the manufacturer.

Postpartum Care After Hospital Dismissal

Clinical care in the postpartum period should be focused on continued care of the mom and baby and not as a single visit. To better facilitate this, the patient should have clinical contact by phone or at appointment with the provider or clinical team in the first 3 weeks. Ongoing care should be provided on an as-needed basis. Ultimately, the postpartum period ends with a comprehensive visit and exam occurring by 12 weeks. This visit should include full physical and psychosocial assessment as well as discussion of interpregnancy spacing and management of any chronic health conditions.

Fever and Infection

Fever greater than 38°C (100.4°F) should be evaluated and a source identified. Box 2 lists the most common causes of postpartum fever. Evaluation should include a physical examination to include the uterus and breasts, with attention to any lacerations or incisions. Laboratory testing should include urinalysis, complete blood count (CBC), and blood cultures if appropriate.

Endometritis, a polymicrobial infection of the endometrium of the uterus, typically causes fever in the first 1 to 2 weeks postpartum. Diagnostic criteria include fever and uterine pain with palpation. Endometritis is treated with IV broad-spectrum antibiotics until fever and uterine pain resolve. If there is no clinical improvement after several days of treatment, imaging with computed tomography (CT) or ultrasound of the pelvis can be used to look for complications, including pelvic abscess and septic pelvic thrombophlebitis.

Mastitis causes fever in breastfeeding mothers. It is caused by the introduction of skin flora through cracks in the nipple and skin and infects milk ducts and surrounding soft tissues in areas of stasis. Treatment includes frequent feeding or pumping to alleviate the stasis. There is inadequate evidence to support antibiotic use, but if symptoms persist after effectively emptying breasts, most practitioners treat with a 10- to 14-day course of oral narrow-spectrum antibiotics. Complications can include breast abscesses, which are usually diagnosed by ultrasound.

Immunization

Immunizations should be updated during the postpartum period. Rubella status is routinely checked during the prenatal period and immunization should be given if indicated. Tdap (tetanus toxoid, reduced diphtheria toxoid, and acellular pertussis vaccine [Adacel, Boostrix]) should be given to the patient and offered to other members of the family if they have not received a pertussis booster to help protect the infant from contracting pertussis. Influenza vaccine should be given if it was not given during pregnancy. Rh(D)-negative mothers should receive anti-D immune globulin if their infants are Rh(D) positive.

BOX 2	Causes of Postpartum Fever

- Mastitis
- Endometritis
- Urinary tract infection
- Wound infection (perineal or abdominal)
- Septic thrombophlebitis
- Deep vein thrombosis

Breastfeeding

Breast milk is universally recognized as the best nutrition for newborns. Infants who are breastfed have fewer ear, lower respiratory, and gastrointestinal infections. They are also less likely to develop asthma, diabetes, and obesity. Contraindications to breastfeeding include human immunodeficiency virus (HIV), active herpetic lesions on breasts, maternal drug abuse, and certain medications. Any medications prescribed during breastfeeding should be checked for safety. It is currently recommended, when possible, for infants to be exclusively breastfed until 6 months and supplemented with foods between the ages of 6 months and 1 year. Clinicians play a crucial role in educating mothers about the importance of breastfeeding and supporting them during breastfeeding.

Contraception

Discussing contraception after delivery is important for healthy birth spacing. Ovulation can occur as early as 3 weeks after delivery. Breastfeeding mothers can use lactational amenorrhea during this period if they are exclusively breastfeeding. They can also use progesterone-only contraception (Micronor, Depo-Provera, Nexplanon) or intrauterine device starting 6 weeks postpartum. Combined estrogen-progesterone formulations can be started as early as 3 weeks postpartum in nonbreastfeeding mothers. Starting estrogen-containing formulations before this can increase the risk for thromboembolism. Intrauterine devices and diaphragms are typically placed at 6 weeks after the uterus has returned to its normal size. Medroxyprogesterone intramuscular (IM) injection (Depo-Provera) and etonogestrel subcutaneous (SC) implant (Nexplanon) may be given in the first 5 days postpartum if a patient is not breastfeeding.

Other Considerations

Close evaluation and continued management of medical conditions that develop during pregnancy, including thyroid disease, gestational diabetes, and preeclampsia, should be continued.

The postpartum period is an important time for new mothers. Open communication with their providers during this time helps support them and helps them to recognize conditions that are important for their health and the health of their newborn.

References

American College of Obstetricians and Gynecologists: *Compendium of selected publications*, Atlanta, 2007, American College of Obstetricians and Gynecologists.

Breastfeeding, Family Physicians Supporting. Available at. http://www.aafp.org/online/en/home/policy/policies/b/breastfeedingpositionpaper.html (accessed February 25, 2020).

Centers for Disease Control: Pertussis (whooping cough) vaccination. Available at http://www.cdc.gov/vaccines/vpd-vac/pertussis/default.htm (accessed February 25, 2020).

French LM, Smaill FM: Antibiotic regimens for endometritis after delivery, *Cochrane Database Syst Rev* (4):CD001067, 2004.

Jahanfar S, Ng C-J, Teng CL: Antibiotics for mastitis in breastfeeding women, *Cochrane Database Syst Rev* 1:CD005458, 2009.

Optimizing postpartum care. ACOG Committee Opinion No. 736: American College of Obstetricians and Gynecologists, *Obstet Gynecol* 131:e140–e150, 2018.

Truitt ST, Fraser AB, Gallo MFet al, et al: Combined hormonal versus nonhormonal versus progestin-only contraception in lacation, *Cochrane Database Syst Rev* (2):CD003988, 2003.

WOMAN Trial Collaborators: Effect of early tranexamic acid administration on mortality, hysterectomy, and other morbidities in women with post-partum haemorrhage (WOMAN): an international, randomised, double-blind, placebo-controlled trial, *Lancet* 389(10084):2105–2116, 2017.

POSTPARTUM DEPRESSION

Method of
Daniel S. Oram, MD; and Lydia U. Lee, MD

CURRENT DIAGNOSIS

- All pregnant and postpartum women should be screened for postpartum depression with a validated tool, such as the Edinburgh Postpartum Depression Scale
- Care should be taken to exclude bipolar disorder

CURRENT THERAPY

- Cognitive behavioral therapy and interpersonal therapy are the most well-studied interventions
- Selective serotonin reuptake inhibitors are modestly effective for postpartum depression and are generally safe, with most data for sertraline (Zoloft)
- A newly approved neuroactive steroid, brexanolone (Zulresso), may prove to be useful in rapidly inducing remission, although use will likely be limited to the inpatient setting

Introduction

Postpartum depression is a common mood disorder that carries the potential for substantial morbidity. There is no universally agreed-upon definition. Increasingly, postpartum- and antepartum-onset depression are being considered together as peripartum depression; the *Diagnostic and Statistical Manual of Mental Disorders*, fifth edition (DSM-5) uses the specifier "with peripartum onset" to refer to an episode of major depression which occurs during pregnancy or within 4 weeks of delivery. Clinically, however, postpartum depression is often identified if onset is within 1 year of delivery. There are considerations in management of mood disorders that are unique to the postpartum period. Therefore this chapter will focus on depressive episodes with postpartum onset, in line with much of the primary literature on this topic.

Epidemiology

In developed countries, postpartum depression has an incidence of about 15% (including both major and minor depression) in the first 3 months of the postpartum period. Worldwide prevalence varies widely by country; estimates using most rigorous methods vary from 0.1% to 26%, with culture influencing both maternal mood and how mood symptoms are communicated.

Risk Factors

The most consistently identified risk factors for depression with postpartum onset include history of mental illness prior to or during the pregnancy (especially prior postpartum depression, recurrent major depression, and bipolar disorder), stressful life events, poor social support, poor partner relationships, and infant medical illness. Abuse is also frequently reported as a risk factor, and includes current or lifetime history of physical, psychological, or sexual abuse by intimate partners or family members. A wide range of other risk factors that have been less consistently cited include infant temperament, negative attitude toward pregnancy, low socioeconomic status, young maternal age, unplanned pregnancy, and obstetric complications. Among women who are identified as having postpartum depression, a recent prospective cohort study predicted risk factors for a severe depressive episode with high accuracy. They found that at-risk women had higher Edinburgh Postpartum Depression Scale (EPDS) scores obtained, higher parity, lower education, and lower Global Assessment of Functioning scores, though this approach will need further validation.

Pathophysiology

While the etiology of postpartum depression has not been fully elucidated, it is best understood through a biopsychosocial model. Sex hormones fall rapidly after delivery and likely precipitate depressive symptoms. In particular, experimental evidence in postpartum women supports the role of low postpartum levels of estrogen and the progesterone metabolite allopregnanolone (which affects GABA signaling) in contributing to the depressed mood. Genetic variants in hormonal and serotonergic pathways likely place some women at increased risk. This genetic risk is likely potentiated by social stressors. Finally, cultural factors affect both norms of social support provided to new mothers, and the language mothers use to express their symptoms.

Prevention

Care teams should identify women at high risk early in pregnancy; this process should include routine use of a mood inventory such as the EPDS. At-risk women should receive multifaceted support throughout pregnancy and the postpartum period. Components can include a longitudinal patient-provider relationship, which may benefit from more frequent visits, social needs assessment, referral to community maternal–infant health resources, and early initiation of therapy. Interpersonal therapy is the best-supported modality for the prevention of postpartum depression. Postpartum home visits and telephone follow-up have been found helpful in decreasing depression incidence. Starting an antidepressant prophylactically has not been effective experimentally in preventing postpartum depression. However, discontinuing antidepressants prescribed prior to pregnancy increases the risk of depression relapse, even in women whose depression is in remission prior to pregnancy.

Clinical Manifestations

In general, postpartum depression is similar to other forms of depression. However, the stresses of feeding and caring for a new infant, changes in partner relationship dynamics, and the sometimes traumatic experiences of childbirth add unique themes to the experience of postpartum depression. Depressive symptoms may arise in part from unmet expectations about childbirth or mothering; a sense of loss is common among women with postpartum depression. Compared to other episodes of depression, postpartum depression episodes are less correlated with sleep or appetite disruption, perhaps because these are common experiences among new mothers. Thoughts of harming the infant are extremely common, though of varying severity. Effects of depression may be visible in a dysfunctional parenting style. Conversely, new moms may experience recurrent worries and intrusive thoughts about harm befalling their newborn, sometimes accompanied by a need to repetitively check the infant, which can be reminiscent of obsessive compulsive disorder.

Diagnosis

Screening should be performed during pregnancy and the postpartum period. The EPDS is the most well-studied inventory, and has been validated for use in the identification of patients with postpartum depression. It has a sensitivity of about 80% and a specificity of about 90%. Scores of 13 or higher are generally interpreted as a positive screen. Alternatively, it is reasonable to employ a lower score of 10 as a threshold for pursuing further investigation to improve sensitivity for detecting potential cases of postpartum depression. A clinical interview supportive of an episode of major depression then confirms the diagnosis (Table 1).

Differential Diagnosis

"Baby blues" is the most common mood disruption of the postpartum period. Though it lacks formal diagnostic criteria, it is considered to be a mild, self-limited condition characterized by frequent mood swings that does not extend beyond 2 weeks postpartum. Depending on how it is defined, it is present in 20% to 80% of postpartum women. Bipolar disorder should be considered any time postpartum depression is diagnosed. It is associated with increased morbidity, and antidepressants may trigger manic episodes in affected women. Further, up to 25% of women who screen positive on the EPDS meet criteria for bipolar disorder in some studies. Clinicians should consider routine screening for bipolar disorder with a validated questionnaire such as the Mood Disorder Questionnaire at the time of identification of a depressive episode. Finally, review of systems should include evaluation for hallucinations, delusions, or disorganized behaviors that would suggest psychosis.

Therapy

Postpartum depression can often be effectively managed in the primary care setting, and should begin with establishing a supportive clinician–patient relationship through frequent visits. Therapy is the cornerstone of treatment. Cognitive–behavioral therapy and interpersonal therapy are the most well-studied interventions. Interpersonal therapy, which focuses on troubleshooting relationships and maximizing social support, may be particularly well-suited to the relational transitions of the postpartum period. However, a wide variety of modalities and settings have been found to be effective. In light of this, brief office interventions can enhance patient's early access to care. For instance, clinicians can use motivational interviewing to support behavioral activation. Similarly, problem-solving interventions can assist patients in working through relationship difficulties, and discussion of mindfulness practices can promote more adaptive responses to stress.

In contrast to other forms of depression, the evidence base for pharmacotherapy is fairly small, and effect sizes are modest. Selective serotonin reuptake inhibitors (SSRIs) are the best-studied drug class, followed by tricyclic antidepressants (Table 2). Limited experimental evidence has not supported concurrent therapy and antidepressant use. However, this remains a clinically reasonable approach. In severe postpartum depression, therapy and medication may be started concurrently, as medication efficacy may be delayed several weeks.

Antidepressant safety is a frequent concern. A detailed discussion of use during pregnancy is outside the scope of this article. The most common class-related adverse effect is neonatal withdrawal, a syndrome of irritability and poor feeding, which affect a minority of infants and is usually self-limited. Inconsistent evidence suggests SSRIs may be associated with

TABLE 1	Abbreviated Diagnostic Criteria for Major Depressive Disorder

Five or more during a 2-week period; must include either depressed mood or anhedonia.

SYMPTOM	ASSESSED IN EPDS?
Depressed mood	Yes
Anhedonia	Yes
Insomnia/hypersomnia	Yes
Weight or appetite decrease or increase	No
Psychomotor agitation or retardation	No
Fatigue or loss of energy	No
Worthlessness or guilt	Yes
Decreased concentration or indecisiveness	No
Thoughts of death, or suicidal plan/attempt	Yes

EPDS, Edinburgh Postpartum Depression Scale.

a small risk of congenital cardiac lesions (possibly higher risk with paroxetine [Paxil]) or persistent pulmonary hypertension. Antidepressants are generally excreted in low levels in breastmilk, and evidence of infant toxicity is limited to case reports. There is limited evidence that antidepressants may transiently decrease breastmilk supply. While sertraline (Zoloft), paroxetine (Paxil), and nortriptyline (Pamelor) are the preferred agents in the postpartum period, in general, breastfeeding is not contraindicated with antidepressants. Consideration should be given to risk for future pregnancy; for instance, paroxetine is generally avoided in pregnancy due to potentially higher risk for cardiac anomalies.

An allopregnanolone analogue, brexanolone (Zulresso), was recently approved for the treatment of postpartum depression. It requires a 60-hour monitored infusion, gradually titrated to a target dose of 90 mcg/kg/h, which, in addition to cost, will likely limit its use to psychiatric hospitalizations. However, administration rapidly induced remission in women with moderate and severe depression, with a number needed to treat for remission at the end of infusion of about 3 to 4 in industry-funded stage 3 clinical trials. Differences from placebo were less pronounced at 30 days. Other allopregnanolone analogues are also undergoing clinical trials.

Among complementary modalities for treating postpartum depression, exercise has most consistently been shown to be beneficial. Yoga may also facilitate recovery. Limited evidence supports light therapy. The use of supplements is generally not evidence-based. For instance, omega-3 fatty acids[7] are the most-studied supplement and have not been clearly shown to alleviate postpartum depression.

Monitoring

Clinicians should monitor for return to function in self-care, child care, and other interpersonal relationships. Re-administering depression inventories, such as the EPDS, can provide further objective evidence of disease course. An EPDS score of less than 10 is often used as evidence of remission. If antidepressants are being used, they should be continued for a minimum of 6 months beyond entrance into remission.

The maternal-infant pair should be assessed in the office for signs of dysfunctional attachment. Women with depression may display decreased responsiveness to infant needs, or conversely

[7]Available as dietary supplement.

TABLE 2 Selected Antidepressant Characteristics for Postpartum Depression

CLASS	MEDICATION	RCT SUPPORTING USE?	PREGNANCY CONSIDER-ATIONS	BREAST-MILK LEVELS	POSSIBLE INFANT ADVERSE EFFECTS?	CLINICAL COMMENTS
SSRIs	Sertraline (Zoloft)[1]	Yes	Preferred SSRI	Very low	None known	Most studied; preferred SSRI during breastfeeding
	Paroxetine (Paxil)[1]	Yes	Possibly higher risk of neonatal symptoms, cardiac malformations	Very low	None known	Well-studied in breastfeeding. Avoid in pregnancy. High risk for maternal withdrawal symptoms
	Fluoxetine (Prozac)[1]	Yes	Delayed infant clearance (long half-life)	Low-medium	Possible: poor weight gain. Case reports: colic, sleep disturbance, GI disturbance.	Metabolite with long half-life may dose-accumulate in infant
	Citalopram (Celexa)[1]/ escitalopram (Lexapro)[1]	No*	Preferred SSRI	Low	Case reports: sleep disturbance, irritability.	Escitalopram is less well-studied than citalopram in breastfeeding, although clinical experience supports a similar safety profile
SNRIs	Venlafaxine (Effexor)[1]	No	Less well-studied than SSRIs	Low	None known	Case reports of higher infant levels of active metabolite. High risk for maternal withdrawal symptoms
	Duloxetine (Cymbalta)[1]	No	Minimal data	Low	None known	Less-studied in breastfeeding. Case reports of galactorrhea
Tricyclics	Nortriptyline (Pamelor)[1]	Yes	Less well-studied than SSRIs	Low	None known	Well-studied in breastfeeding
	Amitriptyline (Elavil)[1]	No		Low	Case report: Oversedation.	
Other	Bupropion (Wellbutrin)[1]	No	Minimal data	Low	Case report: seizure	Case report of galactorrhea
	Mirtazapine (Remeron)[1]	No	Minimal data	Low	None known	Less-studied in breastfeeding. Case reports of galactorrhea

GI, Gastrointestinal; *RCT*, randomized controlled trial; *SNRIs*, serotonin/norepinephrine reuptake inhibitors; *SSRIs*, selective serotonin reuptake inhibitors.
[1]Not FDA approved for this indication.
*Citalopram (Celexa) and escitalopram (Lexapro) were among medications used in a naturalistic open-label RCT.

an anxiety-driven over-responsiveness. Breastfeeding difficulties may be a sign of impaired attachment. Clinicians should offer nonjudgmental support to women regardless of their preference to continue or discontinue breastfeeding, as this can be a significant source of stress for some mothers while providing therapeutic benefit to others.

Risk for suicide and infanticide should be assessed routinely. Suicide is a leading cause of death in the postpartum period, and postpartum women may be more likely than their peers to attempt suicide with high-lethality methods such as use of a weapon. Similarly, thoughts of infanticide are very common, although rarely acted upon. Risk-increasing factors include the presence of psychosis, mania, or severe cognitive distortions.

Management of Complications

Hospitalization is indicated if a woman demonstrates signs of mania, psychosis, or high-risk thoughts of suicide or infanticide. Expert consultation should be considered if depression is refractory to therapy or medication. Electroconvulsive therapy has been shown to be effective for treatment of refractory postpartum depression.

References

Association AP: *Diagnostic and statistical manual of mental disorders (DSM-5®)*, American Psychiatric Pub, 20132013.

Beck CT: Postpartum depression: a metasynthesis, *Qualitative Health Research* 12(4):453–472, 2002.

Buttner MM, O'Hara MW, Watson D: The structure of women's mood in the early postpartum, *Assessment* 19(2):247–256, 2012.

Cohen LS, Altshuler LL, Harlow BL, et al: Relapse of major depression during pregnancy in women who maintain or discontinue antidepressant treatment, *JAMA* 295(5):499–507, 2006.

Dennis CL, Dowswell T: Psychosocial and psychological interventions for preventing postpartum depression, *The Cochrane Database of Systematic Reviews*(2), 2013. Cd001134.

Field T: Postpartum depression effects on early interactions, parenting, and safety practices: a review, *Infant Behavior & Development* 33(1):1–6, 2010.

Fisher SD, Sit DK, Yang A, Ciolino JD, Gollan JK, Wisner KL: Four maternal characteristics determine the 12-month course of chronic severe postpartum depressive symptoms, *Depression and Anxiety* 36(4):375–383, 2019.

Gavin NI, Gaynes BN, Lohr KN, Meltzer-Brody S, Gartlehner G, Swinson T: Perinatal depression: a systematic review of prevalence and incidence, *Obstet Gynecol* 106(5 Pt 1):1071–1083, 2005.

Larsen ER, Damkier P, Pedersen LH, et al: Use of psychotropic drugs during pregnancy and breast-feeding, *Acta Psychiatrica Scandinavica Supplementum*(445)1–28, 2015.

Lindahl V, Pearson JL, Colpe L: Prevalence of suicidality during pregnancy and the postpartum, *Archives of Women's Mental Health* 8(2):77–87, 2005.

Meltzer-Brody S, Colquhoun H, Riesenberg R, et al: Brexanolone injection in post-partum depression: two multicentre, double-blind, randomised, placebo-controlled, phase 3 trials, *The Lancet* 392(10152):1058–1070, 2018.

Molyneaux E, Howard LM, McGeown HR, Karia AM, Trevillion K: Antidepressant treatment for postnatal depression, *Cochrane Database of Systematic Reviews* (9), 2014.

Molyneaux E, Telesia LA, Henshaw C, Boath E, Bradley E, Howard LM: Antidepressants for preventing postnatal depression, *The Cochrane database of systematic reviews* 4, 2018:Cd004363.

Nillni YI, Mehralizade A, Mayer L, Milanovic S: Treatment of depression, anxiety, and trauma-related disorders during the perinatal period: A systematic review, *Clinical Psychology Review* 66:136–148, 2018.

Norhayati MN, Hazlina NH, Asrenee AR, Emilin WM: Magnitude and risk factors for postpartum symptoms: a literature review, *Journal of Affective Disorders* 175:34–52, 2015.

O'Connor E, Rossom RC, Henninger M, Groom HC, Burda BU: Primary Care Screening for and Treatment of Depression in Pregnant and Postpartum Women: Evidence Report and Systematic Review for the US Preventive Services Task Force, *JAMA* 315(4):388–406, 2016.

Rundgren S, Brus O, Bave U, et al: Improvement of postpartum depression and psychosis after electroconvulsive therapy: A population-based study with a matched comparison group, *Journal of Affective Disorders* 235:258–264, 2018.

Sharma V, Doobay M, Baczynski C: Bipolar postpartum depression: An update and recommendations, *Journal of Affective Disorders* 219:105–111, 2017.

Sie SD, Wennink JM, van Driel JJ, et al: Maternal use of SSRIs, SNRIs and NaSSAs: practical recommendations during pregnancy and lactation, *Arch Dis Child Fetal Neonatal Ed* 97(6):F472–476, 2012.

Venkatesh KK, Zlotnick C, Triche EW, Ware C, Phipps MG: Accuracy of brief screening tools for identifying postpartum depression among adolescent mothers, *Pediatrics* 133(1):e45–53, 2014.

Yim IS, Tanner Stapleton LR, Guardino CM, Hahn-Holbrook J, Dunkel Schetter C: Biological and psychosocial predictors of postpartum depression: systematic review and call for integration, *Annual Review of Clinical Psychology* 11:99–137, 2015.

VAGINAL BLEEDING IN PREGNANCY

Method of
Zachary J. Baeseman, MD, MPH

CURRENT DIAGNOSIS

- There are several diagnoses in the differential of dangerous late pregnancy bleeding and management varies based on the etiology.
- Avoid digital vaginal examination in a patient with late pregnancy bleeding until placenta previa has been excluded by ultrasound.
- Uterine tenderness with vaginal bleeding is consistent with a clinical diagnosis of placental abruption.
- Vaginal bleeding with a rupture of membranes should prompt consideration of vasa previa.
- Early pregnancy bleeding in a hemodynamically stable patient is worked up with a complete history and physical, complete blood count, human chorionic gonadotropin, and a transvaginal ultrasound.

CURRENT THERAPY

- Placenta previa requires cesarean delivery; however, with a placental edge of more than 2 cm from the cervical os, a vaginal delivery may be attempted in a stable patient.
- Antenatal diagnosis of vasa previa by ultrasound, appropriate administration of antenatal steroids, and a planned cesarean delivery between 34 and 36 weeks gestation is associated with significantly reduced perinatal morbidity and mortality.
- Definitive management of a patient with late-pregnancy bleeding who is hemodynamically unstable should not be delayed in order to obtain an ultrasound or other diagnostic testing.
- In early and late pregnancy bleeding, attention must be directed to the Rh status of the pregnant woman.

Vaginal Bleeding in Late Pregnancy

Epidemiology

Bleeding in the second half of pregnancy complicates 2% to 5% of pregnancies. Placental previa, placental insertion into the lower uterine segment covering all or part of the internal cervical os, causes 30% of late-pregnancy bleeds and occurs in 0.5% of all pregnancies. Placental abruption, premature separation of the placenta from the uterine wall, causes 20% of antepartum hemorrhages and occurs in 1% of all pregnancies. The diagnosis of placental abruption is typically clinical; ultrasound can be useful to rule in the diagnosis, but notably, it can miss >50% of diagnoses. Other serious causes include uterine rupture (occurs in approximately 0.7% of women with a history of previous low-transverse cesarean section) and vasa previa (0.5% of late-pregnancy bleeding and approximately 0.0002% to 0.0008% of all pregnancies). Vasa previa occurs when fetal blood vessels are present in the membranes, traversing the cervix beneath the fetal presenting part.

Risk Factors

Higher parity and maternal age, smoking or cocaine use, a prior history of placenta previa or placental abruption, and multifetal gestation are risk factors for both placenta previa and abruption. Risk factors for placenta previa also include uterine abnormalities, assisted reproductive technology (ART), and history of uterine surgery, including cesarean section. Additional risk factors for abruption include blunt abdominal trauma, polyhydramnios, hypertensive disorders in pregnancy, and external cephalic version. The greatest risk factor for uterine rupture is a trial of labor after cesarean section (TOLAC), particularly with induction and the use of prostaglandins, which are contraindicated in TOLAC. A uterine scar increases risk; spontaneous uterine rupture is rare on an unscarred uterus. Other risk factors include uterine abnormalities, maternal connective tissue disease, abnormal placentation, and uterine hyperstimulation during labor. Shortened interpregnancy interval (less than 18 to 24 months between pregnancies) can also increase risk. Risk factors for vasa previa include artificial reproductive techniques, bilobed or succenturiate lobed placenta (odds ratio [OR] = 22.11), placenta previa (OR = 22.86), certain fetal anomalies, and a velamentous cord insertion.

Pathophysiology

The cause of placenta previa is unknown but may be related to impaired placental attachment in a uterus with a previous scar. Placental abruption, defined as premature separation of the placenta from the uterus, is caused by hemorrhage where the placenta and decidua meet. Abruption is often preceded by vasospasm (such as that induced by cocaine), thrombosis, or shearing forces. Some cases are acute, but many cases could present a chronic process in which abruption is the end result. Uterine rupture most often occurs in a uterus with a previous scar and is a dehiscence of that scar; often the presenting sign is an abnormal fetal heart rate or a regression of fetal station in labor. The pathophysiology of vasa previa is unknown, although it is theorized to be caused by abnormal development or growth of the umbilical cord secondary to a velamentous insertion or reduced intrauterine space.

Prevention

Previous cesarean section is a risk factor for both placenta previa and uterine rupture, therefore reducing unnecessary cesarean sections can prevent these conditions. Patients who have had a cesarean section should be advised to space out their next pregnancy by 18 to 24 months to mitigate the risk of uterine rupture. Uterine rupture may also be prevented by limiting or avoiding certain agents to induce or augment labor. In women undergoing TOLAC, spontaneous labor is preferred due to the lower risk of uterine rupture. Although vasa previa cannot be prevented, fetal morbidity and mortality are significantly reduced by early diagnosis and delivery. Placental abruption is associated with smoking and cocaine use; counseling directed to cessation theoretically reduces risk. Seat belts are recommended for all pregnant women; trauma sustained during a motor vehicle accident is a potential cause of abruption due to shearing forces. Control of hypertension and treatment of thrombophilia have not been proved to prevent abruption, although both interventions are recommended. Magnesium sulfate given intrapartum to women with preeclampsia can reduce the risk of placental abruption.

Clinical Manifestations

Placenta previa classically manifests with painless vaginal bleeding, whereas placental abruption and uterine rupture are typically associated with pain and bleeding. Because these conditions are not mutually exclusive, it is important to consider the possibility of more than one serious cause of antepartum hemorrhage. Bleeding secondary to placenta previa may be heavy or light, can recur, and is not associated with the degree of previa or prognosis. Thirty percent of women with placental abruption may not present with vaginal bleeding and have a retroplacental clot concealing an abruption. Approximately one half of women with placental abruption present in labor, and 30% of cases are complicated by fetal death. Monitoring can reveal uterine irritability or hypertonicity. Uterine rupture can manifest with abnormal fetal heart tracing, loss of fetal station, or palpable uterine defect. Pain and bleeding might not occur until after uterine rupture, when both maternal and fetal status are compromised. Vasa previa is detectable on ultrasound and color Doppler imaging, but it most commonly presents as vaginal bleeding with rupture of membranes. Placental abruption, uterine rupture, and vasa previa can manifest with concerning fetal heart tracings.

Diagnosis

Ultrasound can reliably detect placenta previa and vasa previa. Transvaginal ultrasonography (TVU) is recommended to establish placental location because transabdominal ultrasonography has a false-positive rate for placenta previa up to 25%. TVU has a sensitivity of 87.5% and a specificity of 98.8% for placenta previa and is safe in the presence of vaginal bleeding. Vasa previa can be diagnosed using TVU and color Doppler. High-risk women may be screened in order to plan for cesarean delivery at 34 to 36 weeks of gestation. Vasa previa may also be detected on magnetic resonance imaging (MRI; rarely used), amnioscopy, palpitation of vessels during reginal examination, or identifying fetal blood cells in vaginal blood, although tests to detect fetal hemoglobin cannot be performed quickly enough to be clinically useful. Placental abruption is primarily a clinical diagnosis; it can be ruled in by ultrasound, but notably >50% of cases of placental abruption are missed on ultrasound. The diagnosis is made clinically in a patient with bleeding and a hard or tender uterus, uterine irritability, and often a nonreassuring fetal heart tracing; bleeding may be absent in 20% to 30% of presentations.

Differential Diagnosis

In addition to placenta previa, placental abruption, uterine rupture, and vasa previa, diagnostic considerations include bloody show, cervical trauma, cervical polyp, cervical cancer, or infection.

Therapy

Women with placenta previa and active bleeding are managed expectantly in the hospital, although outpatient management may be a reasonable approach in women who are not bleeding, have adequate support at home, and are able to get to the hospital quickly. Women with any degree of placental overlap with the cervical os should be delivered by cesarean section.

Treatment of women with placental abruption depends on multiple factors including severity of clinical presentation, gestational age, fetal status, and maternal status. In the most severe cases in which there has been fetal death, vaginal delivery is acceptable if the maternal status is reassuring. Because of risk for disseminated intravascular coagulopathy (DIC) and blood loss, women should be carefully monitored, proceeding to cesarean

section for worsening maternal status or failed vaginal delivery. In mild cases of placental abruption before term, steroids should be administered between 24 and up to 36 6/7 weeks of gestation; preterm birth is the leading reason for perinatal death. With a stable abruption in a preterm patient with reassuring fetal and maternal status, outpatient management may be reasonable after a period of inpatient observation. Antenatal magnesium sulfate in women <32 weeks gestation can reliably decrease cerebral palsy and neonatal gross motor dysfunction, however, tocolysis is not routinely recommended in placental abruption. Labor may progress toward a goal of vaginal delivery if both maternal and fetal status are reassuring, although cesarean section should be performed expeditiously for any fetal or maternal compromise. Longer decision-to-incision intervals are associated with worse perinatal outcomes. When placental abruption is known or suspected in a term patient, delivery should proceed.

Vasa previa is managed with immediate cesarean section if diagnosed during labor and with a planned cesarean section if diagnosed antenatally. Administration of steroids is recommended at 28 to 34 weeks of gestation depending on the timing of planned delivery, and hospitalization should be considered at around 30 to 32 weeks of gestation because approximately 10% of women have premature rupture of membranes and could need an urgent cesarean section. Certain patients are appropriate candidates for outpatient management. Optimal time for planned cesarean section is not definitely established and has been recommended between 34 and 36 weeks gestation. Neonatal resuscitation, including fluid resuscitation or transfusion, may be required and should be anticipated.

Uterine rupture is associated with high perinatal morbidity and mortality. When rupture is clinically recognized or suspected, cesarean delivery should proceed rapidly. Occasionally a uterine window can be seen antenatally within the previous uterine scar on ultrasound. Scheduled cesarean delivery at 37 weeks is recommended for these patients and labor is contraindicated due to the risk of uterine rupture during labor.

Monitoring

In placenta previa, the distance between the placental edge and cervical os is monitored during pregnancy by ultrasound because the placental location can change with advancing pregnancy. After 35 weeks' gestation, women with a placental edge more than 20 mm from the internal cervical os may be offered a trial of labor because they are likely to achieve vaginal delivery. When the placental edge is greater than 0 mm but less than 20 mm from the internal cervical os, vaginal delivery might still be possible, although the likelihood of cesarean section and intrapartum complications are much higher. Women at increased risk of vasa previa should be screened with TVU and color Doppler. When vasa previa is identified, serial ultrasound is indicated because abnormal vessels regress in up to 15% of women. If a woman has an Rh negative blood type and experiences bleeding in pregnancy, she should receive a standard dose of 300 μg Rho(D) human immune globulin to prevent maternal Rh alloimmunization. For massive maternal-fetal hemorrhage a Kleihauer-Betke test should be performed in Rh negative mothers to assist in confirming maternal-fetal hemorrhage and Rho(D) human immune globulin dosing.

Complications

Maternal risks associated with placenta previa include need for cesarean section, postpartum hemorrhage, and blood transfusion. Women who have history of cesarean section and who have placenta previa are at increased risk for placenta accreta. Fetal risks are primarily associated with prematurity. Placental abruption can cause hypovolemic shock, postpartum hemorrhage, and DIC. Perinatal complications include prematurity, intrauterine growth restriction, anemia, coagulopathy, and death. Uterine rupture can be catastrophic for both mother and baby. Maternal risks include surgical risk associated with cesarean section, hypovolemic shock and hemorrhage, and hysterectomy. Perinatal morbidity can include hypoxic-ischemic encephalopathy. Stillbirth and neonatal death are possible as well. When undiagnosed prior to labor vasa previa carries a fetal mortality rate of greater than 60%. Antenatal diagnosis with planned cesarean section decreases fetal mortality to 2% to 3% and reduces the need for transfusion from 60% to 3%. Because the hemorrhage is fetal blood, maternal risk from vasa previa is primarily associated with complications related to cesarean section.

Vaginal Bleeding in Early Pregnancy

Epidemiology

Vaginal bleeding in early pregnancy is common and has been reported in 20% to 40% of pregnant women. A viable intrauterine pregnancy is the most common diagnosis. The two most common complicating diagnoses of early pregnancy bleeding are threatened abortion and ectopic pregnancy. Threatened abortion, an intrauterine pregnancy with bleeding and pain before 20 weeks gestation that has cardiac activity and a closed cervix, is the cause of 12% to 57% of early pregnancy bleeding. The incidence of ectopic pregnancy is 19.7 cases per 1000 pregnancies and is increasing worldwide. Ectopic pregnancy is the leading cause of morbidity and maternal mortality in the first trimester of pregnancy.

It has been suggested that the rate of miscarriage can be as high as 30% to 50% of all fertilized eggs and often goes undetected. The incidence of miscarriage in an intrauterine pregnancy with confirmed fetal cardiac activity is 2.1% in women under 35 years of age and 16.1% in women greater than 35 years of age. Other common causes of early pregnancy bleeding include intercourse, cervicitis, pelvic inflammatory disease, functional placenta hormonal changes, fertilized egg implantation into the uterine wall, and gestational trophoblastic disease.

Pathophysiology

The most common diagnosis of bleeding in early pregnancy is a normal and viable intrauterine pregnancy. Vaginal spotting can commonly occur after implantation of a fertilized egg into the intrauterine wall, usually occurring a few days prior to the expected onset of menstruation (8 to 9 days after ovulation and fertilization). Early pregnancy bleeding may also be caused by the commencement of a hormonally functional placenta, usually at 6 to 7 weeks of gestation. Concerning causes of early pregnancy bleeding are maternal hormonal deficiency, placental dysfunction, subchorionic hemorrhage, extrauterine implantation of the embryo, and nonviability of the pregnancy. The amount of hemorrhage in early pregnancy may be associated with the risk of pregnancy loss.

Management

Early pregnancy bleeding is worked up with a complete set of vital signs, a complete history and physical examination including visualization of the cervix with a speculum, a complete blood count, β-hCG (human chorionic gonadotropin), and a transvaginal ultrasound (TVU) to determine fetal viability and exclude an ectopic pregnancy. Concern for ectopic or early pregnancy loss should be raised if the β-hCG level is greater than the discriminatory level (1500 to 3000 mIU/mL) without intrauterine contents seen on TVU. If the patient is hemodynamically unstable, urgent surgical consultation is paramount as it is possible to have intraabdominal exsanguination from a ruptured ectopic pregnancy. If the patient is hemodynamically stable and the pregnancy is viable, bleeding is most often managed expectantly, provided the fetus has not reached extrauterine viability of 23 to 24 weeks gestation.

If the patient is hemodynamically stable, a miscarriage can be managed expectantly, inducing medical expulsion of the nonviable fetal tissue with a combination of mifepristone and misoprostol, or surgical management with dilation and suction curettage depending on the risk of infection, maternal hemorrhage and

anemia, maternal preference, and medical necessity. Medical management has been proven to increase the effectiveness and decrease the time of complete expulsion compared to expectant management. Due to the risk of alloimmunization, it is recommended that women who are Rh negative blood type have surgical management and receive prophylactic Rho(D) human immune globulin to reduce the risk of alloimmunization. Alloimmunization is a devastating complication where an Rh negative mother can develop antibodies to Rh positive fetal blood, placing future pregnancies at risk.

If a woman has an Rh negative blood type and experiences bleeding in pregnancy, she should receive Rho(D) human immune globulin to prevent maternal Rh alloimmunization. Failure to receive Rho(D) human immune globulin can complicate all subsequent pregnancies and ultimately lead to future severe fetal anemia and hydrops fetalis (severe and life-threatening fetal edema secondary to profound fetal anemia). For early pregnancy bleeding in an Rh negative mother of less than 12 weeks of gestation, 150 μg of Rho(D) is sufficient; greater than 12 weeks of gestation, a standard dose of 300 μg should be given. These dosages provide maternal protection from up to 30 mL of fetal whole blood. For massive maternal-fetal hemorrhage a Kleihauer-Betke test should be performed in Rh negative mothers to assist in confirming maternal-fetal hemorrhage and Rho(D) human immune globulin dosing.

If there is recurrent pregnancy loss, defined as greater than 3 total pregnancy losses, two consecutive pregnancy losses, or a pregnancy loss greater than 20 weeks of gestation, secondary causes should be sought including a workup for antiphospholipid antibody disorder, clotting disorders, and maternal or fetal chromosomal testing. The products of conceptions resulting from gestational trophoblastic disease should undergo chromosomal analysis.

References

Antenatal corticosteroid therapy for fetal maturation. Committee Opinion No. 677. American College of Obstetricians and Gynecologists, *Obstet Gynecol* 128:e187–194, 2016.

Deutchman M, Tubay AT, Turok D: First trimester bleeding, *Am Fam Physician* 79(11):985–994, 2009 Jun 1.

Duley L, Guelmezoglu AM, Henderson-Smart DJ, Chou D: Magnesium sulphate and other anticonvulsants for women with pre-eclampsia, *Cochrane Database Syst Rev* 11, 2010.

Early Pregnancy Loss: Practice Bulletin No. 200. American College of Obstetricians and Gynecologists, *Obstet Gynecol*, August 29, 2018. Interim Update.

Gagnon R, Morin L, Bly S, et al: Guidelines for the management of vasa previa, *J Obstet Gynaecol Can* 31:748–760, 2009.

Hasan R, Baird DD, Herring AH, et al: Patterns and predictors of vaginal bleeding in the first trimester of pregnancy, *Ann Epidemiol* 20(7):524–531, 2010, Available at: https://doi.org/10.1016/j.annepidem.2010.02.006.

Hendricks E, et al: First trimester bleeding: evaluation and management, *Am Fam Physician* 99(3):166–174, 2019 Feb 1.

Krywko DM, Shunkwiler SM: Kleihauer Betke Test. [Updated 2019 Jan 27]. In: StatPearls [Internet]. Treasure Island (FL): StatPearls Publishing; 2019 Jan-. Available from: https://www.ncbi.nlm.nih.gov/books/NBK430876/.

Magann EF, Cummings JE, Niderhauser A: Antepartum bleeding of unknown origin in the second half of pregnancy: A review, *Obstet Gynecol Surv* 60:741–745, 2005.

Management of preterm labor. Practice Bulletin No. 171. American College of Obstetricians and Gynecologists, *Obstet Gynecol* 128:e155–164, 2016.

Oppenheimer L, Armson A, Farine D, et al: Diagnosis and management of placenta previa, *J Obstet Gynaecol Can* 29:261–266, 2007.

Oyelese Y, Ananth C: Placental abruption, *Obstet Gynecol* 108:1005–1016, 2006.

Royal College of Obstetricians and Gynaecologists (RCOG): *Antepartum hemorrhage*, London (UK), November 2011, Royal College of Obstetricians and Gynaecologists (RCOG)November 2011.

Sinha P, Kuruba N: Ante-partum hemorrhage: An update, *J Obstet Gynaecol* 28:377–381, 2008.

Smith JG, Mertz HL, Merrill DC: Identifying risk factors for uterine rupture, *Clin Perinatol* 35:85–99, 2008.

Smith KE, Buyalos RP: The profound impact of patient age on pregnancy outcome after early detection of fetal cardiac activity, *Fertil Steril* 65:35–40, 1996.

Tenore J: *Am Fam Physician* 61(4):1080–1088, 2000 Feb 15.

Zlatnik MG, Cheng YW, Norton ME, et al: Placenta previa and the risk of preterm delivery, *J Matern Fetal Neonatal Med* 20:719–723, 2007.

19 Children's Health

ACUTE LEUKEMIA IN CHILDREN

Method of
Stacy Cooper, MD; and Rachel E. Rau, MD

Leukemias are characterized by a marked proliferation of abnormal blood cells in the bone marrow and blood that may be associated with widespread infiltration in extramedullary sites including the central nervous system (CNS), testes, thymus, liver, spleen, and lymph nodes.

Classification

The first level of classification of leukemia is *acute* versus *chronic*. Acute leukemia is characterized by the predominance of very immature white blood cell precursors, or blasts, and is an aggressive, rapidly fatal disease if left untreated. Conversely, chronic leukemia is characterized by proliferation of relatively mature white blood cells and is typically a more indolent disease. Chronic leukemias are uncommon in pediatrics.

The second level of classification is *lymphoid* versus *myeloid*, depending on whether the leukemic cells display characteristics of lymphocyte precursors or myelocyte (granulocyte, erythrocyte, monocyte, or megakaryocyte) precursors. Acute lymphoblastic leukemia (ALL) and acute myeloid leukemia (AML) account for the overwhelming majority of pediatric leukemias.

ALL and AML are further subclassified by morphology and expression of cell surface antigens using flow cytometry. For ALL, classification is largely based on cell surface and cytoplasmic marker expression (Table 1). AML cases are classified by characteristic chromosomal abnormalities (if present) or by light microscopic morphology in cases where these specific chromosomal changes are absent (Box 1).

Epidemiology

Leukemia accounts for approximately 30% of childhood cancers, making it the most common form of childhood cancer. The distribution of the major forms of leukemia is vastly different in children than in adults (Figure 1). In general, children are far more likely to have acute leukemia, and ALL is much more common than AML. In adults, most cases of leukemia are chronic, and AML is more common than ALL. Specifically, there are approximately 3100 children and adolescents diagnosed with ALL in the United States each year and approximately 700 children and adolescents diagnosed with AML in the United States each year.

The incidence of the various forms of leukemia varies by age in both children and adults (Figure 2). This is especially true for childhood ALL, for which there is a marked incidence peak in the 2- to 4-year-old age group. This ALL age peak is primarily found in children living in industrialized nations, leading to speculation that a common environmental exposure, coupled with age-related immunologic susceptibility, is at least partially responsible for many cases of ALL. Except for a small peak in infants, the incidence of AML is fairly constant in childhood but rises quickly in later adulthood.

Prognosis

One of the most dramatic success stories in modern medicine is the improvement in survival of children with ALL over the past four decades. Leukemia was once a uniformly fatal diagnosis, with less than a 5% to 10% cure rate until the mid- to late 1960s. Today, approximately 90% of children with ALL are cured. The improved prognosis has been built on pioneering observations on the efficacy of multiagent systemic therapy and the importance of CNS treatment in the late 1960s and early 1970s. Further successive, incremental improvements in outcome have been achieved due to clinical trials conducted by large single centers and national and international cooperative groups that have successfully enrolled a high percentage of eligible children.

Similar approaches have unfortunately not been quite so successful in improving the prognosis of children with AML. Although approximately one half of children with AML are cured today, this has been accomplished by intensifying therapy to the point that the toxic death rate in the early phases of therapy is about 10%. Current research in AML is therefore focusing on developing novel molecularly targeted agents that hold the promise of improving efficacy and limiting toxicity.

TABLE 1	Classification of Childhood Acute Lymphoblastic Leukemia					
	PHENOTYPIC MARKER					
ALL SUBTYPE	**CD19**	**CD10**	**CLG**	**SLG**	**%**	**COMMENT**
Pre-pre B	+	–	–	–	5	Mostly infants, poor prognosis, frequent *KMT2A* 11q23 rearrangements
Early pre-B	+	+	–	–	63	Common ALL, young children, good prognosis
Pre-B	+	+	+	–	16	Older children, good prognosis with intense therapy
B-cell	+	+	+	+	4	Burkitt leukemia, *MYC/Ig* fusion genes, good prognosis with lymphoma-type therapy
T-cell	–	–	–	–	12	Adolescents, anterior mediastinal mass, CNS involvement, good prognosis with intense therapy

ALL, Acute myeloid leukemia; *clg,* cytoplasmic immunoglobulin; *CNS,* central nervous system; *slg,* surface immunoglobulin.

Classification of Childhood Acute Myeloid Leukemia (World Health Organization Criteria)

Acute Myeloid Leukemia With Recurrent Genetic Abnormalities

Acute myeloid leukemia with t(8;21)(q22;q22), *(RUNX1/ RUNX1T1)*

Acute myeloid leukemia with abnormal bone marrow eosinophils and inv(16)(p13q22) or t(16;16)(p13;q22), *(CBFβ/MYH11)*

Acute promyelocytic leukemia with t(15;17)(q22;q12), *(PML/ RARA),* and variants

Acute myeloid leukemia with 11q23 *(KMT2A)* abnormalities

Acute Myeloid Leukemia, Not Otherwise Categorized

Acute myeloid leukemia, minimally differentiated (FAB M0)

Acute myeloid leukemia without maturation (FAB M1)

Acute myeloid leukemia with maturation (FAB M2)

Acute myelomonocytic leukemia (FAB M4)

Acute monoblastic/acute monocytic leukemia (FAB M5)

Acute erythroid leukemia (FAB M6)

Acute megakaryoblastic leukemia (FAB M7)

FAB, French–American–British classification.

Etiology

The question "What is the cause of leukemia?" can be considered on a few different levels. First, what is wrong with *this child* that caused the child to develop leukemia? Second, what is wrong with *the leukemia cell* that causes it to behave so badly? Third, what is wrong with *the leukemia cell's genes* that cause the cell to behave that way?

Predispositions

The answer to the first question is unknown in the vast majority of cases. Attempts to correlate various genetic features or environmental or infectious exposures with risk of childhood leukemia have been largely uninformative. It is presumed that children are particularly susceptible to ALL because of the marked expansion and genetic rearrangement of lymphocytes that occurs during early childhood as the result of exposure to a multitude of immunogenic antigens for the first time. The proliferation required to meet the constant demand for granulocytes, erythrocytes, and platelets is likely a setup for the development of AML in children.

Although a number of constitutional and single-gene disorders confer an increased risk of childhood leukemia (Table 2), in total, these are known to be involved in only a minority of cases. However, with a growing list of recognized genetic disorders predisposing to myeloid malignancies in particular, a careful

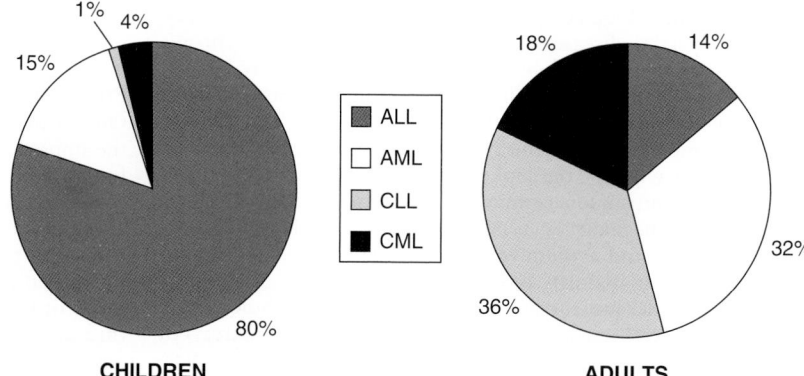

Figure 1 Relative incidence of four major leukemia subtypes in children and adults. *ALL,* Acute lymphoblastic leukemia; *AML,* acute myeloid leukemia; *CLL,* chronic lymphoblastic leukemia; *CML,* chronic myeloid leukemia.

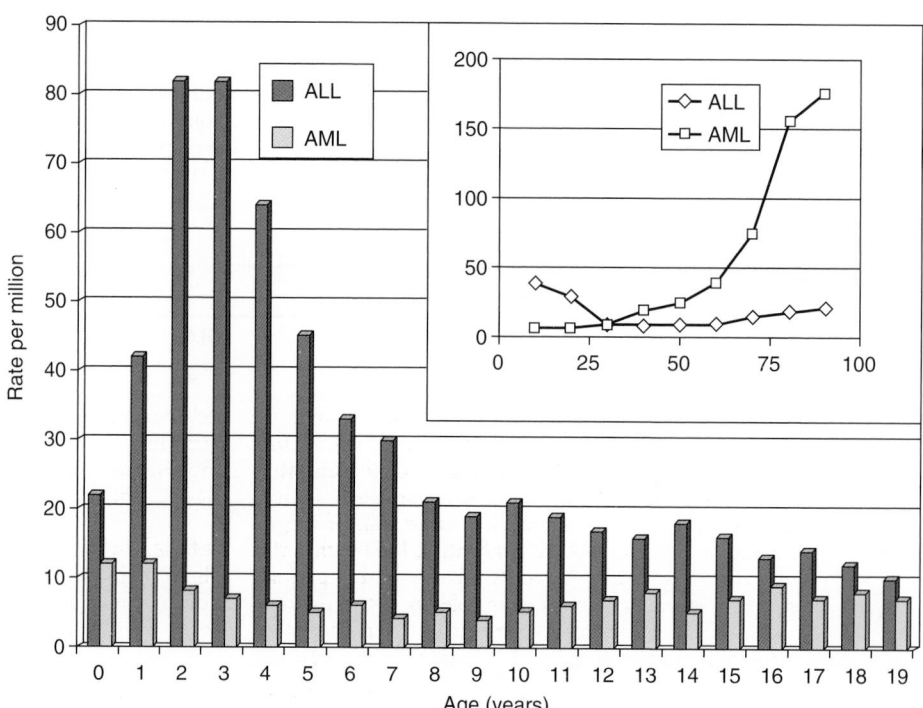

Figure 2 Age-specific incidence of acute lymphoblastic leukemia *(ALL)* and acute myeloid leukemia *(AML)* in children and in adults *(inset).*

TABLE 2 Summary of Known Constitutional and Heritable Childhood Leukemia Predispositions

DISORDER	INHERITANCE	MALIGNANCY TYPE	COMMENTS
Ataxia-telangiectasia	AR	ALL, NHL	*ATM* gene mutations lead to defective DNA repair
Bloom's syndrome	AR	AML, ALL	Chromosomal instability, sister chromatid exchanges
Down syndrome	Sporadic	AML, ALL	See text
Li-Fraumeni syndrome	AD	AML, ALL, many others	*p53* mutations; leukemias less common than solid tumors
Fanconi's anemia	AR	AML	Chromosomal instability, increased sensitivity to DNA damage
Kostmann's syndrome	AR	AML	G-CSF receptor mutations lead to agranulocytosis
Neurofibromatosis type 1	AD	AML, JMML, MPNST	*NF1* gene mutations lead to enhanced *RAS* signaling
Familial platelet disorder with associated myeloid malignancy	AD	MDS, AML, ALL	Loss of function mutations of the myeloid transcription factor RUNX1 lead to abnormal myeloid development Individuals have platelet defects and ~35% risk of myeloid malignancy development
Germline CEBPA mutations	AD	AML	Estimated penetrance of AML development ~90% in affected individuals. Approximately 10% of patients with biallelic *CEBPA* mutant AML have a germline *CEBPA* mutation. AML in those with germline CEBPA mutations are chemosensitive, but individuals have high rates of second primary AMLs.
MonoMAC syndrome; germline *GATA2* mutations	AD	MDS, AML	MonoMAC is an immunodeficiency with risk for mycobacterial, fungal, and human papilloma virus infections with monocytopenia and risk for MDS/AML, often with monosomy of chromosome 7
MIRAGE syndrome, ATXPC/MLSM7 syndrome; Germline mutation of *SAMD9* and *SAMD9L*	Mostly de novo		MIRAGE syndrome (myelodysplasia, infection, restriction of growth, adrenal hypoplasia, genital phenotypes, enteropathy); ATXPC, ataxia-pancytopenia syndrome and MLSM7, myelodysplasia and leukemia syndrome with monosomy 7 caused by gain of function mutation of *SAMD9* or *SAMD9L*
CBL syndrome	AD	JMML	Impaired growth, developmental delay, cryptorchidism, deafness, and predisposition to JMML caused by loss of function mutation of rumor suppressor gene *CBL*. JMML that develops can be self-resolving. Vasculitis risk later in life after JMML resolution.

AD, Autosomal dominant; *ALL,* acute lymphoblastic leukemia; *AML,* acute myeloid leukemia; *AR,* autosomal recessive; *G-CSF,* granulocyte colony-stimulating factor; *JMML,* juvenile myelomonocytic leukemia; *MPNST,* malignant peripheral nerve sheath tumor; *NHL,* non-Hodgkin lymphoma.

past medical history, family history, and examination for dysmorphisms and low threshold for genetic referral is warranted for any child with a myeloid malignancy. The most common of these is Down syndrome. Children with Down syndrome have a 10- to 20-fold increased risk of leukemia, with an approximately equal incidence of ALL and AML. The peak age at onset of leukemia for children with Down syndrome is earlier than for other children. In the newborn period, patients with Down syndrome can present with transient myeloproliferative disease (also known as transient abnormal myelopoiesis), which can manifest with hepatomegaly and peripheral blasts, that appears indistinguishable from congenital AML but usually resolves spontaneously within 3 to 6 months. These children have an increased risk of megakaryoblastic leukemia (AMKL, FAB classification M7) within the first 4 years of life. Children with Down syndrome tend to present with leukemia that is particularly susceptible to chemotherapy agents (e.g., cytarabine [Cytosar], methotrexate), but they also suffer increased toxicity from therapy. On balance, the prognosis of leukemia in Down syndrome patients with ALL is inferior to those without Down syndrome, whereas in AML, children with

Down syndrome have favorable outcomes compared with children without Down syndrome.

The only environmental exposures that are known to predispose to leukemia are ionizing radiation (such as was seen with atomic bomb survivors) and prior exposure to certain chemotherapy drugs (e.g., cyclophosphamide [Cytoxan], etoposide [Toposar, VePesid]). There is also evidence that in utero exposure to maternal diagnostic radiation also increases the risk of childhood cancer (including leukemia), particularly if the exposure is in the first trimester. Other environmental or infectious exposures remain unproven as risk factors for childhood leukemia, including electromagnetic fields from power lines.

Cellular Pathogenesis

Three major characteristics of leukemia cells distinguish them from normal hematopoietic cells. They proliferate rapidly, they do not differentiate, and they have defects in apoptosis. This results in a growth advantage for leukemia cells, leading to progressive replacement of the normal bone marrow with a massive clonal population of poorly differentiated leukemic blasts.

TABLE 3	Summary of Common Leukemogenic Genetic Events

ACUTE LYMPHOBLASTIC LEUKEMIA	ACUTE MYELOID LEUKEMIA
Chimeric Transcription Factors	
t(12;21): *ETV6-RUNX1* fusion	t(8;21): *RUNX1-RUNX1T1* fusion
t(1;19): *TCF3-PBX1* fusion	t(15;17): *PML-RARA* fusion
t(4;11), et al: *KMT2A* fusions	t(9;11), et al: *KMT2A* fusions
t(8;14), t(8;22), t(2;8): *Ig-MYC* fusions	inv(16): MYH11-CBFB
T-cell receptor fusions	
Mutationally Activated Oncogenes	
t(9;22): *BCR-ABL1* fusion	*FLT3* mutation
JAK2 mutation	*RAS* mutation
CRLF2 fusion	*KIT* mutation
Altered Tumor-Suppressor Genes	
CDKN2A deletion	*NPM1* mutation
IKZF1 mutation	*WT1* mutation
TP53 mutation	*CEBPA* mutation

BOX 2	Summary of Clinical Manifestations of Childhood Leukemia*

Bone Marrow
Pancytopenia, bone pain

Reticuloendothelial System
Lymphadenopathy
Hepatosplenomegaly

Thymus
Anterior mediastinal mass (T-cell leukemia)

Bones
Bone pain is common
Fractures and chloromas are rare

Gums
Gingival hypertrophy (M4 and M5 AML)

Skin
Leukemia cutis and chloromas (M2, M4, and M5 AML, infant ALL)

Central Nervous System
Meningitis
Cranial nerve palsies
Rarely intracranial epidural or orbital chloromas (M4 and M5 AML, T-cell ALL)

Kidneys
Often infiltrated or enlarged
Rarely acute renal failure (except in tumor lysis syndrome)

Genitourinary
Testicular enlargement (T-cell ALL)

---
*See Box 1 for descriptions of classifications.
ALL, Acute lymphoblastic leukemia; *AML,* acute myeloid leukemia; *TBSA,* total body surface area.

Another characteristic of leukemia cells is their tendency to spread throughout the body and infiltrate organs other than the bone marrow. This is discussed in more detail in the section on clinical presentation.

Molecular Pathogenesis

As is true of most human cancers, development of leukemia is a multihit process. The initiating mutation (first hit) in childhood ALL often occurs in utero or early infancy, which is the peak of lymphocyte expansion and recombinase activity for the normal immune system.

The initiating events are typically chromosomal rearrangements that activate expression of cellular proto-oncogenes by fusing them to transcriptionally active immunoglobulin or T-cell receptor genes or alternatively by joining two genes from different chromosomes to create a new fusion gene that encodes a chimeric protein with unique functional properties. The most common of these sentinel chromosomal rearrangements are translocations (exchanges of genetic material between chromosomes), which can serve as a unique marker of the malignant clone. Retrospective studies of blood obtained at birth and preserved on filter paper used for diagnosis of genetic disorders (Guthrie cards) of children who developed leukemia in early childhood have shown that leukemia-associated fusion genes were present at birth in a large percentage of children, including some who did not develop leukemia for one or more years.

In ALL, the promotional mutation (second hit) likely occurs during the proliferative stress generated by immune responses to exogenous antigens. Because these are maximal in the 2- to 4-year-old age group, this is thought to explain the age peak of childhood ALL during these years. The lack of such a peak in AML suggests that the promotional mutations can occur at any time or are not necessarily triggered by immune stimulation. Examples of specific genetic hits known to be associated with the development of childhood leukemia are summarized in Table 3.

Clinical Presentation

Most symptoms and signs of childhood leukemia are the result of the propensity of leukemia cells to replace the bone marrow and infiltrate multiple other organs throughout the body. It is estimated that approximately 10^9 (1 trillion) leukemia cells are present in the child's body at diagnosis.

The replacement of normal bone marrow is responsible for the characteristic abnormal blood counts, which in most cases include the triad of neutropenia, anemia, and thrombocytopenia. Depending on the number of circulating leukemic blasts in the peripheral blood, the total white blood cell (WBC) count may be low, normal, or high. The neutropenia is often profound (absolute neutrophil count <500/μL) and is associated with an increased risk of serious infection. Blood cultures and broad-spectrum intravenous antibiotic coverage are indicated in any patient with newly diagnosed leukemia and fever. Anemia is often manifested by fatigue, lethargy, headache, pallor, and, in extreme cases, congestive heart failure that may be precipitated by vigorous transfusion or intravenous hydration. Thrombocytopenia often leads to bruising and petechiae; however, clinically significant hemorrhage is uncommon in industrialized countries. Platelet transfusion is indicated for bleeding or for very low platelet counts (<10,000–20,000/μL).

Infiltration of organs other than the bone marrow with leukemia cells is responsible for additional presenting clinical features. Box 2 summarizes the organ systems most often involved in leukemia and the typical clinical manifestations.

Medical Emergencies in Childhood Leukemia

A child with newly diagnosed leukemia needs to be promptly evaluated for several medical emergencies. There are several potentially life-threatening complications that may be present at diagnosis or can develop within a short time after diagnosis, in addition to the need to diagnose and treat potential infection in patients who are febrile and neutropenic, which was discussed earlier.

Tumor lysis syndrome (TLS) is a complication resulting from the rapid breakdown of large numbers of tumor cells, releasing intracellular contents. Although TLS is seen most often after initial treatment with chemotherapy, it can also be present before therapy is initiated due to spontaneous lysis. Risk factors include high WBC count, lymphadenopathy, hepatosplenomegaly, high mitotic index, and specific diagnoses of ALL (especially Burkitt leukemia or lymphoma and T-cell ALL). TLS is characterized by the triad of hyperuricemia (from breakdown of purines by xanthine oxidase), hyperkalemia, and hyperphosphatemia (with secondary hypocalcemia). Renal insufficiency can develop due to the nephrotoxic effects of precipitated urate crystals in the renal tubules; in severe cases, dialysis may be necessary.

Management consists of aggressive hydration to reduce tubular uric acid concentration. The xanthine oxidase inhibitor allopurinol (Zyloprim) is routinely used to decrease uric acid production. Rasburicase (Elitek) (recombinant urate oxidase) is a new agent used in severe cases of TLS to almost instantaneously convert uric acid to the more soluble allantoin. Frequent electrolyte monitoring with standard management of abnormal levels is essential.

Hyperleukocytosis becomes a potential clinical problem and is usually seen with WBC counts above 100,000/μL. Markedly elevated WBCs lead to increased blood viscosity that can produce sludging of blood in the brain, lungs, kidneys, and other organs, causing clinical features such as depressed level of consciousness, stroke, intracranial hemorrhage, respiratory distress, hypoxia, diffuse pulmonary infiltrates, and renal insufficiency. The risk of hyperviscosity is higher with AML than ALL because myelolasts are generally larger and "stickier" than lymphoblasts (likely due to increased expression of integrins and other mediators of cell–cell adherence on the surface of myeloblasts). Management consists of treating the leukemia as soon as possible. It is also possible to perform exchange transfusion or leukopheresis in cases where symptoms are severe, although this is only a temporizing measure at best.

Life-threatening bleeding is another potential complication of leukemia. Although all patients with thrombocytopenia are at risk, patients with concomitant coagulopathy due to disseminated intravascular coagulation (DIC) are at particularly high risk. The leukemia subtype most commonly complicated by DIC and serious bleeding is acute promyelocytic leukemia (APL). This association results from the release of thromboplastin from the cytoplasmic granules in these promyelocytic blasts. Aggressive blood product support through transfusions and early treatment with the differentiation-inducing agent all-*trans* retinoic acid (ATRA, tretinoin) has been shown to decrease the risk of bleeding in APL. Despite these measures, up to 10% of patients die of bleeding complications during the initial weeks of therapy, and additional patients suffer lasting morbidity from retinal hemorrhages and nonfatal CNS hemorrhages.

Tracheal compression and superior vena cava syndrome can result from large anterior mediastinal masses, which are commonly present in T-cell ALL but are also rarely seen in other forms of leukemia as well. Patients can present with respiratory distress, cough, orthopnea, headaches, syncope, dizziness, facial swelling, or plethora. A chest x-ray should be performed to assess the mediastinum in any patient suspected to have leukemia. If the mediastinum is enlarged, a neck computed tomography (CT) is indicated to assess airway patency. This evaluation must precede any attempts at sedation for diagnostic procedures because even light sedation can precipitate acute airway collapse. Diagnostic material should be obtained by the least invasive method possible before treatment. If necessary, emergent airway compromise can be treated with radiation or steroids, or both, although recognize that the use of steroids prior to diagnostic procedures can impair staging (e.g., CSF involvement at diagnosis, presenting peripheral WBC count).

Differential Diagnosis

Although leukemia should be considered in cases of isolated neutropenia, anemia, or thrombocytopenia, the vast majority of leukemia patients present with decreases in more than one cell line. In suspected cases of immune thrombocytopenic purpura (ITP), for example, a careful review of the peripheral blood smear should be performed to rule out the presence of circulating leukemic blasts or other morphologic abnormalities. Routine bone marrow aspiration is not necessary for children with ITP, but it should be performed in patients with atypical features, such as concomitant anemia or neutropenia, hepatosplenomegaly, bone pain, or significant weight loss. Treatment of ITP with corticosteroids should be instituted only after evaluation by an experienced hematologist.

Pancytopenia can be caused by diseases other than leukemia. Some viral infections have a propensity to suppress bone marrow function and cause low peripheral blood cell counts, including Epstein-Barr virus (EBV), herpes simplex virus (HSV), influenza, hepatitis viruses, and HIV. Infectious mononucleosis from EBV infection can be particularly difficult to differentiate from leukemia because patients often have hepatosplenomegaly and circulating atypical lymphocytes (which can appear very similar to leukemic blasts). Pancytopenia on the basis of bone marrow failure (from acquired aplastic anemia or rare inherited bone marrow failure syndromes) can be distinguished from leukemia by bone marrow biopsy for assessment of overall marrow cellularity. Certain solid tumors have a tendency to metastasize to the bone marrow and cause cytopenias, including neuroblastoma and rhabdomyosarcoma, but it is rare for pancytopenia to be the sole primary presenting feature in these cases.

Joint pain, fever, hepatosplenomegaly, and pallor are common presenting features in both systemic-onset juvenile idiopathic arthritis (JIA) and leukemia. An elevated platelet count should be seen in JIA and can be helpful to distinguish the two, as a low or even normal platelet count is rare in JIA given the inflammation that should cause elevations in acute phase reactants. A bone marrow aspirate should be performed to rule out leukemia before treatment with steroids in suspected cases of systemic-onset JIA.

Risk Stratification

In the last several years, treatment decisions for children with newly diagnosed acute leukemia have been based on the concept of risk stratification. Using factors identified during clinical trials to predict a high or low risk of relapse, patients are separated into risk groups before the start of treatment, at the end of the first month of induction therapy, and at postinduction therapy timepoints for select patients. Based on these features, the treatment plan is tailored to the degree of risk. The desired result is that patients with relatively low-risk disease can be treated with less toxic therapy without compromising cure rates, and patients with high-risk disease receive more-intensive, potentially toxic therapy and/or warrant consideration of experimental options. The risk groups are currently defined based on several criteria and differ for ALL and AML. Different centers and cooperative groups typically employ different risk-stratification strategies.

In ALL, risk assignment is based on a combination of leukemia phenotype (B- versus T-lineage), clinical and genetic features, and early response to therapy. The initial risk assessment for B-ALL is based on two simple clinical parameters that are available immediately at the time of diagnosis (the National Cancer Institute [NCI] or Rome criteria): WBC count (>50,000/μL is high risk), and age (<1 year or >9 years is high risk). Presence or absence of leukemia outside of the bone marrow (extramedullary) including presence and level of disease in the CNS and leukemic involvement of the testes increases the risk of relapse.

For B-ALL, low-risk cytogenetic features include hyperdiploidy (≥50 chromosomes in the leukemia cells) or trisomies of specific chromosomes or the presence of a t(12;21) that results in *TEL/AML1* fusion. High-risk cytogenetic features include hypodiploidy (<44 chromosomes in the leukemia cells), the presence of either an 11q23 (*KMT2A*, formerly *MLL*, gene) rearrangement,

TABLE 4 Summary of Treatment for Childhood Leukemia

CHARACTERISTICS	ACUTE LYMPHOBLASTIC LEUKEMIA	ACUTE MYELOID LEUKEMIA
Remission Induction		
Chemotherapy	4 weeks with prednisone or dexamethasone, vincristine, PEG asparaginase, daunorubicin (not all cases)	Two courses (6–8 weeks) with cytarabine (Ara-C), doxorubicin, others (e.g., etoposide,[1] thioguanine)
Toxic death rate	Low (<3%)	High (>10%)
Remission rate	>98%	75%–85%
CNS Preventive Therapy		
Intrathecal Chemotherapy	Methotrexate	Cytarabine
Cranial irradiation	For high risk only (excessive disease in CSF at diagnosis)	None
Consolidation		
Chemotherapy	Combinations of various drugs (not cross-resistant) Intensity/duration based on risk stratification	Based on cytogenic/molecular risk group and minimal residual disease (MRD) Low risk: 2–3 additional courses Intermediate risk: If MRD-negative, treat as low risk; if MRD positive, treat as high risk High risk: BMT for patients with best available donor
Maintenance		
Chemotherapy	Low-dose oral (6-mercaptopurine)[1] and methotrexate) Total duration of therapy 2–3 years	No maintenance therapy (does not improve survival)

BMT, Bone marrow transplant; *CNS,* central nervous system; *CSF,* cerebrospinal fluid; *HLA,* human leukocyte antigen; *WBC,* white blood cell.
[1]Not FDA approved for this indication.

the presence of intrachromosomal amplification of chromosome 21 at the locus containing the gene, *RUNX1* (iAMP21), or a t(9;22), or Philadelphia chromosome, that creates a *BCR/ABL* fusion gene. For T-ALL, cytogenetic features have not been routinely incorporated into risk stratification.

Early response has historically been measured by the response to a prednisone prophase that includes a single dose of intrathecal methotrexate and 7 days of prednisone, or by the percentage of blast cells remaining in the bone marrow after 7 to 14 days of multiagent therapy. Over the past 15 to 20 years, measures of tumor burden remaining in the marrow at the end of induction therapy (minimal residual disease [MRD]) have been shown to be highly predictive of outcome and have been integrated into risk-stratification schemata of all the major leukemia cooperative groups.

In AML, risk stratification is based largely on cytogenetics. Low-risk features include t(8;21), which results in the *RUNX1-RUNX1T1* (formerly *AML1/ETO)* fusion and either inv(16) or a t(16;16), both of which create the *CBFβ/MYH11* fusion. High-risk features include monosomy 7 and abnormalities in the long arm of chromosome 5. More recently, data suggest other cytogenetic features may portend a poor prognosis, such as certain *KMT2A* fusions, t(3;21)(q26.2;q22) resulting in the *RUNX1-MECOM* fusion, and 11p15 rearrangements involving the gene *NUP98,* among others. Most other cytogenetic abnormalities, as well as normal cytogenetics (which are seen in approximately 60% of cases), are considered intermediate risk by most pediatric leukemia consortia. In addition to cytogenetic features, specific molecular lesions are also prognostically relevant in AML. Mutations of the genes *NPM1* and *CEBPA* are associated with a more favorable outcome. Mutations of the receptor tyrosine kinase, *FLT3,* most commonly as internal tandem duplications (ITD) of the juxtamembrane domain, have been historically associated with a poor prognosis, but this risk appears to be dependent on the constellation of co-occuring mutations, as those with both *FLT3*-ITD mutations and either mutation of *NPM1* or *CEBPA* appear to have favorable outcomes. Thus how such mutations are

incorporated into risk stratification schemas varies among pediatric cancer consortia.

Response to therapy has also been incorporated into the risk stratification of AML. Failure to achieve remission with induction chemotherapy is another high-risk feature in AML. Measurement of MRD at the end of induction is now also routinely used for risk stratification of AML.

Treatment

There are significant differences in the specific treatments for ALL and AML, so they will be discussed separately. Table 4 summarizes the most salient features of the treatment for each.

Acute Lymphoblastic Leukemia

Treatment for ALL generally occurs in three phases: remission induction, consolidation, and maintenance with CNS preventive therapy administered throughout each of these phases. Remission induction in ALL typically lasts 4 to 6 weeks and includes three to five systemic agents. Common to almost all regimens are a corticosteroid (either prednisone [Deltasone] or dexamethasone [Decadron]), vincristine (Vincasar), and PEG asparaginase (pegaspargase [Oncaspar]), which compose the three-drug induction. An anthracycline, typically daunorubicin (Cerubidine), is also included in many regimens (four-drug induction), with other agents such as cyclophosphamide (Cytoxan) or etoposide (Toposar, VePesid)[1] used in a small minority of centers. More than 98% of children enter morphologic remission (defined as <5% blasts in the bone marrow) by the end of 4 weeks of induction therapy, and the mortality rate from toxicity during induction therapy is generally less than 2% to 3% in industrialized countries.

The concept that the CNS could be a sanctuary site for leukemia emerged in the mid-1960s when the introduction of multiagent systemic chemotherapy led to high remission rates,

[1]Not FDA approved for this indication.

but a majority of patients relapsed within 6 to 12 months, with many of these recurrences being limited to the CNS. Routine introduction of presymptomatic CNS radiation in the late 1960s and early 1970s led to substantial increases in cure rates to approximately 50%. Modern CNS preventive therapy includes periodic administration of intrathecal chemotherapy (usually methotrexate) starting at the time of the first diagnostic lumbar puncture. Systemic agents with improved CNS penetration (dexamethasone rather than prednisone, higher doses of intravenous methotrexate) might also play an important role in CNS control. Cranial irradiation is currently reserved for patients at the highest risk for CNS relapse (e.g., those with high diagnostic WBC count or leukemic blasts in CSF at diagnosis). Over time, CNS radiation has been given to fewer and fewer ALL patients; some groups believe that it can be eliminated for all patients. With these modern strategies, the risk of isolated CNS relapse is less than 5%.

Following the induction of remission, patients receive additional chemotherapy designed to consolidate the remission. The intensity and duration of the consolidation phase are risk based, and alternating cycles of non–cross-resistant chemotherapy drugs are typically used. These consolidation or intensification phases typically last about 6 months and often include a reinduction phase similar to the first month of treatment.

It has been clearly demonstrated that the risk of relapse in ALL can be reduced with an extended phase of continuous low-dose chemotherapy (maintenance) that lasts until 2 to 3 years from the time of diagnosis. Oral 6-mercaptopurine (Purixan, Purinethol) and methotrexate are used universally, with variable administration of intrathecal chemotherapy. Some centers or groups also employ periodic doses of vincristine and 5- to 7-day pulses of prednisone or dexamethasone. The optimal frequency of intrathecal chemotherapy treatments and vincristine and steroid pulses is uncertain and might depend on the intensity of therapy delivered during the induction and consolidation phases.

Acute Myeloid Leukemia

Remission induction in AML typically consists of two courses of very intensive chemotherapy with cytarabine (Cytosar, Tarabine) and doxorubicin (Adriamycin), often combined with thioguanine (Tabloid) or etoposide.[1] Remission rates are 75% to 85%, with about one half of the failures due to resistant leukemia and the others to mortality from toxicity (usually infection).

Similar to ALL, CNS preventive therapy in AML begins at diagnosis with intrathecal chemotherapy (usually cytarabine) and continues with additional periodic intrathecal treatments during consolidation. High-dose cytarabine, which is a key component of most AML treatment regimens, also contributes to CNS treatment. Cranial radiation is not typically administered by most groups to children with AML, except for treatment of chloromas (solid masses of leukemia cells) that do not resolve with chemotherapy.

Consolidation in AML is risk dependent. High-risk patients can be identified who have less than a 20% to 25% chance of cure with intensive chemotherapy. Most groups consider these patients to be candidates for bone marrow transplant (BMT). If a matched sibling is unavailable, then alternative donor sources (e.g., matched unrelated bone marrow, umbilical cord blood, or haplo-identical transplant from a parent) are usually offered. For low-risk patients, for whom the cure rate with chemotherapy alone approaches 70%, BMT is usually not offered in first remission, even for patients with a matched sibling donor. In addition, relapses in low-risk patients, unlike relapses in intermediate-risk or high-risk patients, can often be successfully treated with BMT in second remission, justifying reservation of BMT for use as a salvage therapy for low-risk patients. Consolidation in these cases consists of two to three additional chemotherapy courses that are slightly less intense and usually consist of cytarabine combined with drugs not used in induction, such as mitoxantrone (Novantrone) and L-asparaginase (Elspar).[1] For intermediate-risk patients, MRD testing at the end of induction is increasingly being used to determine whether to consolidate with chemotherapy or BMT. Unlike ALL, most groups have found no benefit to extended maintenance therapy in children with AML.

Relapse

The most common site of relapsed leukemia is the bone marrow (with or without concomitant CNS involvement). Less common are isolated extramedullary relapses (CNS or testicular relapse in ALL, chloromas in AML). For both ALL and AML, a critical determinant of outcome following relapse is the time from diagnosis to relapse.

ALL patients who relapse within 18 months of initial diagnosis have a dismal outcome, with only about one half able to attain a second remission and less than 10% overall cure rate; the outcome is marginally better for those who relapse between 18 and 36 months after diagnosis. ALL patients with such early relapses are typically treated with 3 to 4 months of intensive therapy to achieve a second remission and attain further cytoreduction, followed by BMT using a matched sibling or unrelated donor. In contrast, children with ALL who relapse more than 3 years after initial diagnosis have an approximately 95% chance of entering a second remission, and 40% to 70% can be cured with intensive chemotherapy without BMT. Notably, with successful introduction of immunotherapeutic agents such as blinatumomab (Blincyto), the CD19-targeting bispecific T-cell engager and CD19-directed chimeric antigen receptor T-cell (CART) tisagenlecleucel (Kymriah), the therapeutic approach for relapsed B-ALL is evolving. Recent data suggest blinatmomab compared with standard chemotherapy is better tolerated and more likely to achieve an MRD-negative remission prior to hematopoietic stem cell transplant (HSCT) in high-risk relapsed B-ALL. Additionally, emerging evidence suggest CD19 CART can achieve durable remissions in some relapsed B-ALL patients without BMT. Thus the approach for the treatment of relapsed ALL is largely shifting away from intensive standard chemotherapy and BMT to a hybrid of chemotherapy and immunotherapy with or without BMT.

Overall, relapsed AML has a dismal outcome (long-term survival approximately 20%), and the approach is to attempt to reinduce remission and then proceed to BMT or investigational treatments. Even in this setting, there is clearly an improved outcome for patients who relapse after a prolonged initial remission (>12 months from the end of remission-induction therapy) compared with patients who have refractory disease or who relapse after a shorter period of remission.

New treatment strategies are urgently needed for patients with relapsed ALL and AML because the current regimens produce poor results and are associated with a great deal of toxicity. The major clinical trial groups are testing novel and targeted therapies in these patient populations.

Late Effects

Approximately 70% of children with leukemia are cured of their disease. As the numbers of long-term survivors of childhood leukemia have grown, there has been increasing interest in assessing the late effects of leukemic therapy. In childhood ALL, with cure rates of 90%, a major effort is being made in ongoing clinical trials to reduce the intensity of therapy for lower-risk patients, with the hope of reducing late effects of therapy without compromising high cure rates. The most common late effects of leukemia therapy, with the known treatment-related risk factors and recommended diagnostic approach for each, are summarized in Table 5. Many pediatric

---

[1]Not FDA approved for this indication.

[1]Not FDA approved for this indication.

TABLE 5 Summary of Late Effects of Leukemia Treatment

LATE EFFECT	TREATMENT-RELATED RISK FACTORS	DIAGNOSTIC APPROACH
Bone	Avascular necrosis, osteonecrosis	X-ray and/or MRI of major joints for persistent pain
Cardiac dysfunction	Anthracyclines: cardiomyopathy (risk related to cumulative dose, higher risk in AML)	ECG or echocardiogram every 3–5 years (cardiomyopathy can occur decades after treatment)
Cataracts	CNS RT	Yearly eye examination
CNS and psychosocial	CNS RT, IT chemotherapy: learning problems, neurocognitive dysfunction	Yearly educational assessment, neurocognitive testing
Dental abnormalities	CNS RT	Yearly dental examinations
Endocrine and reproductive	CNS RT: pituitary dysfunction Alkylators: primary gonadal failure	Yearly growth curves, TSH, LH, FSH LH, FSH, estradiol or testosterone, semen analysis
Hepatic dysfunction	Methotrexate, 6-mercaptopurine, 6-thioguanine: late hepatic fibrosis	Yearly LFTs
Secondary neoplasms	CNS RT: brain tumors Alkylators or epipodophyllotoxins: secondary AML	MRI for symptoms CBC in symptomatic patients

ALL, Acute lymphoblastic leukemia; *AML,* acute myeloid leukemia; *FSH,* follicle-stimulating hormone; *IT,* intrathecal; *LFT,* liver function test; *LH,* luteinizing hormone; *MRI,* magnetic resonance imaging; *RT,* radiation therapy; *TSH,* thyroid-stimulating hormone.

oncology centers have developed late-effects programs to conduct surveillance for the development of these problems and provide follow-up care to patients who develop late complications of therapy.

References

Special section: cancer in children and adolescents. In: American Cancer Society: cancer Facts and Figures 2014. American Cancer Society, 2014, pp 25-42.

Bolouri H, Farrar JE, Triche T, et al: The molecular landscape of pediatric acute myeloid leukemia reveals recurrent structural alterations and age-specific mutational interactions, *Nat Med* 24(1):103–112, 01 2018, https://doi.org/10.1038/nm.4439.

Brown AL, Arts P, Carmichael CL, et al: RUNX1-mutated families show phenotype heterogeneity and a somatic mutation profile unique to germline predisposed AML, *Blood Adv* 4(6):1131–1144, 03 2020, https://doi.org/10.1182/bloodadvances.2019000901.

Brown PA, Ji L, Xu X, et al: Effect of postreinduction therapy consolidation with blinatumomab vs chemotherapy on disease-free survival in children, adolescents, and young adults with first relapse of B-cell acute lymphoblastic leukemia: a randomized clinical trial, *J Am Med Assoc* 325(9):833–842, 03 2021, https://doi.org/10.1001/jama.2021.0621.

Buitenkamp TD, Izraeli S, Zimmermann M, et al: Acute lymphoblastic leukemia in children with Down syndrome: a retrospective analysis from the Ponte di Legno study group, *Blood* 123(1):70–77, Jan 2, 2014, https://doi.org/10.1182/blood-2013-06-509463.

Creutzig U, Zimmermann M, Reinhardt D, et al: Changes in cytogenetics and molecular genetics in acute myeloid leukemia from childhood to adult age groups, *Cancer* 122(24):3821–3830, Dec 2016, https://doi.org/10.1002/cncr.30220.

Davidsson J, Puschmann A, Tedgård U, Bryder D, Nilsson L, Cammenga J: SAMD9 and SAMD9L in inherited predisposition to ataxia, pancytopenia, and myeloid malignancies, *Leukemia* 32(5):1106–1115, 05 2018, https://doi.org/10.1038/s41375-018-0074-4.

Gaynon PS, Qu RP, Chappell RJ, et al: Survival after relapse in childhood acute lymphoblastic leukemia: Impact of site and time to first relapse—the Children's Cancer Group Experience, *Cancer* 82:1387–1395, 1998.

Gibson BE, Wheatley K, Hann IM, et al: Treatment strategy and long-term results in paediatric patients treated in consecutive UK AML trials, *Leukemia* 19:2130–2138, 2005.

Greaves MF, Wiemels J: Origins of chromosome translocations in childhood leukaemia, *Nat Rev Cancer* 3:639–649, 2003.

Hunger SP, Mullighan CG: Acute lymphoblastic leukemia in children, *N Engl J Med* 373(16):1541–1552, Oct 15, 2015, https://doi.org/10.1056/NEJMra1400972.

Locatelli F, Zugmaier G, Rizzari C, et al: Effect of blinatumomab vs chemotherapy on event-free survival among children with high-risk first-relapse B-cell acute lymphoblastic leukemia: a randomized clinical trial, *J Am Med Assoc* 325(9):843–854, 03 2021, https://doi.org/10.1001/jama.2021.0987.

Loh ML, Sakai DS, Flotho C, et al: Mutations in CBL occur frequently in juvenile myelomonocytic leukemia, *Blood* 114(9):1859–1863, Aug 27, 2009.

Maude SL, Laetsch TW, Buechner J, et al: Tisagenlecleucel in children and young adults with B-cell lymphoblastic leukemia, *N Engl J Med* 378(5):439–448, 02 2018, https://doi.org/10.1056/NEJMoa1709866.

Möricke A, Zimmermann M, Reiter A, et al: Long-term results of five consecutive trials in childhood acute lymphoblastic leukemia performed by the ALL-BFM study group from 1981 to 2000, *Leukemia* 24(2):265–284, Feb 2010, https://doi.org/10.1038/leu.2009.257.

Pui CH, Campana D, Pei D, et al: Treating childhood acute lymphoblastic leukemia without cranial irradiation, *N Engl J Med* 360(26):2730–2741, Jun 2009, https://doi.org/10.1056/NEJMoa0900386.

Pui CH, Cheng C, Leung W, et al: Extended follow-up of long-term survivors of childhood acute lymphoblastic leukemia, *N Engl J Med* 349:640–649, 2003.

Pui CH, Pei D, Sandlund JT, et al: Long-term results of St Jude total therapy studies 11, 12, 13A, 13B, and 14 for childhood acute lymphoblastic leukemia, *Leukemia* 24(2):371–382, Feb 2010, https://doi.org/10.1038/leu.2009.252.

Ries LAG, Melbert D, Krapcho M, et al: *SEER cancer statistics review, 1975–2004*, Bethesda, Md, 2007, National Cancer Institute 2007.

Silverman LB, Stevenson KE, O'Brien JE, et al: Long-term results of Dana-Farber Cancer Institute ALL Consortium protocols for children with newly diagnosed acute lymphoblastic leukemia (1985-2000), *Leukemia* 24(2):320–334, Feb 2010, https://doi.org/10.1038/leu.2009.253.

Stahnke K, Boos J, Bender-Gotze C, et al: Duration of first remission predicts remission rates and long-term survival in children with relapsed acute myelogenous leukemia, *Leukemia* 12:1534–1538, 1998.

Uffmann M, Rasche M, Zimmermann M, et al: Therapy reduction in patients with Down syndrome and myeloid leukemia: the international ML-DS 2006 trial, *Blood* 129(25):3314–3321, 06 2017, https://doi.org/10.1182/blood-2017-01-765057.

Wakeford R, Little MP: Risk coefficients for childhood cancer after intrauterine irradiation: a review, *Int J Radiat Biol* 79:293–309, 2003.

Wlodarski MW, Hirabayashi S, Pastor V, et al: Prevalence, clinical characteristics, and prognosis of GATA2-related myelodysplastic syndromes in children and adolescents, *Blood* 127(11):1387–1397, Mar 2016, https://doi.org/10.1182/blood-2015-09-669937. quiz 1518.

Woods WG, Neudorf S, Gold S, et al: A comparison of allogeneic bone marrow transplantation, autologous bone marrow transplantation, and aggressive chemotherapy in children with acute myeloid leukemia in remission, *Blood* 97:56–62, 2001.

ADOLESCENT HEALTH

Kari R. Harris, MD

CURRENT DIAGNOSIS

- In addition to general medical care, it is important to identify psychosocial health concerns at all adolescent visits.
- The key components of a psychosocial history are addressed in the HEADS private and confidential interview.
- Conducting a Home/Education/Employment/Activities/ Accident Prevention/Diet/Disordered Eating/Drugs/ Depression/Suicide/Self-harm/Sex/Sleep/Social Media (HEADS) interview is standard practice for adolescent care: it should be part of all adolescent well-checks and used, as time permits, in acute visits for teens who have high-risk behaviors or have no regular health care.
- High-acuity areas identified from the HEADS interview include substance use, disordered eating, sexual activity, and mental health.
- Depression screening should be part of well visits for all patients between 12 and 21 years of age.
- Anxiety screening is recommended for girls 13 years and older. Clinical discretion should guide screening frequency.
- Substance use screening should be included in all adolescent well visits.
- HIV universal screening should be completed initially between 15 and 18 years of age and the need for rescreening reassessed annually.
- Immunization status should be assessed at every visit, with routine and catch-up vaccines provided.

CURRENT THERAPY

- Long-acting reversible contraception (LARC) provides safe and effective contraception for teenagers.
- Emergency contraception should be offered within 5 days of unprotected sexual activity.
- Treatment for teens is often multidisciplinary, involving subspecialists, mental health providers, medical or psychiatric inpatient units, and county welfare or health departments.

Setting the Stage for the Adolescent Visit

Comprehensive care for adolescents includes screening for high-risk behaviors in addition to routine medical care. To facilitate open communication, providers should be clear about consent and confidentiality policies in their practices. This can be achieved by discussing policies with patients and parents/caretakers during young adolescent visits (11 to 14 years) and by providing materials documenting the policies and practices, such as a standard letter to parents. Policies can also be displayed in the office, provided in practice newsletters and materials, and made available through patient access portals.

Adolescent visits differ from early childhood visits in several important respects. At the beginning of the visit, time should be spent with both the teen and parent or caregiver clarifying medical history and current concerns. The adolescent should then be offered time without the parent or caregiver present to discuss sensitive issues, including reproductive and mental health. At the end of the visit, the parent/caregiver should be provided with a summary of the visit, limited to the nonconfidential portion, and including recommendations and arrangements for follow-up appointments.

Consent and Confidentiality Laws—Consent Does Not Equal Confidential

Consent and confidentiality laws vary by state. Most states allow minors to consent for reproductive health care, including testing and treatment for sexually transmitted infections (STIs). Most states also allow providers to prescribe contraceptives to minors. Many states have a "mature minor" statute that allows physicians to provide care if they deem the adolescent patient mature and capable of understanding the medical care. These laws give teens autonomy to consent to their own health care and they also enable care to be provided when a parent is unable to attend the appointment.

While consent and confidentiality laws are related, they are separate entities. Many states allow minors to consent for specific health services but do not prohibit a provider from informing the teen's parent/caretaker about that service. Even if allowed by law, expert consensus holds that such disclosures should only be made when in the best interest of the minor patient. The disclosure should not compromise future health care. Many teens will not seek reproductive health care if they have to involve a parent, making confidentiality necessary for comprehensive adolescent health care.

Confidentiality is limited when a minor patient is in direct harm, such as intimate partner violence, sexual coercion or rape, certain pregnancy, suicidality, or self-harm. In such instances, a parent/caretaker should become involved, unless he/she is the perpetrator or some other extraordinary circumstances exist. Local authorities or social welfare agencies may also need to be contacted. These necessary breaches in confidentiality to protect safety must be explained beforehand to the patient and be included in written policies. Any breach of confidentiality must be carried out in a professional manner, explained sensitively to the patient and others, and be well documented. Every attempt must be made not to compromise future care.

Information on consent and confidentiality laws for each state is available at the Guttmacher Institute website (guttmacher.org).

The HEADS Interview

The HEADS acronym provides a structured psychosocial history-taking tool that also screens for high-risk behaviors (Table 1). Although several variations of HEADS have been described, they all cover the most common risk categories for adolescents. Progressing from the least invasive topics to the most sensitive issues, HEADS covers all essential categories (see Table 1).

When using the HEADS interview tool, it is important to build rapport with the patient. The teen deserves explanation of why they are being asked personal questions and every attempt should be made to increase patient comfort and trust. The interview begins with questions regarding hobbies, school, and home life. Once rapport is established, questions proceed to more sensitive issues. Questioning should be open-ended, nonassuming, and nonjudgmental. This allows for honest answers and does not discriminate among patients.

Home/Education/Employment/Activities/Accident Prevention

These topics begin the confidential interview with the least risky activities for adolescents. Although grouped together in this text, each category deserves its own time and questions (see Table 1). All adolescents should have a trusted adult with whom they can discuss concerns. Safety at home and school safety, including any bullying or coercion regardless of site or circumstances, should be discussed and addressed. Current school performance, concerns, grades and post graduation goals should be discussed. After-school employment has benefits but can also negatively impact academic performance, mood, or family dynamics. These should be screened for and addressed if present. Healthy after-school activities should be encouraged. Predictably, adolescent illegal activity, drug use, and sexual activity peak during after-school

TABLE 1	HEADS Acronym with Sample Questions	
H	Home	Who lives with you at home? Tell me about your relationships at home. Are you safe at home? Do you have a trusted adult to confide in at home? Do you have your own space at home? Have there been any changes at home?
E	Education	What grade are you in and what school? Do you feel like you have enough food at home? Are you ever worried you might not get three meals a day because there is not enough food? Is your school safe? Tell me about your friends. Does anyone bother you at school? How are your grades? Do you have any problems with school? How many days of school have you missed this year and why? Do you plan to graduate? What do you want to do after graduation?
	Employment	Are you working? Do you like your job? How do you spend the money you earn from working? Do you feel stressed because of work? Is your family stressed by your work? How many hours a week do you work?
A	Activities	What do you do for fun? Who do you hang out with? Tell me what you do after school. Are you in any organized after-school or summer activities? Tell me about your hobbies. Do you have a religious preference?
	Accident prevention	Tell me about your activities. Do you wear a seatbelt? Do you wear a helmet while biking or using an all-terrain vehicle? Have you ever ridden with someone while they were under the influence of drugs or alcohol, or have you ever driven under the influence? Where is your cell phone while you are driving?
D	Diet/disordered eating	Tell me about your diet. Do you feel like you have enough food at home? Are you ever worried you might not get three meals a day because there is not enough food? Do you eat breakfast daily? How many fruits and vegetables do you eat? How do you feel about your weight? Do you like the way you look? Have you ever not eaten to try to lose weight? Do you ever feel guilty about what you have eaten? Have you ever skipped meals, thrown up on purpose, or exercised excessively after you have eaten?
	Drugs	Have you seen drugs at your school? Do any of your friends smoke, vape, drink alcohol, or use other drugs? Have you ever tried drugs? Have you ever been in trouble because of drug use?
	Depression	Do you ever feel sad, down, or depressed? Have you ever felt like you had nothing to look forward to? Do you still like to do the things you used to do? Do others say you are more irritable than normal?
S	Suicide/self-harm	Have you ever been so upset you have wanted to hurt yourself? Have you ever cut yourself? Have you ever thought about killing yourself or someone else? Who would you talk with if you did have thoughts like this?
	Sex	Are you in a relationship? When is the last time you had sex? Did you use a condom? Are you using anything to prevent pregnancy? Have you ever been tested for STIs? How many partners have you had? Tell me about your partner (age, gender, etc.). Do you feel safe with your partner? Have you ever been forced to have sex or do something you were not comfortable with?
	Sleep	What time do you go to bed? Where is your cell phone when you go to sleep? When do you wake up in the morning?
	Social media	What social media sites do you have profiles on? Are you friends with people you do not know in real life? How much time do you spend on social media? Does this affect your grades? Tell me about your privacy settings. Do you have any trusted adults that can access your social media sites?

STI, Sexually transmitted infections.

Adapted from Klein DA, Goldenring JM: HEEADSSS 3.0: The psychosocial interview for adolescents updated for a new century fueled by media. *Contemporary Pediatrics.* 2014. Available at http://contemporarypediatrics.modernmedicine.com/contemporary-pediatrics/news/probing-scars-how-ask-essential-questions?page=full (Accessed October 13, 2014).

hours. Participation in organized, supervised, extracurricular activities has been shown to decrease these risky behaviors and confer positive health and emotional benefits. Accidents remain the leading cause of death for this age group and prevention should be emphasized. Safety should be assessed at this time, as well as throughout the course of the interview as it applies to each topic.

Diet/Disordered Eating

Nutritional health problems are of concern with adolescents. Many lifestyle habits, especially regarding nutrition, are formedduring this period. Asking the teen to describe his/her typical diet provides insight on potential areas for improvement. Limiting portion sizes, avoiding excessive or late night snacking, and replacing sugary drinks with water is common advice for teens. This portion of the interview provides opportunity to screen for body image distortion or disordered eating. The growth chart should be reviewed and any significant weight changes discussed.

Drugs (Substance Use)

When asking about riskier behaviors, it is important to have rapport and trust. The subject of substance use can be broached by asking if peers use substances. Because alcohol, marijuana, electronic vaping, and tobacco use is so prevalent among high school students (reported by 60%, 35%, 42%, and 29%, respectively), this initial question can make a teen more comfortable moving on to talk about personal use. The CRAFFT acronym is a brief and effective screening tool designed specifically for use with adolescents and helps the provider determine if further conversation or evaluation regarding substance use is warranted. The questions are broken into part A and B. If a patient answers "yes" to any

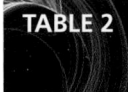

TABLE 2 CRAFFT+N Substance Use Disorder Screening Tool for Adolescents (to be verbally administered by a clinician in a private setting with the teen)

Part A.

During the past 12 months did you:

1. Drink more than a few sips of beer, wine, or any drink containing alcohol? Say "0" if none.
2. Smoked any marijuana (weed, oil, or hash by smoking, vaping, or in food) or "synthetic marijuana" (like "K2", "Spice")? Say "0" if none.
3. Used anything else to get high (like other illegal, prescription, or over-the-counter medications, and things that you sniff, huff, or vape)? Say "0" if none.
4. Use any tobacco or nicotine products (for example, cigarettes, e-cigarettes, hookahs, smokeless tobacco)? Say "0" if none.

If all answers in part A are 0, then ask only "CAR" Part B, then stop.
If any answer to part A is >0, then ask all 6 questions of Part B.

Part B.

C	1. Have you ever ridden in a **CAR** driven by someone (including yourself) who was high or had been using alcohol or other drugs?
R	
A	
F	2. Do you ever use alcohol or other drugs to **RELAX**, feel better about yourself, or fit in?
F	
T	3. Do you ever use alcohol or other drugs while you are by yourself, **ALONE**?
	4. Do you ever **FORGET** things you did while using alcohol or drugs?
	5. Do your **FAMILY** or **FRIENDS** ever tell you that you should cut down on your drinking or drug use?
	6. Have you ever gotten into **TROUBLE** while you were using alcohol or other drugs?

*Two or more YES answers suggest a serious problem and need for further assessment. See http://crafft.org/get-the-crafft/ for further instructions.
The CRAFFT+N 2.1. John R. Knight, MD: The Center for Adolescent Substance Abuse Research (CeASAR); Boston Children's Hospital; Harvard Medical School Teaching Hospital. 2018. Available at: http://crafft.org (Accessed October 4, 2019).

questions in A, then part B questions are asked. If the patient answers "yes" to two or more questions of part B, the screen is positive and further evaluation is recommended (Table 2). If necessary, referral should be made to a qualified mental health provider for treatment. Substance use is a leading cause of morbidity and mortality for teens in the United States, and teens who use substances at an early age are more likely to become addicted. Substance use should not be ignored or minimized by providers. Counseling on prevention should contain a clear message of nonuse.

Depression/Anxiety/Suicide/Self-Harm

Depression screening is recommended at all well visits beginning at age 12. Several screening tools are available. Questions covering loss of interest in normal activities and feeling depressed, down, or hopeless open the door to more specific questions regarding signs and symptoms of depression. In addition to depressive feelings, teens should be explicitly screened for suicidal intention, past attempts, plans, self-harm, and safety. If a teen discloses an unsafe environment, law enforcement should be included in an immediate plan of care. If a teen is actively suicidal, then immediate inpatient treatment is warranted. Anxiety is common in adolescent females, and those 13 and older should be screened. Screening can occur concomitantly with depression screening History should assess social function, somatic symptoms, and coping strategies. Outpatient treatment for mental health disorders in teens includes cognitive behavioral therapy with or withoutmedication. For most teens, parental involvement is necessary when treating mental

health disorders. If the provider feels the teen is unsafe due to their own actions or those of others, then the confidential interview is no longer appropriate and the caretaker must be included in the next stage of management.

Sex

Nearly half of high school students have had sex. Of those, only about a quarter used reliable contraception at their last intercourse. Adolescents and young adults account for the majority of gonorrhea and chlamydia cases each year. Risk factors for morbidity related to sexual activity include early sexual initiation, increasing number of partners, substance use prior to sex, and unprotected sexual acts. Teenagers and men who have sex with men are the population groups at highest risk for STIs. STI screening should be discussed for those at risk. Recommendations are outlined in Table 3.

When discussing the sensitive issue of sex with teens, it is important to use neutral terms and remain nonjudgmental. It is also important to include gender identity in the history. Sexual history should include age of first sexual encounter, age of partner(s), gender of partner, number of partners, type of sexual activities, date of last sexual activity, and contraceptive and barrier use. Quality of relationships should also be assessed, as 7% of high school students report that they have experienced sexual dating violence including sexual coercion and rape. As with substance use, providers should relay a clear message of abstinence as the safest method to prevent morbidity.

Teens should be counseled on contraceptive options, emphasizing that LARC (intrauterine contraception and implants) is safe and the most reliable contraception available for teens. Quick-start contraception (prescribing or providing contraception at the current appointment) should be strongly considered to improve adherence in sexually active teens. The possibility of pregnancy should be reasonably ruled out prior to providing contraception by taking a careful sexual history, including last menstrual period, date of last sex, and method of contraception; lab work may also be considered (see the US Selected Practice Recommendations for Contraceptive Use for guidance on how to reasonably rule out pregnancy, https://www.cdc.gov/reproductivehealth/contraception/contraception_guidance.htm). If a patient has been recently sexually active, most non-intrauterine contraceptives have not been shown to harm an existing pregnancy. Nevertheless, counseling regarding this risk is important prior to initiating contraception, and pregnancy testing should be performed 2 to 4 weeks following contraception initiation. For patients who have had unprotected sex in the past 5 days, emergency contraception should be discussed and offered at the time of quick start contraception. Concurrent barrier contraception should be stressed. Aside from abstinence, male condoms are the most effective way of preventing STIs.

Sleep/Social Media

The conclusion of this format of the HEADS interview concerns less sensitive topics and allows for a comfortable close to the interview. Sleep is problematic for many teens and can usually be improved with better sleep hygiene. Encourage all teens to have a consistent sleep and wake time and 8 to 10 hours of sleep daily. Caffeinated beverages should be limited. Daily exercise should be recommended. The teen's bedroom should be free from distractions, including screened electronic devices.

Social media and cell phones are now integral to popular culture. While these offer benefits to teens, use should be limited. Both social media and cell phones contribute to unintentional injuries, especially with distracted driving. In addition, personal information being shared on the internet through electronic media opens the teen up to vulnerability. Lastly, both can act as significant distractions from academic work, family

TABLE 3 Laboratory Screening and Procedure Recommendations

SCREENING	AGE	TEST/PROCEDURE	COMMENTS
Dyslipidemia	9–11 17–21	Nonfasting lipid profile	Once between 9 and 11 years and again between 17 and 21 years with annual risk assessment (NHLBI, AAP) Insufficient evidence for screening (USPSTF)
Hemoglobin/ hematocrit	11–21	Verbally screen for risk	No routine testing recommended
Human immunodeficiency virus (HIV)	15–18	HIV 1–2 immunoassay	At least once if >15 years with more frequent screening if high-risk (CDC, USPSTF, AAP) Screen MSM at least annually (CDC)
Chlamydia	Females <25	NAAT at site of potential infection	Screen all sexually active women <25 years at risk (USPSTF) or annually and MSM at least annually (CDC)
Gonorrhea	Females <25	NAAT at site of potential infection	Screen all sexually active women <25 years at risk (USPSTF) and MSM at least annually (CDC)
Syphilis*	Adolescents at increased risk	Serology with confirmatory testing if positive	Screen persons at increased risk (USPSTF). Screen MSM at least annually (CDC)
Cervical dysplasia screening	21 years	Pap smear	Other indications for pelvic exam still apply but routine Pap testing <21 years is not recommended (USPSTF, AAP)
Immunizations	All ages	Routine vaccinations per CDC guidelines	Immunization status should be assessed and routine and catch-up vaccines provided at all adolescent visits

AAP, American Academy of Pediatrics; *CDC*, Center for Disease Control and Prevention; *MSM*, Men who have sex with men; *NAAT*, nucleic acid amplification testing; *NIHLB*, National Heart, Lung, and Blood Institute; *Pap smear*, Papanicolaou smear; *USPSTF*, US Preventive Services Task Force.
*Also consider screening high-risk adolescents for hepatitis B infection with HbsAg (USPSTF).

time, and sleep. Discuss safe and appropriate use of electronic devices with patients and summarize to parents.

Pandemic/Post-pandemic Screening

Adolescents have been significantly affected by the COVID-19 pandemic of 2020 and 2021. It is important to acknowledge this and screen for negative effects and for resiliency. Asking teens about safety at home and access to a trusted adult is important. As many families are experiencing extreme financial stress, the questions outlined regarding adolescent employment and food security are also important. Likewise, many families have lost loved ones to the pandemic. These experiences affect the mental health of adolescents, and therefore, screening for bereavement, major depression, and anxiety should be included in all visits for the foreseeable future. Traditional schooling has also been altered during this time; therefore, talking with teens about their learning environment, use of multiple digital devices, and academic performance can shed light on areas to target for behavioral counseling. Last, physicians and clinicians should talk with teens about resiliency and encourage good self-care during adolescent health visits.

Summary

In addition to providing routine health care to teens, providers should focus on the psychosocial history. The HEADS acronym provides a tool for providers to approach these sensitive topics systematically. This interview should take place privately, respecting the teen's ability to consent for certain care, and when able, keeping care confidential. Providers should be familiar with the laws regarding consent and confidentiality of minors in their state. Although teens should be allowed access to confidential health care, providers must be aware that often the best care includes a trusted adult. Parents should be involved in their teen's care when appropriate. Once teens have been assessed for high-risk behaviors, problematic behaviors should be addressed and low-risk behaviors should be commended and encouraged.

References

American Academy of Pediatrics. *Performing preventive services: A bright futures handbook*, 2010, AAP. Available at http://brightfutures.aap.org/pdfs/preventive%20services%20pdfs/physical%20examination.pdf [accessed 10.13.14].

American Academy of Pediatrics Committee on Practice and Ambulatory Medicine: Bright Futures: Recommendations for Preventive Pediatric Health Care, Committee on practice and ambulatory medicine, bright futures periodicity schedule workgroup, *Pediatrics*, 2017. (No. RR-3). Available at https://www.aap.org/en-us/documents/periodicity_schedule.pdf.

Centers for Disease Control and Prevention: Sexually transmitted diseases treatment guidelines, *MMWR Recomm Rep* 64:1–137, 2015. 2015. Available at https://www.cdc.gov/std/tg2015/.

Cohen DA, Farley TA, Taylor SN, et al: When and where do youths have sex? The potential role of adult supervision, Pediatrics 110: Available at http://pediatrics.aappublications.org/content/110/6/e66.long [accessed 02.10.18].

Curtis KM, Jatlaoui TC, Tepper NK, et al: 2016 U.S. Selected Practice Recommendations for Contraceptive Use, *MMWR Recomm Rep* 65(No. RR-4):1–66, 2016, https://doi.org/10.15585/mmwr.rr6504a1. . [Accessed 14 March 2017]. accessed.

Daniels SR, Benuck I, Christakis DA, et al: Expert panel on integrated guidelines for cardiovascular health and risk reduction in children and adolescents: summary report. National Heart, Lung, and Blood Institute. Available at http://www.nhlbi.nih.gov/health-pro/guidelines/current/cardiovascular-health-pediatric-guidelines/summary.htm [accessed 03.10.14].

Gregory KD, Chelmow D, Nelson HD: Screening for anxiety in adolescent and adult women: a recommendation from the Women's Preventive Services Initiative, *Ann Intern Med* 173(1):48–56, 2020.

Guttmacher Institute: *State policies in brief: an overview of minors' consent law*, 2014. Available at https://www.guttmacher.org/statecenter/spibs/spib_OMCL.pdf [accessed 10.13.14].

Kann L, McManus T, Harris WA, et al: Youth risk behavior surveillance—United States, *MMWR Surveill Summ* 67(No. SS-8):1–114, 2017. 2018.

Klein DA, Goldenring JM: HEEADSSS 3.0: the psychosocial interview for adolescents updated for a new century fueled by media, *Contemp Pediatr*, 2014. Available at http://contemporarypediatrics.modernmedicine.com/contemporary-pediatrics/news/probing-scars-how-ask-essential-questions?page=full [accessed 10.13.14].

The CRAFFT+N 2.1. John R. Knight, MD, The Center for Adolescent Substance Abuse Research (CeASAR); Boston Children's Hospital; Harvard Medical School Teaching Hospital. 2018. Available at: http://crafft.org/. Accessed Oct. 4, 2019.

U.S. Preventive Services Task Force. Recommendations for Primary Care Practice. Available at https://www.uspreventiveservicestaskforce.org/Page/Name/recommendations [accessed 02.10.18].

ASTHMA IN CHILDREN

Method of
Susan M. Pollart, MD, MS; Katharine C. DeGeorge, MD, MS; and Amanda Kolb, MD

CURRENT DIAGNOSIS

- Recurrent wheeze, cough, and shortness of breath are typical asthma symptoms.
- A personal or family history of atopy is associated with an increased risk of developing asthma.
- Atopy, allergic rhinitis, eczema, or nasal polyps are common comorbidities in patients with asthma.
- Specifically ask about symptom triggers such as allergens, irritants, exercise, stress, cold, or infection.
- At initial diagnosis, outline symptom frequency, intensity, and timing to classify severity.
- Physical examination of asthmatic children is often normal, but mucosal edema of nasal turbinates, eczematous skin rashes, tachypnea, tachycardia, expiratory wheezes, and lung hyperexpansion may be observed.
- In children older than 5 years, spirometry revealing an obstructive pattern at least partially reversible with bronchodilators confirms the diagnosis. In children younger than 5 years, diagnosis is based on history, physical examination, and a trial of antiasthma medications.
- Chest x-ray, complete blood count (CBC), and IgE levels are not routinely recommended but may be useful in certain situations.

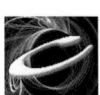

CURRENT THERAPY

- The goal of asthma management is to reduce impairment of activities and decrease risk of exacerbations.
- Initial assessment of asthmatics should focus on symptom frequency, timing, and effect on activities.
- The four central components of management are frequent assessment and monitoring, patient education, controlling environmental triggers, and appropriate use of medication.
- Short-acting inhaled β_2-adrenergic receptor agonists such as albuterol are the mainstay of acute therapy in an episode of bronchoconstriction. Additionally, anticholinergics such as ipratropium bromide[1] and systemic steroids are important components of managing an acute exacerbation. Magnesium sulfate[1], epinephrine[1], and terbutaline[1] are reserved for refractory cases, and terbutaline is only approved for children 12 years and older.
- Inhaled corticosteroids are the most effective daily controller medications for children. Long-acting β_2-agonists, leukotriene-receptor antagonists, and mast cell stabilizers are commonly used adjunctive therapies.
- Visits should be scheduled frequently in the outpatient setting to reassess symptom severity, adjust medications accordingly, and emphasize patient education.
- Consider increasing medication therapy only after assessing the patient's adherence and technique with medications. Consider a step-down in therapy only after 3 months of adequate control of symptoms.
- Involve both children and their caregivers in designing a written asthma action plan to empower patients in recognizing and managing escalating symptoms.
- Refer to a pulmonologist or allergist if there is any question regarding diagnosis or if symptoms are not adequately controlled with standard treatment. Consultation by a pulmonologist is recommended for children aged 5 years or older at ≥step 4 of therapy (or ≥step 3 in children younger than 5 years).

[1]Not FDA approved for this indication.

Epidemiology

Asthma prevalence in the United States has been on the rise since the 1990s. It is currently estimated that 9.6% of children younger than 18 years (7.1 million children) carry the diagnosis of asthma. Male sex, African American or Puerto Rican ethnicity, and lower socioeconomic status are associated with an increased risk of developing asthma. Prevalence estimates for these groups are as high as 11% to 16%.

Although no significant difference in asthma prevalence between urban areas and suburban or rural areas has been found, there do seem to be broader geographic trends with higher prevalence in the Northeast and Midwest. Mortality rates remain low, but preventable deaths attributable to asthma exacerbations persist.

Risk Factors

No clear precipitating factors have been associated with the onset of asthma in children, but multiple risk factors for the development of this disease have been identified. Perhaps the strongest link is that between a family history of atopy, atopic dermatitis in infancy, or elevated serum immunoglobulin (Ig)E levels and subsequent sensitization to aeroallergens at 5 years of age. Recent observational data support an association with both prenatal exposure to acid-suppressive drugs and the use of antibiotics or acid-suppressive drugs in the first 6 months of life. Other identified associations include sensitization to dust mites, preterm birth, exposure to tobacco smoke, and certain respiratory infections such as respiratory syncytial virus (RSV).

Pathophysiology

Asthma is a chronic disease with recurrent episodes of reversible airway obstruction. It is thought to consist of three major pathophysiologic components: bronchoconstriction, airway inflammation, and bronchial hyperresponsiveness. Bronchoconstriction results from bronchial smooth muscle contraction in response to exposure to allergens, irritants, stress, infection, exercise, or certain medications such as aspirin and nonsteroidal antiinflammatory drugs (NSAIDs). Inflammation occurs via the T helper 2-(T_H2) and IgE-mediated pathways. Examination of the airways of asthmatics reveals inflammatory infiltrates consisting of neutrophils, eosinophils, lymphocytes, and activated mast cells. These mast cells release histamine along with other inflammatory mediators, causing airway edema, mucous hypersecretion, and airway hyperresponsiveness to environmental stimuli. Over time, remodeling can occur with airway thickening and smooth muscle hyperplasia, with a resulting decline in lung function and reduced response to therapeutic interventions.

Long-term observational studies have suggested that declining lung function is most commonly seen in children with symptom onset before 3 years of age. It still remains unclear whether older children or adults experience the same reductions in lung function.

Prevention

Primary prevention of asthma is a much-studied topic, yet few studies have successfully identified effective strategies for preventing asthma. The effect of breast-feeding on asthma prevalence has been a focus of extensive research. Much of the literature regarding breast-feeding as primary prevention for asthma suggests a protective effect of breast-feeding, but this has not been borne out consistently. A Cochrane review of 5 trials (952 pregnant or lactating mothers) found no evidence that avoidance of antigens (milk, eggs, nuts) by breast-feeding mothers during pregnancy or lactation decreased asthma or eczema in children through the study period of 18 months.

There is conflicting evidence regarding allergen avoidance to prevent the onset of asthma, although reducing exposure to inhalant allergens such as mites and pet dander can improve symptoms in patients with diagnosed asthma.

Based on the best available evidence, breast-feeding should be encouraged for its many known health benefits and potential protective effect on developing asthma. Avoidance of household dust mite aeroallergen or specific single food allergen exposure during pregnancy, breast-feeding, or first years of life is not routinely

BOX 1 | Asthma Triggers.

Allergens
- Animal dander
- Pollen
- Dust mites
- Mold

Chemical irritants
- Tobacco smoke
- Wood stove smoke
- Air pollution
- Cleaning chemicals
- Gases

Medications
- Aspirin
- Nonsteroidal antiinflammatory drugs
- β-Blockers

Other
- Gastroesophageal reflux
- Exercise
- Respiratory infection
- Extremes of emotion
- Stress
- Changes in weather
- Cold air

BOX 2 | Differential Diagnosis.

Upper Airway
Allergic rhinitis
Sinusitis

Large Airway Obstruction
Vocal cord dysfunction
Laryngotracheomalacia (infants)
Tracheal stenosis (infants)
Vascular rings
Tracheal webs
Inhaled foreign body
Tumor or enlarged lymph nodes compressing airway

Small Airway Obstruction
Viral bronchiolitis
Pneumonia
Obliterative bronchiolitis
Cystic fibrosis
Bronchopulmonary dysplasia
Heart failure

Other
Gastroesophageal reflux disease
Swallowing mechanism dysfunction leading to aspiration

From National Heart, Lung, and Blood Institute, National Asthma Education and Prevention Program. Expert Panel Report 3: Guidelines for the diagnosis and management of asthma. Summary report 2007. http://www.nhlbi.nih.gov/guidelines/asthma/asthgdln.htm. Accessed March 13, 2018.

recommended for primary prevention of asthma. The topic of primary prevention of asthma warrants further study to clearly establish feasible preventive measures.

Clinical Manifestations

Asthma is characterized by recurrent episodes of wheezing, chest tightness, and shortness of breath. Asthma can also manifest as a chronic dry cough, especially if occurring at night. Young children commonly present with chronic cough alone, a form of asthma called cough-variant asthma. Wheezing that recurs in the setting of specific, predictable triggers is also a manifestation of asthma.

Diagnosis

A focused history revealing recurrent episodes of wheezing, shortness of breath, or cough suggests asthma and merits further investigation. In infants, the symptoms of asthma can involve difficulty feeding. Parents might also report intermittent grunting or loud breathing.

When taking the history, it is important to ask about symptom triggers, time course, and frequency of symptoms to assess severity. It is also important to discuss any family history of atopy, asthma, eczema, or nasal polyps. Triggers such as exposure to inhalant allergens (mold, dust, pollen, pet dander), irritants (chemicals, cigarette smoke), weather changes, intense emotion, physical activity, and viral illnesses should be elicited specifically (Box 1).

Begin the physical examination with measurements of height and weight and inspection of the growth chart. Most children do not have a significant growth or height reduction as a result of asthma. If a child's growth chart demonstrates a marked decrease in growth velocity, it is prudent to seriously consider alternative diagnoses.

Owing to the intermittent nature of asthma symptoms, children with asthma often have an entirely normal examination. Upper airway findings can include nasal polyps or mucosal edema of nasal turbinates. The skin examination might reveal signs of atopic dermatoses such as eczema or urticaria. Lung examination may be remarkable for wheezing, hyperexpanded barrel chest, increased respiratory rate, or tachycardia, depending on severity of symptoms. The American Academy of Allergy, Asthma, and Immunology recommends spirometry as a useful means of obtaining objective data on lung function and presence of obstructive disease for the diagnosis of asthma prior to trial of medications in patients over the age of 5 years, a recommendation that is part of the Choosing Wisely campaign.

Spirometry before and after short-acting β-agonist inhalation should show reversibility of obstruction in a patient with asthma. A rise in forced expiratory volume in 1 second (FEV_1) of 200 mL and 12% above baseline after bronchodilator is consistent with reversible obstruction. In children younger than 5 years, such studies might not be feasible. In these cases, diagnosis is based on history and physical. A trial of bronchodilator is helpful in establishing the diagnosis as well as ruling out other possible etiologies of symptoms.

A common presenting symptom of asthma in children is chronic cough. In cough-variant asthma, spirometry may be entirely normal. A trial of antiasthma medication that results in resolution of cough confirms the diagnosis.

Peak flow meters are useful in monitoring symptom severity but should not be used to make a diagnosis owing to wide variations in individual results and normal values.

Chest x-ray should be considered when ruling out alternative diagnoses but is not recommended in routine diagnostic testing for asthma. Allergy skin testing can identify potentially avoidable inhalant indoor allergens and, when appropriate, guide immunotherapy. Finally, checking a complete blood count with differential and serum IgE levels is not clearly indicated in making a diagnosis but may be useful in guiding treatment. Eosinophilia (greater than 4%) can indicate the need for controller medications, and patients with high levels of IgE have been shown to have a particularly good response to inhaled corticosteroids.

Finally, fractional exhalation of nitrous oxide (FeNO) may have an emerging role in diagnosing asthma and monitoring response to treatment. A 2016 Cochrane review of nine randomized controlled trials suggested that using FeNO levels to tailor treatment may decrease exacerbations overall, including severe exacerbations requiring oral corticosteroids.

Differential Diagnosis

The differential diagnosis of recurrent respiratory symptoms is broad and must be considered when initiating diagnostic work-up. When creating a list of other diagnoses, it can be useful to consider the airway from the top down, as is shown in Box 2. Also keep in mind that the age of the patient and the chronicity of symptoms can point to certain diagnoses in your differential.

TABLE 1 Classification of Asthma Severity.

COMPONENTS OF SEVERITY	AGE (YEAR)	INTERMITTENT	PERSISTENT		
			MILD	MODERATE	SEVERE
Impairment					
Symptoms	All	≤2 days/week	>2 day/week but not daily	Daily	Throughout the day
Nighttime awakenings	0–4≥5	0≤2 times /month	1–2 times/month 3–4 times /month	3–4 times /month> 1 times /week but not nightly	>1 times /weekOften 7 times /week
SABA for symptom control	All	≤2 days/week	>2 days/week but not daily	Daily	Several times /day
Interference with normal activity	All	None	Minor limitation	Some limitation	Extremely limited
Lung Function		Normal FEV$_1$ between exacerbations			
FEV$_1$ (predicted) or PEF (personal best)	≥5	>80%	>80%	60%–80%	<60%
FEV$_1$/FVC	5–11≥12	>85%Normal	>80%Normal	75%–80%Reduced 5%	<60%Reduced >5%
Risk					
Exacerbations requiring oral corticosteroids	0–4	≤1/year	≥2 times in 6 months or ≥4 wheezing episodes/year lasting >1 day *and* risk factors for persistent asthma		
	5–11	≤1/year	≥2 times/yearfnlowast*		
	≥12	≤1/year			
Starting Treatment					
Recommended step	0–4	Step 1	Step 2	Step 3	Step 3
	5–11	Step 1	Step 2	Step 3	Step 3 or 4
	≥12	Step 1	Step 2	Step 3	Step 4 or 5
	All			Consider short course of oral corticosteroids	
	All	In 2–6 weeks, evaluate level of asthma control and adjust therapy accordingly. For children 0–4 years, if no clear benefit is observed in 4–6 weeks, stop treatment and consider alternative diagnosis or adjusting therapy			

*Consider severity and interval since last exacerbation. Frequency and severity can fluctuate over time for patients in any severity category. Relative annual risk of exacerbations may be related to FEV1.

FEV1, Forced expiratory volume in 1 second; *FVC*, forced vital capacity; *PEF*, peak expiratory flow; *SABA*, short-acting β$_2$-adrenergic receptor agonist.

From National Heart, Lung, and Blood Institute. National Asthma Education and Prevention Program Expert Panel Report 3: Guidelines for the Diagnosis and Management of Asthma. NIH Publication Number 08-5846. Washington, DC: National Heart, Lung, and Blood Institute; 2007.

Treatment

To treat asthma in children appropriately, the severity of symptoms must first be assessed. This initial evaluation should be followed by an ongoing assessment that monitors response to therapy. The general tenets of asthma treatment are to reduce the functional limitations caused by asthma symptoms and decrease the risk of exacerbations, decline in lung function, and side effects of medications. The Expert Panel Report 3 of the National Asthma Education and Prevention Program describes a patient-oriented and clinically relevant approach to asthma management. Emphasis is placed on organized primary care visits and patient education. It is important to plan routine visits with a child's pediatrician or family physician until symptoms are adequately controlled.

Once the diagnosis of asthma is made in a child, symptom severity should be assessed. To determine severity, the frequency of daytime symptoms, nighttime symptoms, frequency of using short-acting β$_2$-agonists, impairment of activities, frequency of exacerbations requiring oral steroids, and lung function must be considered (Table 1). Once severity has been classified, treatment can be started based on the stepwise approach outlined in Table 2. This stepwise approach is intended to be a guideline only. Clinical judgment is necessary when applying these guidelines to the individual patient. Children 12 years and older may be assessed and treated according to the guidelines described for adults.

Assessing adequacy of symptom control is essential to the management of asthma. At each follow-up visit, discussion should focus on how often the patient is having asthma symptoms and how much those symptoms are interfering with normal activities. Tools such as the Asthma Control Test (ACT) or the Childhood Asthma Control Test are helpful in measuring symptom control in a standardized fashion. Symptom assessment determines adequacy of control and guides changes in treatment, as shown in Tables 2 and 3. Frequency of primary care visits depends on severity of symptoms and can initially occur every 2 to 6 weeks. As control improves, visits may be decreased to every 1 to 6 months. At each visit, medications can be reviewed, doses adjusted, and education reiterated on recognizing symptoms and using medication and spacers.

Only after at least 3 months of adequate control should a decrease in therapy be considered. When stepping down, do so gradually, with frequent reassessment for reemerging symptoms. In the same way, therapy should be increased only after ensuring that the patient has been adherent with medications and is using the inhaler properly and that comorbid conditions have been addressed.

Referral to a pulmonologist or allergist is recommended if there is any question about the accuracy of diagnosis or if symptoms are difficult to control. The National Heart, Lung, and Blood Institute (NHLBI) recommends consultation if a child older than 5 years requires step 4 or higher level of therapy (step 3 or higher therapy in children younger than 5 years).

TABLE 2 Levels of Asthma Control

COMPONENTS OF CONTROL	AGE (YEAR)	WELL CONTROLLED	NOT WELL CONTROLLED	VERY POORLY CONTROLLED
Impairment				
Symptoms	0–4	≤2 day/week but ≤1 times/day	>2 day/week or multiple times on ≤2 day/week	Throughout the day
	5–11			
	≥12	≤2 day/week	>2 day/week	
Nighttime awakenings	0–4	≤1 times/month	>1 times/month	>1 times/week
	5–11	≤1 times/month	≥2 times/month	≥2 times/week
	≥12	≤2 times/month	1–3 times/week	≥4 times/week
Interference with normal activity	All	None	Some limitation	Extremely limited
SABA for symptoms	All	≤2 day/week	>2 day/week	Several times/day
Lung Function				
FEV$_1$ (predicted) or PEF (personal best)	≥5	>80%	60%–80%	<60%
FEV$_1$/FVC	5–11	<80%	75%–80%	<75%
Validated Questionnaires				
ATAQ	≥12	0	1–2	3–4
ACQ	≥12	≤0.75	≥1.5	N/A
ACT	≥12	≥20	16–19	≤15
Risk				
Exacerbations requiring oral corticosteroids	0–4	≤1 times/year	2–3 times/year	>3 times/year
	5–11	≤1 times/year	≤2 times/year	
	≥12	≤1 times/year	Consider severity and interval since last exacerbation	
Reduction in lung growth	5–11	Evaluation requires long-term follow-up care		
Loss of lung function	≥12	Evaluation requires long-term follow-up care		
Treatment-related adverse effects	All	Medication side effects can vary in intensity from none to very troublesome and worrisome		
Recommended Treatment				
Recommended treatment actions	All	Maintain current step Regular follow-up q1–6 months Consider stepping down if well controlled for ≥3 months	Step up 1 step	Step up 1–2 steps and consider short course of oral corticosteroids
			Before stepping up, review adherence to medication, inhaler technique, environmental control, comorbid conditions If an alternative treatment option was used in a step, discontinue and use the preferred treatment for that step	
			Reevaluate the level of asthma control in 2–6 weeks and adjust therapy accordingly	
			For side effects, consider alternative treatment options	

ACQ, Asthma control questionnaire; *ACT*, asthma control test; *ATAQ*, asthma therapy assessment questionnaire; *FEV1*, forced expiratory volume in 1 second; *FVC*, forced vital capacity; *ICS*, inhaled corticosteroid; *PEF*, peak expiratory flow; *SABA*, short-acting β$_2$-adrenergic receptor agonist.
From National Heart, Lung, and Blood Institute: National Asthma Education and Prevention Program Expert Panel Report 3: Guidelines for the Diagnosis and Management of Asthma. NIH Publication Number 08-5846. Washington, DC: National Heart, Lung, and Blood Institute; 2007.

Allergen avoidance is currently recommended in the management of all asthmatics, but there is limited evidence that these interventions are effective. Various studies have analyzed the effects of controlling dust mite exposure with specially designed mattress and pillow covers and the use of air filtration units to reduce the burden of airborne pet dander. None of these studies have demonstrated clear benefits in decreasing symptoms. One nonblinded, randomized controlled trial, however, did suggest that removal of mold and improved ventilation in homes affected by mold can reduce symptoms of wheezing, rhinitis, and need for asthma medications.

Yearly inactivated influenza vaccination is recommended for all children with asthma to reduce the risk of complications due to influenza, although any clinically significant benefit for asthma symptoms

TABLE 3	Stepwise Treatment of Asthma in Children Younger than 12 Years.	
STEP	**0–4 YEARS OLD**	**5–11 YEARS OLD**
Step 1: Intermittent	SABA as needed	SABA as needed
Step 2: Mild persistent	Add low-dose daily ICS or cromolyn or montelukast (Singulair)	Add low-dose daily ICS or cromolyn, LTRA, nedocromil (Tilade)* or theophylline
Step 3: Moderate persistent	Increase ICS to medium dose	Increase ICS to medium dose or continue low-dose ICS plus either LTRA, LABA, or theophylline
Step 4: Severe persistent	Medium-dose ICS plus either LABA or montelukast	Medium-dose ICS plus LABA, or medium-dose ICS plus either LTRA or theophylline
Step 5: Severe persistent	High-dose ICS plus either LABA or montelukast	High-dose ICS plus LABA, or high-dose ICS plus LTRA or theophylline
Step 6: Severe persistent	Step 5 plus oral glucocorticoids	Step 5 plus oral glucocorticoids
Step-Down Therapy	Step-Up Therapy	
If control is adequate for 3 months, may consider gradual decrease in treatment Reassess every 1–3 months	SABA use >2 times /week can indicate inadequate control Check for triggers, medication adherence, medication technique, comorbid disease before increasing therapy	

Children ≥12 years: May be treated according to adult guidelines.
Children 5–11 years: Consider subcutaneous allergen immunotherapy if the child has allergic asthma in steps 2 to 6.
All children: Treat comorbid conditions to improve asthma control.
For exacerbations that occur at all levels:
SABA 2–4 puffs every 4–6 h for 24 h with physician consultation.
Consider 3- to 10-day course of oral glucocorticoids for moderate to severe exacerbation.

*Not available in the United States.
ICS, Inhaled corticosteroid; LABA, long-acting β-agonist; LTRA, leukotriene receptor antagonist; SABA, short-acting β_2-adrenergic receptor agonist.
From National Heart, Lung, and Blood Institute: National Asthma Education and Prevention Program Expert Panel. Report 3: Guidelines for the Diagnosis and Management of Asthma. NIH Publication Number 08-5846. Washington, DC: National Heart, Lung, and Blood Institute; 2007.

TABLE 4	Usual Dosing of Rescue Medications.	
DRUG	**BRONCHOSPASM***	**ACUTE EXACERBATION†**
Albuterol	>4 years old: 2 inhalations q4–6 h prn >2 years old (min 15 kg): 0.083% nebulized soln (AccuNeb) inhaled over 5–15 min 3–4 times daily prn	4–8 inhalations q20 min × 3 doses, then q1–4 h prn; add mask in children <4 years 0.15 mg/kg (min 2.5 mg) q20min × 3 doses, then 0.15–0.3 mg/kg up to 10 mg q1–4 h prn
Levalbuterol	Age 0–4 years: 0.31–1.25 mg nebulized soln q4–6 h prn Age 5–11 years: 0.31–0.63 mg q8h prn	0.075 mg/kg (min 1.25 mg) q20min × 3 doses, then 0.075–0.15 mg/kg up to 5 mg q1–4 h prn

*Symptoms of obstruction, cough, wheeze, breathlessness.
Information from Micromedex Healthcare Series. http://www.micromedex.com.
†Symptoms of obstruction not responsive to initial SABA use.
SABA, Short-acting β_2-adrenergic receptor agonist; soln, solution.

is questionable. The live attenuated influenza vaccine (LAIV, Flu-Mist) is typically not offered to children with asthma due to limited safety data in this population, although one trial of 2229 children and adolescents with asthma demonstrated better prevention of influenza with LAIV than injectable vaccine and no differences in asthma symptoms or exacerbations. Pneumococcal vaccination is recommended for all children and, based on limited data, appears to reduce asthma exacerbations in those with asthma. Finally, management of comorbid conditions has been implicated in improving asthma control. Sinusitis, allergic rhinitis, gastroesophageal reflux disease (GERD), and obesity are thought to contribute to asthma symptoms. Research has shown, however, that treatment of GERD with lansoprazole (Prevacid) in children with poorly controlled asthma not only had no effect on asthma symptoms but also led to a significant increase in respiratory infections.

Medications

Asthma management requires both fast-acting rescue medications and long-term controller medications. The goal of therapy is to find a daily controller medicine that reduces symptoms to such a degree that rescue medications are needed only rarely. Patients and their caretakers must be educated regarding the different roles of these two classes of medication to ensure the best possible outcome and the patient's safety.

Rescue Medications

Fast-acting bronchodilators are important in both the mildest and the most-severe forms of asthma. Short-acting β_2-adrenergic receptor agonists lead to smooth muscle relaxation and airway dilation. Racemic albuterol is a commonly used member of this group, but levalbuterol is an alternative. Initially levalbuterol was thought to have fewer side effects, but studies have shown similar tolerability between racemic albuterol and levalbuterol. There is no significant difference in efficacy between these medications. Short-acting β_2-adrenergic receptor agonists should be reserved for relief of acute symptoms. Frequent use is discouraged and can indicate inadequate control of symptoms. See Table 4 for usual dosing of rescue medications.

Controller Medications

Inhaled corticosteroids are the most effective long-term controller medications. Some commonly used inhaled corticosteroids are fluticasone, budesonide, beclomethasone, mometasone, and flunisolide. No single formulation of inhaled corticosteroid is superior to another. These medications reduce frequency of exacerbations and hospitalizations and are superior to leukotriene receptor antagonists and mast cell stabilizers. They are available as both metered-dose inhalers and dry-powder inhalers. A significant concern related to their use in children, however, is their effect on bone density and growth. High- and medium-dose inhaled corticosteroids have been linked to reduced growth velocity, but several studies have shown that at low doses they do not consistently or significantly affect growth. A systematic review and meta-analysis of effects of asthma and ICS on final adult height concluded that ICS does not significantly affect final adult height. To minimize potential side effects, continuous monitoring, reevaluation, and consideration of step-down treatment is imperative.

Long-acting β-agonists include salmeterol and formoterol. They are an adjunctive therapy to inhaled corticosteroids and should be considered in step 3 of management of symptoms in children aged 5 to 11 years and in step 4 in children 0 to 4 years old. Long-acting β-agonists carry a risk of increased asthma-related deaths, intubations, and hospitalizations when used alone. This risk was most prominent in children 4 to 11 years of age. Long-acting β-agonists should never be used as monotherapy and are not recommended for use during exacerbations. In combination with inhaled corticosteroids, however, long-acting β-agonists have been shown to increase asthma control days and improve lung function, but safety data are unclear based on a systematic review in 2012. For children younger than 5 years, data are lacking.

Leukotriene-receptor antagonists, including montelukast (Singulair) and zafirlukast (Accolate), are another adjunctive therapy to inhaled corticosteroids. They reduce symptoms by blocking the inflammatory cascade initiated by mast cells. In the mildest forms of asthma, they may be used as an alternative to inhaled corticosteroids if the steroids are not well tolerated or there is difficulty with administration. They are also effective in decreasing symptoms of exercise-induced asthma.

Mast cell stabilizers such as cromolyn sodium (Intal) or nedocromil (Tilade)[2] have a role similar to that of the leukotriene-receptor antagonists. They reduce inflammation by preventing mast cells from initiating the inflammatory cascade. They are safe and well tolerated in children, but the efficacy of inhaled sodium cromoglycate (Intal) has been brought into question after a systematic review found insufficient evidence to demonstrate sodium cromoglycate's superiority over placebo. The nedocromil inhaler has been discontinued owing to difficulties with manufacturing inhaler propellant.

Immunotherapy consists of subcutaneous injections of extracts from allergens intended to desensitize a patient to specific allergic triggers. This should occur in consultation with an allergist and may be considered at steps 2 through 6 of asthma treatment in children ages 5 to 11 years if asthma symptoms are predominantly allergic.

Immunomodulators are reserved for the most refractory cases of asthma. Omalizumab (Xolair, an anti-IgE agent) functions by blocking the binding of IgE to mast cells and basophils. It is effective in children with allergic triggers for their asthma but carries a risk of anaphylaxis, and the FDA, as of 2014, has associated its use with an increase in cardiovascular and cerebrovascular events. In 2013, the National Institute for Health and Care Excellence (NICE) issued a recommendation that omalizumab be reserved for children age 6 and older who have frequent need for oral steroids (more than three courses in prior 12 months) and who have failed optimized therapy. Optimized therapy is defined as a full trial of inhaled high-dose corticosteroid, long-acting β2 agonist, leukotriene receptor antagonist, theophyllines, and oral steroids.

Early data from a randomized controlled trial suggests improved FEV_1 in children with severe symptomatic asthma with the addition of the anticholinergic drug tiotropium to an established regimen of medium- or high-dose inhaled steroids plus 1 or 2 other asthma control medications. More studies are needed to determine clinical benefit, however.

Theophylline was previously a mainstay of asthma management but is no longer a first-line medication. With the development of alternative treatments and because of theophylline's risk for toxicity, theophylline now has a lesser role in asthma management. Currently it is used as an alternative treatment in the chronic management of patients with symptoms refractory to or intolerant of standard therapies. Use of this medication requires frequent monitoring of drug serum levels. It can cause nausea, vomiting, or tachyarrhythmias if dosing is too high. See Table 5 for usual dosing of controller medications.

Acute Asthma Exacerbations

Exacerbations consist of worsening wheezing, cough, or shortness of breath. They can vary in severity from mild to life threatening. When deciding how to treat a patient in an exacerbation, use the history and physical examination to determine severity. As in all emergency situations, first assess airway, breathing, and circulation. In a life-threatening exacerbation, the patient can appear confused or obtunded, may be bradycardic, and can have minimal respiratory effort, indicating imminent respiratory arrest. A child in a severe exacerbation can appear short of breath even at rest, may be agitated, and might only be speaking one word at a time. The child is likely tachycardic and tachypneic, with obvious use of accessory muscles. In certain cases, lung examination might not reveal wheezing owing to severe impairment of aeration; only after treatment does the wheezing become audible as air movement improves. In mild to moderate exacerbations, the patient might only be short of breath with walking, might speak in short phrases or full sentences, and can appear anxious but not necessarily agitated. Lung examination can reveal wheezing.

The cornerstone of treatment of asthma exacerbations is rapid recognition of symptoms, correction of hypoxemia, and early initiation of short-acting β2-adrenergic receptor agonists and corticosteroids. Oxygen administration should be employed to maintain oxygen saturation at greater than 94%. Short-acting β-agonists are essential to relieve bronchoconstriction and may be combined with ipratropium[1], especially if the patient is not responsive to initial therapy with a short-acting β2-adrenergic receptor agonist alone. Ipratropium should not be used as single agent, as it is less efficacious than β2 agonists alone as well as combined β2 agonist–ipratropium. Combined anticholinergics and short-acting β-agonists were shown to decrease the rate of hospitalization in children when used during initial treatment for an exacerbation with a NNT of 16; however, benefit did not persist with continuing use during hospitalization. In 2006, a systematic review showed that metered-dose inhalers with a spacer are as effective in administering β-agonists as nebulizers are in children older than 2 years. It was noted in the same study that length of stay in the emergency department was reduced in those using the spacers.

Corticosteroids given systemically are also considered rescue medications, although the onset of action is 1 to 2 hours and duration of action is 18 to 36 hours. They work primarily as antiinflammatories and are an important treatment in exacerbations. Early use of systemic steroids, either oral or intravenous, reduced rates of relapse and decreased admissions to the hospital. The greatest benefit of systemic steroids was seen in patients having a severe attack and those who were not already on a course of steroids. Studies have shown that oral steroids are as effective as intravenous or intramuscular preparations. Even a short course of oral steroids can reduce relapse and decrease the need for rescue inhalers. Systemic corticosteroids should be continued for 3 to 10 days after an exacerbation. A taper is not necessary if the course is less than 1 week or less than 10 days in a patient who is also using an inhaled corticosteroid (ICS). Prolonged use of systemic corticosteroids carries significant risk for side effects such as adrenal suppression, osteoporosis, reduced growth, and

---

[2]Not available in the United States.

[1]Not FDA approved for this indication.

TABLE 5 Usual Dosing of Controller Medications

DRUG	FORMAT	DOSING
Fluticasone	HFA: 44, 110, 220 µg per puff DPI: 50, 100, 250 µg per inhalation	Low: 88–176 µg BID Medium: 176–440 µg BID High: > 440 µg BID
Fluticasone-salmeterol	DPI 100 µg/50 µg MDI 45 µg/25 µg	> 5 y: DPI 100 µg/50 µg BID MDI 90 µg/50 µg BID
Budesonide	DPI 90 or 180 µg/inhalation	Low: 90–180 µg BID Medium: 180–360 µg BID High: 540–720 µg TID-QID
Budesonide-formoterol	HFA MDI 80 µg/4.5 µg per inhalation	80 µg/4.5 µg–160 µg/ 9 µg BID
Beclomethasone HFA	40 or 80 µg per puff	Low: 80–160 µg BID Medium: 160–320 µg BID High: > 320 µg BID
Mometasone aerosol DPI	110, 220 µg per puff	110 µg daily is max per guidelines for 4–11 yR
Flunisolide HFA	80 µg per puff	5–11 y: 80–160 µg BID >12 y: 160–320 µg BID
Montelukast	4 mg or 5 mg chewable tablet 4 mg granule packets	< 5 y: 4 mg hs 6–14 y: 5 mg hs
Zafirlukast	10 mg tablet	Ages 5–11 y: 10 mg BID
Cromolyn sodium	Nebulized soln (20 mg/2 mL), MDI[2] 800 µg	> 2 y: nebulized soln: inhale 20 mg qid Age > 2: MDI: 2 puffs QID
Theophylline	Liquids, sustained-release tablets and capsules	Starting dose: 10 mg/kg/d < 1 y: max dose 0.2 × (age in weeks) + 5 = mg/kg/d ≥ 1 y: max dose 16 mg/kg/day

cap, Capsule; *DPI*, dry powder inhaler; *HFA*, hydrofluoroalkane; *MDI*, metered-dose inhaler; *soln*, solution.
[2]Not available in the United States.
Information from Lexicomp. http://online.lexi.com

cataracts, and thus their use should be minimized. Despite some evidence that use of ICS in acute exacerbations can reduce hospital admission rates, mounting data do not support treatment with increased doses of ICS (2 to 5 times maintenance dose) in children with acute asthma exacerbations, as rates of oral corticosteroid use do not appear to be reduced, yet the magnitude of increased cumulative ICS dose with this practice raises concern for potential height restriction.

Use of intravenous magnesium sulfate[1] (a smooth muscle relaxer) should be reserved for severe exacerbations only. Its use has not been shown to reduce admission rates in milder exacerbations but can improve lung function in those with only a partial response to short-acting β-agonists. Similarly, subcutaneous epinephrine[1] and subcutaneous terbutaline[1] should be reserved for emergency department settings when patients are not responding to short-acting β2-adrenergic receptor agonists, anticholinergics, or corticosteroids, or when air entry is so diminished that inhaled medications are not effective.

Finally, not enough evidence exists to make a recommendation regarding routine use of antibiotics during an acute asthma exacerbation. In some circumstances, when there are findings consistent with bacterial infections (such as consolidation on chest x-ray), their use may be warranted. See Table 6 for usual dosing of medications used in acute exacerbations.

Monitoring

Asthma is a dynamic disease whose symptoms fluctuate based on a number of variables. Routine scheduled appointments with a pediatrician or family physician are essential to monitor symptoms and adjust therapy. Initial management can require visits every 2 to 6 weeks; as control of symptoms improves, the interval may be increased to every 3 to 6 months.

Patient education is essential to successfully controlling this disease. Education should be focused on the theory behind controller and rescue medications, the importance of

TABLE 6 Usual Dosing of Medications Used in Exacerbations

DRUG	DOSING
Chronic Management	
Corticosteroids (methylprednisolone, prednisolone, prednisone)	0.25–2 mg/kg daily or every other day
Acute Exacerbation	
Ipratropium bromide[1]	Age 0–5 years: 250 µg nebulized × 2, then q4h prn Age 5–11: 500 µg nebulized × 2, then q4h prn
Corticosteroids (methylprednisolone, prednisolone, prednisone)	1–2 mg/kg/day (max 60 mg/day) in 2 divided doses × 3–10 days
Severe Acute Exacerbation	
Not Responding to SABAs	
Magnesium sulfate[1]	25–50 mg/kg IV up to 2 g over 10–20 min
Terbutaline[1]	0.01 mg/kg SC q20min for 3 doses, then every 2–6 hr prn
Epinephrine[1]	0.01 mg/kg up to 0.3–0.5 mg SC q20min for 3 doses
Related to Allergic Reaction	
Epinephrine	1:1000: 0.01 mL/kg SC (max 0.3 mL)

[1]Not FDA approved for this indication.
SABA = Short-acting β2-adrenergic receptor agonist.

medication compliance, and how to administer these medications properly. Newer trial data support improved inhaler adherence with the use of electronic reminders such as mobile phone alarms. The National Asthma Education and Prevention Program Expert Panel 3 emphasizes the importance of asthma action plans to empower patients in recognizing and treating escalating symptoms of asthma. Action plans also provide recommendations on reducing exposure to irritants, allergens, and triggers. Some plans are based on peak flow levels, but studies show that symptom-based written action plans are better at decreasing acute care visits. Examples of asthma action plans can be found on the National Heart, Lung, and Blood Institute website.

Complications

The most worrisome complications of asthma include reduced lung function, pneumonia, pneumothorax, and death. More common complications include chronic cough, fatigue due to poor sleep, missed school days and worse academic performance, and limited ability to participate in sports.

References

Brightling CE, Bradding P, Symon FA, et al: Mast-cell infiltration of airway smooth muscle in asthma, *N Engl J Med* 346:1699–1705, 2002.

British Thoracic Society/Scottish Intercollegiate Guidelines Network (BTS/SIGN): *Guideline on the management of asthma Guideline.* Available at http://www.brit-thoracic.org.uk/document-library/clinical-information/asthma/btssign-asthma-guideline-2016. [Accessed 11 March 2018], 2016.

Burr ML, Matthew IP, Arthur RA, et al: Effects on patients with asthma of eradicating visible indoor mould: a randomised controlled trial, *Thorax* 62:767–772, 2007.

Cates CJ, Jefferson T, Rowe BH: Vaccines for preventing influenza in people with asthma, *Cochrane Database Syst Rev*(2), 2008.

Centers for Disease Control and Prevention (CDC): Vital signs: Asthma prevalence, disease characteristics, and self-management education: United States, 2001–2009, *MMWR Morb Mortal Wkly Rep* 60(17):547–552, 2011. Available at: http://www.ncbi.nlm.nih.gov/pubmed/21544044. [Accessed 12 March 2018].

Chen LH, Chen SS, Liang L, Li CC: Effects of asthma and inhaled corticosteroids in children on the final adult height: a systemic review and meta-analysis, *Zhongguo Dang Dai Er Ke Za Zhi* 17(11):1242–1247, 2015.

Courtney U, McCarter D, Pollart S: Childhood asthma: Treatment update, *Am Fam Physician* 71:1959–1968, 2005.

Dicpinigaitis PV: Chronic cough due to asthma: ACCP evidence-based clinical practice guidelines, *Chest* 129:75S–79S, 2006.

Elward K, Pollart S: Medical therapy for asthma: Updates from the NAEPP guidelines, *Am Fam Physician* 82(10):1242–1251, 2010.

Fleming DM, Crovari P, Wahn U, et al: Comparison of the efficacy and safety of live attenuated cold-adapted influenza vaccine, trivalent, with trivalent inactivated influenza virus vaccine in children and adolescents with asthma, *Pediatr Infect Dis J* 25(10):860–869, 2006.

Global Initiative for Asthma (GINA): GINA Report, Global Strategy for Asthma Management and Prevention. Available at: http://ginasthma.org/gina-reports, 2017. [Accessed 11 March 2018].

Holbrook JT, Wise RA, Gold BD: Lansoprazole for children with poorly controlled asthma: a randomized controlled trial, *JAMA* 307(4):373–381, 2012.

Irazuzta JE, Chiriboga N: Magnesium sulfate infusion for acute asthma in the emergency department, *J Pediatr (Rio J)* 93, 2017.

Jackson DJ, Bacharier LB, Mauger DT, et al: Quintupling inhaled glucocorticoids to prevent childhood asthma exacerbations, *N Engl J Med* 378:891–901, 2018.

Kramer MS, Kakuma R: Maternal dietary antigen avoidance during pregnancy or lactation, or both, for preventing or treating atopic disease in the child, *Cochrane Database Syst Rev* (3), CD000133.

Lai T, Wu M, Liu J, et al: Acid-suppressing drug use during pregnancy and the risk of childhood asthma: a meta-analysis, *Pediatrics* 141(2), 2018. e 20170889.

Lemanske RF, Mauger DT, Sorkness CA, Jackson DJ: Step up therapy for children with uncontrolled asthma receiving inhaled corticosteroids, *N Engl J Med* 362(11):975–985, 2010.

Maas T, Kaper J, Sheikh A, et al: Mono and multifaceted inhalant and/or food allergen reduction interventions for preventing asthma in children at high risk of developing asthma, *Cochrane Database Syst Rev* (3), CD006480.

McCowan C, Neville R, Thomas G, et al: Effect of asthma and its treatment on growth: four year follow up of cohort of children from general practices in Tayside, Scotland, *BMJ* 316(7132):668–672, 1998.

McIvor RA, Kaplan A, Koch C: Montelukast as an alternative to low dose inhaled corticosteroids in the management of mild asthma(the SIMPLE trial): an open label effectiveness trial, *Can Respir J* 16:11A–21A, 2009.

Mitre E, Susi A, Kroop LE, et al: Association between use of acid-suppressive medications and antibiotics during infancy and allergic diseases in early childhood, *JAMA Pediatr* 172(6):e180315, 2018.

Morton RW, Elphick HE, Rigby AS, et al: STAAR: a randomised controlled trial of electronic adherence monitoring with reminder alarms and feedback to improve clinical outcomes for children with asthma, *Thorax* 72(4):347–354, 2017.

National Asthma Education and Prevention Program, National Heart, Lung, and Blood Institute (NHLBI). Expert panel report 3: guidelines for the diagnosis and management of asthma. NHLBI website. Available at: https://www.nhlbi.nih.gov/files/docs/guidelines/asthgdln.pdf. [Accessed March 11, 2018].

National Heart Lung, Blood Institute: Asthma action plan. Available at http://www.nhlbi.nih.gov/health/public/lung/asthma/asthma_actplan.pdf. [Accessed 13 March 2018].

Petsky HL, Kew KM, Chang AB: Exhaled nitric oxide levels to guide treatment for children with asthma, *Cochrane database Syst Rev* 11:CD011439, 2016.

Pollart S, Compton R, Elward K: Management of acute asthma exacerbations, *Am Fam Physician* 84:40–47, 2011.

Pollart S, Elward K: Overview of changes to asthma guidelines: Diagnosis and screening, *Am Fam Physician* 79:761–767, 2009.

Prevention strategies for asthma—primary prevention, *CMAJ* 173(Suppl. 6):S20–S24, 2005.

Sheik A, Alves B, Dhami S. *Pneumococcal vaccine for asthma (Cochrane Review).* The Cochrane Library Issue 2. Ed. Chichester, UK, 2009, John Wiley and Sons, Ltd.

Sokol KC, Sharma G, Lin Y-L, Goldblum RM: Choosing wisely: adherence by physicians to recommended use of spirometry in the diagnosis and management of adult asthma, *Am J Med* 128(5):502–508, 2015.

Toelle B, Ng K: Eight year outcomes of the Childhood Asthma Prevention Study, *J Allergy Clin Immunol* 126:388–389, 2010.

ATTENTION-DEFICIT/HYPERACTIVITY DISORDER

Method of
Scott E. Moser, MD

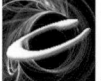

CURRENT DIAGNOSIS

- Diagnosis is clinical and based on DSM-5 criteria for inattentive symptoms, hyperactive/impulsive symptoms, or combined symptoms with onset of some symptoms by age 12 years.
- For the inattentive presentation, symptoms must include six of the following nine (five of nine if age >17 years): fails to give attention to details, has difficulty sustaining attention, does not seem to listen, does not follow through, has difficulty organizing, avoids mental effort, loses things, is easily distracted, and is forgetful in daily activities.
- For hyperactive/impulsive presentation, six of the following nine must be documented (five of nine for age >17 years): fidgets, leaves seat, runs about or climbs excessively, has difficulty playing quietly, is "on the go/driven by a motor," talks excessively, blurts answers before the end of questions, has difficulty awaiting turn/waiting in line, interrupts/intrudes on others.
- Clinical diagnosis should incorporate the use of standardized questionnaires and must account for potential comorbid psychological or learning problems.

CURRENT THERAPY

- For all patients older than age 6 years, stimulants are the primary treatment unless contraindicated.
- Important second-line or adjunctive medications include atomoxetine (Strattera), guanfacine (Intuniv), clonidine (Kapvay), venlafaxine (Effexor),[1] and bupropion (Wellbutrin).[1]
- Behavioral therapies are important adjuncts to medication for best outcomes.

---

[1] Not FDA approved for this indication.

Epidemiology/Pathophysiology

Attention-deficit/hyperactivity disorder (ADHD) is one of the most commonly diagnosed conditions in childhood, affecting at least 5% of school-aged children. It is more commonly diagnosed in boys than girls at a 2:1 ratio, a difference that may be exaggerated by bias inherent in the standardized questionnaires used to detect ADHD.

Risk Factors

DSM-5 categorizes ADHD among the neurodevelopmental disorders based on its heritability of about 75%, chromosomal pattern evidence, and brain metabolism studies in the control centers for attention (prefrontal cortex) and motor activity (temporal lobe). In addition to genetic factors, several environmental factors have been associated: maternal smoking or alcohol use, pregnancy/delivery complications, psychosocial adversity, and exposure to environmental toxins including polychlorinated biphenyls (PCBs) and pesticides. Food additives and television viewing have been studied without consistent evidence that they contribute.

Clinical Manifestations and Diagnosis

ADHD is a clinical diagnosis based on the criteria described in *Diagnostic and Statistical Manual of Mental Disorders,* 5th Edition (DSM-5). Despite growing evidence for characteristic findings in chromosomal and brain metabolism studies, there are no genetic, biochemical, or imaging tests validated for clinical use in making the diagnosis. Thus a clinician considering the diagnosis should review the explicit DSM-5 criteria.

DSM-5 recognizes three presentations: predominantly inattentive, predominantly hyperactive/impulsive, and a combined presentation. The use of the word *presentation* in DSM-5 is a change from the use of the word *type* in DSM-4, recognizing that the predominant symptoms can change modestly over time. ADHD begins in childhood, so to make the diagnosis after age 12, evidence must be found for significant symptoms before that age. At any age, the symptoms must be present in at least two different settings (home, school, work, etc.) and clearly interfere with social, academic, or occupational functioning. The symptoms cannot be better explained by another mental disorder (e.g., mood disorder, anxiety disorder, substance abuse).

To meet criteria for the inattentive presentation, the patient must exhibit age-inappropriate levels of at least six of the following nine symptoms: (1) fails to give attention to details or makes careless mistakes, (2) has difficulty sustaining attention, (3) does not seem to listen when addressed, (4) does not follow through on instructions/fails to finish schoolwork or chores, (5) has difficulty organizing tasks/activities, (6) avoids/refuses to engage in tasks that require sustained mental effort, (7) loses items necessary for tasks or activities, (8) is easily distracted by extraneous stimuli, and (9) is forgetful in daily activities/routines.

To meet criteria for the hyperactive/impulsive presentation, the patient must exhibit age-inappropriate levels of at least six of the following nine symptoms: (1) often fidgets or squirms in seat, (2) leaves seat inappropriately, (3) runs or climbs excessively, (4) is unable to play quietly, (5) is "on the go" or "driven by a motor," (6) talks excessively, (7) blurts out answers before a question is completed, (8) has difficulty waiting turns, and (9) interrupts or intrudes on others.

The combined presentation requires meeting criteria for both the inattentive and hyperactive/impulsive presentations.

Patients aged 17 years and older need to meet only five of the nine criteria in a presentation category. DSM-5 includes examples of adult equivalents of the criteria. For example, inattention criterion (6) reads, "Often avoids, dislikes, or is reluctant to engage in tasks that require sustained mental effort (e.g., schoolwork or homework; for older adolescents and adults, preparing reports, completing forms, reviewing lengthy papers)." Several of the symptoms must have been present before 12 years of age. For most patients, the hyperactivity improves by adolescence, but patients continue to have challenges with inattention and impulsivity as adults unless adequately treated.

The diagnosis of ADHD requires that the patient manifest symptoms in multiple environments, so it is important to obtain information from parents and teachers and as many other observers as is realistic. The use of standardized questionnaires simplifies and systematizes the collection of this information, so their use should be a routine part of the diagnostic process. Each of the commercially available questionnaires has advantages and disadvantages such that clinicians should cooperate with local school and mental health partners regarding which forms to use. Commonly used scales include the Conners, Vanderbilt, Achenbach, and others. In addition to supporting the diagnosis of ADHD, these scales can give clues to comorbid conditions and alternative diagnoses. Also, the scales can be used to monitor treatment response.

When gathering the history, it is important to obtain specific examples of behaviors rather than general labels. For example, "doesn't pay attention" could mean "spends the day staring out the window" or "slumps in his chair and doesn't respond to questions for several minutes." Because there are no specific diagnostic tests for ADHD, ordering laboratory studies and imaging is individualized based on the clinician's suspicion of comorbid or alternative diagnoses as described later.

Making the diagnosis of ADHD is more complicated in adults than in children for several reasons, including the challenges of recall bias by patients, difficulty obtaining information from other observers, less well-validated symptom questionnaires, and potential drug seeking for stimulants. Therefore clinicians should be wary and consider consultation with an experienced mental health colleague in these cases.

Careful evaluation that includes documentation of meeting DSM-5 criteria for ADHD prior to initiating treatment is important for both patients and clinicians. Studies have demonstrated that a lack of adequate documentation by physicians is common. Because the main treatment for ADHD includes use of Drug Enforcement Agency (DEA) Schedule II agents, the stimulants, the clinician is wise to perform a careful evaluation and document findings well.

Differential Diagnosis

Comorbid learning disorders occur in as many as one-third of patients with ADHD, and comorbid oppositional defiant disorder and conduct disorder are also exceedingly common. Thus comorbidity is the rule rather than the exception, implying that when considering the differential diagnosis, clinicians must answer not only, "Could this be ADHD *or* something else?" They must also consider, "Could this be ADHD *and* something else?"

In addition to the potential comorbidities noted, other common and/or important psychological conditions that share manifestations with ADHD or may be comorbid with ADHD include bipolar disorder, depression, anxiety, intellectual disability, and autism spectrum disorder. In adolescents and adults, substance use disorders are also common.

A large number of medical and neurologic conditions share some manifestations with ADHD, including absence seizure disorder, tics, hearing problems, sleep disorders, lead intoxication, allergies, and side effects of medications, particularly those used to treat asthma or allergies. A history of physical or sexual abuse is common. Children who live in a chaotic home environment or attend an unstructured school can exhibit ADHD-like symptoms or have their symptoms of ADHD exacerbated. Parental psychopathology or chemical dependency may complicate symptomatology. Therefore a careful social, developmental, and medical history and physical examination are important to making the diagnosis with individualized testing on the basis of the clinical suspicion of alternative or comorbid conditions. In cases where the clinician suspects complex or comorbid conditions, referral for neuropsychological assessment should be considered.

Treatment

For uncomplicated ADHD, careful medication management, in collaboration with parents and school, and parent education is the core of treatment. Psychosocial interventions are essential for those with comorbidities or if medication management is of limited benefit. This evidence comes primarily from studies of school-aged children. Because of concerns about accurate diagnosis in children younger than 6 years old and less evidence of stimulant efficacy in younger children, guidelines encourage great caution in starting medications before age 6, relying primarily on behavioral therapy in younger children. As soon as ADHD is diagnosed, the clinician should point patients and families to reliable sources of education about the disorder, especially because so much misinformation is circulating among the public (Box 1). Regardless of the treatment plan, it is important to establish communication links between physician, family, school, and mental health partners to address the myriad of complications and consequences that often develop. Because ADHD has a high rate of inheritance, parents of affected children often also have the disorder. The clinician should remain vigilant for ways this can complicate management, including treatment nonadherence, parental denial, or inconsistency with behavioral interventions. Therefore establishment of a medical home and a chronic disease management approach are especially important in the context of parents who have ADHD themselves. Treatment in adolescents and adults is similar to that in children with exceptions noted in the text later and in Table 1, which includes the medications with current Food and Drug Administration (FDA) approval for treatment of ADHD and several that are not approved but are in common use. In general, clinicians should not exceed FDA maximum doses because this practice increases the risk of side effects with little evidence of improved efficacy.

Stimulants

The psychostimulants are first-line treatment for all presentations of ADHD at all ages, age 6 years and older. Their mechanism of action is thought to be primarily caused by inhibition of reuptake of dopamine and norepinephrine in the prefrontal cortex, a key to regulating attention, behavior, and emotion. Children with ADHD who take stimulants have longer attention spans, are less impulsive and distractible, perform better in school, and have better relationships with family and peers than those who do not.

All the stimulants are DEA Schedule II agents because of their abuse potential, which makes prescribing more challenging than nonstimulant alternatives. Despite this, the stimulants remain the medications of first choice because of their strong record of efficacy and safety. The stimulants are grouped into two major categories: methylphenidate and the amphetamines. Both categories of stimulants are available in a variety of dosing options including short-acting, long-acting, and very long-acting preparations (see Table 1). Standard methylphenidate and dextroamphetamine maintain therapeutic levels for only 3 to 4 hours, necessitating multiple doses throughout the day. Therefore the longer-acting preparations have become much more popular. Many of the longer-acting drug choices achieve their prolonged effect because of technological modifications of their surface coating, resulting in slow intestinal release of the active medication. Thus it is important that patients avoid breaking or chewing these pills. For children who have difficulty swallowing pills, several long-acting preparations are now available as suspensions, chewable tablets, or as encapsulated beads or powders that can be emptied into applesauce or other soft food, as noted on Table 1.

The effectiveness of stimulants is great enough that if the initial trial of a stimulant is not effective or is poorly tolerated, evidence-based guidelines generally encourage the trial of a stimulant from the other category before resorting to a nonstimulant. When converting from one class of stimulant to another, 1 mg of amphetamine is roughly equivalent to 2 mg of methylphenidate. At present, pharmacogenetic tools are not able to reliably predict response to category, dose, or timing of stimulants, so their use is not recommended.

Common side effects of stimulants include loss of appetite, abdominal pain, headache, irritability, and weight loss. These side effects are often transient and can be minimized by using a low starting dose and increasing the dosage gradually. Stimulants can exacerbate tics or seizure disorders. A rare but serious side effect is sudden cardiac death. The risk is so rare and unpredictable that current guidelines do not recommend routine electrocardiographic or other screening tests before initiating therapy. However, it is prudent to carefully assess cardiac risk factors prior to initiating treatment.

Apart from the kinetics of short-acting versus longer-acting options and the various routes of administration (e.g., pills, suspensions, transdermal patches), two stimulants have specific niches. Dexmethylphenidate is the active isomer of methylphenidate. Theoretically, this may improve the side effect profile, although clinical evidence for this is lacking. Because it is the active isomer, the therapeutic conversion is 1 mg of dexmethylphenidate approximates 2 mg of methylphenidate. Lisdexamfetamine (Vyvanse) is a prodrug of dextroamphetamine. It was developed to reduce the risk of abuse, but the DEA has maintained its Schedule II designation.

Parents are often concerned about whether the use of a DEA-controlled substance might increase the risk of their child developing a substance use disorder as they mature. Current evidence is reassuring in this regard in that appropriate treatment with stimulants likely decreases that risk.

Stimulants are also first-line treatment for ADHD in adults, though the evidence from controlled studies is not as strong as with children. As indicated in Table 1, for women who clearly benefit from treatment with stimulants and who are pregnant or could become pregnant, methylphenidate is considered the safest choice.

Nonstimulants

All nonstimulants are second-line agents or adjuncts to stimulant treatment. An important agent in this class is atomoxetine (Strattera). It should be titrated up over days to weeks and may require 4 weeks to see the full benefit. Usually, once-daily dosing is effective, but genetically fast metabolizers may require multiple daily doses. Common side effects include loss of appetite, headache, and drowsiness. One benefit of atomoxetine is that it is not a DEA-scheduled agent, so it is more convenient to prescribe than a stimulant. Also, it does not exacerbate tics. A downside to atomoxetine is that it carries a black-box warning of increased risk of suicidality, especially during the first months of treatment. A rare

---

BOX 1	Patient and Parental Resources for the Management of Attention-Deficit/Hyperactivity Disorder

1. www.chadd.org/Resources from the national support group for children and adults with ADHD.
2. www.add.org/Resources from the ADD Association, a national ADHD adult support group.
3. www.nimh.nih.gov/health/topics/attention-deficit-hyperactivity-disorder-adhd/index.shtml Information on ADHD from the National Institutes of Mental Health, including a link to current ADHD clinical trials.
4. *Taking Charge of ADHD, Fourth Edition: The Complete, Authoritative Guide for Parents* by Russell A. Barkley (2020). Book recommending environmental changes to structure the schedule and behavior of children with ADHD.
5. *Smart but Scattered: The Revolutionary Executive Skills Approach to Helping Kids Reach Their Potential,* by Peg Dawson and Richard Guare (2009). Book recommending routines and study skills to maximize functioning in children with ADHD.

TABLE 1   Common ADHD Medications

CATEGORY	GENERIC NAME	SELECTED BRAND NAME EXAMPLES	ONSET	THERAPEUTIC EFFECT	PREGNANCY RISK	COMMENTS
Stimulants						
	Methylphenidate				No known teratogenicity based on animal data	Variety of dosing options as noted
	Short-acting	Ritalin	20 min	3–4 h		Requires multiple doses to last through school day
	Long-acting	Metadate CD	30 min	8 h		Single dose to last through school day but may require afternoon boost for homework; capsule contents may be sprinkled on food
		Quillivant XR	20 min	8–10 h		Liquid suspension
		QuilliChew ER	30 min	8 h		Chewable tablet
	Very long-acting	Concerta	1–2 h	12–14 h		Single dose to last entire day but more likely to interfere with sleep
		Daytrana patch	2–4 h	>20 h		Must be removed before bedtime
	Delayed release	Jornay PM	8 h	24 h		Dose in the evening
	Dexmethylphenidate	Focalin	20 min	3–4 h	Caution in pregnancy because of inadequate data to assess risk	Bioactive isomer may reduce side effects
		Focalin XR	20 min	8 h		Capsule contents may be sprinkled on food
	Amphetamine/ dextroamphetamine				Avoid in pregnancy because of risk of teratogenicity and neonatal complications including premature delivery	
		Adderall	20 min	6 h		
		Adderall XR	30–60 min	12 h		Capsule contents may be sprinkled on food
	d- and l-Amphetamine				Avoid in pregnancy because of risk of teratogenicity and neonatal complications including premature delivery	
	Long-acting	Adzenys ER, Dyanavel XR	20–30 min	12 h		Liquid suspension
		Adzenys XR-ODT, Evekeo ODT	20 min	10–12 h		Tablet dissolves in the mouth
	Very long-acting	Mydayis		12–16 h		ER capsule
	Dextroamphetamine				Avoid in pregnancy because of risk of teratogenicity and neonatal complications including premature delivery	
	Short-acting	(generic)	20 min	3–4 h		Requires multiple doses to last through school day

Continued

TABLE 1	Common ADHD Medications—cont'd					
CATEGORY	GENERIC NAME	SELECTED BRAND NAME EXAMPLES	ONSET	THERAPEUTIC EFFECT	PREGNANCY RISK	COMMENTS
		ProCentra	20 min	4–6 h		Oral suspension
	Long-acting	Dexedrine Spansule		6–8 h		
	Lisdexamfetamine	Vyvanse	30 min	10–12 h	No human data but avoid in pregnancy based on limited human data with amphetamines	Prodrug with theoretically less abuse potential; capsule contents may be sprinkled on food
Nonstimulants						
	Atomoxetine	Strattera	1 h	>10 h	Caution in pregnancy; inadequate human data to assess risk; no known harm	Usually once daily dosing; fast metabolizers may need twice daily dosing
	Clonidine, extended release	Kapvay	30–60 min	10–16 h	Caution in pregnancy; risk of low birth weight; risk of fetal death from animal data	Dose at bedtime
	Guanfacine, extended release	Intuniv	30–60 min	16–24 h	Caution in pregnancy; no known risk of fetal harm	Dose at bedtime
	Viloxazine	Qelbree			Avoid in pregnancy; inadequate human data to determine risk	Capsule may be opened but contents should not be crushed or chewed
	Venlafaxine[1]	Effexor			Caution in pregnancy especially in third trimester because of potential withdrawal or serotonin syndrome	
	Bupropion[1]	Wellbutrin (immediate release, 12 h extended release, 24 h extended release)			Caution in pregnancy; risk of congenital heart defects inconclusive	Extended-release forms not approved for children <12 years old

[1]Not FDA approved for this indication.

but serious potential side effect is hepatotoxicity. Atomoxetine should be considered first-line therapy in patients with a comorbid tic disorder, significant anxiety disorder, or recent substance abuse.

Clonidine (Kapvay) and guanfacine (Intuniv) are alpha-adrenergic agonists that are helpful adjuncts to treating hyperactivity or aggression that does not adequately respond to a stimulant alone. Because a side effect is drowsiness, nighttime dosing can actually improve sleep. Use of extended-release formulations allows for single daily dosing. Patients should be monitored for development of hypotension or bradycardia. Because of the risk of rebound hypertension, these agents should be tapered slowly rather than stopped abruptly.

In controlled trials, the serotonin-norepinephrine reuptake inhibitors (SNRIs) have demonstrated effectiveness for ADHD. Viloxazine (Qelbree), marketed in Europe for many years as an antidepressant, received FDA approval for ADHD in 2021. Venlafaxine (Effexor)[1] is commonly used for ADHD but does not have FDA approval for this indication. SNRIs are particularly useful adjuncts in patients with significant mood instability, common in adolescents. Prescribers should use caution because of the black-box warning regarding potential increased suicide risk.

Bupropion (Wellbutrin)[1] has been shown to be somewhat effective in treating ADHD, and its value is similar to that of the SNRIs as adjuncts in special situations. Like the SNRIs, it has a black-box warning regarding increased suicidality risk.

Several tricyclic antidepressants have demonstrated efficacy for ADHD in controlled trials, but their use is limited because of side effects and lack of FDA approval. Selective serotonin reuptake inhibitors (SSRIs) have not demonstrated effectiveness for ADHD and should only be considered for comorbid mood disorders. Other mood stabilizers and atypical antipsychotics should generally be reserved for use by specialists.

Behavior Therapy and Educational Interventions

For younger children, the emphasis is on behavior training for parents and teachers. All parents should receive instruction in common behavioral mistakes, such as overreliance on

[1]Not FDA approved for this indication.

negative rather than positive reinforcement, and delay in dispensing rewards. Most parents benefit from specific training in parenting techniques or support groups. As children enter adolescence and beyond, cognitive behavior therapies, group therapy with peers, and individual coaching approaches show the most promise. Educational placement and classroom interventions are also important. The diagnosis of ADHD, at the very least, deserves consideration for special classroom accommodations under federal law for this chronic handicapping condition. If the child is still failing in spite of these accommodations, consideration should be given for special education placement. Patients of all ages may benefit from counseling regarding adequate physical activity and good sleep hygiene.

Monitoring

Once satisfactory response to treatment is established, children on stimulants should continue to be seen at least every 6 months for height and weight checks to be sure they are continuing to grow normally and for blood pressure and pulse checks, watching for onset of hypertension or tachycardia. Guidelines typically recommend annual consideration of a medication holiday to evaluate the need for continued treatment. Children typically require gradually increasing doses during the school years, then some tapering of the dose in late adolescence. Regardless of treatment, patients with ADHD may benefit from ongoing monitoring because they remain at increased risk for injuries, suicide, psychiatric comorbidity (especially substance use disorders), lower educational achievement, incarceration, and interpersonal difficulties.

Management of Complications

Children with suspected comorbid psychiatric conditions and those who do not respond to initial treatment should be referred to a specialist.

References

AACAP: Practice parameter for the assessment and treatment of children and adolescents with attention-deficit/hyperactivity disorder, *J Am Acad Child Adolesc Psychiatry* 46(7):894–921, 2007.

American Psychiatric Association: *Diagnostic and statistical manual of mental disorders*, 5 ed, American Psychiatric Association, 2013.

Biederman J, Wilens T, Mick E, Spencer T, Faraone S: Pharmacotherapy of attention-deficit/hyperactivity disorder reduces risk for substance use disorder, *Pediatrics* 104(2):1–5, 1999.

Fabiano GA, Pelham Jr WE, Coles EK, et al: A meta-analysis of behavioral treatments for attention-deficit/hyperactivity disorder, *Clin Psychol Rev* 29:129–140, 2009.

Gould MS, Walsh BT, Munfakh JL, et al: Sudden death and use of stimulant medications in youth, *Am J Psychiatry* 166:992–1001, 2009.

MTA Cooperative Group: A 14-month randomized clinical trial of treatment strategies for attention-deficit/hyperactivity disorder. Multimodal Treatment Study of Children with ADHD, *Arch Gen Psychiatry* 56:1073–1086, 1999.

Wolraich ML, Hagan JF, Allan C, et al: AAP subcommittee on children and adolescents with attention-deficit/hyperactivity disorder. Clinical practice guideline for the diagnosis, evaluation, and treatment of attention-deficit/hyperactivity disorder in children and adolescents, *Pediatrics* 144(4):e20192528 2019.

BRONCHIOLITIS

Method of
Tamara Wagner, MD

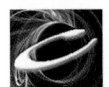

CURRENT DIAGNOSIS

- Clinical diagnosis most commonly associated with respiratory distress in a child less than 2 years of age.
- Symptoms include nasal congestion or rhinorrhea associated with findings of lower respiratory tract involvement, most notably elevated respiratory rate, wheezing, or crackles.
- Diagnostic testing in the form of chest x-ray or viral testing is not recommended.

CURRENT THERAPY

- Standard treatment is supportive care, including clearance of nasal passages, oxygen for saturation less than 90%, fluids for dehydration, and early nutritional support.
- There is no indication for corticosteroids (inhaled or systemic), albuterol, racemic epinephrine, or decongestant drops.
- Nebulized hypertonic saline has recently become a treatment option but clear benefit has not been established.
- Humidified high-flow nasal cannula (HHFNC) oxygen therapy, a new method of respiratory support, is used frequently in patients with increased work of breathing. Systemic reviews support HFNC as safe and well tolerated, but evidence is lacking to show superiority to standard oxygen therapy.

Background

Clinical bronchiolitis remains one of the most significant diseases within the pediatric population. Bronchiolitis is caused by a viral infection, most often the respiratory syncytial virus (RSV). Bronchiolitis as a clinical disease has a long history of applied medical therapies, which initially showed some promise in small studies and then were abandoned later, when larger studies failed to demonstrate benefit. There remains a high variation in care for patients, which persists despite the development of standardized guidelines. Bronchiolitis is a self-limited disease with a good prognosis; recent care guidelines support elimination of therapies without proven benefit.

Epidemiology and Virology

Bronchiolitis follows a seasonal epidemic most closely tied to the spread of the RSV virus. Within the United States the incidence of RSV peaks between November and April with regional variation. Approximately 800,000 children in the United States will require outpatient medical management during the first year of life due to bronchiolitis and approximately 100,000 hospitalizations will occur annually. RSV is the most commonly isolated viral pathogen in patients with bronchiolitis. RSV accounts for 50% to 80% of the all hospitalizations for bronchiolitis. Other viruses associated with bronchiolitis include human rhinovirus, parainfluenza virus, human meta-pneumovirus, coronavirus, adenovirus, influenza virus, and enterovirus.

Risk Factors

The most significant risk factor for bronchiolitis is age. Up to 90% of children will become infected with RSV before the age of 2 and nearly half of those children will experience bronchiolitis. Infants younger than 3 months and those with a history of prematurity have a higher risk of severe bronchiolitis and the complication of apnea. Other risk factors for a severe course include congenital heart disease, chronic lung disease, and patients with poor immune function. Recent studies have demonstrated that environmental factors such as cigarette smoke exposure or air pollution may increase risk for bronchiolitis.

Pathophysiology

The pathophysiology of bronchiolitis is due to the progressive obstruction of the distal airways due to mucous production, airway edema, and direct cellular injury of the bronchiolar epithelium. Following viral infection, increased mucous production, airway edema, and impaired ciliary function result in varying degrees of intraluminal obstruction. This obstruction during the positive pressure phase of expiration may cause an audible wheeze. As the disease progresses further, virus-induced injury to the bronchiolar lining leads to sloughed cells and distortion of the alveolar structure, resulting in air trapping and atelectasis. With the progression of lung atelectasis, mismatching of ventilation and perfusion occur, resulting in increased work of breathing and hypoxemia.

TABLE 1	Guidelines for Use of Palivizumab
DISEASE CONDITION	**PALIVIZUMAB (SYNAGIS) PROPHYLAXIS**
Prematurity	Recommended routinely in first year of life for infants born <29 weeks or <32 weeks with chronic lung disease defined as oxygen therapy for at least 28 days after birth Recommended within second year of life for children with chronic lung disease who continue to require supplemental oxygen, diuretic therapy, or chronic corticosteroid therapy
Congenital heart disease	May be considered in first year of life for infants with hemodynamically significant heart disease
Congenital pulmonary abnormality	May be considered in first year of life for infants with impaired lung physiology
Neuromuscular disease	May be considered in first year of life for infants with impaired ability to clear secretions
Immunodeficiency	May be considered in first 2 years of life for patients with profound immunosuppression

Prevention

Breastfeeding infants (whether exclusive or partial) have demonstrated benefit of breastfeeding in prevention of hospitalization due to bronchiolitis. Additionally, infants receiving breast milk who are hospitalized with bronchiolitis have shorter hospital admissions.

Palivizumab (Synagis) is a human-derived immunoglobulin G monoclonal antibody directed against RSV. Use of Synagis has been shown to reduce the rate of hospitalization in premature infants. In 2014 the American Academy of Pediatrics (AAP) released guidelines for patients who should receive Synagis; these are listed in Table 1. Patients receiving prophylactic therapy should receive 1 shot per month, 15 mg/kg per dose, for a maximum of 5 doses. This should be administered during the regional RSV season.

Clinical Manifestations

Bronchiolitis begins with upper respiratory findings of congestion or rhinorrhea, which then progresses to involve the lower respiratory tract. An increased respiratory rate is the earliest and most sensitive vital sign change. On physical exam the most important observation is the work of breathing. All patients should have the shirt lifted and the chest directly observed for retractions. Retractions may be visible in the subcostal, intercostal or supra costal region. Head bobbing, grunting, "sighing," and "singing" are signs of severe respiratory distress in infants. In very young infants, especially those with a history of prematurity, apnea alone may be the presenting sign, as well as a complication of bronchiolitis. Auscultation can reveal a variety of findings from minimal sounds to a combination of wheezes, crackles, or referred upper airway congestion. The physical exam findings in bronchiolitis are characteristically dynamic, so that the physical exam findings may vary from examiner to examiner. There are no robustly supported physical exam findings that have reliably correlated with clinical outcomes such as severity or disposition. Despite fully validated parameters, many institutions use bronchiolitis scoring tools to align resources with patients with more severe clinical symptoms. Respiratory rate, work of breathing, and hypoxia remain the most clinically significant parameters in determining illness severity.

Diagnosis

Bronchiolitis remains a clinical diagnosis based on physical exam and history. Chest x-rays are not recommended for diagnosis. Patients with bronchiolitis often have abnormal appearing radiographs, with findings of hyperinflation, areas of atelectasis, and small infiltrates. These findings do not correlate with disease severity and do not change management. Obtaining chest x-rays has been associated with increased prescription of antibiotics, although a primary or concurrent bacterial pneumonia is rare in bronchiolitis. Viral testing similarly does not change management in the majority of clinical cases and should not be routinely obtained. There are a few clinical situations when viral testing may aid management. Young infants (<60 days) may present with fever due to bronchiolitis. The risk of a serious bacterial infection (SBI) within these infants is low; viral testing may support the provider in decreased additional testing, decreased administration of empiric antibiotics, and avoidance of unnecessary hospitalization. During the seasonal influenza epidemic influenza testing may identify bronchiolitis secondary to influenza that may benefit from antiviral medications.

Differential Diagnosis

The differential diagnosis for bronchiolitis includes first episode of asthma, virus-induced wheezing, pertussis infection, chronic aspiration, congenital heart disease, and anatomic thoracic abnormalities. Separating clinical bronchiolitis from a primary asthma exacerbation remains particularly challenging even for experienced providers. Epidemiologic data support that there is a large burden of virus-induced wheezing in young children, of this large group only a small percentage will progress to a diagnosis of asthma. It remains unclear whether bronchiolitis causes a lung injury leading to asthma or whether patients with severe bronchiolitis have preexisting differences predisposing them to a severe course and later diagnosis of asthma. Given the high prevalence of viral-induced wheezing in young children a potential asthma diagnosis (and associated use of albuterol or potentially steroids) should only be considered in patients with risk factors for asthma including eczema, food allergies, or family history of atopy and demonstration of bronchospasm reversed by a bronchodilator. As bronchodilators are not recommended for bronchiolitis if a trial is performed the medical team should carefully assess for efficacy. Pertussis should be considered in prolonged or atypical courses, especially if the infant has had contact with adults who have not received a booster vaccination. Children with an abnormal neurologic baseline should prompt consideration of chronic aspiration as an etiology or contributor to a prolonged course. Undiagnosed congenital heart defects may present with similar exam findings to bronchiolitis. Other anatomic abnormalities that may be considered include pulmonary malformations, vascular rings, or aspiration of a foreign body.

Treatment

The treatment for bronchiolitis remains supportive therapy.
- Improve comfort of child by clearance of nasal secretion and administration of antipyretics for fever
- Administration of oxygen to maintain oxygen saturations greater than 90%
- Maintenance of hydration by intravenous fluids or nasogastric tube
- Support adequate nutrition
- Education of caregivers on return-to care-precautions

In 2014 the AAP published "Clinical Practice Guideline: The Diagnosis, Management, and Prevention of Bronchiolitis" and revised version of the 2006 guidelines. A summary of the recommended treatments is given in Table 2.

Outpatient Management

Outpatient management centers on parental education in supportive care that can be provided for the child while sick and emphasis on return-to-care precautions. The typical course for bronchiolitis begins with upper respiratory infection (URI) symptoms that

TABLE 2	Summary of Evidence for Treatment of Bronchiolitis	
MEDICATION	**RECOMMENDATION**	**EVIDENCE QUALITY**
Systemic corticosteroids	Not recommended	Cochrane systematic review shows that corticosteroids do not significantly reduce outpatient admissions when compared with placebo and do not reduce length of stay for inpatient admissions
Epinephrine	Not recommended	Cochrane meta-analysis systematically evaluated the evidence and found no evidence for utility in the inpatient setting
Albuterol	Not recommended	Meta-analyses and systematic reviews have shown that bronchodilators improve clinical symptom scores, but they do not affect disease resolution, need for hospitalization, or length of stay
Hypertonic saline	May consider	May decrease inpatient length of stay (LOS) in settings where LOS is greater than 3 days (typical US LOS is 2.4 days)
Oxygen therapy	Provide supplemental oxygen if oxyhemoglobin saturation is <90%	
Nutrition and hydration	Administer intravenous or nasogastric fluid for infants unable to maintain hydration orally	

Adapted from AAP Clinical Practice Guideline: The Diagnosis, Management and Prevention of Bronchiolitis. 2014.

will progress to lower respiratory symptoms (cough, increased work of breathing) which peak on days 3 to 5. Cough is the last symptom to resolve with the majority of patients having some resolving cough for up to 2 weeks and a minority extending to 4 weeks. Parents should be discouraged from administering over-the-counter cough suppressants. Clearance of the nasal passages by bulb, or a device of parent choice, may increase comfort of breathing as well as support feeding in infants. Fever is an expected complication of bronchiolitis and may be treated with antipyretics. Caregivers should monitor comfort with breathing; if persistent retractions are present, patient is unable to feed, or patient appears to have distress they should be evaluated immediately for inpatient supportive care.

Inpatient Management

Inpatient admission to the hospital should be considered for patients with hypoxia defined as oxygen saturation less than 90% on room air, dehydration, or moderate to severe respiratory distress manifested by tachypnea for age, retractions, grunting, or concern for apnea. Nasal clearance for comfort, oxygen therapy for hypoxia, and nutritional support remain the foundational therapy for inpatient care. Although nasal suction has not been robustly compared with withholding nasal suction it has become standard of care in most hospitals. Deep suction is not recommended and may be associated with longer lengths of stay. Medications including albuterol, corticosteroids, and racemic epinephrine are not recommended. Nebulized hypertonic saline (3%) has been studied as a therapeutic agent with conflicting trial results. These studies have suffered from design variability both within the United States and internationally. Current evidence does not demonstrate clear benefit for patients with bronchiolitis. Patients with concurrent dehydration should have volume replacement with isotonic fluids. Bronchiolitis has been described as an independent stimulus for anti-diuretic hormone release, placing these patients at risk for inappropriate retention of free water and development of hyponatremia. Isotonic fluid should be used in these patients to decrease the risk of iatrogenic hyponatremia. Aggressive nutritional support should be initiated for infants with poor feeding; nasogastric support should be given to any patient who is not able to meet caloric goals. Oxygen should be administered to maintain saturations greater than 90%. Humidified high-flow nasal cannula (HHFNC) oxygen therapy is frequently used as a safe method of increased respiratory support for hospitalized patients with moderate to severe work of breathing. HHFNC

uses blended, humidified, heated air and oxygen at higher flow rates used with nonhumidified oxygen. Systemic reviews support HHFNC as safe and well tolerated, but evidence is lacking to show superiority to standard oxygen therapy. There is high variability in the use and interpretation of pulse oximetry in patients with bronchiolitis. Although pulse oximetry readings are instrumental in determining need for admission, continuous monitoring has been associated with increased length of stay. Patients should be transitioned to intermittent monitoring as soon as possible and providers should focus on the clinical course over transient variations in oximetry. Chest physiotherapy is not recommended when managing hospitalized patients with bronchiolitis. Antibiotic therapy should only be used if there is concern for a secondary bacterial infection. Secondary bacterial infections in mild to moderate bronchiolitis are rare but severe bronchiolitis may have a higher percentage of bacterial co-infection.

Complications

The most common complication of bronchiolitis is acute otitis media, which should be treated according to current guidelines. A small percentage of bronchiolitis patients will progress to respiratory failure requiring intensive care support and mechanical ventilation. These patients may represent a unique cohort with a higher incidence of pre-existing co-morbid conditions, co-infection from multiple viral agents, or bacterial superinfection. Mortality due to RSV in the United States is rare, accounting for fewer than 100 children annually, but worldwide bronchiolitis remains a significant contributor to pediatric mortality in resource-limited countries.

References

American Academy of Pediatrics Committee on Infectious Diseases: American Academy of Pediatrics Bronchiolitis Guidelines Committee: Updated guidance for palivizumab prophylaxis among infants and young children at increased risk of hospitalization for respiratory syncytial virus infection, *Pediatrics* 134:415–420, 2014.

Franklin D, Babl FE, Schlapbach LJ, et al: A randomized trial of high-flow oxygen therapy in infants with bronchiolitis, *N ENgl J Med*, 2018 Mar.

Hall CB, Weinberg GA, Iwane MK, et al: The burden of respiratory syncytial virus infection in young children, *N Engl J Med* 360:588–598, 2009.

Hasegawa K, Tsugawa Y, Brown D, et al: Trends in bronchiolitis hospitalizations in the United States, 2000–2009, *Pediatrics* 132:28–36, 2013.

Meissner HC: Viral bronchiolitis in children, *N Engl J Med* 374:62–72, 2016.

Ralston SL, Lieberthal AS, Meissner HC, et al: Clinical practice guideline: the diagnosis, management and prevention of bronchiolitis, *Pediatrics* 134:1474–1502, 2014.

DIABETES MELLITUS IN CHILDREN

Gregory Goodwin, MD

CURRENT DIAGNOSIS

- Random glucose >200 mg/dL and symptoms (polyuria, polydipsia)
- Fasting glucose >126 mg/dL
- 2-h glucose >200 mg/dL after glucose tolerance test
- Hemoglobin A1c >6.5%
- Diabetic ketoacidosis: pH <7.3, serum bicarbonate <15 mmol/L

CURRENT TREATMENT

Type 1 Diabetes
- Basal/bolus regimen**: rapid-acting insulin* before meals and long-acting insulin‡† at bedtime
- Insulin pump therapy**: continuous infusion of short-acting insulin
- NPH insulin at breakfast and bedtime, rapid-acting insulin before meals
- Premixed insulins (75/25‡ 50/50§) at breakfast and dinner
- Total daily insulin dose (TDD): 0.15–1.2 U/kg per day
  - Basal/bolus: 50% long acting, 50% rapid acting
  - NPH/rapid acting: two-thirds TDD in a.m., one-third TDD in p.m.
  - a.m. and p.m. doses: two-thirds NPH, one-third rapid-acting
  - Premixed insulins: two-thirds a.m., one-third before dinner

Diabetic Ketoacidosis
- Fluids: 10–20 mL/kg normal saline once, repeat if shock/poor perfusion. Ongoing fluids: one-half normal saline with 20 mEq/L K acetate and 20 mEq/L K phosphate at 1.5–2.0 times maintenance fluids
- Regular insulin infusion: 0.05–0.1 U/kg per hour
- Add dextrose (5%–10%) when glucose is below 300 mg/dL
- Urgent consultation with center experienced in treatment of pediatric ketoacidosis (if not available on site)

Type 2 Diabetes
- Aggressive dietary modification: lower total carbohydrates to 25%–40% of total calories
- Metformin (Glucophage): 500–1000 mg bid, titrate up to avoid gastrointestinal side effects
- The first two items on this list plus insulin therapy: either as single long-acting insulin at bed or full basal bolus regimen until stable glucose control
- Glucagon-like peptide-1 (GLP-1) agonist in obese insulin-resistant pediatric patients above 10 years of age

---

**Preferred treatment.
*Rapid-acting insulin: lispro (Humalog, Admelog), aspart (Novolog, Fiasp), glulisine (Apidra).
‡75% intermediate-acting insulin, 25% rapid-acting insulin (Humalog 75/25).
†Long-acting insulin: glargine (Lantus, Toujeo, Basaglar), detemir (Levemir), degludec (Tresiba).
§50% intermediate-acting insulin, 50% rapid-acting insulin (Humalog 50/50).

Type 1 Diabetes: Introduction

Type 1 diabetes mellitus (T1DM) results from progressive autoimmune destruction of insulin-producing cells (β cells) of the pancreatic islets, ultimately leading to insulin deficiency and resulting in hyperglycemia and in some cases ketoacidosis.

The precise cause or causes of T1DM remains elusive, but an association with human lymphocytic antigens (HLAs) has been known for decades. Whole genomewide linkage studies have identified up to 60 genes associated with T1DM, and many are related to the immune response. However, identical twin studies show a concordance rate of only 30% to 60%, suggesting that unidentified environmental factors make up the remaining risk. Environmental factors implicated in T1DM risk include viral infections, toxins (nitrosamines), and dietary factors such as exposure to cow's milk and gluten-containing cereals in early infancy. However, recent prospective studies have shown no advantage of using elemental formulas or delaying the introduction of gluten until 1 year of life in infants at increased risk for development of T1DM. A large meta-analysis of 24 studies of over 4000 participants showed an almost 10-fold risk of reverse transcription polymerase chain reaction (RT-PCR)–determined enteroviral infections in T1DM patients versus controls, whereas the TEDDY study showed an almost 50% conversion of high-risk infants and children to expressing islet cell antibodies when more than five respiratory infections in the preceding 9 months were reported.

Epidemiology

The prevalence of T1DM is about 1 per 300 individuals (0.3%) in the United States, with significant global and racial variations. The presence of a first-degree relative with T1DM, such as a sibling or parent, increases the chances of developing T1DM to 3% to 6%.

The highest incidence rates of T1DM in children are seen in early adolescence (10–14 years), followed by early childhood (5–9 years). The youngest age of onset of T1DM can be seen in infants below 1 year of age, but usually not before 6 months.

The incidence of T1DM has been increasing steadily by 2% to 5% per year over the past several decades in the United States, Europe, and Australia. Interestingly, in some but not all studies, the youngest age group (0–4 years) demonstrates the highest rates of increase.

The onset of T1DM is seasonal. In the northern hemisphere, the highest incidence of onset is in the fall and winter and the fewest are in the summer.

Presentation

The classic symptoms of diabetes are polyuria, polydipsia, and nocturia, which is the result of an osmotic diuresis induced by hyperglycemia. Symptoms can be present for days to months, but the majority of patients present after 1 to 2 weeks of symptoms. Weight loss is a common finding on presentation because insulin plays an important role in the synthesis of protein and fat; therefore insulin deficiency results in the loss of muscle and fat stores. Weight loss also occurs because calorie loss from high concentrations of glucose in the urine can be substantial.

Abdominal pain, nausea, and vomiting are classic signs of ketoacidosis that can often be misdiagnosed as gastroenteritis. Approximately 70% of patients with new-onset diabetes have hyperglycemia without ketoacidosis at presentation, whereas some 25% to 30% of cases present in diabetic ketoacidosis (DKA), although there can be significant variations from various centers internationally.

Diagnosis

A random glucose greater than 200 mg/dL in the presence of classic symptoms of diabetes is diagnostic of diabetes. A fasting glucose greater than 126 mg/dL is also diagnostic of diabetes; however, a fasting glucose or a glucose tolerance test is rarely necessary in the diagnosis of T1DM.

A venous pH below 7.3 or a serum bicarbonate below 15 mmol/L is diagnostic of DKA in the presence of hyperglycemia. Distinguishing type 1 from type 2 diabetes can sometimes be difficult at presentation, particularly in an overweight adolescent. In this circumstance islet cell autoantibodies are useful in making this distinction. Islet cell autoantibodies include anti–glutamic acid decarboxylase (GAD), anti-insulin, anti-insulinoma autoantigen 2 (IA-2), and anti-zinc transporter 8 (ZnT8). These antibodies are available in most commercial laboratories, but results are usually not available until weeks after initial presentation. The safest course of action in most pediatric patients with new-onset diabetes is to treat with insulin until islet antibodies and other parameters such as endogenous insulin production as assessed by c-peptide levels are available.

Treatment of Type 1 Diabetes Mellitus

Type 1 Diabetes Mellitus (Without Ketoacidosis or After Ketoacidosis Has Resolved)

Insulin is the mainstay of treatment for T1DM. Intensive insulin therapy has become the standard of care for patients with T1DM. Typically a long-acting basal insulin—such as glargine (Lantus, Toujeo, Basaglar), detemir (Levemir), or degludec (Tresiba)—along with premeal boluses of rapid-acting insulin—such as lispro (Humalog, Admelog), aspart (NovoLog, Fiasp), or glulisine (Apidra)—is instituted.

Required total daily insulin dosing (TDD) is dependent on age at presentation, pubertal stage, and the presence of acidosis at diagnosis. Total daily insulin requirements range from about 0.25 to 1.0 U/kg per day (Table 1). Long-acting or basal insulin is typically 50% of TDD; the remaining 50% is bolus insulin. Bolus rapid-acting insulin dosing is calculated by the following formulas (Fig. 1):

To cover meal carbohydrates, a *carbohydrate ratio* is derived from the formula

500 divided by total daily insulin dose

To correct hyperglycemia, a *correction factor* is derived from the formula

1500 divided bytotal daily insulin dose

Correction doses should not be given more frequently than every 3 hours.

For new-onset patients, a *target glucose* of 150 mg/dL is assigned, whereas more established patients typically use 120 mg/dL. Correction at bedtime or during the night should be less aggressive and a higher target may be assigned—for example, 150 to 200 mg/dL.

Carbohydrate ratios, correction factors, and targets are adjusted on the basis of fasting and postprandial glucose levels. High postprandial glucose levels would require a lower carbohydrate ratio. High blood glucose levels that do not correct after a correction dose has been given would require a lowering of the correction factor. High morning fasting glucose levels would require an increase in the long-acting insulin dose.

Implicit in these recommended treatment regimen is that (1) the patient or family is able to count carbohydrates correctly, and (2) the family is able to calculate insulin dosing correctly using the carbohydrate ratio, correction factor, and target. If the patient or family is unable or unwilling to perform these calculations a simplified insulin regimen should be devised using fixed doses of intermediate-acting insulin and a sliding scale of rapid-acting insulin.

Less complex insulin regimens include NPH and rapid-acting insulin given at breakfast, dinner, and bedtime (Fig. 2). NPH and rapid-acting insulin are given at breakfast (no insulin at lunch if glucose <200 mg/dL), rapid-acting insulin at dinner, and NPH at bedtime. This regimen can be used to avoid giving insulin at lunchtime. Typically, two-thirds of the daily dose is given in the morning; then two-thirds NPH, one-third rapid-acting insulin, and one-third of the daily dose is given in evening. The evening dose is divided, with one-third rapid-acting before dinner and two-thirds NPH at bedtime. The patient should, however, consume a relatively fixed amount of carbohydrate at each meal. Consistency in meal content and portion size is very important in overall glycemic control. A simplified sliding scale of rapid-acting insulin may be added to the NPH and rapid-acting insulin regimen.

In certain challenging cases where there are significant compliance or cognitive deficits, fixed doses of premixed intermediate- and rapid- or short-acting insulin such as Humalog mix (75/25) can be used before breakfast and before dinner (Fig. 3). Premixed 75/25 insulin preparations come in vials or pens and consist of 75% intermediate-acting neutral protamine hagedorn; (NPH) and 25% rapid-acting (lispro) insulins. Insulin pens are a very convenient way to give insulin, but in some cases, because of patient preference or insurer restrictions, dosing by syringe is preferred or required.

Treatment of Diabetic Ketoacidosis

There are critical differences in the treatment of DKA between children and adults. A major complication of the treatment of DKA in children is cerebral edema, a complication rarely seen in adults. Although a relatively infrequent complication (<1% of DKA episodes), cerebral edema can be associated with serious morbidity and mortality.

Risk factors for the development of cerebral edema include new-onset diabetes, younger age at diagnosis, longer duration of

TABLE 1	Suggested Total Daily Insulin Dosage in New-Onset Type I Diabetes
PATIENT CATEGORY	**INSULIN DOSE (U/KG PER DAY)**
Prepubertal without DKA	0.25–0.5 (<6 years, 0.15-0.25)
Prepubertal with DKA	0.5–0.75
Pubertal without DKA	0.5–0.75
Pubertal with DKA	0.75–1.2

DKA, Diabetic ketoacidosis.

Patient Example 2

- 8 y.o. boy—2 week history of polydipsia, polyuria and vomiting for for the past 24 hours.
- In doctors office: glucose 380 mg/dl and urine ketones are large.
- In emergency room serum HCO3 9, anion gap 25.
- Admitted to ICU for insulin drip, IV fluids, and frequent monitoring.
- At 7 am the following morning: glucose 120, HCO3 20.
- Weight: 25
- Family would like to avoid insulin at lunch as school nurse not available.

- Total daily dose 0.6 X 25 kg = 15 units
- 2/3 am = 10 units
  - 2/3 NPH ~ 6.5 units
  - 1/3 rapid acting 3.5 units
- 1/3 pm = 5 units
  - 1/3 rapid acting ~ 1.5 units before dinner
  - 2/3 NPH 3.5 units at bedtime
- Supplement with sliding scale: 0.5 unit rapid-acting insulin per 50 mg/dl above 200 mg/dl.

Figure 2 An 8-year-old boy who presented in diabetic ketoacidosis. He was treated with an insulin drip overnight and his acidosis had resolved by morning. The parents requested a regimen that would not require insulin at lunch time. The total daily insulin dose is shown in Table 1.

Patient Example 1

- 6 y.o. girl presents with 2 week history of polydipsia and polyuria.
- She is otherwise well with a normal exam.
- Serum glucose in the ER is 425 mg/dl and serum bicarbonate is 20.
- Weight in the ER : 20 kg

- Total daily insulin =
  - 20 kg X 0.3 u/kg/d = 6 units.
- ~50% basal = 3.0 units (glargine, degludec)
- Target = 150
- Carbohydrate ratio: 500/6 = 83~80
- Correction factor: 1500/6 = 250

Figure 1 New-onset type 1 diabetes in a 6-year-old girl who is not in diabetic ketoacidosis (DKA). Total daily insulin dosage is determined by multiplying body weight by recommended dosage requirements for a prepubertal girl who is not in DKA. One-half of the total daily insulin dose is given as long-acting insulin, which is 3.0 units in this example. Carbohydrate ratio and correction factors are calculated using formulas provided in the text. Calculated ratios can be adjusted up to 10% to simplify calculations.

Patient Example 3

- 14 y.o. boy with cognitive delays presents with 3-week history of polydipsia and polyuria and 10 lb weight loss.
- Glucose 625 mg/dl in ER
- Bicarbonate 19 meq/l.
- Tanner 4 on exam
- Weight 44 kg
- Parents also have cognitive impairments

- Total daily dose: 44 kg X 0.6 u/kg/d = 26.4 units per day.
- Medical team decides fixed mixed 75/25 insulin regimen may be best.
- 2/3 TDD given before breakfast = 17 units
- 1/3 before dinner = 9 units
- Sliding scale rapid acting: 1 unit per 50 mg/dl over 200 mg/dl.

Figure 3 A 14-year-old boy with intellectual impairments presents with new-onset type 1 diabetes without diabetic ketoacidosis. Because of cognitive delays in both the patient and his parents, a simplified two-injection regimen was derived using the previously described calculations. This regimen may be supplemented with a sliding scale of rapid-acting insulin.

symptoms before diagnosis, and severity of acidosis—manifested as DKA with hypocapnia, high blood urea nitrogen, bicarbonate boluses, and failure for the corrected serum sodium to rise as treatment for DKA progresses. For these reasons, overly aggressive fluid resuscitation and boluses of bicarbonate are avoided in the treatment of pediatric DKA.

Judicious fluid replacement with a bolus of normal saline—initially 10 mL/kg and, if necessary, a second 10-mL/kg bolus of saline solution—may be given in the first hour of treatment. Thereafter half normal saline with 40 mEq/L of potassium acetate or potassium phosphate at a fluid rate of no more than 1.5 to 2.0 times maintenance is administered (Table 2). Potassium should not be added to intravenous fluid until the K is <5 meq/L. The two-bag system for fluid management of DKA—in which two bags contain identical electrolytes but differ in that one bag contains no dextrose and the second bag contains 10% dextrose—can be useful. The relative contribution of each bag is then titrated depending on the blood glucose level. Although estimates of fluid deficit in DKA are between 5% and 10% of body weight, intravascular volume is often preserved in the hyperosmolar state; hence hypovolemic shock is uncommon in DKA. The goal is to replace the fluid deficit slowly over 24 to 48 hours. Frequent neurologic checks are highly recommended in the first 24 hours of treatment. Altered mental status or the development of a severe headache during treatment for DKA is a potentially serious sign of cerebral edema.

Insulin plays a critical role in the treatment of DKA, not only in lowering serum glucose levels but also in the paramount role of shutting down ketogenesis in the liver. The standard insulin drip for pediatric DKA is 0.1 U/kg per hour; however, treatment with 0.05 U/kg per hour has also been effective. Human regular insulin remains the standard insulin in the intravenous treatment of DKA.

Once the acidosis has resolved, as reflected by a normal anion gap and serum bicarbonate greater than 15 mmol/L and pH greater than 7.35, the insulin drip can be discontinued. Hyperchloremic non–anion gap acidosis (HCO_3 <15 but normal anion gap <12) can occur during the recovery phase of DKA. Hyperchloremic metabolic acidosis is likely due to a large amount of chloride administered in intravenous fluids as both NaCl and KCL supplementation. For this reason many centers typically give 50% of the potassium replacement as potassium phosphate. Once the acidosis is resolved and the patient can tolerate oral intake, subcutaneous insulin can be started per the section, Treatment of Type 1 Diabetes Mellitus, earlier in this chapter. The most convenient time to do so is just before a meal.

Importantly, treatment of pediatric DKA should ideally occur in centers with experienced pediatric intensivists, endocrinologists, and nursing staff. If referral to a pediatric center is not practical, then early contact with a pediatric endocrinologist for treatment guidance is highly recommended.

Finally, the most common causes of pediatric DKA are (1) new-onset diabetes presenting in DKA and (2) infusion site failure in a patient on an insulin pump or missed long-acting insulin injections in a patient on insulin injections. Infections including gastroenteritis and febrile illnesses are infrequently the exclusive cause of DKA in pediatrics.

Diabetes Self-Management Education

Children and adolescents with type 1 diabetes should receive outpatient care by multidisciplinary teams including an endocrinologist, certified diabetes educator, nurse, registered dietician, and licensed clinical social worker. Provision of comprehensive education at the time of diagnosis is essential because this is the time when the patient and family are most receptive and impressionable. Patients who do not receive proper early education often fall into habits of suboptimal diabetes care, which can be hard to undo once established.

Important educational topics that must be rapidly learned by the family and patient (in addition to glucose monitoring and insulin administration) include diet and carbohydrate counting, prevention and treatment of hypoglycemia, emergency glucagon, exercise and hypoglycemia, prevention of ketoacidosis, and sick day management. Learning to count carbohydrates accurately can be a particular challenge.

Mental Health Considerations in Type 1 Diabetes Mellitus

Diabetes "burnout" issues are common in the treatment of youth with diabetes, particularly during the adolescent years. Conflicts between parents and teens can often arise during this time. It is important for the parents to maintain a healthy supporting role with their child or teenager in a manner appropriate to the child's age and level of development. Recognition of relatively common mental health comorbidities—such as depression, anxiety, and eating disorders—is essential to the overall well-being of the pediatric patient with T1DM.

Goals of Therapy for Patients With Type 1 Diabetes Mellitus

The number-one goal of the diabetes health care team is to prevent readmission to the hospital for severe hypoglycemia or ketoacidosis. Resumption of the full range of daily activities, including returning to school and work as well as engaging in essentially all meaningful activities that preceded the diagnosis of diabetes, is to be expected.

Although the goal in the pediatric age group is to reduce hemoglobin A1c to below 7.5%, less than 25% of pediatric patients in the United States are able to achieve that goal. The average hemoglobin A1c in the pediatric population is approximately 8.2%, whereas in 19-year-olds the average hemoglobin A1c is 9.2%.

The Diabetes Control and Complications Trial (DCCT) in 1993 showed convincingly that lowering the hemoglobin A1c from 9% to 7.1% resulted in significantly less diabetes-related retinopathy, nephropathy, and neuropathy. Most patients in the DCCT trial who were randomized to the intensively treated group used insulin pumps to achieve tighter control, but tight control was achieved with injectable insulin regimens as well.

Sick Day Management

Patients with T1DM who have intercurrent infectious illnesses are prone to develop hyperglycemia with ketosis and also hypoglycemia, depending on the nature of the illness. Blood glucose levels should be monitored every 1 to 3 hours during illnesses. Rapid-acting insulin may need to be administered every 2 to 4 hours for hyperglycemia, especially in the presence of serum or urine ketones. Rapid-acting insulin can be dosed at 0.1 to 0.2 U/kg per dose in this setting. Improvement in hyperglycemia and particularly in ketosis using this treatment regimen can be invaluable in preventing ketoacidosis or hospitalization. Patients with persistent vomiting who are unable to keep fluids down need to be referred to the emergency department for intravenous hydration and assessment for DKA.

For patients on an insulin pump, ketosis with nausea and vomiting is often a sign that the insulin infusion set is not properly functioning. Insulin therefore should be given by syringe or pen device until the ketones have cleared and a new infusion set has been placed.

Poor oral intake during a gastrointestinal illness may result in hypoglycemia. Frequent small volumes of sugar-containing fluids such as juice or sports drinks may be necessary to keep the blood glucose above 70 mg/dL, and basal insulin requirements may need to be decreased by 10% to 50%. Low-dose glucagon may be used in the setting of recurrent hypoglycemia and poor oral intake. Glucagon can be dosed at 1 unit on an insulin syringe for every year of age, using a standard 1-mg/mL glucagon preparation. The

TABLE 2	Formulas for the Calculation of Maintenance Fluids for Infants and Children
For infants 3.5–10 kg, daily fluid requirement = 100 mL/kg	
For children 11–20 kg, daily fluid requirement = 1000 mL + 50 mL/kg for every kg over 10 years of age	
For children >20 kg, daily fluid requirement = 1500 mL + 20 mL/kg for every kg over 20, up to a maximum of 2400 mL daily	

dose may be repeated every 15 minutes as needed. In some cases, persistent low glucose levels (<70 mg/dL) in the setting of recurrent vomiting may be best managed in an emergency department or hospital setting where intravenous dextrose-containing fluids are readily available.

Risk for Additional Autoimmune Disorders

Patients with one autoimmune disorder are at increased risk for the development of one or more additional autoimmune conditions. Children and adolescents with T1DM are particularly at risk for thyroid and celiac disorders. Screening for thyroid disorders with serum TSH and free T_4 should occur in the first 6 months after the T1DM diagnosis and every 1 to 2 years thereafter. Celiac disorder should also be screened in the first year after the T1DM diagnosis. Most cases of celiac disorder are detected within the first 5 years after the diagnosis of T1DM, and the majority of cases are asymptomatic. Recent American Diabetes Association recommendations include screening for celiac disorder at diagnosis and again at 2 and 5 years after diagnosis. Elevated serum tissue transglutaminase levels should be referred to a pediatric gastroenterologist. Because celiac disorder is a lifelong condition, it is advised to obtain a small bowel biopsy. Autoimmune adrenal (Addison) disease rarely occurs with T1DM but has the unique presentation of recurrent hypoglycemia, necessitating significant reductions in daily insulin requirements. Sending simultaneous adrenocorticotropic hormone and cortisol levels on a morning blood specimen will usually render the diagnosis of Addison disease.

Screening for Complications of Type 1 Diabetes Mellitus

Microvascular complications of T1DM are infrequent in the pediatric age group, although background retinopathy and microalbuminuria become more prevalent in the late-adolescent and young-adult age ranges. Proactive early screening regimens are advocated to detect diabetes complications early so that medical interventions can prevent more serious diabetes-related complications such as proliferative retinopathy and end-stage renal disease.

Annual screening for microalbuminuria with a random urine specimen should be performed at puberty or at age 10 years and above once the child has had diabetes for 5 years. Elevated urine albumin/urine creatinine (>30 mg/g creatinine) ratios should be repeated two to three times over a 6-month period to confirm the diagnosis because transient microalbuminuria is a common finding. Variables such as exercise or recent illness can lead to microalbuminuria; therefore a repeat study after recovery and on a first morning specimen will often yield a normal result. In addition, individuals with the benign condition of orthostatic albuminuria can be identified by finding completely normal albumin excretion on a first morning voided specimen, whereas a random specimen will often be frankly proteinuric. When urinary albumin/creatinine ratios are found to be consistently elevated, treatment with an angiotensin converting enzyme inhibitor is recommended. Referral to a pediatric nephrologist should be arranged in complex cases.

Annual dilated eye examinations are recommended after age 10 or at pubertal onset (whichever comes first) once the patient has had diabetes for 3 to 5 years. Referral to an eye care professional with expertise in diabetic retinopathy is recommended.

Cardiovascular risk factors including blood pressure and lipid profiles should be monitored in patients with T1DM. Blood pressure should be obtained at each visit.

High blood pressure is defined as systolic or diastolic blood pressure above the 90th percentile, and hypertension is defined as above the 95th percentile for age, sex, and height. Blood pressure measurements should be obtained using an appropriate cuff size, particularly in the overweight patient. White-coat hypertension can be problematic in the adolescent population. Such patients will often demonstrate an elevated heart rate as a clue to stress-induced hypertension. Monitoring blood pressure in a nonthreatening environment, such as at home, using an accurate home blood pressure monitor, may be helpful. When white-coat hypertension is suspected, 24–hour home blood pressure monitoring can be very useful.

Initial management of high blood pressure includes salt restriction and weight-control measures. For persistent hypertension, treatment with an antihypertensive medication (lisinopril) may be necessary.

Shortly after diagnosis and once glucose control has been established, it is important to obtain nonfasting total and high-density lipoprotein cholesterol readings. If total cholesterol is high, a fasting morning lipid panel should be obtained. If low-density lipoprotein (LDL) cholesterol is below 100, it would be reasonable to repeat it in 5 years. For LDL cholesterol above 100, dietary measures are taken, along with efforts to improve metabolic control. For patients beyond 10 years of age with an LDL cholesterol above 130 to 160 in whom lifestyle changes have resulted in inadequate control, statin therapy may be considered. Referral to a pediatric preventive cardiology program would also be appropriate.

Technologic Changes in the Care for Patients With Type 1 Diabetes Mellitus

Technological changes have revolutionized the care of patients with T1DM. Unheralded changes such as the emergence of ultrafine lancet technology coupled with glucose test strips requiring less than 10 µL of blood resulted in rapid, essentially painless fingerstick glucose monitoring. Ultrafine insulin syringes and pen needles helped usher in widespread adoption of intensive insulin regimens with rapid-acting insulin taken before all meals and snacks.

The insulin pump further advanced diabetes care in making insulin dosing before meals and snacks even less challenging, especially for children. The development of a tubeless insulin pump (Omnipod) led to an even wider array of choices.

Continuous glucose monitoring (CGM) has evolved into a very powerful and widely used technology in T1DM. Subcutaneous fluid glucose levels are determined every 5 minutes and the user is provided with meaningful feedback to influence diabetes self-management decisions in real time. Particularly useful are alarm functions for impending low glucose levels; these can be invaluable in the prevention of hypoglycemia. Alarms for hyperglycemia are also used with this technology. The accuracy of glucose determinations by CGM technology is now approaching subcutaneous blood glucose technology, and the improved accuracy has led the US Food and Drug Administration (FDA) to approve insulin-dosing decisions based on CGM data (e.g., the Dexcom G6 products). It is important to remember, however, that subcutaneous glucose levels lag behind whole blood glucose levels by about 15 minutes. This fact is particularly important when glucose levels are changing rapidly, so the user is advised to pay attention to the glucose trend. Alarms for predicting hypoglycemia are very important in this regard.

A drawback to CGM technology had been the need to calibrate the device accurately with periodic fingerstick glucose checks. However, the Dexcom G6, which was released to market in 2018, and the Abbot Libre, are factory-calibrated and do not require consumer calibration. Remarkably, patients using calibration-free CGM devices may no longer be required to check fingerstick glucose levels! A CGM sensor placed on the arm or abdomen will last for 10 to 14 days before having to be changed.

The most remarkable technologic change emerging in the care of patients with T1DM is the coupling of CGM and real-time adjustments to insulin delivery. Thus insulin delivery is suspended when hypoglycemia has occurred or is likely to occur, and basal insulin can be significantly increased when hyperglycemia is predicted to occur or has occurred. *Hybrid closed-loop* refers to the fact that some aspects of management, such as carbohydrate counting and manual bolusing for meals, are still required. The first hybrid closed-loop insulin pump was FDA approved in 2016 (Medtronic 670G). Prevention of postprandial hyperglycemia is particularly problematic, but prebolusing rapid-acting insulin 10 to 30 minutes before eating will help to limit postprandial hyperglycemia. Prebolusing of insulin is often difficult in view of modern lifestyles. Use of the Medtronic 670G insulin pump has proven to be challenging in the real-world setting due to frequent calibration requirements and forced exits from the automatic insulin delivery mode. The Tandem insulin pump with Control IQ technology was FDA approved in 2019. This hybrid closed-loop system is user friendly, with no calibration requirements or forced exits from automated insulin delivery. Hybrid closed-loop technology can be particularly useful for optimizing glycemic control overnight, the time when many patients and families are most fearful of hypoglycemia. Despite the remarkable technological achievements of hybrid closed-loop technology, actual improvements in hemoglobin A1c are modest and are on the order of 0.2% to 0.3% lower hemoglobin A1c. Additional hybrid closed-loop systems are currently in clinical trials or awaiting FDA approval (Omnipod Horizon, Beta Bionic iLet). The community of patients with diabetes can look forward to further refinements and improvements in these technologies in the years to come.

Type 2 Diabetes in Children

Since the 1990s, type 2 diabetes mellitus (T2DM) in patients below 18 years of age has risen dramatically. The increased incidence of type 2 diabetes has coincided with the obesity epidemic. Children from minority populations (non-Hispanic blacks, Hispanics, and Native Americans) and those patients with a positive family history of T2DM are at the greatest risk. The majority of pediatric T2DM is found in adolescents and children above 10 years of age.

Diagnosis of T2DM can be made with a fasting glucose above 126 mg/dL, random glucose above 200 mg/dL, and the 2-hour glucose from an oral glucose tolerance test above 200 mg/dL. A hemoglobin A1c greater than 6.5% is indicative of diabetes as well and is a particularly convenient test in the outpatient setting. An elevated fasting or random glucose and an elevated hemoglobin A1c are diagnostic of T2DM in high-risk patients.

Pediatric patients with T2DM are often symptom free at diagnosis but can present acutely with classic diabetes symptoms and even ketosis or mild ketoacidosis. Distinguishing the latter group from T1DM can be difficult initially, but the absence of β cell antibodies and very stable glycemic control after diagnosis are often telltale signs of T2DM.

In individuals who present with marked hyperglycemia (hemoglobin A1c >8.5%), ketosis, or both, stabilization with insulin initially may be required. Basal bolus regimens using a combination of long- and short-acting insulins can be instituted. Insulin resistance may be quite significant at the time of diagnosis, and relatively high doses of insulin can be required to achieve target glucose levels.

Metformin (Glucophage) is the mainstay of treatment for T2DM in those below 18 years of age. Maximal dosing is 1000 mg bid or 2000 mg/day of the extended-release preparation. Gastrointestinal side effects are relatively common, and metformin should be taken with meals. Initial dosing can be 500 mg bid or 1000 mg extended-release daily; the dose can be titrated upward as needed and tolerated. **Dietary modifications such as weight control and exercise are of fundamental importance in the treatment of T2DM.** Liraglutide (Victoza), a glucagon-like peptide (GLP-1) agonist, was FDA approved in 2019 for the treatment of T2DM for patients above 10 years of age. GLP-1 agonists are associated with early satiety, weight loss, and improved glycemic control in adults with T2DM; however, side effects such as nausea are common, and an increased risk of pancreatitis is well recognized. Adherence to a healthy diet in combination with metformin alone, insulin therapy, or both often results in very stable glycemic control in T2DM in pediatrics. In many cases, bolus short-acting insulin and even long-acting insulin therapy can be withdrawn safely 6 to 12 months after diagnosis. However, resumption of lax dietary and self-care habits can result in significant decline in glycemic control and the need to restart insulin. Therefore patients with T2DM need to be as vigilant as patients with T1DM, in monitoring their glucose levels regularly and following up every 3 to 6 months with their healthcare teams.

Monogenic or Maturity-Onset Diabetes of Youth

Single gene mutations leading to diabetes are referred to as *maturity onset diabetes of youth (MODY) diabetes* or *monogenic diabetes*. More than 30 different genes have been identified that are associated with MODY, although some 80% of cases are due to glucokinase and *HNF1A* and *HNF1B* gene mutations. Patients can be diagnosed at any age but are usually diagnosed before age 35 years. Routine laboratory testing or laboratory testing during an illness may lead to the detection of MODY diabetes incidentally. Patients with MODY are often lean, and the family history may reveal two to three affected generations. Testing for islet cell antibodies is universally negative.

Glucokinase diabetes is a very mild form of MODY diabetes that is nonprogressive and does not require treatment, whereas *HNF1A* and *HNF1B* forms of MODY diabetes are progressive; these patients can develop long-term complications of diabetes. HNF diabetes is uniquely sensitive to sulfonylureas, and hence the diagnosis can be life changing in an individual who has been treated with insulin prior to definitive diagnosis.

Genetic panels for MODY diabetes are available commercially, and genetic testing is increasingly covered by insurance companies in the United States. It is important to test for both mutations and deletions of the most common forms of MODY. A full list of laboratories that offer MODY testing is available at the NCBI Genetic Testing Registry (http://www.ncbi.nlm.nih.gov/gtr/).

Neonatal diabetes can also be due to monogenic forms of diabetes, and these infants are usually diagnosed before 6 to 9 months of age. Testing for monogenetic forms of diabetes should be considered in infants below 9 to 12 months of age whose islet cell autoantibodies are negative. Single gene mutations in the K-ATP channel of the β cell leading to neonatal diabetes can be remarkably responsive to oral sulfonylureas. Transient forms of neonatal diabetes in an infant born with intrauterine growth retardation and macroglossia are often associated with imprinting abnormalities on chromosome region 6q24. This type of diabetes usually resolves by 18 months but can recur at adolescence.

References

American Diabetes Association: Children and adolescents: Standards of medical care in diabetes—2018, *Diabetes Care* 41(Suppl 1):S126–S136, 2018.

Copeland KC, Zeiter P, Geffner M, et al: Characteristics of adolescents and youth with recent-onset type 2 diabetes: the TODAY cohort at baseline, *J Clin Endocrinol Metab* 96:159–167, 2011.

Delli AJ, Lernmark A: Type 1 (insulin-dependent) diabetes mellitus: Etiology, pathogenesis, prediction, and prevention. In *Endocrinology: Adult and Pediatric*, Saunders, 2016.

International Consensus on Use of Continuous Glucose Monitoring. *Diabetes Care* 40:1631–1640, 2017.

Levitsky L, Misra M: Epidemiology, presentation and diagnosis of type 1 diabetes in children and adolescents. Up To Date. Available at Up To Date. Accessed March 3, 2020.

Miller KM, Foster NC, Beck RW, et al: Current state of type 1 diabetes treatment in the US: updated data from the T1D Exchange Clinic Registry, *Diabetes Care* 38:971–978, 2015.

Sperling MA, Tamborlane WR, et al: In *Pediatric Endocrinology*, Philadelphia, 2014, Elsevier, pp 847–900.

The Environmental Determinants of Diabetes Study: Available at: https://teddy.epi.usf.edu/. Accessed 9/3/20.

The National Center for Monogenic Diabetes at the University of Chicago Monogenic Diabetes Registry. Available at Monogenic https://monogenicdiabetes.uchicago.edu/. Accessed 9/3/20.

White NH: Long-term outcomes in youth with diabetes mellitus, *Pediatr Clin North Am* 62:889–909, 2015.

Wolfsdorf JI: The International Society of Pediatric and Adolescent Diabetes guidelines for management of ketoacidosis: do the guidelines need to be modified? *Pediatric Diabetes* 15:277–286, 2014.

Wolfsdorf JI, Garvey K: Diabetes mellitus in children. In Jameson L, DeGroot L, editors: *Endocrinology adult and pediatric*, ed 7, Philadelphia, 2016, Saunders, pp 854–882.

Writing Group for the TRIGR Study Group: Effect of hydrolyzed infant formula vs conventional formula on the risk of type 1 diabetes, *JAMA* 319:38, 2018.

Yeung W, Rawlinson W, Craig M: Enterovirus infection and type 1 diabetes mellitus: Systematic review and meta-analysis of observational molecular studies, *BMJ* 342(7794):421, 2011.

ENCOPRESIS

Method of
Sarah Houssayni, MD

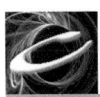

CURRENT DIAGNOSIS

- Voluntary or involuntary passage of stools into inappropriate places at least once a month for 3 consecutive months once a chronologic or developmental age of 4 years has been reached.
- Encopresis can be primary when it persists from infancy onward or secondary when it appears after toilet training.
- The behavior is not due to the direct effects of a substance such as a laxative or a general medical condition except those associated with constipation.
- Distinguishing subtypes is essential because treatment differs:
  - Retentive encopresis: occurs as a result of involuntary leakage of liquid stools due to severe constipation and impaction.
  - Nonretentive encopresis: children pass bowel movements into their underwear due to their refusal to use the toilet.
  - Children occasionally fail to wipe after bowel movements and the secondary soiling should be distinguished from encopresis.

CURRENT THERAPY

Retentive Encopresis
Initial Disimpaction
- Hyperphosphate enemas (Pedia-Lax Enema) (one daily for 2 or 3 days):
  - Less than 1 year old: 60mL.[3]
  - Greater than 1 year old: 6mL/kg, up to 135mL twice.[3]
- Glycerin suppositories (Glycerin Pediatric Suppositories) for infants and toddlers.

Older Children—Slow Disimpaction
- Polyethylene glycol with electrolytes (Golytely, Colyte)[1] ingested over 2–3 days: 25mL/kg/hr up to 1L/hr until stooling clear bowel movements. (This is not approved for bowel cleansing for children.)
- Over 5–7 days:
  - Mineral oil[1] 3mL/kg twice a day for 1 week. (Mineral oil is not approved for use in children younger than 6 years of age.)
  - Lactulose[1] 2mL/kg twice a day for 1 week.
  - Magnesium hydroxide (Milk of Magnesia) 2mL/kg twice a day for 1 week.
  - Polyethylene glycol without electrolyte (MiraLax)[1] 1.5g/kg/day for 3 days.

Maintenance Therapy
- Polyethylene glycol 3350 (MiraLax)[1] age greater than 1 month: 0.7g/kg divided into 1–2 doses daily.
- Lactulose or sorbitol 70% solution age greater than 1 month: 1–3mL/kg/day divided into 1–2 doses daily for 1–3 months.
- Sennosides (Senna, Senna-GRX, Senexon) are habit forming, doses vary greatly in the different available formulations, and they can only be used for short-term treatment. Give at bedtime for a morning bowel movement. Dose is 5mL (1 tablet) for 1-[1] to 5-year-olds and 2 tablets for 5- to 15-year-olds for a maximum of three tablets daily. (Sennosides are not approved for use in children younger than 2 years of age.)
- Glycerin enemas and bisacodyl suppositories (Dulcolax) can be used for short-term constipation treatment.

- Glycerin/saline enema in patients greater than 10 years of age: 20–30mL/day (solution of 1/2 glycerin and 1/2 normal saline).
- Bisacodyl suppositories in patients greater than 10 years of age: 10mg daily.

Nonretentive Encopresis
- **NO** medical treatment.
- Clean up soiling immediately, involve the child.
- Ensure adequate water and dietary fiber intake.
- Avoid use of stool softeners and laxatives.
- **STOP** all reminders, make child responsible for own toilet habits.
- Use rewards when child defecates in toilet.
- Refer to health care professional when refractory (refuses to sit on toilet and older than 5 years of age, refuses to take medication, is older than 8 years of age with nonretentive encopresis).

---

[1]Not FDA approved for this indication.
[3]Exceeds dosage recommended by the manufacturer; manufacturer-recommended doses are: 5–11 y, 1 bottle (60 mL); 2–4 y, half bottle (30 mL); <2 y, do not use.

Encopresis is the voluntary or involuntary passage of stools at least once a month for 3 consecutive months once a chronologic or developmental age of 4 years has been reached. Encopresis is classified as primary when it persists from infancy onward or secondary when it appears after toilet training. Retentive encopresis occurs as a result of involuntary leakage of liquid stools due to severe constipation and fecal impaction. Nonretentive encopresis occurs in children who pass stool into their underwear due to their refusal to use the toilet. It is important to distinguish between the types of encopresis, because treatment differs.

Epidemiology
The prevalence of encopresis is reported to be 4% in 5- to 6-year-olds and 1.5% in 11- to 12-year-olds. Affected boys outnumber girls by a factor of anywhere from 3:1 to 5:1 depending on the source. Encopresis tends to decrease with age. A large number of children with encopresis go unreported due to the shame associated with the condition and underdiagnosis of the condition.

Diagnosis
The diagnosis of encopresis includes the following four criteria: (1) Repeated passage of feces into inappropriate places such as in clothing or on the floor, whether intentional or involuntary. (2) At least one event a month for at least 3 months. (3) A chronologic age of at least 4 years or an equivalent developmental level. (4) The behavior is not due exclusively to the direct physiologic effects of a substance such as a laxative or a general medical condition other than constipation.

Differential Diagnosis
Retentive encopresis is organic in less than 5% of the affected patients. Organic causes include hypothyroidism, hypercalcemia, cerebral palsy, abnormal anatomy of the anus, Hirschsprung's disease, cystic fibrosis, and neuropathy with secondary impaired voiding sensation. Spinal cord conditions such as tethered cord, spina bifida occulta, and spinal cord dysplasia affect stooling through diminished bowel sensation and secondary fecal retention.

Pathophysiology
Patients who are severely constipated hold stools back because of the pain associated with defecation. This becomes a vicious cycle of constipation, rectal dilation, and secondary encopresis. Frequently, emotional problems emerge due to the fear and shame associated with the problem. Control issues with parents trying

TABLE 1	Characteristic Symptoms of Retentive and Nonretentive Encopresis

Retentive Encopresis

- Constipation
- Stained underwear
- Fewer than three bowel movements per week
- Large-caliber or hard stools
- Abdominal pain, reports of bloated sensation
- Odor of feces from leakage onto underwear
- Difficult or painful defecation
- Enuresis
- Overflow incontinence
- Anorexia

Nonretentive Encopresis

- Passage of stools in inappropriate places without presence of constipation
- Refusal to sit on toilet even though old enough to (older than 5 years, even older than 8 years at times)
- Refusal to take medications
- Child may be depressed

to take the stooling issues at hand may worsen the constipation problem.

From 10% to 20% of encopretic patients are not constipated. They are frequently preschoolers or school-age children who are postponing their bowel movements too long because they are distracted or because they associate the bathroom with an unpleasant experience (i.e., fear or disgust).

Clinical Manifestations

History

The history should assess for size and consistency of stools, as well as stooling intervals. Families often confuse soiling with stooling, leading to inaccurate reporting of the frequency of bowel movements. Characteristic symptoms of retentive and nonretentive encopresis differ (Table 1).

In retentive encopresis the physician may elicit a history of difficult or painful defecation, crying with bowel movements, and posturing that suggests the child is deliberately holding back stools due to the pain associated with passage.

Children may suddenly become still or hide during play, cross their legs, grimace, or shift their position in an attempt to retain stools. The physician should assess for a history of enuresis and urinary tract infections, anorexia, sensations of bloating, fullness, and abdominal pain leading to the patient's avoidance of food and weight loss. Obtain a dietary history including fiber, fluid, and dairy intake. The historian needs to inquire about streaks of blood on toilet paper and underwear. With retentive encopresis, when the child does pass stool, it may be of large caliber and hard, indicative of constipation.

With nonretentive encopresis, the history often reveals bowel movements of normal size and consistency passed into the underwear once or twice a day. Symptoms of constipation are usually absent. A history of behavioral problems, child-parent struggles, and history of abuse may be elicited. Toilet avoidance is common.

Patients with encopresis eventually develop secondary emotional problems, which can be elicited from the history taking.

Physical Examination

Retentive Encopresis

In retentive soiling the physical examination should assess for abdominal distention and tenderness on palpation. A mass can be occasionally felt in the midline in the suprapubic area. This mass of hardened fecal matter most commonly involves the rectosigmoid area and can sometimes extend throughout the entire colon. If the patient is anxious or in pain and tightens the rectus abdominis, this mass can be missed. Rectal examination is a must; it can be done with minimal discomfort. Rectal examination assesses the dilation of the rectum, which may be 6 to 10 cm wide. It is usually packed with stools with clay-like consistency. Visually inspect the anal opening for tone, fissure, and hemorrhoids.

Nonretentive Encopresis

The child with nonretentive encopresis typically has a normal abdominal examination, is likely to have a rectal vault that is not dilated, and the stool will be of normal caliber and consistency. The rectal vault may be empty if the child has just passed a bowel movement. The anal opening may reveal protruding fecal material in children who are deliberate stool holders.

Treatment

Encopresis is treated through a multistep approach. First, clearing the colon of fecal material will allow the dilated rectal vault and rectosigmoid colon to return to normal. The rectal cleanout can be achieved in different ways (see Current Therapy). Enemas and stool softeners are often used in combination.

Maintenance is achieved by keeping stools soft and ensuring daily bowel movements with mineral oil and hyperosmolar agents (e.g., Miralax[1]) that are very safe and can be used from a very young age and are not habit forming. The goal is painless stools once or twice a day with no associated withholding behavior.

Education is key for families so that they understand the physiology and process of stool elimination. Frustration is associated with failure, guilt, and depression and should be replaced with a positive attitude if success is to be achieved.

- Patients should sit daily on the toilet for 5 minutes after meals twice a day.
- Families need to keep a record of the events, as well as a record for success.
- Soiled underwear should be changed as soon as noticed and the child should be cleaned and changed in a timely, emotionally neutral fashion.
- As soon as compliance wanes, the problem is expected to return and is sometimes worse than the previous episode.
- The care provider's continued involvement in titrating medication with the patient's symptoms is necessary.
- Pain-related impaction can be cured in the majority of cases with medical management of the initial presentation. The success rate is reported to be about 70% with psychogenic impaction.
- With nonretentive encopresis, behavioral modification is essential. Stress reduction, effective coping techniques, relaxation training, and a combination of individual and family therapy is sometimes indicated.

---

[1]Not FDA approved for this indication.

References

Baker SS, et al: Clinical practice guideline. Evaluation and treatment of constipation in infants and children: recommendations of the North American Society for Pediatric Gastroenterology, Hepatology and Nutrition, *J Pediatr Gastroenterol Nutr* 43:e1–e13, 2006.

Becker A, Ruby M, El Khatib D, et al: Central nervous system processing of emotions with faecal incontinence, *Acta Paediatr* 100:e267–e747, 2011.

Boris NM, Dalton R, et al: Encopresis. *Nelson Textbook of Pediatrics*, ed 19, Philadelphia, 2011, Saunders.

Brazzelli M, Griffiths P: Behavioral and cognitive interventions with or without other treatments for the management of faecal incontinence in children, Art. No. CD002240 *Cochrane Database Syst Rev*(2), 2006. https://doi.org/10.1002/14651858.CD002240.pub3.

Coelho DP: Encopresis. A medical and family approach, *Pediatr Nurs* 37:107–112, 2011.

Har AF, Groffie JM: Encopresis, *Pediatr Rev* 31:368–374, 2010.

Raghumath N, Glassman MS, Halata MS, et al: Anorectal motility abnormalities in children with encopresis and chronic constipation, *J Pediatr* 158:293–296, 2011.

EPILEPSY IN INFANTS AND CHILDREN

Method of
Adam L. Hartman, MD

CURRENT DIAGNOSIS

- At initial diagnosis, determine whether the event was a seizure or a non-epileptic event.
- If appropriate, diagnose an epilepsy *syndrome*.
- Age of onset aids in the development of a differential diagnosis.

CURRENT THERAPY

- Selection of an antiseizure medicine should be made based on the type of seizure.
- General principles include the use of a single agent at the lowest effective dose with the goal of no side effects.
- Epilepsy can be associated with comorbidities, including depression and anxiety. Successful management includes referrals and/or management of these and associated psychosocial issues.

A seizure can be defined as clinical signs or symptoms resulting from abnormal neuronal firing. Epilepsy is defined as either (1) at least two unprovoked seizures occurring >24 hours apart; (2) one unprovoked seizure and a probability of further seizures similar to the general recurrence risk (at least 60%) after two unprovoked seizures, occurring over the next 10 years; or (3) diagnosis of an epilepsy syndrome. There may be associated psychological, social, and cognitive consequences. Approximately 3% to 5% of the US population have had a seizure (mostly febrile seizures). Nearly 1% of the US population are being treated actively for seizures at any given time. Infants and children represent one of the two major peaks in seizure incidence, making this a very common diagnosis in pediatric practice.

Risk Factors
The primary risk factors for epilepsy in any age group include a history of meningitis, encephalitis, brain trauma, complicated perinatal course, and febrile seizures. Other risk factors for seizures include cortical or developmental malformations, certain inborn errors of metabolism or genetic syndromes, congenital infections, stroke, intracranial hemorrhage, acute metabolic abnormalities, and drug withdrawal.

Pathophysiology
Because the primary abnormality is abnormal neuron firing, many different types of pathology can lead to seizures. Abnormalities in neuronal networks (e.g., cortical malformations), structure (e.g., abnormal dendrite structure in trisomy 21), or ion channels (e.g., *KCNQ2*) can lead to seizures. In many cases, an underlying cause of seizures cannot be identified. Some forms of epilepsy have been linked to various genetic mutations, although the exact relationship between specific genotypes and phenotypes is unclear for most.

Clinical Manifestations
Broadly speaking, the clinical manifestations of seizures vary depending on which brain structures are involved. Although most people think of seizures only as generalized tonic–clonic seizures (GTCS), a wide variety of signs and symptoms can be caused by seizures. Furthermore, a GTCS may be the initial manifestation of a seizure (i.e., as seen in primary generalized epilepsy) or it may be the end result of a seizure that started in one brain location and then spread to the rest of the brain (e.g., a focal-onset seizure with spread to other broad cortical regions of the brain). These two broad categories (generalized versus focal onset) are approached somewhat differently from a diagnostic and therapeutic perspective.

Signs of a generalized seizure (i.e., those involving abnormal neuronal firing in both sides of the brain) include loss of interaction or staring (absence seizures), myoclonus, tonic posturing, and/or tonic–clonic seizures. Signs of focal-onset seizures can involve specific regions controlling motor, sensory, or autonomic function, a loss of interaction and/or awareness, or automatisms (chewing, lip smacking, repetitive hand motions), to name a few. Patients with focal seizures might have an aura (a warning sign just prior to the seizure). The aura is an altered sensory function that can include salty or metallic taste, tingling sensations, rising sensation in the abdomen, déjà vu, jamais vu, sense of fear, or a nonspecific feeling that something is about to happen. After a seizure, patients also can have a period of postictal lethargy, confusion, or irritability. The latter can be misinterpreted by bystanders as disruptive behavior and has led to inappropriate interventions, even by law enforcement. This becomes a safety issue for the patient. Education about this type of behavior, if present, is critical.

The initial symptoms or signs of a seizure are the most important in determining whether a seizure is generalized or focal in origin because they often localize the anatomic site of pathology. Thus, it is the beginning of a seizure, rather than its end, that is most useful in making a specific diagnosis.

Diagnosis and Management
History and Physical Examination
A detailed history is usually more valuable than any expensive test in diagnosing a seizure or epilepsy. In addition to a description of the actual event, it is useful to inquire about subtle signs that might not be recognized by observers as a seizure, including staring spells, myoclonic jerks, loss of time, and unexplained nocturnal tongue biting, enuresis, or emesis. The presence of postictal weakness can help localize the hemisphere of onset after a focal seizure, even if secondarily generalized. Making the diagnosis of a specific epilepsy syndrome allows the clinician to develop a plan for further diagnosis and treatment and to counsel about prognosis. On physical examination, any signs of focal neurologic deficits can indicate an underlying lesion. A skin examination might identify a neurophakomatosis, such as tuberous sclerosis complex or Sturge Weber syndrome.

Diagnostic Studies
In selected cases, typical clinical findings in the right clinical context strongly support the diagnosis of epilepsy, but an electroencephalogram (EEG) may be required to confirm the diagnosis. Even if the patient does not have a seizure during the EEG recording, interictal findings (when the patient is not having a seizure) can provide enough evidence to make the diagnosis of epilepsy. Under ideal circumstances, a single EEG can detect epileptiform activity in a patient with untreated generalized epilepsy about 75% of the time, making it a very sensitive test. In contrast, an EEG can detect epileptiform activity in a patient with focal-onset seizures only 50% of the time (although this number increases to about 90% after three EEGs have been done). Conversely, a normal interictal EEG (particularly one that includes sleep and provocative maneuvers such as intermittent photic stimulation and hyperventilation) in an untreated patient suggests, but is not necessarily diagnostic of, a focal rather than generalized onset.

Other ancillary studies can show underlying structural lesions that lead to epilepsy or provide physiologic information. Magnetic resonance imaging (MRI) can be useful in detecting lesions such as tumors, cortical dysgenesis, and strokes (both ischemic and hemorrhagic). Recent advances in image analysis have substantially improved the ability to find subtle regions of cortical dysgenesis that may be the source of seizures. Positron-emission tomography (PET) scans may show regions of abnormal metabolism that might not be evident on MRI. Another nuclear medicine study, single photon emission tomography (SPECT), can be used to identify the region of onset of a seizure. Functional MRI (fMRI) studies show regions involved in a specific task (e.g., motor or language).

Magnetoencephalography, when combined with MRI, can be useful in detecting areas of abnormal electrical activity that might not be evident on a scalp EEG recording. Neuropsychology evaluations can aid in localization of regions of dysfunction and also aid in determining risk for loss of function if surgery is performed. The intracarotid amobarbital (Amytal)[1] test (Wada test) or intracarotid methohexital (Brevital)[1] test is used to lateralize language function and memory; fMRI is being investigated as a replacement for aspects of this invasive test. Some institutions use intracranial electrodes to localize the onset of a seizure prior to a surgical resection and to identify regions of eloquent neurologic function (regions where critical function would be lost if they were resected).

Specific Epilepsy Syndromes

Some of the more common syndromes are described here, listed by typical age at presentation.

Neonatal Seizures

Seizures in neonates can be caused by any type of neurologic pathology, including infections (prenatal or postnatal), strokes, hemorrhages, electrolyte abnormalities, cortical dysgenesis, inborn errors of metabolism (including vitamin B_6 dependency), genetic syndromes, drug (illicit and licit) withdrawal, and medications. Some neonatal seizure syndromes (benign idiopathic neonatal seizures and benign familial neonatal seizures) are benign in terms of resolution of seizures; early infantile epileptic encephalopathy (Ohtahara syndrome) and early myoclonic encephalopathy frequently are refractory to medical treatment and have a poor prognosis for development. Neonatal seizures should be managed in conjunction with specialists.

Febrile Seizures

Febrile seizures are the most common type of seizure, occurring in 3% to 5% of people in the United States. Febrile seizures, even though they can recur, are not diagnostic of epilepsy because they are provoked (i.e., by fever). With an onset between 1 month and 5 years of age (and almost always outgrown by 6 to 7 years of age), these seizures can be generalized or focal in onset. Meningitis and encephalitis also can manifest with seizures and fever and thus are exclusion criteria for febrile seizures because the prognosis and treatment are completely different. Febrile seizures that last longer than 15 minutes, have a focal onset, or occur more than once in a febrile illness are complex febrile seizures (only one of the three criteria are needed to make the diagnosis). Patients with complex febrile seizures are at a higher risk for developing epilepsy, although the overall risk is still low (4%). In patients who lack all three of these factors (i.e., simple febrile seizures), routine imaging, blood work, lumbar puncture, and EEG are not necessary for diagnosing the cause of the seizure. Rather, the workup should be guided by other concerns, such as dehydration, concern for occult bacteremia, or, in the appropriate clinical context, meningitis.

Approximately one-third of patients have a recurrence of a febrile seizure. Factors that increase the recurrence risk include very young age at onset, family history of febrile seizures, low-grade fever at onset of the seizure, frequent febrile illnesses, or the occurrence of the seizure in the first hour of the fever. Febrile seizures always are outgrown, so typically long-term seizure prophylaxis is not used. Oral diazepam (Valium) prophylaxis[1], started at the onset of fever, prevents febrile seizures but can lead to excessive sedation. Patients who have prolonged febrile seizures can benefit from rectal diazepam gel (Diastat) or other benzodiazepines given soon after the onset of a febrile seizure to prevent additional prolonged seizures or febrile status epilepticus.

A similarly good prognosis is seen in infants and children who have febrile seizures in the setting of acute gastroenteritis (whether febrile or not). The risk of epilepsy is increased after a febrile seizure in the setting of a complex febrile seizure, abnormal development, frequent febrile seizures, or a family history of epilepsy.

Infantile Spasms

With an onset typically around 4 to 8 months of age, infantile spasms consist of a triad of typical seizures (head drops and brief flexor and/or extensor spasms occurring in clusters around sleep transitions), a highly disorganized multifocal EEG pattern called hypsarrhythmia, and developmental delays. Between 70% and 90% of patients have identifiable underlying neurologic pathology associated with this syndrome. This is one of the most medically intractable epilepsy syndromes, and the prognosis for seizure control and development is very poor, except in a small subset of patients with no identifiable underlying pathology. Treatment typically is with corticosteroids (prednisolone [Orapred][1] or ACTH [Acthar HP]), or vigabatrin (Sabril), which is commonly the first-line treatment in infants with tuberous sclerosis complex (Box 1).

Dravet Syndrome

The typical presentation for Dravet syndrome is a prolonged febrile seizure involving one side of the body (hemiclonic) or recurrent GTCS in a previously normal infant. After a relatively quiescent period, seizures (including myoclonic, focal, and absence) may appear in the second year of life. Additional features include developmental abnormalities, ataxia, and extrapyramidal signs. Seizures induced by heat (either with fevers or exogenous) may be noted.

Genetic testing for mutations in the *SCN1A* gene is recommended because this eliminates the need for other extensive testing for an underlying diagnosis and allows the clinician to prognosticate. The EEG may be normal initially but later shows generalized spike-and-wave complexes and may show focal abnormalities. Treatment typically is with antiseizure medications; drugs that block sodium channels are typically avoided because they may exacerbate seizures. The ketogenic diet may be useful. Heated environments might need to be avoided and accommodations (e.g., air-conditioned buses and classrooms) may be recommended in some cases.

Lennox–Gastaut Syndrome

Typically occurring between the ages of 1 and 8 years, Lennox–Gastaut syndrome is characterized by mixed seizure types, a markedly abnormal EEG, and abnormal development. Virtually any type of brain pathology can be seen as an antecedent of Lennox–Gastaut syndrome. The syndrome of infantile spasms is a common antecedent. Patients with Lennox–Gastaut syndrome typically have combinations of tonic, atonic, and absence seizures, although focal-onset seizures and GTCS also occur. The EEG shows slow (less than 2.5 Hz) spike-and-wave complexes and occasionally a paroxysmal fast pattern, although background slowing also is very common. The vast majority of patients have developmental delays. Diagnosis is made in the setting of typical findings. Seizures are very difficult to control, but treatment commonly includes medicines and/or nonpharmacologic options (see Box 1). The prognosis for seizure control and development is poor. The differential diagnosis of Lennox–Gastaut syndrome also includes Doose syndrome, which is characterized by myoclonic and astatic seizures (although other seizure types can occur). In Doose syndrome, patients often have normal development and a good prognosis once seizures are controlled.

Childhood and Juvenile Absence Epilepsy

Most clinicians are familiar with childhood and juvenile absence epilepsy. The typical age of onset is 4 to 14 years, and there is a slight female predominance. The most common type of seizure is

---

[1] Not FDA approved for this indication.

[1] Not FDA approved for this indication.

BOX 1   Recommendations for Treatment

Infantile Spasms, West Syndrome
Oral steroids[1]
Adrenocorticotropic hormone
Ketogenic diet
Topiramate (Topamax)[1]
Valproate (Depakote)[1]
Zonisamide (Zonegran)[1]
Pyridoxine[1]
Benzodiazepines[1]
Surgery (if there is a lesion)
Vigabatrin (Sabril) (may use first if patient has tuberous sclerosis)

Dravet Syndrome
Valproate[1]
Topiramate[1]
Stiripentol (Diacomit)
Cannabidiol (Epidiolex)
Fenfluramine (Fintepla)
Ketogenic diet
Benzodiazepines[1]

Lennox–Gastaut Syndrome
Valproate[1]
Clobazam (Onfi)
Lamotrigine (Lamictal)
Topiramate
Benzodiazepines
Rufinamide (Banzel)
Felbamate (Felbatol)
Ketogenic diet
Vagus nerve stimulator
Surgery

Doose Syndrome
Valproate[1]
Ketogenic diet
Lamotrigine[1]
Ethosuximide (Zarontin)[1]
Vagus nerve stimulator

Childhood Absence Epilepsy
Ethosuximide
Valproate
Lamotrigine[1]

Juvenile Absence Epilepsy
Valproate
Ethosuximide
Lamotrigine[1]

Childhood Epilepsy with Centrotemporal Spikes
Levetiracetam (Keppra)
Carbamazepine (Tegretol)
Zonisamide
Oxcarbazepine (Trileptal)
Lacosamide (Vimpat)

Juvenile Myoclonic Epilepsy
Valproate[1]
Levetiracetam
Topiramate
Zonisamide[1]
Lamotrigine

---

[1] Not FDA approved for this indication.
Adapted from Muthugovindan D, Hartman AL: Pediatric epilepsy syndromes. *Neurologist* 2010;16:223–237.

---

an absence seizure, characterized by staring and loss of interaction lasting 5 to 20 seconds, occurring tens to hundreds of times per day. Patients also can have GTCS (particularly if they present later in childhood) and/or myoclonic seizures. There is no aura and there are no postictal behavior changes. Absence seizures can be induced with 3 to 4 minutes of hyperventilation at the bedside. The interictal EEG shows a 3Hz generalized spike-and-wave pattern. Treatment includes ethosuximide (Zarontin) if the patient has not had a GTCS (see Box 1). Valproate (Depakene) is the first choice if the patient has had a GTCS. Nearly two-thirds of patients grow out of their seizures by young adulthood.

Childhood Epilepsy With Centrotemporal Spikes and "Benign" Occipital Epilepsy

One of the more common epilepsies in childhood, childhood epilepsy with centrotemporal spikes (also known commonly as benign rolandic epilepsy), first occurs between the ages of 3 and 13 years. The typical seizure involves the face and/or hand, but GTCS also are common. The most common time for a seizure is within the first few hours of sleep, but a minority of patients only have daytime seizures. The diagnosis is made based on a typical seizure history and EEG (which shows spikes over bilateral central and temporal regions). Learning disabilities, which may be very subtle, are fairly common in patients with this syndrome, so extra vigilance is warranted.

Panayiotopoulos syndrome (also known as "benign" occipital epilepsy) can occur between the ages of 1 and 14 years (with a peak at 4 to 5 years) with autonomic symptoms such as emesis, pallor, flushing, or tachycardia, as well as focal-onset or generalized seizures. Patients also can have visual symptoms. The EEG can show sharp waves in the occipital regions, but abnormal activity has been reported in other brain regions as well.

Because most patients have fewer than six seizures in both syndromes, medicine usually is not prescribed. Seizures typically are outgrown by adolescence. Patients with frequent seizures are treated with medicine. Gastaut occipital epilepsy (not to be confused with Lennox–Gastaut syndrome) occurs in older children and can require medication treatment because of seizure recurrence.

Juvenile Myoclonic Epilepsy

The most common form of generalized seizures in adolescents, juvenile myoclonic epilepsy first occurs between the ages of 12 and 20 years. Most patients have brief myoclonic seizures that tend to cluster in the early morning hours (but may occur at any time of day). Patients often are unaware that these are seizures but on careful questioning report loss of control of a toothbrush or spoon. Many patients also have absence seizures. The interictal EEG typically shows a 4 to 5Hz generalized spike-and-wave pattern. The prognosis for lifelong remission of seizures is poor, although most patients' seizures are controlled easily with medicines (see Box 1). There is a subgroup of patients (many of whom previously had childhood absence epilepsy) whose seizures are very challenging to control.

Other Epilepsy Syndromes With a Poor Prognosis

Landau–Kleffner syndrome and epileptic encephalopathy with continuous spike-and-wave during sleep are syndromes characterized by mild seizures, nearly continuous epileptiform activity during sleep, and neuropsychological deterioration. Progressive myoclonus epilepsy represents a family of disorders characterized by medically intractable epilepsy (commonly including myoclonic seizures) and significant neurologic deterioration. Underlying diagnoses include myoclonus epilepsy with ragged red fibers (MERRF), Unverricht–Lundborg disease, and Lafora disease, among others. Gelastic (laughing) seizures can be caused either by hypothalamic hamartomas or temporal lobe seizures. The prognosis depends on response to medication and/or surgery but is not always bad. Rasmussen syndrome is characterized by medically intractable epilepsy, progressive unilateral neurologic deficits, and cortical atrophy on MRI. Because they are so rare, any suspicion of these diagnoses should prompt referral to a pediatric epilepsy center with expertise in diagnosing and managing these conditions.

Tumors

Brain tumors can manifest with seizures and are covered in a separate chapter. Certain developmental tumors are seen with an increased frequency in pediatric epilepsy clinics, including dysembryoplastic neuroepithelial tumors (DNET) and gangliogliomas. These tumors typically manifest with seizures and can be associated with malformations of cortical development. EEG can show abnormalities over the involved region but can be falsely localizing as well. MRI shows the location of the tumor but can underestimate the extent of surrounding abnormal tissue. If seizures are not controlled with medicine, or if there is progression in tumor size, resection surgery is recommended.

Cortical Dysgenesis

Abnormal brain development can lead to inappropriately wired brain circuitry, which can be the underlying substrate for seizures. Two forms of abnormal cortical development include lissencephaly (abnormally smooth, or simplified, gyral pattern) and polymicrogyria. Another form of cortical dysgenesis, malformations of cortical development, is graded based on both dyslamination of the normal six-layer neocortex and the occurrence of abnormal cell types (including balloon cells). EEG shows epileptiform abnormalities over the involved region. MRI shows the anatomic location of the involved tissue in more severe cases but may be normal if the abnormality is mild. In patients with focal abnormalities, if seizures are not controlled with medicine, resection surgery is an option. Patients with more extensive abnormalities can try nonpharmacologic options if medicines do not work.

Mesial Temporal Lobe Epilepsy With Hippocampal Sclerosis

The mesial temporal structures (particularly the hippocampus) can become scarred, and the remaining neurons develop abnormal connections. This can lead to medically intractable seizures. EEG shows interictal epileptiform activity over the temporal head regions. Imaging studies show atrophic mesial temporal structures with increased signal on T2-weighted FLAIR (fluid-attenuated inversion recovery) images. A temporal lobectomy should be considered as an option for patients who do not respond to two appropriately chosen and tolerated medications for seizure control.

Comorbidities

The definition of epilepsy includes comorbidities, which in turn can have a significant impact on quality of life. Clinicians must actively probe for these underlying conditions in order to optimize outcomes. People with epilepsy have increased rates of depression and anxiety compared to the general population. Developmental disorders and learning disabilities are more common in children with epilepsy, as are attention-deficit/hyperactivity disorder and migraines. Once identified, these conditions should be managed by clinicians experienced with their treatment.

Differential Diagnosis

The differential diagnosis of seizures depends largely on age. In infants, opisthotonic posturing can be seen in gastroesophageal reflux disease (Sandifer syndrome). Some infants have benign myoclonus or shuddering attacks. The EEG in all these disorders is normal, but the diagnosis can be made based on the history. Brief resolved unexplained events can appear to be seizures, although apnea rarely is the only manifestation of a seizure. Hyperekplexia is an exaggerated startle response that can be due to abnormal glycine receptor subunits in the spinal cord. Because of potential involvement of the diaphragm, this disorder can be lethal. In children, stereotypies can be paroxysmal and persistent, but the behaviors during these episodes are typical enough that the diagnosis usually is made based on the history.

Breath-holding spells may be associated with an older infant or toddler who is upset, followed by unresponsiveness and either facial pallor or mild cyanosis, lasting less than 1 to 3 minutes. These episodes are typical enough that the history is all that is usually needed to make the diagnosis. Children with pallid breath-holding spells are at higher risk for vasovagal syncope in the adolescent and young adult ages.

Night terrors, one of the parasomnias, occur in toddlers and young children. Persistent screaming (lasting minutes to 1 hour) and lack of memory of the event are seen commonly; the latter raises a question of whether the child had a seizure. Most commonly, these are outgrown by the late preschool years.

Patients with syncope may have a few mild clonic twitches, but this typically does not represent epilepsy. Screening orthostatic blood pressures should be done to rule out one of the orthostatic syndromes. Consideration also should be given to an electrocardiogram or a cardiology consultation in the appropriate clinical context.

Older children and adolescents can have psychogenic nonepileptic events, also known as psychogenic nonepileptic seizures. Cognitive behavioral therapy is helpful in some patients. This is a very important diagnosis to make so that patients receive appropriate treatment and are not exposed to medicines where the risks outweigh the benefits.

In all age groups, focal lesions such as infarctions, hemorrhages, and infections should be considered in the differential diagnosis, although the diagnostic workup should be guided by the history and physical examination.

Treatment

The goals for treatment are to maximize efficacy and minimize side effects. Medication is the first line of therapy for most patients. Nearly 70% to 80% of children are treated successfully by one of the first two medications tried. Practically speaking, neurologists try to use a single agent at the lowest tolerated dosage. Suggested medicines for the epilepsy syndromes discussed previously are listed in Box 1. Details about specific medicines are listed in Table 1. If one of the first two medicines tried does not work, there are three major options.

1. Trials of Additional Medication

Although the first two medicines might not work, new medicines often are introduced into the market. Clinical trials often show that a modest number of patients respond well to newer medicines, although the positive response to newer medicines is no greater overall than response to older medicines, despite lower rates of adverse effects and drug–drug interactions.

2. Surgery

Any patient who fails to respond to two appropriately-selected medications should be assessed for surgery. In patients with a potentially resectable lesion, surgery offers the greatest chance of seizure freedom. Ideal surgical candidates have identifiable lesions on imaging studies and a seizure onset zone that is distinct from eloquent cortex. Patients without identifiable lesions or those with multifocal or generalized seizures are poor candidates for resection surgery. Options for these patients include the vagus nerve stimulator, which has outstanding compliance and adherence because it is surgically implanted. Although this device significantly decreases seizure frequency in some patients, it only rarely leads to seizure freedom. Neurostimulation devices, some of which also include seizure detectors, are being introduced into clinical practice for adults and will be used in children in the future.

3. Diet Therapy

The concept of fasting to improve seizure control dates back to Hippocrates, but in modern times, dietary management of epilepsy is implemented using a high-fat, low-carbohydrate (adequate protein) ketogenic diet. A modified Atkins diet and a low glycemic index treatment have been used successfully as well. These diets require varying degrees of clinical supervision at centers experienced in their implementation.

TABLE 1 Summary of New Commonly Used Antiseizure Drugs

DRUG	MAINTENANCE DOSAGE*	STARTING DOSAGE*	HALF-LIFE (H)	COMMON SIDE EFFECTS	SERIOUS IDIOSYNCRATIC SIDE EFFECTS
Brivaracetam (Briviact)	> 16y, 25–100mg bid	50mg bid	9	Agitation, behavioral disinhibition, dizziness	Suicidality
Cannabidiol (Epidiolex)	5mg/kg bid (can go up to 10mg/kg bid)	2.5mg/kg bid	56–61	Somnolence, decreased appetite, diarrhea, transaminase elevations (check before initiating therapy), fatigue, rash, sleep disorders, infections	Severe encephalopathy leading to respiratory depression and oversedation, hepatic injury, suicidality
Cenobamate (Xcopri; adults only)	200mg once/day	12.5mg once daily, titrate per manfacturer	50–60	Somnolence, dizziness, aphasia, dysarthria, vertigo, diplopia, vomiting, constipation, diarrhea, transaminase elevations	Hyperkalemia, appendicitis, QTc shortening, DRESS, suicidality
Fenfluramine (Fintepla)	Maintenance >2y, w/o stiripentol: 0.1-0.35 mg/kg/dose bid; >2 y, w/ stiripentol and clobazam, 0.1-0.2 mg/kg/dose bid;	Starting 0.1 mg/kg/dose bid	20	Anorexia, diarrhea, fatigue, echocardiographic abnormalities, weight loss, blood pressure change, behavior changes, tremor, irritability, gastroenteritis, URI, rash	serotonin syndrome, suicidality, hypertension, angle-closure glaucoma
Clobazam (Onfi)	> 2y, < 30kg: 10mg bid > 2y, > 30kg: 20mg bid	> 2y, < 30kg: 5mg/d > 2y, > 30kg: 5mg bid	Parent drug: 36–42 Active metabolite: 71–82	Sedation irritability Needs to be tapered off slowly	Respiratory depression, benzodiazepine withdrawal, Stevens–Johnson syndrome
Eslicarbazepine (Aptiom)	4-17y (11-21kg), 400-600mg once/day 4-17y (22-31kg), 500-800mg once/day 4-17y (32-38kg), 600-900mg once/day 4-17y (>38kg), 800-1200mg once/day >17y, 800–1600mg once/day	4-17y (11-21kg), 200mg once/day 4-17y (22-31kg), 300mg once/day 4-17y (32-38kg), 300mg once/day >4y (>38kg), 400mg once/day	13–20	Somnolence, dizziness, hyponatremia, thyroid dysfunction	Stevens-Johnson, toxic epidermal necrolysis, withdrawal seizures if stopped abruptly
Lacosamide (Vimpat)	4-16y (11-<30kg), 3-6mg/kg bid 4-16y (30-50kg), 2-4mg/kg bid >4y (>50kg), 100–200mg bid	4-16y (<50kg), 1mg/kg bid >4y (≥50kg), 50mg bid	13	Somnolence, fatigue, headache	Cardiac conduction abnormalities, Stevens-Johnson syndrome, cytopenias
Levetiracetam (Keppra)	20–60mg/kg/d	10mg/kg/d, incr in 10-mg/kg increments	6–8	Agitation, behavioral disinhibition, rashes	Suicidal ideation
Oxcarbazepine (Trileptal)	30–60mg/kg/d	8–10mg/kg/d, incr by 10–15mg/kg increments	Parent drug: 2 Metabolite: 9	Hyponatremia, somnolence, lethargy, dizziness, blurred vision	Rash
Perampanel (Fycompa)	> 12y, 8–12mg at bedtime	> 12y, 2–4mg at bedtime	105h	Somnolence, headaches	Serious psychiatric and behavior reactions
Rufinamide (Banzel)	45mg/kg/d	10mg/kg/d	6–10	Nausea, vomiting, somnolence	Seizures, QT shortening
Stiripentol (Diacomit; to be used as a clobazam adjunct)	Up to 3g/day	25mg/kg bid	4.5–13	Somnolence, decreased appetite, agitation, ataxia, tremor, cytopenias, vomiting, weight gain	Suicidality, cytopenias, withdrawal seizures
Vigabatrin (Sabril)	50–150mg/kg/d	50mg/kg/d	7.5 (5.7 in infants)	Headache, dizziness, fatigue, tremor, swallowing problems, T2-weighted or DWI hyperintensities	Vision loss
Zonisamide (Zonegran)	> 16y: 100–600mg/d	> 16y: 100mg once/day	63	Somnolence, irritability, cognitive slowing, weight loss, renal stones, oligohidrosis	Rash

Abbreviations: DWI = diffusion-weighted imaging; incr = increase.
*Dosages should not exceed maximum adult dosages.

Monitoring

Seizure calendars (which can take the form of notebooks or electronic tools) are very useful for tracking frequency of events, especially if they are completed on a daily basis. There has been a recent explosion in wearable devices and other types of biotechnology for monitoring seizures and vital signs during seizures (for home use). Monitoring for medication-related adverse effects and comorbidities should continue during treatment. In addition, some comorbidities can occur even if seizures have stopped; there is good evidence for this in patients with childhood absence epilepsy, which typically is considered a "benign" syndrome because seizures typically resolve by adulthood. Patients taking certain medicines are screened periodically for evidence of renal and/or hepatic abnormalities and abnormal blood cell counts. Scenarios for testing drug levels include the following:
- Assessing adherence to a prescribed drug regimen
- Testing whether symptoms result from drug toxicity
- Determining whether a patient can benefit from higher amounts of medicine when the administered doses are already high (i.e., fast metabolizers)

Reminders about seizure-related safety should be reinforced periodically. GTCS counseling typically includes instructions about safety for the patient, including protecting the head and airway (putting the patient on his or her side to prevent aspiration) and not putting anything in the patient's mouth. Other safety topics include water safety and wearing helmets, as well as discouraging participation in certain sports (e.g., scuba diving). Periodic assessments of bone health should be considered for patients taking enzyme-inducing or enzyme-inhibiting medicines. Patients of an appropriate age should be counseled about local driving laws. Adolescent girls should be counseled about the effect of antiseizure medicines on hormonal forms of contraception (and vice versa). Consideration should be given to prescribing folate in this group, as well.

Complications

Single GTCS can lead to trauma (e.g., from a fall), tongue biting, pneumothorax, fractures of the vertebrae or limbs, and joint dislocations. A brief physical examination can rule out the more serious complications of a single GTCS. Adverse effects of medications are listed in Table 1. Surgical resections can lead to a variety of neurologic deficits, depending on which tissue is involved. Vagus nerve stimulator surgery can lead to hoarseness and coughing. Unsupervised diet therapy also can have adverse effects; such therapy should be undertaken only by centers with experience. Rarely, patients with epilepsy can die unexpectedly from no apparent cause, known as sudden unexplained death in epilepsy (SUDEP). The cause is unknown, but most (not all) patients have epilepsy that is resistant to medications. Counseling about this condition should be provided by an epilepsy expert.

Notice

This material does not represent the official view of the National Institute of Neurological Disorders and Stroke (NINDS), the National Institutes of Health (NIH), or any part of the US Federal Government. No official support or endorsement of this article by the NINDS or NIH is intended or should be inferred.

References

Baldin E, Hauser WA, Buchhalter JR, et al: Yield of epileptiform electroencephalogram abnormalities in incident unprovoked seizures: a population-based study, *Epilepsia* 55:1389–1398, 2014.

Dang LT, Silverstein FS: Drug treatment of seizures and epilepsy in newborns and children, *Pediatr Clin North Am* 64:1291–1308, 2017.

El Achkar CM, Olson HE, Poduri A, et al: The genetics of the epilepsies, *Curr Neurol Neurosci Rep* 15:39, 2015.

Fisher RS, Acevedo C, Arzimanoglou A, et al: ILAE official report: a practical clinical definition of epilepsy, *Epilepsia* 55:475–482, 2014.

Go CY, Mackay MT, Weiss SK, et al: Child Neurology Society, American Academy of Neurology: Evidence-based guideline update: medical treatment of infantile spasms. Report of the Guideline Development Subcommittee of the American Academy of Neurology and the Practice Committee of the Child Neurology Society, *Neurology* 78:1974–1980, 2012.

Muthugovindan D, Hartman AL: Pediatric epilepsy syndromes, *Neurologist* 16:223–237, 2010.

Scheffer IE, Berkovic S, Capovilla G, et al: ILAE classification of the epilepsies: position paper of the ILAE Commission for Classification and Terminology, *Epilepsia* 58:512–521, 2017.

Subcommittee on Febrile Seizures: American Academy of Pediatrics: Neurodiagnostic evaluation of the child with a simple febrile seizure, *Pediatrics* 127:389–394, 2011.

INFANT HYPERBILIRUBINEMIA

Method of
Sheevaun Khaki, MD

CURRENT DIAGNOSIS

- As bilirubin levels rise during the newborn period, jaundice appears and progresses caudally from head to toe.
- Hyperbilirubinemia is classified as conjugated or unconjugated; conjugated hyperbilirubinemia is always considered pathologic.
- Universal screening for hyperbilirubinemia with a total serum bilirubin (TSB) or transcutaneous bilirubin (TcB) should be performed for all newborns within the first 24 hours of life.
- The bilirubin level should be interpreted based on the newborn's hours of age, gestational age, and absence or presence of risk factors for hyperbilirubinemia.
- Standardized nomograms should be used to monitor the newborn's degree of hyperbilirubinemia and to initiate treatment.
- Newborns born to mothers with blood type O should have a blood type and Coombs' test performed to assess for possible ABO incompatibility when the bilirubin is approaching phototherapy threshold.

CURRENT THERAPY

- Newborn feeding should be emphasized to maintain hydration and promote clearance of bilirubin.
- Phototherapy should be initiated when the newborn has met the hour-specific phototherapy threshold.
- Newborns within 2 to 3 mg/dL of the exchange transfusion threshold should be hospitalized for initiation of phototherapy, possible intravenous fluid rehydration, and close monitoring.
- Occasionally, intravenous immunoglobulin (IVIG)[1] is used to manage hemolytic disease of the newborn due to ABO or Rhesus factor (Rh) incompatibility.

[1]Not FDA approved for this indication.

Background

Neonatal hyperbilirubinemia is common during the newborn period, with approximately 50% of term newborns developing jaundice in the first week of age. As bilirubin levels increase, clinical signs of jaundice develop due to deposition of bilirubin in the skin and mucous membranes. For the majority of newborns, this is a transient condition that does not require medical intervention. However, a small portion of late preterm and term newborns will develop hyperbilirubinemia that may require close monitoring and/or medical intervention. The goal of treating neonatal hyperbilirubinemia is to prevent bilirubin-induced neurologic dysfunction, acute bilirubin encephalopathy (ABE), and chronic bilirubin encephalopathy (CBE) or kernicterus. Various screening and monitoring strategies exist to prevent these serious outcomes.

Risk Factors

Prior to hospital discharge, all newborns should be systematically assessed for the risk of hyperbilirubinemia requiring intervention. The American Academy of Pediatrics (AAP) has developed a list of major and minor risk factors for the development of hyperbilirubinemia (Table 1). As part of this risk assessment, all mothers' blood types should be reviewed to determine whether the baby is at risk for hyperbilirubinemia due to ABO or Rhesus factor (Rh) incompatibility. The newborn's gestational age (GA) is particularly important as late preterm infants (GA 34w0d–36w6d) have additional feeding difficulties and relatively immature red blood cells (RBCs) and hepatic cells, which lead to both increased production and decreased clearance of bilirubin. A thorough family history may provide additional information regarding inheritable conditions such as glucose-6-phosphate dehydrogenase (G6PD) deficiency that lead to hemolysis and, therefore, hyperbilirubinemia. Additionally, there are certain factors that decrease the newborn's risk of developing severe hyperbilirubinemia, including GA ≥ 41 weeks, exclusive bottle feeding, black race, and hospital discharge after 72 hours of age.

Pathogenesis

An understanding of bilirubin metabolism is essential in determining the etiology of neonatal hyperbilirubinemia. Bilirubin results from the breakdown of heme, the majority of which comes from catabolism of hemoglobin from RBCs. There are multiple steps involved in the removal of bilirubin from the bloodstream. Initially, bilirubin is bound to albumin and transported to the liver where it is conjugated by uridine diphosphate glucuronosyltransferase (UGT1A1). Conjugated bilirubin is excreted into the biliary system and ultimately the gastrointestinal system. Finally, conjugated bilirubin is either deconjugated in the intestines by bacteria and reabsorbed back into the circulation or excreted as stool. A disturbance in any of the above steps of bilirubin clearance can lead to hyperbilirubinemia. Hyperbilirubinemia is classified into unconjugated (indirect) and conjugated (direct) forms.

Unconjugated Hyperbilirubinemia

Unconjugated hyperbilirubinemia results from either increased production or decreased clearance of indirect (unconjugated) bilirubin. Physiologic jaundice results from a combination of these processes. In this condition, bilirubin levels rise from increased number and turnover of RBCs due to the shorter life span of fetal RBCs, decreased activity of UGT1A1 in the liver, and increased enterohepatic circulation due to poor feeding and relative gut sterility. Breastfeeding jaundice results from increased enterohepatic circulation and mild dehydration as breastfeeding is established. Additionally, there are many pathologic conditions that may result in unconjugated hyperbilirubinemia. Hemolytic diseases such as isoimmune-mediated hemolysis (ABO or Rh incompatibility), RBC membrane defects (hereditary spherocytosis), or RBC enzyme defects (G6PD deficiency) contribute to significant morbidity. Decreased clearance of bilirubin may result from a defect in UGT1A1 (Crigler-Najjar syndrome types I and II, Gilbert syndrome), increased enterohepatic circulation due to impaired intestinal motility and poor milk intake, and breast milk jaundice.

Conjugated Hyperbilirubinemia

Conjugated hyperbilirubinemia is always considered pathologic. It is defined as a direct bilirubin concentration that is ≥20% of the total serum bilirubin (TSB). Direct bilirubin should be measured when the TSB is not responding appropriately to phototherapy or when jaundice persists past 2 weeks of age. Broadly, cholestatic jaundice can be divided into obstructive and hepatocellular etiologies. Obstructive etiologies include biliary atresia and choledochal cysts. Hepatocellular etiologies include endocrinopathies (thyroid abnormalities), metabolic disorders (galactosemia, tyrosinemia), and infection (sepsis, congenital infections). For newborns with jaundice past 2 weeks of age, total and direct bilirubin levels should be obtained to rule out biliary atresia, a diagnosis that deserves prompt identification and treatment.

Prevention

While mild physiologic jaundice cannot be prevented in most instances, more severe cases of indirect hyperbilirubinemia can be avoided. Starting in the prenatal setting, all pregnant women should be tested for ABO and Rh blood types and red blood cell antibodies to identify mothers whose newborns may be at risk of developing isoimmune hemolytic disease. Mothers who are Rh-negative should receive Rho(D) immune globulin (Rho-GAM) to prevent the development of antibodies after exposure to Rh-positive blood. Mothers should receive at least one dose between 26 and 28 weeks of pregnancy and another within 72 hours after delivery if the baby is found to be Rh-positive. All newborns born to Rh-negative mothers should have their blood type tested to allow for timely administration of RhoGAM. Additionally, mothers should receive RhoGAM after maternal or fetal bleeding during pregnancy, abdominal trauma, an invasive procedure, and with each pregnancy, including an ectopic pregnancy. If administered correctly, the risk of hemolytic disease of the fetus and newborn is significantly reduced. Pregnancies where mothers have an O blood type are considered to be a "setup" for ABO incompatibility. Early identification of ABO incompatibility may prevent more severe cases of hyperbilirubinemia.

Postnatally, provision of adequate nutrition helps prevent readmission for phototherapy. During the newborn hospitalization, mothers who intend to breastfeed should receive information and support to establish an adequate milk supply. Early and sustained skin-to-skin contact should be emphasized to promote lactogenesis and maternal-newborn dyads should be assessed for risks of delayed lactogenesis. Serial newborn weights should be obtained to document weight loss as an early sign of inadequate intake. The newborn early weight loss tool, NEWT, (https://www.newbornweight.org) may be used to identify newborns 36 weeks of gestation and greater who have lost an excessive amount of weight and incorporated into the decision

TABLE 1	Major and Minor Risk Factors for the Development of Severe Hyperbilirubinemia	
MAJOR RISK FACTORS	**MINOR RISK FACTORS**	
Pre-discharge TSB or TcB level in the high-risk zone	Pre-discharge TSB or TcB level in the high-intermediate-risk zone	
Jaundice observed in the first 24 hours	Gestational age 37–38 weeks	
Blood group incompatibility with positive direct antiglobulin test, other known hemolytic disease (e.g., G6PD deficiency), elevated end tidal carbon monoxide (ETCO)	Jaundice observed before discharge	
Gestational age 35–36 weeks	Previous sibling with jaundice	
Previous sibling received phototherapy	Macrosomic infant of a diabetic mother	
Cephalohematoma or significant bruising	Maternal age ≥ 25 years	
Exclusive breastfeeding, particularly if nursing is not going well and weight loss is excessive	Male gender	
East Asian race		

TcB, Transcutaneous bilirubin; *TSB*, total serum bilirubin.
From American Academy of Pediatrics, Subcommittee on Hyperbilirubinemia. Management of Hyperbilirubinemia in the Newborn Infant 35 or More Weeks of Gestation. *Pediatrics*. 2004;114:297–316.

to initiate supplemental feeds. Prevention of dehydration in the early newborn period may help prevent clinically significant hyperbilirubinemia.

Diagnosis

During the newborn hospitalization, the newborn should be assessed clinically for visible jaundice with all routine vital sign checks, preferably next to a well-lit window. The newborn who is jaundiced within the first 24 hours of age should have a TSB level drawn immediately as this finding is considered to be pathologic. It should be understood that while visual assessments are important to gauge progression of jaundice as it proceeds caudally from head to toe, they are particularly problematic in estimating the degree of hyperbilirubinemia and should not solely be relied upon. Rather, all newborns should undergo routine bilirubin testing either by TSB or transcutaneous (TcB) measurement within the first 24 hours of life. A TcB screening device offers the ability to estimate the bilirubin level quickly and avoids a painful procedure. However, providers must understand the limitations of their specific device (including decreased accuracy at higher bilirubin levels) and decide on thresholds where a serum level should be obtained.

The current AAP guidelines recommend plotting the measured bilirubin level on an hour-specific nomogram (Figure 1) to designate the newborn's risk for developing hyperbilirubinemia requiring treatment. A newborn's bilirubin level should be interpreted to determine what level of risk—low, low intermediate, high intermediate, high—they have of developing hyperbilirubinemia that requires phototherapy. Newborns in the high-intermediate or high-risk zones deserve additional consideration for the presence of risk factors that may be contributing to hyperbilirubinemia. Specifically, a blood type and direct Coombs' test should be obtained for newborns whose mothers are blood type O. If the baby is blood type A, B, or AB, this is referred to as a "setup" for ABO incompatibility. In this setting, a Coombs' test will evaluate the presence of anti-A or anti-B antibodies on the surface of the newborn's red blood cells that may be causing hemolysis. A positive Coombs' test does not automatically result in hyperbilirubinemia and, equally, a negative Coombs' test may be present in the setting of active hemolysis (e.g., G6PD deficiency).

The bilirubin risk zone can be used to help determine when the newborn should be reassessed for hyperbilirubinemia. As bilirubin levels peak around 3 to 5 days of age, determination of the newborn's risk is especially important for those discharged from the hospital prior to 72 hours of age as this will inform the decision regarding timing of outpatient follow-up. In general, newborns discharged prior to 24 hours of age should be seen by 72 hours, while those discharged between 24 and 48 hours of age should be seen by 96 hours. The majority of newborns will be discharged between 48 to 72 hours of age and they should be reevaluated in the outpatient setting by 120 hours of age. Those who have additional risk factors such as significant weight loss or an elevated bilirubin risk zone should be seen earlier in the outpatient clinic. After discharge, it is important for guardians to monitor their newborns for clinical signs of jaundice that may necessitate earlier medical follow-up care.

Both in the inpatient and outpatient settings, the TcB or TSB should be plotted on the hour-specific nomogram (Figure 2) to determine the level at which phototherapy should be initiated. The nomogram makes use of three separate curves that correspond to various risk factors for ABE, specifically isoimmune hemolytic disease, G6PD deficiency, asphyxia, lethargy, temperature instability, sepsis, acidosis, or albumin < 3.0 g/dL. Those who are defined as lower risk are GA ≥ 38 weeks and well; medium risk are GA ≥ 38 weeks and have risk factors or are GA 35 to 37 6/7 weeks and well; higher risk are GA 35 to 37 6/7 weeks and have risk factors.

Treatment

The treatment of hyperbilirubinemia is focused on effective and efficient removal of bilirubin from the bloodstream to prevent ABE and kernicterus. Guardians should be encouraged to feed their newborns frequently, a minimum of 8 to 12 times per day, especially for those who are breastfed, as frequent feeding will help establish the mother's milk supply. The newborn's weight and urine and stool output should be assessed daily during the

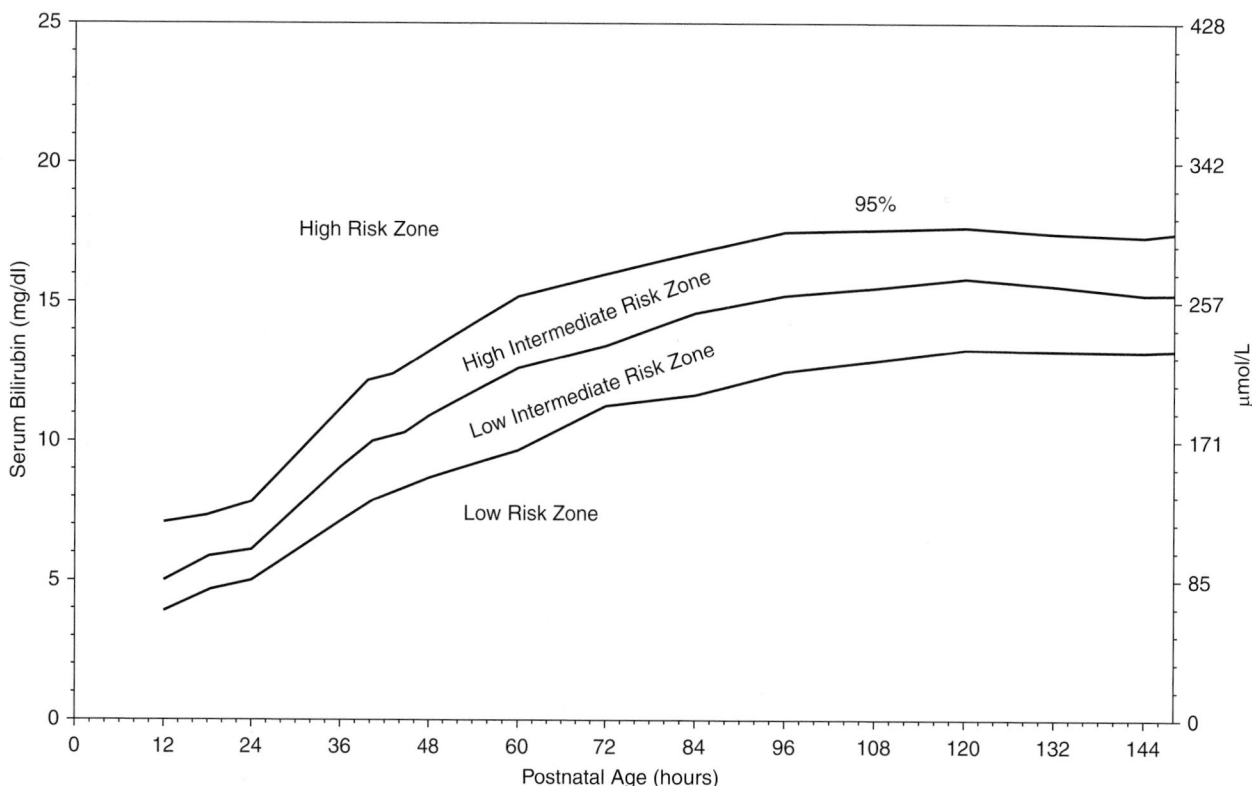

Figure 1 Hour-specific nomogram indicating risk zone for serum bilirubin levels for newborns that predicts the likelihood that a subsequent bilirubin level will exceed the 95th percentile.

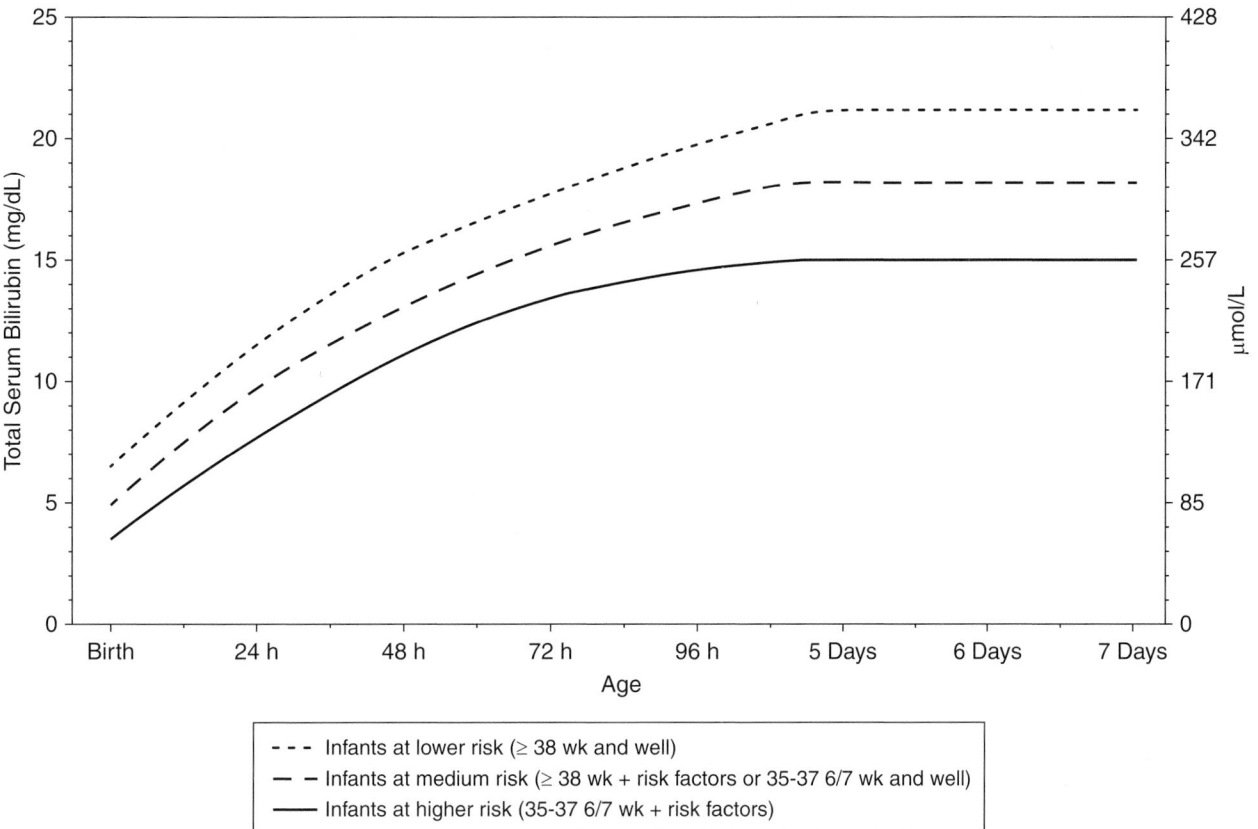

Figure 2 Hour-specific nomogram indicating phototherapy thresholds for various risk categories for newborns ≥35 weeks' gestation.

Legend:
- - - - Infants at lower risk (≥ 38 wk and well)
- – – Infants at medium risk (≥ 38 wk + risk factors or 35-37 6/7 wk and well)
- —— Infants at higher risk (35-37 6/7 wk + risk factors)

inpatient hospitalization to determine adequate milk transfer. Mothers who intend to breastfeed but experience delayed lactogenesis should work with a lactation specialist and provide supplemental feeds (either in the form of formula or human donor milk) at appropriate volumes to decrease the enterohepatic circulation of bilirubin caused by low intake.

Phototherapy

When a newborn's TSB surpasses the phototherapy threshold, phototherapy should be administered. Phototherapy removes bilirubin by converting it into lumirubin, a water-soluble molecule that can bypass the liver and be excreted in urine or stool. Phototherapy can be delivered using overhead lights or fiberoptic blankets that provide light in the 430 to 490 nanometer wavelength, which is most strongly absorbed by the bilirubin molecule. The total body surface area that is exposed to light should be maximized for effective phototherapy. To accomplish this, the newborn should receive phototherapy while only wearing eye protection and a diaper. The newborn's temperature and hydration status should be monitored. The manufacturer's instructions should be followed to safely administer phototherapy. It is important to remember that the clinical appearance of jaundice will be affected by phototherapy and thus cannot be used to estimate the degree of hyperbilirubinemia.

Bilirubin levels should be monitored as the newborn is receiving phototherapy. TcB measurements will not be accurate after phototherapy is initiated and the provider must rely on serum levels. For newborns being admitted for phototherapy after hospital discharge, the provider should obtain a baseline TSB prior to starting treatment. A repeat serum bilirubin level is typically obtained within 12 hours of phototherapy initiation to ensure that it is not continuing to rise. Subsequent checks can be ordered at the discretion of the clinician. For newborns with ongoing hemolysis or whose bilirubin levels are close to the exchange transfusion threshold, consideration should be given to earlier and more frequent TSB checks. A bilirubin level that continues to rise despite appropriate phototherapy should prompt the provider to consider other etiologies for hyperbilirubinemia. The provider should consider verifying a normal metabolic screen with the state lab and additional laboratory evaluation, including a direct bilirubin.

While the newborn is receiving phototherapy, every effort should be made to optimize feeding. For a breastfeeding mother, she may be encouraged to express milk either manually or using a pump as the newborn may be too inactive for effective milk transfer. The expressed milk can be fed back to the baby and additional supplementation may be offered if needed.

The duration of phototherapy will vary based on the newborn's age, presence of hemolysis, and other risk factors. There is no clear guidance as to when phototherapy should be stopped. Some providers will discontinue phototherapy when the TSB is at least 3 mg/dL below the phototherapy threshold. However, for those with ongoing hemolysis, an even lower level may be desirable due to concern for rebound hyperbilirubinemia. Rebound hyperbilirubinemia occurs when the TSB returns to or exceeds the AAP phototherapy threshold within 72 hours of terminating phototherapy. A calculator by Chang et al. has been developed(https://pediatrics.aappublications.org/content/139/3/e20162896)to help determine the probability of rebound hyperbilirubinemia for late preterm or term newborns.

Exchange Transfusion

In the current era of universal screening for hyperbilirubinemia, the need for double volume exchange transfusion is rare for late preterm and full-term newborns. Exchange transfusion should be considered when the serum bilirubin exceeds the hour-specific threshold on the exchange transfusion nomogram (Fig. 3). The AAP recommends that any newborn whose TSB meets the exchange transfusion threshold or is at a level of 25 mg/dL, be admitted directly to the inpatient unit for treatment to avoid delays through the emergency department. A TSB at this level is considered a medical emergency and must be treated aggressively.

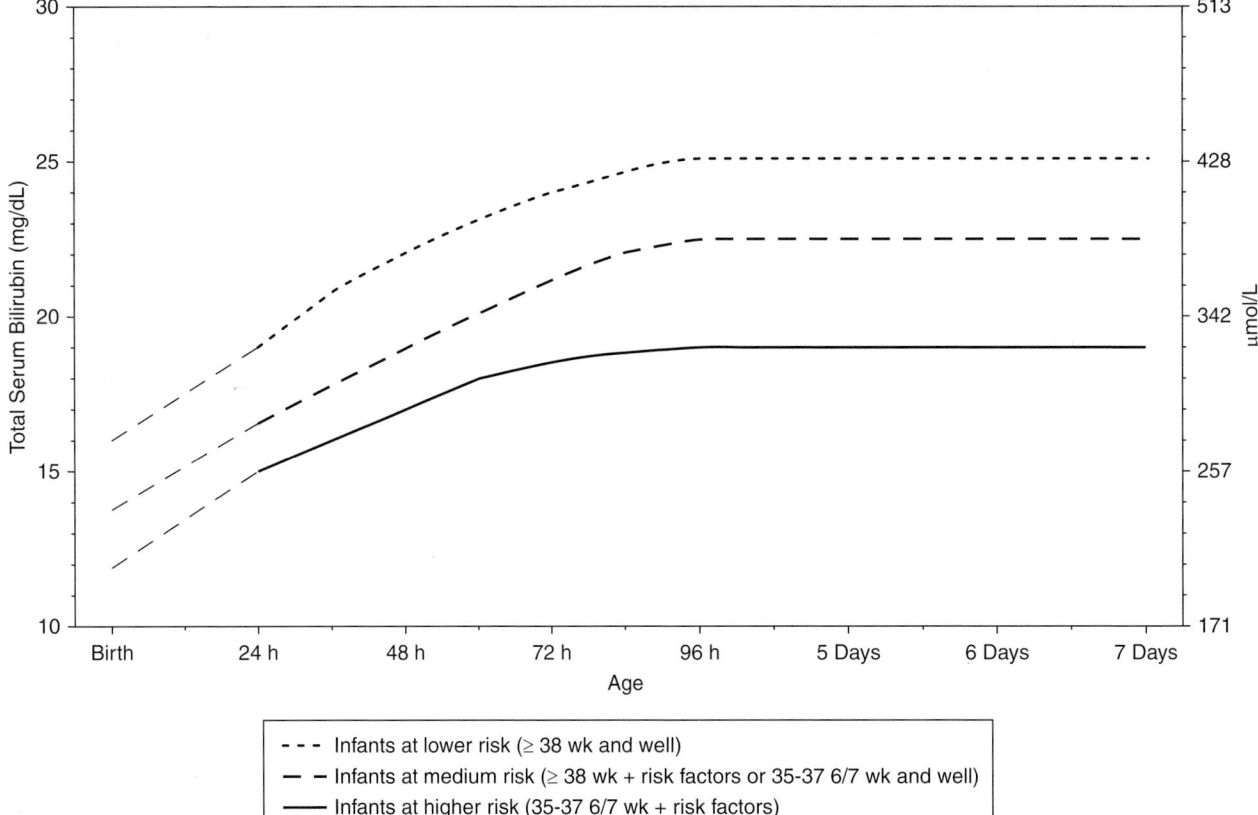

Figure 3 Hour-specific nomogram indicating exchange transfusion thresholds for various risk categories for newborns ≥35 weeks' gestation.

Exchange transfusion is a procedure where small, calculated aliquots of the newborn's blood are removed and replaced with donated reconstituted RBCs with plasma, preferably through two central lines, in an effort to remove the circulating bilirubin and antibodies. The procedure is continued until the total blood volume has been replaced twice. This is a risky procedure that must only be performed in a neonatal intensive care unit. The procedure carries a complication rate of about 12% and includes coagulopathy, infection, electrolyte imbalance, and even death. The newborn requires close monitoring during and after the procedure.

Pharmacologic Treatment
For newborns with ongoing hemolysis due to ABO or Rh incompatibility whose TSB is continuing to rise despite phototherapy or for those approaching the exchange transfusion threshold, intravenous gamma globulin (IVIG, Gammagard)[1] may be administered. IVIG should be administered at 0.5 to 1 g/kg over 2 hours and repeated after 12 hours if necessary. Studies have shown that IVIG for newborns with hemolytic disease may reduce the need for exchange transfusion.

Complications
The spectrum of complications associated with hyperbilirubinemia and its treatments range from mild to severe. Many newborns with hyperbilirubinemia who are approaching the phototherapy threshold may become increasingly tired and not feed effectively. This perpetuates the poor feeding and dehydration that contributed to their hyperbilirubinemia in the first place. Once phototherapy is initiated, efforts are made to maximize exposure to phototherapy, which results in maternal-newborn separation and may also compromise the breastfeeding relationship. Phototherapy has been shown to result in a small reduction in breastfeeding at 12 months and exclusivity at 1, 2, and 4 months.

The feared complications of severe hyperbilirubinemia, formerly termed kernicterus, are ABE and CBE. Bilirubin encephalopathy results from unconjugated bilirubin that crosses the blood-brain

barrier and deposits in the brain tissue. The exact incidence of ABE is unknown, but in a large cohort of around half a million newborns in Northern California, less than 0.001% presented with ABE and all had TSB levels greater than 35. The symptoms of ABE typically progress through three stages: early, intermediate, and advanced. In the early stage, newborns may present with increased sleepiness, hypotonia, and a high-pitched cry. As symptoms progress to the intermediate stage, the newborn may be lethargic, jittery, and develop backward arching of the neck and trunk (retrocollis and opisthotonos). Finally, in the advanced stage, the newborn develops seizures, hypertonicity, and inconsolability. Death often results from seizures or respiratory failure.

CBE refers to the permanent sequelae of bilirubin-induced neurotoxicity and develops during the first year after birth. In the same cohort in Northern California, newborns who developed cerebral palsy all had TSBs that were at least 5 mg/dL above the exchange transfusion threshold. Additional symptoms of CBE include sensorineural hearing loss, gaze abnormalities, and dental enamel hypoplasia.

Recently, reports have been published regarding potential long-term complications associated with phototherapy. In a study analyzing data of nearly half a million patients, an increased risk of epilepsy was seen, though only in boys. Two studies with very large datasets looked at the potential associations between phototherapy and cancer. After accounting for confounding variables, an association persisted for myeloid leukemia, but this was based on two newborns who received higher doses of phototherapy. For newborns with Down syndrome who have a baseline risk of cancer that is 10 times higher than the general population, extra caution when initiating phototherapy is warranted. Mechanical issues related to phototherapy are rare but do include hypothermia. For patients with porphyria, phototherapy can result in a blistering skin reaction and is therefore an absolute contraindication.

References
American Academy of Pediatrics, Subcommittee on Hyperbilirubinemia: Management of Hyperbilirubinemia in the Newborn Infant 35 or More Weeks of Gestation, *Pediatrics* 114:297–316, 2004.

---

[1] Not FDA approved for this indication.

Canadian Paediatric Society, Fetus and Newborn Committee: Guidelines for Detection, Management and Prevention of Hyperbilirubinemia in Term and Late Preterm Newborn Infants (35 or More Weeks' Gestation), *Paediatr Child Health* 12:1B–12B, 2007.

Chang P, Newman T: A Simpler Prediction Rule for Rebound Hyperbilirubinemia, *Pediatrics* 144:e20183712, 2019.

Flaherman VJ, Schaefer EW, Kuzniewicz MW, et al: Early Weight Loss Nomograms for Exclusively Breastfed Newborns, *Pediatrics* 135:e16–e23, 2015.

Harb R, Thomas D: Conjugated Hyperbilirubinemia, *Pediatrics in Review* 28:83–91, 2007.

Kuzniewiicz MW, Wickremasinghe AC, Wu YW, et al: Incidence, Etiology, and Outcomes of Hazardous Hyperbilirubinemia in Newborns, *Pediatrics* 134:504–509, 2014.

Lauer B, Spector N: Hyperbilirubinemia in the Newborn, *Pediatrics in Review* 32:341–349, 2011.

Maisels MJ: Transcutaneous Bilirubinometry, *Neoreviews* 7:e217–225, 2006.

Maisels MJ, Bhutani V, Bogen D, et al: Hyperbilirubinemia in the Newborn Infant > 35 Weeks' Gestation: An Update with Clarifications, *Pediatrics* 124:1193–1198, 2009.

MITOCHONDRIAL DISEASE

Method of
Sonal Sharma, MD; Amy Goldstein; and Marni J. Falk, MD

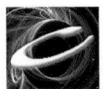

CURRENT DIAGNOSIS

- Mitochondrial disease diagnosis may be a challenge due to their extensive phenotypic and genotypic heterogeneity.
- Biochemical analyses of blood, urine, and cerebrospinal fluid are utilized to evaluate for evidence of mitochondrial dysfunction that may be present in some cases. However, there are no highly specific or sensitive biomarkers applicable for all forms of mitochondrial disease.
- Diagnosis predominantly relies on next generation sequencing molecular analyses for pathogenic variants in hundreds of genes in both nuclear DNA and mitochondrial DNA (mtDNA). Front-line genomic testing is performed in noninvasive tissues (blood, urine, saliva, etc.).
- Invasive tissue-based diagnostic testing may be beneficial when noninvasive tissue genetic and biochemical testing is inconclusive. Muscle, liver, and/or fibroblast histology, immunohistochemistry, electron microscopy, electron transport chain enzyme activity analyses, fatty acid oxidation analysis, biochemical analyte analyses such as coenzyme Q10 level analysis, mtDNA genome sequencing and deletion quantitation, and mtDNA content analysis are specific tests that may be indicated.

CURRENT THERAPY

- No cures exist for mitochondrial disease.
- Symptom management is the mainstay of mitochondrial disease care.
- Clinicians employ a variety of mitochondrial medicine regimens consisting of vitamins, enzyme cofactors, antioxidants, and metabolic modifiers to enhance electron transport chain enzyme function and reduce toxic metabolites. The use of mitochondrial medicine therapies is based on contemporary understanding of mitochondrial disease pathophysiology to improve resiliency and prevent decompensation, although their clinical efficacy has not been proven in randomized clinical trials. In some cases, mitochondrial medicines may alter disease progression, such as oral arginine to prevent recurrent metabolic strokes.
- Targeted treatment therapies for mitochondrial diseases are increasingly being developed for specific molecular subtypes.
- An increasing array of clinical treatment trials evaluating small molecules and genetic therapies are underway or being planned to develop effective treatment strategies that improve health in patients with primary (genetic-based) mitochondrial disease.

Epidemiology

Mitochondrial diseases are a clinically heterogeneous group of genetic disorders that are characterized by impaired energy production. Primary mitochondrial disease are caused by pathogenic variants in nuclear DNA (nDNA) or mitochondrial DNA (mtDNA) genes that play a vital role in mitochondrial structure and function. The prevalence of childhood-onset mitochondrial disease (<16 years of age) has been estimated as 5 to 15 cases per 100,000 individuals. A study in North East of England reported the prevalence of mitochondrial disease per 100,000 individuals in adults due to mtDNA mutations as 9.6 cases and those due to nDNA mutations as 2.9 cases. However, prevalence of some mitochondrial disease subtypes may be higher in regions with specific genetic founder effects.

Pathophysiology

Mitochondria are double membrane-bound organelles present in all nucleated eukaryotic cells. The fundamental function of mitochondria is energy production through the process of oxidative phosphorylation (OXPHOS) that occurs in the respiratory chain. In this aerobic process, reducing equivalence generated through the biochemical processing of cellular nutrients enter the electron transport chain (ETC) that is composed of complexes I, II, III, and IV, with oxygen serving as the final electron acceptor (Figure 1). Electron transfer powers complexes I, III, and IV to generate a proton gradient across the inner mitochondrial membrane, which is dissipated to drive the production of energy by complex V (ATP synthase) in the chemical form of adenosine triphosphate (ATP).

Independent from the nuclear genome, mitochondria have their own mtDNA genome composed of 37 genes. Multiple mitochondria exist per cell, with multiple mitochondrial genome copies in each mitochondrion. Of the 37 genes, 13 encode proteins that are all core structural subunits of ETC complexes, while 22 encode transfer RNAs and two encode ribosomal RNAs to assist in the mitochondrial translation of these 13 protein-coding subunits. Nuclear genes are fundamentally important to mitochondria structure and function, with up to 1500 total proteins comprising mitochondria in different tissues. Thus there exists remarkable heterogeneity in the candidate genes that may directly disrupt mitochondrial dysfunction. Indeed, primary mitochondrial diseases are currently known to result from pathogenic variants in any of the 37 mtDNA genes, single or multiple large-scale deletions of mtDNA involving multiple mtDNA genes, and pathogenic variants in at least 350 nuclear genes. As mtDNA genomes are inherited through the maternal germ cells (oocytes), mtDNA disorders are maternally inherited, or rarely may occur de novo in the affected individual. By contrast, nDNA gene disorders may variably be inherited in an autosomal dominant, autosomal recessive or X-linked pattern. The majority of pathogenic variants cause mitochondrial disease by disrupting OXPHOS, which results in lowered ATP production, increased oxidative stress, and dysfunction of other interlinked metabolic pathways such as fatty acid oxidation. Some nuclear gene pathogenic variants may also cause mitochondrial diseases known as mtDNA depletion syndromes, which result from mtDNA genome instability and reduction in the mtDNA genome content in each mitochondrion.

A pathogenic mtDNA variant is usually present only in a proportion of all mtDNA genomes within a cell or tissue. This phenomenon of harboring healthy or "wild-type" mtDNA genomes as well as affected or "mutant" mtDNA genomes is termed heteroplasmy. Many mtDNA pathogenic variants only cause clinical manifestations when present in a given tissue at a certain level of heteroplasmy, which is known as "threshold effect." The precise threshold for symptom occurrence is not clear for every disease-causing mtDNA pathogenic variant. A general rule-of-thumb is that heteroplasmy levels above 70% are more likely to manifest with severe mitochondrial disease symptoms. However, this depends on the specific pathogenic variant and tissue tested, as some pathogenic variants may cause severe disease at much lower heteroplasmy levels discernible in peripheral tissues, and some may appear at much higher levels even including homoplasmic

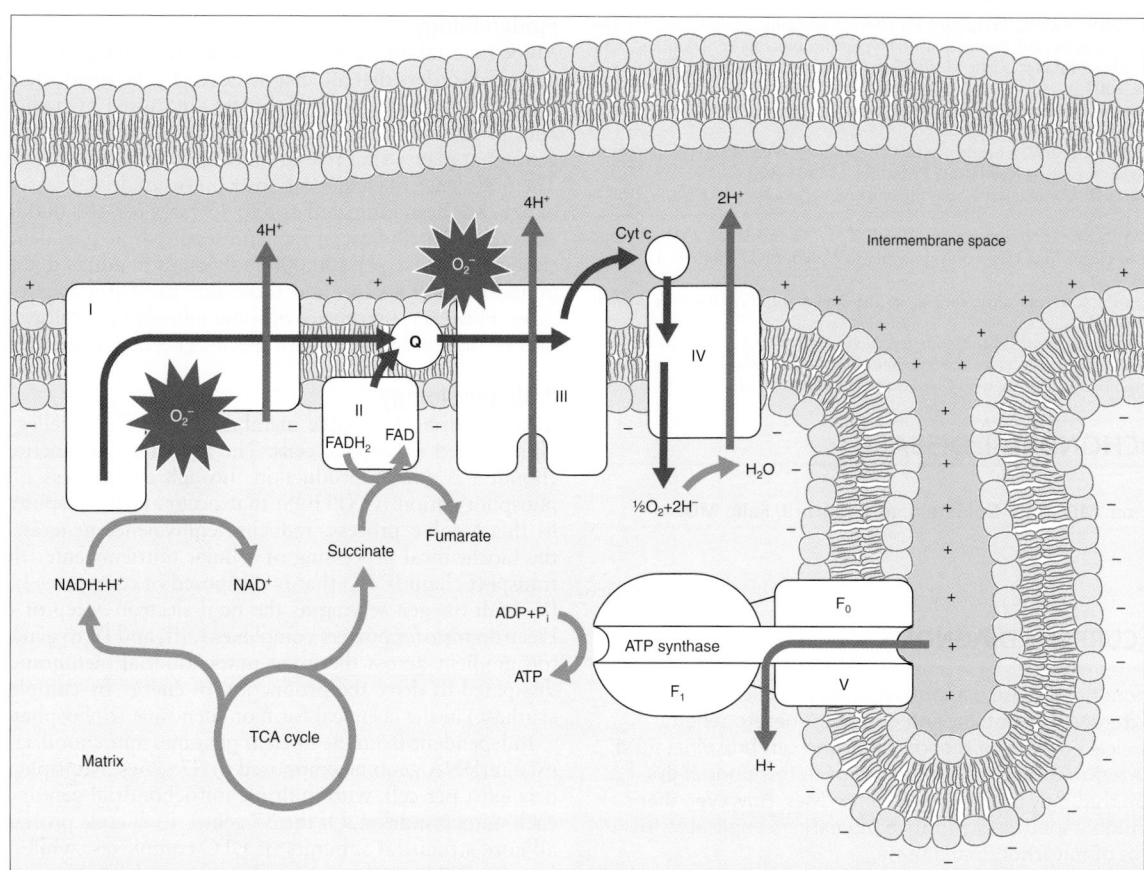

Figure 1 Mitochondrial respiration. The mitochondrial electron transport chain consists of four protein complexes (I–IV) embedded in the inner mitochondrial membrane that are coupled to a fifth (V) unlinked complex, ATP synthase. Reducing equivalents such as NADH and FADH$_2$ generated from other biochemical pathways, mainly the tricarboxylic acid (TCA) cycle and fatty acid oxidation, are oxidized by complex I and II. Electrons from complex I and II are transported to reduce coenzyme Q10 (CoQ10), which transports electrons to complex III, then to cytochrome C and finally to complex IV. The electrons are transferred by complex IV to molecular oxygen in a process that generates water. Complex I, III, and IV pump protons, which result from these reactions from the mitochondrial matrix into the intermembrane space, thereby creating a proton gradient. These protons reenter the matrix through complex V and drive the reaction to synthesize adenosine triphosphate (ATP) from adenosine diphosphate (ADP) and inorganic phosphate. Energy stored in the phosphate bonds of the ATP molecule power multiple cellular reactions. Adapted from Hagberg H, Mallard C, Rousset CI, Thornton C: Mitochondria: hub of injury responses in the developing brain. *Lancet Neurol* 13(2):217–232, 2014.

mutant (with no wild-type copies present) with little to no clinical symptoms. Environmental stressors such as intercurrent infections, fevers, fasting, and lifestyle choices such as nutrition, exercise, and medication or environmental exposures may all influence the onset and progression of clinical symptoms in individuals harboring pathogenic variants in mtDNA.

Clinical Manifestations

Due to impairment of the common pathway of energy production, mitochondrial diseases have wide-ranging variability, even among affected family members, in their age of onset and particular organ system involvement. Secondary mitochondrial dysfunction may also occur in other genetic or complex classes of disease that affect energy production or upon exposure to certain environmental factors and medications. Patients with mitochondrial disease report an average of 16 symptoms involving different organ systems, with a range of 7 to 35 symptoms per patient (Figure 2). Common symptoms include fatigue, exercise intolerance, muscle weakness, developmental delay or regression, poor growth, metabolic strokes, intellectual disability, seizures, dysautonomia, cardiomyopathy, arrhythmia, sensorineural hearing loss, endocrinopathies (diabetes mellitus, thyroid abnormalities, pancreatic, and adrenal dysfunction) as well as impairment of vision, immune, gastrointestinal, liver, and kidney function. It is prudent for primary care physicians to suspect mitochondrial disease in patients who present with typical "red-flag" symptoms of mitochondrial disease or unexplained symptoms involving three or more unrelated organ systems, although in some cases only single organ dysfunction may be present at presentation. It is also

important to recognize that disease onset in a given individual may occur at any age from prenatal to adult, and the severity of symptoms tends to worsen in a nonlinear, progressive manner. There can be episodes of acute decline triggered by infection or other stressors, followed by periods of stability.

Emergencies in mitochondrial disease include acute decompensation that may result from increased metabolic demand secondary to physiologic stressors including ongoing infection, systemic illness, fasting, dehydration, surgery, and/or anesthesia. The presence of neurologic regression, focal neurologic deficits, altered mental status, or seizures should raise concern for acute metabolic stroke. It is also vital to recognize signs of severe metabolic acidosis in patients with primary mitochondrial disease, which include altered mental status, hyperpnea, bradycardia, arrhythmia, hypotension, nausea, vomiting, and severe lethargy.

An additional challenge to the recognition of mitochondrial disease is the complex relationship between genotype and clinical phenotype. A specific gene pathogenic variant can result in different clinical symptoms. A clear example is the m.3243A>G pathogenic variant in *MT-TL1*, which can cause chronic progressive external ophthalmoplegia (CPEO), mitochondrial encephalopathy, lactic acidosis and stroke-like episodes (MELAS), or maternally inherited diabetes and deafness (MIDD). Similarly, a specific syndrome can result from numerous genetic etiologies such as Leigh syndrome (subacute necrotizing encephalomyelopathy), which can be caused by pathogenic variants in approximately 100 nuclear and mtDNA genes. The clinical symptoms of common mitochondrial diseases are described in Table 1.

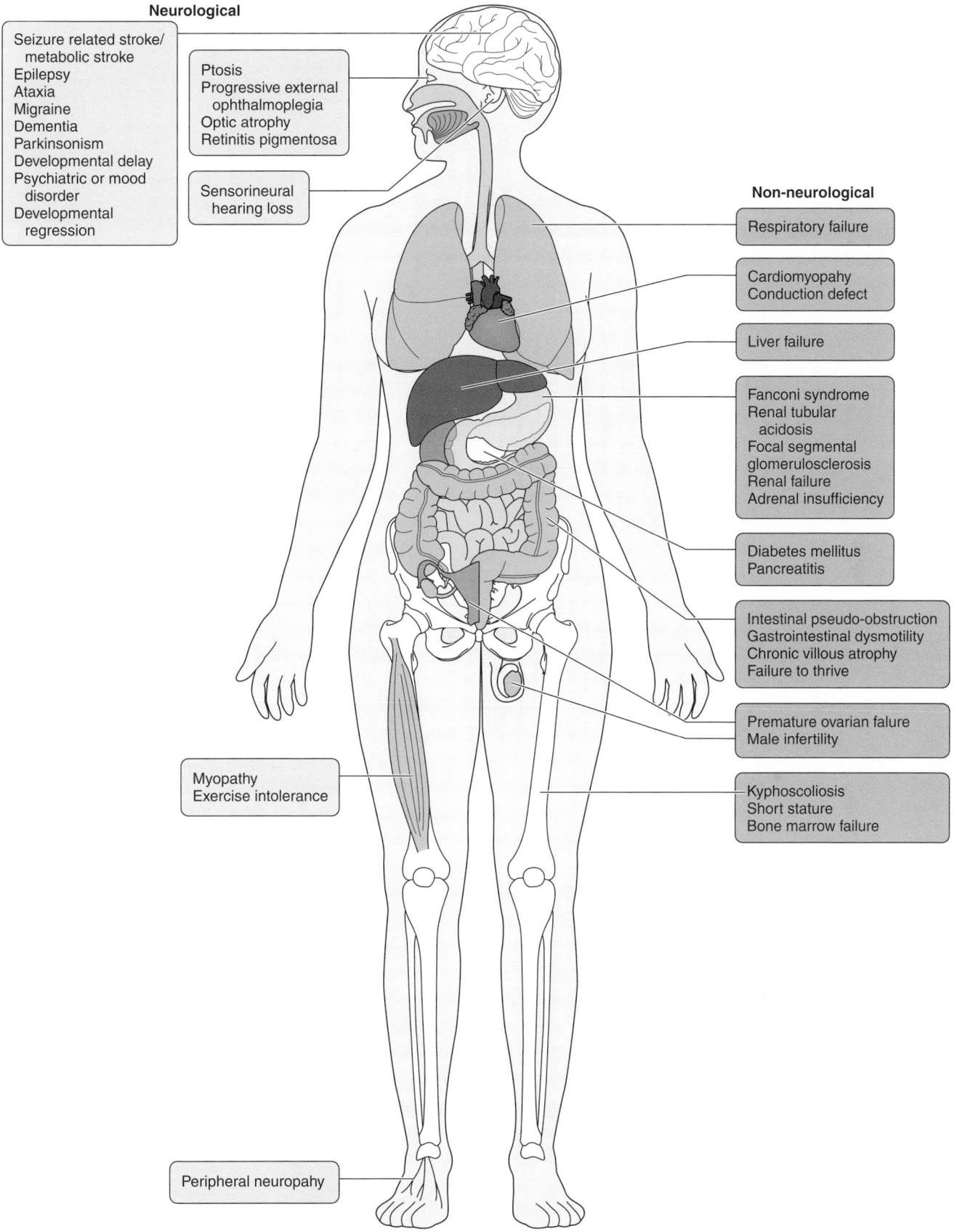

Neurological

Seizure related stroke/
  metabolic stroke
Epilepsy
Ataxia
Migraine
Dementia
Parkinsonism
Developmental delay
Psychiatric or mood
  disorder
Developmental
  regression

Ptosis
Progressive external
  ophthalmoplegia
Optic atrophy
Retinitis pigmentosa

Sensorineural
hearing loss

Non-neurological

Respiratory failure

Cardiomyopahy
Conduction defect

Liver failure

Fanconi syndrome
Renal tubular
  acidosis
Focal segmental
glomerulosclerosis
Renal failure
Adrenal insufficiency

Diabetes mellitus
Pancreatitis

Intestinal pseudo-obstruction
Gastrointestinal dysmotility
Chronic villous atrophy
Failure to thrive

Premature ovarian falure
Male infertility

Kyphoscoliosis
Short stature
Bone marrow failure

Myopathy
Exercise intolerance

Peripheral neuropahy

Figure 2 Clinical symptoms in mitochondrial disease are variable and usually involve multiple high-energy demand organ systems. Gorman GS, Chinnery PF, DiMauro S, et al: Mitochondrial diseases. *Nat Rev Dis Primers* 2:16080, 2016.

Diagnosis

Noninvasive Biochemical Analysis

The diagnosis of mitochondrial disease requires a thoughtful, stepwise approach (Figure 3). Noninvasive laboratory screening using blood and urine samples involves chemistry and biochemistry tests to determine the patient's metabolic stability as well as other organ involvement. Standard biochemistry profiling tests include comprehensive metabolic profile, plasma lactate, plasma pyruvate, lactate to pyruvate ratio, quantitative plasma amino acid analysis, plasma carnitine levels and acylcarnitine profile, ammonia, plasma

TABLE 1 Presentation Overview of Common Mitochondrial Disease Clinical Syndromes

DISEASE	GENETIC ETIOLOGY	CLINICAL FEATURES	OTHER FINDINGS	NEUROIMAGING	SPECIFIC TREATMENT
Mitochondrial encephalomyopathy, lactic acidosis and stroke-like episodes (MELAS)	80%: m.3243A>G variant in MT-TL1; <10%: variants in MT-ND5; less common—15 other mitochondrial disease genes	Seizures, recurrent headaches, stroke-like episodes, cortical vision loss, muscle weakness, recurrent vomiting, short stature, hearing impairment, impaired thinking, diabetes mellitus (type 1 or 2), developmental delay	Lactic acidemia or acidosis in blood and cerebrospinal fluid (CSF), elevated CSF protein, Muscle biopsy: Ragged red fibers, ETC: Low complex I and/or complex IV activities	MRI: asymmetric, T2 hyperintensity not corresponding to specific vascular distribution during stroke-like episodes with predominant posterior cerebrum involvement, slow spreading of stroke-like lesion over weeks; MRA: usually normal; MRS: elevated N-acetylaspartate (NAA) and lactate; CT: basal ganglia calcification	Acute or subacute stroke episode: intravenous (IV) arginine[1] 500 mg/kg/day over 60 min for 3–5 days; Prevention of recurrent stroke: oral arginine[7] 150–300 mg/kg/day
Leigh syndrome (subacute necrotizing encephalomyelopathy)	>80 nuclear genes (most common SURF1, in up to 10% of Leigh syndrome cases) 14 mtDNA genes (MT-ATP6 associated with ~50% of all mtDNA-based Leigh syndrome)	Psychomotor retardation or regression, usually provoked by a period of illness followed by a period of stabilization, hypotonia, spasticity, movement disorders, cerebellar ataxia, peripheral neuropathy, hypertrophic cardiomyopathy	Lactic acidosis in blood and CSF during intercurrent illness, ratio of lactate to pyruvate is normal to low in pyruvate dehydrogenase (PDH) deficiency, increased alanine on plasma amino acids reflective of persistent hyperlactic acidemia, respiratory chain complex I, II, III, IV, or V deficiency depending on genetic etiology	MRI: bilateral symmetric T2 signal hyperintensities in the basal ganglia and/or brainstem; spinal cord involvement can appear as demyelinating lesions involving white matter or ischemic/infectious lesions involving gray matter MRS: elevated lactate	Biotin-thiamine responsive basal ganglia disease associated with mutation of SLC19A3: oral biotin[7] (5–10 mg/kg/day) and thiamine[1] (in doses ranging from 300–900 mg/day); Biotinidase deficiency: oral biotin 5–10 mg/day; Coenzyme Q10 (CoQ10) deficiency: ubiquinOL[7] (reduced) formulation preferred, at dose up to 8 mg/kg/day If ubiquinONE[7] (oxidized) formulation is used, oral CoQ10 10–30 mg/kg/day in children, 1,200–3,000 mg/kg/day in adults
Neuropathy, Ataxia, and Retinitis Pigmentosa (NARP)	MT-ATP6	Continuum of clinical spectrum of Leigh syndrome, muscle weakness, neuropathy, ataxia, seizures, retinitis pigmentosa or optic atrophy, learning difficulty	Electromyography (EMG)/Nerve Conduction Velocity (NCV) studies: sensory or sensorimotor axonal polyneuropathy	MRI: cerebral and/or cerebellar atrophy	
Myoclonic Epilepsy associated with Ragged Red Fibers (MERRF)	>80%: m.8344A>G variant in MT-TK, 7 other mtDNA genes also associated with MERRF phenotype	Myoclonus is often the first symptom followed by generalized epilepsy, ataxia, weakness, exercise intolerance, dementia, peripheral neuropathy, hearing loss, short stature, optic atrophy, ptosis, ophthalmoplegia, retinitis pigmentosa, cardiomyopathy, dysrhythmias such as Wolff-Parkinson-White syndrome, multiple lipomas	Lactic acidemia or acidosis in blood and CSF, lactate and pyruvate are elevated at rest and increase excessively after moderate activity, elevated CSF protein, Electron transport chain (ETC) enzyme activity studies: deficiency of respiratory complexes I, III, or IV with mtDNA-encoded subunits Muscle biopsy: ragged red fibers, hyperactive fibers with succinate dehydrogenase stain	MRI: brain atrophy, basal ganglia lesions, bilateral putaminal necrosis, brainstem and cerebellum atrophy	

Disease	Genetics	Clinical features	Diagnostic findings	MRI	Treatment
Leber's Hereditary Optic Neuropathy (LHON)	>90%: m.3460G>A in *MT-ND1*, m.11778G>A in *MT-ND4*, or m.14484T>C in *MT-ND6*. Six other mtDNA genes may also be causal	Bilateral, painless, subacute visual failure (starts as central visual field blurring in one eye followed by involvement of other eye 2–3 months later), males are four–five times more likely to be affected than females, penetrance 15% in females and 50% in males, with penetrance exacerbated by smoking and alcohol exposure, visual acuity is reduced to counting fingers or worse, optic disc atrophy after acute phase, ataxia, peripheral neuropathy, myopathy, movement disorders, multiple sclerosis-like illness, cardiac arrhythmias	ECG: pre-excitation syndrome, Visual field testing; enlarging dense central or centroceccal scotoma, ETC enzyme activity analysis: m.3460G>A in *MT-ND1* associated with severe complex I deficiency	MRI: white matter lesions and/or a high signal within the optic nerves	Treatment of raised intraocular pressure Idebenone (available in Europe, not in the United States) and/or antioxidant vitamin supplementation (N-Acetylcysteine,[1] vitamin E, B12, and C) may be tried to stabilize visual loss and/or accelerate visual recovery to improve final visual outcome
Chronic Progressive External Ophthalmoplegia (CPEO)	Single, large scale mtDNA deletion syndrome (single large-scale deletion ranging in size from 1.1–10 kilobase); can be identified in skeletal muscle, and multiple mtDNA deletions may be seen in *POLG*	Ptosis, ophthalmoplegia, oropharyngeal weakness, proximal limb weakness, exercise intolerance		MRI: leukoencephalopathy, cerebral or cerebellar atrophy, basal ganglia and brainstem lesions (Leigh syndrome pattern)	Eyelid slings and/or ptosis repair for severe ptosis, eyeglass prisms for diplopia, eye drops for dry eye
Kearns-Sayre syndrome (KSS)	Single large-scale mtDNA deletion syndrome can be identified in blood leukocytes, buccal sample, urine sediment, or muscle	Pigmentary retinopathy, progressive ophthalmoplegia, cerebellar ataxia, impaired intellect, sensorineural hearing loss, oropharyngeal and esophageal dysfunction, muscle weakness, exercise intolerance, cardiac conduction block, endocrinopathy (diabetes mellitus, hypothyroidism, hypoparathyroidism, adrenal insufficiency), renal impairment	Lactic acidemia or acidosis in blood and CSF, elevated CSF protein, Muscle biopsy: ragged red fibers, ETC enzyme activity analysis: reduced activity of complexes I, III, and/or IV	MRI: Leukoencephalopathy, cerebral or cerebellar atrophy, basal ganglia and brainstem lesions (Leigh syndrome pattern)	Prophylactic placement of cardiac pacemakers in individuals with cardiac conduction block, Folinic acid supplementation[1] in individuals with KSS with low CSF 5-methyltetrahydrofolate, Pancreatic enzyme replacement Hearing aids and/or cochlear implants for sensorineural hearing loss
Pearson syndrome	Single large scale mtDNA deletion syndrome can be identified in blood leukocytes	Infancy or early childhood onset, sideroblastic anemia typically transfusion-dependent until resolution in early childhood, growth failure, and exocrine pancreatic dysfunction	Macrocytic, sideroblastic anemia with a variable degree of neutropenia and thrombocytopenia (pancytopenia), normocellular bone marrow, hemosiderosis, and ringed sideroblasts	MRI: white matter involvement	Pancreatic enzyme replacement, Transfusion therapy for sideroblastic anemia

[1]Not FDA approved for this indication.

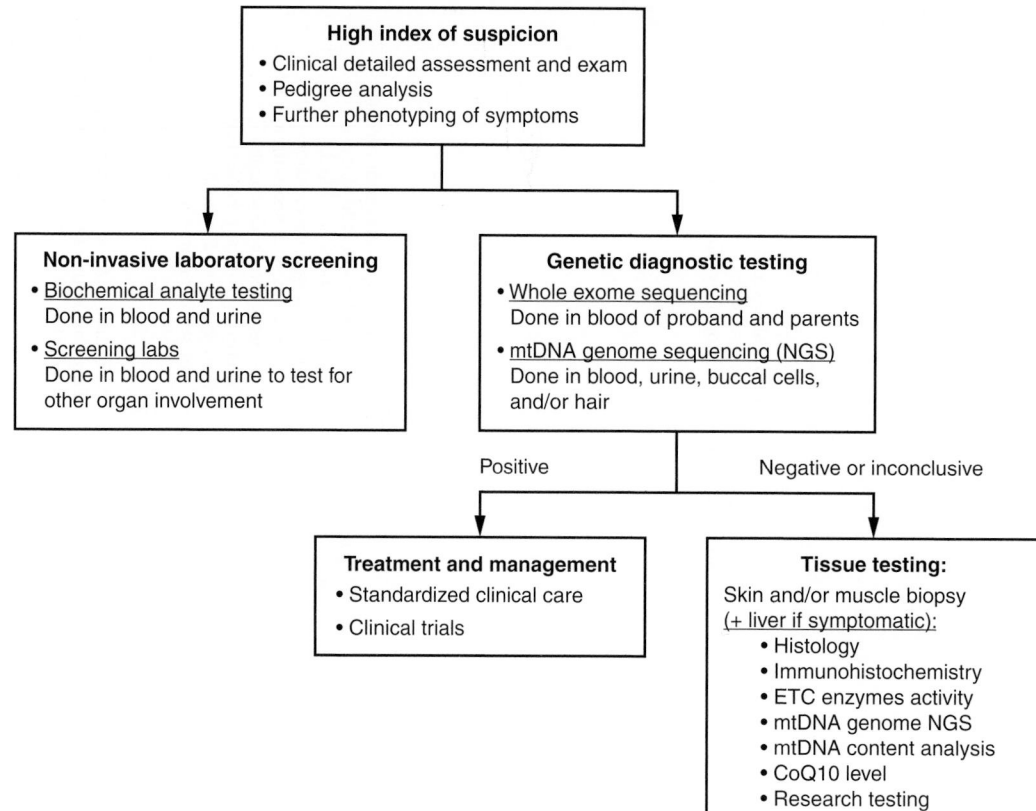

Figure 3 Algorithm for clinical diagnostic evaluation of mitochondrial disease. Muraresku CC, McCormick EM, Falk MJ: Mitochondrial disease: Advances in clinical diagnosis, management, therapeutic development, and preventative strategies. *Curr Genet Med Rep* 6(2):62–72, 2018.

glutathione level, GDF-15 level, and quantitative urine organic acid analysis. Tests for secondary organ involvement may include complete blood count with differential, creatine kinase, hemoglobin A1c, lipoprotein profile, iron profile and ferritin, thyroid screen, cortisol, adrenocorticotropic hormone, parathyroid hormone, amylase, lipase, fecal elastase, immunoglobulin levels, and urinalysis. However, these tests are not specific for mitochondrial disease and none have sufficiently high sensitivity and specificity to be useful as a biomarker sufficient to confirm or refute the diagnosis of mitochondrial disease. For example, elevated plasma lactate may occur in mitochondrial disease, but levels may also be normal or only intermittently increased under some scenarios or in certain disease subtypes. Further, elevated lactate results in individuals without primary mitochondrial disease from poor tissue perfusion, stroke, sepsis, seizures, or improper handling of the sample.

Neuroimaging

Mitochondrial disease patients with clinical CNS involvement may have nonspecific brain and spine magnetic resonance imaging (MRI) abnormalities. Bilateral, symmetric involvement of deep gray structures in the absence of hypoxia, ischemia, or infection should raise suspicion for mitochondrial dysfunction. However, patients with CNS involvement can have a normal MRI depending on the timing of the scan, as some findings may fluctuate, both resolving or newly occurring over time. Certain mitochondrial disease syndromes can be associated with hallmark neuroimaging findings. Leigh syndrome is associated with progressive signal abnormality (T2 hyperintensity, T1 hypointensity) most commonly in the lentiform nuclei (putamen and globus pallidus) and caudate nuclei of the basal ganglia. Signal abnormalities in Leigh syndrome may also involve the thalamus, periaqueductal gray, tegmentum, red nuclei, and dentate nuclei. In some cases, there can also be extensive gliosis and cystic degeneration of white matter and marked global atrophy as the disease

progresses. MELAS syndrome is associated with landmark MRI affecting gray matter and not confined to any specific vascular territory. While any cortical location may be involved in MELAS, a predilection for the occipital lobes exists, with clinical correlate of vision loss during a stroke-like episode. Diffuse white matter involvement, particularly in the periventricular and centrum semiovale region, may also occur in multiple mitochondrial disease clinical syndromes such as MELAS, Kearns-Sayre syndrome, and mitochondrial neurogastrointestinal encephalomyopathy (MNGIE) syndrome.

Genetic Diagnostic Testing

Over the past decade, substantial advancements have occurred in the accessibility, affordability, clinical utility, and diagnostic yield of whole exome sequencing (WES) for mitochondrial disease diagnosis. WES is now considered to be the first-line genetic test, with demonstrated improved performance over gene panel-based approaches due to the rapid pace of gene discovery that requires frequent updating of gene panels, as well as the clinically heterogenous nature of mitochondrial disorders that would otherwise require sequential use of multiple different gene panels. Trio-based WES testing is preferred, as this incorporates analysis of proband and both parental samples to allow accurate segregation analysis of multiple variants identified in a proband as well as determination of autosomal dominant disorders with de novo occurrence in the proband. An important application of WES raw data is reanalysis at a future date, which may identify novel gene disorders that were previously not recognized by the diagnostic laboratory at the time of the initial WES report. This is particularly important in pediatric patients, in whom nDNA mutations are the underlying cause of 75% of mitochondrial disease. Appropriate use of WES in the clinical setting requires genetic counselor support for completing informed consent, to understand testing limitations and choices in the type of results that will be returned. Lack of insurance coverage may limit the ability to pursue WES for a specific patient, which may often require insurance preauthorization and escalated coverage requests and justification by the clinician. WES has limitations in the types of genetic errors that may be found, as it may miss certain gene regions not targeted and analyzed, is unable to detect genomic copy number variation, and is unable to be used for triple repeat size analysis. For these reasons, whole genome sequencing (WGS) is emerging as a new clinical test that is able to provide a more comprehensive "exome" than WES, as well as evaluate for these other types of genetic mutations. Further, while WES does not include the mtDNA genome unless it is specifically targeted for capture and analysis, WGS coverage inherently does include the entire mtDNA genome.

Commonly, mtDNA genome sequencing is performed by next-generation sequencing (NGS) methodologies, which can be performed in a stand-alone fashion or in many cases ordered concurrently with WES. Approximately 75% of mitochondrial disease among adults result from pathogenic variants in the mtDNA genome. NGS-based tests may accurately detect single nucleotide variants as well as single or multiple large-scale deletions or duplications down in many cases to 1% heteroplasmy levels. NGS testing detects the breakpoints of large-scale rearrangements in mtDNA but is not reliable for their heteroplasmy quantitation due to polymerase chain reaction (PCR)-based overamplification of deleted genomes; thus performance of additional clinical tests such as digital droplet PCR is required to accurately quantify the mtDNA deletion(s) heteroplasmy level in a given tissue. While most mtDNA mutations are detectable in blood, saliva, or urinary sediment, it is important to note that some mutations, such as single large-scale deletions and other mtDNA single nucleotide variants may only be discernible in postmitotic or symptomatic tissues like muscle; thus a normal mtDNA genome sequence test in a peripheral tissue may need to be followed by symptomatic tissue-based mtDNA genome sequencing if clinical suspicion remains. Additionally, the blood heteroplasmy level of some mtDNA point mutations may decline with age, as is known to commonly occur at a rate of 1% per year for the m.3243A>G mutation. mtDNA genome depletion detectable on PCR-based mtDNA content analysis of muscle or liver may also occur, which when found is indicative that any of dozens of known nuclear gene etiology are present that underlies imbalance in the mtDNA genome and nucleotide pools.

If a mtDNA mutation of uncertain significance is identified, heteroplasmy levels of that variant should be tested by ordering clinical testing in as many tissues as possible (e.g., blood, buccal or saliva, fibroblast cells, urine sediment, muscle, etc.). Commonly, pathogenic variants have higher heteroplasmy levels found in clinically symptomatic but are only rarely homoplasmic. Measuring levels of heteroplasmy of the suspected pathogenic variant in tissues of both affected and unaffected maternal relatives may also be beneficial to aide in its pathogenicity assertion determination. The presence of the same or higher heteroplasmy level of a specific mutation in unaffected maternal relatives decreases its likelihood of being pathogenic in the proband.

Invasive Tissue Testing

When genetic diagnostic testing in noninvasive tissues is unrevealing or identifies variants of uncertain significance, tissue biopsies may be useful to obtain sample in which to perform extensive histologic, immunohistochemical, electron microscopy, genetic, and biochemical analysis. Ideally, the most profoundly affected tissue in a patient is the best option. Muscle is commonly affected in mitochondrial disease patients and can be obtained by open biopsy or percutaneous needle biopsy; the right leg vastus lateralis tissue is the standard sample in which normative values have been obtained for biochemical testing of mitochondrial function. While skin is a less metabolically active tissue, skin-derived primary fibroblast cell lines are readily obtainable without general anesthesia and have been widely demonstrated to have utility for a wide array of biochemical analyses that may be informative about mitochondrial function. Liver biopsy can be beneficial in select patients with hepatic involvement.

All three tissues can be clinically tested for respiratory chain enzyme activity spectrophotometric analyses and (where available) high-resolution respirometry studies of integrated OXPHOS capacity. Histologic and immunohistochemical analysis of muscle can reveal evidence of myopathy or lipid or glycogen storage. Ragged-red fibers on modified Gomori trichrome staining may also be seen as red granular deposits of mitochondria in the subsarcolemmal space, which are suggestive of a mitochondrial proliferative response often occurring in response to mtDNA-based disorder. Immunohistochemical analysis of muscle involves several stains to screen mitochondrial enzymatic activities such as NADH dehydrogenase for evaluation of complex I activity, succinate dehydrogenase (SDH) for complex II activity, and cytochrome c oxidase (COX) for complex IV activity. COX-deficient fibers are a nonspecific finding that may be indicative of a mtDNA disorder. Stains are also used to evaluate for a host of other muscle diseases that may aid in the differential diagnosis of mitochondrial disease. Electron microscopy study of muscle in patients with mitochondrial disease may reveal increased mitochondrial number and size, distorted or absent cristae, and paracrystalline or "parking lot" inclusions. Liver histology may reveal microvesicular or macrovesicular steatosis as well as eosinophilic granulations, representing proliferation of mitochondria. Additional biochemical analysis may include quantification of coenzyme Q10 that plays an important role in ETC; while the concentration of coenzyme Q10 varies greatly in tissues, leukocyte Q10 levels have been shown to be most indicative of tissue coenzyme Q10 deficiency.

Quantitative PCR analysis of mtDNA content in liver or muscle tissue is important to identify mtDNA depletion syndromes. mtDNA genome sequencing is also informative, as above, to complete the evaluation for a suspected mtDNA disorder.

Treatment

Acute Symptom Management

Maintenance of adequate hydration through enteral or intravenous (IV) fluids with dextrose to prevent a catabolic state is an important intervention to consider during an episode of acute decompensation. If a stroke-like lesion is identified on brain MRI, treatment should be pursued with IV arginine[1] to aid in vasodilation through its conversion to nitric oxide mediated by nitric oxide synthase. Arginine has proven effective in decreasing severity of stroke like symptoms, reducing frequency of stroke-like episodes, and reducing tissue injury in patients with MELAS and also found to be effective in pediatric Leigh syndrome, particularly those with hemiplegic symptoms, with 50% of patients in a recent study at our center back to their neurologic baseline by hospital discharge. High-dose steroids may also be considered for treatment of vasogenic edema, which can be associated with stroke-like lesions. If severe metabolic acidosis is identified, subspecialty consultation with metabolic medicine, intensive care, or nephrology should be pursued and buffers such as sodium bicarbonate[1] therapy should be considered.

Additional acute symptoms should be managed by organ-based specialists, such as neurology for acute epilepsy or stroke, nephrology for acute renal failure, ophthalmology for acute visual changes, gastroenterology for obstruction or dysmotility, and cardiology for arrhythmia or cardiac failure.

Chronic Management

Unfortunately, no FDA approved treatments exist for mitochondrial disease at this time. Consensus expert opinion has guided the therapeutic dosing of mitochondrial supplemental medicines, colloquially referred to as a "cocktail," based on underlying known pathophysiology of mitochondrial disease, animal or cellular experimental studies, and expert clinical experience.

---

[1]Not FDA approved for this indication.

Vitamins and nonvitamin cofactor serve essential roles for several cellular reactions. These include vitamin B1 (thiamine, a cofactor for the pyruvate dehydrogenase complex), vitamin B2 (riboflavin, promotes assembly of complex I), vitamin B3 (niacin or nicotinic acid, a precursor of nicotinamide adenine dinucleotide that serves as the primary electron donor to complex I), vitamin B7 (biotin, cofactor for mitochondrial carboxylases), and vitamin B9 (folic acid, where cerebral folate deficiency is associated with white matter changes in mitochondrial disease that may be responsive to folinic acid that crosses the blood–brain barrier). Antioxidants are empirically used to reduce oxidative stress both in the mitochondria and throughout the cell that occurs commonly in mitochondrial disease, including vitamin E, alpha-lipoic acid,[1] coenzyme Q10,[1] taurine,[1] and N-acetylcysteine (Acetadote).[1] Amino acid therapies commonly used to prevent stroke-like episodes in mitochondrial disease patients include arginine,[1] citrulline,[1] and/or taurine. High-dose biotin[1] and thiamine[1] may be indicated in biotin-thiamine-responsive basal ganglia disease. L-creatine[1] may be helpful in myopathy to improve phosphocreatine energy stores. Lutein[1] is commonly recommended in individuals with pigmentary retinopathy.

While L-carnitine (Carnitor)[1] has historically been widely used in mitochondrial disease, its use is associated with long-term risk of coronary artery disease in the general population, so is not used in mitochondrial disease patients only for documented carnitine deficiency or in specific fatty acid oxidation disorders. As the molecular basis for specific patient's symptoms are increasingly recognized, additional therapies may be rationally considered to address their unique cellular pathophysiology. Additional, optimizing nutrition, hydration, and exercise are key components of optimizing long-term management and health outcomes in mitochondrial disease.

Preventative Therapies

Preimplantation genetic diagnosis is available for nuclear gene causes of primary mitochondrial disease when the causal gene pathogenic variant(s) are known in advance in a given family. Preimplantation genetic diagnosis for mtDNA pathogenic variants has become increasingly available and reliably performed in several European countries but remains limited in the United States at the time of this writing. Utilizing mitochondrial replacement therapies (MRT) to not just diagnose but actively reduce the heteroplasmy level for a known pathogenic mtDNA variant in oocytes or early-stage embryos remains legally prohibited in the United States at the time of this writing but is being performed under strict government oversight for select patients in the United Kingdom.

Future Therapies

Therapies under active development for mitochondrial diseases include gene-editing techniques to correct specific pathogenic variants in nuclear and mtDNA genes, intramitochondrial RNA or protein delivery (to replace mutated mitochondrial proteins), cellular therapies to shift mtDNA heteroplasmy levels (selectively damaging mutated mtDNA to increase proportion of wild type mtDNA), and a host of pharmacologic drug therapies for a wide range of mitochondrial disease molecular causes, clinical subtypes, and health outcomes. Clinical trials for mitochondrial disease can be explored on https://clinicaltrials.gov.

Monitoring

Annual monitoring with cardiology, audiology, ophthalmology, and endocrinology is recommended to evaluate for the development of often-treatable organ-specific manifestations of mitochondrial disease. Growth and development should be closely monitored in children.

Specialists commonly needed to care for mitochondrial disease patients include a complex care coordinating primary care physician, geneticist or mitochondrial medicine clinician, neurologist, gastroenterologist, cardiologist, ophthalmologist, physiatrist, and therapists with expertise in physical, occupational, and speech/swallowing therapy. Other specific evaluations such as nephrology, neuropsychology, psychiatry, or exercise physiology

evaluation may be helpful to pursue based on symptoms present. Laboratory measurement of certain analytes such as glutathione[1] (to support administration and dose optimization of n-acetylcysteine), leukocyte CoQ10 (for dosing of coenzyme Q10), and plasma amino acids (for dosing of arginine or citrulline) is helpful for management of mitochondrial supplements.

Considerations

There are few absolute medication prohibitions in mitochondrial disease, with careful consideration of the health status and potential benefit and risk of each medication the most prudent course. However, some medications are contraindicated in specific mitochondrial disease disorder, such as valproic acid that may induce fulminant liver failure in POLG-related disease and aminoglycosides, which can cause ototoxicity in certain mitochondrial diseases (m.1555A > G and m.1494C > T). Further, statins may induce or exacerbate myopathy by impairing coenzyme Q10 synthesis and inducing mtDNA depletion that may be reversible over time when statin therapy is discontinued. Prolonged use of certain anesthetics such as propofol (Diprivan) (for longer than 30–60 minutes) and volatile anesthetics (sevoflurane [Ultane], isoflurane [Forane, Terrell], etc.) should be carefully administered by knowledgeable clinicians or avoided as they can inhibit complex I activity. Indeed, a recent consortium review found that many medications previously "contraindicated" were being needlessly avoided by the mitochondrial disease patient population and rather, should each be discussed thoroughly with the individual treating clinicians.

Conflicts of Interest

SS and AG have no relevant conflicts of interest to declare. MJF is coinventor on International Patent Application No. PCT/US19/39631 entitled "Compositions and Methods for Treatment of Mitochondrial Respiratory Chain Dysfunction and Other Mitochondrial Disorders and Methods for Identifying Efficacious Agents for the Alleviating Symptoms of the Same," filed in the name of The Children's Hospital of Philadelphia on June 27, 2019. MJF is a scientific advisory board member with equity interest in RiboNova, Inc., and scientific board member as paid consultant with Khondrion and with Larimar Therapeutics.

MJF has previously been or is currently engaged with several companies involved in mitochondrial disease therapeutic preclinical and/or clinical stage development as a paid consultant (Astellas [formerly Mitobridge] Pharma, Inc., Casma Therapeutics, Cyclerion Therapeutics, Imel Therapeutics, Minovia Therapeutics, NeuroVive Pharmaceutical, Reneo Therapeutics, Stealth BioTherapeutics, Zogenix, Inc.) and/or a sponsored research collaborator (AADI Therapeutics, Astellas [formerly Mitobridge] Pharma, Inc., Cyclerion Therapeutics, Epirium Therapeutics, Khondrion, Imel Therapeutics, Minovia Therapeutics Inc., Mission Therapeutics, NeuroVive Pharmaceutical, Raptor Therapeutics, REATA, Inc., RiboNova, Inc., Standigm Therapeutics, and Stealth BioTherapeutics), and has served as a paid speaker on mitochondrial disease (Platform Q).

Key Web Resources

Mitochondrial Disease Genes Compendium is a print and/or electronic reference for clinicians on mitochondrial disease from a gene-based perspective. (www.elsevier.com/books/mitochondrial-disease-genes-compendium/falk/978-0-12-820029-2).

Mitochondrial Disease Expert Panel Leigh Syndrome Gene Curation(https://search.clinicalgenome.org/kb/affiliate/10027?page=1&size=25&search=).

Mitochondrial Disease Sequence Resource (MSeqDR) is a publicly accessible bioinformatics resource that provides access to curated knowledge and tools designed to help evaluate nuclear and mtDNA related mitochondrial disease genes and variants(www.mseqdr.org).

Mitochondrial Medicine at Children's Hospital of Philadelphia\(www.chop.edu/centers-programs/mitochondrial-disease-clinical-center).

Mitochondrial Medicine Society(www.mitosoc.org/toolkit).

Mitomap is an online database of mitochondrial DNA variants reported to date.

United. Mitochondrial Disease Foundation. (www.umdf.org).

---

[1]Not FDA approved for this indication.

References

Alves CAPF, Teixeira SR, Martin-Saavedra JS, et al: Pediatric leigh syndrome: neuroimaging features and genetic correlations, *Ann Neurol* 88(2):218–232, 2020.

Barcelos I, Shadiack E, Ganetzky RD, Falk MJ: Mitochondrial medicine therapies: rationale, evidence, and dosing guidelines, *Curr Opin Pediatr* 32(6):707–718, 2020.

Falk M: In Kliegman R St, Geme J, editors: *Nelson textbook of pediatrics*, ed 21, Elsevier, pp 807–811, 2020.

Genetics of mitochondrial respiratory chain disease. In Ganetzky R, Falk M, Pyeritz R, Korf B, Korf B, Grody W, editors: *Emery and Rimoin's principles and practice of medical genetics and genomics*, 7 ed, Elsevier, pp 709–737, 2021.

Gorman GS, Chinnery PF, DiMauro S, et al: Mitochondrial diseases, *Nat Rev Dis Primers* 2:16080, 2016.

Muraresku CC, McCormick EM, Falk MJ: Mitochondrial Disease: advances in clinical diagnosis, management, therapeutic development, and preventative strategies, *Curr Genet Med Rep* 6(2):62–72, 2018.

Parikh S, Goldstein A, Koenig MK, et al: Diagnosis and management of mitochondrial disease: a consensus statement from the Mitochondrial Medicine Society, *Genet Med* 17(9):689–701, 2015.

Rahman S, Thorburn D. Nuclear Gene-Encoded Leigh Syndrome Spectrum Overview. 2015 Oct 1 [Updated 2020 Jul 16]. In: Adam MP, Ardinger HH, Pagon RA, et al., editors. GeneReviews® [Internet]. Seattle (WA): University of Washington, Seattle; 1993-2021. Available from: https://www.ncbi.nlm.nih.gov/books/NBK320989/

Schaefer A, Lim A, Gorman GM, Mancuso T: In Klopstock, editor: *Diagnosis and management of mitochondrial disorders*, Springer Nature, pp 63–74, 2019.

Zolkipli-Cunningham Z, Xiao R, Stoddart A, et al: Mitochondrial disease patient motivations and barriers to participate in clinical trials, *PLoS One* 13(5):e0197513, 2018.

NOCTURNAL ENURESIS

Method of
Alexander K.C. Leung, MBBS

Note: This chapter has been published in part in *Common Problems in Ambulatory Pediatrics: Specific Clinical Problems*, volume 1, with permission from Nova Science Publishers, Inc.

CURRENT DIAGNOSIS

- Nocturnal enuresis is defined as involuntary nighttime bedwetting in a child at least 5 years of age.
- Primary nocturnal enuresis is present when the child has never achieved a period of nighttime dryness greater than 6 consecutive months. Secondary nocturnal enuresis is present when the child has experienced a period of nighttime dryness of at least 6 consecutive months.
- The most common causes of primary nocturnal enuresis are a deep sleep pattern, nocturnal polyuria, and a small-capacity bladder or nocturnal detrusor overactivity.
- A urinalysis is warranted to rule out urinary tract infection, glycosuria, and a defect in the ability to concentrate urine.
- Ultrasound examination of the bladder (prevoid and postvoid) can be used to evaluate bladder dysfunction and functional bladder capacity.

CURRENT THERAPY

- Desmopressin (DDAVP, 1-deamino-8-arginine vasopressin) is indicated as a first-line therapy for children with monosymptomatic nocturnal enuresis associated with nocturnal polyuria and normal bladder function.
- Enuretic alarm is indicated as a first-line therapy for children with monosymptomatic nocturnal enuresis associated with a small bladder capacity or in children with severe enuretic symptoms refractory to desmopressin therapy.
- Behavioral therapy such as encouraging the child to urinate frequently during the daytime, emptying the bladder before bedtime, and restricting fluid in the evening may increase the success rate of pharmacologic therapy or enuretic alarm therapy.

Nocturnal enuresis is defined as involuntary nighttime bedwetting in a child at least 5 years of age. Primary nocturnal enuresis is present when the child has never achieved a period of nighttime dryness greater than 6 consecutive months. Secondary nocturnal enuresis is present when the child has experienced a period of nighttime dryness of at least 6 consecutive months. For the majority of children with secondary nocturnal enuresis, the pathogenesis is no different from that of primary nocturnal enuresis.

Nocturnal enuresis is a common problem that is frustrating for children, parents, and physicians alike. The condition may affect the child's self-esteem and may lead to reduced social interaction and behavioral problems.

Epidemiology

It has been estimated that 15% to 25% of 5-year-old children and 5% to 10% of 7-year-old children have nocturnal enuresis. Without specific treatment, approximately 15% of affected children become dry each year. The male-to-female ratio is approximately 3:1.

Risk Factors

Encopresis, daytime wetting (diurnal enuresis), and male gender are significant risk factors. Constipation, emotional stress, developmental delay, bladder dysfunction, sleep deprivation, adenotonsillar hypertrophy, and attention-deficit/hyperactivity disorder also play a role.

Pathogenesis

The most common causes of primary nocturnal enuresis are a high arousal threshold, nocturnal polyuria, and a small-capacity bladder or nocturnal detrusor overactivity. Although these causes may overlap, it is important to conceptualize them separately, because this differentiation will help the physician to understand the problem, to educate both the parents and child, and to plan an appropriate treatment program.

It has been shown that enuretic children have a high arousal threshold and a reduced prepulse inhibition of startle. In most children, arousability from sleep improves with maturation of the central nervous system.

In most circumstances, the rate of secretion of antidiuretic hormone from the posterior pituitary gland is increased at night. This circadian variation is usually established when the child is 3 to 4 years old. Some children with primary nocturnal enuresis have a lack of this circadian variation with an abnormally low nocturnal secretion of antidiuretic hormone with resultant nocturnal polyuria. Other causes of nocturnal polyuria include fluid and solute overload in the evening.

Children with a small-capacity bladder or nocturnal detrusor overactivity often have primary nocturnal enuresis. Conditions that may reduce the functional bladder capacity include cystitis and constipation.

There is a strong genetic component to nocturnal enuresis. The child of parents who were both enuretic has a 77% chance of developing enuresis. If one parent was enuretic, there is up to a 44% occurrence rate. If neither parent was enuretic, the occurrence rate is only 15%. Twin studies also support a genetic basis for nocturnal enuresis: the concordance rate is much higher in monozygotic twins (68%) when compared with dizygotic twins (36%). Linkage studies have suggested possible genetic markers for primary nocturnal enuresis located on chromosomes 12, 13, and 22.

A neurogenic bladder is one of the few anatomic abnormalities that can cause primary nocturnal enuresis. Congenital urethral obstruction is another infrequent anatomic cause of primary nocturnal enuresis. The enuresis in these children is due to an overflow phenomenon from a poorly compliant bladder. The most common cause of urethral obstruction in the male is posterior urethral valves. Girls and boys with significant congenital urethral stenosis may also present with this problem. An ectopic ureter or vesicovaginal fistula is an infrequent anatomic cause of primary nocturnal enuresis in girls.

A defect in the ability of the kidney to concentrate urine can cause primary nocturnal enuresis. The causes of concentrating defects include any cause of chronic renal failure and diabetes insipidus.

Diagnosis
History
Onset and Frequency
The timing of the onset and the frequency of nocturnal enuresis are important historical clues to the etiology. Secondary nocturnal enuresis and intermittent nocturnal enuresis are not usually associated with structural abnormalities in the urinary tract. Nocturnal enuresis due to a structural abnormality of the urinary tract is usually present from birth and is not associated with periods of remission.

Timing, Frequency, and Volume per Episode
A history of soaking absorbent underpants in the morning suggests nocturnal polyuria. Parents of children with nocturnal polyuria often remark that the volume of urine associated with the enuretic episode or the first morning void is very large. Frequent episodes of nocturnal enuresis with a small volume of urine suggest bladder dysfunction such as may occur with a urethral obstruction or a neurogenic bladder. Several episodes of nocturnal enuresis with a large volume suggest diabetes mellitus or diabetes insipidus. Constant wetting suggests an ectopic ureter or vesicovaginal fistula.

Associated Symptoms
Nocturnal enuresis associated with daytime urinary frequency, urgency, incontinence, and difficulties in initiating the urinary stream suggests urethral obstruction. Daytime urinary frequency, urgency, incontinence, squatting behavior, constipation, encopresis, gait disturbance, and a history of spina bifida or spinal trauma suggest a neurogenic bladder. Constant dampness in the underwear by day and night in a female suggests an ectopic ureter or vesicovaginal fistula. Secondary nocturnal enuresis associated with dysuria, urinary frequency, urgency, fever, suprapubic/loin pain, or cloudy, foul-smelling urine suggests a urinary tract infection. Polyuria, polydipsia, polyphagia, and weight loss suggest diabetes mellitus. Polyuria, polydipsia, and episodes of dehydration in a child with a history of central nervous system disease suggest diabetes insipidus. A history of constipation is important because the condition is associated with a reduced functional bladder capacity.

Volume of First Morning Void
Most children with nocturnal enuresis void only a small or average amount of urine in the morning after an enuretic episode. A large volume of urine voided following a significant episode of nocturnal enuresis may be a clue to the presence of low nocturnal secretion of antidiuretic hormone.

Soundness of Sleep
Children with nocturnal enuresis often sleep more deeply than other family members. Some children only wet when they are overtired. Conversely, children who are usually enuretic may be continent during periods of wakeful sleep such as during intercurrent illnesses.

Past Health
A child with a history of a structural abnormality of the urinary tract or neurogenic bladder may have nocturnal enuresis due to these causes. A history of spinal trauma may indicate a neurogenic bladder as a cause of enuresis. A history of central nervous system disorder may indicate neurogenic diabetes insipidus. Certain medications such as methylxanthines and caffeine may be associated with nocturnal enuresis.

Family History
A family history of nocturnal enuresis should be sought because nocturnal enuresis tends to run in the family. A family history of diabetes mellitus, diabetes insipidus, or kidney disease suggests the corresponding disorder. Any stressful events in the family such as birth of a sibling and parental disharmony should be explored, especially in children with secondary nocturnal enuresis.

Physical Examination
Height and weight should be measured and plotted onto standard growth charts. All children should have their blood pressure checked, which, if elevated, might indicate renal disease. A thorough physical examination should include examination of the abdomen and genitalia and a complete neurologic examination. In chronic constipation, fecal masses are often palpable in the left lower quadrant of the abdomen and in the suprapubic area.

In the majority of children with primary nocturnal enuresis, the physical examination is unremarkable. An abnormal physical examination is only present when primary nocturnal enuresis is due to a structural cause. A myelomeningocele is usually obvious at birth; however, subtle spinal defects may also be associated with primary nocturnal enuresis. A midline tuft of hair, an exaggerated dimple, or a birthmark in the area of the lumbosacral spine; a gait abnormality; absence of anal wink; or abnormal motor power, tone, reflexes, or sensation in the lower extremities suggests a neurogenic bladder. A palpably enlarged bladder or kidney and a weak or dribbling urinary stream suggests urinary obstruction, such as may result from posterior urethral valves.

Laboratory and Imaging Studies
A urinalysis is warranted to rule out urinary tract infection, diabetes mellitus, and a defect in the ability to concentrate urine. Ultrasound examination of the bladder (prevoid and postvoid) can be used to evaluate bladder dysfunction and functional bladder capacity.

Treatment
One essential part of the treatment plan of every child with primary nocturnal enuresis should be compassion and support from both the family and physician. It is important to clarify to parents that the child is not at fault and to specify that punishment for bedwetting is inappropriate. The child and family can be reassured that in the absence of structural defect, primary nocturnal enuresis tends to resolve with time.

Simple behavioral strategies such as encouraging the child to urinate frequently during the daytime, emptying the bladder before bedtime, and limiting fluid and solute intake in the evening are often recommended. Caffeinated beverages should be avoided, particularly in the evening. Some authors recommend waking the child 1.5 to 2 hours after bedtime to go to the bathroom. Star charts and reward systems need to reinforce positive behavior. Behavioral therapy may increase the success rate of pharmacologic therapy or enuretic alarm therapy.

Desmopressin (DDAVP, 1-deamino-8-arginine vasopressin) is an analogue of vasopressin that has a profound antidiuretic activity without pressor activity. The medication acts on the V2 receptors of the renal tubules and increases the reabsorption of fluid from the renal tubules, thereby decreasing the amount of urine produced. The medication is indicated as a first-line therapy for children with monosymptomatic nocturnal enuresis associated with nocturnal polyuria and normal bladder function. Desmopressin is available in a sublingual lyophilisate (melt) preparation,[2] as well as a tablet. The bioavailability of the lyophilisate (melt) preparation is approximately 60% greater than that of the tablet formulation. The recommended dose of desmopressin is 120 to 240 μg melt and 200 to 400 μg tablet. The former is usually given 30 minutes to 1 hour before bedtime, and the latter is usually given 1 hour before bedtime. Side effects are rare and include symptomatic hyponatremia with water intoxication. When desmopressin is prescribed, patients should be instructed to avoid high fluid intake in the evening.

---

[1] Not FDA approved for this indication.

Imipramine (Tofranil), a tricyclic agent with antimuscarinic property, may be helpful in children who have not responded to desmopressin alone. Presumably, the medication decreases the amount of time spent in rapid eye movement sleep, stimulates antidiuretic hormone secretion, and relaxes the detrusor muscle. The recommended starting dose is 25 mg for children 6 to 12 years of age and 50 mg for those older than 12 years, given 1 to 2 hours before bedtime. If necessary, the dose may be increased gradually to a maximum of 50 mg in children 6 to 12 years of age and 75 mg for those older than 12 years. However, potential side effects (anxiety, depression, dizziness, headache, drowsiness, lethargy, sleep disturbance, dry mouth, anorexia, vomiting, skin rashes) and serious adverse effects (hepatotoxicity, cardiotoxicity) with overdose limit their use.

Monotherapy with oxybutynin (Ditropan),[1] an anticholinergic and antispasmodic agent that decreases uninhibited bladder contraction, is not effective in treating monosymptomatic nocturnal enuresis. The medication can be added, however, as a second-line drug in the treatment of children with both diurnal and nocturnal enuresis. The dose is 5 mg administered 1 hour before bedtime.

Enuretic alarm is indicated as a first-line therapy for children with monosymptomatic nocturnal enuresis associated with a small bladder capacity or nocturnal detrusor overactivity. Randomized controlled trials have demonstrated that the enuretic alarm has greater efficacy than other forms of treatment. The enuretic alarm is triggered when a sensor in the sheets or night clothes gets wet; a bell or buzzer is thereby activated. Presumably, alarm therapy startles the child and improves arousal from sleep either by classical conditioning or avoidance conditioning. A disadvantage of alarm therapy is that it takes a couple of weeks to take effect. As such, alarms should be used for at least 6 weeks in children who do not respond before discontinuing their use. Because success depends on a cooperative, motivated child, conditioning therapy with an alarm device is generally used in children over 6 years of age.

It has been shown that combination of alarm and desmopressin works better than either treatment alone. Such treatment may be considered for children with refractory nocturnal enuresis.

When an anatomic abnormality or defect in urinary concentration ability is present, the underlying problem may require specific dietary, pharmacologic, or surgical treatment. Any underlying constipation should also be treated.

[2] Not available in the United States.

References

Brown ML, Pope AW, Brown EJ: Treatment of primary nocturnal enuresis in children: a review, *Child Care Health Dev* 37:153–160, 2011.
Glazener CM, Evans JH: Desmopressin for nocturnal enuresis in children, *Cochrane Database Syst Rev* 3:CD002112, 2002.
Glazener CM, Evans JH, Pero RE: Alarm interventions for nocturnal enuresis in children, *Cochrane Database Syst Rev* 2:CD002911, 2005.
Kamperis K, Hagstroem S, Rittig S, et al: Combination of the enuresis alarm and desmopressin: Second line treatment for nocturnal enuresis, *J Urol* 179:1128–1131, 2008.
Leung AK: Nocturnal enuresis. In Leung AK, editor: Common Problems in Ambulatory Pediatrics: Specific Clinical Problems, vol 1. New York, 2011, Nova Science Publishers, pp 161–171.
Lottmann H, Froeling F, Alloussi S, et al: A randomized comparison of oral desmopressin lyophilisate (MELT) and tablet formulations in children and adolescents with primary nocturnal enuresis, *Int J Clin Pract* 61:1454–1460, 2007.
Nevéus T: Nocturnal enuresis—theoretic background and practical guidelines, *Pediatr. Nephrol* 26:1207–1214, 2011.
Robson WL: Evaluation and management of enuresis, *N Engl J Med* 360:1429–1436, 2009.
Robson WL, Leung AK, van Howe R: Primary and secondary nocturnal enuresis: similarities in presentation, *Pediatrics* 115:956–959, 2005.
Robson WL, Leung AK, Norgaard JP: The comparative safety of oral versus intranasal desmopressin in the treatment of children with nocturnal enuresis, *J Urol* 178:24–30, 2007.
Van de Walle J, Rittig S, Bauer S, et al: Practical consensus guidelines for the management of enuresis, *Eur J Pediatr* 171:971–983, 2012.

NORMAL INFANT FEEDING

Method of
Amy Seery, MD

CURRENT THERAPY

- Breast milk is considered the best nutritional source for all infants including preterm infants.
- Breast-feeding is strongly encouraged, but many mothers require support from a multidisciplinary medical team to achieve success.
- There are few absolute contraindications to breast-feeding but these include maternal HIV, infant galactosemia, herpetic lesions on the breast, maternal use of illicit drugs, and mothers undergoing some types of chemotherapy.
- Maternal medications should be individually reviewed for safety during breast-feeding.
- Newborns should be fed at least every 3 hours during the day and every 4 hours during the night.
- Breast-fed infants can go up to 10 days between stools. This is a normal stooling pattern so long as the infant shows no signs of distress or illness.

The newborn period is defined as birth through the 28th day of life. During this time, newborns primarily feed, grow, and sleep. Therefore adequate nutrition carries special significance during this phase of life. This chapter focuses on available options for newborn nutrition (e.g., breast milk and commercial formulas), information medical caregivers can use when counseling families, definitions of adequate quality and quantity of nutritional sources, and assessing for appropriate intake in terms of growth.

Breast-feeding and Breast Milk

Breast-feeding is the nutritional source of choice as recommended by the American Academy of Pediatrics (AAP), the Canadian Pediatric Society, and the American Academy of Family Physicians. Caregivers should always respect the choice of the mother and support her during her bonding period with her newborn infant. However, because many misconceptions exist regarding breast-feeding, it is practical for caregivers to inquire about a mother's reasons if she chooses to use formula to feed her infant. She may have several concerns about breast-feeding including returning to work, the logistics of pumping, or her modesty, or she may consider breast-feeding to be "antiquated." Breast-feeding may be contrary to cultural and ethnic beliefs of the mother. For example, some Hispanic women are concerned that when breast-feeding they might inadvertently pass on negative emotions to their newborn. Because Somalian mothers attribute special powers to Western medicine and infant formulas, they often breast-feed but supplement with formula to ensure their infant gets everything that modern medicine can offer. With proper education and support, many mothers find breast-feeding to be a more reasonable option than they first thought.

Thanks to the efforts of several organizations promoting the health benefits of breast-feeding, even mothers who choose to formula feed recognize breast milk as the best nutritional option for their infant. But even after making the decision to breast-feed, some mothers continue to struggle with the actual undertaking of breast-feeding. There remains in our culture the inaccurate belief that something so "natural" must be easy to do. Many first-time mothers are easily frustrated and discouraged during the first few attempts at breast-feeding because they have unreasonable expectations based on the media and popular culture. With more and more women willing to try breast-feeding after delivery, adequate support and teaching should be provided by the entire medical team.

Thanks to multiple initiatives and ongoing education efforts, breast-feeding rates have been increasing in the US and are currently at their highest rates since World War II. Healthy People 2020 has a goal for a national breast-feeding initiation rate of 81.9%, and the actual rate of breast-feeding initiation in 2012 was 80.0%. Targets for exclusive breast-feeding at 3 months and 6 months are 46% and 25% respectively. The actual rate reported at 3 months is 43.3% and at 6 months is 21.9%. The rate for any breast-feeding at 12 months old is 29.2% though the goal is 34.1%. While significant progress has been made, especially in the last decade, there is still substantial room for further improvement. The biggest disparities in breast-feeding rates are among racial and ethnic minorities. Special attention should be made by medical teams to provide sufficient support and education to these women.

Breast milk is considered the ideal source of nutrition for all newborns, including premature infants, in a large part owing to its contents. There is a greater ratio of whey to casein in breast milk than in formula. Whey is associated with better absorption and digestion, as well as faster gastrointestinal transit times. There are also several specific proteins found only in breast milk, such as lactoferrin, lysozyme, and secretory immunoglobulin A, that aid in immune defense in the gut. Breast milk also contains long-chain polyunsaturated fatty acids (PUFAs) that aid in neural and visual development. Infants given formulas that contain long-chain PUFAs have serum concentrations that never match those of breast milk–fed infants, but there is also no known minimum amount needed to achieve benefit.

There is also a difference in the intestinal microflora seen in infants fed breast milk versus those fed formula. Larger percentages of *Lactobacillus* and *Bifidobacterium* species are found in infants fed breast milk, whereas *Bacteroides* spp and enterobacteria are in more abundance in formula-fed counterparts. Newer evidence suggests this difference in the diversity of gut microflora accounts for the stronger immune systems seen in breast-fed infants.

Breast milk has the benefit of containing several nonnutritive substances that are advantageous for young infants including maternal antibodies, growth regulators, digestive enzymes, and hormones. Breast milk has been associated with a reduced risk for many chronic illnesses including asthma, food and environmental allergies, diabetes mellitus, eczema, cardiovascular disease, and obesity. There is a reduction in the number of short-term illnesses of childhood including acute respiratory and gastrointestinal illnesses, as well as otitis media.

Newer research shows an association between being fed breast milk and having higher IQ scores later in childhood.

The act of breast-feeding offers several benefits to the infant. There is a sense of security and closeness that comes from skin-to-skin contact and the resultant interaction between infant and mother. Nursing can also reduce the opportunities and risk for bottle-propping and overfeeding. Breast-feeding allows nutrition to be more immediately available with minimal preparation work compared to the mixing and warming of formula. Breast milk is a much cheaper alternative to supplemental formulas. Breast-feeding can also lead to health benefits for the mother such as decreased risk of ovarian and breast cancers, as well as diabetes mellitus type II.

There are very few contraindications to breast-feeding. Contraindications include maternal HIV, active herpetic lesions on the breast (herpetic lesions elsewhere are not a contraindication), maternal use of illicit drugs, women undergoing chemotherapy with antimetabolite agents, and mothers with active tuberculosis. Nearly all over-the-counter medications are safe to take during breast-feeding. Some prescription medications are contraindicated, although safe substitutes are usually available. Providers can use the online National Library of Medicine's Drugs and Lactation Database (LactMed) to check safety and provide up-to-date counseling. Infants with galactosemia should not be breast-fed or bottle fed with milk products.

Infant Formulas

Commercially available infant formulas became widely used during World War II when there was a large influx of women into the national workforce. Since that time, infant formulas have been continuously improved upon and contain all the necessary energy and nutrient requirements for full-term infants up to the age of 6 months. According to the AAP there are three indications for the use of formulas:

- An alternative primary nutritional source for infants whose mothers choose not to or are unable to breast-feed
- A supplementary nutritional source for mothers with an inadequate supply of breast milk
- A nutritional source in infants with a medical condition in which breast-feeding is contraindicated (e.g., galactosemia)

Commercial formulas usually come in three distinct preparations, including ready-to-feed, concentrated liquid, and powder. All three preparations yield 20 kcal per fluid ounce when prepared correctly, the same amount of energy per volume found in breast milk. Powder preparations are generally the least expensive. An advantage to formulas over breast-feeding is the ability to increase caloric density for an infant with increased metabolic needs (e.g., infants with congenital heart defects). Breast-feeding mothers have the option to breast pump and add a fortifier if needed to achieve similar increases in caloric density.

Formulas carry the risk of improper preparation, whether intentional or accidental. Caregivers might choose to dilute the formula secondary to financial pressures or to concentrate formula preparations in a desire to have a larger infant, because some cultures equate larger infant size and weight with better health. Either change can be dangerous to the infant. Diluting leads to an excess of free water with an insufficient solute load (e.g., hyponatremia) and concentrating can conversely lead to hypernatremia. Nevertheless, formulas remain an appropriate alternative when desired by the infant's mother or when medically indicated (Table 1).

Micronutrients

Both breast milk and formula contain most of the micronutrients needed by infants. Calcium and phosphorus are found in lower concentrations in breast milk but are more bioavailable than the minerals present in formulas. Therefore there is no difference in bone mineral concentrations in both sets of infants. Iron, zinc, and copper serum levels are sufficient during the first 6 months of life in breast-fed infants, although tissue stores are gradually depleted. After 6 months breast-feeding should be supplemented with complementary foods to prevent outcomes such as iron deficiency anemia.

Vitamin K, necessary to prevent hemorrhagic disease, is produced by the digestive actions of intestinal flora. For this reason, most infants at the time of birth are given a single intramuscular dose to provide adequate amounts until intestinal flora concentrations are more mature and dietary supplementation with solid food begins at 6 months.

Vitamin D needs historically have been achieved with adequate sunlight exposure. However, with appropriate use of sunscreens and sunlight avoidance, most infants are at risk for vitamin D deficiency. Vitamin D is not passed in sufficient quantities in breast milk, and the content in formulas is so low that the daily recommended amount of 400 IU is only achieved when infants are consuming a volume typical of a 6-month old. Therefore supplementation should be recommended for all infants regardless of skin color and nutritional source to help prevent rickets. The recommendation is 400 IU of vitamin D for all pediatric age groups beginning after the first 2 weeks of life.

Neither formula-fed nor breast-fed infants usually require supplementation with water. In fact, providing infants with excess free water can lead to hyponatremia, seizures, and death. If there is concern that the infant is constipated or overheated, caregivers can provide up to a tablespoon of water daily to infants younger than 4 months old.

Defining Adequate Intake

To determine whether a newborn is receiving adequate nutrition, physicians should ask the caregiver how often feedings are

TABLE 1 | Infant Formulas and their Indications

CLASS	BRAND NAMES	CALORIES (KCAL PER OZ)	CARBOHYDRATE SOURCE	PROTEIN SOURCE	INDICATIONS
Breast milk	—	20	Lactose	Human milk	Preferred for all infants
Term formula	Gerber Good Start Gentle	20	Lactose	Cow's milk	Appropriate for most infants
Term formula with DHA and ARA	Enfamil Premium Infant; Good Start Protect; Similac Advanced	20	Lactose	Cow's milk	Marketed to promote eye and brain development
Preterm formula	Enfamil Premature; Similac Special Care 24 with Iron	24	Lactose	Cow's milk	<34 wk gestational age Weight <1800 g
Enriched formula	Enfacare; Similac Neosure	22	Lactose	Cow's milk	34–36 wk gestational age Weight ≥1800 g
Soy formula	Enfamil Prosobee; Good Start Soy; Similac Isomil	20	Corn-based	Soy	Congenital lactase deficiency, galactosemia
Lactose-free formula	Similac Sensitive	20	Corn-based	Cow's milk	Congenital lactase deficiency, primary lactase deficiency, galactosemia
Hypoallergenic formula	Similac Alimentum; Enfamil Nutramigen; Enfamil Pregestimil	20	Corn or Sucrose	Hydrolyzed proteins	Milk protein allergy
Nonallergenic formula	Elecare; Neocate Infant; Nutramigen AA	20	Corn or Sucrose	Amino acids	Milk protein allergy
Antireflex formula	Enfamil AR; Similac Sensitive for Spit-Up	20	Lactose (thickened with rice starch)	Cow's milk	Gastroesophageal reflux

Abbreviations: ARA=arachidonic acid; DHA=docosahexaenoic acid.
Adapted from O'Connor NR. Infant formula. Am Fam Physician 2009;79:565–70.

TABLE 2 | Expected Growth Velocities during Infancy

AGE	WEIGHT GAIN (g/d)	LENGTH (cm/mo)	HEAD CIRCUMFERENCE (cm/wk)
0–3 mo	25–30	2.5	0.5
3–6 mo	15–20	2.5	0.5
6–12 mo	10	1.25	0.25

occurring, for how long (for breast-fed infants), and how much is eaten (for formula-fed infants) and should assess the number of wet diapers and stools daily. Initially infants should consume 10 to 15 mL per feeding for the first 24 to 36 hours, gradually increasing to 30 to 45 mL by the fourth day of life. Breast-fed infants should feed 15 to 20 minutes each side. At the time of discharge to home, all newborns should be feeding 8 to 12 times a day, or every 2 to 3 hours. This interval can be increased to every 4 hours at night, and parents should be encouraged to wake any infants who sleep for longer than this duration. If an infant has lost more than 10% of his or her birth weight, the care team should consider delaying discharge to review the infant's nutritional status and feeding habits. Caregivers should be attentive to infant cues of hunger and satiety to provide an ideal feeding pattern for each infant.

Voiding and stooling patterns change with age and can also be influenced by the infant's diet. All newborns should have at least one wet diaper and one stool within the first 24 hours of life. If this does not occur, close observation and further workup are indicated to rule out structural or metabolic abnormalities. During the first week of life, infants usually void and stool with every feeding or even more often. Beyond the first week, infants should have at least 4 to 6 voids daily regardless of diet.

Formula-fed infants might have one stool every other day up to 2 to 3 stools daily. Because of the higher percentage of protein that is absorbed in breast milk, breast-fed infants can go up to 10 days between stools. Physicians should review with families the signs and symptoms (emesis, refusal to feed, lethargy, inconsolability, and abdominal distention) that indicate an infant with infrequent stooling should be medically evaluated. Breast-fed infants also have stools that are described as loose, yellow, and seedy. Caregivers should be educated that this is a normal stool color and consistency and is not considered diarrhea.

Medical providers can also calculate an infant's nutritional needs and compare to the actual intake. Nutritional needs are represented as kcal/kg per day (KKD). The following formula can be used:

$$KKD = \frac{Volume\ in\ mL\ consumed\ in\ 24h}{Weight\ in\ kg} \times \frac{20\ kcal/oz}{30}$$

During the first 3 months of life, infants should consume an intake that equals 90 to 135 kcal/kg per day. This intake goal should lead to a weight gain of approximately 25 to 30 g daily. From 3 to 6 months of age, infants gain at a slightly slower rate of approximately 15 to 20 g per day (Table 2). For example, a

2-month-old who weighs 6 kg should consume between 810 mL to 1215 mL daily.

At subsequent visits an infant can be assessed for adequate growth using standardized, gender-specific growth curves. Attention should be paid to growth parameters including weight, length, head circumference, and weight-for-length. Weight-for-length charts are used during the first 2 years of life as a gross equivalent to body-mass-index charts used for children older than 2 years. For years, practices defined adequate weight gain using growth charts as designed by the National Center for Health Statistics (NCHS), a branch of the Centers for Disease Control and Prevention (CDC). These charts were last updated in 2000 and unfortunately still reflect means for a population with a predominance of formula-fed infants. The World Health Organization (WHO) has since completed the Multi-Centre Growth Reference Study to better establish growth norms for infants and children who are breast-fed throughout the first year of life. A provider who is uncertain whether an exclusively breast-fed infant is meeting minimum growth requirements should refer to these charts before automatically encouraging caregivers to begin formula supplementation. Growth failure is usually considered a weight less than the third percentile or a drop of two or more percentiles in a short time (Figures 1 to 8, available on Expert Consult).

Overfeeding of newborns is unfortunately common, although bottle-fed infants are at a greater risk compared with breast-fed infants. Several factors can contribute to overfeeding, including lack of caregiver experience and support, as well as cultural biases such as the desire to have a chubbier infant. Many caregivers are unable to recognize infant cues for hunger and satiety and misinterpret cries or other vocalizations as a request for food. Medical providers should teach families about the rooting and sucking reflex and explain that some forms of sucking provide the infant with a means for self-soothing and are not signals that the infant is hungry (non-nutritive vs nutritive sucking).

Introduction of Complementary Foods

It remains controversial when solid foods should be added to the diet of an infant. The WHO recommends waiting until 6 months old. The AAP encourages waiting until an infant is 4 months old before adding solids and encourages continued breast-feeding until at least 1 year of age. However, some families want to start solids sooner than 4 months of age for a variety of reasons. A common explanation is "helping the baby sleep better at night." Only by 4 months will infants have attained sufficient muscle strength and coordination to keep their head upright when seated and to protect their own airway during feedings that contain solid foods. Families should be encouraged to wait at least until 4 months old before introducing solids, usually starting with rice cereal. Introduction of solids should not be delayed for much longer than 6 months, especially for breast-fed infants, because this is typically when micronutrient stores have been depleted and dietary supplementation with solid foods is needed. Only one new solid should be introduced every 3 to 5 days so infants can be monitored for adverse food reactions.

Either formula or breast milk should continue to be offered until 12 months old, at which time infants can be transitioned to whole-fat cow's milk. Low-fat milk does not provide toddlers with sufficient lipid concentrations for adequate brain development or the required caloric density for general growth. Large quantities of fruit juices should be avoided throughout infancy and childhood because they provide little nutritional value.

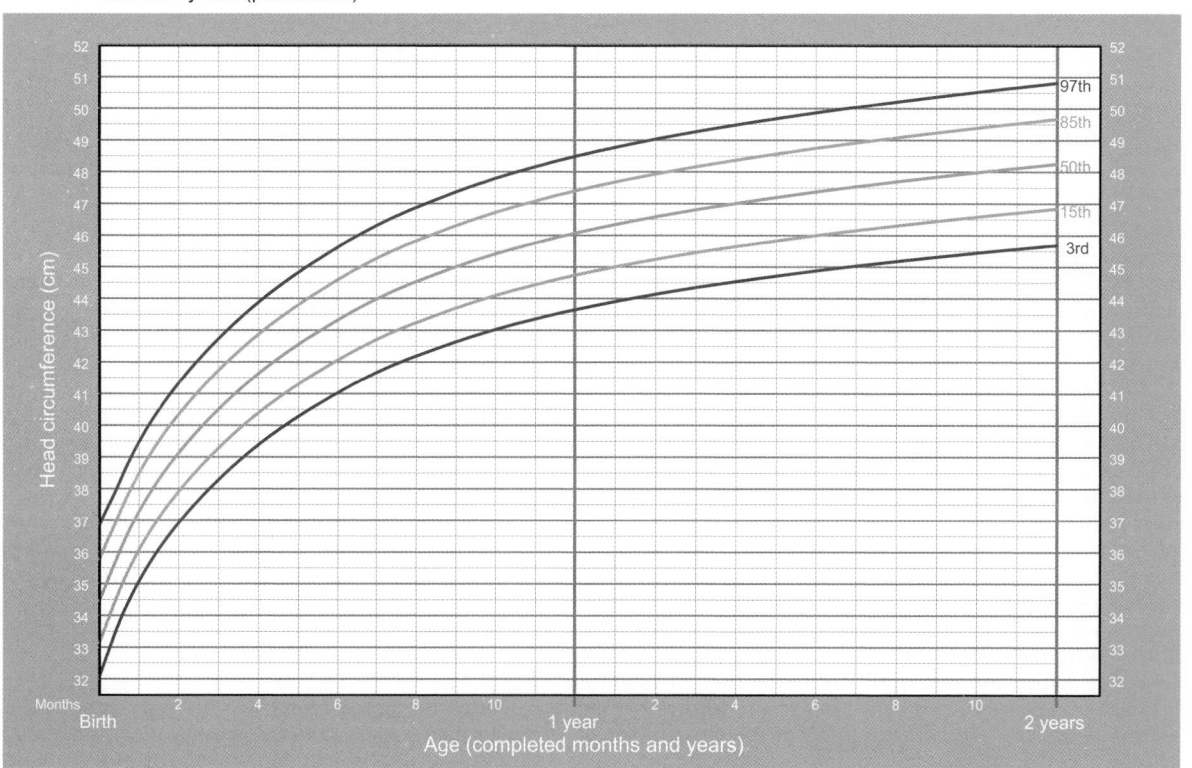

WHO Child Growth Standards

Figure 1 Head circumference for age: boys.

Length-for-age BOYS
Birth to 2 years (percentiles)

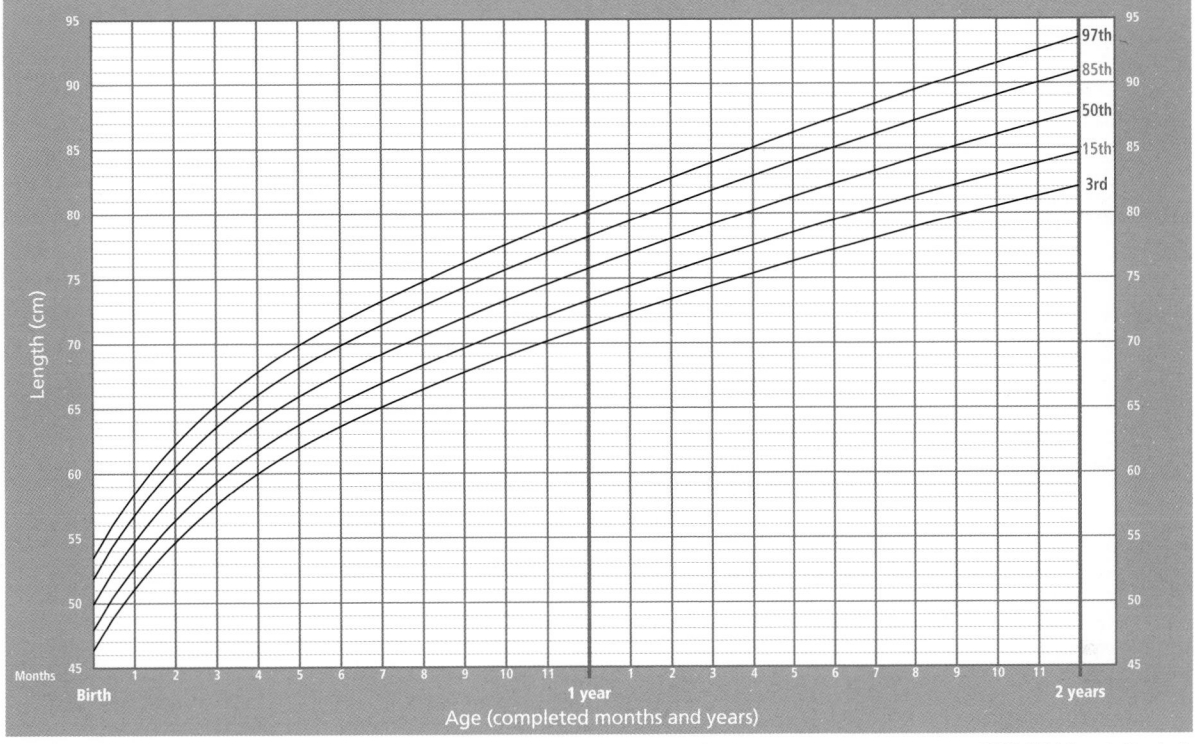

WHO Child Growth Standards

Figure 2 Length for age: boys.

Weight-for-age GIRLS
Birth to 2 years (percentiles)

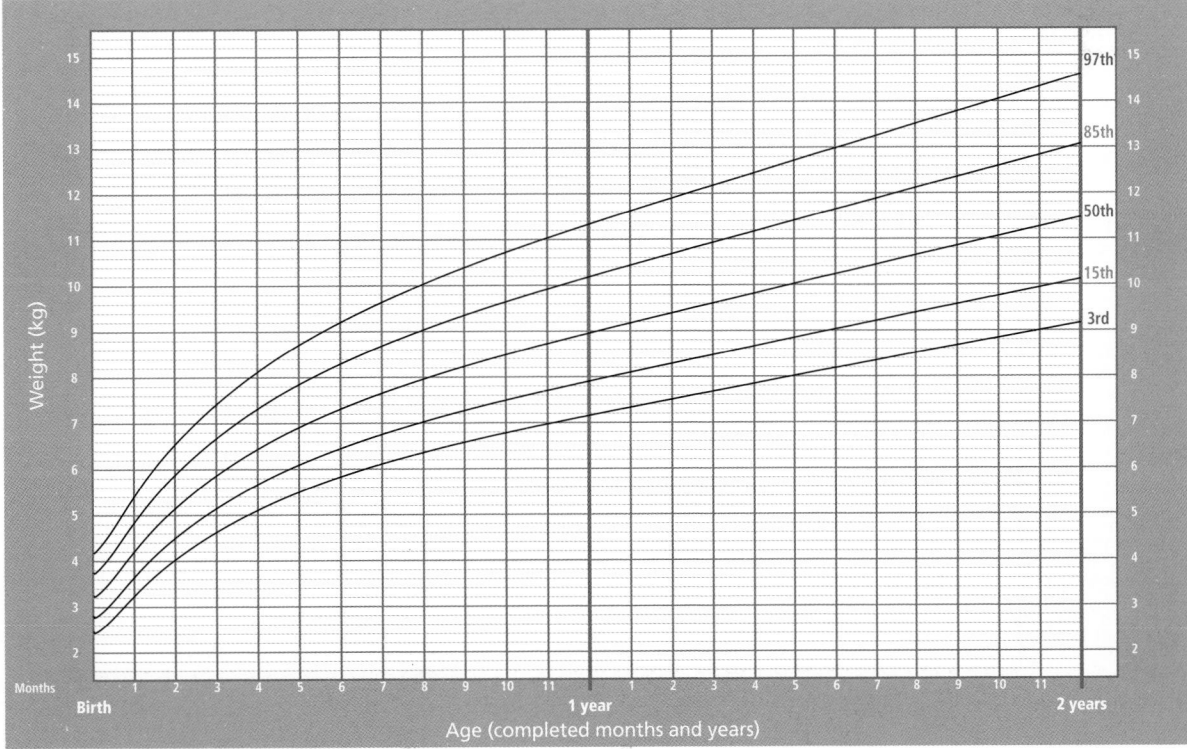

WHO Child Growth Standards

Figure 3 Weight for age: girls.

Weight-for-length GIRLS

Birth to 2 years (percentiles)

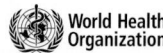
World Health
Organization

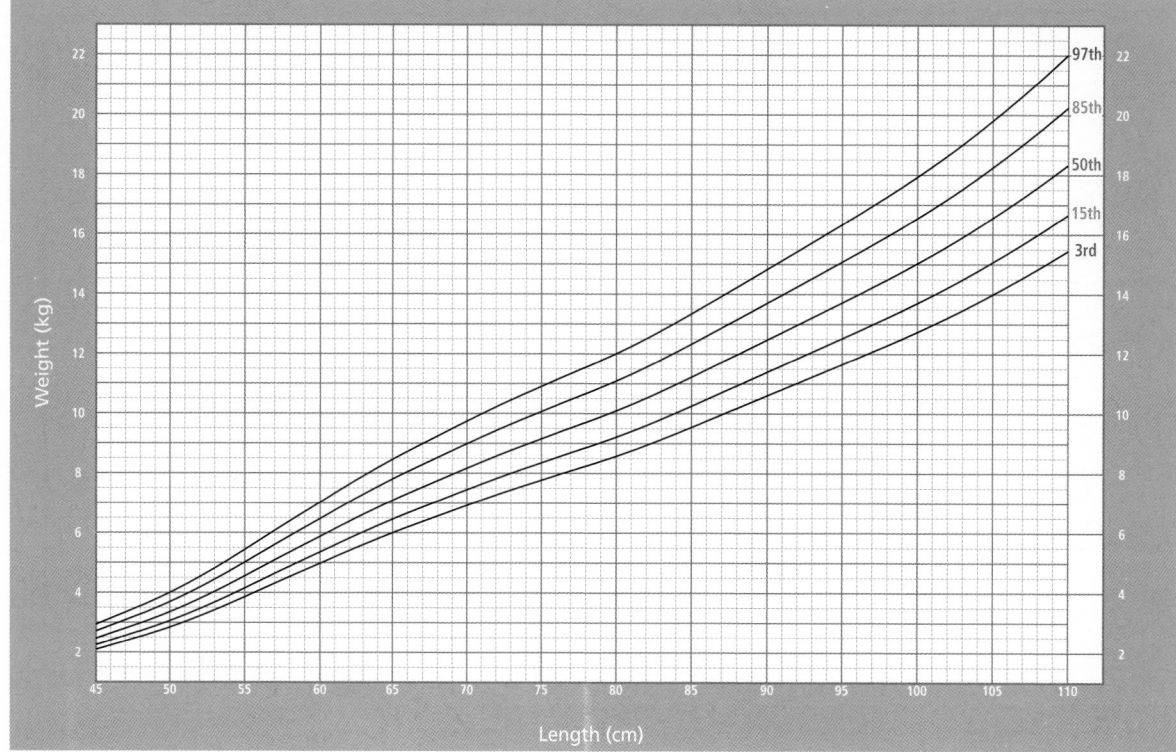

WHO Child Growth Standards

Figure 4 Weight for length: girls.

Head circumference-for-age GIRLS

Birth to 2 years (percentiles)

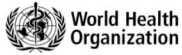
World Health
Organization

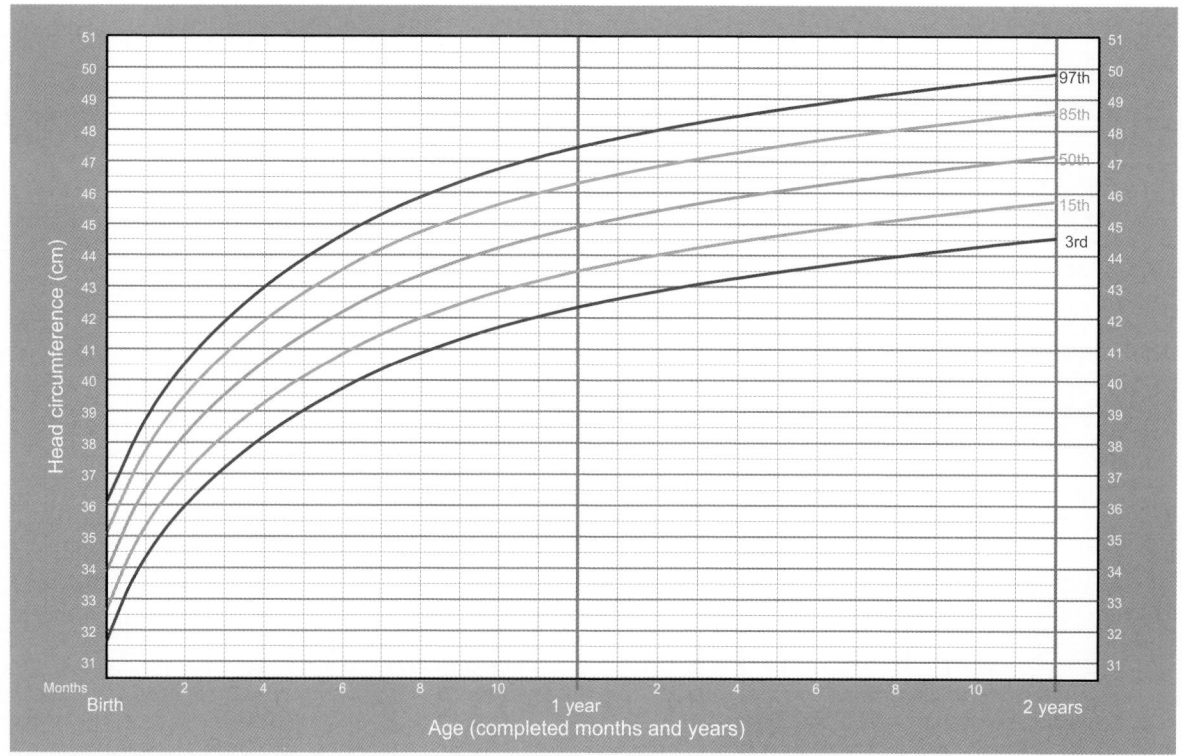

WHO Child Growth Standards

Figure 5 Head circumference for age: girls.

Weight-for-length BOYS

Birth to 2 years (percentiles)

World Health Organization

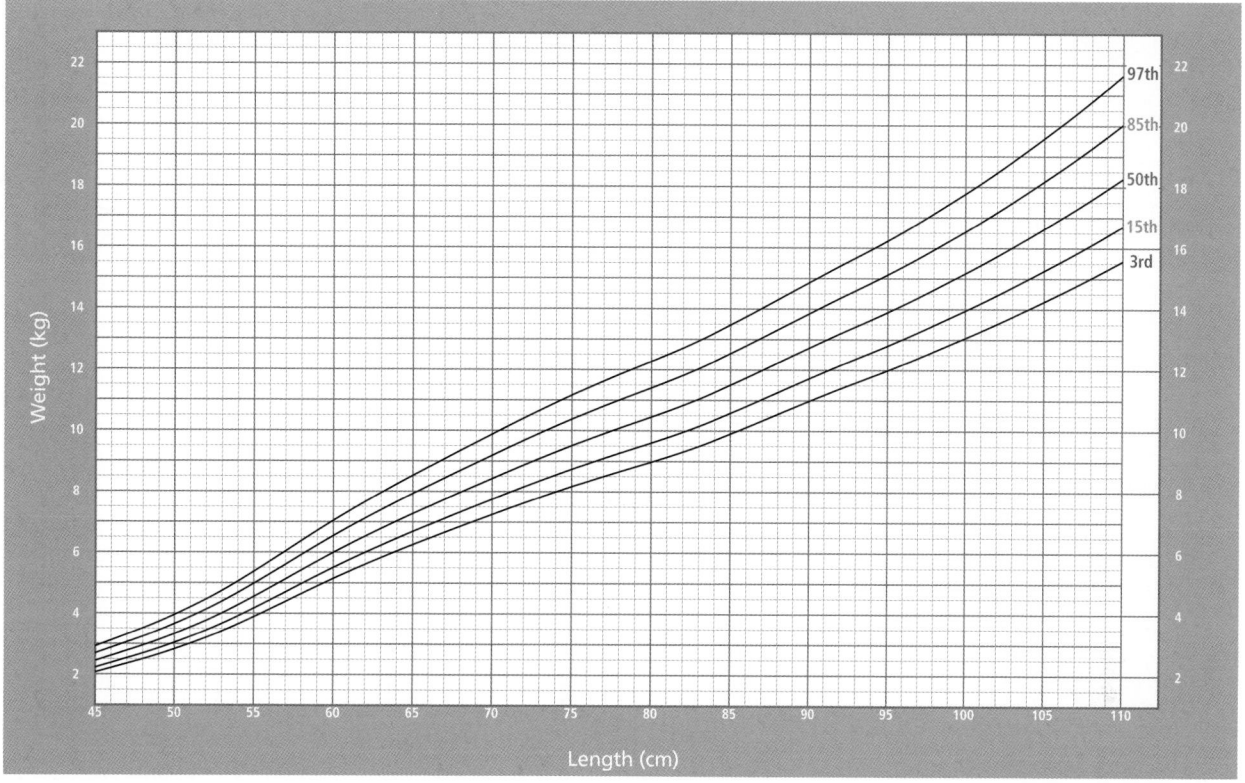

Length (cm)

WHO Child Growth Standards

Figure 6 Weight for length: boys.

Weight-for-age BOYS

Birth to 2 years (percentiles)

World Health Organization

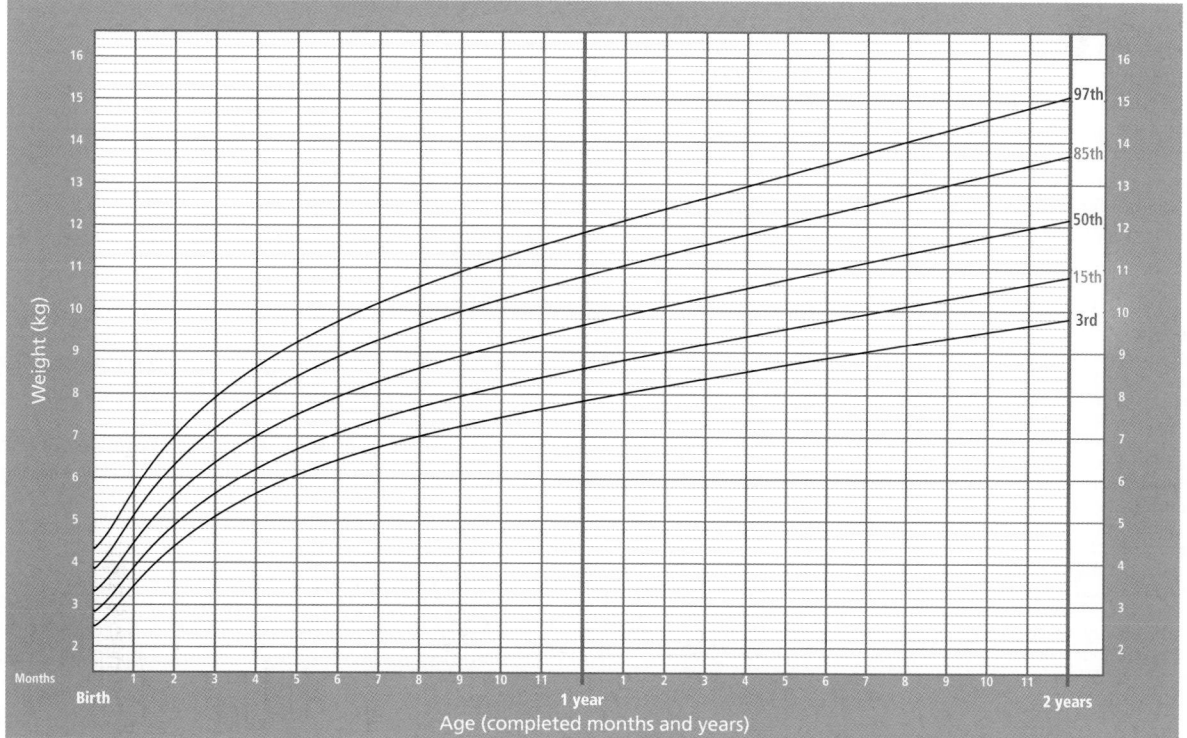

Age (completed months and years)

WHO Child Growth Standards

Figure 7 Weight for age: boys.

Length-for-age GIRLS
Birth to 2 years (percentiles)

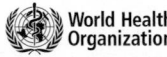

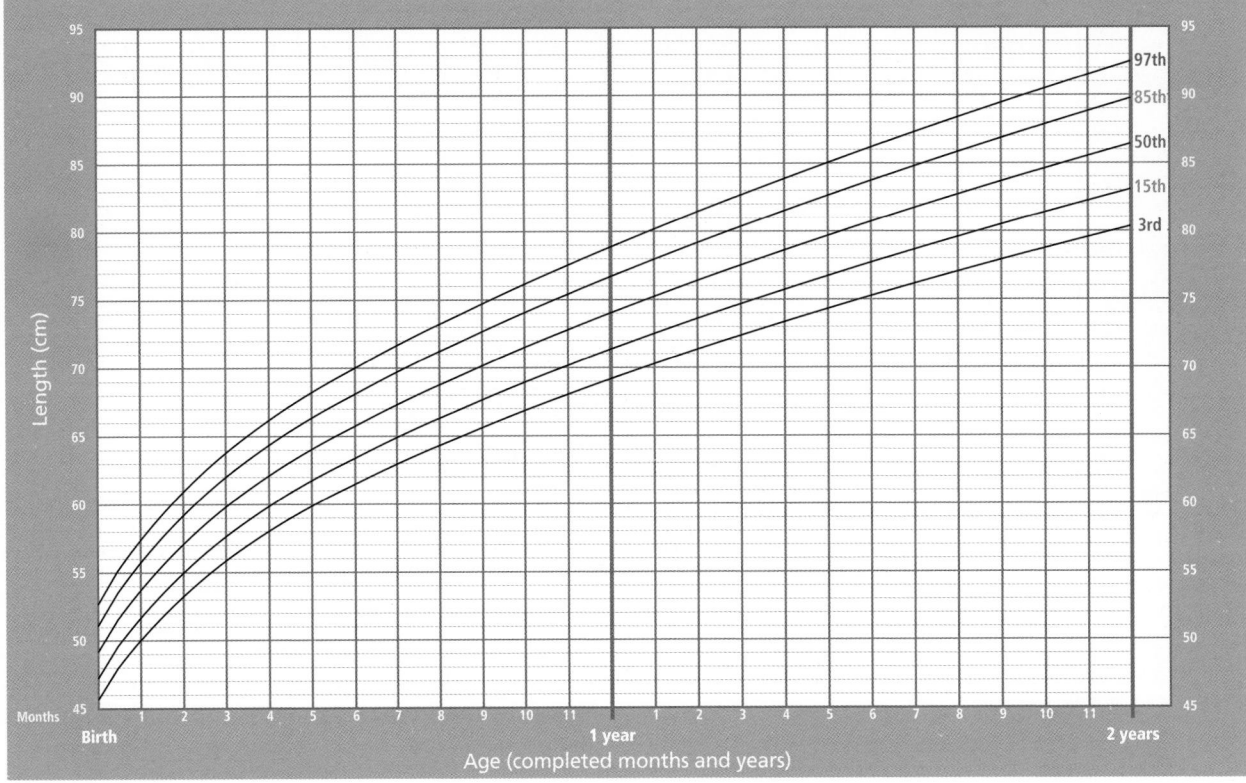

Figure 8 Length for age: girls.

Summary

The majority of term infants are born ready and able to begin feeding, but it is up to providers to know available nutritional options, normal feeding patterns, and means for measuring adequate intake and growth. Providers and other members of the care team also need to be able to counsel caregivers about best practices when feeding infants. When infants are suspected to be overfed or underfed, it may take a multidisciplinary approach by physicians, nurses, dieticians, speech therapists, lactation counselors, and social workers to help patients and their families.

References

American Academy of Family Physicians. Breastfeeding, Family Physicians Supporting (Position Paper). Available at http://www.aafp.org/online/en/home/policy/policies/b/breastfeedingpositionpaper.htm; [accessed August 17, 2017].

American Academy of Pediatrics, HealthyChildren.Org. Feeding and Nutrition, 0 to 12 Months. Available at http://www.healthychildren.org/English/ages-stages/baby/feeding-nutrition/Pages/default.aspx; [accessed August 17, 2017].

Duncan P: *Bright Futures: Guidelines for Health Supervision of Infants, Children, and Adolescents*, 3rd ed., Elk Grove Village, IL, 2007, American Academy of Pediatrics.

Kleinmann RE: *Pediatric Nutrition Handbook*, ed 6, Elk Grove Village, IL, 2008, American Academy of Pediatrics.

McInerny TK: *AAP Textbook of Pediatric Care*, ed 1, Elk Grove Village, IL, 2009, American Academy of Pediatrics.

National Library of Medicine. Drugs and Lactation Database. Available at http://toxnet.nlm.nih.gov/cgi-bin/sis/htmlgen?LACT; [accessed August 17, 2017].

O'Connor NR: Infant formula, *Am Fam Physician* 79:565–570, 2009.

USPSTF.: Primary care interventions to support breastfeeding- USPSTF recommendation statement, *JAMA* 316(16):1688–1693, 2016.

World Health Organization. The WHO Multicentre Growth Reference Study. Available at http://www.who.int/childgrowth/mgrs/en/; [accessed August 17, 2017].

OBESITY IN CHILDREN

Method of
Casey R. Johnson, MD, MS; and Seema Kumar, MD

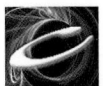

CURRENT DIAGNOSIS

- Body mass index (BMI) is calculated as weight in kilograms divided by height (or length) in meters squared (kg/m²). BMI is currently the standard measure for classifying the weight status of a child.
- A child ≥2 years of age is diagnosed as overweight if the BMI is ≥85th percentile and <95th percentile for age and sex, as obese if the BMI is ≥95th percentile, and as severely obese if the BMI is ≥120% of the 95th percentile or ≥35 kg/m² (whichever is lower).
- The Centers for Disease Control and Prevention (CDC) recommends using growth curves based on the World Health Organization (WHO) reference standards for infants and toddlers <2 years of age and using the CDC/National Center for Health Statistics growth reference standards for children ≥2 years of age.

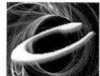
CURRENT THERAPY

- Lifestyle modifications including dietary changes, increased physical activity, and decreased sedentary time remain first-line for prevention and treatment of childhood obesity.
- Family-based lifestyle interventions and a multidisciplinary team approach are key components of effective management of childhood obesity.
- Pharmacotherapy should be considered for carefully selected children with obesity; however, there is limited data on long-term efficacy and safety of weight-loss medications in children.
- Bariatric surgery has been shown to result in significant weight loss and should be considered for children with severe obesity and those that have significant obesity-related comorbidities.

Introduction

Childhood obesity has emerged as an important public health problem in the United States and across the globe. The increasing prevalence of childhood obesity, severe obesity, and weight-related comorbidities places great risk on affected individuals, societies, and healthcare infrastructures. Moreover, childhood obesity tracks closely with obesity in adulthood, especially those with severe obesity and/or a strong family history of obesity, a relationship that foreshadows bigger problems for future generations. Childhood obesity and evidence-based treatment guidelines are discussed in this chapter.

Diagnosis

Childhood obesity is marked by excess accumulation of body fat. Body mass index (BMI) is considered the most practical method for evaluation of obesity. BMI is calculated from weight in kilograms and the square of the height (or length) in meters, as shown below:

$$BMI = \frac{Weight}{Height^2}$$

Normal growth and development during childhood results in dynamic changes in weight and height, which vary based on age and sex. Childhood growth parameters, including BMI, may then be plotted against growth curves created from standardized reference populations, normalized by age and sex. The World Health Organization (WHO) has developed growth standards for infants and children up to 5 years of age, and the Centers for Disease Control and Prevention (CDC) has similarly published reference standards for children between ages 2 and 20 years. The CDC recommends using the WHO standards from infancy until a child's second birthday, and the CDC/National Center for Health Statistics standards for children 2 years of age and older.

Weight status categories for children are generally segregated by BMI percentile by age and sex. Weight status in childhood is categorized as follows: underweight, normal weight, overweight, obese, and severe obesity. Obesity can be further classified as follows: class I obesity, defined as BMI at or above the 95th percentile to less than 120% of the 95th percentile; class II obesity, defined as BMI ≥120% to less than 140% of the 95th percentile, or BMI ≥35 kg/m² and <40 kg/m²; and class III obesity, defined as BMI at or above 140% of the 95th percentile, or BMI ≥40 kg/m².

Epidemiology

The prevalence of obesity among children has more than tripled over the last four decades. However, it has stabilized in recent years (Figure 1A). The prevalence of severe obesity in childhood, on the other hand, continues to increase. According to the 2015 to 2016 National Health and Nutrition Examination Survey (NHANES), one-third of US children are overweight and one in five is obese. Overweight affects 26% of preschool aged children,

34% of school-aged children, and 40% of adolescents. Obesity and severe obesity affect 14% and 2% of preschool aged children, 19% and 5% of school-aged children, and 21% and 8% of adolescents, each, respectively (Figure 1B). Childhood obesity is more common among Black populations, Mexican Americans, and American Indians than in non-Hispanic White populations and Asians. Presence of parental obesity increases the risk of obesity in children. Additionally, higher prevalence of obesity is associated with lower socioeconomic status.

Pathophysiology

Childhood obesity develops as a result of a complex interaction between genetic, metabolic, environmental, and behavioral factors. As such, our historical understanding of "weight equals calories in minus calories out" is a gross oversimplification of obesity and its pathophysiology. Environmental factors such as family socio-economic status, wealth, and access to food; neighborhood safety and available community activities; and family dietary patterns are all critical components. Approximately 40% to 85% of variability in adipose tissue deposition may be contributed to heritable factors (polygenic and largely unidentified genetic changes). Having one obese parent increases the risk of childhood obesity by two-to threefold; having two obese parents increases that risk by up to 15-fold. Obesity can rarely (<1% of childhood obesity) result from single gene mutations (e.g., melanocortin 4 receptor deficiency, leptin deficiency, leptin receptor deficiency) and congenital syndromes (e.g., Prader-Willi, Bardet-Biedel, Cohen) (Table 1). As children age and gain more control over their surroundings, individual factors such as lifestyle and dietary choices may also play a role. A host of other etiologic factors include endocrine disorders, neurologic and hypothalamic disorders, and medications.

Environmental factors affecting childhood obesity are diverse and complex. Specific dietary factors that portend risk of childhood obesity include sugar-sweetened beverages, sweet snacks, fast foods, large portion sizes, and maladaptive coping strategies such as eating to suppress negative emotions. Adverse childhood events and emotion and psychological distress increase the risk of childhood obesity. Intrauterine growth restriction and birth size, as well as antibiotic use, may also be predictive factors. Children, adolescents, and adults are also now spending less time being physically active. Time is increasingly spent in sedentary activities such as use of electronic devices: cellular phones, television, tablets, and computers. Evidence suggests that shortened sleep duration and/or decreased quality of sleep also contribute to development of obesity. Certain epigenetic factors, affected by environment, also influence risk of obesity such as nutrition and microbiome.

Clinical Manifestations and Associated Comorbidities

Obesity is categorized as a complex chronic disease by the American Medical Association. Obesity affects essentially every organ system, most notably, the endocrine, gastrointestinal, pulmonary, cardiovascular, musculoskeletal, and psychological systems. Importantly, comorbid conditions once thought to be "adult onset"—type 2 diabetes mellitus (T2DM), dyslipidemia, obstructive sleep apnea (OSA), steatohepatitis—are now commonly encountered in children with obesity.

Cardiometabolic and Cardiovascular

Children with obesity have increased risk of developing prediabetes and T2DM, an association that varies with age and ethnicity. Children with T2DM tend to have higher rates of poor response to metformin therapy and more rapid progression of complications of diabetes, compared with those who present with T2DM later in life. Children with obesity also have a high prevalence of cardiometabolic risk factors including hypertension (approximately 50% of obese children and adolescents) and associated echocardiographic left ventricular hypertrophy, low levels of high-density lipoprotein cholesterol, and elevated triglycerides. Obesity during childhood is associated with an increased risk for cardiovascular disease during adult life, even after adjusting for BMI during adulthood.

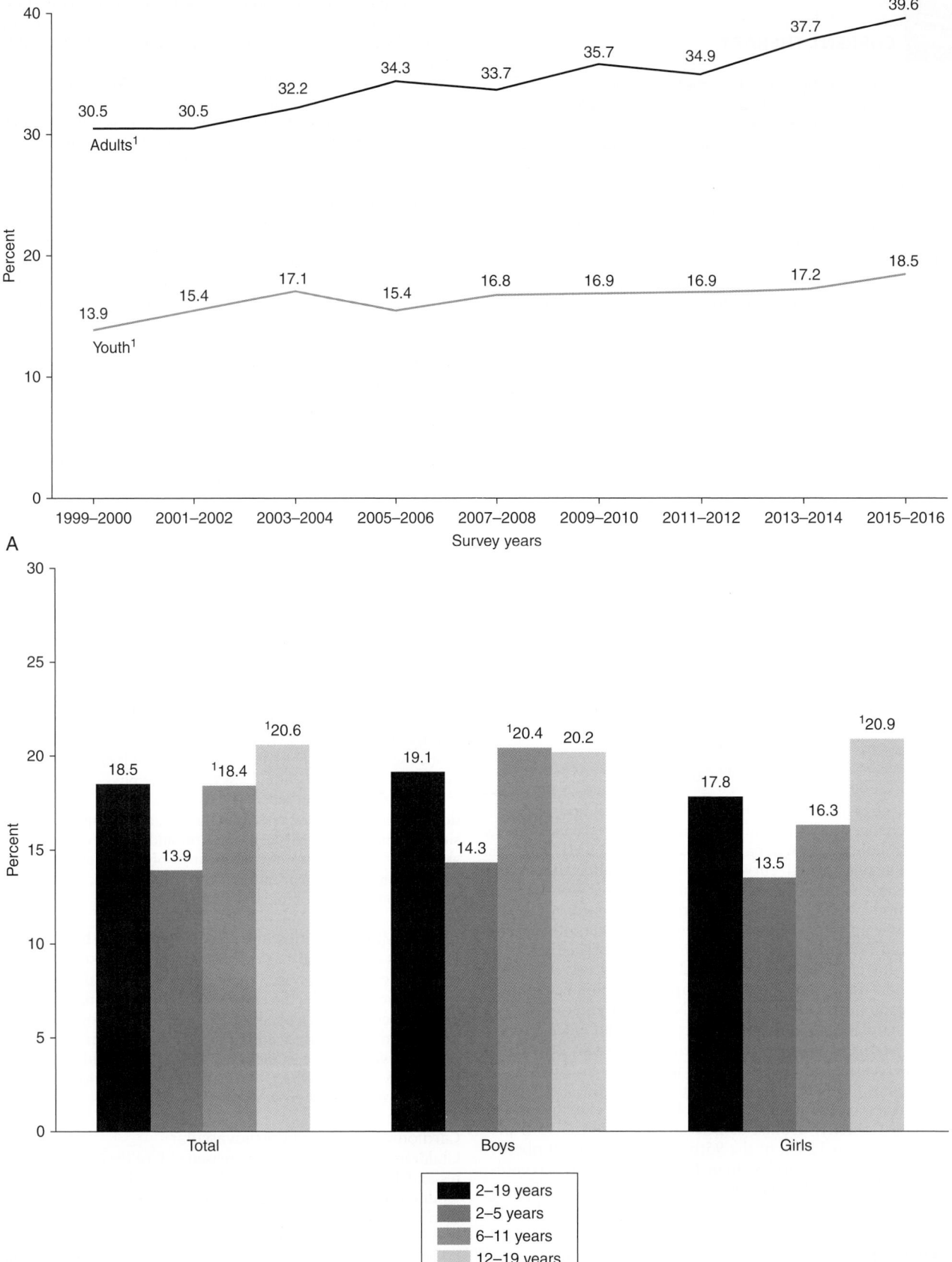

A

B

Figure 1 (A) Trends in obesity prevalence among adults aged 20 and over (adjusted age) and youth aged 2 to 19 years: United States, 1999 to 2000 through 2015 to 2016.
Reproduced with permission from: https://www.cdc.gov/nchs/data/databriefs/db288.pdf.
B, Prevalence of obesity among youth aged 2 to 19 years, by sex and age: United States, 2015 to 2016. Reproduced with permission from: https://www.cdc.gov/nchs/data/databriefs/db288.pdf.

TABLE 1	Secondary Causes of Pediatric Obesity
Monogenic Disorders	
Leptin deficiency	
Leptin dysfunction	**Endocrine**
Leptin receptor deficiency	Hypothyroidism
Proopiomelanocortin deficiency	Glucocorticoid excess (Cushing syndrome)
Melanocortin 4 receptor haploinsufficiency	Growth hormone deficiency
Melanocortin receptor accessory protein 2	Pseudohypoparathyroidism
Proconvertase 1 deficiency	**Drug Induced**
Syndromes	Tricyclic antidepressants
Prader-Willi	Steroid hormones (e.g., glucocorticoids, birth control pills)
Bardet-Biedl	Antipsychotic drugs
Cohen	Antiepileptic drugs
Alström	Diabetic medications (e.g., sulfonylureas, insulin, thiazolidinediones)
Albright hereditary osteodystrophy	Antidepressants (e.g., tricyclic antidepressants, SSRIs)
Beckwith-Wiedemann	Beta blockers
Carpenter	**Hypothalamic Causes**
Neurologic	Tumor
Brain injury	After brain surgery/radiation (craniopharyngioma)
Brain tumor	ROHHAD/ROHHADNET syndrome

SSRIs, Selective serotonin reuptake inhibitors.
Adapted from Kumar S, Kelly AS. Review of childhood obesity: from epidemiology, etiology, and comorbidities to clinical assessment and treatment. *Mayo Clinic Proceedings* 92(2):251–265, 2017.

Endocrine
Children with obesity may experience accelerated linear growth and skeletal maturation. Postpubertal females with obesity are also at greater risk of developing hyperandrogenism and polycystic ovarian syndrome, commonly associated with menstrual irregularities, hirsutism, acne, and acanthosis nigricans.

Pulmonary
Obesity during childhood is a significant risk factor for OSA. The severity of OSA and its prevalence are directly related to the severity of obesity. Children with obesity are also at risk for alveolar hypoventilation syndrome, which can result in significant blood-oxygen desaturation and carbon dioxide retention. Childhood obesity is also associated with asthma.

Gastrointestinal
Childhood obesity is associated with a spectrum of liver abnormalities known as nonalcoholic fatty liver disease (NAFLD). This disease spectrum—progressing from nonalcoholic fatty liver to nonalcoholic steatohepatitis (NASH) to NASH cirrhosis—is the most common cause of liver disease in children in the United States. Children with obesity also are at increased risk for gastroesophageal reflux disease (GERD).

Musculoskeletal
Limited mobility, lower extremity joint pain and back pain, genu valgum, lower extremity malalignment, and fractures are more common among obese children than nonobese children. Obesity during childhood is also a predisposing factor to unilateral or bilateral slipped capital femoral epiphysis and tibia vara (Blount disease).

Psychosocial
Psychosocial consequences of childhood obesity are numerous and include poor self-esteem, depression, anxiety, alienation, distorted body image, and low self-reported quality of life. Psychosocial disturbances increase in prevalence and severity with age and are more common in females. Children with obesity are more likely to experience bullying and discrimination. Adult women who were obese during childhood years completed fewer years of advanced education and had greater rates of poverty and lower rates of marriage compared with normal-weight peers. Obesity has also been associated with disordered eating patterns. Overweight or obese adolescents are more likely to engage in self-induced vomiting or laxative use. Weight talk by family members and healthcare providers, and especially weight teasing, are related to disordered eating patterns.

Dermatologic
Obesity is associated with several dermatologic conditions, including acanthosis nigricans, intertrigo, hidradenitis suppurativa, furunculosis, and stretch marks.

Neurologic
Idiopathic intracranial hypertension (pseudotumor cerebri) is rare in childhood but more prevalent among obese children. This risk is further increased among children with severe obesity. Symptoms include headache, vomiting, visual disturbances, and retroocular eye pain. Retinal examination is significant for papilledema.

Clinical Evaluation of the Child With Obesity
Initial evaluation of a pediatric patient with obesity should include a thorough history and physical examination. These components are generally sufficient to determine the cause of the obesity and help the clinician in selecting the children that need further evaluation with laboratory and radiologic testing.

Obtaining an effective history requires identifying factors contributing to obesity and screening for obesity-related comorbid conditions. Dietary history should detail eating habits including frequency, content, and location of meals and snacks. Identifying intake of both calorie-dense foods, such as fruit juices and soda, as well as healthy foods such as fresh vegetables and fruits, is helpful with dietary recommendations and with motivational interviewing. Physical activity assessment should detail time spent in unstructured play, organized sports, school recess, physical education, and recreational screen time. Identifying interest in specific physical activities, regardless of current participation, can be incorporated into motivational interviewing techniques. Medical history should include height, weight, and BMI growth trajectories and use of medications that may cause weight gain such as steroids, antipsychotic drugs, and antiepileptic drugs. Identification of developmental delay during a careful developmental history may suggest genetic or chromosomal causes for obesity. A complete review of systems may be helpful in determining secondary causes of obesity (Table 1) and screening for obesity-related comorbidities such as OSA, musculoskeletal problems, and idiopathic intracranial hypertension. Psychosocial screening should evaluate for bullying, depression, disordered eating habits, and family support and other social support.

Physical examination should include accurate measurement of weight and height and evaluation for dysmorphic features that could represent monogenic or syndromal obesity. Children with obesity and short stature are more likely to have a genetic or syndromic form of obesity. Weight gain in a child with poor linear growth can be indicative of an endocrine cause for obesity such as Cushing syndrome. Physical examination should include evaluation for comorbid features of obesity. A few examples include skin examination for acanthosis nigricans, funduscopic examination to evaluate for papilledema, and musculoskeletal examination for bowing of the legs. Laboratory evaluation to identify comorbid conditions in children with obesity is recommended by several expert societies. These recommendations include obtaining fasting lipid profile for all children who are obese or overweight, and the frequency of follow-up testing should be every 1 to 3 years depending on the child's risk profile. Measurement of serum alanine aminotransferase (ALT) is recommended for screening for fatty liver disease in children who are obese with retesting every 2 to 3 years if initial ALT is normal. Screening for T2DM with fasting glucose or hemoglobin A1c is recommended in overweight or obese children with one or more risk factors for T2DM. These risk factors include family history of T2DM in a first- or second-degree relative; high-risk race/ethnicity (Native American, African American, Hispanic, Asian American, Pacific Islander); maternal history of diabetes or gestational diabetes mellitus during the child's gestation; small for gestational age; signs of insulin resistance on physical examination such as acanthosis nigricans; and conditions associated with insulin resistance (hypertension, polycystic ovary syndrome, dyslipidemia). Screening for T2DM is recommended starting at 10 years of age or sooner if onset of puberty occurs before age 10. Rescreening should occur every 1 to 3 years depending on the weight trajectory and risk factor profile.

Children in whom a genetic, syndromic, or endocrine cause of obesity is suspected need to undergo specific testing. Children with signs and symptoms of OSA should be evaluated with overnight polysomnography. Children with features suggestive of idiopathic intracranial hypertension require head imaging and referral to appropriate experts.

Treatment: A Staged Approach to Prevention, Clinical Interventions, and Monitoring

Managing childhood overweight and obesity is challenging but, when conducted properly, can be both effective and rewarding. A staged approach to weight management in children (Box 1) has been recommended by the Expert Committee on Assessment, Prevention, and Treatment of Child and Adolescent Overweight and Obesity. The four stages progress in a stepwise fashion and involve primary care providers and, subsequently, a multidisciplinary team—primary care providers, dietitians, behavior counselors, exercise specialists, and occasionally surgical specialists. The stages encompass primary and secondary prevention; clinical interventions such as lifestyle modifications, pharmacotherapy, and bariatric procedures; and ongoing monitoring.

Lifestyle Interventions

Weight Management Goals

The goals for weight management are dependent on the child's age and severity of obesity. In children with mild obesity that are continuing to grow, maintenance of weight or slower rate of weight gain compared with previous is sufficient as that itself will lead to a decrease in BMI percentile. On the other hand, weight loss is recommended for children with severe obesity. A weight loss of up to 1 lb per month is safe for children between 2 and 11 years of age with obesity and comorbidities. More weight loss (up to 1–2 pounds per week) is safe in adolescents with obesity and comorbidities, although a weight loss of 1 to 2 pounds per month is more realistic in this age group.

Stage I

Stage I (Prevention Plus) focuses on prevention and encouraging healthy habits: emphasizing the importance of five or more servings of fruits and vegetables per day; minimizing (or eliminating) consumption of sugar-containing beverages; limiting screen time to less than 2 hours per day; and encouraging at least 1 hour of physical activity per day. This stage may be implemented in the outpatient setting by a primary care provider. Recommendations from this stage may be applied in well-child visits, regardless of weight status. Goals of treatment for children with obesity at this stage may include weight maintenance rather than weight loss, taking into account

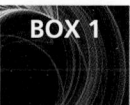

BOX 1 Staged Approach to Weight Management in Children and Adolescents as Recommended by the American Academy of Pediatrics

- Stage I (Prevention Plus) guidelines include five or more servings of fruits and vegetables per day, minimizing or eliminating consumption of sugar-containing beverages, limiting screen time to 2 hours (none for children <2 years old), and >1 hour of physical activity per day. These interventions can be implemented in a primary care office setting.
- Stage II (Structured Weight Management) includes stage I guidelines plus increased structure of meals and snacks with attention to energy density of foods. These interventions can be implemented in a primary care office with a dietitian.
- Stage III (Comprehensive Multidisciplinary Intervention) includes stage II guidelines with additional increased structured physical activity and dietary program. These interventions can be implemented in a primary care office with a multidisciplinary team and outside facilities for structured physical activity, or, alternatively, in a pediatric weight management center.
- Stage IV (Tertiary Care Intervention) includes stage III guidelines with use of medications, rigorously structured dietary regimens, or bariatric surgery in select adolescents. These interventions can be ideally implemented in a pediatric weight management center with a multidisciplinary team with expertise in pediatric obesity.

Adapted from Barlow SE and the Expert Committee. Expert committee recommendations regarding the prevention, assessment, and treatment of child and adolescent overweight and obesity: summary report. *Pediatrics* 120 (Suppl)2007:S164–S192, 2007.

normal growth changes. Frequency of follow-up visits should be individualized for each child and family. The follow-up schedule should be guided by patient/family readiness to change and severity of obesity. Recognizing risk factors and protective factors in this stage and counseling appropriately is crucial. There may be financial, cultural, behavioral, or family barriers that can significantly impact treatment planning and follow through. Family involvement and participation in this stage and subsequent stages are essential for effective implementation of dietary and lifestyle changes. Helping children and their parents to identify their own lifestyle or dietary goals empowers children to be involved in their management and can be very effective. Goals should be "SMART": specific, measurable, attainable, realistic, and timely.

Dietary recommendations center on increasing consumption of low energy-density foods such as fruits and vegetables and decreasing high energy-density foods such as sugar-added food products and refined carbohydrates. The Dietary Guidelines for Americans suggest that half of each meal should comprise fruits and vegetables, with preference for whole fruits and dark green vegetables such as leafy greens and broccoli (https://www.myplate.gov/). Some weight management programs use a "traffic light" dietary format, labeling foods as red, yellow, or green on the basis of energy density (red foods indicate high calorie density, green foods indicate low calorie density). Children are encouraged to eat green foods frequently and red foods more sparingly, such as on special occasions.

Motivational interviewing is a counseling technique that may be helpful in this and subsequent stages. This nonjudgmental method helps people to resolve ambivalent feelings to find inner motivation to make lifestyle changes. The process involves reflective listening and helps children realize their own strengths, values, and motivation to change. This tool has been shown to be useful in treatment of childhood obesity.

Stage II

If the child is being managed for obesity as indicated in *stage I (Prevention Plus)* and there is no improvement in BMI within 3 to 6 months, progression to *stage II (Structured Weight Management)* should be considered. *Stage II* includes physical activity of at least 1 hour per day; a more structured dietary approach focusing on low energy-dense foods, balanced diet, and structured meal times; and no more than 1 hour of screen time per day. At this stage, referral to a provider with additional training in nutrition or behavioral counseling such as a dietitian is warranted. Explicit behavior goals are set and eating and physical activity logs are encouraged in order to monitor diet and activity. Strategies used in previous clinic visits, such as motivational interviewing and family involvement, should be continued. Positive reinforcement techniques are recommended in order to achieve weight loss. Interventions should be tailored to the individual child and family. Monthly contact between the patient and providers is recommended in order to monitor progress and facilitate continued involvement of the family and child.

Stage III

If improvements in BMI, or significant improvements in lifestyle habits, are not achieved after 3 to 6 months of stage II treatment, *stage III (Comprehensive Multidisciplinary Intervention)* should be considered. *Stage III* further increases the intensity of behavioral intervention by addition of more specialists and increase in frequency of the visits. The intervention is aimed at creating a negative energy balance and goal setting for diet and physical activity. This stage requires a multidisciplinary team with expertise in childhood obesity that includes a behavioral counselor (e.g., social worker, psychologist, trained nurse practitioner, or other mental health provider), registered dietitian, and exercise specialist, and a primary care provider who oversees the intervention and manages medical issues. This type of intervention may be implemented in a primary care office provided an appropriate multidisciplinary team and resources are available within the medical center or community, otherwise referral to a pediatric weight management center may be necessary. Primary care offices may require partnerships with community programming: public health programs, local schools, Head Start, Young Men's Christian Association, and Boys and Girls Club. Stage III requires more intensive follow-up, with frequent provider-patient contact. Weekly office visits for the first 8 to 12 weeks are recommended, followed by monthly visits once the patient and family are able to take more responsibility for the treatment plan. Involvement of the parents and extended family is crucial for children younger than 12 years of age, though even in older children, parental involvement is helpful for improvement of the home environment.

Stage IV

Children with severe obesity that have attempted *stage III* recommendations and have not met their weight loss goals should be considered for *stage IV (Tertiary Care Intervention)*. Patients should be motivated and be able to understand the risks and benefits of intervention in this stage. *Stage IV* requires referral to a pediatric weight management center, where a multidisciplinary team with significant expertise in childhood obesity, including clinical and research protocols for assessment of outcomes and risks, help coordinate and individualize patient care. This stage builds on recommendations from *stage III* and also incorporates the use of meal replacements, low-energy diets, medications, and/or bariatric procedures.

The success of weight loss interventions in children is related to the intensity of interventions. Behavioral interventions of moderate or high intensity (defined as 26–75 hours and >75 hours of provider contact, respectively) have been shown to be effective in achieving weight loss. Interventions of moderate or high intensity often are not available or feasible in the majority of primary care settings.

Pharmacologic Therapy

Pharmacologic treatment options for children and adolescents with obesity are limited (Table 2). Several medications are currently being used off-label for pediatric obesity. Use of medications for weight loss in children should be done under the care of a multidisciplinary team, and regular monitoring for efficacy and side effects is essential. Some experts suggest consideration of pharmacotherapy in adolescents with BMI ≥95th percentile and with at least one obesity-related comorbidity, or with BMI ≥120% of the 95th percentile or BMI ≥35 kg/m² (whichever is lower), irrespective of comorbidities. Experts emphasize that patients should have attempted lifestyle interventions prior to initiation of pharmacologic therapy. Continuation of pharmacotherapy is recommended only if the medication is felt to be effective, as demonstrated by ≥5% BMI reduction from baseline within 12 weeks on the optimal dose, or if slowing down/arrest of weight gain is considered satisfactory due to linear growth in adolescence. Weight-loss medications should be discontinued in the presence of side effects that persist despite adjustment of the dose. Adolescence is defined as age 10 to 19 years by the World Health Organization and 11 to 21 years by the American Academy of Pediatrics. There is scarcity of data on the long-term safety or efficacy of weight-loss medications (orlistat or any of the other medications used off-label) in children and adolescents.

Orlistat (Xenical) is approved by the United States Food and Drug Administration (FDA) for treatment of obesity in children 12 years of age and older. It is a lipase inhibitor that, when taken at the recommended dose of 120 mg three times a day with meals, blocks absorption of about one-third of fat digested in a meal. Lower doses of 60 mg three times per day with meals are available over-the-counter (Alli).[1] Side effects include flatulence, oily spotting, fatty stools, diarrhea, and potential for micronutrient deficiencies. Moreover, long-term safety data are lacking. The efficacy of orlistat over placebo for treatment of childhood obesity is modest, decreasing BMI by less than 1 kg/m² after 1 year of therapy.

Phentermine (Adipex-P) is a sympathomimetic drug (class IV controlled substance) that is approved by the FDA for short-term use (up to 12 weeks) in adolescents 17 years of age and older. It is approved in adults for long-term treatment of obesity in combination with topiramate (Qsymia). Doses in adults have ranged between 15 and 37.5 mg (phentermine) per day. One pediatric study found that the drug resulted in a 4.1% decrease in BMI at 6 months. Adverse effects noted in adults include insomnia, restlessness, euphoria, palpitations, hypertension, cardiac arrhythmias, headache, dizziness, visual disturbances, and ocular irritation. Adolescents should be screened for congenital heart disease and other cardiac pathology and also have baseline assessment of blood pressure and heart rate before initiation of this drug. Long-term safety data are lacking. Phentermine is contraindicated in patients with hyperthyroidism, glaucoma, cardiovascular disease, or history of drug abuse. Phentermine use is not recommended for treatment of childhood obesity in primary care due to its risk factor profile and lack of data on long-term use.

Liraglutide (Saxenda) is a glucagon-like 1 receptor (GLP-1) agonist that is FDA approved for weight management in children and adolescents 12 years and older. A recent randomized, double-blind, controlled trial in adolescents 12 to <18 years of age showed placebo-subtracted BMI reduction of −0.22 kg/m² at 56 weeks; 43% of subjects achieved a BMI reduction of at least 5%. Adverse effects include nausea, vomiting, abdominal pain, diarrhea, and potential hypoglycemia. Long-term safety data are lacking. Exenatide (Bydureon, Byetta),[1] another GLP-1 agonist, has been used off-label for treatment of childhood obesity in small studies and the effect has been modest with a BMI reduction of 3.4% in one study at 3 months. Long-term safety data for use of GLP-1 agonists for weight loss in children are lacking. GLP-1 agonists may

---

[1]Not FDA approved for this indication.

DRUG NAME	MECHANISM OF ACTION	FDA INDICATION	SIDE EFFECTS	ADOLESCENT WEIGHT-LOSS OUTCOMES DATA
FDA Approved				
Orlistat (Xenical)	Pancreatic and gastric lipase inhibitor	Obesity ≥12 years	Flatulence, diarrhea, oily spotting, fatty stools, micronutrient deficiencies	Weight loss of 2.6 kg more than placebo at 1 year. Placebo subtracted BMI reduction of −0.7 kg/m^2 at 1 year.
Phentermine (Adipex-P)	Sympathomimetic amine	Obesity >16 years of age for short-term treatment	Dry mouth, insomnia, irritability increased heart rate, blood pressure, constipation, anxiety	BMI decreased by 4.1% at 6 months.
Liraglutide (Saxenda)	GLP-1 agonist	Obesity in ≥12 years	Nausea, vomiting, abdominal pain, diarrhea, potential hypoglycemia	Placebo subtracted BMI reduction of −0.22 kg/m^2 at 56 weeks. BMI reduction of at least 5% was achieved by 43% of subjects.
Setmelanotide (Imcivree)	Melanocortin 4 receptor agonist	Obesity at age ≥6 years due to genetically confirmed proopiomelanocortin (POMC), proprotein convertase subtilisin/kexin type 1 (PCSK1), or leptin receptor (LEPR) deficiency	Injection site reaction, skin hyperpigmentation, nausea, vomiting, skin discoloration	80% of participants with POMC deficiency and 45% of participants with LEPR deficiency achieved at least 10% weight loss at approximately 1 year.
Not FDA Indicated for Obesity				
Metformin (Glucophage)	Activation of protein kinase pathway	≥10 years of age for type 2 diabetes mellitus	Epigastric discomfort, diarrhea, flatulence	BMI z-score decreased by 0.10 and BMI 0.86.
Topiramate (Topamax)	Modulation of various neurotransmitters	Treatment of epilepsy ≥2 years and migraines prevention ≥12 years of age	Cognitive dysfunction, metabolic acidosis, kidney stones, teratogenicity	BMI decreased by 4.9% on topiramate 75 mg daily for at least 3 months.
Exenatide (Bydureon, Byetta)	GLP-1 agonist	Type 2 diabetes mellitus in adults	Bloating, nausea/vomiting, abdominal pain, elevation of pancreatic amylase and lipase	BMI decreased by 3.4% at 3 months

Adapted from Srivastava G, Fox CK, Kelly AS, et al. Clinical considerations regarding the use of obesity pharmacotherapy in adolescents with obesity. *Obesity* 27(2): 190–204, 2019.
BMI, Body mass index; *FDA,* US Food and Drug Administration; *GLP-1,* glucagon-like 1 receptor.

have a potential role in syndromic and hypothalamic obesity with hyperphagia. Both liraglutide and exenatide are contraindicated in patients with a personal or family history of medullary thyroid cancer or multiple endocrine neoplasia 2A or 2B.

Setmelanotide (Imcivree), a melanocortin 4 receptor agonist, has been recently approved for adults and children at age ≥6 years with obesity due to genetically confirmed proopiomelanocortin (POMC), proprotein convertase subtilisin/kexin type 1 (PCSK1), or leptin receptor (LEPR) deficiency. In a single-arm, open-label, multicenter phase III trial, 80% (8/10) of participants with POMC deficiency and 45% (5/11) of participants with LEPR deficiency achieved at least 10% weight loss at approximately 1 year. Adverse events include injection site reaction, skin hyperpigmentation, nausea, vomiting, and skin discoloration.

Metformin (Glucophage, Glumetza, Riomet) is approved by the FDA for treatment of T2DM in children 10 years of age and older. Use of metformin for weight loss is considered off-label; however, it is the initial drug of choice for weight loss in adolescents with prediabetes,[1] metabolic syndrome,[1] polycystic ovary syndrome,[1] and insulin resistance.[1] Metformin may be helpful in children with weight gain secondary to treatment with antipsychotic drugs.[1] The dose may be gradually increased as tolerated to a maximum of 2000 mg/day. Improvements in BMI have been

modest with a meta-analysis finding BMI z-score reduction of 0.10 and BMI reduction of 0.86 mg/kg^2. Adverse effects include abdominal discomfort, diarrhea, flatulence, vitamin B2 deficiency, and lactic acidosis.

Topiramate (Topamax) is another medication that is used off-label for treatment of obesity in children. The weight-loss effect is likely mediated through modulation of various neurotransmitters. This drug is FDA approved for treatment of epilepsy in children aged 2 years and older and for migraine prophylaxis in children 12 years of age and older. Adverse effects include cognitive dysfunction, paresthesia, metabolic acidosis, kidney stones, and teratogenicity. Adolescents must be counseled against pregnancy because of decreased efficacy of oral contraceptives with treatment. Topiramate also has modest efficacy for treatment of obesity. In a small randomized placebo-controlled pilot clinical trial of 30 adolescents, 2% reduction in BMI was noted on topiramate 75 mg at 6 months.

Bariatric Procedures

Bariatric procedures, including bariatric surgery, should be considered for adolescents with severe obesity and, often, with significant health comorbidities (Table 3). Severe obesity in childhood is a unique subset which has outpaced less severe forms of childhood obesity in prevalence. Importantly, lifestyle modifications—a cornerstone of pediatric obesity therapy—have not demonstrated significant and lasting weight loss in children with severe obesity.

[1]Not FDA approved for this indication.

Eligibility criteria for bariatric surgery include the following:
1. BMI ≥120% of the 95th percentile for age and gender or BMI ≥35 kg/m², whichever is lower, and a severe comorbidity having significant effects on health (e.g., moderate to severe OSA; apnea-hypopnea index >15), T2DM, idiopathic intracranial hypertension, or severe and progressive steatohepatitis

or

BMI ≥140% of the 95th percentile for age and gender or BMI ≥40 kg/m², whichever is lower, with any obesity-related comorbidity or self-reported impaired quality of life;
2. History of previous sustained efforts to lose weight through changes in diet and physical activity;
3. Commitment from the patient and family to adhere to recommended pre- and postoperative treatments, including vitamin and mineral supplementation; and
4. Patient and family understanding of the risks and benefits of bariatric surgery.

The most recent expert guidelines do not recommend withholding surgery in those that have not completed puberty or physical maturity as determined by Tanner stage or skeletal maturation. Contraindications for bariatric surgery include the following:
1. Medically correctable cause of obesity;
2. An ongoing substance abuse problem (within the preceding year);
3. A medical, psychiatric, psychosocial, or cognitive condition that prevents adherence to postoperative dietary and medication regimens or impairs decisional capacity;
4. Current or planned pregnancy within 12 to 18 months of the procedure; and
5. Inability on the part of the patient or parent to comprehend the risks and benefits of the surgical procedure.

Types of Bariatric Procedures

The sleeve gastrectomy (SG; Figure 2A) is the most commonly performed procedure among adolescents with obesity. SG involves resecting the majority of the greater curvature of the stomach, leaving a tubular structure that serves as the new stomach. SG was initially performed as the first stage of a two stage procedure in high-risk adults with extreme obesity. The SG procedure is attractive during adolescence and particularly for adolescents with cognitive deficits. The procedure is less complex and can be converted to gastric bypass in the future if there is weight regain. The risk of micronutrient deficiencies is theoretically lower, as it is a purely restrictive procedure.

TABLE 3	Indications for Bariatric Surgery in Adolescents
WEIGHT CRITERIA	**COMORBID CONDITIONS PRESENT**
BMI ≥120% to <140% of the 95th percentile or BMI ≥35 kg/m² and <40 kg/m²	Moderate-severe obstructive sleep apnea, T2DM, idiopathic intracranial hypertension, NASH, Blount disease, slipped capital femoral epiphysis, hypertension, gastroesophageal reflux disease
BMI ≥140% of the 95th percentile or BMI ≥40 kg/m².	None required, though commonly present

Adapted from Armstrong SC, Bolling CF, Michalsky MP, Reichard KW. Pediatric metabolic and bariatric surgery: evidence, barriers, and best practices. *Pediatrics* 144(6), 2019.
NASH, Nonalcoholic steatohepatitis; *T2DM*, type 2 diabetes mellitus.

Roux-en-Y gastric bypass (RYGB; Figure 2B) was previously considered the gold standard of bariatric procedures among adolescents with severe obesity but is now performed less frequently than the SG. The surgery involves creation of a small proximal gastric pouch (<30 mL) and separation of the pouch from the distal stomach and anastomosis to a Roux-limb of small bowel that measures 75 to 150 cm in length. Though it is primarily considered a restrictive surgery, some degree of malabsorption does occur that leads to weight loss and places patients at risk for micronutrient deficiencies.

Both bariatric procedures have been shown to result in significant decreases in body weight and body mass index in the majority of adolescents undergoing those procedures. In the largest prospective study of bariatric surgery in adolescents (Teen-LABS), 26% reduction in BMI following SG and 28% reduction following RYGB was noted at 3 years. BMI reduction of 29.2% was noted at 5 years in 58 individuals undergoing RYGB. Both procedures have been shown to result in improvement of various comorbid conditions including T2DM, prediabetes, hypertension, dyslipidemia, and renal disease.

Long-term adverse effects include deficiencies of iron, vitamin D, thiamine, and vitamin B12. Adolescents undergoing bariatric surgery need long-term monitoring, as long-term safety and efficacy data in this particular age group are limited.

Common bariatric procedures

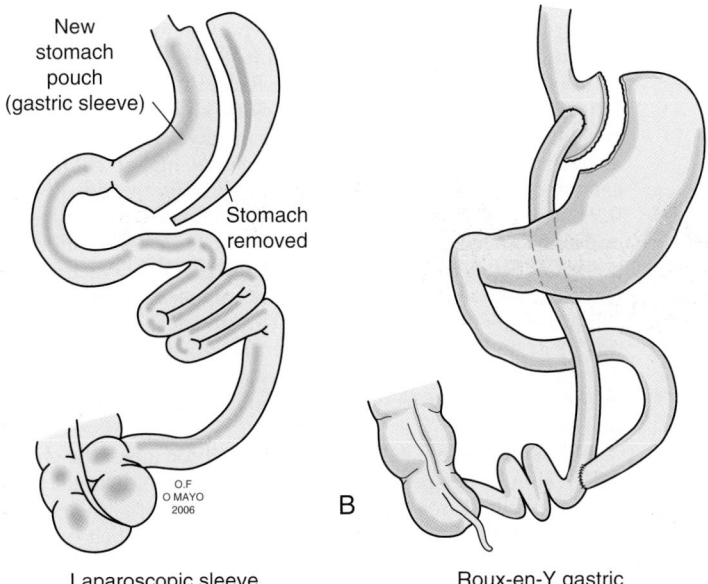

New stomach pouch (gastric sleeve)

Stomach removed

O.F O MAYO 2006

A

Laparoscopic sleeve gastrectomy

B

Roux-en-Y gastric bypass

Figure 2 Bariatric surgical procedures commonly used for the surgical treatment of childhood obesity. (A) Laparoscopic sleeve gastrectomy. (B) Roux-en-Y gastric bypass.

Conclusion

Childhood obesity presents a growing public health concern in the United States and globally. Weight-related comorbid conditions are common among children with obesity, conferring significant health risks, and such children should undergo routine clinical and laboratory screening. Treatment of obesity in childhood should follow a staged approach, focusing heavily on environment and lifestyle interventions. Children with severe obesity and those with weight-related comorbid conditions should be considered for pharmacotherapy and/or bariatric surgery. Bariatric surgery in adolescents has been associated with significant weight loss and improvement in weight-related comorbid conditions in the short and intermediate term.

References

Armstrong SC, Bolling CF, Michalsky MP, Reichard KW: Pediatric metabolic and bariatric surgery: evidence, barriers, and best practices, *Pediatrics* 144(6), 2019.

Barlow SE, the Expert Committee: Expert committee recommendations regarding the prevention, assessment, and treatment of child and adolescent overweight and obesity: summary report, *Pediatrics* 120(Supplement):S164–S192, 2007.

Golden NH, Schneider M, Wood C: Preventing obesity and eating disorders in adolescents, *Pediatrics* 138(3):e20161649, 2016.

Inge TH, Courcoulas AP, Jenkins TM, et al: Weight loss and health status 3 Years after bariatric surgery in adolescents, *N Engl J Med* 374(2):113–123, 2016.

Kelly AS, Barlow SE, Rao G, et al: Severe obesity in children and adolescents: identification, associated health risks, and treatment approaches: a scientific statement from the American Heart Association, *Circulation* 128(15):1689–1712, 2013.

Kumar S, Kelly AS: Review of childhood obesity: from epidemiology, etiology, and co-morbidities to clinical assessment and treatment, *Mayo Clin Proc* 92(2):251–265, 2017.

Skinner AC, Ravanbakht SN, Skelton JA, Perrin EM, Armstrong SC: Prevalence of obesity and severe obesity in US children, 1999–2016, *Pediatrics* 141(3):e20173459, 2018.

Srivastava G, Fox CK, Kelly AS, et al: Clinical considerations regarding the use of obesity pharmacotherapy in adolescents with obesity, *Obesity* 27(2):190–204, 2019.

PARENTERAL FLUID THERAPY FOR INFANTS AND CHILDREN

Method of
Alan M. Hall, MD; Jimmy Chen, MD; Deval Patel, MD; and Michael L. Moritz, MD

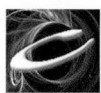

CURRENT DIAGNOSIS

- Maintenance intravenous fluids are used continuously to maintain extracellular volume and electrolyte homeostasis when enteral fluid (oral or via feeding tube) intake is insufficient.
- Resuscitation intravenous fluids are used for the rapid restoration of intravascular volume.
- Replacement fluids are required to prevent hypovolemia and electrolyte abnormalities when continued excessive fluid losses are present.

CURRENT THERAPY

- Intravenous fluids should be utilized only when enteral intake is inadequate and discontinued as soon as safely possible.
- Intravenous fluids should be individualized to each patient with isotonic fluids recommended for most acutely ill hospitalized patients when maintenance or resuscitation fluids are indicated.
- Balanced intravenous fluids should be considered, especially in the setting of resuscitation.
- While a patient is receiving intravenous fluids, continuous reassessment is needed including of vital signs, clinical exam, intake/output, daily weights, and consideration of lab monitoring, especially sodium levels.

Introduction

Intravenous fluid therapy is an integral component in the care of the acutely ill child. Intravenous fluids may be required as a bolus infusion for resuscitation, as a continuous infusion when sufficient fluids cannot be ingested orally, and to replace excessive ongoing losses from the gastrointestinal (GI) tract or urinary tract or from serous drains. The ultimate goal of fluid therapy is to provide sufficient fluids to maintain tissue perfusion and normal serum electrolytes. Choosing the appropriate volume and composition requires great care in order to prevent a disorder in volume or electrolyte balance, as acutely ill patients frequently have disorders that impair normal water and electrolyte homeostasis.

Maintenance Intravenous Fluid Therapy

Maintenance intravenous fluids (MIVFs) are infused continuously to maintain extracellular volume and electrolyte homeostasis when enteral fluid (oral or via feeding tube) intake is insufficient to meet daily requirements. Crystalloid intravenous fluids used for maintenance are categorized as isotonic (approximately equal to the plasma sodium concentration) or hypotonic (less than the plasma sodium concentration). Table 1 shows the composition of commonly used intravenous fluids.

In 1957, Holliday and Segar proposed a theoretical approach to MIVF prescribing; they recommended that hypotonic MIVFs approximating the sodium and potassium concentration of breast or cow's milk could provide the water and electrolyte needs foracutely ill children. This led to widespread use of hypotonic MIVFs; however, the first reports of the syndrome of antidiuretic hormone (SIADH) did not appear until after this publication. SIADH occurs when excess free water is retained, leading to hyponatremia secondary to the nonosmotic and nonhemodynamic triggered release of antidiuretic hormone (ADH). Virtually all acutely ill hospitalized children have a potential hemodynamic or nonhemodynamic stimulus for ADH production, placing them at risk for hyponatremia (Fig. 1). The administration of hypotonic fluids increases their risk for developing hyponatremia, in particular from SIADH, which is the most common cause of hospital-acquired hyponatremia.

Multiple randomized controlled trials and meta-analyses have demonstrated a lower risk of hyponatremia when hospitalized children receive isotonic fluids as compared with hypotonic fluids, with an approximate number needed to treat of 7.5. As aresult, the American Academy of Pediatrics' Clinical Practice Guideline (AAP CPG) on MIVFs recommends isotonic MIVFs for most patients between 28 days and 18 years of age. In children less than 28 days of age, the evidence is less clear on the choice between hypotonic and isotonic fluids. We tend to extrapolate the evidence from older children and use isotonic fluids in neonates given that they are also at risk for hyponatremia.

Isotonic fluids can be separated into balanced and unbalanced solutions. Balanced fluids include Ringer's lactate and Plasma-Lyte 148; they contain a buffer with chloride concentrations close to serum concentrations. The prime example of an unbalanced solution that contains significantly higher chloride concentrations as compared with serum without an added buffer is 0.9% saline. Evidence is lacking on the choice between balanced and unbalanced solutions for maintenance in both children and adults. When MIVFs are used for short periods, which is typical for most pediatric patients, either a balanced solution or 0.9% saline is likely reasonable. If MIVFs are needed for long periods or at high doses, it is possible that 0.9% saline could cause a hyperchloremic metabolic acidosis, which, as detailed below in the resuscitation section, could have the potential for adverse outcomes.

Although isotonic MIVFs are indicated for most, the choice of MIVF should be specifically tailored to each individual patient. Hypotonic fluids may be indicated in a subset of patients, including those with hypernatremia and a free water deficit or ongoing free water losses from a renal concentrating defect such as diabetes insipidus or voluminous watery diarrhea. Dextrose should be added to the MIVF for most children to prevent ketosis. Dextrose

TABLE 1 Composition of Commonly Used Intravenous Fluids

IV FLUID	SODIUM	CHLORIDE	POTASSIUM	CALCIUM	MAGNESIUM	BUFFER	OSMOLARITY (mOsm/L)
			mmol/L				
Human plasma	135–144	95–105	3.5–5.3	2.2–2.6	0.8–1.2	23–30 bicarbonate	308
Isotonic/Near Isotonic Solutions							
0.9% saline	154	154	0	0	0	0	308
Plasma-Lyte 148	140	98	5	0	1.5	27 acetate and 23 gluconate	294
Ringer lactate	130	109	4	1.5	0	28 lactate	273
Hypotonic Solutions							
0.45% saline	77	77	0	0	0	0	154
0.2% saline	34	34	0	0	0	0	78

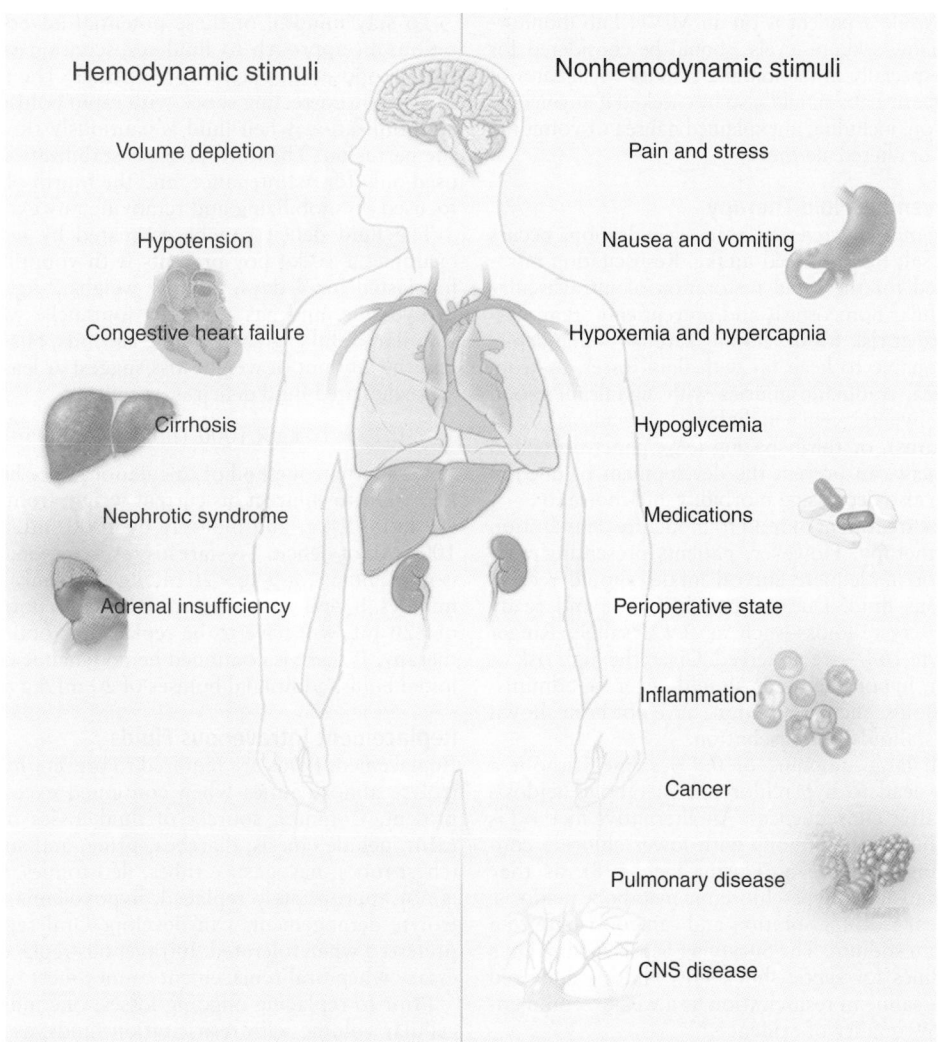

Figure 1 Nonosmotic states of antidiuretic hormone (ADH) excess. From Moritz ML, Ayus JC: Maintenance intravenous fluids in acutely ill patients. *N Engl J Med* 373:1350–1360, 2015. ©2015 Massachusetts Medical Society. Reprinted with permission.

is rapidly metabolized upon infusion and does not contribute to the tonicity of the MIVF except in those with uncontrolled diabetes mellitus. There is little guiding evidence, but based on the AAP CPG, it is also recommended to add a potassium additive, typically 20 mEq/L, which can be in the form of potassium chloride. When MIVFs are used for only a short time, a potassium additive may not be needed except in patients with hypokalemia or risk factors for hypokalemia, including severe malnutrition

and diuretic use. Hyperkalemia is a potentially serious complication of intravenous fluids, and potassium should be withheld from fluids if there is any concern for abnormal renal function or decreased or unknown urinary output.

The rate of infusion for MIVFs should be customized to each patient. There is no robust evidence to guide infusion rates, but this can be estimated by body surface area (1500 mL per 1.73 m² of body surface area per 24 hours) or weight (the Holliday-Segar formula). With the Holliday-Segar formula, fluids are calculated as follows:

- 100 mL/kg per 24 hours for the first 10 kg of body weight plus
- 50 mL/kg per 24 hours for weight between 10 and 20 kg plus
- 20 mL/kg per 24 hours for weight above 20 kg

This formula is estimated by what is known as the "4-2-1 rule." It provides an estimate for the hourly MIVF infusion rate as follows:

- 4 mL/kg per hour for the first 10 kg of body weight
- 2 mL/kg per hour for weight between 10 and 20 kg
- and 1 mL/kg per hour for weight above 20 kg

MIVF infusion rates may have to be increased from those estimates in patients with polyuria from renal concentrating defects. Additionally, MIVFs may have to be avoided or used at lower rates of infusion in patients with volume overload states, including oliguric acute kidney injury, chronic kidney disease, cirrhosis, and congestive heart failure. Close monitoring—with daily weights, frequent vital signs, strict measurements of intake and output, and serial physical exams—is necessary while a patient is on an MIVF. Lab monitoring, specifically to follow sodium levels, should be considered for patients on MIVFs, especially in the initial 24 hours when rates of hyponatremia are highest. Labs should also be checked if any neurologic symptoms develop, including unexplained nausea or vomiting, headache, confusion, or altered alertness.

Resuscitation Intravenous Fluid Therapy

Volume depletion, commonly referred to as dehydration, occurs whenever water and salt losses exceed intake. Resuscitation intravenous fluids are used for the rapid restoration of intravascular volume to ensure cellular homeostasis and prevent end-organ dysfunction. Children are at risk for developing severe volume depletion when they are unable to keep up with fluid losses, as from vomiting and diarrhea, traumatic injuries with significant blood loss, renal losses (e.g., hyperglycemia in diabetic ketoacidosis), cutaneous losses (e.g., burns), or third spacing (e.g., pancreatitis and sepsis). Rapid treatment can prevent the development of uncompensated shock while also decreasing morbidity and mortality.

The mainstay in the treatment of mild to moderate dehydration is oral rehydration therapy. However, patients presenting with severe dehydration or inadequate enteral intake should receive boluses of intravenous fluid. Due to their low cost and ready availability, isotonic crystalloids—such as 0.9% saline, Ringer lactate, or Plasma-Lyte 148—are preferred. Given the high risk of severe hyponatremia, hypotonic fluids should never be administered as boluses. Colloids, such as albumin, have not been shown to be superior to crystalloids in resuscitation.

Resuscitation with large amounts of 0.9% saline without a base equivalent may lead to hyperchloremic metabolic acidosis with potentially negative consequences. An alternative method is to use balanced or buffered solutions with lower chloride concentrations (e.g., Ringer lactate or Plasma-Lyte 148), as they pose a lesser risk of causing a hyperchloremic metabolic acidosis. Ringer lactate is a near isotonic solution and can contribute to a mild decrease in serum sodium. The Surviving Sepsis Campaign's International Guidelines for septic shock now endorse buffered fluid instead of 0.9% saline in resuscitation as a weak recommendation with a very low quality of evidence.

The clinical signs of dehydration are a manifestation of extracellular volume depletion. Signs of extracellular volume depletion in children include an elevation in heart rate, delayed capillary refill, diminished tearing, dry mucous membranes, a sunken fontanel, poor skin turgor, decreased peripheral pulses, cool extremities, and ultimately a fall in blood pressure when volume depletion is severe. Three factors determine the amount of extracellular volume depletion and therefore the severity of dehydration: (1) the fluid deficit, (2) the electrolyte deficit, and (3) the speed at which dehydration occurs. Given the same volume loss, hyponatremic dehydration is clinically more severe than hypernatremic dehydration because in hyponatremic dehydration fluid shifts intracellularly. This is the basis for classifying dehydration according to the serum sodium as hyponatremic, isonatremic, or hypernatremic.

To restore intravascular volume rapidly and provide adequate perfusion to vital organs, resuscitation fluid is given in rapid aliquots of 20 mL/kg followed by clinical reassessment. Patients with preexisting conditions, such as cardiac and renal disease, may require using smaller volumes of fluid (e.g., 5 to 10 mL/kg). In septic shock, up to 40 to 60 mL/kg may be given with vasopressors quickly added if hemodynamics are not restored based on frequent clinical reassessments.

Potential harm is associated with excessive fluid resuscitation. Severe illness has been associated with damage to the glycocalyx, which lines the vascular endothelium. Damage to the glycocalyx can contribute to increased permeability of the endothelium and resultant increased risk of interstitial edema and fluid overload with intravenous fluid administration. Fluid overload has been associated with increased mortality, specifically in patients with acute kidney injury. Additionally, a large randomized controlled trial showed increased mortality when African children were given fluid boluses when they presented with a febrile illness and signs of shock.

To stay mindful of these potential adverse effects of resuscitation, an approach to fluid resuscitation with four phases has been proposed in critical care settings. The first phase, rescue, is focused on correcting shock with rapid boluses. The second phase is optimization when fluid is cautiously titrated to optimize tissue perfusion. The third phase is stabilization with minimal fluid used only for maintenance, and the fourth phase is de-escalation, focused on mobilizing and removing any excess fluid.

The fluid deficit can be estimated by using Table 2. As an example, a 10-kg boy presents with vomiting and diarrhea that has lasted for 3 days; he now weighs 9 kg. He is lethargic and tachycardic, and has a sunken fontanelle with cool extremities. Capillary refill is greater than 3 seconds. His clinical presentation and the amount of weight loss suggest at least 10% dehydration. His calculated fluid deficit is as follows:

$$0.10 \times 10 \text{ kg} \times 1000 \text{ (mL/kg)} = 1000 \text{ mL (fluid deficit)}$$

An alternate method of calculation, since his preillness weight is known, is to subtract his current weight from his preillness weight (10 kg to 9 kg) and multiply by 1000 (mL/kg), also resulting in 1000 mL of deficit. To start his resuscitation, a 20 mL/kg bolus of isotonic fluids (or 9 kg × 20 mL/kg = 180 mL) is then given over 30 minutes. If vital signs are restored back to normal, a residual deficit of 820 mL will have to be replaced as oral or intravenous fluid therapy. If there is continued hemodynamic compromise after the initial bolus, additional boluses of 20 mL/kg are given.

Replacement Intravenous Fluids

Replacement fluids are required to prevent hypovolemia and electrolyte abnormalities when continued excessive fluid losses are present. Common sources of fluid losses necessitating replacement include emesis, diarrhea, urine, and surgical drain outputs (chest tubes, nasogastric tubes, ileostomies, fistulas). If this fluid is not appropriately replaced, hypovolemia and significant electrolyte derangements can develop. Oral replacement of fluid is preferred when tolerated. Intravenous replacement of fluid is necessary when oral replacement cannot meet ongoing losses.

Prior to replacing ongoing losses, one must first restore extracellular volume with resuscitation fluids, as outlined previously. Once euvolemia is restored, ongoing fluid losses must be closely replaced. It is important to note that this fluid replacement is in addition to the volume of required maintenance fluid. Replacement fluid therapy should be individually tailored for each patient, with inputs and outputs closely monitored. Existing guidelines recommend using 0.9% sodium chloride containing potassium as the initial fluid for replacement therapy. If fluid loss is ongoing and excessive, serial measurement of serum electrolytes is required to adjust the intravenous fluid prescription. The measurement of electrolyte concentrations may be helpful, as the electrolyte composition varies between sites of fluid loss. When measurement of electrolyte composition is not feasible, one must

| TABLE 2 | Clinical Signs to Estimate Dehydration |

Older Child

	3% (30 mL/kg)	6% (60 mL/kg)	9% (90 mL/kg)

Infant

	5% (50 mL/kg)	10% (100 mL/kg)	15% (150 mL/kg)
Dehydration	Mild	Moderate	Severe
Skin turgor	Normal	Tenting	None
Skin (touch)	Normal	Dry	Clammy
Buccal mucosa/lips	Dry	Dry	Dry/cracked
Eyes	Normal	Slightly sunken	Sunken
Tears	Present	Decreased	None
Fontanelle	Flat	Soft	Sunken
Mental status	Alert	Alert/altered	Lethargic/obtunded
Pulse rate	Normal	Slightly increased	Increased
Pulse quality	Normal	Weak	Weak/very weak
Capillary refill	Normal	2–3 s	>3 s
Urine output	Normal/mild oliguria	Mild oliguria	Severe oliguria

| TABLE 3 | Electrolyte Composition of Body Fluids |

FLUID	Na+ (mmol/L)	K+ (mmol/L)	Cl− (mmol/L)	HCO3−
Gastric	20–60	14	140	60–80
Biliary drain	145	5	105	30
Pancreatic drain	125–138	8	56	85
Diarrhea/colostomy	30–140	30–70	—	20–80
Ileostomy	45–140	4–5	25–125	0–30

be familiar with the electrolyte contents of the fluid loss in varying disease processes in order to maintain the correct balance of electrolytes. The electrolyte composition of some of the common sites of fluid loss is shown in Table 3.

In GI losses from infectious gastroenteritis, the electrolyte content varies based on the type of infection. A typical rotavirus enteritis can lead to a mean sodium loss of 50 mmol/L and up to 50 mmol/L of bicarbonate. Secretory diarrheal illnesses, such as cholera, can cause massive loss of fluid, with sodium losses as high as 140 mmol/L and bicarbonate losses several times that of other GI illnesses. If either hypernatremia or a metabolic acidosis is developing, a hypotonic replacement fluid or a buffered solution may be required. In the loss of other bodily fluids, such as emesis, a large amount of chloride is lost (90 to 150 mmol/L) instead of bicarbonate, and buffered solutions should not be used for replacement. Potassium and magnesium may also have to be replaced in diseases such as renal tubulopathies. In understanding the composition of the fluid lost, the appropriate type of intravenous fluid can be prescribed (see Table 1).

The management of ongoing fluid losses is a labor-intensive process that requires meticulous monitoring of the patient's total input and output. Close clinical assessment of the patient, daily weight measurements, and routine monitoring of electrolytes are necessary to ensure euvolemia and electrolyte homeostasis.

Sodium Disorders

Disorders in serum sodium are the most frequent electrolyte abnormality in hospitalized patients and can occur on presentation or be hospital acquired. Hyponatremia and hypernatremia are both associated with potential neurologic and systemic complications and increased hospital morbidity and mortality. Careful fluid therapy is needed for both prevention and treatment.

Hyponatremia

Hyponatremia is defined as a serum sodium less than 135 mEq/L. The body's primary defense against developing hyponatremia is the kidney's ability to generate dilute urine and excrete free water. In most cases of hyponatremia there is a stimulus for ADH production that results in impaired free water excretion. There are numerous stimuli for ADH production (see Fig. 1) that place virtually all hospitalized children at risk for hyponatremia. A particularly common cause of hyponatremia is SIADH. SIADH refers to euvolemic hyponatremia due to nonphysiologic stimuli for ADH production in the absence of renal or endocrine dysfunction. SIADH can be difficult to diagnose, as volume status is difficult to assess accurately and there are no specific biochemical tests for diagnosing SIADH. Before SIADH can be diagnosed, diseases causing decreased effective circulating volume, renal impairment, adrenal insufficiency, and hypothyroidism must be excluded. The hallmarks of SIADH are (1) mild volume expansion with low to normal plasma concentrations of creatinine, urea, uric acid, and potassium; (2) impaired free water excretion with normal sodium excretion, which reflects sodium intake; and (3) hyponatremia that is relatively unresponsive to sodium administration in the absence of fluid restriction. The biochemical parameters most suggestive of SIADH in adults are a spot urine sodium concentration greater than 30 mEq/L, fractional excretion of sodium greater than 0.5%, fractional excretion of urea greater than 55%, fractional excretion of urate greater than 11%, and plasma uric acid less than 4 mg/dL. These parameters may not apply to young children.

The most serious complication of hyponatremia is hyponatremic encephalopathy, which is a medical emergency that can be fatal or can lead to irreversible brain injury if inadequately treated. The primary symptoms of hyponatremia are those of cerebral edema. The most consistent symptoms are nonspecific and can easily be overlooked: headache, nausea, vomiting, and generalized weakness. Advanced symptoms include seizures, respiratory arrest, noncardiogenic pulmonary edema, and decorticate posturing. Children are at particularly high risk for developing hyponatremic encephalopathy as they have a relatively larger brain-to-intracranial volume compared with adults. There is evidence to suggest that even mild and seemingly asymptomatic hyponatremia has deleterious consequences, being an independent risk factor for mortality.

Hyponatremic encephalopathy is a medical emergency that requires immediate therapy with 3% sodium chloride (3% NaCl, 513 mEq/L). The consensus treatment for hyponatremic encephalopathy is to give repeated boluses of 3% NaCl (2 mL/kg, maximum 150 mL) in order to raise the serum sodium acutely by approximately 5 mEq/L. Fluid restriction is the cornerstone of treatment in asymptomatic hyponatremia. Isotonic saline is effective in treating hypovolemic hyponatremia, although it can aggravate hyponatremia due to SIADH. SIADH is usually of short duration and resolves with treatment of the underlying disorder or discontinuation of the offending medication. For more chronic forms of SIADH, therapies include oral sodium supplementation, oral urea (Ure-Na)[1], or vasopressin V2-receptor antagonist.

Overcorrection of severe and chronic hyponatremia can result in brain injury from cerebral demyelination. Cerebral demyelination is primarily seen in chronically hyponatremic patients of greater than 48 hours' duration with a serum sodium of less than 115 mEq/L. Other risk factors that increase the likelihood of cerebral demyelination independent of the degree of hyponatremia or rate of correction are hypokalemia, thiazide diuretic use, severe liver disease, malnutrition, hypophosphatemia, and hypoxia. Excessive increases in serum sodium should be avoided under all circumstances, not just with hyponatremia. In patients with severe and chronic hyponatremia, the serum sodium should not be corrected by greater than 20 mEq/L in the first 48 hours of therapy.

Hypernatremia

Hypernatremia is defined as a serum sodium >145 mEq/L. Hypernatremia occurs in children in the presence of restricted access to water, such as infants, debilitation by an acute or a chronic illness, neurologic impairment, or in the critically ill. Contributing factors for hypernatremia in the intensive care setting are excess sodium administration, renal concentrating defects, GI fluid losses, increased insensible water losses, restricted access to oral fluids, and dialysis-related complications.

If the thirst mechanism is intact and there is unrestricted access to free water, it is rare for someone to develop sustained hypernatremia from either excess sodium ingestion or a renal concentrating defect. The cause of hypernatremia is usually multifactorial. Measuring urine osmolality and electrolyte concentration can help to determine whether the renal concentrating ability is appropriate and to quantify the urinary free water losses. Less than maximally concentrated urine (<800 mOsm/kg) in the face of hypernatremia associated with signs of dehydration is a sign of a renal concentrating defect, as hypernatremia is a maximal stimulus for ADH release. A relatively new and useful clinical lab test for distinguishing central from nephrogenic diabetes insipidus is plasma copeptin testing. Copeptin, the C-terminal segment of the prehormone for arginine vasopressin, can be used as a surrogate marker of ADH as it is easier and more reliable to measure than ADH.

Hypernatremia results in an efflux of fluid from the intracellular space to the extracellular space to maintain osmotic equilibrium. This leads to transient cerebral dehydration with cell shrinkage. Children with hypernatremia are usually agitated and irritable but can progress to lethargy, listlessness, and coma. On neurologic examination they frequently have increased tone, nuchal rigidity, and brisk reflexes. Myoclonus, asterixis, and chorea can be present; tonic-clonic and absence seizures have been described.

The cornerstone of hypernatremia management is providing adequate free water to correct the serum sodium concentration but doing this at a rate that limits the risk of brain injury. Hypernatremia is frequently accompanied by volume depletion; if hemodynamic instability is present, fluid resuscitation with an isotonic solution should be instituted to establish more normal hemodynamics prior to slowly correcting the free-water deficit. Following initial volume expansion, composition of parenteral fluid therapy largely depends on the etiology of the hypernatremia. Patients with sodium overload or a renal concentrating defect require a more hypotonic fluid than those with volume depletion and intact renal concentrating ability. Oral hydration should be instituted as soon as it can be safely tolerated. Plasma electrolytes should be checked frequently until adequate correction is achieved.

A simple way of estimating the minimum amount of fluid necessary to correct the serum sodium is by the following equation:

$$\text{Free water deficit (mL)} = 4 \text{ mL} \times \text{lean body weight (kg)} \times (\text{Desired change in serum Na mEq/L})$$

The rate of correction of hypernatremia is largely dependent on the severity of the hypernatremia and the etiology. Due to the brain's relative inability to extrude unmeasured organic substances (idiogenic osmoles), rapid correction of hypernatremia can lead to cerebral edema. Although there are no definitive studies documenting the optimal rate of correction without causing cerebral edema to develop, empiric data have shown that a rate of correction of 0.5 mEq/h or 12 mEq/24 h is reasonable. Sodium chloride 0.45% with appropriate amounts of potassium is usually the most suitable composition of IVF to treat hypernatremia in children with hypovolemic hyponatremia and intact renal function.

References

Antequera Martín AM, Barea Mendoza JA, Muriel A, et al: Buffered solutions versus 0.9% saline for resuscitation in critically ill adults and children, *Cochrane Database of Systematic Reviews* (7), 2019. Art. No. CD012247.

Holliday MA, Segar WE: The maintenance need for water in parenteral fluid therapy, *Pediatrics* 19:823–832, 1957.

Feld LG, Neuspiel DR, Foster BA, et al: Clinical practice guideline: maintenance intravenous fluids in children, *Pediatrics* 142:e20183083, 2018.

Moritz ML, Ayus JC: Maintenance intravenous fluids in acutely ill patients, *N Engl J Med* 373:1350–1360, 2015.

Moritz ML, Ayus JC: Preventing neurological complications from dysnatremias in children, *Pediatr Nephrol* 20:1687–1700, 2005.

Moritz ML: Syndrome of Inappropriate Antidiuresis, *Pediatr Clin N Am* 66:209–226, 2019.

National Clinical Guideline Centre (UK): *IV Fluids in Children: Intravenous Fluid Therapy in Children and Young People in Hospital*, London, United Kingdom, 2015, National Clinical Guideline Centre. https://www.ncbi.nlm.nih.gov/pubmed/26741016. Accessed 13 April 2020.

Weiss S, Peters M, Alhazzani W, et al: Surviving Sepsis Campaign International Guidelines for the Management of Septic Shock and Sepsis-Associated Organ Dysfunction in Children, *Pediatric Critical Care Medicine* 21:e52–e106, 2020.

[1] Not FDA approved for this indication.

PEDIATRIC FAILURE TO THRIVE

Method of
Gretchen Homan, MD

CURRENT DIAGNOSIS

- Pediatric failure to thrive (PFTT), also known as weight faltering, refers to failure to gain weight at an appropriate rate over time.
- History taking, physical examination, and growth chart data are used to identify PFTT.
- Weight below the fifth percentile with a negative growth trend over time indicates potential PFTT.
- Weight measurements declining across two major percentiles may indicate PFTT.
- Failure to gain or maintain weight is the earliest indication of PFTT, but length and head circumference may be impacted and should always be monitored.

CURRENT THERAPY

- Successful treatment includes addressing all causes, including underlying medical problems.
- Hospitalization is generally not indicated, and serial clinic visits can be used to monitor weight gain and maintenance.
- Growth chart parameters can help set a goal weight. Daily weight gain goals can be identified to monitor treatment over weeks to months.
- The majority of patients respond to generalized techniques for increased calories combined with frequent outpatient monitoring of progress.
- Consulting with a dietitian or using detailed nutrition calculations can provide specific guidance for protein and calorie goals in complicated cases.

In pediatric failure to thrive (PFTT), also known as weight faltering, the child fails to gain weight at an appropriate rate; this failure is documented over time. The concept has been recognized for over a century, but there is still no consensus on terminology or a definition. Historically, the terms *organic* and *nonorganic* were used to identify PFTT, and they were attributed to medical conditions and psychosocial causes, respectively. Insufficient usable nutrition is now regarded as the underlying cause of PFTT. It can be due to problems with calorie intake or absorption or both. Approximately 80% of children with PFTT are diagnosed by age 18 months. For older children, the preferred term is *poor weight gain*.

Epidemiology

In the United States, PFTT occurs in approximately 5% to 10% of children seen in primary care and in up to 5% of children admitted to the hospital. An estimated 20% to 30% of cases are undiagnosed. PFTT is a condition rather than a specific diagnosis, and imprecise diagnostic criteria complicate estimating its incidence and prevalence. Some children show a decrease in their weight curves followed by weight maintenance on the new curve; although this occurs in approximately 25% of children, it is not considered weight faltering.

Risk Factors

Risk factors for PFTT can be medical and/or psychosocial. In up to 80% of cases, no obvious medical etiology is identified. Any disease process has the potential to cause PFTT. Prenatal predisposing factors include exposure to toxins, intrauterine growth retardation, and poor maternal nutrition. Infants born

prematurely are at high risk for PFTT. Premature infants need to catch up in growth over months to years and should not be expected to reach normal peer percentiles too quickly, as this could have negative implications for healthy weight in adult life. Any medical problem that interferes with or inhibits calorie intake and absorption of nutrients can cause PFTT, as can any condition that creates increased caloric demand. Leading medical causes include development delay, congenital anomalies such as cleft lip and/or palate, genetic conditions such as cystic fibrosis or celiac disease, and childhood cancers and related treatments.

Poverty is the most powerful psychosocial risk factor for PFTT, as it limits access to appropriate nutrition. Healthcare providers should be aware of "food deserts" in their communities as well as families within their practice that are food insecure. Children of families with increased life stresses, social isolation, poor parenting skills, or substance abuse are at increased risk for PFTT. Personal nutritional beliefs and practices can also limit nutrition, leading to PFTT. Examples include prolonged exclusive breast feeding or avoidance of multiple food categories for cultural or religious reasons or real or perceived food allergy.

Pathophysiology

Inadequate caloric intake, malabsorption, or increased metabolic demand, either as isolated entities or concurrently, can lead to PFTT. Caloric intake may be impaired by use of diluted formula, poor feeding habits, neglect, or mechanical feeding difficulties. Inadequate nutrient absorption can be caused by a range of diseases or conditions that affect the gastrointestinal tract, including celiac disease, cystic fibrosis and other pancreatic diseases, milk protein allergy, inborn errors of metabolism, and chronic infections. Increased energy needs and potential caloric deficit leading to PFTT can occur in children with chronic infections, congenital heart or lung disease, hyperthyroidism, malignancy, renal failure, inflammatory conditions, and HIV.

Prevention

Prevention of PFTT begins with prenatal care and maternal health, especially limiting potential exposure to toxins, optimizing maternal nutrition, and conducting routine pregnancy screenings. Being aware of potential genetic conditions facilitates planning appropriate support for the family. State-mandated newborn screening tests provide opportunities for early intervention in patients at risk for PFTT. Routine well-child visits in the first 2 years of life provide surveillance for growth and anticipatory guidance regarding nutrition to support development. Connecting families with appropriate community resources can help provide high-risk children and families with access to nutritional resources. Supporting overall good health with patient education and general preventive services, including oral health and immunization, is essential to reducing the risk of FTT.

Clinical Manifestations

PFTT is defined by problems with weight as a documented trend over time. The Centers for Disease Control and Prevention (CDC) recommend that the World Health Organization growth charts be used to document growth for children under age 2 years and that the CDC growth charts be used for children ages 2 years and older. The majority of PFTT patients show at least one of three characteristics: weight below the 5th percentiles for age and sex, weight drop of two major percentiles, or weight less than the 80th percentile of ideal body weight. Some infants may benefit from a PFTT evaluation when their daily weight gain is less than expected for age and sex but does not yet meet these criteria. If weight faltering persists, length and then head circumference are impacted, and these indicate severe PFTT.

Patients with PFTT can generally be diagnosed as outpatients. Laboratory evaluation or imaging is not generally required. Detailed history taking and physical examination, along with the growth chart information, are sufficient to identify PFTT. A delay in development coupled with weight faltering noted on the growth chart comprise the clinical presentation of severe or prolonged PFTT. The aim of the physical examination is to identify any underlying or contributing medical condition that could impair nutrition and/or increase metabolic demands. The clinician should observe for any dysmorphic features and look for signs of abuse or neglect. Signs of malnutrition may become evident when PFTT is allowed to persist. The most severely affected children show edema, wasting, hepatomegaly, rash, or skin and hair changes.

Differential Diagnosis

Prematurely born infants and those with intrauterine growth retardation may be mistaken for patients with PFTT. These infants and children may meet the diagnostic criteria for delay on standard growth charts (values less than the 5th percentile) for age and sex. Ongoing monitoring for underlying medical conditions, regular developmental assessments, and evaluation of the social support network for each patient can provide reassurance that the child does not have PFTT and is expected to "catch up" in growth parameters within 18 to 36 months.

Genetic short stature and constitutional growth delay should be ruled out by reviewing the midparental height and growth patterns for delays. Radiologic testing for bone age may be helpful when confirming constitutional growth delay. Children with autism may have behaviorally restricted diets combined with medical complexities that predispose them to malnutrition and thus should be monitored carefully.

Therapy

PFTT can have one or multiple causes or complicating factors. Each issue should be addressed in the context of the overall health of the child and family. Any underlying medical condition must be diagnosed and treated. Children with a history of choking or oral motor dysfunction may benefit from a speech therapist evaluation and treatment program. Hospitalization is rarely indicated but may be helpful if there are complicating medical or social problems or if outpatient treatment has failed. Outpatient therapy is centered on increasing calorie intake with appropriate food options (Table 1). Equations can be used to calculate estimated calorie and protein needs by age and sex for both normal and catch-up growth. To simplify this process, a generalized list of targets is provided in Table 2. When available, a dietitian can define the required protein and calorie goals for catch-up growth initially and over the remaining treatment period. Alternatively, the primary care physician can use the growth chart to determine the desired weight goal for age and plan for a daily weight gain goal over weeks or months. The techniques described in Table 1 can be used to initiate treatment. Frequent visits are necessary. At each visit, the child's measurements should be done on the same well-calibrated scale to provide reliable data for clinical decision making about appropriate weight gain and maintenance. Patients who are unable to grow with these interventions may benefit from either short-term nasogastric tube feedings or more long-term gastric tube feedings.

Monitoring

Children with PFTT may require more frequent monitoring than the scheduled routine well-child visits. Young infants can be seen weekly or monthly and older patients every 2 to 4 months. At these visits, patients should be weighed and measured, preferably without clothing, by trained staff using routinely calibrated devices and standardized techniques to ensure the most accurate measurements. The clinician should review the patient's growth charts, diet and activity history, any changes in the social and medical history, and perform a physical examination. Recent acute illness may slow or reverse growth progress and should be addressed. It may take months for malnourished patients to show and maintain growth recovery. Patients who were born prematurely or with intrauterine growth retardation may require years to catch up. Depending on the underlying cause of PFTT, relapse is possible.

Complications

Weight loss or deceleration is the earliest clinical indicator for PFTT; if allowed to persist, height and length can be affected.

TABLE 2	Estimated Calorie Needs by Age
AGE	KCAL/KG/DAY
Preterm infant	115–130; up to 150 for very low birth weight infants
Full-term infant • 0–2 months • 3 months • 4–35 months	• 104–107 • 95 • 82
Toddler	70–80

Add 5–20 kcal/kg/day for catch-up growth, depending on tolerance and desired rate of recovery.

TABLE 1	Techniques to Increase Calories	
AGE	CALORIE SOURCE ADJUSTMENT	FEEDING TECHNIQUE
Infant – breast fed	• Increase feeds up to 12 in 24 hours • Pump after feeds and use expressed breast milk (EBM) to supplement nursing; add formula powder to expressed breast milk	• Evaluate and ensure proper latch/position • Feed both breasts with each feeding • Work to keep baby awake for complete feeding • Do not allow feeds to persist beyond 30 minutes total
Infant – formula fed	• Increase calorie concentration by mixing formula powder with less water, from 19/20 to 24/26 kcal; monitor for tolerance • Evaluate feeding volume and frequency to avoid over- or underfeeding; rule of thumb feeds average 1 oz/h (e.g., 3 oz/3 h)	• Evaluate for intolerance and change formula if needed; consider predigested proteins • Use proper bottle nipple speed • Avoid bottle propping
Toddler	• Add butter, dips such as ranch or mayonnaise, and cheese to foods • Use high-calorie foods and offer proteins such as cheese, peanut butter, avocados, and high-fat yogurts • Encourage a variety of healthy foods such as fruits, vegetables, proteins, and grains • Consider supplement drinks or shake powders to mix 1–2 times/day	• Structured mealtimes in a high chair with adult supervision and without distractions (e.g., television, other children) • Evaluate toddler's ability to self-feed effectively; intervene and teach if needed • Aim for 3 meals with 3 snacks daily • Minimize fruit juices • Offer water with meals and offer foods before milk or supplement drinks

Eventually, head size and brain growth can be impaired. At this level of severity, PFTT puts cognitive development and achievement of milestones in jeopardy. Immune system function may be impaired during a malnourished state, thus putting affected patients at risk for infections. Social and emotional health may also be impacted. Research is ongoing to understand the long-term effects of PFTT.

References

Black MM, Dubowitz H, Krishnakumar A, Starr Jr RH: Early intervention and recovery among children with failure to thrive: follow-up at age 8, *Pediatrics* 120:59–69, 2007.

Cole SZ, Lanham JS: Failure to thrive: an update, *Am Fam Physician* 83:829–834, 2011.

Emond AM, Blair PS, Emmett PM, Drewett RF: Weight faltering in infancy and IQ levels at 8 years in the Avon Longitudinal Study of Parents and Children, *Pediatrics* 120:e1051–8, 2007.

Engorn B, Flerlage J, editors: *The Harriet Lane Handbook: A Manual for Pediatric House Officers*, 20th ed., Philadelphia, 2014, Elsevier Saunders.

Kleinman RE, Greer FR: Failure to thrive. In *Pediatric Nutrition*, Elk Grove Village, IL, 2014, American Academy of Pediatrics, pp 663–700.

Olsen EM, Petersen J, Skovgaard AM, et al: Failure to thrive: the prevalence and concurrence of anthropometric criteria in a general infant population, *Arch Dis Child* 92:109–114, 2007.

Rybak A: Organic and nonorganic feeding disorders, *Ann Nutr Metab* 66(suppl 5):16–22, 2015.

Shields B, Wacogne I, Wright CM: Weight faltering and failure to thrive in infancy and early childhood, *BMJ* 345:e5931, 2012.

Wright CM, Parkinson KN, Drewett RF: How does maternal and child feeding behavior relate to weight gain and failure to thrive? Data from a prospective birth cohort, *Pediatrics* 117:1262–1269, 2006.

Yoo SD, Hwang EH, Lee YJ, Park JH: Clinical characteristics of failure to thrive in infant and toddler: organic vs. nonorganic, *Pediatr Gastroenterol Hepatol Nutr* 16:261–268, 2013.

PEDIATRIC SLEEP DISORDERS

Method of
Julie M. Baughn, MD

CURRENT DIAGNOSIS

- Sleep disorders are common in children.
- Evaluation of pediatric sleep disorders in children begins with a thorough sleep history.
- Overnight polysomnography is most commonly used to evaluate for sleep-disordered breathing
- Other diagnostic tools include the multiple sleep latency test (MSLT), oximetry, sleep logs, and actigraphy.
- Common sleep disorders in children include obstructive sleep apnea, insomnia, restless legs syndrome, and delayed sleep phase syndrome.

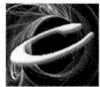

CURRENT THERAPY

- For most children tonsillectomy and adenoidectomy are an effective treatment for obstructive sleep apnea.
- Behavioral therapy is essential to treating insomnia.
- Only in select circumstances are medications used to treat children with sleep disorders.

Introduction

Pediatric sleep medicine has grown as the importance of sleep in the developing child has been recognized along with the impact that insufficient or disrupted sleep can have on cognitive development and behavior. The American Academy of Sleep Medicine (AASM) and the American Academy of Pediatrics (AAP) have recently published guidelines and practice parameters addressing several aspects of pediatric sleep medicine. Pediatric sleep disorders have unique societal impact; both the child's and the family's sleep can be affected when a disorder is present. The aim of this chapter is to offer a practical approach to the diagnosis and treatment of the most common pediatric sleep disorders, discuss diagnostic tools available, and discuss recommended treatment.

Developmental Aspects of Sleep

Pediatric sleep disorders also have the unique challenge of dealing with sleep issues that are subject to change based on the child's developmental age. The amount of sleep required by age has been described in a recent AASM consensus statement (Table 1). The sleep architecture of the child characteristically changes as he or she develops. The portion of rapid eye movement (REM) sleep declines from 50% at birth to 25% to 30% in adolescence. The proportion of slow-wave sleep is highest in early childhood and continues to decline throughout life. The pattern of sleep and sleep requirement also change. Neonates may not develop a regular sleep-wake pattern until about 3 months of age. Most infants are capable of sleeping through the night by about 6 months of age, but many may continue to waken. Naps are typically given up somewhere between 3 and 5 years of age. Most adolescents, due to many societal and social constraints, do not get a requisite 8 to 10 hours of sleep at night.

Clinical Approach
Taking a Sleep History

There are several key elements to obtaining a sleep history in children. The mnemonic BEARS (*B*edtime problems, *E*xcessive daytime sleepiness, *A*wakenings during the night, *R*egularity and duration of sleep, and *S*leep-disordered breathing) has been offered as a practical starting point for obtaining a history, tailoring questions to both parent and child where appropriate (Table 2).

The primary sleep complaint should be obtained in the child's or parent's own words. Once the primary complaint is detailed, the presence/absence of snoring, the presence of restlessness at sleep initiation and during sleep, and the child's sleep-wake patterns during school should be gathered. The presence or absence of a bedtime routine and the details of that routine should be noted. A child's sleep environment should be carefully queried. A child who shares his or her bedroom, sleeps in his or her parents' bed, or ends up sleeping on a couch in front of the television may lead to specific sleep complaints. A history of whether there is more than one household involved (i.e., shared custody) is particularly important.

Sleepiness in children can be a particularly challenging symptom to evaluate. It is normal physiologically for children to nap until age 5. Other clues to daytime sleepiness that can be obtained in children include behavior issues, hyperactivity,

TABLE 1	Sleep Requirements in Children by Age
AGE	**AVERAGE SLEEP DURATION IN 24 HOURS (OVERNIGHT AND NAPS)**
Infants (4 to 12 months)	12 to 16 hours
Children (1-2 years)	11-14 hours
Children (3-5 years)	10–13 hours Most give up naps between 3 and 5 years
Children (6-12 years)	9–12 hours
Teenagers (> 12 years13-18 years)	9 hours8-10 hours

Paruthi S, Brooks LJ, D'Ambrosio C, et al. Consensus Statement of the American Academy of Sleep Medicine on the Recommended Amount of Sleep for Healthy Children: Methodology and Discussion, *J Clin Sleep Med* 2016; 12(11):1549-1561.

TABLE 2 | BEARS Mnemonic: A Screening Tool for Sleep Disorders in Children

	PRESCHOOL (2–5 YEARS)	SCHOOL-AGE (6–12 YEARS)	ADOLESCENT (13–18 YEARS)
Bedtime problems	Does your child have any problems going to bed? Falling asleep?	Does your child have any problems at bedtime? (P) Do you have any problems going to bed? (C)	Do you have any problems falling asleep at bedtime? (C)
Excessive daytime sleepiness	Does your child seem overly tired or sleepy during the day? Does your child still take naps?	Does your child have difficulty waking in the morning, seem sleepy during the day, or take naps? (P) Do you feel tired a lot? (C)	Do you feel sleepy a lot during the day? In school? While driving? (C)
Awakenings during the night	Does your child wake up a lot at night?	Does your child seem to wake up a lot at night? Any sleepwalking or nightmares? (P) Do you wake up a lot at night? Have trouble getting back to sleep? (C)	Do you wake up a lot at night? Have trouble getting back to sleep? (C)
Regularity and duration of sleep	Does your child have a regular bedtime and wake time? What are they?	What time does your child go to bed and get up on school days? Weekends? Do you think your child is getting enough sleep? (P)	What time do you usually go to bed on school nights? Weekends? How much sleep do you usually get? (C)
Sleep-disordered breathing	Does your child snore a lot or have difficulty breathing at night?	Does your child have loud or nightly snoring or any breathing difficulties at night? (P)	Does your teenager snore loudly or nightly? (P)

Abbreviations: C = child; P = parent.
From Owens JA, Dalzell V: Use of the "BEARS" sleep screening tool in a pediatric residents' continuity clinic: A pilot study. Sleep Med 2005;6:63–69.

TABLE 3 | Principles of Sleep Hygiene in Children

The child's bedroom should be dark and quiet.
Bedtime routines should be strictly enforced. Routines should be relaxing and only 20 to 30 minutes in length.
The time of morning awakening should be firmly and consistently structured.
Bedroom temperatures should be kept comfortably cool (< 75 °F).
Environmental noise should be minimized as much as possible. Background music and/or white noise may inhibit extraneous noise.
Children should not go to bed hungry and may have a snack before bedtime.
Excessive fluids before bedtime may result in bladder distention and arousal and disrupt sleep.
Children should learn to fall asleep alone (i.e., without their parents' presence in the room).
Vigorous activity should be avoided before bedtime.
A bath is often a stimulating activity for children. If bedtime struggles are present after a child's bath, it may be moved to the morning or separated from the child's bedtime by at least 2 hours.
Methylxanthine-containing beverages and food (e.g., caffeinated beverages/colas, tea, chocolate) should be avoided several hours before bedtime.
Parents should read labels on all over-the-counter and prescription medications. Some may contain alcohol or caffeine and may disrupt sleep.
Naps should be developmentally appropriate. Brief naps may be refreshing, but prolonged naps or napping too frequently may result in significant accumulation of sleep during the day and make it more difficult to fall asleep at night.

Modified from Sheldon SH, Ferber R, Kryger M (eds): Principles and Practice of Pediatric Sleep Medicine. Philadelphia: Elsevier Saunders, 2005.

excessive napping, or napping after age 5 years (intentionally or unintentionally). School-age children often display symptoms of behavioral problems or inattentiveness rather than sleepiness. Sleep-wake patterns on school days, weekends, and vacations need to be detailed. Often the child's most natural sleep pattern will emerge over the summer months.

Determining the child's sleep hygiene or good sleep practices is important in diagnosing and treating sleep disorders. Principles of good sleep hygiene are listed in Table 3.

Past Medical History/Family History

A history of prematurity, trisomy 21, velopharyngeal cleft palate repair, or hypotonia is each associated with an increased risk of sleep-disordered breathing. A past history of adenotonsillectomy for snoring is important information to obtain. Chronic nasal obstruction can cause maxillary hypoplasia. Arnold-Chiari malformation, myelomeningocele, or a brainstem lesion can predispose to central sleep apnea due to impaired central respiratory drive. Chronic health issues can also be associated with sleep disruption and consequently with behavioral problems associated with sleep.

A family history of obstructive sleep apnea (OSA), insomnia, or restless legs syndrome (RLS) is important; a family history of RLS can be used to support a diagnosis of RLS in the child. In particular, questioning the mother if she had symptoms of RLS during any of her pregnancies can be helpful because this is a common time for RLS to present or worsen. Morning or evening preferences (i.e., "night-owl" or "lark" tendencies) can also have a familial element. In addition, sleepwalking can be found to occur in families.

Focused Physical Examination

The physical examination in a child presenting with a sleep complaint should include a general assessment. Presence/absence of sleepiness, fatigue, and irritability/hyperactivity are all important. Height, weight, and body mass index (BMI) should be recorded. Children with OSA can have poor growth and even failure to thrive. Obesity is a risk factor for OSA. Special attention to a child's craniofacial features is important because these may make a child more at risk for sleep-disordered breathing.

Assessment of tonsil size, oropharyngeal crowding (using the Mallampati or Friedman classification systems can be useful), and presence of maxillary/mandibular hypoplasia can all offer clues to an airway that may predispose to OSA. The practitioner should evaluate for evidence of nasal obstruction by noting mouth breathing and signs of allergy (i.e., allergic shiners, nasal crease).

Diagnostic Tools
Polysomnography
The AASM has published practice parameters on both the respiratory and nonrespiratory indications for polysomnography (PSG) in pediatric patients. In this chapter, a sleep study or PSG will refer only to an in-laboratory attended study, because home monitoring currently has not been sufficiently evaluated in the pediatric population. PSG in children entails spending the night at a sleep center. A parent or caregiver must also spend the night. During the night, the child's sleep characteristics, respiratory function, and movement are analyzed. This is done by the following measures: electroencephalography (EEG), electromyography (EMG) of chin and limbs, airflow by thermistor and nasal pressure, end-tidal or transcutaneous carbon dioxide measurements, and induction plethysmography to measure respiratory effort. Scoring of a PSG performed on a child is done using pediatric scoring rules set forth by the AASM.

The most common indication for a sleep study in children is OSA. PSG can be used to both diagnose OSA and treat sleep apnea with continuous positive airway pressure (CPAP). PSG can also be used to evaluate for elevated periodic limb movements of sleep, and in rare cases to characterize abnormal nocturnal behavior such as evaluation of parasomnias or nocturnal seizures.

Overnight Oximetry
The gold standard for diagnosis of pediatric OSA is PSG. Overnight oximetry has been suggested as an alternative screening tool for pediatric sleep-disordered OSA. Although an abnormal oximetry will suggest OSA, a normal oximetry does not rule out OSA. Children can have sleep apnea that is severe and still maintain normal oxygenation. In a study by Brouillette and colleagues (2000), when a positive oximetry graph was present (defined by three or more desaturation clusters and at least three desaturations < 90%) in a referred population, the positive predictive value for OSA on PSG was 97%. A negative or inconclusive oximetry by this definition did not rule out OSA and there was still a 47% chance OSA was present on PSG.

Sleep Logs/Actigraphy
Sleep logs can be effective in demonstrating a child's sleep-wake patterns. Actigraphy is often done in conjunction with a sleep log. Actigraphy is a portable wristband that measures movement. The absence of movement over a certain time period is used as a surrogate marker of sleep, and the presence of movement over a certain time period is used as a surrogate for wakefulness. Some devices also measure ambient light exposure. Used in conjunction with actigraphy sleep logs can be extremely helpful in demonstrating discrepancies between perceived and actual sleep, and are helpful in demonstrating insufficient sleep and circadian rhythm disorders. Those that measure light as well can aid in uncovering sleep hygiene issues.

Multiple Sleep Latency Test
The multiple sleep latency test (MSLT) is a daytime study used to objectively measure sleepiness. It is often used to aid in the diagnosis of narcolepsy or hypersomnia. It is a set of four to five scheduled naps that typically occur the day after an overnight sleep study. Often 2 weeks of actigraphy are done before the MSLT to determine sleep-wake patterns.

Common Pediatric Sleep Diagnoses and Treatment
Obstructive Sleep Apnea
Epidemiology
Up to one-fifth of children can have intermittent snoring. Prevalence rates of OSA range from 1.2% to 5.7%. OSA is most common in children 2 to 8 years of age corresponding to the peak age of adenotonsillar hypertrophy. Due to the rise in childhood obesity there is now a corresponding rise in older children diagnosed with OSA.

Pathophysiology
The pharynx has many roles, including swallowing, speaking, and maintaining airway patency. Pharyngeal size is determined by the bones and soft tissue. The soft tissue is affected by the size of the tonsils and adenoids, as well as adipose tissue. Airway patency is maintained during wakefulness; a small airway can become vulnerable during sleep resulting in partial or total closure of the airway, hypoxemia, hypercapnia, and an arousal that results in opening of the airway and termination of the obstructive event. This leads to sleep disruption and daytime consequences. OSA in children likely results from a combination of narrowing of the upper airway, abnormal upper airway tone, and genetic factors.

Clinical Manifestation
OSA in adults is typically associated with daytime sleepiness. Associations have been made with hypertension, stroke, and metabolic syndrome. In children, OSA may not present with daytime sleepiness. Children may present with daytime inattention and/or neurocognitive and behavioral issues. Symptoms include snoring with or without apneic pauses or gasps. Restless sleep or secondary enuresis may also be noted. Parents may comment on increased work of breathing while sleeping. Other associations include poor growth, obesity, hypertension, and systemic inflammation.

Diagnosis
The gold standard for diagnosis of pediatric OSA is an in-laboratory attended PSG by an accredited sleep laboratory. History and physical examination lack sensitivity and specificity in predicting which children with snoring have OSA. However, a history of loud snoring, tonsillar hypertrophy, and abnormal oximetry is strongly suggestive of the diagnosis of OSA (see above). History alone cannot distinguish children with OSA from those with primary snoring. Criteria for the diagnosis of OSA in children are met when there is one or more apnea or hypopnea events per hour identified using scoring criteria by the AASM.

Differential Diagnosis
Other forms of sleep-disordered breathing are not as common as OSA. Sleep-related hypoventilation can occur in patients with neuromuscular weakness. Central hypoventilation syndromes are rare, but should be considered in children with persistent gas exchange abnormalities without additional explanation. Sleep-related hypoxemia can be present in pediatric patients with chronic lung disease. Central sleep apnea should be thought of in patients with brainstem abnormalities or Arnold-Chiari malformation. Sleep-related seizures may be difficult to differentiate from OSA in infants and an extended EEG montage may be necessary during their sleep study. Normal breathing patterns of infants and children should also be identified; brief (less than 10 seconds), central respiratory pauses that are self-resolving (and without significant desaturation) are common in normal children in either REM sleep or post-arousal/post-sigh.

Treatment

Treatment of OSA in most children is adenotonsillectomy. Recent guidelines from the AAP recommend an overnight sleep study in children where the practitioner had a clinical suspicion of OSA before adenotonsillectomy. Children with mild OSA preoperative can be monitored clinically postoperatively. Children with moderate to severe OSA, as well as children with craniofacial abnormalities, neurologic disorders, and obesity, should have a follow-up PSG to demonstrate resolution of OSA after surgery. Recent randomized controlled trials have shown that some children may outgrow their OSA, particularly if it is mild. Children who are not candidates for adenotonsillectomy may be treated with CPAP and use may have an impact on neurobehavioral outcomes. Treatment with CPAP therapy in children requires close follow-up because pressure needs may change with growth. In certain children, treatment with intranasal corticosteroids and/or montelukast may be considered with close follow-up.

Difficulty with Sleep Initiation and Night Wakings
Epidemiology
Bedtime problems and night wakings occur in up to 30% of children.

Clinical Manifestations
The diagnosis of insomnia includes difficulty going to sleep and/or staying asleep, the complaint that sleep is not of good quality, and the report of poor daytime functioning. The sleep complaints of infants and young children are often in the words of their parent or caregiver.

In preschool-age children both bedtime problems and night wakings are common and characterized by two types of behavioral insomnia of childhood: sleep-onset association type and limit-setting type. The definition of the *sleep-onset association type*, as defined in the ICSD-3, includes the following: sleep initiation is an extended process, associations are demanding, if the associations are not present sleep onset is delayed, and awakenings require caregiver intervention. The *limit-setting type* involves difficulty initiating or maintaining sleep, there is bedtime stalling or refusal, and the caregiver does not set sufficient and appropriate limits around this behavior. Children with frequent and prolonged night wakings have the sleep-onset association type. They often require an intervention by the caretaker to reinitiate sleep. Both problems can be present at once. Children who have difficulty going to sleep and provide resistance to bedtime have the limit-setting type. Parents of these children may complain of daytime behavioral issues due to the parent's inability to set limits during the day as well.

Diagnosis
Diagnosis is made from the history in the majority of cases. An overnight sleep study may be indicated in cases where another sleep disorder is suspected.

Differential Diagnosis
The differential diagnosis of insomnia or behavioral insomnia of childhood includes sleep disorders such as OSA, RLS, or nocturnal seizures. These disorders can prompt nocturnal awakenings or make sleep initiation difficult. If there is clinical suspicion of one of these disorders, an overnight sleep study may be indicated.

Treatment
Behavioral interventions have been shown to be effective in treating all forms of insomnia. In older children, primary and secondary insomnia can be effectively treated with cognitive-behavioral therapy. This often includes stimulus control and sleep restriction. Stimulus control includes maintaining a regular sleep-wake pattern and using the bed and bedroom only for sleeping. It involves getting out of bed if sleep is not initiated within about 20 minutes. Sleep restriction includes minimizing the time in bed to be only sleeping. It often includes delaying bedtime to the child's actual sleep onset, and then over time gradually advancing the bedtime. Sleep hygiene should be effectively addressed, including development of a relaxing bedtime routine, maintaining a regular sleep-wake pattern, and eliminating electronic use before bedtime.

There are several treatments of behavioral insomnia of childhood sleep-onset association type. No one treatment has been found to be superior. The goal of all of these methods is for the child to fall asleep in his or her crib or bed on the child's own. These include extinction (i.e., "cry it out"), which is often not palatable to caregivers. There is the graduated extinction method, which has parents ignoring crying or protests for specified periods of increasingly longer intervals. Some prefer an even more gradual approach of sitting next to the child's bed in a chair and over several days to weeks moving that chair across the room and out of the room. A consistent bedtime routine should also be implemented. Use of a transitional object can be helpful. Treatment of the limit-setting type includes firm limit setting. Positive reinforcement and limiting negative reinforcement should be used. The use of a reward system can be helpful. Effectively addressing behavioral treatment of sleep issues can be challenging for the primary care provider because of time constraints.

Restless Legs Syndrome/Willis Ekbom Disease
Epidemiology
Prevalence rates for pediatric RLS/WED have ranged from 1% to 6%.

Risk Factors
Risk factors include a family history and a history of anemia or iron deficiency. Attention-deficit/hyperactivity disorder (ADHD) is associated with RLS.

Pathophysiology
Decreased dopamine has been suggested in the pathophysiology of RLS/WED. Iron is a cofactor in the synthesis of dopamine and treatment of iron deficiency or low ferritin, if present, may improve symptoms.

Diagnosis
Diagnosis of pediatric RLS/WED is a clinical diagnosis. It is made using the adult criteria set forth in the ICSD-3 but with some modification for children due to developmental issues. It consists of the child reporting an urge to move the legs, usually accompanied by an uncomfortable sensation; this urge or sensation worsens during rest or inactivity; the sensations are improved or resolved by movement; the sensations are present or worsen in the evening or night. If a child cannot express a description in his or her own words, diagnosis can be made using two out of the following three criteria: a sleep disturbance for age, a family history of RLS, and a periodic limb movement index on PSG of > 5 per hour. Because of this last criterion, a sleep study can be helpful in children to make this diagnosis. There can be an association with sleep initiation and maintenance difficulties.

Differential Diagnosis
Differential diagnosis of RLS should include insomnia, sleep-disordered breathing, or neurologic or musculoskeletal etiologies for the discomfort.

Treatment
Nonpharmacologic treatment of RLS includes good sleep hygiene, moderate exercise a few hours before bedtime, and avoidance of

substances that are associated with worsening of RLS symptoms, including caffeine, alcohol, antihistamines, and antiemetics. A serum ferritin should be drawn in all children with RLS and if < 50 ng/mL, treatment with 6 mg/kg/day of oral elemental iron should be considered. Oral iron absorption is enhanced by vitamin C and impaired by calcium. Gastrointestinal upset and constipation can be common side effects. Compliance can be difficult. A serum ferritin should be rechecked at 3 months to evaluate therapy. Referral to a sleep medicine specialist should be made if lifestyle and oral iron therapy have been unsuccessful. There are no FDA-approved medications for the treatment of RLS in children. Dopamine agonists, gabapentin (Neurontin),[1] clonazepam (Klonopin)[1], and clonidine (Catapres)[1] have been used to treat pediatric RLS.

Delayed Sleep Phase Syndrome
Epidemiology
Delayed sleep phase syndrome (DSPS) occurs most commonly in adolescents and young adults.

Clinical Manifestations
Symptoms usually present in adolescents but can occur in younger children. Adolescents with DSPS consistently have sleep onset at a later time, typically after midnight. They have difficulty initiating sleep earlier. They do not have difficulty maintaining sleep. They have difficulty waking in the morning unless able to sleep until their preferred time, which is typically after 10 AM. They may have sleepiness during the daytime if forced to rise early (i.e., for school); however, during long vacations or summer breaks when allowed to sleep to preferred wake time they feel refreshed. Children who already have a preferred evening preference may find this exacerbated in adolescence. Poor school performance can be present.

Diagnosis
Diagnosis is made from history; actigraphy and sleep logs are also useful. An overnight sleep study may be indicated if another sleep disorder is suspected (e.g., OSA).

Differential Diagnosis
The differential diagnosis includes insomnia, poor sleep hygiene, insufficient sleep, mood disorder, OSA, and RLS.

Treatment
Treatment is typically behavioral and includes good sleep hygiene. Typically either the patient's sleep-wake schedule is advanced (if there is less than 3 hours between actual and desired bedtime) by 15 minutes every 2 to 3 days until the goal bedtime is achieved. Rise time is advanced as well and if set at the desired wake time initially it should facilitate the advancement of the bedtime by increasing sleep drive. If the desired bedtime of the adolescent is greater than 3 hours from the current bedtime, phase delay can be considered. Bedtime is delayed by 2 to 3 hours each day until the target bedtime is reached. Timing of this therapy should be considered, because it will interfere with school or other daytime activities. Parental or caregiver support is necessary, as well as commitment by the adolescent.

Once the new pattern is established weekends must not differ from weekdays by more than 1 to 2 hours. This is particularly important for the rise time. Relapse is common if strict sleep-wake patterns are not adhered to, a problem common on vacations.

Both bright light exposure and melatonin have been used to help reset the circadian rhythm. Exposure to bright light in the morning is encouraged and can be as simple as increasing sun exposure in the morning. Light boxes using 2500 to 10,000 lux can be used in the morning for 20 to 30 minutes. Exposure to light in the evening should be limited. A small dose of melatonin[7] (0.5 mg) can be used in the early evening (about 5 hours before desired bedtime) to attempt to physiologically advance sleep onset. If the timing is not optimal for both light and melatonin, the phase delay can be worsened; consultation with a sleep physician should be considered.

Parasomnias
Parasomnias can occur out of both non-REM (NREM) and REM sleep. Those occurring out of NREM sleep include sleepwalking, sleep terrors, and confusional arousals. They typically occur in the first one-third of the night, when NREM-3 sleep is most prevalent, and are not recalled the next day. They can be part of normal development, but depending on their nature, they can be distressing to caregiver and child. Parasomnias occurring out of REM sleep include nightmares and REM-sleep behavior disorder (RBD). Nightmares are commonly recalled and have been associated with anxiety in children. Nightmares typically peak in the school-age child. RBD is rare in children but has been reported; it involves the loss of atonia that occurs in REM sleep and consequently dreams are "acted out."

Risk Factors
Poor sleep hygiene, insufficient sleep, irregular sleep-wake patterns, and a positive family history are all risk factors. Sleep disruption from sleep-disordered breathing or periodic limb movements of sleep can exacerbate parasomnias.

Differential Diagnosis
The differential diagnosis should include nocturnal seizures. In addition, if another sleep disorder is present, parasomnias can be exacerbated.

Treatment
Safety is most important in children with parasomnias, and it is important that the child's sleep environment is kept clear of things that could cause injury. Door alarms can be effective. The child should not be awakened during the episode. The event should not be referred to the next morning because this can cause distress for the child. Maintaining good sleep hygiene and regular sleep-wake patterns is important. If the events occur at a predictable time each night, the caregiver can do planned awakenings 30 minutes before the event typically occurs for several weeks. This may abolish the episodes. It can also have the effect of pushing the episode to later in the night. Pharmacologic treatment with a small dose of a benzodiazepine (e.g., 0.5 mg of clonazepam [Klonopin][1] at bedtime) may be indicated in severe cases with the drug tapered slowly after episodes are suppressed.

Hypersomnias
A full discussion of primary hypersomnias (including narcolepsy) in children is beyond the scope of this chapter. Consideration for a primary hypersomnia should be made in a child who is sleepy after common causes of sleepiness such as insufficient sleep and obstructive sleep apnea have been ruled out. Symptoms of narcolepsy include disrupted nocturnal sleep, hallucinations on going to sleep or waking up, and sleep paralysis. Daytime sleepiness is present with "sleep attacks" both during quiet activities and while active. Cataplexy may also be present and is defined by loss of muscle tone without loss of consciousness. It should be noted that onset of narcolepsy is often in adolescence or as a young adult.

---

[1]Not FDA approved for this indication.

[1]Not FDA approved for this indication.
[7]Available as dietary supplement.

Diagnosis is often delayed because the symptoms are attributed to other conditions. Treatment of pediatric hypersomnia is done under the supervision of a sleep specialist and often involves use of stimulants.

References

Aurora RN, Lamm CI, Zak RS, et al: Practice parameters for the non-respiratory indications for polysomnography and multiple sleep latency testing for children, *Sleep* 35:1467–1473, 2012.

Aurora RN, Zak RS, Karippot A, et al: Practice parameters for the respiratory indications for polysomnography in children, *Sleep* 34:379–388, 2011.

Berry RB, Brooks R, Gamaldo C, et al: *The AASM Manual for the Scoring of Sleep and Associated Events*, Westchester, Illinois, 2012, American Academy of Sleep Medicine2012.

Brouillette RT, Morielli A, Leimanis A, et al: Nocturnal pulse oximetry as an abbreviated testing modality for pediatric obstructive sleep apnea, *Pediatrics* 105:405–412, 2000.

Fehrm J, Nerfeldt P, Browaldh N, Friberg D: Effectiveness of adenotonsillectomy vs watchful waiting in young children with mild to moderate obstructive sleep apnea: A randomized clinical trial, *JAMA Otolaryngol Head Neck Surg* 146(7):647–654, 2020.

Kaditis A, Kheirandish-Gozal L, Gozal D: Algorithm for the diagnosis and treatment of pediatric OSA: a proposal of two pediatric sleep centers, *Sleep Med* 13:217–227, 2012.

Kheirandish-Gozal L, Bhattacharjee R, Bandla HP, Gozal D: Antiinflammatory therapy outcomes for mild OSA in children, *Chest* 146(1):88–95, 2014.

Kirk V, Baughn J, D'Andrea L, et al: American Academy of Sleep Medicine Position Paper for the Use of a Home Sleep Apnea Test for the Diagnosis of OSA in Children, *J Clin Sleep Med* 13(10):1099–1203.

Kotagal S, Nichols CD, Grigg-Damberger MM, et al: Non-respiratory indications for polysomnography and related procedures in children: an evidence-based review, *Sleep* 35:1451–1466, 2012.

Kuhle S, Hoffmann DU, Mitra S, Urschitz MS: Anti-inflammatory medications for obstructive sleep apnoea in children, *Cochrane Database Syst Rev* 1(1):Cd007074, 2020.

Lloyd R, Tippmann-Peikert M, Slocumb N, et al: Characteristics of REM sleep behavior disorder in childhood, *J Clin Sleep Med* 8:127–131, 2012a.

Marcus CL, Brooks LJ, Draper KA, et al: Diagnosis and management of childhood obstructive sleep apnea syndrome, *Pediatrics* 130:576–584, 2012b.

Marcus CL, Brooks LJ, Draper KA, et al: Diagnosis and management of childhood obstructive sleep apnea syndrome, *Pediatrics* 130:e714–e755, 2012.

Marcus CL, Moore RH, Rosen CL, et al: A randomized trial of adenotonsillectomy for childhood sleep apnea, *N Engl J Med* 368(25):2366–2376, 2013.

Marcus CL, Radcliffe J, Konstantinopoulou S, et al: Effects of positive airway pressure therapy on neurobehavioral outcomes in children with obstructive sleep apnea, *Am J Respir Crit Care Med* 185:998–1003, 2012.

Mindell JA, Barrett KM: Nightmares and anxiety in elementary-aged children: is there a relationship? *Child Care Health Dev* 28:317–322, 2002.

Mindell JA, Owens J: *A clinical guide to pediatric sleep: diagnosis and management of sleep problems*, Philadelphia, 2003, Lippincott Williams & Wilkins.

Mindell JA, Owens J: *A clinical guide to pediatric sleep: diagnosis and management of sleep problems*, ed 2, Philadelphia, 2010, Lippincott Williams & Wilkins.

Morgenthaler T, Alessi C, Friedman L, et al: Practice parameters for the use of actigraphy in the assessment of sleep and sleep disorders: an update for 2007, *Sleep* 30:519–529, 2007.

Morgenthaler T, Kramer M, Alessi C, et al: Practice parameters for the psychological and behavioral treatment of insomnia: an update. An American Academy of Sleep Medicine report, *Sleep* 29:1415–1419, 2006.

Owens JA, Dalzell V: Use of the "BEARS" sleep screening tool in a pediatric residents' continuity clinic: a pilot study, *Sleep Med* 6:63–69, 2005.

Paruthi S, Brooks LJ, D'Ambrosio C, et al: Consensus Statement of the American Academy of Sleep Medicine on the Recommended Amount of Sleep for Healthy Children: Methodology and Discussion, *J Clin Sleep Med* 12(11):1549–1561, 2016.

Picchietti D, Allen RP, Walters AS, et al: Restless legs syndrome: prevalence and impact in children and adolescents—the Peds REST study, *Pediatrics* 120:253–266, 2007.

Sateia MJ, editor: *The International Classification of Sleep Disorders*, 3rd ed, Westchester, Illinois, 2014, American Academy of Sleep Medicine.

Sheldon SH, Ferber R, Kryger M, editors: *Principles and Practice of Pediatric Sleep Medicine*, Philadelphia, 2005, Elsevier Saunders.

St Louis EK, Morgenthaler TI: Sleep disorders. In Bope E, Kellerman R, editors: *Conn's Current Therapy 2013*, Philadelphia, 2013, Saunders Elsevier.

RESUSCITATION OF THE NEWBORN

Method of
David S. Gregory, MD

CURRENT DIAGNOSIS

- The transition from intrauterine to extrauterine life at birth requires effective breathing by the infant to expand the lungs and oxygenate the blood. All newborn infants are at risk for delays in this process, prompting a need for resuscitation.
- The fetal and newborn response to hypoxia is to develop apnea. If primary apnea is diagnosed, it can be corrected by gentle stimulation and oxygen delivery. If hypoxia persists, secondary apnea will occur. It is not readily apparent whether a newborn has primary or secondary apnea, and the approach to resuscitation therefore requires that any apneic event be treated using the same sequence of interventions.
- The initial steps of newborn resuscitation include drying the infant, providing warmth, using gentle stimulation, and clearing the airway if needed. Infants who do not respond to these interventions need more assistance. Establishment of effective ventilation spontaneously by the newborn or with assistance by positive-pressure ventilation is the most important step in newborn resuscitation.
- Reassessment of the infant's heart rate, respiratory effort, pulse oximeter reading or color, and tone every 30 seconds during resuscitation is crucial to determine the next appropriate intervention. Apgar scoring should *not* be used to guide newborn resuscitation. Electrocardiographic (ECG) monitoring is the best method for assessing heart rate. Pulse oximetry in the delivery room should be used to guide oxygen therapy. Temperature of the infant should be monitored.
- If application of positive-pressure ventilation does not improve the infant's heart rate, chest compressions or drug therapy, or both, may be required. A team approach is needed to coordinate these interventions, and ongoing reassessment is necessary to determine cardiorespiratory and hemodynamic status. Subsequent assessment and treatment should be performed in an intensive care setting.

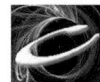

CURRENT THERAPY

- Term gestation infants who are breathing and crying with good muscle tone do not need newborn resuscitation.
- Most newborns do not require immediate cord clamping and can be monitored during skin-to-skin contact with their mothers.
- Initial resuscitation includes drying the infant, providing warmth, giving gentle stimulation, and clearing the mouth and nose, if needed.
- If the infant is apneic, breathing slowly, or gasping, positive-pressure ventilation (PPV) with a mask and bag should be administered. A rise in heart rate is the best indicator of effective ventilation and response to resuscitation.
- When oxygen therapy is needed during resuscitation, pulse oximetry should be used to guide oxygen concentration.
- If the heart rate does not improve with ventilation efforts, endotracheal intubation should be considered.
- When the infant's heart rate drops below 60 beats/min, chest compressions should be initiated using the two-thumb technique. Heart rate should be monitored using ECG.
- If the heart rate remains less than 60 beats/min despite PPV and chest compressions, IV epinephrine (Adrenalin) may be given using an umbilical venous catheter or via intraosseous catheter.
- Infants who do not improve with epinephrine and have a history consistent with blood loss may improve with fluid expansion.
- Reassessment of the newborn every 30 seconds during resuscitation is required to adjust therapy as indicated. The best indicator of successful resuscitation is an increase in heart rate.

The changes that occur in the transition from fetus to newborn are unmatched in any other time of life. Most newborns manage to make this transition on their own, but about 10% require some assistance. Approximately 1% of newborns require extensive resuscitative measures to survive. The approach to resuscitation in infants is similar to that in adults, consisting of evaluation and intervention when needed for the infant's airway, breathing, and circulation. Every birth should be attended by personnel trained in neonatal resuscitation. Specific training and certification are offered by the American Academy of Pediatrics/American Heart Association's Neonatal Resuscitation Provider (NRP) course. This chapter has been updated based on the American Heart Association 2020 Guidelines and the 8th edition of the NRP June 2021 (Box 1). Ongoing training and a team-based approach are vital components of newborn resuscitation.

Transition From Fetal to Extrauterine Life

The environment of the fetus differs greatly from that of the infant after birth. The fetus depends on receiving oxygen and nutrients from the mother through the placental circulation. The fetus experiences relative hypoxia and almost constant body temperature in the amniotic fluid. The fetal lungs are filled with fluid and do not participate in the exchange of oxygen and carbon dioxide. Several adaptations in the fetus permit survival in this environment.

Oxygenated blood from the mother enters the fetus by means of the placenta through the umbilical vein. Most of this oxygenated blood bypasses the liver through the ductus venosus and enters the inferior vena cava. On entering the right atrium, this oxygenated blood is directed toward the patent foramen ovale into the left atrium, bypassing the fetal lungs. Fetal blood also passes through the right atrium into the right ventricle and then into the pulmonary artery. The vascular resistance and blood pressure of the pulmonary vessels in the fetal lung are higher than in the aorta and systemic circulation; most of the blood is therefore shunted away from the lungs through the ductus arteriosus into the ascending aorta. Only a small amount of fetal blood passes through the lungs to the left atrium and then to the left ventricle. The umbilical arteries branch off from the internal iliac arteries and return fetal blood to the placenta. The functional organ for gas exchange of oxygen and carbon dioxide in the fetus is the placenta.

At birth, the newborn is no longer connected to the placenta, and the lungs become the only source of oxygen. The first breaths of the infant cause the fluid in the lung alveoli to be replaced with air. The umbilical arteries and veins constrict at birth and are eventually clamped. This increases the vascular resistance and blood pressure of the systemic circulation. As the oxygen level in the alveoli increases, the blood vessels in the lung start to relax, decreasing pulmonary vascular resistance. Blood in the pulmonary artery travels toward the lung and away from the ductus arteriosus because the blood pressure in the systemic circulation is higher than that in the pulmonary circulation. Increased blood flow to the lungs allows the oxygen from the alveoli to enter the infant's blood, increasing the Po_2. Oxygenated blood enters the left heart through the pulmonary vein and is delivered to the rest of the infant's tissues through the aorta.

Although the initial steps in this transition occur within a few minutes of birth, the entire process may not be completed for several hours to days. The ductus venosus, foramen ovale, and ductus arteriosus remain potentially patent and do not completely involute for days or weeks. Changes in the infant's systemic and pulmonary pressures can result in blood flow through these channels in the infant.

Transition can be prevented or delayed in several circumstances. The infant may not breathe adequately, in which case the lung fluid is not forced out of the alveoli. Material such as meconium may block air from entering the alveoli. If the lungs do not fill with air, hypoxia will quickly develop. Systemic hypotension caused by excessive blood loss, poor cardiac function, or bradycardia prevents the change in the direction of blood flow that is necessary to promote blood flow into the lungs. Failure of the lungs to expand or hypoxia can prevent relaxation of the pulmonary blood vessels, resulting in a high pulmonary vascular resistance. This leads to decreased blood flow to the lungs and worsening of hypoxia.

Risk Factors for Newborn Resuscitation

A number of prenatal and intrapartum factors are associated with a higher chance that the infant will have a delay in transition and require resuscitation (Table 1). A recent multicenter review of risk factors for resuscitation at gestation age 34 weeks or greater found that the following risk factors were significantly associated with a need for advanced resuscitation: 34 to 37 weeks gestation, intrauterine growth retardation (IUGR), gestational diabetes, meconium-stained amniotic fluid, vacuum or forceps assisted delivery, clinical chorioamnionitis, fetal bradycardia, placenta abruption, general anesthesia, and emergency cesarean section. In preparation for labor and delivery, staff should ask the following questions: (1) What is the expected gestational age of the infant? (2) Is the amniotic fluid clear? (3) Are there additional risk factors? and (4) What is the umbilical cord management plan? However, some infants *with no risk factors* need resuscitation; therefore preparations for neonatal resuscitation should be made during all deliveries.

Reaction to Hypoxia and Asphyxia

Normally at birth, the newborn makes vigorous efforts to breathe. The process of leaving the warm, dark, and liquid environment in utero is replaced by cold air, dryness, and bright lights. Drying the infant with towels and wiping the mouth and nose are

---

| **BOX 1** | **Summary of Key Points for Newborn Resuscitation Based on Neonatal Resuscitation Program, 8th Edition** |

1. Individual providers and neonatal resuscitative teams should train, prepare, brief and check equipment as a team prior to resuscitative efforts.
2. Vigorous newborn infants—whether term or preterm—do not require immediate cord clamping with resuscitative efforts, but rather can be evaluated and monitored while providing skin-to-skin contact with their mother and 30 seconds of delayed cord clamping.
3. Ventilation of a newborn's lungs is the priority when support is required.
4. Routine intubation and tracheal suctioning is not recommended for infants born in meconium stained amniotic fluid (including those who may be nonvigorous).
5. Effective ventilation and proper response to resuscitative efforts is first indicated by a rise in newborn heart rate.
6. After initial use of room air for ventilation efforts in term infants, pulse oximetry monitoring guides oxygen concentration adjustment to meet goals at specific minute-based intervals after birth.
7. In cases of insufficient heart rate response to ventilation of a newborn's lungs (including corrective steps, such as endotracheal intubation), chest compressions are indicated.
8. Electrocardiographic monitoring is necessary to assess the heart rate response to chest compressions and medication.
9. When chest compressions do not result in an adequate increase in heart rate, epinephrine, preferably via the intravenous route, is indicated.
10. Infants with history or examination consistent with blood loss, and having poor response to epinephrine, may require volume expansion.
11. Following effective resuscitation, if no heart rate is attained by 20 minutes, cessation of resuscitative efforts should be discussed with team and family.

TABLE 1 Risk Factors for Newborn Resuscitation

PRENATAL FACTORS	INTRAPARTUM FACTORS

• Maternal
  • Diabetes, preexisting
  • Chronic hypertension
  • Infection
  • Cardiac, renal, pulmonary, thyroid, or neurologic disease
  • Drug therapy
  • Substance use
  • Lack of prenatal care
  • Age <16 or >35 years
  • Previous fetal or neonatal death
• Pregnancy
  • Bleeding in second or third trimester
  • Pregnancy-induced hypertension
  • Toxemia
  • Gestational diabetes
  • Fetal anemia or isoimmunization
  • Polyhydramnios
  • Oligohydramnios
  • Fetal hydrops
  • Postterm gestation
  • Multiple gestation
  • Size-date discrepancy
  • Diminished fetal activity
  • Fetal malformation or abnormality
	• Placental
	  • Placenta previa
	  • Abruption of the placenta
	  • Premature or prolonged rupture of membranes
	  • Chorioamnionitis
	• Fetal
	  • Macrosomia
	  • Low birth weight
	  • Breech or other abnormal presentation
	  • Persistent fetal bradycardia
	  • Nonreassuring fetal heart rate patterns
	• Labor
	  • Premature labor
	  • Precipitous labor
	  • Prolonged labor (>24h)
	  • Prolonged second stage of labor (>2h)
	  • Prolapsed cord
	  • Emergency cesarean section
	  • Forceps or vacuum-assisted delivery
	• Other
	  • Meconium-stained amniotic fluid
	  • General anesthesia
	  • Narcotics given within 4h of delivery
	  • Uterine hyperstimulation
	  • Severe intrapartum bleeding

all the assistance that most newborns require. The end result of any mechanism that delays transition is a period of hypoxia for the fetus or newborn infant. Laboratory studies have shown that the first sign of oxygen deprivation in the newborn is a change in the breathing pattern. After an initial period of rapid breathing attempts, cessation of breathing occurs. This is called *primary apnea*. Stimulation by drying the infant or slapping the feet can cause breathing to resume. If hypoxia continues after primary apnea has occurred, the infant will make attempts at gasping and then stop breathing. This is called *secondary apnea*. Stimulation does not affect secondary apnea. Assisted ventilation is necessary to provide breaths to the newborn to reverse the hypoxia. The infant's heart rate starts to decrease when primary apnea occurs. The heart rate increases with stimulation if the infant has primary apnea, and blood pressure is maintained. With continued hypoxia, the heart rate continues to drop, and hypotension develops. If assisted ventilation is not adequate to increase the infant's heart rate, chest compressions will be required.

When a newborn becomes apneic, it is not readily apparent whether the infant has primary or secondary apnea. The approach to resuscitation therefore requires that any apneic event in a newborn be treated using the same sequence of interventions. If the apneic infant responds to simple stimulation, the diagnosis is primary apnea, and no further intervention is required. If the infant does not improve with stimulation, secondary apnea has occurred, and more intensive intervention is needed.

Unlike adults, the progression from primary apnea to secondary apnea in newborns results in the cessation of respiratory activity before the onset of cardiac failure. For this reason, neonatal resuscitation should begin with PPV rather than with chest compressions. Delays in initiating adequate ventilation in newly born infants increase the risk of death.

Preparation for Newborn Resuscitation

The neonatal resuscitation team, prior to resuscitative efforts, should attempt to perform a team brief and check all necessary equipment. The team brief should include answers to questions that should be asked of the delivery team to clarify neonatal needs, including gestational age, amniotic fluid color and clarity, known risk factors for cardiopulmonary dysfunction (such as congenital heart disease) or infection (such as chorioamnionitis), and any concern for delayed cord clamping. The team brief allows the neonatal team to refocus and organize their team response, while checking all equipment ensures that needed instruments, devices, and medications are at their disposal for the resuscitative efforts.

Sequence of Newborn Resuscitation
Initial Steps and Basic Resuscitation

Resuscitation of the newborn starts with the rapid assessment of three characteristics: Is the infant at term gestation, does the infant have good tone, and is the infant crying and breathing? The answers to these questions will affect the approach to care. Resuscitation when fluid is meconium stained is discussed later in this chapter. The information presented here refers to term infants with clear amniotic fluid. More information regarding the care of premature infants is discussed in a later section.

The infant at term who is crying and breathing with good muscle tone does not need resuscitation and should not be separated from the mother. Current evidence suggests cord clamping should be delayed for at least 30 seconds for most vigorous term and preterm infants unless there is evidence of placental abruption or bleeding. The baby should be dried, placed skin-to-skin with the mother, and covered with dry linen to maintain temperature. Ongoing observation for breathing, activity, and color should continue while the infant is with the mother. If the infant is not term, is not crying and breathing, or does not have good muscle tone, newborn resuscitation should begin with the initial steps: providing warmth, drying and stimulating the infant, then positioning and clearing (if needed) the airway,

The newborn should be placed under a radiant warmer to prevent heat loss and allow easy observation. Although warm blankets or towels can be used to dry the infant, they should not be left in place to cover the infant. Drying the infant, slapping the feet, and rubbing the back are appropriate forms of stimulation. More forceful methods of stimulation can harm the infant. Primary apnea, if present, will respond to stimulation in less than 30 seconds. Prolonged apnea will require positive-pressure ventilation (PPV).

The newborn should be placed on the back with the neck slightly extended in the "sniffing" position (Figure 1). This facilitates air entry into the lungs by lining up the posterior pharynx, larynx, and trachea. Hyperextension or hyperflexion of the neck can obstruct air entry into the lungs.

If the newborn is crying vigorously, secretions can be removed by wiping the nose and the mouth with a towel. Routine suctioning should be avoided. Gentle suctioning of the mouth and nose with a bulb syringe or suction catheter is *only* indicated when there is obvious obstruction to spontaneous breathing or when there is a need for positive-pressure ventilation. Deep or vigorous suctioning can be detrimental to the infant because of stimulation of the vagus nerve, causing bradycardia or apnea. The mouth should be suctioned before the nose to prevent aspiration if the infant gasps during suctioning.

Evaluating the infant's response to resuscitation is essential. The Apgar score is a traditional method for evaluating newborn status at 1 and 5 minutes after delivery. However, effective resuscitation demands that evaluation of the newborn's status not be delayed until 1 minute of age, and Apgar scores therefore should *not* be used to guide resuscitative efforts. Within 30 seconds of delivery, the infant's need for PPV must be assessed. Establishment of effective ventilation spontaneously by the newborn or with assistance by PPV is the most important step in newborn resuscitation. The respiratory status, heart rate, and color or oximetry reading should be determined. The chest wall should move with each breath, and the newborn should be breathing spontaneously. Although heart rate can be assessed by feeling for a pulse at the base of the umbilical cord, this method can be unreliable. Auscultation with

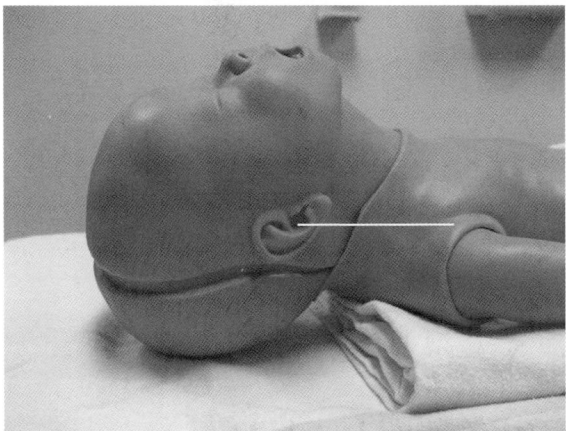

Figure 1 The sniffing position. Positioning the infant on the back with the neck slightly extended brings the posterior pharynx, larynx, and trachea in line (*white line*) to facilitate air entry into the lungs.

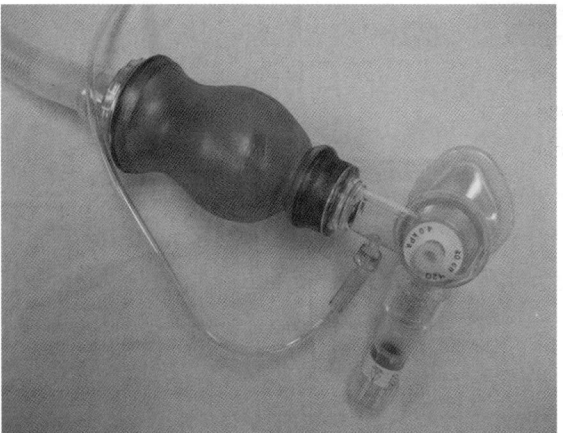

Figure 2 Self-inflating bag with infant mask and reservoir. This type of device is available in most delivery rooms.

a stethoscope is the preferred method during initial resuscitation. The heart rate should be greater than 100 beats/min. Placement of 3-lead ECG (electrocardiograph) as soon as possible to monitor the infant's heart rate during resuscitation may be beneficial. Monitoring of heart rate using ECG is more reliable than palpation and auscultation and is faster than using the pulse oximeter. Peripheral cyanosis (i.e., blueness of the hands and feet) is acceptable in the initial period after delivery. Central cyanosis in which the lips and trunk are blue indicates hypoxemia and the need for more resuscitation efforts. Pulse oximetry should be used to confirm the perception of central cyanosis. A pulse oximeter can provide continuous assessment of the oxygen saturation and is the optimal method for monitoring the infant's state of oxygenation. The oximeter probe should be placed on the newborn's right wrist or hand to detect preductal saturation. Temperature should be monitored during newborn resuscitation. The normal range is an axillary temperature of 36.5°C to 37.5°C. The initial steps of stabilization, reassessment, and establishing ventilation should be completed within the first minute of life (the "Golden Minute").

Respiratory Support and Positive-Pressure Ventilation

If the infant is breathing with a heart rate higher than 100 beats/min but has central cyanosis, free-flowing oxygen delivery is indicated. This can be administered with a facemask or by holding oxygen tubing or a flow-inflating bag and mask close to the infant's face. *A self-inflating bag and mask cannot be used to give free-flowing oxygen.* If the newborn is apneic, not breathing effectively, or has a heart rate less than 100 beats/min, PPV using a self-inflating bag, flow-inflating (or anesthesia) bag, or a T-piece resuscitator is required. Use of a flow-inflating bag requires a compressed gas source and considerable practice to be used effectively. A T-piece resuscitator needs special equipment and a compressed gas source. Most delivery rooms are equipped with self-inflating bags (Figure 2) because they are easy to use and can be fitted with a pressure-release valve to decrease overinflation. A reservoir must be used with a self-inflating bag to provide 100% oxygen. For free-flow oxygen or PPV, the flow meter on the oxygen source should be set to 10 liters/minute.

PPV should begin using room air for term newborns. The facemask should cover the infant's nose, mouth, and tip of chin, but not the eyes (Figure 3). Multiple sizes should be available. A tight seal between the infant's skin and the facemask is needed, but excessive pressure can bruise the face. The mask can be held in place using the thumb and index finger in a C-shaped position on top of the mask, with the remaining fingers in an E-shaped position below the infant's chin (Figure 4). Inspiratory pressures of 20 to 25 cm H_2O are usually needed when squeezing the bag to make the infant's chest rise; peak inspiratory pressures in a term newborn of 30 cm H_2O may be required. A pressure gauge can be connected to the self-inflating bag for monitoring inspiratory

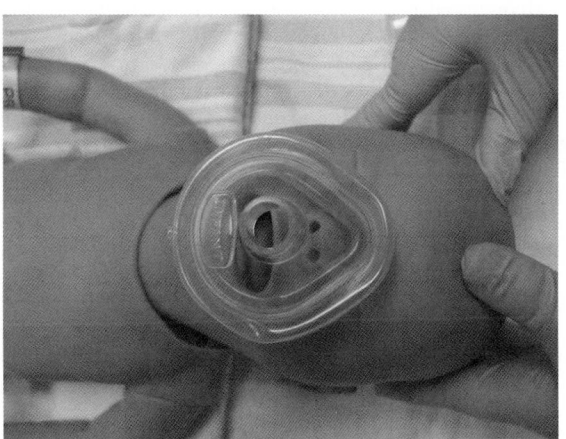

Figure 3 Facemask. Choose a size that covers the infant's mouth and nose.

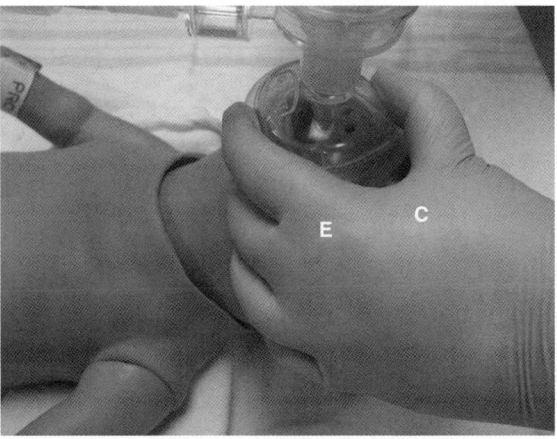

Figure 4 Facemask placement. The thumb and index finger are held in a C-shaped position on top of the mask, and the remaining fingers are held in an E-type position under the chin.

pressure. The heart rate and color of the infant should rapidly improve if enough pressure is being given. An assistant can also use a stethoscope to listen to breath sounds for air movement. Breaths should be given at a rate of 40 to 60 breaths/min.

Traditionally, 100% oxygen has been used in newborn resuscitation. However, several randomized, controlled studies enrolling term and near-term infants have shown that room air can be used initially with oxygen as a backup if room air fails. A meta-analysis of these trials showed a benefit for the use of room air. Providing oxygen at concentrations between room air and 100%

TABLE 2	Titrated Oxygen Saturations After Birth
1 minute	60–65%
2 minutes	65–70%
3 minutes	70–75%
4 minutes	75–80%
5 minutes	80–85%
10 minutes	85–95%

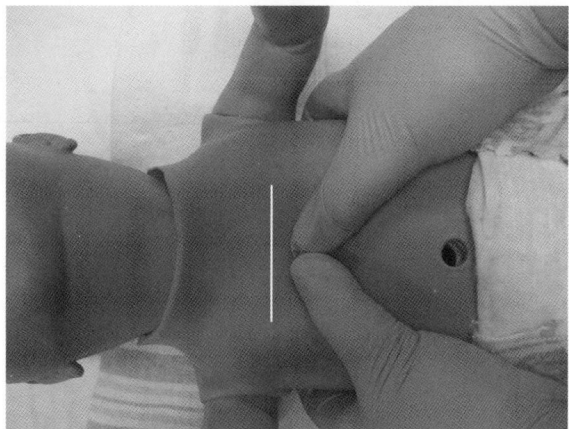

Figure 5 Two-thumb technique. The hands encircle the torso, and the thumbs are placed on top of the lower sternum above the xyphoid process and below a line drawn between the nipples (white line).

requires the use of compressed air, oxygen, and blenders by experienced personnel. A pulse oximeter with a probe designed for use in newborns can be used to guide oxygen administration during newborn resuscitation. It will take 1 to 2 minutes to apply the pulse oximeter probe to the infant's right palm or wrist (preductal site) and get a consistent reading. Pulse oximetry often displays lower-than-actual heart rate readings during the first 2 minutes of life. The pulse oximeter may not function during states of very poor cardiac output or perfusion. In these situations, observation for central cyanosis will be necessary. The infant's oxygen saturation may remain in the 70% to 80% range for several minutes after birth. Oxygen may be titrated to the interquartile range of preductal saturations measured in healthy babies following vaginal birth at sea level (Table 2). If blended oxygen is not available, room air should be used for resuscitation. If the infant's heart rate does not respond to positive pressure ventilation with room air after 90 seconds, 100% oxygen should then be used.

After 30 seconds of PPV, the infant should be reevaluated. Once PPV is started, an electronic cardiac monitor (ECG) is the preferred method to measure heart rate. Ventilation with a bag and mask can be stopped when the newborn has a heart rate higher than 100 beats/min, spontaneous breathing, improved color, and good muscle tone. Supplemental oxygen should still be given to the infant. If the newborn is not improving, use the acronym MR SOPA to correct the technique of PPV: M = mask adjustment to check seal, R = reposition head in sniffing position, S = suction mouth and nose, O = open mouth with infant's jaw lifted forward, P = increase pressure up to 30 to 40 cm H_2O, and A = consider using an alternative airway such as endotracheal (ET) intubation.

ET intubation is a technical skill that must be learned and practiced to maintain competency. Effective ventilation can be given with a bag and mask approach to most newborns. This skill is easily mastered and maintained. If an infant is responding well to bag and mask ventilation, it can be continued for longer periods; however, some air may escape into the esophagus and into the stomach. This may cause gastric distention, which can prevent full expansion of the lungs and cause vomiting and aspiration. An orogastric tube can be placed in the stomach and left open to air to vent any air introduced into the infant's stomach during bag and mask ventilation.

Chest Compressions

Before beginning chest compressions, intubation is strongly recommended to provide effective ventilation. After 30 seconds of effective PPV, the heart rate should be assessed. If the heart rate dips below 60 beats/min, chest compressions are needed to support the circulation. The two-thumb technique (Figure 5) is recommended. The two-thumb technique generates higher blood pressure and coronary perfusion with less rescuer fatigue. It can also be continued with the rescuer at the head of the bed if access to the abdomen is needed. If chest compressions are required, 100% oxygen should be given by PPV. Two people are required to give PPV and chest compressions effectively. To coordinate the breaths and chest compressions, three compressions are given followed by one breath, and this sequence is repeated to give the infant 90 compressions and 30 breaths/min. The thumbs are placed on the lower third of the infant's sternum but above the xyphoid process. The sternum is depressed to a depth of one third of the infant's anteroposterior chest diameter. The purpose of chest compressions is to squeeze the heart between the sternum and the spine, forcing blood in and out of the heart and to the body. The direction of the compressions should be perpendicular to the chest surface, and the thumbs should not be lifted off of the chest after the correct placement is obtained. Incorrect methods during chest compressions can cause rib fracture and liver laceration.

After 60 seconds of chest compressions, the infant's heart rate, breathing, pulse oximeter reading or color, and tone are reassessed. If the heart rate is higher than 60 beats/min, chest compressions can be stopped, although PPV may still be needed. If the heart rate is not improving, the following problems must be considered: ventilation is not adequate, 100% oxygen concentration is not being given, or the compressions may not be deep enough or well- coordinated with the breaths. If the arrest is suspected to be of primary cardiac etiology, a compression ratio of 15 compressions to 2 breaths may be more effective.

Medications for Newborn Resuscitation

If the newborn heart rate remains below 60 beats/min despite 30 seconds of effective PPV and 60 seconds of chest compressions, epinephrine (Adrenalin) can be used to stimulate the newborn heart. Fewer than 2 of 1000 infants will require this step in resuscitation. *IV administration of epinephrine is preferred.*

In the delivery room, a catheter can be quickly inserted into the umbilical vein for intravenous access. A 3.5 or 5F catheter prefilled with saline and connected to a 3-way stopcock is inserted about 2 to 4 cm into the umbilical vein using sterile technique. After blood is aspirated, insertion of the catheter is stopped, and the epinephrine is given rapidly, followed by a 3 mL saline flush. The concentration of epinephrine used in neonatal resuscitation is 1:10,000 (0.1 mg/mL). The intravenous dose is 0.01 to 0.03 mg/kg (0.1–0.3 mL/kg) (Table 3). The 8th edition of NRP recommends an initial dose of epinephrine as 0.02 mg/kg (0.2 mL/kg). The intraosseous route can be used if needed. A dose of epinephrine may be considered through the ET tube during the umbilical vein catheterization process but there is no evidence of benefit. The ET dose of epinephrine is 0.05 to 0.1 mg/kg (0.5–1 mL/kg).[1] The 8th edition of NRP recommends giving 0.1 mg/kg (1 mL/kg) via the ET tube if needed while establishing vascular access. *These higher doses are for ET use only.* Because lung absorption of epinephrine varies, the intravenous route using the umbilical vein or intraosseous catheter is preferred.

During umbilical vein cannulation, PPV and chest compressions are continued. More personnel will be needed to place the catheter and draw up the medications and saline flushes. After an intravenous dose of epinephrine, the infant's heart rate, respirations, color or oximeter reading, and tone are reevaluated. The heart rate should increase to more than 60 beats/min. If the heart rate does

---

[1]Not FDA approved for this indication.

TABLE 3	Drugs for Newborn Resuscitation			
DRUG	**CONCENTRATION**	**DOSE**	**INDICATIONS**	**COMMENTS**
Epinephrine	1:10,000 (0.1 mg/mL)	0.01–0.03 mg/kg IV = 0.1–0.3 mL/kg IV route preferred initial dose: 0.02 mg/kg = 0.2 mL/kg* ETT dose: 0.05–0.1 mg/kg recommended: 0.1 mg/kg = 1 mL/kg*,[1]	Asystole Bradycardia that does not improve with PPV and chest compressions Shock	May repeat every 3–5min. No evidence for giving epinephrine via ETT.
Volume expanders	Normal saline O negative blood	10 mL/kg IV	Hypovolemia	Crossmatch blood to mother if possible Repeat if needed
Glucose	10% Dextrose	2–5 mL/kg IV	Hypoglycemia	Monitor glucometer or venous glucose levels

Abbreviations: ETT = endotracheal tube; IV = intravenous.
[1]Not FDA approved for this indication.
*8th edition Neonatal Resuscitation Program (NRP) 2021

not respond, the dose of epinephrine can be repeated every 3 to 5 minutes. The effectiveness of ventilation and compressions should be reassessed. If the infant appears pale, has delayed capillary refill, or has decreased pulses, shock may be present. Infant blood loss might have occurred during delivery from placental problems or other sources. Administration of an isotonic crystalloid solution such as normal saline or type O negative blood at 10 mL/kg over 5 to 10 minutes can improve circulation. Ringer's lactate is no longer recommended for newborns. Volume expansion should be used cautiously because there is evidence from animal studies for poorer outcomes when it is used in the absence of hypovolemia. Rapid infusion of large volumes has been associated with intraventricular hemorrhage in premature infants.

Hypoglycemia is common in newborns who have required resuscitation. Blood from the infant's heel or the umbilical vein can be tested at the bedside and intravenous 10% dextrose (2–5 mL/kg) given for low blood glucose. No specific glucose level has been associated with a poorer outcome. There is no evidence that use of sodium bicarbonate benefits the neonate, and its use during resuscitation in the delivery room is not recommended.

After resuscitation, newborns should be monitored in an intensive care setting. These infants are at risk for several complications, such as infection, metabolic abnormalities, and seizures. Infants of 36 weeks' gestation or older with moderate to severe hypoxic-ischemic encephalopathy may benefit from induced hypothermia under clearly defined protocols.

Special Considerations
Some newborns do not respond to resuscitation because of specific problems. Infants with upper airway obstruction from micrognathia can be helped by a nasopharyngeal airway and placement of the infant in the prone position. Choanal atresia can be treated by placing an oral airway. Absence of breath sounds on one side of the chest can indicate a pneumothorax, requiring needle aspiration of the chest. An infant with a scaphoid abdomen and decreased breath sounds may have a diaphragmatic hernia. These infants should be intubated, and PPV by mask and bag should not be used. If the mother has received narcotics shortly before the delivery, the narcotic may be the cause of respiratory depression in the infant. These infants need PPV and respiratory support. Naloxone is no longer recommended as part of initial resuscitative efforts in the delivery room. Heart rate and oxygenation should be supported by PPV.

Endotracheal Intubation
During neonatal resuscitation, endotracheal intubation may be indicated in the following circumstances: cases in which bag and mask ventilation is ineffective or prolonged, in which chest compressions are performed, and in special situations such as congenital diaphragmatic hernia or extremely low birth weight infants. Intubation of the newborn requires preparation that can be performed while the infant is being ventilated by bag and mask. The

ET tube should not be placed unless the glottis is visualized by direct laryngoscopy. To ensure that the tube is in the trachea, a carbon dioxide (CO_2) detector should be used. Listening for equal breath sounds and looking for vapor condensation in the ET tube during exhalation can help, but an increase in the infant's heart rate or a positive detection of CO_2 is most reliable. It should be noted that poor or absent pulmonary blood flow may result in the absence of CO_2 detection despite tube placement in the trachea. The best indicator for effective ventilation is an increase in the newborn's heart rate.

Intubation should be performed as quickly as possible, with a goal of 30 seconds from insertion of the laryngoscope to the connection of the ET tube to the resuscitation bag. Complications of intubation include worsening of hypoxia and bradycardia, pneumothorax, contusions, perforation of the trachea or esophagus, and infection. After the infant has been intubated, deterioration in the infant's status should prompt an organized sequence to assess the adequacy of ventilation using the mnemonic DOPE:

- *Dislodged* (D): Is the tube in the right bronchus or out of the trachea?
- *Obstructed* (O): Is the tube obstructed by secretions or blood?
- *Pneumothorax* (P)
- *Esophagus* (E): Is the tube in the esophagus?

An alternative to intubation for infants ≥34 weeks gestation and ≥2000 grams is placement of a laryngeal mask airway. This type of airway does not require laryngoscopy. A soft inflatable mask that is attached to a flexible airway tube is placed in the hypopharynx such that the air in the tube is directed into the larynx and away from the esophagus. However, this type of airway cannot be used to suction the trachea nor to give endotracheal drugs. Its use has not been evaluated during chest compressions. For infants who require an alternative airway, cardiac monitoring (ECG) is recommended to assess the heart rate and whether chest compressions are needed or not.

Premature Infants
Infants born before 37 weeks' gestation are at increased risk for complications and the need for resuscitation. Premature lungs may lack surfactant, making ventilation difficult. Very-low-birth-weight (less than 1500 g) infants will need additional warming techniques such as prewarming the delivery room, covering the baby in plastic wrapping, and placing the baby under a radiant warmer and/or an exothermic mattress; however, iatrogenic hyperthermia (axillary temperature >38°C) should be avoided. Immature brain development may decrease the drive to breathe. Weak muscles make respiratory efforts less effective. Thin skin and decreased subcutaneous fat make temperature regulation a challenge. Premature infants often have infections such as pneumonia or sepsis. The blood vessels in their brains are fragile and can easily bleed during periods of blood pressure variation. The lower birth weights of premature newborns also require smaller sizes of equipment for resuscitation such

as facemasks, suction catheters, endotracheal tubes, and umbilical catheters. Initial oxygen concentrations between room air and 30% should be used to protect premature infants <35 weeks gestation from oxygen toxicity. The use of continuous positive airway pressure (CPAP) in premature infants who are breathing spontaneously but with difficulty following birth may reduce the need for intubation, mechanical ventilation, and surfactant use. If PPV is needed, it is preferable to use a device that can deliver positive end expiratory pressure (PEEP). More than one person trained in newborn resuscitation should be present at the delivery of a high-risk premature infant.

Meconium Staining of the Amniotic Fluid

Meconium is formed in the newborn gastrointestinal system during gestation. Intrauterine stress can cause release of meconium into the amniotic fluid. Aspiration of meconium-stained amniotic fluid into the lungs can result in severe pneumonitis and lung injury. The approach to resuscitation for an infant born in meconium-stained amniotic fluid (MSAF) has been revised. There is no evidence that the consistency of meconium-stained fluid (i.e., thick or thin) has an effect on the outcome of the newborn.

Crying and Vigorous Infant

If the newborn born in MSAF has normal respiratory effort and muscle tone with a heart rate higher than 100 beats/min, routine care including delayed cord clamping and skin to skin time with the mother is appropriate. Secretions can be wiped from the baby's mouth and nose. *Gentle* mouth and nose suctioning can be performed using a bulb syringe or suction catheter *only if needed*. Deep and prolonged suctioning should be avoided. ET intubation is not required for vigorous infants with meconium-stained amniotic fluid.

Nonvigorous Infant

Routine endotracheal intubation and tracheal suctioning is no longer recommended for nonvigorous newborns born in MSAF; however, the resuscitation team should include someone skilled in endotracheal intubation. If the newborn is gasping or apneic and has poor muscle tone, the initial steps of routine resuscitation should be started: provide warmth, dry the infant, position the airway, and clear the mouth and nose. Tactile stimulation should be limited to drying the infant and rubbing the back and soles of the feet. If there is visible fluid obstructing the airway or a concern about obstructed breathing, the mouth and nose may be suctioned. If there is no response, PPV should be started using a bag and mask. Suction may also be considered if there is evidence of airway obstruction during PPV. If bag and mask ventilation is not effective, intubation should be performed. There is no evidence that suctioning the trachea of nonvigorous newborns born in MSAF prevents morbidity or mortality. It is possible that the main cause of meconium aspiration into the lungs is caused by intrauterine fetal gasping.

Newborn Resuscitation Outside of the Delivery Room

Resuscitation of infants born at home, in an emergency room, in an ambulance, or otherwise outside of a delivery room setting should proceed according to the same principles as in the delivery room. Providing warmth with stimulation and wiping the airway are usually adequate measures. Establishing effective ventilation using a bag and mask is the most important step if the infant fails to breathe on its own. Emergency providers should be familiar with resuscitation of the newborn, and basic equipment (Table 4) should be available.

Withholding and Withdrawing Newborn Resuscitation

Newborns should be offered resuscitation at delivery except in extreme circumstances. Newborn resuscitation should not be used if the infant has a condition that is incompatible with survival, such as a confirmed gestational age of less than 22 completed weeks, birth weight less than 400g, or congenital anomalies associated with certain death or extreme morbidity.

In most situations, initial resuscitation can provide time to observe the infant's response to interventions and to discuss the infant's condition with the parents. Techniques for obstetric

TABLE 4	Equipment for Newborn Resuscitation
TYPE OF USE	**EQUIPMENT**
General	Warmed towels Radiant warmer or heat lamps Pulse oximeter Cardiorespiratory monitor Sterile gowns, gloves
Airway	Bulb syringe Suction catheters (5, 8, 10, 12, 14F) Suction source with manometer Oral and nasopharyngeal airways (newborn sizes) Laryngoscope and straight blades sizes 0 and 1 Endotracheal tubes (sizes 2.5, 3.0, 3.5)
Ventilation	Face masks (premature, newborn, and infant sizes) Self-inflating bag (450–750 mL) with oxygen reservoir and manometer Oxygen source Orogastric tubes (8, 10F) Carbon dioxide (CO_2) indicator Chest tubes (8 and 10F)
Circulation	Umbilical catheters (3.5 and 5F) Umbilical catheter tray (sterile scissors, scalpel, forceps, umbilical tape) Three-way stopcock Syringes (1, 3, 5, 10 mL) Normal saline Epinephrine 1:10,000 10% Dextrose

dating of pregnancies are accurate only to ±1 to 2 weeks, and estimates of fetal weight are accurate only to ±100 to 200 g. Care must be taken before deciding to withhold resuscitation from a newborn. Ongoing conversation between parents and medical caregivers allows mutual decision making. Withdrawal of care is indicated if continued support is futile. After 20 minutes of asystole (heart rate of 0), newborns are very unlikely to survive, at which point cessation of resuscitative efforts may be considered, based upon patient specific factors.

References

Neonatal Resuscitation 2020 American Heart Association Guidelines for Cardiopulmonary Resuscitation and Emergency Cardiovascular Care, *Pediatrics* 147:number s1, January 2021:e2020038505E, Downloaded from www.aappublications.org/news on February 18, 2021.

American Academy of Pediatrics Committee on Fetus and Newborn: EF Bel: Noninitiation or withdrawal of intensive care for high-risk newborns, *Pediatrics* 119:401, 2007.

Aschner JL, Poland RL: Sodium bicarbonate: basically useless therapy, *Pediatrics* 122:831, 2008.

Chettri S, Adhisivam B, Bhat V: Endotracheal suction for nonvigorous neonate born through meconium stained amniotic fluid: a randomized controlled trial, *J Pediatr* 166:1208–1213, 2015.

Berazategui JP, Aguilar A, Escobedo M, et al: Risk factors for advanced resuscitation in term and near-term infants: a case-control study, *Arch Dis Child Fetal Neonatal Ed* 102:F44–F50, 2017.

Field DJ, Dorling JS, Manktelow BN, et al: Survival of extremely premature babies in a geographically defined population: prospective cohort study of 1994–99 compared with 2000–05, *BMJ* 336:1221, 2008.

Halling C, Sparks JE, Christie L, Wyckoff MH: Efficacy of intravenous and endotracheal epinephrine during neonatal cardiopulmonary resuscitation in the delivery room, *J Pediatr* 185:232–236, 2017, https://doi.org/10.1016/j.jpeds.2017.02.024.

Weiner GM, Zaichkin J, Kattwinkel J, editors: *Textbook of neonatal resuscitation*, ed 7, Elk Grove Village, IL, 2016, American Academy of Pediatrics and American Heart Association.

Weiner GM, Zaichkin J, editors: *Textbook of neonatal resuscitation*, ed 8, Elk Grove Village, IL, 2021, American Academy of Pediatrics and American Heart Association.

Welsford M, Nishiyama C, Shortt C, et al: Room air for initiating term newborn resuscitation: a systematic review with meta-analysis, *Pediatrics* 143(1):e20181825 2019.

Wiswell TE, Gannon CM, Jacob J, et al: Delivery room management of the apparently vigorous meconium-stained neonate: results of the multicenter, international collaborative trial, *Pediatrics* 105(1), 2000.

URINARY TRACT INFECTIONS IN INFANTS AND CHILDREN

Method of
Ellen R. Wald, MD

The urinary tract is the most common site for serious bacterial infections in infants and young children. Urinary tract infections (UTIs) are more common than bacterial meningitis, bacterial pneumonia, and bacteremia.

Infection of the urinary tract may involve only the bladder, or only the kidney, or both. In general, infections of the bladder (cystitis), while causing substantial morbidity, are not regarded as serious bacterial infections. In contrast, infections that involve the kidney (pyelonephritis) can cause acute morbidity and lead to scarring with rare consequences of hypertension, preeclampsia, and chronic renal disease.

Diagnosis

The diagnosis of UTI may be suggested by certain signs and symptoms, but culture of the urine is the gold standard. Because culture results are not available for at least 24 hours, there has been considerable interest in evaluating tests that may predict the results of urine culture, so that appropriate therapy can be initiated at the first encounter with the symptomatic patient. The tests that have received the most attention are urine microscopy for white blood cells and bacteria and biochemical analysis of leukocyte esterase and nitrite, which can be assessed rapidly by dipstick.

Several studies have concluded that both the presence of any bacteria on Gram staining of an uncentrifuged urine sample and dipstick analysis for leukocyte esterase perform similarly in children from birth through 12 years of age and are helpful in identifying individuals with UTI. Other recent studies done involving young infants (<2 months of age) and older infants (<12 months and 1–24 months) concluded that a hemocytometer white blood cell count of 10 or more cells/μL provides the most valuable cutoff point for identifying infants for whom urine culture is warranted.

The definition of a positive urine culture depends on the method used to collect the specimen. This variable definition reflects the fact that urine that has passed through the urethra may be contaminated by bacteria present in the distal urethra. If the urine is obtained by the clean-catch method, a positive culture is defined as equal to or greater than 10^5 colony-forming units (CFU)/mL. If the specimen is obtained by catheterization of the urethra, a positive culture is defined as equal to or greater than 5×10^4 CFU/mL. Finally, if a urine culture is obtained by suprapubic aspiration, a method that bypasses the potential source of contamination, a positive culture is defined as recovery of any bacteria from the urine.

Imaging

Imaging studies have been the standard of care for young children with a first UTI for the past decade. Commonly, a renal ultrasound study is performed to evaluate the gross anatomy of the urinary tract (size and shape of the kidneys, duplication or dilatation of the ureters). A voiding cystourethrogram (VCUG) is done to determine whether vesicoureteral reflux is present. This practice has rested on the assumption that continuous prophylactic antimicrobial therapy is effective in reducing the incidence of reinfection of the kidney and renal scarring that may occur in children with vesicoureteral reflux. The 2011 guidelines on diagnosis and management of urinary tract infection in infants and children 2–24 months of age issued by the American Academy of Pediatrics recommend postponing performance of the VCUG until the second infection (unless there is a major abnormality of the renal ultrasound).

Treatment

In general, there are many choices for the antibiotic treatment of UTIs in children. If a child is toxic in appearance or vomiting (thereby precluding oral antimicrobials), admission to the hospital for parenteral therapy is appropriate. Many would recommend a third-generation cephalosporin, such as ceftriaxone (Rocephin) 50 mg/kg/d given once daily or ceftazidime (Fortaz) 50 mg/kg/dose every 8 hours, until the emesis has resolved and the patient can be treated orally. Otherwise, children, even those with presumed pyelonephritis, do well on oral therapy.

For the child who is to receive oral therapy, the choices are amoxicillin potassium clavulanate (Augmentin) 30 mg/kg/dose given every 12 hours[3]; a second- or third-generation cephalosporin such as cefuroxime (Ceftin) 50 mg/kg/dose twice daily,[3] cefpodoxime (Vantin)[1] 5 mg/kg/dose given twice daily, cefdinir (Omnicef)[1] 7 mg/kg/dose given twice daily, or cefixime (Suprax) 10 mg/kg/dose once daily[3]; or sulfamethoxazole-trimethoprim (Bactrim) 6 mg/kg/day of trimethoprim given once daily. There has been a tendency during the past several years for the prevalence of antimicrobial resistance to increase. The overall resistance to antibiotics varies geographically, and it is essential for the practitioner to be familiar with local antibiotic resistance patterns. In patients with suspected acute pyelonephritis, amoxicillin (Amoxil), cephalexin (Keflex), and sulfamethoxazole-trimethoprim should be avoided as presumptive therapy because of the potentially high rate of antibiotic resistance.

The optimal duration of therapy for children with UTI has been somewhat controversial. If the diagnosis of pyelonephritis is known or suspected, 10 days of treatment is conventional. Shorter courses of therapy have been successful in adult women with infection of the lower urinary tract. A recent meta-analysis conducted by the Cochrane Database of Systematic Reviews evaluated 10 trials (652 children) with lower-tract UTI. There was no significant difference in frequency of positive urine cultures between short-term (2–4 days) and standard (7–14 days) duration of oral antibiotic therapy for cystitis in children, either early after treatment or at 1 to 15 months after treatment. Furthermore, there was no difference between groups in the development of resistant organisms at the end of treatment or in the incidence of recurrent UTIs. Accordingly, in cases in which the diagnosis of cystitis is assured, 4 days of antimicrobial therapy is sufficient.

Voiding Dysfunction

Voiding dysfunction is a broad term indicating a voiding pattern that is abnormal for the child's age. This is a condition that should be considered in all children who are diagnosed as having a UTI after toilet training has been accomplished. Constipation plays a significant role in some children with voiding dysfunction, and attention to this comorbidity sometimes results in resolution of recurrent UTIs.

Prophylaxis

For children who are thought to be at very high risk for recurrent UTIs and potential scarring, prophylactic treatment with sulfamethoxazole-trimethoprim or nitrofurantoin (Macrodantin) should be considered. These groups include children with high degrees of vesicoureteral reflux (grades 4 and 5), those with frequent and closely spaced UTIs without reflux, and, occasionally, those who have urologic abnormalities.

The RIVUR study, Randomized Intervention for Children with Vesicoureteral Reflux (VUR), was undertaken in 2007 to determine whether antimicrobial prophylaxis with SMX-TMP is effective in preventing recurrent UTI in infants and children with reflux of any grade. The study showed a modest benefit of prophylaxis with regard to febrile episodes of UTI but no difference in scarring. There is no question of the biologic plausibility of prophylactic antimicrobial therapy in preventing recurrent UTI; however, adverse effects, emergence of antimicrobial resistance, and difficulties with long-term adherence to prophylactic strategies present barriers to effectiveness.

---

[3] Exceeds dosage recommended by the manufacturer.
[1] Not FDA approved for this indication.

References

Gorelick MH, Shaw KN: Screening tests for urinary tract infection: A meta-analysis, *Pediatrics* 104:e54, 1999.

Hellerstein S, Linebarger JS: Voiding dysfunction in pediatric patients, *Clin Pediatr* 42:43–49, 2003.

Hoberman A, Charron M, Hickey RW, et al: Imaging studies after a first febrile urinary tract infection in young children, *N Engl J Med* 348:195–202, 2003.

Hoberman A, Wald ER, Hickey RW, et al: Oral versus initial intravenous therapy for urinary tract infections in young febrile children, *Pediatrics* 104:79–86, 1999.

Hoberman A, Wald ER, Reynolds EA, et al: Pyuria and bacteriuria in urine specimens obtained by catheter from young children with fever, *J Pediatr* 124:513–519, 1994.

Huicho L, Campos-Sanchez M, Alamo C: Metaanalysis of urine screening tests for determining the risk of urinary tract infection in children, *Pediatr Infect Dis J* 21:1–11, 2002.

Michael M, Hodson EM, Craig JC, et al: Short versus standard duration oral antibiotic therapy for acute urinary tract infection in children, *Cochrane Database Syst Rev* 1:CD003966, 2009. [First published in 2003].

RIVUR Trial Investigators, Hoberman A, Greenfield SP, Mattoo TK, et al: Antimicrobial prophylaxis for children with vesicoureteral reflux, *N Engl J Med* 370:2367–2376, 2014.

Subcommittee on Urinary Tract Infection: Steering Committee on Quality Improvement and Management, Roberts KB. Urinary tract infection: clinical practice guideline for the diagnosis and management of the initial UTI in febrile infants and children 2 to 24 months, *Pediatrics* 128:595–610, 2011.

Subcommittee on Urinary Tract Infection: Reaffirmation of AAP clinical practice guideline: The diagnosis and management of the initial urinary tract infection in febrile infants and young children 2-24 months of age, *Pediatrics* 138(6):e20163026, 2016.

Williams G, Craig JC: Long-term antibiotics for preventing recurrent urinary tract infection in children, *Cochrane Database Rev*, 2019.

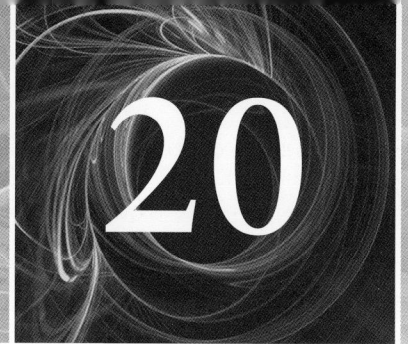

20 Physical and Chemical Injuries

BURNS

Method of
Allyson M. Briggs, MD; and Bradley E. Barth, MD

CURRENT DIAGNOSIS

- Perform primary and secondary survey to assess for concomitant injuries.
- Calculate percentage of burns—use a diagram.
- Chemical burns—be aware of treatment difference based on the substance involved.
- Ocular injury—assess for injury and consult ophthalmology.
- Carbon monoxide—check CO-oximetry on burn patients from enclosed fires or with prolonged smoke exposure.

CURRENT THERAPY

- The first, immediate treatment is to stop the burning.
- Use cool water irrigation (NOT ice or ice water); avoid hypothermia.
- Perform standard airway, breathing, and circulation (ABC) resuscitation.
- Calculate resuscitation fluids on the basis of surface area of deep partial and deeper burns—do not include superficial burns.
- Update tetanus vaccination if needed.
- Consult poison control center for chemical injuries.
- Hyperoxia is the treatment of choice for carbon monoxide exposure.
- Hydroxocobalamin (CYANOKIT) is the treatment of choice for cyanide exposure.
- Develop transfer relationship with burn center.

Epidemiology

Annually in the United States there are nearly 500,000 burns that are significant enough to require emergency treatment with 40,000 hospital admissions. The vast majority of the injuries that require admission are treated at a specialized burn center. Fire and fire-related inhalations injuries are responsible for nearly 3300 deaths. Worldwide incidence of burn death from all causes of burns is difficult to estimate due to a lack of centralized reporting, but 180,000 deaths occur annually from fire alone, with 95% of these occurring in low- and middle-income countries.

Risk Factors

Burns are distributed across the spectrum of age, although their types and mechanisms vary. Overall, burn injury tends to be more common in males. Males tend to get burned by flames, while females are more likely to sustain scald or heat contact wounds. Older and pediatric patients are more likely to sustain injury due to inability to get away from heat sources or flame. Use of alcohol and other substances is associated with increased risk of burn injury. Burns tend to have higher incidence in lower socioeconomic groups and are much more common in countries with lower incomes.

Prevention

Public safety initiatives have decreased the risk of burn injury in the developed world. Patient visits provided opportunities for educational interventions, especially if a patient is seen for a minor burn. Campaigns to decrease hot water heater temperatures in homes have helped reduce scald injuries. Safety plugs for electrical outlets decrease the risk of electrical injury in children. Smoke detectors and planned and practiced escape routes increase the likelihood of escaping from structure fires. Reminders to check smoke detectors and to change the batteries with the seasonal clock change ensure that devices are functional. Child-resistant lighters and safety matches increase fire safety, especially when stored out of reach of children. Keeping screens or safety devices around fireplaces and fire pits may decrease injuries as well. Avoiding activities with potential fuel sources and flames, especially while intoxicated, will also decrease fire injuries.

Pathophysiology

The injuries that result from burns are due to a combination of immediate tissue injury and resulting inflammation. This includes the activation of an inflammatory cascade, immediate and delayed cellular and humoral effects, and the delayed effects of changes in gene expression induced by the earlier injuries. The immediate injury is classically divided into three zones. The most severely injured is the central zone of necrosis; this area is surrounded by the zone of stasis, which is surrounded by the zone of hyperemia (Figure 1). The zone of necrosis is composed of coagulated tissue that will progress to rapid cell death and eschar formation. The outer zone of hyperemia has increased blood flow and minimal tissue damage and will almost certainly heal. The middle zone of stasis is the region where blood flow has ceased within the capillary bed. Depending on subsequent actions over the next 24 to 48 hours, this area either will worsen to necrotic tissue or may reepithelialize to healing. The immediate postinjury efforts are focused on salvaging this area.

Burning Tissue

As heat transfers to tissue, damage begins to occur as cellular temperature rises above 44°C. Once the internal cellular temperature reaches 60°C, the cell will die. Generally, once the heat source is removed from the skin, the tissue temperature rapidly returns to normal, but the tissue injury does not stop at that point. Within seconds of the injury, arterioles begin to spasm, and red blood cells aggregate within the tissues. Histologic changes are visible within 15 minutes, and tissue edema begins. Tissue edema typically peaks 6 to 12 hours postinjury.

It is much easier for a burn injury to penetrate through the dermal layers in thin skin than in thick skin, leading to more severe injury in the former with a similar degree of heat transfer. These injuries pose a particular risk in infants and children as well as the elderly.

Shortly after the burning stops, processes of both inflammation and healing begin. There is a complex interplay of inflammatory mediators, immune cell action, and changes in gene expression that will continue over the following weeks to months and will play a role in how the wound heals.

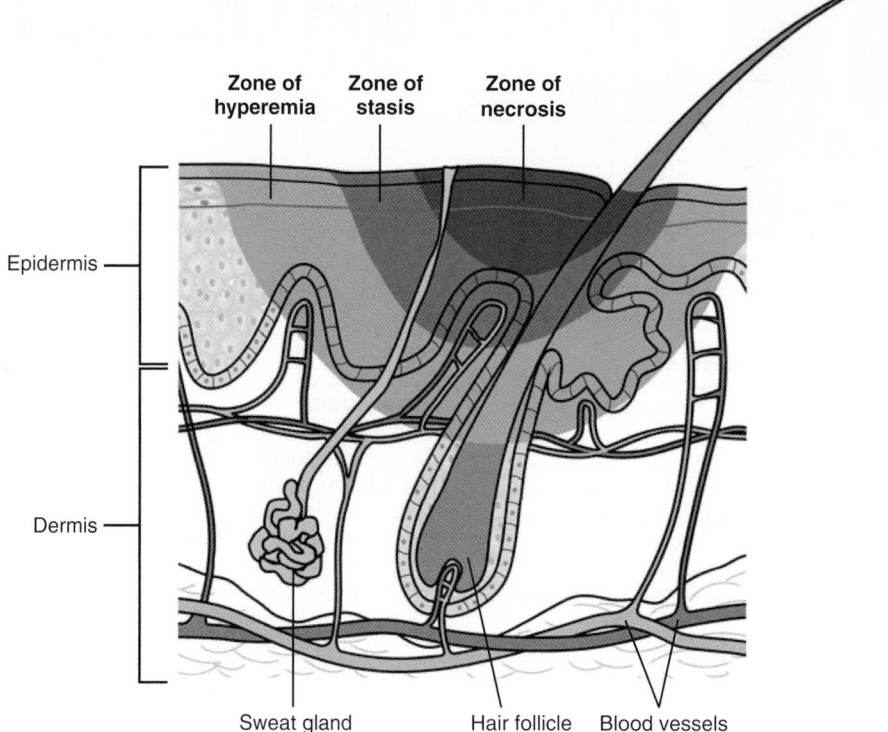

Zone of hyperemia   Zone of stasis   Zone of necrosis

Epidermis

Dermis

Sweat gland   Hair follicle   Blood vessels

Figure 1 Burn injury.

TABLE 1	Types of Burns				
DEPTH	**ANATOMY**	**APPEARANCE**	**SENSATION**	**TIME**	**TREATMENT**
Superficial	Epidermis only	Pink or red and dry, blanches	Painful	Days	Topical
Superficial partial thickness	Epidermis and upper papillary dermis	Pink, clear blisters, moist surface, blanches	Painful	14–21 days	Debride and topical medication
Deep partial thickness	Epidermis, papillary dermis, and lower reticular dermis	Pink or red, moist surface, blisters, may be hemorrhagic, does not blanch	Painful, may have decreased sensation	Weeks or may progress to full thickness	Debride, topical medication, possible surgery
Full thickness	Epidermis, dermis, and into underlying tissue	White or brown, dry, leathery, does not blanch	Insensate	Weeks, and heals by contraction and scarring	Surgical

Clinical Manifestations

Descriptions of burns are based on the depth of the injury and the extent of coverage. They are divided into superficial partial, which is further characterized as superficial partial or deep partial, and full thickness (Table 1). Superficial burns involve the epidermis alone. These injuries are typically painful and erythematous, and they will heal without scarring. These injuries are not included in calculations of the percentage total body surface area (TBSA) burned. Superficial partial thickness burns involve the entire epidermis and extend down to the papillary region of the upper dermis. These injuries are painful, erythematous, and moist, and they form blisters. Deep partial thickness burns involve the entire epidermis and extend deeper into the lower reticular dermis. These wounds are typically painful and whitish, and they have less weeping and blanching than superficial partial thickness wounds. These may have less pain than expected depending on the extent of damage to nerve endings in the skin. Full-thickness burns extend through the epidermis and entire dermis and destroy nerves and other deep structures. These wounds are insensate, stiff, white or tan in color, and they do not blanch. Wounds of this depth cannot heal spontaneously

and will have significant scarring and contracture if not surgically managed.

Areas of burn that have extensive or circumferential deep partial thickness or full-thickness burns are at risk for development of restrictive eschars. Eschars can restrict circulation, leading to compartment syndrome in extremities and can decrease respiration if on the chest or neck. Ideally, burn patients can reach burn centers before these complications arise, but an escharotomy could be required urgently in some cases.

Inhalation injury is a source of significant morbidity in burn patients. The initial injury may not seem particularly severe, but edema can develop rapidly in the airway, which makes delayed airway management perilous. Early intubation may be necessary.

Special Situations
Ocular Injuries

Patients with any signs of burns to the face, complaints of eye pain, or inability to communicate should undergo eye examinations with fluorescein staining. If corneal burns are identified, appropriate antibiotic ointment should be started, and consultation with an eye specialist should be obtained.

Nonaccidental Trauma

Clinicians should have a high index of suspicion for nonaccidental trauma (NAT) in burns occurring in pediatric patients. NAT has been shown to be present in up to 25% of pediatric burn cases. Burns caused by NAT are more likely to occur in males and children with developmental delays and may result in a delay in seeking care. Other concerning findings are burns that have clear lines of demarcation (e.g., cigarette burns, dunking, radiator, grill, curling iron), that are symmetric on both extremities, or spare the flexor creases with deep surrounding burns. If NAT is suspected, it must be reported, and the child must be kept in a safe place until authorities have cleared the child to go home.

Chemical Burns

The risk and degree of injury caused by chemical burns vary greatly, depending on the substance involved as well as on the concentration of the material and the duration of exposure. The Centers for Disease Control and Prevention has a website that provides information on treatment for chemical injuries: https://emergency.cdc.gov/chemical/mmg.asp. General precautions for chemical burns are to decontaminate as quickly as possible while avoiding rescuer contamination or injury. For dry or powdered chemicals, remove as much chemical as possible while it is still in the dry form by brushing or other mechanical removal. After mechanical removal, or for liquid contamination, dilute the chemical and continue the removal process by using water. Water should be used via copious, high-flow, low-pressure irrigation for at least 20 minutes. If feasible, check the pH of the contaminated area and continue irrigation until it returns to normal. In most cases, removal and irrigation are more important to neutralizing the chemical because using neutralizing agents can make the injury worse. Evaluate the patient for possible inhalation or ocular injury as well. Ocular chemical exposures should be irrigated with water or lactated Ringer's solution, starting as early as possible after exposure, until a normal pH is obtained. There are important exceptions to typical management, some of which are listed in Table 2.

Electrical Injuries

Injuries with electrical sources vary based on the type of circuit (alternating vs. direct current), amperage, voltage, tissue resistance, duration of exposure, and path of current through the body. High voltage (≥1000V) tends to cause more thermal tissue injury and often causes concomitant traumatic injuries. Depending on the path of electricity, there may be significant internal injuries beneath normal-appearing skin, especially in high-voltage cases. Significant injuries should be treated more like crush injuries, as the extent of the internal injuries is difficult to assess. Cutaneous burns due to electrical injury can be treated similarly to thermal burns. During the initial evaluation of electrical injury, patients should undergo assessment for other injuries, electrocardiography, and cardiac monitoring. In patients with injury from high-voltage sources, obtaining serum levels of electrolytes, renal function studies, creatine kinase, troponin, and coagulation studies should be considered.

Special circumstances include multivictim injuries and oral commissure burns. In cases of multiple victims of a lightning strike, a reverse triage process occurs whereby care is provided first to the patients who appear to be in cardiac arrest, as cardiopulmonary resuscitation and defibrillation may save their lives if applied early enough. Oral commissure burns occur most often in young children who have chewed through electrical cords. Caregivers should be warned about delayed bleeding from the labial artery that can occur during wound healing. Due to risk of scar contracture and concern for aesthetic outcomes, these patients should be referred to a plastic or oral surgeon.

Therapy and Treatment

First Aid and Office Management

The initial management for burn injuries consists of stopping further injury by removing the heat source and providing cooling. Remove the patient from the burning area in the event of flame injury. If the patient's clothing is on fire, it is important to stop the burning and remove hot clothing as quickly as possible. Hot liquid or scald injuries especially require prompt removal of overlying clothing, as the clothing will trap the heat, which can continue the tissue damage. After the heat source is removed, copious cool water should be used to irrigate the injured area, and any constricting jewelry should be removed immediately. The ideal temperature for cool water irrigation is not clear, but it is likely between 15°C and 25°C (59°F–77°F); colder temperatures can be damaging. The cooling irrigation should be continued for 20 minutes. Early wound cooling decreases the temperature of the injured area quickly to halt the burning process, but irrigation has

TABLE 2	Chemical Burns*	
CHEMICAL	**TREATMENT**	**SPECIAL NOTES**
Dry chemical	Brush or remove as much chemical as possible, then copious irrigation	Obtain material safety data sheet information on exposure
Liquid chemical	Copious irrigation	
Ocular injury	Copious irrigation with lactated Ringer's solution, measure pH early and repeat frequently	
Elemental metals (e.g., sodium, magnesium)	Cover with mineral oil if available, physically remove as soon as possible, irrigate with water if no other options	Water causes an intense exothermic reaction, but tissue damage occurs with continued contact
Strong alkalis (pH 10–12; e.g., lye, bleach, cement [calcium oxide], ammonia)	Copious irrigation, continue until pH normalizes but at least 1 hour; may require 12 or more hours	Current recommendations are not to try to neutralize, but research is continuing
Petroleum	Irrigation, mild soap solution	May be seen in vehicle trauma patients
Hydrofluoric acid	Irrigation, topical calcium gluconate (Calgonate)[1] mixed with water-based lubricant (e.g., K-Y jelly), intradermal or intravenous calcium gluconate[1]	Associated with pain out of proportion to appearance, fluoride ion can cause hypocalcemia and death
Phenol	Polyethylene glycol (PEG) (Miralax)[1] stops phenol burn more quickly than water; if PEG is not available, use high-flow, low-pressure, copious irrigation	

*Consider contacting a burn center or poison control center for assistance with chemical injury treatment.
[1]Not FDA approved for this indication.

been shown to be beneficial even after the wound has returned to a normal temperature. Cooling the wound is thought to be effective up to 3 hours after the injury. It is unclear why cool water irrigation improves burn outcomes; heat removal and edema prevention play a role, but it may also lead to alterations in gene expression that decrease injury and improve healing. After cooling the injured area, the initial treatment is to cover the wounds with a clean, thin cloth or sterile sheets while the patient awaits further care. Ensure that the patient's tetanus vaccination is up to date. Check the patient's temperature and provide warm blankets or a warm air environment to avoid hypothermia.

Superficial burns or superficial partial thickness burns can generally be treated on an outpatient basis, with important exceptions: >10% TBSA, extremes of age, circumferential injury, or burns on the head, face, or genital areas. Debride any ruptured blister tissue. Clean the wounds with mild soap and water or dilute antiseptic solutions and dress the wound. Topical bacitracin or triple-antibiotic ointment with an occlusive dressing is often used. Silver sulfadiazine cream 1% (Silvadene) is now generally discouraged as it may delay healing and can lead to pigmented scarring. Wound dressings may include topical antibiotic cream or ointment, silver impregnated nylon, bismuth tribromophenate and petrolatum impregnated gauze (Xeroform), or various specialized products to form occlusive dressings (including polyurethane films and foams, hydrocolloid, hydrogel, alginate, and chitin in various forms). The management of intact blisters is controversial; however, if a blister appears fragile or likely to rupture, unroof and debride the wound before dressing the wound. If the blister is in thicker skin or appears stable, most recommendations are to aspirate the blister fluid and dress the wound.

Burns are painful injuries and often require early, aggressive pain control, such as with nonsteroidal antiinflammatory drugs (NSAIDs), opioid medications, and acetaminophen. It is important to remember to provide additional analgesia as needed for dressing changes and wound care. Pruritus and neuropathic pain may occur as the wound heals. These are often treated with adjunct pain medications such as gabapentin (Neurontin),[1] and diphenhydramine (Benadryl).[1]

Deep partial thickness or deeper wounds usually require some form of surgical management and should be referred for specialized care. Early surgical management has been demonstrated to be beneficial. Prophylactic antibiotics should not be used for burn management, as they have been shown to be harmful. If burns have not healed within 2 weeks, they should be referred to a specialist.

Initial Hospital Management

For patients with more severe injuries, follow the traditional algorithm of assessing and stabilizing the respiratory and circulatory system first, then proceeding with a complete history and physical examination, including comorbid conditions, allergies, medications, and other past medical history. If possible, identify the mechanisms and circumstances surrounding the injury, including agents involved, duration of exposure, and situation, including possibility of inhalation injury or enclosed space involvement. Assess whether there are chemical or electrical burns and any associated trauma. The social history may play an important role in disposition and management decisions.

Management of Inhalation Injury

Patients who were in an enclosed space or structure fire or who were otherwise exposed to high levels of smoke or toxins should be assessed for carbon monoxide and cyanide injuries. Lactate, troponin, and carboxyhemoglobin levels should be checked in patients at risk for carbon monoxide or cyanide exposure. Patients at risk for cyanide exposure with decreased level of consciousness, hypotension, or a lactate level greater than 9 should receive 5 g (or 70 mg/kg to a maximum of 5 g) of hydroxocobalamin

---

[1]Not FDA approved for this indication.

(Cyanokit) intravenously. If the patient is in cardiac arrest or does not improve with the initial dose, a total of 10 g should be given.

A patient with carbon monoxide exposure should have a carboxyhemoglobin level obtained and be placed on 100% oxygen as soon as possible, typically delivered via a nonrebreather face mask. Carbon monoxide binds tightly to hemoglobin, and by increasing the oxygen concentration in the lungs and blood, the half-life of carboxyhemoglobin is greatly reduced. With oxygen levels typically delivered by nonrebreather face mask, the half-life of carboxyhemoglobin is 74 minutes. After 6 hours on 100% oxygen, if the patient is asymptomatic, treatment can be stopped. It is unnecessary to use arterial blood or to repeat carboxyhemoglobin levels. Patients with carbon monoxide poisoning may experience delayed neurologic sequelae. Hyperbaric oxygen therapy may reduce the risk of delayed neurologic sequelae in appropriately selected patients. Although controversial, this therapy is thought to be most helpful if it occurs within 12 hours after the end of the patient's exposure, but patients may benefit up to 24 hours after exposure. If possible, consult with a physician capable of providing hyperbaric oxygen therapy or with a poison control center for patients with carboxyhemoglobin levels greater than 10, symptoms consistent with carbon monoxide exposure, or pregnant patients (Box 1).

Patients with inhalation injuries can develop rapidly progressing airway swelling. The initial evaluation of burn patients should include assessment for perioral injury, singed facial or nasal hair, and soot or swelling in the oral or hypopharyngeal cavities. These findings, extensive neck burns, other indications of airway swelling, or difficulty breathing should prompt early placement of a definitive airway. Delay may make placement of an endotracheal tube difficult or impossible.

Burn Management

After evaluation and stabilization of the respiratory and circulatory status of the patient, and after stabilizing acute traumatic injuries, the next step is to evaluate the extent of the burn injuries. Removing the heat source and cooling the injured areas remain a priority. Burned areas can be cooled with cool water irrigation or saline-soaked gauze. Because patients with extensive wounds can be at risk of developing hypothermia during this phase, it is important to raise the ambient temperature in the resuscitation room or use warm blankets to maintain normothermia. The extent of the burns should be determined. The "rule of nines" diagram is an accepted mechanism for approximating the percentage of TBSA burned in adults, but it tends to overestimate. Because children have a proportionally larger head and torso, diagrams have been adapted for use in pediatric populations. The Lund-Browder chart can be utilized with patients of all ages (Figure 2). It can also be useful to diagram the areas of burn by estimated depth. For determination of burn severity, calculation of transfer criteria, and fluid resuscitation, only the areas of deep partial thickness and deeper burns are added together to determine TBSA. Use of a diagram is recommended because TBSA is frequently overestimated when providers

BOX 1	Symptoms of Carbon Monoxide Exposure*

Headache
Dizziness
Nausea
Vomiting
Confusion
Fatigue
Chest pain
Shortness of breath
Loss of consciousness

---

*It is important to note that carboxyhemoglobin levels do not correlate well with symptoms or with severity of exposure.
Arterial blood gas samples are not superior to venous blood samples.

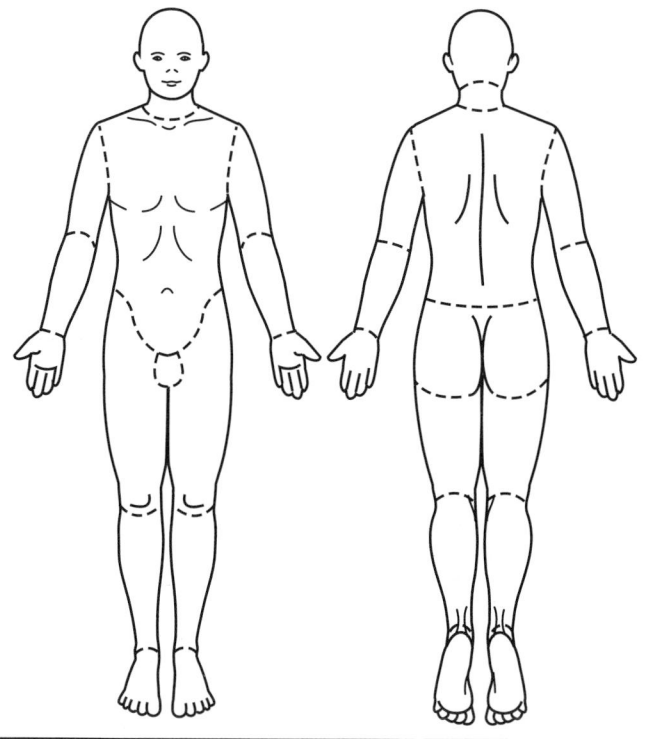

	Birth 1 yr.	1–4 yrs.	5–9 yrs.	10–14 yrs.	15 yrs.	Adult	Burn size estimate
Head	19	17	13	11	9	7	
Neck	2	2	2	2	2	2	
Anterior trunk	13	13	13	13	13	13	
Posterior trunk	13	13	13	13	13	13	
Right buttock	2.5	2.5	2.5	2.5	2.5	2.5	
Left buttock	2.5	2.5	2.5	2.5	2.5	2.5	
Genitalia	1	1	1	1	1	1	
Right upper arm	4	4	4	4	4	4	
Left upper arm	4	4	4	4	4	4	
Right lower arm	3	3	3	3	3	3	
Left lower arm	3	3	3	3	3	3	
Right hand	2.5	2.5	2.5	2.5	2.5	2.5	
Left hand	2.5	2.5	2.5	2.5	2.5	2.5	
Right thigh	5.5	6.5	8	8.5	9	9.5	
Left thigh	5.5	6.5	8	8.5	9	9.5	
Right leg	5	5	5.5	6	6.5	7	
Left leg	5	5	5.5	6	6.5	7	
Right foot	3.5	3.5	3.5	3.5	3.5	3.5	
Left foot	3.5	3.5	3.5	3.5	3.5	3.5	

Total BSAB ——————————

Figure 2 Lund-Browder classification of burn size.

estimate the extent of burned areas. Overestimating TBSA burned leads to excessive fluid administration and the complications that accompany fluid overload.

Fluid Resuscitation and Monitoring

Critically ill burn patients should be monitored in an intensive care setting while awaiting transfer to a burn center. In addition to monitoring respiratory and circulatory status, a Foley catheter should be placed to monitor urinary output and for intermittent assessment of bladder pressure to evaluate for the development of intraabdominal compartment syndrome.

Because burned tissue increases insensible fluid losses, burn victims have increased fluid requirements. Various formulas are available for calculating approximate fluid requirements, but all require careful monitoring of the results and progress of fluid resuscitation. Patients who receive more than 250 mL/kg in the first 24 hours are at increased risk of developing fluid-related complications. The American Burn Association Consensus Statement formula is used to guide initial fluid management. The starting fluid requirements are 2 to 4 mL/kg of lactated Ringer's solution per TBSA percent value, with half given in the first 8 hours and the rest over the next 16 hours (Box 2). Urine output should be monitored hourly and maintained between 0.5 and 1 mL/kg/h. If a patient's urine output is greater than 1 mL/kg/h, the rate of fluid administration should be decreased by 20% and continued to be monitored hourly. If the urine output is less than 0.5 mL/kg/h, the rate of fluid administration should be increased by 20% and continued to be monitored.

> **BOX 2**   Fluid Administration and Calculation
>
> 80-kg male patient with a burn of 35% TBSA full-thickness and partial thickness burns:
>
> 80 kg × 35 × 3 mL/kg = 8400 mL in first 24 hours
>
> 8400 mL/24 hours ÷ 2 = 4200 mL in first 8 hours, 4200 mL in next 16 hours
>
> Initial rate of 525 mL/h over first 8 hours, then switching to a rate of 265 mL/h over next 16 hours
>
> Expected urine output is 0.5–1 mL/kg/h
>
> 80 kg × 0.5 mL/kg/h = 40 mL/h
>
> 80 kg × 1 mL/kg/h = 80 mL/h
>
> So, for our 80-kg patient, we would expect 40–80 mL of urine every hour. In hours 1 and 2 of resuscitation, the patient has 65 mL of urine per hour. In hour 3 of resuscitation, the patient has 90 mL of urine per hour. We would then decrease the fluid administration rate by 20%, or
>
> 525 mL/h−(0.20 × 525) = 420 mL/h
>
> Thus, the rate of administration of lactated Ringer's solution would change from 525 mL/h to 420 mL/h and continue to be monitored and recorded hourly, with continued adjustments based on hourly urine output.
>
> ---
>
> *TBSA*, Total body surface area.

> **BOX 3**   Burn Center Referral Criteria
>
> Partial thickness burns greater than 10% TBSA
>
> Full-thickness burns
>
> Burns to high-risk areas, such as the face, hands, feet, genitals, perineum, or major joints
>
> Circumferential burns
>
> Electrical burns, including lightning strikes
>
> Chemical burns
>
> Inhalation injury
>
> Preexisting conditions known to impair healing and increase risk of mortality
>
> Burns in combination with traumatic injury (e.g., fracture, traumatic brain injury) whereby the burn is the leading risk for patient mortality
>
> Burn injury in patients who will require special social, emotional, or long-term rehabilitative intervention
>
> Burns in a setting unequipped (personnel, equipment, or unit) to care for critically ill children
>
> ---
>
> *TBSA*, Total body surface area.
>
> Available from https://ameriburn.org/public-resources/burn-center-referral-criteria/. Accessed May 1, 2021.

Unfortunately, ensuring adequate urine output does not necessarily guarantee adequate fluid resuscitation. In addition to using urine output as an indicator of resuscitation adequacy, other modes of monitoring can be used to help guide fluid resuscitation (hemodynamic monitoring, echocardiography, gastric tonometry, or other devices). Whether they lead to any increased improvement or survivability is not clear, however.

Burn Center Referral Criteria and Transfer

It is important to identify the regional burn referral center and to establish a line of communication with it before a burn patient is encountered in order to know of the center's suggested criteria for transfer (Box 3). Burn centers typically manage more than 200 burn patients annually and have specially trained physicians, nurses, and ancillary personnel who are focused on treating burn patients. Severely burned patients who are treated at specialized centers have better outcomes. It is recommended that hospitals and clinics have agreements with burn centers for the management of complicated patients and patients who meet criteria for burn center transfer.

In general, the following criteria are recommended for transfer to a burn center: burns greater than 10% of TBSA; inhalation injury; burns with significant associated mechanical injury; burns of the face, hands, feet, perineum, or genitalia or across major joints; full-thickness burns of any size; and circumferential burns. Burns that warrant a discussion with a burn center for possible transfer or outpatient follow-up include burns in children; patients with comorbid conditions that will impact healing; and patients with special social, emotional, psychological, or rehabilitative needs.

Complications

Pain management for burns may require multiple modalities because the type of pain varies, depending on where the patient is in the cycle of treatment and healing. There are four types of pain that need to be treated during the care of a burn patient: background pain, breakthrough pain, procedural pain, and long-term pain. Background pain is present from the onset of the injury, and the pain is typically intensified during procedures. There will also be episodes of breakthrough pain. Depending on the severity of the injury, initial pain and background pain may be treated with multimodal therapy including acetaminophen, NSAIDs (e.g., ibuprofen, naproxen sodium), or opioids. Low-dose ketamine (Ketalar)[1] is increasingly used in addition to opioids for background and breakthrough pain. Procedural pain may require bolus dosing of opioids or other adjunctive medications such as ketamine (0.1–0.2 mg/kg IV). Long-term pain may respond to medications such as gabapentin (Neurontin),[1] clonidine (Catapres),[1] or others.

Psychosocial recovery from burns is impacted by the preexisting conditions and the resilience of the patient. Preexisting mental health, substance abuse, and other medical and psychosocial issues complicate the patient's recovery from burns. Risk factors for burn injury include poverty, a history of abuse or neglect, substance abuse, serious mental illness, and risk for suicide or assault. Psychiatric recovery is negatively affected by posttraumatic stress disorder, depression, learning disorders, substance abuse, stigma, and disability. Individual resilience, social support, and education or occupation also impact patient outcomes.

The patient's age and stage of life at the time of injury impact recovery as well. Younger victims have a longer remaining lifespan to live with persistent scarring and disfigurement. Pediatric patients often have fewer comorbid medical conditions, which can speed their recovery and limit disability, and they tend to heal more quickly. However, their injuries may have a significant impact on their body image development, self-confidence, and interpersonal relationship building. The family may be of assistance in recovery from the injury, but family members, too, may experience stress and psychological concerns related to the child's injury. Adults and older patients have to deal with the impact of the injury on their identity and their ability to return to their preinjury roles.

Some patients and caregivers may develop posttraumatic stress disorder related to the injury or to postinjury treatment. It is thought that early multidisciplinary interventions may decrease this risk, but the research is unclear. Some patients will require long-term, continued outpatient treatment.

Hypertrophic scarring is the most common complication related to healing of burn wounds, but scar contracture and pruritus are common complications as well. It is thought that hypertrophic scarring may be decreased with early, appropriate surgical repair, but it still can occur. The development of hypertrophic scarring is multifactorial; it is likely a result of a complex interplay of humoral and cellular immunity causing an inappropriate response to healing tissue. Multiple host and injury factors contribute, but protracted healing of a partial thickness injury is a common theme. There are some experimental therapies for manipulating different components of the host response, but none has clearly proven to be beneficial.

---

[1]Not FDA approved for this indication.

Scar contracture results from tissue loss at the time of injury and tissue-healing properties. Burn injuries are more complicated than other traumatic wounds because the destroyed tissue is surrounded by profoundly damaged tissue. As a result of this tissue injury, there is increased collagen deposition resulting from changes in inflammation, proliferation, and remodeling at the cellular and extracellular matrix levels. Hypertrophic scars tend to form within the first month after injury and may improve over the first 6 months but then tend not to show significant changes after that time. Burn treatment and scar prevention consist of tissue replacement, tissue rehabilitation, and tension release. Early and existing scars are often treated with compression garments and silicone sheets. It is thought that these may alter and improve remodeling of the extracellular matrix and thereby improve scarring. In some cases, surgical release of tension may be necessary.

References

Akelma H, Karahan ZA: Rare chemical burns: review of the literature, *Int Wound J* 16(6):1330–1338, 2019, https://doi.org/10.1111/iwj.13193.

Barrett W, Buxhoeveden M, Dhillon S: Ketamine: a versatile tool for anesthesia and analgesia, *Curr Opin Anaesthesiol* 33(5):633–638, 2020, https://doi.org/10.1097/aco.0000000000000916.

Bitter CC, Erickson TB: Management of burn injuries in the wilderness: lessons from low-resource settings, *Wilderness Environ Med* 27(4):519–525, 2016, https://doi.org/10.1016/j.wem.2016.09.001.

Bizrah M, Yusuf A, Ahmad S: An update on chemical eye burns, *Eye* 33(9):1362–1377, 2019, https://doi.org/10.1038/s41433-019-0456-5.

Burn Incidence and Treatment in United States: 2016, American Burn Association, 2016.

Carboni RM, Santos GL, Carboni Júnior IC, et al: Therapy for patients with burns —an integrating review, *Rev Assoc Med Bras* 65:1405–1412, 2019.

Cartotto R, Greenhalgh DG, Cancio C: Burn state of the science: fluid resuscitation, *J Burn Care Res* 38(3):e596–e604, 2017, https://doi.org/10.1097/bcr.0000000000000541.

Culnan DM, Craft-Coffman B, Bitz GH, et al: Carbon monoxide and cyanide poisoning in the burned pregnant patient: an indication for hyperbaric oxygen therapy, *Ann Plast Surg* 80(3 Suppl 2):S106–S112, 2018, https://doi.org/10.1097/sap.0000000000001351.

Culnan DM, Farner K, Bitz GH, et al: Volume resuscitation in patients with high-voltage electrical injuries, *Ann Plast Surg* 80(3 Suppl 2):S113–s118, 2018, https://doi.org/10.1097/sap.0000000000001374.

Dyamenahalli K, Garg G, Shupp JW, Kuprys PV, Choudhry MA, Kovacs EJ: Inhalation injury: unmet clinical needs and future research, *J Burn Care Res* 40(5):570–584, 2019, https://doi.org/10.1093/jbcr/irz055.

Friedstat J, Brown D, Levi B: Chemical, electrical, and radiation injuries, *Clin Plast Surg* 44(3):657–659, 2017, https://doi.org/10.1016/j.cps.2017.02.021.

Gigengack RK, Cleffken BI, Loer SA: Advances in airway management and mechanical ventilation in inhalation injury, *Curr Opin Anaesthesiol* 33(6):774–780, 2020, https://doi.org/10.1097/aco.0000000000000929.

Griggs C, Goverman J, Bittner EA, Levi B: Sedation and pain management in burn patients, *Clin Plast Surg* 44(3):535–540, 2017, https://doi.org/10.1016/j.cps.2017.02.026.

Hall AH, Mathieu L, Maibach HI: Acute chemical skin injuries in the United States: a review, *Crit Rev Toxicol* 48(7):540–554, 2018, https://doi.org/10.1080/10408444.2018.1493085.

ISBI Practice guidelines for burn care, Part 2, *Burns* 44(7):1617–1706, 2018, https://doi.org/10.1016/j.burns.2018.09.012.

Jeschke MG, Peck MD: Burn care of the elderly, *J Burn Care Res* 38(3):e625–e628, 2017, https://doi.org/10.1097/bcr.0000000000000535.

Jeschke MG, Shahrokhi S, Finnerty CC, Branski LK, Dibildox M: Wound coverage technologies in burn care: established techniques, *J Burn Care Res* 39(3):313–318, 2018, https://doi.org/10.1097/BCR.0b013e3182920d29.

Jeschke MG, van Baar ME, Choudhry MA, Chung KK, Gibran NS, Logsetty S: Burn injury, *Nat Rev Dis Primers* 6(1):11, 2020, https://doi.org/10.1038/s41572-020-0145-5.

Kim DE, Pruskowski KA, Ainsworth CR, Linsenbardt HR, Rizzo JA, Cancio LC: A review of adjunctive therapies for burn injury pain during the opioid crisis, *J Burn Care Res* 40(6):983–995, 2019, https://doi.org/10.1093/jbcr/irz111.

Partain KP, Fabia R, Thakkar RK: Pediatric burn care: new techniques and outcomes, *Curr Opin Pediatr* 32(3):405–410, 2020a, https://doi.org/10.1097/mop.0000000000000902.

Porter C, Tompkins RG, Finnerty CC, Sidossis LS, Suman OE, Herndon DN: The metabolic stress response to burn trauma: current understanding and therapies, *Lancet* 388(10052):1417–1426, 2016, https://doi.org/10.1016/s0140-6736(16)31469-6.

Shah A, Pedraza I, Mitchell C, Kramer GC: Fluid volumes infused during burn resuscitation 1980–2015: a quantitative review, *Burns* 46(1):52–57, 2020, https://doi.org/10.1016/j.burns.2019.11.013.

Shpichka A, Butnaru D, Bezrukov EA, et al: Skin tissue regeneration for burn injury, *Stem Cell Res Ther* 10(1), 2019, https://doi.org/10.1186/s13287-019-1203-3.

Smolle C, Cambiaso-Daniel J, Forbes AA, et al: Recent trends in burn epidemiology worldwide: a systematic review, *Burns* 43(2):249–257, 2017, https://doi.org/10.1016/j.burns.2016.08.013.

Sofia J, Ambardekar A: Pediatric burn resuscitation, management, and recovery for the pediatric anesthesiologist, *Curr Opin Anaesthesiol* 33(3):360–367, 2020, https://doi.org/10.1097/aco.0000000000000859.

Soussi S, Dépret F, Benyamina M, Legrand M: Early hemodynamic management of critically ill burn patients, *Anesthesiology* 129(3):583–589, 2018, https://doi.org/10.1097/aln.0000000000002314.

Stapelberg F: Challenges in anaesthesia and pain management for burn injuries, *Anaesth Intensive Care* 48(2):101–113, 2020, https://doi.org/10.1177/0310057x20914908.

Walls R, Hockberger R, Gausche-Hill M: *Rosen's emergency medicine—concepts and clinical practice E-Book*, Vol 2, 9 ed, Elsevier Health Sciences, 2018.

Yeroshalmi F, Sidoti EJ, Adamo AK, Lieberman BL, Badner VM: Oral electrical burns in children—a model of multidisciplinary care, *J Burn Care Res* 32(2):e25–e30, 2011, https://doi.org/10.1097/bcr.0b013e31820ab393.

Yoshino Y, Ohtsuka M, Kawaguchi M, et al: The wound/burn guidelines—6: guidelines for the management of burns, *J Dermatol* 43(9):989–1010, 2016, https://doi.org/10.1111/1346-8138.13288.

DISTURBANCES DUE TO COLD[a]

Method of
Jerrold B. Leikin, MD; Scott Leikin, DO; Frederick K. Korley, MD; and Ernest Wang, MD

CURRENT DIAGNOSIS

- Accidental hypothermia may be classified as mild, moderate, or severe.
- The measured temperature should be the core body temperature.
- The method of rewarming depends on the severity of the temperature drop.
- The complications of rewarming include arrhythmias, rewarming-related hypotension, core temperature after drop, and rhabdomyolysis.
- Patients can be declared dead only after they are warm.

CURRENT THERAPY

Mild Hypothermia: 32.2°C (90°F) to 35°C (95°F)
- Start passive external rewarming; remove wet clothing.
- Ambient temperature should exceed 21.0°C (70.0°F).
- Cover patient with insulating material.

Moderate Hypothermia: 28°C (82.4°F) to 32.2°C (90°F)
- Start active external rewarming; use radiant heat.
- Use thermal mattresses and electric heating blankets.
- Use forced-air heating blankets.
- Perform active core rewarming; use warmed humidified oxygen.
- Give warmed intravenous saline.
- Give bladder, colonic, and gastric irrigation.
- Start pleural cavity lavage.
- Avoid alcohol, caffeine, and nicotine (tobacco).

Severe Hypothermia: Less than 28°C (82.4°F)
- Begin aggressive active core rewarming; use warmed, humidified oxygen.
- Give warmed intravenous saline.
- Give bladder, colonic, and gastric irrigation.
- Start pleural cavity lavage.
- Perform peritoneal lavage or dialysis.
- Perform extracorporeal warming or heated cardiopulmonary bypass.

---

[a]Portions of this chapter have been previously printed in *Conn's Current Therapy* 2009–2012. The content of this chapter has also appeared in *Disease-a-Month* 2012;58(1):6–32.

Frostnip
- Gentle rewarming, generally in a water bath of 104°F to 108°F (40°C to 42°C).
- It is usually self-resolving.

Frostbite
- Immerse in warm (not hot) water.
- Débride broken vesicles.
- Do not débride hemorrhagic or intact blisters.
- Apply topical aloe vera[7] or antibiotic ointment.
- Use nonsteroidal antiinflammatory drugs (NSAIDs) for pain.
- Update tetanus status.
- Do not rub or massage the affected area.
- Do not use a heating pad or heat lamp; affected areas can be easily burned.
- Avoid alcohol and tobacco products.

Chilblain
- Rewarm gently.
- Nifedipine (Procardia)[1] may be useful.

Trench foot
- Dry the foot.
- Rewarm gently.
- Use NSAIDs for pain.

[1]Not FDA Approved for this indication.
[7]Available as dietary supplement.

Accidental Systemic Hypothermia

Hypothermia is classically defined as a reduction in the body's core temperature below 95.0°F (35.0°C). Most reported cases of hypothermia are due to environmental exposure to low ambient temperatures (accidental hypothermia). Other causes of hypothermia include sepsis, severe hypothyroidism (myxedema coma), acute spinal cord injury, diabetic ketoacidosis, multisystem trauma, and prolonged cardiac arrest. Episodic hypothermia can be encountered in patients with advanced secondary progressive multiple sclerosis, subarachnoid hemorrhage, HIV-1 infections, and brain contusion. Shapiro syndrome is episodic hypothermia associated with hyperhydrosis due to ageness or lesions of the corpus callosum.

Epidemiology

Risk factors for developing hypothermia include extremes of age (elderly people might not be able to remove themselves from cold environments, and young children lose heat more rapidly because of their increased total body surface area), major trauma, homelessness, psychiatric illness, and drug and alcohol abuse (Box 1). Cold-related deaths also are reported in military combatants and outdoor winter sports participants. Several drugs and chemicals can predispose to hypothermia (Box 2). Alcohol is the most common intoxicant associated with hypothermia because of its ability to cause cutaneous vasodilation, impairment of shivering, and impairment of adaptive behavior.

Between 1979 and 2002, 16,555 deaths in the United States, an average of 689 per year, were attributed to exposure to low environmental temperatures. In 2002, of the 646 hypothermia-related deaths reported, 66% occurred in male patients, 52% of all decedents were aged 65 years or younger, 45% of the deaths occurred among white male patients, and 14% occurred among black male patients. The states of Alaska, New Mexico, North Dakota, and Montana had the largest overall death rates from hypothermia in 2002. The lowest recorded core temperature in a pediatric survivor of accidental hypothermia is 57.9°F (14.4°C) and the lowest in an adult survivor is 56.7°F (13.7°C).

Pathophysiology

The normal range of human core temperature is 97.5°F (36.4°C) to 99.5°F (37.5°C). Humans are thus warm-blooded and are normally able to maintain their body temperature by heat-generating mechanisms and heat-conserving behavior. These compensatory responses,

---

BOX 1 — Factors Predisposing to Hypothermia or Frostbite

Physiologic
Decreased heat production
Age extremes (infants, elderly)
Dehydration or malnutrition
Diaphoresis or hyperhidrosis
Endocrinologic insufficiency
Hypoxia
Insufficient fuel
Overexertion
Physical conditioning
Prior cold injury
Trauma (multisystem or extremity)

Increased heat loss
Burns
Dermatologic malfunction
Cold infusions
Emergency resuscitation
Poor acclimatization or conditioning
Shock
Vascular diseases

Impaired thermoregulation
Central nervous system trauma or disease
Metabolic disorders
Pharmacologic or toxicologic agents
Sepsis
Spinal cord injury

Psychological
Fatigue
Fear or panic
Hunger
Intense concentration on tasks
Intoxicants
Mental status or attitude
Peer pressure

Environmental
Altitude with or without associated conditions
Ambient temperature or humidity
Duration of exposure
Heat loss (conductive, evaporative, radiative, convective)
Quantity of exposed surface area
Wind chill factor

Mechanical
Constricting or wet clothing or boots
Inadequate insulation
Immobility or cramped positioning

---

however, can be overwhelmed under extreme environmental conditions, leading to hypothermia.

The anterior hypothalamus coordinates the nonshivering heat conservation and dissipation mechanisms, and the posterior hypothalamus coordinates shivering thermogenesis. Heat loss usually occurs by four mechanisms: About 55% to 65% of heat is lost by radiation, 25% to 30% by evaporation from the skin and respiratory tract, and 10% to 15% by conduction and convection. The amount of heat lost via conduction is markedly increased in cold-water immersion (by about 32-fold). Each organ system is affected uniquely by hypothermia.

Skin

Cutaneous blood flow is regulated by the individual's thermoregulatory needs, modulated by neural control through the arteriovenous anastomoses located in the extremities. Sympathetic tone is increased, which leads to arteriovenous constriction, which is maximum at 59°F (15°C). Cold-induced dermal vasodilatation can occur at 50°F (10°C).

BOX 2 Drugs and Chemicals That Can Cause Hypothermia

Medicinals

Acetaminophen (Tylenol)
N-Acetylcysteine (Mucomyst)
β-Adrenergic blocking agents
Alprostadil (Caverject, Muse)
Amphotericin B (Fungizone)
Atropine
Azithromycin (Zithromax)
Baclofen (Lioresal)
Barbiturates
Benzodiazepines
Bethanechol (Urecholine)
Biperiden (Akineton)
Bromocriptine (Parlodel)
Carbamazepine (Tegretol)
Chloral hydrate (Noctec)
Chlorpromazine (Thorazine)
Clobazam (Onfi)
Clonidine (Catapres)
Clozapine (Clozaril)
Colchicine (Colcrys)
Delorazepam (Dadumir)[2]
Diazepam (Valium)
Diltiazem (Cardizem)
Enflurane
Erythromycin
Ethchlorvynol (Placidyl)[2]
Ethyl alcohol
Fenoprofen (Nalfon)
Fluphenazine (Prolixin)
Fosphenytoin (Cerebyx)
Gallium nitrate (Ganite)
Glutethimide (Doriden)[2]
Guanabenz (Wytensin)
Guanfacine (Tenex)
Haloperidol (Haldol)
Halothane (Fluothane)
Heroin
γ-Hydroxybutyrate (as sodium salt [Xyrem])
Ibuprofen (Advil, Motrin)
Immune globulin
Insulin preparations
Interferon β-1b (Betaseron)
Iobitridol (Xenetix)[2]
Iopanoic acid (Telepaque)
Ipsapirone
Isoflurane (Forane)
Lincomycin (Lincocin)
Lithium (Eskalith, Lithobid)
Lormetazepam
Loxapine (Loxitane)
Magnesium sulfate
Maprotiline (Ludiomil)
Mefenamic acid (Ponstel)
Melatonin
Methyldopa (Aldomet)
Methyprylon (Noludar)[2]
Moricizine (Ethmozine)

Morphine sulfate
Naphazoline (Naphcon)
Nitrofurantoin (Macrodantin)
Nitrous oxide
Olanzapine (Zyprexa)
Omeprazole (Prilosec)
Oseltamivir (Tamiflu)
Oxcarbazepine (Trileptal)
Oxymetazoline (Afrin)
Paliperidone (depot injection) (Invega Sustenna, Invega Trinza)
Penicillin V
Phencyclidine (PCP)
Phenol
Phenytoin (Dilantin)
Pilocarpine (Salagen)
Pipamperone
Prazosin (Minipress)
Propoxyphene (Darvon)[2]
Procarbazine (Matulane)
Propylthiouracil (PTU)
Quinine (Quinamm)
Rauwolfia serpentine
Reserpine
Risperidone (Risperdal)
Salicylate
Spectinomycin (Trobicin)[2]
Terazosin (Hytrin)
Tetracycline (Sumycin)
Tetrahydrozoline (Visine, Opti-Clear)
Thioridazine (Mellaril)
Topiramate (Topamax)
Tretinoin (topical) (Retin-A)
Triazolam (Halcion)
Tricyclic antidepressants
Valproic acid and derivatives (Depakene)
Zinc sulfate

Nonmedicinals

Acrylamide
Aldicarb
Amitraz
Ashwagandha
Barium
Bis(chloromethyl) ether
Boron hydrides
Bromophos
Cadmium oxide
Cannabis (pediatric overdose)*
Carbon disulfide
Carbon monoxide
Castor pornace
Chloralose
Chlorfenvinphos
Chlorpyrifos
Copper fumes
Coumaphos
Cyanide
Diazinon Dichlorvos
Dicrotophos

Dioxathion
Disulfoton
Ethanol
Ether
Ethion
Fensulfothion
Fenthion
Hexachlorobenzene
Hyaluronidase (Hylenex)
Hydrochloric acid
Hydrogen sulfide
Isopropyl alcohol
Lewisite
Lobelia
Mace
Malathion
Mephedrone
Metal fume fever
Methidathion
Methiocarb
Methomyl
Methyl bromide
Methylene chloride
Methylparathion
Mitragynine (Kratom)[7]
Nickel carbonyl
Parathion
Profenofos
Pyrimidifen
Sarin
Sodium azide
Terbufos
Tetraethyl pyrophosphate
Tetrafluoroethylene
Thiocyanates
Vacor
Zinc fumes (zinc oxide)

Biologicals

Ackee fruit poisoning
Brown recluse spider
Ciguatera food poisoning
Clostridium perfringens
Clupeotox
Copperhead envenomation
Cotton mouth envenomation
Delphinium
Grayanotoxin ("Mad Honey")
Lobelia
Marijuana (Cannabis)
Monkshood
Nutmeg
Salmonella food poisoning
Selenious acid fume
Star of Bethlehem (Hippobroman longiflora)
Streptococcus food poisoning
Tetrodotoxin food poisoning
White chameleon

[2]Not available in the United States.
*Available in marijuana dispensary.
[7]Available as dietary supplement.

Cardiovascular System

One of the initial heat-conserving mechanisms is peripheral vasoconstriction to decrease blood flow to the skin. There are also initial increases in heart rate and blood pressure owing to a catecholamine surge. At core temperatures below 82.4°F (28.0°C), bradycardia can result from a decrease in spontaneous depolarization of the pacemaker cell firing. The myocardium also becomes irritable, predisposing it to bradyarrhythmias and hypotension. Cardiac output decreases to approximately 45% at 77°F (25°C).

Atrial arrhythmias can occur with a slow ventricular response, and they can precede ventricular arrhythmias and asystole at core temperatures below 77.0°F (25.0°C). Moderate hypothermia (82.4°F or 28.0°C) does not significantly alter ventricular conduction but can result in prolongation of repolarization leading to arrhythmia. The characteristic Osborn or J waves (a hump seen at the QRS-ST junction) may be seen on the electrocardiogram (ECG) at core temperatures below 89.6°F (32.0°C). The development of the Osborn wave appears to be related to lower blood pH, low serum bicarbonate, and higher serum creatinine levels. Orthostasis also commonly occurs. Risk factors for development of cardiac arrest include core temperature under 82.4°F (28°C), ventricular arrhythmia development, and systolic blood pressure under 90 mm Hg.

Renal System
Renal blood flow is affected by peripheral vasoconstriction, causing the glomerular filtration rate to fall and contributing to metabolic acidosis. Antidiuretic hormone activity is usually inhibited. This can result in intravascular volume depletion, subsequent vasodilation, increased renal blood flow, and, ultimately, acute renal failure. Urinary output can increase three-fold, and this may be accentuated with concomitant ethanol use.

Respiratory System
At core temperatures below 82.4°F (28°C), minute ventilation, tidal volume, respiratory rate, and thoracic elasticity all are reduced; bronchorrhea can occur, with a loss of cough and gag reflexes leading to an increased risk for aspiration. Carbon dioxide production drops by one-half for every 14°F (8°C) drop in temperature, and oxygen consumption is reduced by 75% at 72°F (22°C). Apnea can then result.

Central Nervous System
Cerebral metabolism is depressed 6% to 7% per 1°C decrease in core temperature. Cerebrovascular autoregulation remains intact until below 77.0°F (25.0°C), which helps maintain cortical blood flow. Electroencephalographic activity is clearly not prognostic, but it is abnormal below 92°F (33°C); burst suppression can occur at 71.6°F (22°C) and it silences around 66.2°F to 68.0°F (19.0°C to 20.0°C). Most patients are unconscious at a core temperature of 82.4°F to 86°F (28°C to 30°C).

Coagulation
Because of depression of enzymatic activity of the activated clotting factors, clotting time (particularly partial thromboplastin time [PTT]) is prolonged. At 84°F (29°C), a 50% increase of PTT can be expected. Thrombocytopenia also commonly occurs due to bone marrow suppression along with splenic and hepatic platelet sequestration, which can be exacerbated by cryoglobinemia.

Clinical Presentation
Accidental hypothermia is classified as mild at body temperatures of 90°F (32.2°C) to 95°F (35°C), moderate at body temperatures of 82.4°F (28.0°C) to 90°F (32.2°C), or severe at body temperatures less than 82.4°F (28°C).

In general, a patient's symptoms depend on the severity of the temperature drop. Patients with mild hypothermia can develop vigorous shivering and cold diuresis. Those with moderate hypothermia can have a paradoxical decrease in shivering, slurred speech, hyporeflexia, and confusion. They are also at risk for intravascular thrombosis. Splanchnic vasoconstriction, gastric erosions, hepatic necrosis, and pancreatitis can occur. Prominent laboratory abnormalities include leukopenia (from splenic sequestration), thrombocytopenia (during rewarming), hypoglycemia, respiratory or metabolic acidosis, and hyperkalemia. In pregnant patients, fetal bradycardia can occur in

response to maternal hypothermia, but long-term sequelae are unknown.

During severe hypothermia, shivering gives way to rigor, minute ventilation decreases, and heart rate and cardiac output decrease. Cardiac instability can be seen at this stage and can manifest in the form of arrhythmias, heart blocks, and eventually asystole. Neurologically, the patient's mental status declines. The patient might attempt to undress (paradoxical undressing) and might respond only to painful stimuli, have decreased gag reflexes, and eventually become apneic. Generally, at about 68.0°F (20.0°C), patients become totally neurologically unresponsive, lose corneal and ocular reflexes, and can have a flat electroencephalogram (EEG).

Emergency Department Evaluation
Typically, the source of hypothermia is revealed from the patient's history; however, it is very important to rule out secondary causes of hypothermia, such as sepsis, hypothyroidism, central nervous system lesions, and hypoglycemia, among others. All patients arriving in the emergency department with hypothermia need a complete evaluation to rule out traumatic injuries and drug or toxin ingestion or overdose.

As in all resuscitation, attention should be paid to the ABCs (airway, breathing, and circulation). Successful neurologic recovery has been documented following 5 hours of cardiopulmonary resuscitation (CPR) in the setting of profound accidental hypothermia (62.4°F or 16.9°C). Ideally, in patients in cardiac arrest, CPR should be maintained throughout the prehospital period. In a patient with a core temperature of under 28°C, evidence supports alternating 5 minutes of CPR with less than or equal to 5 minutes without CPR, if feasible. With a core temperature under 20°C, data supports alternating 5 minutes of CPR with less than or equal to 10 minutes without CPR. Respiratory failure should be treated with endotracheal intubation and mechanical ventilation. Hypotension can be treated initially with warmed fluids. Placing the patient in a warm environment, removing all cold and wet clothes, and remembering to cover up the patient after he or she has been exposed should help prevent further heat loss.

The temperature should be confirmed by checking a core temperature (e.g., rectal, bladder, or esophageal), using a thermometer capable of recording very low temperatures. Patients should be placed on a cardiac monitor and an ECG should be obtained. Laboratory testing is especially useful in the postresuscitative period, when complications begin. Laboratory tests should include a complete blood count (CBC), a chemistry panel with liver function tests, creatine phosphokinase (CPK) to evaluate for rhabdomyolysis, a coagulation profile, blood type and screen, an arterial blood gas, and a drug screen. A Foley catheter should be placed to assess urinary output.

Rewarming Strategies
There are several methods of rewarming. The method of choice usually depends on the severity of hypothermia. During rewarming, the patient should be placed on a cardiac monitor with frequent measurements of blood pressure and temperature (via a rectal probe) for easy detection of complications of rewarming, such as rewarming-related hypotension, arrhythmias, and core temperature after-drop. It should be noted that the human body is capable of raising the body temperature through heat generation by approximately 1°C/h.

Passive External Warming
Passive external warming is ideal for patients with mild hypothermia (greater than 93°F or 34°C) who are otherwise healthy. It uses the patient's endogenous heat production for rewarming and it involves simple, logical passive maneuvers that minimize heat dissipation. When using this method, all wet clothing should be removed and the patient should be covered with insulating materials. Patients warmed easily using this method can be safely discharged.

Active External Rewarming

Active external rewarming should be considered for patients with core temperatures between 86°F and 92°F (30°C to 34°C). It involves exposing the patient's skin to exogenous heat sources. Radiant heat, thermal mattresses, electric heating blankets, and forced-air heating blankets are some of the available techniques. Heat applied externally is most effective if concentrated on the axillae, chest, and back which exhibits the greatest potential for conductive heat transfer. Additionally, heat can be applied to the neck region to prevent heat loss. Extremity placement of heat should be avoided. Also, localized pressure to skin that is cold should be avoided. Chemical heat packs do not provide sufficient heat transfer to increase core temperature and should not be used. The rate of temperature rise is approximately 2.7°F to 7.2°F (1.5°C to 4°C) per hour.

This method has several disadvantages. First, burn injuries can occur to the vasoconstricted skin. Second, any sort of immersion can hinder monitoring and other resuscitative activities. Finally and most important, active external rewarming produces a phenomenon called *core-temperature after-drop*. This refers to a drop in core temperature resulting from sudden peripheral vasodilation. This causes cold, acidic blood to return to the core. Hypotension and potentially fatal dysrhythmias can result. Focusing on rewarming the trunk only (rather than the trunk and extremities) can prevent these temperature gradients. In general, active external rewarming is used in conjunction with active core rewarming.

Active Core Rewarming

Active core rewarming involves techniques to deliver direct heat internally. It should be used in patients with moderate to severe hypothermia (under 86°F or 30°C). The simplest method entails the administration of heated, humidified oxygen at 107.6°F to 114.8°F (42.0°C to 46.0°C), which can be used as adjunctive therapy, and intravenous saline solution warmed to 109.4°F (43.0°C). Saline should be administered via a central line at 150 to 200 mL/h. Gastric, bladder, and colonic irrigations have been used, but their relatively small surface areas usually limit their effect. Urinary bladder or gastric lavage (which is rarely used due to aspiration potential and electrolyte shifts) can rewarm at an hourly rate of 0.9°F to 1.8°F (0.5°C to 1°C).

Another method of active core rewarming is pleural irrigation using two large-bore (36°F or greater) thoracostomy tubes. One tube is placed at the midclavicular line and is connected to saline at 107.6°F (42.0°C). The other tube is placed at the posterior axillary line and connected to a chest tube drainage kit.

A more-aggressive method of active core rewarming is via peritoneal lavage and dialysis. This can be accomplished using a standard diagnostic peritoneal lavage kit and introducing an 8-F catheter into the peritoneum using the Seldinger technique. The crystalloid dialysate should be warmed at 104.0°F to 113.0°F (40.0°C to 45.0°C). This method affords the added advantage of allowing the serum potassium level to be adjusted.

The most efficient and physiologic active core rewarming method is via extracorporeal warming or heated cardiopulmonary bypass. This is the method of choice for the most-severe cases, patients with severe rhabdomyolysis, and patients who require CPR. Survival rates with no chronic neurological sequelae as high as 75% have been documented. Excellent recovery has been documented from a nasopharyngeal temperature of 13.8°C (and a serum potassium of 11.3 mmol/L) due to drowning with a submersion time of at least 83 minutes in icy sea water with slow rewarming with extracorporeal membrane oxygenation. Extracorporeal life support can be an effective rewarming tool in patients with prolonged cardiac arrest from accidental hypothermia, particularly in the absence of asphyxia, trauma, or severe hyperkalemia. Venoarterial extracorporeal membrane oxygenation (VA-ECMO) is increasingly utilized for its ability to gradually increase core

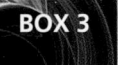

BOX 3	Drugs Displaying Reduced Metabolism or Clearance in Hypothermia

Atropine
Digoxin
Fentanyl (Sublimaze, Duragesic)
Gentamicin (Garamycin)
Lidocaine (Xylocaine)
Phenobarbital
Procaine
Propranolol (Inderal)
Sulfanilamide (AVC cream)
Suxamethonium (succinylcholine, Anectine)
D-Tubocurarine
Brain natriuretic peptide

body temperature while providing respiratory and hemodynamic support. It should be considered, especially in pediatric patients or in individuals requiring prolonged support. Survival rates as high as 40% (with good neurologic outcome) have been documented.

Most arrhythmias are corrected by rewarming. Atrial dysrhythmias often occur during rewarming and generally resolve without treatment. Atropine is typically ineffective for cold-associated bradydysrhythmias. Ventricular tachycardia and fibrillation require electrocardioversion; automated external defibrillator (AED) devices can be used as directed for pulseless ventricular tachycardia or ventricular fibrillation. Dopamine, epinephrine[1], and vasopressin (Pitressin)[1] may be effective vasopressors for core temperatures above 30°C (86°F). External pacing may be ineffective. Empiric antibiotics may be given. However, the empiric use of levothyroxine (Synthroid)[1] and corticosteroids may be hazardous. Phenytoin (Dilantin)[1] might have cardiac-depressant qualities in the moderately hypothermic patient. Box 3 demonstrates drugs with possible decreased metabolism or clearance with resultant increase in toxicity in hypothermia.

For hypothermia due to myxedema coma, levothyroxine (Synthroid) should be administered intravenously (at a dose of 250 to 500 μg over 30 to 60 seconds). Daily intravenous injections of 100 μg may be required for up to 7 days. Hydrocortisone (Solu-Cortef)[1] (200 to 400 mg IV daily) administration should also be considered. Other active core rewarming techniques are usually not required. Treatment of episodic, spontaneous hyperhydrosis hyperthermia or Shapiro's syndrome often respond to clonidine (Catapres)[1] (up to 0.6 mg daily) through its actions on hypothalmic thermoregulation.

Indicators of grave prognosis include development of profound hyperkalemia (serum potassium greater than 10 mEq/L), elevated serum creatinine, serum sodium, serum lactate concentration, or lower prothrombin time, underlying medical conditions, intravascular thrombosis (fibrinogen less than 59 mg/dL), pH less than 6.5, and a core temperature less than 82.4°F (28.0°C). Elevated serum potassium in a hypothermic patient may indicate that hypoxia preceded the onset of hypothermia. Submersion in cold water for over 10 minutes is associated with a poor prognosis; if the water is less than 43°F (6°C), survival is unlikely to occur if submerged for over 90 minutes.

Peripheral Cold Injuries

Peripheral cold injuries span a spectrum ranging from minimal to severe tissue damage. Freezing and nonfreezing syndromes can cause these injuries. About 500 patients with frostbite are hospitalized yearly in the United States, with about an 80% male demographic and lower extremity predominance. The average

[1]Not FDA approved for this indication.

length of stay in critical care units and total hospital stay is approximately 7 and 10 days, respectively. Frostnip and frostbite are caused by exposure to freezing temperatures. *Frostnip* refers to the numbness and blue-white discoloration of the face and extremities that occur during exposure to freezing temperatures. It is a precursor to frostbite. It is characterized by reversible skin changes, including blanching and numbness with no permanent tissue damage, unlike frostbite. Nonfreezing injuries depend on whether the ambient environment during exposure was wet (trench or immersion foot) or dry (pernio or chilblain).

Pathophysiology

During exposure to cold temperatures, the core body temperature is preserved to the detriment of the extremities. Frostbite occurs in four stages: prefreeze, freeze–thaw, vascular stasis, and late ischemic stages. The prefreeze phase occurs when the temperature of the extremities falls below 50.0°F (10.0°C) and cutaneous sensation is lost. Vasoconstriction also occurs along with leakage of intracellular fluid into the interstitium.

The freeze–thaw phase begins at the freezing point of water (32.0°F or 0°C) with the formation of ice crystals extracellularly. This further enhances the exit of water from the intracellular space under osmotic forces, resulting in cell shrinkage and, ultimately, damage. During the vascular stasis phase, plasma leakage and formation of ice crystals continue. Arachidonic acid breakdown products are then released from underlying damaged tissue. Both prostaglandin $F_{2\alpha}$ and thromboxane A_2 produce platelet aggregation, leukocyte immobilization, and vasoconstriction.

Endothelial cells are sensitive to cold injury, and the microvasculature becomes distorted and clogged, leading to tissue ischemia. The late ischemic phase is characterized by ischemia, thrombosis, continued shunting, gangrene, autonomic dysfunction, and denaturation of tissue proteins. The tissue can eventually mummify and demarcate more than 60 to 90 days later.

Clinical Presentation of Local Extremity Issues

Frostnip and Frostbite

The face and ears are the most common sites prone to cold injury, followed by the hands and feet. Patients with frostnip usually have blanching and numbness of their fingertips. The skin has a firm or waxy texture. Often the patient is unaware of these changes. Frostnip is usually reversible. Frostbite has been classified as superficial, affecting the skin and subcutaneous tissue, or deep, affecting the bones, joints, and tendons. When a superficial frostbite is rewarmed, the skin can form a clear blister; however, when a deep frostbite is rewarmed, it can form a hemorrhagic blister. This classification, however, has no therapeutic or prognostic value given that frostbites can initially appear benign. Many weeks can pass before the demarcation between viable and nonviable tissues becomes apparent. Facial frostbite, with skin blistering, can also occur following halogenated (especially fluorinated) hydrocarbon inhalation abuse. This can appear initially as angioneurotic edema if it involves the oral mucosa membranes. Acute compartment syndrome of the foot and ankle, associated with gangrenous toe changes, have been described.

Although no prognostic factors can be entirely predictive, favorable factors include retained sensation, normal skin color, and clear rather than cloudy fluid in the blisters, if present. Poor prognostic features include nonblanching cyanosis, firm skin, and dark, fluid-filled blisters. Patients can present with pain, numbness, and a clumsy "chunk of wood" sensation in the affected extremity. The pain is initially described as a dull ache and evolves to become a throbbing sensation in about 48 to 72 hours.

Chilblain

Chilblain, also referred to as perniosis, results from repetitive exposure to cold, dry air. It manifests as painful erythematous nodules or cyanotic lesions often referred to as cold sores. These lesions usually develop on exposed surfaces after a delay of 12 to 14 hours and are characterized by pruritus and burning

paresthesias. Young women, especially those with Raynaud phenomenon and/or a low body mass index, are at risk.

Chilblains are located on acral skin associated with cold exposure. They are usually located on the dorsum of the fingers, toes, and thighs, where blisters or ulcerations can develop in very severe cases. Perivascular lymphocytic infiltration with vacuolation of the basal layer is often seen on histologic analysis, especially when it is associated with an autoimmune disease (particularly lupus erythematosus).

Susceptibility to chilblains increases when the ambient temperature is less than 10°C and relative humidity is 60%.

Trench Foot and Immersion Foot

Trench foot occurs as a result of prolonged exposure (about 10 to 15 hours) to a damp, cold, nonfreezing environment (with temperature as high as 15°C or 59°F). It has been classically described among soldiers in World War I, many of whom were confined to cold and damp trenches for prolonged periods. Symptoms include numbness and painful paresthesias that can progress to a throbbing and burning sensation. Initial evaluation reveals a cold, pale extremity, with or without vesicles or bullae. Inflammatory serum markers, such as erythrocyte sedimentation rate (ESR) or C-reactive protein (CRP), may be elevated.

Immersion foot may be considered the sailor's counterpart to trench foot. It occurs after prolonged immersion in cold water at temperatures above freezing.

Treatment

Treatment of frostbite should begin with removing all wet or frozen clothing. For patients with moderate or severe hypothermia, initial resuscitative efforts should be geared toward raising their core temperature. The patient should be moved to a warm environment and all wet clothing should be removed. The frozen extremity should be rewarmed by immersion in circulation water at 98.6°F to 102.2°F (37.0°C to 39.0°C) for about 15 to 30 minutes. Given the risks of thermal injury, the frozen parts should not be exposed to direct or dry heat (such as hair dryers, heating pads, or heat lamps). Do not rub or massage the affected area. The process should be continued until the extremity appears warm and well perfused. Following rewarming, the extremity should be air dried and elevated. Because of the pain associated with reperfusion, there may be the temptation to abruptly abort the rewarming process. This can, however, promote further tissue damage.

Oral or intravenous fluid administration should be administered to prevent dehydration and vascular stasis. Because the pain is usually prominent at night, amitriptyline (Elavil)[1] at an initial dosage of 10 to 25 mg and a maximum of 100 mg may be helpful. Gabapentin (Neurontin)[1] also may be an alternative therapy. Parenteral analgesic medications—nonsteroidal antiinflammatory drugs (NSAIDs) and opioids—may be administered as needed to make this process more tolerable. Ibuprofen at a dose of 12 mg/kg twice daily (400 mg in adults twice daily, which can be increased to a maximum of 2400 mg daily) may be helpful for its analgesic and antiinflammatory effects.

Almost all authors agree that hemorrhagic blisters should not be débrided because of the risk of secondary desiccation of deep dermal layers, extending the injury. Débriding broken vesicles or bullae is also widely accepted; however, clear, intact vesicles may be broken and débrided or left intact. Topical aloe vera ointment (Dermaide Aloe)[7] or topical antibiotic ointments may be applied. Cold extremity wounds are not considered tetanus prone.

The injured tissue should be loosely covered with sterile, dry, bulky, nonadherent dressing. If possible, elevate the extremity above the cardiac level to decrease dependent edema. Hands and feet may be splinted and elevated to reduce edema. Because the damaged tissue is tetanus prone, patients

---

[1]Not FDA approved for this indication.

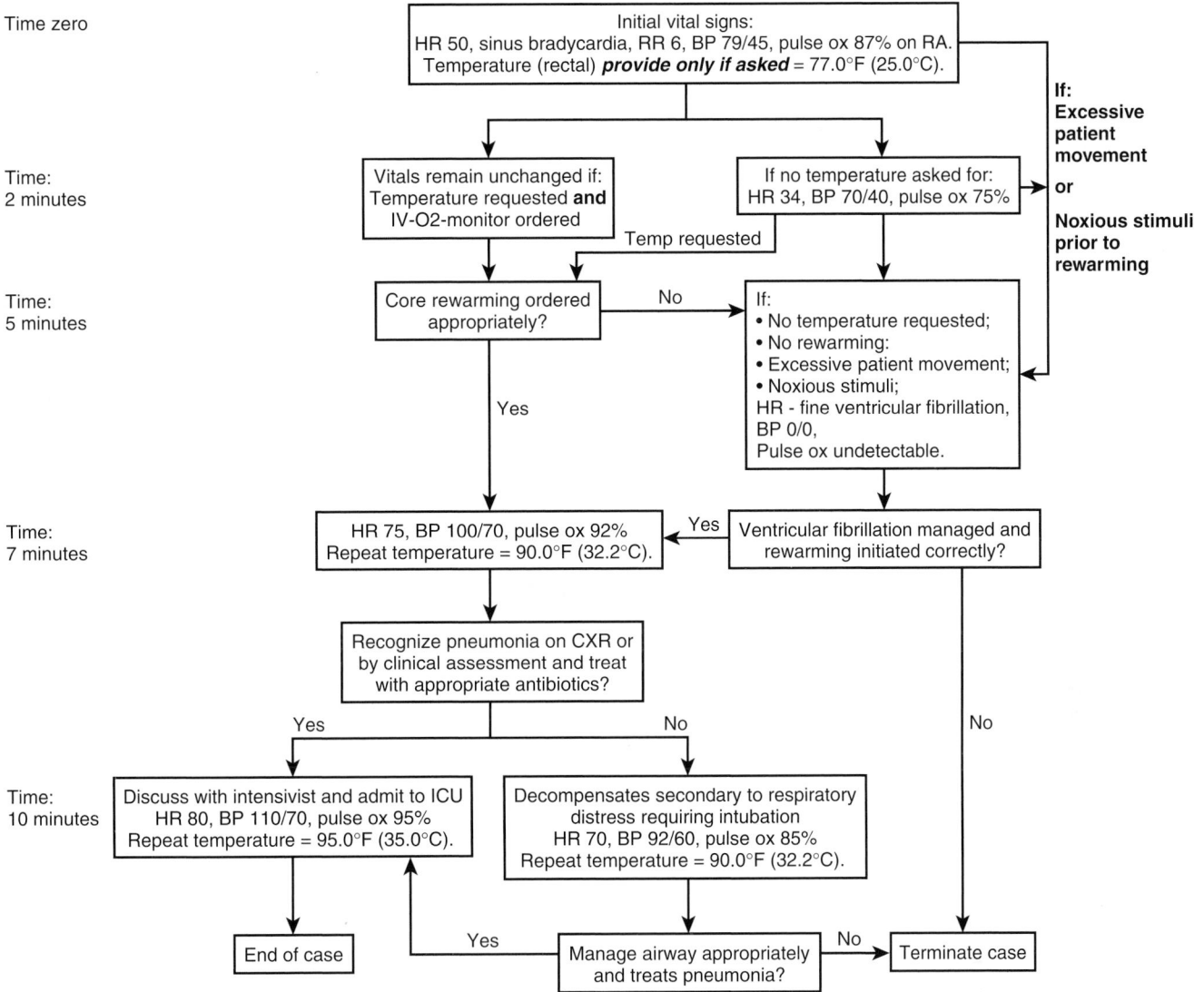

Figure 1 Hypothermia simulation flow diagram.

whose tetanus status has not been updated may require a tetanus booster (Td).

Adjunctive agents that have been used for their antithrombotic and vasodilative properties with varying success include heparin[1], steroids[1], NSAIDs[1], dimethylsulfoxide (DMSO, Rimso-50)[1], nonionic detergents[1], dipyridamole (Persantine)[1], calcium channel blockers[1], thrombolytics, pentoxifylline (Trental)[1], and phenoxybenzamine (Dibenzyline)[1]. Iloprost (Ventavis) is a prostacyclin analogue that is a potent vasodilator that can inhibit aggregation of platelets. It may also have fibrinolytic activity. The intravenous dosing is 0.5 ng/kg/min, which can be increased by 0.5 ng/kg/min at 30-minute intervals to a maximum dose of 2 ng/kg/min for up to 8 days. Although not yet approved by the U.S. FDA, it has been suggested for severe frostbite within 72 hours of injury. Hyperbaric oxygen with thrombolytic therapy has been used to treat severe frostbite of the hand. Negative pressure wound therapy, following blister excision, has been demonstrated to be beneficial in treating infant frostbite hand injures. Following rewarming, intravenous tissue plasminogen activator (TPA, Activase)[1] with an initial 3 mg bolus followed by a 6- to 12-hour infusion of 1 mg/ml (10 ml/hour) heparin at a dose of 500 units per hour administered concurrently has been utilized effectively with systemic anticoagulation and/or anti-platelet therapy to follow. Intra-arterial TPA (Activase)[1] has also been utilized. Surgical consultation is appropriate for guiding long-term management, because some patients might need débridement of infections or skin grafts for nonhealing wounds. A sympathetic nerve block (sympathectomy) can relieve painful and refractory vasospasms.

A familial association of chilblain (associated with contractual arachnodactyly) has been described in Italy. Chilblain (pernio) may be treated with nifedipine[1] at an oral dose of 20 mg three times daily. Oral prednisolone (Millipred)[1], 0.5 mg/kg in two divided doses over 2 weeks, and topical glucocorticoids have been used to treat perniosis; pentoxyfylline[1] (1200 mg/day in three divided doses for 2 weeks) has also been demonstrated to be effective. Acupuncture treatment (once weekly for 12 weeks) has been used to decrease cold sensitivity due to second-degree frostbite in the fingertips.

Sequelae

Late sequelae of frostbite include cold hypersensitivity, arthritis, numbness, chronic pain, ulceration, decreased sensation, and functional loss of the extremity. This is a result of early neuronal damage and abnormal sympathetic tone. Patients with chronic symptoms should be advised to avoid nicotine and cold exposure while using NSAIDs. Tissue demarcation can occur 60 to 90 days after initial injury. Amputation decisions should be deferred unless there is supervening sepsis or gangrene. The ultimate tissue salvage after a spontaneous slough usually far exceeds the most optimistic initial estimates. A medical simulation flow diagram is presented in Figure 1.

---

[7]Available as dietary supplement.

References

Albright JT, Lebovitz BL, Lipson R, et al: Upper aerodigestive tract frostbite complicating volatile substance abuse, *Int J Pediatr Otorhinolaryngol* 1:63–67, 1999.

Boada A, Bielsa I, Frenandez-Figueras MT, et al: Perniosis: clinical and histopathological analysis, *Am J Dermatopathol* 32(1):19–23, 2010.

Bottie Y, Lavolaine J, Bouzat P, et al: Neurologic recovery from profound accidental hypothermia after 5 hours of cardiopulmonary resuscitation, *Crit Care Med* 42:e167–e170, 2014.

Brandao RA, St John JM, Langan TM, et al: Acute compartment syndrome of the foot due to frostbite: literature review and case report, *Journal of Foot and Ankle Surgery* 57(2):382–387, 2018.

Bright F, Gilbert JD, Winskog C, Byard RW: Additional risk factors for lethal hypothermia, *J Forensic Leg Med* 20(6):595–597, 2013.

Bush JS, Watson S: Trench foot (updated 2018 Jan 12). In *Stat Pearls (Internet)*, Treasure Island, FL, 2018 Jan, Stat Pearls Publishing. Available from http://www./ncbi.nim.nih.gov/books/NBK482364/.

Centers for Disease Control and Prevention (CDC): Hypothermia-related deaths—United States, 2003–2004, *MMWR Morb Mortal Wkly Rep* 54:173–175, 2005.

Danzl D: Hypothermia, *Semin Respir Crit Care Med* 23:57–68, 2002.

Danzl DF: Accidental hypothermia. In Auerbach PS, editor: *Wilderness Medicine*, 5th ed, St. Louis, 2007, Mosby, pp 125–160.

Darku B, Kalra P, Prasad C, et al: Episodic hyperhydrosis with corpus callosum agenesis: a rare case of Shapiro syndrome, *Neurol India* 59(1):130–131, 2011.

Dietrichs ES, McGlynn K, Allan A, et al: Moderate but Not Severe Hypothermia Causes Pro-Arrythmic Changes in Cardiac Electrophysiology, *Cardiovasc Res* 2020 Feb 7;cvz309. Online ahead of print.

Dow J, Glesbrecht GG, Danzl DF, et al: Wilderness Medical Society Clinical Practice Guidelines for the out-of-hospital evaluation and treatment of accidental hypothermia: 2019 update, *Wilderness Environ Med* 30(4):S47–S69, 2019.

Eroglu O, Serbest S, Kufeciler T, Kalkan A: Osborn wave in hypothermia and relation to mortality, *Am J Emerg Med* 37(6):1065–1068, 2019.

Fudge J: Exercise in the cold. Preventing and managing hypothermia and frostbite injury, *Sports Health* 8(2):133–139, 2016.

Gilbert M, Busund R, Skagseth A, et al: Resuscitation from accidental hypothermia of 13.7°C with circulatory arrest, *Lancet* 355:375–376, 2000.

Gomez CR: Disorders of body temperature, *Handbook of Clinical Neurology* 120:947–957, 2014.

Handford C, Thomas O, Imray CHE: Frostbite, *Emerg Clin N Am* 35:281–299, 2017.

Hemelsoet DM, DeBleecker JL: Post-traumatic spontaneous recurrent hypothermia: a variant of Shapiro's syndrome, *Eur J Neurol* 14(2):224–227, 2007.

Herzog E, Shapiro J, Aziz EF, et al: Pathway for the management of survivors of out-of-hospital cardiac arrest, *Crit Pathw Cardiol* 9:49–54, 2010.

Higginson R: Causes of hypothermia and the use of patient-rewarming techniques, *Br J Nursing* 27(21):1222–1224, 2018.

Imray CH, Richards P, Greeves J, et al: Nonfreezing cold-induced injuries, *J R Army Med Corps* 157:79–84, 2011.

Jones LM, Coffey RA, Natwa MP, Bailey JK: The use of intravenous TPA for the treatment of severe frostbite, *Burns* 43(5):1088–1096, 2017.

Kurbat RS, Pollack Jr. CV: Facial injury and airway threat from inhalant abuse: a case report, *J Emerg Med* 16(2):167–169, 1998.

Linford A, Valtonen J, Hult M, et al: The evolution of the Helsinki frostbite management protocol, *Burns* 43:1455–1463, 2017.

Lloyd EL: Accidental hypothermia, *Resuscitation* 32:111–124, 1996.

Lorentzen AK, Davis C, Penninga L: Interventions for frostbite injuries, *Cochrane Database Syst Rev*(3), 2018. Available from: https://doi.org/10.1002/14651858.CD012980,2018.

Mazur P, Kosinski S, Podsiadlo P, et al: Extracorporeal membrane oxygenation of accidental deep hypothermia - current challenges and future perspectives, *Ann Cardiothoracic Surg* 8(1):137–142, 2019.

McCauley RD, Killyon GW, Smith Jr. DJ, et al: Frostbite and other cold-induced injuries. In Auerbach PS, editor: *Wilderness Medicine*, 5th ed, St. Louis, 2007, Mosby, pp 195–210.

McIntosh SE, Freer L, Grisson SK, et al: Wilderness Medical Society Practice Guidelines for the Prevention and Treatment of Frostbite: 2019 update, *Wilderness Environ Med* 30(4):S15–S532, 2019.

Mommse P, Andruszkow H, Fromke C, et al: Effects of accidental hypothermia on posttraumatic complications and outcome in multiple trauma patients, *Injury* 44:86–90, 2013.

Monti M, Mommi V, Forte MB, et al: Olazapine-associated hypothermia: a case report of a rare event, *Italian Journal of Medicine* 12:67–69, 2018.

Noaimi AA, Fadheel BM: Treatment of perniosis with oral pentoxyfilline in comparison with oral prednisolone plus topical clobetasol ointment in Iraqi patients, *Saudi Med J* 29:1762–1764, 2008.

Norheim AJ, Alraek T: Acupuncture for frostbite sequel—a case report, *European Journal of Integrative Medicine* 17:102–106, 2018.

Nygaard RM, Endorf FW. Frostbite in the United States: an examination of the national burn repository and national trauma data back, *J Burn Care Res* 39(5):780–785, 2018.

Paal P, Gordon L, Strapazzon G, et al: Accidental hypothermia-an update, *Scandivavian Journal of Trauma, Resuscitation and Emergency Medicine* 24(1):111, 2016. 10-1186/S13049-016-0303-7.

Parna SL, Wisco OJ: What is your diagnosis? Perniosis (chilblain), *Cutis* 84:27–29, 2009.

Piga M, Vacca A, Cauli A, et al: Familial chilbain and late contractual arachnodactyly: a novel association? *Joint Bone Spine* 7:205–208, 2009.

Plumb J, Thomas RG, Corneli HM: Facial frostbite associated with intentional inhalation of a commercial dusting product, *Clin Toxicol* 49:529, 2011.

Pratsinis A, Devuyst O, Leroux JC: Peritoneal dialysis beyond kidney failure? *J Control Release* 282:3–12, 2018.

Raza N, Sajid MD, Suhail M: et al: Onset of chilblains in relation to weather conditions, *J Ayub Med Coll Abbottabad* 20:17–20, 2008.

Saczkowski RS, Brown DJA, Abu-Laban RB, et al: Prediction of survival in accidental hypothermia requiring extracorporeal life support: an individual patient meta analysis, *Resuscitation* 127:51–57, 2018.

Toledano M, Weinshenker BG, Kaufmann TJ, et al: Demographics and clinical characteristics of episodic hypothermia in multiple sclerosis, *Mult Scler J* 25(5):709–714, 2019.

Ulrich AS, Rathlev NK: Hypothermia and localized cold injuries, *Emerg Med Clin North Am* 22:281–298, 2004.

Urbanic RC, Mazzaferri EL: Thyrotoxic crisis and myxedema coma, *Heart Lung* 7:435–447, 1978.

Walker BR, Anderson J, Edwards CRW: Clonidine therapy for Shapiro's syndrome, *QJM* 82(3):235–245, 1992.

Wexler A, Zavala S: The use of thrombolytic therapy in the treatment of frostbite injury, *Journal of Burn Care and Research* 38(5):e877–e881, 2017.

Wiersinga WM: Myxedema and coma (Severe Hypothyroidism) [Updated 2018 Apr 25]. In Feingold KR, Anawalt B, Boyce A, et al: *Endotext [Internet]*. South Dartmouth (MA), MDText.com, Inc., 2000. Available from: https://www.ncbi.nlm.nih.gov/books/NBK279007/.

HEAT-RELATED ILLNESS

Method of
Paul Cleland, MD

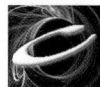

CURRENT DIAGNOSIS

- Heat illness is a spectrum of illness which is usually seen among athletes in hot and humid environments.
- Children, elderly and poorly acclimatized individuals are at increased risk for developing exertional heat illness (EHI).
- Exercise-associated cramps are intense, prolonged, painful muscle spasms that occur during physical activity.
- Heat exhaustion is an elevation in core temperature (<104°F) without central nervous system (CNS) dysfunction resulting in a collapse or difficulty continuing activity.
- Heat stroke is a life-threatening illness characterized by elevation in core temperature (≥104°F) with CNS dysfunction (altered consciousness, seizure, coma) and usually end-organ damage.

CURRENT THERAPY

- Acclimatization is key for prevention of EHI.
- Heat illness is most effectively managed by immediate recognition of the signs and symptoms and proper diagnosis.
- Core temperature measurement MUST be done with a rectal thermometer.
- Exercise-Associated Collapse
  - Continue walking after race to prevent development.
  - Position the patient in a Trendelenburg position and start fluid administration.
- Heat exhaustion
  - Rapid cooling with ice bags to areas adjacent to large vasculature (groin, neck, axilla).
  - Oral or intravenous (IV) fluid administration to correct for hydration deficit.
- Heat stroke
  - Ensure the ability to maintain adequate circulation, airway, and breathing.
  - Rapid cooling with ice-water immersion is the most effective way to cool.
  - Goal of cooling is to reduce and maintain temperature below 101°F.
  - May require transport to hospital if patient does not reduce temperature effectively or return to normal mental status after 30 minutes of medical treatment.

Heat illness is a continuum of disease that can affect a wide array of individuals including athletes, firefighters, construction workers, military, and others. Exertional heat illness (EHI) is a leading cause of death among young athletes and may be on the rise with possible climate change and increasing popularity of mass events such as marathons. Knowledge of the risk factors presented by the patient and the environment can provide clinicians with a better understanding toward prevention of heat illness. Early recognition and treatment of EHI can lead to significant reduction in the morbidity and mortality associated with this disease.

In the United States, most cases of EHI occur in summer months. Elevations in the ambient temperature and humidity as well as athletic deconditioning are predominant contributing factors. There is a rising incidence of heat illness associated with decreased heat acclimation and an increase in the wet-bulb globe temperature (WBGT). High school and collegiate athletic programs that have protocols in place to stop practice or reduce duration or frequency in certain heat situations have shown a decreased incidence of heat illness compared to those that do not.

It is important to understand the pathophysiology of the regulation of heat within the body to gain an accurate picture of heat illness. The human body has a great capacity to withstand drastic reductions in temperature to tolerate cold. However, only mild increases in core temperature can results in severe consequences. Heat is generated by normal metabolic processes that occur continuously in our bodies and is also absorbed from the environment. Exercise generates additional heat from the skeletal muscles. As a core temperature rise is detected in the hypothalamus, signals are sent out to induce sweating and cutaneous vasodilation. Blood is then shunted to the skin and exercising skeletal muscle. Under normal conditions, the body can dissipate heat through evaporation, radiation, convection, and conduction. Evaporation is the primary means of heat dissipation and occurs as water is converted from its liquid to its vapor form but becomes ineffective above a relative humidity of 75%. Radiation, convection, and conduction are also methods to dissipate heat but are decreasingly effective as the ambient temperature approaches the skin's temperature. When the physiologic cooling mechanisms fail, heat is continually produced, and the core temperature increases. As the temperature rises, cell damage occurs and a systemic inflammatory response ensues, releasing cytokines throughout the body. Blood is shunted to the peripheral circulation leading to organ hypoperfusion and ischemia. Organ failure and disseminated intravascular coagulation (DIC) will develop and eventually result in death.

The injury that occurs as a result of heat illness can be mitigated by acclimatization of the patient and is the most important factor to thrive in hot and humid conditions. Acclimatization occurs as the body is repeatedly exposed to certain levels of stress and then makes compensatory changes to allow for better performance the next time the body is under duress. This process occurs over 1 to 2 weeks of exposure to new conditions and appears to be lost with re-exposure to the previous climate for about the same time period. There are several key changes that occur as the body is exposed to heat, including: production of heat shock proteins which give cells the ability to resist heat-stress, decreased sweat temperature threshold, increased sweat production, decreased salt concentration in sweat, and increased skin blood flow. These factors all serve to aid the athlete under high-risk heat conditions to improve performance and alleviate potential heat illness. It is recommended that the athlete spend at least 2 weeks acclimatizing to the environment mimicking both temperature and humidity for maximal outcome. If an athlete returns to a more temperate environment after training, such as an air-conditioned room, they would not see the same benefit as they would with exposure to the conditions for 24 hours a day. If possible, air-conditioning should be restricted to nighttime only when the athlete is resting.

Risk Factors

Although each person has unique genetic traits that determine how their body reacts to specific conditions, there are known congenital and acquired risk factors that may preclude an individual toward development of EHI. Exposure to a hot and humid environment may be the most obvious risk factor as ambient heat is transferred to the body and elevated humidity impairs the body's ability to dissipate heat. Poor conditioning, lack of acclimatization, obesity, and dehydration are all contributors that have been shown to increase the incidence of EHI. The use of prescription medications, supplements, and recreational drugs (Table 1) may cause disturbances in the capacity to dissipate heat or cause a production of heat. Creatine supplementation does not appear to impair heat dissipation or cause a negative impact on hydration.

Children are at increased risk of developing heat illness for several physiologic reasons. A larger surface area to mass ratio allows for more heat absorption from the environment. Children also produce more heat compared to their adult counterparts due to higher basal metabolic rates. Fluid is conserved more efficiently than adults and consequently children have lower sweat rates, as they depend more on non-evaporative forms of heat transfer for cooling. Children can make the same physiologic changes of acclimatization that adults can, though it appears to occur at a slower rate.

Environmental characteristics such as heat and humidity may play the largest role in development of heat illness. The wet bulb globe temperature index (WBGT) is a tool that assesses the overall environmental conditions and can accurately predict the development of EHI in a particular setting and allows for modification of work or athletic events. The WBGT is a measurement of temperature, relative humidity, and radiant heat from the sun and ground and is recommended over the use of the heat index. A dangerous clinical situation is likely to develop when activities are performed with an elevated WBGT. It is recommended that endurance events be adjusted when the WBGT exceeds 82°F (28°C) and that only events where adequate rest and recovery is observed may continue.

Heat Edema

Heat edema is caused by vasodilation of blood vessels resulting in swelling that is typically observed in the hands and feet. The core temperature of the body is not elevated. Treatment begins with removal from the hot environment, elevation of the extremities, and may involve use of compression with stockings or wrapping. Diuretics are not recommended.

Heat Cramps

Also known as exercise-associated cramps, heat cramps present as intense pain, spasm, and prolonged muscle contraction as athletes undergo high intensity activity. Although they are termed "heat cramps," they are known to occur in cool settings as well, such as swimming and winter sports. The pathophysiology has not been entirely agreed upon but seems to stem from a neurogenic response to muscle fatigue in conjunction with fluid and electrolyte losses. To make the diagnosis, no signs of other illness may be present such as rhabdomyolysis, sickle cell disease or trait, or heat stroke, and it is important to remember to take a thorough medical history to avoid pitfalls in the diagnosis.

Management consists of stretching and massaging the affected muscle and oral replacement of fluid and electrolytes. IV fluids and benzodiazepines may be used for refractory cases. One study has shown that ingestion of pickle juice at 1 mL/kg may cause a faster recovery from electrically induced muscle cramps when compared to deionized water. This would owe to the theory of a neurogenic-mediated process, as the recovery occurred before the contents of the pickle juice had time to reach the sites of action in the cramping skeletal muscle with discontinuation of cramping seen at an average of 85 seconds compared to deionized water at 134 seconds.

TABLE 1	Substances That May Increase Risk of Heat Illness

- Amphetamines
- Anticholinergic agents
- Antiepileptic agents
- Antihistamines
- Benzodiazepines
- Beta blockers
- Calcium channel blockers
- Cocaine
- Decongestants
- Diuretics
- Ergogenic stimulants
- Ethanol
- Laxatives
- Lithium
- Phenothiazines
- Tricyclic antidepressants

Data from Bouchama, Wexler

Exercise-Associated Collapse

Also termed Exercise-Associated Postural Hypotension, exercise-associated collapse (EAC) is an inability of the athlete to maintain a standing posture due to hypotension that develops commonly *after* an endurance event. Blood in circulation pools in the lower extremities as the athlete finishes the event and discontinues exercising. The skeletal muscles in the lower extremities normally exert a pressure on the corresponding vasculature, but as exercise ceases, the blood pools cause an unexpected drop in cranial blood pressure, triggering collapse. Heat may play an indirect role in the development of EAC, but the terms "heat syncope" and "heat collapse" are incorrect because there is no elevation in the athlete's core temperature. Athletes may develop dizziness, nausea, and vomiting as a result of the rapid drop in blood pressure.

Athletes should be encouraged to continue activity such as walking or light activity at the end of events (rather than abrupt cessation or standing in place) to continue normal blood flow to avoid a sudden collapse, risking injury. If an athlete does collapse, treatment should begin with laying the patient supine in a Trendelenburg position, keeping the legs and pelvis elevated. Administration of oral fluids containing glucose and electrolytes is helpful. Intravenous fluid administration should be reserved for those with elevated pulse (>100 bpm) or hypotension (<110 SBP) and not responding to oral fluid intake. Generally, these athletes will respond favorably within 10 to 30 minutes, and should be allowed to leave under their own power.

Heat Exhaustion

Heat exhaustion occurs when the cardiovascular system is unable to provide adequate output to the body to continue to perform activity as a result of fatigue produced by exercise and environmental heat stress. This is clinically manifested most often by collapse or difficulty continuing activity that occurs *before* the event has finished. Core body temperature (rectal) is commonly elevated between 98.6°F and 104°F. It may be accompanied by nausea, vomiting, diarrhea, headache, muscle cramping, tachycardia, hypotension, weakness, dehydration, and electrolyte depletion. Dehydration can be difficult to judge clinically as the only reliable assessment of dehydration is measurement of water loss that occurs through pre-weight and post-weight measurements. A clear distinction between heat exhaustion and heat stroke is the development of CNS dysfunction such as an altered level of consciousness, delirium, or seizure. Confusion may be present but should be mild and resolve quickly with treatment measures.

Athletes with heat exhaustion should be removed from the heat and placed in a cool, shaded, or air-conditioned environment. Vital signs including a rectal temperature should be measured to ensure the proper diagnosis is made and to be able to monitor cooling status. Any excess clothing should be removed, and the athlete should be placed in a Trendelenburg position or supine with feet elevated. Cooling may be performed initially with placement of ice bags over the groin, axilla, and neck, and water or ice-soaked towels over the head, trunk, and extremities. Immersion in an ice bath, tub of cold water, or simply running cold water from a hose over the athlete may be necessary, but these measures tend to be more for comfort as heat exhaustion is not life threatening. Oral administration of an electrolyte-containing solution is helpful to restore adequate hydration and assists in returning the cardiac output to normal. Intravenous fluid would be beneficial to individuals who do not respond or are not able to take oral fluids. Athletes who do not respond to these measures should be transported to a hospital to monitor for other developing conditions.

Heat Stroke and Heat Injury

Heat stroke is defined as a core body temperature elevated above 104°F associated with central nervous system dysfunction and end-organ damage. The CNS dysfunction can be observed in several ways, including: confusion, delirium, aggression or irritability, seizures, altered consciousness, and coma. Heat stroke can occur as classic heat stroke (non-exertional) or exertional heat stroke. Classic heat stroke usually afflicts the elderly population in the summer season and can be related to a lack of access to adequate air-conditioning. Heat is continually absorbed from the environment and may be poorly dissipated secondary to other medical conditions and medications that preclude cooling. Exertional heat stroke is seen in a younger and more athletic population and does not necessarily occur in hot and humid environments. Other signs and symptoms are similar to those seen in heat exhaustion, but vital sign abnormalities are more likely to be present. The presence or absence of sweating does not make a diagnosis of heat stroke. Examining a collapsed individual can be difficult and the differential diagnosis can extend beyond heat exhaustion and heat stroke to include cardiac arrhythmia and exercise-associated hyponatremia. It is important to maintain a degree of suspicion for those athletes who present with collapse but do not have an elevated core temperature.

The term heat injury is not currently recognized by the World Health Organization as a diagnosis but was created by the US military physicians to further categorize patients suffering from heat illness. Heat injury is diagnosed as an elevation in core temperature above 104°F with associated end-organ damage but lacks the CNS dysfunction seen in heat stroke. Organs most commonly affected with heat stroke or injury include the liver, kidneys, and skeletal muscle (rhabdomyolysis).

Individuals who present with heat stroke should be assessed beginning with basic life support measures. Secure the airway and make sure adequate circulation and breathing are maintained. An initial set of vital signs including a rectal temperature should be performed and repeated throughout the course of treatment. If a rectal thermometer is not available, do not use other methods to determine temperature, as these are inaccurate to measure core temperature in athletes who have been exercising. If available, rapid assessment of serum electrolytes including sodium and glucose should be done, especially with longer endurance events such as marathons. Rapid cooling should commence as soon as possible after the diagnosis is made, as the prognosis worsens the longer the core temperature is elevated. The most effective cooling measure is ice-water immersion and expected cooling rates are about 1°F per 3 minutes or 1°C per 5 minutes of immersion. Measurement with a rectal thermistor allows for continuous monitoring but if this is not available, measurement by a rectal thermometer should be done approximately once every 10 minutes. Cooling should continue until the core temperature reaches 101°F. If no rectal thermometer is available, cool until the athlete begins to shiver or about 15 to 20 minutes. If other interventions need to be performed (intubation, administration of IV medications or fluid) and ice-water immersion is not practical, other cooling tactics such as ice bags to the groin, axilla, and neck, and placement of ice or water-soaked towels to the rest of the body should be performed. Fluid resuscitation should be performed but careful attention should be paid to fluid overload as pulmonary edema can develop with rapid administration of IV fluids. Despite rapid reduction in core temperature, these individuals are still at risk for organ damage and transport to the hospital is usually necessary, where appropriate monitoring and lab evaluation can be performed. Transport to the hospital is always required in patients who do not regain consciousness within 30 minutes of appropriate cooling and medical intervention, or if appropriate response to cooling is not achieved.

Return to Play

The prognosis for returning to physical activity after an episode of EHI is dependent upon the individual and the severity of the illness incurred. Athletes who develop heat cramps or EAC should be allowed to return to activity as soon as they feel capable. Decisions about returning those who develop heat exhaustion or heat stroke are more complicated. These athletes should avoid physical activity for at least 7 days. All lab abnormalities should be corrected, and the athlete should feel physically and psychologically capable of returning. Once these conditions are met, a gradual progression of activity can begin in a cool or temperate environment. Acclimatization occurs over a period of approximately 2 weeks as activity is increased in duration and intensity and the individual is gradually reexposed to heat. Once the athlete can perform full-intensity workouts for 2 to 4 weeks in the heat, they may be returned to competition. For individuals who fail to acclimatize at 4 weeks or who have had multiple episodes of EHI, an exercise-heat tolerance test should be performed.

References

American College of Sports Medicine, Armstrong LE, Casa DJ, et al: American College of Sports Medicine Position Stand. Exertional heat illness during training and competition, *Medicine & Science in Sports & Exercise* 39:556–572, 2007.

Asplund CA, O'Connor FG: Challenging return to play decisions: heat stroke, exertional rhabdomyolysis, and exertional collapse associated with sickle cell trait, *Sports Health* 8(2):117–125, 2016 Mar-Apr.

Boeckmann M, Rohn I: Is planned adaptation to heat reducing heat-related mortality and illness? A systematic review, *BMC Public Health* 14:1112, 2014 Oct 28.

Bouchama A, Knochel JP: Heat Stroke, *New England Journal of Medicine* 346(25):1978–1988, 2002. June 20.

Brukner P, Karim K, Noakes T: *Exercise in the Heat. In Brukner & Khan's Clinical Sports Medicine*, 4th ed., Sydney, 2012, McGraw-Hill, pp 1132–1143.

Cooper ER, Ferrara MS, Casa DJ, et al: Exertional heat illness in american football players: when is the risk greatest? *Journal of Athletic Training* 51(8):593–600, 2016.

Gaudio FG, Grissom CK: Cooling methods in heat stroke, *Journal of Emergency Medicine* 50(4):607–616, 2016 Apr.

Ishimine, P. Heat Stroke in Children. *UpToDate*. N.p., 26 Oct. 2016. Web. 1 Jan. 2017.

Lopez RM, Casa DJ, McDermott BP, et al: Does creatine supplementation hinder exercise heat tolerance or hydration status? A systematic review with meta-analyses, *J Athl Train.* 44(2):215–223, 2009 Mar.

Maron BJ, Doerer JJ, Haas TS, et al: Sudden deaths in young competitive athletes: analysis of 1866 deaths in the United States, 1980-2006, *Circulation* 119(8):1085–1092, 2009.

Miller KC, Mack GW, Knight KL, et al: Reflex inhibition of electrically induced muscle cramps in hypohydrated humans, *Medicine & Science in Sports & Exercise* 42(5):953–961, 2010. May.

O'Connor FG, Casa DJ. Exertional heat illness in adolescents and adults: epidemiology, thermoregulation, risk factors, and diagnosis. *UpToDate*. N.p., 12 Nov 2018. Web. 22 July 2019.

Wexler RK: Evaluation and treatment of heat-related illnesses, *American Family Physician* 65:2307–2314, 2002.

Yeargin SW, Kerr ZY, Casa DJ, et al: Epidemiology of exertional heat illnesses in youth, high school, and college football, *Medicine & Science in Sports & Exercise* 48(8):1523–1529, 2016 Aug.

Zurawlew MJ, Walsh NP, et al: Post-exercise hot water immersion induces heat acclimation and improves endurance exercise performance in the heat, *Scandinavian Journal of Medicine & Science in Sports* 26(7):745–754, 2016 Jul.

HIGH ALTITUDE ILLNESS

Method of
Adrienne N. Kovalsky, DO, MPH; and Ryan M. Commins, MD

CURRENT DIAGNOSIS

Acclimatization
- Symptoms include exertional dyspnea, increased respiratory rate, polyuria, peripheral edema, and insomnia.

High Altitude Headache (HAH)
- New-onset headache that fulfills at least two of the following:
  - Develops in temporal relation to altitude gain above 2500 m (8000 ft)
  - Worsens in conjunction with continued ascent and/or resolves within 24 hours of descent below 2500 m (8000 ft)
  - Includes at least two of the following characteristics: bilateral; mild or moderate intensity; aggravated by exertion, movement, straining, coughing, and/or bending

Acute Mountain Sickness (AMS)
- New-onset headache occurs within 12 hours of altitude gain above 2500 m (8000 ft), and
- Anorexia, nausea, vomiting, fatigue, weakness, dizziness, or lightheadedness (see Box 3).

High Altitude Cerebral Edema (HACE)
- Mental status changes or ataxia with preexisting AMS, or
- Mental status changes and ataxia without a prodrome of AMS

High Altitude Pulmonary Edema (HAPE)
- Relative hypoxemia in the setting of at least two signs or symptoms from each of the following lists:
  - Resting dyspnea, cough, weakness, decreased exercise performance, and chest tightness or congestion
  - Wheezing, rales, tachypnea, tachycardia, or central cyanosis

CURRENT THERAPY

Insomnia or Sleep Disturbance
- Acetazolamide (Diamox)[1] 125 mg PO at bedtime is recommended.
- Consider diphenhydramine (Benadryl) 50 mg at bedtime, zolpidem (Ambien) 5–10 mg at bedtime, or temazepam (Restoril) 15 mg at bedtime for patients with no history of altitude illness.

High Altitude Headache
- Medications for headache include ibuprofen (Advil) 600–800 mg PO every 8 hours, acetaminophen (Tylenol) 650–1000 mg PO every 6 hours, enteric-coated aspirin (Ecotrin) 325–650 mg PO every 4 hours, oxygen by nasal cannula at 1–2 L/min, or acetazolamide[1] 125 mg PO twice daily.

Acute Mountain Sickness, Mild
- Avoid respiratory depressants, strenuous activity, or further ascent until the patient is asymptomatic.
- Acetazolamide 125–250 mg PO twice daily may be tried.
- Symptomatic treatment as for headache and nausea.

Acute Mountain Sickness, Moderate to Severe
- Stop ascent and rest until asymptomatic AND:

- Administer acetazolamide 250 mg PO twice daily.
- Oxygen (1–2 L) or hyperbaric chamber 2–4 psi may be used if available.
- Consider dexamethasone (Decadron)[1] 4 mg PO or IM every 6 hours as an adjunct or if acetazolamide is contraindicated.
- Monitor for mental status changes, confusion, or ataxia and descend immediately at onset.
- If symptoms are severe, or if there is no response to 24 hours of therapy, immediate descent of at least 500 m or to last asymptomatic altitude is the definitive treatment.

High Altitude Cerebral Edema
- Prepare for evacuation or emergent descent of at least 1000 m (3,280 ft).
- Administer dexamethasone[1] 8 mg PO, IM, or IV once followed by 4 mg every 6 hours.
- Consider adding acetazolamide[1] 250 mg PO twice daily as an adjunct.
- Early recognition and treatment are essential.

High Altitude Pulmonary Edema
- Bed rest with oxygen 4–6 L by nasal cannula.
- If the patient is not improving or if HAPE is severe, descend at least 500 m, avoiding exertion.
- Use a hyperbaric chamber at 2–4 psi if oxygen is unavailable or the patient is unable to descend.
- If oxygen is unavailable or the patient is unable to descend, or if the patient is not responding to either:
  - Give nifedipine (Procardia)[1] 10 mg PO once and 30 mg extended-release PO every 12 to 24 hours[3] (contraindicated in HACE).
  - Consider adding tadalafil (Cialis)[1] 10 mg PO twice daily[3], sildenafil (Viagra)[1] 50 mg PO thrice daily[3], or salmeterol (Serevent)[1] 125 μg inhaled twice daily[3].
  - It is not advisable to use both nifedipine and a phosphodiesterase inhibitor; if this becomes necessary, carefully monitor blood pressure and stagger doses to prevent potential cerebral hypoperfusion.

Concurrent High Altitude Pulmonary and Cerebral Edema
- As always, immediate descent and supplemental oxygen therapy are critical.
- Treatment as for HAPE with the addition of dexamethasone.[1]

[1]Not FDA approved for this indication.
[3]Exceeds dosage recommended by the manufacturer.

The appeal of travel to high altitude is vast. For many it is tourism, skiing, or mountaineering, but for others it is far more fundamental, as many travel to high altitudes for work. The number of people residing at elevations higher than 1500 m has risen significantly in the last two decades, and is approximately 440 million worldwide. While elevation greater than 1500 m (5000 ft) is generally considered high altitude (Denver, for example, is 1609 m or 5,278 ft), most high altitude illness occurs above 2500 m or 8000 ft. It is at these altitudes that the effects of hypoxia and decreasing barometric pressure start to be seen. Elevation greater than 5500 m (18,000 ft) is considered extreme altitude. Many persons become symptomatic during the adaptive process known as acclimatization, and some develop acute high altitude syndromes, including acute mountain sickness (AMS), high altitude cerebral edema (HACE), and high altitude pulmonary edema (HAPE). These syndromes are often preventable, but they have the potential to cause significant morbidity and mortality for the patient and for those involved in risky rescue efforts by land or air.

Epidemiology and Risk Factors
The incidence of altitude illnesses is highly variable and commonly idiosyncratic. At 3000 m (~10,000 ft) the incidence of AMS ranges from 4% to 58%, whereas the incidence of HAPE and HACE generally is less than 1%. The occurrence of altitude illness depends on the rate of ascent, altitude of residence, exertion, prior history of altitude illness, and individual susceptibility. For each 1000 m (3,280 ft) above 2500 m (8,000 ft) the rate of AMS increases 13%. The most predictive risk factor for AMS is previous AMS, and the risk of recurrence in similar elevations is as high as 60%. Physical fitness does not alter susceptibility, whereas obesity is a risk factor. Tobacco smoking, asthma, and diabetes do not confer any additional risk. Certain medical conditions including chronic obstructive pulmonary disease, pulmonary hypertension, congestive heart failure, coronary artery disease, sickle cell disease, and sleep apnea increase risk of developing altitude illness. Stable and well-controlled conditions such as hypertension and diabetes do not appear to increase the risk for altitude illness. A more detailed discussion of some of these diseases is included later in the text.

Physiologic Adaptation and Pathophysiology
Hypoxia inducible factors (HIFs) are a family of transcription regulators that respond to level of oxygenation and ultimately control the physiologic response to hypoxia. In hypoxic conditions, they are able to increase transcription of hypoxia-responsive genes. The HIFs have a wide range of effects including increasing glycolysis and angiogenesis, stimulating erythropoiesis, regulating endothelial nitric oxide synthase, and controlling ventilation.

The physiologic response to altitude rests along one end of a spectrum of compensatory mechanisms that can evolve into high altitude syndromes. The pathophysiology of AMS and HACE is incompletely understood, but hypoxemia and changes in the brain itself have been implicated. Hypoxemia is thought to increase cerebral blood flow though it is unclear whether there is a true difference in cerebral blood flow in patients with and without AMS. Hypoxemia may also increase vascular permeability through various mechanisms. Changes that occur in the brain include edema, increased ICP, vascular distention due to increased intravascular pressure, and release of nociceptive chemicals or substances. The development of HAPE is usually preceded by an excessive rise in the pulmonary artery pressure in response to hypoxic vasoconstriction. However, other factors including alveolar inflammation, impaired sodium and water reabsorption by the alveolar epithelium and uneven hypoxic vasoconstriction may also play a role.

In the first few hours at high altitude, peripheral chemoreceptors are activated by hypoxia, leading to an increased respiratory rate. The increased minute ventilation reduces the dilutional effects of CO_2 in the alveolar air and causes a respiratory alkalosis. This subsequent alkalosis also improves oxygen binding in the lung but ultimately slows respiration. After 24 to 48 hours the kidneys excrete excess bicarbonate, normalizing the elevated pH that would otherwise prevent an adequate increase in respiration. This is the basis for acclimatization.

Periodic breathing is also more likely to occur at higher elevations owing to hypoxia and the resulting respiratory alkalosis. Altitude-dependent diuresis causes transient hemoconcentration in the first 1 to 2 days, with true erythropoiesis starting at 4 to 5 days. Long-term residence at altitude can cause polycythemia, increasing the risk for tissue infarction. With permanent residence at high altitude there is evidence that cognitive development may be slowed in children and that neuropsychological function is impaired in adults. Permanent residents will see improved maximal oxygen consumption at lower elevations. The most complex effects of hypobaric hypoxia are seen in the lung and the brain and are not completely understood.

Prevention
High altitude illness is a morbid and potentially fatal disease, and preventive measures should be employed. The most reliable way to prevent altitude illness is through graded ascent, thereby allowing sufficient time for acclimatization. A conservative guideline for activities above 2500 m (8,000 ft) is increasing sleep altitude by no more than 300 m (1000 ft) in a 24-hour period and

BOX 1	Prevention of High Altitude Sickness

Ascent above 2500 m (8,000 ft) should be at a gradual rate of 300 m per 24 hours, with an additional rest day for every 1000 m (3,280 ft) gain

With rapid ascent above 2500 m (8,000 ft), light activity may be helpful with acclimatization, but strenuous activity should be avoided for at least 48 hours.

Avoid respiratory depressants such as alcohol until acclimatized.

Five days of comparable altitude exposure should be undertaken within 2 months of ascent.

For AMS or HACE, begin prophylaxis 1 or 2 days before starting ascent:

- Acetazolamide 125 mg PO bid
- Dexamethasone[1] 2 mg q6 or 4 mg q12 h for patients with sulfa allergy
- Prophylaxis is strongly recommended for patients with a history of AMS or HACE or for rapid ascent.

For persons with a history of HAPE, begin prophylaxis 1 day before starting ascent:

- Nifedipine[1] 30 mg BID[3]
- Salmeterol[1] (adjust) 125 μg inhaled bid[3]
- Dexamethasone[1] 8 mg PO bid
- Tadalafil (Cialis)[1] 10 mg PO bid[3]
- Sildenafil (Viagra)[1] 50 mg PO tid[3]

Stop ascent with onset of even mild AMS to prevent evolution to HACE.

Abbreviations: AMS = acute mountain sickness; HACE = high altitude cerebral edema; HAPE = high altitude pulmonary edema.

[1]Not FDA approved for this indication.

[3]Exceeds dosage recommended by the manufacturer.

BOX 2	Medications for AMS, HACE, and HAPE

Acetazolamide

Acetazolamide (Diamox) is a central-acting respiratory stimulant that causes a metabolic acidosis and ultimately facilitates acclimatization. It is effective in preventing and treating AMS and HACE.[1] Patients should be warned about side effects, including paresthesias, flat taste of carbonated beverages, and polyuria, particularly at night. Persons with a history of asthma, sulfonamide allergy, anaphylaxis, or penicillin allergy should try this medication under the supervision of a medical professional prior to departure. It should not be used in type 1 diabetics due to the risk for ketoacidosis. It also should not be used in chronic lung disease if FEV_1 is less than 25% predicted, in patients on potassium-wasting diuretics, or on long-term high doses of aspirin.

Dexamethasone

Dexamethasone (Decadron)[1] is also effective in the prevention and treatment of AMS and HACE, though its mechanism is not completely understood. Unlike with acetazolamide, symptoms can recur after stopping treatment, and it does not facilitate acclimatization. It is not recommended for prophylaxis of AMS unless acetazolamide is contraindicated, though it is the drug of choice for treatment of HACE. Use is cautioned in diabetics due to hyperglycemia and in patients at risk for amebiasis or strongyloides.

Nifedipine

Nifedipine (Procardia)[1] is a calcium channel blocker that inhibits pulmonary vasoconstriction secondary to hypoxia at high altitude and is used in treatment and prevention of HAPE. Caution should be used with other antihypertensives due to risk for hypotension. Medications that inhibit the cytochrome P450 3A4 pathway, including macrolides, doxycycline, and azoles, may increase plasma concentrations and also precipitate hypotension. Ginkgo biloba[7] may also increase levels of nifedipine and cause hypotension and should be avoided.

Tadalafil (Cialis) and sildenafil (Viagra)

These are phosphodiesterase inhibitors[1] that cause pulmonary vasodilation and are used in preventing HAPE. They should not be used in conjunction with nitrates due to risk for significant hypotension, nor with alpha-blockers due to orthostatic hypotension. Medications that inhibit the cytochrome P450 3A4 pathway, including macrolides, doxycycline, and azoles, may increase plasma concentrations and also precipitate hypotension.

Abbreviations: AMS = acute mountain sickness; HACE = high altitude cerebral edema; HAPE = high altitude pulmonary edema

[1]Not FDA approved for this indication.

[7]Available as a dietary supplement.

---

with an additional rest day every 1000 m (3,280 ft). If symptoms of AMS are noted, no further ascent should be attempted until they resolve in order to prevent more severe illness or evolution of HACE or HAPE. Additional preventive measures should be taken and are of particular importance for persons planning rapid ascent, whether on foot or flying directly into altitudes of 2500 m (8,000 ft) or greater. Light activity can accelerate acclimatization, but strenuous exertion should be avoided in the first 2 days. Pre-exposure of 5 days of comparable altitude within 2 months of ascent is protective. CNS depressants such as alcohol are thought to worsen effects of altitude, particularly overnight when respiration is already more depressed, and they should be avoided. Abrupt cessation of caffeine intake in chronic users may provoke withdrawal symptoms that can mimic AMS. If available, residing and working in an oxygen-enriched environment may also help reduce the incidence of AMS. Refer to Box 1 for a summary.

Medical prophylaxis should be considered when graded ascent is not possible, whether on foot or flying directly into altitudes of 2500 m (8,000 ft) or greater, and for persons with any history of prior altitude illness returning to the same elevation. Prophylaxis is also advised for ascent profiles that are considered moderate to high risk in patients with unknown susceptibility, including planned ascent to more than 3000 m (10,000 ft) in one day, rapid ascent greater than 500 m (1,640 ft) per day above 3000 m (10,000 ft), or very rapid ascent to a final altitude greater than 4000 m (13,000 ft). This should be started the day prior to beginning ascent and continue until at a stable altitude for at least 2 to 4 days. If further ascent is undertaken, or if symptoms recur, prophylaxis can be restarted at any point.

The most effective medication for prophylaxis of AMS and HACE is acetazolamide (Diamox) 125 mg PO twice daily starting 1–2 days before ascent. This is a central-acting respiratory stimulant that causes a metabolic acidosis and ultimately facilitates acclimatization. Patients should be warned about side effects

and possible allergy (Box 2). Dexamethasone (Decadron)[1] 2 mg every 6 hours or 4 mg every 12 hours also is effective, though its mechanism is not completely understood. Unlike with acetazolamide, symptoms can recur after stopping dexamethasone, and it does not facilitate acclimatization. It is not recommended for prophylaxis unless acetazolamide is contraindicated, and it is best saved for treatment of severe AMS or HACE. Ginkgo biloba[7] is no better than placebo at preventing AMS. Ibuprofen (Advil)[1] has not been shown to prevent AMS but does prevent high altitude headache.

Prophylaxis of HAPE has been studied in preventing recurrence in persons with a history of HAPE, though it also would be prudent to consider prophylaxis for anyone undertaking very rapid ascent. Numerous agents have been evaluated in patients with

---

[1]Not FDA approved for this indication.

[7]Available as a dietary supplement.

history of HAPE and are listed in Box 1. Nifedipine (Procardia)[1] is the preferred medication for prevention, with salmeterol (Serevent)[1] as a potential adjunct if there is significant history of HAPE and anticipated rapid ascent profile.

Symptomatic Acclimatization and Disrupted Sleep

Many people experience symptoms of normal adaptation that do not always herald illness, but they should nonetheless always be completely evaluated. Expected symptoms include exertional dyspnea, polyuria, peripheral and facial edema, and nocturnal awakenings and insomnia. The most common side effects of normal acclimatization are disrupted sleep and mild peripheral edema. Acetazolamide[1] 125 mg at bedtime has been shown to decrease nocturnal oxygen saturation and lessen awakenings (see Box 2). Diphenhydramine (Benadryl)[1] 25 to 50 mg may also be used, but it does not have the same benefits. Studies have shown that zolpidem (Ambien)[1] 10 mg and temazepam (Restoril)[1] 15 mg are probably safe, but because studies have been small and targeted, these medications probably should be avoided whenever possible, particularly in persons with a history of altitude illness.

High Altitude Headache

Headache is a common occurrence and does not always evolve into AMS. The headache is generally bilateral, and throbbing is exacerbated with coughing, bending, straining, and exertion, and is often worst early in the morning. There should be no other associated symptoms. Onset can occur within 1 hour but usually begins within 6 to 10 hours. Numerous medications are effective for treatment, including analgesics and medications used in prophylaxis of AMS. See the Current Therapy box for a complete listing.

High Altitude Syndromes

Acute Mountain Sickness

In the setting of a recent gain in altitude, AMS is defined as headache with at least one of the following: anorexia, nausea, or vomiting; fatigue or weakness; or dizziness or lightheadedness. Clinically, a lack of headache with otherwise suggestive symptoms should not rule out AMS. As with high altitude headache, onset can occur within 1 hour but usually begins within 6 to 10 hours. Other symptoms can include decreased urine output, lassitude, and ataxia. All symptoms typically resolve within 2 to 3 days, though on occasion at higher altitudes symptoms can persist for days or weeks without progression or resolution. Examination is normal and no diagnostic studies are indicated. The differential includes dehydration, exhaustion, hangover, viral illness, carbon monoxide poisoning, caffeine withdrawal, migraine, and meningitis. Early recognition of AMS is essential in order to begin appropriate measures that might help prevent evolution to the potentially fatal HACE, which exists along the same spectrum.

If mild, AMS can be monitored at a stable altitude with no further ascent undertaken. Analgesics and antiemetics are effective for managing symptoms. Acetazolamide may be considered for mild AMS and is recommended for moderate to severe symptoms. Dexamethasone[1] may be added, or used in substitution if intolerant of or allergic to acetazolamide, for a short course (less than 5 days) while acclimatizing. Low-flow supplemental oxygen and hyperbaric chambers can be used as an adjunct for moderate to severe symptoms. Descent is advised for symptoms that progress after 24 hours of rest or treatment or for symptoms that are severe or stable but prolonged in order to prevent evolution to HACE, but graded ascent can be resumed once symptoms resolve. Immediate descent should be undertaken for ataxia, altered mental status, or any signs or symptoms of pulmonary edema. Refer to the Current Therapy box for dosing and summary.

High Altitude Cerebral Edema

In the setting of a recent gain in altitude, HACE is defined as a change in mental status and/or ataxia in a person with AMS, or both mental status changes and ataxia in a person without AMS. There may be changes in mood or hallucinations. It generally progresses over 1 to 3 days, but it can also cause loss of consciousness within 12 hours. Examination has nonfocal neurologic findings with confusion. Papilledema may be seen, and rales are often present from concurrent HAPE. If computed tomography (CT) or magnetic resonance imaging (MRI) is available acutely, findings would be consistent with vasogenic edema. If a lumbar puncture is performed, increased opening pressure is usually present.

Differential diagnosis is similar to that for AMS but should be expanded to include diabetic ketoacidosis, hypoglycemia, electrolyte imbalances, brain tumor, stroke, acute psychosis, and seizure. After a long term at altitude or any length of time at very high altitudes blood can become hyperviscous and increasingly thrombogenic, so in these circumstances stroke should rise on the differential.

Early recognition is crucial in management of HACE to prevent evolution to irreversible disease. The most important element of treatment is descent of at least 1000 m (3,280 ft). Supplemental oxygen and hyperbaric bags may be used during descent and are imperative if descent is not possible. Dexamethasone[1] should be initiated, and should be continued after descent if symptoms persist. Acetazolamide[1] may be added. Dosages are listed in the Current Therapy box.

High Altitude Pulmonary Edema

In the setting of a recent gain in altitude, HAPE is diagnosed with at least two of resting dyspnea, cough, weakness or decreased exercise performance, and chest tightness or congestion and two of wheezing or rales, tachypnea, tachycardia, or central cyanosis. There may also be an associated low-grade temperature elevation. Cough is initially dry but in late stages is productive of pink or bloody sputum. Onset often occurs during sleep, usually the second night at altitude, and often after the use of sleep aids that cause respiratory depression. It rarely occurs after 4 or 5 days at a stable altitude and should resolve within 48 hours of descent.

Examination is significant for rales that can begin in the right axilla and progress diffusely and for low-grade temperature elevation. Hypoxia, often very pronounced, is noted on pulse oximetry; oxygen levels will be disproportionately low for a given elevation. If available, chest radiography typically demonstrates bilaterally diffuse patchy opacities without pulmonary vascular changes, though initially they may be seen in the right middle lobe. Computed tomography of the chest typically shows a patchy peripheral and nodular distribution of edema. Ultrasound may be more readily available than radiography in remote locations and through the use of the comet-tail technique may be helpful in identifying HAPE and differentiating from pneumonia or other conditions.

HAPE can occur in conjunction with severe AMS or HACE. Differential includes heart failure, acute myocardial ischemia, pulmonary embolus, asthma, bronchitis, and pneumonia. Among the altitude illnesses, HAPE is associated with the highest rate of mortality but, unlike HACE, it is unlikely to cause long-term sequelae if treated appropriately. As with all altitude illness, removing the hypoxic stimulus is the central principle in management, and with HAPE it is also the most effective. This can be done with descent, supplemental oxygen, or a hyperbaric chamber. If available, supplemental oxygen and bed rest may be sufficient. If the pulmonary edema is severe, descent is the definitive treatment and should be undertaken without delay. Exertion and cold stress should be avoided during descent. Nifedipine (Adalat, Procardia)[1] and salmeterol (Serevent)[1] may be of benefit in treatment of HAPE, but they are not as effective as oxygen or descent and should be used as an adjunct or if no other alternatives exist.

---

[1] Not FDA approved for this indication.

---

[1] Not FDA approved for this indication.

Dual vasodilating agent use (nifedipine[1] and a phosphodiesterase inhibitor[1]) is not recommended, but if attempted when no alternatives exist, doses should be staggered and blood pressure carefully monitored to prevent potentially disastrous hypotension and cerebral hypoperfusion. Refer to the Current Therapy box for dosing. Reascent may be considered 2 to 3 days after resolution, but risk of recurrence is significantly higher.

Other High Altitude Disorders
Upper Respiratory Disorders
Rhinorrhea, chronic cough, and noninfectious pharyngitis and bronchitis are commonly seen at high altitude and very prevalent at extreme altitude. Sputum is often purulent. Onset of high altitude bronchitis and chronic cough is generally after strenuous activity, and use of a balaclava to increase humidification of inhaled air may help prevent this. Symptoms may become severe enough to cause rib fracture. Comprehensive studies on the most effective treatment are lacking, but symptomatic therapies may be helpful, including decongestant nasal sprays, inhaled corticosteriods and beta agonists, and codeine-based cough medications; the latter should never be used in the pediatric population or in combination with other opiate medications or benzodiazepines. Infectious upper respiratory syndromes should remain in the differential; however, viral etiologies are most common with judicious consideration of antibiotic therapy.

High Altitude Retinopathy (HAR)
Hypoxia is known to cause hyperemia and engorgement of the retinal vessels at any elevation, and will be seen above 2500 meters (8,000 ft) in the setting of hypobaric hypoxia. Evolution to retinal hemorrhage indicates the presence of high altitude retinopathy (HAR) and may occur above 4000 meters (13,000 ft). Macular or vitreous hemorrhage, disc edema, and cotton wool spots can be seen in more severe HAR. There may be a delay between ascent and onset of hemorrhage. The retinopathy is generally asymptomatic; however, scotomas and visual field deficits may occur, particularly with macular hemorrhage.

Lower oxygen saturation, higher ascent, strenuous exertion, and longer duration at high altitude are associated with HAR. Higher baseline intraocular pressure, hypercoagulable disorders, and aspirin and NSAID use also appear to be risk factors. Slower ascent and improved acclimatization are protective. Acetazolamide does not appear to affect incidence. Recent research has not shown a definitive correlation between HAR and AMS or HACE.

Most HAR will resolve within days to weeks of descent. Rarely visual deficits have persisted longer. Descent is recommended for any premacular hemorrhage due to higher risk to central vision and unclear long-term prognosis, as well as any new visual deficits. Given the potential risk of worsening retinopathy, diabetics and other patients with risk for or preexisting retinopathy should avoid travel to elevations greater than 4000 meters (13,000 ft), and consult with their ophthalmologist if such travel is unavoidable or if any travel is intended above 2500 meters (8,000 ft).

Chronic High Altitude Diseases
Residence above 2500 meters (8,000 ft) in the United States is rising, and numbers in the hundreds of millions worldwide. Prevalence is dependent on many factors, most notably residence altitude and ethnicity. Ethnic groups with longer history of high altitude residence, such as Tibetans, have improved adaptation and lower prevalence compared to other ethnic groups at the same elevation. Prevalence increases with increasing altitude, even among more adapted ethnic groups.

Chronic Mountain Sickness (CMS). Symptoms include headache, dizziness, dyspnea, palpitations, insomnia, fatigue, arthralgias, myalgias, distal peripheral paresthesias, anorexia, and cognitive dysfunction. Diagnosis is made by excessive erythrocytosis (hemoglobin greater than 19 g/dL in women or 21 g/dL in men) in the setting of severe hypoxemia (there is not yet consensus on threshold value, but less than <85% is highly suggestive),

normal pulmonary function tests, and chronic residence above 2500 meters (8,000 ft). Pulmonary hypertension and heart failure may also be present. Patients with a history of antecedent chronic pulmonary disease such as COPD or other medical condition that may account for hypoxia are excluded from this diagnosis, as the presentation cannot be fully attributed to altitude, though consideration for a diagnosis of secondary CMS may be made. Phlebotomy, optimally with isovolemic hemodilution, provides temporary benefit and may result in more significant recurrence and is not recommended as a long-term solution. Consideration may be made for severe symptoms or as a short-term bridge to permanent resettlement at lower elevation. Supplemental oxygen, slow breathing technique, a supervised mild to moderate exercise regimen, and intermittent pulses of acetazolamide[1] 250 mg per day for three weeks have all been found to help. Other medications are still being studied. Strenuous activity should be avoided. Definitive therapy is migration to lower elevations, upon which CMS will slowly resolve, but will reappear upon return to high altitude. Periodic travel to lower altitude is recommended if permanent migration is not possible.

High Altitude Pulmonary Hypertension (HAPH). Symptoms include cough, dyspnea, cyanosis, and insomnia, and may include physical findings of right heart failure. Diagnosis is made by a mean pulmonary artery pressure greater than 30 mmHg or systolic pulmonary artery pressure greater than 50 mmHg measured at altitude of residence with moderate hypoxemia, absence of excessive erythrocytosis, and chronic residence above 2500 meters (8,000 ft) after the exclusion of chronic lung disease and other causes of pulmonary hypertension. Screening diagnosis should be made by echocardiography and confirmed via invasive measurement. As with CMS, definitive therapy is migration to low altitude. If this is not feasible, calcium channel blockers and phosphodiesterase inhibitors may be of benefit. Early referral to a pulmonary hypertension specialist is recommended.

Additional Considerations
Traveling to high altitude with children, during pregnancy or in the setting of chronic medical conditions includes additional considerations, some of which are summarized below. Patients should include consultation with the patient's pediatrician, obstetrician, or specialist prior to travel. Complete medication list, including as-needed prescriptions for travel, such as antibiotics, should be carefully reviewed for interactions, contraindications, and dose adjustments prior to prescribing medications for prevention or treatment of altitude illness. Refer to Box 2 for a limited summary.

Children
Susceptibility of the pediatric population to altitude illness is comparable to that of the adult population. Travel to high altitude should not be undertaken in first 4 to 6 weeks or in prematurity. It should also be avoided in any children with history of cardiopulmonary conditions, Down syndrome, at increased risk for pulmonary hypertension, or a recent upper respiratory illness. Presentation will generally mimic that in adults; however, assessment of nonverbal children is more complicated with criteria including fussiness, decreased playfulness, decreased appetite, and sleep disturbance. Physical findings are similar to the adult population and may also include agitation, productive cough, cyanosis, and tachycardia. Management and prevention are comparable with the following dosage adjustments: acetazolamide* 2.5 mg/kg every 12 hours can be used for prevention and treatment of both AMS and HACE[1]. Dexamethasone[1] 0.15 mg/kg every 6 hours should be used for treatment of severe AMS and HACE, in conjunction with descent. Medications to prevent and treat HAPE have not been adequately studied in the pediatric population.

---

[1] Not FDA approved for this indication.
*Acetazolamide is approved for use in children aged 12 years and older only.

Pregnant Women

Women who travel to high altitude during pregnancy are at higher risk for preterm labor, but the rate of complications does not appear to be significantly changed in the setting of uncomplicated low-risk pregnancy, and travel to 2500 meters (8,000 ft) is likely safe. While exercise during pregnancy is associated with better outcome, it should be minimized the first few days at high altitude while acclimatizing, and strenuous exertion should be avoided. Most medications used for the treatment of high altitude illness are rated category C for pregnancy, and priority should be made for descent rather than medical management of altitude illness. Travel to high altitude should be avoided in any pregnancy that is complicated or not low risk. Residence at high altitude during pregnancy is associated with a decrease in birth rate in proportion to the increase in altitude, as well as increased complications, although highland ancestry is protective.

Hypertension

Blood pressure response to high altitude is variable. Adequately controlled hypertension should not confer any additional risk for altitude illness. Any patient requiring more than one medication or maximum dose of one medication should travel with a blood pressure cuff and monitor their blood pressure. These patients should also develop an algorithm with their physician for how to manage elevated blood pressure and when to decrease or hold doses.

Coronary Artery Disease (CAD)

All patients with known history or antecedent symptoms should undergo risk stratification, cardiac stress testing, and consult with their cardiologist. Patients with stable CAD who are able to exercise will likely tolerate travel to high altitude. It is advisable to avoid exertion until acclimatized, or for at least 4 to 5 days. Subsequent exertion should be below tolerated exertion at their elevation of residence, and strenuous exercise should be avoided. Other patients, including those with abnormal stress tests, angina, or acute coronary syndrome within six months without revascularization, should not travel to altitude.

Heart Failure

High altitude may increase risk for decompensation of chronic heart failure, and patients with poorly compensated heart failure should avoid travel. If heart failure is stable and controlled, patients may tolerate travel to altitude less than 3000 meters, but physical activity should remain below what is tolerated at their altitude of residence. These patients should monitor their body weight and develop an algorithm with their physician for how to adjust diuretics for increasing edema or weight gain.

Respiratory Conditions

Asthma. Allergic asthma will likely improve at high altitude, but asthma that is exercise- or cold-induced may be made worse. An optimized pre-travel medical regimen should be continued, and these patients should travel with additional rescue medications, including bronchodilators and corticosteroids. Patients should travel with an up-to-date asthma action plan and know where to seek medical attention for an exacerbation that cannot be managed independently. Travel should be avoided in moderate persistent or severe asthma, history of hospitalization, or recent exacerbation.

Chronic Obstructive Pulmonary Disease (COPD). Studies evaluating patients with COPD at high altitude are limited, and data from commercial flights assess exposure of insufficient duration to evaluate risk for high altitude illness. Those who are chronically hypoxemic may have some tolerance to hypobaric hypoxia due to their adaptations to chronic hypoxia. Data is more limited on patients with chronic carbon dioxide retention, and these patients should avoid travel to high altitude. Those with an $FEV_1 < 1$ liter should travel with supplemental oxygen. If FEV_1 is 1–1.5 liters, patients should be assessed by their pulmonologist for possible initiation of supplemental oxygen after arrival at altitude. If supplemental oxygen is already being utilized, the anticipated increase in flow rate may be estimated by the ratio of higher to lower barometric pressure. Patients who have dyspnea at rest or with minimal exertion should not travel to altitudes higher than residence. High-altitude travel also should be avoided if there is a history of frequent recurrent exacerbations or hospitalizations. The home medical regimen should be optimized, and patients should travel with additional rescue medications and inhalers. All patients should travel with a pulse oximeter and seek medical attention for new persistent respiratory symptoms, hypoxia, or fatigue. Acetazolamide should not be used in patients with severe COPD or history of CO_2 retention.

Pulmonary Hypertension. Patients with pulmonary hypertension are at increased risk for developing HAPE and should be educated about the clinical presentation and treatment of HAPE. If mean pulmonary arterial pressure is 35 mm Hg or greater, or if systolic pulmonary arterial pressure is 50 mm Hg or greater, patients should travel with supplemental oxygen. If not on vasodilator therapy, these patients should also be started on nifedipine[1] 30mg SR BID. Those with milder pulmonary hypertension should monitor oxygen saturation and consider prophylaxis with nifedipine[1] 30mg SR BID. Pre-travel evaluation by a pulmonary hypertension specialist is recommended.

Sleep Apnea. Patients with obstructive sleep apnea tend to do better at high altitudes than those with central sleep apnea, but both of these populations should continue CPAP while at altitude. Older machines may lack pressure-compensating features and thus need intended CPAP pressure adjusted at high altitude. In patients not using CPAP, acetazolamide prophylaxis is recommended.

Other Considerations. Travel to high altitude should be avoided in patients with obesity hypoventilation or bilateral carotid body resection. If such travel is unavoidable, supplemental oxygen should be used and any home use of CPAP should be continued while at altitude.

Diabetes Mellitus

Patients with controlled type 1 diabetes do not appear to be at higher risk for AMS. Those with type II diabetes may be at higher risk for AMS, possibly related to other underlying risk factors and the metabolic syndrome. The elevated risk for cerebrovascular accident in diabetics may be further increased at high altitude. The prevalence of diabetes is lower at higher altitudes.

Metabolism and glucose control will change at altitude. Basal metabolic rate will increase, appetite may be suppressed, and absorption may be slowed, but hypoxia also causes hyperglycemia. Close glucose monitoring is imperative. Glucose-monitoring devices may lose accuracy, though glucose dehydrogenase-based glucometers may have more reliable performance. Malfunction risk is decreased if devices are kept warm. Acetaminophen may cause hyperglycemia, and care should be taken in use for HAH. Hydration is also particularly important for diabetic patients, particularly type 1, which can be self monitored by urine output and color.

Despite the above changes at altitude that suggest later administration of prandial insulin, there may also be a delay in the effects of rapid-acting insulin with increasing elevation, which may require earlier administration. This will also be affected by rate of ascent, acclimatization, exertion, and of course diet. Given this variability and individual response, patients should track their specific responses upon ascent and factor this in during descent, particularly if rapid, as is often the case. Glucose should be checked at a greater frequency to assess response, and any insulin administration should be adjusted accordingly. Continuous glucose monitoring may help track trends but, given the lag time compared to capillary testing and lack of studies at high altitude, probably only be used in conjunction with capillary testing.

---

[1] Not FDA approved for this indication.

In Type 1 diabetes, travel to altitude induces hyperglycemia initially and with any acute hypoxia or further ascent. After acclimatization there is a decrease in fasting glucose, and a further drop with exertion. The initial hypoxia-induced hyperglycemia may contribute to ketonuria as well as ketoacidosis, particularly with rapid ascent. This is particularly notable at very high to extreme elevations, and increased exertion and decreased appetite at these elevations may not be adequate to compensate for this hyperglycemia. Risk for DKA is increased due to these metabolic effects of altitude as well as the increased risk infectious diarrhea in some high-altitude regions, changes in diet, and certain medications. As symptoms of AMS, HACE, and diarrheal illness may mimic DKA, onset of symptoms of AMS or HACE, diarrhea in the setting of hyperglycemia, or suspected DKA warrants immediate descent.

Use of an insulin pump at altitude in controlled type 1 diabetics appears safe without significant pump dysfunction, though with rapid pressure changes such as cabin pressurization during air travel there have been reports of bubble formation affecting insulin delivery. It is advisable to also carry injectable insulin in case of pump failure. Use of acetazolamide is not advisable for type 1 diabetics due to increased risk for acidosis and diuresis increasing risk for dehydration. Dexamethasone should also be avoided due to the risk for hyperglycemia. This should be reserved for treatment of severe AMS, HACE, or if descent is not possible but emergent descent is a priority.

Type 2 diabetics do not appear to have the same extent of glycemic changes, though they may also experience hyperglycemia with initial ascent and hypoxia. Once acclimatized, they may need to decrease doses of sulfonylurea medications and insulin due to increased basal metabolic rate. It may be safe to use acetazolamide with caution in type 2 diabetes if not on insulin. Dexamethasone will cause hyperglycemia.

All travel companions should be educated on the signs and symptoms of hyper- and hypoglycemia, diabetic ketoacidosis (DKA) if applicable, overlap between these and AMS, HACE, and gastrointestinal illness, and how these conditions should be managed. Patients with poorly controlled or brittle diabetes should not travel to high altitude. Sedentary patients are advised to discuss cardiac stress testing with their physician.

References

Antony KM, Ehrenthal D, Evensen A, et al: Travel during pregnancy: considerations for the obstetric provider, *Obstet Gynecol Surv* 72(2):97–115, 2017.
Barthelmes D, Bosch MM, Merz TM, et al: Delayed appearance of high altitude retinal hemorrhages, *PLoS ONE* 6(2):1–7, 2011.
Bartsch P, Maggiorini M, Ritter M, et al: Prevention of high-altitude pulmonary edema by nifedipine, *N Engl J Med* 325:1284–1289, 1991.
Butler FK, Harris DJ, Reynolds RD: Altitude retinopathy on Mount Everest, *Ophthalmology* 99(5):739–746, 1992.
Campbell AD, McIntosh SE, Nyberg A, et al: Risk stratification for athletes and adventurers in high-altitude environments: recommendations for preparticipation evaluation, *Wilderness Environ Med* 26:S30–S39, 2015.
Ghofrani HA, Reichenberger F, Kohstall M, et al: Sildenafil increased exercise capacity during hypoxia at low altitudes and at Mount Everest base camp: a randomized, double-blind, placebo-controlled crossover trial, *Ann Intern Med* 141:169–177, 2004.
Hackett PH, Roach RC: High-altitude medicine and physiology. In Auerbach PS, editor: *Wilderness Medicine*, 6th ed., Philadelphia, 2012, Mosby, pp 2–33.
Ho TY, Kao WF, Lee SM, et al: High-altitude retinopathy after climbing Mount Aconcagua in a group of experienced climbers, *Retina* 31(8):1650–1655, 2011.
Joy E, Van Baak K, Dec KL, et al: Wilderness preparticipation evaluation and considerations for special populations, *Wild Env Med* 26:576–591, 2015.
Leon-Velarde F, Maggiorini M, Reeves JT, et al: Consensus statement on chronic and subacute high altitude diseases, *High Alt Med Biol* 6(2):147–157, 2005.
Luks AM: Should travelers with hypertension adjust their medications when traveling to high altitude, *High Alt Med Biol* 10:11–15, 2009.
Luks AM, Hackett PH: High altitude and common medical problems. In Swenson ES, Bartsch P, editors: *High Altitude: Human Adaptation to Hypoxia*, New York, 2014, Springer, pp 449–477.
Luks AM, Swenson ER: Medication and dosage considerations in the prophylaxis and treatment of high-altitude illness, *Chest* 133:744–755, 2008.
Luks AM, Swenson ER, Bärtsch P: Acute high-altitude sickness, *Eur Respir Rev* 26(143):214–220, 2017.
Maggiorini M, Brunner-La Rocca HP, Peth S, et al: Both tadalafil and dexamethasone may reduce the incidence of high-altitude pulmonary edema, *Ann Intern Med* 145:497–506, 2006.
Matejko B, Gawrecki A, Wrobel M, et al: Type 1 diabetes at high altitude: performance of personal insulin pumps and patient metabolic control, *Diabetes Technol Ther* 19(10):600–602, 2017.
McFadden DM, Houston CS, Sutton JR, et al: High-altitude retinopathy, *JAMA* 245(6):581–586, 1981.
del Mol P, de Vries ST, de Koning EJ, et al: Physical activity at altitude: challenges for people with diabetes: a review, *Diabetes Care* 37(8):2404–2413, 2014.
Oelz O, Maggiorini M, Ritter M, et al: Nifedipine for high altitude pulmonary oedema, *Lancet* 2:1241–1244, 1989.
Richards P, Hillebrandt D: Clinicians corner. The practical aspects of insulin at high altitude, *High Alt Med Biol* 14:197–204, 2013.
Roach RC, Hackett PH, Oelz O, et al: The 2018 Lake Louise Acute Mountain Sickness Score, *High Alt Med Biol.* 19:1–4, 2018.
Schneider M, Bernasch D, Weymann J, et al: Acute mountain sickness: influence of susceptibility, pre-exposure and ascent rate, *Med Sci Sports Exerc* 34:1886–1891, 2002.
West JB: Physiological effects of chronic hypoxia, *N Engl J Med* 376(20):1965–1971, 2017.
Woolcott OO, Adler M, Bergman RN: Glucose homeostasis during short tern and prolonged exposure to high altitudes, *Endocr Rev* 36(2):149–173, 2015 (for elevation ref.
Zafren K, Reeves JT, Schoene R: Treatment of high-altitude pulmonary edema by bed rest and supplemental oxygen, *Wilderness Environ Med* 7(2):127–132, 1996.

MARINE POISONINGS, ENVENOMATIONS, AND TRAUMA

Method of
Allen Perkins, MD, MPH

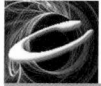

CURRENT DIAGNOSIS

- History of exposure is necessary for diagnosis.
- Ingested toxins can cause unusual symptoms, predominately gastrointestinal.
- Jellyfish envenomation is very painful but almost always self-limited.
- Trauma management follows principles of dirty wounds.
- Specific marine pathogens should be covered if contamination is suspected.

CURRENT THERAPY

Ingestions
- Avoidance is the best strategy.
- Early decontamination with activated charcoal (Actidose-Aqua) can reduce duration of symptoms.
- Symptomatic care is generally sufficient.

Jellyfish
- Remove visible stingers.
- Control pain with topical analgesia.

Trauma
- Avoiding water at feeding time can help avoid injury.
- If envenomation is suspected, consider hot water immersion.
- Tetanus status should be checked.
- Antibiotic coverage should take marine pathogens into account.

The United States has more than 80,000 miles of coastline, and more people are enjoying water-dependent recreation activities such as scuba diving, snorkeling, and surfing. As a consequence, people are more likely to suffer trauma, envenomation, or poisoning related to an encounter with a marine creature, which will come to the attention of a physician. The science of marine medicine is limited; hence, treatment of these conditions is largely based on case reports and expert opinion; very few randomized, controlled studies are

---

BOX 1 Symptom Patterns Associated With Ciguatera Fish Poisoning

Gastrointestinal Pattern
Onset 15 minutes to 24 hours, typically worsens, lasts 1–2 days and resolves
- Nausea and/or vomiting
- Profuse, watery diarrhea
- Abdominal pain

Neurologic Pattern
Onset up to 24 hours after ingestion, commonly nonphysiologic pattern, can last several months
- Numbness and paresthesias
- Vertigo
- Ataxia
- Severe weakness or lethargy
- Severe myalgia
- Decreased vibration and pain sensations
- Diffuse pain pattern
- Cold sensation reversal
- Coma

Cardiovascular Pattern
Onset up to 24 hours after ingestion is uncommon but occurs rapidly
- Bradycardia
- Hypotension
- Cardiovascular collapse

---

available. Misdiagnosis is common, especially when the patient has returned from vacationing or when the patient has been poisoned by improperly handled seafood. This article describes common ailments and injuries occurring as a consequence of direct contact with sea creatures and discusses management and prevention.

Ingestions
Ciguatera Fish Poisoning
Epidemiology

Ciguatera fish poisoning (CFP) is the most commonly reported marine toxin disease in the world. It is caused by human ingestion of reef fish that have bioaccumulated sufficient amounts of the dinoflagellate *Gambierdiscus toxicus*, either through direct ingestion or through ingestion of smaller reef fish. Although limited to tropical regions, it is heat and cold tolerant, is lipid soluble, and can survive transport to other areas. The toxin becomes more concentrated as it passes up the food chain; fish such as amberjack, grouper, and snapper pose less of a risk than predatory fish such as barracuda and moray eel. Ciguatera fish poisoning affects at least 50,000 people worldwide annually, and there are several thousand cases of poisoning in Puerto Rico, the U.S. Virgin Islands, Hawaii, and Florida each year.

Clinical Features

Patients can exhibit a primarily gastrointestinal (diarrhea, abdominal cramps, and vomiting), neurologic (parasthesias, diffuse pain, blurred vision), cardiac (bradycardia), or mixed pattern of symptoms. Additionally, a cold sensation reversal, in which a patient perceives the cold temperatures as a hot sensation and vice versa, occurs in 80% of patients and is considered pathognomonic for ciguatera poison (Box 1).

The attack rate is high. As many as 80% to 100% of people who ingest affected fish develop symptoms depending on the size of the fish and the toxin load. Ingestion of internal organs where the toxin accumulates (e.g., liver, roe) is associated with more severe symptoms, but avoiding these organs is not protective. The symptoms are also related to the number of exposures over time, and patients typically have more severe symptoms with subsequent exposures. There is no age-related susceptibility, and no immunity is acquired through exposure.

Symptoms typically begin 1 to 6 hours after ingestion, although a delay of 12 to 24 hours can occur. Duration is 7 to 14 days, and neurologic symptoms occasionally persist for months to years. Chronic ciguatera syndrome can also occur as a constellation of symptoms such as general malaise, depression, headaches, muscle aches, and dysesthesias in the extremities. Patients with chronic disease report recurrences with ingestion of fish, ethanol, caffeine, and nuts up to 6 months after the acute illness resolves.

Diagnosis

The diagnosis should be entertained in any patient who has neurologic, gastrointestinal, or cardiac symptoms and a history of ingesting predatory fish within the past 24 hours. The symptom constellation can be similar to other ingestions, such as certain shellfish toxins, and differentiation requires knowledge of the patient's diet for the previous day. Additionally, scombroid and type E botulinum poisoning should be considered, but these are unlikely if the patient did not ingest ill-appearing game. Other poisonings, such as organophosphates, can produce a similar symptom complex. There are no currently available clinical assays to assist in making the diagnosis, which is based on clinical suspicion and knowledge of the patient's diet history.

Treatment

If CFP is suspected soon after ingestion, I would consider gut decontamination with activated charcoal (Actidose-Aqua) because it can reduce the toxin load and subsequent symptoms. Initial symptomatic treatment typically consists of fluid replacement to replace gastrointestinal losses.

Atropine (AtroPen) is used in patients who have bradycardia. Temporary electrical pacing may be used for refractory symptoms, and pressors may be needed in cases of severe hypotension. Neurologic symptoms are problematic because of their extended course as well as their severity. Mannitol (Osmitrol)[1] is often cited as effective in reducing the duration of neurologic symptoms, but I would use it with caution because the only double-blind trial failed to show any benefit. There are many local remedies used throughout the world that are said to be successful, which likely attests to the self-limited course of the ingestion in most cases. Table 1 offers more details regarding treatments currently used for CFP.

Prevention

Prevention is difficult except by avoiding ingestion of affected reef fish. The toxin is not deactivated by cooking, freezing, smoking, or salting. There are no outward signs of ciguatera: The fish look, taste, and smell normal. Although several commercial assays are available, they are neither sensitive nor specific enough to be relied on to prevent CFP.

To decrease the risk of CFP, I recommend the following steps: Avoid warm-water reef fish, especially those caught where ciguatera poisoning is known to occur; avoid moray eel injection; avoid ingesting large game fish; avoid consuming the internal organs; and limit the amount of initial ingestion if you are in an area where ciguatera is known to occur. Additionally, patients travelling to distant locales should be made aware that, although the vast majority of cases result from direct ingestion, there have been cases of CFP passed through sexual contact and through breast milk, so they should be wary of body fluid contact if ciguatoxin is endemic to the area, if for no other reasons.

Scombroid
Epidemiology

Scombroid poisoning (also known as histamine fish poisoning) results from improper handling of certain fish between the time the fish is caught and the time it is cooked. In the United States it is most common in Hawaii and California. Improper preservation and refrigeration lead to histamine and histamine-like substances being produced in the dark meat of certain fish through a conversion of histidine to histamine by bacterial decarboxylases. Members of the family Scombridae, such as tuna and mackerel, contain the highest amounts of this substance, but both scombroid

---

[1] Not FDA approved for this indication.

TABLE 1 Treatment for Ciguatera Fish Poisoning

DRUG	DOSE	INDICATION
Activated charcoal (Actidose-Aqua)	Children <1 y: 1 g/kg	Gut emptying and decontamination
	Children 1–12 y: 25–50 g	
	Adults: 25–100 g	More effective in first hour
Antiemetics (no preference)	Administer per dosing recommendations	Intractable nausea and/or vomiting
Intravenous fluid bolus and infusion (normal saline or lactated Ringer's as initial)	Per volume replacement protocols	Hypovolemia
Atropine (AtroPen)	0.5–1.0 mg IV every 3–5 min to a maximum dose of 0.04 mg/kg per episode	Bradycardia
	Maximum total dose: 3 mg for adults, 2 mg for adolescents, 1 mg for young children	
Pressors: Dopamine (Intropin), dobutamine (Dobutrex), epinephrine	Varies with clinical response	Hypotension, shock
Antihistamines (no preference)	Administer per dosing recommendations	Pruritus
Mannitol (Osmitrol)[1]	1 g/kg of a 20% solution given IV over several h	Neurologic symptoms, double-blind study did not show benefit
	Adult dose: 25–100 g, titrate to urinary output of 100 mL/h	
Amitriptyline (Elavil)[1]	25–75 mg PO bid for patients >25 kg	Pruritus, dysesthesias

[1]Not FDA approved for this indication.

and nonscombroid fish have been associated with the disease. The production of toxins requires the introduction of bacteria during the handling process, primarily during storage at high temperatures. It is the total amount of histamine, the presence of other biogenic amines, and individual susceptibility that determine the severity of the symptoms.

Clinical Features
The patient develops a histamine reaction 20 to 30 minutes after ingestion. Symptoms can be cutaneous, gastrointestinal, neurologic, or hemodynamic, or any combination of these. Cutaneous symptoms include flushing, urticaria and conjunctival injection, and localized edema; gastrointestinal symptoms include dry mouth, nausea, vomiting, diarrhea, and abdominal cramping; neurologic symptoms include severe headache and dizziness; and hemodynamic symptoms include palpitations and hypotension. In severe cases there can be bronchospasm and respiratory distress. These symptoms typically come on rapidly (within several minutes) and last less than 6 to 8 hours. Flushing is the most consistent clinical sign, occurring on exposed areas so it typically resembles sunburn. Diarrhea is also very common, occurring in 75% of symptomatic patients.

Diagnosis
As with ciguatera, the diagnosis is one of history. If the time between ingestion and illness is short and the patient has ingested a type of fish previously implicated in scombroid, then a tentative diagnosis can be made. The diagnosis is often confused with an allergic reaction. It can be distinguished from allergy by the lack of a previous allergic reaction as well as by testing the remaining fish for histamine, although testing is rarely warranted.

Treatment
Treatment is the same as for any histamine reaction, the cornerstone of which is antihistamine. Diphenhydramine (Benadryl) 50 mg for adults and 0.5–1 mg/kg/dose for children, repeated every 4 hours until symptoms abate, is delivered either intravenously or intramuscularly in severe cases and orally for milder cases. For severe cases, cimetidine (Tagamet)[1] 300 mg for adults, 20 mg/kg for children, either orally or intravenously, might be

added for more complete histamine-receptor blockade. In cases where ingestion was recent, consider induced emesis using syrup of ipecac: 15 mL for children younger than 12 years or 30 mL otherwise. Most patients require only reassurance, and pharmacologic treatment will be unnecessary. It should be stressed to the patient that this is not an *allergic* reaction to fish, because the histamine is exogenous. Prevention is possible in regions where food storage and preparation are monitored through identification and removal of suspect fish.

Other Ingested Toxins
In addition to the toxins just discussed, ingestion of certain other marine creatures can lead to problems.

Ingestion of bivalves harvested from contaminated waters has been associated with hepatitis A, Norwalk virus, *Vibrio parahaemolyticus* and *Vibrio vulnificans* infections, the latter two particularly problematic and occasionally fatal in immunocompromised patients. I counsel patients likely to be immunocompromised, including diabetics and those with known liver disease, to avoid uncooked bivalves.

Shellfish are occasionally known to contain one or more of several toxins acquired through bioaccumulation of certain algae. These dinoflagellates tend to bloom in summer months. The symptoms occur immediately after ingestion and last several hours and are typically neurologic or gastrointestinal, or both. The shellfish poisoning syndromes are known as paralytic, neurologic, diarrheal, or amnestic depending on the predominant symptom. The care is typically supportive. Public health officials typically monitor local mollusk populations fairly carefully and alert the public to possible hazards.

Ingestion of the flesh of certain puffer fish has been associated with tetrodotoxin poisoning. The flesh of the fish (fugu) is considered a delicacy. The toxin builds up in internal organs such as the liver and the roe. If the toxin is ingested, it is likely to be fatal, but there are certified chefs who are trained in avoiding the toxin when preparing the dish. Despite this precaution, as many as 50 deaths occur in Japan annually from exposure to this toxin. Avoiding this puffer fish and avoiding the ingestion of certain other exotic animals (such as the blue-ringed octopus) eliminate the risk of acquiring this toxin.

[1]Not FDA approved for this indication.

Envenomations

Many marine creatures are venomous, and beachgoers experience clinically significant envenomations with some regularity. Jellyfish and related creatures (Cnidarians), sea urchins (Echinodermata), and stingrays (Chondrichthyes) are some of the more commonly identified marine animals involved with envenomations.

Jellyfish

These invertebrates have stinging cells called *nematocytes*, which carry nematocysts that continue to function when separated from the larger organism. For example, jellyfish nematocysts can sting if the tentacle is separated and after the jellyfish is dead. The venom is antigenic and causes a reaction of a dermatonecrotic, hemolytic, cardiopathic, or neurotoxic nature. The severity of the reaction depends on several variables, including the number of nematocysts that discharge, the toxicity of the coelenterate involved, and each patient's unique antigenic response.

Clinical Features

Although occasionally fatal as a consequence of an anaphylactic response in the United States and Caribbean, the primary concern in these areas with contact is pain, which is almost always self-limiting. Other, less common symptoms include parasthesias, nausea, headaches, and chills. The symptoms may last up to 2 to 3 days. Certain Pacific jellyfish primarily found in the waters around Australia have a more potent toxin and are much more likely to cause death (which is still very uncommon). Additionally, the Irukandji syndrome, which occurs in the Pacific, is a suite of symptoms including muscle spasms, vomiting, hypertension, incessant coughing, and occasionally heart failure and brain hemorrhage. Almost all exposed people, regardless of the geographic location, do not have a severe reaction, and the principles of first aid are primarily the same throughout the world.

Treatment

In my experience, treatment is mostly concerned with limiting pain and neurologic symptoms, because anaphylaxis and other severe reactions are rare, and the following general guidelines can be applied. In the field, either the victim or a companion should remove any visible tentacles. To do so requires using care, with gloves or forceps being optimal to prevent further stings. If a towel is used, any nematocysts remaining on the towel can still discharge. Salt water can be used to wash off the nematocysts. Urine, household vinegar, fresh water, and rubbing with sand should be avoided.

Should the victim present to the physician's office or emergency department, topical lidocaine (4%)[1] should be liberally applied for 30 minutes or until the pain subsides, followed by removal of the nematocysts, usually through use of the gloved hand or with forceps. Another method for removing the nematocysts is to apply shaving cream or baking soda slurry to the area and scrape off the nematocysts with a razor. Applications of cold, in the form of an ice pack, and immersion in hot water have variously been shown to improve pain, but because of the self-limited nature of the discomfort, it is hard to gauge an optimum therapy. Either is probably acceptable until the patient is comfortable. Meat tenderizer has been found to be ineffective. Local anesthetics, antihistamines, and steroids are all used to control prolonged symptoms, based on anecdotal experience. Antibiotics are not generally necessary. In the rare cases of cardiovascular collapse, supportive care and principles of treatment of anaphylaxis should be followed. A delayed hypersensitivity reaction can occur 1 to 3 days out, which will almost certainly be self-limited and can be treated with oral antihistamines and topical steroids if symptoms are severe.

Sea bather's itch is a form of jellyfish sting caused by the larvae of the thimble jellyfish. It is characterized by a painful, itchy rash under the edges of the bathing suit or wet suit. It can occasionally progress to a papular rash. Topical steroids can be used to relieve symptoms.

Prevention

Prevention is mostly a matter of common sense. Staying away from the organism (the tentacles can extend several meters from the body of the organism) and staying out of the water when jellyfish are known to be present are the most effective. There is a commercially available product, Safe Sea, which has been shown to reduce the number of nematocyst discharges and thus the severity of the sting should a swimmer need to be in the water when jellyfish are present. Wetsuits and other protective gear are ineffective.

Echinoderms

The Echinoderm family includes sea urchins. Urchins have toxin-coated spines that break off, leaving calcareous material in the wound, which can potentially cause infection. Symptoms include local pain, burning, and local discoloration. The discoloration is thought to be a temporary tattooing of the skin resulting from dye in the spines; absence of a spine is indicated if the discoloration spontaneously resolves within 48 hours. Theoretically, hot water disables the toxin, although there is no evidence in humans that it is effective. If a spine is present and easily accessible, it should be removed with fingers or forceps. If it is close to a joint or neurovascular structure, it should be surgically removed. If the spines do not cause symptoms, retained pieces will likely reabsorb into the skin.

Stingrays

Although many fish are venomous, stingrays are the most clinically important, accounting for an estimated 1500 mostly minor injuries in the United States annually. These creatures partially bury themselves in the shallow, sandy bottom of the ocean, leading water enthusiasts to accidentally step on them or grab at what they think is a seashell.

Clinical Features

Stingrays have a spine at the base of their tail, which contains a venom gland. The spine, including the venom gland, is broken off and may be left in the resulting wound. The venom has vasoconstrictive properties that can lead to cyanosis and necrosis with poor wound healing and infection. Symptoms can include immediate and intense pain, salivation, nausea, vomiting, diarrhea, muscle cramps, dyspnea, seizures, headaches, and cardiac arrhythmias. Fatalities are rare and mostly a consequence of exsanguination at the scene or penetration of a vital organ.

Treatment

Home care should include rinsing the area thoroughly with fresh water if available (salt water if not) and removing any foreign body. If the damage is minimal, the victim may soak the wound in warm water at home. The victim should watch for signs of infection and seek care for excessive bleeding, retained foreign body, or infection.

For severe wounds that lead the victim to seek medical attention, treatment should include achieving hemostasis followed by submersion of the affected region in hot but not scalding water (42–45 °C, 108–113 °F) for 30 to 90 minutes or until the pain resolves. Spines and stingers are typically radiopaque, so radiographs or an ultrasound should be obtained if a retained spine is suspected. The wound should be thoroughly cleansed, and delayed closure should be allowed. Tetanus immunization status should be reviewed and updated as appropriate. Surgical exploration may be necessary to remove residual foreign bodies. Prophylactic antibiotics are typically not necessary unless there is a residual foreign body or if the patient is immunosuppressed. If the wound becomes infected, *Staphylococcus* and *Streptococcus* species are the most common pathologic organisms. Unique to the marine environment are *Vibrio vulnificus* and *Mycobacterium marinum*, and antibiotic coverage should include coverage for all of these (Table 2).

Other Venomous Sea Creatures

Seasnakes are venomous creatures found most commonly in the Indo-Pacific area. Bites are uncommon (and envenomation is even less common), but should they occur, the toxin is very potent. The care is supportive. There is antivenom, which may be available in areas where the snakes are endemic.

Certain other fish and octopi have been associated with envenomation and occasional death. Most are tropical such as the stonefish, scorpionfish, and rabbitfish and the blue-ringed octopus. Certain varieties of catfish have venom as well. Envenomations are rare, and if they occur, treatment is based on good first-aid principles and antivenom where available (mostly in tropical areas).

---

[1] Not FDA approved for this indication.

TABLE 2 Antibiotic Choices in Marine Injuries

| | DOSAGE | |
DRUG	PEDIATRIC	ADULT
Outpatient Management		
Ciprofloxacin (Cipro)[1]	20–30 mg/kg/day PO × 14 d[1]	500 mg PO bid × 14 d
Levofloxin (Levaquin)[1]		750 mg PO qd × 14 d
Doxycycline (Vibramycin, Doryx)[1]	>8 y: 2.2 mg/kg PO qd × 14 d	100 mg bid × 14 d
Inpatient Management		
	Preferred	
Ceftazidime (Fortaz, Tazicef)[1] *plus*	150 mg/kg/d q8h	1 g IV q8h
PO or IV quinolone or doxycycline	See outpatient dosing above	See outpatient dosing above
Alternative		
Clindamycin[1] *plus* PO or IV quinalone or doxycycline	25 to 40 mg/kg per day See outpatient dosing	600 mg IV q 8 hours See outpatient dosing

[1]Not FDA approved for this indication.
Abbreviation: TMP-SMX = trimethoprim-sulfamethoxazole.

Certain cone shells contain a toxin that can be fatal. This toxin is injected by the mollusk into the victim from a proboscis, which it extends from the small end of the cone. Treatment is primarily supportive.

Trauma

Abrasions, bites, and lacerations are usually the result of a marine animal's instinct to protect itself against a perceived danger. The most commonly involved marine animals are octopi, sharks, moray eels, and barracuda. The trauma alone creates problems for patients, but the trauma can be further complicated by envenomation. It is often difficult to identify the marine animal involved in the attack. Treatment is for the most part symptomatic, with local cleansing and topical dressing usually sufficing. If the wound becomes infected, antibiotics should cover common organisms (see Table 2).

Environmental Hazards

Abrasions from the ambient environment are also common. These wounds should be thoroughly cleansed with soap and water and a topical antibiotic applied, because the wounds can contain toxins and are commonly contaminated with bacteria. Coral contains nematocysts and also has very sharp edges. Scuba divers in particular suffer from coral cuts in the course of their recreational diving. If these wounds become infected, coverage for *Vibrio* species should be included as well.

Sharks

Although shark attacks receive a lot of publicity, there are only around 50 such attacks worldwide annually and they result in fewer than 10 deaths. The majority of the deaths are in South Africa. Typically these attacks involve the tiger, great white, gray reef, and bull sharks. Attacks occur in shallow water within 100 feet of shore during the evening hours when sharks tend to feed. Common sense dictates avoiding areas where aggressive shark feeding has been noted.

Sequelae of a shark attack range from abrasions to death from hemorrhage. Abrasions and lacerations can occur when sharks brush or aggressively investigate humans. Soft tissue damage, fractures, and neurovascular damage result from such attacks. The majority of attacks result in minor injuries that require simple suturing. Morbidity increases in wounds that are greater than 20 cm or where more than one myofascial compartment is lost. General principles of first aid in marine animal injuries are found in Box 2. Although it would seem self-evident, practices such as urinating on the injury, applying oil or gasoline to injuries, and application of any strong oxidizing agents, such as strong bases or acids, should be counseled against when doing patient education regarding self-care.

BOX 2

Management of Marine Trauma
Remove the victim from the water.
Ensure airway control.
Control bleeding.
Do not remove the wet suit if the victim is wearing one.
Attempt to identify the animal involved in the injury.
If the injury is severe, transport the victim to a hospital.
If envenomation is suspected, consider hot water immersion.
Irrigate the wound with normal saline.
Perform surgical débridement of the wound as appropriate.
If sutures must be placed, place them loosely and allow drainage. Primary suturing should be avoided in puncture wounds, crush injuries, and wounds in the distal extremities.
Start appropriate antibiotics if indicated.

References

Birsa L, Verity P, Lee R: Evaluation of the effects of various chemicals on discharge of and pain caused by jellyfish nematocysts, *Comp Biochem and Physiol Part C: Toxicology & Pharmacology* 151:426–430, 2010.
Centers for Disease Control and Prevention. *Vibrio vulnificans* after a disaster. Available at http://emergency.cdc.gov/disasters/vibriovulnificus.asp (accessed August 19, 2015).
Edmonds C: Marine animal injuries. In Bove AA, editor: *Bove and Davis' Diving Medicine*, ed 4, Philadelphia, 2004, Saunders, pp 287–318.
Fleming LE: Ciguatera fish poisoning. In *National Institute of Environmental Health Sciences, Marine and Freshwater Biomedical Sciences Center*, 2006.
Isbister GK: Venomous fish stings in tropical northern Australia, *Am J Emerg Med* 19:561–565, 2001.
Lahey T: Invasive *Mycobacterium marinum* infections, *Emerg Infect Dis [serial online]* 2003. November; Available at http://wwwnc.cdc.gov/eid/article/9/11/03-0192_article.htm (accessed August 19, 2015).
Lehane L, Olley J: *Histamine (scombroid) fish poisoning: A review in a risk-assessment framework*, Canberra, Australia, 1999, National Office of Animal and Plant Health.
Lynch PR, Bove AA: Marine poisonings and intoxications. In Bove AA, editor: *Bove and Davis' Diving Medicine*, ed 4, Philadelphia, 2004, Saunders, pp 287–318.
Perkins A, Morgan S: Poisonings, envenomations, and trauma from marine creatures, *Am Fam Physician* 69:885–890, 2004.
Thomas C, Scott SA: *All Stings Considered: First Aid and Medical Treatment of Hawaii's Marine Injuries*, Honolulu, 1997, University of Hawaii Press.
Thomas CS, Scott SA, Galanis DJ, Goto RS: Box jellyfish *Carybdea alata* in Waikiki. The analgesic effect of Sting-Aid, Adolph's meat tenderizer and fresh water on their stings: a double-blinded, randomized, placebo-controlled clinical trial, *Hawaii Med J* 60:205–210, 2001.
Thomas CS, Scott SA, Galanis DJ, Goto RS: Box jellyfish *Carybdea alata* in Waikiki. Their influx cycle plus the analgesic effect of hot and cold packs on their stings to swimmers at the beach: a randomized, placebo-controlled, clinical trial, *Hawaii Med J* 60:100–107, 2001.

MEDICAL TOXICOLOGY

Method of
Howard C. Mofenson, MD; Thomas R. Caraccio, PharmD; Michael McGuigan, MD; and Joseph Greensher, MD

Introduction and Epidemiology

According to the national Toxic Exposure Surveillance System (TESS), over 2.4 million potentially toxic exposures were reported last year to Poison Control Centers throughout the United States. Poisonings were responsible for 1183 deaths and more than 500,000 hospitalizations. Poisoning accounts for 2% to 5% of pediatric hospital admissions, 10% of adult admissions, 5% of hospital admissions in the elderly (>65 years of age), and 5% of ambulance calls. In one urban hospital, drug-related emergencies accounted for 38% of the emergency department visits. An evaluation of a medical intensive care unit and step-down unit over a 3-month period indicated that poisonings accounted for 19.7% of admissions.

The largest number of fatalities resulting from poisoning reported to the TESS are caused by analgesics. The other principal toxicologic causes of fatalities are antidepressants, sedative hypnotics/antipsychotics, stimulants/street drugs, cardiovascular agents, and alcohols. Less than 1% of overdose cases reaching the hospitals result in fatality. However, patients presenting in deep coma to medical care facilities have a fatality rate of 13% to 35%. The largest single cause of coma of inapparent etiology is drug poisoning.

Pharmaceutical preparations are involved in 50% of poisonings. The number one pharmaceutical agent involved in exposures is acetaminophen. The severity of the manifestations of acute poisoning exposures varies greatly depending on whether the poisoning was intentional or unintentional. Unintentional exposures make up 85% to 90% of all poisoning exposures. The majority of cases are acute, occurring in children younger than 5 years of age, in the home, and resulting in no or minor toxicity. Many are actually ingestions of relatively nontoxic substances that require minimal medical care. Intentional poisonings, such as suicides, constitute 10% to 15% of exposures and may require the highest standards of medical and nursing care and the use of sophisticated equipment for recovery. Intentional ingestions are often of multiple substances and frequently include ethanol, acetaminophen, and aspirin. Suicides make up 54% of the reported fatalities. About 25% of suicides are attempted with drugs. Sixty percent of patients who take a drug overdose use their own medication and 15% use drugs prescribed for close relatives. The majority of the drug-related suicide attempts involve a central nervous system (CNS) depressant, and coma management is vital to the treatment.

Assessment and Maintenance of the Vital Functions

The initial assessment of all patients in medical emergencies follows the principles of basic and advanced cardiac life support. The adequacy of the patient's airway, degree of ventilation, and circulatory status should be determined. The vital functions should be established and maintained. Vital signs should be measured frequently and should include body core temperature. The assessment of vital functions should include the rate numbers (e.g., respiratory rate) and indications of effectiveness (e.g., depth of respirations and degree of gas exchange). Table 1 gives important measurements and vital signs.

Level of consciousness should be assessed by immediate AVPU (Alert, responds to Verbal stimuli, responds to Painful stimuli, and Unconscious). If the patient is unconscious, one must assess the severity of the unconsciousness by the Glasgow Coma Scale (Table 2).

If the patient is comatose, management requires administering 100% oxygen, establishing vascular access, and obtaining blood for pertinent laboratory studies. The administration of glucose, thiamine, and naloxone, as well as intubation to protect the airway, should be considered. Pertinent laboratory studies include arterial blood gases (ABG), electrocardiography (ECG), determination of blood glucose level, electrolytes, renal and liver tests, and acetaminophen plasma concentration in all cases of intentional ingestions. Radiography of the chest and abdomen may be useful. The severity of a stimulant's effects can also be assessed and should be documented to follow the trend.

The examiner should completely expose the patient by removing clothes and other items that interfere with a full evaluation. One should look for clues to etiology in the clothes and include the hat and shoes.

Prevention of Absorption and Reduction of Local Damage
Exposure

Poisoning exposure routes include ingestion (76.8%), dermal (8%), ophthalmologic (5%), inhalation (6%), insect bites and stings (4%), and parenteral injections (0.5%). The effect of the toxin may be local, systemic, or both.

Local effects (skin, eyes, mucosa of respiratory or gastrointestinal tract) occur where contact is made with the poisonous substance. Local effects are nonspecific chemical reactions that depend on the chemical properties (e.g., pH), concentration, contact time, and type of exposed surface.

Systemic effects occur when the poison is absorbed into the body and depend on the dose, the distribution, and the functional reserve of the organ systems. Shock and hypoxia are part of systemic toxicity.

Delayed Toxic Action

Therapeutic doses of most pharmaceuticals are absorbed within 90 minutes. However, the patient with exposure to a potential toxin may be asymptomatic at this time because a sufficient amount has not yet been absorbed or metabolized to produce toxicity at the time the patient presents for care.

Absorption can be significantly delayed under the following circumstances:

1. Drugs with anticholinergic properties (e.g., antihistamines, belladonna alkaloids, diphenoxylate with atropine [Lomotil], phenothiazines, and tricyclic antidepressants).
2. Modified release preparations such as sustained-release, enteric-coated, and controlled-release formulations have delayed and prolonged absorption.
3. Concretions may form (e.g., salicylates, iron, glutethimide, and meprobamate [Equanil]) that can delay absorption and prolong the toxic effects. Large quantities of drugs tend to be absorbed more slowly than small quantities.

Some substances must be metabolized into a toxic metabolite (acetaminophen, acetonitrile, ethylene glycol, methanol, methylene chloride, parathion, and paraquat). In some cases, time is required to produce a toxic effect on organ systems (*Amanita phalloides* mushrooms, carbon tetrachloride, colchicine, digoxin [Lanoxin], heavy metals, monoamine oxidase inhibitors, and oral hypoglycemic agents).

Initial Management

1. Stabilization of airway, breathing, and circulation and protection of same.
2. Identification of specific toxin or toxic syndrome.
3. Initial treatment: D50W; consider thiamine, naloxone (Narcan), oxygen, and antidotes if needed.
4. Physical assessment.
5. Decontamination: Gastrointestinal tract, skin, eyes.

Decontamination

In the asymptomatic patient who has been exposed to a toxic substance, decontamination procedures should be considered if the patient has been exposed to potentially toxic substances in toxic amounts.

Ocular exposure should be immediately treated with water irrigation for 15 to 20 minutes with the eyelids fully retracted. One should not use neutralizing chemicals. All caustic and corrosive injuries should be evaluated with fluorescein dye and by an ophthalmologist.

TABLE 1 — Important Measurements and Vital Signs

AGE	BODY SURFACE AREA (M²)	WEIGHT (KG)	HEIGHT (CM)	PULSE (BPM) RESTING	HYPOTENSION	HYPERTENSION SIGNIFICANT	HYPERTENSION SEVERE	RESPIRATORY RATE (RPM)
Newborn	0.19	3.5	50	70–190	<60/40	>96	>106	30–60
1 mo–6 mo	0.30	4–7	50–65	80–160	<70/45	>104	>110	30–50
6 mo–1 y	0.38	7–10	65–75	80–160	<70/45	>104	>110	20–40
1–2 y	0.50–0.55	10–12	75–85	80–140	<74/47	>112/74	>118/82	20–40
3–5 y	0.54–0.68	15–20	90–108	80–120	<80/52	>116/76	>124/84	20–40
6–9 y	0.68–0.85	20–28	122–133	75–115	<90/60	>122/82	>130/86	16–25
10–12 y	1.00–1.07	30–40	138–147	70–110	<90/60	>126/82	>134/90	16–25
13–15 y	1.07–1.22	42–50	152–160	60–100	<90/60	>136/86	>144/92	16–20
16–18 y	1.30–1.60	53–60	160–170	60–100	<90/60	>142/92	>150/98	12–16
Adult	1.40–1.70	60–70	160–170	60–100	<90/60	>140/90	>210/120	10–16

Data from Nadas A: Pediatric Cardiology, 3rd ed. Philadelphia, WB Saunders, 1976; Blumer JL (ed): A Practice Guide to Pediatric Intensive Care. St Louis, Mosby, 1990; AAP and ACEP: Respiratory Distress in APLS Pediatric Emergency Medicine Course, 1993; Second Task Force: Blood pressure control in children–1987, Pediatr 79:1, 1987; Linakis JG: Hypertension. In Fliesher GR, Ludwig S (eds); Textbook of Pediatric Emergency Medicine, 3rd ed. Baltimore, Williams & Wilkins, 1993.

TABLE 2 — Glasgow Coma Scale

SCALE	ADULT RESPONSE	SCORE	PEDIATRIC, 0–1 YEARS
Eye opening	Spontaneous	4	Spontaneous
	To verbal command	3	To shout
	To pain	2	To pain
	None	1	No response
Motor response			
To verbal command	Obeys	6	
To painful stimuli	Localized pain	5	Localized pain
	Flexion withdrawal	4	Flexion withdrawal
	Decorticate flexion	3	Decorticate flexion
	Decerebrate extension	2	Decerebrate flexion
	None	1	None
Verbal response: adult	Oriented and converses	5	Cries, smiles, coos
	Disoriented but converses	4	Cries or screams
	Inappropriate words	3	Inappropriate sounds
	Incomprehensible sounds	2	Grunts
	None	1	Gives no response
Verbal response: child	Oriented	5	
	Words or babbles	4	
	Vocal sounds	3	
	Cries or moans to stimuli	2	
	None	1	

Data from Teasdale G, Jennett B: Assessment of coma impaired consciousness. Lancet 2:83, 1974; Simpson D, Reilly P: Pediatric coma scale. Lancet 2:450, 1982; Seidel J: Preparing for pediatric emergencies. Pediatr Rev 16:470, 1995.

Dermal exposure is treated immediately with copious water irrigation for 30 minutes, not a forceful flushing. Shampooing the hair, cleansing the fingernails, navel, and perineum, and irrigating the eyes are necessary in the case of an extensive exposure. The clothes should be specially bagged and may have to be discarded. Leather goods can become irreversibly contaminated and must be abandoned. Caustic (alkali) exposures can require hours of irrigation. Dermal absorption can occur with pesticides, hydrocarbons, and cyanide.

Injection exposures (e.g., snake envenomation) can be treated with venom extractors. Venom extractors can be used within minutes of envenomation, and proximal lymphatic constricting bands or elastic wraps can be used to delay lymphatic flow and immobilize the extremity. Cold packs and tourniquets should not be used and incision is generally not recommended. Substances of abuse may be injected intravenously or subcutaneously. In these cases, little decontamination can be done.

Inhalation exposure to toxic substances is managed by immediate removal of the victim from the contaminated environment by protected rescuers.

Gastrointestinal exposure is the most common route of poisoning. Gastrointestinal decontamination historically has been done by gastric emptying: induction of emesis, gastric lavage, administration of activated charcoal, and the use of cathartics or whole bowel irrigation. No procedure is routine; it should be individualized for each case. If no attempt is made to decontaminate the patient, the reason should be clearly documented on the medical record (e.g., time elapsed, past peak of action, ineffectiveness, or risk of procedure).

Gastric Emptying Procedures

The gastric emptying procedure used is influenced by the age of the patient, the effectiveness of the procedure, the time of ingestion (gastric emptying is usually ineffective after 1 hour postingestion), the patient's clinical status (time of peak effect has passed or the patient's condition is too unstable), formulation of the substance ingested (regular release versus modified release), the amount ingested, and the rapidity of onset of CNS depression or stimulation (convulsions). Most studies show that only 30% (range, 19% to 62%) of the ingested toxin is removed by gastric emptying under optimal conditions. It has not been demonstrated that the choice of procedure improved the outcome.

A mnemonic for gathering information is STATS:
S—substance
T—type of formulation
A—amount and age
T—time of ingestion
S—signs and symptoms

The examiner should attempt to obtain AMPLE information about the patient:
A—age and allergies
M—available medications
P—past medical history including pregnancy, psychiatric illnesses, substance abuse, or intentional ingestions
L—time of last meal, which may influence absorption and the onset and peak action
E—events leading to present condition

The intent of the patient should also be determined.

The Regional Poison Center should be consulted for the exact ingredients of the ingested substance and the latest management. The treatment information on the labels of products are notoriously inaccurate.

Ipecac Syrup

Syrup of ipecac–induced emesis has virtually no use in the emergency department. Although at one time it was considered most useful in young children with a recent witnessed ingestion, it is no longer advised in most cases. Current guidelines from the American Association of Poison Control Centers have significantly limited the indications for inducing emesis because the risk most often exceeds the benefit derived from this procedure. The Poison Control Center should be called if inducting emesis is being considered.

Contraindications or situations in which induction of emesis is inappropriate include the following:
• Ingestion of caustic substance
• Loss of airway protective reflexes because of ingestion of substances that can produce rapid onset of CNS depression (e.g., short-acting benzodiazepines, barbiturates, nonbarbiturate sedative-hypnotics, opioids, tricyclic antidepressants) or convulsions (e.g., camphor [Ponstel], chloroquine [Aralen], codeine, isoniazid [Nydrazid], mefenamic acid, nicotine, propoxyphene [Darvon], organophosphate insecticides, strychnine, and tricyclic antidepressants)
• Ingestion of low-viscosity petroleum distillates (e.g., gasoline, lighter fluid, kerosene)
• Significant vomiting prior to presentation or hematemesis
• Age under 6 months (no established dose, safety, or efficacy data)
• Ingestion of foreign bodies (emesis is ineffective and may lead to aspiration)

• Clinical conditions including neurologic impairment, hemodynamic instability, increased intracranial pressure, and hypertension
• Delay in presentation (more than 1 hour postingestion)

The dose of syrup of ipecac in the 6- to 9-month-old infant is 5 mL; in the 9- to 12-month-old, 10 mL; and in the 1- to 12-year-old, 15 mL. In children older than 12 years and in adults, the dose is 30 mL. The dose can be repeated once if the child does not vomit in 15 to 20 minutes. The vomitus should be inspected for remnants of pills or toxic substances, and the appearance and odor should be documented. When ipecac is not available, 30 mL of mild dishwashing soap (not dishwasher detergent) can be used, although it is less effective.

Complications are very rare but include aspiration, protracted vomiting, rarely cardiac toxicity with long-term abuse, pneumothorax, gastric rupture, diaphragmatic hernia, intracranial hemorrhage, and Mallory-Weiss tears.

Gastric Lavage

Gastric lavage should be considered only when life-threatening amounts of substances were involved, when the benefits outweigh the risks, when it can be performed within 1 hour of the ingestion, and when no contraindications exist.

The contraindications are similar to those for ipecac-induced emesis. However, gastric lavage can be accomplished after the insertion of an endotracheal tube in cases of CNS depression or controlled convulsions. The patient should be placed with the head lower than the hips in a left-lateral decubitus position. The location of the tube should be confirmed by radiography, if necessary, and suctioning equipment should be available.

Contraindications to gastric lavage include the following:
• Ingestion of caustic substances (risk of esophageal perforation)
• Uncontrolled convulsions, because of the danger of aspiration and injury during the procedure
• Ingestion of low-viscosity petroleum distillate products
• CNS depression or absent protective airway reflexes, without endotracheal protection
• Significant cardiac dysrhythmias
• Significant emesis or hematemesis prior to presentation
• Delay in presentation (more than 1 hour postingestion)

Size of Tube. The best results with gastric lavage are obtained with the largest possible orogastric tube that can be reasonably passed (nasogastric tubes are not large enough to remove solid material). In adults, a large-bore orogastric Lavacuator hose or a No. 42 French Ewald tube should be used; in young children, orogastric tubes are generally too small to remove solid material and gastric lavage is not recommended.

The amount of fluid used varies with the patient's age and size. In general, aliquots of 50 to 100 mL per lavage are used in adults. Larger amounts of fluid may force the toxin past the pylorus. Lavage fluid is 0.9% saline.

Complications are rare and may include respiratory depression, aspiration pneumonitis, cardiac dysrhythmias as a result of increased vagal tone, esophageal-gastric tears and perforation, laryngospasm, and mediastinitis.

Activated Charcoal

Oral activated charcoal adsorbs the toxin onto its surface before absorption. According to recent guidelines set forth by the American Academy of Clinical Toxicology, activated charcoal should not be used routinely. Its use is indicated only if a toxic amount of substance has been ingested and is optimally effective within 1 hour of the ingestion. Because of the slow absorption of large quantities of toxin, activated charcoal may be beneficial after 1 hour postingestion.

Activated charcoal does not effectively adsorb small molecules or molecules lacking carbon (Table 3). Activated charcoal adsorption may be diminished by milk, cocoa powder, and ice cream.

TABLE 3	Substances Poorly Adsorbed by Activated Charcoal
C	Caustics and corrosives
H	Heavy metals (arsenic, iron, lead, mercury)
A	Alcohols (ethanol, methanol, isopropanol) and glycols (ethylene glycols)
R	Rapid onset of absorption (cyanide and strychnine)
C	Chlorine and iodine
O	Others insoluble in water (substances in tablet form)
A	Aliphatic hydrocarbons (petroleum distillates)
L	Laxatives (sodium, magnesium, potassium, and lithium)

There are a few relative contraindications to the use of activated charcoal:

1. Ingestion of caustics and corrosives, which may produce vomiting or cling to the mucosa and falsely appear as a burn on endoscopy.
2. Comatose patient, in whom the airway must be secured prior to activated charcoal administration.
3. Patient without presence of bowel sounds.

Note: Activated charcoal was shown not to interfere with effectiveness of N-acetylcysteine in cases of acetaminophen overdose, so it is no longer contraindicated as was thought in the past.

The usual initial adult dose is 60 to 100 g and the dose for children is 15 to 30 g. It is administered orally as a slurry mixed with water or by nasogastric or orogastric tube. *Caution:* Be sure the tube is in the stomach. Cathartics are not necessary.

Although repeated dosing with activated charcoal may decrease the half-life and increase the clearance of phenobarbital, dapsone, quinidine, theophylline, and carbamazepine (Tegretol), recent guidelines indicate there is insufficient evidence to support the use of multiple-dose activated charcoal unless a life-threatening amount of one of the substances mentioned is involved. At present there are no controlled studies that demonstrate that multiple-dose activated charcoal or cathartics alter the clinical course of an intoxication. The dose varies from 0.25 to 0.50 g/kg every 1 to 4 hours, and continuous nasogastric tube infusion of 0.25 to 0.5 g/kg/h has been used to decrease vomiting.

Gastrointestinal dialysis is the diffusion of the toxin from the higher concentration in the serum of the mesenteric vessels to the lower levels in the gastrointestinal tract mucosal cell and subsequently into the gastrointestinal lumen, where the concentration has been lowered by intraluminal adsorption of activated charcoal.

Complications of treatment with activated charcoal include vomiting in 50% of cases, desorption (especially with weak acids in intestine), and aspiration (at least a dozen cases of aspiration have been reported). There are many cases of unreported pulmonary aspirations and "charcoal lungs," intestinal obstruction or pseudoobstruction (three case reports with multiple dosing, none with a single dose), empyema following esophageal perforation, and hypermagnesemia and hypernatremia, which have been associated with repeated concurrent doses of activated charcoal and saline cathartics. Catharsis was used to hasten the elimination of any remaining toxin in the gastrointestinal tract. There are no studies to demonstrate the effectiveness of cathartics, and they are no longer recommended as a form of gastrointestinal decontamination.

Whole-Bowel Irrigation

With whole-bowel irrigation, solutions of polyethylene glycol (PEG) with balanced electrolytes are used to cleanse the bowel without causing shifts in fluids and electrolytes. The procedure is not approved by the US Food and Drug Administration (FDA) for this purpose.

Indications. The procedure has been studied and used successfully in cases of iron overdose when abdominal radiographs reveal incomplete emptying of excess iron. There are additional indications for other types of ingestions, such as with body-packing of illicit drugs (e.g., cocaine, heroin).

The procedure is to administer the solution (GoLYTELY or Colyte), orally or by nasogastric tube, in a dose of 0.5 L per hour in children younger than 5 years of age and 2 L per hour in adolescents and adults for 5 hours. The end point is reached when the rectal effluent is clear or radiopaque materials can no longer be seen in the gastrointestinal tract on abdominal radiographs.

Contraindications. These measures should not be used if there is extensive hematemesis, ileus, or signs of bowel obstruction, perforation, or peritonitis. Animal experiments in which PEG was added to activated charcoal indicated that activated charcoal-salicylates and activated charcoal-theophylline combinations resulted in decreased adsorption and desorption of salicylate and theophylline and no therapeutic benefit over activated charcoal alone. Polyethylene solutions are bound by activated charcoal in vitro, decreasing the efficacy of activated charcoal.

Dilutional treatment is indicated for the immediate management of caustic and corrosive poisonings but is otherwise not useful. The administration of diluting fluid above 30 mL in children and 250 mL in adults may produce vomiting, reexposing the vital tissues to the effects of local damage and possible aspiration.

Neutralization has not been proven to be either safe or effective.

Endoscopy and surgery have been required in the case of body-packer obstruction, intestinal ischemia produced by cocaine ingestion, and iron local caustic action.

Differential Diagnosis of Poisons on the Basis of Central Nervous System Manifestations

Neurologic parameters help to classify and assess the need for supportive treatment as well as provide diagnostic clues to the etiology. Table 4 lists the effects of CNS depressants, CNS stimulants, hallucinogens, and autonomic nervous system anticholinergics and cholinergics.

CNS depressants are cholinergics, opioids, sedative-hypnotics, and sympatholytic agents. The hallmarks are lethargy, sedation, stupor, and coma. In exception to the manifestations listed in Table 4, (a) barbiturates may produce an initial tachycardia; (b) convulsions are produced by codeine, propoxyphene (Darvon), meperidine (Demerol), glutethimide, phenothiazines, methaqualone, and tricyclic and cyclic antidepressants; (c) benzodiazepines rarely produce coma that will interfere with cardiorespiratory functions; and (d) pulmonary edema is common with opioids and sedative-hypnotics.

The CNS stimulants are anticholinergic, hallucinogenic, sympathomimetic, and withdrawal agents. The hallmarks of CNS stimulants are convulsions and hyperactivity.

There is considerable overlapping of effects among the various hallucinogens, but the major hallmark manifestation is hallucinations.

Guidelines for In-Hospital Disposition

Classification of patients as high risk depends on clinical judgment. Any patient who needs cardiorespiratory support or has a persistently altered mental status for 3 hours or more should be considered for intensive care.

Guidelines for admitting patients older than 14 years of age to an intensive care unit, after 2 to 3 hours in the emergency department, include the following:

1. Need for intubation
2. Seizures

TABLE 4	Agents with Central Nervous System (CNS) Effects			
AGENTS	**GENERAL MANIFESTATIONS**		**AGENTS**	**GENERAL MANIFESTATIONS**

CNS Depressants

Agents	General Manifestations
Alcohols and glycols (S–H)	Bradycardia
Anticonvulsants (S–H)	Bradypnea
Antidysrhythmics (S–H)	Shallow respirations
Antihypertensives (S–H)	Hypotension
Barbiturates (S–H)	Hypothermia
Benzodiazepines (S–H)	Flaccid coma
Butyrophenones (Syly)	Miosis
β-Adrenergic blockers (Syly)	Hypoactive bowel sounds
Calcium channel blockers (Syly)	
Digitalis (Syly)	
Opioids	
Lithium (mixed)	
Muscle relaxants	
Phenothiazines (Syly)	
Nonbarbiturate/benzodiazepine glutethimide, methaqualone, methyprylon, sedative–hypnotics (chloral hydrate, ethchlorvynol, bromide)	
Tricyclic antidepressants (late Syly)	

CNS Stimulants

Agents	General Manifestations
Amphetamines (Sy)	Tachycardia
Anticholinergics*	Tachypnea and dysrhythmias
Cocaine (Sy)	Hypertension
Camphor (mixed)	Convulsions
Ergot alkaloids (Sy)	Toxic psychosis
Isoniazid (mixed)	Mydriasis (reactive)
Lithium (mixed)	Agitation and restlessness
Lysergic acid diethylamide (H)	Moist skin
Hallucinogens (H)	Tremors
Mescaline and synthetic analogues	
Metals (arsenic, lead, mercury)	
Methylphenidate (Ritalin) (Sy)	
Monoamine oxidase inhibitors (Sy)	
Pemoline (Cylert) (Sy)	
Phencyclidine (H)†	
Salicylates (mixed)	
Strychnine (mixed)	
Sympathomimetics (Sy) (phenylpropanolamine, theophylline, caffeine, thyroid)	
Withdrawal from ethanol, β-adrenergic blockers, clonidine, opioids, sedative–hypnotics (W)	

Hallucinogens

Agents	General Manifestations
Amphetamines‡	Tachycardia and dysrhythmias
Anticholinergics	Tachypnea
Cardiac glycosides	Hypertension
Cocaine	Hallucinations, usually visual
Ethanol withdrawal	Disorientation
Hydrocarbon inhalation (abuse)	Panic reaction
Mescaline (peyote)	Toxic psychosis
Mushrooms (psilocybin)	Moist skin
Phencyclidine	Mydriasis (reactive)
	Hyperthermia
	Flashbacks

Anticholinergics

Agents	General Manifestations
Antihistamines	Tachycardia, dysrhythmias (rare)
Antispasmodic gastrointestinal preparations	Tachypnea
Antiparkinsonian preparations	Hypertension (mild)
Atropine	Hyperthermia
Cyclobenzaprine (Flexeril)	Hallucinations ("mad as a hatter")
Mydriatic ophthalmologic agents	Mydriasis (unreactive) ("blind as a bat")
Over-the-counter sleep agents	Flushed skin ("red as a beet")
Plants (*Datura* spp.)/mushrooms	Dry skin and mouth ("dry as a bone")
Phenothiazines (early)	Hypoactive bowel sounds
Scopolamine	Urinary retention
Tricyclic/cyclic antidepressants (early)	Lilliputian hallucinations ("little people")

Cholinergics

Agents	General Manifestations
Bethanechol (Urecholine)	Bradycardia (muscarinic)
Carbamate insecticides (Carbaryl)	Tachycardia (nicotinic effect)
Edrophonium	Miosis (muscarinic)
Organophosphate insecticides (Malathion, parathion)	Diarrhea (muscarinic)
Parasympathetic agents (physostigmine, pyridostigmine)	Hypertension (variable)
Toxic mushrooms (*Clitocybe* spp.)	Hyperactive bowel sounds
	Excess urination (muscarinic)
	Excess salivation (muscarinic)
	Lacrimation (muscarinic)
	Bronchospasm (muscarinic)
	Muscle fasciculations (nicotinic)
	Paralysis (nicotinic)

Abbreviations: H = hallucinogen; S–H = sedative–hypnotic; Sy = sympathomimetic; Syly = sympatholytic; W = withdrawal.

*Anticholinergics produce dry skin and mucosa and decreased bowel sounds.

†Phencyclidine may produce miosis.

‡The amphetamine hybrids are methylene dioxymethamphetamine (MDMA, ecstasy, "Adam") and methylene dioxyamphetamine (MDA, "Eve"), which are associated with deaths.

3. Unresponsiveness to verbal stimuli
4. Arterial carbon dioxide pressure greater than 45 mm Hg
5. Cardiac conduction or rhythm disturbances (any rhythm except sinus arrhythmia)
6. Close monitoring of vital signs during antidotal therapy or elimination procedures
7. The need for continuous monitoring
8. QRS interval greater than 0.10 second, in cases of tricyclic antidepressant poisoning
9. Systolic blood pressure less than 80 mm Hg
10. Hypoxia, hypercarbia, acid-base imbalance, or metabolic abnormalities
11. Extremes of temperature
12. Progressive deterioration or significant underlying medical disorders

Use of Antidotes

Antidotes are available for only a relatively small number of poisons. An antidote is not a substitute for good supportive care. Table 5 summarizes the commonly used antidotes, their indications, and their methods of administration. The Regional Poison Control Center can give further information on these antidotes.

Enhancement of Elimination

The acceptable methods for elimination of absorbed toxic substances are dialysis, hemoperfusion, exchange transfusion, plasmapheresis, enzyme induction, and inhibition. Methods of increasing urinary excretion of toxic chemicals and drugs have been studied extensively, but the other modalities have not been well evaluated.

In general, these methods are needed in only a minority of cases and should be reserved for life-threatening circumstances when a definite benefit is anticipated.

Dialysis

Dialysis is the extrarenal means of removing certain substances from the body, and it can substitute for the kidney when renal failure occurs. Dialysis is not the first measure instituted; however, it may be lifesaving later in the course of a severe intoxication. It is needed in only a minority of intoxicated patients.

Peritoneal dialysis uses the peritoneum as the membrane for dialysis. It is only 1/20 as effective as hemodialysis. It is easier to use and less hazardous to the patient but also less effective in removing the toxin; thus it is rarely used except in small infants.

Hemodialysis is the most effective dialysis method but requires experience with sophisticated equipment. Blood is circulated past a semipermeable extracorporeal membrane. Substances are removed by diffusion down a concentration gradient. Anticoagulation with heparin is necessary. Flow rates of 300 to 500 mL/min can be achieved, and clearance rates may reach 200 or 300 mL/min.

Dialyzable substances easily diffuse across the dialysis membrane and have the following characteristics: (a) a molecular weight less than 500 daltons and preferably less than 350; (b) a volume of distribution less than 1 L/kg; (c) protein binding less than 50%; (d) high water solubility (low lipid solubility); and (e) high plasma concentration and a toxicity that correlates reasonably with the plasma concentration. Considerations for hemodialysis and hemoperfusion are cases of serious ingestions (the nephrologist should be notified immediately), and cases involving a compound that is ingested in a potentially lethal dose and the rapid removal of which may improve the prognosis. Examples of the latter are ethylene glycol 1.4 mL/kg 100% solution or equivalent and methanol 6 mL/kg 100% solution or equivalent. Common dialyzable substances include alcohol, bromides, lithium, and salicylates.

The patient-related criteria for dialysis are (a) anticipated prolonged coma and the likelihood of complications; (b) renal compromise (toxin excreted or metabolized by kidneys and dialyzable chelating agents in heavy metal poisoning); (c) laboratory confirmation of lethal blood concentration; (d) lethal dose poisoning with an agent with delayed toxicity or known to be metabolized into a more toxic metabolite (e.g., ethylene glycol, methanol); and (e) hepatic impairment when the agent is metabolized by the liver, and clinical deterioration despite optimal supportive medical management. Table 6 gives plasma concentrations above which removal by extracorporeal measures should be considered.

The contraindications to hemodialysis include the following: (a) substances are not dialyzable; (b) effective antidotes are available; (c) patient is hemodynamically unstable (e.g., shock); and (d) presence of coagulopathy because heparinization is required.

Hemodialysis also has a role in correcting disturbances that are not amenable to appropriate medical management. These are easily remembered by the "vowel" mnemonic:
A—refractory acid-base disturbances
E—refractory electrolyte disturbances
I—intoxication with dialyzable substances (e.g., ethanol, ethylene glycol, isopropyl alcohol, methanol, lithium, and salicylates)
O—overhydration
U—uremia

Complications of dialysis include hemorrhage, thrombosis, air embolism, hypotension, infections, electrolyte imbalance, thrombocytopenia, and removal of therapeutic medications.

Hemoperfusion

Hemoperfusion is the parenteral form of oral activated charcoal. Heparinization is necessary. The patient's blood is routed extracorporeally through an outflow arterial catheter with a filter-adsorbing cartridge (charcoal or resin) and returned through a venous catheter. Cartridges must be changed every 4 hours. The blood glucose, electrolytes, calcium, and albumin levels; complete blood cell count; platelets; and serum and urine osmolarity must be carefully monitored. This procedure has extended extracorporeal removal to a large range of substances that were formerly either poorly dialyzable or nondialyzable. It is not limited by molecular weight, water solubility, or protein binding, but it is limited by a volume distribution greater than 400 L, plasma concentration, and rate of flow through the filter. Activated charcoal cartridges are the primary type of hemoperfusion currently available in the United States.

The patient-related criteria for hemoperfusion are (a) anticipated prolonged coma and the likelihood of complications; (b) laboratory confirmation of lethal blood concentrations; (c) hepatic impairment when an agent is metabolized by the liver; and (d) clinical deterioration despite optimally supportive medical management.

The contraindications are similar to those for hemodialysis.

Limited data are available as to which toxins are best treated with hemoperfusion. Hemoperfusion has proved useful in treating glutethimide intoxication, phenobarbital overdose, and carbamazepine, phenytoin, and theophylline intoxication.

Complications include hemorrhage, thrombocytopenia, hypotension, infection, leukopenia, depressed phagocytic activity of granulocytes, decreased immunoglobulin levels, hypoglycemia, hypothermia, hypocalcemia, pulmonary edema, and air and charcoal embolism.

Hemofiltration

Continuous arteriovenous or venovenous hemodiafiltration (CAVHD or CVVHD, respectively) has been suggested as an alternative to conventional hemodialysis when the need for rapid removal of the drug is less urgent. These procedures, like peritoneal dialysis, are minimally invasive, have no significant impact on hemodynamics, and can be carried out continuously for many hours. Their role in the management of acute poisoning remains uncertain, however.

TABLE 5 Initial Doses of Antidotes for Common Poisonings

ANTIDOTE	USE	DOSE	ROUTE	ADVERSE REACTIONS/COMMENTS
N-Acetyl Cysteine (NAC, Mucomyst): Stock level to treat 70kg adult for 24h: 25 vials, 20%, 30mL	Acetaminophen, carbon tetrachloride (experimental)	140mg/kg loading, followed by 70mg/kg q4h for 17 doses 150mg/kg in 200mL of D_5W over 1h, then 50mg/kg in 1 liter D_5W over 16h	PO IV	Nausea, vomiting. Dilute to 5% with sweet juice or flat cola. Useful for those who cannot tolerate oral route.
Atropine: Stock level to treat 70kg adult for 24h: 1g (1mg/mL in 1, 10mL)	Organophosphate and carbamate pesticides: bradydysrhythmics, β-adrenergics, calcium channel blockers/nerve agents	*Child:* 0.02–0.05 mg/kg repeated q5–10min to max of 2mg as necessary until cessation of secretions *Adult:* 1–2 mg q5–10min as necessary. Dilute in 1–2mL of 0.9% saline for ET instillation. *IV infusion dose:* Place 8mg of atropine in 100mL D_5W or saline. Conc. = 0.08 mg/mL; dose range = 0.02–0.08 mg/kg/h or 0.25–1 mL/kg/h. Severe poisoning may require supplemental doses of IV atropine intermittently in doses of 1–5 mg until drying of secretions occurs.	IV/ET	Tachycardia, dry mouth, blurred vision, and urinary retention. Ensure adequate ventilation before administration.
Calcium Chloride (10%): Stock level to treat 70kg adult for 24h: 10 vials 1g (1.35 mEq/mL)	Hypocalcemia, fluoride, calcium channel blockers, β-blockers, oxalates, ethylene glycol, hypermagnesemia	0.1–0.2 mL/kg (10–20 mg/kg) slow push q10min up to max 10mL (1g). Since calcium response lasts 15 min, some may require continuous infusion 0.2 mL/kg/h up to maximum of 10mL/h while monitoring for dysrhythmias and hypotension.	IV	Administer slowly with BP and ECG monitoring and have magnesium available to reverse calcium effects. Tissue irritation, hypotension, dysrhythmias from rapid injection. Contraindications: digitalis glycoside intoxication.
Calcium Gluconate (10%): Stock level to treat 70kg adult for 24h: 20 vials 1g (0.45 mEq/mL)	Hypocalcemia, fluoride, calcium channel blockers, hydrofluoric acid; black widow envenomation	0.3–0.4 mL/kg (30–40 mg/kg) slow push; repeat as needed to max dose 10–20mL (1–2g).	IV	Same comments as calcium chloride.
Infiltration of Calcium Gluconate	Hydrofluoric acid skin exposure	Dose: Infiltrate each square cm of affected dermis/subcutaneous tissue with about 0.5 mL of 10% calcium gluconate using a 30-gauge needle. Repeat as needed to control pain.	Infiltrate	
Intra-arterial Calcium Gluconate	Hydrofluoric acid skin exposure	Infuse 20mL of 10% calcium gluconate (not chloride) diluted in 250mL D_5W via the radial or brachial artery proximal to the injury over 3–4h.		Alternatively, dilute 10mL of 10% calcium gluconate with 40–50mL of D_5W.
Calcium Gluconate Gel: Stock level: 3.5g	Hydrofluoric acid skin exposure	2.5 g USP powder added to 100mL water-soluble lubricating jelly, e.g., K-Y jelly or Lubifax (or 3.5 mg into 150mL). Some use 6g of calcium carbonate in 100g of lubricant. Place injured hand in surgical glove filled with gel. Apply q4h. If pain persists, calcium gluconate injection may be needed (above).	Dermal	Powder is available from Spectrum Pharmaceutical Co. in California: 800-772-8786. Commercial preparation of Ca gluconate gel is available from Pharmascience in Montreal, Quebec: 514-340-1114.
Cyanide Antidote Kit: Stock level to treat 70kg adult for 24h: 2 Lilly Cyanide Antidote kits	Cyanide Hydrogen sulfide (nitrites are given only) Do not use sodium thiosulfate for hydrogen sulfide Individual portions of the kit can be used in certain circumstances (consult PCC)	Amyl nitrite: 1 crushable ampule for 30sec of every min. Use new amp q3min. May omit step if venous access is established.	Inhalation	If methemoglobinemia occurs, do not use methylene blue to correct this because it releases cyanide.

Continued

Antidote	Indication	Dose	Route	Comments
	Cyanide Hydrogen sulfide (nitrites are given only) Do not use sodium thiosulfate for hydrogen sulfide Individual portions of the kit can be used in certain circumstances (consult PCC)	Sodium nitrite: *Child*: 0.33 mL/kg of 3% solution if hemoglobin level is not known, otherwise based on tables with product. *Adult*: up to 300 mL (10 mL). Dilute nitrite in 100 mL 0.9% saline, administer slowly at 5 mL/min. Slow infusion if fall in BP.	IV	If methemoglobinemia occurs, do not use methylene blue to correct this because it releases cyanide.
	Do not use sodium thiosulfate for hydrogen sulfide Individual portions of the kit can be used in certain circumstances (consult PCC)	Sodium thiosulfate: *Child*: 1.6 mL/kg of 25% solution, may be repeated q30–60min to a maximum of 12.5 or 50 mL in adult. Administer over 20 min.	IV	Nausea, dizziness, headache. Tachycardia, muscle rigidity, and bronchospasm (rapid administration).
Dantrolene Sodium (Dantrium): Stock level to treat 70 kg adult for 24 h: 700 mg, 35 vials (20 mg vial)	Malignant hyperthermia	2–3 mg/kg IV rapidly. Repeat loading dose every 10 min. If necessary up to a maximum total dose of 10 mg/kg. When temperature and heart rate decrease, slow the infusion 1–2 mg/kg q6h for 24–28 h until all evidence of malignant hyperthermia syndrome has subsided. Follow with oral doses 1–2 mg/kg four times a day for 24 h as necessary.	IV/PO	Hepatotoxicity occurs with cumulative dose of 10 mg/kg. Thrombophlebitis (best given in central line). Available as 20 mg lyophilized dantrolene powder for reconstruction, which contains 3 g mannitol and sodium hydroxide in 70-mL vial. Mix with 60 mL sterile distilled water without a bacteriostatic agent and protect from light. Use within 6 hours after reconstituting.
Deferoxamine (Desferal): Stock level to treat 70 kg adult for 24 h: 17 vials (500 mg/amp)	Iron	IV infusion of 15 mg/kg/h (3 mL/kg/h: 500 mg in 100 mL D_5W) max 6 g/d Rates of >45 μg/kg/h if cone >1000 μg/dL.	Preferred IV: avoid therapy >24 h	Hypotension (minimized by avoiding rapid infusion rates) DFO challenge test 50 mg/kg is unreliable if negative.
Diazepam (Valium): Stock level to treat 70 kg adult for 24 h: 200 mg, 5 mg/mL; 2, 10 mL	Any intoxication that provokes seizures when specific therapy is not available (e.g., amphetamines, PCP, barbiturate and alcohol withdrawal) Chloroquine poisoning	*Adult*, 5–10 mg IV (max 20 mg) at a rate of 5 mg/min until seizure is controlled. May be repeated 2 or 3 times. *Child*, 0.1–0.3 mg/kg up to 10 mg IV slowly over 2 min.	IV	Confusion, somnolence, coma, hypotension. Intramuscular absorption is erratic. Establish airway and administer 100% oxygen and glucose.
Digoxin-Specific Fab Antibodies (Digibind): Stock level to treat 70 kg adult for 24 h: 20 vials	Digoxin, digitoxin, oleander tea with the following: (1) Imminent cardiac arrest or shock (2) Hyperkalemia >5.0 mEq/L (3) Serum digoxin >5 ng/mL (child) at 8–12 h post ingestion in adults (4) Digitalis delirium (5) Ingestion over 10 mg in adults or 4 mg in child (6) Bradycardia or second- or third-degree heart block unresponsive to atropine (7) Life-threatening digitoxin or oleander poisoning	(1) If amount ingested is known total dose × bioavailability (0.8) = body burden. The body burden ÷ 0.6 (0.5 mg of digoxin is bound by 1 vial of 38 mg of Fab) = # vials needed. (2) If amount is unknown but the steady state serum concentration is known in ng/mL: Digoxin: ng/mL: (5.6 L/kg Vd) × (wt kg) = μg body burden. Body burden ÷ 100 = mg body burden/0.5 = # vials needed. Digitoxin body burden = ng/mL × (0.56 L/kg Vd) × (wt kg) Body burden ÷ 1000 = mg body burden/0.5 = # vials needed. (3) If the amount is not known, it is administered in life-threatening situations as 10 vials (400 mg) IV in saline over 30 min in adults. If cardiac arrest is imminent, administer 20 vials (adult) as a bolus.	IV	Allergic reactions (rare), return of condition being treated with digitalis glycoside. Administer by infusion over 30 min through a 0.22-μ filter. If cardiac arrest is imminent, may administer by bolus. Consult PCC for more details.

TABLE 5 Initial Doses of Antidotes for Common Poisonings—cont'd

ANTIDOTE	USE	DOSE	ROUTE	ADVERSE REACTIONS/COMMENTS
Dimercaprol (BAL in Peanut Oil): Stock level to treat 70 kg adult for 24 h: 1200 mg (4 amps—100 mg/mL 10% in oil in 3 mL amp)	Chelating agent for arsenic, mercury, and lead	3–5 mg/kg q4h usually for 5–10 d	Deep IM	Local infection site pain and sterile abscess, nausea, vomiting, fever, salivation, hypertension, and nephrotoxicity (alkalinize urine).
2,3 Dimercaptosuccinic Acid (DMSA Succimer): 100 mg/capsule:20 capsules	Used as a chelating agent for lead, especially blood lead levels >45 μg/dL. May also be used for symptomatic mercury exposure	10 mg/kg 3 × daily for 5 days followed by 10 mg/kg 2 × daily for 14 days	PO	Precautions: monitor AST/ALT; use with caution in G6PD-deficient patients. Avoid concurrent iron therapy. Relatively safe antidote, rarely severe, uncommon minor skin rashes may occur.
Diphenhydramine (Benadryl): Antiparkinsonian action. Stock level to treat a 70 kg adult for 24 h: 5 vials (10 mg/mL, 10 mL each)	Used to treat extrapyramidal symptoms and dystonia induced by phenothiazines, phencyclidine, and related drugs	*Children:* 1–2 mg/kg IV slowly over 5 min up to maximum 50 mg followed by 5 mg/kg/24 h orally divided every 6 h up to 300 mg/24 h *Adults:* 50 mg IV followed by 50 mg orally four times daily for 5–7 d. *Note:* Symptoms abate within 2–5 min after IV.	IV	Fatal dose: 20–40 mg/kg. Dry mouth, drowsiness.
Ethanol (Ethyl Alcohol): Stock level to treat 70 kg adult for 24 h: 3 bottles 10% (1 L each)	Methanol, ethylene glycol	10 mL/kg loading dose concurrently with 1.4 mL/kg (average) infusion of 10% ethanol (consult PCC for more details)	IV	Nausea, vomiting, sedation. Use 0.22-μ filter if preparing from bulk 100% ethanol.
Flumazenil (Romazicon): Stock level to treat 70 kg adult for 24 h: 4 vials (0.1 mg/mL, 10 mL)	Benzodiazepines (may also be beneficial in the treatment of hepatic encephalopathy)	Administer 0.2 mg (2 mL) IV over 30 sec (pediatric dose not established, 0.01 mg/kg), then wait 3 min for a response, then if desired consciousness is not achieved, administer 0.3 mg (3 mL) over 30 sec, then wait 3 min for response, then if desired consciousness is not achieved, administer 0.5 mg (5 mL) over 30 sec at 60-sec intervals up to a maximum cumulative dose of 3 mg (30 mL) (1 mg in children). Because effects last only 1–5 h, if patient responds, monitor carefully over next 6 h for resedation. If multiple repeated doses, consider a continuous infusion of 0.2–1 mg/h.	IV	Nausea, vomiting, facial flushing, agitation, headache, dizziness, seizures, and death. It is not recommended to improve ventilation. Its role in CNS depression needs to be clarified. It should not be used routinely in comatose patients. It is **contraindicated** in cyclic antidepressant intoxications, stimulant overdose, long-term benzodiazepine use (may precipitate life-threatening withdrawal), if benzodiazepines are used to control seizures, in head trauma.
Folic Acid (Folvite): Stock level to treat 70 kg adult for 24 h: 4 100-mg vials	Methanol/ethylene glycol (investigational)	1 mg/kg up to 50 mg q4h for 6 doses	IV	Uncommon
Fomepizole (4-MP, Antizol): Stock level to treat 70 kg adult: 4 1.5-mL vials (1 g/mL)	Ethylene glycol Methanol	Loading dose: 15 mg/kg (0.015 mL/kg) IV followed by maintenance dose of 10 mg/kg (0.01 mL/kg) q12h for 4 doses, then 15 mg/kg q12h until ethylene glycol levels are <20 mg/dL. Fomepizole can be given to patients undergoing hemodialysis (dose q4h).	IV	Suggested: co-administer folate 50 mg IV (child 1 mg/kg), thiamine 100 mg/d (child 50 mg), and pyridoxine 50 mg IV/IM q6h until intoxication is resolved. Monitor for urinary oxalate crystals. Adverse reactions include headache, nausea, and dizziness. Antizole should be diluted in 100 mL 0.9% saline or D₅W and mixed well. Antizole should not be given undiluted.

Drug	Indication	Dose	Route	Comments
Glucagon: Stock level to treat 70 kg adult for 24 h: 10 vials, 10 units	β-Blocker, calcium channel blocker	3–10 mg in adult, then infuse 2–5 mg/h (0.05–0.1 mg/kg in child, then infuse 0.07 mg/kg/h) Large doses up to 100 mg/24 h used	IV	Use D$_5$W, not 0.9% saline, to reconstitute the glucagon (rather than diluent of Eli Lilly, which contains phenol). Vomiting precautions.
Magnesium Sulfate: Stock level to treat 70 kg adult for 24 h: approx 2.5 g (50 mL of 50% or 200 mL of 12.5%)	Torsades de pointes	*Adult:* 2 g (20 mL or 20%) over 20 min. If no response in 10 min, repeat and follow by continuous infusion 1 g/h. *Children:* 25–50 mg/kg initially and maintenance is 30–60 mg/kg/24 h (0.25–0.5 mEq/kg/24 h) up to 1000 mg/24 h. (Dose not studied in controlled fashion.)	IV	Use with caution if renal impairment is present.
Methylene Blue: Stock level to treat 70 kg adult for 24 h: 5 amps (10 mg/10 mL)	Methemoglobinemia	0.1–0.2 mL/kg of 1% solution, slow infusion, may be repeated q30–60 min	IV	Nausea, vomiting, headache, dizziness.
Naloxone (Narcan): Stock level to treat 70 kg adult for 24 h: 3 vials (1 mg/mL, 10 mL)	Comatose patient; decreased respirations <12; opioids	In postoperative opioid depression reversal, IV 0.1–0.5 µg/kg q2 min as needed and may repeat up to a total dose of 1 µg/kg. In **suspected overdose**, administer IV 0.1 mg/kg in a child younger than 5 years of age up to 2 mg; in older children and adults administer 2 mg every 2 min up to a total of 10–20 mg. Can also be administered into the endotracheal tube. If no response by 10 mg, a pure opioid intoxication is unlikely. If **opioid abuse** is suspected, **restraints** should be in place before administration; **initial dose** 0.1 mg to avoid withdrawal and violent behavior. The initial dose is then doubled every minute progressively to a total of 10 mg. A **continuous infusion** has been advocated because many opioids outlast the short half-life of naloxone (30–60 min). The **naloxone infusion hourly rate** to produce a response is equal to the effective dose required (improvement in ventilation and arousal). An additional dose may be required in 15–30 min as a bolus.	IV, ET	**Larger doses** of naloxone may be required for more poorly antagonized synthetic opioid drugs: buprenorphine (Buprenex), codeine, dextromethorphan, fentanyl, pentazocine (Talwin), propoxyphene (Darvon), diphenoxylate, nalbuphine (Nubain), new potent "designer" drugs, or long-acting opioids such as methadone (Dolophine). **Complications.** Although naloxone is safe and effective, there are rare reports of complications (<1%) of pulmonary edema, seizures, hypertension, cardiac arrest, and sudden death. The infusions are titrated to avoid respiratory depression and opioid withdrawal manifestations. Tapering of infusions can be attempted after 12 h and when the patient is stable.
Physostigmine (Antilirium): Stock level to treat 70 kg adult for 24 h: 2–4 mg (2 mL each)	Anticholinergic agents (not routinely used, only indicated if life-threatening complications)	*Child:* 0.02 mg/kg slow push to max 2 mg q30–60 min *Adult:* 1–2 mg q5 min to max 6 mg.	IV	Bradycardia, asystole, seizures, bronchospasm, vomiting, headaches. Do not use for cyclic antidepressants.
Pralidoxime (2PAM, Protopam): Stock level to treat 70 kg adult for 24 h: 12 vials (1 g per 20 mL)	Organophosphates/nerve agents	Child ≤12 y, 25–50 mg/kg max (4 mg/min); >12 y, 1–2 g/dose in 250 mL of 0.9% saline over 5–10 min. Max 200 mg/min. Repeat q6–12h for 24–48h. Max adult 6 g/d. Alternative: Maintenance infusion 1 g in 100 mL of 0.9% saline at 5–20 mg/kg/h (0.5–12 mL/kg/h) up to max 500 mg/h or 50 mL/h. Titrate to desired response. End point is absence of fasciculations and return of muscle strength.	IV	Nausea, dizziness, headache; tachycardia, muscle rigidity, bronchospasm (rapid administration).
Pyridoxine (Vitamin B$_6$): Stock level to treat 70 kg adult for 24 h: 100 mg/mL 10% solution. For a 70 kg patient, 10 g = 10 vials	Seizures from isoniazid or *Gyromitra* mushrooms, ethylene glycol	*Isoniazid: Unknown amount ingested:* 5 g (70 mg/kg) in 50 mL D$_5$W over 5 min + diazepam 0.3 mg/kg IV at rate of 1 mg/min in child or 10 mg dose at rate up to 5 mg/min in adults. Use different site (synergism). May repeat q5–20 min until seizure controlled. Up to 375 mg/kg have been given (52 g). *Known amount:* 1 g for each gram isoniazid ingested over 5 min with diazepam (dose above) *Gyromitra mushroom:* Child 25 mg/kg or 2–5 g, adults IV over 15–30 min to max 20 g	IV	After seizure is controlled, administer remainder of pyridoxine 1 g/1 g isoniazid total 5 g as infusion over 60 min. Adverse reactions uncommon; do not administer in same bottle as sodium bicarbonate. For *Gyromitra* mushrooms, some use PO 25 mg/kg/d early when mushroom ingestion is suspected.

Continued

Medical Toxicology

1381

TABLE 5   Initial Doses of Antidotes for Common Poisonings—cont'd

ANTIDOTE	USE	DOSE	ROUTE	ADVERSE REACTIONS/COMMENTS
Sodium Bicarbonate (NaHCO3): Stock level to treat 70kg adult for 24h: 10 ampules or syringes (500 mEq)	Tricyclic antidepressant cardiotoxicity (QRS >0.12 sec; ventricular tachycardia, severe conduction disturbances); metabolic acidosis: phenothiazine toxicity Salicylate: to keep blood pH 7.5–7.55 (not >7.55) and urine pH 7.5–8.0. Alkalinization recommended if salicylate conc. >40mg/dL in acute poisoning and at lower levels if symptomatic in chronic intoxication, 2 mEq/kg will raise blood pH 0.1 unit	*Ethylene glycol:* 100mg IV daily. 1–2mEq/kg undiluted as a bolus. If no effect on cardiotoxicity, repeat twice a few minutes apart *Adult* with clear physical signs and laboratory findings of acute moderate or severe salicylism: Bolus 1–2mEq/kg followed by infusion of 100–150 mEq NaHCO3 added to 1L of 5% dextrose at rate of 200–300mL/h *Child:* Bolus same as adult followed by 1–2 mEq/kg in infusion of 20mL/kg/h 5% dextrose in 0.45% saline Add potassium when patient voids Rate and amount of the initial infusion, if patient is volume depleted: 1h to achieve urine output of 2 mL/kg/h and urine pH 7–8 In mild cases without acidosis and urine pH >6, administer 5% dextrose in 0.9% saline with 50mEq/L or 1 mEq/kg NaHCO3 as maintenance to replace ongoing renal losses. If acidemia is present and pH <7.2, add 2mEq/kg as loading dose followed by 2mEq/kg q3–4h to keep pH at 7.5–7.55. If acidemia is present, recommend isotonic NaHCO3, 3 ampules to 1L of D5W at 10–15 mL/kg/h or sufficient to produce normal urine flow and a urine pH of 7.5 or higher	IV	Monitor sodium, potassium, and blood pH because fatal alkalemia and hyponatremia have been reported. Monitor both urine and blood pH. Do not use the urine pH alone to assess the need for alkalinization because of the paradoxical aciduria that may occur. Adjust the urine pH to 7.5–8 by NaHCO3 infusion. After urine output established, add potassium 40mEq/L.
	Long-acting barbiturates: Phenobarbital and primidone (Mysoline). *Note:* Alkalinization is ineffective for the short- or intermediate-acting barbiturates	NaHCO3: 2 mEq/kg during the first hour or 100mEq in 1L of D5W with 40mEq/L potassium at a rate of 100mL/h in adults Adequate potassium is necessary to accomplish alkalinization	IV	Additional sodium bicarbonate and potassium chloride may be needed. Adjust the urine pH to 7.5–8 by NaHCO3 infusion.
Thiamine: 100 mg/mL, 2 vials	Thiamine deficiency, ethylene glycol poisoning, alcoholism	100 mg IV followed with 100 mg V/IM for 5–7 days in an alcoholic and followed by 100mg/d orally	IV/IM	
Vitamin K1 (Aqua Mephyton): 10 mg/1–5 mL; 5-mg tablets	Warfarin anticoagulant or rodenticide toxicity	Oral 0.4 mg/kg/dose child, 10–25 mg adults. If evidence of bleeding, administer vitamin K1 SC, IV 0.6 mg/kg/ dose child and up to 25–50 mg adults for 6 hours depending on severity	PO/SC, IV	Give vitamin K daily until PT/INR are normal. Examine stools and urine for evidence of bleeding.

Abbreviations: ALT = alanine aminotransferase; amp = ampule; AST = aspartate aminotransferase; BAL = British anti-Lewisite; BP = blood pressure; conc. = concentration; ECG = electrocardiogram; ET = endotracheal; G6PD = glucose-6-phosphate dehydrogenase; IM = intramuscular; IV = intravenous; PCC = poison control center; PO = oral; PT = prothrombin time; SC = subcutaneous.

TABLE 6 Plasma Concentrations Above Which Removal by Extracorporeal Measures Should Be Considered

DRUG	PLASMA CONCENTRATION	PROTEIN BINDING (%)	VOLUME DISTRIBUTION (L/KG)	METHOD OF CHOICE
Amanitin	NA	25	1.0	HP
Ethanol	500–700 mg/dL	0	0.3	HD
Ethchlorvynol	150 µg/mL	35–50	3–4	HP
Ethylene glycol	25–50 µg/mL	0	0.6	HD
Glutethimide	100 µg/mL	50	2.7	HP
Isopropyl alcohol	400 mg/dL	0	0.7	HD
Lithium	4 mEq/L	0	0.7	HD
Meprobamate (Equanil)	100 µg/mL	0	NA	HP
Methanol	50 mg/dL	0	0.7	HD
Methaqualone	40 µg/dL	20–60	6.0	HP
Other barbiturates	50 µg/dL	50	0–1	HP
Paraquat	0.1 mg/dL	poor	2.8	HP > HD
Phenobarbital	100 µg/dL	50	0.9	HP > HD
Salicylates	80–100 mg/dL	90	0.2	HD > HP
Theophylline		0	0.5	
Chronic	40–60 µg/mL			HP
Acute	80–100 µg/mL			HP
Trichlorethanol	250 µg/mL	70	0.6	HP

Abbreviations: HD = hemodialysis; HP = hemoperfusion; HP > HD = hemoperfusion preferred over hemodialysis.
Data from Winchester JF: Active methods for detoxification. In Haddad LM, Winchester JF (eds). Clinical Management of Poisoning and Drug Overdose, 2nd ed. Philadelphia, WB Saunders, 1990; Balsam L, Cortitsidis GN, Fienfeld DA: Role of hemodialysis and hemoperfusion in the treatment of intoxications. Contemp Manage Crit Care 1:61, 1991.
Note: Cartridges for charcoal hemoperfusion are not readily available anymore in most locations. So hemodialysis may be substituted in these situations. In mixed or chronic drug overdoses, extracorporeal measures may be considered at lower drug concentrations.

Plasmapheresis

Plasmapheresis consists of removal of a volume of blood. All the extracted components are returned to the blood except the plasma, which is replaced with a colloid protein solution. There are limited clinical data on guidelines and efficacy in toxicology. Centrifugal and membrane separators of cellular elements are used. It can be as effective as hemodialysis or hemoperfusion for removing toxins that have high protein binding, and it may be useful for toxins not filtered by hemodialysis and hemoperfusion.

Plasmapheresis has been anecdotally used in treating intoxications with the following agents: paraquat (removed 10%), propranolol (removed 30%), quinine (removed 10%), L-thyroxine (removed 30%), and salicylate (removed 10%). It has been shown to remove less than 10% of digoxin, phenobarbital, prednisolone, and tobramycin. Complications include infection; allergic reactions including anaphylaxis; hemorrhagic disorders; thrombocytopenia; embolus and thrombus; hypervolemia and hypovolemia; dysrhythmias; syncope; tetany; paresthesia; pneumothorax; acute respiratory distress syndrome; and seizures.

Supportive Care, Observation, and Therapy for Complications

Altered Mental Status

If airway protective reflexes are absent, endotracheal intubation is indicated for a comatose patient or a patient with altered mental status. If respirations are ineffective, ventilation should be instituted, and if hypoxemia persists, supplemental oxygen is indicated. If a cyanotic patient fails to respond to oxygen, the practitioner should consider methemoglobinemia.

Hypoglycemia

Hypoglycemia accompanies many poisonings, including with ethanol (especially in children), clonidine (Catapres), insulin, organophosphates, salicylates, sulfonylureas, and the unripe fruit or seed of a Jamaican plant called ackee. If hypoglycemia is present or suspected, glucose should be administered immediately as an intravenous bolus. Doses are as follows: in a neonate, 10% glucose (5 mL/kg); in a child, 25% glucose 0.25 g/kg (2 mL/kg); and in an adult, 50% glucose 0.5 g/kg (1 mL/kg).

A bedside capillary test for blood glucose is performed to detect hypoglycemia, and the sample is sent to the laboratory for confirmation. If the glucose reagent strip visually reads less than 150 mg/dL, one administers glucose. Venous blood should be used rather than capillary blood for the bedside test if the patient is in shock or is hypotensive. Large amounts of glucose given rapidly to nondiabetic patients may cause a transient reactive hypoglycemia and hyperkalemia and may accentuate damage in ischemic cerebrovascular and cardiac tissue. If focal neurologic signs are present, it may be prudent to withhold glucose, because hypoglycemia causes focal signs in less than 10% of cases.

Thiamine Deficiency Encephalopathy

Thiamine is administered to avoid precipitating thiamine deficiency encephalopathy (Wernicke-Korsakoff syndrome) in alcohol abusers and in malnourished patients. The overall incidence of thiamine deficiency in ethanol abusers is 12%. Thiamine 100 mg intravenously should be administered around the time of the glucose administration but not necessarily before the glucose. The clinician should be prepared to manage the anaphylaxis that sometimes is caused by thiamine, although it is extremely rare.

Opioid Reactions

Naloxone (Narcan) reverses CNS and respiratory depression, miosis, bradycardia, and decreased gastrointestinal peristalsis caused by opioids acting through μ, κ, and δ receptors. It also affects endogenous opioid peptides (endorphins and enkephalins), which accounts for the variable responses reported in patients with intoxications from ethanol, benzodiazepines, clonidine (Catapres), captopril (Capoten), and valproic acid (Depakote) and in patients with spinal cord injuries. There is a high sensitivity for predicting a response if pinpoint pupils and circumstantial evidence of opioid abuse (e.g., track marks) are present.

In cases of suspected overdose, naloxone 0.1 mg/kg is administered intravenously initially in a child younger than 5 years of age. The dose can be repeated in 2 minutes, if necessary up to a total dose of 2 mg. In older children and adults, the dose is 2 mg every 2 minutes for five doses up to a total of 10 mg. Naloxone can also be administered into an endotracheal tube if intravenous access is unavailable. If there is no response after 10 mg, a pure opioid intoxication is unlikely. If opioid abuse is suspected, restraints should be in place before the administration of naloxone, and it is recommended that the initial dose be 0.1 to 0.2 mg to avoid withdrawal and violent behavior. The initial dose is then doubled every minute progressively to a total of 10 mg. Naloxone may unmask concomitant sympatho-mimetic intoxication as well as withdrawal.

Larger doses of naloxone may be required for more poorly antagonized synthetic opioid drugs: buprenorphine (Buprenex), codeine, dextromethorphan, fentanyl and its derivatives, pentazocine (Talwin), propoxyphene (Darvon), diphenoxylate, nalbuphine (Nubain), and long-acting opioids such as methadone (Dolophine).

Indications for a continuous infusion include a second dose for recurrent respiratory depression, exposure to poorly antagonized opioids, a large overdose, and decreased opioid metabolism, as with impaired liver function. A continuous infusion has been advocated because many opioids outlast the short half-life of naloxone (30 to 60 minutes). The hourly rate of naloxone infusion is equal to the effective dose required to produce a response (improvement in ventilation and arousal). An additional dose may be required in 15 to 30 minutes as a bolus. The infusions are titrated to avoid respiratory depression and opioid withdrawal manifestations. Tapering of infusions can be attempted after 12 hours and when the patient's condition has been stabilized.

Although naloxone is safe and effective, there are rare reports of complications (less than 1%) of pulmonary edema, seizures, hypertension, cardiac arrest, and sudden death.

Agents Whose Roles Are Not Clarified

Nalmefene (Revex), a long-acting parenteral opioid antagonist that the FDA has approved, is undergoing investigation, but its role in the treatment of comatose patients and patients with opioid overdose is not clear. It is 16 times more potent than naloxone, and its duration of action is up to 8 hours (half-life 10.8 hours, versus naloxone 1 hour).

Flumazenil (Romazicon) is a pure competitive benzodiazepine antagonist. It has been demonstrated to be safe and effective for reversing benzodiazepine-induced sedation. It is not recommended to improve ventilation. Its role in cases of CNS depression needs to be clarified. It should not be used routinely in comatose patients and is not an essential ingredient of the coma therapeutic regimen. It is contraindicated in cases of co-ingestion of cyclic antidepressant intoxication, stimulant overdose, and long-term benzodiazepine use (may precipitate life-threatening withdrawal) if benzodiazepines are used to control seizures. There is a concern about the potential for seizures and cardiac dysrhythmias that may occur in these settings.

Laboratory and Radiographic Studies

An electrocardiogram (ECG) should be obtained to identify dysrhythmias or conduction delays from cardiotoxic medications. If aspiration pneumonia (history of loss of consciousness, unarousable state, vomiting) or noncardiac pulmonary edema is suspected, a chest radiograph is needed. Electrolyte and glucose concentrations in the blood, the anion gap, acid-base balance, the arterial blood gas (ABG) profile (if patient has respiratory distress or altered mental status), and serum osmolality should be measured if a toxic alcohol ingestion is suspected. Table 7 lists appropriate testing on the basis of clinical toxicologic presentation. All laboratory specimens should be carefully labeled, including time and date. For potential legal cases, a "chain of custody" must be established. Assessment of the laboratory studies may provide a clue to the etiologic agent.

Electrolyte, Acid-Base, and Osmolality Disturbances

Electrolyte and acid-base disturbances should be evaluated and corrected. Metabolic acidosis (usually low or normal pH with a low or normal/high $PaCO_2$ and low HCO_3) with an increased anion gap (AG) is seen with many agents in cases of overdose.

The AG is an estimate of those anions other than chloride and HCO_3 necessary to counterbalance the positive charge of sodium. It serves as a clue to causes, compensations, and complications. The AG is calculated from the standard serum electrolytes by subtracting the total CO_2 (which reflects the actual measured bicarbonate) and chloride from the sodium: $(Na - [Cl + HCO_3]) = AG$. The potassium is usually not used in the calculation because it may be hemolyzed and is an intracellular cation. The lack of anion gap does not exclude a toxic etiology.

The normal gap is usually 7 to 11 mEq/L by flame photometer. However, there has been a "lowering" of the normal AG to 7 ± 4 mEq/L by the newer techniques (e.g., ion selective electrodes or colorimetric titration). Some studies have found AGs to be relatively insensitive for determining the presence of toxins.

It is important to recognize anion gap toxins, such as salicylates, methanol, and ethylene glycol, because they have specific antidotes, and hemodialysis is effective in management of cases of overdose with these agents.

Table 8 lists the reasons for increased AG, decreased anion gap, or no gap. The most common cause of a decreased AG is

TABLE 7	Patient Condition/Systemic Toxin and Appropriate Tests
CONDITION	**TESTS**
Comatose	Toxicologic tests (acetaminophen, sedative-hypnotic, ethanol, opioids, benzodiazepine), glucose.
Respiratory toxicity	Spirometry, FEV_1, arterial blood gases, chest radiograph, monitor O_2 saturation
Cardiac toxicity	ECG 12-lead and monitoring, echocardiogram, serial cardiac enzymes (if evidence or suspicion of a myocardial infarction), hemodynamic monitoring
Hepatic toxicity	Enzymes (AST, ALT, GGT), ammonia, albumin, bilirubin, glucose, PT, PTT, amylase
Nephrotoxicity	BUN, creatinine, electrolytes (Na, F, Mg, Ca, PO_4), serum and urine osmolarity, 24-hour urine for heavy metals if suspected, creatine kinase, serum and urine myoglobin, urinalysis and urinary sodium
Bleeding	Platelets, PT, PTT, bleeding time, fibrin split products, fibrinogen, type and match

Abbreviations: ALT = alanine transaminase; AST = aspartate transaminase; BUN = blood urea nitrogen; ECG = electrocardiogram; FEV_1 = forced expiratory volume in 1 second; GGT = γ-glutamyltransferase; PT = prothrombin time; PTT = partial thromboplastin time.

TABLE 8	Etiologies of Metabolic Acidosis	
NORMAL ANION GAP HYPERCHLOREMIC	**INCREASED ANION GAP NORMOCHLOREMIC**	**DECREASED ANION GAP**
Acidifying agents	Methanol	Laboratory error[†]
Adrenal insufficiency	Uremia*	Intoxication—bromine, lithium
Anhydrase inhibitors	Diabetic ketoacidosis*	Protein abnormal
Fistula	Paraldehyde,* phenformin	Sodium low
Osteotomies	Isoniazid	
Obstructive uropathies	Iron	
Renal tubular acidosis	Lactic acidosis[†]	
Diarrhea, uncomplicated*	Ethanol,* ethylene glycol*	
Dilutional	Salicylates, starvation solvents	
Sulfamylon		

*Indicates hyperosmolar situation. Studies have found that the anion gap may be relatively insensitive for determining the presence of toxins.
[†]Lactic acidosis can be produced by intoxications of the following: carbon monoxide, cyanide, hydrogen sulfide, hypoxia, ibuprofen, iron, isoniazid, phenformin, salicylates, seizures, theophylline.

laboratory error. Lactic acidosis produces the largest AG and can result from any poisoning that results in hypoxia, hypoglycemia, or convulsions.

Table 9 lists other blood chemistry derangements that suggest certain intoxications.

Serum osmolality is a measure of the number of molecules of solute per kilogram of solvent, or mOsm/kg water. The osmolarity is molecules of solute per liter of solution, or mOsm/L water at a specified temperature. Osmolarity is usually the calculated value and osmolality is usually a measured value. They are considered interchangeable where 1 L equals 1 kg. The normal serum osmolality is 280 to 290 mOsm/kg. The freezing point serum osmolarity measurement specimen and the serum electrolyte specimens for calculation should be drawn simultaneously.

The serum osmolal gap is defined as the difference between the measured osmolality determined by the freezing point method and the calculated osmolarity. It is determined by the following formula (BUN is blood urea nitrogen):

$$(Sodium \times 2) + (BUN/3) + (Glucose/20)$$

This gap estimate is normally within 10 mOsm of the simultaneously measured serum osmolality. Ethanol, if present, may be included in the equation to eliminate its influence on the osmolal gap (the ethanol concentration divided by 4.6; Table 10).

The osmolal gap is not valid in cases of shock and postmortem state. Metabolic disorders such as hyperglycemia, uremia, and dehydration increase the osmolarity but usually do not cause gaps greater than 10 mOsm/kg. A gap greater than 10 mOsm/mL suggests that unidentified osmolal-acting substances are present: acetone, ethanol, ethylene glycol, glycerin, isopropyl alcohol, isoniazid, ethanol, mannitol, methanol, and trichloroethane. Alcohols and glycols should be sought when the degree of obtundation exceeds that expected from the blood ethanol concentration or when other clinical conditions exist: visual loss (methanol), metabolic acidosis (methanol and ethylene glycol), or renal failure (ethylene glycol).

A falsely elevated osmolar gap can be produced by other low molecular weight un-ionized substances (dextran, diuretics, sorbitol, ketones), hyperlipidemia, and unmeasured electrolytes (e.g., magnesium).

Note: A normal osmolal gap may be reported in the presence of toxic alcohol or glycol poisoning, if the parent compound is already metabolized. This situation can occur when the osmolar gap is measured after a significant time has elapsed since the ingestion. In cases of alcohol and glycol intoxication, an early osmolar gap is a result of the relatively nontoxic parent drug and delayed metabolic acidosis, and an anion gap is a

TABLE 9	Blood Chemistry Derangements in Toxicology
DERANGEMENT	**TOXIN**
Acetonemia without acidosis	Acetone or isopropyl alcohol
Hypomagnesemia	Ethanol, digitalis
Hypocalcemia	Ethylene glycol, oxalate, fluoride
Hyperkalemia	β-Blockers, acute digitalis, renal failure
Hypokalemia	Diuretics, salicylism, sympathomimetics, theophylline, corticosteroids, chronic digitalis
Hyperglycemia	Diazoxide, glucagon, iron, isoniazid, organophosphate insecticides, phenylurea insecticides, phenytoin (Dilantin), salicylates, sympathomimetic agents, thyroid vasopressors
Hypoglycemia	β-Blockers, ethanol, insulin, isoniazid, oral hypoglycemic agents, salicylates
Rhabdomyolysis	Amphetamines, ethanol, cocaine, or phencyclidine, elevated creatine phosphokinase

TABLE 10	Conversion Factors for Alcohols and Glycols		
ALCOHOLS/ GLYCOLS	**1 MG/DL IN BLOOD RAISES OSMOLALITY MOSM/L**	**MOLECULAR WEIGHT**	**CONVERSION FACTOR**
Ethanol	0.228	40	4.6
Methanol	0.327	32	3.2
Ethylene glycol	0.190	62	6.2
Isopropanol	0.176	60	6.0
Acetone	0.182	58	5.8
Propylene glycol	NA	72	7.2

Example: Methanol osmolality. Subtract the calculated osmolality from the measured serum osmolarity (freezing point method) = osmolar gap × 3.2 (one-tenth molecular weight) = estimated serum methanol concentration.
Note: This equation is often not considered very reliable in predicting the actual measured blood concentration of these alcohols or glycols.

result of the more toxic metabolites. The serum concentration is calculated as

$$mg/dL = mOsm\ gap \times MW\ of\ substance\ divided\ by\ 10.$$

Radiographic Studies

Chest and neck radiographs are useful for suspected pathologic conditions such as aspiration pneumonia, pulmonary edema, and foreign bodies and to determine the location of the endotracheal tube. Abdominal radiographs can be used to detect radiopaque substances.

The mnemonic for radiopaque substances seen on abdominal radiographs is CHIPES:
C—chlorides and chloral hydrate
H—heavy metals (arsenic, barium, iron, lead, mercury, zinc)
I—iodides
P—PlayDoh, Pepto-Bismol, phenothiazine (inconsistent)
E—enteric-coated tablets
S—sodium, potassium, and other elements in tablet form (bismuth, calcium, potassium) and solvents containing chlorides (e.g., carbon tetrachloride)

Toxicologic Studies

Routine blood and urine screening is of little practical value in the initial care of the poisoned patient. Specific toxicologic analyses and quantitative levels of certain drugs may be extremely helpful. One should always ask oneself the following questions: (a) How will the result of the test alter the management? and (b) Can the result of the test be returned in time to have a positive effect on therapy?

Owing to long turnaround time, lack of availability, factors contributing to unreliability, and the risk of serious morbidity without supportive clinical management, toxicology screening is estimated to affect management in less than 15% of cases of drug overdoses or poisonings. Toxicology screening may look specifically for only 40 to 50 drugs out of more than 10,000 possible drugs or toxins and more than several million chemicals. To detect many different drugs, toxic screens usually include methods with broad specificity, and sensitivity may be poor for some drugs, resulting in false-negative or false-positive findings. On the other hand, some drugs present in therapeutic amounts may be detected on the screen, even though they are causing no clinical symptoms. Because many agents are not sought or detected during a toxicologic screening, a negative result does not always rule out poisonings. The specificity of toxicologic tests is dependent on the method and the laboratory. The presence of other drugs, drug metabolites, disease states, or incorrect sampling may cause erroneous results.

For the average toxicologic laboratory, false-negative results occur at a rate of 10% to 30% and false-positives at a rate of 0% to 10%. The positive screen predictive value is approximately 90%. A negative toxicology screen does not exclude a poisoning. The negative predictive value of toxicologic screening is approximately 70%. For example, the following benzodiazepines may not be detected by some routine immunoassay benzodiazepine screening tests: alprazolam (Xanax), clonazepam (Klonopin), temazepam (Restoril), and triazolam (Halcion).

The "toxic urine screen" is generally a qualitative urine test for several common drugs, usually substances of abuse (cocaine and metabolites, opioids, amphetamines, benzodiazepines, barbiturates, and phencyclidine). Results of these tests are usually available within 2 to 6 hours. Because these tests may vary with each hospital and community, the physician should determine exactly which substances are included in the toxic urine screen of his or her laboratory. Tests for ethylene glycol, red blood cell cholinesterase, and serum cyanide are not readily available.

For cases of ingestion of certain substances, quantitative blood levels should be obtained at specific times after the ingestion to avoid spurious low values in the distribution phase, which result from incomplete absorption. The detection time for drugs is influenced by many variables, such as type of substance, formulation, amount, time since ingestion, duration of exposure, and half-life. For many drugs, the detection time is measured in days after the exposure.

Common Poisons

Acetaminophen (Paracetamol, *N*-Acetyl-Paraaminophenol)

Toxic Mechanism

At therapeutic doses of acetaminophen, less than 5% is metabolized by P450-2E1 to a toxic reactive oxidizing metabolite, *N*-acetyl-p-benzoquinoneimine (NAPQI). In a case of overdose, there is insufficient glutathione available to reduce the excess NAPQI into nontoxic conjugate, so it forms covalent bonds with hepatic intracellular proteins to produce centrilobular necrosis. Renal damage is caused by a similar mechanism.

Toxic Dose

The therapeutic dose of acetaminophen is 10 to 15 mg/kg, with a maximum of five doses in 24 hours for a maximum total daily dose of 4 g. An acute single toxic dose is greater than 140 mg/kg, possibly greater than 200 mg/kg in a child younger than age 5 years. Factors affecting the P450 enzymes include enzyme inducers such as barbiturates and phenytoin (Dilantin), ingestion of isoniazid, and alcoholism. Factors that decrease glutathione stores (alcoholism, malnutrition, and HIV infection) contribute to the toxicity of acetaminophen. Alcoholics ingesting 3 to 4 g/d of acetaminophen for a few days can have depleted glutathione stores and require *N*-acetylcysteine therapy at 50% below hepatotoxic blood acetaminophen levels on the nomogram.

Kinetics

Peak plasma concentration is usually reached 2 to 4 hours after an overdose. Volume distribution is 0.9 L/kg, and protein binding is less than 50% (albumin).

Route of elimination is by hepatic metabolism to an inactive nontoxic glucuronide conjugate and inactive nontoxic sulfate metabolite by two saturable pathways; less than 5% is metabolized into reactive metabolite NAPQI. In patients younger than 6 years of age, metabolic elimination occurs to a greater degree by conjugation via the sulfate pathway.

The half-life of acetaminophen is 1 to 3 hours.

Manifestations

The four phases of the intoxication's clinical course may overlap, and the absence of a phase does not exclude toxicity.
- Phase I occurs within 0.5 to 24 hours after ingestion and may consist of a few hours of malaise, diaphoresis, nausea, and vomiting or produce no symptoms. CNS depression or coma is not a feature.
- Phase II occurs 24 to 48 hours after ingestion and is a period of diminished symptoms. The liver enzymes, serum aspartate aminotransferase (AST) (earliest), and serum alanine aminotransferase (ALT) may increase as early as 4 hours or as late as 36 hours after ingestion.
- Phase III occurs at 48 to 96 hours, with peak liver function abnormalities at 72 to 96 hours. The degree of elevation of the hepatic enzymes generally correlates with outcome, but not always. Recovery starts at about 4 days unless hepatic failure develops. Less than 1% of patients with a history of overdose develop fulminant hepatotoxicity.
- Phase IV occurs at 4 to 14 days, with hepatic enzyme abnormalities resolving. If extensive liver damage has occurred, sepsis and disseminated intravascular coagulation may ensue.

Transient renal failure may develop at 5 to 7 days with or without evidence of hepatic damage. Rare cases of myocarditis and pancreatitis have been reported. Death can occur at 7 to 14 days.

Laboratory Investigations

The therapeutic reference range is 10 to 20 µg/mL. For toxic levels, see the nomogram presented in Figure 1.

Appropriate and reliable methods for analysis are radioimmunoassay, high-pressure liquid chromatography, and gas

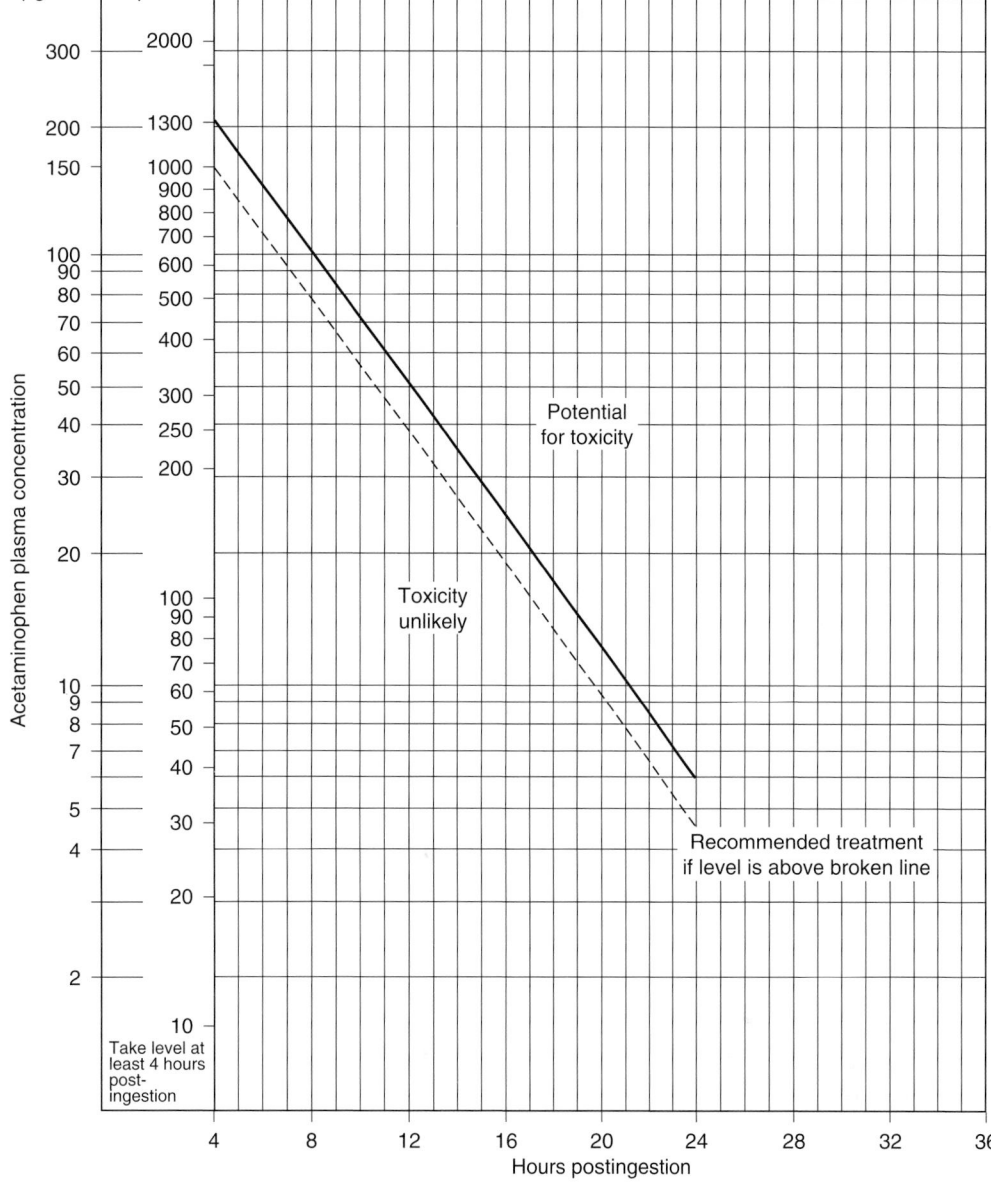

Figure 1 Nomogram for acetaminophen intoxication. *N*-acetylcysteine therapy is started if levels and time coordinates are above the lower line on the nomogram. Continue and complete therapy even if subsequent values fall below the toxic zone. The nomogram is useful only in cases of acute single ingestion. Levels in serum drawn before 4 hours may not represent peak levels. From Rumack BH, Matthew H: Acetaminophen poisoning and toxicity. *Pediatrics* 55:871, 1975.

Labels within figure:
- µg/mL / µmo/L (vertical axes)
- Acetaminophen plasma concentration (y-axis)
- Potential for toxicity
- Toxicity unlikely
- Recommended treatment if level is above broken line
- Take level at least 4 hours postingestion
- Hours postingestion (x-axis)

TABLE 11	Protocol for *N*-Acetylcysteine Administration			
ROUTE	**LOADING DOSE**	**MAINTENANCE DOSE**	**COURSE**	**FDA APPROVAL**
Oral	140 mg/kg	70 mg/kg every 4 h	72 h	Yes
Intravenous	150 mg/kg over 15 min	50 mg/kg over 4 h followed by 100 mg/kg over 16 h	20 h	Yes

chromatography. Spectroscopic assays often give falsely elevated values: bilirubin, salicylate, salicylamide, diflunisal (Dolobid), phenols, and methyldopa (Aldomet) increase the acetaminophen level. Each 1 mg/dL increase in creatinine increases the acetaminophen plasma level 30 µg/mL.

If a toxic acetaminophen level is reached, liver profile (including AST, ALT, bilirubin, and prothrombin time), serum amylase, and blood glucose must be monitored. A complete blood cell count (CBC); platelet count; phosphate, electrolytes, and bicarbonate level measurements; ECG; and urinalysis are indicated.

Management

Gastrointestinal Decontamination. Although ipecac-induced emesis may be useful within 30 minutes of ingestion of the toxic substance, we do not advise it because it could result in vomiting of the activated charcoal. Gastric lavage is not necessary. Studies

have indicated that activated charcoal is useful within 1 hour after ingestion. Activated charcoal does adsorb *N*-acetylcysteine (NAC) if given together, but this is not clinically important. However, if activated charcoal needs to be given along with NAC, separate the administration of activated charcoal from the administration of NAC by 1 to 2 hours to avoid vomiting.

N-Acetylcysteine (Mucomyst). NAC (Table 11), a derivative of the amino acid cysteine, acts as a sulfhydryl donor for glutathione synthesis, as surrogate glutathione, and may increase the nontoxic sulfation pathway resulting in conjugation of NAPQI. Oral NAC should be administered within the first 8 hours after a toxic amount of acetaminophen has been ingested. NAC can be started while one awaits the results of the blood test for acetaminophen plasma concentration, but there is no advantage to giving it before 8 hours. If the acetaminophen concentration result after 4 hours following ingestion is above the upper line on the modified Rumack-Matthew nomogram (see Figure 1), one should continue with a maintenance course. Repeat blood specimens should be obtained 4 hours after the initial level is measured if it is greater than 20 mg/mL, which is below the therapy line, because of unexpected delays in the peak by food and co-ingestants. Intravenous NAC (see Table 11) is approved in the United States.

There have been a few cases of anaphylactoid reaction and death by the intravenous route.

Variations in Therapy

In patients with chronic alcoholism, it is recommended that NAC treatment be administered at 50% below the upper toxic line on the nomogram.

If emesis occurs within 1 hour after NAC administration, the dose should be repeated. To avoid emesis, the proper dilution from 20% to 5% NAC must be used, and it should be served in a palatable vehicle, in a covered container through a straw. If this administration is unsuccessful, a slow drip over 30 to 60 minutes through a nasogastric tube or a fluoroscopically placed nasoduodenal tube can be used. Antiemetics can be used if necessary: metoclopramide (Reglan) 10 mg per dose intravenously 30 minutes before administration of NAC (in children, 0.1 mg/kg; maximum, 0.5 mg/kg/d) or ondansetron (Zofran) 32 mg (0.15 mg/kg) by infusion over 15 minutes and repeated for three doses if necessary. The side effects of these antiemetics include anaphylaxis and increases in liver enzymes.

Some investigators recommend variable durations of NAC therapy, stopping the therapy if serial acetaminophen blood concentrations become nondetectable and the liver enzyme levels (ALT and AST) remain normal after 24 to 36 hours.

There is a loss of efficacy if NAC is initiated 8 or 10 hours postingestion, but the loss is not complete, and NAC may be initiated 36 hours or more after ingestion. Late treatment (after 24 hours) decreases the rates of morbidity and mortality in patients with fulminant liver failure caused by acetaminophen and other agents.

Extended relief formulations (ER embossed on caplet) contain 325 mg of acetaminophen for immediate release and 325 mg for delayed release. A single 4-hour postingestion serum acetaminophen concentration can underestimate the level because ER formulations can have secondary delayed peaks. In cases of overdose of the ER formulation, it is recommended that additional acetaminophen levels be obtained at 4-hour intervals after the initial level is measured. If any level is in the toxic zone, therapy should be initiated.

It is recommended that pregnant patients with toxic plasma concentrations of acetaminophen be treated with NAC to prevent hepatotoxicity in both fetus and mother. The available data suggest no teratogenicity to NAC or acetaminophen.

Indications for NAC therapy in cases of chronic intoxication are a history of ingestion of 3 to 4 g for several days with elevated liver enzyme levels (AST and ALT). The acetaminophen blood concentration is often low in these cases because of the extended time lapse since ingestion and should not be plotted on the Rumack-Matthew nomogram. Patients with a history of chronic alcoholism or those on chronic enzyme inducers may also present with elevated liver enzyme levels and should be considered for NAC therapy if they have a history of taking acetaminophen on a chronic basis, because they are considered to be at a greater risk for hepatotoxicity despite a low acetaminophen blood concentration.

Specific support care may be needed to treat liver failure, pancreatitis, transient renal failure, and myocarditis.

Liver transplantation has a definite but limited role in patients with acute acetaminophen overdose. A retrospective analysis determined that a continuing rise in the prothrombin time (4-day peak, 180 seconds), a pH of less than 7.3 2 days after the overdose, a serum creatinine level of greater than 3.3 mg/dL, severe hepatic encephalopathy, and disturbed coagulation factor VII/V ratio greater than 30 suggest a poor prognosis and may be indicators for hepatology consultation for consideration of liver transplantation.

Extracorporeal measures are not expected to be of benefit.

Disposition

Adults who have ingested more than 140 mg/kg and children younger than 6 years of age who have ingested more than 200 mg/kg should receive therapy within 8 hours postingestion or until the results of the 4-hour postingestion acetaminophen plasma concentration are known.

Amphetamines

The amphetamines include illicit methamphetamine ("Ice"), diet pills, and formulations under various trade names. Analogues include MDMA (3,4 methylenedioxymethamphetamine, known as "ecstasy," "XTC," or "Adam") and MDA (3,4-methylenedioxyamphetamine, known as "Eve"). MDA is a common hallucinogen and euphoriant "club drug" used at "raves," which are all-night dances. Use of methamphetamine and designer analogues is on the rise, especially among young people between the ages of 12 and 25 years. Other similar stimulants are phenylpropanolamine and cocaine.

Toxic Mechanism

Amphetamines have a direct CNS stimulant effect and a sympathetic nervous system effect by releasing catecholamines from α- and β-adrenergic nerve terminals but inhibiting their reuptake.

Hallucinogenic MDMA has an additional hazard of serotonin effect (refer to serotonin syndrome in the SSRI section). MDMA also affects the dopamine system in the brain. Because of its effects on 5-hydroxytryptamine, dopamine, and norepinephrine, MDMA can lead to serotonin syndrome associated with malignant hyperthermia and rhabdomyolysis, which contributes to the potentially life-threatening hyperthermia observed in several patients who have used MDMA.

Phenylpropanolamine stimulates only the β-adrenergic receptors.

Toxic Dose

In children, the toxic dose of dextroamphetamine is 1 mg/kg; in adults, the toxic dose is 5 mg/kg. The potentially fatal dose of dextroamphetamine is 12 mg/kg.

Kinetics

Amphetamine is a weak base with pKa of 8 to 10. Onset of action is 30 to 60 minutes, and peak effects are 2 to 4 hours. The volume distribution is 2 to 3 L/kg.

Through hepatic metabolism, 60% of the substance is metabolized into a hydroxylated metabolite that may be responsible for psychotic effects.

The half-life of amphetamines is pH dependent—8 to 10 hours in acid urine (pH <6.0) and 16 to 31 hours in alkaline urine (pH >7.5). Excretion is by the kidney—30% to 40% at alkaline urine pH and 50% to 70% at acid urine pH.

Manifestations

Effects are seen within 30 to 60 minutes following ingestion.

Neurologic manifestations include restlessness, irritation and agitation, tremors and hyperreflexia, and auditory and visual hallucinations. Hyperpyrexia may precede seizures, convulsions, paranoia, violence, intracranial hemorrhage, psychosis, and self-destructive behavior. Paranoid psychosis and cerebral vasculitis occur with chronic abuse.

MDMA is often adulterated with cocaine, heroin, or ketamine, or a combination of these, to create a variety of mood alterations. This possibility must be taken into consideration when one manages patients with MDMA ingestions, as the symptom complex may reflect both CNS stimulation and CNS depression.

Other manifestations include dilated but reactive pupils, cardiac dysrhythmias (supraventricular and ventricular), tachycardia, hypertension, rhabdomyolysis, and myoglobinuria.

Laboratory Investigations

The clinician should monitor ECG and cardiac readings, ABG and oxygen saturation, electrolytes, blood glucose, BUN, creatinine, creatine kinase, cardiac fraction if there is chest pain, and liver profile. Also, one should evaluate for rhabdomyolysis and check urine for myoglobin, cocaine and metabolites, and other substances of abuse. The peak plasma concentration of amphetamines is 10 to 50 ng/mL 1 to 2 hours after ingestion of 10 to 25 mg. The toxic plasma concentration is 200 ng/mL. When the rapid immunoassays are used, cross-reactions can occur with amphetamine derivatives (e.g., MDA, "ecstasy"), brompheniramine (Dimetane), chlorpromazine (Thorazine), ephedrine, phenylpropanolamine, phentermine (Adipex-P), phenmetrazine, ranitidine (Zantac), and Vicks Inhaler (L-desoxyephedrine). False-positive results may occur.

Management

Management is similar to management for cocaine intoxication. Supportive care includes blood pressure and temperature control, cardiac monitoring, and seizure precautions. Diazepam (Valium) can be administered. Gastrointestinal decontamination can be undertaken with activated charcoal administered up to 1 hour after ingestion.

Anxiety, agitation, and convulsions are treated with diazepam. If diazepam fails to control seizures, neuromuscular blockers can be used and the electroencephalogram (EEG) monitored for nonmotor seizures. One should avoid neuroleptic phenothiazines and butyrophenone, which can lower the seizure threshold.

Hypertension and tachycardia are usually transient and can be managed by titration of diazepam. Nitroprusside can be used for hypertensive crisis at a maximum infusion rate of 10 µg/kg/min for 10 minutes followed with a lower infusion rate of 0.3 to 2 mg/kg/min. Myocardial ischemia is managed by oxygen, vascular access, benzodiazepines, and nitroglycerin. Aspirin and thrombolytics are not routinely recommended because of the danger of intracranial hemorrhage. It is important to distinguish between angina and true ischemia. Delayed hypotension can be treated with fluids and vasopressors if needed. Life-threatening tachydysrhythmias may respond to an α-blocker such as phentolamine (Regitine) 5 mg IV for adults or 0.1 mg/kg IV for children and a short-acting β-blocker such as esmolol (Brevibloc) 500 µg/kg IV over 1 minute for adults, or 300 to 500 µg/kg over 1 minute for children. Ventricular dysrhythmias may respond to lidocaine or, in a severely hemodynamically compromised patient, immediate synchronized electrical cardioversion.

Rhabdomyolysis and myoglobinuria are treated with fluids, alkaline diuresis, and diuretics. Hyperthermia is treated with external cooling and cool 100% humidified oxygen. More extensive therapy may be needed in severe cases. If focal neurologic symptoms are present, the possibility of a cerebrovascular accident should be considered and a CT scan of the head should be obtained.

Paranoid ideation and threatening behavior should be treated with rapid tranquilization using a benzodiazepine. One should observe for suicidal depression that may follow intoxication and may require suicide precautions.

Extracorporeal measures are of no benefit.

Disposition

Symptomatic patients should be observed on a monitored unit until the symptoms resolve and then observed for a short time after resolution for relapse.

Anticholinergic Agents

Drugs with anticholinergic properties include antihistamines (H_1 blockers), neuroleptics (phenothiazines), tricyclic antidepressants, antiparkinsonism drugs (trihexyphenidyl [Artane], benztropine [Cogentin]), ophthalmic products (atropine), and a number of common plants.

The antihistamines are divided into the sedating anticholinergic types and the nonsedating single daily dose types. The sedating types include ethanolamines (e.g., diphenhydramine [Benadryl], dimenhydrinate [Dramamine], and clemastine [Tavist]), ethylenediamines (e.g., tripelennamine [Pyribenzamine]), alkyl amines (e.g., chlorpheniramine [Chlor-Trimeton], brompheniramine [Dimetane]), piperazines (e.g., cyclizine [Marezine], hydroxyzine [Atarax], and meclizine [Antivert]), and phenothiazine (e.g., Phenergan). The nonsedating types include astemizole (Hismanal), terfenadine (Seldane), loratadine (Claritin), fexofenadine (Allegra), and cetirizine (Zyrtec).

The anticholinergic plants include jimsonweed (*Datura stramonium*), deadly nightshade (*Atropa belladonna*), henbane (*Hyoscyamus niger*), and antispasmodic agents for the bowel (atropine derivatives).

Toxic Mechanism

By competitive inhibition, anticholinergics block the action of acetylcholine on postsynaptic cholinergic receptor sites. The toxic mechanism primarily involves the peripheral and CNS muscarinic receptors. H_1 sedating-type agents also depress or stimulate the CNS, and in large overdoses some have cardiac membrane–depressant effects (e.g., diphenhydramine [Benadryl]) and α-adrenergic receptor blockade effects (e.g., promethazine [Phenergan]). Nonsedating agents produce peripheral H_1 blockade but do not possess anticholinergic or sedating actions. The original agents terfenadine (Seldane) and astemizole (Hismanal) were recently removed from the market because of the severe cardiac dysrhythmias associated with their use, especially when used in combination with macrolide antibiotics and certain antifungal agents such as ketoconazole (Nizoral), which inhibit hepatic metabolism or excretion. The newer nonsedating agents, including loratadine (Claritin), fexofenadine (Allegra), and cetirizine (Zyrtec), have not been reported to cause the severe drug interactions associated with terfenadine and astemizole.

Toxic Dose

The estimated toxic oral dose of atropine is 0.05 mg/kg in children and more than 2 mg in adults. The minimal estimated lethal dose of atropine is more than 10 mg in adults and more than 2 mg in children. Other synthetic anticholinergic agents are less toxic, and the fatal dose varies from 10 to 100 mg.

The estimated toxic oral dose of diphenhydramine (Benadryl) in a child is 15 mg/kg, and the potential lethal amount is 25 mg/kg. In an adult, the potential lethal amount is 2.8 g. Ingestion of five times the single dose of an antihistamine is toxic.

For the nonsedating agents, an overdose of 3360 mg of terfenadine was reported in an adult who developed ventricular tachycardia and fibrillation that responded to lidocaine and defibrillation. A 1500-mg overdose produced hypotension. Cases of delayed serious dysrhythmias (torsades de pointes) have been reported with doses of more than 200 mg of astemizole. The toxic doses of fexofenadine (Allegra), cetirizine, and loratadine (Claritin) need to be established.

Kinetics

The onset of absorption of intravenous atropine is in 2 to 4 minutes. Peak effects on salivation after intravenous or intramuscular administration are at 30 to 60 minutes.

Onset of absorption after oral ingestion is 30 to 60 minutes, peak action is 1 to 3 hours, and duration of action is 4 to 6 hours, but symptoms are prolonged in cases of overdose or with sustained-release preparations.

The onset of absorption of diphenhydramine is in 15 minutes to 1 hour, with a peak of action in 1 to 4 hours. Volume distribution is 3.3 to 6.8 L/kg, and protein binding is 75% to 80%. Ninety-eight percent of diphenhydramine is metabolized via the liver by *N*-demethylation. Interactions with erythromycin, ketoconazole (Nizoral), and derivatives produce excessive blood levels of the antihistamine and ventricular dysrhythmias.

The half-life of diphenhydramine is 3 to 10 hours.

The chemical structure of nonsedating agents prevents their entry into the CNS. Absorption begins in 1 hour, with peak effects in 4 to 6 hours. The duration of action is greater than 24 hours.

These agents are metabolized in the gastrointestinal tract and liver. Protein binding is greater than 90%. The plasma half-life is 3.5 hours. Only 1% is excreted unchanged; 60% of that is excreted in the feces and 40% in the urine.

Manifestations
Anticholinergic signs are hyperpyrexia ("hot as a hare"), mydriasis ("blind as a bat"), flushing of skin ("red as a beet"), dry mucosa and skin ("dry as a bone"), "Lilliputian type" hallucinations and delirium ("mad as a hatter"), coma, dysphagia, tachycardia, moderate hypertension, and rarely convulsions and urinary retention. Other effects include jaundice (cyproheptadine [Periactin]), dystonia (diphenhydramine [Benadryl]), rhabdomyolysis (doxylamine), and, in large doses, cardiotoxic effects (diphenhydramine).

Overdose with nonsedating agents produces headache and confusion, nausea, and dysrhythmias (e.g., torsades de pointes).

Laboratory Investigations
Monitoring of ABG (in cases of respiratory depression), electrolytes, glucose, and the ECG should be undertaken. Anticholinergic drugs and plants are not routinely included on screens for substances of abuse.

Management
For patients in respiratory failure, intubation and assisted ventilation should be instituted. Gastrointestinal decontamination can be instituted. Caution must be taken with emesis in cases of diphenhydramine (Benadryl) overdose because of the drug's rapid onset of action and risk of seizures. If bowel sounds are present for up to 1 hour after ingestion, activated charcoal can be given. Seizures can be controlled with benzodiazepines (diazepam [Valium] or lorazepam [Ativan]).

The administration of physostigmine (Antilirium) is not routine and is reserved for life-threatening anticholinergic effects that are refractory to conventional treatments. It should be administered with adequate monitoring and resuscitative equipment available. The use of physostigmine should be avoided if a tricyclic antidepressant is present because of increased toxicity. Urinary retention should be relieved by catheterization to avoid reabsorption of the drug and additional toxicity.

Supraventricular tachycardia should be treated only if the patient is hemodynamically unstable. Ventricular dysrhythmias can be controlled with lidocaine or cardioversion. Sodium bicarbonate 1 to 2 mEq/kg IV may be useful for myocardial depression and QRS prolongation. Torsades de pointes, especially when associated with terfenadine and astemizole ingestion, has been treated with magnesium sulfate 4 g or 40 mL 10% solution intravenously over 10 to 20 minutes and countershock if the patient fails to respond.

Hyperpyrexia is controlled by external cooling. Hemodialysis and hemoperfusion are not effective.

Disposition
Antihistamine H$_1$ Antagonists. Symptomatic patients should be observed on a monitored unit until the symptoms resolve, then observed for a short time (3 to 4 hours) after resolution for relapse.

Nonsedating Agents. All asymptomatic children who acutely ingest more than the maximum adult dose and all symptomatic children should be referred to a health care facility for a minimum of 6 hours' observation as well as cardiac monitoring. Asymptomatic adults who acutely ingest more than twice the maximum adult daily dose should be monitored for a minimum of 6 hours. All symptomatic patients should be monitored for as long as there are symptoms present.

Barbiturates
Barbiturates have been used as sedatives, anesthetic agents, and anticonvulsants, but their use is declining as safer, more effective drugs become available.

Toxic Mechanism
Barbiturates are γ-aminobutyric acid (GABA) agonists (increasing the chloride flow and inhibiting depolarization). They enhance the CNS depressant effect of GABA and depress the cardiovascular system.

Toxic Dose
The shorter-acting barbiturates (including the intermediate-acting agents) and their hypnotic doses are as follows: amobarbital (Amytal), 100 to 200 mg; aprobarbital (Alurate), 50 to 100 mg; butabarbital (Butisol), 50 to 100 mg; butalbital, 100 to 200 mg; pentobarbital (Nembutal), 100 to 200 mg; secobarbital (Seconal), 100 to 200 mg. They cause toxicity at lower doses than long-acting barbiturates and have a minimum toxic dose of 6 mg/kg; the fatal adult dose is 3 to 6 g.

The long-acting barbiturates and their doses include mephobarbital (Mebaral), 50 to 100 mg, and phenobarbital, 100 to 200 mg. Their minimum toxic dose is greater than 10 mg/kg, and the fatal adult dose is 6 to 10 g. A general rule is that an amount five times the hypnotic dose is toxic and an amount 10 times the hypnotic dose is potentially fatal. Methohexital and thiopental are ultrashort-acting parenteral preparations and are not discussed.

Kinetics
The barbiturates are enzyme inducers. Short-acting barbiturates are highly lipid-soluble, penetrate the brain readily, and have shorter elimination times. Onset of action is in 10 to 30 minutes, with a peak at 1 to 2 hours. Duration of action is 3 to 8 hours. The volume distribution of short-acting barbiturate is 0.8 to 1.5 L/kg; pKa is about 8. Mean half-life varies from 8 to 48 hours.

Long-acting agents have longer elimination times and can be used as anticonvulsants. Onset of action is in 20 to 60 minutes, with a peak at 1 to 6 hours. In cases of overdose, the peak can be at 10 hours. Usual duration of action is 8 to 12 hours. Volume distribution is 0.8 L/kg, and half-life is 11 to 120 hours. The pKa of phenobarbital is 7.2. Alkalinization of urine promotes its excretion.

Manifestations
Mild intoxication resembles alcohol intoxication and includes ataxia, slurred speech, and depressed cognition. Severe intoxication causes slow respirations, coma, and loss of reflexes (except pupillary light reflex).

Other manifestations include hypotension (vasodilation), hypothermia, hypoglycemia, and death by respiratory arrest.

Laboratory Investigations
Most barbiturates are detected on routine drug screens and can be measured in most hospital laboratories. Investigation should include barbiturate level; ABG; toxicology screen, including acetaminophen; glucose, electrolyte, BUN, creatinine, and creatine kinase levels; and urine pH. The minimum toxic plasma levels are greater than 10 μg/mL for short-acting barbiturates and greater than 40 μg/dL for long-acting agents. Fatal levels are 30 μg/mL for short-acting barbiturates and 80 to 150 μg/mL for long-acting agents. Both short-acting and long-acting agents can be detected in urine 24 to 72 hours after ingestion, and long-acting agents can be detected up to 7 days.

Management
Vital functions must be established and maintained. Intensive supportive care including intubation and assisted ventilation should dominate the management. All stuporous and comatose patients should have glucose (for hypoglycemia), thiamine (if chronically alcoholic), and naloxone (Narcan) (in case of an opioid ingestion) intravenously and should be admitted to the intensive care unit. Emesis should be avoided especially in cases of ingestion of the shorter-acting barbiturates. Activated charcoal followed by MDAC (0.5 g/kg) every 2 to 4 hours has been shown to reduce the serum half-life of phenobarbital by 50%, but its effect on clinical course is undetermined.

Fluids should be administered to correct dehydration and hypotension. Vasopressors may be necessary to correct severe hypotension, and hemodynamic monitoring may be needed. The patient must be observed carefully for fluid overload. Alkalinization (ion trapping) is used only for phenobarbital (pKa 7.2) but not for short-acting barbiturates. Sodium bicarbonate, 1 to 2 mEq/kg IV in 500 mL of 5% dextrose in adults or 10 to 15 mL/kg in children during the first hour, followed by sufficient bicarbonate to keep the urinary pH at 7.5 to 8.0, enhances excretion of phenobarbital and shortens the half-life by 50%. Diuresis is not advocated because of the danger of cerebral or pulmonary edema.

Hemodialysis shortens the half-life to 8 to 14 hours, and charcoal hemoperfusion shortens the half-life to 6 to 8 hours for long-acting barbiturates such as phenobarbital. Both procedures may be effective in patients with both long-acting and short-acting barbiturate ingestion. If the patient does not respond to supportive measures or if the phenobarbital plasma concentration is greater than 150 µg/mL, both procedures may be tried to shorten the half-life.

Bullae are treated as a local second-degree skin burn. Hypothermia should be treated.

Disposition

All comatose patients should be admitted to the intensive care unit. Awake and oriented patients with an overdose of short-acting agents should be observed for at least 6 asymptomatic hours; overdose of long-acting agents warrants observation for at least 12 asymptomatic hours because of the potential for delayed absorption. In the case of an intentional overdose, psychiatric clearance is needed before the patient can be discharged. Chronic use can lead to tolerance, physical dependency, and withdrawal and necessitates follow-up.

Benzodiazepines

Benzodiazepines are used as anxiolytics, sedatives, and relaxants.

Toxic Mechanism

The GABA agonists produce CNS depression and increase chloride flow, inhibiting depolarization.

Flunitrazepam (Rohypnol; street name "roofies") is a long-acting benzodiazepine agonist sold by prescription in more than 60 countries worldwide, but it is not legally available in the United States.

Toxic Dose

The long-acting benzodiazepines (half-life >24 hours) and their maximum therapeutic doses are as follows: chlordiazepoxide (Librium), 50 mg; clorazepate (Tranxene), 30 mg; clonazepam (Klonopin), 20 mg; diazepam (Valium), 10 mg in adults or 0.2 mg/kg in children; flurazepam (Dalmane), 30 mg; and prazepam, 20 mg.

The short-acting benzodiazepines (half-life 10 to 24 hours) and their doses include the following: alprazolam (Xanax), 0.5 mg, and lorazepam (Ativan), 4 mg in adults or 0.05 mg/kg in children, which act similar to the long-acting benzodiazepines.

The ultrashort-acting benzodiazepines (half-life <10 hours) are more toxic and include temazepam (Restoril), 30 mg; triazolam (Halcion), 0.5 mg; midazolam (Versed), 0.2 mg/kg; and oxazepam (Serax), 30 mg.

In cases of overdose of short- and long-acting agents, 10 to 20 times the therapeutic dose (>1500 mg diazepam or 2000 mg chlordiazepoxide) have been ingested with resulting mild coma but without respiratory depression. Fatalities are rare, and most patients recover within 24 to 36 hours after overdose. Asymptomatic unintentional overdoses of less than five times the therapeutic dose can be seen. Ultrashort-acting agents have produced respiratory arrest and coma within 1 hour after ingestion of 5 mg of triazolam (Halcion) and death with ingestion of as little as 10 mg. Midazolam (Versed) and diazepam (Valium) by rapid intravenous injection have produced respiratory arrest.

Kinetics

Onset of CNS depression is usually in 30 to 120 minutes; peak action usually occurs within 1 to 3 hours when ingestion is by the oral route. The volume distribution varies from 0.26 to 6 L/kg (LA, 1.1 L/kg); protein binding is 70% to 99%. For flunitrazepam, the onset of action is in 0.5 to 2 hours, oral peak is in 2 hours, and duration 8 hours or more. The half-life of flunitrazepam is 20 to 30 hours, volume distribution is 3.3 to 5.5 L/kg, and 80% is protein bound. Flunitrazepam can be identified in urine 4 to 30 days after ingestion.

Manifestations

Neurologic manifestations include ataxia, slurred speech, and CNS depression. Deep coma leading to respiratory depression suggests the presence of short-acting benzodiazepines or other CNS depressants. In elderly persons, the therapeutic doses can produce toxicity and can have an additive effect with other CNS depressants. Chronic use can lead to tolerance, physical dependency, and withdrawal.

Laboratory Investigations

Most benzodiazepines can be detected in urine drug screens. Quantitative blood levels are not useful. Some of the immunoassay urinary screens cannot detect all of the new benzodiazepines currently available. A consultation with the laboratory analyst is warranted if a specific case occurs in which the test result is negative but benzodiazepine use is suspected by the patient's history. Situations in which benzodiazepines may not be detected include ingestion of a low dose (e.g., <10 mg), rapid elimination, and a different or no metabolite. Some immunoassay methods can produce a false-positive finding for the benzodiazepines when nonsteroidal antiinflammatory drugs (tolmetin [Tolectin], naproxen [Aleve], etodolac [Lodine], and fenoprofen [Nalfon]) are used. If this is a concern, the laboratory analyst should be consulted.

In cases in which "date rape" drugs such as flunitrazepam are suspected, a police crime or reference laboratory should be consulted for testing.

Management

Emesis and gastric lavage should be avoided. Activated charcoal can be useful only if given early before the peak time of absorption occurs. Supportive treatment should be instituted but rarely requires intubation or assisted ventilation.

Flumazenil (Romazicon) is a specific benzodiazepine receptor antagonist that blocks the chloride flow and inhibitor of GABA neurotransmitters. It reverses the sedative effects of benzodiazepines, zolpidem (Ambien), and endogenous benzodiazepines associated with hepatic encephalopathy. It is not recommended to reverse benzodiazepine-induced hypoventilation. The manufacturer advises that flumazenil be used with caution in cases of overdose with possible benzodiazepine dependency (because it can precipitate life-threatening withdrawal), if cyclic antidepressant use is suspected, or if a patient has a known seizure disorder.

Disposition

If the patient is comatose, he or she must be admitted to the intensive care unit. If the overdose was intentional, psychiatric clearance is needed before the patient can be discharged.

β-Adrenergic Blockers (β-Blockers)

β-Blockers are used in the treatment of hypertension and of a number of systemic and ophthalmologic disorders. Properties of β-blockers include the factors listed in Table 12.

Lipid-soluble drugs have CNS effects, active metabolites, longer duration of action, and interactions (e.g., propranolol). Cardioselectivity is lost in overdose. Intrinsic partial agonist agents (e.g., pindolol) may initially produce tachycardia and hypertension. Cardiac membrane depressive effect (quinidine-like) occurs in cases of overdose but not at therapeutic doses (e.g., with metoprolol or sotalol). α-Blocking effect is weak (e.g., with labetalol or acebutolol).

TABLE 12 Pharmacologic and Toxic Properties of β-Blockers

B-BLOCKER	MAXIMUM SOLUBILITY	THERAPEUTIC PLASMA LEVEL	LIPID SOLUBILITY	INTRINSIC SYMPATHOMIMETIC ACTIVITY (PARTIAL AGONIST)	MEMBRANE STABILIZING EFFECT B-SELECTIVE		CARDIAC SELECTIVITY
					B_1	B_2	A-SELECTIVE
Acebutolol (Sectral)	800 mg	200–2000 ng/mL	Moderate	+	+	+	+
Alprenolol[2]	800 mg	50–200 ng/mL	Moderate	2+	+	–	–
Atenolol (Tenormin)	100 mg	200–500 ng/mL	Low	–	–	2+	–
Betaxolol (Kerlone)	20 mg	NA	Low	+	–	+	–
Carteolol (Cartrol)	10 mg	NA	No	+	–	–	–
Esmolol (Brevibloc) (Class II antidysrhythmic, IV only)			Low	–	–	+	–
Labetalol (Trandate)	800 mg	50–500 ng/mL	Low	+	+/–	–	+
Levobunolol (AKBeta eyedrop) (Eye drops 0.25% and 0.5%)	20 mg	NA	No	–	–	–	–
Metoprolol (Lopressor)			Moderate	–	–	2+	–
Nadolol (Corgard)	320 mg	20–40 ng/mL	Low	–	–	–	–
Oxyprenolol[2]	480 mg	80–100 ng/mL	Moderate	2+	+	–	–
Pindolol (Visken)	60 mg	50–150 ng/mL	Moderate	3+	+/–	–	–
Propranolol (Inderal) (Class II antidysrhythmic)	360 mg	50–100 ng/mL	High	–	2+	–	–
Sotalol (Betapace) (Class II antidysrhythmic)	480 mg	500–4000 ng/mL	Low	–	–	–	–
Timolol (Blocadren)	60 mg	5–10 ng/mL	Low	–	+/–	–	–

[2]Not available in the United States.

Toxic Mechanism

β-Blockers compete with the catecholamines for receptor sites and block receptor action in the bronchi, the vascular smooth muscle, and the myocardium.

Toxic Dose

Ingestions of greater than twice the maximum recommended daily therapeutic dose are considered toxic (see Table 12). Ingestion of 1 mg/kg propranolol in a child may produce hypoglycemia. Fatalities have been reported in adults with 7.5 g of metoprolol. The most toxic agent is sotalol, and the least toxic is atenolol.

Kinetics

Regular-release formulations usually cause symptoms within 2 hours. Propranolol's onset of action is 20 to 30 minutes and peak is at 1 to 4 hours, but it may be delayed by co-ingestants. The onset of action with sustained-release preparations may be delayed to 6 hours and the peak to 12 to 16 hours. Volume distribution is 1 to 5.6 L/kg. Protein binding is variable, from 5% to 93%.

Metabolism

Atenolol (Tenormin), nadolol (Corgard), and sotalol (Betapace) have enterohepatic recirculation. The duration of action for regular-acting agents is 4 to 6 hours, but in cases of overdose it may be 24 to 48 hours. The duration of action for sustained-release agents is 24 to 48 hours.

The regular preparation with the longest half-life is nadolol, at 12 to 24 hours, and the one with the shortest half-life is esmolol, at 5 to 10 minutes.

Manifestations

See "Toxic Properties" and Table 12.

Highly lipid soluble agents produce coma and seizures. Bradycardia and hypotension are the major cardiac symptoms and may lead to cardiogenic shock. Intrinsic partial agonists initially may cause tachycardia and hypertension. ECG changes include atrioventricular conduction delay or asystole. Membrane-depressant effects produce prolonged QRS and QT interval, which may result in torsades de pointes. Sotalol produces a very prolonged QT interval. Bronchospasm may occur in patients with reactive airway disease with any β-blocker because the selectivity is lost in overdose. Other manifestations include hypoglycemia (because β-blockers block catecholamine counter-regulatory mechanisms) and hyperkalemia.

Laboratory Investigations

Measurements of blood levels are not readily available or useful. ECG and cardiac monitoring should be maintained, and blood glucose and electrolytes, BUN, and creatinine levels should be monitored, as well as ABG if there are respiratory symptoms.

Management

Vital functions must be established and maintained. Vascular access, baseline ECG, and continuous cardiac and blood pressure monitoring should be established. A pacemaker must be available. Gastrointestinal decontamination can be undertaken initially with activated charcoal up to 1 hour after ingestion. MDAC is no longer recommended, based on the latest guidelines. Whole-bowel irrigation can be considered in cases of large overdoses with sustained-release preparations, but there are no studies evaluating the efficacy of intervention.

If there are cardiovascular disturbances, a cardiac consultation should be obtained. Class IA antidysrhythmic agents (procainamide, quinidine) and III (bretylium) are not recommended. Hypotension is treated with fluids initially, although it usually does not respond. Frequently, glucagon and cardiac pacing are needed. Bradycardia in asymptomatic, hemodynamically stable patients requires no therapy. It is not predictive of the future course of the disease. If the patient is unstable (has hypotension or a high-degree atrioventricular block), atropine 0.02 mg/kg (up to 2 mg) in adults, glucagon, and a pacemaker can be used. In case of ventricular tachycardia, overdrive pacing can be used. A wide QRS interval may respond to sodium bicarbonate. Torsades de pointes (associated with sotalol) may respond to magnesium sulfate and overdrive pacing. Prophylactic magnesium for prolonged QT interval has been suggested, but there are no data. Epinephrine must not be used because an unopposed α effect may occur.

Hypotension and myocardial depression are managed by correction of dysrhythmias, Trendelenburg position, fluids, glucagon, or amrinone (Inocor), or a combination of these. Hemodynamic monitoring with a Swan-Ganz catheter or arterial line may be necessary to manage fluid therapy.

Glucagon is the initial drug of choice. It works through adenyl cyclase and bypasses catecholamine receptors; therefore, it is not affected by β-blockers. Glucagon increases cardiac contractility and heart rate. It is given as an intravenous bolus of 5 to 10 mg[3] over 1 minute and followed by a continuous infusion of 1 to 5 mg/h (in children, 0.15 mg/kg followed by 0.05 to 0.1 mg/kg/h). In large doses and in infusion therapy D_5W, sterile water, or saline should be used as a diluant to reconstitute glucagon in place of the 0.2% phenol diluent provided with some drugs. Effects are seen within minutes. It can be used with other agents such as amrinone.

Amrinone (Inocor) inhibits phosphodiesterase enzyme, which metabolizes cyclic AMP. It is administered as a bolus of 0.15 to 2 mg/kg (0.15 to 0.4 mL/kg) intravenously, followed by infusion of 5 to 10 μg/kg/min.

Hypoglycemia should be treated with intravenous glucose. Life-threatening hyperkalemia is treated with calcium (avoid if digoxin is present), bicarbonate, and glucose or insulin. Convulsions can be controlled with diazepam or phenobarbital. If bronchospasm is present, β_2 nebulized bronchodilators are given.

Extraordinary measures such as intra-aortic balloon pump support can be instituted. Extracorporeal measures can be undertaken. Hemodialysis for cases of atenolol, acebutolol, nadolol, and sotalol (low volume distribution, low protein binding) ingestion may be helpful, particularly when there is evidence of renal failure. Hemodialysis is not effective for propranolol, metoprolol, and timolol.

Prenalterol[2] has successfully reversed both bradycardia and hypotension but is not currently available in the United States.

Disposition

Asymptomatic patients with history of overdose require baseline ECG and continuous cardiac monitoring for at least 6 hours with regular-release preparations and for 24 hours with sustained-release preparations. Symptomatic patients should be observed with cardiac monitoring for 24 hours. If seizures or abnormal rhythm or vital signs are present, the patient should be admitted to the intensive care unit.

Calcium Channel Blockers

Calcium channel blockers are used in the treatment of effort angina, supraventricular tachycardia, and hypertension.

Toxic Mechanism

Calcium channel blockers reduce influx of calcium through the slow channels in membranes of the myocardium, the atrioventricular nodes, and the vascular smooth muscles and result in peripheral, systemic, and coronary vasodilation, impaired cardiac conduction, and depression of cardiac contractility. All calcium channel blockers have vasodilatory action, but only bepridil, diltiazem, and verapamil depress myocardial contractility and cause atrioventricular block.

Toxic Dose

Any ingested amount greater than the maximum daily dose has the potential of severe toxicity. The maximum oral daily doses in adults and toxic doses in children of each are as follows: amlodipine (Norvasc), 10 mg for adults and more than 0.25 mg/kg for children; bepridil (Vascor), 400 mg for adults and more than 5.7 mg/kg for children; diltiazem (Cardizem), 360 mg for adults (toxic dose >2 g) and more than 6 mg/kg for children; felodipine (Plendil), 40 mg for adults and more than 0.56 mg/kg for children; isradipine (DynaCirc), 40 mg for adults and more than 0.4 mg/kg for children; nicardipine (Cardene), 120 mg for adults and more than 0.85 mg/kg for children; nifedipine (Procardia), 120 mg for adults and more than 2 mg/kg for children; nimodipine (Nimotop), 360 mg for adults and more than 0.85 mg/kg for children; nitrendipine (Baypress),[1] 80 mg for adults and more than 1.14 mg/kg for children; and verapamil (Calan), 480 mg for adults and 15 mg/kg for children.

Kinetics

Onset of action of regular-release preparations varies: for verapamil it is 60 to 120 minutes, for nifedipine 20 minutes, and for diltiazem 15 minutes after ingestion. Peak effect for verapamil is 2 to 4 hours, for nifedipine 60 to 90 minutes, and for diltiazem 30 to 60 minutes, but the peak action may be delayed for 6 to 8 hours. Duration of action is up to 36 hours. The onset of action for sustained-release preparations is usually 4 hours but may be delayed, and peak effect is at 12 to 24 hours. In cases of massive overdose, concretions and prolonged toxicity can develop.

Volume distribution varies from 3 to 7 L/kg. Hepatic elimination half-life varies from 3 to 7 hours. Patients receiving digitalis and calcium channel blockers run the risk of digitalis toxicity, because calcium channel blockers increase digitalis levels.

Manifestations

Cardiac manifestations include hypotension, bradycardia, and conduction disturbances occurring 30 minutes to 5 hours after ingestion. A prolonged PR interval is an early finding and may occur at therapeutic doses. Torsades de pointes has been reported. All degrees of blocks may occur and may be delayed up to 16 hours. Lactic acidosis may be present. Calcium channel blockers do not affect intraventricular conduction, so the QRS interval is usually not affected.

Hypocalcemia is rarely present. Hyperglycemia may be present because of interference in calcium-dependent insulin release. Mental status changes, headaches, seizures, hemiparesis, and CNS depression may occur.

Laboratory Investigations

Specific drug levels are not readily available and are not useful. Monitor blood sugar, electrolytes, calcium, ABG, pulse oximetry, creatinine, and BUN, and also use hemodynamic monitoring, ECG, and cardiac monitoring.

---

[2] Not available in the United States.
[3] Exceeds dosage recommended by the manufacturer.

[1] Not FDA approved for this indication.

Management

Vital functions must be established and maintained. Baseline ECG readings should be obtained and continuous cardiac and blood pressure monitoring maintained. A pacemaker should be available. Cardiology consultation should be sought.

Gastrointestinal decontamination with activated charcoal is recommended. If a large dose of a sustained-release preparation was ingested, whole-bowel irrigation can be considered, but its effectiveness has not been investigated.

If the patient is symptomatic, immediate cardiology consult must be obtained, because a pacemaker and hemodynamic monitoring may be needed. In the case of heart block, atropine is rarely effective and isoproterenol (Isuprel) may produce vasodilation. The use of a pacemaker should be considered early.

Hypotension and bradycardia can be treated with positioning, fluids, and calcium gluconate or chloride, glucagon, amrinone (Inocor), and ventricular pacing. Calcium salts must be avoided if digoxin is present. Calcium usually reverses depressed myocardial contractility but may not reverse nodal depression or peripheral vasodilation. Calcium chloride can be given in a 10% solution, 0.1 to 0.2 mL/kg up to 10 mL in an adult, or calcium gluconate in a 10% solution 0.3 to 0.4 mL/kg up to 20 mL in an adult. Administration is intravenous, over 5 to 10 minutes. One should monitor for dysrhythmias, hypotension, and the serum ionized calcium. The aim is to increase calcium 4 mg/dL to a maximum of 13 mg/dL. The calcium response lasts 15 minutes and may require repeated doses or a continuous calcium gluconate infusion 0.2 mL/kg/h up to maximum of 10 mL/h.

If calcium fails, glucagon can be tried for its positive inotropic and chronotropic effect, or both. Amrinone (Inocor), an inotropic agent, may reverse the effects of calcium channel blockers. An effective dose is 0.15 mg to 2 mg/kg (0.15–0.4 mL/kg) by intravenous bolus followed by infusion of 5 to 10 µg/kg/min.

In case of hypotension, fluids, norepinephrine (Levophed), and epinephrine may be required. Amrinone and glucagon have been tried alone and in combination. Dobutamine and dopamine are often ineffective.

Extracorporeal measures (e.g., hemodialysis and charcoal hemoperfusion) are not useful, but extraordinary measures such as intra-aortic balloon pump and cardiopulmonary bypass have been used successfully.

For cases of calcium channel blocker toxicity that fail to respond to aggressive management, recent studies demonstrate that insulin and glucose have therapeutic value. The suggested dose range for insulin is to infuse regular insulin at 0.5 IU/kg/h with a simultaneous infusion of glucose 1 g/kg/h, with glucose monitoring every 30 minutes for at least the first 4 hours of administration and subsequent glucose adjustment to maintain euglycemia (70 to 100 mg/dL). Potassium levels should be monitored regularly, as they may shift in response to the insulin.

Disposition

Patients who have ingested regular-release preparations should be monitored for at least 6 hours and those who have ingested sustained-release preparations should be monitored for 24 hours after the ingestion. Intentional overdose necessitates psychiatric clearance. Symptomatic patients should be admitted to the intensive care unit.

Carbon Monoxide

Carbon monoxide is an odorless, colorless gas produced from incomplete combustion; it is also an in vivo metabolic breakdown product of methylene chloride used in paint removers.

Toxic Mechanism

Carbon monoxide's affinity for hemoglobin is 240 times greater than that of oxygen. It shifts the oxygen dissociation curve to the left, which impairs hemoglobin release of oxygen to tissues and inhibits the cytochrome oxidase enzymes.

Toxic Dose and Manifestations

Table 13 describes the manifestations of carbon monoxide toxicity. Exposure to 0.5% for a few minutes is lethal. Sequelae correlate with the patient's level of consciousness at presentation. ECG abnormalities may be noted. Creatine kinase is often elevated, and rhabdomyolysis and myoglobinuria may occur.

The carboxyhemoglobin (CoHB) expresses in percentage the extent to which carbon monoxide has bound with the total hemoglobin. This may be misleadingly low in the anemic patient with less hemoglobin than normal. The patient's presentation is a more reliable indicator of severity than the CoHB level. The manifestations listed in Table 13 for each level are in addition to those listed at the level above. The CoHB may not correlate reliably with the severity of the intoxication, and linking symptoms to specific levels of CoHB frequently leads to inaccurate conclusions. A level of carbon monoxide greater than 40% is usually associated with obvious intoxication.

Kinetics

The natural metabolism of the body produces small amounts of CoHB, less than 2% for nonsmokers and 5% to 9% for smokers.

Carbon monoxide is rapidly absorbed through the lungs. The rate of absorption is directly related to alveolar ventilation. Elimination also occurs through the lungs. The half-life of CoHB in room air (21% oxygen) is 5 to 6 hours; in 100% oxygen, it is 90 minutes; in hyperbaric pressure at 3 atmospheres oxygen, it is 20 to 30 minutes.

Laboratory Investigations

An ABG reading may show metabolic acidosis and normal oxygen tension. In cases of significant poisoning, the ABG, electrolytes, blood glucose, serum creatine kinase and cardiac enzymes, renal function tests, and liver function tests should be monitored. A urinalysis and test for myoglobinuria should be obtained. Chest radiograph can be useful in cases of smoke inhalation or if the patient is being considered for hyperbaric chamber. ECG monitoring should be maintained, especially if the patient is older than 40 years, has a history of cardiac disease, or has moderate to severe symptoms. Which toxicology studies are used is based on symptoms and circumstances. CoHB should be monitored during and at the end of therapy. The pulse oximeter has two wavelengths and overestimates oxyhemoglobin saturation in carbon monoxide poisoning. The true oxygen saturation is determined

TABLE 13	Carbon Monoxide Exposure and Possible Manifestations
COHB SATURATION (%)	**MANIFESTATIONS**
3.5	None
5	Slight headache, decreased exercise tolerance
10	Slight headache, dyspnea on vigorous exertion, may impair driving skills
10–20	Moderate dyspnea on exertion, throbbing, temporal headache
20–30	Severe headache, syncope, dizziness, visual changes, weakness, nausea, vomiting, altered judgment
30–40	Vertigo, ataxia, blurred vision, confusion, loss of consciousness
40–50	Confusion, tachycardia, tachypnea, coma, convulsions
50–60	Cheyne-Stokes, coma, convulsions, shock, apnea
60–70	Coma, convulsions, respiratory and heart failure, death

by blood gas analysis, which measures the oxygen bound to hemoglobin. The co-oximeter measures four wavelengths and separates out CoHB and the other hemoglobin binding agents from oxyhemoglobin. Fetal hemoglobin has a greater affinity for carbon monoxide than adult hemoglobin and may falsely elevate the CoHB as much as 4% in young infants.

Management
The first step is to adequately protect the rescuer. The patient must be removed from the contaminated area, and his or her vital functions must be established.

The mainstay of treatment is 100% oxygen via a non-rebreathing mask with an oxygen reservoir or endotracheal tube. All patients receive 100% oxygen until the CoHB level is 5% or less. Assisted ventilation may be necessary. ABG and CoHB should be monitored and the present CoHB level determined. *Note:* A near-normal CoHB level does not exclude significant carbon monoxide poisoning, especially if the measurement is taken several hours after termination of exposure or if oxygen has been administered prior to obtaining the sample.

The exposed pregnant woman should be kept on 100% oxygen for several hours after the CoHB level is almost 0, because carbon monoxide concentrates in the fetus and oxygen is needed longer to ensure elimination of the carbon monoxide from fetal circulation. The fetus must be monitored, because carbon monoxide and hypoxia are potentially teratogenic.

Metabolic acidosis should be treated with sodium bicarbonate only if the pH is below 7.2 after correction of hypoxia and adequate ventilation. Acidosis shifts the oxygen dissociation curve to the right and facilitates oxygen delivery to the tissues.

The decision to use the hyperbaric oxygen chamber must be made on the basis of the ability to handle other acute emergencies that may coexist in the patient and of the severity of the poisoning. The standard of care for persons exposed to carbon monoxide has yet to be determined, but most authorities recommend using the hyperbaric oxygen chamber under any of the following conditions:

- If the patient is in a coma or has a history of loss of consciousness or seizures
- If there is cardiovascular dysfunction (clinical ischemic chest pain or ECG evidence of ischemia)
- If the patient has metabolic acidosis
- If symptoms persist despite 100% oxygen therapy
- In a child, if the initial CoHB is greater than 15%
- In symptomatic patients with preexisting ischemia
- If there are signs of maternal or fetal distress regardless of CoHB level (infants and fetus are a special problem because fetal hemoglobin has greater affinity for carbon monoxide)

Although controversial, a neurologic-cognitive examination has been used to help determine which patients with low carbon monoxide levels should receive more aggressive therapy. Testing should include the following: general orientation memory testing involving address, phone number, date of birth, and present date; and cognitive testing, involving counting by 7s, digit span, and forward and backward spelling of three-letter and four-letter words. Patients with delayed neurologic sequelae or recurrent symptoms up to 3 weeks may benefit from hyperbaric oxygen chamber treatment.

Seizures and cerebral edema must be treated.

Disposition
Patients with no or mild symptoms who become asymptomatic after a few hours of oxygen therapy, have a carbon monoxide level less than 10%, and have normal physical and neurologic-cognitive examination findings can be discharged, but they should be instructed to return if any signs of neurologic dysfunction appear. Patients with carbon monoxide poisoning requiring treatment need follow-up neuropsychiatric examinations.

Caustics and Corrosives
The terms *caustic* and *corrosive* are used interchangeably and can be divided into acids and alkalis. The U.S. Consumer Product Safety Commission Labeling Recommendations on containers for acids and alkalis indicate the potential for producing serious damage, as follows:

- Caution—weak irritant
- Warning—strong irritant
- Danger—corrosive

Some common acids with corrosive potential include acetic acid, formic acid, glycolic acid, hydrochloric acid, mercuric chloride, nitric acid, oxalic acid, phosphoric acid, sulfuric acid (battery acid), zinc chloride, and zinc sulfate. Some common alkalis with corrosive potential include ammonia, calcium carbide, calcium hydroxide (dry), calcium oxide, potassium hydroxide (lye), and sodium hydroxide (lye).

Toxic Mechanism
Acids produce mucosal coagulation necrosis and may be absorbed systemically; they do not penetrate deeply. Injury to the gastric mucosa is more likely, although specific sites of injury for acids and alkalis are not clearly defined.

Alkalis produce liquefaction necrosis and saponification and penetrate deeply. The esophageal mucosa is likely to be damaged. Oropharyngeal and esophageal damage is more frequently caused by solids than by liquids. Liquids produce superficial circumferential burns and gastric damage.

Toxic Dose
The toxicity is determined by concentration, contact time, and pH. Significant injury is more likely with a substance that has a pH of less than 2 or greater than 12, with a prolonged contact time, and with large volumes.

Manifestations
The absence of oral burns does not exclude the possibility of esophageal or gastric damage. General clinical findings are stridor; dysphagia; drooling; oropharyngeal, retrosternal, and epigastric pain; and ocular and oral burns. Alkali burns are yellow, soapy, frothy lesions. Acid burns are gray-white and later form an eschar. Abdominal tenderness and guarding may be present if perforation has happened.

Laboratory Investigations
If acid ingestion has taken place, the patient's acid-base balance and electrolyte status should be determined. If pulmonary symptoms are present, a chest radiograph, ABG measurement, and pulse oximetry are called for.

Management
It is recommended that the container be brought to the examination, as the substance must be identified and the pH of the substance, vomitus, tears, or saliva tested.

If the acid or alkali has been ingested, all gastrointestinal decontamination procedures are contraindicated except for immediate rinse, removal of substance from the mouth, and dilution with small amounts (sips) of milk or water. The examiner should check for ocular and dermal involvement. Contraindications to oral dilution are dysphagias, respiratory distress, obtundation, or shock. If there is ocular involvement one should immediately irrigate the eye with tepid water for at least 30 minutes, perform fluorescein stain of eye, and consult an ophthalmologist. If there is dermal involvement, one should immediately remove contaminated clothes and irrigate the skin with tepid water for at least 15 minutes. Consultation with a burn specialist is called for.

In cases of acid ingestion, some authorities advocate a small flexible nasogastric tube and aspiration within 30 minutes after ingestion.

Patients should receive only intravenous fluids following dilution until endoscopic consultation is obtained. Endoscopy is valuable to predict damage and risk of stricture. The indications are controversial, with some authorities recommending it in all cases of caustic ingestions regardless of symptoms, and others selectively using clinical features such as vomiting, stridor, drooling, and oral or facial lesions as criteria. We recommend endoscopy for all symptomatic patients or patients with intentional ingestions. Endoscopy may be performed immediately if the patient is symptomatic, but it is usually done 12 to 48 hours postingestion.

The use of corticosteroids is considered controversial. Some feel they may be useful for patients with second-degree circumferential burns. They recommend starting with hydrocortisone sodium succinate (Solu-Cortef) intravenously 10 to 20 mg/kg/d within 48 hours and changing to oral prednisolone 2 mg/kg/d for 3 weeks before tapering the dose. We do not usually recommend using corticosteroids because they have not been shown to be effective.

Tetanus prophylaxis should be provided if the patient requires it for wound care. Antibiotics are not useful prophylactically. Contrast studies are not useful in the first few days and may interfere with endoscopic evaluation; later, they can be used to assess the severity of damage.

Emergency medical therapy includes agents to inhibit collagen formation and intraluminal stents. Esophageal and gastric outlet dilation may be needed if there is evidence of stricture. Bougienage of the esophagus, however, has been associated with brain abscess. Interposition of the colon may be necessary if dilation fails to provide an adequate-sized passage.

Management of inhalation cases requires immediate removal from the environment, administration of humid supplemental oxygen, and observation for airway obstruction and noncardiac pulmonary edema. Radiographic and ABG evaluation should be obtained when appropriate. Intubation and respiratory support may be required.

Certain caustics produce systemic disturbances. Formaldehyde causes metabolic acidosis, hydrofluoric acid causes hypocalcemia and renal damage, oxalic acid causes hypocalcemia, phenol causes hepatic and renal damage, and picric acid causes renal injury.

Disposition

Infants and small children should be medically evaluated and observed. All symptomatic patients should be admitted. If they have severe symptoms or danger of airway compromise, they should be admitted to the intensive care unit. After endoscopy, if no damage is detected, the patient may be discharged when he or she can tolerate oral feedings. Intentional exposures require psychiatric evaluation before the patient can be discharged.

Cocaine (Benzoylmethylecgonine)

Cocaine is derived from the leaves of *Erythroxylum coca* and *Truxillo coca*. "Body packing" refers to the placement of many small packages of contraband cocaine for concealment in the gastrointestinal tract or other areas for illicit transport. "Body stuffing" refers to spontaneous ingestion of substances for the purpose of hiding evidence.

Toxic Mechanism

Cocaine directly stimulates the CNS presynaptic sympathetic neurons to release catecholamines and acetylcholine, while it blocks the presynaptic reuptake of the catecholamines; it blocks the sodium channels along neuronal membranes; and it increases platelet aggregation. Long-term use depletes the CNS of dopamine.

Toxic Dose

The maximum mucosal local anesthetic therapeutic dose of cocaine is 200 mg or 2 mL of a 10% solution. Although CNS effects can occur at relatively low local anesthetic doses (50 to 95 mg), they are more common with doses greater than 1 mg/kg; cardiac effects can occur with doses greater than 1 mg/kg. The potential fatal dose is 1200 mg intranasally, but death has occurred with 20 mg parenterally.

Kinetics

Cocaine is well absorbed by all routes, including nasal insufflation, and oral, dermal, and inhalation routes (Table 14). Protein binding is 8.7%, and volume distribution is 1.5 L/kg.

Cocaine is metabolized by plasma and liver cholinesterase to the inactive metabolites ecgonine methyl ester and benzoylecgonine. Plasma pseudocholinesterase is congenitally deficient in 3% of the population and decreased in fetuses, young infants, the elderly, pregnant people, and people with liver disease. These enzyme-deficient individuals are at increased risk for life-threatening cocaine toxicity.

Ten percent of cocaine is excreted unchanged. Cocaine and ethanol undergo liver synthesis to form cocaethylene, a metabolite with a half-life three times longer than that of cocaine. It may account for some of cocaine's cardiotoxicity and appears to be more lethal than cocaine or ethanol alone.

Manifestations

The CNS manifestations of cocaine ingestion are euphoria, hyperactivity, agitation, convulsions, and intracranial hemorrhage. Mydriasis and septal perforation can occur, as well as cardiac dysrhythmias, hypertension, and hypotension (with severe overdose). Chest pain is frequent, but only 5.8% of patients have true myocardial ischemia and infarction. Other manifestations include vasoconstriction, hyperthermia (because of increased metabolic rate), ischemic bowel perforation if the substance is ingested, rhabdomyolysis, myoglobinuria, and renal failure. In pregnant users, premature labor and abruptio placentae can occur.

Body cavity packing should be suspected in cases of prolonged toxicity.

Mortality can result from cerebrovascular accidents, coronary artery spasm, myocardial injury, or lethal dysrhythmias.

Laboratory Investigations

Monitoring of the ECG and cardiac rhythms, ABG, oxygen saturation, electrolytes, blood glucose, BUN, creatinine, and creatine kinase levels should be maintained. One should monitor cardiac fraction if the patient has chest pain, as well as the liver profile, and the urine for myoglobin. Intravenous drug users should have HIV and hepatitis virus testing.

Urine should be tested for cocaine and metabolites and other substances of abuse, and abdominal radiographs or ultrasonogram should be ordered for body packers. If the urine sample was collected more than 12 hours after cocaine intake, it will contain little or no cocaine. If cocaine is present, cocaine has been used within the past 12 hours. Cocaine's metabolite benzoylecgonine may be detected within 4 hours after a single nasal insufflation and for up to 114 hours. Cross-reactions with some herbal

TABLE 14	Routes and Kinetics of Cocaine				
TYPE	**ROUTE**	**ONSET**	**PEAK (MIN)**	**HALF-LIFE (MIN)**	**DURATION (MIN)**
Cocaine leaf	Oral, chewing	20–30 min	45–90	—	240–360
Hydrochloride	Insufflation	1–3 min	5–10	78	60–90
	Ingestion	20–30 min	50–90	54	Sustained
	Intravenous	30–120 sec	5–11	36	60–90
Freebase/crack	Smoking	5–10 sec	5–11	—	Up to 20
Coca paste	Smoking	Unknown	—	—	—

teas, lidocaine, and droperidol (Inapsine) may give false-positive results by some immunoassay methods.

Management

Supportive care includes blood pressure, cardiac, and thermal monitoring and seizure precautions. Diazepam (Valium) is the drug of choice for treatment of cocaine toxicity agitation, seizures, and dysrhythmias; doses are 10 to 30 mg intravenously at 2.5 mg per minute for adults and 0.2 to 0.5 mg/kg at 1 mg per minute up to 10 mg for a child.

Gastrointestinal decontamination should be instituted, if the cocaine was ingested, by administration of activated charcoal. MDAC may adsorb cocaine leakage in body stuffers or body packers. Whole-bowel irrigation with polyethylene glycol solution (PEG) has been used in body packers and stuffers if the contraband is in a firm container. If the packages are not visible on plain radiographs of the abdomen, a contrast study or CT scan can help to confirm successful passage. Cocaine in the nasal passage can be removed with an applicator dipped in a non–water-soluble product (lubricating jelly) if this is done within a few minutes after application.

In body packers and stuffers, venous access must be secured, and drugs must be readily available for treating life-threatening manifestations until the contraband is passed in the stool. Surgical removal may be indicated if the packet does not pass the pylorus, in an asymptomatic body packer, or in the case of intestinal obstruction.

Hypertension and tachycardia are usually transient and can be managed by careful titration of diazepam. Nitroprusside may be used for severe hypertension. Myocardial ischemia is managed by oxygen, vascular access, benzodiazepines, and nitroglycerin. Aspirin and thrombolysis are not routinely recommended because of the danger of intracranial hemorrhage.

Dysrhythmias are usually supraventricular (SVT) and do not require specific management. Adenosine is ineffective. Life-threatening tachydysrhythmias may respond to phentolamine (Regitine) 5 mg IV bolus in adults or 0.1 mg/kg in children at 5- to 10-minute intervals. Phentolamine also relieves coronary artery spasm and myocardial ischemia. Electrical synchronized cardioversion should be considered for patients with hemodynamically unstable dysrhythmias. Lidocaine is not recommended initially but may be used after 3 hours for ventricular tachycardia. Wide complex QRS ventricular tachycardia may be treated with sodium bicarbonate 2 mEq/kg as a bolus. β-Adrenergic blockers are not recommended.

Anxiety, agitation, and convulsions can be treated with diazepam. If diazepam fails to control seizures, neuromuscular blockers can be used. The EEG should be monitored for nonmotor seizure activity. For hyperthermia, external cooling and cool humidified 100% oxygen should be administered. Neuromuscular paralysis to control seizures will reduce temperature. Dantrolene and antipyretics are not recommended. Rhabdomyolysis and myoglobinuria are treated with fluids, alkaline diuresis, and diuretics.

If the patient is pregnant, the fetus must be monitored and the patient observed for spontaneous abortion.

Paranoid ideation and threatening behavior should be treated with rapid tranquilization. The patient should be observed for suicidal depression that may follow intoxication and may require suicide precautions. If focal neurologic manifestations are present, one should consider the possibility of a cerebrovascular accident and obtain a CT scan.

Extracorporeal clearance techniques are of no benefit.

Disposition

Patients with mild intoxication or a brief seizure that does not require treatment who become asymptomatic may be discharged after 6 hours with appropriate psychosocial follow-up. If cardiac or cerebral ischemic manifestations are present, the patient should be monitored in the intensive care unit. Body packers and stuffers require care in the intensive care unit until passage of the contraband.

Cyanide

Hydrogen cyanide is a byproduct of burning plastic and wools in residential fires. Hydrocyanic acid is the liquefied form of hydrogen cyanide. Cyanide salts can be found in ore extraction. Nitriles, such as acetonitrile (artificial nail removers), are metabolized in the body to produce cyanide. Cyanogenic glycosides are present in some fruit seeds (such as amygdalin in apricots, peaches, and apples). Sodium nitroprusside, the antihypertensive vasodilator, contains five cyanide groups.

Toxic Mechanism

Cyanide blocks the cellular electron transport mechanism and cellular respiration by inhibiting the mitochondrial ferricytochrome oxidase system and other enzymes. This results in cellular hypoxia and lactic acidosis. *Note:* Citrus fruit seeds form cyanide in the presence of intestinal β-glucosidase (the seeds are harmful only if the capsule is broken).

Toxic Dose

The ingestion of 1 mg/kg or 50 mg of hydrogen cyanide can produce death within 15 minutes. The lethal dose of potassium cyanide is 200 mg. Five to 10 mL of 84% acetonitrile is lethal. Infusions of sodium nitroprusside in rates above 2 μg/kg per minute may cause cyanide to accumulate to toxic concentrations in critically ill patients.

Kinetics

Cyanide is rapidly absorbed by all routes. In the stomach, it forms hydrocyanic acid. Volume distribution is 1.5 L/kg. Protein binding is 60%. Cyanide is detoxified by metabolism in the liver via the mitochondrial thiosulfate-rhodanase pathway, which catalyzes the transfer of sulfur donor to cyanide, forming the less toxic irreversible thiocyanate that is excreted in the urine. Cyanide is also detoxified by reacting with hydroxocobalamin (vitamin B_{12a}) to form cyanocobalamin (vitamin B_{12}).

The cyanide elimination half-life from the blood is 1.2 hours. The elimination route is through the lungs.

Manifestations

Hydrogen cyanide has the distinctive odor of bitter almonds or silver polish. Manifestations of cyanide intoxication include hypertension, cardiac dysrhythmias, various ECG abnormalities, headache, hyperpnea, seizures, stupor, pulmonary edema, and flushing. Cyanosis is absent or appears late.

Laboratory Investigations

The examiner should obtain and monitor ABGs, oxygen saturation, blood lactate, hemoglobin, blood glucose, and electrolytes. Lactic acidemia, a decrease in the arterial-venous oxygen difference, and bright red venous blood occurs. If smoke inhalation is the possible source of cyanide exposure, CoHB and methemoglobin (MetHb) concentrations should be measured.

Cyanide levels in whole blood, red blood cells, or serum are not useful in the acute management because the determinations are not readily available. Specific cyanide blood levels are as follows: smokers have less than 0.5 μg/mL; a patient with flushing and tachycardia has 0.5 to 1.0 μg/mL, one with obtundation has 1.0 to 2.5 μg/mL, and one in coma or who has died has more than 2.5 μg/mL.

Management

If the cyanide was inhaled, the patient must be removed from the contaminated atmosphere. Attendants should not administer mouth-to-mouth resuscitation. Rescuers and attendants must be protected. Immediate administration of 100% oxygen is called for and oxygen should be continued during and after the administration of the antidote. The clinician must decide whether to use any or all components of the cyanide antidote kit.

The mechanism of action of the antidote kit is twofold: to produce methemoglobinemia and to provide a sulfur substrate for the detoxification of cyanide. The nitrites make methemoglobin, which has a greater affinity for cyanide than does the cytochrome oxidase enzymes. The combination of methemoglobin and cyanide forms cyanomethemoglobin. Sodium thiosulfate provides a sulfur substrate for the rhodanese enzyme, which converts cyanide into the relatively nontoxic sodium thiocyanate, which is excreted by the kidney.

The procedure for using the antidote kit is as follows:

Step 1: Amyl nitrite inhalant perles is only a temporizing measure (forms only 2% to 5% methemoglobin) and it can be omitted if venous access is established. Alternate 100% oxygen and the inhalant for 30 seconds each minute. Use a new perle every 3 minutes.

Step 2: Sodium nitrite ampule is indicated for cyanide exposures, except for cases of residential fires, smoke inhalation, and nitroprusside or acetonitrile poisonings. It is administered intravenously to produce methemoglobin of 20% to 30% at 35 to 70 minutes after administration. A dose of 10 mL of 3% solution of sodium nitrite for adults and 0.33 mL/kg of 3% solution for children is diluted to 100 mL 0.9% saline and administered slowly intravenously at 5 mL/min. If hypotension develops, the infusion should be slowed.

Step 3: Sodium thiosulfate is useful alone in cases of smoke inhalation, nitroprusside toxicity, and acetonitrile toxicity and should not be used at all in cases of hydrogen sulfide poisoning. The administration dose is 12.5 g of sodium thiosulfate or 50 mL of 25% solution for adults and 1.65 mL/kg of 25% solution for children intravenously over 10 to 20 minutes.

If cyanide symptoms recur, further treatment with nitrites or the perles is controversial. Some authorities suggest repeating the antidotes in 30 minutes at half of the initial dose, but others do not advise this for lack of efficacy. The child dosage regimen on the package insert must be carefully followed.

One hour after antidotes are administered, the methemoglobin level should be obtained and should not exceed 20%. Methylene blue should not be used to reverse excessive methemoglobin.

Gastrointestinal decontamination of oral ingestion by activated charcoal is recommended but is not very effective because of the rapidity of absorption. Seizures are treated with intravenous diazepam. Acidosis should be treated with sodium bicarbonate if it does not rapidly resolve with therapy. There is no role for hyperbaric oxygen or hemodialysis or hemoperfusion.

Other antidotes include hydroxocobalamin (vitamin B_{12a}) (Cyanokit), which has proven effective when given immediately after exposure in large doses of 4 g (50 mg/kg) or 50 times the amount of cyanide exposure with 8 g of sodium thiosulfate. Hydroxocobalamin has FDA orphan drug approval.

Disposition

Asymptomatic patients should be observed for a minimum of 3 hours. Patients who ingest nitrile compounds must be observed for 24 hours. Patients requiring antidote administration should be admitted to the intensive care unit.

Digitalis

Cardiac glycosides are found in cardiac medications, common plants, and the skin of the Bufo toad.

Toxic Mechanism

Cardiac glycosides inhibit the enzyme sodium/potassium-adenosine triphosphatase ($Na^+,K^+,ATPase$), leading to intracellular potassium loss and increased intracellular sodium, and producing phase 4 depolarization, increased automaticity, and ectopy. There is increased intracellular calcium and potentiation of contractility. Pacemaker cells are inhibited, and the refractory period is prolonged, leading to atrioventricular blocks. There is increased vagal tone.

Toxic Dose

Digoxin total digitalizing dose, the dose required to achieve therapeutic blood levels of 0.6 to 2.0 ng/mL, is 0.75 to 1.25 mg or 10 to 15 µg/kg for patients older than 10 years of age; 40 to 50 µg/kg for patients younger than 2 years of age; and 30 to 40 µg/kg for patients 2 to 10 years of age.

The acute single toxic dose is greater than 0.07 mg/kg or greater than 2 or 3 mg in an adult, but 2 mg in a child or 4 mg in an adult usually produces only mild toxicity. One to 3 mg or more may be found in a few leaves of oleander or foxglove. Serious and fatal overdoses are more than 4 mg in a child and more than 10 mg in an adult.

Acute digitoxin ingestion of 10 to 35 mg has produced severe toxicity and death. Digitoxin therapeutic steady state is 15 to 25 ng/mL. In cases of chronic or acute-on-chronic ingestions in patients with cardiac disease, more than 2 mg may produce toxicity; however, toxicity can develop within therapeutic range on chronic therapy.

Patients at greatest risk of overdose include those with cardiac disease, those with electrolyte abnormalities (low potassium, low magnesium, low T_4, high calcium), those with renal impairment, and those on amiodarone (Cordarone), quinidine, erythromycin, tetracycline, calcium channel blockers, and β-blockers.

Kinetics

Digoxin is a metabolite of digitoxin. In cases of oral overdose, the typical onset is 30 minutes, with peak effects in 3 to 12 hours. Duration is 3 to 4 days. Intravenous onset is in 5 to 30 minutes; peak level is immediate, and peak effect is at 1.5 to 3 hours.

Volume distribution is 5 to 6 L/kg. The cardiac-to-plasma ratio is 30:1. After an acute ingestion overdose, the serum concentration is not reflective of tissue concentration for at least 6 hours or more, and steady state is 12 to 16 hours after last dose.

Sixty percent to 80% of the parent compound is excreted unchanged in the urine. The elimination half-life is 30 to 50 hours.

Manifestations

Onset of manifestations is usually within 2 hours but may be delayed up to 12 hours.

Gastrointestinal effects of nausea and vomiting are frequently present in cases of acute ingestion but may also occur in cases of chronic ingestion. The "digitalis effect" on ECG is scooped ST segments and PR prolongation; in cases of overdose, any dysrhythmia or block is possible but none are characteristic. Bradycardia occurs in patients with acute overdose with healthy hearts; supraventricular tachycardia occurs in patients with existing heart disease or chronic overdose. Ventricular tachycardia is seen only in cases of severe poisoning.

The CNS effects include headaches, visual disturbances, and colored halo vision. Hyperkalemia occurs following acute overdose and correlates with digoxin level and outcome. Among patients with serum potassium levels of less than 5.0 mEq/L, all survive. If the level is 5 to 5.5, 50% survive, and if the level is greater than 5.5, all die. Hypokalemia is commonly seen with chronic intoxication. Patients with normal digitalis levels may have toxicity in the presence of hypokalemia.

Chronic intoxications are more likely to produce scotoma, color perception disturbances, yellow vision, halos, delirium, hallucinations or psychosis, tachycardia, and hypokalemia.

Laboratory Investigations

Continuous monitoring of ECG, pulse, and blood pressure is called for. Blood glucose, electrolytes, calcium, magnesium, BUN, and creatinine levels should also be monitored. An initial digoxin level should be measured on patient presentation and repeated thereafter. Levels should be measured more than 6 hours postingestion because earlier values do not reflect tissue distribution. Digoxin clinical toxicity is usually associated with serum digoxin levels of greater than 3.5 ng/mL in adults.

An endogenous digoxin-like substance cross-reacts in most common immunoassays (not with high-pressure liquid chromatography) and values as high as 4.1 ng/mL have been reported in newborns, patients with chronic renal failure, patients with abnormal immunoglobulins, and women in the third trimester of pregnancy.

Management

A cardiology consult should be obtained and a pacemaker should be readily available.

In undertaking gastrointestinal decontamination, excessive vagal stimulation should be avoided (e.g., emesis and gastric lavage). Activated charcoal should be administered, and if a nasogastric tube is required for the activated charcoal, pretreatment with atropine (0.02 mg/kg in children and 0.5 mg in adults) should be considered.

Digoxin-specific antibody fragments (Fab, Digibind) 38 mg binds 0.5 mg digoxin and then is excreted through the kidneys. The onset of action is within 30 minutes. Problems associated with Fab therapy are mainly from withdrawal of digoxin and worsening heart failure, hypokalemia, decrease in glucose (if the patient has low glycogen stores), and allergic reactions (very rare). Digitalis administered after Fab therapy is bound and may be inactivated for 5 to 7 days.

Absolute indications for Fab therapy include the following:
- Life-threatening malignant (hemodynamically unstable) dysrhythmias
- Ventricular dysrhythmias, unstable severe bradycardia, or second- or third-degree blocks unresponsive to atropine or rapid deterioration in clinical status
- Life-threatening digitoxin and oleander poisonings

Relative indications for Fab therapy include the following:
- Ingestions greater than 4 mg in a child and 10 mg in an adult
- Serum potassium level greater than 5.0 mEq/L
- Serum digoxin level greater than 10 ng/mL in adults or greater than 5 ng/mL in children 6 hours after an acute ingestion
- Digitalis delirium and thrombocytopenia response

Digoxin-specific Fab fragments therapy can be administered as a bolus through a 22-μm filter if the case is a critical emergency. If the case is less urgent, then it can be administered over 30 minutes. An empiric dose is 10 vials in adults and 5 vials in a child for an unknown amount ingested in a symptomatic patient with history of a digoxin overdose.

To calculate the dose in the case of a known ingestion, the following equation is used:

$$\text{Amount (total mg)} \times (0.8) \text{ body burden}$$

If liquid capsules were taken or the substance was given intravenously the 80% bioavailability figure is not used. Instead, the body burden divided by 0.5 (0.5 mg digoxin is bound by 1 vial of 38 mg of Fab) equals the number of vials needed.

If the amount is unknown but the steady state serum concentration is known, the following equations are used:

For digoxin:

$$\text{Digitoxin ng/mL} \times (5.6 \text{ L/kg Vd}) \times (\text{wt kg}) = \text{mg body burden}$$
$$\text{Body burden} \div 1000 = \text{mg body burden}$$
$$\text{Body burden}/0.5 = \text{number of vials needed}$$

For digitoxin:

$$\text{Digitoxin ng/mL} \times (0.56 \text{ L/kg Vd}) \times (\text{wt kg}) = \text{mg body burden}$$
$$\text{Body burden} \div 1000 = \text{mg body burden}$$
$$\text{Body burden}/0.5 = \text{number of vials needed}$$

Antidysrhythmic agents or a pacemaker should be used only if Fab therapy fails. For ventricular tachydysrhythmias, electrolyte disturbances should be corrected by the administration of lidocaine or phenytoin. For torsades de pointes, magnesium sulfate 20 mL 20% IV can be given slowly over 20 minutes (or 25 to 50 mg/kg in a child), titrated to control the dysrhythmia. Magnesium should be discontinued if hypotension, heart block, or decreased deep tendon reflexes are present. Magnesium is used with caution if the patient has renal impairment.

Unstable bradycardia and second-degree and third-degree atrio-ventricular block should be treated by Fab first. A pacemaker should be available if necessary. Isoproterenol should be avoided because it causes dysrhythmias. Cardioversion is used with caution, starting at a setting of 5 to 10 joules. The patient should be pretreated with lidocaine, if possible, because cardioversion may precipitate ventricular fibrillation or asystole.

Potassium disturbances are caused by a shift, not a change, in total body potassium. Hyperkalemia (>5.0 mEq/L) is treated with Fab only. Calcium must never be used, and insulin/glucose and sodium bicarbonate should not be used concomitantly with Fab because they may produce severe life-threatening hypokalemia. Sodium polystyrene sulfonate (Kayexalate) should not be used. Hypokalemia must be treated with caution because it may be cardioprotective. Treatment can be administered if the patient has ventricular dysrhythmias or a serum potassium level less than 3.0 mEq/L and atrioventricular block.

Extracorporeal procedures are ineffective. Hemodialysis is used for severe or refractory hyperkalemia.

One must never use antidysrhythmic types Ia (procainamide, quinidine, disopyramide [Norpace], amiodarone [Cordarone]), Ic (propafenone [Rythmol], flecainide [Tambocor]), II (β-blockers), or IV (calcium channel blockers). Class Ib drugs (lidocaine, phenytoin [Dilantin], mexiletine [Mexitil], and tocainide [Tonocard]) can be used.

Disposition

Consultation with a poison control center and a cardiologist experienced with digoxin-specific Fab fragments is warranted. All patients with significant dysrhythmias, symptoms, elevated serum digoxin concentration, or elevated serum potassium level should be admitted to the intensive care unit.

Ethanol

Table 15 lists the features of alcohols and glycols.

Toxic Mechanism

Ethanol has CNS depressant and anesthetic effects. Ethanol stimulates the γ-aminobutyric acid (GABA) system. It promotes cutaneous vasodilation (contributes to hypothermia), stimulates secretion of gastric juice (gastritis), inhibits the secretion of the antidiuretic hormone, inhibits gluconeogenesis (hypoglycemia), and influences fat metabolism (lipidemia).

Toxic Dose

A dose of 1 mL/kg of absolute ethanol (100% ethanol, or 200 proof) gives a blood ethanol concentration of 100 mg/dL. A potentially fatal dose is 3 g/kg for children or 6 g/kg for adults. Children are more prone to developing hypoglycemia than adults.

Kinetics

Onset of action is 30 to 60 minutes after ingestion; peak action is 90 minutes on empty stomach. Volume distribution is 0.6 L/kg. The major route of elimination (>90%) is by hepatic oxidative metabolism. The first step is by the enzyme alcohol dehydrogenase, which converts ethanol to acetaldehyde. Alcohol dehydrogenase metabolizes ethanol at a constant rate of 12 to 20 mg/dL/h (12 to 15 mg/dL/h in nondrinkers, 15 to 30 mg/dL/h in social drinkers, 30 to 50 mg/dL/h in heavy drinkers, and 25 to 30 mg/dL/h in children). At very low blood ethanol concentration (>30 mg/dL), the metabolism is by first-order kinetics. In the second step, acetaldehyde is metabolized by acetaldehyde dehydrogenase to acetic acid, which is metabolized by the Krebs cycle to carbon dioxide and water. The enzyme steps are nicotinamide adenine dinucleotide-dependent, which interferes with gluconeogenesis. Less than 10% of ethanol is excreted unchanged by the kidneys. The relationship between blood ethanol concentration (BEC) and dose (amount ingested) can be calculated as follows:

$$\text{BEC (mg/dL)} = \text{amount ingested (mL)} \times$$
$$\% \text{ ethanol product} \times \text{SG (0.79)}/\text{Vd (0.6 L/kg)} \times \text{body wt (kg)}$$
$$\text{Dose (amount ingested)} = \text{BEC (mg/dL)} \times$$
$$\text{Vd (0.6)} \times \text{body wt (kg)}/\% \text{ ethanol} \times$$
$$\text{specific gravity (0.79)}$$

TABLE 15 Summary of Alcohol and Glycol Features

	METHANOL	ISOPROPANOL	ETHANOL	ETHYLENE GLYCOL
Principal uses	Gas line antifreeze, Sterno, windshield de-icer	Solvent jewelry cleaner, rubbing alcohol	Beverage, solvent	Radiator antifreeze, windshield de-icer
Specific gravity	0.719	0.785	0.789	1.12
Fatal dose	1 mL/kg 100%	3 mL/kg 100%	5 mL/kg 100%	1.4 mL/kg
Inebriation	±	2+	2+	1+
Metabolic change		Hyperglycemia	Hypoglycemia	Hypocalcemia
Metabolic acidosis	4+	0	1+	2+
Anion gap	4+	±	2+	4+
Ketosis	Ketobutyric	Acetone	Hydroxybutyric	None
Gastrointestinal tract	Pancreatitis	Hemorrhagic gastritis	Gastritis	
Osmolality*	0.337	0.176	0.228	0.190

*1 mL/dL of substances raises freezing point osmolarity of serum. The validity of the correlation of osmolality with blood concentrations has been questioned.

Manifestations

Table 16 lists the clinical signs of acute ethanol intoxication.

Chronic alcoholic patients tolerate higher blood ethanol concentration, and correlation with manifestations is not valid. Rapid interview for alcoholism is the CAGE questions:

- C—Have you felt the need to Cut down?
- A—Have others Annoyed you by criticism of your drinking?
- G—Have you felt Guilty about your drinking?
- E—Have you ever had a morning Eye-opening drink to steady your nerves or get rid of a hangover?

Two affirmative answers indicate probable alcoholism.

Laboratory Investigations

The blood ethanol concentration should be specifically requested and followed. Gas chromatography or a breathalyzer test gives rapid reliable results if no belching or vomiting is present. Enzymatic methods do not differentiate between the alcohols. ABG, electrolytes, and glucose should be measured, the anion and osmolar gaps determined (measure by freezing point depression, not vapor pressure), and a check for ketosis made.

Management

The examiner should inquire about trauma and disulfiram use. The patient must be protected from aspiration and hypoxia. Vital functions must be established and maintained. The patient may require intubation and assisted ventilation.

Gastrointestinal decontamination plays no role in the management of ethanol intoxication.

If the patient is comatose, glucose should be administered intravenously, 1 mL/kg 50% glucose in adults and 2 mL/kg 25% glucose in children. Thiamine, 100 mg intravenously, is administered if the patient has a history of chronic alcoholism, malnutrition, or suspected eating disorders to prevent Wernicke-Korsakoff syndrome. Naloxone (Narcan) has produced a partial inconsistent response but is not recommended for known alcoholics.

General supportive care includes administration of fluids to correct hydration and hypotension and correction of electrolyte abnormalities and acid-base imbalance. Vasopressors and plasma expanders may be necessary to correct severe hypotension. Hypomagnesemia is frequent in chronic alcoholics. In case of hypomagnesemia, a loading dose of 2 g magnesium sulfate 10% is administered by intravenous solution over 5 minutes in the intensive care unit with blood pressure and cardiac monitoring and calcium chloride 10% on hand in case of overdose. This is followed with constant infusion of 6 g of 10% solution over 3 to 4 hours. Caution must be taken with the use of magnesium if renal failure is present.

TABLE 16 Clinical Signs in the Nontolerant Ethanol Drinker

ETHANOL BLOOD CONCENTRATION (MG/DL)*	MANIFESTATIONS
>25	Euphoria
>47	**Mild incoordination,** sensory and motor impairment
>50	Increased risk of motor vehicle accidents
>100	Ataxia (legal toxic level in many localities)
>150	**Moderate incoordination,** slow reaction time
>200	Drowsiness and confusion
>300	Severe incoordination, stupor, blurred vision
>500	**Flaccid coma,** respiratory failure, hypotension; may be fatal

*Ethanol concentrations sometimes reported in %.
Note: mg% is not equivalent to mg/dL because ethanol weighs less than water (specific gravity 0.79). A 1% ethanol concentration is 790 mg/dL and 0.1% is 79 mg/dL. There is great variation in individual behavior at different blood ethanol levels. Behavior is dependent on tolerance and other factors.

Hypothermic patients should be warmed. See the section on disturbances caused by cold.

Hemodialysis can be used in severe cases when conventional therapy is ineffective (rarely needed).

Repeated or prolonged seizures should be treated with diazepam (Valium). The brief "rum fits" do not need long-term anticonvulsant therapy. Repeated seizures or focal neurologic findings may warrant skull radiographs, lumbar puncture, and CT scan of the head, depending on the clinical findings. Withdrawal is treated with hydration and large doses of chlordiazepoxide (Librium) 50 to 100 mg or diazepam (Valium) 2 to 10 mg intravenously; these doses may be repeated in 2 to 4 hours. Very large doses of benzodiazepines may be required for delirium tremens. Withdrawal can occur in presence of elevated blood ethanol concentration and can be fatal if left untreated.

Chest radiograph is warranted to determine whether aspiration pneumonia is present. Renal and liver function tests and bilirubin level measurement should be made.

Disposition

Clinical severity (e.g., intubation, assisted ventilation, aspiration pneumonia) should determine the level of hospital care needed. Young children with significant unintentional exposure to ethanol (calculated to reach a blood ethanol concentration of 50 mg/dL) should have blood ethanol concentration obtained and blood glucose levels monitored for hypoglycemia frequently for 4 hours after ingestion. Patients with acute ethanol intoxication seldom require admission unless a complication is present. However, intoxicated patients should not be discharged until they are fully functional (can walk, talk, and think independently), have suicide potential evaluated, have proper disposition environment, and have a sober escort.

Ethylene Glycol

Ethylene glycol is found in solvents, de-icers, radiator antifreeze (95%), and air-conditioning units. Ethylene glycol is a sweet-tasting, colorless, water-soluble liquid with a sweet aromatic fragrance.

Toxic Mechanism

Ethylene glycol is oxidized by alcohol dehydrogenase to glycolaldehyde, which is metabolized to glycolic acid and glyoxylic acid. Glyoxylic acid is metabolized to oxalic acid via a pyridoxine-dependent pathway to glycine and by thiamine and magnesium-dependent pathways to α-hydroxy-ketoadipic acid. The metabolites of ethylene glycol produce a profound metabolic acidosis, increased anion gap, hypocalcemia, and oxalate crystals, which deposit in tissues (particularly the kidney).

Toxic Dose

The ingestion of 0.1 mL/kg 100% ethylene glycol can result in a toxic serum ethylene glycol concentration of 20 mg/dL. Ingestion of 3.0 mL (less than 1 teaspoonful or swallow) of a 100% solution in a 10-kg child or 30 mL of 100% ethylene glycol in an adult produces a serum ethylene glycol concentration of 50 mg/dL, a concentration that requires hemodialysis. The fatal amount is 1.4 mL/kg of 100% solution.

Kinetics

Absorption is via dermal, inhalation, and ingestion routes. Ethylene glycol is rapidly absorbed from the gastrointestinal tract. Onset is usually in 30 minutes but may be delayed by co-ingestion of food and ethanol. The usual peak level is at 2 hours. Volume distribution is 0.65 to 0.8 L/kg.

For metabolism, see *Toxic Mechanism*.

The half-life of ethylene glycol without ethanol is 3 to 8 hours; with ethanol, it is 17 hours, and with hemodialysis it is 2.5 hours. Renal clearance is 3.2 mL/kg/min. About 20% to 50% is excreted unchanged in the urine. The relationship between serum ethylene glycol concentration (SEGC) and dose (amount ingested) can be calculated as follows:

$$0.12 \text{ mL/kg of } 100\% = \text{SEGC } 10 \text{ mg/dL}$$

Manifestations

Phase I. The onset of manifestations is 30 minutes to several hours longer after ingestion with concomitant ethanol ingestion. The patient may be inebriated. Hypocalcemia, tetany, and calcium oxalate and hippuric acid crystals in urine can be seen within 4 to 8 hours but are not always present. Early, before metabolism of ethylene glycol, an osmolal gap may be present (see *Laboratory Investigations*). Later, the metabolites of ethylene glycol produce changes starting 4 to 12 hours following ingestion, including an anion gap, metabolic acidosis, coma, convulsions, cardiac disturbances, and pulmonary and cerebral edema. Because fluorescein is added to some antifreeze, the presence of fluorescence may be a clue to ethylene glycol exposure. However, it has been shown that fluorescent urine is not a reliable indicator of ethylene glycol ingestion and should not be used as a screen.

Phase II. After 12 to 36 hours, cardiopulmonary deterioration occurs, with pulmonary edema and congestive heart failure.

Phase III. Phase III occurs 36 to 72 hours after ingestion, with pulmonary edema and oliguric renal failure from oxalate crystal deposition and tubular necrosis predominating.

Phase IV. Neurologic sequelae may occur rarely, especially in patients who fail to receive early antidotal therapy. The onset ranges from 6 to 10 days after ingestion. Findings include facial diplegia, hearing loss, bilateral visual disturbances, elevated cerebrospinal fluid pressure with or without elevated protein levels and pleocytosis, vomiting, hyperreflexia, dysphagia, and ataxia.

Laboratory Investigations

Blood glucose and electrolytes should be monitored. Urinalysis should look for oxalate ("envelope") and monohydrate ("hemp seed") crystals. Urine fluorescence is not reliable as a screen. ABG, ethylene glycol, and ethanol levels, plasma osmolarity (using freezing point depression method), calcium, BUN, and creatinine should be measured. A serum ethylene glycol concentration of 20 mg/dL is toxic (ethylene glycol levels are very difficult to obtain). If possible, a glycolate level should be obtained. Cross-reactions with propylene glycol, a vehicle in many liquids and intravenous medications (phenytoin [Dilantin], diazepam [Valium]), other glycols, and triglycerides, may produce spurious ethylene glycol levels. False-positive ethylene glycol values may occur with colorimetric or gas chromatography using an OV-17 column in the presence of propylene glycol.

The following equations can be used to calculate the osmolality, osmolal gap, and ethylene glycol level:

$$2(\text{Na} + \text{mEq/L}) + (\text{Blood glucose mg/dL})/20 + (\text{BUN mg/dL})/3 =$$
$$\text{Total calculated osmolality(mOsm/L)}$$
$$\text{Osmolar Gap} = \text{measured osmolality (by freezing point depression}$$
$$\text{method)} - \text{calculate osmolality}$$

A gap greater than 10 is abnormal. *Note:* if ethanol is involved, add ethanol level/4.6 to the calculated equation.

An increased osmolal gap is produced by the following common substances: acetone, dextran, dimethyl sulfoxide, diuretics, ethanol, ethyl ether, ethylene glycol, isopropanol, paraldehyde, mannitol, methanol, sorbitol, and trichloroethane. Table 10 gives the conversion factors for these substances.

Although a specific blood level of ethylene glycol in milligrams per deciliter can be estimated using the equation below, this is not considered to be a reliable method and should not take the place of obtaining a measured ethylene glycol blood concentration.

$$\text{Osmolar gap} \times \text{conversion factor} = \text{serum concentration}$$

Caution: The accuracy of the ethylene glycol estimated decreases as the ethylene glycol levels decrease. The toxic metabolites are not osmotically active, and patients presenting late may show signs of severe toxicity without an elevated osmolar gap.

The anion gap can be calculated using the following equation:

$$\text{Na} - (\text{Cl} + \text{HCO}_3) = \text{anion gap}$$

The normal gap is 8 to 12. Potassium is not used because it is a small amount and may be hemolyzed. Table 8 lists factors that may account for an increased or a decreased anion gap.

Management

Vital functions should be established and maintained. The airway must be protected, and assisted ventilation can be used, if necessary. Gastrointestinal decontamination has a limited role. Only gastric aspiration can be used within 60 minutes after ingestion. Activated charcoal is not effective.

Baseline measurements of serum electrolytes and calcium, glucose, ABGs, ethanol, serum ethylene glycol concentration (may be difficult to obtain readily in some institutions), and methanol concentrations should be obtained. In the first few hours, the measured serum osmolality should be determined and compared to calculated osmolality (see osmolality equation, earlier). If seizures occur, one should measure serum calcium (preferably ionized calcium) and treat with intravenous diazepam. If the patient has hypocalcemic seizures, he or she should also be treated with 10 to 20 mL 10% calcium gluconate (0.2 to 0.3 mL/kg in children) slowly intravenously, with the dose repeated as needed. Metabolic acidosis should be corrected with intravenous sodium bicarbonate.

Ethanol therapy should be initiated immediately if fomepizole (Antizol) is unavailable (see next paragraph). Alcohol dehydrogenase has a greater affinity for ethanol than ethylene glycol. Therefore, ethanol blocks the metabolism of ethylene glycol. Ethanol therapy is called for if there is a history of ingestion of 0.1 mL/kg of 100% ethylene glycol, serum ethylene glycol concentration is greater than 20 mg/dL, there is an osmolar gap not accounted for by other alcohols or factors (e.g., hyperlipidemia), metabolic acidosis is present with an increased anion gap, or there are oxalate crystals in the urine. Ethanol should be administered intravenously (the oral route is less reliable) to produce a blood ethanol concentration of 100 to 150 mg/dL. The loading dose is 10 mL/kg of 10% ethanol intravenously, administered concomitantly with a maintenance dose of 10% ethanol of 1.0 mL/kg/h. This dose may need to be increased to 2 mL/kg/h in patients who are heavy drinkers. The blood ethanol concentration should be measured hourly and the infusion rate should be adjusted to maintain a blood ethanol concentration of 100 to 150 mg/dL.

Fomepizole (Antizol, 4-methylpyrazole) inhibits alcohol dehydrogenase more reliably than ethanol and it does not require constant monitoring of ethanol levels and adjustment of infusion rates. Fomepizole is available in 1 g/mL vials of 1.5 mL. The loading dose is 15 mg/kg (0.015 mL/kg) IV; maintenance dose is 10 mg/kg (0.01 mL/kg) every 12 hours for four doses, then 15 mg/kg every 12 hours until the ethylene glycol levels are less than 20 mg/dL. The solution is prepared by being mixed with 100 mL of 0.9% saline or D_5W (5% dextrose in water). Fomepizole can be given to patients requiring hemodialysis but should be dosed as follows:

Dose at the beginning of hemodialysis:
- If <6 hours since last Antizol dose, do not administer dose
- If >6 hours since last dose, administer next scheduled dose

Dosing during hemodialysis:
- Dose every 4 hours

Dosing at the time hemodialysis is completed:
- If <1 hour between last dose and end of dialysis, do not administer dose at end of dialysis
- If 1 to 3 hours between last dose and end of dialysis, administer one half of next scheduled dose
- If >3 hours between last dose and end of dialysis, administer next scheduled dose

Maintenance dosing off hemodialysis:
- Give the next scheduled dose 12 hours from the last dose administered

Hemodialysis is indicated if the ingestion was potentially fatal; if the serum ethylene glycol concentration is greater than 50 mg/dL (some recommend at levels of >25 mg/dL); if severe acidosis or electrolyte abnormalities occur despite conventional therapy; or if congestive heart failure or renal failure is present. Hemodialysis reduces the ethylene glycol half-life from 17 hours on ethanol therapy to 3 hours. Therapy (fomepizole and hemodialysis) should be continued until the serum ethylene glycol concentration is less than 10 mg/dL, the glycolate level is nondetectable (not readily available), the acidosis has cleared, there are no mental disturbances, the creatinine level is normal, and the urinary output is adequate. This may require 2 to 5 days.

Adjunct therapy involving thiamine, 100 mg/d (in children, 50 mg), slowly over 5 minutes intravenously or intramuscularly and repeated every 6 hours and pyridoxine, 50 mg IV or IM every 6 hours, has been recommended until intoxication is resolved, but these agents have not been extensively studied. Folate, 50 mg IV (child 1 mg/kg), can be given every 4 hours for 6 doses.

Disposition

All patients who have ingested significant amounts of ethylene glycol (calculated level above 20 mg/dL), have a history of a toxic dose, or are symptomatic should be referred to the emergency department and admitted. If the serum ethylene glycol concentration cannot be obtained, the patient should be followed for 12 hours, with monitoring of the osmolal gap, acid-base parameters, and electrolytes to exclude development of metabolic acidosis with an anion gap. Transfer should be considered for fomepizole therapy or hemodialysis.

Hydrocarbons

The lower the viscosity and surface tension of hydrocarbons or the greater the volatility, the greater the risk of aspiration. Volatile substance abuse has produced the "Sudden Sniffing's Death Syndrome," most likely caused by dysrhythmias.

Toxicologic Classification and Toxic Mechanism

All systemically absorbed hydrocarbons can lower the threshold of the myocardium to dysrhythmias produced by endogenous and exogenous catecholamines.

Aliphatic hydrocarbons are branched straight chain hydrocarbons. A few aspirated drops are poorly absorbed from the gastrointestinal tract and produce no systemic toxicity by this route. However, aspiration of very small amounts can produce chemical pneumonitis. Examples of aliphatic hydrocarbons are gasoline, kerosene, charcoal lighter fluid, mineral spirits (Stoddard's solvent), and petroleum naphtha. Mineral seal oil (signal oil), found in furniture polishes, is a low-viscosity and low-volatility oil with minimum absorption that never warrants gastric decontamination. It can produce severe pneumonia if aspirated.

Aromatic hydrocarbons are six carbon ring structures that are absorbed through the gastrointestinal tract. Systemic toxicity includes CNS depression and, in cases of chronic abuse, multiple organ effects such as leukemia (benzene) and renal toxicity (toluene). Examples are benzene, toluene, styrene, and xylene. The seriously toxic ingested dose is 20 to 50 mL in adults.

Halogenated hydrocarbons are aliphatic or aromatic hydrocarbons with one or more halogen substitutions (Cl, Br, Fl, or I). They are highly volatile and are abused as inhalants. They are well absorbed from the gastrointestinal tract, produce CNS depression, and have metabolites that can damage the liver and kidneys. Examples include methylene chloride (may be converted into carbon monoxide in the body), dichloroethylene (also causes a disulfiram [Antabuse] reaction known as "degreaser's flush" when associated with consumption of ethanol), and 1,1,1-trichloroethane (Glamorene Spot Remover, Scotchgard, typewriter correction fluid). An acute lethal oral dose is 0.5 to 5 mL/kg.

Dangerous additives to the hydrocarbons can be summed up with the mnemonic CHAMP: C, camphor (demothing agent); H, halogenated hydrocarbons; A, aromatic hydrocarbons; M, metals (heavy); and P, pesticides. Ingestion of these substances may warrant gastric emptying with a small-bore nasogastric tube.

Heavy hydrocarbons have high viscosity, low volatility, and minimal gastrointestinal absorption, so gastric decontamination is not necessary. Examples are asphalt (tar), machine oil, motor oil (lubricating oil, engine oil), home heating oil, and petroleum jelly (mineral oil).

Laboratory Investigations

The ECG, ABG, pulmonary function, serum electrolytes, and serial chest radiographs should be continuously monitored. Liver and renal function should be monitored in cases of inhalation of aromatic hydrocarbons.

Management

Asymptomatic patients who ingested small amounts of aliphatic petroleum distillates can be followed at home by telephone for development of signs of aspiration (cough, wheezing, tachypnea, and dyspnea) for 4 to 6 hours. Inhalation of any hydrocarbon vapors in a closed space can produce intoxication. The victim must be removed from the environment, have oxygen administered, and receive respiratory support.

Gastrointestinal decontamination is not advised in cases of hydrocarbon ingestion that usually do not cause systemic toxicity (aliphatic petroleum distillates, heavy hydrocarbons). In cases of ingestion of hydrocarbons that cause systemic toxicity in small amounts (aromatic hydrocarbons, halogenated hydrocarbons), the clinician should pass a small-bore nasogastric tube and aspirate if the ingestion was within 2 hours and if spontaneous vomiting has not occurred. Some toxicologists advocate ipecac-induced emesis under medical supervision instead of small-bore nasogastric gastric lavage; we do not.

Patients with altered mental status should have their airway protected because of concern about aspiration. The use of activated charcoal has been suggested, but there are no scientific data as to effectiveness and it may produce vomiting. Activated charcoal may, however, be useful in adsorbing toxic additives such as pesticides or co-ingestants.

The symptomatic patient who is coughing, gagging, choking, or wheezing on arrival has probably aspirated. The clinician should provide supportive respiratory care and supplemental oxygen, while monitoring pulse oximetry, ABG, chest radiograph, and ECG. The patient should be admitted to the intensive care unit. A chest radiograph for aspiration may be positive as early as 30 minutes after ingestion, and almost all are positive within 6 hours. Negative chest radiographs within 4 hours do not rule out aspiration.

Bronchospasm is treated with a nebulized β-adrenergic agonist and intravenous aminophylline if necessary. Epinephrine should be avoided because of susceptibility to dysrhythmias. Cyanosis in the presence of a normal arterial Pao$_2$ may be a result of methemoglobinemia that requires therapy with methylene blue. Corticosteroids and prophylactic antimicrobial agents have not been shown to be beneficial. (Fever or leukocytosis may be produced by the chemical pneumonitis itself.)

Most infiltrations resolve spontaneously in 1 week; lipoid pneumonia may last up to 6 weeks. It is not necessary to surgically treat pneumatoceles that develop because they usually resolve. Dysrhythmias may require α- and β-adrenergic antagonists or cardioversion.

There is no role for enhanced elimination procedures.

Methylene chloride is metabolized over several hours to carbon monoxide. See treatment of carbon monoxide poisoning. Halogenated hydrocarbons are hepatorenal toxins; therefore, hepatorenal function should be monitored. N-acetylcysteine therapy may be useful if there is evidence of hepatic damage.

Extracorporeal membrane oxygenation (ECMO) has been used successfully for a few patients with life-threatening respiratory failure. Surfactant used for hydrocarbon aspiration was found to be detrimental.

Disposition

Asymptomatic patients with small ingestions of petroleum distillates can be managed at home. Symptomatic patients with abnormal chest radiographic, oxygen saturation, or ABG findings should be admitted. Patients who become asymptomatic and have normal oxygenation and a normal repeat radiograph can be discharged.

Iron

There are more than 100 iron over-the-counter preparations for supplementation and treatment of iron deficiency anemia.

Toxic Mechanism

Toxicity depends on the amount of elemental iron available in various salts (gluconate 12%, sulfate 20%, fumarate 33%, lactate 19%, chloride 21% of elemental iron), not the amount of the salt. Locally, iron is corrosive and may cause fluid loss, hypovolemic shock, and perforation. Excessive free unbound iron in the blood is directly toxic to the vasculature and leads to the release of vasoactive substances, which produces vasodilation. In cases of overdose, iron deposits injure mitochondria in the liver, the kidneys, and the myocardium. The exact mechanism of cellular damage is not clear but is thought to be related to free radical formation.

Toxic Dose

The therapeutic dose is 6 mg/kg/d of elemental iron. An elemental iron dose of 20 to 40 mg/kg may produce mild self-limited gastrointestinal symptoms, 40 to 60 mg/kg produces moderate toxicity, more than 60 mg/kg produces severe toxicity and is potentially lethal, and more than 180 mg/kg is usually fatal without treatment. Children's chewable vitamins with iron have between 12 and 18 mg of elemental iron per tablet or 0.6 mL of liquid drops. These preparations rarely produce toxicity unless very large quantities are ingested and have never caused death.

Kinetics

Absorption occurs chiefly in the upper small intestine. Ferrous (+2) iron is absorbed into the mucosal cells, where it is oxidized to the ferric (+3) state and bound to ferritin. Iron is slowly released from ferritin into the plasma, where it binds to transferrin and is transported to specific tissues for production of hemoglobin (70%), myoglobin (5%), and cytochrome. About 25% of iron is stored in the liver and spleen. In cases of overdose, larger amounts of iron are absorbed because of direct mucosal corrosion. There is no mechanism for the elimination of iron (elimination is 1 to 2 mg/d) except through bile, sweat, and blood loss.

Manifestations

Serious toxicity is unlikely if the patient remains asymptomatic for 6 hours and has a negative abdominal radiograph. Iron intoxication can produce five phases of toxicity. The phases may not be distinct from one another.

Phase I. Gastrointestinal mucosal injury occurs 30 minutes to 12 hours postingestion. Vomiting starts within 30 minutes to 1 hour of ingestion and is persistent; hematemesis and bloody diarrhea may occur; abdominal cramps, fever, hyperglycemia, and leukocytosis may occur. Enteric-coated tablets may pass through the stomach without causing symptoms. Acidosis and shock can occur within 6 to 12 hours.

Phase II. A latent period of apparent improvement occurs over 8 to 12 hours postingestion.

Phase III. Systemic toxicity phase occurs 12 to 48 hours postingestion with cardiovascular collapse and severe metabolic acidosis.

Phase IV. Two to 4 days postingestion, hepatic injury associated with jaundice, elevated liver enzymes, and prolonged prothrombin time occur. Kidney injury with proteinuria and hematuria occur. Pulmonary edema, disseminated intravascular coagulation, and *Yersinia enterocolitica* sepsis can occur.

Phase V. Four to 8 weeks postingestion, pyloric outlet or intestinal stricture may cause obstruction or anemia secondary to blood loss.

Laboratory Investigations

Iron poisoning produces anion gap metabolic acidosis. Monitoring should include complete blood cell counts, blood glucose level, serum iron, stools and vomitus for occult blood, electrolytes, acid-base balance, urinalysis and urinary output, liver function tests, and BUN and creatinine levels. Blood type and match should be obtained.

Serum iron measurements taken at the proper time correlate with the clinical findings. The lavender top Vacutainer tube contains EDTA, which falsely lowers serum iron. One must obtain the serum iron measurement before administering deferoxamine. Serum iron levels of less than 350 μg/dL at 2 to 6 hours predict an asymptomatic course; levels of 350 to 500 μg/dL are usually associated with mild gastrointestinal symptoms; those greater than 500 μg/dL have a 20% risk of shock and serious iron toxicity. A follow-up serum iron measurement after 6 hours may not be elevated even in cases of severe poisoning, but a serum iron measurement taken at 8 to 12 hours is useful to exclude delayed absorption from a bezoar or sustained-release preparation. The total iron-binding capacity is not necessary.

Adult iron tablet preparations are radiopaque before they dissolve by 4 hours postingestion. A "negative" abdominal radiograph more than 4 hours postingestion does not exclude iron poisoning.

Patients who develop high fevers and signs of sepsis following iron overdose should have blood and stool cultures checked for *Yersinia enterocolitica*.

Management

Gastrointestinal decontamination should involve immediate induction of emesis in cases of ingestions of elemental iron of greater than 40 mg/kg if vomiting has not already occurred. Activated charcoal is ineffective. An abdominal radiograph should be obtained after emesis to determine the success of gastric emptying. Children's chewable vitamins and liquid iron preparations are not radiopaque. If radiopaque iron is still present, whole-bowel irrigation with polyethylene glycol solution should be considered. In extreme cases, removal by endoscopy or surgery may be necessary because coalesced iron tablets produce hemorrhagic infarction in the bowel and perforation peritonitis.

Deferoxamine (Desferal) in a dose of about 100 mg binds 8.5 to 9.35 mg of free iron in the serum. The deferoxamine infusion should not exceed 15 mg/kg/h or 6 g daily, but faster rates (up to 45 mg/kg) and larger daily amounts have been administered and tolerated in extreme cases of iron poisoning (>1000 mg/dL). The deferoxamine-iron complex is hemodialyzable if renal failure develops.

Indications for chelation therapy are any of the following:

- Very large, symptomatic ingestions
- Serious clinical intoxication (severe vomiting and diarrhea [often bloody], severe abdominal pain, metabolic acidosis, hypotension, or shock)
- Symptoms that persist or progress to more serious toxicity
- Serum iron level greater than 500 mg/dL

Chelation should be performed as early as possible within 12 to 18 hours to be effective. One should start the infusion slowly and gradually increase to avoid hypotension.

Adult respiratory distress syndrome has developed in patients with high doses of deferoxamine for several days; infusions longer than 24 hours should be avoided.

The end point of treatment is when the patient is asymptomatic and the urine clears if it was originally a positive "vin rosö" color.

For supportive therapy, intravenous bicarbonate may be needed to correct the metabolic acidosis. Hypotension and shock treatment may require volume expansion, vasopressors, and blood transfusions. The physician should attempt to keep the urinary output at greater than 2 mL/kg/h. Coagulation abnormalities and overt bleeding require blood products or vitamin K. Pregnant patients are treated in a fashion similar to any other patient with iron poisoning.

Hemodialysis and hemoperfusion are ineffective. Exchange transfusion has been used in single cases of massive poisonings in children.

Disposition

The asymptomatic or minimally symptomatic patient should be observed for persistence and progression of symptoms or development of toxicity signs (gastrointestinal bleeding, acidosis, shock, altered mental state). Patients with mild self-limited gastrointestinal symptoms who become asymptomatic or have no signs of toxicity for 6 hours are unlikely to have a serious intoxication and can be discharged after psychiatric clearance, if needed. Patients with moderate or severe toxicity should be admitted to the intensive care unit.

Isoniazid

Isoniazid is a hydrazide derivative of vitamin B_3 (nicotinamide) and is used as an antituberculosis drug.

Toxic Mechanism

Isoniazid produces pyridoxine deficiency by increasing the excretion of pyridoxine (vitamin B_6) and by inhibiting pyridoxal 5-phosphate (the active form of pyridoxine) from acting with L-glutamic acid decarboxylase to form γ-aminobutyric acid (GABA), the major CNS neurotransmitter inhibitor, resulting in seizures. Isoniazid also blocks the conversion of lactate to pyruvate, resulting in profound and prolonged lactic acidosis.

Toxic Dose

The therapeutic dose is 5 to 10 mg/kg (maximum 300 mg) daily. A single acute dose of 15 mg/kg lowers the seizure threshold; 35 to 40 mg/kg produces spontaneous convulsions; more than 80 mg/kg produces severe toxicity. A fatal dose in adults is 4.5 to 15 g. The malnourished patients, those with a previous seizure disorder, alcoholic patients, and slow acetylators are more susceptible to isoniazid toxicity. In cases of chronic intoxication, 10 mg/kg/d produces hepatitis in 10% to 20% of patients but less than 2% at doses of 3 to 5 mg/kg/d.

Kinetics

Absorption from intestine occurs in 30 to 60 minutes, and onset is in 30 to 120 minutes, with peak levels of 5 to 8 μg/mL within 1 to 2 hours. Volume distribution is 0.6 L/kg, with minimal protein binding.

Elimination is by liver acetylation to a hepatotoxic metabolite, acetyl-isoniazid, which is then hydrolyzed to isonicotinic acid. In slow acetylators, isoniazid has a half-life of 140 to 460 minutes (mean 5 hours), and 10% to 15% is eliminated unchanged in the urine. Most (45% to 75%) whites and 50% of African blacks are slow acetylators, and, with chronic use (without pyridoxine supplements), they may develop peripheral neuropathy. In fast acetylators, isoniazid has a half-life of 35 to 110 minutes (mean 80 minutes), and 25% to 30% is excreted unchanged in the urine. About 90% of Asians and patients with diabetes mellitus are fast acetylators and may develop hepatitis on chronic use.

In patients with overdose and hepatic disease, the serum half-life may increase. Isoniazid inhibits the metabolism of phenytoin (Dilantin), diazepam, phenobarbital, carbamazepine (Tegretol), and prednisone. These drugs also interfere with the metabolism of isoniazid. Ethanol may decrease the half-life of isoniazid but increase its toxicity.

Manifestations

Within 30 to 60 minutes, nausea, vomiting, slurred speech, dizziness, visual disturbances, and ataxia are present. Within 30 to 120 minutes, the major clinical triad of severe overdose includes refractory convulsions (90% of overdose patients have one or more seizures), coma, and resistant severe lactic acidosis (secondary to convulsions), often with a plasma pH of 6.8.

Laboratory Investigations

Isoniazid produces anion gap metabolic acidosis. Therapeutic levels are 5 to 8 μg/mL and acute toxic levels are greater than 20 μg/mL. These levels are not readily available to assist in making decisions in acute overdose situations. One should monitor the blood glucose (often hyperglycemia), electrolytes (often hyperkalemia), bicarbonate, ABGs, liver function tests (elevations occur with chronic exposure), BUN, and creatinine.

Management

Seizures must be controlled. Pyridoxine and diazepam should be administered concomitantly through different IV sites. Pyridoxine (vitamin B_6) is given in a dose of 1 g for each gram of isoniazid ingested. If the dose ingested is unknown, at least 5 g of pyridoxine should be given intravenously. Pyridoxine is administered in 50 mL D_5W or 0.9% saline over 5 minutes intravenously. It must not be administered in the same bottle as sodium bicarbonate. Intravenous pyridoxine is repeated every 5 to 20 minutes until the seizures are controlled. Total doses of pyridoxine up to 52 g have been safely administered; however, patients given 132 and 183 g of pyridoxine have developed a persistent crippling sensory neuropathy.

Diazepam is administered concomitantly with pyridoxine but at a different site. They work synergistically. Diazepam should be administered intravenously slowly, 0.3 mg/kg at a rate of 1 mg/min in children or 10 mg at a rate of 5 mg/min in adults. After the seizures are controlled, the remainder of the pyridoxine is administered (1 g/1 g isoniazid) or a total dose of 5 g.

Phenobarbital or phenytoin is ineffective and should not be used.

In asymptomatic patients or patients without seizures, pyridoxine has been advised by some toxicologists prophylactically in gram-for-gram doses in cases of large overdoses (<80 mg/kg per dose) of isoniazid, although there are no studies to support this recommendation. In comatose patients, pyridoxine administration may result in the patient's rapid regaining of consciousness. Correction of acidosis may occur spontaneously with pyridoxine administration and correction of the seizures. Sodium bicarbonate should be administered if acidosis persists.

Hemodialysis is rarely needed because of antidotal therapy and the short half-life of isoniazid, but it may be used as an adjunct for cases of uncontrollable acidosis and seizures. Hemoperfusion has not been adequately evaluated. Diuresis is ineffective.

Disposition
Asymptomatic or mildly symptomatic patients who become asymptomatic can be observed in the emergency department for 4 to 6 hours. Larger amounts of isoniazid may warrant pyridoxine administration and longer periods of observation. Intentional ingestions necessitate psychiatric evaluation before the patient is discharged. Patients with convulsions or coma should be admitted to the intensive care unit.

Isopropanol (Isopropyl Alcohol)
Isopropanol can be found in rubbing alcohol, solvents, and lacquer thinner. Coma has occurred in children sponged for fever with isopropanol. See Table 10 for ethanol features of alcohols and glycols.

Toxic Mechanism
Isopropanol is a gastric irritant. It is metabolized to acetone, a CNS and myocardial depressant. It inhibits gluconeogenesis. Normal propyl alcohol is related to isopropyl alcohol but is more toxic.

Toxic Dose
A toxic dose of 0.5 to 1 mg/kg of 70% isopropanol (1 mL/kg of 70%) produces a blood isopropanol plasma concentration of 70 mg/dL. The CNS depressant potency is twice that of ethanol.

Kinetics
Onset of action is within 30 to 60 minutes, and peak is 1 hour postingestion. Volume distribution is 0.6 kg/L. Isopropyl alcohol metabolizes to acetone. Its excretion is renal.

Note: The serum isopropyl concentration and amount ingested can be estimated using the same equation as is used in ethanol kinetics and substituting the specific gravity of 0.785 for isopropyl alcohol.

Manifestations
Ethanol-like inebriation occurs, with an acetone odor to the breath, gastritis, occasionally with hematemesis, acetonuria, and acetonemia without systemic acidosis.

Depression of the CNS occurs: lethargy at blood isopropyl alcohol levels of 50 to 100 mg/dL, coma at levels of 150 to 200 mg/dL, potentially death in adults at levels greater than 240 mg/dL.

Hypoglycemia and seizures may occur.

Laboratory Investigation
Monitoring of blood isopropyl alcohol levels (not readily available in all institutions), acetone, glucose, and ABG should be maintained. The osmolal gap increases 1 mOsm per 5.9 mg/dL of isopropyl alcohol and 1 mOsm per 5.5 mg/dL of acetone. The absence of excess acetone in the blood (normal is 0.3 to 2 mg/dL) within 30 to 60 minutes or excess acetone in the urine within 3 hours excludes the possibility of significant isopropanol exposure.

Management
The airway must be protected with intubation, and assisted ventilation administered if necessary. If the patient is hypoglycemic,

TABLE 17	Occupations Associated With Lead Exposure
Lead production or smelting	Demolition of ships and bridges
Production of illicit whiskey	Battery manufacturing
Brass, copper, and lead foundries	Machining/grinding lead alloys
Radiator repair	Welding of old painted metals
Scrap handling	Thermal paint stripping of old buildings
Sanding of old paint	
Lead soldering	Ceramic glaze/pottery mixing
Cable stripping	
Worker or janitor at a firing range	

Modified from Rempel D: The lead-exposed worker. *JAMA* 262:533, 1989.

glucose should be administered. Supportive treatment is similar to that for ethanol ingestions.

Gastrointestinal decontamination has no role in the treatment of isopropanol ingestion. Hemodialysis is warranted in cases of life-threatening overdose but is rarely needed. A nephrologist should be consulted if the blood isopropanol plasma concentration is greater than 250 mg/dL.

Disposition
Symptomatic patients with concentrations greater than 100 mg/dL require at least 24 hours of close observation for resolution and should be admitted. If the patient is hypoglycemic, hypotensive, or comatose, he or she should be admitted to the intensive care unit.

Lead
Acute lead intoxication is rare and usually occurs by inhalation of lead, resulting in severe intoxication and often death. Lead fumes can be produced by burning of lead batteries or use of a heat gun to remove lead paint. Acute lead intoxication also occurs from exposure to high concentrations of organic lead (e.g., tetraethyl lead).

Chronic lead poisoning occurs most often in children 6 months to 6 years of age who are exposed in their environment and in adults in certain occupations (Table 17). In the United States, the prevalence in children aged 1 to 5 years with a venous blood lead greater than 10 μg/dL decreased from 88.2% in a 1976–1980 survey to 8.9% in a 1988–1991 survey as a consequence of measures to reduce lead in the environment, particularly leaded gasoline. However, an estimated 1.7 million children between 1 and 5 years of age and more than 1 million workers in over 100 different occupations still have blood lead levels greater than 10 μg/dL.

Toxic Dose
In cases of chronic lead poisoning, a daily intake of more than 5 μg/kg/d in children or more than 150 μg/d in adults can give a positive lead balance. In 1991, the Centers for Disease Control and Prevention (CDC) recommended routine screening for all children younger than 6 years of age. In children a venous blood level greater than 10 μg/dL was determined to be a threshold of concern. The average venous blood level in the United States is 4 μg/dL. In cases of occupational exposure (see Table 17), a venous blood level greater than 40 μg/dL is indicative of increased lead absorption in adults.

Toxic Mechanism
Lead affects the sulfhydryl enzyme systems, the immature CNS, the enzymes of heme synthesis, vitamin D conversion, the kidneys, the bones, and growth. Lead alters the tertiary structure of cell proteins by denaturing them and causing cell death. Risk factors are mouthing behavior of infants and children and excessive oral behavior (pica), living in the inner city, a poorly maintained home, and poor nutrition (e.g., low calcium and iron). The CDC

questionnaire given in Table 18 is recommended at every pediatric visit. If any answers to the CDC questionnaire are "positive," a blood screening test for lead should be administered. To be more accurate, however, identifying lead exposure studies have suggested that the questionnaire will have to be modified for each individual community because it has had poor sensitivity (40%) and specificity (60%) as it stands.

Table 19 lists sources of lead. The number one source is deteriorating lead-based paint, which forms leaded dust. Lead concentrations in indoor paint were not reduced to safer (0.06%) levels until 1978. Lead can also be produced by improper interior or exterior home renovation (scraping or demolition). It is found in pre-1960 built homes. The use of leaded gasoline (limited in 1973) resulted in residue from leaded motor vehicle emissions. Lead persists in the soil near major highways and in deteriorating homes and buildings. Vegetables grown in contaminated soil may contain lead.

Oil refineries and lead-processing smelters produce lead residue. Food cans produced in Mexico contain lead solder (95% do not in the United States). Lead water pipes (until 1950) and lead solder (until 1986) deliver lead-containing drinking water (calcium deposits, however, may offer some protection). Water at a consumer's tap should contain less than 15 parts per billion (ppb) of lead (Table 20).

For occupational exposure, see Table 17. The Occupational Safety and Health Administration (OSHA) standards require employers to provide showering and clothes changing facilities for personnel working with lead; however, businesses with fewer than 25 employees are exempt from the regulation. The OSHA lead standard of 1978 set a limit of 60 μg/dL for occupational exposure to lead. At a blood lead level of 60 μg/dL, a worker should be removed from lead exposure and not allowed back until his or her lead level is below 40 μg/dL. Many authorities believe that this level should be lower. The lead residue on the clothes of the workers may represent a hazard to the family. Other occupations that are potential sources of lead exposure include plumbers, pipe fitters, lead miners, auto repairers, shipbuilders, printers, steel welders and cutters, construction workers, and rubber product manufacturers.

Leaded pots to make molds for "kusmusha" tea represent lead exposure. Imported pottery lined with ceramic glaze can leach large amounts of lead into acids (e.g., citrus fruit juices).

Hobbies associated with lead exposure are listed in Box 1. Some "traditional" folk remedies or cosmetics that contain lead include the following:

TABLE 18 · CDC Questionnaire: Priority Groups for Lead Screening

1. Children age 6–72 months (was 12–36 months) who live in or are frequent visitors to older, deteriorated housing built before 1960.

2. Children age 6–72 months who live in housing built prior to 1960 with recent, ongoing, or planned renovation or remodeling.

3. Children age 6–72 months who are siblings, housemates, or playmates of children with known lead poisoning.

4. Children age 6–72 months whose parents or other household members participate in a lead-related industry or hobby.

5. Children age 6–72 months who live near active lead smelters, battery recycling plants, or other industries likely to result in atmospheric lead release.

TABLE 19 · Sources of Lead

PRODUCT	LEAD CONTENT (%) BY DRY WEIGHT
Paint	0.06
Solder	0.6
Plastic additives	2.0
Priming inks	2.0
Plumbing fixtures	2.0
Pesticides	0.1
Stained glass panes	0.1
Wine bottle foils	0.1
Construction material	0.1
Fertilizers	0.1
Glazes, enamels	0.06
Toys/recreational games	0.1
Curtain weights	0.1
Fishing weights	0.1

TABLE 20 · Agency Regulations and Recommendations Concerning Lead Content

AGENCY	SPECIMEN	LEVEL	COMMENTS
CDC	Blood (child)	10 μg/dL	Investigate community
OSHA	Blood (adult)	60 μg/dL	Medical removal from work
OSHA	Air	50 μg/m³	PEL*
	Air	0.75 μg/m³	Tetraethyl or tetramethyl
ACGIH	Air	150 μg/m³	TWA†
EPA	Air	1.5 μg/m³	Three-month average
EPA	Water	15 μg/L (ppb)	5 ppb circulating
EPA	Food	100 μg/d	Advisory
FDA	Wine	300 ppm	Plan to reduce to 200 ppm
EPA	Soil/dust	50 ppm	
CPSC	Paint	600 ppm (0.06%) by dry weight	

*PEL = permissible exposure limit (highest level over an 8-hour workday).
†TWA = time-weighted average (air concentration for 8-hour workday and 40-hour workweek).
Abbreviations: ACGIH = American Conference of Governmental Industrial Hygienists; CDC = Centers for Disease Control and Prevention; CPSC = Consumer Product Safety Commission; EPA = Environmental Protection Agency; FDA = Food and Drug Administration; OSHA = Occupational Safety and Health Administration.

- "Azarcon por empacho" ("Maria Louisa" 90% to 95% lead trioxide): a bright orange powder used in Hispanic culture, especially Mexican, for digestive problems and diarrhea.
- "Greta" (4% to 90% lead): a yellow powder "por empacho" ("empacho" refers to a variety of gastrointestinal symptoms), used in Hispanic cultures, especially Mexican.
- "Pay-loo-ah": an orange-red powder used for rash and fever in Southeast Asian cultures, especially among Northern Laos Hmong immigrants.

BOX 1	Hobbies Associated With Lead Exposure

Casting of ammunition
Collecting antique pewter
Collecting/painting lead toys (e.g., soldiers and figures)
Ceramics or glazed pottery
Refinishing furniture
Making fishing weights
Home renovation
Jewelry making, lead solder
Glass blowing, lead glass
Bronze casting
Print making and other fine arts (when lead white, flake white, chrome yellow pigments are involved)
Liquor distillation
Hunting and target shooting
Painting
Car and boat repair
Burning/engraving lead-painted wood
Making stained leaded glass
Copper enameling

- "Alkohl" (Al-kohl, kohl, suma 5% to 92% lead): a black powder used in Middle Eastern, African, and Asian cultures as a cosmetic and an umbilical stump astringent.
- "Farouk": an orange granular powder with lead used in Saudi Arabian culture.
- "Bint Al Zahab": used to treat colic in Saudi Arabian culture.
- "Surma" (23% to 26% lead): a black powder used in India as a cosmetic and to improve eyesight.
- "Bali goli": a round black bean that is dissolved in "grippe water," used by Asian and Indian cultures to aid digestion.

Cases of substance abuse involving lead poisoning have been reported, in which the patient sniffs leaded gasoline or uses improperly synthesized amphetamines.

Kinetics

Absorption of lead is 10% to 15% of the ingested dose in adults; in children, up to 40% is absorbed, especially in cases of iron deficiency anemia. With inhalation of fumes, absorption is rapid and complete. Volume distribution in blood (0.9% of total body burden) is 95% in red blood cells. Lead passes through the placenta to the fetus and is present in breast milk.

Organic lead is metabolized in the liver to inorganic lead. Its half-life is 35 to 40 days in blood; in soft tissue, the half-life is 45 days and in bone (99% of the lead), the half-life is 28 years. The major elimination route is the stool, 80% to 90%, and then renal 10% (80 g/d) and hair, nails, sweat, and saliva. Nine percent of organic lead is excreted in the urine per day.

Manifestations

Adverse health effects are given in Table 21 and include the following.

TABLE 21	Summary of Lead-Induced Health Effects in Adults and Children

BLOOD LEAD LEVEL (MG/DL)	AGE GROUP	HEALTH EFFECT
>100	Adult	Encephalopathic signs and symptoms
>80	Adult	Anemia
	Child	Encephalopathy Chronic nephropathy (e.g., aminoaciduria)
>70	Adult	Clinically evident peripheral neuropathy
	Child	Colic and other gastrointestinal symptoms
>60	Adult	Female reproductive effects CNS disturbance symptoms (i.e., sleep disturbances, mood changes, memory and concentration problems, headaches)
>50	Adult	Decreased hemoglobin production Decreased performance on neurobehavioral tests
	Adult	Altered testicular function Gastrointestinal symptoms (i.e., abdominal pain, constipation, diarrhea, nausea, anorexia)
	Child	Peripheral neuropathy*
>40	Adult	Decreased peripheral nerve conduction Hypertension, age 40–59 years Chronic neuropathy*
>25	Adult	Elevated erythrocyte protoporphyrin in males
15–25	Adult	Elevated erythrocyte protoporphyrin in females
>10	Child	Decreased intelligence and growth Impaired learning Reduced birth weight* Impaired mental ability
	Fetus	Preterm delivery

From Anonymous: Implementation of the Lead Contamination Control Act of 1988. *MMWR Morb Mortal Wkly Rep* 41:288, 1992.
*Controversial.

Hematologic. Lead inhibits γ-aminolevulinic acid dehydratase (early in the synthesis of heme) and ferrochelatase (transfers iron to ferritin for incorporation of iron into protoporphyrin to produce heme). Anemia is a late finding. Decreased heme synthesis starts at >40 µg/dL. Basophilic stippling occurs in 20% of severe lead poisoning.

Neurologic. Segmental demyelination and peripheral neuropathy, usually of the motor type (wrist and ankle drop), occurs in workers. A venous blood level of lead greater than 70 µg/dL (usually >100 µg/dL), produces encephalopathy in children (symptom mnemonic "PAINT": P, persistent forceful vomiting and papilledema; A, ataxia; I, intermittent stupor and lucidity; N, neurologic coma and refractory convulsions; T, tired and lethargic). Decreased cognitive abilities have been reported with a venous blood level of lead greater than 10 µg/dL, including behavioral problems, decreased attention span, and learning disabilities. IQ scores may begin to decrease at 15 µg/dL. Encephalopathy is rare in adults.

Renal. Nephropathy as a result of damaged capillaries and glomerulus can occur at a venous blood level of lead greater than 80 µg/dL, but recent studies show renal damage and hypertension with low venous blood levels. A direct correlation between hypertension and venous blood level over 30 µg/dL has been reported. Lead reduces excretion of uric acid, and high-level exposure may be associated with hyperuricemia and "saturnine gout," Fanconi's syndrome (aminoaciduria and renal tubular acidosis), and tubular fibrosis.

Reproductive. Spontaneous abortion, transient delay in the child's development (catch up at age 5 to 6 years), decreased sperm count, and abnormal sperm morphology can occur with lead exposure. Lead crosses the placenta and fetal blood levels reach 75% to 100% of maternal blood levels. Lead is teratogenic.

Metabolic. Decreased cytochrome P450 activity alters the metabolism of medication and endogenously produced substances. Decreased activation of cortisol and decreased growth are caused by interference in vitamin conversion (25-hydroxyvitamin D to 1,25-hydroxyvitamin D) at venous blood levels of 20 to 30 µg/dL.

Other Manifestations. Abnormalities of thyroid, cardiac, and hepatic function occur in adults. Abdominal colic is seen in children at doses greater than 50 µg/dL. "Lead gum lines" at the dental border of the gingiva can occur in cases of chronic lead poisoning.

Laboratory Investigations

Serial venous blood lead measurements are taken on days 3 and 5 during treatment and 7 days after chelation therapy, then every 1 to 2 weeks for 8 weeks, and then every month for 6 months. Intravenous infusion should be stopped at least 1 hour before blood lead levels are measured. Table 22 gives a classification of blood lead concentrations in children.

One should evaluate CBC, serum ferritin, erythrocyte protoporphyrin (>35 µg/dL indicates lead poisoning as well as iron deficiency and other causes), electrolytes, serum calcium and phosphorus, urinalysis, BUN, and creatinine. Abdominal and long bone radiographs may be useful in certain circumstances to identify radiopaque material in bowel and "lead lines" in proximal tibia (which occur after prolonged exposure in association with venous blood lead levels greater than 50 µg/dL).

Neuropsychological tests are difficult to perform in young children but should be considered at the end of treatment, especially to determine auditory dysfunction.

Management

The basis of treatment is removal of the source of lead. Cases of poisoning in children should be reported to local health department and cases of occupational poisoning should be reported to OSHA. The source must be identified and abated and dust controlled by wet mopping. Cold water should be let to run for 2 minutes before being used for drinking. Planting shrubbery (not vegetables) in contaminated soil will keep children away.

TABLE 22 Classification of Blood Lead Concentrations in Children

BLOOD LEAD (MG/DL)	RECOMMENDED INTERVENTIONS
<9	None
10–14	Community intervention Repeat blood lead in 3 months
15–19	Individual case management Environmental counseling Nutritional counseling Repeat blood lead in 3 months
20–44	Medical referral Environmental inspection/abatement Nutritional counseling Repeat blood lead in 3 months
45–69	Environmental inspection/abatement Nutritional counseling Pharmacologic therapy DMSA succimer oral or CaNa₂EDTA parenteral Repeat every 2 weeks for 6–8 weeks, then monthly for 4–6 months
>70	Hospitalization in intensive care unit Environmental inspection/abatement Pharmacologic therapy Dimercaprol (BAL in oil) IM initial alone Dimercaprol IM and CaNa₂EDTA together Repeat every week

Abbreviations: BAL = British anti-Lewisite; CaNa₂EDTA = edetate calcium disodium; DMSA = dimercaptosuccinic acid; IM = intramuscular.

Supportive care should be instituted, including measures to deal with refractory seizures (continued antidotal therapy, diazepam, and possibly neuromuscular blockers), with the hepatic and renal failure, and intravascular hemolysis in severe cases. Seizures are treated with diazepam followed by neuromuscular blockers if needed.

Lead does not bind to activated charcoal. One must not delay chelation therapy for complete gastrointestinal decontamination in severe cases. Whole-bowel irrigation has been used prior to treatment. Some authorities recommend abdominal radiographs followed by gastrointestinal decontamination if necessary before switching to oral therapy. Chelation therapy can be used for patients in whom venous blood level of lead is greater than 45 µg/dL in children and greater than 80 µg/dL in adults or in adults with lower levels who are symptomatic or who have a "positive" lead mobilization test result (not routinely performed at most centers) (Table 23).

Succimer (dimercaptosuccinic acid, DMSA, Chemet), a derivative of British anti-Lewisite (BAL), is an oral agent for chelation in children with a venous blood level of greater than 45 µg/dL. The recommended dose is 10 mg/kg every 8 hours for 5 days, then every 12 hours for 14 days. DMSA is under investigation to determine its role in children with a venous blood level less than 45 µg/dL. Although not approved for adults, it has been used in the same dosage. Monitoring should be maintained by CBC, liver transaminases, and urinalysis for adverse effects.

D-Penicillamine (Cuprimine) is another oral chelator that is given in doses of 20 to 40 mg/kg/d not to exceed 1 g/d. However, it is not FDA approved and has a 10% adverse reaction rate. Nevertheless, D-penicillamine has been used infrequently in adults and children with elevated venous blood lead levels.

Edetate calcium disodium (ethylene diaminetetra-acetic acid or CaNa₂EDTA Versenate) is a water-soluble chelator given intramuscularly (with 0.5% procaine) or intravenously. The calcium in the compound is displaced by divalent and trivalent heavy metals, forming a soluble complex, which is stable at physiologic pH (but not at acid pH) and enhances lead clearance in the urine. EDTA

TABLE 23 Pharmacologic Chelation Therapy of Lead Poisoning

DRUG	ROUTE	DOSE	DURATION	PRECAUTIONS	MONITOR
Dimercaprol (BAL in oil)	IM	3–5 mg/kg q4–6h	3–5 days	G6PD deficiency Concurrent iron therapy	AST/ALT enzymes
CaNa$_2$EDTA (calcium disodium versenate)	IM/IV	50 mg/kg per day	5 days	Inadequate fluid intake Renal impairment Penicillin allergy	Urinalysis, BUN Creatinine Urinalysis, BUN
D-Penicillamine (Cuprimine)	PO	10 mg/kg per day increase 30 mg/kg over 2 weeks	6–20 weeks	Concurrent iron therapy; lead exposure Renal impairment	Creatinine, CBC
2,3-Dimercaptosuccinic acid (DMSA; succimer)	PO	10 mg/kg per dose 3 times daily 10 mg/kg per dose twice daily for 14 days	19 days	AST/ALT Concurrent iron therapy G6PD deficiency lead exposure	AST/ALT

Abbreviations: ALT = alanine aminotransferase; AST = aspartate transaminase; BAL = British anti-Lewisite; bid = twice daily; BUN = blood urea nitrogen; CBC = complete blood count; G6PD = glucose-6-phosphate dehydrogenase; IM = intramuscular; IV = intravenous; PO = oral; tid = three times daily.

usually is administered intravenously, especially in severe cases. It must not be administered until adequate urine flow is established. It may redistribute lead to the brain; therefore, BAL may be given first at a venous blood lead level of greater than 55 µg/dL in children and greater than 100 µg/dL in adults. Phlebitis occurs at a concentration greater than 0.5 mg/mL. Alkalinization of the urine may be helpful. CaNa$_2$EDTA should not be confused with sodium EDTA (disodium edetate), which is used to treat hypercalcemia; inadvertent use may produce severe hypocalcemia.

Dimercaprol (BAL) is a peanut oil–based dithiol (two sulfhydryl molecules) that combines with one atom of lead to form a heterocyclic stable ring complex. It is usually reserved for patients in whom venous blood lead is greater than 70 µg/dL, and it chelates red blood cell lead, enhancing its elimination through the urine and bile. It crosses the blood-brain barrier. Approximately 50% of patients have adverse reactions, including bad metallic taste in the mouth, pain at the injection site, sterile abscesses, and fever.

A venous blood lead level greater than 70 µg/dL or the presence of clinical symptoms suggesting encephalopathy in children is a potentially life-threatening emergency. Management should be accomplished in a medical center with a pediatric intensive care unit by a multidisciplinary team including a critical care specialist, a toxicologist, a neurologist, and a neurosurgeon. Careful monitoring of neurologic status, fluid status, and intracranial pressure should be undertaken if necessary. These patients need close monitoring for hemodynamic instability. Hydration should be maintained to ensure renal excretion of lead. Fluids, renal and hepatic function, and electrolyte levels should be monitored.

While waiting for adequate urine flow, therapy should be initiated with intramuscular dimercaprol (BAL) only (25 mg/kg/d divided into 6 doses). Four hours later, the second dose of BAL should be given intramuscularly, concurrently with CaNa$_2$EDTA 50 mg/kg/d as a single dose infused over several hours or as a continuous infusion. The double therapy is continued until the venous blood level is less than 40 µg/dL.

As long as the venous blood level is greater than 40 µg/dL, therapy is continued for 72 hours and followed by two alternatives: either parenteral therapy with two drugs (CaNa$_2$EDTA and BAL) for 5 days or continuation of therapy with CaNa$_2$EDTA alone if a good response is achieved and the venous blood level of lead is less than 40 µg/dL. If one cannot get the venous blood lead report back, one should continue therapy with both BAL and EDTA for 5 days. In patients with lead encephalopathy, parenteral chelation should be continued with both drugs until the patient is clinically stable before changing therapy. Mannitol and dexamethasone can reduce the cerebral edema, but their role in lead encephalopathy is not clear. Surgical decompression is not recommended to reduce cerebral edema in these cases.

If BAL and CaNa$_2$EDTA are used together, a minimum of 2 days with no treatment should elapse before another 5-day course of therapy is considered. The 5-day course is repeated with CaNa$_2$EDTA alone if the blood lead level rebounds to greater than 40 µg/dL or in combination with BAL if the venous blood level is greater than 70 µg/dL. If a third course is required, unless there are compelling reasons, one should wait at least 5 to 7 days before administering the course.

Following chelation therapy, a period of equilibration of 10 to 14 days should be allowed and a repeat venous blood lead concentration should be obtained. If the patient is stable enough for oral intake, oral succimer 30 mg/kg/d in three divided doses for 5 days followed by 20 mg/kg/d in two divided doses for 14 days has been suggested, but there are limited data to support this recommendation. Therapy should be continued until venous blood lead level is less than 20 µg/dL in children or less than 40 µg/dL in adults.

Chelators combined with lead are hemodialyzable in the event of renal failure.

Disposition

All patients with a venous blood lead level of greater than 70 µg/dL or who are symptomatic should be admitted. If a child is hospitalized, all lead hazards must be removed from the home environment before allowing the child to return. The source must be eliminated by environmental and occupational investigations. The local health department should be involved in dealing with children who are lead poisoned, and OSHA should be involved with cases of occupational lead poisoning. Consultation with a poison control center or experienced toxicologist is necessary when chelating patients. Follow-up venous blood lead concentrations should be obtained within 1 to 2 weeks and followed every 2 weeks for 6 to 8 weeks, then monthly for 4 to 6 months if the patient required chelation therapy. All patients with venous blood level greater than 10 µg/dL should be followed at least every 3 months until two venous blood lead concentrations are 10 µg/dL or three are less than 15 µg/dL.

Lithium (Eskalith, Lithane)

Lithium is an alkali metal used primarily in the treatment of bipolar psychiatric disorders. Most intoxications are cases of chronic overdose. One gram of lithium carbonate contains 189 mg (5.1 mEq) of lithium; a regular tablet contains 300 mg (8.12 mEq) and a sustained-release preparation contains 450 mg or 12.18 mEq.

Toxic Mechanism

The brain is the primary target organ of toxicity, but the mechanism is unclear. Lithium may interfere with physiologic functions by acting as a substitute for cellular cations (sodium and potassium), depressing neural excitation and synaptic transmission.

Toxic Dose

A dose of 1 mEq/kg (40 mg/kg) of lithium will give a peak serum lithium concentration about 1.2 mEq/L. The therapeutic serum lithium concentration in cases of acute mania is 0.6 to 1.2 mEq/L, and for maintenance it is 0.5 to 0.8 mEq/L. Serum lithium concentration levels are usually obtained 12 hours after the last dose. The toxic dose is determined by clinical manifestations and serum levels after the distribution phase.

Acute ingestion of twenty 300-mg tablets (300 mg increases the serum lithium concentration by 0.2 to 0.4 mEq/L) in adults may produce serious intoxication. Chronic intoxication can be produced by conditions listed below that can decrease the elimination of lithium or increase lithium reabsorption in the kidney.

The risk factors that predispose to chronic lithium toxicity are febrile illness, impaired renal function, hyponatremia, advanced age, lithium-induced diabetes insipidus, dehydration, vomiting and diarrhea, and concomitant use of other drugs, such as thiazide and spironolactone diuretics, nonsteroidal antiinflammatory drugs, salicylates, angiotensin-converting enzyme inhibitors (e.g., captopril), serotonin reuptake inhibitors (e.g., fluoxetine [Prozac]), and phenothiazines.

Kinetics

Gastrointestinal absorption of regular-release preparations is rapid; serum lithium concentration peaks in 2 to 4 hours and is complete by 6 to 8 hours. The onset of toxicity may occur at 1 to 4 hours after acute overdose but usually is delayed because lithium enters the brain slowly. Absorption of sustained-release preparations and the development of toxicity may be delayed 6 to 12 hours.

Volume distribution is 0.5 to 0.9 L/kg. Lithium is not protein bound. The half-life after a single dose is 9 to 13 hours; at steady state, it may be 30 to 58 hours. The renal handling of lithium is similar to that of sodium: glomerular filtration and reabsorption (80%) by the proximal renal tubule. Adequate sodium must be present to prevent lithium reabsorption. More than 90% of lithium is excreted by the kidney, 30% to 60% within 6 to 12 hours.

Manifestations

The examiner must distinguish between side effects, acute intoxication, acute or chronic toxicity, and chronic intoxications. Chronic is the most common and dangerous type of intoxication.

Side effects include fine tremor, gastrointestinal upset, hypothyroidism, polyuria and frank diabetes insipidus, dermatologic manifestations, and cardiac conduction deficits. Lithium is teratogenic.

Patients with acute poisoning may be asymptomatic, with an early high serum lithium concentration of 9 mEq/L, and deteriorate as the serum lithium concentration falls by 50% and the lithium distributes to the brain and the other tissues. Nausea and vomiting may occur within 1 to 4 hours, but the systemic manifestations are usually delayed several more hours. It may take as long as 3 to 5 days for serious symptoms to develop. Acute toxicity and acute on chronic toxicity are manifested by neurologic findings, including weakness, fasciculations, altered mental state, myoclonus, hyperreflexia, rigidity, coma, and convulsions with limbs in hypertension. Cardiovascular effects are nonspecific and occur at therapeutic doses, flat T or inverted T waves, atrioventricular block, and prolonged QT interval. Lithium is not a primary cardiotoxin. Cardiogenic shock occurs secondary to CNS toxicity. Chronic intoxication is associated with manifestations at lower serum lithium concentrations. There is some correlation with manifestations, especially at higher serum lithium concentrations. Although the levels do not always correlate with the manifestations, they are more predictive in cases of severe intoxication. A serum lithium concentration greater than 3.0 mEq/L with chronic intoxication and altered mental state indicates severe toxicity. Permanent neurologic sequelae can result from lithium intoxication.

Laboratory Investigations

Monitoring should include CBC (lithium causes significant leukocytosis), renal function, thyroid function (chronic intoxication), ECG, and electrolytes. Serum lithium concentrations should be determined every 2 to 4 hours until levels are close to therapeutic range. Cross-reactions with green-top Vacutainer specimen tubes containing heparin will spuriously elevate serum lithium concentration 6 to 8 mEq/L.

Management

Vital function must be established and maintained. Seizure precautions should be instituted and seizures, hypotension, and dysrhythmias treated. Evaluation should include examination for rigidity and hyperreflexia signs, hydration, renal function (BUN, creatinine), and electrolytes, especially sodium. The examiner should inquire about diuretic and other drug use that increase serum lithium concentration, and the patient must discontinue the drugs. If the patient is on chronic therapy, the lithium should be discontinued. Serial serum lithium concentrations should be obtained every 4 hours until serum lithium concentration peaks and there is a downward trend toward almost therapeutic range, especially in sustained-release preparations. Vital signs should be monitored, including temperature, and ECG and serial neurologic examinations should be undertaken, including mental status and urinary output. Nephrology consultation is warranted in case of a chronic and elevated serum lithium concentration (>2.5 mEq/L), a large ingestion, or altered mental state.

An intravenous line should be established and hydration and electrolyte balance restored. Serum sodium level should be determined before 0.9% saline fluid is administered in patients with chronic overdose because hypernatremia may be present from diabetes insipidus. Although current evidence supports an initial 0.9% saline infusion (200 mL/h) to enhance excretion of lithium, once hydration, urine output, and normonatremia are established, one should administer 0.45% saline and slow the infusion (100 mL/h) for all patients.

Gastric lavage is often not recommended in cases of acute ingestion because of the large size of the tablets, and it is not necessary after chronic intoxication. Activated charcoal is ineffective. For sustained-release preparations, whole-bowel irrigation may be useful but is not proven. Sodium polystyrene sulfonate (Kayexalate), an ion exchange resin, is difficult to administer and has been used only in uncontrolled studies. Its use is not recommended.

Hemodialysis is the most efficient method for removing lithium from the vascular compartment. It is the treatment of choice for patients with severe intoxication with an altered mental state, those with seizures, and anuric patients. Long runs are used until the serum lithium concentration is less than 1 mEq/L because of extensive re-equilibration. Serum lithium concentration should be monitored every 4 hours after dialysis for rebound. Repeated and prolonged hemodialysis may be necessary. A lag in neurologic recovery can be expected.

Disposition

An acute asymptomatic lithium overdose cannot be medically cleared on the basis of single lithium level. Patients should be admitted if they have any neurologic manifestations (altered mental status, hyperreflexia, stiffness, or tremor). Patients should be admitted to the intensive care unit if they are dehydrated, have renal impairment, or have a high or rising lithium level.

Methanol (Wood Alcohol, Methyl Alcohol)

The concentration of methanol in Sterno fuel is 4% and it contains ethanol, in windshield washer fluid it is 30% to 60%, and in gas-line antifreeze it is 100%.

Toxic Mechanism

Methanol is metabolized by alcohol dehydrogenase to formaldehyde, which is metabolized to formate. Formate inhibits cytochrome oxidase, producing tissue hypoxia, lactic acidosis, and optic nerve edema. Formate is converted by folate-dependent enzymes to carbon dioxide.

Toxic Dose

The minimal toxic amount is approximately 100 mg/kg. Serious toxicity in a young child can be produced by the ingestion of 2.5 to 5.0 mL of 100% methanol. Ingestion of 5-mL 100% methanol by a 10-kg child produces estimated peak blood methanol of 80 mg/dL. Ingestion of 15 mL 40% methanol was lethal for a 2-year-old child in one report. A fatal adult oral dose is 30 to 240 mL 100% (20 to 150 g). Ingestion of 6 to 10 mL 100% causes blindness in adults. The toxic blood concentration is greater than 20 mg/dL; very serious toxicity and potential fatality occur at levels greater than 50 mg/dL.

Kinetics

Onset of action can start within 1 hour but may be delayed up to 12 to 18 hours by metabolism to toxic metabolites. It may be delayed longer if ethanol is ingested concomitantly or in infants. Peak blood methanol concentration is 1 hour. Volume distribution is 0.6 L/kg (total body water).

For metabolism, see *Toxic Mechanism*.

Elimination is through metabolism. The half-life of methanol is 8 hours; with ethanol blocking it is 30 to 35 hours; and with hemodialysis 2.5 hours.

Manifestations

Metabolism creates a delay in onset for 12 to 18 hours or longer if ethanol is ingested concomitantly. Initial findings are as follows:

- 0 to 6 hours: Confusion, ataxia, inebriation, formaldehyde odor on breath, and abdominal pain can be present, but the patient may be asymptomatic. *Note:* Methanol produces an osmolal gap (early), and its metabolite formate produces the anion gap metabolic acidosis (see later). Absence of osmolar or anion gap does not always exclude methanol intoxication.
- 6 to 12 hours: Malaise, headache, abdominal pain, vomiting, visual symptoms, including hyperemia of optic disc, "snow vision," and blindness can be seen.
- More than 12 hours: Worsening acidosis, hyperglycemia, shock, and multiorgan failure develop, with death from complications of intractable acidosis and cerebral edema.

Laboratory Investigation

Methanol can be detected on some chromatography drug screens if specified. Methanol and ethanol levels, electrolytes, glucose, BUN, creatinine, amylase, and ABG should be monitored every 4 hours. Formate levels correlate more closely than blood methanol concentration with severity of intoxication and should be obtained if possible.

Management

One should protect the airway by intubation to prevent aspiration and administer assisted ventilation as needed. If needed, 100% oxygen can be administered. A nephrologist should be consulted early regarding the need for hemodialysis.

Gastrointestinal decontamination procedures have no role.

Metabolic acidosis should be treated vigorously with sodium bicarbonate 2 to 3 mEq/kg intravenously. Large amounts may be needed.

Antidote therapy is initiated to inhibit metabolism if the patient has a history of ingesting more than 0.4 mL/kg of 100% with the following conditions:

- Blood methanol level is greater than 20 mg/dL
- The patient has osmolar gap not accounted for by other factors
- The patient is symptomatic or acidotic with increased anion gap and/or hyperemia of the optic disc.

The ethanol or fomepizole therapy outlined below can be used.

Ethanol Therapy. Ethanol should be initiated immediately if fomepizole is unavailable (see *Fomepizole Therapy*). Alcohol dehydrogenase has a greater affinity for ethanol than ethylene glycol. Therefore, ethanol blocks the metabolism of ethylene glycol.

Ethanol should be administered intravenously (oral administration is less reliable) to produce a blood ethanol concentration of 100 to 150 mg/dL. The loading dose is 10 mL/kg of 10% ethanol administered intravenously concomitantly with a maintenance dose of 10% ethanol at 1.0 mL/kg/h. This dose may need to be increased to 2 mL/kg/h in patients who are heavy drinkers. The blood ethanol concentration should be measured hourly and the infusion rate should be adjusted to maintain a concentration of 100 to 150 mg/dL.

Fomepizole Therapy. Fomepizole (Antizol, 4-methylpyrazole) inhibits alcohol dehydrogenase more reliably than ethanol and it does not require constant monitoring of ethanol levels and adjustment of infusion rates. Fomepizole is available in 1 g/mL vials of 1.5 mL. The loading dose is 15 mg/kg (0.015 mL/kg) IV, maintenance dose is 10 mg/kg (0.01 mL/kg) every 12 hours for 4 doses, then 15 mg/kg every 12 hours until the ethylene glycol levels are less than 20 mg/dL. The solution is prepared by being mixed with 100 mL of 0.9% saline or D_5W. Fomepizole can be given to patients requiring hemodialysis but should be dosed as follows:

Dose at the beginning of hemodialysis:
- If less than 6 hours since last Antizol dose, do not administer dose
- If more than 6 hours since last dose, administer next scheduled dose

Dosing during hemodialysis:
- Dose every 4 hours

Dosing at the time hemodialysis is completed:
- If less than 1 hour between last dose and end dialysis, do not administer dose at end of dialysis
- If 1 to 3 hours between last dose and end dialysis, administer one half of next scheduled dose
- If more than 3 hours between last dose and end dialysis, administer next scheduled dose

Maintenance dosing off hemodialysis:
- Give the next scheduled dose 12 hours from the last dose administered

Hemodialysis increases the clearance of both methanol and formate 10-fold over renal clearance. A blood methanol concentration greater than 50 mg/dL has been used as an indication for hemodialysis, but recently some toxicologists from the New York City Poison Center recommended early hemodialysis in patients with blood methanol concentration greater than 25 mg/dL because it may be able to shorten the course of intoxication if started early. One should continue to monitor methanol levels and/or formate levels every 4 hours after the procedure for rebound. Other indications for early hemodialysis are significant metabolic acidosis and electrolyte abnormalities despite conventional therapy and if visual or neurologic signs or symptoms are present.

A serum formate level greater than 20 mg/dL has also been used as a criterion for hemodialysis, although this is often not readily available through many laboratories. If hemodialysis is used, the infusion rate of 10% ethanol should be increased 2.0 to 3.5 mL/kg/h. The blood ethanol concentration and glucose level should be obtained every 2 hours.

Therapy is continued with both ethanol and hemodialysis until the blood methanol level is undetectable, there is no acidosis, and the patient has no neurologic or visual disturbances. This may require several days.

Hypoglycemia is treated with intravenous glucose. Doses of folinic acid (Leucovorin) and folic acid have been used successfully in animal investigations to enhance formate metabolism to carbon dioxide and water. Leucovorin 1 mg/kg up to 50 mg IV is administered every 4 hours for several days.

An initial ophthalmologic consultation and follow-up are warranted.

Disposition

All patients who have ingested significant amounts of methanol should be referred to the emergency department for evaluation and blood methanol concentration measurement. Ophthalmologic follow-up of all patients with methanol intoxications should be arranged.

Monoamine Oxidase Inhibitors

Nonselective monoamine oxidase inhibitors (MAOIs) include the hydrazines phenelzine (Nardil) and isocarboxazid (Marplan), and the nonhydrazine tranylcypromine (Parnate). Furazolidone (Furoxone) and pargyline (Eutonyl) are also considered nonselective MAOIs. Moclobemide,[22] which is available in many countries but not the United States, is a selective MAO-A inhibitor. MAO-B inhibitors include selegiline (Eldepryl), an antiparkinsonism agent, which does not have similar toxicity to MAO-A and is not discussed. Selectivity is lost in an overdose. MAOIs are used to treat severe depression.

Toxic Mechanism

Monoamine oxidase enzymes are responsible for the oxidative deamination of both endogenous and exogenous catecholamines such as norepinephrine. MAO-A in the intestinal wall also metabolizes tyramine in food. MAOIs permanently inhibit MAO enzymes until a new enzyme is synthesized after 14 days or longer. The toxicity results from the accumulation, potentiation, and prolongation of the cate-cholamine action followed by profound hypotension and cardiovascular collapse.

Toxic Dose

Toxicity begins at 2 to 3 mg/kg and fatalities occur at 4 to 6 mg/kg. Death has occurred after a single dose of 170 mg of tranylcypromine in an adult.

Kinetics

Structurally, MAOIs are related to amphetamines and catecholamines. The hydrazine peak levels are at 1 to 2 hours; metabolism is hepatic acetylation; and inactive metabolites are excreted in the urine. For the nonhydrazines, peak levels occur at 1 to 4 hours, and metabolism is via the liver to active amphetamine-like metabolites.

The onset of symptoms in a case of overdose is delayed 6 to 24 hours after ingestion, peak activity is 8 to 12 hours, and duration is 72 hours or longer. The peak of MAO inhibition is in 5 to 10 days and lasts as long as 5 weeks.

Manifestations

Manifestations of an acute ingestion overdose of MAO-A inhibitors are as follows:

Phase I. An adrenergic crisis occurs, with delayed onset for 6 to 24 hours, and may not reach peak until 24 hours. The crisis starts as hyperthermia, tachycardia, tachypnea, dysarthria, transient hypertension, hyperreflexia, and CNS stimulation.

Phase II. Neuromuscular excitation and sympathetic hyperactivity occur with increased temperature greater than 40°C (104°F), agitation, hyperactivity, confusion, fasciculations, twitching, tremor, masseter spasm, muscle rigidity, acidosis, and electrolyte abnormalities. Seizures and dystonic reactions may occur. The pupils are mydriatic, sometimes nonreactive with "ping-pong gaze."

Phase III. CNS depression and cardiovascular collapse occur in cases of severe overdose as the catecholamines are depleted. Symptoms usually resolve within 5 days but may last 2 weeks.

Phase IV. Secondary complications occur, including rhabdomyolysis, cardiac dysrhythmias, multiorgan failure, and coagulopathies.

Biogenic interactions usually occur while the patient is on therapeutic doses of MAOI or shortly after they are discontinued (30 to 60 minutes), before the new MAO enzyme is synthesized. The following substances have been implicated: indirect acting sympathomimetics such as amphetamines, serotonergic drugs, opioids (e.g., meperidine, dextromethorphan), tricyclic antidepressants, specific serotonin reuptake inhibitors (SSRIs; e.g., fluoxetine [Prozac], sertraline [Zoloft], paroxetine [Paxil]), tyramine-containing foods (e.g., wine, beer, avocados, cheese, caviar, chocolate, chicken liver), and L-tryptophan. SSRIs should not be started for at least 5 weeks after MAOIs have been discontinued.

In mild cases, usually caused by foods, headache and hypertension develop and last for several hours. In severe cases, malignant hypertension and severe hyperthermia syndromes consisting of hypertension or hyperthermia, altered mental state, skeletal muscle rigidity, shivering (often beginning in the masseter muscle), and seizures may occur.

The serotonin syndrome, which may be a result of inhibition of serotonin metabolism, has similar clinical findings to those of malignant hyperthermia and may occur with or without hyperthermia or hypertension.

Chronic toxicity clinical findings include tremors, hyperhidrosis, agitation, hallucinations, confusion, and seizures and may be confused with withdrawal syndromes.

Laboratory Investigations

Monitoring of the ECG, cardiac monitoring, CPK, ABG, pulse oximeter, electrolytes, blood glucose, and acid-base balance should be maintained.

Management

In the case of MAOI overdose, ipecac-induced emesis should not be used. Only activated charcoal alone should be used.

If the patient is admitted to the hospital and is well enough to eat, a nontyramine diet should be ordered.

Extreme agitation and seizures can be controlled with benzodiazepines and barbiturates. Phenytoin is ineffective. Nondepolarizing neuromuscular blockers (not depolarizing succinylcholine) may be needed in severe cases of hyperthermia and rigidity. If the patient has severe hypertension (catecholamine mediated), phentolamine (Regitine), a parenteral β-blocking agent, 3 to 5 mg intravenously, or labetalol (Normodyne), a combination of an α-blocking agent and a β-blocker, 20-mg intravenous bolus, should be given. If malignant hypertension with rigidity is present, a short-acting nitroprusside and benzodiazepine can be used. Hypertension is often followed by severe hypotension, which should be managed by fluid and vasopressors. *Caution:* Vasopressor therapy should be administered at lower doses than usual because of exaggerated pharmacologic response. Norepinephrine is preferred to dopamine, which requires release of intracellular amines.

Cardiac dysrhythmias are treated with standard therapy but are often refractory, and cardioversion and pacemakers may be needed.

For malignant hyperthermia, dantrolene (Dantrium), a nonspecific peripheral skeletal relaxing agent, is administered, which inhibits the release of calcium from the sarcoplasm. Dantrolene is reconstituted with 60 mL sterile water without bacteriostatic agents. Glass equipment must not be used, and the drug must be protected from light and used within 6 hours. Loading dose is 2 to 3 mg/kg intravenously as a bolus, and the loading dose is repeated until the signs of malignant hyperthermia (tachycardia, rigidity, increased end-tidal CO_2, and temperature) are controlled. Maximum total dose is 10 mg/kg to avoid hepatotoxicity.

When malignant hyperthermia has subsided, 1 mg/kg IV is given every 6 hours for 24 to 48 hours, then orally 1 mg/kg every 6 hours for 24 hours to prevent recurrence. There is a danger of thrombophlebitis following peripheral dantrolene, and it should be administered through a central line if possible. In addition one should administer external cooling and correct metabolic acidosis and electrolyte disturbances. Benzodiazepine can be used for sedation. Dantrolene does not reverse central dopamine blockade; therefore, bromocriptine mesylate (Parlodel) 2.5 to 10 mg should be given orally or through a nasogastric tube three times a day.

Rhabdomyolysis and myoglobinuria are treated with fluids. Urine alkalinization should also be treated.

Hemodialysis and hemoperfusion are of no proven value.

Biogenic amine interactions are managed symptomatically, similar to cases of overdose. For the serotonin syndrome cyproheptadine (Periactin), a serotonin blocker, 4 mg orally every hour for three doses, or methysergide (Sansert), 2 mg orally every 6 hours for three doses, should be considered. The effectiveness of these drugs has not been proven.

Disposition

All patients who have ingested more than 2 mg/kg of an MAOI should be admitted to the hospital for 24 hours of observation and monitoring in the intensive care unit because the life-threatening manifestations may be delayed. Patients with drug or dietary interactions that are mild may not require admission if symptoms subside within 4 to 6 hours and the patients remain asymptomatic. Patients with symptoms that persist or require active intervention should be admitted to the intensive care unit.

Opioids (Narcotic Opiates)

Opioids are used for analgesia, as antitussives, and as antidiarrheal agents and are illicit agents (heroin, opium) used in substance abuse. Tolerance, physical dependency, and withdrawal may develop.

Toxic Mechanism

At least four main opioid receptors have been identified. The μ receptor is considered the most important for central analgesia and CNS depression. The κ and δ receptors predominate in spinal analgesia. The σ receptors may mediate dysphoria. Death is a consequence of dose-dependent CNS respiratory depression or secondary to pulmonary aspiration or noncardiac pulmonary edema. The mechanism of noncardiac pulmonary edema is unknown.

Dextromethorphan can interact with MAOIs, causing severe hyperthermia, and may cause the serotonin syndrome (see *Selective Serotonin Reuptake Inhibitors*). Dextromethorphan inhibits the metabolism of norepinephrine and serotonin and blocks the reuptake of serotonin. It is found as a component of a large number of non-prescription cough and cold remedies.

Toxic Dose

The toxic dose depends on the specific drug, route of administration, and degree of tolerance. For therapeutic and toxic doses, see Table 24. In children, respiratory depression has been produced by 10 mg of morphine or methadone, 75 mg of meperidine, and 12.5 mg of diphenoxylate. Infants younger than 3 months of age are more susceptible to respiratory depression. The dose should be reduced by 50%.

Kinetics

Oral onset of analgesic effect of morphine is 10 to 15 minutes; the action peaks in 1 hour and lasts 4 to 6 hours. With sustained-release preparations, the duration is 8 to 12 hours. Opioids are 90% metabolized in the liver by hepatic conjugation and 90% excreted in the urine as inactive compounds. Volume distribution is 1 to 4 L/kg. Protein binding is 35% to 75%. The typical plasma half-life of opiates is 2 to 5 hours, but that of methadone is 24 to 36 hours. Morphine metabolites include morphine-3-glucuronide (inactive) and morphine-6-glucuronide (active) and normorphine (active). Meperidine (Demerol) is rapidly hydrolyzed by tissue esterases into the active metabolite normeperidine, which has twice the convulsant activity of meperidine. Heroin (diacetylmorphine) is deacetylated within minutes to 6-monacetylmorphine and morphine. Propoxyphene (Darvon) has a rapid onset of action, and death has occurred within 15 to 30 minutes after a massive overdose. Propoxyphene is metabolized to norpropoxyphene, an active metabolite with convulsive, cardiac dysrhythmic,

TABLE 24	Doses and Onset and Duration of Action of Common Opioids					
DRUG	**ADULT ORAL DOSE**	**CHILD ORAL DOSE**	**ONSET OF ACTION**	**DURATION OF ACTION**	**ADULT FATAL DOSE**
Camphored tincture of opium	25 mL	0.25–0.50 mL/kg (0.4 mg/mL)	15–30 min	4–5 h	NA
Codeine	30–180 mg	0.5–1 mg/kg	15–30 min	4–6 h	800 mg
	>1 mg/kg is toxic in a child, above 200 mg in adult >5 mg/kg fatal in a child				
Dextromethorphan	15 mg 10 mg/kg is toxic	0.25 mg/kg	15–30 min	3–6 h	NA
Diacetylmorphine; street heroin is less than 10% pure	60 mg	NA	15–30 min	3–4 h	100 mg
Diphenoxylate atropine (Lomotil)	5–10 mg	NA	120–240 min	14 h	300 mg
	7.5 mg is toxic in a child, 300 mg is toxic in adult				
Fentanyl (Duragesic)	0.1–0.2 mg	0.001–0.002 mg/kg	7–8 min	Intramuscular: ½–2 h	1.0 mg
Hydrocodone with APAP (Lortab)	5–30 mg	0.15 mg/kg	30 min	3–4 h	100 mg
Hydromorphone (Dilaudid)	4 mg	0.1 mg/kg	15–30 min	3–4 h	100 mg
Meperidine (Demerol)	100 mg	1–1.5 mg/kg	10–45 min	3–4 h	350 mg
Methadone (Dolophine)	10 mg	0.1 mg/kg	30–60 min	4–12 h	120 mg
Morphine	10–60 mg	0.1–0.2 mg/kg	<20 min	4–6 h	200 mg
	Oral dose is 6 times parenteral dose, MS Contin sustained-release prep				
Oxycodone APAP (Percocet)	5 mg	NA	15–30 min	4–5 h	NA
Pentazocine (Talwin)	50–100 mg	NA	15–30 min	3–4 h	NA
Propoxyphene (Darvon)	65–100 mg	NA	30–60 min	2–4 h	700 mg

and heart block properties. Symptoms of diphenoxylate overdose appear within 1 to 4 hours. It is metabolized into the active metabolite difenoxin, which is five times more active as a regular respiratory depressant agent. Death has been reported in children after ingestion of a single tablet.

Manifestations

Initially, mild intoxication produces miosis, dull face, drowsiness, partial ptosis, and "nodding" (head drops to chest then bobs up). Larger amounts produce the classic triad of miotic pupils (exceptions below), respiratory depression, and depressed level of consciousness (flaccid coma). The blood pressure, pulse, and bowel activity are decreased.

Dilated pupils do not exclude opioid intoxication. Some exceptions to the miosis effect include dextromethorphan (paralyzes iris), fentanyl, meperidine, and diphenoxylate (rarely). Physiologic disturbances including acidosis, hypoglycemia, hypoxia, and postictal state, or a co-ingestant may also produce mydriasis.

Usually, the muscles are flaccid, but increased muscle tone can be produced by meperidine and fentanyl (chest rigidity). Seizures are rare but can occur with ingestion of codeine, meperidine, propoxyphene, and dextromethorphan. Hallucinations and agitation have been reported.

Pruritus and urticaria are caused by histamine release by some opioids or by sulfite additives.

Noncardiac pulmonary edema may occur after an overdose, especially with intravenous heroin abuse. Cardiac effects include vasodilation and hypotension. A heart murmur in an intravenous addict suggests endocarditis. Propoxyphene can produce delayed cardiac dysrhythmias.

Fentanyl is 100 times more potent than morphine and can cause chest wall muscle rigidity. Some of its derivatives are 2000 times more potent than morphine.

Laboratory Investigations

For patients with overdose, one should obtain and monitor ABG, blood glucose, and electrolyte levels; chest radiographs; and ECG. For drug abusers, one should consider testing for hepatitis B, syphilis, and HIV antibody (HIV testing usually requires consent). Blood opioid concentrations are not useful. They confirm diagnosis (morphine therapeutic dose, 65 to 80 ng/mL; toxic, <200 ng/mL), but are not useful for making a therapeutic decision. Cross-reactions can occur with Vick's Formula 44, poppy seeds, and other opioids (codeine and heroin are metabolized to morphine). Naloxone 4 mg IV was not associated with a positive enzyme multiplied immunoassay technique urine screen at 60 minutes, 6 hours, or 48 hours.

Management

Supportive care should be instituted, particularly an endotracheal tube and assisted ventilation. Temporary ventilation can be provided by a bag-valve mask with 100% oxygen. The patient should be placed on a cardiac monitor, have intravenous access established, and have specimens for ABG, glucose, electrolytes, BUN, and creatinine levels, CBC, coagulation profile, liver function, toxicology screen, and urinalysis taken.

For gastrointestinal decontamination, emesis should not be induced, but activated charcoal can be administered if bowel sounds are present.

If it is suspected that the patient is an addict, he or she should be restrained first and then 0.1 mg of naloxone (Narcan) should be administered. The dose should be doubled every 2 minutes until the patient responds or 10 to 20 mg has been given. If the patient is not suspected to be an addict, then 2 mg every 2 to 3 minutes to total of 10 to 20 mg is administered.

It is essential to determine whether there is a complete response to naloxone (mydriasis, improvement in ventilation), because it is a diagnostic therapeutic test. A continuous naloxone infusion may be appropriate, using the "response dose" every hour. Repeat doses of naloxone may be necessary because the effects of many opioids can last much longer than naloxone does (30 to 60 minutes). Methadone ingestions may require a naloxone infusion for 24 to 48 hours. Half of the response dose may need to be repeated in 15 to 20 minutes, after the infusion has been started.

Acute iatrogenic withdrawal precipitated by the administration of naloxone to a dependent patient should not be treated with morphine or other opioids. Naloxone's effects are limited to 30 to 60 minutes (shorter than most opioids) and withdrawal will subside in a short time.

Nalmefene (Revex), an FDA-approved long-acting (4 to 8 hours) pure opioid antagonist, is being investigated, but its role in cases of acute intoxication is unclear and it could produce prolonged withdrawal. It may have a role in place of naloxone infusion.

Noncardiac pulmonary edema does not respond to naloxone, and the patient needs intubation, assisted ventilation, positive end-expiratory pressure, and hemodynamic monitoring. Fluids should be given cautiously in patients with opioid overdose because opioids stimulate the antidiuretic hormone.

If the patient is comatose, 50% glucose (3% to 4% of comatose opioid overdose patients have hypoglycemia) and thiamine should be given prior to naloxone. If the patient has seizures that are unresponsive to naloxone, one administers diazepam and examines for metabolic (hypoglycemia, electrolyte disturbances) causes and structural disturbances.

Hypotension is rare and should direct a search for another etiology. If the patient is agitated, hypoxia and hypoglycemia must be excluded before opioid withdrawal is considered as a cause. Complications to consider include urinary retention, constipation, rhabdomyolysis, myoglobinuria, hypoglycemia, and withdrawal.

Disposition

If a patient responds to intravenous naloxone, careful observation for relapse and the development of pulmonary edema is required, with cardiac and respiratory monitoring for 6 to 12 hours. Patients requiring repeated doses of naloxone or an infusion, or those who develop pulmonary edema, require intensive care unit admission and cannot be discharged from the intensive care unit until they are symptom free for 12 hours. Intravenous overdose complications are expected to be present within 20 minutes after injection, and discharge after 4 symptom-free hours has been recommended. Adults with oral overdose have delayed onset of toxicity and require 6 hours of observation. Children with oral opioid overdose should be admitted to the hospital for observation because of delayed toxicity. Some toxicologists advise restraining a patient who attempts to sign out against medical advice after treatment with naloxone, at least until the patient receives psychiatric evaluation.

Organophosphates and Carbamates

Cholinergic intoxication sources are insecticides (organophosphates or carbamates), some medications, and some mushrooms. Examples of organophosphate insecticides are malathion (low toxicity, median lethal dose [LD_{50}] 2800 mg/kg), chlorpyrifos, which has been removed from market (moderate toxicity), and parathion (high toxicity, LD_{50} 2 mg/kg). Carbamate insecticides include carbaryl (low toxicity, LD_{50} 500 mg/kg), propoxur (moderate toxicity, LD_{50} 95 mg/kg), and aldicarb (high toxicity, LD_{50} 0.9 mg/kg). Pharmaceuticals with carbamate properties include neostigmine (Prostigmin) and physostigmine (Antilirium). Cholinergic compounds also include the "G" nerve war weapons tabun (GA), sarin (GB), soman (GB), and venom X (VX).

Toxic Mechanism

Organophosphates phosphorylate the active site on red cell acetylcholinesterase and pseudocholinesterase in the serum, neuromuscular and parasympathetic neuroeffector junctions, and in the major synapses of the autonomic ganglia, causing irreversible inhibition. There are two types of organophosphate intoxication: (a) direct action by the parent compound (e.g., tetraethylpyrophosphate), or (b) indirect action by the toxic metabolite (e.g., parathoxon or malathoxon).

Carbamates (esters of carbonic acid) cause reversible carbamylation of the active site of the enzymes. When a critical amount, greater than 50%, of cholinesterase is inhibited, acetylcholine accumulates and causes transient stimulation at cholinergic synapses and sympathetic terminals (muscarinic effect), the somatic nerves, the autonomic ganglia (nicotinic effect), and CNS synapses. Stimulation of conduction is followed by inhibition of conduction.

The major differences between the carbamates and the organophosphates are as follows: (a) carbamate toxicity is less and the duration is shorter; (b) carbamates rarely produce overt CNS effects (poor CNS penetration); (c) carbamate inhibition of the acetylcholinesterase enzyme is reversible and activity returns to normal rapidly; (d) pralidoxime, the enzyme regenerator, may not be necessary in the management of mild carbamate intoxication (e.g., carbaryl).

Toxic Dose

Parathion's minimum lethal dose is 2 mg in children and 10 to 20 mg in adults. The lethal dose of malathion is greater than 1375 mg/kg and that of chlorpyrifos is 25 g; the latter compound is unlikely to cause death.

Kinetics

Absorption is by all routes. The onset of acute ingestion toxicity occurs as early as 3 hours, usually before 12 hours and always before 24 hours. Lipid-soluble agents absorbed by the dermal route (e.g., fenthion) may have a delayed onset of more than 24 hours. Inhalation toxicity occurs immediately after exposure. Massive ingestion can produce intoxication within minutes.

Metabolism is via the liver. With some pesticides (e.g., parathion, malathion), the effects are delayed because they undergo hepatic microsomal oxidative metabolism to their toxic metabolites, the -oxons (e.g., paroxon, malaoxon).

The half-life of malathion is 2.89 hours and that of parathion is 2.1 days. The metabolites are eliminated in the urine and the presence of p-nitrophenol in the urine is a clue up to 48 hours after exposure.

Manifestations

Many organophosphates produce a garlic odor on the breath, in the gastric contents, or in the container. Diaphoresis, excessive salivation, miosis, and muscle twitching are helpful clues to diagnosis.

Early, a cholinergic (muscarinic) crisis develops that consists of parasympathetic nervous system activity. DUMBELS is the mnemonic for defecation, cramps, and increased bowel motility; urinary incontinence; miosis (mydriasis may occur in 20%); bronchospasm and bronchorrhea; excess secretion; lacrimation; and seizures. Bradycardia, pulmonary edema, and hypotension may be present.

Later, sympathetic and nicotinic effects occur, consisting of MATCH: muscle weakness and fasciculation (eyelid twitching is often present), adrenal stimulation and hyperglycemia, tachycardia, cramps in muscles, and hypertension. Finally, paralysis of the skeletal muscles ensues.

The CNS effects are headache, blurred vision, anxiety, ataxia, delirium and toxic psychosis, convulsions, coma, and respiratory depression. Cranial nerve palsies have been noted. Delayed hallucinations may occur.

Delayed respiratory paralysis and neurologic and neurobehavioral disorders have been described following certain organophosphate ingestions or dermal exposure. The "intermediate syndrome" is paralysis of proximal and respiratory muscles developing 24 to 96 hours after the successful treatment of organophosphate poisoning. A delayed distal polyneuropathy has been described with ingestion of certain organophosphates, such as triorthocresyl phosphate, bromoleptophos, and methomidophos.

Complications include aspiration, pulmonary edema, and acute respiratory distress syndrome.

Laboratory Investigations

Monitoring should include chest radiograph, blood glucose (nonketotic hyperglycemia is frequent), ABG, pulse oximetry, ECG, blood coagulation status, liver function, hyperamylasemia (pancreatitis reported), and urinalysis for the metabolite alkyl phosphate paranitrophenol. Blood should be drawn for red blood cell cholinesterase determination before pralidoxime is given. The red blood cell cholinesterase activity roughly correlates with clinical severity. Mild poisoning is 20% to 50% of normal, moderate poisoning is 10% to 20% of normal, and severe poisoning is 10% of normal (>90% depressed). A postexposure rise of 10% to 15% in the cholinesterase level determined at least 10 to 14 days after the exposure confirms the diagnosis.

Management

Protection of health care personnel with clothing (masks, gloves, gowns, goggles) and respiratory equipment or hazardous material suits, as necessary, is called for. General decontamination consists of isolation, bagging, and disposal of contaminated clothing and other articles. Vital functions should be established and maintained. Cardiac and oxygen saturation monitoring are needed. Intubation and assisted ventilation may be needed. Secretions should be suctioned until atropinization drying is achieved.

Dermal decontamination involves prompt removal of clothing and cleansing of all affected areas of skin, hair, and eyes. Ocular decontamination involves irrigation with copious amounts of tepid water or 0.9% saline for at least 15 minutes. Gastrointestinal decontamination, if the ingestion was recent, involves the administration of activated charcoal.

Atropine sulfate can be given as an antidote. It is both a diagnostic and a therapeutic agent. Atropine counteracts the muscarinic effects but is only partially effective for the CNS effects (seizures and coma). Preservative-free atropine (no benzyl alcohol) should be used. If the patient is symptomatic (bradycardia or bronchorrhea), a test dose should be administered, 0.02 mg/kg in children or 1 mg in adults, intravenously. If no signs of atropinization are present (tachycardia, drying of secretions, and mydriasis), atropine should be administered immediately, 0.05 mg/kg in children or 2 mg in adults, every 5 to 10 minutes as needed to dry the secretions and clear the lungs. Beneficial effects are seen within 1 to 4 minutes and maximum effect in 8 minutes. The average dose in the first 24 hours is 40 mg, but 1000 mg or more has been required in severe cases. Glycopyrrolate (Robinul) can be used if atropine is not available. The maximum dose should be maintained for 12 to 24 hours, then tapered and the patient observed for relapse. Poisoning, especially with lipophilic agents (e.g., fenthion, chlorfenthion), may require weeks of atropine therapy. An alternative is a continuous infusion of atropine 8 mg in 100 mL 0.9% saline at rate of 0.02 to 0.08 mg/kg/h (0.25 to 1.0 mL/kg/h) with additional 1 to 5 mg boluses as needed to dry the secretions.

Pralidoxime chloride (Protopam) has both antinicotinic and antimuscarinic effects and possibly also CNS effects. Successful treatment with pralidoxime chloride may allow a reduction in the dose of atropine. Pralidoxime acts to reactivate the phosphorylated cholinesterases by binding the phosphate moiety on the esteritic site and displacing it. It should be given early before "aging" of phosphate bond produces tighter binding. However, recent reports indicate that pralidoxime chloride is beneficial even several days after the poisoning. Improvement is seen within 10 to 40 minutes. The initial dose of pralidoxime chloride is 1 to 2 g in 250 mL 0.89% saline over 5 to 10 minutes, maximum 200 mg/min, in adults or 25 to 50 mg/kg, maximum 4 mg/kg/min, in children younger than 12 years of age. The dose can be repeated every 6 to 12 hours for several days. An alternative is a continuous infusion of 1 g in 100 mL 0.89% saline at 5 to 20 mg/kg/h (0.5 to 12 mL/g/h) up to 500 mg/h and titrated to desired response. Maximum adult daily dose is 12 g. Cardiac and blood pressure monitoring is advised during and for several hours after the infusion. The end point is absence of fasciculations and return of muscle strength.

Contraindicated drugs include morphine, aminophylline, barbiturates, opioids, phenothiazine, reserpine-like drugs, parasympathomimetics, and succinylcholine.

Noncardiac pulmonary edema may require respiratory support. Seizures may respond to atropine and pralidoxime chloride but often require anticonvulsants. Cardiac dysrhythmias may require electrical cardioversion or antidysrhythmic therapy if the patient is hemodynamically unstable. Extracorporeal procedures are of no proven value.

Disposition
Asymptomatic patients with normal examination findings after 6 to 8 hours of observation may be discharged. In cases of intentional poisoning, the patients require psychiatric clearance for discharge. Symptomatic patients should be admitted to the intensive care unit. Observation of milder cases of carbamate poisoning, even those requiring atropine, for 6 to 8 hours symptom-free may be sufficient to exclude significant toxicity. In cases of workplace exposure, OSHA should be notified.

Phencyclidine (Angel Dust)
Phencyclidine is an arylcyclohexylamine related to ketamine and chemically related to the phenothiazines. Originally a "dissociative" anesthetic banned in United States since 1979, it is now an illicit substance, with at least 38 analogues. It is inexpensively manufactured by "kitchen chemists" and is mislabeled as other hallucinogens. Improper phencyclidine synthesis may release cyanide when heated or smoked and can cause explosions.

Toxic Mechanism
The mechanism of phencyclidine is complex and not completely understood. It inhibits some neurotransmitters and causes a loss of pain sensation without depressing the CNS respiratory status. It stimulates α-adrenergic receptors and may act as a "false neurotransmitter." The effects are sympathomimetic, cholinergic, and cerebellar.

Toxic Dose
The usual dose of phencyclidine mixed with marijuana joints is 100 to 400 mg of phencyclidine. Joints or leaf mixtures contain 0.24% to 7.9% of PCP, 1 mg of PCP/150 leaves. Tablets contain 5 mg (the usual street dose). CNS effects at doses of 1 to 6 mg include hallucinations and euphoria, 6 to 10 mg produces toxic psychosis and sympathetic stimulation, 10 to 25 mg produces severe toxicity, and more than 100 mg has resulted in fatalities.

Kinetics
Phencyclidine is a lipophilic weak base, with a pKa of 8.5 to 9.5. It is rapidly absorbed when smoked and snorted, poorly absorbed from the acid stomach, and rapidly absorbed from the alkaline middle small intestine. It has an enterogastric secretion and is reabsorbed in the small intestine. The onset of action when smoked is 2 to 5 minutes, with a peak in 15 to 30 minutes. With oral ingestion, the onset is in 30 to 60 minutes and when taken intravenously it is immediate. Most adverse reactions in cases of overdose begin within 1 to 2 hours. Its duration of action at low doses is 4 to 6 hours and normality returns in 24 hours; in large overdoses, fluctuating coma may last 6 to 10 days.

Volume distribution is 6.2 L/kg. Phencyclidine concentrates in brain and adipose tissue. Protein binding is 70%. The route of elimination is by gastric secretion, liver metabolism, and 10% urinary excretion of conjugates and free phencyclidine. Renal excretion may be increased 50% with urinary acidification. The half-life is 1 hour (in cases of overdose, it is 11 to 89 hours).

Manifestations
The classic picture is bursts of horizontal, vertical, and rotary nystagmus, which is a clue to diagnosis (occurs in 50% of cases), miosis, hypertension, and fluctuating altered mental state. There is a wide spectrum of clinical presentations.

Mild intoxication with 1 to 6 mg produces drunken and bizarre behavior, agitation, rotary nystagmus, and blank stare. Violent behavior and sensory anesthesia make these patients insensitive to pain, self-destructive, and dangerous. Most are communicative within 1 to 2 hours, are alert and oriented in 6 to 8 hours, and recover completely in 24 to 48 hours.

Moderate intoxication with 6 to 10 mg produces excess salivation, hypertension, hyperthermia, muscle rigidity, myoclonus, and catatonia. Recovery of consciousness occurs in 24 to 48 hours and complete recovery in 1 week.

Severe intoxication with 10 to 25 mg results in opisthotonus, decerebrate rigidity, convulsions, prolonged fluctuating coma, and respiratory failure. Patients in this category have a high rate of medical complications. Recovery of consciousness occurs in 24 to 48 hours, with complete normality in a month. Medical complications include apnea, aspiration pneumonia, cardiac arrest, hypertensive encephalopathy, hyperthermia, intracerebral hemorrhage, psychosis, rhabdomyolysis and myoglobinuria, and seizures. Loss of memory and "flashbacks" last for months. Phencyclidine-induced depression and suicide have been reported.

Fatalities occur with ingestions of greater than 100 mg and with serum levels greater than 100 to 250 ng/mL.

Laboratory Investigations
Marked elevation of creatine kinase level may occur. Values greater than 20,000 units have been reported. Urinalysis should be monitored and urine tested for myoglobin. One should monitor the blood for creatine kinase, uric acid (an early clue to rhabdomyolysis), BUN, creatinine, electrolytes (hyperkalemia), blood glucose (20% of patients have hypoglycemia), urinary output, liver function tests, ECG, and ABG if the patient has any respiratory manifestations. Measurement of phencyclidine in the gastric juice is called for because concentrations are 10 to 50 times higher than in blood or urine. Phencyclidine blood concentrations are not helpful. Phencyclidine may be detected in the urine of the average user for 10 days to 3 weeks after the last dose. In chronic users, it can be detected for over 1 month. The analogues of phencyclidine may not produce positive test results for phencyclidine in the urine. Cross-reactions with bleach and dextromethorphan may cause false-positive urine test results on immunoassay, and cross-reaction with doxylamine may produce a false-positive finding on gas chromatography.

Management
The patient should be observed for violent, self-destructive, bizarre behavior, and paranoid schizophrenia. Patients should be placed in a low sensory environment and dangerous objects should be removed from the area.

Gastrointestinal decontamination is not effective because phencyclidine is rapidly absorbed from intestines. Overtreating the mild intoxication should be avoided. There is insufficient evidence to support the use of MDAC. In cases of severe toxicity (stupor or coma), continuous gastric suction can be tried (with protection of the airway) because the drug is secreted into the gastric juice. The value of this procedure is controversial because of limited data.

The patient must be protected from harming himself or herself or others. Physical restraints may be necessary, but they should be used sparingly and for the shortest time possible because they increase risk of rhabdomyolysis. Metal restraints such as handcuffs should be avoided. For behavioral disorders and toxic psychosis, diazepam is the agent of choice. Pharmacologic intervention includes diazepam (Valium) 10 to 30 mg orally or 2 to 5 mg intravenously initially and titrated upward to 10 mg; however, up to 30 mg may be required. "Talk down" technique is usually ineffective and dangerous. Phenothiazines and butyrophenones should be avoided in the acute phase because they lower the convulsive threshold; however, they may be needed later for psychosis. Haloperidol (Haldol) administration has been reported to produce catatonia.

Seizures and muscle spasm are managed with diazepam, from 2.5 mg up to 10 mg. Hyperthermia (>38.5°C [101.3°F]) is treated with external cooling measures. Hypertension is usually transient and does not require treatment. In the case of emergent hypertensive crisis (blood pressure >200/115 mm Hg) nitroprusside can be used in a dose of 0.3 to 2 µg/kg/min. Maximum infusion rate is 10 µg/kg/min for only 10 minutes.

Acid ion trapping diuresis is not recommended because of the danger of myoglobin precipitation in the renal tubules. Rhabdomyolysis and myoglobinuria are treated by correcting volume depletion and ensuring a urinary output of greater than 2 mL/kg/h. Alkalinization is controversial because of reabsorption of phencyclidine.

Hemodialysis is beneficial if renal failure occurs; otherwise, the extracorporeal procedures are not beneficial.

Disposition

All patients with coma, delirium, catatonia, violent behavior, aspiration pneumonia, sustained hypertension greater than 200/115 mm Hg, and significant rhabdomyolysis should be admitted to the intensive care unit until asymptomatic for at least 24 hours. If patients with mild intoxication are mentally and neurologically stable and become asymptomatic (except for nystagmus) for 4 hours, they may be discharged in the company of a responsible adult. All patients must be assessed for suicide risk before discharge. Drug counseling and psychiatric follow-up should be arranged. Patients should be warned that episodes of disorientation and depression may continue intermittently for 4 weeks or more.

Phenothiazines and Nonphenothiazines (Neuroleptics)

Toxic Mechanism

Neuroleptics have complex mechanisms of toxicity, including (a) block of the postsynaptic dopamine receptors; (b) block of peripheral and central α-adrenergic receptors; (c) block of cholinergic muscarinic receptors; (d) quinidine-like antidysrhythmic and myocardial depressant effect in cases of large overdose; (e) lowering of the convulsive threshold; (f) effect on hypothalamic temperature regulation (Table 25).

Toxic Dose

Extrapyramidal reactions, anticholinergic effects, and orthostatic hypotension may occur at therapeutic doses. The toxic amount is not established, but the maximum daily therapeutic dose may result in significant side effects, and twice this amount may be potentially fatal. Chlorpromazine (Thorazine), the prototype, may produce serious hypotension and CNS depression at doses greater than 200 mg (17 mg/kg) in children and 3 to 5 g in an adult. Fatalities have been reported after 2.5 g of loxapine (Loxitane) and mesoridazine (Serentil) and 1.5 g of thioridazine (Mellaril).

Kinetics

These agents are lipophilic and have unpredictable gastrointestinal absorption. Peak levels occur 2 to 6 hours postingestion and have enterohepatic recirculation.

The mean serum half-life in phase 1 is 1 to 2 hours and the biphasic half-life is 20 to 40 hours. Volume distribution is 10 to 40 L/kg; protein binding is 92% to 98%. Chlorpromazine taken

COMPOUND	ANTIPSYCHOTIC	ANTICHOLINERGIC	EXTRAPYRAMIDAL	HYPOTENSIVE AND CARDIOTOXIC	SEDATIVE
Phenothiazine					
Aliphatic	1+	3+	2+	2+	3+
Chlorpromazine (Thorazine)					
Promethazine (Phenergan)					
Piperazine	3+	1+	3+	1+	1+
Fluphenazine (Prolixin)					
Perphenazine (Trilafon)					
Prochlorperazine (Compazine)					
Trifluoperazine (Stelazine)					
Piperidine	1+	2+	1+	3+	3+
Mesoridazine (Serentil)					
Thioridazine (Mellaril)					
Nonphenothiazine					
Butyrophenone	3+	1+	3+	1+	1+
Haloperidol (Haldol)					
Dibenzoxazepine	3+	1+	3+	1+	2+
Loxapine (Loxitane)					
Dihydroindolone	3+	1+	3+	1+	1+
Molindone (Moban)					
Thioxanthenes	3+	1+	3+	3+	1+
Thiothixene (Navane)					
Chlorprothixene (Taractan)					

TABLE 25 Neuroleptics and Properties

1+ = very low activity; 2+ = moderate activity; 3+ = very high activity.

orally has an onset of action in 30 to 60 minutes, peak in 2 to 4 hours, and duration of 4 to 6 hours. With sustained-release preparations, the onset is in 30 to 60 minutes and duration is 6 to 12 hours.

Elimination is by hepatic metabolism, which results in multiple metabolites (some are active). Metabolites can be detected in urine months after chronic therapy. Only 1% to 3% is excreted unchanged in the urine.

Manifestations

In cases of phenothiazine overdose, anticholinergic symptoms may be present early but are not life-threatening. Miosis is usually present (80%) if the phenothiazine has strong α-adrenergic blocking effect (e.g., chlorpromazine), but anticholinergic activity mydriasis may occur. Agitation and delirium rapidly progress into coma. Major problems are cardiac toxicity and hypotension. The cardiotoxic effects are seen more commonly with thioridazine and its metabolite mesoridazine. These agents have produced the largest number of fatalities in patients with phenothiazine overdose. Cardiac conduction disturbances include prolonged PR, QRS, and QTc intervals, U- and T-wave abnormalities, and ventricular dysrhythmias, including torsades de pointes. Seizures occur mainly in patients with convulsive disorders or with administration of loxapine. Sudden death in children and adults has been reported.

Idiosyncratic dystonic reactions are most common with the piperidine group. Reactions are not dose-dependent and consist of opisthotonos, torticollis, orolingual dyskinesia, or oculogyric crisis (painful upward gaze). These reactions are more frequent in children and women. Neuroleptic malignant syndrome occurs in patients on chronic therapy and is characterized by hyperthermia, muscle rigidity, autonomic dysfunction, and altered mental state. There is one case reported with acute overdose. The loxapine syndrome consists of seizures, rhabdomyolysis, and renal failure.

Laboratory Investigations

Monitoring should include arterial blood gases, renal and hepatic function, electrolytes, blood glucose, and creatine kinase and myoglobinemia in neuroleptic malignant syndrome. Most of these agents are detected on routine screening. Quantitative serum levels are not useful in management. Cross-reactions with enzyme multiplied immunoassay technique tests occur with cyclic antidepressants. Phenothiazines give false-negative results on pregnancy urine tests using human chorionic gonadotropin as an indicator, and give false-positive results for urine porphyrins, indirect Coombs test, urobilinogen, and amylase.

Management

Vital functions must be established and maintained. All overdose patients require venous access, 12-lead ECG (to measure intervals), cardiac and respiratory monitoring, and seizure precautions. One should monitor core temperature to detect poikilothermic effect. If the patient is comatose, intubation and assisted ventilation may be required, as well as 100% oxygen, intravenous glucose, naloxone (Narcan), and thiamine.

Emesis is not recommended. Activated charcoal can be administered if ingestion was within 1 hour. MDAC has not been proven beneficial. A radiograph of the abdomen may be useful, if the phenothiazine is radiopaque. Haloperidol (Haldol) and trifluoperazine (Stelazine) are most likely to be radiopaque. Whole-bowel irrigation may be useful when a large number of pills are visualized on radiograph or if sustained-release preparations were taken, but whole-bowel irrigation has not been evaluated in patients with phenothiazine overdose.

Convulsions are treated with diazepam or lorazepam (Ativan). Loxapine (Loxitane) overdose may result in status epilepticus. If nondepolarizing neuromuscular blockade is required, pancuronium (Pavulon) or vecuronium (Norcuron) should be used (not succinyl-choline [Anectine], which may cause malignant hyperthermia), and EEG should be monitored during paralysis.

Patients with dysrhythmias should be monitored with serial ECGs. Unstable rhythms can be treated with electrical cardioversion. Class 1a antidysrhythmics (procainamide, quinidine, and disopyramide [Norpace]) must be avoided.

Hypokalemia predisposes to dysrhythmias and should be corrected aggressively. Supraventricular tachycardia with hemodynamic instability is treated with electrical cardioversion. The role of adenosine has not been defined. Calcium channel and β-blockers should be avoided.

Prolongation of the QRS interval is treated with sodium bicarbonate 1 to 2 mEq/kg by intravenous bolus over a few minutes. Torsades de pointes is treated with magnesium sulfate IV 20% solution 2 g over 2 to 3 minutes. If there is no response in 10 minutes, the dose is repeated and followed by a continuous infusion of 5 to 10 mg/min or given as an infusion of 50 mg/min for 2 hours followed by 30 mg/min for 90 minutes twice a day for several days, as needed. The dose in children is 25 to 50 mg/kg initially and maintenance dose is 30 to 60 mg/kg per 24 hours (0.25 to 0.50 mEq/kg per 24 hours) up to 1000 mg per 24 hours. Serum magnesium levels should be monitored.

To treat ventricular tachydysrhythmias in a stable patient, lidocaine is used. If the patient is unstable, electrical cardioversion is used. Patients with heart block with hemodynamic instability should be managed with temporary cardiac pacing.

Hypotension is treated with the Trendelenburg position and 0.9% saline. If the condition is refractory to treatment or there is a danger of fluid overload, vasopressors are administered. The vasopressor of choice is α-adrenergic agonist norepinephrine (Levophed), titrated to response. Epinephrine and dopamine should not be used because β-receptor stimulation in the presence of α-receptor blockade may provoke dysrhythmias and phenothiazines are antidopaminergic.

Hypothermia and hyperthermia are treated with external warming and cooling measures, respectively. Antipyretic drugs must not be used.

Management of the neuroleptic malignant syndrome includes the following actions:

- Immediately discontinuing the offending agent
- Hyperventilating the patient, using 100% humidified, cooled oxygen at high gas flows (at least 10 L/min) because of rapid breathing
- Administering a benzodiazepine to control convulsions and facilitate cooling measures
- Initiating appropriate mechanical cooling measures, which may include intravenous cold saline (not lactated Ringer's), ice baths, cold lavage of the stomach, bladder, and rectum, and a hypothermic blanket
- Correcting acid-base and electrolyte disturbances and treating significant hyperkalemia with hyperventilation, calcium, sodium bicarbonate, intravenous glucose, and insulin; hemodialysis may be necessary

In addition, dysrhythmias usually respond to correction of the underlying acid-base disturbances and hyperkalemia. If antidysrhythmic agents are required, calcium channel blockers must be avoided because they may precipitate hyperkalemia and cardiovascular collapse. Dantrolene sodium (Dantrium), which is a phenytoin derivative, inhibits calcium release from the sarcoplasmic reticulum and results in decreased muscle contraction. Dantrolene acts peripherally and does not reverse the rigidity or psychomotor disturbances resulting from the central dopamine blockade; it therefore is often used in combination with bromocriptine. Bromocriptine mesylate (Parlodel) acts centrally as a dopamine agonist, as does amantadine hydrochloride (Symmetrel). Bromocriptine and dantrolene have been reported to be successful in combination with cooling and good supportive measures in malignant hyperthermia.

Dosing for these agents is as follows: dantrolene sodium at 2 to 3 mg/kg IV as a bolus, then 1 mg/kg/min to a maximum of 10 mg/kg or until the tachycardia, rigidity, increased end-tidal CO_2, and temperature elevation are controlled. *Note:* Hepatotoxicity occurs with doses greater than 10 mg/kg. To prevent symptom recurrence, 1 mg/kg should be administered every 6 hours for 24 to 48 hours after the episode. After that time, oral dantrene can be used at a dose of 1 mg/kg every 6 hours for 24 hours as necessary. The patient should be observed for thrombophlebitis following intravenous dantrolene. It is best administered via a central line. Bromocriptine mesylate at 2.5 to 10 mg orally or via a nasogastric tube, three times a day, should be used in combination with dantrolene.

Idiosyncratic dystonic reaction can be treated with diphenhydramine (Benadryl) 1 to 2 mg/kg/dose intravenously over 5 minutes up to maximum of 50 mg intravenously; a response is noted within 2 to 5 minutes. This can be followed with oral doses for 4 to 6 days to prevent recurrence.

Extracorporeal measures (hemodialysis, hemoperfusion) are not effective in removing these agents.

Disposition

Asymptomatic patients should be observed for at least 6 hours after gastric decontamination. Symptomatic patients with cardiotoxicity, hypotension, and convulsions should be admitted to the intensive care unit and monitored for 48 hours.

Salicylates (Acetylsalicylic Acid, Salicylic Acid)

Toxic Mechanism

The primary toxic mechanisms include (a) direct stimulation of the medullary chemoreceptor trigger zone and respiratory center; (b) uncoupling oxidative phosphorylation; (c) inhibition of the Krebs cycle enzymes; (d) inhibition of vitamin K dependent and independent clotting factors; (e) alteration of platelet function; and (f) inhibition of prostaglandin synthesis.

Toxic Dose

Acute mild intoxication occurs at a dose of 150 to 200 mg/kg, moderate intoxication at 200 to 300 mg/kg, and severe intoxication at 300 to 500 mg/kg. Acute salicylate plasma concentration greater than 30 mg/dL (usually >40 mg/dL) may be associated with clinical toxicity. Chronic intoxication occurs at ingestions greater than 100 mg/kg/d for more than 2 days because of accumulation kinetics. Methyl salicylate (oil of wintergreen) is the most toxic form of salicylate. A dose of 1 mL of 98% contains 1.4 g of salicylate. Fatalities have occurred with ingestion of 1 teaspoonful in children and 1 ounce in adults. It is found in topical ointments and liniments (18% to 30%).

Kinetics

Acetylsalicylic acid and salicylic acid are weak acids with a pKa of 3.5 and 3.0, respectively. Acetylsalicylic acid is absorbed from the stomach, from the small bowel, and dermally. Onset of action is within 30 minutes. Methyl salicylate and effervescent tablets are absorbed more rapidly. Salicylate plasma concentration is detectable within 15 minutes after ingestion and peaks in 30 to 120 minutes. The peak may be delayed 6 to 12 hours in cases of large overdose, overdose with enteric-coated or sustained-release preparations, and development of concretions. The therapeutic duration of action is 3 to 4 hours but is markedly prolonged in cases of overdose.

Volume distribution is 0.13 L/kg for salicylic acid but increases as the salicylate plasma concentration increases. Protein binding is greater than 90% for salicylic acid at pH 7.4 and a salicylate plasma concentration of 20 to 30 mg/dL, 75% at a salicylate plasma concentration greater than 40 mg/dL, 50% at a salicylate plasma concentration of 70 mg/dL, and 30% at a salicylate plasma concentration of 120 mg/dL.

The half-life for salicylic acid is 3 hours after a 300 mg dose, 6 hours after a 1 g overdose, and greater than 10 hours after a 10 g overdose. Elimination includes Michaelis-Menten hepatic metabolism by three saturable pathways: (a) glycine conjugation to salicyluric acid (75%); (b) glucuronyl transferase to salicyl phenol glucuronide (10%); and (c) salicyl aryl glucuronide (4%). Nonsaturable pathways are hydrolysis to gentisic acid (<1%). Ten percent is excreted unchanged.

Acidosis increases the severity of the intoxication by increasing the non-ionized salicylate that can cross membranes and enter the brain cells. In kidneys, the unionized salicylic acid undergoes glomerular filtration, and the ionized portion undergoes tubular secretion in proximal tubules and passive reabsorption in the distal tubules. Renal excretion of salicylate is enhanced by alkaline urine.

Manifestations

The ingestion of concentrated topical salicylic acid preparations (e.g., wart remover) can cause mucosal caustic injury to the gastrointestinal tract. Occult salicylate overdose should be considered in any patient with unexplained acid-base disturbance.

The manifestations of acute overdose of salicylates are as follows:

Minimal Symptoms. Tinnitus, dizziness, and deafness may occur at high therapeutic salicylate plasma concentrations of 20 to 30 mg/dL. Nausea and vomiting may occur immediately because of local gastric irritation.

Phase I. Mild manifestations occur at 1 to 12 hours after ingestion with a 6-hour salicylate plasma concentration of 45 to 70 mg/dL. Nausea and vomiting followed by hyperventilation are usually present within 3 to 8 hours after acute overdose. Hyperventilation, an increase in both rate (tachypnea) and depth (hyperpnea), is present but it may be subtle. It results in a mild respiratory alkalosis with a serum pH greater than 7.4 and urine pH greater than 6.0. Some patients may have lethargy, vertigo, headache, and confusion. Diaphoresis may be noted.

Phase II. Moderate manifestations occur at 12 to 24 hours after ingestion with a 6-hour salicylate plasma concentration of 70 to 90 mg/dL. Serious metabolic disturbances, including a marked respiratory alkalosis with anion gap metabolic acidosis, dehydration, and urine pH less than 6.0, may occur. Other metabolic disturbances include hypoglycemia or hyperglycemia, hypokalemia, decreased ionized calcium, and increased BUN, creatinine, and lactate. Mental disturbances (confusion, disorientation, hallucinations) may occur. Hypotension and convulsions have been reported.

Phase III. Severe intoxication occurs more than 24 hours after ingestion with a 6-hour salicylate plasma concentration of 90 to 130 mg/dL. In addition to the above clinical findings, coma and seizures develop and indicate severe intoxication. Pulmonary edema may occur. Metabolic disturbances include metabolic acidemia (pH <7.4) and aciduria (pH <6.0). In adults, alkalosis may persist until terminal respiratory failure.

In children younger than 4 years of age, a mixed metabolic acidosis and respiratory alkalosis develop earlier (within 4 to 6 hours) than in adults because children have less respiratory reserve and accumulate lactate and other organic acids. Hypoglycemia is more common in children.

Fatalities occur at 6-hour salicylate plasma concentrations greater than 130 to 150 mg/dL and result from CNS depression, cardiovascular collapse, electrolyte imbalance, and cerebral edema.

Chronic salicylism is more serious than acute intoxication and the 6-hour salicylate plasma concentration does not correlate well with the manifestations in both acute and chronic cases of intoxication. Chronic intoxication usually occurs with therapeutic errors in young children or the elderly with underlying illness, and the diagnosis is delayed because it is not recognized. Noncardiac pulmonary edema is a frequent complication in the elderly. The mortality rate is about 25%. Chronic salicylate poisoning in children may mimic Reye syndrome. It is associated with exaggerated CNS findings (hallucinations, delirium, dementia, memory loss, papilledema, bizarre behavior, agitation, encephalopathy, seizures, and coma). Hemorrhagic manifestations, renal failure, and pulmonary and cerebral edema may occur. The metabolic picture is hypoglycemia and mixed acid-base derangements. A chronic salicylate plasma concentration greater than 60 mg/dL with metabolic acidosis and an altered mental state is very serious.

Laboratory Investigations

All patients with intentional salicylate overdoses should have acetaminophen plasma level measured after 4 hours.

One should continuously monitor ECG, urine output, urine pH, and specific gravity. Every 2 to 4 hours in cases of severe intoxication, salicylate plasma concentration, glucose (in a case of salicylism, CNS hypoglycemia may be present despite normal serum glucose), electrolytes, ionized calcium, magnesium and phosphorus, anion gap, ABGs, and pulse oximeter should be monitored. Daily monitoring of BUN, creatinine, liver function tests, and prothrombin time should take place.

The therapeutic salicylate plasma concentration is less than 10 mg/dL for analgesia and 15 to 30 mg/dL for antiinflammatory effect. Cross-reaction with diflunisal (Dolobid) will give a falsely high salicylate plasma concentration. The Done nomogram is not considered accurate in evaluating acute or chronic salicylate intoxications.

Management

Treatment is based on clinical and metabolic findings, not on salicylate levels. Continuous monitoring of the urine pH is essential for successful alkalinization treatment. One should always obtain an acetaminophen plasma level.

Vital functions must be established and maintained. If the patient is in an altered mental state, glucose, naloxone, and thiamine are administered in standard doses. Depending on the severity, the initial studies include an immediate and a 6-hour postingestion salicylate plasma concentration, ECG and cardiac monitoring, pulse oximeter, urine (analysis, pH, and specific gravity), chest radiograph, ABGs, blood glucose, electrolytes and anion gap calculation, calcium (ionized), magnesium, renal and liver profiles, and prothrombin time. Gastric contents and stool should be tested for occult blood. Bismuth and magnesium salicylate preparations may be radiopaque on radiographs. Consultation with a nephrologist is warranted in cases of moderate, severe, or chronic intoxication.

For gastrointestinal decontamination, activated charcoal is useful (each gram of activated charcoal binds 550 mg of salicylic acid) if a toxic dose was ingested up to 4 hours postingestion. MDAC is not recommended for salicylate intoxication.

Concretions may occur with massive (usually >300 mg/kg) ingestions. If blood levels fail to decline, prompt contrast radiography of the stomach may reveal concretions that have to be removed by repeated lavage, whole-bowel irrigation, endoscopy, or gastrostomy.

Fluids and electrolyte treatment of salicylate poisonings is given in Table 26. For shock, perfusion and vascular volume should be established with 5% dextrose in 0.9% saline, then the treatment can proceed with correction of dehydration and alkalinization.

For cases of acute moderate or severe salicylism (see Table 26), adults should receive a bolus of 1 to 2 mEq/kg of sodium bicarbonate (NaHCO₃) followed by an infusion of 100 to 150 mEq NaHCO₃ added to 500 to 1000 mL of 5% dextrose and administered over 60 minutes. Children should receive a bolus of 1 to 2 mEq/kg of NaHCO₃ followed by an infusion of 1 to 2 mEq/kg added to 20 mL/kg of 5% dextrose administered over 60 minutes. Potassium is added after the patient voids. The goal is to achieve a urine output of greater than 2 mL/kg/h and a urine pH of greater than 8. The initial infusion is followed by subsequent infusions (two to three times normal maintenance) of 200 to 300 mL/h in adults or 10 mL/kg/h in children. If the patient is acidotic and has a serum pH of less than 7.15, an additional 1 to 2 mEq/kg of NaHCO₃ is given over 1 to 2 hours; persistent acidosis may require 1 to 2 mEq/kg of bicarbonate every 2 hours. The infusion rate, the amount of bicarbonate, and the electrolytes should be adjusted to correct serum abnormalities and to maintain the targeted urine output and urinary pH. Diuresis is not as important as the alkalinization. Careful monitoring for fluid overload should take place for patients at risk of pulmonary and cerebral edema (e.g., the elderly) and because of inappropriate secretion of the antidiuretic hormone.

In patients with mild intoxication who are not acidotic and have a urine pH greater than 6, 5% dextrose in 0.45% saline should be administered as maintenance to replace ongoing fluid loss. Some toxicologists may consider adding sodium bicarbonate 50 mEq/L or 1 mEq/kg in some cases.

To achieve alkalinization, sodium bicarbonate is administered to produce a serum pH 7.4 to 7.5 and a urine pH greater than 8. Carbonic anhydrase inhibitors (acetazolamide [Diamox]) should not be used. If the patient is acidotic, additional bicarbonate may be required. About 2 mEq/kg raises the blood pH 0.1. In children, alkalinization may be a difficult problem because of the organic acid production and hypokalemia. Hypokalemic and fluid-depleted patients cannot be adequately alkalinized. Alkalinization is usually discontinued in asymptomatic patients with

| TABLE 26 | Fluid and Electrolyte Treatment of Salicylate Poisoning |

TYPE OF SALICYLISM	METABOLIC DISTURBANCE	BLOOD PH	URINE PH	HYDRATING SOLUTION	AMOUNT OF NAHCO₃ (MEQ/L)	AMOUNT OF POTASSIUM (MEQ/L)
Mild	Respiratory alkalosis	>7.4	>6.0	5% Dextrose, 0.45% saline	50 (adult) 1 mEq/kg (child)	20
Moderate Chronic Child <4 years	Respiratory alkalosis Metabolic acidosis	>7.4	<6.0	5% Dextrose in water	100 (adult) 1–2 mEq/kg (child)	40
Severe Chronic Child <4 years	Metabolic acidosis Respiratory alkalosis	<7.4	<6.0	5% Dextrose in water	150 (adult) 2 mEq/kg (child)	60
CNS Depressant Co-ingestant	Respiratory acidosis	<7.4	<6.0	5% Dextrose in water	100–150*	60

*Correct hypoventilation.

Modified from Linden CH, Rumack BH: The legitimate analgesics, aspirin and acetaminophen. In Hansen Jr W (ed): *Toxic Emergencies*. New York, Churchill Livingstone, 1984.

a salicylate plasma concentration less than 30 to 40 mg/dL but is continued in symptomatic patients regardless of the salicylate plasma concentration. A decreased serum bicarbonate but normal or high blood pH indicates respiratory alkalosis predominating over metabolic acidosis, and the bicarbonate should be administered cautiously. An alkalemic pH of 7.40 to 7.50 is not a contraindication to bicarbonate therapy because these patients have a significant base deficit in spite of elevated blood pH.

Potassium is added, 20 to 40 mEq/L, to the infusion after the patient voids. In cases of severe, late, and chronic salicylism, 60 mEq/L of potassium may be needed. When the serum potassium is below 4.0 mEq/L, 10 mEq/L should be added over the first hour. If the patient has hypokalemia less than 3 mEq/L and flat T waves and U waves, 0.25 to 0.5 mEq/kg up to 10 mEq/h is administered. Potassium should be administered under ECG monitoring. Serum potassium is rechecked after each rapidly administered dose. A paradoxical urine acidosis (alkaline serum pH and acid urine pH) indicates that potassium is probably needed.

Convulsions are treated with diazepam or lorazepam, but hypoglycemia, low ionized calcium, cerebral edema, and hemorrhage should first be excluded with a CT scan. If tetany develops, the NaHCO$_3$ therapy is discontinued and calcium gluconate 0.1 to 0.2 mL/kg 10% administered.

Pulmonary edema management consists of fluid restriction, high FiO$_2$, mechanical ventilation, and positive end-expiratory pressure.

Cerebral edema management consists of fluid restriction, elevation of the head, hyperventilation, osmotic diuresis, and administration of dexamethasone. Vitamin K$_1$ is administered parenterally to correct an increased prothrombin time (>20 seconds) and coagulation abnormalities. If the patient has active bleeding, fresh plasma and platelets are administered as needed. Hyperpyrexia is managed by external cooling measures, not antipyretics.

Hemodialysis is the choice for removal of salicylates because it corrects the acid-base, electrolyte, and fluid disturbances as well. The indications for hemodialysis include the following:

- Acute poisoning with salicylate plasma concentration greater than 100 mg/dL without improvement after 6 hours of appropriate therapy
- Chronic poisoning with cardiopulmonary disease and a salicylate plasma concentration as low as 40 mg/dL with refractory acidosis, severe CNS manifestations (coma and seizures), and progressive deterioration, especially in elderly patients
- Impairment of vital organs of elimination
- Clinical deterioration in spite of good supportive care and alkalinization
- Severe refractory acid-base or electrolyte disturbances despite appropriate corrective measures

Disposition

There are limitations of salicylate plasma levels and patients are treated on the basis of clinical and laboratory findings. Patients who are asymptomatic should be monitored for a minimum of 6 hours, and longer if enteric-coated tablets or massive overdose was taken or if there is suspicion of concretions. Those who remain asymptomatic with a salicylate plasma concentration less than 35 mg/dL may be discharged following psychiatric evaluation, if indicated. Chronic salicylate-intoxicated patients with acidosis and an altered mental state should be admitted to the intensive care unit. Patients with acute ingestion and a salicylate plasma concentration less than 60 mg/dL and mild symptoms may be able to be treated in the emergency department. Patients with moderate and severe intoxications should be admitted to the intensive care unit.

Selective Serotonin Reuptake Inhibitors

Selective serotonin reuptake inhibitors (SSRIs) are primarily prescribed as antidepressants. SSRIs include fluoxetine (Prozac), paroxetine (Paxil), and sertraline (Zoloft).

Toxic Mechanism

The SSRIs interfere with the neuron reuptake of serotonin (5-hydroxytryptamine) at the presynaptic ganglia sites in the brain, increasing the activity of serotonin. SSRIs should not be used within 5 weeks of when a MAOI is given, nor should MAOI therapy be initiated or discontinued within 5 weeks of SSRI therapy.

Toxic Dose

The therapeutic oral dose of fluoxetine is 20 to 80 mg/d. No toxicity is seen in children with up to 3.5 mg/kg/dose orally. A fatal dose for adults is 6 g. The therapeutic dose for paroxetine is 20 to 50 mg/d. In 35 adult patients, none developed serious side effects after the ingestion of 10 to 1000 mg, and a study involving 35 children failed to demonstrate serious adverse effects at doses less than 180 mg. The therapeutic dose for sertraline is 50 mg to 200 mg/d. Patients have ingested up to 2.6 g without serious side effects. Overdose involving children who ingested less than 100 mg failed to cause adverse events.

Kinetics

Fluoxetine is well absorbed from the gastrointestinal tract and has a peak plasma concentration at 6 to 8 hours. Volume distribution is 20 to 42 L/kg; 95% is protein bound. The half-life is 4 days (for the demethylated active metabolite norfluoxetine, the half-life is 7 to 15 days). Elimination is 80% renal. Fluoxetine and other serotonin inhibitors are inhibitors of the cytochrome P450, CYP2D6 enzyme. Therefore interactions may occur with many other medications, such as antidysrhythmic class IC drugs (quinidine), phenytoin (Dilantin), haloperidol, lithium, tricyclic antidepressants (TCAs), β-blockers, codeine, and carbamazepine (Tegretol).

Paroxetine is almost completely absorbed from the gastrointestinal tract, with a peak in 2 to 8 hours. Protein binding is greater than 90%; volume distribution is 13 L/kg. Paroxetine undergoes extensive first-pass liver metabolism by oxidation and methylation to inactive metabolites. It inhibits the P450 system (see fluoxetine metabolism). The average half-life is 21 hours.

Sertraline peaks in 8 to 12 hours. Its volume distribution is 20 L/kg and protein binding is 98%. The average half-life of sertraline is 26 hours. It is metabolized to form a less-active metabolite, N-desmethylsertraline (half-life of 62 to 104 hours).

Manifestations

All SSRIs may cause serotonin syndrome, a potentially life-threatening reaction, if they are administered concurrently with an MAOI. Serotonin syndrome is caused by cerebral serotonergic stimulation and can cause severe hyperthermia, myoclonus, rhabdomyolysis, confusion, tremors, and a variety of psychological disturbances. In addition, cardiovascular complications and extrapyramidal side effects, including akathisia, dyskinesia, and Parkinson-like syndromes may occur. Also, increased suicidal ideation, seizures, sexual disorders, and hematologic disorders (platelet serotonin activity blockade leading to prolonged bleeding times) may develop. Inappropriate secretion of antidiuretic hormone resulting in hyponatremia may occur when SSRIs are administered to the elderly. This effect is usually seen within the first week of therapy.

Overdose effects are similar to the serotonin syndrome.

Laboratory Investigations

One should obtain a complete blood count (CBC), electrolytes, glucose levels, a coagulation profile, liver function tests, creatine kinase level, and an ECG.

Management

There is no specific antidote to SSRI intoxication.

Initial management consists of stabilizing vital functions, including thermoregulation. Supportive therapy and anticipation of potential life-threatening manifestations (hypotension, hyperthermia, seizures, coma, disseminated intravascular coagulation, ventricular tachycardia, and metabolic acidosis) are essential. Vital signs, EEG, creatine kinase, and blood chemistry should be monitored.

Benzodiazepines are administered to prevent and control muscle hyperactivity (diazepam [Valium] for seizures, clonazepam [Klonopin] for myoclonus). If benzodiazepine therapy fails to control muscle activity or seizures, anesthesia or nondepolarizing neuromuscular blockade may be necessary.

Electrolyte abnormalities and acid-base balance should be corrected. Fluids are used to maintain a urine output of greater than 2 mL/kg/h if there is a risk of myoglobinuria.

There are no data to support the use of gastrointestinal decontamination, although activated charcoal may be used if an ingestion has occurred within 1 hour. Hemodialysis and charcoal hemoperfusion are unlikely to be beneficial. Haloperidol (Haldol), phenothiazines, and other highly protein-bound drugs are to be avoided.

Benzodiazepine and cooling therapy can be used for hyperthermia. Serotonin antagonists, such as cyproheptadine (Periactin), may be useful in treating serotonin syndrome, although there are no controlled data. Dantrolene (Dantrium) and bromocriptine (Parlodel) are not recommended and may actually precipitate serotonin syndrome.

Disposition

Cases of ingestions in children up to 5 years of age of less than 180 mg of paroxetine (Paxil), less than 3.5 mg/kg of fluoxetine (Prozac), or less than 100 mg of sertraline (Zoloft) can be observed at home. Symptomatic patients should be admitted to the intensive care unit until asymptomatic for 24 hours. Asymptomatic patients should be observed for 6 hours. All patients should be assessed for risk of suicide before discharge. When taken chronically, SSRIs may increase cholesterol and triglycerides and decrease uric acid, so these test results should be followed.

Theophylline

Theophylline (Slo-Phyllin) is a methylxanthine alkaloid similar to caffeine and theobromine. Aminophylline is 80% theophylline. Theophylline is used in the acute treatment of asthma, pulmonary edema, chronic obstructive pulmonary disease, and neonatal apnea.

Toxic Mechanism

The proposed mechanisms of action include phosphodiesterase inhibition, adenosine receptor antagonism, inhibition of prostaglandins, and increase in serum catecholamines. Theophylline stimulates the central nervous, respiratory, and emetic centers and reduces the seizure threshold. It has positive cardiac inotropic and chronotropic effects, acts as a diuretic, relaxes smooth muscle, and causes peripheral vasodilation but cerebral vasoconstriction. Gastric secretions, gastrointestinal motility, lipolysis, glycogenolysis, and gluconeogenesis are all increased.

Toxic Dose

A single dose of 1 mg/kg produces a theophylline plasma concentration of approximately 2 μg/mL. The therapeutic range usually is 10 to 20 μg/mL. An acute, single dose greater than 10 mg/kg causes mild toxicity, a dose greater than 20 mg/kg causes moderate toxicity, and a dose greater than 50 mg/kg causes serious, possibly fatal toxicity. Fatalities occur at lower doses in patients with chronic toxicity, especially those with risk factors (see *Kinetics*).

Kinetics

The pKa is 9.5. Absorption from the stomach and upper small intestine is complete and rapid, with onset in 30 to 60 minutes.

TABLE 27	Theophylline Blood Concentrations and Acute Toxicity	
PLASMA CONCENTRATION (MG/ML)	**TOXICITY DEGREE**	**MANIFESTATIONS**
8–10	None	Bronchodilation
10–20	Mild	Therapeutic range: nausea, vomiting, nervousness, respiratory alkalosis, tachycardia
15–25		35% have mild manifestations of toxicity
20–40	Moderate	Gastrointestinal complaints and central nervous system stimulation Transient hypertension, tachypnea, tachycardia; 80% will have some manifestations of toxicity
60–100	Severe	Convulsions, dysrhythmias Hypokalemia, hyperglycemia Ventricular dysrhythmias, protracted convulsions, hypotension, acid-base abnormalities

Reprinted and modified from Linden CH, Rumack BH: In Hansen Jr W (ed): *Toxic Emergencies*. New York, Churchill Livingstone, 1984. With permission from Elsevier.

Peak theophylline plasma concentration occurs within 1 to 2 hours after ingestion of liquid preparations, 2 to 4 hours after ingestion of regular tablets, and 7 to 24 hours after ingestion of slow-release formulations. Volume distribution is 0.3 to 0.7 L/kg. Protein binding is 40% to 60% in adults, mainly to albumin (low albumin increases free active theophylline).

Elimination is 90% by hepatic metabolism to an active metabolite, 2-methyl xanthine. The half-life is 3.5 hours in a child and 4 to 6 hours in an adult. The half-life is shorter in smokers and patients taking enzyme-inducing drugs. Only 8% to 10% of the drug is excreted unchanged in the urine.

Risk factors that produce a longer half-life include age younger than 6 months or older than 60 years, use of enzyme-inhibitor drugs (calcium channel blockers, oral contraceptives, cimetidine [Tagamet], ciprofloxacin [Cipro], erythromycin, macrolide antibiotics, isoniazid), illness (persistent fever >38.9°C [>102°F]), viral illness, liver impairment, heart failure, chronic obstructive pulmonary disease, and influenza vaccination.

Manifestations

Acute toxicity generally correlates with blood levels; chronic toxicity does not (Table 27).

In the case of an acute, single, regular-release overdose, vomiting and occasionally hematemesis occur at low theophylline plasma concentrations. CNS stimulation includes restlessness, muscle tremors, and protracted tonic–clonic seizures, but coma is rare. Convulsions are a sign of severe toxicity and usually are preceded by gastrointestinal symptoms (except with sustained-release and chronic intoxications). Cardiovascular disturbances include cardiac dysrhythmias (supraventricular tachycardia) and transient hypertension with mild overdoses, but hypotension and ventricular dysrhythmias with severe intoxications. Rhabdomyolysis and renal failure are occasionally seen. Children tolerate higher serum levels, and cardiac dysrhythmias and seizures occur at theophylline plasma concentrations greater than 100 μg/mL. Possible metabolic disturbances include hyperglycemia, pronounced hypokalemia, hypocalcemia, hypomagnesemia, hypophosphatemia, increased serum amylase, and elevation of uric acid.

Chronic intoxication, defined as multiple doses of theophylline over 24 hours, or cases in which interacting drugs or illness interfere with theophylline metabolism are more serious and difficult to treat. Cardiac dysrhythmias and convulsions may occur at theophylline plasma concentrations of 40 to 60 μg/mL and there is no correlation with TPC. The seizures occur without warning and are protracted and repetitive and may produce status epilepticus. Vomiting and typical metabolic disturbances do not occur.

Differences with slow-release preparations are that few or no gastrointestinal symptoms occur, peak concentrations and convulsions may be delayed 12 to 24 hours postingestion, and convulsions occur without warning.

Laboratory Investigations
Monitoring includes vital signs, pulse oximeter, ABG, hemoglobin, hematocrit (for gastrointestinal hemorrhage), ECG and cardiac monitor, renal and hepatic function, electrolytes, blood glucose, acid-base balance, and serum albumin. Gastric contents and stools should be tested for occult blood. Samples for theophylline plasma concentration measurement should be drawn within 1 to 2 hours after ingestion of liquid preparations, 2 to 4 hours after ingestion of regular-release formulations, and 4 hours after ingestion of slow-release formulations. One should check the serum albumin level because a decrease in albumin levels may cause manifestations of toxicity despite normal theophylline plasma concentration. A single theophylline plasma concentration reading may be misleading; therefore, theophylline plasma concentration measurement should be repeated every 2 to 4 hours to determine the trend until a declining trend is reached and then monitored every 4 to 6 hours until it is below 20 μg/mL.

Management
Vital functions must be established and maintained. If the patient is in a coma or has convulsions or vomiting, he or she should be intubated immediately. The theophylline plasma concentration is obtained and repeated every 2 to 4 hours to determine peak absorption, and a theophylline bezoar should be considered if the theophylline plasma concentration fails to decline. Consultation with a nephrologist about charcoal hemoperfusion is recommended.

Gastrointestinal decontamination is warranted in the case of an acute overdose, but emesis must not be induced. Activated charcoal is the choice decontamination procedure in a dose of 1 g/kg to all patients, followed with MDAC 0.5 g/kg every 2 to 4 hours until the theophylline plasma concentration is less than 20 μg/mL. MDAC is effective in treating acute, chronic, and intravenous overdoses. Activated charcoal shortens the half-life of theophylline by about 50% and may be indicated up to 24 hours following ingestion.

Whole-bowel irrigation with polyethylene-electrolyte solution has been recommended for cases of massive overdose, possible concretions, and ingestion of sustained-release preparations. If intractable vomiting occurs, the antiemetic metoclopramide (Reglan) (0.1 mg/kg adult dose), droperidol (Inapsine) (2.5 to 10 mg IV), or ondansetron (Zofran) (8 to 32 mg IV) is administered. Ondansetron, however, inhibits metabolism of theophylline after a few doses.

Convulsions are controlled with lorazepam (Ativan) or diazepam (Valium) and phenobarbital. Phenytoin (Dilantin) is ineffective. The convulsions in patients with chronic intoxication are often refractory and may require, in addition to anticonvulsants, neuromuscular paralyzing agents, sedation, assisted ventilation, and EEG monitoring.

Hypotension is treated with fluids and vasopressors, if necessary. Norepinephrine (Levophed) 0.05 μg/kg/min is preferred as the vasopressor over dopamine.

Supraventricular tachycardia with hemodynamic instability requires cardioversion. Low-dose β-blockers may be used but should not be used in patients with reactive airway disease or hypotension. Adenosine (Adenocard) is ineffective. For ventricular dysrhythmias, electrolyte disturbances should be corrected. Lidocaine is the treatment of choice but has the potential to cause seizures at toxic concentrations. Cardioversion may be needed.

Hematemesis is managed with sucralfate (Carafate) 1 g four times daily and/or Maalox TC 30 mL every 2 hours and blood replacement, if necessary. H₂ antihistamine blockers that are enzyme inhibitors are not used.

Fluid and metabolic disturbances should be corrected. Hyperglycemia does not require insulin therapy. Hypokalemia should be corrected cautiously, as it may be largely an intracellular shift and not total body loss. Usually adding 40 mEq potassium to a liter of fluid will suffice. The serum potassium level must be monitored closely.

Charcoal hemoperfusion is the management of choice for patients with serious intoxications. Hemoperfusion can increase the clearance twofold to threefold over hemodialysis, but hemodialysis can be used if hemoperfusion is not available. Criteria for charcoal hemoperfusion are as follows:
- Life-threatening events such as convulsions or dysrhythmias
- Intractable vomiting refractory to antiemetics
- Acute intoxications with a theophylline plasma concentration greater than 80 μg/mL or greater than 70 μg/mL 4 hours after overdose with a sustained-release formulation and greater than 40 μg/mL in the case of chronic intoxication
- Acute or chronic overdoses with a theophylline plasma concentration greater than 40 μg/mL, especially if the patient has risk factors that lengthen the half-life of the drug (see Kinetics).

Disposition
Patients with mild symptoms and a theophylline plasma concentration less than 20 μg/mL can be treated in emergency department and discharged when asymptomatic for a few hours. Any patient with acute ingestion and a theophylline plasma concentration greater than 35 μg/mL should be admitted to a monitored bed with seizure precautions and suicide precautions, if needed. If neurologic or cardiotoxic effects or a theophylline plasma concentration greater than 50 μg/mL is present, the patient should be admitted to the intensive care unit. A patient with an overdose of a sustained-release preparation, regardless of symptoms or initial theophylline plasma concentration, requires admission, monitoring, activated charcoal, and MDAC. In patients on chronic therapy, toxicity may occur at a lower theophylline plasma concentration, and these patients should not be discharged until they are asymptomatic for several hours.

Tricyclic and Cyclic Antidepressants
Historically, tricyclic antidepressants are an important cause of pharmaceutical overdose fatalities. The mortality rate was reduced from 15% in the 1970s to less than 1% in the 1990s because of a better understanding of the pathophysiology of these agents and improvements in management (Table 28).

Toxic Mechanism
The major mechanisms of toxicity of the tricyclic antidepressants are (a) central and peripheral anticholinergic effects; (b) peripheral α-adrenergic blockade; (c) quinidine-like cardiac membrane stabilizing action blockade of the fast inward sodium channels; and (d) inhibition of synaptic neurotransmitter reuptake in the CNS presynaptic neurons. The tetracyclics, monocyclic aminoketones, and dibenzoxazepines possess convulsive activity and less cardiac toxicity in overdose than the older tricyclic antidepressants. Triazolopyridine has less serious cardiac and CNS toxicity.

TABLE 28 Cyclic Antidepressants: Daily Dose and Their Major Properties

GENERIC NAME (TRADE NAME)	ADULT DAILY DOSE (MG)	THERAPEUTIC RANGE (NG/ML)	HALF-LIFE (HOURS)	TOXICITY		
				ANTICHOL	CNS	CARDIAC
Tertiary Amines						
Amitriptyline (Elavil)	75–300	120–250	31–46	3+	3+	3+
Imipramine (Tofranil)	75–300	125–250	9–24	3+	3+	2+
Doxepin (Sinequan)	75–300	30–150	8–24	3+	3+	2+
Trimipramine (Surmantil)	75–200	10–240	16–18	3+	3+	2+
Secondary Amines						
Nortriptyline (Pamelor)	75–150	50–150	18–93	2+	3+	3+
Desipramine (Norpramin)	75–200	75–160	14–62	1+	3+	3+
Protriptyline (Vivactil)	20–60	70–250	54–198	2+	3+	3+
Newer Cyclic Antidepressants						
Teracyclic			30–60	1+	2+	3+
Maprotiline (Ludiomil)	75–300	—	30–60	1+	2+	3+
Trizolopyridine, a noncyclic, produces less serious cardiac and CNS toxicity						
Trazodone (Desyrel)	50–600	700	4–7	1+	1+	1+
Monocyclic Aminoketones						
Bupropion (Wellbutrin)	200–400	—	8–24	1+	3+	1+
Dibenzazepine						
Clomipramine (Anafranil)	100–250	200–500	21–32	2+	2+	2+
Dibenoxazepine						
Amoxapine (Ascendin)	150–300	200–500	6–10	1+	3+	2+

Abbreviations: Antichol = anticholinergic effect; CNS = central nervous system effect primarily seizures; cardiac = cardiac effect.
Other drugs with similar structures are cyclobenzaprine, a muscle relaxant (similar to amitriptyline), and carbamazepine, an anticonvulsant (similar to imipramine); however, they cause less cardiac toxicity.

Toxic Dose

The therapeutic dose of imipramine (Tofranil) is 1.5 to 5 mg/kg; a dose greater than 5 mg/kg may be mildly toxic; 10 to 20 mg/kg may be life threatening, although less than 20 mg/kg has produced few fatalities; greater than 30 mg/kg carries a 30% mortality rate; and at a dose greater than 70 mg/kg, patients rarely survive. In children 375 mg and in adults as little as 500 mg have been fatal. In adults, five times the maximum daily dose is toxic and 10 times is potentially fatal. Although major overdose symptoms are associated with plasma concentrations greater than 1 μg/mL (>1000 ng/mL), plasma tricyclic levels do not correlate well with toxicity; clinical signs and symptoms should guide therapy.

The relative dosage or potency equivalents are as follows: amitriptyline (Elavil) 100 mg = amoxapine (Asendin) 125 mg = desipramine (Norpramin) 75 mg = doxepin (Sinequan) 100 mg = imipramine (Tofranil) 75 mg = maprotiline (Ludiomil) 75 mg = nortriptyline (Pamelor) 50 mg = trazodone (Desyrel) 200 mg. This allows one to determine an equivalent dosage of an agent compared with another (see Table 28).

Kinetics

The tricyclic and cyclic antidepressants are lipophilic. They are rapidly absorbed from the alkaline small intestine, but absorption may be prolonged and delayed in cases of massive overdose owing to anticholinergic action. Onset varies from less than 1 hour (30 to 40 minutes) to, rarely, 12 hours. The peak serum levels are reached in 2 to 8 hours and the peak effect is in 6 hours but may be delayed 12 hours because of erratic absorption. The clinical effects correlate poorly with plasma levels.

Cyclic antidepressants are highly protein-bound to plasma glycoproteins, 98% at a pH 7.5 and 90% at 7.0. Volume distribution is 10 to 50 L/kg. The elimination route is by hepatic metabolism. The tertiary amines are metabolized into active demethylated secondary amine metabolites. The active secondary amine metabolites undergo a 15% enterohepatic recirculation and are metabolized over a period of days into nonactive metabolites. The intestinal bacterial flora may reconstitute the metabolites, which are active.

The half-life varies from 10 hours for imipramine to 81 hours for amitriptyline and 100 hours for nortriptyline. The active metabolites have longer half-lives.

Only 3% of the ingested dose is excreted in the urine unchanged.

Manifestations

There are reports of asymptomatic patients who, upon arrival to an emergency department, suddenly have a seizure, develop hemodynamically unstable dysrhythmias, and die shortly thereafter from ingestion of a tricyclic antidepressant. Most patients with severe toxicity develop symptoms within 1 to 2 hours, but symptoms may be delayed 6 hours after overdose.

Small overdoses produce early anticholinergic effects, agitation, and transient hypertension, which are not life-threatening. Large overdoses produce depression of the CNS and myocardium, convulsions, and hypotension. Death can occur within the first 2 to 6 hours following ingestion.

Some ECG screening tools for predicting cardiac or neurologic toxicity from ingestion of a tricyclic antidepressant have been developed: (a) a QRS greater than 0.10 second may produce seizures, and if greater than 0.16 second, 50% of patients may develop ventricular dysrhythmias (20% of these may be life-threatening) and seizures; (b) a terminal 40 msec of the QRS axis greater than 120 degrees in the right frontal plane may be associated with toxicity; or (c) a large R wave greater than 3 mm in ECG lead aVR may predispose the patient to toxicity. The quinidine cardiac membrane stabilizing effect produces depression of myocardium, conduction, and ECG changes. The peripheral α-adrenergic blockade produces hypotension.

The secondary amines are metabolized to inactive metabolites. The tetracyclics produce a high incidence of cardiovascular disturbances and seizures. Monocyclic aminoketones produce seizures in doses greater than 600 mg. Dibenzoxazepines produce a syndrome of convulsions, rhabdomyolysis, and renal failure.

Laboratory Investigations
If the patient has altered mental status or ECG abnormalities, ABG, ECG, chest radiograph, blood glucose, serum electrolytes, calcium, magnesium, blood urea nitrogen, and creatinine levels, liver profile, creatine kinase level, urine output, and, in severe cases, hemodynamic monitoring are indicated. Levels of the tricyclic and cyclic antidepressants less than 300 ng/mL are therapeutic; levels greater than 500 ng/mL indicate toxicity, and levels greater than 1000 ng/mL indicate serious poisoning and are associated with QRS widening.

Management
Vital functions must be established and maintained. Even if the patient is asymptomatic, intravenous access should be established, vital signs and neurologic status monitored, and baseline 12-lead ECG and continuous cardiac monitoring obtained for at least 6 hours from admission or 8 to 12 hours postingestion. QRS interval should be measured on a limb lead ECG every 15 minutes for 6 hours postingestion.

For gastrointestinal decontamination, emesis should not be induced and gastric lavage should not be used. Activated charcoal is preferable. If the patient is in an altered mental state, the airway must be protected. Activated charcoal 1 g/kg is recommended up to 1 hour postingestion. Benefit from MDAC has not been demonstrated.

Alkalinization does not control seizures; diazepam or lorazepam should be used. Status epilepticus may require high-dose barbiturates or neuromuscular blockers with intravenous diazepam. If not successful, the patient can be paralyzed with short-term nondepolarizing neuromuscular blockers such as vecuronium (Norcuron), intubation, and assisted ventilation. A bolus of sodium bicarbonate is recommended as an adjunct to correct the acidosis produced by the seizures.

Sodium bicarbonate is administered in a dose of 1 to 2 mEq/kg undiluted as a bolus and repeated twice a few minutes apart, if needed, for "sodium loading" and alkalinization, which may increase protein binding from 90% to 98%. The sodium loading overcomes the sodium channel blockage and is more important than the alkalinization. Indications include (a) a QRS complex greater than 0.12 second, (b) ventricular tachycardia, (c) severe conduction disturbances, (d) metabolic acidosis, (e) coma, and (f) seizures. A continuous infusion of sodium bicarbonate is of limited usefulness for controlling dysrhythmias. Bolus therapy should be used as needed.

Hyperventilation alone has been recommended, but the pH elevation is not as instantaneous and there is compensatory renal excretion of bicarbonate; therefore, we do not recommend it. The combination of hyperventilation and sodium bicarbonate has produced fatal alkalemia and is not recommended. One should monitor serum potassium level (the sudden increase in blood pH can aggravate or precipitate hypokalemia), serum sodium, and ionized calcium levels (hypocalcemia may occur with alkalinization) and blood pH.

Specific cardiovascular complications should be treated as follows: Hypotension is treated with norepinephrine, a predominantly α-adrenergic drug, which is preferred over dopamine. Hypertension that occurs early rarely requires treatment. Sinus tachycardia usually does not require treatment. Supraventricular tachycardia in a patient who is hemodynamically unstable requires synchronized electrical cardioversion, starting at 0.25 to 1.0 watt-second per kilogram, after sedation. Ventricular tachycardia that persists after alkalinization requires intravenous lidocaine or countershock if the patient is hemodynamically unstable. Ventricular fibrillation should be treated with defibrillation. Torsades de pointes is treated with magnesium sulfate IV 20% solution, 2 g over 2 to 3 minutes, followed by a continuous infusion of 1.5 mL 10% solution or 5 to 10 mg per minute. For the treatment of bradydysrhythmias, atropine is contraindicated because of the anticholinergic activity. Isoproterenol 0.1 μg/kg/min, used with caution, may produce hypotension. If the patient is hemodynamically unstable, a pacemaker is used.

Extraordinary measures, such as aortic balloon pump and cardiopulmonary bypass, have been successful.

Investigational treatments include FAB fragments specific for tricyclic antidepressant, which have been successful in animals. Prophylactic $NaHCO_3$ to prevent dysrhythmias is also being investigated.

Physostigmine has produced asystole, and flumazenil has produced seizures. Both are contraindicated.

Disposition
A patient with an antidepressant overdose who meets any of the following criteria should be admitted to the intensive care unit for 12 to 24 hours: (a) ECG abnormalities except sinus tachycardia, (b) altered mental state, (c) seizures, (d) respiratory depression, and (e) hypotension. Low-risk patients include those in whom the above symptoms are absent at 6 hours postingestion, those who present with minor transient manifestations such as sinus tachycardia who subsequently become and remain asymptomatic for a 6-hour period, and asymptomatic patients who remain asymptomatic for 6 hours. These patients may be discharged if the ECG remains normal, they have normal bowel sounds, and they undergo psychiatric disposition.

Even if the patient is asymptomatic upon presentation to the health care facility, intravenous access should be established, vital signs and neurologic status monitored, a baseline 12-lead ECG obtained, and cardiac monitoring continued for at least 6 hours. *Caution:* In 25% of fatal cases, the patients were initially alert and awake at presentation. However, in most cases of fatality initially deemed as sudden cardiac death, the patient, upon reexamination, actually had symptoms that were missed.

Children younger than 6 years of age with non-intentional (accidental) exposures to amitriptyline (Elavil), desipramine (Norpramin), doxepin (Sinequan), imipramine (Tofranil), or nortriptyline (Aventyl) in a dose less than 5 mg/kg, who are asymptomatic and have what are deemed reliable caregivers, can be observed at home, with close poison control follow-up for 6 hours. Parents or caregivers should be given instructions regarding signs and symptoms to be alert for. Children who are symptomatic, or who ingested greater than 5 mg/kg, should be referred to the emergency department for monitoring, observation, and activated charcoal treatment.

SPIDER BITES AND SCORPION STINGS

Method of
Anne-Michelle Ruha, MD

CURRENT DIAGNOSIS

Black Widow Bite
- Target lesion, not always present
- Generalized pain and muscle cramps
- Hypertension, regional diaphoresis

Brown Recluse Bite
- Unlikely to occur outside of endemic areas
- Cyanotic or blistering wound within area of pallor surrounded by erythema
- Systemic loxoscelism associated with rash, fever, hemolysis, renal failure

Bark Scorpion Sting
- Absence of lesion or local inflammatory reaction
- Painful paresthesias
- Disconjugate, roving eye movements are characteristic
- Restlessness, agitation, and involuntary jerking of muscles

CURRENT THERAPY

Black Widow Bite
- Opioid analgesics to control pain
- Benzodiazepines to control muscle cramping and anxiety
- Anti-*Latrodectus* antivenom (Antivenin) for persistent severe symptoms

Brown Recluse Bite
- General wound care
- If surgical excision is required, perform after 6 to 8 weeks
- Antibiotics only if infected

Bark Scorpion Sting
- Close attention to airway
- Opioid analgesics to control pain
- Benzodiazepines to control agitation
- *Centruroides* (scorpion) Immune F(ab')₂

Spider Bites

The majority of spiders native to the United States are incapable of envenomating humans. Important exceptions are *Latrodectus* and *Loxosceles* spiders, which produce clinical envenomations that, on rare occasion, are life-threatening.

Brown Recluse Spider

The most famous and abundant *Loxosceles* spider in the United States is *Loxosceles reclusa*, known as the brown recluse or fiddleback spider, due to the violin-shaped marking on its cephalothorax. The brown recluse inhabits the midwestern United States, with a range extending from east Texas to west Georgia and reaching north to southern Iowa. Bites from this nonaggressive spider are defensive, and they generally occur when spiders become trapped in clothes or bedsheets. The risk of a bite, even in heavily infested homes, appears to be very small. Most diagnoses of brown recluse bites, including many published in the medical literature, are likely erroneous, occurring in nonendemic areas without identification of the spider. Other *Loxosceles* species found in the United States are even less likely to bite because they avoid human dwellings. Evidence supporting an association between other native spider species and necrotic wounds is weak.

Although the majority of brown recluse bites do not produce significant injury, some result in loxoscelism, which ranges from minor dermonecrosis to, very rarely, life-threatening illness. The venom component thought responsible for loxoscelism is sphingomyelinase D, which affects platelets and cell membranes and activates inflammatory mediators. The first signs of dermonecrosis are often erythema, pruritus, and pain at the bite site. Over hours the site becomes pale and edematous. Erythema can progress and spread gravitationally. A vesicle can develop, form an eschar, and slough over days to weeks. In the first days after the bite, a sunken bluish wound surrounded by a ring of pallor and then erythema is characteristic. Some patients develop a generalized maculopapular rash. Although most necrotic lesions are not serious, some can enlarge to 40 cm and leave a significant scar. Obese persons are at risk for more-severe lesions.

Very rarely, systemic loxoscelism develops within 48 hours of the bite, characterized by fever, myalgias, and hemolysis. Vomiting and diarrhea can occur, and some patients develop a diffuse erythroderma. Renal failure, disseminated intravascular coagulation, and death can result. Death from massive hemolysis is rare and is more likely to occur in children.

Diagnosis of loxoscelism depends on recognition of signs and symptoms in combination with positive identification of the spider when possible. Alternative etiologies for necrotic wounds are much more common than necrotic arachnidism, especially in nonendemic areas. The differential diagnosis of brown recluse bite is large and includes infectious causes, neoplastic disease, and vascular disease.

Treatment is supportive. Most wounds heal without intervention, although a scar might remain. Early surgical excision, dapsone,[1] hyperbaric oxygen, or prophylactic antibiotics cannot be recommended owing to lack of convincing evidence. Patients should receive tetanus prophylaxis (Td) and general wound care. In severe cases, healing can take months and require surgical intervention, which should occur 6 to 8 weeks following the bite after the wound is fully demarcated.

Black Widow Spiders

Latrodectus, or widow, spiders are, medically, the most important group of spiders in the world. Native black widow spiders are shiny black with a red hourglass pattern on their ventral surface. They can reside in or near human structures, leading to contact with humans and subsequent bites.

α-Latrotoxin in venom causes neurotransmitters to be released from synaptic vesicles. This results in a combination of neuromuscular and autonomic effects unique to *Latrodectus* bites, termed *latrodectism*. Bites are inconsistently felt, and they might or might not leave visible puncture marks and a target-like lesion. Pain can progress locally or become generalized within several hours. Severe muscle pain, particularly involving the abdomen and back, is common. Other findings include hypertension, tachycardia, tremor, localized or diffuse diaphoresis, periorbital edema, and urinary retention. Less commonly, vomiting, fever, priapism, paresthesias, and fasciculations occur. Rhabdomyolysis can result from increased muscle activity. Rarely, acute cardiomyopathy, cardiac ischemia, and pulmonary edema occur. Deaths are uncommon but reported.

Diagnosis of latrodectism is based on history of a spider bite and consistent clinical findings. In the absence of a witnessed bite, diagnosis can be difficult. Sudden onset and rapid progression of symptoms should raise suspicion. Infectious and surgical etiologies must be considered in a febrile or vomiting patient. Similar neuromuscular and autonomic findings might also be seen with intoxication by stimulant drugs and scorpion envenomations, and these should be considered in the differential.

Latrodectism typically resolves within 2 to 7 days. Opioid analgesics are often required to treat pain. Severe symptoms require intravenous opioids for adequate pain control and benzodiazepines for muscle spasms and anxiety. If symptoms are life-threatening or not controlled with these therapies, antivenom (Antivenin [*Latrodectus mactans*, equine origin], Merck, Boston, Mass.) should be considered. One vial reverses symptoms of envenomation. This

---

[1]Not FDA approved for this indication.

whole-immunoglobulin product can produce acute hypersensitivity and should be administered in a monitored setting. Risks and benefits must be weighed before using this product. If antivenom is not an option or the patient is critically ill, care is supportive, including oxygen and airway support as needed, antihypertensives, antiemetics, and other symptomatic treatment.

Tarantulas

Tarantulas are common pets and are generally harmless. Bites may be painful, but envenomation by native species has not been reported. Most injury to humans resulting from interaction with tarantulas is secondary to trauma and inflammation caused by barbed abdominal hairs that the spiders eject defensively when threatened. If the hairs embed in the skin, a rash and pruritus can result. They can also embed in the cornea or be transferred there by rubbing the eyes after handling a tarantula. Ophthalmia nodosa, iritis, and keratouveitis have all been reported following exposure to tarantula hairs.

Treatment of embedded corneal hairs entails referral to an ophthalmologist and removal of the hairs if possible. Topical steroids are generally recommended, and some authors also recommend topical antibiotics.

Scorpion Stings

The bark scorpion, *Centruroides sculpturatus*, is the only native scorpion capable of producing a life-threatening envenomation. This small (<3 inches), yellowish-brown scorpion is found throughout Arizona and in bordering areas of surrounding states.

The scorpion seeks cool, dark environments and commonly enters homes. It injects venom by thrusting its stinger, located at the tip of its tail, toward the victim. The neurotoxic venom increases release of neurotransmitters that act at the neuromuscular junction and autonomic nerve endings.

Most stings are minor, producing local pain and paresthesias. Less than 5% of stings result in neurotoxicity, and the majority of these occur in children. Stings typically do not produce a visible skin lesion, although on rare occasion a small red mark is noted. Pain is immediate, and in a grade 1 envenomation remains local and resolves quickly. Grade 2 envenomations involve pain and paresthesias distal from the sting site, which can persist for days to weeks.

Most severe envenomations affect children younger than 5 years. Symptoms develop within 5 to 45 minutes and can progress for 4 hours. Infants and toddlers can exhibit sudden agitation and crying and transient vomiting, and they might rub their face and ears in response to paresthesias. If the child is verbal, complaints of burning pain and sensation of tongue swelling are common. Sinus tachycardia, hypertension, low-grade fever, and hypersalivation are common, and some children develop stridor. Restlessness, agitation, and twisting of the trunk with thrashing of the extremities is typical, as are tongue fasciculations and dysconjugate eye movements, or opsoclonus. Patients are conscious but often keep their eyes closed owing to diplopia. Presence of cranial nerve findings or neuromuscular agitation constitute a grade 3 envenomation; both are present in grade 4 envenomation. Severe envenomation may be associated with pulmonary edema, rhabdomyolysis, and aspiration pneumonia. Respiratory failure can occur due to several factors, including loss of tongue and respiratory muscle control, hypersalivation, and use of respiratory depressant medications.

Diagnosis often relies on recognition of symptoms, because children might not report a sting. Characteristic findings in regions inhabited by this scorpion usually make diagnosis straightforward. Differential diagnosis includes seizures or amphetamine toxicity. If a suspected envenomation does not follow the expected clinical course, a urine drug screen should be obtained.

Patients with grade 4 envenomation must be monitored for respiratory compromise in an emergency department or intensive care unit. If available, treatment with the antivenom Centruroides (Scorpion) Immune F(ab')2 (Equine) Injection (Anascorp) should be considered. Anascorp reverses neurotoxicity within hours and often allows discharge home from the emergency department. In clinical trials Anascorp had an excellent safety profile; however, acute hypersensitivity reactions are possible, so antihistamines

and epinephrine (Adrenalin) must be accessible. Serum sickness can also develop up to 3 weeks after receiving antivenom.

If antivenom is not an option, longer-acting medications (morphine and lorazepam [Ativan][1]) may be used to control pain and agitation. Intubation and mechanical ventilation is sometimes necessary owing to venom effects and respiratory depression from the medications used to control symptoms. While the patient is intubated, continuous infusion of sedative, analgesic, and muscle relaxing agents may be necessary until signs and symptoms of envenomation resolve. This typically occurs within 24 hours, although residual medication effects can require prolonged observation.

References

Anascorp package insert: http://www.fda.gov/downloads/BiologicsBloodVaccines/BloodBloodProducts/ApprovedProducs/LicensedProductsBLAs/FractionatedPlasmaProducts/UCM266725.pdf.
Bernardino CR, Rapuano C: Ophthalmia nodosa caused by casual handling of a tarantula, *CLAO* 26(2):111–112, 2000.
Boyer LV, Theodorou AA, Berg RA, et al: Antivenom for critically ill children with neurotoxicity from scorpion stings, *N Engl J Med* 360(20):2090–2098, 2009.
Clark RF, Wethern-Kestner S, Vance MV, Gerkin R: Clinical presentation and treatment of black widow spider envenomation: A review of 163 cases, *Ann Emerg Med* 21(7):782–787, 1992.
Curry SC, Vance MV, Ryan PJ, et al: Envenomation by the scorpion *Centruroides sculpturatus*, *J Toxicol Clin Toxicol* 21(4–5):417–449, 1983-1984.
Furbee RB, Kao LW, Ibrahim D: Brown recluse spider envenomation, *Clin Lab Med* 26:211–226, 2006.
Vetter RS: Spiders of the genus *Loxosceles (Araneae, Sicariidae)*: A review of biological, medical and psychological aspects regarding envenomations, *J Arachnol* 36:150–163, 2008.
Vetter RS, Isbister GK: Medical aspects of spider bites, *Annu Rev Entomol* 53:409–429, 2008.
Vetter RS, Isbister GK: Do hobo spider bites cause dermonecrotic injuries? *Ann Emerg Med* 44(6):605–607, 2004.
Watts P, Mcpherson R, Hawksworth NR: Tarantula keratouveitis, *Cornea* 19(3):393–394, 2000.

VENOMOUS SNAKEBITE

Method of
Steven A. Seifert, MD

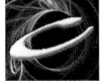

CURRENT DIAGNOSIS

Crotalinae (rattlesnake, copperhead, cottonmouth) bite
- One or two fang puncture marks
- Dry bites (nonenvenomation) may occur in up to 20%; if no local effects, no envenomation, but patients should be observed for at least 8 to 10 hours
- Envenomation produces pain and progressive swelling, often with an active, proximal leading edge, usually finished progressing by 24 hours
- Edema and functional deficits may take many weeks to completely resolve
- May include clear or hemorrhagic blisters
- May include ecchymosis
- Tissue necrosis and infection are rare and usually late (>2 days) complications
- Abnormalities in hematologic clotting elements (platelets, fibrinogen, PT/INR) are variable, may result in significant bleeding, and may persist for more than 2 weeks
- Typical findings in an endemic area may be sufficient as an indication for antivenom treatment

Coral snake bite
- One or two fang puncture marks
- Dry bites (non-envenomation) may occur in up to 50%; patients should be observed for 24 hours
- Local effects, even with significant systemic envenomation, may be minimal to nil
- Neurologic effects (progressive, descending paralysis) predominate and may require airway support
- Motor effects may be poorly reversible once established and may persist for many weeks

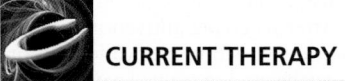
Two families of significantly venomous snakes are native to the United States. The Viperidae family (viperids) is composed of three genera and more than 30 species of rattlesnakes, copperheads, and cottonmouths. The Elapidae family (elapids) is composed of two genera and several species of coral snakes.

Each year, there are more than 6500 venomous snakebites by native species reported to United States' poison centers, with fewer than 5 deaths. Ninety-eight percent of these bites are from viperids. Currently, there are two antivenoms that are effective against viperid species. Crotalidae Polyvalent Immune Fab (Ovine) antivenom (CroFab, Boston Scientific/BTG, Farnham, UK) is effective and indicated for all native species in this family. A second F(ab')₂ antivenom, Crotalidae Immune F(ab')₂ (Equine) (Anavip; Rare Disease Therapeutics, Inc., Franklin, TN) is specifically indicated for all North American rattlesnake envenomations. There is also a single antivenom (Antivenin [*Micrurus fulvius*], equine origin, Pfizer/Wyeth Laboratories, New York, NY) against coral snakes, which are usually easily recognized by their distinctive markings.

There are approximately 50 additional bites per year from a wide variety of nonnative venomous species of snakes housed in zoos, academic institutions, serpentariums, and private collections. Identification of the biting species in these cases is usually not an issue.

Diagnostic and Management Overview

Taking Action

There are only a few actions that can be undertaken in the field to reduce morbidity or mortality from a venomous snakebite. Most "treatments" that have been advocated—cutting or sucking, or applying tourniquets, heat, cold, or electricity—have no proven efficacy and are much more likely to result in additional tissue injury and delay of definitive therapy. Appropriate local injury management—removal of jewelry, splinting of the extremity, and measures to slow venom entry into central circulation until definitive therapy can be undertaken *in carefully selected cases*—and expeditious transport to a healthcare facility can produce optimal outcomes.

Definitive management for native venomous snakes in the United States is achieved with appropriate local wound care and antivenom, which is composed of antibodies raised in a host animal (horses or sheep) against snake venom components. Because native viperids inhabit every state except Maine, every hospital should stock or have ready access to one or both antivenoms.

No US Food and Drug Administration (FDA)–approved elapid antivenom is currently being manufactured in the United States. Older stocks of a previously produced antivenom ("Antivenin") are still available at many hospitals in endemic areas (e.g., Florida,

Georgia, Alabama, Louisiana, Texas), but they are rapidly being depleted, and existing stocks will eventually be consumed or pass their expiration dates. An experimental antivenom has completed a Phase 3 clinical trial but is not currently available. Foreign-produced antivenoms against related coral snake species may also have efficacy against United States' snakes but should be used only in the unavailability of an FDA-approved drug and, ideally, with prior FDA approval.

An even more difficult situation results from exotic envenomations, for which the appropriate antivenom (if one exists) is certain to be a non-FDA-approved product and may be located at a zoo or other non-healthcare source quite distant from the location of the envenomation.

Antivenom, local wound care, and symptomatic and supportive care are the mainstays of envenomation management. A regional poison center should be contacted for information and assistance in managing any venomous snake exposure, including locating an appropriate antivenom. Poison centers have personnel who are experienced at assessing and managing envenomations and have access to a database, the Antivenom Index, which lists sources of antivenoms for nonnative species. Poison centers can be contacted from anywhere in the United States by calling 1-800-222-1222.

Snake Identification

Beyond determining whether the victim has been bitten by a coral snake or a viperid, it may be useful to distinguish a rattlesnake bite from a copperhead or cottonmouth bite for the selection of the antivenom. A photo may be of some value to the treating physician, but it should be obtained only if it can be done safely and without causing a delay in transporting the patient. Viperid snakes are easily differentiated from coral snakes by virtue of the latter's distinctive color pattern of red, yellow, and black bands. It can be difficult to differentiate a coral snake from nonvenomous snakes that have similar markings. The rhyme "red touches yellow, kills a fellow; red touches black, venom lack," which describes the red band being surrounded on either side by yellow or black, is accurate only for North American coral snakes. South American coral snakes may have the opposite pattern.

As all viperid envenomations are currently treated with a single product and the physical findings or laboratory evaluation is all that is required to determine that the snake is venomous, attempting to kill or capture the snake is unlikely to add additional information to treatment decisions but is likely to result in the individual being bitten a second time or other individuals becoming bite victims. Differences in the appearance of the bite wound (e.g., fang punctures, swelling, ecchymosis) and the observation of signs and symptoms are usually sufficient to determine whether the biting snake was venomous and to guide therapy.

Since approximately half of envenomations are associated with intentional interactions with snakes, remember this advice: "Red touches yellow, leave it alone. Red touches black, leave it alone. Slithers on the ground, LEAVE IT ALONE."

Factors Affecting Toxicity and the Severity of Envenomation

Many factors govern whether an envenomation occurs after a bite, the signs and symptoms that develop, and the overall severity of the effects. Up to 25% of viperid bites and up to 50% of elapid bites do not result in an envenomation. Barriers to fang penetration and other factors may result in no venom being injected. Patients must be watched for a sufficient length of time (i.e. 8 to 10 hours for a viperid bite and 24 hours for a coral snakebite) to ensure that this is the case.

If an envenomation has occurred, the family and species of snake generally determines the spectrum of symptoms and signs. The amount of venom, specific venom components, and underlying health status of the victim determine severity.

Viperid Envenomations

Epidemiology and Recognition

Viperid snakes are distributed throughout North America, with the exception of Maine. Bites are more common in southern states and during summer months, but they occur year-round and may occur at any time and in any location with captive collections. The various genera and species of viperids in the United States have relatively stable geographic ranges, with much overlap. Many different species of venomous snakes may inhabit any given area. Nonvenomous or mildly venomous colubrid snakes are also native to the United States. Viperids, also called pit vipers (i.e., rattlesnakes, copperheads, and cottonmouths), may be recognized, in general, by a triangular-shaped head, with the so-called pit (an infrared heat-detection organ) located approximately midway between the nostril and the eye, and pupils shaped like those of a cat (not round).

Pit vipers have large, movable fangs through which venom is injected into the victim. Because the fangs are curved, venom is usually injected subcutaneously rather than into deeper muscle compartments. Because of anatomic and other physical factors, bite wounds may appear as scratches or as one or more punctures. Envenomation may occur with any break in the skin.

Viperid venom is complex, consisting of dozens of proteolytic enzymes, small peptides, phospholipases, and other elements responsible for the spectrum of clinical effects seen. There is a great variability in this complex poison between species, within species, and even within a single specimen over the course of a season and its entire life span.

Clinical Effects

The spectrum of clinical effects is based on the specific genus or species of viperid and is unpredictable, ranging from non-envenomation (a "dry bite"; up to 25% of bites) to life-threatening reactions. Viperid snake envenomation invariably results in tissue injury, manifested by pain and progressive swelling, and it may include ecchymosis, elevated tissue and compartment pressures, tissue necrosis, and tissue loss. The complete absence of local effects can be used as a reliable marker of nonenvenomation in a viperid bite as long as a sufficient period (8 to 10 hours) of observation has occurred.

Systemic effects may occur, including hematologic, neurologic, cardiovascular, and nonspecific findings. Rattlesnake envenomations are more likely to result in hematologic effects, such as thrombocytopenia, hypofibrinogenemia, or prolongation of the prothrombin time (PT) or activated partial thromboplastin time (aPTT) and are more likely to produce neurologic effects, such as muscle fasciculation or weakness, compared with copperhead or cottonmouth envenomations; however, these effects can be seen with any viperid snake. Hypotension reactions from direct myocardial depression or from type 1 hypersensitivity (i.e., anaphylactic or anaphylactoid) may occur with any viperid exposure. Nausea, vomiting, diaphoresis, anxiety, and other nonspecific effects may be seen.

Duration of Clinical Effects

Local effects may develop rapidly or may not be apparent for many hours. Progression may occur for 24 to 36 hours, with resolution of tissue injury occurring over 3 to 6 weeks. Complications of tissue necrosis or infection have their own time frame of resolution. Hematologic effects usually begin within 1 to 2 hours of envenomation. If antivenom is given within this time frame, the detection of those effects may be masked and become apparent only after unbound antivenom has been eliminated from the body, usually within a week after treatment. Hematologic effects may persist for 1 to 3 weeks after an envenomation. Neurologic and other systemic effects tend to occur within a few hours of envenomation and resolve over 24 to 36 hours.

Severity of Envenomation

Untreated, local injury worsens over time, with proximal progression of tissue injury. Hematologic effects can be profound, resulting in spontaneous hemorrhage. Hypotension may be profound and can result in death. Neurologic and other systemic effects are rarely life-threatening events. Owing to changes in basic medical care and healthcare systems, it is not directly applicable to compare case-fatality rates before the introduction of antivenom

| BOX 1 | Prehospital Management of Viperid Envenomation |

- Remove jewelry.
- Splint the extremity and position just below heart level.
- Expeditiously transport to a healthcare facility.
- Consider use of a lymphatic constriction band (blood pressure cuff at 50 mm Hg in upper extremities, 70 mm Hg in lower extremities) *for life-threatening effects only.*
- Obtain intravenous access if possible.
- Do not use cutting, sucking, heat, cold, or other local "therapies."

(1950) with what can be expected today. Currently, there are fewer than five deaths from viperid snakebites per year in the United States.

Management

Determining Whether Envenomation Has Occurred and Its Severity

Owing to the unpredictability of envenomation and the variability of possible clinical effects, each viperid bite must be assessed and responded to individually (Box 1). It is important to determine whether an envenomation has occurred. If there are no signs or symptoms of envenomation, there is no indication for antivenom or other specific treatment. The severity of the envenomation helps to determine the amount of antivenom required to counter and neutralize venom effects, but this may not be immediately apparent because envenomations tend to progress over time, and what may at first appear to be mild venom effects may progress to a severe envenomation.

Initial Hospital Management

On arrival at the hospital, jewelry should be removed and the bitten extremity loosely splinted. The wound should be cleaned and explored, and a radiograph or ultrasound should be performed to rule out the presence of a foreign body (Box 2). Tetanus status should be updated if required. In the absence of other factors, the extremity should be positioned slightly below heart level until antivenom is started and it should then be elevated. If there are immediate life-threatening effects (e.g., anaphylaxis, hypotension), the extremity should be placed in an inferior position and consideration given to impeding venom entry into central circulation by means of a lymphatic constriction band or pressure immobilization bandage, weighing the potential benefit against the possible risk of increased local tissue injury from increasing venom concentration and duration in the tissues. Patients often require opioid-level pain relief.

At least one large intravenous line should be initiated and crystalloid infused as required. Initial hospital therapy, including a first dose of antivenom, should be provided in an area capable of close monitoring of vital signs and capable of managing life-threatening reactions; this usually is an emergency department. Whether an intensive care unit or similar patient care area is used for subsequent management depends on the clinical situation.

Indications for Antivenom

Owing to the safety of the current FDA-approved antivenoms and their ability to stop proximal progression of local tissue injury, all patients with signs of progressive local envenomation effects as well as those with significant systemic effects are candidates for treatment with antivenom. In areas where the ranges of rattlesnakes, copperheads, and/or cottonmouths overlap, CroFab is the only antivenom specifically indicated for the latter two snakes, if the biting species cannot be definitively determined. Aside from the benefit in managing systemic venom effects, a recent study of Fab antivenom in the treatment of copperhead envenomation demonstrated that antivenom improved limb function at 14 days post envenomation.

BOX 2 Hospital Diagnosis and Initial Management for Viperid Envenomation

- Remove jewelry.
- If an arterial or venous tourniquet has been placed, convert to a lymphatic constriction band.
- Obtain intravenous access, and use crystalloid as indicated.
- Obtain CBC with platelet count, PT or INR, aPTT, and fibrinogen level q 6–12 h for 1 day and then daily if values are abnormal. An initial D-dimer value (or fibrin degradation products) should be obtained to detect fibrinogenolytic activity that may not yet have produced hypofibrinogenemia. Multiple D-dimer determinations are not required beyond 2 h of envenomation and an elevated D-dimer is not an independent indication for antivenom. It is an indication of fibrinogenolytic activity and indicates the potential for late hypofibrinogenemia.
- Determine whether an envenomation has occurred.
- Determine severity based on the family or species of snake, age and health status of the victim, and development and rate of progression of signs and symptoms (e.g., local injury, hematologic abnormalities, hypotension, and other systemic effects).
- Determine the tetanus vaccination status and update if necessary.
- Seek consultation from a poison center: 1-800-222-1222.
- If a pressure immobilization or lymphatic constriction band was placed before arriving at the hospital, determine whether antivenom is indicated, and remove the band after the antivenom infusion has started.
- If there are minimal or no signs of envenomation or if the bands are placed inappropriately, remove them under close observation.
- Determine whether antivenom is indicated and administered per protocol.
- Provide basic wound care (i.e., cleaning and radiograph), and determine whether local injury requires specific management.
- Determine whether hematologic or other systemic effects require specific management.

aPTT, Activated partial thromboplastin time; *CBC,* complete blood cell count; *INR,* international normalized ratio; *PT,* prothrombin time.

Depending on the original indication for treatment (local effects, systemic effects, or both), initial control of envenomation effects is the goal of the loading dose of antivenom. Currently, there are two FDA-approved viperid antivenoms for North American pit viper envenomation: CroFab and Anavip. The incidence of type 1 reactions with CroFab and Anavip are low and generally mild and were found to be similar between products in the comparative trial. Pretreatment sensitivity testing is not required or recommended. There are rare reports of IgE-mediated type 1 hypersensitivity reactions on repeat exposure in individuals who were previously treated with CroFab, but most people who have been previously treated do not develop an adverse reaction to subsequent administrations. The incidence of type 3 hypersensitivity reactions ("serum sickness") with both antivenoms was approximately 2.5% in the comparative trial. In a recent study with a structured interview at 21 days post-envenomation, and liberal attribution of symptoms as possible type 3 effects, rates were 36% and 44% with Anavip and CroFab, respectively. All effects were mild and rarely required treatment.

The half-life of CroFab is approximately 18 to 24 hours, which is considerably shorter than IgG or F(ab')₂ antivenoms, and it is believed to be responsible for the recurrence of hematologic effects in 50% to 70% of patients with an initial coagulopathy. Anavip has a longer half-life (approximately 133 hours) and a lower risk of subacute coagulopathy. In a study during Anavip's first year of commercial marketing, none of the 11 patients (6 with initial coagulopathy) developed recurrence or late, new-onset hematological effects. In comparison, 6 of 22 (27%) patients treated with CroFab developed recurrent or late, new-onset effects and 50% of those had an early hematologic effect.

For confirmed and progressive envenomations, antivenom is administered as an intravenous solution, with 4 to 6 vials of Cro-Fab, or 10 vials of Anavip diluted into 250 mL of normal saline. The infusion should be started at 25 to 50 mL/h over the first 5 to 10 minutes and then the rate increased to finish by 1 hour if there is no reaction. Type 1 reactions are usually anaphylactoid (rate-related, not IgE-mediated) in nature or reflect true anaphylaxis (IgE-mediated). Anaphylaxis is usually, but not always, more severe and distinguishing between them is mostly based on a history of prior exposure or reaction.

If a type 1 reaction occurs, the infusion should be slowed or stopped, depending on the severity, and appropriate symptomatic treatment should be started with H₁- and H₂-blockers, epinephrine, corticosteroids, and other supportive measures, as required. It should be determined whether antivenom is still required, and if so, it should be restarted at a slower rate or higher dilution, or both, and consideration should be given to using an antivenom from a different source animal. CroFab is raised in sheep and Anavip in horses.

Treatment of Local Tissue Injury

Monitoring of the proximal extent of the active leading edge of edema, an indication for antivenom usually seen as a raised, tender, and perhaps erythematous margin, is usually sufficient to document progressive local injury. There is little to no value in circumferential measurements of extremities, although comparisons between right and left in large fleshy areas (e.g., the thigh) may be helpful in detecting a deeper envenomation. If the antivenom is given exclusively for local findings, the syndromic response to envenomation is deemed to be controlled if there is cessation of proximal progression of edema at the end of the infusion. There is often some redistribution of existing tissue edema, but uncontrolled proximal progression is usually seen as an active leading edge of edema. If antivenom is being given for hematologic effects, cessation of worsening or reversal should be seen. Often, thrombocytopenia rebounds dramatically. Hypofibrinogenemia may not rebound as quickly or merely stabilize because the liver must manufacture new fibrinogen. Although an elevated D-dimer value indicates fibrinogenolytic activity, it is not an independent indicator for antivenom treatment.

Other systemic effects may serve as indicators for antivenom use, and they should show control by the end of the initial infusion. If initial control is not deemed to have occurred, additional doses of antivenom should be administered until initial control is determined to have occurred. Most patients achieve initial control with 4 to 12 vials of Fab antivenom and 10 to 20 vials of F(ab')₂AV.

Maintenance Doses

Because of the rapid decline of antivenom levels resulting from the larger volume of distribution of CroFab, a Fab antivenoms, after initial control is achieved, maintenance dosing of 2 vials every 6 hours for three doses is commenced. This usually maintains adequate antivenom serum levels to prevent recurrence of local tissue injury progression. If progression of local effects does recur, an additional 2 vials of antivenom are usually sufficient to control local worsening. Routine maintenance dosing with Anavip, a F(ab'2 antivenom, is not recommended. In the comparative clinical trial of Anavip versus CroFab, additional antivenom was not required in any of the 38 patients who received placebo maintenance doses following initial control with Anavip. In a two-year post-marketing study, neither maintenance nor rescue doses were required with Anavip. If required, however, 4 vials should be used. Tissue pressures may be increased and elevated muscle compartment pressures may be identified when measured directly. My colleagues and I do not routinely measure tissue or compartment pressures. When pressures are measured and demonstrated to be elevated, it should be remembered that the mechanisms of these phenomena are different from muscle compartment syndromes. For example, extensive edema in the subcutaneous space circumferentially in an extremity may elevate compartment pressures by extrinsic compression. Case reports and series suggest that additional antivenom and extremity elevation result in reduced tissue and compartment pressures. Intracompartmental injection of venom can result in a true compartment syndrome; however, there is no evidence that fasciotomy is beneficial in this setting, and there are animal data to suggest that it may result in worse clinical outcomes.

Bleb formation at the site of a bite is not an important sign in and of itself, although it may suggest significantly elevated tissue pressures resulting in dermal-epidermal separation or the presence of tissue necrosis. Bleb fluid may contain unneutralized venom. It is reasonable to unroof blebs at or near the bite site and to debride obviously necrotic tissue, which usually becomes apparent several days after the bite.

Antibiotics

The incidence of culture-proven infection in the United States, viperid bites is low, probably less than 5%. There are no data to support the use of prophylactic antibiotics, and it is best to limit the opportunities for adverse drug effects. It is often difficult to distinguish inflammatory venom effects from infection starting on the second day after an envenomation. If antibiotics are prescribed, a first-generation, broad-spectrum agent should be used.

Long-Term Local Tissue Effects

The edema and tissue injury produced by most North American viperid envenomations usually resolves within one to two months, and a return to normal function can be anticipated; however, tissue necrosis or deep tissue injury may result in longer-term or even permanent structural and functional disability. Loss of tissue may occur, including digits and other parts of extremities, although this is rare and may be associated with pre-hospital application of tourniquets or other imprudent surgical interventions, delayed care, or complications such as infections. Some victims engage in behaviors that result in multiple envenomations, and this may increase the risks of long-term tissue injury. Although the use of and time to antivenom do not seem to change the incidence of tissue necrosis, this is rare in North American viperid envenomations. Early antivenom treatment is associated with faster recovery and antivenom administration associated with decreased opioid use. In a study of 45 patients with copperhead envenomations, those treated within 5.47 hours had a significantly shorter time to full recovery. In another study of 74 patients with copperhead envenomations, the proportion of patients who used opioids post-treatment was decreased in FabAV-treated patients compared with those given a placebo (OR 5.67 times increased opioid use in placebo-treated patients).

Hematologic Abnormalities and Bleeding

One or more hematologic abnormalities may occur with native viperid envenomation (Box 3). Significant decreases in platelet count or fibrinogen concentrations are independent indications for antivenom treatment. Isolated, mild prolongations of PT or aPTT may not require antivenom treatment; however, these effects may be progressive or indicate an impending hypofibrinogenemia, and early antivenom treatment may prevent severe abnormalities. Even if platelets, fibrinogen, and intrinsic and extrinsic clotting systems are involved, the end result is not a true disseminated intravascular coagulopathy because there is no true intravascular coagulation. Sufficient platelets, fibrinogen, and thrombin are usually available for hemostasis, and clinically significant bleeding is rarely seen; however, severe depletion of individual clotting elements or a combination of hematologic abnormalities can result in bleeding.

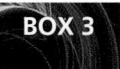

BOX 3 | Management of Hematologic Effects and Recurrence in Viperid Envenomation

- CroFab
  - Administer 4–6 vials of antivenom (Crotalidae Polyvalent Immune Fab [Ovine, CroFab]) in rattlesnake, copperhead, or cottonmouth envenomations for significant abnormalities of platelet count, PT or INR, aPTT, or fibrinogen.
- Anavip
  - Administer 10 vials of antivenom Crotalidae Immune F(ab')₂ ([Equine], Anavip) in rattlesnake envenomations for significant abnormalities of platelet count, PT or INR, aPTT, or fibrinogen.
- An elevated D-dimer value indicates accelerated fibrinogen breakdown and should prompt close monitoring of the fibrinogen concentrations, but it is not an independent indication to treat with antivenom. A single D-dimer should be obtained at >4 h post-envenomation.
- Administer additional antivenom in 4–6-vial (CroFab) or 10-vial (Anavip) increments until there is reversal of hematologic abnormalities. Replacement of platelets, clotting factors, or fibrinogen may be gradual, and a positive trend indicates neutralization of venom or replacement in excess of venom effect.
- Patients with initial hematologic effects or who were treated within 1–2 h of envenomation are at risk for recurrent effects 2–4 days after treatment and should be followed closely, every other day, until no recurrence at 7 days or daily for declining parameters.
- Consider treating recurrent hematologic abnormalities with additional antivenom. Indications include platelets < 25,000/mm³; fibrinogen < 50 mg/dL; INR > 5; aPTT >150 seconds; and lesser abnormalities involving more than one parameter.
- Consider readmission for severe abnormalities, other risk factors (e.g., uncontrolled hypertension, advanced age, other bleeding diatheses), or clinically significant bleeding.
- Administer blood products *plus* additional antivenom for significant bleeding.

aPTT, Activated partial thromboplastin time; *INR*, international normalized ratio; *PT*, prothrombin time.

The management of initial or persistent laboratory abnormalities is achieved with additional antivenom. Administration of blood products (e.g., fresh-frozen plasma, platelet concentrates, other blood products) should be reserved for clinically significant bleeding and given in conjunction with additional antivenom because transfused elements are similarly likely to be consumed by venom activity. Ecchymosis in damaged tissues, expansion of the vascular volume from crystalloid administration, and red blood cell hemolysis from hemolytic venom factors may produce an anemia that may rarely require a red blood cell transfusion.

Recurrence of Hematologic Effects

Approximately 70% of patients who develop an initial hematologic effect will have a recurrence of those effects, usually beginning several days after initial treatment, which may not manifest for up to 1 week. The incidence of recurrence of hematologic abnormalities was 5% to 10% with Anavip and 30% with CroFab in the comparative trial. One likely mechanism is recurrent unneutralized venomemia after elimination of unbound antivenom. Because Anavip has a longer half-life, it remains in circulation longer and thus provides longer protection against recurrence. Post-discharge hematologic abnormalities may be severe, or even appear to be occurring de novo if the patient was treated soon after envenomation, blunting the acute effects of the venom and masking the true severity of the envenomation.

In the first two years of post-marketing experience, in one study of persistent, recurrent, or late hematological effects in rattlesnake envenomations, there were significantly fewer such events with Anavip than with CroFab antivenom (4% v 22%; p = .04848). There were similar rates of Type 1 reactions, bleeding complications and readmissions.

In patients treated with CroFab, those who present with severe early hematologic effects, an elevated D-dimer, or an increase in the platelet count of more than 20% within 4 hours of the initial antivenom dose, or who are treated with antivenom within 1 to 2 hours of envenomation, are at risk for severe recurrent effects and should be followed closely after discharge. Although the incidence of significant bleeding is low, even with profound laboratory abnormalities, it seems prudent to administer additional antivenom if the platelet count is less than 25,000, the fibrinogen level is less than 50 mg/dL, the PT or aPTT values indicate nonclotting, there is a combination of significant defects in coagulation, or there are underlying medical conditions that make hemorrhage more likely, such as advanced age, hypertension, or a bleeding diathesis. Additional antivenom may be given for severe hematologic effects or abnormalities associated with significant bleeding. In patients who have been discharged and who are not actively bleeding, additional CroFab antivenom has been given in an outpatient setting and the patients followed daily. Such additional doses may be needed for more than 2 weeks. For patients who remain hospitalized or are readmitted, CroFab antivenom has been given by continuous IV infusion in a number of individual cases and small case series. An infusion initiated at 3 vials over 24 hours and titrated to clinical effect (up to 4 vials per 24 hours) was successful in reversing recurrent hematologic effects in all five cases reported in one series. Sterility and stability data for this product during prolonged administration are not currently available, however. If used in this way, sterile reconstitution and infusing 1 vial continuously over no more than 8 hours (3 vials per 24 hours) would be prudent. All patients treated in this way were able to discontinue antivenom administration within 14 days and most were able to discontinue it within 7 to 10 days post-envenomation.

Disposition

Patients whose local effects are regressing and do not have complications, such as infection or necrosis, and whose hematologic and other systemic effects are controlled, may be discharged. Typically, this occurs between 36 and 48 hours after envenomation but may be delayed for up to a week. Patients with any venom-related hematologic abnormality during hospitalization (thrombocytopenia, hypofibrinogenemia, elevated D-dimer, or prolonged PT/international normalized ratio [PT/INR] or aPTT) should have at least one repeat set of labs within 7 days of treatment because there is a risk of recurrent effects or late, new onset of hematologic abnormalities. In my practice, I obtain one set of labs at 3 to 4 days in high-risk patients and a second at 5 to 7 days. Ongoing pain relief may be required, with an effort to transition to nonopioid agents during the first week, and the patient should be warned to watch for signs of serum sickness. In patients considered at low risk for late, new onset or recurrent coagulopathy and thrombocytopenia, nonsteroidal antiinflammatory drugs (NSAIDs) and acetaminophen are reasonable first-line agents. Occupational or physical therapy should be arranged to maximize return of function, and follow-up for local and systemic effects should be arranged.

Elapid Envenomations
Epidemiology and Recognition

The US coral snakes can be recognized by their distinctive band pattern, with a red band seeming to be placed on top of a larger yellow band. This color pattern applies only to North American coral snakes. Each year, there are approximately 75 to 100 bites by coral snakes in the United States. Two genera and several species inhabit the United States, with the *Micrurus* genus responsible for most bites in Florida, Texas, Georgia, Louisiana, Alabama, and some neighboring states. A smaller genus, *Micruroides*, is found

in Arizona and New Mexico, but it is responsible for very few bites, and there have been no reports of serious envenomations in recent years. Bites are more common during the warmer months.

Elapids have fixed, relatively short fangs, which may decrease the rate of envenomation. More than one puncture, deep punctures, and this type of snake being one that tends to hold on are all factors that increase the risk of envenomation.

Clinical Effects

Envenomation by the coral snake primarily produces neurologic toxicity from presynaptic toxins, initially producing bulbar muscle weakness, ptosis, diplopia, and dysphagia. These effects can begin within 15 to 30 minutes or may be delayed up to 24 hours after an envenomation. Muscle weakness and paralysis progress to include respiratory muscles, and they can result in respiratory arrest and death. Typical of presynaptic toxins, effect progression can be arrested with the use of antivenom, but the effects are not rapidly reversed. Typically, there is little or no local tissue injury, and the absence of local injury cannot be used to exclude envenomation. Likewise, there is usually no effect on hematologic function, and other systemic effects are rare. Patients cannot be assumed to have eluded envenomation by a coral snake because they lack these symptoms and should be observed for at least 24 hours before concluding that an envenomation has not occurred.

Because of changes in basic medical care and healthcare systems, it is not directly applicable to compare case-fatality rates before the introduction of antivenom (1967) with what can be expected today; however, at that time, the case-fatality rate was approximately 10%.

Management

Because of the potential for rapid progression of motor paralysis and respiratory compromise, the difficulty of reversing paralysis after it is established, and the lack of local effects, it is reasonable to attempt to slow the venom's progression into the circulation until a decision regarding antivenom can be made. A pressure immobilization band (i.e., elastic bandage wrapped from an extremity's tip to the trunk with the degree of tension used for sprains) is used for this purpose for elapid envenomations elsewhere in the world (Boxes 4 and 5). In Australian studies, a pressure immobilization bandage has been shown to slow venom absorption and in those studies, bandage pressures have been between 40 and 70 mm Hg in the upper extremity and 55 to 70 mm Hg in the lower extremity. However, the proper technique requires training, and the infrequency of these bites makes teaching and retention of such skills problematic. A blood pressure cuff inflated to similar pressures may also slow venom entry into circulation, and it can be a more reliable and easily taught technique, although it has not been validated in clinical studies.

Standard wound care should be performed, including cleansing the wound, obtaining a radiograph, and updating the tetanus status, if required. Wound infection is uncommon, and prophylactic antibiotics are not recommended.

As the first signs of envenomation can be rapidly progressive neurotoxicity and because of the difficulty of reversing paralysis, some authorities have proposed administering antivenom in cases in which an envenomation is possible before the appearance of any clinical symptoms. Others have pointed to the infrequency of respiratory muscle paralysis, resulting in the need for intubation and respiratory support, and to possible geographic differences in snake toxicity, and they have counseled observation and antivenom treatment only after envenomation has been confirmed by progressive symptoms. Recent analysis of the national database has not demonstrated a significant difference in clinical severity between Florida and Texas coral snake envenomations, which supports early treatment when envenomation is suspected. As of February 2020, Pfizer has new, in-date coral snake antivenom listed as in stock and available for shipment (ordering phone number: 844-646-4398). Poison centers will also have information on antivenom availability in their regions. When paralysis has progressed to

---

BOX 4   Prehospital Management of Elapid Envenomation

- Remove jewelry.
- Splint the extremity and position just below heart level.
- Expeditiously transport to a healthcare facility.
- Apply a pressure immobilization bandage (i.e., 3–4-inch crepe bandage at lymphatic pressure from the tip of the extremity to the trunk) or a lymphatic constriction band (i.e., wide rubber band or blood pressure cuff at 15–25 mm Hg) proximal to the bite site.
- Obtain intravenous access if possible.
- Do not use cutting, sucking, heat, cold, or other local "therapies."

BOX 5   Hospital Diagnosis and Initial Management of Elapid Envenomation

- Remove jewelry.
- If an arterial or a venous tourniquet has been placed, convert to a lymphatic constriction band.
- Obtain intravenous access, and use crystalloid as indicated.
- Determine whether an envenomation has occurred.
- Determine severity based on the family or species of snake, the age and health status of the victim, and the rate of progression of signs or symptoms (i.e., paralysis and other neurologic effects).
- Determine the tetanus vaccination status and update if necessary.
- Seek consultation from a poison center: 1-800-222-1222.
- If a pressure immobilization band or lymphatic constriction band has been placed before arrival at the hospital, determine whether antivenom is required, and begin antivenom infusion before removing the band.
- Determine whether antivenom is indicated, and administer per protocol.
- Provide basic wound care (i.e., cleaning and radiograph), and determine whether local injury requires specific management.
- Determine whether other systemic effects require specific management.

---

significant airway compromise, complete or partial reversal with antivenom may not be possible and aggressive and meticulous respiratory support, including intubation and ventilation, may be needed for days or weeks. If an FDA-approved coral snake antivenom is not readily available, there are reports of coral snake antivenoms from Mexico, Costa Rica, and Brazil, and of tiger snake antivenom from Australia, reversing the neurotoxicity of *M. tener*. The use of foreign, non-FDA-approved antivenoms should be reserved for circumstances where an FDA-approved product is not available in a timely manner and, if possible, with prior FDA Office of Biologics approval (240-402-8010; 800-835-4709; after-hours emergency: 866-300-4374; 301-796-8240; industry.biologics@fda.gov). Since these drugs are imported into the United States as Investigational New Drugs, institutional Investigational Review Boards will also have notification requirements.

Exotic Snakebite
Epidemiology and Clinical Effects
In the United States, most exotic snake envenomations occur in private collections. These are not usually known to authorities or healthcare providers until an envenomation occurs, and they may involve the collection owner or family members, including children. They may occur in any locale, and victims may present to any healthcare facility.

Viperid and elapid snakes, which account for the bulk of venomous bites worldwide, have patterns of venom activity similar to those of their North American counterparts, with some variation and with generally greater toxicity for some non-US species. Some nonnative elapids, such as cobras, mambas, black snakes, or taipans, produce much higher rates of respiratory paralysis and may produce much greater local tissue injury than US coral snakes. Similarly, envenomation from some nonnative viperids, such as *Bothrops*, *Echis*, or *Bitis* species, or from an African colubrid, such as the boomslang, results in a greater risk of bleeding. Some of these species may directly activate prothrombin (e.g., *Echis* species, *Bothrops* species) and factor X (e.g., *Vipera* species, *Dispholidus* species), leading to a venom-induced consumptive coagulopathy with intravascular thrombosis, marked organ dysfunction, and, potentially, death.

Management
The specific management of exotic envenomations is beyond the scope of this chapter. Not all venomous exotic snakes have antivenoms, and even for snakes with antivenoms, they may not be available in the United States, although zoos stock antivenoms for snakes in their collections. An updatable online database, the Antivenom Index, lists these antivenoms and is accessible to regional poison centers. For information on exotic antivenoms and assistance in managing an exotic snake envenomation, the regional poison center should be contacted.

References
Anderson VE, Gerardo CJ, Rapp-Olsson M, et al: Early administration of Fab antivenom resulted in faster limb recovery in copperhead snake envenomation patients, *Clin Toxicol (Phila)* 57(1):25–30, 2019. https://doi.org/10.1080/15563650.2018.1491982.Epub.2018.Sep.3.

Boyer LV, Seifert SA, Cain JS: Recurrence phenomena after immunoglobulin therapy for snake envenomations. Part 2. Guidelines for clinical management with Crotaline Fab antivenom, *Ann Emerg Med* 37:196–201, 2001.

Boyer LV, Seifert SA, Clark RF, et al: Recurrent and persistent coagulopathy following pit viper envenomation, *Arch Intern Med* 159(7):706–710, 1999.

Bush SP, Ruha AM, Seifert SA: Comparison of F(ab')2 versus Fab antivenom for pit viper envenomation: a prospective, blinded, multicenter, randomized clinical trial, *Clin Toxicol (Phila)* 53(1):37–45, 2015. https://doi.org/10.3109/15563650.2014.974263. Epub 2014 Oct 31.

Bush SP, Seifert SA, Oakes J, et al: Continuous IV crotalidae polyvalent immune fab (ovine) (FabAV) for selected North American rattlesnake bite patients, *Toxicon* 69:29–37, 2013. https://doi.org/10.1016/j.toxicon.2013.02.008. Epub 2013 Mar 6.

Extension of Expiration Date of Coral Snake Antivenin: https://www.fda.gov/vaccines-blood-biologics/safety-availability-biologics/expiration-date-extension-north--american-coral-snake-antivenin-micrurus-fulvius-equine-origin-lot-1.

Freiermuth CE, Lavonas EJ, Anderson VE, Kleinschmidt KC, Sharma K, Rapp-Olsson M, Gerardo C, Copperhead Recovery Workgroup: Antivenom treatment is associated with fewer patients using opioids after copperhead envenomation, *West J Emerg Med* 20(3):497–505, 2019. https://doi.org/10.5811/westjem.2019.3.42693. Epub 2019 Apr 26.

Gerardo CJ, Quackenbush E, Lewis B: The efficacy of crotalidae polyvalent immune fab (ovine) antivenom versus placebo plus optional rescue therapy on recovery from copperhead snake envenomation: a randomized, double-blind, placebo-controlled, clinical trial, *Ann Emerg Med* 70(2):233–244, 2017.

Gold BS, Barish RA, Dart RC: North American snake envenomation: Diagnosis, treatment, and management, *Emerg Med Clin North Am* 22(2):423–443, 2004. ix.

Kitchens CS, Van Mierop LH: Envenomation by the Eastern coral snake (*Micrurus fulvius fulvius*). A study of 39 victims, *JAMA* 258(12):1615–1618, 1987.

McAninch SA, Morrissey RP, Rosen P, Meyer TA, Hessel MM, Vohra MH: Snake eyes: coral snake neurotoxicity associated with ocular absorption of venom and successful treatment with exotic antivenom, *J Emerg Med* 56(5):519–522, 2019. https://doi.org/10.1016/j.jemermed.2019.01.019. Epub 2019 Mar 14.

Pham HX, Mullins ME. Safety of nonsteroidal anti-inflammatory drugs in copperhead snakebite patients. *Clin Toxicol*, 1121–1127, 2018.

Seifert SA, Boyer LV: Recurrence phenomena after immunoglobulin therapy for snake envenomations. Part 1. Pharmacokinetics and pharmacodynamics of immunoglobulin antivenoms and related antibodies, *Ann Emerg Med* 37(2):189–195, 2001.

Seifert SA, Boyer LV, Dart RC, et al: Relationship of venom effects to venom antigen and antivenom serum concentrations in a patient with *Crotalus atrox* envenomation treated with a Fab antivenom, *Ann Emerg Med* 30(1)49–53, 1997.

Seifert SA, Kirschner RI, Martin N: Recurrent, persistent, or late, new-onset hematologic abnormalities in crotaline snakebite, *Clin Toxicol (Phila)* 49:324–329, 2011. https://doi.org/10.3109/15563650.2011.566883.

Seifert SA, Oakes JA, Boyer LV: Toxic Exposure Surveillance System (TESS)-based characterization of U.S. non-native venomous snake exposures, 1995–2004, *Clin Toxicol(Phila)* 45(5):571–578, 2007.

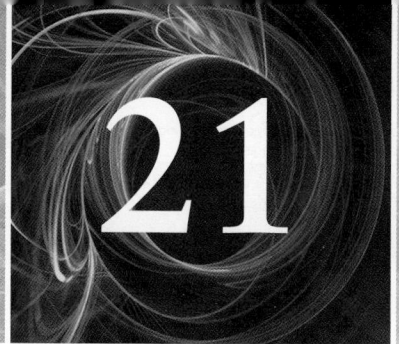

21 Preventive Health

IMMUNIZATION PRACTICES

Method of
Beth A. Damitz, MD

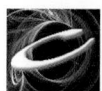

CURRENT DIAGNOSIS

- Single-agent and poly-agent variety vaccines are available in the United States.
- Vaccine-preventable diseases are occurring in the United States despite efforts.
- Vaccine registries and office-based strategies can increase vaccination rates.

CURRENT THERAPY

- Vaccination schedules are available through various sources such as the Centers for Disease Control and Prevention (CDC), including catch-up dosing.
- Vaccines can prevent diseases that are still occurring in the United States.
- Vaccination registry participation can increase vaccination rates.
- Each office visit should be used as an opportunity to review and offer vaccines.
- Providers need to be aware of special populations such as breast-feeding and pregnant women, immunosuppressed persons, and healthcare workers who could need different vaccines.

Definitions and Background

Vaccination is one of the most successful and cost-effective ways to prevent infectious diseases. Immunization is the process of inducing immunity artificially by either active immunization or passive immunization. It also occurs naturally through transplacental transmission of antibodies to a fetus, which provides protection against many infectious diseases for the first few months of life.

Physiology of Vaccines

Vaccines prevent disease in the people who receive them and protect those who come into contact with unvaccinated individuals such as children too young to receive vaccines, those who cannot be immunized for medical reasons, and those who cannot make an adequate response to vaccination. Vaccines are preparations of proteins, polysaccharides, or nucleic acids of pathogens that are delivered to the immune system as single entities, as part of complex particles, or by live, attenuated agents to induce specific responses that inactivate, destroy, or suppress the pathogen.

Immunization Recommendations

The Advisory Committee on Immunization Practices (ACIP) sponsored by the Centers for Disease Control and Prevention

(CDC; https://www.cdc.gov/vaccines/schedules/hcp/index.html), the American Academy of Pediatrics (AAP), and the American Academy of Family Physicians (AAFP) work together to issue a national schedule for routinely recommended vaccinations. They recommend routine vaccination to prevent 17 vaccine-preventable diseases that occur in infants, children, adolescents, or adults. These recommendations are reviewed and revised periodically. These immunization schedules give ranges of target ages for vaccines to be given (Figures 1–4). They include single and combination vaccine products. Catch-up dosing and special-population schedules are also available (updated immunization schedules are available at https://www.cdc.gov/vaccines/schedules/index.html).

Disease Prevention

Since the development of vaccines, we have seen a dramatic decrease in both cases and deaths from vaccine-preventable diseases. For example, in 1950, there were 319,124 cases and 468 deaths from measles. This dramatically decreased to 43 cases and zero deaths in 2007. Obviously, decrease in disease and death is paramount, but it is also important to decrease the cost burden to our healthcare system. For every $1 spent on measles, mumps, and rubella (MMR) vaccine, $21 is saved in direct medical costs of treating a case of measles.

COVID-19 Vaccines

COVID-19 is a respiratory disease caused by SARS-CoV-2, a virus in the Coronavirus family, that was discovered first in China in December of 2019. It spread rapidly across the world, causing a pandemic. Pharmaceutical companies immediately pursued the development of vaccines to COVID-19. Within the next year, several COVID-19 vaccines were approved for emergency use. Currently, three vaccines are available in the United States from these manufacturers: Pfizer-BioNTech, Moderna, and Johnson & Johnson/Janssen. The Pfizer and Moderna vaccines are mRNA-derived vaccines. The Pfizer vaccine is approved for ages 12 and older and is delivered in a two-shot series 21 days apart. The Moderna vaccine is approved for ages 18 and older and is delivered in a two-shot series 28 days apart. The Johnson & Johnson vaccine is a viral vector–derived vaccine. It is approved for ages 18 and older and is a one-shot regimen. All three vaccines can have side effects. Common side effects are minor and include injection site redness, swelling and pain, fever, headaches, fatigue, muscle pain, and nausea. More severe reactions are rare. There have been reports of thrombosis with thrombocytopenia syndrome with the Johnson & Johnson vaccine. Women under the age of 50 seem to be at a higher risk. In addition, there have been reports of myocarditis and pericarditis after the second doses of the mRNA vaccines (Pfizer and Moderna). These reactions are rare, and the CDC has recommended to continue to offer these vaccines as the benefits outweigh the risks. As with many viruses, COVID-19 can and does mutate. At this time there have been several variants identified. Studies demonstrate that the available vaccines are effective against them. Of note, since COVID-19 is evolving, new information is constantly being obtained. It is advised to explore other resources such as https://www.cdc.gov for the most up-to-date information.

Immunization Responsibility

Appropriate vaccination is the responsibility of the healthcare team and patient (and parents). Education is critical. This can be

Recommended child and adolescent immunization schedule for ages 18 years or younger, United States, 2021

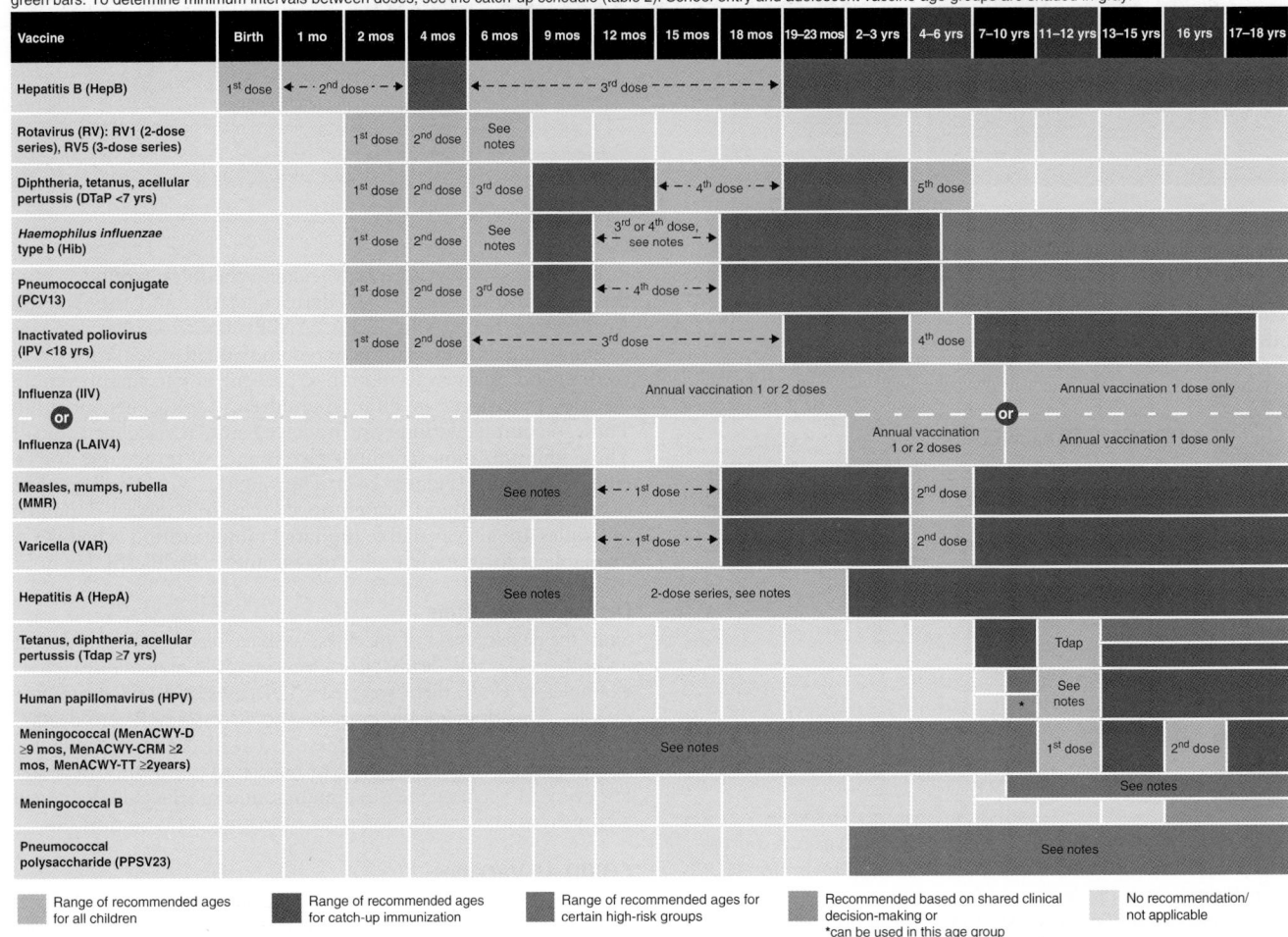

Figure 1 Recommended immunization schedule for children and adolescents aged 18 years or younger–United States, 2021. All notes may be accessed at: https://www.cdc.gov/vaccines/schedules/hcp/imz/child-adolescent.html. From the Centers for Disease Control and Prevention.

done through various dissemination techniques such as one-on-one counseling, posters in the office, health fairs, and handouts at school and work. An office-based strategy consists of nursing and physician education of updates and changes in vaccines, the ability to track patient immunization records through registries, sending reminder letters to patients that there are recommended vaccines, and adopting standing orders to take advantage of appropriate office visits to maximize vaccination opportunities.

There are many sources for keeping current on immunizations and vaccines including the CDC's *Morbidity and Mortality Weekly Report* (MMWR). For parents and patients, the vaccine information statement (VIS), which is made available by the CDC to inform patients about the risks and benefits of immunizations, is very helpful and by law must be distributed before administering any vaccine. After the patient reads the VIS, the physician can then give any further information or answer questions before administering the vaccine. This discussion should be documented in the patient's medical record, including the refusal to receive certain vaccines (i.e., informed refusal).

General Principles for Vaccine Scheduling
Optimal response to a vaccine depends on several factors, including the type of vaccine, age of the recipient, and immune status of the recipient. Simultaneous administration of vaccines increases the probability that a patient will be vaccinated fully by the appropriate age. Simultaneous administration of all age-appropriate doses of vaccines is recommended by the MMWR for children for whom no specific contraindications exist at the

time of the visit. The use of combination vaccine preparations greatly reduces the overall number of injections a child or patient will receive. However, care must be taken to ensure that the individual vaccine entities are not administered too early and too many are not administered at once. This can be a challenge when patients switch clinics or in times of vaccine shortages.

More often, dosing intervals longer than recommended are encountered in the office. With the exception of oral live typhoid vaccine (Vivotif Berna), an interruption in the vaccination schedule does not require restarting the entire series of a vaccine or toxoid or addition of extra doses. When an unknown or uncertain vaccination status is encountered, every effort should be made to access records. If this cannot be done in a reasonable amount of time, these persons should be considered susceptible and started on the age-appropriate vaccination schedule. Serologic testing for immunity is an alternative to vaccination; however, commercial serologic testing might not always be sufficiently sensitive or standardized for detection of vaccine-induced immunity, and research laboratory testing might not be readily available.

Route of Administration
There are three orally administered vaccines in the United States: rotavirus, cholera (Vaxchora), and typhoid vaccines. Rotavirus (Rotarix, RotaTeq) is licensed for infants and does not need to be repeated if the vaccine is spit up or vomited. Typhoid vaccine capsules (Vivotif) should be taken as directed by the manufacturer. Live, attenuated influenza vaccine (LAIV4, FluMist) is the only intranasal vaccine available. It does not need to be repeated

Recommended adult immunization schedule by age group, United States, 2021

Vaccine	19–26 years	27–49 years	50–64 years	≥65 years
Influenza inactivated (IIV) or **Influenza recombinant** (RIV4)		1 dose annually		
Influenza live, attenuated (LAIV4)	1 dose annually			
Tetanus, diphtheria, pertussis (Tdap or Td)	1 dose Tdap each pregnancy; 1 dose Td/Tdap for wound management (see notes)			
	1 dose Tdap, then Td or Tdap booster every 10 years			
Measles, mumps, rubella (MMR)	1 or 2 doses depending on indication (if born in 1957 or later)			
Varicella (VAR)	2 doses (if born in 1980 or later)		2 doses	
Zoster recombinant (RZV)			2 doses	
Human papillomavirus (HPV)	2 or 3 doses depending on age at initial vaccination or condition	27 through 45 years		
Pneumococcal conjugate (PCV13)	1 dose			1 dose
Pneumococcal polysaccharide (PPSV23)	1 or 2 doses depending on indication			1 dose
Hepatitis A (HepA)	2 or 3 doses depending on vaccine			
Hepatitis B (HepB)	2 or 3 doses depending on vaccine			
Meningococcal A, C, W, Y (MenACWY)	1 or 2 doses depending on indication, see notes for booster recommendations			
Meningococcal B (MenB)	19 through 23 years	2 or 3 doses depending on vaccine and indication, see notes for booster recommendations		
***Haemophilus influenzae* type b** (Hib)	1 or 3 doses depending on indication			

Recommended vaccination for adults who meet age requirement, lack documentation of vaccination, or lack evidence of past infection ▪ Recommended vaccination for adults with an additional risk factor or another indication ▪ Recommended vaccination based on shared clinical decision-making ▪ No recommendation/ not applicable

Figure 2 Recommended immunization schedule for adults aged 19 years and older–United States, 2021. All notes may be accessed at: https://www.cdc.gov/vaccines/schedules/hcp/imz/child-adolescent.html. From the Centers for Disease Control and Prevention.

if the person coughs or sneezes immediately after administration. Except for bacille Calmette-Guerin (BCG) vaccine and smallpox vaccine,[a] injectable vaccines are administered by the intramuscular or subcutaneous route.

Storage

In general, vaccines need to be stored in a refrigerator or freezer. When vaccines are inappropriately stored, they can lose potency. Refrigerator and freezer storage units must be properly monitored and maintained to ensure vaccine integrity. Temperature logs should be maintained for 3 years unless state or local authorities require a longer time. Vaccines that have been stored at inappropriate temperatures should not be administered. An office protocol should be established for handling inappropriately stored vaccines, procedures for follow-up when these vaccines are inadvertently given, emergency vaccine retrieval and storage, handling vaccine shipments, maintaining a vaccine inventory log, and rotating vaccine stock to avoid expiration. Care should be taken to store similar vaccine products (sound-alike or look-alike) away from each other (on different shelves) or by color-coding labels. Diphtheria toxoid-, tetanus toxoid-, and acellular pertussis-containing vaccines are easily confused.

Vaccine Safety

Vaccines in the United States undergo extensive safety and efficacy evaluations through the FDA licensing process. Despite this rigorous process, adverse reactions can and do occur. Adverse reactions are reportable to the Vaccine Adverse Event Reporting System (VAERS). VAERS is a national reporting system created in 1990 to unify the collection of all reports of adverse events after vaccination. Its primary purpose is detecting new or rare vaccine adverse events, increases in rates of known side effects, and risk factors for particular types of adverse events.

In 1986, the National Childhood Vaccine Injury Act established the Vaccine Injury Compensation Program (VICP). It is a no-fault program that covers all routinely recommended childhood vaccines. Those claims may be based on a vaccine injury table, which lists the adverse events associated with vaccines and provides a rebuttable presumption of causation, or by proving by preponderant evidence that the vaccine caused an injury not on the table. The table was created to provide swift compensation to those possibly injured by vaccines.

The provider's role to help ensure safety of vaccination includes proper vaccine storage and administration, timing and spacing of vaccine doses, observation of contraindications and precautions, and reporting adverse events to the VAERS.

Contraindications and Adverse Events

A contraindication is a condition in a recipient that increases the chance of a *serious* adverse reaction. A precaution is a condition in a recipient that *might* increase the chance or severity of an adverse reaction or compromise the ability of the vaccine to produce immunity. Situations do arise when the benefits outweigh the risks of a side effect. The only contraindication applicable to all vaccines is a history of a severe allergic reaction (anaphylaxis) after a previous dose of vaccine or to a vaccine component unless the recipient has been desensitized. Children who experienced encephalopathy within 7 days after administration of a previous dose of DTP,[2] DTaP

[a]Available in the United States from the Centers for Disease Control and Prevention.

[2]Not available in the United States.

Recommended adult immunization schedule by medical condition and other indications, United States, 2021

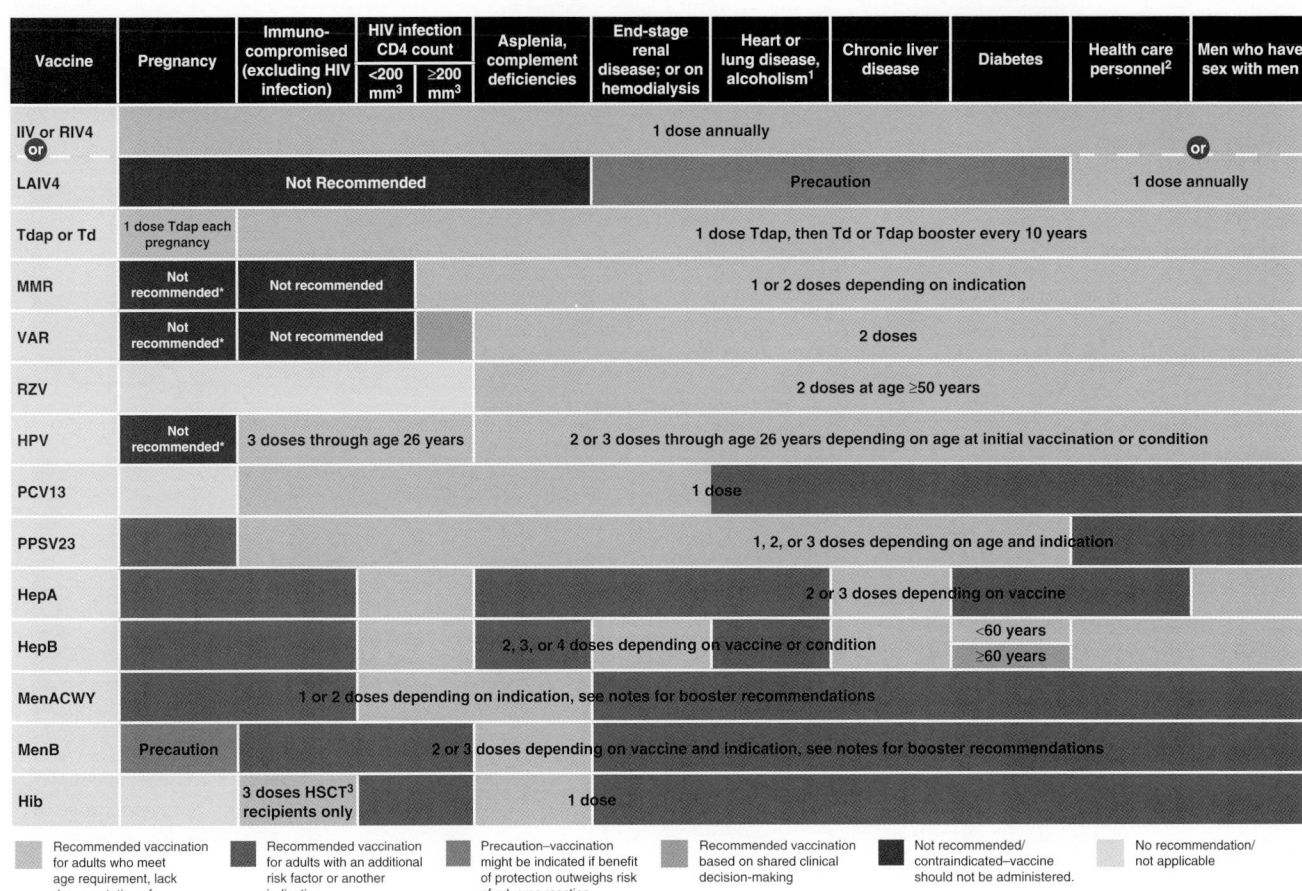

Vaccine	Pregnancy	Immuno-compromised (excluding HIV infection)	HIV infection CD4 count <200 mm³	HIV infection CD4 count ≥200 mm³	Asplenia, complement deficiencies	End-stage renal disease; or on hemodialysis	Heart or lung disease, alcoholism¹	Chronic liver disease	Diabetes	Health care personnel²	Men who have sex with men
IIV or RIV4 or	1 dose annually										or
LAIV4	Not Recommended					Precaution				1 dose annually	
Tdap or Td	1 dose Tdap each pregnancy	1 dose Tdap, then Td or Tdap booster every 10 years									
MMR	Not recommended*	Not recommended		1 or 2 doses depending on indication							
VAR	Not recommended*	Not recommended		2 doses							
RZV				2 doses at age ≥50 years							
HPV	Not recommended*	3 doses through age 26 years		2 or 3 doses through age 26 years depending on age at initial vaccination or condition							
PCV13		1 dose									
PPSV23		1, 2, or 3 doses depending on age and indication									
HepA		2 or 3 doses depending on vaccine									
HepB		2, 3, or 4 doses depending on vaccine or condition						<60 years			
								≥60 years			
MenACWY	1 or 2 doses depending on indication, see notes for booster recommendations										
MenB	Precaution	2 or 3 doses depending on vaccine and indication, see notes for booster recommendations									
Hib		3 doses HSCT³ recipients only	1 dose								

Recommended vaccination for adults who meet age requirement, lack documentation of vaccination, or lack evidence of past infection		Recommended vaccination for adults with an additional risk factor or another indication		Precaution–vaccination might be indicated if benefit of protection outweighs risk of adverse reaction		Recommended vaccination based on shared clinical decision-making	Not recommended/contraindicated–vaccine should not be administered. · No recommendation/not applicable · *Vaccinate after pregnancy.

1. Precaution for LAIV4 does not apply to alcoholism. 2. See notes for influenza; hepatitis B; measles, mumps, and rubella; and varicella vaccinations. 3. Hematopoietic stem cell transplant.

Figure 3 Recommended immunization schedule for adults aged 19 years or older by medical condition and other indications, United States, 2021. All notes may be accessed at: https://www.cdc.gov/vaccines/schedules/hcp/imz/adult-conditions.htm. From the Centers for Disease Control and Prevention.

(Daptacel, Infanrix), or Tdap (Adacel, Boostrix) not attributable to another identifiable cause should not receive additional doses of a vaccine that contains pertussis. The following are *not* contraindications to vaccination:

- Minor illness
- Diarrhea
- Mild or moderate local reaction or fever following a prior dose
- Antimicrobial therapy
- Disease exposure or convalescence
- Pregnant or immunosuppressed person in the household
- Premature birth
- Breast-feeding

Vaccination should be deferred for persons with a moderate or severe acute illness. This precaution avoids causing diagnostic confusion between manifestations of the underlying illness and possible adverse effects of vaccination or superimposing adverse effects of the vaccine on the underlying illness.

Vaccine adverse reactions are classified as local, systemic, or allergic. Allergic reactions might be caused by the vaccine antigen, residual animal protein, antimicrobial agents, preservatives, stabilizers, or other vaccine components. Anaphylaxis is rare and usually begins within minutes of vaccine administration. Children who have had an apparent severe allergic reaction to a vaccine should be evaluated by an allergist to determine the responsible allergen and to make recommendations regarding future vaccination.

Barriers

Barriers to appropriate and timely vaccination include patients' misconceptions, false contraindications, complexity of the immunization schedules, religious or philosophic beliefs, and cost. The Vaccines for Children Program (VCP) is a federally funded program that provides free ACIP-recommended vaccines to adolescents and children younger than 19 years old. This program has reduced the barrier of cost.

Recording Vaccinations

Healthcare providers who administer vaccines covered by the National Childhood Vaccine Injury Act are required to ensure that the permanent medical record of the recipient indicates the date the vaccine was administered, the vaccine manufacturer, the vaccine lot number, and the name, address, and title of the person administering the vaccine. In addition, the provider is required to record the edition date of the VIS distributed and the date those materials were provided. Patients should also keep a record of the immunizations they receive, when they were received, and at what facility they received them. A permanent vaccination record card should be established for each newborn infant and maintained by the parent or guardian.

Immunization information systems (IIS), formerly referred to as immunization registries, are confidential population-based computerized information systems that collect and consolidate vaccination data from multiple healthcare providers within a geographic area. The CDC oversees a network of 64 IIS programs distributed throughout all 50 states, the District of Columbia, and eight US territories. A fully operational IIS can prevent duplicate vaccinations, provide a complete record of immunizations if the patient has received vaccines from multiple sites, and offer catch-up and needed vaccine information. Although participation of a provider is voluntary, it is highly encouraged.

Special Populations

Children
Although infants are born with some level of immunoglobulin (Ig) G that is contributed from the mother via passive immunity, these levels generally decrease by 9 months of age, leaving them vulnerable to many infectious diseases. Infants begin developing IgG shortly after birth and continue to increase these levels throughout the first year of life, but they remain generally susceptible to infection until they achieve adult levels of IgG at 10 years of age. Therefore this age group is especially important to vaccinate.

Breast-Feeding
Neither inactivated nor live virus vaccines administered to a lactating woman affect the safety of breast-feeding for women or their infants. Breast-feeding is a contraindication for smallpox vaccination of the mother because of the theoretical risk for contact transmission from mother to infant. Yellow fever vaccine (YF-VAX) should be avoided. Breast-fed infants should be vaccinated according to the recommended schedule.

Pregnancy
No evidence exists of risk to the fetus from vaccinating pregnant women with inactivated virus or bacterial vaccines or toxoids. Live vaccines, such as smallpox, MMR, and varicella (Varivax), pose a theoretical risk to the fetus and therefore are generally contraindicated during pregnancy. New recommendations from ACIP advise to give all pregnant women a Tdap in every pregnancy. New data indicate that maternal antipertussis antibodies are short-lived; therefore Tdap vaccination in one pregnancy will not provide high levels of antibodies to protect newborns during subsequent pregnancies. Alternatively, if Tdap is not administered during pregnancy, the woman should receive a dose of Tdap as soon as possible after delivery to ensure pertussis immunity and reduce the risk for transmission to the newborn regardless of when she last received a tetanus booster. Routine influenza vaccination is recommended for all women who are or will be pregnant (in any trimester) during influenza season, which usually occurs early October through late March.

Altered Immunocompetence
Persons with altered immunocompetence include those with primary and secondary causes of immunodeficiency as well as those with asplenia, chronic kidney disease, treatments with therapeutic monoclonal antibodies, and prolonged administration of high-dose corticosteroids. In general, they should receive inactivated influenza virus (Afluria, Fluad, Fluarix, Fluzone) and age-appropriate polysaccharide-based vaccines (pneumococcal conjugate vaccine [PCV, Prevnar], pneumococcal polyvalent [PPSV, Pneumovax 23], meningococcal conjugate [MCV4, Menactra], meningococcal polysaccharide [MPSV4, Menomune], and haemophilus B conjugate [Hib, ActHib, PedvaxHib]). Persons with most forms of altered immunocompetence should not receive live vaccines (MMR, varicella, MMRV [ProQuad], LAIV, zoster [Zostavax], yellow fever, oral typhoid, BCG, and rotavirus).

Healthcare Personnel
Healthcare personnel are at substantial risk for acquiring or transmitting hepatitis B, influenza, measles, mumps, rubella, pertussis, and varicella and should be counseled on appropriate vaccinations.

TRAVEL MEDICINE

Method of
Kristine Matson, MD, MPH; and Dawd S. Siraj, MD, MPH&TM

The affordability and ease of cross-border travel, combined with the growing world population, is increasing the number of individuals traveling internationally. In 2018, the number of arriving international tourists in all countries exceeded 1.4 billion persons and the number of arrivals to countries with emerging markets has surpassed the number of arrivals to developed countries (UN World tourism paper. https://www.e-unwto.org/doi/pdf/10.18111/9789284419876). This increase in international travel has created a need for the specialty of Travel Medicine, which focuses on the unique and location-dependent health related needs of travelers.

An estimated 22% to 64% of travelers report some type of illness while abroad. Most of these illnesses are mild and self-limited, requiring minimal intervention. Approximately 4% of travelers who seek medical help have an acute, potentially life-threatening disease and about 1/100,000 of those travelers die from complications related to their travels.

The goal of a Travel Medicine visit is to maximize health and prevent illness while traveling by offering travelers specific structured advice, malaria prophylaxis, and immunization recommendations. Disease risks, current outbreaks, and local health conditions are destination-dependent and constantly change, thus the use of current, up-to-date resources is essential for providing Travel Medicine care. See Table 1. Unfortunately, 20% to 80% international travelers do not undergo a health consultation or receive location-specific pre-travel advice before traveling. Travelers visiting friends and relatives in their country of origin (VFR), pregnant mothers, children, and travelers who are staying abroad for a long period of time are at particularly high risk for morbidity and mortality during their trip, requiring special attention to pre-trip medical planning. Ideally pre-travel health consultations should take place 4 to 6 weeks prior to departure to give travelers adequate time to complete required vaccine series. Pre-travel health consultations should be structured and comprehensive. Table 2 lists items that require consideration and discussion during the consultation, as appropriate to the type of travel and destination. Patients should arrive to their consultation with documentation of their vaccination history. A useful "Travel History Form" is available on the Shoreland Travax website (www.travax.com).

Vaccinations
Travel clinics often provide travelers the opportunity to update routine vaccinations that they missed. Additionally, Travel Medicine provides vaccines that are recommended or required due to country- or ongoing outbreak-specific risks. When deciding which vaccination to recommend, several factors must be considered, including any specific potential risks associated with the travel itinerary, length of stay, and activities. For each vaccine-preventable disease (VPD), one should consider the prevalence and impact of the disease in question.

Routine Vaccinations
Routine vaccines are those that are administered at a regular interval for all individuals regardless of travel plans. As the risk of acquisition of these diseases increase during international travel, Travel Medicine providers should confirm that travelers are up to date on their routine vaccinations prior to departure. The recent importation of diseases such as measles and mumps, which have resulted in outbreaks of these diseases in the travelers' country of origin, are reminders of the importance of updating routine vaccinations prior to travel. Travelers are advised to bring documentation of all prior vaccinations to confirm vaccination status and determine the need for booster doses.

TABLE 1	List of Information Resources for Risk Assessment of Travel	
Centers for Disease Control and Prevention	Comprehensive travel reports and travel vaccination and preparation information including the Yellow Book with information on country-specific risks and travel advice	www.cdc.gov/travel/
Travax (Shoreland)	Commercial software–generated reports combining itinerary-specific recommendations on recommended travel vaccines and risks. Requires a fee.	www.shoreland.com
U.S. Department of State	Travel warnings	https://travel.state.gov/content/passports/en/alertswarnings.html
World Health Organization	General travel health information and access to its international travel guide and alerts	www.who.int/ith/en/

TABLE 2	Checklist of Items to Address in the Pretravel Consultation
CATEGORY	**ISSUES THAT SHOULD BE ADDRESSED**
Patient risk assessment	Obtain history: itinerary, type of travel, personal medical history, age, underlying diseases, allergies, current medications, pregnancy status, previous vaccination status
Immunizations	Update routine immunization Provide routine travel immunization Provide destination-specific immunization
Malaria prophylaxis	If indicated: Provide malaria education and advice; discuss bite avoidance measures Prescribe antimalaria prophylaxis
Travelers' diarrhea	Prescribe oral rehydration therapy and loperamide (Imodium) 4 mg initially and 2 mg after each loose stool not to exceed 16 mg/day Prescribe appropriate antibiotic (see Table 4)
Prevention against mosquito bites	Give advice regarding mosquito-borne disease Discuss personal protection measures
Rabies prevention	Give advice regarding behavior near animals Discuss measures to be taken if bitten or scratched by an animal—seek urgent medical advice Administer vaccine where indicated
Altitude sickness	Provide education Prescribe acetazolamide (Diamox) 125 mg orally twice a day, for 1 day before ascent, continuing for 2–3 days on arrival at maximum altitude
Prevention of sexually transmitted diseases	Provide education regarding safe sex
Zika	Discuss potential risk of congenital Zika syndrome for pregnant women or women/men planning to conceive following return from an endemic area
Others	Deep venous thrombosis prevention Accident prevention Motion sickness

Some of the recommendations are indicated only for specific destinations or specific at-risk groups.

Measles–Mumps–Rubella Vaccine

Measles remains a serious cause of morbidity and mortality in the non-Western world. Importation of measles by unvaccinated travelers from regions that report endemic disease, such as Europe, Africa, and parts of Asia, remains a concern for countries where disease transmission has been interrupted (like the Americas). Indeed, several cases have been associated with exposure during air travel itself. All travelers born after 1957 (USA) and 1970 (Canada and UK) must have two documented vaccines or evidence of immunity as confirmed by antibody titer. Infants of 6 to 11 months who are traveling to a measles-endemic area should be given one dose of measles–mumps–rubella (MMR) vaccine prior to departure. Individuals who have no documented vaccination and a negative antibody titer should receive two doses of MMR vaccine at least 4 weeks apart. Those who have two documented doses are considered immune for at least 20 years.

Poliovirus Vaccine

Owing to successful efforts to eradicate poliomyelitis, most of the world is now polio-free. As of 2019, a few developing countries, particularly Afghanistan and Pakistan report endemic wild-type poliovirus (WPV) outbreaks. In addition, a small number of developing countries continue to report cases of circulating vaccine-derived poliovirus (cVDPV; www.polioeradication.org, last accessed on February 18, 2021).

The injectable, inactivated poliovirus vaccine (IPV, IPOL) is the only polio vaccine available in the United States. All children must have four doses of IPV. Travelers who are traveling to countries with WPV or VDPV circulation and who have completed the age-appropriate series are recommended to receive a single life-time adult booster dose prior to travel. The recommendation also applies to travelers to bordering countries and have high risk of exposure, such as those working in health care, refugee camps or humanitarian aid settings (CDC health information for international travel 2019). As the list of countries with WPV or VDPV circulation and recommendation for vaccine is dynamic, providers are encouraged to refer to the CDC Traveler's web page (wwwnc.cdc.gov/travel/news-announcements/polio-guidance-new-requirements/) for up-to-date advice.

A small number of countries require proof of polio vaccination upon entry or prior to departure and, thus administration should be documented on a vaccination certificate.

Tetanus–Diphtheria–Pertussis Vaccine

Unvaccinated or inadequately vaccinated travelers are at risk of contracting diphtheria in developing countries, as well as tetanus and pertussis anywhere in the world. The potential risk of exposure to pertussis is worldwide, with the highest rates of disease in developing countries where vaccine coverage is low. In recent decades, countries with high vaccination rates, including the United States, have seen resurgence of pertussis despite adequate vaccination programs. Immunity from natural disease or childhood vaccination wanes over time and thus adolescent and adult travelers who have completed their childhood series should receive a booster dose of Tdap (Adacel, Boostrix). Once one documented Tdap booster is given, subsequent booster can be Td or Tdap. If more than 5 years have elapsed since the last booster dose, a tetanus-containing booster should be considered for persons going to remote areas where tetanus boosters may not be readily available after a contaminated trauma.

Varicella Vaccine

Varicella infection remains prevalent worldwide. Infection can occur via inhalation of aerosols or contact of vesicular fluid from a skin lesion. Exposure to active herpes zoster lesion poses a risk of varicella infection to a susceptible traveler. In children, disease is generally mild and self-limited. However serious complications can occur in infants, adults, and immunocompromised individuals. Travelers who have not completed age-appropriate vaccination or do not have laboratory evidence of immunity should receive the varicella vaccination (Varivax) prior to travel. Those over the age of 13 should get two doses at least 4 weeks apart.

Influenza Vaccine

Influenza is the most common VPD among travelers. Travelers aged 6 months and older should receive the most up-to-date influenza vaccine available in their countries annually if they are traveling to an area where influenza is circulating at the time of their travel (year round in tropical and subtropical areas and winter months in temperate areas). Travelers who are over 65 years of age should receive the high-dose influenza vaccine (Fluzone High-Dose) to elicit higher levels of antibody response.

Pneumococcal Vaccine

The prevalence of pneumococcal disease is highest in developing countries. Since 2014, the Advisory Committee of Immunization Practices (ACIP) of the Centers for Disease Control and Prevention (CDC) recommends administration of pneumococcal conjugate vaccine (PCV13; Prevnar13) to all individuals 65 years or older who did not receive a pneumococcal vaccine in the past, followed by a dose of pneumococcal polysaccharide vaccine (PPSV23; Pneumovax) given 1 or more years later for immunocompetent individuals and 8 or more weeks later for immunocompromised patients.

Recommended Travel Vaccination

Hepatitis A Vaccine

Hepatitis A through ingestion of contaminated food or water. Hepatitis A virus remains viable in ice and frozen foods. Travelers who are visiting rural areas, trek in the backcountry and often eat in a poor sanitary environment are at high risk of infection. Outbreaks have been reported among men who have sex with men (MSM) traveling to endemic areas. Hepatitis A vaccine is recommended for travel to any developing country and some industrialized countries where sanitary conditions are variable.

Two hepatitis A vaccine preparations are available (Havrix, Vaqta), which are approved for administration in those aged 12 months or older. It should be administered to infants aged 6 to 11 months who are traveling to high-risk countries. A combination of hepatitis A and B vaccines (Twinrix) is also available and is approved for people aged 18 years or older, with accelerated schedules available to provide protection for those traveling with short notice. A single dose of hepatitis A vaccine given any time before travel will provide complete protection for healthy persons. A booster dose is generally recommended at 6 to 12 months after the first dose to ensure lifetime protection. Infants who received one dose prior to travel should receive two more doses of the vaccine for long-term protection. Immunoglobulin for hepatitis A virus prophylaxis (GamaSTAN S/D), which can be administered to travelers who are not immune and traveling in less than 2 weeks' time, is rarely recommended considering the immunogenicity of the vaccine and long incubation period of hepatitis A. A study comparing hepatitis A vaccine with immunoglobulin to prevent post-exposure hepatitis A infection did not show a difference between the two, suggesting the efficacy of the vaccine as an alternate considering the ease and safety of vaccine compared to immunoglobulin

Typhoid Vaccine

Although hepatitis A and typhoid are both transmitted by contaminated food and water, hepatitis A is 100 times more common than typhoid in travelers. The Indian subcontinent seems to be a key focus of typhoid in travelers, accounting for more than 80% of travel-related typhoid cases in the United States. The efficacy of typhoid vaccines ranges from 50% to 80% in various published studies.

Typhoid vaccine is protective against *Salmonella enterica* serotype *typhi*, but not against paratyphoid fever, which is caused by strains of *S. enterica* paratyphi A, B, and C. Typhoid vaccine is recommended to long-term travelers to developing countries and short-term travelers to South Asia, as well as other destinations for high-risk groups such as travelers VFR and food adventurers.

Two unconjugated vaccines are available in the United States: the oral live, attenuated typhoid vaccine (Ty21A, Vivotif Berna), which is approved for all travelers over 6 years of age and the injectable typhoid Vi polysaccharide vaccine (Typhim Vi) for those over 2 years age. The oral vaccine, which consists of four capsules (one taken every other day) is protective for 5 years while the injectable vaccine is only effective for 2 years. Ideally, either vaccine should be given at least 2 weeks before departure.

Hepatitis B

Hepatitis B (HBV) is transmitted by contact with blood, blood products, and body fluids and as such, poses limited risk to most travelers; however, health care professionals traveling to endemic area are at high risk. HBV is endemic worldwide, with high prevalence in Asia and sub-Saharan Africa.

Travelers should be counseled on HBV transmission and minimizing exposure. All travelers traveling to intermediate-to-high-prevalence countries (>2% prevalence of HBV surface antigen) should receive the vaccine. The vaccines (Engerix-B, Recombivax HB, Twinrix) are approved as a series of three doses given at day 0, 1 month, and 6 months. For those traveling on short notice, Twinrix is approved for an accelerated schedule of day 0, 7, and 21 to 30 days. For long-term immunity, a booster dose of Twinrix is recommended at 12 months. Two doses of this regimen completed in a 1-week interval gives adequate immediate protection for travel. A new conjugate (adjuvanted) vaccine (Heplisav-B) with two doses 1 month apart has been approved for all travelers aged 18 and above. Protective immunity of Heplisav-B is robust with over 95% of those who complete the series achieving immunity and it will likely replace the vaccines that are currently available.

Cholera

Most cases of cholera are reported from sub-Saharan Africa, Asia, and the island of Hispanola (Haiti and the Dominican Republic). The risk of cholera to an average traveler is extremely low. The vaccine is indicated for emergency relief workers, health care workers traveling to an endemic area, and travelers going to an area with a declared outbreak. The vaccine is not required for entry to any country. In 2016, a single dose, oral, live-attenuated vaccine (Vaxchora) was approved for adults over 18 years old.

Japanese Encephalitis

Japanese encephalitis (JE) is a mosquito-borne neurologic disease endemic to China, Korea, the Indian subcontinent, Southeast Asia, and the Western Pacific. The risk varies according to destination, length of stay, season, and activities being undertaken. The risk is highest for travelers to rural areas, especially with nighttime outdoor activities. The overall incidence of JE among persons from non-endemic countries traveling to Asia is estimated to be less than 1 case per 1 million, though this could be much higher depending on the type, time, and duration of travel. Vaccination should be considered for all frequent travelers and those who are planning to stay over 1 month in an endemic country.

An inactivated, cell culture-derived vaccine (IXIARO) is licensed in the United States for use in persons aged 2 months or older. Children 2 months to 2 years old are given half the dose used for adults. The vaccine is given as a two-dose series at 0 and 28 days. An accelerated vaccine schedule of two doses 1 week apart has been approved for travelers who do not have enough time to complete the series before departure.

Rabies

Rabies is a fatal viral infection that is transmitted through exposure to saliva of a rabid animal. The virus is neurotropic and results in progressive encephalomyelitis that is often fatal. It has a worldwide distribution with highest prevalence in Asia, Africa, and South and Central America. Dog bite remains the primary source of infection, though bat exposure is increasingly identified as a common risk factor for disease acquisition. From 1990 to 2013, 66 cases of rabies were documented in travelers—40% from Asia, and 85% following canine exposure.[2,3] Animal bites are common during travel. Approximately 2700 travelers received care for animal-related exposures and required rabies post-exposure prophylaxis at GeoSentinel clinics during a 15-year period (1997–2012). Clinical illness follows variable incubation period ranging in days to months from exposure. Early symptoms include pain and paresthesia at the site of the bite, invariably followed by paresis, paralysis, and fatal encephalitis. Hydrophobia, delirium, and convulsions are classic presentations that often are followed by coma and death. Symptomatic and supportive care, including aggressive wound care and post-exposure prophylaxis may improve survival to this uniformly fatal disease.

A three-dose pre-exposure course of rabies vaccine (Imovax Rabies, RabAvert) is recommended for travelers based on length of stay, country of destination, and risk of exposure. Veterinarians, animal handlers, field biologists, laboratory workers who handle animals, and children are at high risk and require pre-exposure vaccination.

In the event of an exposure, vaccinated individuals require two additional doses of vaccine 3 days apart while unvaccinated travelers require four doses of vaccine and additional human rabies immune globulin (HRIG [HyperRab, Imogam Rabies]), which may be expensive, unavailable, or unreliable in the traveler's locale. In light of the devastating consequences of rabies, the fact that animal bites, scratches, or licks over mucous membranes are common among travelers even during short trips; the difficulties in receiving rabies immune globulin in the developing world; and the fact that a one-time pre-exposure course of vaccine is "for life" suggest that the threshold for recommending rabies vaccine to travelers to the developing world should be low.

Tick-Borne Encephalitis

Tick-borne encephalitis (TBE) is an arboviral zoonosis transmitted primarily through the bite of *Ixodes* species ticks. It is endemic in many popular tourist destinations in Europe, Eastern Europe, and parts of Asia including China, Japan, Russia, and Siberia. Symptoms include fever body ache, headache, and arthralgia. Up to 20% to 30% of those infected might develop encephalitis. Human infections usually are seen in the spring and summer months in temperate zones and in fall and winter in the Mediterranean region. A TBE vaccine (TicoVac) is available in Europe and Canada but not in the USA and is considered immunogenic and safe.[2] Vaccination is recommended for travelers with extensive outdoor exposures such as camping in endemic regions during the transmission season. In addition, travelers should be advised to use insect repellants and avoid tick bite to protect themselves from TBE.

Required Vaccines

Yellow Fever Vaccine

Yellow fever (YF) is a mosquito-borne disease endemic to parts of sub-Saharan Africa and tropical South America. Though most patients with YF are asymptomatic, about 15% develop severe disease with a reported case fatality rate of 20% to 60%. YF vaccine (YF-VAX) is a live-attenuated vaccine that travelers should receive at least 10 days prior to arriving in an endemic country. A large YF outbreak was documented in eastern Brazil in 2016–2018, which expanded the previously known endemic area within Brazil. World Health Organization (WHO) and CDC are now recommending YF vaccination for all travelers to eastern and southeastern states of Brazil. The risk of a traveler acquiring YF varies with season, location, activities, and duration of travel. Since January 2018, 10 travel-related cases of YF, including 4 deaths, have been reported in travelers returning from Brazil. None of the 10 travelers had YF vaccination.

The vaccine is recommended for personal protection of travelers to endemic areas. In addition, under WHO rules, any given country may routinely require YF vaccination for entry into its territory. The aim of the regulation is to protect countries that have the mosquito vector, which could be introduced to the virus by blood meal from a viremic traveler.

Yellow fever vaccine (YF-VAX) is rarely associated with severe and fatal adverse reactions, which generally follow the first dose to the individual. The overall rate of serious adverse reaction is about 1 event per 250,000 doses. The likelihood of serious adverse events increases with age, with patients older than age 60 years having a much higher risk for severe adverse reaction.

A change in the IHR in July 2016 now considers a valid YF vaccination to be effective for life, with no need for booster vaccines at 10-year intervals. This also applies retrospectively to YF vaccines given any time before 2016. The new policy extends to the validity of the vaccine for personal protection, with no need for booster doses among healthy, immune-competent individuals. Per this recommendation, countries cannot require proof of vaccination (booster) against YF as a condition of entry to travelers whose YF vaccination was over 10 years prior. A booster vaccine after 10 years is still recommended for specific high-risk individuals: long-term travelers, travelers to West Africa, and travelers to an area where there is a current outbreak.

Meningococcal Vaccine

Meningitis is caused by the bacteria *Neisseria meningitidis*. It is acquired by nasopharyngeal droplets during close contact. Disease spectrum ranges from fever and bacteremia to meningitis. There are eight serogroups of meningococci, but most travel-related disease is caused by A, C, X and W135 serogroups. Disease is endemic worldwide, but the highest risk area is the sub-Saharan region loosely named the "meningitis belt." There is seasonality to disease incidence with seasonal epidemics occurring during the dry season (December–June).

Meningococcal disease is rare in travelers (1:100,000 to <1:1,000,000 per month of travel). A quadrivalent conjugated

---

[2] Not available in the United States.

TABLE 3 FDA-approved Medication Options for Chemoprophylaxis of Malaria

DRUG	USE IN PROPHYLAXIS	ADULT DOSE	LENGTH OF TREATMENT
Chloroquine	Areas with chloroquine sensitive *Plasmodium falciparum*	500 mg (300 mg base) weekly	Start 1–2 weeks prior to exposure. Continue weekly while in the malaria zone and for 4 weeks after leaving
Mefloquine (Lariam)	Areas with mefloquine sensitive *P. falciparum*	250 mg weekly	Start ≥ 2 weeks prior to exposure. Continue weekly while in the malaria zone and for 4 weeks after leaving
Atovaquone-proguanil (Malarone)	All malaria zones	250 mg/100 mg once daily	Start 1–2 days prior to exposure. Continue daily while in the malaria zone and for 7 days after leaving
Doxycycline	All malaria zones	100 mg daily	Start 1–2 days prior to exposure. Continue daily while in the malaria zone and for 4 weeks after leaving
Tafenoquine (Arakoda)	All malaria zones	200 mg	A loading dose is 200 mg taken daily for 3 days prior to exposure. Then continue 200 mg weekly while in the malaria zone, and for 1 week after leaving

vaccine is recommended for travelers that protects against serogroups A, C, X, and W135 (Menactra, Menveo, and Nimenrix[1]). Travelers to countries in the meningitis belt who anticipate close contact with crowds or the local population and aid workers in refugee camps are recommended to get the vaccine prior to travel. Vaccination is required for entry to Saudi Arabia during Hajj or Umrah seasons. Travelers returning to Saudi Arabia or high-risk zones need a booster vaccine every 5 years.

Malaria

Reports of malaria cases in the USA have been steadily increasing over the last few decades, mainly as a result of infection in travelers to areas of the world with ongoing malaria transmission. In 2016, there were 2078 cases of malaria reported in the USA. Only 26.3% of US residents who developed malaria that year reported taking a malaria prophylaxis and 94% did not complete an appropriate chemoprophylactic regimen. Of those who reported a reason for travel, the majority of cases were in travelers VFR (69.4%).

Prior to travel, a risk assessment should be performed to determine if malaria chemoprophylaxis is indicated. Malaria transmission can vary greatly, even within a country, based on the region and season of travel. The traveler's specific itinerary should be reviewed for the cities visited, type of accommodations (bed nets, window screens, air-conditioning), reason for travel, and special activities while traveling. Mosquito avoidance measures should be recommended in addition to chemoprophylaxis.

The life cycle of malaria in humans involves an initial asymptomatic liver stage, followed by a later symptomatic erythrocytic stage. Malaria chemoprophylaxis is used to prevent the development of clinical malaria if a person is infected. Certain chemoprophylactic agents (chloroquine [Aralen], mefloquine [Lariam], and doxycycline [Vibramycin]) only work on the later erythrocytic stage of malaria parasites and, are therefore, recommended to be taken for a longer time (4 weeks) after leaving a malaria-endemic area. Atovaquone-proguanil (Malarone) can act on the earlier non-dormant liver parasite stage and, therefore, a shorter duration post-travel is recommended (1 week). Unlike other *Plasmodium* species, *P. vivax* and *P. ovale* have dormant liver stages known as hypnozoites, which are responsible for relapse of disease with these species months or years after an acute infection. Tafenoquine (Arakoda, Krintafel) and primaquine[2] are the only available medications effective against the liver hypnozoites of *P. vivax* and *P. ovale*.

Malaria Chemoprophylaxis

All malaria chemoprophylactic options should be started prior to travel, taken throughout travel, and continued for a period of time post-travel (Table 3). When choosing a chemoprophylactic agent, things to consider include the traveler's age and medical history, pregnancy status, length of the trip, cost of the drug, drug allergies, drug interactions, and drug resistance at the destination.

Chloroquine (Aralen) may only be used for malaria prophylaxis in areas of the world with chloroquine-sensitive *Plasmodium falciparum*. Resistance is found worldwide except in Central America west of the Panama Canal, Haiti, and the Dominican Republic. Chloroquine is used once a week for prophylaxis. It should be started 1 to 2 weeks prior to travel, taken weekly during travel, and continued for 4 weeks after leaving the malaria zone. The most common side effects are gastrointestinal discomfort, nausea, vomiting, or headache. Serious adverse effects are rare, and are more likely to occur with prolonged and high doses of therapy. Retinopathy is associated with high doses, and when used for more than 5 years. An overdose of chloroquine could be fatal, and the medication should be stored in childproof containers. If a traveler is already taking hydroxychloroquine (Plaquenil) chronically for a rheumatological condition, they may not have to take additional malaria prophylaxis.

There are four potential FDA-approved options for malaria chemoprophylaxis in areas with chloroquine-resistant malaria: Atovaquone/proguanil (Malarone), doxycycline, mefloquine (Lariam), and tafenoquine (Arakoda). Primaquine may be used off-label (not FDA approved) for malaria chemoprophylaxis in areas of the world with predominantly *P. vivax* malaria.

Mefloquine should only be used for malaria prophylaxis in areas of the world with mefloquine-sensitive *P. falciparum*. Mefloquine-resistant *P. falciparum* malaria is found in parts of Southeast Asia (along the borders of Thailand with Cambodia and Burma, western Cambodia, eastern Burma, and southern Vietnam), and mefloquine should not be used for malaria prophylaxis in these areas. Mefloquine is used once a week for prophylaxis. It should be started ≥2 weeks prior to travel, taken weekly during travel, and continued for 4 weeks after leaving the malaria zone. Adverse effects tend to be noted within the first weeks of mefloquine initiation, and therefore the medication can be started 2 to 4 weeks prior to travel to help ensure the medication will be tolerated during travel. Mefloquine may be associated with sleep disturbance, strange dreams and insomnia. The FDA also has issued a boxed warning that mefloquine may cause neuropsychiatric adverse effects that can persist after mefloquine has been discontinued. Mefloquine is contraindicated in those with neurologic and psychiatric disorders and should be avoided in travelers with a significant family history of seizures or major psychiatric

[1] Not available in the United States.
[2] Not FDA approved for this indication.

disorders. It is also recommended to avoid mefloquine in travelers with cardiac conduction abnormalities. A traveler who is prescribed mefloquine must receive a copy of its FDA medication guide found at www.accessdata.fda.gov/drugsatfda_docs/label/2008/019591s023lbl.pdf.

Atovaquone-progaunil can be used for malaria prophylaxis in any malaria zone worldwide. Atovaquone-progaunil is a daily prophylactic drug. It should be started 1 to 2 days prior to travel, taken daily during travel, and continued for 7 days after leaving a malaria zone. The drug is usually well-tolerated, with the most common adverse effect being gastrointestinal upset.

Doxycycline can be used for malaria prophylaxis in any malaria zone worldwide. Doxycycline is a daily prophylactic drug. It should be started 1 to 2 days prior to travel, taken daily during travel, and continued for 4 weeks after leaving a malaria zone. An added benefit of doxycycline is that it may also provide some protections against rickettsial infections and leptospirosis. However, photosensitivity is a common adverse effect of doxycycline.

Tafenoquine (Arakoda) can be used for malaria prophylaxis in any malaria zone worldwide. Tafenoquine is used once a week for prophylaxis. It should be started 1 to 2 weeks prior to travel, taken weekly during travel, and continued for 1 week after leaving the malaria zone. G6PD deficiency must be ruled out by laboratory testing prior to prescribing this medication because fatal hemolysis could occur in individuals with G6PD deficiency. Tafenoquine should be avoided in those with a history of a psychotic disorder since rare psychiatric events have been observed. The most common adverse events include nonsignificant decreases in hemoglobin, gastrointestinal discomfort, and headache. Tafenoquine is the only FDA-approved medication for malaria prophylaxis that has activity on the hypnozoite stage of the malaria parasite. Note that another tafenoquine-based antimalarial (Krintafel) is approved for radical cure of *P. vivax* infections in those over 16 years of age.

Post-travel

No prophylaxis is 100% effective. Travelers should be advised to seek medical attention during travel if malaria symptoms occur. They should also be told to notify their physician of their travel history if they develop a febrile illness for up to 1-year post-travel.

COVID-19

A novel coronavirus was identified in Wuhan, China, in late 2019, and subsequently spread worldwide. In February 2020, the WHO officially named the novel coronavirus-associated disease coronavirus disease 2019, abbreviated COVID-19. The virus is spread mainly person to person through respiratory droplets, and spread is most likely to occur when individuals are within approximately 6 feet of one another. By the end of July 2021, the COVID-19 pandemic had resulted in more than 200 million cases worldwide, and nearly 4.25 million deaths.

It is recommended that both domestic and international travelers delay travel until they can be fully vaccinated. Masks are required on planes, buses, trains and other forms of public transportation traveling into, within, or out of the United States and while indoors at United States transportation hubs such as airports and stations. Passengers should not travel if they are sick, have been exposed to COVID-19, or have recently tested positive for COVID-19.

Since January 26, 2021, all air passengers 2 years of age and older arriving into the United States have been required to have a negative COVID-19 test result (nucleic acid amplification or antigen test) obtained no more than 3 days before travel into the United States. Air passengers who have recently recovered from COVID-19 may travel if they provide documentation of their positive viral test result, along with a letter from a healthcare provider stating the passenger has been cleared to end isolation. Travelers to other countries should also be aware of travel health notices and arrival restrictions at their destinations.

After international travel, it is recommended that all travelers get a COVID-19 viral test within 3–5 days. Unvaccinated travelers should also stay home and self-quarantine for a full 7 days after travel if this COVID-19 viral test is negative, or for 10 days if a COVID-19 viral test is not obtained.

More information on international travel during COVID-19 can be found at the CDC Travel Recommendations by Destination website: https://www.cdc.gov/coronavirus/2019-ncov/travelers/map-and-travel-notices.html.

Personal Protection Measures

Risk for vector borne disease depends on many factors, including the traveler's destination, season of travel, and length of stay. Viral diseases that may be of concern include JE, Zika, dengue, and chikungunya. Rickettsial diseases are found worldwide on all continents with the exception of Antarctica. Malaria is the parasite of greatest concern, but leishmaniasis, trypanosomiasis, and filariasis are other potential parasitic diseases spread by arthropod vectors.

The type of accommodation can affect the traveler's risk of vector borne diseases. An air conditioned room for sleeping, effective window screens, and/or bednets are protective. Wearing long-sleeved shirts, long pants, and socks can also decrease risk. For added protection, a clothing insect repellent, such as permethrin, is recommended. Permethrin activity is maintained on treated clothes despite several wash cycles.

Insect repellants for use on skin have variable efficacy depending on the repellant type and form, concentration, frequency of application, and vector. Typically, a higher concentration of insecticide will provide a longer duration of protection. However, there is a peak at which no further protection is seen, and more toxicity could result. DEET, at a concentration of 20% to 25%, has efficacy against all mosquito species and some tick species, biting flies, chiggers, and fleas. Concentrations above DEET 50% do not appear to provide added benefit. Products containing picaridin (icaridin outside the USA) are also good options. Potential benefits of picaridin over DEET are that it is odorless and does not damage plastic. Products containing IR3535 are another option, and appear to have particularly good activity against *Ixodes scapularis* ticks (commonly known as deer ticks or black-legged ticks).

Traveler's Diarrhea

During a 2-week trip, traveler's diarrhea has an incidence between 10% and 40%. Higher risk areas include parts of Asia and Central/West Africa. Certain behaviors may affect the risk of developing diarrhea. Practicing hand hygiene measures prior to eating has been shown to reduce the incidence of diarrhea. Other potentially beneficial measures include avoiding food that has not been properly cooked, avoiding ice, and drinking only bottled or treated water in resource-poor settings.

Traveler's diarrhea is predominantly caused by bacterial pathogens. However, antibiotic prophylaxis to prevent traveler's diarrhea is rarely indicated, given both the cost and potential for adverse events. Bismuth subsalicylate (BSS [Pepto-Bismol])[1] has shown efficacy in decreasing the risk of traveler's diarrhea, and may be considered for prevention. However, BSS requires frequent dosing, causes blackening of the tongue, and has the potential for drug-drug interactions.

Treatment

Treatment recommendations for traveler's diarrhea depend on the severity of illness. Ensuring adequate hydration is always a mainstay of treatment. In the case of severe diarrhea, WHO recommends oral rehydration therapy (ORS) which is available at most pharmacies. An anti-motility agent, such as loperamide (Imodium), can also provide symptomatic benefit for mild to severe traveler's diarrhea. Loperamide is not recommended to be used alone in travelers with dysentery.

---

[1] Not FDA approved for this indication.

TABLE 4   Treatment Options for Empiric Treatment of Traveler's Diarrhea

ANTIBIOTIC	ADULT DOSE	DURATION	COMMENTS
Rifaximin (Xifaxan)	200 mg TID	3 days	Not recommend in patients with fever or bloody diarrhea
Rifamycin SV (Aemcolo)	388 mg BID	3 days	Not recommend in patients with fever or bloody diarrhea
Azithromycin (Zithromax)[1]	1000 mg	Single dose (or 2 divided doses on the same day to reduce nausea)	Preferred empiric option in SE Asia, and preferred treatment for dysentery
	500 mg daily	3 days	
Ciprofloxacin (Cipro)[1]	750 mg	Single dose	
	500 mg BID	3 days	
Levofloxacin (Levaquin)[1]	500 mg daily	1–3 days	

[1]Not FDA approved for this indication.

When antibiotics are used for self-treatment of traveler's diarrhea, they may reduce the duration of diarrhea by 1 to 3 days. Several effective antibiotic options are available (Table 4). A combination of an antibiotic with loperamide further shortens the duration of diarrhea. However, the benefits of antimicrobial treatment of traveler's diarrhea must be weighed against the potential risks. Each antibiotic option has the potential for specific side effects, such as tendinopathies in the case of fluoroquinolones. Antibiotic use also increases the risk of developing *Clostridioides difficile* diarrhea. Further, multiple studies have shown that antibiotic use for the self-treatment of traveler's diarrhea increases a traveler's risk of developing colonization with antibiotic-resistant bacteria, including extended-spectrum B-lactamase-producing *Enterobacteriaceae* and carbapenemase-producing *Enterobacteriaceae*.

Given the potential risks, antimicrobial therapy is not recommended for acute diarrhea that is tolerable and does not interfere with planned activities. Loperamide or BSS can be used alone for these mild cases. Loperamide, with or without an antibiotic, may be used in the case of moderate diarrhea that is distressing or interferes with planned activities. An antibiotic is recommended to treat severe travelers' diarrhea, which includes all dysentery cases, as well as diarrhea that is incapacitating or prevents planned activities. Single-dose antibiotic treatment regimens are as effective as 3-day regimens for most cases of traveler's diarrhea.

Fluoroquinolones, such as ciprofloxacin (Cipro)[1] and levofloxacin (Levaquin)[1], have long been used to treat traveler's diarrhea. However, there has been increasing resistance to fluoroquinolones among diarrheal pathogens, especially *Campylobacter* isolates in South and Southeast Asia. In this area of the world, azithromycin (Zithromax) is preferred for empiric treatment of travelers' diarrhea. Azithromycin is also the preferred treatment for dysentery. Rifaximin (Xifaxan) is approved to treat traveler's diarrhea caused by non-invasive strains of *Escherichia coli*. Rifamycin SV (Aemcolo) is a non-absorbable antibiotic with an enteric coating, and has the same mechanism of action as rifaximin. Since rifamycin SV and rifaximin are not recommended for treatment of invasive diarrhea, their role in the self-treatment of diarrhea is limited.

High-Altitude Illness

High-altitude illnesses (HAI)s due to hypoxia can occur during travel to high-elevation areas, typically greater than 8000 feet above sea level. There are three syndromes that may comprise altitude illness: acute mountain sickness (AMS), high-altitude cerebral edema (HACE), and high-altitude pulmonary edema (HAPE).

AMS is the most common form of HAI, and symptoms may include headache, nausea, and fatigue. If left untreated, AMS can progress to HACE, which is a more serious condition. Manifestations of HACE can include ataxia, drowsiness, confusion, and even death. Acute hypoxia may also lead to HAPE. The pathophysiology of HAPE is different than that of AMS/HACE, and is presumably due to pulmonary vasoconstriction that leads to pulmonary edema. Cough, dyspnea on exertion, and pulmonary congestion can progress to death if ascent is continued.

Prevention of High-Altitude Illnesses

Certain individuals are more susceptible to HAI, but it is not possible to reliably predict who may develop symptoms. Rate of ascent, ultimate elevation, underlying medical conditions and degree of physical exertion are all potential factors in determining risk of developing HAI. The body's ability to acclimate to a high elevation typically takes 3 to 5 days. A slow ascent that allows time for acclimatization is helpful in preventing the development of all forms of HAI; however, this is not always possible. There are several popular high-altitude tourist destinations that may be reached via direct flights from areas of low elevation. Examples include Cuzco, Peru located at 11,000 feet, La Paz, Bolivia at 12,000 feet, and Lhasa, Tibet at 12,000 feet.

Acetazolamide (Diamox) is a nonantibiotic sulfonamide that was developed as a diuretic to treat hypertension. Its efficacy for that purpose was limited. However multiple studies have since shown the preemptive use of acetazolamide can decrease the risk of developing AMS. Acetazolamide is able to block carbonic anhydrase, primarily in the kidney. This decreases reabsorption of bicarbonate and leads to the development of metabolic acidosis, compensating for the respiratory alkalosis associated with high elevations. Acetazolamide is associated with increased risk of paresthesia and diuresis. The recommended dose of acetazolamide, to prevent AMS while minimizing adverse effects, is 125 mg orally twice a day. It is generally recommended to start 1 day prior to ascent, and continue through the first 2 days at peak elevation.

A number of other medications have been studied to prevent AMS, but the benefits of alternative therapies are less clear. Dexamethasone (Decadron)[1] is one of the more commonly used alternatives. The typical dose for prophylaxis is 2 mg every 6 hours or 4 mg every 12 hours. Inhaled budesonide (Pulmicort)[1] was found to be ineffective in preventing AMS in a recent randomized controlled study and is not recommended.

Treatment

Symptomatic travelers should not continue to ascend further until all symptoms resolve, and should descend to a lower elevation immediately if symptoms progress. Acetazolamide can be considered for treatment of AMS, but it is better at preventing than treating this disorder. Dexamethasone is more reliable for treatment of moderate to severe AMS. However, descent is often needed as well, and should occur immediately in cases of HACE or HAPE.

Summary

A pre-travel consultation should include a health assessment, interventions and counseling to decrease travel-related risks and improve the likelihood of a safe and enjoyable travel experience.

References

Air Passenger Forecasts. Global Report. https://www.iata.org/publications/Documents/global-report-sample1.pdf. Accessed on 01.09.2017.

Centers for Disease Control and Prevention: *CDC Yellow Book 2020: Health Information for International Travel*, New York, 2017, Oxford University Press.

Cullen KA, Mace KE, Arguin PM: Malaria surveillance - United States, 2013, *MMWR Surveill Summ* 65:1–22, 2016.

Freedman DO: Protection of travelers. In Bennett JE, Raphael D, Blaser MJ, editors: *Mandell, Douglas, and Bennett's Principles and Practice of Infectious Diseases*, 8th ed., Philadelphia, 2015, Saunders Elsevier, pp 3559–3567.

Freedman DO, Chen LH, Kozarsky PE: Medical considerations before international travel, *N Engl J Med* 375:247–260, 2016.

Freedman DO, Weld LH, Kozarsky PE: Spectrum of disease and relation to place of exposure among ill returned travelers, *N Engl J Med* 354:119–130, 2006.

Gautret P, Harvey K, Pandey P: Animal-associated exposure to rabies virus among travelers, 1997-2012, *Emerg Infect Dis* 21:569–577, 2015.

Gautret P, Parola P: Rabies in travelers, *Curr Infect Dis Rep* 16:394, 2014.

Giddings SL, Stevens AM, Leung DT: Traveler's Diarrhea, *Med Clin North Am* 100(2):317–330, 2016.

Grobusch MP: Malaria chemoprophylaxis with atovaquone-proguanil: Is a shorter regimen fully protective? *J Travel Med* 21(2):79–81, 2014.

Jelinek T, Burchard GD, Dieckmann S, et al: Short-term immunogenicity and safety of an accelerated pre-exposure prophylaxis regimen with Japanese encephalitis vaccine in combination with a rabies vaccine: a phase III, multicenter, observer-blind study, *J Travel Med* 22:225–231, 2015.

Jensenius M, Han PV, Schlagenhauf P, et al: Acute and potentially life-threatening tropical diseases in western travelers–A GeoSentinel multicenter study, 1996-2011, *Am J Trop Med Hyg* 88:397–404, 2013.

Kantele A, Laaveri T, Mero S: Antimicrobials increase travelers' risk of colonization by extended-spectrum betalactamase-producing Enterobacteriaceae, *Clin Infect Dis* 60:837–846, 2015.

Kantele A, Mero S, Kirveskari J: Increased risk for ESBL-producing bacteria from co-administration of loperamide and antimicrobial drugs for travelers' diarrhea, *Emerg Infect Dis* 22(1):117–120, 2016.

Leshem E, Meltzer E, Stienlauf S: Effectiveness of short prophylactic course of atovaquone-proguanil in travelers to sub-Saharan Africa, *J Travel Med* 21(2):82–85, 2014.

Leshem E, Pandey P: Clinical features of patients with severe altitude illness in Nepal, *J Travel Med* 15:315–322, 2008.

Luks AM, Auerbach PS, Freer L: Wilderness medical society clinical practice guidelines for the prevention and treatment of acute altitude illness: 2019 Update, *Wilderness Environ Med* 30(4S):S3–S18, 2019.

Lupi E, Hatz C, Schlagenhauf P: The efficacy of repellents against Aedes, Anopheles, Culex and Ixodes spp.—a literature review, *Travel Med Infect Dis* 11(6):374–411, 2013.

Mace KE, Arguin PM, Lucchi NW, Tan KR: Malaria Surveillance – United States, 2016, *MMWR Surveill Summ* 68(No. SS-5):1–31, 2019.

Meltzer E, Paran Y, Lustig Y: Travel-related tick-borne encephalitis, Israel, 2006-2014, *Emerg Infect Dis* 23:119–121, 2017.

Menachem M, Grupper M, Paz A: Assessment of rabies exposure risk among Israeli travelers, *Travel Med Infect Dis* 6:12–16, 2008.

Novitt-Moreno A, Ransom J, Dow G, Smith B, Read LT, Toovey S: Tafenoquine for malaria prophylaxis in adults: an integrated safety analysis, *Travel Med Infect Dis* 17:19–27, 2017.

Riddle MS, Connor BA, Beeching NJ, et al: Guidelines for the prevention and treatment of travelers' diarrhea, *J Travel Med* 24:S63–S80, 2017.

Shlim David R: The use of acetazolamide for the prevention of high-altitude illness, *J Travel Med* 1–6, 2020.

Steffen R: Epidemiology of tick-borne encephalitis (TBE) in international travellers to Western/Central Europe and conclusions on vaccination recommendations, *J Travel Med* 23(4).

Steffen R, Hill DR, DuPont HL: Traveler's diarrhea: A clinical review, *JAMA* 313:71–80, 2015.

Victor JC, Monto AS, Surdina TY, et al: Hepatitis A vaccine versus immune globulin for postexposure prophylaxis, *N Engl J Med* 357(17):1685, 2007.

Yezli S, Alotaibi B: Meningococcal disease during the Hajj and Umrah mass gatherings: A, C, W, Y may be covered but don't forget the B and X factors, *Travel Med Infect Dis* 15:5–7, 2017.

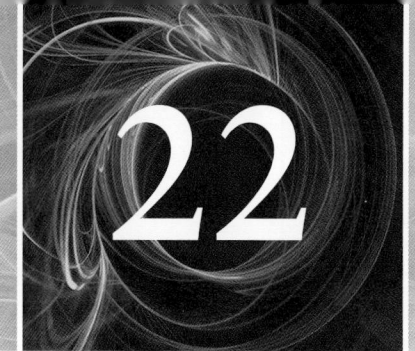

22 Emerging Therapies

STEM CELL THERAPY

Method of
Sunil Abhyankar, MD; and Rupal Soder, PhD

The two words "stem cell" evoke a vision of a multipotent cell that can develop into different kinds of tissue cells. Only *embryonic stem cells* fit this definition and they are guided in their development by external growth factors and environmental events in their final path to form a particular tissue and ultimately a body organ.

The progeny of the embryonic stem cells function as *differentiated stem cells* that are capable of forming new cells for the tissue in which they reside. These are *tissue-specific stem cells*. Such is the case, for example, with hematopoietic stem cells, which reside in the bone marrow (BM) space and are responsible for producing all the cells that make up the blood components. Most of the tissue stem cells have the capacity to regenerate tissue and, under certain growth conditions, can be coaxed to produce related tissues. An example of the latter is the *mesenchymal stem cell* (MSC), also located in the bone marrow, which under certain growth conditions can form cartilage, bone, and other connective tissue cells.

Another category of stem cell is the one artificially produced in the laboratory termed the *induced pluripotent stem cell* (iPSC). These are generally derived from tissue cells (e.g., fibroblasts) and made to grow in selective conditions into the cell of interest, hence the term induced pluripotent cells. iPSCs are finding increasing uses in cellular therapy in the cancer arena.

This review will focus on the committed stem cells that harbor in our tissues and are responsible for healing and replenishing cells of that tissue that are naturally dying (Figure 1).

In the United States, the US Food and Drug Administration (FDA) has the authority to approve cellular therapies. The FDA lists approved cellular and gene therapy products on their website, https://www.fda.gov/vaccines-blood-biologics/cellular-gene-therapy-products/approved-cellular-and-gene-therapy-products. The list includes cellular therapies with chimeric antigen receptor technology utilized in cancer therapy, autologous cultured chondrocytes on a porcine collagen membrane, and mesenchymal cells used in treatment of severe nasolabial folds defects. The stem cell-based products that are FDA-approved for use in the United States consist of blood-forming stem cells (hematopoietic progenitor cells) derived from cord blood. The blood stem cells are approved for use in patients with disorders that affect the body system that is involved in the production of blood (i.e., the hematopoietic and the immune system). Bone marrow also is used for these treatments but is generally not regulated by the FDA for this use and is considered "grandfathered" for FDA approval. The use of bone marrow–derived MSC has been approved for use in Canada and Japan for the treatment of graft versus host disease in pediatric patients who have undergone a bone marrow transplant.

Transplantation of Hematopoietic Stem Cells

The first report of the use of a hematopoietic stem cells from the bone marrow for transplant was in 1957 by E. Donell Thomas, when he and colleagues performed a bone marrow transplant (BMT) in monozygotic twins, one of whom had acute leukemia.

This is considered a *syngeneic* (i.e., genetically identical) transplant. Although the procedure was successful, the patient subsequently relapsed. Dr. Thomas continued his pioneering work in BMT and was the recipient of the Nobel Prize in Medicine in 1990.

Utilization of *allogeneic* (genetically dissimilar) bone marrow stem cells in transplant was first described in the 1960s in pediatric patients with congenital immune deficiency (SCID). Subsequently allogeneic BMT has been used to treat a host of hematologic and immunologic conditions including aplastic anemia, hemoglobinopathies (sickle cell anemia and thalassemia), acute and chronic leukemias, and myelodysplastic syndromes. Success of allogeneic BMT has improved over the past decades as shown by data from the Center for International Blood and Marrow Transplant Research registry (CIBMTR). This has been due to several factors including improvements in human leukocyte antigen (HLA) typing resulting in better matched donors, improved supportive care, and an improved understanding of the immune process at play in allogeneic BMT. Thus young patients with idiopathic aplastic anemia can expect a 90% or higher long-term survival with an HLA matched related bone marrow stem cell donor. Despite these advances, the long-term success after an allogeneic BMT in adults is typically in the 50% range; survival is higher in younger compared with older adult patients. A major cause of the lower success in older patients is due to the risk of relapse of the underlying malignancy as well as acute and chronic graft versus host disease (GvHD) occurring after transplantation and the risk of opportunistic infections, usually viral and fungal. Newer approaches to mitigate and treat GvHD (e.g., the use of MSC in acute GvHD), measures to prevent relapse after transplant (e.g., use of targeted chemotherapeutic agents for maintenance therapy after transplant), and the use of viral specific T cells to treat viral infections post-BMT are being investigated. The outcomes of allogeneic BMT continue to improve.

Hematopoietic stem cells can be obtained from the bone marrow, the peripheral blood, and from umbilical cord blood. BM stem cells to be used in transplantation can be harvested surgically from the donor's bone marrow under general anesthesia or from the peripheral blood when stem cells can be mobilized from the BM with high doses of granulocyte colony-stimulating factor (G-CSF). These peripheral blood stem cells are BM stem cells isolated from the blood, making it easier on the donor. Umbilical cord blood (UCB) is also rich in hematopoietic stem cells and can be easily obtained after the birth of the baby after the cord has been cut. The leftover blood from the umbilical cord and placenta can be banked for use in transplantation.

Which source of stem cells is to be used in hematopoietic transplantation? This is dependent on the patient diagnosis and age. In patients who have malignant hematologic diseases, stem cells obtained from the peripheral blood of the donor are often preferred as these stem cell collections are accompanied by a higher number of T lymphocytes, which can improve a patient's ability to fight off their cancerous cells. In contrast, in patients with aplastic anemia or sickle cell anemia, bone marrow harvested stem cells are preferred due to the lower amount of T cells in this product causing less GvHD.

With advances in hematopoietic transplantation, almost every person who will benefit from an allogeneic transplant will be able

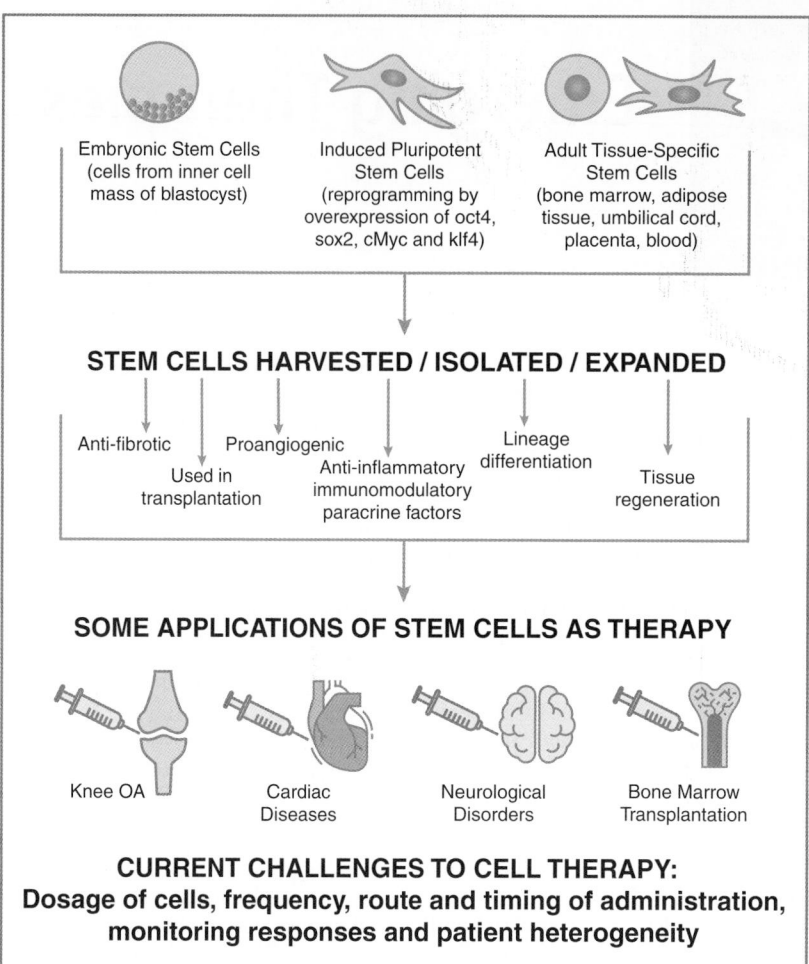

Figure 1 Current stem cell therapies.

to find a donor. The choice for finding a donor includes searching for sibling matches and donors in the National Marrow Donor Program (NMDP) database, which contains the HLA typing results of more than 25 million volunteers. For those patients with rare HLA genotypes or for whom a matched donor is not readily available, a half (haplo) matched donor from a family member (e.g., sibling, parent, child, nephew, niece) can often be identified. The use of haploidentical donors in transplantation has been pioneered in the last decade from the BMT team at Johns Hopkins University.

UCB can also serve as the donor source for hematopoietic cells with the advantage that they are readily available and do not need a complete HLA matching for the transplant. BMT teams in Minnesota and Memorial Sloan Kettering have pioneered the use of UCB for transplant. UCB as a source of hematopoietic stem cells for transplant is more often used in the pediatric age group than in adults due to the paucity of the stem cells in UCB samples, which is adequate for engraftment in a child but insufficient for an adult who will either need two cord blood units or the use of UCB stem cells that are expanded by growing them in the laboratory.

In contrast to allogeneic BMT, *autologous* hematopoietic stem cell transplantation uses the patient's own BM stem cells collected from their blood to treat myeloma, lymphoma, and certain autoimmune conditions like severe systemic sclerosis, lupus, certain types of multiple sclerosis, and diabetes. In autologous transplant the stem cells are harvested from the patient's own blood and cryopreserved. The cells are then infused after high-dose chemotherapy to "rescue" the patient. In this situation the benefit from the procedure is mainly due to the effect of the high-dose chemotherapy on the underlying malignancy or autoimmune lymphocytes. In the future it is likely that chimeric antigen receptor

(CAR) cell therapy may supplant the need for the high-dose chemotherapy and autologous stem cell rescue.

Stem Cell Therapy in Knee Osteoarthritis (OA)

Knee osteoarthritis (OA), the most common form of arthritis, is characterized by loss of articular cartilage, osteophyte formation, and inflammation of the synovial membrane. The main therapeutic approach for knee OA is to improve joint function by cartilage repair, reduction of inflammation, and control of pain. Using cartilage tissue or chondrocytes to replace damaged articular cartilage is one of the potential therapeutic approaches in treating knee OA. In 1997 the FDA approved implantation of autologous chondrocytes, which are allowed to divide and proliferate in vitro, in a process known as expansion, and then injected into the defective cartilage tissue.

Currently, the third generation of this technology, matrix-induced autologous cultured chondrocytes implantation on porcine collagen membrane (MACI), is used where chondrocytes are amplified on a three-dimensional scaffold system before introduction into the joint for the repair of symptomatic cartilage defects of the knee in adult patients. This technology has demonstrated positive results in a 20-year follow-up compared with bone cartilage transplantation. However for autologous chondrocyte transplantation, the number of healthy chondrocytes that can be harvested from older adults are limited in number, and cartilage repair takes a long time after the implantation of chondrocytes. Hence for cartilage repair, several cell sources are under investigation.

Based on the in vivo and in vitro potential of the MSC to differentiate into chondrocytes and osteocytes and their immunomodulatory and immunosuppressive potential, the employment of MSCs for the treatment of OA is a rapidly growing area of clinical research. The use of MSC therapies in the treatment of OA has been determined to be feasible and safe in several different studies; however, there are differences in types of cells used, harvesting techniques, cell yield, and chondrogenic potential. The most used MSCs for the clinical use of the treatment of OA are bone marrow–derived mesenchymal stem cells (BMMSC) and adipose-derived stem cells (ASCs), with bone marrow being the gold standard source for musculoskeletal tissue engineering approaches. Various preclinical animal experiments revealed that MSCs, when injected intraarticularly into joints, inhibited synovial lining thickening, inhibited induction of ligament damage, and protected the joint from destruction by both anabolic and metabolic mediators.

Clinical feasibility, safety, and efficacy of allogenic human BMMSC was studied in a randomized controlled trial of 30 patients with chronic knee OA. Patients who received intraarticular injection of 40 million cells displayed improved cartilage quality posttreatment based on MRI imaging and reported improved knee function and a significant decrease in knee pain. There were no adverse events reported. The clinical application of BMMSC is limited due to their low numbers of stem cells on harvesting and differentiation capacity based on donor age. A multinational meta-analysis report of use of MSC therapy in knee OA involving 582 patients suggested that MSC therapy is safe with low rates of adverse events and improved pain and functional scores after 24-month follow-up compared with controls. ASCs have also been studied in the treatment of OA. Intraarticular injection of ASC exhibited a dose-response effect with significant improvement in knee pain and function in the patients who received a higher dose (i.e., 1×10^8 cells).

Due to invasiveness of harvesting procedures for BMMSC and ASCs, various allogeneic MSC products are now available commercially. Park et al. reported the results of a first-in human clinical trial utilizing a stem cell–based product called Cartistem, a composite of allogenic human UCB-derived MSCs and HA hydrogel. A single dose of Cartistem was demonstrated to be safe with no detectable immunologic issues, improved joint function, and improved quality of life over 7 years of follow-up. The South Korean government approved the sale of Cartistem produced by Medipost Inc. in 2012, as the world's first allogenic, off-the-shelf stem cell drug for the treatment of degenerative arthritis and knee cartilage defects. Though current clinical trials have demonstrated the safety of allogeneic MSCs, there is still a debate about whether there is benefit. Larger randomized controlled trials with large sample sizes utilizing standardized and established outcome scores are required. A number of clinical studies are underway to understand the mechanism of action of stem cells and to explore the cell infusion mechanisms, best cell type, dosage size, dosing frequency, and timing of intervention for MSC therapy. The combination of MSCs with scaffolds, platelet rich plasma (PRP), and growth factors is also being investigated to determine the optimal therapeutic effect.

Overall, for OA of the knee, there is limited availability of strong clinical effectiveness data, a lack of study comparability, and a lack of standardization associated with patient selection and assessment parameters, making it difficult to justify recommendation for the use of this therapy.

Stem Cell Therapy for Cardiac Diseases

Cardiovascular diseases are the most common cause of death, accounting for approximately one-third of deaths worldwide. It has been nearly two decades since the first encouraging preclinical studies reported the repair of infarcted cardiac tissue utilizing bone marrow stem cell transplantation in a model of myocardial infarction. Various studies over the years hypothesize multiple mechanisms by which transplanted cells contribute to repair. The proposed modes of actions include differentiation of cells into cardiomyocytes and paracrine signaling via secretion of cytokines, growth hormones, exosomes, and mitochondrial transfer.

Fueled by the preclinical findings, randomized clinical studies were conducted utilizing BMMSCs and demonstrated safety and improved left ventricular function in patients with acute myocardial infarction. The POSEIDON-DCM study was designed to test the safety and efficacy of allogenic versus autologous BMMSCs in patients with nonischemic dilated cardiomyopathy. The data indicated that allogenic BMMSCs were superior at providing a greater magnitude of clinical efficacy, improved endothelial function, and reduction in the proinflammatory cytokine tumor necrosis factor (TNF)-α in the study population. A recent meta-analysis report that included data between 2017 and 2019 in patients with advanced heart failure suggested that stem cell therapy was safe and was associated with moderate improvement in cardiac function. BOOST, REPAIR-AMI, and REEGENERATE-AMI are some of the other trials that aimed to investigate BMMSC therapy for myocardial infarction (MI) and reported significant improvements in left ventricle (LV) function and emphasized the importance of the timing of cell delivery post-MI.

In contrast to these findings, the SWISS-AMI, Late TIME, and TIME trial showed no improvement in LV function, LV volumes, or infarct size in the treatment group leading to discordant conclusions. These inconsistencies can be attributed to patient variability, heterogenous population of bone marrow–derived cells, different processing procedures, timing of cell delivery, study endpoints, and the unpredictable dynamic course of MI. BioCardia is currently conducting the Phase III CardiAMP Heart Failure (HF) trial using autologous bone marrow cells in patients who developed heart failure post-MI. The study is designed to apply a personalized medicine approach by selecting patients and tailoring treatment to those who are most likely to benefit.

ASCs have been evaluated for their usability, safety, and beneficial effects in a few clinical trials in patients with chronic ischemic heart disease and refractory angina. The initial results from the Precise Trial showed improved left ventricular mass and improved exercise capacity at 18-month follow-up. Intracardiac infusion of two doses of autologous ASCs (40 million and 80 million) were assessed in the Athena trial. While the findings supported the feasibility, safety, and scalability for the treatment of ischemic cardiomyopathy, the efficacy was limited with benefits observed on symptoms, quality of life, and VO₂max. There were no differences observed in left ventricular ejection fraction (LVEF) or LV volumes. These findings clearly require confirmation in additional trials.

Safety and efficacy of Wharton's jelly (WJ) MSC was evaluated for the first time in 2015 in patients with ST-elevation MI (STEMI). In this randomized multicenter trial with 116 patients, Gao et al. reported reductions in scar size, improved LVEF, and increased cardiac function after intracoronary infusion of WJ MSCs in patients with ST-elevation acute MI.

Cardiac stem cells (CSCs), a heterogenous cell population in the heart representing multipotent, self-replicating, c-kit+ cells expressing cardiac markers, have an effective capacity to differentiate into cardiomyocytes. CSCs were first tested in humans in the SCIPIO phase I clinical trial in which c-kit+ CSCs were isolated from biopsies obtained from patients with ischemic cardiomyopathy undergoing coronary artery bypass grafting and administered via intracoronary infusion 4 months later. The results showed improved LVEF and decreased infarct size at 12-month follow-up. Similarly, the CADUCEUS trial reported that intracoronary infusion of autologous CDCs after MI led to scar reduction, an increase in viable heart mass, and improved cardiac contractility. Advantages and disadvantages of stem cells evaluated for the treatment of cardiovascular disorders is outlined in Table 1.

Whereas lessons learned from more than 200 trials of cardiovascular diseases demonstrated the safety and feasibility of the addition of various stem cell types to the routine of care, efficacy studies only showed marginal improvements in cardiac function. The disappointing clinical success of stem cell therapy in heart disease has been attributed to the low retention and poor survival of transplanted cells. Large scale, randomized, placebo controlled clinical trials with strategies to improve stem cell survival and engraftment need to be conducted to unearth these details. In addition, the cell type that would result in maximal benefit is yet to be determined.

TABLE 1 Advantages and Disadvantages of Stem Cells Evaluated for the Treatment of Cardiovascular Disorders

CELL TYPES	ADVANTAGES	DISADVANTAGES
Bone marrow mononuclear cells (BMMNCs)	Extensively studied in clinical trials; safe; some trials showed improved LV functions and contractility.	Heterogenous cell population; inconsistent results regarding therapeutic action; lack of standard methodologies between trials; recent trials showing no improvement.
Mesenchymal stem cells (MSCs)	Autologous and allogeneic sources used; safe; no evidence of tumorigenicity; low risk of rejection; ease of isolation and expansion; immunomodulatory and immunoprivileged ability.	Lack standard study methodologies; limited differentiation potential; inconsistent reports of efficacy; need long-term follow-up.
Cardiac stem cells (CSCs)	Autologous transplantation; safe; immunomodulatory and immunosuppressive ability.	Invasive isolation procedure; limited cell quantity; poor cell quality from older donors; costly expansion.
Embryonic stem cells (ESCs)	Pluripotent; off-the-shelf products; differentiate into cardiomyocytes that can integrate with cardiac muscle.	Ethical concerns; tumorigenic potential; genetic instability; risk of immune rejection; availability issues.
Induced pluripotent stem cells (iPSCs)	Pluripotent; derived from adult somatic cells; no ethical concerns; unlimited quantity; superior functional integration into host cardiac tissue.	Tumorigenic potential; genetic instability; possible risk of immune rejection; lack of efficient procedures to induce pluripotency; no clinical translation yet.

Stem Cell Therapy for Neurologic Disorders

Several clinical trials have been conducted to evaluate the safety and efficacy of stem cell therapy for central nervous system disorders. MSCs were shown to be able to cross the blood–brain barrier through paracellular pathways despite the presence of tight junctions. Stem cells can be transplanted into the brain directly intracerebrally or intrathecally or can be delivered by blood infusion. Several mechanisms by which stem cell therapy may offer therapeutic potential in patients with neurologic disorders include:

- Transplantation of stem cells and differentiated neuronal or glial cells to replace damaged neural cells with new, viable cells
- Transplanted cells may promote angiogenesis and neuroprotection by secreting several neurotropic and growth factors
- Induction of neurogenesis by activating endogenous stem cells accelerating new nerve growth in proliferative niches
- Immunomodulation by reducing the local inflammatory response and promoting remyelination in damage nervous system

Over the past few decades, safety and feasibility of stem cell therapy have been demonstrated in experimental animal models and in phase I/II clinical trials of neurologic diseases such as Alzheimer's disease, stroke, spinal cord injury, amyotrophic lateral sclerosis, multiple sclerosis, traumatic brain injury, cerebral infarction, and Parkinson's disease. Cell sources for these studies include autologous or allogeneic umbilical cord blood, autologous bone marrow, fetal neural stem cells, embryonic stem cells, and mesenchymal stromal cells derived from adipose tissue or umbilical cord tissue. Most of these trials are registered for stroke, multiple sclerosis, and spinal cord injury. Use of MSCs in early stage clinical trials (phase I/II) for ischemic stroke and multiple sclerosis has demonstrated improvements in motor impairment scales and signs of clinical stabilization. Intrathecal and/or intravenous infusion of MSCs following expansion in patients with spinal cord injury demonstrated that MSC administration is safe and well tolerated, with apparent and subtle improvements in sensory (e.g., light touch and pin prick) and bladder functions. However, relative to rehabilitation therapy, no significant improvements in motor function were reported. Japanese authorities have recently granted approval of stem cell therapy (Stemirac) for spinal cord injury based on positive outcomes of a 13-patient study, which was not placebo controlled. Independent researchers warn of the premature nature of this approval and that the trial design cannot claim definitive efficacy.

Bone marrow stem cells have been used in an autologous stem cell transplant setting after high-dose chemotherapy for select patients with multiple sclerosis as reported by Burt and colleagues from Chicago. This needs to be validated by other centers before being accepted as the standard.

Whereas the future of stem cell therapy for neurologic disease appears to be promising, the variables to be determined include the optimal type of stem cell, dosage, route and timing of administration, and the stage of the patient's disease. Evidence is also accumulating on advantages of combined administration of different stem cells/progenitor cells along with various scaffolds. Since complex disease requires complex therapies, it is unlikely that stem cell therapy could be administered as a monotherapy but rather will form part of a more holistic approach that aims to significantly improve the quality of life of affected patients.

Other Promising Indications for Stem Cell Therapy

The future of stem cell therapies looks promising with ongoing clinical research trials for macular degeneration, Crohn disease, rheumatoid arthritis, muscular dystrophy, wound healing, and baldness. Currently there are no approved cell therapies for these indications.

References

Beltrami AP, et al: Adult cardiac stem cells are multipotent and support myocardial regeneration, *Cell* 114(6):763–776, 2003.

Burt RK, et al: Effect of nonmyeloablative hematopoietic stem cell transplantation vs continued disease-modifying therapy on disease progression in patients with relapsing-remitting multiple sclerosis: a randomized clinical trial, *J Am Med Assoc* 321(2):165–174, 2019.

Center for International Blood and Marrow Transplant Research: https://www.cibmtr.org/ReferenceCenter/SlidesReports/SummarySlides/pages/index.aspx.

Chen SL, et al: Effect on left ventricular function of intracoronary transplantation of autologous bone marrow mesenchymal stem cell in patients with acute myocardial infarction, *Am J Cardiol* 94(1):92–95, 2004.

Chugh AR, et al: Administration of cardiac stem cells in patients with ischemic cardiomyopathy: the SCIPIO trial: surgical aspects and interim analysis of myocardial function and viability by magnetic resonance, *Circulation* 126(11 suppl 1):S54–S64, 2012.

Cyranoski D: Japan's approval of stem-cell treatment for spinal-cord injury concerns scientists, *Nature* 565(7741):544–545, 2019.

FDA: https://www.fda.gov/vaccines-blood-biologics/cellular-gene-therapy-products/approved-cellular-and-gene-therapy-products, F.a.s.c.t.

Fisher SA, et al: Stem cell therapy for chronic ischaemic heart disease and congestive heart failure, *Cochrane Database Syst Rev* (4):CD007888, 2014.

Gao LR, et al: Intracoronary infusion of Wharton's jelly-derived mesenchymal stem cells in acute myocardial infarction: double-blind, randomized controlled trial, *BMC Med* 13:162, 2015.

Hare JM, et al: Randomized comparison of allogeneic versus autologous mesenchymal stem cells for nonischemic dilated cardiomyopathy: POSEIDON-DCM trial, *J Am Coll Cardiol* 69(5):526–537, 2017.

Henry TD, et al: The Athena trials: autologous adipose-derived regenerative cells for refractory chronic myocardial ischemia with left ventricular dysfunction, *Catheter Cardiovasc Interv* 89(2):169–177, 2017.

Henry TD, Moye L, Traverse JH: Consistently inconsistent-bone marrow mononuclear stem cell therapy following acute myocardial infarction: a decade later, *Circ Res* 119(3):404–406, 2016.

Jayaraj JS, et al: Efficacy and safety of stem cell therapy in advanced heart failure patients: a systematic review with a meta-analysis of recent trials between 2017 and 2019, *Cureus* 11(9):e5585, 2019.

Jo CH, et al: Intra-articular injection of mesenchymal stem cells for the treatment of osteoarthritis of the knee: a proof-of-concept clinical trial, *Stem Cell* 32(5):1254–1266, 2014.

Lee JW, et al: A randomized, open-label, multicenter trial for the safety and efficacy of adult mesenchymal stem cells after acute myocardial infarction, *J Korean Med Sci* 29(1):23–31, 2014.

Makkar RR, et al: Intracoronary cardiosphere-derived cells for heart regeneration after myocardial infarction (CADUCEUS): a prospective, randomised phase 1 trial, *Lancet* 379(9819):895–904, 2012.

Orlic D, et al: Bone marrow cells regenerate infarcted myocardium, *Nature* 410(6829):701–705, 2001.

Park YB, et al: Cartilage regeneration in osteoarthritic patients by a composite of allogeneic umbilical cord blood-derived mesenchymal stem cells and Hyaluronate hydrogel: results from a clinical trial for safety and proof-of-concept with 7 Years of extended follow-up, *Stem Cells Transl Med* 6(2):613–621, 2017.

Pelletier JP, Martel-Pelletier J, Abramson SB: Osteoarthritis, an inflammatory disease: potential implication for the selection of new therapeutic targets, *Arthritis Rheum* 44(6):1237–1247, 2001.

Perin EC, et al: Adipose-derived regenerative cells in patients with ischemic cardiomyopathy: the PRECISE Trial, *Am Heart J* 168(1):88–95.e2, 2014.

Richter DL, et al: Knee articular cartilage repair and restoration techniques: a review of the literature, *Sports Health* 8(2):153–160, 2016.

Robinton DA, Daley GQ: The promise of induced pluripotent stem cells in research and therapy, *Nature* 481(7381):295–305, 2012.

Schachinger V, et al: Intracoronary bone marrow-derived progenitor cells in acute myocardial infarction, *N Engl J Med* 355(12):1210–1221, 2006.

Soder RP, et al: A phase I study to evaluate two doses of Wharton's jelly-derived mesenchymal stromal cells for the treatment of De Novo high-risk or Steroid-refractory acute graft versus host disease, *Stem Cell Rev Rep* 16(5):979–991, 2020.

Stamm C, et al: Autologous bone-marrow stem-cell transplantation for myocardial regeneration, *Lancet* 361(9351):45–46, 2003.

ter Huurne M, et al: Antiinflammatory and chondroprotective effects of intraarticular injection of adipose-derived stem cells in experimental osteoarthritis, *Arthritis Rheum* 64(11):3604–3613, 2012.

Thomas ED, et al: Intravenous infusion of bone marrow in patients receiving radiation and chemotherapy, *N Engl J Med* 257(11):491–496, 1957.

Thomson JA, et al: Embryonic stem cell lines derived from human blastocysts, *Science* 282(5391):1145–1147, 1998.

Wollert KC, et al: Intracoronary autologous bone-marrow cell transfer after myocardial infarction: the BOOST randomised controlled clinical trial, *Lancet* 364(9429):141–148, 2004.

Yubo M, et al: Clinical efficacy and safety of mesenchymal stem cell transplantation for osteoarthritis treatment: a meta-analysis, *PloS One* 12(4):e0175449, 2017.

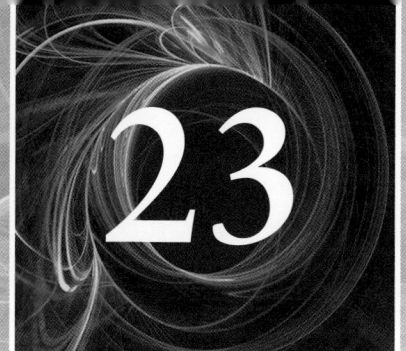

Appendices and Index

BIOLOGIC AGENTS REFERENCE CHART

Method of
Laurie A.M. Hommema, MD; and Kevin Hommema, BSME

Biological weapons are devices used intentionally to cause disease or death through dissemination of microorganisms or toxins in food and water, by insect vectors, or by aerosols. Potential targets include human beings, food crops, livestock, and other resources essential for national security, economy, and defense. Unlike nuclear, chemical, and conventional weapons, the onset of a biological attack will probably be insidious. For some infectious agents, secondary and tertiary transmission could continue for weeks or months after the initial attack. In the United States, anthrax has been used in 2001 and ricin in 2003, 2004, and 2013 to target individuals. The Department of Homeland Security leads a national strategy to prevent, detect, respond to, and recover from acts of bioterrorism.

Initial detection of an unannounced biological attack will likely occur when an astute health professional notices an unusual case or disease cluster and reports his or her concerns to local public health authorities. Due to the incubation period of most biologic agents, subjects may have traveled from site of exposure to other geographic locations. Physicians and other health professionals should be alert to the following:

- Unusual temporal or geographic clustering of illnesses in humans, as well as animals
- Increase in specific lab testing or prescription drugs
- Sudden increase of illness in previously healthy persons
- Sudden increase in nonspecific illnesses such as pneumonia; flulike illness; bleeding disorders; unexplained rashes, particularly in adults; neuromuscular illnesses; and gastrointestinal syndromes

To enhance detection and treatment capabilities, physicians and other health professionals in acute care settings should be familiar with the clinical manifestations, diagnostic techniques, isolation precautions, treatment, and prophylaxis for likely causative agents (e.g., smallpox, pneumonic plague, anthrax, viral hemorrhagic fevers). Table 1 provides a quick summary of diagnostic and treatment considerations for various infectious and toxic biological agents. For some of these agents, delay in medical response could result in a potentially devastating number of casualties. To mitigate such consequences, early identification and intervention are imperative. Frontline physicians must have an increased level of suspicion regarding the possible intentional use of biological agents as well as an increased sensitivity to reporting those suspicious to public health authorities, who, in turn, must be willing to evaluate a predictable increase in false-positive reports.

Medical response efforts require coordination and planning with emergency management agencies, law enforcement, health care facilities, and social services agencies. Due to the criminal nature of the act, samples need to be collected and handled as evidence. Healthcare agencies should ensure that physicians know whom to call with reports of suspicious cases and clusters of infectious diseases, and they should work to build a good relationship with the local medical community. Resource integration is absolutely necessary to:

- Establish adequate capacity to initiate rapid investigation of an outbreak
- Establish and ensure decontamination protocols are in place
- Educate and protect healthcare workers and the public
- Coordinate mass distribution of antibiotics and vaccines
- Address psychological consequences

In an epidemic, overwhelming numbers of critically ill patients will require acute and follow-up medical care. Both infected persons and the worried well will seek medical attention, with a corresponding need for medical supplies, diagnostic tests, and hospital beds. The impact—or even the threat—of an attack can elicit widespread panic and civil disorder, overwhelm hospital resources, and disrupt social services.

Any suspicious or confirmed exposure to a biological weapons agent should be reported immediately to the local health department, local Federal Bureau of Investigation office, National Response Center (800-424-8802), and the Centers for Disease Control and Prevention Operation's Center (770-488-7100).

TABLE 1 Quick Reference Chart on Biological Weapon Agents

DISEASE AND AGENT	DIAGNOSTIC CONSIDERATIONS			TREATMENT CONSIDERATIONS*			
	SIGNS AND SYMPTOMS	INCUBATION PERIOD	DIAGNOSIS	LETHALITY	TREATMENT	PROPHYLAXIS	COMMENTS
Bacteria							
Anthrax *Bacillus anthracis* (all forms)		1–6 days (perhaps ≤60 days)[†]	Gram stain and culture of blood, pleural fluid, cerebrospinal fluid, ascitic fluid, vesicular fluid, or lesion exudate. Confirmatory serologic and PCR tests are available through public health laboratory network.		Steroids may be considered for severe edema and for meningitis. Penicillin G should be considered if strain is susceptible and does not possess inducible β-lactamases.	Ciprofloxacin or doxycycline with or without vaccination. If strain is susceptible, penicillin VK[1] or amoxicillin[1] (Amoxil) should be considered. Anthrax Vaccine Adsorbed (BioThrax) Preexposure (PrEP): 5 IM injections given at day 0, 1 month, and 6 months, then 12 and 18 months; and annually thereafter for persons who remain at risk. Postexposure (PEP): SC injection given at 0, 2, and 4 weeks combined with po ciprofloxacin or doxycycline for up to 60 days. Raxibacumab (ABthrax) is approved for PEP if no other options are available.	If meningitis is suspected, doxycycline may be less optimal because of poor CNS penetration. Sporicidal decontamination is necessary, such as sodium hypochlorite (chlorine bleach).
Cutaneous	Evolving *painless* skin lesion (face, neck, arms), progresses to vesicle, depressed ulcer, eschar with edema and regional lymphadenopathy		Gram stain and culture of unroofed vesicle, or under eschar	20% if untreated, otherwise rarely fatal	Ciprofloxacin[1] or doxycycline		
Gastrointestinal	Oropharyngeal: fever, severe pharyngitis, oral ulcers with patches and pseudo-membranes. Intestinal: Nausea, vomiting, abdominal pain, bloody diarrhea, sepsis. Widened mediastinum on chest radiograph is occasionally seen‡.		Gram stain and culture of throat lesions or stool culture	Approaches 100% if untreated, but data are limited. Rapid, aggressive treatment can reduce mortality.			

TABLE 1 Quick Reference Chart on Biological Weapon Agents—cont'd

DISEASE AND AGENT	DIAGNOSTIC CONSIDERATIONS				TREATMENT CONSIDERATIONS*			
	SIGNS AND SYMPTOMS	INCUBATION PERIOD	DIAGNOSIS	LETHALITY	TREATMENT	PROPHYLAXIS	COMMENTS	
Inhalational	Abrupt onset of flulike symptoms, fever with or without chills, sweats, fatigue or malaise, non- or minimally productive cough, nausea, vomiting, dyspnea, headache, chest pain, followed in 2–5 days by severe respiratory distress, mediastinitis, hemorrhagic meningitis, sepsis, shock§ Widened mediastinum on chest radiograph or CT is characteristic‡.		Routine blood culture, CSF, and pleural effusions. Sputum is rarely positive.	Once respiratory distress develops, mortality rates approach 90%. Begin treatment when inhalational anthrax is suspected; do not wait for confirmatory testing¶.	Combination therapy of ciprofloxacin[1] or doxycycline plus one or two other antimicrobials should be considered¶. Raxibacumab (a human monoclonal antibody) and Anthrasil (an anthrax immune globulin IV [AIGIV]) are also available as FDA-approved drugs to treat inhalational anthrax.			
Brucellosis *Brucella abortus, B. canis, B. melitensis, B. suis*	Nonspecific flulike symptoms, fever, headache, profound weakness, profuse sweats, chills, weight loss, malaise. Abdominal pain, nausea, vomiting, and diarrhea are common. Hepatomegaly and splenomegaly may be found on exam, as well as osteoarticular findings.	5–60 days, usually 1–2 months	Blood and bone marrow culture (can require 6 weeks to grow *Brucella*) Confirmatory culture and serologic testing	Fatality is rare; morbidity is often significant.	Doxycycline plus rifampin[1] *Alternative therapies:* Ofloxacin[1] plus rifampin[1] Doxycycline plus gentamicin (Garamycin)[1] TMP-SMX[1] plus gentamicin	Doxycycline plus rifampin[1] for high-risk exposure. No approved human vaccine; livestock vaccines are available.	Osteoarticular complications are common, including sacroiliitis, bursitis, tenosynovitis, paravertebral abscess, or discitis.	
Glanders *Burkholderia mallei* Melioidosis *Burkholderia pseudomallei*	Fever, sweats, myalgias, headaches, cough, lymphadenopathy. Can progress to hepatosplenomegaly with pustular eruptions. CXR with infiltrates, cavitation, abscess, or miliary lesions. Imaging with splenic or hepatic abscesses.	Glanders: days to weeks Melioidosis: days to decades	Gram stain, culture, and PCR	Fatal if untreated	IV ceftazidime (Fortaz)[1], meropenem (Merrem)[1] or imipenem (+ cilastatin [Primaxin][1] and prolonged oral TMP-SMX[1]	No approved PEP or vaccines available. TMP-SMX[1] can be considered.	One of the first bacterial agents to be weaponized. Prostatic abscess may be seen. Life-long follow-up for melioidosis as risk of relapse is 10%.	

Continued

Biologic Agents Reference Chart

TABLE 1 Quick Reference Chart on Biological Weapon Agents—cont'd

DISEASE AND AGENT	DIAGNOSTIC CONSIDERATIONS			TREATMENT CONSIDERATIONS*			
	SIGNS AND SYMPTOMS	INCUBATION PERIOD	DIAGNOSIS	LETHALITY	TREATMENT	PROPHYLAXIS	COMMENTS
Typhoidal tularemia *Francisella tularensis*	Sudden onset of acute febrile illness, weakness, chills, headache, generalized body aches, elevated WBCs Pulmonary symptoms such as dry cough, chest pain, or tightness with or without objective signs of pneumonia Progressive weakness, malaise, anorexia, and weight loss, potentially leading to sepsis and organ failure. Temperature/pulse mismatch may be seen.	3–5 days' range, 1–21 days	Largely clinical Culture of blood, sputum, biopsies, pleural fluid, bronchial washings; notify laboratory if suspected as culturing poses risk in standard lab.	~30%–60% Fatal if untreated	Streptomycin or gentamicin[1] *Alternative therapies:* Ciprofloxacin[1] Doxycycline Chloramphenicol (Chloromycetin)[1]	Tetracycline Doxycycline Ciprofloxacin[1] Live, attenuated vaccine (USAMRIID, IND) given by scarification; currently under FDA review, limited availability	Ulceroglandular forms with regional lymphadenopathy may also be seen.
Pneumonic plague *Yersinia pestis*	Acute onset of flulike prodrome: fever, myalgia, weakness, headache; within 24 h of prodrome, chest discomfort, cough with bloody sputum, and dyspnea By day 2–4 of illness, symptoms progressing to cyanosis, respiratory distress, shock, and bleeding diathesis.	1–6 days	Gram stain and culture of blood, CSF, sputum, lymph node aspirates, bronchial washings Confirmatory serologic and bacteriologic tests available through public health laboratory network	Almost 100% if untreated 20%–60% if appropriately treated within 18–24 h of symptoms	Streptomycin, gentamicin[1] *Alternative therapies:* Doxycycline Tetracycline Ciprofloxacin[1] Chloramphenicol (Chloromycetin) is first choice for meningitis except for pregnant women.	Tetracycline Doxycycline Ciprofloxacin[1] Previous licensed vaccine not effective against aerosol exposure	Pneumonic plague is expected outcome of biological agent attack, as opposed to the presentation of Bubonic plague with swollen lymph nodes. Begin treatment when diagnosis of plague is suspected; do not wait for confirmatory testing.
Rickettsia Q-fever *Coxiella burnetii*	Nonspecific febrile disease, chills, cough, weakness and fatigue, pleuritic chest pain Pneumonia is possible.	10–17 days, up to 5 weeks	Isolation of organism may be difficult; IgG antibody testing by IFA is gold standard. Confirmatory testing via serology or PCR available through public health laboratory network.	1%–3% Fatalities are uncommon, except in cases of endocarditis. Pregnancy loss if infected in first trimester.	Tetracycline Doxycycline	Tetracycline doxycycline, not endorsed by CDC. Inactivated whole-cell vaccine (Q-Vax) is available in Australia and Europe, but only available in USA for investigational basis (IND).	Chronic disease may occur, including endocarditis. Skin test to determine prior exposure to *C. burnetii* is recommended before vaccination.

TABLE 1 Quick Reference Chart on Biological Weapon Agents—cont'd

DISEASE AND AGENT	DIAGNOSTIC CONSIDERATIONS				TREATMENT CONSIDERATIONS*		
	SIGNS AND SYMPTOMS	INCUBATION PERIOD	DIAGNOSIS	LETHALITY	TREATMENT	PROPHYLAXIS	COMMENTS
Viruses							
Smallpox Variola major virus	Prodrome of high fever, malaise, prostration, headache, vomiting, delirium followed in 2–3 days by maculopapular rash uniformly progressing to pustules and scabs, mostly on extremities and face	7–17 days	Clinical pharyngeal swab, vesicular fluid, biopsies, scab material for electron microscopy and PCR testing through public health laboratory network	30% in unvaccinated persons	Supportive care Tecovirimat (Tpoxx) was approved for the treatment of smallpox under the FDA's Animal Rule; however, its efficacy in humans has not been determined. Other IND products are available including cidofovir (Vistide).	Live, attenuated vaccinia vaccine (ACAM2000) derived from calf lymph; given by scarification (licensed, restricted supply) New vaccine being developed from tissue culture Vaccination given within 3–4 days following exposure can prevent or decrease the severity of disease.	Requires astute clinical evaluation; may be confused with chickenpox, erythema multiforme with bullae, or allergic contact dermatitis. Strict airborne and contact precautions. Notify CDC Poxvirus Section at 404-639-2184.
Viral Encephalitis							
All forms	Systemic febrile illness, with encephalitis developing in some populations Generalized malaise, spiking fevers, headache, myalgia		Clinical and epidemiologic diagnosis WBC count can show striking leukopenia and lymphopenia. Confirmatory test and viral isolation available through public health laboratory network.		Supportive care Analgesics, anticonvulsants as needed	No accepted PEP. Several IND vaccines available.	Incidence of seizures and/or focal neurologic deficits may be higher after biological attack.
Eastern equine encephalitis		5–15 days		50%–75%			
Western equine encephalitis		5–10 days		10%			
Venezuelan equine encephalitis		2–6 days		<10%			

Continued

Biologic Agents Reference Chart

TABLE 1 Quick Reference Chart on Biological Weapon Agents—cont'd

DISEASE AND AGENT	DIAGNOSTIC CONSIDERATIONS				TREATMENT CONSIDERATIONS*			
	SIGNS AND SYMPTOMS	INCUBATION PERIOD	DIAGNOSIS	LETHALITY	TREATMENT	PROPHYLAXIS	COMMENTS	

Viral Hemorrhagic Fevers

DISEASE AND AGENT	SIGNS AND SYMPTOMS	INCUBATION PERIOD	DIAGNOSIS	LETHALITY	TREATMENT	PROPHYLAXIS	COMMENTS
Arenaviruses (Lassa, Junin, and related viruses) Bunyaviruses (Hanta, Congo–Crimean, Rift Valley) Filoviruses (Ebola, Marburg) Flaviviruses (yellow fever, dengue, various tick-borne disease viruses)	Fever with facial flushing, mucous membrane bleeding, petechiae, thrombocytopenia, and hypotension. Malaise, myalgias, headache, vomiting, diarrhea possible	4–21 days	Clinical diagnosis. Confirmatory testing and viral isolation available through BSL-4 laboratories.	Variable depending on viral strain; 15%–25% with Lassa fever to ≤90% with Ebola	Supportive therapy Ribavirin (Virazole)[1] may be effective for Lassa fever, Rift Valley fever, Argentine hemorrhagic fever, and Congo–Crimean hemorrhagic fever.	Ribavarin (Virazole)[1] is suggested for Arenaviruses and Bunyaviruses. Yellow fever vaccine (YF-VAX) is the only licensed vaccine available for yellow fever prevention. Vaccines for some of the other VHFs exist but are for investigational use only.	Strict airborne, droplet, and contact precautions. Call CDC Special Pathogens Office at 404-639-1115.

Biological Toxins

DISEASE AND AGENT	SIGNS AND SYMPTOMS	INCUBATION PERIOD	DIAGNOSIS	LETHALITY	TREATMENT	PROPHYLAXIS	COMMENTS
Botulism *Clostridium botulinum* toxin	Cranial nerve palsies including diplopia, dry mouth, ptosis, dysphagia. As disease progresses, acute bilateral descending flaccid paralysis, respiratory paralysis resulting in death	1–5 days, typically 12–36 h	Clinical Serum and stool should be assayed for toxin by mouse neutralization bioassay, which can take several days. NCV or EMG.	60% without ventilatory support	Intensive and prolonged supportive care; ventilation may be necessary. Heptavalent Botulism Antitoxin (HBAT) is available.	Pentavalent toxoid (A–E), no longer available. Antitoxin may be sufficient to prevent illness following exposure but is not recommended until patient is showing symptoms.	Anaphylaxis and serum sickness are potential complications of antitoxin. Aminoglycosides and clindamycin (Cleocin) must not be used.
Enterotoxin B *Staphylococcus aureus*	Inhaled: acute onset of fever, chills, headache, nonproductive cough Ingested: nausea, vomiting, cramps diarrhea	3–12 h inhaled, 1–6 h ingested	Clinical Normal chest radiograph Serology on acute and convalescent serum can confirm diagnosis.	Probably low (few data available for respiratory exposure)	Supportive care	No vaccine available. Use of mask to prevent inhalation.	
Ricin toxin *Ricinus communis*	Weakness, nausea, chest tightness, fever, cough, pulmonary edema, respiratory failure, circulatory collapse, hypoxemia resulting in death (usually within 36–72 h)	≤6–24 h	Clinical and epidemiologic Confirmatory serological testing available through public health laboratory network.	Mortality data are not available, but likely to be high with extensive exposure.	Supportive care Treatment for pulmonary edema Gastric decontamination if toxin is ingested. NSAIDs.	No vaccine or antitoxin available. Use of mask to prevent inhalation.	Hypochlorite inactivates.

TABLE 1 Quick Reference Chart on Biological Weapon Agents—cont'd

DISEASE AND AGENT	DIAGNOSTIC CONSIDERATIONS			TREATMENT CONSIDERATIONS*			
	SIGNS AND SYMPTOMS	INCUBATION PERIOD	DIAGNOSIS	LETHALITY	TREATMENT	PROPHYLAXIS	COMMENTS
T-2 Mycotoxins *Fusarium* *Myrothecium* *Trichoderma* *Stachybotrys*	Skin pain, pruritis, erythema, vesiculation, and sloughing. Throat pain, rhinorrhea, cough, and hemoptysis. Weakness, ataxia, shock can occur in severe exposure.	Minutes to hours	Suspect if "yellow rain" with oily pigmented fluids staining close and environment.	Can be seen in severe exposures.	Clinical support	No vaccine available.	Soap and water washing within 4–6 h reduces dermal toxicity; washing within 1 h can eliminate toxicity entirely.
Other filamentous fungi			Confirmation requires testing blood, tissue, and environmental samples.	Severe exposure can cause death in hours to days.			Consult with local health department regarding specimen collection and diagnostic testing procedures.

[1]Not FDA approved for this indication.

*Different situations can require different dosage and treatment regimens. Please consult other references and an infectious disease specialist for definitive dosage information, especially dosages for pregnant women and children.

†Data from 22 patients infected with anthrax in October and November 2001 indicate a median incubation period of 4 days (range, 4–7 days) for inhalational anthrax and a mean incubation of 5 days (range, 1–10 days) for cutaneous anthrax.

‡Chest radiograph abnormalities include paratracheal and hilar fullness and may be subtle. Consider chest computed tomography if diagnosis is uncertain.

§Limited data from the October and November 2001 anthrax infections indicate hemorrhagic pleural effusions to be strongly associated with inhalational anthrax; rhinorrhea was present in only 1/10 patients.

‖Limited data from the 2001 terrorist-related anthrax infections indicate that early treatment significantly decreased the mortality rate.

¶Other agents with in vitro activity suggested for use in conjunction with ciprofloxacin or doxycycline for treatment of inhalational anthrax include rifampin[1], vancomycin (Vancocin)[1], imipenem (Primaxin)[1], chloramphenicol (Chloromycetin)[1], penicillin G and ampicillin[1], clindamycin (Cleocin)[1], and clarithromycin (Biaxin)[1].

CDC, Centers for Disease Control and Prevention; *CNS,* central nervous system; *CSF,* cerebrospinal fluid; *GI,* gastrointestinal; *IND,* investigational new drug; *PEP,* post-exposure prophylaxis; *PCR,* polymerase chain reaction; *TMP-SMX,* trimethoprim-sulfamethoxazole; *USAMRIID,* U.S. Army Medical Research Institute of Infectious Diseases; *VHF,* viral hemorrhagic fever; *WBC,* white blood cell.

Adapted from "Blue Book" USAMRIID's Medical Management of Biological Casualties, 8th edition, September 2014; and Lyznicki JL: AMA quick reference guide: exposure to toxic chemical agents. In: American Medical Association: Management of Public Health Emergencies, *A Resource Guide for Physicians and Other Community Responders,* Chicago, American Medical Association, 2005.

Popular Herbs and Nutritional Supplements

HERB OR NUTRITIONAL SUPPLEMENT	COMMON USES	REASONABLE ADULT ORAL DOSAGE*	PRECAUTIONS AND DRUG INTERACTIONS
Aloe vera	Commonly found in skin products as a moisturizer Used topically to treat burns, wounds, skin infections, and inflammation Approved in Germany to use orally as a laxative Used orally for a variety of conditions, including diabetes, asthma, epilepsy, and osteoarthritis	For external use, apply aloe gel on the skin tid to qid For constipation, 40–170 mg of dried aloe juice or latex (corresponds to 10–30 mg hydroxyanthracene derivatives) taken in the evening For other conditions, no established dosage documented	Aloe gel is generally well tolerated and safe when used topically Aloe gel taken orally can cause hypoglycemia in patients who are concomitantly taking antidiabetic drugs Aloe juice or latex contains anthraquinone, a cathartic laxative and should not be taken by people with intestinal obstruction, acute intestinal inflammation, and ulcers Pregnant women should not take aloe latex because it may cause uterine contractions Oral use of aloe latex can cause abdominal cramps and diarrhea. Long-term use or abuse can cause electrolyte imbalances, albuminuria, hematuria, and pseudomelanosis coli. Prolonged use of high doses (≥ 1 g/d) can cause nephritis, acute renal failure, and death In 2002, the FDA banned the sale of aloe-containing laxative products in the United States because of the lack of safety data Aloe can decrease platelet aggregation and should be avoided at least 2 weeks before surgery
Astragalus	Used in combination with other herbs to support and enhance the immune system Used to prevent and treat common colds and upper respiratory infections Used for heart disease Widely used in China for chronic hepatitis and as an adjunctive therapy in cancer	Extract: 250–500 mg tid to qid standardized to 0.4% 4-hydroxy-3-methoxyisoflavone 7-sug Powdered root: 500–1000 mg tid Tincture (1:5) in 30% ethanol: 3–5 mL tid Decoction: 3–6 g of dried root per 12 oz water tid	Avoid using astragalus in organ transplant patients and those with autoimmune disorders Side effects include mild stomach upset and allergic reactions Astragalus can decrease the effects of cyclophosphamide and other immunosuppressants
Bilberry fruit	Often used orally to improve visual acuity and to treat degenerative retinal conditions Used orally to treat chronic venous insufficiency, varicose veins, and hemorrhoids Approved in Germany to use orally for acute diarrhea and topically for mild inflammation of the mucous membranes of mouth and throat	For eye conditions and circulation, 80–160 mg tid of the extract standardized to at least 25% anthocyanosides For diarrhea, 20–60 g/d of the dried, ripe berries or as a tea preparation (5–10 g of crushed dried berries in 150 mL water, brought to a boil for 10 min, then strained) For external use, 10% decoction	No known side effects reported with bilberry fruit and extract However, bilberry leaf taken in large quantities or used long term has been shown to cause wasting, anemia, jaundice, acute excitation, disturbances of tonus, and death in animals The anthocyanidin extracts from bilberry can increase the risk of bleeding in those taking warfarin or other blood thinners
Black cohosh root	Commonly used to relieve hot flashes and other menopausal symptoms Used to treat premenstrual discomfort and dysmenorrhea	20 mg bid of the rhizome extract standardized to triterpene glycosides Remifemin is the proprietary brand used in a number of clinical trials The German guidelines do not recommend its use for > 6 months	Black cohosh may have an estrogen-like effect and should be avoided in women with breast cancer Large doses may induce miscarriage and it is contraindicated during pregnancy It may cause GI disturbances, headache, and hypotension International case reports of liver dysfunction suspected to be associated with its use
Black haw	To relieve uterine cramps and painful periods To prevent miscarriage and ease pain that follows childbirth	For menstrual pain, 5 mL of tincture in water, taken 3–5 times daily For prevention of miscarriage, 1–2 cups of tea per day (1 tsp of dried herb in 1 cup of boiling water, steeped for 10 min)	Black haw should not be used in pregnancy because of its uterine relaxant effects The salicylate constituent in black haw could trigger allergic reactions in individuals with aspirin allergies or asthma Black haw may aggravate tinnitus Large doses of black haw can prolong bleeding time The oxalic acid component of black haw can increase kidney stone formation in susceptible individuals Black haw can interact with warfarin and increase risk of bleeding

HERB OR NUTRITIONAL SUPPLEMENT	COMMON USES	REASONABLE ADULT ORAL DOSAGE*	PRECAUTIONS AND DRUG INTERACTIONS
Cat's claw	Used primarily to reduce pain in osteoarthritis and rheumatoid arthritis Used for a variety of health conditions, including viral infections (e.g., herpes, HIV), Alzheimer disease, and cancer Used to support the immune system and promote kidney health Used to prevent and abort pregnancy	For osteoarthritis, 100 mg/d of the dry encapsulated extract For rheumatoid arthritis, 20 mg tid of the dry extract standardized to 1.3% pentacyclic oxindole alkaloids free of tetracyclic oxindole alkaloids For general uses, 1–3 cups of tea per day (1 g root bark boiled for 15 min in 250 mL of water) or 1 mL of tincture 2–3 times/d	Avoid using cat's claw during pregnancy or breastfeeding People with autoimmune diseases and transplant recipients should avoid cat's claw because of its immune stimulating effects Side effects include headaches, dizziness, and vomiting Cat's claw can lower blood pressure and cause hypotension when used with antihypertensive drugs Cat's claw can inhibit CYP3A4 enzyme and increase levels of drugs metabolized by this enzyme
Cannabidiol (CBD) (A cannabinoid extracted from the hemp plant and often made into an oil for use)	For relieving anxiety, insomnia, chronic pain, and many common ailments Epidiolex, a purified CBD solution, is the only prescription CBD approved by the FDA to treat Lennox-Gastaut syndrome, Dravet syndrome, or tuberous sclerosis complex in patients aged 1 year and older A variety of CBD products (oral, sublingual, inhaling, topical) are marketed and sold as dietary supplements and CBD-infused foods While the 2018 Farm Bill legalized CBD oil derived from the hemp plant containing ≤ 0.3% tetrahydrocannabinol (THC) at the federal level, all 50 states have laws legalizing CBD with varying degrees of restriction. CBD products are readily obtainable in most parts of the United States and have become the hot new products in states that have legalized medical marijuana Currently, the FDA does not allow CBD to be added in foods and it does not approve CBD to be sold as dietary supplements	No established dosage documented for CBD supplement There are concerns about the quality and purity of CBD products. Many have shown to be mislabeled and contain THC (>3%) and other contaminants (e.g., toxic chemicals including heavy metals and pesticides). Consumers should look for the US Hemp Authority seal that certifies the quality of CBD products. A product's certificate of analysis (COA) if available can also be used to determine labeling accuracy and presence of contaminants	Marijuana contains THC and CBD. Unlike THC, pure CBD does not cause a "high" CBD may cause nausea, diarrhea, fatigue, and irritability High CBD doses are linked to elevated liver function tests Effects of cumulative CBD exposure are unknown Avoid CBD in infants and children, and in pregnant or breastfeeding women Many potential drug interactions: Worsening sedation when combining with CNS depressants CBD inhibits CYP2C8, 2C9, and 2C19 enzymes and can increase levels of drugs such as carbamazepine, warfarin, amitriptyline, citalopram, phenytoin, and valproic acid CBD levels can be increased by CYP3A4 inhibitors, such as clarithromycin, ritonavir, and verapamil Increased sedation when CBD is taken with herbal supplements, including kava, melatonin, and St. John's wort
Chamomile flower	Used orally to calm nerves and treat GI spasms and inflammatory diseases of the GI tract Used topically to treat wounds, skin infections, and skin or mucous membrane inflammation	1 cup of freshly made tea 3–4 times daily (1 tbsp or 3 g of dried flower in 150 mL boiling water for 5–10 min)	Chamomile can cause an allergic reaction, especially in people with severe allergies to ragweed or other members of the daisy family (e.g., echinacea, feverfew, and milk thistle) It should not be taken concurrently with other sedatives, such as alcohol or benzodiazepines
Chaste tree berry (Chasteberry, Vitex)	For normalizing irregular menstrual periods and relieving premenstrual complaints For relieving menopausal symptoms For restoring fertility in women For treating acne associated with menstrual cycles For increasing breast milk production in lactating women	For menstrual irregularities and premenstrual complaints, 30–40 mg/d of the dried berries or an equivalent amount of aqueous-alcoholic extracts (50%–70% v/v) Dried fruit extract, standardized to 0.6% agnusides, is used in doses of 175–225 mg/d For other conditions, no established dosage documented	Chaste tree berry can have uterine stimulant properties and should be avoided in pregnancy Women with hormone-dependent conditions (e.g., breast, uterine, and ovarian cancers, and endometriosis and uterine fibroids) and men with prostate cancer should avoid chaste tree berry because it contains progestins Side effects include intramenstrual bleeding, dry mouth, headache, nausea, rash, alopecia, and tachycardia High doses (≥480 mg/d extract) can paradoxically decrease lactation Chaste tree berry is thought to have dopaminergic effects and can interact with dopamine antagonists, such as antipsychotics and metoclopramide Chaste tree berry can decrease the effects of oral contraceptives and hormone therapy

HERB OR NUTRITIONAL SUPPLEMENT	COMMON USES	REASONABLE ADULT ORAL DOSAGE*	PRECAUTIONS AND DRUG INTERACTIONS
Chondroitin	Orally, used frequently in combination with glucosamine for osteoarthritis Topically, in combination with sodium hyaluronate, as a viscoelastic agent in cataract surgery	Oral: 200–400 mg tid	Occasional mild side effects include nausea, indigestion, and allergic reactions Chondroitin derived from bovine cartilage carries a potential risk of contamination with diseased animals
Chromium	For diabetes For hypercholesterolemia Commonly found in weight-loss products Also promoted for body building	For diabetes, 100 µg bid for ≤4 months or 500 µg bid for 2 months For hypercholesterolemia, 200 µg tid or 500 µg bid for 2–4 months For body building, 200–400 µg/d Chromium picolinate has been used in most studies, even though the chloride form is also available	Adverse effects are rare, but they include headaches, insomnia, sleep disturbances, irritability, and mood changes; some patients may also experience cognitive, perceptual, and motor dysfunction Long-term use of high doses (600–2400 µg/d) can cause anemia, thrombocytopenia, hemolysis, hepatic dysfunction, and renal failure Interstitial nephritis has been reported A few studies suggest that chromium can cause DNA damage Chromium competes with iron for binding to transferrin and can cause iron deficiency Antacids, H_2 blockers, and proton pump inhibitors can decrease the absorption of chromium
Coenzyme Q10	As adjunctive treatment for congestive heart failure, angina, hypertension, and diabetes Used for reducing cardiotoxicity associated with doxorubicin Used to treat statin-induced myopathy	For heart failure, 100 mg/d in 2 or 3 divided doses For angina, 50 mg tid For hypertension, 60 mg bid For diabetes, 100–200 mg/d	Mild adverse events include gastric distress, nausea, vomiting, and hypotension Doses >300 mg/d can cause elevated liver enzyme levels Coenzyme Q10 can reduce the anticoagulation effects of warfarin Oral hypoglycemic agents and HMG-CoA reductase inhibitors can reduce serum coenzyme Q10 levels
Cranberry	To prevent and treat UTIs or *Helicobacter pylori* infections that can lead to stomach ulcers To prevent dental plaque As an antioxidant to prevent cardiovascular disease and cancer	For UTIs, 150–600 mL of cranberry juice daily or 300–400 mg of standardized extract bid For other conditions, no dosage determined	Drinking excessive amounts of juice could cause GI upset or diarrhea Prolonged use of cranberry juice in large doses increases the risk of kidney stone formation because of its high oxalate content Cranberry can interact with warfarin and cause an increase in INR The effectiveness of proton pump inhibitors can be reduced by cranberry because of its acidity
Creatine	To enhance muscle performance, especially during short-duration, high-intensity exercise	Loading dose of 20 g/d for 5–7 d followed by a maintenance dose of ≥2 g/d An alternative dosing of 3 g/d for 28 d has been suggested	Creatine can cause gastroenteritis, diarrhea, heat intolerance, muscle cramps, and elevated serum creatinine levels Creatine is contraindicated in patients taking diuretics Concurrent use with cimetidine, probenecid, or nonsteroidal antiinflammatory drugs increases the risk of adverse renal effects Caffeine can decrease creatine's ergogenic effects
Dehydroepian-drosterone (DHEA)	Replace low serum DHEA levels in adrenal insufficiency Treat SLE Reverse aging Used in many other conditions, including Alzheimer disease, depression, diabetes, menopause, osteoporosis, impotence, and AIDS Used to promote weight loss Used by bodybuilders to increase muscle mass	For replacement therapy, 25–50 mg/d For SLE, 200 mg/d For antiaging and osteoporosis, 50 mg/d For other conditions, no established dosage documented	Most common side effects are androgenic in nature and include acne, hair loss, hirsutism, and deepening of the voice Cases of hepatitis have been reported When used in high doses, DHEA can cause insomnia, manic symptoms, and palpitations DHEA at physiologic doses increases circulating androgens in women, but not in men; it also increases circulating estrogens in both men and women Avoid use of DHEA in individuals with a history of sex hormone–dependent malignancy Safety of DHEA in individuals aged < 30 years is unknown DHEA inhibits CYP3A4 enzyme and could increase serum concentrations of drugs metabolized by this enzyme (e.g., lovastatin, ketoconazole, itraconazole, and triazolam)

HERB OR NUTRITIONAL SUPPLEMENT	COMMON USES	REASONABLE ADULT ORAL DOSAGE*	PRECAUTIONS AND DRUG INTERACTIONS
Dong quai root	Commonly used for the relief of premenstrual and menopausal symptoms Used as a "blood tonic" and a strengthening treatment for the heart, spleen, liver, and kidneys	For premenstrual and menopausal symptoms, 3–4 g/d in 3 divided doses For other conditions, no established dosage documented	Dong quai should not be used in pregnant women because of its uterine stimulant and relaxant effects Women with hormone sensitive conditions (e.g., breast, uterine, and ovarian cancers, and endometriosis and uterine fibroids) should avoid dong quai because of its estrogenic effects Drinking the essential oil of dong quai is not recommended because it contains a small amount of carcinogenic constituents Dong quai contains psoralens that can cause photosensitivity and photodermatitis Dong quai contains natural coumarin derivatives that can increase the risk of bleeding in those who are taking anticoagulant or antiplatelet drugs
Echinacea	As an immune stimulant, particularly for the prevention and treatment of the common cold and influenza Supportive therapy for lower urinary tract infections Used topically to treat skin disorders and promote wound healing	300 mg tid of *Echinacea pallida* root or 2–3 mL tid of expressed juice of *Echinacea purpurea* herb Do not use for >8 weeks because echinacea may suppress immunity if used long term	Echinacea should not be used in transplant patients and those with autoimmune disease or liver dysfunction Allergic reactions have been reported Adverse events are rare and include mild GI effects It should be discontinued as far in advance of surgery as possible Echinacea can decrease effectiveness of the immunosuppressants
Ephedra (ma huang)	For diseases of the respiratory tract with mild bronchospasm Promoted for weight loss and performance enhancement	1 tsp or 2 g of dried herb (15–30 mg of ephedrine) in 240 mL boiling water for 10 min In Canada, the maximum allowable dosage of ephedrine is 8 mg per dose or 32 mg/d	Ephedra contains ephedrine, which has sympathomimetic activities; consequently, it should not be used in patients who have cardiovascular disease, diabetes, glaucoma, hypertension, hyperthyroidism, prostate enlargement, psychiatric disorders, or seizures Serious adverse effects, including seizures, arrhythmias, heart attack, stroke, and death, have been associated with the use of ephedra; as a result, the FDA banned the sale of ephedra-containing products in the United States. The ban does not apply to traditional Chinese herbal remedies Because of the cardiovascular effects of ephedrine, patients taking ephedra should discontinue use at least 24 h before surgery Concurrent use of ephedra and digitalis, guanethidine, monoamine oxidase inhibitors, or other stimulants, including caffeine, is not recommended
Evening primrose oil	For PMS, especially if mastalgia is present For treatment of atopic eczema Used for other medical conditions, including rheumatoid arthritis, menopausal symptoms, Raynaud phenomenon, Sjögren syndrome, and diabetic neuropathy	For PMS, 2–4 g/d For atopic eczema, 6–8 g/d For rheumatoid arthritis, 2.8 g/d These doses are based on products standardized to 9% γ-linolenic acid Daily dose can be given in divided doses	Evening primrose oil can increase the risk of pregnancy complications Side effects include indigestion, nausea, soft stools, and headache Seizures have been reported in patients with schizophrenia who were taking phenothiazines and evening primrose oil concomitantly Evening primrose oil can interact with anesthesia and cause seizures Concomitant use of evening primrose oil with anticoagulant and antiplatelet drugs can increase the risk of bleeding
Fenugreek seed	For diabetes and hypercholesterolemia For constipation, dyspepsia, gastritis, and kidney ailments Approved in Germany for use orally for loss of appetite and topically as a poultice for local inflammation	For loss of appetite, 1–2 g of the seed tid or 1 cup of tea (500 mg seed in 150 mL cold water for 3 h) several times a day Maximum 6 g/d For other conditions, no established dosage documented For topical use, 50 g powdered seed in 0.25 L of hot water to form a paste	Fenugreek can cause uterine contractions and should be avoided in pregnancy Individuals who have allergies to peanuts or soybeans might also be allergic to fenugreek Fenugreek can cause diarrhea and flatulence; it can also make urine smell like maple syrup Hypoglycemia can occur if fenugreek is taken in large amounts Repeated external applications can result in undesirable skin reactions Fenugreek contains small amounts of coumarins and can interact with anticoagulants and antiplatelet drugs High mucilage content of fenugreek can affect the absorption of oral drugs; therefore, fenugreek should not be taken within 2 h of other drugs

HERB OR NUTRITIONAL SUPPLEMENT	COMMON USES	REASONABLE ADULT ORAL DOSAGE*	PRECAUTIONS AND DRUG INTERACTIONS
Feverfew	For migraine headache prophylaxis For treatment of fever, menstrual problems, and arthritis	Migraine prevention: 25–75 mg bid of the encapsulated dried leaf extract standardized to 0.2% parthenolide, for up to 4 months 2.08–18.75 mg tid for MIG-99 preparation (a carbon dioxide extract enriched with parthenolide) for 3–4 months For other conditions, no established dosage documented	Feverfew can induce menstrual bleeding and is contraindicated in pregnancy Fresh leaves can cause oral ulcers and GI irritation Sudden discontinuation of feverfew can precipitate rebound headache Feverfew can interact with anticoagulants and potentiate the antiplatelet effect of aspirin
Fish oils (omega-3 fatty acids)	Commonly used in the treatment of hypertriglyceridemia Used to prevent CHD and stroke Used in many noncardiac conditions, including depression, diabetes, dysmenorrhea, rheumatoid arthritis, and IgA nephropathy Used to reduce the risk of developing age-related maculopathy, Alzheimer disease, and cancer Promotes visual and mental development in children	For hypertriglyceridemia, 3–5 g/d For cardioprotection, 1 g/d for patients with CHD; oily fish at least twice a week, or about 0.5 g/d for people with no known heart disease For other conditions, no established dosage documented Fish oils are composed of EPA and DHA; fish oil capsules vary widely in amounts and ratios of EPA and DHA; the most common fish oil capsules in the United States provide 180 mg of EPA and 120 mg DHA per capsule, and three capsules will provide about 1 g/d of omega-3 fatty acids	Common side effects include fishy aftertaste, GI disturbances, belching, halitosis, and heartburn High doses can cause nausea and loose stools Doses > 3 g/d can inhibit platelet aggregation, suppress immune function, worsen glycemic control, and raise LDL cholesterol levels Long-term use may be associated with weight gain Less well-controlled preparations can contain appreciable amount of organochloride contaminants Fish oil can increase the risk of bleeding in patients taking warfarin, an antiplatelet agent, or herbs that have antiplatelet constituents (e.g., garlic, ginkgo, and red clover) Fish oils can lower blood pressure and can have additive effects with antihypertensive agents Oral contraceptives can interfere with the triglyceride lowering effects of fish oils
Flaxseed	Orally, approved in Germany for chronic constipation, irritable bowel, and other colon disorders Often used orally for hypercholesterolemia and atherosclerosis Topically, approved in Germany for painful skin inflammation	For constipation, 1 tbsp (5 g) of whole or "bruised" seeds (not ground) in 150 mL of liquid 2–3 times daily For bowel inflammation, 2–3 tbsp of milled flaxseed soaked in 200–300 mL water and strain after 30 min For hypercholesterolemia, 1–2 tbsp flaxseed oil daily Topical: 30–50 g flaxseed flour as poultice or compress for a moist-heat direct application directly to the skin	Flaxseed should be taken with plenty of water to prevent possible intestinal blockage Patients with ileus should not take flaxseed High mucilage content of flaxseed can delay absorption of other drugs taken at the same time
Garlic	To lower blood pressure and serum cholesterol To prevent atherosclerosis	Fresh clove: one 4 g clove per day Tablet: 300 mg bid to tid standardized to 0.6%–1.3% allicin	Intake of large quantities can lead to stomach complaints Garlic has antiplatelet effects, so patients should discontinue use of garlic at least 7 d before surgery Concomitant use of garlic and anticoagulants can increase the risk of bleeding
Ginger root	As an antiemetic For prevention of motion sickness	Fresh rhizome: 2–4 g/d Powdered ginger: 250 mg 3–4 times daily Tea: 1 cup of tea tid (0.5–1 g dried root in 150 mL boiling water for 5–10 min)	Ginger should not be used by patients with gallstones because of its cholagogic effect It can inhibit platelet aggregation; cases of postoperative bleeding have been reported Large doses of ginger can increase bleeding time in patients taking antiplatelet agents
Ginkgo biloba leaf	To slow cognitive deterioration in dementia To increase peripheral blood flow in claudication To treat sexual dysfunction associated with the use of SSRIs	60–120 mg bid of extract Egb761 standardized to 24% flavonoids and 6% terpenoids	Adverse effects are rare and can include mild stomach or intestinal upset, headache, or allergic skin reaction Ginkgo can inhibit platelet aggregation; reports of spontaneous bleeding have been published Patients should discontinue ginkgo at least 36 h before surgery Concurrent use of ginkgo and anticoagulants, antiplatelet agents, vitamin E, or garlic can increase the risk of bleeding

HERB OR NUTRITIONAL SUPPLEMENT	COMMON USES	REASONABLE ADULT ORAL DOSAGE*	PRECAUTIONS AND DRUG INTERACTIONS
Ginseng root	As a tonic during times of stress, fatigue, disability, and convalescence To improve physical performance and stamina	Root: 1–2 g/d Tablet: 100 mg bid of extract standardized to 4%–7% ginsenosides A 2- to 3-week period of using ginseng followed by a 1- to 2-week "rest" period is generally recommended Ginseng is commonly adulterated, especially Siberian ginseng (eleuthero) products	Ginseng has a mild stimulant effect and should be avoided in patients with cardiovascular disease Tachycardia and hypertension can occur Overdosages can lead to ginseng abuse syndrome, characterized by insomnia, hypotonia, and edema Ginseng has estrogenic effects and can cause vaginal bleeding and breast tenderness Ginseng has been shown to inhibit platelets, so patients should discontinue ginseng use at least 7 d before surgery Ginseng should not be used with other stimulants Patients taking antidiabetic agents and ginseng should be monitored to avoid the hypoglycemic effects of ginseng Ginseng can interact with warfarin and cause a decreased INR Siberian ginseng can increase digoxin levels Ginseng can interact with phenelzine (a MAOI) resulting in insomnia, headache, tremulousness, and manic-like symptoms
Glucosamine	For osteoarthritis	500 mg tid with meals Glucosamine is available in the form of sulfate, hydrochloride, or N-acetyl salt; glucosamine sulfate is the form that has been used in most clinical studies	Side effects are generally limited to mild GI symptoms, including stomach upset, heartburn, diarrhea, nausea, and indigestion Glucosamine derived from marine exoskeletons may cause reactions in people allergic to shellfish Glucosamine may raise blood glucose level in patients with diabetes
Goldenseal	Often combined with echinacea to treat colds and other upper respiratory infections Used for diarrhea, dyspepsia, and gastritis Used topically as an eyewash, mouthwash, feminine cleansing product, and skin remedy	Oral: 0.5–1 g of the dried rhizome/root or 2–4 mL tincture (1:10, 60% ethanol) or 0.3–1 mL fluid extract (1:1, 60% ethanol) tid Eyewash: For trachoma infections, 2 drops of a 0.2% aqueous berberine solution tid × 3 week	Avoid using goldenseal during pregnancy and breast feeding; berberine, the principle constituent in goldenseal, can cause uterine contractions and neonatal jaundice Avoid using goldenseal in kidney failure because of inadequate urinary excretion of its alkaloids High dosages or long-term usage can lead to nausea, vomiting, headache, hypotension, bradycardia, leucopenia, and mucosal irritation Berberine can increase the risk of bleeding in patients taking warfarin or an antiplatelet agent Be aware that other herbs containing berberine, including Chinese goldthread and Oregon grape, are sometimes substituted for goldenseal
Grape seed	For conditions related to the heart and blood vessels, such as atherosclerosis, high blood pressure, high cholesterol, and poor circulation For vision problems, diabetic neuropathy or retinopathy, and swelling after an injury or surgery For cancer prevention and wound healing	For general health purposes, 100–300 mg daily of a standardized extract (95% oligomeric proanthocyanidin complexes)	Side effects include headache, dizziness, nausea, and dry, itchy scalp Concomitant use with warfarin or antiplatelet agents can increase risk of bleeding because of the tocopherol content of grape seed oil
Hawthorn leaf with flower	Commonly used in Germany to increase cardiac output in patients with New York Heart Association stage I and II heart failure	160–900 mg water-ethanol extract (30–169 mg procyanidins or 3.5–19.8 mg flavonoids) divided into 2–3 doses	Side effects include GI upset, palpitations, hypotension, headache, dizziness, and insomnia Concomitant use with CNS depressants can have additive CNS effects Hawthorn can potentiate effects of digoxin and vasodilators
Hops	For mood disturbances such as restlessness and anxiety For sleep disturbances Commonly found in combination products with other herbal sedatives	0.5 g of cut or powdered strobile in a single dose; can be taken as tea (0.5 g in 150 mL water), fluid extract 1:1 (0.5 mL), tincture 1:5 (2.5 mL), or dry extract 6–8:1 (60–80 mg) The preparation contains at least 0.35% (v/w) essential oil	Side effects are rare but include drowsiness and allergic reactions Hops is not recommended for use during pregnancy and lactation It can potentiate the sedative effect of CNS depressants (e.g., benzodiazepines, alcohol) and other herbal tranquilizers

HERB OR NUTRITIONAL SUPPLEMENT	COMMON USES	REASONABLE ADULT ORAL DOSAGE*	PRECAUTIONS AND DRUG INTERACTIONS
Horse chestnut seed	To relieve symptoms of chronic venous insufficiency	250 mg bid of extract standardized to 50 mg aescin in delayed-release form Unsafe to ingest the raw seed, which contains significant amounts of the most toxic constituent, esculin	Mild GI symptoms, headache, dizziness, and pruritis have been reported Ingestion of high doses can cause renal, hepatic, and hematologic toxicity Concomitant use with anticoagulants can increase the risk of bleeding Horse chestnut can potentiate the effects of hypoglycemic drugs
Kava kava	As an anxiolytic for nervous anxiety, stress, and restlessness As a sedative to induce sleep	Herb and preparations equivalent to 60–120 mg/d of kava pyrones Most clinical trials have used 100 mg tid of extract standardized to 70% kava pyrones for anxiety disorders	Kava should not be used by patients with depression Kava should be avoided in pregnant or nursing women Kava can affect motor reflexes and judgment, so it should not be taken while driving and/or operating heavy machinery Accommodative disturbances have been reported; kava can exacerbate Parkinson disease Extended use can cause a temporary yellow discoloration of skin, hair, and nails Reports have linked kava use to at least 25 cases of severe liver toxicity; sale of products containing kava has been banned in Canada and several European countries Kava has been shown to have additive CNS depressant effects with benzodiazepines, alcohol, and herbal tranquilizers Kava can potentiate the sedative effects of anesthetics, so kava should be discontinued at least 24 h before surgery
Lutein	Commonly used to prevent AMD and cataracts Used to prevent skin cancer, breast cancer, and colon cancer Used to protect against cardiovascular disease	For AMD and cataracts, 6–20 mg/d of lutein from diet For other uses, no established dosage documented Foods containing high concentrations of lutein include kale, spinach, broccoli, and romaine lettuce Not known if supplemental lutein is as effective as natural lutein Supplemental lutein in the form of esters might require a higher fat intake for effective absorption than purified lutein	No major adverse effects and drug interactions have been reported
Lycopene	Commonly used to prevent and treat prostate cancer Used for cancer prevention, arthrosclerosis prevention, and reduction of asthma symptoms	For decreasing the growth of prostate cancer, 15 mg supplement bid For prostate cancer prevention, at least 6 mg/d from tomato products (or ≥10 servings/wk) For other uses, no established dosage documented Heat processing converts lycopene in fresh tomatoes from the *trans-* to the *cis*-configuration. The *cis* isomer has better bioavailability Lycopene supplements usually do not specify the type and amount of isomers in their product labeling	Lycopene, when consumed in amounts found in foods, is generally considered to be safe Concomitant ingestion of beta-carotene can increase lycopene absorption Lycopene may reduce cholesterol levels and potentiate the effects of statins
Melatonin	For jet lag, insomnia, shift-work disorder, and circadian rhythm disorders For other medical conditions, including depression, multiple sclerosis, tinnitus, headache, and cancer	For jet lag, 5 mg at bedtime for 2–5 d beginning the day of return For sleep disorders, 0.3–5 mg taken 2 h before bedtime Avoid melatonin from animal pineal gland because of the possibility of contamination.	Avoid use in pregnancy because melatonin decreases serum luteinizing hormone concentrations and increases serum prolactin levels The common adverse reactions include headache, transient depressive symptoms, daytime fatigue and drowsiness, dizziness, abdominal cramps, irritability, and reduced alertness Concomitant use of melatonin with alcohol, benzodiazepines, or other CNS depressants can cause additive sedation Melatonin can affect immune function and may interfere with immunosuppressive therapy Concomitant use with other herbs that have sedative properties (e.g., chamomile, goldenseal, hop, kava, valerian) can produce additive CNS-impairing effects

HERB OR NUTRITIONAL SUPPLEMENT	COMMON USES	REASONABLE ADULT ORAL DOSAGE*	PRECAUTIONS AND DRUG INTERACTIONS
Milk thistle fruit	As a hepatoprotectant and antioxidant, particularly for treatment of hepatitis, cirrhosis, and toxic liver damage Used in Europe for the treatment of hepatotoxic mushroom poisoning from *Amanita phalloides*	Average daily dose is 12–15 g of crude drug or formulations equivalent to 200–400 mg of silymarin	Adverse effects are rare but include diarrhea and allergic reactions Milk thistle can potentiate the hypoglycemic effect of antidiabetic agents
Peppermint	Commonly used for indigestion and irritable bowel syndrome (IBS) Used externally for myalgia and neuralgia	Indigestion: 1 tsp dried leaves in 1 cup of boiling water, steeped for 10 min; drink 4–5 times/d between meals IBS: 1–2 enteric coated cap (0.2 mL of peppermint oil/cap) 2–3 times/d. Take peppermint ≥2 h before or after an acid-reducing drug to ensure adequate absorption	Peppermint, in amounts normally found in food, is likely to be safe Larger supplemental amounts can cause side effects including heartburn, flushing, headache, and mouth sores Hypersensitivity reactions, contact dermatitis, and exacerbations of asthma may occur Peppermint can exacerbate symptoms in patients with gastroesophageal reflux disease (GERD) because it can relax the lower esophageal sphincter Peppermint tea has been shown to reduce free testosterone levels in men Peppermint can decrease the blood levels of cyclosporine and drugs that metabolized by the CYP3A4 isoenzyme
Probiotics	Prevent and treat antibiotic-associated diarrhea and acute infectious diarrhea Relieve symptoms of IBS Treat atopic dermatitis for at-risk infants	Dosage varies based on preparations *Lactobacillus* sp., *Bifidobacterium* sp., *Saccharomyces boulardii* are the most widely used organisms For *Lactobacillus* sp., 10 billion CFUs/d For *Lactobacillus* sp./*Bifidobacterium* sp., 100 million to 35 billion CFUs/d For *Saccharomyces boulardii*, 250–500 mg/d Quality of products varies among brands Refrigeration is required to maintain potency	Avoid use in short-gut syndrome and severe immuno-compromised condition Common adverse effects include flatulence, mild abdominal discomfort, and, rarely, septicemia
Red clover flower	Commonly used for conditions associated with menopause, such as hot flashes, cardiovascular health, and osteoporosis Used for PMS, benign prostate hyperplasia, and cancer prevention Used topically to treat psoriasis, eczema, and other rashes	For hot flashes, 40 mg/d of the isoflavones extract (Promensil) For other conditions, no established dosage documented	Red clover has estrogenic activity and should be avoided during pregnancy and lactation Women with hormone-dependent conditions (e.g., breast, uterine, and ovarian cancer, and endometriosis and uterine fibroids) and men with prostate cancer should also avoid taking red clover Side effects include headache, myalgia, nausea, and rash Red clover contains coumarin derivatives and can increase the risk of bleeding in those who are taking anticoagulants or antiplatelet drugs Preliminary report suggests that red clover might antagonize the effects of tamoxifen Some evidence suggests that red clover can increase the levels of drugs that metabolized by the cytochrome P450 3A4 isoenzyme (e.g., lovastatin, ketoconazole, itraconazole, fexofenadine, and triazolam)
SAMe (S-adenosyl-L-methionine)	For treatment of osteoarthritis, depression, fibromyalgia, and liver disease	For osteoarthritis, 200 mg tid For depression and fibromyalgia, 800 mg bid For liver disease, 600–800 mg bid	Common side effects include flatulence, nausea, vomiting, and diarrhea SAMe can cause anxiety in people with depression and hypomania in people with bipolar disorder Concurrent use of SAMe and other antidepressants can cause serotonin syndrome
Saw palmetto berry	To treat symptomatic benign prostatic hyperplasia and irritable bladder	160 mg bid of extract standardized to 85%–95% fatty acids and sterols	Adverse effects are rare but include headache, nausea, and upset stomach High doses can cause diarrhea

HERB OR NUTRITIONAL SUPPLEMENT	COMMON USES	REASONABLE ADULT ORAL DOSAGE*	PRECAUTIONS AND DRUG INTERACTIONS
Soy	Commonly used for cholesterol reduction in combination with a low-fat diet Used for menopausal symptoms and for prevention of osteoporosis and cardiovascular disease in postmenopausal women	For lowering cholesterol, 25–50 g/d of soy protein For hot flashes, 20–60 g/d of soy protein For osteoporosis, 40 g/d of soy protein containing 90 mg isoflavones	Soy, when consumed as whole foods (e.g., tofu or soy milk), has minimal adverse effects Consumption of large amounts of soy can cause gastric complaints such as constipation, bloating, and nausea Long-term use of soy tablets containing isoflavones (150 mg/d for 5 years) has been shown to cause endometrial hyperplasia
St. John's wort	Used for treatment of mild to moderate depression May have antiinflammatory and antiinfective activities	300 mg tid of hypericum extract standardized to 0.3% hypericin	St. John's wort should not be used in pregnancy Side effects include dry mouth, GI upset, dizziness, fatigue, and constipation St. John's wort can induce photosensitivity, especially in fair-skinned individuals It can cause serotonin syndrome if used with other antidepressants, including SSRIs, or other serotonergic drugs It has been shown to induce CYP3A4 and decrease blood levels of many drugs such as indinavir, nevirapine, cyclosporine, digoxin, theophylline, simvastatin, oral contraceptive pills, and warfarin St. John's wort should be discontinued at least 5 d before surgery to avoid any potential drug interactions
Stinging nettle root	Approved in Germany for difficulty in urination in BPH stage 1 and 2	4–6 g/d of cut root; can be taken as tea (1.5 g in 150 mL boiling water for 10–20 min, tid), fluid extract 1:1 (1.5 mL tid), tincture 1:5 (5–7.5 mL tid), or dry extract 5.4–6.6:1 (0.22–0.33 g tid)	Occasionally, mild GI upsets may occur No known interactions with drugs
Turmeric root	Approved by the German Commission E for dyspeptic conditions Used extensively in Ayurveda medicine for its antiinflammatory and antiarthritic effects Other uses include allergic rhinitis, depression, nonalcoholic fatty liver disease, osteoarthritis and cancer	For dyspeptic conditions: 1.5–3 g/d of cut root as tea infusion or equivalent preparations (e.g., powder, extract, tincture) The Commission E monograph requires turmeric to contain not less than 3% curcuminoids, calculated as curcumin and not less than 3% volatile oil	Side effects are uncommon and are generally limited to mild stomach distress Topical curcumin can cause allergic contact dermatitis Individuals with bile duct obstruction or gallstones should avoid curcumin due to its stimulating effects on the gallbladder
Valerian root	Used as a mild sedative for insomnia and anxiety	2–3 g of dried root or 1–3 mL of tincture, qd to several times per day Two clinical trials found 400–450 mg of the root extract effective for insomnia	Valerian has a bad odor and can cause morning drowsiness Long-term administration can lead to paradoxical stimulation, including restlessness and palpitations Because of the risk of benzodiazepine-like withdrawal, valerian should be tapered over a period of several weeks before surgery It can potentiate the sedative effect of CNS depressants (e.g., benzodiazepines, alcohol) and other herbal tranquilizers

*Doses presented in the table are adapted from the German Commission E Monographs and/or data from clinical trials. Products from different manufacturers vary considerably. A reliable product should have a label clearly stating the botanical name of the herb and milligram amount contained in the product. Standardized extracts should be used whenever possible and are often disclosed on the label of quality products.

AMD, Age-related macular degeneration; *BPH*, benign prostatic hyperplasia; *CFU*, colony-forming unit; *CHD*, coronary heart disease; *CNS*, central nervous system; *CYP3A4*, cytochrome P450 3A4; *DHA*, docosahexaenoic acid; *EPA*, eicosapentaenoic acid; *FDA*, Food and Drug Administration; *GI*, gastrointestinal; *HMG-CoA*, 3-hydroxy-3-methylglutaryl coenzyme A; *INR*, international normalized ratio; *LDL*, low-density lipoprotein; *MAOI*, monoamine oxidase inhibitor; *PMS*, premenstrual syndrome; *SLE*, systemic lupus erythematosus; *SSRIs*, selective serotonin reuptake inhibitors; *UTIs*, urinary tract infections.

References

Ang-Lee MK, Moss J, Yuan C: Herbal medicines and perioperative care, *JAMA* 286:208–216, 2001.

Bent S: Herbal medicine in the United States: Review and efficacy, safety, and regulation, *J Gen Intern Med* 23:854–859, 2008.

Blumenthal M, editor: *Herbal Medicines: Expanded Commission E monographs*, Austin, TX, 2000, American Botanical Council.

Blumenthal M, editor: *The ABC Clinical Guide to Herbs*, Austin, TX, 2003, American Botanical Council.

Ernst E: The risk-benefit profile of commonly used herbal therapies: Ginkgo, St John's wort, ginseng, Echinacea, saw palmetto, and kava, *Ann Intern Med* 136:42–53, 2002.

Gregory PJ, Worthington M, Shkayeva M, et al, editors: Natural Medicines (database online), Stockton, CA: 2018 Therapeutic Research Center. Available at https://naturalmedicines.therapeuticresearch.com/. (Assessed July 7, 2019).

Holland S, Silberstein SD, Freitag F, et al: Evidence-based guideline update: NSAIDs and other complementary treatments for episodic migraine prevention in adults: report of the Quality Standards Subcommittee of the American Academy of Neurology and the American Headache Society, *Neurology* 78(17):1346–1353, 2012.

Kligler B, Cohrssen A: Probiotics, *Am Fam Physician* 78:1073–1078, 2008.

Kronenberg F, Fugh-Berman A: Complementary and alternative medicine for menopausal symptoms: A review of randomized controlled trials, *Ann Intern Med* 137:805–813, 2002.

National Center for Complementary and Integrative Health: Herbs at a Glance. Available at https://nccih.nih.gov/health/herbsataglance.htm. Accessed 19 March 2018.

Smet P: Herbal remedies, *N Engl J Med* 347:2046–2056, 2002.

TOXIC CHEMICAL AGENTS REFERENCE CHART

Method of
Laurie A.M. Hommema, MD; and Kevin Hommema, BSME

Toxic chemical agents are poisonous vapors, aerosols, gases, liquids, or solids that have toxic effects on people, animals, or plants. Most of these agents are liquid at room temperature and are disseminated as vapors and aerosols. They may be released as bombs, sprayed from aerosolizing devices, through ventilation systems or introduced to food or water supply. Some of these agents are highly toxic and persistent, features that can render a site uninhabitable and require costly and potentially hazardous decontamination and remediation. Health effects range from irritation and burning of skin and mucous membranes to rapid cardiopulmonary collapse and death.

Efficient deployment of hazardous materials (HazMat) teams is critical to control a chemical agent attack. Although all major cities and emergency medical systems have plans and equipment in place to address this situation, physicians and other health professionals must be aware of principles involved in managing a patient or multiple patients exposed to these agents. Chemical weapon agents have a high potential for secondary contamination from victims to responders. This requires that medical treatment facilities have clearly defined procedures for handling contaminated casualties, many of whom will transport themselves to the facility. Precautions must be used until thorough decontamination has been performed or the specific chemical agent is identified. Healthcare professionals must first protect themselves (e.g., by using protective suits, respiratory protection, and chemical-resistant gloves) because secondary contamination with even small amounts of these substances (particularly nerve agents such as VX) may be lethal.

Primary detection of exposure to chemical agents is based on the signs and symptoms of the potential victim (Table 1). Confirmation of a chemical agent, using detection equipment or laboratory analyses, takes considerable time and will not likely contribute to the early management of mass casualty victims. Several patients presenting with the same symptoms should alert physicians and hospital staff to the possibility of a chemical attack. If a chemical attack occurs, most victims will likely arrive within a short time. This situation differentiates a chemical attack from a biological attack involving infectious microorganisms, which can take days for symptom onset. Additional diagnostic clues include the following:
- Unusual temporal or geographic clustering of illness
- Any sudden increase in illness in previously healthy persons
- Sudden increase in nonspecific syndromes (e.g., sudden unexplained weakness in previously healthy persons; dimmed or blurred vision; hypersecretion, inhalation, or burn-like syndrome)

A coordinated communication network is critical for transmitting reliable information from the incident scene to treatment facilities. Any suspicious or confirmed exposure to a chemical weapons agent should be reported to the local health department, local Federal Bureau of Investigation office, National Response Center (800-424-8802), and the Centers for Disease Control and Prevention (770-488-7100).

TABLE 1   Quick Reference Chart on Chemical Weapon Agents

	DIAGNOSTIC CONSIDERATIONS				TREATMENT CONSIDERATIONS*			
CHEMICAL AGENT	SIGNS AND SYMPTOMS	SYMPTOM ONSET	ODOR	ACTION	TESTING	TREATMENT	ANTIDOTE	COMMENTS
Cyanides—Asphyxiant/Blood								
Cyanogen chloride (CK) Hydrogen cyanide (AC)	"Cherry red" skin Resp: SOB, chest tightness, hyperventilation, resp arrest GI: nausea, vomiting CV: ventricular arrhythmias, hypotension, cardiac arrest, shock CNS: anxiety, headache, drowsiness, weakness, apnea, convulsions, seizure, coma Metabolic acidosis and increased concentration of venous oxygen (possibly also cyanosis)	Rapid, seconds to minutes	Bitter almond, musty, or chlorine-like	Binds cellular cytochrome oxidase, causing chemical asphyxia	Cyanide, thiocyanate, serum lactate levels Venous and arterial partial oxygen pressure	Immediate treatment of symptomatic patients is critical. Hydroxocobalamin (vitamin B₁₂ₐ [Cyanokit]) administered IV with sodium thio sulfate⁵,†; Activated charcoal¹ for oral exposure Mechanical ventilation as needed Circulatory support with crystalloids and vasopressors Metabolic acidosis corrected with IV sodium bicarbonate Seizures controlled with benzodiazepines	Sodium nitrite and sodium thiosulfate (Nithiodote); repeat one-half initial doses of both agents in 30 min if inadequate clinical response; amyl nitrite¹ capsules are available for first aid until intravenous access is achieved. Hydroxocobalamin (vitamin B₁₂ₐ, Cyanokit)	Cyanide antidote kits are commercially available. CNS effects may be confused with carbon monoxide and hydrogen sulfide poisoning. Nonpersistent, not contact hazard.
Incapacitating Agents								
Agent 15 3-quinuclidinyl benzilate (BZ)	May appear as drug intoxication with erratic behaviors, hallucinations. Mydriasis, blurred vision, dry mouth, dry skin, possible atropine-like flush, initial rise in heart rate, hyperthermia, decreased level of consciousness, confusion, disorientation, impaired memory.	Hours—up to 36 h if only on skin 0–4 h: parasympathetic blockade and mild CNS effects 4–20 h: stupor with ataxia and hyperthermia 20–96 h: full-blown delirium Resolution phase: paranoia, deep sleep, reawakening, crawling, climbing automatisms, eventual reorientation	Odorless	Competitive inhibitor of acetylcholine muscarinic receptor		Support, intravenous fluids	Physostigmine salicylate (Antilirium)¹	Persistent in soil and water and on contact surfaces. Contact hazard.

TABLE 1 Quick Reference Chart on Chemical Weapon Agents—cont'd

	DIAGNOSTIC CONSIDERATIONS					TREATMENT CONSIDERATIONS*			
CHEMICAL AGENT	SIGNS AND SYMPTOMS	SYMPTOM ONSET	ODOR	ACTION	TESTING	TREATMENT	ANTIDOTE	COMMENTS

Nerve Agents

Cyclohexyl sarin (GF) Sarin (GB) Soman (GD) Tabun (GA) VX	Most toxic of known chemical agents May be confused with organophosphate and carbamate pesticide poisoning Eyes: excessive lacrimation, miosis may be present and blurred vision Resp: rhinorrhea, bronchospasm, resp failure GI: hypersalivation, nausea, vomiting, diarrhea Skin: localized sweating Cardiac: sinus bradycardia Skeletal muscles: fasciculations followed by weakness, flaccid paralysis CNs: loss of consciousness, convulsions, apnea, seizures	Vapor: seconds Liquid: minutes or hours Symptom onset may be delayed up to 18 h, particularly for localized exposures.	GB, VX: none GA: fruity GD: camphor-like	Irreversible acetylcholinesterase inhibitors	Erythrocyte or serum cholinesterase activity to confirm exposure	Rapid establishment of patent airway Early administration of 2-PAM (pralidoxime [Protopam]) is critical to minimize permanent agent inactivation of acetylcholinesterase (i.e., "aging"). Benzodiazepines to control nerve agent–induced seizures Airway and ventilatory support as needed	Atropine and 2-PAM Additional doses until bronchial secretions are cleared and ventilation improved	Atropine, 2-PAM, and diazepam[1] are available in autoinjector kits through the US military. VX is a contact hazard.

Continued

Toxic Chemical Agents Reference Chart

TABLE 1   Quick Reference Chart on Chemical Weapon Agents—cont'd

| CHEMICAL AGENT | DIAGNOSTIC CONSIDERATIONS | | | | TREATMENT CONSIDERATIONS* | | | |
	SIGNS AND SYMPTOMS	SYMPTOM ONSET	ODOR	ACTION	TESTING	TREATMENT	ANTIDOTE	COMMENTS
Pulmonary or Choking Agents								
Acrolein Ammonia (NH₃) Chlorine (Cl) Chloropicrin (PS) Diphosgene (DP) Nitrogen oxides (NO$_x$) Perfluoroisobutylene (PFIB) Phosgene (CG) Sulfur dioxide (SO₂)	Degree of water solubility of the agent influences onset and severity of respiratory injury. Eye and airway irritation, dyspnea, chest tightness, rhinorrhea, hypersalivation, cough, wheezing High-dose inhalation can cause laryngospasm, pneumonitis, and acute lung injury with delayed onset (≤ 48 h) of acute resp distress syndrome. Chest radiograph: hyperinflation, noncardiogenic pulmonary edema	Rapid or delayed 1–24 h; rarely up to 72 h	CG: freshly mown hay or grass			Supportive measures Specific treatment depends on the agent IV fluids for hypotension; no diuretics Ventilation with or without positive airway pressure Bronchodilators for bronchospasm Methylprednisolone[1] may be effective in preventing noncardiogenic pulmonary edema.	No specific antidote	Easily absorbed via mucous membranes of eyes, nose, oropharynx. May be confused with inhalation exposure to industrial chemicals (e.g., HCl, Cl₂, NH₃). Not contact hazard.
Riot Control Agents								
Mace (CN) Tear gas (CS)	Metallic taste Burning and pain on mucosal membranes and skin Eyes: irritation, pain, tearing, blepharospasm Airways: burning in nose and mouth, respiratory discomfort, bronchospasm (may be delayed 36 h) Skin: tingling, erythema	Immediate	CN: apple blossom CS: pepper	SN2 alkylating agents	No specific laboratory tests	Supportive care Irrigation as necessary Persons with asthma, emphysema might need oxygen, inhaled bronchodilators, steroids, assisted ventilation. Lotions, such as calamine[1] for persistent erythema		Not contact hazard

TABLE 1 Quick Reference Chart on Chemical Weapon Agents—cont'd

CHEMICAL AGENT	DIAGNOSTIC CONSIDERATIONS				TREATMENT CONSIDERATIONS*			COMMENTS
	SIGNS AND SYMPTOMS	SYMPTOM ONSET	ODOR	ACTION	TESTING	TREATMENT	ANTIDOTE	
	Nausea and vomiting are common. CN can cause corneal opacification.							
Vesicant or Blister Agents								
General	Clinical effects depend on extent and route of exposure.	Effects may be delayed, appearing hours after exposure		Intracellular enzyme and DNA alkylating agents		Immediate decontamination within 2 min if able Supportive care Thermal burn-type treatment Symptomatic management of lesions		Primary liquid hazard. May be confused with skin exposure to caustic irritants (e.g., NaOH, NH$_3$). Persistent contact hazard.
Sulfur mustard (H) Distilled mustard (HD)	Skin: erythema and blisters (may be delayed ≤ 8 h), pruritus Eye: irritation, conjunctivitis, corneal damage, lacrimation, pain, blepharospasm Resp: mild to marked acute airway damage, pneumonitis within 1–3 days, respiratory failure GI effects (nausea, vomiting diarrhea) may be present Bone marrow stem cell suppression leading to pancytopenia and increased susceptibility to infection Fever, sputum production	Delayed 2–48 h	Garlic, horseradish, or mustard			Skin: silver sulfadiazine[1] Eye: homatropine[1] ophthalmic ointment Pulmonary: antibiotics, bronchodilators, steroids Colony-stimulating factor may be helpful for leukopenia. Systemic analgesic and antipruritics Early use of PEEP or CPAP Maintain fluid and electrolyte balance (do not excessively fluid resuscitate as in thermal burns).	No specific antidote	Combination with lewisite (called mustard-Lewisite or HL) results in rapid effects of lewisite and delayed effects of mustard agents.

Toxic Chemical Agents Reference Chart

Continued

TABLE 1 Quick Reference Chart on Chemical Weapon Agents—cont'd

CHEMICAL AGENT	DIAGNOSTIC CONSIDERATIONS					TREATMENT CONSIDERATIONS*			
	SIGNS AND SYMPTOMS	SYMPTOM ONSET	ODOR	ACTION	TESTING	TREATMENT	ANTIDOTE	COMMENTS	
Lewisite (L)	Skin: gray area of dead skin within 5 min, erythema within 30 min, blistering 2–3 h, immediate irritation or burning pain on contact, severe tissue necrosis. Eye: pain, blepharospasm, conjunctival and lid edema. Airway: pseudomembrane formation, nasal irritation. Intravascular fluid loss, hypovolemia, shock, organ congestion, leukocytosis	Immediate	Fruity or geranium				British anti-lewisite (BAL or dimercaprol)	More volatile than mustard. Damages eyes, skin, and airways by direct contact.	
Phosgene oxime (CX)	Burning, irritation, wheal-like skin lesions, eye and airway damage, conjunctivitis, lacrimation, lid edema, blepharospasm	Immediate	Freshly mown hay	Urticant, nonvesicant agent	No distinctive laboratory findings	Parenteral methylprednisolone[1] may be effective in preventing noncardiogenic pulmonary edema. Experimental: aerosolized dexamethasone[1] and theophylline[1] for pulmonary involvement	No antidote	Vapor extremely irritating; vapor and liquid cause tissue damage upon contact.	

	DIAGNOSTIC CONSIDERATIONS				TREATMENT CONSIDERATIONS*			
CHEMICAL AGENT	SIGNS AND SYMPTOMS	SYMPTOM ONSET	ODOR	ACTION	TESTING	TREATMENT	ANTIDOTE	COMMENTS
Vomiting (Arsine-Based) Agents								
Adamsite (DM) Diphenylchlor-arsine (DA) Diphenylcyano-arsine (DC)	Eyes: conjunctival irritation, tearing, and blepharospasm Airways: sneezing, mucosal lung irritation, edema, progressive cough, wheezing Cardiac: tachypnea, tachycardia GI: intestinal cramps, emesis, diarrhea Skin: erythema, edema at the site of dermal contact CNS: depression, syncope	All rapidly acting within minutes	DA: none DC: garlic DM: burning fireworks	Arsine gas depletes erythrocyte glutathione and causes hemolysis.	Chest radiograph to rule out chemical pneumonitis	Supportive care Monitor for hemolysis Wheezing or dyspnea: may need albuterol inhalation Eye irrigation (water, normal saline, lactated Ringer's) in patients with ocular exposure Treat repetitive emesis with IV hydration and antiemetics. Blood transfusion may be required. Exchange transfusion may be required. Hemodialysis may be useful in decreasing arsenic level and treating renal failure.		Primary route of absorption is through respiratory system.

*Different situations can require different treatment and dosage regimens. Please consult other references as well as a regional poison control center (800-222-1222), medical toxicologist, clinical pharmacologist, or other drug information specialist for definitive dosage information, especially dosages for pregnant women and children.

†Available in Europe.

‡Not FDA approved for this indication.

§Investigational drug in the United States.

CNS, Central nervous system; *CPAP*, continuous positive airway pressure; *CV*, cardiovascular; *GI*, gastrointestinal; *2-PAM*, pralidoxime (2-pyridine aldoxime methyl chloride); *PEEP*, positive end-expiratory pressure; *resp*, respiratory; *SOB*, shortness of breath.

Adapted from Lyznicki JL: AMA quick reference guide: Exposure to toxic chemical agents. In American Medical Association: Management of Public Health Emergencies *A Resource Guide for Physicians and Other Community Respond-ers*, Chicago, American Medical Association, 2005.

U.S. Department of Health and Human Services Chemical Hazards Emergency Medical Management Acute Patient Care Guidelines. 2020. https://chemm.nlm.nih.gov/mmghome.htm

Toxic Chemical Agents Reference Chart

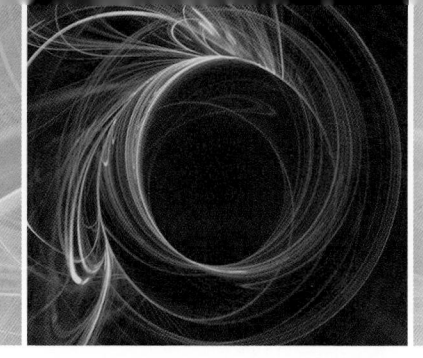

Index

Note: Page numbers followed by "f" indicate figures and "t" indicate tables.

Index

1482

Index

1538

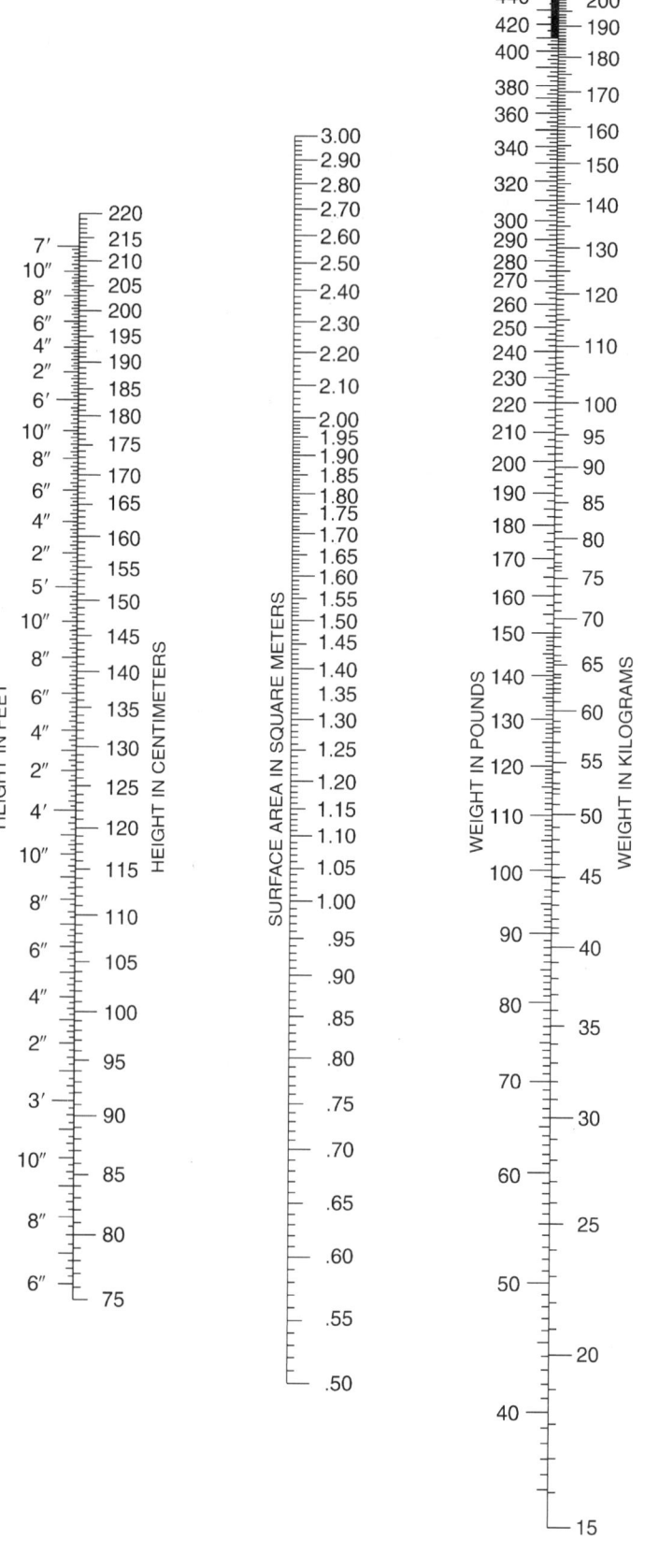

HEIGHT IN FEET

7'
10"
8"
6"
4"
2"
6'
10"
8"
6"
4"
2"
5'
10"
8"
6"
4"
2"
4'
10"
8"
6"
4"
2"
3'
10"
8"
6"

HEIGHT IN CENTIMETERS

220
215
210
205
200
195
190
185
180
175
170
165
160
155
150
145
140
135
130
125
120
115
110
105
100
95
90
85
80
75

SURFACE AREA IN SQUARE METERS

3.00
2.90
2.80
2.70
2.60
2.50
2.40
2.30
2.20
2.10
2.00
1.95
1.90
1.85
1.80
1.75
1.70
1.65
1.60
1.55
1.50
1.45
1.40
1.35
1.30
1.25
1.20
1.15
1.10
1.05
1.00
.95
.90
.85
.80
.75
.70
.65
.60
.55
.50

WEIGHT IN POUNDS

440
420
400
380
360
340
320
300
290
280
270
260
250
240
230
220
210
200
190
180
170
160
150
140
130
120
110
100
90
80
70
60
50
40
15

WEIGHT IN KILOGRAMS

200
190
180
170
160
150
140
130
120
110
100
95
90
85
80
75
70
65
60
55
50
45
40
35
30
25
20